Quick Contents

PORTH'S

Pathophysiology

Concepts of Altered Health States

TENTH EDITION

PORTH'S

Pathophysiology

Concepts of Altered Health States

TENTH EDITION

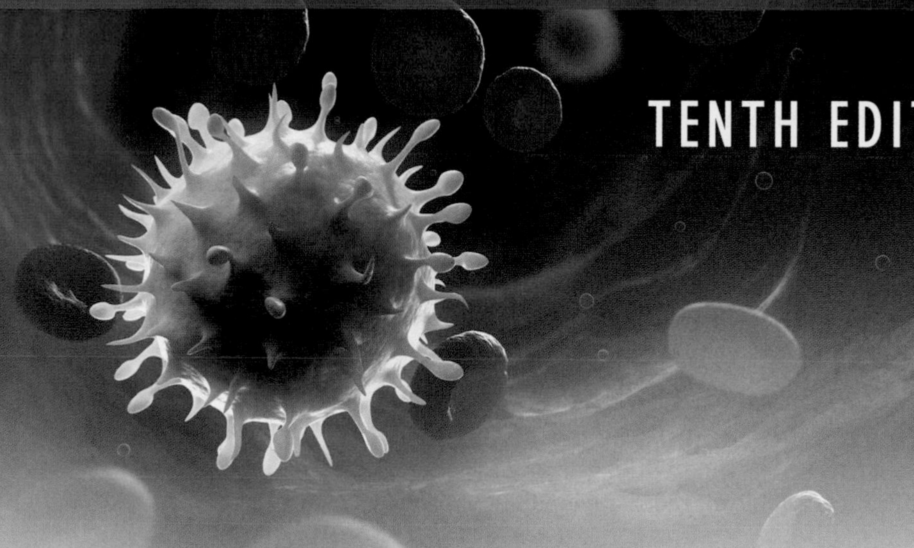

TOMMIE L. NORRIS, DNS, RN
AACN Leadership for Academic Nursing Fellow
Dean, School of Nursing
Miami Dade College
Miami, Florida

Subject Matter Expert Reviewer:
RUPA LALCHANDANI TUAN, PhD
Assistant Professor
Notre Dame de Namur University
Belmont, California

Wolters Kluwer

Philadelphia • Baltimore • New York • London
Buenos Aires • Hong Kong • Sydney • Tokyo

Not authorised for sale in United States, Canada, Australia, New Zealand, Puerto Rico, and U.S. Virgin Islands.

Vice President and Publisher: Julie K. Stegman
Executive Editor: Kelley Squazzo
Director of Product Development: Jennifer K. Forestieri
Senior Development Editor: Meredith L. Brittain
Editorial Coordinator: Tim Rinehart
Marketing Manager: Brittany Clements
Editorial Assistant: Leo Gray
Design Coordinator: Steve Druding
Art Director, Illustration: Jennifer Clements
Production Project Manager: Linda Van Pelt
Manufacturing Coordinator: Karin Duffield
Prepress Vendor: SPi Global

Tenth Edition

9 8 7 6 5 4 3 2 1

Printed in China

Cataloging-in-Publication Data available on request from the Publisher

ISBN: 978-1-4963-7759-3

shop.lww.com

RRS1808

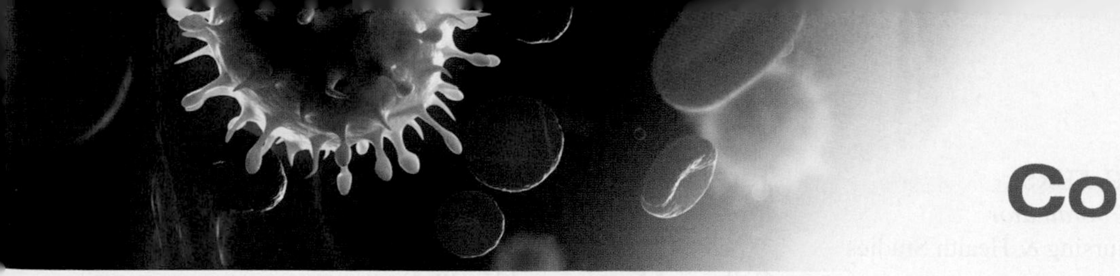

Contributors

Contributors to the Tenth Edition*

Sawsan Abuhammad, PhD
Assistant Professor, Maternal and Child Health
Jordan University of Science and Technology
Irbid, Jordan
Chapter 42: Structure and Function of the Male Genitourinary System

Maeghan Arnold, MNSc, APRN, AGACNP-BC
Clinical Instructor
College of Nursing, Practice Department
University of Arkansas for Medical Sciences
Little Rock, Arkansas
Chapter 20: Disorders of Hearing and Vestibular Function

Michele R. Arwood, DNP, MSN, BSN, CNS-BC, NE-BC, CJCP
System Director, Quality and Accreditation
Baptist Memorial Health Care Corporation
Memphis, Tennessee
Chapter 8: Disorders of Fluid and Electrolyte and Acid Base Balance
Chapter 29: Structure and Function of the Respiratory System

Trina Barrett, DNP, RN, CNE, CCRN
Assistant Professor
College of Nursing
University of Tennessee Health Science Center
Memphis, Tennessee
Chapter 3: Cellular Adaptation, Injury, and Death

Cynthia Bautista, PhD, CCRN, SCRN, CCNS, ACNS-BC, FNCS
Associate Professor
Marion Peckham Egan School of Nursing and Health Studies
Fairfield University
Fairfield, Connecticut
Chapter 13: Organization and Control of Neural Function
Chapter 14: Somatosensory Function, Pain, Headache, and Temperature
Chapter 15: Disorders of Motor Function
Chapter 16: Disorders of Brain Function

*For a list of the contributors and reviewers for this title's online ancillaries, go to thepoint.lww.com/Porth10e.

Hallie Bensinger, DNP, APN, FNP-BC
Kaplan Nurse Consultant
New York, New York
Chapter 44: Structure and Function of the Female Reproductive System
Chapter 45: Disorders of the Female Reproductive System

Jami S. Brown, DHEd, RN, CNN
Assistant Professor
College of Nursing
University of Tennessee Health Science Center
Memphis, Tennessee
Chapter 34: Acute Kidney Injury and Chronic Kidney Disease

Melissa Brown, MS, RN
Instructional Academic Staff
College of Nursing
University of Wisconsin–Milwaukee
Milwaukee, Wisconsin
Chapter 43: Disorders of the Male Reproductive System

Jacqueline Rosenjack Burchum, DNSc, FNP-BC, CNE
Associate Professor
College of Nursing
University of Tennessee Health Science Center
Memphis, Tennessee
Chapter 21: Blood Cells and Hematopoietic System
Chapter 23: Disorders of Red Blood Cells

Kathy Diane Butler, DNP, APRN, FNP/GNP-BC, NP-C
Clinical Associate Professor
College of Nursing
University of Memphis
Memphis, Tennessee
Chapter 49: Disorders of Musculoskeletal Function: Developmental and Metabolism Disorders, Activity Intolerance, and Fatigue

Freddy W. Cao, MD, PhD
Clinical Associate Professor
College of Nursing
University of Wisconsin–Milwaukee
Milwaukee, Wisconsin
Chapter 36: Structure and Function of the Gastrointestinal System
Chapter 37: Disorders of Gastrointestinal Function
Chapter 38: Disorders of Hepatobiliary and Exocrine Pancreas Function

Jaclyn Conelius, PhD, FNP-BC, FHRS
Associate Professor & FNP Track Coordinator
Marion Peckham Egan School of Nursing & Health Studies
Fairfield University
Fairfield, Connecticut
Chapter 28: Disorders of Cardiac Conduction and Rhythm

Herodotos Ellinas, MD, FAAP/FACP
Associate Professor, Department of Anesthesiology
Residency Program Director
Medical College of Wisconsin
Milwaukee, Wisconsin
Chapter 27: Disorders of Cardiac Function, and Heart Failure and Circulatory Shock

Deena Garner, DNP, RN
Clinical Instructor
College of Nursing, Practice Department
University of Arkansas for Medical Sciences
Little Rock, Arkansas
Chapter 20: Disorders of Hearing and Vestibular Function

Sandeep Gopalakrishnan, PhD
Assistant Professor
College of Nursing
University of Wisconsin–Milwaukee
Milwaukee, Wisconsin
Chapter 7: Stress and Adaptation
Chapter 9: Inflammation, Tissue Repair, and Wound Healing
Chapter 12: Disorders of the Immune Response

Lisa Hight, EdD
Professor of Biology
General Education - Biomedical Sciences - Biology
Baptist College of Health Sciences
Memphis, Tennessee
Chapter 51: Structure and Function of the Skin
Chapter 52: Disorders of Skin Integrity and Function

Deborah L. Hopla, DNP, APRN-BC, FAANP
Associate Professor
Director MSN/FNP and DNP Programs
Amy V. Cockcroft Leadership Fellow
Department of Nursing
School of Health Sciences
Francis Marion University
Florence, South Carolina
Chapter 46: Sexually Transmitted Infections

Teresa Kessler, PhD, RN, ACNS-BC, CNE
Professor, Kreft Endowed Chair for the Advancement of Nursing Science
College of Nursing and Health Professions
Valparaiso University
Valparaiso, Indiana
Chapter 8: Disorders of Fluid, Electrolyte, and Acid–Base Balance

Christine Paquin Kurtz, DNP
Associate Professor
Nursing and Health Professions
Valparaiso University – College of Nursing
Valparaiso, Indiana
Chapter 17: Sleep and Sleep-Wake Disorders

Elizabeth M. Long, DNP, APRN-BC, CNS
Assistant Professor
School of Nursing
Lamar University
Beaumont, Texas
Chapter 18: Disorders of Thought, Emotion, and Memory

Tracy McClinton, DNP, AG-ACNP, BC
Assistant Professor
College of Nursing
University of Tennessee Health Science Center
Memphis, Tennessee
Chapter 30: Respiratory Tract Infections, and Neoplasms
Chapter 31: Disorders of Ventilation and Gas Exchange

Linda C. Mefford, PhD, MSN, APRN, NNP-BC, RNC-NIC
Associate Professor of Nursing
Lansing School of Nursing and Clinical Sciences
Bellarmine University
Louisville, Kentucky
Chapter 26: Disorders of Blood Flow and Blood Pressure Regulation
Chapter 32: Structure and Function of the Kidney
Chapter 33: Disorders of Renal Function
Chapter 40: Mechanisms of Endocrine Control
Chapter 41: Disorders of Endocrine Control

Sarah Morgan, PhD, RN
Clinical Associate Professor
College of Nursing
University of Wisconsin–Milwaukee
Milwaukee, Wisconsin
Chapter 47: Structure and Function of the Musculoskeletal System
Chapter 48: Disorders of Musculoskeletal Function: Trauma, Infection, Neoplasms
Chapter 50: Disorders of Musculoskeletal Function: Rheumatic Disorders

Nancy A. Moriber, PhD, MSN, BSN, CRNA, APRN
Assistant Professor
School of Nursing; Nurse Anesthesia
Fairfield University
Fairfield, Connecticut
CHAPTER 11: INNATE AND ADAPTIVE IMMUNITY

Emma Murray, DNP, APRN, ACNP-BC
Assistant Professor
College of Nursing
University of Tennessee Health Science Center
Memphis, Tennessee
CHAPTER 30: RESPIRATORY TRACT INFECTIONS, NEOPLASMS, AND CHILDHOOD DISORDERS
CHAPTER 31: DISORDERS OF VENTILATION AND GAS EXCHANGE

Cheryl Neudauer, PhD, MEd
Faculty
Department of Biology
Minneapolis Community and Technical College
Minneapolis, Minnesota
CHAPTER 2: CELL AND TISSUE CHARACTERISTICS

Stephanie Nikbakht, DNP, PPCNP-BC
Assistant Professor
College of Nursing
University of Tennessee Health Science Center
PNP, Division of Genetics
Le Bonheur Children's Hospital
Memphis, Tennessee
CHAPTER 30: RESPIRATORY TRACT INFECTIONS, NEOPLASMS, AND CHILDHOOD DISORDERS

Alyssa Norris, MS, RD, LDN, CLC
Clinical Dietitian II
Nutrition Therapy
Le Bonheur Children's Hospital
Memphis, Tennessee
CHAPTER 39: ALTERATIONS IN NUTRITIONAL STATUS

Keevia Porter, DNP, NP-C
Assistant Professor
College of Nursing
University of Tennessee Health Science Center
Memphis, Tennessee
CHAPTER 35: DISORDERS OF THE BLADDER AND LOWER URINARY TRACT

Michelle Rickard, DNP, CPNP-AC
Assistant Professor
College of Nursing
University of Tennessee Health Science Center
Memphis, Tennessee
CHAPTER 6: NEOPLASIA

Archie Sims, MSN
Nurse Practitioner
Hospitalist
Palmetto Health Tuomey
Sumter, South Carolina
CHAPTER 1: CONCEPTS OF HEALTH AND DISEASE

Diane Smith, DNP, FNP-BC
Clinical Professor
University of Wisconsin–Milwaukee
Milwaukee, Wisconsin
CHAPTER 19: DISORDERS OF VISUAL FUNCTION

Ansley Grimes Stanfill, PhD, RN
Assistant Professor
College of Nursing
University of Tennessee Health Science Center
Memphis, Tennessee
CHAPTER 4: GENETIC CONTROL OF CELL FUNCTION AND INHERITANCE
CHAPTER 5: GENETIC AND CONGENITAL DISORDERS

Sharon Stevenson, DNP, APRN, PPCNP-BC
Clinical Assistant Professor
College of Nursing, Practice Department
University of Arkansas for Medical Sciences
Little Rock, Arkansas
CHAPTER 20: DISORDERS OF HEARING AND VESTIBULAR FUNCTION

James Mark Tanner, DNP, RN
Assistant Clinical Professor
BSN Program Director
UAMS College of Nursing
University of Arkansas for Medical Sciences
Little Rock, Arkansas
CHAPTER 25: STRUCTURE AND FUNCTION OF THE CARDIOVASCULAR SYSTEM

Janet Tucker, PhD, RNC-OB
Assistant Professor
Loewenberg College of Nursing
University of Memphis
Memphis, Tennessee
CHAPTER 39: ALTERATIONS IN NUTRITIONAL STATUS

Reba A. Umberger, PhD, RN, CCRN-K
Assistant Professor
College of Nursing
University of Tennessee Health Science Center
Memphis, Tennessee
CHAPTER 10: MECHANISMS OF INFECTIOUS DISEASE
CHAPTER 32: STRUCTURE AND FUNCTION OF THE KIDNEY
CHAPTER 33: DISORDERS OF RENAL FUNCTION

Melody Waller, PhD, RN
Assistant Professor
College of Nursing
University of Tennessee Health Science Center
Memphis, Tennessee
Chapter 44: Structure and Function of the Female Reproductive system
Chapter 45: Disorders of the Female Reproductive System

Paige Wimberley, PhD, APRN, CNS-BC, CNE
Associate Professor
College of Nursing and Health Professions
Arkansas State University
Jonesboro, Arkansas
Chapter 22: Disorders of Hemostasis
Chapter 24: Disorders of White Blood Cells and Lymphoid Tissues

Sachin Yende, MD, MS
Professor
Department of Critical Care Medicine and Clinical and Translational Sciences
University of Pittsburgh
Pittsburgh, Pennsylvania
Chapter 10: Mechanisms of Infectious Disease

Contributors to the Ninth Edition

Cynthia Bautista, PhD, RN, CNRN, CCNS, ACNS-BC
Neuroscience Clinical Nurse Specialist
Yale New Haven Hospital
New Haven, Connecticut
(Chapters 17, 18, 19, 20)

Jaclyn Conelius, PhD, APRN, FNP-BC
Assistant Professor
Fairfield University School of Nursing
Fairfield, Connecticut
(Chapters 29, 30, 31, 32, 33, 34)

Sally O. Gerard, DNP, RN, CDE
Assistant Professor of Nursing and Coordinator, Nursing Leadership Track
Fairfield University School of Nursing
Fairfield, Connecticut
(Chapters 48, 50)

Lisa Grossman, MD, MPH
Administrative Chief Resident
Obstetrics/Gynecology
Columbia University Medical Center
New York, New York
(Chapters 6, 7, 53, 54, 55)

Theresa Kessler, PhD, RN, ACNS-BC, CNE
Professor
Valparaiso University
Valparaiso, Indiana
(Chapters 21, 40)

Melissa Kramps, DNP, APRN
Nurse Practitioner
Memory Disorders Center
New York, New York
(Chapter 3)

Zachary Krom, MSN, RN, CCRN
Service Line Educator: Adult Surgery
Yale New Haven Hospital
New Haven, Connecticut
(Chapters 44, 45, 46)

Christine Kurtz, DNP, PMHCNS-BC
Adjunct Assistant Professor
Valparaiso University College of Nursing
Valparaiso, Indiana
(Chapter 21)

Jessie Moore, MS, APRN
Program Coordinator, Weight Loss Surgery
Yale New Haven Hospital – Saint Raphael Campus
New Haven, Connecticut
(Chapter 47)

Nancy A. Moriber, PhD, CRNA, APRN
Visiting Assistant Professor and Director, Nurse Anesthesia Track
Fairfield University School of Nursing
Fairfield, Connecticut
(Chapters 13, 15)

Martha Burke O'Brien, MS, ANP-BC, APRN
Director of Student Health Services
Trinity College
Hartford, Connecticut
(Chapter 23)

Eileen O'Shea, PhD
Assistant Professor
Fairfield University School of Nursing
Fairfield, Connecticut
(Chapter 2)

Kathleen Wheeler, PhD, APRN, PMHNP-BC, FAAN
Professor
Fairfield University School of Nursing
Fairfield, Connecticut
(Chapter 22)

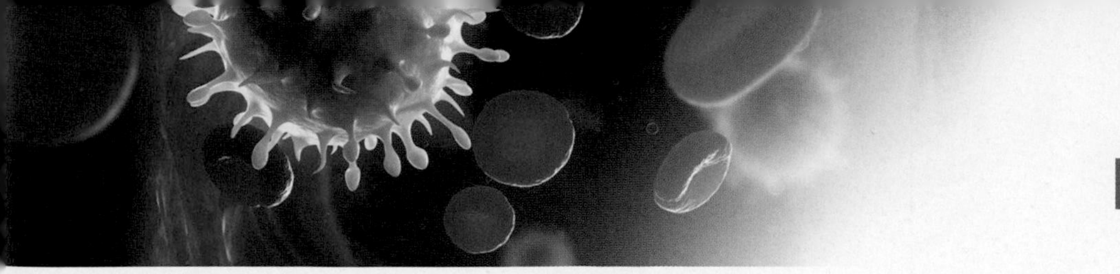

Reviewers

Brittny Chabalowski, RN, MSN, CEN, CNE, CHSE
Program Director
University of South Florida College of Nursing
Tampa, Florida

Susan Dentel
Professional Faculty
Washtenaw Community College
Ann Arbor, Michigan

Dr. Christi Jo Emerson, EdD, MSN, RN
Associate Professor
University of Mary Hardin-Baylor
Belton, Texas

Jill Guttormson, RN
Assistant Professor
Marquette University
Milwaukee, Wisconsin

Gina Hale, PhD, RN, CNE
Director of Recruitment and Retention
Lamar University
Beaumont, Texas

Lori Juza, RN, MSN
Instructor
Northeast Wisconsin Technical College
Green Bay, Wisconsin

Leslie Reifel, RN, MSN, CPNP, CNE
Associate Professor
Sentara College of Health Sciences
Chesapeake, Virginia

Michelle Roa, PhD, RN
Dean of Academic Affairs/Nursing
Good Samaritan College of Nursing and Health Science
Cincinnati, Ohio

Scott Seamans
Lecturer
Penn State University
Centre County, Pennsylvania

Jennifer Sofie, DNP, FNP-C, ANP-BC, RN
Associate Clinical Professor
Montana State University in Bozeman
Bozeman, Montana

Rupa Lalchandani Tuan, PhD
Assistant Professor
Notre Dame de Namur University
Belmont, California

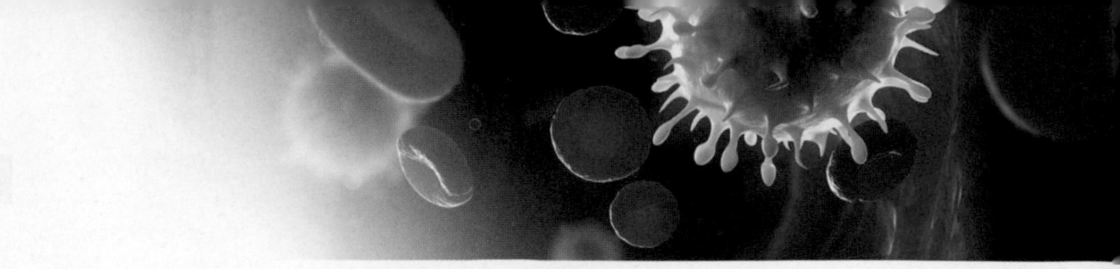

Preface

Since its first edition in 1982, *Porth's Pathophysiology* has grown to become a trusted and definitive resource for students, instructors, and health care professionals. The goal for each edition has been to develop a text that is current, accurate, and comprehensive, and presented in a logical manner. This book was written with the intent of making the subject of pathophysiology an exciting exploration that relates normal body functioning to the physiologic changes that occur as a result of disease, as well as the body's remarkable ability to compensate for these changes. Indeed, it is these changes that represent the signs and symptoms of disease.

Although this book's vision and objectives have remained consistent, this edition considers the many technological advances allowing health care providers to diagnose earlier and with more accuracy. Contributors from around the world and from diverse disciplines provided the expertise to make the information applicable to a broad audience. A strong foundation in pathophysiology is essential to give health care providers the clinical reasoning tools to critically analyze complex patient situations—both those that are common and those that are rare.

This text focuses on the scientific basis upon which the practice components of the health professions are based. The evidenced-based information garnered from the text provides practitioners with the knowledge for effective clinical decision-making within a dynamic profession.

A holistic conceptual framework uses body systems as an organizing structure and demonstrates how the systems are interrelated. Selection of content was based on common causes of morbidity and mortality across the life span, and recent advances in the fields of genetics, epigenetics, immunology, microbiology, and molecular biology are included. Concepts are presented in a manner that is logical and understandable for students. One goal of the new edition is to provide critical information needed to understand complex health alterations while delivering the content in a reader-friendly format. The chapters are arranged so that fundamental concepts such as cellular adaptation, inflammation and repair, genetic control of cell function and inheritance, and immunologic processes appear in the early chapters before the specific discussions of particular disease states.

Proven strengths of the text include the expanded chapters on health and disease; nutrition; sleep and sleep disorders; pediatrics; gerontology; and thought, emotion, and mood disorders. Advances in health care are presented through the inclusion of international studies, World Health Organization guidelines, updated standards, and the health variants of diverse populations.

ORGANIZATION

The units in this book identify broad areas of content, such as alterations in the circulatory system. Many of the units have an introductory chapter that contains essential information about the structure and function of the body systems that are being discussed in the unit. Each such chapter provides the foundation for understanding the pathophysiology content presented in the subsequent chapters. The chapter outline that appears at the beginning of each chapter provides an overall view of the chapter content and organization.

FEATURES OF THIS BOOK

This book includes the following special features to help you master the essential content.

Case Studies

Each unit opens with a case study that introduces a patient's case history and symptoms. Throughout some of the chapters in that unit, more information is added to the case as it relates to the information being presented, showing students an example of a real-life application of the content.

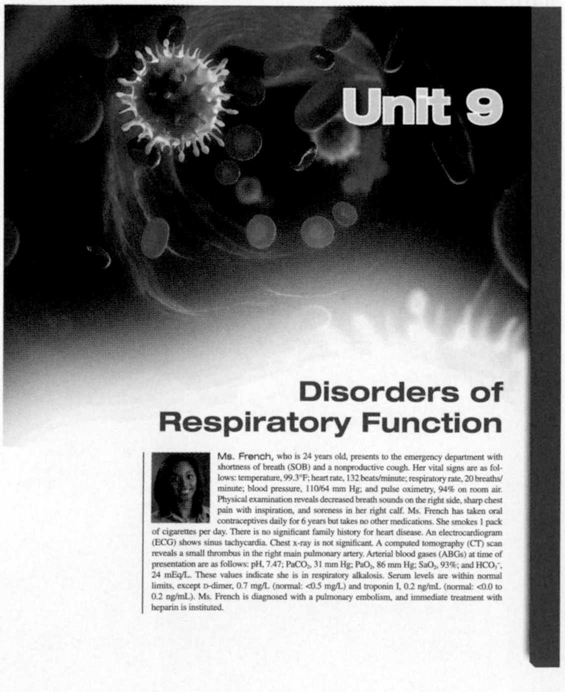
Unit 9

Disorders of Respiratory Function

Ms. French, who is 24 years old, presents to the emergency department with shortness of breath (SOB) and a nonproductive cough. Her vital signs are as follows: temperature, 99.3°F; heart rate, 132 beats/minute; respiratory rate, 20 breaths/minute; blood pressure, 110/64 mm Hg; and pulse oximetry, 94% on room air. Physical examination reveals decreased breath sounds on the right side, sharp chest pain with inspiration, and soreness in her right calf. Ms. French has taken oral contraceptives daily for 6 years but takes no other medications. She smokes 1 pack of cigarettes per day. There is no significant family history for heart disease. An electrocardiogram (ECG) shows sinus tachycardia. Chest x-ray is not significant. A computed tomography (CT) scan reveals a small thrombus in the right main pulmonary artery. Arterial blood gases (ABGs) at time of presentation are as follows: pH, 7.47; $PaCO_2$, 31 mm Hg; PaO_2, 86 mm Hg; SaO_2, 93%; and HCO_3^-, 24 mEq/L. These values indicate she is in respiratory alkalosis. Serum levels are within normal limits, except D-dimer, 0.7 mg/L (normal: <0.5 mg/L) and troponin I, 0.2 ng/mL (normal: <0.0 to 0.2 ng/mL). Ms. French is diagnosed with a pulmonary embolism, and immediate treatment with heparin is instituted.

Objectives

Objectives appear at the beginning of each major section of content to provide a focus for your study. After you have finished each of these areas of content, you may want to go back and make sure that you have met each of the objectives.

CELL INJURY AND DEATH

After completing this section of the chapter, the learner will be able to meet the following objectives:

- Describe the mechanisms whereby physical agents such as blunt trauma, electrical forces, and extremes of temperature produce cell injury.
- Differentiate between the effects of ionizing and nonionizing radiation in terms of their ability to cause cell injury.
- State the mechanisms and manifestations of cell injury associated with lead poisoning.
- Relate free radical formation and oxidative stress to cell injury and death.

Key Terms and Glossary

It is essential for any professional to use and understand the vocabulary of his or her profession. Throughout the text, you will encounter key terms in bold purple. This is a signal that a word and the ideas associated with it are important to learn. In addition, a glossary is provided to help you expand your vocabulary and improve your comprehension of what you are reading. The glossary contains concise definitions of frequently encountered terms. If you are unsure of the meaning of a term you encounter in your reading, check the glossary in the back of the book before proceeding.

Normally, sleep and wakefulness occur in a cyclic manner, integrated into the 24-hour light–dark solar day. The term **circadian**, from the Latin *circa* ("about") and *dies* ("day"), is used to describe these 24-hour diurnal rhythms. The function of the circadian time system is to provide a temporal organization for physiologic processes and behaviors as a means of promoting effective adaptation to the environment. At the behavioral level, this is expressed in regular cycles of sleep and waking and body functions such as temperature regulation and hormone secretion based on changes in the 24-hour light–dark solar day.

Boxes

Boxes are used throughout the text to summarize and highlight key information.

"Key Points" Boxes

One of the ways to approach learning is to focus on the major ideas or concepts rather than trying to memorize a list of related and unrelated bits of information. Health care providers must apply these concepts in the clinical setting, which requires an understanding of the underlying etiology, histology, symptoms, risk factors, and hallmark features of a particular disease. As you have probably already discovered, it is impossible to memorize everything that is in a particular section or chapter of the book. Not only does your brain have a difficult time trying to figure out where to store all the different bits of information, your brain does not know how to retrieve the information when you need it. Most important of all, memorized lists of content can seldom, if ever, be applied directly to an actual clinical situation. The "Key Points" boxes guide you in identifying the major ideas or concepts that form the foundation for truly understanding the major areas of content. When you understand the concepts in the "Key Points" boxes, you will have a framework for remembering and using the facts given in the text.

KEY POINTS

FUNCTIONS OF THE SKIN

- The skin prevents body fluids from leaving the body, protects the body from potentially damaging environmental agents, and serves as an area for heat exchange. In addition, cells of the skin immune system provide protection against invading microorganisms.
- Receptors in the skin relay touch, pressure, temperature, and pain sensation to the central nervous system for localization and discrimination.

"In Summary" Boxes

The "In Summary" boxes at the end of each main section provide a review and a reinforcement of the important content that has been covered. Use the summaries to ensure that you have covered and understood what you have read.

IN SUMMARY

Physiologic and psychological adaptation involves the ability to maintain the constancy of the internal environment (homeostasis) and behavior in the face of a wide range of changes in the internal and external environments. It involves control and negative feedback systems that regulate cellular function, control life's processes, regulate behavior, and integrate the function of the different body systems.

"Understanding" Boxes

"Understanding" boxes focus on the physiologic processes and phenomena that form the basis for understanding disorders presented in the text. This feature breaks a process or phenomenon down into its component parts and presents it in a sequential manner, providing an insight into the many opportunities for disease processes to disrupt the sequence.

Understanding **The Hemodynamics of Blood Flow** *(Continued)*

Vessel Radius

In addition to pressure and resistance, the rate of blood flow through a vessel is affected by the fourth power of its radius (the radius multiplied by itself four times). Thus, blood flow in vessel B with a radius of 2 mm will be 16 times greater than in vessel A with a radius of 1 mm.

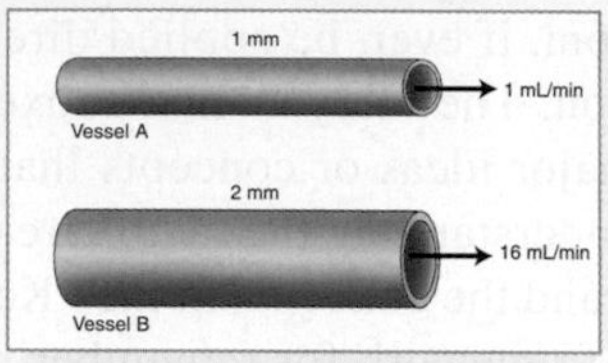

Cross-Sectional Area and Velocity of Flow

The velocity or rate of forward movement of the blood is affected by the cross-sectional area of a blood vessel. As the cross-sectional area of a vessel increases (sections 1 and 3), blood must flow laterally as well as forward to fill the increased area. As a result, the mean forward velocity decreases. In contrast, when the cross-sectional area is decreased (section 2), the lateral flow decreases and the mean forward velocity is increased.

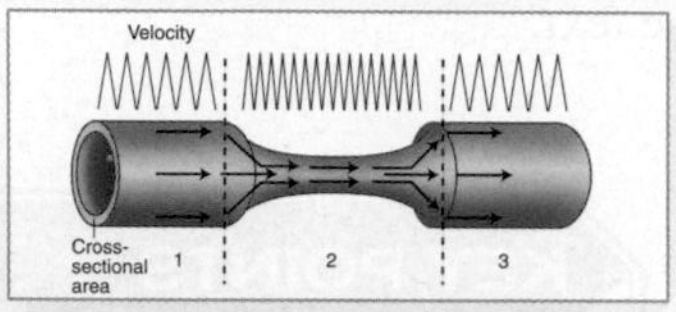

"Geriatric Considerations" and "Pediatric Considerations" Boxes

"Geriatric Considerations" and "Pediatric Considerations" boxes at the end of each chapter provide insight on how the content of the chapter is reflected in these two populations. These life span considerations highlight variations that can be attributed to age—for example, the immaturity of the immune system of newborns and the decreased phagocytic action in older adults, both of which increase the risk for disease.

GERIATRIC Considerations

- Hematocrit levels in both men and women are lower after age 60 because of a decreased production of RBCs by the bone marrow, leading to fatigue.[19]
- The most common hematologic system disorder in aging is anemia, which can be attributed to decreased production of RBCs and chronic illnesses or infections.[20]
- Anemia in the elderly should be investigated; it is never normal.[20]
- Nutrient deficiencies lead to alteration in RBCs. Folate, vitamin B_{12} (pernicious anemia), and vitamin C deficiencies are more common in older adults because of altered absorption, interference by medications, and malabsorption.[20]

PEDIATRIC Considerations

- Children are at risk for infectious disease because their immune systems are still developing and they tend to place hands and potentially infected objects in the mouth.[48]
- Vaccines, both old and new, have led to a significant decrease in the number and severity of infections.[48]
- Pediatric daycare and schoolrooms have common rooms, placing children at risk for transmission of infectious agents.[48]
- The presence of a rash is common in many infections that are a challenge to identify. A thorough description and history from the caregiver are the key to assessment.[48]
- Although most infections in children manifest with fever, neonates may be hypothermic with an infection, and other children may have no fever.[49]

Tables and Charts

Tables and charts are designed to present complex information in a format that makes it more meaningful and facilitates recall of the information. Tables, which have two or more columns, are often used for the purpose of comparing or contrasting information. Charts, which have one column, are used to summarize information.

TABLE 20.1 COMMON DISORDERS AFFECTING THE VESTIBULAR SYSTEM

TYPE OF DISORDER	PATHOLOGY
Acoustic neuroma	A noncancerous growth or tumor on the vestibulocochlear nerve
Benign paroxysmal positional vertigo (BPPV)	Disorder of otoliths
Ménière disease	Dislodgement of otoliths that participate in the receptor function of the vestibular system
Motion sickness	Repeated stimulation of the vestibular system such as during car, air, and boat travel
Labyrinthitis	Acute viral or bacterial infection of the vestibular pathways
Vestibular migraine	Dizziness or vertigo occurs with or without headache; related to the neurotransmitter serotonin

Illustrations and Photos

The detailed, full-color illustrations will help you to build your own mental image of the content that is being presented. Each drawing has been developed to fully support and build upon the ideas in the text. Some illustrations are used to help you picture the complex interactions of the multiple phenomena that are involved in the development of a particular disease; others can help you to visualize normal function or understand the mechanisms that enable the disease processes to exert their effects. In addition, photographs provide a realistic view of selected pathologic processes and lesions.

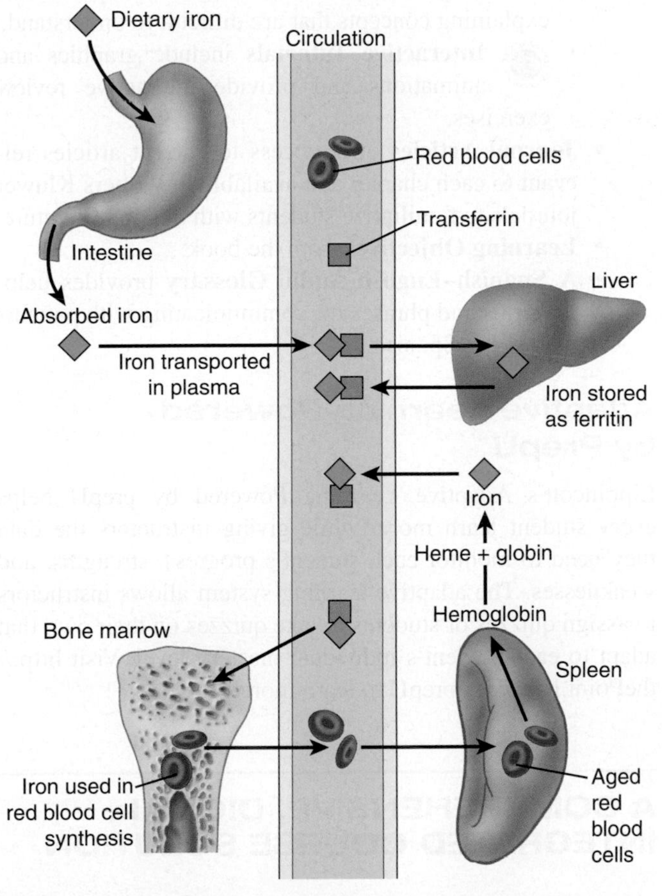

Figure 23.3 • Diagrammatic representation of the iron cycle, including its absorption from the gastrointestinal tract, transport in the circulation, storage in the liver, recycling from aged red cells destroyed in the spleen, and use in the bone marrow synthesis of red blood cells.

Concept Mastery Alerts

Concept Mastery Alerts clarify fundamental nursing concepts to improve the reader's understanding of potentially confusing topics, as identified by Misconception Alerts in Lippincott's Adaptive Learning Powered by prepU.

Concept Mastery Alert

The electricity in nonsynchronized defibrillation depolarizes the entire heart, interrupting the chaotic rhythm and allowing the SA node to take control.

Interactive Learning Resources

Interactive learning tools available online enrich learning and are identified with icons in the text.

- **Concepts in Action Animations** bring physiologic and pathophysiologic concepts to life, explaining concepts that are difficult to understand.
- **Interactive Tutorials** include graphics and animations and provide interactive review exercises.

Review Exercises

The Review Exercises at the end of each chapter are designed to help integrate and synthesize material and to help you verify your understanding of the material presented. If you are unable to answer a question, reread the relevant section in the chapter. (Answers are available for instructors at http://thepoint.lww.com/Porth10e.)

REVIEW EXERCISES

1. A 75-year-old woman with a history of congestive heart failure presents to the clinic complaining of feeling tired. Her heart rate is 121 beats/minute, and the rhythm is irregular.
   A. *What type of arrhythmia do you think she might be having? What would it look like if you were to obtain an ECG?*
   B. *What causes this irregularity?*
   C. *Why do you think she is feeling tired?*
   D. *What are some of the concerns with this type of arrhythmia?*
2. A 45-year-old man appears at the urgent care center with complaints of chest discomfort, shortness of breath, and generally not feeling well. You assess vital signs and find that his temperature is 99.2°F, blood pressure 180/90, pulse 90 and slightly irregular, and respiratory rate 26. You do an ECG, and the readings from the anterior leads indicate that he is experiencing an ischemic episode.
   A. *You attach him to a cardiac monitor and see that his underlying rhythm is normal sinus rhythm, but he is having frequent premature contractions that are more than 0.10 second in duration. What type of premature contractions do you suspect?*
   B. *What would you expect his pulse to feel like?*
   C. *What do you think the etiology of this arrhythmia might be? How might it be treated?*

Appendix

The appendix, "Lab Values," provides rapid access to normal values for many laboratory tests, as well as a description of the prefixes, symbols, and factors (*e.g.,* micro, μ, 10^{-6}) used for describing these values. Knowledge of normal values can help you to put abnormal values in context.

A COMPREHENSIVE PACKAGE FOR TEACHING AND LEARNING

To further facilitate teaching and learning, a carefully designed ancillary package has been developed to assist faculty and students.

Instructor Resources

Tools to assist you with teaching your course are available upon adoption of this text on thePoint® at http://thepoint.lww.com/Porth10e.

- A **Test Generator** features NCLEX-style questions mapped to chapter learning objectives.
- An extensive collection of materials is provided for each book chapter:
  - **Pre-lecture Quizzes** (and answers) allow you to check students' reading.
  - **PowerPoint Presentations** provide an easy way to integrate the textbook with your students' classroom experience; multiple-choice and true/false questions are included to promote class participation.
  - **Guided Lecture Notes** walk you through the chapter, learning objective by learning objective, with integrated references to the PowerPoint presentations.
  - **Discussion Topics** (and suggested answers) can be used in the classroom or in online discussion boards to facilitate interaction with your students.
  - **Assignments** (and suggested answers) include group, written, clinical, and Web assignments to engage students in varied activities and assess their learning.
  - **Case Studies** with related questions (and suggested answers) give students an opportunity to apply their knowledge to a client case similar to one they might encounter in practice.
  - **Answers to the Review Exercises** in the book facilitate review of student responses to these exercises.
- Sample **Syllabi** are provided for 14-week and 28-week courses.
- An **Image Bank** lets you use the photographs and illustrations from this textbook in your course materials.
- An **ebook** serves as a handy resource.
- **Strategies for Effective Teaching** provides general tips for instructors related to preparing course materials and meeting student needs.
- **Dosage Calculation Quizzes** and **Drug Monographs** are convenient references.
- Access to all **Student Resources** is provided so that you can understand the student experience and use these resources in your course as well.

Student Resources

An exciting set of free learning resources is available on thePoint® to help students review and apply vital concepts. Multimedia engines have been optimized so that students can access many of these resources on mobile devices. Students can access all these resources at http://thepoint.lww.com/Porth10e using the codes printed in the front of their textbooks.

- **NCLEX-Style Review Questions** for each chapter help students review important concepts and practice for NCLEX.
- **Interactive learning resources** appeal to a variety of learning styles. As mentioned previously in this preface, icons in the text direct readers to relevant resources:
  - **Concepts in Action Animations** bring physiologic and pathophysiologic concepts to life, explaining concepts that are difficult to understand.
  - **Interactive Tutorials** include graphics and animations and provide interactive review exercises.
- **Journal Articles** offer access to current articles relevant to each chapter and available in Wolters Kluwer journals to familiarize students with nursing literature.
- **Learning Objectives** from the book.
- **A Spanish–English Audio Glossary** provides helpful terms and phrases for communicating with patients who speak Spanish.

Adaptive Learning Powered by PrepU

Lippincott's Adaptive Learning Powered by prepU helps every student learn more, while giving instructors the data they need to monitor each student's progress, strengths, and weaknesses. The adaptive learning system allows instructors to assign quizzes or students to take quizzes on their own that adapt to each student's individual mastery level. Visit http://thePoint.lww.com/prepU to learn more.

A COMPREHENSIVE, DIGITAL, INTEGRATED COURSE SOLUTION

Lippincott CoursePoint is an integrated digital learning solution designed for the way students learn. It is the only nursing education solution that integrates:

- **Leading content in context:** Content provided in the context of the student learning path engages students and encourages interaction and learning on a deeper level.
  - The interactive ebook features content updates based on the latest evidence-based practices and provides students with anytime, anywhere access on multiple devices.
  - Multimedia resources, including animations and interactive tutorials, walk students through knowledge application and address multiple learning styles.
  - Full online access to *Stedman's Medical Dictionary for Health Professions and Nursing* ensures students work with the best medical dictionary available.

- **Powerful tools to maximize class performance:** Course-specific tools, such as adaptive learning powered by prepU, provide a personalized learning experience for every student.
- **Real-time data to measure students' progress:** Student performance data provided in an intuitive display lets you quickly spot which students are having difficulty or which concepts the class as a whole is struggling to grasp.
- **Training services and personalized support:** To ensure your success, our dedicated educational consultants and training coaches will provide expert guidance every step of the way.

ACKNOWLEDGMENTS

The history of the text is rich, and I would be remiss if I didn't thank the original and long-time editor, Dr. Carol Porth, who forged the "nurse–physiologist" approach that is still the hallmark signature of the book; this text is built on her insights. The expertise of the contributors, both current and previous, keeps the book at the forefront of advances in science and medicine. Their attention to detail and desire to share current, relevant, and essential information with learners is to be applauded. For the 10th edition, several chapters were merged to improve flow of content, requiring both extra time and talent of the contributors. Thanks also to Dr. Rupa Lalchandani Tuan for her diligence in ensuring the accuracy of the information contained in the book.

I would like to thank Kelley Squazzo, Executive Editor, for allowing me to serve as editor for this project. Many thanks go to Meredith Brittain, Senior Development Editor, for her many suggestions, revisions, and reminders of due dates. Tim Rinehart, who tracked our progress and encouraged contributors to submit their chapters, kept the entire team informed.

I would also like to thank my peers, who shared my enthusiasm. Lastly, I want to thank my family for understanding when so much of my time was devoted to the project and for allowing me to share my excitement about the impact the book will have on learners as they strive to apply the evidenced-based information to improve patient outcomes.

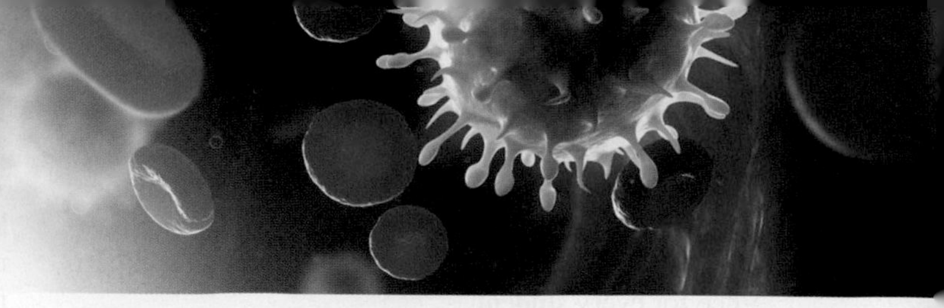

Contents

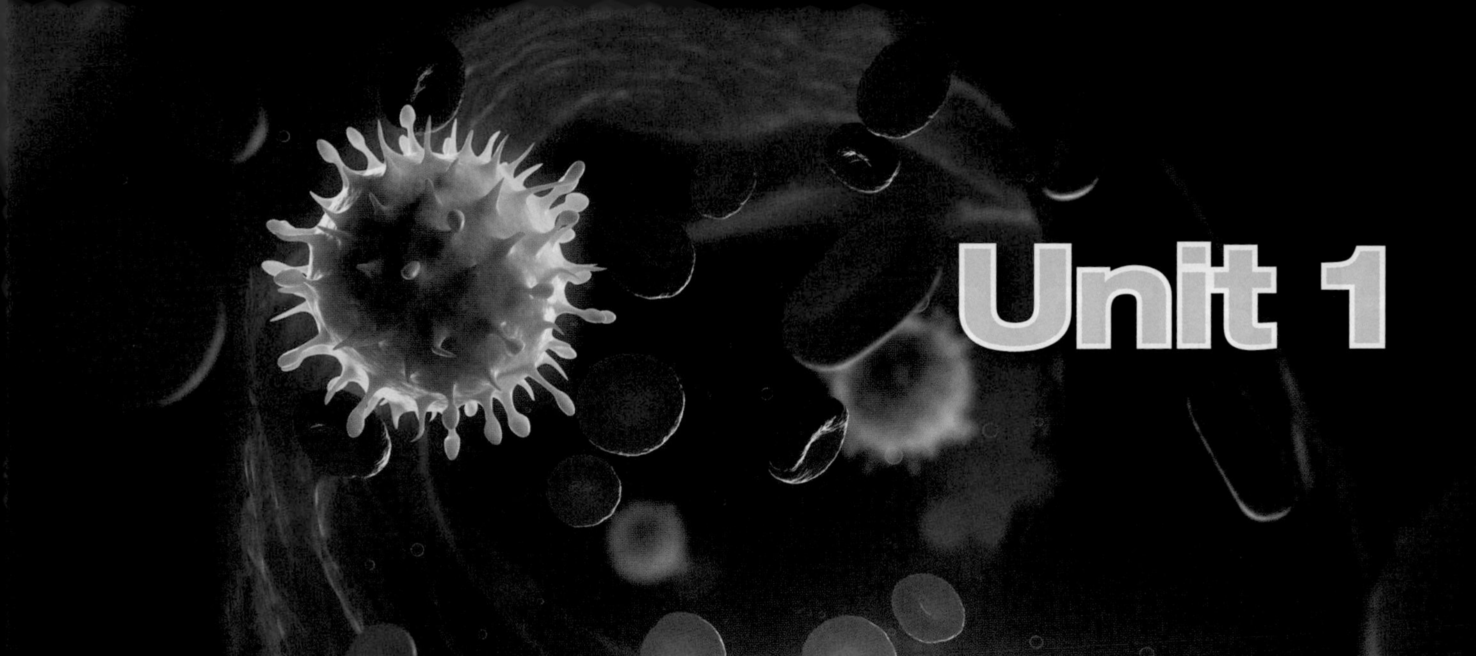

Unit 1

Concepts of Health and Disease

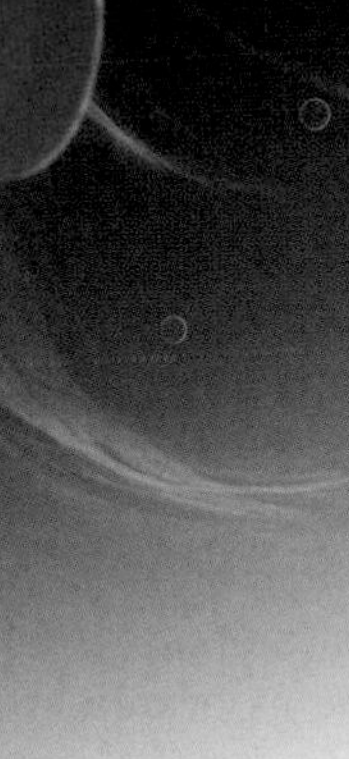

Mrs. Sora, 85 years old, was born during the Great Depression. She is a widow who has recently moved in with her daughter because her only income is social security. She presents with soreness and back pain, describing "a tingling and burning feeling on the left side of my back just above my waist." The discomfort started about 2 days ago, and she thought it would go away. However, it has increased in intensity, and this morning, she noticed a rash over the painful region.

Her daughter suspects that her mother's vision has declined, because she has had a few recent falls in the evenings. The daughter is also concerned about her mother's loss of hearing acuity and appetite and her growing fatigue. The daughter adds that her mom was hospitalized for pneumonia about 4 months ago and became very confused during the course of the illness.

Mrs. Sora's vital signs are all within normal limits (blood pressure = 122/68 mm Hg, pulse = 77, respiratory rate = 14/minute, and temperature = 98.8°F). Physical examination of the rash on Mrs. Sora's back reveals grouped vesicular papules over the T7 left side dermatome. Discomfort is felt with light palpation. Upon further questioning, Mrs. Sora says, "Yes, I had chicken pox when I was in first grade." The rash is diagnosed as varicella-zoster virus (VZV).

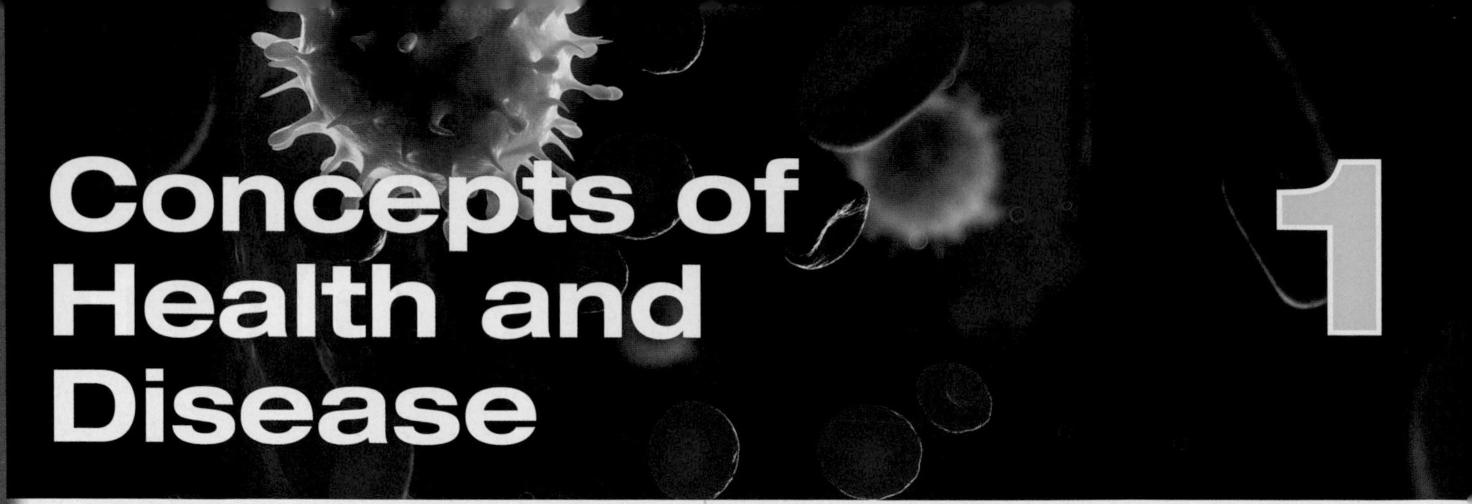

Concepts of Health and Disease

1

Archie Sims

CONCEPTS OF HEALTH AND DISEASE
- Health
- Disease
  - *Etiology*
  - *Pathogenesis*
  - *Morphology and Histology*
  - *Clinical Manifestations*
  - *Diagnosis*
  - *Clinical Course*

HEALTH AND DISEASE IN POPULATIONS
- Epidemiology and Patterns of Disease
  - *Incidence and Prevalence*
  - *Morbidity and Mortality*
- Determination of Risk Factors
  - *Cross-Sectional and Case–Control Studies*
  - *Cohort Studies*
- Natural History
- Preventing Disease
- Evidence-Based Practice and Practice Guidelines

The term *pathophysiology*, which is the focus of this book, may be defined as the physiology of altered health. The term combines the words *pathology* and *physiology*. Pathology (from the Greek *pathos*, meaning "disease") deals with the study of the structural and functional changes in cells, tissues, and organs of the body that cause or are caused by disease. Physiology deals with the functions of the human body. Thus, pathophysiology deals not only with the cellular and organ changes that occur with disease but also with the effects that these changes have on total body function (Fig. 1.1). Examples of atrophy of the brain (Fig. 1.1A) and hypertrophy of the myocardium (Fig. 1.1B) illustrate pathophysiologic changes from a cerebrovascular accident to long-standing unmanaged hypertension and how this impacts the myocardium. Pathophysiology also focuses on the mechanisms of the underlying disease and provides information to assist with planning preventive as well as therapeutic health care measures and practices such as following a healthy diet, exercising, and being compliant with prescribed medications. This chapter is intended to orient the reader to the concepts of health and disease, various terms that are used throughout the book, the sources of data and what they mean, and the broader aspects of pathophysiology in terms of the health and well-being of populations.

CONCEPTS OF HEALTH AND DISEASE

After completing this section of the chapter, the learner will be able to meet the following objectives:

- State the World Health Organization definition of health.
- Define *pathophysiology*.
- Explain the meaning of reliability, validity, sensitivity, specificity, and predictive value as it relates to observations and tests used in the diagnosis of disease.

What constitutes health and disease often is difficult to determine because of the way different people view the topic. What is defined as health is determined by many factors,

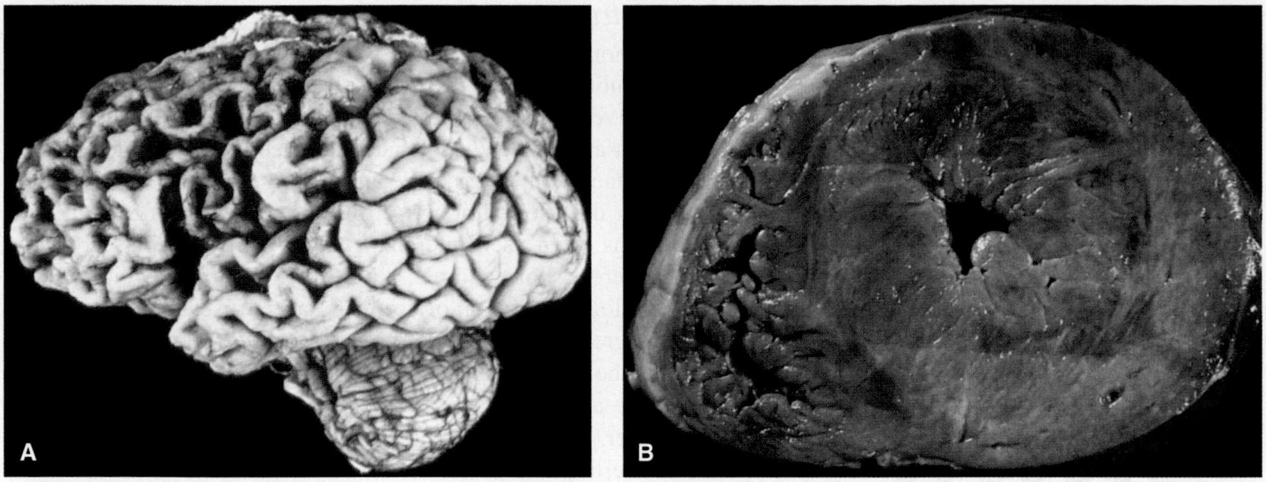

Figure 1.1 • **(A)** Atrophy of the frontal lobe of the brain. The gyri are thin and the sulci are extremely wide. **(B)** Myocardial hypertrophy. This cross-section of the heart illustrates left ventricular hypertrophy because of long-standing hypertension. (From Strayer D. S., Rubin R. (2015). *Rubin's pathology: Clinicopathologic foundations of medicine* (7th ed., p. 16). Philadelphia, PA: Lippincott Williams & Wilkins.)

including genetics, age, gender, cultural, and ethnic differences, as well as individual, group, and governmental expectations.

Health

In 1948, the Preamble to the Constitution of the World Health Organization (WHO) defined health as a "state of complete physical, mental, and social well-being and not merely the absence of disease and infirmity," a definition that has not been amended since that time.[1] Although ideal for many people, this was an unrealistic goal. The U.S. Department of Health and Human Services in *Healthy People 2020* describes the determinants of health as

1. Attain lives free of preventable disease, disability, injury, and premature death.
2. Achieve health equity and eliminate disparities.
3. Promote good health for all.
4. Promote healthy behaviors across the life span.[2]

Every decade, the U.S. Department of Health and Human Services spearheads initiatives to facilitate the goals of the new decade in their report such as the current *Healthy People 2020*. These consensus reports are developed to specifically assist in preventing some health problems and to offer advice to promote health as defined by the WHO.

Disease

A disease is considered an acute or chronic illness that one acquires or is born with that causes physiologic dysfunction in one or more body system. Each disease generally has specific signs and symptoms that characterize its pathology and identifiable etiology. The aspects of the disease process include etiology, pathogenesis, morphologic changes, clinical manifestations, diagnosis, and clinical course.

Etiology

The causes of disease are known as *etiologic factors*. Among the recognized etiologic agents are biologic agents (*e.g.*, bacteria, viruses), physical forces (*e.g.*, trauma, burns, radiation), chemical agents (*e.g.*, poisons, alcohol), one's genetic inheritance, and nutritional excesses or deficits.

Most disease-causing agents are nonspecific, and many different agents can cause disease of a single organ. On the other hand, a single agent or traumatic event can lead to disease of a number of organs or systems. For example, in cystic fibrosis, sickle cell anemia, and familial hypercholesterolemia, a single amino acid, transporter molecule, or receptor protein produces widespread pathology. Although a disease agent can affect more than a single organ and a number of disease agents can affect the same organ, most disease states do not have a single cause. Instead, the majority of diseases are multifactorial in origin. This is particularly true of diseases such as cancer, heart disease, and diabetes. This is illustrated in Figure 1.2, which traces the five causes of cancer and the pathophysiology that evolves from the disease mechanisms triggered by the causes. The multiple factors that predispose to a particular disease often are referred to as *risk factors*.

One way to view the factors that cause disease is to group them into categories according to whether they were present at birth or acquired later in life. *Congenital conditions* are defects that are present at birth, although they may not be evident until later in life or may never manifest. Congenital conditions may be caused by genetic influences, environmental factors (*e.g.*, viral infections in the mother, maternal drug use, irradiation, or gestational position in utero), or a combination of genetic and environmental factors. *Acquired defects* are those that are caused by events that occur after birth. These include injury, exposure to infectious agents, inadequate nutrition, lack of oxygen, inappropriate immune responses, and neoplasia. Many diseases are thought to be

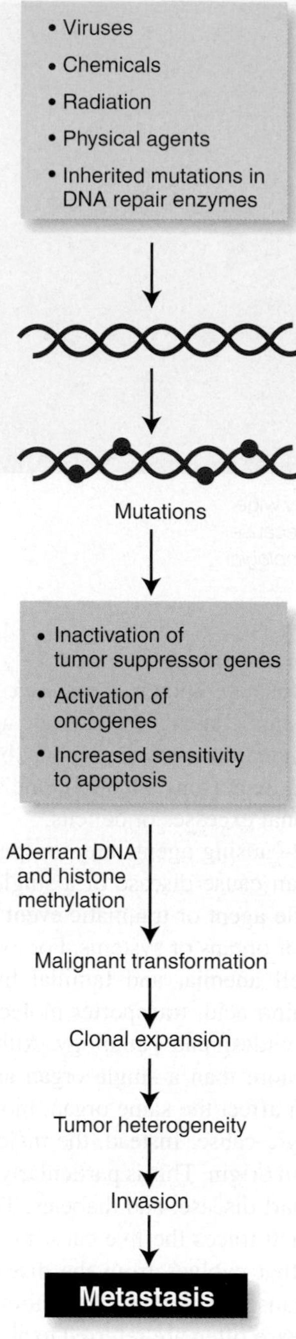

Figure 1.2 • Summary of the general mechanisms of cancer. (From Strayer D. S., Rubin R. (2015). *Rubin's pathology: Clinicopathologic foundations of medicine* (7th ed., p. 231). Philadelphia, PA: Lippincott Williams & Wilkins.)

the result of a genetic predisposition and an environmental event or events that serve as a trigger to initiate disease development. There are 35,000 genes in the human genome, 1 to 10 million proteins, and 2 to 3000 metabolites of the human metabolome.[3] Huge advances in molecular biology and the wide variability of people have led to evolution in systems biology and personalized medicine. This will assist in identifying etiology of disease and in the development of individualized interventions.[3]

Pathogenesis

Although etiology describes what sets the disease process in motion, *pathogenesis* explains how the disease process evolves. In other words, pathogenesis is the sequence of cellular and tissue events that take place from the time of initial contact with an etiologic agent until the ultimate expression of a disease. Although etiology and pathogenesis are two terms often used interchangeably, their meanings are quite different. For example, atherosclerosis often is cited as the etiology (or cause) of coronary artery disease. In reality, the progression of the inflammatory process from a fatty streak to the occlusive vessel lesion seen in people with coronary artery disease represents the pathogenesis of the disorder. The true etiology of atherosclerosis remains largely uncertain.

Morphology and Histology

Morphology refers to the fundamental structure or form of cells or tissues. *Morphologic changes* are concerned with both the gross anatomic and microscopic changes that are characteristic of a disease. **Histology** deals with the study of the cells and extracellular matrix of body tissues. The most common method used in the study of tissues is the preparation of histologic sections—thin, translucent sections of human tissues and organs—that can be examined with the aid of a microscope. Histologic sections play an important role in the diagnosis of many types of cancer. A **lesion** represents a pathologic or traumatic discontinuity of a body organ or tissue. Descriptions of lesion size and characteristics often can be obtained through the use of radiographs, ultrasonography, and other imaging methods. Lesions also may be sampled by biopsy and the tissue samples subjected to histologic study. Diagnostic pathology has evolved greatly in the last few years to include immunologic and molecular biologic tools for studying disease states[4] (Fig. 1.3).

Clinical Manifestations

Diseases can manifest in a number of ways. Sometimes, the condition produces manifestations, such as fever, that make it evident that the person is sick. In other cases, the condition is silent at the onset and is detected during examination for other purposes or after the disease is far advanced.

Signs and *symptoms* are terms used to describe the structural and functional changes that accompany a disease. A *symptom* is a subjective complaint that is noted by the person with a disorder, whereas a *sign* is a manifestation that is noted by an observer. Pain, difficulty in breathing, and dizziness are symptoms of a disease. An elevated temperature, a swollen extremity, and changes in pupil size are objective signs that can be observed by someone other than the person with the disease. Signs and symptoms may be related to the primary disorder, or they may represent the body's attempt to compensate for the altered function caused by the pathologic condition. Many pathologic states are not observed directly. For example, one cannot see that a person is hemorrhaging or

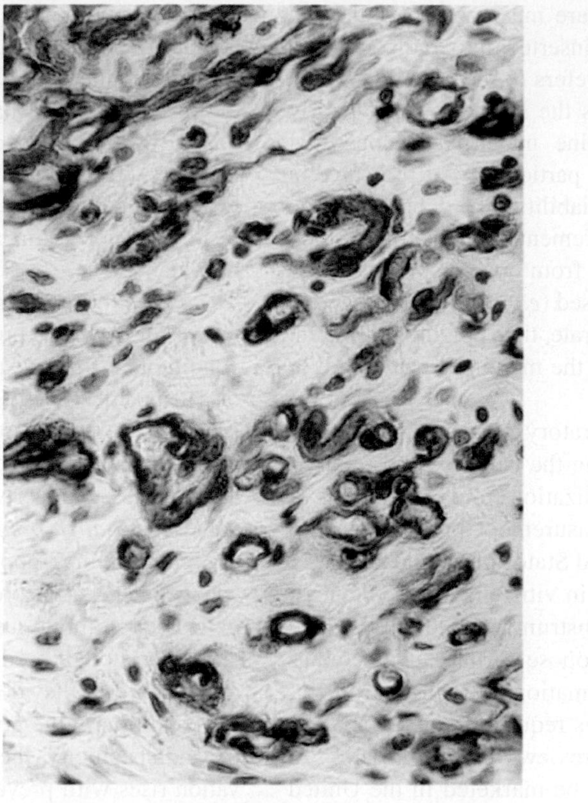

Figure 1.3 • Granulation tissue. A photomicrograph of granulation tissue shows thin-walled capillary spouts immunostained to highlight the basement membrane collagens. The infiltrating capillaries penetrate a loose connective tissue matrix containing mesenchymal cells and occasional inflammatory cells. (From Rubin R., Strayer D. S. (2015). *Rubin's pathology: Clinicopathologic foundations of medicine* (7th ed., p. 113. Figure 3-9). Philadelphia, PA: Lippincott Williams & Wilkins.)

that he or she has decreased pulmonary gas exchange. Instead, what can be observed is the body's attempt to compensate for changes in function brought about by the disease, such as the tachycardia that accompanies blood loss or the increased respiratory rate that occurs with pneumonia.

A **syndrome** is a compilation of signs and symptoms (*e.g.*, chronic fatigue syndrome) that are characteristic of a specific disease state. *Complications* are possible adverse extensions of a disease or outcomes from treatment. *Sequelae* are lesions or impairments that follow or are caused by a disease.

Diagnosis

A *diagnosis* is the designation as to the nature or cause of a health problem (*e.g.*, bacterial pneumonia or hemorrhagic stroke). The diagnostic process requires a careful history, physical examination (PE), and diagnostic tests. The history is used to obtain a person's account of his or her symptoms and their progression and the factors that contribute to a diagnosis. The PE is done to observe for signs of altered body structure or function. The diagnostic tests are ordered to validate what is thought to be the problem. They are also performed to determine other possible health problems that were not obtained from the history and PE, but may be present given the signs and symptoms identified.

The development of a diagnosis involves weighing competing possibilities and selecting the most likely one from among the conditions that might be responsible for the person's clinical presentation. The clinical probability of a given disease in a person of a given age, gender, race, lifestyle, genetic background, and locality often is influential in arrival at a presumptive diagnosis. Laboratory tests and imaging are used to confirm a diagnosis.

An important factor when interpreting diagnostic test results is the determination of whether they are normal or abnormal. Is a blood count above normal, within the normal range, or below normal? What is termed a *normal* value for a laboratory test is established statistically from test results obtained from a selected sample of people. A normal value represents the test results that fall within the bell curve or the 95% distribution. Thus, the normal levels for serum sodium (136 to 145 mEq/L) represent the mean serum level for the reference population ±2 standard deviations. The normal values for some laboratory tests are adjusted for gender, other comorbidities, or age. For example, the normal hemoglobin range for women is 12.0 to 16.0 g/dL and for men, 14.0 to 17.4 g/dL.[5] Serum creatinine level often is adjusted for age in the elderly, and normal values for serum phosphate differ between adults and children.

Laboratory parameters are interpreted based on the reliability, validity, sensitivity, and specificity of the measurement.[5,6] *Validity* refers to the extent to which a measurement tool measures what it is intended to measure. For example, the validity of blood pressure measurements obtained by a sphygmomanometer might be compared with those obtained by intra-arterial findings, which are measurements obtained from invasive arterial catheters inserted into radial arteries of acutely ill people. *Reliability* refers to the extent to which an observation, if repeated, gives the same result. A poorly calibrated blood pressure machine may give inconsistent measurements of blood pressure, particularly of pressures in either the high or low range. Reliability also depends on the person's skill in taking the measurements. For example, blood pressure measurements may vary from one person to another because of the technique that is used (*e.g.*, different observers may deflate the cuff at a different rate, thus obtaining different values), the way the numbers on the manometer are read, or differences in hearing acuity.

In the field of clinical laboratory measurements, *standardization* is aimed at increasing the trueness and reliability of measured values. Standardization relies on the use of written standards, reference measurement procedures, and reference materials.[7] In the United States, the Food and Drug Administration (FDA) regulates in vitro diagnostic devices, including clinical laboratory instruments, test kits, and reagents. Manufacturers who propose to market new diagnostic devices must submit information on their instrument, test kit, or reagent to the FDA, as required by existing statutes and regulations. The FDA reviews this information to decide whether the product may be marketed in the United States.

Measures of sensitivity and specificity are concerned with determining how likely or how well the test or observation will identify people with the disease and people without the disease[5,6] (Fig. 1.4). *Sensitivity* refers to the proportion of people with a disease who are positive for that disease on a given test or observation (called a *true positive* result). If the result of a very sensitive test is negative, it tells us the person does not have the disease and the disease has been excluded or "ruled out." *Specificity* refers to the proportion

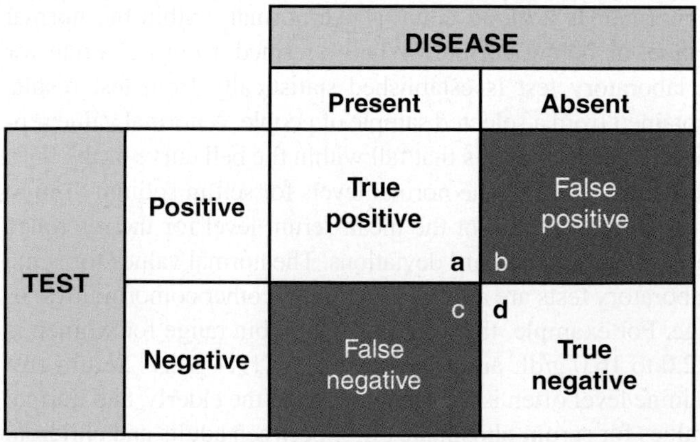

Figure 1.4 • The relationship between a diagnostic test result and the occurrence of disease. There are two possibilities for the test result to be correct (true positive and true negative) and two possibilities for the result to be incorrect (false positive and false negative). (From Fletcher R. H., Fletcher S. W. (2014). *Clinical epidemiology: The essentials* (5th ed., p. 109). Philadelphia, PA: Lippincott Williams & Wilkins.)

of people without the disease who are negative on a given test or observation (called a *true negative* result). Specificity can be calculated only from among people who do not have the disease. A test that is 95% specific correctly identifies 95 of 100 normal people. The other 5% are *false-positive* results. A false-positive test result can be unduly stressful for the person being tested, whereas a *false-negative* test result can delay diagnosis and jeopardize the outcome of treatment.

Predictive value is the extent to which an observation or test result is able to predict the presence of a given disease or condition.[8] A *positive predictive value* refers to the proportion of true positive results that occurs in a given population. In a group of women found to have "suspect breast nodules" in a cancer screening program, the proportion later determined to have breast cancer would constitute the positive predictive value. A *negative predictive value* refers to the true negative observations in a population. In a screening test for breast cancer, the negative predictive value represents the proportion of women without suspect nodules who do not have breast cancer. Although predictive values rely in part on sensitivity and specificity, they depend more heavily on the prevalence of the condition in the population. Despite unchanging sensitivity and specificity, the positive predictive value of an observation rises with prevalence, whereas the negative predictive value falls.

Clinical Course

The clinical course describes the evolution of a disease. A disease can have an acute, subacute, or chronic course. An *acute disorder* is one that is relatively severe, but self-limiting. *Chronic disease* implies a continuous, long-term process. A chronic disease can run a continuous course or can present with exacerbations (aggravation of symptoms and severity of the disease) and remissions (a period during which there is a decrease in severity and symptoms). *Subacute disease* is intermediate or between acute and chronic. It is not as severe as an acute disease and not as prolonged as a chronic disease.

The spectrum of disease severity for infectious diseases, such as hepatitis B, can range from preclinical to persistent chronic infection. During the *preclinical stage*, the disease is not clinically evident but is destined to progress to clinical disease. As with hepatitis B, it is possible to transmit a virus during the preclinical stage. *Subclinical disease* is not clinically apparent and is not destined to become clinically apparent. It is diagnosed with antibody or culture tests. Most cases of tuberculosis are not clinically apparent, and evidence of their presence is established by skin tests. *Clinical disease* is manifested by signs and symptoms. A persistent chronic infectious disease persists for years, sometimes for life. *Carrier status* refers to a person who harbors an organism but is not infected, as evidenced by antibody response or clinical manifestations. This person still can infect others. Carrier status may be of limited duration or it may be chronic, lasting for months or years.

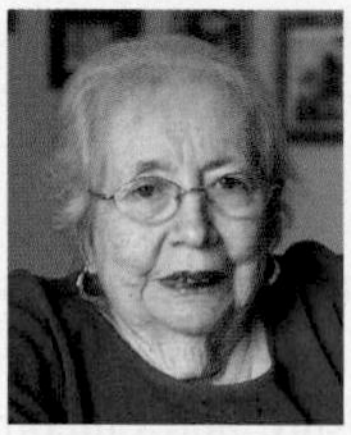

You may recall Mrs. Sora, the 85-year-old woman introduced at the beginning of the unit. Mrs. Sora was born during the Great Depression and recently moved two states away to live with her daughter. Mrs. Sora has had a burning sensation on the left side of her back, where a rash developed a few days later. This combination of a tingling/burning feeling (**Symptom ,which is subjective**) on one side of the body followed by a rash of small fluid-filled blisters (**Sign, which can be observed**) is known as herpes zoster, or shingles (**Diagnosis**), and is commonly seen in older people **(Cohort)**. It is a reactivation of the chicken pox virus (varicella zoster virus) (**Etiology**) and occurs along a nerve pathway. What makes it unique is that it only occurs on one side of the body. Some people are left with pain in the area of the rash long after it has healed (**Clinical Course**). The reason for reactivation of the virus is not clear, but it seems to be linked to stress and immune suppression **(Risk Factors)**.

IN SUMMARY

The term *pathophysiology*, which is the focus of this book, may be defined as the physiology of altered health. A *disease* has been defined as any deviation from or interruption of the normal structure or function of any part, organ, or system of the body that is manifested by a characteristic set of symptoms or signs and whose etiology, pathology, and prognosis may be known or unknown. The causes of disease are known as *etiologic factors. Pathogenesis* describes how the disease process evolves. *Morphology* refers to the structure or form of cells or tissues; *morphologic changes* are changes in structure or form that are characteristic of a disease.

A disease can manifest in a number of ways. A *symptom* is a subjective complaint, such as pain or dizziness, whereas a *sign* is an observable manifestation, such as an elevated temperature or a reddened, sore throat. A *syndrome* is a compilation of signs and symptoms that are characteristic of a specific disease state.

A *diagnosis* is the designation as to the nature and cause of a health problem. Health care providers need to perform comprehensive histories and PEs and validate their findings with diagnostic tests, including laboratory tests, imaging studies (*e.g.*, CT scans), and other tests. The value of many diagnostic tests is based on their reliability and validity, as well as their sensitivity and specificity. Having a comprehensive understanding of pathophysiology will assist the health care provider to best identify problems during the history and PE and to use laboratory data as further validation.[5]

The *clinical course* of a disease describes its evolution. It can be acute (relatively severe, but self-limiting), chronic (continuous or episodic, but taking place over a long period), or subacute (not as severe as acute or as prolonged as chronic). Within the disease spectrum, a disease can be designated preclinical, or not clinically evident; subclinical, not clinically apparent and not destined to become clinically apparent; or clinical, characterized by signs and symptoms.

HEALTH AND DISEASE IN POPULATIONS

After completing this section of the chapter, you should be able to meet the following objectives:

- Define the term *epidemiology*.
- Compare the meaning of the terms *incidence* and *prevalence* as they relate to measures of disease frequency.
- Differentiate primary, secondary, and tertiary levels of prevention.

The health of people is closely linked to the health of the community and to the population it encompasses. The ability to traverse continents in a matter of hours has opened the world to issues of populations at a global level. Diseases that once were confined to local areas of the world now pose a threat to populations throughout the world.

As we move through the 21st century, we are continually reminded that the health care system and the services it delivers are targeted to particular populations. Managed care systems are focused on a population-based approach to planning, delivering, providing, and evaluating health care. The focus of health care also has begun to emerge as a partnership in which people are asked to assume greater responsibility for their own health.

Epidemiology and Patterns of Disease

Epidemiology is the study of disease occurrence in human populations.[8] It was initially developed to explain the spread of infectious diseases during epidemics and has emerged as a science to study risk factors for multifactorial diseases, such as heart disease and cancer. Epidemiology looks for patterns of people affected with a particular disorder, such as age, race, dietary habits, lifestyle, or geographic location. In contrast to biomedical researchers who study the mechanisms of disease production, epidemiologists are more concerned with whether something happens than how it happens. For example, the epidemiologist is more concerned with whether smoking itself is related to cardiovascular disease and whether the risk of heart disease decreases when smoking ceases. On the other hand, the biomedical researcher is more concerned about the causative agent in cigarette smoke and the pathway by which it contributes to heart disease.

Much of our knowledge about disease comes from epidemiologic studies. Epidemiologic methods are used to determine how a disease is spread, how to control it, how to prevent it, and how to eliminate it. Epidemiologic methods also are used to study the natural history of disease, to evaluate new preventive and treatment strategies, to explore the impact of different patterns of health care delivery, and to predict future health care needs. As such, epidemiologic studies serve as a basis for clinical decision making, allocation of health care dollars, and development of policies related to public health issues.

Incidence and Prevalence

Measures of disease frequency are an important aspect of epidemiology. They establish a means for predicting what diseases are present in a population and provide an indication of the rate at which they are increasing or decreasing. A *disease case* can be either an existing case or the number of new episodes of a particular illness that is diagnosed within a given period. **Incidence** reflects the number of new cases arising in a population at risk during a specified time. The population at risk is considered to be people without the disease but who are at risk for developing it. It is determined by dividing the number of new cases of a disease by the population at risk for development of the disease during the same period (*e.g.*, new cases per 1000 or 100,000 people in the population who are at risk). The cumulative incidence estimates the risk of developing the disease during that period of time. **Prevalence** is a measure of existing disease in a population at a given point in time (*e.g.*, number of existing cases divided by the current population).[8] The prevalence is not an estimate of risk of developing a disease because it is a function of both new cases and how long the cases remain in the population. Incidence and prevalence are always reported as rates (*e.g.*, cases per 100 or cases per 100,000).

Morbidity and Mortality

Morbidity and mortality statistics provide information about the functional effects (morbidity) and death-producing (mortality) characteristics of a disease. These statistics are useful in terms of anticipating health care needs, planning of public education programs, directing health research efforts, and allocating health care dollars.

Morbidity describes the effects an illness has on a person's life. Many diseases, such as arthritis, have low death rates but a significant impact on a person's life. Morbidity is concerned not only with the occurrence or incidence of a disease but with persistence and the long-term consequences of the disease.

Mortality statistics provide information about the causes of death in a given population. In most countries, people are legally required to record certain facts such as age, gender, and cause of death on a death certificate. Internationally agreed on classification procedures (the International Classification of Diseases [ICD] by the WHO) are used for coding the cause of death, and the data are expressed as death rates.[1] Crude mortality rates (*i.e.*, number of deaths in a given period) do not account for age, gender, race, socioeconomic status, and other factors. For this reason, mortality often is expressed as death rates for a specific population, such as the infant mortality rate. Mortality also can be described in terms of the leading causes of death according to age, gender, race, and ethnicity. For example, among all people 65 years of age and older, leading causes of death in the United States are heart disease, cancer, chronic lower respiratory disease, and cerebrovascular diseases.[9]

Determination of Risk Factors

Conditions suspected of contributing to the development of a disease are called *risk factors*. They may be inherent to the person (high blood pressure or overweight) or external (smoking or drinking alcohol). There are different types of studies used to determine risk factors, including cross-sectional studies, case–control studies, and cohort studies.

Cross-Sectional and Case–Control Studies

Cross-sectional studies use the simultaneous collection of information necessary for classification of exposure and outcome status. They can be used to compare the prevalence of a disease in those with the factor (or exposure) with the prevalence of a disease in those who are unexposed to the factor, for example, by comparing the prevalence of coronary heart disease in smokers and nonsmokers. *Case–control studies* are designed to compare people known to have the outcome of interest (*cases*) and those known not to have the outcome of interest (*controls*).[8] Information on exposures or characteristics of interest is then collected from people in both groups. For example, the characteristics of maternal alcohol consumption in infants born with fetal alcohol syndrome (cases) can be compared with those in infants born without the syndrome (controls).

Cohort Studies

A *cohort* is a group of people who were born at approximately the same time or share some characteristics of interest.[8] People enrolled in a cohort study (also called a *longitudinal study*) are followed over a period of time to observe a specific health outcome. A cohort may consist of a single group of people chosen because they have or have not been exposed to suspected risk factors. For example, two groups specifically selected because one has been exposed and the other has not or a single exposed group in which the results are compared with the general population.

Framingham Study. One of the best-known examples of a cohort study is the Framingham Study, which was carried out in Framingham, MA.[10] Framingham was selected because of the size of the population, the relative ease with which the people could be contacted, and the stability of the population in terms of moving into and out of the area. This longitudinal study, which began in 1950, was set up by the U.S. Public Health Service to study the characteristics of people who would later develop coronary heart disease. The study consisted of 5000 persons, between 30 and 59 years of age, selected at random and followed for an initial period of 20 years. During this time, it was predicted that 1500 of them would develop coronary heart disease. The advantage of such a study is that it can explore a number of risk factors at the same time and determine the relative importance of each. Another advantage is that the risk factors can be related later to other diseases such as stroke.

Nurses' Health Study. Another well-known cohort study is the Nurses' Health Study, which was developed by Harvard University and Brigham and Women's Hospital. The study began in 1976 with a cohort of 121,700 female caregivers, 30 to 55 years of age, living in the United States.[11] The study expanded in 1989 to include a group of 238,000 female caregiver participants.[11] Initially designed to explore the relationship between oral contraceptives and breast cancer, caregivers in the study have provided answers to detailed questions about their menstrual cycle, smoking habits, diet, weight and waist measurements, activity patterns, health problems, and medication use. They have collected urine and blood samples and even provided researchers with their toenail clippings. In selecting the cohort, it was reasoned that caregivers would be well organized, accurate, and observant in their responses and that physiologically they would be no different from other groups of women. It also was anticipated that their child-bearing, eating, and smoking patterns would be similar to those of other working women.

Natural History

The *natural history* of a disease refers to the progression and projected outcome of the disease without medical intervention. By studying the patterns of a disease over time in populations, epidemiologists can better understand its natural history. Knowledge of the natural history can be used to determine disease outcome, establish priorities for health care services, determine the effects of screening and early detection programs on disease outcome, and compare the results of new treatments with the expected outcome without treatment.

There are some diseases for which there are no effective treatment methods available, or the current treatment measures are effective only in certain people. In this case, the natural history of the disease can be used as a predictor of outcome. For example, the natural history of hepatitis C indicates that 75% to 85% of people who become infected with the virus fail to clear the virus and progress to chronic infection.[12] Information about the natural history of a disease and the availability of effective treatment methods provides directions for preventive measures. In the case of hepatitis C, careful screening of blood donations and education of intravenous drug abusers can be used to prevent transfer of the virus. At the same time, scientists are striving to develop a vaccine that will prevent infection in people exposed to the virus. The development of vaccines to prevent the spread of infectious diseases such as polio and hepatitis B undoubtedly has been motivated by knowledge about the natural history of these diseases and the lack of effective intervention measures. With other diseases, such as breast cancer, early detection through the use of breast self-examination and mammography increases the chances for a cure.

Prognosis refers to the probable outcome and prospect of recovery from a disease. It can be designated as chances for full recovery, possibility of complications, or anticipated survival time. Prognosis often is presented in relation to treatment options, that is, the expected outcomes or chances for survival with or without a certain type of treatment. The prognosis associated with a given type of treatment usually is presented along with the risk associated with the treatment.

Preventing Disease

Basically, leading a healthy life contributes to the prevention of disease. There are three fundamental types of prevention—primary prevention, secondary prevention, and tertiary

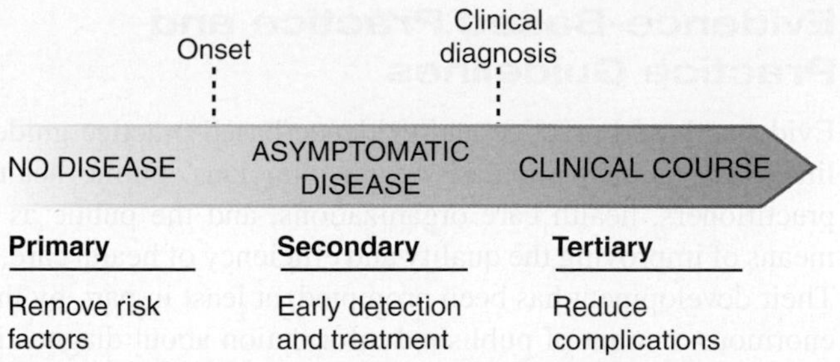

Figure 1.5 • Levels of prevention. Primary prevention prevents disease from occurring. Secondary prevention detects and cures disease in the asymptomatic phase. Tertiary prevention reduces complications of disease. (From Fletcher R. H., Fletcher S. W. (2014). *Clinical epidemiology: The essentials* (5th ed., p. 153). Philadelphia, PA: Lippincott Williams & Wilkins.)

prevention[8] (Fig. 1.5). It is important to note that all three levels are aimed at prevention.

Primary prevention is directed at keeping disease from occurring by removing all risk factors. Examples of primary prevention include the administration of folic acid to pregnant women and women who may become pregnant to prevent fetal neural tube defects, giving immunizations to children to prevent communicable disease, and counseling people to adopt healthy lifestyles as a means of preventing heart disease.[8] Primary prevention is often accomplished outside the health care system at the community level. Some primary prevention measures are mandated by law (*e.g.*, wearing seat belts in automobiles and helmet use on motorcycles). Other primary prevention activities (*e.g.*, use of earplugs or dust masks) occur in specific occupations.

Secondary prevention detects disease early when it is still asymptomatic and treatment measures can effect a cure or stop the disease from progressing. The use of a Papanicolaou (Pap) smear for early detection of cervical cancer is an example of secondary prevention. Screening also includes history taking (asking if a person smokes), PE (blood pressure measurement), laboratory tests (cholesterol level determination), and other procedures (colonoscopy) that can be "applied reasonably rapidly to asymptomatic people."[8] Most secondary prevention is done in clinical settings. All types of health care professionals (*e.g.*, physicians, caregivers, dentists, audiologists, optometrists) participate in secondary prevention.

Tertiary prevention is directed at clinical interventions that prevent further deterioration or reduce the complications of a disease once it has been diagnosed. An example is the use of β-adrenergic drugs to reduce the risk of death in people who have had a heart attack. The boundaries of tertiary prevention go beyond treating the problem with which the person presents. In people with diabetes, for example, tertiary prevention requires more than good glucose control. It also includes provision for regular ophthalmologic examinations for early detection of retinopathy, education for good foot care, and treatment for other cardiovascular risk factors such as hyperlipidemia.[8] Tertiary prevention measures also include measures to limit physical impairment and the social consequences of an illness. Most tertiary prevention programs are located within health care systems and involve the services of a number of different types of health care professionals.

Evidence-Based Practice and Practice Guidelines

Evidence-based practice and evidence-based practice guidelines have gained popularity with clinicians, public health practitioners, health care organizations, and the public as a means of improving the quality and efficiency of health care.[13] Their development has been prompted, at least in part, by the enormous amount of published information about diagnostic and treatment measures for various disease conditions as well as demands for better and more cost-effective health care.

Evidence-based practice refers to making decisions in health care based on scientific data that has shown a specific way of managing a disease, patient symptoms, and complaints. Using evidence-based practice mandates that health care providers cannot practice according to only "their" way or according to "how it has always been done before." Evidence-based practice is based on the integration of the individual clinical expertise of the practitioner with the best external clinical evidence from systematic research.[13]

The term *clinical expertise* implies the proficiency and judgment that individual clinicians gain through clinical experience and clinical practice. The best external clinical evidence relies on the identification of clinically relevant research, often from the basic sciences, but especially from patient-centered clinical studies that focus on the accuracy and precision of diagnostic tests and methods, the power of prognostic indicators, and the effectiveness and safety of therapeutic, rehabilitative, and preventive regimens.

Clinical practice guidelines are systematically developed statements intended to inform practitioners and people in making decisions about health care for specific clinical circumstances.[6,13] Providers not only should review but must weigh various outcomes, both positive and negative, and make recommendations. Guidelines are different from systematic reviews. They can take the form of algorithms, which are step-by-step methods for solving a problem, written directives for care, or a combination thereof.

The development of evidence-based practice guidelines often uses methods such as meta-analysis to combine evidence from different studies to produce a more precise estimate of the accuracy of a diagnostic method or the effects of an intervention method.[14] Development of evidence-based practice guidelines requires review. Those who should review the guidelines include practitioners with expertise in clinical content, who can verify the completeness of the literature review and ensure clinical sensibility, experts in guideline development who can examine the method by which the guideline was developed, and potential users of the guideline.[13]

Once developed, practice guidelines must be continually reviewed and changed to keep pace with new research findings and new diagnostic and treatment methods. For example, both the Guidelines for the Prevention, Evaluation, and Treatment of High Blood Pressure, first developed in 1972 by the Joint National Committee, and the Guidelines for the Diagnosis and Management of Asthma,[15] first developed in 1991 by the Expert Panel, have undergone multiple revisions as new evidence from research has evolved.

Evidence-based practice guidelines, which are intended to direct patient care, are also important in directing research into the best methods of diagnosing and treating specific health problems. For example, health care providers use the same criteria for diagnosing the extent and severity of a particular condition such as hypertension with the proven guidelines for hypertension (the 8th Report of the Joint National Committee on Prevention, Detection, and Evaluation, and Treatment of High Blood Pressure [JNC 8]). Providers also use the same protocols for treatment of people with hypertension until new data support a change such as the use of new pharmacologic agents.

IN SUMMARY

Epidemiology refers to the study of disease in populations. It looks for patterns such as age, race, and dietary habits of people who are affected with a particular disorder. These patterns are used to determine under what circumstances the particular disorder will occur. *Incidence* is the number of new cases arising in a given population during a specified time. *Prevalence* is the number of people in a population who have a particular disease at a given point in time or period. Incidence and prevalence are reported as proportions or rates (*e.g.*, cases per 100 or 100,000 population). *Morbidity* describes the effects an illness has on a person's life. It is concerned with the incidence of disease as well as its persistence and long-term consequences. *Mortality*, or death, statistics provide information about the causes of death in a given population.

Conditions suspected of contributing to the development of a disease are called *risk factors*. Studies used to determine risk factors include cross-sectional studies, case–control studies, and cohort studies. The *natural history* refers to the progression and projected outcome of a disease without medical intervention. *Prognosis* is the term used to designate the probable outcome and prospect of recovery from a disease.

The three fundamental types of prevention are primary prevention, secondary prevention, and tertiary prevention. *Primary prevention*, such as immunizations, is directed at removing risk factors so disease does not occur. *Secondary prevention*, such as a Pap smear, detects disease when it still is asymptomatic and curable with treatment. *Tertiary prevention*, such as use of β-adrenergic drugs to reduce the risk of death in persons who have had a heart attack, focuses on clinical interventions that prevent further deterioration or reduce the complications of a disease.

Evidence-based practice and *evidence-based practice guidelines* are mechanisms that use the current best evidence to make decisions about the health care of people. They are based on the expertise of the individual practitioner integrated with the best clinical evidence from systematic review of credible research studies. Practice guidelines may take the form of algorithms, which are step-by-step methods for solving a problem, written directives, or a combination thereof.

GERIATRIC Considerations

- Individuals age because their cells age. Age is one of the strongest independent risk factors for many chronic diseases. Cellular aging is not acute; rather, it is progressive in nature as a result of environmental damage such as free radical damage, fixed **cellular senescence**, genetic influences, and decline in function.[4]
- Leading causes of death in persons age 65 and older include heart disease, malignant neoplasms, cerebrovascular disease, pneumonia and influenza, and chronic obstructive pulmonary disease.[16]
- Special needs of elderly persons must be considered when preparing the older adult person for obtaining laboratory specimens. Normal values may vary, for example, the normal range of lipase for the adult is 10 to 140 U/L compared to 18 to 180 U/L in persons over 65 years.[5]

PEDIATRIC Considerations

Of the 5.9 million children under the age of 5 who died in 2015, more than half were preventable or treatable.[16]

- Cells from children have the capacity to undergo more rounds of replication than do cells of older people.[4]
- Globally, malnutrition is the contributing factor for 45% of all child deaths making children susceptible to serious diseases.[17]
- The five leading causes of death in children aged 1 to 4 years include (1) unintentional injuries, (2) congenital malformations/deformities and chromosomal abnormalities, (3) cancer, (4) diseases of the heart, and (5) homicide. For children aged 5 to 14, the leading causes of death are (1) unintentional injuries, (2) cancer, and (3) congenital anomalies, homicide, and diseases of the heart.[16]
- The Federal Interagency Forum on Child and Family Statistics published national indicators for America's children. Key health conditions such as obesity, asthma, and emotional difficulties impact the health of children.[18]
- Normal ranges for laboratory values are much more complex in the pediatric population (Fischbach & Dunning, p. 17).[5] It is critical for health care professionals to access, plan, implement, and evaluate care based on normal laboratory value ranges appropriate for age.

References

1. World Health Organization. (2003). *About WHO: Definition of health; disease eradication/elimination goals. [Online].* Available: www.who.int/about/definition/en/. Accessed January 12, 2011.
2. U.S. Department of Health and Human Services. (2010). *Healthy People 2020—The mission, vision, and goals of 2020 [Online].* Available: http://www.healthypeople.gov/2020/TopicsObjectives2020/pdfs/HP2020_brochure.pdf. Accessed January 22, 2011.
3. Carlsten C., Brauer M., Brinkman F., et al. (2014). Genes, the environment and personalized medicine: We need to harness both environmental and genetic data to maximize personal and population health. *EMBO Reports* 15(7), 736–739.
4. Kumar V., Abbas A., Aster J. C. (2014). *Robbins and Cotran pathologic basis of disease* (9th ed., p. 40). Philadelphia, PA: Elsevier Saunders.
5. Fischbach F., Dunning M. B. (2014). *A manual of laboratory and diagnostic tests* (9th ed., pp. 12–13, 96). Philadelphia, PA: Lippincott Williams & Wilkins.
6. Benjamin I. J., Griggs R. C., Wing E. J., et al. (2016). *Andreoli and Carpenter's Cecil essentials of medicine* (9th ed., pp. 266–270). Philadelphia, PA: Elsevier Saunders.
7. American Association for Clinical Chemistry. (2017). *How reliable is laboratory testing?* Available: https://labtestsonline.org/understanding/features/reliability/start1/. Accessed October 8, 2017.
8. Fletcher R. H., Fletcher S. W., Fletcher G. S. (2012). *Clinical epidemiology: The essentials* (5th ed.). Philadelphia, PA: Lippincott Williams & Wilkins.
9. Centers for Disease Control and Prevention. (2017). *FastStats. Older persons' health.* Available: https://www.cdc.gov/nchs/fastats/older-american-health.htm. http://www.cdc.gov/nchs/fastats/lcod.htm. Accessed October 8, 2017.
10. Framingham Heart Study. (2001). *Framingham Heart Study: Design, rationale, objectives, and research milestones. [Online].* Available: www.nhlbi.nih.gov/about/framingham/design.htm. Accessed January 6, 2011.
11. Channing Laboratory. (2008). *The Nurse's Health Study. [Online].* Available: http://www.channing.harvard.edu/nhs/. Accessed January 29, 2011.
12. Center for Disease Control and Prevention. (2017). *Hepatitis c faqs for health professionals.* Available: https://www.cdc.gov/hepatitis/hcv/hcvfaq.htm. Accessed October 8, 2017.
13. Duke University Medical Center. (2017). *What is evidenced-based practice?* Available: http://guides.mclibrary.duke.edu/ebmtutorial. Accessed October 8, 2017.
14. Berlin J. A., Golulb R. M. (2014). Meta-analysis as evidence building a better pyramid. *JAMA* 312(6), 603–606. doi:10.1001/jama.2014.8167.
15. National Asthma Education and Prevention Program. (2007). *Expert Panel Report 3: Guidelines for the diagnosis and management of asthma. [Online].* Available: http://www.aanma.org/advocacy/guidelines-for-the-diagnosis-and-management-of-asthma/#Guidelines. Accessed May 22, 2013.
16. Center for Disease Control. (2016). Available: https://www.cdc.gov/nchs/data/hus/hus16.pdf#020 (Table 20, pp. 131–132). Accessed October 11, 2017.
17. World Health Organization. (2017). *Fact sheets: Child health.* Available: http://www.who.int/topics/child_health/factsheets/en/. Accessed October 11, 2017.
18. Federal Interagency Forum on Child and Family Statistics. (2017). *Welcome to America's children: Key national indicators of well-being.* Available: https://www.childstats.gov/index.asp. Accessed October 11, 2017.

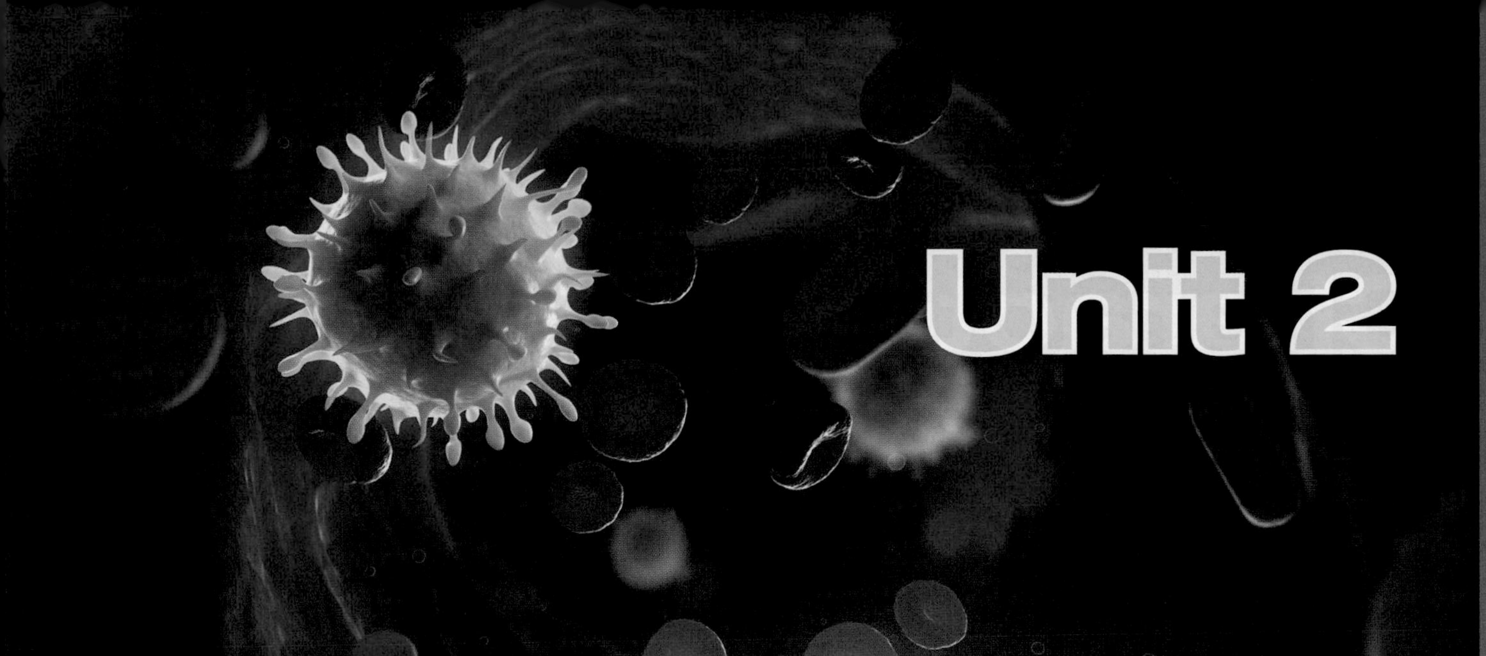

Unit 2

Cell Function and Growth

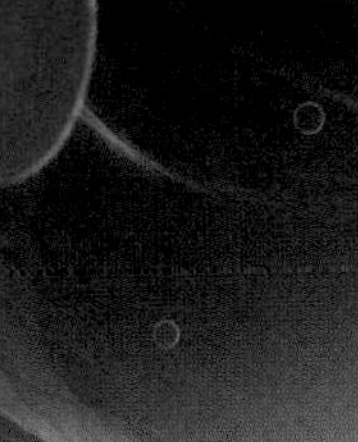

Jennifer is a 1-day-old infant born after an uncomplicated vaginal delivery to a 46-year-old primipara. She is noted to have poor muscle tone and irregular facies, including up-slanting almond-shaped eyes and a flat facial profile with a depressed nasal bridge. Additionally, she has a heart murmur, and there is concern about a potential heart condition. The pediatrician believes she may have Down syndrome (trisomy 21). A blood sample is drawn for karyotype and sent to the laboratory. Results indicate 47, XX, +21, meaning that Jennifer has 47 chromosomes, including two X chromosomes and an extra copy of chromosome 21.

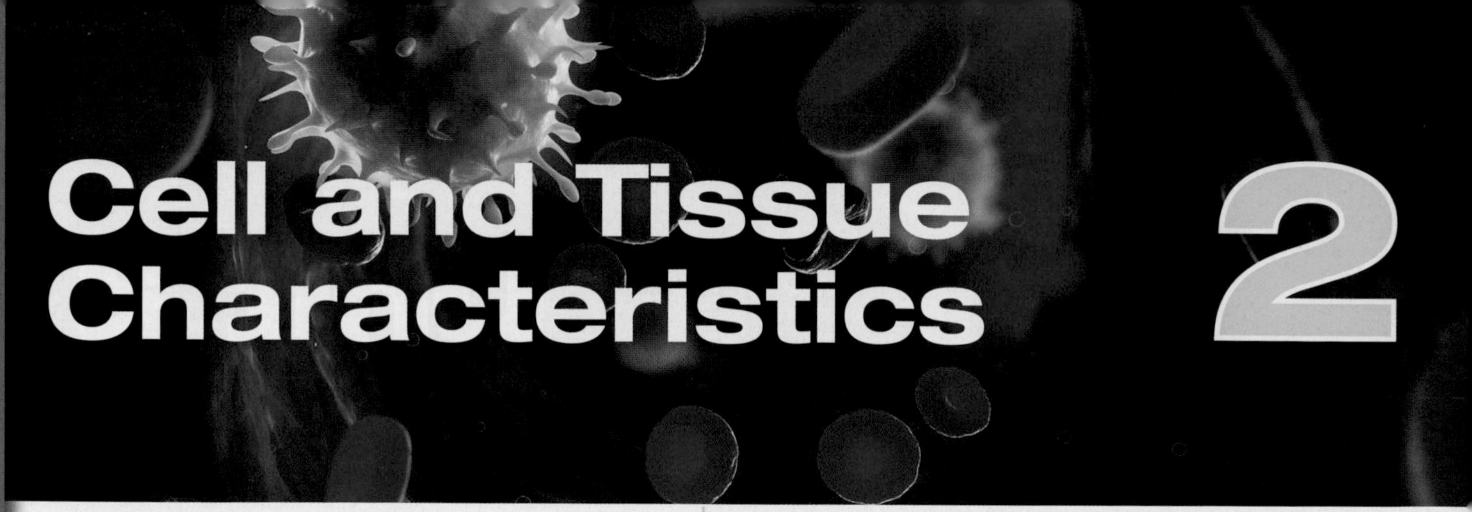

Cell and Tissue Characteristics 2

Cheryl Neudauer

In most organisms, the **cell** is the smallest functional unit that has the characteristics necessary for life. Cells combine to form **tissues** based on their embryonic origin. These tissues combine to form organs. Although cells of different tissues and organs vary in structure and function, certain characteristics are common to all cells. Cells are able to exchange materials with their environment, obtain energy from nutrients, and make complex molecules, and some can replicate themselves. Because most disease processes start at the cellular level, we need to understand cell function to understand disease processes. Some diseases affect the cells of one tissue type, some diseases affect the cells of one organ, and other diseases affect the cells of the entire organism. This chapter discusses the structural parts of cells, cell functions and growth, movement of substances such as ions across the cell membrane, and tissue types.

FUNCTIONAL COMPONENTS OF THE CELL

After completing this section of the chapter, you should be able to meet the following objectives:

- Describe why the cell nucleus is called the "control center" of the cell.
- Predict the effects of dysfunction in each cellular organelle.
- Differentiate the four functions of the cell membrane.

Most organisms, including humans, contain eukaryotic cells that are made up of internal membrane-bound compartments called organelles ("small organs" within cells); an example of an organelle is the nucleus. This is in contrast to prokaryotes, such as bacteria, that do not contain membrane-bound organelles. Although diverse in their organization, all eukaryotic cells have common structures that perform unique functions. When seen under a microscope, three major components of a eukaryotic cell become evident—the nucleus, the cytoplasm, and the cell membrane (Fig. 2.1).

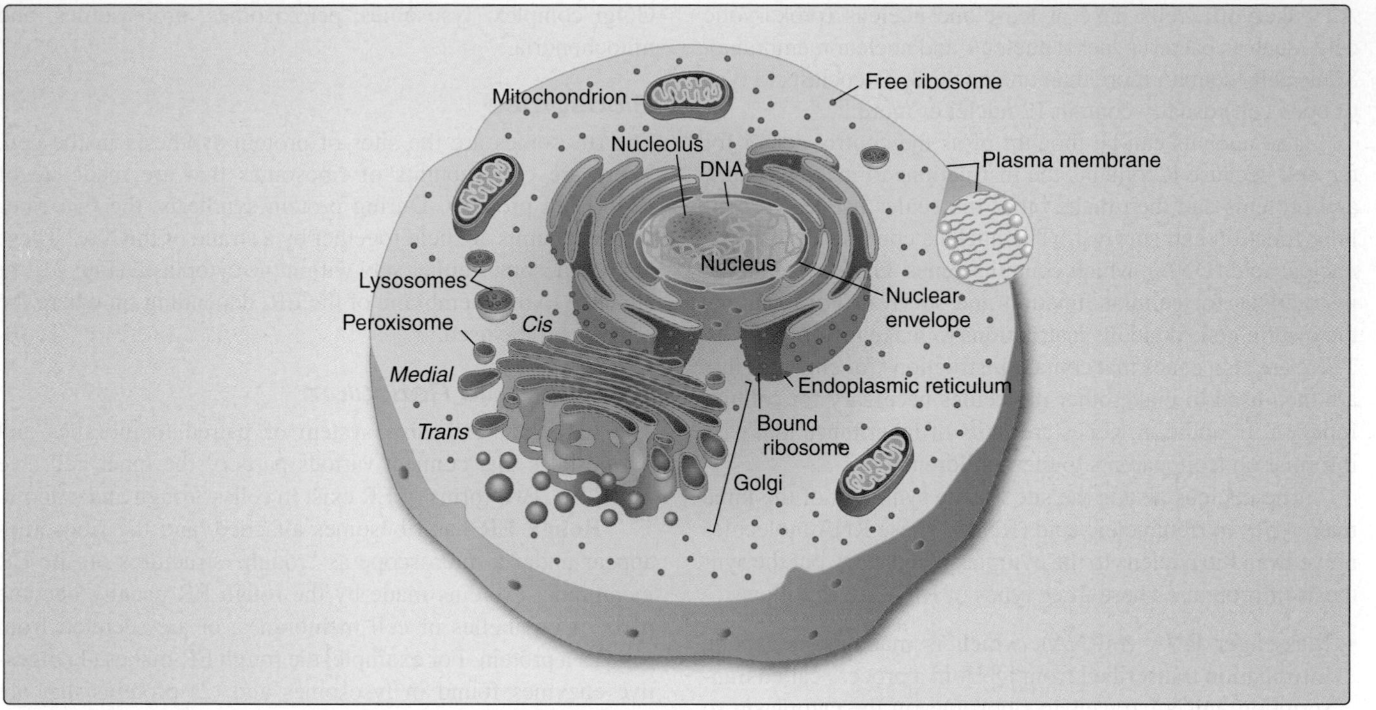

Figure 2.1 • Cell organelles. (Reprinted from Leeper-Woodford. (2016). *Lippincott illustrated reviews: Integrated systems* (Fig. 2.1, p. 39). Philadelphia, PA: Wolters Kluwer, with permission.)

Protoplasm

Biologists call the intracellular fluid **protoplasm**. Protoplasm is composed of water, proteins, lipids, carbohydrates, and electrolytes.[1]

- Water makes up 70% to 85% of the cell's protoplasm.[1]
- Proteins make up 10% to 20% of the protoplasm. Proteins are polar and hydrophilic (water loving), making them soluble in water. Examples of proteins include enzymes necessary for cellular reactions, structural proteins, ion channels, and receptors.[1] Proteins can be bound to other substances to form nucleoproteins, glycoproteins, and lipoproteins.
- Lipids make up 2% to 3% of the protoplasm. Lipids are nonpolar and hydrophobic (water fearing), making them insoluble in water. They are the main parts of cell membranes surrounding the outside and inside of cells. Examples of lipids include phospholipids and cholesterol. Some cells also contain large quantities of triglycerides. In fat cells, triglycerides can make up as much as 95% of the total cell mass.[1] This is stored energy, which can be broken down for use wherever it is needed in the body.
- Carbohydrates make up approximately 1% of the protoplasm. These serve primarily as a rapid source of energy.[1]
- The major intracellular electrolytes include potassium, magnesium, phosphate, sulfate, and bicarbonate ions. Small quantities of the electrolytes sodium, chloride, and calcium ions are also present in cells. These electrolytes participate in reactions that are necessary for the cell's metabolism, and they help generate and send signals in neurons, muscle cells, and other cells.

Two distinct regions of protoplasm exist in the cell:

- The **karyoplasm** or **nucleoplasm** is inside the nucleus.
- The **cytoplasm** is outside the nucleus. The **cytosol** is the fluid of the cytoplasm (cytoplasm = cytosol + organelles).

KEY POINTS

THE FUNCTIONAL ORGANIZATION OF THE CELL

- Organelles in the cytoplasm perform functions within cells similar to how organs in the body perform functions within the organism.
- The nucleus is the largest and most visible organelle in the cell. The nucleus is the control center for the cell. In eukaryotic cells, it contains genetic information. The DNA that we inherit is from our parents (there is also DNA in the mitochondria that we inherit from our mothers.)[1]
- Other organelles include the mitochondria, which help to make energy molecules cells can use, and the lysosomes and proteasomes, which function as the cell's digestive system. Ribosomes, which are not surrounded by membranes, are the cellular structures that make proteins; those proteins may help to make other molecules needed for cell function.

The Nucleus

The cell nucleus (singular; plural is nuclei) is a rounded or elongated structure near the center of the cell (see Fig. 2.1).

All eukaryotic cells have at least one nucleus (prokaryotic cells, such as bacteria, lack a nucleus, and nuclear membrane). Some cells contain more than one nucleus; osteoclasts (a type of bone cell) usually contain 12 nuclei or more.[1]

The nucleus can be thought of as the control center for the cell because it contains the instructions to make proteins, and proteins can then make other molecules needed for cellular function and survival.[1] The nucleus contains deoxyribonucleic acid (DNA), which contains genes. Genes contain the instructions for cellular function and survival. For example, the insulin gene contains instructions to make insulin protein. There are also genes that contain instructions for enzymes that are then used to make other molecules necessary for cellular function. In addition, genes are units of inheritance that pass information from parents to their children.

The nucleus also is the site for the synthesis of the three main types of ribonucleic acid (RNA). These RNA molecules move from the nucleus to the cytoplasm and carry out the synthesis of proteins. These three types of RNA are as follows:

- Messenger RNA (mRNA), which is made from genetic information transcribed from DNA in a process called transcription. mRNA travels to ribosomes in the cytoplasm so these instructions can be used to make proteins.
- Ribosomal RNA (rRNA) is the RNA component of ribosomes, the site of proteins production.
- Transfer RNA (tRNA) transports amino acids to ribosomes so that mRNA can be turned into a sequence of amino acids. This process, known as translation, uses the mRNA template to link amino acids to synthesize proteins.[1]

The nucleoplasm inside the nucleus is separated from the cytoplasm outside of the nucleus by the **nuclear envelope** that surrounds the nucleus.[1] The nuclear envelope contains many nuclear pores.[1] Fluids, electrolytes, RNA, some proteins, and some hormones move in both directions through the nuclear pores, and this exchange between the nucleoplasm and cytoplasm appears to be regulated.[1]

The Cytoplasm and Its Organelles

The cytoplasm includes the fluid and organelles outside the nucleus but within the cell membrane surrounding the cell. Cytoplasm is a solution that contains water, electrolytes, proteins, fats, and carbohydrates.[1] Pigments may also accumulate in the cytoplasm. Some pigments are normal parts of cells. One example is melanin, which gives skin its color. Some pigments are not normal parts of cells. For example, when the body breaks down old red blood cells, pigments in red blood cells are changed to the pigment bilirubin, which the body can excrete; some conditions cause bilirubin to build up in cells to cause *jaundice,* which is seen clinically by a yellowish discoloration of the skin and sclera (normally the white part of the eye).

Embedded in the cytoplasm are various organelles that function as the organs of the cell. In addition to the nucleus, which was discussed in the previous section, these organelles include the ribosomes, the endoplasmic reticulum (ER), the Golgi complex, lysosomes, peroxisomes, proteasomes, and mitochondria.[1]

Ribosomes

The ribosomes are the sites of protein synthesis in the cell. There are two subunits of ribosomes that are made up of rRNA and proteins. During protein synthesis, the two ribosomal subunits are held together by a strand of mRNA.[1] These active ribosomes either stay within the cytoplasm (Fig. 2.2) or attached to the membrane of the ER, depending on where the protein will be used.[1]

Endoplasmic Reticulum

The ER is an extensive system of paired membranes and flat vesicles that connect various parts of the inner cell (see Fig. 2.2).[1] Two forms of ER exist in cells—rough and smooth.

Rough ER has ribosomes attached, and the ribosomes appear under a microscope as "rough" structures on the ER membrane. Proteins made by the rough ER usually become parts of organelles or cell membranes, or are secreted from cells as a protein. For example, the rough ER makes (1) digestive enzymes found in lysosomes and (2) proteins that are secreted, such as the protein hormone insulin.

The **smooth ER** is free of ribosomes and has a smooth structure when viewed through a microscope. Because it does not have ribosomes attached, the smooth ER does not participate in protein synthesis. Instead, the smooth ER is involved

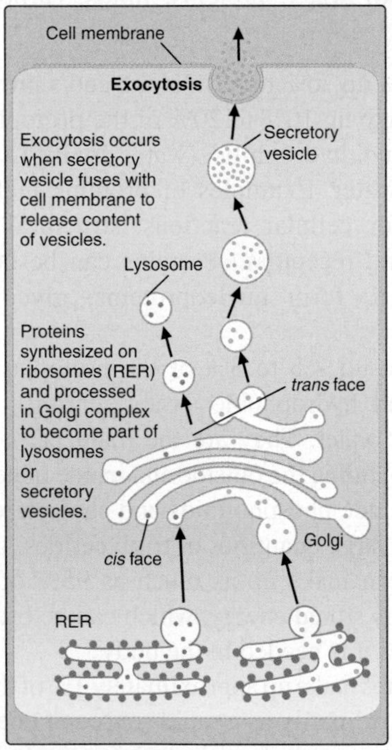

Figure 2.2 • Endoplasmic reticulum (ER), ribosomes, and Golgi apparatus. The rough ER consists of intricately folded membranes studded with ribosomes. Ribosomes are made of protein and rRNA organized together. Golgi apparatus process proteins synthesized on ribosomes. (Reprinted from Leeper-Woodford. (2016). *Lippincott illustrated reviews: Integrated systems* (Fig. 2.3, p. 41). Philadelphia, PA: Wolters Kluwer, with permission.)

in the synthesis of lipids including steroid hormones. The sarcoplasmic reticulum of muscle cells is a form of smooth ER; calcium ions are stored in and then released from the sarcoplasmic reticulum to stimulate muscle contraction. The smooth ER of the liver is involved in storage of extra glucose as glycogen as well as metabolism of some hormone drugs.

If proteins build up in the ER faster than they can be removed, the cell is said to experience "ER stress." The cell responds by slowing down protein synthesis and restoring homeostasis. Abnormal responses to ER stress, which can cause inflammation and even cell death, have been implicated in inflammatory bowel disease,[2] a genetic form of diabetes mellitus,[3] and a disorder of skeletal muscle known as myositis,[4] as well as many other diseases.

Golgi Complex

The Golgi apparatus, sometimes called the **Golgi complex**, consists of four or more stacks of thin, flattened vesicles or sacs (see Fig. 2.3).[1] Substances produced in the ER are carried to the Golgi complex in small, membrane-covered transfer vesicles. The Golgi complex modifies these substances and packages them into secretory granules or vesicles. For example, insulin is synthesized as a large, inactive proinsulin protein that is cut apart to make smaller, active insulin proteins within the Golgi complex of the beta cells in the pancreas. Insulin is then packaged into vesicles ready for secretion from the cell when blood sugar is increased (*e.g.*, after a meal).

In addition to making secretory granules, the Golgi complex is thought to make large carbohydrate molecules that combine with proteins produced in the rough ER to form glycoproteins. Recent data suggest that the Golgi apparatus has yet another function: it can receive proteins and other substances from the cell surface by a retrograde transport mechanism. Several bacterial toxins, such as Shiga and cholera toxins, and plant toxins, such as ricin, that have cytoplasmic targets have exploited this retrograde pathway.[1]

Lysosomes and Peroxisomes

Lysosomes can be thought of as the digestive system or the stomach of the cell. These small, membrane-enclosed sacs contain powerful enzymes that can break down excess and worn-out cell parts as well as foreign substances that are taken into the cell (*e.g.*, bacteria taken in by phagocytosis). All of the lysosomal enzymes require an acidic environment, and the lysosomes maintain a pH of approximately 5 in their interior (similar to how the stomach maintains a low pH). The pH of the cytoplasm, which is approximately 7.2, protects other cellular structures from being broken down by these enzymes if they were to leak from the lysosome. **Primary lysosomes** are membrane-bound intracellular organelles that contain a variety of enzymes that have not yet entered the digestive process. They receive their enzymes as well as their membranes from the Golgi apparatus. Primary lysosomes become **secondary lysosomes** after they fuse with membrane-bound vacuoles that contain material to be digested. Lysosomes break down phagocytosed material by either heterophagy or autophagy (Fig. 2.3).

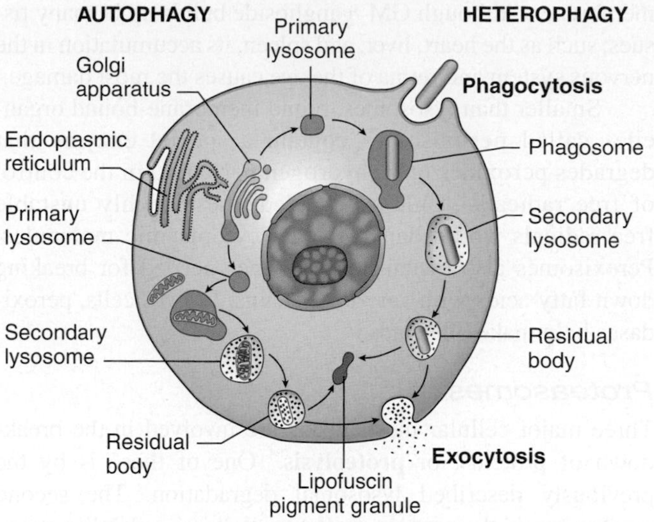

Figure 2.3 • The processes of autophagy and heterophagy, showing the primary and secondary lysosomes, residual bodies, extrusion of residual body contents from the cell, and lipofuscin-containing residual bodies.

Heterophagy (*hetero*, different; *phagy*, eat) refers to digestion of a substance phagocytosed from the cell's external environment.[5] An infolding of the cell membrane takes external materials into the cell to form a surrounding phagocytic vesicle, or **phagosome**. Primary lysosomes then fuse with phagosomes to form secondary lysosomes. Heterophagocytosis is most common in phagocytic white blood cells such as neutrophils and macrophages.

Autophagy involves the digestion of damaged cellular organelles, such as mitochondria or ER, which the lysosomes must remove if the cell's normal function is to continue.[5] Autophagocytosis is most common in cells undergoing atrophy (cell degeneration).

Although enzymes in the secondary lysosomes can break down most proteins, carbohydrates, and lipids to their basic constituents, some materials remain undigested. These undigested materials may stay in the cytoplasm as **residual bodies** or are removed from the cell by exocytosis. In some long-lived cells, such as neurons and heart muscle cells, large amounts of residual bodies accumulate as lipofuscin granules or age pigment. Other indigestible pigments, such as inhaled carbon particles and tattoo pigments, also accumulate and may remain in residual bodies for decades.

Lysosomes play an important role in the normal metabolism of certain substances in the body. In some inherited diseases known as **lysosomal storage disorders**, a specific lysosomal enzyme is absent or inactive, and the digestion of certain cellular substances does not occur.[6] As a result, these substances build up in cells. There are approximately 50 lysosomal storage disorders, each caused by a lack of activity of one or more lysosomal enzymes, and each disorder is rare.

In Tay-Sachs disease, an autosomal recessive disorder, cells do not make hexosaminidase A, a lysosomal enzyme needed for degrading the GM_2 ganglioside found in nerve cell membranes. Although GM_2 ganglioside builds up in many tissues, such as the heart, liver, and spleen, its accumulation in the nervous system and retina of the eye causes the most damage.[6]

Smaller than lysosomes, round membrane-bound organelles called **peroxisomes** contain a special enzyme that degrades peroxides (*e.g.*, hydrogen peroxide) in the control of free radicals.[6] Unless degraded, these highly unstable free radicals would damage other cytoplasmic molecules. Peroxisomes also contain the enzymes needed for breaking down fatty acids with very long chains. In liver cells, peroxidases help make bile acids.[5]

Proteasomes

Three major cellular mechanisms are involved in the breakdown of proteins, or **proteolysis**.[5] One of these is by the previously described lysosomal degradation. The second mechanism is the **caspase pathway** that is involved in apoptotic cell death. The third method of proteolysis occurs within an organelle called the **proteasome**. Proteasomes are small organelles made up of protein complexes in the cytoplasm and nucleus. These organelles recognize misformed and misfolded proteins that have been targeted for degradation. It has been suggested that as much as one third of the newly formed polypeptide chains are selected for proteasome degradation because of quality control mechanisms in the cell.

Mitochondria

The mitochondria are the "power plants" of the cell because they contain enzymes that can change carbon-containing nutrients into energy that is easily used by cells. This multistep process is often referred to as **cellular respiration** because it requires oxygen.[1] Cells store most of this energy as high-energy phosphate bonds in substances such as adenosine triphosphate (ATP) and use the ATP as energy in various cellular activities. Mitochondria are found close to the site of energy use in the cell (*e.g.*, near the myofibrils in muscle cells). The number of mitochondria in a given cell type varies by the type of activity the cell performs and the energy needed for this activity.[1] For example, a large increase in mitochondria occurs in skeletal muscle repeatedly stimulated to contract.

Mitochondria (plural) are made up of two membranes: an outer membrane around the mitochondrion and an inner membrane that forms shelflike projections, called **cristae** (Fig. 2.4). The narrow space between the outer and inner membranes is called the **intermembrane space**, whereas the large space inside the inner membrane is termed the **matrix space**.[5] The outer mitochondrial membrane contains a large number of transmembrane porins, through which water-soluble substances (including proteins) may pass. The inner membrane contains the respiratory chain enzymes and transport proteins needed to make ATP. In certain regions, the outer and inner membranes contact each other; these contact points serve as pathways for proteins and small substances to enter and leave the matrix space.

Mitochondria contain their own DNA and ribosomes and are self-replicating. Mitochondrial DNA (mtDNA) is

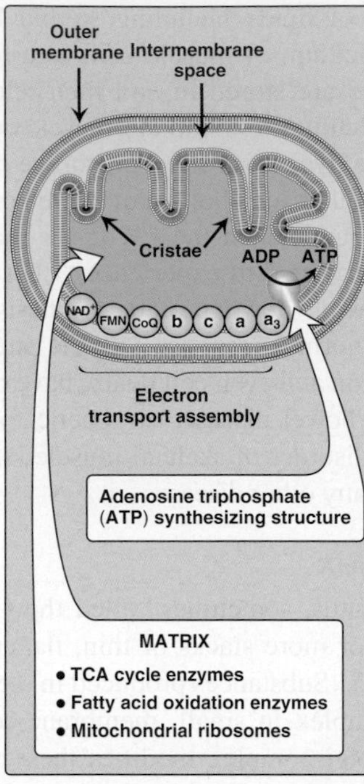

Figure 2.4 • Mitochondrion. The inner membrane forms transverse folds called *cristae*, where the enzymes needed for the final step in adenosine triphosphate (ATP) production (*i.e.*, oxidative phosphorylation) are located. (Reprinted from Leeper-Woodford. (2016). *Lippincott illustrated reviews: Integrated systems* (Fig. 2.4, p. 41). Philadelphia, PA: Wolters Kluwer, with permission.)

found in the mitochondrial matrix and is different from the chromosomal DNA found in the nucleus. Also known as the "other human genome," mtDNA is a double-stranded, circular molecule that contains the instructions to make 13 of the proteins needed for mitochondrial function. The DNA of the nucleus contains the instructions for the structural proteins of the mitochondria and other proteins needed for cellular respiration.[5,7]

mtDNA is inherited from the mother and is used to study inheritance from the mother's lineage. Mutations have been found in each of the mitochondrial genes, and an understanding of the role of mtDNA in certain diseases and aging is beginning to emerge. Most cells in the body can be affected by mtDNA mutations.[5]

Mitochondria also function as key regulators of apoptosis, or programmed cell death. Too little or too much apoptosis has been implicated in a wide range of diseases, including cancer, in which there is too little apoptosis (*i.e.*, less cell death leads to increased cell numbers), and neurodegenerative diseases, in which there is too much apoptosis.

The Cytoskeleton

In addition to its organelles, the cytoplasm contains a *cytoskeleton*, or the skeleton of the cell. The cytoskeleton is a network of microtubules, microfilaments, intermediate filaments, and thick filaments (Fig. 2.5).[5] The cytoskeleton controls cell shape and movement.

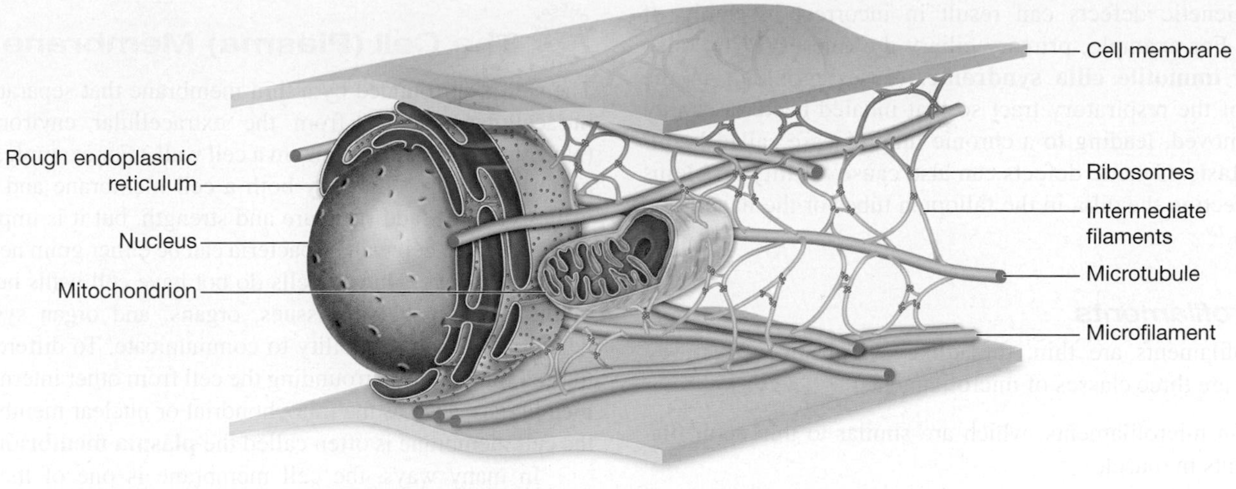

Figure 2.5 • Cytoskeleton. The cytoskeleton is made up of microfilaments, microtubules, and intermediate filaments. (Reprinted with permission from Wingerd B. (2014). *The human body* (3rd ed., Fig. 3.10, p. 55). Philadelphia, PA: Wolters Kluwer.)

Microtubules

Microtubules are formed from protein subunits called **tubulin**. Microtubules are long, stiff, hollow structures shaped like cylinders.[7] Microtubules can rapidly disassemble in one location (in the cytoplasm, from microtubules into free tubulin) and reassemble in another location (from free tubulin into microtubules). This constant reassembling forms elements of the cytoskeleton by continuously shortening and lengthening the tubulin dimers, a process known as dynamic instability.[6]

Microtubules function in the development and maintenance of cell formation. Microtubules participate in transport mechanisms inside cells, including transport of materials in the long axons of neurons and melanin in skin cells. Microtubules are also part of other cell structures such as cilia and flagella[7] (Fig. 2.6).

Another important role of microtubules is participating in mitosis (cell division). Some cancer drugs (e.g., vinblastine and vincristine) bind to microtubules and inhibit cell division.[8]

Cilia and Flagella. Flagella and cilia (*plural*) are microtubule-filled cellular extensions surrounded by a membrane that is continuous with the cell membrane. Eukaryotic flagellated cells are generally classified as having only one flagellum (*singular*), whereas ciliated cells typically have a large number of cilia.[7] In humans, sperm cells are the only cell type with flagella. Cilia are found on surfaces of many epithelial linings, including the nasal sinuses and bronchi in the upper respiratory system. Here, cilia function in the mucus escalator, where the cilia beat like the oars on a boat to help bring substances trapped in mucus (such as bacteria and dust) up from the airways into the mouth so they can be swallowed. Damage to cilia or ciliated cells causes a cough, which is then used to help remove these substances from airways.

Cilia also play roles in sensory tissues in the eye, olfactory epithelium, the inner ear, and during embryonic development, and cilia are essential for the normal functioning of many tissues, including the kidney. A condition called **polycystic kidney disease** is linked to a genetic defect in the cilia of the renal tubular cells.

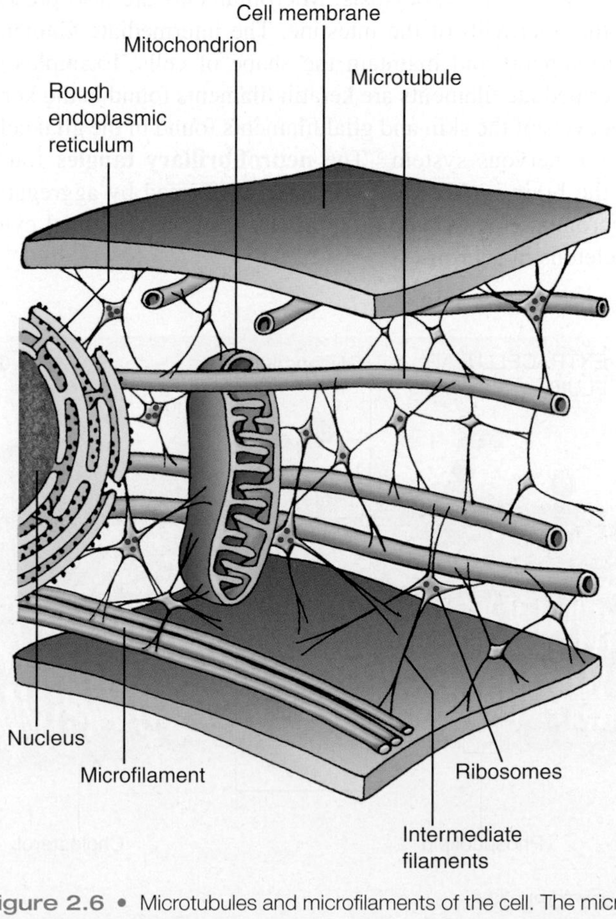

Figure 2.6 • Microtubules and microfilaments of the cell. The microfilaments are associated with the inner surface of the cell and aid in cell motility. The microtubules form the cytoskeleton and maintain the position of the organelles.

Genetic defects can result in incorrect assembly of cilia.[7] For example, primary ciliary dyskinesia (PCD), also called **immotile cilia syndrome**, causes problems in the cilia of the respiratory tract so that inhaled bacteria cannot be removed, leading to a chronic lung disease called **bronchiectasis**. Genetic defects can also cause fertility problems by affecting the cilia in the fallopian tubes or the flagella on sperm.[7,9]

Microfilaments

Microfilaments are thin, threadlike cytoplasmic structures. There are three classes of microfilaments:

1. Thin microfilaments, which are similar to thin actin filaments in muscle
2. Intermediate filaments, which are a group of filaments with diameter sizes between those of the thick and thin filaments
3. Thick myosin filaments, which are in muscle cells but may also exist temporarily in other cells.[5]

Muscle contraction depends on the interaction between the thin actin filaments and thick myosin filaments. Contractile activities involving the microfilaments and thick myosin filaments help the cytoplasm and cell membrane move during endocytosis and exocytosis. Microfilaments are also present in the microvilli of the intestine. The intermediate filaments help support and maintain the shape of cells. Examples of intermediate filaments are keratin filaments found in the keratinocytes of the skin and glial filaments found in the glial cells of the nervous system.[5] The **neurofibrillary tangles** found in the brain in Alzheimer disease are formed by aggregated microtubule-associated proteins and result in abnormal cytoskeletons in neurons.

The Cell (Plasma) Membrane

The cell is surrounded by a thin membrane that separates the intracellular contents from the extracellular environment. (Note that this is different from a cell wall.) For example, some bacteria are surrounded by both a cell membrane and a cell wall. Cell walls add structure and strength, but it is important to note that the cell wall of bacteria can be either gram negative or gram positive. Human cells do not have cell walls because of the development of tissues, organs, and organ systems, which must have the ability to communicate. To differentiate the cell membrane surrounding the cell from other internal cell membranes, such as the mitochondrial or nuclear membranes, the cell membrane is often called the **plasma membrane**.

In many ways, the cell membrane is one of the most important parts of the cell. It acts as a semipermeable structure that helps determine what can and cannot enter and exit cells. The cell membrane contains receptors for hormones, neurotransmitters, and other chemical signals, as well as transporters that allow ions to cross the membrane during electrical signaling in cells (such as neurons and muscle cells). It also helps regulate cell growth and division.

The cell membrane is a dynamic and fluid structure made up of organized lipids, carbohydrates, and proteins (Fig. 2.7). The main part of the membrane is the lipid bilayer, made up mostly of phospholipids, with glycolipids and cholesterol.[7] This lipid bilayer is a mostly impermeable barrier to all but lipid-soluble substances.

Phospholipid molecules are arranged so their hydrophilic, water-loving heads face outward on each side of the membrane, where there is watery extracellular or intracellular fluid, and their hydrophobic tails project toward the middle of the membrane (think of this as a peanut butter sandwich,

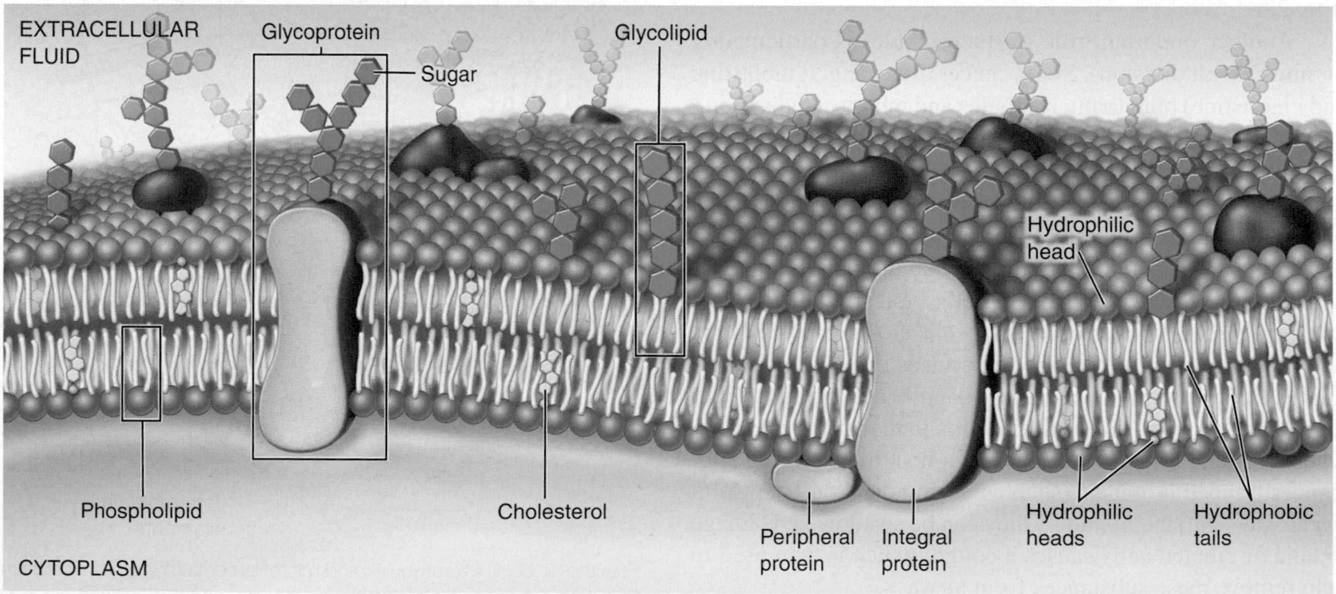

Figure 2.7 • Structure of the cell membrane showing the hydrophilic (polar) heads and the hydrophobic (fatty acid) tails. (From McConnell T. H., Hull K. L. (2011). *Human form, human function: Essentials of anatomy & physiology* (p. 67). Philadelphia, PA: Lippincott Williams & Wilkins.)

where the two slices of bread are the hydrophilic heads, and the peanut butter is the lipophilic tails).

Although the lipid bilayer provides the basic structure of the cell membrane, proteins carry out most of the functions. The way proteins are associated with the cell membrane often determines their function. The **integral proteins** cross the entire lipid bilayer and are also called **transmembrane proteins**. Transmembrane proteins can function on both sides of the membrane or transport molecules across it. For example, many transmembrane proteins form ion channels and are selective for which substances move through them. Mutations in channel proteins, often called **channelopathies**, can cause genetic disorders.[10] For example, **cystic fibrosis** involves an abnormal chloride channel, which causes the epithelial cell membrane to be impermeable to the chloride ion. The defective chloride secretion with excessive sodium and water causes abnormally thick and viscid respiratory secretions, blocking the airways. Water channels or pores called **aquaporins** are also transmembrane proteins in the cell membrane. Changes in water transport through aquaporin can cause diseases, including diabetes insipidus. Carriers are another type of transmembrane protein that allows substances to cross membranes. Glucose transporters (GLUT) are examples of carriers, and changes in the movement of glucose through these carriers are involved in diabetes mellitus.[8]

The **peripheral proteins** are temporarily bound to one side or the other of the membrane and do not pass into the lipid bilayer, and they have functions involving the inner or outer side of the membrane where they are found. Several peripheral proteins are receptors for chemical signals or are involved in intracellular signaling systems.

IN SUMMARY

The cell is a self-sufficient structure that functions similarly to the total organism. In most cells, a single nucleus controls cell function. It contains DNA, which provides the information necessary to make the various proteins the cell needs to stay alive and to transmit genetic information from one generation to another. The nucleus also is where RNA is made. The three types of RNA (mRNA, rRNA, tRNA) move to the cytoplasm to make proteins.

The cytoplasm contains the cell's organelles and cytoskeleton. Ribosomes are sites for protein synthesis in the cell. The ER transports substances from one part of the cell to another and makes proteins (rough ER), carbohydrates, and lipids (smooth ER). Golgi bodies modify substances made in the ER and package them into secretory granules for transport within the cell or for export from the cell. Lysosomes, which are viewed as the digestive system of the cell, contain enzymes that digest worn-out cell parts and foreign materials. The proteasome digests misformed and misfolded proteins. The mitochondria serve as power plants for the cell because they change nutrient energy into ATP to power cell activities. Mitochondria contain their own DNA, which is important for making mitochondrial RNAs and proteins used in oxidative metabolism. The cytoplasm also contains microtubules, microfilaments, intermediate filaments, and thick filaments. Microtubules help determine cell shape, provide a means of moving organelles through the cytoplasm, and help move cilia and chromosomes during cell division. Actin microfilaments and myosin thin filaments interact so that muscle cells can contract.

The cell membrane is a lipid bilayer that surrounds the cell and separates it from its surrounding external environment. Although the lipid bilayer provides the basic structure of the cell membrane, proteins carry out most of the specific functions of the cell membrane. Peripheral proteins often function as receptor sites for signaling molecules, and transmembrane proteins frequently form transporters for ions and other substances.

INTEGRATION OF CELL FUNCTION AND REPLICATION

After completing this section of the chapter, you should be able to meet the following objectives:

- Order the pathway for cell communication, from the receptor to the response, and explain why the process is often referred to as *signal transduction*.
- Link the phases of the cell cycle to cell replication.
- Predict how changes in oxygen delivery to cells changes cellular respiration and levels of ATP and carbon dioxide.

Cell Communication

Cells in multicellular organisms need to communicate with each other to coordinate their function and control their growth. The human body has several ways of sending information between cells. These include direct communication between neighboring cells through gap junctions, autocrine and paracrine signaling, and endocrine or synaptic signaling.[7] In some parts of the body, the same chemical messenger can function as a neurotransmitter, a paracrine mediator, and a hormone secreted by neurons into the bloodstream.

- **Autocrine signaling** (*auto*: self) occurs when a cell releases a chemical into the extracellular fluid that affects its own activity (Fig. 2.8).
- **Paracrine signaling** acts mainly on nearby cells.
- **Endocrine signaling** relies on hormones carried in the bloodstream to cells throughout the body.
- **Synaptic signaling** occurs in the nervous system, where neurotransmitters are released from neurons to act only on neighboring cells at **synapses**.

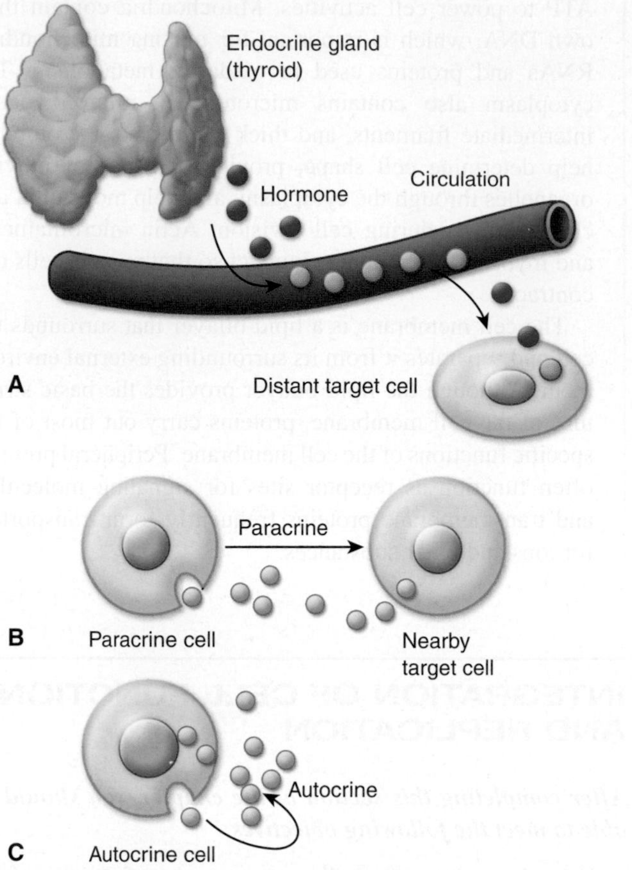

Figure 2.8 • Examples of endocrine **(A)**, paracrine **(B)**, and autocrine **(C)** secretions.

KEY POINTS

CELL COMMUNICATION

- Cells communicate with each other and with the internal and external environments in a number of ways; for example, electrical and chemical signaling systems control electrical potentials, the overall function of a cell, and gene activity needed for cell division and cell replication.
- Chemical messengers bind to protein receptors on the cell surface or inside of cells in a process called **signal transduction.**
- Cells can regulate their responses to chemical messengers by increasing or decreasing the number of receptors.

Cell Receptors

Signaling systems include receptors found either in the cell membrane (cell surface receptors) or within the cells (intracellular receptors). Receptors are activated by a variety of extracellular chemical signals or **first messengers**, including neurotransmitters, hormones and growth factors, and other chemical messengers. Receptors are proteins, and the chemical that bind to them are called ligands.

Hydrophilic (water-loving) chemicals do not easily enter cells, so they usually bind to cell surface receptors. Lipophilic (lipid-loving) substances can cross the lipophilic center of the membrane and can bind to receptors in cytoplasm or nucleus receptors.

Signaling systems also include transducers and effectors that are involved in changing the signal into a response. The pathway may include additional intracellular molecules called **second messengers.**[7] Many molecules involved in signal transduction are proteins because proteins can change their shape or conformation, thereby changing their function and consequently the functions of the cell. Often during signal transduction, enzymes called **protein kinases** catalyze the addition of a phosphate to proteins, and this changes their structure and function.[7]

Cell Surface Receptors

Each cell type in the body contains a unique set of surface receptors that allow the cell to respond to a set of signaling molecules in a specific way. These proteins can increase or decrease in number according to the needs of the cell. When excess chemical signals are present, the number of active receptors decreases in a process called **down-regulation**. When there are decreased chemical signals, the number of active receptors increases through **up-regulation**. The three classes of cell surface receptor proteins are G-protein linked, ion channel linked, and enzyme linked.[5]

G-Protein–Linked Receptors. With more than 1000 members, G-protein–linked receptors are the largest family of cell surface receptors.[5] These receptors rely on the activity of membrane-bound, intracellular regulatory proteins to convert external signals (first messengers) into internal signals (second messengers). Because these regulatory proteins bind to guanine diphosphate (GDP) and guanine triphosphate (GTP), they are called **G-proteins**. G-protein–linked receptors participate in cellular responses for many types of first messengers.[5]

Although there are differences between the G-protein–linked receptors, all share a number of features.[7] They all have an extracellular receptor part that binds to the chemical signal (first messenger). They all undergo shape changes when the receptor binds to a signal, and the shape change activates the intracellular G-protein. The G-proteins use a **GTPase cycle**, which functions as a molecular switch. In its activated (on) state, the G-protein binds GTP, and in its inactivated (off) state, it binds GDP.[5]

At the molecular level, G-proteins are heterotrimeric, meaning they have three (tri) different (hetero) subunits (see Fig. 2.9)[1]: alpha (α), beta (β), and gamma (γ) (Fig. 2.9). The α subunit can bind either GDP or GTP and contains the GTPase activity.[1] When GTP is bound, the G-protein is

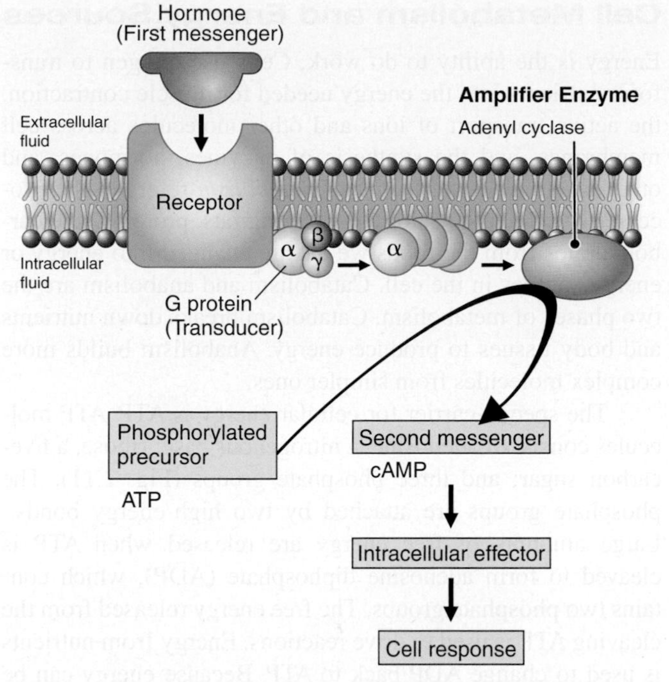

Figure 2.9 • Activation of a G-protein–linked receptor and production of cyclic adenosine monophosphate (cAMP). Binding of a hormone (the first messenger) causes the activated receptor to interact with the inactive, GDP-bound G-protein. This results in activation of the G-protein and dissociation of the G-protein α, β, and γ subunits. The activated α subunit of the G-protein can then interact with and activate the membrane protein adenylyl cyclase to catalyze the conversion of adenosine triphosphate (ATP) to the second messenger cAMP. The second messenger then activates an internal effector, which leads to the cell response.

active. The activated G-protein has GTPase activity, which changes the bound GTP (with three phosphate groups) to GDP (with two phosphate groups), and the G-protein changes to its inactive state. Receptor activation causes the α subunit to separate from the receptor and the β and γ subunits and to send the signal from the first messenger to its effector protein.

Often, the effector is an enzyme that converts an inactive precursor molecule into a second messenger, which diffuses into the cytoplasm and carries the signal beyond the cell membrane. A common second messenger is cyclic adenosine monophosphate (cAMP). It is activated by the enzyme **adenylyl cyclase**, which generates cAMP by transferring phosphate groups from ATP to other proteins.[1] This transfer changes the shape and function of these proteins. Such changes eventually produce the cell response to the first messenger, whether it is a secretion, muscle contraction or relaxation, a change in metabolism, or the opening of ion channels.

Enzyme-Linked Receptors. Like G-protein–linked receptors, enzyme-linked receptors are transmembrane proteins, with their ligand-binding site on the outer surface of the cell membrane.[5] Instead of having an intracellular part that associates with a G-protein, their intracellular part either has enzyme activity or binds directly with an enzyme.

There are several classes of enzyme-linked receptors, including those that activate or have tyrosine kinase activity. Enzyme-linked receptors stimulate cellular responses such as calcium entry into cells, increased sodium–potassium exchange across the cell membrane, and stimulation of glucose and amino acid entry into cells. Insulin, for example, acts by binding to a surface receptor with tyrosine kinase activity.

The intracellular signaling cascades stimulated by the activation of tyrosine kinase receptors are also involved in the function of growth factors. As their name implies, many growth factors are important messengers in signaling cell replacement and cell growth. Most of the growth factors belong to one of three groups:

- Factors that stimulate the division and development of various cell types (*e.g.*, epidermal growth factor and vascular endothelial growth factor)
- Cytokines, which are important in the regulation of the immune system
- Colony-stimulating factors, which regulate the division and maturation of white and red blood cells.

All growth factors function by binding to specific receptors that deliver signals to target cells. These signals have two general effects: (1) they stimulate protein synthesis from many genes that were silent in resting cells, and (2) they stimulate cells to enter the cell cycle for cell division.

Ion Channel–Linked Receptors. Ion channel–linked receptors are involved in the rapid signaling between electrically excitable cells such as neurons and muscle cells.[5] Remember that ions have charge, and when ions move through the membrane, they change local charges, or voltages, and there is an electrical signal in cells. Many neurotransmitters stimulate this type of signaling by opening or closing ion channels in the cell membrane.

Intracellular Receptors

Some signals, such as thyroid hormone and steroid hormones, do not bind to cell surface receptors but move across the cell membrane and bind to intracellular receptors, and they influence DNA activity. Many of these hormones bind to a cytoplasmic receptor, and the receptor–hormone complex enters the nucleus. In the nucleus, the receptor–hormone complex binds to DNA to change protein synthesis.[1]

The Cell Cycle and Cell Division

The life cycle of a cell is called the **cell cycle**. It is usually divided into five phases (Fig. 2.10):

1. G_0 is when the cell may leave the cell cycle and either remain in a state of inactivity or reenter the cell cycle at another time.

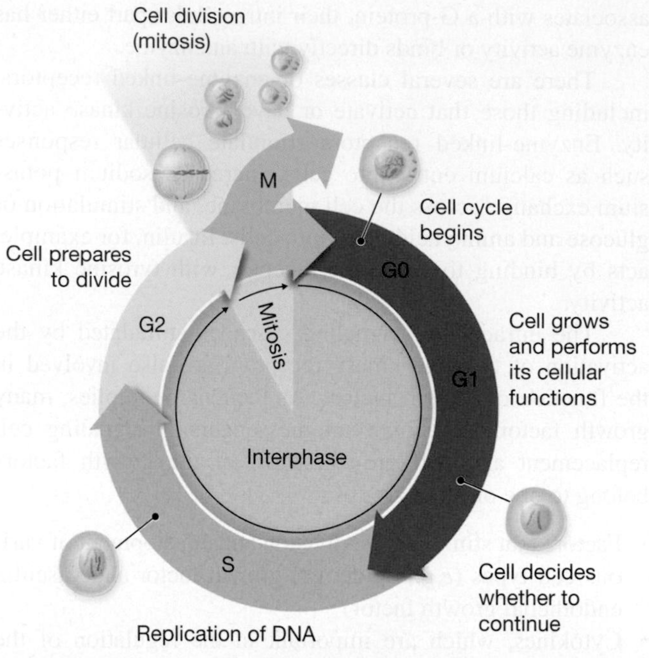

Figure 2.10 • The cell cycle. G_0, nondividing cell; G_1, cell growth; S, DNA replication; G_2, protein synthesis; and M, mitosis. (From Wingerd B. (2014). *The human body. Concepts of anatomy and physiology* (3rd ed.). Philadelphia, PA: Lippincott Williams & Wilkins.)

2. G_1 is when the cell begins to prepare for mitosis by increasing proteins, organelles, and cytoskeletal elements.
3. S phase is the synthesis phase, when DNA synthesis or replication occurs and the centrioles begin to replicate.
4. G_2 is the premitotic phase and is similar to G_1 in terms of RNA activity and protein synthesis.
5. M phase is when cell mitosis occurs.[7]

Tissues may be made up mostly of cells in G_0, but most tissues contain a combination of cells that are continuously moving through the cell cycle and cells that occasionally enter the cell cycle. Nondividing cells, such as neurons and skeletal and cardiac muscle cells, have left the cell cycle and are not capable of mitotic division in postnatal life.[7]

Cell division, or mitosis, is the process during which a parent cell divides and each daughter cell receives chromosomes identical to the parent cell.[7] Cell division gives the body a means of replacing cells that have a limited life span such as skin and blood cells, increasing tissue mass during periods of growth, and providing for tissue repair and wound healing.

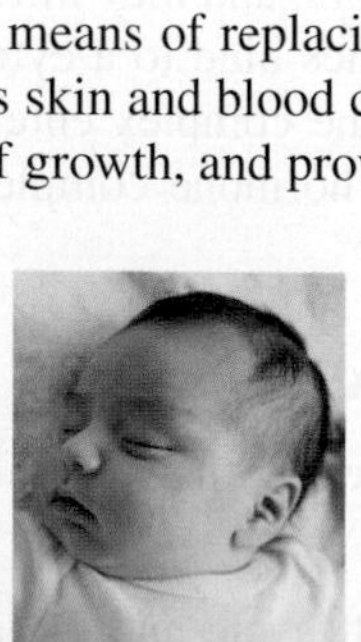

Remember **Jennifer,** the newborn from the unit opener case study? When children are born with specific characteristics, such as poor muscle tone, depressed nasal bridge, a flat facial profile, and upslanting almond-shaped eyes, a genetic analysis called a karyotype is performed. The karyotype results indicate a positive trisomy 21, or three copies of chromosome 21.

Cell Metabolism and Energy Sources

Energy is the ability to do work. Cells use oxygen to transform nutrients into the energy needed for muscle contraction, the active transport of ions and other molecules across cell membranes, and the synthesis of enzymes, hormones, and other macromolecules. *Energy metabolism* refers to the processes by which the calorie-containing fats, proteins, and carbohydrates from the foods we eat are changed into energy or energy sources in the cell. Catabolism and anabolism are the two phases of metabolism. Catabolism breaks down nutrients and body tissues to produce energy. Anabolism builds more complex molecules from simpler ones.

The special carrier for cellular energy is ATP. ATP molecules consist of adenosine, a nitrogenous base; ribose, a five-carbon sugar; and three phosphate groups (Fig. 2.11). The phosphate groups are attached by two high-energy bonds.[7] Large amounts of free energy are released when ATP is cleaved to form adenosine diphosphate (ADP), which contains two phosphate groups. The free energy released from the cleaving ATP is used to drive reactions. Energy from nutrients is used to change ADP back to ATP. Because energy can be "saved or spent" using ATP, ATP is often called the *energy currency* of the cell.

Energy transformation takes place within the cell through two types of energy production pathways:

- The **anaerobic** (*i.e.*, without oxygen) glycolytic pathway occurs in the cytoplasm.
- The **aerobic** (*i.e.*, with oxygen) pathway occurs in the mitochondria.

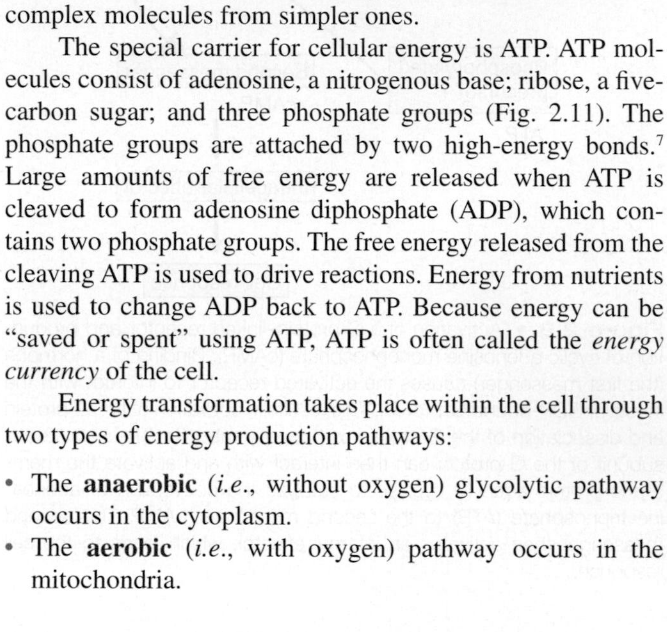

Figure 2.11 • ATP is the major source of cellular energy. **(A)** Each molecule of ATP contains two high-energy bonds, each containing about 12 kcal of potential energy. **(B)** The high-energy ATP bonds are in constant flux. They are generated by substrate (glucose, amino acid, and fat) metabolism and are consumed as the energy is expended.

Understanding Cell Metabolism

Cell metabolism is the process that changes the calorie-containing nutrients (carbohydrates, proteins, and fats) into ATP, which provides for the energy needs of the cell. ATP is formed through three major pathways: (1) the glycolytic pathway, (2) the citric acid cycle, and (3) the electron transport chain. Without oxygen, cells will use the glycolytic pathway in the cytosol and make two molecules of ATP from one glucose molecule. With oxygen and mitochondria, cells will make much more ATP per glucose molecule.

Cells start the energy metabolism process with the anaerobic glycolytic pathway in the cytoplasm, and if oxygen is present, the pathway moves into the mitochondria for the aerobic pathway. Both pathways involve oxidation–reduction reactions involving an electron donor, which is oxidized in the reaction, and an electron acceptor, which is reduced in the reaction. In energy metabolism, the breakdown products of carbohydrate, fat, and protein metabolism donate electrons and are oxidized, and the coenzymes nicotinamide adenine dinucleotide (NAD^+) and flavin adenine dinucleotide (FAD) accept electrons and are reduced.[7]

Anaerobic Metabolism

Glycolysis (*glycol*, sugar; *lysis*, breaking down) is the process by which energy is released from glucose. It is an important energy provider for cells that lack mitochondria, the cell organelles where aerobic metabolism occurs. Glycolysis also provides energy in situations when delivery of oxygen to the cell is delayed or impaired (*e.g.*, in skeletal muscle during the first few minutes of exercise).

Glycolysis, which occurs in the cytoplasm of the cell, involves the splitting of the six-carbon glucose molecule into two three-carbon molecules of pyruvic acid. Because the reaction that splits glucose requires two molecules of ATP, there is a net gain of only two molecules of ATP from each molecule of glucose that is metabolized. The process is anaerobic and does not require oxygen (O_2) or produce carbon dioxide (CO_2). When O_2 is present, pyruvic acid moves into the mitochondria, where it enters the aerobic citric acid cycle. Under anaerobic conditions, such as cardiac arrest or circulatory shock, pyruvate is converted to lactic acid, allowing glycolysis to continue as a means of supplying cells with ATP when O_2 is lacking.

Converting pyruvate to lactic acid is reversible, and after the oxygen supply has been restored, lactic acid is converted back to pyruvate and used for energy or to make glucose.

The liver and a few other tissues remove lactic acid from the bloodstream and convert it to glucose in a process called **gluconeogenesis** (*gluco*, glucose; *neo*, new; *genesis*, to generate or make; this process generates new glucose). This glucose is released into the bloodstream to be used again by cells. Heart muscle is also efficient in changing lactic acid to pyruvate and then using the pyruvate for energy. Pyruvate is a particularly important source of energy for the heart during heavy exercise when the skeletal muscles are producing large amounts of lactic acid and releasing it into the bloodstream.

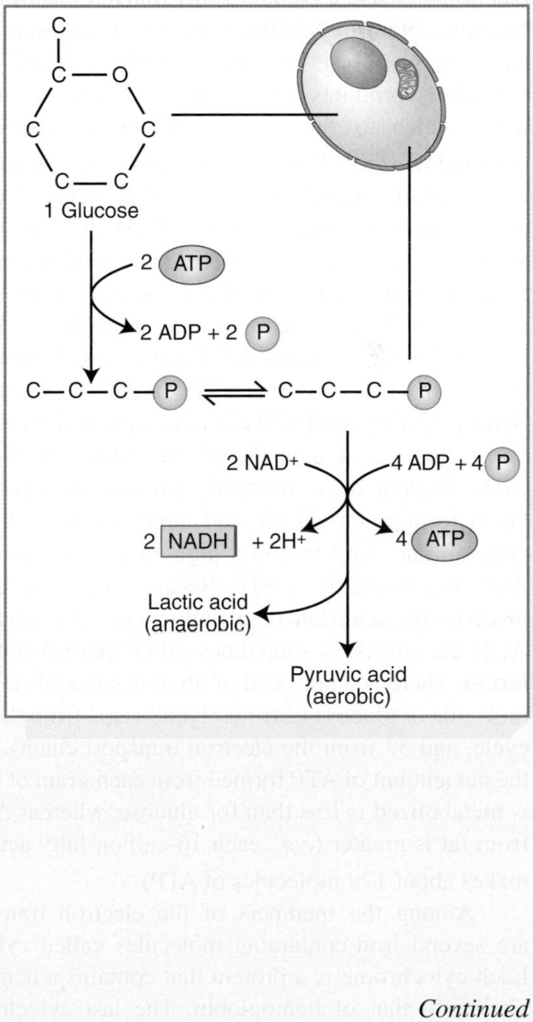

Continued

Understanding Cell Metabolism *(Continued)*

Aerobic Metabolism

Aerobic metabolism occurs in the cell's mitochondria and involves the citric acid cycle and the electron transport chain. It is here that the carbon compounds from the fats, proteins, and carbohydrates in our diet are broken down and their electrons combined with oxygen to form carbon dioxide, water, and ATP. Unlike lactic acid, which is an end product of anaerobic metabolism, carbon dioxide and water are generally harmless and easily eliminated from the body.[7]

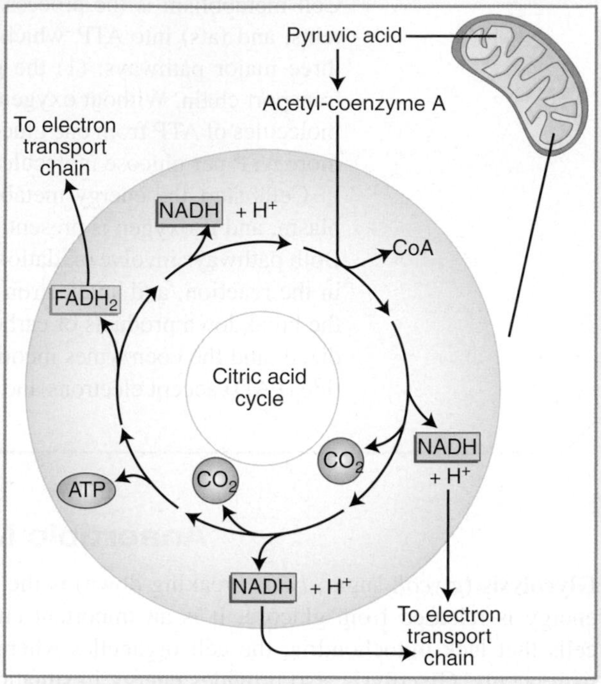

Under aerobic conditions, both of the pyruvate molecules formed by the glycolytic pathway enter the mitochondria, where pyruvate combines with acetyl-coenzyme to form acetyl-coenzyme A (acetyl-CoA). The formation of acetyl-CoA begins the reactions in the citric acid cycle, also called the **tricarboxylic acid** (TCA) or **Krebs cycle**. Some reactions release CO_2, and some transfer electrons from the hydrogen atom to NADH or FADH. In addition to pyruvate from the glycolysis of glucose, fatty acid and amino acid breakdown products can also enter the citric acid cycle. Fatty acids, which are the major source of fuel in the body, are oxidized to acetyl-CoA for entry into the citric acid cycle.[1,6,7]

Oxidative metabolism takes place in the electron transport chain in the mitochondria.[1,6,7] At the end of the citric acid cycle, each glucose molecule has yielded four new molecules of ATP (two from glycolysis and two from the citric acid cycle). In fact, the main function of these earlier stages is to make the electrons (e^-) from glucose and other nutrients available for oxidation. Oxidation of the electrons carried by NADH and $FADH_2$ is accomplished through a series of enzyme reactions in the mitochondrial electron transport chain. During these reactions, protons (H^+) combine with O_2 to form water (H_2O), and large amounts of energy are released and used to add a high-energy phosphate bond to ADP, converting it to ATP. Because the formation of ATP involves the addition of a high-energy phosphate bond to ADP, the process is sometimes called **oxidative phosphorylation**. There is a net yield of 36 molecules of ATP from one molecule of glucose (2 from glycolysis, 2 from the citric acid cycle, and 32 from the electron transport chain). In general, the net amount of ATP formed from each gram of protein that is metabolized is less than for glucose, whereas ATP formed from fat is greater (*e.g.*, each 16-carbon fatty acid molecule makes about 129 molecules of ATP).

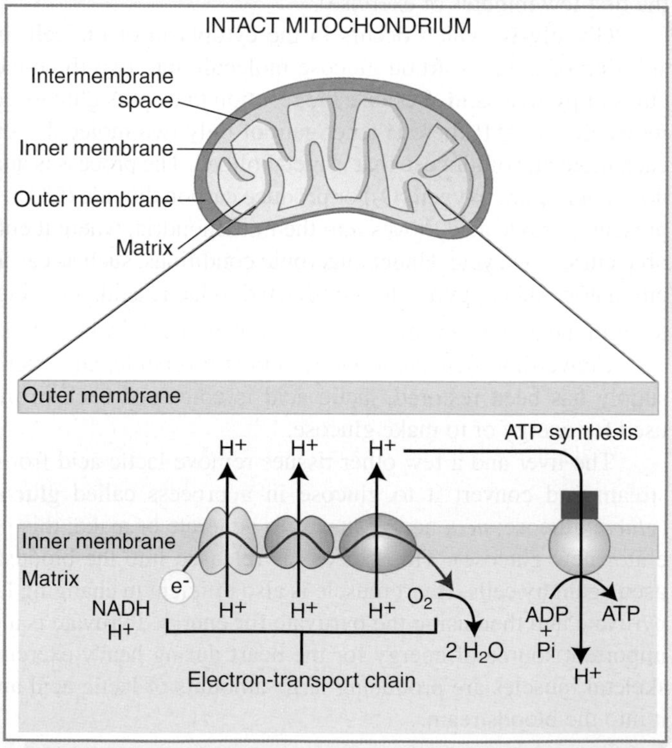

Among the members of the electron transport chain are several iron-containing molecules called **cytochromes**. Each cytochrome is a protein that contains a heme structure similar to that of hemoglobin. The last cytochrome complex is cytochrome oxidase, which passes electrons from cytochrome c to oxygen. Cytochrome oxidase has a lower

Understanding Cell Metabolism *(Continued)*

binding affinity for oxygen than myoglobin (the intracellular heme-containing oxygen carrier) or hemoglobin (the heme-containing oxygen transporter in erythrocytes in the blood). Thus, oxygen is pulled from red blood cells to myoglobin and from myoglobin to cytochrome oxidase, where it is reduced to H_2O.[6,7] Although iron deficiency anemia is characterized by decreased levels of hemoglobin, the iron-containing cytochromes in the electron transport chain in tissues such as skeletal muscle are affected as well. Thus, the fatigue that develops in iron deficiency anemia results, in part, from impaired function of the electron transport chain.

IN SUMMARY

Cells communicate with each other by chemical messenger systems. In some tissues, chemical messengers move from cell to cell through gap junctions without entering the extracellular fluid. Other types of chemical messengers bind to cell surface or intracellular receptors. Three classes of cell surface receptor proteins are G-protein linked, ion channel linked, and enzyme linked. G-protein–linked receptors rely on molecules called **G-proteins** that work like an on–off switch to change external signals (first messengers) into internal signals (second messengers). Ion channel–linked signaling opens or closes ion channels formed in the cell membrane. Enzyme-linked receptors activate intracellular enzymes. Intracellular receptors bind to DNA to change protein synthesis.

The life cycle of a cell is called the **cell cycle**. It is usually divided into five phases: G_0, or the resting phase; G_1, during which the cell begins to prepare for division; the S or synthetic phase, during which DNA replication occurs; G_2, which is the premitotic phase and is similar to G_1; and the M phase, during which cell division occurs. Cell division, or mitosis, is the process during which a parent cell divides into two daughter cells, each receiving an identical pair of chromosomes.

Metabolism is the process whereby carbohydrates, fats, and proteins from the foods we eat are broken down and then changed into the energy needed for cell function. Energy is converted to ATP, the energy currency of the cell. Two sites of energy conversion are present in cells: the anaerobic glycolytic pathway in the cytoplasm and the aerobic pathways in the mitochondria. The most efficient of these pathways is the aerobic citric acid cycle and electron transport chain in the mitochondria. This pathway requires oxygen and produces carbon dioxide and water as end products. The glycolytic pathway in the cytoplasm involves the breakdown of glucose to form ATP. This pathway can function without oxygen by producing lactic acid.

MOVEMENT ACROSS THE CELL MEMBRANE AND MEMBRANE POTENTIALS

After completing this section of the chapter, you should be able to meet the following objectives:

- Compare and contrast membrane transport mechanisms: diffusion, osmosis, active transport, endocytosis, and exocytosis.
- Predict changes in membrane potentials based on diffusion of ions.

The cell membrane serves as a barrier that controls which substances enter and leave the cell. This barrier allows substances that are essential for cellular function to enter the cell while keeping out substances that are harmful. Most cell membranes are semipermeable, meaning that some substances such as water can cross the membrane (the membranes are *permeable* to these substances), but other substances cannot cross the membrane (the membranes are *impermeable* to these substances).

The cell membrane is responsible for differences in the composition of intracellular and extracellular fluids. For example, the extracellular fluid usually has higher concentrations of sodium, calcium, and chloride ions compared to the intracellular fluid, and the intracellular fluid usually has higher concentrations of potassium compared to the extracellular fluid.

Movement of Substances across the Cell Membrane

Movement through the cell membrane occurs in essentially three ways:

- By simple diffusion following the concentration gradient
- By carrier proteins, which are responsible for transporting only one type of molecule and may be involved in active transport
- By channel proteins, which transfer water-soluble molecules and serve as the ion selectivity filter (Fig. 2.12).

Vesicular transport allows the cell membrane to remain intact while allowing molecules to pass through. This process is achieved by endocytosis, which brings materials into the cell, and exocytosis, which removes substances from the cell (Fig. 2.13). The cell membrane can also engulf a particle, forming a membrane-bound vesicle; this membrane-coated vesicle is moved into the cell by endocytosis. Substances can also leave the cell when a membrane-bound vesicle fuses with the membrane during exocytosis.[5]

Passive Transport

Passive transport of substances across the cell membrane is influenced by chemical or electrical gradients and does not require an input of energy. A difference in the number of particles on either side of the membrane creates a chemical gradient, and a difference in charged particles or ions creates an electrical gradient. Chemical and electrical gradients are often linked and are called *electrochemical gradients*.[1] For example, positively charged sodium is higher outside the cell compared to inside, and this creates both a chemical gradient (higher concentration) and an electrical gradient (higher charge).

Diffusion. Diffusion is the process by which substances become widely dispersed and reach a uniform concentration because of the energy from their spontaneous kinetic movements (Fig. 2.14A). Substances move from an area of higher to an area of lower concentration. An example of diffusion is when odorant molecules move from a pot of soup to your nose when you are cooking.[1] Lipophilic (lipid-loving) substances such as oxygen, carbon dioxide, alcohol, and steroid hormones can diffuse through the lipid layer of the cell membrane. Hydrophilic (water-loving) substances cannot pass through the lipids of the membrane; instead, they diffuse through water-filled passages in the cell membrane (*i.e.*, the integral proteins discussed previously such as ion channels, aquaporins, and carriers).

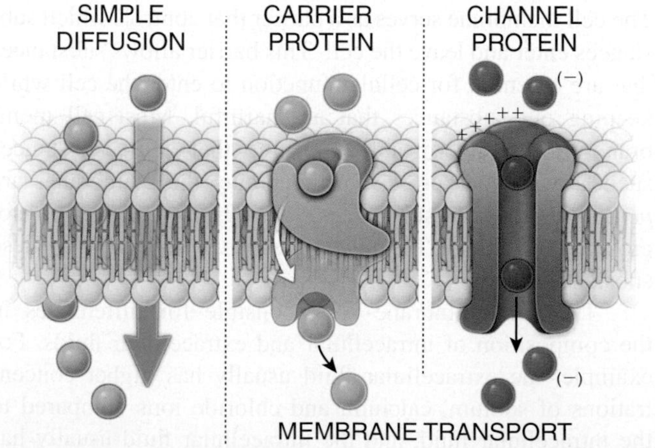

Figure 2.12 • Movement of molecules through the plasma membrane. (Reprinted from Pawlina W. *Histology: A text and atlas with correlated cell and molecular biology* (7th ed., Fig. 2.7, p. 31). Philadelphia, PA: Wolters Kluwer, with permission.)

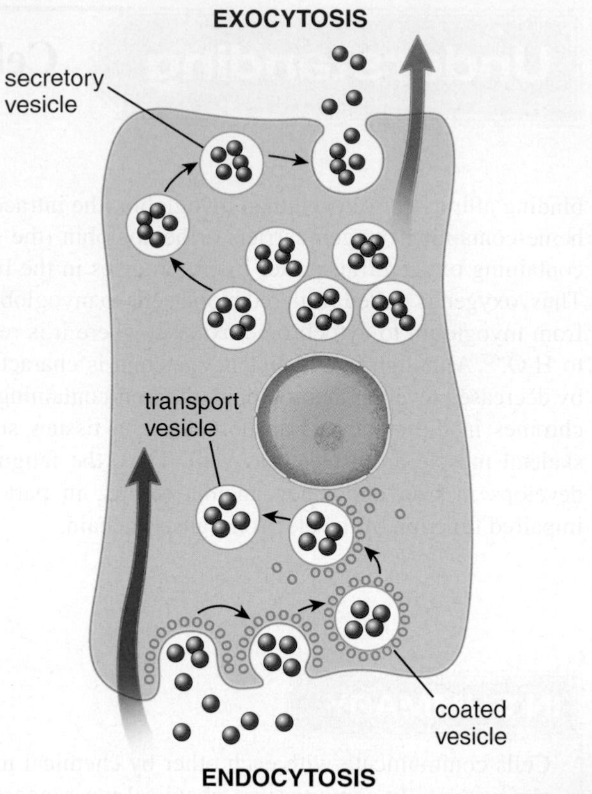

Figure 2.13 • Endocytosis and exocytosis are two major forms of vesicular transport. (Reprinted from Pawlina W. *Histology: A text and atlas with correlated cell and molecular biology* (7th ed., Fig. 2.8, p. 32). Philadelphia, PA: Wolters Kluwer, with permission).

The rate of movement depends on:

- How many particles are available for diffusion
- The kinetic movement of the particles
- The number of openings in the cell membrane through which the particles can move
- Temperature, which changes the motion of the particles—that is, the greater the temperature, the greater the thermal motion of the molecules

Facilitated Diffusion. As described above, small, lipophilic substances can pass through the lipids in cell membranes. Some substances, such as glucose, cannot pass through the cell membrane because they are not lipophilic or are too large to pass through the membrane. These substances need help to cross the membrane, and protein-assisted diffusion is assisted by a transport protein.

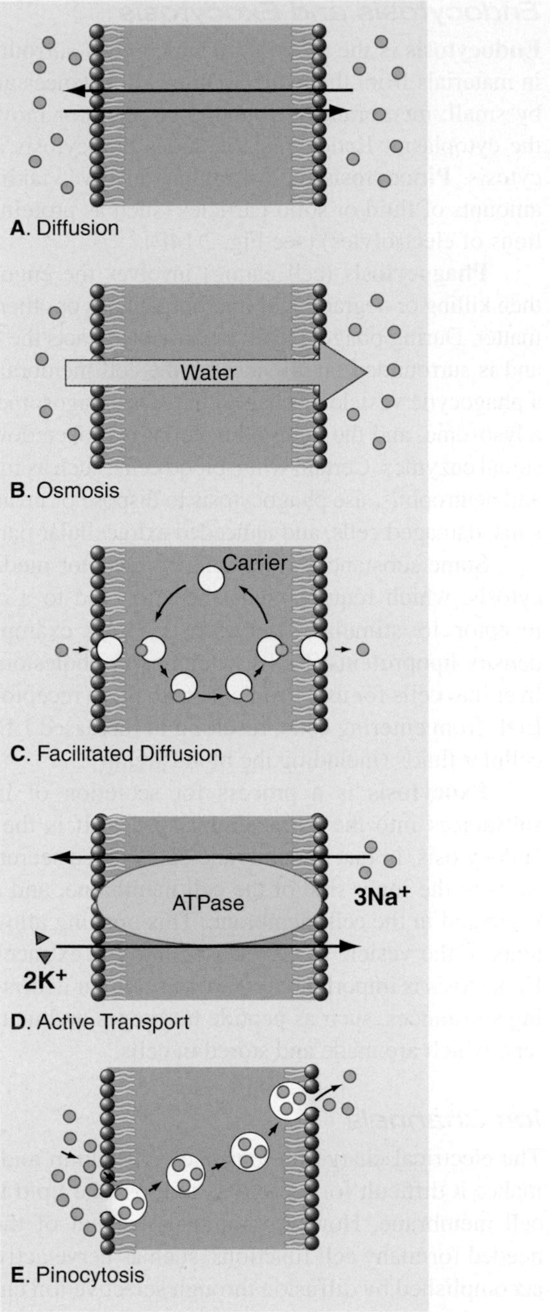

Figure 2.14 • Mechanisms of membrane transport. **(A)** In diffusion, particles move freely to become equally distributed across the membrane. **(B)** In osmosis, osmotically active particles regulate the flow of water. **(C)** Facilitated diffusion uses a carrier system. **(D)** In active transport, selected molecules are transported across the membrane using the energy-driven (Na^+/K^+–ATPase) pump. **(E)** In pinocytosis, the membrane forms a vesicle that engulfs the particle and transports it across the membrane, where it is released.

Substances move from areas of higher concentration to areas of lower concentration, and this does not require an input of energy (see Fig. 2.14C). For example, sodium ions can diffuse through ion channels from outside the cells, where sodium ions have higher concentration, to the inside of cells, where sodium ions have lower concentration.

Substances can move through protein channels (such as ion channels or aquaporins) or through carriers. When substances move through carriers, they bind to the carrier on the membrane's outer surface, are carried across the membrane attached to the carrier, and are then released on the inside of the membrane.

The rate at which a substance moves across the membrane depends on the difference in concentration between the two sides of the membrane. Also important are the availability of transport proteins and how long it takes the substance to cross the membrane. Insulin, which stimulates the transport of glucose into cells, acts by increasing the number of glucose carriers in cell membranes.[1] If a person does not make insulin, or if cells do not respond to insulin, there are fewer GLUT in cell membranes, and less glucose moves from outside the cells from the extracellular fluid (which includes the bloodstream). This results in **hyperglycemia** (*hyper*, high; *gly*, sugar; *emia*, in the blood) and occurs in diabetes mellitus.

Osmosis. Water usually crosses membranes through water channels (aquaporins) down the concentration gradient for water, moving from an area of higher water concentration to areas of lower water concentration (see Fig. 2.12B). This process is called osmosis and is driven by **osmotic pressure.**[1]

Osmosis is regulated by the concentration of substances (besides water) on either side of a membrane that cannot diffuse across the membrane (*e.g.*, if there are no open sodium channels, sodium cannot diffuse across the membrane). When there is a difference in the concentration of impermeable substances across a membrane, water can move via aquaporins from the side with the lower concentration of particles to the side with the higher concentration of particles (and, in effect, moving from the side with higher water concentration to the side with lower water concentration). The movement of water continues until the concentration of substances on either side of the membrane is equally diluted, or until the osmotic pressure opposes the flow of water.

Active Transport and Cotransport

Active transport mechanisms involve the input and use of energy. As we have learned, diffusion moves substances from an area of higher concentration to one of lower concentration, resulting in an equal distribution across the cell membrane. Sometimes, however, different concentrations of a substance are needed in the intracellular and extracellular fluids. For example, to function, a cell requires a much higher intracellular concentration of potassium ions than is present in the extracellular fluid while maintaining a much lower intracellular concentration of sodium ions than the extracellular fluid. In these situations, energy is required to pump the ions "uphill" or against their concentration gradient. When cells use an input of energy to move substances against an electrical or chemical gradient, the process is called **active transport.**[1,7]

The active transport system studied in the greatest detail is the sodium–potassium (Na^+/K^+)–ATPase pump (see Fig. 2.14D). This pump moves three sodium ions from inside the cell to outside the cell and moves two potassium ions from the outside of the cell to the inside of the cell. The Na^+/K^+–ATPase pump moves both of these ions against their concentration gradients.[7] Energy used to do so comes from splitting and releasing energy from the high-energy phosphate bond in ATP by the enzyme ATPase, which is part of the Na^+/K^+–ATPase transport protein. If there is decreased activity of the Na^+/K^+–ATPase pump, the sodium ions will increase in the cell, increasing the osmotic pressure. Water will then diffuse into the cell, causing swelling. If this continues, the cell can burst and die. This can occur in heart attacks and some types of stroke, when blood flow is reduced to some cells. Without blood flow, oxygen cannot be delivered to the cells, causing cells to switch to anaerobic metabolism and make much less ATP. With decreased ATP, the activity of the Na^+/K^+–ATPase pump decreases, sodium ions increase in cells, water diffuses into cells, and cells in the heart or brain die.

There are two types of active transport systems: primary active transport and secondary active transport. In **primary active transport**, the source of energy (*e.g.*, ATP) is used directly in the transport of a substance. **Secondary active transport** mechanisms use the energy from the transport of one substance for the cotransport of a second substance. For example, when sodium ions diffuse into cells, the energy of this movement is used to drive the transport of a second substance against its concentration gradient. Similar to protein-assisted diffusion, secondary active transport mechanisms use membrane transport proteins. Secondary transport systems are classified into two groups: **cotransport** or **symport** systems, in which substances are transported in the same direction, and **countertransport** or **antiport** systems, in which substances are transported in the opposite direction (Fig. 2.15).[7] An example of cotransport occurs in the intestine, where the absorption of glucose and amino acids are linked to sodium transport.

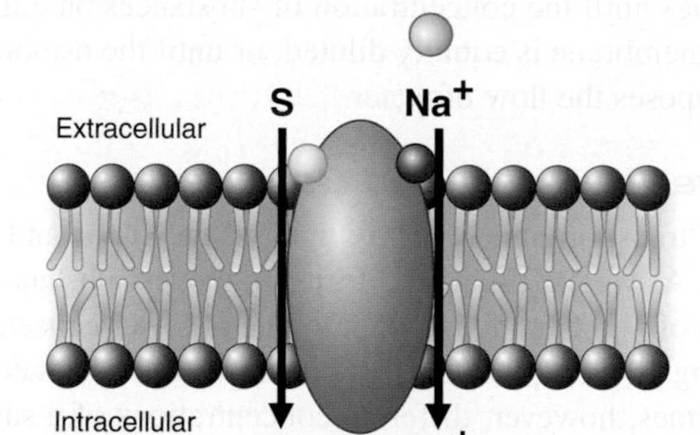

Figure 2.15 • Secondary active transport systems. **(A)** Symport or cotransport carries the transported solute (S) in the same direction as the sodium (Na^+) ion. **(B)** Antiport or countertransport carries the solute and Na^+ in the opposite direction.

Endocytosis and Exocytosis

Endocytosis is the process by which cells surround and take in materials from their surroundings. Substances are engulfed by small, membrane-surrounded vesicles for movement into the cytoplasm. Endocytosis includes pinocytosis and phagocytosis. **Pinocytosis** (cell drinking) involves taking in small amounts of fluid or solid particles (such as proteins and solutions of electrolytes) (see Fig. 2.14E).[5]

Phagocytosis (cell eating) involves the engulfment and then killing or degrading of microorganisms or other particulate matter. During phagocytosis, a particle contacts the cell surface and is surrounded on all sides by the cell membrane, forming a phagocytic vesicle or phagosome. The phagosome fuses with a lysosome, and the ingested material is broken down by lysosomal enzymes. Certain white blood cells, such as macrophages and neutrophils, use phagocytosis to dispose of invading organisms, damaged cells, and unneeded extracellular parts.[5]

Some substances enter cells by receptor-mediated endocytosis, which requires substances to bind to a cell surface receptor to stimulate endocytosis.[5,7] An example is low-density lipoproteins (LDL), which carry cholesterol from the liver into cells for use. Problems with these receptors can keep LDL from entering cells, resulting in increased LDL in extracellular fluids (including the bloodstream).

Exocytosis is a process for secretion of intracellular substances into the extracellular spaces. It is the reverse of endocytosis, in that a membrane-surrounded secretory vesicle fuses to the inner side of the cell membrane, and an opening is created in the cell membrane. This opening allows the contents of the vesicle to be released into the extracellular fluid. Exocytosis is important in removing cellular debris and releasing substances, such as peptide hormones and neurotransmitters, which are made and stored in cells.[5]

Ion Channels

The electrical charge on ions such as sodium and potassium makes it difficult for these ions to cross the lipid layer of the cell membrane. However, rapid movement of these ions is needed for many cell functions, such as nerve activity. This is accomplished by diffusion through selective ion channels. Ion channels are highly selective: Some channels allow only for passage of sodium ions, and other channels are selective for potassium ions, calcium ions, or chloride ions.[7]

Channels are proteins that span the cell membrane with a watery (aqueous) center so that ions and other hydrophilic substances can remain in contact with the aqueous solution that fills the channel. Channels that remain open are called leak channels. Other channels are gated channels, and specific stimuli cause the channels to undergo shape changes from one form to another form. Gated channels can be closed and stimulated to open, or they can be open and stimulated to close (Fig. 2.16).[7]

Three main types of gated channels are present in cell membranes:

- **Voltage-gated channels**, which open or close with changes in the membrane potential

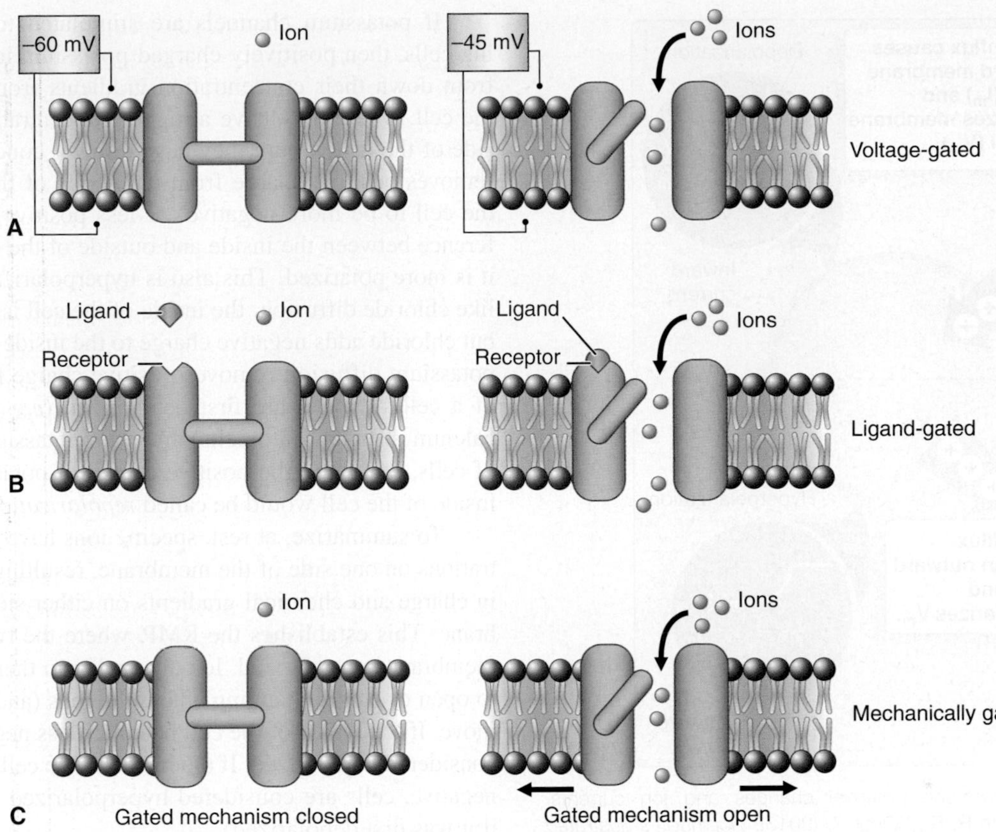

Figure 2.16 • Gated ion channels that open in response to a specific stimulus. **(A)** Voltage-gated channels are controlled by a change in membrane potential. **(B)** Ligand-gated channels are controlled by binding of a ligand to a receptor. **(C)** Mechanically gated channels, which are controlled by mechanical stimuli such as stretching, often have links that connect to the cytoskeleton.

- **Ligand-gated channels** or *chemically gated channels*, which open or close when chemicals bind to the channels; these channels are also receptors, and the chemicals that bind to receptors are called ligands (*e.g.*, the neurotransmitter acetylcholine)
- **Mechanically gated**, which open or close in response to such mechanical stimulations such as vibrations, tissue stretching, temperature, or pressure (see Fig. 2.16).[7]

The gates are what open or close ion channels. Once channels are open, specific ions may move through them, similar to how your key can open a specific gate, allowing you to move through it. In the case of gated channels in cell membranes, the key can be voltage changes, ligand binding, or mechanical stimulations. The ultimate result of the opening of these gates is the movement of ions.

Membrane Potentials

As mentioned above, the concentrations of ions are often different on the two sides of the cell membrane, and this leads to differences in charge on the two sides of a cell membrane. These differences create electrical potentials across the cell membranes of most cells in the body, and these are called **membrane potentials**.[5]

In nerve or muscle cells, changes in the membrane potential are needed for nerve impulses and muscle contraction. In other types of cells, such as glandular cells, changes in the membrane potential stimulate hormone secretion and other functions (*e.g.*, the secretion of insulin from beta cells in the pancreas).

Electrical potentials are measured in volts (V) or millivolts (mV; see below). Electrical potentials describe the ability of separated electrical charges of opposite polarity (+ and –) to do work. The potential difference is the difference between the separated charges. The terms *potential difference* and *voltage* are synonymous.[5]

Voltage is always measured by comparing two points in a system. For example, the voltage in a car battery (6 or 12 V) is the potential difference between the two battery terminals. Because the total amount of charge that can be separated by a cell membrane is small, the potential differences in cells are small and are measured in millivolts (mV) or 1/1000 of a volt (Fig 2.17).

Potential differences across the cell membrane can be measured by inserting a very fine electrode into the cell and another into the extracellular fluid surrounding the cell and connecting the two electrodes to a voltmeter. The voltmeter is set so that the outside is 0 mV, and then the difference in voltage inside the cell is measured. For example, the inside of neurons is –70 mV because there are more negative charges

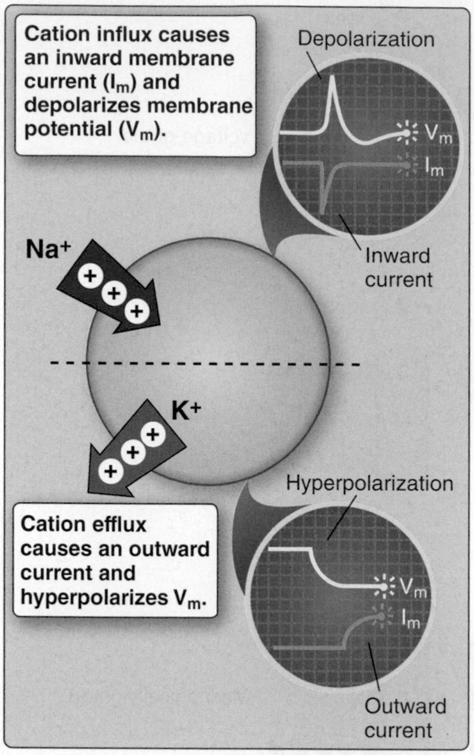

Figure 2.17 • Membrane potential changes and ion currents. (Reprinted from Preston R. R., Wilson T. (2013). *Lippincott's illustrated reviews: Physiology* (Fig. 2.8, p. 20). Philadelphia, PA: Wolters Kluwer, with permission.)

inside of these cells. If cells are not stimulated and at rest, this difference is called the *resting membrane potential* (RMP). The cell is said to be polarized at rest because the two sides of the membrane have different voltages (think of being polarized on an issue, where the two sides have different opinions). In most resting cells, sodium, calcium, and chloride ions are higher outside the cell, and potassium is higher inside the cell.

If sodium or calcium channels are stimulated to open in resting cells, then these positively charged ions will diffuse down their concentration gradients from the outside of the cell, where they have a higher concentration, to the inside of the cell, where they have a lower concentration. This brings positive charge into the cell, causing the cell to be less negative (or more positive). Now, the difference between the inside and outside of the cell is less, so it is less polarized. This is called **depolarization**. (Think again of being polarized on an issue; if your friend changes his or her opinions to be more like your opinions, the two of you would be less polarized, or depolarized, on this issue.)

If chloride channels are stimulated to open in resting cells, then negatively charged chloride ions will also diffuse from the outside of the cell to the inside of the cell. However, this brings negative charge into the cell, causing the cell to be more negative (or less positive). Now, the difference between the inside and outside of the cell is more, so it is more polarized. This is called **hyperpolarization**. (To continue our example: Now, if your friend changes his or her opinions to be less like your opinions, you would be more polarized, or hyperpolarized, on this issue).

If potassium channels are stimulated to open in resting cells, then positively charged potassium ions will diffuse from down their concentration gradients from the inside of the cell, where they have a higher concentration, to the outside of the cell, where they have a lower concentration. This removes positive charge from the inside of the cell, causing the cell to be more negative (or less positive). Now the difference between the inside and outside of the cell is more, so it is more polarized. This also is hyperpolarization (note that like chloride diffusion, the inside of the cell is more negative, but chloride adds negative charge to the inside of the cell, and potassium diffusion removes positive charge from the inside of a cell). If cells are first depolarized (*e.g.*, by sodium or calcium diffusing into cells) and then potassium diffuses out of cells, removing the positive charge of potassium from the inside of the cell would be called *repolarization*.

To summarize, at rest, specific ions have higher concentrations on one side of the membrane, resulting in differences in charge and chemical gradients on either side of the membrane. This establishes the RMP, where the two sides of the membrane are polarized. Ion channels can then be stimulated to open or close, changing where the ions (and their charges) move. If the inside of the cell becomes less negative, cells are considered depolarized. If the inside of the cell becomes more negative, cells are considered hyperpolarized (or repolarized if it was first depolarized).

Graded Potentials

In neurons, dendrites receive signals that change which ion channels are open. If sodium or calcium channels are opened, then the dendrites and cell body are depolarized, because this would result in positive charge traveling into the cell. This is called a graded potential because it is graded to the strength of the signal (stronger signals results in greater depolarization). If there is enough signal and depolarization, then an action potential is stimulated in the axon so that this signal can be passed to the next cell. For example, if someone pokes you in the arm, in your body mechanically gated sodium and/or calcium channels will open, and your neurons will send a signal that will result in your body responding (*i.e.*, pulling your arm away).

If chloride or potassium channels are stimulated to open in dendrites, the inside of the cell becomes more negative. This is called hyperpolarizing graded potential and is inhibitory. As a result of hyperpolarizing graded potentials, even more depolarizing signal is needed to stimulate an action potential and to send the response to the next cell. Drugs such as barbiturates and alcohol can have a profound effect by inhibiting neurotransmitters such as gamma-aminobutyric acid (GABA).

Action Potential

In neurons, if a graded potential is strong enough, then an action potential is generated in the axon of the neuron. The ion movement in graded potentials causes changes in voltage, and this stimulates voltage-gated sodium channels to open in the axon. Sodium ions diffuse into the axon, causing depolarization. This stimulates nearby voltage-gated potassium channels

Understanding Membrane Potentials

Electrochemical potentials are present across the membranes of virtually all cells in the body. Some cells, such as nerve and muscle cells, are capable of generating rapidly changing electrical impulses, and these impulses are used to transmit signals along their membranes. In other cells, such as glandular cells, membrane potentials are used to signal the release of hormones or activate other functions of the cell. Generation of membrane potentials relies on (1) diffusion of current-carrying ions, (2) development of an electrochemical equilibrium, (3) establishment of a RMP, and (4) triggering of action potentials.

Diffusion Potentials

A diffusion potential is a potential difference generated across a membrane when a current-carrying ion, such as the potassium (K^+) ion, diffuses down its concentration gradient. Two conditions are necessary for this to occur: (1) the membrane must be selectively permeable to a particular ion, and (2) the concentration of the diffusible ion must be greater on one side of the membrane than the other.

The magnitude of the diffusion potential, measured in millivolts, depends on the size of the concentration gradient. The sign (+ or –) or polarity of the potential depends on the diffusing ion. It is negative on the inside when a positively charged ion such as K^+ diffuses from the inside to the outside of the membrane, carrying its charge with it.

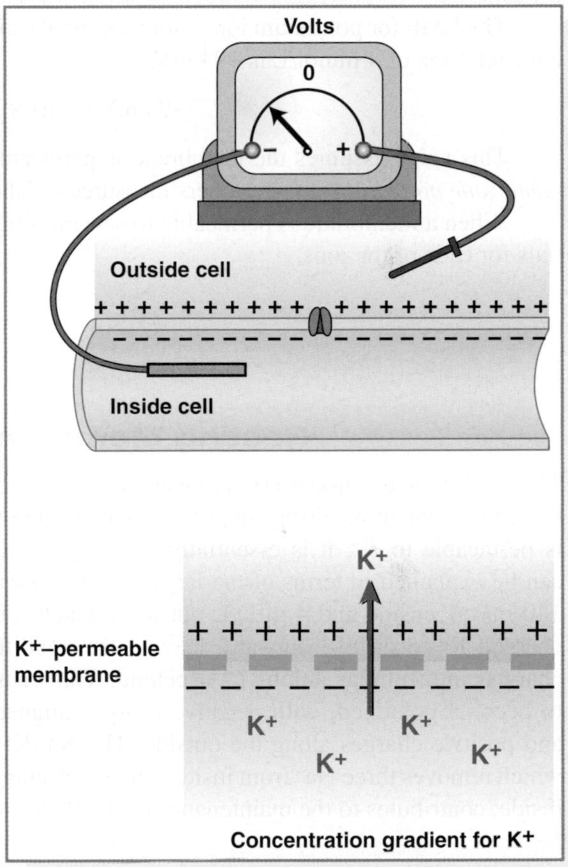

Equilibrium Potentials

An equilibrium potential is the membrane potential that exactly balances and opposes the net diffusion of an ion down its concentration gradient. As a cation diffuses down its concentration gradient, it carries its positive charge across the membrane, thereby generating an electrical force that will eventually retard and stop its diffusion. An electrochemical equilibrium is one in which the *chemical forces driving* diffusion and the *repelling electrical forces* are exactly balanced so that no further diffusion occurs. The equilibrium potential (EMF, electromotive force) can be calculated by inserting the inside and outside ion concentrations into the Nernst equation.

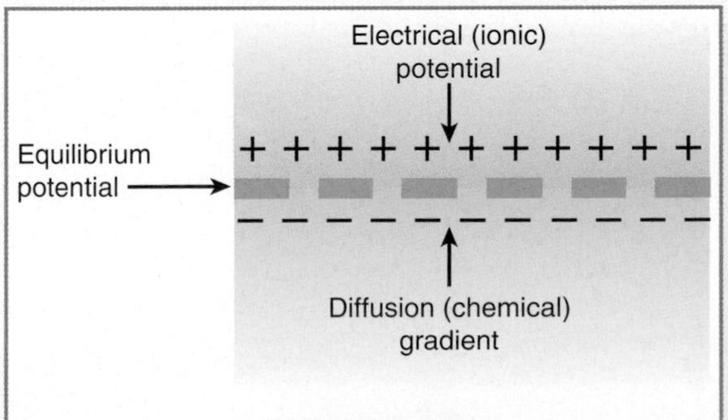

Nernst equation

$$\text{EMF (mV)} = -61 \times \log_{10} (\text{ion concentration inside/ion concentration outside})$$

Continued

Understanding Membrane Potentials (Continued)

The Nernst Equation for Calculating an Equilibrium Potential

The following equation, known as the *Nernst equation*, can be used to calculate the equilibrium potential (electromotive force [EMF] in millivolts [mV] of a univalent ion at body temperature of 37°C).

$$\text{EMF (mV)} = -61 \times \log_{10} \text{(ion concentration inside/ion concentration outside)}$$

For example, if the concentration of an ion inside the membrane is 100 mmol/L and the concentration outside the membrane is 10 mmol/L, the EMF (mV) for that ion would be $-61 \times \log_{10}$ (100/10 [$\log_{10}$ of 10 is 1]). Therefore, it would take 61 mV of charge inside the membrane to balance the diffusion potential created by the concentration difference across the membrane for the ion.

The EMF for potassium ions using a normal estimated intracellular concentration of 140 mmol/L and a normal extracellular concentration of 4 mmol/L is −94 mV:

$$-94 \text{ mV} = -61 \times \log_{10} \text{(140 mmol inside/4 mmol outside)}$$

This value assumes the membrane is permeable only to potassium. This value approximates the −70 to −90 mV *resting membrane potential* for nerve fibers measured in laboratory studies.

When a membrane is permeable to several different ions, the diffusion potential reflects the sum of the equilibrium potentials for each of the ions.

Resting Membrane Potential

The RMP, which is necessary for electrical excitability, is present when the cell is not transmitting impulses. Because the resting membrane is permeable to K^+, it is essentially a K^+ equilibrium potential. This can be explained in terms of the large K^+ concentration gradient (*e.g.*, 140 mEq/L inside and 4 mEq/L outside), which causes the positively charged K^+ to diffuse outward, leaving the nondiffusible, negatively charged intracellular anions (A^-) behind. This causes the membrane to become polarized, with negative charges aligned along the inside and positive charges along the outside. The Na^+/K^+ membrane pump, which removes three Na^+ from inside while returning only two K^+ to the inside, contributes to the maintenance of the RMP.

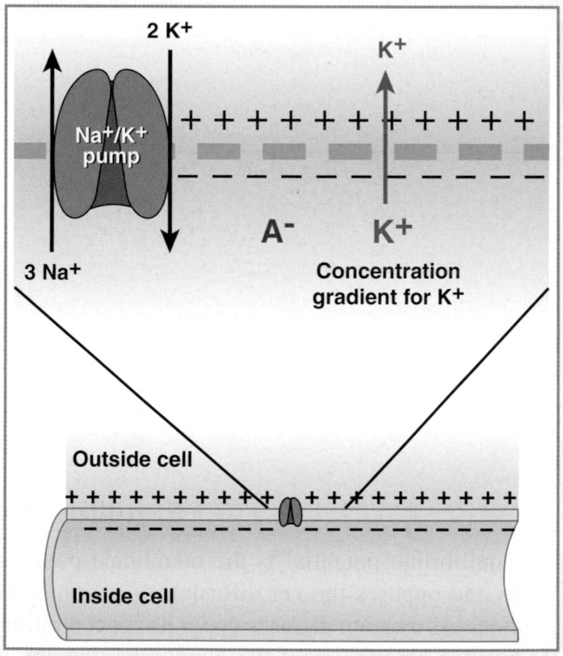

Understanding Membrane Potentials (Continued)

Action Potentials

Action potentials involve rapid changes in the membrane potential. Each action potential begins with a sudden change from the negative RMP to a positive threshold potential, causing an opening of the membrane channels for Na^+ (or other ions of the action potential). Opening of the Na^+ channels allows large amounts of the positively charged Na^+ ions to diffuse to the interior of the cell, causing the membrane potential to undergo depolarization or a rapid change to positive on the inside and negative on the outside. This is quickly followed by closing of Na^+ channels and opening of the K^+ channels, which leads to a rapid efflux of K^+ from the cell and re-establishment of the RMP.

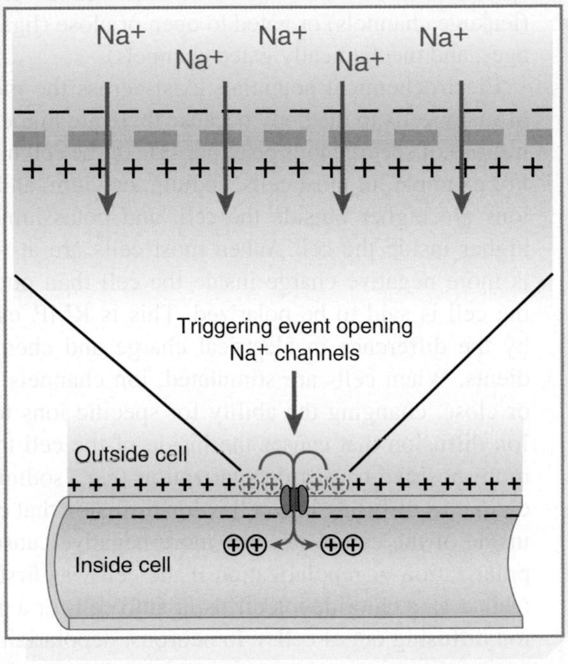

to open, and potassium ions diffuse out of the axon, causing repolarization. This sequence continues until the signal reaches the axon terminal. Some neurons in the central nervous system (CNS) have gap junctions with target neurons, and ions diffuse into the target neuron to stimulate the neuron. Most neurotransmitters are released from neurons by exocytosis, and the neurotransmitters bind to and stimulate target cells. At the axon terminal, the depolarization from the action potential causes calcium channels to open. Calcium diffuses in to stimulate a chain of reactions that stimulates exocytosis of neurotransmitter.

Action potentials are also generated in cardiac muscle cells and skeletal muscle cells. However, ions are involved in different ways compared to neurons. Changes in membrane potential are also involved in other cell types. For example, beta cells in the pancreas respond to increased blood sugar by closing potassium channels, which decreases potassium diffusion out of cells, increasing positive charge inside of beta cells, leading to depolarization. Like in axon terminals of neurons, this depolarization causes calcium channels to open. Calcium diffuses in to cause a chain of reactions that stimulates exocytosis of insulin into the bloodstream to respond to the increase in blood glucose. Many drugs used to treat type II diabetes mellitus target these steps to increase insulin secretion.

IN SUMMARY

Movement of materials across the cell's membrane is needed for survival of the cell. Diffusion is a process by which substances such as ions move down a concentration gradient, from an area of greater concentration to an area of lower concentration. Osmosis is the diffusion of only water molecules through a membrane down the concentration gradient for water, from where water is more concentrated (where there are fewer solutes) to where water is less concentrated (where there are more solutes). Protein-assisted diffusion allows small, hydrophilic (water-loving) substances such as ions or glucose to cross the cell's membrane with the assistance of a transport protein that spans the membrane (a channel or a carrier protein). Another type of transport, called **active transport**, requires the cell to input energy to move substances against a concentration gradient, from an area of lower concentration to an area of higher concentration. Two types of active transport exist, primary and secondary, both of which require carrier proteins. The Na^+/K^+–ATPase pump is the best-known active transporter. **Endocytosis** is a process by which cells engulf materials from the surrounding medium. Small particles are ingested by a process called pinocytosis and larger particles by **phagocytosis**. Some particles require bonding with a ligand, and this process is called **receptor-mediated endocytosis. Exocytosis** involves the removal of large particles from the cell and is essentially the reverse of endocytosis.

Ion channels are integral transmembrane proteins that span the width of the cell membrane and are either open (leakage channels) or gated to open or close (ligand-, voltage-, and mechanically gated channels).

Electrochemical potentials exist across the membranes of many cells in the body because there are higher concentrations of specific ions on either side of the cell membrane. For example, in most cells, sodium, calcium, and chloride ions are higher outside the cell, and potassium ions are higher inside the cell. When most cells are at rest, there is more negative charge inside the cell than outside, and the cell is said to be polarized. This is RMP, established by the difference in electrical charge and chemical gradients. When cells are stimulated, ion channels can open or close, changing the ability for specific ions to diffuse. Ion diffusion that causes the inside of the cell to become more positive causes depolarization (*e.g.*, sodium or calcium ions diffusing into cells). Ion diffusion that causes the inside of the cell to become more negative causes hyperpolarization or repolarization if the cell was first depolarized (*e.g.*, a chloride ion diffusing into cells or a potassium ion diffusing out of cells). In neurons, depolarizing graded potentials can stimulate action potentials to send signals to other cells; hyperpolarizing graded potentials can inhibit action potentials and signaling. Changes in diffusion of ions across a membrane also stimulates electrical signaling in other cells, such as muscles and glands.

BODY TISSUES

After completing this section of the chapter, you should be able to meet the following objectives:

- Link the process of cell differentiation to the development of organ systems in the embryo and the regeneration of tissues in postnatal life.
- Compare and contrast the characteristics of the four different tissue types.

Earlier in this chapter, we discussed the individual cell, its metabolic processes, and ways cells communicate and replicate. Although all cells share certain characteristics, their structures and functions are specialized depending on where they are found in the body. For example, muscle, skin, and nervous cells are structurally distinct from one another and perform vastly different functions. Groups of cells that work together are called tissues. Four categories of tissue exist:

1. Epithelial tissue
2. Connective (supportive) tissue
3. Muscle tissue
4. Nervous tissue

These tissues do not exist in isolated units but combine with other tissues to form the organs of the body. This section provides a brief overview of the cells in each of these four tissue types, the structures that hold these cells together, and the extracellular matrix in which they live.

Cell Differentiation

After conception, the fertilized egg undergoes a series of cell divisions, leading to approximately 200 different cell types. The formation of different types of cells and the placement of these cells into tissue types is called **cell differentiation**, a process controlled by a system that switches genes on (to increase transcription) and switches genes off (to decrease transcription).

Embryonic cells must differentiate (become different) to develop into all of the various cell types and organ systems. Cells must then remain different after the signal that initiated cell differentiation is gone. The process of cell differentiation is controlled by cell memory, which is maintained by proteins in the individual cells of a particular cell type. This means that after differentiation has occurred, the tissue type does not change back to an earlier stage of differentiation. The process of cell differentiation normally moves forward, producing cells that are more specialized than their predecessors.[1] Usually, highly differentiated cell types, such as skeletal muscle and nervous tissue, lose their ability to undergo cell division in postnatal life. You can think of stem cells as the trees from which blocks of wood are used to make furniture items with specific functions. Once items such as chairs and tables are made, the process cannot be reversed so the furniture is turned back into a tree.

Although most cells differentiate into specialized cell types, many tissues contain a few partially differentiated **stem cells.**[1] These stem cells, which are still capable of cell division, serve as a reserve source for specialized cells throughout the life of the organism and make regeneration possible in some tissues. Stem cells have varying abilities to differentiate. For example, skeletal muscle tissue lacks enough undifferentiated cells and has limited ability to regenerate. Hematopoietic (blood) stem cells have the greatest potential for differentiation, and these stem cells can potentially remake all of the blood and immune cells (and are the main cells in bone marrow transplants). Other stem cells, such as those that replace epithelial cells lining the gastrointestinal tract, are less general but can still differentiate.

KEY POINTS

ORGANIZATION OF CELLS INTO TISSUES

- Cells are organized into larger functional units called *tissues*. Tissues associate with other tissues to form the various organs of the body.

Embryonic Origin of Tissue Types

All of the approximately 200 different types of body cells can be classified into four basic or primary tissue types: (1) epithelial, (2) connective, (3) muscle, and (4) nervous (Table 2.1). These basic tissue types are often described by their embryonic origin. The embryo is essentially a three-layered tubular structure (Fig. 2.18):

1. The outer layer of the tube is called the ectoderm.
2. The middle layer of the tube is called the mesoderm.
3. The inner layer of the tube is called the endoderm.

All of the adult body tissues develop from these three cellular layers. Epithelial tissues develop from all three embryonic layers, connective tissue and muscle tissue develop mainly from the mesoderm, and nervous tissue develops from the ectoderm.

Epithelial Tissue

Epithelial tissue covers the body's outer surface and lines the internal closed cavities (including blood vessels) and body tubes that connect with the exterior of the body (gastrointestinal, respiratory, and genitourinary tracts). Epithelial tissue also forms the secretory portion of glands and their ducts.

Origin and Characteristics

Epithelial tissue develops from all three embryonic layers.[5]

Most epithelia of the skin, mouth, nose, and anus develop from the outer ectoderm.

TABLE 2.1 CLASSIFICATION OF TISSUE TYPES

TISSUE TYPE	LOCATION
Epithelial Tissue	
Covering and lining of body surfaces	
Simple epithelium	
Squamous	Lining of blood vessels, body cavities, alveoli of the lungs
Cuboidal	Collecting tubules of the kidney; covering of the ovaries
Columnar	Lining of the intestine and gallbladder
Stratified epithelium	
Squamous keratinized	Skin
Squamous nonkeratinized	Mucous membranes of the mouth, esophagus, and vagina
Cuboidal	Ducts of the sweat glands
Columnar	Large ducts of the salivary and mammary glands; also found in the conjunctiva
Transitional	Bladder, ureters, renal pelvis
Pseudostratified	Tracheal and respiratory passages
Glandular	
Endocrine	Pituitary gland, thyroid gland, adrenal and other glands
Exocrine	Sweat glands and glands in the gastrointestinal tract
Neuroepithelium	Olfactory mucosa, retina, tongue
Reproductive epithelium	Seminiferous tubules of the testis; cortical portion of the ovary
Connective Tissue	
Embryonic connective tissue	
Mesenchymal	Embryonic mesoderm
Mucous	Umbilical cord (Wharton jelly)
Adult connective tissue	
Loose or areolar	Subcutaneous areas
Dense regular	Tendons and ligaments
Dense irregular	Dermis of the skin
Adipose	Fat pads, subcutaneous layers
Reticular	Framework of lymphoid organs, bone marrow, liver
Specialized connective tissue	
Bone	Long bones, flat bones
Cartilage	Tracheal rings, external ear, articular surfaces
Hematopoietic	Blood cells, myeloid tissue (bone marrow)
Muscle Tissue	
Skeletal	Skeletal muscles
Cardiac	Heart muscles
Smooth	Gastrointestinal tract, blood vessels, bronchi, bladder, and others
Nervous Tissue	
Neurons	Central and peripheral neurons and nerve fibers
Supporting cells	Glial and ependymal cells in the CNS; Schwann and satellite cells in the PNS

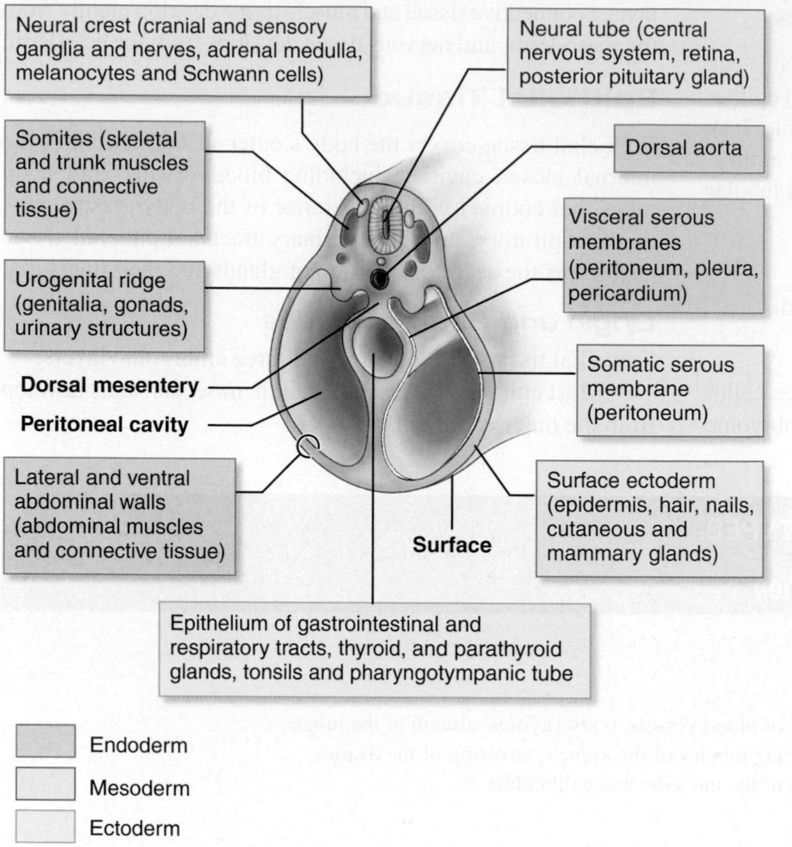

Figure 2.18 • Cross-section of human embryo illustrating the development of the somatic and visceral structures.

1. The endothelial lining of blood vessels develops from the middle mesoderm.
2. Linings of the respiratory tract, gastrointestinal tract, and glands of the digestive system develop from the inner endoderm.
3. Many types of epithelial tissue retain the ability to differentiate and undergo rapid proliferation for replacing injured cells.

The cells that make up epithelial tissue have three general characteristics:

- They have three distinct surfaces: (1) a free surface or apical surface, (2) a lateral surface (on the sides of cells), and (3) a basal surface (at the base of the tissue).
- The basal surface of epithelial cells is attached to a basement membrane (below the epithelial cells, like a basement is below a house)
- Cells in epithelial tissues are close to neighboring cells and are joined to neighboring cells by cell-to-cell adhesion molecules (CAMs) (Fig. 2.19).[5]

The characteristics and arrangement of the cells in epithelial tissues determine their function.

1. The free or apical surface is always directed toward the exterior surface or lumen of an enclosed cavity or tube (*e.g.*, the inside or lumen of the intestines or blood vessels).
2. The lateral surface communicates with neighboring cells and is characterized by specialized attachment areas.
3. The basal surface rests on the basement membrane and attaches or anchors the cell to the surrounding connective tissue.

Epithelial tissue is **avascular** (*a*, without; *vascular*, refers to blood vessels). Therefore, epithelial tissues receive oxygen and nutrients from the capillaries of the connective tissue on which the epithelial tissue rests (see Fig. 2.19).

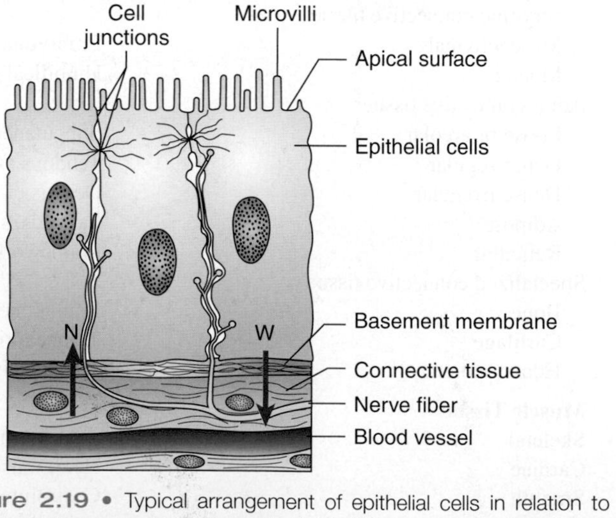

Figure 2.19 • Typical arrangement of epithelial cells in relation to underlying tissues and blood supply. Epithelial tissue has no blood supply of its own but relies on the blood vessels in the underlying connective tissue for nutrition (N) and elimination of wastes (W).

To survive, epithelial tissue must be kept moist. Even the skin epithelium, which seems dry, is kept moist by a waterproof layer of skin cells called **keratinocytes**, which make **keratin**; keratin prevents evaporation of moisture from deeper skin cells.

Basement Membrane. Underneath all types of epithelial tissue is an extracellular matrix, called the **basement membrane**. A basement membrane consists of (1) the basal lamina and (2) an underlying reticular layer. The terms **basal lamina** and **basement membrane** are often used interchangeably.[6]

Cell Junctions and Cell-to-Cell Adhesions. Cells of epithelial tissue are tightly joined together by specialized junctions. These specialized junctions enable the cells to form barriers to prevent the movement of water, solutes, and cells from one body compartment to the next. Three basic types of intercellular junctions are observed in epithelial tissues (Fig. 2.20):

1. **Continuous tight** or **occluding junctions** (*i.e.*, zonula occludens), which are found only in epithelial tissue, bind neighboring cells together. This type of intercellular junction prevents materials such as macromolecules in the intestines from passing between cells and entering the bloodstream or body cavities.[5]
2. **Adhering junctions** are sites of strong adhesion between neighboring cells. The main role of adhering junctions is to prevent cells from separating from each other. Adhering junctions are found in epithelial tissue and between cardiac muscle cells.
3. **Gap junctions** are sites of strong adhesion between neighboring cells with channels that link the cytoplasm of the two neighboring cells (like a tunnel between cells). Gap junctions are found in epithelial tissue and in many other types of cell-to-cell communication. For example, gap junctions allow ions to move between cells as part of electrical signals (*e.g.*, in smooth muscle or cardiac muscle).[5,7]

Types of Epithelial Tissues

Epithelial tissues are classified according to the:

1. Shape of the cells: **squamous** (thin and flat), **cuboidal** (cube shaped), and **columnar** (resembling a column)
2. Number of layers that are present: **simple**, **stratified**, and **pseudostratified** (Fig. 2.21).[6]

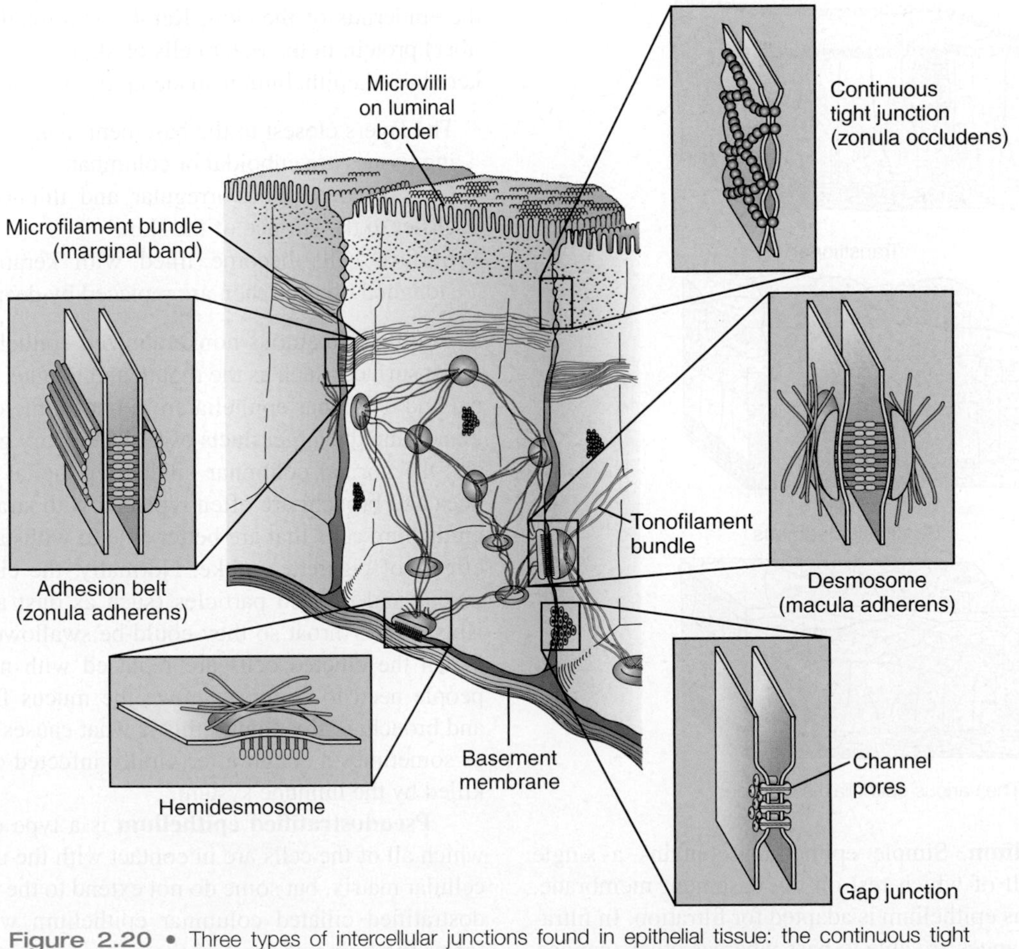

Figure 2.20 • Three types of intercellular junctions found in epithelial tissue: the continuous tight junction (zonula occludens); the adhering junction, which includes the adhesion belt (zonula adherens), desmosomes (macula adherens), and hemidesmosomes; and the gap junction.

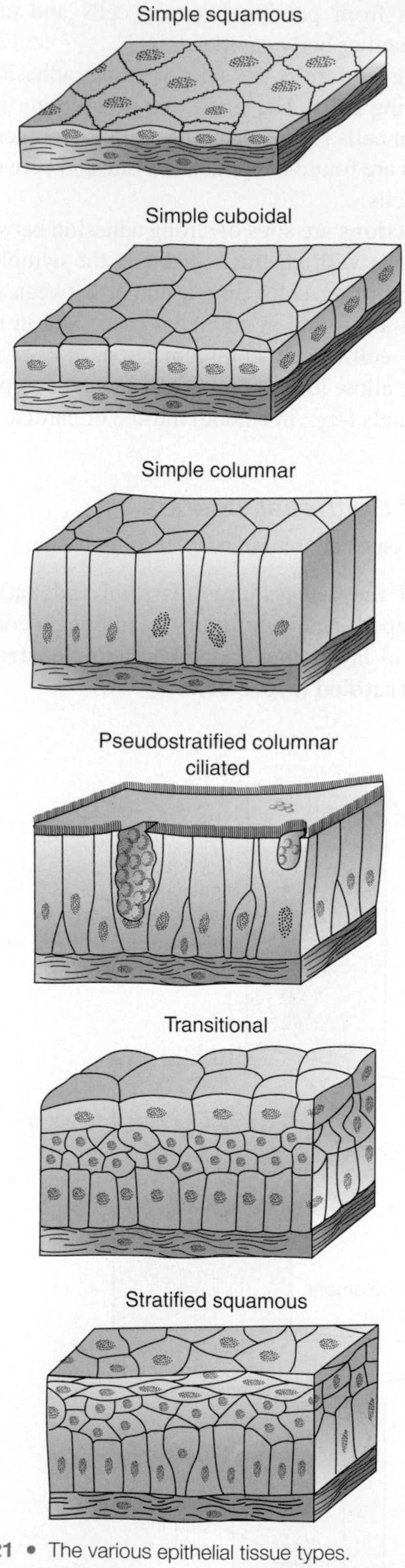

Figure 2.21 • The various epithelial tissue types.

Simple Epithelium. Simple epithelium contains a single layer of cells, all of which rest on the basement membrane. Simple squamous epithelium is adapted for filtration. In filtration, some substances are able to pass whereas others cannot. Filtration is used when making coffee: the water and dissolved substances pass through the coffee filter (similar to the simple epithelium), but the coffee grounds cannot pass through this layer.

- Simple epithelium lines the blood vessels, lymph nodes, and alveoli of the lungs.
- A single layer of squamous (thin and flat) epithelium lines the heart and blood vessels and is called the **endothelium**.
- A similar type of layer forms the serous membranes that line the pleural, pericardial, and peritoneal cavities and cover the organs of these cavities. This type of layer is called the **mesothelium**.
- **Simple cuboidal epithelium** is found on the surface of the ovary and in the thyroid.
- **Simple columnar epithelium** lines the intestine.
- One specialized form of a simple columnar epithelium has hairlike projections called **cilia**, often with mucus-secreting cells called **goblet cells**. This form of simple columnar epithelium lines the airways of the respiratory tract.[5]

Stratified and Pseudostratified Epithelia. Stratified epithelium contains more than one layer of cells, with only the deepest layer resting on the basement membrane. It is designed to protect body surfaces.

Stratified squamous keratinized epithelium makes up the epidermis of the skin. Keratin is a tough, fibrous (like a fiber) protein in the outer cells of skin. A stratified squamous keratinized epithelium is made up of many layers.

- The layers closest to the basement membrane and underlying tissues are cuboidal or columnar.
- Cells become more irregular and thinner as they move closer to the surface of the skin.
- Surface cells become filled with keratin and die, are sloughed off, and then are replaced by deeper cells.

A stratified squamous nonkeratinized epithelium is found on moist surfaces such as the mouth and tongue. Stratified cuboidal and columnar epithelia are found in the ducts of salivary glands and the larger ducts of the mammary glands.[5] In smokers, the normal columnar ciliated epithelial cells of the trachea and bronchi are often replaced with stratified squamous epithelium cells that are better able to withstand the irritating effects of cigarette smoke. Normally, the cilia would move mucus and trapped particles (such as dust and microorganisms) to the throat so they could be swallowed and digested. When the ciliated cells are replaced with nonciliated cells, people need to cough to move the mucus from the trachea and bronchi to the mouth; this is what causes smoker's cough or sometimes a cough after virally infected ciliated cells are killed by the immune system.

Pseudostratified epithelium is a type of epithelium in which all of the cells are in contact with the underlying intercellular matrix, but some do not extend to the surface. A pseudostratified ciliated columnar epithelium with goblet cells forms the lining of most of the upper respiratory tract. All of the tall cells reaching the surface of this type of epithelium are either ciliated cells or mucus-producing goblet cells. The basal cells that do not reach the surface serve as stem cells for ciliated and goblet cells.[5] **Transitional epithelium** is a stratified epithelium characterized by cells that can change shape and become thinner when the tissue is stretched. Such tissue can be stretched without pulling the superficial cells apart. Transitional epithelium is well adapted for the lining of organs that are constantly changing their volume, such as the urinary bladder.

Glandular Epithelium. Glandular epithelial tissue is formed by cells specialized to produce a fluid secretion.[5] This process usually occurs with the intracellular synthesis of macromolecules (which macromolecules are synthesized varies depending on the cell type and location in the body). The macromolecules are usually stored in the cells in small, membrane-bound vesicles called **secretory granules**. For example, glandular epithelial cells can make, store, and secrete proteins (*e.g.*, insulin), lipids (*e.g.*, adrenocortical hormones, secretions of the sebaceous glands), and complexes of carbohydrates and proteins (*e.g.*, saliva).

Exocrine glands use ducts to secrete substances outside of the body or into body cavities, such as the sweat glands and lactating mammary glands. **Endocrine glands** are ductless and secrete hormones directly into the bloodstream.

Connective or Supportive Tissue

Connective or supportive tissue is the most common tissue in the body. As its name suggests, it connects and binds or supports the various tissues.[5] Connective tissue is unique in that its cells produce the extracellular matrix that supports and holds tissues together. The capsules that surround organs of the body are composed of connective tissue. Adult connective tissue can be divided into two types (1): connective tissue proper, which includes loose (areolar), adipose, reticular, and dense connective tissue, and (2) specialized connective tissue that functions to support the soft tissues of the body and store fat (cartilage, bone, and blood cells), which is discussed in other chapters (47).

Muscle Tissue

Muscle tissue, whose main function is contraction, is responsible for movement of the body and its parts and for changes in the size and shape of internal organs. Muscle tissue contains two types of fibers that are responsible for contraction: thin and thick filaments. The thin filaments are made of actin, and the thick filaments are made of myosin. These two types of myofilaments make up most of the cytoplasm, which in muscle cells is called the sarcoplasm.[7]

There are three types of muscle tissues: **skeletal**, **cardiac**, and **smooth**. Skeletal and cardiac muscles are striated muscles, in which the actin and myosin filaments are arranged in large, parallel sarcomeres, giving the muscle fibers a striped or striated appearance when seen with a microscope. **Smooth muscle** does not have striations and is found in the iris of the eye, the walls of blood vessels, surrounding hollow organs (*e.g.*, the stomach and urinary bladder), and hollow tubes (*e.g.*, the ureters and common bile duct).[7]

Neither skeletal nor cardiac muscle can divide to replace injured cells. Smooth muscle, however, can divide. Some increases in smooth muscle are normal, as occurs in the uterus during pregnancy. Other increases are pathologic, such as the increase in smooth muscle that occurs in the arteries of people with chronic hypertension.

Skeletal Muscle

Skeletal muscle is the most abundant tissue in the body, making up 40% to 45% of the total body weight.[7] Most skeletal muscles are attached to bones, and skeletal muscle contractions are responsible for movements of the skeleton. Each skeletal muscle is a separate organ made up of hundreds or thousands of muscle fibers (skeletal muscle cells are also called muscle fibers). Although muscle fibers are the main cell type, connective tissue, blood vessels, and nerve fibers are also present.

Organization and Structure. The structures of skeletal muscle fibers/cells often start with the prefix *sarco-*. For example, the cytoplasm is called the sarcoplasm and is contained within the **sarcolemma** (the cell membrane). Skeletal muscle cells have many nuclei. Throughout the sarcoplasm are the contractile proteins actin and myosin, which are arranged in parallel bundles called **myofibrils** (Fig. 2.22A). These contain actin thin filaments and myosin thick filaments. Each myofibril consists of regularly repeating units along the length of the myofibril, called **sarcomeres** (see Fig. 2.22B).[7] Sarcomeres are the structural and functional units of cardiac and skeletal muscle. Sarcomeres appear as striations (stripes) under the microscope.

The **sarcoplasmic reticulum**, which is comparable to the smooth ER (see Fig. 2.22C & D), stores calcium that is released during muscle contraction. Concentration levels of calcium ions in the sarcoplasmic reticulum are 10,000 times higher than in the sarcoplasm.

The **transverse** or **T tubules** are extensions of the cell membrane and run perpendicular to the muscle fiber. The hollow portion or lumen of the transverse tubule is continuous with the extracellular fluid compartment. Action potentials are rapidly conducted over the surface of the muscle fiber and into the T tubules to the sarcoplasmic reticulum. The sarcoplasmic reticulum then releases calcium, starting muscle contraction. The membrane of the sarcoplasmic reticulum also has an active transport mechanism for pumping calcium back into the sarcoplasmic reticulum to stop muscle contraction.

Skeletal Muscle Contraction. Myosin makes up thick filaments. Myosin has (1) a thin tail, which provides the structural backbone for the filament, and (2) a globular (globelike) head. Each myosin head has a binding site for actin and a separate active site that catalyzes the breakdown of ATP to provide the energy to move the myosin head so it can pull on the actin filament during muscle contraction.

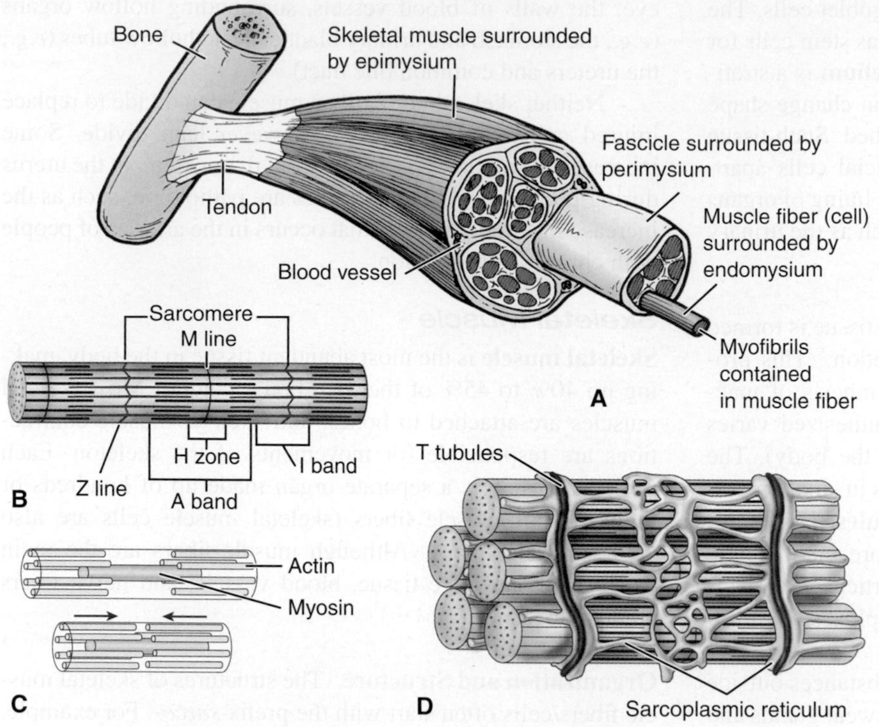

Figure 2.22 • Connective tissue components of a skeletal muscle (A). Striations of the myofibril showing the overlap of contractile proteins and the A and I bands, the H zone, and the Z and M lines (B). The relaxed and contracted states of the myofibril showing the position of actin filaments (*blue*) between the myosin filaments (*pink*) in the relaxed muscle (*top*) and pulling of the Z membranes toward each other (*bottom*) as the muscle contracts (C). The sarcoplasmic reticulum with T tubules (D).

Actin makes up the thin filaments. Actin is a globular (globe-like) protein that lines up in two rows that coil around each other to form a long helical strand. Two regulatory proteins associate with actin: (1) tropomyosin and (2) troponin (see Fig. 2.23A).

In the noncontracted state, **tropomyosin** blocks the myosin-binding sites on the actin filaments.

During an action potential, calcium ions released from the sarcoplasmic reticulum into the sarcoplasm can bind to

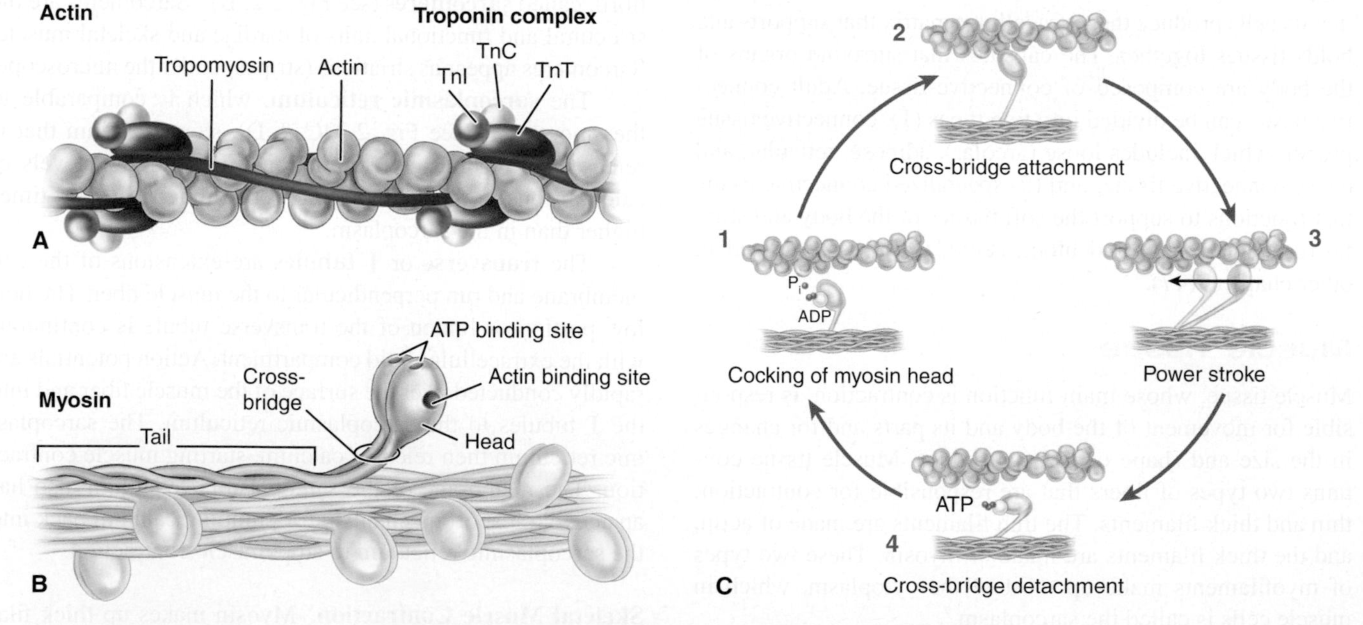

Figure 2.23 • Molecular structure of the thin actin filament (A) and the thicker myosin filament (B) of striated muscle. The thin filament is a double-stranded helix of actin molecules with tropomyosin and troponin molecules lying along the grooves of the actin strands. (C) Sequence of events involved in sliding of adjacent actin and myosin filaments: (*1*) Cocking of the myosin head occurs as ATP is split to ADP, (*2*) cross-bridge attachment, (*3*) power stroke during which the myosin head bends as it moves the actin forward, and (*4*) cross-bridge detachment occurs as a new ATP attaches to the myosin head.

troponin (Fig. 2.23B). Binding of calcium to troponin moves the tropomyosin so that the myosin can bind to actin.[5]

When activated by ATP, the myosin–actin cross-bridges swivel, like the oars of a boat, as they become attached to the actin filament. During contraction, myosin binds and releases actin over and over again, moving down an actin filament. This pulls the thin and thick filaments past each other to shorten the sarcomeres, which shortens muscle fibers, which in turn shortens muscles (see Fig. 2.22C).

When stimulation of muscles stops, the concentration of calcium in the sarcoplasm decreases as calcium is actively transported into the sarcoplasmic reticulum by a membrane pump that uses energy from ATP.

The basis of **rigor mortis** can be explained by the binding of actin and myosin. As the muscle begins to break down after death, the sarcoplasmic reticulum releases calcium ions, which allow myosin heads to bind actin. As ATP supplies decrease, energy is not available for normal interaction between actin and myosin, and the muscle is in a state of rigor until further breakdown destroys the cross-bridges between actin and myosin.[5]

Cardiac Muscle

Cardiac muscle is the main part of the heart. Like skeletal muscle cells, the actin and myosin filaments and associated proteins are arranged into sarcomeres, and these appear striated (striped) under a microscope.

Also visible under the microscope are intercalated disks (if you clasp your hands together with your fingers between one another, you will have intercalated your fingers). Intercalated disks are where cardiac muscle cells join, and these contain gap junctions that allow ions to pass between cardiac muscle cells for coordinated contraction of the heart.

Cardiac muscle cells are also called cardiac muscle fibers or cardiomyocytes. There are two types of cardiac muscle cells:

1. Autorhythmic cells or pacemaker cells make up about 1% of cardiac muscle cells and are found in the SA and AV nodes. These cells automatically go through action potentials without stimulation by the nervous system (these cells allow the heart to beat outside of the body). The rate of these action potentials can be increased by sympathetic stimulation or decreased by parasympathetic stimulation.
2. Cardiac contractile cells make up the rest of the cardiac muscle cells and are responsible for the contraction of the heart. Contraction of the chambers of the heart increases the pressure within the chambers so that blood flows from these higher-pressure areas into lower-pressure areas (*e.g.*, from the left ventricle to the aorta).

Cardiac muscle cells also contain troponin, and this is important clinically. During a heart attack, blood vessels to cardiac muscle cells are blocked, decreasing oxygen delivery to these cells. With decreased oxygen, ATP decreases, and the pumping of sodium out of cells decreases. As sodium increases in cardiac muscle cells, osmolarity increases and water diffuses in osmosis to try to dilute the sodium. If blood flow (and oxygen and ATP) is not quickly returned to the cardiac muscle cells, the cells can burst from the increased water. When the cells burst, they release their contents into the blood. Increases in troponin and cardiac enzymes in blood tests are used to help diagnose a heart attack.

Smooth Muscle

Smooth muscle is often called **involuntary muscle** because its activity is spontaneous or is stimulated by the autonomic nervous system (the sympathetic or parasympathetic nervous systems). Smooth muscle contractions are slower and longer than skeletal or cardiac muscle contractions.

Organization and Structure. Smooth muscle cells do not contain sarcomeres and therefore do not appear striated under a microscope. The bundles of filaments are not parallel to each other but instead crisscross through the cell. In smooth muscles, actin filaments are attached to structures called *dense bodies* (Fig. 2.24). Some dense bodies are attached to the cell membrane, and others are throughout the cell and linked together by structural proteins.[5,10]

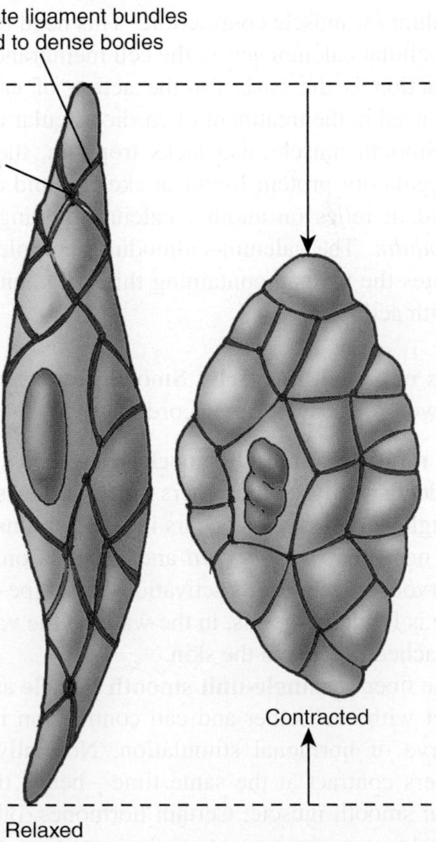

Figure 2.24 • Structure of smooth muscle showing the dense bodies. In smooth muscle, the force of contraction is transmitted to the cell membrane by bundles of intermediate fibers.

The lack of regular overlapping of contractile filaments provides a greater range of tension development in smooth muscle. This is important in hollow organs that undergo changes in volume, with resulting changes in the length of the smooth muscle fibers in their walls. Even with the distention of a hollow organ, the smooth muscle fiber retains some ability to develop tension, whereas such distention would stretch skeletal muscle beyond the area where the thick and thin filaments overlap.

Smooth muscle is usually arranged in sheets or bundles. In hollow organs, such as the intestines, the bundles are organized into the two-layered muscularis externa consisting of an outer, longitudinal layer and an inner, circular layer. A thinner muscularis mucosae often lies between the muscularis externa and the endothelium lining blood vessels. In blood vessels, the bundles are arranged circularly or helically around the vessel wall.

Smooth Muscle Contraction. As with cardiac and skeletal muscle, smooth muscle contraction is started by an increase in intracellular calcium. However, smooth muscle differs from skeletal muscle in the way its cross-bridges are formed. The sarcoplasmic reticulum of smooth muscle is less developed than in skeletal muscle, and no transverse tubules are present. Smooth muscle cells rely on extracellular calcium entering cells and the release of calcium from the sarcoplasmic reticulum for muscle contraction.[5] This need for movement of extracellular calcium across the cell membrane during muscle contraction is the basis for the action of calcium-blocking drugs used in the treatment of cardiovascular disease.

Smooth muscle also lacks troponin, the calcium-binding regulatory protein found in skeletal and cardiac muscle. Instead, it relies on another calcium-binding protein called *calmodulin*. The calcium–calmodulin complex binds to and activates the myosin-containing thick filaments, which interact with actin.

Types of Smooth Muscle. Smooth muscle may be divided into two broad categories according to how it is activated:

1. In **multiunit smooth muscle**, each unit operates almost independently of the others and is often stimulated by a single nerve, such as occurs in skeletal muscle. It has little or no activity on its own and depends on the autonomic nervous system for its activation. This type of smooth muscle is found in the iris, in the walls of the vas deferens, and attached to hairs in the skin.
2. The fibers in **single-unit smooth muscle** are in close contact with each other and can contract on its own without nerve or hormonal stimulation. Normally, most muscle fibers contract at the same time—hence the term *single-unit* smooth muscle. Certain hormones, other agents, and local factors can increase or decrease smooth muscle activity. Smooth muscle cells found in the uterus and small-diameter blood vessels are also single-unit smooth muscle.

Nervous Tissue

Nervous tissue is distributed throughout the body as a communication system. Anatomically, the nervous system is divided into (1) the CNS, which consists of the brain and spinal cord, and (2) the peripheral nervous system (PNS), which consists of nervous tissue outside the CNS. Nerve cells are highly differentiated and most are not capable of regeneration in postnatal life. Structurally, nervous tissue consists of two cell types: (1) nerve cells, called neurons, and (2) glial or supporting cells.

Most neurons consist of these parts:

1. The soma, or cell body, which contains the nucleus and most organelles
2. Dendrites, which are multiple elongated extensions that receive and carry stimuli from the environment, from sensory epithelial cells, and from other neurons to the cell
3. The axons, which are specialized for generating and conducting action potentials away from the cell body to other nerve cells, muscle cells, and glandular cells
4. Axon terminals where neurotransmitters are stored in vesicles for release onto neighboring cells after an action potential

Peripheral neurons can be classified as afferent and efferent neurons according to their function:

1. Afferent or sensory neurons carry information toward the CNS; they are involved in the reception of sensory information from the external environment and from within the body.
2. Efferent or motor neurons carry information away from the CNS; they are needed for control of muscle fibers and endocrine and exocrine glands. There are two divisions of the efferent PNS: (1) somatic motor neurons, which stimulate skeletal muscle contractions (*soma*, body; *motor*, move; somatic motor neurons make your body move), and (2) autonomic neurons, which stimulate the other two types of muscle (cardiac and smooth), glands, and adipose tissues (autonomic neurons are automatic; they stimulate mostly involuntary/automatic functions). The autonomic nervous system is further divided into the (a) sympathetic (fight or flight) neurons and the (b) parasympathetic (rest and digest) neurons.

Communication between neurons and other cells, such as other neurons or muscle cells, occurs at specialized structures called *synapses*. A chemical synapse contains (1) the axon terminal of one neuron, (2) the area of the cell membrane that contains receptors on the target cell, and (3) the space between these two cells. At the chemical synapse, neurotransmitters bind to receptor on target cells such as another neuron or muscle cell. In addition, electrical synapses exist where neurons are linked through gap junctions that allow ions to pass from one cell to another.

Neuroglia (glia means "glue") or glial cells are the cells that support neurons. Examples of glial cells found in the CNS include the following:

1. Astrocytes, the most common glial cells, have many long extensions that surround blood vessels in the CNS. They provide structural support for neurons, and their extensions form a sealed barrier that protects the CNS.
2. Oligodendrocytes wrap around axons of CNS neurons to form myelin, which insulates neurons and speeds up action potentials.
3. Microglia are phagocytic cells.
4. Ependymal cells line the cavities of the brain and spinal cord and are in contact with the cerebrospinal fluid.

Examples of glial cells in the PNS include the following:

1. Schwann cells (like oligodendrocytes in the CNS) wrap around axons of PNS neurons to form myelin, which insulates neurons and speeds up action potentials.
2. Satellite cells enclose and protect the dorsal root ganglia and autonomic ganglion cells.

Extracellular Matrix

The discussion so far has focused on the cells in the different tissue types. Within tissues, cells are held together by cell junctions; the space between cells is filled with an extracellular matrix; and adhesion molecules form intercellular contacts.

Tissues are not made up only of cells. A large part of tissue volume is made up of an extracellular matrix. This matrix is made up of a variety of proteins and polysaccharides (*poly*, many; *saccharide*, sugar; a polysaccharide is a molecule made up of many sugars).[6] These proteins and polysaccharides are secreted by cells into the tissues and are organized into a supporting mesh in close association with the cells that made them. The amount and makeup of the matrix vary with the different tissues and their functions. For example, in bone, there are more matrices than the cells that surround it; in the brain, there are more cells, and the matrix is only a minor part.[5]

Two main classes of extracellular macromolecules make up the extracellular matrix:

1. Polysaccharide chains of a class called **glycosaminoglycans** (GAGs), which are usually found linked to protein as proteoglycans (protein + sugar).
2. Fibrous (fiber-like) proteins (collagen, elastin, fibronectin, and laminin) that are found in the basement membrane.

Collagen is the most common protein in the body. It is a tough, nonliving, white fiber that gives structure to skin, ligaments, tendons, and many other structures. **Elastin** acts like a rubber band; after being stretched, it returns to its original form. There are many elastin fibers in structures that are stretched frequently, such as the aorta and some ligaments.[5]

IN SUMMARY

Body cells are organized into four basic tissue types: epithelial, connective, muscle, and nervous.

1. Epithelial tissue covers and lines the body surfaces and forms the functional components of glandular structures. Epithelial tissue is classified into three types (squamous, cuboidal, and columnar) according to the shape of the cells and the number of layers that are present. The cells in epithelial tissue are held together by three types of intercellular junctions: tight, adhering, and gap junctions.
2. Connective tissue supports and connects body structures; it forms the bones and skeletal system, joint structures, blood cells, and intercellular substances. Connective tissue can be divided into four types: loose or areolar, which fills body spaces and is characterized by plenty of ground substance; adipose, which stores fat; reticular, which forms the architectural framework in many structures of the body; and dense—regular and irregular—which forms structures such as tendons and ligaments (and the dermis of the skin).
3. Muscle tissue is a specialized tissue that can contract. There are three types of muscle tissue: skeletal, cardiac, and smooth. Skeletal and cardiac muscle cells have actin, myosin, and other proteins arranged into sarcomeres, which appear as striations (stripes) under the microscope. Cardiac muscle cells are connected by gap junctions, which allow ions to pass between cells for coordinated contraction. Smooth muscles have actin and myosin in a different arrangement and so are not striated (and appear smooth). Actin and myosin filaments interact to shorten muscles, a process activated by the presence of calcium. In skeletal muscle, calcium is released from the sarcoplasmic reticulum in response to an action potential. Smooth and cardiac muscles are often called *involuntary muscle* because they contract spontaneously or through activity of the autonomic nervous system. The sarcoplasmic reticulum is less defined and depends on the entry of extracellular calcium ions for muscle contraction.
4. Nervous tissue consists of two cell types: nerve cells, called neurons, and glial cells, which are the supporting cells. Nervous tissue is found throughout the body and is part of the body's communication system. The nervous system is divided anatomically into the CNS, which consists of the brain and spinal cord, and the PNS, which is composed of nerve tissue outside the CNS.

Nervous tissue which is made up of neurons and glial cells reacts to external and internal changes and communicates these in the body.

The extracellular matrix is made up of a variety of proteins and polysaccharides. The amount and makeup of matrix vary with the different tissues and their function.

GERIATRIC Considerations

- Theories attempt to explain the biology of aging. However, scientists remain unable to come to a unanimous conclusion.[10]
  - The fundamental limitation theory supports the "wear and tear" of vital cell molecules, such as mitochondrial DNA damage.
  - The nonprogrammed aging theory suggests tissue damage accumulates, resulting in aging.
  - The programmed aging theory, also referred to as the nonstochastic theory, postulates we are genetically programmed to suicide through nonrenewal of some cells.
- Heart disease, the leading cause of morbidity and mortality in the United States, starts at the molecular level, known as cardiovascular senescence, leading to weakening of cellular process in aging cells.[11]

PEDIATRIC Considerations

- Cellular senescence takes place during normal embryonic development.[12]
- Cystic fibrosis, an inherited disease, results in the absence of chloride ion pumps damaging the structural proteins of cells. The advanced study of genetics has led to improvements in treating children with this disease.[13]
- Cord blood of the fetus and blood of the newborn infant contain many cells such as stem, red and white blood cells, and T cells. There is debate about whether the use of these cells to prevent certain illness treated with stem cells can be successful.[14]

REVIEW EXERCISES

1. Tattoos consist of pigments that have been injected into the skin.
   A. *Explain what happens to the dye once it has been injected and why it does not eventually wash away.*
2. People who drink sufficient amounts of alcohol show rapid changes in CNS function, including both motor and behavioral changes, and the odor of alcohol can be detected on their breath.
   A. *Use the concepts related to the lipid bilayer structure of the cell membrane to explain these observations.*
3. The absorption of glucose from the intestine involves a cotransport mechanism in which the active primary transport of sodium ions is used to provide for the secondary transport of glucose.
   A. *Hypothesize how this information might be used to design an oral rehydration solution for someone who is suffering from diarrhea.*

References

1. Hall J. E. (2016). *Guyton and Hall textbook of medical physiology* (13th ed.). Philadelphia, PA: Saunders.
2. Luo K., Cao S. S. (2015). Endoplasmic reticulum stress in intestinal epithelial cell function and inflammatory bowel disease. *Gastroenterology Research and Practice* 2015, Article 328791, 6 pages.
3. Hasnain S. Z., Prins J. B., McGuckin M. A. (2016). Oxidative and endoplasmic reticulum stress in β-cell dysfunction in diabetes. *Journal of Molecular Endocrinology* 56, R33–R54.
4. Manole E., Bastian A. E., Butoianu N., et al. (2017). Myositis non-inflammatory mechanisms: An up-dated review. *Journal of Immunoassay and Immunochemistry* 38(2), 115–126.
5. Boron W. F., Boulpaep E. L. (2017). *Medical physiology* (3rd ed.). Philadelphia, PA: Saunders.
6. Ross M. H., Pawina W. (2015). *Histology: A text and atlas* (7th ed.). Philadelphia, PA: Lippincott Williams & Wilkins.
7. Strayer D. S., Rubin E. (2014). *Rubin's pathology: Clinicopathologic foundations of medicine* (7th ed.). Philadelphia, PA: Lippincott Williams & Wilkins.
8. Horani A., Brody S. L., Feerkol T. W. (2014). Picking up speed: Advances in the genetics of primary cilia dyskinesia. *Pediatric Research* 75(1–2), 158–164.
9. Spillane J., Kullmann D. M., Hanna M. G. (2016). Genetic neurological channelopathies: Molecular genetics and clinical phenotypes. *Journal of Neurology, Neurosurgery, and Psychiatry* 87(1), 37–48.
10. Goldsmith T. S. (2014). *The evolution of aging*. Crownsville, MD: Azinet Press.
11. Iop L., Dal Sasso E., Schirone L., et al. (2017). The light and shadow of senescence and inflammation in cardiovascular pathology and regenerative medicine. *Mediators of Inflammation* 2017, Article ID 7953486, 13 pages. doi: 10.1155/2017/7953486.
12. Munoz-Espin D., Serrano M. (2014). *Cellular senescence: From physiology to pathology. Nature Reviews. Molecular Cell Biology* 15(7), 482–496. doi: 10.1038/nrm3823.
13. Patton K. T., Thibodeau K. T. (2014). *The human body in health and disease* (6th ed.). MO: Elsevier.
14. Mohora R., Hudita D., Stoicescu S.-M. (2017). The mirage of long term vital benefice—Risk for the beginning of life? *Mædica* 12(1), 13–18.

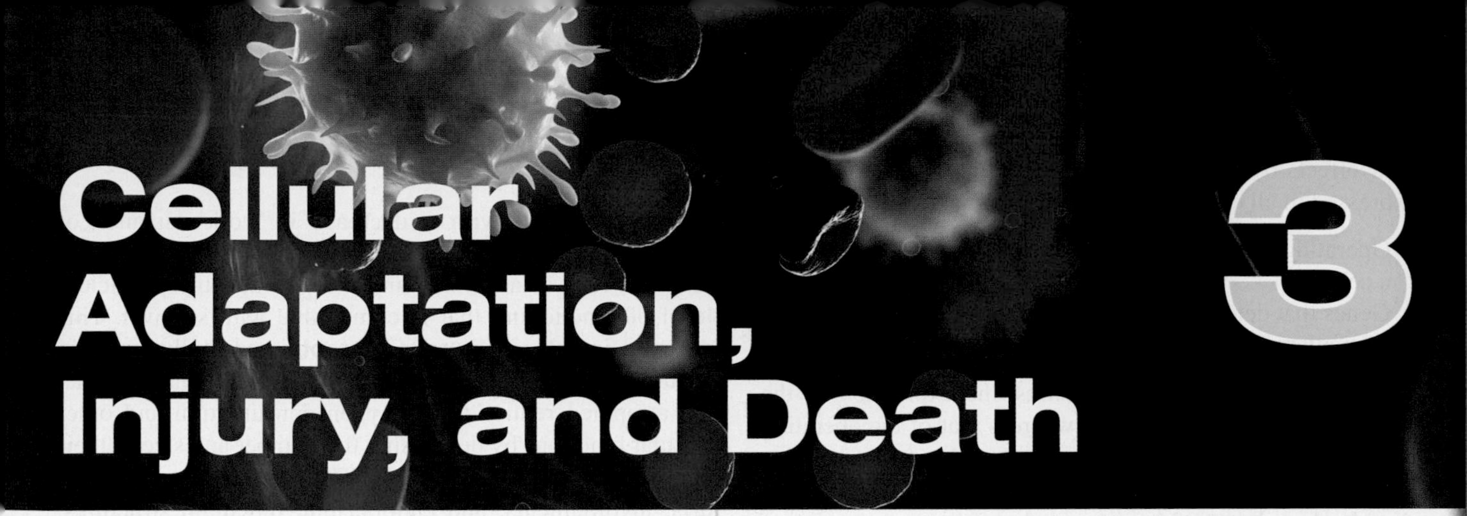

Cellular Adaptation, Injury, and Death

3

Trina Barrett

When confronted with stresses that endanger its normal structure and function, the cell undergoes adaptive changes that permit survival and maintenance of function. It is only when the stress is overwhelming or adaptation is ineffective that cell injury and death occur. This chapter focuses on cellular adaptation, injury, and death.

CELLULAR ADAPTATION

After completing this section of the chapter, the learner will be able to meet the following objectives:

- Cite the general purpose of changes in cell structure and function that occur as the result of normal adaptive processes.
- Describe cell changes that occur with atrophy, hypertrophy, hyperplasia, metaplasia, and dysplasia, and state general conditions under which the changes occur.
- Compare the pathogenesis and effects of dystrophic and metastatic calcifications.

Cells adapt to changes in the internal environment, just as the total organism adapts to changes in the external environment. Cells may adapt by undergoing changes in size, number, and type. These changes, occurring singly or in combination, may lead to

- Atrophy
- Hypertrophy
- Hyperplasia
- Metaplasia
- Dysplasia

Adaptive cellular responses also include intracellular accumulations and storage of products in abnormal amounts.[1]

There are numerous molecular mechanisms mediating cellular adaptation, including factors produced by other cells or by the cells themselves. These mechanisms depend largely on signals transmitted by chemical messengers that exert their effects by altering gene function. In general, the genes expressed in all cells fall into two categories:

- Operating genes that are necessary for normal function of a cell
- Genes that determine the differentiating characteristics of a particular cell type

In many adaptive cellular responses, the expression of the differentiation genes is altered, whereas that of the operating genes remains unaffected. Thus, a cell is able to change size or form without compromising its normal function. Once the stimulus for adaptation is removed, the effect on expression of the differentiating genes is removed and the cell resumes its previous state of specialized function. Whether adaptive cellular changes are normal or abnormal depends on whether the response was mediated by an appropriate stimulus. Normal adaptive responses occur in response to need and an appropriate stimulus. After the need has been removed, the adaptive response ceases.

KEY POINTS

CELLULAR ADAPTATIONS

- Cells are able to adapt to increased work demands or threats to survival by changing their size (atrophy and hypertrophy), number (hyperplasia), and form (metaplasia).
- Normal cellular adaptation occurs in response to an appropriate stimulus and ceases once the need for adaptation has ceased.

Atrophy

When confronted with a decrease in work demands or adverse environmental conditions, most cells are able to revert to a smaller size and a lower and more efficient level of functioning that is compatible with survival. This decrease in cell size is called **atrophy** and is illustrated in Figure 3.1 regarding atrophy of the endometrium. Cells that are atrophied reduce their oxygen consumption and other cellular functions by decreasing the number and size of their organelles and other structures. There are fewer mitochondria, myofilaments, and endoplasmic reticulum structures. When a sufficient number of cells are involved, the entire tissue or muscle atrophies.

Cell size, particularly in muscle tissue, is related to workload. As the workload of a cell declines, oxygen consumption and protein synthesis decrease. Furthermore, proper muscle mass is maintained by sufficient levels of insulin and insulin-like growth factor-1 (IGF-1).[2] When insulin and IGF-1 levels are low or catabolic signals are present, muscle atrophy occurs by mechanisms that include reduced synthetic processes, increased proteolysis by the ubiquitin–proteasome system, and apoptosis or programmed cell death.[3] In the ubiquitin–proteasome system, intracellular proteins destined for destruction are covalently bonded to a small protein called *ubiquitin* and then degraded by small cytoplasmic organelles called *proteasomes*.[4]

The general causes of atrophy can be grouped into five categories:

1. Disuse
2. Denervation
3. Loss of endocrine stimulation
4. Inadequate nutrition
5. Ischemia or decreased blood flow

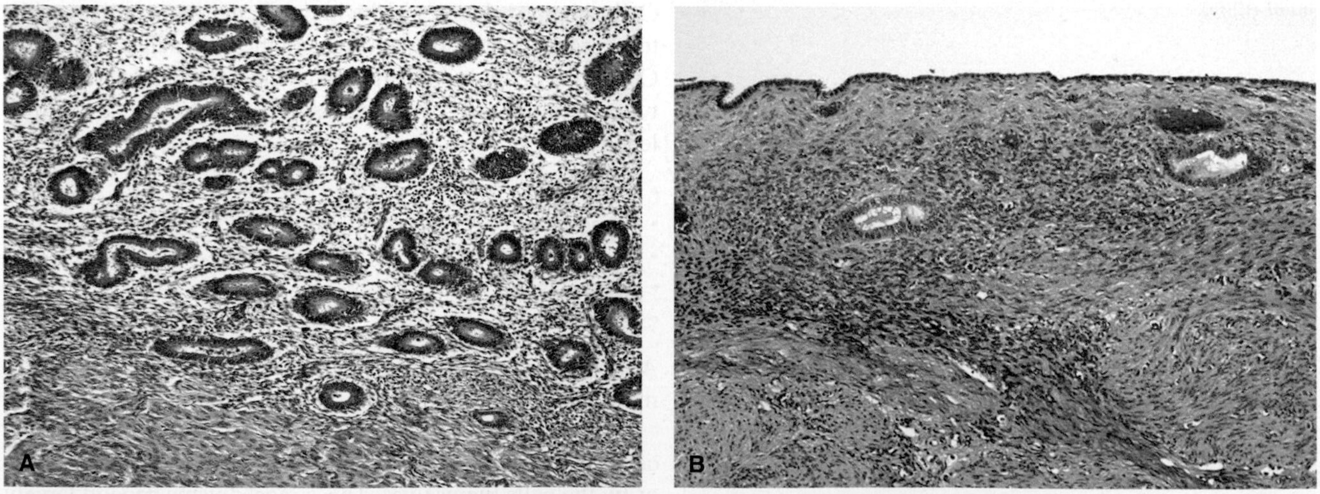

Figure 3.1 • Atrophy of cells in endometrium. **(A)** This section illustrates a piece of a woman of reproductive age who has a normal thick endometrium. **(B)** This section of endometrium is of a 75-year-old woman and shows atrophic cells and cystic glands. (Both slides are taken at the same magnification.) (From Rubin R., Strayer D. (2015). *Rubin's pathology: Clinicopathologic foundations of medicine* (7th ed., Fig. 1-19, p. 17). Philadelphia, PA: Lippincott Williams & Wilkins.)

Disuse atrophy occurs when there is a reduction in skeletal muscle use. An extreme example of disuse atrophy is seen in the muscles of extremities that have been encased in plaster casts. Because atrophy is adaptive and reversible, muscle size is restored after the cast is removed and muscle use is resumed. Denervation atrophy is a form of disuse atrophy that occurs in the muscles of paralyzed limbs.[3,5] Lack of endocrine stimulation produces a form of disuse atrophy. In women, the loss of estrogen stimulation during menopause results in atrophic changes in the reproductive organs. With malnutrition and decreased blood flow, cells decrease their size and energy requirements as a means of survival.

Hypertrophy

Hypertrophy represents an increase in cell size and with it an increase in the amount of functioning tissue mass (Fig. 3.2). It results from an increased workload imposed on an organ or body part and is commonly seen in cardiac and skeletal muscle tissue, which cannot adapt to an increase in workload through mitotic division and formation of more cells.[1] Hypertrophy involves an increase in the functional components of the cell that allows it to achieve equilibrium between demand and functional capacity. For example, as muscle cells hypertrophy, additional actin and myosin filaments, cell enzymes, and adenosine triphosphate (ATP) are synthesized.[1,5]

Hypertrophy may occur as the result of normal physiologic or abnormal pathologic conditions. The increase in muscle mass associated with exercise is an example of physiologic hypertrophy. Pathologic hypertrophy occurs as the result of disease conditions and may be adaptive or compensatory. Examples of adaptive hypertrophy are the thickening of the urinary bladder from long-continued obstruction of urinary outflow and the myocardial hypertrophy that results from valvular heart disease or hypertension. Compensatory hypertrophy is the enlargement of a remaining organ or tissue after a portion has been surgically removed or rendered inactive.

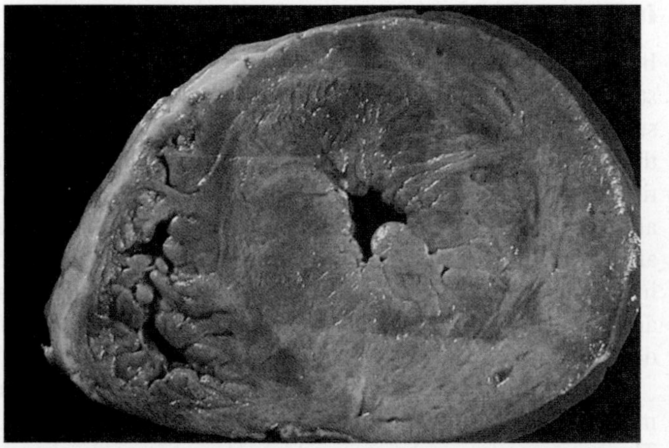

Figure 3.2 • Myocardial hypertrophy. Cross-section of the heart with left ventricular hypertrophy. (From Rubin R., Strayer D. (2015). *Rubin's pathology: Clinicopathologic foundations of medicine* (7th ed., p. 16). Philadelphia, PA: Lippincott Williams & Wilkins.)

For instance, if one kidney is removed, the remaining kidney enlarges to compensate for the loss.

The initiating signals for hypertrophy appear to be complex and related to ATP depletion, mechanical forces such as stretching of the muscle fibers, activation of cell degradation products, and hormonal factors.[5] An example of hormonal changes in the hypertrophied heart is increased glycolysis. Therefore, with an accelerated glycolytic rate, the potential for adaptations in the hypertrophied heart is increased.[6] In the case of the heart, initiating signals can be divided into two broad categories[6]:

1. Biomechanical stress
2. Neurohumoral factors

Signaling events regulating cardiac plasticity constitute a network that integrates a multitude of signals to activate a limited number of responses. Research shows intracellular signaling cascades promote protein synthesis and protein stability in which both can increase cardiomyocyte size. The exact mechanisms of how biomechanical signals are transduced across the cell membrane are unclear. The literature suggests the mechanisms involve stretch-sensitive ion channels, integrins, and other structural proteins. The complex network links the extracellular matrix, cytoskeleton, sarcomere, Ca^{2+}–handling proteins, and the nucleus.[6] A limit is eventually reached beyond which further enlargement of the tissue mass can no longer compensate for the increased work demands. The limiting factors for continued hypertrophy might be related to limitations in blood flow. In hypertension, for example, the increased workload required to pump blood against an elevated arterial pressure in the aorta results in a progressive increase in left ventricular muscle mass and need for coronary blood flow.

There continues to be interest in the signaling pathways that control the arrangement of contractile elements in myocardial hypertrophy. Research suggests that certain signal molecules can alter gene expression controlling the size and assembly of the contractile proteins in hypertrophied myocardial cells. For example, the hypertrophied myocardial cells of well-trained athletes have proportional increases in width and length. This is in contrast to the hypertrophy that develops in dilated cardiomyopathy, in which the hypertrophied cells have a relatively greater increase in length than width. In pressure overload, as occurs with hypertension, the hypertrophied cells have greater width than length.[6] It is anticipated that further elucidation of the signal pathways that determine the adaptive and nonadaptive features of cardiac hypertrophy will lead to new targets for treatment.

Hyperplasia

Hyperplasia refers to an increase in the number of cells in an organ or tissue. It occurs in tissues with cells that are capable of mitotic division, such as the epidermis, intestinal epithelium, and glandular tissue.[1] Certain cells, such as neurons, rarely divide and therefore have little capacity, if any, for hyperplastic growth. There is evidence that hyperplasia involves activation of genes controlling cell proliferation and the presence of intracellular messengers that control cell replication and growth. As with other normal adaptive cellular responses, hyperplasia is a controlled process that occurs in response to an appropriate stimulus and ceases after the stimulus has been removed.

The stimuli that induce hyperplasia may be physiologic or nonphysiologic. There are two common types of physiologic hyperplasia: hormonal and compensatory. Breast and uterine enlargements during pregnancy are examples of a physiologic hyperplasia that results from estrogen stimulation. The regeneration of the liver that occurs after partial hepatectomy (*i.e.*, partial removal of the liver) is an example of compensatory hyperplasia. Hyperplasia is also an important response of connective tissue in wound healing, during which proliferating fibroblasts and blood vessels contribute to wound repair. Although hypertrophy and hyperplasia are two distinct processes, they may occur together and are often triggered by the same mechanism.[1] For example, the pregnant uterus undergoes both hypertrophy and hyperplasia as the result of estrogen stimulation.

Most forms of nonphysiologic hyperplasia are due to excessive hormonal stimulation or the effects of growth factors on target tissues.[2] The public seems to appreciate that a laboratory finding including the term hyperplasia generally is something to take seriously. For example, excessive estrogen production can cause endometrial hyperplasia and abnormal menstrual bleeding. Endometrial hyperplasia is considered a high risk for developing endometrial cancer and is a condition that is monitored carefully.[7] Benign prostatic hyperplasia (BPH), which is a common disorder of men older than 50 years of age, is related to the action of androgens. BPH is a nonmalignant condition that causes lower urinary tract symptoms. BPH sometimes develops into prostate cancer.[8] Women with atypical hyperplasia of the breast are also monitored carefully because they have a fourfold higher risk of developing ductal carcinoma in situ or invasive breast cancer.[9] Skin warts are another example of hyperplasia caused by growth factors produced by certain viruses, such as the papillomaviruses.

Metaplasia

Metaplasia represents a reversible change in which one adult cell type (epithelial or mesenchymal) is replaced by another adult cell type. Metaplasia is thought to involve the reprogramming of undifferentiated stem cells that are present in the tissue undergoing the metaplastic changes.[1]

Metaplasia usually occurs in response to chronic irritation and inflammation and allows for substitution of cells that are better able to survive under circumstances in which a more fragile cell type might succumb. However, the conversion of cell types never oversteps the boundaries of the primary tissue type (*e.g.*, one type of epithelial cell may be converted to another type of epithelial cell, but not to a connective tissue cell). An example of metaplasia is the adaptive substitution of stratified squamous epithelial cells for the ciliated columnar epithelial cells in the trachea and large airways of a habitual cigarette smoker.

Chronic inflammation during gastroesophageal acid reflux disease (GERD) is a primary risk factor of Barrett esophagus (BE) and esophageal carcinogenesis. The literature defines BE as the presence of a metaplastic columnar-lined esophagus induced by GERD. People with BE have a 30% to 40% risk of developing Barrett esophageal adenocarcinoma (BEA).[10]

Dysplasia

Dysplasia is characterized by deranged cell growth of a specific tissue that results in cells that vary in size, shape, and organization. Minor degrees of dysplasia are associated with chronic irritation or inflammation. The pattern is most frequently encountered in areas of metaplastic squamous epithelium of the respiratory tract and uterine cervix. Although dysplasia is abnormal, it is adaptive in that it is potentially reversible after the irritating cause has been removed. Dysplasia is strongly implicated as a precursor of cancer.[1] In cancers of the respiratory tract and the uterine cervix, dysplastic changes have been found adjacent to the foci of cancerous transformation. Through the use of the Papanicolaou (Pap) smear, it has been documented that cancer of the uterine cervix develops in a series of incremental epithelial changes ranging from severe dysplasia to invasive cancer.[7] However, dysplasia is an adaptive process and as such does not necessarily lead to cancer.

Preterm babies who are ventilated for long periods of time because of their prematurity and lack of surfactant, and term infants who require intubation and ventilated oxygen in the first month of life, often develop bronchopulmonary dysplasia (BPD). Research shows that children with BPD are significantly more likely to have persistent respiratory symptoms at school age such as airway obstruction and hyperinflation and use asthma medications at school age. The literature defines BPD as the need for oxygen supplementation at 36 weeks' gestational age and predicts greater lung dysfunction and increased respiratory morbidity at school age.[11]

Intracellular Accumulations

Intracellular accumulations represent the buildup of substances that cells cannot immediately use or eliminate. The substances may accumulate in the cytoplasm (frequently in the lysosomes) or in the nucleus. In some cases, the accumulation may be an abnormal substance that the cell has produced, and in other cases, the cell may be storing exogenous materials or products of pathologic processes occurring elsewhere in the body. An example would be the accumulation of beta-amyloid fragments, which progress to a skeletal muscle disorder called myositis.[12]

These substances may accumulate transiently or permanently, and they may be harmless or, in some cases, toxic. These substances can be grouped into three categories:

1. Normal body substances, such as lipids, proteins, carbohydrates, melanin, and bilirubin, that are present in abnormally large amounts

2. Abnormal endogenous products, such as those resulting from inborn errors of metabolism
3. Exogenous products, such as environmental agents and pigments, that cannot be broken down by the cell[1]

The accumulation of normal cellular constituents occurs when a substance is produced at a rate that exceeds its metabolism or removal. An example of this type of process is fatty changes in the liver due to intracellular accumulation of triglycerides. Liver cells normally contain some fat, which is either oxidized and used for energy or converted to triglycerides. This fat is derived from free fatty acids released from adipose tissue. Abnormal accumulation occurs when the delivery of free fatty acids to the liver is increased, as in starvation and diabetes mellitus, or when the intrahepatic metabolism of lipids is disturbed, as in alcoholism.

Intracellular accumulation can result from genetic disorders that disrupt the metabolism of selected substances. A normal enzyme may be replaced with an abnormal one, resulting in the formation of a substance that cannot be used or eliminated from the cell, or an enzyme may be missing, so that an intermediate product accumulates in the cell. For example, there are at least 10 genetic disorders that affect glycogen metabolism, most of which lead to the accumulation of intracellular glycogen stores. In the most common form of this disorder, von Gierke disease, large amounts of glycogen accumulate in the liver and kidneys because of a deficiency of the enzyme glucose-6-phosphatase. Without this enzyme, glycogen cannot be broken down to form glucose. The disorder leads not only to an accumulation of glycogen but also to a reduction in blood glucose levels. In Tay-Sachs disease, another genetic disorder, abnormal lipids accumulate in the brain and other tissues, causing motor and mental deterioration beginning at approximately 6 months of age, followed by death at 2 to 5 years of age. In a similar manner, other enzyme defects lead to the accumulation of other substances.

Pigments are colored substances that may accumulate in cells. They can be endogenous (*i.e.*, arising from within the body) or exogenous (*i.e.*, arising from outside the body). Icterus, also called *jaundice*, is characterized by a yellow discoloration of tissue due to the retention of bilirubin, an endogenous bile pigment. This condition may result from increased bilirubin production from red blood cell destruction, obstruction of bile passage into the intestine, or toxic diseases that affect the liver's ability to remove bilirubin from the blood. Lipofuscin is a yellow-brown pigment that results from the accumulation of the indigestible residues produced during normal turnover of cell structures (Fig. 3.3). The accumulation of lipofuscin increases with age, and it is sometimes referred to as the *wear-and-tear pigment*. It is more common in heart, nerve, and liver cells than other tissues and is seen more often in conditions associated with atrophy of an organ.

One of the most common exogenous pigments is carbon in the form of coal dust. In coal miners or people exposed to heavily polluted environments, the accumulation of carbon dust blackens the lung tissue and may cause serious lung disease. The formation of a blue lead line along the margins of the gum is one of the diagnostic features of lead poisoning. Tattoos are the result of insoluble pigments introduced into the skin, where they are engulfed by macrophages and persist for a lifetime.

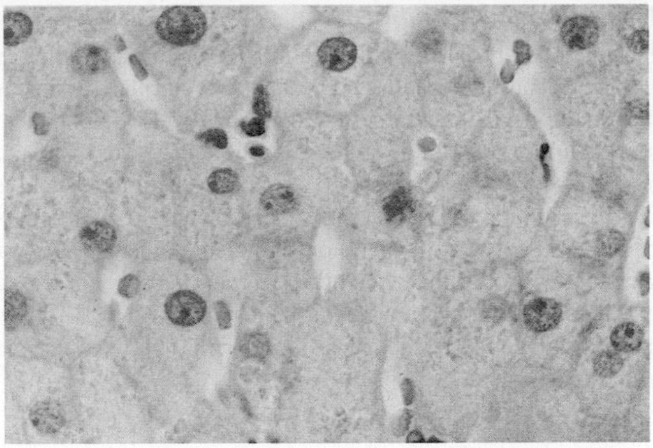

Figure 3.3 • Accumulation of intracellular lipofuscin. A photomicrograph of the liver of an 80-year-old man shows golden cytoplasmic granules, which represent lysosomal storage of lipofuscin. (From Rubin R., Strayer D. (2015). *Rubin's pathology: Clinicopathologic foundations of medicine* (7 ed., p. 11). Philadelphia, PA: Lippincott Williams & Wilkins.)

The significance of intracellular accumulations depends on the cause and severity of the condition. Many accumulations, such as lipofuscin and mild fatty change, have no effect on cell function. Some conditions, such as the hyperbilirubinemia that causes jaundice, are reversible. Other disorders, such as glycogen storage diseases, produce accumulations that result in organ dysfunction and other alterations in physiologic function.

Pathologic Calcifications

Pathologic calcification involves the abnormal tissue deposition of calcium salts, together with smaller amounts of iron, magnesium, and other minerals. It is known as *dystrophic calcification* when it occurs in dead or dying tissue and as *metastatic calcification* when it occurs in normal tissue.

Dystrophic Calcification

Dystrophic calcification represents the macroscopic deposition of calcium salts in injured tissue.[13] It is often visible to the naked eye as deposits that range from gritty, sandlike grains to firm, hard rock material. The pathogenesis of dystrophic calcification involves the intracellular or extracellular formation of crystalline calcium phosphate. The components of the calcium deposits are derived from the bodies of dead or dying cells as well as from the circulation and interstitial fluid.

Dystrophic calcification is commonly seen in atheromatous lesions of advanced atherosclerosis, areas of injury in the aorta and large blood vessels, and damaged heart valves.[13] Dystrophic calcifications are seen in human tissues in the absence of known calcium or phosphate imbalances—for example, in necrotic tissues or atherosclerotic plaques—and, when found, are used for long-term management of chronic venous insufficiency.[14]

Metastatic Calcification

In contrast to dystrophic calcification, which occurs in injured tissues, metastatic calcification occurs in normal tissues as the result of increased serum calcium levels (hypercalcemia). Almost any condition that increases the serum calcium level can lead to calcification in inappropriate sites such as the lung, renal tubules, and blood vessels.[13] The major causes of hypercalcemia are hyperparathyroidism, either primary or secondary to phosphate retention in renal failure; increased mobilization of calcium from bone as in Paget disease, cancer with metastatic bone lesions, or immobilization; and vitamin D intoxication.[14]

IN SUMMARY

Cells adapt to changes in their environment and in their work demands by changing their size, number, and characteristics. These adaptive changes are consistent with the needs of the cell and occur in response to an appropriate stimulus. The changes are usually reversed after the stimulus has been withdrawn.[1]

When confronted with a decrease in work demands or adverse environmental conditions, cells atrophy or reduce their size and revert to a lower and more efficient level of functioning. Hypertrophy results from an increase in work demands and is characterized by an increase in tissue size brought about by an increase in cell size and functional intracellular components. An increase in the number of cells in an organ or tissue that is still capable of mitotic division is called *hyperplasia*.[13,15] Metaplasia occurs in response to chronic irritation and represents the substitution of cells of a type that is better able to survive under circumstances in which a more fragile cell type might succumb. Dysplasia is characterized by deranged cell growth of a specific tissue that results in cells that vary in size, shape, and appearance. It is often a precursor of cancer.

Under some circumstances, cells may accumulate abnormal amounts of various substances. If the accumulation reflects a correctable systemic disorder, such as the hyperbilirubinemia that causes jaundice, the accumulation is reversible.[14] If the disorder cannot be corrected, as often occurs in many inborn errors of metabolism, the cells become overloaded, causing cell injury and death.

Pathologic calcification involves the abnormal tissue deposition of calcium salts. Dystrophic calcification occurs in dead or dying tissue. Although the presence of dystrophic calcification may only indicate the presence of previous cell injury, it is also a frequent cause of organ dysfunction (*e.g.*, when it affects the heart valves). Metastatic calcification occurs in normal tissues as the result of elevated serum calcium levels. Almost any condition that increases the serum calcium level can lead to calcification in inappropriate sites such as the lung, renal tubules, and blood vessels.

CELL INJURY AND DEATH

After completing this section of the chapter, the learner will be able to meet the following objectives:

- Describe the mechanisms whereby physical agents such as blunt trauma, electrical forces, and extremes of temperature produce cell injury.
- Differentiate between the effects of ionizing and nonionizing radiation in terms of their ability to cause cell injury.
- State the mechanisms and manifestations of cell injury associated with lead poisoning.
- Relate free radical formation and oxidative stress to cell injury and death.

Cells can be injured in many ways. The extent to which any injurious agent can cause cell injury and death depends in large measure on the intensity and duration of the injury and the type of cell that is involved. Cell injury is usually reversible up to a certain point, after which irreversible cell injury and death occur. Whether a specific stress causes irreversible or reversible cell injury depends on the severity of the insult and on variables such as blood supply, nutritional status, and regenerative capacity. Cell injury and death are ongoing processes, and in the healthy state, they are balanced by cell renewal.

KEY POINTS

CELL INJURY

- Cells can be damaged in a number of ways, including physical trauma, extremes of temperature, electrical injury, exposure to damaging chemicals, radiation damage, injury from biologic agents, and nutritional factors.
- Most injurious agents exert their damaging effects through uncontrolled free radical production, impaired oxygen delivery or utilization, or the destructive effects of uncontrolled intracellular calcium release.

Causes of Cell Injury

Cell damage can occur in many ways. For purposes of discussion, the ways by which cells are injured have been grouped into five categories:

1. Injury from physical agents
2. Radiation injury
3. Chemical injury
4. Injury from biologic agents
5. Injury from nutritional imbalances

Injury from Physical Agents

Physical agents responsible for cell and tissue injury include mechanical forces, extremes of temperature, and electrical forces. They are common causes of injuries due to environmental exposure, occupational and transportation accidents, and physical violence and assault.

Mechanical Forces. Injury or trauma due to mechanical forces occurs as the result of body impact with another object. The body or the mass can be in motion or, as sometimes happens, both can be in motion at the time of impact. These types of injuries split and tear tissue, fracture bones, injure blood vessels, and disrupt blood flow.

Extremes of Temperature. Extremes of heat and cold cause damage to the cell, its organelles, and its enzyme systems. Exposure to low-intensity heat (43–46°C), such as occurs with partial-thickness burns and severe heat stroke, causes cell injury by inducing vascular injury, accelerating cell metabolism, inactivating temperature-sensitive enzymes, and disrupting the cell membrane. With more intense heat, coagulation of blood vessels and tissue proteins occurs. Exposure to cold increases blood viscosity and induces vasoconstriction by direct action on blood vessels and through reflex activity of the sympathetic nervous system. The resultant decrease in blood flow may lead to hypoxic tissue injury, depending on the degree and duration of cold exposure. Injury from freezing probably results from a combination of ice crystal formation and vasoconstriction. The decreased blood flow leads to capillary stasis and arteriolar and capillary thrombosis. Edema results from increased capillary permeability.

Electrical Injuries. Electrical injuries can affect the body through extensive tissue injury and disruption of neural and cardiac impulses. Voltage, type of current, amperage, pathway of the current, resistance of the tissue, and interval of exposure determine the effect of electricity on the body.[16]

Alternating current (AC) is usually more dangerous than direct current (DC) because it causes violent muscle contractions, preventing the person from releasing the electrical source and sometimes resulting in fractures and dislocations. In electrical injuries, the body acts as a conductor of the electrical current.[16] The current enters the body from an electrical source, such as an exposed wire, and passes through the body and exits to another conductor, such as the moisture on the ground or a piece of metal the person is holding. The pathway that a current takes is critical because the electrical energy disrupts impulses in excitable tissues. Current flow through the brain may interrupt impulses from respiratory centers in the brain stem, and current flow through the chest may cause fatal cardiac arrhythmias.

The resistance to the flow of current in electrical circuits transforms electrical energy into heat. This is why the elements in electrical heating devices are made of highly resistive metals. Much of the tissue damage produced by electrical injuries is caused by heat production in tissues that have the highest electrical resistance. Resistance to electrical current varies from the greatest to the least in bone, fat, tendons, skin, muscles, blood, and nerves. The most severe tissue injury usually occurs at the skin sites where the current enters and leaves the body (Fig. 3.4). After electricity has penetrated the skin, it passes rapidly through the body along the lines of least resistance—through body fluids and nerves. Degeneration of vessel walls may occur, and thrombi may form as current flows along the blood vessels. This can cause extensive muscle and deep tissue injury. Thick, dry skin is more resistant to the flow of electricity than thin, wet skin. It is generally believed that the greater the skin resistance, the greater is the amount of local skin burn, and the less the resistance, the greater are the deep and systemic effects.

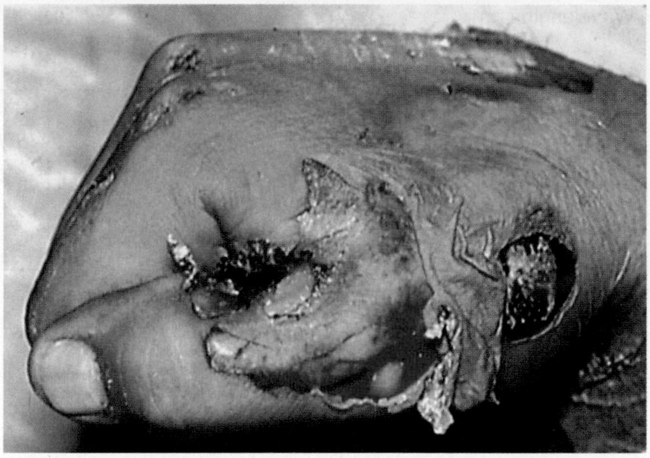

Figure 3.4 • Electrical burn of the skin. The victim was electrocuted after attempting to stop a fall from a ladder by grasping a high-voltage electrical line. (From Strayer D. S., Rubin E. (2015). Cell injury. In Rubin R., Strayer D. S. (Eds.), *Rubin's pathology: Clinicopathologic foundations of medicine* (7th ed., Fig. 8-21, p. 352). Philadelphia, PA: Lippincott Williams & Wilkins.)

Radiation Injury

Electromagnetic radiation comprises a wide spectrum of wave-propagated energy, ranging from ionizing gamma rays to radiofrequency waves (Fig. 3.5). A photon is a particle of radiation energy. Radiation energy above the ultraviolet (UV) range is called *ionizing radiation* because the photons have enough energy to knock electrons off atoms and molecules. *Nonionizing radiation* refers to radiation energy at frequencies below those of visible light. *UV radiation* represents the portion of the spectrum of electromagnetic radiation just above the visible range.[16] It contains increasingly energetic rays that are powerful enough to disrupt intracellular bonds and cause sunburn.

Ionizing Radiation. Ionizing radiation impacts cells by causing ionization of molecules and atoms in the cell. This is accomplished by releasing free radicals that destroy cells and by directly hitting the target molecules in the cell.[17] It can immediately kill cells, interrupt cell replication, or cause a variety of genetic mutations, which may or may not be lethal. Most radiation injury is caused by localized irradiation that is used in the treatment of cancer. Except for unusual circumstances such as the use of high-dose irradiation that precedes bone marrow transplantation, exposure to whole-body irradiation is rare.

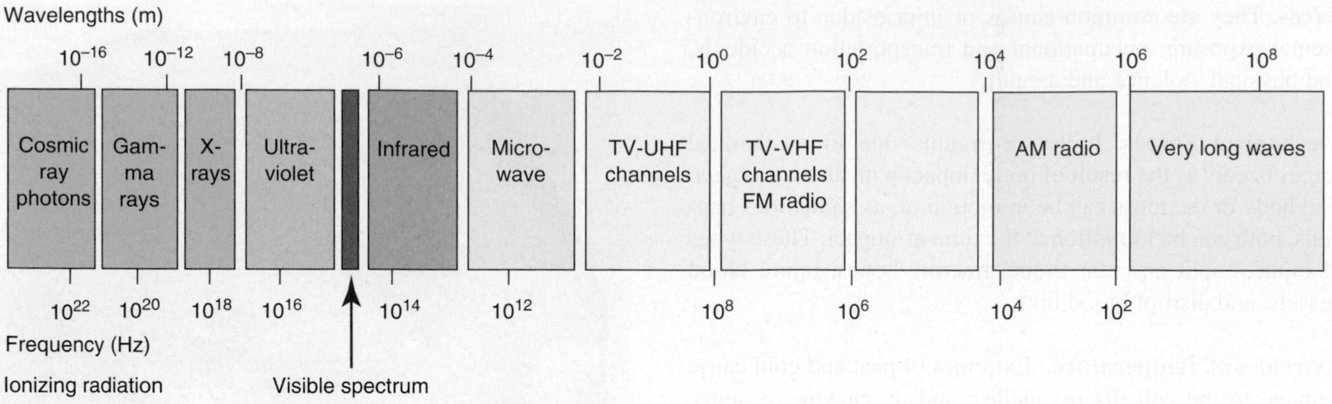

Figure 3.5 • Spectrum of electromagnetic radiation.

The injurious effects of ionizing radiation vary with the dose, dose rate (a single dose can cause greater injury than divided or fractionated doses), and the differential sensitivity of the exposed tissue to radiation injury. Because of the effect on deoxyribonucleic acid (DNA) synthesis and interference with mitosis, rapidly dividing cells of the bone marrow and intestine are much more vulnerable to radiation injury than tissues such as bone and skeletal muscle. Over time, occupational and accidental exposure to ionizing radiation can result in increased risk for the development of various types of cancers, including skin cancers, leukemia, osteogenic sarcomas, and lung cancer. This is especially true when the person is exposed to radiation during childhood.[17]

Many of the clinical manifestations of radiation injury result from acute cell injury, dose-dependent changes in the blood vessels that supply the irradiated tissues, and fibrotic tissue replacement. The cell's initial response to radiation injury involves swelling, disruption of the mitochondria and other organelles, alterations in the cell membrane, and marked changes in the nucleus. The endothelial cells in blood vessels are particularly sensitive to irradiation. During the immediate postirradiation period, only vessel dilation is apparent (*e.g.*, the initial erythema of the skin after radiation therapy). Later or with higher levels of radiation, destructive changes occur in small blood vessels such as the capillaries and venules. Acute reversible necrosis is represented by such disorders as radiation cystitis, dermatitis, and diarrhea from enteritis. More persistent damage can be attributed to acute necrosis of tissue cells that are not capable of regeneration and chronic ischemia. Chronic effects of radiation damage are characterized by fibrosis and scarring of tissues and organs in the irradiated area (*e.g.*, interstitial fibrosis of the heart and lungs after irradiation of the chest). Because the radiation delivered in radiation therapy inevitably travels through the skin, radiation dermatitis is common. There may be necrosis of the skin, impaired wound healing, and chronic radiation dermatitis.

Ultraviolet Radiation. Ultraviolet radiation causes sunburn and increases the risk of skin cancers. The degree of risk depends on the type of UV rays, the intensity of exposure, and the amount of protective melanin pigment in the skin. Skin damage produced by UV radiation is thought to be caused by reactive oxygen species (ROS) and by damage to melanin-producing processes in the skin.[18] UV radiation also damages DNA, resulting in the formation of pyrimidine dimers (*i.e.*, the insertion of two identical pyrimidine bases into replicating DNA instead of one). Other forms of DNA damage include the production of single-stranded breaks and formation of DNA–protein cross-links. Normally, errors that occur during DNA replication are repaired by enzymes that remove the faulty section of DNA and repair the damage. The importance of DNA repair in protecting against UV radiation injury is evidenced by the vulnerability of people who lack the enzymes needed to repair UV-induced DNA damage. In a genetic disorder called *xeroderma pigmentosum*, an enzyme needed to repair sunlight-induced DNA damage is lacking. This autosomal recessive disorder is characterized by extreme photosensitivity and an increased risk of skin cancer in sun-exposed skin.[18]

Nonionizing Radiation. Nonionizing radiation includes infrared light, ultrasound, microwaves, and laser energy. Unlike ionizing radiation, which can directly break chemical bonds, nonionizing radiation exerts its effects by causing vibration and rotation of atoms and molecules.[16] All of this vibrational and rotational energy is eventually converted to thermal energy. Low-frequency nonionizing radiation is used widely in radar, television, industrial operations (*e.g.*, heating, welding, melting of metals, processing of wood and plastic), household appliances (*e.g.*, microwave ovens), and medical applications (*e.g.*, diathermy). Isolated cases of skin burns and thermal injury to deeper tissues have occurred in industrial settings and from improperly used household microwave ovens. Injury from these sources is mainly thermal and, because of the deep penetration of the infrared or microwave rays, tends to involve dermal and subcutaneous tissue injury.

Chemical Injury

Chemicals capable of damaging cells are everywhere around us. Air and water pollution contains chemicals capable of tissue injury, as does tobacco smoke and some processed or preserved foods. Some of the most damaging chemicals exist in our environment, including gases such as carbon monoxide, insecticides, and trace metals such as lead.

Chemical agents can injure the cell membrane and other cell structures, block enzymatic pathways, coagulate cell proteins, and disrupt the osmotic and ionic balance of the cell. Corrosive substances such as strong acids and bases destroy cells as the substances come into contact with the body. Other chemicals may injure cells in the process of metabolism or elimination. Carbon tetrachloride (CCl_4), for example, causes little damage until it is metabolized by liver enzymes to a highly reactive free radical ($CCl_3\bullet$). Carbon tetrachloride is extremely toxic to liver cells.[17]

Drugs. Many drugs—alcohol, prescription drugs, over-the-counter drugs, and street drugs—are capable of directly or indirectly damaging tissues. Ethyl alcohol can harm the gastric mucosa, liver, developing fetus, and other organs. Antineoplastic and immunosuppressant drugs can directly injure cells. Other drugs produce metabolic end products that are toxic to cells. Acetaminophen, a commonly used over-the-counter analgesic drug, is detoxified in the liver, where small amounts of the drug are converted to a highly toxic metabolite. This metabolite is detoxified by a metabolic pathway that uses a substance (*i.e.*, glutathione) normally present in the liver. When large amounts of the drug are ingested, this pathway becomes overwhelmed and toxic metabolites accumulate, causing massive liver necrosis.

Lead Toxicity. Lead is a particularly toxic metal. Small amounts accumulate to reach toxic levels. There are innumerable sources of lead in the environment, including flaking paint, lead-contaminated dust and soil, lead-contaminated root vegetables, lead water pipes or soldered joints, pottery glazes, newsprint, and toys made in foreign countries. Adults often encounter lead through occupational exposure. Children are exposed to lead through ingestion of peeling lead paint, by breathing dust from lead paint, or from playing in contaminated soil. There has been a decline in blood lead levels of both adults and children since the removal of lead from gasoline and from soldered food cans.[19] High lead blood levels continue to be a problem, however, particularly among children. Research has found that low levels of lead in the blood can have devastating cognitive and intellectual deficits, as well as neurobehavioral problems in children. This finding led to the 2012 ACCLPP reference for blood lead to decrease from 10 to 5 μg/dL.[19]

Lead is absorbed through the gastrointestinal tract or the lungs into the blood. A deficiency in calcium, iron, or zinc increases lead absorption. In children, most lead is absorbed through the lungs. Although children may have the same or a lower intake of lead, the absorption in infants and children is greater; thus, they are more vulnerable to lead toxicity.[19,20] Lead crosses the placenta, exposing the fetus to levels of lead that are comparable with those of the mother. Lead is stored in the bone and eliminated by the kidneys. Although the half-life of lead is hours to days, bone deposits serve as a repository from which blood levels are maintained. In a sense, bone protects other tissues, but the slow turnover maintains blood levels for months to years.

The toxicity of lead is related to its multiple biochemical effects. It has the ability to inactivate enzymes, compete with calcium for incorporation into bone, and interfere with nerve transmission and brain development. The major targets of lead toxicity are the red blood cells, the gastrointestinal tract, the kidneys, and the nervous system.

Anemia is a cardinal sign of lead toxicity. Lead competes with the enzymes required for hemoglobin synthesis and with the membrane-associated enzymes that prevent hemolysis of red blood cells. The resulting red cells are coarsely stippled and hypochromic, resembling those seen in iron-deficiency anemia. The life span of the red cell is also decreased. The gastrointestinal tract is the main source of symptoms in the adult. This is characterized by "lead colic," a severe and poorly localized form of acute abdominal pain. A lead line formed by precipitated lead sulfite may appear along the gingival margins. The lead line is seldom seen in children. The kidneys are the major route for excretion of lead. Lead can cause diffuse kidney damage, eventually leading to renal failure. Even without overt signs of kidney damage, lead toxicity leads to hypertension.

In the nervous system, lead toxicity is characterized by demyelination of cerebral and cerebellar white matter and death of cortical cells. When this occurs in early childhood, it can affect neurobehavioral development and result in lower IQ levels and poorer classroom performance.[20] Peripheral demyelinating neuropathy may occur in adults. The most serious manifestation of lead poisoning is acute encephalopathy. It is manifested by persistent vomiting, ataxia, seizures, papilledema, impaired consciousness, and coma. Acute encephalopathy may manifest suddenly, or it may be preceded by other signs of lead toxicity such as behavioral changes or abdominal complaints.

Because of the long-term neurobehavioral and cognitive deficits that occur in children with even moderately elevated lead levels, the Centers for Disease Control and Prevention have issued recommendations for childhood lead screening.[19,20] A safe blood level of lead is still uncertain. At one time, 25 μg/dL was considered safe. Surveys have shown abnormally low IQs in children with lead levels as low as 10 to 15 μg/dL.

Screening for lead toxicity involves the use of capillary blood obtained from a finger stick to measure free erythrocyte protoporphyrin (EP). Elevated levels of EP result from the inhibition by lead of the enzymes required for heme synthesis in red blood cells. The EP test is useful in detecting high lead levels but usually does not detect levels below 20 to 25 μg/dL. Thus, capillary screening test values greater than 10 μg/dL should be confirmed with those from a venous blood sample. Because the symptoms of lead toxicity usually are vague, diagnosis is often delayed. Anemia may provide the first clues to the disorder. Laboratory tests are necessary to establish a diagnosis. Treatment involves removal of the lead source and, in cases of severe toxicity, administration of a chelating agent. Asymptomatic children with blood levels of 45 to 69 µg/dL usually are treated.[20,21] A public health team should evaluate the source of lead because meticulous removal is needed.

Mercury Toxicity. Mercury has been used for industrial and medical purposes for hundreds of years. Mercury is toxic, and the hazards of mercury-associated occupational and accidental exposures are well known. Currently, mercury and lead are the most toxic metals. Mercury is toxic in four primary forms: mercury vapor, inorganic divalent mercury, methyl mercury, and ethyl mercury.[20] Depending on the form of mercury exposure, toxicity involving the central nervous system and kidney can occur.[20]

In the case of dental fillings, the concern involves mercury vapor being released into the mouth. However, the amount of mercury vapor released from fillings is very small. The main source of methyl mercury exposure is from consumption of long-lived fish, such as tuna and swordfish. Fish concentrate mercury from sediment in the water. Only certain types of fish pose potential risk, however, and types such as salmon have miniscule amounts or no mercury. Because the developing brain is more susceptible to mercury-induced damage, it is recommended that young children and pregnant and nursing women avoid consumption of fish known to contain high mercury content. Thimerosal is an ethyl mercury–containing preservative that helps prevent microorganism growth in vaccines. Because of the concern of this preservative, it is hardly ever used in the United States.

Injury from Biologic Agents

Biologic agents differ from other injurious agents in that they are able to replicate and can continue to produce their injurious effects. These agents range from submicroscopic viruses to the larger parasites. Biologic agents injure cells by diverse mechanisms. Viruses enter the cell and become incorporated into its DNA synthetic machinery. Certain bacteria elaborate exotoxins that interfere with cellular production of ATP. Other bacteria, such as the gram-negative bacilli, release endotoxins that cause cell injury and increased capillary permeability.

Injury from Nutritional Imbalances

Nutritional excesses and nutritional deficiencies predispose cells to injury. Obesity and diets high in saturated fats are thought to predispose people to atherosclerosis. The body requires more than 60 organic and inorganic substances in amounts ranging from micrograms to grams. These nutrients include minerals, vitamins, certain fatty acids, and specific amino acids. Dietary deficiencies can occur in the form of starvation, in which there is a deficiency of all nutrients and vitamins, or because of a selective deficiency of a single nutrient or vitamin. Iron-deficiency anemia, scurvy, beriberi, and pellagra are examples of injury caused by the lack of specific vitamins or minerals. The protein and calorie deficiencies that occur with starvation cause widespread tissue damage.

Mechanisms of Cell Injury

The mechanisms by which injurious agents cause cell injury and death are complex. Some agents, such as heat, produce direct cell injury. Other factors, such as genetic derangements, produce their effects indirectly through metabolic disturbances and altered immune responses.[16] There seem to be at least three major mechanisms whereby most injurious agents exert their effects:

- Free radical formation
- Hypoxia and ATP depletion
- Disruption of intracellular calcium homeostasis (Fig. 3.6)

Free Radical Injury

Many injurious agents exert damaging effects through reactive chemical species known as *free radicals*.[22] Free radicals are highly reactive chemical species with an unpaired electron in the outer orbit (valence shell) of the molecule.[16] In the literature, the unpaired electron is denoted by a dot, for example, •NO. The unpaired electron causes free radicals to be unstable and highly reactive, so that they react nonspecifically with molecules in the vicinity. Moreover, free radicals can establish chain reactions consisting of many events that generate new free radicals. In cells and tissues, free radicals react with proteins, lipids, and carbohydrates, thereby damaging cell membranes; inactivate enzymes; and damage nucleic acids that make up DNA. The actions of free radicals may disrupt and damage cells and tissues.

Reactive oxygen species (ROS) are oxygen-containing molecules that include free radicals such as superoxide O_2^- and hydroxyl radical (OH•) and nonradicals such as hydrogen peroxide (H_2O_2).[16] These molecules are produced endogenously by normal metabolic processes or cell activities, such as the metabolic burst that accompanies phagocytosis. However, exogenous causes, including ionizing and UV radiation, can cause ROS production in the body. *Oxidative stress* is a condition that occurs when the generation of ROS exceeds the ability of the body to neutralize and eliminate ROS.[16] Oxidative stress can lead to oxidation of cell components, activation of signal transduction pathways, and changes in gene and protein expression. DNA modification and damage can occur as a result of oxidative stress. Although ROS and oxidative stress are clearly associated with cell and tissue damage, evidence shows that ROS do not always act in a random and damaging manner. Current studies have found that ROS are also important signaling molecules that are used in healthy cells to regulate and maintain normal activities and functions such as vascular tone and insulin and vascular endothelial growth factor signaling.[22] Oxidative damage has been implicated in many diseases. Mutations in the gene for SOD are linked with amyotrophic lateral sclerosis (ALS; so-called Lou Gehrig

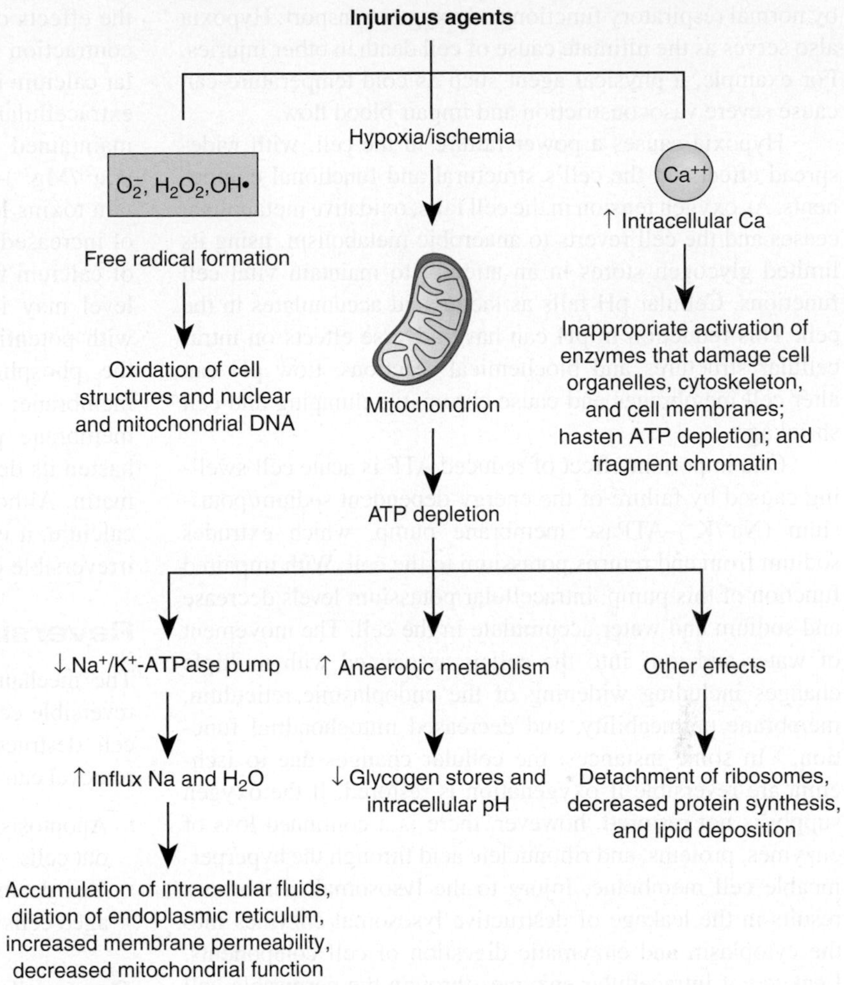

Figure 3.6 • Mechanisms of cell injury. The injurious agents tend to cause hypoxia/ischemia (see *middle arrow*, which illustrates the manifestations that trigger anaerobic metabolism to develop and cellular injury). Also, on the left aspect of the figure, the free radical formation causes oxidation of cell structures leading to decreased ATP, and on the right side, the increased intracellular calcium damages many aspects of the cell that also causes ATP depletion. These three paths illustrate how injurious agents cause cell injury and death.

disease).[23] Oxidative stress is thought to play an important role in the development of cancer.[16] Reestablishment of blood flow after loss of perfusion, as occurs during heart attack and stroke, is associated with oxidative injury to vital organs.[24] The endothelial dysfunction that contributes to the development, progression, and prognosis of cardiovascular disease is thought to be caused in part by oxidative stress.[24] In addition to the many diseases and altered health conditions associated with oxidative damage, oxidative stress has been linked with the age-related functional declines that underlie the process of aging.[25]

Antioxidants are natural and synthetic molecules that inhibit the reactions of ROS with biologic structures or prevent the uncontrolled formation of ROS. Antioxidants include enzymatic and nonenzymatic compounds.[16] Catalase can catalyze the reaction that forms water from hydrogen peroxide. Nonenzymatic antioxidants include carotenes (*e.g.*, vitamin A), tocopherols (*e.g.*, vitamin E), ascorbate (vitamin C), glutathione, flavonoids, selenium, and zinc.[16]

Hypoxic Cell Injury

Hypoxia deprives the cell of oxygen and interrupts oxidative metabolism and the generation of ATP. The actual time necessary to produce irreversible cell damage depends on the degree of oxygen deprivation and the metabolic needs of the cell. Some cells, such as those in the heart, brain, and kidney, require large amounts of oxygen to provide energy to perform their functions. Brain cells, for example, begin to undergo permanent damage after 4 to 6 minutes of oxygen deprivation. A thin margin can exist between the time involved in reversible and irreversible cell damage. During hypoxic conditions, hypoxia-inducible factors (HIFs) cause the expression of genes that stimulate red blood cell formation, produce ATP in the absence of oxygen, and increase angiogenesis[23,24] (*i.e.*, the formation of new blood vessels).

Hypoxia can result from an inadequate amount of oxygen in the air, respiratory disease, ischemia (*i.e.*, decreased blood flow due to vasoconstriction or vascular obstruction), anemia, edema, or inability of the cells to use oxygen. Ischemia is characterized by impaired oxygen delivery and impaired removal of metabolic end products such as lactic acid. In contrast to pure hypoxia, which depends on the oxygen content of the blood and affects all cells in the body, ischemia commonly affects blood flow through limited numbers of blood vessels and produces local tissue injury. In some cases of edema, the distance for diffusion of oxygen may become a limiting factor in the delivery of oxygen.[24] In hypermetabolic states, cells may require more oxygen than can be supplied by normal respiratory function and oxygen transport. Hypoxia also serves as the ultimate cause of cell death in other injuries. For example, a physical agent such as cold temperature can cause severe vasoconstriction and impair blood flow.

Hypoxia causes a power failure in the cell, with widespread effects on the cell's structural and functional components. As oxygen tension in the cell falls, oxidative metabolism ceases and the cell reverts to anaerobic metabolism, using its limited glycogen stores in an attempt to maintain vital cell functions. Cellular pH falls as lactic acid accumulates in the cell. This reduction in pH can have adverse effects on intracellular structures and biochemical reactions. Low pH can alter cell membranes and cause chromatin clumping and cell shrinkage.

One important effect of reduced ATP is acute cell swelling caused by failure of the energy-dependent sodium/potassium (Na^+/K^+)–ATPase membrane pump, which extrudes sodium from and returns potassium to the cell. With impaired function of this pump, intracellular potassium levels decrease and sodium and water accumulate in the cell. The movement of water and ions into the cell is associated with multiple changes including widening of the endoplasmic reticulum, membrane permeability, and decreased mitochondrial function.[16] In some instances, the cellular changes due to ischemia are reversible if oxygenation is restored. If the oxygen supply is not restored, however, there is a continued loss of enzymes, proteins, and ribonucleic acid through the hyperpermeable cell membrane. Injury to the lysosomal membranes results in the leakage of destructive lysosomal enzymes into the cytoplasm and enzymatic digestion of cell components. Leakage of intracellular enzymes through the permeable cell membrane into the extracellular fluid provides an important clinical indicator of cell injury and death.

Impaired Calcium Homeostasis

Calcium functions as an important second messenger and cytosolic signal for many cell responses. Various calcium-binding proteins, such as troponin and calmodulin, act as transducers for the cytosolic calcium signal. Calcium-/calmodulin-dependent kinases indirectly mediate the effects of calcium on responses such as smooth muscle contraction and glycogen breakdown. Normally, intracellular calcium ion levels are kept extremely low compared with extracellular levels. The low intracellular calcium levels are maintained by membrane-associated calcium/magnesium (Ca^{2+}/Mg^{2+})–ATPase exchange systems. Ischemia and certain toxins lead to an increase in cytosolic calcium because of increased influx across the cell membrane and the release of calcium from intracellular stores. The increased calcium level may inappropriately activate a number of enzymes with potentially damaging effects. These enzymes include the phospholipases, responsible for damaging the cell membrane; proteases that damage the cytoskeleton and membrane proteins; ATPases that break down ATP and hasten its depletion; and endonucleases that fragment chromatin. Although it is known that injured cells accumulate calcium, it is unknown whether this is the ultimate cause of irreversible cell injury.

Reversible Cell Injury and Cell Death

The mechanisms of cell injury can produce sublethal and reversible cellular damage or lead to irreversible injury with cell destruction or death (Fig. 3.7). Cell destruction and removal can involve one of two mechanisms:

- Apoptosis, which is designed to remove injured or worn-out cells
- Cell death or necrosis, which occurs in irreversibly damaged cells[1]

Reversible Cell Injury

Reversible cell injury, although impairing cell function, does not result in cell death. Two patterns of reversible cell injury can be observed under the microscope: cellular swelling and fatty change. Cellular swelling occurs with impairment of the energy-dependent Na^+/K^+–ATPase membrane pump, usually as the result of hypoxic cell injury.

Fatty changes are linked to intracellular accumulation of fat. When fatty changes occur, small vacuoles of fat disperse throughout the cytoplasm. The process is usually more

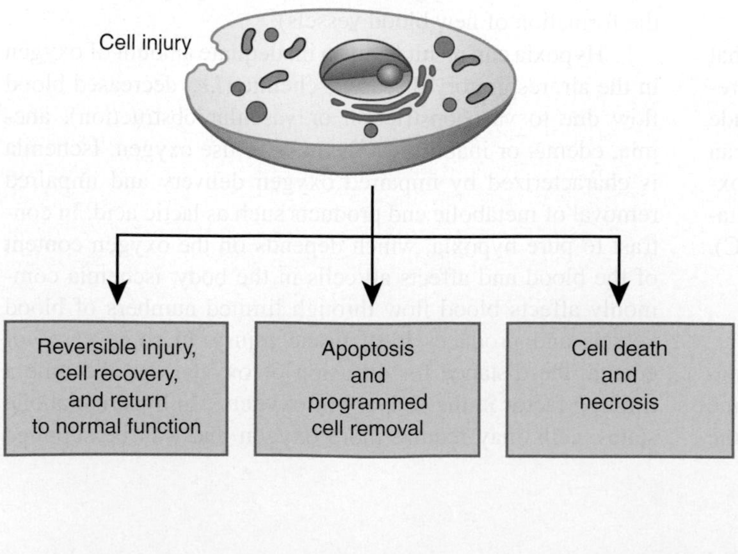

Figure 3.7 • Outcomes of cell injury: reversible cell injury, apoptosis and programmed cell removal, and cell death and necrosis.

ominous than cellular swelling, and although it is reversible, it usually indicates severe injury. These fatty changes may occur because normal cells are presented with an increased fat load or because injured cells are unable to metabolize the fat properly. In obese people, fatty infiltrates often occur within and between the cells of the liver and heart because of an increased fat load. Pathways for fat metabolism may be impaired during cell injury, and fat may accumulate in the cell as production exceeds use and export. The liver, where most fats are synthesized and metabolized, is particularly susceptible to fatty change, but fatty changes may also occur in the kidney, the heart, and other organs.

Programmed Cell Death

In most normal nontumor cells, the number of cells in tissues is regulated by balancing cell proliferation and cell death. Cell death occurs by necrosis or a form of programmed cell death called apoptosis.[1]

Apoptosis is a highly selective process that eliminates injured and aged cells, thereby controlling tissue regeneration. Cells undergoing apoptosis have characteristic morphologic features as well as biochemical changes. As shown in Figure 3.8, shrinking and condensation of the nucleus and cytoplasm occur. The chromatin aggregates at the nuclear envelope, and DNA fragmentation occurs. Then, the cell becomes fragmented into multiple apoptotic bodies in a manner that maintains the integrity of the plasma membrane and does not initiate inflammation. Changes in the plasma membrane induce phagocytosis of the apoptotic bodies by macrophages and other cells, thereby completing the degradation process.

Apoptosis is thought to be responsible for several normal physiologic processes, including the programmed destruction of cells during embryonic development, hormone-dependent involution of tissues, death of immune cells, cell death by cytotoxic T cells, and cell death in

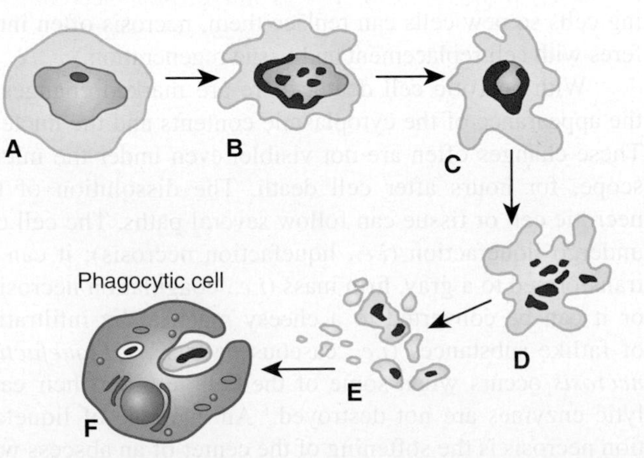

Figure 3.8 • Apoptotic cell removal: shrinking of the cell structures (*A*), condensation and fragmentation of the nuclear chromatin (*B* and *C*), separation of nuclear fragments and cytoplasmic organelles into apoptotic bodies (*D* and *E*), and engulfment of apoptotic fragments by phagocytic cell (*F*).

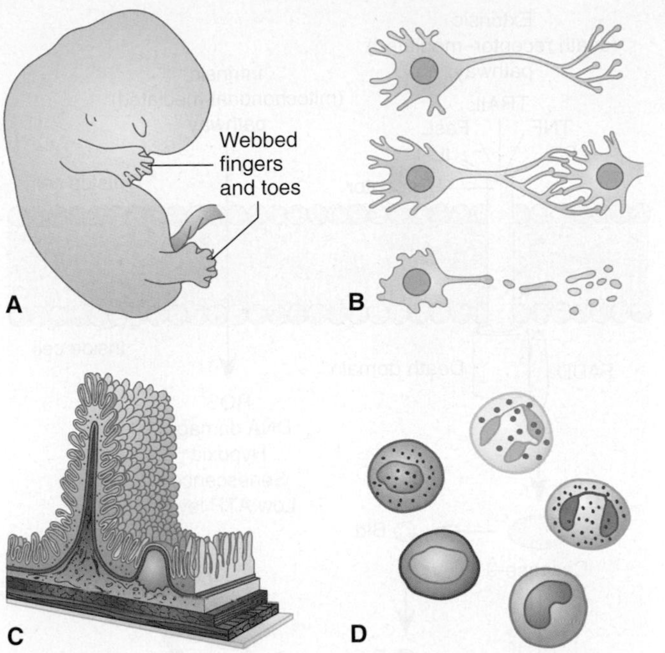

Figure 3.9 • Examples of apoptosis: **(A)** separation of webbed fingers and toes in embryo; **(B)** development of neural connections; neurons that do not establish synaptic connections and receive survival factors may be induced to undergo apoptosis; **(C)** removal of cells from intestinal villi; new epithelial cells continuously form in the crypt, migrate to the villus tip as they age, and undergo apoptosis at the tip at the end of their life span; and **(D)** removal of senescent blood cells.

proliferating cell populations. During embryogenesis, in the development of a number of organs such as the heart, which begins as a pulsating tube and is gradually modified to become a four-chambered pump, apoptotic cell death allows for the next stage of organ development. It also separates the webbed fingers and toes of the developing embryo (Fig. 3.9). Apoptotic cell death occurs in the hormone-dependent involution of endometrial cells during the menstrual cycle and in the regression of breast tissue after weaning from breastfeeding. The control of immune cell numbers and destruction of autoreactive T cells in the thymus have been credited to apoptosis. Cytotoxic T cells and natural killer cells are thought to destroy target cells by inducing apoptotic cell death.

Concept Mastery Alert

The involution that occurs in hormone-dependent cells, such as in breast tissue after weaning, occurs as a result of programmed cell death or apoptosis.

Apoptosis is linked to many pathologic processes and diseases. For example, interference with apoptosis is known to be a mechanism that contributes to carcinogenesis.[26] Apoptosis may also be implicated in neurodegenerative disorders such as Alzheimer disease, Parkinson disease, and ALS. However, the exact mechanisms involved in these diseases remain under investigation.

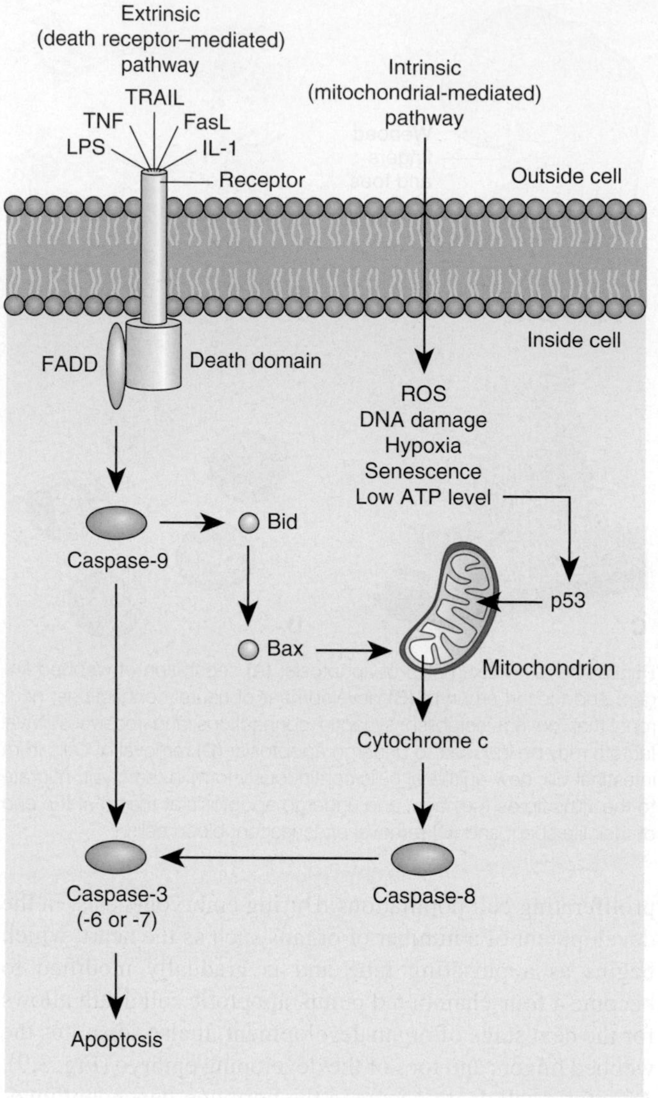

Figure 3.10 • Extrinsic and intrinsic pathways of apoptosis. The extrinsic pathway is activated by signals such as Fas ligand (FasL) that on binding to the Fas receptor form a death-inducing complex by joining the Fas-associated death domain (FADD) to the death domain of the Fas receptor. The intrinsic pathway is activated by signals, such as ROS and DNA damage that induce the release of cytochrome *c* from mitochondria into the cytoplasm. Both pathways activate caspases to execute apoptosis.

Two basic pathways for apoptosis have been described (Fig. 3.10). These are the extrinsic pathway, which is death receptor dependent, and the intrinsic pathway, which is death receptor independent. The execution phase of both pathways is carried out by proteolytic enzymes called *caspases*, which are present in the cell as *procaspases* and are activated by cleavage of an inhibitory portion of their polypeptide chain.

The *extrinsic pathway* involves the activation of receptors such as tumor necrosis factor (TNF) receptors and the Fas ligand receptor.[25] Fas ligand may be expressed on the surface of certain cells such as cytotoxic T cells or appear in a soluble form. When Fas ligand binds to its receptor, proteins congregate at the cytoplasmic end of the Fas receptor to form a death-initiating complex. The complex then converts procaspase-8 to caspase-8. Caspase-8, in turn, activates a cascade of caspases that execute the process of apoptosis.[2,25] The end result includes activation of endonucleases that cause fragmentation of DNA and cell death. In addition to TNF and Fas ligand, primary signaling molecules known to activate the extrinsic pathway include TNF-related apoptosis-inducing ligand (TRAIL), the cytokine interleukin-1 (IL-1), and lipopolysaccharide (LPS), the endotoxin found in the outer cell membrane of gram-negative bacteria.

The *intrinsic pathway*, or *mitochondrion-induced pathway*, of apoptosis is activated by conditions such as DNA damage, ROS, hypoxia, decreased ATP levels, cellular senescence, and activation of the p53 protein by DNA damage.[25] It involves the opening of mitochondrial membrane permeability pores with release of cytochrome c from the mitochondria into the cytoplasm. Cytoplasmic cytochrome c activates caspases, including caspase-3. Caspase-3 activation is a common step to both the extrinsic and intrinsic pathways. Furthermore, activation or increased levels of proapoptotic proteins, such as Bid and Bax, after caspase-8 activation in the extrinsic pathway can lead to mitochondrial release of cytochrome *c*, thereby bridging the two pathways for apoptosis. Many inhibitors of apoptosis within cells are known and thought to contribute to cancer and autoimmune diseases.[2] The therapeutic actions of certain drugs may induce or facilitate apoptosis. Apoptosis continues to be an active area of investigation to better understand and treat a variety of diseases.

Necrosis

Necrosis refers to cell death in an organ or tissue that is still part of a living organism.[16] Necrosis differs from apoptosis because it causes loss of cell membrane integrity and enzymatic breakdown of cell parts and triggers the inflammatory process.[1] In contrast to apoptosis, which functions in removing cells so new cells can replace them, necrosis often interferes with cell replacement and tissue regeneration.

With necrotic cell death, there are marked changes in the appearance of the cytoplasmic contents and the nucleus. These changes often are not visible, even under the microscope, for hours after cell death. The dissolution of the necrotic cell or tissue can follow several paths. The cell can undergo liquefaction (*i.e.*, liquefaction necrosis); it can be transformed to a gray, firm mass (*i.e.*, coagulation necrosis); or it can be converted to a cheesy material by infiltration of fatlike substances (*i.e.*, caseous necrosis).[1] *Liquefaction necrosis* occurs when some of the cells die but their catalytic enzymes are not destroyed.[1] An example of liquefaction necrosis is the softening of the center of an abscess with discharge of its contents. During *coagulation necrosis*, acidosis develops and denatures the enzymatic and structural proteins of the cell. This type of necrosis is characteristic of hypoxic injury and is seen in infarcted areas.[1] Infarction (*i.e.*, tissue death) occurs when an artery supplying an organ or part of the body becomes occluded and no other source of blood supply exists. As a rule, the shape of the infarction is conical and corresponds to the distribution of the artery and its branches. An artery may be occluded by an embolus, a thrombus, disease of the arterial wall, or pressure from outside the vessel.

Caseous necrosis is a distinctive form of coagulation necrosis in which the dead cells persist indefinitely.[1] It is most commonly found in the center of tuberculosis granulomas or tubercles.[1]

Gangrene. The term *gangrene* is applied when a considerable mass of tissue undergoes necrosis. Gangrene may be classified as dry or moist. In dry gangrene, the part becomes dry and shrinks, the skin wrinkles, and its color changes to dark brown or black. The spread of dry gangrene is slow, and its symptoms are not as marked as those of wet gangrene. The irritation caused by the dead tissue produces a line of inflammatory reaction (*i.e.*, line of demarcation) between the dead tissue of the gangrenous area and the healthy tissue. Dry gangrene usually results from interference with the arterial blood supply to a part without interference with venous return and is a form of coagulation necrosis.

In moist or wet gangrene, the area is cold, swollen, and pulseless. The skin is moist, black, and under tension. Blebs form on the surface, liquefaction occurs, and a foul odor is caused by bacterial action. There is no line of demarcation between the normal and diseased tissues, and the spread of tissue damage is rapid. Systemic symptoms are usually severe, and death may occur unless the condition can be arrested. Moist or wet gangrene primarily results from interference with venous return from the part. Bacterial invasion plays an important role in the development of wet gangrene and is responsible for many of its prominent symptoms. Dry gangrene is confined almost exclusively to the extremities, but moist gangrene may affect the internal organs or the extremities. If bacteria invade the necrotic tissue, dry gangrene may be converted to wet gangrene.

Gas gangrene is a special type of gangrene that results from infection of devitalized tissues by one of several *Clostridium* bacteria, most commonly *Clostridium perfringens*.[1] These anaerobic and spore-forming organisms are widespread in nature, particularly in soil. Gas gangrene is prone to occur in trauma and compound fractures in which dirt and debris are embedded. Some species have been isolated in the stomach, gallbladder, intestine, vagina, and skin of healthy people. Characteristic of this disorder are the bubbles of hydrogen sulfide gas that form in the muscle. Gas gangrene is a serious and potentially fatal disease. Antibiotics are used to treat the infection and surgical methods are used to remove the infected tissue. Amputation may be required to prevent spreading infection involving a limb. Hyperbaric oxygen therapy has been used, but clinical data supporting its efficacy have not been rigorously assessed.

Cellular Aging

Like adaptation and injury, aging is a process that involves the cells and tissues of the body. A number of theories have been proposed to explain the cause of aging. These theories are not mutually exclusive, and aging is most likely complex with multiple causes. The main theories of aging can be categorized based on evolutionary, molecular, cellular, and systems-level explanations.[1]

The *evolutionary theories* focus on genetic variation and reproductive success. After the reproductive years have passed, it is not clear that continued longevity contributes to the fitness of the species. Thus, "antiaging" genes would not necessarily be selected, preserved, and prevalent in the gene pool.

The *molecular theories* of cellular aging focus more on mutations or changes in gene expression. Because the appearance, properties, and function of cells depend on gene expression, this aspect is likely to be involved in aging at some level. Recent attention is being given to the so-called aging genes identified in model systems.

There are a number of *cellular theories of senescence* that are currently under investigation, including those that focus on telomere shortening, free radical injury, and apoptosis. It has been known since the mid-1960s that many cells in culture exhibit a limit in replicative capacity, the so-called Hayflick limit of about 50 population doublings. This limit seems to be related to the length of the telomeres, which are DNA sequences at the ends of chromosomes. Each time a cell divides, the telomeres shorten until a critical minimal length is attained, senescence ensues, and further cell replication does not occur. Some cells have telomerase, an enzyme that "rebuilds" telomeres and lessens or prevents shortening. Cancer cells have high levels of telomerase, which prevents senescence and contributes to the cellular immortality that characterizes cancer. Telomere shortening appears to be related to other theories of cellular causes of aging. For example, free radicals and oxidative damage can kill cells and hasten telomere shortening. Caloric restriction, which appears to increase longevity, may be related to reduced mitochondrial free radical generation owing to reduced methionine or other dietary amino acid intake.[27–29]

Systems-level theories center on a decline in the integrative functions of organ systems such as the immunologic and neuroendocrine systems, which are necessary for overall control of other body systems. The immune system may decline with age and be less effective in protecting the body from infection or cancer. In addition, mutations and manipulations of genes such as *daf*-2, which is similar to human insulin/IGF-1 receptor genes, in the aging worm model *Caenorhabditis elegans* cause significant changes in longevity.[30] Pathways related to *daf*-2 may be responsible for relationships between caloric restriction and prolonged life span in rodents and other animals. The mechanisms that regulate aging are likely to be complex and multifactorial, as will be any interventions to prolong aging.[31]

IN SUMMARY

Cell injury can be caused by a number of agents, including physical agents, chemicals, biologic agents, and nutritional factors. Among the physical agents that generate cell injury are mechanical forces that produce tissue trauma, extremes of temperature, electricity, radiation, and nutritional disorders. Chemical agents can cause cell injury through several mechanisms: they can block enzymatic pathways, cause coagulation of tissues, or disrupt the osmotic or ionic balance of the cell. Biologic agents differ from other injurious agents in that they are able to replicate and continue to produce injury. Among the nutritional factors that contribute to cell injury are excesses and deficiencies of nutrients, vitamins, and minerals.

Injurious agents exert their effects largely through generation of free radicals, production of cell hypoxia, or dysregulation of intracellular calcium levels. Partially reduced oxygen species called *free radicals* are important mediators of cell injury in many pathologic conditions. They are an important cause of cell injury in hypoxia and after exposure to radiation and certain chemical agents. Lack of oxygen underlies the pathogenesis of cell injury in hypoxia and ischemia. Hypoxia can result from inadequate oxygen in the air, cardiorespiratory disease, anemia, or the inability of the cells to use oxygen. Increased intracellular calcium activates a number of enzymes with potentially damaging effects.

Injurious agents may produce sublethal and reversible cellular damage or may lead to irreversible cell injury and death. Cell death can involve two mechanisms: apoptosis or necrosis. Apoptosis involves controlled cell destruction and is the means by which the body removes and replaces cells that have been produced in excess, developed improperly, have genetic damage, or are worn out. Necrosis refers to cell death that is characterized by cell swelling, rupture of the cell membrane, and inflammation.

Like adaptation and injury, aging is a process that involves the cells and tissues of the body. A number of theories have been proposed to explain the complex causes of aging, including those based on evolutionary mechanisms that explain aging as a consequence of natural selection, in which traits that maximize the reproductive capacity of an individual are selected over those that maximize longevity; molecular theories, such as those that explain aging as a result of changes in gene expression; cellular theories that explain cellular senescence in relation to telomere length or molecular events, free radical damage, accumulated wear and tear, or apoptosis; and systems theories that attribute cellular aging to a decline in the integrative functions of organ systems such as the neuroendocrine and immunologic systems.

GERIATRIC Considerations

- Most organs do not continue to regenerate new cells; this is a universal cause of atrophy in aging.[1]
- Age-related sarcopenia, the loss of muscle mass, is due to loss of type II fibers. This is different from cachexia, which is associated with loss of type I fibers.[1]
- Macroautophagy, a process in which damaged cytoplasmic is delivered to lysosomes for digestion, decreases with age, contributing to chronic inflammation, Alzheimer disease, and changes in the central nervous system and heart.[32]

PEDIATRIC Considerations

- Secondhand smoke and environmental tobacco smoke prevent amino acids that are needed for fetal growth from being absorbed by the cells in the placenta.[33]
- Substance abuse such as ingestion of alcohol, cocaine, and methamphetamines, which cross the placenta, cause cellular damage and birth defects.[33]
- Puberty is associated with cellular hypertrophy due to rapid increases in androgens and growth hormones.[1]

REVIEW EXERCISES

1. A 30-year-old man sustained a fracture of his leg 2 months ago. The leg has been encased in a cast, and he has just had it removed. He is amazed at the degree to which the muscles in his leg have shrunk.
   A. *Would you consider this to be a normal adaptive response? Explain.*
   B. *Will these changes have an immediate and/or long-term effect on the function of the leg?*
   C. *What types of measures can be taken to restore full function to the leg?*
2. A 45-year-old woman has been receiving radiation therapy for breast cancer.
   A. *Explain the effects of ionizing radiation in eradicating the tumor cells.*
   B. *Why is the radiation treatment given in smaller divided, or fractionated, doses rather than as a single large dose?*
   C. *Partway through the treatment schedule, the woman notices that her skin over the irradiated area has become reddened and irritated. What is the reason for this?*

3. People who have had a heart attack may experience additional damage once blood flow has been restored, a phenomenon referred to as *reperfusion injury*.
   A. *What is the proposed mechanism underlying reperfusion injury?*
   B. *What factors might influence this mechanism?*
4. Every day, blood cells in our body become senescent and die without producing signs of inflammation, yet massive injury or destruction of tissue, such as occurs with a heart attack, produces significant signs of inflammation.
   A. *Explain.*

References

1. Rubin R., Strayer D. (Eds.). (2015). *Rubin's pathology: Clinicopathologic foundations of medicine* (7th ed.). Philadelphia, PA: Lippincott Williams & Wilkins.
2. Rawlings D., Metzler G., Dutra M. W., et al. (2017). Altered B cell signalling in autoimmunity. *Nature Reviews Immunology* 17, 670–678. http://dx.doi.org/10.1038/nri.2017.24
3. Bodine S. C. (2013). Disuse-induced muscle wasting. *The International Journal of Biochemistry* 45, 2200–2208. https://doi.org/http://dx.doi.org/10.1016/j.biocel.2013.06.011
4. Chowdhury M., Enenkel C. (2015). Intracellular dynamics of the ubiquitin-proteasome-system [version 2; referees: 3 approved] F100Research. *F100Research* 4(367), 1–16. https://doi.org/10.12688/f1000research.6835.2
5. Schiaffino S., Dyar K. A., Cicilio S., et al. (2013). Mechanisms regulating skeletal muscle growth and atrophy. *Feb Journal* 280, 4294–4314. https://doi.org/doi:10.1111/febs.12253
6. Kundu B. K., Zhong M., Sen S., et al. (2015). Remodeling of glucose metabolism precedes pressure overload-induced left ventricular hypertrophy: Review of a hypothesis. *Cardiology* 130, 211–220. https://doi.org/10.1159/000369782
7. Baker J., Obermair A., Gebski V., et al. (2012). Efficacy of oral or intrauterine device-delivered progestin in patients with complex endometrial hyperplasia with atypia or early endometrial adenocarcinoma: A meta-analysis and systematic review of the literature. *Gynecologic Oncology* 125, 263–270. https://doi.org/10.1016/j.ygyno.2011.11.043
8. Gandaglia G., Briganti A., Gontero P., et al. (2013). The role of chronic prostatic inflammation in the pathogenesis and progression of benign prostatic hyperplasia (BPH). *BJU International* 112, 432–441. https://doi.org/10.1111/bju.12118
9. Hartmann L. C., Degnim A. C., Santen R. J., et al. (2015). Atypical hyperplasia of the breast: Risk assessment and management options. *The New England Journal of Medicine* 372(1), 78–89. https://doi.org/10.1056/NEJMsr140716
10. Thanan R., Ma N., Hiraku Y., et al. (2016). DNA damage in CD133-positive cells in Barrett's esophagus and esophageal adenocarcinoma. *Mediators of Inflammation* 2016, 1–8. http://dx.doi.org/http://dx.doi.org/10.1155/2016/7937814
11. Hove M. V., Prenzel F., Uhlig H. H., et al. (2014). Pulmonary outcome in former preterm, very low birth weight children with bronchopulmonary dysplasia: A case control follow up at school age. *The Journal of Pediatrics* 164(1), 40–45. http://dx.doi.org/http://dx.doi.org/10.1016/j.jpeds.2013.07.045
12. Askanas V., Engel K., Nogalska A. (2012). Pathogenic considerations in sporadic inclusion-body myositis, a degenerative muscle disease associated with aging and abnormalities of myoproteostasis. *Journal of Neuropathology & Experimental Neurology* 71(8), 680–693.
13. Mohiuddin S. A., Badal S., Doiphode A., et al. (2012). Multiple supramassetric dystrophic calcinosis. *Annals of Maxillofacial Surgery* 2(1), 74–76. https://doi.org/10.4103/2231-0746.95328
14. Smith E. R. (2016). Vascular calcification in uremia: new-age concepts about an old-age problem vascular calcification in uremia: new-age concepts about an old-age problem. In T. Hewitson E. Smith, S. Holt (Eds.), *Methods in molecular biology*. https://doi.org/https://doi.org/10.1007/978-1-4939-3353-2_13
15. Kim H. Y., Park J. H., Lee J. B., et al. (2017). A case of dystrophic calcification in the masseter muscle. *Maxillofacial Plastic and Reconstructive Surgery* 39(31), 1–5. https://doi.org/10.1186/s40902-017-0130-4
16. McConnell T. H., Hull K. L. (2011). *Human form human function: Essentials of anatomy & physiology*. Philadelphia, PA: Lippincott Williams & Wilkins.
17. Wu S., Powers S., Zhu W., et al. (2016). Substantial contribution of extrinsic risk factors to cancer development. *Nature* 529, 43–57. https://doi.org/10.1038/nature16166
18. Naik S. M., Shenoy A. M., Nanjundappa A., et al. (2013). Cutaneous malignancies in xeroderma pigmentosum: Earlier management improves survival. *Indian Journal of Otolaryngology and Head & Neck Surgery* 65(2), 162–167. https://doi.org/10.1007/s12070-012-0614-6
19. Schnur J., John R. M. (2013). Childhood lead poisoning and the new Centers for Disease Control and Prevention guidelines for lead exposure. *Journal of the American Association of Nurse Practitioners*, 26, 283–247. https://doi.org/10.1002/2327-6924.12112
20. Centers for Disease Control and Prevention. (2014). Lead. [Online]. Available: http://www.cdc.gov/nceh/lead/. Accessed January 28, 2018.
21. Centers for Disease Control and Prevention. (2014). *Lead prevention tips*. [Online]. Available: http://www.cdc.gov/nceh/lead/tips.htm. Accessed January 28, 2018.
22. Ma Q. (2013). Role of Nrf2 in oxidative stress and toxicity. *Annual Review of Pharmacology and Toxicology* 53, 401–426. http://doi.org/10.1146/annurev-pharmtox-011112-140320
23. Niki E. (2014). Biomarkers of lipid peroxidation in clinical material. *Biochimica et Biophysica Acta* 1840, 809–817. https://doi.org/http://dx.doi.org/10.1016/j.bbagen.2013.03.020
24. Semenza G. L. (2012). Hypoxia-inducible factors in physiology and medicine. *Cell* 148, 399–408. https://doi.org/10.1016/j.cell.2012.01.021
25. Wang J., Gao J., Li Y., et al. (2013). Functional polymorphisms in FAS and FASL contribute to risk of squamous cell carcinoma of the larynx and hypopharynx in a Chinese population. *Gene* 524, 193–196. https://doi.org/http://dx.doi.org/10.1016/j.gene.2013.04.034
26. Okuda H., Xing F., Pandey P. R., et al. (2013). miR-7 Suppresses brain metastasis of breast cancer stem-like cells by modulating KLF4. *Cancer Research* 73(4), 1434–1445. https://doi.org/10.1158/0008-5472.CAN-12-2037
27. Brandhorst S., Choi I. Y., Min M., et al. (2015). A periodic diet that mimics fasting promotes multi-system regeneration, enhanced cognitive performance, and health span. *Cell Metabolism* 22, 86–99. https://doi.org/http://dx.doi.org/10.1016/j.cmet.2015.05.012
28. Mendell J. T., Olson E. N. (2012). MicroRNAs in stress signaling and human disease. *Cell* 1172–1187. https://doi.org/10.1016/j.cell.2012.02.005
29. Saifan C., Saad M., Charabaty E. E., et al. (2013). Warfarin-induced calciphylaxis: A case report and review of literature. *International Journal of General Medicine* 6, 665–669. https://doi.org/http://dx.doi.org/10.2147/IJGM.S47397
30. Gems D., Partridge L. (2013). Genetics of longevity in model organisms: Debates and paradigm shifts. *The Annual Review of Physiology* 75, 621–644. https://doi.org/10.1146/annurev-physiol-030212-183712
31. Eggermont A. M., Spatz A., Robert C. (2013). Cutaneous melanoma. *Seminar* 383, 816–827. https://doi.org/http://dx.doi.org/10.1016/
32. Oishi Y., Manabe I. (2016). Macrophages in age-related chronic inflammatory diseases. *Nature Partner Journals*. doi: 10.1038/npjamd.2016.18.
33. Bowden V. R., Greenberg C. S. (2014). *Children and their families the continuum of nursing care*. Philadelphia, PA: Wolters Kluwer.

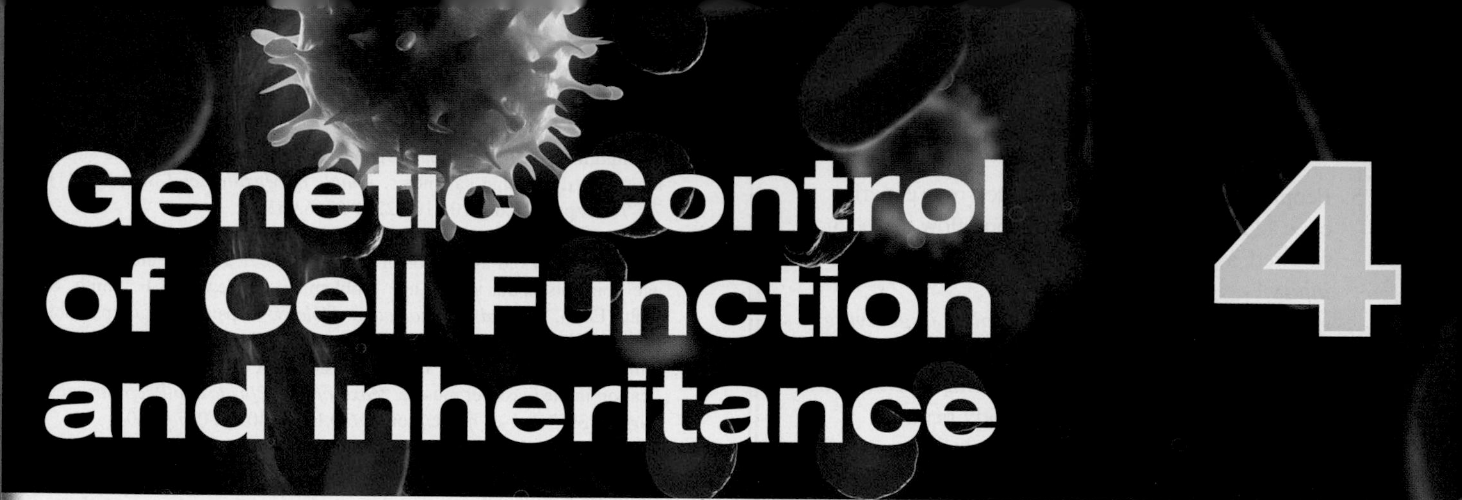

Genetic Control of Cell Function and Inheritance

4

Ansley Grimes Stanfill

Our genetic information is stored within the structure of *deoxyribonucleic acid* (DNA), an extremely stable macromolecule. Genetic information directs the function of our cells, determines our appearance and how we respond to our environment, and serves as the unit of inheritance passed on from generation to generation. Genes also determine our disease susceptibility and how we react to drugs.

An understanding of the role that genetics plays in pathogenesis of disease has expanded greatly over the past century. This is due to the completion of the Human Genome Project in 2003, in which the entire human genome was sequenced. Building upon this information, researchers have shown us that many common diseases, including cancer, diabetes, and cardiovascular disease, have a genetic component. In the case of cancer, recent genetic advances have led to new methods for early detection and more effective treatment. Advances in recombinant DNA technology have provided the methods for producing human insulin, growth hormone, and clotting factors. This chapter includes discussions of genetic control of cell function, chromosomes, patterns of inheritance, and gene technology.

GENETIC CONTROL OF CELL FUNCTION

After completing this section of the chapter, the learner will be able to meet the following objectives:

- Compare and contrast the structure and function of DNA and RNA.
- Explain how the DNA code is transcribed into RNA and translated into protein.
- Describe ways in which gene expression is regulated.

The DNA that contains our genetic information is an extremely stable molecule. Because of its stable structure, the genetic information carried in DNA can survive the many stages of cell division and the day-to-day process of cell renewal and tissue growth. Its stable structure also allows the information to survive the many processes of reduction division involved in gamete (*i.e.*, ovum and sperm) formation, the fertilization process, and the mitotic cell divisions involved in the formation of a new organism from the single-celled fertilized ovum called the *zygote*.

A second type of nucleic acid, *ribonucleic acid* (RNA), is involved in the actual synthesis of cellular proteins. The information contained in a given gene is first transcribed from DNA into RNA, processed in the nucleus, and then carried to the cytoplasm where it is translated and synthesized into proteins.

Although DNA and RNA have received a lot of attention, it is the proteins that the genes encode that make up the majority of cellular structures and perform most life functions. Proteins are responsible for the functional diversity of cells, they perform most biologic functions, and it is at the protein level that many regulatory processes take place, many disease processes occur, and most drug targets are found.

Concept Mastery Alert

The term *proteome* defines the complete set of proteins encoded by a genome. *Proteomics*, the study of the proteome, uses highly sophisticated technologic methods to examine the molecular and biochemical events in a cell.

KEY POINTS

THE ROLE OF DNA IN CONTROLLING CELL FUNCTION

- The information needed for the control of cell structure and function is embedded in the genetic information encoded within the DNA molecule.
- Although every cell in the body contains the same genetic information, each cell type uses only a portion of the information, depending on its specific function in the body.

DNA Structure and Function

The DNA molecule that stores the genetic information in the nucleus is a long, double-stranded, helical structure. DNA is composed of *nucleotides*, which consist of phosphoric acid, a five-carbon sugar called *deoxyribose*, and one of four nitrogenous bases (Fig. 4.1). These nitrogenous bases carry the genetic information and are divided into two groups: the *pyrimidine bases*, thymine (T) and cytosine (C), which have one nitrogen ring, and the *purine bases*, adenine (A) and guanine (G), which have two. The backbone of DNA consists of alternating groups of sugar and phosphate, with the paired bases projecting inward from the sides of the sugar molecule.

Double Helix and Base Pairing

The structure of DNA, as first described by James Watson and Frances Crick in 1953, is that of a spiral staircase, with the paired bases representing the steps (see Fig. 4.1). A precise and complementary pairing of purine and pyrimidine bases occurs in the double-stranded DNA molecule. Adenine is paired with thymine (A-T) and guanine is paired with cytosine (G-C). The paired bases on opposite DNA strands are bound together by stable hydrogen bonds. The double-stranded structure of DNA molecules allows them to replicate precisely by separation of the two strands and also allows efficient and correct repair of damaged DNA molecules.

Before cell division, the two strands of the helix separate and a complementary strand is duplicated next to each original strand such that the two strands become four strands. During cell division, the newly duplicated double-stranded molecules are separated into pairs made up of one old strand and one new strand. One pair is placed into each of the two daughter cells by the mechanics of mitosis. In 1958, Meselson and Stahl first characterized this process of replication of DNA

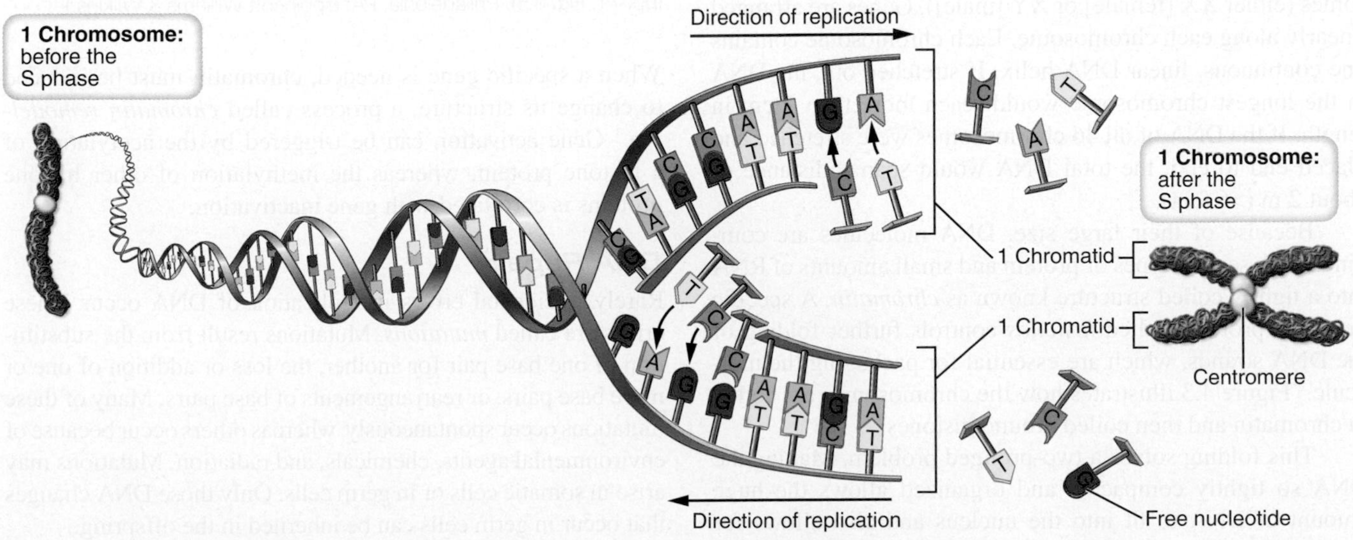

Figure 4.1 • A replicating DNA helix. The DNA helix is unwound, and base pairing rules (A with T and G with C) operate to assemble a new DNA strand on each original strand. After DNA replication is complete, each DNA molecule (chromatid) consists of an old strand and a new synthesized strand. They are joined together at the centromere. (From McConnell T., Hull K. (2011). *Human form human function: Essentials of anatomy & physiology* (pp. 78). Philadelphia, PA: Lippincott Williams & Wilkins.)

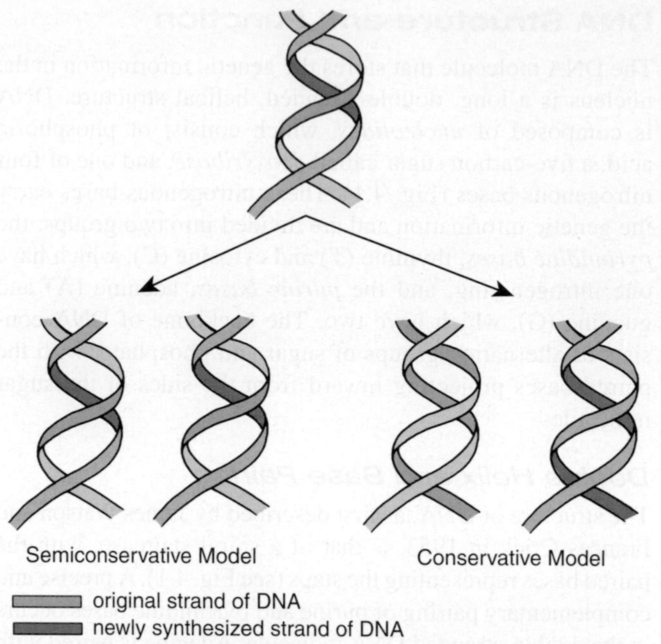

Figure 4.2 • Semiconservative versus conservative models of DNA replication as proposed by Meselson and Stahl in 1958. In semiconservative DNA replication, the two original strands of DNA unwind and a complementary strand is formed along each original strand.

as *semiconservative*, as opposed to conservative replication in which the original parental strands reassociate when the two strands are brought together (Fig. 4.2).[1]

Packaging of DNA

The genome (total genetic content) is distributed in chromosomes. Each human somatic cell (cells other than the gametes [sperm and ovum]) has 23 pairs of different chromosomes, one pair derived from the individual's mother and the other from the individual's father. Twenty-two of these pairs are autosomes, whereas the last pair is made up of the sex chromosomes (either XX [female] or XY [male]). Genes are arranged linearly along each chromosome. Each chromosome contains one continuous, linear DNA helix. If stretched out, the DNA in the longest chromosome would reach more than 7 cm in length. If the DNA of all 46 chromosomes were stretched and placed end to end, the total DNA would span a distance of about 2 m (>6 feet).

Because of their large size, DNA molecules are combined with several types of protein and small amounts of RNA into a tightly coiled structure known as *chromatin*. A specific group of proteins called *histones* controls further folding of the DNA strands, which are essential for packaging the molecule.[2] Figure 4.3 illustrates how the chromosomes are coiled in chromatin and then coiled around histones.

This folding solves a two-pronged problem. Making the DNA so tightly compacted and organized allows the huge amount of DNA to fit into the nucleus and also allows for faithful replication during cell division. The coiling and packaging can also work (alongside other mechanisms) to prevent certain genes from being accessed when they are not needed.

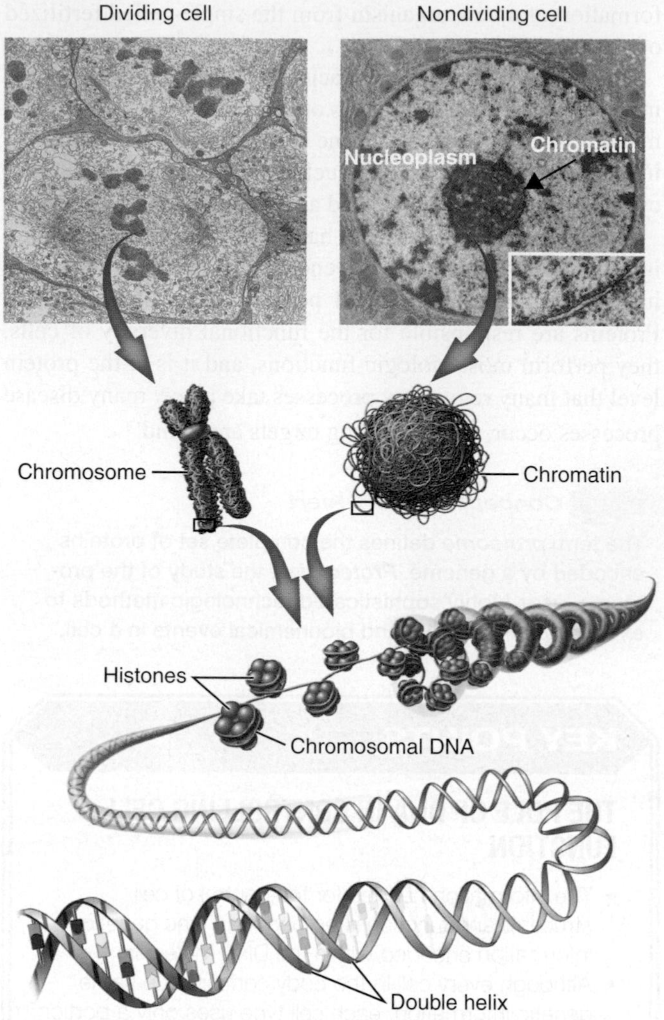

Figure 4.3 • DNA strand organization. The DNA strands are shown in chromosomes for dividing cells and in chromatin for nondividing cells and are coiled around histones. (From McConnell T. H., Hull K. L. (2011). *Human form human function: Essentials of anatomy & physiology* (pp. 71, Fig. 3.5). Philadelphia, PA: Lippincott Williams & Wilkins.)

When a specific gene is needed, chromatin must be induced to change its structure, a process called *chromatin remodeling*.[3] Gene activation can be triggered by the acetylation of a histone protein, whereas the methylation of other histone proteins is correlated with gene inactivation.

DNA Repair

Rarely, accidental errors in replication of DNA occur. These errors are called *mutations*. Mutations result from the substitution of one base pair for another, the loss or addition of one or more base pairs, or rearrangements of base pairs. Many of these mutations occur spontaneously, whereas others occur because of environmental agents, chemicals, and radiation. Mutations may arise in somatic cells or in germ cells. Only those DNA changes that occur in germ cells can be inherited in the offspring.

Fortunately, most of these defects are corrected by DNA repair mechanisms. Several types of repair mechanisms exist, and each depends on specific enzymes called *endonucleases* that recognize local distortions of the DNA helix, cleave the abnormal chain, and remove the distorted region.[6] The gap is then filled when the correct deoxyribonucleotides, created by a DNA polymerase using the intact complementary strand as a template, are added to the cleaved DNA. The newly synthesized end of the segment is then joined to the remainder of the DNA strand by a DNA ligase. Specific DNA repair genes control the regulation of these mechanisms. Changes to these genes can potentially render the DNA susceptible to accumulation of mutations, and cancer may result.

Genetic Variability

The human genome sequence is almost exactly (99.9%) the same in all people. It is the small variation (0.01%) in gene sequence that is thought to account for the individual differences in physical traits, behaviors, and disease susceptibility. These normal variations are sometimes referred to as *polymorphisms* (from the existence of more than one morphologic or body form in a population). An international effort has been organized to develop a map (HapMap) of these variations with the intent of providing a link between specific genetic variations and common complex diseases.[4]

From Genes to Proteins

Although DNA determines the type of biochemical product needed by the cell and directs its synthesis, it is RNA that is responsible for the actual assembly of the products. The RNA assembles the amino acids into functional protein by the process of translation.

RNA Structure and Function

RNA, like DNA, is a large molecule made up of a long string of nucleotides. However, it differs from DNA in three aspects of its structure. First, RNA is a single-stranded rather than a double-stranded molecule. Second, the sugar in each nucleotide of RNA is ribose instead of deoxyribose. Third, the pyrimidine base thymine in DNA is replaced by uracil in RNA.

Here, we will discuss messenger RNA (mRNA), ribosomal RNA (rRNA), and transfer RNA (tRNA). All three types of RNA are synthesized in the nucleus by RNA polymerase enzymes and then moved into the cytoplasm, where protein synthesis takes place. *Messenger RNA* carries the instructions for protein synthesis, obtained from the DNA molecule, into the cytoplasm. *Transfer RNA* reads the instructions and delivers the appropriate amino acids to the ribosome, and *ribosomal RNA* translates the instructions and provides the machinery needed for protein synthesis.

Messenger RNA. Messenger RNA is the template for protein synthesis. It is a long molecule containing several hundred to several thousand nucleotides. As mentioned before, four bases—guanine, adenine, cytosine, and thymine (in DNA) or uracil (in RNA)—make up the alphabet of the genetic code. A sequence of three of these bases in RNA forms the fundamental triplet code used in transmitting the genetic information needed for protein synthesis. This triplet code is called a *codon* (Table 4.1). An example is the nucleotide sequence UGG (uracil, guanine, guanine), which is the triplet RNA code for the amino acid tryptophan. The genetic code is a

TABLE 4.1 TRIPLET CODES FOR AMINO ACIDS

AMINO ACID	RNA CODONS					
Alanine	GCU	GCC	GCA	GCG		
Arginine	CGU	CGC	CGA	CGG	AGA	AGG
Asparagine	AAU	AAC				
Aspartic acid	GAU	GAC				
Cysteine	UGU	UGC				
Glutamic acid	GAA	GAG				
Glutamine	CAA	CAG				
Glycine	GGU	GGC	GGA	GGG		
Histidine	CAU	CAC				
Isoleucine	AUU	AUC	AUA			
Leucine	CUU	CUC	CUA	CUG	UUA	UUG
Lysine	AAA	AAG				
Methionine	AUG					
Phenylalanine	UUU	UUC				
Proline	CCU	CCC	CCA	CCG		
Serine	UCU	UCC	UCA	UCG	AGC	AGU
Threonine	ACU	ACC	ACA	ACG		
Tryptophan	UGG					
Tyrosine	UAU	UAC				
Valine	GUU	GUC	GUA	GUG		
Start (CI)	AUG					
Stop (CT)	UAA	UAG	UGA			

universal language used by most living cells (*i.e.*, the code for the amino acid tryptophan is the same in a bacterium, a plant, and a human being). Mathematically, the four bases can be arranged in 64 different combinations. Sixty-one of the triplets correspond to particular amino acids, and three are *stop codons*, which signal the end of a protein molecule.[5] But only 20 amino acids are used in protein synthesis in humans. Several of the possible triplets code for the same amino acid; therefore, the genetic code is said to be *redundant* or *degenerate*. For example, the codons AAA and AAG both code for the amino acid lysine. Codons that specify the same amino acid are called *synonyms*. Synonyms usually have the same first two bases but differ in the third base, defined as *wobble*. An example of wobble is in the codons for the amino acid leucine: if the first two bases are CU, it does not matter what the third base is.

Messenger RNA is formed from DNA by a process called *transcription*. In this process, the weak hydrogen bonds of the DNA nucleotides are temporarily broken so that free RNA nucleotides can pair with their exposed DNA counterparts of the DNA molecule (see Fig. 4.4). As with the base pairing of the DNA strands, complementary RNA bases pair with the DNA bases. Again in RNA, uracil (U) replaces thymine and pairs with adenine. As with DNA, guanine pairs with cytosine.

Ribosomal RNA. The ribosome is the physical structure in the cytoplasm where protein synthesis takes place. Ribosomal RNA forms a little over half of the ribosome, with the remainder of the ribosome composed of the structural proteins and enzymes needed for protein synthesis. As with the other types of RNA, rRNA is synthesized in the nucleus. Unlike the two other types of RNA, rRNA is produced in a specialized nuclear structure called the *nucleolus*. The formed rRNA combines with ribosomal proteins in the nucleus to produce the ribosome, which is then transported into the cytoplasm. On reaching the cytoplasm, most ribosomes become attached to the endoplasmic reticulum and begin the task of protein synthesis.

Transfer RNA. *Transfer RNA* is a clover-shaped molecule and works to deliver the activated form of an amino acid to the protein that is being synthesized in the ribosomes. At least 20 different types of tRNA are known, each of which recognizes and binds to only one type of amino acid. Each tRNA molecule has two recognition sites: the first is complementary to the mRNA codon, and the second is complementary to the amino acid itself. Each type of tRNA carries its own specific amino acid to the ribosomes, where protein synthesis is taking place; there it recognizes the appropriate codon on the mRNA and delivers the amino acid to the newly forming protein molecule.

Transcription

Transcription occurs in the cell nucleus and is the process in which RNA is synthesized from the DNA template (Fig. 4.4). Genes are transcribed by enzymes called *RNA polymerases* that generate a single-stranded RNA identical in sequence (with the exception of U in place of T) to one of the strands of DNA. It is initiated by the assembly of a transcription complex composed of RNA polymerase and other associated factors. This complex binds to the double-stranded DNA at a specific site called the *promoter region*. Within the promoter region, there is a crucial thymine–adenine–thymine–adenine nucleotide sequence (called the TATA box) that RNA polymerase recognizes and binds to. This binding also requires transcription factors, a transcription initiation site, and other proteins. Transcription continues to copy the meaningful

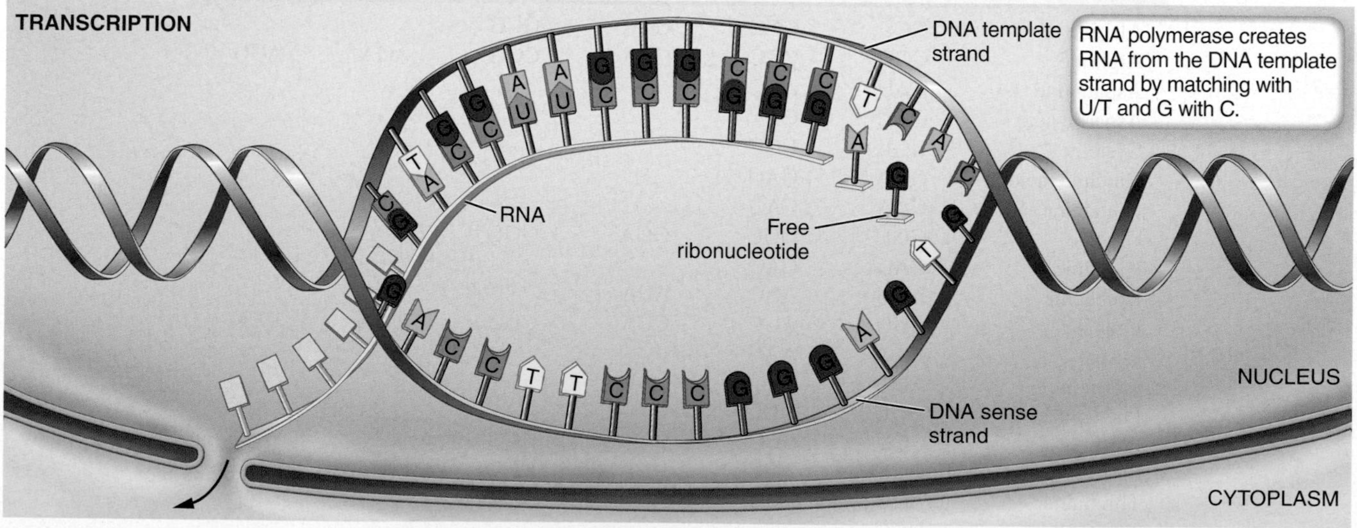

Figure 4.4 • The DNA helix and transcription of messenger RNA (mRNA). The DNA helix unwinds and a new mRNA strand is built on the template strand of the DNA. The mRNA contains the same base sequence as the DNA strand except that T bases are replaced with U bases. The mRNA leaves the nucleus through pores in the nuclear envelope. (From McConnell T., Hull K. (2011). *Human form human function: Essentials of anatomy & physiology* (pp. 83). Philadelphia, PA: Lippincott Williams & Wilkins.)

strand into a single strand of RNA as it travels along the length of the gene, continuing until it reaches the stop codon. On reaching the stop signal, the RNA polymerase enzyme leaves the gene and releases the RNA strand. The RNA strand then is processed into a mature mRNA molecule.

Processing involves the addition of certain nucleic acids at the ends of the RNA strand and cutting and splicing of certain internal sequences. Splicing involves the removal of stretches of RNA. Because of the splicing process, the final mRNA sequence is different from the original DNA template. The retained protein-coding regions of the mRNA sequences are called *exons,* and the regions between exons are called *introns*. Although they are not used in making the protein product, introns are still important.

Splicing permits a cell to produce a variety of mRNA molecules from a single gene. By varying the splicing segments of the initial mRNA, different mRNA molecules are formed. For example, in a muscle cell, the original tropomyosin mRNA is spliced in as many as 10 different ways, yielding distinctly different protein products. This permits different proteins to be expressed from a single gene and reduces how much DNA must be contained in the genome.

Translation

After the mRNA is processed (adding nucleic acids to the ends and splicing out the exons), it is a mature molecule and is passed into the cytoplasm of the cell, where translation occurs. Translation is the synthesis of a protein using the mRNA template. All proteins are made from amino acids, which are joined end to end to form the long polypeptide chains of protein molecules. Each polypeptide chain may have more than 300 amino acids in it. Translation requires the coordinated actions of mRNA, rRNA, and tRNA to make such a complex molecule (Fig. 4.5). The mRNA provides the information needed for placing the amino acids in their proper order for each specific type of protein. During protein synthesis, mRNA contacts and passes through the ribosome (binding to rRNA), during which it "reads" the directions for protein synthesis. As mRNA passes through the ribosome, tRNA delivers the appropriate amino acids for attachment to the growing polypeptide chain. Each of the 20 different tRNA molecules transports its specific amino acid to the ribosome for incorporation into the developing protein molecule.

Next, this new polypeptide chain must fold up into its unique three-dimensional conformation. The folding of many proteins is made more efficient by special classes of proteins called *molecular chaperones.*[6] These proteins also assist in the transport to the site in the cell where the protein will carry out its function and help to prevent misfolding of existing proteins. Disruption of these chaperoning mechanisms causes intracellular molecules to become denatured and insoluble. These denatured proteins tend to stick to one another, precipitate, and form inclusion bodies, which is a pathologic process that occurs in Parkinson, Alzheimer, and Huntington diseases.

During folding, other modifications can occur. A newly synthesized polypeptide chain may also need to combine with one or more polypeptide chains from the same or an adjacent chromosome, bind small cofactors for its activity, or undergo

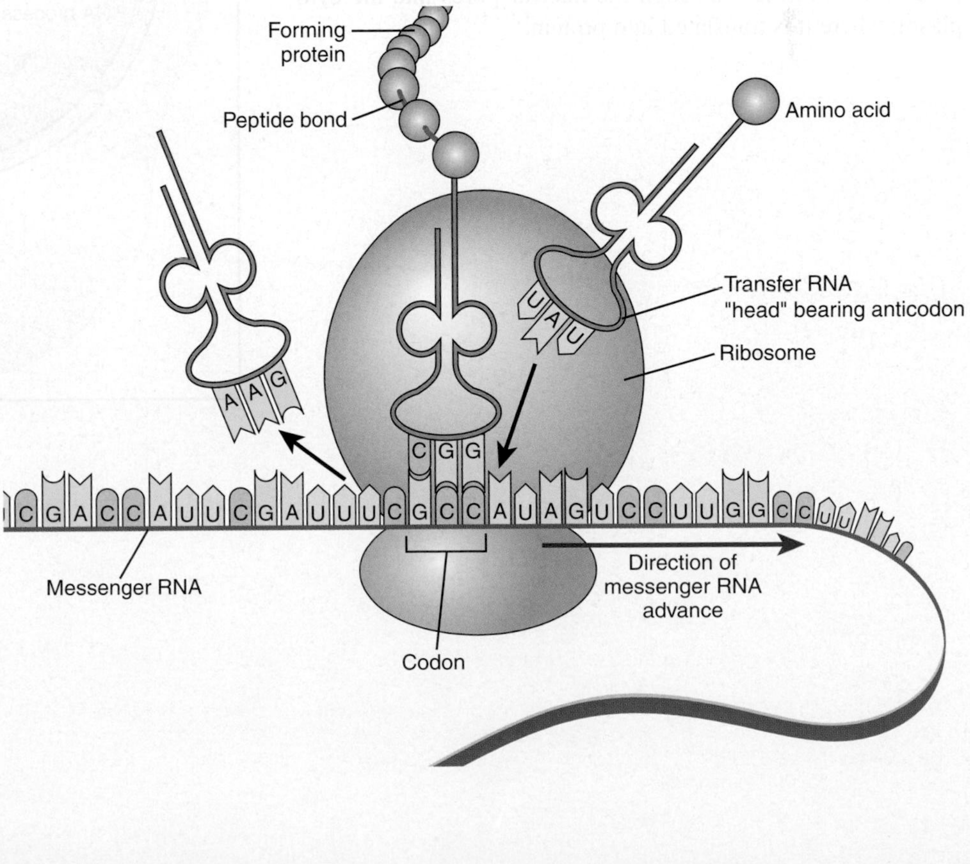

Figure 4.5 • Protein synthesis. A messenger RNA (mRNA) strand is shown moving along a small ribosomal subunit in the cytoplasm. As the mRNA codon passes along the ribosome, a new amino acid is added to the growing peptide chain by the transfer RNA (tRNA). As each amino acid is bound to the next by a peptide bond, its tRNA is released.

Understanding DNA-Directed Protein Synthesis

Deoxyribonucleic acid (DNA) contains the information to direct the synthesis of the many thousands of proteins that are contained in the different cells of the body. A second type of nucleic acid—ribonucleic acid (RNA)—participates in the actual assembly of the proteins.

There are three types of RNA: messenger RNA (mRNA), ribosomal RNA (rRNA), and transfer RNA (tRNA) that participate in (1) the transcription of the DNA instructions for protein synthesis and (2) the translation of those instructions into the assembly of the polypeptides that make up the various proteins.

The genetic code is a triplet of four bases (adenine [A], thymine [T], guanine [G], and cytosine [C], with thymine in DNA being replaced with uracil [U] in RNA) that control the sequence of amino acids in a protein molecule that is being synthesized. The triplet RNA code is called a *codon*.

Transcription

Transcription occurs when the DNA is copied into a complementary strand of mRNA. Transcription is initiated by an enzyme called *RNA polymerase*, which binds to a promoter site on DNA. Many other proteins, including transcription factors, function to increase or decrease transcriptional activity of the genes. After mRNA has been transcribed, it detaches from DNA and is processed by adding nucleotide sequences to the beginning and end of the molecule, and introns are spliced out. Changes to the splicing allow the production of a variety of mRNA molecules from a single gene. Once mRNA has been processed, it diffuses through the nuclear pores into the cytoplasm, where it is translated into protein.

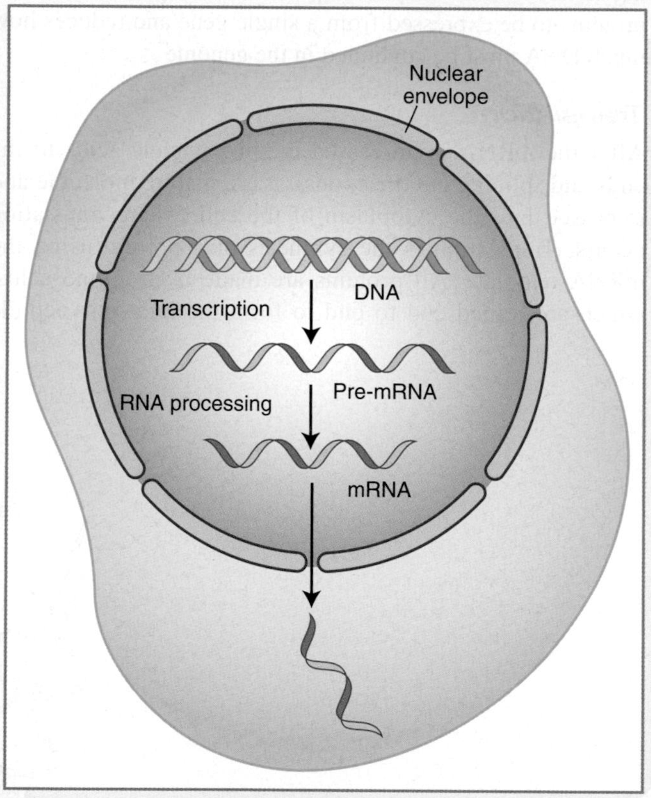

Understanding DNA-Directed Protein Synthesis *(Continued)*

Translation

Translation begins when the mRNA carrying the instructions for a particular protein comes in contact with a ribosome and binds to a small subunit of the rRNA. It then travels through the ribosome while the tRNA delivers and transfers the correct amino acid to its proper position on the growing peptide chain. There are 20 types of tRNA, one for each of the 20 different types of amino acid. In order to be functional, the newly synthesized protein must be folded into its functional form, modified further, and then routed to its final position in the cell.

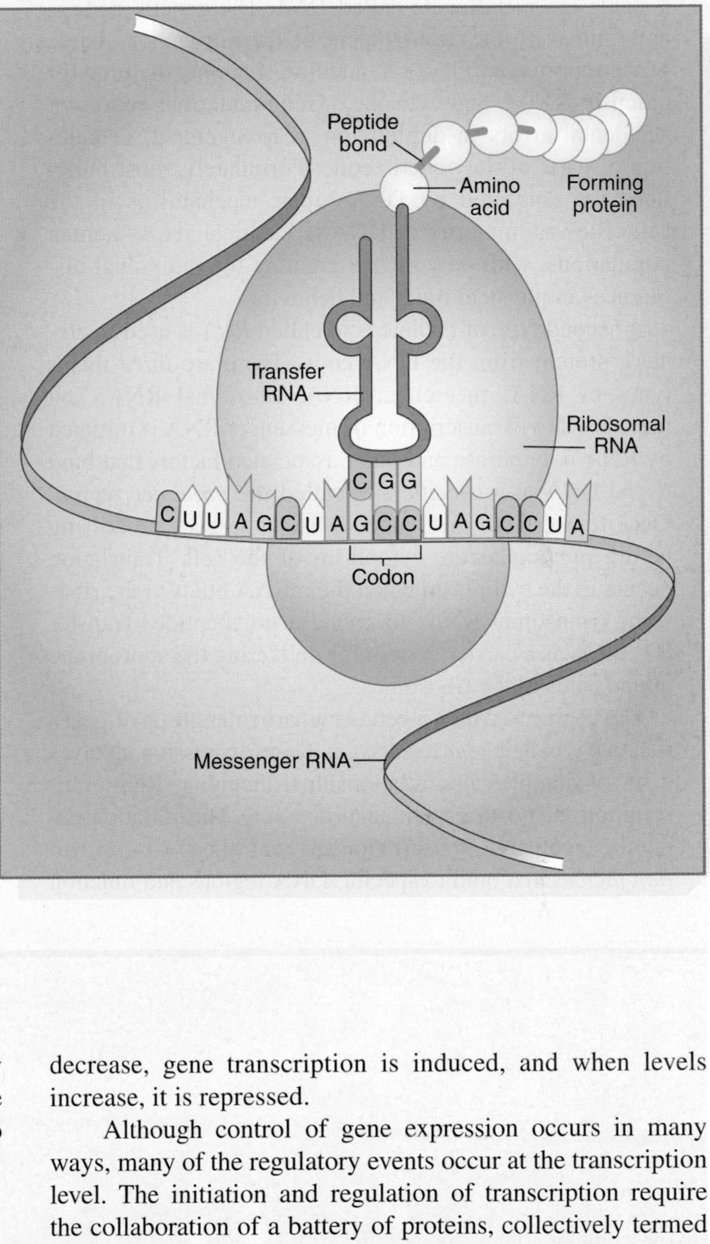

appropriate enzyme modification. Other modifications may involve cleavage of the protein, which can happen to remove a specific amino acid sequence or to split the molecule into smaller chains.

Regulation of Gene Expression

Only about 2% of the genome encodes instructions for synthesis of proteins; the remainder consists of noncoding regions that are structural or serve to determine where, when, and in what quantity proteins are made. The degree to which a gene or particular group of genes are actively being transcribed is called *gene expression*. A phenomenon termed *induction* is an important process by which gene expression is increased. *Gene repression* is a process by which a regulatory gene acts to reduce or prevent gene expression. Activator and repressor sites commonly monitor levels of the synthesized product and regulate gene transcription through a negative feedback mechanism. Whenever product levels decrease, gene transcription is induced, and when levels increase, it is repressed.

Although control of gene expression occurs in many ways, many of the regulatory events occur at the transcription level. The initiation and regulation of transcription require the collaboration of a battery of proteins, collectively termed *transcription factors*.[7] Transcription factors are a class of proteins that bind to their own specific DNA region and function to increase or decrease transcriptional activity of the genes. Transcription factors are one component that allows neurons and liver cells to use the same DNA yet still have completely different structures and functions. Some of these, referred to as *general transcription factors*, are required for transcription of all genes. Others, termed *specific transcription factors*, have more specialized roles, activating genes only at specific stages of development. For example, the PAX family of transcription factors is involved in the development of such embryonic tissues as the eye and portions of the nervous system.[8]

IN SUMMARY

Genes determine the types of proteins and enzymes made by the cell and therefore control both inheritance and day-to-day cell function. Genetic information is stored in a stable macromolecule called *DNA*. The genetic code is determined by the arrangement of the nitrogenous bases of the four nucleotides (*i.e.*, adenine, guanine, thymine [or uracil in RNA], and cytosine). Gene mutations represent accidental errors in duplication, rearrangement, or deletion of parts of the genetic code. Fortunately, most mutations are corrected by DNA repair mechanisms in the cell. The vast majority of DNA is identical across human populations, with only 0.01% creating the individual differences in physical traits and behavior.

A second type of nucleic acid called *RNA* is used to create a protein from the DNA code. There are three major types of RNA: messenger RNA, ribosomal RNA, and transfer RNA. Transcription of messenger RNA is initiated by RNA polymerase and other associated factors that bind to the DNA at a specific site called the *promoter region*. Once transcribed, messenger RNA undergoes processing before moving to the cytoplasm of the cell. Translation occurs in the cytoplasm when the mRNA binds to the ribosome (ribosomal RNA) to create a polypeptide. Transfer RNA acts as a carrier system for delivering the appropriate amino acids to the ribosomes.

The degree to which a gene or a particular group of genes is active is called *gene expression*. Gene expression involves a set of complex interrelationships, including RNA transcription and posttranslational processing. The initiation and regulation of RNA transcription are controlled by *transcription factors* that bind to specific DNA regions and function to regulate gene expression of the many different types of cells in the body. Posttranslational processing involves the proper folding of the newly synthesized polypeptide chain into its unique three-dimensional conformation. Special classes of proteins called *molecular chaperones* make the folding of many proteins more efficient. Posttranslational processing may also involve the combination of polypeptide chains from the same or an adjacent chromosome, the binding of small cofactors, or enzyme modification.

CHROMOSOMES

After completing this section of the chapter, the learner will be able to meet the following objectives:

- List the specific parts of the chromosome.
- Describe the processes of mitosis and meiosis.
- Explain what a karyotype might be used for.

Most of the genetic information in a cell is organized, stored, and retrieved in structures called *chromosomes*. Although the chromosomes are visible only in dividing cells, they retain their integrity between cell divisions. The chromosomes are arranged in pairs where one member of the pair is inherited from the father and the other member is inherited from the mother. Each species has a characteristic number of chromosomes. In the human, 46 chromosomes are present, and these are arranged into 23 pairs. Of the 23 pairs of human chromosomes, 22 are called *autosomes*, and each has been given a numeric designation for classification purposes (Fig. 4.6). The pairs of autosomal chromosomes each contain similar genes and have similar sequences and are therefore called *homologous chromosomes*. They are not identical, however, because one comes from the father and one comes from the mother.

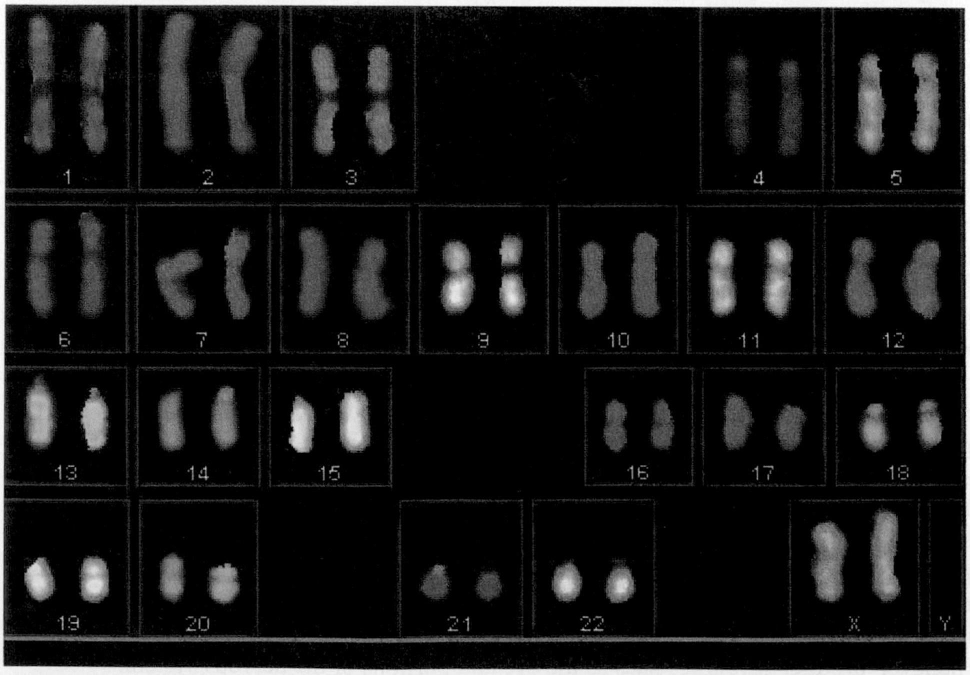

Figure 4.6 • Karyotype of human chromosomes. (From Rubin R., Strayer D. (Eds.) (2012). *Rubin's pathology: Clinicopathologic foundations of medicine* (6th ed., pp. 221). Philadelphia, PA: Lippincott Williams & Wilkins.)

The sex chromosomes, which make up the 23rd pair of chromosomes, determine the sex of a person. Human males have an X and Y chromosome (*i.e.*, an X chromosome from the mother and a Y chromosome from the father); human females have two X chromosomes (*i.e.*, one from each parent). The much smaller Y chromosome contains the *male-specific region* (MSY) that determines male sex.[9] But only one X chromosome in the female is active in controlling the expression of genetic traits. Whether the active X chromosome is derived from the mother or father is determined within a few days after conception. The selection of either X is random for each possible cell line. Thus, the tissues of normal women have on average 50% maternally derived and 50% paternally derived active X chromosomes. This is known as the *Lyon principle.*[10]

Cell Division

Two types of cell division occur in humans and many other animals: mitosis and meiosis. **Mitosis** involves the replication of DNA to duplicate somatic cells in the body and is represented by the cell cycle (Fig. 4.7). Each of the two resulting cells should have an identical set of 23 pairs of chromosomes. **Meiosis** is limited to replicating germ cells (Fig. 4.8). It results in the formation of gametes or reproductive cells (*i.e.*, ovum and sperm), each of which has only a single set of 23 chromosomes. Meiosis is typically divided into two distinct phases, meiosis I and meiosis II. As in mitosis, the first step of meiosis I is to replicate the DNA during interphase. During metaphase I, all homologous autosomal chromosomes pair up, forming a tetrad of *bivalents*. The X and Y chromosomes are not homologs and do not form bivalents. Because the bivalents are lined up, an interchange of chromatid segments can occur in metaphase I. This process is called *crossing-over* (Fig. 4.9). Crossing-over allows for new combinations of genes, increasing genetic variability. After telophase I, each of the two daughter cells contains one member of each homologous pair of chromosomes and a sex chromosome (23 double-stranded chromosomes). During anaphase of meiosis II, the 23 double-stranded chromosomes (two chromatids) divide at their centromeres. Each subsequent daughter cell will then receive 23 single-stranded chromatids.

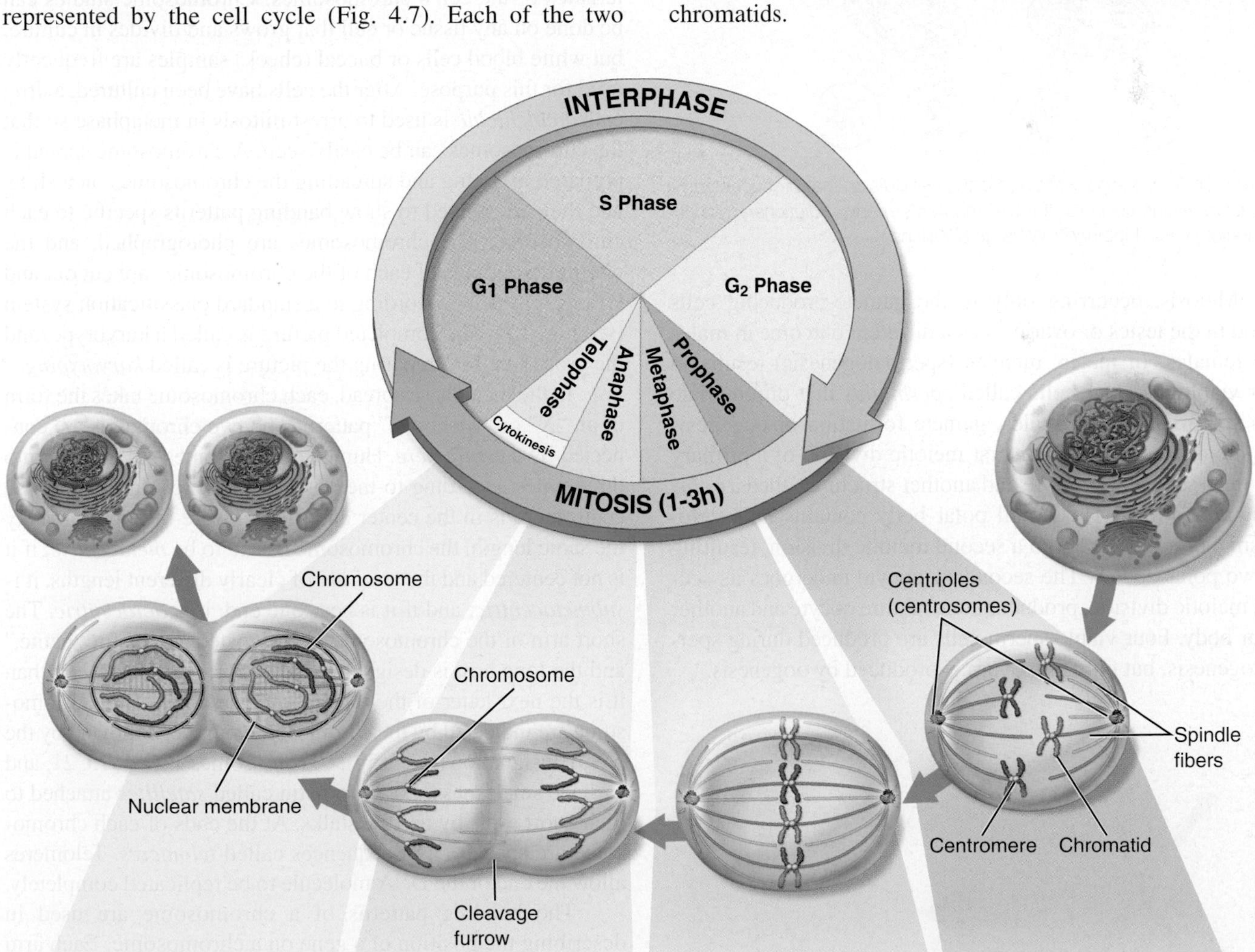

Figure 4.7 • Mitosis. Mitosis consists of division of the nucleus and is made up of four steps: telophase, anaphase, metaphase, and prophase. (From McConnell T. H., Hull K. L. (2011). *Human form human function: Essentials of anatomy & physiology* (pp. 79, Fig. 3.12). Philadelphia, PA: Lippincott Williams & Wilkins.)

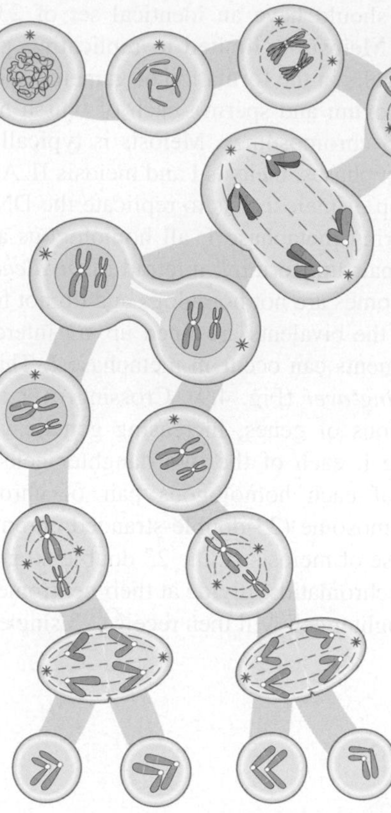

Figure 4.8 • Meiosis. Meiosis is the cell division that produces gametes or reproductive cells. (From *Stedman's medical dictionary* (2015). Philadelphia, PA: Lippincott Williams & Wilkins.)

Meiosis, occurring only in the gamete-producing cells found in the testes or ovaries, has a different outcome in males and females. In males, meiosis (spermatogenesis) results in four viable daughter cells called *spermatids* that differentiate into sperm cells. In females, gamete formation or oogenesis is quite different. After the first meiotic division of a primary oocyte, a secondary oocyte and another structure called a *polar body* are formed. This small polar body contains little cytoplasm, but it may undergo a second meiotic division, resulting in two polar bodies. The secondary oocyte undergoes its second meiotic division, producing one mature oocyte and another polar body. Four viable sperm cells are produced during spermatogenesis, but only one ovum is produced by oogenesis.

Figure 4.9 • Crossing-over of DNA at the time of meiosis.

KEY POINTS

CHROMOSOMES

- DNA is organized into 23 pairs of chromosomes. There are 22 pairs of autosomes, which are alike for males and females, and one pair of sex chromosomes, with XX pairing in females and XY pairing in males.
- Cell division requires the duplication of chromosomes. Duplication of chromosomes in a somatic cell line is completed by the process of mitosis, in which each daughter cell receives 23 pairs of chromosomes. Meiosis is limited to replicating germ cells and results in daughter cells that each have a single set of 23 chromosomes.

Chromosome Structure

Cytogenetics is the study of the structure and numeric characteristics of the cell's chromosomes. Chromosome studies can be done on any tissue or cell that grows and divides in culture, but white blood cells or buccal (cheek) samples are frequently used for this purpose. After the cells have been cultured, a drug called *colchicine* is used to arrest mitosis in metaphase so that the chromosomes can be easily seen. A chromosome spread is prepared by fixing and spreading the chromosomes on a slide, and they are stained to show banding patterns specific to each chromosome. The chromosomes are photographed, and the photomicrographs of each of the chromosomes are cut out and arranged in pairs according to a standard classification system (see Fig. 4.7). The completed picture is called a karyotype, and the procedure for preparing the picture is called *karyotyping*.

In the metaphase spread, each chromosome takes the form of an "X" or "wishbone" pattern. The two chromatids are connected by a *centromere*. Human chromosomes are divided into three types according to the position of the centromere. If the centromere is in the center and the arms are of approximately the same length, the chromosome is said to be *metacentric*; if it is not centered and the arms are of clearly different lengths, it is *submetacentric*; and if it is near one end, it is *acrocentric*. The short arm of the chromosome is designated as "p" for "petite," and the long arm is designated as "q" for no other reason than it is the next letter of the alphabet.[14] The arms of the chromosome are indicated by the chromosome number followed by the p or q designation (*e.g.*, 15p). Chromosomes 13, 14, 15, 21, and 22 have small masses of chromatin called *satellites* attached to their short arms by narrow stalks. At the ends of each chromosome are special DNA sequences called *telomeres*. Telomeres allow the end of the DNA molecule to be replicated completely.

The banding patterns of a chromosome are used in describing the position of a gene on a chromosome. Each arm of a chromosome is divided into regions, which are numbered from the centromere outward (*e.g.*, 1, 2). The regions are further divided into bands, which are also numbered (Fig. 4.10). These numbers are used in designating the position of a gene on a chromosome. For example, Xp22 refers to band 2, region 2 of the short arm (p) of the X chromosome.

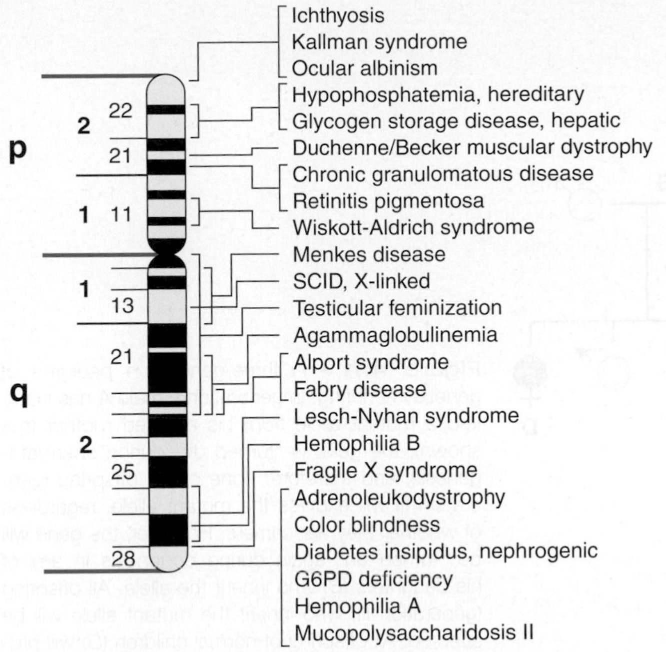

Figure 4.10 • Localization of representative inherited diseases on the X chromosome. G6PD, glucose-6-phosphate dehydrogenase; SCED, severe combined immunodeficiency (syndrome). (From Rubin R., Strayer D. (Eds.) (2015). *Rubin's pathology: Clinicopathologic foundations of medicine* (7th ed., Fig. 6.32, pp. 282). Philadelphia, PA: Lippincott Williams & Wilkins.)

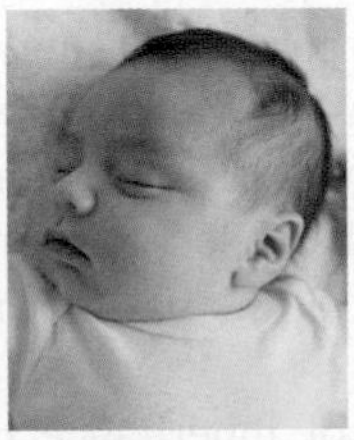

Recall from the unit-opening case study that Jennifer's karyotype revealed an additional chromosome 21. This additional chromosome resulted from an act of nondisjunction. This event has been found to occur more frequently as a woman ages. Therefore, women 35 years of age and older are particularly encouraged to undergo prenatal screening, as will be described in Chapter 5.

IN SUMMARY

The genetic information in a cell is organized in structures called *chromosomes*. In humans, the 46 chromosomes are arranged into 23 pairs. Twenty-two of these pairs are autosomes. The 23rd pair are the sex chromosomes. Two types of cell division occur, meiosis and mitosis. Mitotic division occurs in somatic cells and results in two daughter cells, each with 23 pairs of chromosomes. Meiosis is limited to replicating germ cells and results in the formation of gametes or reproductive cells (ovum and sperm), each of which has only a single set of 23 chromosomes. A karyotype is a photographic arrangement of a person's chromosomes. It is prepared by special laboratory techniques in which cells are cultured, fixed, and stained to display identifiable banding patterns.

PATTERNS OF INHERITANCE

After completing this section of the chapter, the learner will be able to meet the following objectives:

- Contrast genotype and phenotype.
- Define the terms *allele, locus, homozygote, and heterozygote*.
- Explain why an individual might be a "carrier" of a particular trait.

The characteristics inherited from a person's parents are carried within genes found along the length of the chromosomes. Alternate forms of the same gene are possible, and each may produce a different aspect of a trait.

Definitions

Genetics has its own set of definitions. The genotype of a person is the genetic information stored in the sequence of base pairs. The phenotype refers to the recognizable traits, physical or biochemical, that are associated with a specific genotype. But more than one genotype may have the same phenotype. Some brown-eyed people are carriers of the code for blue eyes, and other brown-eyed people are not. Phenotypically, these two types of brown-eyed people appear the same, but genotypically they are different.

The position of a gene on a chromosome is called its *locus*, and alternate forms of a gene at the same locus are called *alleles*. When only one pair of genes is involved in the transmission of information, the term *single-gene trait* is used. Single-gene traits follow the mendelian laws of inheritance.

Polygenic inheritance involves multiple genes at different loci, with each gene exerting a small effect in determining a trait. Multiple pairs of genes, many with alternate codes, determine most human traits. Polygenic traits are predictable, but with less reliability than single-gene traits. *Multifactorial* inheritance is similar to polygenic inheritance in that multiple alleles at different loci affect the outcome; the difference is that multifactorial inheritance also includes environmental effects on the genes.

Many other gene–gene interactions are known. These include *epistasis*, in which one gene masks the phenotypic effects of another gene; *multiple alleles*, in which more than one allele affects the same trait (*e.g.*, ABO blood types); *complementary genes*, in which each gene is mutually dependent on the other; and *collaborative genes*, in which two different genes influencing the same trait interact to produce a phenotype neither gene alone could produce.

Genetic Imprinting

Certain genes exhibit a "parent of origin" type of transmission in which the parental genomes do not always contribute equally in the development of a person (Fig. 4.11). The transmission of this phenomenon is called *genetic imprinting*.

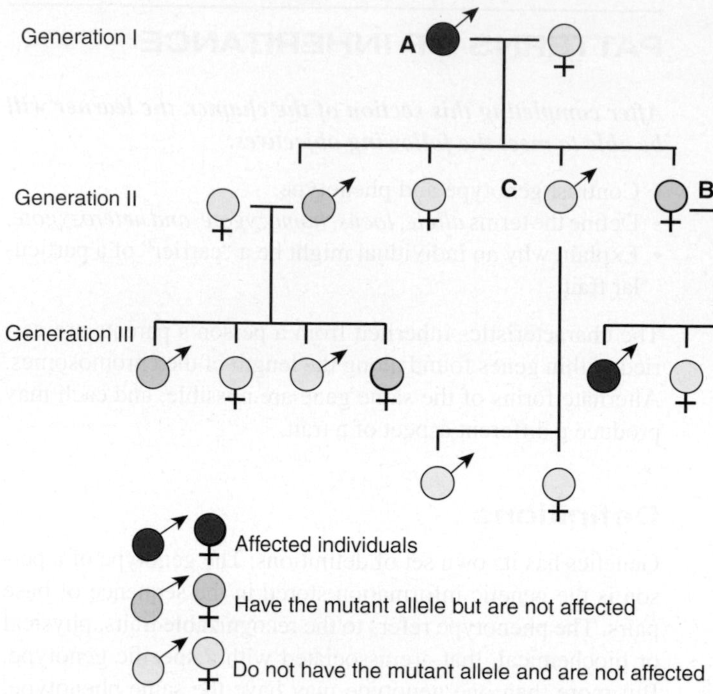

Figure 4.11 • A three-generation pedigree of genetic imprinting. In generation I, male *A* has inherited a mutant allele from his affected mother (not shown); the gene is "turned off" during spermatogenesis, and therefore, none of his offspring (generation II) will express the mutant allele, regardless of whether they are carriers. However, the gene will be "turned on" again during oogenesis in any of his daughters (*B*) who inherit the allele. All offspring (generation III) who inherit the mutant allele will be affected. All offspring of normal children (*C*) will produce normal offspring. Children of female *D* will all express the mutation if they inherit the allele.

Although rare, it is estimated that approximately 100 genes exhibit genetic imprinting.

Well-known examples of genomic imprinting are the transmission of the mutations in Prader-Willi and Angelman syndromes.[11] Both syndromes exhibit mental retardation as a common feature. It was also found that both disorders had the same deletion in chromosome 15. When the deletion is inherited from the mother, the infant presents with Angelman ("happy puppet") syndrome. When the same deletion is inherited from the father, Prader-Willi syndrome results.

A related chromosomal disorder is *uniparental disomy*. This occurs when two chromosomes of the same number are inherited from one parent. Normally, this is not a problem except in cases where a chromosome has been imprinted by a parent. In this case, the offspring will have only one working copy of the chromosome, resulting in possible problems.

KEY POINTS

TRANSMISSION OF GENETIC INFORMATION

- The transmission of information from one generation to the next is vested in genetic material transferred from each parent at the time of conception.
- Mendelian, or single-gene, patterns of inheritance are transmitted from parents to their offspring in a predictable manner. Polygenic inheritance, which involves multiple genes, and multifactorial inheritance, which involves multiple genes as well as environmental factors, are less predictable.

Mendel Laws

A main feature of inheritance is predictability: given certain conditions, the likelihood of the occurrence or recurrence of a specific trait in the offspring is remarkably predictable. The units of inheritance are the genes, and the pattern of single-gene transmission can often be predicted using Mendel laws of genetic transmission. Since Gregor Mendel original work was published in 1865, new discoveries have led to some modification of the original laws, but many of the basic principles still hold true.

Mendel discovered the basic pattern of inheritance by conducting carefully planned experiments with simple garden peas. Experimenting with several phenotypic traits in peas, Mendel proposed that inherited traits are transmitted from parents to offspring by means of independently inherited factors—now known as genes—and that these factors are transmitted as recessive and dominant traits. Mendel labeled dominant factors (his round peas) "A" and recessive factors (his wrinkled peas) "a." Geneticists continue to use capital letters to designate dominant traits and lowercase letters to identify recessive traits. The possible combinations that can occur with transmission of single-gene dominant and recessive traits can be described by constructing a figure called a *Punnett square* using capital and lowercase letters (Fig. 4.12).

The observable traits of single-gene inheritance are inherited by the offspring from the parents. The germ cells (*i.e.*, sperm and ovum) of both parents undergo meiosis, in which the number of chromosomes is divided in half (from 46 to 23) and each germ cell receives only one allele from each pair (*i.e.*, Mendel first law). According to Mendel second law, the alleles from the different gene loci segregate independently and recombine randomly in the offspring.

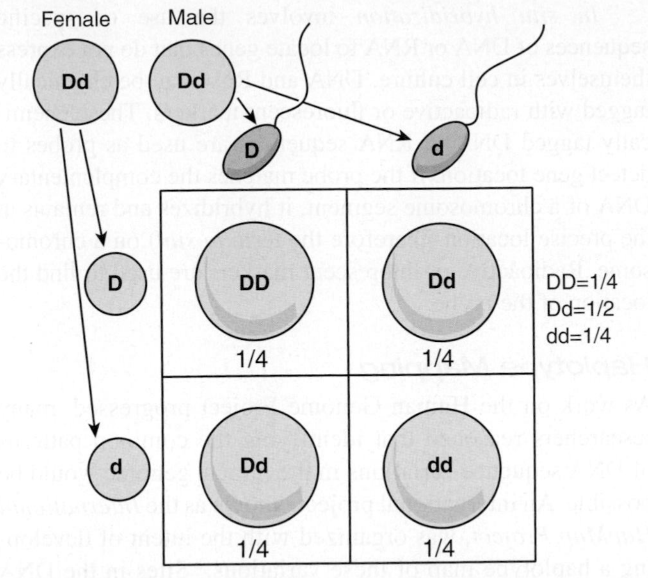

Figure 4.12 • The Punnett square showing all possible combinations for transmission of a single-gene trait (dimpled cheeks). The example shown is when both parents are heterozygous (Dd) for the trait. The alleles carried by the mother are on the left, and those carried by the father are on the top. The D allele is dominant, and the d allele is recessive. The DD and Dd offspring have dimples, and the dd offspring does not.

People in whom the two alleles of a given pair are the same (AA or aa) are called *homozygotes*. *Heterozygotes* have different alleles (Aa) at a gene locus. A *recessive trait* is one expressed only in a homozygous (aa) pairing; a *dominant trait* is one expressed in either a homozygous (AA) or a heterozygous (Aa) pairing. If the trait follows simple Mendelian inheritance, then all people with a dominant allele in either one or two copies will show the phenotype for that trait. For example, the genes for blond hair are recessive and those for brown hair are dominant. Therefore, only people with a genotype having two alleles for blond hair would be blond; people with either one or two brown alleles would have brown hair.

Sometimes, the person that is heterozygous for a recessive trait (Aa) is called a *carrier*. That individual will not exhibit the phenotype for the recessive trait, but they "carry" the allele for the recessive trait. If they have offspring with someone that exhibits and is homozygous for the recessive trait, or with someone who is also a carrier, then that offspring could also exhibit the recessive trait. Such a situation might occur when two people that have a phenotype of brown eyes have a child with blue eyes. Brown (B) eyes are dominant to blue eyes (b), so both parents had to be genotypically heterozygous (Bb).

Pedigree

A pedigree is a graphic method (see Figs. 4.11 and 4.12) for portraying a family history for an inherited trait. It is constructed from a carefully obtained family history and is useful for tracing the pattern of inheritance for a particular trait.

IN SUMMARY

Inheritance patterns can calculate the likelihood of the occurrence or recurrence of a specific genetic trait. The genotype refers to information stored in the genetic code of a person, whereas the phenotype represents the recognizable traits, physical and biochemical, associated with the genotype. The specific region of the DNA molecule where a particular gene is located is called a *gene locus*. Alternate forms of a gene are called *alleles*. Traits can be either recessive or dominant. A recessive trait is one expressed only when two copies (homozygous) of the recessive allele are present. Dominant traits are expressed when either one (heterozygous) or two (homozygous) copies of the dominant allele is present. A pedigree is a graphic method for portraying a family history of an inherited trait.

GENE TECHNOLOGY

After completing this section of the chapter, the learner will be able to meet the following objectives:

- Briefly describe the methods used in linkage and hybridization studies.
- Describe the process of recombinant DNA technology.
- Characterize the process of RNA interference.

The past several decades have seen phenomenal advances in the field of genetics. These advances have included the completion of the Human Genome Project, the establishment of the International HapMap Project to map the haplotypes of variations in the human genome, and the development of methods for applying the technology of these projects to the diagnosis and treatment of disease. Many health care professions also have established clinical competencies for their specific professions regarding genetics, because the application of genetic technology is becoming more evident in all areas of disease screening and management. There are multiple new genetic diagnostics being used that are able to assess people for various genetic alterations. Information obtained from these technologies greatly assists in planning the care and pharmacologic management of many types of diseases. Health care professionals need to be able to answer questions and explain to people and families the results of testing and how this knowledge may or may not influence the course of one's health.

Genetic Mapping

Genetic mapping is the assignment of genes to a specific locus or to specific parts of the chromosome. Another type of mapping strategy, the *haplotype* map, focuses on identifying the slight variations in the human genome that affect a person's susceptibility to disease and responses to environmental factors such as microbes, toxins, and drugs.

The Human Genome Project

The Human Genome Project, initiated in 1990 and completed in 2003, sought to identify all the genes in the human genome. The international project was charged with both determining the precise locations of genes and also exploring technologies that would enable the sequencing of large amounts of DNA with high accuracy and low cost. Some of what was discovered was quite unexpected, including the revelation that humans have a mere 30,000 genes, rather than the 100,000 that were initially predicted from the number of different proteins in our body. Another surprising finding was mentioned earlier in this chapter. On average, any two unrelated people will still share 99.9% of their DNA sequence, indicating that the remarkable diversity among people is carried in about 0.1% of our DNA.

Genetic Mapping Methods

Many methods have been used for developing genetic maps. The most important ones are family linkage studies, gene dosage methods, and hybridization studies. Often, the specific assignment of a gene locus is made using information from several mapping techniques.

Linkage Studies. Linkage studies assume that genes occur in a linear array along the chromosomes. During meiosis, the paired chromosomes of the germ cells sometimes exchange genetic material because of crossing-over (see Fig. 4.8). This exchange usually involves more than one gene; large blocks of genes (representing large portions of the chromosome) are usually exchanged. Although the point at which one block separates from another occurs randomly, the closer together two genes are on the same chromosome, the greater the chance is that they will be passed on together to the offspring. When two inherited traits occur together at a rate greater than would occur by chance alone, they are said to be *linked*. Linkage analysis can be used clinically to identify affected people in a family with a known genetic defect.

Hybridization Studies. A recent biologic discovery revealed that two somatic cells from different species, when grown together in the same culture, occasionally fuse to form a new hybrid cell. Two types of hybridization methods are used in genomic studies: somatic cell hybridization and in situ hybridization.

Somatic cell hybridization involves the fusion of human somatic cells with those of a different species (typically, the mouse) to yield a cell containing the chromosomes of both species. Because these hybrid cells are unstable, they begin to lose chromosomes of both species during subsequent cell divisions. This makes it possible to obtain cells with different partial combinations of human chromosomes. The proteins of these cells are then studied with the understanding that for a protein to be produced, a certain chromosome must be present and, therefore, the coding for that protein must be located on that chromosome.

In situ hybridization involves the use of specific sequences of DNA or RNA to locate genes that do not express themselves in cell culture. DNA and RNA can be chemically tagged with radioactive or fluorescent markers. These chemically tagged DNA or RNA sequences are used as probes to detect gene location. If the probe matches the complementary DNA of a chromosome segment, it hybridizes and remains at the precise location (therefore the term *in situ*) on a chromosome. Radioactive or fluorescent markers are used to find the location of the probe.

Haplotype Mapping

As work on the Human Genome Project progressed, many researchers reasoned that identifying the common patterns of DNA sequence variations in the human genome would be possible. An international project, known as the *International HapMap Project*, was organized with the intent of developing a haplotype map of these variations.[4] Sites in the DNA sequence where people differ at a single DNA base are called *single nucleotide polymorphisms* (SNPs, pronounced "snips"). A haplotype consists of the many closely linked SNPs on a single chromosome that generally are passed as a block from one generation to another in a particular population. One of the motivating factors behind the HapMap Project was the realization that the identification of a few SNPs was enough to uniquely identify the haplotypes in a block. The specific SNPs that identify the haplotypes are called *tagging SNPs*. This approach reduces the number of SNPs required to examine an entire genome and makes genome scanning methods much more efficient in finding regions with genes that contribute to disease development. Much attention has focused on the use of SNPs indicating disease susceptibility in one population versus another, as well as determining appropriate medications and therapies based upon genotype.

Recombinant DNA Technology

The term *recombinant DNA* refers to a combination of DNA molecules that are not found together in nature. Recombinant DNA technology makes it possible to identify the DNA sequence in a gene and produce the protein product encoded by a gene. The specific nucleotide sequence of a DNA fragment can often be identified by analyzing the amino acid sequence and mRNA codon of its protein product. Short sequences of base pairs can be synthesized, radioactively labeled, and subsequently used to identify their complementary sequence. In this way, identifying both normal and abnormal gene structures is possible.

Gene Isolation and Cloning

The gene isolation and cloning methods used in recombinant DNA technology rely on the fact that the genes of all organisms, from bacteria through mammals, are based on a similar molecular organization. *Gene cloning* requires cutting a DNA molecule apart, modifying and reassembling its fragments, and producing copies of the modified DNA, its mRNA, and its gene product. The DNA molecule is cut apart by using a bacterial enzyme, called a *restriction enzyme*, that binds to DNA wherever a particular short sequence of base pairs is found and cleaves the molecule at a specific nucleotide site. In this way, a long DNA molecule can be broken down into smaller, discrete fragments, one of which contains the gene of interest. Many restriction enzymes are commercially available that cut DNA at different recognition sites.

The fragments of DNA can then often be replicated through insertion into a unicellular organism, such as a bacterium. To do this, a cloning vector such as a bacterial virus or a small DNA circle that is found in most bacteria, called a *plasmid*, is used. Viral and plasmid vectors replicate autonomously in the host bacterial cell. During gene cloning, a bacterial vector and the DNA fragment are mixed and joined by a special enzyme called a *DNA ligase*. The recombinant vectors formed are then introduced into a suitable culture of bacteria, and the bacteria are allowed to replicate and express the recombinant vector gene.

Pharmaceutical Applications

The methods of recombinant DNA technology can also be used in the treatment of disease. For example, recombinant DNA technology is used in the manufacture of human insulin that is used to treat diabetes mellitus. Recombinant DNA corresponding to the A chain of human insulin was isolated and inserted into plasmids that were in turn used to transform *Escherichia coli*. The bacteria then synthesized the insulin chain. A similar method was used to obtain the B chains. The A and B chains were then mixed and allowed to fold and form disulfide bonds, producing active insulin molecules. Human growth hormone has also been produced in *E. coli*. More complex proteins are produced in mammalian cell culture using recombinant DNA techniques. These include erythropoietin, which is used to stimulate red blood cell production; factor VIII, which is used to treat hemophilia; and tissue plasminogen activator (tPA), which is frequently administered after a heart attack to dissolve thrombi.

DNA Fingerprinting

The technique of DNA fingerprinting also uses recombinant DNA technology, as well as basic principles of medical genetics.[12] Using restriction enzymes, DNA is first cleaved at specific regions (Fig. 4.13). The DNA fragments are separated according to size by electrophoresis and denatured (by heating or treating chemically) so that all the DNA is single stranded. The single-stranded DNA is then transferred to nitrocellulose paper, baked to attach the DNA to the paper, and treated with series of radioactive probes. After the radioactive probes have been allowed to bond with the denatured DNA, radiography is used to reveal the labeled DNA fragments.

When used in forensic pathology, this procedure is applied to specimens from the suspect and the forensic specimen. This can be done with even very small samples of DNA

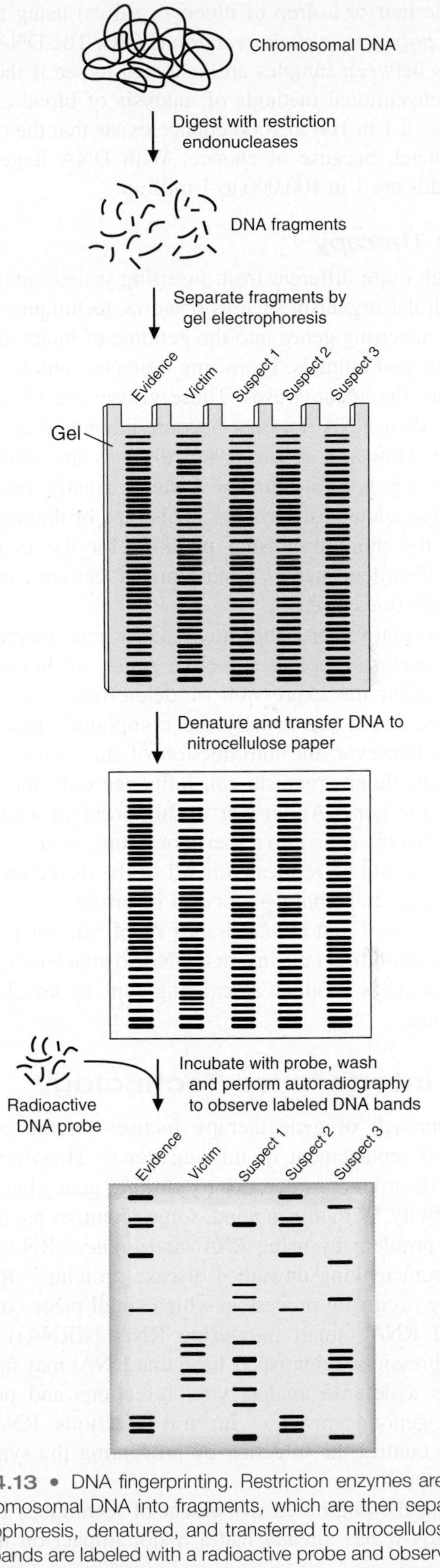

Figure 4.13 • DNA fingerprinting. Restriction enzymes are used to break chromosomal DNA into fragments, which are then separated by gel electrophoresis, denatured, and transferred to nitrocellulose paper; the DNA bands are labeled with a radioactive probe and observed using autoradiography. (Modified from Smith C., Marks A. D., Lieberman M. (2005). *Marks' basic medical biochemistry* (2nd ed., pp. 309). Philadelphia, PA: Lippincott Williams & Wilkins.)

(a single hair or a drop of blood or saliva) using amplification by *polymerase chain reaction* (PCR). The DNA banding patterns between samples are analyzed to see if they match. With conventional methods of analysis of blood and serum enzymes, a 1 in 100 to 1000 chance exists that the two specimens match because of chance. With DNA fingerprinting, these odds are 1 in 100,000 to 1 million.

Gene Therapy

Although quite different from inserting genetic material into a unicellular organism such as bacteria, techniques are available for inserting genes into the genome of intact multicellular plants and animals. Promising delivery vehicles for these genes are the adenoviruses. These viruses are ideal vehicles because their DNA does not become integrated into the host genome. However, repeated inoculations are often needed because the body's immune system usually targets cells expressing adenovirus proteins. This type of therapy remains one of the more promising methods for the treatment of genetic disorders such as cystic fibrosis, certain cancers, and many infectious diseases.

Two main approaches are used in gene therapy: transferred genes can replace defective genes, or they can selectively inhibit the expression of deleterious genes. Cloned DNA sequences are usually the compounds used in gene therapy. However, the introduction of the cloned gene into the multicellular organism can influence only the few cells that get the gene. An answer to this problem would be the insertion of the gene into a sperm or ovum; after fertilization, the gene would be replicated in all of the differentiating cell types. Even so, techniques for cell insertion are limited. Not only are moral and ethical issues involved, but these techniques cannot direct the inserted DNA to attach to a particular chromosome or supplant an existing gene by knocking it out of its place.

RNA Interference Technology

One approach of gene therapy focuses on the previously described replacement of missing genes. However, several genetic disorders are due not to missing genes but to faulty gene activity. With this in mind, some scientists are approaching the problem by using *RNA interference* (RNAi) to stop genes from making unwanted disease proteins.[13] RNAi is a naturally occurring process in which small pieces of double-stranded RNA (small interfering RNA [siRNA]) suppress gene expression. Scientists believe that RNAi may have originated as a defense against viral infections and potentially harmful genomic invaders. In viral infections, RNAi would serve to control the infection by preventing the synthesis of viral proteins.

With the continued refinement of techniques to silence genes, RNAi has already had a major impact on molecular biology. For example, it has given scientists the ability to practice reverse genomics, in which a gene's function can be inferred through silencing its expression. Increasingly, pharmaceutical companies are using RNAi to identify disease-related drug targets. There also is considerable interest in harnessing RNAi for therapeutic purposes, including the treatment of human immunodeficiency virus (HIV) infection and hepatitis C. Before this can occur, however, the therapeutic methods must be shown to be safe and effective, and obstacles to delivering the RNAi into targeted cells must be overcome. It is difficult for RNA to cross the cell membrane, and enzymes in the blood quickly break it down.

IN SUMMARY

Genomic mapping is a method used to assign genes to particular chromosomes or parts of a chromosome. Linkage studies assign a chromosome location to genes based on their close association with other genes of known location or their tendency to be inherited together. A haplotype consists of the many closely linked SNPs on a single chromosome that generally are passed as a block from one generation to another in a particular population. The International HapMap Project has been developed to map the SNPs on the human genome with the anticipation that it may be useful in the prediction and management of disease.

Genetic engineering has provided the methods for manipulating nucleic acids and recombining genes (recombinant DNA) into hybrid molecules that can be inserted into unicellular organisms and reproduced many times over. As a result, proteins that formerly were available only in small amounts can now be made in large quantities once their respective genes have been isolated. DNA fingerprinting, which relies on recombinant DNA technologies and those of genetic mapping, is often used in forensic investigations. A newer strategy for management of genetic disorders focuses on gene silencing by using RNAi to stop genes from making unwanted disease proteins.

GERIATRIC Considerations

- Genetic influences on aging are evident by a substantially longer life (up to 65%) when single-gene mutations occur in specific signaling pathways.[14]
- The shortening or erosion of telomeres contributes to organismal aging.[14]

PEDIATRIC Considerations

- 1 of 150 live births have a chromosomal anomaly causing cognitive impairment and birth defects. Chromosomal abnormalities are even more prevalent among still births and spontaneous abortions.
- Inborn errors of metabolism, caused by gene mutations, may be lethal if not treated, thus prompting many states to require mandatory newborn screening.[15]
- Creation of a family pedigree helps families to identify genetic disorders and is useful when going for genetic counseling.[15]

REVIEW EXERCISES

1. The Human Genome Project has revealed that humans have only 30,000 to 35,000 genes. Only about 2% of the genome encodes instructions for protein synthesis, whereas 50% consists of repeat sequences that do not code proteins.
   A. *Use this information to explain how this small number of protein-encoding genes is able to produce the vast array of proteins needed for organ and structural development in the embryo, as well as those needed for normal function of the body in postnatal life.*
2. A child about to undergo surgery is typed for possible blood transfusions. His parents are told that he is type O positive. Both his mother and father are type A positive.
   A. *How would you explain this variation in blood type to the parents?*
3. More than 100,000 people die of adverse drug reactions each year; another 2.2 million experience serious reactions, whereas others fail to respond at all to the therapeutic actions of drugs.
   A. *Explain how the use of information about single nucleotide polymorphisms (SNPs) might be used to map individual variations in drug responses.*
4. Human insulin, prepared by recombinant DNA technology, is used for the treatment of diabetes mellitus.
   A. *Explain the techniques used for the production of a human hormone with this technology.*

References

1. Meselson M., Stahl F. W. (1958). The replication of DNA in Escherichia coli. *Proceedings of the National Academy of Sciences of the United States of America* 44(7), 671–682.
2. Biterge B., Schneider R. (2014). Histone variants: Key players of chromatin. *Cell and Tissue Research* 356(3), 457–466. doi:10.1007/s00441-014-1862-4.
3. Clapier C. R., Iwasa J., Cairns B. R., et al. (2017). Mechanisms of action and regulation of ATP-dependent chromatin-remodelling complexes. *Nature Reviews Molecular Cell Biology* 18(7), 407–422. doi:10.1038/nrm.2017.26.
4. International HapMap C. (2003). The International HapMap Project. *Nature* 426(6968), 789–796. doi:10.1038/nature02168.
5. Brown A., Shao S., Murray J., et al. (2015). Structural basis for stop codon recognition in eukaryotes. *Nature* 524(7566), 493–496. doi:10.1038/nature14896.
6. Brandvold K. R., Morimoto R. I. (2015). The chemical biology of molecular chaperones—Implications for modulation of proteostasis. *Journal of Molecular Biology* 427(18), 2931–2947. doi:10.1016/j.jmb.2015.05.010.
7. Spitz F., Furlong E. E. (2012). Transcription factors: From enhancer binding to developmental control. *Nature Reviews Genetics* 13(9), 613–626. doi:10.1038/nrg3207.
8. Blake J. A., Ziman M. R. (2014). Pax genes: Regulators of lineage specification and progenitor cell maintenance. *Development* 141(4), 737–751. doi:10.1242/dev.091785.
9. Hughes J. F., Rozen S. (2012). Genomics and genetics of human and primate y chromosomes. *Annual Review of Genomics and Human Genetics* 13, 83–108. doi:10.1146/annurev-genom-090711-163855.
10. Rubin R., Strayer D. (Eds.) (2012). *Rubin's pathology: Clinicopathologic foundations of medicine*. Philadelphia, PA: Lippincott Williams & Wilkins.
11. Kalsner L., Chamberlain S. J. (2015). Prader-Willi, Angelman, and 15q11-q13 duplication syndromes. *Pediatric Clinics of North America* 62(3), 587–606. doi:10.1016/j.pcl.2015.03.004.
12. Thompson R., Zoppis S., McCord B. (2012). An overview of DNA typing methods for human identification: Past, present, and future. *Methods in Molecular Biology* 830, 3–16. doi:10.1007/978-1-61779-461-2_1.
13. Fischer S. E. (2015). RNA interference and microRNA-mediated silencing. *Current Protocols in Molecular Biology* 112(26), 1–5. doi:10.1002/0471142727.mb2601s112.
14. Strayer D. S., Rubin E. (2015). *Rubin's pathology clinicopathologic foundations of medicine* (7th ed.). Philadelphia, PA: Wolter Kluwers.
15. Kyle T., Carman S. (2017). Nursing care of the child with an alteration in genetics. In *Essentials of pediatric nursing* (3rd ed.). Philadelphia, PA: Wolter Kluwers.

Genetic and Congenital Disorders

5

Ansley Grimes Stanfill, PhD, RN

GENETIC AND CHROMOSOMAL DISORDERS
- Single-Gene Disorders
  - *Autosomal Dominant Disorders*
  - *Autosomal Recessive Disorders*
  - *X-Linked Recessive Disorders*
  - *X-Linked Dominant Disorders*
  - *Fragile X Syndrome*
- Inherited Multifactorial Disorders
  - *Cleft Lip and Cleft Palate*
- Chromosomal Disorders
  - *Structural Chromosomal Abnormalities*
  - *Numeric Disorders Involving Autosomes*
  - *Numeric Disorders Involving Sex Chromosomes*
- Mitochondrial Gene Disorders

DISORDERS DUE TO ENVIRONMENTAL INFLUENCES
- Period of Vulnerability
- Teratogenic Agents
  - *Radiation*
  - *Chemicals and Drugs*
  - *Infectious Agents*
- Folic Acid Deficiency

DIAGNOSIS AND COUNSELING
- Genetic Assessment
- Prenatal Screening and Diagnosis
  - *Ultrasonography*
  - *Maternal Serum Markers*
  - *Amniocentesis*
  - *Chorionic Villus Sampling*
  - *Percutaneous Umbilical Cord Blood Sampling*
  - *Cytogenetic and DNA Analyses*

Congenital defects, sometimes called birth defects, are abnormalities of a body structure, function, or metabolism that are present at birth. They affect more than 185,000 infants discharged from the hospital in the United States each year and are the leading cause of infant death.[1] Congenital defects may be caused by genetic factors (*i.e.*, single-gene or multifactorial inheritance or chromosomal aberrations) or environmental factors that are active during embryonic or fetal development (*e.g.*, maternal disease, infections, or drugs taken during pregnancy). Although congenital defects caused by genetic factors are present at birth, they may not make their appearance until later in life. This chapter provides an overview of genetic and congenital disorders and is divided into three parts:

1. Genetic and chromosomal disorders
2. Disorders due to environmental agents
3. Diagnosis and counseling

GENETIC AND CHROMOSOMAL DISORDERS

After completing this section of the chapter, the learner will be able to meet the following objectives:

- Describe three types of single-gene disorders and their patterns of inheritance.
- Contrast disorders due to multifactorial inheritance with those caused by single-gene inheritance.

Most genetic disorders are caused by changes in the deoxyribonucleic acid (DNA) sequence that alters the synthesis of a single gene product. Other genetic disorders are a result of chromosomal aberrations such as deletion or duplication errors, or are due to an abnormal number of chromosomes.

The genes on each chromosome are arranged in strict order, with each gene occupying a specific location or *locus*. The two members of a gene pair, one inherited from the mother and the other from the father, are called *alleles*. If the members of a gene pair are identical (*i.e.*, code the exact same gene product), the person is homozygous, and if the two members are different, the person is heterozygous. The genetic composition of a person is called a genotype, whereas the phenotype is the observable expression of a genotype in terms of physical or biochemical traits. If the trait is phenotypically seen in the heterozygote, the allele is said to be *dominant*. If it is phenotypically seen only in the homozygote, the allele is *recessive*. Many genes have more than one normal allele (alternate forms) at the same locus. This is called a *polymorphism*. Although most traits follow a dominant or recessive pattern, it is possible for both alleles of a gene pair to be phenotypically seen in the heterozygote, a condition called *codominance*. Blood group inheritance (*e.g.*, AO, BO, AB) is an example of both codominance and polymorphism.

A gene *mutation* is a biochemical event such as nucleotide change, deletion, or insertion that produces a new allele for a particular gene. A single mutant gene may be expressed in many different parts of the body. Marfan syndrome, for example, is a single gene defect in a connective tissue protein that has widespread effects involving skeletal, eye, and cardiovascular structures. The disorder may be inherited as a family trait or arise as a sporadic case because of a new mutation.

Single-Gene Disorders

Single-gene disorders are caused by a defective or mutant allele at a single gene locus and follow Mendelian patterns of inheritance. Single-gene disorders are characterized by their patterns of transmission, which usually are obtained through a family genetic history. The patterns of inheritance depend on whether the phenotype is dominant or recessive and whether the gene of concern is located on an autosomal or sex chromosome. In addition to disorders caused by mutations of genes located on the chromosomes located within the nucleus, another (but more rare) class of disorders involves the mitochondrial genome and shows a maternal pattern of inheritance.

Virtually all single-gene disorders lead to formation of an abnormal protein or the decreased production of a gene product. These changes can result in many different types of systemic alterations. Table 5.1 lists some of the common single-gene disorders and their manifestations.

Autosomal Dominant Disorders

In autosomal dominant disorders, a single mutant allele from an affected parent is transmitted to an offspring regardless of sex. The affected parent has a 50% chance of transmitting the

TABLE 5.1 SOME DISORDERS OF MENDELIAN OR SINGLE-GENE INHERITANCE AND THEIR SIGNIFICANCE

DISORDER	SIGNIFICANCE
Autosomal Dominant	
Achondroplasia	Short-limb dwarfism
Adult polycystic kidney disease	Chronic kidney disease
Huntington chorea	Neurodegenerative disorder
Familial hypercholesterolemia	Premature atherosclerosis
Marfan syndrome	Connective tissue disorder with abnormalities in the skeletal, ocular, cardiovascular systems
Neurofibromatosis (NF)	Neurogenic tumors: fibromatous skin tumors, pigmented skin lesions, and ocular nodules in NF-1; bilateral acoustic neuromas in NF-2
Osteogenesis imperfecta	Brittle bone disease due to defects in collagen synthesis
Spherocytosis	Disorder of red blood cells
von Willebrand disease	Bleeding disorder
Autosomal Recessive	
Cystic fibrosis	Disorder of membrane transport of chloride ions in exocrine glands causing lung and pancreatic disease
Glycogen storage diseases	Excess accumulation of glycogen in the liver and hypoglycemia (von Gierke disease); glycogen accumulation in striated muscle in myopathic forms
Oculocutaneous albinism	Hypopigmentation of skin, hair, eyes as a result of inability to synthesize melanin
Phenylketonuria (PKU)	Lack of phenylalanine hydroxylase with hyperphenylalaninemia and impaired brain development
Sickle cell disease	Red blood cell defect
Tay-Sachs disease	Deficiency of hexosaminidase A; severe mental and physical deterioration beginning in infancy
X-Linked Recessive	
Bruton-type hypogammaglobulinemia	Immunodeficiency
Hemophilia A	Bleeding disorder
Duchenne dystrophy	Muscular dystrophy
Fragile X syndrome	Intellectual disability

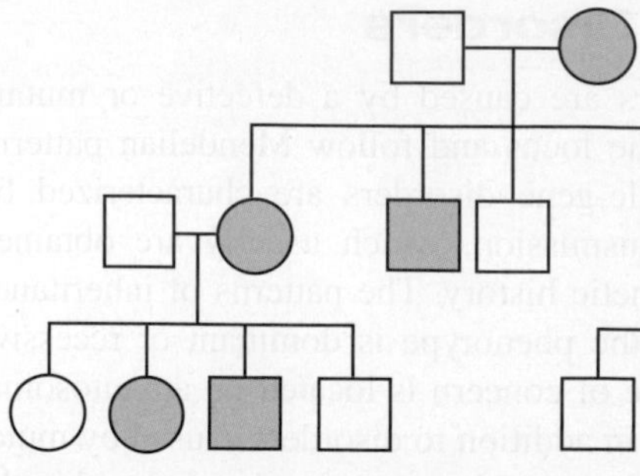

Figure 5.1 • Simple pedigree for inheritance of an autosomal dominant trait. *Squares* represent males, *circles* represent females. The *shaded symbols* represent an affected parent with a mutant gene. An affected parent with an autosomal dominant trait has a 50% chance of passing the mutant gene on to each child regardless of sex.

disorder to each offspring (Fig. 5.1). The unaffected relatives of the parent or unaffected siblings of the offspring do not transmit the disorder. In many conditions, the age of onset is delayed, and the signs and symptoms of the disorder do not appear until later in life (as in Huntington disease).

Autosomal dominant disorders also may manifest as a new mutation. Whether the mutation is passed on to the next generation depends on the affected person's reproductive capacity. Many autosomal dominant mutations are accompanied by reduced reproductive capacity; therefore, the defect is not perpetuated in future generations. If an autosomal defect is accompanied by a total inability to reproduce, essentially all new cases of the disorder will be due to new mutations. If the defect does not affect reproductive capacity, it is more likely to be inherited from a parent.

Although there is a 50% chance of inheriting a dominant genetic disorder from an affected parent, there can be wide variation in gene penetrance and expression. When a person inherits a dominant mutant gene but fails to exhibit the associated phenotype, the trait is described as having *reduced penetrance*. Penetrance is expressed in mathematical terms: a 50% penetrance indicates that a person who inherits the defective gene has a 50% chance of expressing the disorder. The person who has a mutant gene but does not express it is an important exception to the rule that unaffected persons do not transmit an autosomal dominant trait. These people can transmit the gene to their descendants and so produce a "skipped generation" in their family history. Autosomal dominant disorders also can display *variable expressivity*, meaning that they can be expressed differently in people that carry the mutant gene. Polydactyly or supernumerary digits, for example, may be expressed in either the fingers or the toes.[2] Other disorders of autosomal inheritance, Marfan syndrome and neurofibromatosis (NF), are described here.

Marfan Syndrome. Marfan syndrome is an autosomal dominant disorder of the connective tissue, which gives shape and structure to other tissues in the body and holds them in place. The basic biochemical abnormality in Marfan syndrome affects *fibrillin I*, a major component of microfibrils found in the extracellular matrix.[3] Fibrillin I is coded by the *FBNI* gene, which maps to chromosome 15q21. The prevalence of Marfan syndrome is estimated to be 1 per 5000. Approximately 70% to 80% of cases are familial and the remainder are sporadic, arising from new mutations in the germ cells of the parents.[3]

Marfan syndrome affects several organ systems, including the eyes; the cardiovascular system; and the skeletal system (bones and joints).[3] There is a wide range of variation in the phenotype for the disorder. People may have abnormalities of one, two, or more systems. The skeletal deformities, which are the most obvious features of the disorder, include a long, thin body with exceptionally long extremities and long, tapering fingers, sometimes called *arachnodactyly* or *spider fingers;* hyperextensible joints; and a variety of spinal deformities, including kyphosis and scoliosis (Fig. 5.2). Chest deformities, pectus excavatum (*i.e.*, deeply depressed sternum) or pigeon chest deformity, often are present and may require surgery. The most common eye disorder is bilateral dislocation of the lens because of weakness of the suspensory ligaments. Myopia and predisposition to retinal

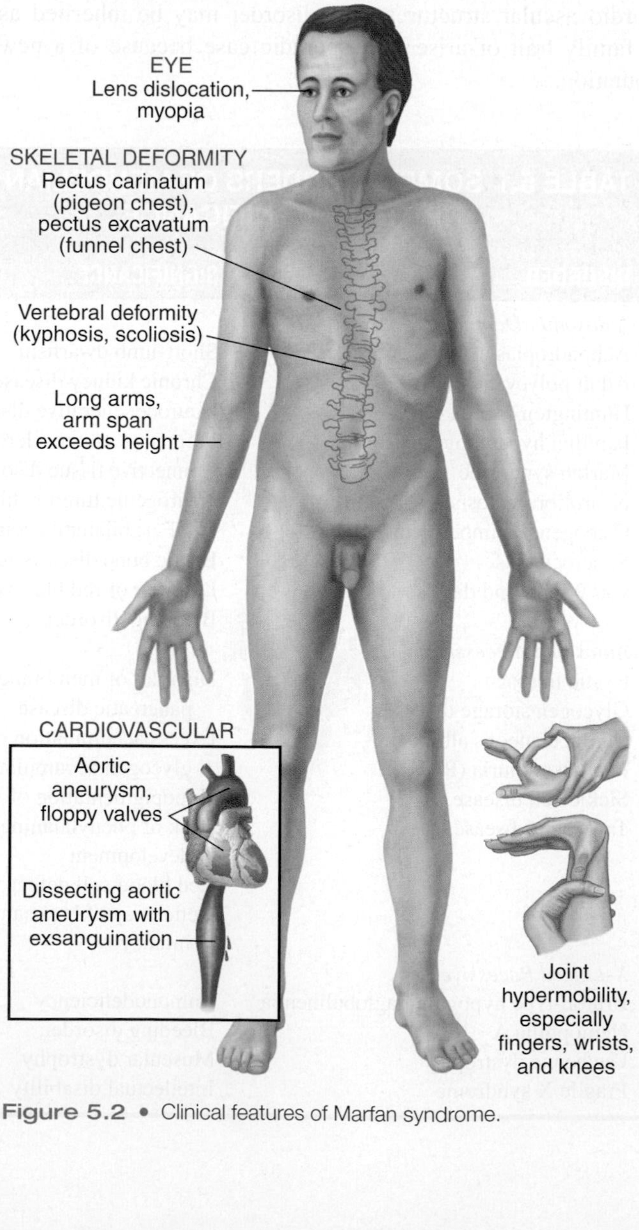

Figure 5.2 • Clinical features of Marfan syndrome.

detachment also are common. However, the most life-threatening aspects of the disorder are the cardiovascular defects, which include mitral valve prolapse, progressive dilation of the aortic valve ring, and weakness of the aorta and other arteries. Dissection and rupture of the aorta may lead to premature death.

Since over 100 mutations have been associated with the disease, the diagnosis of Marfan syndrome is based on major and minor diagnostic criteria that include skeletal, cardiovascular, and ocular deformities. There is currently no cure for Marfan syndrome. Treatment plans include echocardiograms and electrocardiograms to assess the status of the cardiovascular system, periodic eye examinations, and evaluation of the skeletal system, especially in children and adolescents.

Neurofibromatosis. Neurofibromatosis is a condition that causes tumors to develop from the Schwann cells of the neurologic system.[4] There are at least two genetically and clinically distinct forms of the disorder:

1. Type 1 NF (NF-1), also known as *von Recklinghausen disease*.
2. Type 2 bilateral acoustic NF (NF-2).[4,9]

Both of these disorders result from a genetic defect in a tumor suppressor gene that regulates cell differentiation and growth. The gene for NF-1 has been mapped to the long arm of chromosome 17 and the gene for NF-2 to chromosome 22.[4,5]

Type 1 NF is a common disorder, characterized by cutaneous and subcutaneous neurofibromas develop in late childhood or adolescence.[4] The cutaneous neurofibromas, which vary in number from a few to many hundreds, manifest as soft, pedunculated lesions that project from the skin. They are the most common type of lesion, often are not apparent until puberty, and are present in greatest density over the trunk (Fig. 5.3). The subcutaneous lesions grow just below the skin. They are firm and round and may be painful. Plexiform neurofibromas involve the larger peripheral nerves. They tend to form large tumors that cause severe disfigurement of the face, overgrowth of an extremity, or skeletal deformities such as scoliosis. Pigmented nodules of the iris (Lisch nodules), which are specific for NF-1, usually are present after 6 years of age.[6] They do not present any clinical problem but are useful in establishing a diagnosis.

A second major component of NF-1 is the presence of large (usually ≥15 mm in diameter), flat cutaneous pigmentations, known as *café au lait spots*. They are usually a uniform light brown in whites and darker brown in people of color, with sharply demarcated edges. Although small single lesions may be found in normal children, larger lesions or six or more spots larger than 1.5 cm in diameter suggest NF-1.[7] The skin pigmentations become more evident with age as the melanosomes in the epidermal cells accumulate melanin.

Children with NF-1 are also susceptible to neurologic complications. There is an increased incidence of learning disabilities, attention deficit disorders, and abnormalities of speech among affected children. Complex partial and generalized tonic–clonic seizures are a frequent complication.

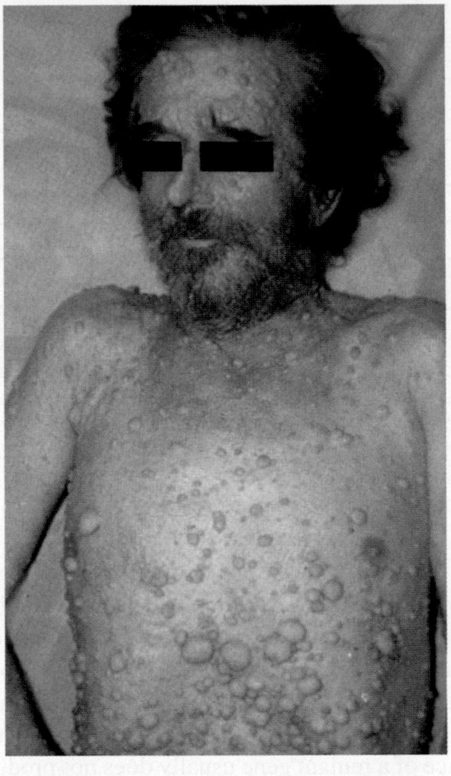

Figure 5.3 • Neurofibromatosis type 1. Multiple cutaneous neurofibromas are noted on the face and trunk. (From Strayer D. S., Rubin E. (Eds.) (2015). *Rubin's pathology: Clinicopathologic foundations of medicine* (7th ed., Fig. 6-20C, p. 269). Philadelphia, PA: Lippincott Williams & Wilkins.)

Malignant neoplasms are also a significant problem in people with NF-1. One of the major complications of NF-1, occurring in 3% to 5% of people, is the appearance of a neurofibrosarcoma in a neurofibroma, usually a larger plexiform neurofibroma.[4] NF-1 is also associated with increased incidence of other neurogenic tumors, including meningiomas, optic gliomas, and pheochromocytomas.

Type 2 NF is characterized by tumors of the acoustic nerve. Most often, the disorder is asymptomatic through the first 15 years of life. This type of NF occurs less frequently, at a rate of 1 in 50,000 people. The most frequent symptoms are headaches, hearing loss, and tinnitus. There may be associated intracranial and spinal meningiomas. Surgery may be indicated for debulking or removal of the tumors.[5]

Autosomal Recessive Disorders

Autosomal recessive disorders are manifested only when both members of the gene pair are affected (homozygous). In this case, both parents may be unaffected but are carriers of the defective gene. Autosomal recessive disorders affect both sexes. The occurrence risks in each pregnancy are one in four for an affected child, two in four for a carrier child, and one in four for a normal (noncarrier, unaffected), homozygous child (Fig. 5.4). *Consanguineous mating* (mating of two related people), or inbreeding, increases the chance that two people who mate will be carriers of an autosomal recessive disorder.

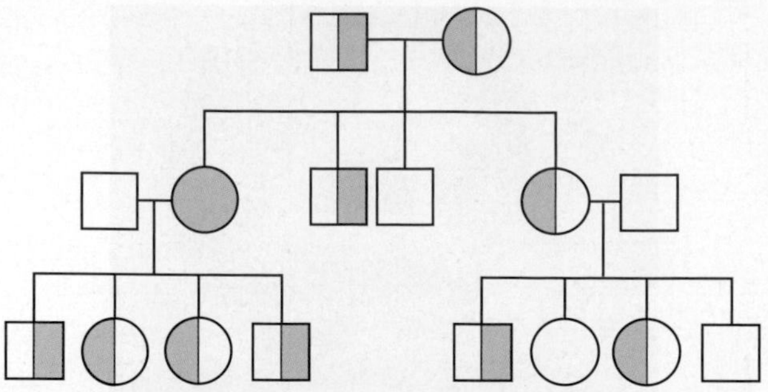

Figure 5.4 • Sample pedigree for inheritance of an autosomal recessive trait. *Squares* represent males, *circles* represent females. When the symbols are *half shaded*, then that parent is a carrier of an autosomal recessive trait. When both parents are carriers, on each conception, there is a 25% chance of having an affected child (*full-shaded circle* or *square*), a 50% chance of a carrier child, and a 25% chance of a nonaffected or noncarrier child, regardless of sex.

With autosomal recessive disorders, the age of onset is frequently early in life. In addition, the symptomatology tends to be more uniform than with autosomal dominant disorders. Autosomal disorders are characteristically caused by loss-of-function mutations, many of which impair or eliminate the function of an enzyme. In the case of a heterozygous carrier, the presence of a mutant gene usually does not produce symptoms because equal amounts of normal and defective enzymes are synthesized. This "margin of safety" ensures that cells with half their usual amount of enzyme function normally. By contrast, the inactivation of both alleles in a homozygote results in complete loss of enzyme activity. Autosomal recessive disorders include almost all inborn errors of metabolism. Enzyme disorders that impair catabolic pathways result in an accumulation of dietary substances (*e.g.*, phenylketonuria [PKU]) or cellular constituents (*e.g.*, lysosomal storage diseases). Other disorders result from a defect in the enzyme-mediated synthesis of an essential protein (*e.g.*, the cystic fibrosis transmembrane conductance regulator in cystic fibrosis). Two examples of autosomal recessive disorders that are not covered elsewhere in this book are PKU and Tay-Sachs disease.

Phenylketonuria. PKU is a rare autosomal recessive metabolic disorder that affects approximately 1 in every 10,000 to 15,000 infants in the United States. The disorder is caused by a deficiency of the liver enzyme phenylalanine hydroxylase, which allows toxic levels of the amino acid, phenylalanine, to accumulate in tissues and the blood.[8] If untreated, the disorder results in mental retardation, microcephaly, delayed speech, and other signs of impaired neurologic development.

Because the symptoms of PKU develop gradually and are difficult to assess, policies have been in place for quite some time to screen all infants for abnormal levels of serum phenylalanine.[9] Infants with the disorder are treated with a special diet that restricts phenylalanine intake. The diet can prevent mental retardation as well as other neurodegenerative effects of untreated PKU. However, dietary treatment must be started early in neonatal life to prevent brain damage. Infants with elevated phenylalanine levels should begin treatment by 7 to 10 days of age, indicating the need for early diagnosis.[8]

Tay-Sachs Disease. Tay-Sachs disease is a variant of a class of lysosomal storage diseases, known as the *gangliosidoses*, in which there is failure to break down the GM2 gangliosides of cell membranes.[10] Tay-Sachs disease is inherited as an autosomal recessive trait and occurs ten times more frequently in offspring of Eastern European (Ashkenazi) Jews as compared to the general population, although targeted carrier screening efforts have shown success in reducing rates for this population.[11]

The GM2 ganglioside accumulates in the lysosomes of all organs in Tay-Sachs disease, but is most prominent in the brain neurons and retina.[10] Microscopic examination reveals neurons ballooned with cytoplasmic vacuoles, each of which constitutes a markedly distended lysosome filled with gangliosides.[10] In time, there is progressive destruction of neurons, including in the cerebellum, basal ganglia, brain stem, spinal cord, and autonomic nervous system. Involvement of the retina is detected by ophthalmoscopy as a cherry-red spot on the macula.[10]

Infants with Tay-Sachs disease appear normal at birth but begin to manifest progressive weakness, muscle flaccidity, and decreased responsiveness at approximately 6 to 10 months of age.[10] This is followed by rapid deterioration of motor and mental function, often with development of generalized seizures. Retinal involvement leads to visual impairment and eventual blindness. Death usually occurs before 4 to 5 years of age.[10] Analysis of the blood serum for the lysosomal enzyme, hexosaminidase A, which is deficient in Tay-Sachs disease, allows for accurate identification of genetic carriers for the disease so that they may make educated and informed decisions about having a child.[11]

X-Linked Recessive Disorders

Sex-linked disorders are almost always associated with the X chromosome, and the inheritance pattern is predominantly recessive. Remember that the sex chromosomes for human females are XX and human males are XY. Because of the presence of a normal X, female heterozygotes (carriers) rarely experience the effects of a recessive defective gene, whereas all males who receive the gene are typically affected as they only have the mutant copy.

The common pattern of inheritance in a family is one in which an unaffected mother is a carrier of the mutant allele. She is not affected herself because she has one normal X that is dominant over the mutant recessive X. Because she will contribute one of these two X chromosomes to each of her offspring, she has a 50% chance of transmitting the mutant gene to her sons (who only have one X and will be affected), and her daughters have a 50% chance of being carriers of the mutant gene (who have two X chromosomes and so will not be affected because of the presence of a normal X) (Fig. 5.5).

When the affected son procreates, he only has his mutant X or a normal Y to pass on to the next generation. In order to have a daughter, the father donates his only X chromosome, which combines with one of the mother's two X chromosomes, resulting in a XX child. Because his X is mutated, he transmits the mutant gene to 100% of his daughters, who then become carriers. Because the genes of the Y chromosome are unaffected, the affected male does not transmit the defect to

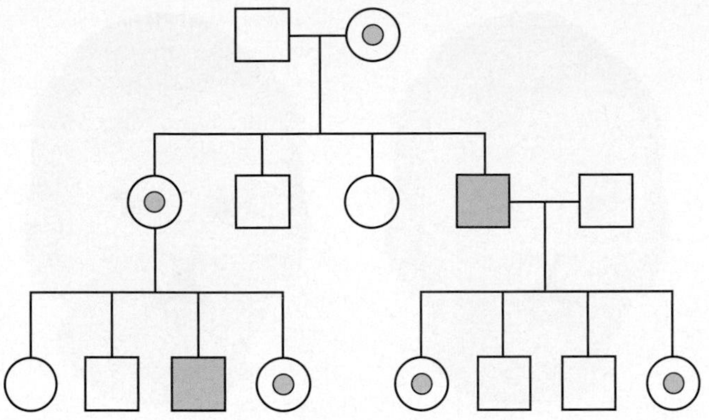

Figure 5.5 • Sample pedigree for inheritance of an X-linked recessive trait. X-linked recessive traits are expressed phenotypically in the male offspring, whereas females are typically carriers for the trait. A *small shaded circle* represents a carrier female and the *larger shaded square*, the affected male. A carrier female will transmit her carrier status to 50% of her daughters and 50% of her sons will be affected. The affected male passes the mutant gene to all of his daughters, who become carriers of the trait. The affected male will have no affected sons.

any of his sons, and they will not be carriers or transmit the disorder to their children.

Although rare, females can be affected with an X-linked recessive disorder. In order for this to happen, an affected male would need to have a child with a carrier female. In this case, 50% of the sons would be affected, and 50% of the daughters would be affected. The remaining daughters would be carriers like their mother. X-linked recessive disorders include color blindness, glucose-6-phosphate dehydrogenase deficiency, hemophilia A, and X-linked agammaglobulinemia.

X-Linked Dominant Disorders

X-linked dominant disorders are not as common as X-linked recessive disorders. In X-linked dominant disorders, the disease will affect both males and females that inherit a copy of the mutated X chromosome. For the females, the mutant X chromosome is dominant to the normal X chromosome. Although both sexes are affected, many times the mutation will be embryonic lethal for males (who only have the mutated X and a normal Y) or for homozygous mutant females. Affected females that are heterozygous with one mutant X chromosome and one normal X chromosome will transmit the disorder to 50% of their offspring regardless of sex. Affected males will have 100% affected daughters or 100% normal sons. This is explained because all sons inherited their father's Y chromosome, but the daughters inherited the mutated X chromosome from their father. Examples of X-linked dominant disorders include fragile X syndrome and Rett syndrome.

Fragile X Syndrome

Fragile X syndrome is a single-gene disorder that causes intellectual disability.[12] The mutation occurs at the Xq27 on the fragile site and is characterized by amplification of a cytosine, guanine, guanine (CGG) repeat.[13] The disorder, which affects approximately 1 in 1250 males and 1 in 2500 females, is the most common form of inherited intellectual disability.[12]

Pathogenesis. The fragile X gene has been mapped to the long arm of the X chromosome, designated the *FMR1* (fragile X mental retardation 1) site.[13] The gene product, the fragile X mental retardation protein (FMRP), is a widely expressed cytoplasmic protein. It is most abundant in the brain and testis, the organs most affected by the disorder. Each gene contains a promoter region and an instruction region that carries the directions for protein synthesis. The promoter region of the *FMR1* gene contains repeats of a specific CGG triplet code that, when normal, controls gene activity. Once the repeat exceeds a threshold length for the disease, no FMRP is produced, resulting in the fragile X phenotype. People without fragile X syndrome have between 6 and 40 repeats. A gene with 55 to 200 repeats is generally considered a permutation and one with more than 200 repeats, a full mutation.[13]

Clinical Manifestations and Diagnosis. Affected boys are intellectually disabled and share a common physical phenotype that includes a long face with large mandible and large, everted ears. Hyperextensible joints, a high-arched palate, and mitral valve prolapse, which are observed in some cases, mimic a connective tissue disorder.[12] Some physical abnormalities may be subtle or absent. Because girls have two X chromosomes, they are more likely to have relatively normal cognitive development, or they may show a learning disability in a particular area.

Diagnosis of fragile X syndrome is based on mental and physical characteristics. DNA tests can be done to confirm the presence of an abnormal *FMR1* gene. Because the manifestations of fragile X syndrome may resemble those of other learning disorders, it is recommended that people with intellectual disability of unknown cause, developmental delay, learning disabilities, autism, or autism-like behaviors be evaluated for the disorder.[12] Fragile X screening is now often offered along with routine prenatal screening to determine if the woman is a carrier.

KEY POINTS

SINGLE-GENE DISORDERS

- Genetic disorders can be inherited as autosomal dominant disorders, in which the phenotype is seen in both the homozygous dominant or heterozygous genotype, or as autosomal recessive disorders, in which the phenotype is only seen in the homozygous recessive genotype.
- Sex-linked disorders almost always are associated with the X chromosome and are predominantly recessive.

Inherited Multifactorial Disorders

Multifactorial disorders are caused by the influence of multiple genes along with environmental factors. These traits do not follow the same clear-cut pattern of inheritance as do single-gene disorders because the appearance of the disorder phenotype will be dependent on environmental changes in addition to genetic mutations. Disorders of multifactorial inheritance can be present at birth, or they may be expressed later in life. Congenital disorders that are thought to arise through multifactorial inheritance include cleft lip or palate, clubfoot, congenital dislocation of the hip, congenital heart disease, pyloric stenosis, and urinary tract malformation. Environmental factors are thought to play an even greater role in disorders of multifactorial inheritance that develop in adult life, such as coronary artery disease, diabetes mellitus, hypertension, and cancer.

Although multifactorial traits cannot be predicted with the same degree of accuracy as mendelian single-gene mutations, characteristic patterns do exist for congenital disorders. First, multifactorial congenital malformations tend to involve a single organ or tissue derived from the same embryonic developmental field. Second, the risk of recurrence in future pregnancies is high for the same or a similar defect. For instance, this means that parents of a child with a cleft palate defect have an increased risk of having another child with a cleft palate defect. Third, first-degree relatives of an affected person have an increased risk (as compared with the general population) of having a child with the disease. The risk increases with increasing numbers of the incidence of the defect among relatives.

Cleft Lip and Cleft Palate

Cleft lip with or without cleft palate is one of the most common birth defects, occurring in about 0.1% of all pregnancies.[14] It is also one of the more conspicuous birth defects, resulting in an abnormal facial appearance and defective speech.

Developmentally, the defect has its origin at about the 35th day of gestation when the frontal prominences of the craniofacial structures fuse with the maxillary process to form the upper lip.[14] This process is under the control of many genes, and disturbances in these (whether hereditary or environmental) at this time may result in cleft lip with or without cleft palate (Fig. 5.6). The defect may also be caused by teratogens (*e.g.*, rubella, anticonvulsant drugs) and is often encountered in children with chromosomal abnormalities.

Cleft lip and palate defects may vary from a small notch in the vermilion border of the upper lip to complete separation involving the palate and extending into the floor of the nose. The clefts may be unilateral or bilateral and may involve the alveolar ridge. The condition may be accompanied by deformed, supernumerary, or absent teeth. Isolated cleft palate occurs in the midline and may involve only the uvula or may extend into or through the soft and hard palates.

A child with cleft lip or palate may require years of special treatment by medical and dental specialists, including a plastic surgeon, pediatric dentist, orthodontist, and speech therapist. The immediate problem in an infant with cleft palate is feeding. Nursing at the breast or nipple depends on suction developed by pressing the nipple against the hard palate with the tongue. Although infants with cleft lip usually have no problems with feeding, those with cleft palate usually require specially constructed, soft artificial nipples with large openings and a squeezable bottle. As the child ages, speech may be impaired because of these issues.

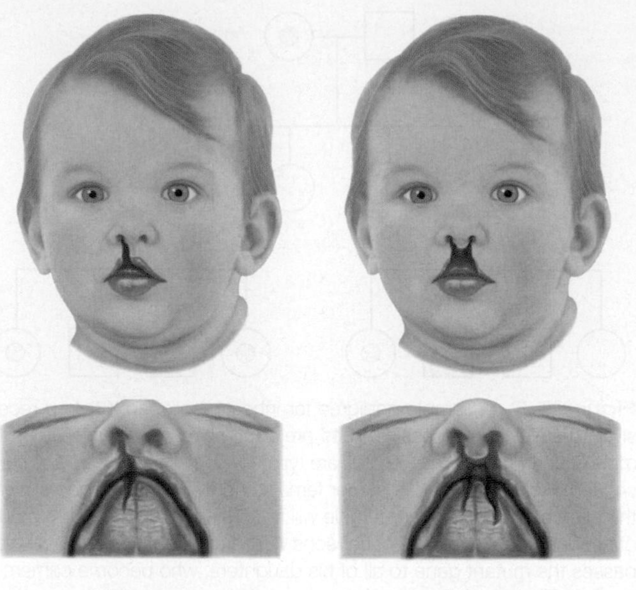

Figure 5.6 • Cleft lip and cleft palate.

Major advances in the care of children born with cleft lip and palate have occurred within the last quarter of the 20th century.[15] Surgical closure of the lip is usually performed by 3 months of age, with closure of the palate usually done before 1 year of age. Depending on the extent of the defect, additional surgery may be required as the child grows. In some situations, the palate is repaired prior to the cleft lip, and results indicate that the palate surgery is easier when done prior to the cleft lip repair.[15] Also, the time between surgeries when cleft palate is repaired prior to lip repair is shorter.[15] Displacement of the maxillary arches and malposition of the teeth usually require orthodontic correction.

Chromosomal Disorders

Chromosomal disorders form a major category of genetic disease, accounting for a large proportion of early miscarriages, congenital malformations, and intellectual disability. The study of chromosomal disorders is called *cytogenetics*.

During mitosis in human somatic cells, the chromosomes replicate so that each cell receives a total of 23 pairs of chromosomes. But in germ cells undergoing meiosis, these pairs are reduced so that each daughter cell only receives 23 individual chromosomes. At the time of conception, the set of 23 individual chromosomes in the ovum and the set of 23 individual chromosomes in the sperm join to produce an offspring with 23 pairs, or 46 total chromosomes.

Chromosomal abnormalities are commonly described according to the shorthand description of the karyotype. In this system, the total number of chromosomes is given first, followed by the sex chromosome complement, and then the description of any abnormality. For example, a male with trisomy 21 is designated 47,XY,+21.

Structural Chromosomal Abnormalities

The aberrations underlying chromosomal disorders can be an abnormal number of chromosomes, but there can also be alterations to the structure of one or more chromosomes. Structural changes in chromosomes usually result from breakage in one or more of the chromosomes during meiosis followed by rearrangement or deletion of chromosome parts. Among the factors believed to cause chromosome breakage are exposure to radiation sources, such as x-rays; influence of certain chemicals; extreme changes in the cellular environment; and viral infections.

Several patterns of chromosome breakage and rearrangement can occur (Fig. 5.7). There can be a *deletion* of the broken portion of the chromosome. When one chromosome is involved, the broken parts may be *inverted*. *Isochromosome formation* occurs when the centromere of the chromosome separates horizontally instead of vertically. *Ring formation* results when deletion is followed by uniting of the chromatids to form a ring. *Translocation* occurs when there are simultaneous breaks in two chromosomes from different pairs, with exchange of chromosome parts. With a balanced reciprocal translocation, no genetic information is lost; therefore, persons with translocations usually are normal.

A special form of translocation called a *centric fusion* or *robertsonian translocation* involves two acrocentric chromosomes in which the centromere is near the end, most commonly chromosomes 13 and 14, or 14 and 21. Typically, the break occurs near the centromere affecting the short arm in one chromosome and the long arm in the other. Transfer of the chromosome fragments leads to one long and one extremely short fragment. The short fragment is usually lost during subsequent divisions. In this case, the person has only 45 chromosomes, but the amount of genetic material that is lost is so small that it often goes unnoticed. Difficulty, however, arises during meiosis; the result is gametes with an unbalanced number of chromosomes. The chief clinical importance of this type of translocation is that carriers of a robertsonian translocation involving chromosome 21 are at high risk for producing a child with Down syndrome.

The manifestations of aberrations in chromosome structure depend to a great extent on the amount of genetic material that is lost or displaced. Many cells sustaining major unrestored breaks are eliminated within the next few replication cycles because of deficiencies that may in themselves be fatal. This is beneficial because it prevents the damaged cells from becoming a permanent part of the organism or, if it occurs in the gametes, from giving rise to grossly defective zygotes.

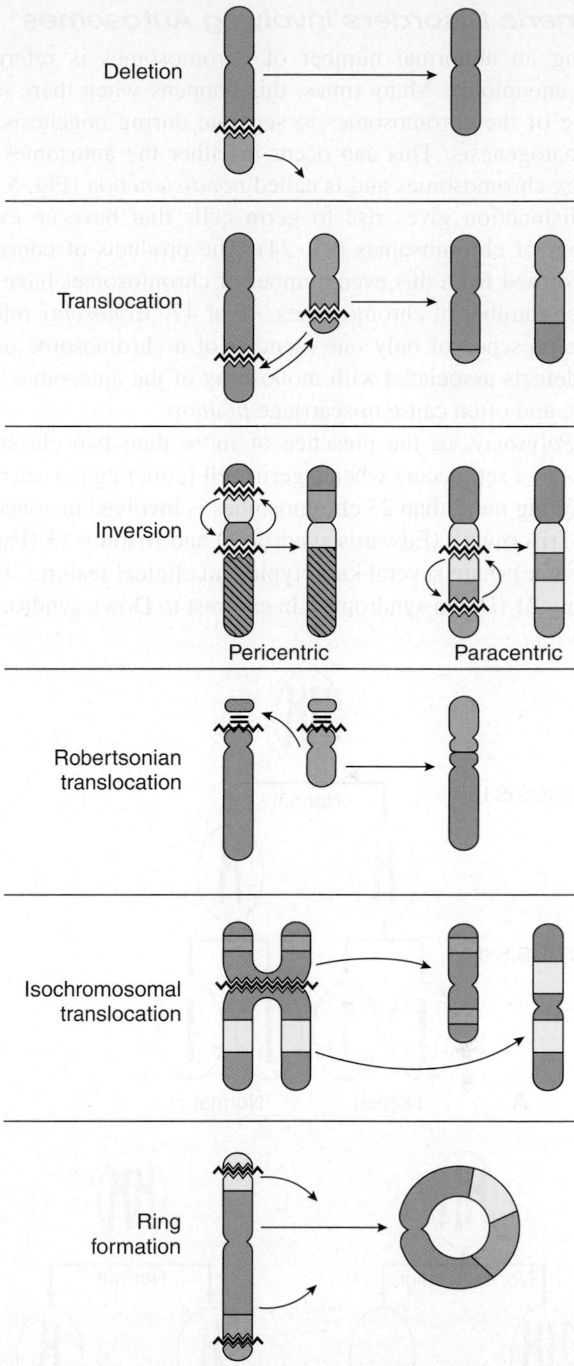

Figure 5.7 • Structural abnormalities in the human chromosome. The deletion of a portion of a chromosome leads to loss of genetic material and shortening of the chromosome. A **reciprocal translocation** involves breaks on two nonhomologous chromosomes, with exchange of the acentric segment. An **inversion** requires two breaks in a single chromosome. If the breaks are on opposite sides of the centromere, the inversion is **pericentric**; it is **paracentric** if the breaks are on the same arm. A **robertsonian translocation** occurs when two nonhomologous acrocentric chromosomes break near their centromeres, after which the long arms fuse to form one large metacentric chromosome. **Isochromosomes** arise from faulty centromere division, which leads to duplication of the long arm and deletion of the short arm, or the reverse (iso p). Ring chromosomes form with breaks in both telomeric portions of a chromosome, deletion of the acentric fragments, and fusion of the remaining centric portion. (From Rubin R, Strayer D. S., (Eds.) (2015). *Rubin's pathology: Clinicopathologic foundations of medicine* (7th ed., Fig. 6-8, p. 253). Philadelphia, PA: Lippincott Williams & Wilkins.)

Numeric Disorders Involving Autosomes

Having an abnormal number of chromosomes is referred to as aneuploidy. Many times, this happens when there is a failure of the chromosomes to separate during oogenesis or spermatogenesis. This can occur in either the autosomes or the sex chromosomes and is called *nondisjunction* (Fig. 5.8). Nondisjunction gives rise to germ cells that have an even number of chromosomes (22, 24). The products of conception formed from this even number of chromosomes have an uneven number of chromosomes, 45 or 47. *Monosomy* refers to the presence of only one member of a chromosome pair. The defects associated with monosomy of the autosomes are severe and often cause miscarriage *in utero*.

Polysomy, or the presence of more than two chromosomes to a set, occurs when a germ cell (either egg or sperm) containing more than 23 chromosomes is involved in conception. Trisomy 18 (Edwards syndrome) and trisomy 13 (Patau syndrome) share several karyotypic and clinical features with trisomy 21 (Down syndrome). In contrast to Down syndrome, however, the first two malformations are much more severe. As a result, these infants rarely survive beyond the first years of life.[5]

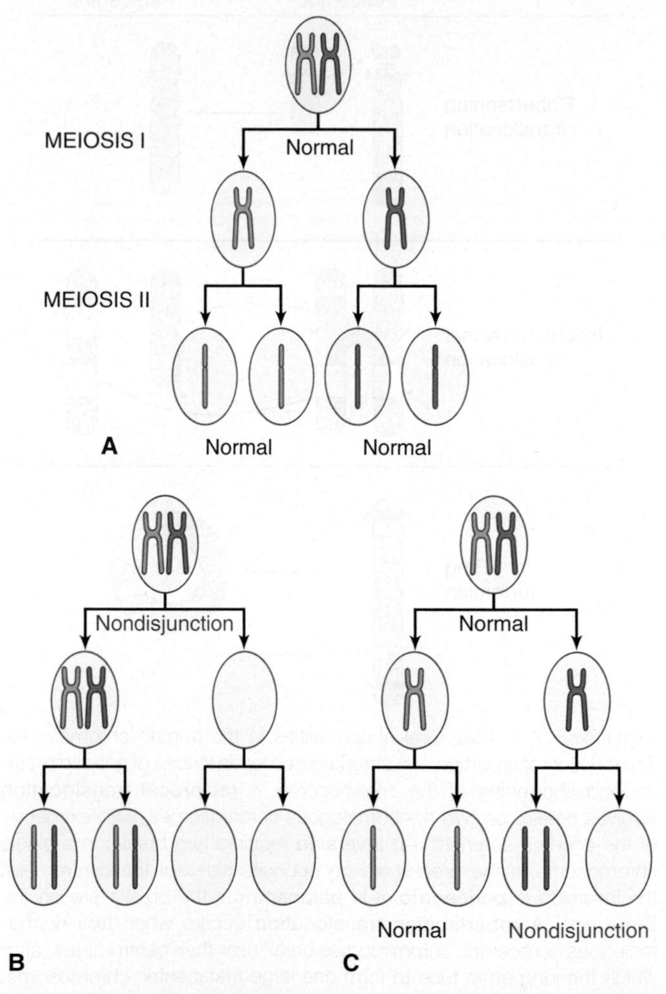

Figure 5.8 • Nondisjunction as a cause of disorders of chromosomal numbers. **(A)** Normal distribution of chromosomes during meiosis I and II. **(B)** If nondisjunction occurs at meiosis I, the gametes contain either a pair of chromosomes or a lack of chromosomes. **(C)** If nondisjunction occurs at meiosis II, the affected gametes contain two of copies of one parenteral chromosome or a lack of chromosomes.

Down Syndrome. First described in 1866 by John Langdon Down, trisomy 21, or Down syndrome, causes a combination of birth defects including some degree of intellectual disability, characteristic facial features, and other health problems. It is the most common chromosomal disorder.

Approximately 95% of cases of Down syndrome are caused by nondisjunction or an error in cell division during meiosis, resulting in a trisomy of chromosome 21. A rare form of Down syndrome can occur in the offspring of people in whom there has been a robertsonian translocation (see Fig. 5.7) involving the long arm of chromosome 21q and the long arm of one of the acrocentric chromosomes (most often 14 or 22). The translocation adds to the normal long arm of chromosome 21. Therefore, the person with this type of Down syndrome has 46 chromosomes, but a trisomy of the long arm of chromosome 21 (21q).[16]

The risk of having a child with Down syndrome increases with maternal age. The reason for the correlation between maternal age and nondisjunction is unknown, but is thought to reflect some aspect of aging of the oocyte. Although men continue to produce sperm throughout their reproductive life, women are born with all the oocytes they ever will have. These oocytes may change as a result of the aging process and are likely to have chromosomal abnormalities.

A child with Down syndrome has specific physical characteristics that are evident at birth. These features include a small and rather square head. There is a flat facial profile, with a small nose and somewhat depressed nasal bridge; small folds on the inner corners of the eyes (epicanthal folds) and upward slanting of the eyes; small, low-set, and malformed ears; a fat pad at the back of the neck; an open mouth; and a large, protruding tongue (Fig. 5.9). The child's hands usually are short and stubby, with fingers that curl inward, and there usually is only a single palmar (*i.e.*, simian) crease. There is excessive space between the large and second toes. There often are accompanying congenital heart defects and an increased risk of gastrointestinal malformations. In addition, there is an increased risk of Alzheimer disease among older people with Down syndrome.

There are several prenatal screening tests that can be done to determine the risk of having a child with Down syndrome.[18] The most commonly used are blood tests that measure maternal serum levels of α-fetoprotein (AFP), human chorionic gonadotropin (hCG), unconjugated estriol, inhibin A, and pregnancy-associated plasma protein A (PAPP-A) (see section on Diagnosis and Counseling). The results of three or four of these tests, together with the woman's age, often are used to determine the probability of a pregnant woman having a child with Down syndrome. Between 10 and 13 weeks, women can have an ultrasound that assesses for nuchal translucency (sonolucent space on the back of the fetal neck). The fetus with Down syndrome tends to have a greater area of

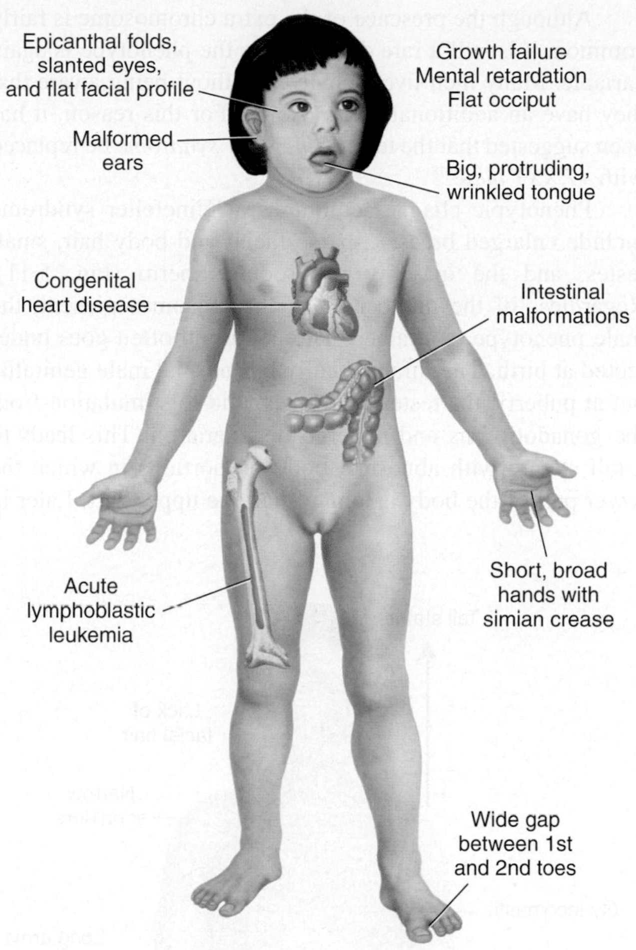

Figure 5.9 • Clinical features of a child with Down syndrome.

translucency as compared to a chromosomally normal infant. But the definitive diagnosis of Down syndrome in the fetus is through chromosome analysis using chorionic villus sampling, amniocentesis, or percutaneous umbilical blood sampling, which is discussed later in this chapter.

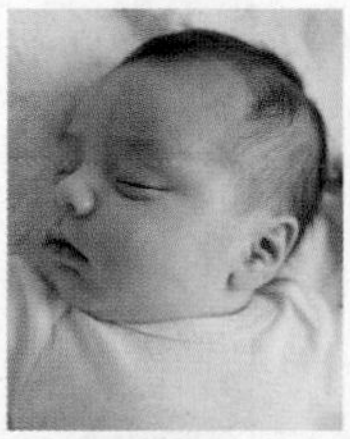

Remember **Jennifer,** the newborn born with Down syndrome in the unit opener case study? Her disorder could have been diagnosed prenatally. Her mother was 46, which is considered an advanced maternal age and these pregnancies are associated with an increased risk of aneuploidy, such as trisomy 21. The mother was offered first trimester screening at her first sonogram at 12 weeks and accepted. An increased nuchal translucency was seen on sonogram, and her trisomy 21 risk calculated from her first trimester screen indicated a 1:20 risk for trisomy 21. She declined invasive testing, such as amniocentesis, because she stated that positive results from further testing would not change her decision to continue with the pregnancy. On her anatomy sonogram and follow-up sonograms, the fetus was noted to have an absent nasal bone, echogenic bowel, short long bones, and an echogenic focus in the heart, which are all markers for possible Down syndrome. Women with abnormal first trimester screens, abnormal second trimester screens, abnormal sonogram findings, a personal or family history of genetic conditions, or who are of advanced maternal age should be referred to a genetic counselor during their pregnancy for further discussion and management.

Numeric Disorders Involving Sex Chromosomes

Chromosomal disorders associated with the sex chromosomes are much more common than those related to the autosomes, except for trisomy 21. Furthermore, imbalances in the number (either excesses or deletions) are much better tolerated than those chromosomal abnormalities involving the autosomes. This is related in a large part to two factors that are peculiar to the sex chromosomes:

1. All but one X chromosome is inactivated
2. There are very few genes that are carried on the Y chromosome

Although females normally receive both a paternal and a maternal X chromosome, the clinical manifestations of X chromosome abnormalities can be quite variable because of the process of X inactivation. In somatic cells of females, only one X chromosome is transcriptionally active and creates protein from the DNA template. The other chromosome is inactive. The process of X inactivation, which is random, occurs early in embryonic life and is usually complete at about the end of the first week of development. After one X chromosome has become inactivated in a cell, all cells descended from that cell will have the same active and inactive X chromosome. Although much of one X chromosome is inactivated in females, several regions do contain genes that escape inactivation and can continue to be expressed by both X chromosomes. These genes may explain some of the variations in clinical symptoms seen in cases of numeric abnormalities of the X chromosome.

Turner Syndrome. Turner syndrome describes an absence of all (45,X/0) or part of the X chromosome. Some women with Turner syndrome may have part of the X chromosome, and some may display a mosaicism where one or more additional cell lines are active. This disorder affects approximately 1 of every 2500 live births and is the most frequently occurring genetic disorder in women.[17]

Characteristically, a female with Turner syndrome is short in stature, but her body proportions are normal (Fig. 5.10). Females with Tuner syndrome lose the majority of their oocytes by the age of 2 years. Therefore, they do not menstruate and show no signs of secondary sex characteristics. There are variations in the syndrome, with abnormalities ranging from essentially a normal phenotype to cardiac abnormalities such as bicuspid aortic valve and coarctation of the aorta, and a small webbed neck.[17]

Because the phenotype can be somewhat variable, the diagnosis of Turner syndrome often is delayed until late

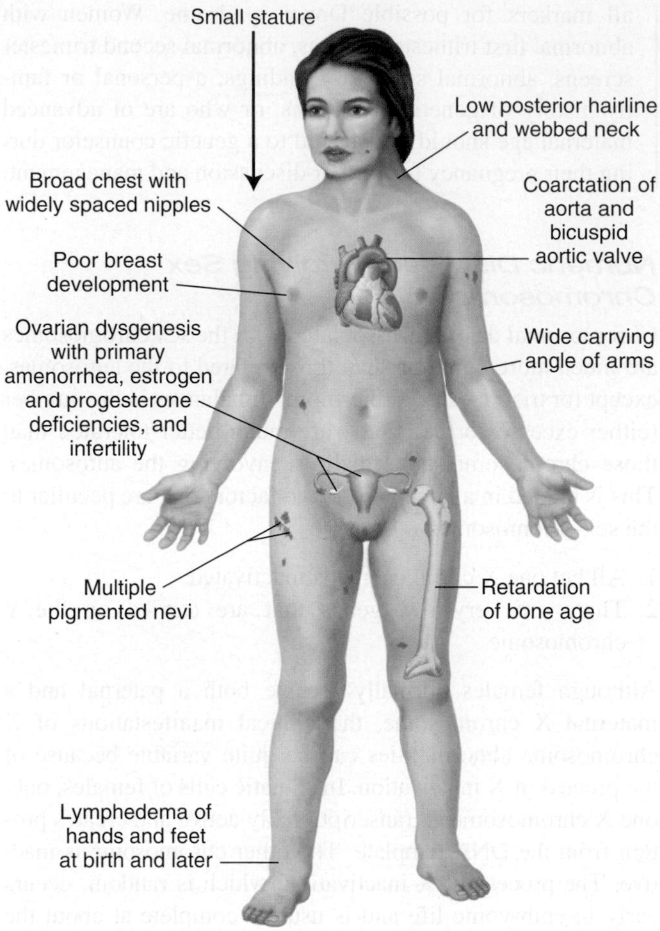

Figure 5.10 • Clinical features of Turner syndrome.

childhood or early adolescence in girls who do not present with all of the classic features of the syndrome. It is important to diagnose girls with Turner syndrome as early as possible so treatment plans can be implemented and managed throughout their lives. The management of Turner syndrome begins during childhood and requires ongoing assessment and treatment. Growth hormone therapy generally can result in a gain of 6 to 10 cm in final height. Estrogen therapy, which is instituted around the normal age of puberty, is used to promote development and maintenance of secondary sexual characteristics.[17]

Klinefelter Syndrome. Klinefelter syndrome is a condition of testicular dysgenesis accompanied by the presence of one or more extra X chromosomes in excess of the normal male XY complement.[18] Most males with Klinefelter syndrome have one extra X chromosome (47,XXY). In rare cases, there may be more than one extra X chromosome (48,XXXY). The presence of the extra X chromosome in the 47,XXY male results from nondisjunction during meiotic division in one of the parents, but the cause of the nondisjunction is unknown. Advanced maternal age increases the risk, but only slightly. Klinefelter syndrome occurs in approximately 1 per 700 newborn male infants.[18]

Although the presence of the extra chromosome is fairly common, it is still a rare diagnosis as the phenotype is again variable. Many men live their lives without being aware that they have an additional chromosome. For this reason, it has been suggested that the term *Klinefelter syndrome* be replaced with *47,XXY male*.[18]

Phenotypic changes common to Klinefelter syndrome include enlarged breasts, sparse facial and body hair, small testes, and the inability to produce sperm (Fig. 5.11). Regardless of the number of X chromosomes present, the male phenotype is retained. The condition often goes undetected at birth. The infant usually has normal male genitalia, but at puberty, the testes do not respond to stimulation from the gonadotropins and undergo degeneration. This leads to a tall stature with abnormal body proportions in which the lower part of the body is longer than the upper part. Later in

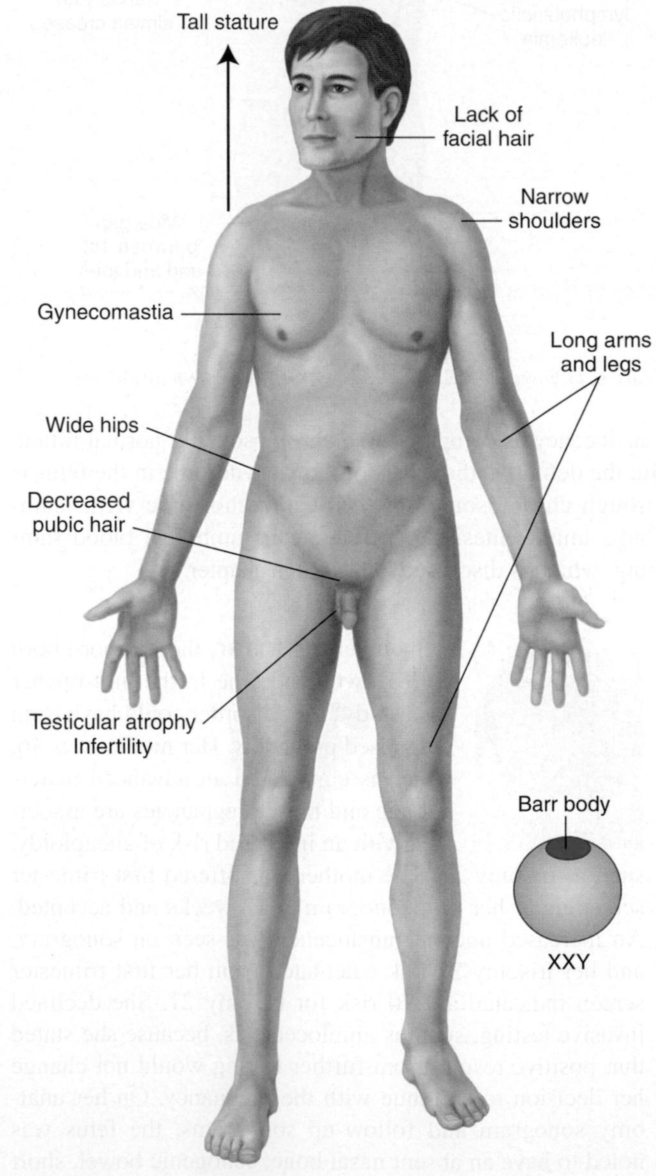

Figure 5.11 • Clinical features of Klinefelter syndrome.

life, the body build may become heavy, with a female distribution of subcutaneous fat and variable degrees of breast enlargement. There may be deficient secondary male sex characteristics, such as a voice that remains feminine in pitch and sparse beard and pubic hair. Although the intellect usually is normal, most 47,XXY males have some degree of language impairment.[18]

Adequate management of Klinefelter syndrome requires a comprehensive neurodevelopmental evaluation. In infancy and early childhood, this often includes a multidisciplinary approach to determine appropriate treatments such as physical therapy, infant stimulation programs, and speech therapy. Males with Klinefelter syndrome have congenital hypogonadism, which results in an inability to produce normal amounts of testosterone accompanied by an increase in hypothalamic gonadotrophic hormones. Androgen therapy is usually initiated when there is evidence of a testosterone deficit. Infertility is common in men with Klinefelter syndrome because of a decreased sperm count. If sperm are present, cryopreservation may be useful for future family planning.[18] However, genetic counseling is advised because of the increased risk of autosomal and sex chromosomal abnormalities.

Mitochondrial Gene Disorders

The mitochondria contain their own DNA, which is distinct from the DNA contained in the cell nucleus. Although the majority of inherited disorders come from nuclear DNA abnormalities, there are multiple disease causing rearrangements and mutations that can occur in mitochondrial DNA (mtDNA). This DNA is packaged in a double-stranded circular chromosome and contains 37 genes: 2 ribosomal RNA (rRNA) genes, 22 transfer RNA (tRNA) genes, and 13 structural genes encoding subunits of the mitochondrial respiratory chain enzymes, which participate in oxidative phosphorylation and generation of adenosine triphosphate.

Because mtDNA is inherited only from the mother, all disorders of mtDNA are also inherited on the maternal line. Maternal inheritance is explained by the processes occurring during conception. Ova contain numerous mitochondria in their abundant cytoplasm, whereas spermatozoa contain few, if any, mitochondria. Thus, the mtDNA in the zygote is derived solely from the mother. The zygote and its daughter cells have many mitochondria, each of which contains multiple copies of the maternally derived mtDNA. During growth of the fetus or later, it is likely that some cells will contain only normal or mutant mtDNA (a situation called *homoplasmy*), whereas others receive a mixture of normal and mutant DNA (*heteroplasmy*). In turn, the clinical expression of a disease produced by a given mutation of mtDNA depends on the total content of mitochondrial genes and the proportion that is mutant. The fraction of mutant mtDNA must exceed a critical value for a mitochondrial disease to become symptomatic. This threshold varies in different organs and is presumably related to the energy requirements of the cells.

Mitochondrial DNA mutations generally affect tissues that are dependent on oxidative phosphorylation to meet their high needs for metabolic energy. Thus, mtDNA mutations frequently affect the neuromuscular system and produce disorders such as encephalopathies, myopathies, retinal degeneration, loss of extraocular muscle function, and deafness. The range of mitochondrial diseases is broad, however, and may include liver dysfunction, bone marrow failure, and pancreatic islet cell dysfunction and diabetes, among other disorders. Table 5.2 describes representative examples of disorders due to mutations in mtDNA.

TABLE 5.2 SOME DISORDERS OF ORGAN SYSTEMS ASSOCIATED WITH MITOCHONDRIAL DNA MUTATIONS

DISORDER	MANIFESTATIONS
Chronic progressive external ophthalmoplegia	Progressive weakness of the extraocular muscles
Deafness	Progressive sensorineural deafness, often associated with aminoglycoside antibiotics
Kearns-Sayre syndrome	Progressive weakness of the extraocular muscles of early onset with heart block, retinal pigmentation
Leber hereditary optic neuropathy	Painless, subacute, bilateral visual loss, with central blind spots (scotomas) and abnormal color vision
Leigh disease	Proximal muscle weakness, sensory neuropathy, developmental delay, ataxia, seizures, dementia, and visual impairment due to retinal pigment degeneration
MELAS	*M*itochondrial *e*ncephalomyopathy (cerebral structural changes), *l*actic *a*cidosis, and *s*trokelike syndrome, seizures, and other clinical and laboratory abnormalities; may manifest only as diabetes mellitus
MERRF	*M*yoclonic *e*pilepsy, *r*agged *r*ed *f*ibers in muscle, ataxia, sensorineural deafness
Myoclonic epilepsy with ragged red fibers	Myoclonic seizures, cerebellar ataxia, mitochondrial myopathy (muscle weakness, fatigue)

IN SUMMARY

Genetic disorders can affect a single gene (mendelian inheritance) or several genes (polygenic inheritance). Single-gene mutations may be present on an autosome or on the X chromosome, and they may be expressed as a dominant or recessive trait. In autosomal dominant disorders, the affected parent has a 50% chance of transmitting the disorder to each offspring. Autosomal recessive disorders are manifested only when both members of the gene pair are affected. Usually, both parents are unaffected but are carriers of the defective gene. Their chances of having an affected child are one in four; of having a carrier child, two in four; and of having a noncarrier, unaffected child, one in four. X-linked recessive disorders, which are associated with the X chromosome, are typically transmitted by an unaffected carrier mother, who carries one normal X chromosome and one mutant X chromosome. She has a 50% chance of transmitting the defective gene to her sons, who are affected, and her daughters have a 50% chance of being carriers of the mutant gene. Because of a normal paired gene, female heterozygotes rarely experience the effects of a defective gene. X-linked dominant disorders are less common than X-linked recessive, but do exist. Multifactorial inheritance disorders are caused by multiple genes and, in many cases, environmental factors.

Chromosomal disorders result from a change in chromosome number or structure. A change in chromosome number is called *aneuploidy. Monosomy* involves the presence of only one member of a chromosome pair; it is seen in Turner syndrome, in which there is monosomy of the X chromosome. *Polysomy* refers to the presence of more than two chromosomes in a set. Klinefelter syndrome involves polysomy of the X chromosome. Trisomy 21 (*i.e.*, Down syndrome) is the most common form of chromosome disorder. Alterations in chromosome structure involve deletion or addition of genetic material, or a translocation of genetic material from one chromosome pair to another.

The mitochondria contain their own DNA, which is distinct from nuclear DNA. This mtDNA is only inherited maternally. Disorders of mitochondrial genes interfere with oxidative phosphorylation and the production of cellular energy. The range of mitochondrial gene disorders is diverse, with neuromuscular disorders predominating.

DISORDERS DUE TO ENVIRONMENTAL INFLUENCES

After completing this section of the chapter, the learner will be able to meet the following objectives:

- Cite the most susceptible period of intrauterine life for development of defects because of environmental agents.
- State the cautions that should be observed when considering use of drugs during pregnancy, including the possible effects of alcohol abuse, vitamin A derivatives, and folic acid deficiency on fetal development.

The developing embryo is subject to many nongenetic influences. After conception, development is influenced by the environmental factors that the embryo shares with the mother. The physiologic status of the mother—her hormone balance, her general state of health, her nutritional status, and the drugs she takes undoubtedly influences the development of the unborn child. For example, maternal smoking is associated with lower than normal neonatal weight. Maternal use of alcohol is known to cause fetal abnormalities. Various drugs can cause early miscarriage. Measles and other infectious agents cause congenital malformations. Other agents, such as radiation, can cause chromosomal and genetic defects and produce developmental disorders.

Period of Vulnerability

The embryo's development is most easily disturbed during the period when differentiation and development of the organs are taking place. This time interval, which is often referred to as the period of *organogenesis*, extends from day 15 to day 60 after conception. Environmental influences during the first 2 weeks after fertilization may interfere with implantation and result in abortion or early resorption of the products of conception. Each organ has a critical period during which it is highly susceptible to environmental derangements (Fig. 5.12).

Teratogenic Agents

A teratogenic agent is a chemical, physical, or biologic agent that produces abnormalities during embryonic or fetal development. Maternal disease or altered metabolic state also can affect the development of the embryo or fetus. Theoretically, teratogenic agents can cause birth defects in three ways:

1. By direct exposure of the pregnant female and the embryo or fetus to the agent.
2. Through exposure of the soon to be pregnant female to an agent that has a slow clearance rate, such that a teratogenic dose is retained during early pregnancy.
3. As a result of mutagenic effects of an environmental agent that occur before pregnancy, causing permanent damage to a female's or a male's reproductive cells.

For discussion purposes, teratogenic agents have been divided into three groups: radiation, drugs and chemical substances, and infectious agents. Chart 5.1 lists commonly identified agents in each of these groups.

Radiation

Heavy doses of ionizing radiation are teratogenic and mutagenic and have the capacity to effect inheritable changes in genetic materials. Specifically, excessive levels of radiation have been shown to cause microcephaly, skeletal malformations, and mental retardation. There is no evidence that *diagnostic* levels of radiation (*e.g.*, from a chest x-ray) cause congenital abnormalities, but all efforts to shield the fetus are taken when possible.

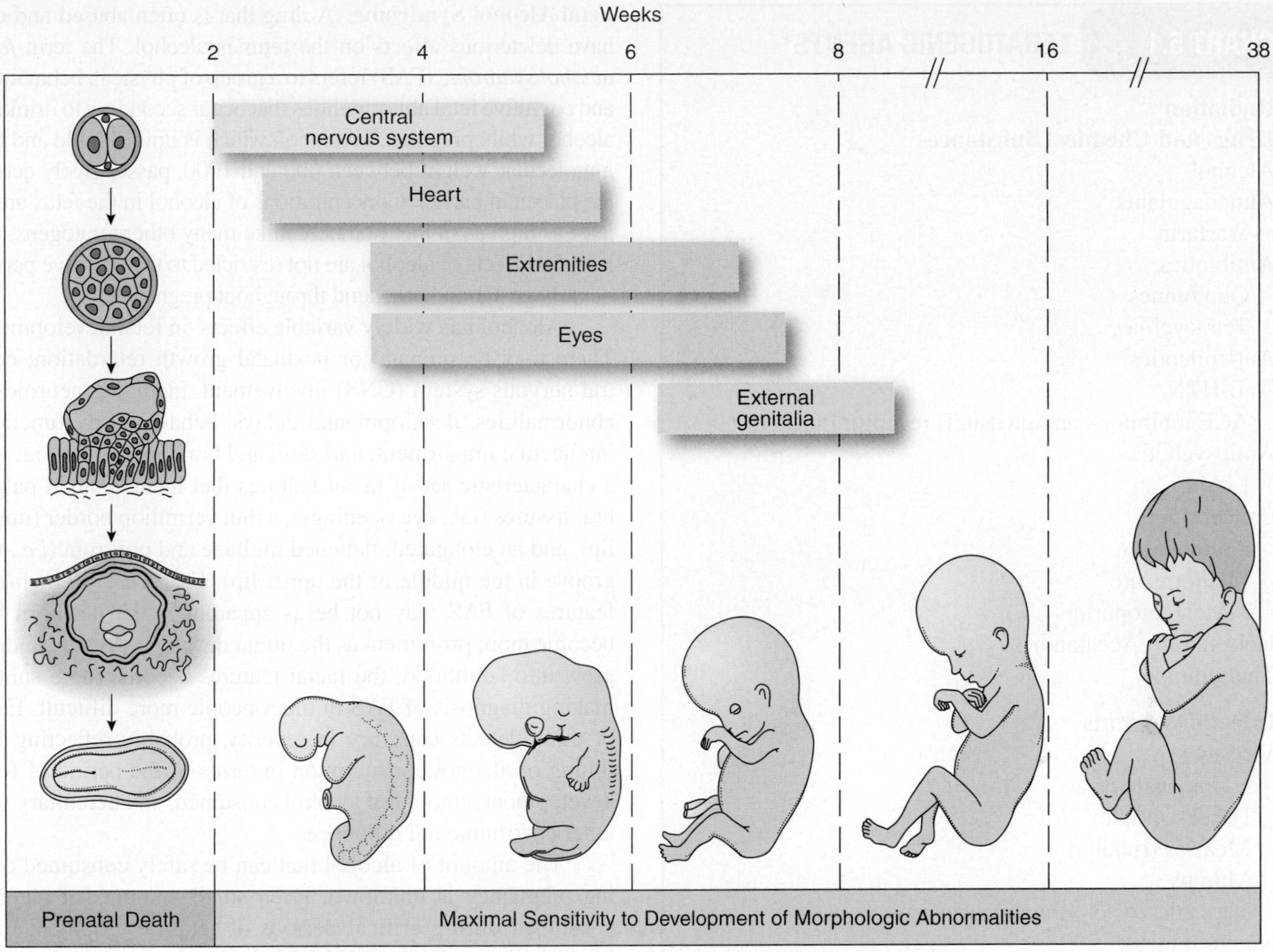

Figure 5.12 • Sensitivity of specific organs to teratogenic agents at critical periods in embryogenesis. Exposure to adverse influences in the preimplantation and early postimplantation stages of development (*far left*) leads to prenatal death. Periods of maximal sensitivity to teratogens (*horizontal bars*) vary for different organ systems, but overall are limited to the first 8 weeks of pregnancy. (From Strayer D. S., Rubin E. (Eds.) (2015). *Rubin's pathology: Clinicopathologic foundations of medicine* (7th ed., Fig. 6-2, p. 246). Philadelphia, PA: Lippincott Williams & Wilkins.)

In situations where a study is necessary for the woman's health, the benefits to her of having proper diagnostic imaging must outweigh potential theoretical risks to the fetus.

Chemicals and Drugs

Environmental chemicals and drugs can cross the placenta and cause damage to the developing embryo and fetus. Some of the best-documented environmental teratogens are the organic mercurials, which cause neurologic deficits and blindness. Certain fish and water sources may be contaminated by mercury. The precise mechanisms by which chemicals and drugs exert their teratogenic effects are largely unknown. They may produce cytotoxic (cell killing), antimetabolic, or growth-inhibiting effects to the embryonic and fetal development.

Drugs top the list of chemical teratogens. Many drugs can cross the placenta and expose the fetus to both the pharmacologic and teratogenic effects. Factors that affect placental drug transfer and drug effects on the fetus include the rate at which the drug crosses the placenta, the duration of exposure, and the stage of placental and fetal development at the time of exposure.[19] Lipid-soluble drugs tend to cross the placenta more readily and enter the fetal circulation. The molecular weight of a drug also influences the rate and amount of drug transferred across the placenta.

Several medications have been considered teratogenic. However, perhaps the best known of these drugs is thalidomide, which has been shown to give rise to a full range of malformations, including phocomelia (*i.e.*, short, flipper-like appendages) of all four extremities. Other drugs known to cause fetal abnormalities are those used in the treatment of cancer, the anticoagulant drug warfarin, several of the anticonvulsant drugs, ethyl alcohol, and cocaine. Some drugs affect a single developing structure; for example, propylthiouracil can impair thyroid development and tetracycline can interfere with the mineralization phase of tooth development. More recently, vitamin A and its derivatives (the retinoids)

CHART 5.1 TERATOGENIC AGENTS*

Radiation
Drugs and Chemical Substances
Alcohol
Anticoagulants
  Warfarin
Antibiotics
  Quinolones
  Tetracycline
Antiepileptics
Anti-HTN
  ACE inhibitors, angiotensin II receptor blockers
Antipsychotics
  Lithium
Cancer drugs
  Aminopterin
  Methotrexate
  6-Mercaptopurine
Isotretinoin (Accutane)
Thalidomide

Infectious Agents
Viruses
  Cytomegalovirus
  Herpes simplex virus
  Measles (rubella)
  Mumps
  Varicella-zoster virus (chickenpox)
Nonviral factors
  Syphilis
  Toxoplasmosis

*Not inclusive.

have been targeted for concern because of their teratogenic potential. Concern over the teratogenic effects of vitamin A derivatives arose with the introduction of the acne drug isotretinoin (Accutane).

In 1983, the U.S. Food and Drug Administration established a system for classifying drugs according to probable risks to the fetus. According to this system, drugs are put into five categories: A, B, C, D, and X. Drugs in category A are the least dangerous, and categories B, C, and D are increasingly more dangerous. Those in category X are contraindicated during pregnancy because of proven teratogenicity.[19]

Because many drugs are suspected of causing fetal abnormalities, and even those that were once thought to be safe are now being viewed critically, it is recommended that women in their childbearing years avoid unnecessary use of drugs. This pertains to nonpregnant women as well as pregnant women because many developmental defects occur early in pregnancy. As happened with thalidomide, the damage to the embryo may occur before pregnancy is suspected or confirmed.

Fetal Alcohol Syndrome. A drug that is often abused and can have deleterious effects on the fetus is alcohol. The term *fetal alcohol syndrome* (FAS) refers to a group of physical, behavioral, and cognitive fetal abnormalities that occur secondary to drinking alcohol while pregnant.[20] Alcohol, which is lipid soluble and has a molecular weight between 600 and 1000, passes freely across the placental barrier. Concentrations of alcohol in the fetus are at least as high as in the mother. Unlike many other teratogens, the harmful effects of alcohol are not restricted to the sensitive period of early gestation but extend throughout pregnancy.

Alcohol has widely variable effects on fetal development. There may be prenatal or postnatal growth retardation; central nervous system (CNS) involvement, including neurologic abnormalities, developmental delays, behavioral dysfunction, intellectual impairment, and skull and brain malformation; and a characteristic set of facial features that include small palpebral fissures (*i.e.*, eye openings), a thin vermilion border (upper lip), and an elongated, flattened midface and philtrum (*i.e.*, the groove in the middle of the upper lip) (Fig. 5.13).[20] The facial features of FAS may not be as apparent in the newborn but become more prominent as the infant develops. As the children grow into adulthood, the facial features become more subtle, making diagnosis of FAS in older people more difficult. Each of these defects can vary in severity, probably reflecting the timing of alcohol consumption in terms of the period of fetal development, amount of alcohol consumed, and hereditary and other environmental influences.

The amount of alcohol that can be safely consumed during pregnancy is unknown. Even small amounts of alcohol consumed during critical periods of fetal development may be teratogenic. For example, if alcohol is consumed during the period of organogenesis, a variety of skeletal and organ defects may result. If alcohol is consumed later in gestation, when the brain is undergoing rapid development, there may be behavioral and cognitive disorders in the absence of physical abnormalities. Chronic alcohol consumption throughout

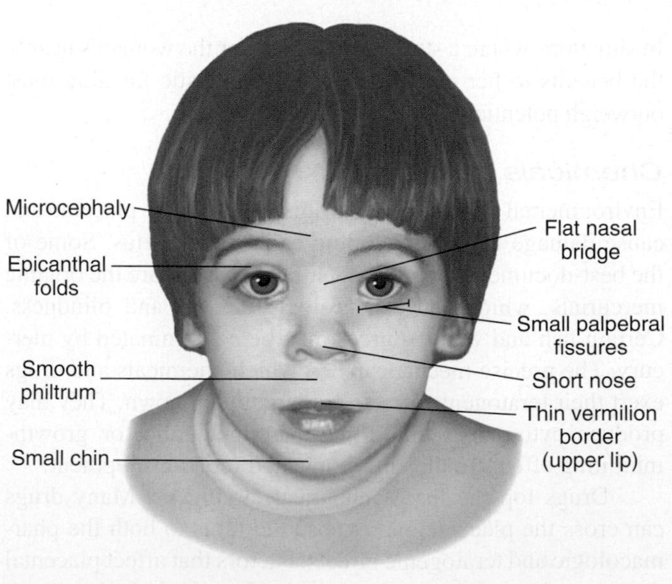

Figure 5.13 • Clinical features of fetal alcohol syndrome.

pregnancy may result in a variety of effects, ranging from physical abnormalities to growth retardation and compromised CNS functioning. Evidence suggests that short-lived high concentrations of alcohol, such as those that occur with binge drinking, may be particularly significant, with abnormalities being unique to the period of exposure.[20] Because of the possible effect on the fetus, it is recommended that women abstain completely from alcohol during pregnancy.

KEY POINTS

TERATOGENIC AGENTS

- Teratogenic agents such as radiation, chemicals and drugs, and infectious organisms are agents that produce abnormalities in the developing embryo.
- The stage of development of the embryo determines the susceptibility to teratogens. The period during which the embryo is most susceptible to teratogenic agents is the time during which rapid differentiation and development of body organs and tissues are taking place, usually from days 15 to 60 postconception.

Infectious Agents

Many microorganisms cross the placenta and enter the fetal circulation, often producing multiple malformations. The acronym TORCH stands for *t*oxoplasmosis, *o*ther, *r*ubella (*i.e.*, German measles), *c*ytomegalovirus, and *h*erpes, which are the agents most frequently implicated in fetal anomalies.[21] Other infections that can cause fetal anomalies include varicella-zoster virus infection, listeriosis, leptospirosis, Epstein-Barr virus infection, tuberculosis, and syphilis.[21] Human immunodeficiency virus (HIV) and human parvovirus (B19) have been suggested as other potential additions to the list. Common clinical and pathologic manifestations include growth retardation and abnormalities of the brain (microcephaly, hydrocephalus), eye, ear, liver, hematopoietic system (anemia, thrombocytopenia), lungs (pneumonitis), and heart (myocarditis, congenital heart disorders).[21] These manifestations will vary among symptomatic newborns, however, and only a few present with multisystem abnormalities.

Folic Acid Deficiency

Although most birth defects are related to exposure to a teratogenic agent, deficiencies of nutrients and vitamins also may be a factor. Folic acid deficiency has been implicated in the development of neural tube defects (NTDs) (*e.g.*, anencephaly, spina bifida, encephalocele). Studies have shown a significant decrease in NTDs when folic acid was taken long term by women of reproductive age.[22] Therefore, it is recommended that all women of childbearing age receive 400 μg (0.4 mg) of folic acid daily and then continue upon becoming pregnant.

IN SUMMARY

A teratogenic agent is one that produces abnormalities during embryonic or fetal life. It is during the early part of pregnancy (15 to 60 days after conception) that environmental agents are most apt to produce their deleterious effects on the developing embryo. A number of environmental agents can be damaging to the unborn child, including radiation, drugs and chemicals, and infectious agents. Because many drugs have the potential for causing fetal abnormalities, often at an early stage of pregnancy, it is recommended that women of childbearing age avoid unnecessary use of drugs.

DIAGNOSIS AND COUNSELING

After completing this section of the chapter, the learner will be able to meet the following objectives:

- Describe the process of genetic assessment.
- Describe methods used in arriving at a prenatal diagnosis, including ultrasonography, amniocentesis, chorionic villus sampling, percutaneous umbilical fetal blood sampling, and laboratory methods to determine the biochemical and genetic makeup of the fetus.

The birth of a child with a congenital defect is a traumatic event in any parent's life. Usually, two issues must be resolved. The first deals with the immediate and future care of the affected child and the second with the possibility of future children in the family having a similar defect. Genetic assessment and counseling can help to determine whether the defect was inherited and the risk of recurrence. Prenatal diagnosis provides a means of determining whether an unborn child has certain types of abnormalities. It is important that the parents are aware of the potential complications of acquiring more information from these genetic tests.

Genetic Assessment

Effective genetic counseling requires accurate diagnosis and communication of the findings and of the risks of recurrence to the parents and other family members who need such information. Counseling may be provided after the birth of an affected child, or it may be offered to people that are at higher risk for having an affected child. A team of trained counselors can help the family to understand the problem and can support educated decisions about whether or not to have more children.

Assessment of genetic risk and prognosis usually is directed by a clinical geneticist, often with the aid of laboratory and clinical specialists. A detailed family history (*i.e.*, pedigree), a pregnancy history, and detailed accounts of the birth process and postnatal health and development are included. A careful physical examination of the affected child and often of the parents and siblings usually is needed. Laboratory tests, including chromosomal analysis and biochemical studies, often precede a definitive diagnosis.

Prenatal Screening and Diagnosis

The purpose of prenatal screening and diagnosis is not just to detect fetal abnormalities but also to allay anxiety and provide assistance to prepare for a child with a specific disability. Prenatal screening cannot be used to rule out all possible fetal abnormalities. It is limited to determining whether the fetus has (or probably has) predesignated conditions as indicated by late maternal age, family history, or well-defined risk factors.

There are multiple methods that can assist in diagnosing a fetus regarding genetic disorders, including ultrasonography, maternal serum (blood) screening tests, amniocentesis, chorionic villus sampling, and percutaneous umbilical fetal blood sampling (Fig. 5.14). Prenatal diagnosis can also provide the information needed for prescribing prenatal treatment for the fetus or making appropriate plans for the birth of a child with a known disease.

Ultrasonography

Ultrasonography is a noninvasive diagnostic method that uses reflections of high-frequency sound waves to visualize soft tissue structures. Since its introduction in 1958, it has been used during pregnancy to determine the number of fetuses, fetal size and position, amount of amniotic fluid, and placental location. But improved resolution and real-time units have enhanced the ability of ultrasound scanners to detect congenital anomalies. Ultrasonography makes possible the in utero diagnosis of cardiac defects, hydrocephalus, spina bifida, facial defects, congenital heart defects, congenital diaphragmatic hernias, disorders of the gastrointestinal tract, skeletal anomalies, and various other defects. Three-dimensional (3D) sonography has become useful in better assessing facial profiles and abdominal wall defects. A fetal echocardiogram can be done as follow-up for possible cardiac anomalies. Fetal magnetic resonance imaging (MRI) can be done to better assess skeletal, neurologic, and other anomalies. Intrauterine diagnosis of congenital abnormalities permits better monitoring, further workup and planning with appropriate specialties, preterm delivery for early correction, selection of cesarean section to reduce fetal injury, and, in some cases, intrauterine therapy.

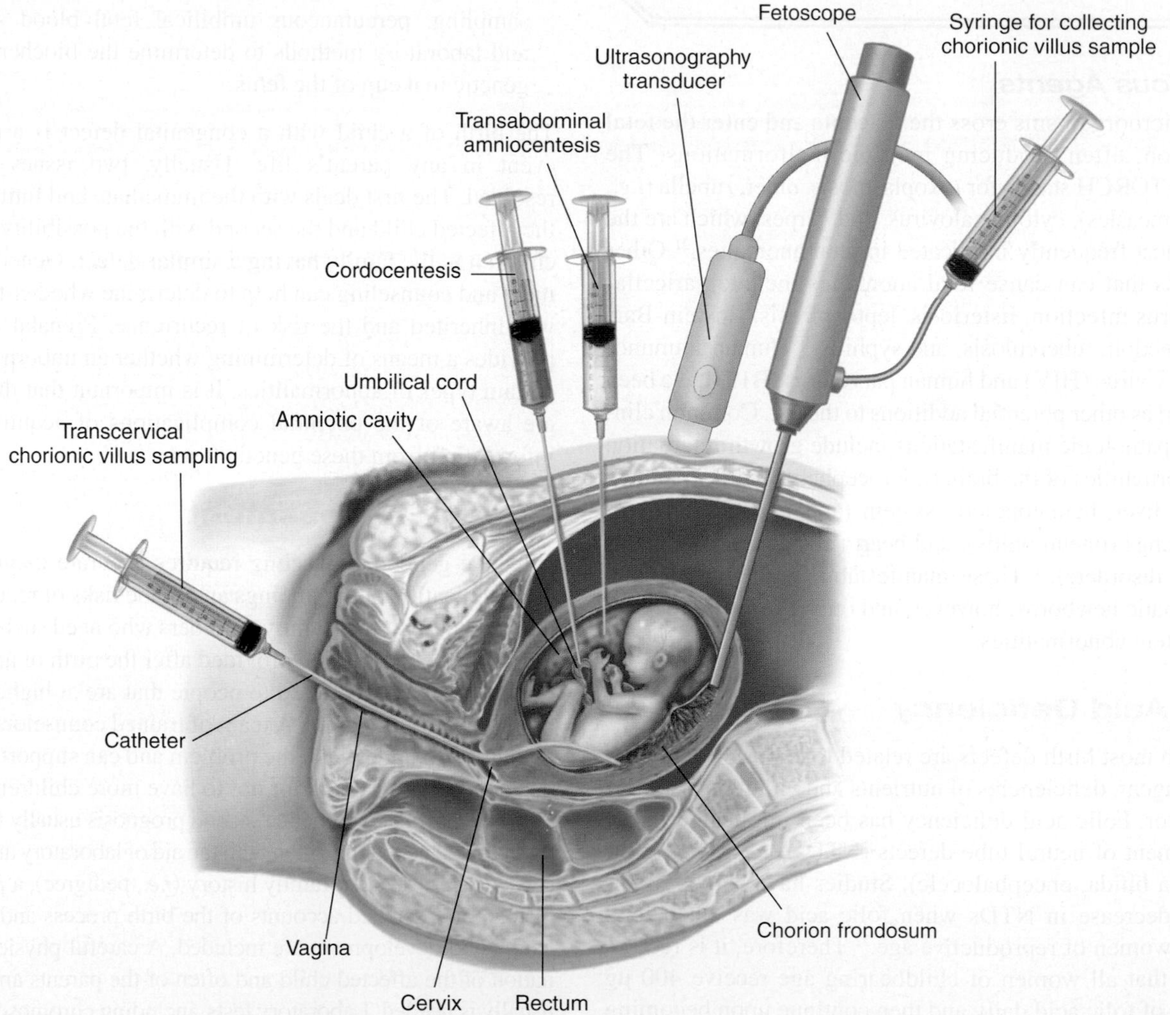

Figure 5.14 • Methods of prenatal screening.

Maternal Serum Markers

Maternal blood testing began in the early 1980s. Since that time, a number of serum factors have been studied as screening tests for fetal anomalies.

Current maternal testing favors first trimester screening for all women between 11 and 13 weeks combining nuchal translucency seen on sonogram with PAPP-A level, hCG level, and maternal age to determine a risk for trisomy 21, 13, and 18. PAPP-A, which is secreted by the placenta, has been shown to play an important role in promoting cell differentiation and proliferation in various body systems. In complicated pregnancies, the PAPP-A concentration increases with gestational age until term. Decreased PAPP-A levels in the first trimester (between 10 and 13 weeks) are associated with Down syndrome. When used along with maternal age, free β-hCG, and ultrasonographic measurement of nuchal translucency, serum PAPP-A levels can reportedly detect 85% to 95% of affected pregnancies with a false-positive rate of approximately 5%.

AFP is a major fetal plasma protein and has a structure similar to the albumin found in postnatal life. AFP is made initially by the yolk sac, gastrointestinal tract, and liver. Fetal plasma levels of AFP peak at approximately 10 to 13 weeks' gestation and decrease until the third trimester when the level peaks again. Maternal and amniotic fluid levels of AFP are elevated in pregnancies where the fetus has an NTD (*i.e.*, anencephaly and open spina bifida) or certain other malformations such as an anterior abdominal wall defect in which the fetal integument is not intact. Although NTDs have been associated with elevated levels of AFP, decreased levels have been associated with Down syndrome.

A complex glycoprotein, hCG, is produced exclusively by the outer layer of the trophoblast shortly after implantation in the uterine wall. It increases rapidly in the first 8 weeks of gestation, declines steadily until 20 weeks, and then plateaus. The single maternal serum marker that yields the highest detection rate for Down syndrome is an elevated level of hCG. Inhibin A, which is secreted by the corpus luteum and fetoplacental unit, is also a maternal serum marker for fetal Down syndrome.

Unconjugated estriol is produced by the placenta from precursors provided by the fetal adrenal glands and liver. It increases steadily throughout pregnancy to a higher level than that normally produced by the liver. Unconjugated estriol levels are decreased in Down syndrome and trisomy 18.

KEY POINTS

DIAGNOSIS AND COUNSELING

- Sonography, first trimester screening, quad screening, amniocentesis, chorionic villi sampling, and percutaneous umbilical cord blood sampling (PUBS) are important procedures that allow prenatal diagnosis and management.

Amniocentesis

Amniocentesis is an invasive diagnostic procedure that involves the withdrawal of a sample of amniotic fluid from the pregnant uterus usually using a transabdominal approach (see Fig. 5.14). The procedure is useful in women with elevated risk on first trimester screen or quad screen, abnormal fetal findings on sonogram, or in parents who are carriers or with a strong family history of an inherited disease. Ultrasonography is used to gain additional information and to guide the placement of the amniocentesis needle. The amniotic fluid and cells that have been shed by the fetus are studied. Amniocentesis can be performed on an outpatient basis starting at 15 weeks. For chromosomal analysis, the fetal cells are grown in culture and the result is available in 10 to 14 days.

Chorionic Villus Sampling

Chorionic villus sampling is an invasive diagnostic procedure that obtains tissue that can be used for fetal chromosome studies, DNA analysis, and biochemical studies. Sampling of the chorionic villi usually is done after 10 weeks of gestation. Performing the test before 10 weeks is not recommended because of the danger of limb reduction defects in the fetus. The chorionic villi are the site of exchange of nutrients between the maternal blood and the embryo—the chorionic sac encloses the early amniotic sac and fetus, and the villi are the primitive blood vessels that develop into the placenta. The sampling procedure can be performed using either a transabdominal or transcervical approach (see Fig. 5.14).

Percutaneous Umbilical Cord Blood Sampling

PUBS is an invasive diagnostic procedure that involves the transcutaneous insertion of a needle through the uterine wall and into the umbilical artery. It is performed under ultrasonographic guidance and can be done any time after 16 weeks of gestation. It is used for prenatal diagnosis of hemoglobinopathies, coagulation disorders, metabolic and cytogenetic disorders, and immunodeficiencies. Fetal infections such as rubella and toxoplasmosis can be detected through measurement of immunoglobulin M antibodies or direct blood cultures. Because the procedure carries a greater risk of pregnancy loss compared to amniocentesis, it usually is reserved for situations in which rapid cytogenetic analysis is needed or in which diagnostic information cannot be obtained by other methods.

Cytogenetic and DNA Analyses

Amniocentesis and chorionic villus sampling yield cells that can be used for cytogenetic and DNA analyses. Cytogenetic studies are used for fetal karyotyping to detect abnormalities of chromosome number and structure in the fetus. Karyotyping also reveals the sex of the fetus. This may be useful when an inherited defect is known to affect only one sex.

Analysis of DNA can be done on cells extracted from the amniotic fluid, chorionic villi, or fetal blood from percutaneous umbilical sampling. These analyses are used to detect genetic defects that cause inborn errors of metabolism, such as Tay-Sachs disease, glycogen storage diseases, and familial hypercholesterolemia. Prenatal diagnoses are possible for more than 70 inborn errors of metabolism.

The newest realm of fetal diagnosis involves looking at fetal DNA in the maternal blood. Some private companies and many research institutions are exploring the efficacy of looking at fetal DNA for sex determination and other genetic testing. More research is needed before this will be offered to all women.

IN SUMMARY

Genetic and prenatal diagnosis and counseling are done in an effort to determine the risk of having a child with a genetic or chromosomal disorder. They often involve a detailed family history (*i.e.*, pedigree), examination of any affected and other family members, and laboratory studies including chromosomal analysis and biochemical studies. These exams are usually done by a genetic counselor and a specially prepared team of health care professionals. Prenatal screening and diagnosis are used to detect fetal abnormalities. Ultrasonography is used for fetal anatomic imaging. It is used for determination of fetal size and position and for the presence of structural anomalies. Maternal serum screening is used to identify pregnancies that are at increased risk for some disorders. Amniocentesis and chorionic villus sampling may be used to obtain specimens for cytogenetic and biochemical studies.

GERIATRIC Considerations

- Aging is an important risk factor for development of Parkinson's disease.
- Parkinson disease has been found to have a genetic component. Mutations in certain genes (such as LRRK2, PARK7, PINK1, PRKN, SNCA) are strongly associated with the development of Parkinson's disease; whereas, alterations in other genes (GBA, UCHL1) only increase the lifetime risk for developing the condition.[23]
- Genetic risks associated with normal cognitive aging and Alzheimer disease, AD, interact to predict susceptibility for dementia.[24]

PEDIATRIC Considerations

- In more than 67% of birth defects, the exact cause is not immediately known.[21]
- For comparison, the majority of morbidities in infants and children from developed countries are caused by genetic defects; whereas, 95% of infant deaths in underdeveloped countries are due to infection, malnutrition, and other environmental causes.[21]
- Mitochondrial disorders are passed from the mother to all her children due to mutations in the mitochondrial DNA. Prognosis depends on the number of organ systems involved.[25]

REVIEW EXERCISES

1. A 23-year-old woman with sickle cell disease and her husband want to have a child but worry that the child will be born with the disease.
   A. *What is the mother's genotype in terms of the sickle cell gene? Is she heterozygous or homozygous?*
   B. *If the husband is found not to have the sickle cell gene, what is the probability of their child having the disease or being a carrier of the sickle cell trait?*
2. A couple has a child who was born with a congenital heart disease.
   A. *Would you consider the defect to be the result of a single gene or a polygenic trait?*
   B. *Would these parents be at greater risk of having another child with a heart defect or would they be at equal risk of having a child with a defect in another organ system, such as cleft palate?*
3. A couple has been informed that their newborn child has the features of Down syndrome, and it is suggested that genetic studies be performed.
   A. *The child is found to have trisomy 21. Use Figure 5.8, which describes the events that occur during meiosis, to explain the origin of the third chromosome 21.*
   B. *If the child had been found to have the robertsonian chromosome, how would you explain the origin of the abnormal chromosome?*
4. An 8-year-old boy has been diagnosed with mitochondrial myopathy. His major complaints are those of muscle weakness and exercise intolerance. His mother gives a report of similar symptoms, but to a much lesser degree.
   A. *Explain the cause of this boy's symptoms.*
   B. *Mitochondrial disorders follow a nonmendelian pattern of inheritance. Explain.*

5. A 26-year-old woman is planning to become pregnant.
   A. *What information would you give her regarding the effects of medications and drugs on the fetus? What stage of fetal development is associated with the greatest risk?*
   B. *What is the rationale for ensuring that she has an adequate intake of folic acid before conception?*

References

1. Centers for Disease C. (2007). Birth defects and congenital abnormalities. Available: https://www.cdc.gov/nchs/fastats/birth-defects.htm Accessed November 15, 2017.
2. Malik S. (2014). Polydactyly: Phenotypes, genetics and classification. *Clinical Genetics* 85(3), 203–212. doi: 10.1111/cge.12276.
3. Verstraeten A., Alaerts M., Van Laer L., et al. (2016). Marfan syndrome and related disorders: 25 years of gene discovery. *Human Mutation* 37(6), 524–531. doi: 10.1002/humu.22977.
4. Hirbe A. C., Gutmann D. H. (2014). Neurofibromatosis type 1: A multidisciplinary approach to care. *Lancet Neurology* 13(8), 834–843. doi: 10.1016/S1474-4422(14)70063-8.
5. Kresak J. L., Walsh M. (2016). Neurofibromatosis: A review of NF1, NF2, and schwannomatosis. *Journal of Pediatric Genetics* 5(2), 98–104. doi: 10.1055/s-0036-1579766.
6. Abdolrahimzadeh B., Piraino D. C., Albanese G., et al. (2016). Neurofibromatosis: An update of ophthalmic characteristics and applications of optical coherence tomography. *Clinical Ophthalmology* 10, 851–860. doi: 10.2147/OPTH.S102830.
7. Bernier A., Larbrisseau A., Perreault S. (2016). Cafe-au-lait macules and neurofibromatosis type 1: A review of the literature. *Pediatric Neurology* 60, 24–29 e1. doi: 10.1016/j.pediatrneurol.2016.03.003.
8. Al Hafid N., Christodoulou J. (2015). Phenylketonuria: A review of current and future treatments. *Translational Pediatrics* 4(4), 304–317. doi: 10.3978/j.issn.2224-4336.2015.10.07.
9. Berry S. A., Brown C., Grant M., et al. (2013). Newborn screening 50 years later: Access issues faced by adults with PKU. *Genetics in Medicine* 5(8), 591–599. doi: 10.1038/gim.2013.10.
10. Patterson M. C. (2013). Gangliosidoses. *Handbook of Clinical Neurology* 113, 1707–1708. doi: 10.1016/B978-0-444-59565-2.00039-3.
11. Lew R. M., Burnett L., Proos A. L., et al. (2015). Ashkenazi Jewish population screening for Tay-Sachs disease: The international and Australian experience. *Journal of Paediatrics and Child Health* 51(3), 271–279. doi: 10.1111/jpc.12632.
12. Kidd S. A., Lachiewicz A., Barbouth D., et al. (2014). Fragile X syndrome: A review of associated medical problems. *Pediatrics* 134(5), 995–1005. doi: 10.1542/peds.2013-4301.
13. Bagni C, Oostra B. A. (2013). Fragile X syndrome: From protein function to therapy. *American Journal of Medical Genetics. Part A* 161A(11), 2809–2821. doi: 10.1002/ajmg.a.36241.
14. Seto-Salvia N., Stanier P. (2014). Genetics of cleft lip and/or cleft palate: Association with other common anomalies. *European Journal of Medical Genetics* 57(8), 381–393. doi: 10.1016/j.ejmg.2014.04.003.
15. Smith D. M., Losee J. E. (2014). Cleft palate repair. *Clinics in Plastic Surgery* 41(2), 189–210. doi: 10.1016/j.cps.2013.12.005.
16. Asim A., Kumar A., Muthuswamy S., et al. (2015). Down syndrome: An insight of the disease. *Journal of Biomedical Science* 22, 41. doi: 10.1186/s12929-015-0138-y.
17. Milbrandt T., Thomas E. (2013). Turner syndrome. *Pediatrics in Review* 34(9), 420–421. doi: 10.1542/pir.34-9-420.
18. Groth K. A., Skakkebaek A., Host C., et al. (2013). Clinical review: Klinefelter syndrome—A clinical update. *Journal of Clinical Endocrinology and Metabolism* 98(1), 20–30. doi: 10.1210/jc.2012-2382.
19. Burkey B. W., Holmes A. P. (2013). Evaluating medication use in pregnancy and lactation: What every pharmacist should know. *Journal of Pediatric Pharmacology and Therapeutics* 18(3), 247–258. doi: 10.5863/1551-6776-18.3.247.
20. Memo L., Gnoato E., Caminiti S. (2013). Fetal alcohol spectrum disorders and fetal alcohol syndrome: The state of the art and new diagnostic tools. *Early Human Development* 89(Suppl 1), S40–S43. doi: 10.1016/S0378-3782(13)70013-6.
21. Strayer D. S., Rubin E. (Eds.) (2015). *Rubin's pathology: Clinicopathologic foundations of medicine* (7th ed). Philadelphia, PA: Wolters Kluwer.
22. Burdge G. C., Lillycrop K. A. 2012. Folic acid supplementation in pregnancy: Are there devils in the detail? *British Journal of Nutrition* 108(11), 1924–1930. doi: 10.1017/S0007114512003765.
23. NIH. (2018). Parkinson disease. Retrieved July 18, 2018. Available: https://ghr.nlm.nih.gov/condition/parkinson-disease#inheritance.
24. Sapkota S., Dixon, R. A. (2018). A network of genetic effects on non-demented cognitive aging: Alzheimer's genetic risk (CLU + CR1+PICALM) intensifies cognitive aging genetic risk (COMT + BDNF) selectively for APOEε4 carriers. *Journal of Alzheimer's Disease* 62(2), 887–900. doi: 10.3233/JAD-170909.
25. Goodhue C. J. (2014). The child with an inborn error of metabolism. In Bowden V. R., Greenberg, C. S. (Eds). *Children and their families the continuum of nursing care*. Philadelphia, PA: Wolters Kluwer.

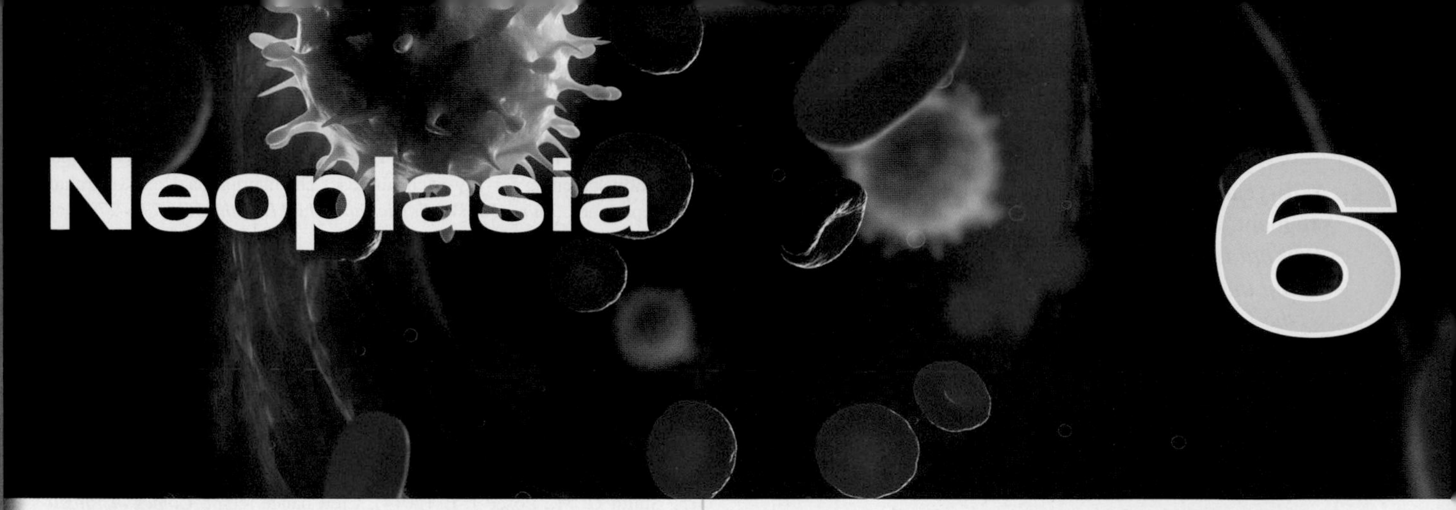

Neoplasia 6

Michelle Rickard

Cancer is a leading cause of death in adults worldwide, second only to cardiovascular disease.[1] It is the second leading cause of death in school-aged children in the United States.[2] Exposure to external factors such as tobacco, ultraviolet radiation, unhealthy diet, infectious agents, and carcinogens as well as internal factors such as gender, ethnicity, and genetics affect incidence of cancer.[3] Research has led to an enhanced understanding of the causes of cancer and improved screening tools and prevention modalities.[3] Survival rates are affected by the type of cancer, stage at diagnosis, and what or if treatment is available.[4]

This chapter is divided into six sections:

- Concepts of cell differentiation and growth
- Characteristics of benign and malignant neoplasms
- Etiology of cancer
- Clinical manifestations
- Diagnosis and treatment
- Childhood cancers

CONCEPTS OF CELL DIFFERENTIATION AND GROWTH

After completing this section of the chapter, the learner will be able to meet the following objectives:

- Define *neoplasm* and explain how neoplastic growth differs from the normal adaptive changes seen in atrophy, hypertrophy, and hyperplasia.
- Describe the phases of the cell cycle.

Cancer is a disorder of altered cell differentiation and growth. The resulting process is called *neoplasia*, which means "new growth." Unlike changes in tissue growth that occur with hypertrophy and hyperplasia, the growth of a neoplasm tends to be uncoordinated and relatively autonomous in that it lacks normal regulatory controls over cell growth and division.

Normal tissue renewal and repair involves two components: cell proliferation and differentiation. **Proliferation**, or the process of cell division, is an adaptive process for new cell growth to replace old cells or when additional cells are needed.[5,6] Differentiation describes the mechanism by which cells become increasingly more specialized with each mitotic division.[5,6] Apoptosis is a form of programmed cell death that eliminates senescent cells, cells with deoxyribonucleic acid (DNA) damage, or unwanted cells.[5,6]

The Cell Cycle

The cell cycle is an orderly sequence of events that occur as a cell duplicates its contents and divides (Fig. 6.1). During the cell cycle, genetic information is duplicated and the duplicated chromosomes are appropriately aligned for distribution between two genetically identical daughter cells.

The cell cycle is divided into four phases, referred to as G_1, S, G_2, and M. *G_1 (gap 1)* occurs after the postmitosis phase when DNA synthesis stops and ribonucleic acid (RNA) and protein synthesis and cell growth take place.[5,6] During the *S phase*, DNA synthesis occurs, causing two separate sets of chromosomes to develop, one for each daughter cell. *G_2 (gap 2)* is the premitotic phase and is similar to G_1 in that DNA synthesis stops, but RNA and protein synthesis continue. The phases, G_1, S, and G_2 are referred to as *interphase*. The *M phase* is the phase of nuclear division, or mitosis, and cytoplasmic division. Continually dividing cells, such as the skin's stratified squamous epithelium, continue to cycle from one mitotic division to the next. When environmental conditions are adverse, such as nutrient or growth factor unavailability, or when cells are highly specialized, cells may leave the cell cycle, becoming mitotically quiescent, and reside in a resting state known as *G_0*. Cells in G_0 may re-enter the cell cycle in response to extracellular nutrients, growth factors, hormones, and other signals such as blood loss or tissue injury that trigger cell growth.[7] Highly specialized and terminally differentiated cells, such as neurons, may permanently stay in G_0.

Within the cell cycle, pauses can be made if the specific events of the cell cycle phases have not been completed. For example, mitosis is prevented until DNA is properly replicated. In addition, chromosome separation in mitosis is delayed until all spindle fibers have attached to the chromosomes. These are opportunities for checking the accuracy of DNA replication. These DNA damage checkpoints allow for any defects to be identified and repaired, thereby ensuring that each daughter cell receives a full complement of genetic information, identical to that of the parent cell.[6]

The cyclins are a group of proteins that control the entry and progression of cells through the cell cycle. Cyclins bind to proteins called *cyclin-dependent kinases* (CDKs). Kinases are enzymes that phosphorylate proteins. The CDKs phosphorylate specific target proteins and are expressed continuously during the cell cycle but in an inactive form, whereas the cyclins are synthesized during specific phases of the cell cycle

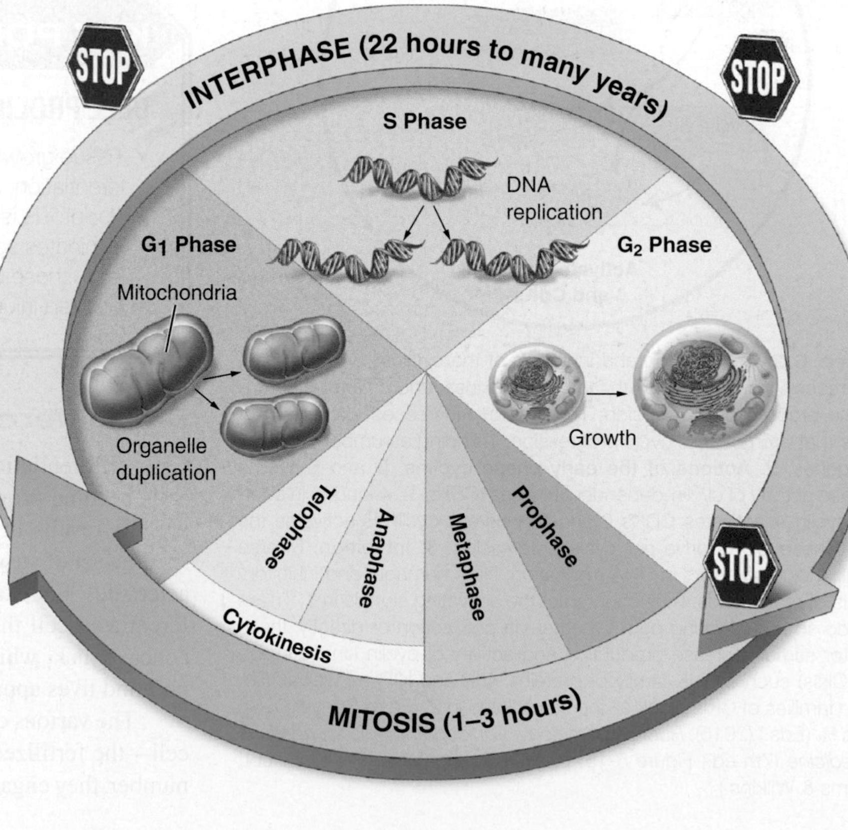

Figure 6.1 • Cell cycle. The cell cycle's four steps are illustrated beginning with G_1 and proceeding to M. The first growth phase (G_1), DNA synthesis phase (S), second growth phase (G_2), and mitosis (M) are illustrated. (From McConnell T. H., Hull K. L. (2011). *Human form, human function: Essentials of anatomy & physiology* (p. 77, Figure 3.10). Philadelphia, PA: Lippincott Williams & Wilkins.)

and then degraded by ubiquitination once their task is completed.[7] Although each phase of the cell cycle is monitored carefully, the transition from G_2 to M is considered to be one of the most important checkpoints in the cell cycle. In addition to the synthesis and degradation of the cyclins, the cyclin–CDK complexes are regulated by the binding of CDK inhibitors (CKIs). The CKIs are particularly important in regulating cell cycle checkpoints during which mistakes in DNA replication are repaired.[8] Manipulation of cyclins, CDKs, and CKIs is the basis for development of newer forms of drug therapy that can be used in cancer treatment (Fig. 6.2).[9]

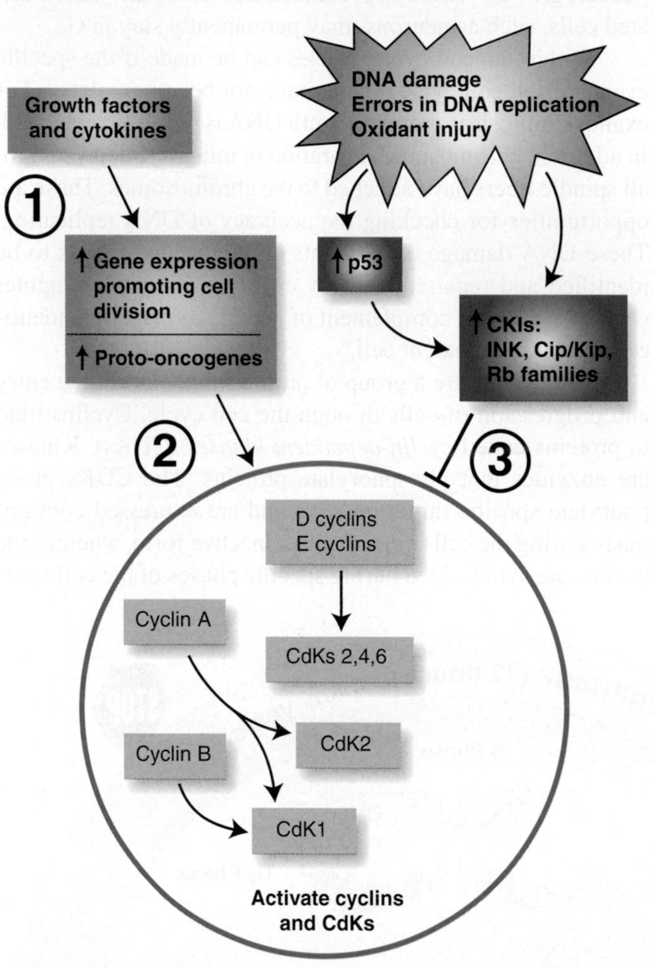

Figure 6.2 • Activation and inhibition of the cyclins. **1. Activation.** Cells receive signals via growth factors, cytokines, and so forth that trigger the process of cell division. This leads to increased expression of genes that promote cell cycle progression, including a number of proto-oncogenes. **2. Actions of the early-phase cyclins.** D and E cyclins increase activity of cyclin-dependent kinases (CDKs) 2, 4, and 6. In addition, cyclin A activates CDKs 2 and 1, whereas cyclin B activates the latter. These CDKs drive cell cycle progression. **3. Inhibition.** Diverse stimuli, including errors in DNA replication, DNA damage, and inhibitory signals of many kinds, may counteract the activating signals in **1**. These may do so by activating p53. Whether via p53 action or directly, these inhibitor stimuli increase production and activity of cyclin kinase inhibitors (CKIs) such as INK family of proteins, CIP and KIP, as well as Rb. These families of CKIs block all the steps listed in **2**. (From Strayer D. S., Rubin R. (Eds.) (2015). *Rubin's pathology: Clinicopathologic foundations of medicine* (7th ed., Figure 5-15, p. 179). Philadelphia, PA: Lippincott Williams & Wilkins.)

Cell Proliferation

Cell proliferation is the process of increasing cell numbers by mitotic cell division. In normal tissue, cell proliferation is regulated so that the number of cells actively dividing is equivalent to the number dying or being shed. In humans, there are two major categories of cells: gametes and somatic cells. The *gametes* (ovum and sperm) are *haploid*, having only one set of chromosomes from one parent, and are designed specifically for sexual fusion. After fusion, a diploid cell containing both sets of chromosomes is formed. This cell is the *somatic cell* that goes on to form the rest of the body.

In terms of cell proliferation, the 200 various cell types of the body can be divided into three large groups: (1) the well-differentiated neurons and cells of skeletal and cardiac muscle cells that rarely divide and reproduce; (2) the progenitor or parent cells that continue to divide and reproduce, such as blood cells, skin cells, and liver cells; and (3) the undifferentiated stem cells that can be triggered to enter the cell cycle and produce large numbers of progenitor cells if needed.[2] The rates of reproduction of cells vary greatly. White blood cells and cells that line the gastrointestinal tract live several days and must be replaced constantly. In most tissues, the rate of cell reproduction is greatly increased when tissue is injured or lost. Bleeding, for example, stimulates reproduction of the blood-forming cells of the bone marrow. In some types of tissue, the genetic program for cell replication normally is suppressed but can be reactivated under certain conditions. The liver, for example, has extensive regenerative capabilities under certain conditions.

KEY POINTS

CELL PROLIFERATION AND GROWTH

- Tissue growth and repair involve cell proliferation, differentiation, and apoptosis.
- Apoptosis is a form of programmed cell death that eliminates senescent and some types of injured cells (*e.g.*, those with DNA damage or hydrogen peroxide–induced injury).

Cell Differentiation

Cell differentiation is the process whereby proliferating cells become progressively more specialized cell types. This process results in a fully differentiated, adult cell that has a specific set of structural, functional, and life expectancy characteristics. For example, the red blood cell is a terminally differentiated cell that has been programmed to develop into a concave disk, which functions as a vehicle for oxygen transport and lives approximately 3 months.

The various cell types of the body originate from a single cell—the fertilized ovum. As the embryonic cells increase in number, they engage in a coordinated process of differentiation

Understanding The Cell Cycle

A cell reproduces by performing an orderly sequence of events called the *cell cycle*. The cell cycle is divided into four phases of unequal duration that include the (1) synthesis (S) and mitosis (M) phases that are separated by (2) two gaps (G_1 and G_2). There is also (3) a dormant phase (G_0) during which the cell may leave the cell cycle. Movement through each of these phases is mediated at (4) specific checkpoints that are controlled by specific enzymes and proteins called *cyclins*.

Synthesis and Mitosis

Synthesis (S) and mitosis (M) represent the two major phases of the cell cycle. The S phase, which takes about 10 to 12 hours, is the period of DNA synthesis and replication of the chromosomes. The M phase, which usually takes less than an hour, involves formation of the mitotic spindle and cell division with formation of two daughter cells.

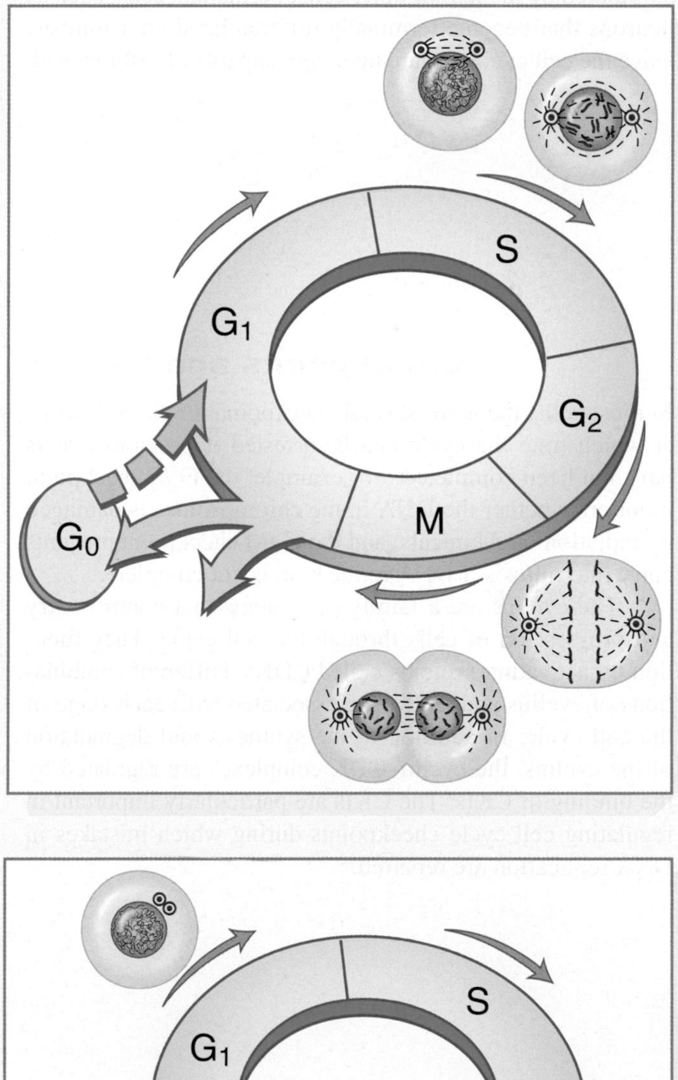

Gaps 1 and 2

Because most cells require time to grow and double their mass of proteins and organelles, extra gaps (G) are inserted into the cell cycle. G_1 is the stage during which the cell is starting to prepare for DNA replication and mitosis through protein synthesis and an increase in organelle and cytoskeletal elements. G_2 is the premitotic phase. During this phase, enzymes and other proteins needed for cell division are synthesized and moved to their proper sites.

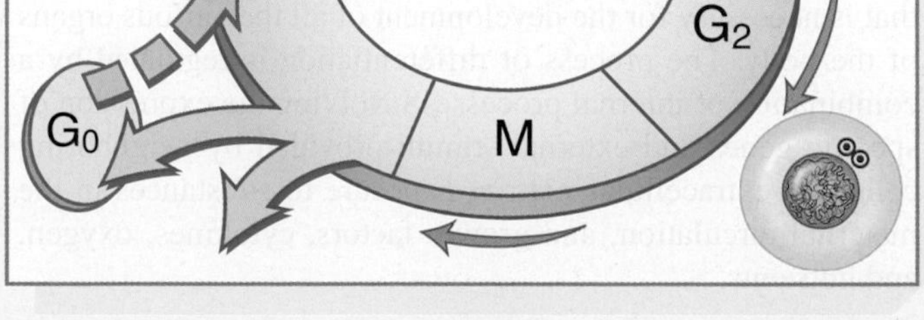

Continued

Understanding The Cell Cycle *(Continued)*

Gap O

G_0 is the stage after mitosis during which a cell may leave the cell cycle and either remain in a state of inactivity or re-enter the cell cycle at another time. Labile cells, such as blood cells and those that line the gastrointestinal tract, do not enter G_0 but continue cycling. Stable cells, such as hepatocytes, enter G_0 after mitosis but can re-enter the cell cycle when stimulated by the loss of other cells. Permanent cells, such as neurons that become terminally differentiated after mitosis, leave the cell cycle and are no longer capable of cell renewal.

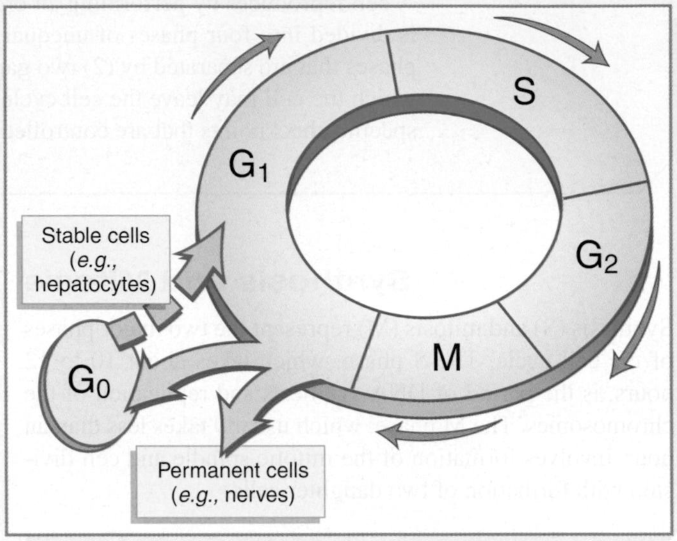

Checkpoints and Cyclins

In most cells, there are several checkpoints in the cell cycle, at which time the cycle can be arrested if previous events have not been completed. For example, the G_1/S checkpoint monitors whether the DNA in the chromosomes is damaged by radiation or chemicals, and the G_2/M checkpoint prevents entry into mitosis if DNA replication is not complete.

The cyclins are a family of proteins that control entry and progression of cells through the cell cycle. They function by activating proteins called CDKs. Different combinations of cyclins and CDKs are associated with each stage of the cell cycle. In addition to the synthesis and degradation of the cyclins, the cyclin–CDK complexes are regulated by the binding of CKIs. The CKIs are particularly important in regulating cell cycle checkpoints during which mistakes in DNA replication are repaired.

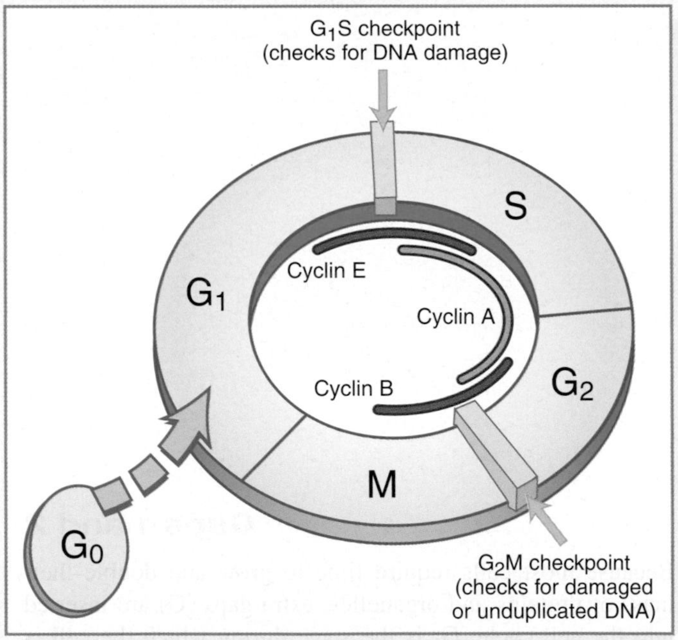

that is necessary for the development of all the various organs of the body. The process of differentiation is regulated by a combination of internal processes involving the expression of specific genes and external stimuli provided by neighboring cells, the extracellular matrix, exposure to substances in the maternal circulation, and growth factors, cytokines, oxygen, and nutrients.

What make the cells of one organ different from those of another organ are the specific genes that are expressed and the particular pattern of gene expression. Although all cells have the same complement of genes, only a small number of these genes are expressed in postnatal life. When cells, such as those of the developing embryo, differentiate and give rise to committed cells of a particular tissue type, the appropriate genes are maintained in an active state, whereas the rest remain inactive. Normally, the rate of cell reproduction and the process of cell differentiation are precisely controlled in prenatal and postnatal life so that both of these mechanisms cease once the appropriate numbers and types of cells are formed.

The process of differentiation occurs in orderly steps. With each progressive step, increased specialization is exchanged for a loss of ability to develop different cell characteristics and different cell types. As a cell becomes more highly specialized, the stimuli that are able to induce mitosis become more limited. Neurons, which are highly specialized cells, lose their ability to divide and reproduce once development of the nervous system is complete. More importantly, there are very few remaining precursor cells to direct their replacement. However, appropriate numbers of these cell types are generated in the embryo that loss of a certain percentage of cells does not affect the total cell population and specific functions.

In some tissues, such as the skin and mucosal lining of the gastrointestinal tract, a high degree of cell renewal continues throughout life. Even in these continuously renewing cell populations, the more specialized cells are unable to divide. These cell populations rely on *progenitor* or *parent cells* of the same lineage that have not yet differentiated to the extent that they have lost their ability to divide. These cells are sufficiently differentiated so that their daughter cells are limited to the same cell line, but they are insufficiently differentiated to preclude the potential for active proliferation. However, their cell renewal properties are restricted by growth factors required for cell division.

Another type of cell, called a *stem cell*, remains incompletely differentiated throughout life. Stem cells are reserve cells that remain dormant until there is a need for cell replacement, in which case they divide, producing other stem cells and cells that can carry out the functions of the differentiated cell. When a stem cell divides, one daughter cell retains the stem cell characteristics, and the other daughter cell becomes a progenitor cell that proceeds through a process that leads to terminal differentiation (Fig. 6.3). The progeny of each progenitor cell follows more restricted genetic programs, with the differentiating cells undergoing multiple mitotic divisions in the process of becoming a mature cell type and with each generation of cells becoming more specialized. In this way, a single stem cell can give rise to the many cells needed for normal tissue repair or blood cell production. When the dividing cells become fully differentiated, the rate of mitotic division is reduced. In the immune system, for example, appropriately stimulated B lymphocytes become progressively more differentiated as they undergo successive mitotic divisions, until they become mature plasma cells that no longer can divide but are capable of secreting large amounts of antibody.

Stem cells have two important properties, that of self-renewal and potency. *Self-renewal* means that the stem cells can undergo numerous mitotic divisions while maintaining

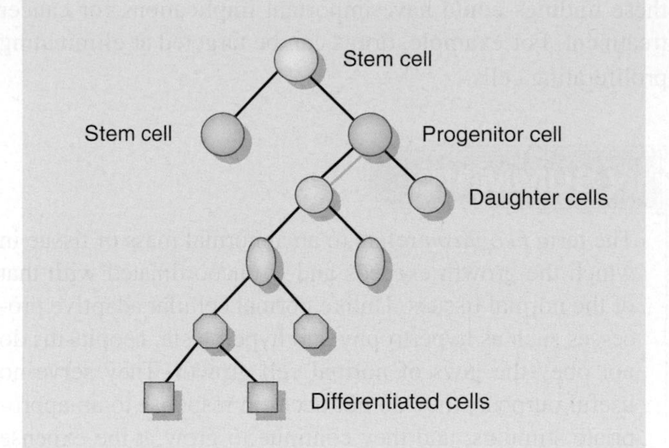

Figure 6.3 • Mechanism of stem cell–mediated cell replacement. Division of a stem cell with an unlimited potential for proliferation results in one daughter cell, which retains the characteristics of a stem cell, and a second daughter cell that differentiates into a progenitor or parent cell, with a limited potential for differentiation and proliferation. As the daughter cells of the progenitor cell proliferate, they become more differentiated, until they reach the stage where they are fully differentiated.

an undifferentiated state.[6,10] The term *potency* is used to define the differentiation potential of stem cells. *Totipotent stem cells* are those produced by fertilization of the egg. The first few cells produced after fertilization are totipotent and can differentiate into embryonic and extraembryonic cells. Totipotent stem cells give rise to *pluripotent stem cells* that can differentiate into the three germ layers of the embryo. *Multipotent stem cells* are cells such as hematopoietic stem cells that give rise to only a few cell types. Finally, *unipotent stem cells* produce only one cell type but retain the property of self-renewal.

It has become useful to categorize stem cells into two basic categories: embryonic stem cells and adult stem cells (sometimes called *somatic stem cells*).[6,10] *Embryonic stem cells* are pluripotent cells derived from the inner cell mass of the blastocyst stage of the embryo. These give rise to the three embryonic germ cell layers. As development progresses, the embryo forms germline stem cells for reproduction and somatic stem cells for organogenesis. Both the germline stem cells and the somatic stem cells retain the property of self-renewal. *Adult stem cells* reside in specialized microenvironments that differ depending on tissue type. These stem cells have important roles in homeostasis as they contribute to tissue regeneration and replacement of cells lost to cell death.[11]

An important role of stem cells in the pathogenesis of cancer has been identified, and it continues to be studied.[11] Cancer stem cells (called *tumor-initiating cells* [TICs]) have been identified in breast, prostate, acute myeloid leukemia (AML), and other cancers.[12] To maintain their self-renewing properties, these stem cells express cell cycle inhibitors. There is also strong experimental support for the idea that, in certain cancers, cancer stem cells are the initial target for malignant transformation.[12] If confirmed, identifying these findings could have important implications for cancer treatment. For example, drugs can be targeted at eliminating proliferating cells.

IN SUMMARY

The term *neoplasm* refers to an abnormal mass of tissue in which the growth exceeds and is uncoordinated with that of the normal tissues. Unlike normal cellular adaptive processes such as hypertrophy and hyperplasia, neoplasms do not obey the laws of normal cell growth. They serve no useful purpose, they do not occur in response to an appropriate stimulus, and they continue to grow at the expense of the host.

The process of cell growth and division is called the *cell cycle*. It is divided into four phases: G_1, the postmitotic phase, during which protein synthesis and cell growth take place; S, the phase during which DNA synthesis occurs, giving rise to two separate sets of chromosomes; G_2, the premitotic phase, during which RNA and protein synthesis continues; and M, the phase of cell mitosis or cell division. The G_0 phase is a resting or inactive phase in which nondividing cells reside. The entry into and progression through the various stages of the cell cycle are controlled by cyclins, CDKs, and CKIs.

Normal tissue renewal and repair involves cell proliferation, differentiation, and apoptosis. Proliferation, or the process of cell division, is a natural adaptive mechanism for cell replacement when old cells die or additional cells are needed. Differentiation is the process of specialization whereby new cells acquire the structure and function of the cells they replace. Apoptosis is a form of programmed cell death that eliminates senescent cells, cells with damaged DNA, or unwanted cells. Body cells can be divided into two large groups: the well-differentiated neurons and cells of skeletal and cardiac muscle that rarely divide and reproduce, and the progenitor or parent cells that continue to divide and reproduce, such as blood cells, skin cells, and liver cells.

A third category of cells are the stem cells that remain dormant until there is a need for cell replenishment, in which case they divide, producing other stem cells and cells that can carry out the functions of differentiated cells. Stem cells have two important properties, those of self-renewal and potency. Self-renewal means that the stem cells can undergo numerous mitotic divisions while maintaining an undifferentiated state. The term *potency* is used to define the differentiation potential of stem cells. There are two main categories of stem cells. Embryonic stem cells are pluripotent cells derived from the inner cell mass of the blastocyst stage of the embryo. Adult stem cells reside in specific microenvironments and have significant roles in homeostasis as they contribute to tissue regeneration and replacement of cells lost to apoptosis. Cancer stem cells have been identified in breast, prostate, AML, and other cancers.

CHARACTERISTICS OF BENIGN AND MALIGNANT NEOPLASMS

After completing this section of the chapter, the learner will be able to meet the following objectives:

- Relate the properties of cell differentiation to the development of a cancer cell clone and the behavior of the tumor.
- Trace the pathway for hematologic spread of a metastatic cancer cell.
- Use the concepts of growth fraction and doubling time to explain the growth of cancerous tissue.

Body organs are composed of two types of tissue: parenchymal tissue and stromal or supporting tissue. The *parenchymal tissue cells* represent the functional components of an organ. The parenchymal cells of a tumor determine its behavior and are the component for which a tumor is named. The *supporting tissue* includes the extracellular matrix and connective tissue that surround the parenchymal cells. The lymphatic and blood vessels provide nourishment and support for the parenchymal cells.

Terminology

Traditionally, by definition, a *tumor* is a swelling that can be caused by a number of conditions, including inflammation and trauma. In addition, the term has been used to define a mass of cells that arises because of overgrowth. Although not synonymous, the terms *tumor* and *neoplasm* often are used interchangeably. Neoplasms usually are classified as benign or malignant. Neoplasms that contain well-differentiated cells that are clustered together in a single mass are considered to be benign. These tumors usually do not cause death unless their location or size interferes with vital functions. In contrast, *malignant neoplasms* are less well differentiated and have the ability to break loose, enter the circulatory or lymphatic system, and form secondary malignant tumors at other sites.

Tumors usually are named by adding the suffix *-oma* to the parenchymal tissue type from which the growth originated.[6] Thus, a benign tumor of glandular epithelial tissue is called an *adenoma*, and a benign tumor of bone tissue is called an *osteoma*. The term *carcinoma* is used to designate a malignant tumor of epithelial tissue origin. In the case of a malignant tumor of glandular epithelial tissue, the term *adenocarcinoma* is used. Malignant tumors of mesenchymal origin are called *sarcomas* (*e.g.*, osteosarcoma). *Papillomas* are benign, microscopic or macroscopic finger-like projections that grow on any surface. A polyp is a growth that projects from a mucosal surface, such as the intestine. Although the term usually implies a benign neoplasm, some malignant tumors also appear as polyps.[6] Adenomatous polyps are considered precursors to adenocarcinomas of the colon. *Oncology* is the study of tumors and their treatment. Table 6.1 lists the names of selected benign and malignant tumors according to tissue types.

TABLE 6.1 NAMES OF SELECTED BENIGN AND MALIGNANT TUMORS ACCORDING TO TISSUE TYPES

TISSUE TYPE	BENIGN TUMORS	MALIGNANT TUMORS
Epithelial		
Surface	Papilloma	Squamous cell carcinoma
Glandular	Adenoma	Adenocarcinoma
Connective		
Fibrous	Fibroma	Fibrosarcoma
Adipose	Lipoma	Liposarcoma
Cartilage	Chondroma	Chondrosarcoma
Bone	Osteoma	Osteosarcoma
Blood vessels	Hemangioma	Hemangiosarcoma
Lymph vessels	Lymphangioma	Lymphangiosarcoma
Lymph tissue		Lymphosarcoma
Muscle		
Smooth	Leiomyoma	Leiomyosarcoma
Striated	Rhabdomyoma	Rhabdomyosarcoma
Neural Tissue		
Nerve cell	Neuroma	Neuroblastoma
Glial tissue	Glioma	Glioblastoma, astrocytoma, medulloblastoma, oligodendroglioma
Nerve sheaths	Neurilemmoma	Neurilemmal sarcoma
Meninges	Meningioma	Meningeal sarcoma
Hematologic		
Granulocytic		Myelocytic leukemia
Erythrocytic		Erythrocytic leukemia
Plasma cells		Multiple myeloma
Lymphocytic		Lymphocytic leukemia or lymphoma
Monocytic		Monocytic leukemia
Endothelial Tissue		
Blood vessels	Hemangioma	Hemangiosarcoma
Lymph vessels	Lymphangioma	Lymphangiosarcoma

Benign and malignant neoplasms usually are distinguished by the following:

- Cell characteristics
- Rate of growth
- Manner of growth
- Capacity to invade and metastasize to other parts of the body
- Potential for causing death

The characteristics of benign and malignant neoplasms are summarized in Table 6.2.

TABLE 6.2 CHARACTERISTICS OF BENIGN AND MALIGNANT NEOPLASMS

CHARACTERISTICS	BENIGN	MALIGNANT
Cell characteristics	Well-differentiated cells that resemble cells in the tissue of origin	Cells are undifferentiated, with anaplasia and atypical structure that often bears little resemblance to cells in the tissue of origin
Rate of growth	Usually progressive and slow; may come to a standstill or regress	Variable and depends on level of differentiation; the more undifferentiated the cells, the more rapid the rate of growth
Mode of growth	Grows by expansion without invading the surrounding tissues; usually encapsulated	Grows by invasion, sending out processes that infiltrate the surrounding tissues
Metastasis	Does not spread by metastasis	Gains access to blood and lymph channels to metastasize to other areas of the body

Benign Neoplasms

Benign tumors are composed of well-differentiated cells that resemble the cells of the tissues of origin and are characterized by a slow, progressive rate of growth that may come to a standstill or regress.[12] For unknown reasons, benign tumors have lost the ability to suppress the genetic program for cell proliferation but have retained the program for normal cell differentiation. They grow by expansion and remain localized to their site of origin, lacking the capacity to infiltrate, invade, or metastasize to distant sites. Because they expand slowly, they develop a surrounding rim of compressed connective tissue called a *fibrous capsule*.[6] The capsule is responsible for a sharp line of demarcation between the benign tumor and the adjacent tissues, a factor that facilitates surgical removal.

Benign tumors are usually much less of a threat to health and well-being than malignant tumors, and they usually do not cause death unless they interfere with vital functions because of their anatomic location. For instance, a benign tumor growing in the cranial cavity can eventually cause death by compressing brain structures. Benign tumors also can cause disturbances in the function of adjacent or distant structures by producing pressure on tissues, blood vessels, or nerves. Some benign tumors are also known for their ability to cause alterations in body function by abnormally producing hormones.

KEY POINTS

BENIGN AND MALIGNANT NEOPLASMS

- A neoplasm, benign or malignant, represents a new growth.
- Benign neoplasms are well-differentiated tumors that resemble the tissues of origin but have lost the ability to control cell proliferation. They grow by expansion, are enclosed in a fibrous capsule, and do not cause death unless their location is such that it interrupts vital body functions.
- Malignant neoplasms are less well-differentiated tumors that have lost the ability to control both cell proliferation and differentiation. They grow in a disorganized and uncontrolled manner to invade surrounding tissues, have cells that break loose and travel to distant sites to form metastases, and inevitably cause suffering and death unless their growth can be controlled through treatment.

Malignant Neoplasms

Malignant neoplasms, which invade and destroy nearby tissue and spread to other parts of the body, tend to grow rapidly and spread widely and have the potential to cause death. Because of their rapid rate of growth, malignant tumors may compress blood vessels and outgrow their blood supply, causing ischemia and tissue injury. Some malignancies secrete hormones or cytokines, release enzymes and toxins, or induce an inflammatory response that injures normal tissue as well as the tumor itself.

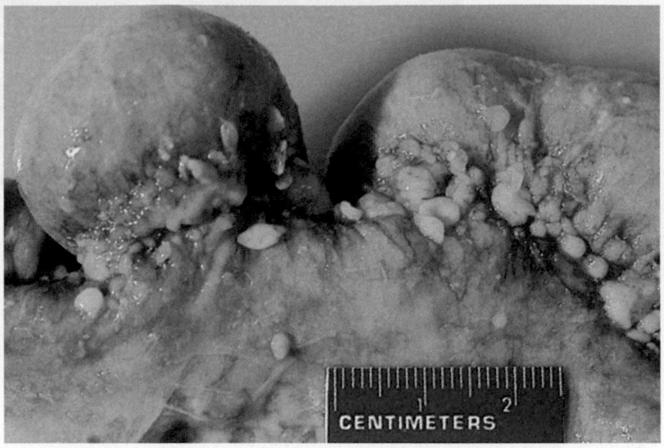

Figure 6.4 • Peritoneal carcinomatosis. The mesentery attached to a loop of small bowel is studded with small nodules of metastatic ovarian carcinoma. (From Strayer D. S., Rubin R. (Eds.) (2015). *Rubin's pathology: Clinicopathologic foundations of medicine* (7th ed., Figure 5-8, p. 175). Philadelphia, PA: Lippincott Williams & Wilkins.)

There are two categories of malignant neoplasms—solid tumors and hematologic cancers. Solid tumors initially are confined to a specific tissue or organ. As the growth of the primary solid tumor progresses, cells detach from the original tumor mass, invade the surrounding tissue, and enter the blood and lymph systems to spread to distant sites, a process termed metastasis (Fig. 6.4). Hematologic cancers involve cells normally found in the blood and lymph, thereby making them disseminated diseases from the beginning (Fig. 6.5).

Carcinoma in situ is a localized preinvasive lesion (Fig. 6.6). As an example, in breast ductal carcinoma in situ,

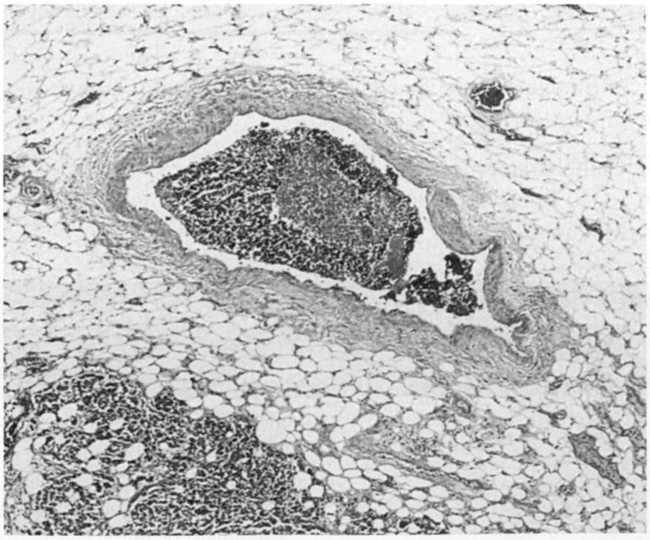

Figure 6.5 • Hematogenous spread of cancer. A malignant tumor **(bottom)** has attached to adipose tissue and penetrated into a vein. (From Strayer D. S., Rubin R., (Eds.) (2015). *Rubin's pathology: Clinicopathologic foundations of medicine* (7th ed., Figure 5-9, p. 175). Philadelphia, PA: Lippincott Williams & Wilkins.)

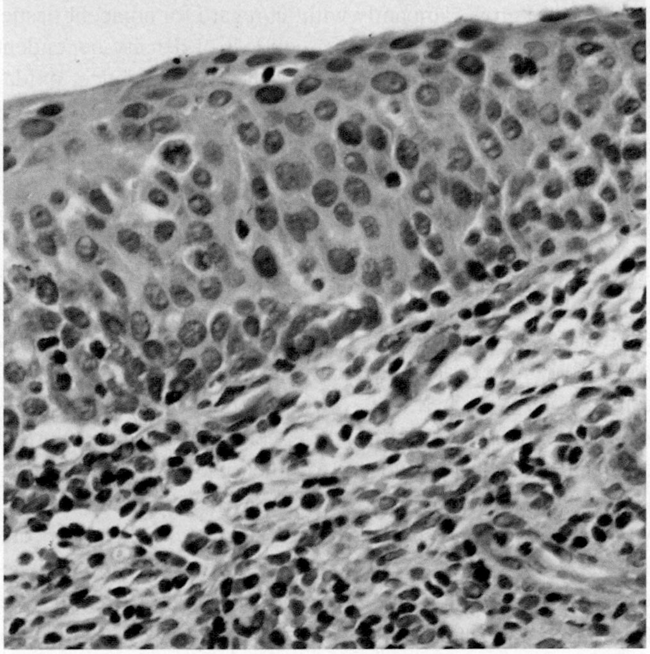

Figure 6.6 • Carcinoma in situ. A section of the uterine cervix shows neoplastic squamous cells occupying the full thickness of the epithelium and confined to the mucosa by the underlying basement membrane. (From Strayer D. S., Rubin R. (Eds.) (2015). *Rubin's pathology: Clinicopathologic foundations of medicine* (7th ed., Figure 5-6, p. 174). Philadelphia, PA: Lippincott Williams & Wilkins.)

the cells have not crossed the basement membrane. Depending on its location, in situ lesions usually can be removed surgically or treated so that the chances of recurrence are small. For example, carcinoma in situ of the cervix is essentially 100% curable.

Cancer Cell Characteristics

Cancer cells are characterized by two main features—abnormal and rapid proliferation and loss of differentiation. Loss of differentiation means that they do not exhibit normal features and properties of differentiated cells and hence are more similar to embryonic cells.

The term anaplasia describes the loss of cell differentiation in cancerous tissue.[6] Undifferentiated cancer cells are marked by a number of morphologic changes. The cells of undifferentiated tumors usually display greater numbers of cells in mitosis because of their high rate of proliferation. They also display atypical, bizarre mitotic figures, sometimes producing tripolar, tetrapolar, or multipolar spindles (Fig. 6.7B). Highly anaplastic cancer cells, whatever their tissue of origin, begin to resemble undifferentiated or embryonic cells more than they do their tissue of origin. Some cancers display only slight anaplasia, whereas others display marked anaplasia. The cytologic/histologic grading of tumors is based on the degree of differentiation and the number of proliferating cells. The closer the tumor cells resemble comparable normal tissue cells, both morphologically and functionally, the lower the grade. Accordingly, on a scale ranging from grades I to IV, grade I neoplasms are well differentiated and grade IV are poorly differentiated and display marked anaplasia.[6]

The characteristics of altered proliferation and differentiation are associated with a number of other changes in cell characteristics and function that distinguish cancer cells from their normally differentiated counterparts. These changes are listed in Table 6.3.

Genetic Instability. Most cancer cells exhibit a characteristic called *genetic instability* that is often considered to be a hallmark of cancer. The concept arose after the realization that uncorrected mutations in normal cells are rare because of the numerous cellular mechanisms to prevent them. To account for

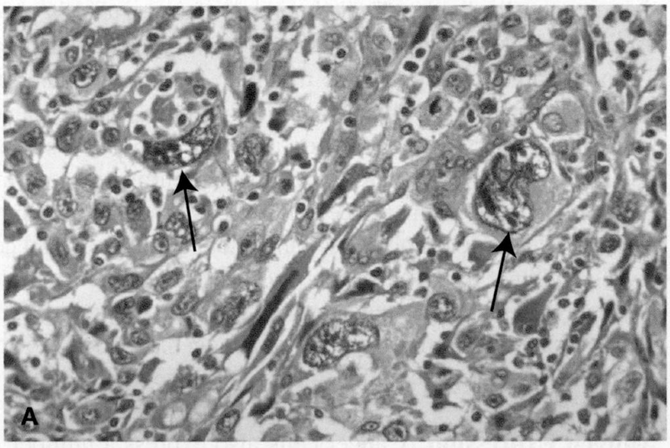

Figure 6.7 • Anaplastic features of malignant tumors. **(A)** The cells of this anaplastic carcinoma are highly pleomorphic (*i.e.*, they vary in size and shape). The nuclei are hyperchromatic and are large relative to the cytoplasm. Multinucleated tumor giant cells are present (*arrows*). **(B)** A malignant cell in metaphase exhibits an abnormal mitotic figure. (From Strayer D. S., Rubin R., (Eds.) (2015). *Rubin's pathology: Clinicopathologic foundations of medicine* (7th ed., Figure 5-2, p. 171). Philadelphia, PA: Lippincott Williams & Wilkins.)

TABLE 6.3 COMPARISON OF NORMAL CELL CHARACTERISTICS WITH THOSE OF CANCER CELLS

CHARACTERISTICS	NORMAL CELLS	CANCER CELLS
Growth	Regulated	Unregulated
Differentiation	High	Low
Genetic stability	Stable	Unstable
Growth factor dependence	Dependent	Independent
Density dependent	High	Low inhibition
Cell-to-cell adhesion	High	Low
Anchorage dependence	High	Low
Cell-to-cell communication	High	Low
Cell life span	Limited	Unlimited
Antigen expression	Absent	May be present
Substance production (*e.g.*, proteases, hormones)	Normal	Abnormal
Cytoskeletal composition and arrangement	Normal	Abnormal

the high frequency of mutations in cancer cells, it is thought that cancer cells have a "mutation phenotype" with genetic instability that contributes to the development and progression of cancer.[6] Characteristics of genetic instability include aneuploidy, in which chromosomes are lost or gained; intrachromosomal instability, which includes insertions, deletions, and amplifications; microsatellite instability, which involves short, repetitive sequences of DNA; and point mutations.

Growth Factor Independence. Another characteristic of cancer cells is the ability to proliferate even in the absence of growth factors. This characteristic is often observed when cancer cells are propagated in cell culture—the addition of serum, which is rich in growth factors, is unnecessary for the cancers to proliferate. Normal cells grown in culture often die without serum or growth factor addition. In some cases, this is because the cancer cells can rapidly divide without growth factor binding to its receptor. Breast cancer cells that do not express estrogen receptors are an example. These cancer cells grow even in the absence of estrogen, which is the normal growth stimulus for breast duct epithelial cells. Some cancer cells may produce their own growth factors and secrete them into the culture medium, whereas others have abnormal receptors or signaling proteins that may inappropriately activate growth signaling pathways in the cells.

Cell Density–Dependent Inhibition. Cancer cells often lose *cell density–dependent inhibition*, which is the cessation of growth after cells reach a certain density. This is sometimes referred to as *contact inhibition* because cells often stop growing when they come into contact with each other. In wound healing, contact inhibition causes tissue growth to cease at the point where the edges of the wound come together. Cancer cells, however, tend to grow rampantly without regard for adjacent tissue. Possible explanations for cancer cell loss of density-dependent contact inhibition include growth factor independence, oxidative mechanisms,[13,14] and alterations in interactions between cell adhesion and cell growth signaling pathways (*e.g.*, surface integrin receptors, mitogen-activated protein [MAP] kinase, and focal adhesion kinase [FAK] phosphorylation).[15]

Anchorage Dependence. Cancer cells also differ from their normal counterparts in attaining anchorage independence. Normal epithelial cells must be anchored to either neighboring cells or the underlying extracellular matrix to live and grow. If normal cells become detached, they often undergo a type of apoptosis known as *anoikis*, a term from the Greek for "homeless." Normal epithelial cells must be attached to either other cells or extracellular matrix to stay alive. Cancer cells, however, frequently remain viable and multiply without normal attachments to other cells and the extracellular matrix. Cancer cells often survive in microenvironments different from those of normal cells. Although the process of anchorage independence is complex and incompletely understood, recent studies have made progress in understanding the genes and mechanistic pathways involved.[16]

Cell-to-Cell Communication. Another characteristic of cancer cells is faulty cell-to-cell communication, a feature that may in turn contribute to other characteristics of cancer cells. Impaired cell-to-cell communication may interfere with formation of intercellular connections and responsiveness to membrane-derived signals. For example, changes in gap junction proteins, which enable cytoplasmic continuity and communication between cells, have been described in some types of cancer.[17]

Life Span. Cancer cells differ from normal cells by being *immortal*, with an unlimited life span. If normal, noncancerous cells are harvested from the body and grown under culture conditions, most cells divide a limited number of times, usually about 50 population doublings, and then become senescent and fail to divide further. In contrast to the limited life span of normal cells, cancer cells may divide an infinite number of times, hence achieving immortality. Telomeres are short, repetitive nucleotide sequences at outermost extremities of chromosome arms. Telomeres shorten with each cell division. When length is diminished sufficiently, chromosomes can no longer replicate, and cell division will not occur. Most cancer cells maintain high levels of telomerase, an enzyme that prevents telomere shortening. This keeps telomeres from aging and attaining the critically short length that is associated with cellular replicative senescence.

Antigen Expression. Cancer cells also express a number of cell surface molecules or antigens that are immunologically identified as foreign. The genes of a cell code these *tissue antigens*. Many transformed cancer cells revert to embryonic patterns of gene expression and produce antigens that are immunologically distinct from the antigens that are expressed by cells of the well-differentiated tissue from which the cancer originated. Some cancers express fetal antigens that are not produced by comparable cells in the adult. Tumor antigens may be clinically useful as markers to indicate the presence, recurrence, or progressive growth of a cancer.

Production of Enzymes, Hormones, and Other Substances. Cancer cells may produce substances that normal cells of the tissue of origin either do not produce or secrete in lesser amounts. They may also secrete degradative enzymes that enable invasion and metastatic spread. Cancer cells may also assume hormone synthesis or production and secretion of procoagulant substances that affect clotting mechanisms.

Cytoskeletal Changes. Finally, cancer cells may show cytoskeletal changes and abnormalities. These may involve the appearance of abnormal intermediate filament types or changes in actin filaments and microtubules that facilitate invasion and metastasis. Actin, microtubules, and their regulatory proteins remain the focus of many cancer-related investigations.

Invasion and Metastasis

Unlike benign tumors, which grow by expansion and usually are surrounded by a capsule, cancer spreads by direct invasion and extension, seeding of cancer cells in body cavities, and metastatic spread through the blood or lymph pathways. The word *cancer* is derived from the Latin word meaning "crablike" because cancers grow and spread by sending crablike projections into the surrounding tissues. Most cancers synthesize and secrete enzymes that break down proteins and contribute to the infiltration, invasion, and penetration of the surrounding tissues. The lack of a sharp line of demarcation separating them from the surrounding tissue makes the complete surgical removal of malignant tumors more difficult than removal of benign tumors. Often, it is necessary for the surgeon to excise portions of seemingly normal tissue bordering the tumor for the pathologist to establish that cancer-free margins are present around the excised tumor and to ensure that the remaining tissue is cancer-free.

The *seeding* of cancer cells into body cavities occurs when a tumor sheds cells into these spaces. Most often, the peritoneal cavity is involved, but other spaces such as the pleural cavity, pericardial cavity, and joint spaces may be involved. Seeding into the peritoneal cavity is particularly common with ovarian cancers. Similar to tissue culture, tumors in these sites grow in masses and are often associated with fluid accumulation (*e.g.*, ascites, pleural effusion).[6] Seeding of cancers into other areas of the body is often a complication postoperatively after removal of a cancer. The term *metastasis* is used to describe the development of a secondary tumor in a location distant from the primary tumor.[6] Metastatic tumors frequently retain many of the characteristics of the primary tumor from which they were derived. This enables determination of the primary site of the tumor based on cellular characteristics of the metastatic tumor. Some tumors tend to metastasize early in their developmental course, whereas others do not metastasize until later. Occasionally, a metastatic tumor will be advanced before the primary tumor becomes clinically detectable. Malignant tumors of the kidney, for example, may go completely undetected and be asymptomatic until a metastatic lesion is found in the lung.

Metastasis occurs through the lymph channels (*i.e.*, lymphatic spread) and the blood vessels (*i.e.*, hematogenic spread).[6] In many types of cancer, the first evidence of disseminated disease is the presence of tumor cells in the lymph nodes that drain the tumor area. When metastasis occurs by the lymphatic route, the tumor cells lodge first in the initial lymph node that receives drainage from the tumor site. Once in this lymph node, the cells may die because of the lack of a proper environment, grow into a discernible mass, or remain dormant for unknown reasons. If they survive and grow, the cancer cells may spread from more distant lymph nodes to the thoracic duct and then gain access to the vasculature.

The term *sentinel node* is used to describe the initial lymph node to which the primary tumor drains.[6] Because the initial metastasis in breast cancer is almost always lymphatic, lymphatic spread and therefore extent of disease may be determined through lymphatic mapping and sentinel lymph node biopsy. This is done by injecting a radioactive tracer and/or blue dye into the tumor to determine the first lymph node in the route of lymph drainage from the cancer. Once the sentinel lymph node has been identified, it is examined to determine the presence or absence of cancer cells. The procedure is also used to map the spread of melanoma and other cancers that have their initial metastatic spread through the lymphatic system.

With hematologic spread, the blood-borne cancer cells may enter the venous flow that drains the site of the primary neoplasm. Cancer cells may also enter tumor-associated blood vessels that either infiltrate the tumor or are found at the periphery of the tumor. Before entering the general circulation, venous blood from the gastrointestinal tract, pancreas, and spleen is routed through the portal vein to the liver. The liver is therefore a common site for metastatic spread of cancers that originate in these organs. Although the site of hematologic spread usually is related to vascular drainage of the primary tumor, some tumors metastasize to distant and unrelated sites. One explanation is that cells of different tumors tend to metastasize to specific target organs that provide suitable microenvironments containing substances such as cytokines or growth factors that are needed for their survival.[6] For example, transferrin, a growth-promoting substance isolated from lung tissue, has been found to stimulate the growth of malignant cells that typically metastasize to the lungs. Other organs that are preferential sites for metastasis contain particular cytokines, growth factors, and other microenvironmental characteristics that facilitate metastatic tumor survival and growth.

The selective nature of hematologic spread indicates that metastasis is a finely orchestrated, multistep process, and only a small, select clone of cancer cells has the right combination of gene products to perform all of the steps needed for establishment of a secondary tumor. To metastasize, a cancer cell must be able to break loose from the primary tumor, invade the surrounding extracellular matrix, gain access to a blood vessel, survive its passage in the bloodstream, emerge from the bloodstream at a favorable location, invade the surrounding tissue, begin to grow, and establish a blood supply (Fig. 6.8). However, there is also growing evidence for the significant role of the

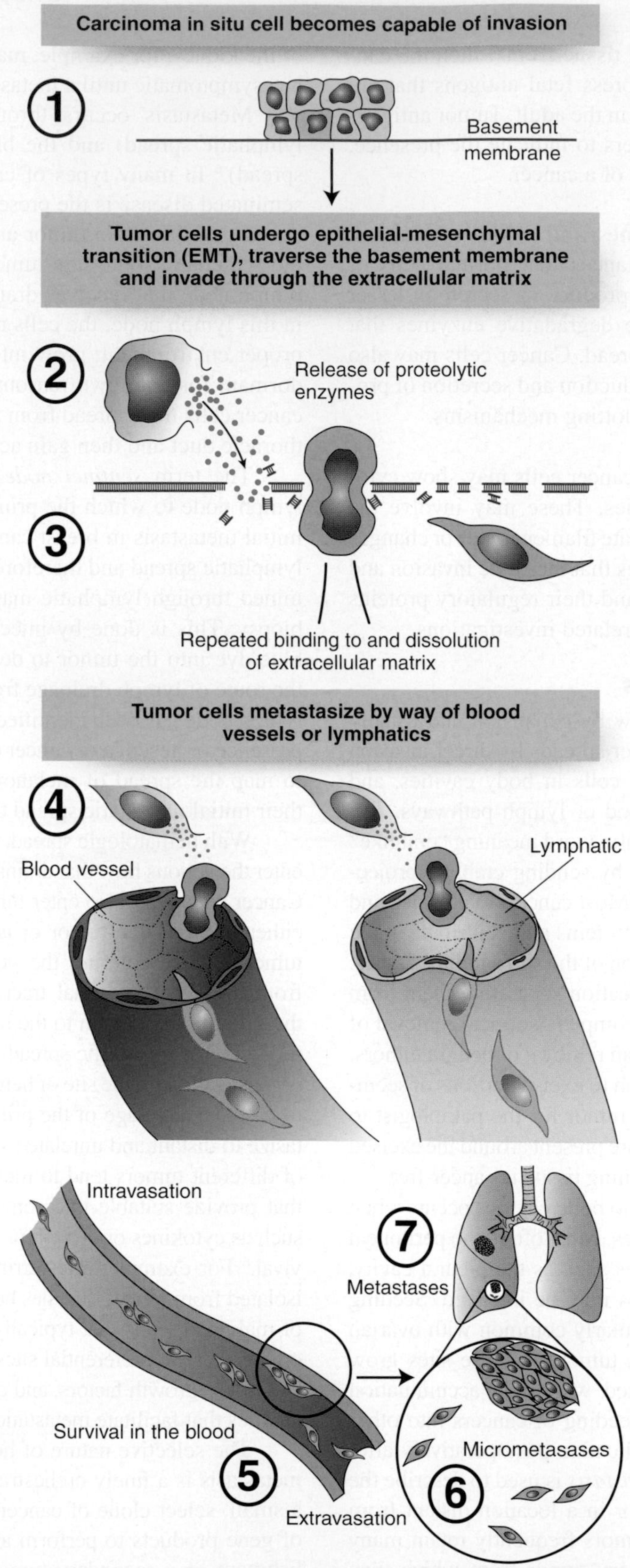

Figure 6.8 • Mechanisms of tumor invasion and metastasis. The mechanism by which a malignant tumor initially penetrates a confining basement membrane and then invades the surrounding extracellular environment involves several steps. **1.** The tumor first acquires the ability to bind components of the extracellular matrix. These interactions are mediated by the expression of a number of adhesion molecules. **2.** The tumor undergoes epithelial–mesenchymal transition (EMT) and traverses the basement membrane. **3.** Proteolytic enzymes are then released from the tumor cells, and the extracellular matrix is degraded. **4.** After moving through the extracellular environment, the invading cancer penetrates blood vessels and lymphatics by the same mechanisms. **5.** After survival in blood vessels or lymphatics, the tumor exits the vascular system. **6.** It establishes micrometastases at the site where it leaves the vasculature. **7.** These micrometastases grow into gross masses of metastatic tumor. (From Strayer D. S., Rubin R. (Eds.) (2015). *Rubin's pathology: Clinicopathologic foundations of medicine* (7th ed., Figure 5-31, p. 196). Philadelphia, PA: Lippincott Williams & Wilkins.)

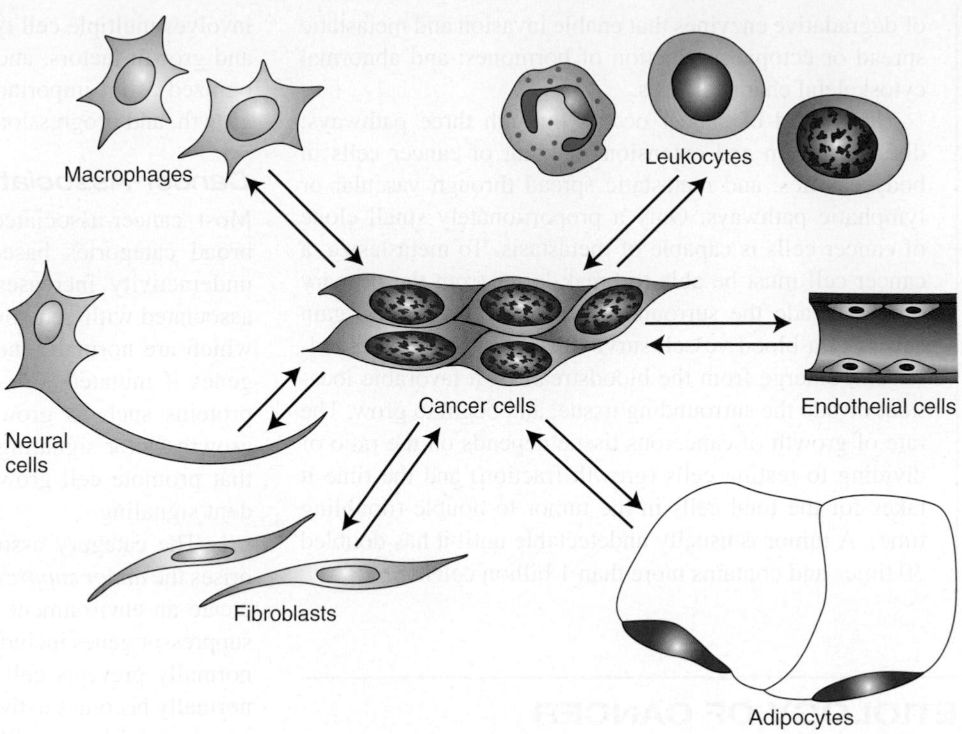

Figure 6.9 • The cancer cell ecosystem. The developing tumor cells interact with the nonmalignant cells in their environment, via production of soluble and other mediators. (From Strayer D. S., Rubin R., (Eds.) (2015). *Rubin's pathology: Clinicopathologic foundations of medicine* (7th ed., Figure 5-32, p. 197). Philadelphia, PA: Lippincott Williams & Wilkins.)

cancer cell ecosystem—which includes, but is not limited to, the extracellular matrix, neural cells, leukocytes, endothelial cells, adipocytes, fibroblasts, and macrophages—in enabling cancer cells to establish metastatic sites[6] (Fig. 6.9).

Tumor Growth

Once cells have an adequate blood supply, the rate of tissue growth in normal and cancerous tissue depends on three factors:

1. The number of cells that are actively dividing or moving through the cell cycle.
2. The duration of the cell cycle.
3. The number of cells that are being lost relative to the number of new cells being produced.

One of the reasons cancerous tumors often seem to grow so rapidly relates to the size of the cell pool that is actively engaged in cycling. It has been shown that the cell cycle time of cancerous tissue cells is not necessarily shorter than that of normal cells. Rather, cancer cells do not die on schedule and growth factors prevent cells from exiting the cycle cell and entering the G_0 phase. Thus, a greater percentage of cells are actively engaged in cycling than occurs in normal tissue.

The ratio of dividing cells to resting cells in a tissue mass is called the *growth fraction*. The *doubling time* is the length of time it takes for the total mass of cells in a tumor to double. As the growth fraction increases, the doubling time decreases. When normal tissues reach their adult size, equilibrium between cell birth and cell death is reached. Cancer cells, however, continue to divide until limitations in blood supply and nutrients inhibit their growth.

IN SUMMARY

Neoplasms may be either benign or malignant. Benign and malignant tumors differ in terms of cell characteristics, manner of growth, rate of growth, potential for metastasis, ability to produce generalized effects, tendency to cause tissue destruction, and capacity to cause death. The growth of a benign tumor is restricted to the site of origin, and the tumor usually does not cause death unless it interferes with vital functions. Malignant neoplasms grow in a poorly controlled fashion that lacks normal organization, spreads to distant parts of the body, and causes death unless tumor growth and metastasis are inhibited or stopped by treatment. There are two basic types of cancer: solid tumors and hematologic tumors. In solid tumors, the primary tumor is initially confined to a specific organ or tissue, whereas hematologic cancers are disseminated from the onset.

Cancer is a disorder of cell proliferation and differentiation. The term *anaplasia* is used to describe the loss of cell differentiation in cancerous tissue. Undifferentiated cancer cells are marked by a number of morphologic changes, including variations in size and shape, a condition referred to a *pleomorphism*. The characteristics of altered proliferation and differentiation are associated with a number of other changes in cell characteristics and cell function, including genetic instability; growth factor independence; loss of cell density–dependent inhibition, cohesiveness and adhesion, and anchorage dependence; faulty cell-to-cell communication; indefinite cell life span (immortality); expression of altered tissue antigens; abnormal secretion of degradative enzymes that enable invasion and metastatic spread or ectopic production of hormones; and abnormal cytoskeletal characteristics.

The spread of cancer occurs through three pathways: direct invasion and extension, seeding of cancer cells in body cavities, and metastatic spread through vascular or lymphatic pathways. Only a proportionately small clone of cancer cells is capable of metastasis. To metastasize, a cancer cell must be able to break loose from the primary tumor, invade the surrounding extracellular matrix, gain access to a blood vessel, survive its passage in the bloodstream, emerge from the bloodstream at a favorable location, invade the surrounding tissue, and begin to grow. The rate of growth of cancerous tissue depends on the ratio of dividing to resting cells (growth fraction) and the time it takes for the total cells in the tumor to double (doubling time). A tumor is usually undetectable until it has doubled 30 times and contains more than 1 billion cells.

ETIOLOGY OF CANCER

After completing this section of the chapter, the learner will be able to meet the following objectives:

- Describe various types of cancer-associated genes and cancer-associated cellular and molecular pathways.
- Describe genetic events and epigenetic factors that are important in tumorigenesis.
- State the importance of cancer stem cells, angiogenesis, and the cell microenvironment in cancer growth and metastasis.

The causes of cancers are very diverse and complex. It is useful to discuss causation in terms of:

1. The genetic and molecular mechanisms that are involved and that characterize the transformation of normal cells to cancer cells.
2. The external and more contextual factors such as age, heredity, and environmental agents that contribute to the development and progression of cancer.

Together, both mechanisms contribute to a multidimensional web of causation by which cancers develop and progress over time.

Genetic and Molecular Basis of Cancer

The molecular pathogenesis of most cancers is thought to originate with genetic damage or mutation with resultant changes in cell physiology that transform a normally functioning cell into a cancer cell. Epigenetic factors that involve silencing of a gene or genes may also be involved in the molecular pathogenesis of cancer. In recent years, an important role of cancer stem cells in the pathogenesis of cancer has been identified. Finally, the cellular microenvironment, which involves multiple cell types, the complex milieu of cytokines and growth factors, and the extracellular matrix, is now recognized as an important contributor to cancer development, growth, and progression.

Cancer-Associated Genes

Most cancer-associated genes can be classified into two broad categories based on whether gene overactivity or underactivity increases the risk for cancer. The category associated with gene overactivity involves *proto-oncogenes*, which are normal genes that become cancer-causing oncogenes if mutated. Proto-oncogenes encode for normal cell proteins such as growth factors, growth factor receptors, growth factor signaling molecules, and transcription factors that promote cell growth or increase growth factor–dependent signaling.

The category associated with gene underactivity comprises the *tumor suppressor genes*, which, by being less active, create an environment in which cancer is promoted. Tumor suppressor genes include the retinoblastoma (*RB*) gene, which normally prevents cell division, and the *TP53* gene, which normally becomes activated in DNA-damaged cells to initiate apoptosis.[6,18] Loss of *RB* activity may accelerate the cell cycle and lead to increased cell proliferation,[18] whereas inactivity of *TP53* may increase the survival of DNA-damaged cells. The TP53 gene has become a reliable prognostic indicator.[19] There are a number of genetic events that can lead to oncogene formation or loss of tumor suppressor gene function.

Genetic Events Leading to Oncogene Formation or Activation. Chromosomal translocations have traditionally been associated with cancers such as Burkitt lymphoma and chronic myelogenous leukemia (CML). In Burkitt lymphoma, the *myc* proto-oncogene, which encodes a growth signal protein, is translocated from its normal position on chromosome 8 to chromosome 14[6] (Fig. 6.10C). The outcome of the translocation in CML is the appearance of the so-called *Philadelphia chromosome* involving chromosomes 9 and 22 and the formation of an abnormal fusion protein, a hybrid oncogenic protein (bcr–abl) that promotes cell proliferation (Fig. 6.10A and B). Biotechnology and genomics are enabling the identification of gene translocations and an increased understanding of how these translocations, even within the same chromosome, contribute to tumorigenesis by the creation of abnormal fusion proteins that promote cell proliferation.

Another genetic event common in cancer is gene amplification. Multiple copies of certain genes may lead to overexpression, with higher-than-normal levels of proteins that increase cell proliferation. For example, the human epidermal growth factor receptor-2 (*HER-2/neu*) gene is amplified in many breast cancers; its presence indicates an aggressive tumor with a poor prognosis.[20] One of the agents used in treatment of *HER-2/neu*–overexpressing breast cancers is trastuzumab (Herceptin), a monoclonal antibody that selectively binds to HER-2, thereby inhibiting the proliferation of tumor cells that overexpress HER-2.

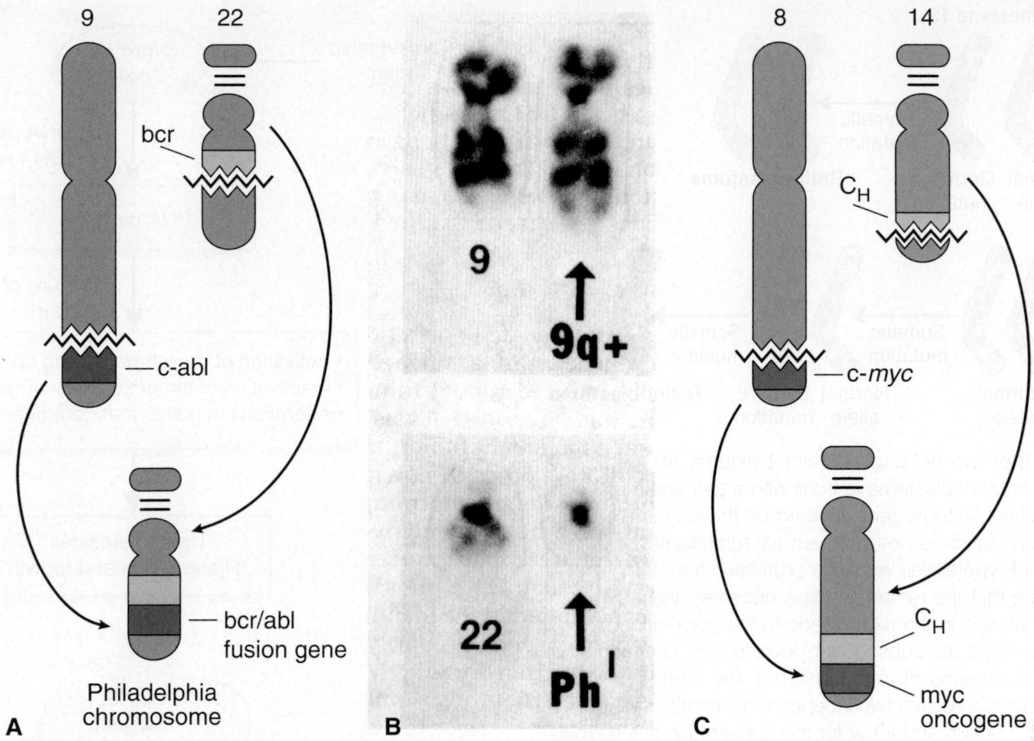

Figure 6.10 • Oncogene activation by chromosomal translocation. **(A)** Chronic myelogenous leukemia. Reciprocal translocation occurs at the breaks at the ends of the long arms of chromosomes 9 and 22. This results in the Philadelphia chromosome (Ph^1), which contains a new fusion gene coding for a hybrid oncogenic protein (bcr–abl), presumably involved in the pathogenesis of chronic myelogenous leukemia. **(B)** Karyotypes of a person with CML showing the results of reciprocal translocations between chromosomes 9 and 22. The Philadelphia chromosome is recognized by a smaller-than-normal chromosome 22 (22q−). One chromosome 9 (9q+) is larger than its normal counterpart. **(C)** Burkitt lymphoma. Chromosomal breaks involve the long arms of chromosomes 8 and 14. The c-*myc* gene on chromosome 8 is translocated to a region on chromosome 14 adjacent to the gene coding for the constant region of an immunoglobulin heavy chain (C_H). (From Rubin R., Strayer D. S. (Eds.) (2012). *Rubin's pathology: Clinicopathologic foundations of medicine* (6th ed., p. 174). Philadelphia, PA: Lippincott Williams & Wilkins.)

Genetic Events Leading to Loss of Tumor Suppressor Gene Function. Tumor suppressor genes inhibit the proliferation of cells in a tumor. When this type of gene is inactivated, a genetic signal that normally inhibits cell proliferation is removed, thereby causing unregulated growth to begin. Multiple tumor suppressor genes have been found that connect with various types of cancer.[6] Of particular interest in this group is the *TP53* gene, which is on the short arm of chromosome 17 and codes for the p53 protein. Mutations in the *TP53* gene have been associated with lung, breast, and colon cancer.[19] The *TP53* gene also appears to initiate apoptosis in radiation- and chemotherapy-damaged tumor cells.

Although a single mutation generally plays an important role in oncogene activation, the malfunction of tumor suppressor genes may require "two hits" to contribute to total loss of function, as suggested by the *two-hit hypothesis* of carcinogenesis[6] (Fig. 6.11). The first "hit" may be a point mutation in an allele of a particular chromosome; later, a second "hit" occurs that involves the companion allele of the gene. In hereditary cases, the first hit is inherited from an affected parent and is therefore present in all somatic cells of the body. In RB, the second hit occurs in one of many retinal cells (all of which already carry the mutated gene). In sporadic (noninherited) cases, both mutations (hits) occur in a single somatic cell, whose progeny then forms the cancer. In people carrying an inherited mutation, such as a mutated *RB* allele, all somatic cells are perfectly normal, except for the increased risk of developing cancer. That person is said to be heterozygous at the gene locus. Cancer develops when a person becomes homozygous for the mutant allele, a condition referred to as *loss of heterozygosity*, which confers a poor prognosis.[6] For example, loss of heterozygosity is known to occur in hereditary cancers, in which a mutated gene is inherited from a parent, and other conditions (*e.g.*, radiation exposure) are present that make people more susceptible to cancer.

Epigenetic Mechanisms

In addition to mechanisms that involve DNA and chromosomal structural changes, there are molecular and cellular mechanisms, termed *epigenetic mechanisms*, which involve changes in the patterns of gene expression without a change in the DNA. Epigenetic mechanisms may "silence" genes, such

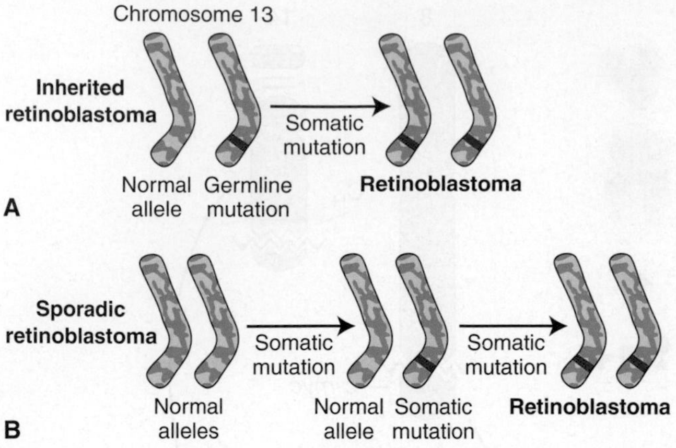

Figure 6.11 • The "two-hit" origin of retinoblastoma. **(A)** A child with the inherited form of retinoblastoma is born with a germline mutation in one allele of the retinoblastoma gene located on the long arm of chromosome 13. This mutation is not sufficient for tumorigenesis, but the absence of two wild-type alleles weakens protection from tumor development in the event that the remaining allele becomes altered. Then, a second somatic mutation in the retina leads to the inactivation of the y functioning *RB* allele and the subsequent development of a retinoblastoma. **(B)** In sporadic cases of retinoblastoma, the child is born with two normal *RB* alleles. It requires two independent somatic mutations to inactivate *RB* gene function and allow for the appearance of a neoplastic clone. (From Strayer D., Rubin R. (Eds.) (2015). *Rubin's pathology: Clinicopathologic foundations of medicine* (7th ed., Figure 5-40, p. 208). Philadelphia, PA: Lippincott Williams & Wilkins.)

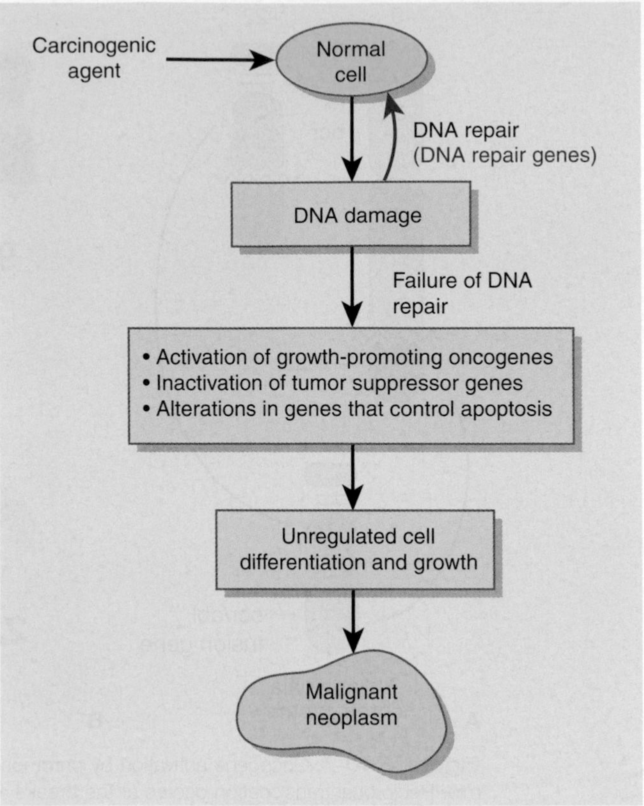

Figure 6.12 • Flowchart depicting the stages in the development of a malignant neoplasm resulting from exposure to an oncogenic agent that produces DNA damage. When DNA repair genes are present (*red arrow*), the DNA is repaired and gene mutation does not occur.

as tumor suppressor genes, so that even though the gene is present, it is not expressed and a cancer-suppressing protein is not made. One such mechanism of epigenetic silencing is by methylation of the promoter region of the gene, a change that prevents transcription and causes gene inactivity. The epigenetic mechanisms that alter expression of genes associated with cancer are still under investigation. The two hypomethylating agents available to treat myelodysplastic syndrome (MDS) and AML are azacitidine and decitabine.[5]

Molecular and Cellular Pathways

There are numerous molecular and cellular mechanisms with a myriad of associated pathways and genes that are known or suspected to facilitate the development of cancer. Genes that increase susceptibility to cancer or facilitate cancer include defects in DNA repair mechanisms, defects in growth factor signaling pathways, evasion of apoptosis, avoidance of cellular senescence, development of sustained angiogenesis, and metastasis and invasion. In addition, associated genetic mutations are involved that enable invasion of and survival in neighboring tissue, as well as evasion of immune detection and attack.

DNA Repair Defects. Genetic mechanisms that regulate repair of damaged DNA have been implicated in the process of oncogenesis (Fig. 6.12). The DNA repair genes affect cell proliferation and survival indirectly through their ability to repair damage in proto-oncogenes, genes impacting apoptosis, and tumor suppressor genes.[6] Genetic damage may be caused by the action of chemicals, radiation, or viruses, or it may be inherited in the germline. Significantly, it appears that the acquisition of a single-gene mutation is not sufficient to transform normal cells into cancer cells. Instead, cancerous transformation appears to require the activation of multiple independently mutated genes.

Defects in Growth Factor Signaling Pathways. A relatively common way in which cancer cells gain autonomous growth is through mutations in genes that control growth factor signaling pathways. These signaling pathways connect the growth factor receptors to their nuclear targets.[6] Under normal conditions, cell proliferation involves the binding of a growth factor to its receptor on the cell membrane, activation of the growth factor receptor on the inner surface of the cell membrane, transfer of the signal across the cytosol to the nucleus by signal-transducing proteins that function as second messengers, induction and activation of regulatory factors that initiate DNA transcription, and entry of the cell into the cell cycle (Fig. 6.13). Many of the proteins involved in the signaling pathways that control the action of growth factors exert their effects through *kinases*, enzymes that phosphorylate proteins. In some types of cancer such as CML, mutation in a proto-oncogene controlling tyrosine kinase activity occurs, causing unregulated cell growth and proliferation.

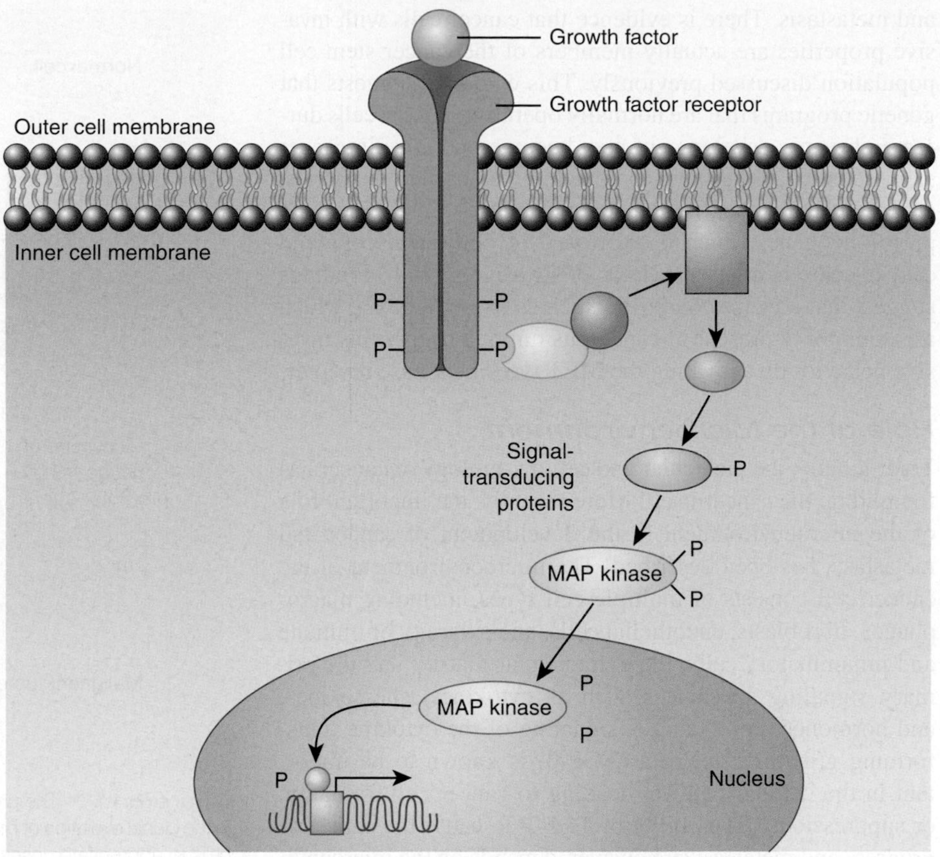

Figure 6.13 • Pathway for genes regulating cell growth and replication. Stimulation of a normal cell by a growth factor results in activation of the growth factor receptor and signaling proteins that transmit the growth-promoting signal to the nucleus, where it modulates gene transcription and progression through the cell cycle. Many of these signaling proteins exert their effects through enzymes called *kinases* that phosphorylate proteins. MAP, mitogen-activated protein.

Evasion of Apoptosis. Faulty apoptotic mechanisms have an important role in cancer. The failure of cancer cells to undergo apoptosis in a normal manner may be due to a number of problems. There may be altered cell survival signaling, overly active Ras proteins, *TP53* mutations, downregulation of death receptors (*e.g.*, TRAIL), stabilization of the mitochondria, inactivation of proapoptotic proteins (*e.g.*, methylation of caspase-8), overactivity of nuclear factor kappa B (NF-κB), heat-shock protein production, or failure of immune cells to induce cell death.[25] Alterations in apoptotic and antiapoptotic pathways, genes, and proteins have been found in many cancers.

Evasion of Cellular Senescence. Another normal cell response to DNA damage is cellular senescence. As stated earlier, cancer cells are characterized by immortality because of high levels of telomerase that prevent cell aging and senescence. High levels of telomerase and prevention of telomere shortening may also contribute to cancer and its progression because senescence is considered to be a normal response to DNA damage in cells as well as a tumor suppressor mechanism, and in model systems, short telomeres limit cancer growth.[21]

Development of Sustained Angiogenesis. Even with all the aforementioned genetic abnormalities, tumors cannot enlarge unless angiogenesis occurs and supplies them with the blood vessels necessary for survival. Angiogenesis is required not only for continued tumor growth but for metastasis. The molecular basis for the angiogenic switch is unknown, but it appears to involve increased production of angiogenic factors or loss of angiogenic inhibitors. The normal *TP53* gene seems to inhibit angiogenesis by inducing the synthesis of an antiangiogenic molecule called *thrombospondin 1*.[6] With mutational inactivation of both *TP53* alleles (as occurs in many cancers), the levels of thrombospondin 1 drop precipitously, tilting the balance in favor of angiogenic factors. Angiogenesis is also influenced by hypoxia and release of proteases that are involved in regulating the balance between angiogenic and antiangiogenic factors. Because of the crucial role of angiogenic factor in tumor growth, bevacizumab, a monoclonal antibody, has been approved to treat metastatic colorectal and renal cell carcinomas, non–small cell lung cancer, and some brain tumors.[6] Antiangiogenesis therapy is showing synergistic antitumor actions when combined with conventional forms of chemotherapy in the treatment of these cancers. It is being studied in other cancers as well.

Furthermore, antiangiogenesis therapy may have more broad-based actions. For example, it is now thought that cancer cells are a heterogeneous population of cells that include a cancer stem cell population characterized by mitotic quiescence and an increased ability to survive chemotherapy agents, which make cancer stem cells particularly difficult to treat. Cancer stem cells may reside close to blood vessels, where they receive signals for self-renewal.

Invasion and Metastasis. Finally, multiple genes and molecular and cellular pathways are known to be involved in invasion and metastasis. There is evidence that cancer cells with invasive properties are actually members of the cancer stem cell population discussed previously. This evidence suggests that genetic programs that are normally operative in stem cells during embryonic development may become operative in cancer stem cells, enabling them to detach, cross tissue boundaries, escape death by anoikis, and colonize new tissues.[22] The *MET* proto-oncogene, which is expressed in both stem cells and cancer cells, is a key regulator of invasive growth. Findings suggest that adverse conditions such as tissue hypoxia, which are commonly present in cancerous tumors, trigger this invasive behavior by activating the MET tyrosine kinase receptor.

Role of the Microenvironment

Traditionally, the molecular and cellular biology of cancer has focused on the cancer itself. More recently, the important role of the microenvironment in the development of cancer and metastasis has been described. The microenvironment of the cancer cell consists of multiple cell types, including macrophages, fibroblasts, endothelial cells, and a variety of immune and inflammatory cells; the extracellular matrix; and the primary signaling substances such as cytokines, chemokines, and hormones. For example, signaling of the cytokine transforming growth factor-beta (TGF-β) is known to be important in the cellular pathway leading to cancer cell formation or suppression.[29] The ability of TGF-β to cause the cancer to progress and metastasize, however, depends on the microenvironment of various cell types and cross talk of signals among the cell types. In some cases, the phenotype of a cancer cell can actually normalize when it is removed from the tumor microenvironment and placed in a normal environment and vice versa. Finally, essential steps needed for tumor growth and metastasis, such as angiogenesis and metastatic tumor survival, depend on the microenvironment.

Carcinogenesis

The process by which carcinogenic (cancer-causing) agents cause normal cells to become cancer cells is hypothesized to be a multistep mechanism that can be divided into three stages: initiation, promotion, and progression (Fig. 6.14). *Initiation* is the first step and describes the exposure of cells to a carcinogenic agent that causes them to be vulnerable to cancer transformation.[6] The carcinogenic agents can be chemical, physical, or biologic and produce irreversible changes in the genome of a previously normal cell. Because the effects of initiating agents are irreversible, multiple divided doses may achieve the same effects as a single exposure to the same total dose or to small amounts of highly carcinogenic substances. The cells most susceptible to mutagenic alterations are those that are actively synthesizing DNA.

Promotion is the second step that allows for prolific growth of cells triggered by multiple growth factors and chemicals.[6] Promotion is reversible if the promoter substance is removed. Cells that have been irreversibly initiated may be promoted even after long latency periods. The latency period varies with the type of agent, the dosage, and the characteristics of the target cells. Many chemical carcinogens are called *complete carcinogens* because they can initiate and promote neoplastic transformation. *Progression* is the last step of the process that manifests when tumor cells acquire malignant phenotypic changes that promote invasiveness, metastatic competence, autonomous growth tendencies, and increased karyotypic instability.

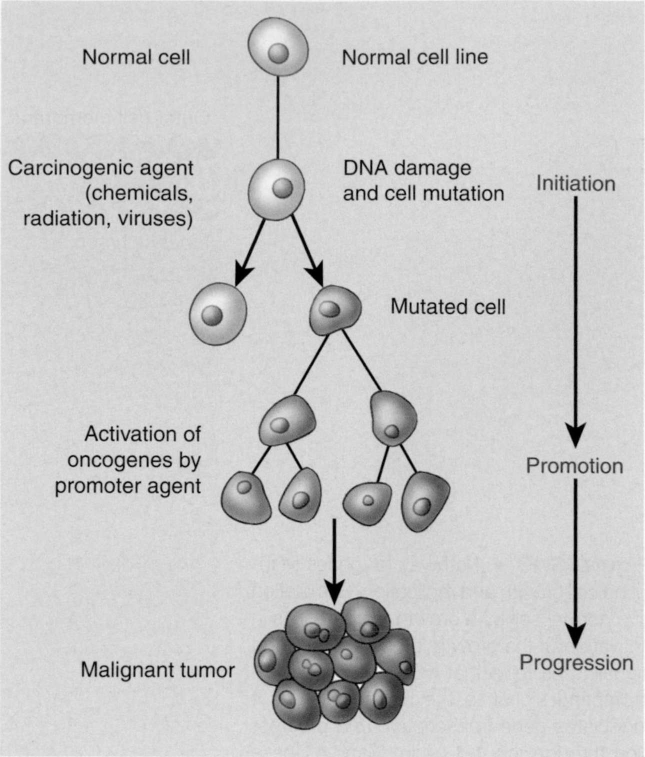

Figure 6.14 • The processes of initiation, promotion, and progression in the clonal evolution of malignant tumors. Initiation involves the exposure of cells to appropriate doses of a carcinogenic agent; promotion, the unregulated and accelerated growth of the mutated cells; and progression, the acquisition of malignant characteristics by the tumor cells.

Host and Environmental Factors

Because cancer is not a single disease, it is reasonable to assume that it does not have a single cause. More likely, cancer occurs because of interactions among multiple risk factors or repeated exposure to a single carcinogenic agent. Among the traditional risk factors that have been linked to cancer are heredity, hormonal factors, immunologic mechanisms, and environmental agents such as chemicals, radiation, and cancer-causing viruses. More recently, there has been interest in obesity as a risk factor for cancer. A strong and consistent relationship has been reported between obesity and mortality from all cancers among men and women.[23] Obese people tend to produce increased amounts of androgens, a portion of which is converted to the active form of estrogen in adipose tissue, causing a functional state of hyperestrogenism. Because of the association of estrogen with postmenopausal breast cancer and endometrial cancer, the relation is stronger among women than among men.[24]

Heredity

A hereditary predisposition to approximately 50 types of cancer has been observed in families. Breast cancer, for example, occurs more frequently in women whose grandmothers, mothers, aunts, or sisters also have experienced a breast malignancy. A genetic predisposition to the development of cancer has been documented for a number of cancerous and precancerous lesions that follow mendelian inheritance patterns. Two tumor suppressor genes, called *BRCA1* (breast carcinoma 1) and *BRCA2* (breast carcinoma 2), have been identified in genetic susceptibility to breast and ovarian cancer.[2] People carrying a *BRCA* mutation have a lifetime risk (if they live to the age of 85 years) of 80% for developing breast cancer. The lifetime risk for developing ovarian cancer is 10% to 20% for carriers of *BRCA2* mutations and 40% to 60% for *BRCA1* mutations.[6] These genes have also been associated with an increased risk of prostate, pancreatic, colon, and other cancers.

Several cancers exhibit an autosomal dominant inheritance pattern that greatly increases the risk of developing a tumor.[6] The inherited mutation is usually a point mutation occurring in a single allele of a tumor suppressor gene. People who inherit the mutant gene are born with one normal and one mutant copy of the gene.[25,26] For cancer to develop, the normal gene must be inactivated, usually through a somatic mutation. RB, a rare childhood tumor of the retina, is an example of a cancer that follows an autosomal dominant inheritance pattern. About 1/3 of RBs are inherited, and carriers of the mutant *RB* tumor suppressor gene have a significantly increased risk for developing RB, usually with bilateral involvement.[27] Familial adenomatous polyposis of the colon also follows an autosomal dominant inheritance pattern. It is caused by mutation of another tumor suppressor gene, the *APC* gene.[28] In people who inherit this gene, hundreds of adenomatous polyps may develop, and a percentage may become cancerous.[28]

Hormones

Hormones have received considerable research attention with respect to cancer of the breast, ovary, and endometrium in women and of the prostate and testis in men. Although the link between hormones and the development of cancer is unclear, it has been suggested that it may reside with the ability of hormones to drive the cell division of a malignant phenotype. Because of the evidence that endogenous hormones affect the risk of these cancers, concern exists regarding the effects on cancer risk if the same or closely related hormones are administered for therapeutic purposes.

Immunologic Mechanisms

There is substantial evidence for the immune system's participation in resistance against the progression and spread of cancer. The central concept, known as the *immune surveillance hypothesis*, first proposed in 1909, postulates that the immune system plays a central role in resistance against the development of tumors.[6,29] In addition to cancer–host interactions as a mechanism of cancer development, immunologic mechanisms provide a means for the detection, classification, and prognostic evaluation of cancers and as a potential method of treatment. *Immunotherapy* is a cancer treatment modality designed to heighten the person's general immune responses in order to increase tumor destruction.

It has been suggested that the development of cancer might be associated with impairment or decline in the surveillance capacity of the immune system. For example, increases in cancer incidence have been observed in people with immunodeficiency diseases and in those with organ transplants who are receiving immunosuppressant drugs. The incidence of cancer also is increased in older adults, in whom there is a known decrease in immune activity. The association of Kaposi sarcoma with acquired immunodeficiency syndrome (AIDS) further emphasizes the role of the immune system in preventing malignant cell proliferation.

It has been shown that most tumor cells have molecular configurations that can be specifically recognized by immune T cells or by antibodies and hence are termed *tumor antigens*. The most relevant tumor antigens fall into two categories: unique, tumor-specific antigens found only on tumor cells and tumor-associated antigens found on tumor cells and normal cells.

Virtually all of the components of the immune system have the potential for eradicating cancer cells, including T lymphocytes, B lymphocytes and antibodies, macrophages, and natural killer (NK) cells. The T-cell response is undoubtedly one of the most important host responses for controlling the growth of antigenic tumor cells. It is responsible for direct killing of tumor cells and for activation of other components of the immune system. The T-cell immunity to cancer cells reflects the function of two subsets of T cells: the $CD4^+$ helper T cells and $CD8^+$ cytotoxic T cells. The finding of tumor-reactive antibodies in the serum of people with cancer supports the role of the B cell as a member of the immune surveillance team. Antibodies can destroy cancer cells through complement-mediated mechanisms or through antibody-dependent cellular cytotoxicity, in which the antibody binds the cancer cell to another effector cell, such as the NK cell, that does the actual killing of the cancer cell. NK cells do not require antigen recognition and can lyse a wide variety of target cells. The cytotoxic activity of NK cells can be augmented by the cytokines interleukin (IL)-2 and interferon, and its activity can be amplified by immune T-cell responses. Macrophages are important in tumor immunity as antigen-presenting cells to initiate the immune response and as potential effector cells to participate in tumor cell lysis.

Chemical Carcinogens

A carcinogen is an agent capable of causing cancer. Chemical carcinogens can be divided into two groups: (1) direct-reacting agents, which do not require activation in the body to become carcinogenic, and (2) indirect-reacting agents, called *procarcinogens or initiators*, which become active only after metabolic conversion. Direct- and indirect-acting initiators form highly reactive species (*i.e.*, electrophiles and free radicals) that bind with the nucleophilic residues on DNA, RNA, or cellular proteins. The action of these reactive species tends to cause cell mutation or alteration in synthesis of cell enzymes and structural proteins in a manner that alters cell replication and interferes with cell regulatory controls. The carcinogenicity of some chemicals is augmented by agents called *promoters* that, by themselves, have little or no cancer-causing ability. It is believed that promoters exert their effect by changing the expression of genetic material in a cell, increasing DNA synthesis, enhancing gene amplification (*i.e.*, number of gene copies that are made), and altering intercellular communication.

Exposure to many chemical carcinogens is associated with lifestyle risk factors, such as smoking, dietary factors, and alcohol consumption. Cigarette smoke contains both procarcinogens and promoters. It is directly associated with lung and laryngeal cancer and has also been linked with multiple other types of cancer. Chewing tobacco or tobacco products increases the risk of cancers of the oral cavity and esophagus. It has been estimated that 40% of all cancer diagnosed in the United States are linked to tobacco use.[30] Not only is the smoker at risk, but others passively exposed to cigarette smoke are at risk. Environmental tobacco smoke has been classified as a "group A" carcinogen based on the U.S. Environmental Protection Agency's system of carcinogen classification.

There is also strong evidence that certain elements in the diet contain chemicals that contribute to cancer risk. Many dietary carcinogens occur either naturally in plants (*e.g.*, aflatoxins) or are used to preserve foods.[31] For example, benzo[*a*] pyrene and other polycyclic hydrocarbons are converted to carcinogens when foods are fried in fat that has been reused multiple times. Among the most potent of the procarcinogens are the polycyclic aromatic hydrocarbons. The polycyclic aromatic hydrocarbons are of particular interest because they are produced from animal fat in the process of charcoal-broiling meats and are present in smoked meats and fish. They also are produced in the combustion of tobacco and are present in cigarette smoke. Cancer of the colon has been associated with high dietary intake of fat and red meat and a low intake of dietary fiber. A high-fat diet was thought to be carcinogenic because it increases the flow of primary bile acids that are converted to secondary bile acids in the presence of anaerobic bacteria in the colon, producing carcinogens. Studies have identified obesity and lowered physical activity with an increased risk of colon cancer.[23,32]

Alcohol is associated with a variety of cancers; the causative mechanisms are very complex. The first and most toxic metabolite of ethanol is acetaldehyde that can cause point mutations in some cells.[6] In addition, ethanol can alter DNA methylation and interfere with retinoid metabolism, which is important in antioxidant mechanisms. The carcinogenic effect of cigarette smoke can be enhanced by concomitant consumption of alcohol; people who smoke and drink considerable amounts of alcohol are at increased risk for development of cancer of the oral cavity, larynx, and esophagus.

The effects of carcinogenic agents usually are dose dependent—the larger the dose or the longer the duration of exposure, the greater the risk that cancer will develop. Some chemical carcinogens may act in concert with other carcinogenic influences, such as viruses or radiation, to induce neoplasia. There usually is a time delay ranging from 5 to 30 years from the time of chemical carcinogen exposure to the development of overt cancer. This is unfortunate because many people may have been exposed to the agent and its carcinogenic effects before the association was recognized. This occurred, for example, with the use of diethylstilbestrol, which was widely used in the United States from the mid-1940s to 1970 to prevent miscarriages. But it was not until the late 1960s that many cases of vaginal adenosis and adenocarcinoma in young women were found to be the result of their exposure in utero to diethylstilbestrol.[33]

See Chart 6.1 for a list of chemical and environmental agents known to be carcinogenic to humans.

Radiation

The effects of *ionizing radiation* in carcinogenesis have been well documented in atomic bomb survivors, in people diagnostically exposed, and in industrial workers, scientists, and physicians who were exposed during employment. Malignant epitheliomas of the skin and leukemia were significantly elevated in these populations. Between 1950 and

CHART 6.1 CHEMICAL AND ENVIRONMENTAL AGENTS KNOWN TO BE CARCINOGENIC IN HUMANS

Polycyclic Hydrocarbons
Soots, tars, and oils
Cigarette smoke

Industrial Agents
Aniline and azo dyes
Arsenic compounds
Asbestos
β-Naphthylamine
Benzene
Benzo[*a*]pyrene
Carbon tetrachloride
Insecticides, fungicides
Nickel and chromium compounds
Polychlorinated biphenyls
Vinyl chloride

Food and Drugs
Smoked foods
Nitrosamines
Aflatoxin B_1
Diethylstilbestrol
Anticancer drugs (*e.g.*, alkylating agents, cyclophosphamide, chlorambucil, nitrosourea)

1970, the death rate from leukemia alone in the most heavily exposed population groups of atomic bomb survivors in Hiroshima and Nagasaki was 147 per 100,000 people, 30 times the expected rate.[34]

The type of cancer that developed depended on the dose of radiation, the person's gender, and the age at which exposure occurred. For instance, approximately 25 to 30 years after total body or trunk irradiation, there were increased incidences of leukemia and cancers of the breast, lung, stomach, thyroid, salivary gland, gastrointestinal system, and lymphoid tissues. The length of time between exposure and the onset of cancer is related to the age of the person. For example, children exposed to ionizing radiation in utero have an increased risk for developing leukemias and childhood tumors, particularly 2 to 3 years after birth. This latency period for leukemia extends to 5 to 10 years if the child was exposed after birth and to 20 years for certain solid tumors.[39] As another example, the latency period for the development of thyroid cancer in infants and small children who received radiation to the head and neck to decrease the size of the tonsils or thymus was as long as 35 years after exposure.

The association between sunlight and the development of skin cancer has been reported for more than 100 years. *Ultraviolet radiation* consists of relatively low-energy rays that do not deeply penetrate the skin. The evidence supporting the role of ultraviolet radiation in the cause of skin cancer includes skin cancer that develops primarily on the areas of skin more frequently exposed to sunlight (*e.g.*, the head and neck, arms, hands, and legs), a higher incidence in light-complexioned people who lack the ultraviolet-filtering skin pigment melanin, and the fact that the intensity of ultraviolet exposure is directly related to the incidence of skin cancer, as evidenced by higher rates occurring in Australia and the American Southwest.[35] Some studies also suggest that intense, episodic exposure to sunlight, particularly during childhood, is more connected to the development of melanoma than prolonged, low-intensity exposure. As with other carcinogens, the effects of ultraviolet radiation usually are additive, and there usually is a long delay between the time of exposure and detection of the cancer.

Oncogenic Viruses

An oncogenic virus is one that can induce cancer. It has been suspected for some time that viruses play an important role in the development of certain forms of cancer, particularly leukemia and lymphoma. Interest in the field of viral oncology, particularly in human populations, has burgeoned with the discovery of reverse transcriptase and the development of recombinant DNA technology and, more recently, with the discovery of oncogenes and tumor suppressor genes.

Viruses, which are small particles containing genetic material (DNA or RNA), enter a host cell and become incorporated into its chromosomal DNA, taking control of the cell's machinery for the purpose of producing viral proteins. A large number of DNA and RNA viruses (*i.e.*, retroviruses) have been shown to be oncogenic in animals. However, only a few viruses have been linked to cancer in humans.

Four DNA viruses have been identified in human cancers: the human papillomavirus (HPV), Epstein-Barr virus (EBV), hepatitis B virus (HBV), and human herpesvirus-8 (HHV-8),[2] which causes Kaposi sarcoma in people with AIDS. There are over 60 genetically different types of HPV. Some types (*i.e.*, types 1, 2, 4, 7) have been shown to cause benign squamous papillomas (*i.e.*, warts). HPVs also have been implicated in squamous cell carcinoma of the cervix and anogenital region. HPV types 16 and 18, which are considered the most highly related to cervical cancer, and, less commonly, HPV types 31, 33, 35, and 51 are found in approximately 85% of squamous cell carcinomas of the cervix and presumed precursors (*i.e.*, severe cervical dysplasia and carcinoma in situ).[2] Two vaccines to protect against specific HPV types are now available for young women and men.

EBV is a member of the herpesvirus family. It has been implicated in the pathogenesis of four human cancers: Burkitt lymphoma; nasopharyngeal cancer; B-cell lymphomas in immunosuppressed people, such as those with AIDS; and in some cases of Hodgkin lymphoma. Burkitt lymphoma, a tumor of B lymphocytes, is endemic in parts of East Africa and occurs sporadically in other areas worldwide. In people with normal immune function, the EBV-driven B-cell proliferation is readily controlled, and the person becomes asymptomatic or experiences a self-limited episode of infectious mononucleosis. In regions of the world where Burkitt lymphoma is endemic, concurrent malaria or other infections cause impaired immune function, allowing sustained B-lymphocyte proliferation. An increased risk of B-cell lymphomas is seen in people with drug-suppressed immune systems, such as people with transplanted organs.

HBV is the etiologic agent in the development of hepatitis B, cirrhosis, and hepatocellular carcinoma. A significant correlation between elevated rates of hepatocellular carcinoma worldwide and the prevalence of HBV carriers has been found.[6] Other etiologic factors also may contribute to the development of liver cancer. The precise mechanism by which HBV induces hepatocellular cancer has not been determined, although it has been suggested that it may be the result of prolonged HBV-induced liver damage and regeneration.

Although there are a number of retroviruses (RNA viruses) that cause cancer in animals, human T-cell leukemia virus-1 (HTLV-1) is the only known retrovirus to cause cancer in humans. HTLV-1 is associated with a form of T-cell leukemia that is endemic in parts of Japan and found sporadically in some other areas of the world.[40] Similar to the human immunodeficiency virus (HIV) responsible for AIDS, HTLV-1 is attracted to $CD4^+$ T cells, and this subset of T cells is therefore the major target for cancerous transformation. The virus requires transmission of infected T cells through sexual intercourse, infected blood, or breast milk.

IN SUMMARY

The causes of cancer are highly complex and can be viewed from two perspectives: (1) the molecular and cellular origins and mechanisms and (2) the external and contextual causative factors, including age, heredity, and environmental agents, that influence its inception and growth. In most cases, the molecular pathogenesis of cancer is thought to have its origin in genetic damage or mutation that changes cell physiology and transforms a normally functioning cell into a cancer cell. However, the complexity of the causation and pathogenesis of cancer is becoming increasingly apparent as more is learned about the roles of epigenetic mechanisms, cancer stem cells, and the microenvironment in tumorigenesis.

The types of genes involved in cancer are numerous, with the two main categories being the proto-oncogenes, which control cell growth and replication, and tumor suppressor genes, which are growth-inhibiting regulatory genes. Genetic and molecular mechanisms that increase susceptibility to cancer or facilitate cancer include defects in DNA repair mechanisms, defects in growth factor signaling pathways, evasion of apoptosis, development of sustained angiogenesis, and invasion and metastasis. Because cancer is not a single disease, it is likely that multiple factors interact at the molecular and cellular levels to transform normal cells into cancer cells. Genetic and epigenetic damage may be the result of interactions between multiple risk factors or repeated exposure to a single carcinogen. Among the risk factors that have been linked to cancer are heredity, hormonal factors, immunologic mechanisms, and environmental agents such as chemicals, radiation, and cancer-causing viruses.

CLINICAL MANIFESTATIONS

After completing this section of the chapter, the learner will be able to meet the following objectives:

- Characterize the mechanisms involved in the anorexia and cachexia, fatigue and sleep disorders, anemia, and venous thrombosis experienced by people with cancer.
- Define the term *paraneoplastic syndrome* and explain its pathogenesis and manifestations.

There probably is not a single body function left unaffected by the presence of cancer. Because tumor cells replace normally functioning parenchymal tissue, the initial manifestations of cancer usually reflect the primary site of involvement. For example, cancer of the lung initially produces impairment of respiratory function; as the tumor grows and metastasizes, other body structures become affected. Cancer also produces generalized manifestations such as fatigue, anorexia and cachexia, anemia, decreased resistance to infections, and symptoms unrelated to the tumor site (paraneoplastic syndromes; see Table 6.4). Many of these manifestations are compounded by the side effects of methods used to treat the disease. In its late stages, cancer often causes pain. Pain is one of the most dreaded aspects of cancer, and pain management is one of the major treatment concerns for persons with incurable cancers.

Tissue Integrity

Cancer disrupts tissue integrity. As cancers grow, they compress and erode blood vessels, causing ulceration and necrosis along with frank bleeding and sometimes hemorrhage. One of the early warning signals of colorectal cancer is blood in the stool. Cancer cells also may produce enzymes and metabolic toxins that are destructive to the surrounding tissues. Usually, tissue damaged by cancerous growth does not heal normally. Instead, the damaged area persists and often continues to grow; a sore that does not heal is another warning signal of cancer. Cancer has no regard for normal anatomic boundaries; as it grows, it invades and compresses adjacent structures. Abdominal cancer, for example, may compress the viscera and cause bowel obstruction.

The development of effusions or fluid in the pleural, pericardial, or peritoneal spaces is often the presenting sign of some tumors.[6] Direct involvement of the serous surface seems to be the most significant inciting factor, although many other mechanisms, such as obstruction of lymphatic flow, may play a role. It has been reported that almost 50% of undiagnosed effusions in people not known to have cancer turn out to be due to malignancy. Lung cancers, breast cancers, and lymphomas are the most common causes of malignant pleural effusion (MPE).[6,36] Most people with pleural effusions are symptomatic at presentation, with chest pain, shortness of breath, and cough. More than any other malignant neoplasms, ovarian cancers are associated with the accumulation of fluid in the peritoneal cavity. Abdominal discomfort, swelling and a feeling of heaviness, and increase in abdominal girth, which reflect the presence of peritoneal effusions or ascites, shortness of breath, and increased urinary urgency or frequency are common presenting symptoms in ovarian cancer.[37]

Systemic Manifestations

Many of the clinical manifestations of cancer, including anorexia and cachexia, fatigue and sleep disorders, and anemia, are not directly related to the presence of a tumor mass but to altered metabolic pathways and the presence of circulating cytokines and other mediators. Although research has produced amazing insights into the causes and cures for cancer, much still is needed regarding management of the associated side effects of the disease.[6]

Anorexia and Cachexia

Many cancers are associated with weight loss and wasting of body fat and muscle tissue, accompanied by profound weakness, anorexia, and anemia. This wasting syndrome is often referred to as the *cancer anorexia–cachexia syndrome*.[38] It is a common manifestation of most solid tumors, with the exception of breast cancer. It has been estimated that it is a significant cause of morbidity and mortality in 50% to 80% of

TABLE 6.4 COMMON PARANEOPLASTIC SYNDROMES

TYPE OF SYNDROME	ASSOCIATED TUMOR TYPE	PROPOSED MECHANISM
Endocrinologic		
Syndrome of inappropriate ADH	Small cell lung cancer, others	Production and release of ADH by tumor
ACTH–Cushing syndrome	Small cell lung cancer, bronchial carcinoid cancers	Production and release of adrenocorticotropic hormone (ACTH) by tumor
Humoral hypercalcemia	Squamous cell cancers of the lung, head, neck, ovary	Production and release of polypeptide factor with close relationship to parathyroid hormone (PTH)
Hematologic		
Venous thrombosis	Pancreatic, lung, most solid tumor metastatic cancers	Production of procoagulation factors
Nonbacterial thrombolytic endocarditis and anemia of malignancy	Advanced cancers	
Neurologic		
Eaton-Lambert syndrome	Small cell lung cancer	Autoimmune production of antibodies to motor end-plate structures
Myasthenia gravis	Thymoma	Autoimmune generating abnormal neuron transmission
Dermatologic		
Cutaneous syndromes	Gastric carcinoma and other	Possibly caused by production of growth factors (epidermal) by tumor cells
Acanthosis nigricans	Cancers	Sometimes occur prior to cancer
Pemphigus		
Ichthyosis		
Extramammary Paget		Damage to renal glomerulus
Renal		
Nephrotic syndrome	Renal cancers	

people with advanced cancer and is responsible for death in up to 20% of cases.[43] The condition is more common in children and older adults and becomes more pronounced as the disease progresses. People with cancer cachexia also respond less well to chemotherapy and are more prone to toxic side effects.

Although anorexia, reduced food intake, and abnormalities of taste are common in people with cancer and often are accentuated by treatment methods, the extent of weight loss and protein wasting cannot be explained in terms of diminished food intake alone. In contrast to starvation because of lack of food intake, where weight is preferentially lost from the fat compartment, in cachexia, it is lost from both the fat and skeletal muscle compartments.[38] Furthermore, the protein loss that occurs with starvation is divided equally between skeletal muscle and visceral proteins, whereas in cachexia, visceral proteins are relatively well preserved. Thus, there is a loss of liver mass in starvation, but an increase in cachectic people because of hepatic recycling of nutrients and the acute-phase response. Finally, and more important, weight loss that occurs with starvation is usually reversed by refeeding, whereas oral or parenteral nutritional supplementation does not reverse cachexia.

The mechanisms of cancer cachexia appear to reside in a hypermetabolic state and altered nutrient metabolism that are specific to the tumor-bearing state. Tumors tend to consume large amounts of glucose, with a resultant increase in lactate formation because the tumor oxygen levels are too low to support the citric acid cycle and mitochondrial oxidative phosphorylation. The lactate that is produced then circulates to the liver, where it is converted back to glucose. The production of glucose (gluconeogenesis) from lactate uses adenosine triphosphate (ATP) and is very energy inefficient, contributing to the hypermetabolic state of cachectic people. Another mechanism for the increasing energy expenditure in cachectic people is the increased expression of mitochondrial uncoupling proteins that uncouple the oxidative phosphorylation process, so that energy is lost as heat. Abnormalities in fat and protein metabolism have also been reported. During starvation in people without cancer, ketones derived from fat replace the glucose normally used by the brain, leading to decreased gluconeogenesis from amino acids with conservation of muscle mass, whereas in people with cancer cachexia, amino acids are not spared and there is depletion of lean body mass, a condition thought to contribute to decreased survival time.

Although the mechanisms of the cancer anorexia–cachexia syndrome remain incompletely understood, they are probably multifactorial, resulting from a persistent inflammatory response in conjunction with production of specific cytokines and catabolic factors by the tumor. The syndrome shows similarities to that of the acute-phase response seen with tissue injury, infection, or inflammation, in which liver protein synthesis changes from synthesis of albumin to acute-phase proteins such as C-reactive protein, fibrinogen, and α_1-antitrypsin.

The acute-phase response is known to be activated by cytokines such as tumor necrosis factor-α (TNF-α) and IL-1 and IL-6, suggesting that they may also play a role in cancer cachexia.[39] High serum levels of these cytokines have been observed in people with cancer, and their levels appear to correlate with progression of the tumor. TNF-α, secreted primarily by macrophages in response to tumor cell growth or gram-negative bacterial infections, was the first cytokine associated with cachexia and wasting to be identified. It causes anorexia by suppressing satiety centers in the hypothalamus and increasing the synthesis of lipoprotein lipase, an enzyme that facilitates the release of fatty acids from lipoproteins so that they can be used by tissues. IL-1 and IL-6 share many of the features of TNF-α in terms of the ability to initiate cachexia.

Fatigue and Sleep Disorders

Fatigue and sleep disturbances are two of the most frequent side effects experienced by people with cancer.[40] Cancer-related fatigue is characterized by feelings of tiredness, weakness, and lack of energy and is distinct from the normal tiredness experienced by healthy people in that it is not relieved by rest or sleep. It occurs both as a consequence of the cancer itself and as a side effect of cancer treatment. Cancer-related fatigue may be an early symptom of malignant disease and has been reported by more than a third of people at the time of diagnosis.[40] Furthermore, the symptom often remains for months or even years after treatment.

Although cancer-related fatigue and sleep disorders are distinct conditions, they are closely linked in terms of prevalence and symptoms.[40] People with cancer report poor sleep quality, disturbed initiation and maintenance of sleep, insufficient sleep, nighttime awakening, and restless sleep. As with fatigue, precipitating factors include the diagnosis of cancer, type and stage of cancer, pain, and side effects of treatment (*e.g.*, nausea, vomiting). Once it begins, insomnia is often self-perpetuating because of the natural tendency to compensate for sleep loss by napping, going to bed earlier, and getting out of bed later. It may also be that the fatigue that occurs with cancer or anticancer therapy may, in fact, prompt people to extend their sleep opportunity and thus becomes a contributing factor to ongoing insomnia. Correlations have also been noted between fatigue and daytime symptoms of sleep problems, such as daytime sleepiness and napping.

Anemia

Anemia is common in people with various types of cancers. It may be related to blood loss, hemolysis, impaired red blood cell production, or treatment effects.[6] For example, drugs used in treatment of cancer are cytotoxic and can decrease red blood cell production. Also, there are many mechanisms through which erythrocyte production can be impaired in people with malignancies, including nutritional deficiencies, bone marrow failure, and a blunted erythropoietin response to hypoxia. Inflammatory cytokines generated in response to tumors decrease erythropoietin production, resulting in a decrease in erythrocyte production.

Cancer-related anemia is associated with reduced treatment effectiveness, increased mortality, increased transfusion requirements, and reduced performance and quality of life. Hypoxia, a characteristic feature of advanced solid tumors, has been recognized as a critical factor in promoting tumor resistance to radiation therapy and some chemotherapeutic agents. Severe anemia may delay surgical interventions when preoperative transfusions are required. Similarly, low hemoglobin levels before or during chemotherapy may require dose reductions or delays in administration, resulting in a decrease in overall treatment effectiveness. Cancer-related anemia is often treated with recombinant human erythropoietin.

IN SUMMARY

There probably is no single body function left unaffected by the presence of cancer. Because tumor cells replace normally functioning parenchymal tissue, the initial manifestations of cancer usually reflect the primary site of involvement. Cancer compresses blood vessels, obstructs lymph flow, disrupts tissue integrity, invades serous cavities, and compresses visceral organs. It may result in development of effusion (*i.e.*, fluid) in the pleural, pericardial, or peritoneal spaces and generalized manifestations such as anorexia and cachexia, fatigue and sleep disorders, and anemia. Many of these manifestations are compounded by the side effects of methods used to treat the disease.

SCREENING, DIAGNOSIS, AND TREATMENT

After completing this section of the chapter, the learner will be able to meet the following objectives:

- Compare the different screening mechanisms for cancer.
- Differentiate among the three types of cancer treatment (curative, control, and palliative), considering the risks and benefits of each approach.

Screening

Screening represents a secondary prevention measure for the early recognition of cancer in an otherwise asymptomatic population.[2] Screening can be achieved through observation (*e.g.*, skin, mouth, external genitalia), palpation (*e.g.*, breast, thyroid, rectum and anus, prostate, lymph nodes), and laboratory tests and procedures (*e.g.*, Papanicolaou [Pap] smear, colonoscopy, mammography). It requires a test that will specifically detect early cancers or premalignancies, is cost-effective, and results in improved therapeutic outcomes.[6] For most cancers, stage at presentation is related to curability, with the highest rates reported when the tumor is small and there is no evidence of metastasis. For some tumors, however, metastasis tends to occur early, even from a small primary tumor. More sensitive screening methods such as tumor markers are being developed for forms of cancer. Lung cancer guidelines were developed by the American Cancer Society and recommend the initiation of discussions with healthy people aged 55 years to 74 years who have a minimum of 30-pack/year smoking history and who have stopped smoking in the last 15 years or continue to smoke.[41]

Cancers for which current screening or early detection has led to improvement in outcomes include cancers of the breast (mammography), cervix (Pap smear), colon and rectum (rectal examination, fecal occult blood test, and colonoscopy), prostate (prostate-specific antigen [PSA] testing and transrectal ultrasonography), and malignant melanoma (self-examination). Although not as clearly defined, it is recommended that screening for other types of cancers such as cancers of the thyroid, testicles, ovaries, lymph nodes, and oral cavity be done at the time of periodic health examinations.

Diagnostic Methods

The methods used in the diagnosis and staging of cancer are determined largely by the location and type of cancer suspected. A number of procedures are used in the diagnosis of cancer, including blood tests for tumor markers, cytologic studies and tissue biopsy, endoscopic examinations, ultrasonography, x-ray studies, MRI, computed tomography (CT), and positron emission tomography (PET).

Tumor Markers

Tumor markers are antigens expressed on the surface of tumor cells or substances released from normal cells in response to the presence of tumor.[6,42] Some substances, such as hormones and enzymes, that are produced normally by the involved tissue become overexpressed as a result of cancer. Other tumor markers, such as oncofetal proteins, are produced during fetal development and are induced to reappear later in life as a result of benign and malignant neoplasms. Tumor markers are used for screening, establishing prognosis, monitoring treatment, and detecting recurrent disease.[42] Table 6.5 identifies some of the more commonly used tumor markers and summarizes their source and the cancers associated with them.

The serum markers that have proved most useful in clinical practice are human chorionic gonadotropin (hCG), CA 125, PSA, α-fetoprotein (AFP), carcinoembryonic antigen (CEA), and CD blood cell antigens.[6] A hormone normally produced by the placenta, hCG, is used as a marker for diagnosing, prescribing treatment, and following the disease course in

TABLE 6.5 TUMOR MARKERS

MARKER	SOURCE	ASSOCIATED CANCERS
Antigens		
AFP	Fetal yolk sac and gastrointestinal structures early in fetal life	Primary liver cancers; germ cell cancer of the testis
CA 15-3	Breast tissue protein	Tumor marker for tracking breast cancer; liver, lung
CA 27-29	Breast tissue protein	Breast cancer recurrence and metastasis
CEA	Embryonic tissues in gut, pancreas, liver, and breast	Colorectal cancer and cancers of the pancreas, lung, and stomach
Hormones		
hCG	Hormone normally produced by placenta	Gestational trophoblastic tumors; germ cell cancer of testis
Calcitonin	Hormone produced by thyroid parafollicular cells	Thyroid cancer
Catecholamines (epinephrine, norepinephrine) and metabolites	Hormones produced by chromaffin cells of the adrenal gland	Pheochromocytoma and related tumors
Specific Proteins		
Monoclonal immunoglobulin	Abnormal immunoglobulin produced by neoplastic cells	Multiple myeloma
PSA	Produced by the epithelial cells lining the acini and ducts of the prostate	Prostate cancer
Mucins and Other Glycoproteins		
CA 125	Produced by müllerian cells of ovary	Ovarian cancer
CA 19-9	Produced by alimentary tract epithelium	Cancer of the pancreas, colon
Cluster of Differentiation		
CD antigens	Present on leukocytes	Used to determine the type and level of differentiation of leukocytes involved in different types of leukemia and lymphoma

people with high-risk gestational trophoblastic tumors. PSA is used as a marker in prostate cancer, and CA 125 is used as a marker in ovarian cancer. Markers for leukemia and lymphomas are grouped by so-called *cluster of differentiation* (CD) antigens. The CD antigens help to distinguish among T and B lymphocytes, monocytes, granulocytes, and NK cells and immature variants of these cells.[6]

Some cancers express fetal antigens that are normally present only during embryonal development.[6] The two that have proved most useful as tumor markers are AFP and CEA. AFP is synthesized by the fetal liver, yolk sac, and gastrointestinal tract and is the major serum protein in the fetus. Elevated levels are encountered in people with primary liver cancers and have also been observed in some testicular, ovarian, pancreatic, and stomach cancers. CEA normally is produced by embryonic tissue in the gut, pancreas, and liver and is elaborated by a number of different cancers. Depending on the serum level adopted for significant elevation, CEA is elevated in approximately 60% to 90% of colorectal carcinomas, 50% to 80% of pancreatic cancers, and 25% to 50% of gastric and breast tumors.[6] As with most other tumor markers, elevated levels of CEA and AFP are found in other, noncancerous conditions, and elevated levels of both depend on tumor size, so that neither is useful as an early screening test for cancer.

As diagnostic tools, tumor markers have limitations. Nearly all markers can be elevated in benign conditions, and most are not elevated in the early stages of malignancy. Hence, tumor markers have limited value as screening tests. Furthermore, they are not in themselves specific enough to permit a diagnosis of a malignancy, but once a malignancy has been diagnosed and shown to be associated with elevated levels of a tumor marker, the marker can be used to assess response to therapy. Examples of tumor markers that assist in evaluating peoples' response to therapy, and if a recurrence of breast cancer may be occurring, are CA 15-3 and CA 27-29, both antigens that are found in breast tissue.[3] Extremely elevated levels of a tumor marker can indicate a poor prognosis or the need for more aggressive treatment. Perhaps the greatest value of tumor markers is in monitoring therapy in people with widespread cancer. The level of most cancer markers tends to decrease with successful treatment and increase with recurrence or spread of the tumor.

Cytologic and Histologic Methods

Histologic and cytologic studies are laboratory methods used to examine tissues and cells. Several sampling approaches are available, including cytologic smears, tissue biopsies, and needle aspiration.[6]

Papanicolaou Test. The Pap test is a cytologic method used for detecting cancer cells. It consists of a microscopic examination of a properly prepared slide by a cytotechnologist or pathologist for the purpose of detecting the presence of abnormal cells. The usefulness of the Pap test relies on the fact that the cancer cells lack the cohesive properties and intercellular junctions that are characteristic of normal tissue. Without these characteristics, cancer cells tend to exfoliate and become mixed with secretions surrounding the tumor growth. Although the Pap test is widely used as a screening test for cervical cancer, it can be performed on other body secretions, including nipple drainage, anal washings, pleural or peritoneal fluid, and gastric washings.

Tissue Biopsy. Tissue biopsy, which is of critical importance in diagnosing the correct cancer and histology, involves the removal of a tissue specimen for microscopic study. Biopsies are obtained in a number of ways, including needle biopsy; endoscopic methods, such as bronchoscopy or cystoscopy, which involve the passage of an endoscope through an orifice and into the involved structure; or laparoscopic methods. In some instances, a surgical incision is made from which biopsy specimens are obtained. Excisional biopsies are those in which the entire tumor is removed. The tumors usually are small, solid, palpable masses. If the tumor is too large to be completely removed, a wedge of tissue from the mass can be excised for examination. Appropriate preservation of the specimen includes prompt immersion in a fixative solution such as formalin, with preservation of a portion of the specimen in a special fixative for electron microscopy, or prompt refrigeration to permit optimal hormone, receptor, and other types of molecular analysis. A quick frozen section may be done to determine the nature of a mass lesion or evaluate the margins of an excised tumor to ascertain that the entire neoplasm has been removed.[6]

Fine needle aspiration is another approach that is widely used. The procedure involves aspirating cells and attendant fluid with a small-bore needle. The method is most commonly used for assessment of readily palpable lesions in sites such as the thyroid, breast, and lymph nodes. Modern imaging techniques have also enabled the method to be extended to deeper structures such as the pelvic lymph nodes and pancreas.

Immunohistochemistry. Immunohistochemistry involves the use of antibodies to facilitate the identification of cell products or surface markers.[6] For example, certain anaplastic carcinomas, malignant lymphomas, melanomas, and sarcomas look very similar under the microscope, but must be accurately identified because their treatment and prognosis are quite different. Antibodies against intermediate filaments have proved useful in such cases because tumor cells often contain intermediate filaments characteristic of their tissue of origin.[6] Immunohistochemistry can also be used to determine the site of origin of metastatic tumors. Many people with cancer present with metastasis. In cases in which the origin of the metastasis is obscure, immunochemical detection of tissue-specific or organ-specific antigens can often help to identify the tumor source. Immunohistochemistry can also be used to detect molecules that have prognostic or therapeutic significance. For example, detection of estrogen receptors on breast cancer cells is of prognostic and therapeutic significance because these tumors respond to antiestrogen therapy.

Microarray Technology. Microarray technology uses "gene chips" that can simultaneously perform miniature assays to detect and quantify the expression of large numbers of genes.[6]

The advantage of microarray technology is the ability to analyze a large number of changes in cancer cells to determine overall patterns of behavior that could not be assessed by conventional means. DNA arrays are now commercially available to assist in making clinical decisions regarding breast cancer treatment. In addition to identifying tumor types, microarrays have been used for predicting prognosis and response to therapy, examining tumor changes after therapy, and classifying hereditary tumors.[6]

Staging and Grading of Tumors

The two basic methods for classifying cancers are *grading* according to the histologic or cellular characteristics of the tumor and *staging* according to the clinical spread of the disease. Both methods are used to determine the course of the disease and aid in selecting an appropriate treatment or management plan. Grading of tumors involves the microscopic examination of cancer cells to determine their level of differentiation and the number of mitoses. Cancers are classified as grades I, II, III, and IV with increasing anaplasia or lack of differentiation. Staging of cancers uses methods to determine the extent and spread of the disease. Surgery may be used to determine tumor size and lymph node involvement.

The clinical staging of cancer is intended to group people according to the extent of their disease. It is useful in determining the choice of treatment for individual people, estimating prognosis, and comparing the results of different treatment regimens. The TNM system of the American Joint Committee on Cancer (AJCC) is used by most cancer facilities.[43] This system, which is briefly described in Chart 6.2, classifies the disease into stages using three tumor components:

- *T* stands for the size and local spread of the primary tumor.
- *N* refers to the involvement of the regional lymph nodes.
- *M* describes the extent of the metastatic involvement.

The time of staging is indicated as postsurgical resection–pathologic staging (pTNM), surgical–evaluative staging (sTNM), retreatment staging (rTNM), and autopsy staging (aTNM).[44]

CHART 6.2 TNM CLASSIFICATION SYSTEM

T (Tumor)

Tx	Tumor cannot be adequately assessed
T0	No evidence of primary tumor
Tis	Carcinoma in situ
T1–4	Progressive increase in tumor size or involvement

N (Nodes)

Nx	Regional lymph nodes cannot be assessed
N0	No evidence of regional node metastasis
N1–3	Increasing involvement of regional lymph nodes

M (Metastasis)

Mx	Not assessed
M0	No distant metastasis
M1	Distant metastasis present, specify sites

Cancer Treatment

The goals of cancer treatment methods fall into three categories: curative, control, and palliative. The most common modalities are surgery, radiation therapy, chemotherapy, hormonal therapy, and biotherapy. The treatment of cancer involves the use of a carefully planned program that combines the benefits of multiple treatment modalities and the expertise of an interdisciplinary team of specialists, including medical, surgical, and radiation oncologists; clinical nurse specialists; nurse practitioners; pharmacists; and a variety of ancillary personnel.

Surgery

Surgery is the oldest treatment for cancer and is used for diagnosis, staging of cancer, tumor removal, and palliation (*i.e.*, relief of symptoms) when a cure cannot be achieved. The type of surgery to be used is determined by the extent of the disease, the location and structures involved, the tumor growth rate and invasiveness, the surgical risk to the person, and the quality of life the person will experience after the surgery. Surgery often is the first treatment used with solid tumors. If the tumor is small and has well-defined margins, the entire tumor often can be removed. If, however, the tumor is large or involves vital tissues, surgical removal may be difficult, if not impossible.

Surgery provides several approaches for cancer treatment. For example, it can be the primary, curative treatment for cancers that are locally or regionally contained, have not metastasized, or have not invaded major organs. It also is used as a component of adjuvant therapy in combination with chemotherapy or radiation therapy in other types of cancers. Surgical techniques also may be used to control oncologic emergencies such as gastrointestinal hemorrhages. Another approach includes using surgical techniques for cancer prophylaxis in families that have a high genetically confirmed risk for developing cancer. For instance, a total colectomy with a colostomy may be suggested for a person with familial adenomatous polyposis coli because of the increased risk for developing cancer by 40 years of age.

Surgical techniques have expanded to include cryosurgery, chemosurgery, laser surgery, and laparoscopic surgery. *Cryosurgery* involves the instillation of liquid nitrogen into the tumor through a probe. It is used in treating cancers of the liver and prostate. *Chemosurgery* is used in skin cancers. It involves the use of a corrosive paste in combination with multiple frozen sections to ensure complete removal of the tumor. *Laser surgery* uses a laser beam to resect a tumor. It has been used effectively in retinal and vocal cord surgery. *Laparoscopic surgery* involves the performance of abdominal surgery through two small incisions—one for viewing within the cavity and the other for insertion of the instruments to perform the surgery.

Cooperative efforts among cancer centers throughout the world have helped to standardize and improve surgical procedures, determine which cancers benefit from surgical intervention, and establish in what order surgical and other treatment modalities should be used. Increased emphasis also has been placed on the development of surgical techniques that preserve body image and form without compromising essential function. Nerve- and tissue-sparing surgeries are the primary method used if at all possible even if complete removal of the tumor is the goal.

Radiation Therapy

Radiation therapy is one of the most commonly used methods of cancer treatment.[6] It can be used alone as a primary method of therapy or as an adjuvant treatment with surgery, chemotherapy, or both. It can also be used as a palliative treatment to reduce symptoms such as bone pain resulting from metastasis in people with advanced cancers. Radiation is used to treat oncologic emergencies such as superior vena cava syndrome, spinal cord compression, or bronchial obstruction.

Radiation therapy uses high-energy particles or waves to destroy or damage cancer cells. The absorption of energy from radiation in tissue leads to the ionization of molecules or creation of free radicals. Radiation can also produce effects indirectly by interacting with water (which makes up approximately 80% of a cell's volume) to produce free radicals, which damage cell structures. Radiation can interrupt the cell cycle process, kill cells, or damage DNA in the cells.[6] Radiation must produce double-stranded breaks in DNA to kill a cell, owing to the high capacity of cells for repairing single-stranded breaks.

The therapeutic effects of radiation therapy derive from the fact that the rapidly proliferating and poorly differentiated cells of a cancerous tumor are more likely to be injured than are the more slowly proliferating cells of normal tissue. To some extent, however, radiation is injurious to all rapidly proliferating cells, including those of the bone marrow and the mucosal lining of the gastrointestinal tract. Normal tissue usually is able to recover from radiation damage more readily than cancerous tissue. In addition to its lethal effects, radiation also produces sublethal injury. Recovery from sublethal doses of radiation occurs in the interval between the first dose of radiation and subsequent doses.[6,45] This is why large total doses of radiation can be tolerated when they are divided into multiple, smaller fractionated doses.[53]

The radiation dose that is chosen for treatment of a particular cancer is determined by factors such as the radiosensitivity of the tumor type, the size of the tumor, and, more important, the tolerance of the surrounding tissues.[6,46] The term *radiosensitivity* describes the inherent properties of a tumor that determine its responsiveness to radiation. It varies widely among the different types of cancers and is thought to vary as a function of their position in the cell cycle. Fast-growing cancers have cells that typically are more radiosensitive than slow-growing cancers. The combination of selected cytotoxic drugs with radiation has demonstrated a radiosensitizing effect on tumor cells by altering the cell cycle distribution, increasing DNA damage, and decreasing DNA repair. Radiosensitizers include 5-fluorouracil, capecitabine, paclitaxel, and cisplatin.[47,48]

Radiation responsiveness describes the manner in which a radiosensitive tumor responds to irradiation. One of the major determinants of radiation responsiveness is tumor oxygenation because oxygen is a rich source of free radicals that form and destroy essential cell components during irradiation.[49] Many rapidly growing tumors outgrow their blood supply and become deprived of oxygen. The hypoxic cells of these tumors are more resistant to radiation than normal or well-oxygenated tumor cells. Methods of ensuring adequate oxygen delivery, such as adequate hemoglobin levels, are important.

Dose–response curves, which express the extent of lethal tissue injury in relation to the dose of radiation, are determined by the number of cells that survive graded, fractional doses of radiation. The use of more frequent fractionated doses increases the likelihood that the cancer cells will be dividing and in the vulnerable period of the cell cycle during radiation administration. This type of dose also allows time for normal tissues to repair the radiation damage. An important focus of research has been the search for drugs to reduce the biologic effects of radiation on normal tissue. These drugs, known as *radioprotectants*, would preferentially protect normal cells from the cytotoxic effects of radiation. One drug, amifostine, is poorly understood and has had varying degrees of success in protecting cells from the cytotoxic effects of radiation.[50,51] Therefore, although there have been some promising developments, more research is necessary regarding radioprotectants.

Administration. Therapeutic radiation can be delivered in one of three ways: external beam or teletherapy, with beams generated at a distance and aimed at the tumor in a person; brachytherapy, in which a sealed radioactive source is placed close to or directly in the tumor site; and systemic therapy, when radioisotopes are given orally or injected into the tumor site.[6] Radiation from any source decreases in intensity as a function of the square of the distance from the source. Teletherapy, which is the most commonly used form of radiation therapy, maintains intensity over a large volume of tissue by increasing the source to surface distance. In brachytherapy, the source to surface distance is small; therefore, the effective treatment volume is small.

External beam radiation is most frequently used with a linear accelerator or a cobalt-60 machine.[6] The linear accelerator is the preferred machine because of its versatility and precision of dose distribution, as well as the speed with which treatment can be given. Linear accelerators produce ionizing radiation through a process in which electrons are accelerated at a very high rate, strike a target, and produce high-energy x-rays (photons). The linear accelerator can vary the level of radiation energy that is delivered so that different depths can be treated. Various beam-modifying approaches are used to define and shape the beam, thereby increasing the radiation damage to the tumor site while sparing the normal surrounding tissues. The person is fitted with a plastic mold or cast to keep the body still, whereas radiation beams are delivered to the body from several directions. Intensity-modulated radiation therapy (IMRT) and three-dimensional conformal radiation therapy (3DCRT) are advanced forms of external radiation therapy. As with 3DCRT, computer imaging techniques are used to calculate the most efficient dosages and combinations of radiation treatment. This precise mapping of the tumor allows for the delivery of radiation beams that conform to the contours of the tumor, reducing the dose and therefore the toxicity to adjacent normal tissue. Because of its precision, it is even more important that the person remain in the right place and perfectly still during the treatment. This usually requires fabricating a special cast or mold before treatment to keep the body in place.

Brachytherapy involves the insertion of sealed radioactive sources into a body cavity (intracavitary) or directly into body tissues (interstitial). *Brachytherapy* means "short therapy," implying that the radiation effect is limited to areas close to the radiation source.[52] Brachytherapy can be subdivided into high-dose radiation (HDR) and low-dose radiation (LDR) according to the rate at which the radiation is delivered. HDR uses a single highly radioactive source that is attached to a cable and housed in a robotic machine referred to as an HDR remote afterloader. When the treatment is delivered, the radiation source is pushed from the remote afterloader through a tube to a location near the tumor site. Remote afterloading machines make it possible to insert a radioactive material (*e.g.*, cesium-137, iridium-192) into a tumor area for a specific time and remove it while oncology personnel are outside the treatment room. This minimizes staff radiation exposure and decreases treatment times by allowing use of intermediate- and high-dose radioactive sources.[52] In contrast, the radiation source for LDR brachytherapy may be packed into catheter devices or sealed radiation sources (*e.g.*, beads, seeds) and placed directly in or near the area being treated. LDR therapy can be temporary or permanent. Temporary LDR brachytherapy can be accomplished as an inpatient procedure, with radiation applicators and sources remaining in the person for a few days. Radioactive materials with a relatively short half-life, such as iodine-125 or palladium-103, are commonly encapsulated and used in permanent implants (*e.g.*, seed implants used to treat prostate cancer).

Unsealed internal radiation sources are injected intravenously or administered by mouth. Iodine-131, which is given by mouth, is used in the treatment of thyroid cancer. Stereotactic radiosurgery is a method of destroying brain tumors and brain metastases by delivering a single large dose of radiation through stereotactically directed narrow beams. Gamma Knife radiosurgery allows the application of focused radiation for limited brain metastasis and is associated with fewer long-term complications, such as cognitive dysfunction, compared to whole-brain radiation.

Adverse Effects. Radiation therapy negatively effects normal tissue that is rapidly proliferative similar to malignant cells. Tissues within the treatment fields that are most frequently affected are the skin, the mucosal lining of the gastrointestinal tract, and bone marrow. Anorexia, nausea, emesis, and diarrhea are common with abdominal and pelvic irradiation. These symptoms are usually controlled by medication and dietary measures. The primary systemic effect is fatigue. Most of these side effects are temporary and reversible.

Radiation can also cause bone marrow suppression, particularly when it is delivered to the bone marrow in skeletal sites. Subsequently, the complete blood count is affected, resulting in an initial decrease in the number of the leukocytes, followed by a decrease in thrombocytes (platelets) and red blood cells. This predisposes the person to infection, bleeding, and anemia, respectively.

External beam radiation must first penetrate the skin, and depending on the total dose and type of radiation used, skin reactions may develop. With moderate doses of radiation, the hair falls out spontaneously or when being combed after the 10th to the 14th day. With larger doses, erythema develops (much like sunburn) and may turn brown, and at higher doses, patches of dry or moist desquamation may develop. Mucositis or desquamation of the oral and pharyngeal mucous membranes, which sometimes may be severe, may occur as a predictable side effect in people receiving head and neck irradiation. Pain and difficulty eating and drinking can negatively affect the person's nutritional status. Pelvic radiation can cause impotence or erectile dysfunction in men and vaginal irritation, dryness, and discharge, dyspareunia, and, as a late effect, vaginal stenosis in women.

Chemotherapy

Cancer chemotherapy has evolved as one of the major systemic treatment modalities for cancer. Unlike surgery and radiation, chemotherapy is a systemic treatment that enables drugs to reach the site of the tumor as well as other distant sites. Chemotherapeutic drugs may be the primary form of treatment, or they may be used as part of a multimodal treatment plan. It is the primary treatment for most hematologic and some solid tumors. In people with widespread disseminated disease, chemotherapy may provide only palliative rather than curative therapy.

Chemotherapeutic drugs exert their effects through several mechanisms. At the cellular level, they exert their lethal action by targeting processes that prevent cell growth and replication. Chemotherapy kills cancer cells by stopping DNA, RNA, and protein synthesis; influencing enzyme production; and generally preventing cell mitosis.[6] Under ideal conditions, anticancer drugs would eradicate cancer cells without damaging normal tissues. Although in the process of development, targeted cancer agents are not available without toxic effects.

For most chemotherapy drugs, the relationship between tumor cell survival and drug dose is exponential, with the number of cells surviving being proportional to the drug dose and the number of cells at risk for exposure being proportional to the destructive action of the drug. Chemotherapeutic drugs are most effective in treating tumors that have a high growth fraction because of their ability to kill rapidly dividing cells.

A major problem in cancer chemotherapy is the development of cellular resistance. Experimentally, drug resistance can be highly specific to a single agent and is usually based on genetic changes in a given tumor cell. In other instances, a multidrug-resistant phenomenon encompassing anticancer drugs with differing structures occurs. This type of resistance often involves the increased expression of transmembrane transporter genes involved in drug efflux.

Chemotherapy drugs are commonly classified according to their site and mechanism of action. Chemotherapy drugs that have similar structures and effects on cell function usually are grouped together, and these drugs usually have similar side effect profiles. Direct DNA-interacting and indirect DNA-interacting agents are two major categories of chemotherapy drugs.[6] Other systemic agents include hormonal and molecularly targeted agents. Cancer chemotherapy drugs may also be classified as either cell cycle specific or cell cycle nonspecific. Drugs are cell cycle specific if they exert their action during a specific phase of the cell cycle. For example, methotrexate, an antimetabolite, acts by interfering with DNA synthesis and thereby interrupts the S phase of the cell cycle. Drugs that are cell cycle nonspecific exert their effects throughout all phases of the cell cycle. The alkylating agents are cell cycle nonspecific and act by disrupting DNA when the cells are in the resting state as well as when they are dividing. Because chemotherapy drugs differ in their mechanisms of action, cell cycle–specific and cell cycle–nonspecific agents are often combined to treat cancer.

Direct DNA-Interacting Agents. The direct DNA-interacting agents include the alkylating agents, antitumor antibiotics, and topoisomerase inhibitors. As a class, the alkylating agents exert their cytotoxic effects by transferring their alkyl group to many cellular constituents.[53] Alkylation of DNA within the cell nucleus is probably the major interaction that causes cell death. Alkylating agents have direct vesicant effects and can damage tissues at the site of injection as well as produce systemic toxicity. Toxicities are generally dose related and occur particularly in rapidly proliferating tissues such as bone marrow, the gastrointestinal tract, and reproductive tissues.

The *antitumor antibiotics* are substances produced by bacteria that in nature appear to provide protection against hostile microorganisms. As a class, they bind directly to DNA and frequently undergo electron transfer reactions to generate free radicals in close proximity to DNA, resulting in DNA damage in the form of single breaks or cross-links. Approximately 75% of all anticancer antibiotics in clinical use are originally isolated by the soil microbe, *Streptomyces*.[54] These include the anthracyclines, dactinomycin, bleomycin, and mitomycin. The anthracycline antibiotics (*e.g.*, doxorubicin and daunorubicin) are among the most widely used cytotoxic cancer drugs.[54] The main dose-limiting toxicity of all anthracyclines is cardiotoxicity and myelosuppression, with neutropenia more commonly observed than thrombocytopenia. Two forms of cardiotoxicity can occur—acute and chronic. The acute form occurs within the first 2 to 3 days of therapy and presents with arrhythmias, conduction disorders, other electrocardiographic changes, pericarditis, and myocarditis.[54,55] This form is usually transient and in most cases asymptomatic. The chronic form of cardiotoxicity results in a dose-dependent dilated cardiomyopathy. Efforts to minimize the toxicity profile of the antitumor antibiotics have resulted in the development of analog compounds (*e.g.*, idarubicin, epirubicin). Liposome technology has been used with two antitumor antibiotics (*i.e.*, doxorubicin and daunorubicin) to develop chemotherapy drugs that are encapsulated by coated liposomes.

The DNA *topoisomerase inhibitors* block cell division by interfering with the action of the topoisomerase enzymes that break and rejoin phosphodiester bonds in the DNA strands to prevent them from tangling during separation and unwinding of the double helix.[56] Topoisomerase I produces single-strand breaks (nicks) and topoisomerase II double-strand breaks. The epipodophyllotoxins (etoposide and teniposide) are topoisomerase II inhibitors that block cell division in the late S to G2 phase of the cell cycle. The camptothecins (topotecan, irinotecan) inhibit the action of topoisomerase I, the enzyme responsible for cutting and rejoining single DNA strands. Inhibition of this enzyme interferes with resealing of the breaks and DNA damage.

Indirect DNA-Interacting Agents. The indirect DNA-interacting agents include the antimetabolites and mitotic spindle inhibitors. The antimetabolites (folic acid antagonists and purine and pyrimidine antagonists) interrupt the biochemical pathways relating to nucleotide and nucleic acid synthesis. Antimetabolites can cause DNA damage indirectly through misincorporation into DNA or abnormal timing of DNA synthesis or by causing abnormal functioning of purine and pyrimidine biosynthetic enzymes.[56] They tend to convey their greatest effect during the S phase of the cell cycle. Because of their S-phase specificity, the antimetabolites have been shown to be more effective when given as a prolonged infusion. Common side effects include stomatitis, diarrhea, and myelosuppression.

The plant alkaloids, including the vinca alkaloids and taxanes, are drugs affecting the microtubule structures required for formation of the cytoskeleton and mitotic spindle.[57] Although each group of drugs affects the microtubule, their mechanism of action differs. The vinca alkaloids (*e.g.*, vinblastine, vincristine) inhibit tubulin polymerization, which disrupts assembly of microtubules. This inhibitory effect results in mitotic arrest in metaphase, bringing cell division to a stop, which then leads to cell death. Vinblastine is a potent vesicant and care must be taken in its administration. Toxicities include nausea and vomiting, bone marrow suppression, and alopecia. Despite similarities in their mechanisms of action, vincristine has a different spectrum of actions and toxicities than vinblastine. The main dose-limiting toxicity is neurotoxicity, usually expressed as a peripheral sensory neuropathy, although autonomic nervous system dysfunction (*e.g.*, orthostatic hypotension, sphincter problems, paralytic ileus), cranial nerve palsies, ataxia, seizures, and coma have been observed. The taxanes (*e.g.*, paclitaxel, docetaxel) differ from the vinca alkaloids in that they stabilize the microtubules against depolymerization. The stabilized microtubules are unable to undergo the normal changes necessary for cell cycle completion. These drugs are administered intravenously and require the use of a vehicle that can cause hypersensitivity reactions. In addition to hypersensitivity reactions, their side effect profile includes myelosuppression and peripheral neurotoxicity in the form of glove-and-stocking numbness and paresthesia.

Combination Chemotherapy. Combination chemotherapy has been found to be more effective than treatment with a single drug. Combination chemotherapy creates a more hostile environment for tumor cell growth through higher drug concentrations and prevents the development of resistant clones of cancer cells. With this method, several drugs with different mechanisms of action, metabolic pathways, times of onset of action and recovery, side effects, and times of onset of side effects are used. Drugs used in combination must be individually effective against the tumor and may be synergistic with each other. Routes of administration and dosage schedules are carefully designed to ensure optimal delivery of the active forms of the drugs to a tumor during the sensitive phase of the cell cycle.

Administration. Many of the cancer chemotherapy drugs are administered intravenously. Venous access devices (VADs) often are used for people with poor venous access and those who require frequent or continuous intravenous therapy. The VAD can be used for home administration of chemotherapy drugs, blood sampling, and administration of blood components. These systems access the venous circulation either through an externalized catheter or an implanted catheter with access ports. In some cases, the drugs are administered by continuous infusion using an ambulatory infusion pump that allows the person to remain at home and maintain his or her activities.

Adverse Effects. Chemotherapy is administered on a dose–response basis (*i.e.*, the more drug administered, the greater the number of cancer cells killed). Chemotherapeutic drugs affect neoplastic cells and the rapidly proliferating cells of normal tissue. The nadir (*i.e.*, lowest point) is the point of maximal toxicity for a given adverse effect of a drug and is stated in the time it takes to reach that point. Because many toxic effects of chemotherapeutic drugs persist for some time after the drug is discontinued, the nadir times and recovery rates are useful guides in evaluating the effects of cancer therapy. Some side effects appear immediately or after a few days (acute), some within a few weeks (intermediate), and others months to years after chemotherapy administration (long term).

Most chemotherapeutic drugs cause pancytopenia because of bone marrow suppression, resulting in neutropenia (causing infections), anemia (resulting in fatigue), and thrombocytopenia (increasing risk for bleeding). The availability of hematopoietic growth factors (*e.g.*, granulocyte colony-stimulating factor [G-CSF] and IL-11, a cytokine, which stimulates platelet production) has shortened the period of myelosuppression, thereby reducing the need for hospitalizations because of infection and bleeding. The growth factor epoetin alfa, a form of the protein erythropoietin manufactured by the kidneys to help produce red blood cells, is used with a select population of people. The drug has been under scrutiny since 2004 when it was found that it could promote tumor progression and shorten survival. The risk–benefit of epoetin needs to be weighed carefully before the drug is given for chemotherapy-induced anemia.[58]

Anorexia, nausea, and vomiting are common problems associated with cancer chemotherapy.[6] The severity of the vomiting is related to the emetic potential of the particular drug. These symptoms can occur within minutes or hours of drug administration and are thought to be due to stimulation of the chemoreceptor trigger zone in the medulla that initiates vomiting. The chemoreceptor trigger zone responds to levels of chemicals circulating in the blood. The acute symptoms usually subside within 24 to 48 hours and often can be relieved by antiemetics. The pharmacologic approaches to prevent chemotherapy-induced nausea and vomiting have greatly improved over the past several decades. Serotonin receptor (5-HT_3) antagonists (*e.g.*, ondansetron, granisetron, dolasetron, palonosetron) facilitate the use of highly emetic chemotherapy drugs by more effectively reducing the nausea and vomiting induced by these drugs. These antiemetics are effective when given by both the oral and intravenous routes.

Alopecia or hair loss results from impaired proliferation of the hair follicles and is a side effect of a number of cancer drugs. It usually is temporary, and the hair tends to regrow when treatment is stopped. The rapidly proliferating structures of the reproductive system are particularly sensitive to the action of cancer drugs. Women may experience changes in menstrual flow or have amenorrhea. Men may have a decreased sperm count (*i.e.*, oligospermia) or absence of sperm (*i.e.*, azoospermia). Teratogenic or mutagenic effects can also occur from taking chemotherapy.

Chemotherapy drugs are toxic to all cells. The mutagenic, carcinogenic, and teratogenic potential of these drugs has been strongly supported by both animal and human studies. Because of these potential risks, special care is required when handling or administering the drugs. Drugs, drug containers, and administration equipment require special disposal as hazardous waste. The Occupational Safety and Health Administration (OSHA), the Oncology Nursing Society (ONS), and the American Society of Hospital Pharmacists (ASHP) have created chemotherapy guidelines dedicated to their safe administration.

Epidemiologic studies have shown an increased risk for second malignancies such as acute leukemia after long-term use of alkylating agents. These second malignancies are thought to result from direct cellular changes produced by the drug or from suppression of the immune response.

Hormonal Therapy

Hormonal therapy consists of administration of drugs designed to disrupt the hormonal environment of cancer cells. The actions of hormones and antihormones depend on the presence of specific receptors in the tumor. Among the tumors that are known to be responsive to hormonal manipulation are those of the breast, prostate, and endometrium. Additionally, other cancers, such as Kaposi sarcoma and renal, liver, ovarian, and pancreatic cancer, can be treated with hormonal therapy. The theory behind the majority of hormone-based cancer treatments is to deprive the cancer cells of the hormonal signals that otherwise would stimulate them to divide.

The therapeutic options for altering the hormonal environment in the woman with breast cancer or the man with prostate cancer include surgical and pharmacologic measures. Surgery involves the removal of the organ responsible for the hormone production that is stimulating the target tissue (*e.g.*, oophorectomy in women or orchiectomy in men). Pharmacologic methods focus largely on reducing circulating hormone levels or changing the hormone receptors so that they no longer respond to the hormone.

Pharmacologic suppression of circulating hormone levels can be effected through pituitary desensitization, as with the administration of androgens, or through the administration of *gonadotropin-releasing hormone* (GnRH) analogues that act at the level of the hypothalamus to inhibit gonadotropin production and release. Another class of drugs, the *aromatase inhibitors*, is used to treat some forms of early-stage breast cancer. These drugs act by interrupting the biochemical processes that convert the adrenal androgen androstenedione to estrone.[59] Aromatization of an androgenic precursor into an estrogen occurs in body fat. Because estrogen promotes the growth of breast cancer, estrogen synthesis in adipose tissue can be an important factor in breast cancer growth in postmenopausal women.

Hormone receptor function can be altered by the administration of pharmacologic doses of exogenous hormones that act by producing a decrease in hormone receptors or by antihormone drugs (*i.e.*, antiestrogens [tamoxifen, fulvestrant] and antiandrogens [flutamide, bicalutamide, nilutamide]) that bind to hormone receptors, making them inaccessible to hormone stimulation. Initially, people often respond favorably to hormonal treatments, but eventually, the cancer becomes resistant to hormonal manipulation, and other approaches must be sought to control the disease.

Biotherapy

Biotherapy involves the use of immunotherapy and biologic response modifiers as a means of changing the person's own immune response to cancer.[60] The major mechanisms by which biotherapy exerts its effects are modifications of host responses or tumor cell biology.

Immunotherapy. The use of immunotherapy has proven to be an effective treatment strategy of malignancy and has less toxicity than chemotherapy regimens.[61] Immunotherapy is a treatment that uses one's own immune system to treat cancer by either stimulating the immune system to attack cancer cells or improving the individual's immune system.[62] Immunotherapy may be used as a single-agent treatment or used in conjunction with other treatment modalities.[62]

Types of cancer immunotherapy include monoclonal antibodies, immune inhibitors, cancer vaccines, and nonspecific immunotherapies.[62] *Monoclonal antibodies* are made in the laboratory and target specific proteins or antigens often found on cancer cells allowing for an attack on specific cells.[62] *Immune inhibitors* allow the body to recognize molecules on specific immune cells in order to create an immune response.[62] *Cancer vaccines* are one of the latest biologic response modifiers that act by stimulating the immune system to fight a specific infection or disease, most often cancer-causing viruses such as hepatitis B and HPV.[63,64]

Biologic Response Modifiers. Biologic response modifiers can be grouped into three types: cytokines, which include the interferons and ILs; monoclonal antibodies (MoAbs); and hematopoietic growth factors. Some agents, such as interferons, have more than one biologic function, including antiviral, immunomodulatory, and antiproliferative actions. The *interferons* are endogenous polypeptides that are synthesized by a number of cells in response to a variety of cellular or viral stimuli. The three major types of interferons are alpha (α), beta (β), and gamma (γ), each group differing in terms of their cell surface receptors.[5,65] The interferons appear to inhibit viral replication and also may be involved in inhibiting tumor protein synthesis and in prolonging the cell cycle, increasing the percentage of cells in the G_0 phase. Interferons stimulate NK cells and T-lymphocyte killer cells. Interferon-γ has been approved for the treatment of hairy cell leukemia, AIDS-related Kaposi sarcoma, and CML and as adjuvant therapy for people at high risk for recurrent melanoma.[6,65]

The ILs are cytokines that affect communication between cells by binding to receptor sites on the cell surface membranes of the target cells. Of the 18 known ILs, IL-2 has been the most widely studied. A recombinant human IL-2 (rIL-2, aldesleukin) has been approved by the FDA and is being used for the treatment of metastatic renal cell and melanoma.[65]

IN SUMMARY

The methods used in the diagnosis of cancer vary with the type of cancer and its location. Because many cancers are curable if diagnosed early, health care practices designed to promote early detection are important. Histologic studies are done in the laboratory using cells or tissue specimens. There are two basic methods of classifying tumors: grading according to the histologic or tissue characteristics and clinical staging according to spread of the disease. The TNM system for clinical staging of cancer takes into account tumor size, lymph node involvement, and presence of metastasis.

Treatment plans that use more than one type of therapy, often in combination, are providing cures for a number of cancers that a few decades ago had a poor prognosis and are increasing the life expectancy in other types of cancer. Surgical procedures are more precise and less invasive, preserving organ function and resulting in better quality-of-life outcomes. Newer radiation equipment and novel radiation techniques permit greater and more controlled destruction of cancer cells while sparing normal tissues. Cancer chemotherapy has evolved as one of the major systemic treatment modalities for cancer. Unlike surgery and radiation, chemotherapy is a systemic treatment that enables drugs to reach the site of the tumor as well as other distant sites. The major classifications of chemotherapy drugs are the direct DNA-interacting (alkylating agents, antitumor antibiotics, and topoisomerase inhibitors) and indirect DNA-interacting agents (antimetabolites and mitotic spindle inhibitors). Cancer chemotherapeutic drugs may also be classified as either cell cycle specific or cell cycle nonspecific depending on whether they exert their action during a specific phase of the cell cycle. Other systemic agents include hormonal and molecularly targeted agents that block specific enzymes and growth factors involved in cancer cell growth.

CHILDHOOD CANCERS

After completing this section of the chapter, the learner will be able to meet the following objectives:

- Cite the most common types of cancer affecting infants, children, and adolescents.
- Describe how cancers that affect children differ from those that affect adults.
- Discuss possible long-term effects of radiation therapy and chemotherapy on adult survivors of childhood cancer.

Cancer in children is relatively rare, accounting for about 1% of all malignancies in the United States.[1] Although rare, cancer remains the second leading cause of death among school-age children in the United States.[1] Common cancers that occur in children include leukemia, non-Hodgkin and Hodgkin lymphomas, and bone cancers (osteosarcoma and Ewing sarcoma). The overall survival rate for children is 85%.[2]

Incidence and Types

The spectrum of cancers that affect children differs markedly from those that affect adults. Although most adult cancers are of epithelial cell origin (*e.g.*, lung cancer, breast cancer, colorectal cancers), childhood cancers differ in that they generally involve the hematopoietic system, nervous system, soft tissues, bone, and kidneys.[66]

During the first year of life, embryonal tumors such as Wilms tumor, RB, and neuroblastoma are among the most common types of tumors. Embryonal tumors along with acute leukemia, non-Hodgkin lymphoma, and gliomas have a peak incidence in children 2 to 5 years of age. As children age, especially after they pass puberty, bone malignancies, Hodgkin lymphoma, gonadal germ cell tumors (testicular and ovarian carcinomas), and various carcinomas such as thyroid cancer and malignant melanoma increase in incidence.

Embryonal Tumors

A number of the tumors of infancy and early childhood are embryonal in origin, meaning that they exhibit features of organogenesis similar to that of embryonic development. Because of this characteristic, these tumors are frequently designated with the suffix “blastoma” (*e.g.*, nephroblastoma [Wilms tumor], RB, and neuroblastoma).[2] Wilms tumor and neuroblastoma are particularly illustrative of this type of childhood tumor.

Neuroblastoma. Neuroblastomas arise from the primordial neural crest tissue in the sympathetic nervous system and adrenal medulla.[67] It is the second most common solid malignancy in childhood after brain tumors. About 40% of neuroblastomas arise in the adrenal gland, with the remainder occurring anywhere along the sympathetic chain, most commonly in the paravertebral region of the abdomen and posterior mediastinum. Tumors may arise in numerous other sites, including the pelvis, neck, and within the brain. Clinical manifestations vary with the primary site and neuroendocrine function of the tumor. In children younger than 2 years of age, neuroblastoma generally presents with large abdominal masses, fever, and possibly weight loss. Bone pain suggests metastatic disease. About 90% of the tumors, regardless of location, secrete catecholamines, which is an important diagnostic feature (*i.e.*, elevated blood levels of catecholamines and elevated urine levels of catecholamine metabolites).[67]

Neuroblastoma is also an extremely malignant neoplasm, particularly in children with advanced disease.[67] Although the 5-year survival rate has improved, neuroblastoma continues to account for approximately 15% of all childhood cancer deaths. Infants tend to have a better prognosis than older children. Almost all children with neuroblastoma are diagnosed before 5 years of age, and the younger the child is diagnosed, the more positive the prognosis is.[67]

Biology of Childhood Cancers

As with adult cancers, there probably is no single cause of childhood cancer. Although a number of genetic conditions are associated with childhood cancer, such conditions are relatively rare, suggesting an interaction between genetic susceptibility and environmental exposures. There are some inheritable conditions that increase susceptibility to childhood and even adult cancer. An example is Down syndrome, which actually increases the risk of acute lymphoblastic leukemia (ALL) and AML.[2,68]

Although constituting only a small percentage of childhood cancers, the biology of a number of these tumors illustrates several important biologic aspects of neoplasms, such as the two-hit theory of recessive tumor suppressor genes (*e.g.*, *RB* gene mutation in RB); defects in DNA repair; and the histologic similarities between organogenesis and oncogenesis. Syndromes associated with defects in DNA repair include xeroderma pigmentosa, in which there is increased risk of skin cancers owing to defects in repair of DNA damaged by ultraviolet light. The development of childhood cancers has also been linked to genomic imprinting. The inactivation is determined by whether the gene is inherited from the mother or father. For example, the maternal allele for the insulin-like growth factor-2 (IGF-2) gene normally is inactivated (imprinted). In some Wilms tumors, loss of imprinting (re-expression of the maternal allele) can be demonstrated by overexpression of the IGF-2 protein, which is an embryonal growth factor.[69]

Diagnosis and Treatment

Early detection often leads to less therapy and improved outcomes. Because of generalized symptoms experienced by children such as prolonged fever, fatigue, and bone pain, diagnosis is often delayed. When these symptoms are experienced in the setting of persistent lymphadenopathy, unexplained weight loss, growing masses (especially in association with weight loss), and abnormalities of CNS function, they should be viewed as warning signs of cancer in children. Because these signs and symptoms of cancer are often similar to those of common childhood diseases, it is easy to miss a cancer diagnosis in the early stages.

Diagnosis of childhood cancers involves many of the same methods used in adults. Histologic examination is usually an essential part of the diagnostic procedure. Accurate disease staging is especially beneficial in childhood cancers, in which the potential benefits of treatment must be carefully weighed against potential long-term effects.

The treatment of childhood cancers is complex, intensive, prolonged, and continuously evolving. It usually involves appropriate multidisciplinary and multimodal therapies, as well as the evaluation for recurrent disease and late effects of the disease and therapies used in its treatment.

Two modalities are frequently used in the treatment of childhood cancer, with chemotherapy being the most widely used, followed, in order of use, by surgery, radiation therapy, and biologic agent therapy. Chemotherapy is more widely used in treatment of children with cancer than in adults because children better tolerate the acute adverse effects and, in general, pediatric tumors are more responsive to chemotherapy than adult cancers.[70]

With improvement in treatment methods, the number of children who survive childhood cancer continues to increase. However, therapy may produce late sequelae, such as impaired growth, neurologic dysfunction, hormonal dysfunction, cardiomyopathy, pulmonary fibrosis, and risk for second malignancies. Thus, one of the growing challenges is providing appropriate health care to survivors of childhood and adolescent cancers.[71]

Radiation Therapy

Radiation therapy poses the risk of long-term effects for survivors of childhood cancer. The late effects of radiation therapy are influenced by the organs and tissues included in the treatment field, type of radiation administered, daily fractional and cumulative radiation dose, and age at treatment. There is increased risk for melanoma, squamous cell carcinoma, and basal cell carcinoma. Musculoskeletal changes are also common after radiation. Even with current methods, survivors may have changes leading to pain and altered musculoskeletal function.

Cranial radiation therapy (CRT) has been used to treat brain tumors, ALL, head and neck soft tissue tumors, and RB. The most common late effect of moderate- to high-dose whole-brain radiation is diminished intellectual function.[71] Brain tumor survivors treated at a younger age are particularly susceptible. Cranial radiation is also associated with neuroendocrine disorders, particularly growth hormone deficiency. Thus, children reaching adulthood after CRT may have reduced physical stature. The younger the age and the higher the radiation dose, the greater the deviation from normal growth. Growth hormone deficiency in adults is associated with increased prevalence of dyslipidemia, insulin resistance, and cardiovascular mortality. Moderate doses of CRT are also associated with obesity, particularly in female patients.[71] For many years, whole-brain radiation or CRT was the primary method of preventing CNS relapse in children with ALL. Recognition of cognitive dysfunction associated with CRT has led to the use of other methods of CNS prophylaxis.[71]

Radiation to the chest or mantle field (lymph nodes of neck, subclavicular, axillary, and mediastinal areas) is often used in treatment of Hodgkin and non-Hodgkin lymphomas and metastases to the lung. This field exposes the developing breast tissue, heart, and lungs to ionizing radiation. Female survivors who were treated with this type of radiation face significant risk for development of breast cancer.[71] Much of the heart is exposed in chest and mantle radiation fields, resulting in subsequent premature coronary artery, valvular, and pericardial disease. Exposure of the lungs to radiation therapy can result in a reduction in pulmonary function. Thyroid disease, particularly hypothyroidism, is common after mantle or neck radiation.

Childhood cancer survivors treated with abdominal or pelvic radiation are also at risk for a variety of late health problems involving the gastrointestinal tract, liver, spleen, kidneys, and genitourinary tract structures, including the gonads.[71] Gastrointestinal tract complications include chronic mucosal inflammation that interferes with absorption and digestion of nutrients. Chronic radiation injury to the kidneys may interfere with glomerular or tubular function, and fibrosis from pelvic radiation may adversely affect bladder capacity and function. The adverse effects of radiation on gonadal function vary by age, sex, and cumulative dose. Delayed sexual maturation in boys and girls can result from irradiation of the gonads. In boys, sperm production is reduced in a dose-dependent manner. In girls, radiation to the abdomen, pelvis, and spine is associated with increased risk of ovarian failure, especially if the ovaries are in the treatment field.

Chemotherapy

Chemotherapy also poses the risk of long-term effects for survivors of childhood cancer. Potential late effects of alkylating agents include dose-related gonadal injury (hypogonadism, infertility, and early menopause).[71] Alkylating agent therapy has also been linked to dose-related secondary acute myelogenous leukemia, pulmonary fibrosis, kidney disease, and bladder disorders. Anthracyclines, including doxorubicin and daunomycin, which are widely used in treatment of childhood cancers, can result in cardiomyopathy and eventual congestive heart failure.[71] The late effects of cisplatin and carboplatin, the most frequently used nonclassic alkylators, are nephrotoxicity, ototoxicity, and neurotoxicity. Although combination chemotherapy increases the effectiveness of treatment, it may also be associated with increased risk of side effects if the agents have a similar spectrum of toxicity. Intrathecal combination chemotherapy to prevent relapse of ALL in the CNS, which is a sanctuary for ALL cells, is known to cause significant and persistent cognitive impairment in many children.

IN SUMMARY

Although most adult cancers are of epithelial cell origin, most childhood cancers usually involve the hematopoietic system, nervous system, or connective tissue. Heritable forms of cancer tend to have an earlier age of onset, a higher frequency of multifocal lesions in a single organ, and bilateral involvement of paired organs or multiple primary tumors. The early diagnosis of childhood cancers often is missed because the signs and symptoms mimic those of other childhood diseases. With improvement in treatment methods, the number of children who survive childhood cancer is continuing to increase. As these children approach adulthood, there is continued concern that the lifesaving therapy they received during childhood may produce late effects, such as impaired growth, cognitive dysfunction, hormonal dysfunction, cardiomyopathy, pulmonary fibrosis, and risk for second malignancies.

GERIATRIC Considerations

- The occurrence of new cases for the four major cancers (colon/rectum, lung/bronchus, breast [female], prostate) increases with age.[72]
- Geriatric oncology, a multidisciplinary/multidimensional approach, arose from the growing number of persons age 65 and older with cancer.[73]
- Comorbidities, polypharmacy, and lack of inclusion in clinical trials limit the understanding of chemotherapy in this age group.[73]
- Recovery from cancer and cancer treatment is often delayed because of slower tissue healing and function of pulmonary and cardiovascular systems.[73]

PEDIATRIC Considerations

- Cancer is the leading cause of death by disease in children older than 1 year.[74]
- Developmental tasks during adolescence may be delayed because of isolation from peers and may be accompanied by inferior school performance.[74]
- A change in blood cell production is a warning sign of cancer in children, leading to more frequent and severe infections, fatigue, and paleness.[74]
- Treatment choices may depend on long-term effects, especially the impact on growth and development.[74]

REVIEW EXERCISES

1. A 30-year-old woman has experienced heavy menstrual bleeding and is told she has a uterine tumor called a *leiomyoma*. She is worried she has cancer.
   A. *What is the difference between a leiomyoma and leiomyosarcoma?*
   B. *How would you explain the difference to her?*
2. Among the characteristics of cancer cells are lack of cell differentiation, impaired cell-to-cell adhesion, and loss of anchorage dependence.
   A. *Explain how each of these characteristics contributes to the usefulness of the Pap smear as a screening test for cervical cancer.*
3. A 12-year-old boy is seen at the pediatric cancer clinic with osteosarcoma. His medical history reveals that his father had been successfully treated for RB as an infant.
   A. *Relate the genetics of the RB gene and the "two-hit" hypothesis to the development of osteosarcoma in the son of the man who had RB.*
4. A 48-year-old man presents at his health care clinic with complaints of leg weakness. He is a heavy smoker and has had a productive cough for years. Subsequent diagnostic tests reveal he has a small cell lung cancer with brain metastasis. His proposed plan of treatment includes chemotherapy and radiation therapy.
   A. *What is the probable cause of the leg weakness, and is it related to the lung cancer?*
   B. *Relate this man's smoking history to the development of lung cancer.*
   C. *Explain the mechanism of cancer metastasis.*
   D. *Explain the mechanisms whereby chemotherapy and irradiation are able to destroy cancer cells while having a lesser or no effect on normal cells.*

5. A 17-year-old-girl is seen by a guidance counselor at her high school because of problems in keeping up with assignments in her math and science courses. She tells the counselor that she had leukemia when she was 2 years old and was given radiation treatment to the brain. She confides that she has always had more trouble with learning than her classmates and thinks it might be due to the radiation. She also relates that she is shorter than her classmates, and this has been bothering her.
   A. *Explain the relationship between cranial radiation therapy (CRT) and decreased cognitive function and short stature.*
   B. *What other neuroendocrine problems might this girl have as a result of the radiation treatment?*

References

1. Centers for Disease Control and Prevention. (2016). Deaths and mortality. [Online]. Available: https://www.cdc.gov/nchs/fastats/deaths.htm. Accessed October 26, 2017.
2. Center for Disease Control and Prevention. (2014). Child health. [Online]. Available: https://www.cdc.gov/nchs/fastats/child-health.htm. Accessed October 20, 2017.
3. American Cancer Society. (2017). Cancer facts & figures: 2017. [Online]. Available: https://www.cancer.org/content/dam/cancer-org/research/cancer-facts-and-statistics/annual-cancer-facts-and-figures/2017/cancer-facts-and-figures-2017.pdf. Accessed November 8, 2017.
4. American Cancer Society. (2015). *Global cancer facts & figures (3rd ed). [Online].* Available: https://www.cancer.org/content/dam/cancer-org/research/cancer-facts-and-statistics/global-cancer-facts-and-figures/global-cancer-facts-and-figures-3rd-edition.pdf. Accessed November 14, 2017.
5. Dominguez-Brauer C., Thu K. L., Mason J. M. (2015). Targeting mitosis in cancer: Emerging strategies. *Molecular Cell* 60(4), 524–536.
6. Rubin R., Strayer D. S. (Eds). (2014). *Rubin's pathology: Clinicopathologic foundations of medicine* (7th ed). Philadelphia, PA: Lippincott Williams & Wilkins.
7. Yarbro C. H., Wujcik D., Gobel B. H. (Eds.). (2018). *Cancer nursing: Principles & practice* (8th ed.). Sudbury, MA: Jones & Bartlett Publishers.
8. Ross M. H., Pawlina W. (2015). *Histology: A test and atlas with correlated cell and molecular biology* (7th ed.). Philadelphia, PA: Lippincott Williams & Williams.
9. Asghar U., Witkiewicz A. K., Turner N. C., et al. (2015). The history and future of targeting cyclin-dependent kinases in cancer therapy. *Nature Reviews Drug Discovery* 14(2), 130–146.
10. Guo G., von Meyenn F., Santos F., et al. (2016). Naïve pluripotent stem cells derived directly from isolated cells of the human inner cell mass. *Stem Cell Reports* 6, 437–446.
11. Islam F., Gopalan V., Smith R. A., et al. (2015). Translational potential of cancer stem cells: A review of the detection of cancer stem cells and their roles in cancer recurrence and cancer treatment. *Experimental Research* 335(1), 135–147.
12. Cermeno E. A., Garcia A. J. (2016). Tumor-initiating cells: Emerging biophysical methods of isolation. *Current Stem Cell Reports* 2(1), 21-32
13. Mori M., Triboulet R., Mohseni M., et al. (2013). Hippo signaling regulates microprocessor and links cell-density-dependent miRNA biogenesis to cancer. *Cell* 156, 893–906.
14. Hafner M. Niepel M., Chung M., et al. (2016). Growth rate inhibition metrics correct for confounders in measuring sensitivity to cancer drugs. *Nature Methods* 13(6), 521–526.
15. Aksamitiene E., Kiyatkin A., Kholodenko B. N. (2012). Cross-talk mitogenic Ras/MAPK and survival P13K/AKT pathways: A fine balance. *Biochemical Society Transactions* 40(1), 139–146.
16. Paoli P., Giannoni E., Chiarugi P. (2013). Anoikis molecular pathways and its role in cancer progression. *Biochemica et Biophysica Acta* 1833, 3481–3498.
17. Herve' J. C., Derangeon M. (2013). Gap-junction-mediated cell-to-cell communication. *Cell and Tissue Research* 352(1), 21–31.
18. Manning A. L., Dyson N. J. (2012). RB: Mitotic implications of a tumor suppressor. *Nature Reviews Cancer* 12(3), 220–226.
19. Aloni-Grinstein R., Shetzer Y., Kaufman T., et al. (2014). P53: The barrier to cancer stem cell formation. *FEBS Letters* 588(16), 2580–2589.
20. Zhou H., Wang H., Yu G., et al. (2017). Synergistic inhibitory effects of an engineered antibody-like modecult ATF-Fc and trastuzumab on tumor growth and invasion in a human breast cancer xenograft mouse model. *Oncology Letters* 14, 5189–5196.
21. Maclejowski J., deLange T. (2017). Telomeres in cancer: Tumour suppression and genome stability. *Nature Reviews. Molecular Cell Biology* 18(3), 175–186.
22. Scheel C., Weinberg R. A. (2012). Cancer stem cells and epithelial-mesenchymal transition: Concepts and molecular links. *Seminars in Cancer Biology* 22, 396–403.
23. Flegal K. M., Kit B. K., Orpana H., et al. (2013). Association of all-cause mortality with overweight and obesity using standard body mass index categories: A systematic review and meta-analysis. *Journal of the American Medical Association* 309(1), 71–82.
24. Brown S. B., Hankinson S. E. (2015). Endogenous estrogens and the risk of breast, endometrial and ovarian cancers. *Steroids* 99, 8–10.
25. Rahman N. (2014). Realizing the promise of cancer predisposition genes. *Nature* 505, 302–308.
26. Campbell C. D., Eichler E. E. (2013). Properties and rates of germline mutation in humans. *Trends in Genetics* 29(10), 575–584.
27. Kleinerman R. A., Schonfeld S. J., Tucker M. A. (2012). Sarcomas in hereditary retinoblastoma. *Clinical Sarcoma Research* 2(15), 1–7.
28. Plawski A., Banasiewicz T., Borun P., et al. (2013). Familial adenomatous polyposis of the colon. *Hereditary Cancer in Clinical Practice* 11(1), 15.
29. Ribatti D. (2017). The concept of immune surveillance against tumors: The first theories. *Oncotarget* 8(4), 7175–7180.
30. Center for Disease Control. (2016). *Cancers linked to tobacco use make up 40% of all cancers diagnosed in the United States.* Available: https://www.cdc.gov/media/releases/2016/p1110-vital-signs-cancer-tobacco.html
31. Hemeryck L. Y., Vanhaecke L. (2016). Diet-related DNA adduct formation in relation to carcinogenesis. *Nutrition Reviews* 74(8), 475–489.
32. Moore S. C., Lee M., Weiderpass E. L., et al. (2016). Association of leisure-time physical activity with risk of 26 types of cancer in 1.44 million adults. *Journal of the American Medical Association* 176(6), 816–825.
33. Poskanzer D. C., Herbst A. (1977). Epidemiology of vaginal adenosis and adenocarcinoma associated with exposure to stilbestrol in utero. *Cancer* 39, 1892–1895.
34. Jablon S., Kato H. (1972). Studies of the mortality of A-bomb survivors: Radiation dose and mortality, 1950-1970. *Radiation Research* 50, 649–698.
35. Ruddon R. W. (Ed). (1995). *Cancer biology*. New York: Oxford University Press.
36. Morgensztern D., Waqar S., Subramanian J., et al. (2012). Prognostic impact of malignant pleural effusion at presentation in patients with metastatic non-small-cell lung cancer. *Journal of Thoracic Oncology* 7, 1485–1489.
37. Gilbert L., Sampalis J., Karp I., et al. (2012). Assessment of symptomatic women for early diagnosis of ovarian cancer: Results from the prospective DOvE pilot project. *Lancet* 13, 285–291.
38. Muliawati Y., Haroen H., Rotty L. (2012). Cancer anorexia – cachexia syndrome. *The Indonesian Journal of Internal Medicine* 44(2), 154–162.
39. Aoyagi T., Terracina K. P., Matsubara H., et al. (2015). Cancer cachexia, mechanism and treatment. *World Journal of Gastrointestinal Oncology* 7(4), 17–29.

40. Bower J. E. (2014). Cancer-related fatigue-mechanisms, risk factors, and treatments. *National Review of Clinical Oncology* 11, 597–609.
41. Wender R., Fontham E. T., Barrera E., et al. (2013). American Cancer Society lung cancer screening guidelines. *A Cancer Journal for Clinicians* 63, 106–117.
42. Duffy M. J. (2013). Tumor markers in clinical practice: A review focusing on common solid cancers. *Medial Principles and Practice* 22, 4–11.
43. Mirsadraee S., Oswal D., Alizadeh Y., et al. (2012). The 7th lung cancer TNM classification and staging system: Review of the changes and implications. *World Journal of Radiology* 4(4), 128–134.
44. Liang J., Gao P., Wang Z, et al. (2012), The integration of macroscopic tumor invasion of adjacent organs into TNM staging system for colorectal cancer. *PLoS ONE* 7(12), e52269
45. Ramroth J., Cutter D. J., Darby S. C., et al. (2016). Dose and fractionation in radiation therapy of curative intent for non-small cell lung cancer: Meta-analysis of randomized trials. *International Journal of Radiation Oncology* 96(4), 736–747.
46. Willers H., Gheorghiu L., Liu Q., et al. (2015). DNA damage response assessments in human tumor samples provide functional biomarkers of radiosensitivity. *Seminars in Radiation Oncology* 25, 237–250.
47. Gabikian P., Tyler B. M., Zhang I., et al. (2014). Radiosensitization of malignant gliomas following intracranial delivery of paclitaxel biodegradable polymer microspheres laboratory investigation. *Journal of Neurosurgery* 120(5), 1078–1085.
48. Saif M. W., Garcon M. C., Rdriguez G., et al. (2013). Bolus 5-Fluorouracil as an alternative in patients with cardiotoxicity associated with infusion 5-Fluorouracil and Capecitabine: A case series. *In Vivo* 27, 531–534.
49. Maas A. L., Carter S. L., Wileyto E. P., et al. (2012). Tumor vascular microenvironment determines responsiveness to photodynamic therapy. *Cancer Research* 72(8), 2079–2088.
50. Ormsby R. J., Lawrence M. D., Blyth B. J., et al. (2014). Protection from radiation-induced apoptosis by radioprotector amifostine (WR-2721) is radiation dose dependent. *Cell Biology and Toxicology* 30, 55–66.
51. Koukourakis M. I., Giatromanolaki A., Zois C., et al. (2016). Normal tissue radioprotection by amifostine via Warburg-type effects. *Scientific Reports* 6, 1–14
52. Kamrava M. (2014). Potential role of ultrasound imaging in interstitial image based cervical cancer brachytherapy. *Journal of Contemporary Brachytherapy* 6(2), 223–230.
53. Fu D., Calvo J. A., Samson L. D. (2012). Balancing repair and tolerance of DNA damage caused by alkylating agents. *Nature* 12, 104–120.
54. Lucas X., Senger C., Erxleben A., et al. (2013). StreptomeDB:A resource for natural compounds isolated from Streptomyces species. *Nucleic Acids Research* 31, 1130–1136.
55. Tacar O., Sriamornsak P., Dass C. R. (2013). Doxorubicin: An update on anticancer molecular action, toxicity and novel drug delivery systems. *Journal of Pharmacy and Pharmacology* 65, 157–170.
56. Yang F., Teves S. S., Kemp C. J., et al. (2014). Doxorubicin, DNA torsion, and chromatin dynamics. *Biochimica et Biophysica Acta* 1845, 84–89.
57. Mukhtar E., Adhami V. M. Kukhtar H. (2016). Targeting microtubules by natural agents for cancer therapy. *Molecular Cancer Therapeutics* 13(2), 275–284.
58. Glaspy J. (2012). Update on safety of ESAs in cancer-induced anemia. *Journal of the National Cancer Network* 10(5), 659–667.
59. Renoir J. M., Marsaud V., Lazennec G. (2013). Estrogen receptor signaling as a target for novel breast cancer therapeutics. *Biochemical Pharmacy* 85, 449–465
60. Kuroki M., Miyamoto S., Morisaki T., et al. (2012) Biological response modifiers used in cancer biotherapy. *Anticancer Research* 32, 2229–2234.
61. Myint Z. W., Goil G. (2017). Role of modern immunotherapy in gastrointestinal malignancies: A review of current clinical progress. *Journal of Hematology & Oncology* 10, 86–98.
62. American Cancer Society (2017). Treatment and support (online). Available at https://www.cancer.org/treatment.html. Retrieved November 18, 2017.
63. Ott P. A., Fritsch E. F., Wu C. J., et al. (2014). Vaccines and melanoma. *Hematology Oncology Clinics of North America* 28 559–569.
64. Joura E. A., Giuliano A. R., Iversen E. E., et al. (2015). A 9-valent HPV vaccine against infection and intraepithelial neoplasia in women. *The New England Journal of Medicine* 372(8), 711–723.
65. Lin F. Young H. (2014). Interferons: Success in anti-viral immunotherapy. *Cytokine & Growth Factor Reviews* 25, 369–376.
66. Siegel R. L., Miller K. D., Jemal A. (2018). Cancer statistics, 2018. *CA: A Cancer Journal for Clinicians* 68, 7–30.
67. Cheung N. V. Dyer M. A. (2013). Neuroblastoma: Developmental biology, cancer genomics and immunotherapy. *Nature Reviews. Cancer* 13, 397–411.
68. Bruwier A. Chantrain C. F. (2012). Hematological disorders and leukemia in children with Down syndrome. *European Journal of Pediatrics* 171, 1301–1307.
69. Harris L. K. Westwood M. (2012). Biology and significance of signaling pathways activated by IGF-II. *Growth Factors* 30(1), 1–12.
70. American Cancer Society. (2016). What are the differences between cancers in adults and children? [Online]. Available: https://www.cancer.org/cancer/childhood-non-hodgkin-lymphoma/about/differences-children-adults.html. Accessed March 2, 2018.
71. Robinson L. L. Hudson M. M. (2014). Survivors of childhood and adolescent cancer: Life-long risks and responsibilities. *Nature Reviews Cancer* 14, 61–70
72. Siegel R. L. , Miller K. D., Jemal A. (2017). Cancer statistics, 2017. *CA: A Cancer Journal for Clinicians.* https://doi.org/10.3322/caac.21387
73. Stern C. (2018). Management of patients with oncologic disorders. In Hinkle J. L., Kj H. *Cheever Brunner & Suddarth's textbook of medical-surgical nursing* (14 ed.). Philadelphia: Wolters Kluwer.
74. Kyle T., Carman S. (2017). *Essentials of pediatric nursing* (3rd ed.). Philadelphia: Wolters Kluwer.

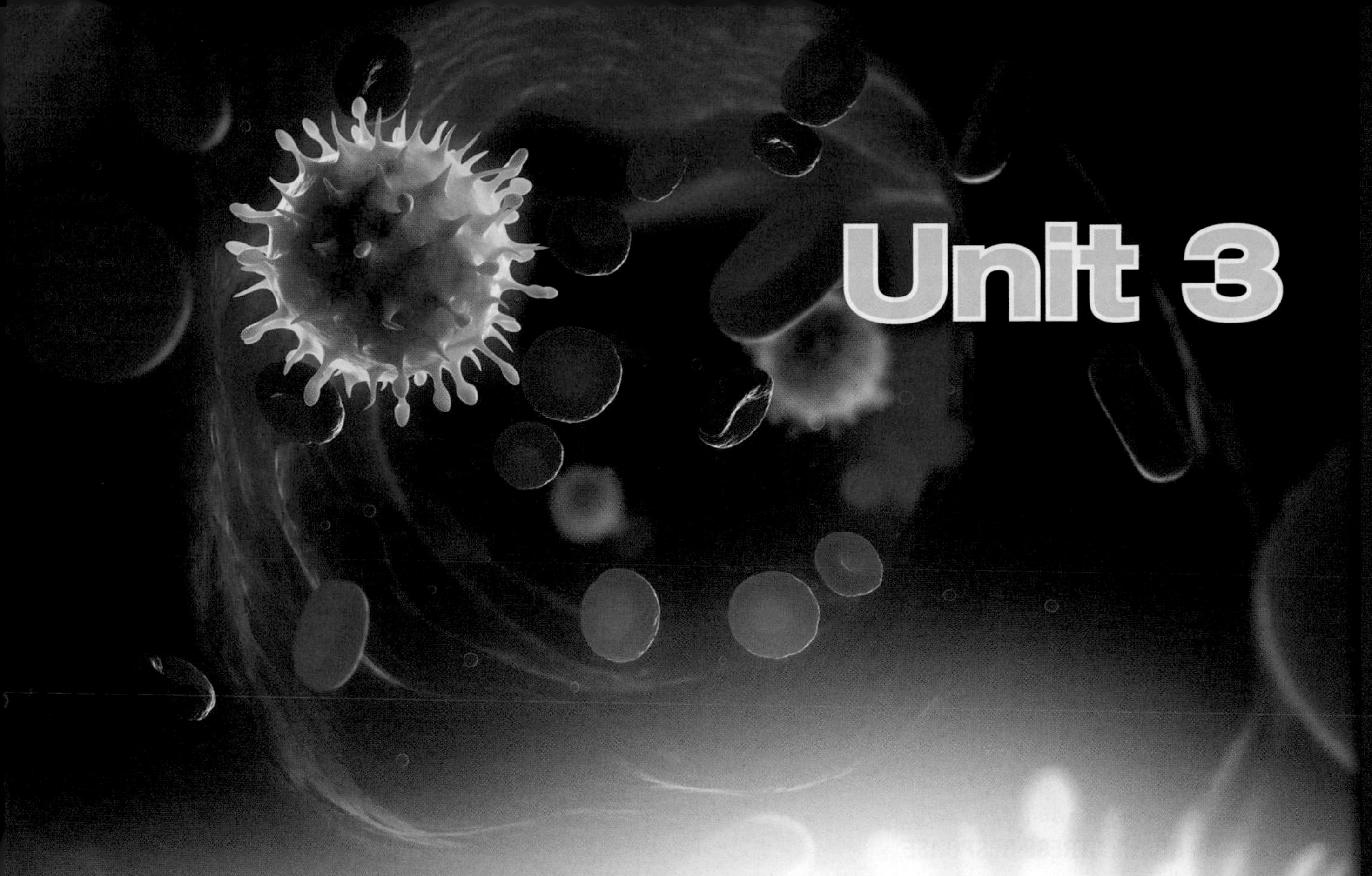

Unit 3

Disorders of Integrative Function

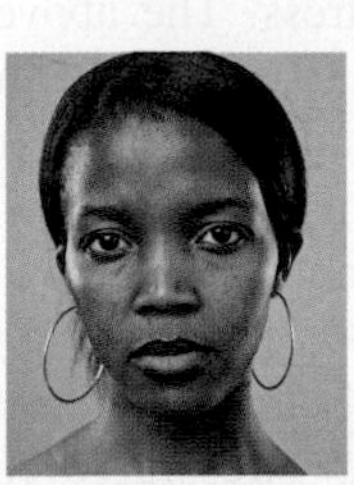

Mrs. Iona Smith, 38 years old, presents with a malar (butterfly) rash, generalized joint discomfort, fatigue, and intense photosensitivity. She is worked up for systemic lupus erythematosus (SLE). Mrs. Smith states that she has experienced these symptoms intermittently for about 9 months and is under considerable stress. Her extended family (parents, sister, two brothers, and grandmother) were all killed in a motor vehicle accident about 1 year ago when they were traveling to her home for Christmas. She and her husband have a child with Asperger autism, and her husband recently lost his job. Lacking health care insurance, she has delayed going to a doctor. Upon questioning, she has no personal or family history of SLE.

The clinic health care provider completes some blood work and schedules a return appointment in 3 weeks. The blood work indicates an elevated white blood cell count and lymphocytes count, a decreased platelet count, and hemolytic anemia. Serologic testing identifies three autoantibodies in Mrs. Smith's blood sample that are strongly indicative of SLE: antinuclear antibody (ANA), lupus anticoagulant, and anti-Smith antibody. She also has significant amounts (+2) of protein in her urine, indicating that she is already experiencing some degree of renal disease. Her symptoms and clinical results lead to the diagnosis of SLE.

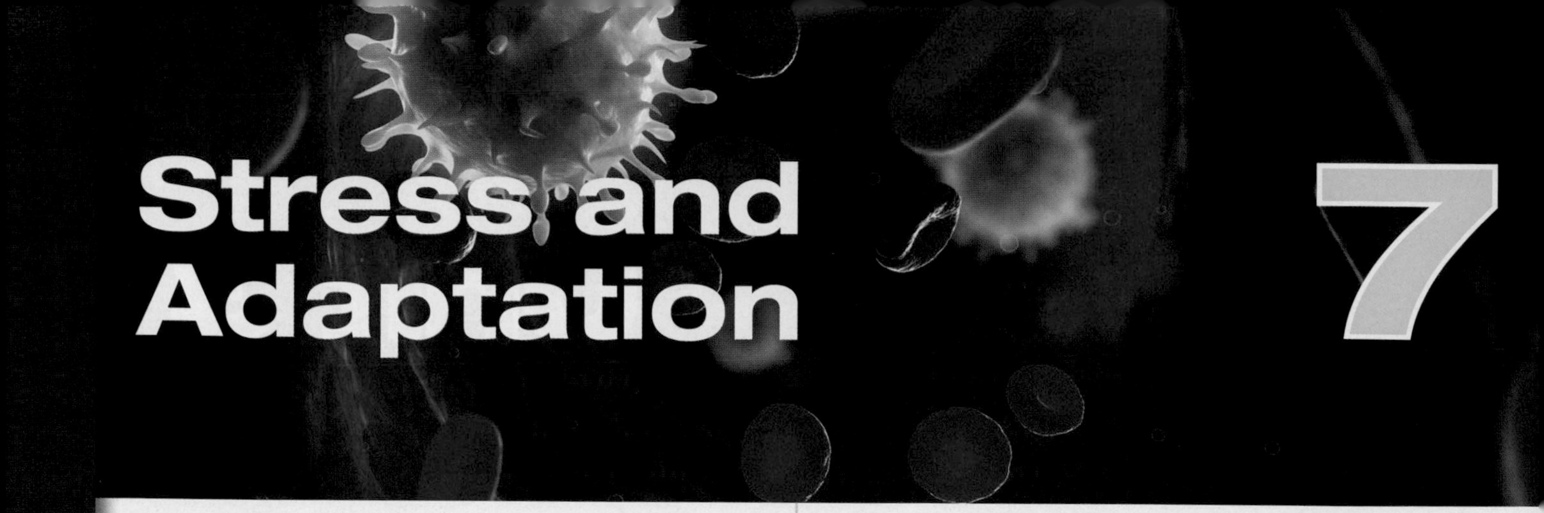

Stress and Adaptation

7

Sandeep Gopalakrishnan

Stress has become an increasingly discussed topic in today's world. The concept is discussed extensively in the health care fields and is found in economics, political science, business, and education. In the popular press, the physiologic response to stress is often implicated as a contributor to a variety of individual physical and mental challenges and societal problems. The 2017 American Psychological Association's (APA) Stress in America™ survey identified various sources of stress and its effect on the overall health and well-being of Americans living in the Unites States. Interestingly, it identified that 57% of Americans reported that the current political climate is a significant source of stress. Other significant stressors included stress related to personal safety and future, police violence toward minorities, work and economy, terrorism, mass shootings, and gun violence. Technology and social media have changed the way people around the world access information. According to the APA, 8 in 10 Americans are attached to their devices on any typical day and are considered as constant checkers of information on their personal electronic devices, and this activity with technology is considered as a source of stress. The above-mentioned stressors affect the health of our society, and the percentage of Americans reported to have at least one symptom of stress (headache, anxiety, depression, etc.) increased from 71 percent in August 2016 to 80% in January 2017.[1]

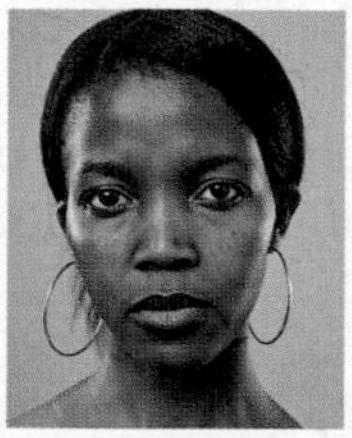

Iona has been living with extremely stressful events, including the death of multiple family members, possibly some guilt because the family members were traveling to her home for the holidays, and dealing with her son who has Asperger autism. Now she also has the added stress of her husband losing his job. Iona will need to gain skills in managing stress and resources to assist her with her son as well as her own health. She should be referred to a psychologist and social worker who will be able to assist her in stress management. Otherwise, these added stresses in her life will cause her to experience multiple exacerbations of her disease.

In 1910, when Sir William Osler delivered his Lumleian Lectures on "angina pectoris," he described the relationship of stress and strain to angina pectoris.[2] Approximately 15 years later, Walter Cannon, well known for his work in physiology, began to use the word *stress* in relation to his laboratory experiments on the "fight-or-flight" response. It seems possible that the term emerged from his work on the homeostatic features of living organisms and their tendency to "bound back" and "resist disruption" when acted on by an "external force."[3] At about the same time, Hans Selye, who became known for his research and publications on stress, began using the term *stress* in a very special way to mean an orchestrated set of bodily responses to any form of noxious stimulus.[4]

The content in this chapter has been organized into three sections: homeostasis, the stress response and adaptation to stress, and disorders of the stress response.

HOMEOSTASIS

After completing this section of the chapter, the learner will be able to meet the following objectives:

- Describe the concept of homeostasis.
- Describe the components of a control system, including the function of a negative feedback system.

The concepts of stress and adaptation have their origin in the complexity of the human body and the interactions between its cells and its many organ systems. These interactions require that a level of homeostasis or constancy be maintained during the many changes that occur in the internal and external environments. In effecting a state of constancy, homeostasis requires feedback control systems that regulate cellular function and integrate the function of the different body systems.

Constancy of the Internal Environment

Claude Bernard, a 19th century physiologist, was the first to describe clearly the central importance of a stable internal environment, which he termed the *milieu intérieur*.[5] Bernard recognized that body fluids surrounding the cells (extracellular fluids) and the various organ systems provide the means for exchange between the external and the internal environments. It is from this internal environment that body cells receive their nourishment, and it is into this fluid that they secrete their wastes. Even the contents of the gastrointestinal tract and lungs do not become part of the internal environment until they have been absorbed into the extracellular fluid. A multicellular organism is able to survive only as long as the composition of the internal environment is compatible with the survival needs of the individual cells. For example, even a small change in the pH of the body fluids can disrupt the metabolic processes of the individual cells.

The concept of a stable internal environment was supported by Walter Bradford Cannon, who proposed that this kind of stability, which he called *homeostasis*, was achieved through a system of carefully coordinated physiologic processes that oppose change.[6] Cannon pointed out that these processes were largely automatic and emphasized that homeostasis involves resistance to both internal and external disturbances.

In his book *Wisdom of the Body*, published in 1939, Cannon presented four tentative propositions to describe the general features of homeostasis.[6] With this set of propositions, Cannon emphasized that when a factor is known to shift homeostasis in one direction, it is reasonable to expect the existence of mechanisms that have the opposite effect. In the homeostatic regulation of blood sugar, for example, mechanisms that both raise and lower blood sugar would be expected to play a part. As long as the responding mechanism to the initiating disturbance can recover homeostasis, the integrity of the body and the status of normality are retained.

Control Systems

The ability of the body to function and maintain homeostasis under conditions of change in the internal and external environment depends on the thousands of physiologic *control systems* that regulate body function. A homeostatic control system consists of a collection of interconnected components that function to keep a physical or chemical parameter of the body relatively constant. The body's control systems regulate cellular function, control life processes, and integrate functions of the different organ systems.

Of recent interest have been the neuroendocrine control systems that influence behavior. Biochemical messengers that exist in our brain serve to control nerve activity, regulate information flow, and, ultimately, influence behavior.[7] These control systems mediate the physical, emotional, and behavioral reactions to stressors that, taken together, are called the *stress response*.

Just like any control system, each stress response involves a *sensor* to detect the change, an *integrator* to sum all incoming data and compare them with "normal," and *effector(s)* to try to reverse the change. For instance, a hiker's eyes (sensor) see a snake (stressor), and the cerebral cortex (integrator) of the individual determines that the snake is a threat and activates the heart, respiratory muscles, and many other organs (effectors) to assist in escape.

More complex stressors invoke more complex control systems, and sometimes, the stress response cannot restore balance and homeostasis. For instance, adverse physical and psychological experiences early in life (prenatal and childhood periods) can impact one's adult health.[8] The impact may appear decades later, in the form of mental health issues, immune dysregulations, cardiovascular diseases, cancer, and so on.[8] Therefore, it is important to identify early negative experiences and treat them, not only for the current health of the child but also for the future health of the adult.[9]

Some data suggest that it is beneficial to actively create a feeling of balance by, for example, keeping a reflective journal of interactions with individuals who may ordinarily stress them. In writing down how to apply new methods of communication with these individuals, one may create a less stressful image of their daily interactions with stressful individuals. This activity may facilitate some physiologic benefits.[10] Some data suggest that in playing an active role in maintaining a sense of balance, the brain may attempt to reorganize itself for the future.[10] This increased neuroplasticity in the brain could potentially improve emotional balance, flexibility, immune and cardiac function and increase the ability to empathize.[9] Other studies suggest that assisting people in trying to remember previous experiences and taking time to imagine possible future scenarios helps them be more prepared to manage future stressful experiences.[11]

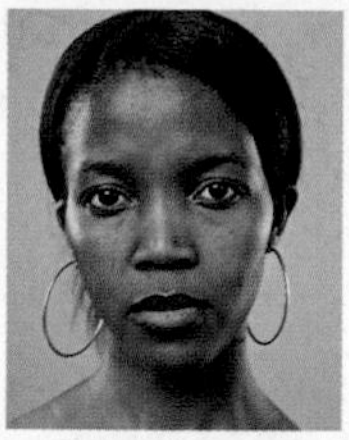

These studies validate the need for Iona to meet with a psychologist and a social worker who can assist her in stress management and possibly help her identify some past experience(s) that may need to be discussed. Working with these professionals may help her brain reorganize itself to deal more effectively with her son and his autism as well as managing appropriate rest times for herself.

KEY POINTS

HOMEOSTASIS

- Homeostasis is the purposeful maintenance of a stable internal environment by coordinated physiologic processes that oppose change.
- The physiologic control systems that oppose change operate by negative feedback mechanisms consisting of a sensor that detects a change, an integrator/comparator that sums and compares incoming data with a set point, and an effector system that returns the sensed function to within the range of the set point.

Feedback Systems

Most control systems in the body operate by *negative feedback mechanisms*, which function in a manner similar to the thermostat on a heating system. When the monitored function or value decreases below the set point of the system, the feedback mechanism causes the function or value to increase. When the function or value is increased above the set point, the feedback mechanism causes it to decrease (Fig. 7.1). For example, in the negative feedback mechanism that controls blood glucose levels, an increase in blood glucose stimulates an increase in insulin, which enhances the removal of glucose from the blood. When glucose has been taken up by cells and blood glucose levels fall, insulin secretion is inhibited and glucagon and other counterregulatory mechanisms stimulate the release of glucose from the glycogen stores of liver, which causes the blood glucose to return to normal. The same is true for all endocrine hormones that are connected to the pituitary for their stimulating hormone and the hypothalamus for their

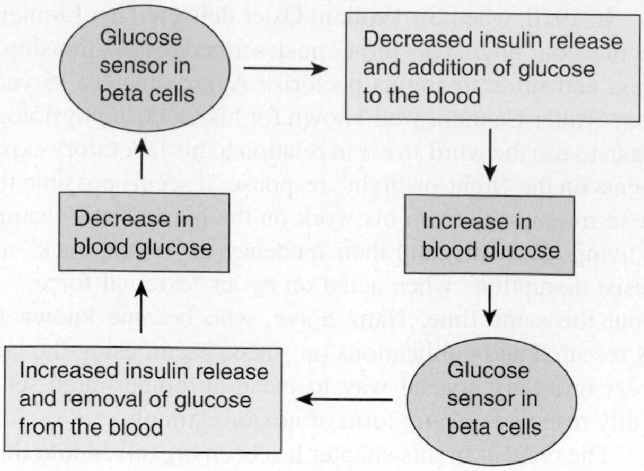

Figure 7.1 • Illustration of negative feedback control mechanisms using blood glucose as an example.

releasing hormone. For example, when thyroxine (T4) in the thyroid is low, it triggers the pituitary to increase thyroid-stimulating hormone (TSH), which then increases T4 secretion from the thyroid.

The reason most physiologic control systems function under negative rather than *positive feedback mechanisms* is that a positive feedback mechanism interjects instability rather than stability into a system. It produces a cycle in which the initiating stimulus produces more of the same. For example, in a hypothetical positive feedback system, exposure to an increase in environmental temperature would invoke compensatory mechanisms designed to increase rather than decrease body temperature.

IN SUMMARY

Physiologic and psychological adaptation involves the ability to maintain the constancy of the internal environment (homeostasis) and behavior in the face of a wide range of changes in the internal and external environments. It involves control and negative feedback systems that regulate cellular function, control life's processes, regulate behavior, and integrate the function of the different body systems.

STRESS AND ADAPTATION

After completing this section of the chapter, the learner will be able to meet the following objectives:

- State Selye's definition of stress.
- Explain the interactions among components of the nervous system in mediating the stress response.
- Describe the stress responses of the autonomic nervous system, the endocrine system, the immune system, and the musculoskeletal system.
- Explain adaption and its physiologic purpose.
- Discuss the *general adaptation syndrome* (GAS).

The increased focus on health promotion has heightened interest in the roles of stress and biobehavioral stress responses in the development of disease. Stress may contribute directly to the production or exacerbation of a disease, or it may contribute to the development of behaviors such as smoking, overeating, and drug abuse that increase the risk of disease.[11]

The Stress Response

In the early 1930s, the world-renowned endocrinologist Hans Selye was the first to describe a group of specific anatomic changes that occurred in rats that were exposed to a variety of different experimental stimuli. He came to an understanding that these changes were manifestations of the body's attempt to adapt to stimuli. Selye described *stress* as "a state manifested by a specific syndrome of the body developed in response to any stimuli that made an intense systemic demand on it."[12] As a young medical student, Selye noticed that people with diverse disease conditions had many signs and symptoms in common. He observed, "whether a man suffers from a loss of blood, an infectious disease, or advanced cancer, he loses his appetite, his muscular strength, and his ambition to accomplish anything. Usually the patient also loses weight and even his facial expression betrays that he is ill."[13] Selye referred to this as the "syndrome of just being sick."

In his early career as an experimental scientist, Selye noted that a triad of adrenal enlargement, thymic atrophy, and gastric ulcers appeared in rats he was using for his studies. These same three changes developed in response to many different or nonspecific experimental challenges. He assumed that the hypothalamic–pituitary–adrenal (HPA) axis played a pivotal role in the development of this response. To Selye, the response to stressors was a process that enabled the rats to resist the experimental challenge by using the function of the system best able to respond to it. He labeled the response the *general adaptation syndrome* (GAS): *general* because the effect was a general systemic reaction, *adaptive* because the response was in reaction to a stressor, and **syndrome** because the physical manifestations were coordinated and dependent on each other.[12]

According to Selye, the GAS involves three stages: the alarm stage, the resistance stage, and the exhaustion stage. The *alarm stage* is characterized by a generalized stimulation of the sympathetic nervous system and the HPA axis, resulting in the release of catecholamines and cortisol. During the *resistance stage*, the body selects the most effective and economic channels of defense. During this stage, the increased cortisol levels, which were present during the first stage, drop because they are no longer needed. If the stressor is prolonged or overwhelms the ability of the body to defend itself, the *exhaustion stage* ensues, during which resources are depleted and signs of "wear and tear" or systemic damage appear.[14] Selye contended that many ailments, such as various emotional disturbances, mildly annoying headaches, insomnia, upset stomach, gastric and duodenal ulcers, certain types of rheumatic disorders, and cardiovascular and kidney diseases, appear to be initiated or encouraged by the "body itself because of its faulty adaptive reactions to potentially injurious agents."[13]

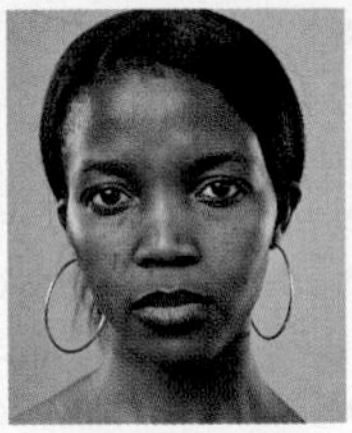

With a new diagnosis of SLE, Iona is manifesting the last stage of the stress response. She has certainly depleted many of her body's resources and is experiencing "wear and tear" and systemic damage, such as renal disease and some type of joint inflammatory disorder.

The events or environmental agents responsible for initiating the stress response were called *stressors*. According to Selye, stressors could be endogenous, arising from within the body, or exogenous, arising from outside the body.[13] In explaining the stress response, Selye proposed that two factors determine the nature of the stress response—the properties of the stressor and the conditioning of the person being stressed. Selye indicated that not all stress was detrimental; hence, he coined the terms *eustress* and *distress*.[14] He suggested that mild, brief, and controllable periods of stress could be perceived as positive stimuli to emotional and intellectual growth and development. It is the severe, protracted, and uncontrolled situations of psychological and physical distress that are disruptive of health.[13] For example, the joy of becoming a new parent and the sorrow of losing a parent are completely different experiences, yet their stressor effect—the nonspecific demand for adjustment to a new situation—can be similar.

It is increasingly clear that the physiologic stress response is far more complicated than can be explained fully by a classic stimulus–response mechanism. Stressors tend to produce different responses in different people or in the same person at different times, indicating the influence of the adaptive capacity of the person, or what Selye called *conditioning factors*. These conditioning factors may be internal (*e.g.*, genetic predisposition, age, sex) or external (*e.g.*, exposure to environmental agents, life experiences, dietary factors, level of social support).[13] The relative risk for development of a stress-related pathologic process seems, at least in part, to depend on these factors.

Richard Lazarus, a well-respected psychologist who devoted his career to the study of stress and emotions, considered "meanings and values to be at the center of human life and to represent the essence of stress, emotion and adaptation."[15] There is evidence that the hypothalamic–pituitary–adrenocortical axis, the adrenomedullary hormonal system, and the sympathetic nervous system are differentially activated depending on the type and intensity of the stressor.[16]

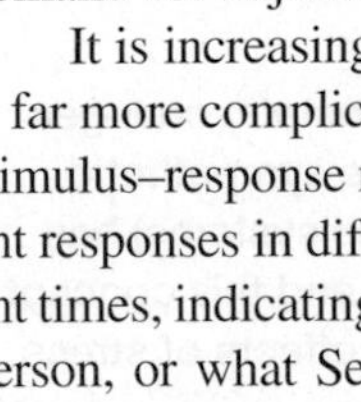

Iona has two internal conditioning factors for SLE, such as being female and in her late thirties. She also has external conditioning factors, such as life experiences and level of social support. With so many stressors in her life, she is most vulnerable for the stress response to go awry.

Neuroendocrine Responses

The manifestations of the stress response are strongly influenced by both the nervous and endocrine systems. The neuroendocrine systems integrate signals received along neurosensory pathways and from circulating mediators that are carried in the bloodstream. In addition, the immune system both affects and is affected by the stress response. Table 7.1 summarizes the action of hormones involved in the neuroendocrine responses to stress. The results of the coordinated release of these neurohormones include the mobilization of energy, a sharpened focus and awareness, increased cerebral blood flow and glucose utilization, enhanced cardiovascular and respiratory functioning, redistribution of blood flow to the brain and muscles, modulation of the immune response, inhibition of reproductive function, and a decrease in appetite.[16]

The stress response is a normal, coordinated physiologic system meant to increase the probability of survival, but also designed to be an acute response—turned on when necessary to bring the body back to a stable state and turned off when the challenge to homeostasis abates. Therefore, under normal circumstances, the neural responses and the hormones that are released during the response do not persist long enough to cause damage to vital tissues. Since the early 1980s, the term *allostasis* has been used by some investigators to describe the physiologic changes in the neuroendocrine, autonomic, and immune systems that occur in response to either real or perceived challenges to homeostasis.

Concept Mastery Alert

The persistence or accumulation of the allostatic changes (*e.g.*, immunosuppression, activation of the sympathetic nervous and renin–angiotensin–aldosterone systems) has been called an *allostatic load or overload*, and this concept has been used to measure the cumulative effects of stress on humans.[17]

The integration of the components of the stress response, which occurs at the level of the central nervous system (CNS), is complex and not completely understood. It relies on communication along neuronal pathways of the cerebral cortex, the limbic system, the thalamus, the hypothalamus, the pituitary gland, and the reticular activating system (RAS; Fig. 7.2). The cerebral cortex is involved with vigilance, cognition, and focused attention and the limbic system with the emotional components (*e.g.*, fear, excitement, rage, anger) of the stress response. The thalamus functions as the relay center and is important in receiving, sorting out, and distributing sensory input. The hypothalamus coordinates the responses of the endocrine and autonomic nervous systems (ANS). The RAS modulates mental alertness, ANS activity, and skeletal muscle tone, using input from other neural structures. The musculoskeletal tension that occurs during the stress response reflects increased activity of the RAS and its influence on the reflex circuits that control muscle tone. Adding to the complexity of this system is the fact that the individual brain circuits that participate in the mediation of the stress response interact and regulate the activity of each other. For example, reciprocal connections exist between neurons in the hypothalamus that initiate release of corticotropin-releasing factor (CRF) and neurons in the locus coeruleus (LC) associated with release of norepinephrine (NE). Thus, NE stimulates the secretion of CRF, and CRF stimulates the release of NE.[17]

Locus Coeruleus. Central to the neural component of the neuroendocrine response to stress is an area of the brain stem called the *locus coeruleus (LC)*.[17] The LC is densely populated with neurons that produce NE and is thought to be the central integrating site for the ANS response to stressful stimuli

TABLE 7.1 HORMONES INVOLVED IN THE NEUROENDOCRINE RESPONSES TO STRESS

HORMONES ASSOCIATED WITH THE STRESS RESPONSE	SOURCE OF THE HORMONE	PHYSIOLOGIC EFFECTS
Catecholamines (NE, epinephrine)	LC, adrenal medulla	Produces a decrease in insulin release and an increase in glucagon release resulting in increased glycogenolysis, gluconeogenesis, lipolysis, proteolysis, and decreased glucose uptake by the peripheral tissues; an increase in heart rate, cardiac contractility, and vascular smooth muscle contraction; and relaxation of bronchial smooth muscle
Corticotropin-releasing factor (CRF)	Hypothalamus	Stimulates ACTH release from the anterior pituitary and increased activity of the LC neurons
Adrenocorticotropic hormone (ACTH)	Anterior pituitary	Stimulates the synthesis and release of cortisol
Glucocorticoid hormones (*e.g.*, cortisol)	Adrenal cortex	Potentiates the actions of epinephrine and glucagon; inhibits the release and/or actions of the reproductive hormones and thyroid-stimulating hormone; and produces a decrease in immune cells and inflammatory mediators
Mineralocorticoid hormones (*e.g.*, aldosterone)	Adrenal cortex	Increases sodium absorption by the kidney
Antidiuretic hormone (ADH, vasopressin)	Hypothalamus, posterior pituitary	Increases water absorption by the kidney; produces vasoconstriction of blood vessels; and stimulates the release of ACTH

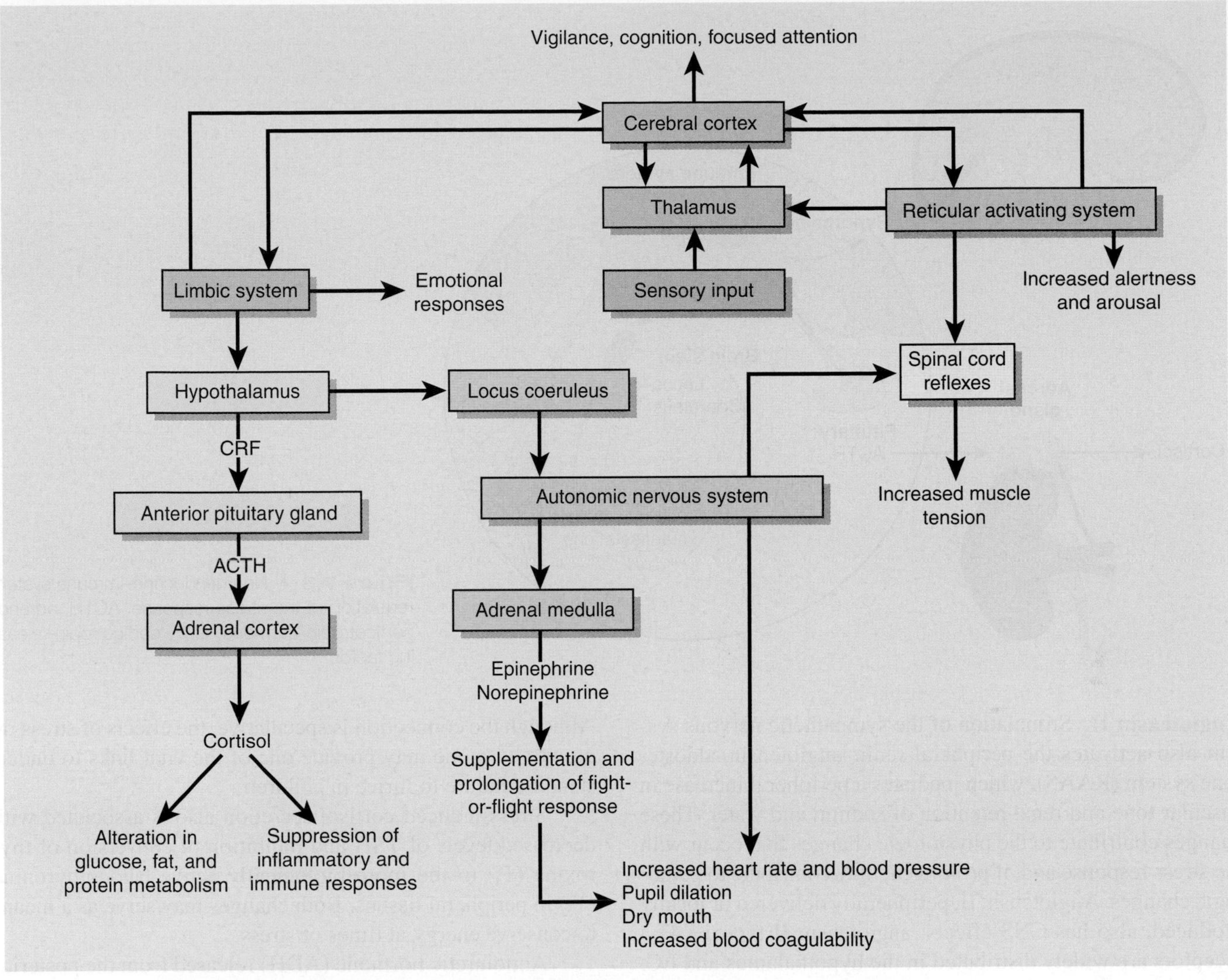

Figure 7.2 • Neuroendocrine pathways and physiologic responses to stress. ACTH, adrenocorticotropic hormone; CRF, corticotropin-releasing factor.

(Fig. 7.3). The LC–NE system has afferent pathways to the hypothalamus, the limbic system, the hippocampus, and the cerebral cortex.

The LC–NE system confers an adaptive advantage during a stressful situation. The sympathetic nervous system manifestation of the stress reaction has been called the *fight-or-flight response*. This is the most rapid of the stress responses and represents the basic survival response of our primitive ancestors when confronted with the perils of the wilderness and its inhabitants. The increase in sympathetic activity in the brain increases attention and arousal and thus may intensify memory. The heart and respiratory rates increase, the hands and feet become moist, the pupils dilate, the mouth becomes dry, and the activity of the gastrointestinal tract decreases.

Corticotropin-Releasing Factor. CRF is central to the endocrine component of the neuroendocrine response to stress (see Fig. 7.3). CRF is a small peptide hormone secreted by the paraventricular nucleus (PVN) of the hypothalamus. It is both an important endocrine regulator of pituitary and adrenal activity and a neurotransmitter involved in ANS activity, metabolism, and behavior.[17] Receptors for CRF are distributed throughout the brain as well as in many peripheral sites. CRF secreted from the hypothalamus in response to stress stimulus induces secretion of adrenocorticotropic hormone (ACTH) from the anterior pituitary gland. ACTH, in turn, stimulates the adrenal gland to synthesize and secrete the glucocorticoid hormones (*e.g.*, cortisol).

The glucocorticoid hormones have a number of direct or indirect physiologic effects that mediate the stress response, enhance the action of other stress hormones, or suppress other components of the stress system. In this regard, cortisol acts not only as a mediator of the stress response but as an inhibitor, such that overactivation of the stress response does not occur.[17] Cortisol maintains blood glucose levels by antagonizing the effects of insulin and enhances the effect of catecholamines on the cardiovascular system. It also suppresses osteoblast activity, hematopoiesis, collagen synthesis, and immune responses. All of these functions are meant to protect the organism against the effects of a stressor and to focus energy on regaining balance in the face of an acute challenge to homeostasis.

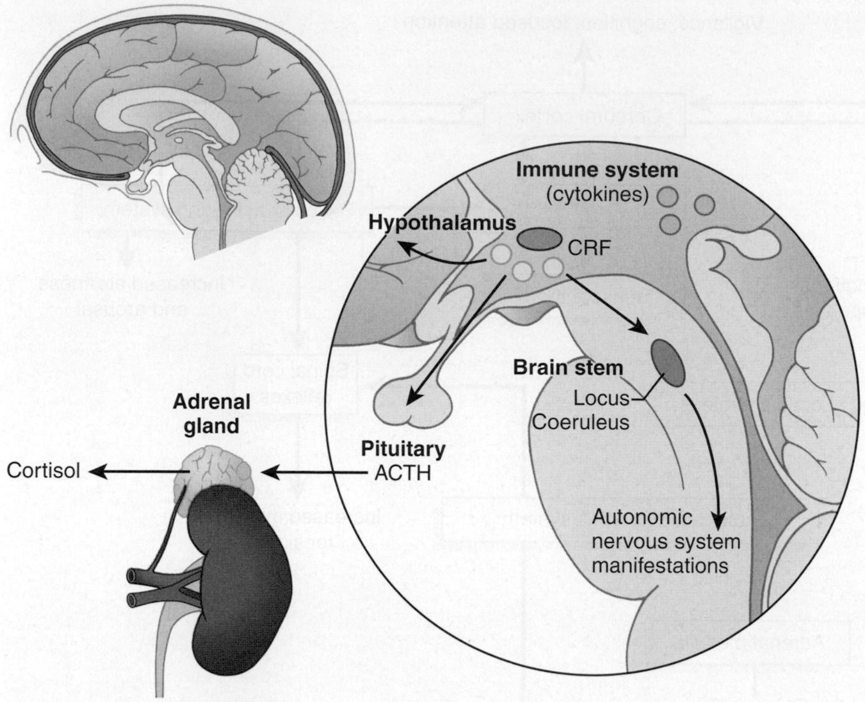

Figure 7.3 • Neuroendocrine–immune system regulation of the stress response. ACTH, adrenocorticotropic hormone; CRF, corticotropin-releasing factor.

Angiotensin II. Stimulation of the sympathetic nervous system also activates the peripheral renin–angiotensin–aldosterone system (RAAS), which mediates a peripheral increase in vascular tone and renal retention of sodium and water. These changes contribute to the physiologic changes that occur with the stress response and, if prolonged, may contribute to pathologic changes. Angiotensin II, peripherally delivered or locally produced, also has CNS effects; angiotensin II type 1 (AT_1) receptors are widely distributed in the hypothalamus and LC. Through these receptors, angiotensin II enhances CRF formation and release, contributes to the release of ACTH from the pituitary, enhances stress-induced release of vasopressin from the posterior pituitary, and stimulates the release of NE from the LC.[17]

Other Hormones. A wide variety of other hormones, including growth hormone, thyroid hormone, and the reproductive hormones, also are responsive to stressful stimuli. Systems responsible for reproduction, growth, and immunity are directly linked to the stress system, and the hormonal effects of the stress response profoundly influence these systems. Studies have shown that in females, stress and severe trauma can cause menstrual irregularities, anovulation, and amenorrhea.[16] In males, stress can induce decreased spermatogenesis, ejaculatory disorders, decreased levels of testosterone, and infertility.[18]

Although growth hormone is initially elevated at the onset of stress, the prolonged presence of cortisol leads to suppression of growth hormone, insulin-like growth factor 1 (IGF-1), and other growth factors, exerting a chronically inhibitory effect on growth. In addition, CRF directly increases somatostatin, which in turn inhibits growth hormone secretion. Although the connection is speculative, the effects of stress on growth hormone may provide one of the vital links to understanding failure to thrive in children.

Stress-induced cortisol secretion also is associated with decreased levels of TSH and inhibition of conversion of thyroxine (T_4) to the more biologically active triiodothyronine (T_3) in peripheral tissues. Both changes may serve as a means to conserve energy at times of stress.

Antidiuretic hormone (ADH) released from the posterior pituitary is also involved in the stress response, particularly in hypotensive stress or stress due to fluid volume loss. ADH, also known as *vasopressin*, increases water retention by the kidneys and produces vasoconstriction of blood vessels. In addition, vasopressin synthesized in parvocellular neurons of the hypothalamus and transported to the anterior pituitary appears to synergize the capacity of CRF to stimulate the release of ACTH.

The neurotransmitter serotonin or 5-hydroxytryptamine (5-HT) also plays a role in the stress response through neurons that innervate the hypothalamus, amygdala, and other limbic structures. Administration of 5-HT receptor agonists to laboratory animals was shown to increase the secretion of several stress hormones. Other hormones that have a possible role in the stress response include vasoactive intestinal peptide (VIP), neuropeptide Y, cholecystokinin (CCK), and substance P. These hormones have well characterized physiologic roles in periphery, but they are also found in the CNS, and literature supports that they are involved in the stress response.[19]

Oxytocin is a neuropeptide/neurohormone produced in the PVN and supraoptic (SON) of the hypothalamus. A large body of literature suggests that oxytocin plays a significant role in reducing stress-related physiologic consequences.

Exogenous delivery of oxytocin via intranasal route has shown reduction in psychosocial stress reactivity, fear and anxiety, and increases reward processing.[20]

Immune Responses

The hallmark of the stress response, as first described by Selye, are the endocrine–immune interactions (*i.e.*, increased corticosteroid production and atrophy of the thymus) that are known to suppress the immune response. In concert, these two components of the stress system, through endocrine and neurotransmitter pathways, produce the physical and behavioral changes designed to adapt to acute stress. Much of the literature regarding stress and the immune response focuses on the causal role of stress in immune-related diseases. It has also been suggested that the reverse may occur. That is, emotional and psychological manifestations of the stress response may be a reflection of alterations in the CNS resulting from the immune response (see Fig. 7.3). Immune cells such as monocytes and lymphocytes can penetrate the blood–brain barrier and take up residence in the brain, where they secrete chemical messengers called *cytokines* that influence the stress response.

The exact mechanism by which stress produces its effect on the immune response is unknown and probably varies from person to person, depending on genetic and environmental factors. The most significant arguments for interaction between the neuroendocrine and immune systems derive from evidence that the immune and neuroendocrine systems share common signal pathways (*i.e.*, messenger molecules and receptors), that hormones and neuropeptides can alter the function of immune cells, and that the immune system and its mediators can modulate neuroendocrine function.[17] Receptors for a number of CNS-controlled hormones and neuromediators reportedly have been found on lymphocytes. Among these are receptors for glucocorticoids, insulin, testosterone, prolactin, catecholamines, estrogens, acetylcholine, and growth hormone, suggesting that these hormones and neuromediators influence lymphocyte function. For example, cortisol is known to suppress immune function, and pharmacologic doses of cortisol are used clinically to suppress the immune response. It has been observed that the HPA axis is activated by cytokines such as interleukin-1, interleukin-6, and tumor necrosis factor-α (TNFα) that are released from immune cells.

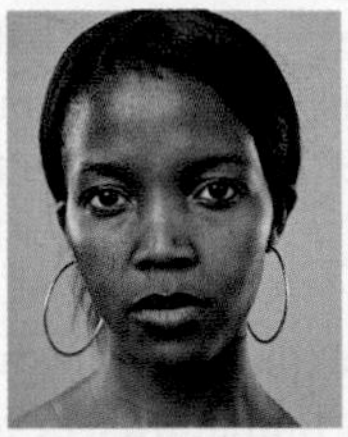

With SLE, there is an increase in lymphocytes, and these can migrate to the brain where they secrete cytokines, which trigger inflammation. Also the immunologic system can be modulated to recognize one's own cells as antigens and destroy their own cells. This is seen in the autoimmune disorder, SLE (Iona's diagnosis).

A second possible route for neuroendocrine regulation of immune function is through the sympathetic nervous system and the release of catecholamines. The lymph nodes, thymus, and spleen are supplied with ANS nerve fibers. Centrally acting CRF activates the ANS through multisynaptic descending pathways, and circulating epinephrine acts synergistically with CRF and cortisol to inhibit the function of the immune system.

Not only is the quantity of immune expression changed because of stress, but the quality of the response is changed as well. Stress hormones differentially stimulate the proliferation of subtypes of T lymphocyte helper cells. Because these T helper cell subtypes secrete different cytokines, they stimulate different aspects of the immune response. One subtype tends to stimulate T lymphocytes and the cellular-mediated immune response, whereas a second type tends to activate B lymphocytes and humoral-mediated immune responses.[17]

KEY POINTS

STRESS AND ADAPTATION

- Stress is a state manifested by symptoms that arise from the coordinated activation of the neuroendocrine and immune systems, which Selye called the general adaptation syndrome.
- The hormones and neurotransmitters (catecholamines and cortisol) are released during the stress response function to alert the individual to a threat or challenge to homeostasis, to enhance cardiovascular and metabolic activity in order to manage the stressor, and to focus the energy of the body by suppressing the activity of other systems that are not immediately needed.
- Adaptation is the ability to respond to challenges of physical or psychological homeostasis and to return to a balanced state.
- The ability to adapt is influenced by previous learning, physiologic reserve, time, genetic endowment, age, health status and nutrition, sleep–wake cycles, and psychosocial factors.

Coping and Adaptation to Stress

The ability to adapt to a wide range of environments and stressors is not peculiar to humans. According to René Dubos (a microbiologist noted for his study of human responses to the total environment), "adaptability is found throughout life and is perhaps the one attribute that distinguishes most clearly the world of life from the world of inanimate matter."[21] Living organisms, no matter how primitive, do not submit passively to the impact of environmental forces. They attempt to respond adaptively, each in its own unique and most suitable manner. The higher the organism is on the evolutionary scale, the larger its repertoire of adaptive mechanisms and its ability to select and limit aspects of the environment to which it responds. The most fully evolved mechanisms are the social responses through which people or groups modify their environments, their habits, or both to achieve a way of life that is best suited to their needs.

Adaptation

Human beings, because of their highly developed nervous system and intellect, usually have alternative mechanisms for adapting and have the ability to control many aspects of their environment. Air conditioning and central heating limit the need to adapt to extreme changes in environmental temperature. The availability of antiseptic agents, immunizations, and antibiotics eliminates the need to respond to common infectious agents. At the same time, modern technology creates new challenges for adaptation and provides new sources of stress, such as noise and air pollution, increased exposure to harmful chemicals, changes in biologic rhythms imposed by shift work and global travel, and exposure to electronic gadgets.

Of particular interest are the differences in the body's response to events that threaten the integrity of the body's physiologic environment and those that threaten the integrity of the person's psychosocial environment. Many of the body's responses to physiologic disturbances are controlled on a moment-by-moment basis by feedback mechanisms that limit their application and duration of action. For example, the baroreflex-mediated rise in heart rate that occurs when a person moves from the recumbent to the standing position is almost instantaneous and subsides within seconds. Furthermore, the response to physiologic disturbances that threaten the integrity of the internal environment is specific to the threat; the body usually does not raise the body temperature when an increase in heart rate is needed. In contrast, the response to psychological disturbances is not regulated with the same degree of specificity and feedback control. Instead, the effect may be inappropriate and sustained.

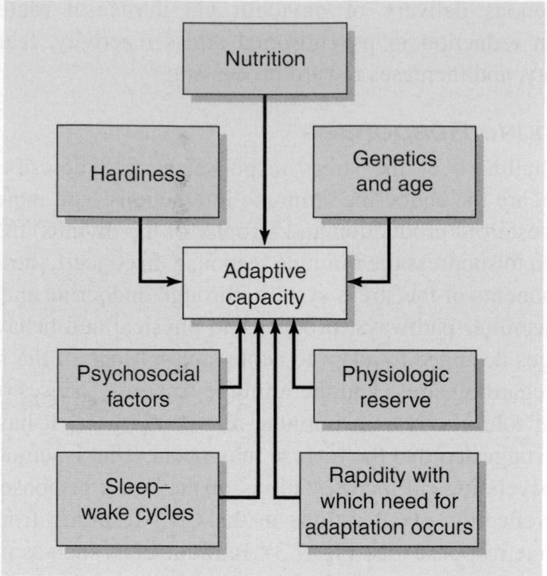

Figure 7.4 • Factors affecting adaptation.

Factors Affecting the Ability to Adapt

Adaptation implies that an individual has successfully created a new balance between the stressor and the ability to deal with it. The means used to attain this balance are called *coping strategies* or *coping mechanisms*. Coping mechanisms are the emotional and behavioral responses used to manage threats to our physiologic and psychological homeostasis. According to Lazarus, how we cope with stressful events depends on how we perceive and interpret the event.[22] Is the event perceived as a threat of harm or loss? Is the event perceived as a challenge rather than a threat? Physiologic reserve, time, genetics, age, health status, nutrition, sleep–wake cycles, hardiness, and psychosocial factors influence a person's appraisal of a stressor and the coping mechanisms used to adapt to the new situation (Fig. 7.4).

Physiologic and Anatomic Reserve. The trained athlete is able to increase cardiac output six- to sevenfold during exercise. The safety margin for adaptation of most body systems is considerably greater than that needed for normal activities. The red blood cells carry more oxygen than the tissues can use, the liver and fat cells store excess nutrients, and bone tissue stores calcium in excess of that needed for normal neuromuscular function. The ability of body systems to increase their function given the need to adapt is known as the *physiologic reserve*. Many of the body organs, such as the lungs, kidneys, and adrenals, are paired to provide anatomic reserve as well. Both organs are not needed to ensure the continued existence and maintenance of the internal environment. Many people function normally with only one lung or one kidney. In kidney disease, for example, signs of renal failure do not occur until approximately 80% of the functioning nephrons have been destroyed.

Time. Adaptation is most efficient when changes occur gradually rather than suddenly. It is possible, for instance, to lose a liter or more of blood through chronic gastrointestinal bleeding over a week without manifesting signs of shock. However, a sudden hemorrhage that causes rapid loss of an equal amount of blood is likely to cause hypotension and shock.

Genetics. Adaptation is further affected by the availability of adaptive responses and flexibility in selecting the most appropriate and economical response. The greater the number of available responses, the more effective is the capacity to adapt. Genetics can ensure that the systems that are essential to adaptation function adequately. Even a gene that has deleterious effects may prove adaptive in some environments. In Africa, the gene for sickle cell anemia persists in some populations because it provides some resistance to infection with the parasite that causes malaria.

Age. The capacity to adapt is decreased at the extremes of age. The ability to adapt is impaired by the immaturity of an infant, much as it is by the decline in functional reserve that occurs with age. For example, the infant has difficulty concentrating urine because of immature renal structures and therefore is less able than an adult to cope with decreased water intake or exaggerated water losses. A similar situation exists in the elderly owing to age-related changes in renal function.

Gender. Within the last decade, primarily because females have been included in basic science and clinical investigations, differences between the sexes in cardiovascular, respiratory, endocrine, renal, and neurophysiologic function have been found, and it has been hypothesized that sex hormones are the basis of these biologic differences. Technologic advances in cellular and molecular biology have made it clear, however, that there are fundamental differences in the locale and regulation of individual genes in the male and female genome. These differences have general implications for the prevention, diagnosis, and treatment of disease and specific implications for our understanding of the sex-based differences in response to life's stressors.

Given the nature of sex-based differences, it is not surprising that there are differences in the physiologic stress response in both the HPA axis and in the ANS. Premenopausal women tend to have a lower activation of the sympathetic nervous system than men in response to stressors. Gender-based differences in activation of the stress response may partially explain differences in susceptibility to diseases in which the stress response may play a causal role. These research results are not definitive but are intriguing and can serve as a springboard for further research.

Health Status. Physical and mental health status determines physiologic and psychological reserves and is a strong determinant of the ability to adapt. For example, people with heart disease are less able to adjust to stresses that require the recruitment of cardiovascular responses. Severe emotional stress often produces disruption of physiologic function and limits the ability to make appropriate choices related to long-term adaptive needs. Those who have worked with acutely ill people know that the will to live often has a profound influence on survival during life-threatening illnesses.

Nutrition. There are 50 to 60 essential nutrients, including minerals, lipids, certain fatty acids, vitamins, and specific amino acids. Deficiencies or excesses of any of these nutrients can alter a person's health status and impair the ability to adapt. The importance of nutrition to enzyme function, immune response, and wound healing is well known. On a worldwide basis, malnutrition may be one of the most common causes of immunodeficiency.

Among the problems associated with dietary excess are obesity and alcohol abuse. Obesity is a common problem. It predisposes a person to a number of health problems, including atherosclerosis and hypertension. Alcohol is commonly used in excess. It acutely affects brain function and, with long-term use, can seriously impair the function of the liver, brain, and other vital structures.

Circadian Rhythm. Sleep is considered to be a restorative function in which energy is restored and tissues are regenerated.[23] Sleep occurs in a cyclic manner, alternating with periods of wakefulness and increased energy use. Biologic rhythms play an important role in adaptation to stress, development of illness, and response to medical treatment. Many rhythms such as rest and activity, work and leisure, and eating and drinking oscillate with a frequency similar to that of the 24-hour light–dark solar day. The term circadian, from the Latin *circa* ("about") and *dies* ("day"), is used to describe these 24-hour diurnal rhythms.

Sleep disorders and alterations in the sleep–wake cycle have been shown to alter immune function, the normal circadian pattern of hormone secretion, and physical and psychological functioning.[23,24] The two most common manifestations of an alteration in the sleep–wake cycle are insomnia and sleep deprivation or increased somnolence. In some people, stress may produce sleep disorders, and in others, sleep disorders may lead to stress. Acute stress and environmental disturbances, loss of a loved one, recovery from surgery, and pain are common causes of transient and short-term insomnia. Air travel and jet lag constitute additional causes of altered sleep–wake cycles, as does shift work.

Hardiness. Studies by social psychologists have focused on individuals' emotional reactions to stressful situations and their coping mechanisms to determine those characteristics that help some people remain healthy despite being challenged by high levels of stressors. For example, the concept of *hardiness* describes a personality characteristic that includes a sense of having control over the environment, a sense of having a purpose in life, and an ability to conceptualize stressors as a challenge rather than a threat.[25] Many studies by nurses and social psychologists suggest that hardiness is correlated with positive health outcomes.[26]

Psychosocial Factors. Several studies have related social factors and life events to illness. Scientific interest in the social environment as a cause of stress has gradually broadened to include the social environment as a resource that modulates the relation between stress and health. Presumably, people who can mobilize strong supportive resources from within their social relationships are better able to withstand the negative effects of stress on their health. Studies suggest that social support has direct and indirect positive effects on the health and well-being and serves as a buffer or modifier of the physical and psychosocial effects of stress.[27] Social support has been viewed in terms of the number of relationships a person has and the person's perception of these relationships. Close relationships with others can involve positive effects as well as the potential for conflict and may, in some situations, leave the person less able to cope with life stressors.

IN SUMMARY

The stress response involves the activation of several physiologic systems (sympathetic nervous system, the HPA axis, and the immune system) that work in a coordinated fashion to protect the body against damage from the intense demands made on it. Selye called this response the *general adaptation syndrome*. The stress response is divided into three stages: the *alarm stage*, with activation of the sympathetic nervous system and the HPA axis; the *resistance stage*, during which the body selects the most effective defenses; and the *exhaustion stage*, during which physiologic resources are depleted and signs of systemic damage appear.

The activation and control of the stress response are mediated by the combined efforts of the nervous and endocrine systems. The neuroendocrine systems integrate signals received along neurosensory pathways and from circulating mediators that are carried in the bloodstream. In addition, the immune system both affects and is affected by the stress response.

Adaptation is affected by a number of factors, including experience and previous learning, the rapidity with which the need to adapt occurs, genetic endowment and age, health status, nutrition, sleep–wake cycles, hardiness, and psychosocial factors.

DISORDERS OF THE STRESS RESPONSE

After completing this section of the chapter, the learner will be able to meet the following objectives:

- Describe the physiologic and psychological effects of a chronic stress response.
- Describe the characteristic of posttraumatic stress disorder.
- List five nonpharmacologic methods of treating stress.

For the most part, the stress response is meant to be acute and time limited. The time-limited nature of the process renders the accompanying catabolic and immunosuppressive effects advantageous. It is the chronicity of the response that is thought to be disruptive to physical and mental health.

Stressors can assume a number of patterns in relation to time. They may be classified as acute time limited, chronic intermittent, or chronic sustained. An acute time-limited stressor is one that occurs over a short time and does not recur. A chronic intermittent stressor is one to which a person is chronically exposed. The frequency or chronicity of circumstances to which the body is asked to respond often determines the availability and efficiency of the stress responses. The response of the immune system, for example, is more rapid and efficient on second exposure to a pathogen than it is on first exposure. However, chronic exposure to a stressor can fatigue the system and impair its effectiveness.

Effects of Acute Stress

The reactions to acute stress are those associated with the ANS, the fight-or-flight response. The manifestations of the stress response—a pounding headache; a cold, moist skin; and a stiff neck—are all part of the acute stress response. Centrally, there is facilitation of neural pathways mediating arousal, alertness, vigilance, cognition, and focused attention, as well as appropriate aggression. The acute stress response can result from either psychologically or physiologically threatening events. In situations of life-threatening trauma, these acute responses may be lifesaving in that they divert blood from less essential to more essential body functions. Increased alertness and cognitive functioning enable rapid processing of information and arrival at the most appropriate solution to the threatening situation.

However, for people with limited coping abilities, either because of physical or mental health, the acute stress response may be detrimental (Chart 7.1). This is true of people with preexisting heart disease in whom the overwhelming sympathetic behaviors associated with the stress response can lead to arrhythmias. For people with other chronic health problems, such as headache disorder, acute stress may precipitate a recurrence. In healthy people, the acute stress response can redirect attention from behaviors that promote health, such as attention to proper meals and getting adequate sleep. For those with health problems, it can interrupt compliance with medication regimens and exercise programs. In some situations, the acute arousal state actually can be life-threatening, physically immobilizing the person when movement would avert catastrophe (*e.g.*, moving out of the way of a speeding car).

Effects of Chronic Stress

The stress response is designed to be an acute self-limited response in which activation of the ANS and the HPA axis is controlled in a negative feedback manner. As with all negative feedback systems, pathophysiologic changes can occur in the stress response system. Function can be altered in several ways, including when a component of the system fails; when

CHART 7.1 POSSIBLE STRESS-INDUCED HEALTH PROBLEMS

- Mood disorders
- Anxiety
- Depression
- PTSD
- Eating disorders
- Sleep disorders
- Diabetes type 2
- Hypertension
- Infection
- Exacerbation of autoimmune disorders
- Gastrointestinal problems
- Pain
- Obesity
- Eczema
- Cancer
- Atherosclerosis
- Migraine

the neural and hormonal connections among the components of the system are dysfunctional; and when the original stimulus for the activation of the system is prolonged or of such magnitude that it overwhelms the ability of the system to respond appropriately. In these cases, the system may become overactive or underactive.

Chronicity and excessive activation of the stress response can result from chronic illnesses as well as contribute to the development of long-term health problems. Chronic activation of the stress response is an important public health issue from both a health and a cost perspective. Stress is linked to a myriad of health disorders, such as diseases of the cardiovascular, gastrointestinal, immune, and neurologic systems, as well as depression, chronic alcoholism and drug abuse, eating disorders, accidents, and suicide.

Posttraumatic Stress Disorder

Posttraumatic Stress Disorder (PTSD) is a disabling syndrome caused by the chronic activation of the stress response as a result of experiencing a significant traumatic event. The person may remember the traumatic event, or PTSD may occur with no recollection of an earlier stressful experience. PTSD that is manifested 6 months after the traumatic event is called PTSD with delayed onset.[28] PTSD was formerly called *battle fatigue* or *shell shock* because it was first characterized in soldiers returning from combat. Although war is still a significant cause of PTSD, other major catastrophic events, such as weather-related disasters (hurricanes, earthquakes, and floods), airplane crashes, terrorist bombings, and rape or child abuse, also may result in development of the disorder. In the United States, the most frequently reported traumatic events include physical and sexual assaults (with 52% prevalence) and accidents (with 50% prevalence).[28] People who are exposed to traumatic events are also at risk for development of major depression, panic disorder, generalized anxiety disorder, and substance abuse.[28] They may also have physical symptoms and illnesses (*e.g.*, hypertension, asthma, and chronic pain syndromes).

PTSD is characterized by a constellation of symptoms that are experienced as states of intrusion, avoidance, and hyperarousal. *Intrusion* refers to the occurrence of "flashbacks" during waking hours or nightmares in which the past traumatic event is relived, often in vivid and frightening detail. *Avoidance* refers to the emotional numbing that accompanies this disorder and disrupts important personal relationships. Because a person with PTSD has not been able to resolve the painful feelings associated with the trauma, depression is commonly a part of the clinical picture. Survivor guilt also may be a product of traumatic situations in which the person survived the disaster but loved ones did not. *Hyperarousal* refers to the presence of increased irritability, difficulty concentrating, an exaggerated startle reflex, and increased vigilance and concern over safety. In addition, memory problems, sleep disturbances, and excessive anxiety are commonly experienced by people with PTSD.

For a diagnosis of PTSD to be made, the person must have experienced, witnessed, or confronted a traumatic event, which caused a response in the person involving horror and fear. The triad of symptoms of intrusion, avoidance, and hyperarousal that characterize PTSD must be present together for at least 1 month, and the disorder must have caused clinically significant distress.[28] Although the pathophysiology of PTSD is not completely understood, the revelation of physiologic changes related to the disorder has shed light on why some people recover from the disorder, whereas others do not. It has been hypothesized that the intrusive symptoms of PTSD may arise from exaggerated sympathetic nervous system activation in response to the traumatic event. People with chronic PTSD have been shown to have increased levels of NE and increased activity of α_2-adrenergic receptors.

Recent neuroanatomic studies have identified alterations in neural systems that are part of the amygdala and hippocampus that play a significant role in fear learning, threat detection, executive function and emotion regulation, and contextual processing.[28] Positron emission tomography and functional magnetic resonance imaging have shown increased reactivity of the amygdala and hippocampus and decreased reactivity of the anterior cingulate and orbitofrontal areas. These areas of the brain are involved in fear responses. The hippocampus also functions in memory processes. Differences in hippocampal function and memory processes suggest a neuroanatomic basis for the intense problems suffered by people diagnosed with PTSD. People with PTSD demonstrate decreased cortisol levels, increased sensitivity of cortisol receptors, and an enhanced negative feedback inhibition of cortisol release with the dexamethasone suppression test. Dexamethasone is a synthetic glucocorticoid that mimics the effects of cortisol and directly inhibits the action of CRF and ACTH. The hypersuppression of cortisol observed with the dexamethasone test suggests that people with PTSD do not exhibit a classic stress response as described by Selye. Because this hypersuppression has not been described in other psychiatric disorders, it may serve as a relatively specific marker for PTSD.

Little is known about the risk factors that predispose people to the development of PTSD. Statistics indicate there is a need for studies to determine risk factors for PTSD as a means of targeting people who may need intensive therapeutic measures after a life-threatening event. Research also is needed to determine the mechanisms by which the disorder develops so that it can be prevented or, if that is not possible, so that treatment methods can be developed to decrease the devastating effects of this disorder on affected people and their families.[29]

Health care professionals need to be aware that people who present with symptoms of depression, anxiety, and alcohol or drug abuse may in fact be suffering from PTSD. The patient history should include questions concerning the occurrence of violence, major loss, or traumatic events in the person's life.

Debriefing, or talking about the traumatic event at the time it happens, often is an effective therapeutic tool. Crisis teams are often among the first people to attend to the emotional needs of those caught in catastrophic events. Some people may need continued individual or group therapy. Often concurrent pharmacotherapy with antidepressant and antianxiety agents is useful and helps the person participate more fully in therapy.

Most importantly, the person with PTSD should not be made to feel responsible for the disorder or that it is evidence of a so-called character flaw. It is not uncommon for people with this disorder to be told to "get over it" or "just get on with it, because others have." There is ample evidence to suggest that there is a biologic basis for the individual differences in responses to traumatic events, and these differences need to be taken into account.

Treatment and Research of Stress Disorders

The change that occurs in the biochemical stress response system of people who have experienced some type of mistreatment as a child so that they are not able to respond effectively to stressors in the future is called the traumatic stress response.[30] Evidence supports that early intervention can assist the person in adapting new and effective coping mechanisms to better manage stress in the future.[30] Additionally, a study conducted with caregivers of a spouse or family member demonstrates that those who reported higher levels of caregiver stress also had poorer self-perceived health. When early interventions for stress management were given to these caregivers, there were less negative self-identified behaviors.[31] Several studies have supported the use of early interventions to assist in managing stress. In fact, one study describes how resilience development was conducted with oncology nurses to decrease their burnout. Findings of the study indicated the program was successful and recommended to be implemented for all nurses.[31]

Treatment

The treatment of stress should be directed toward helping people avoid coping behaviors that impose a risk to their health and providing them with alternative stress-reducing strategies. People who are overwhelmed by the number of life stressors to which they have been exposed can use purposeful priority setting and problem solving. Other nonpharmacologic methods used for stress reduction are relaxation techniques, guided imagery, music therapy, massage, and biofeedback.

Relaxation. Practices for evoking the relaxation response are numerous. They are found in virtually every culture and are credited with producing a generalized decrease in sympathetic system activity and musculoskeletal tension. Herbert Benson, a physician who worked in developing the technique, described four elements integral to the various relaxation techniques: a repetitive mental device, a passive attitude, decreased mental tonus, and a quiet environment. He developed a noncultural method that is commonly used for achieving relaxation.[32]

Progressive muscle relaxation is one method of relieving tension. Tension can be defined physiologically as the inappropriate contraction of muscle fibers. Progressive muscle relaxation, which has been modified by a number of therapists, consists of systematic contraction and relaxation of major muscle groups. As the person learns to relax, the various muscle groups are combined. Eventually, the person learns to relax individual muscle groups without first contracting them.

Imagery. Guided imagery is another technique that can be used to achieve relaxation. One method is scene visualization, in which the person is asked to sit back, close the eyes, and concentrate on a scene narrated by the therapist. Whenever possible, all five senses are involved. The person attempts to see, feel, hear, smell, and taste aspects of the visual experience. Other types of imagery involve imagining the appearance of each of the major muscle groups and how they feel during tension and relaxation.

Music Therapy. Music therapy is used for both its physiologic and psychological effects. It involves listening to selected pieces of music as a means of ameliorating anxiety or stress, reducing pain, decreasing feelings of loneliness and isolation, buffering noise, and facilitating expression of emotion. Music usually is selected based on a person's musical preference and past experiences with music. Depending on the setting, headphones may be used to screen out other distracting noises. Radio and television music is inappropriate for music therapy because of the inability to control the selection of pieces that are played, the interruptions that occur (*e.g.*, commercials and announcements), and the quality of the reception.

Biofeedback. Biofeedback is a technique in which a person learns to control physiologic functioning. It involves electronic monitoring of one or more physiologic responses to stress with immediate feedback of the specific response to the person undergoing treatment. Several types of responses are used: electromyography (EMG), electrothermal, and electrodermal.[33] The EMG response involves the measurement of electrical potentials from muscles, usually the forearms extensor or frontalis. This is used to gain control over the contraction of skeletal muscles that occurs with anxiety and tension. The electrodermal sensors monitor skin temperature in the fingers or toes. The sympathetic nervous system exerts significant control over blood flow in the distal parts of the body such as the digits of the hands and feet. Consequently, anxiety often is manifested by a decrease in skin temperature in the fingers and toes. Electrodermal sensors measure conductivity of skin (usually the hands) in response to anxiety.

Massage Therapy. Massage is the manipulation of the soft tissues of the body to promote relaxation and relief of muscle tension. The technique that is used may involve a soft stroking along the length of the muscle (effleurage), application of pressure across the width of a muscle (petrissage), deep massage movement applied by a circular motion of the thumbs or fingertips (friction), squeezing across the width of a muscle (kneading), or use of light slaps or chopping actions (hacking).[34]

Research

Research in stress has focused on personal reports of the stress situation and the physiologic responses to stress. A number of interview guides and written instruments are available for measuring the personal responses to stress and coping in adults.

Measurements of vital signs, ACTHs, glucocorticoids (cortisol) and glucose levels, and immunologic counts are all part of current research studies involving stress.

People who are critically ill and on ventilators were assigned to listen to music or not were studied regarding their vital signs and sedation levels (Ramsay Sedation Scale). All were medicated with the same sedative and dosed according to weight. The experimental group (those who were given music) had higher levels of sedation as evidenced by higher Ramsay scores than those in the control group, although there was no difference in vital signs.[35] Having maintained higher levels of sedation on the Ramsay Sedation Scale was deemed to be a positive outcome for preventing stress.[35] A study conducted with Puerto Rican women living in the United States showed that many experienced stress as evidenced by increased respiratory rate, heart rate, and blood pressure.[36] These women were found to have a statistically significantly higher chance to develop cardiovascular disease, arthritis, abdominal obesity, hypertension, and diabetes mellitus in the future.[36] Evidence from another study illustrates that Ecuadorian women with high stress are developing SLE, which is an autoimmune disorder that causes systemic inflammation.[37]

Research that attempts to establish a link between the stress response and disease needs to be interpreted with caution owing to the influence that individual differences have in the way people respond to stress. Not everyone who experiences stressful life events develops a disease. The evidence for a link between the stress response system and the development of disease in susceptible people is compelling but not conclusive. No study has established a direct cause-and-effect relationship between the stress response and disease occurrence. For example, depressive illness often is associated with an increase in both plasma cortisol and cerebrospinal fluid concentrations of CRF. The question that arises is whether this increased plasma cortisol is a cause or an effect of the depressive state. Although health care professionals continue to question the role of stressors and coping skills in the pathogenesis of disease states, we must resist the temptation to suggest that any disease is due to excessive stress or poor coping skills.

IN SUMMARY

Stress in itself is neither negative nor deleterious to health. The stress response is designed to be time limited and protective, but in situations of prolonged activation of the response because of overwhelming or chronic stressors, it could be damaging to health. PTSD is an example of chronic activation of the stress response as a result of experiencing a severe trauma. In this disorder, memory of the traumatic event seems to be enhanced. Flashbacks of the event are accompanied by intense activation of the neuroendocrine system.

Treatment of stress should be aimed at helping people avoid coping behaviors that can adversely affect their health and providing them with other ways to reduce stress. Nonpharmacologic methods used in the treatment of stress include relaxation techniques, guided imagery, music therapy, massage techniques, and biofeedback.

Research in stress has focused on personal reports of the stress situation and the physiologic responses to stress. A number of interview guides and written instruments are available for measuring the personal responses to acute and chronic stressors. Methods used for studying the physiologic manifestations of the stress response include electrocardiographic recording of heart rate, blood pressure measurement, electrodermal measurement of skin resistance associated with sweating, and biochemical analyses of hormone levels.

GERIATRIC Considerations

- A sense of coherence may help caregivers of frail elderly individuals cope with their chronic stress. (Coherence is defined as a reliable feeling focusing on factors rather than disease that helps with understanding life events and how to deal with them, knowing they have meaning.)[38]
- Stressors associated with aging include financial concerns, death of loved ones, difficulty with self-care independence, and retirement.[39]
- Good nutrition can reduce the negative effects of stress on the immune system.[39]
- Chronic stress is thought to accelerate biologic aging; increased levels of interleukin-6 linked with stress indicates the presence of subclinical stress.[40]

PEDIATRIC Considerations

- Stress in children can be due to normal developmental issues or atypical events including sickness, violence, or trauma. Resilience (coping skills to effectively deal with stress) will help the child to achieve balance.[41]
- Infants deal with stress by sucking. Regression back to a pacifier or bottle may occur during times of stress, and allowing these provides a sense of safety.[42]
- Tai chi, an alternative or complementary therapy, has been shown to offer muscle relaxation, which promotes self-control in children.[43]

REVIEW EXERCISES

1. A 21-year-old college student notices that she frequently develops "cold sores" during the stressful final exam week.
   A. What is the association between stress and the immune system?
   B. One of her classmates suggests that she listen to music or try relaxation exercises as a means of relieving stress. Explain how these interventions might work in relieving stress.
2. A 75-year-old woman with congestive heart failure complains that her condition gets worse when she worries and is under stress.
   A. Relate the effects stress has on the neuroendocrine control of cardiovascular function and its possible relationship to a worsening of the woman's congestive heart failure.
   B. She tells you that she dealt with much worse stresses when she was younger and never had any problems. How would you explain this?
3. A 30-year-old woman who was rescued from a collapsed building has been having nightmares recalling the event, excessive anxiety, and loss of appetite and is afraid to leave her home for fear something will happen.
   A. Given her history and symptoms, what is the likely diagnosis?
   B. How might she be treated?

References

1. American Psychological Association. (2017). *Stress in America: Coping with change. Stress in America™ Survey.*
2. Osler W. (1910). The Lumleian lectures in angina pectoris. *Lancet* 1, 696–700, 839–844, 974–977.
3. Cannon W. B. (1935). Stresses and strains of homeostasis. *American Journal of Medical Science* 189, 1–5.
4. Selye H. (1946). The general adaptation syndrome and diseases of adaptation. *Journal of Clinical Endocrinology* 6, 117–124.
5. Bernard C. (1878). *Leçons sur les phénomènes de la vie communs aux animaux et aux vegetaux*. Paris: Bailliere JB.
6. Cannon W. B. (1939). *The wisdom of the body* (pp. 299–300). New York: WW Norton.
7. Understanding the stress response. Chronic activation of this survival mechanism impairs health. (2016). *Harvard Medical School*. Harvard Health Publishing. Available: https://www.health.harvard.edu/staying-healthy/understanding-the-stress-response. Accessed February 24, 2018.
8. Momen N. C., Olsen J., Gissler M., et al. (2013). Early life bereavement and childhood cancer: a nationwide follow-up study in two countries. *BMJ Open* 3(5).
9. Finkelhor D., Shattuck A., Turner H., et al. (2013). Improving the adverse childhood experiences study scale. *Journal of the American Medical Association Pediatrics* 167(1), 70–75.
10. Siegel D. J. (2007). *The mindful brain: Reflection and attunement in the cultivation of well-being*. New York: WW Norton.
11. Schacter D. L., Gaesser B., Addis D. R. (2013). Remembering the past and imagining the future in the elderly. *Gerontology* 59(2), 143-151.
12. Selye H. (1976). *The stress of life* (rev. ed.). New York: McGraw-Hill.
13. Selye H. (1973). The evolution of the stress concept. *American Scientist* 61, 692–699.
14. Selye H. (1974). *Stress without distress* (p. 6). New York: New American Library.
15. Lazarus R. (2006). *Stress and emotion: A new synthesis* (p. 6). New York: Springer.
16. Herman J. P., McKlveen J. M., Ghosal S., et al. (2016). Regulation of the hypothalamic-pituitary-adrenocortical stress response. *Comprehensive Physiology* 6(2), 603–621.
17. Hall J. E. (2015). *Guyten and Hall textbook of medical physiology* (13th ed.). Philadelphia, PA: Saunders.
18. Sengupta P., Dutta S., Krajewska-Kulak E. (2017). The disappearing sperms: Analysis of reports published between 1980 and 2015. *American Journal of Men's Health* 11(4), 1279–1304.
19. Yam K. Y., Naninck E. F., Schmidt M. V., et al. (2015). Early-life adversity programs emotional functions and the neuroendocrine stress system: The contribution of nutrition, metabolic hormones and epigenetic mechanisms. *Stress* 18(3), 328–342.
20. Sippel L. M., Allington C. E., Pietrzak R. H., et al. (2017). Oxytocin and stress-related disorders: Neurobiological mechanisms and treatment opportunities. *Chronic Stress (Thousand Oaks)* 1. doi:10.1177/2470547016687996.
21. Dubos R. (1965). *Man adapting* (pp. 256, 258, 261, 264). New Haven, CT: Yale University.
22. Lazarus R. (2011). Evolution of a model of stress, coping, and discrete emotions. In Rice V. H. (Ed.), *Handbook of stress, coping, and health* (2nd ed., pp. 195–222). Thousand Oaks, CA: Sage.
23. Buysse D. J. (2014). Sleep health: Can we define it? Does it matter? *Sleep* 37(1), 9–17.
24. Sollars P. J., Pickard G. E. (2015). The neurobiology of circadian rhythms. *Psychiatric Clinics of North America* 38(4), 645–665.
25. Hague A., Leggat S. G. (2010). Enhancing hardiness among health care workers: The perceptions of senior managers. *Health Services Management Research* 23(2), 54–59.
26. Jordan T. R., Khubchandani J., Wiblishauser M. (2016). The impact of perceived stress and coping adequacy on the health of nurses: A pilot investigation. *Nursing Research and Practice* 2016, 5843256.
27. Ozbay F., Johnson D. C., Dimoulas E., et al. (2007). Social support and resilience to stress: From neurobiology to clinical practice. *Psychiatry (Edgmont)* 4(5), 35–40.
28. Shalev A., Liberzon I., Marmar C. (2017). Post-traumatic stress disorder. *The New England Journal of Medicine* 376(25), 2459–2469.
29. Lehrner A., Yehuda R. (2018). Trauma across generations and paths to adaptation and resilience. *Psychological Trauma: Theory, Research, Practice, and Policy* 10(1), 22–29.
30. De Bellis M. D., Woolley D. P., Hooper S. R. (2013). Neuropsychological findings in pediatric maltreatment: Relationship of PTSD, dissociative symptoms, and abuse/neglect indices to neurocognitive outcomes. *Child Maltreatment* 18(3), 171–183.
31. Kelley D. E., Lewis M. A., Southwell B. G. (2017). Perceived support from a caregiver's social ties predicts subsequent care-recipient health. *Preventive Medicine Reports* 8, 108–111.
32. Benson H. (1977). Systemic hypertension and the relaxation response. *The New England Journal of Medicine* 296, 1152–1154.
33. Strada E. A., Portenoy R. K. Psychological rehabilitative, and integrative therapies for cancer pain. In D. M. F. Savarese (Ed.). *UpToDate*. Available: https://www-uptodate-com./contents/psychological-rehabilitative-and-integrative-therapies-for-cancer-pain?search=Biofeedback:%20An%20overview%20in%20the%20context%20%20of%20heart-brain%20medicine&source=search_result&selectedTitle=3~150&usage_type=default&display_rank=3. Accessed February 24, 2018.
34. Salvo S. G. (2015). *Massage therapy: Principles and practice* (5th ed.). St. Louis, MO: Saunders.
35. Lee C. H., Lee C. Y., Hsu M. Y., et al. (2017). Effects of music intervention on state anxiety and physiological indices in patients undergoing mechanical ventilation in the intensive care unit. *Biological Research for Nursing* 19(2), 137–144.

36. Mattei J., Demissie S., Falcon L. M., et al. (2010). Allostatic load is associated with chronic conditions in the Boston Puerto Rican Health. *Social Science & Medicine* 70(12), 1988–1996.
37. Miles A. (2011). Emerging chronic illness: Women and lupus erythematosus in Ecuador. *Health Care for Women International* 32(8), 651–668.
38. Potier F., Degryse J., Henrard S., et al. (2018). A high sense of coherence protects from the burden of caregiving in older spousal caregivers. *Archives of Gerontology & Geriatrics* 75, 76–82. doi: 10.1016/j.archger.2017.11.013.
39. Eliopoulos C. (2018). *Gerontological nursing* (9th ed.). Philadelphia, PA: Wolters Kluwer.
40. American Institute of Stress. (n.d.). Seniors. *Transforming stress through awareness, education, and collaboration*. Available: https://www.stress.org/seniors/. Accessed February 24, 2018.
41. Kyle T., Carman S. (2017). *Essentials of pediatric nursing* (3rd ed.). Philadelphia, PA: Wolters Kluwer.
42. Bowden V. R., Greenberg C. S. (2014). *Children and their families the continuum of nursing care*. Philadelphia, PA: Wolters Kluwer.
43. McClafferty H. (2018). Mind-body therapies in pediatrics. *Alternative & Complementary Therapies* 24(1), 29-31. doi: 10.1089/act.2017.29143.hm.

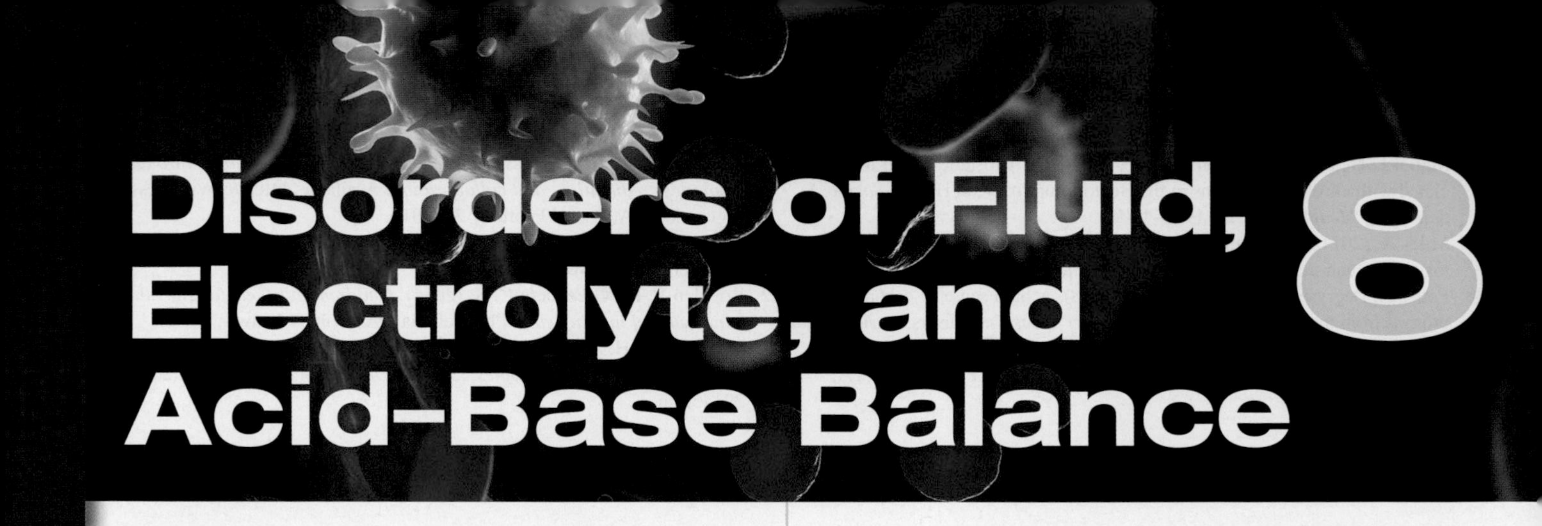

Disorders of Fluid, Electrolyte, and Acid–Base Balance

8

Michele R. Arwood and
Theresa Kessler

This chapter discusses disorders of fluid and electrolyte and acid–base balances. Electrolytes significantly affect all cell functions and are maintained within a narrow range primarily by the kidneys. Hydrogen (H^+) concentration is controlled by buffers, and an imbalance results in either acidosis or alkalosis. Fluids and electrolytes are present in body cells, in the tissue spaces between the cells, and in the blood that fills the vascular compartment. Body fluids transport gases, nutrients, and wastes; help generate the electrical activity needed to power body functions; take part in the transforming of food into energy; and otherwise maintain the overall function of the body. Although fluid volume and composition remain relatively constant in the presence of a wide range of changes in intake and output, conditions such as environmental stresses and disease can impair intake, increase losses, and interfere with mechanisms that regulate fluid volume, composition, and distribution. This chapter discusses the composition and compartmental distribution of body fluids; sodium and water balance; potassium balance; and calcium, phosphorus, and magnesium balance, and disorders of fluid and electrolyte balance.

The need for precise regulation of hydrogen ion (H^+) balance is similar in many ways to that of other ions in the body. Membrane excitability, enzyme systems, and chemical reactions all depend on the H^+ concentration being regulated within a narrow physiologic range to function in an optimal way. Many conditions, pathologic or otherwise, can alter H^+ concentration and acid–base balance. The content related to H+ balance has been organized into two sections: Mechanisms of acid–base balance and disorders of acid–base balance.

COMPOSITION AND COMPARTMENTAL DISTRIBUTION OF BODY FLUIDS

After completing this section of the chapter, the learner will be able to meet the following objectives:

- Differentiate the intracellular from the extracellular fluid compartments in terms of distribution and composition of water, electrolytes, and other osmotically active solutes.
- Relate the concept of a concentration gradient to the processes of diffusion and osmosis.
- Describe the control of cell volume and the effect of isotonic, hypotonic, and hypertonic solutions on cell size.

Body fluids are distributed between the intracellular fluid (ICF) and extracellular fluid (ECF) compartments. The *ICF compartment* consists of fluid contained within all of the billions of cells in the body. It is the larger of the two compartments, with approximately two thirds of the body water in healthy adults. The remaining one third of body water is in the *ECF compartment*, which contains all the fluids outside the cells, including those in the interstitial or tissue spaces and blood vessels (Fig. 8.1).

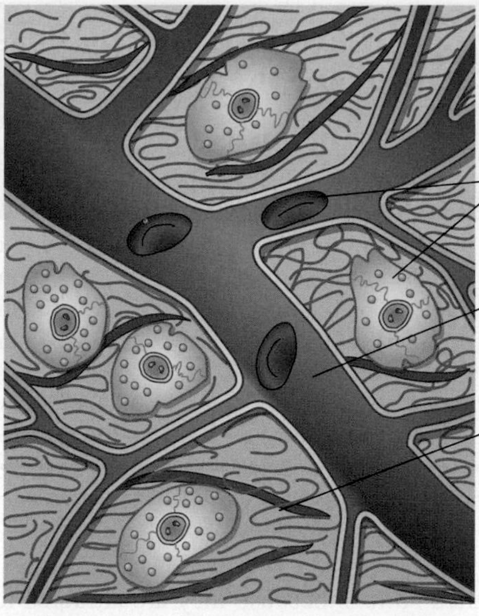

Figure 8.1 • Distribution of body water. The extracellular space includes the vascular compartment and the interstitial spaces.

The ECF, including blood plasma and interstitial fluids, contains large amounts of sodium and chloride and moderate amounts of bicarbonate but only small quantities of potassium, magnesium, calcium, and phosphorus. In contrast to the ECF, the ICF contains almost no calcium; small amounts of sodium, chloride, bicarbonate, and phosphorus; moderate amounts of magnesium; and large amounts of potassium (Table 8.1). It is the ECF levels of electrolytes in the blood or blood plasma that are measured clinically. Although blood levels usually are representative of the total-body levels of an electrolyte, this is not always the case, particularly with potassium, which has only about 2% in the ECF.[1] Potassium is the most abundant intracellular electrolyte.

The cell membrane serves as the primary barrier to the movement of substances between the ECF and ICF compartments. Lipid-soluble substances (*e.g.*, oxygen [O_2] and carbon dioxide [CO_2]), which dissolve in the lipid bilayer of the cell membrane, pass directly through the membrane, whereas many ions (*e.g.*, sodium [Na^+] and potassium [K^+]) rely on transport mechanisms such as the Na^+/K^+ pump located in the cell membrane for movement across the membrane.[2] Because the Na^+/K^+ pump relies on adenosine triphosphate (ATP) and the enzyme ATPase for energy, it is often referred to as the Na^+/K^+-ATPase membrane pump. Water crosses the cell membrane by osmosis using special transmembrane protein channels that are called *aquaporins.*[3]

Dissociation of Electrolytes

Body fluids contain water and electrolytes. Electrolytes are substances that dissociate in solution to form charged particles, or *ions.* For example, a sodium chloride (NaCl) molecule dissociates to form a positively charged Na^+ and a negatively charged Cl^- ion. Particles that do not dissociate into ions such as glucose and urea are called *nonelectrolytes.* Positively

TABLE 8.1 CONCENTRATIONS OF EXTRACELLULAR AND INTRACELLULAR ELECTROLYTES IN ADULTS

	EXTRACELLULAR CONCENTRATION*		INTRACELLULAR CONCENTRATION*	
ELECTROLYTE	**CONVENTIONAL UNITS**	**SI UNITS**	**CONVENTIONAL UNITS**	**SI UNITS**
Sodium	135–145 mEq/L	135–145 mmol/L	10–14 mEq/L	10–14 mmol/L
Potassium	3.5–5.0 mEq/L	3.5–5.0 mmol/L	140–150 mEq/L	140–150 mmol/L
Chloride	98–106 mEq/L	98–106 mmol/L	3–4 mEq/L	3–4 mmol/L
Bicarbonate	24–31 mEq/L	24–31 mmol/L	7–10 mEq/L	7–10 mmol/L
Calcium	8.5–10.5 mg/dL	2.1–2.6 mmol/L	<1 mEq/L	<0.25 mmol/L
Phosphorus	2.5–4.5 mg/dL	0.8–1.45 mmol/L	Variable	Variable
Magnesium	1.8–3.0 mg/dL	0.75–1.25 mmol/L	40 mEq/kg†	20 mmol/L

*Values may vary among laboratories, depending on the method of analysis used.
†Values vary among various tissues and with nutritional status.

charged ions are called *cations* because they are attracted to the cathode of a wet electric cell, and negatively charged ions are called *anions* because they are attracted to the anode. The ions found in body fluids carry one charge (*i.e.*, monovalent ion) or two charges (*i.e.*, divalent ion). Because of their attraction forces, positively charged cations are always accompanied by negatively charged anions. Thus, all body fluids contain equal amounts of anions and cations. However, cations and anions may be exchanged one for another, providing they carry the same charge. For example, a positively charged H^+ ion may be exchanged for a positively charged K^+ ion, and a negatively charged HCO_3^- ion may be exchanged for a negatively charged Cl^- ion.

Diffusion and Osmosis

Diffusion

Diffusion is the movement of charged or uncharged particles along a concentration gradient. All molecules and ions, including water and dissolved molecules, are in constant random motion. It is the motion of these particles, each colliding with one another, that supplies the energy for diffusion. Because there are more molecules in constant motion in a concentrated solution, particles move from an area of higher concentration to one of lower concentration. Measurement units used to describe the amount of electrolytes and solutes in body fluids are discussed in Chart 8.1.

Osmosis

Osmosis is the movement of water across a semipermeable membrane (*i.e.*, one that is permeable to water but impermeable to most solutes). As with particles, water diffuses down its concentration gradient, moving from the side of the membrane with the lesser number of particles and greater concentration of water to the side with the greater number of particles and lesser concentration of water (Fig. 8.2). As water moves across the semipermeable membrane, it generates a pressure called the *osmotic pressure*. The magnitude of the osmotic pressure represents the hydrostatic pressure (measured in millimeters of mercury [mm Hg]) needed to oppose the movement of water across the membrane.

CHART 8.1 MEASUREMENT UNITS

The amount of electrolytes and solutes in body fluids is expressed as a concentration or amount of solute in a given volume of fluid, such as milligrams per deciliter (mg/dL), milliequivalents per liter (mEq/L), or millimoles per liter (mmol/L). The *milligrams per deciliter* measurement unit expresses the weight of the solute in one tenth of a liter (dL) or 100 mL of solution. The concentration of electrolytes, such as calcium, phosphate, and magnesium, is often expressed in mg/dL.

The *milliequivalent* is used to express the charge equivalency for a given weight of an electrolyte. Electroneutrality requires that the total number of cations in the body equals the total number of anions. When cations and anions combine, they do so according to their ionic charge, not according to their atomic weight. Thus, 1 mEq of sodium has the same number of charges as 1 mEq of chloride, regardless of molecular weight (although sodium is positive and chloride is negative). The number of milliequivalents of an electrolyte in a liter of solution can be derived from the following equation:

$$\text{mEq} = \frac{\text{mg/100 mL} \times 10 \times \text{valence}}{\text{atomic weight}}$$

The Système Internationale (SI) units express electrolyte content of body fluids in *millimoles per liter* (mmol/L). A millimole is one thousandth of a mole, or the molecular weight of a substance expressed in milligrams. The number of millimoles of an electrolyte in a liter of solution can be calculated using the following equation:

$$\text{mmol/L} = \frac{\text{mEq/L}}{\text{valence}}$$

For monovalent electrolytes such as sodium and potassium, the mmol and mEq values are identical. For example, 140 mEq is equal to 140 mmol of sodium.

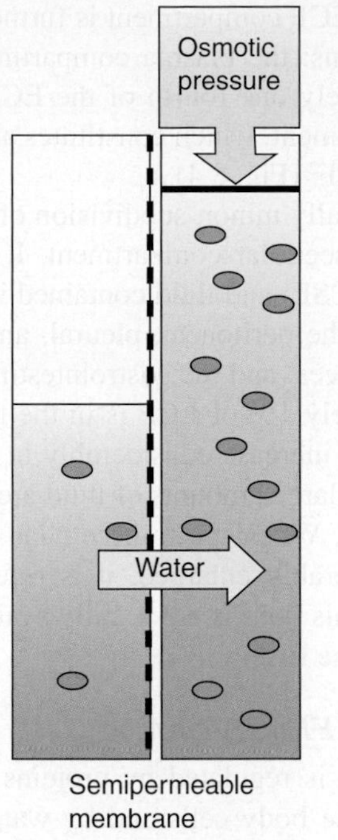

Figure 8.2 • Movement of water across a semipermeable membrane. Water moves from the side that has fewer nondiffusible particles to the side that has more. The osmotic pressure is equal to the hydrostatic pressure needed to oppose water movement across the membrane.

The osmotic activity that nondiffusible particles exert in pulling water from one side of the semipermeable membrane to the other is measured by a unit called an *osmole*. The osmole is derived from the gram molecular weight of a substance (*i.e.*, 1 g molecular weight of a nondiffusible and nonionizable substance is equal to 1 osmole). In the clinical setting, osmotic activity usually is expressed in milliosmoles (one thousandth of an osmole) per liter. Each nondiffusible particle, large or small, is equally effective in its ability to pull water through a semipermeable membrane. Thus, it is the number, rather than the size, of the nondiffusible particles that determines the osmotic activity of a solution.

The osmotic activity of a solution may be expressed in terms of either its osmolarity or osmolality. Osmolarity refers to the osmolar concentration in 1 L of solution (mOsm/L) and osmolality to the osmolar concentration in 1 kg of water (mOsm/kg of H_2O). Osmolarity is usually used when referring to fluids outside the body and osmolality for describing fluids inside the body. Because 1 L of water weighs 1 kg, the terms *osmolarity* and *osmolality* are often used interchangeably.

The predominant osmotically active particles in the ECF are Na^+ and its attendant anions (Cl^- and HCO_3^-), which together account for 90% to 95% of the osmotic pressure. Blood urea nitrogen (BUN) and glucose, which also are osmotically active, account for less than 5% of the total osmotic pressure in the extracellular compartment.[2] This can change, however, as when blood glucose levels are elevated in people with diabetes mellitus or when BUN levels change rapidly in people with chronic kidney disease. Serum osmolality, which normally ranges between 275 and 295 mOsm/kg, can be calculated using the following equation[4]:

$$\text{Osmolality (mOsm/kg)} = 2[\text{Na}^+\ (\text{mEq/L})] + \frac{\text{glucose (mg/dL)}^*}{18} + \frac{\text{BUN (mg/dL)}^*}{2.8}$$

$$^*1\ \text{mOsm of glucose} = 180\ \text{mg/L}$$

$$\text{and } 1\ \text{mOsm of urea} = 28\ \text{mg/L}$$

Ordinarily, the calculated and measured osmolality are within 10 mOsm of one another. The difference between the calculated and measured osmolality is called the *osmolar gap*. An osmolar gap larger than 10 mOsm suggests the presence of an unmeasured, osmotically active substance such as alcohol, acetone, or mannitol. Urine osmolality is discussed in Chart 8.2.

Concept Mastery Alert

Urine osmolality reflects the kidneys' ability to produce a concentrated or diluted urine based on serum osmolality and the need for water conservation or excretion.

Tonicity

A change in water content causes cells to swell or shrink. The term *tonicity* refers to the tension or effect that the effective osmotic pressure of a solution with impermeable solutes exerts on cell size because of water movement across the cell membrane. An effective osmole is one that exerts an osmotic force and cannot permeate the cell membrane, whereas an ineffective osmole is one that exerts an osmotic force but crosses the cell membrane. Tonicity is determined solely by effective

CHART 8.2 URINE OSMOLALITY

The ratio of urine osmolality to serum osmolality in a 24-hour urine sample normally exceeds 1:1, and after a period of overnight water deprivation, it should be greater than 3:1. A dehydrated person (one who has a loss of water) may have a urine–serum ratio that approaches 4:1. In these persons, urine osmolality may exceed 1000 mOsm/kg H_2O. In those who have difficulty concentrating their urine (*e.g.*, those with DI or chronic renal failure), the urine–serum ratio often is less than or equal to 1:1.

Urine specific gravity compares the weight of urine with that of water, providing an index for solute concentration. Water is considered to be 1.000. A change in specific gravity of 1.010 to 1.020 is an increase of 400 mOsm/kg H_2O. In the sodium-depleted state, the kidneys usually try to conserve sodium, urine specific gravity is normal, and urine sodium and chloride concentrations are low.

solutes such as glucose that cannot penetrate the cell membrane, thereby producing an osmotic force that pulls water out of the cell. In contrast, urea, which is osmotically active but lipid soluble, tends to distribute equally across the cell membrane. Therefore, when ECF levels of urea are elevated, ICF levels also are elevated. Urea is therefore considered to be an ineffective osmole. It is only when extracellular levels of urea change rapidly, as during hemodialysis treatment, that urea affects tonicity.

Solutions to which body cells are exposed can be classified as isotonic, hypotonic, or hypertonic depending on whether they cause cells to swell or shrink (Fig. 8.3). Cells placed in an isotonic solution, which has the same effective osmolality as the ICF (*i.e.*, 280 mOsm/L), neither shrink nor swell. An example of an isotonic solution is 0.9% NaCl. When cells are placed in a hypotonic solution, which has a lower effective osmolality than the ICF, they swell as water moves into the cell, and when they are placed in a hypertonic solution, which has a greater effective osmolality than the ICF, they shrink as water is pulled out of the cell. However, an isoosmotic solution is not necessarily isotonic. For example, the intravenous administration of a solution of 5% dextrose in water, which is isoosmotic, is equivalent to the infusion of a hypotonic solution of distilled water because the glucose is rapidly metabolized to CO_2 and water.

Compartmental Distribution of Body Fluids

Body water in the average adult male is about 60% of body weight (or about 42 L of water). Because adult females have more adipose tissue, approximately 50% of their body weight is made up of body water.[2] Body water is distributed between the ICF and ECF compartments. In the adult, the fluid in the ICF compartment constitutes approximately 40% of body weight, and fluid in the ECF constitutes approximately 20%.[2]

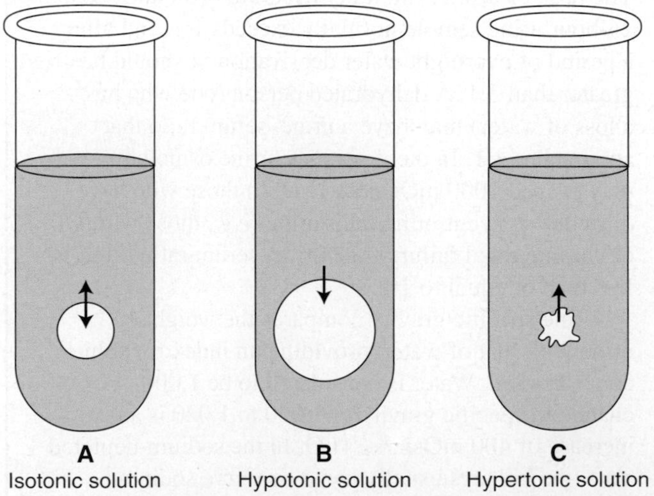

Figure 8.3 • Osmosis. **(A)** Red cells undergo no change in size in isotonic solutions. **(B)** They increase in size in hypotonic solutions and **(C)** decrease in size in hypertonic solutions.

The fluid in the ECF compartment is further divided into two major subdivisions: the plasma compartment, which constitutes approximately one fourth of the ECF, and the interstitial fluid compartment, which constitutes approximately three fourths of the ECF[2] (Fig. 8.4).

A third, usually minor, subdivision of the ECF compartment is the transcellular compartment. It includes the cerebrospinal fluid (CSF) and fluid contained in the various body spaces, such as the peritoneal, pleural, and pericardial cavities; the joint spaces; and the gastrointestinal tract. Normally, only approximately 1% of ECF is in the transcellular space. This amount can increase considerably in conditions such as ascites, in which large amounts of fluid are sequestered in the peritoneal cavity. When the transcellular fluid compartment becomes considerably enlarged, it is referred to as a *third space*, because this fluid is not readily available for exchange with the rest of the ECF.

Intracellular Fluid Volume

The ICF volume is regulated by proteins and organic compounds within the body cells and by water and solutes that move between the ECF and ICF. The membrane in most cells is freely permeable to water. Therefore, water moves between the ECF and ICF as a result of osmosis. In contrast, osmotically active proteins and other organic compounds cannot pass through the membrane. Water entry into the cell is regulated by these osmotically active substances as well as by solutes such as sodium and potassium that pass through the cell membrane. Many of the intracellular proteins are negatively charged and attract positively charged ions such as K^+, accounting for its higher concentration in the ICF. Na^+, which has a greater concentration in the ECF than the ICF, tends to enter the cell by diffusion. Na^+ is osmotically active, and, if left unchecked, its entry would pull water into the cell until it ruptured. The reason this does not occur is because the Na^+/K^+-ATPase membrane pump continuously removes three Na^+ ions from the cell for every two K^+ ions that are moved back

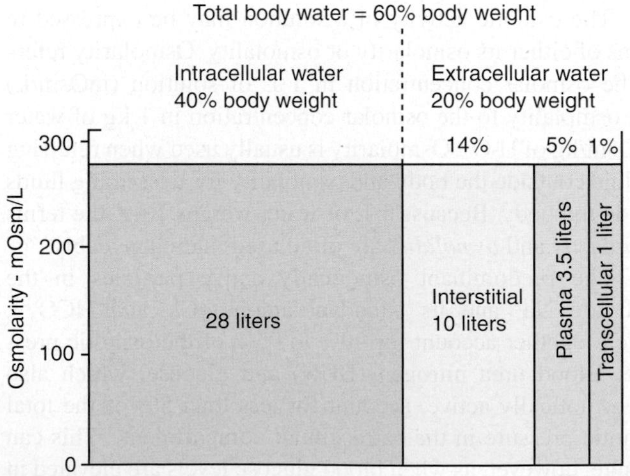

Figure 8.4 • Approximate sizes of body compartments in a 70-kg adult.

into the cell. Situations that impair the function of the Na^+/K^+-ATPase pump, such as hypoxia, cause cells to swell because of an accumulation of Na^+ ions.

The ICF volume is also affected by the concentration of osmotically active substances in the ECF that cannot cross the cell membrane. In diabetes mellitus, for example, glucose cannot enter the cell, and its increased concentration in the ECF pulls water out of the cell. Some cells, such as those in the central nervous system (CNS), defend against significant shifts in fluid volume through a change in osmotically active intracellular molecules. As an initial compensatory mechanism to preserve cell volume, there is a rapid shift of sodium, potassium, chloride, and water out of brain cells in response to a decrease in ECF osmolality and into brain cells in response to an increase in ECF osmolality. After 48 to 72 hours, a slower adaptive process takes place, during which brain cells mobilize organic osmolytes, composed mainly of amino acids, in an effort to maintain a normal cellular volume.

Extracellular Fluid Volume

The ECF is divided between the vascular, interstitial, and transcellular fluid compartments. The vascular compartment contains blood, which is essential to the transport of substances such as electrolytes, gases, nutrients, and waste products throughout the body. The fluid in the interstitial spaces acts as a transport vehicle for gases, nutrients, wastes, and other materials that move between the vascular compartment and body cells. Interstitial fluid also provides a reservoir from which the vascular volume can be maintained during periods of hemorrhage or loss of vascular fluid. A tissue gel, which is a spongelike material composed of large quantities of proteoglycan filaments, fills the tissue spaces and aids in even distribution of interstitial fluid[2] (see Fig. 8.1). Normally, most of the fluid in the interstitium is in gel form. The tissue gel is supported by collagen fibers that hold the gel in place. The tissue gel, which has a firmer consistency than water, opposes the outflow of water from the capillaries and helps to prevent the accumulation of free water in the interstitial spaces.

Capillary–Interstitial Fluid Exchange

The transfer of water between the vascular and interstitial compartments occurs at the capillary level. Four forces control the movement of water between the capillary and interstitial spaces:

1. The capillary filtration pressure, which pushes water out of the capillary into the interstitial spaces
2. The capillary colloidal osmotic pressure, which pulls water back into the capillary
3. The interstitial hydrostatic pressure, which opposes the movement of water out of the capillary
4. The tissue colloidal osmotic pressure, which pulls water out of the capillary into the interstitial spaces.[2]

Normally, the combination of these four forces is such that only a small excess of fluid remains in the interstitial compartment. This excess fluid is removed from the interstitium by the lymphatic system and returned to the systemic circulation.

Capillary filtration refers to the movement of water through capillary pores because of a mechanical, rather than an osmotic, force. The capillary filtration pressure (about 30 to 40 mm Hg at the arterial end, 10 to 15 mm Hg at the venous end, and 25 mm Hg in the middle), sometimes called the *capillary hydrostatic pressure*, is the pressure pushing water out of the capillary into the interstitial spaces. It reflects the arterial and venous pressures, the precapillary (arterioles) and postcapillary (venules) resistances, and the force of gravity.[2] A rise in arterial or venous pressure increases capillary pressure. The force of gravity increases capillary pressure in the dependent parts of the body. In a person who is standing absolutely still, the weight of blood in the vascular column causes an increase of 1 mm Hg in pressure for every 13.6 mm of distance from the heart.[2] This pressure results from the weight of water and is therefore called *hydrostatic pressure*. In the adult who is standing absolutely still, the pressure in the veins of the feet can reach 90 mm Hg. This pressure is then transmitted to the capillaries.

The *capillary colloidal osmotic pressure* (about 28 mm Hg) is the osmotic pressure generated by the plasma proteins that are too large to pass through the pores of the capillary wall.[2] The term *colloidal osmotic pressure* differentiates this type of osmotic pressure from the osmotic pressure that develops at the cell membrane from the presence of electrolytes and nonelectrolytes. Because plasma proteins do not normally penetrate the capillary pores and because their concentration is greater in the plasma than in the interstitial fluids, it is the capillary colloidal osmotic pressure that pulls fluids back into the capillary.

The interstitial fluid pressure (about −3 mm Hg) and the tissue colloidal osmotic pressure (about 8 mm Hg) contribute to movement of water into and out of the interstitial spaces.[2] The interstitial fluid pressure, which is normally negative, contributes to the outward movement of water into the interstitial spaces. The tissue colloidal osmotic pressure, which reflects the small amount of plasma proteins that normally escape into the interstitial spaces from the capillary, also pulls water out of the capillary into the tissue spaces.

The lymphatic system represents an accessory route whereby fluid from the interstitial spaces can return to the circulation. More important, the lymphatic system provides a means for removing plasma proteins and osmotically active particulate matter from the tissue spaces, neither of which can be reabsorbed into the capillaries.

Edema

Edema can be defined as palpable swelling produced by expansion of the interstitial fluid volume. In fact, the interstitial fluid spaces can actually contract to hold an additional 10 to 30 L of fluid.[2] The physiologic mechanisms that contribute to edema formation include factors that increase the capillary filtration pressure; decrease the capillary colloidal osmotic pressure; increase capillary permeability; or produce obstruction to lymph flow.[2] The causes of edema are summarized in Chart 8.3.

CHART 8.3 CAUSES OF EDEMA

Increased Capillary Pressure
Increased vascular volume
- Heart failure
- Kidney disease
- Premenstrual sodium retention
- Pregnancy
- Environmental heat stress
- Thiazolidinedione (*e.g.*, pioglitazone, rosiglitazone) therapy

Venous obstruction
- Liver disease with portal vein obstruction
- Acute pulmonary edema
- Venous thrombosis (thrombophlebitis)

Decreased arteriolar resistance
- Calcium channel–blocking drug responses

Decreased Colloidal Osmotic Pressure
Increased loss of plasma proteins
- Protein-losing kidney diseases
- Extensive burns

Decreased production of plasma proteins
- Liver disease
- Starvation, malnutrition

Increased Capillary Permeability
Inflammation
Allergic reactions (*e.g.*, hives)
Malignancy (*e.g.*, ascites, pleural effusion)
Tissue injury and burns

Obstruction of Lymphatic Flow
Malignant obstruction of lymphatic structures
Surgical removal of lymph nodes

Increased Capillary Filtration Pressure. As the capillary filtration pressure rises, the movement of vascular fluid into the interstitial spaces increases. Among the factors that increase capillary pressure are (1) increased arterial pressure or decreased resistance to flow through the precapillary sphincters, (2) an increase in venous pressure or increased resistance to outflow at the postcapillary sphincter, and (3) capillary distention because of increased vascular volume.

Edema can be either localized or generalized. The localized edema that occurs with urticaria (*i.e.*, hives) or other allergic or inflammatory conditions results from the release of histamine and other inflammatory mediators that cause dilation of the precapillary sphincters and arterioles that supply the swollen lesions. Thrombophlebitis obstructs venous flow, producing an elevation of venous pressure and edema of the affected part, usually one of the lower extremities.

Generalized body edema (termed *anasarca*) is frequently the result of increased vascular volume. The swelling of hands and feet that occurs in healthy people during hot weather is an example of edema that is caused by the vasodilation of superficial blood vessels along with sodium and water retention. Generalized edema is common in conditions such as congestive heart failure that produce fluid retention and venous congestion. In right-sided heart failure, blood pools throughout the entire venous system, causing organ congestion and edema of the dependent extremities.

Because of the effects of gravity, edema resulting from increased capillary pressure commonly causes fluid to accumulate in the dependent parts of the body, a condition referred to as *dependent edema*. For example, edema of the ankles and feet becomes more pronounced during prolonged periods of standing.

Decreased Capillary Colloidal Osmotic Pressure. Plasma proteins exert the osmotic force needed to pull fluid back into the capillary from the tissue spaces. The plasma proteins constitute a mixture of proteins, including albumin, globulins, and fibrinogen. Albumin, the smallest of the plasma proteins, has a molecular weight of 69,000; globulins have molecular weights of approximately 140,000; and fibrinogen has a molecular weight of 400,000.[2] Because of its lower molecular weight, 1 g of albumin has approximately twice as many osmotically active molecules as 1 g of globulin and almost six times as many osmotically active molecules as 1 g of fibrinogen. Also, the concentration of albumin (approximately 4.5 g/dL) is greater than that of the globulins (2.5 g/dL) and fibrinogen (0.3 mg/dL).

Edema because of decreased capillary colloidal osmotic pressure usually is the result of inadequate production or abnormal loss of plasma proteins, mainly albumin. The plasma proteins are synthesized in the liver. In people with severe liver failure, the impaired synthesis of albumin results in a decrease in colloidal osmotic pressure. In starvation and malnutrition, edema develops because there is a lack of amino acids for plasma protein synthesis.

The most common site of plasma protein loss is the kidney. In kidney diseases such as glomerulonephritis, the glomerular capillaries become permeable to the plasma proteins, particularly albumin, which is the smallest of the proteins. When this happens, large amounts of albumin are filtered out of the blood and lost in the urine. An excessive loss of plasma proteins also occurs when large areas of skin are injured or destroyed. Edema is a common problem during the early stages of a burn, resulting from capillary injury and loss of plasma proteins.[1]

Because the plasma proteins are evenly distributed throughout the body and are not affected by the force of gravity, edema because of a decrease in capillary colloidal osmotic pressure tends to affect tissues in nondependent as well as dependent parts of the body. There is swelling of the face as well as the legs and feet.

Increased Capillary Permeability. When the capillary pores become enlarged or the integrity of the capillary wall is damaged, capillary permeability is increased. When this occurs, plasma proteins and other osmotically active particles leak into the interstitial spaces, increasing the tissue colloidal osmotic pressure and thereby contributing to the accumulation of interstitial fluid. Among the conditions that increase capillary permeability are burn injury, capillary congestion, inflammation, and immune responses.

Obstruction of Lymph Flow. Osmotically active plasma proteins and other large particles that cannot be reabsorbed through the pores in the capillary membrane rely on the lymphatic system for movement back into the circulatory system. Edema because of impaired lymph flow caused by a disruption or malformation of the lymphatic system develops as a result of high protein swelling in an area of the body is referred to as *lymphedema*.[5] Malignant involvement of lymph structures and removal of lymph nodes at the time of cancer surgery are common causes of lymphedema.[6] Another cause of lymphedema is infection and trauma involving the lymphatic channels and lymph nodes.

Clinical Manifestations. The effects of edema are determined largely by its location. Edema of the brain, larynx, or lungs is an acute, life-threatening condition. Although not life threatening, edema may interfere with movement, limiting joint motion. Swelling of the ankles and feet often is insidious in onset and may or may not be associated with disease. At the tissue level, edema increases the distance for diffusion of O_2, nutrients, and wastes. Edematous tissues usually are more susceptible to injury and development of ischemic tissue damage, including pressure ulcers. Edema can also compress blood vessels. The skin of a severely swollen finger can act as a tourniquet, shutting off the blood flow to the finger. Edema can also be disfiguring, causing psychological effects and disturbances in self-concept. It can also create problems with obtaining proper-fitting clothing and shoes.

Pitting edema occurs when the accumulation of interstitial fluid exceeds the absorptive capacity of the tissue gel. In this form of edema, the tissue water becomes mobile and can be translocated with pressure exerted by a finger. *Nonpitting edema* usually reflects a condition in which plasma proteins have accumulated in the tissue spaces and coagulated. It is seen most commonly in areas of localized infection or trauma. The area often is firm and discolored.

Assessment and Treatment. Methods for assessing edema include daily weight, visual assessment, measurement of the affected part, and application of finger pressure to assess for pitting edema. Daily weight performed at the same time each day with the same amount of clothing provides a useful index of water gain (1 L of water weighs 1 kg [2.2 lb]) because of edema. Visual inspection and measurement of the circumference of an extremity can also be used to assess the degree of swelling. This is particularly useful when swelling is due to thrombophlebitis. Finger pressure can be used to assess the degree of pitting edema. If an indentation remains after

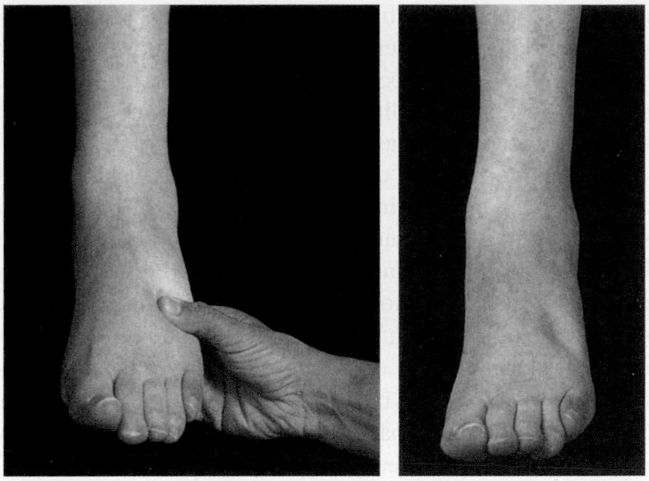

Figure 8.5 • 3+ pitting edema. (Adapted from Bickley L. S. (2017). *Bates' guide to physical examination and history taking* (12th ed., Figs. 12-24 and 12-25, p. 529). Philadelphia, PA: Wolter Kluwer.)

the finger has been removed, pitting edema is identified. It is evaluated on a scale of +1 (minimal) to +4 (severe) (Fig. 8.5).

Distinguishing lymphedema from other forms of edema can be challenging, especially early in its course. Papillomatosis, a characteristic honeycomb appearance of the skin because of dilated lymph vessels that are enveloped in fibrotic tissue, distinguishes lymphedema from other edemas. Computed tomography (CT) or magnetic resonance imaging (MRI) may be used to confirm the diagnosis.[5,6]

Treatment of edema usually is directed toward maintaining life when the swelling involves vital structures, correcting or controlling the cause, and preventing tissue injury. Edema of the lower extremities may respond to simple measures such as elevating the feet. Diuretic therapy commonly is used to treat edema associated with an increase in ECF volume. Serum albumin levels can be measured, and albumin may be administered intravenously to raise the plasma colloidal osmotic pressure when edema is caused by hypoalbuminemia.

Elastic support stockings and sleeves increase interstitial fluid pressure and resistance to outward movement of fluid from the capillary into the tissue spaces. These support devices typically are prescribed for people with conditions such as lymphatic or venous obstruction and are most efficient if applied before the tissue spaces have filled with fluid—in the morning, for example, before the effects of gravity have caused fluid to move into the ankles. Moderate to severe lymphedema is usually treated with light-pressure massage designed to increase lymph flow by encouraging opening and closing of lymph vessel valves; compression garments or pneumatic compression pumps; range-of-motion exercises; and scrupulous skin care to prevent infection.[5,6]

Third-Space Accumulation

Third spacing represents the loss or trapping of ECF into the transcellular space. The serous cavities are part of the transcellular compartment (*i.e.*, third space) located in strategic body areas where there is continual movement of body structures—the pericardial sac, the peritoneal cavity, and the pleural cavity. The exchange of ECF between the capillaries, the interstitial spaces, and the transcellular space of the serous cavity uses the same mechanisms as capillaries elsewhere in the body. The serous cavities are closely linked with lymphatic drainage systems. The milking action of the moving structures, such as the lungs, continually forces fluid and plasma proteins back into the circulation, keeping these cavities empty. Any obstruction to lymph flow causes fluid accumulation in the serous cavities. As with edema fluid, third-space fluids represent an accumulation or trapping of body fluids that contribute to body weight but not to fluid reserve or function. Some causes of third spacing include systemic inflammatory response syndrome or leaky capillary syndrome in pancreatitis; hypoalbuminemia, which occurs with severe liver failure; and third-degree burns.[7]

The prefix *hydro-* may be used to indicate the presence of excessive fluid, as in *hydrothorax*, which means excessive fluid in the pleural cavity. The accumulation of fluid in the peritoneal cavity is called ascites. The transudation of fluid into the serous cavities is also referred to as effusion. Effusion can contain blood, plasma proteins, inflammatory cells (*i.e.*, pus), and ECF.

IN SUMMARY

Body fluids, which contain water and electrolytes, are distributed between the ICF and ECF compartments of the body. Two thirds of body fluid is contained in the body cells of the ICF compartment, and one third is contained in the vascular compartment, interstitial spaces, and third-space areas of the ECF compartment. The ICF has high concentrations of potassium, calcium, phosphorus, and magnesium and the ECF high concentrations of sodium, chloride, and bicarbonate.

Electrolytes and nonelectrolytes move by diffusion across cell membranes that separate the ICF and ECF compartments. Water crosses the cell membrane by osmosis, using special protein channels called *aquaporins*. It moves from the side of the membrane that has the lesser number of particles and greater concentration of water to the side that has the greater number of particles and lesser concentration of water. The osmotic tension or effect that a solution exerts on cell volume in terms of causing the cell to swell or shrink is called *tonicity*.

Edema represents an increase in interstitial fluid volume. The physiologic mechanisms that contribute to the development of edema include factors that (1) increase capillary filtration pressure, (2) decrease capillary colloidal osmotic pressure, (3) increase capillary permeability, and (4) obstruct lymphatic flow. The effect that edema exerts on body function is determined by its location. Edema of the brain, larynx, or lungs is an acute, life-threatening situation, whereas swelling of the ankles and feet can be a normal discomfort that accompanies hot weather. Fluid can also accumulate in the transcellular compartment—the joint spaces, the pericardial sac, the peritoneal cavity, and the pleural cavity. Because this fluid is not easily exchanged with the rest of the ECF, it is often referred to as third-space fluid.

SODIUM AND WATER BALANCE

After completing this section of the chapter, the learner will be able to meet the following objectives:

- State the functions and physiologic mechanisms controlling body water levels and sodium concentration, including the effective circulating volume, sympathetic nervous system, renin–angiotensin–aldosterone system, and antidiuretic hormone.
- Describe the relationship between antidiuretic hormone and aquaporin-2 channels in reabsorption of water by the kidney.
- Compare the pathology, manifestations, and treatment of diabetes insipidus and the syndrome of inappropriate antidiuretic hormone.

The movement of body fluids between the ICF and ECF compartments occurs at the cell membrane and depends on ECF levels of water and sodium. Almost 93% of body fluids are made up of water, and sodium salts account for approximately 90% to 95% of ECF solutes.[2] Normally, equivalent changes in sodium and water are such that the volume and osmolality of ECF are maintained within a normal range. Because it is the concentration of sodium that controls ECF osmolality, changes in sodium are usually accompanied by proportionate changes in water volume.

Body Water Balance

Total body water (TBW) varies with sex and weight. These differences can be explained by differences in body fat, which is essentially water free (*i.e.*, fat is approximately 10% water by composition, compared with 75% for skeletal muscle). In young adult males, TBW approximates 60% of body weight, whereas TBW is approximately 50% for young adult females.[1] The TBW tends to decrease with old age because of more adipose tissue and less muscle.[1] Obesity produces further decreases in TBW because adipose tissue only contains about 10% water.[1]

Infants normally have more TBW than older children or adults. TBW constitutes approximately 75% of body weight in full-term infants and an even greater proportion in premature infants.[1] In addition to having proportionately more body water than adults, infants have relatively more water in their ECF compartment. Infants have more than half of their TBW in the ECF compartment. The greater ECF water content of an infant can be explained in terms of its higher metabolic rate,

Understanding Capillary Fluid Exchange

Movement of fluid between the vascular compartment and the interstitial fluid compartment surrounding the body cells occurs at the capillary level. The direction and amount of fluid that flows across the capillary wall are determined by (1) the hydrostatic pressure of the two compartments, (2) the colloidal osmotic pressures of the two compartments, and (3) the removal of excess fluid and osmotically active particles from the interstitial spaces by the lymphatic system.

Hydrostatic Pressure

The hydrostatic pressure is the pushing force exerted by a fluid. Inside the capillaries, the hydrostatic pressure is the same as the capillary filtration pressure, about 30 mm Hg at thc arterial end and 10 mm Hg at the venous end. The interstitial fluid pressure is the force of fluid in the interstitial spaces pushing against the outside of the capillary wall. Evidence suggests that the interstitial pressure is slightly negative (–3 mm Hg), contributing to the outward movement of fluid from the capillary.

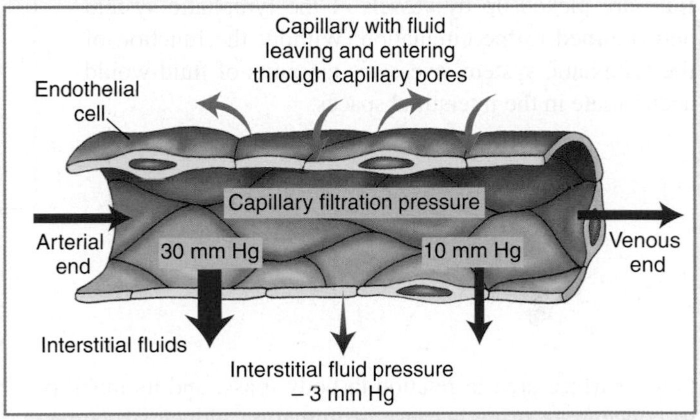

Colloidal Osmotic Pressure

The colloidal osmotic pressure is the pulling force created by the presence of evenly dispersed particles, such as the plasma proteins, that cannot pass through the pores of the capillary membrane. The capillary colloidal osmotic pressure is normally about 28 mm Hg throughout the length of the capillary bed. The interstitial colloidal osmotic pressure (about 8 mm Hg) represents the pulling pressure exerted by the small amounts of plasma proteins that leak through the pores of the capillary wall into the interstitial spaces. The capillary colloidal osmotic pressure, which is greater than both the hydrostatic pressure at the venous end of the capillary and the interstitial colloidal osmotic pressure, is largely responsible for the movement of fluid back into the capillary.

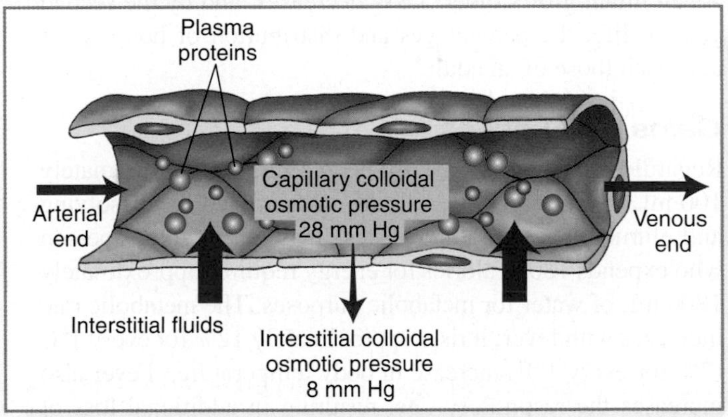

Continued

Understanding Capillary Fluid Exchange *(Continued)*

Lymph Drainage

The lymphatic system represents an accessory system by which fluid can be returned to the circulatory system. Normally the forces moving fluid out of the capillary into the interstitium are greater than those returning fluid to the capillary. Any excess fluids and osmotically active plasma proteins that may have leaked into the interstitium are picked up by vessels of the lymphatic system and returned to the circulation. Without the function of the lymphatic system, excessive amounts of fluid would accumulate in the interstitial spaces.

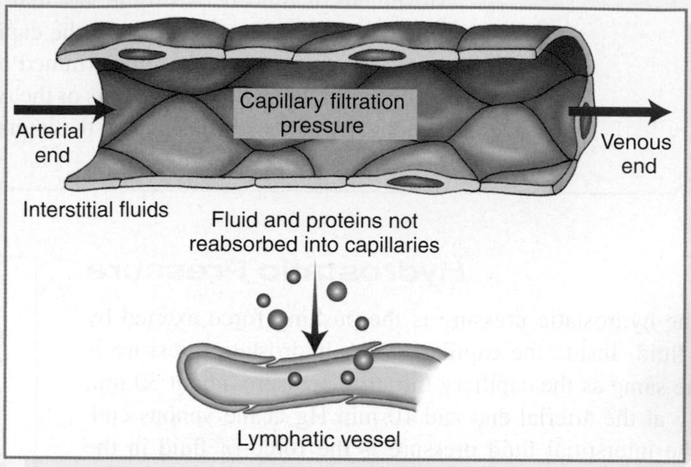

larger surface area in relation to body mass, and its inability to concentrate urine because of immature kidney structures. Because ECFs are more readily lost from the body, infants are more vulnerable to fluid deficit than older children and adults. As an infant grows older, TBW decreases, and by the second year of life, the percentages and distribution of body water approach those of an adult.[8]

Gains and Losses

Regardless of age, all healthy people require approximately 100 mL of water per 100 calories metabolized for dissolving and eliminating metabolic wastes. This means that a person who expends 1800 calories for energy requires approximately 1800 mL of water for metabolic purposes. The metabolic rate increases with fever; it rises approximately 12% for every 1°C (7% for every 1°F) increase in body temperature.[2] Fever also increases the respiratory rate, resulting in additional loss of water vapor through the lungs.

The main source of water gain is through oral intake and metabolism of nutrients. Water, including that obtained from liquids and solid foods, is absorbed from the gastrointestinal tract. Tube feedings and parenterally administered fluids are also sources of water gain. Metabolic processes also generate a small amount of water.

Normally, the largest loss of water occurs through the kidneys, with lesser amounts being lost through the skin, lungs, and gastrointestinal tract. Even when oral or parenteral fluids are withheld, the kidneys continue to produce urine as a means of ridding the body of metabolic wastes. The urine output that is required to eliminate these wastes is called the *obligatory urine output.* The obligatory urine loss is approximately 300 to 500 mL/day. Water losses that occur through the skin and lungs are referred to as *insensible water losses.* The gains and losses of body water are summarized in Table 8.2.

Sodium Balance

Sodium is the most abundant cation in the body, averaging approximately 60 mEq/kg of body weight.[1] Most of the body's sodium is in the ECF compartment (135 to 145 mEq/L [135 to 145 mmol/L]), with only a small amount (10 to 14 mEq/L [10 to 14 mmol/L]) located in the ICF compartment. The resting cell membrane is relatively impermeable to sodium; sodium that enters the cell is transported out of the cell against an electrochemical gradient by the Na^+/K^+-ATPase membrane pump.

TABLE 8.2 SOURCES OF BODY WATER GAINS AND LOSSES IN THE ADULT

GAINS		LOSSES	
Oral intake		Urine	1500 mL
As water	1000 mL	Insensible losses	
In food	1300 mL	Lungs	300 mL
Water of oxidation	200 mL	Skin	500 mL
		Feces	200 mL
Total	2500 mL	Total	2500 mL

KEY POINTS

SODIUM AND WATER BALANCE

- It is the amount of water and its effect on sodium concentration in the ECF that serves to regulate the distribution of fluid between the ICF and the ECF compartments.
- Hyponatremia or hypernatremia that is brought about by disproportionate losses or gains in sodium or water exerts its effects on the ICF compartment, causing water to move in or out of body cells. Many of the manifestations of changes in sodium concentration reflect changes in the intracellular volume of cells, particularly those in the nervous system.

Sodium functions mainly in regulating the ECF volume. As the major cation in the ECF compartment, Na^+ and its attendant anions (Cl^- and HCO_3^-) account for approximately 90% to 95% of the osmotic activity in the ECF. Because sodium is part of the sodium bicarbonate molecule, it is important in regulating acid–base balance. As a current-carrying ion, Na^+ contributes to the function of the nervous system and other excitable tissue.

Gains and Losses

Sodium normally enters the body through the gastrointestinal tract and is eliminated by the kidneys or lost from the gastrointestinal tract or skin. Sodium intake normally is derived from dietary sources. Body needs for sodium usually can be met by as little as 500 mg/day. The average salt intake is approximately 6 to 15 g/day, or 12 to 30 times the daily requirement. Dietary intake, which frequently exceeds the amount needed by the body, is often influenced by culture and food preferences rather than need. As package labels indicate, many commercially prepared foods and soft drinks contain considerable amounts of sodium. Other sources of sodium are intravenous saline infusions and medications that contain sodium.

Most sodium losses occur through the kidneys. The kidneys are extremely efficient in regulating sodium output, and when sodium intake is limited or conservation of sodium is needed, the kidneys are able to reabsorb almost all the sodium that has been filtered by the glomerulus. This results in essentially sodium-free urine. Conversely, urinary losses of sodium increase as intake increases.

Usually less than 10% of sodium intake is lost through the gastrointestinal tract and skin. Although the sodium concentration of fluids in the upper part of the gastrointestinal tract approaches that of the ECF, sodium is reabsorbed as the fluids move through the lower part of the bowel, so that the concentration of sodium in the stool is only approximately 40 mEq/L (40 mmol/L). Sodium losses increase with conditions such as vomiting, diarrhea, fistula drainage, and gastrointestinal suction that remove sodium from the gastrointestinal tract. Irrigation of gastrointestinal tubes with distilled water removes sodium from the gastrointestinal tract, as do repeated tap water enemas.

Sodium leaves the skin through the sweat glands. Sweat is a hypotonic solution containing both sodium and chloride. Although sodium losses because of sweating are usually negligible, they can increase greatly during exercise and periods of exposure to a hot environment. A person who sweats profusely can lose up to 15 to 30 g of salt each day for first few days of exposure to a hot environment. This amount usually drops to less than 3 to 5 g a day after 4 to 6 weeks of acclimatization.[2]

Mechanisms of Regulation

The major regulator of sodium and water balance is the maintenance of the *effective circulating volume* also called the *effective arterial blood volume*. This is the vascular bed that perfuses the body. A low effective circulating volume activates feedback mechanisms that produce an increase in renal sodium and water retention, and a high effective circulating volume triggers feedback mechanisms that decrease sodium and water retention.

The effective circulating volume is monitored by a number of sensors that are located in both the vascular system and the kidney. These sensors are the *baroreceptors* because they respond to pressure-induced stretch of the vessel walls.[1] There are baroreceptors located in the low-pressure side of the circulation (walls of the cardiac atria and large pulmonary vessels) that respond primarily to fullness of the circulation. Baroreceptors are also present in the high-pressure arterial side of the circulation (aortic arch and carotid sinus) that respond primarily to changes in the arterial pressure. The activity of both types of receptors regulates water elimination by modulating sympathetic nervous system outflow and antidiuretic hormone (ADH) secretion.[1] The sympathetic nervous system responds to changes in arterial pressure and blood volume by adjusting the glomerular filtration rate and thus the rate at which sodium is filtered from the blood. Sympathetic activity also regulates tubular reabsorption of sodium and renin release. An additional mechanism related to renal sodium excretion is atrial natriuretic peptide (ANP), which is released from cells in the atria of the heart. ANP, which is released in response to atrial stretch and overfilling, increases sodium excretion by the kidney, which in turn pulls out more water.[1]

Pressure-sensitive receptors in the kidney, particularly in the afferent arterioles, respond directly to changes in arterial pressure through stimulation of the sympathetic nervous system and release of renin with activation of the renin–angiotensin–aldosterone system (RAAS).[1] The RAAS exerts its action through angiotensin II and aldosterone. Renin is a small protein enzyme that is released by the kidney in response to changes in arterial pressure, the glomerular filtration rate, and the amount of sodium in the tubular fluid. Most of the renin that is released leaves the kidney and enters the bloodstream, where it interacts enzymatically to convert a circulating plasma protein called *angiotensinogen* to angiotensin I.

Angiotensin I is rapidly converted to angiotensin II by the angiotensin-converting enzyme (ACE) in the small blood vessels of the lung. Angiotensin II acts directly on the renal tubules to increase sodium reabsorption. It also acts to constrict renal blood vessels, thereby decreasing the glomerular filtration rate and slowing renal blood flow so that less sodium is filtered and more is reabsorbed.

Angiotensin II is also a powerful regulator of *aldosterone*, a hormone secreted by the adrenal cortex. Aldosterone acts at the level of the cortical collecting tubules of the kidneys to increase sodium reabsorption while increasing potassium elimination. The sodium-retaining action of aldosterone can be inhibited by blocking the actions of aldosterone with potassium-sparing diuretics (*e.g.*, spironolactone, amiloride, and triamterene), by suppressing renin release (*e.g.*, β-adrenergic blocking drugs), by inhibiting the conversion of angiotensin I to angiotensin II (*i.e.*, ACE inhibitors), or by blocking the action of angiotensin II on the angiotensin receptor (*i.e.*, angiotensin II receptor blockers [ARBs]).[1]

Thirst and Antidiuretic Hormone

Two other mechanisms that contribute directly to the regulation of body water and indirectly to the regulation of sodium are thirst and ADH. Thirst is primarily a regulator of water intake and ADH a regulator of water output. Both thirst and ADH are responsive to changes in extracellular osmolality and the resultant effective circulating volume (Fig. 8.6).[1]

Disorders of Thirst

Thirst is the conscious sensation of the need to obtain and drink fluids high in water content. Drinking of water or other fluids often occurs as the result of habit or for reasons other than those related to thirst. Most people drink without being thirsty, and water is consumed before it is needed. As a result, thirst is basically an emergency response. It usually occurs only when the need for water has not been anticipated.

Thirst is controlled by the thirst center in the hypothalamus. There are two stimuli for true thirst based on water need: (1) cellular dehydration caused by an increase in ECF osmolality and (2) a decrease in blood volume, which may or may not be associated with a decrease in serum osmolality. Sensory neurons, called *osmoreceptors*, which are located in or near the thirst center in the hypothalamus, respond to changes in ECF osmolality by swelling or shrinking (see Fig. 8.7). Thirst normally develops when there is as little as a 1% to 2% change in serum osmolality.[9] The previously described stretch receptors in the vascular system that monitor the effective circulating volume also aid in the regulation of thirst. Thirst is one of the earliest symptoms of hemorrhage and is often present before other signs of blood loss appear.

A third important stimulus for thirst is angiotensin II, levels of which increase in response to low blood volume and low blood pressure. The renin–angiotensin mechanism

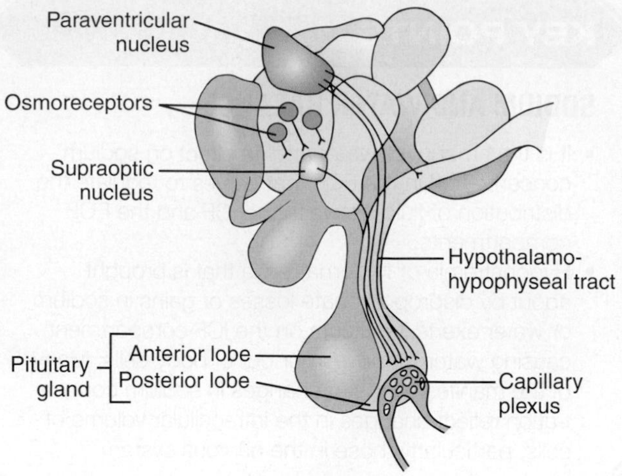

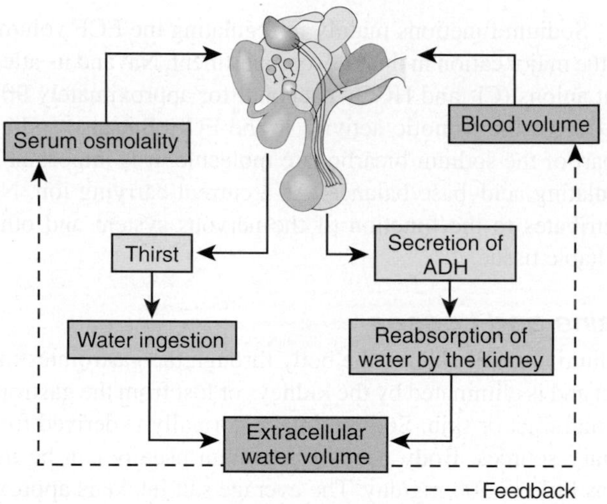

Figure 8.6 • Effect of isotonic fluid excess and deficit and of hyponatremia and hypernatremia on movement of water between the extracellular (ECF) and intracellular fluid (ICF) compartments.

contributes to nonosmotic thirst. This system is considered a backup system for thirst should other systems fail. Because it is a backup system, it probably does not contribute to the regulation of normal thirst. However, elevated levels of angiotensin II may lead to thirst in conditions, such as chronic kidney disease and congestive heart failure, in which renin levels may be elevated.

Dryness of the mouth, such as the thirst a lecturer experiences during speaking, produces a sensation of thirst that is not necessarily associated with the body's hydration status. Thirst sensation also occurs in those who breathe through their mouths, such as smokers and people with chronic respiratory disease or hyperventilation syndrome.

Hypodipsia. Hypodipsia represents a decrease in the ability to sense thirst. It is commonly associated with lesions in the area of the hypothalamus (*e.g.*, head trauma, meningiomas, occult hydrocephalus, subarachnoid hemorrhage). There is also evidence that thirst is decreased and water intake reduced

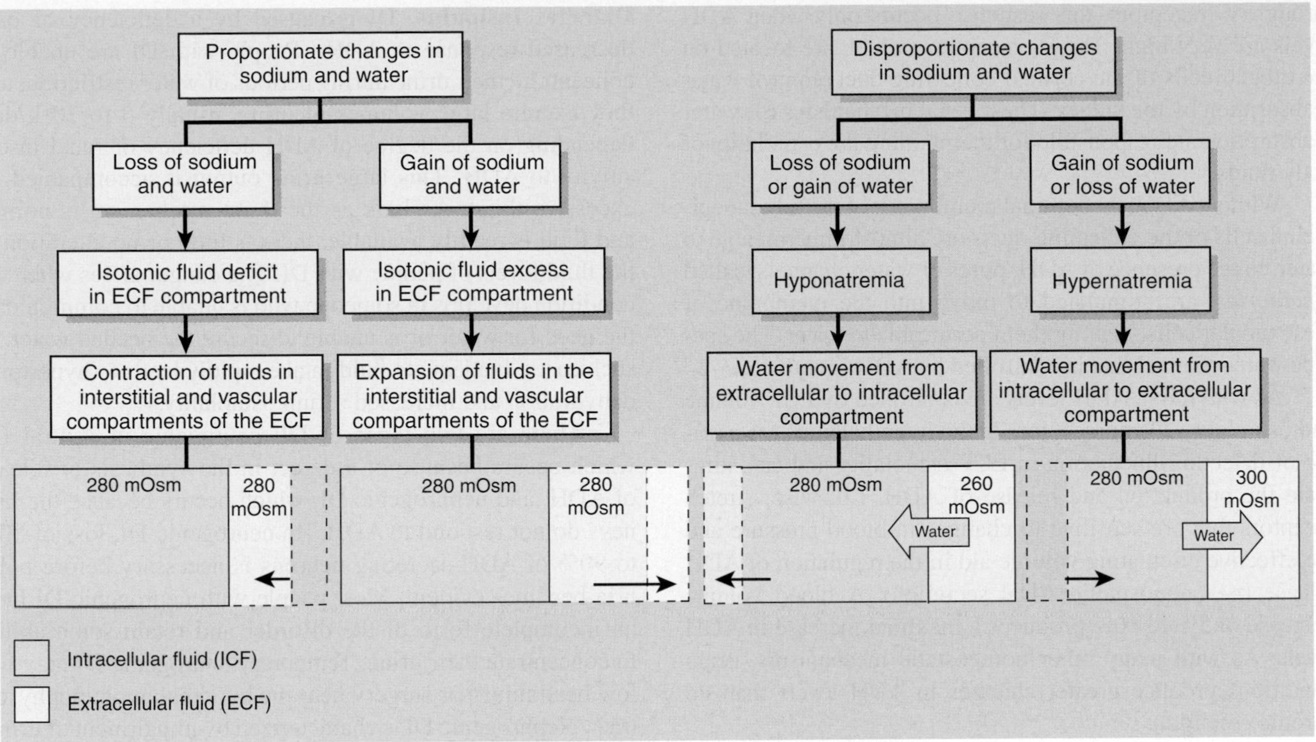

Figure 8.7 • (*Top*) Sagittal section through the pituitary and anterior hypothalamus. Antidiuretic hormone (ADH) is formed primarily in the supraoptic nucleus and to a lesser extent in the paraventricular nucleus of the hypothalamus. It is then transported down the hypothalamohypophyseal tract and stored in secretory granules in the posterior pituitary, where it can be released into the blood. (*Bottom*) Pathways for regulation of extracellular water volume by thirst and ADH.

in oldest older adults (age >80 years), despite higher plasma sodium and osmolality levels.[10] The inability to perceive and respond to thirst is compounded in older adults who have had a stroke and may be further influenced by confusion, sensory deficits, and motor disturbances.

Polydipsia. Polydipsia, or excessive thirst, is normal when it accompanies conditions of water deficit. Increased thirst and drinking behavior can be classified into three categories: (1) symptomatic or true thirst, (2) inappropriate or false thirst that occurs despite normal levels of body water and serum osmolality, and (3) compulsive water drinking. *Symptomatic thirst* develops when there is a loss of body water and resolves after the loss has been replaced. Among the most common causes of symptomatic thirst are water losses associated with diarrhea, vomiting, diabetes mellitus, and diabetes insipidus (DI). *Inappropriate or excessive thirst* may persist despite adequate hydration. It is a common complaint in people with congestive heart failure, diabetes mellitus, and chronic kidney disease. Although the cause of thirst in these people is unclear, it may result from increased angiotensin levels. Thirst is also a common complaint in people with dry mouth caused by decreased salivary function or treatment with drugs with an anticholinergic action (*e.g.*, antihistamines, atropine) that leads to decreased salivary flow.

Psychogenic polydipsia involves compulsive water drinking and is usually seen in people with psychiatric disorders, most commonly schizophrenia.[11] People with the disorder drink large amounts of water and excrete large amounts of urine. The cause of excessive water drinking in these people is uncertain. The condition may be compounded by antipsychotic medications that increase ADH levels and interfere with water excretion by the kidneys. Cigarette smoking, which is common among people with psychiatric disorders, also stimulates ADH secretion. Excessive water ingestion coupled with impaired water excretion (or rapid ingestion at a rate that exceeds renal excretion) in people with psychogenic polydipsia can lead to water intoxication. Treatment usually consists of water restriction and behavioral measures aimed at decreasing water consumption.

Disorders of Antidiuretic Hormone

The reabsorption of water by the kidneys is regulated by ADH, also known as *vasopressin.* ADH is synthesized by cells in the supraoptic and paraventricular nuclei of the hypothalamus and then transported along a neural pathway (*i.e.*, hypothalamohypophyseal tract) to the posterior pituitary gland, where it is stored. When the supraoptic and paraventricular nuclei in the hypothalamus are stimulated by increased serum osmolality or other factors, nerve impulses travel down the hypothalamohypophyseal tract to the posterior pituitary gland, causing the stored ADH to be released into the circulation[12] (see Fig. 8.7).

ADH exerts its effects through two types of vasopressin (V) receptors—V_1 and V_2. V_1 receptors, which are located in vascular smooth muscle, cause vasoconstriction—hence the name *vasopressin*. Although ADH can increase blood pressure through V_1 receptors, this response occurs only when ADH levels are very high. The V_2 receptors, which are located on the tubular cells of the cortical collecting duct, control water reabsorption by the kidney. These renal mechanisms for water reabsorption are responsible for maintaining the osmolality of body fluids.[2]

Without ADH, the luminal membranes of the tubular epithelial cells of the collecting ducts are almost impermeable to water. In the presence of ADH, pores or water channels, called *aquaporins*, are stimulated to move into the membrane of these tubular cells, making them permeable to water. The specific water channel that is controlled by ADH is aquaporin-2.[2]

As with thirst, ADH levels are controlled by ECF volume and osmolality. Osmoreceptors in the hypothalamus are capable of detecting fluctuation in ECF osmolality and can stimulate the production and release of ADH. Likewise, stretch receptors that are sensitive to changes in blood pressure and the effective circulating volume aid in the regulation of ADH release (*i.e.*, nonosmotic ADH secretion). A blood volume decrease of 5% to 10% produces a maximal increase in ADH levels. As with many other homeostatic mechanisms, acute conditions produce greater changes in ADH levels than do chronic conditions.

The abnormal synthesis and release of ADH occurs in a number of stress situations. Severe pain, nausea, trauma, surgery, certain anesthetic agents, and some narcotics (*e.g.*, morphine and meperidine) increase ADH levels.[2] Among the drugs that affect ADH are nicotine, which stimulates its release, and alcohol, which inhibits it (Table 8.3). Two important conditions alter ADH levels: DI and inappropriate secretion of ADH.

TABLE 8.3 DRUGS THAT AFFECT ANTIDIURETIC HORMONE LEVELS*

DRUGS THAT DECREASE ADH LEVELS/ACTION	DRUGS THAT INCREASE ADH LEVELS/ACTION
Amphotericin B	Anticancer drugs (vincristine and cyclophosphamide)
Demeclocycline	Carbamazepine
Ethanol	Chlorpropamide
Foscarnet	Clofibrate
Lithium	General anesthetics (most)
Morphine antagonists	Narcotics (morphine and meperidine)
	Nicotine
	Nonsteroidal anti-inflammatory drugs
	Phenothiazine antipsychotic drugs
	Selective serotonin reuptake inhibitors
	Thiazide diuretics (chlorothiazide)
	Thiothixene (antipsychotic drug)
	Tricyclic antidepressants

*List not inclusive.
ADH, antidiuretic hormone.

Diabetes Insipidus. DI is caused by a deficiency of or a decreased response to ADH.[2] People with DI are unable to concentrate their urine during periods of water restriction, and they excrete large volumes of urine, usually 3 to 20 L/day, depending on the degree of ADH deficiency or renal insensitivity to ADH. This large urine output is accompanied by excessive thirst. As long as the thirst mechanism is normal and fluid is readily available, there is little or no alteration in the fluid levels of people with DI. The danger arises when the condition develops in someone who is unable to communicate the need for water or is unable to secure the needed water. In such cases, inadequate fluid intake rapidly leads to hypertonic dehydration and increased serum osmolality.

There are two types of DI: neurogenic or central DI, which occurs because of a defect in the synthesis or release of ADH, and nephrogenic DI, which occurs because the kidneys do not respond to ADH.[2] In neurogenic DI, loss of 80% to 90% of ADH-secreting neurons is necessary before polyuria becomes evident. Most people with neurogenic DI have an incomplete form of the disorder and retain some ability to concentrate their urine. Temporary neurogenic DI may follow head injury or surgery near the hypothalamohypophyseal tract. Nephrogenic DI is characterized by impairment of urine-concentrating ability and free-water conservation. It may be because of a genetic trait that affects the V_2 receptor that binds ADH or the aquaporin-2 protein that forms the water channels in the collecting tubules.[2] Other, acquired causes of nephrogenic DI are drugs such as lithium and electrolyte disorders such as potassium depletion or chronic hypercalcemia. Lithium and the electrolyte disorders are thought to interfere with the postreceptor actions of ADH on the permeability of the collecting ducts.

Diagnosis of DI usually starts by attempting to document the total 24-hour urine output. Also, it must be documented that an osmotic diuresis is not caused by glucose or such disorders as kidney disease. Further evaluation is based on measurement of ADH levels along with plasma and urine osmolality before and after a period of fluid deprivation or hypertonic saline infusion. Persons with neurogenic DI do not increase their ADH levels in response to increased plasma osmolality. Another diagnostic approach is to conduct a carefully monitored trial of a pharmacologic form of ADH. People with nephrogenic DI do not respond to pharmacologic preparations of the hormone. When central DI is suspected, diagnostic methods such as MRI studies of the pituitary–hypothalamic area are used to determine the cause of the disorder. MRI studies localize the normal posterior pituitary as a high-intensity signal on T1-weighted images. Research reports indicate the "bright spot" is related to the content of stored ADH. This high-intensity signal is present in most (but not all) normal subjects and is absent in most (but not all) people with DI.[13]

The management of central DI depends on the cause and severity of the disorder. Many people with incomplete neurogenic DI maintain near-normal water balance when permitted to ingest water in response to thirst. Pharmacologic preparations of ADH are available for people who cannot be managed by conservative measures. The preferred drug for treating chronic DI is desmopressin acetate (DDAVP). It usually is given orally, but is also available in parenteral and nasal forms. The oral antidiabetic agent chlorpropamide may be used to stimulate ADH release in partial neurogenic DI. It usually is reserved for special cases because of its ability to cause hypoglycemia. Both neurogenic and nephrogenic forms of DI respond partially to the thiazide diuretics (*e.g.*, hydrochlorothiazide). These diuretics are thought to act by increasing sodium excretion by the kidneys, leading to ECF volume contraction, a decrease in the glomerular filtration rate (along with filtered load of sodium), and an increase in sodium and water reabsorption. It also has been postulated that the thiazide diuretics increase water permeability in the collecting tubules.[13]

Syndrome of Inappropriate Antidiuretic Hormone. The syndrome of inappropriate ADH (SIADH) results from a failure of the negative feedback system that regulates the release and inhibition of ADH.[2] In people with this syndrome, ADH secretion continues even when serum osmolality is decreased, causing marked water retention and dilutional hyponatremia.

SIADH may occur as a transient condition, as in a stress situation, or, more commonly, as a chronic condition, resulting from disorders such as lung or brain tumors. Stimuli such as surgery, pain, stress, and temperature changes are capable of triggering ADH release through action of the CNS. Drugs induce SIADH in different ways. Some drugs are thought to increase hypothalamic production and release of ADH, and others are believed to act directly on the renal tubules to enhance the action of ADH. More chronic forms of SIADH may result from lung tumors, chest lesions, and CNS disorders. Tumors, particularly bronchogenic carcinomas and cancers of the lymphoid tissue, prostate, and pancreas, are known to produce and release ADH independent of normal hypothalamic control mechanisms. Other intrathoracic conditions, such as advanced tuberculosis, severe pneumonia, and positive-pressure breathing, also cause SIADH. The suggested mechanism for SIADH in positive-pressure ventilation is activation of baroreceptors (*e.g.*, aortic baroreceptors, cardiopulmonary receptors) that respond to marked changes in intrathoracic pressure. Disease and injury to the CNS can cause direct pressure on or direct involvement of the hypothalamic–posterior pituitary structures.[14] Examples include brain tumors, hydrocephalus, head injury, meningitis, and encephalitis. Human immunodeficiency virus (HIV) infection is an established cause of SIADH (*e.g.*, related to associated infections, tumors, drugs).

The manifestations of SIADH are those of dilutional hyponatremia. Urine osmolality is high and serum osmolality is low. Urine output decreases despite adequate or increased fluid intake. Hematocrit and the plasma sodium and BUN levels are all decreased because of the expansion of the ECF volume. The diagnosis of SIADH should be considered only if the five cardinal features are fulfilled: (1) hypotonic hyponatremia, (2) natriuresis (>20 mEq/L [20 mmol/L]), (3) urine osmolality in excess of plasma osmolality, (4) absence of edema and volume depletion, and (5) normal renal, thyroid, and adrenal function.[2]

The treatment of SIADH depends on its severity. In mild cases, treatment consists of fluid restriction. If fluid restriction is not sufficient, diuretics such as mannitol and furosemide (Lasix) may be given to promote diuresis and free-water clearance. Lithium and the antibiotic demeclocycline inhibit the action of ADH on the renal collecting ducts and sometimes are used in treating the disorder. In cases of severe water intoxication, a hypertonic (*e.g.*, 3%) NaCl solution may be administered intravenously. The recently developed antagonists to the antidiuretic action of ADH (aquaretics) offer a new therapeutic approach to the treatment of euvolemic hyponatremia.[15] These agents (*e.g.*, conivaptan) are specific ADH V_2 receptor antagonists and result in aquaresis (*i.e.*, the electrolyte-sparing excretion of free water).

Disorders of Sodium and Water Balance

Disorders of sodium and water balance can be divided into two main categories:

1. Isotonic contraction or expansion of ECF volume
2. Hypotonic dilution (hyponatremia) or hypertonic concentration (hypernatremia) of extracellular sodium brought about by changes in extracellular water (Fig. 8.6)

Isotonic disorders usually are confined to the ECF compartment, producing a contraction (fluid volume deficit) or expansion (fluid volume excess) of the interstitial and vascular fluids. Disorders of sodium concentration produce a change in the osmolality of the ECF, with movement of water from the ECF compartment into the ICF compartment (hyponatremia) or from the ICF compartment into the ECF compartment (hypernatremia).

Isotonic Fluid Volume Deficit

Fluid volume deficit is characterized by a decrease in the ECF, including the circulating blood volume. The term *isotonic fluid volume deficit* is used to differentiate the type of fluid deficit in which there are proportionate losses in sodium and water from water deficit and the hyperosmolar state associated with hypernatremia. Unless other fluid and electrolyte imbalances are present, the concentration of plasma electrolytes remains essentially unchanged. When the effective circulating blood volume is compromised, the condition is often referred to as *hypovolemia.*

Etiology. Isotonic fluid volume deficit results when water and electrolytes are lost in isotonic proportions (Table 8.4). It is almost always caused by a loss of body fluids and is often accompanied by a decrease in fluid intake. It can occur because of a loss of gastrointestinal fluids, polyuria, or sweating because of fever and exercise. Fluid intake may be reduced because of a lack of access to fluids, impaired thirst,

TABLE 8.4 CAUSES AND MANIFESTATIONS OF ISOTONIC FLUID VOLUME DEFICIT

CAUSES	MANIFESTATIONS
Inadequate Fluid Intake	**Acute Weight Loss (% Body Weight)**
Oral trauma or inability to swallow	Mild fluid volume deficit: 2%
Inability to obtain fluids (*e.g.*, impaired mobility)	Moderate fluid volume deficit: 2%–5%
Impaired thirst sensation	Severe fluid deficit: 8% or greater
Therapeutic withholding of fluids	**Compensatory Increase in Antidiuretic Hormone**
Unconsciousness or inability to express thirst	Decreased urine output
	Increased osmolality and specific gravity
Excessive Gastrointestinal Fluid Losses	**Increased Serum Osmolality**
Vomiting	Thirst
Diarrhea	Increased hematocrit and BUN
Gastrointestinal suction	**Decreased Vascular Volume**
Draining gastrointestinal fistula	Postural hypotension
Excessive Renal Losses	Tachycardia, weak and thready pulse
Diuretic therapy	Decreased vein filling and increased vein refill time
Osmotic diuresis (hyperglycemia)	Hypotension and shock
Adrenal insufficiency (Addison disease)	**Decreased ECF Volume**
Salt-wasting kidney disease	Depressed fontanel in an infant
Excessive Skin Losses	Sunken eyes and soft eyeballs
Fever	**Impaired Temperature Regulation**
Exposure to hot environment	Elevated body temperature
Burns and wounds that remove skin	
Third-Space Losses	
Intestinal obstruction	
Edema	
Ascites	
Burns (first several days)	

unconsciousness, oral trauma, impaired swallowing, or neuromuscular problems that prevent fluid access.

In a single day, 8 to 10 L of ECF is secreted into the gastrointestinal tract. Most of it is reabsorbed in the ileum and proximal colon, and only approximately 150 to 200 mL/day is eliminated in the feces. Vomiting and diarrhea interrupt the reabsorption process and, in some situations, lead to increased secretion of fluid into the intestinal tract. In Asiatic cholera, death can occur within a matter of hours as the cholera organism causes excessive amounts of fluid to be secreted into the bowel. These fluids are then lost as vomitus or excreted as diarrheal fluid. Gastrointestinal suction, fistulas, and drainage tubes can remove large amounts of fluid from the gastrointestinal tract.

Excess sodium and water losses also can occur through the kidney. Certain forms of kidney disease are characterized by salt wasting because of impaired sodium reabsorption. Fluid volume deficit also can result from osmotic diuresis or injudicious use of diuretic therapy. Glucose in the urine filtrate prevents reabsorption of water by the renal tubules, causing a loss of sodium and water. In Addison disease, a condition of chronic adrenocortical insufficiency, there is unregulated loss of sodium in the urine with a resultant loss of ECF. This is accompanied by increased potassium retention.

The skin acts as an exchange surface for heat and as a vapor barrier to prevent water from leaving the body. Body surface losses of sodium and water increase when there is excessive sweating or when large areas of skin have been damaged. Hot weather and fever increase sweating. In hot weather, water losses through sweating may be increased by as much as 1 to 3 L/hour, depending on acclimatization.[2] The respiratory rate and sweating usually are increased as body temperature rises. As much as 3 L of water may be lost in a single day as a result of fever. Burns are another cause of excess fluid loss. Evaporative losses can increase 10-fold with severe burns, up to 3 to 5 L/day.[2]

Third-space losses cause sequestering of ECF in the serous cavities, extracellular spaces in injured tissues, or lumen of the gut.[7] Because the fluid remains in the body, fluid volume deficit caused by third spacing does not usually cause weight loss.

Clinical Manifestations. The manifestations of fluid volume deficit reflect a decrease in ECF volume. They include thirst, loss of body weight, signs of water conservation by the kidney, impaired temperature regulation, and signs of reduced interstitial and vascular volume (see Table 8.4).

A loss in fluid volume is accompanied by a decrease in body weight. One liter of water weighs 1 kg (2.2 lb). A mild ECF deficit exists when weight loss equals 2% of body weight. In a person who weighs 68 kg (150 lb), this percentage of weight loss equals 1.4 L of water. To be accurate, weight must be measured at the same time each day with the person wearing the same amount of clothing. Because the ECF is trapped in the body in people with third-space losses, their body weight may not decrease.

Thirst is a common symptom of fluid deficit, although it is not always present in the early stages of isotonic fluid deficit. It develops as the effective circulatory volume decreases to a point sufficient to stimulate the thirst mechanism. Urine output decreases and urine osmolality and specific gravity increase as ADH levels rise because of a decrease in vascular volume. Although there is an isotonic loss of fluid from the vascular compartment, the other blood components such as red blood cells (RBCs) and BUN become more concentrated.

The fluid content of body tissues decreases as fluid is removed from the interstitial spaces. The eyes assume a sunken appearance and feel softer than normal as the fluid content in the anterior chamber of the eye is decreased. Fluids add resiliency to the skin and underlying tissues that is referred to as *skin* or *tissue turgor*. Tissue turgor is assessed by pinching a fold of skin between the thumb and forefinger. The skin should immediately return to its original configuration when the fingers are released.[16] If 3% to 5% of body water is lost in children, there is fairly normal turgor, whereas with 6%to 9% loss of body water, there is poor turgor and a sunken anterior fontanel.[8] Decreased tissue turgor is less predictive of fluid deficit in older persons (>65 years) because of the loss of tissue elasticity. In infants, fluid deficit may be evidenced by depression of the anterior fontanel because of a decrease in CSF.

Arterial and venous volumes decline during periods of fluid deficit, as does filling of the capillary circulation. As the volume in the arterial system declines, the blood pressure decreases, the heart rate increases, and the pulse becomes weak and thready. Postural hypotension (a drop in blood pressure on standing) is an early sign of fluid deficit. On the venous side of the circulation, the veins become less prominent. When volume depletion becomes severe, signs of hypovolemic shock and vascular collapse appear.

Diagnosis and Treatment. Diagnosis of fluid volume deficit is based on a history of conditions that predispose to sodium and water losses, weight loss, and observations of altered physiologic function indicative of decreased fluid volume. Intake and output measurements afford a means for assessing fluid balance. However, these measurements may not represent actual losses and gains, largely because accurate measurements of intake and output often are difficult to obtain and insensible losses are difficult to estimate.

Measurement of heart rate and blood pressure provides useful information about vascular volume. A simple test to determine venous refill time consists of compressing the distal end of a vein on the dorsal aspect of the hand when it is not in the dependent position. The vein is then emptied by "milking" the blood toward the heart. The vein should refill almost immediately when the occluding finger is removed. In the case of decreased venous volume, as occurs in fluid deficit, venous refill time increases. Capillary refill time is also increased. Capillary refill can be assessed by applying pressure to a fingernail for 5 seconds and then releasing the pressure and observing the time (normally 1 to 2 seconds) it takes for the color to return to normal.[17]

Treatment of fluid volume deficit consists of fluid replacement and measures to correct the underlying cause. Usually, isotonic electrolyte solutions are used for fluid replacement. Acute hypovolemia and hypovolemic shock can cause renal damage. Therefore, prompt assessment of the degree of fluid deficit and adequate measures to resolve the deficit and treat the underlying cause are essential.

Isotonic Fluid Volume Excess

Fluid volume excess represents an isotonic expansion of the ECF compartment with increases in both interstitial and vascular volumes. Although increased fluid volume is usually the result of a disease condition, this is not always true. For example, a compensatory isotonic expansion of body fluids can occur in healthy people during hot weather as a mechanism for increasing body heat loss.

Etiology. Isotonic fluid volume excess almost always results from an increase in total body sodium that is accompanied by a proportionate increase in body water. Although it can occur as the result of excessive sodium intake, it is most commonly caused by a decrease in sodium and water elimination by the kidney.

Among the causes of decreased sodium and water elimination are disorders of renal function, heart failure, liver failure, and corticosteroid excess (Table 8.5). Heart failure produces a decrease in the effective circulating volume and renal blood flow and a compensatory increase in sodium and water retention. People with severe congestive heart failure maintain a precarious balance between sodium and water intake and output. Even small increases in sodium intake can precipitate a state of fluid volume excess and a worsening of heart failure. A condition called *circulatory overload* results from an increase in blood volume; it can occur during infusion of intravenous fluids or transfusion of blood if the amount or rate of administration is excessive. Liver failure (*e.g.*, cirrhosis of the liver) impairs aldosterone metabolism and decreases effective circulating volume and renal perfusion, leading to increased salt and water retention. The corticosteroid hormones increase sodium reabsorption by the kidneys. People taking corticosteroid medications and those with Cushing disease often have problems with sodium retention.

Clinical Manifestations. Isotonic fluid volume excess is manifested by an increase in interstitial and vascular fluids. It is characterized by weight gain over a short period of time. Mild fluid volume excess represents a 2% gain in weight; moderate

TABLE 8.5 CAUSES AND MANIFESTATIONS OF ISOTONIC FLUID VOLUME EXCESS

CAUSES	MANIFESTATIONS
Inadequate Sodium and Water Elimination	**Acute Weight Gain (% Body Weight)**
Congestive heart failure	Mild fluid volume excess: 2%
Renal failure	Moderate fluid volume excess: 5%
Increased corticosteroid levels	Severe fluid volume excess: 8% or greater
Hyperaldosteronism	
Cushing disease	**Increased Interstitial Fluid Volume**
Liver failure (*e.g.*, cirrhosis)	Dependent and generalized edema
Excessive Sodium Intake in Relation to Output	**Increased Vascular Volume**
Excessive dietary intake	Full and bounding pulse
Excessive ingestion of sodium-containing medications or home remedies	Venous distention
Excessive administration of sodium-containing parenteral fluids	Pulmonary edema
	Shortness of breath
	Crackles
	Dyspnea
Excessive Fluid Intake in Relation to Output	Cough
Ingestion of fluid in excess of elimination	
Administration of parenteral fluids or blood at an excessive rate	

fluid volume excess, a 5% gain in weight; and severe fluid volume excess, a gain of 8% or more in weight[8] (see Table 8.5). The presence of edema is characteristic of isotonic fluid excess. When the excess fluid accumulates gradually, as often happens in debilitating diseases and starvation, edema fluid may mask the loss of tissue mass. There may be a decrease in BUN and hematocrit as a result of dilution because of expansion of the plasma volume. An increase in vascular volume may be evidenced by distended neck veins, slow-emptying peripheral veins, a full and bounding pulse, and an increase in central venous pressure. When excess fluid accumulates in the lungs (*i.e.*, pulmonary edema), there are complaints of shortness of breath and difficult breathing, respiratory crackles, and a productive cough. Ascites and pleural effusion may occur with severe fluid volume excess.

Diagnosis and Treatment. Diagnosis of fluid volume excess is usually based on a history of factors that predispose to sodium and water retention, weight gain, and manifestations such as edema and cardiovascular symptoms indicative of an expanded ECF volume.

The treatment of fluid volume excess focuses on providing a more favorable balance between sodium and water intake and output. A sodium-restricted diet is often prescribed as a means of decreasing extracellular sodium and water levels. Diuretic therapy is commonly used to increase sodium elimination. When there is a need for intravenous fluid administration or transfusion of blood components, the procedure requires careful monitoring to prevent fluid overload.

Hyponatremia

The normal plasma concentration of sodium ranges from 135 to 145 mEq/L (135 to 145 mmol/L). Plasma sodium values reflect the sodium concentration expressed in milliequivalents or millimoles per liter, rather than an absolute amount. Because sodium and its attendant anions account for 90% to 95% of the osmolality of ECF, serum osmolality (normal range, 275 to 295 mOsm/kg) usually changes with changes in plasma sodium concentration.

Hyponatremia represents a plasma sodium concentration below 135 mEq/L (135 mmol/L). It is one of the most common electrolyte disorders seen in general hospital patients and is also common in the outpatient population, particularly in older adults. A number of age-related events make the older adult population more vulnerable to hyponatremia, including a decrease in renal function accompanied by limitations in sodium conservation. Although older people maintain body fluid homeostasis under most circumstances, the ability to withstand environmental, drug-related, and disease-associated stresses becomes progressively limited.

Types and Etiology. Because of the effects of osmotically active particles such as glucose, hyponatremia can present as a hypotonic or hypertonic state.[2] *Hypertonic (translocational) hyponatremia* results from an osmotic shift of water from the ICF to the ECF compartment, such as that occurring in hyperglycemia (the correction for hyperglycemia is a 1.6-mEq/L [1.6 mmol/L] increase in plasma sodium for every 100 mg/dL rise in plasma glucose above the normal 100 mg/dL [5.5 mmol/L]). In this case, the sodium in the ECF becomes diluted as water moves out of cells in response to the osmotic effects of the elevated blood glucose level. *Hypotonic (dilutional) hyponatremia*, by far the most common type of hyponatremia, is caused by water retention. It can be classified as hypovolemic, euvolemic, or hypervolemic based on accompanying ECF fluid volumes.[2,12] Because of its effect on both sodium and water elimination, diuretic therapy can cause either hypovolemic or euvolemic hyponatremia.

Hypovolemic hypotonic hyponatremia occurs when water is lost along with sodium resulting in low plasma level, but to a lesser extent.[18] Among the causes of hypovolemic hyponatremia are excessive sweating in hot weather, particularly during heavy exercise, which leads to loss of salt and water. Hyponatremia develops when water, rather than electrolyte-containing liquids, is used to replace fluids lost in sweating. Another potential cause of hypovolemic hyponatremia is the loss of sodium from the gastrointestinal tract caused by frequent gastrointestinal irrigations with distilled water. Isotonic fluid loss, such as that occurring in vomiting or diarrhea, does not usually lower plasma sodium levels unless these losses are replaced with disproportionate amounts of orally ingested or parenterally administered water. Gastrointestinal fluid loss and ingestion of excessively diluted formula are common causes of acute hyponatremia in infants and children. Hypovolemic hyponatremia is also a common complication of adrenal insufficiency and is attributable to a decrease in aldosterone levels. A lack of aldosterone increases renal losses of sodium, and a cortisol deficiency leads to increased release of ADH with water retention.

Euvolemic or *normovolemic hypotonic hyponatremia* represents retention of water with dilution of sodium while maintaining the ECF volume within a normal range. It is the most common, accounting for up to 60% of all hyponatremia cases, and is usually a result of SIADH.[18] The risk of normovolemic hyponatremia is increased during the postoperative period. During this time ADH levels are often high, producing an increase in water reabsorption by the kidney. Although these elevated levels usually resolve in about 72 hours, they can persist for as long as 5 days. The hyponatremia becomes exaggerated when electrolyte-free fluids (*e.g.*, 5% glucose in water) are used for fluid replacement.

Hypervolemic hypotonic hyponatremia is seen when hyponatremia is accompanied by edema-associated disorders such as decompensated heart failure, advanced liver disease, and renal disease. Although the total body sodium is increased in heart failure, the effective circulating volume is often sensed as inadequate by the baroreceptors (*i.e.*, relative arterial underfilling), resulting in increased ADH levels (nonosmotic ADH secretion).[18]

Abuse of the drug, methylenedioxymethamphetamine (MDMA), also known as "ecstasy," can lead to severe neurologic symptoms, including seizures, brain edema, and herniation because of severe hyponatremia.

Clinical Manifestations. The manifestations of hypotonic hyponatremia are largely related to sodium dilution (Table 8.6). Serum osmolality is decreased, and cellular swelling occurs owing to the movement of water from the ECF to the ICF compartment. The manifestations of hyponatremia depend on the rapidity of onset and the severity of the sodium dilution. The signs and symptoms may be acute (*i.e.*, onset within 48 hours), as in severe water intoxication, or more insidious in onset and less severe, as in chronic hyponatremia. Because of water movement, hyponatremia produces an increase in intracellular water, which is responsible for many of the clinical manifestations of the disorder. Fingerprint edema is a sign of excess intracellular water. This phenomenon is demonstrated by pressing the finger firmly over the bony surface of the sternum for 15 to 30 seconds. Fingerprint edema exists if an indented fingerprint remains in the sternum where the pressure was applied.

Muscle cramps, weakness, and fatigue reflect the effects of hyponatremia on skeletal muscle function and are often early signs of hyponatremia. These effects commonly are observed in persons with hyponatremia that occurs during heavy exercise in hot weather. Gastrointestinal manifestations such as nausea and vomiting, abdominal cramps, and diarrhea may develop.

Concept Mastery Alert

The cells of the brain and nervous system are the most seriously affected by increases in intracellular water. Symptoms include apathy, lethargy, and headache, which can progress to disorientation, confusion, gross motor weakness, and depression of deep tendon reflexes.

Seizures and coma occur when plasma sodium levels reach extremely low levels. These severe effects, which are caused by brain swelling, may be irreversible. If the condition develops slowly, signs and symptoms do not develop until plasma sodium levels approach 120 mEq/L (120 mmol/L) (*i.e.*, severe hyponatremia).[2] The term *water intoxication* is often used to describe the neurologic effects of acute hypotonic hyponatremia.

Diagnosis and Treatment. Diagnosis of hyponatremia is based on laboratory reports of a decreased plasma sodium concentration, plasma and urine osmolality, and urine sodium concentration; assessment of the person's volume status; presence of conditions that predispose to sodium loss or water retention; and signs and symptoms indicative of the disorder.

The treatment of hyponatremia with water excess focuses on the underlying cause. When hyponatremia is caused by water intoxication, limiting water intake or discontinuing medications that contribute to SIADH may be sufficient. The administration of a saline solution orally or intravenously may be needed when hyponatremia is caused by sodium deficiency. Symptomatic hyponatremia (*i.e.*, neurologic manifestations) is often treated with hypertonic saline solution and a loop diuretic, such as furosemide, to increase water elimination. This combination allows for correction of plasma sodium levels while ridding the body of excess water. New, specific ADH V_2 receptor antagonists to the antidiuretic action of ADH (aquaretics) offer a new therapeutic approach to the treatment of euvolemic hyponatremia.[16]

There is concern about the rapidity with which plasma sodium levels are corrected, particularly in people with chronic

TABLE 8.6 CAUSES AND MANIFESTATIONS OF HYPONATREMIA

CAUSES	MANIFESTATIONS
Hypotonic Hyponatremia	**Laboratory Values**
Hypovolemic (Decreased Serum Sodium with Decreased ECF Volume)	Serum sodium levels below 135 mEq/L (135 mmol/L)
Use of excessively diluted infant formula	Hypotonic hyponatremia
Administration of sodium-free parenteral solutions	Serum osmolality 280 mOsm/kg
Gastrointestinal losses	Dilution of blood components, including hematocrit, BUN
Vomiting, diarrhea	Hypertonic hyponatremia
Sweating, with sodium-free fluid replacement	Serum osmolality > 280 mOsm/kg
Repeated irrigation of body cavities with sodium-free solutions	**Signs Related to Hypo-Osmolality of ECFs and Movement of Water into Brain Cells and Neuromuscular Tissue**
Irrigation of gastrointestinal tubes with distilled water	Muscle cramps
Tap water enemas	Weakness
Use of nonelectrolyte irrigating solutions during prostate surgery	Headache
Third spacing (paralytic ileus, pancreatitis)	Depression
Diuretic use	Apprehension, feeling of impending doom
Mineralocorticoid deficiency (Addison disease)	Personality changes
Salt-wasting nephritis	Lethargy
Euvolemic (Decreased Serum Sodium with Normal ECF Volume)	Stupor, coma
Increased ADH levels	**Gastrointestinal Manifestations**
Trauma, stress, pain	Anorexia, nausea, vomiting
SIADH	Abdominal cramps, diarrhea
Use of medications that increase ADH	**Increased ICF**
Diuretic use	Fingerprint edema
Glucocorticoid deficiency	
Hypothyroidism	
Psychogenic polydipsia	
Endurance exercise	
MDMA ("ecstasy") abuse	
Hypervolemic (Decreased Serum Sodium with Increased ECF Volume)	
Decompensated heart failure	
Advanced liver disease	
Kidney failure without nephrosis	
Hypertonic Hyponatremia (Osmotic Shift of Water from the ICF to the ECF Compartment)	Manifestations largely related to hyperosmolality of ECFs
Hyperglycemia	

symptomatic hyponatremia. Cells, particularly those in the brain, tend to defend against changes in cell volume caused by changes in ECF osmolality by increasing or decreasing their concentration of organic osmolytes.[16] In the case of prolonged water intoxication, brain cells reduce their concentration of osmolytes as a means of preventing an increase in cell volume. It takes several days for brain cells to restore the osmolytes lost during hyponatremia. Thus, treatment measures that produce rapid changes in serum osmolality may cause a dramatic change in brain cell volume. One of the reported effects of rapid treatment of hyponatremia is an osmotic demyelinating condition called *central pontine myelinolysis*, which produces serious neurologic sequelae and sometimes causes death.[16] This complication occurs more commonly in premenopausal women and in people with hypoxia.

Hypernatremia

Hypernatremia implies a plasma sodium level above 145 mEq/L (145 mmol/L) and a serum osmolality greater than 295 mOsm/kg. Because sodium is functionally an impermeable solute, it contributes to tonicity and induces movement of water across cell membranes. Hypernatremia is characterized by hypertonicity of ECF and almost always causes cellular dehydration.[2]

Etiology. Hypernatremia represents a deficit of water in relation to the body's sodium stores. It can be caused by net loss of water or sodium gain. Net water loss can occur through the urine, gastrointestinal tract, lungs, or skin. A defect in thirst or inability to obtain or drink water can interfere with water replacement. Rapid ingestion or infusion of sodium with insufficient time or opportunity for water ingestion can produce a disproportionate gain in sodium (Table 8.7). This can occur with critically ill people who present with multiple needs for fluid resuscitation and electrolyte balance. In fact hypernatremia is an independent risk factor linked highly with increased mortality.[18]

Hypernatremia almost always follows a loss of body fluids that have a lower-than-normal concentration of sodium, so that water is lost in excess of sodium. This can result from increased losses from the respiratory tract during fever or strenuous exercise, from watery diarrhea, or when osmotically active tube feedings are given with inadequate amounts of water. With pure water loss, each body fluid compartment loses an equal percentage of its volume. Because approximately one third of the water is in the ECF compartment, compared with the two thirds in the ICF compartment, more actual water volume is lost from the ICF than the ECF compartment.[2]

Normally, water deficit stimulates thirst and increases water intake. Therefore, hypernatremia is more likely to occur in infants and in people who cannot express their thirst or obtain water to drink. With hypodipsia, or impaired thirst, the need for fluid intake does not activate the thirst response. Hypodipsia is particularly prevalent among older adults. In people with DI, hypernatremia can develop when thirst is impaired or access to water is impeded.

The therapeutic administration of sodium-containing solutions may also cause hypernatremia. Hypertonic saline solution intended for intra-amniotic instillation for therapeutic abortion may inadvertently be injected intravenously, causing hypernatremia. Rarely, salt intake occurs rapidly, as in taking excess salt tablets or during near-drowning in salt water.

Clinical Manifestations. The clinical manifestations of hypernatremia caused by water loss are largely those of ECF loss and cellular dehydration (see Table 8.7). The severity of signs and symptoms is greatest when the increase in plasma sodium is large and occurs rapidly. Body weight is decreased in proportion to the amount of water that has been lost. Because blood plasma is roughly 90% to 93% water, the concentrations of blood cells and other blood components increase as ECF water decreases.

TABLE 8.7 CAUSES AND MANIFESTATIONS OF HYPERNATREMIA

CAUSES	MANIFESTATIONS
Excessive Water Losses Watery diarrhea Excessive sweating Increased respirations because of conditions such as tracheobronchitis Hypertonic tube feedings Diabetes insipidus	**Laboratory Values** Serum sodium level above 145 mEq/L (145 mmol/L) Increased serum osmolality Increased hematocrit and BUN
Decreased Water Intake Unavailability of water Oral trauma or inability to swallow Impaired thirst sensation Withholding water for therapeutic reasons Unconsciousness or inability to express thirst	**Thirst and Signs of Increased ADH Levels** Polydipsia Oliguria or anuria High urine specific gravity **Intracellular Dehydration** Dry skin and mucous membranes Decreased tissue turgor Tongue rough and fissured Decreased salivation and lacrimation
Excessive Sodium Intake Rapid or excessive administration of sodium-containing parenteral solutions Near-drowning in salt water	**Signs Related to Hyperosmolality of ECFs and Movement of Water Out of Brain Cells** Headache Agitation and restlessness Decreased reflexes Seizures and coma **Extracellular Dehydration and Decreased Vascular Volume** Tachycardia Weak and thready pulse Decreased blood pressure Vascular collapse

Thirst is an early symptom of water deficit, occurring when water losses are equal to 0.5% of body water. Urine output is decreased and urine osmolality increased because of renal water-conserving mechanisms. Body temperature frequently is elevated, and the skin becomes warm and flushed. The vascular volume decreases, the pulse becomes rapid and thready, and the blood pressure drops. Hypernatremia produces an increase in serum osmolality and results in water being pulled out of body cells. As a result, the skin and mucous membranes become dry, and salivation and lacrimation are decreased. The mouth becomes dry and sticky, and the tongue becomes rough and fissured. Swallowing is difficult. The subcutaneous tissues assume a firm, rubbery texture. Most significantly, water is pulled out of the cells in the CNS, causing decreased reflexes, agitation, headache, and restlessness. Coma and seizures may develop as hypernatremia progresses.

Diagnosis and Treatment. The diagnosis of hypernatremia is based on history, physical examination findings indicative of dehydration, and results of laboratory tests. The treatment of hypernatremia includes measures to treat the underlying cause of the disorder and fluid replacement therapy to treat the accompanying dehydration. Replacement fluids can be given orally or intravenously. The oral route is preferable. Oral glucose–electrolyte replacement solutions are available for the treatment of infants with diarrhea.[19] Until recently, these solutions were used only early in diarrheal illness or as a first step in reestablishing oral intake after parenteral replacement therapy. These solutions are now widely available in grocery stores and pharmacies for use in the treatment of diarrhea and other dehydrating disorders in infants and young children.

One of the serious aspects of fluid volume deficit is dehydration of brain and nerve cells. Serum osmolality should be corrected slowly in cases of chronic hypernatremia. If hypernatremia is corrected too rapidly before the osmolytes have had a chance to dissipate, the plasma may become relatively hypotonic in relation to brain cell osmolality. When this occurs, water moves into the brain cells, causing cerebral edema and potentially severe neurologic impairment.

IN SUMMARY

Body fluids are distributed between the ICF and ECF compartments. Regulation of fluid volume, solute concentration, and distribution between the two compartments depends on water and sodium balance. Water provides approximately 90% to 93% of fluid volume, and sodium salts approximately 90% to 95% of extracellular solutes. Both water and sodium are absorbed from the gastrointestinal tract and eliminated by the kidneys. The main regulator of sodium and water is the maintenance of the effective circulating blood volume, which is monitored by stretch receptors in the vascular system, which exert their effects through ADH and the sympathetic nervous system, and those in the kidney, which exert their effects through the sympathetic nervous system and the RAAS. Body water and serum osmolality are also regulated by thirst, which controls water intake, and ADH, which controls urine concentration and renal output.

Isotonic fluid disorders result from contraction or expansion of ECF volume brought about by proportionate losses of sodium and water. *Isotonic fluid volume deficit* is characterized by a decrease in ECF volume. It causes thirst, decreased vascular volume and circulatory function, decreased urine output, and increased urine specific gravity. *Isotonic fluid volume excess* is characterized by an increase in ECF volume. It is manifested by signs of increased vascular volume and edema.

Alterations in extracellular sodium concentration are brought about by a disproportionate gain (hyponatremia) or loss (hypernatremia) of water. As the major cation in the ECF compartment, sodium controls the ECF osmolality and its effect on cell volume. Hyponatremia can present as a *hypertonic (translocational) hyponatremia* in which water moves out of the cell in response to elevated blood glucose levels or as a *hypotonic (dilutional) hyponatremia* that is caused by retention of water by the body in excess of sodium. Hypotonic hyponatremia, which can present as a hypovolemic, euvolemic, or hypervolemic state, is characterized by water being pulled into the cell from the ECF compartment, causing cells to swell. It is manifested by muscle cramps and weakness; nausea, vomiting, abdominal cramps, and diarrhea; and CNS signs such as headache, lethargy, depression of deep tendon reflexes, and in severe cases seizure and coma.

Hypernatremia represents a disproportionate loss of body water in relation to sodium. It is characterized by intracellular water being pulled into the ECF compartment, causing cells to shrink. It is manifested by thirst and decreased urine output; dry mouth and decreased tissue turgor; signs of decreased vascular volume (tachycardia, weak and thready pulse); and CNS signs, such as decreased reflexes, agitation, headache, and in severe cases seizures and coma.

POTASSIUM BALANCE

After completing this section of the chapter, the learner will be able to meet the following objectives:

- Characterize the distribution of potassium in the body and explain how extracellular potassium levels are regulated in relation to body gains and losses.
- Relate the functions of potassium to the manifestations of hypokalemia and hyperkalemia.

Regulation of Potassium Balance

Potassium is the second most abundant cation in the body and the major cation in the ICF compartment. Approximately 98% of body potassium is contained within body cells, with an intracellular concentration of 140 to 150 mEq/L (140 to 150 mmol/L).[2] The potassium content of the ECF (3.5 to 5 mEq/L [3.5 to 5 mmol/L]) is considerably lower. Because potassium is an intracellular ion, total body stores of potassium are related to body size and muscle mass. In adults, total body potassium is approximately 50 mEq/kg of body weight.[2]

Gains and Losses

Potassium intake is normally derived from dietary sources. In healthy people, potassium balance usually can be maintained by a daily dietary intake of 50 to 100 mEq. Additional amounts of potassium are needed during periods of trauma and stress. The kidneys are the main source of potassium loss. Approximately 90% to 95% of potassium losses occur in the urine, with the remainder being lost in stools or sweat.[2]

Mechanisms of Regulation

Normally, the ECF concentration of potassium is precisely regulated at about 4.2 mEq/L (4.2 mmol/L). The precise control is necessary because many cell functions are sensitive to even small changes in ECF potassium levels. An increase in potassium of as small an amount as 0.3 to 0.4 mEq/L (0.3 to 0.4 mmol/L) can cause serious cardiac dysrhythmias and even death. A single meal may contain as much as 50 mEq, which means the daily intake can be as high as 200 mEq/L. Therefore, it is important for the kidneys to rapidly remove this extracellular potassium to avoid serious complications.[2]

Plasma potassium is largely regulated through two mechanisms: (1) renal mechanisms that conserve or eliminate potassium and (2) a transcellular shift between the ICF and ECF compartments.

Renal Regulation. The major route for potassium elimination is the kidney. Unlike other electrolytes, the regulation of potassium elimination is controlled by secretion from the blood into the tubular filtrate rather than through reabsorption from the tubular filtrate into the blood. Potassium is filtered in the glomerulus, reabsorbed along with sodium and water in the proximal tubule and with sodium and chloride in the thick ascending loop of Henle, and then secreted into the late distal and cortical collecting tubules for elimination in the urine. The latter mechanism serves to "fine-tune" the concentration of potassium in the ECF.

Aldosterone plays an essential role in regulating potassium elimination by the kidney. The effects of aldosterone on potassium elimination are mediated through an Na^+/K^+ exchange mechanism located in the late distal and cortical collecting tubules of the kidney. In the presence of aldosterone, Na^+ is transported back into the blood and K^+ is secreted in the tubular filtrate for elimination in the urine. The rate of aldosterone secretion by the adrenal gland is strongly controlled by plasma potassium levels. For example, an increase of less than 1 mEq/L (1 mmol/L) of potassium causes aldosterone levels to triple.[2] The effect of plasma potassium on aldosterone secretion is an example of the powerful feedback regulation of potassium elimination. In the absence of aldosterone, as occurs in people with Addison disease, renal elimination of potassium is impaired, causing plasma potassium levels to rise to dangerously high levels. Aldosterone is often referred to as a *mineralocorticoid hormone* because of its effect on sodium and potassium. The term *mineralocorticoid activity* is used to describe the aldosterone-like actions of other adrenocortical hormones, such as cortisol.

There is also a K^+/H^+ exchange mechanism in the cortical collecting tubules of the kidney. When plasma potassium levels are increased, K^+ is secreted into the urine and H^+ is reabsorbed into the blood, producing a decrease in pH and metabolic acidosis. Conversely, when potassium levels are low, K^+ is reabsorbed and H^+ is secreted in the urine, leading to metabolic alkalosis.

Extracellular–Intracellular Shifts. To avoid an increase in extracellular potassium levels, excess potassium is temporarily shifted into RBCs and other cells such as those of muscle, liver, and bone. This movement is controlled by the function of the Na^+/K^+-ATPase membrane pump and the permeability of the ion channels in the cell membrane.

Among the factors that alter the intracellular–extracellular distribution of potassium are serum osmolality, acid–base disorders, insulin, and β-adrenergic stimulation. Acute increases in serum osmolality cause water to leave the cell. The loss of cell water produces an increase in intracellular potassium, causing it to move out of the cell into the ECF.

The H^+ and K^+ ions, which are positively charged, can be exchanged between the ICF and ECF in a cation shift (Fig. 8.8). In metabolic acidosis, for example, H^+ moves into body cells for buffering, causing K^+ to leave and move into the ECF.[8] Both insulin and the catecholamines (*e.g.*, epinephrine) increase cellular uptake of K^+ by increasing the activity of the Na^+/K^+-ATPase membrane pump.[1] Insulin produces an increase in cellular uptake of potassium after a meal.

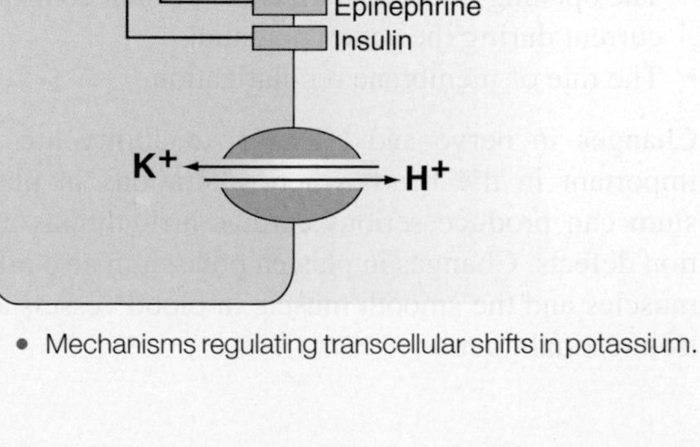

Figure 8.8 • Mechanisms regulating transcellular shifts in potassium.

The catecholamines, particularly epinephrine, facilitate the movement of potassium into muscle tissue during periods of physiologic stress. β-Adrenergic agonist drugs, such as pseudoephedrine and albuterol, have a similar effect on potassium distribution.

Exercise also produces compartmental shifts in potassium. Repeated muscle contraction releases potassium into the ECF. Although the increase usually is small with modest exercise, it can be considerable during exhaustive exercise. Even the repeated clenching and unclenching of the fist during a blood draw can cause potassium to move out of cells and artificially elevate plasma potassium levels.

KEY POINTS

POTASSIUM BALANCE

- Potassium is mainly an intracellular ion with only a small, but vital, amount being present in the ECFs.
- The distribution of potassium between the intracellular and extracellular compartments regulates electrical membrane potentials controlling the excitability of nerve and muscle cells as well as contractility of skeletal, cardiac, and smooth muscle tissue.
- Two major mechanisms function in the control of serum potassium: (1) renal mechanisms that conserve or eliminate potassium and (2) transcellular buffer systems that remove potassium from and release it into the serum as needed. Conditions that disrupt the function of either mechanisms can result in a serious alteration in serum potassium levels.

Disorders of Potassium Balance

As the major intracellular cation, potassium is critical to many body functions. It is involved in a wide range of body functions, including the maintenance of the osmotic integrity of cells, acid–base balance, and the kidney's ability to concentrate urine. Potassium is necessary for growth and it contributes to the intricate chemical reactions that transform carbohydrates into energy, change glucose into glycogen, and convert amino acids to proteins. Potassium also plays a critical role in conducting nerve impulses and the excitability of skeletal, cardiac, and smooth muscle. It does this by regulating the following:

- The resting membrane potential
- The opening of the sodium channels that control the flow of current during the action potential
- The rate of membrane repolarization

Changes in nerve and muscle excitability are particularly important in the heart, where alterations in plasma potassium can produce serious cardiac arrhythmias and conduction defects. Changes in plasma potassium also affect skeletal muscles and the smooth muscle in blood vessels and the gastrointestinal tract.

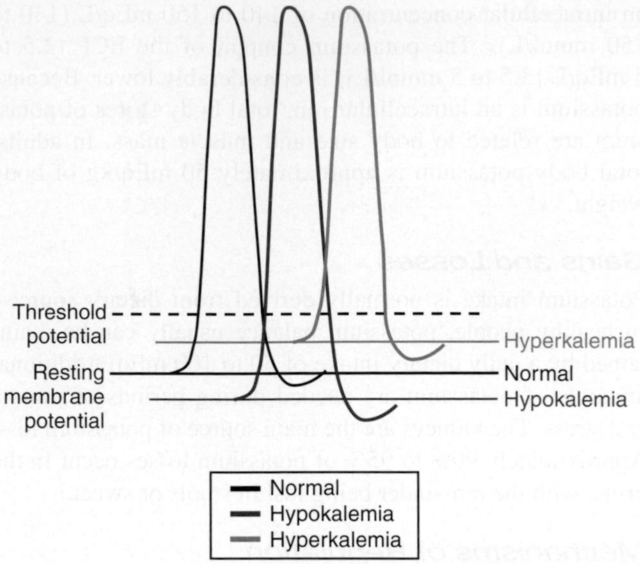

Figure 8.9 • Effect of changes in plasma hypokalemia (*red*) and hyperkalemia (*blue*) on the resting membrane potential, activation and opening of the sodium channels at threshold potential, and the rate of repolarization during a nerve action potential.

The *resting membrane potential* is determined by the ratio of ICF to ECF potassium concentration (Fig. 8.9). A decrease in plasma potassium causes the resting membrane potential to become more negative, moving it further from the threshold for excitation. Thus, it takes a greater stimulus to reach threshold and open the sodium channels that are responsible for the action potential. An increase in plasma potassium has the opposite effect; it causes the resting membrane potential to become more positive, moving it closer to threshold. With severe hyperkalemia, there may be prolonged depolarization that can decrease excitability. The *rate of repolarization* varies with plasma potassium levels. It is more rapid in hyperkalemia and delayed in hypokalemia. Both the inactivation of the sodium channels and the rate of membrane repolarization are important clinically because they predispose to cardiac arrhythmias or conduction defects. Hyperkalemia is one of the most life-threatening electrolyte disturbances especially with children.[20]

Hypokalemia

Hypokalemia refers to a decrease in plasma potassium levels below 3.5 mEq/L (3.5 mmol/L). Because of transcellular shifts, temporary changes in plasma potassium may occur as the result of movement between the ICF and ECF compartments.

Etiology. The causes of potassium deficit can be grouped into three categories: (1) inadequate intake; (2) excessive gastrointestinal, renal, and skin losses; and (3) redistribution between the ICF and ECF compartments (Table 8.8).[2]

Inadequate Intake. Inadequate intake is a frequent cause of hypokalemia. A potassium intake of at least 40 to 50 mEq/day is needed daily. Insufficient dietary intake may

TABLE 8.8 CAUSES AND MANIFESTATIONS OF HYPOKALEMIA

CAUSES	MANIFESTATIONS
Inadequate Intake	**Laboratory Values**
Diet deficient in potassium	Serum potassium level below 3.5 mEq/L (3.5 mmol/L)
Inability to eat	**Impaired Ability to Concentrate Urine**
Administration of potassium-free parenteral solutions	Polyuria
Excessive Renal Losses	Urine with low osmolality and specific gravity
Diuretic therapy (except potassium- sparing diuretics)	Polydipsia
Diuretic phase of renal failure	**Gastrointestinal Manifestations**
Increased mineralocorticoid levels	Anorexia, nausea, vomiting
Primary hyperaldosteronism	Constipation
Treatment with corticosteroid drugs	Abdominal distention
Excessive Gastrointestinal Losses	Paralytic ileus
Vomiting	**Neuromuscular Manifestations**
Diarrhea	Muscle flabbiness, weakness, and fatigue
Gastrointestinal suction	Muscle cramps and tenderness
Draining gastrointestinal fistula	Paresthesias
Transcompartmental Shift	Paralysis
Administration of β-adrenergic agonist (*e.g.*, albuterol)	**Cardiovascular Manifestations**
Administration of insulin for treatment of diabetic ketoacidosis	Postural hypotension
Alkalosis, metabolic or respiratory	Increased sensitivity to digitalis toxicity
	Changes in electrocardiogram
	Cardiac dysrhythmias
	CNS Manifestations
	Confusion
	Depression
	Acid–Base Disorders
	Metabolic alkalosis

result from the inability to obtain or ingest food or from a diet that is low in potassium-containing foods. Potassium intake is often inadequate in persons on fad diets and those who have eating disorders. Older adults are particularly likely to have potassium deficits. Many have poor eating habits as a consequence of living alone; they may have limited income, which makes buying foods high in potassium difficult; they may have difficulty chewing many foods that have high potassium content because of dental problems; or they may have problems with swallowing.

Excessive Losses. The kidneys are the main source of potassium loss. Approximately 80% to 90% of potassium losses occur in the urine, with the remaining losses occurring in the stool and sweat. The kidneys do not have the homeostatic mechanisms needed to conserve potassium during periods of insufficient intake. After trauma and in stress situations, urinary losses of potassium are generally increased and can cause a serious hypokalemia.[2] This means that a potassium deficit can develop rather quickly if intake is inadequate. Renal losses also can be increased by medications such as thiazides, metabolic alkalosis, magnesium depletion, and increased levels of aldosterone. Some antibiotics, particularly amphotericin B and gentamicin, are impermeable anions that require the presence of positively charged cations for elimination in the urine; this causes potassium wasting.

Diuretic therapy, with the exception of potassium-sparing diuretics, is the most common cause of hypokalemia. Both thiazide and loop diuretics increase the loss of potassium in the urine. The degree of hypokalemia is directly related to diuretic dose and is greater when sodium intake is higher.[2] Magnesium depletion causes renal potassium wasting. Magnesium deficiency often coexists with potassium depletion because of diuretic therapy or disease processes such as diarrhea. Importantly, the ability to correct potassium deficiency is impaired when magnesium deficiency is present.

Renal losses of potassium are accentuated by aldosterone and cortisol. Increased potassium losses occur in situations such as trauma and surgery that produce a stress-related increase in these hormones. Primary aldosteronism, caused by either a tumor or hyperplasia of the cells of the adrenal cortex that secrete aldosterone, produces severe potassium losses and a decrease in plasma potassium levels.[2] Cortisol binds to aldosterone receptors and exerts aldosterone-like effects on potassium elimination.

Other rare, genetic disorders that can also result in hypokalemia are the Bartter, Gitelman, and Liddle syndromes. *Bartter syndrome*, which involves the $Na^+/K^+/2Cl^-$ cotransporter in the thick loop of Henle, is manifested by metabolic alkalosis, hypercalciuria or excessive loss of calcium in the urine, and *normal* blood pressure.[2] Because the loop diuretics act at the same site in the kidney, these features are identical to those seen with chronic loop diuretic ingestion. The manifestations of *Gitelman syndrome*, which involves the Na^+/Cl^- transporter in the distal tubule, are similar to those of Bartter syndrome, but with hypocalciuria and hypomagnesemia because of renal magnesium wasting.[2] Because this is the site where the thiazide diuretics exert their action, these manifestations are identical to those seen with chronic thiazide diuretic ingestion. *Liddle syndrome* has manifestations similar to Bartter syndrome, but with *high* blood pressure because of excessive sodium reabsorption.[2]

Although potassium losses from the skin and the gastrointestinal tract usually are minimal, these losses can become excessive under certain conditions. For example, burns increase surface losses of potassium. Losses because of sweating increase in persons who are acclimated to a hot climate, partly because increased secretion of aldosterone during heat acclimatization increases the loss of potassium in urine and sweat. Gastrointestinal losses also can become excessive; this occurs with vomiting and diarrhea and when gastrointestinal suction is being used. The potassium content of liquid stools, for example, is approximately 40 to 60 mEq/L (40 to 60 mmol/L).

Transcellular Shifts. Because of the high ratio of intracellular to extracellular potassium, conditions that produce a redistribution of potassium from the ECF to the ICF compartment can cause a marked decrease in plasma potassium levels (see Fig. 8.8). Insulin increases the movement of glucose and potassium into cells; therefore, potassium deficit often develops during treatment of diabetic ketoacidosis. A wide variety of β_2-adrenergic agonist drugs (*e.g.*, decongestants and bronchodilators) shift potassium into cells and cause transient hypokalemia.

Clinical Manifestations. The manifestations of hypokalemia include alterations in renal, gastrointestinal, cardiovascular, and neuromuscular function (see Table 8.8). These manifestations reflect both the intracellular functions of potassium as well as the body's attempt to regulate ECF potassium levels within the very narrow range needed to maintain the normal electrical activity of excitable tissues such as nerve and muscle cells. The signs and symptoms of potassium deficit seldom develop until plasma potassium levels have fallen to levels below 3 mEq/L (3 mmol/L). They are typically gradual in onset, and therefore the disorder may go undetected for some time.

The renal processes that conserve potassium during hypokalemia interfere with the kidney's ability to concentrate urine. Urine output and plasma osmolality are increased, urine specific gravity is decreased, and complaints of polyuria, nocturia, and thirst are common (an example of nephrogenic DI). Metabolic alkalosis and renal chloride wasting are signs of severe hypokalemia.[2]

There are numerous signs and symptoms associated with gastrointestinal function, including anorexia, nausea, and vomiting. Atony of the gastrointestinal smooth muscle can cause constipation, abdominal distention, and, in severe hypokalemia, paralytic ileus. When gastrointestinal symptoms occur gradually and are not severe, they often impair potassium intake and exaggerate the condition.

The most serious effects of hypokalemia are those affecting cardiovascular function. Postural hypotension is common. Most people with plasma potassium levels below 3 mEq/L (3 mmol/L) demonstrate electrocardiographic (ECG) changes typical of hypokalemia. These changes include prolongation of the PR interval, depression of the ST segment, flattening of the T wave, and appearance of a prominent U wave (Fig. 8.10). Normally, potassium leaves the cell during the repolarization phase of the action potential, returning the membrane

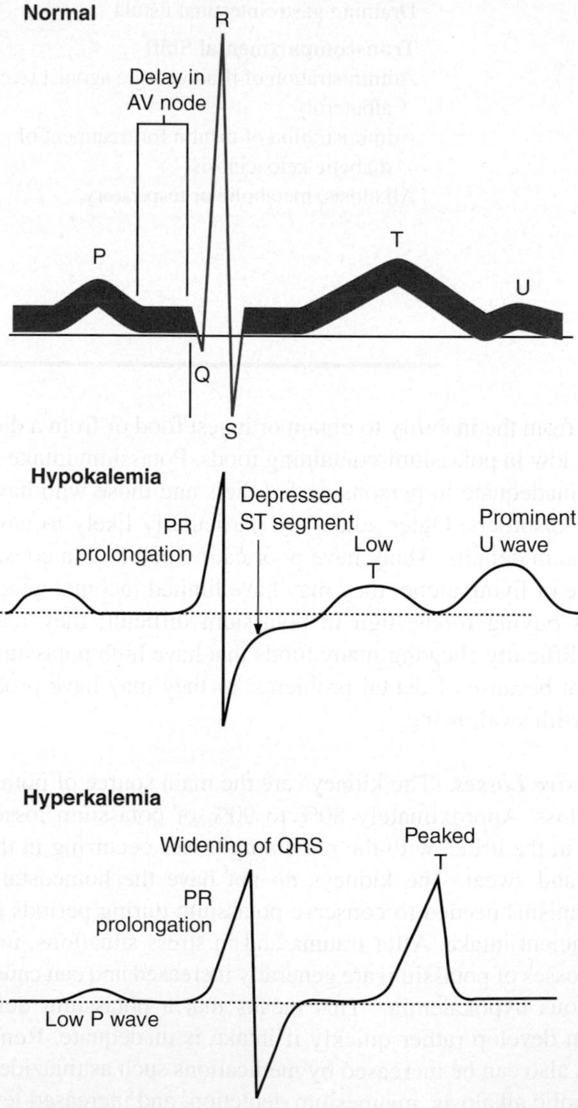

Figure 8.10 • ECG changes with hypokalemia and hyperkalemia.

potential to its normal resting value. Hypokalemia reduces the permeability of the cell membrane to potassium and thus produces a decrease in potassium efflux that prolongs the rate of repolarization and lengthens the relative refractory period. The U wave normally may be present on the ECG but should be of lower amplitude than the T wave. With hypokalemia, the amplitude of the T wave decreases as the U-wave amplitude increases. Although these changes in electrical activity of the heart usually are not serious, they may predispose to sinus bradycardia and ectopic ventricular arrhythmias. Digitalis toxicity can be provoked in people treated with this drug, and there is an increased risk of ventricular arrhythmias, particularly in people with underlying heart disease. The dangers associated with digitalis toxicity are compounded in people who are receiving diuretics that increase urinary losses of potassium.

Complaints of weakness, fatigue, and muscle cramps, particularly during exercise, are common in moderate hypokalemia (plasma potassium 3 to 2.5 mEq/L [3 to 2.5 mmol/L]). Muscle paralysis with life-threatening respiratory insufficiency can occur with severe hypokalemia (plasma potassium <2.5 mEq/L [2.5 mmol/L]). Leg muscles, particularly the quadriceps, are most prominently affected. Some people complain of muscle tenderness and paresthesias rather than weakness. In chronic potassium deficiency, muscle atrophy may contribute to muscle weakness.

In a rare genetic condition called *hypokalemic familial periodic paralysis*, episodes of hypokalemia cause attacks of severe muscle weakness and flaccid paralysis that last 6 to 48 hours if untreated.[21] The paralysis may be precipitated by situations that cause severe hypokalemia by producing an intracellular shift in potassium, such as ingestion of a high-carbohydrate meal or administration of insulin, epinephrine, or glucocorticoid drugs. The paralysis often can be reversed by potassium replacement therapy.

Treatment. When possible, hypokalemia caused by potassium deficit is treated by increasing the intake of foods high in potassium content—meats, dried fruits, fruit juices (particularly orange juice), and bananas. Oral potassium supplements are prescribed for persons whose intake of potassium is insufficient in relation to losses. This is particularly true of people who are receiving diuretic therapy and those who are taking digitalis.

Potassium may be given intravenously when the oral route is not tolerated or when rapid replacement is needed. It is necessary to consistently measure serum magnesium levels because if a person has hypokalemia they often also have magnesium deficiency. The rapid infusion of a concentrated potassium solution can cause death from cardiac arrest. Health personnel who assume responsibility for administering intravenous solutions that contain potassium should be fully aware of all the precautions pertaining to their dilution and flow rate.

Hyperkalemia

Hyperkalemia refers to an increase in plasma levels of potassium in excess of 5 mEq/L (5 mmol/L). It seldom occurs in healthy people because the body is extremely effective in preventing excess potassium accumulation in the ECF.

Etiology. The three major causes of potassium excess are (1) decreased renal elimination, (2) excessively rapid administration, and (3) movement of potassium from the ICF to ECF compartment[22] (Table 8.9). A pseudohyperkalemia can occur secondary to release of potassium from intracellular stores after a blood sample has been collected, hemolysis of RBCs from excessive agitation of a blood sample, traumatic venipuncture, or prolonged application of a tourniquet during venipuncture.[23]

The most common cause of hyperkalemia is decreased renal function. Chronic hyperkalemia is almost always

TABLE 8.9 CAUSES AND MANIFESTATIONS OF HYPERKALEMIA

CAUSES	MANIFESTATIONS
Excessive Intake	**Laboratory Values**
Excessive oral intake	Serum potassium level above 5.0 mEq/L (5.0 mmol/L)
Treatment with oral potassium supplements	**Gastrointestinal Manifestations**
Excessive or rapid infusion of potassium-containing parenteral fluids	Nausea and vomiting
Release from Intracellular Compartment	Intestinal cramps
Tissue trauma	Diarrhea
Burns	**Neuromuscular Manifestations**
Crushing injuries	Paresthesias
Extreme exercise or seizures	Weakness, dizziness
Inadequate Elimination by Kidneys	Muscle cramps
Renal failure	**Cardiovascular Manifestations**
Adrenal insufficiency (Addison disease)	Changes in electrocardiogram
Treatment with potassium-sparing diuretics	Risk of cardiac arrest with severe excess
Treatment with ACE inhibitors or ARBs	

associated with renal failure. Usually, the glomerular filtration rate must decline to less than 10 mL/minute before hyperkalemia develops. Some renal disorders, such as sickle cell nephropathy, lead nephropathy, and systemic lupus nephritis, can selectively impair tubular secretion of potassium without causing renal failure. Acidosis further diminishes potassium elimination by the kidney and needs to be treated. People with acute renal failure accompanied by lactic acidosis or ketoacidosis are at increased risk for development of hyperkalemia.

Aldosterone acts at the level of the distal tubular Na^+/K^+ exchange system to increase potassium excretion while facilitating sodium reabsorption. A decrease in aldosterone-mediated potassium elimination can result from adrenal insufficiency (*i.e.*, Addison disease), depression of aldosterone release because of a decrease in renin or angiotensin II, or impaired ability of the kidneys to respond to aldosterone. Potassium-sparing diuretics (*e.g.*, spironolactone, amiloride, triamterene) can produce hyperkalemia by means of the latter mechanism. Because of their ability to decrease aldosterone levels, the ACE inhibitors and ARBs can also produce an increase in plasma potassium levels.

Potassium excess can result from excessive oral ingestion or intravenous administration of potassium. It is difficult to increase potassium intake to the point of causing hyperkalemia when renal function is adequate and the aldosterone Na^+/K^+ exchange system is functioning. An exception to this rule is the intravenous route of administration. In some cases, severe and fatal incidents of hyperkalemia have occurred when intravenous potassium solutions were infused too rapidly. Because the kidneys control potassium elimination, intravenous solutions that contain potassium should never be started until urine output has been assessed and renal function has been deemed to be adequate.

The movement of potassium out of body cells into the ECF also can lead to elevated plasma potassium levels. Tissue injury causes release of intracellular potassium into the ECF compartment. For example, burns and crushing injuries cause cell death and release of potassium into the ECF. The same injuries often diminish renal function, which contributes to the development of hyperkalemia. Transient hyperkalemia may be induced during extreme exercise or seizures, when muscle cells are permeable to potassium. In a rare autosomal dominant disorder called *hyperkalemic periodic paralysis*, hyperkalemia may cause transient periods of muscle weakness and paralysis after exercise, cold exposure, or other situations that cause potassium to move out of the cells. These hyperkalemic-induced periods of paralysis tend to be short in duration.[24]

Clinical Manifestations. The signs and symptoms of potassium excess are closely related to a decrease in neuromuscular excitability (see Table 8.9). The neuromuscular manifestations of potassium excess usually are absent until the plasma concentration exceeds 6 mEq/L (6 mmol/L). The first symptom associated with hyperkalemia typically is paresthesia. There may be complaints of generalized muscle weakness or dyspnea secondary to respiratory muscle weakness.

The most serious effect of hyperkalemia is on the heart. As potassium levels increase, disturbances in cardiac conduction occur. The earliest changes are peaked, narrow T waves and widening of the QRS complex. If plasma levels continue to rise, the PR interval becomes prolonged, followed by disappearance of P waves (see Fig. 8.10). The heart rate may be slow. Ventricular fibrillation and cardiac arrest are terminal events. Detrimental effects of hyperkalemia on the heart are most pronounced when the plasma potassium level rises rapidly. It is important to realize that multiple transfusions of RBCs can cause hyperkalemia and, if the transfusions are given rapidly, this is potentially life threatening.[25]

Diagnosis and Treatment. Diagnosis of hyperkalemia is based on complete history, physical examination to detect muscle weakness and signs of volume depletion, plasma potassium levels, and ECG findings. The history should include questions about dietary intake, use of potassium-sparing diuretics, history of kidney disease, and recurrent episodes of muscle weakness.

The treatment of potassium excess varies with the degree of increase in plasma potassium and whether there are ECG and neuromuscular manifestations. Calcium antagonizes the potassium-induced decrease in membrane excitability, restoring excitability toward normal. The protective effect of calcium administration is usually short-lived (15 to 30 minutes), and it must be accompanied by other therapies to decrease the ECF potassium concentration. The administration of sodium bicarbonate, β-adrenergic agonists (*e.g.*, nebulized albuterol), or insulin distributes potassium into the ICF compartment and rapidly decreases the ECF concentration. Intravenous infusions of insulin and glucose are often used for this purpose.

Less emergent measures focus on decreasing or curtailing intake or absorption, increasing renal excretion, and increasing cellular uptake. Decreased intake can be achieved by restricting dietary sources of potassium. The major ingredient in most salt substitutes is potassium chloride, and such substitutes should not be given to people with renal problems. Increasing potassium output often is more difficult. People with renal failure may require hemodialysis or peritoneal dialysis to reduce plasma potassium levels. Sodium polystyrene sulfonate, a cation exchange resin, also may be used to remove K^+ ions from the colon. The Na^+ ions in the resin are exchanged for K^+ ions, and the potassium-containing resin is eliminated in the stool.

IN SUMMARY

Potassium is the major ICF cation. It contributes to the maintenance of intracellular osmolality; plays a critical role in conducting nerve impulses and in the excitability of skeletal, cardiac, and smooth muscle; and influences acid–base balance. Potassium is ingested in the diet and eliminated through the kidney. Because potassium is poorly conserved by the kidney, an adequate daily intake is needed. A transcellular shift can produce a redistribution of potassium between the ECF and ICF compartments, causing blood levels to increase or decrease.

Hypokalemia represents a decrease in plasma potassium to levels below 3.5 mEq/L (3.5 mmol/L). It can result from inadequate intake, excessive losses, or redistribution between the ICF and ECF compartments. The manifestations of potassium deficit include alterations in renal, skeletal muscle, gastrointestinal, and cardiovascular function, reflecting the crucial role of potassium in cell metabolism and neuromuscular function.

Hyperkalemia represents an increase in plasma potassium to levels plasma greater than 5 mEq/L (5 mmol/L). It seldom occurs in healthy people because the body is extremely effective in preventing excess potassium accumulation in the ECF. The major causes of potassium excess are decreased elimination of potassium by the kidney, excessively rapid intravenous administration of potassium, and a transcellular shift of potassium out of the cell to the ECF compartment. The most serious effect of hyperkalemia is cardiac arrest.

CALCIUM, PHOSPHORUS, AND MAGNESIUM BALANCE

After completing this section of the chapter, the learner will be able to meet the following objectives:

- Describe the associations among intestinal absorption, renal elimination, bone stores, and the functions of vitamin D and parathyroid hormone in regulating calcium, phosphorus, and magnesium levels.
- State the difference between ionized and bound or chelated forms of calcium in terms of physiologic function.

Mechanisms Regulating Calcium, Phosphorus, and Magnesium Balance

Calcium, phosphorus, and magnesium are the major cations in the body. They are ingested in the diet, absorbed from the intestine, filtered in the glomerulus of the kidney, reabsorbed in the renal tubules, and eliminated in the urine. Approximately 99% of calcium, 85% of phosphorus, and 50% to 60% of magnesium are found in bone. Most of the remaining calcium (approximately 1%), phosphorus (approximately 14%), and magnesium (approximately 40% to 50%) are located inside cells. Only a small amount of these three ions is present in ECF. This small, but vital, amount of ECF calcium, phosphorus, and magnesium is directly or indirectly regulated by vitamin D and parathyroid hormone (PTH). Calcitonin, a hormone produced by C cells in the thyroid, is thought to act on the kidney and bone to remove calcium from the extracellular circulation.

Vitamin D

Although classified as a vitamin, vitamin D functions as a hormone. It acts to sustain normal plasma levels of calcium and phosphorus by increasing their absorption from the intestine, and it also is necessary for normal bone formation. Vitamin D is synthesized by ultraviolet irradiation of 7-dehydrocholesterol, which is present in the skin or obtained from foods in the diet, many of which are fortified with vitamin D. The synthesized or ingested forms of vitamin D are essentially prohormones that lack biologic activity and must undergo metabolic transformation to achieve potency. Once vitamin D enters the circulation from the skin or intestine, it is concentrated in the liver. There it is hydroxylated to form 25-hydroxyvitamin D [25-$(OH)D_3$], also called *calcidiol.* It is then transported to the kidney, where it is transformed into active 1,25-$(OH)_2D_3$. The major action of the activated form of vitamin D, also called *calcitriol*, is to increase the absorption of calcium from the intestine. Calcitriol also sensitizes bone to the resorptive actions of PTH. There is evidence that vitamin D controls parathyroid gland growth and suppresses the synthesis and secretion of PTH.[26] The formation of 1,25-$(OH)_2D_3$ in the kidneys is regulated in feedback fashion by plasma calcium and phosphate levels. Low calcium levels lead to an increase in PTH, which then increases vitamin D activation. A lowering of plasma phosphate also augments vitamin D activation. Additional control of renal activation of vitamin D is exerted by a negative feedback loop that monitors 1,25-$(OH)_2D_3$ levels.

Parathyroid Hormone

PTH, a major regulator of plasma calcium and phosphorus, is secreted by the parathyroid glands. There are four parathyroid glands located on the dorsal surface of the thyroid gland. The dominant regulator of PTH is the plasma calcium concentration. A unique calcium receptor on the parathyroid cell membrane (extracellular calcium-sensing receptor) responds rapidly to changes in plasma calcium levels.[2] When the plasma calcium level is high, PTH is inhibited and the calcium is deposited in the bones. When the level is low, PTH secretion is increased and calcium is mobilized from the bones. The response to a decrease in plasma calcium is prompt, occurring within seconds. Phosphorus does not exert a direct effect on PTH secretion. Instead, it acts indirectly by forming a complex with calcium, thereby decreasing the plasma calcium concentration.

The secretion, synthesis, and action of PTH are also influenced by magnesium. Magnesium serves as a cofactor in the generation of cellular energy and is important in the function of second messenger systems. Magnesium's effects on the synthesis and release of PTH are thought to be mediated through these mechanisms. Because of its function in regulating PTH release, severe and prolonged hypomagnesemia can markedly inhibit PTH levels.

The main function of PTH is to maintain the calcium concentration of the ECF. It performs this function by promoting the release of calcium from bone, increasing the activation of vitamin D as a means of enhancing intestinal absorption of calcium, and stimulating calcium conservation by the kidney while increasing phosphate excretion (Fig. 8.11). PTH acts on bone to accelerate the mobilization and transfer of calcium to

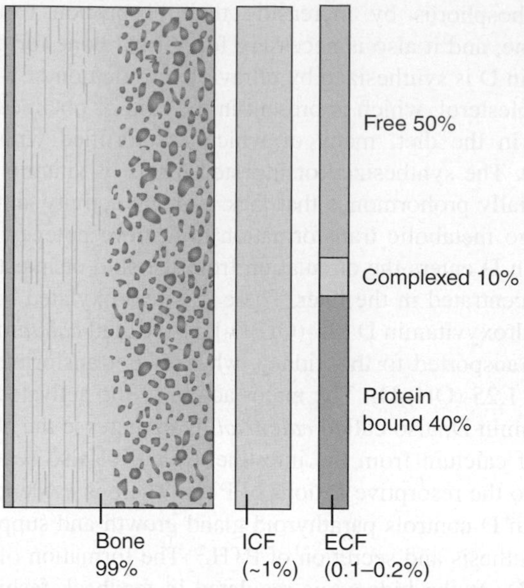

Figure 8.11 • Distribution of body calcium between bone and the intracellular fluid (ICF) and extracellular fluid (ECF) compartments. The percentages of free, complexed, and protein-bound calcium in ECFs are indicated.

the ECF. The skeletal response to PTH is a two-step process. There is an immediate response in which calcium that is present in bone fluid is released into the ECF and a second, more slowly developing response in which completely mineralized bone is resorbed, resulting in the release of both calcium and phosphorus. The actions of PTH in terms of bone resorption require normal levels of both vitamin D and magnesium. The activation of vitamin D by the kidney is enhanced by the presence of PTH; it is through the activation of vitamin D that PTH increases intestinal absorption of calcium and phosphorus as well as acting on the kidney to increase tubular reabsorption of calcium and magnesium while increasing phosphorus elimination. The accompanying increase in phosphorus elimination ensures that the phosphorus released from bone does not produce hyperphosphatemia and increases the risk of soft tissue deposition of calcium phosphate crystals.

Hypoparathyroidism. Hypoparathyroidism reflects deficient PTH secretion, resulting in hypocalcemia. PTH deficiency may be caused by a congenital absence of all of the parathyroid glands, as in DiGeorge syndrome. An acquired deficiency of PTH may occur after neck surgery, particularly if the surgery involves removal of a parathyroid adenoma, thyroidectomy, or bilateral neck resection for cancer. A transient form of PTH deficiency, occurring within 1 to 2 days and lasting up to 5 days, may occur after thyroid surgery owing to parathyroid gland suppression.[2] Hypoparathyroidism also may have an autoimmune origin. Antiparathyroid antibodies have been detected in some persons with hypoparathyroidism, particularly those with multiple autoimmune disorders such as type 1 diabetes, Graves disease, Hashimoto disease, and vitiligo (autoimmune destruction of melanocytes resulting in the development of totally white areas of skin). Other causes of hypoparathyroidism include heavy metal damage such as that occurring in Wilson disease, metastatic tumors, and surgery. Functional impairment of parathyroid function occurs with magnesium deficiency. Correction of the hypomagnesemia results in rapid disappearance of the condition.

Manifestations of acute hypoparathyroidism, which result from a decrease in plasma calcium, include tetany with muscle cramps, carpopedal spasm, and convulsions. Paresthesias, such as tingling of the circumoral area and the hands and feet, are almost always present. Low calcium levels may cause prolongation of the QT interval, resistance to digitalis, hypotension, and refractory heart failure. Symptoms of chronic PTH deficiency include lethargy, anxiety state, and personality changes. There may be blurring of vision because of cataracts, which develop over a number of years. Extrapyramidal signs, such as those seen with Parkinson disease, may occur because of calcification of the basal ganglia. Successful treatment of the hypocalcemia may improve the disorder and is sometimes associated with a decrease in basal ganglia calcification on radiography. Teeth may be defective if the disorder occurs during childhood.

Diagnosis of hypoparathyroidism is based on low plasma calcium levels, high plasma phosphate levels, and low plasma PTH levels. Plasma magnesium levels usually are measured to rule out hypomagnesemia as a cause of the disorder. Acute hypoparathyroid tetany is treated with intravenous calcium gluconate followed by oral administration of calcium salts and vitamin D. Magnesium supplementation is used when the disorder is caused by magnesium deficiency. Persons with chronic hypoparathyroidism are treated with oral calcium and vitamin D. Plasma calcium levels are monitored at regular intervals (at least every 3 months) as a means of maintaining plasma calcium within a slightly low but asymptomatic range. Maintaining plasma calcium within this range helps to prevent hypercalciuria and kidney damage.

Pseudohypoparathyroidism is a rare familial disorder characterized by target tissue resistance to PTH. It is characterized by hypocalcemia, increased parathyroid function, and a variety of congenital defects in the growth and development of the skeleton, including short stature and short metacarpal and metatarsal bones. There are variants in the disorder, with some persons having pseudohypoparathyroidism with the congenital defects and others having the congenital defects with normal calcium and phosphate levels. The manifestations of the disorder are due primarily to chronic hypocalcemia. Treatment is similar to that for hypoparathyroidism.

Hyperparathyroidism. Hyperparathyroidism is caused by hypersecretion of PTH. Hyperparathyroidism can manifest as a primary disorder caused by hyperplasia (15%), an adenoma (85%), and rarely carcinoma of the parathyroid glands, or as a secondary disorder seen in people with chronic renal failure or chronic malabsorption of calcium. Parathyroid adenomas and hyperplasia can occur in several distinct familial diseases (including multiple endocrine neoplasia [MEN] types 1 and 2a).

Primary hyperparathyroidism is seen more commonly after 50 years of age and is more common in women than men.[22] Primary hyperparathyroidism causes hypercalcemia and an increase in calcium in the urine filtrate, resulting in hypercalciuria and the potential for development of kidney stones. Chronic bone resorption may produce diffuse demineralization, pathologic fractures, and cystic bone lesions. A dual-energy x-ray absorptiometry (DEXA) bone scan may be used to assess bone mineral density (BMD). Signs and symptoms of the disorder are related to skeletal abnormalities, exposure of the kidney to high calcium levels, and elevated plasma calcium levels. At present, most people with primary hyperparathyroidism manifest an asymptomatic disorder that is discovered in the course of routine biochemical testing.

Diagnostic procedures, which include plasma calcium levels and intact PTH levels, are used to differentiate between the two most common causes of hypercalcemia: primary hyperparathyroidism and hypercalcemia of malignancy (HCM). Assays of intact PTH use two antibodies that bind to different sites on PTH and are designed to measure the intact, biologically active hormone, specifically. In primary hyperparathyroidism, the intact PTH levels are elevated in 75% to 90% of affected persons or are inappropriately "normal" in the face of hypercalcemia, when they should be suppressed. In HCM, the intact PTH levels are suppressed. Imaging studies of the parathyroid area may be used to identify a parathyroid adenoma. However, the role of imaging studies before and during surgery is the topic of much debate.[2] Parathyroid surgery is usually the treatment of choice.

Secondary hyperparathyroidism involves hyperplasia of the parathyroid glands and occurs primarily in persons with renal failure.[2] In early renal failure, an increase in PTH results from decreased plasma calcium and activated vitamin D levels. As the disease progresses, there is a decrease in vitamin D and calcium receptors, making the parathyroid glands more resistant to feedback regulation by plasma calcium and vitamin D level. At this point, elevated plasma phosphate levels induce hyperplasia of the parathyroid glands independent of calcium and activated vitamin D. The bone disease seen in people with secondary hyperparathyroidism because of renal failure is known as *chronic kidney disease–mineral bone disorder (CKD–MBD)*. This disorder has three major pathophysiologic manifestations including abnormal metabolism of calcium, phosphate, vitamin D, or PTH; calcification of soft tissue or vessels; and abnormalities in bone turnover.[27] CKD–MBD was formerly called renal osteodystrophy.[28] Evidence suggests that with CKD–MBD, the increased phosphorus levels cause atherosclerosis by increasing the thickness of the carotid intima–media.[28]

Treatment of hyperparathyroidism includes resolving the hypercalcemia with increased fluid intake. People with mild disease are advised to keep active and drink adequate fluids. They also are advised to avoid calcium-containing antacids, vitamin D, and thiazide diuretics, which increase reabsorption of calcium by the kidney. Parathyroidectomy may be indicated in people with symptomatic hyperparathyroidism, kidney stones, or bone disease. Avoiding hyperphosphatemia may lessen the problems of CKD–MBD caused by secondary hyperparathyroidism in renal failure. Calcium acetate or a calcium-free agent (sevelamer HCl [Renagel]) can be given with meals to bind phosphate.[29] Calcitriol, the activated form of vitamin D, may be used to control parathyroid hyperplasia and suppress the synthesis and secretion of PTH. However, because of its potent effect on intestinal absorption and bone mobilization, calcitriol can cause hypercalcemia. Newer analogs of activated vitamin D are being developed that retain the ability to suppress parathyroid function while having minimal effects on calcium or phosphorus reabsorption.

KEY POINTS

CALCIUM BALANCE

- ECF calcium levels are made up of free (ionized), complexed, and protein-bound fractions. Only the ionized Ca^{2+} plays an essential role in neuromuscular and cardiac excitability.
- Serum calcium levels are regulated by PTH and by renal mechanisms in which serum levels of calcium and phosphate are reciprocally regulated to prevent the damaging deposition of calcium phosphate crystals in the soft tissues of the body.

Disorders of Calcium Balance

Calcium enters the body through the gastrointestinal tract, is absorbed from the intestine under the influence of vitamin D, stored in bone, and excreted by the kidney. Approximately 99% of body calcium is found in bone, where it provides strength and stability for the skeletal system and serves as an exchangeable source to maintain extracellular calcium levels. Most of the remaining calcium (approximately 1%) is located inside cells, and only approximately 0.1% to 0.2% (approximately 8.5 to 10.5 mg/dL [2.1 to 2.6 mmol/L]) of the remaining calcium is present in the ECF.

The ECF calcium exists in three forms: (1) protein bound, (2) complexed, and (3) ionized (Fig. 8.11). Approximately 40% of ECF calcium is bound to plasma proteins, mostly albumin, and cannot diffuse or pass through the capillary wall to leave the vascular compartment. Another 10% is complexed (*i.e.*, chelated) with substances such as citrate, phosphate, and sulfate. This form is not ionized. The remaining 50% of ECF calcium is present in the ionized form. It is the ionized form of calcium that is free to leave the vascular compartment and participate in cellular functions. The total plasma calcium level fluctuates with changes in plasma albumin and pH. Ionized calcium serves a number of functions.[2,30] It participates in many enzyme reactions; exerts an important effect on membrane potentials and neuronal excitability; is necessary for contraction in skeletal, cardiac, and smooth muscle; participates in the release of hormones, neurotransmitters, and other chemical messengers; influences cardiac contractility and automaticity through the slow calcium channels; and is essential for blood clotting. The use of calcium channel–blocking drugs in circulatory disorders demonstrates the importance of Ca^{2+} ions in the normal functioning of the heart and blood vessels. Calcium is required for all but the first two steps of the intrinsic pathway for blood coagulation. Because of its ability to bind calcium, citrate often is used to prevent clotting in blood that is to be used for transfusions. Studies indicate that admission ionized calcium (iCa) levels in people who are critically ill because of trauma are predictors for the need for multiple blood transfusions and also the low iCa levels predict mortality.[2,30]

Gains and Losses

The major dietary sources of calcium are milk and milk products. Only 30% to 50% of dietary calcium is absorbed from the duodenum and upper jejunum; the remainder is eliminated in the stool. There is a calcium influx of approximately 150 mg/day into the intestine from the blood. Net absorption of calcium is equal to the amount that is absorbed from the intestine less the amount that moves into the intestine. Calcium balance can become negative when dietary intake (and calcium absorption) is less than intestinal secretion.

Calcium is stored in bone and excreted by the kidney. Approximately 60% to 65% of filtered calcium is passively reabsorbed in the proximal tubule, driven by the reabsorption of NaCl; 15% to 20% is reabsorbed in the thick ascending loop of Henle, driven by the $Na^+/K^+/2Cl^-$ cotransport system; and 5% to 10% is reabsorbed in the distal convoluted tubule. The distal convoluted tubule is an important regulatory site for controlling the amount of calcium that enters the urine. PTH and possibly vitamin D stimulate calcium reabsorption in this segment of the nephron. Thiazide diuretics, which exert their effects in the distal convoluted tubule, enhance calcium reabsorption. Other factors that may influence calcium reabsorption in the distal convoluted tubule are phosphate levels and glucose and insulin levels.

Hypocalcemia

Hypocalcemia represents a plasma calcium level of less than 8.5 mg/dL (2.1 mmol/L). Hypocalcemia occurs in many forms of critical illness and has affected as much 70% of people in intensive care units.[31]

Etiology. The causes of hypocalcemia can be divided into four categories: (1) impaired ability to mobilize calcium from bone stores, (2) abnormal losses of calcium from the kidney, (3) increased protein binding or chelation such that greater proportions of calcium are in the nonionized form, and (4) soft tissue sequestration (Table 8.10). A pseudohypocalcemia is caused by hypoalbuminemia. In this case, a malnourished person may indicate a low serum total calcium level, but have no symptoms.

Plasma calcium exists in a dynamic equilibrium with calcium in bone. The ability to mobilize calcium from bone

TABLE 8.10 CAUSES AND MANIFESTATIONS OF HYPOCALCEMIA

CAUSES	MANIFESTATIONS
Impaired Ability to Mobilize Calcium from Bone Hypoparathyroidism Resistance to the actions of PTH Hypomagnesemia **Decreased Intake or Absorption** Malabsorption Vitamin D deficiency Failure to activate Liver disease Kidney disease Medications that impair activation of vitamin D (*e.g.*, phenytoin) **Abnormal Renal Losses** Renal failure and hyperphosphatemia **Increased Protein Binding or Chelation** Increased pH Increased fatty acids Rapid transfusion of citrated blood **Increased Sequestration** Acute pancreatitis	**Laboratory Values** Serum calcium level below 8.5 mg/dL (2.1 mmol/L) **Neuromuscular Manifestations (Increased Neuromuscular Excitability)** Paresthesias, especially numbness and tingling Skeletal muscle cramps Abdominal spasms and cramps Hyperactive reflexes Carpopedal spasm Tetany Laryngeal spasm Positive Chvostek and Trousseau signs **Cardiovascular Manifestations** Hypotension Signs of cardiac insufficiency Failure to respond to drugs that act by calcium-mediated mechanisms Prolongation of QT interval predisposes to ventricular dysrhythmias **Skeletal Manifestations (Chronic Deficiency)** Osteomalacia Bone pain, deformities, fracture

depends on adequate levels of PTH. Decreased levels of PTH may result from primary or secondary forms of hypoparathyroidism. Suppression of PTH release may also occur when vitamin D levels are elevated. The activated form of vitamin D (calcitriol) can be used to suppress the secondary hyperparathyroidism that occurs in persons with chronic kidney disease. Magnesium deficiency inhibits PTH release and impairs the action of PTH on bone resorption. This form of hypocalcemia is difficult to treat with calcium supplementation alone and requires correction of the magnesium deficiency.

There is an inverse relation between calcium and phosphate excretion by the kidneys. Phosphate elimination is impaired in chronic kidney disease, causing plasma calcium levels to decrease. Hypocalcemia and hyperphosphatemia occur when the glomerular filtration rate falls below 59 mL/minute (normal values, which are related to age, sex, and body size, are approximately 120 mL/minute in young women and 130 mL/minute in young men).

Only the ionized form of calcium is able to leave the capillary and participate in body functions. A change in pH alters the proportion of calcium that is in the bound and ionized forms. An acid pH decreases binding of calcium to protein, causing a proportionate increase in ionized calcium, whereas total plasma calcium remains unchanged. An alkaline pH has the opposite effect. As an example, hyperventilation sufficient to cause respiratory alkalosis can produce tetany because of increased protein binding of calcium. Free fatty acids also increase binding of calcium to albumin, causing a reduction in ionized calcium. Elevations in free fatty acids sufficient to alter calcium binding may occur during stressful situations that cause elevations of epinephrine, glucagon, growth hormone, and adrenocorticotropic hormone levels. Heparin, β-adrenergic drugs (*i.e.*, epinephrine, isoproterenol, and norepinephrine), and alcohol can also produce elevations in free fatty acid levels sufficient to increase calcium binding.

Citrate, which complexes with calcium, is often used as an anticoagulant in blood transfusions. Theoretically, excess citrate in donor blood could combine with the calcium in a recipient's blood, producing a sharp drop in ionized calcium. This normally does not occur because the liver removes the citrate within a matter of minutes. When blood transfusions are administered at a slow rate, there is little danger of hypocalcemia caused by citrate binding.[2]

Hypocalcemia is a common finding in people with acute pancreatitis. Inflammation of the pancreas causes release of proteolytic and lipolytic enzymes. It is thought that the Ca^{2+} combines with free fatty acids released by lipolysis in the pancreas, forming soaps and removing calcium from the circulation.

Calcium deficit because of dietary deficiency exerts its effects on bone stores rather than extracellular calcium levels. A dietary deficiency of vitamin D is still seen today despite many foods being fortified with vitamin D. Vitamin D deficiency is more likely to occur in malabsorption states, such as biliary obstruction, pancreatic insufficiency, and celiac disease, in which the ability to absorb fat and fat-soluble vitamins is impaired. Failure to activate vitamin D is another cause of hypocalcemia. Anticonvulsant medications, particularly phenytoin, can impair initial activation of vitamin D in the liver. The final step in activation of vitamin D is impaired in people with chronic kidney disease. Fortunately, the activated form of vitamin D, calcitriol, has been synthesized and is available for use in the treatment of calcium deficit in persons with chronic kidney disease.

Clinical Manifestations. Hypocalcemia can manifest as an acute or chronic condition. The manifestations of acute hypocalcemia reflect the increased neuromuscular excitability and cardiovascular effects of a decrease in ionized calcium (see Table 8.10). Ionized calcium stabilizes neuromuscular excitability, thereby making nerve cells less sensitive to stimuli. Nerves exposed to low ionized calcium levels show decreased thresholds for excitation, repetitive responses to a single stimulus, and, in extreme cases, continuous activity. The severity of the manifestations depends on the underlying cause, rapidity of onset, accompanying electrolyte disorders, and extracellular pH. Increased neuromuscular excitability can manifest as paresthesias (*i.e.*, tingling around the mouth and in the hands and feet) and tetany (*i.e.*, spasms of the muscles of the face, hands, and feet).[32] Severe hypocalcemia can lead to laryngeal spasm, seizures, and even death.

Cardiovascular effects of acute hypocalcemia include hypotension, cardiac insufficiency, cardiac dysrhythmias (particularly heart block and ventricular fibrillation), and failure to respond to drugs such as digitalis, norepinephrine, and dopamine that act through calcium-mediated mechanisms.

The Chvostek and Trousseau tests can be used to assess for an increase in neuromuscular excitability and tetany.[32] The Chvostek sign is elicited by tapping the face just below the temple at the point where the facial nerve emerges. Tapping the face over the facial nerve causes spasm of the lip, nose, or face when the test result is positive. An inflated blood pressure cuff is used to test for the Trousseau sign. The cuff is inflated 10 mm Hg above systolic blood pressure for 3 minutes. Contraction of the fingers and hands (*i.e.*, carpopedal spasm) indicates the presence of tetany.

Chronic hypocalcemia is often accompanied by skeletal manifestations and skin changes. There may be bone pain, fragility, deformities, and fractures. The skin may be dry and scaling, the nails brittle, and hair dry. Development of cataracts is common.

Treatment. Acute hypocalcemia is an emergency, requiring prompt treatment. An intravenous infusion containing calcium (*e.g.*, calcium gluconate, calcium chloride) is used when tetany or acute symptoms are present or anticipated because of a decrease in the plasma calcium level.[33]

Chronic hypocalcemia is treated with oral intake of calcium. One glass of milk contains approximately 300 mg of calcium. Oral calcium supplements of carbonate, gluconate, or lactate salts may be used. Long-term treatment may require the use of vitamin D preparations, especially in persons with hypoparathyroidism and chronic kidney disease. The active form of vitamin D is administered when the liver or kidney mechanisms needed for hormone activation are impaired. Synthetic PTH (1-34) can be administered by subcutaneous injection as replacement therapy in hypoparathyroidism.

Hypercalcemia

Hypercalcemia represents a total plasma calcium concentration greater than 10.5 mg/dL (2.6 mmol/L). Falsely elevated levels of calcium can result from prolonged drawing of blood with an excessively tight tourniquet. Increased plasma proteins (*e.g.*, hyperalbuminemia, hyperglobulinemia) may elevate the total plasma calcium but not affect the ionized calcium concentration.

Etiology. A plasma calcium excess (*i.e.*, hypercalcemia) results when calcium movement into the circulation overwhelms the calcium regulatory hormones or the ability of the kidney to remove excess calcium ions (Table 8.11). The two most common causes of hypercalcemia are increased bone resorption because of neoplasms and hyperparathyroidism.[2] These two etiologies account for the majority of all people with hypercalcemia. Hypercalcemia is a common complication of malignancy, occurring in approximately 10% to 20% of people with advanced disease and is called HCM.[34] A number of malignant tumors, including carcinoma of the lungs, have been associated with hypercalcemia. Some tumors destroy the bone, whereas others produce humoral agents that stimulate osteoclastic activity, increase bone resorption, or inhibit bone formation. The majority of people with HCM produce PTH-related protein (PTHrP), which is designated the major humoral factor responsible for HCM.[34] PTH and PTHrP have marked homology, or structural similarity, at their amino terminal ends. This homology results in both PTH and PTHrP binding to the same receptor (PTH/PTHrP receptor). PTHrP is detected in people with many types of solid organs and also with adult T cell leukemia/lymphoma.[34]

Less frequent causes of hypercalcemia are prolonged immobilization, increased intestinal absorption of calcium, excessive doses of vitamin D, or the effects of drugs such as lithium and thiazide diuretics. Children with hypercalcemia will need to expedite urinary excretion of calcium, which

TABLE 8.11 CAUSES AND MANIFESTATIONS OF HYPERCALCEMIA

CAUSES	MANIFESTATIONS
Increased Intestinal Absorption	**Laboratory Values**
Excessive vitamin D	Serum calcium level above 10.5 mg/dL (2.6 mmol/L)
Excessive calcium in the diet	**Impaired Ability to Concentrate Urine and Exposure of Kidney to Increased Concentration of Calcium**
Milk-alkali syndrome	
Increased Bone Resorption	
Increased levels of PTH	Polyuria
Malignant neoplasms	Polydipsia
Prolonged immobilization	Flank pain
Decreased Elimination	Signs of acute and chronic renal insufficiency
Thiazide diuretics	Signs of kidney stones
Lithium therapy	**Gastrointestinal Manifestations**
	Anorexia
	Nausea, vomiting
	Constipation
	Neuromuscular Manifestations (Decreased Neuromuscular Excitability)
	Muscle weakness and atrophy
	Ataxia, loss of muscle tone
	Skeletal Manifestations
	Osteopenia
	Osteoporosis
	CNS Manifestations
	Lethargy
	Personality and behavioral changes
	Stupor and coma
	Cardiovascular Manifestations
	Hypertension
	Shortening of the QT interval
	Atrioventricular block on electrocardiogram

is the main treatment goal.[35] Prolonged immobilization and lack of weight bearing cause demineralization of bone and release of calcium into the bloodstream. Intestinal absorption of calcium can be increased by excessive doses of vitamin D or as a result of a condition called the *milk-alkali syndrome*. The milk-alkali syndrome is caused by excessive ingestion of calcium (often in the form of milk) and absorbable antacids. Because of the availability of nonabsorbable antacids, the condition is seen less frequently than in the past, but it may occur in women who are overzealous in taking calcium preparations for osteoporosis prevention. Discontinuance of the antacid repairs the alkalosis and increases calcium elimination.

A variety of drugs elevate calcium levels. The use of lithium to treat bipolar disorders has caused hypercalcemia and hyperparathyroidism. The thiazide diuretics increase calcium reabsorption in the distal convoluted tubule of the kidney. Although the thiazide diuretics seldom cause hypercalcemia, they can unmask hypercalcemia from other causes such as underlying bone disorders and conditions that increase bone resorption.

Clinical Manifestations. The signs and symptoms associated with calcium excess reflect (1) changes in neural excitability, (2) alterations in smooth and cardiac muscle function, and (3) exposure of the kidneys to high concentrations of calcium (see Table 8.11). Neural excitability is decreased in people with hypercalcemia. There may be a dulling of consciousness, stupor, weakness, and muscle flaccidity. Behavioral changes may range from subtle alterations in personality to acute psychoses. The heart responds to elevated levels of calcium with increased contractility and ventricular arrhythmias. Digitalis accentuates these responses. Gastrointestinal symptoms reflect a decrease in smooth muscle activity and include constipation, anorexia, nausea, and vomiting. High calcium concentrations in the urine impair the ability of the kidneys to concentrate urine by interfering with the action of ADH (an example of nephrogenic DI). This causes salt and water diuresis and an increased sensation of thirst. Hypercalciuria also predisposes to the development of renal calculi. Pancreatitis is another potential complication of hypercalcemia and is probably related to stones in the pancreatic ducts.

Hypercalcemic crisis describes an acute increase in the plasma calcium level.[8] Malignant disease and hyperparathyroidism are the major causes of hypercalcemic crisis. In hypercalcemic crisis, cardiac dysrhythmias, oliguria, excessive thirst, volume depletion, fever, altered levels of consciousness, and a disturbed mental state accompany other signs of calcium excess.[8] Symptomatic hypercalcemia is associated with a high mortality rate; death often is caused by cardiac arrest.

Treatment. Treatment of calcium excess usually is directed toward rehydration and use of measures to increase urinary excretion of calcium.[2,8] Fluid replacement is needed in situations of volume depletion. The excretion of sodium is accompanied by calcium excretion. Diuretics and NaCl can be administered to increase urinary elimination of calcium after the ECF volume has been restored. Loop diuretics commonly are used rather than thiazide diuretics, which increase calcium reabsorption. Initial lowering of calcium levels is followed by measures to inhibit bone reabsorption. Drugs that are used to inhibit calcium mobilization include bisphosphonates, calcitonin, corticosteroids, mithramycin, and gallium nitrate. The bisphosphonates (*e.g.*, pamidronate, zoledronate), which act mainly by inhibiting osteoclastic activity, provide a significant reduction in calcium levels with relatively few side effects. Calcitonin inhibits osteoclastic activity, thereby decreasing resorption. The corticosteroids and mithramycin inhibit bone resorption and are used to treat hypercalcemia associated with cancer. The long-term use of mithramycin, an antineoplastic drug, is limited because of its potential for nephrotoxicity and hepatotoxicity. Gallium nitrate is highly effective in the treatment of severe hypercalcemia associated with malignancy. It is a chemical compound that inhibits bone resorption, although the precise mechanism of action is unclear. Dialysis can be used in people with hypercalcemia with renal failure and in people with heart failure in whom fluid overload is a concern.

Disorders of Phosphorus Balance

Phosphorus is mainly an intracellular anion. Approximately 85% of phosphorus is contained in bone, and most of the remainder (14%) is located in cells. Only approximately 1% is in the ECF compartment, and of that, only a minute proportion is in the plasma. In the adult, the normal plasma phosphorus level ranges from 2.5 to 4.5 mg/dL (0.8 to 1.45 mmol/L). These values are slightly higher in infants (3.7 to 8.5 mg/dL, 01.2 to 02.7 mmol/L) and children (4 to 5.4 mg/dL, 1.3 to 1.7 mmol/L), probably because of increased growth hormone and decreased gonadal hormones.

Phosphorus exists in two forms within the body—inorganic and organic. The inorganic form (phosphate [$H_2PO_4^-$ or HPO_4^{2-}]) is the principal circulating form of phosphorus and is the form that is routinely measured (and reported as phosphorus) for laboratory purposes.[2] Most of the intracellular phosphorus (approximately 90%) is in the organic form (*e.g.*, nucleic acids, phospholipids, ATP). Entry of phosphorus into cells is enhanced after glucose uptake because phosphorus is incorporated into the phosphorylated intermediates of glucose metabolism. Cell injury or atrophy leads to a loss of cell components that contain organic phosphate; regeneration of these cellular components results in withdrawal of inorganic phosphate from the ECF compartment.

Phosphorus is essential to many bodily functions. It plays a major role in bone formation; is essential to certain metabolic processes, including the formation of ATP and the enzymes needed for metabolism of glucose, fat, and protein; is a necessary component of several vital parts of the cell, being incorporated into the nucleic acids of DNA and RNA and the phospholipids of the cell membrane; and serves as an acid–base buffer in the ECF and in the renal excretion of hydrogen ions. Delivery of O_2 by the RBC depends on organic phosphorus in ATP and 2,3-diphosphoglycerate (2,3-DPG).

Phosphorus is also needed for normal function of other blood cells, including the white blood cells and platelets.

Gains and Losses

Phosphorus is ingested in the diet and eliminated in the urine. Phosphorus is derived from many dietary sources, including milk and meats. Approximately 80% of ingested phosphorus is absorbed in the intestine, primarily in the jejunum. Absorption is diminished by concurrent ingestion of substances that bind phosphorus, including calcium, magnesium, and aluminum.

Phosphate is not bound to plasma proteins, and essentially all of the phosphate that is present in the plasma is filtered in the glomerulus.[2] Renal elimination of phosphate is then regulated by an overflow mechanism in which the amount of phosphate lost in the urine is directly related to phosphate concentrations in the blood. Essentially all the filtered phosphate is reabsorbed when phosphate levels are low; when plasma phosphate levels rise above a critical level, the excess phosphate is eliminated in the urine. Phosphate is reabsorbed from the filtrate into the proximal tubular epithelial cells through the action of a sodium–phosphate cotransporter (NPT2). PTH can play a significant role in regulating phosphate reabsorption by inhibiting the synthesis and expression of the NPT2 transporter. Thus, whenever PTH is increased, tubular reabsorption of phosphate is decreased, and more phosphate is lost in the urine. NPT2 is also inhibited by the hormones called *phosphatonins*.[36] There are two most significant phosphatonins including fibroblast growth factor 23 (FGF 23) and secreted frizzled-related protein 4 (sFRP4).[37] When these hormones are overproduced, as in tumor-induced osteomalacia, marked hypophosphatemia occurs because of decreased intestinal phosphate absorption. In addition, increased phosphatonin causes excessive calcitriol (active vitamin D) degradation, resulting in osteomalacia or rickets.[36]

Hypophosphatemia

Hypophosphatemia is commonly defined by a plasma phosphorus level of less than 2.5 mg/dL (0.8 mmol/L) in adults; it is considered severe at concentrations of less than 1 mg/dL (0.32 mmol/L).[2] Hypophosphatemia may occur despite normal body phosphate stores as a result of movement from the ECF into the ICF compartment. Serious depletion of phosphorus may exist with low, normal, or high plasma concentrations.

Etiology. The most common causes of hypophosphatemia are depletion of phosphorus because of insufficient intestinal absorption, transcompartmental shifts, and increased renal losses (Table 8.12). Often, more than one of these mechanisms is active. Unless food intake is severely restricted, dietary intake and intestinal absorption of phosphorus are usually adequate. Intestinal absorption may be inhibited by administration of glucocorticoids, high dietary levels of magnesium, and hypothyroidism. Prolonged ingestion of antacids may also interfere with intestinal absorption. Antacids that contain aluminum hydroxide, aluminum carbonate, and calcium carbonate bind with phosphate, causing increased phosphate losses in the stool. Because of their ability to bind phosphate, calcium-based antacids are sometimes used therapeutically to decrease plasma phosphate levels in people with chronic kidney disease.

TABLE 8.12 CAUSES AND MANIFESTATIONS OF HYPOPHOSPHATEMIA

CAUSES	MANIFESTATIONS
Decreased Intestinal Absorption	**Laboratory Values**
Antacids (aluminum and calcium)	Serum level below 2.5 mg/dL (0.8 mmol/L) in adults and 4.0 mg/dL (1.3 mmol/L) in children
Severe diarrhea	
Lack of vitamin D	**Neural Manifestations**
Increased Renal Elimination	Intention tremor
Alkalosis	Ataxia
Hyperparathyroidism	Paresthesias
Diabetic ketoacidosis	Confusion, stupor, coma
Renal tubular absorption defects	Seizures
Malnutrition and Intracellular Shifts	**Musculoskeletal Manifestations**
Alcoholism	Muscle weakness
Total parenteral hyperalimentation	Joint stiffness
Recovery from malnutrition	Bone pain
Administration of insulin during recovery from diabetic ketoacidosis	Osteomalacia
	Blood Disorders
	Hemolytic anemia
	Platelet dysfunction with bleeding disorders
	Impaired white blood cell function

Alcoholism is a common cause of hypophosphatemia. The mechanisms underlying hypophosphatemia in the person addicted to alcohol may be related to malnutrition, increased renal excretion rates, or hypomagnesemia. Malnutrition and diabetic ketoacidosis increase phosphate excretion and phosphorus loss from the body. Refeeding of people who are malnourished increases the incorporation of phosphorus into nucleic acids and phosphorylated compounds in the cell.[38] The same thing happens when diabetic ketoacidosis is reversed with insulin therapy. Urinary losses of phosphate may be caused by drugs, such as theophylline, corticosteroids, and loop diuretics, which increase renal excretion.

Hypophosphatemia also can occur during prolonged courses of glucose administration or hyperalimentation. Glucose administration causes insulin release, with transport of glucose and phosphorus into the cell. The catabolic events that occur with diabetic ketoacidosis also deplete phosphorus stores. Usually the hypophosphatemia does not become apparent, however, until insulin and fluid replacement have reversed the dehydration and glucose has started to move back into the cell. Administration of hyperalimentation solutions without adequate phosphorus can cause a rapid influx of phosphorus into the body's muscle mass, particularly if treatment is initiated after a period of tissue catabolism. Because only a small amount of total body phosphorus is in the ECF compartment, even a small redistribution between the ECF and ICF compartments can cause hypophosphatemia, even though total phosphorus levels have not changed.

Respiratory alkalosis because of prolonged hyperventilation can produce hypophosphatemia through decreased levels of ionized calcium from increased protein binding, increased PTH release, and increased phosphate excretion.

Clinical Manifestations. The manifestations of phosphorus deficiency result from a decrease in cellular energy stores because of deficiency in ATP and impaired O_2 transport because of a decrease in RBC 2,3-DPG. Hypophosphatemia results in altered neural function, disturbed musculoskeletal function, and hematologic disorders (see Table 8.12).

RBC metabolism is impaired by phosphorus deficiency; the cells become rigid, undergo increased hemolysis, and have diminished ATP and 2,3-DPG levels. The chemotactic and phagocytic functions of white blood cells and the hemostatic functions of the platelets are also impaired. Acute severe hypophosphatemia (0.1 to 0.2 mg/dL) can lead to acute hemolytic anemia with increased erythrocyte fragility, increased susceptibility to infection, and platelet dysfunction with petechial hemorrhages. Anorexia and dysphagia can occur. Neural manifestations (intention tremors, paresthesias, hyporeflexia, stupor, coma, and seizures) are uncommon but serious manifestations. Respiratory insufficiency resulting from impaired function of the respiratory muscles can develop in people with severe hypophosphatemia.

Chronic phosphorus depletion interferes with mineralization of newly formed bone matrix. In growing children, this process causes abnormal endochondral growth and clinical manifestations of rickets. In adults, the condition leads to joint stiffness, bone pain, and skeletal deformities consistent with osteomalacia.

Treatment. The treatment of hypophosphatemia is usually directed toward prophylaxis. This may be accomplished with dietary sources high in phosphorus (one glass of milk contains approximately 250 mg of phosphorus) or with oral or intravenous replacement solutions. Phosphorus supplements usually are contraindicated in hyperparathyroidism, chronic kidney disease, and hypercalcemia because of the increased risk of extracellular calcifications.

Hyperphosphatemia

Hyperphosphatemia represents a plasma phosphorus concentration in excess of 4.5 mg/dL (1.45 mmol/L) in adults. Growing children normally have plasma phosphate levels higher than those of adults.

Etiology. Hyperphosphatemia results from failure of the kidneys to excrete excess phosphate, rapid redistribution of intracellular phosphate to the ECF compartment, and excessive intake of phosphorus.[2] The most common cause of hyperphosphatemia is impaired renal function (Table 8.13).

Hyperphosphatemia is a common electrolyte disorder in people with chronic kidney disease. The increase in phosphate levels in people with chronic kidney disease occurs despite compensatory increases in PTH. Evidence illustrates an increase in cardiovascular calcification and mortality with people with CKD and high phosphorous levels.[2] Release of intracellular phosphorus can result from conditions such as massive tissue injury, rhabdomyolysis, heat stroke, potassium deficiency, and seizures. Chemotherapy can raise plasma phosphate levels because of the rapid destruction of tumor cells (tumor lysis syndrome).

The administration of excess phosphate-containing antacids, laxatives, or enemas can be another cause of hyperphosphatemia, especially when there is a decrease in vascular volume and a reduced glomerular filtration rate. Phosphate-containing laxatives and enemas predispose to hypovolemia and a decreased glomerular filtration rate by inducing diarrhea, thereby increasing the risk of hypophosphatemia.

Clinical Manifestations. Hyperphosphatemia is accompanied by a decrease in plasma calcium. Many of the signs and symptoms of a phosphate excess are related to a calcium deficit (see Table 8.13). Inadequately treated hyperphosphatemia in chronic disease can lead to secondary hyperparathyroidism, renal osteodystrophies or mineral bone disorders, and extraosseous calcifications in soft tissues.

Treatment. The treatment of hyperphosphatemia is directed at the cause of the disorder. Dietary restriction of foods that are high in phosphorus may be used. Calcium-based phosphate binders are useful in chronic hyperphosphatemia. Sevelamer, a calcium- and aluminum-free phosphate binder,

TABLE 8.13 CAUSES AND MANIFESTATIONS OF HYPERPHOSPHATEMIA

CAUSES	MANIFESTATIONS
Acute Phosphate Overload	**Laboratory Values**
Laxatives and enemas containing phosphorus	Serum level above 4.5 mg/dL (1.45 mmol/L) in adults and 5.4 mg/dL (1.7 mmol/L) in children
Intravenous phosphate supplementation	
Intracellular-to-Extracellular Shift	**Neuromuscular Manifestations (Reciprocal Decrease in Serum Calcium)**
Massive trauma	Paresthesias
Heat stroke	Tetany
Seizures	**Cardiovascular Manifestations**
Rhabdomyolysis	Hypotension
Tumor lysis syndrome	Cardiac arrhythmias
Potassium deficiency	
Impaired Elimination	
Kidney failure	
Hypoparathyroidism	

is as effective as a calcium-based binder, but lacks its adverse manifestations such as elevation of the calcium × phosphate product, hypercalcemia, and vascular and cardiac calcifications.[29] Hemodialysis is used to reduce phosphate levels in people with chronic kidney disease.

KEY POINTS

PHOSPHORUS BALANCE

- Approximately 85% of the phosphorus is contained in bone. Most of the remaining phosphorus is incorporated into organic compounds such as nucleic acids, high-energy compounds (*e.g.*, ATP), and coenzymes that are critically important for cell function.
- Serum phosphorus levels are regulated by the kidneys, which eliminate or conserve phosphate as serum levels change. Serum levels of calcium and phosphate are reciprocally regulated to prevent the damaging deposition of calcium phosphate crystals in the soft tissues of the body. Many of the manifestations of hyperphosphatemia reflect a decrease in serum calcium levels.

Disorders of Magnesium Balance

Magnesium is the fourth most abundant cation in the body and the second most abundant intracellular cation after potassium. Of the total magnesium content, approximately 50% to 60% is stored in bone, 8% to 49% is contained in the body cells, and the remaining 1% is dispersed in the ECF.[2] Approximately 20% to 30% of ECF magnesium is protein bound, and only a small fraction of ICF magnesium (15% to 30%) is exchangeable with the ECF. The normal plasma concentration of magnesium is 1.8 to 3.0 mg/dL (0.75 to 1.25 mmol/L).

Only recently has the importance of magnesium to the overall function of the body been recognized. Magnesium acts as a cofactor in many intracellular enzyme reactions, including the transfer of high-energy phosphate groups in the generation of ATP from adenosine diphosphate (ADP). It is essential to all reactions that require ATP, for every step related to replication and transcription of DNA, and for the translation of messenger RNA. It is required for cellular energy metabolism, functioning of the Na^+/K^+-ATPase membrane pump, membrane stabilization, nerve conduction, ion transport, and potassium and calcium channel activity.[2] Potassium channels, including the acetylcholine-sensitive potassium channel, depend on adequate intracellular magnesium levels. Magnesium blocks the outward movement of potassium in cardiac cells. When magnesium levels are low, the channel permits outward flow of potassium, resulting in low levels of intracellular potassium. Many calcium channels are also magnesium dependent. Higher ICF magnesium concentrations inhibit calcium transport into the cell and its release from the sarcoplasmic reticulum. Therefore, magnesium tends to act as a smooth muscle relaxant by altering calcium levels that are responsible for muscle contraction. Magnesium does have an anticonvulsant effect. The suggested mechanism of action is cerebral vasodilation or prevention of ischemic neuronal damage by blockade of *N*-methyl-D-aspartate (NMDA) receptors in the brain. Magnesium is the first-line drug in the treatment of eclampsia in pregnant women.[39] In addition, magnesium is commonly used as a neuroprotective agent for infants. In fact, evidence suggests that approximately 1000 cases per year of cerebral palsy in the United States could be prevented if magnesium was consistently used during labor.[39]

Gains and Losses

Magnesium is ingested in the diet, absorbed from the intestine, and excreted by the kidneys. Intestinal absorption is not closely regulated, and approximately 25% to 65% of dietary magnesium is absorbed. Magnesium is contained in all green vegetables, grains, nuts, meats, and seafood. Magnesium is also present in much of the groundwater in North America.

The kidney is the principal organ of magnesium regulation. The kidneys filter about 70% to 80% of the plasma magnesium and excrete about 6%, although this amount can be influenced by other conditions and medications.[2] Magnesium is a unique electrolyte in that only approximately 12% to 20% of the filtered amount is reabsorbed in the proximal tubule.[2] The greatest quantity, 65%, is passively reabsorbed in the thick ascending loop of Henle.[2] The major driving force for magnesium absorption in the thick ascending loop of Henle is the positive voltage gradient created in the tubular lumen by the $Na^+/K^+/2Cl^-$ cotransport system. Inhibition of this transport system by loop diuretics lowers magnesium reabsorption. Active reabsorption of magnesium takes place in the distal convoluted tubule and accounts for about 10% of the filtered load. Magnesium reabsorption is stimulated by PTH and is decreased in the presence of increased plasma levels of magnesium and calcium.

Hypomagnesemia

Magnesium deficiency refers to depletion of total body stores, whereas hypomagnesemia describes a plasma magnesium concentration below 1.8 mg/dL (0.75 mmol/L).[40] It is seen in conditions that limit intake or increase intestinal or renal losses, and it is a common finding in emergency departments and intensive care units.

Etiology. Magnesium deficiency can result from insufficient intake, excessive losses, or movement between the ECF and ICF compartments (Table 8.14). It can result from conditions that directly limit intake, such as malnutrition, starvation, or prolonged maintenance of magnesium-free parenteral nutrition. Other conditions, such as diarrhea, malabsorption syndromes, prolonged nasogastric suction, or laxative abuse, decrease intestinal absorption. Another common cause of magnesium deficiency is chronic alcoholism. Many factors contribute to hypomagnesemia in alcoholism, including low intake and gastrointestinal losses from diarrhea. The effects of hypomagnesemia are exaggerated by other electrolyte disorders, such as hypokalemia, hypocalcemia, and metabolic acidosis.

Although the kidneys are able to defend against hypermagnesemia, they are less able to conserve magnesium and prevent hypomagnesemia. Urine losses are increased in diabetic ketoacidosis, hyperparathyroidism, and hyperaldosteronism. Some drugs increase renal losses of magnesium, including both loop and thiazide diuretics and nephrotoxic drugs such as aminoglycoside antibiotics, cyclosporine, cisplatin, and amphotericin B. Several rare, genetic disorders can also result in hypomagnesemia (*i.e.*, Gitelman and Bartter syndromes).

Relative hypomagnesemia may also develop in conditions that promote movement of magnesium between the ECF and ICF compartments, including rapid administration of glucose, insulin-containing parenteral solutions, and alkalosis. Although transient, these conditions can cause serious alterations in body function.

Clinical Manifestations. Magnesium deficiency usually occurs in conjunction with hypocalcemia and hypokalemia, producing a number of related neurologic and cardiovascular manifestations (see Table 8.14). Hypocalcemia is typical of severe hypomagnesemia. Most persons with hypomagnesemia-related hypocalcemia have decreased PTH levels, probably as a result of impaired magnesium-dependent mechanisms that control PTH release and synthesis. There is also evidence that hypomagnesemia decreases both the PTH-dependent and PTH-independent release of calcium

TABLE 8.14 CAUSES AND MANIFESTATIONS OF HYPOMAGNESEMIA

CAUSES	MANIFESTATIONS
Impaired Intake or Absorption	**Laboratory Values**
Alcoholism	Serum magnesium level below 1.8 mg/dL (0.75 mmol/L)
Malnutrition or starvation	**Neuromuscular Manifestations**
Malabsorption	Personality change
Small bowel bypass surgery	Athetoid or choreiform movements
Parenteral hyperalimentation with inadequate amounts of magnesium	Nystagmus
High dietary intake of calcium without concomitant amounts of magnesium	Tetany
Increased Losses	Positive Babinski, Chvostek, Trousseau signs
Diuretic therapy	**Cardiovascular Manifestations**
Hyperparathyroidism	Tachycardia
Hyperaldosteronism	Hypertension
Diabetic ketoacidosis	Cardiac arrhythmias
Magnesium-wasting kidney disease	

from bone. In hypomagnesemia, magnesium ions (Mg^{2+}) are released from bone in exchange for increased uptake of calcium from the ECF.

Hypomagnesemia leads to a reduction in intracellular potassium and impairs the ability of the kidney to conserve potassium. When hypomagnesemia is present, hypokalemia is unresponsive to potassium replacement therapy.

Magnesium is vital to carbohydrate metabolism and the generation of both aerobic and anaerobic metabolisms. Many of the manifestations of magnesium deficit are because of related electrolyte disorders such as hypokalemia and hypocalcemia. Hypocalcemia may be evidenced by personality changes and neuromuscular irritability along with tremors, athetoid or choreiform movements, and positive Chvostek or Trousseau signs. Cardiovascular manifestations include tachycardia, hypertension, and ventricular dysrhythmias. There may be ECG changes such as widening of the QRS complex, appearance of peaked T waves, prolongation of the PR interval, T-wave inversion, and appearance of U waves. Ventricular arrhythmias, particularly in the presence of digitalis, may be difficult to treat unless magnesium levels are normalized.

Persistent magnesium deficiency has been implicated as a risk factor for osteoporosis and osteomalacia, particularly in people with chronic alcoholism, diabetes mellitus, and malabsorption syndrome.

Treatment. Hypomagnesemia is treated with magnesium replacement. The route of administration depends on the severity of the condition. Symptomatic, moderate to severe magnesium deficiency is treated by parenteral administration. Treatment must be continued for several days to replace stored and plasma levels. In conditions of chronic intestinal or renal loss, maintenance support with oral magnesium may be required. Magnesium often is used therapeutically to treat cardiac arrhythmia, myocardial infarct, angina, bronchial asthma, and pregnancy complicated by preeclampsia or eclampsia. Caution to prevent hypermagnesemia is essential; it is important to carefully monitor people with any degree of renal failure to prevent magnesium excess.

KEY POINTS

MAGNESIUM BALANCE

- Most of the body's magnesium is located within cells, where it functions in regulation of enzyme activity, generation of ATP, and calcium transport. Magnesium is necessary for PTH function, and hypomagnesemia is a common cause of hypocalcemia.
- Elimination of magnesium occurs mainly through the kidney, which adjusts urinary excretion as a means of maintaining serum magnesium levels. Diuretics tend to disrupt renal regulatory mechanisms and increase urinary losses of magnesium.

Hypermagnesemia

Hypermagnesemia represents an increase in total body magnesium and a plasma magnesium concentration in excess of 3.0 mg/dL (1.25 mmol/L). Because of the ability of the normal kidney to excrete magnesium, hypermagnesemia is rare.

Etiology. When hypermagnesemia does occur, it usually is related to renal insufficiency and the injudicious use of magnesium-containing medications such as antacids, mineral supplements, or laxatives (Table 8.15). Older adults are particularly at risk because they have age-related reductions in renal function and tend to consume more magnesium-containing medications, including antacids and laxatives. Magnesium sulfate is used to treat toxemia of pregnancy and premature labor; in these cases, careful monitoring for signs of hypermagnesemia is essential.

TABLE 8.15 CAUSES AND MANIFESTATIONS OF HYPERMAGNESEMIA

CAUSES	MANIFESTATIONS
Excessive Intake	**Laboratory Values**
Intravenous administration of magnesium for treatment of preeclampsia	Serum magnesium level above 3.0 mg/dL (1.25 mmol/L)
Excessive use of oral magnesium-containing medications	**Neuromuscular Manifestations**
Decreased Excretion	Lethargy
Kidney disease	Hyporeflexia
Glomerulonephritis	Confusion
Tubulointerstitial kidney disease	Coma
Acute renal failure	**Cardiovascular Manifestations**
	Hypotension
	Cardiac arrhythmias
	Cardiac arrest

Clinical Manifestations. Hypermagnesemia affects neuromuscular and cardiovascular function (see Table 8.15). Because magnesium tends to suppress PTH secretion, hypocalcemia may accompany hypermagnesemia. The signs and symptoms usually occur only when plasma magnesium levels exceed 4.8 mg/dL (2 mmol/L).[40]

Hypermagnesemia diminishes neuromuscular function, causing hyporeflexia, muscle weakness, and confusion. Magnesium decreases acetylcholine release at the myoneural junction and may cause neuromuscular blockade and respiratory paralysis. Cardiovascular effects are related to the calcium channel–blocking effects of magnesium. Blood pressure is decreased, and the ECG shows shortening of the QT interval, T-wave abnormalities, and prolongation of the QRS and PR intervals. Severe hypermagnesemia (>12 mg/dL) is associated with muscle and respiratory paralysis, complete heart block, and cardiac arrest.

Treatment. The treatment of hypermagnesemia includes cessation of magnesium administration. Calcium is a direct antagonist of magnesium, and intravenous administration of calcium may be used. Peritoneal dialysis or hemodialysis may be required.

IN SUMMARY

Calcium, phosphorus, and magnesium are major divalent ions in the body. Calcium is a major divalent cation. Approximately 99% of body calcium is found in bone; less than 1% is found in the ECF compartment. The calcium in bone is in dynamic equilibrium with ECF calcium. Of the three forms of ECF calcium (*i.e.*, protein bound, complexed, and ionized), only the ionized form can cross the cell membrane and contribute to cellular function. Ionized calcium has a number of functions. It contributes to neuromuscular function, plays a vital role in the blood clotting process, and participates in a number of enzyme reactions. Alterations in ionized calcium levels produce neural effects; neural excitability is increased in hypocalcemia and decreased in hypercalcemia.

Phosphorus is largely an ICF anion. It is incorporated into the nucleic acids and ATP. The most common causes of altered levels of ECF phosphate are alterations in intestinal absorption, transcompartmental shifts, and disorders of renal elimination. Phosphorus deficit causes signs and symptoms of neural dysfunction, disturbed musculoskeletal function, and hematologic disorders. Most of these manifestations result from a decrease in cellular energy stores because of a deficiency in ATP and O_2 transport by 2,3-DPG in the RBC. Phosphorus excess occurs with renal failure and PTH deficit. It is associated with decreased plasma calcium levels.

Magnesium is the second most abundant ICF cation. It acts as a cofactor in many intracellular enzyme reactions and is required for cellular energy metabolism, functioning of the Na^+/K^+-ATPase membrane pump, nerve conduction, ion transport, and potassium and calcium channel activity. Magnesium blocks the outward movement of potassium in cardiac cells; when magnesium levels are low, the channel permits outward flow of potassium, resulting in low levels of intracellular potassium. It acts on calcium channels to inhibit the movement of calcium into cells. More than half of the body's magnesium can be found in the bones.[2] Magnesium deficiency can result from insufficient intake, excessive losses, or movement between the ECF and ICF compartments. Hypomagnesemia impairs PTH release and the actions of PTH; it leads to a reduction in ICF potassium and impairs the ability of the kidney to conserve potassium. Hypermagnesemia usually is related to renal insufficiency and the injudicious use of magnesium-containing medications such as antacids, mineral supplements, or laxatives. It can cause neuromuscular dysfunction with hyporeflexia, muscle weakness, and confusion. Magnesium decreases acetylcholine release at the myoneural junction and may cause neuromuscular blockade and respiratory paralysis.

MECHANISMS OF ACID–BASE BALANCE

After completing this section of the chapter, the learner will be able to meet the following objectives:

- Describe the three forms of carbon dioxide transport and their contribution to acid–base balance.
- Describe the intracellular and extracellular mechanisms for buffering changes in body pH.
- Compare the roles of the kidneys and respiratory system in regulation of acid–base balance.

Normally, the concentration of body acids and bases is regulated so that the pH of extracellular body fluids is maintained within a very narrow range of 7.35 to 7.45. This balance is maintained through mechanisms that generate, buffer, and eliminate acids and bases. This section of the chapter focuses on acid–base chemistry, the production and regulation of metabolic acids and bicarbonate, calculation of pH, and laboratory tests of acid–base balance.

Acid–Base Chemistry

An *acid* is a molecule that can release an H^+, and a *base* is an ion or molecule that can accept or combine with an H^+.[44–46] For example, hydrochloric acid (HCl) dissociates in water to form hydrogen (H^+) and chloride (Cl^-) ions. A base, such as the bicarbonate ion (HCO_3^-), is a base because it can combine with H^+ to form carbonic acid (H_2CO_3). Most of the body's acids and bases are weak acids and bases, the most important being *carbonic acid* (H_2CO_3), which is a weak acid derived from carbon dioxide (CO_2), and *bicarbonate* (HCO_3^-), which is a weak base.

Acids and bases exist as buffer pairs or systems—a mixture of a weak acid and its conjugate base or a weak base and its conjugate acid. When an acid (HA) is added to water, it dissociates reversibly to form H^+ and its conjugate anion (A^-). The degree to which an acid dissociates and acts as an H^+ donor determines whether it is a strong or weak acid.[1] *Strong acids*, such as sulfuric acid, dissociate completely. *Weak acids*, such as acetic acid, dissociate only to a limited extent. The same is true of a base and its ability to dissociate and accept an H^+.

The concentration of H^+ in body fluids is low compared with other ions.[1] For example, the sodium ion (Na^+) is present at a concentration approximately 3.5 million times that of H^+. Because it is cumbersome to work with such a small number, the H^+ concentration is commonly expressed in terms of the *pH*. Specifically, pH represents the negative logarithm ($\log_{10}$) of the H^+ concentration expressed in milliequivalents per liter (mEq/L).[1,3] Thus, a pH value of 7.0 implies an H^+ concentration of 10^{-7} (0.0000001 mEq/L). Because the pH is inversely related to the H^+ concentration, a low pH indicates a high concentration of H^+, and a high pH indicates a low concentration.

The *dissociation constant* (K) is used to describe the degree to which an acid or base in a buffer system dissociates.[1,2] The symbol pK refers to the negative $\log_{10}$ of the dissociation constant for an acid and represents the pH at which an acid is 50% dissociated.[3] Use of a negative $\log_{10}$ for the dissociation constant allows pH to be expressed as a positive value. Each acid in an aqueous solution has a characteristic pK that varies slightly with temperature and pH. At normal body temperature, the pK for the bicarbonate buffer system of the ECF compartment is 6.1.[44,46]

Overall, there are three ways to assess changes in acid–base balance: (1) the more traditional method of the Henderson-Hasselbalch (physiologic) approach, which looks at the relationship between HCO_3^- and PCO_2; (2) the standard base excess (SBE) approach; and (3) the Stewart (quantitative) approach, which looks at strong ion differences and total weak acids.[47,48]

KEY POINTS

MECHANISMS OF ACID–BASE BALANCE

- The pH is regulated by extracellular (carbonic acid [H_2CO_3]/bicarbonate [HCO_3^-]) and intracellular (proteins) systems that buffer changes in pH that would otherwise occur because of the metabolic production of volatile (CO_2) and nonvolatile (*i.e.*, sulfuric and phosphoric) acids.

Metabolic Acid and Bicarbonate Production

Acids are continuously generated as by-products of metabolic processes (Fig. 8.12). Physiologically, these acids fall into two groups: the *volatile acid* H_2CO_3 and all other *nonvolatile* or *fixed acids*. The difference between the two types of acids arises because H_2CO_3 is in equilibrium with CO_2 ($H_2CO_3 \leftrightarrow CO_2 + H_2O$), which is volatile and leaves the body by way of the lungs. Therefore, the lungs and their capacity to exhale CO_2 determine H_2CO_3 concentration. The lungs do not eliminate fixed or *nonvolatile acids* (*e.g.*, sulfuric, hydrochloric, phosphoric). Instead, they are buffered by body proteins or extracellular buffers, such as HCO_3^-, and then eliminated by the kidney.

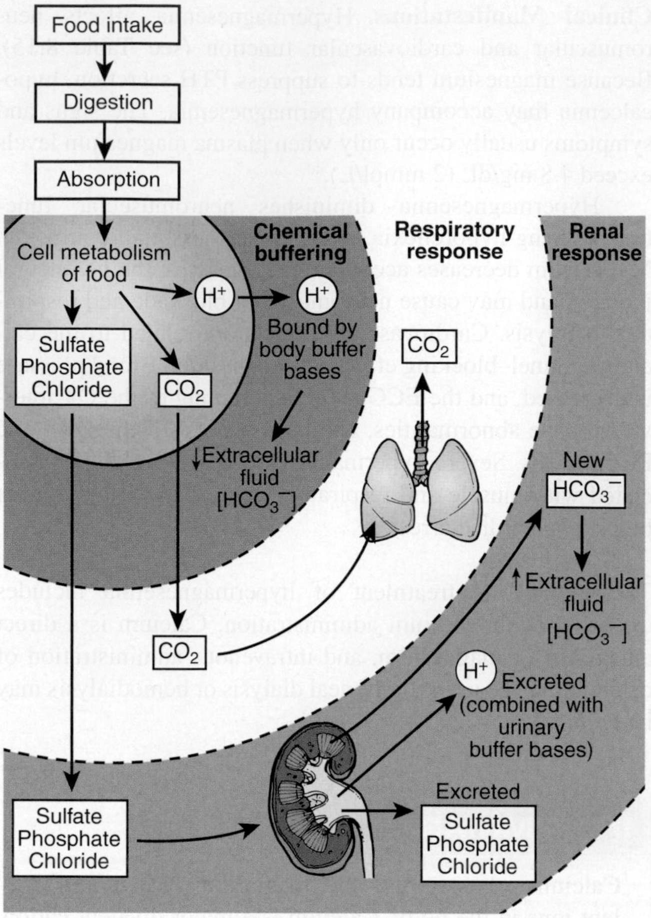

Figure 8.12 • The maintenance of normal blood pH by chemical buffers, the respiratory system, and the kidneys. On a mixed diet, pH is threatened by the production of strong acids (sulfuric, hydrochloric, and phosphoric) mainly as the result of protein metabolism. These strong acids are buffered in the body by chemical buffer bases, such as extracellular fluid (ECF) bicarbonate (HCO_3^-). The kidneys eliminate hydrogen ions (H^+) combined with urinary buffers and anions in the urine. At the same time, they add new HCO_3^- to the ECF, to replace the HCO_3^- consumed in buffering strong acids. The respiratory system disposes of carbon dioxide (CO_2). (From Rhodes R. A., Bell D. R. (2017). *Medical physiology principles for clinical medicine* (5th ed., Fig. 24.2, p. 488). Philadelphia, PA: Wolters Kluwer.)

Carbon Dioxide and Bicarbonate Production

Body metabolism results in the production of approximately 15,000 mmol of CO_2 each day.[49] Carbon dioxide is transported in the circulation in three forms:

1. As a dissolved gas
2. As bicarbonate
3. As carbaminohemoglobin (see "Understanding: Carbon Dioxide Transport")

Understanding Carbon Dioxide Transport

Body metabolism results in a continuous production of carbon dioxide (CO_2). As CO_2 is formed during the metabolic process, it diffuses out of body cells into the tissue spaces and then into the circulation. It is transported in the circulation in three forms: (1) dissolved in the plasma, (2) as bicarbonate, and (3) attached to hemoglobin.

Plasma

A small portion (about 10%) of the CO_2 that is produced by body cells is transported in the dissolved state to the lungs and then exhaled. The amount of dissolved CO_2 that can be carried in plasma is determined by the partial pressure of the gas (PCO_2) and its solubility coefficient (0.03 mL/100 mL plasma for each 1 mm Hg PCO_2). Thus, each 100 mL of arterial blood with a PCO_2 of 40 mm Hg would contain 1.2 mL of dissolved CO_2. It is the carbonic acid (H_2CO_3) formed from hydration of dissolved CO_2 that contributes to the pH of the blood.

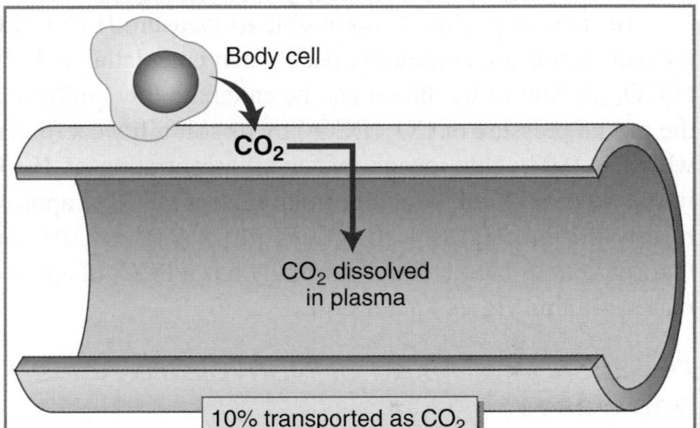

10% transported as CO_2 dissolved in plasma

Bicarbonate

Carbon dioxide in excess of that which can be carried in the plasma moves into the red blood cells, where the enzyme carbonic anhydrase (CA) catalyzes its conversion to carbonic acid (H_2CO_3). The H_2CO_3, in turn, dissociates into hydrogen (H^+) and bicarbonate (HCO_3^-) ions. The H^+ combines with hemoglobin and the HCO_3^- diffuses into plasma, where it participates in acid–base regulation. The movement of HCO_3^- into the plasma is made possible by a special transport system on the red blood cell membrane in which HCO_3^- ions are exchanged for chloride ions (Cl^-). Ventilation and the kidney handling of bicarbonate determines plasma bicarbonate concentrations.[7]

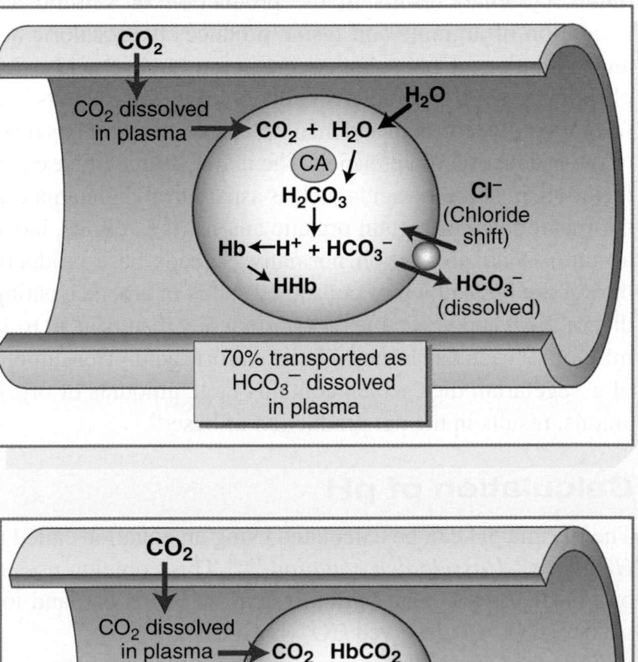

70% transported as HCO_3^- dissolved in plasma

Hemoglobin

The remaining CO_2 in the red blood cells combines with hemoglobin to form carbaminohemoglobin ($HbCO_2$).[2] The combination of CO_2 with hemoglobin is a reversible reaction characterized by a loose bond, so that CO_2 can be easily released in the alveolar capillaries and exhaled from the lung.

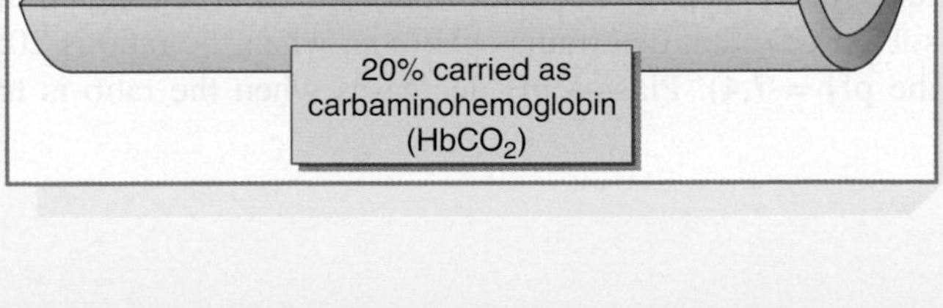

20% carried as carbaminohemoglobin ($HbCO_2$)

Collectively, dissolved CO_2 and HCO_3^- account for approximately 77% of the CO_2 that is transported in the ECF; the remaining CO_2 travels as carbaminohemoglobin (CO_2 bound to amino acids in hemoglobin).[44] Although CO_2 is a gas and not an acid, a small percentage of the gas combines with water to form H_2CO_3. The reaction that generates H_2CO_3 from CO_2 and water is catalyzed by an enzyme called *carbonic anhydrase*, which is present in large quantities in RBCs, renal tubular cells, and other tissues in the body. The rate of the reaction between CO_2 and water is increased approximately 5000 times by the presence of CA. Were it not for this enzyme, the reaction would occur too slowly to be of any significance in maintaining acid–base balance.

Because it is almost impossible to measure H_2CO_3, CO_2 measurements are commonly used when calculating pH. The H_2CO_3 content of the blood can be calculated by multiplying the partial pressure of CO_2 (PCO_2) by its solubility coefficient, which is 0.03. This means that the concentration of H_2CO_3 in the arterial blood, which normally has a PCO_2 of approximately 40 mm Hg, is 1.20 mEq/L ($40 \times 0.03 = 1.20$), and that for venous blood, which normally has a PCO_2 of approximately 45 mm Hg, is 1.35 mEq/L.

Production of Fixed or Nonvolatile Acids and Bases

The metabolism of dietary proteins and other nutrients results in the generation of fixed or nonvolatile acids and bases.[46,50] Oxidation of the sulfur-containing amino acids (*e.g.*, methionine, cysteine) results in the production of sulfuric acid. Oxidation of arginine and lysine produces hydrochloric acid, and oxidation of phosphorus-containing nucleic acids yields phosphoric acid. Incomplete oxidation of glucose results in the formation of lactic acid and incomplete oxidation of fats results in the production of ketoacids. The major source of base is the metabolism of amino acids such as aspartate and glutamate and the metabolism of certain organic anions (*e.g.*, citrate, lactate, acetate). Acid production normally exceeds base production during the breakdown of consumed foods in a person eating a diet of meat and vegetables.[3] A normal diet results in 50 to 100 mEq of H^+ each day as nonvolatile sulfuric acid.[6] Consumption of a vegetarian diet, which contains large amounts of organic anions, results in the net production of base.[46]

Calculation of pH

The plasma pH can be calculated using an equation called the *Henderson-Hasselbalch equation.*[44–46] This equation uses the pK_a of the bicarbonate buffer system, which is 6.1, and $\log_{10}$ of the HCO_3^- to dissolved CO_2 (H_2CO_3) ratio[46]:

$$pH = 6.1 + \log_{10}(HCO_3^- / PCO_2 \times 0.03)$$

The pH designation was created to express the low value of H+ more easily.[2] It should be noted that it is the ratio rather than the absolute values for bicarbonate and dissolved CO_2 that determines pH (*e.g.*, when the ratio is 20:1, the pH = 7.4). Plasma pH decreases when the ratio is less than 20:1, and it increases when the ratio is greater than 20:1 (Fig. 8.13). Because it is the ratio rather than the absolute values of HCO_3^- or CO_2 that determines pH, the pH can remain within a relatively normal range as long as changes in HCO_3^- are accompanied by similar changes in CO_2, or vice versa. For example, the pH will remain at 7.4 when plasma HCO_3^- has increased from 24 to 48 mEq/L as long as CO_2 levels have also doubled. Likewise, the pH will remain at 7.4 when plasma HCO_3^- has decreased from 24 to 12 mEq/L as long as CO_2 levels have also been reduced by one half. Plasma pH only indicates the balance or ratio and not where problems originate.[9]

Regulation of pH

The pH of body fluids (or change in H^+ concentration) is regulated by three major mechanisms:

1. Chemical buffer systems of the body fluids, which immediately combine with excess acids or bases to prevent large changes in pH
2. The lungs, which control the elimination of CO_2
3. The kidneys, which eliminate H^+ and both reabsorb and generate new HCO_3^-

Chemical Buffer Systems

The moment-by-moment regulation of pH depends on chemical buffer systems of the ICF and ECF. As previously discussed, a *buffer system* consists of a weak base and its conjugate acid pair or a weak acid and its conjugate base pair. In the process of preventing large changes in pH, the system trades a strong acid for a weak acid or a strong base for a weak base.

The three major buffer systems that protect the pH of body fluids are

1. The bicarbonate buffer system
2. Proteins
3. The transcellular H^+/K^+ exchange system[44,46]

These buffer systems act immediately to combine with excess acids or bases and prevent large changes in pH from occurring during the time it takes for the respiratory and renal mechanisms to become effective. Even though these buffer systems act immediately, they have a limited effect on pH and cannot correct large or long-term changes.

Bone represents an additional source of acid–base buffering.[10] Excess H^+ ions can be exchanged for Na^+ and K^+ on the bone surface, and dissolution of bone minerals with release of compounds such as sodium bicarbonate ($NaHCO_3$) and calcium carbonate ($CaCO_3$) into the ECF can be used for buffering excess acids. It has been estimated that as much as 40% of buffering of an acute acid load takes place in bone. The role of bone buffers is even greater in the presence of chronic acidosis. The consequences of bone buffering include demineralization of bone and predisposition to development of kidney stones because of increased urinary excretion of

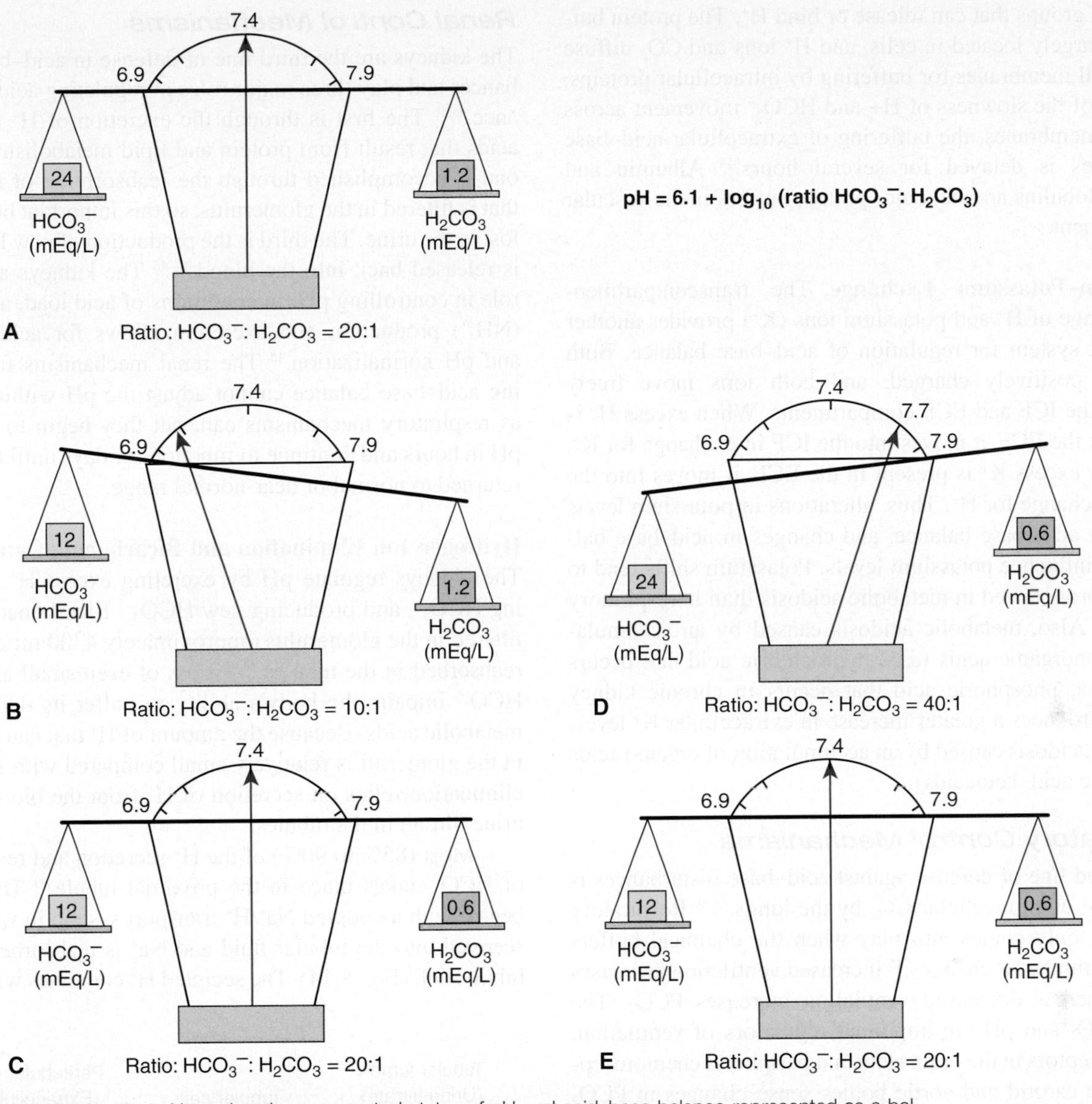

Figure 8.13 • Normal and compensated states of pH and acid–base balance represented as a balance scale. **(A)** When the ratio of bicarbonate (HCO_3^-) to carbonic acid (H_2CO_3, arterial $CO_2 \times 0.03$) = 20:1, the pH = 7.4. **(B)** Metabolic acidosis with a HCO_3^-:H_3CO_3 ratio of 10:1 and a pH of 7.1. **(C)** Respiratory compensation lowers the H_3CO_3 to 0.6 mEq/L and returns the HCO_3^-:H_3CO_3 ratio to 20:1 and the pH to 7.4. **(D)** Respiratory alkalosis with a HCO_3^-:H_3CO_3 ratio of 40:1 and a pH of 7.7. **(E)** Renal compensation eliminates HCO_3^-, reducing serum levels to 12 mEq/L, returning the HCO_3^-:H_3CO_3 ratio to 20:1 and the pH to 7.4. Normally, these compensatory mechanisms are capable of buffering large changes in pH but do not return the pH completely to normal as illustrated here.

calcium. People with chronic kidney disease are at particular risk for reduction in bone calcium because of acid retention.

Bicarbonate Buffer System. The HCO_3^- buffer system, which is the most powerful ECF buffer, uses H_2CO_3 as its weak acid and a bicarbonate salt such as sodium bicarbonate ($NaHCO_3$) as its weak base.[44,45] It substitutes the weak H_2CO_3 for a strong acid such as hydrochloric acid ($HCl + NaHCO_3 \times H_2CO_3 + NaCl$) or the weak bicarbonate base for a strong base such as sodium hydroxide ($NaOH + H_2CO_3 \times NaHCO_3 + H_2O$). The bicarbonate buffer system is a particularly efficient system because its components can be readily added or removed from the body.[44–46] Metabolism provides an ample supply of CO_2, which can replace any H_2CO_3 that is lost when excess base is added, and CO_2 can be readily eliminated when excess acid is added. Likewise, the kidney can conserve or form new HCO_3^- when excess acid is added, and it can excrete HCO_3^- when excess base is added.

Protein Buffer Systems. Proteins are the largest buffer system in the body.[44,45] Proteins are amphoteric, meaning that they can function either as acids or bases. They contain many ionizable groups that can release or bind H^+. The protein buffers are largely located in cells, and H^+ ions and CO_2 diffuse across cell membranes for buffering by intracellular proteins. Because of the slowness of H+ and HCO_3^- movement across the cell membranes, the buffering of extracellular acid–base imbalances is delayed for several hours.[44] Albumin and plasma globulins are the major protein buffers in the vascular compartment.

Hydrogen–Potassium Exchange. The transcompartmental exchange of H^+ and potassium ions (K^+) provides another important system for regulation of acid–base balance. Both ions are positively charged, and both ions move freely between the ICF and ECF compartments. When excess H^+ is present in the ECF, it moves into the ICF in exchange for K^+, and when excess K^+ is present in the ECF, it moves into the ICF in exchange for H^+. Thus, alterations in potassium levels can affect acid–base balance, and changes in acid–base balance can influence potassium levels. Potassium shifts tend to be more pronounced in metabolic acidosis than in respiratory acidosis.[3] Also, metabolic acidosis caused by an accumulation of nonorganic acids (*e.g.*, hydrochloric acid that occurs in diarrhea, phosphoric acid that occurs in chronic kidney disease) produces a greater increase in extracellular K^+ levels than does acidosis caused by an accumulation of organic acids (*e.g.*, lactic acid, ketoacids).

Respiratory Control Mechanisms

The second line of defense against acid–base disturbances is the control of extracellular CO_2 by the lungs.[45,49] Respiratory regulation only comes into play when the chemical buffers do not minimize H^+ changes.[45] Increased ventilation decreases PCO_2, whereas decreased ventilation increases PCO_2. The blood PCO_2 and pH are important regulators of ventilation. Chemoreceptors in the brain stem and peripheral chemoreceptors in the carotid and aortic bodies sense changes in PCO_2 and pH and alter the ventilation rate.

When the H+ concentration is above normal, the respiratory system is stimulated resulting in increased ventilation. This control of pH is rapid, occurring within minutes, and is maximal within 12 to 24 hours. Although the respiratory response is rapid, it does not completely return the pH to normal. It is only about 50% to 75% effective as a buffer system.[44,45] This means that if the pH falls from 7.4 to 7.0, the respiratory system can return the pH to a value of about 7.2 to 7.3.[44] In acting rapidly, however, it prevents large changes in pH from occurring while waiting for the much more slowly reacting kidneys to respond.

Although CO_2 readily crosses the blood–brain barrier, there is a lag for entry of HCO_3^-. Thus, blood levels of HCO_3^- change more rapidly than CSF levels. In metabolic acidosis, for example, there is often a primary decrease in pH of the cerebral fluids and a slower decrease in HCO_3^-. When metabolic acid–base disorders are corrected rapidly, the respiratory response may persist because of a delay in adjustment of CSF HCO_3^- levels.

Renal Control Mechanisms

The kidneys are the third line of defense in acid–base disturbances and play three major roles in regulating acid–base balance.[45,46] The first is through the excretion of H^+ from fixed acids that result from protein and lipid metabolism. The second is accomplished through the reabsorption of the HCO_3^- that is filtered in the glomerulus, so this important buffer is not lost in the urine. The third is the production of new HCO_3^- that is released back into the blood.[44–46] The kidneys also play a role in controlling pH: in conditions of acid load, ammonium (NH_4^+) production and excretion allows for acid secretion and pH normalization.[45] The renal mechanisms for regulating acid–base balance cannot adjust the pH within minutes, as respiratory mechanisms can, but they begin to adjust the pH in hours and continue to function for days until the pH has returned to normal or near-normal range.

Hydrogen Ion Elimination and Bicarbonate Conservation. The kidneys regulate pH by excreting excess H^+, reabsorbing HCO_3^-, and producing new HCO_3^-. Bicarbonate is freely filtered in the glomerulus (approximately 4300 mEq/day) and reabsorbed in the tubules.[44,46] Loss of even small amounts of HCO_3^- impairs the body's ability to buffer its daily load of metabolic acids. Because the amount of H^+ that can be filtered in the glomeruli is relatively small compared with HCO_3^-, its elimination relies on secretion of H^+ from the blood into the urine filtrate in the tubules.

Most (85% to 90%) of the H^+ secretion and reabsorption of HCO_3^- takes place in the proximal tubule.[49] The process begins with a coupled Na^+/H^+ transport system in which H^+ is secreted into the tubular fluid and Na^+ is reabsorbed into the tubular cell (Fig. 8.14). The secreted H^+ combines with filtered

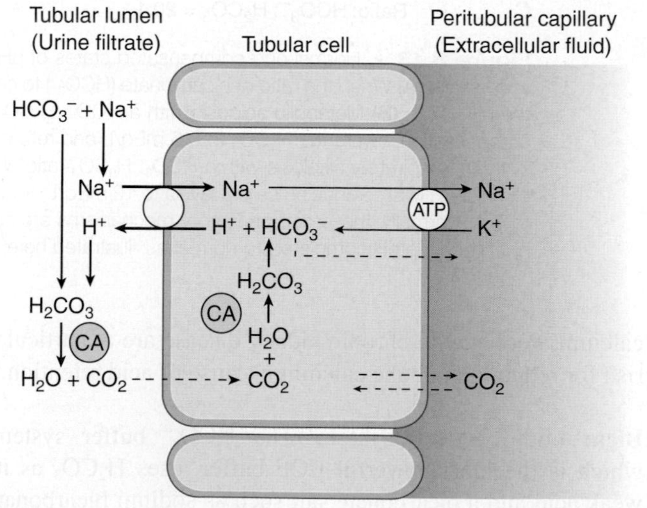

Figure 8.14 • Hydrogen ion (H^+) secretion and bicarbonate ion (HCO_3^-) reabsorption in a renal tubular cell. Carbon dioxide (CO_2) diffuses from the blood or urine filtrate into the tubular cell, where it combines with water in a carbonic anhydrase (CA)–catalyzed reaction that yields carbonic acid (H_2CO_3). The H_2CO_3 dissociates to form H^+ and HCO_3^-. The H^+ is secreted into the tubular fluid in exchange for Na^+. The Na^+ and HCO_3^- enter the ECF. ATP, adenosine triphosphate.

HCO_3^- to form H_2CO_3. The H_2CO_3 then decomposes into CO_2 and H_2O, catalyzed by a brush border CA. The CO_2 and H_2O that are formed readily cross the luminal membrane and enter the tubular cell. Inside the cell, the reactions occur in reverse. The CO_2 and H_2O combine to form a new H_2CO_3 molecule in a CA-mediated reaction. The H_2CO_3, in turn, is dissociated into HCO_3^- and H^+. The HCO_3^- is then reabsorbed into the blood along with Na^+, and the newly generated H^+ is secreted into the tubular fluid to begin another cycle. Normally, only a few of the secreted H^+ ions remain in the tubular fluid because the secretion of H^+ is roughly equivalent to the number of HCO_3^- ions filtered in the glomerulus.

Tubular Buffer Systems. Because an extremely acidic urine filtrate would be damaging to structures in the urinary tract, the minimum urine pH is about 4.5.[44,45] Once the urine pH reaches this level of acidity, H^+ secretion ceases. This limits the amount of unbuffered H^+ that can be eliminated by the kidney. When the amount of free H^+ secreted into the tubular fluid threatens to cause the pH of the urine to become too acidic, it must be carried in another form. This is accomplished by combining H^+ ions with intratubular buffers before they are excreted in the urine. There are two important intratubular buffer systems: the phosphate and ammonia buffer systems.[44,50] The HCO_3^- that is generated by these two buffer systems is new bicarbonate, demonstrating one of the ways that the kidney is able to replenish the ECF stores of HCO_3^-.

The *phosphate buffer system* uses HPO_4^{2-} and $H_2PO_4^-$ that are present in the tubular filtrate. Both forms of phosphate become concentrated in the tubular fluid because of their relatively poor absorption and because of reabsorption of water from the tubular fluid. Another factor that makes phosphate so effective as a urinary buffer is the fact that urine pH is close to the pK of the phosphate buffer system. The process of H^+ secretion in the tubules is the same as that used for reabsorption of HCO_3^-. As long as there is excess HCO_3^- in the tubular fluid, most of the secreted H^+ combines with HCO_3^-. However, once all the HCO_3^- has been reabsorbed and is no longer available to combine with H^+, any excess H^+ combines with HPO_4^{2-} to form $H_2PO_4^-$ (Fig. 8.15). After H^+ combines with HPO_4^{2-}, it can be excreted as NaH_2PO_4, carrying the excess H^+ with it.

Another important but more complex buffer system is the *ammonia buffer system*. The excretion of H^+ and generation of HCO_3^- by the ammonia buffer system occurs in three major steps:

1. The synthesis of ammonium (NH_4^+) from the amino acid glutamine in the proximal tubule
2. The reabsorption and recycling of NH_4^+ within the medullary portion of the kidney
3. The buffering of H^+ ions by NH_3 in the collecting tubules[44,46]

The metabolism of glutamate in the proximal tubule results in the formation of two NH_4^+ and two HCO_3^- ions[1,3] (Fig. 8.16). The two NH_4^+ ions are secreted into the tubular fluid by a countertransport mechanism in exchange for Na^+. The two HCO_3^- ions move out of the tubular cell along with the reabsorbed

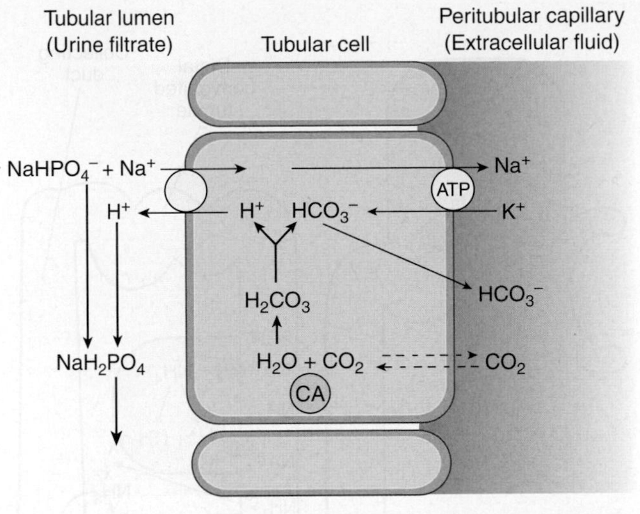

Figure 8.15 • The renal phosphate buffer system. The monohydrogen phosphate ion (HPO_4^{2-}) enters the renal tubular fluid in the glomerulus. An H^+ combines with the HPO_4^{2-} to form $H_2PO_4^-$ and is then excreted into the urine in combination with Na^+. The HCO_3^- moves into the ECF along with the Na^+ that was exchanged during secretion of the H^+. ATP, adenosine triphosphate; CA, carbonic anhydrase.

Na^+ to enter the peritubular capillary system. Thus, for each molecule of glutamine metabolized in the proximal tubule, two NH_4^+ ions are secreted into the tubular filtrate, and two HCO_3^- ions are reabsorbed into the blood. The HCO_3^- generated by this process constitutes new HCO_3^-.

A significant portion of the NH_4^+ secreted by the proximal tubular cells is reabsorbed in the thick ascending loop of Henle, where the NH_4^+ substitutes for K^+ on the $Na^+/K^+/2Cl^-$ cotransporter.[50] The NH_4^+ that is reabsorbed by the thick ascending loop of Henle accumulates in the medullary interstitium of the kidney, where it exists in equilibrium with NH_3 (see Fig. 8.16). Although both NH_4^+ and NH_3 are present in the medullary interstitial fluid, only NH_3 is lipid soluble and can diffuse across the collecting duct cells into the tubular fluid. Once in the tubular fluid, NH_3 combines with secreted H^+ to form NH_4^+. NH_4^+ is not lipid soluble, and thus is trapped in the tubular fluid and excreted in urine. Note that the source of the H^+ secreted by the cells of the collecting tubules is CO_2 and H_2O. Thus, for each H^+ that is produced in the cells and secreted, an additional new HCO_3^- is generated and added to the blood.

One of the most important features of the ammonia buffer system is that it is subject to physiologic control. Under normal conditions, the amount of H^+ eliminated by the ammonia buffer system is about 50% of the acid excreted and 50% of new HCO_3^- regenerated.[44] However, with chronic acidosis, it can become the dominant mechanism for H^+ excretion and new HCO_3^- generation. The urine anion gap (AG), which is an indirect method for assessing urine NH_4^+ levels, can be used to assess kidney function in terms of H^+ elimination.

Potassium–Hydrogen Exchange. Plasma K^+ levels influence renal elimination of H^+ and vice versa. Hypokalemia is a potent stimulus for H^+ secretion and HCO_3^- reabsorption.

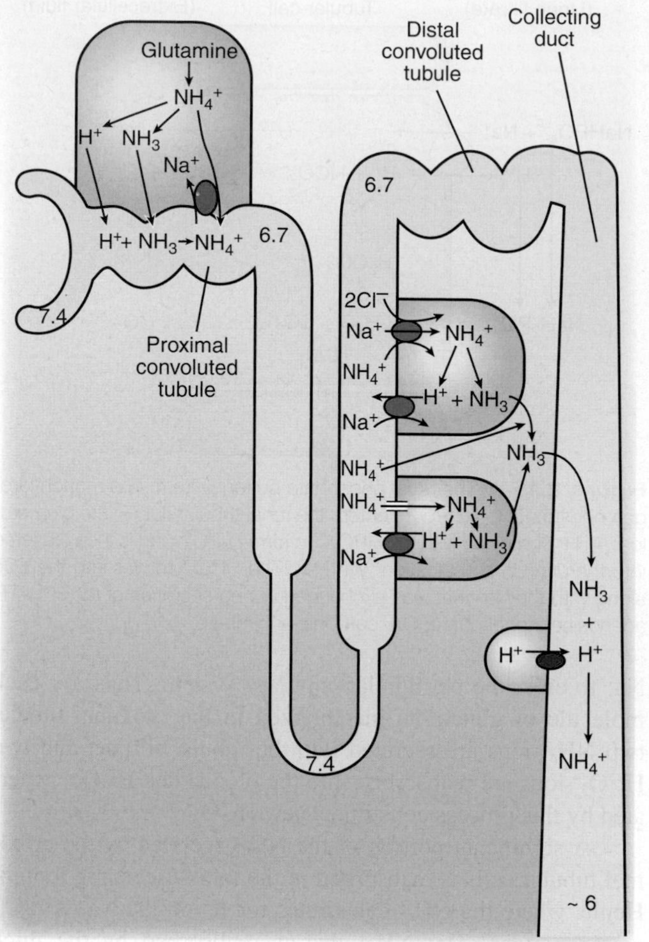

Figure 8.16 • Acidification along the nephron. The pH of tubular urine decreases along the proximal convoluted tubule, rises along the descending limb of the Henle loop, falls along the ascending limb, and reaches its lowest values in the collecting ducts. Ammonia (NH_3 + NH_4) is chiefly produced in proximal tubule cells and is secreted into the tubular urine. NH_4 is reabsorbed in the thick ascending limb and accumulates in the kidney medulla. NH_3 diffuses into acidic collecting duct urine, where it is trapped as NH_4. (From Rhodes R. A., Bell D. R. (2017). *Medical physiology: Principles for clinical medicine* (5th ed., Fig. 24.5, p. 492). Philadelphia, PA: Wolters Kluwer.)

When plasma K^+ levels fall, there is movement of K^+ from the ICF into the ECF compartment and a reciprocal movement of H^+ from the ECF into the ICF compartment. A similar process occurs in the distal tubules of the kidney, where the H^+/K^+-adenosine triphosphatase (ATPase) exchange pump actively reabsorbs K^+ as well as secretes H^+.[44,46] An elevation in plasma K^+ levels has the opposite effect. Plasma K^+ levels are similarly altered by acid–base balance. Thus, acidosis tends to increase H^+ elimination and decrease K^+ elimination, with a resultant increase in plasma potassium levels, whereas alkalosis tends to decrease H^+ elimination and increase K^+ elimination, with a resultant decrease in plasma K^+ levels.[45]

Aldosterone also influences H^+ elimination by the kidney. It acts in the collecting duct to stimulate H^+ secretion indirectly, while increasing Na^+ reabsorption and K^+ secretion. Thus, hyperaldosteronism tends to lead to a decrease in plasma K^+ levels and an increase in pH because of increased H^+ secretion, whereas hypoaldosteronism has the opposite effect.

Chloride–Bicarbonate Exchange. Another mechanism that the kidneys use in regulating HCO_3^- is the chloride–bicarbonate anion exchange that occurs in association with Na^+ reabsorption. Normally, Cl^- is absorbed along with Na^+ throughout the tubules. In situations of volume depletion because of vomiting and chloride depletion, the kidneys are forced to substitute HCO_3^- for the Cl^- anion, thereby increasing its absorption of HCO_3^-. *Hypochloremic alkalosis* refers to an increase in pH induced by excess HCO_3^- reabsorption because of a decrease in Cl^- levels, and *hyperchloremic acidosis* refers to a decrease in pH because of decreased HCO_3^- reabsorption because of an increase in Cl^- levels.

Laboratory Tests

Laboratory tests that are used in assessing acid–base balance include arterial blood gases and pH, CO_2 content and HCO_3^- levels, base excess or deficit, and blood and urine AGs. Although useful in determining whether acidosis or alkalosis is present, measurements of the blood pH provide little information about the cause of an acid–base disorder.

Carbon Dioxide and Bicarbonate Levels

The PCO_2 of the arterial blood gas measurement provides a means of assessing the respiratory component of acid–base balance. Arterial blood gases are used because venous blood gases are highly variable, depending on metabolic demands of the various tissues that empty into the vein from which the sample is being drawn. The H_2CO_3 levels can be determined from arterial blood gas measurements using the PCO_2 and the solubility coefficient for CO_2 (normal arterial PCO_2 is 35 to 45 mm Hg). Arterial blood gases also provide a measure of blood oxygen (PO_2) levels. This measure can be important in assessing respiratory function.

The CO_2 content refers to the total CO_2 in the blood, including dissolved CO_2, that is contained in HCO_3^-, and that attached to hemoglobin (carbaminohemoglobin [CO_2HHb]). The normal range of values for venous HCO_3^- concentration is 24 to 31 mEq/L (24 to 31 mmol/L), and arterial is 22 to 26 mEq/L.

Base Excess or Deficit

The total base excess or deficit, also referred to as the *whole blood buffer base*, measures the level of all the buffer systems of the blood—hemoglobin, protein, phosphate, and HCO_3^-. The base excess or deficit describes the amount of a fixed acid or base that must be added to a blood sample to achieve a pH of 7.4 (normal ± 2 mEq/L). For clinical purposes, base excess or deficit can be viewed as a measurement of bicarbonate excess or deficit and indicates a nonrespiratory change in acid–base balance. A base excess indicates metabolic alkalosis, and a base deficit indicates metabolic acidosis.

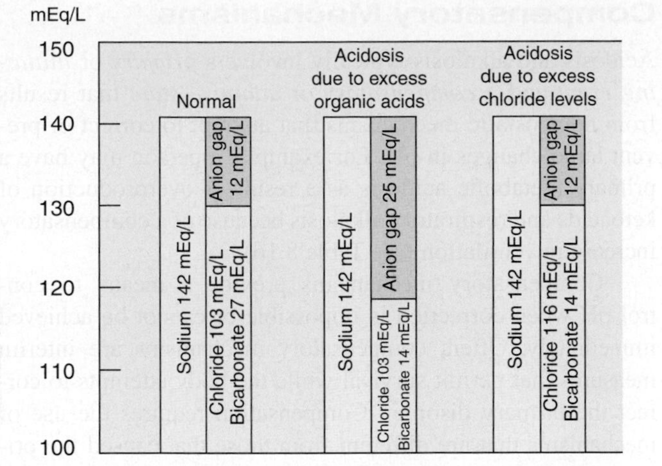

Figure 8.17 • The anion gap in acidosis because of excess metabolic acids and excess plasma chloride levels. Unmeasured anions such as phosphates, sulfates, and organic acids increase the anion gap because they replace bicarbonate. This assumes there is no change in sodium content.

Anion Gap

The AG, a diagnostic concept, describes the difference between the plasma concentration of the major measured cation (Na^+ and K+) and the sum of the measured anions (Cl^- and HCO_3^-).[44,51] This difference represents the concentration of unmeasured anions, such as phosphates, sulfates, organic acids, and proteins (Fig. 8.17). Normally, the AG measured by flame atomic emission spectrometry (FAES) ranges between 8 and 16 mEq/L[1] (a value range of 12 to 20 mEq/L is normal when potassium is included in the calculation).[52] Because albumin is an anion, it is often measured and used in determining the AG in people with decreased albumin levels. For every 1 g/dL decline in plasma albumin concentration, a correction factor should be added to the gap that is calculated from the formula: $AG = Na^+ - (Cl^- + HCO_3^-)$.[53] The AG is used typically in diagnosing causes of metabolic acidosis.[46,54,55] An increased level is found in conditions such as lactic acidosis, alcoholic acidosis, poisoning by substances such as salicylate and ethylene glycol (antifreeze), and ketoacidosis that result from elevated levels of metabolic acids.[44,51] A low AG is found in conditions that produce a fall in unmeasured anions (primarily albumin) or rise in unmeasured cations. The latter can occur in hyperkalemia, hypercalcemia, hypermagnesemia, lithium intoxication, or multiple myeloma, in which an abnormal immunoglobulin is produced.[51]

The AG of urine can be useful as a diagnostic tool in critically ill people.[11,13,15] Urine electrolyte determinations do not include bicarbonate. Instead, the urine AG uses the difference between the measurable cations (Na^+ and K^+) and anions (Cl^-) to provide an estimate of ammonium (NH_4^+) excretion.[55,56] Because ammonium is a cation, the value of the AG becomes more negative as the ammonium level increases. In normal persons secreting 20 to 40 mmol of ammonium per liter, the urine AG is close to zero representing electroneutrality. In metabolic acidosis, the amount of unmeasured NH_4^+ should increase if renal excretion of H^+ is intact; as a result, the urine AG should become more negative.

IN SUMMARY

Normal body function depends on the precise regulation of acid–base balance. The pH of the ECF is normally maintained within the narrow physiologic range of 7.35 to 7.45. Metabolic processes produce volatile and fixed or nonvolatile metabolic acids that must be buffered and eliminated from the body. The volatile acid, H_2CO_3, is in equilibrium with dissolved CO_2, which is eliminated through the lungs. The nonvolatile metabolic acids, which are derived mainly from protein metabolism and incomplete carbohydrate and fat metabolism, are excreted by the kidneys. It is the ratio of the HCO_3^- concentration to dissolved CO_2 (H_2CO_3 concentration) that determines the pH of the ECFs. When this ratio is 20:1, the pH is 7.4.

The ability of the body to maintain pH within the normal physiologic range depends on respiratory and renal mechanisms and on chemical buffers in the ICF and ECF, the most important of which is the HCO_3^- buffer system. The respiratory regulation of pH is rapid but does not return the pH completely to normal. The kidneys aid in regulation of pH by eliminating H^+ ions, conserving HCO_3^- ions, and producing new HCO_3^- ions. In the process of eliminating H^+, it uses the phosphate and ammonia buffer systems. Body pH is also affected by the distribution of exchangeable cations (K^+ and H^+) and anions (Cl^- and HCO_3^-).

Laboratory tests used in assessing acid–base balance include arterial blood gas measurements, CO_2 content and HCO_3^- levels, base excess or deficit, and the AG. The base excess or deficit describes the amount of a fixed acid or base that must be added to a blood sample to achieve a pH of 7.4. The AG describes the difference between the plasma concentration of the major measured cations (Na^+ and K+) and the sum of the anions (Cl^- and HCO_3^-). This difference represents the concentration of unmeasured anions, such as phosphates, sulfates, and organic acids, which are present. The urine AG uses the difference between the measurable cations (Na^+ and K^+) and anions (Cl^-) to provide an estimate of ammonium (NH_4^+) excretion and the ability of the kidney to rid the body of excess H^+.

DISORDERS OF ACID–BASE BALANCE

After completing this section of the chapter, the learner will be able to meet the following objectives:

- Define metabolic acidosis, metabolic alkalosis, respiratory acidosis, and respiratory alkalosis.
- Describe the common causes of metabolic and respiratory acidosis and metabolic and respiratory alkalosis.
- Contrast and compare the clinical manifestations and treatments of metabolic and respiratory acidosis and of metabolic and respiratory alkalosis.

The terms *acidosis* and *alkalosis* describe the clinical conditions that arise as a result of changes in dissolved CO_2 and HCO_3^- concentrations. An alkali represents a combination of one or more alkali metals such as sodium or potassium with a highly basic ion such as a hydroxyl ion (OH^-). Sodium bicarbonate is the main alkali in the ECF. Although the definitions differ somewhat, the terms *alkali* and *base* are often used interchangeably.[44] Hence, the term *alkalosis* has come to mean the opposite of *acidosis*. *Alkalosis* is removal of excess H+ ions from body fluids, whereas *acidosis* is the addition of excess H+ ions. Typically, imbalances in acid–base result in acidosis. Alkalosis is usually compensatory.

Metabolic Versus Respiratory Acid–Base Disorders

There are two types of acid–base disorders: metabolic and respiratory (Table 8.16). *Metabolic disorders* produce an alteration in the plasma HCO_3^- concentration and result from the addition to or loss from the ECF of nonvolatile acid or alkali. A reduction in pH because of a decrease in HCO_3^- is called *metabolic acidosis*, and an elevation in pH because of increased HCO_3^- levels is called *metabolic alkalosis. Respiratory disorders* involve an alteration in the PCO_2, reflecting an increase or decrease in alveolar ventilation. *Respiratory acidosis* is characterized by a decrease in pH, reflecting a decrease in ventilation and an increase in PCO_2. *Respiratory alkalosis* involves an increase in pH, resulting from an increase in alveolar ventilation and a decrease in PCO_2.

Compensatory Mechanisms

Acidosis and alkalosis typically involve a *primary* or *initiating event* and a *compensatory* or *adaptive state* that results from homeostatic mechanisms that attempt to correct or prevent large changes in pH. For example, a person may have a primary metabolic acidosis as a result of overproduction of ketoacids and respiratory alkalosis because of a compensatory increase in ventilation (see Table 8.16).

Compensatory mechanisms provide a means to control pH when correction is impossible or cannot be achieved immediately. Often, compensatory mechanisms are interim measures that permit survival while the body attempts to correct the primary disorder. Compensation requires the use of mechanisms that are different from those that caused the primary disorder. For example, the lungs cannot compensate for respiratory acidosis that is caused by lung disease, nor can the kidneys compensate for metabolic acidosis that occurs because of chronic kidney disease. The body can, however, use renal mechanisms to compensate for respiratory-induced changes in pH, and it can use respiratory mechanisms to compensate for metabolically induced changes in acid–base balance. Because compensatory mechanisms become more effective with time, there are often differences between the level of pH change that is present in acute and chronic acid–base disorders. There is a distinction between acute and chronic respiratory acid–base disorders but not for metabolic acid–base disorders.[46] This difference is because of the fact that renal compensation for a respiratory disorder may take days, but the respiratory compensation for a metabolic disorder is within minutes to hours.[46]

TABLE 8.16 SUMMARY OF SINGLE ACID–BASE DISTURBANCES AND THEIR COMPENSATORY RESPONSES

ACID–BASE IMBALANCE	PRIMARY DISTURBANCE	RESPIRATORY COMPENSATION AND PREDICTED RESPONSE*	RENAL COMPENSATION AND PREDICTED RESPONSE*,†
Metabolic acidosis	↓pH and HCO_3^- HCO_3^- < 22 mEq/L	↑ventilation and ↓PCO_2 *1 mEq/L ↓HCO_3^- → 1–1.2 mm Hg ↓PCO_2*	↑H^+ excretion and ↑HCO_3^- reabsorption if no renal disease
Metabolic alkalosis	↑pH and HCO_3^- HCO_3^- > 26 mEq/L	↓ventilation and ↑PCO_2 *1 mEq/L ↑HCO_3^- → 0.7 mm Hg ↑PCO_2*	↓H^+ excretion and ↓HCO_3^- reabsorption if no renal disease
Respiratory acidosis	↓pH and ↑PCO_2 PCO_2 > 45 mm Hg	None	↑H^+ excretion and ↑HCO_3^- reabsorption *Acute: 1 mm Hg ↑PCO_2 → 0.1 mEq/L ↑HCO_3^-* *Chronic: 1 mm Hg ↑PCO_2 → 0.3 mEq/L ↑HCO_3^-*
Respiratory alkalosis	↑pH and ↓PCO_2 PCO_2 < 35 mm Hg	None	↓H^+ excretion and ↓HCO_3^- reabsorption *Acute: 1 mm Hg ↓PCO_2 → 0.2 mEq/L ↓HCO_3^-* *Chronic: 1 mm Hg ↓PCO_2 → 0.4 mEq/L ↓HCO_3^-*

Note: Predicted compensatory responses are in *italics*.

*If blood values are the same as predicted compensatory values, a single acid–base disorder is present; if values are different, a mixed acid–base disorder is present.[1]

†Acute renal compensation refers to duration of minutes to several hours; chronic renal compensation refers to a duration of several days.[1]

Single Versus Mixed Acid–Base Disorders

Thus far, we have discussed acid–base disorders as if they existed as a single primary disorder such as metabolic acidosis, accompanied by a predicted compensatory response (*i.e.*, hyperventilation and respiratory alkalosis). It is not uncommon, however, for people to present with more than one primary disorder or a mixed disorder.[46] For example, a person may present with a low plasma HCO_3^- concentration because of metabolic acidosis and a high PCO_2 because of chronic lung disease. Values for the predicted renal or respiratory compensatory responses can be used in the diagnosis of these mixed acid–base disorders[46] (see Table 8.16). If the values for the compensatory response fall outside the predicted plasma values, it can then be concluded that more than one disorder (*i.e.*, a mixed disorder) is present. Because the respiratory response to changes in HCO_3^- occurs almost immediately, there is only one predicted compensatory response for primary metabolic acid–base disorders. This is in contrast to the primary respiratory disorders, which have two ranges of predicted values, one for the acute and one for the chronic response. Renal compensation takes several days to become fully effective. The acute compensatory response represents the HCO_3^- levels before renal compensation has occurred, and the chronic response after it has occurred. Thus, the values for the plasma pH tend to be more normal in the chronic phase.

KEY POINTS

METABOLIC ACID–BASE IMBALANCE

- Metabolic acidosis can be defined as a decrease in plasma HCO_3^- and pH that is caused by an excess of production or accumulation of fixed acids or loss of HCO_3^- ion. Compensatory responses include an increase in ventilation and elimination of CO_2 and the reabsorption and generation of bicarbonate by the kidney.
- Metabolic alkalosis can be defined as an increase in plasma HCO_3^- and pH that is initiated by excess H^+ ion loss or HCO_3^- ion gain and maintained by conditions that impair the ability of the kidney to excrete the excess HCO_3^- ion. Compensatory responses include a decreased respiratory rate with retention of PCO_2 and increased elimination of HCO_3^- by the kidney.

Metabolic Acidosis

Metabolic acidosis involves a decreased plasma HCO_3^- concentration along with a decrease in pH. It is the most common acid–base disorder. In metabolic acidosis, the body compensates for the decrease in pH by increasing the respiratory rate in an effort to decrease PCO_2 and H_2CO_3 levels. The PCO_2 can be expected to fall on average by 1.3 mm Hg for each 1-mEq/L fall in HCO_3^{-3} with a range of 1 to 1.5 mm Hg for each 1-mEq/L fall in HCO_3^-.

Etiology

Metabolic acidosis can be caused by one or more of the following four mechanisms:

1. Increased production of fixed metabolic acids or ingestion of fixed acids such as salicylic acid
2. Inability of the kidneys to excrete the fixed acids produced from normal metabolism
3. Excessive loss of bicarbonate through the kidneys or gastrointestinal tract
4. Increased plasma Cl^- concentration[44,53]

The AG is often useful in determining the cause of the metabolic acidosis (Chart 8.4). The presence of excess metabolic acids produces an increase in the AG as sodium salt of the offending acid (*e.g.*, sodium lactate) replaces sodium bicarbonate. Diarrhea is a frequent cause of a normal AG metabolic acidosis.[1] When the acidosis results from an increase in plasma Cl^- levels (*e.g.*, hyperchloremic acidosis), the AG also remains within normal levels. The pneumonic "MUDPILES" can be used to remember the most common etiologies of a high AG acidosis (Methanol, Uremia, Diabetic ketoacidosis,

CHART 8.4 THE ANION GAP IN DIFFERENTIAL DIAGNOSIS OF METABOLIC ACIDOSIS

Decreased Anion Gap (<8 mEq/L)[52]
Hypoalbuminemia (decrease in unmeasured anions)
Multiple myeloma (increase in unmeasured cationic IgG paraproteins)
Increased unmeasured cations (hyperkalemia, hypercalcemia, hypermagnesemia, lithium intoxication)

Increased Anion Gap (>16 mEq/L)[52]
Presence of unmeasured metabolic anion
- Diabetic ketoacidosis
- Alcoholic ketoacidosis
- Lactic acidosis
- Starvation
- Renal insufficiency

Presence of drug or chemical anion
- Salicylate poisoning
- Methanol poisoning
- Ethylene glycol poisoning

Normal Anion Gap (8 to 16 mEq/L)[52]
Loss of bicarbonate
- Diarrhea
- Pancreatic fluid loss
- Ileostomy (unadapted)

Chloride retention
- Renal tubular acidosis
- Ileal loop bladder
- Parenteral nutrition (arginine, histidine, and lysine)

TABLE 8.17 CAUSES AND MANIFESTATIONS OF METABOLIC ACIDOSIS

CAUSES	MANIFESTATIONS
Excess Metabolic Acids (Increased Anion Gap)	**Blood pH, HCO_3^-, CO_2**
Excessive production of metabolic acids	pH decreased
Lactic acidosis (*e.g.*, strenuous exercise)	HCO_3^- (primary) decreased
Diabetic ketoacidosis	PCO_2 (compensatory) decreased
Alcoholic ketoacidosis	**Gastrointestinal Function**
Fasting and starvation	Anorexia
Poisoning (*e.g.*, isoniazid, salicylate, methanol, paraldehyde, ethylene glycol)	Nausea and vomiting
Impaired elimination of metabolic acids	Abdominal pain
Kidney failure or dysfunction	**Neural Function**
Uremic acidosis (*e.g.*, severe renal failure)	Weakness
Excessive Bicarbonate Loss (Normal Anion Gap)	Lethargy
Loss of intestinal secretions	General malaise
Diarrhea (severe)	Confusion
Intestinal suction	Stupor
Intestinal or biliary fistula	Coma
Increased renal losses	Depression of vital functions
Renal tubular acidosis	**Cardiovascular Function**
Treatment with carbonic anhydrase inhibitors	Peripheral vasodilation
Hypoaldosteronism	Decreased heart rate
Increased Chloride Levels (Normal Anion Gap)	Cardiac arrhythmias
Excessive reabsorption of chloride by the kidney	**Skin**
Sodium chloride infusions	Warm and flushed
Treatment with ammonium chloride	**Skeletal System**
Parenteral hyperalimentation	Bone disease (*e.g.*, chronic acidosis)
	Signs of Compensation
	Increased rate and depth of respiration (*i.e.*, Kussmaul breathing)
	Hyperkalemia
	Acid urine
	Increased ammonia in urine

Paraldehyde, Isoniazid, Lactic acid, Ethanol [ethylene glycol], and Salicylates [starvation]). The causes of metabolic acidosis are summarized in Table 8.17.[58] Non–AG acidosis is most often caused by loss of large quantities of base because of profuse diarrhea or the administration of large amounts of solutions that contain chloride, causing the AG to fall within normal limits.[44]

Lactic Acidosis. Acute lactic acidosis is a common type of metabolic acidosis in people who are hospitalized and develops when there is excess production or diminished removal of lactic acid from the blood. Lactic acid is produced by the anaerobic metabolism of glucose. Most cases of lactic acidosis are caused by inadequate oxygen delivery, or hypoxia, as in shock or cardiac arrest.[59] Such conditions not only increase lactic acid production, but they tend to impair lactic acid clearance because of poor liver and kidney perfusion. Mortality rates are high for people with lactic acidosis because of shock and tissue hypoxia.[60] Severe sepsis is also commonly associated with lactic acidosis, and hyperlactatemia can be a strong predictor of mortality for people with sepsis.[61] Lactic acidosis can occur during periods of intense exercise in which the metabolic needs of the exercising muscles outpace their aerobic capacity for production of ATP, causing them to revert to anaerobic metabolism and the production of lactic acid.[60]

Lactic acidosis is associated with disorders in which tissue hypoxia does not appear to be present. It has been reported in people with leukemia, lymphomas, and other cancers; those with poorly controlled diabetes; and in people with severe liver failure. Mechanisms causing lactic acidosis in these conditions are poorly understood. Some conditions such as neoplasms may produce local increases in tissue metabolism and lactate production, or they may interfere with blood flow to noncancerous cells. Drugs can produce life-threatening lactic acidosis by inhibiting mitochondrial function predominantly in the liver. These drugs include the biguanide antidiabetic drugs (metformin).[56,62] Metformin-associated lactic acidosis (MALA) occurs as a result of the medication's effect on cells following an overdose of the drug; however, the reported incidence of acidosis has been low.[62,63] A relatively rare form of lactic acidosis, called D-lactic acidosis, can occur in people with intestinal disorders that involve the generation and absorption of D-lactic acid (L-lactic acid is the usual cause of lactic acidosis).[7,53] It most commonly occurs in people with jejunoileal bypass surgery for the treatment of obesity or who have short bowel syndrome, in which there is impaired absorption of carbohydrate in the small intestine. In these cases, the unabsorbed carbohydrate is delivered to the colon, where it is converted to D-lactic acid by an overgrowth of gram-positive anaerobes. People with D-lactic acidosis experience episodic periods of metabolic acidosis often brought on by eating a meal high in carbohydrates. Neurologic manifestations include confusion, cerebellar ataxia, slurred speech, and loss of memory. They may complain of feeling (or appear) intoxicated. Treatment includes use of antimicrobial agents to decrease the number of D-lactic acid–producing microorganisms in the bowel along with a low-carbohydrate diet.

Ketoacidosis. Ketoacids (*i.e.*, acetoacetic and β-hydroxybutyric acid), produced in the liver from fatty acids, are the source of fuel for many body tissues. An overproduction of ketoacids occurs when carbohydrate stores are inadequate or when the body cannot use available carbohydrates as a fuel. Under these conditions, fatty acids are mobilized from adipose tissue and delivered to the liver, where they are converted to ketones. Ketoacidosis develops when ketone production by the liver exceeds tissue use.[49]

A common cause of ketoacidosis is uncontrolled diabetes mellitus, in which an insulin deficiency leads to the release of fatty acids from adipose cells with subsequent production of excess ketoacids. Ketoacidosis may also develop as the result of fasting or food deprivation, during which the lack of carbohydrates produces a self-limited state of ketoacidosis.[64]

Ketones are formed during the oxidation of alcohol, a process that occurs in the liver. A condition called *alcoholic ketoacidosis* can develop in people who engage in excess alcohol consumption and can be fatal clinically.[64,65] It usually follows prolonged alcohol ingestion, particularly if accompanied by decreased food intake and vomiting: conditions that result in using fatty acids as an energy source. Ketone formation may be further enhanced by the hypoglycemia that results from alcohol-induced inhibition of glucose synthesis (*i.e.*, gluconeogenesis) by the liver and impaired ketone elimination by the kidneys because of dehydration. An ECF volume deficit caused by vomiting and decreased fluid intake often contributes to the acidosis. Numerous other factors, such as elevations in cortisol, growth hormone, glucagon, and catecholamines, mediate free fatty acid release and thereby contribute to the development of alcoholic ketoacidosis. Diagnosis is difficult because of a variety of nonspecific clinical manifestations; however, the condition is treatable if recognized early and managed appropriately.[65]

Salicylate Toxicity. Salicylates are another potential source of metabolic acids. Acetylsalicylic acid (Aspirin) is readily absorbed in the stomach and small bowel and then rapidly converted to salicylic acid in the body. Although aspirin is the most common cause of salicylate toxicity, other salicylate preparations such as methyl salicylate, sodium salicylate, and salicylic acid may produce similar effects. Salicylate overdose produces serious toxic effects, including death. Serum salicylate levels along with clinical findings are important in predicting morbidity and mortality following ingestion.[66]

A variety of acid–base disturbances occur with salicylate toxicity. The salicylates cross the blood–brain barrier and directly stimulate the respiratory center, causing hyperventilation and respiratory alkalosis. The kidneys compensate by secreting increased amounts of HCO_3^-, K^+, and Na^+, thereby contributing to the development of metabolic acidosis. Salicylates also interfere with carbohydrate metabolism, which results in increased production of metabolic acids.

One of the treatments for salicylate toxicity is *alkalinization* of the plasma. Salicylic acid, which is a weak acid, exists in equilibrium with the alkaline salicylate anion. It is the salicylic acid that is toxic because of its ability to cross cell membranes and enter brain cells. The salicylate anion crosses membranes poorly and is less toxic. With alkalinization of the ECF, the ratio of salicylic acid to salicylate is greatly reduced. This allows salicylic acid to move out of cells into the ECF along a concentration gradient. The renal elimination of salicylates follows a similar pattern when the urine is alkalinized.

Methanol and Ethylene Glycol Toxicity. Ingestion of methanol and ethylene glycol results in the production of metabolic acids and causes metabolic acidosis. Both produce an osmolar gap because of their small size and osmotic properties. Methanol (wood alcohol) is a component of shellac, varnish, deicing solutions, and other commercial products. A person addicted to alcohol sometimes consumes it as a substitution for ethanol.[49] Methanol can be absorbed through the skin or gastrointestinal tract or inhaled through the lungs. A dose as small as one ounce can be toxic. In addition to metabolic acidosis, methanol produces severe optic nerve and CNS toxicity. Organ system damage occurs after a 24-hour period in which methanol is converted to formaldehyde and formic acid.

Ethylene glycol is a solvent found in products ranging from antifreeze and deicing solutions to carpet and fabric cleaners. It tastes sweet and is intoxicating. These factors contribute to its abuse potential in adults as it can serve as a substitute for ethanol, but toxicity is most commonly found in children because of its bright colors and sweet taste.[67,68] It is rapidly absorbed from the intestine, making treatment with gastric lavage and syrup of ipecac ineffective. Acidosis occurs as ethylene glycol is converted to oxalic and lactic acid. Manifestations of ethylene glycol toxicity occur in three stages:

1. Neurologic symptoms within the CNS ranging from drunkenness to coma, which appear during the first 12 hours
2. Metabolic acidosis and cardiopulmonary symptoms such as tachycardia and pulmonary edema

3. Flank pain and acute renal failure caused by plugging of the tubules with oxalate crystals (from excess oxalic acid production) which results in oliguria/anuria[67]

The enzyme *alcohol dehydrogenase* metabolizes methanol and ethylene glycol into their toxic metabolites. This is the same enzyme that is used in the metabolism of ethanol. Because alcohol dehydrogenase has a greater affinity for ethanol than its affinity for methanol or ethylene glycol, intravenous or oral ethanol is used as an antidote for methanol and ethylene glycol poisoning. Extracellular volume expansion and hemodialysis are also used. Fomepizole (Antizol) is approved by The U.S. Food and Drug Administration as an antidote for methanol and ethylene glycol poisoning.[67,68] Fomepizole is thought to act as an inhibitor of alcohol dehydrogenase, thereby preventing the formation of the toxic ethylene glycol metabolites.

Decreased Renal Function. Chronic kidney disease is the most common cause of chronic metabolic acidosis. The kidneys normally conserve HCO_3^- and secrete H^+ ions into the urine as a means of regulating acid–base balance. In chronic kidney disease, there is loss of both glomerular and tubular function, with retention of nitrogenous wastes and metabolic acids. The most prominent effect of these changes is on the musculoskeletal system. In a condition called *renal tubular acidosis*, glomerular function is normal or mildly impaired, but the tubular secretion of H^+ or reabsorption of HCO_3^- is abnormal.[69]

Increased Bicarbonate Losses. Increased HCO_3^- losses occur with the loss of bicarbonate-rich body fluids or with impaired conservation of HCO_3^- by the kidney. Intestinal secretions have a high HCO_3^- concentration. Consequently, excessive loss of HCO_3^- occurs with severe diarrhea; small bowel, pancreatic, or biliary fistula drainage; ileostomy drainage; and intestinal suction. In diarrhea of microbial origin, HCO_3^- is also secreted into the bowel as a means of neutralizing the metabolic acids produced by the microorganisms causing the diarrhea. Creation of an ileal bladder, which is done for conditions such as neurogenic bladder or surgical removal of the bladder because of cancer, involves the implantation of the ureters into a short, isolated loop of ileum that serves as a conduit for urine collection. With this procedure, contact time between the urine and ileal bladder is normally too short for significant anion exchange, and HCO_3^- is lost in the urine.[70]

Hyperchloremic Acidosis. Hyperchloremic acidosis occurs when Cl^- levels are increased out of proportion to sodium.[53] Because Cl^- and HCO_3^- are exchangeable anions, the plasma HCO_3^- decreases when there is an increase in Cl^-. Hyperchloremic acidosis can occur as the result of abnormal absorption of Cl^- by the kidneys or as a result of treatment with chloride-containing medications (*i.e.*, sodium chloride, amino acid–chloride hyperalimentation solutions, and ammonium chloride). Ammonium chloride is broken down into NH_4^+ and Cl^-. The ammonium ion is converted to urea in the liver, leaving the Cl^- free to react with H^+ to form HCl. The administration of intravenous sodium chloride or parenteral hyperalimentation solutions that contain an amino acid–chloride combination can cause acidosis in a similar manner.[12] With hyperchloremic acidosis, the AG remains within the normal range, whereas plasma Cl^- levels are increased and plasma HCO_3^- levels are decreased.

Clinical Manifestations

Metabolic acidosis is characterized by a decrease in pH (<7.35) and HCO_3^- levels (<22 mEq/L) because of a gain in H^+ or a loss of HCO_3^-. Acidosis typically produces a compensatory increase in respiratory rate with a decrease in PCO_2.

The manifestations of metabolic acidosis fall into three categories:

1. Signs and symptoms of the disorder causing the acidosis
2. Changes in body function related to recruitment of compensatory mechanisms
3. Alterations in cardiovascular, neurologic, and musculoskeletal function resulting from the decreased pH (see Table 8.17)

The signs and symptoms of metabolic acidosis usually begin to appear when the plasma HCO_3^- concentration falls to 20 mEq/L or less. A fall in pH to less than 7.1 to 7.2 can reduce cardiac output and predispose to potentially fatal cardiac arrhythmias.

Metabolic acidosis is seldom a primary disorder. It usually develops during the course of another disease.[49] The manifestations of metabolic acidosis frequently are superimposed on the symptoms of the contributing health problem. With diabetic ketoacidosis, which is a common cause of metabolic acidosis, there is an increase in blood and urine glucose and a characteristic smell of ketones to the breath. In the metabolic acidosis that accompanies chronic kidney disease, BUN levels are elevated and other tests of renal function yield abnormal results.

Clinical manifestations related to respiratory and renal compensatory mechanisms usually occur early in the course of metabolic acidosis. In situations of acute metabolic acidosis, the respiratory system compensates for a decrease in pH by increasing ventilation to reduce PCO_2. This is accomplished through deep and rapid respirations. In diabetic ketoacidosis, this breathing pattern is referred to as *Kussmaul breathing.* For descriptive purposes, it can be said that Kussmaul breathing resembles the hyperpnea of exercise—the person breathes as though he or she had been running. There may be complaints of difficulty breathing or dyspnea with exertion. With severe acidosis, dyspnea may be present even at rest. Respiratory compensation for acute acidosis tends to be somewhat greater than for chronic acidosis. When kidney function is normal, H^+ excretion increases promptly in response to acidosis, and the urine becomes more acidic.

Changes in pH have a direct effect on body function that can produce signs and symptoms common to most types of metabolic acidosis, regardless of cause. People with metabolic acidosis often complain of weakness, fatigue, general malaise, and a dull headache. They also may have anorexia, nausea, vomiting, and abdominal pain. Tissue turgor is impaired, and the skin is dry when fluid deficit accompanies acidosis. In people with undiagnosed diabetes mellitus, the nausea, vomiting, and abdominal symptoms may be misinterpreted as being caused by gastrointestinal flu or other abdominal disease, such as appendicitis. Acidosis depresses neuronal excitability, and it decreases binding of calcium to plasma proteins, so that more free calcium is available to decrease neural activity. As acidosis progresses, the level of consciousness declines, and stupor and coma develop. The skin is often warm and flushed because blood vessels in the skin become less responsive to sympathetic nervous system stimulation and lose their tone.

When the pH falls to 7.1 to 7.2, cardiac contractility and cardiac output decrease, the heart becomes less responsive to catecholamines (*i.e.*, epinephrine and norepinephrine), and arrhythmias, including fatal ventricular arrhythmias, can develop. A decrease in ventricular function may be particularly important in perpetuating shock-induced lactic acidosis, and partial correction of the acidemia may be necessary before tissue perfusion can be restored.

Chronic acidemia, as in chronic kidney disease, can lead to a variety of musculoskeletal problems, some of which result from the release of calcium and phosphate during bone buffering of excess H^+ ions.[46] Of particular importance is impaired growth in children. In infants and children, acidemia may be associated with a variety of nonspecific symptoms such as anorexia, weight loss, muscle weakness, and listlessness. Muscle weakness and listlessness may result from alterations in muscle metabolism.

Treatment

The treatment of metabolic acidosis focuses on correcting the condition that caused the disorder and restoring the fluids and electrolytes that have been lost from the body. The use of supplemental sodium bicarbonate ($NaHCO_3$) has been the mainstay of treatment for some forms of normal AG acidosis.[56] In most people with circulatory shock, cardiac arrest, or sepsis, impaired oxygen delivery is the primary cause of lactic acidosis. In these situations, the administration of large amounts of $NaHCO_3$ does not improve oxygen delivery nor the underlying metabolic problem.[46] With lactic acidosis, treatment measures to improve tissue perfusion are necessary, and with sepsis-related acidosis, treatment of the infection is essential.

Metabolic Alkalosis

Metabolic alkalosis is a systemic disorder caused by an increase in plasma pH because of a primary excess in HCO_3^-.[44,54] It can result from a variety of situations including ingestion of antacids, vomiting, and renal loss of H+.

Etiology

Metabolic alkalosis can be caused by factors that generate a loss of fixed acids or a gain of bicarbonate and those that maintain the alkalosis by interfering with excretion of the excess bicarbonate (Table 8.18). They include

TABLE 8.18 CAUSES AND MANIFESTATIONS OF METABOLIC ALKALOSIS

CAUSES	MANIFESTATIONS
Excessive Gain of Bicarbonate or Alkali	**Blood pH, HCO_3^-, CO_2**
Ingestion or administration of $NaHCO_3$	pH increased
Administration of hyperalimentation solutions containing acetate	HCO_3^- (primary) increased
Administration of parenteral solutions containing lactate	PCO_2 (compensatory) increased
Administration of citrate-containing blood transfusions	**Neural Function**
Excessive Loss of Hydrogen Ions	Confusion
Vomiting	Hyperactive reflexes
Gastric suction	Tetany
Binge–purge syndrome	Convulsions
Potassium deficit (severe)	**Cardiovascular Function**
Diuretic therapy	Hypotension
Hyperaldosteronism	Arrhythmias
Milk-alkali syndrome	**Respiratory Function**
Increased Bicarbonate Retention	Respiratory acidosis because of decreased respiratory rate
Loss of chloride with bicarbonate retention	**Signs of Compensation**
Volume Contraction	Decreased rate and depth of respiration
Loss of body fluids	Increased urine pH
Diuretic therapy	

1. A gain of base through the oral or intravenous route
2. Loss of fixed acids from the stomach
3. Maintenance of the increased bicarbonate levels by contraction of the ECF volume, hypokalemia, and hypochloremia

Excess Base Loading. Because the normal kidney is extremely efficient at excreting bicarbonate, excess base intake is rarely a cause of significant chronic metabolic alkalosis. Transient acute alkalosis, on the other hand, is a rather common occurrence during or immediately after excess oral ingestion of bicarbonate-containing antacids (*e.g.*, Alka-Seltzer) or intravenous infusion of $NaHCO_3$ or base equivalent (*e.g.*, acetate in hyperalimentation solutions, lactate in Ringer lactate, and citrate in blood transfusions). A condition called the *milk-alkali syndrome* occurs when chronic ingestion of milk or calcium carbonate antacids leads to hypercalcemia and metabolic alkalosis. This condition was more common at the beginning of the last century. Nowadays, the condition is called calcium–alkali syndrome (CAS).[13,56] In this case, the antacids raise the plasma HCO_3^- concentration, whereas the hypercalcemia prevents the urinary excretion of HCO_3^-. The most common cause at present is the chronic administration of calcium carbonate for dyspepsia and gastroesophageal reflux disease (GERD) as well as a supplement with vitamin D for postmenopausal women and older adults for the prevention of osteoporosis.[71]

Loss of Fixed Acid. The loss of fixed acids occurs mainly through the loss of acid from the stomach and the loss of chloride in the urine. Vomiting and removal of gastric secretions by nasogastric suction are common causes of metabolic alkalosis in acutely ill or hospitalized people. Gastric secretions contain high concentrations of HCl and lesser concentrations of potassium chloride (KCl). As Cl^- is taken from the blood and secreted into the stomach, it is replaced by HCO_3^-. Thus, the loss of gastric secretions through vomiting or gastric suction is a common cause of metabolic alkalosis. The accompanying ECF volume depletion, hypochloremia, and hypokalemia serve to maintain the metabolic alkalosis by increasing HCO_3^- reabsorption by the kidneys (Fig. 8.18).

The loop (*e.g.*, furosemide [Lasix]) and thiazide (*e.g.*, hydrochlorothiazide) diuretics are commonly associated with metabolic alkalosis, the severity of which varies directly with the degree of diuresis. The volume contraction and loss of H^+ in the urine contribute to the problem. The latter is primarily because of the enhanced H^+ secretion in the distal tubule that results from an interplay between the diuretic-induced increase in Na^+ delivery to the distal tubule and collecting duct, where an accelerated excretion of H^+ and K^+ takes place, and an increase in aldosterone secretion resulting from the volume contraction. Although aldosterone blunts the loss of Na^+, it also accelerates the secretion of K^+ and H^+. The resulting loss of K^+ also accelerates HCO_3^- reabsorption.

Metabolic alkalosis can also occur with abrupt correction of respiratory acidosis in people with chronic respiratory acidosis. Chronic respiratory acidosis is associated with a compensatory loss of H^+ and Cl^- in the urine along with HCO_3^- retention. When respiratory acidosis is corrected abruptly, as with mechanical ventilation, a "posthypercapneic" metabolic alkalosis may develop because although the PCO_2 drops rapidly, the plasma HCO_3^-, which must be eliminated through the kidney, remains elevated.

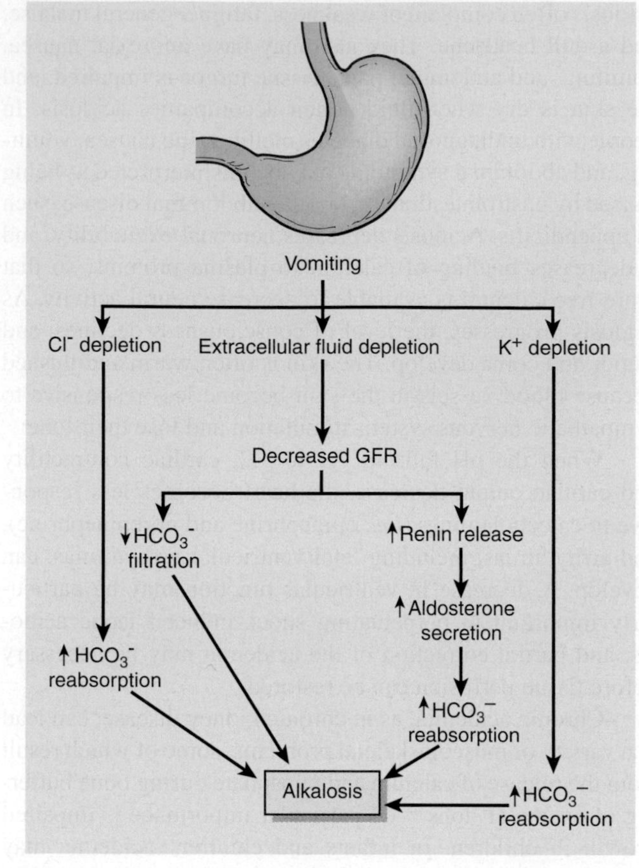

Figure 8.18 • Renal mechanisms for bicarbonate (HCO_3^-) reabsorption and maintenance of metabolic alkalosis after depletion of ECF volume, chloride (Cl^-), and potassium (K^+) because of vomiting. GFR, glomerular filtration rate.

Maintenance of Metabolic Alkalosis. Maintenance of metabolic alkalosis resides within the kidney and its inability to rid the body of excess HCO_3^-. Many of the conditions that accompany the development of metabolic alkalosis, such as contraction of the ECF volume, hypochloremia, and hypokalemia, also increase reabsorption of HCO_3^- by the kidney, thereby contributing to its maintenance.

Depletion of the ECF causes a decline in the glomerular filtration rate with a subsequent increase in Na^+ and H_2O reabsorption. When there is Cl^- depletion from loss of HCl, the available anion for reabsorption with Na^+ is HCO_3^-. Hypokalemia, which generally accompanies metabolic alkalosis, also contributes to its maintenance. This is due partly to the direct effect of alkalosis on potassium excretion by the kidney and partly to a secondary hyperaldosteronism resulting from volume depletion. In hypokalemia, the distal tubular reabsorption of K^+ is accompanied by an increase in H^+

secretion. The secondary hyperaldosteronism, in turn, promotes extensive reabsorption of Na^+ from the distal and collecting tubules and at the same time stimulates the secretion of H^+ from cells in the collecting tubules. Hypokalemia induced in this manner further worsens the metabolic alkalosis by increasing HCO_3^- reabsorption in the proximal tubule and H^+ secretion in the distal tubule.

Clinical Manifestations

Metabolic alkalosis is characterized by a pH above 7.45, HCO_3^- above 26 mEq/L (26 mmol/L), and base excess above 2 mEq/L (2 mmol/L; see Table 8.18). People with metabolic alkalosis often are asymptomatic or have signs related to ECF volume depletion or hypokalemia. Neurologic signs and symptoms (*e.g.*, hyperexcitability) occur less frequently with metabolic alkalosis than with other acid–base disorders because HCO_3^- enters the CSF more slowly than CO_2. When neurologic manifestations do occur, as in acute and severe metabolic alkalosis, they include mental confusion, hyperactive reflexes, tetany, and carpopedal spasm. Metabolic alkalosis also leads to a compensatory hypoventilation with development of various degrees of hypoxemia and respiratory acidosis. Significant morbidity occurs with severe metabolic alkalosis (pH > 7.55), including respiratory failure, cardiac arrhythmias, seizures, and coma.

Treatment

The treatment of metabolic alkalosis usually is directed toward correcting the cause of the condition. A chloride deficit requires correction. Potassium chloride usually is the treatment of choice when there is an accompanying K^+ deficit. When KCl is used as a therapy, the Cl^- anion replaces the HCO_3^- anion and the K^+ corrects the potassium deficit, allowing the kidneys to retain H^+ while eliminating K^+. Fluid replacement with normal saline or one-half normal saline often is used in treatment of volume contraction alkalosis.

Respiratory Acidosis

Respiratory acidosis occurs in conditions that impair alveolar ventilation and cause an increase in plasma PCO_2, also known as hypercapnia, along with a decrease in pH. Respiratory acidosis can occur as an acute or chronic disorder, but occurs most often as a result of decreased ventilation.[54] Acute respiratory failure is associated with a rapid rise in arterial PCO_2 with a minimal increase in plasma HCO_3^- and large decrease in pH. Chronic respiratory acidosis is characterized by a sustained increase in arterial PCO_2, resulting in renal adaptation with a more marked increase in plasma HCO_3^- and a lesser decrease in pH.

Etiology

Respiratory acidosis occurs in acute or chronic conditions that impair effective alveolar ventilation and cause an accumulation of PCO_2 (Table 8.19). Impaired ventilation can occur as the result of decreased respiratory drive, lung disease, or disorders of chest wall and respiratory muscles. Less commonly, it results from excess CO_2 production.

TABLE 8.19 CAUSES AND MANIFESTATIONS OF RESPIRATORY ACIDOSIS

CAUSES	MANIFESTATIONS
Depression of Respiratory Center	**Blood pH, CO_2, HCO_3^-**
Drug overdose	pH decreased
Head injury	PCO_2 (primary) increased
	HCO_3^- (compensatory) increased
Lung Disease	**Neural Function**
Bronchial asthma	Dilation of cerebral vessels and depression of neural function
Emphysema	Headache
Chronic bronchitis	Weakness
Pneumonia	Behavior changes
Pulmonary edema	Confusion
Respiratory distress syndrome	Depression
Airway Obstruction, Disorders of Chest Wall and Respiratory Muscles	Paranoia
Paralysis of respiratory muscles	Hallucinations
Chest injuries	Tremors
Kyphoscoliosis	Paralysis
Extreme obesity	Stupor and coma
Treatment with paralytic drugs	
Breathing Air with High CO_2 Content	**Skin**
	Skin warm and flushed
	Signs of Compensation
	Acid urine

Acute Disorders of Ventilation. Acute respiratory acidosis can be caused by impaired function of the respiratory center in the medulla (as in narcotic overdose), lung disease, chest injury, weakness of the respiratory muscles, or airway obstruction. Almost all people with acute respiratory acidosis are hypoxemic if they are breathing room air. In many cases, signs of hypoxemia develop before those of respiratory acidosis because CO_2 diffuses across the alveolar capillary membrane 20 times more rapidly than oxygen.[44]

Chronic Disorders of Ventilation. Chronic respiratory acidosis is a relatively common disturbance in people with chronic obstructive lung disease. In these people, the persistent elevation of PCO_2 stimulates renal H^+ secretion and HCO_3^- reabsorption. The effectiveness of these compensatory mechanisms can often return the pH to near-normal values as long as oxygen levels are maintained within a range that does not unduly suppress chemoreceptor control of respirations.

An acute episode of respiratory acidosis can develop in people with chronic lung disease who receive oxygen therapy at a flow rate that is sufficient to raise their PO_2 to a level that produces a decrease in ventilation. In these people, the medullary respiratory center has adapted to the elevated levels of CO_2 and no longer responds to increases in PCO_2. Instead, a decrease in the PO_2 becomes the major stimulus for respiration. If oxygen is administered at a flow rate that is sufficient to suppress this stimulus, the rate and depth of respiration decrease, and the PCO_2 increases. Any person who is in need of additional oxygen should have it administered, albeit at a flow rate that does not depress the respiratory drive.

Increased Carbon Dioxide Production. Carbon dioxide is a product of the body's metabolic processes, generating a substantial amount of acid that must be excreted by the lungs or kidneys to prevent acidosis. An increase in CO_2 production can result from numerous processes, including exercise, fever, sepsis, and burns. Nutrition also affects the production of carbon dioxide. A carbohydrate-rich diet produces larger amounts of CO_2 than one containing reasonable amounts of protein and fat. Although excess CO_2 production can lead to an increase in PCO_2, it seldom does. In healthy people, an increase in CO_2 is usually matched by an increase in CO_2 elimination by the lungs. In contrast, people with respiratory diseases may be unable to eliminate the excess CO_2.

Clinical Manifestations

Respiratory acidosis is associated with a pH below 7.35 and a PCO_2 above 45 mm Hg (see Table 8.19). The clinical manifestations of respiratory acidosis depend on the rapidity of onset and whether the condition is acute or chronic. Because respiratory acidosis often is accompanied by hypoxemia, the manifestations of respiratory acidosis often are intermixed with those of oxygen deficit. Carbon dioxide readily crosses the blood–brain barrier, exerting its effects by changing the pH of brain fluids. Elevated levels of CO_2 produce vasodilation of cerebral blood vessels, causing headache, blurred vision, irritability, muscle twitching, and psychological disturbances. If the condition is severe and prolonged, it can cause an increase in CSF pressure and papilledema. Impaired consciousness, ranging from lethargy to coma, develops as the PCO_2 rises to extreme levels. Paralysis of the extremities may occur, and there may be respiratory depression. Less severe forms of acidosis often are accompanied by warm and flushed skin, weakness, and tachycardia.

Treatment

The treatment of acute and chronic respiratory acidosis is directed toward improving ventilation. In severe cases, mechanical ventilation may be necessary.

KEY POINTS

RESPIRATORY ACID–BASE IMBALANCE

- Respiratory acidosis, or hypercapnia, represents an increase in PCO_2 and a decrease in plasma pH, resulting from a decrease in effective alveolar ventilation. Compensatory mechanisms include increased conservation and generation of HCO_3^- and elimination of H^+ by the kidney.
- Respiratory alkalosis, or hypocapnia, represents a decrease in PCO_2 and an increase in plasma pH, resulting from increased alveolar ventilation. Compensatory mechanisms include increased elimination of HCO_3^- and conservation of H^+ by the kidney.

Respiratory Alkalosis

Respiratory alkalosis is a systemic acid–base disorder characterized by a primary decrease in plasma PCO_2, also referred to as hypocapnia, which produces an elevation in pH and a subsequent decrease in HCO_3^-. Because respiratory alkalosis can occur suddenly, a compensatory decrease in bicarbonate level may not occur before respiratory correction has taken place.

Etiology

Respiratory alkalosis is caused by hyperventilation or a respiratory rate in excess of that needed to maintain normal plasma PCO_2 levels (Table 8.20). It may occur as the result of central stimulation of the medullary respiratory center or stimulation of peripheral (*e.g.*, carotid chemoreceptor) pathways to the medullary respiratory center, but rarely does it occur as a result of a physical pathologic condition.[44]

Mechanical ventilation may produce respiratory alkalosis if the rate and tidal volume are set, so that CO_2 elimination exceeds CO_2 production. Carbon dioxide crosses the alveolar capillary membrane 20 times more rapidly than oxygen. Therefore, increased minute ventilation may be necessary to maintain adequate oxygen levels while producing a concomitant decrease in CO_2 levels. Respiratory alkalosis is seen as a treatment with the ventilator with intubated people

TABLE 8.20 CAUSES AND MANIFESTATIONS OF RESPIRATORY ALKALOSIS

CAUSES	MANIFESTATIONS
Excessive Ventilation	**Blood pH, CO_2, HCO_3^-**
Anxiety and psychogenic hyperventilation	pH increased
Hypoxia and reflex stimulation of ventilation	PCO_2 (primary) decreased
Lung disease that causes a reflex stimulation of ventilation	HCO_3^- (compensatory) decreased
Stimulation of respiratory center	**Neural Function**
Elevated blood ammonia level	Constriction of cerebral vessels and increased neuronal excitability
Salicylate toxicity	Dizziness, panic, light-headedness
Encephalitis	Tetany
Fever	Numbness and tingling of fingers and toes
Mechanical ventilation	Positive Chvostek and Trousseau signs
	Seizures
	Cardiovascular Function
	Cardiac arrhythmias

experiencing high intracranial pressure (ICP) in order to attempt to lower the ICP.

Central stimulation of the medullary respiratory center occurs with anxiety, pain, pregnancy, febrile states, sepsis, encephalitis, and salicylate toxicity. Respiratory alkalosis has long been recognized as an acid–base disorder in people who are critically ill, and is a consistent finding in pulmonary embolism and congestive heart failure.

One of the most common causes of respiratory alkalosis is hyperventilation, which is characterized by recurring episodes of over-breathing often associated with voluntary effort, anxiety, direct stimulation of the respiratory center by an abnormality such as fever and salicylate intoxication, and hypoxia from severe anemia.[46] People experiencing panic attacks frequently present in the emergency department with manifestations of acute respiratory alkalosis.

A physiologic type of respiratory alkalosis can occur when a person climbs to high altitudes.[46] The lower oxygen content in the air stimulates the respiratory rate. This increased rate causes loss of CO_2 and results in a mild form of respiratory alkalosis. Typically, the body will compensate for this through the kidneys to increase HCO_3^- excretion.[44,46]

Hypoxemia exerts its effect on pH through the peripheral chemoreceptors in the carotid bodies. Stimulation of peripheral chemoreceptors occurs in conditions that cause hypoxemia with relatively unimpaired CO_2 transport, such as exposure to high altitudes.

Clinical Manifestations

Respiratory alkalosis manifests with a decrease in PCO_2 and a deficit in H_2CO_3 (see Table 8.20). In respiratory alkalosis, the pH is above 7.45, PCO_2 is below 35 mm Hg, and HCO_3^- levels usually are below 22 mEq/L (22 mmol/L).

The signs and symptoms of respiratory alkalosis are associated with hyperexcitability of the nervous system and a decrease in cerebral blood flow. Alkalosis increases protein binding of extracellular calcium. This reduces ionized calcium levels, causing an increase in neuromuscular excitability. A decrease in the CO_2 content of the blood causes constriction of cerebral blood vessels. Because CO_2 crosses the blood–brain barrier rather quickly, the manifestations of acute respiratory alkalosis are usually of sudden onset. The person often experiences light-headedness, dizziness, tingling, and numbness of the fingers and toes. Sweating, palpitations, panic, air hunger, and dyspnea may accompany these manifestations. Chvostek and Trousseau signs may be positive and tetany and convulsions may occur. Because CO_2 provides the stimulus for short-term regulation of respiration, short periods of apnea may occur in people with acute episodes of hyperventilation.

Treatment

Because respiratory alkalosis is typically a compensatory state, it is should not be treated directly. Thus, the treatment of respiratory alkalosis focuses on measures to correct the underlying cause. Hypoxia may be corrected by administration of supplemental oxygen. Changing ventilator settings may be used to prevent or treat respiratory alkalosis in persons who are being mechanically ventilated. People with hyperventilation may benefit from reassurance, rebreathing from a paper bag during symptomatic attacks, and attention to the psychological stress.

IN SUMMARY

Acidosis describes a decrease in pH and alkalosis an increase in pH. Acid–base disorders may be caused by alterations in the body's volatile acids (*i.e.*, respiratory acidosis or respiratory alkalosis) or nonvolatile or fixed acids (*i.e.*, metabolic acidosis or metabolic alkalosis). Acidosis and alkalosis typically involve a primary or initiating event and a compensatory or adaptive state that results from homeostatic mechanisms that attempt to prevent or correct large changes in pH. A mixed acid–base disorder is one in which there is both a primary and a compensatory change in acid–base balance.

Metabolic acidosis is defined as a decrease in pH because of a decrease in the HCO_3^- level, and metabolic alkalosis as an increase in pH because of an increase in the HCO_3^- level. Metabolic acidosis is caused by an increased production of nonvolatile metabolic acids such as lactic acid or ketoacids, decreased acid excretion by the kidney, excessive loss of HCO_3^- as in diarrhea, or an increase in Cl^-. Metabolic acidosis may present with an increased AG in which sodium bicarbonate is replaced by the sodium salt of the offending anion, or with a normal AG when HCO_3^- is replaced by Cl^-. Metabolic alkalosis involves generation of the increased pH and HCO_3^- levels through a loss of H^+ or gain of HCO_3^-, and the maintenance of the alkalotic state because of the kidney's failure to eliminate the excess HCO_3^- owing to an accompanying ECF volume contraction, increased aldosterone levels, and decreased Cl^- and K^+ levels.

Respiratory acidosis reflects an increase in PCO_2 levels and is caused by conditions that impair alveolar ventilation. It can occur as an acute disorder in which there is a rapid rise in PCO_2, a minimal increase in plasma HCO_3^-, and a large decrease in pH. Respiratory alkalosis is caused by conditions that cause hyperventilation and a reduction in PCO_2 levels. Because respiratory alkalosis often occurs suddenly, a compensatory decrease in HCO_3^- levels may not occur before corrections have been accomplished.

The signs and symptoms of acidosis and alkalosis reflect alterations in body function associated with the disorder causing the acid–base disturbance, the effect of the change of pH on body function, and the body's attempt to correct and maintain the pH within a normal physiologic range. In general, neuromuscular excitability is decreased in acidosis and increased in alkalosis.

GERIATRIC Considerations

- Dehydration can be life-threatening in older adults because they already have a reduced amount of body fluid. Skin turgor, concentrated urine, and elevated blood urea nitrogen (greater than 60 mg/dL) are clinical signs of dehydration. Confusion often accompanies dehydration in older adults.[72]
- Electrolyte replacements may have an increased bitter taste because of loss of taste buds for sweetness that occurs with age.[72]
- Older adults are at high risk for fluid and electrolyte imbalances because of inability to easily compensate for imbalances associated with impaired renal and pulmonary function. Polypharmacy and certain medications (*e.g.*, diuretics, antacids) increase this risk.
- Recoding intake and output for elderly (especially frail elderly) is a preventative measure to prevent fluid and electrolyte imbalances.[72]

PEDIATRIC Considerations

- The normally increased basal metabolic rate of children results in a throughput of electrolytes and water that is more than two to three times that of an adult.[73]
- Fluid deficits occur in infants because of an exchange of 50% of the ECF daily.[73]
- Hypotension because of fluid deficit in children is a late sign and critical finding.[73]
- Normal values for fluid, electrolytes, and acid–base vary according to age of the infant or child and when compared to the adult. Consult a reference that is specific to the pediatric population when evaluating these values.[73]
- Acidosis paired with hypotension in a child is life threatening and places child at risk for failure of the cardiovascular and pulmonary systems. Acidosis also depletes the potassium level.[73]
- Adequate urine production is necessary prior to administering potassium supplements to prevent buildup of potassium that places child at risk for cardiac death or dysrhythmias.[73]
- Increased mobilization can prevent hypercalcemia from resorption of calcium from the child's bones.[73]

REVIEW EXERCISES

1. A 40-year-old man with advanced acquired immunodeficiency syndrome (AIDS) presents with an acute chest infection. Investigations confirm a diagnosis of *Pneumocystis jirovecii* (formerly *P. carinii*) pneumonia. Although he is being treated appropriately, his plasma sodium level is 118 mEq/L (118 mmol/L). Results of adrenal function tests are normal.
   A. *What is the likely cause of his electrolyte disturbance?*
   B. *What are the five cardinal features of this condition?*
2. A 70-year-old woman who is taking furosemide (a loop diuretic) for congestive heart failure complains of weakness, fatigue, and cramping of the muscles in her legs. Her plasma potassium is 2 mEq (2 mmol/L), and her plasma sodium is 140 mEq/L (140 mmol/L). She also complains that she notices a "strange heartbeat" at times.
   A. *What is the likely cause of this woman's symptoms?*
   B. *An ECG shows depressed ST segment and low T-wave changes. Explain the physiologic mechanism underlying these changes.*
   C. *What would be the treatment for this woman?*

3. A 50-year-old woman presents with symptomatic hypercalcemia. She has a recent history of breast cancer treatment.
   A. How do you evaluate this person with increased plasma calcium levels?
   B. What is the significance of the recent history of malignancy?
   C. What further tests may be indicated?
4. A 34-year-old woman with diabetes is admitted to the emergency department in a stuporous state. Her skin is flushed and warm, her breath has a sweet odor, her pulse is rapid and weak, and her respirations are rapid and deep. Her initial laboratory tests indicate a blood sugar of 320 mg/dL, serum HCO_3^- of 12 mEq/L (normal, 22 to 26 mEq/L), and a pH of 7.1 (normal, 7.35 to 7.45).
   A. What is the most likely cause of her lowered pH and bicarbonate levels?
   B. How would you account for her rapid and deep respirations?
   C. Using the Henderson-Hasselbalch equation and the solubility coefficient for CO_2 given in this chapter, what would you expect her PCO_2 to be?
   D. How would you explain her warm, flushed skin and stuporous mental state?
5. Explain the use of the urine anion gap to determine the kidney's ability to compensate for acid–base disorders by secreting and eliminating H^+ ions.
6. A 16-year-old girl is seen by her primary care provider because of her parents' concern over her binge eating and their recent discovery that she engages in self-induced vomiting. A tentative diagnosis of bulimia nervosa is made. Initial laboratory tests reveal a plasma K^+ of 3 mEq/L (normal, 3.5 to 5.0 mEq/L) and a Cl^- of 93 mEq/L (normal, 98 to 106 mEq/L).
   A. Explain her low K^+ and Cl^-.
   B. What type of acid–base abnormality would you expect her to have?
7. A 65-year-old man with chronic obstructive lung disease has been using low-flow oxygen therapy because of difficulty in maintaining adequate oxygenation of his blood. He has recently had a severe respiratory tract infection and has had difficulty breathing. He is admitted to the emergency department because he became increasingly lethargic and his wife has had trouble arousing him. His respirations are 12 breaths/minute. She relates that he had "turned his oxygen way up" because of difficulty breathing.
   A. What is the most likely cause of this man's problem?
   B. How would you explain the lethargy and difficulty in arousal?
   C. Arterial blood gases, drawn on admission to the emergency department, indicated a PO_2 of 85 mm Hg (normal, 90 to 95 mm Hg) and a PCO_2 of 90 mm Hg (normal, 40 mm Hg). His serum HCO_3^- was 34 mEq/L (normal, 22 to 26 mEq/L). What is his pH?
   D. What would be the main goal of treatment for this man in terms of acid–base balance?

References

1. Rhoades R. A., Bell D. R. (Eds.). (2017). Acid–base homeostasis. In *Medical physiology: Principles for clinical medicine* (5th ed., pp. 485–507). Baltimore, MD: Wolters Kluwer.
2. Hall J. E. (2016). *Guyton and Hall textbook of medical physiology* (13th ed.). Philadelphia, PA: Elsevier Saunders.
3. Noda Y. (2014) Dynamic regulation and dysregulation of the water channel aquaporin-2: A common cause of and promising therapeutic target for water balance disorders. *Clinical and Experimental Nephrology* 18(4), 558–570.
4. Rennke H. G., Denker B. M. (2014). *Renal pathophysiology: The essentials* (4th ed.). Philadelphia, PA: Lippincott Williams & Wilkins.
5. Chance-Hetzler J., Armer J., Van Loo M., et al. (2015). Prospective lymphedema surveillance in a clinic setting. *Journal of Personalized Medicine* 5(3), 311–325.
6. Zuther J. E. (2013). *Lymphedema management: The comprehensive guide for practitioners* (3rd ed.). New York: Thieme Medical Publishers.
7. Morton P. G., Fontaine D. K. (2013). *Critical care nursing: A holistic approach* (10th ed.). Philadelphia, PA: Lippincott Williams & Wilkins.
8. Ball J., Bindler R., Cowen K., et al. (2017). *Principles of pediatric nursing: Caring for children* (12th ed.). Boston, MA: Pearson.
9. Sterns R. (2018) Etiology and evaluation of hypernatremia in adults. In Emmet M. (Ed.), *Uptodate*. Available: https://www-uptodate-com.ezproxy.uu.edu/contents/etiology-and-evaluation-of-hypernatremia-in-adults?search=The%20physiological%20regulation%20of%20thirst%20and%20fluid%20intake,%20thirst&source=search_result&selectedTitle=3~150&usage_type=default&display_rank=3. Accessed March 12, 2018.
10. Shah M. K., Workeneh B. M., Taffet G. E. (2014). Hypernatremia in the geriatric population. *Clinical Interventions of Aging*, 2014(9), 1987–1992.
11. Martin L. M., Higueras P. H. (2016). Psychogenic polydipsia and schizophrenia. *European Psychiatry* 33, S722–S723.
12. Sterns R. H. General principles of disorders of water balance (hyponatremia and hypernatremia) and sodium balance (hypovolemia and edema). In Emmett M. (Ed.), *UpToDate*. Available: https://www-uptodate-com.ezproxy.uu.edu/contents/general-principles-of-disorders-of-water-balance-hyponatremia-and-hypernatremia-and-sodium-balance-hypovolemia-and-edema?search=Disorders%20of%20water%20imbalance&source=search_result&selectedTitle=1~150&usage_type=default&display_rank=1. Accessed March 12, 2018.
13. Rondon-Berrios H. (2016). Vasopressin receptor and clinical role. *Best Practice & Research Clinical Endocrinology & Metabolism* 30(2), 289–303.
14. Bichet D. G. (2017). Clinical manifestations and causes of central diabetes insipidus. In Sterns R. (Ed.), *UpToDate*. Available: https://www-uptodate-com.ezproxy.uu.edu/contents/clinical-manifestations-and-causes-of-central-diabetes-insipidus?search=MRI%20diabetes%20insipidus&source=search_result&selectedTitle=1~150&usage_type=default&display_rank=1. Accessed March 14, 2018.
15. Sterns R. (2018). Pathophysiology and etiology of the syndrome of inappropriate antidiuretic hormone secretion (SIADH). In Emmett M. (Ed.), *UpToDate*. Available: https://www-uptodate-com.ezproxy.uu.

edu/contents/pathophysiology-and-etiology-of-the-syndrome-of-inappropriate-antidiuretic-hormone-secretion-siadh?search=syndrome%20of%20inappropriate%20antidiuretic%20hormone%20secretion&source=search_result&selectedTitle=1~150&usage_type=default&display_rank=8. Accessed March 14, 2018.

16. Sterns H. (2018). Etiology, clinical manifestations, and diagnosis of volume depletion in adults. In Emmett M. (Ed.), *UpToDate.* Available: https://www-uptodate-com.ezproxy.uu.edu/contents/etiology-clinical-manifestations-and-diagnosis-of-volume-depletion-in-adults?search=decreased%20skin%20turgor&source=search_result&selectedTitle=1~44&usage_type=default&display_rank=1#H11.
17. Jensen S. (2015). *Nursing health assessment: A best practice approach* (2nd ed.). Philadelphia, PA: Lippincott Williams & Wilkins.
18. Sahay M., Sahay R. (2014). Hyponatremia: A practical approach. *Indian Journal of Endocrinology and Metabolism* 18(6), 760–771.
19. Freedman S. (2017). Oral rehydration therapy. In Mattoo T. (Ed.), *Up ToDate.* Available: https://www.uptodate.com/contents/oral-rehydration-therapy.
20. Daly K., Farrington E. (2013). Hypokalemia and hyperkalemia in infants and children: Pathophysiology and treatment. *Journal of Pediatric Healthcare* 27(6), 486–496.
21. Braun M. M., Barstow C. H. (2015). Diagnosis and management of sodium disorders: Hyponatremia and hypernatremia. *American Family Physicians* 1(5), 299–307.
22. Gutmann L., Conwit R. (2014). Hypokalemic periodic paralysis. In Sheffner J. (Ed.), *UpToDate.* Available: https://www-uptodate-com.ezproxy.uu.edu/contents/hypokalemic-periodic-paralysis?search=hypokalemic%20familial%20periodic%20paralysis&source=search_result&selectedTitle=1~104&usage_type=default&display_rank=1. Accessed March 14, 2018.
23. Marcocci C., Bollerslev J., Kahn A. A., et al. (2014). Medical management of primary hyperparathyroidism: Proceedings of the fourth international workshop on the management of asymptomatic primary hyperparathyroidism. *The Journal of Clinical Endocrinology and Metabolism* 99(10), 3607–3618.
24. Meng Q. H., Wagar E. A. (2015). Pseudohyperkalemia: A new twist on an old phenomenon. *Critical Reviews of Clinical Laboratory Sciences* 52(2), 45–55.
25. Charles G., Zheng C., Lehmann-Horn F., et al. (2013). Characterization of hyperkalemic periodic paralysis: A survey of genetically diagnosed individuals. *Journal of Neurology* 260(10), 2606–2613.
26. Rizos C. V., Milionis H. J., Elisaf M. S. (2017). Severe hyperkalemia following blood transfusions: Is there a link? *World Journal of Nephrology* 6(1), 53–56.
27. Ross M. H., Pawlina W. (2016). *Histology: A text and atlas with correlated cell and molecular biology* (7th ed.). Philadelphia, PA: Lippincott Williams & Wilkins.
28. Caulley L., Johnson-Obaseki S., Luo L., et al. (2017). Risk factors for postoperative complications in total thyroidectomy: A retrospective, risk-adjusted analysis from the National Surgical Quality Improvement Program. *Medicine* 96(5), e5752.
29. Verdelli C., Corbett S. (2017). Mechanisms in endocrinology. Kidney involvement in patients with primary hyperparathyroidism: An update on clinical and molecular aspects. *European Journal of Endocrinology* 176, R39–R52.
30. Moschella C. (2016). Chronic kidney disease-mineral and bone disorder: Guidelines for diagnosis, treatment, and management. *Journal of American Academy of Physician Assistants* 29(7), 21-29.
31. Moorthi R. N., Moe S. M. (2013). Recent advances in the non-invasive diagnosis of renal osteodystrophy. *Kidney International* 84(5), 886–894.
32. Yuen N. K., Ananthakrishnan S., Campbell M. J. (2016). Hyperparathyroidism of renal disease. *The Permanente Journal* 20(3), 78–83.
33. Webster S., Todd S. J. H., Wright C. R. (2015). A retrospective cohort analysis of ionised calcium levels in major trauma patients who have received early blood product transfusion in the Emergency Department. *Scandinavian Journal of Trauma, Resuscitation and Emergency Medicine* 23(2), 03–08.
34. Steele T., Kolamunnage-Dona R., Downey C., et al. (2013). Assessment and clinical course of hypocalcemia in critical illness. *Critical Care* 4(17), 1365–1385.
35. Dunphy L. M., Winland-Brown J. E., Porter B. O., et al. (2015). *Primary care: The art and science of advanced practice nursing* (4th ed.). Philadelphia, PA: FA Davis.
36. Burchum J., Rosenthal L. (2015). *Pharmacology for nursing care* (9th ed.). St. Louis, MO: Elsevier.
37. Yarbro C. H., Wujcik D., Gobel B. H. (Eds.) (2018). *Oncology nursing: Principles and practice* (8th ed.). Sudbury, MA: Jones & Bartlett Publishers.
38. Crowley R., Gittoes N. (2013). *Clinical Medicine* 13(3), 287–290.
39. Boulding R., McCann P. (2014). Hypercalcemic crisis treated with calcium-free hemodialysis with subsequent parathyroidectomy and postsurgical hypocalcemia. *Journal of Acute Medicine* 4, 135–137.
40. Hogan J., Goldfarb S. (2018). Regulation of calcium and phosphate balance. In Sterns R. (Ed.), *UpToDate.* Available: https://www-uptodate-com.ezproxy.uu.edu/contents/regulation-of-calcium-and-phosphate-balance?search=phosphatonins%20sodium-phosphate%20cotransporter&source=search_result&selectedTitle=2~20&usage_type=default&display_rank=2. Accessed March 14, 2018.
41. Windpessi M., Mayrbaeurl B., Baldinger C. M., et al. (2017). Refeeding syndrome in oncology: Report of four cases. *World Journal of Oncology* 8(1), 25–29.
42. Smith J. M., Lowe R. F., Fullerton J., et al. (2013). An integrative review of the side effects related to the use of magnesium sulfate for pre-eclampsia and eclampsia management. *BioMedCentral Pregnancy and Childbirth* 13(1), 34–36.
43. Grober U., Schmidt J., Kisters K. (2015). Magnesium in prevention and therapy. *Nutrients* 7(9), 8199–8226.
44. Hall J. E. (2016). *Guyton and Hall textbook of medical physiology* (13th ed., pp. 409–426). Philadelphia, PA: Saunders Elsevier.
45. Sherwood L. (2016). *Human physiology: From cells to systems* (9th ed., pp. 547–562). Boston, MA: Cengage Learning.
46. Tanner G. A. (2018). Acid-base homeostatis. In Rhoades R. A., Bell D. R. (Eds.) Medical physiology principles for clinical medicine (5th ed., pp. 458–507). Philadelphia, PA: Wolters Kluwer.
47. Gomez H., Kellum J. A. (2015). Understanding acid base disorders. *Critical Care Clinics* 31, 849–860. http://dx.doi.org/10.1016/j.ccc.2015.06.016.
48. Antonogiannaki E., Mitrouska I., Amargianitakis V., et al. (2015). Evaluation of acid-base status in patients admitted to ED-physiocochemical vs traditional approaches. *American Journal of Emergency Medicine* 33(2105), 378–382. http://dx.doi.org/10.1016/j.ajem.2014.12.010.
49. Hamm L. L., Nakhoul N., Hering-Smith K. S. (2015). Acid-base homeostasis. *Clinical Journal of the American Society of Nephrology* 10(12), 2232–2242. doi:10.2215/CJN.07400715.
50. Fischbach F., Dunning M. B. (2015). *A manual of laboratory and diagnostic tests* (9th ed.). Philadelphia, PA: Wolters Kluwer/Lippincott Williams & Wilkins.
51. Berend K., deVries A. P. J., Gans, R.O. B. (2014). Physiological approach to assessment of acid-base disturbances. *New England Journal of Medicine* 371, 1434–1445. doi:10.1056/NEJMra1003327.
52. Rice M., Ismail B., Pillow M. T. (2014). Approach to metabolic acidosis in the emergency department. *Emergency Medicine Clinics of North America* 32, 403–420. http://dx.doi.org/10.1016/j.emc.2014.01.002.
53. Adeva-Andany M. M., Carneiro-Freire N., Donapetry-Garcia C., et al. (2014). The importance of the ionic product for water to understand the physiology of the acid-base balance in humans. *BioMed Research International* 2014, 1–16. Available: http://dx.doi.org/10.1155/2014/695281.
54. Kitterer D., Schwab M., Alscher M. D., et al. (2015). Drug-induced acid–base disorders. *Pediatric Nephrology* 30, 1407–1423. doi:10.1007/s00467-014-2958-5.
55. DeFronzo R., Fleming G. A., Chen K., Bicsak T. A. (2016). Metformin-associated lactic acidosis: Current perspectives on causes and risk. *Metabolism Clinical and Experimental* 65, 20–29. Available: http://dx.doi.org/10.1016/j.metabol.2015.10.014.

56. Berend K., deVries A. P. J., Gans R. O. B. (2015). Correspondence physiological approach to assessment of acid-base disturbances. *New England Journal of Medicine* 372, 193–195. doi:10.1056/NELMc1413880.
57. Glasmacher S. A., Stone W. (2016). Anion gap as a prognostic tool for risk stratification in critically ill patients—A systematic review and meta-analysis. *BMC Anesthesiology* 16(68), 1–13. doi:10.1186/s12871-016-0241-y.
58. Rastegar M., Nagami G. T. (2017). Non-anion gap metabolic acidosis: A clinical approach to evaluation. *American Journal of Kidney Disease* 69(2), 296–301. Available: http://dx.doi.org/10.1053/j.ajkd.2016.09.013.
59. Ferreruela M. Raurich J. M., Ayerstaran L., et al. (2017). Hyperlactatemia in ICU patients: Incidence, causes, and associated mortality. *Journal of Critical Care* 42, 200–205. https://dx.doi.org/10.1016/jere.2017.07.039.
60. Bakker J., Nijsten M., Jansen T. C. (2013). Clinical use of lactate monitoring in critically ill patients. *Annals of Intensive Care* 3(12), 1–8. Available: http://www.annalsofintensivecare.com/content/3/1/12.
61. Garcia-Alvarez M., Marik P., Bellomo R. (2014). Sepsis-associated hyperlactatemia. *Critical Care* 18(503), 1–11. Available: http://ccforum.co/content/18/4/503.
62. McNamara K., Isbister G. K. (2015). Hyperlactatemia and clinical severity of acute metformin overdose. *Internal Medicine Journal* 45(4), 402–408. doi:10.1111/imj.12713.
63. Fabian E., Kramer L., Siebert F., et al. (2017). D-Lactic acidosis—case report and review of the literature. *Zeitschrift für Gastroenterologie* 55(1), 75–82. doi:10.1055/s-0042-117647.
64. Palmer B. F., Clegg D. J. (2015). Electrolyte and acid–base disturbances in patients with diabetes mellitus. *New England Journal of Medicine* 373, 548–559. doi:10.1056/NEJMra1503102.
65. Noor N. M., Basavaraju K., Sharpstone D. (2016). Alcoholic ketoacidosis: A case report and review of the literature. *Oxford Medical Case Reports* 3, 31–33. doi:10.1093/omcr/omw006.
66. Shivley R. M., Hoffman R. S., Manini A. F. (2017). Acute salicylate poisoning: Risk factors for severe outcome. *Clinical Toxicology* 55(3), 175–180. doi:10.1080/15563650.2016.1271127.
67. Agency for Toxic Substances and Disease Registry. (2014). *Medical management guidelines for ethylene glycol*. Available: https://www.atsdr.cdc.gov/MHMI/mmg96.pdf.
68. Singh R., Arain E., Buth A., et al. (2016). Ethylene glycol poisoning: An unusual cause of altered mental status and the lessons learned from management of the disease in the acute setting. *Case Reports in Critical Care* 2016, 1–6. Available: http://dx.doi.org/10.1155/20126/9157393.
69. Santos F., Ordonez F. A., Claramunt-Taberner D., et al. (2015). Clinical and laboratory approaches in the diagnosis of renal tubular acidosis. *Pediatric Nephrology* 30, 2099–2107. doi:10.1007/s00467-015-3083-9.
70. Van der A. F., Joniau S., Van Den Braden M., et al. (2011). Metabolic changes after urinary diversion. *Advances in Urology* 2011, 1–5. doi:10.1155/2011/764325.
71. Malcolm O. T. (2015). Identification, treatment, and prevention of calcium-alkali syndrome in elderly patients. *The Consultant Pharmacist* 30(8), 444–454. doi:10.4140/TCP.n.2015.444.
72. Eliopoulos C. (2018). *Gerontological nursing* (9th ed.). Philadelphia, PA: Wolters Kluwer.
73. Bowden V. R., Greenberg C. S. (2014). *Children and their families: The continuum of nursing care* (3rd ed.). Philadelphia, PA: Wolters Kluwer.

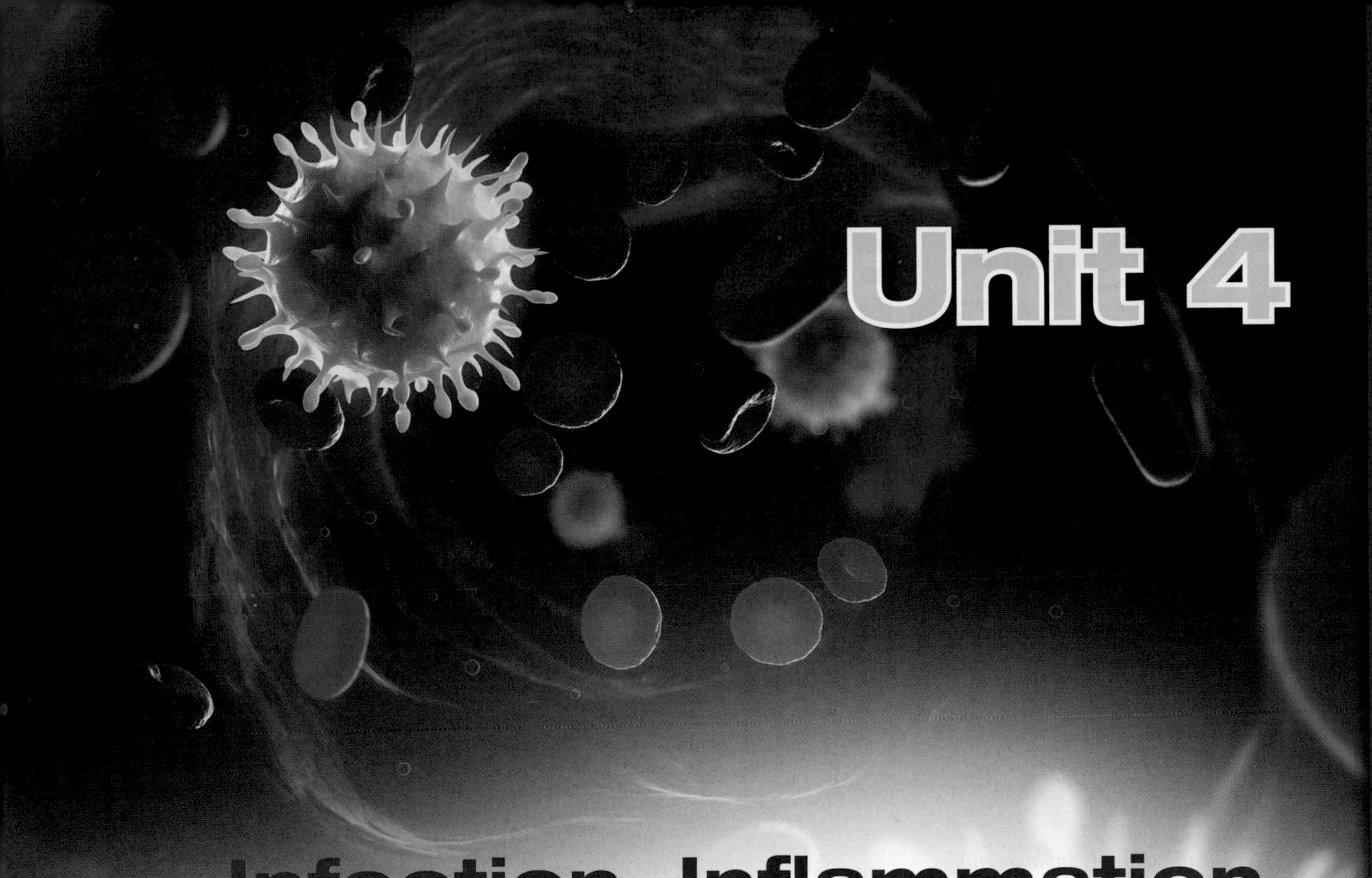

Unit 4

Infection, Inflammation, and Immunity

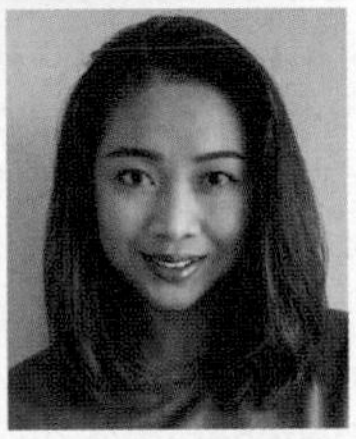

Sue Roon, 19 years old, presented at her primary care provider's office with a swollen left ankle about twice the ankle's normal size. She explains that she has had this same swelling occur spontaneously without injury or trauma about five times over the last 18 months. The swelling usually lasts approximately 36 hours and then resolves on its own. Her primary care provider has had it x-rayed, and it shows no fracture or abnormal findings. She also shares that her right wrist has swelled up similarly about three times over the last 18 months (spontaneously, without any injury, and resolves on its own). She generally takes two tablets of ibuprofen (Advil) twice daily, applies ice, uses a compression bandage, and tries to forget about the swelling.

She explains that, in addition to the unusual swelling, she has started to feel more tired than usual. She can think of no reason for this given she has not had any strenuous activity or stress lately. She also reports a slight headache that comes and goes and just began again about 2 days ago when the latest swelling began. Her vital signs are all normal but she has a temperature of 100.2°F. She has no other complaints and perceives herself to be in "good health." She has no family history of autoimmune disorders such as Sjögren syndrome or rheumatoid arthritis. She also has no personal history of any neurologic or muscle disorders or current muscle discomfort or tenderness at the fibromyalgia classic anatomical sites. She states she does do a good amount of hiking and gardening but denies being bitten by a tick. She says she did not have any skin rash or feel that any insects had bitten her over the last 2 years. However, because she lives in New Jersey (which is a high-risk area for infection with Lyme disease), and she spends a lot of time outdoors, her primary care provider decides she should be worked up for Lyme disease (*Borrelia burgdorferi*). A complete blood count (CBC) with differential, sedimentation rate, and Lyme enzyme immunoassay come back positive. She then is retested with a Western blot test, which is also positive for *B. burgdorferi* reactive antibodies. She is diagnosed with Lyme disease and given doxycycline 100 mg BID for 21 days. Her primary care provider refers her to an infectious disease physician because it is thought she may have had Lyme disease for 18 months.

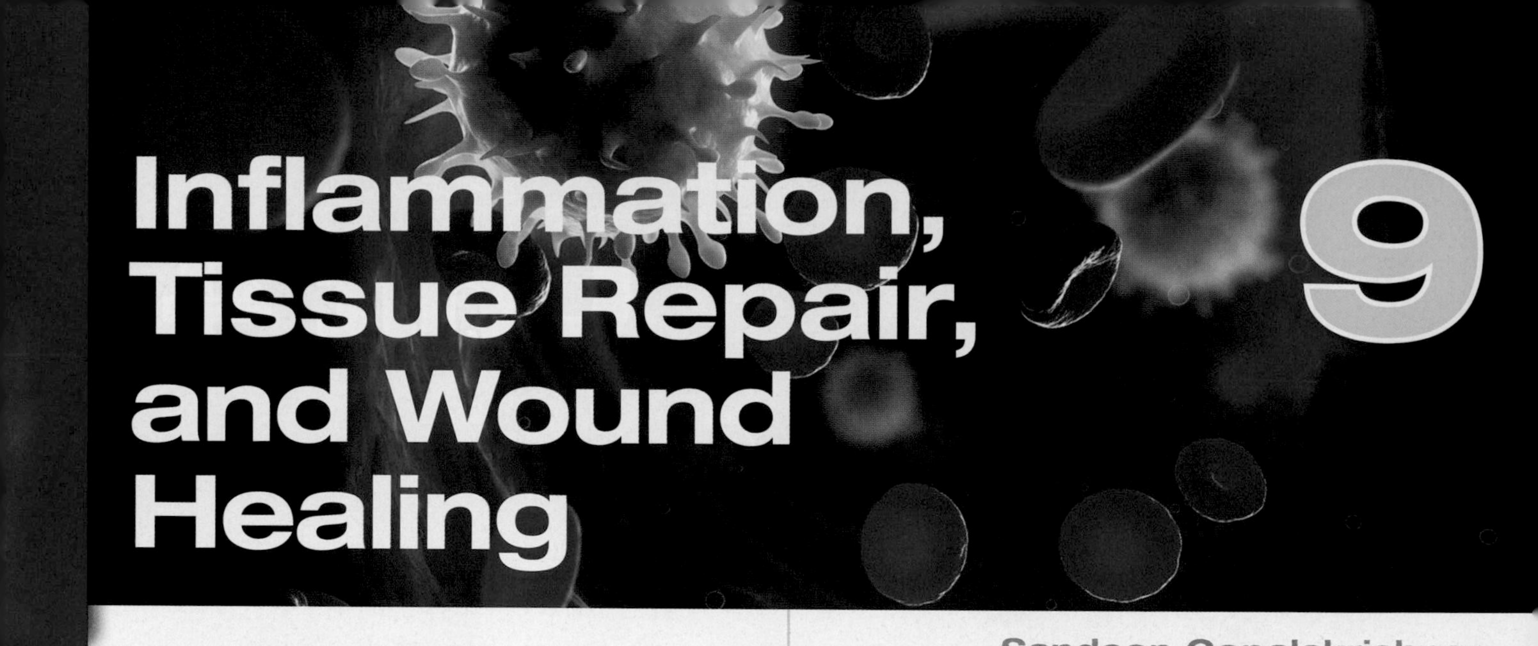

Inflammation, Tissue Repair, and Wound Healing

9

Sandeep Gopalakrishnan

Inflammation involves a wide variety of physiologic and pathologic responses intended to eliminate the initial cause of cell injury, remove the damaged tissue, and generate new tissue. It accomplishes this by destroying, enzymatically digesting, walling off, or otherwise neutralizing the harmful agents such as toxins, foreign agents, or infectious organisms.[1] These processes set the stage for the events that will eventually heal the damaged tissue. Thus, inflammation is intimately interwoven with the repair processes that replace damaged tissue or fill in the residual defects with fibrous scar tissue.

Although first described over 2000 years ago, the inflammatory response has evoked renewed interest during the past several years. As a result, the pathogeneses of multiple diseases are now known to be linked to a dysregulated inflammatory response.[2–4] For example, the inflammatory response is attributed to the production of incapacitating bronchial asthma, the generation of atherosclerotic plaques that lead to myocardial infarction, and the crippling effects of diabetes, autoimmune, and neurodegenerative disorders. This chapter focuses on the morphologic and functional manifestations of acute and chronic inflammation, tissue repair, and wound healing.

THE INFLAMMATORY RESPONSE

After completing this section of the chapter, the learner will be able to meet the following objectives:

- Identify and state the physiologic reasons behind five cardinal signs of acute inflammation.
- Describe the vascular changes in an acute inflammatory response.
- Characterize the interaction of adhesion molecules, chemokines, and cytokines in leukocyte adhesion, migration, and phagocytosis, which are part of the cellular phase of inflammation.
- List four types of inflammatory mediators and state their function.

- Contrast acute and chronic inflammation.
- Define the systemic manifestation of inflammation, including the characteristics of an acute-phase response.

Inflammation is the reaction of vascularized tissues to injury. It is characterized by inflammatory mediators, such as complement, tumor necrosis factor-α (TNF-α), vascular endothelial growth factor (VEGF), neutrophils, and serum amyloid, and the movement of fluid, either within the cells or the interstitial fluid. Inflammation generally localizes and eliminates microbes, foreign particles, and abnormal cells and paves the way for repair of the injured tissue.[5] Inflammatory conditions are commonly named by adding the suffix *-itis* to the affected organ or system. For example, *appendicitis* refers to inflammation of the appendix, *pericarditis* to inflammation of the pericardium, and *neuritis* to inflammation of a nerve. More descriptive expressions of the inflammatory process might indicate whether the process is acute or chronic.

The classic description of inflammation has been handed down through the ages. In the first century AD, the Roman physician Celus described the local reaction of injury in terms that are now known as the *cardinal signs* of inflammation.[1] These signs are *rubor* (redness), *tumor* (swelling), *calor* (heat), and *dolor* (pain). In the second century AD, the Greek physician Galen described a fifth cardinal sign, *functio laesa* (loss of function). In addition to the cardinal signs that appear at the site of injury, systemic or constitutional manifestations (*e.g.*, fever) may occur as chemical mediators (*e.g.*, cytokines) produced at the site of inflammation gain entrance to the circulatory system. The constellation of systemic manifestations that may occur during acute inflammation is known as the *acute-phase response*.

The degree of the inflammatory response is impacted by multiple factors, such as the duration of the insult, the type of foreign agent, the degree of injury, and the microenvironment.[1] Inflammation can be divided into acute and chronic types.[1] *Acute inflammation* is of relatively short duration, lasting from a few minutes to several days, and is characterized by the exudation of fluid and plasma components and emigration of leukocytes, predominantly neutrophils, into the extravascular tissues. *Chronic inflammation* is of a longer duration, lasting for days to years, and is associated with the presence of lymphocytes and macrophages, proliferation of blood vessels, fibrosis, and tissue necrosis. These basic forms of inflammation often overlap, and many factors may influence their course.

Acute Inflammation

Acute inflammation is the early (appearing within minutes to hours) host protective response of local tissues and their blood vessels to injury and is critical for restoration of tissue homeostasis.[6] It typically occurs before adaptive immunity becomes established and is aimed primarily at removing the injurious agent and limiting the extent of tissue damage. Acute inflammation can be triggered by a variety of stimuli, including infections, immune reactions, blunt and penetrating trauma, physical or chemical agents (*e.g.*, burns, frostbite, irradiation, caustic chemicals), and tissue necrosis from any cause.

Cells of Inflammation

Acute inflammation involves two major components: the vascular and cellular stages.[6] Many tissues and cells are involved in these reactions, including the endothelial cells that line blood vessels, circulating white blood cells, connective tissue cells (mast cells, fibroblasts, tissue macrophages, and lymphocytes), and components of the extracellular matrix (ECM) (Fig. 9.1). The ECM consists of fibrous proteins

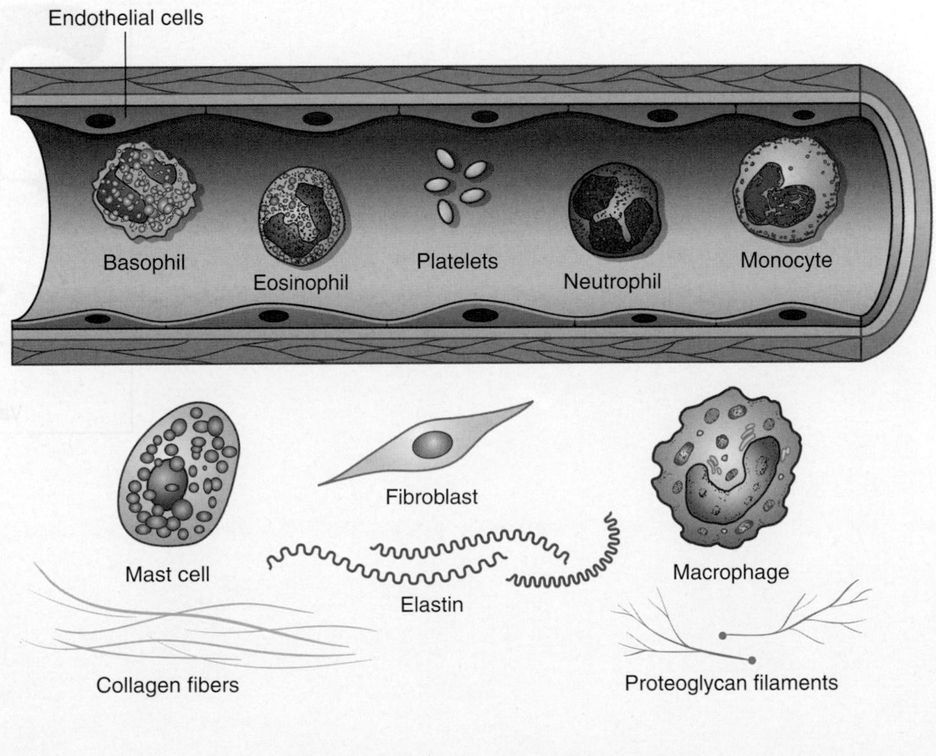

Figure 9.1 • Cells of acute inflammation.

Understanding Acute Inflammation

Acute inflammation is the immediate and early response to an injurious agent, which is critical for the restoration of tissue homeostasis. The response, which is a highly coordinated program to control and eliminate altered cells, microorganisms, and antigens, occurs in two phases: (1) the vascular phase, which leads to an increase in blood flow and changes in the small blood vessels of the microcirculation, and (2) the cellular phase, which leads to the migration of leukocytes from the circulation and their activation to eliminate the injurious agent. The primary function of inflammatory response is to limit the injurious effect of the pathologic agent and remove the injured tissue components, thereby allowing tissue repair to take place.

Vascular Phase

The vascular phase of acute inflammation is characterized by changes in the small blood vessels at the site of injury, which is marked by tissue edema. It begins with momentary vasoconstriction followed rapidly by vasodilation mediated in part by lipid mediators and vasoactive products.[6] Vasodilation involves the arterioles and venules with a resultant increase in capillary blood flow, causing heat and redness, which are two of the cardinal signs of inflammation. This is accompanied by an increase in vascular permeability with outpouring of protein-rich fluid (exudate) into the extravascular spaces. The loss of proteins reduces the capillary osmotic pressure and increases the interstitial osmotic pressure. This, coupled with an increase in capillary pressure, causes a marked outflow of fluid and its accumulation in the tissue spaces, producing the swelling, pain, and impaired function that represent the other cardinal signs of acute inflammation. As fluid moves out of the vessels, stagnation of flow and clotting of blood occur. This aids in localizing the spread of infectious microorganisms.

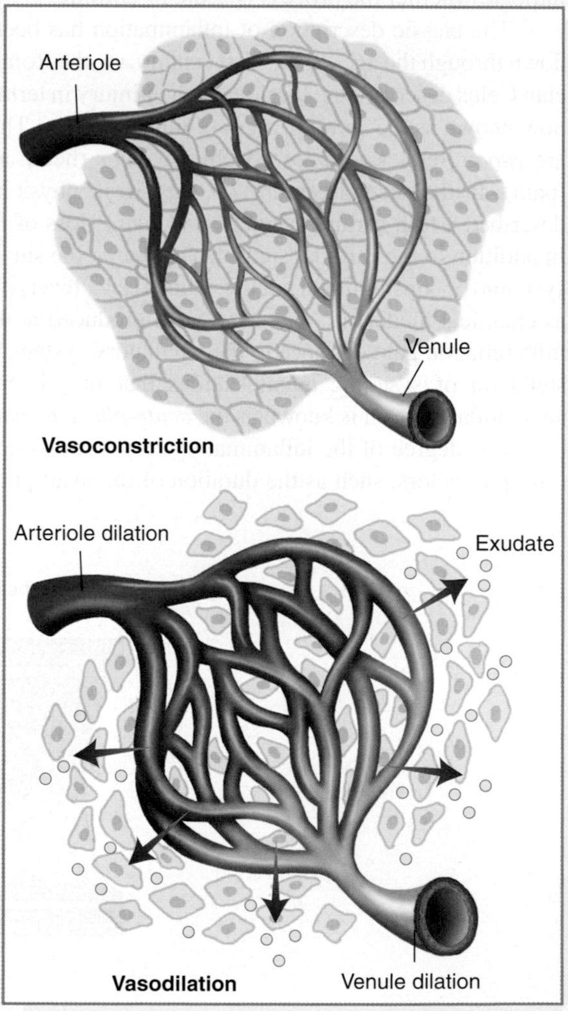

Understanding Acute Inflammation *(Continued)*

Cellular Phase: Leukocyte Margination, Adhesion, and Transmigration

The cellular phase of acute inflammation involves the delivery of leukocytes, mainly polymorphonuclear neutrophils (PMNs), to the site of injury so they can perform their normal functions of host defense through phagocytosis. The delivery and activation of leukocytes can be divided into the following steps: endothelial activation, adhesion and margination, transmigration, and chemotaxis. The recruitment of leukocytes to the precapillary venules, where they exit the circulation, is facilitated by the slowing of blood flow and margination along the vessel surface. Leukocyte adhesion and transmigration from the vascular space into the extravascular tissue is facilitated by complementary adhesion molecules (*e.g.*, selectins, integrins) on the leukocyte and endothelial surfaces. After extravasation, leukocytes migrate in the tissues toward the site of injury by chemotaxis or locomotion oriented along a chemical gradient.

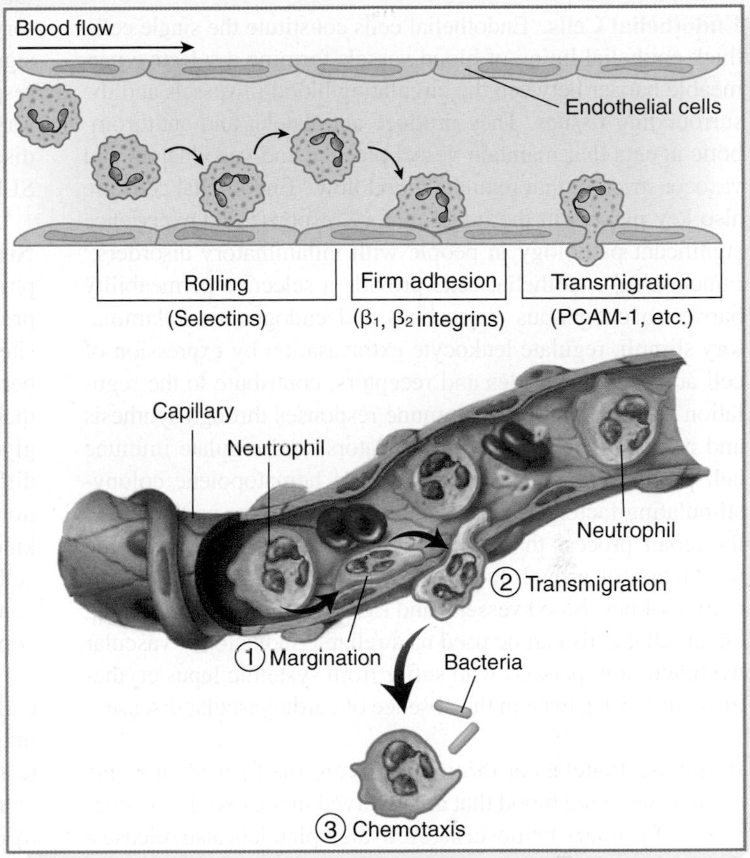

Leukocyte Activation and Phagocytosis

Once at the sight of injury, the products generated by tissue injury trigger a number of leukocyte responses, including phagocytosis and cell killing. Opsonization of microbes by complement factor C3b and antibody facilitates recognition by neutrophil C3b and the antibody Fc receptor. Receptor activation triggers intracellular signaling and actin assembly in the neutrophil, leading to formation of pseudopods that enclose the microbe within a phagosome. The phagosome then fuses with an intracellular lysosome to form a phagolysosome into which lysosomal enzymes and oxygen free radicals are released to kill and degrade the microbe.[6,7]

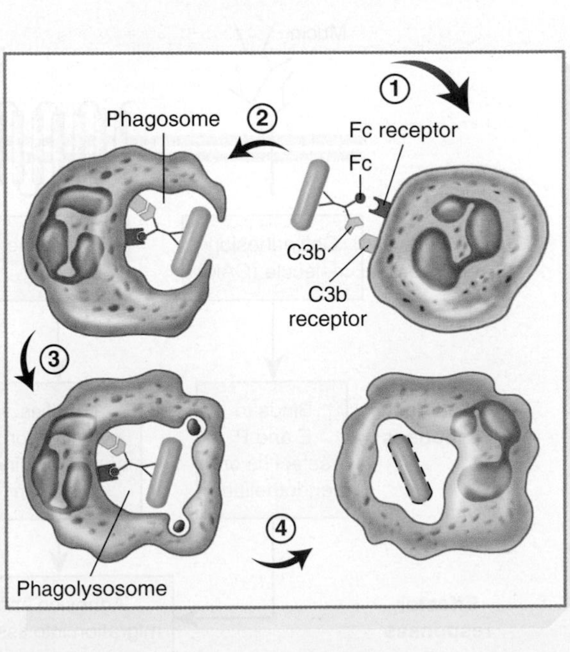

(collagen and elastin), adhesive glycoproteins, and proteoglycans. At the biochemical level, the inflammatory mediators, acting together or in sequence, amplify the initial response and influence its evolution by regulating the subsequent vascular and cellular responses.

Endothelial Cells. Endothelial cells constitute the single cell–thick epithelial lining of blood vessels forming a selective permeable barrier between the circulating blood in vessels and the surrounding tissues. They produce antiplatelet and antithrombotic agents that maintain vessel patency and vasodilators and vasoconstrictors that regulate blood flow.[8] Endothelial cells are also key players in the inflammatory response and experience significant pathology in people with inflammatory disorders.[9] Functioning endothelial cells provide a selective permeability barrier to exogenous (microbial) and endogenous inflammatory stimuli, regulate leukocyte extravasation by expression of cell adhesion molecules and receptors, contribute to the regulation and modulation of immune responses through synthesis and release of inflammatory mediators, and regulate immune cell proliferation through secretion of hematopoietic colony-stimulating factors (CSFs). Endothelial cells also participate in the repair process that accompanies inflammation through the production of growth factors that stimulate angiogenesis (formation of new blood vessels) and ECM synthesis.[8,9] Circulating endothelial cells can be used as a reliable indicator of vascular dysfunction in persons who suffer from systemic lupus erythematosus (SLE), even in the absence of cardiovascular disease.[10]

Platelets. Platelets or thrombocytes are the formed elements circulating in the blood that are involved in the cellular mechanisms of primary hemostasis. Activated platelets also release a number of potent inflammatory mediators, thereby increasing vascular permeability and altering the chemotactic, adhesive, and proteolytic properties of the endothelial cells.[11] When a platelet undergoes activation, over 300 proteins are released. Although only a relatively small proportion of these have been identified, it appears that a significant number are inflammatory mediators. There is growing evidence suggesting the significant role of platelets in inflammatory and immune responses.[11] The association between platelets and inflammatory diseases is highlighted by the number of inflammatory disease processes (*e.g.*, atherosclerosis, migraine headache, SLE) shown to be associated with platelet activation.[11]

Neutrophils and Monocytes/Macrophages. The neutrophils and macrophages are phagocytic leukocytes that are present in large numbers and are evident within hours at the site of inflammation. Both types of leukocytes express a number of surface receptors and molecules that are involved in their activation. They include mannose receptors that bind glycoproteins of bacteria; toll-like receptors that respond to different types and components of microbes; cell communication receptors that recognize specific cytokines and chemokines produced in response to infections and tissue injury; cell adhesion molecules that affect leukocyte adhesion; and complement receptors that recognize degraded fragments of complement deposited on the microbial surface (Fig. 9.2).

The *neutrophil* is the primary phagocyte that arrives early at the site of inflammation, usually within 90 minutes of injury.[1] These leukocytes have nuclei that are divided into three to five lobes. Therefore, they often are referred to as *PMNs* or *segmented neutrophils (segs)*. A white blood cell identified by distinctive cytoplasmic granules is called a granulocyte.

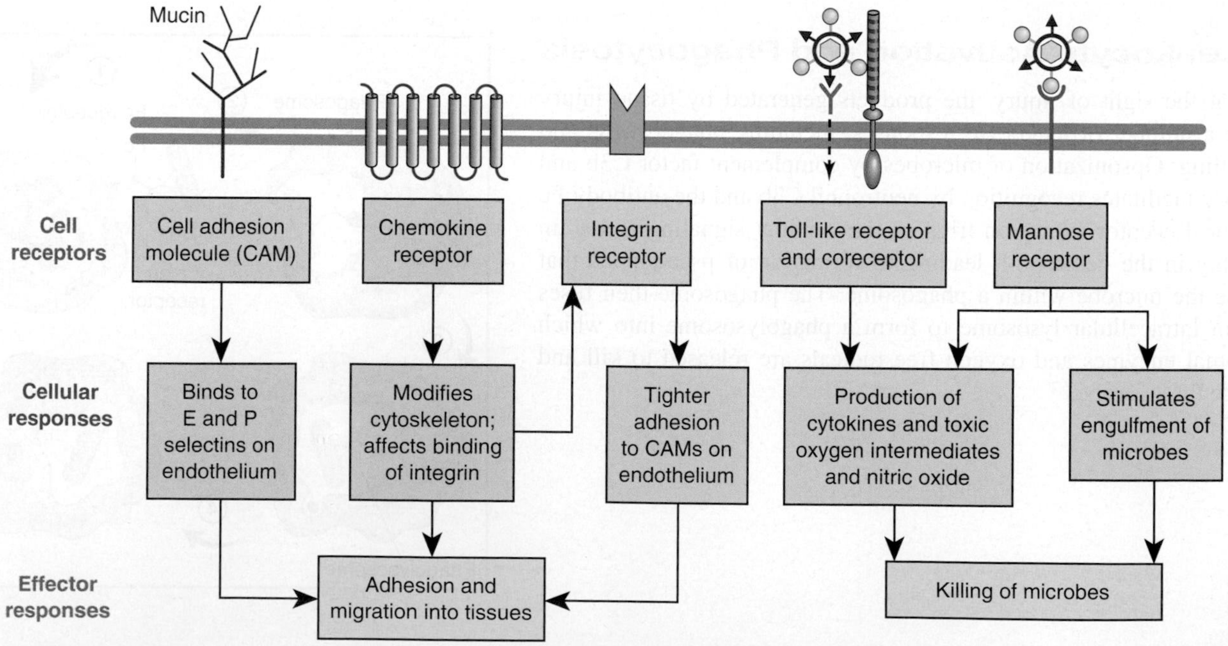

Figure 9.2 • Leukocyte activation. Different classes of leukocyte cell surface receptors recognize different stimuli. The receptors initiate responses that mediate the functions of the leukocytes.

The cytoplasmic granules of the granulocytes, which resist staining and remain a neutral color, contain enzymes and antibacterial material that are used in destroying engulfed microbes and dead tissue.[12] Neutrophils are able to generate oxygen (hydrogen peroxide) and nitrogen products (nitric oxide [NO]) that assist in destroying the engulfed debris.[12]

The neutrophil count in the blood often increases greatly during an inflammatory process, especially with bacterial infections. After being released from the bone marrow, circulating neutrophils have a life span of only approximately 10 hours and therefore must be constantly replaced if their numbers are to remain adequate. This requires an increase in circulating white blood cells, a condition called *leukocytosis*, which is frequently elevated with bacterial infections and tissue injury.[1] With excessive demand for phagocytes, immature forms of neutrophils are released from the bone marrow. These immature cells often are called *bands* because of the horseshoe shape of their nuclei.

Circulating monocytes, which have a single kidney-shaped nucleus and are the largest of the circulating leukocytes, constitute 3% to 8% of the white blood cell count. The monocytes are released from the bone marrow to act as macrophages.[1,12] Mononuclear cells arrive at the inflammatory site shortly after the neutrophils and perform their phagocytic functions for several days.[1]

Monocytes and macrophages produce potent vasoactive mediators, including prostaglandins and leukotrienes (LT), platelet-activating factor (PAF), inflammatory cytokines, and growth factors that promote regeneration of tissues. The macrophages engulf larger and greater quantities of foreign material than the neutrophils. These longer-lived phagocytes help to destroy the causative agent, aid in the signaling processes of immunity, serve to resolve the inflammatory process, and contribute to initiation of the healing processes. They also play an important role in chronic inflammation, where they can surround and wall off foreign material that cannot be digested.

Eosinophils, Basophils, and Mast Cells. Eosinophils, basophils, and mast cells produce lipid mediators and cytokines that induce inflammation. Although all three cell types have unique characteristics, they all contain cytoplasmic granules that induce inflammation. They are particularly important in inflammation associated with immediate hypersensitivity reactions and allergic disorders.

Eosinophils circulate in the blood and are recruited to tissues, similar to neutrophils. These granulocytes increase in the blood during allergic reactions and parasitic infections. The granules of eosinophils, which stain red with the acid dye eosin, contain a protein that is highly toxic to large parasitic worms that cannot be phagocytized. They also play an important role in allergic reactions by controlling the release of specific chemical mediators.

Basophils are blood granulocytes with structural and functional similarities to mast cells of the connective tissue. They are derived from bone marrow progenitors and circulate in blood. The granules of the *basophils*, which stain blue with a basic dye, contain histamine and other bioactive mediators of inflammation. Both basophils and mast cells bind an antibody, immunoglobulin E (IgE), secreted by plasma cells through receptors on their cell surface.[13] Binding of IgE triggers release of histamine and vasoactive agents from the basophil granules.

Mast cells derive from the same hematopoietic stem cells as basophils but do not develop until they leave the circulation and lodge in tissue sites. Activation of mast cells results in release of preformed contents of their granules (histamine, proteoglycans, proteases, and cytokines such as TNF-α and interleukin [IL]-16), synthesis of lipid mediators derived from cell membrane precursors (arachidonic acid metabolites, such as prostaglandins, and PAF), and stimulation of cytokine and chemokine synthesis by other inflammatory cells such as monocytes and macrophages. Mast cells are involved in IgE-triggered reactions and with helminth infections.[14]

Vascular Stage

The vascular changes that occur with inflammation involve the arterioles, capillaries, and venules of the microcirculation. These changes begin soon after injury and are characterized by vasodilation, changes in blood flow, increased vascular permeability, and leakage of fluid into the extravascular tissues.[1]

> Vasodilation, which is one of the earliest manifestations of inflammation, follows a transient constriction of the arterioles, lasting a few seconds. Vasodilation first involves the arterioles and then results in opening of capillary beds in the area. As a result, the area becomes congested, causing the redness (erythema) and warmth associated with acute inflammation. Vasodilation is induced by the action of several mediators, such as histamine and NO.[6]

Vasodilation is quickly followed by increased permeability of the microvasculature, with the outpouring of a protein-rich fluid (exudate) into the extravascular spaces. The loss of fluid results in an increased concentration of blood constituents (red cells, leukocytes, platelets, and clotting factors), stagnation of flow, and clotting of blood at the site of injury. This aids in localizing the spread of infectious microorganisms. The loss of plasma proteins reduces the intracapillary osmotic pressure and increases the osmotic pressure of the interstitial fluid, causing fluid to move into the tissues and produce the swelling (*i.e.*, edema), pain, and impaired function that are the cardinal signs of acute inflammation. The exudation of fluid into the tissue spaces also serves to dilute the offending agent.[6,8]

The increased permeability characteristic of acute inflammation results from formation of endothelial gaps in the venules of the microcirculation. Binding of the chemical mediators to endothelial receptors causes contraction of endothelial cells and separation of intercellular junctions. This is the most common mechanism of vascular leakage and is elicited by histamine, bradykinin, LT, and many other classes of chemical mediators.[1]

Vascular Response Patterns. Depending on the severity of injury, the vascular changes that occur with inflammation follow one of three patterns of responses.[15] The first pattern is an *immediate transient response*, which occurs with minor injury. It develops rapidly after injury and is usually reversible and of short duration (15 to 30 minutes). Typically, this type of leakage affects venules 20 to 60 μm in diameter, leaving capillaries and arterioles unaffected.[15] Although the precise mechanism for restriction of this effect to the venules is unknown, it may reflect the greater density of receptors in the endothelium of the venules. It has also been suggested that the later leukocyte events of inflammation (*i.e.*, adhesion and emigration) also occur predominantly in the venules of most organs.

The second pattern is *an immediate sustained response*, which occurs with more serious types of injury and continues for several days. It affects arterioles, capillaries, and venules and is generally because of direct damage of the endothelium. Neutrophils that adhere to the endothelium may also injure endothelial cells.

The third pattern is a *delayed hemodynamic response*, in which the increased permeability occurs in the venules and capillaries. A delayed response often accompanies injuries due to radiation, such as sunburn. The mechanism of the leakage is unknown, but it may result from the direct effect of the injurious agent, leading to delayed endothelial cell damage.

Cellular Stage

The cellular stage of acute inflammation is marked by changes in the endothelial cells lining the vasculature and movement of phagocytic leukocytes into the area of injury or infection. Although attention has been focused on the recruitment of leukocytes from the blood, a rapid response also requires the release of chemical mediators from tissue cells (mast cells and macrophages) that are prepositioned in the tissues. The sequence of events in the cellular response to inflammation includes leukocyte

1. Margination and adhesion to the endothelium
2. Transmigration across the endothelium
3. Chemotaxis
4. Activation and phagocytosis

Margination, Adhesion, and Transmigration. During the early stages of the inflammatory response, the leukocytes are concentrated along the endothelium wall. Cross talk between the blood leukocytes and the vascular endothelium defines a definite inflammatory event and ensures secure adhesion and arrest of the leukocytes along the endothelium.[5,8,15] As a consequence, the leukocytes slow their migration, adhere tightly to the endothelium, and begin to move along the periphery of the blood vessels. This process of leukocyte accumulation is called *margination*. The subsequent release of cell communication molecules called *cytokines* causes the endothelial cells lining the vessels to express cell adhesion molecules, such as *selectins*, that bind to carbohydrate residues on the leukocyte surface.[13] This interaction slows their flow and causes the leukocytes to move along the endothelial cell surface with a rolling movement, finally coming to rest and adhering strongly to intercellular adhesion molecules (ICAMs), thus, attaching on the endothelium.[1,13] The adhesion causes the endothelial cells to separate, allowing the leukocytes to extend pseudopodia and *transmigrate* through the vessel wall and then, under the influence of chemotactic factors, migrate into the tissue spaces.

Several families of adhesion molecules, including selectins, integrins (VLA-5, a fibronectin receptor), and the immunoglobulin superfamily, are involved in leukocyte recruitment.[5,8,15] The selectins are a family of three closely related proteins (P-selectin, E-selectin, and L-selectin) that differ in their cellular distribution but all function in adhesion of leukocytes to endothelial cells. The integrin superfamily consists of 30 structurally similar proteins that promote cell-to-cell and cell-to-ECM interactions. The name *integrin* derives from the hypothesis that they coordinate (integrate) signals of extracellular ligands with cytoskeleton-dependent motility, shape change, and phagocytic responses of immune cells. Adhesion molecules of the immunoglobulin superfamily include ICAM-1, ICAM-2, and vascular adhesion molecule (VCAM)-1, all of which interact with integrins on leukocytes to mediate their recruitment.

Chemotaxis. Chemotaxis is the dynamic and energy-directed process of directed cell migration.[1] Once leukocytes exit the capillary, they wander through the tissue guided by a gradient of secreted chemoattractants, such as chemokines, bacterial and cellular debris, and protein fragments generated from activation of the complement system (*e.g.*, C3a, C5a). Chemokines, an important subgroup of chemotactic cytokines, are small proteins that direct the trafficking of leukocytes during the early stages of inflammation or injury.[16] Several immune (*e.g.*, macrophages) and nonimmune cells secrete these chemoattractants to ensure the directed movement of leukocytes to the site of infection.

Leukocyte Activation and Phagocytosis. During the final stage of the cellular response, monocytes, neutrophils, and tissue macrophages are activated to engulf and degrade the bacteria and cellular debris in a process called phagocytosis.[1] Phagocytosis involves three distinct steps: (1) recognition and adherence, (2) engulfment, and (3) intracellular killing. Phagocytosis is initiated by the recognition and binding of particles by specific receptors on the surface of phagocytic cells. This binding is essential for trapping the agent, which triggers engulfment and activates the killing potential of the cell. Microbes can be bound directly to the membrane of phagocytic cells by several types of pattern recognition receptors (*e.g.*, toll-like and mannose receptors) or indirectly by receptors that recognize microbes coated with carbohydrate-binding lectins, antibody, or complement. The coating of an antigen with antibody or complement to enhance binding is called *opsonization*. Receptor-mediated endocytosis is triggered by opsonization and binding of the agent to phagocyte cell surface receptors. Endocytosis is accomplished through cytoplasmic extensions (pseudopods) that surround and enclose the particle in a membrane-bounded phagocytic vesicle or *phagosome*. Once inside the cell cytoplasm, the phagosome merges with a cytoplasmic lysosome containing antibacterial molecules and enzymes that can kill and digest the microbe.

Intracellular killing of pathogens is accomplished through several mechanisms, including toxic oxygen and nitrogen products, lysozymes, proteases, and defensins. The metabolic burst pathways that generate toxic oxygen and nitrogen products (*i.e.*, NO, hydrogen peroxide, and hypochlorous acid) require oxygen and metabolic enzymes such as myeloperoxidase, nicotinamide adenine dinucleotide phosphate (NADPH) oxidase, and NO synthetase. Oxygen-independent pathways generate several types of digestive enzymes and antimicrobial molecules (*e.g.*, defensins). Individuals born with genetic defects in some of these enzymes have immunodeficiency conditions that make them susceptible to repeated bacterial infection.

Inflammatory Mediators

Although inflammation is precipitated by infection and injury, its signs and symptoms are produced by chemical mediators. Mediators can originate either from the plasma or from cells (Fig. 9.3). The plasma-derived mediators, which are synthesized in the liver, include the coagulation factors and the complement proteins. These mediators are present in the plasma in a precursor form that must be activated by a series of proteolytic processes to acquire their biologic properties. Cell-derived mediators are normally sequestered in intracellular granules that need to be secreted (*e.g.*, histamine from mast cells) or are newly synthesized (*e.g.*, cytokines) in response to a stimulus. Although the major sources of these mediators are platelets, neutrophils, monocytes/macrophages, and mast cells, endothelial cells, smooth muscle, fibroblasts, and most epithelial cells can be induced to produce some of the mediators.[17,18]

The production of active mediators is triggered by microbes or host proteins, such as those of the complement, kinin, or coagulation systems, that are themselves activated by microbes or damaged tissues. Mediators can act on one or a few target cells, have diverse targets, or have differing effects on different types of cells. Once activated and released from the cell, most mediators are short-lived. They may be transformed into inactive metabolites, inactivated by enzymes, or otherwise scavenged or degraded.

Inflammatory mediators can be classified by function: (1) those with vasoactive and smooth muscle–constricting properties such as histamine, arachidonic acid metabolites (prostaglandins and LT), and PAF; (2) plasma proteases that activate members of the complement system, coagulation factors of the clotting cascade, and vasoactive peptides of the

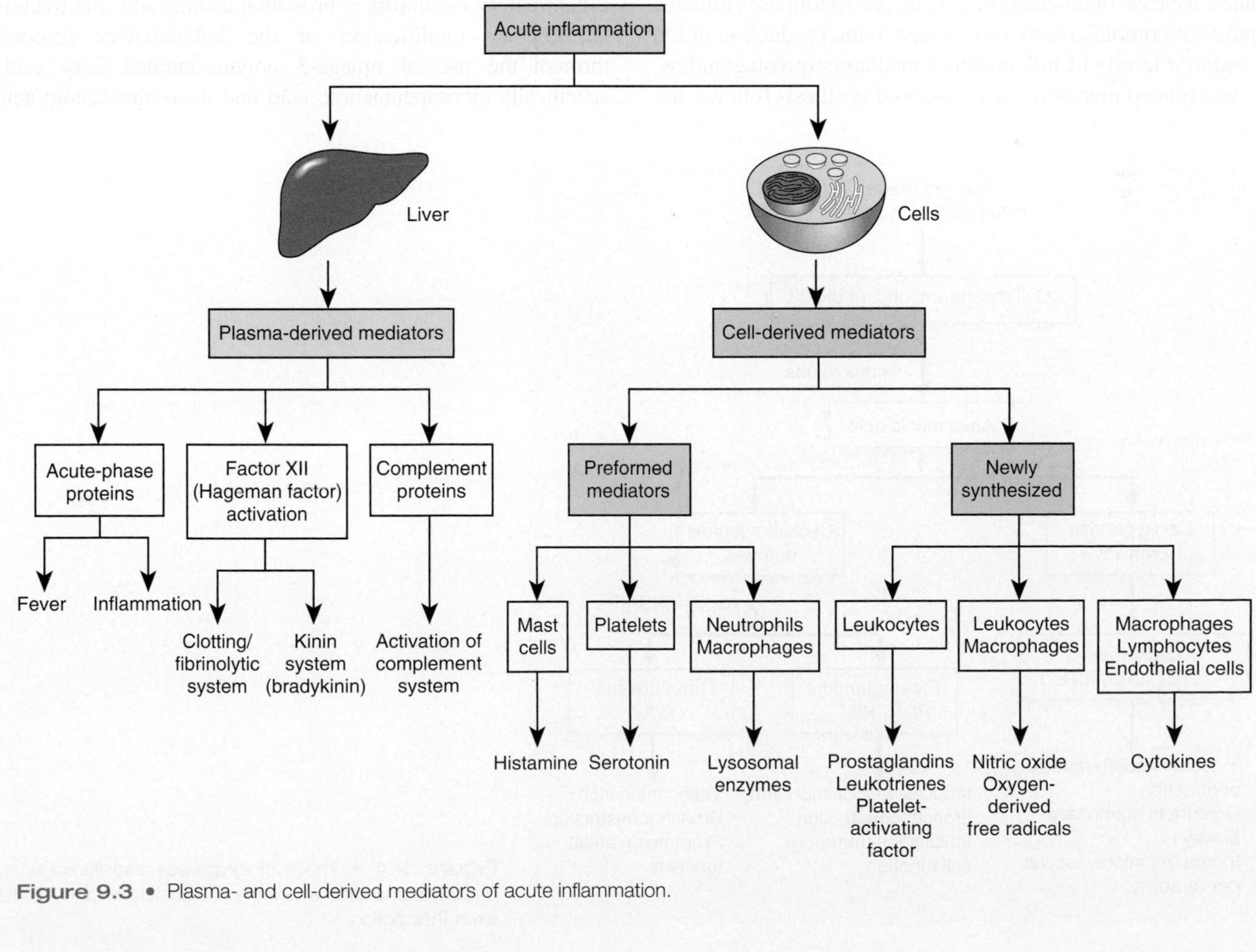

Figure 9.3 • Plasma- and cell-derived mediators of acute inflammation.

kinin system; (3) chemotactic factors such as complement fragments and chemokines; and (4) reactive molecules and cytokines liberated from leukocytes, which when released into the extracellular environment can affect the surrounding tissue and cells.

Histamine. Histamine is present in preformed stores in cells and is therefore among the first mediators to be released during an acute inflammatory reaction. Preformed histamine is widely distributed in tissues, the highest concentrations being found in the connective tissues adjacent to blood vessels. It is also found in circulating blood platelets and basophils. Preformed histamine is found in mast cell granules and is released in response to a variety of stimuli, including trauma and immune reactions involving binding of IgE antibodies. Histamine causes dilation of arterioles and increases the permeability of venules. It acts at the level of the microcirculation by binding to histamine type 1 (H_1) receptors on endothelial cells and is considered the principal mediator of the immediate transient phase of increased vascular permeability in the acute inflammatory response. Antihistamine drugs (H_1 receptor antagonists), which bind to the H_1 receptors, act competitively to antagonize many of the effects of the immediate inflammatory response.

Arachidonic Acid Metabolites. Arachidonic acid is a 20-carbon unsaturated fatty acid found in phospholipids of cell membranes. Release of arachidonic acid by phospholipases initiates a series of complex reactions that lead to the production of the *eicosanoid* family of inflammatory mediators (prostaglandins, LT, and related metabolites). Eicosanoid synthesis follows one of two pathways: the cyclooxygenase pathway, which culminates in the synthesis of prostaglandins and thromboxane, collectively termed prostanoids, and the lipoxygenase pathway, which culminates in the synthesis of the LT (Fig. 9.4).[19–21]

Through the cyclooxygenase metabolic pathway, many prostaglandins are synthesized from arachidonic acid.[1] The prostaglandins (*e.g.*, prostaglandin D_2 [PGD_2], prostaglandin [PG] E_2 [PGE_2], prostaglandin F2α [PGF2α], and prostacyclin [PGI_2]) induce inflammation and potentiate the effects of histamine and other inflammatory mediators. The prostaglandins and thromboxane A_2 promotes platelet aggregation and vasoconstriction. Aspirin and the nonsteroidal anti-inflammatory drugs (NSAIDs) reduce inflammation by inactivating the first enzyme in the cyclooxygenase pathway for prostaglandin synthesis.

Like the prostaglandins, the LT are formed from arachidonic acid, but through the lipoxygenase pathway. Histamine and LT are complementary in action in that they have similar functions. Histamine is produced rapidly and transiently while the more potent LT are being synthesized. The LT also have been reported to affect the permeability of the postcapillary venules, the adhesion properties of endothelial cells, and the extravasation and chemotaxis of neutrophils, eosinophils, and monocytes. LTC_4, LTD_4, and LTE_4, collectively known as the *slow-reacting substance of anaphylaxis* (SRS-A), cause slow and sustained constriction of the bronchioles and are important inflammatory mediators in bronchial asthma and anaphylaxis.

Dietary modification of the inflammatory response through the use of omega-3 polyunsaturated fatty acids, specifically eicosapentaenoic acid and docosahexaenoic acid,

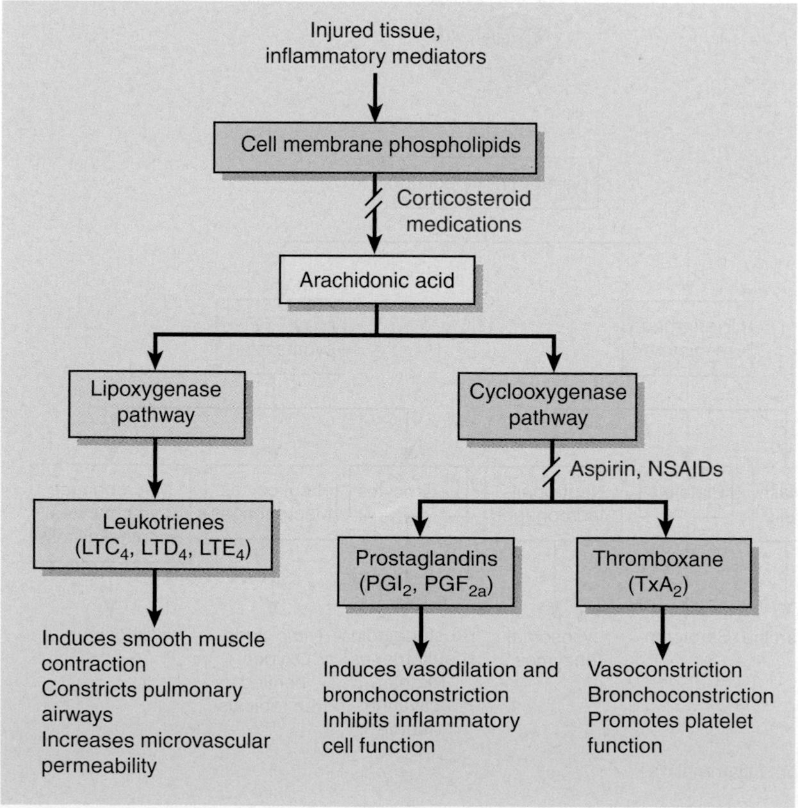

Figure 9.4 • The cyclooxygenase and lipoxygenase pathways and sites where the corticosteroids and NSAIDs exert their action.

which are present in the fish oil, may be effective in preventing some negative manifestations of inflammation.[22–24] Alpha-linolenic acid, which is present in flaxseed, canola oil, green leafy vegetables, walnuts, and soybeans, is another source of omega-3 fatty acid. The omega-3 polyunsaturated fatty acids, which are considered antithrombotic and anti-inflammatory, are structurally different from the prothrombotic and proinflammatory omega-6 polyunsaturated fatty acids, which are present in most seeds, vegetable oils, and meats. Typically, the cell membranes of inflammatory cells contain high proportions of omega-6 arachidonic acid, which is the source of prostaglandin and leukotriene inflammatory mediators. Consuming fish oil and other foods that are high in omega-3 fatty acids results in partial replacement of arachidonic acid in inflammatory cell membranes by eicosapentaenoic acid, a change that leads to decreased production of arachidonic acid–derived inflammatory mediators. This response alone is a potentially beneficial effect of omega-3 fatty acids. However, omega-3 fatty acids have a number of other effects that might occur downstream of altered eicosanoid production or might be independent of this function. For example, animal and human research has shown that dietary fish oil results in suppressed production of proinflammatory cytokines and decreased expression of adhesion molecules that participate in the inflammatory response.[25]

Platelet-Activating Factor. PAF, which is generated from a complex lipid stored in cell membranes, affects a variety of cell types and induces platelet aggregation. It activates neutrophils and is a potent eosinophil chemoattractant. When injected into the skin, PAF causes a wheal-and-flare reaction and the leukocyte infiltrate characteristic of immediate hypersensitivity reactions. When inhaled, PAF causes bronchospasm, eosinophil infiltration, and nonspecific bronchial hyperreactivity.

Plasma Proteins. A number of phenomena in the inflammatory response are mediated by plasma proteins that belong to three interrelated systems, the clotting, complement, and kinin systems.

The clotting system contributes to the vascular phase of inflammation, mainly through fibrinopeptides that are formed during the final steps of the clotting process. The protease thrombin, which binds to receptors called *protease-activated receptors* (PARs), provides the final link between the coagulation system and inflammation.[26] Engagement of the so-called type 1 receptor (PAR-1) by proteases, particularly thrombin, triggers several responses that induce inflammation, including production of chemokines, expression of endothelial adhesion molecules, induction of prostaglandin synthesis, and production of PAF.

The complement system consists of 20 component proteins (and their cleavage products) that are found in greatest concentration in the plasma. The complement proteins are present in inactive forms in the plasma. Many of them are activated to become proteolytic enzymes that degrade other complement proteins, thus forming a cascade that plays an important role in both immunity and inflammation.[27–29] The complement proteins assist the inflammatory cascade by increasing vascular permeability, improving phagocytosis, and causing vasodilation.

The kinin system generates vasoactive peptides from plasma proteins called *kininogens*, by the action of proteases called *kallikreins*.[30] Activation of the kinin system results in release of bradykinin, which increases vascular permeability and causes contraction of smooth muscle, dilation of blood vessels, and pain when injected into the skin. These effects are similar to those of histamine. The action of bradykinin is short-lived, because it is quickly inactivated by an enzyme called *kininase*. Any bradykinin that escapes inactivation by the kininase enzyme is degraded by the angiotensin-converting enzyme in the lung.[30]

Cytokines and Chemokines. Cytokines are proteins produced by many cell types (principally activated macrophages and lymphocytes but also endothelium, epithelium, and connective tissue types) that modulate the function of other cells.[1] Although well known for their role in immune responses, these products also play important roles in both acute and chronic inflammation.

TNF-α and IL-1 are two of the major cytokines that mediate inflammation. The major cellular source of TNF-α and IL-1 is activated macrophages (Fig. 9.5). IL-1 is also

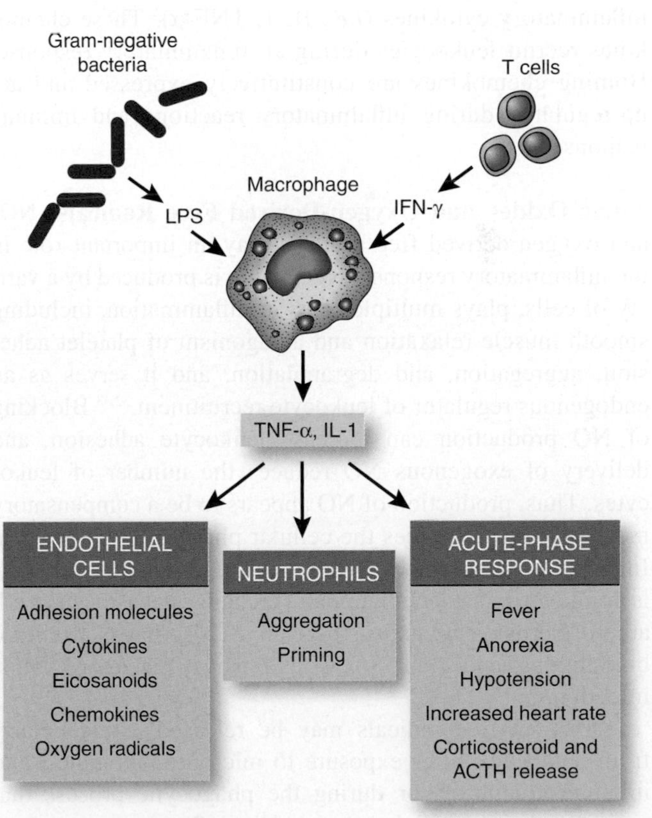

Figure 9.5 • Central role of IL-1 and TNF-α in the acute inflammatory response. Lipopolysaccharide (LPS) and IFN-γ activate macrophages to release inflammatory cytokines, principally IL-1 and TNF-α, responsible for directing both local and systemic inflammatory responses. ACTH, adrenocorticotropic hormone. (From Rubin E., Strayer D. S. (Eds.) (2015). *Rubin's pathology: Clinicopathologic foundations of medicine* (7th ed., Figure 2-14, p. 68). Philadelphia, PA: Lippincott Williams & Wilkins.)

produced by many cell types other than macrophages, including neutrophils, endothelial cells, and epithelial cells (*e.g.*, keratinocytes). The secretion of TNF-α and IL-1 can be stimulated by endotoxin and other microbial products, immune cells, injury, and a variety of inflammatory stimuli. TNF-α and IL-1 induce endothelial cells to express adhesion molecules and release cytokines, chemokines, and reactive oxygen species. TNF-α induces priming and aggregation of neutrophils, leading to augmented responses of these cells to other mediators. IL-1 and TNF-α are also mediators of the acute-phase responses associated with infection or injury. Features of these systemic responses include fever, hypotension and increased heart rate, anorexia, release of neutrophils into the circulation, and increased levels of corticosteroid hormones.

Chemotactic cytokines, or *chemokines*, are a family of small proteins that act primarily as chemoattractants to recruit and direct the migration of immune and inflammatory cells.[31] Chemokines generate a chemotactic gradient by binding to proteoglycans on the surface of endothelial cells or in the ECM. As a result, high concentrations of chemokines persist at sites of tissue injury or infection. Two classes of chemokines have been identified: inflammatory chemokines and homing chemokines. Inflammatory chemokines are produced in response to bacterial toxins and inflammatory cytokines (*i.e.*, IL-1, TNF-α). These chemokines recruit leukocytes during an inflammatory response. Homing chemokines are constitutively expressed and are up-regulated during inflammatory reactions and immune responses.[31]

Nitric Oxide– and Oxygen-Derived Free Radicals. NO- and oxygen-derived free radicals play an important role in the inflammatory response. NO, which is produced by a variety of cells, plays multiple roles in inflammation, including smooth muscle relaxation and antagonism of platelet adhesion, aggregation, and degranulation, and it serves as an endogenous regulator of leukocyte recruitment.[32,33] Blocking of NO production can increase leukocyte adhesion, and delivery of exogenous NO reduces the number of leukocytes. Thus, production of NO appears to be a compensatory mechanism that reduces the cellular phase of inflammation. Impaired production of NO by vascular endothelial cells is implicated in the inflammatory changes that occur with atherosclerosis. NO and its derivatives also have antimicrobial actions, and thus, NO is also a host mediator against infection.

Oxygen free radicals may be released extracellularly from leukocytes after exposure to microbes, cytokines, and immune complexes or during the phagocytic process that occurs during the cellular phase of the inflammatory process. The superoxide radical, hydrogen peroxide, and the hydroxyl radical are the major species produced in the cell. These species can combine with NO to form other reactive nitrogen intermediates, which can increase the inflammatory process and cause more tissue injury.

Local Manifestations

Although all acute inflammatory reactions are characterized by vascular changes and leukocyte infiltration, the severity of the reaction, its specific cause, and the site of involvement introduce variations in its manifestations and clinical correlates. These manifestations can range from swelling and the formation of exudates to abscess formation or ulceration.

Characteristically, the acute inflammatory response involves the production of exudates. These exudates vary in terms of fluid type, plasma protein content, and the presence or absence of cells. They can be serous, hemorrhagic, fibrinous, membranous, or purulent. Often the exudate is composed of a combination of these types. *Serous exudates* are watery fluids low in protein content that result from plasma entering the inflammatory site. *Hemorrhagic exudates* occur when there is severe tissue injury that damages blood vessels or when there is significant leakage of red cells from the capillaries. *Fibrinous exudates* contain large amounts of fibrinogen and form a thick and sticky meshwork, much like the fibers of a blood clot. *Membranous* or *pseudomembranous exudates* develop on mucous membrane surfaces and are composed of necrotic cells enmeshed in a fibropurulent exudate.

A *purulent* or *suppurative exudate* contains pus, which is composed of degraded white blood cells, proteins, and tissue debris. Certain microorganisms, such as *Staphylococcus*, are more likely to induce localized suppurative inflammation than others. An abscess is a localized area of inflammation containing a purulent exudate that may be surrounded by a neutrophil layer (Fig. 9.6). Fibroblasts may eventually enter the area and wall off the abscess. Because antimicrobial agents cannot penetrate the abscess wall, surgical incision and drainage may be required to effect a cure.

An *ulceration* refers to a site of inflammation where an epithelial surface (*e.g.*, skin or gastrointestinal epithelium) has become necrotic and eroded, often with associated subepithelial inflammation. Ulceration may occur as the result of traumatic injury to the epithelial surface (*e.g.*, peptic ulcer) or because of vascular compromise (*e.g.*, foot ulcers associated with diabetes).

KEY POINTS

THE INFLAMMATORY RESPONSE

- The manifestations of an acute inflammatory response can be attributed to the immediate vascular changes that occur (vasodilation and increased capillary permeability), the influx of inflammatory cells such as neutrophils, and, in some cases, the widespread effects of inflammatory mediators, which produce fever and other systemic signs and symptoms.
- The manifestations of chronic inflammation are due to infiltration with macrophages, lymphocytes, and fibroblasts, leading to persistent inflammation, fibroblast proliferation, and scar formation.

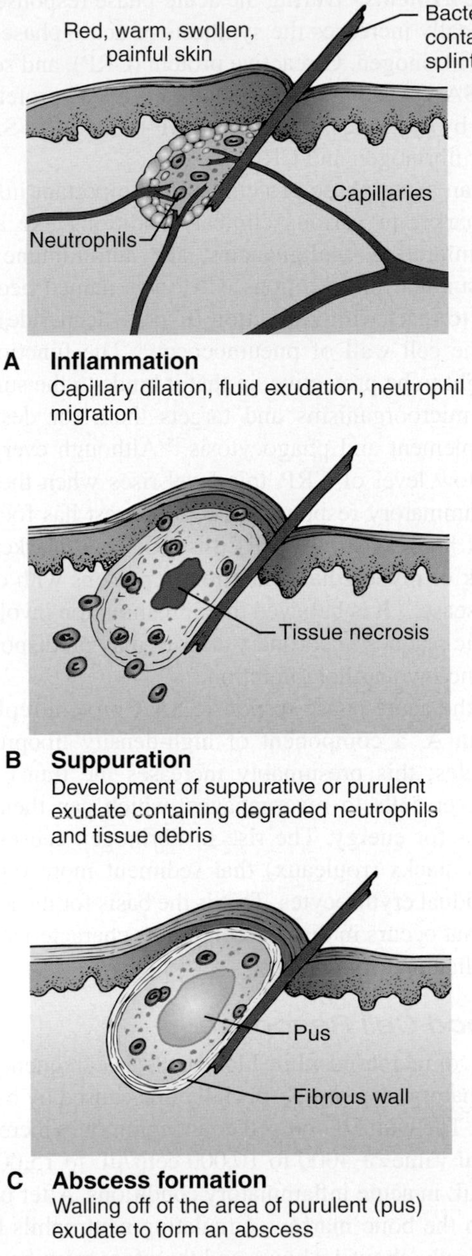

Figure 9.6 • Abscess formation. **(A)** Bacterial invasion and development of inflammation. **(B)** Continued bacterial growth, neutrophil migration, liquefaction tissue necrosis, and development of a purulent exudate. **(C)** Walling off of the inflamed area and its purulent exudate to form an abscess.

Chronic Inflammation

In contrast to acute inflammation, which is usually self-limited and of short duration, chronic inflammation is self-perpetuating and may last for weeks, months, or even years. It may develop as the result of a recurrent or progressive acute inflammatory process or from low-grade, smoldering responses that fail to evoke an acute response.

Characteristic of chronic inflammation is an infiltration by mononuclear cells (macrophages) and lymphocytes instead of the influx of neutrophils commonly seen in acute inflammation. Chronic inflammation also involves the proliferation of fibroblasts instead of exudates. As a result, the risk of scarring and deformity usually is greater than in acute inflammation. Agents that evoke chronic inflammation typically are low-grade, persistent infections or irritants that are unable to penetrate deeply or spread rapidly.[34] Among the causes of chronic inflammation are foreign bodies such as talc, silica, asbestos, and surgical suture materials. Many viruses provoke chronic inflammatory responses, as do certain bacteria, fungi, and larger parasites of moderate to low virulence. Examples are the tubercle bacillus and the treponeme of syphilis. The presence of injured tissue such as that surrounding a healing fracture also may incite chronic inflammation. Immunologic mechanisms are thought to play a key role in chronic inflammation. The two patterns of chronic inflammation are a nonspecific chronic inflammation and granulomatous inflammation.

Nonspecific Chronic Inflammation

Nonspecific chronic inflammation involves a diffuse accumulation of macrophages and lymphocytes at the site of injury. Ongoing chemotaxis causes macrophages to infiltrate the inflamed site, where they accumulate owing to prolonged survival and immobilization. These mechanisms lead to fibroblast proliferation, with subsequent scar formation that in many cases replaces the normal connective tissue or the functional parenchymal tissues of the involved structures. For example, scar tissue resulting from chronic inflammation of the bowel causes narrowing of the bowel lumen.[35]

Granulomatous Inflammation

A granulomatous lesion is a distinctive form of chronic inflammation. A granuloma typically is a small, 1- to 2-mm lesion in which there is a massing of macrophages surrounded by lymphocytes. These modified macrophages resemble epithelial cells and sometimes are called *epithelioid cells*.[1] Like other macrophages, the epithelioid cells are derived originally from blood monocytes. Granulomatous inflammation is associated with foreign bodies such as splinters, sutures, silica, and asbestos and with microorganisms that cause tuberculosis, syphilis, sarcoidosis, deep fungal infections, and brucellosis. These types of agents have one thing in common: they are poorly digested and usually are not easily controlled by other inflammatory mechanisms.[36] The epithelioid cells in granulomatous inflammation may clump in a mass or coalesce, forming a multinucleated giant cell that attempts to surround the foreign agent (Fig. 9.7). A dense membrane of connective tissue eventually encapsulates the lesion and isolates it. These cells are often referred to as *foreign body giant cells*.

Systemic Manifestations of Inflammation

Under optimal conditions, the inflammatory response remains confined to a localized area. In some cases, however, local injury can result in prominent systemic manifestations as inflammatory mediators are released into the circulation. The most prominent systemic manifestations of inflammation

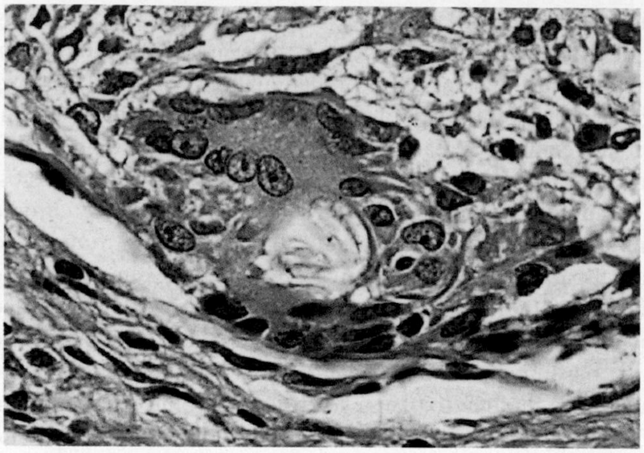

Figure 9.7 • Types of granulomas. Foreign body giant cell with numerous nuclei randomly arranged in the cytoplasm and foreign material in the center. (From Rubin E., Farber J. L. (Eds.) (2015). *Rubin's pathology: Clinicopathologic foundations of medicine* (7th ed., Figure 2-42C, p. 92). Philadelphia, PA: Lippincott Williams & Wilkins.)

include the acute-phase response, alterations in white blood cell count, and fever. Localized acute and chronic inflammation may extend to the lymphatic system and lead to a reaction in the lymph nodes that drain the affected area.

Acute-Phase Response

Along with the cellular responses that occur during the inflammatory response, a constellation of systemic effects called the *acute-phase response* occurs. The acute-phase response, which usually begins within hours or days of the onset of inflammation or infection, includes changes in the concentrations of plasma proteins (*i.e.*, acute-phase proteins), skeletal muscle catabolism, negative nitrogen balance, elevated erythrocyte sedimentation rate (ESR), and increased numbers of leukocytes. These responses are generated by the release of cytokines, particularly IL-1, IL-6, and TNF-α. These cytokines affect the thermoregulatory center in the hypothalamus to produce fever, the most obvious sign of the acute-phase response. IL-1 and other cytokines induce an increase in the number of circulating neutrophils by stimulating their production in the bone marrow. Other manifestations of the acute-phase response include anorexia, somnolence, and malaise, probably because of the actions of IL-1 and TNF-α on the central nervous system. The metabolic changes, including skeletal muscle catabolism, provide amino acids that can be used in the immune response and for tissue repair. In general, the acute-phase response serves to coordinate the various changes in body function to enable an optimal host response.

In severe bacterial infections (sepsis), the large quantities of microorganisms in the blood result in an uncontrolled inflammatory response with the production and release of enormous quantities of inflammatory cytokines (most notably IL-1 and TNF-α) and development of what is referred to as the *systemic inflammatory response syndrome*.[37] These cytokines cause generalized vasodilation, increased vascular permeability, intravascular fluid loss, myocardial depression, and circulatory shock.

Acute-Phase Proteins. During the acute-phase response, the liver dramatically increases the synthesis of acute-phase proteins such as fibrinogen, C-reactive protein (CRP), and serum amyloid A (SAA) protein.[1] The synthesis of these proteins is up-regulated by cytokines, especially TNF-α, IL-1 (for SAA), and IL-6 (for fibrinogen and CRP).

CRP is an acute-phase protein and an important inflammatory biomarker in various clinical conditions like acute myocardial infarction, malignancies, and autoimmune disorders, and surgical interventions. CRP was named because of its ability to react with C fraction (C-polysaccharide) isolated from the cell wall of pneumococci.[38] The function of CRP is thought to be protective, in that it binds to the surface of invading microorganisms and targets them for destruction by complement and phagocytosis.[38] Although everyone maintains a low level of CRP, this level rises when there is an acute inflammatory response. Recent interest has focused on the use of high-sensitivity CRP (hsCRP) as a marker for increased risk of myocardial infarction in persons with coronary heart disease.[39] It is believed that inflammation involving atherosclerotic plaques in coronary arteries may predispose to thrombosis and myocardial infarction.[39]

During the acute-phase response, SAA protein replaces apolipoprotein A, a component of high-density lipoprotein (HDL) particles; this presumably increases the transfer of HDL from liver cells to macrophages, which can then use these particles for energy. The rise in fibrinogen causes red cells to form stacks (rouleaux) that sediment more rapidly than do individual erythrocytes. This is the basis for the accelerated ESR that occurs in disease conditions characterized by a systemic inflammatory response.

White Blood Cell Response

Leukocytosis, or increased white blood cells, is a frequent sign of an inflammatory response, especially one caused by bacterial infection. The white blood cell count commonly increases from a normal value of 4000 to 10,000 cells/μL to 15,000 to 20,000 cells/μL in acute inflammatory conditions. After being released from the bone marrow, circulating neutrophils have a life span of only about 10 hours and therefore must be constantly replaced if their numbers are to be adequate. With excessive demand for phagocytes, immature forms of neutrophils (bands) are released from the bone marrow.

Bacterial infections produce a relatively selective increase in neutrophils (neutrophilia), whereas parasitic and allergic responses induce eosinophilia. Viral infections tend to produce a decrease in neutrophils (neutropenia) and an increase in lymphocytes (lymphocytosis). A decrease in white blood cells (leukopenia) may occur with overwhelming infections or an impaired ability to produce white blood cells.

Lymphadenitis

Localized acute and chronic inflammation may lead to a reaction in the lymph nodes that drain the affected area. This response represents a nonspecific response to mediators released from the injured tissue or an immunologic response to a specific antigen. Painful palpable nodes are more commonly associated with inflammatory processes, whereas nonpainful lymph nodes are more characteristic of neoplasms.

IN SUMMARY

Inflammation describes a local response to tissue injury and can present as an acute or chronic condition. The classic signs of an acute inflammatory response are redness, swelling, local heat, pain, and loss of function. Acute inflammation is orchestrated by the endothelial cells that line blood vessels, phagocytic leukocytes (mainly neutrophils and monocytes) that circulate in the blood, and tissue cells (macrophages, mast cells) that direct the tissues responses. Acute inflammation involves a hemodynamic phase during which blood flow and capillary permeability are increased and a cellular phase during which phagocytic white blood cells move into the area to engulf and degrade the inciting agent. The inflammatory response is orchestrated by chemical mediators such as cytokines and chemokines, histamine, prostaglandins, PAF, complement fragments, and reactive molecules liberated by leukocytes. Acute inflammation may involve the production of exudates containing serous fluid (serous exudate), red blood cells (hemorrhagic exudate), fibrinogen (fibrinous exudate), or tissue debris and white blood cell breakdown products (purulent exudate).

In contrast to acute inflammation, which is self-limiting, chronic inflammation is prolonged and usually is caused by persistent irritants, most of which are insoluble and resistant to phagocytosis and other inflammatory mechanisms. Chronic inflammation involves the presence of mononuclear cells (lymphocytes and macrophages) rather than granulocytes.

The systemic manifestations of inflammation include the systemic effects of the acute-phase response, such as fever and lethargy; increased ESR and levels of hsCRP and other acute-phase proteins; leukocytosis or, in some cases, leukopenia; and enlargement of the lymph nodes that drain the affected area.

TISSUE REPAIR AND WOUND HEALING

After completing this section of the chapter, the learner will be able to meet the following objectives:

- Compare labile, stable, and permanent cell types in terms of their capacity for regeneration.
- Trace the wound-healing process through the inflammatory, proliferative, and remodeling phases.
- Explain the effects of malnutrition; ischemia and oxygen deprivation; impaired immune and inflammatory responses; and infection, wound separation, and foreign bodies on wound healing.
- Discuss the effects of age on wound healing.

Tissue Repair

Tissue repair, which overlaps the inflammatory process, is a response to tissue injury and represents an attempt to maintain normal body structure and function. It can take the form of regeneration in which the injured cells are replaced with cells of the same type, sometimes leaving no residual trace of previous injury, or it can take the form of replacement by connective tissue, which leaves a permanent scar. Both regeneration and repair by connective tissue replacement are determined by similar mechanisms involving cell migration, proliferation, and differentiation, as well as interaction with the ECM.[40]

Tissue Regeneration

Body organs and tissues are composed of two types of structures: parenchymal and stromal. The parenchymal tissues contain the functioning cells of an organ or body part (*e.g.*, hepatocytes, renal tubular cells). The stromal tissues consist of the supporting connective tissues, blood vessels, ECM, and nerve fibers.

Tissue regeneration involves replacement of the injured tissue with cells of the same type, leaving little or no evidence of the previous injury. The capacity for regeneration varies with the tissue and cell type. Body cells are divided into three types according to their ability to undergo regeneration: labile, stable, or permanent cells.[40] *Labile cells* are those that continue to divide and replicate throughout life, replacing cells that are continually being destroyed. They include the surface epithelial cells of the skin, oral cavity, vagina, and cervix; the columnar epithelium of the gastrointestinal tract, uterus, and fallopian tubes; the transitional epithelium of the urinary tract; and bone marrow cells. *Stable cells* are those that normally stop dividing when growth ceases. However, these cells are capable of undergoing regeneration when confronted with an appropriate stimulus and are thus capable of reconstituting the tissue of origin. This category includes the parenchymal cells of the liver and kidney, smooth muscle cells, and vascular endothelial cells. *Permanent* or *fixed cells* cannot undergo mitotic division. The fixed cells include nerve cells, skeletal muscle cells, and cardiac muscle cells. These cells do not normally regenerate; once destroyed, they are replaced with fibrous scar tissue that lacks the functional characteristics of the destroyed tissue.

Fibrous Tissue Repair

Severe or persistent injury with damage to both the parenchymal cells and ECM leads to a situation in which the repair cannot be accomplished with regeneration alone. Under these conditions, repair occurs by replacement with connective tissue, a process that involves generation of granulation tissue and formation of scar tissue.

Granulation tissue is a glistening red, moist connective tissue that contains newly formed capillaries, proliferating fibroblasts, and residual inflammatory cells. The development of granulation tissue involves the growth of new capillaries (angiogenesis), fibrogenesis, and involution to the formation of scar tissue. Angiogenesis involves the generation and sprouting of new blood vessels from preexisting vessels. These sprouting capillaries tend to protrude from the surface of the wound as minute red granules, imparting the name *granulation tissue*. Eventually, portions of the new capillary bed differentiate into arterioles and venules.

Fibrogenesis involves the influx of activated fibroblasts. Activated fibroblasts secrete ECM components, including fibronectin, hyaluronic acid, proteoglycans, and collagen. Fibronectin and hyaluronic acid are the first to be deposited in the healing wound, and proteoglycans appear later. Because the proteoglycans are hydrophilic, their accumulation contributes to the edematous appearance of the wound. The initiation of collagen synthesis contributes to the subsequent formation of scar tissue.

Scar formation builds on the granulation tissue framework of new vessels and loose ECM. The process occurs in two phases: (1) emigration and proliferation of fibroblasts into the site of injury and (2) deposition of ECM by these cells. As healing progresses, the number of proliferating fibroblasts and new vessels decreases, and there is increased synthesis and deposition of collagen. Collagen synthesis is important to the development of strength in the healing wound site. Ultimately, the granulation tissue scaffolding evolves into a scar composed of largely inactive spindle-shaped fibroblasts, dense collagen fibers, fragments of elastic tissue, and other ECM components. As the scar matures, vascular degeneration eventually transforms the highly vascular granulation tissue into a pale, largely avascular scar.

Regulation of the Healing Process

Tissue healing is regulated by the actions of chemical mediators and growth factors that mediate the healing process as well as orchestrate the interactions between the extracellular and cell matrix.[40–43]

Chemical Mediators and Growth Factors. Considerable research has contributed to the understanding of chemical mediators and growth factors that orchestrate the healing process. These chemical mediators and growth factors are released in an orderly manner from many of the cells that participate in tissue regeneration and the healing process. The chemical mediators include the ILs, interferons (IFNs), TNF-α, and arachidonic acid derivatives (prostaglandins and LT) that participate in the inflammatory response.[19] The growth factors are hormone-like molecules that interact with specific cell surface receptors to control processes involved in tissue repair and wound healing.[44] They may act on adjacent cells or on the cell producing the growth factor. The growth factors are named for their tissue of origin (*e.g.*, platelet-derived growth factor [PDGF], fibroblast growth factor [FGF]), their biologic activity (*e.g.*, transforming growth factor [TGF]), or the cells on which they act (*e.g.*, epithelial growth factor [EGF] or connective tissue growth factor beta [TGF-β] or VEGF).[44] The growth factors control the proliferation, differentiation, and metabolism of cells during wound healing. For example, the VEGF stimulates wound healing by way of collagen deposition, angiogenesis, and epithelialization.[44] The growth factors assist in regulating the inflammatory process; serve as chemoattractants for neutrophils, monocytes (macrophages), fibroblasts, and epithelial cells; stimulate angiogenesis; and contribute to the generation of the ECM.

Extracellular Matrix. The understanding of tissue regeneration and repair has expanded over the past several decades to encompass the complex environment of the ECM. The ECM is secreted locally and assembles into a network of spaces surrounding tissue cells. There are three basic components of the ECM: fibrous structural proteins (*e.g.*, collagen and elastin fibers), water-hydrated gels (*e.g.*, proteoglycans and hyaluronic acid) that permit resilience and lubrication, and adhesive glycoproteins (*e.g.*, fibronectin and laminin) that connect the matrix elements to each other and to cells. The ECM occurs in two basic forms: (1) the *basement membrane* that surrounds epithelial, endothelial, and smooth muscle cells and (2) the *interstitial matrix*, which is present in the spaces between cells in connective tissue and between the epithelium and supporting cells of blood vessels.

The ECM provides turgor to soft tissue and rigidity to bone; it supplies the substratum for cell adhesion; it is involved in the regulation of growth, movement, and differentiation of the cells surrounding it; and it provides for the storage and presentation of regulatory molecules that control the repair process. The ECM also provides the scaffolding for tissue renewal. Although the cells in many tissues are capable of regeneration, injury does not always result in restoration of normal structure unless the ECM is intact. The integrity of the underlying basement membrane, in particular, is critical to the regeneration of tissue. When the basement membrane is disrupted, cells proliferate in a haphazard way, resulting in disorganized and nonfunctional tissues.

Critical to the process of wound healing is the transition from granulation tissue to scar tissue, which involves shifts in the composition of the ECM. In the transitional process, the ECM components are degraded by proteases (enzymes) that are secreted locally by a variety of cells (fibroblasts, macrophages, neutrophils, synovial cells, and epithelial cells). Some of the proteases, such as the collagenases, are highly specific, cleaving particular proteins at a small number of sites.[45] This allows for the structural integrity of the ECM to be retained while cell migration occurs. Because of their potential to produce havoc in tissues, the actions of the proteases are tightly controlled. They are typically elaborated in an inactive form that must be activated by chemical mediators that are present at the site of injury, and they are rapidly inactivated by tissue inhibitors. Research has focused on the unregulated action of the proteases in disorders such as cartilage matrix breakdown in arthritis and neuroinflammation in multiple sclerosis, and arterial stiffness causing increased peripheral resistance.[45] Evidence from an animal study shows that a lack of tissue inhibitor of metalloproteinase 2 (MMP2) can lead to left ventricular heart dysfunction and poor EMC remodeling in response to biomechanical stress.[46]

Understanding Wound Healing

Wound healing involves the restoration of the integrity of injured tissue. The healing of skin wounds, which are commonly used to illustrate the general principles of wound healing, is generally divided into three phases: (1) the inflammatory phase, (2) the proliferative phase, and (3) the wound contraction and remodeling phase. Each of these phases is mediated through cytokines and growth factors.

Inflammatory Phase

The inflammatory phase begins at the time of injury with the formation of a blood clot and the migration of phagocytic white blood cells into the wound site. The first cells to arrive, the neutrophils, ingest and remove bacteria and cellular debris. After 24 hours, the neutrophils are joined by macrophages, which continue to ingest cellular debris and play an essential role in the production of growth factors for the proliferative phase.

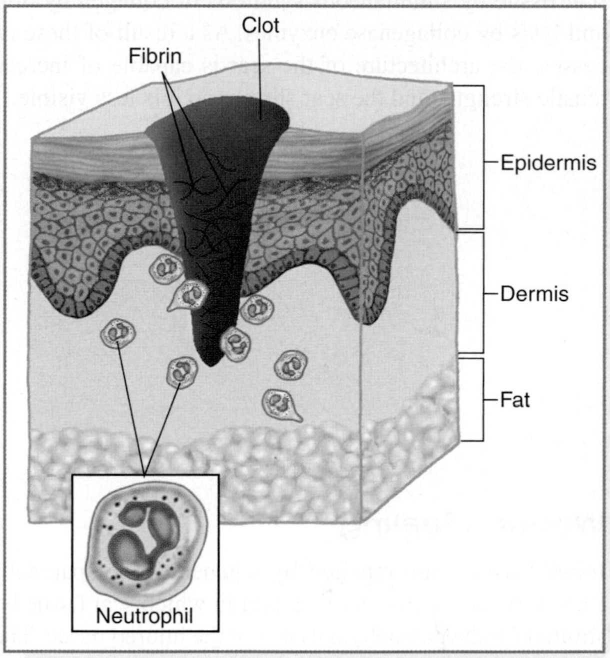

Proliferative Phase

The primary processes during this phase focus on the building of new tissue to fill the wound space. The key cell during this phase is the *fibroblast*, a connective tissue cell that synthesizes and secretes the collagen, proteoglycans, and glycoproteins needed for wound healing. Fibroblasts also produce a family of growth factors that induce angiogenesis (growth of new blood vessels) and endothelial cell proliferation and migration. The final component of the proliferative phase is epithelialization, during which epithelial cells at the wound edges proliferate to form a new surface layer that is similar to that which was destroyed by the injury.

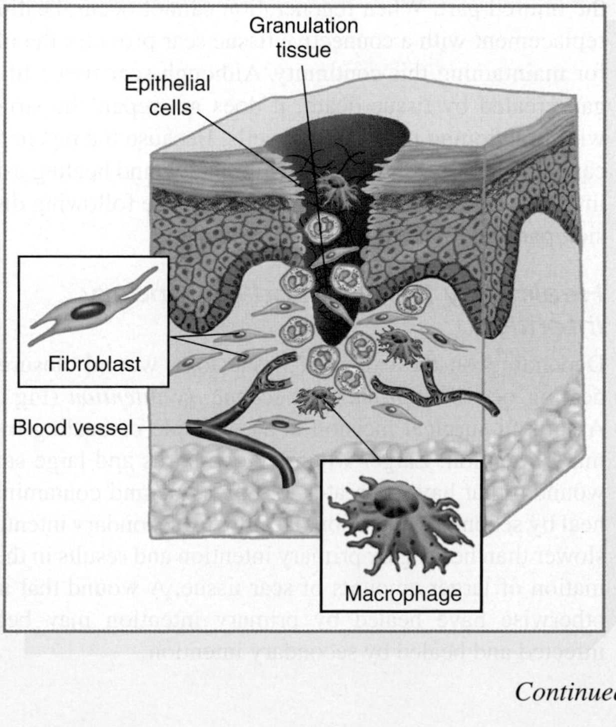

Continued

Understanding Wound Healing *(Continued)*

Wound Contraction and Remodeling Phase

This phase begins approximately 3 weeks after injury with the development of the fibrous scar and can continue for 6 months or longer, depending on the extent of the wound. During this phase, there is a decrease in vascularity and continued remodeling of scar tissue by simultaneous synthesis of collagen by fibroblasts and lysis by collagenase enzymes. As a result of these two processes, the architecture of the scar is capable of increasing its tensile strength, and the scar shrinks so it is less visible.

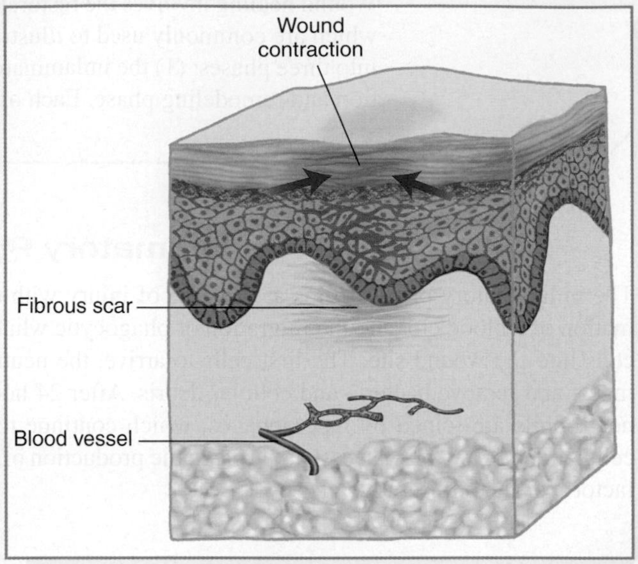

Wound Healing

Injured tissues are repaired by regeneration of parenchymal cells or by connective tissue repair in which scar tissue is substituted for the parenchymal cells of the injured tissue. The primary objective of the healing process is to fill the gap created by tissue destruction and to restore the structural continuity of the injured part. When regeneration cannot occur, healing by replacement with a connective tissue scar provides the means for maintaining this continuity. Although scar tissue fills the gap created by tissue death, it does not repair the structure with functioning parenchymal cells. Because the regenerative capabilities of most tissues are limited, wound healing usually involves some connective tissue repair. The following discussion particularly addresses skin wounds.

Healing by Primary and Secondary Intention

Depending on the extent of tissue loss, wound closure and healing occur by *primary* or *secondary intention* (Fig. 9.8). A sutured surgical incision is an example of healing by primary intention. Larger wounds (*e.g.*, burns and large surface wounds) that have a greater loss of tissue and contamination heal by secondary intention. Healing by secondary intention is slower than healing by primary intention and results in the formation of larger amounts of scar tissue. A wound that might otherwise have healed by primary intention may become infected and healed by secondary intention.

Phases of Wound Healing

Wound healing is commonly divided into three phases: (1) the inflammatory phase, (2) the proliferative phase, and (3) the maturational or remodeling phase.[1,28] The duration of the

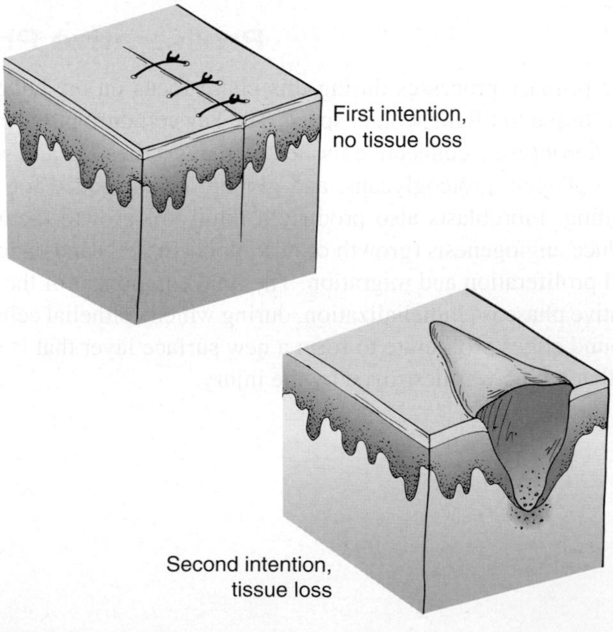

Figure 9.8 • Healing of a skin wound by primary and secondary intention.

phases is fairly predictable in wound healing by primary intention. In wound healing by secondary intention, the process depends on the extent of injury and the healing environment.

Inflammatory Phase. The inflammatory phase of wound healing begins at the time of injury and is a critical period because it prepares the wound environment for healing. It includes hemostasis and the vascular and cellular phases of inflammation. Hemostatic processes are activated immediately at the time of injury. There is constriction of injured blood vessels and initiation of blood clotting through platelet activation and aggregation. After a brief period of constriction, the same vessels dilate and capillaries increase their permeability, allowing plasma and blood components to leak into the injured area. In small surface wounds, the clot loses fluid and becomes a hard, desiccated scab that protects the area.

The cellular phase of inflammation follows and is evidenced by the migration of phagocytic white blood cells that digest and remove invading organisms, fibrin, extracellular debris, and other foreign matter. The neutrophils are the first cells to arrive and are usually gone by day 3 or 4. They ingest bacteria and cellular debris. After approximately 24 hours, macrophages, which are larger phagocytic cells, enter the wound area and remain for an extended period. These cells, arising from blood monocytes, are essential to the healing process. Their functions include phagocytosis and release of growth factors that stimulate epithelial cell growth and angiogenesis and attract fibroblasts. When a large defect occurs in deeper tissues, neutrophils and macrophages are required to remove the debris and facilitate wound closure. Although a wound may heal in the absence of neutrophils, it cannot heal in the absence of macrophages.

Proliferative Phase. The proliferative phase of healing usually begins within 2 to 3 days of injury and may last as long as 3 weeks in wound healing by primary intention. The primary processes during this time focus on the building of new tissue to fill the wound space. The key cell during this phase is the *fibroblast*. The fibroblast is a connective tissue cell that synthesizes and secretes collagen and other intercellular elements needed for wound healing. Fibroblasts also produce a family of growth factors that induce angiogenesis and endothelial cell proliferation and migration.

As early as 24 to 48 hours after injury, fibroblasts and vascular endothelial cells begin proliferating to form the granulation tissue that serves as the foundation for scar tissue development. This tissue is fragile and bleeds easily because of the numerous, newly developed capillary buds. Wounds that heal by secondary intention have more necrotic debris and exudate that must be removed, and they involve larger amounts of granulation tissue. The newly formed blood vessels are semipermeable and allow plasma proteins and white blood cells to leak into the tissues.

The final component of the proliferative phase is epithelialization, which is the migration, proliferation, and differentiation of the epithelial cells at the wound edges to form a new surface layer that is similar to the one destroyed by the injury. In wounds that heal by primary intention, these epidermal cells proliferate and seal the wound within 24 to 48 hours.[41] Because epithelial cell migration requires a moist vascular wound surface and is impeded by a dry or necrotic wound surface, epithelialization is delayed in open wounds until a bed of granulation tissue has formed. When a scab has formed on the wound, the epithelial cells migrate between it and the underlying viable tissue; when a significant portion of the wound has been covered with epithelial tissue, the scab lifts off.

At times, excessive granulation tissue, sometimes referred to as *proud flesh*, may form and extend above the edges of the wound, preventing reepithelialization from taking place. Surgical removal or chemical cauterization of the defect allows healing to proceed.

As the proliferative phase progresses, there is continued accumulation of collagen and proliferation of fibroblasts. Collagen synthesis reaches a peak within 5 to 7 days and continues for several weeks, depending on wound size. By the second week, the white blood cells have largely left the area, the edema has diminished, and the wound begins to blanch as the small blood vessels become thrombosed and degenerate.

Remodeling Phase. The third phase of wound healing, the remodeling process, begins approximately 3 weeks after injury and can continue for 6 months or longer, depending on the extent of the wound. As the term implies, there is continued remodeling of scar tissue by simultaneous synthesis of collagen by fibroblasts and lysis by collagenase enzymes. As a result of these two processes, the architecture of the scar becomes reoriented to increase the tensile strength of the wound.

Most wounds do not regain the full tensile strength of unwounded skin after healing is completed. Carefully sutured wounds immediately after surgery have approximately 70% of the strength of unwounded skin, largely because of the placement of the sutures. This allows people to move about freely after surgery without fear of wound separation. When the sutures are removed, usually at the end of the first week, wound strength is approximately 10%. It increases rapidly over the next 4 weeks and then slows, reaching a plateau of approximately 70% to 80% of the tensile strength of unwounded skin at the end of 3 months.[41]

An injury that heals by secondary intention undergoes wound contraction during the proliferative and remodeling phases. As a result, the scar that forms is considerably smaller than the original wound. Cosmetically, this may be desirable because it reduces the size of the visible defect. However, contraction of scar tissue over joints and other body structures tends to limit movement and cause deformities. As a result of loss of elasticity, scar tissue that is stretched fails to return to its original length.

An abnormality in healing by scar tissue repair is *keloid* formation. Keloids are tumor-like masses caused by excess

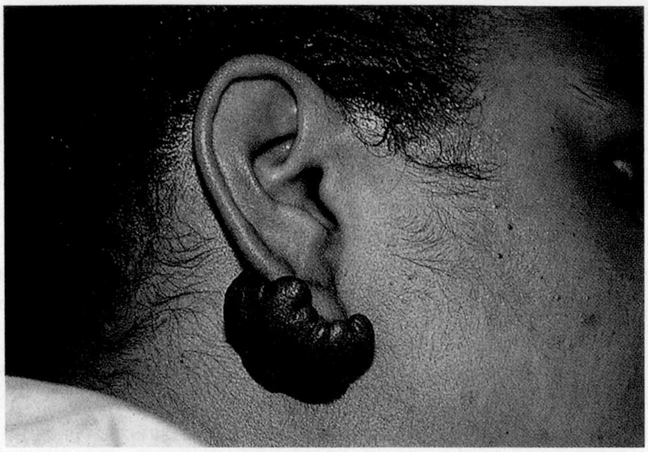

Figure 9.9 • Keloid. A light-skinned black woman developed a keloid as a reaction to having her earlobe pierced. (From Strayer D. E., Rubin R. (Eds.) (2015). *Rubin's pathology: Clinicopathologic foundations of medicine* (7th ed., Figure 3-18A, p. 129). Philadelphia, PA: Lippincott Williams & Wilkins.)

production of scar tissue (Fig. 9.9). The tendency toward development of keloids is more common in African-Americans and seems to have a genetic basis.

KEY POINTS

TISSUE REPAIR AND WOUND HEALING

- Injured tissues can be repaired by regeneration of the injured tissue cells with cells of the same tissue or parenchymal type or by connective repair processes in which scar tissue is used to effect healing.
- Wound healing is impaired by conditions that diminish blood flow and oxygen delivery, restriction of nutrients essential for healing, and depression of inflammatory and immune responses by infection, wound separation, the presence of foreign bodies, and aging.

Factors That Affect Wound Healing

Many local and systemic factors influence wound healing. Among the causes of impaired wound healing are malnutrition; impaired blood flow and oxygen delivery; impaired inflammatory and immune responses; infection, wound separation, and foreign bodies; and age effects.[40,42] Specific disorders that slow wound healing include diabetes mellitus, peripheral artery disease, venous insufficiency, and nutritional disorders. Although there are many factors that impair healing, science has found few ways to hasten the normal process of wound repair.

Malnutrition. Successful wound healing depends in part on adequate stores of proteins, carbohydrates, fats, vitamins, and minerals. Malnutrition has been identified as a significant factor that slows, or even prevents, wound healing.[47] Protein deficiencies prolong the inflammatory phase of healing and impair fibroblast proliferation, collagen and protein matrix synthesis, angiogenesis, and wound remodeling. Carbohydrates are needed as an energy source for white blood cells. Carbohydrates also have a protein-sparing effect and help to prevent the use of amino acids for fuel when they are needed for the healing process. Fats are essential constituents of cell membranes and are needed for the synthesis of new cells.

Although most vitamins are essential cofactors for the daily functions of the body, vitamins A and C play an essential role in the healing process. Vitamin C is needed for collagen synthesis. In vitamin C deficiency, improper sequencing of amino acids occurs, proper linking of amino acids does not take place, the by-products of collagen synthesis are not removed from the cell, new wounds do not heal properly, and old wounds may fall apart. Administration of vitamin C rapidly restores the healing process to normal. Vitamin A functions in stimulating and supporting epithelialization, capillary formation, and collagen synthesis. Vitamin A also has been shown to counteract the anti-inflammatory effects of corticosteroid drugs and can be used to reverse these effects in people who are on chronic steroid therapy. The B vitamins are important cofactors in enzymatic reactions that contribute to the wound-healing process. All are water soluble and, with the exception of vitamin B_{12}, which is stored in the liver, almost all must be replaced daily. Vitamin K plays an indirect role in wound healing by preventing bleeding disorders that contribute to hematoma formation and subsequent infection.

The role of minerals in wound healing is less clearly defined. The macrominerals including sodium, potassium, calcium, and phosphorus, as well as the microminerals (trace minerals), such as copper and zinc, must be present for normal cell function. Zinc is a cofactor in a variety of enzyme systems responsible for cell proliferation. In animal studies, zinc has been found to aid in reepithelialization.

Blood Flow and Oxygen Delivery. For healing to occur, wounds must have adequate blood flow to supply the necessary nutrients and to remove the resulting waste, local toxins, bacteria, and other debris. Impaired wound healing due to poor blood flow may occur as a result of wound conditions (*e.g.*, swelling) or preexisting health problems. Arterial disease and venous pathology are well-documented causes of impaired wound healing. In situations of trauma, a decrease in blood volume may cause a reduction in blood flow to injured tissues.

Molecular oxygen is required for collagen synthesis. Hypoxia is a serious factor in preventing wound healing because it has been shown to decrease fibroblast growth, collagen production, and angiogenesis.[48,49] Wounds in ischemic tissue become infected more frequently than wounds in well-vascularized tissue. PMNs and macrophages require oxygen for destruction of microorganisms that have invaded the area. Although these cells can accomplish phagocytosis in a relatively anoxic environment, they cannot digest bacteria.

Hyperbaric oxygen is a treatment that has demonstrated improved wound healing in multiple types of injuries. This therapy delivers 96% to 100% oxygen at greater than twice the normal atmospheric pressure at sea level.[48] The goal is to increase oxygen delivery to tissues by increasing the partial pressure of oxygen dissolved in the plasma. An increase in tissue oxygen tension by hyperbaric oxygen enhances wound healing by a number of mechanisms, including the increased killing of bacteria by neutrophils, impaired growth of anaerobic bacteria, and the promotion of angiogenesis and fibroblast activity. Hyperbaric oxygen is generally reserved for the treatment of problem wounds in which hypoxia and infection interfere with healing.

Impaired Inflammatory and Immune Responses. Inflammatory and immune mechanisms function in wound healing. Inflammation is essential to the first phase of wound healing, and immune mechanisms prevent infections that impair wound healing. Among the conditions that impair inflammation and immune function are disorders of phagocytic function, diabetes mellitus, and therapeutic administration of corticosteroid drugs.

Phagocytic disorders may be divided into extrinsic and intrinsic defects. Extrinsic disorders are those that reduce the total number of phagocytic cells (*e.g.*, immunosuppressive agents), impair the attraction of phagocytic cells to the wound site, interfere with the engulfment of bacteria and foreign agents by the phagocytic cells (*i.e.*, opsonization), or suppress the total number of phagocytic cells (*e.g.*, immunosuppressive agents). Intrinsic phagocytic disorders are the result of enzymatic deficiencies in the metabolic pathway for destroying the ingested bacteria by the phagocytic cell. The intrinsic phagocytic disorders include chronic granulomatous disease, an X-linked inherited disease in which there is a deficiency of the myeloperoxidase or NADPH oxidase enzymes. Deficiencies of these compounds prevent generation of superoxide and hydrogen peroxide needed for killing bacteria.

Many people with diabetes mellitus who have wounds do not respond well to traditional methods of wound treatment because of their high blood glucose levels.[49] Evidence shows delayed wound healing and complications such as prolonged infections in people with diabetes.[49] Of particular importance is the effect of hyperglycemia on phagocytic function. Neutrophils, for example, have diminished chemotactic and phagocytic function, including engulfment and intracellular killing of bacteria, when exposed to altered glucose levels. Small blood vessel disease is also common among people with diabetes, impairing the delivery of inflammatory cells, oxygen, and nutrients to the wound site.

The therapeutic administration of corticosteroid drugs decreases the inflammatory process and may delay the healing process. These hormones decrease capillary permeability during the early stages of inflammation, impair the phagocytic property of the leukocytes, and inhibit fibroblast proliferation and function.

Infection, Wound Separation, and Foreign Bodies. Wound contamination, wound separation, and foreign bodies delay wound healing. Infection impairs all dimensions of wound healing.[50] It prolongs the inflammatory phase, impairs the formation of granulation tissue, and inhibits proliferation of fibroblasts and deposition of collagen fibers. All wounds are contaminated at the time of injury. Although body defenses can handle the invasion of microorganisms at the time of wounding, badly contaminated wounds can overwhelm host defenses. Trauma and existing impairment of host defenses also can contribute to the development of wound infections.

Approximation of the wound edges (*i.e.*, suturing of an incision type of wound) greatly enhances healing and prevents infection. Epithelialization of a wound with closely approximated edges occurs within 1 to 2 days. Large, gaping wounds tend to heal more slowly because it is often impossible to effect wound closure with this type of wound. Mechanical factors such as increased local pressure or torsion can cause wounds to pull apart, or *dehisce*. Foreign bodies tend to invite bacterial contamination and delay healing. Fragments of wood, steel, glass, and other compounds may have entered the wound at the site of injury and can be difficult to locate when the wound is treated. Sutures are also foreign bodies, and although needed for the closure of surgical wounds, they are an impediment to healing. This is why sutures are removed as soon as possible after surgery. Wound infections are of special concern in people with implantation of foreign bodies such as orthopedic devices (*e.g.*, pins, stabilization devices), cardiac pacemakers, and shunt catheters. These infections are difficult to treat and may require removal of the device. New topical therapeutics regarding debridement and diagnostic methods have been successful in breaking down the microbial biofilm that develops on wound surfaces.[50]

Bite Wounds. Animal and human bites are particularly troublesome in terms of infection.[51] The animal inflicting the bite, the location of the bite, and the type of injury are all important determinants of whether the wound becomes infected. Cat bites (30% to 50%) are more apt to become infected with *Pasteurella multocida* compared to human bites.[51] Dog bites, for unclear reasons, become infected only approximately 5% of the time and generally either with *P. multocida* or *Capnocytophaga canimorsus*.[51] Bites inflicted by children are usually superficial and seldom become infected, whereas bites inflicted by adults have a much higher rate of infection. Puncture wounds are more likely to become infected than lacerations, probably because lacerations are easier to irrigate and debride.

Treatment of bite wounds involves vigorous irrigation and cleansing as well as debridement or removal of necrotic tissue. Whether bite wounds are closed with sutures to promote healing by primary intention depends on the location of the bite and whether the wound is already infected. Wounds that are not infected and require closure for mechanical or cosmetic reasons may be sutured. Wounds of the hand are not usually sutured because closed-space infection of the hand can produce loss of function. Antibiotics are usually administered prophylactically to people with high-risk bites (*e.g.*, cat bites in any location and human or animal bites to the hand). All people with bites should be evaluated to determine if tetanus or rabies prophylaxis is needed.

The Effect of Age on Wound Healing

Wound Healing in Neonates and Children. Wound healing in children is similar to that in the adult population.[52] The child has a greater capacity for repair than the adult but may lack the reserves needed to ensure proper healing. A lack in reserves is evidenced by an easily upset electrolyte balance, a sudden change in temperature, and rapid spread of infection. The neonate and small child may have an immature immune system with no antigenic experience with organisms that contaminate wounds. The younger the child, the more likely the immune system is not fully developed.

Successful wound healing also depends on adequate nutrition. Children need sufficient calories to maintain growth and wound healing. The premature infant is often born with immature organ systems and minimal energy stores but high metabolic requirements—a condition that predisposes to impaired wound healing.

Children with certain comorbidities such as diabetes and malabsorption problems will be at higher risk for wound complication. Likewise, these children will be more apt to develop a skin breakdown or pressure sore. The Braden Q Scale is used to assess children's skin breakdown and is designed specifically for use with children.[53]

Wound Healing in Older Adults. A number of structural and functional changes occur in aging skin, including a decrease in dermal thickness, a decline in collagen content, and a loss of elasticity.[54] The observed changes in skin that occur with aging are complicated by the effects of sun exposure. Because the effects of sun exposure are cumulative, older adults show more changes in skin structure.

Wound healing is thought to be progressively impaired with aging. Older adults have reduced collagen and fibroblast synthesis, impaired wound contraction, and slower reepithelialization of open wounds.[55] Although wound healing may be delayed, most wounds heal, even in the debilitated older adult undergoing major surgical procedures.

Older adults are more vulnerable to chronic wounds, especially pressure, diabetic, and ischemic ulcers, compared to younger people, and these wounds heal more slowly. However, these wounds are more likely because of other disorders such as immobility, diabetes mellitus, or vascular disease, rather than aging.[55] New disease-specific formulas for older adults with slow healing wounds are being studied, and pharmacoeconomic evaluations are being considered.[55] Evidence suggests that older adults should have their nutritional formula assessed to make sure it correlates with each older adult's needs and that it specifically includes arginine, zinc, protein, and vitamin C.[55]

IN SUMMARY

The ability of tissues to repair damage because of injury depends on the body's ability to replace the parenchymal cells and to organize them as they were originally. Regeneration describes the process by which tissue is replaced with cells of a similar type and function. Healing by regeneration is limited to tissue with cells that are able to divide and replace the injured cells. Body cells are divided into types according to their ability to regenerate: labile cells, such as the epithelial cells of the skin and gastrointestinal tract, which continue to regenerate throughout life; stable cells, such as those in the liver, which normally do not divide but are capable of regeneration when confronted with an appropriate stimulus; and permanent or fixed cells, such as nerve cells, which are unable to regenerate. Scar tissue repair involves the substitution of fibrous connective tissue for injured tissue that cannot be repaired by regeneration.

Wound healing occurs by primary and secondary intention and is commonly divided into three phases: the inflammatory phase, the proliferative phase, and the maturational or remodeling phase. In wound healing by primary intention, the duration of the phases is fairly predictable. In wound healing by secondary intention, the process depends on the extent of injury and the healing environment. Wound healing can be impaired or complicated by factors such as malnutrition; restricted blood flow and oxygen delivery; diminished inflammatory and immune responses; and infection, wound separation, and the presence of foreign bodies. With infants and young children, wound healing is generally not impaired unless there is a hygiene issue and adolescents tend to have dry skin that can decrease the rate of wound healing.[56] Older adults experience dry skin and decreased subcutaneous fat that can lead to increased time with wound healing.[55]

GERIATRIC Considerations

- Because the risk for pressure wounds due to changes in the skin composition increase with age (discussed earlier in the chapter), to prevent pressure wounds, pressure tolerance should be assessed by inspecting for redness after individual has been in a position for 30 minutes—if redness is present, avoid leaving the individual in the same position for longer than 30 minutes. If no redness occurs, time between repositioning can be incrementally increased until redness appears or up to 2 hours. Simple shifting of weight when sitting can reduce pressure.[54]
- Unrelieved pressure greater than 6 hours leads to ulceration and even with antibiotics may take weeks to months to completely heal.[54]

- Stasis ulcers increase the risk for infection and skin necrosis in older adults. Prevention is key—adding protein to the diet, elevating legs when sitting, massaging bony prominences, use of support stockings, and patting rather rubbing skin dry are recommended.[54]
- Inflammation often has a different presentation than with younger adults—low-grade fever, minimal pain, and increased proinflammatory cytokines increase with age.[54]

PEDIATRIC Considerations

- Increased water content in the skin and laxity of the epidermis' attachment to the dermis place children at risk for wounds.[56]
- Obese children have an increased number of inflammation-related molecules, including TNF-α, IL 6, and cardiotrophin-1, linked to certain comorbidities such as cardiovascular risk factors.[57]
- Shorter leukocyte telomere length is associated with chronic inflammation and stress in children.[58]

REVIEW EXERCISES

1. A 15-year-old boy presents with abdominal pain, a temperature of 38°C (100.5°F), and an elevated white blood cell count of 13,000/μL, with an increase in neutrophils. A tentative diagnosis of appendicitis is made.
   A. *Explain the significance of pain as it relates to the inflammatory response.*
   B. *What is the cause of the fever and elevated white blood cell count?*
   C. *What would be the preferred treatment for this boy?*
2. Aspirin and other nonsteroidal anti-inflammatory drugs (NSAIDs) are used to control the manifestations of chronic inflammatory disorders such as arthritis.
   A. *Explain their mechanism of action in terms of controlling the inflammatory response.*
3. After a myocardial infarction, the area of heart muscle that has undergone necrosis because of a lack of blood supply undergoes healing by replacement with scar tissue.
   A. *Compare the functioning of the heart muscle that has been replaced by scar tissue with that of the normal surrounding heart muscle.*
4. A 35-year-old man presents with a large abscess on his leg. He tells you he injured his leg while doing repair work on his house and he thinks there might be a wood sliver in the infected area.
   A. *Explain the events that participate in formation of an abscess.*
   B. *He is told that incision and drainage of the lesion will be needed so healing can take place. Explain.*
   C. *He is reluctant to have the procedure done and asks whether an antibiotic would work as well. Explain why antibiotics alone are usually not effective in eliminating the microorganisms contained in an abscess.*

References

1. Rubin E., Strayer D. S. (2015). *Rubin's Pathology: Clinicopathologic Foundations of Medicine* (7th ed.). Philadelphia, PA: Walters Kluwer Health.
2. Kidane D., Chae W. J., Czochor J., et al. (2014). Interplay between DNA repair and inflammation, and the link to cancer. *Critical Reviews in Biochemistry and Molecular Biology* 49(2), 116–139.
3. Baune B. T. (2015). Inflammation and neurodegenerative disorders: is there still hope for therapeutic intervention? *Current Opinion in Psychiatry* 28(2), 148–154.
4. Leonard B. E. (2015). Pain, depression and inflammation: Are interconnected causative factors involved? *Modern Trends in Pharmaco psychiatry* 30, 22–35.
5. Netea M. G., Balkwill F., Chonchol M., et al. (2017). A guiding map for inflammation. *Nature Immunology* 18(8), 826–831.
6. Sansbury B. E., Spite M. (2016). Resolution of acute inflammation and the role of resolvins in immunity, thrombosis, and vascular biology. *Circulation Research* 119(1), 113–130.
7. Lillico D. M., Zwozdesky M. A., Pemberton J. G., et al. (2015). Teleost leukocyte immune-type receptors activate distinct phagocytic modes for target acquisition and engulfment. *Journal of Leukocyte Biology* 98(2), 235–248.
8. Shoda T., Futamura K., Orihara K., et al. (2016). Recent advances in understanding the roles of vascular endothelial cells in allergic inflammation. *Allergology International* 65(1), 21–29.
9. Xiao L., Liu Y., Wang N. (2014). New paradigms in inflammatory signaling in vascular endothelial cells. *American Journal of Physiology: Heart and Circulatory Physiology* 306(3), H317–H325.
10. Henrot P., Foret J., Barnetche T., et al. (2018). Assessment of subclinical atherosclerosis in systemic lupus erythematosus: A systematic review and meta-analysis. *Joint, Bone, Spine* 85(2), 155–163.
11. Thomas M. R., Storey R. F. (2015). The role of platelets in inflammation. *Thrombosis and Haemostasis* 114(3), 449–458.
12. Hall J. E. (2011). *Guyton and Hall Textbook of Medical Physiology* (12th ed.). Philadelphia, PA: Lippincott Williams & Wilkins.
13. Ross M. H., Pawlina W. (2011). *Histology: A Text and Atlas with Correlated Cell and Molecular Biology* (6th ed.). Philadelphia, PA: Lippincott Williams & Wilkins.
14. Theoharides T. C., Alysandratos K. D., Angelidou A., et al. (2012). Mast cells and inflammation. *Biochimica et Biophysica Acta* 1822(1), 21–33.
15. Pober J. S., Sessa W. C. (2014). Inflammation and the blood microvascular system. *Cold Spring Harbor Perspectives in Biology* 7(1), a016345.
16. Griffith J. W., Sokol C. L., Luster A. D. (2014). Chemokines and chemokine receptors: Positioning cells for host defense and immunity. *Annual Review of Immunology* 32, 659–702.

17. Rahmati M., Mobasheri A., Mozafari M. (2016). Inflammatory mediators in osteoarthritis: A critical review of the state-of-the-art, current prospects, and future challenges. *Bone* 85, 81–90.
18. Zanini M., Meyer E., Simon S. (2017). Pulp inflammation diagnosis from clinical to inflammatory mediators: A systematic review. *Journal of Endodontics* 43(7), 1033–1051.
19. Chen C., Wang D. W. (2015). Cytochrome P450-CYP2 family-epoxygenase role in inflammation and cancer. *Advances in Pharmacology* 74, 193–221.
20. Korotkova M., Lundberg I. E. (2014). The skeletal muscle arachidonic acid cascade in health and inflammatory disease. *Nature Reviews Rheumatology* 10(5), 295–303.
21. Stenson W. F. (2014). The universe of arachidonic acid metabolites in inflammatory bowel disease: Can we tell the good from the bad? *Current Opinion in Gastroenterology* 30(4), 347–351.
22. Gerber P. A., Gouni-Berthold I., Berneis K. (2013). Omega-3 fatty acids: Role in metabolism and cardiovascular disease. *Current Pharmaceutical Design* 19(17), 3074–3093.
23. Jain A. P., Aggarwal K. K., Zhang P. Y. (2015). Omega-3 fatty acids and cardiovascular disease. *European Review for Medical and Pharmacological Sciences* 19(3), 441–445.
24. Mori T. A. (2014). Omega-3 fatty acids and cardiovascular disease: Epidemiology and effects on cardiometabolic risk factors. *Food & Function* 5(9), 2004–2019.
25. Skarke C., Alamuddin N., Lawson J. A, et al. (2015). Bioactive products formed in humans from fish oils. *The Journal of Lipid Research* 56(9), 1808–1820.
26. van der Poll T., Herwald H. (2014). The coagulation system and its function in early immune defense. *Thrombosis and Haemostasis* 112(4), 640–648.
27. Morgan B. P., Harris C. L. (2015). Complement, a target for therapy in inflammatory and degenerative diseases. *Nature Reviews Drug Discovery* 14(12), 857–877.
28. Roos D. (2015). Complement and phagocytes – A complicated interaction. *Molecular Immunology* 68(1), 31–34.
29. Xu H., Chen M. (2016). Targeting the complement system for the management of retinal inflammatory and degenerative diseases. *The European Journal of Pharmacology* 787, 94–104.
30. Kalinska M., Meyer-Hoffert U., Kantyka T., Potempa J. (2016). Kallikreins—The melting pot of activity and function. *Biochimie* 122, 270–282.
31. Turner M. D., Nedjai B., Hurst T., Pennington D. J. (2014). Cytokines and chemokines: At the crossroads of cell signalling and inflammatory disease. *Biochimica et Biophysica Acta* 1843(11), 2563–2582.
32. Lee M. Y., Sun K. H., Chiang C. P., et al. (2015). Nitric oxide suppresses LPS-induced inflammation in a mouse asthma model by attenuating the interaction of IKK and Hsp90. *Experimental Biology and Medicine (Maywood, NJ)* 240(4), 498–507.
33. Sardon O., Corcuera P., Aldasoro A., et al. (2014). Alveolar nitric oxide and its role in pediatric asthma control assessment. *BMC Pulmonary Medicine* 14, 126.
34. Minihane A. M., Vinoy S., Russell W. R., et al. (2015). Low-grade inflammation, diet composition and health: Current research evidence and its translation. *The British Journal of Nutrition* 114(7), 999–1012.
35. Huang Y., Chen Z. (2016). Inflammatory bowel disease related innate immunity and adaptive immunity. *American Journal of Translational Research* 8(6), 2490–2497.
36. Rose C. D., Neven B., Wouters C. (2014). Granulomatous inflammation: The overlap of immune deficiency and inflammation. *Best Practice & Research: Clinical Rheumatology* 28(2), 191–212.
37. Sprung C. L., Dellinger R. P. (2015). Systemic inflammatory response syndrome criteria for severe sepsis. *The New England Journal of Medicine* 373(9), 880.
38. Kaur M. (2017). C-reactive protein: A prognostic indicator. *International Journal of Applied and Basic Medical Research* 7(2), 83–84.
39. Xu W., Chen B., Guo L., Li Z., Zhao Y., Zeng H. (2015). High-sensitivity CRP: Possible link between job stress and atherosclerosis. *American Journal of Industrial Medicine* 58(7), 773–779.
40. Takeo M., Lee W., Ito M. (2015). Wound healing and skin regeneration. *Cold Spring Harbor Perspectives in Medicine* 5(1), a023267.
41. Janis J., Harrison B. (2014). Wound healing: Part II. Clinical applications. *Plastic and Reconstructive Surgery* 133(3), 383e–392e.
42. Kasuya A., Tokura Y. (2014). Attempts to accelerate wound healing. *Journal of Dermatological Science* 76(3), 169–172.
43. Martin P., Nunan R. (2015). Cellular and molecular mechanisms of repair in acute and chronic wound healing. *British Journal of Dermatology* 173(2), 370–378.
44. Barrientos S., Brem H., Stojadinovic O., Tomic-Canic M. (2014). Clinical application of growth factors and cytokines in wound healing. *Wound Repair and Regeneration* 22(5), 569–578.
45. Tseng C. C., Chang S. J., Tsai W. C., et al. (2016). Increased incidence of rheumatoid arthritis in multiple sclerosis: A nationwide cohort study. *Medicine (Baltimore)* 95(26), e3999.
46. Zitta K., Meybohm P., Bein B., et al. (2014). Activities of cardiac tissue matrix metalloproteinases 2 and 9 are reduced by remote ischemic preconditioning in cardiosurgical patients with cardiopulmonary bypass. *Journal of Translational Medicine* 12, 94.
47. Quain A. M., Khardori N. M. (2015). Nutrition in wound care management: A comprehensive overview. *Wounds* 27(12), 327–335.
48. de Smet G. H. J., Kroese L. F., Menon A. G., et al. (2017). Oxygen therapies and their effects on wound healing. *Wound Repair and Regeneration* 25(4), 591–608.
49. Sidaway P. (2015). Diabetes: Epigenetic changes lead to impaired wound healing in patients with T2DM. *Nature Reviews Endocrinology* 11(2), 65.
50. Worster B., Zawora M. Q., Hsieh C. (2015). Common questions about wound care. *American Family Physician* 91(2), 86–92.
51. Rothe K., Tsokos M., Handrick W. (2015). Animal and human bite wounds. *Deutsches Ärzteblatt International* 112(25), 433–442; quiz 443.
52. Ball J., Bindler R., Cowen K. (2012). *Principles of Pediatric Nursing: Caring for Children* (5th ed.). Boston, MA: Pearson.
53. Willock J., Habiballah L., Long D., Palmer K., Anthony D. (2016). A comparison of the performance of the Braden Q and the Glamorgan paediatric pressure ulcer risk assessment scales in general and intensive care paediatric and neonatal units. *Journal of Tissue Viability* 25(2), 119–126.
54. Newton V. L., McConnell J. C., Hibbert S. A., Graham H. K., Watson R. E. (2015). Skin aging: Molecular pathology, dermal remodelling and the imaging revolution. *Giornale Italiano di Dermatologia e Venereologia* 150(6), 665–674.
55. Gould L., Abadir P., Brem H., et al. (2015). Chronic wound repair and healing in older adults: Current status and future research. *Wound Repair and Regeneration* 23(1), 1–13.
56. Kyle T., Carman S. (2017). *Essentials of Pediatric Nursing* (3rd ed.). Philadelphia, PA: Wolters Kluwer.
57. Marti A., Morell-Azanza L., Azcona-San Julián M., et al. (2018). Serum and gene expression levels of CT-1, IL-6, and TNF-α after a lifestyle intervention in obese children *Pediatric Diabetes* 19(2), 217–222. Available from: CINAHL Complete, Ipswich, MA. Accessed March 27, 2018.
58. Verstraete S., Vanhorebeek I., Verstraete S., et al. (2018). Leukocyte telomere length in paediatric critical illness: Effect of early parenteral nutrition *Critical Care* 22, 1. Available from: CINAHL Complete, Ipswich, MA. Accessed March 27, 2018.

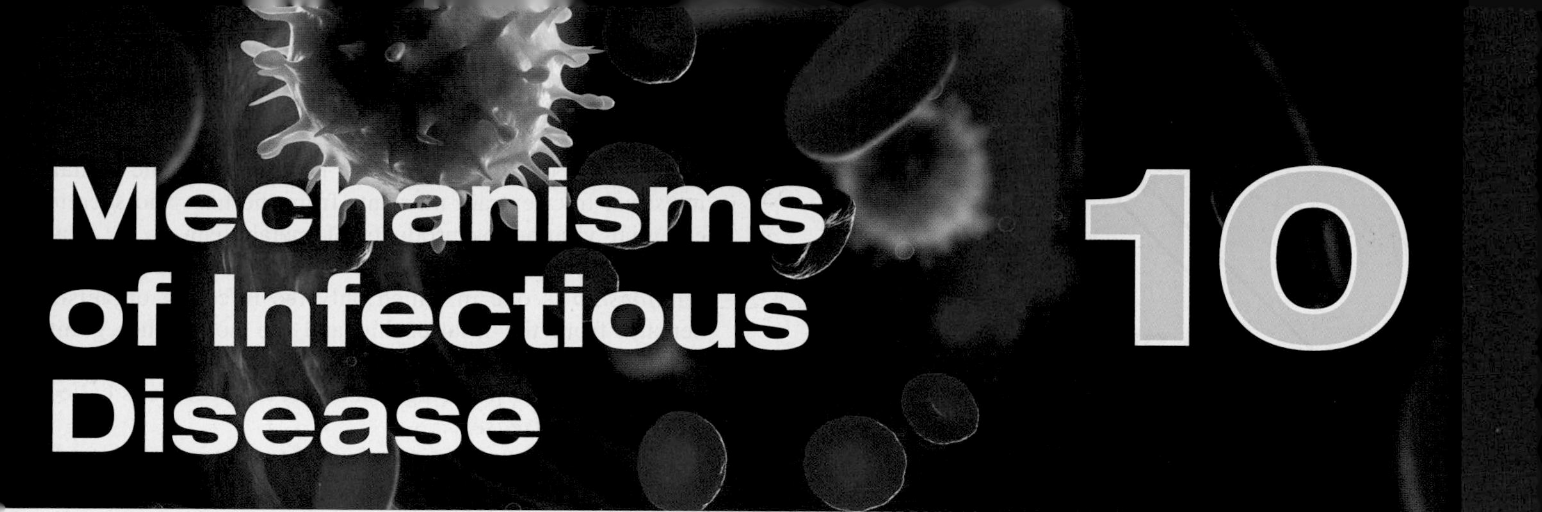

Mechanisms of Infectious Disease 10

Reba A. Umberger and
Sachin Yende

All living organisms share two basic objectives in life: survival and reproduction. This principle applies equally to all members of the living world, including bacteria, viruses, fungi, and protozoa. To meet these objectives, organisms must extract essential nutrients for growth and proliferation from the environment. For countless microscopic organisms, their environment includes the human body, which is inhabited by trillions of organisms living in a symbiotic relationship in an intricate ecosystem.[1] The majority of the organisms found in the human body live in the gastrointestinal tract (over 300 different species) and are usually referred to as normal microflora. We now understand that microbial diversity plays a role in immune response and development of some immune-mediated diseases.[2] There is a continual balance of the immune response to eradicate potential pathogenic organisms and to tolerate self-flora. When pathogenic organisms surpass the barriers of our host defenses (*e.g.*, skin and mucous membranes), and the immune system is unable to eradicate them, they can produce harmful and potentially lethal consequences. The consequences of these invasions are collectively called *infectious diseases.*

INFECTIOUS DISEASES

After completing this section of the chapter, the learner will be able to meet the following objectives:

- Define the terms *host*, *agent*, *infectious disease*, *colonization*, *microflora*, *virulence*, *pathogen*, and *saprophyte*.
- Describe the concept of host–microorganism interaction using the concepts of commensalism, mutualism, and parasitic relationships.
- Describe the triad of infectious disease model.

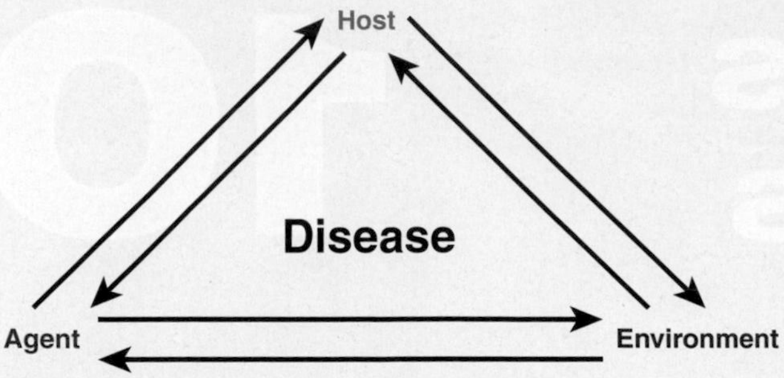

Figure 10.1 • Triad of infectious disease model. Infectious diseases result from the interaction of an agent, a susceptible host, and environmental conditions that promote infection.

Infectious Disease Concepts

The study of infectious diseases is closely intertwined with the disciplines of microbiology, immunology, and epidemiology. Each of these disciplines (although there is an overlap) focuses on an aspect of the well-known triad of disease model (Fig. 10.1), which depicts the relationship between the agent, host, and environment. This model was first used in the study of infectious diseases. We will begin with a discussion of agents that may lead to infectious diseases. The host's immune response (covered in detail in the following chapter) and environmental factors involved in development of infectious disease will be described within the "Mechanisms of Infection" section later in this chapter.

All *scientific* disciplines evolve with a distinct knowledge and use of vocabulary, and the study of infectious diseases is no exception. The most appropriate way to approach this subject is with a brief discussion of the terminology used to characterize interactions between humans and microbes.

Any organism capable of supporting the nutritional and physical growth requirements of another is called a *host*. Throughout this chapter, the term *host* most often refers to humans supporting the growth of microorganisms. Occasionally, *infection* and *colonization* are used interchangeably. However, the term *infection* describes the presence and multiplication within a host of another living organism, with subsequent injury to the host, whereas *colonization* describes the act of establishing a presence, a step required in the multifaceted process of infection.

One common misconception is that all interactions between microorganisms and humans are detrimental. The internal and external exposed surfaces of the human body are normally and harmlessly inhabited by a multitude of bacteria, collectively referred to as the normal *microflora*. Although the colonizing bacteria acquire nutrition, the host is not adversely affected by the relationship. This interaction is called *commensalism*, and the colonizing microorganisms are often referred to as *commensal flora*. The term *mutualism* is applied to an interaction in which both the microorganism and the host derive benefits from the interaction. For example, certain inhabitants of the human intestinal tract extract nutrients from the host and secrete essential vitamin by-products of metabolism (*e.g.*, vitamin K) that are absorbed and used by the host. A *parasitic relationship* is one in which only the infecting organism benefits from the relationship and the host either gains nothing or sustains injury from the interaction. If the host sustains injury or pathologic damage, the process is called an *infectious disease*.

The severity of an infectious disease can range from mild to life threatening. Severity depends on many variables, including the health of the host at the time of infection, the *virulence* (disease-producing potential) of the microorganism, and environmental conditions. Microorganisms capable of causing disease are called *pathogens.* Some microorganisms are highly virulent and frequently cause disease when a host is exposed to the microorganism. Table 10.1 includes a list of common pathogens that cause infectious disease in humans. Fortunately, there are few human pathogens in the microbial world. Most microorganisms are harmless *saprophytes*, free-living organisms obtaining their growth from dead or decaying organic material in the environment. All microorganisms, even saprophytes and members of the normal flora, can be *opportunistic pathogens*, capable of producing an infectious disease when the health and immunity of the host are weakened by illness, malnutrition, or medical therapy.

Agents of Infectious Disease

The agents of infectious disease include prions, viruses, bacteria (*i.e.*, *Rickettsiaceae* and *Chlamydiaceae*), fungi, and parasites. A summary of the relevant characteristics of these human microbial pathogens is presented in Table 10.2.

Prions

In the past, *microbiologists* have assumed that all infectious agents must possess a genetic master plan (a genome of either ribonucleic acid [RNA] or deoxyribonucleic acid [DNA]) that codes to produce the essential proteins and enzymes necessary for survival and reproduction. However, we now know that infection can be transmitted solely by proteins without nucleic acid or genomic material.[3] Prions, discovered in 1982 and once believed to be slow-growing viruses, are protein particles that are able to transmit infection by self-propagating.[3,4] A number of prion-associated diseases have been identified, including Creutzfeldt-Jakob disease and kuru in humans, scrapie in sheep, chronic wasting disease in deer and elk, bovine spongiform encephalopathy (BSE or mad cow disease) in cattle, and recently multiple system atrophy (MSA) in humans.[5] The various prion-associated diseases produce very similar pathologic processes and symptoms in the hosts and are collectively called *transmissible*

TABLE 10.1 COMMON PATHOGENS

PATHOGEN	STRUCTURAL CHARACTERISTICS	FUNCTIONAL CHARACTERISTICS	TREATMENT	COMMON DISEASES
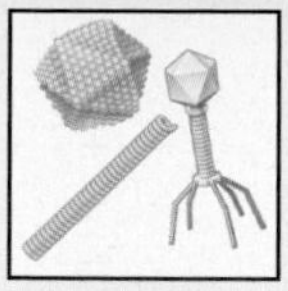 Viruses	DNA/RNA and protein coat	Cannot reproduce outside of cells	Antivirals, which slow viral replication	Influenza, the common cold, measles, HIV/AIDS
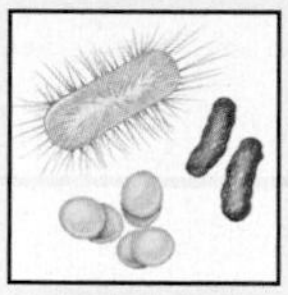 Bacteria	Microscopic cell without nucleus	Common on keyboards, water fountains, toilets, etc.	Antibiotics, which slow bacterial reproduction	Strep throat, some sinus and lung infections, some food poisoning
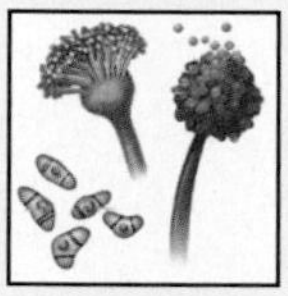 Fungi	Microscopic, unicellular (yeasts) or multicellular (molds)	Usually infect body surfaces and openings	Antifungals, which destroy the cell walls	Athlete's foot, yeast infections
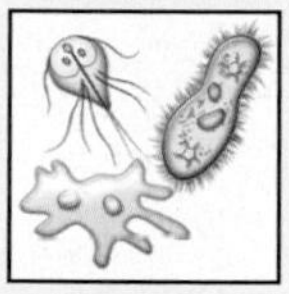 Protozoa	Microscopic, unicellular	Common in water supplies of developing countries	Antiprotozoan drugs, which interfere with protozoan metabolism	Malaria, sleeping sickness
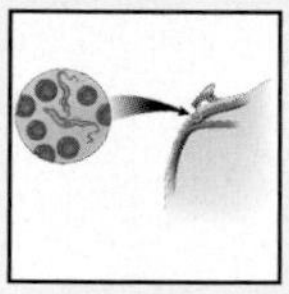 Worms	Multicellular	Prefer to live within body spaces and cells	Antihelminthics, which interfere with the worm's metabolism	Roundworms, tapeworms (helminths)
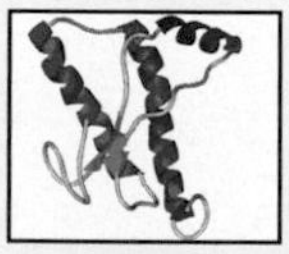 Prion	The protein (PrP) is found throughout the body; however, the PrP^{SC} in infectious materials is misfolded	Protein found in infected animals	Current research for effective treatment	Creutzfeldt-Jakob disease (associated with other neurodegenerative conditions)

Adapted with permission from McConnell T. H., Hull K. L. (2011). *Human form, human function: Essentials of anatomy & physiology*. Philadelphia, PA: Lippincott Williams & Wilkins. Prion image from Knipe, D. M., Howley, P. M., (2013). *Fields virology* (6th ed., Fig. 76.6, p. 2426). Philadelphia, PA: Lippincott Williams & Wilkins.

neurodegenerative diseases (see Fig. 10.2). All are characterized by a slowly progressive, noninflammatory neuronal degeneration, leading to loss of coordination (ataxia), dementia, and death over a period ranging from months to years. The conversion of a cellular precursor protein (PrP^{C}) into an abnormally folded protein (PrP^{SC}) involves modification/refolding of the protein structure, such that it contains many beta pleated sheets. The posttranslational structural modification causes the protein to behave differently. The PrP^{SC} is resistant to the action of proteases (enzymes that degrade excess or deformed proteins). Accumulation of these misfolded proteins becomes toxic to cells; however, as they aggregate, they become less toxic to the cell and can then be captured in plaques, tangles, or inclusion bodies.[4] There is increasing evidence that prion-like proteins are more common than previously known. In fact, the discovery of functional prion-like proteins with normal physiologic function in their aggregated state is leading to speculation that prion-like aggregation may actually serve as a protective factor for the host against viral mechanisms.[4]

Prion diseases present significant challenges for management because of the pathogenic structure of PrP^{SC}. It is

TABLE 10.2 COMPARISON OF CHARACTERISTICS OF HUMAN MICROBIAL PATHOGENS

ORGANISM	DEFINED NUCLEUS	GENOMIC MATERIAL	SIZE*	INTRACELLULAR OR EXTRACELLULAR	MOTILITY
Prions	No	Unknown	55 kDa	E	–
Viruses	No	DNA or RNA	0.02–0.3	I	–
Bacteria	No	DNA	0.5–15	I/E	±
Mycoplasmas	No	DNA	0.2–0.3	E	–
Spirochetes	No	DNA	6–15	E	+
Rickettsiaceae	No	DNA	0.2–2	I	–
Chlamydiaceae	No	DNA	0.3–1	I	–
Yeasts	Yes	DNA	2–60	I/E	–
Molds	Yes	DNA	2–15 (hyphal width)	E	–
Protozoans	Yes	DNA	1–60	I/E	+
Helminths	Yes	DNA	2 mm to >1 m	E	+

*Micrometers unless indicated.

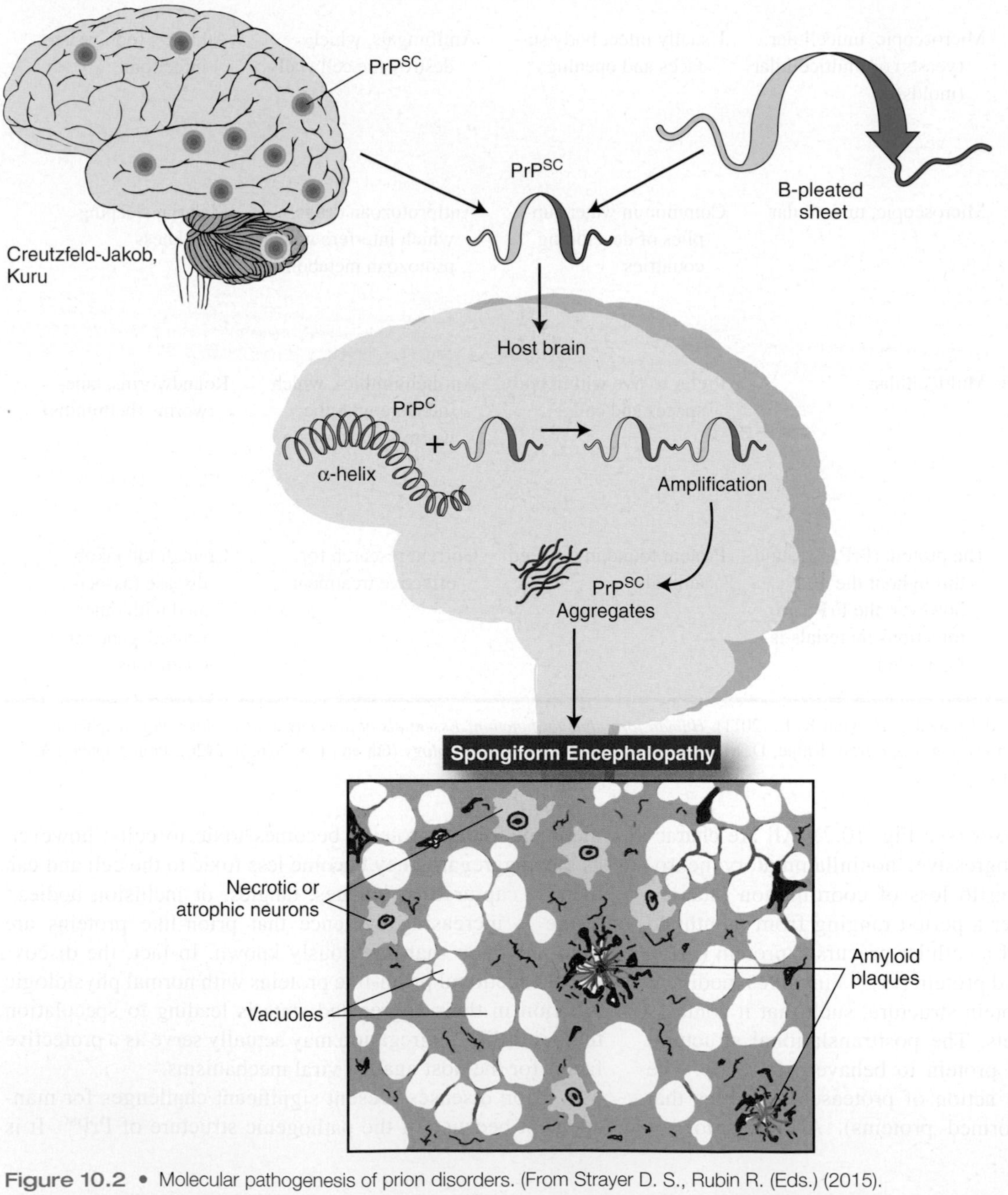

Figure 10.2 • Molecular pathogenesis of prion disorders. (From Strayer D. S., Rubin R. (Eds.) (2015). *Rubin's pathology: Clinicopathologic foundations of medicine* (7th ed., Figure 32.71, p. 1452). Philadelphia, PA: Wolters Kluwer Health.)

very stable and, therefore, is resistant to treatment. Studies investigating transmission of prion diseases in animals clearly demonstrate that prions replicate, leading researchers to investigate how proteins can reproduce in the absence of genetic material.[3] Based on current models, it is believed that PrP^{SC} binds to the normal PrP^{C} on the cell surface, causing it to be processed into PrP^{SC}, which is released from the cell and then aggregates into amyloid-like plaques in the brain. The cell then replenishes the PrP^{C} and the cycle continues. As PrP^{SC} accumulates, it spreads within the axons of the nerve cells, causing progressively greater damage of host neurons and the eventual incapacitation of the host. Because antimicrobial agents attack reproductive or metabolic functions, which prions lack, antimicrobial agents are ineffective against them. Human transmission occurs primarily from eating infected meat or receiving an infected transplant organ or cornea. Two recent case reports indicate possible transmission from infected plasma, but causality has not been confirmed.[6] Because of possible misdiagnosis of MSA cases as Parkinson disease, it is recommended that only single-use surgical electrodes/probes be used for deep brain stimulation in Parkinson disease to prevent possible transmission.[5]

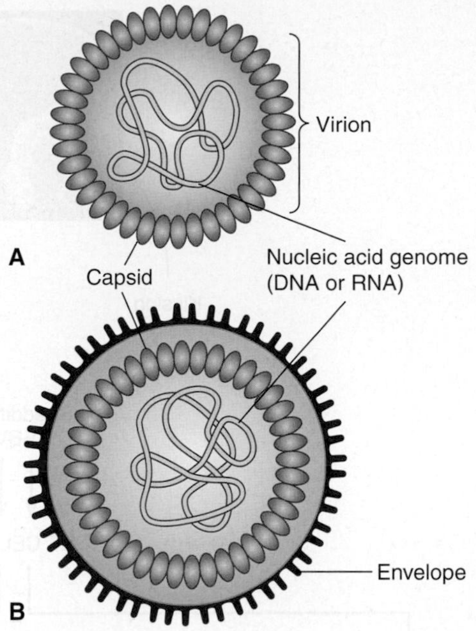

Figure 10.3 • **(A)** The basic structure of a virus includes a protein coat surrounding an inner core of nucleic acid (DNA or RNA). **(B)** Some viruses may also be enclosed in a lipoprotein outer envelope.

Viruses

Viruses are the smallest obligate intracellular pathogens. They have no organized cellular structures but instead consist of a protein coat, or capsid, surrounding a nucleic acid core, or genome, of RNA *or* DNA—never both (Fig. 10.3). Some viruses are enclosed within a lipoprotein envelope derived from the cytoplasmic membrane of the parasitized host cell. Enveloped viruses include members of the herpesvirus group and paramyxoviruses (*e.g.*, influenza and poxviruses). Certain enveloped viruses are continuously shed from the infected cell surface enveloped in buds pinched from the cell membrane.

The viruses of humans and animals have been categorized according to various characteristics. These include the type of viral genome (single-stranded or double-stranded DNA or RNA), physical characteristics (*e.g.*, size, presence or absence of a membrane envelope), the mechanism of replication (*e.g.*, retroviruses), the mode of transmission (*e.g.*, arthropod-borne viruses, enteroviruses), target tissue, and the type of disease produced (*e.g.*, hepatitis A, B, C, D, and E viruses), to name a few.

Viruses are incapable of replication outside of a living cell. They must penetrate a susceptible living cell and use the biosynthetic structure of the cell to replicate.[3] The process of viral replication is shown in Figure 10.4. Not every viral agent causes lysis and death of the host cell during the course of replication. Some viruses enter the host cell and insert their genome into the host cell chromosome, where it remains in a latent, nonreplicating state for long periods without causing disease. Under the appropriate stimulation, the virus undergoes active replication and produces symptoms of disease months to years later. Members of the herpesvirus group and adenovirus are examples of latent viruses. Herpesviruses include the viral agents of chickenpox and zoster (varicella zoster or herpes zoster, also known as shingles), cold sores (herpes simplex virus [HSV] type 1), genital herpes (HSV type 2), cytomegalovirus infections, roseola (human herpesvirus 6), infectious mononucleosis (IM) (Epstein-Barr virus [EBV], herpesvirus 4) (see Fig. 10.5), and Kaposi sarcoma (herpesvirus 8). The resumption of the latent viral replication may produce symptoms of primary disease (*e.g.*, genital herpes) or cause

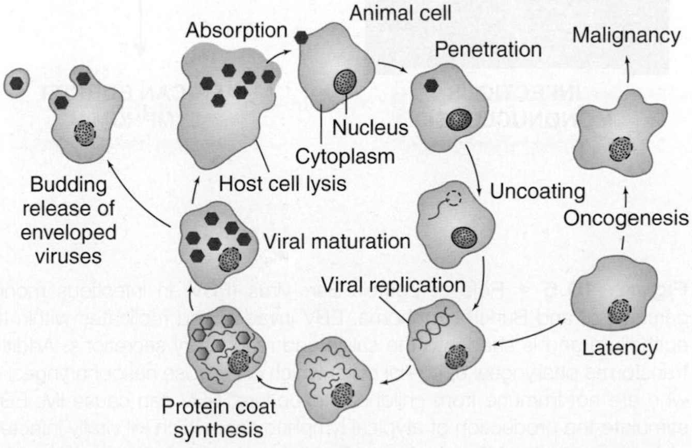

Figure 10.4 • Schematic representation of the many possible consequences of viral infection of host cells, including cell lysis (poliovirus), continuous release of budding viral particles, or latency (herpesviruses) and oncogenesis (papovaviruses).

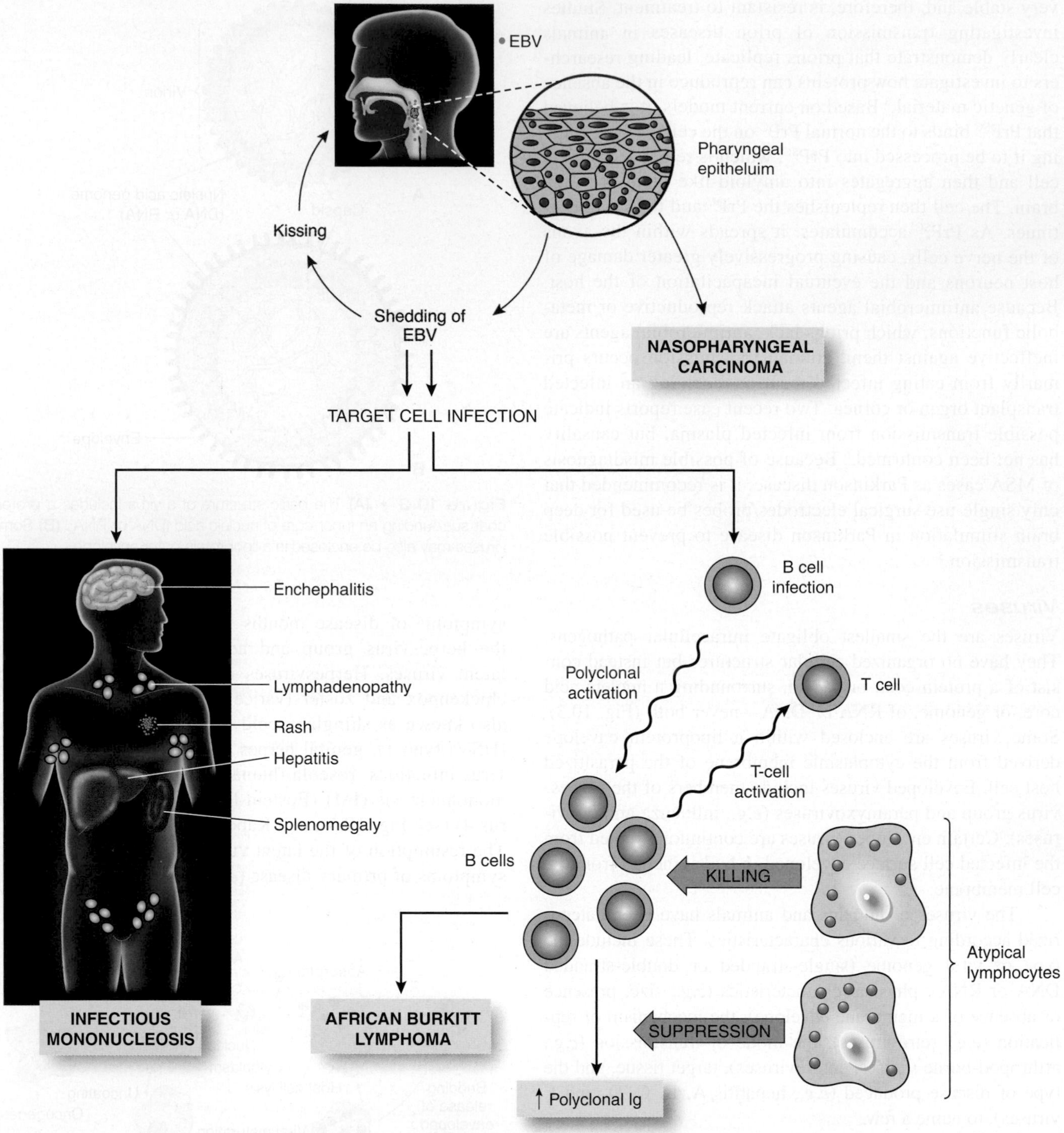

Figure 10.5 • Role of Epstein-Barr virus (EBV) in infectious mononucleosis (IM), nasopharyngeal carcinoma, and Burkitt lymphoma. EBV invades and replicates within the salivary glands or pharyngeal epithelium and is shed into the saliva and respiratory secretions. Additionally, in some people, the virus transforms pharyngeal epithelial cells, which can cause nasopharyngeal carcinoma. Then in some people who are not immune from childhood exposure, EBV can cause IM. EBV can infect B lymphocytes and stimulate the production of atypical lymphocytes, which kill virally infected B cells and suppress immunoglobulin production. Some infected B cells can transform into malignant lymphocytes of Burkitt lymphoma. (From Strayer D. S., Rubin R. (Eds.) (2015). *Rubin's pathology: Clinicopathologic foundations of medicine* (7th ed., Figure 9.9, p. 383). Philadelphia, PA: Wolters Kluwer Health.)

an entirely different symptomatology (*e.g.*, shingles instead of chickenpox).

A family of viruses that has gained a great deal of attention is the *Orthomyxoviridae* or flu viruses. There has been attention focused on the hemagglutinin (H) subtype 5 and neuraminidase (N) subtype 1 or H5N1 variant, commonly known as the *avian influenza virus*, and the H1N1 variant, commonly known as *swine flu*. The avian influenza viruses differ from the usual human influenza viruses by the hosts they normally infect. Avian influenza viruses typically infect wild birds. However, influenza viral antigens change often, and herd immunity rarely develops to protect humans from prior flu epidemics.[2] The human population is susceptible because the virus is unfamiliar to our immune systems. There was a global pandemic caused by H1N1 (or swine flu) in 2009, resulting in more than 30,000 cases in over 70 counties.[7] The CDC recommends rapid influenza diagnostic tests using real-time polymerase chain reaction (PCR) by trained personnel.[7] The antiviral agents oseltamivir and zanamivir are more effective when started within 48 hours of symptom development; thus, a careful history as to the onset of symptoms is very important. Resources must be considered in an epidemic. Supportive care in an intensive care may require mechanical ventilation and vasopressor therapy. Early infection control practices are important to prevent the spread of influenza.[7]

Since the early 1980s, members of the retrovirus group have received considerable attention after identification of the human immunodeficiency viruses (HIV) as the causative agent of acquired immunodeficiency syndrome (AIDS). The retroviruses have a unique mechanism of replication. After entry into the host cell, the viral RNA genome is first translated into DNA by a viral enzyme called *reverse transcriptase*. The viral DNA copy is then integrated into the host chromosome where it exists in a latent state, similar to the herpesviruses. Reactivation and replication require a reversal of the entire process. Some retroviruses lyse the host cell during the process of replication. In the case of HIV, when infected cells (CD4+ T cells) become activated, they release free virus by budding or cell–cell fusion. Lysis of CD4+ cells also releases HIV into the bloodstream, resulting in reduced CD4+ count and suppression of the immune response.[3]

In addition to causing infectious diseases, certain viruses also can transform normal host cells into malignant cells during the replication cycle. This group of viruses is referred to as *oncogenic* and includes certain retroviruses and DNA viruses, such as the herpesviruses, adenoviruses, and papovaviruses. Human papillomaviruses (HPVs), members of the papovavirus family, cause cutaneous and genital warts, and several genotypes are associated with cervical cancer. The first vaccine (Gardasil®) to prevent cervical cancer, precancerous genital lesions, genital warts, and anal and oropharyngeal cancers because of HPV was developed in 2006, and the vaccine coverage has been expanded to be effective against nine HPV types (6, 11, 16, 18, 31, 33, 45, 52, and 58).[8]

Bacteria

Bacteria are autonomously replicating unicellular organisms known as *prokaryotes* because they lack an organized nucleus. Compared with nucleated eukaryotic cells, the bacterial cells are small and structurally primitive.[3] They are the smallest of all living cells and contain no organized intracellular organelles, and the genome consists of only a single double-stranded circular chromosome of DNA, which is associated with RNA and proteins.[3] Many bacteria transiently harbor smaller extrachromosomal pieces of circular DNA called *plasmids*. Occasionally, plasmids contain genetic information that increases the virulence or antibiotic resistance of the organism.

The prokaryotic cell is organized into an internal compartment called the *cytoplasm*, which contains the reproductive and metabolic machinery of the cell. The cytoplasm is surrounded by a flexible lipid membrane, called the *cytoplasmic membrane*.[3] This is in turn usually enclosed within a rigid cell wall. The structure and synthesis of the cell wall determine the microscopic shape of the bacterium (*e.g.*, spherical [cocci], helical [spirilla], or elongate [bacilli]). Further, bacteria can be divided into two types (gram-positive and gram-negative) based on their gram staining properties. Gram-positive bacteria produce a cell wall composed of a distinctive polymer known as *peptidoglycan*. This polymer is produced only by prokaryotes and is used as a target for some antibacterial therapies. Gram-negative bacteria produce an outer membrane composed of lipopolysaccharide (LPS), which can induce shock in the host.[3] Several bacteria synthesize an extracellular capsule composed of protein or polysaccharide. The capsule protects the organism from environmental hazards such as the immunologic defenses of the host.[3] Figure 10.6 shows a variety of bacterial morphologies.

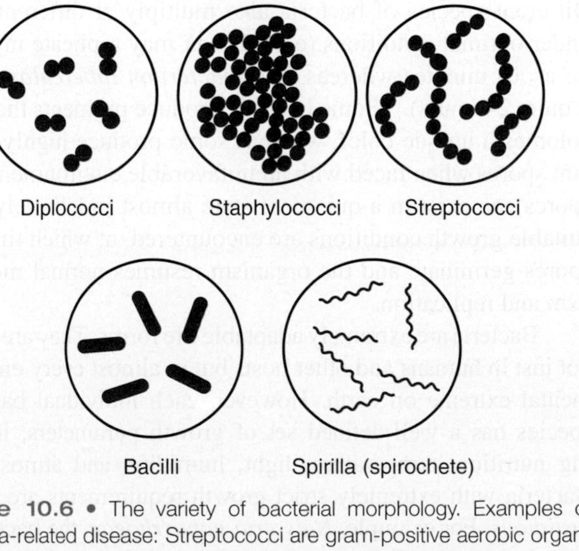

Figure 10.6 • The variety of bacterial morphology. Examples of bacteria-related disease: Streptococci are gram-positive aerobic organisms that cause skin infections such as impetigo, scarlet fever, pharyngitis, endocarditis, pneumonia, and potentially fatal toxic shock and sepsis. Salmonella and *E. coli* are gram-negative, rod-shaped bacteria that cause food-borne illnesses. Spirilla bacteria are gram-negative bacteria that cause bacterial diarrhea and peptic ulcers. (From Houser H. J., Sesser J. R. (2016). *LWW's medical assisting exam review for CMA, RMA, and CMAS certification*. Philadelphia, PA: Wolters Kluwer.)

Certain bacteria are motile as the result of external whiplike appendages called *flagella*. The flagella rotate like a propeller, transporting the organism through a liquid environment. Bacteria can also produce hairlike structures projecting from the cell surface called pili or *fimbriae*, which enable the organism to adhere to surfaces such as mucous membranes or other bacteria.

Most prokaryotes reproduce asexually by simple cellular division. The manner in which an organism divides can influence the microscopic morphology. For instance, when the cocci divide in chains, they are called *streptococci*; in pairs, *diplococci*; and in clusters, *staphylococci*.[3] The growth rate of bacteria varies significantly among different species and depends greatly on physical growth conditions and the availability of nutrients. In the laboratory, a single bacterium placed in a suitable growth environment, such as an agar plate, reproduces to the extent that it forms a visible colony composed of millions of bacteria within a few hours.

In nature, bacteria rarely exist as single cells floating in an aqueous environment. Rather, bacteria prefer to stick to and colonize environmental surfaces, producing structured communities called *biofilms*.[9] The organization and structure of biofilms permit access to available nutrients and elimination of metabolic waste. Within the biofilm, individual organisms use chemical signaling as a form of primitive intercellular communication to represent the state of the environment. This is known as *quorum sensing*. These signals inform members of the community when sufficient nutrients are available for proliferation or when environmental conditions warrant dormancy or evacuation. Examples of biofilms abound in nature and are found on surfaces of aquatic environments and on humans.

The physical appearance of a colony of bacteria grown on an agar plate can be quite distinctive for different species. Different species of bacteria also multiply at different rates under optimal conditions (e.g., *E. coli* may replicate in as little as 10 minutes whereas *Mycobacterium tuberculosis* may require 24 hours).[10] Some bacteria produce pigments that give colonies a unique color, whereas some produce highly resistant spores when faced with an unfavorable environment. The spores can exist in a quiescent state almost indefinitely until suitable growth conditions are encountered, at which time the spores germinate and the organism resumes normal metabolism and replication.

Bacteria are extremely adaptable life forms. They are found not just in humans and other hosts but in almost every environmental extreme on earth. However, each individual bacterial species has a well-defined set of growth parameters, including nutrition, temperature, light, humidity, and atmosphere. Bacteria with extremely strict growth requirements are called *fastidious*. For example, *Neisseria gonorrhoeae*, the bacterium that causes gonorrhea, cannot live for extended periods outside the human body.[10] Some bacteria require oxygen for growth and metabolism and are called *aerobes*. Others cannot survive in an oxygen-containing environment and are called *anaerobes*. An organism capable of adapting its metabolism to aerobic or anaerobic conditions is called *facultatively anaerobic*.

In the laboratory, bacteria are generally classified according to the microscopic appearance and staining properties of the cell. The gram stain is the most widely used staining procedure. Bacteria are designated as *gram-positive* organisms if they are stained purple by a primary basic dye (usually crystal violet). Those that are not stained by the crystal violet but are counterstained red by a second dye (safranin) are called *gram-negative* organisms. Staining characteristics and microscopic morphology are used in combination to describe bacteria. For example, *Streptococcus pyogenes*, the causative agent of scarlet fever and rheumatic fever, is a gram-positive streptococcal organism that is spherical, grows in chains, and stains purple by gram stain. *Legionella pneumophila*, the bacterium responsible for Legionnaire disease, is a gram-negative rod.

Another means of classifying bacteria according to microscopic staining properties is the *acid-fast stain*. Because of their unique cell membrane fatty acid content and composition, certain bacteria are resistant to the decolorization of a primary stain (either carbol-fuchsin or a combination of auramine and rhodamine) when treated with a solution of acid alcohol. These organisms are termed *acid fast* and include a number of significant human pathogens, most notably *Mycobacterium tuberculosis* and other mycobacteria.[10]

For purposes of taxonomy (*i.e.*, identification and classification), each member of the bacterial kingdom is categorized into a small group of biochemically and genetically related organisms called the *genus* and further subdivided into distinct individuals within the genus called *species*. The genus and species assignment of the organism is reflected in its name (*e.g.*, *Staphylococcus* [genus] *aureus* [species]).

Spirochetes. The *spirochetes* are an eccentric category of bacteria that are mentioned separately because of their unusual cellular morphology and distinctive mechanism of motility. Technically, the spirochetes are gram-negative rods but are unique in that the cell's shape is helical and the length of the organism is many times its width. A series of filaments are wound about the cell wall and extend the entire length of the cell. These filaments propel the organism through an aqueous environment in a corkscrew motion.

Spirochetes are anaerobic organisms and comprise three genera: *Leptospira*, *Borrelia*, and *Treponema*. Each genus has saprophytic and pathogenic strains. The pathogenic leptospires infect a wide variety of wild and domestic animals. Infected animals shed the organisms into the environment through the urinary tract. Transmission to humans occurs by contact with infected animals or urine-contaminated surroundings. Leptospires gain access to the host directly through mucous membranes or breaks in the skin and can produce a severe and potentially fatal illness called *Weil syndrome*. In contrast, the borreliae are transmitted from infected animals to humans through the bite of an arthropod vector such as lice or ticks. Included in the genus *Borrelia* are the agents of relapsing fever (*Borrelia recurrentis*) and Lyme disease (*B. burgdorferi*).

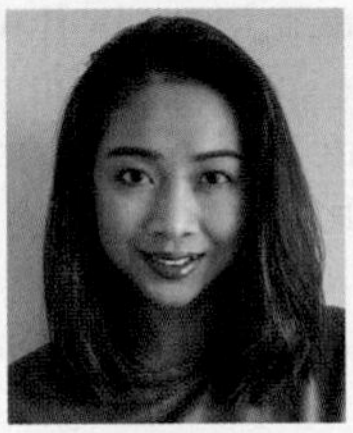

Ms. Roon, the woman diagnosed with Lyme disease introduced in the unit opener case study, has no memory of being bitten by a tick, and she did not experience a bull's eye or erythema migrans rash (52% of people do not experience rash). However, the ticks that carry Lyme disease (*B. burgdorferi*) are less than 2 mm in size. Therefore, it is likely that she didn't notice the attached tick. Ms. Roon has had evident central nervous system and musculoskeletal clinical manifestations, including headaches, fatigue, joint pain, and swelling. Ms. Roon definitely fits the "classic" picture of someone infected with Lyme disease.

Pathogenic *Treponema* species require no intermediates and are spread from person to person by direct contact. The most important member of the genus is *Treponema pallidum*, the causative agent of syphilis.

Mycoplasmas. The mycoplasmas are unicellular prokaryotes capable of independent replication. These organisms are less than one third the size of bacteria at approximately 0.3 μm at their largest diameter and contain a small DNA genome approximately one half the size of the bacterial chromosome. The cell is composed of cytoplasm surrounded by a membrane, but unlike bacteria, the mycoplasmas do not produce a rigid peptidoglycan cell wall. As a consequence, the microscopic appearance of the cell is highly variable, ranging from coccoid forms to filaments, and the mycoplasmas are resistant to cell wall–inhibiting antibiotics, such as penicillins and cephalosporins.

The mycoplasmas affecting humans are divided into three genera: *Mycoplasma*, *Ureaplasma*, and *Acholeplasma*. The first two require cholesterol from the environment to produce the cell membrane; the acholeplasmas do not. In the human host, mycoplasmas are commensals. However, a number of species are capable of producing serious diseases, including pneumonia (*Mycoplasma pneumoniae*), genital infections (*Mycoplasma hominis* and *Ureaplasma urealyticum*), maternally transmitted respiratory infections to infants with low birth weight (*U. urealyticum*), and potential complications during pregnancy.[10,11]

KEY POINTS

AGENTS OF INFECTIOUS DISEASE

- Microorganisms can be separated into eukaryotes (*e.g.*, fungi and parasites), which contain a membrane-bound nucleus, and prokaryotes (*e.g.*, bacteria), which do not have a defined nucleus.
- Eukaryotes and prokaryotes are organisms because they contain all the enzymes and biologic equipment necessary for replication and exploiting metabolic energy.

Rickettsiaceae, Anaplasmataceae, Chlamydiaceae, *and* Coxiella

This interesting group of organisms combines the characteristics of viral and bacterial agents to produce disease in humans. All are obligate intracellular pathogens, like the viruses, but produce a rigid peptidoglycan cell wall, reproduce asexually by cellular division, and contain RNA and DNA, similar to the bacteria.[2]

The *Rickettsiaceae* depend on the host cell for essential vitamins and nutrients, but the *Chlamydiaceae* appear to scavenge intermediates of energy metabolism such as adenosine triphosphate (ATP). The *Rickettsiaceae* infect but do not produce disease in the cells of certain arthropods such as mites, fleas, ticks, and lice.[10] The organisms are transmitted to humans through the bite of the arthropod (*i.e.*, the vector) and produce a number of potentially lethal diseases, including Rocky Mountain spotted fever and epidemic typhus. Rocky Mountain spotted fever (transmitted to humans through a tick vector) is a reportable disease that has increased in frequency over the last decade from 2 cases in 1 million people to 11 cases in 1 million people in 2014.[12] However, the death rate has decreased below 0.50%.[12]

The *Chlamydiaceae* are slightly smaller than the *Rickettsiaceae* and are structurally similar; however, they are transmitted directly between susceptible vertebrates without an intermediate arthropod vector. Transmission and replication of *Chlamydiaceae* occur through a defined life cycle. The infectious form, called an *elementary body*, attaches to and enters the host cell, where it transforms into a larger *reticulate body.*[13] This undergoes active replication into multiple elementary bodies, which are then shed into the extracellular environment to initiate another infectious cycle. Transmission occurs by close person-to-person contact. *Chlamydia trachomatis* is transmitted sexually (it is a leading cause of sexually transmitted disease in men and women) and can cause conjunctivitis in newborns.[10] *Chlamydophila pneumonia* is transmitted via airborne droplets or spread through hands in contact with mucous membranes and causes atypical bacterial pneumonia.[13] *Chlamydophila psittaci* can be transmitted from birds to humans that cause pneumonia.[14] Approximately 1% of community-acquired pneumonia cases are caused by *C. psittaci.*[14]

Organisms within the family *Anaplasmataceae* (including the reorganized genera *Ehrlichia*, *Anaplasma*, *Neorickettsia*, and *Wolbachia*) are also obligate intracellular organisms that resemble the *Rickettsiaceae* in structure and produce a variety of veterinary and human diseases, some of which have a tick vector. These organisms target host mononuclear and polymorphonuclear white blood cells for infection and, similar to the *Chlamydiaceae*, multiply in the cytoplasm of infected leukocytes within vacuoles called *morulae*. Unlike the *Chlamydiaceae*, however, the *Anaplasmataceae* do not have a defined life cycle and are independent of the host cell for energy production. *Ehrlichia sennetsu*, which is primarily restricted to Japan, produces a disease called *sennetsu fever* that resembles IM. Disease caused by this organism differs from other *Anaplasmataceae* because it is associated with eating raw fish infested with *E. sennetsu*–infected parasites. The most common infections caused by *Anaplasmataceae* are human monocytic and granulocytic ehrlichiosis. Human monocytic ehrlichiosis is a disease caused by *Ehrlichia chaffeensis* and *E. canis* that can easily be confused with Rocky Mountain spotted fever.

Clinical disease severity in ehrlichiosis ranges from mild to life threatening.[15] Manifestations include generalized malaise, anorexia and nausea, fever, chills, headache, and body aches. Symptom onset occurs 1 to 2 weeks after a tick bite. A rash may occur (more often in children) as well as gastrointestinal symptoms. Decreases in white blood cells (leukopenia) and platelets (thrombocytopenia) often occur. Severe sequelae may include acute respiratory distress syndrome, severe sepsis, and septic shock (which may lead to acute renal failure) as well as meningitis and meningoencephalitis.[15] The disease is usually more severe in older adults and people with compromised immune function. Evidence validates the importance of empirical antibiotic treatment when one suspects ehrlichiosis because a fulminant and life-threatening infection is likely with immunocompromised people.[16] Human granulocytic ehrlichiosis, which is caused by two species (*Anaplasma phagocytophilum* and *Ehrlichia ewingii*), is also transmitted by ticks. The symptoms are similar to those seen with human monocytotropic ehrlichiosis.

The genus *Coxiella* contains only one species, *C. burnetii*. Like its rickettsial counterparts, it is a gram-negative intracellular organism that infects a variety of animals, including cattle, sheep, and goats.[17] In humans, *Coxiella* infection produces a disease called *Q fever*, characterized by a nonspecific febrile illness often accompanied by headache, retroorbital pain, chills, and mild pneumonia-like symptoms. The organism produces a highly resistant sporelike stage that is transmitted to humans when contaminated animal tissue is aerosolized (*e.g.*, during meat processing) or by ingestion of contaminated milk. It can also be transmitted by exposure to infected animals.[17]

Fungi

The fungi are free-living, eukaryotic saprophytes found in every habitat on earth. Some are members of the normal human microflora. Fortunately, few fungi are capable of causing diseases in humans, and most of these are incidental, self-limited infections of the skin and subcutaneous tissue. Serious fungal infections are rare and usually initiated through puncture wounds or inhalation. Despite their normally harmless nature, fungi can cause life-threatening opportunistic diseases when host defense capabilities have been disabled.

The fungi can be separated into two groups, yeasts and molds, based on rudimentary differences in their morphology. The yeasts are single-celled organisms, approximately the size of red blood cells, which reproduce by a budding process. The buds separate from the parent cell and mature into identical daughter cells. Molds produce long, hollow, branching filaments called *hyphae*. Some molds produce cross walls, which segregate the hyphae into compartments, and others do not. A limited number of fungi are capable of growing as yeasts at one temperature and as molds at another. These organisms are called *dimorphic fungi* and include a number of human pathogens such as the agents of blastomycosis (*Blastomyces dermatitidis*), histoplasmosis (*Histoplasma capsulatum*), and coccidioidomycosis (*Coccidioides immitis*).

The appearance of a fungal colony tends to reflect its cellular composition. Colonies of yeast are generally smooth with a waxy or creamy texture. Molds tend to produce cottony or powdery colonies composed of mats of hyphae collectively called a *mycelium*. The mycelium can penetrate the growth surface or project above the colony like the roots and branches of a tree. Yeasts and molds produce a rigid cell wall layer that is chemically unrelated to the peptidoglycan of bacteria and is therefore not susceptible to the effects of penicillin-like antibiotics.

Most fungi are capable of sexual or asexual reproduction. The former process involves the fusion of zygotes with the production of a recombinant zygospore. Asexual reproduction involves the formation of highly resistant spores called *conidia* or *sporangiospores*, which are borne by specialized structures that arise from the hyphae. Molds are identified in the laboratory by the characteristic microscopic appearance of the asexual fruiting structures and spores.

Like the bacterial pathogens of humans, fungi can produce disease in the human host only if they can grow at the temperature of the infected body site. For example, a number of fungal pathogens called *dermatophytes* are incapable of growing at core body temperature (37°C), and the infection is limited to the cooler cutaneous surfaces. Diseases caused by these organisms, including ringworm, athlete's foot, and jock itch—all examples of tinea—are collectively called *superficial mycoses*.[3] Fungal infections can also be cutaneous, subcutaneous, deep-seated, and invasive infections. Systemic mycoses are serious fungal infections of deep tissues and, by definition, are caused by organisms capable of growth at 37°C. Yeasts such as *Candida albicans* are commensal flora of the skin, mucous membranes, and gastrointestinal tract and are capable of growth at a wider range of temperatures. Candida is considered an opportunistic infection in immunocompromised persons; however, it is a cause of infection in nonneutropenic people. Candida in the blood (*candidemia*) and in the abdomen (intra-abdominal candidiasis) are common causes of infection in the intensive care unit.[18] In addition, aspergillosis is a lethal form of pneumonia.[18] Intact immune mechanisms and competition for nutrients provided by the bacterial flora normally keep colonizing fungi in check. Alterations in either of these components by disease states or antibiotic therapy can upset the balance, permitting fungal overgrowth and setting the stage for opportunistic infections.

Parasites

In a strict sense, any organism that derives benefits from its biologic relationship with another organism is a parasite. In the study of clinical microbiology, however, the term *parasite* has evolved to designate members of the animal kingdom that infect and cause disease in other animals and includes protozoa, helminths, and arthropods. Intestinal microbiota exerts an immunoregulatory effect on the host's immune response in the setting of intestinal parasites.[19]

The protozoa are unicellular animals with a complete complement of eukaryotic cellular machinery, including a well-defined nucleus and organelles. Reproduction may be sexual or asexual, and life cycles may be simple or complicated, with several maturation stages requiring more than one host for completion. Most are saprophytes, but a few have adapted to the accommodations of the human environment and produce a variety of diseases, including malaria, amebic dysentery, and giardiasis.[3] Protozoan infections can be passed directly from host to host such as through sexual contact, indirectly through contaminated water or food, or by way of an arthropod vector. Direct or indirect transmission results from the ingestion of highly resistant cysts or spores that are shed in the feces of an infected host. When the cysts reach the intestine, they mature into vegetative forms called *trophozoites*, which are capable of asexual reproduction or cyst formation. Most trophozoites are motile by means of flagella, cilia, or ameboid motion.

The helminths are a collection of wormlike parasites that include the nematodes or roundworms, cestodes or tapeworms, and trematodes or flukes. The helminths reproduce sexually within the definitive host, and some require an intermediate host for the development and maturation of an offspring. Humans can serve as the definitive or intermediate host and, in certain diseases such as trichinosis, as both. Transmission of helminth diseases occurs primarily through the ingestion of fertilized eggs (ova) or the penetration of infectious larval stages through the skin—directly or with the aid of an arthropod vector. Helminth infections can involve many organ systems and sites, including the liver and lung, urinary and intestinal tracts, circulatory and central nervous systems, and muscle. Although most helminth diseases have been eradicated from the United States, they are still a major health concern of developing nations.

The parasitic arthropods of humans and animals include the vectors of infectious diseases (*e.g.*, ticks, mosquitoes, biting flies) and the ectoparasites. The ectoparasites infest external body surfaces and cause localized tissue damage or inflammation secondary to the bite or burrowing action of the arthropod. The most prominent human ectoparasites are mites (scabies), chiggers, lice (head, body, and pubic), and fleas.[3] Transmission of ectoparasites occurs directly by contact with immature or mature forms of the arthropod or its eggs found on the infested host or the host's clothing, bedding, or grooming articles such as combs and brushes. Many of the ectoparasites are vectors of other infectious diseases, including endemic typhus and bubonic plague (fleas) and epidemic typhus (lice).

IN SUMMARY

Throughout life, humans are continuously and harmlessly exposed to and colonized by a multitude of microscopic organisms. This relationship is kept in check by the intact defense mechanisms of the host (*e.g.*, mucosal and cutaneous barriers, normal immune function) and the innocuous nature of most environmental microorganisms. Those factors that weaken the host's resistance or increase the virulence of colonizing microorganisms can disturb the equilibrium of the relationship and cause disease. The degree to which the balance is shifted in favor of the microorganism determines the severity of illness.

There is an extreme diversity of prokaryotic and eukaryotic microorganisms capable of causing infectious diseases in humans. Immunosuppression (related to underlying medical conditions or immunosuppressive therapy or aging [known as *immunosenescence*]) increases the risk of infections related to opportunistic and other pathogens. However, most infectious illnesses in humans continue to be caused by only a small fraction of the organisms that compose the microscopic world.

MECHANISMS OF INFECTION

After completing this section of the chapter, the learner will be able to meet the following objectives:

- Discuss modes of infectious disease transmission.
- Describe the stages of an infectious disease.
- Discuss clinical manifestations of a dysregulated host defense response to infection.

Epidemiology of Infectious Diseases

Epidemiology is the study of the patterns and determinants of health with the goal of controlling disease and health problems.[20] The principles of epidemiology were first applied to the study of infectious diseases. Whereas descriptive epidemiology focuses on the pattern of disease, analytic epidemiology examines factors associated with disease.[21] In order to interrupt or eliminate the spread of an infectious agent, factors related to the host, agent, and environment—the well-known triad of disease (see Fig. 10.1)—as well as modes of transmission must be considered.

To understand the epidemiology of a disease, cases must be defined and carefully counted so that gradual or abrupt changes in frequency can be observed. The term *incidence* is used to describe the number of new cases of an infectious disease that occur within a defined population (*e.g.*, per 100,000 people) over an established period of time (*e.g.*, monthly, quarterly, yearly). Disease *prevalence* indicates the number of active cases at any given time in a population. A disease is considered to be *endemic* in a particular geographic region if the incidence and prevalence are relatively stable. An *epidemic* describes an abrupt and unexpected increase in the incidence of disease over endemic rates. A *pandemic* refers to the spread of disease beyond continental boundaries. Rapid worldwide travel increases the risk of pandemic transmission of pathogenic microorganisms during outbreaks.

As an illustration of these principles, an outbreak of a suspected respiratory viral illness—subsequently identified as severe acute respiratory syndrome (SARS)—was recognized in the Guangdong province in southern China in November 2002.[22,23] The illness was highly transmissible, as evidenced by the first recognized occurrence in Taiwan. Four days after returning to Taiwan from work in the Guangdong province, a businessman developed a febrile illness and was admitted to a local hospital. Within 1 month, a large outbreak of SARS was documented to have affected approximately 3000 people in Taipei City, Taiwan. Once the SARS outbreak had crossed continental borders for the first time, its classification was changed from an epidemic to pandemic.[22,23]

Modes of Transmission

Modes of transmission include direct and indirect mechanisms. The *portal of entry* refers to the process by which a pathogen enters the body, gains access to susceptible tissues, and causes disease. Among the potential *modes of transmission* are penetration, direct contact, ingestion, and inhalation. The portal of entry does not dictate the site of infection. Ingested pathogens may penetrate the intestinal mucosa, disseminate through the circulatory system, and cause diseases in other organs such as the lung or liver. Whatever the mechanisms of entry, the transmission of infectious agents is directly related to the number of infectious agents absorbed by the host.

Penetration

Any disruption in the integrity of the body's surface barrier—skin or mucous membranes—is a potential site for invasion of microorganisms. The break may be the result of an accidental injury causing abrasions, burns, or penetrating wounds; medical procedures such as surgery or catheterization; or a primary infectious process that produces surface lesions such as chickenpox or impetigo. Translocation of bacteria from the gastrointestinal tract may also occur. Direct inoculation from intravenous drug use or an animal or arthropod bite also can occur.

Direct Contact

Some pathogens are transmitted directly from infected tissue or secretions to exposed, intact mucous membranes. This is especially true of certain sexually transmitted infections (STIs), such as gonorrhea, syphilis, chlamydia, and genital herpes, for which exposure of uninfected membranes to pathogens occurs during intimate contact.

The transmission of STIs is not limited to sexual contact. *Vertical transmission* of these agents, from mother to child, can occur across the placenta or during birth when the mucous membranes of the child contact infected vaginal secretions of the mother. When an infectious disease is transmitted from mother to child during gestation or birth, it is classified as a *congenital infection*. The most frequently observed congenital infections include toxoplasmosis (caused by the parasite *Toxoplasma gondii*), syphilis, rubella, cytomegalovirus infection, and HSV infections (the TORCH infections), varicella zoster (chickenpox), parvovirus B19, group B streptococci (*Streptococcus agalactiae*), and HIV. Of these, cytomegalovirus is a common cause of congenital infection in the United States, occurring in 0.5% to 22% of all live births.[24]

The severity of congenital defects associated with these infections depends greatly on the gestational age of the fetus when transmission occurs, but most of these agents can cause profound mental retardation and neurosensory deficits, including blindness and hearing loss. HIV rarely produces overt signs and symptoms in the infected newborn, and it sometimes takes years for the effects of the illness to manifest.

Ingestion

The entry of pathogenic microorganisms or their toxic products through the oral cavity and gastrointestinal tract represents one of the more efficient means of disease transmission in humans. Many bacterial, viral, and parasitic infections, including cholera, typhoid fever, dysentery (amebic and bacillary), food poisoning, traveler's diarrhea, cryptosporidiosis, and hepatitis A, are initiated through the ingestion of contaminated food and water. This mechanism of transmission necessitates that an infectious agent survive the low pH and enzyme activity of gastric secretions and the peristaltic action of the intestines in numbers sufficient to establish infection, deemed an *infectious dose*. For organisms such as *Vibrio cholerae*, gastric acid secretions reduce the infectious dose; however, some agents such as *Shigella* and *Giardia* cysts cause infections at a lower dose because of their resistance to gastric acid.[24] Ingested pathogens also must compete successfully with the normal bacterial flora of the bowel for nutritional needs. People with reduced gastric acidity because of disease or medication are more susceptible to infection by this route because the number of ingested microorganisms surviving the gastric environment is greater.

Inhalation

The respiratory tract of healthy people is equipped with a multiple-tiered defense system to prevent potential pathogens from entering the lungs. The surface of the respiratory tree is lined with a layer of mucus that is continuously swept up and away from the lungs and toward the mouth by the beating motion of ciliated epithelial cells. Humidification of inspired air increases the size of aerosolized particles, which are effectively filtered by the mucous membranes of the upper respiratory tract. Coughing also aids in the removal of particulate matter from the lower respiratory tract. Respiratory secretions contain antibodies and enzymes capable of inactivating infectious agents. Particulate matter and microorganisms that ultimately reach the lung are cleared by phagocytic cells.

Despite this impressive array of protective mechanisms, a number of pathogens can invade the human body through the respiratory tract, including agents of bacterial pneumonia (*Streptococcus pneumoniae*, *Legionella pneumophila*), meningitis (*Neisseria meningitidis*, *Haemophilus influenzae*), and tuberculosis, as well as the viruses responsible for measles, mumps, chickenpox, influenza, and the common cold. Defective pulmonary function or mucociliary clearance caused by noninfectious processes such as cystic fibrosis, emphysema, or smoking can increase the risk of inhalation-acquired diseases.

Concept Mastery Alert

Chickenpox is spread through the air.

KEY POINTS

EPIDEMIOLOGY OF INFECTIOUS DISEASES

- Epidemiology focuses on the incidence (number of new cases) and prevalence (number of active cases at any given time) of an infectious disease; the source of infection and its portal of entry, site of infection, and virulence factors of the infecting organism; and the signs and symptoms of the infection and its course.
- The ultimate goals of epidemiologic studies are the interruption of the spread of infectious diseases and their eradication.

Source

The source of an infectious disease refers to the location, host, object, or substance from which the infectious agent was acquired: essentially the "who, what, where, and when" of disease transmission. The source may be endogenous (acquired from the host's own microbial flora, as would be the case in an opportunistic infection) or exogenous (acquired from sources in the external environment, such as the water, food, soil, or air). The source of the infectious agent can also be another human being, as from mother to child during gestation (congenital infections); an inanimate object; an animal; or a biting arthropod (*vector*). Inanimate objects that carry an infectious agent are known as *fomites*. For example, rhinoviruses and many other nonenveloped viruses can be spread by contact with contaminated fomites such as handkerchiefs and toys. Zoonoses are a category of infectious diseases passed from other animal species to humans. When a disease originates in humans and moves to animals, it is known as "reverse zoonoses."[24] Zoonoses account for a large percentage (up to 70% of emerging viral diseases) of emerging infectious diseases. Examples of zoonoses include cat-scratch disease, HIV, rabies, plague, and influenza.[24] The spread of infectious diseases (such as Lyme disease or West Nile virus [WNV]) through biting arthropod vectors is another route.

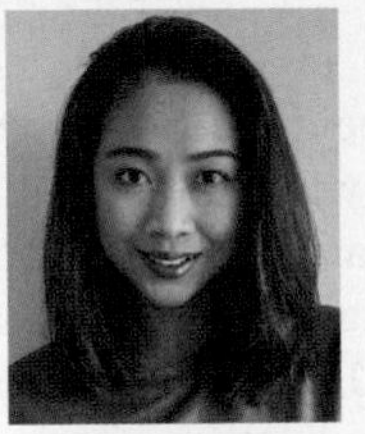

Ms. Roon acquired Lyme disease through the biting arthropod vector route (spread from other animal species to a human). The organism most likely responsible for her infection is the *Borrelia burgdorferi sensu stricto*, which is a bacterial spirochete passed to her by the *Ixodes scapularis* tick (deer tick) that feeds and mates on deer. Because these deer ticks are less than 2 mm, it is easy to miss seeing them attached to one's body. It takes up to 36 hours of tick attachment for the transfer of borreliae from the infected tick to the person.

Source can denote a place. For instance, infections that develop in people while they are hospitalized are called *nosocomial* or *health care–associated infection* and those that are acquired outside of health care facilities are called *community acquired*. The definitions used to distinguish between health care acquired and community acquired involve the timing of infection (development in less than 48 hours defines community acquired) as well as prior hospitalization, dialysis, and wound care. The source may also pertain to the body substance that is the most likely a vehicle for transmission, such as feces, blood, body fluids, respiratory secretions, and urine. Infections can be transmitted from person to person through shared inanimate objects (fomites) contaminated with infected body fluids. An example of this mechanism of transmission would include the spread of the HIV and hepatitis B virus through the use of shared syringes by intravenous drug users. Infection can also be spread through a complex combination of source, portal of entry, and vector. Source control is an important aspect of prevention and treatment.

Clinical Manifestations

The term *clinical manifestations* refers to the collection of signs and symptoms expressed by the host during the disease course. This is also known as the *clinical picture*, or *disease presentation*, and can be characteristic of any given infectious agent. In terms of pathophysiology, symptoms are the outward expression of the struggle between invading organisms and the retaliatory inflammatory and immune responses of the host. The symptoms of an infectious disease may be specific and reflect the site of infection (*e.g.*, diarrhea, rash, convulsions, hemorrhage, and pneumonia). Conversely, symptoms such as fever, myalgia, headache, and lethargy are relatively nonspecific and can be shared by a number of diverse infectious diseases. The symptoms of a diseased host can be obvious, as in the case of chickenpox or measles. Other, covert symptoms, such as an increased white blood cell count, may require laboratory testing to detect. Accurate recognition and documentation of symptomatology can aid in the diagnosis of an infectious disease.

Disease Course

The course of any infectious disease can be divided into several distinguishable stages after the *point* when the potential pathogen enters the host. These stages are the incubation period, the prodromal stage, the acute stage, the convalescent stage, and the resolution stage (Fig. 10.7). The stages are based on the progression and intensity of the host's symptoms, which reflect the host's response to infection over time. The duration of each phase and the pattern of the overall illness can be specific for different pathogens, thereby aiding in the diagnosis of an infectious disease.

The *incubation period* is the phase during which the pathogen begins active replication without producing recognizable symptoms in the host. The incubation period may be short, as in the case of cholera (up to 24 hours), or prolonged, such as that of hepatitis B (up to 180 days) or HIV (months to years).[3] The duration of the incubation period can be influenced by additional factors, including the general health of the host, the portal of entry, and the degree of the infectious dose of the pathogen.

The hallmark of the *prodromal stage* is the initial appearance of symptoms in the host, although the clinical presentation during this time may be only a vague sense of malaise. The host may experience mild fever, myalgia, headache, and fatigue. These are constitutional changes shared by a great number of disease processes. The duration of the prodromal stage can vary considerably from host to host.

The *acute stage* is the period during which the host experiences the maximum impact of the infectious process corresponding to rapid proliferation and dissemination of the pathogen. During this phase, toxic by-products of microbial metabolism, cell lysis, and the immune response mounted by the host combine to produce tissue damage and inflammation.

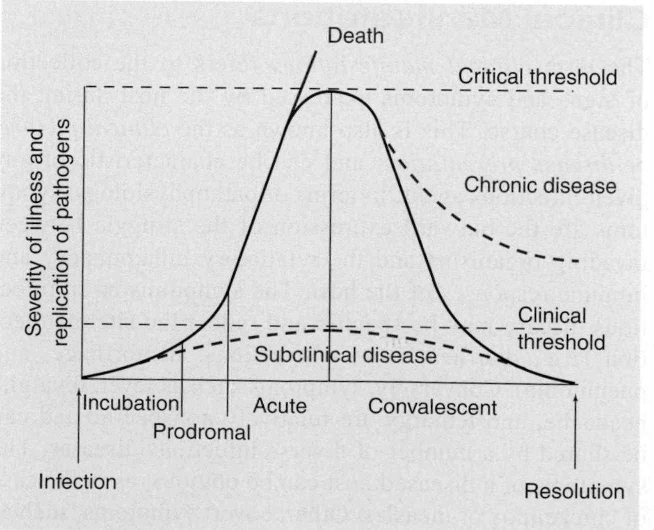

Figure 10.7 • Stages of a primary infectious disease as they appear in relation to the severity of symptoms and numbers of infectious agents. The clinical threshold corresponds with the initial expression of recognizable symptoms, whereas the critical threshold represents the peak of disease intensity.

The symptoms of the host are pronounced and more specific than in the prodromal stage, usually typifying the pathogen and sites of involvement.

The *convalescent period* is characterized by the containment of infection, progressive elimination of the pathogen, repair of damaged tissue, and resolution of associated symptoms. Similar to the incubation period, the time required for complete convalescence may be days, weeks, or months, depending on the type of pathogen and the voracity of the host's immune response. The *resolution* is the total elimination of a pathogen from the body without residual signs or symptoms of disease. Sometimes, infections may lead to a *chronic* infectious state.

Several notable exceptions to the classic presentation of an infectious process have been recognized. Chronic infectious diseases have a markedly protracted and sometimes irregular course. The host may experience symptoms of the infectious process continuously or sporadically for months or years without a convalescent phase. In contrast, *subclinical* or *subacute illness* progresses from infection to resolution without clinically apparent symptoms. A disease is called *insidious* if the prodromal phase is protracted; a fulminant illness is characterized by abrupt onset of symptoms with little or no prodrome. Fatal infections are variants of the typical disease course.

Site of Infection

Inflammation of an anatomic location is usually designated by adding the suffix *-itis* to the name of the involved tissue (*e.g.*, bronchitis, infection of the bronchi and bronchioles; encephalitis, brain infection; endocarditis, infection of the heart valves). These are general terms, however, and they apply equally to inflammation from infectious and noninfectious causes. The suffix *-emia* is used to designate the presence of a substance in the blood (*e.g.*, *bacteremia*, *viremia*, and *fungemia* describe the presence of these infectious agents in the bloodstream). The term *sepsis*, or *septicemia*, has been used to refer to the presence of microbial toxins in the blood. For the past three decades, the definition of sepsis focused on specific clinical manifestations of systemic inflammation (fever/hypothermia, tachycardia, tachypnea, and leukocytosis/leukopenia/bandemia) in the setting of a confirmed or suspected infection. The term *severe sepsis* was used for sepsis with organ failure, and the term *septic shock* was used when the organ failure was hypotension not responsive to fluid resuscitation. The definition will continue to evolve. We now understand that sepsis is a dysregulated host response infection accompanied by life-threatening organ dysfunction.[25]

The type of pathogen, the portal of entry, and the competence of the host's immunologic defense system ultimately determine the site of an infectious disease. Many pathogenic microorganisms are restricted in their capacity to invade the human body. *Mycoplasma pneumoniae*, influenza viruses, and *Legionella pneumophila* rarely cause disease outside the respiratory tract; infections caused by *Neisseria gonorrhoeae* are generally confined to the genitourinary tract; and shigellosis and giardiasis seldom extend beyond the gastrointestinal tract.[3] These are considered localized infectious diseases. The bacterium *Helicobacter pylori* is an extreme example of a site-specific pathogen. *Helicobacter pylori* is a significant cause of gastric ulcers but has not been implicated in disease processes elsewhere in the human body. Bacteria, such as *Neisseria meningitidis causes meningococcal disease*, a prominent pathogen of children and young adults; *Salmonella typhi*, the cause of typhoid fever; and *Borrelia burgdorferi*, the agent of Lyme disease, tend to disseminate from the primary site of infection to involve other locations and organ systems. These are all examples of systemic pathogens disseminated throughout the body by the circulatory system. *Staphylococcal aureus* can lead to many different types of infection (*e.g.*, pneumonia, urinary tract infection, endocarditis, cellulitis).

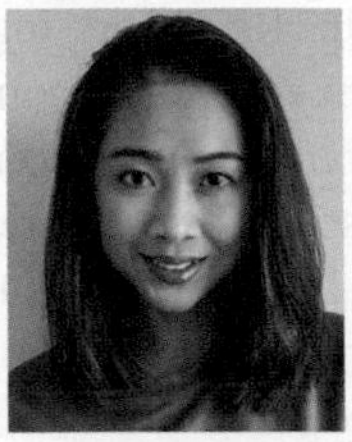

Ms. Roon experienced recurring swelling and aching of two joints over the last 18 months (with no apparent injury). She experiences headaches when her joints are swollen and has felt very tired. In addition, she had a low-grade fever 100° F today at the primary care provider's office. All of these symptoms are examples of the systemic characteristics of Lyme disease. Some of the symptoms may be a result of the inflammatory cascade, which is triggered when she experiences a flare-up. Cytokines and complement trigger some tissue injury as they attempt to fight against the Lyme disease. There is no vaccine for Lyme disease, so there is no way to absolutely prevent this disease. Ms. Roon had developed antibodies to the disease as evidenced from her positive diagnostic tests. For a positive test, one would need 2 out of 3 of the bands[20,23,38,40] for an IgM immunoglobulin to be positive for Lyme.[26] And Ms. Roon would need five of the following bands (18, 21, or 24, 28, 30, 39, 41, 45, 58, 66, or 93) to have a positive IgG titer for Lyme disease.[26]

An abscess is a localized pocket of infection composed of devitalized tissue, microorganisms, and the host's phagocytic white blood cells. In this case, the dissemination of the pathogen has been contained by the host, but white cell function within the toxic environment of the abscess is hampered, and the elimination of microorganisms is slowed if not actually stopped. Abscesses usually must be surgically drained to obtain a complete cure, depending on the location and size. Similarly, infections of biomedical implants such as catheters, artificial heart valves, and prosthetic bone implants are seldom cured by the host's immune response and antimicrobial therapy. The infecting organism colonizes the surface of the implant, producing a dense matrix of cells, host proteins, and capsular material—a biofilm—necessitating the removal of the device.

Virulence Factors

Virulence factors are substances or products generated by infectious agents that enhance their ability to cause disease. Although a large number of microbial products fit this description, they can be grouped generally into four categories: toxins, adhesion factors, evasive factors, and invasive factors (Table 10.3).

Toxins

Toxins are substances that alter or destroy the normal function of the host or host's cells. Toxin production is a trait chiefly monopolized by bacterial pathogens, although certain fungal and protozoan pathogens also elaborate substances toxic to humans. Bacterial toxins have a diverse spectrum of activity and exert their effects on a wide variety of host target cells. For classification purposes, however, the bacterial toxins can be divided into two main types: *exotoxins* and *endotoxins*.

TABLE 10.3 EXAMPLES OF VIRULENCE FACTORS PRODUCED BY PATHOGENIC MICROORGANISMS

FACTOR	CATEGORY	ORGANISM	EFFECT ON HOST
Cholera toxin	Exotoxin	*Vibrio cholerae* (bacterium)	Secretory diarrhea
Diphtheria toxin	Exotoxin	*Corynebacterium diphtheriae* (bacterium)	Inhibits protein synthesis
Lipopolysaccharide	Endotoxin	Many gram-negative bacteria	Fever, hypotension, shock
Toxic shock toxin	Enterotoxin	*Staphylococcus aureus* (bacterium)	Rash, diarrhea, vomiting, hepatitis
Hemagglutinin	Adherence	Influenza virus	Establishment of infection
Pili	Adherence	*Neisseria gonorrhoeae* (bacterium)	Establishment of infection
Leukocidin	Evasive	*S. aureus*	Kills phagocytes
IgA protease	Evasive	*Haemophilus influenzae* (bacterium)	Inactivates antibody
Capsule	Evasive	*Cryptococcus neoformans* (yeast)	Prevents phagocytosis
Collagenase	Invasive	*Pseudomonas aeruginosa* (bacterium)	Penetration of tissue
Protease	Invasive	*Aspergillus* (mold)	Penetration of tissue
Phospholipase	Invasive	*Clostridium perfringens* (bacterium)	Penetration of tissue
Botulinum toxin	Exotoxin	*Clostridium botulinum* (bacterium)	Neuroparalysis, inhibits acetylcholine release
Pneumolysin	Exotoxin	*Streptococcus pneumoniae* (bacterium)	Inhibition of respiratory ciliated and phagocytic cell function

Exotoxins. Exotoxins are proteins released from the bacterial cell during growth that may damage cells. Bacteria toxins have evolved several different strain-specific mechanisms to escape the immune system.[27] *Neurotoxins, enterotoxins, and cytotoxins* are common terms used to describe exotoxins acting on neurons, the gastrointestinal system, and cells, respectively.[3] Although these exotoxins were first described based on their activity, we now know that many are superantigens.[28] Superantigens elicit a response by interaction with both the innate and adaptive immune system. They interact with major histocompatibility antigens on antigen-presenting cells as well as T cells to induce a potent inflammatory response that can act locally or systemically.[27] Bacterial exotoxins enzymatically inactivate or modify key cellular constituents, leading to cell death or dysfunction. Diphtheria toxin, for example, inhibits cellular protein synthesis; botulism toxin decreases the release of neurotransmitter from cholinergic neurons, causing flaccid paralysis; tetanus toxin decreases the release of neurotransmitter from inhibitory neurons, producing spastic paralysis; and cholera toxin induces fluid secretion into the lumen of the intestine, causing diarrhea.

There are five different superantigen groups (I to V), with groups I and II being responsible for serious human disease.[28] *Streptococcus pyogenes* (group A beta-hemolytic streptococci) produces up to 11 different superantigens known as streptococcal pyrogenic exotoxins (SPEs). Some of these SPEs were once called scarlet fever toxins. There are about 10 million cases of pharyngitis each year caused by *Streptococcus pyogenes*, which is capable of producing toxic shock, myositis, autoimmune disease, and acute glomerulonephritis.[28] *Staphylococcus aureus* produces up to 24 different superantigens. Examples are superantigen toxic shock syndrome toxin-1 (TSST-1), which produces a life-threatening toxic shock–like syndrome (similar to the disease associated with tampon use), and staphylococcal enterotoxins (SEs), which are known for their emetic effect. Both of these organisms may cause colonization and lead to carrier states, demonstrating how they have used their virulence factors to evade the host's immune system.[28] Other examples of exotoxin-induced diseases include pertussis (whooping cough), anthrax, traveler's diarrhea, toxic shock syndrome, and a host of food-borne illnesses (*i.e.*, food poisoning).[29]

Endotoxins. In contrast to exotoxins, endotoxins do not contain protein, are not actively released from the bacterium during growth, and have no enzymatic activity. Rather, endotoxins are complex molecules composed of lipid and polysaccharides found in the cell wall of gram-negative bacteria. Studies of different endotoxins have indicated that the lipid portion of the endotoxin confers the toxic properties to the molecule. Endotoxins are potent activators of a number of regulatory systems in humans. A small amount of endotoxin in the circulatory system (endotoxemia) can induce clotting, bleeding, inflammation, hypotension, and fever. The sum of the physiologic reactions to endotoxins is sometimes called *endotoxic shock*.[29]

Adhesion Factors

No interaction between microorganisms and humans can progress to infection or disease if the pathogen is unable to attach to and colonize the host. The process of microbial attachment may be site specific (*e.g.*, mucous membranes, skin surfaces), cell specific (*e.g.*, T lymphocytes, respiratory epithelium, intestinal epithelium), or nonspecific (*e.g.*, moist areas, charged surfaces). In any of these cases, adhesion requires a positive interaction between the surfaces of host cells and the infectious agent.

The site to which microorganisms adhere is called a *receptor*, and the reciprocal molecule or substance that binds to the receptor is called a ligand or adhesin. Receptors may be proteins, carbohydrates, lipids, or complex molecules composed of all three. Similarly, ligands may be simple or complex molecules and, in some cases, highly specific structures. Ligands that bind to specific carbohydrates are called *lectins*. After initial attachment, a number of bacterial agents become embedded in a gelatinous matrix of polysaccharides called a *slime* or *mucous layer*. The slime layer serves two purposes: it anchors the agent firmly to host tissue surfaces, and it protects the agent from the immunologic defenses of the host.[30]

Many viral agents, including influenza, mumps, measles, and adenovirus, produce filamentous appendages or spikes called *hemagglutinins* that recognize carbohydrate receptors on the surfaces of specific cells in the upper respiratory tract of the host.

Evasive Factors

A number of factors produced by microorganisms enhance virulence by evading various components of the host's immune system. Extracellular polysaccharides, including capsules, slime, and mucous layers, discourage engulfment and killing of pathogens by the host's phagocytic white blood cells (*i.e.*, neutrophils and macrophages). Encapsulated organisms such as *S. agalactiae*, *S. pneumoniae*, *N. meningitidis*, and *H. influenzae* type b (before the vaccine) are a cause of significant morbidity and mortality in neonates and children who lack protective anticapsular antibodies. Certain bacterial, fungal, and parasitic pathogens avoid phagocytosis by excreting leukocidin C toxins, which cause specific and lethal damage to the cell membrane of host neutrophils and macrophages. Other pathogens, such as the bacterial agents of salmonellosis, listeriosis, and Legionnaire disease, are adapted to survive and reproduce within phagocytic white blood cells after ingestion, avoiding or neutralizing the usually lethal products contained within the lysosomes of the cell. *Helicobacter pylori*, the infectious cause of gastritis and gastric ulcers, produces a urease enzyme on its outer cell wall.[3] The urease converts gastric urea into ammonia, thus neutralizing the acidic environment of the stomach and allowing the organism to survive in this hostile environment.

Other unique strategies used by pathogenic microbes to evade immunologic surveillance have evolved solely to avoid recognition by host antibodies. Strains of *S. aureus* produce a surface protein (protein A) that immobilizes immunoglobulin G (IgG), holding the antigen-binding region harmlessly away from the organisms. This pathogen also secretes a unique enzyme called *coagulase*. Coagulase converts soluble human coagulation factors into a solid clot, which envelops and protects the organism from phagocytic host cells and antibodies. *H. influenzae* and *N. gonorrhoeae* secrete enzymes that cleave and inactivate secretory IgA, neutralizing the primary defense of the respiratory and genital tracts at the site of infection. *Borrelia* species, including the agents of Lyme disease and relapsing fever, alter surface antigens during the disease course to avoid immunologic detection. It appears that the capability to devise strategic defense systems and stealth technologies is not limited to humans.

Some viruses, such as HIV, impair the function of immunoregulatory cells. Although this property increases the virulence of these agents, it is not considered a virulence factor in the true sense of the definition.

Invasive Factors

Invasive factors are products produced by infectious agents that facilitate the penetration of anatomic barriers and host tissue. Most invasive factors are enzymes capable of destroying cellular membranes (*e.g.*, phospholipases), connective tissue (*e.g.*, elastases, collagenases), intercellular matrices (*e.g.*, hyaluronidase), and structural protein complexes (*e.g.*, proteases).[29] It is the combined effects of invasive factors, toxins, and antimicrobial and inflammatory substances released by host cells to counter infection that mediate the tissue damage and pathophysiology of infectious diseases.

IN SUMMARY

Epidemiology is the study of factors, events, and circumstances that influence the transmission of disease. *Incidence* refers to the number of new cases of an infectious disease that occur in a defined population, and *prevalence* refers to the number of active cases that are present at any given time. Infectious diseases are considered endemic in a geographic area if the incidence and prevalence are expected and relatively stable. An epidemic refers to an abrupt and unexpected increase in the incidence of a disease over endemic rates, and a pandemic refers to the spread of disease beyond continental boundaries.

The ultimate goal of epidemiology and epidemiologic studies is to devise strategies to interrupt or eliminate the spread of infectious disease. To accomplish this, infectious diseases are classified according to incidence, portal of entry, source, symptoms, disease course, site of infection, and virulence factors.

DIAGNOSIS AND TREATMENT OF INFECTIOUS DISEASES

After completing this section of the chapter, the learner will be able to meet the following objectives:

- Explain the different detection methods for diagnosis of infectious disease.
- Cite three general intervention methods that can be used in treatment of infectious illnesses.

Diagnosis

The diagnosis of an infectious disease requires two criteria: the recovery of a probable pathogen or some evidence of its presence from the infected sites of a diseased host and accurate documentation of clinical signs and symptoms compatible with an infectious process. In the laboratory, the diagnosis of an infectious agent is accomplished using three basic techniques: culture, serology, and the detection of characteristic antigens, genomic sequences, or metabolites produced by the pathogen.

Culture

Culture refers to the growth of a microorganism outside of the body, usually on or in artificial growth media such as agar plates or broth. The specimen from the host is inoculated into broth or onto the surface of an agar plate, and the culture is placed in a controlled environment such as an incubator until the growth of microorganisms becomes detectable. In the case of a bacterial pathogen, identification is based on microscopic appearance and gram stain reaction, shape, texture, and color (*i.e.*, morphology) of the colonies and by a panel of biochemical reactions that fingerprint salient biochemical characteristics of the organism. Certain bacteria such as *Mycobacterium leprae*, the agent of leprosy, and *T. pallidum*, the syphilis spirochete, do not grow on artificial media and require additional methods of identification. Fungi and mycoplasmas are cultured in much the same way as bacteria but with more reliance on microscopic and colonial morphology for identification. Some fungi are very slow growing and may take weeks to identify by culture.

Chlamydiaceae, *Rickettsiaceae*, and all human viruses are obligate intracellular pathogens.[3] As a result, the propagation of these agents in the laboratory requires the inoculation of eukaryotic cells grown in culture (cell cultures). A cell culture consists of a flask containing a single layer, or monolayer, of eukaryotic cells covering the bottom and overlaid with broth containing essential nutrients and growth factors. When a virus infects and replicates within cultured eukaryotic cells, it produces pathologic changes in the appearance of the cell called the *cytopathic effect* (CPE). See Figure 10.8. The CPE can be detected microscopically, and the pattern and extent of cellular destruction are often characteristics of a particular virus.

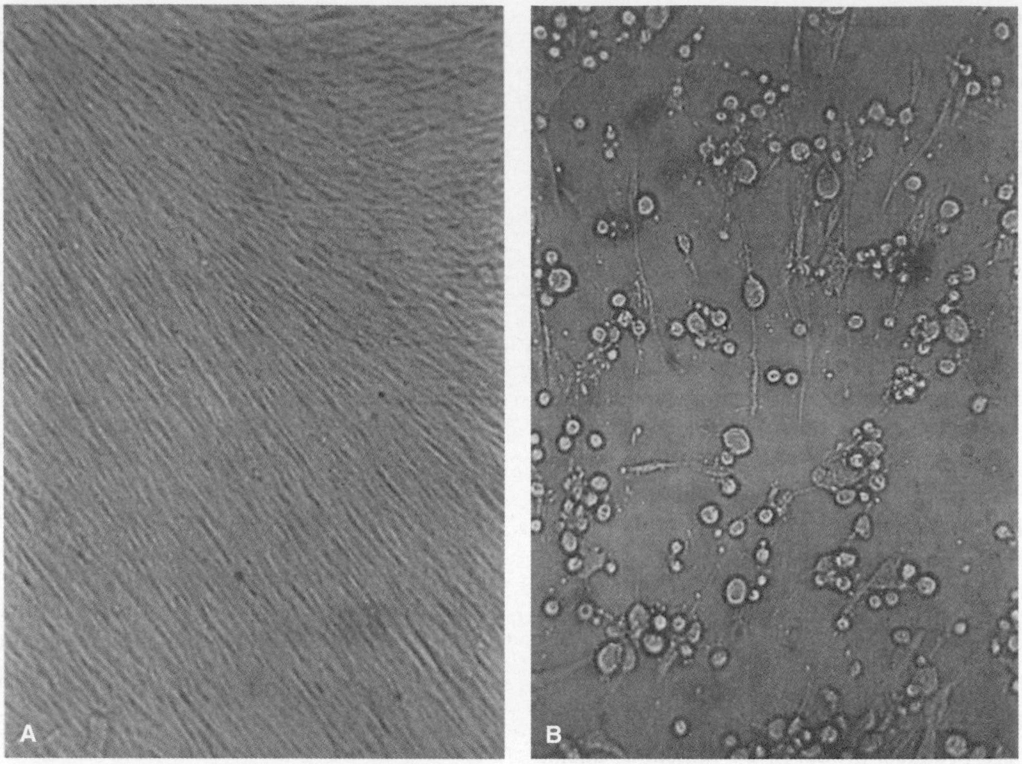

Figure 10.8 • The microscopic appearance of a monolayer of uninfected human fibroblasts grown in cell culture **(A)** and the same cells after infection with HSV **(B)**, demonstrating the CEP caused by viral replication and concomitant cell lysis.

Although culture media have been developed for the growth of certain human-infecting protozoa and helminths in the laboratory, the diagnosis of parasitic infectious diseases has traditionally relied on microscopic or, in the case of worms, visible identification of organisms, cysts, or ova directly from infected patient specimens.

In the setting of acute infection, it is important that cultures are obtained prior to antibiotic administration. The timing, quality, transport, and processing of specimen are all important in obtaining accurate results. The causative organism cannot be identified by culture in up to 33% of people presenting with sepsis.[31] It is unknown how many of these culture results are falsely negative. There are several possible reasons this may occur (*e.g.*, the organism may be fastidious and difficult to culture, the sample may contain a low number of organisms, or antibiotic may have been administered prior to the culture).[32]

Serology

Serology is an indirect means of identifying infectious agents by measuring serum antibodies in the diseased host. A tentative diagnosis can be made if the antibody level, also called *antibody titer*, against a specific pathogen rises during the acute phase of the disease and falls during convalescence. Serologic identification of an infectious agent is not as accurate as culture, but it may be a useful adjunct, especially for the diagnosis of diseases caused by pathogens such as the hepatitis B virus that cannot be cultured. The measurement of antibody titers has another advantage in that specific antibody types, such as IgM and IgG, are produced by the host during different phases of an infectious process. IgM-specific antibodies generally rise and fall during the acute phase of the disease, whereas the synthesis of the IgG class of antibodies increases during the acute phase and remains elevated until or beyond resolution.[26] Measurements of class-specific antibodies are also useful in the diagnosis of congenital infections. IgM antibodies do not cross the placenta, but certain IgG antibodies are transferred passively from mother to child during the final trimester of gestation. Consequently, an elevated level of pathogen-specific IgM antibodies in the serum of a neonate must have originated from the child and therefore indicates congenital infection. A similarly increased IgG titer in the neonate does not differentiate congenital from maternal infection.[26]

The technology of *antigen detection* has evolved rapidly over the past decade and in the process has revolutionized the diagnosis of certain infectious diseases. Antigen detection incorporates features of culture and serology but reduces to a fraction the time required for diagnosis. In principle, this method relies on purified antibodies to detect antigens of infectious agents in specimens obtained from the diseased host. The source of antibodies used for antigen detection can be animals immunized against a particular pathogen or *hybridomas*. Fusing normal antibody-producing spleen cells from an immunized animal with malignant myeloma cells creates hybridomas. The resulting hybrid synthesizes large quantities of antibody. An antibody produced by a hybridoma is called a *monoclonal antibody* and is highly specific for a single antigen and a single pathogen.[33] Regardless of the source, the antibodies are labeled with a substance that allows microscopic or overt detection when bound to the pathogen or its products. In general, the three types of labels used for this purpose are fluorescent dyes, enzymes, and particles such as latex beads. Fluorescent antibodies allow visualization of an infectious agent with the aid of fluorescence microscopy. Depending on the type of fluorescent dye used, the organism may appear bright green or orange against a black background, making detection extremely easy. Enzyme-labeled antibodies function in a similar manner. The enzyme is capable of converting a colorless compound into a colored substance, thereby permitting detection of antibody bound to an infectious agent without the use of a fluorescent microscope. Particles coated with antibodies clump together, or agglutinate, when the appropriate antigen is present in a specimen. Particle agglutination is especially useful when examining infected body fluids such as urine, serum, or spinal fluid. In addition, newer technologies allow for simultaneous analysis of multiple antigens in a small sample volume by using antibody-coated beads, a fluorescent detection system, and software for quantification.

DNA and RNA Sequencing

Methods for identifying infectious agents through the detection of DNA or RNA sequences unique to a single agent have increasingly been used over the past decade. Several techniques have been devised to accomplish this goal, each having different degrees of sensitivity regarding the number of organisms that need to be present in a specimen for detection. The first of these methods is called *DNA probe hybridization*. Small fragments of DNA are cut from the genome of a specific pathogen and labeled with compounds (photoemitting chemicals or antigens) that allow detection. The labeled DNA probes are added to specimens from an infected host. If the pathogen is present, the probe attaches to the complementary strand of DNA on the genome of the infectious agent, permitting rapid diagnosis. The use of labeled probes has allowed visualization of particular agents within and around individual cells in histologic sections of a tissue.

A second and more sensitive method of DNA detection is called the *polymerase chain reaction* (PCR; Fig. 10.9).[26] This method incorporates two unique reagents: a specific pair of oligonucleotides (usually less than 25-nucleotide long) called *primers* and a heat-stable DNA polymerase. To perform the assay, the primers are added to the specimen containing the suspect pathogen, and the sample is heated to melt the DNA in the specimen and then allowed to cool. The primers locate and bind only to the complementary target DNA of the pathogen in question. The heat-stable polymerase begins to replicate the DNA from the point at which the primers attached, similar to two trains approaching one another on separate but converging tracks. After the initial cycle, DNA polymerization ceases at the point where the primers were located, producing a strand of DNA with a distinct size, depending on the distance separating the two primers. The specimen is heated again, and the process starts anew. After many cycles of heating, cooling, and polymerization, a large number of uniformly sized DNA fragments are produced only if the specific pathogen (or its DNA) is present in the specimen. The polymerized DNA fragments are separated by electrophoresis and visualized with a dye or identified by hybridization with a specific probe.

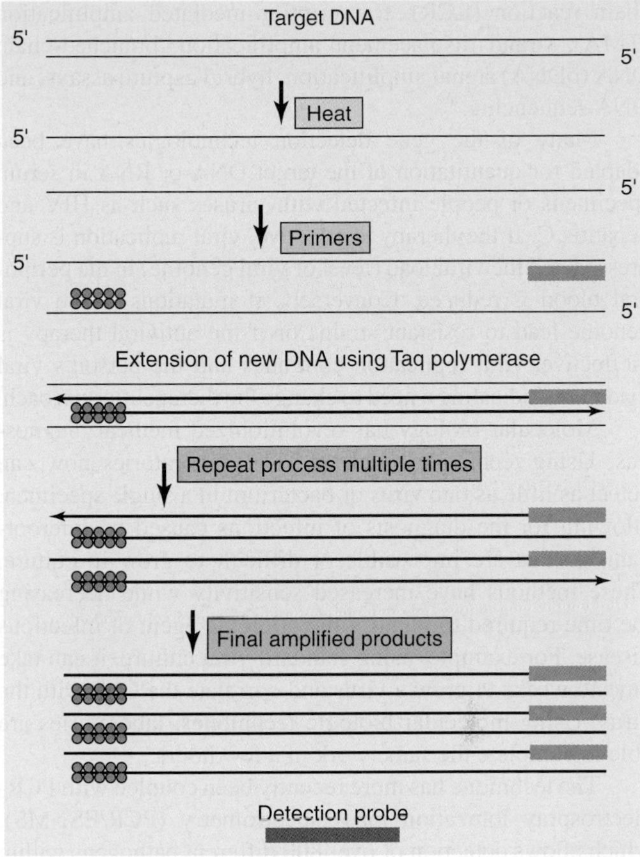

Figure 10.9 • Polymerase chain reaction. The target DNA is first melted using heat (generally around 94°C) to separate the strands of DNA. Primers that recognize specific sequences in the target DNA are allowed to bind as the reaction cools. Using a unique, thermostable DNA polymerase called Taq and an abundance of deoxynucleoside triphosphates, new DNA strands are amplified from the point of the primer attachment. The process is repeated many times (called *cycles*) until millions of copies of DNA are produced, all of which have the same length defined by the distance (in base pairs) between the primer binding sites. These copies are then detected by electrophoresis and staining or through the use of labeled DNA probes that similar to the primers recognize a specific sequence located in the amplified section of DNA.

A modification of PCR, known as real-time PCR, continues to revolutionize medical diagnostics. Real-time PCR uses the same principles as PCR but includes a fluorescence-labeled probe that specifically binds a target DNA sequence between the oligonucleotide primers. As the DNA is replicated by the DNA polymerase, the level of fluorescence in the reaction is measured. If fluorescence increases beyond a minimum threshold, the PCR is considered positive and indicates the presence of the target DNA in a specimen. Real-time PCR is very effective in determining the diagnosis of *Clostridium difficile*. It is quicker, more sensitive, and more specific and can assist the physician/provider in administering antibiotics more efficiently for people with diarrhea secondary to *C. difficile*.[34]

Several variations of molecular gene detection techniques in addition to PCR have been developed and incorporated into diagnostic kits for use in the clinical laboratory, including ligase chain reaction (LCR), transcription-mediated amplification (TMA), strand displacement amplification, branched-chain DNA (bDNA) signal amplification, hybrid capture assays, and DNA sequencing.[30]

Many of the gene detection technologies have been adapted for quantitation of the target DNA or RNA in serum specimens of people infected with viruses such as HIV and hepatitis C. If the therapy is effective, viral replication is suppressed and the viral load (level of viral genome) in the peripheral blood is reduced. Conversely, if mutations in the viral genome lead to resistant strains or if the antiviral therapy is ineffective, viral replication continues and the person's viral load rises, indicating a need to change the therapeutic approach.

Molecular biology has revolutionized medical diagnostics. Using techniques such as PCR, laboratories now can detect as little as one virus or bacterium in a single specimen, allowing for the diagnosis of infections caused by microorganisms that are impossible or difficult to grow in culture. These methods have increased sensitivity while decreasing the time required to identify the etiologic agent of infectious disease. For example, using standard viral culture, it can take days to weeks to grow a virus and correlate the CPE with the virus. Using molecular biologic techniques, laboratories are able to complete the same work in a few hours.

The technique has more recently been coupled with PCR-electrospray ionization mass spectrometry (PCR/ESI-MS), which allows detection of over 800 different pathogens within approximately 6 hours.[35] Antibiotic sensitivity testing is not possible using this technique, but it can detect antibiotic resistance markers. PCR/ESI-MS is a highly sensitive technique for detecting pathogens rapidly, with a sensitivity that is three times higher than standard culture.[35]

KEY POINTS

DIAGNOSIS AND TREATMENT OF INFECTIOUS DISEASES

- The definitive diagnosis of an infectious disease requires recovery and identification of the infecting organism by microscopic identification of the agent in stains of specimens or sections of tissue, culture isolation and identification of the agents, demonstration of antibody- or cell-mediated immune responses to an infectious agent, or DNA or RNA identification of infectious agents.
- Treatment of infectious disease is aimed at eliminating the infectious organism and promoting recovery of the infected person. Treatment is provided by controlling/eradicating the infectious source through the use of antimicrobial agents, immunotherapy, and, when necessary, surgical intervention (*e.g.*, abscess drainage). Supportive care such as adequate hydration is also an important aspect of care to maintain organ perfusion. Adequate sleep and nutrition are also important. Prevention of infectious disease is accomplished with immunization methods.

Treatment

The goal of treatment for an infectious disease is complete removal of the pathogen from the host and the restoration of normal physiologic function to damaged tissues. Most infectious diseases of humans are self-limiting in that they require little or no medical therapy for a complete cure. When an infectious process overcomes the body's defenses, therapeutic intervention is essential. The choice of treatment may be medical through the use of antimicrobial agents; immunologic with antibody preparations, vaccines, or substances that stimulate and improve the host's immune function; or surgical by removing infected tissues. The decision about which therapeutic modality or combination of therapies to use is based on the extent, urgency, and location of the disease process, the pathogen, and the availability of effective antimicrobial agents.

Antimicrobial Agents

It was not until the advent of World War II, after the introduction of sulfonamides and penicillin, that the development of antimicrobial compounds matured into a science of great consequence. Today, the comprehensive list of effective anti-infective agents is burgeoning. Most antimicrobial compounds can be categorized roughly according to mechanism of anti-infective activity, chemical structure, and target pathogen (*e.g.*, antibacterial, antiviral, antifungal, or antiparasitic agents). Guidelines are reviewed and updated by professional societies on a regular basis. We refer readers to review guidelines provided by the Infectious Disease Society of America.[36] In addition to the guidelines, treatment is informed by local antibiotic resistance patterns and institutional antibiograms. Biomarkers (C-reactive protein or procalcitonin levels) are often helpful in monitoring response to treatment along with typical clinical findings (*e.g.*, temperature, heart rate).

Antibacterial Agents. Antibacterial agents are generally called *antibiotics*. Most antibiotics are actually produced by other microorganisms, primarily bacteria and fungi, as by-products of metabolism. Antibiotics usually are effective only against other prokaryotic organisms. An antibiotic is considered *bactericidal* if it causes irreversible and lethal damage to the bacterial pathogen and *bacteriostatic* if its inhibitory effects on bacterial growth are reversed when the agent is eliminated. Antibiotics can be classified into families of compounds with related chemical structure and activity (Table 10.4).

Not all antibiotics are effective against all pathogenic bacteria. Some agents are effective only against gram-negative bacteria, and others are specific for gram-positive organisms (*e.g.*, vancomycin). The so-called broad-spectrum antibiotics, such as the newest class of cephalosporins, are active against a wide variety of gram-positive and gram-negative bacteria. Members of the *Mycobacterium* genus, including *M. tuberculosis*, are extremely resistant to the effects of the major classes of antibiotics and require an entirely different

TABLE 10.4 CLASSIFICATION AND ACTIVITY OF ANTIBACTERIAL AGENTS (ANTIBIOTICS)

FAMILY	EXAMPLE	TARGET SITE	SIDE EFFECTS
Penicillins	Ampicillin	Cell wall	Allergic reactions
Cephalosporins	Cephalexin	Cell wall	Allergic reactions
Monobactams	Aztreonam	Cell wall	Rash
Carbapenem	Imipenem	Cell wall	Nausea, diarrhea
Aminoglycosides	Tobramycin	Ribosomes (protein synthesis)	Hearing loss Nephrotoxicity
Tetracyclines	Doxycycline	Ribosomes (protein synthesis)	Gastrointestinal irritation Allergic reactions Teeth and bone dysplasia
Macrolides	Clarithromycin	Ribosomes (protein synthesis)	Colitis Allergic reactions
Glycopeptides	Vancomycin	Ribosomes (protein synthesis)	Allergic reactions Hearing loss Nephrotoxicity
Quinolones	Ciprofloxacin	DNA synthesis	Gastrointestinal irritation Tendon rupture
Miscellaneous	Chloramphenicol	Ribosomes (protein synthesis)	Anemia
	Rifampin	Ribosomes (protein synthesis)	Hepatotoxicity
	Trimethoprim	Folic acid synthesis	Allergic reactions Same as sulfonamides
Sulfonamides	Sulfadiazine	Folic acid synthesis	Allergic reactions Anemia Gastrointestinal irritation
Oxazolidinone	Linezolid	Ribosomes (protein synthesis)	Diarrhea, thrombocytopenia
Streptogramin	Quinupristin/dalfopristin	Ribosomes (protein synthesis)	Muscle and joint aches
Glycylcycline	Tigecycline	Ribosomes	Nausea, vomiting, diarrhea
Polymyxins	Colistin	Membrane	Confusion, visual disturbances, vertigo, kidney damage
Lipopeptide	Daptomycin	Membrane depolarization	Nausea, vomiting, constipation, diarrhea, headache

spectrum of agents for therapy. The four basic mechanisms of the antibiotic action are interference with a specific step in bacterial cell wall synthesis (*e.g.*, penicillins, cephalosporins, glycopeptides, monobactams, carbapenems), inhibition of bacterial protein synthesis (*e.g.*, aminoglycosides, macrolides, ketolides, tetracyclines, chloramphenicol, oxazolidinones, streptogramins, and rifampin), interruption of nucleic acid synthesis (*e.g.*, fluoroquinolones, nalidixic acid), and interference with normal metabolism (*e.g.*, sulfonamides, trimethoprim).[34]

Despite lack of antibiotic activity against eukaryotic cells, many agents cause unwanted or toxic side effects in humans, including allergic responses (penicillins, cephalosporins, sulfonamides, glycopeptides), hearing and kidney impairment (aminoglycosides), and liver or bone marrow toxicity (chloramphenicol, fluoroquinolones, vancomycin). Of greater concern is the increasing prevalence of bacteria resistant to the effects of antibiotics. The ways in which bacteria acquire resistance to antibiotics are becoming as numerous as the types of antibiotics. Bacterial resistance mechanisms include the production of enzymes that inactivate antibiotics, such as β-lactamases, genetic mutations that alter antibiotic binding sites, alternative metabolic pathways that bypass antibiotic activity, and changes in the filtration qualities of the bacterial cell wall that prevent access of antibiotics to the target site in the organism. Antibiotic stewardship involves judicious use to help prevent the development of antibiotic resistance. When broad-spectrum antibiotics are required, therapy should be narrowed as soon as possible to specific antibiotics based on sensitivity testing.

Antiviral Agents. Until recently, few effective antiviral agents were available for treating human infections. The reason for this is host toxicity. Viral replication requires the use of eukaryotic host cell enzymes, and the drugs that effectively interrupt viral replication are likely to interfere with host cell reproduction as well. However, in response to the AIDS epidemic, there has been massive, albeit delayed, development of antiretroviral agents. Almost all antiviral compounds are synthetic, and with few exceptions, the primary target of antiviral compounds is viral RNA or DNA synthesis. Agents such as acyclovir, ganciclovir, vidarabine, and ribavirin mimic the nucleoside building blocks of RNA and DNA.[34] During active viral replication, the nucleoside analogs inhibit the viral DNA polymerase, preventing duplication of the viral genome and spread of infectious viral progeny to other susceptible host cells. Similar to the specificity of antibiotics, antiviral agents may be active against RNA viruses only, DNA viruses only, or occasionally both. Other nucleoside analogs, such as zidovudine, lamivudine, didanosine, stavudine, and zalcitabine, and nonnucleoside inhibitors, including nevirapine, efavirenz, and delavirdine, were developed specifically for the treatment of AIDS by targeting the HIV-specific enzyme, reverse transcriptase, for inhibition.[34] This key enzyme is essential for viral replication and has no counterpart in the infected eukaryotic host cells.

Another class of antiviral agents developed solely for the treatment of HIV infections is the *protease inhibitors* (*e.g.*, indinavir, ritonavir, saquinavir, tipranavir, atazanavir, nelfinavir). These drugs inhibit an HIV-specific enzyme that is necessary for late maturation events in the virus life cycle.[34]

Experimental approaches to antiviral therapy include compounds that inhibit viral attachment to susceptible host cells, drugs that prevent uncoating of the viral genome once inside the host cell, and agents that directly inhibit viral DNA polymerase. A class of antiviral agents that specifically inhibits influenza virus neuraminidase B, which is an essential enzyme for viral replication, has also been effective with influenza. Two agents in this class, zanamivir and oseltamivir, are used for treatment of both influenza A and B.

Although the treatment of viral infections with antimicrobial agents is a relatively recent endeavor, reports of viral mutations resulting in resistant strains are very common. This is especially troubling in the case of HIV, in which resistance to relatively new antiviral agents, including nucleoside analogs and protease inhibitors, has already been described, prompting the need for combination or alternating therapy with multiple antiretroviral agents.

Antifungal Agents. The target *site* of the two most important families of antifungal agents is the cytoplasmic membranes of yeasts or molds. Fungal membranes differ from human cell membranes in that they contain the sterol ergosterol instead of cholesterol. The polyene family of antifungal compounds (*e.g.*, amphotericin B, nystatin) preferentially binds to ergosterol and forms holes in the cytoplasmic membrane, causing leakage of the fungal cell contents and, eventually, lysis of the cell.[34] The imidazole class of drugs (*e.g.*, fluconazole, itraconazole, voriconazole, posaconazole) inhibits the synthesis of ergosterol, thereby damaging the integrity of the fungal cytoplasmic membrane.[34] Both types of drugs bind to a certain extent to the cholesterol component of host cell membranes and elicit a variety of toxic side effects in treated people. The nucleoside analog 5-fluorocytosine (5-FC) disrupts fungal RNA and DNA synthesis but without the toxicity associated with the polyene and imidazole drugs. Unfortunately, 5-FC demonstrates little or no antifungal activity against molds or dimorphic fungi and is primarily reserved for infections caused by yeasts.

A novel class of antifungal compounds called *echinocandins* has received considerable attention because these drugs inhibit the synthesis of β-1,3-glucan, a major cell wall polysaccharide found in many fungi, including *C. albicans*, *Aspergillus* species, and *Pneumocystis carinii.*[34] The drugs included in this class are caspofungin, micafungin, and anidulafungin. These inhibitors are available for treatment of people with fungal infections, such as candidiasis or invasive aspergillosis, which are refractory to treatment with other antifungal agents.

Antiparasitic Agents. Because of the extreme diversity of human parasites and their growth cycles, a review of antiparasitic therapies and agents would be highly impractical and lengthy. Similar to other infectious diseases caused by eukaryotic microorganisms, treatment of parasitic illnesses is based on exploiting essential components of the parasite's metabolism or cellular anatomy that are not shared by the host. Any relatedness between the target site of the parasite and the cells of the host increases the likelihood of toxic reactions in the host.

Resistance among human parasites to standard, effective therapy is a major concern. In Africa, Asia, and South America, the incidence of chloroquine-resistant malaria (*Plasmodium falciparum*) is on the rise. Resistant strains require more complicated, expensive, and potentially toxic therapy with a combination of agents.

Immunotherapy

An exciting approach to the treatment of infectious diseases is immunotherapy. This strategy involves supplementing or stimulating the host's immune response so that the spread of a pathogen is limited or reversed. Several products are available for this purpose, including intravenous immunoglobulin (IVIG) and cytokines. IVIG is a pooled preparation of antibodies obtained from normal, healthy immune human donors that is infused as an intravenous solution. In theory, pathogen-specific antibodies present in the infusion facilitate neutralization, phagocytosis, and clearance of infectious agents above and beyond the capabilities of the diseased host. Hyperimmune immunoglobulin preparations, which are also commercially available, contain high titers of antibodies against specific pathogens, including hepatitis B virus, cytomegalovirus, rabies, and varicella zoster virus.

Cytokines are substances produced by various cells that, in small quantities, stimulate white cell replication, phagocytosis, antibody production, and the induction of fever, inflammation, and tissue repair—all of which counteract infectious agents and hasten recovery. With the advent of genetic engineering and cloning, many cytokines, including interferons and interleukins, have been produced in the laboratory and are being evaluated experimentally as anti-infective agents. As we learn more about the action of cytokines, it becomes evident that some of the adverse reactions associated with infectious processes result from the body's own inflammatory response. Several experimental agents to block one or more inflammatory cytokine pathways have been tested over the past 30 years, but no agent that blocks a single pathway is currently approved by the U.S Food and Drug Administration for sepsis. Hydrocortisone (which blocks many pathways) has been used to broadly target an overzealous inflammatory response; however, it is only recommended as replacement therapy in the setting of adrenal insufficiency.[37] It is likely that therapies based on the regulation of the inflammatory response will eventually be approved.

One of the most efficient but often overlooked means of preventing infectious diseases is immunization. Proper and timely adherence to recommended vaccination schedules in children and booster immunizations in adults effectively reduces the senseless spread of vaccine-preventable illnesses such as measles, mumps, pertussis, and rubella, which still occur with alarming frequency. New strategies for the development of vaccines carried by harmless viral vectors are currently being developed that someday might lead to inexpensive and effective oral immunization against HIV, hepatitis C, malaria, and other potentially lethal infectious diseases.

Surgical Intervention

Before the discovery of antimicrobial agents, surgical removal of infected tissues, organs, or limbs was occasionally the only option available to prevent the demise of the infected host. Today, medical therapy with antibiotics and other anti-infective agents is an effective solution for most infectious diseases. However, surgical intervention is still an important option for cases in which the pathogen is resistant to available treatments. Surgical interventions may be used to hasten the recovery process by providing access to an infected site by antimicrobial agents (drainage of an abscess), cleaning the site (debridement), or removing infected organs or tissue (*e.g.*, appendectomy). In some situations, surgery may be the only means of affecting a complete cure, as in the case of endocarditis resulting in an infected heart valve, in which the diseased valve must be replaced with a mechanical or biologic valve to restore normal function. In other situations, surgical containment of a rapidly progressing infectious process such as gas gangrene may be the only means of saving a person's life.

Long-Term Outcomes

Infectious disease may persist for prolonged periods (*e.g.*, mycobacterium) with few consequences until reactivated when the immune system begins to fail with advanced age or other forms of immunosuppression. Scientific advances have allowed for an infection with human immunodeficiency virus (HIV), which was once a disease that would always progress to acquired immunodeficiency syndrome (AIDS) with a high risk of death by opportunistic infections, to become a chronic disease with successful pharmacologic management.

As the management of acute life-threatening infections such as sepsis has continued to improve, the number of persons surviving sepsis during hospitalization has increased.[38] Survivors of sepsis have a very high morbidity and mortality rate, with more than 50% requiring rehospitalization in the first year. Infections are the most common reason for rehospitalization,[38] and immunosuppression following sepsis is still not well understood.[39] In addition, survivors of sepsis may experience cognitive impairment, psychological impairment (*e.g.*, depression), functional impairment, and high risk of cardiovascular events, and decreased quality of life has been reported for up to 5 years.[38] Much more work is needed to understand the underlying pathophysiology influencing long-term effects caused by sepsis.

IN SUMMARY

The ultimate outcome of any interaction between microorganisms and the human host is decided by a complex and ever-changing set of variables that consider the overall health and physiologic function of the host and the virulence and infectious dose of the microbe. In many instances, disease is an inevitable consequence, but with continuing advances in science and technology, the majority of cases can now be eliminated or rapidly cured with appropriate therapy. It is the intent of those who study infectious diseases to understand thoroughly the pathogen, the disease course, the mechanisms of transmission, and the host response to infection. This knowledge will lead to the development of improved diagnostic techniques, revolutionary approaches to anti-infective therapy, and eradication or control of microscopic agents that cause frightening devastation and loss of life throughout the world.

BIOTERRORISM AND EMERGING GLOBAL INFECTIOUS DISEASES

After completing this section of the chapter, the learner will be able to meet the following objectives:

- List the infectious agents considered to pose the highest level of bioterrorism threat.
- State an important concept in containment of infections because of bioterrorism and global travel.

Bioterrorism

In October of 2001, less than 1 month after the tragedy of September 11, the world became instantly acquainted with the term *bioterrorism*. By the end of November of that year, 22 cases of human anthrax (11 cutaneous and 11 inhalation) had been identified, resulting in five deaths, and all cases were associated with exposure to four intentionally contaminated envelopes delivered through the U.S. Postal Service. The reality of the 2001 outbreak brought a new sense of awareness concerning the use of microorganisms as weapons.[40]

Anthrax is an ancient disease caused by the cutaneous inoculation, inhalation, or ingestion of the spores of *Bacillus anthracis*, a gram-positive bacillus. Anthrax is more commonly known as a disease of herbivores that can be transmitted to humans through contact with infected secretions, soil, or animal products. It is a rare disease in the United States, and so the sudden increase in cases over a short time was a chilling indication that the spread of the organism had been intentional. Fortunately, the number of deaths was limited, thanks to prompt recognition of cases by physicians and public health personnel and rapid institution of antimicrobial prophylaxis to exposed people.

To prepare for the possibility of bioterrorist attacks, the CDC along with other federal, state, and local agencies has created the Laboratory Response Network (LRN). The LRN is a four-tiered structure consisting of laboratories with ever-increasing expertise, responsibility, and biocontainment facilities that allow for the rapid and coordinated detection and identification of bioterrorism events under safe working conditions.[41,42]

Potential agents of bioterrorism have been categorized into three levels (A, B, C) based on risk of use, transmissibility, invasiveness, and mortality rate. The agents placed in the highest bioterrorism threat level include *B. anthracis*, *Yersinia pestis* (the cause of bubonic plague), *Francisella tularensis* (the cause of tularemia), variola major virus (the cause of smallpox), and several hemorrhagic fever viruses (Ebola, Marburg, Lassa, and Junin). The toxin of the anaerobic gram-positive organism *Clostridium botulinum*, which causes the neuromuscular paralysis termed *botulism*, is also listed as a category A agent. Interestingly, purified *C. botulinum* toxins A and B are finding increasing use under the trade names Botox, Myobloc, and NeuroBloc for various medicinal and cosmetic purposes. The category B agents include agents of food-borne and waterborne diseases (*Salmonella*, *Shigella*, *Vibrio cholerae*, *E. coli* O157:H7), zoonotic infections (*Brucella* species, *C. burnetii*, *Burkholderia mallei*), and viral encephalitides (Venezuelan, Western, and Eastern equine encephalitis viruses), as well as toxins from *S. aureus*, *Clostridium perfringens*, and *Ricinus communis* (the castor bean). Category C agents are defined as emerging pathogens and potential risks for the future, even though many of these organisms are causes of ancient diseases. Category C agents include *M. tuberculosis*, Nipah virus, hantavirus, tick-borne and yellow fever viruses, and, the only protozoan of the group, *Cryptosporidium parvum*. An excellent Web site available through the CDC is the "CDC Public Health Emergency Preparedness and Response Site," which provides detailed information on agents of bioterrorism, emergency contacts, and contingency plans in the event of an outbreak (https://emergency.cdc.gov/bioterrorism/index.asp).[43] In addition, the American Society for Microbiology has been at the forefront of the response effort, providing resources and guidelines for sentinel laboratories to facilitate bioterrorism preparedness.[40]

Global Infectious Diseases

Aided by a global market and the ease of international travel, the first years of the 21st century have witnessed the importation or emergence of a host of novel infectious diseases. During the late summer and early fall of 1999, WNV (an arthropod-borne flavivirus) was identified as the cause of an epidemic involving 56 people in the New York City area.[44] This outbreak, which led to seven deaths (primarily in older adults), marked the first time that WNV had been recognized in the Western Hemisphere since its discovery in Uganda nearly 60 years earlier. Because WNV is a mosquito-borne disease and is transmitted to a number of susceptible avian (*e.g.*, blue jays, crows, and hawks) and equine hosts, the potential for rapid and sustained spread of the disease across the United States was recognized early. By the fall of 2002, a national surveillance network had detected WNV activity in 2289 counties from 44 states, including Los Angeles County, and had identified more than 3000 human cases. The disease ranges in intensity from a nonspecific febrile illness to fulminant meningoencephalitis. In 2002 alone, 3389 cases of WNV-associated illness were identified in the United States with 201 deaths, making this the largest arboviral meningoencephalitis outbreak ever described in the Western Hemisphere. Efforts to prevent further spread of the disease are currently centered on surveillance of WNV-associated illness in birds, humans, and other mammals, as well as mosquito control.[44]

In the winter of 2002, SARS emerged as a global threat. The first inkling of the impending threat was when the Chinese Ministry of Health reported 305 cases of a mysterious and virulent respiratory tract illness that had appeared in Guangdong province in southern China in a 4-month period of time.[22,23] The spread of the disease to household contacts of sick people and medical personnel caring for people with the disease identified it as highly transmissible. In a very short time, people with compatible symptoms were recognized in Hong Kong and Vietnam. The World Health Organization (WHO) promptly issued a global alert and started international surveillance for people with typical symptomatology who had a history of travel to the endemic region. As of June 2003, more than 8000 cases of SARS from 29 countries and 809 deaths were reported to the WHO. In a remarkable feat of molecular technology, the etiology of SARS was quickly determined to be a novel coronavirus, possibly of mammalian or avian origin, and its entire genome was sequenced by the end of May 2003.

The Zika virus is a flavivirus transmitted by mosquitoes. It was first detected in 1947 among rhesus monkeys in Uganda. Human cases were first reported in Africa in the 1960s; however, in 2015, a cluster of cases of congenital microcephaly was linked to Zika.[45,46] Many who had the virus had mild symptoms and might be unlikely to seek care, so the number of persons who contracted Zika is unknown. The WHO declared a public health emergency of international concern on February 1, 2016. Investigation revealed the following cases suspected to be associated with Zika: 3000 suspected in the general population, 22 pregnant women, 13 with Guillain-Barre syndrome, and 29 infants with microcephaly. The public health response provided testing, vector control, and prevention messages (*e.g.*, mosquito netting, DEET, clothing that covers extremities). Zika has been detected in several body fluids and may also be sexually transmitted.[45] More work is needed to understand the impact of Zika on transmission cycles and disease burden in both human and nonhuman populations.

These three scenarios highlight the rapidity with which novel or exotic diseases can be introduced into nonindigenous regions of the world and to a susceptible population. Although great strides in molecular microbiology have allowed for the rapid identification of new or rare microorganisms, the potential devastation in terms of human life and economic loss is great, underscoring the need to maintain resources for public health surveillance and intervention. For more details on these and other intriguing cases of infectious disease detective work, refer to this excellent Web site: www.who.int/en/ and www.cdc.gov. The International Society for Infectious Diseases maintains a LISTSERV known as ProMED-mail that provides early warning and rapid dissemination about infectious disease outbreaks: http://www.promedmail.org/.

IN SUMMARY

The challenges associated with maintaining health throughout a global community are becoming increasingly apparent. Aided by a global market and the ease of international travel, the past decade has witnessed the importation and emergence of a host of novel infectious diseases. There is also the potential threat of the deliberate use of microorganisms as weapons of bioterrorism.

GERIATRIC Considerations

- Aging exposes people to viral infections such as human papillomavirus, hepatitis B, and Epstein-Barr virus, which are linked to cancers worldwide.[47]
- Age-related structural changes causing thinning of the mucous membranes in the larynx that result in tremulous sounds and decreased projection of voice must be differentiated from infectious diseases such as an upper respiratory infection.[47]
- 14.1% of people over age 65 have chronic rhinosinusitis because of changes in the structure of the nose with aging as the tip droops, restricting airflow.[47]

PEDIATRIC Considerations

- Children are at risk for infectious disease because their immune systems are still developing and they tend to place hands and potentially infected objects in the mouth.[48]
- Vaccines, both old and new, have led to a significant decrease in the number and severity of infections.[48]
- Pediatric daycare and schoolrooms have common rooms, placing children at risk for transmission of infectious agents.[48]
- The presence of a rash is common in many infections that are a challenge to identify. A thorough description and history from the caregiver are the key to assessment.[48]
- Although most infections in children manifest with fever, neonates may be hypothermic with an infection, and other children may have no fever.[49]

REVIEW EXERCISES

1. Newborn infants who have not yet developed an intestinal flora are routinely given an intramuscular injection of vitamin K to prevent bleeding because of a deficiency in vitamin K–dependent coagulation factors.
   A. *Use the concept of mutualism to explain why this is done.*
2. People with human granulocytic ehrlichiosis may be coinfected with Lyme disease.
   A. *Explain.*
3. People with chronic lung disease are often taught to contact their health care provider when they notice a change in the color of their sputum (*i.e.*, from white or clear to yellow- or brown-tinged) because it might be a sign of a bacterial infection.
   A. *Explain.*
4. Microorganisms are capable of causing infection only if they can grow at the temperature of the infected body site.
   A. *Using this concept, explain the different sites of fungal infections because of the dermatophyte fungal species that cause tinea pedis (athlete's foot) and Candida albicans which causes infections of the mouth (thrush) and female genitalia (vulvovaginitis).*
5. The threat of global infections, such as SARS and HIV, continues to grow.
   A. *What would you propose to be one of the most important functions of health care professionals in terms of controlling the spread of such infections?*

References

1. Lloyd-Price J., Abu-Ali G., Huttenhower C. (2016). The healthy human microbiome. *Genome Medicine* 8, 51. doi: 10.1186/s13073-016-0307-y.
2. Petersen C., Round J. L. (2014). Defining dysbiosis and its influence on host immunity and disease. *Cellular Microbiology* 16(7), 1024–1033. doi: 10.1111/cmi.12308.
3. Strayer D. S., Rubin R. (Eds.) (2015). *Rubin's pathology: Clinicopathologic foundations of medicine* (7th ed.). Philadelphia, PA: Wolters Kluwer Health.
4. Rayman J. B., Kandel E. R. (2017). Functional prions in the Brain. *Cold Spring Harbor Perspectives in Biology* 9(1), 1–14. doi: 10.1101/cshperspect.a023671.
5. Prusiner S. B., Woerman A. L., Mordes D. A., et al. (2015). Evidence for alpha-synuclein prions causing multiple system atrophy in humans with parkinsonism. *Proceedings of the National Academy of Sciences of the United States of America* 112(38), E5308–E5317. doi: 10.1073/pnas.1514475112.
6. Urwin P., Thanigaikumar K., Ironside J. W., et al. (2017). Sporadic Creutzfeldt-Jakob disease in 2 plasma product recipients, United Kingdom. *Emerging Infectious Diseases* 23(6), 893–897. doi: 10.3201/eid2306.161884.
7. Rewar S., Mirdha D., Rewar P. (2015). Treatment and Prevention of Pandemic H1N1 Influenza. *Annals of Global Health* 81(5), 645–653. doi: 10.1016/j.aogh.2015.08.014.

8. Zhang Z., Zhang J., Xia N., et al (2017). Expanded strain coverage for a highly successful public health tool: prophylactic 9-valent human papillomavirus vaccine. *Human Vaccines & Immunotherapeutics* 13(10), 2280–2291. doi: 10.1080/21645515.2017.1346755.
9. Solano C., Echeverz M., Lasa I. (2014). Biofilm dispersion and quorum sensing. *Current Opinion in Microbiology* 18, 96–104. doi: 10.1016/j.mib.2014.02.008.
10. Goering R. V., Dockrell H. M., Zuckerman M., et al (2013). *Mim's Medical Microbiology* (5th ed.). Philadelphia, PA: Elsevier Saunders.
11. Donders G. G. G., Ruban K., Bellen G., et al. (2017). Mycoplasma/ureaplasma infection in pregnancy: to screen or not to screen. *Journal of Perinatal Medicine* 45(5), 505–515. doi: 10.1515/jpm-2016-0111.
12. Centers for Disease Control and Prevention. (2017). *Rocky mountain spotted fever*. Available http://www.cdc.gov/rmsf/stats/index.html. Accessed November 30, 2017.
13. Centers for Disease Control and Prevention. (2017). *Disease specifics: Chlamydia pneumoniae*. Available https://www.cdc.gov/pneumonia/atypical/cpneumoniae/hcp/disease.html Accessed November 30, 2017.
14. Hogerwerf L., De Gier B., Baan B., et al. (2017). Chlamydia psittaci (psittacosis) as a cause of community-acquired pneumonia: A systematic review and meta-analysis. *Epidemiology and Infection* 145(15), 3096–3105. doi: 10.1017/S0950268817002060.
15. Snowden J., Simonsen K. A. (2017). Ehrlichiosis. In: *StatPearls [Internet]*. Treasure Island, FL: StatPearls Publishing. Available: https://www.ncbi.nlm.nih.gov/books/NBK441966/. Accessed June, 2017.
16. Yachoui R. (2013). Multiorgan failure related to human monocytic ehrlichiosis. *BMJ Case Reports* 2013. doi: 10.1136/bcr-2013-008716.
17. Eldin C., Melenotte C., Mediannikov O., et al. (2017). From Q fever to coxiella burnetii infection: a paradigm change. *Clinical Microbiology Reviews* 30(1), 115–190. doi: 10.1128/CMR.00045-16.
18. Colombo A. L., de Almeida Junior J. N., Slavin M. A., et al. (2017). Candida and invasive mould diseases in non-neutropenic critically ill patients and patients with haematological cancer. *Lancet Infectious Diseases* 17(11), e344–e356. doi: 10.1016/S1473-3099(17)30304-3.
19. Partida-Rodriguez O., Serrano-Vazquez A., Nieves-Ramirez M. E., et al. (2017). Human intestinal microbiota: Interaction between parasites and the host immune response. *Archives of Medical Research*, 1–2. doi: 10.1016/j.arcmed.2017.11.
20. World Health Organization. (2017). *Health topics: Epidemiology*. Available: http://www.who.int/topics/epidemiology/en/ Accessed November 12, 2017.
21. Gordis L. (2014). *Epidemiology* (5th ed.). Philadelphia, PA: Elsevier Saunders.
22. Hui D. S., Chan P. K. (2010). Severe acute respiratory syndrome and coronavirus. *Infectious Disease Clinics* 24(3), 619–638.
23. Hsueh P. R., Yang P. C. (2005). Severe acute respiratory syndrome epidemic in Taiwan, 2003. *Journal of Microbiology, Immunology and Infection* 38, 82–88.
24. Bennett J. E., Dolin R., Blaser, M. J. (Eds.) (2015). *Mandell, Douglas, and Bennett's principles and practice of infectious diseases* (8th ed.). Philadelphia, PA: Elsevier, Saunders.
25. Singer M., Deutschman C. S., Seymour C. W., et al. (2016). The third international consensus definitions for sepsis and septic shock (sepsis-3). *JAMA* 315(8), 801–810. doi: 10.1001/jama.2016.0287.
26. Fischbach F., Dunning M. B. (2015). *A manual of laboratory and diagnostic tests* (9th ed.). Philadelphia, PA: Wolters Kluwer Health | Lippincott Williams & Wilkins.
27. Sastalla I., Monack D. M., Kubatzky K. F. (2016). Editorial: Bacterial exotoxins: how bacteria fight the immune system. *Frontiers in Immunology* 7, 300. doi: 10.3389/fimmu.2016.00300.
28. Spaulding A. R., Salgado-Pabon W., Kohler P. L., et al. (2013). Staphylococcal and streptococcal superantigen exotoxins. *Clinical Microbiology Reviews* 26(3), 422–447. doi: 10.1128/CMR.00104-12.
29. Hall J. (2015). *Guyton and Hall textbook of medical physiology* (13th ed.). Philadelphia, PA: Saunders.
30. Shetty N. (2009). *Infectious disease: Pathogenesis, prevalence and case studies*. Chichester, UK: John Wiley & Sons.
31. Rhodes A., Evans L. E., Alhazzani W., et al. (2017). Surviving sepsis campaign: international guidelines for management of sepsis and septic shock: 2016. *Critical Care Medicine* 45(3), 486–552. doi: 10.1097/CCM.0000000000002255.
32. Opota O., Jaton K., Greub G. (2015). Microbial diagnosis of bloodstream infection: towards molecular diagnosis directly from blood. *Clinical Microbiology and Infection* 21(4), 323–331. doi: 10.1016/j.cmi.2015.02.005.
33. Geskin L. J. (2015). Monoclonal antibodies. *Dermatologic Clinics* 33(4), 777–786. doi: 10.1016/j.det.2015.05.015.
34. Woo T. M., Robinson M. V. (2016). *Pharmacotherapeutics for nurse practitioner prescribers*. Philadelphia, PA: F. A. Davis.
35. Vincent J. L., Brealey D., Libert N., et al. (2015). Rapid diagnosis of infection in the critically ill, a multicenter study of molecular detection in bloodstream infections, pneumonia, and sterile site infections. *Critical Care Medicine*, 43(11), 2283–2291. doi: 10.1097/CCM.0000000000001249.
36. Infectious Disease Society of America. (2017). *IDSA practice guidelines*. Available: http://www.idsociety.org/PracticeGuidelines/
37. Annane D., Pastores S. M., Rochwerg B., et al. (2017). Guidelines for the diagnosis and management of critical illness-related corticosteroid insufficiency (CIRCI) in critically ill patients (part I): Society of Critical Care Medicine (SCCM) and European Society of Intensive Care Medicine (ESICM) 2017. *Critical Care Medicine* 45(12), 2078–2088. doi: 10.1097/CCM.0000000000002737.
38. Shankar-Hari M., Rubenfeld G. D. (2016). Understanding long-term outcomes following sepsis: Implications and challenges. *Current Infectious Disease Reports* 18(11), 37. doi: 10.1007/s11908-016-0544-7.
39. Angus D. C., Opal S. (2016). Immunosuppression and secondary infection in sepsis: part, not all, of the story. *JAMA* 315(14), 1457–1459. doi: 10.1001/jama.2016.2762.
40. Adalja A. A., Toner E., Inglesby T. V. (2015). Clinical management of potential bioterrorism-related conditions. *New England Journal of Medicine* 372(10), 954–962. doi: 10.1056/NEJMra1409755.
41. Wagar E. (2016). Bioterrorism and the role of the clinical microbiology laboratory. *Clinical Microbiology Reviews* 29(1), 175–189. doi: 10.1128/CMR.00033-15.
42. Center for Disease Control and Prevention. (2014). *Laboratory response network*. Available: https://emergency.cdc.gov/lrn/ Accessed December 13, 2017.
43. Center for Disease Control and Prevention. (2017). *Emergency preparedness and response*. Available: https://emergency.cdc.gov/bioterrorism/index.asp Accessed December 13, 2017.
44. Center for Disease Control and Prevention. (2017). *West Nile virus*. Available: http://www.cdc.gov/ncidod/dvbid/westnile/index.htm Accessed December 13, 2017.
45. Waddell L. A., Greig J. D. (2016). Scoping review of the zika virus literature. *PLoS One* 11(5), e0156376. doi: 10.1371/journal.pone.0156376.
46. Journel I., Andrecy L. L., Metellus D., et al. (2017). Transmission of Zika Virus—Haiti, October 12, 2015 to September 10, 2016. *Morbidity and Mortality Weekly Report* 66(6), 172–176. doi: 10.15585/mmwr.mm6606a4.
47. Hinkle J. L. (2018). *Brunner & Suddarth's textbook of medical-surgical nursing*. (14th ed). Philadelphia, PA: Wolters Kluwer.
48. Kyle T., Carman S. (2017). *Essentials of pediatric nursing*. (3rd ed.). Philadelphia, PA: Wolters Kluwer.
49. Smitherman H. F., Macias C. G. (2017). Febrile Infant (younger than 90 days of age): Outpatient evaluation. *UpToDate*. Available: https://www.uptodate.com/contents/febrile-infant-younger-than-90-days-of-age-outpatient-evaluation Accessed February 15, 2018.

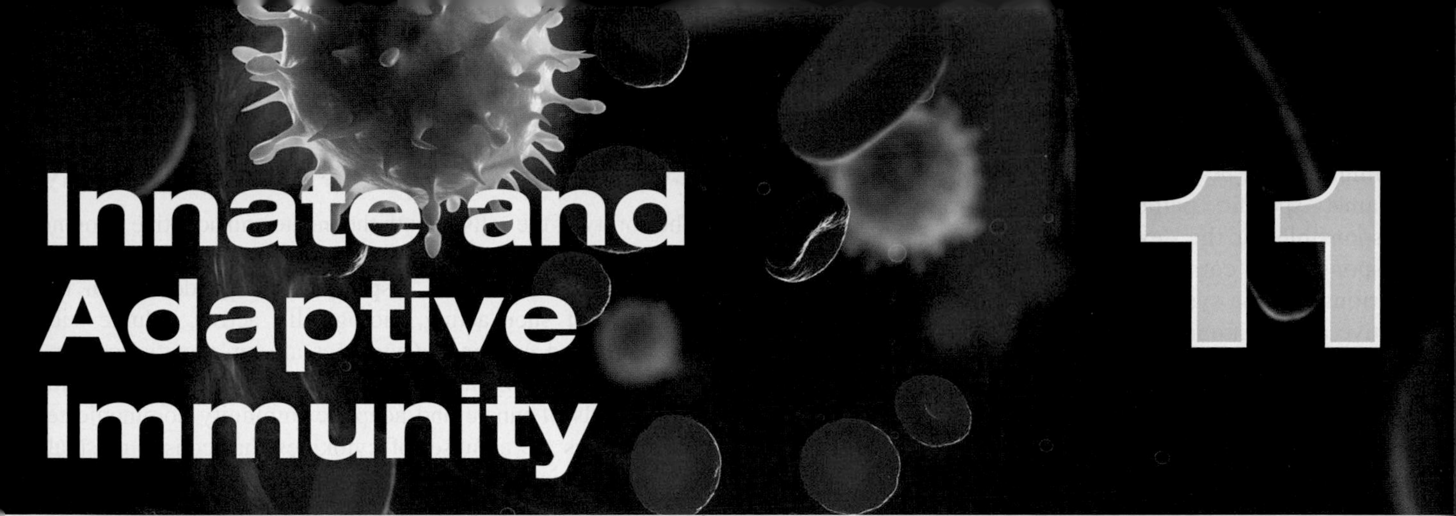

11 Innate and Adaptive Immunity

Nancy A. Moriber

The human body is constantly exposed to potentially harmful microorganisms and foreign substances. Therefore, it has evolved a complete system composed of complementary and interrelated mechanisms that defend against invasion by bacteria, viruses, and other foreign substances. Through recognition of specific patterns found on the surface of organisms and toxins, the body's immune system can distinguish itself from these foreign substances and tell the difference between potentially harmful and nonharmful agents. In addition, the immune system can defend against abnormal cells and molecules that periodically develop within the body. The skin and its epithelial layers in conjunction with the body's normal inflammatory processes make up the first line of the body's defense and confer *innate or natural immunity* to the host. Once these protective barriers have been crossed, the body relies upon a second line of defense known as the *adaptive immune response* to eradicate infection by invading organisms. The adaptive immune response develops slowly over time but results in the development of antibodies that can rapidly target specific microorganisms and foreign substances when a second exposure occurs.

This chapter covers immunity and the immune system, including a complete discussion of innate and adaptive immunity. Concepts related to key cellular processes, recognition systems, and effector responses integral to the immune system are also presented. In addition, developmental aspects of the immune system are discussed.

THE IMMUNE RESPONSE

After completing this section of the chapter, the learner will be able to meet the following objectives:

- Discuss the function of the immune system.
- Compare and contrast the innate and adaptive immune response.
- Understand the role of the chemical mediators that orchestrate the immune response.

Immunity can be defined as the body's ability to defend against specific pathogens and/or foreign substances responsible for the development of disease. The immune response is a complex response initiated by the body's various defense systems. Some of these responses become active almost immediately, whereas others develop slowly over time. It is the coordinated interaction of these mechanisms that allows the body to maintain normal internal homeostasis. However, when these mechanisms are either depressed or become overactive, illness and disease can occur.

Innate immunity and adaptive immunity are complementary processes that work to protect the body. *Innate immunity*, the body's first line of defense, occurs early and more rapidly in response to foreign substances, whereas adaptive immunity is usually delayed unless the host has been exposed before (Table 11.1).

Intact innate immune mechanisms are essential for the initiation of the adaptive immune response. Therefore, a successful immune response requires communication between the two systems. Dendritic cells (DCs) are an essential component of both innate and adaptive immunity and serve as the communication link between the two immune responses through the release of cytokines and chemokines.[1] As a result, innate immune cells are capable of communicating important information about the invading microorganism or foreign substance to the B and T lymphocytes, which are the key cells involved in adaptive immunity. These immune cells in turn recruit and activate additional phagocytes and molecules of the innate immune system to defend the host. Both innate and adaptive immunity are therefore essential for an effective immune response and work together in the fight against infection.

Cytokines and Their Role in Immunity

The ability of the cells of both the innate and adaptive immune systems to communicate critical information with each other and initiate effector cell responses is dependent upon the secretion of short-acting, biologically active, soluble substances called *cytokines*. Cytokines are an essential component of host defense mechanisms and the primary means with which cells of innate and adaptive immunity communicate. Chemokines are a subset of cytokines that consist of small protein molecules involved in both immune and inflammatory responses.[2] They are responsible for directing the migration of leukocytes to both areas of injury and locations where immune responses have been activated such as lymph nodes, the spleen, Peyer patches, and the tonsils.[2] Chemokines can work together to antagonize or activate chemokine receptors. The source and function of the main cytokines that participate in innate and adaptive immunity are summarized in Table 11.2.

General Properties of Cytokines

Cytokines are low molecular weight, pro- or anti-inflammatory proteins that are secreted by cells of the innate and adaptive immune systems and that regulate many of the actions of these cells. The majority of the major cytokines are the interleukins (ILs), interferons (IFNs), and tumor necrosis factor alpha (TNF-α). Cytokines work by binding to specific receptors on the cells that they target and then activating intracellular processes.[3]

Interleukins (ILs) are produced by both the macrophages and lymphocytes in the presence of an invading microorganism or when the process of inflammation is initiated. Their primary function is to enhance the acquired immune

TABLE 11.1 FEATURES OF INNATE AND ADAPTIVE IMMUNITY

FEATURE	INNATE	ADAPTIVE
Time of response	Immediate (minutes/hours)	Dependent upon exposure (first, delayed; second, immediate d/t production antibodies)
Diversity	Limited to classes or groups of microbes	Very large; specific for each unique antigen
Microbe recognition	General patterns on microbes; nonspecific	Specific to individual microbes and antigens (antigen/antibody complexes)
Nonself recognition	Yes	Yes
Response to repeated infection	Similar with each exposure	Immunologic memory; more rapid and efficient with subsequent exposure
Defense	Epithelium (skin, mucous membranes), phagocytes, inflammation, fever	Cell killing; tagging of antigen by antibody for removal
Cellular components	Phagocytes (monocytes/macrophages, neutrophils), NK cells, DCs	T and B lymphocytes, macrophages, DCs, NK cells
Molecular components	Cytokines, complement proteins, acute-phase proteins, soluble mediators	Antibodies, cytokines, complement system

TABLE 11.2 CYTOKINES AND CHEMOKINES OF INNATE AND ADAPTIVE IMMUNITY

CYTOKINES	SOURCE	FUNCTION
Interleukin-1 (IL-1)	Macrophages, endothelial cells, some epithelial cells	Wide variety of biologic effects; activates endothelium in inflammation; induces fever and acute-phase response; stimulates neutrophil production
Interleukin-2 (IL-2)	$CD4^+$, $CD8^+$ T cells	Growth factor for activated T cells; induces synthesis of other cytokines; activates cytotoxic T lymphocytes and NK cells
Interleukin-3 (IL-3)	$CD4^+$ T cells	Growth factor for progenitor hematopoietic cells
Interleukin-4 (IL-4)	$CD4^+$ T_2H cells, mast cells	Promotes growth and survival of T, B, and mast cells; causes T_2H cell differentiation; activates B cells and eosinophils; and induces IgE-type responses
Interleukin-5 (IL-5)	$CD4^+$ T_2H cells	Induces eosinophil growth and development
Interleukin-6 (IL-6)	Macrophages, endothelial cells, T lymphocytes	Stimulates the liver to produce mediators of acute-phase inflammatory response; also induces proliferation of antibody-producing cells by the adaptive immune system
Interleukin-7 (IL-7)	Bone marrow stromal cells	Primary function in adaptive immunity; stimulates pre-B cells and thymocyte development and proliferation
Interleukin-8 (IL-8)	Macrophages, endothelial cells	Primary function in adaptive immunity; chemoattracts neutrophils and T lymphocytes; regulates lymphocyte homing and neutrophil infiltration
Interleukin-10 (IL-10)	Macrophages, some T-helper cells	Inhibitor of activated macrophages and DCs; decreases inflammation by inhibiting T_1H cells and release of IL-12 from macrophages
Interleukin-12 (IL-12)	Macrophages, DCs	Enhances NK cell cytotoxicity in innate immunity; induces T_1H cell differentiation in adaptive immunity
Type I interferons (IFN-α, IFN-β)	Macrophages, fibroblasts	Inhibit viral replication; activate NK cells; and increase expression of MHC-I molecules on virus-infected cells
Interferon-γ (IFN-γ)	NK cells, $CD4^+$ and $CD8^+$ T lymphocytes	Activates macrophages in both innate immune responses and adaptive cell-mediated immune responses; increases expression of MHC-I and MHC-II and antigen processing and presentation
Tumor necrosis factor-α (TNF-α)	Macrophages, T cells	Induces inflammation, fever, and acute-phase response; activates neutrophils and endothelial cells; kills cells through apoptosis
Chemokines	Macrophages, endothelial cells, T lymphocytes	Large family of structurally similar cytokines that stimulate leukocyte movement and regulate the migration of leukocytes from the blood to the tissues
Granulocyte-monocyte CSF (GM-CSF)	T cells, macrophages, endothelial cells, fibroblasts	Promotes neutrophil, eosinophil, and monocyte maturation and growth; activates mature granulocytes
Granulocyte CSF (G-CSF)	Macrophages, fibroblasts, endothelial cells	Promotes growth and maturation of neutrophils consumed in inflammatory reactions
Monocyte CSF (M-CSF)	Macrophages, activated T cells, endothelial cells	Promotes growth and maturation of mononuclear phagocytes

CSF, colony-stimulating factor; MHC, major histocompatibility complex; NK, natural killer; T_1H, T-helper type 1; T_2H, T-helper type 2.

response or regulate through suppression or enhancement the inflammatory process. IFNs are cytokines that primarily protect the host against viral infections and play a role in the modulation of the inflammatory response. Each type of IFN is produced by a specific cell of the immune response. IFN-α and IFN-β are produced primarily by macrophages, and IFN-γ is produced primarily by T lymphocytes. TNF-α is a cytokine that acts as one of the most important mediators of the inflammatory response. TNF-α is produced by macrophages when surface toll-like receptors (TLRs), which play a critical role in the detection of microorganisms, recognize what are known as pathogen-associated molecular patterns (PAMPs) on the surface of the cells.[4] TNF-α acts as an endogenous pyogen (fever producer) that stimulates the synthesis of proinflammatory substances in the liver. With prolonged exposure, it has the ability to cause intravascular coagulation and clot formation.

Despite the diverse functions of the cytokines, they all share certain important properties. All cytokines are secreted in a brief, self-limited manner. They are rarely stored as preformed molecules but instead are synthesized when the cells that produce them are activated. Some of the cytokines exhibit pleiotropism, which means they can act on many different cell types. For example, IL-17 is produced by the T-helper 17 ($T_{17}H$) cells and acts on leukocytes, epithelial cells, mesothelial cells, vascular endothelial cells, and fibroblasts. As a result, IL-17 plays a critical role in host defense against pathogens that can infiltrate skin and mucus membranes.[5] When these defenses malfunction, disease processes that originate in these tissues, such as asthma and psoriasis, can arise. Cytokines also exhibit redundancy, which refers to the ability of different cytokines to stimulate the same or overlapping biologic functions. Because of this redundancy, inhibition of a single cytokine will have minimal or no impact on the integrity of the immune response because other cytokines may compensate.

Concept Mastery Alert

Cytokines have the ability to act on different cell types so they are pleiotropic, not cell specific. They also have the ability to stimulate the same biologic factors as other cytokines or to overlap their effects. This is known as redundancy.

In addition to being pleiotropic and redundant, several different cell types are capable of producing the same cytokine. This allows cytokines to have a broader spectrum of activity. For example, IL-1 is a proinflammatory cytokine that is primarily produced by macrophages but can be produced by virtually all leukocytes, endothelial cells, and fibroblasts. Finally, cytokines can also function to initiate cascade reactions with one cytokine influencing the synthesis and actions of other cytokines, which ultimately produce the desired action. These effects may be localized, acting on a single cell or group of cells in the area surrounding the effector cell, or the effects can be systemic with the cytokines secreted into the bloodstream and transported to their site of action. TNF-α is an example of a cytokine with wide-reaching systemic effects.

Colony-stimulating factors (CSFs) are a unique subset of cytokines that participate in hematopoiesis and stimulate the production of large numbers of mature platelets, erythrocytes, lymphocytes, neutrophils, monocytes, eosinophils, basophils, and DCs. The CSFs were named according to the type of target cell on which they act (see Table 11.2). Although CSF is necessary for normal blood cell production, excess CSF is associated with several disease processes such as chronic obstructive pulmonary disease (COPD).[6] Impaired macrophage function and subsequent impairment of G-CSF activity have been associated with the development of neutrophilia in animal studies.[7] In clinical practice, recombinant CSF is being used to increase the success rates of bone marrow transplantations. The availability of recombinant CSFs and cytokines offers the possibility of several clinical therapies where stimulation or inhibition of the immune response or cell production is desirable.

Chemokines

Chemokines are small protein molecules (70 to 130 amino acids) that are involved in immune and inflammatory cellular responses and function to control the migration of leukocytes to their primary site of action in the immune response.[2] The four distinct classes of chemokines are designated C, CC, CXC, and CX_3C.[8] Currently, 48 distinct chemokine molecules have been identified within the four different classes. The vast majority of these are classified as either CC or CXC chemokines. The CC chemokines attract monocytes, lymphocytes, and eosinophils to sites of chronic inflammation. The CXC chemokines attract neutrophils to sites of acute inflammation.

Chemokines communicate with their target cells by activating G-protein–coupled receptors in the cells. As a result, they are capable of activating different populations of leukocytes based upon the needs of the situation.[8] Most of the G-protein–coupled receptors recognize more than one chemokine, and most chemokines recognize more than one receptor. Binding of a chemokine to a receptor can result in inhibition or activation with the same chemokine acting as an activator at one type of receptor and as an inhibitor at another. Chemokines are implicated in the development of a number of acute and chronic diseases, including atherosclerosis, rheumatoid arthritis, inflammatory bowel disease (Crohn disease, ulcerative colitis), allergic asthma and chronic bronchitis, multiple sclerosis, systemic lupus erythematosus, and HIV infection. They also play a role in the body's immune response against cancer cells through the enhancement of chemokines by activated T cells and other tumor-derived proteins.[9,10]

Understanding Innate and Adaptive Immunity

The innate and adaptive immune systems mediate the body's defenses through an integrated system in which numerous cells and molecules function cooperatively to protect the host against foreign invaders. The innate immune system stimulates adaptive immunity and influences the nature of the adaptive immune responses to make them more effective. Although they use different mechanisms to recognize invading pathogens, both types of immunity use many of the same mechanisms, including destruction of the pathogen by phagocytosis and the complement system, to clear the organism from the body.

Innate Immunity

Innate immunity (also called *natural immunity*) consists of the cellular and biochemical defenses that are normally in place before an encounter with an infectious agent and provide rapid protection against infection. The major effector components of innate immunity include epithelial cells, which block the entry of infectious agents and secrete antimicrobial enzymes, proteins, and peptides; phagocytic neutrophils and macrophages, which engulf and digest microbes; natural killer (NK) cells, which kill intracellular microbes and foreign agents; and the complement system, which amplifies the inflammatory response and uses the membrane attack response to lyse microbes. The cells of the innate immune system also produce chemical messengers that stimulate and influence the adaptive immune response.

The innate immune system uses PRRS, which recognize microbial structures (*e.g.*, sugars, lipid molecules, proteins) that are shared by microbes and are often necessary for their survival, but are not present on human cells. Thus, the innate immune system is able to distinguish between self and nonself, but it does not distinguish between invading agents.

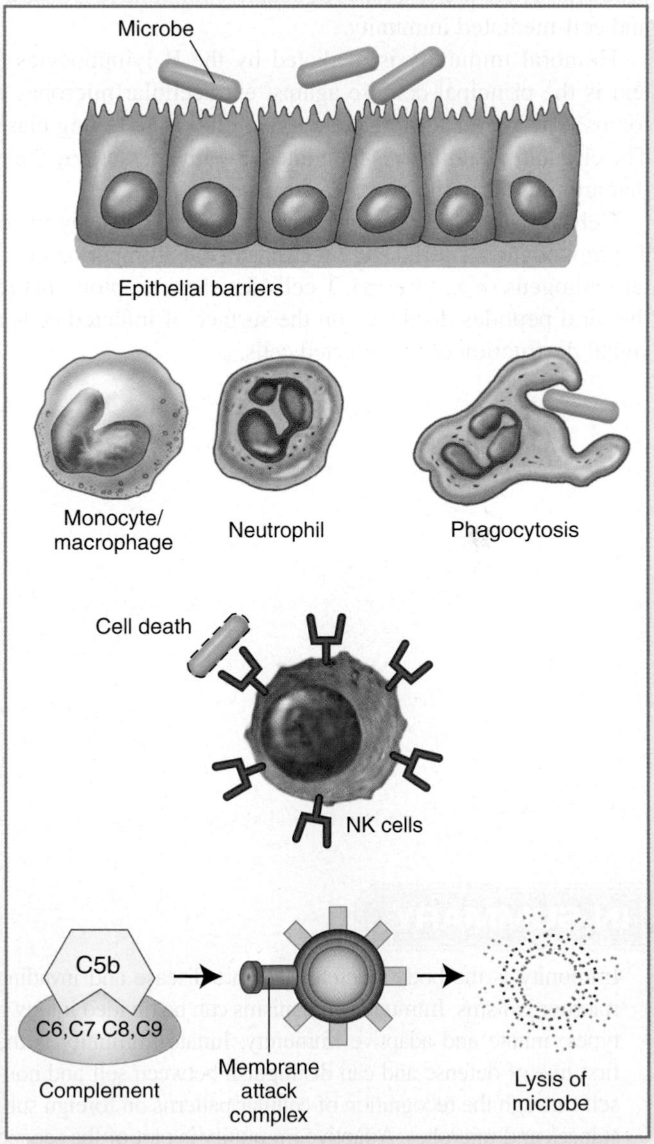

Continued

Understanding Innate and Adaptive Immunity *(Continued)*

Adaptive Immunity

Adaptive immunity (also called *acquired immunity*) refers to immunity that is acquired through previous exposure to infectious and other foreign agents. A defining characteristic of adaptive immunity is the ability not only to distinguish self from nonself but to recognize and destroy specific foreign agents based on their distinct antigenic properties. Therefore, the adaptive immune response is capable of distinguishing between different organisms or substances. The components of the adaptive immune system are the T and B lymphocytes and their products. There are two types of adaptive immune responses, humoral and cell-mediated immunity.

Humoral immunity is mediated by the B lymphocytes (B cells) and is the principal defense against extracellular microbes and their toxins. The B cells differentiate into antibody-secreting plasma cells. The circulating antibodies then interact with and destroy the microbes that are present in the blood or mucosal surfaces.

Cell-mediated, or cellular, immunity is mediated by the cytotoxic T lymphocytes (T cells) and functions in the elimination of intracellular pathogens (*e.g.*, viruses). T cells develop receptors that recognize the viral peptides displayed on the surface of infected cells and then signal destruction of the infected cells.

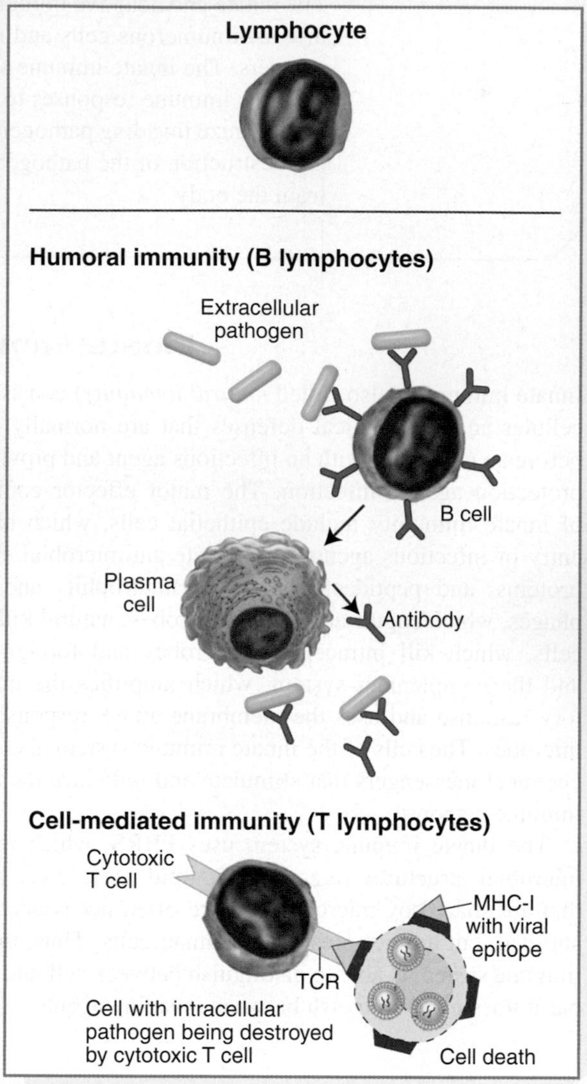

IN SUMMARY

Immunity is the body's defense against disease and invading microorganisms. Immune mechanisms can be divided into two types: innate and adaptive immunity. Innate immunity is the first line of defense and can distinguish between self and nonself through the recognition of cellular patterns on foreign substances and microbes. Adaptive immunity is part of the second line of defense and involves both humoral and cellular mechanisms that respond to cell-specific substances known as antigens. The adaptive immune response is capable of amplifying and sustaining its responses, of distinguishing self from nonself, and finally of memory in that it can recognize the antigen on repeat exposure in order to quickly produce a heightened response on subsequent encounters with the same microorganism. The innate and adaptive immune responses work in concert with one another to ensure that the homeostasis is maintained.

Although cells of both the innate and adaptive immune systems communicate critical information about the invading microbe or pathogen by cell-to-cell contact, many interactions and cellular responses depend on the secretion of chemical mediators in the form of cytokines, chemokines, and CSFs. Cytokines are soluble proteins secreted by cells of both the innate and adaptive immune systems that mediate many of the functions of these cells. Chemokines are cytokines that stimulate the migration and activation of various immune and inflammatory cells. CSFs stimulate the growth and differentiation of bone marrow progenitors of immune cells and play a key role in hematopoiesis.

INNATE IMMUNITY

After completing this section of the chapter, the learner will be able to meet the following objectives:

- Describe the cellular components of the innate immune response and their functions.
- Understand the recognition systems for pathogens in innate immunity.
- Describe the functions of the various cytokines involved in innate immunity.
- Define the role of the complement system in immunity and inflammation.

> **KEY POINTS**
>
> **INNATE IMMUNITY**
>
> - Innate immunity consists of physical, chemical, cellular, and molecular defenses that are ready for activation and mediate rapid, initial protection against infection.
> - The innate immune response relies on the body's ability to distinguish structures present on the surface of pathogens known as PAMPs from structures on human cells.
> - The phagocytic cells of the innate immune response express PRRs that bind with broad patterns shared by groups of microbes but that are not present on mammalian cells. TLRs, a major type of PRR, are expressed on phagocytes and are potent activators of innate immune system cells and molecules.
> - Cytokines and chemokines that are released from activated leukocytes regulate the activities of innate immunity, stimulate the inflammatory process, and initiate the adaptive immune response.

Epithelial Barriers

Physical, mechanical, and biochemical barriers against microbial invasion are found in all common portals of entry into the body, including the skin, respiratory, gastrointestinal, and urogenital tracts. The intact skin is by far the most formidable physical barrier available to infection because of its design. It is comprised of closely packed cells that are organized in multiple layers that are continuously shed. In addition, a protective layer of protein, known as keratin, covers the skin. The skin has simple chemicals that create a nonspecific, salty, acidic environment and antibacterial proteins, such as the enzyme lysozyme, that inhibit the colonization of microorganisms and aid in their destruction. The complexity of the skin becomes evident in cases of contact dermatitis where increased susceptibility to cutaneous infection occurs as the result of abnormalities of the innate immune response including defects in the epithelial layer itself and defects in both signaling and or expression of innate responses.[11]

Sheets of tightly packed epithelial cells line and protect the gastrointestinal, respiratory, and urogenital tracts and physically prevent microorganisms from entering the body. These cells destroy the invading organisms by secreting antimicrobial enzymes, proteins, and peptides. Specialized cells in these linings, such as the goblet cells in the gastrointestinal tract, secrete a viscous material comprised of high molecular weight glycoproteins known as mucin, which when hydrated form *mucus*. The mucins bind to pathogens, thereby trapping them and washing away potential invaders. In the lower respiratory tract, hairlike, mobile structures called cilia protrude through the epithelial cells and move microbes trapped in the mucus up the tracheobronchial tree and toward the throat. The physiologic responses of coughing and sneezing further aid in their removal from the body.

Microorganisms that are trapped by mucus are then subjected to various chemical defenses present throughout the body, including lysozymes and the complement system. Lysozyme is a hydrolytic enzyme found in tears, saliva, and human milk, which is capable of breaking down bacterial cell walls. The complement system is found in the blood and is essential for the activity of antibodies. It is composed of 20 different enzyme precursors, which when activated by antigen–antibody complexes cause bacteria to clump together so that they are more susceptible to phagocytic immune cells (Fig. 11.1). In addition, recent research has shown that complement plays a key role in bridging the innate–adaptive immune responses through the release of C3 complement protein.[12] In the stomach and intestines, death of microbes results from the action of digestive enzymes, acidic conditions, and the secretion of *defensins*, small positively charged peptides that quickly kill both gram-positive and gram-negative microorganisms by disrupting the microbial membrane.

When pathogens are able to breach the epithelial defenses, the innate immune response is initiated by the body's leukocytes, which recognize common surface receptors present on the invading microorganisms.

Cells of Innate Immunity

The cells of the innate immune response recognize microbes that share characteristics common to all of their surface receptors. Once recognized, the innate immune cells initiate a broad spectrum of responses that target the invading microorganisms. The key cells of innate immunity include neutrophils, macrophages, DCs, NK cells, and intraepithelial lymphocytes. The innate immune cells work together to recognize broadly expressed molecules derived from pathogens or apoptotic cells. They have both proinflammatory and anti-inflammatory effects on their targets and play an important role in priming adaptive immune responses.[13,14]

Neutrophils and Macrophages

The leukocytes involved in the innate immune response are derived from myeloid stem cells and subdivided into two distinct groups based upon the presence or absence of specific staining granules in their cytoplasm. Leukocytes that contain granules are classified as granulocytes and include neutrophils, eosinophils,

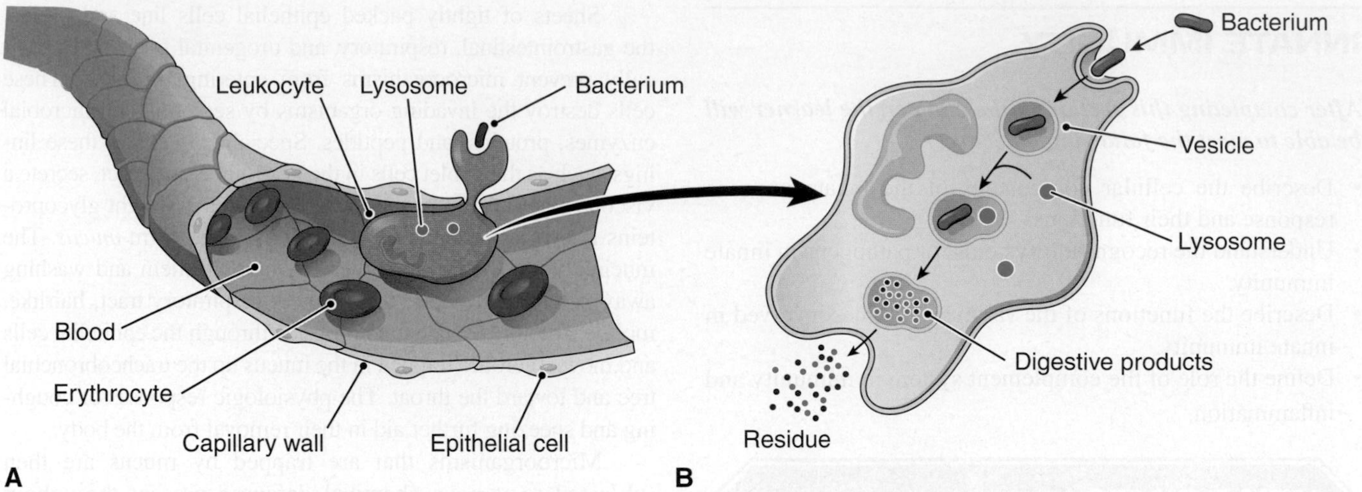

Figure 11.1 • Phagocytosis. **(A)** A phagocytic white blood cell moves through a capillary that is in an infected area and engulfs the bacteria. **(B)** The lysosome digests the bacteria that were in a vesicle. (From Cohen B. J. (2013). *Memmler's the human body in health and disease* (12th ed.). Philadelphia, PA: Lippincott Williams & Wilkins.)

and basophils. Cells that lack granules are classified as agranulocytes and include lymphocytes, monocytes, and macrophages. However, lymphocytes are derived from lymphoid precursors and are not part of the innate immune response.

Neutrophils, which are named for their neutral-staining granules, are the most abundant granulocytes found in the body and make up approximately 55% of all white blood cells. They are also known as polymorphonuclear neutrophils (PMNs). They are phagocytic cells and are capable of amoeboid-like movement, which allows them to migrate throughout the body. They function as early responder cells in innate immunity. They are rare in the tissues and in body cavities and lay predominantly dormant in the blood and bone marrow until they are needed in the immune response.[15] Eosinophils have large coarse granules and normally comprise only 1% to 4% of the total white cell count. In contrast to neutrophils, these cells do not ingest cellular debris but rather antigen–antibody complexes and viruses. They frequently become active in parasitic infections and allergic responses. Basophils make up less than 1% of the total white cell count and contain granules that release a multitude of substances including histamine and proteolytic enzymes. There function is not completely understood, but they are believed to play a role in allergy and parasitic infection as well.

The agranulocytes involved in innate immunity are part of the mononuclear phagocyte system (MPS) and include the monocytes and macrophages. Monocytes are the largest in size of all the white blood cells but make up only 3% to 7% of the total leukocyte count. They are released from the bone marrow into the bloodstream where they migrate into tissues and mature into macrophages and DCs so that they can participate in the inflammatory response and phagocytize foreign substances and cellular debris. Macrophages have a long life span, reside in the tissues, and act as the first phagocyte that invading organisms encounter upon entering the host.[15]

Macrophages are essential for the clearance of bacteria that breach the epithelial barrier in the intestine and other organ systems. They have remarkable plasticity that allows them to alter their phenotype and change their functional characteristics so that they can efficiently respond to environmental signals.[14] This makes them more efficient phagocytic cells than the more abundant neutrophils. Once activated, these cells engulf and digest microbes that attach to their cell membrane. The ability of these phagocytic cells to initiate this response is dependent upon the recognition of microorganism derived surface structures pathogenic surface structures known as PAMPs or PRRs. Phagocytosis of invading microorganisms helps to limit the spread of infection until adaptive immune responses can become fully activated.

In addition to phagocytosis, macrophages and DCs process and present antigens in the initiation of the immune response acting as a major initiator of the adaptive immune response.[1] These cells secrete substances that initiate and coordinate the inflammatory response or activate lymphocytes. Macrophages can also remove antigen–antibody complexes and, under the influence of T cells, destroy malignant host or virus-infected cells.

Dendritic Cells

DCs are specialized, bone marrow–derived leukocytes found in lymphoid tissue and are the bridge between the innate and adaptive immune systems. DCs take their name from the dendrites within the central nervous system because they have surface projections that give them a similar appearance. DCs are relatively rare cells that are found mainly in tissues exposed to external environments such as the respiratory and gastrointestinal systems.[1] They are present primarily in an immature form that is available to directly sense pathogens, capture foreign agents, and transport them to secondary lymphoid tissues.[1] Once activated DCs undergo a complex maturation process in order to function as key antigen-presenting cells (APCs) capable of initiating adaptive immunity.[1] They are responsible for the processing and presentation of antigens to the lymphocytes. DCs, like macrophages, also release several communication molecules that direct the nature of adaptive immune responses.

Natural Killer Cells and Intraepithelial Lymphocytes

NK cells and intraepithelial cells (IELs) are two other cell types involved in the innate immune response. NK cells have the innate ability to spontaneously kill target organisms. Both types of cells rely on the recognition of specific PAMPs on the cell surface of the microorganism.

NK cells are a heterogeneous population of lymphocytes that mediate spontaneous cytotoxicity against infected cells.[16] Because they have the unique ability to target microorganisms without previous exposure, they are considered to be part of the innate immune response despite being of lymphoid origin. They resemble large granular lymphocytes and are capable of killing some types of tumor and/or infected cells without previous exposure to surface antigens. However, they have been shown to play an equally important role in limiting the spread of infection and assisting in the development of adaptive immune responses through the production of cytokines.[16] NK cells can be excitatory or inhibitory, which ensures that only foreign cells are destroyed (see Fig. 11.2).[16] In addition to their role as phagocytes, NK cells assist in T-cell polarization, DC maturation, and innate immune control of viral infection through the secretion of immune modulators and antiviral cytokines. NK cells comprise approximately 10% to 15% of peripheral blood lymphocytes but do not bear T-cell receptors (TCR) or cell surface immunoglobulins (Igs).

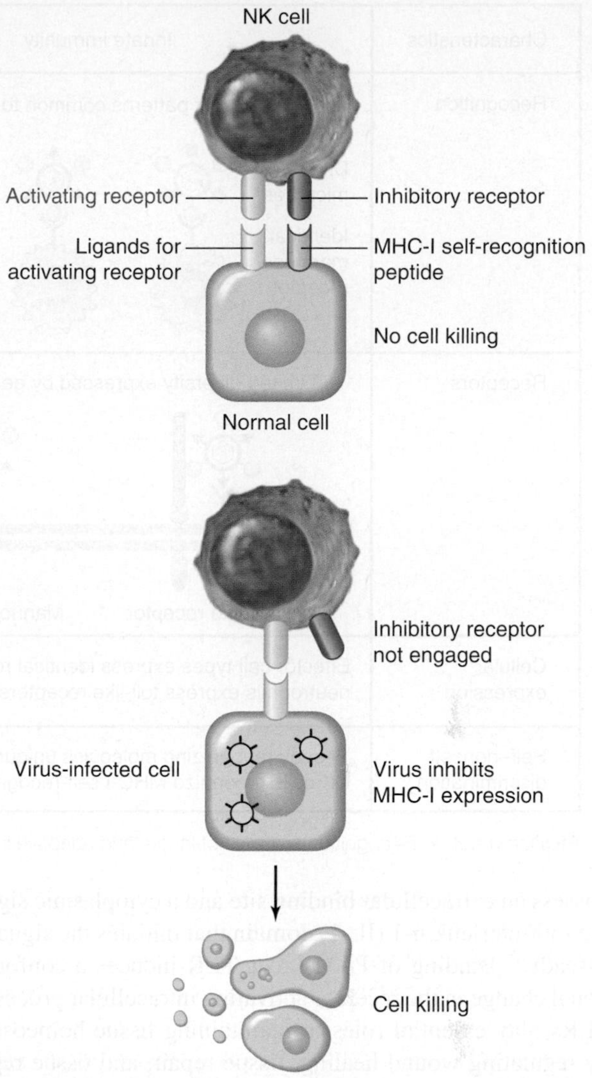

Figure 11.2 • Natural killer (NK) cell receptors. **(A)** NK cells express activating receptors that respond to ligands from virus-infected or injured cells and inhibiting receptors that bind to the class I major histocompatibility complex (MHC-I) self-recognition molecules expressed by normal cells. Normal cells are not killed because inhibitory signals from normal MHC-I molecules override activating signals. **(B)** In virus-infected or tumor cells, increased expression of ligands for activating receptors and reduced expression or alteration of MHC molecules interrupts the inhibitory signals, allowing activation of NK cells and lysis of target cells.

Pathogen Recognition

The innate immune response plays a crucial role in the proinflammatory response to infection and relies upon the ability of host defenses to differentiate self from nonself so that only invading organisms are targeted. The leukocytes involved in this response recognize certain evolutionarily retained patterns present on the surface of pathogens and in response bind to its membrane and destroy the invading organism through the process of phagocytosis (Fig. 11.3).

Pattern Recognition

Invading pathogens contain structures in their cell membranes termed *PAMPs*, which are recognized by the cells of the innate immune system because these cells possess receptors known as *PRRs*. Upon PAMP recognition, PRRs come in contact with the cell surface and/or send intracellular signals to the host that trigger proinflammatory and antimicrobial responses including the synthesis and release of cytokines, chemokines, and cell adhesion molecules.[17] The PAMPs recognized by the host PRRs are made up of a combination of sugars, lipid molecules, proteins, or patterns of modified nucleic acids and are essential to the functioning and infectivity of the pathogen. Because the PAMPs are essential for the functioning of the microorganism, mutation cannot help it avoid immune recognition. The human complement of PRRs is very extensive (approximately 1,000), so the classes of pathogens recognized by them are very diverse.

The ability of the innate immune response to limit microbes early in the infectious process results from the binding of pathogens to the PRRs on leukocytes, which in turn initiates the signaling events that lead to complement activation, phagocytosis, and autophagy. Once initiated, white blood cells, neutrophils, and monocytes migrate from the blood to the tissues, along with other body fluids causing peripheral edema. Blood monocytes mature into macrophages as they traverse the tissues and join the macrophages and DCs already present in the tissues. PRRs present on these cells become activated as well, amplifying the inflammatory response.

Toll-like Receptors

The most studied PRRs associated with the innate immune response are the *TLRs*. TLRs derive their name from the study of the *Drosophila melanogaster* toll protein, which is responsible for the resistance of *Drosophila* to bacterial and fungal infections.[17] Structurally, TLRs are integral glycoproteins that

Characteristics	Innate immunity	Adaptive immunity
Recognition	Molecular patterns common to microbes Different microbes Identical mannose receptor 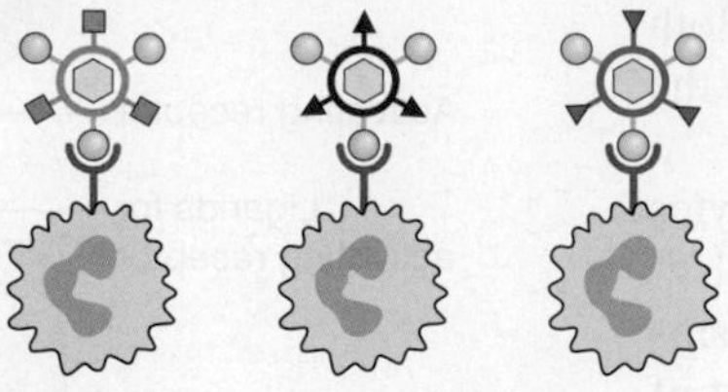	Specific microbial molecules Different microbes Distinct antibodies 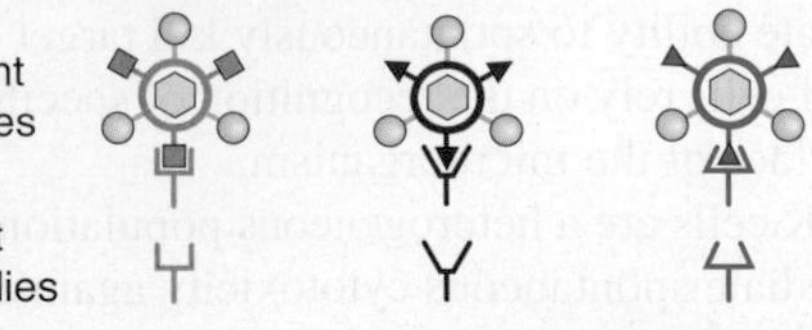
Receptors	Limited diversity expressed by germline genes 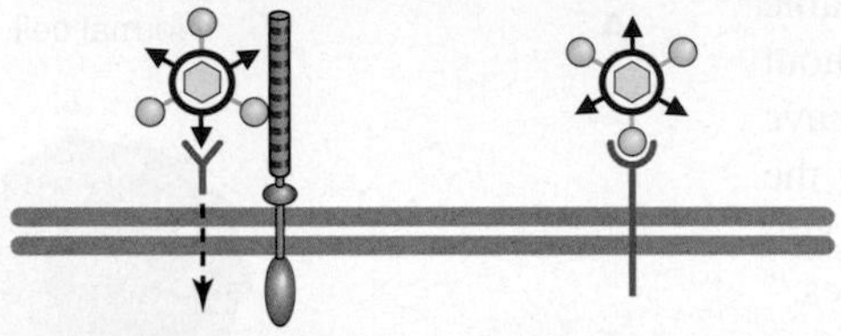 Toll-like receptor Mannose receptor	Great diversity expressed through recombination of somatic genes 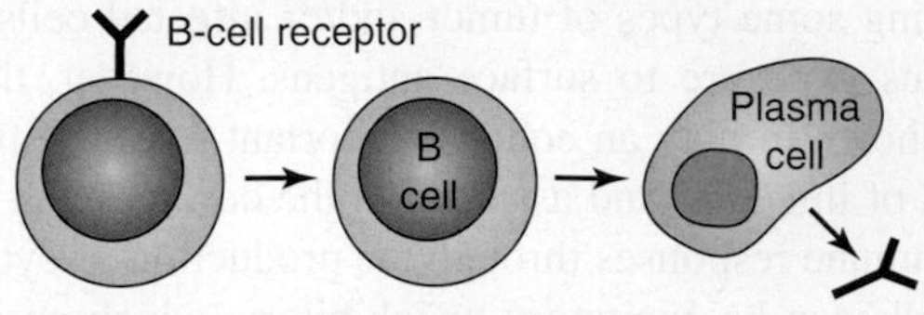 B-cell receptor B cell Plasma cell Antibody
Cellular expression	Effector cell types express identical receptors (*e.g.,* neutrophils express toll-like receptors).	Each clone of lymphocytes expresses unique receptors.
Self–nonself discrimination	Yes, by recognizing molecules unique to pathogen, NK cells recognize MHC-I self-recognizing molecules.	Yes, lymphocytes use MHC-I and -II and foreign peptides (*e.g.,* microbial peptides in recognition).

Figure 11.3 • Recognition systems of innate and adaptive immunity.

possess an extracellular binding site and a cytoplasmic signaling toll/interleukin-1 (IL-1) domain that initiates the signaling cascade.[17] Binding of PAMP to a TLR induces a conformational change in the receptor activating intracellular processes. TLRs play essential roles in maintaining tissue homeostasis by regulating wound healing, tissue repair, and tissue regeneration. TLRs can be found in most of the bone marrow cells including the macrophages, DCs, neutrophils, T cells, B cells, and non-bone marrow cells including epithelial and fibrocytes. Ten different TLRs have been identified in humans, and they each recognize distinct PAMPs derived from various microorganisms including bacteria, viruses, fungi, and protozoa.[18]

Soluble Mediators of Innate Immunity

Although cells of the innate immune system communicate critical information about invading microorganisms and self–nonself recognition through cell-to-cell contact, soluble mediators are also essential for many other aspects of the innate immune response. Development of innate immune response is very much dependent upon the secretion of soluble molecules such as opsonins, cytokines, and acute-phase proteins.

Opsonins

Opsonins are molecules that coat negatively charged particles on cell membranes and as a result enhance the recognition and binding of phagocytic cells to microorganisms. The process by which the cellular particles on microbes are coated is called opsonization. Once the opsonin binds to the microbe, it is able to activate the phagocyte after attachment to a PRR on the phagocytic cell. There are several opsonins important in innate immunity and the acute inflammatory process including acute-phase proteins, lectins, and complement. Components of the adaptive immune response can also act as opsonins. For example, when the humoral response is activated, IgG and IgM antibodies can coat cellular particles on pathogens and bind to Fc receptors on neutrophils and macrophages, enhancing the phagocytic function of innate cells.

Inflammatory Cytokines

Cytokines are low molecular weight proteins that serve as soluble chemical messengers and that mediate the interaction between immune and tissue cells. They are part of an integrated signaling network with extensive functions in both the innate (nonspecific) and adaptive immune defenses. The cytokines involved in innate immunity include TNF-α and lymphotoxin; interferons (IFN-γ, IFN-α, IFN-β); the interleukins IL-1, IL-6, and IL-12; and chemokines (see Table 11.2). These substances modulate innate immunity by stimulating the development of cells involved in both innate and adaptive immunity, producing chemotaxis within leukocytes, and inhibiting viral replication. Once an innate immune phagocyte is activated by PRR–PAMP binding with a pathogen, cytokines are released into the surrounding tissues where they exert their effect. If large numbers of cells are activated, then cytokines may be able to stimulate inflammatory processes in tissues far from the initial site of infection. Under normal circumstances, the duration of activity of cytokines is relatively short so that a prolonged immune response does not occur.

TNF-α and lymphotoxins are cytokines that are structurally related and that have similar cytotoxic activities.[19] The two cytokines differ in that TNF-α can be secreted by a variety of immune cells, but the lymphotoxins are predominantly secreted by activated lymphocytes and NK cells. These cytokines regulate development of the lymphoid tissues and the inflammatory process by enhancing adhesion of immune cells to pathogens and stimulating the release of other cytokines/chemokines.[19] The IFNs are another family of cytokines that are critically involved in initiating and enhancing the cellular immune response to viral infection of host cells. In addition, they play a key role in amplifying the presentation of antigens to specific T cells forming the chemical bridge between the innate and adaptive immune response.[19] Type I interferons (IFN-α and IFN-β) are secreted by virus-infected cells, whereas type II, immune or gamma interferons (IFN-γ), are mainly secreted by T cells, NK cells, and macrophages.[19] IFNs activate macrophages, induce B cells to switch Ig type, alter T-helper response, inhibit cell growth, promote apoptosis, and induce an antiviral state in uninfected cells. Finally, ILs help to regulate the immune response by increasing the expression of adhesion molecules on endothelial cells, stimulating migration of leukocytes into infected tissues, and stimulating the production of antibodies by the cells of the adaptive immune response.

Acute-Phase Proteins

Two acute-phase proteins that are involved in the defense against infections are the mannose-binding ligand (MBL) and C-reactive protein (CRP). MBL and CRP are produced in the liver and released in response to tissue injury and inflammation.[20,21] MBL binds specifically to mannose sugar residues, and CRP binds to both phospholipids and sugars that are found on the surface of microbes. These substances enhance the binding of phagocytic cells to suboptimally opsonized invading microorganisms. They also act as activators of the alternative complement pathway.

The Complement System

The complement system is a powerful effector mechanism of both innate and adaptive immunity that allows the body to localize infection and destroy invading microorganisms. The complement system is composed of group of proteins found in the circulation and in various extracellular fluids. The proteins of the complement system normally circulate as inactive precursors. When activated by components of the immune response, a series of proteolytic and protein–protein interactions is initiated that ultimately culminates in opsonization of invading pathogens, migration of leukocytes to the site of invasion, initiation of a localized inflammatory reaction, and ultimately lysis of the pathogen.[22] The proteins of the complement system are mainly proteolytic enzymes and make up approximately 10% to 15% of the plasma proteins. For a complement reaction to occur, the complement components must be activated in the proper sequence. Inhibitor proteins and the instability of the activated complement proteins at each step of the process prevent uncontrolled activation of the complement system.

There are three parallel but independent activation pathways of the complement system during the innate immune response: the classical, the lectin, and the alternative pathways. The reactions of the complement systems can be divided into three phases:

1. Initiation or activation
2. Amplification of inflammation
3. Late-stage membrane attack response

The three pathways differ in the proteins used in the early stage of activation, but all ultimately converge on the key complement protein C3, which is essential for the amplification stage. Activated C3 then activates all subsequent complement molecules (C5 through C9) resulting in the ultimate lysis of cells.

The classic pathway is initiated by an antigen–antibody complex (either IgG or IgM mediated), which causes a specific reactive site on the antibody to be "uncovered" so that it can bind directly to the C1 molecule in the complement system.[23] Once C1 is activated, a "cascade" of sequential reactions is set in motion. Initially, a small amount of enzyme is produced, but with activation of successive complement proteins successively increasing, concentrations of proteolytic enzymes are produced. This process is known as *amplification*. In the lectin or alternative complement pathway, inactive circulating complement proteins are activated when they are exposed to microbial surface polysaccharides, MBL, CRP, and other soluble mediators that are integral to innate immunity.[24] Like the classic pathway, the lectin and alternative pathways create a series of enzymatic reactions that cleave successive complement proteins in the pathway.

During the activation phase of the complement cascade, cleavage of C3 produces C3a and C3b. C3b is a key opsonin that coats bacteria and allows them to be phagocytized after binding to complement receptor on leukocytes. The presence of C3a triggers the migration of neutrophils into the tissues to enhance the inflammatory response. Production of C3a, C4a, and C5a also leads to activation of mast cells and basophils causing them to release histamine, heparin, and other substances. These mediators of the inflammatory response increase tissue blood flow and increase localized capillary permeability allowing leakage of fluids and protein into the area. In addition, they stimulate changes in the endothelial cells in order to stimulate chemotaxis of neutrophils and macrophages to the site of inflammation.

During the late-phase membrane attack response of the complement cascade, cleavage of C5 triggers the assembly of a membrane attack complex from the C5 to C9 proteins. The resulting complex creates a tubelike structure, which penetrates the microbial cell membrane allowing the passage of ions, small molecules, and water into the cell, causing the cell to ultimately burst. The multiple and complementary functions of the complement system make it an integral component of innate immunity and inflammation. It also serves as an essential bridge between the innate and humoral responses. Pathophysiologic manifestations associated with deficiencies of complement range from increased susceptibility to infection to inflammatory tissue and autoimmune disorders that are the result of impaired activated complement clearance.

IN SUMMARY

The innate immune system is a complex system that works in an organized, rapid, yet nonspecific fashion as the body's first line of defense against invasion. It is comprised of the epithelial cells of the skin and mucus membranes; phagocytic cells such as the neutrophils, macrophages, and NK cells; and a series of plasma proteins including cytokines, chemokines, and the proteins of the complement system. These defenses exist before the body encounters an invading microorganism and are activated independent of the adaptive humoral response. The epithelial cells of the skin and mucous membranes block the entry of infectious agents and secrete antimicrobial enzymes, proteins, and peptides in an attempt to prevent microorganisms from invading the internal environment.

The phagocytes of the innate immune response engulf and digest infectious agents. They use PRRs, which are present on their membranes to recognize and bind broad patterns of molecules (PAMPs) shared by microbes and that are essential for their survival. TLRs are the most studied of all PRRs and are expressed on many of the cells of the innate immune system. TLRs are involved in responses to widely divergent types of molecules that are commonly expressed by microbial but not mammalian cell types.

Development of a healthy innate immune response is dependent not only upon the coordinated activity of the leukocytes but on the secretion of chemical mediators and soluble molecules, such as opsonins, cytokines, acute-phase proteins, and complement proteins. Opsonins bind to and tag microorganisms for more efficient recognition by phagocytes. Activated leukocytes release cytokines that stimulate the migration of leukocytes to the site of inflammation, stimulate production of acute-phase proteins, and enhance phagocytosis.

The complement system is a primary effector system that functions as part of both the innate and adaptive immune responses. It is comprised of a group of proteins that are activated by three distinct but convergent pathways: the classical, the lecithin, and the alternative pathways. The primary function of the complement system is the promotion of inflammation and destruction of the microbes.

ADAPTIVE IMMUNITY

After completing this section of the chapter, the learner will be able to meet the following objectives:

- Characterize the significance and function of major histocompatibility complex (MHC) molecules.
- Compare and contrast the development and function of the T and B lymphocytes.
- Differentiate between the processes of cellular and humoral immunity.
- Describe the function of the five classes of immunoglobulins.
- Describe the function of cytokines involved in the adaptive immune response.

The adaptive immune system is the final line of defense against infection and is activated once the innate immune response initiates the inflammatory process. In contrast to innate immunity, the adaptive immune response is capable of targeting specific cells or organisms that it recognizes as foreign to the body through activation of various lymphocytes and their products, including antibodies. The lymphocytes involved in adaptive immunity have the unique ability to remember specific pathogen and mount a heightened immune response during repeat exposures. Each exposure results in a more rapid and aggressive response. Substances present on the surface of pathogens or other foreign substances that elicit adaptive immune responses are called *antigens*. Adaptive immunity involves two distinct but interconnected mechanisms: humoral and cell-mediated responses. *Humoral immunity* is mediated by *B-lymphocyte* activation and subsequent antibody production. It is the primary defense against extracellular microbes and toxins. In contrast, *cell-mediated immunity* involves the activation of specific *T lymphocytes* (T-helper and T-cytotoxic lymphocytes), which are responsible for the body's defense against intracellular microbes such as viruses.

KEY POINTS

ADAPTIVE IMMUNITY

- The adaptive immune response involves a complex series of interactions between components of the immune system and the antigens of a foreign pathogen. It is able to distinguish between self and nonself, recognize and specifically react to large numbers of different microbes and pathogens, and remember the specific agents.
- Humoral immunity consists of protection provided by the B-lymphocyte–derived plasma cells, which produce antibodies that travel in the blood and interact with circulating and cell surface antigens.
- Cell-mediated immunity provides protection through cytotoxic T lymphocytes, which protect against virus-infected or cancer cells.

Antigens

Antigens, or *immunogens*, are substances or molecules that are foreign to the body but when introduced trigger the production of antibodies by B lymphocytes leading to the ultimate destruction of the invader. Antigens are usually large macromolecules (greater than 10,000 Da) such as proteins, polysaccharides, lipids, and free nucleic acids. Antigens are recognized by specific receptors present on the surface of lymphocytes and by the *antibodies* or *immunoglobulins* secreted in response to the presence of the antigen. Antigens can take the form of any foreign substance including bacteria, fungi, viruses, protozoa, parasites, and nonmicrobial agents such as plant pollens, insect venom, and transplanted organs.

Understanding The Complement System

The complement system provides one of the major effector mechanisms of both humoral and innate immunity. The system consists of a group of proteins (complement proteins C1 through C9) that are normally present in the plasma in an inactive form. Activation of the complement system is a highly regulated process, involving the sequential breakdown of the complement proteins to generate a cascade of cleavage products capable of proteolytic enzyme activity. This allows for tremendous amplification because each enzyme molecule activated by one step can generate multiple activated enzyme molecules at the next step. Complement activation is inhibited by proteins that are present on normal host cells; thus, its actions are limited to microbes and other antigens that lack these inhibitory proteins.

The reactions of the complement system can be divided into three phases: (1) the initial activation phase, (2) the early-step inflammatory responses, and (3) the late-step membrane attack responses.

Initial Activation Phase

There are three pathways for recognizing microbes and activating the complement system: (1) the alternative pathway, which is activated on microbial cell surfaces in the absence of antibody and is a component of innate immunity; (2) the classical pathway, which is activated by certain types of antibodies bound to antigen and is part of humoral immunity; and (3) the lectin pathway, which is activated by a plasma lectin that binds to mannose on microbes and activates the classical system pathway in the absence of antibody.

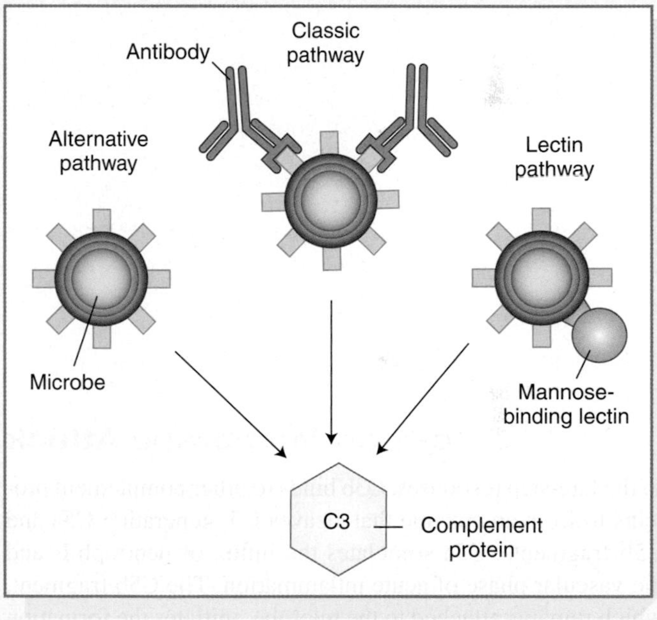

Continued

Understanding The Complement System *(Continued)*

Early-Step Inflammatory Responses

The central component of complement for all three pathways is the activation of the complement protein C3 and its enzymatic cleavage into a larger C3b fragment and a smaller C3a fragment. The smaller 3a fragment stimulates inflammation by acting as a chemoattractant for neutrophils. The larger 3b fragment becomes attached to the microbe and acts as an opsonin for phagocytosis. It also acts as an enzyme to cleave C5 into two components: a C5a fragment, which produces vasodilation and increases vascular permeability, and a C5b fragment, which leads to the late-step membrane attack responses.

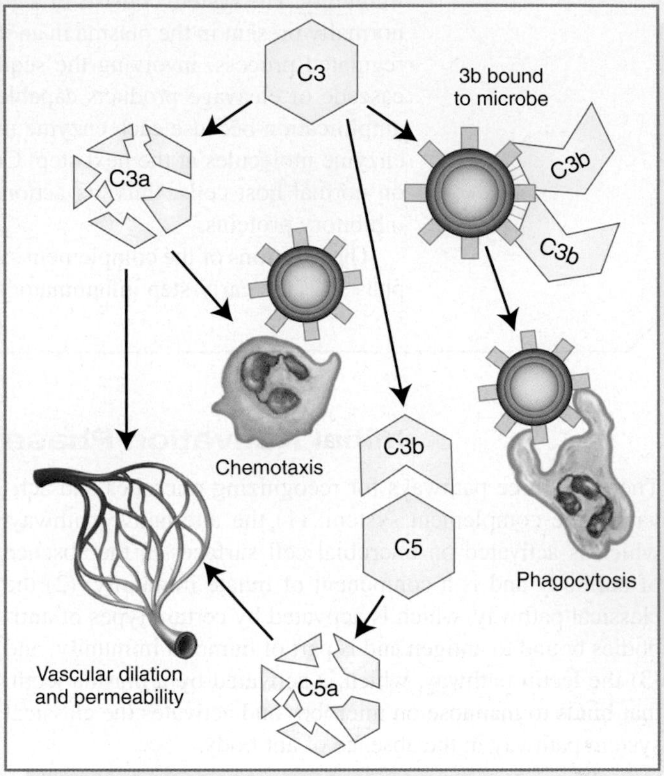

Late-Step Membrane Attack

In the late-step responses, C3b binds to other complement proteins to form an enzyme that cleaves C5, generating C5a and C5b fragments. C5a stimulates the influx of neutrophils and the vascular phase of acute inflammation. The C5b fragment, which remains attached to the microbe, initiates the formation of a complex of complement proteins C6, C7, C8, and C9 into a membrane attack complex protein, or pore, that allows fluids and ions to enter and cause cell lysis.

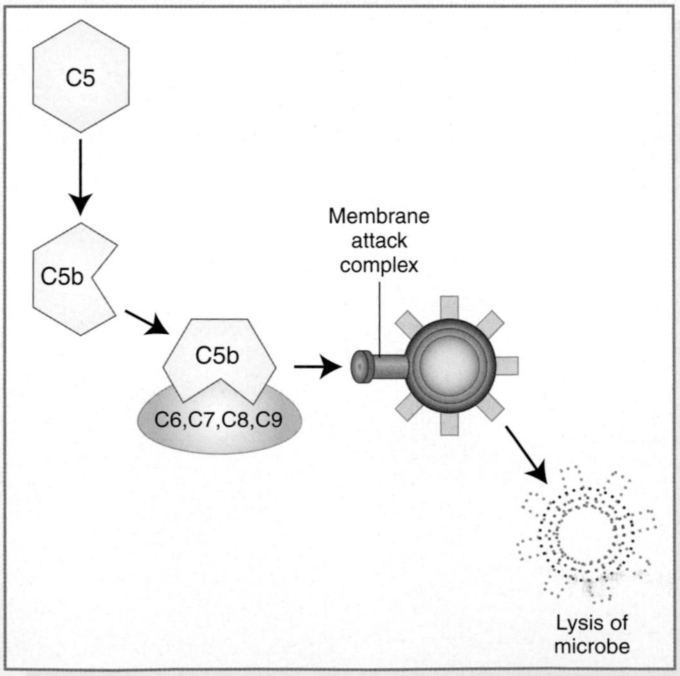

Antigens possess immunologically active sites called *antigenic determinants*, or epitopes. These are smaller, discrete components of the antigen that have a unique molecular shape, which can be recognized by and bound to a specific immunoglobulin (Ig) receptor found on the surface of the lymphocyte or by an antigen-binding site of a secreted antibody (Fig. 11.4). It is not unusual for a single antigen to possess several antigenic determinants and, therefore, be capable of stimulating several different T and B lymphocytes. For example, different proteins that comprise the influenza virus may function as unique antigens (A, B, C, H, and N antigens), each of which contains several antigenic determinants.[25] Hundreds of antigenic determinants are found on structures such as the bacterial cell wall.

Low molecular weight molecules (less than 10,000 Da) may contain antigenic determinants but alone are usually unable to stimulate an immune response. These molecules are known as haptens. When they combine with an immunogenic carrier (usually a protein), they are able to function as antigens. Many haptens exist in nature and frequently create problems for humans. Urushiol is a toxin found in the oils on poison ivy that is responsible for initiating an allergic reaction.[26] An allergic response to the antibiotic penicillin is an example of a medically important reaction because of hapten–carrier complexes. The penicillin molecule is very small (350 Da) and usually nonantigenic. However, in susceptible people, it can complex with carrier proteins in the body, which are then recognized as "foreign" and capable of initiating an antigen–antibody reaction.

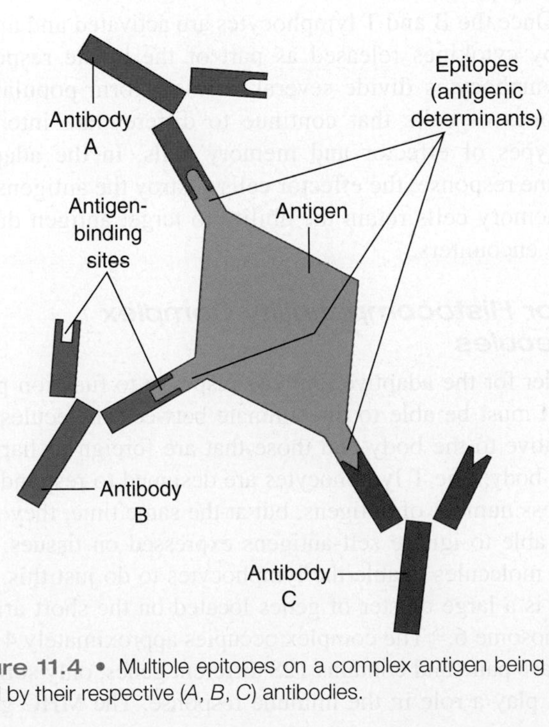

Figure 11.4 • Multiple epitopes on a complex antigen being recognized by their respective (*A*, *B*, *C*) antibodies.

Cells of Adaptive Immunity

The principal cells of the adaptive immune system are the lymphocytes, APCs, and effector cells.

Lymphocytes

Lymphocytes make up approximately 36% of the total white cell count and are the primary cells of the adaptive immune response. They arise from the lymphoid stem cell line in the bone marrow and differentiate into two distinct but interrelated cell types: B lymphocytes and T lymphocytes. B lymphocytes are responsible for forming the antibodies that provide humoral immunity, whereas T lymphocytes provide cell-mediated immunity. T and B lymphocytes are unique in that they are the only cells in the body capable of recognizing organism-specific antigens present on the surfaces of microbial cells and other pathogens. As a result, adaptive immune processes are organism specific and possess the capacity for memory.

The recognition of specific surface antigens by lymphocytes is made possible because of the presence of specific receptors or antibodies on the surface of B and T lymphocytes. Scientists have been able to identify these specific proteins and correlate them with a specific cellular function. This has led to the development of a classification system for these surface molecules known as the "cluster of differentiation" (CD). The nomenclature for the surface proteins uses the letters "CD" followed by a number that specifies the surface proteins that define the cell type or stage of cell differentiation and are recognized by a cluster or group of antibodies. The utilization of this nomenclature has spread to other immune cells and cytokines all of which contribute to the acquired immune response.

Leukocytes involved in the innate immune response, such as macrophages and DCs, also play a key role in adaptive immunity because they function as APCs. They are capable of processing complex antigens into epitopes, which are then displayed on their cell membranes in order to activate the appropriate lymphocytes. Functionally, there are two types of immune cells: regulatory cells and effector cells. The *regulatory cells* assist in orchestrating and controlling the immune response, whereas effector cells carry out the elimination of the antigen (microbial, nonmicrobial, or toxin). In the body, helper T lymphocytes activate other lymphocytes and phagocytes, whereas regulatory T cells (T_{REGS}) keep these cells in check so that an exaggerated immune response does not occur. Cytotoxic T lymphocytes, macrophages, and other leukocytes function as effector cells in different immune responses.

Although T and B lymphocytes are generated from lymphoid stem cells in the bone marrow, they do not stay there to mature. Undifferentiated, immature lymphocytes migrate to lymphoid tissues, where they develop into distinct types of mature lymphocytes (Fig. 11.5). The T lymphocytes first migrate to the thymus gland where they divide

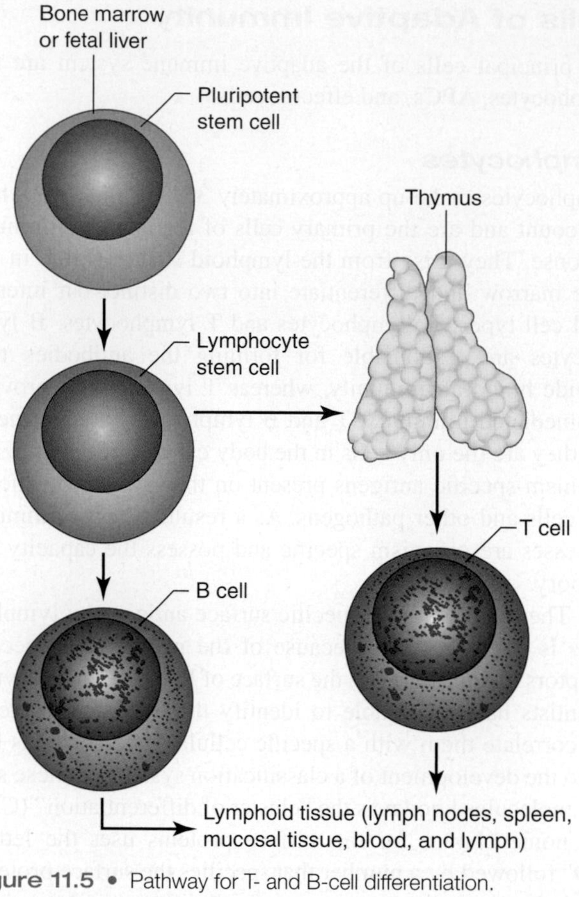

Figure 11.5 • Pathway for T- and B-cell differentiation.

rapidly and develop extensive diversity in their ability to react against different antigens.[27] Each T lymphocyte develops specificity against a specific antigen. Once this differentiation occurs, the lymphocytes leave the thymus gland and migrate via the bloodstream to peripheral lymphoid tissue. At this time, they have been preprogrammed not to attack the body's own tissues. Unfortunately, in many autoimmune diseases it is believed that this process goes astray. In contrast, the *B lymphocytes* mature primarily in the bone marrow and are essential for humoral, or *antibody-mediated, immunity*. Unlike the T lymphocytes, where the entire cell is involved in the immune response, B lymphocytes secrete antibodies, which then act as the reactive agent in the immune process. Therefore, the lymphocytes are distinguished by their function and response to antigens, their cell membrane molecules and receptors, their types of secreted proteins, and their tissue location. High concentrations of mature lymphocytes are found in the lymph tissue throughout the body including the lymph nodes, spleen, skin, and mucosal tissues.

T and B lymphocytes possess all of the processes necessary for the adaptive immune response—specificity, diversity, memory, and self–nonself recognition. When antigens come in contact with the lymphocytes in the lymphoid tissues of the body, specific T cells become activated and specific B cells are stimulated to produce antibodies. Once the first encounter occurs, these cells can exactly recognize a particular microorganism or foreign molecule because each lymphocyte is capable of targeting a specific antigen and differentiating the invader from self or from other substances that may be similar to it. Cell-mediated and humoral immunity is capable of responding to millions of antigens each day because there is an enormous variety of lymphocytes that have been programmed and selected during cellular development. Once the invading substance or organism has been removed from the body, the lymphocytes "remember" the presenting antigen and can respond rapidly during the next encounter. These lymphocytes are called "memory" T and B lymphocytes. They remain in the body for a longer period of time than their predecessors and as a result can respond more rapidly on repeat exposure. The immune system usually can respond to commonly encountered microorganisms so efficiently that we are unaware of the response.

B- and T-lymphocyte activation is triggered by antigen presentation to unique surface receptors (Fig. 11.6). The antigen receptor present on the B lymphocyte consists of membrane-bound Ig molecules that can bind a specific epitope. However, in order for B lymphocytes to produce antibodies, they require the help of specific T lymphocytes, called *helper T cells*. Although the B lymphocytes bind to one determinant (or hapten) on an antigen molecule, the antigen-specific helper T cell recognizes and binds to another determinant known as the "carrier." The carrier is an APC, which has previously picked up the specified antigen. This interaction (B cell–T cell–APC) is restricted by the presence of self-recognition proteins known as a MHC molecules. This allows the lymphocyte to differentiate between self and foreign peptides.

Once the B and T lymphocytes are activated and amplified by cytokines released as part of the innate response, the lymphocytes divide several times to form populations or clones of cells that continue to differentiate into several types of effector and memory cells. In the adaptive immune response, the effector cells destroy the antigens and the memory cells retain the ability to target antigen during future encounters.

Major Histocompatibility Complex Molecules

In order for the adaptive immune response to function properly, it must be able to discriminate between molecules that are native to the body and those that are foreign or harmful to the body. The T lymphocytes are designed to respond to a limitless number of antigens, but at the same time, they need to be able to ignore self-antigens expressed on tissues. The MHC molecules enable the lymphocytes to do just this. The MHC is a large cluster of genes located on the short arm of chromosome 6.[28] The complex occupies approximately 4 million base pairs and contains 128 different genes, only some of which play a role in the immune response. The MHC genes

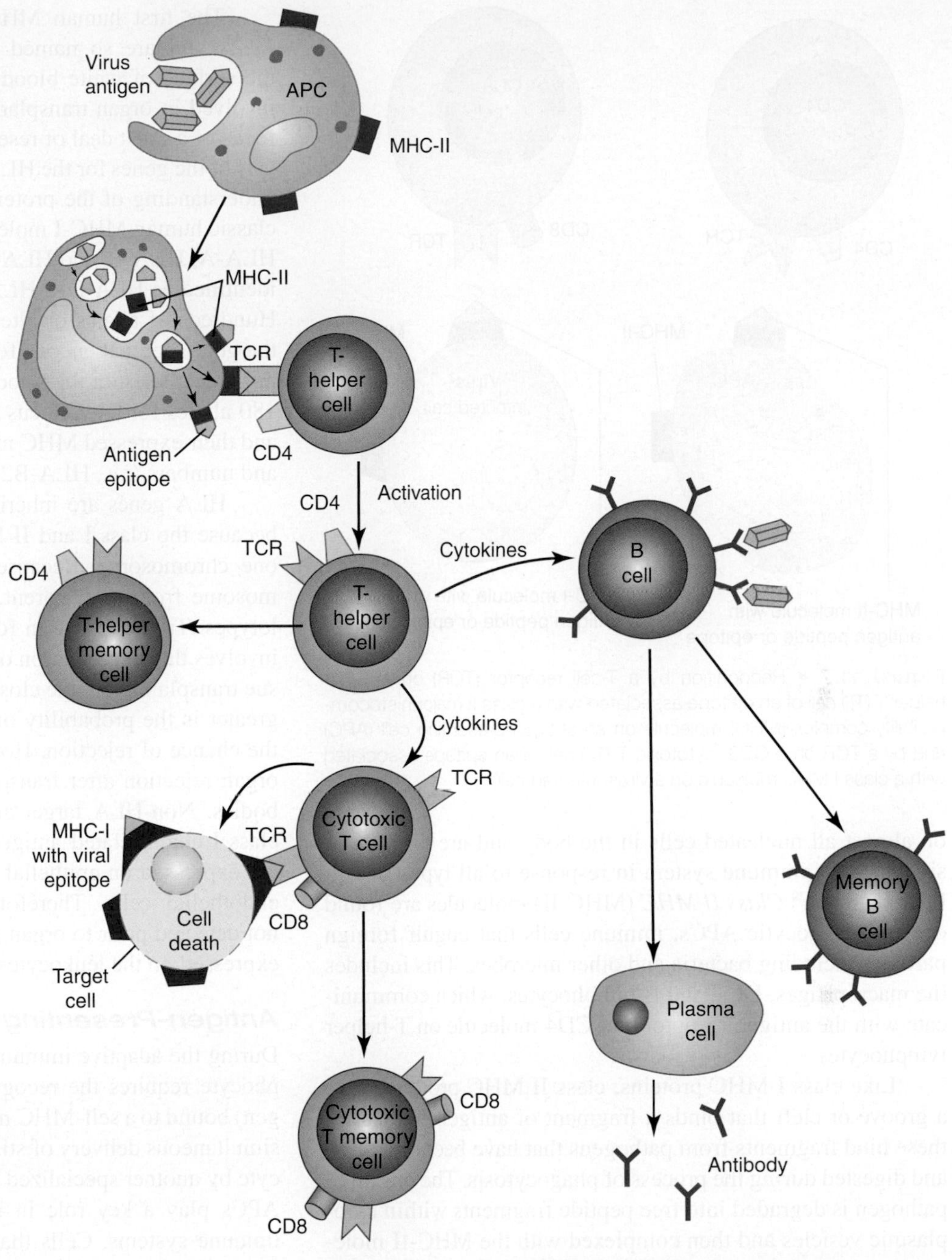

Figure 11.6 • Pathway for immune cell participation in an immune response. (APC, antigen-presenting cell; MHC, major histocompatibility complex; TCR, T-cell receptor.)

are divided in three classes: I, II, and III, based upon their underlying function (Fig. 11.7).

The class I and II MHC genes are responsible for encoding human leukocyte antigens (HLAs), which are proteins found on cell surfaces and define the person's tissue type. These molecules are present on the cell surface glycoproteins that form the basis for human tissue typing. Each person has a unique collection of MHC proteins that affect immune responses as well as susceptibility to a number of diseases. Because of the number of MHC genes and the possibility of several alleles for each gene, it is almost impossible for any two people to have an identical MHC profile.

The class I and II MHC genes also encode proteins that play an important role in antigen presentation. Protein fragments from inside the cell are displayed by MHC complex on the cell surface, allowing the immune system to differentiate between the body's own tissues and foreign substances. Cells, which present unfamiliar peptide fragments on the cell surface, are attacked and destroyed by the B and T lymphocytes. Class III MHC genes encode for many of the components of the complement system and play an important role in the innate immune process.

The MHC-I complexes are cell surface glycoproteins that contain a groove, which is able to accommodate a peptide fragment. MHC-I molecules interact with T-cytotoxic cells and activate them when presented with a foreign antigen peptide. MHC-I complexes may also present degraded viral protein fragments from infected cells. They are found

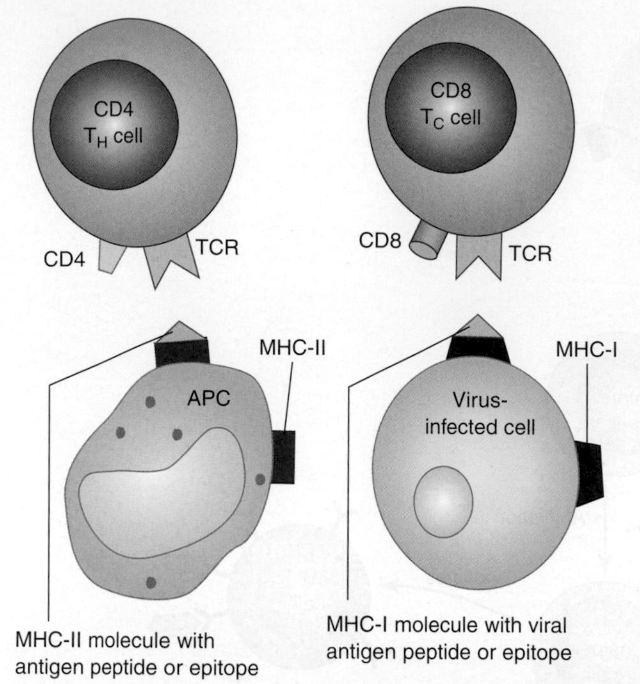

Figure 11.7 • Recognition by a T-cell receptor (TCR) on a $CD4^+$ helper T (T_H) cell of an epitope associated with a class II major histocompatibility complex (MHC) molecule on an antigen-presenting cell (APC) and by a TCR on a $CD8^+$ cytotoxic T (T_C) cell of an epitope associated with a class I MHC molecule on a virus-infected cell.

on almost all nucleated cells in the body and are capable of signaling the immune system in response to all types of cellular changes.[29] *Class II MHC* (MHC-II) molecules are found only on phagocytic APCs, immune cells that engulf foreign particles including bacteria and other microbes. This includes the macrophages, DCs, and B lymphocytes, which communicate with the antigen receptor and CD4 molecule on T-helper lymphocytes.

Like class I MHC proteins, class II MHC proteins have a groove or cleft that binds a fragment of antigen. However, these bind fragments from pathogens that have been engulfed and digested during the process of phagocytosis. The engulfed pathogen is degraded into free peptide fragments within cytoplasmic vesicles and then complexed with the MHC-II molecules on the surface of the cells. T-helper cells recognize these complexes on the surface of APCs and become activated.

The first human MHC proteins discovered are called *HLAs* and are so named because they were identified on the surface of white blood cells. HLAs are the major target involved in organ transplant rejection and as a result are the focus of a great deal of research in immunology. Recent analysis of the genes for the HLA molecules has allowed for better understanding of the proteins involved in this response. The classic human MHC-I molecules are divided into types called HLA-A, HLA-B, and HLA-C, and the MHC-II molecules are identified as HLA-DR, HLA-DP, and HLA-DQ (Table 11.3). Hundreds of alleles or alternative genes can occupy each of the gene loci that encode for HLA molecules. More than 350 possible alleles for the A locus, 650 alleles for the B locus, and 180 alleles for the C locus have been identified. These genes and their expressed MHC molecules are designated by a letter and numbers (*i.e.*, HLA-B27).

HLA genes are inherited as a unit, called a *haplotype*, because the class I and II MHC genes are closely linked on one chromosome. Because each person inherits one chromosome from each parent, each person has two HLA haplotypes. Tissue typing in forensics and organ transplantation involves the identification of these haplotypes. In organ or tissue transplantation, the closer the matching of HLA types, the greater is the probability of identical antigens and the lower the chance of rejection. However, not all people that develop organ rejection after transplantation develop anti-HLA antibodies. Non-HLA target antigens exist including the MHC class I chain-related antigens A (MICA).[30,31] These antigens are expressed on epithelial cells, monocytes, fibroblasts, and endothelial cells. Therefore, donor-specific antibodies are not detected prior to organ tissue typing because they are not expressed on the leukocytes tested.[30]

Antigen-Presenting Cells

During the adaptive immune response, activation of a T lymphocyte requires the recognition of a foreign peptide (antigen) bound to a self-MHC molecule. This process requires the simultaneous delivery of stimulatory signals to the T lymphocyte by another specialized cell known as an *APC*. Therefore, APCs play a key role in bridging the innate and adaptive immune systems. Cells that function as APCs must be able to express both classes of MHC molecules and include the DCs, monocytes, macrophages, and B lymphocytes. Under

TABLE 11.3 PROPERTIES OF CLASS I AND II MHC MOLECULES

PROPERTIES	HLA ANTIGENS	DISTRIBUTION	FUNCTIONS
Class I MHC	HLA-A, HLA-B, HLA-C	Virtually all nucleated cells	Present processed antigen to cytotoxic $CD8^+$ T cells; restrict cytolysis to virus-infected cells, tumor cells, and transplanted cells
Class II MHC	HLA-DR, HLA-DP, HLA-DQ	Immune cells, antigen-presenting cells, B cells, and macrophages	Present processed antigenic fragments to $CD4^+$ T cells; necessary for effective interaction among immune cells

HLA, human leukocyte antigen; MHC, major histocompatibility complex.

certain conditions, endothelial cells are also able to function as APCs. APCs have been shown to play a key role in the development of autoimmune diseases and atherosclerosis. Activated T lymphocytes appear to promote the formation of atherosclerosis, and in experimental models, APC and T-cell deficiency have been associated with up to an 80% reduction in plaque formation.[32]

Macrophages function as the principal APC. They are key cells of the mononuclear phagocytic system and engulf and digest microbes and other foreign substances that gain access to the body. Because macrophages arise from monocytes in the blood, they can move freely throughout the body to the appropriate site of action. Tissue macrophages are scattered in connective tissue or clustered in organs such as the lung (*i.e.*, alveolar macrophages), liver (*i.e.*, Kupffer cells), spleen, lymph nodes, peritoneum, central nervous system (*i.e.*, microglial cells), and other areas. Macrophages are activated during the innate immune response where they engulf and break down complex antigens into peptide fragments. These fragments can then be associated with MHC-II molecules for presentation to cells of the "cell-mediated" response so that self–nonself recognition and activation of the immune response can occur.

DCs are also responsible for presenting processed antigen to activated T lymphocytes. The starlike structure of the DCs provides an extensive surface area rich in MHC-II molecules important for initiation of adaptive immunity. DCs are found in tissues where antigen enters the body and in the peripheral lymphoid tissues. Both DCs and macrophages are capable of "specialization" depending upon their location in the body. For example, Langerhans cells are specialized DCs in the skin, whereas follicular DCs are found in the lymph nodes. Langerhans cells transport antigens found on the skin to nearby lymph nodes for destruction. They are also involved in the development of cell-mediated immune reactions such as allergic type IV contact dermatitis. Finally, DCs are found in the mucosal lining of the bowel and have been implicated in the development of inflammatory bowel diseases such as Crohn disease and ulcerative colitis.

B Lymphocytes and Humoral Immunity

The humoral immune response is mediated by antibodies, which are produced by the B lymphocytes. The primary functions of the B lymphocytes are the elimination of extracellular microbes and toxins and subsequent "memory" for a heightened response during future encounters. Humoral immunity is more important than cellular immunity in defending against microbes with capsules rich in polysaccharides and lipid toxins because only the B lymphocytes are capable of responding to and producing antibodies specific for many types of these molecules. The T cells, which are the mediators of cellular immunity, respond primarily to surface protein antigens.

B lymphocytes are produced in the bone borrow and are classified according to the MHC-II proteins, Ig, and complement receptors expressed on the cell membrane. At each stage of development, a cell-specific pattern of Ig gene is expressed, which then serves to designate the antibody-producing cell type. The B-lymphocyte progenitors are known as pro-B and pre-B cells and develop into both mature and naive B lymphocytes in the bone marrow. Naïve (or immature) B lymphocytes display IgM on the cell surface. These immature cells respond to antigen differently from a mature B cell. They can be functionally removed from the body as a result of interaction with a self-antigen, by undergoing programmed cell death (apoptosis) or by becoming nonresponsive in the presence of the antigen. Naïve B lymphocytes can leave the bone marrow and migrate to peripheral or secondary lymphoid tissues such as the spleen and lymph nodes where they can fully mature. Once they complete the process, they become capable of expressing IgD, in addition to the IgM on the cell membrane surface. Mature B lymphocytes can respond to all antigens and are capable of interacting with T cells.

B-cell lines become committed to a specific antigen when they encounter antigens that match their encoded surface Ig receptor. In the presence of T-helper cell antigen presentation, they undergo a series of conformational changes that transform them into antibody-secreting plasma cells or into memory B cells (Fig. 11.8). Both cell types are necessary

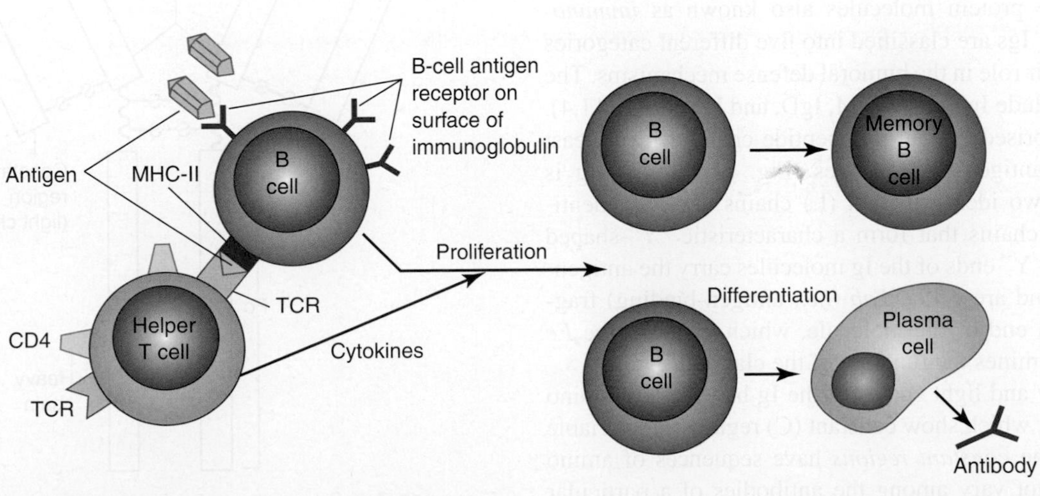

Figure 11.8 • Pathway for B-cell differentiation.

TABLE 11.4 CLASSES AND CHARACTERISTICS OF IGS

FIGURE	CLASS	PERCENTAGE OF TOTAL	CHARACTERISTICS
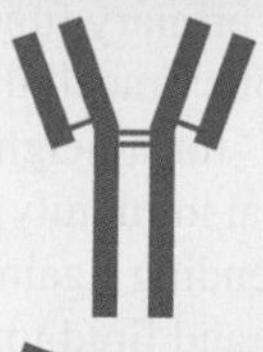	IgG	75.0	Displays antiviral, antitoxin, and antibacterial properties; only Ig that crosses the placenta; responsible for protection of newborn; activates complement and binds to macrophages
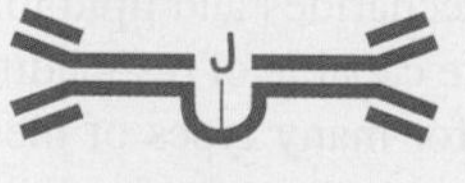	IgG	15.0	Predominant Ig in body secretions, such as saliva, nasal and respiratory secretions, and breast milk; protects mucous membranes
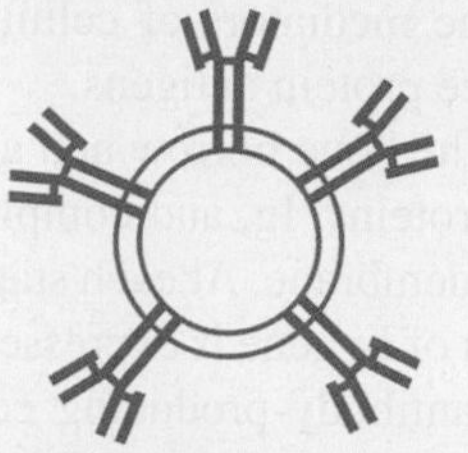	IgG	10.0	Forms the natural antibodies such as those for ABO blood antigens; prominent in early immune responses; activates complement
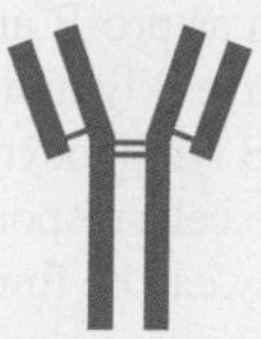	IgG	0.2	Found on B lymphocytes; needed for maturation of B cells
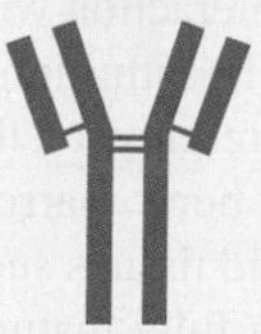	IgG	0.004	Binds to mast cells and basophils; involved in parasitic infections, allergic and hypersensitivity reactions

for the ultimate success of the humoral response. The antibodies produced by the plasma cells are released into the lymph and blood, where they can then bind and remove their specific antigen with the help of other immune effector cells and molecules. The memory B lymphocytes have a longer life span and are distributed to the peripheral tissues in preparation for subsequent antigen exposure.

Immunoglobulins

Antibodies are protein molecules also known as *immunoglobulins* (Igs). Igs are classified into five different categories based upon their role in the humoral defense mechanisms. The five classes include IgG, IgA, IgM, IgD, and IgE (Table 11.4). The Ig is comprised of four-polypeptide chains with at least two identical antigen-binding sites (Fig. 11.9). Each Ig is composed of two identical light (L) chains and two identical heavy (H) chains that form a characteristic "Y"-shaped molecule. The "Y" ends of the Ig molecules carry the antigen-binding sites and are called *Fab* (*i.e.*, antigen-binding) fragments. The tail end of the molecule, which is called the *Fc* fragment, determines the function of the class of Igs.

The heavy and light chains of the Ig have certain amino acid sequences, which show constant (C) regions and variable (V) regions. The *constant regions* have sequences of amino acids that do not vary among the antibodies of a particular class of Ig and determine the classification of the particular

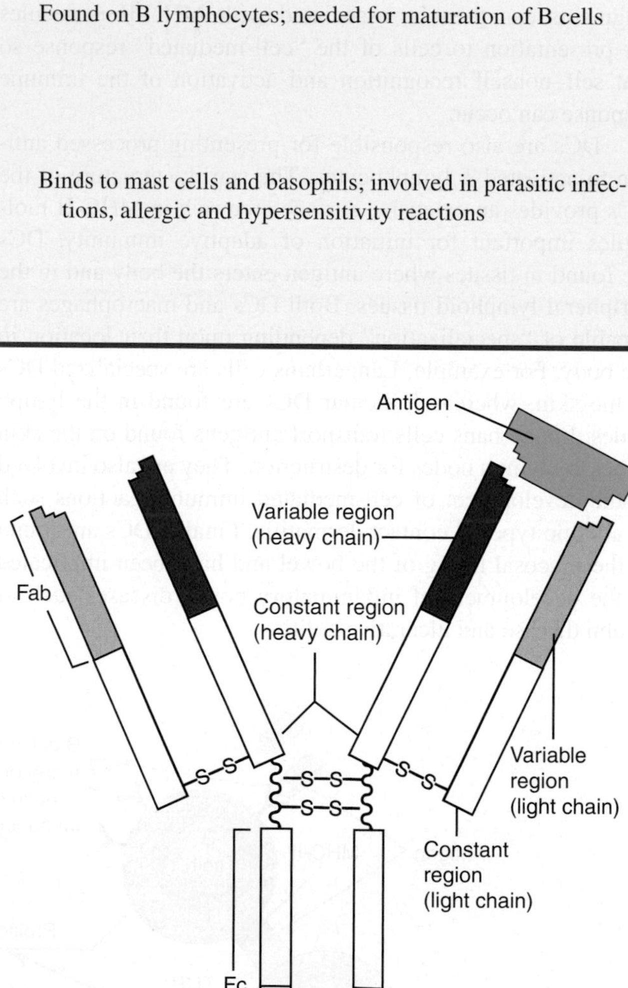

Figure 11.9 • Schematic model of an immunoglobulin G (IgG) molecule showing the constant and variable regions of the light and heavy chains.

Ig (*e.g.*, IgG, IgE). The constant regions, therefore, determine the end function of the particular antibody. In contrast, the amino acid sequences of the *variable regions* differ from antibody to antibody. They also contain the antigen-binding sites of the particular molecule. The different amino acid sequences found in these binding sites allow this region of the antibody to recognize its complementary epitope (antigen). The variable amino acid sequence determines the shape of the binding site, forming a three-dimensional pocket that fits the specific antigen. When B lymphocytes divide, they form clones that produce antibodies with identical antigen-binding regions. During the course of the immune response, however, class switching (*e.g.*, from IgM to IgG) can occur, causing the B-cell clone to produce one of the different Ig types.

IgG (gamma globulin) is the most abundant of the Igs making up 75% of the total circulating antibodies. It is a large molecule and is composed of two different kinds of polypeptide chain. IgG possesses antiviral, antibacterial, and antitoxin properties. It is present in all body fluids, readily enters the tissues, and is capable of crossing the placenta where it confers passive immunity upon the fetus. With the help of APCs, *IgG* binds to target cells as well as Fc receptors on NK cells and macrophages, leading to lysis of the target cell. There are four subclasses of IgG (*i.e.*, IgG1, IgG2, IgG3, and IgG4) with specificity for certain types of antigens. For example, IgG2 appears to target bacteria that are encapsulated with a lipopolysaccharide layer, such as *Streptococcus pneumoniae.*[33,34]

IgA is composed of two identical molecules and is the second most common Ig found in serum accounting for approximately 15% of all antibodies. It is primarily a secretory Ig that is found in saliva, tears, colostrum (*i.e.*, first milk of a nursing mother), and bronchial, gastrointestinal, prostatic, and vaginal secretions. Because it is primarily found in secretions, its primary function is in local immunity on mucosal surfaces. IgA prevents the attachment of viruses and bacteria to epithelial cells.

IgM accounts for approximately 10% of all circulating antibodies. It is a five-membered macromolecule with identical heavy and light chains. Because of its structure, it is an efficient complement fixing Ig and is instrumental in the ultimate lysis of microorganisms. It also functions as an effective *agglutinating* antibody, stimulating clumping of organisms for eventual lysis and elimination. IgM is the first antibody to be produced by the developing fetus and by immature B lymphocytes.

IgD is found primarily on the cell membranes of B lymphocytes where it functions as a receptor for antigen. It circulates in the serum in extremely low levels where its function is essentially unknown but may play a role in B-cell differentiation.

IgE is the least common serum IgE because it binds very tightly to the Fc receptors on basophils and mast cells. It is involved in inflammation and allergic responses by causing mast cell degranulation and release of chemical mediators including histamine. IgE is also essential for combating parasitic infections.

Humoral Immunity

Humoral immunity requires the presence of mature B lymphocytes capable of recognizing antigen and differentiating into antibody-secreting plasma cells. The ultimate response of the antigen–antibody complex formation can take several forms including antigen–antibody complex precipitation, agglutination of pathogens, neutralization of toxins, phagocytosis or lysis of invading organisms, immune cell activation, and complement activation.

Two separate but interrelated responses occur in the development of humoral immunity: a primary and a secondary response (Fig. 11.10). A *primary immune response* develops when the body first encounters the antigen. The antigen comes in contact with various APCs, is processed by these cells in association with the MHC-II molecules on the cells surface, and is then presented to the lymphocytes (*i.e.*, $CD4^+$ T-helper cells) to initiate the immune process. APCs such as macrophages also secrete ILs, which are essential for activating the cell-mediated response via the $CD4^+$ helper T cells. The activated $CD4^+$ helper T cells trigger B cells to proliferate and differentiate into plasma cells that produce antibody. The primary immune response takes 1 to 2 weeks, but once generated, detectable antibody continues to rise for several more weeks even though the infectious process has resolved. The *memory phase or secondary immune response* occurs on subsequent exposure to the antigen. During the secondary response, the rise in antibody occurs sooner and reaches a higher level because of available memory cells.

During the primary response, B lymphocytes proliferate and differentiate into antibody-secreting plasma cells. A fraction of the activated B cells remain intact in order to form a pool of memory B lymphocytes that then become available to efficiently respond to invasion during subsequent exposure. Activated T cells can also generate primary and secondary cell-mediated immune responses and the concurrent development of T memory cells.

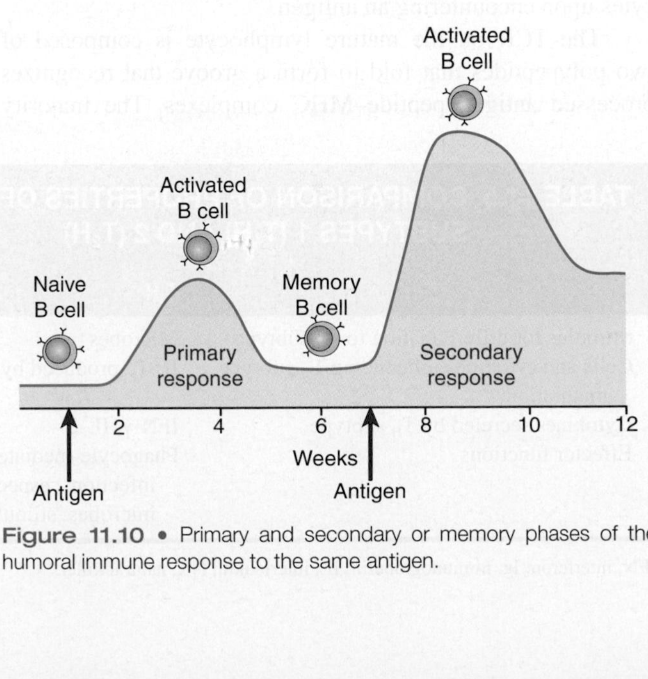

Figure 11.10 • Primary and secondary or memory phases of the humoral immune response to the same antigen.

The immunization process makes use of the primary and secondary phases of the humoral immune responses. The initial vaccination causes production of both plasma cells and memory cells. The plasma cells destroy the invading organism or toxin, and the memory cells provide defense against future exposure. "Booster" immunizations produce an immediate antigen–antibody response that simulates an immediate rise in antibody levels.

T Lymphocytes and Cellular Immunity

T lymphocytes serve many functions in the immune system including the activation of other T cells and B cells, control of intracellular viral infections, rejection of foreign tissue grafts, activation of autoimmune processes, and activation of delayed hypersensitivity reactions. These processes make up the body's *cell-mediated* or *cellular immunity*. The effector phase of cell-mediated immunity is carried out by T lymphocytes and macrophages.

T lymphocytes arise from lymphoid stem cells in the bone marrow, but unlike B lymphocytes, they migrate to the thymus gland to undergo the process of maturation. The thymus gland is richly innervated and produces several peptide hormones such as *thymulin* and *thymopoietin*, which are believed to be involved in T-cell maturation. T-cell precursors are attracted to the thymus by *thymotaxin,* a chemotactic factor secreted by the epithelial cells of the gland. Once the T-cell precursors enter the cortex of the thymus, they undergo rearrangement of their alpha- and beta-chain gene segments so that they can express a unique T-cell antigen receptor (TCR). The beta segment is expressed first resulting in the formation of a TCR. This halts further gene rearrangement and causes full maturation and expression of $CD4^+$ (helper) and $CD8^+$ (cytotoxic) lymphocytes. These are the predominant lymphocytes in the body. Mature T lymphocytes leave the thymus and migrate to peripheral lymphoid tissues, where they multiply and differentiate into memory T cells and various other mature lymphocytes upon encountering an antigen.

The TCR on the mature lymphocyte is composed of two polypeptides that fold to form a groove that recognizes processed antigen peptide–MHC complexes. The majority of TCRs recognize antigens that are bound to MHC-derived molecules. The TCR is associated with several surface molecules such as CD4 and CD8. CD4 is associated with the helper T cell, and CD8 is associated with the cytotoxic T cell. CD4 and CD8 help stabilize the TCR–antigen–MHC complex during T-cell activation. The TCR is also associated with other surface molecules known as the *CD3 complex*, which also aid in cell signaling.

Helper T Cells and Cytokines in Adaptive Immunity

The activation of helper T cells is the central event in the initiation of the humoral and cell-mediated immune response. $CD4^+$ helper T cells (T_H) serve as master regulators for the immune system. They become activated when their TCRs interact with antigens that are complexed with class II MHC on the surface of APCs. Once $CD4^+$ cells are activated, the cytokines they secrete in response influence the function of nearly all other cells of the immune system. Depending upon the specific cytokine that is released by the $CD4^+$ T cell, the subsequent immunologic response will be activated. These cytokines are able to activate and regulate B cells, cytotoxic T lymphocytes, NK cells, macrophages, and other immune cells. The first cytokine to be produced by $CD4^+$ T cells after activation is IL-2. IL-2 plays a major role in cell-mediated immunity and is necessary for the proliferation and function of helper T cells, cytotoxic T cells, B cells, and NK cells. There are other cytokines that are not produced by $CD4^+$ cells, but are essential for its function. IL-1 is produced by inflammatory cells and is responsible for increasing the expression of adhesion molecules on endothelial cells, activating leukocyte migration, and stimulating antibody production.[19]

The activated $CD4^+$ helper T cell can differentiate into two distinct subpopulations of helper T cells (*i.e.*, T_1H or T_2H) based on the cytokines secreted by the APCs at the site of activation (Table 11.5). Macrophages and DCs produce IL-12, which directs $CD4^+$ helper T cells to become the T_1H subtype, whereas mast cells and T cells produce IL-4, which induces differentiation toward the T_2H subtype. The T_2H cells present antigen to the B lymphocytes stimulating the differentiation

TABLE 11.5 COMPARISON OF PROPERTIES OF HELPER T-CELL SUBTYPES 1 (T_1H) AND 2 (T_2H)

	T_1H	T_2H
Stimulus for differentiation to T_H subtype	Microbes	Allergens and parasitic worms
Cells and cytokines influencing T_H subtype maturation	IL-12 produced by macrophages and DCs	IL-4 produced by mast cells and T cells
Cytokines secreted by T_H subtype	IFN-γ, IL-2	IL-4, IL-5
Effector functions	Phagocyte-mediated defense against infections, especially intracellular microbes; stimulates production of IgG	IgE-mediated and eosinophil/mast cell–mediated immune reactions; stimulates production of IgE

IFN, interferon; Ig, immunoglobulin; IL, interleukin; NK, natural killer.

into antibody-producing plasma cells. As part of the allergic or hypersensitivity response, T_2H cells direct B lymphocytes to switch class and produce the IgE antibodies.

The distinct pattern of cytokine secreted by mature T_1H and T_2H cells determines whether a humoral or cell-mediated response will ultimately occur. Activated T_1H cells produce the cytokines IL-2 and IFN-γ, whereas T_2H cells produce IL-4 and IL-5. IL-5 is an activator of eosinophils that, along with IgE, functions in the control of helminth (intestinal parasite) infections. Some of the cytokines (*e.g.*, IL-10) made by T_2H cells are anti-inflammatory and inhibit macrophage activation and suppress other T_1H responses. In most immune responses, a balance between T_1H and T_2H cell activation will occur.

Regulatory T Cells

T_{REGS} are a subset of T lymphocytes that function to control immune system responses. Different populations of T_{REGS} cells produced in the thymus have been identified including those that express CD4 and CD25 on their surface. These cells represent a subset of $CD4^+$ cells that act as "negative regulators" of the immune process because they suppress immune cell activities.[35] T_{REGS} inhibit the proliferation of other potentially harmful self-reactive lymphocytes in order to limit inflammation and tissue damage. Production of T_{REGS} is highly dependent upon the presence of antigen, activation of a TCR by the antigen, and the release of cytokines. There is also recent evidence of the existence of regulatory $CD8^+$ T cells that can selectively downregulate T cells activated by either self or foreign antigens. These cells differentiate into regulatory cells during the primary immune response and function to suppress the secondary immune response. The $CD8^+$ regulators are, therefore, primarily involved in self–nonself discrimination. The ability of the T_{REGS} to control many aspects of the immune response has significant implications for clinical practice. Promise has been shown in the control of inflammatory bowel disease, experimental allergic encephalitis, and autoimmune diabetes.

Cytotoxic T Cells

The primary function of cytotoxic T ($CD8^+$) cells is to monitor the activity of all cells in the body and destroy any that threaten the integrity of the body. $CD8^+$ T cells recognize antigens that are presented on the cell surface by MHC class I–derived molecules that sample protein degradation productions from inside cells infected by viruses or transformed by cancer[36] (Fig. 11.11). The ability of $CD8^+$ cells to recognize the class I MHC–antigen complexes on infected target cells ensures that neighboring uninfected host cells, which express class I MHC molecules alone, are not indiscriminately destroyed. The $CD8^+$ cytotoxic T lymphocytes destroy target cells by a variety of mechanisms including the release of cytolytic enzymes or by triggering membrane molecules and intracellular apoptosis. Apoptosis is a normal biologic process that eliminates excessive, dangerous, or damaged cells from the body. The $CD8^+$ T cells play a large role in controlling

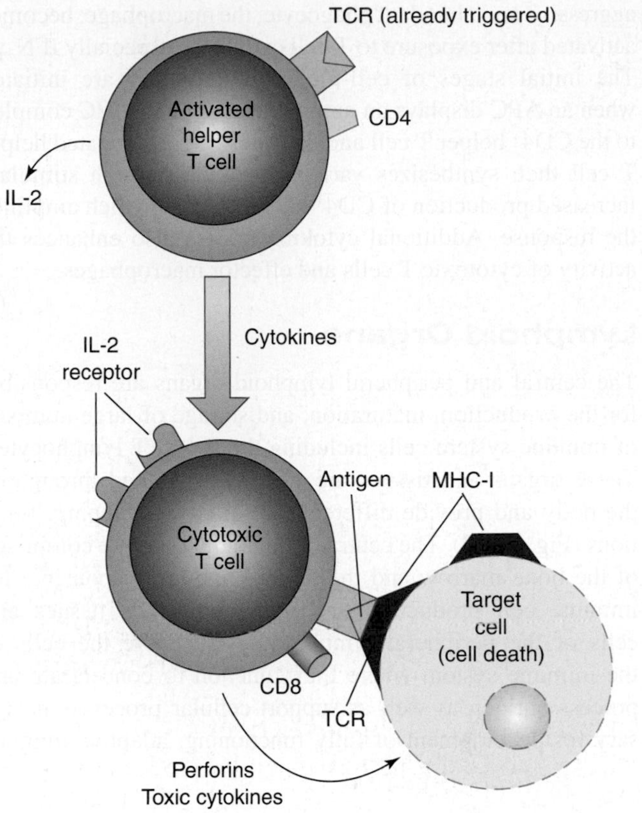

Figure 11.11 • Destruction of target cell by cytotoxic T cell. Cytokines released from the activated helper T cell enhance the potential of the cytotoxic T cell in destruction of the target cell.

replicating viruses and intracellular bacteria because antibody cannot readily penetrate the membrane of living cells.

Cell-Mediated Immunity

In order for the cell-mediated immune response to carry out its function, healthy $CD4^+$ and $CD8^+$ T lymphocytes are required. Activated $CD4^+$ helper T cells release various cytokines (*i.e.*, IFN-γ) that recruit and activate other $CD8^+$ cytotoxic T cells, macrophages, and inflammatory cells. Cytokines (*e.g.*, chemokines) stimulate migration types of inflammatory cells, which further enhance the phagocytic, metabolic, and enzymatic functions of the cell-mediated immune response. This results in a more rapid and more efficient destruction of infected cells. This type of defense is important against many intracellular pathogens such as *Mycobacterium* species and *Listeria monocytogenes* but unfortunately plays a role in delayed hypersensitivity reactions. Allergic contact dermatitis (delayed hypersensitivity type IV) results from the activation of both $CD4^+$ and $CD8^+$ T-cell precursors in the lymph nodes draining the site where antigen was encountered. These "haptenated peptides" stimulate the recruitment of T cells at the site of antigen presentation, inducing inflammatory signals and apoptosis of epidermal cells, leading to the development of inflammation, the release of chemical mediators, and the development of clinical symptoms.

In cell-mediated immune responses, the actions of T lymphocytes and effector macrophages predominate. The most aggressive and abundant phagocyte, the macrophage, becomes activated after exposure to T-cell cytokines, especially IFN-γ.[3] The initial stages of cell-mediated immunity are initiated when an APC displays an antigen–class I or II MHC complex to the $CD4^+$ helper T cell and activates it. The activated helper T cell then synthesizes various cytokines, which stimulate increased production of $CD4^+$ helper T cells, which amplifies the response. Additional cytokine release also enhances the activity of cytotoxic T cells and effector macrophages.

Lymphoid Organs

The central and peripheral lymphoid organs are responsible for the production, maturation, and storage of large numbers of immune system cells including the B and T lymphocytes. These organs and tissues are widely distributed throughout the body and provide different, but often overlapping, functions (Fig. 11.12). The central lymphoid organs are comprised of the bone marrow and the thymus and are responsible for immune cell production and maturation. The tissues and cells of the peripheral lymphoid system store the cells of the immune system where they function to concentrate and process antigen as well as support cellular processes necessary for development of fully functioning, adaptive immune responses. The peripheral lymphoid tissues are comprised of the lymph nodes, spleen, tonsils, appendix, Peyer patches in the intestine, and mucosa-associated lymphoid tissues in the respiratory, gastrointestinal, and reproductive systems. Networks of lymph channels, blood vessels, and capillaries connect the lymphoid organs and transport immune cells, antigens, and cellular debris throughout the body.

Thymus

The thymus is an elongated, bilobed structure located in the mediastinum above the heart and serves as a specialized immune system organ. Each lobe is surrounded by a connective tissue capsule layer and is divided into lobules. The lobules can be divided into an outer cortex and a central medulla, which play different roles in the process of T-lymphocyte maturation. The outer cortex contains densely packed immature T lymphocytes (thymocytes). The inner medulla is a less dense area of tissue that contains fewer but more mature lymphocytes. The medulla is comprised of Hassall corpuscles but also stores DCs and macrophages (Fig. 11.13). The function of the Hassall corpuscles is unclear but does serve as a potent source of cytokines.

The thymus is essential to the development of the immune system because it is responsible for the production of mature, immunocompetent T lymphocytes. The thymus is a fully developed organ at birth, weighing approximately 15 to 20 g. It is most active during the neonatal and preadolescent

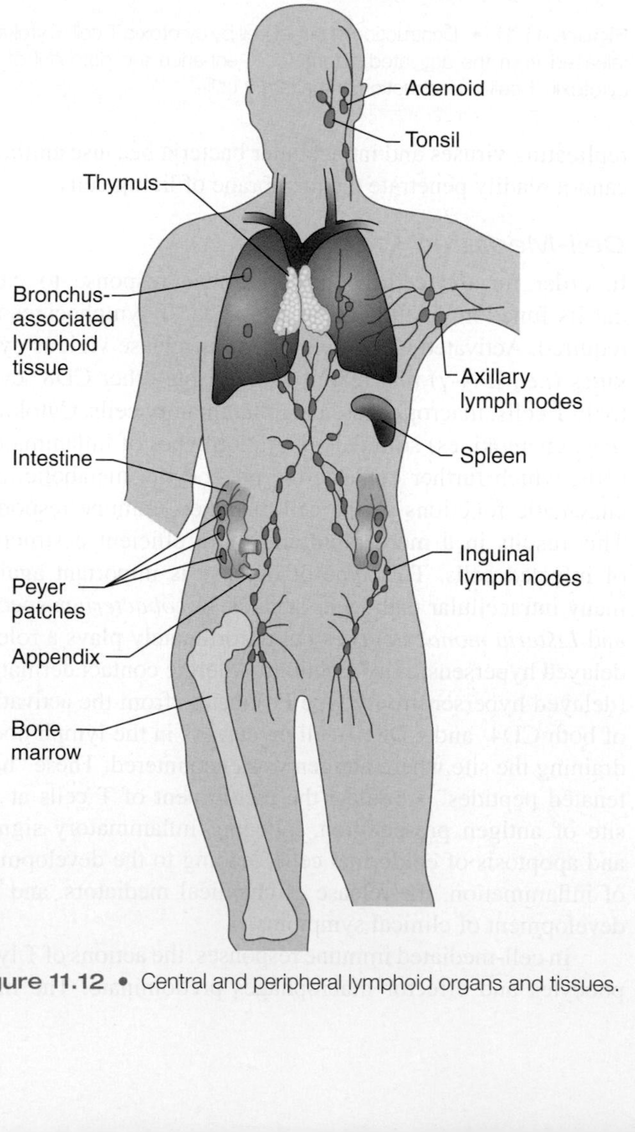

Figure 11.12 • Central and peripheral lymphoid organs and tissues.

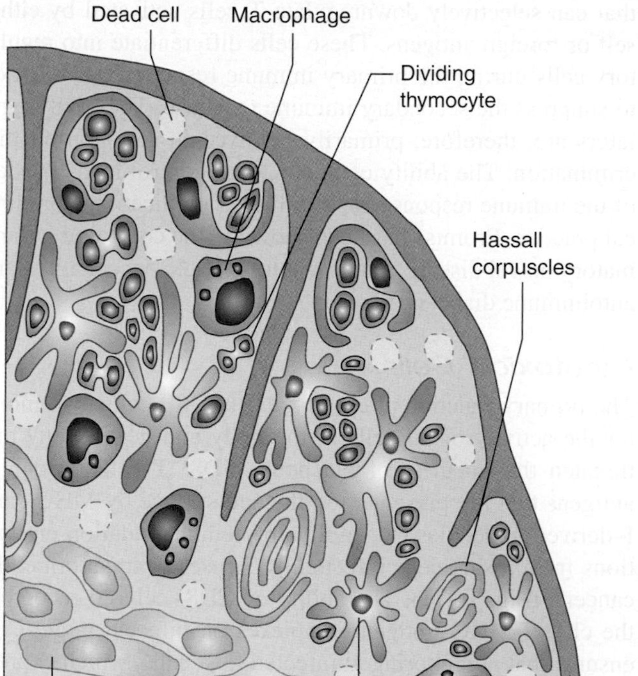

Figure 11.13 • Structural features of the thymus gland. The thymus gland is divided into lobules containing an outer cortex densely packed with dividing thymocytes or premature T cells and an inner medulla that contains mature T lymphocytes, macrophages, dendritic cells, and Hassall corpuscles.

periods. At puberty, when the immune cells are well established in peripheral lymphoid tissues, the thymus begins to atrophy and is replaced by adipose tissue. Nevertheless, residual T-lymphocyte production continues throughout adult life. Precursor T (pre-T) cells enter the thymus as functionally and phenotypically immature T cells. They then mature during different cycles and move from the cortex to the medulla until they are released into the peripheral lymphoid tissues. Rapid cell division, maturation, and selection occur in the cortex under the influence of thymic hormones and cytokines. As the T cells mature, they develop the TCRs that differentiate them from other types of T cells. The majority of the thymocytes die in the cortex during the process of gene rearrangement and maturation because they fail to develop the appropriate receptor types on their cell membranes. Only those T cells capable of recognizing foreign antigen displayed by self-MHC are allowed to mature. This process is called *thymic selection*. Mature, immunocompetent T-helper and T-cytotoxic cells leave the thymus in 2 to 3 days and enter the peripheral lymphoid tissues through the bloodstream.

Lymph Nodes

Lymph nodes are small aggregates of lymphoid tissue located along lymphatic vessels throughout the body. The lymphatic vessels carry lymph, which is a clear sometimes yellow-tinged fluid that contains a variety of white blood cells (predominantly lymphocytes) and transports cellular debris and organisms to the lymph nodes to be removed from the body. Each lymph node processes lymph from a discrete, adjacent anatomic site. Lymph nodes are congregated in the axillae and groin and along the great vessels of the neck, thorax, and abdomen. The lymph nodes receive lymph from the collecting ducts, which ultimately drain into the thoracic duct located in the left side of the chest at the level of the subclavian vein. Lymph nodes have two functions: removal of foreign material from lymph before it enters the bloodstream and serving as centers for proliferation and response of immune cells.

Lymph nodes are bean-shaped, encapsulated tissues, approximately 0.5 to 1 cm in diameter. Lymph enters the node through afferent lymph channels and leaves through the efferent lymph vessels located deep in the node. Lymphocytes and macrophages move slowly through the lymph nodes so that they have adequate time to engulf microorganisms and interact with circulating antigen. The lymphatic system provides a large surface upon which macrophages and DCs can more easily present antigens to T lymphocytes.

Lymph nodes are divided into three distinct and specialized areas—an outer cortex, a paracortex, and an inner medulla (Fig. 11.14). The T lymphocytes predominate in the paracortex and the B lymphocytes predominate in the follicles and germinal centers of the outer cortex. The T lymphocytes proliferate when antigens enter the paracortex of the lymph

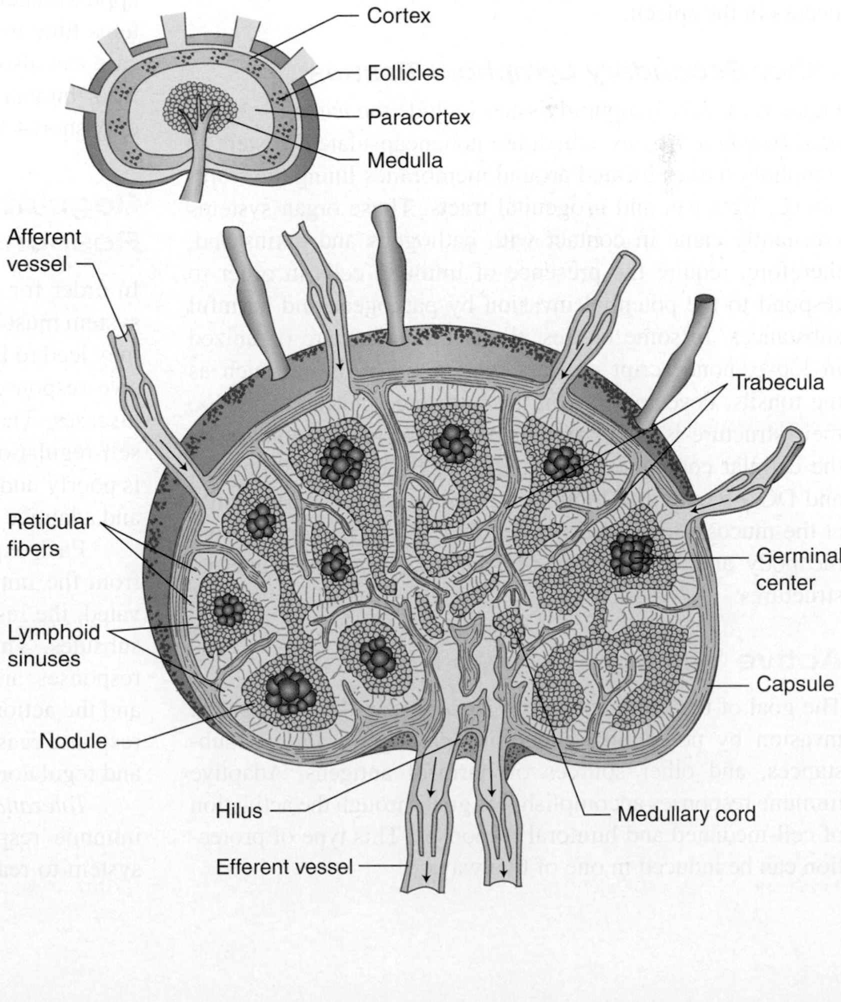

Figure 11.14 • Structural features of a lymph node. Bacteria that gain entry to the body are filtered out of the lymph as it flows through the node.

node. They then migrate to the outer cortex so that they can interact with B lymphocytes that are stored there. Within the follicles the lymphocytes continue to mature, replicate, and interact with the APCs present in the nodes (macrophages and follicular DCs). Activated B cells then migrate to the medulla of the lymph node, where they complete their maturation into plasma cells. Large quantities of antibodies are then released into the systemic circulation.

Spleen

The spleen is a large, ovoid secondary lymphoid organ located high in the left upper quadrant of the abdominal cavity between the diaphragm and the stomach. The spleen filters antigens from the blood and is important in the response to systemic infections. It is divided into two systems: the white pulp and the red pulp. The *red pulp* is well supplied with arteries and venous sinusoids and is the area where senescent (biologically aged) and injured red blood cells are removed. The *white pulp* contains lymphatic nodules and diffuse lymphoid tissue where concentrated areas of B and T lymphocytes, macrophages, and DCs exist. The lymphocytes (primarily T cells) that surround the central arterioles form the area called the *periarterial lymphoid sheath*. There is also a diffuse marginal zone that contains the follicles and germinal centers and is rich in B cells. This separates the white pulp from the red pulp and allows lymphocytes to move easily between the blood and the lymphatic tissue. A sequence of activation events similar to that seen in the lymph nodes occurs in the spleen.

Other Secondary Lymphoid Tissues

Other secondary lymphoid tissues include the *mucosa-associated lymphoid tissues*, which are nonencapsulated clusters of lymphoid tissues located around membranes lining the respiratory, digestive, and urogenital tracts. These organ systems constantly came in contact with pathogens and toxins and, therefore, require the presence of immune cells in order to respond to the potential invasion by pathogens and harmful substances. In some tissues, the lymphocytes are organized in loose, nondescript clusters, but in other tissues such as the tonsils, Peyer patches in the intestine, and the appendix, their structure is better organized. These tissues contain all the cellular components (*i.e.*, T cells, B cells, macrophages, and DCs) required to mount an immune response. Immunity at the mucosal layers helps to exclude many pathogens from the body and, as a result, protects the more vital internal structures.

Active Versus Passive Immunity

The goal of the immune system is to protect the host against invasion by potentially dangerous pathogens, foreign substances, and other sources of harmful antigens. Adaptive immune responses accomplish this goal through the activation of cell-mediated and humoral responses. This type of protection can be induced in one of two ways:

1. After exposure to the offending substance and activation of B and T lymphocytes by the host (active immunity)
2. Through the transfer of antibodies against an antigen directly to the host (passive immunity)

Active immunity is acquired when the host mounts an immune response to an antigen either through the process of vaccination or from environmental exposure. It is called *active immunity* because it requires the host's own immune system to develop an immunologic response including the development of memory. Active immunity is usually long lasting but requires a few days to weeks after a first exposure to sufficiently develop an appropriate immunologic response that culminates in the destruction of the presenting antigen. However, with subsequent exposure, the immune system rapidly becomes fully activated because of the presence of memory B and T lymphocytes and circulating antibodies. The process by which active immunity is acquired through the administration of a vaccine is termed *immunization*. An acquired immune response can improve on repeated exposures to an injected antigen (booster vaccines) or a natural infection.

Passive immunity is immunity transferred from another source. The most common form of passive immunity is that conferred from mother to fetus. During fetal development, maternal IgG antibodies are transferred to the fetus via the placenta. After birth, the neonate also receives IgG antibodies from the mother in breast milk or colostrum. Therefore, infants are provided with some degree of protection from infection for approximately 3 to 6 months, giving their own immune systems time to mature. Some protection against infectious disease can also be provided by the administration of Igs pooled from human or animal sources. Passive immunity produces only short-term protection that lasts weeks to months.

Regulation of the Adaptive Immune Response

In order for a host organism to remain healthy, the immune system must function properly. A weakened immune response may lead to immunodeficiency, but an inappropriate or excessive response can cause allergic reactions and autoimmune diseases. Therefore, the immune system must be capable of self-regulation. The process by which the body regulates itself is poorly understood but must involve all aspects of the innate and adaptive immune responses to be effective.

Each exposure to an antigen elicits a predictable response from the immune system. Once the immune system is activated, the response is amplified until it peaks and eventually subsides. This occurs because the body's normal immune responses are self-limiting. Once the antigen is destroyed and the action of chemical mediators terminated, the immune response ceases. It is believed that anti-inflammatory cytokines and regulatory T lymphocytes play a role in this process.[37]

Tolerance also plays a role in the self-regulation of the immune response. Tolerance is the ability of the immune system to react to foreign antigens but remain nonreactive to self-antigens. Tolerance to self-antigens protects the body from harmful autoimmune responses. This is exquisitely important in vital organs such as the brain, testes, ovaries, and eyes where immunologic damage could be lethal to the organism.

Many autoimmune diseases such as Hashimoto thyroiditis and insulin-dependent diabetes mellitus are caused by impairment in both B and T lymphocyte (specifically cytotoxic lymphocytes) functions resulting in direct cellular damage because the body immune system is no longer capable of distinguishing "self" from "nonself."[38,39]

IN SUMMARY

Adaptive immunity is comprised of two distinct but interrelated processes: cell-mediated and humoral immunity. Together, they respond to foreign antigens, amplify and sustain immunologic responses, distinguish self from nonself, and confer "memory" so that a heightened response can be initiated on subsequent exposure to an organism. Antigens are usually substances foreign to the host that can stimulate an immune response. Antigens possess specific antigenic binding sites for the cells of the immune system known as epitopes. Epitopes allow the adaptive immune system to distinguish foreign antigens from normal cellular substances whose destruction would be detrimental to the organism. Adaptive immunity can be acquired actively or passively. Active immunity develops through immunization or by having a disease, whereas passive immunity develops when the host receives antibodies or immune cells from another source. An acquired immune response can improve with repeated exposure to an injected antigen or a natural infection.

The principal cells of the adaptive immune system are the B and T lymphocytes, APCs, and effector cells that are responsible for the elimination of antigens. The lymphocytes are produced and undergo maturation in the central lymphoid organs (bone marrow and thymus) and are subsequently stored in the peripheral lymphoid tissues. B lymphocytes differentiate into plasma cells that produce antibodies and provide for the elimination of microbes in the extracellular fluid (humoral immunity) as well as memory cells, which are responsible for the rapid immune response with repeat exposure. T lymphocytes differentiate into regulatory (helper T and T_{REGS}) and effector (cytotoxic T cells) cells. APCs consist of macrophages and DCs that process and present antigen peptides to $CD4^+$ helper T cells.

During cellular maturation, T lymphocytes express specific molecules on the cellular surfaces that distinguish between the different cell types and that help determine the cells' functionality. Regulatory $CD4^+$ helper T cells help to modulate the immune response and are essential for the differentiation of B cells into antibody-producing plasma cells and the differentiation of T lymphocytes into effector $CD8^+$ cytotoxic T cells. The $CD8^+$ cytotoxic cells eliminate intracellular microbes, such as viruses and other pathogens. Cells of both the innate and adaptive immune responses produce cytokines that influence adaptive immune responses. These cytokines function as communication molecules for the B and T lymphocytes, stimulate cellular proliferation and differentiation, and ensure the appropriate development of cytotoxic effector and memory cells.

People who are immunocompromised must be closely evaluated to determine the risk-to-benefit ratio when administering vaccines. Killed or inactive vaccines usually are safe, and booster may be required. For people who are immunocompromised not associated with HIV or planned immunosuppression, such as congenital immunodeficiency, live virus vaccines are not generally administered. Immunosuppression affects B and/or T cells causing a decreased or absent antibody response to vaccine. People who are HIV infected need evaluation and testing before live virus vaccines are administered.[40]

DEVELOPMENTAL ASPECTS OF THE IMMUNE SYSTEM

After completing this section of the chapter, the learner will be able to meet the following objectives:

- Explain the transfer of passive immunity from mother to fetus and from mother to infant during breast-feeding.
- Characterize the development of active immunity in the infant and small child.
- Describe the changes in the immune response that occur during the normal aging process.

Development of the immune system begins early in fetal life at approximately 5 to 6 weeks gestation when the fetal liver actively begins hematopoiesis. At about the same time (6 weeks gestation), the thymus arises from the third branchial arch with the cortex arising from its ectodermal layer and the medulla from the endoderm.[41] Over the next 2 to 3 weeks, lymphoid cells initially migrate from the yolk sac and fetal liver and then from the bone marrow to colonize the fetal thymus.[41] Development of the secondary lymphoid organs (*i.e.*, spleen, lymph nodes, and mucosa-associated lymphoid tissues) begins soon after. The secondary lymphoid organs are rather small but well developed at birth and mature rapidly after exposure to microbes during the postnatal period. The thymus is the largest lymphoid tissue in the neonate relative to body size and normally reaches its mature weight by 1 year of age.

Transfer of Immunity from Mother to Infant

The neonate's immune system is functionally immature at birth so protection against infection and toxic substances occurs through transfer of maternal IgG antibodies. Maternal IgG antibodies readily cross the placenta during fetal development and remain functional in the newborn for the first few months of life providing passive immunity until Ig production is well established in the newborn. IgG is the only class of Igs able to cross the placenta. Maternally transmitted IgG is effective against most microorganisms and viruses that a neonate encounters. Maternal vaccination may therefore offer fetal and neonatal passive immunity against common infections such as influenza or herpes zoster.[42] The largest amount of IgG crosses the placenta during the last weeks of pregnancy and is stored in fetal tissues. Infants born prematurely may be deficient in maternal antibodies and, therefore, more susceptible to infection. Because of transfer of IgG antibodies to the fetus, an infant born to a mother infected with HIV has a positive HIV antibody test result, although the child may not be infected with the virus.

Cord blood does not normally contain IgM or IgA. If present, these antibodies are of fetal origin and represent exposure to intrauterine infection because maternal IgM and IgA antibodies do not readily cross the placenta. Normally, the neonate begins producing IgM antibodies shortly after birth, as a result of exposure to the immense number of antigens normally found in the surrounding environment. However, this IgM is of lower binding affinity and effective against a limited range of antigens. It has also been demonstrated that premature infants can produce IgM as well as term infants. At approximately 6 days of age, the IgM rises sharply, and this rise continues until approximately 1 year of age, when the adult level is achieved.

Serum IgA normally is not present at birth but detected in the neonate approximately 13 days after birth. The levels of IgA increase during early childhood and reach between 6 and 7 years of age. Although maternal IgA is not transferred in utero, it is transferred to the breast-fed infant in colostrum. Because IgA antibodies are associated with mucosal members, these antibodies provide local immunity for the intestinal system during early life.

Immune Response in the Older Adult

As we age, the ability of the immune system to protect the body from pathogenic organisms and environmental toxins declines as a result of an overall decline in immune responsiveness. This results from changes in both cell-mediated and humoral immune responses. As a result, older adults are more susceptible to infections, have more evidence of autoimmune and immune complex disorders, and have a higher incidence of cancer than do younger people. In addition, the immune system of older adults is less likely to respond appropriately to immunization. As a result, older adults have a weakened response to vaccination. Older adults also frequently have many comorbid conditions that impair normal immune function and compromise the immune response.

The cause of the altered response in older adults is multifactorial. There is a continued decrease in the size of the thymus gland, which begins during puberty and affects overall T-cell production and function. The size of the thymus diminishes to 15% or less of its maximum size. There may also be a decrease in the number of the lymphocytes in the peripheral lymphoid tissue. The most common finding is a slight decrease in the proportion of T cells to other lymphocytes and a decrease in $CD4^+$ and $CD8^+$ cells.

Aging also produces qualitative changes in lymphocyte function. Lymphocytes seem to exhibit altered responses to antigen stimulation including unresponsiveness to activation. It appears that the $CD4^+$ T lymphocyte is most severely affected because there is a decreased rate of synthesis of cytokines that stimulate the proliferation of lymphocytes and expression of the specific receptors that interact with the circulating cytokines. Specifically, IL-2, IL-4, and IL-12 levels decrease in older adults. Although actual B-cell function is compromised with age, the range of antigens that can be recognized by the B cells does not change.

IN SUMMARY

Neonates are protected against antigens in early life as a result of passive transfer of maternal IgG antibodies through the placenta and IgA antibodies in colostrum and breast milk. Many changes occur with aging, but the exact mechanisms are not completely understood. However, the elderly population is more prone to infection and autoimmune disorders secondary to altered response in both innate and adaptive immune function.

GERIATRIC Considerations

- The immune system begins to decline with age secondary to a decline in the responsiveness of both the innate and adaptive systems. The cause is multifactorial but renders the elderly more susceptible to infection and autoimmune disorders.[43]
- The lack of fever cannot be used to eliminate the diagnosis of infection in the elderly person because of the delayed immune response associated with aging.[43]

PEDIATRIC Considerations

- Cellular immunity is functional at birth, and with exposure to antigens, humoral immunity develops.[44]
- It is not uncommon for young children to have localized enlarged lymph nodes because of numerous exposures to viral illnesses.[44]
- Newborns and infants have decreased phagocytic response when stressed because of the immature complement system.[44]
- Because immunoglobulins (Ig) do not cross the placenta (with the exception of IgG), an exposure to an antigen is needed for production of IgA, IgD, IgE, and IgM.[44]
- Biomarkers (biologic measures that can be evaluated to indicate normal biologic processes, pathologic conditions, or even response to treatment) are an important component of the pediatric immune system that identify defense mechanisms and physiologic function of the immune system used to monitor and predict health states.[45]

REVIEW EXERCISES

1. The systemic manifestations (*e.g.*, generalized muscle aches, chills and fever, loss of appetite) that accompany a severe sore throat or acute respiratory infection are stimulated by reactions to cytokines of the innate immune system rather than by the antibodies or cell-mediated responses of the adaptive immune response.
   A. *Explain.*
2. A nursing student is working in a community clinic as a volunteer. Each time she enters the clinic, she suffers bouts of sneezing and runny nose. She has a history of mold allergy and her younger brother has asthma. Analysis at the allergy clinic indicates a strong reaction to latex. She is advised to avoid exposure to all forms of latex.
   A. *What class of immunoglobulin and what type of mediator cells are responsible for the symptoms expressed in this person?*
   B. *What type of T-helper cell and cytokines direct the expression of this humoral immune response?*
   C. *Is this an example of active or passive immunity? Is this likely to be a primary or secondary immune response?*
3. A child of 5 months of age presents with thrush, a yeast infection of the mouth. In the last 2 months, he has had recurrent bouts of otitis media. His tonsils are very small. Laboratory analysis indicates a low lymphocyte count and no T lymphocytes. Further analysis indicates a genetic mutation in the T-cell receptor molecule complex (TCR–CD3) that affects maturation of all T cells. The final diagnosis is severe combined immunodeficiency disease. A bone marrow transplant is being pursued with cells from his HLA-matched sibling.
   A. *Why were infections not present in the first few months of this child's life?*
   B. *What would be the impact of an absence of T cells on both humoral and cell-mediated immunity?*
   C. *Why would it not be advisable to administer a live virus vaccine in this child?*

References

1. Breedveld A., Groot Kormelink T., van Egmond M., et al. (2017). Granulocytes as modulators of dendritic cell function. *Journal of Leukocyte Biology* 102, 1003–1016.
2. Cecchinato V., D'Agostino G., Raeli L, et al. (2016). Chemokine interaction with synergy-inducing molecules: Fine tuning modulation of cell trafficking. *Journal of Leukocyte Biology* 99, 851–855.
3. Tangye S. G., Pelham S. J., Deenick M. K., et al. (2017). Cytokine-mediated regulation of human lymphocyte development and function: Insights from primary immunodeficiencies. *Journal of Immunology* 199, 1949–1958.
4. Leifer C. A., Medvedev A. E. (2016). Molecular mechanisms of regulation of Toll-like receptor signaling. *Journal of Leukocyte Biology* 100, 927–941.
5. Hoffman M. A., Kiecker F., Zuberbier T. (2016). A systematic review of the role of interleukin-17 and the interleukin-20 family in inflammatory skin diseases. *Current Opinion in Allergy & Clinical Immunology* 16, 451–457.
6. Fan V. S., Gharib S. A., Martin T. R., et al. (2016). COPD disease severity and innate immune response to pathogen-associated molecular patterns. *International Journal of COPD* 111, 467-477.
7. Kruger K., Dischereit G., Seimetz M., et al. (2016). Time course of cigarette smoke-induced changes in systemic inflammation and muscle structure. *American Journal of Physiology-Lung Cellular & Molecular Physiology* 309, 119–128.
8. Nagarsheth, N., Wicha, M. S., Zou, W. (2017). Chemokines in the cancer microenvironment and their relevance in cancer immunotherapy. *Nature Reviews Immunology* 17(9). 559-572. doi: 10.1038/nri2017.49.
9. Massara M., Bonavita O., Mantovani A, et al. (2016). Atypical chemokine receptors in cancer: Friends or foes? *Journal of Leukocyte Biology* 99, 927–933.
10. Yadava K., Bollyky P., Lawson M. A. (2016). The formation and function of tertiary lymphoid follicles in chronic pulmonary inflammation. *Immunology* 149, 262–269.
11. Martin S. F. (2015). New concepts in cutaneous allergy. *Contact Dermatitis* 72, 2–10.
12. Erdei A., Sandor N., Macsik-Valent B., et al. (2016). The versatile functions of complement C3-derived ligands. *Immunological Reviews* 274, 127–140.
13. Spahn J. H., Li W., Kreisel D. (2014). Innate immune cells in transplantation. *Current Opinion in Organ Transplantation* 19, 14–19.
14. Isidro R. A., Appleyard C. B. (2016). Colonic macrophage polarization in homeostasis, inflammation and cancer. *American Journal of Physiology-Gastrointestinal & Liver Physiology* 311, G59–G73.
15. Liszewski, M. K., Elvington, M., Kulkarni, H. S., et al (2017), Complement's hidden arsenal: New insights and novel functions inside the cell. *Molecular Immunology* 84, 2–9. doi: 10.1016/j.molimm2017.01.004.
16. Adams N. M., O'Sullivan T. E. Geary C. D., et al. (2016). NK cell responses redefine immunological memory. *Journal of Immunology* 197, 2963–2970.
17. Shi M., Chen X., Ye K., et al. (2016). Application potential of toll-like receptors in cancer immunotherapy. *Medicine* 95, e3951.
18. Gao Y., Xiao M. D., Wang Y., et al. (2017). Association of single-nucleotide polymorphisms in toll-like receptor 2 gene with asthma susceptibility: A meta-analysis. *Medicine* 96, e6822.
19. De Paepe B., Creus K., De Bleecker J. L. (2009). Role of cytokines and chemokines in idiopathic inflammatory myopathies. *Current Opinion in Rheumatology* 21, 610–616.
20. Li J., Jiao Z., Qui H., et al. (2017). C-reactive protein and risk of ovarian cancer: A systematic review & meta-analysis. *Medicine* 96, e7822.
21. Nelson B., Zhou X., White M., et al. (2014). Recombinant human mannose-binding lectin dampens human alveolar macrophage inflammatory responses to influenza A virus in vitro. *Journal of Leukocyte Biology* 95, 7150722.
22. Kouser L., Madhukaran S. P., Shastri A., et al. (2015). Emerging and novel functions of complement protein C1q. *Frontiers in Immunology* 7, 317, doi: 10.3389/fimmu.2015.00317.
23. Stites E., Le Quintrec M., Thurman J. M. (2015). The complement system and antibody-mediated transplant rejection. *Journal of Immunology* 195, 5525–5531.
24. Garred P., Genster N., Pilely K., et al. (2016). A journey through the lectin pathway of complement-MBL and beyond. *Immunological Reviews* 274, 74–97.

25. Guo C., Xie X., Li H., et al. (2015). Prediction of common epitopes on hemagglutinin of the Influenza A virus (H1 subtype). *Experimental & Molecular Pathology* 98, 79–84.
26. Kim J. H., Hu Y., Yongqing T., et al. (2016). CD1a on Langerhans cells controls inflammatory skin disease. *Nature Immunology* 17, 1159–1166.
27. Lucas B., James K. D., Cosway E. J. et al. (2016). Lymphotoxin beta receptor controls T cell progenitor entry to the thymus. *Journal of Immunology* 197, 2665–2672.
28. Zack E. (2014). Emerging therapies for autoimmune disorders. *Journal of Infusion Nursing* 37, 109–119.
29. Brzostek J., Gascoigne N. R. J. (2017). Thymic origins of T cell receptor alloreactivity. *Transplantation* 101, 1535–1541.
30. Cai, J., Terasaki, P. I., Zhu, D., et al. (2016). Complement-fixing antibodies against denatured HLA and MICA antigens are associated with antibody mediated rejection. *Experimental and Molecular Pathology* 100(1), 45–50. doi: 10.1016/j.yexmp.2015.11.023.
31. Irure J., Lopez-Hoyos M., Rodrigo E., et al. Antibody-mediated rejection in kidney transplantation without evidence of anti-HLA antibodies? *Transplantation Proceedings* 48, 2888-2890.
32. Koltsova E. K., Garcia Z., Chodaczek, G., et al. (2012). Dynamic T cell-APC interactions sustain chronic inflammation in atherosclerosis. *Journal of Clinical Investigation* 122, 3114–3126.
33. Yamasaki R., Yabe U., Kataoka C., et al. (2010). The oligosaccharide of gonococcal lipooligosaccharide contains several epitopes that are recognized by human antibodies. *Infection and Immunity* 78, 3247–3257.
34. De la Torre M. C., Palomera E., Serra-Prat M., et al. (2016). IgG2 as an independent risk factor for mortality in patients with community-acquired pneumonia. *Journal of Critical Care* 35, 115–119.
35. Furukawa A., Wisel S. A., Tang Q. (2016). Impact of immune-modulatory drugs on regulatory T cell. *Transplantation* 100, 2288–2300.
36. Bedoui S., Heath W. R. Mueller S. N. (2016). CD4(=) T-cell help amplifies innate signals for primary CD8(+) T-cell immunity. *Immunological Reviews* 272, 52-64.
37. Chen X., Oppenheim J. J. (2014). Th17 and T_{regs}: Unlikely allies. *Journal of Leukocyte Biology* 95, 723–731.
38. Ajjan R. A., Weetman A. P. (2015). The pathogenesis of Hashimoto's thyroiditis: Further developments in our understanding. *Hormone & Metabolic Research* 47, 702–710.
39. Li M., Song L. J., Qin X. Y. (2014). Advances in the cellular immunological pathogenesis of type 1 diabetes. *Journal of Cellular & Molecular Medicine* 18, 749–758.
40. Rubin, L. G., Levin, M. J., Ljungman, P., et al. (2014). 2013 IDSA clinical practice guideline for vaccination of the immunocompromised host. *Clinical Infectious Diseases* 58, 44–100.
41. Holt P. G., Jones C. A. (2000). The development of the immune system during pregnancy and early life. *Allergy* 55, 688–697.
42. Swamy G. K., Beigi R. H. (2015). Maternal benefits of immunization during pregnancy. *Vaccine* 33, 6436–6440.
43. Eliopoulos, C. (2018). *Gerontological nursing* (9th ed.), Philadelphia: Wolters Kluwer.
44. Kyle, T. (2017). Nursing care of the child with an alteration in immunity or immunologic disorder. In *Essentials of pediatric nursing* (3rd ed). Philadelphia: Wolters Kluwer.
45. Frieri, M., Kumar, K., Boutin, A. (2016). Biomarkers, trauma, and sepsis in pediatrics: A review. *Journal of Pediatrics Review*, 4(1), e4767. doi: 10.17795/jpr-4767

Disorders of the Immune Response, Including HIV/AIDS

12

Sandeep Gopalakrishnan

DISORDERS OF THE IMMUNE RESPONSE

The human immune system is a complex, multidimensional system designed to protect the host against invasion by foreign substances, microorganisms, and toxins. In addition, it helps to protect against the proliferation of neoplastic cells and plays a key role in the process of inflammation and wound healing. Unfortunately, under certain circumstances, the immune system can become inefficient or hyperactive, causing the development of debilitating and/or life-threatening diseases. These disease processes can take the form of immunodeficiency disorders, allergic or hypersensitivity reactions, transplant rejection, and autoimmune disorders. Regardless of the manifestation, the underlying cause can be traced back to an abnormality to one of the cellular or chemical components of the innate and adaptive immune responses.

IMMUNODEFICIENCY DISORDERS

After completing this section of the chapter, the learner will be able to meet the following objectives:

- Identify the differences between primary and secondary immunodeficiency disorders.
- Compare and contrast the pathology and clinical manifestations of humoral (B-cell), cellular (T-cell), and combined T- and B-cell immunodeficiency disorders.
- Discuss the pathophysiology and clinical manifestations of complement disorders including hereditary angioneurotic edema
- Discuss the pathophysiology of phagocytosis disorders.

Immunodeficiency is defined as an abnormality in one or more parts of the immune system that results in an increased susceptibility to disease states normally eradicated by a properly functioning immune response including infection by invading microorganisms or the development of neoplastic syndromes. Immunodeficiency syndromes can be classified as primary or secondary (acquired later in life). Primary immunodeficiency disorders are either congenital or inherited as sex-linked, autosomal dominant, or autosomal recessive traits. Secondary immunodeficiency disorders develop later in life because of other pathophysiologic states such as malnutrition; disseminated cancers; infection of the cells of the immune system, most notably with human immunodeficiency virus (HIV); and treatment with immunosuppressive drugs, such as chemotherapeutic agents, corticosteroids, or transplant rejection medications. The clinical manifestations and the impact on the client's day-to-day function are dependent upon the specific immunodeficiency disorder and the degree of immune system dysfunction. The various categories of immunodeficiency disorders are summarized in Chart 12.1.

The immune system is made up of two distinct but interrelated systems: the innate and adaptive immune systems. These two systems work in concert to protect the body from infection and disease. The innate immune system is the body's first line of defense against infection. It employs rapid yet nonspecific cellular and chemical responses. These include phagocytic leukocytes (*i.e.*, neutrophils, macrophages); natural killer (NK) cells; chemical mediators, such as chemokines and cytokines; and the complement system. The adaptive immune system differs from the innate immune system in its ability to exhibit "memory" for invading organisms and toxic substances. The adaptive immune response develops more

CHART 12.1 IMMUNODEFICIENCY STATES

Humoral (B-Cell) Immunodeficiency
Primary
X-linked hypogammaglobulinemia
Common variable immunodeficiency
Selective deficiency of IgG, IgA, and IgM
Secondary
Increased loss of immunoglobulin (nephrotic syndrome)

Cellular (T-Cell) Immunodeficiency
Primary
Congenital thymic aplasia (DiGeorge syndrome)
Hyper-IgM syndrome
Secondary
Malignant disease (Hodgkin disease and others)
Transient suppression of T-cell production and function due to acute viral infection
HIV/AIDS

Combined B-Cell and T-Cell Immunodeficiency
Primary
Severe combined immunodeficiency syndrome
X-linked
Autosomal recessive (ADA deficiency, Jak3 deficiency)
Wiskott-Aldrich syndrome
Ataxia–telangiectasia
Combined immunodeficiency syndrome
Secondary
Irradiation
Immune suppression and cytotoxic drugs

Complement System Disorders
Primary
Hereditary deficiency of complement proteins
Hereditary deficiency of C1 inhibitor (angioneurotic edema)
Secondary
Acquired disorders that consume complement factors

Disorders of Phagocytosis
Primary
Chronic granulomatous disease
Chédiak-Higashi syndrome
Secondary
Drug induced (corticosteroid and immunosuppressive therapy)
Diabetes mellitus

slowly but with a great deal of specificity. The T and B lymphocytes of the innate immune system possess the ability to express their receptors (T cells) and produce immunoglobulins (Igs) (B cells) in billions of different combinations, which enables them to target billions of different epitopes, viruses, and microorganisms.

The ability of the adaptive immune system to function effectively is dependent upon the interaction of two distinct but intimately connected mechanisms, the humoral (B cell–mediated) and cell-mediated (T cell–mediated) responses. The humoral immune response relies upon the ability of B lymphocytes to produce antigen-specific Igs and "memory" cells. In contrast, the cell-mediated response relies upon the ability of the T lymphocytes to produce various cytokines, to present antigen to B lymphocytes for destruction, and, in the case of cytotoxic T cells, to kill cells infected with intracellular organisms. It is essential that the cells of the humoral and cell-mediated responses work together in defense against invading microorganism and disease processes. For example, B-lymphocyte activation and subsequent Ig production (*i.e.*, IgG versus IgA) are dependent upon the presence of certain cytokines, which are specifically produced by helper T cells. Conversely, cytotoxic T lymphocytes depend on the presence of specific Igs produced by B cells (plasma cells) in order to destroy virally infected cells and cell-free viral particles before they spread to other cellular targets.

Primary immunodeficiency diseases (PIDDs) are caused by genetic abnormalities of the immune system; this group consists of more than 130 distinct disorders.[1] Recent estimates put the overall prevalence of PIDD in the United States at 1:2000.[2] Approximately 65% of these cases present as a primary antibody deficiency syndrome. The incidence has risen from 2.4 per 100,000 for the years 1976 to 1980 to 10.3 per 100,000 from 2001 to 2006.[1] This increase has been attributed to an increased awareness and, therefore, diagnoses of PIDD, not to an increase in the number of actual new cases.[3] In recent years, there has been an abundance of research conducted in order to identify the genetic and biochemical defects that cause the development of the PIDD. This has led to the development of improved treatments and therapies for people with PIDD decreasing the incidence of life-threatening infections. Most of these disorders are inherited as autosomal recessive traits, several are sex linked and caused by mutations in the X chromosome, and the causes of some have yet to be identified.[3] The root cause of many of the PIDD involves mutations that affect the signaling pathways (*e.g.*, cytokines and cytokine signaling, receptor subunits, and metabolic pathways) that dictate immune cell development and function. Autoimmunity is frequently associated with the PIDD because the ability of the immune system to differentiate self from nonself is also affected.[1,3]

Many PIDD have severely debilitating and life-threatening consequences. Although early detection is possible, pediatricians do not normally conduct regular screening. For infants born with severe combined T- and B-cell immunodeficiency, early diagnosis is essential before the development of severe infections and the administration of live attenuated virus vaccines (*e.g.*, measles, mumps, rubella, varicella, bacillus Calmette-Guérin), which could have devastating and life-threatening consequences.[4] Children with PIDD often present with a history of recurrent, severe infections that are resistant to treatment. In fact, the average age of referral for immune testing after recurrent severe infection is about 6 months of age.[4] The infections frequently involve the respiratory tract and are the result of organisms not traditionally seen in this population. These include recurrent bouts of ear infections, sinus infections, and pneumonia within a 1-year period that are unresponsive to a long course (1 to 2 months) of antibiotics, failure to thrive in infancy, persistent thrush or fungal infections, recurrent skin or organ abscesses, and a positive family history of primary immunodeficiency. Because these disorders are frequently inherited, a positive family history may help in the diagnosis. Areas of the world with high consanguinity (descended from the same ancestor) rates have been shown to have a much higher prevalence rate than that in the general population. In addition, identification of the infectious organism can help in the diagnosis of the specific form of PIDD. Bacterial infections (*Streptococcus pneumoniae* and *Haemophilus influenzae*) are frequently seen cases of antibody deficiency, whereas severe viral, fungal, and opportunistic infections most often characterize T-cell deficiencies.[5,6] Recurrent infections with encapsulated bacteria, particularly *S. pneumoniae*, characterize people with complement deficiencies. Recurrent infections with staphylococcal and other catalase-positive organisms are common in people with disorders primarily affecting phagocytosis.[7] Table 12.1 summarizes types of infections that occur with the different types of primary immunodeficiency disorders.

Humoral (B-Cell) Immunodeficiencies

Humoral immunodeficiencies are primarily associated with B-cell dysfunction and decreased Ig production. Because the B lymphocytes are essential for normal defense against bacterial invasion, people with humoral immunodeficiencies are at increased risk for recurrent infections by *S. pneumoniae*, *H. influenzae*, *Staphylococcus aureus*, and several gram-negative organisms, including *Pseudomonas*.[5,6] Humoral immunity usually is not as important in defending against intracellular bacteria (mycobacteria), fungi, and protozoa, so recurrent infection with these organisms is usual. Because T-cell function is not affected, the body's response to viral infection is normal.

Transient Hypogammaglobulinemia of Infancy

At birth, infants are protected from infection by maternal IgG antibodies that have crossed the placenta during fetal development. They are normally deficient in IgA, IgM, IgD, and IgE because these Igs do not normally cross the placenta. During the first 6 months of life, maternal antibody levels gradually

TABLE 12.1 INFECTIOUS ORGANISMS FREQUENTLY ASSOCIATED WITH MAJOR CATEGORIES OF IMMUNODEFICIENCY DISORDERS

IMMUNODEFICIENCY DISORDER	VIRUSES	BACTERIA	FUNGI	PROTOZOA
B-cell (humoral) immunodeficiency	Enteroviruses, *poliovirus*	*Streptococcus pneumoniae, Staphylococcus aureus, Haemophilus influenzae*	No	*Giardia lamblia*
T-cell (cell-mediated) immunodeficiency	Herpesvirus	*Salmonella typhi*, all mycobacteria	*Candida albicans, Coccidioides immitis, Histoplasma capsulatum, Aspergillus fumigatus*	
Combined T-cell and B-cell immunodeficiency	All	*S. pneumoniae, S. aureus, H. influenzae, Neisseria meningitidis, Mycoplasma hominis*, enteric flora	*C. albicans, Pneumocystis jirovecii* (formerly *carinii*)	*Toxoplasma gondii*
Complement system disorders		*S. pneumoniae, S. aureus, H. influenzae*		
Phagocytosis (neutrophils and monocytes) disorders		*S. aureus*, enteric flora, *P. aeruginosa*, all mycobacteria	*A. fumigatus, C. albicans, Nocardia asteroides*	

Source: Alder R., Kalumuck K. (2013). Immunodeficiency disorders. *Magill's medical guide (online edition)* [serial online]. Available from: Research Starters, Ipswich, MA. Accessed May 4, 2018; Nazi N., Ladomenou F. (2018). Gastrointestinal manifestations of primary immune deficiencies in children. *International Reviews of Immunology*, 37(2), 111–118; Preston R. R., Wilson T. (2013). *Lippincott's illustrated reviews: Physiology*. Philadelphia, PA: Wolters Kluwer; Rhoades R. A., Bell D. R. (2018). *Medical physiology* (5th ed.). Philadelphia, PA: Wolter Kluwers.

decline as the infant's humoral immune system gradually takes over antibody production, reaching adult levels by 1 to 2 years of age.

In infants with transient hypogammaglobulinemia of infancy (THI), there is a reduction in one or more serum Ig levels resulting in recurrent infection.[8,9] Most commonly, infants are deficient in both IgG and IgA, but cases of decreased IgA alone or decreased IgG, IgA, and IgM have been reported. Symptoms of THI usually manifest as maternal IgG antibody levels decline during the first 6 months of life and the infant's immune system is unable to synthesize adequate Ig on its own. The most frequently occurring clinical manifestations include upper respiratory tract infections, lower respiratory tract infections (including pneumonia), allergies, and allergic asthma.[9] Treatment of THI is usually with prophylactic antibiotics, but some evidence exists that intravenous immunoglobulin (IVIG) may play a role in improving quality of life and stopping the cycle of infection often seen in these children.[10] Most cases of THI resolve spontaneously by 3 years of age, but some persist into adolescence and are often associated with other primary immunodeficiency syndromes.

Primary Humoral Immunodeficiency Disorders

Primary immunodeficiency disorders that affect B-cell differentiation and antibody production are the most common and are the result of impaired differentiation and maturation of lymphoid stem cells in the bone marrow. Immature or naive B cells expressing surface IgM (IgM+) leave the bone marrow and migrate into the peripheral lymphoid tissues. After antigen and T-cell stimulation, they undergo "class switching" where they lose surface IgM and express other Ig types such as IgG, IgA, or IgE secreting plasma B cells (Fig. 12.1).[11] Primary humoral immunodeficiency disorders can interrupt the production of one or all of the immunoglobulins at any point along the differentiation and maturation cycle.

X-Linked Agammaglobulinemia. X-linked agammaglobulinemia (XLA) is an inherited, sex-linked, recessive disorder that affects 1 in 250,000 males. XLA is a primary humoral immunodeficiency that is caused by a defect in early B-cell development leading to a severe decrease in the production, maturation, and survival of mature B lymphocytes. The end result is a profound hypogammaglobulinemia and severe susceptibility to infection. Affected males are prone to infections with encapsulated bacteria, such as *S. pneumoniae*, *H. influenzae* type b, *Giardia lamblia*, meningococcus, and various enteroviruses.[12,13]

In 1993, the gene mutation for XLA was found to be on Xq21.3-Xq22, which encodes for an intracellular signaling kinase, named Bruton tyrosine kinase (Btk).[14] Btk is expressed during all stages of B-cell development but has its primary function in early maturation where it plays a role in pre–B cell receptor signaling pathways.[14] The absence of Btk causes an arrest in B-cell development. Mutation in the *Btk* gene results in an absence of mature circulating B cells and plasma cells. T lymphocytes, however, are normal in number and function.

Most boys with XLA are asymptomatic at birth because of the presence of circulating maternal antibodies. Once these levels start to drop, affected males develop

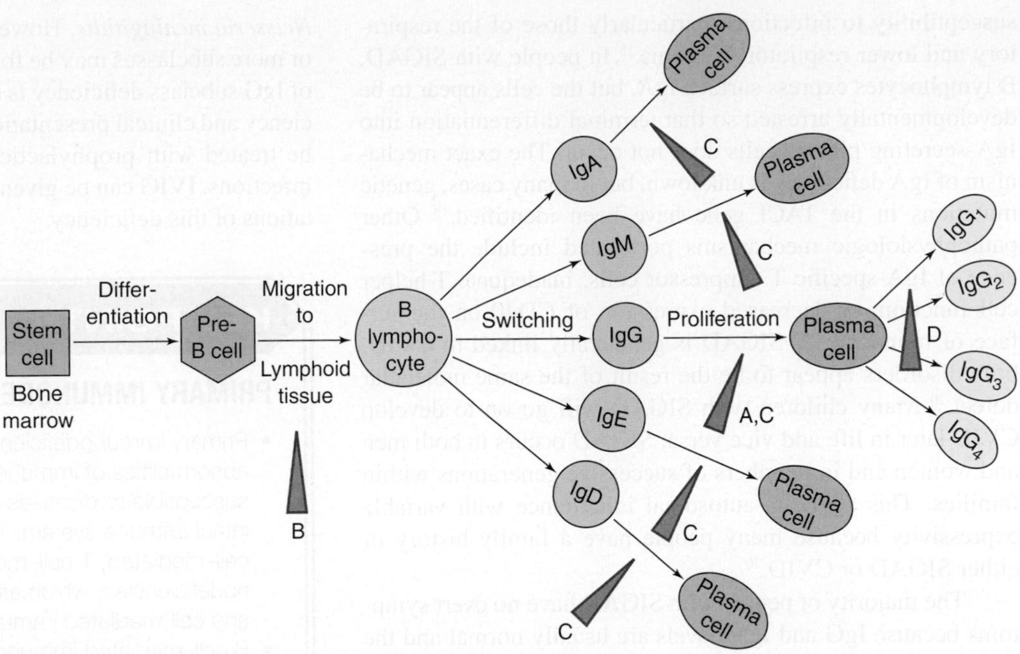

Figure 12.1 • Stem cells to mature Ig-secreting plasma cells. *Arrows* indicate the stage of the maturation process that is interrupted in (*A*) transient hypogammaglobulinemia, (*B*) XLA, (*C*) CVID, and (*D*) IgG subclass deficiency.

life-threatening infections that are unresponsive to antibiotic therapy. Diagnosis is based on demonstration of low or absent serum Igs. Current therapy, which includes chronic administration of IVIG and prophylactic antibiotics, is only partially effective, expensive, and associated with severe long-term complications. New treatments are being tested that utilize gene therapy to promote B-lineage–specific Btk expression; these treatments have had some success.[15]

Common Variable Immunodeficiency. Another form of humoral primary immunodeficiency associated with impaired B-cell differentiation and antibody production is *common variable immunodeficiency* (CVID). All people have low serum IgG levels, but some present with low IgA and/or low IgM as well, resulting in impaired antibody response to specific infections and vaccine challenge.[16] CVID is a heterogeneous disorder, affecting males and females equally, and no one specific gene mutation has been identified. People with this disorder may present with inducible T-cell costimulator (ICOS) deficiency, CD19 deficiency, and polymorphisms of *Escherichia coli* MutS, or transmembrane activator and calcium modulator and cyclophilin ligand interactor (TACI) deficiency result of these mutations is a failure of class switching in naive B cells in the late maturation process.[16] Normally, circulating B cells express surface IgM and IgD and, after antigen and T-cell stimulation in lymphoid tissues, lose these markers and express IgG, IgA, or IgE. Memory B cells will also express the surface marker CD27 or tumor necrosis factor [TNF] receptor subfamily, member 7 (TNFRSF7).[17] Thus, people with CVID have a relatively normal number of nonfunctioning B lymphocytes. CD4 and/or CD8 T lymphocytes are usually not affected, but in many people, overall T-cell counts may be diminished, particularly as a result of loss of $CD4^+$ naive T cells.[17]

Clinical manifestations of CVID can begin at any time of life (from very young to very old) and most commonly include recurrent bacterial and viral infections of the respiratory tract.[16] Autoimmune disease (27%) is frequently seen in people with CVID and is associated with both a reduction in overall T regulatory cell counts and impaired function.[16,17] The most frequently seen autoimmune disorders diagnosed are immune thrombocytopenic purpura and autoimmune hemolytic anemia (AIHA), but cases of aseptic nonerosive seronegative inflammatory arthritis, inflammatory bowel disease, and vasculitis have been reported. Approximately 10% of people will present with a lymphoproliferative disorder at some point in their lives including splenomegaly, lymphadenopathy, interstitial lung disease, and, at its worst, lymphoma, most commonly of the non-Hodgkin type.[17]

Treatment methods for CVID are similar to those used for other primary humoral immunodeficiencies, with IVIG being the mainstay of therapy. Anaphylaxis to IgA in the IVIG has been reported in people with CVID who are deficient in IgA. IgA-depleted IVIG is available, and its use has greatly reduced this risk.

Selective Immunoglobulin A Deficiency. Selective IgA deficiency (SIGAD) is the most common primary immunodeficiency disorder, which was first described in children with ataxia–telangiectasia (AT); the worldwide incidence varies with the ethnic background.[18] The syndrome is characterized by moderate to marked reduction in levels of serum and secretory IgA. In the body, secretory IgA binds to and neutralizes intestinal pathogens and their toxic products, so IgA antibodies are normally not found in the bloodstream unless bacterial flora invasion has occurred. In most cases of SIGAD, clinical manifestations are mild to absent. However, in the fulminant form, the deficiency leads to an increased susceptibility to infections, particularly those of the respiratory and lower respiratory systems.[18] In people with SIGAD, B lymphocytes express surface IgA, but the cells appear to be developmentally arrested so that terminal differentiation into IgA-secreting plasma cells does not occur. The exact mechanism of IgA deficiency is unknown, but in many cases, genetic mutations in the TACI gene have been identified.[19] Other pathophysiologic mechanisms postulated include the presence of IgA-specific T suppressor cells, inadequate T-helper cell function, or decreased expression of CD40 on the surface of monocytes.[19] SIGAD is genetically linked to CVID; both disorders appear to be the result of the same molecular defect.[20] Many children with SIGAD will go on to develop CVID later in life and vice versa. SIGAD occurs in both men and women and in members of successive generations within families. This suggests autosomal inheritance with variable expressivity because many people have a family history of either SIGAD or CVID.[20]

The majority of people with SIGAD have no overt symptoms because IgG and IgM levels are usually normal and the humoral response to infection is usually adequate. At least 50% of affected children overcome the deficiency by the age of 14 years. People with severe deficiencies often experience repeated respiratory and gastrointestinal infections and have an increased incidence of allergy and other autoimmune diseases. In people diagnosed with SIGAD, the frequency of circulating anti-IgA antibodies has been reported to be from 20% to 40%, so anaphylaxis and allergic reactions to blood products are of real concern to practitioners.[20] Therefore, only specially washed erythrocytes from normal donors or erythrocytes from IgA-deficient donors should be used.

There is no definitive treatment available for SIGAD unless there is a concomitant reduction in IgG levels. Administration of IgA Ig is of little benefit because IgA has a short half-life and is normally confined to the mucosal layers. There also is the significant risk of anaphylaxis in people who have circulating anti-IgA present in the bloodstream.

Immunoglobulin G Subclass Deficiency. IgG antibodies can be divided into four subclasses designated as IgG1 through IgG4, based upon their underlying structure and function. People may present with deficiencies in one or more of the IgG subtypes, despite normal levels of overall serum IgG. Deficiencies of IgG1 and IgG2 are most common and are more likely to be associated with low serum IgG levels because they are the major components of IgG antibodies.[21] Most circulating IgG belongs to the IgG1 (70%) and IgG2 (20%) subclasses. In general, antibodies directed against antigenic protein belong to the IgG1 and IgG3 subclasses, whereas antibodies directed against carbohydrate and polysaccharide antigens are primarily of the IgG2 subclass. As a result, people who are deficient in IgG2 subclass antibodies may be at greater risk for development of sinusitis, otitis media, and pneumonia caused by polysaccharide-encapsulated microorganisms such as *S. pneumoniae*, *H. influenzae* type b, and *Neisseria meningitidis*. However, decreased antibodies of one or more subclasses may be found in healthy people. Treatment of IgG subclass deficiency is dependent upon the specific deficiency and clinical presentation. Children with mild forms can be treated with prophylactic antibiotics to prevent repeated infections. IVIG can be given to children with severe manifestations of this deficiency.

KEY POINTS

PRIMARY IMMUNODEFICIENCY DISORDERS

- Primary immunodeficiency disorders are inherited abnormalities of immune function that render a person susceptible to diseases normally prevented by an intact immune system. They can be classified as B cell–mediated, T cell–mediated, or combined immunodeficiencies, which affect all aspects of the humoral and cell-mediated immune response.
- B cell–mediated immunodeficiency disorders affect antibody production and inhibit the ability of the immune system to defend against bacterial infections and toxins that circulate in body fluids (IgM and IgG) or enter the body through the mucosal surface of the respiratory or gastrointestinal tract (IgA).
- T cell–mediated immunodeficiency disorders result from defective expression of the T-cell receptor (TCR) complex, defective cytokine production, and defects in T-cell activation. They impair the ability of the immune system to protect against fungal, protozoan, viral, and intracellular bacterial infections ($CD8^+$ cytotoxic T cells).
- Combined T- and B-cell immunodeficiency disorders affect all aspects of immune system and its function.

Secondary Humoral Immunodeficiency Disorders

There are numerous causes of secondary hypogammaglobulinemia, including malnutrition, burns, gastrointestinal loss, nephrotic syndrome, and malignancy and as a side effect of certain medications.[22] These conditions can result in an increase in Ig loss and/or a decrease in Ig production. For example, nephrotic syndrome is associated with loss of serum IgG as a result of abnormal glomerular filtration and subsequent urinary loss. Serum IgA and IgM remain normal or are slightly elevated because they are large molecular weight molecules that cannot be filtered by the glomerulus.[22] In contrast, several malignancies such as leukemias and lymphomas are associated with antibody deficiencies because they decrease overall antibody production. Many commonly used medications can impair antibody levels by either mechanism and include several of the antiepileptics, antihypertensives, and glucocorticoids. The effects can usually be reversed by withdrawal of the medication.

Cell-Mediated (T-Cell) Immunodeficiencies

Cell-mediated immunodeficiencies are a heterogeneous group of disorders that arise from defects in one or more components of the cell-mediated immune response. Whereas B lymphocytes undergo a definitive path of differentiation that culminates in antibody production, the functions of mature T lymphocytes are immunologically diverse. T lymphocytes are made up of two distinct subpopulations: $CD4^+$ helper T cells and $CD8^+$ cytotoxic T cells. The subpopulations of T lymphocytes work collectively to protect against fungal, protozoan, viral, and intracellular bacterial infections; control malignant cell proliferation; and coordinate the overall immune response. Therefore, defects in different components of the system can result in a wide range of immunologic responses.

Primary Cell-Mediated Immunodeficiency Disorders

Of all the primary immunodeficiencies, the T cell–mediated disorders are considered to be the most severe. Those affected succumb to serious viral, fungal, and opportunistic infections within the first few months of life.[23] The presence of maternal antibodies offers no immunologic advantage against these cell-mediated disorders. Children with the most severe T cell–mediated defects, such as *severe combined immunodeficiency disorder* (SCID), rarely survive beyond infancy or childhood because they are prone to both opportunistic and nonopportunistic infections.[23] Newly identified T-cell defects, such as the X-linked hyper-IgM syndrome, have a more favorable outcome with minimal to no treatment.

Primary T-cell immunodeficiency disorders result from defective expression of the TCR complex, defective cytokine production, and defects in T-cell activation. People are usually diagnosed based upon their clinical presentation and family history. In the most severe types of cell-mediated immunodeficiency, immunologic evaluation reveals reduced numbers of lymphocyte subsets including T, B, and NK cells in peripheral blood smears and a depressed T-cell response to antigen stimulation.[24]

Traditionally, bone marrow transplantation has been the treatment of choice in children with the most severe forms of T-cell immunodeficiency. However, in more recent years, immunologic restoration of the immune system through allogeneic hematopoietic stem cell transplantation (HSCT)[23] and gene therapy[25] is becoming increasingly popular for the treatment of specific T-cell disorders including Wiskott-Aldrich syndrome (WAS), X-linked SCID, and adenosine deaminase (ADA) deficiency. The major risk to recipients of bone marrow and stem cell transplantation is that of graft versus host disease (GVHD).

DiGeorge Syndrome. DiGeorge syndrome or velocardiofacial syndrome is an embryonic developmental defect associated with chromosome 22q11.2 deletion.[26,27] It occurs in approximately 1:4000 births. The incidence of this disorder is increasing because many of those now affected go on to give birth to affected children. The defect is thought to occur before the 12th week of gestation, when the thymus gland, parathyroid gland, and parts of the head, neck, and heart are developing. Children with DiGeorge syndrome present with a wide complex of defects including mild to moderate immunodeficiency resulting from a congenitally absent thymus, cardiac and renal anomalies, palatal abnormalities, hypoparathyroidism, skeletal defects, and developmental delays. The disorder affects both sexes.

The phenotypic expression of the chromosomal abnormality associated with DiGeorge syndrome is extremely variable. Infants born with this defect usually have partial or complete failure of development of the thymus and parathyroid glands and have congenital defects of the head, neck, palate, and heart. In some children, the thymus is not absent but is extremely small and located outside of the mediastinum. In these children, growth and development of the thymus may occur with normal stimulation of the immune system. The facial disorders can include hypertelorism (*i.e.*, increased distance between the eyes); micrognathia (*i.e.*, abnormally small jaw); low-set, posteriorly angulated ears with associated hearing loss; split uvula; a high-arched or cleft palate; and oro- and nasopharyngeal muscle weakness.[27] In the majority of affected children, the palatal defects are associated with poor feeding, impaired speech quality, and delayed speech acquisition. Renal abnormalities affect approximately one third of children with DiGeorge syndrome. Fortunately, renal dysplasia and agenesis are rare consequences requiring immediate dialysis. Hypocalcemia and tetany may develop within 24 hours of birth as a result of absent or hypoplastic parathyroid glands.

The immune system is affected in 75% of children with DiGeorge syndrome as a result of thymic hypoplasia.[27] However, the size of the thymus does correlate directly with circulating T-cell counts because of the presence of a limited number of thymic cells in aberrant locations. As a result, the severity of T-cell dysfunction ranges from no circulating T cells to normal counts. Children with severe T-cell dysfunction are more prone to recurrent or chronic viral, fungal, and intracellular bacterial infections. Impaired helper T-cell function affects antigen presentation to B cells and subsequent antibody production. This phenomenon appears to be limited to children as there is no clinical evidence that adults have an increased risk of infection.

Treatment of DiGeorge syndrome is dependent upon the presenting symptoms. Cardiac anomalies are usually repaired shortly after birth. In children with true thymic aplasia and congenitally absent T cells, a thymus transplant or fully matched T-cell transplant is the treatment of choice to reconstitute T-cell immunity. As with any primary immunodeficiency, autoimmunity is a potential problem. Therefore, precautions must be taken during transplantation or transfusion therapy to prevent GVHD.

X-Linked Immunodeficiency with Hyper-IgM. The hyper-immunoglobulin M (HIGM) syndromes are a heterogeneous group of primary immunodeficiency disorders resulting from defective Ig class switch recombination during B-cell maturation leading to a deficiency in IgG, IgA, and IgE but elevated levels of IgM.[28] This X-linked disorder is found only in males. Under normal conditions, class switch recombination is dependent upon antigen presentation to B-cell receptors, which is mediated through direct T-cell interaction and signaling via the CD40 ligand/CD40 receptor.[29,30] The disorder results from the inability of T cells to signal B cells to undergo isotype switching to IgG and IgA. Thus, they continue to express only the IgM subclass of Igs. In most cases, it is the result of a genetic mutation resulting in a CD40 ligand deficiency. Although the disorder was identified on the basis of an antibody defect, its primary cause is a defect in cell-mediated immunity.

Clinical manifestations of HIGM occur early in life with a median age of onset at less than 12 months.[31] Children usually present with recurrent sinopulmonary infections that may progress to bronchiectasis and pneumonia. In approximately 40% of cases, the presenting symptom is an opportunistic infection such as *Pneumocystis jiroveci* pneumonia (PJP).[32] Unfortunately, these children are at particular risk for the development of autoimmune disorders and malignancies of the biliary tree, intestine, and neuroendocrine system because of defects in CD40 signaling. Treatment is usually with Ig replacement and prophylactic antibiotic treatment.

Secondary Cell-Mediated Immunodeficiency Disorders

Secondary cell-mediated immunodeficiencies are more prevalent than primary deficiencies and are frequently associated with acute viral infections (*e.g.*, measles virus, cytomegalovirus) and with certain malignancies such as Hodgkin disease and other lymphomas. Viral infections frequently impair cell immunity via direct infection of specific T-lymphocyte subpopulations (*e.g.*, helper cells). Lymphotropic viruses such as HIV and human herpesvirus (HSV) type 6 selectively deplete the cell subtype that they invade, resulting in a concomitant loss of immunologic function associated with that subtype. People with malignancies can have impaired T-cell function because of either unregulated proliferation or depletion of a particular cell type. Some cases of T-cell immunodeficiency have no known etiology but are acquired later in life. Idiopathic $CD4^+$ T-cell lymphocytopenia is a rare disorder characterized by a profound and persistent $CD4^+$ T-cell defect that predisposes to the development of severe opportunistic infections in the absence of other immune defects.[33] Regardless of the etiology, people with secondary cell-mediated immune dysfunction may display an increased susceptibility to infections caused by normally harmless pathogens (*i.e.*, opportunistic infections) or may be unable to mount delayed hypersensitivity reactions (*i.e.*, anergy). People with anergy have a diminished or absent reaction to antigen even in the presence of known infection.

Combined T-Cell and B-Cell Immunodeficiencies

Combined T-cell and B-cell lymphocyte disorders manifest with defects in both the humoral and cell-mediated immune responses. Collectively, these disorders are known as combined immunodeficiency syndrome (CIDS), but they are a diverse group caused by mutations in a multitude of genes that influence lymphocyte development or response, including lymphocyte receptors, cytokines, or major histocompatibility complex (MHC) antigens, that could lead to combined immunodeficiency. The end result is a disruption in the communication pathways between the cells of the humoral and cell-mediated immune systems and failure of the adaptive immune response. The spectrum of disease resulting from combined immunodeficiency disorders (CIDs) ranges from mild to severe to, ultimately, fatal forms.

Severe Combined Immunodeficiency Disorders

SCIDs are a group of genetically diverse disorders characterized by profound deficiencies of T and B lymphocytes, and in some forms NK, with the subsequent loss of both humoral and cellular immunities.[23] The reported incidence of SCIDs is 1:100,000 live births, and they collectively account for approximately 20% of primary immunodeficiency disorders.[34] Affected infants are lymphophenic and lack T cells, which normally constitute 70% of the total circulating lymphocytes. They have a disease course that resembles that of acquired immunodeficiency syndrome (AIDS), with failure to thrive, chronic diarrhea, and the development of severe opportunistic infections. SCID is usually fatal within the first 2 years of life unless reconstitution of the immune system through bone marrow or HSCT can be accomplished. Early diagnosis is essential because the chances of successful treatment are better in infants who have not experienced severe opportunistic infections.[34] Therefore, pediatricians and neonatologists are now advocating screening for SCIDs. Early receipt of HSCT is associated with the greatest degree of long-term success.[35] Enzyme replacement therapy and gene therapy are being investigated and have been met with some success in children with certain SCID subtypes.[36,37]

To date, 13 different mutations have been linked to SCID. X-linked mutations account for almost 45% of all cases as a result of defects in the common gamma chain of the cytokine receptor.[29] Mutations inherited as autosomal recessive traits account for the majority of the remaining cases of SCID including mutations in the genes that code for ADA gene, Janus kinase 3 (JAK3) gene, the α chain of the interleukin-7 receptor (IL-7Rα chain [also known as CD127]), and recombination-activating genes 1 and 2 (RAG1 and RAG2).[34]. Many of these mutations result in defects that impair T-cell maturation including defects in cytokine receptor control of T-cell differentiation, antigen gene receptor arrangement on T and B cells, or any other component of T-cell antigen receptor function necessary for normal T-cell development.

The most common form of SCID is X-linked and is therefore more prevalent in males. It is caused by a genetic mutation in interleukin (IL)-2 receptor gamma chain (IL-2Rγ) gene that codes for the common gamma-chain subunit (γc) of cytokine receptors.[29] This transmembrane receptor is a shared element of several IL receptors, including the IL-7 receptor, which is responsible for proliferation of T-lymphocyte precursors. Impaired receptor function results in defective T-lymphocyte differentiation and production. Although the B-cell production is unaffected, antibody production is impaired because of a lack of T-cell help.

ADA deficiency SCID is one of the most common forms of SCID inherited as an autosomal recessive trait. It accounts for 15% to 20% of all SCID cases, with reported prevalence rates ranging from 1:375,000 to 1:660,000 live births.[30] ADA is a key enzyme in the purine pathway that catalyzes the irreversible deamination of adenosine and deoxyadenosine. Defects in the ADA gene cause an accumulation or toxic purine metabolites in the plasma and ultimate destruction of T cells. Soon after birth, infants present with profound lymphopenia (total count <500/mm),[3] an absence of cell-mediated and humoral immunity, recurrent infections, and failure to thrive. The systemic accumulation of toxic purine metabolites causes other end-organ effects in the lung, musculoskeletal and central nervous systems (CNSs), the gastrointestinal tract, and the liver.[30] Bone marrow transplantation from an HLA-identical sibling donor is the treatment of choice for children with ADA-SCID but is feasible in only a minority of cases. Enzyme replacement therapy with pegylated bovine (PEG-ADA) has been proven to be effective in approximately 70% to 80% of people but is frequently associated with incomplete immunologic reconstitution because many people develop anti-ADA antibodies.[38]

The other less common causes of SCID are due to recombinase-activating gene (RAG) deficiencies, JAK3 deficiency, and mutations that impair the expression of class II MHC molecules.[38] Defects in RAG activity are the result of mutations encoded on chromosome 11p13 and impair the somatic gene rearrangements necessary for the somatic rearrangement of antigen receptors on T and B cells.[39] JAK3 is essential for signal transduction through the common γc. This is similar to the defect in X-linked SCID, and therefore, the two disorders share many of the same underlying molecular defects. MHC II defects prevent the development of normal CD4$^+$ helper T cells.

Combined Immunodeficiency Disorders

CIDs are less severe than those categorized as SCIDs because they present with diminished, rather than absent, T-cell function and B-cell antibody production. Like SCID, the CIDs are a heterogeneous group of disorders with diverse genetic causes. They are often associated with other disorders such as AT and WAS.[39]

Like all primary immunodeficiencies, children with CID are prone to development of recurrent infections including pulmonary, skin, and urinary tract infections. They also have a higher incidence of chronic diarrhea and other gastrointestinal disorders, as well as gram-negative sepsis. Although they usually survive longer than do children with SCID, without treatment, they fail to thrive and often have a shortened life span.

Ataxia–Telangiectasia. AT is a rare autosomal recessive disorder caused by a gene mutation (ATM, ataxia–telangiectasia mutated) mapped to chromosome 11q22-23 with a worldwide prevalence estimated to be between 1 in 40,000 and 1 in 100,000 live births.[40] ATM is a large serine/threonine kinase that is involved in the cellular response to breakage in the double strand of the DNA helix. It is a complex, multisystem disorder characterized by neurodegeneration, primarily of the cerebellum, and oculocutaneous telangiectasia. Ataxia is the predominant neurodegenerative feature, which usually goes undiagnosed until the child begins to walk. It is associated with immune deficiencies including lymphopenia, hypogammaglobulinemia, and cell-mediated immune dysfunction that result in recurrent sinopulmonary infections. People with this disorder have an increased risk of cancer and radiation sensitivity. The most common malignancies that occur with this condition are lymphoid in origin, but solid tumors of the kidney (Wilms tumor) are frequently reported.[40]

Cognitive development is normal early in the disease process but levels off during childhood and ceases by 10 years of age. Children with AT have deficiencies of both cellular and humoral immunity. Overall, lymphocyte counts are decreased, and there is a decrease in the ratio of CD4$^+$ helper T cells to CD8$^+$ suppressor T cells as well. Current research indicates that the primary defect in T-cell function is quantitative, not qualitative, because the existing T lymphocytes appear to be functionally intact. The majority of people display Ig deficiencies in IgA, IgE, and IgG, with the IgG2 and IgG4 subclasses being most affected. Ninety-five percent of all affected children demonstrate elevated serum α-fetoprotein (AFP) levels.[40]

Wiskott-Aldrich Syndrome. WAS is a severe, rare, and complex X-linked disorder characterized by the triad of thrombocytopenia, recurrent infections, and eczema, with an increased risk for the development of autoimmune disorders and lymphomas. The syndrome affects approximately one to four cases per 1,000,000 live male births and is caused by mutations in the WAS gene.[41] For children lacking WAS protein (WASp) expression, life expectancy is approximately 15 years. WASp is a key regulator of actin assembly in all hematopoietic cells (including platelets) in response to signals arising at the cell membrane. Hemorrhage, ranging from mild to life threatening, is common and occurs in over 80% of cases. Abnormalities of humoral immunity include decreased serum levels of IgM and markedly elevated serum IgA and IgE concentrations. This may be due to loss of T cell–mediated stimulation and an intrinsic inability of B cells to produce antibodies to T-independent polysaccharide antigens. T-cell dysfunction is initially limited but increases over time resulting in greater susceptibility to infection and the development of malignancies of the mononuclear phagocytic system, including Hodgkin lymphoma and leukemia.[41,42]

Management of people with WAS focuses on treatment of eczema, control of infections, and management of bleeding episodes. Currently, the only definitive treatment is allogenic HSC transplantation, but this is associated with considerable risk of complications including death and transplant rejection. HSC gene therapy is emerging as a promising therapeutic strategy because WASp expression is confined to hematopoietic cells. In clinical trials, people infused with autologous $CD34^+$ cells transduced with WASp-expressing retrovirus have demonstrated immunologic reconstitution.[43]

Disorders of the Complement System

The complement system is an integral part of the innate immune response and essential to the integrity of the immune system, including the adaptive immune response. Activation of the complement system occurs via one of three ways: the classic, lectin-mediated, or alternative pathways. Regardless of the pathway, activation of the complement system promotes chemotaxis, opsonization, and phagocytosis of invasive pathogens and bacteriolysis. Alterations in any component of the complement system can lead to enhanced susceptibility to infectious diseases and to the development of a host of autoimmune processes.

Primary Disorders of the Complement System

Primary disorders of the complement system can be transmitted as autosomal recessive, autosomal dominant, or autosomal codominant traits. In the case of codominance, heterozygotes usually have one functioning gene, and complement levels in most cases are sufficient to prevent disease. The majority of disorders associated with the complement system are the result of inappropriate activation and regulation of complement proteins, not necessarily deficiencies of complement proteins themselves.[44] In fact, protein deficiencies of the classical and alternative pathways are rarely seen. Protein deficiencies of the lectin pathway, although more common, are not a major cause of primary complement disorders.

Primary disorders of the complement system can involve one or more proteins, receptors, and/or control molecules at any point along the complement cascade. However, the clinical presentation is dependent upon the component affected. For example, defects in the classical pathway result in an increased of autoimmunity and infection with high-grade pathogens, whereas defects in the lectin pathway are associated with an increased risk of infection from unusual pathogens such as *Cryptosporidium* and *Aspergillus*.[45] Because all three pathways converge at the activation of C3, defects that impact C3 or late-acting proteins affect activation of complement by all three pathways and are associated with marked increases in infection with high-grade pathogens, including *Neisseria gonorrhoeae* and *N. meningitides* infection, hemolytic uremic syndrome, and adult-onset macular degeneration.[46]

It is now known that the complement system plays a key role in the control of the adaptive immune response. Subjects deficient in complement proteins frequently have significant defects in the adaptive immune response. C1q, C3, and C4 deficiencies are associated with a diminished immune response especially to T cell–dependent antigens.[45] In addition, they have poor germinal center activity and poor immunologic memory. In the C1 subunit, C1q is essential for the binding of immune complexes and apoptotic cells, promoting their eventual removal from the circulation.[44] These people, therefore, have an increased risk of infection from encapsulated bacteria, particularly *S. pneumoniae*. In addition, they are at increased risk for the development of autoimmune disease processes, particularly systemic lupus erythematosus (SLE) and other forms of vasculitis.

Defects in the lectin pathway have just recently been defined to involve the essential protein mannose-binding lectin (MBL). MBL does not require antibody presentation for activation, as does C1 in the classic pathway. MBL possesses a central core and radiating arms with an intertwined, chained collagen structure capable of binding bacterial surface polysaccharides. A single-gene defect that is carried as an autosomal dominant trait results in improper winding of the MBL molecule and abnormally low plasma concentrations (<2 μg/mL).[44]

The majority of the complement disorders are the result of defects in complement control receptors and molecules. Because tight regulation of C3 is essential to prevent host tissue damage, a host of substances and receptors play a role in the process. Deficiency or improper activation can cause significant disease despite normal circulating complement protein levels. Under normal circumstances, the binding of C3b to a target serves two functions, continuation of the complement cascade and opsonization. Factor H and factor I are essential for the inactivation of C3b in the plasma and on erythrocytes. Factor H is a cofactor for the cleavage of C3, and complete deficiencies are associated with glomerulonephritis, atypical hemolytic uremic syndrome (aHUS), age-related macular degeneration, and HELLP (hemolytic anemia, elevated liver enzymes, low platelets) syndrome during pregnancy.[47] Factor 1 is a cofactor for the cleavage of both C4 and C3. Complete deficiency is associated with low circulating C3 and opportunistic infection.[48]

Hereditary Angioneurotic Edema. Hereditary angioedema (HAE), a rare, life-threatening complement disorder that affects 1 in 10,000 to 1 in 150,000 persons, results from a quantitative (type I) or qualitative (type II) deficiency of C1-inhibitor (HAE-C1-INH).[49] HAE is inherited as an autosomal dominant trait that causes mutations in the SERPING1 gene located in the q12-q13.1 region of chromosome 11.[50] In the complement system, C1-INH normally inhibits activated C1r and C1s in the classic pathway as well as the early steps in the lectin pathway. It also functions as an inhibitor of the coagulation, fibrinolysis, and kinin-generating pathways through the inactivation of plasma kallikrein and factor XIIa. Deficiencies in C1-INH result in the uncontrolled release of various vasoactive substances that promote vascular permeability. The net result is the development of spontaneous episodes of deep localized tissue swelling in the subcutaneous tissues of the extremities, face, and torso or the submucosal tissues of the upper airway and gastrointestinal tracts.[50]

Laryngeal edema is a life-threatening manifestation that can lead to complete airway obstruction and death without intervention. Swelling of the structures of the gastrointestinal mucosa is associated with severe nausea, vomiting, and diarrhea. In some people, attacks may be preceded by the development of *erythema marginatum*, a macular, nonpruritic erythematous rash. HAE usually manifests during early childhood and progresses in severity into adolescence. Symptoms usually peak in 1.5 days and then resolve over the same time frame. Management of the disorder involves emergency management in cases of severe airway obstruction including emergency intubation or tracheotomy, C1-INH concentrate, bradykinin receptor B2 antagonists, or kallikrein inhibitor. Preventative treatment usually involves the avoidance of precipitating influences, the administration of attenuated androgens and antifibrinolytics, or C1-INH concentration.[51]

Secondary Disorders of the Complement System

Secondary complement deficiencies occur as a result of rapid activation or turnover of complement components in the face of normal complement levels as seen in immune complex disease. They are also seen in cases of chronic liver disease and malnutrition where complement protein production is negatively impacted. Regardless of the cause, the manifestations of secondary disorders are dependent upon the components of the complement pathways affected.

Disorders of Phagocytosis

The phagocytic system is composed primarily of polymorphonuclear leukocytes (*i.e.*, neutrophils and eosinophils) and mononuclear phagocytes (*i.e.*, circulating monocytes and tissue and fixed macrophages). These cells are primarily responsible for the removal of microorganisms, toxins, and cellular debris from the body. When activated by chemotaxic factors, phagocytic cells migrate to the site of action and envelope the invading microorganisms or foreign substances. In addition, they produce microbicidal substances such as enzymes and metabolic byproducts that kill or ingest pathogens. Following resolution of an infection process, phagocytic cells (*e.g.*, neutrophils) undergo programmed cell death or apoptosis, in order to prevent damage to host cells as a result of exposure to activated microbicidal proteases and chemotaxic substances.[52] A defect in any of these functions or a reduction in the absolute number of available cells can disrupt the ability of phagocytic system to function effectively. People with phagocytic disorders are exquisitely susceptible to bacterial and fungal infections including *Candida*. However, the exact pathogen varies with the particular disease process. As with other alterations in immune function, defects in phagocytosis can be primary or secondary disorders.

Primary Disorders of Phagocytosis

Primary disorders of phagocytosis affect leukocyte adhesion (*e.g.*, leukocyte adhesion deficiency or LAD), microbicidal production and activity (*e.g.*, chronic granulomatous disease [CGD]), and the process of cellular degranulation (*e.g.*, Chédiak-Higashi syndrome [CHS]).

LADs are a group of rare genetic disorders (≤1: 1,000,000 births) that share a common defect in neutrophil adhesion. Currently, three distinct genetic mutations in chromosome 21q22.3 have been linked to the development of LAD. These mutations alter neutrophil CD18 expression resulting in defective chemotaxis, margination, and adherence. In addition, there is a decrease in NK cell and cytotoxic T-cell function.[53] During early stages of an infection, neutrophil adherence to postcapillary endothelium is weak because of rolling selectin interactions. As the immune response mounts, β-integrin interactions strengthen the adherence and allow neutrophils to migrate into surrounding tissues. Clinically relevant defects can occur at any point in this process.

LAD-1 is the most common form of the disorder resulting from deficiencies in the CD18 integrin necessary for surface expression of CD11/CD18. People with LAD-1 typically present with one of two phenotypes, but all present with recurrent, life-threatening bacterial infections and nonhealing ulcers that are often misdiagnosed as ulcerative colitis.[54] People with the most severe forms of the disease have less than 1% of normal CD18, and approximately 75% die before the age of 2 unless they undergo stem cell transplantation. LAD-II results from a defect in fucose metabolism, which is responsible for the absence of fucosylated glycans on cell surface membranes and selectin-mediated adhesion. LAD-III appears to be the result of failed activation of several of the integrins necessary for CD18 expression.[54]

CGD is one of the most common forms of primary phagocyte dysfunction affecting approximately 1: 200,000 births. It results in an increased susceptibility to both bacterial and fungal infections as well as the development of granulomatous lesions. CGD is characterized by defects in microbicidal oxidant production, specifically the superoxide-generating phagocyte oxidases known as *phox* that render affected individuals unable to phagocytize microorganisms. Six different subunits derived from nicotinamide adenine dinucleotide phosphate (NADPH) complex make up the *phox* oxidase molecule.[55] Each is found separately in the cytoplasm or in membrane vesicles in resting neutrophils. Upon neutrophil stimulation, these subunits normally come together to form active oxidases at the phagosome membranes, creating an intracellular environment capable of killing ingested microbes. In people with CGD, mutations exist in the genes that encode for essential components of the *phox* subunits that result in the production of inactive *phox*. Four different genetic forms of CGD exist with 75% of cases inherited as an X-linked trait (mutations is the $gp91^{phox}$ subunit).[56] Therefore, the majority of cases are diagnosed in males.

Children with CGD are subject to chronic and acute infections including pneumonia, subcutaneous and organ abscesses, cellulitis, osteomyelitis, sepsis, and suppurative adenitis despite aggressive prophylactic and therapeutic antibiotic therapy.[57] These infections usually begin during the first 2 years of life. A wide range of fungi and bacteria are responsible for the infections including *S. aureus*, *Burkholderia cepacia*, *Burkholderia pseudomallei*, *Serratia marcescens*, *Escherichia coli*, *Candida albicans*, *Granulibacter bethesdensis*, and *Aspergillus* species. Chronic infection and inflammation result in the development of fibrotic granulomatous masses that may eventually require surgical excision or that cause end-organ damage. Cognitive defects are also associated with CGD, but the exact mechanism is unknown. Bone marrow transplantation is the only known cure for CGD. Supportive care includes the use of recombinant interferon-gamma and prophylactic antibiotic therapy.[56,57]

CHS is a rare (<500 cases) autosomal recessive disorder characterized by severe immunodeficiency, increased susceptibility to infection, bleeding tendency, partial oculocutaneous albinism, and progressive neurologic dysfunction.[58] Abnormally large, dysfunctional granules are readily seen in blood and bone marrow granulocytes and other cells including melanocytes, fibroblasts, endothelial cells, Schwann cells, and neurons. CHS is caused by mutations in a single gene located on chromosome 1q42-43, which encodes for the lysosomal trafficking regulator (LYST).[58] Affected cells exhibit defective chemotaxis, reduced mobilization and microtubular activity, and decreased bactericidal activity.

CHS manifests itself during infancy and early childhood, and few people survive into their teenage years. Sometime after the initial onset of infection, 50% to 85% of people enter into an "accelerated phase," which is characterized by lymphocytic infiltration of the major organs of the body.[59] Although the organisms responsible for the infections seen in CHS are usually bacterial, the trigger for the accelerated phase appears to be a reaction to a viral infection, probably with the Epstein-Barr virus (EBV). People with CHS are unable to clear the EBV infection, which leads to a state of constant lymphoproliferation, end-organ failure, and death. Prophylactic treatment of CHS is symptomatic and includes antibiotics, but unfortunately does not prevent any of the complications from developing. Allogeneic hematopoietic cell transplantation continues to be the treatment of choice to restore hematologic and immunologic function, but does not prevent or reverse any of the other associated complications.[59]

Secondary Disorders of Phagocytosis

Secondary deficiencies of the phagocytic system can result from a multitude of disorders including leukemia, malnutrition, viral infections, or diabetes mellitus. People with diabetes mellitus are more prone to develop poor phagocytic function because of altered cellular chemotaxis. The exact mechanism of the dysfunction is not known, but it does not appear to be associated with age or the severity of the endocrine disorder. There is some evidence that phagocytic dysfunction is coinherited at a higher rate in people with diabetes. Drugs that impair or prevent inflammation and T-cell function, such as corticosteroids or cyclosporine, also alter phagocytic response through modulation of cytokines.

Stem Cell Transplantation

For most of the primary immunodeficiency disorders, HSCT from allogeneic human leukocyte antigen (HLA)-compatible sibling donors is the treatment of choice because it results in effective immunologic reconstitution and improved survival in approximately 90% of people.[60] However, in less than 20% of cases can HLA compatible (*i.e.*, matched for at least three of the six HLA loci) donors be found. For these people, transplants are performed utilizing mismatched family or matched unrelated donor (MUD) cells.[61] However, a significant fraction of these people go on to develop delayed, suboptimal, or short-term immunologic reconstitution. They are also more prone to complications of HSCT such as GVHD, autoimmunity, chronic inflammation, and persistent infection. This had led to the development of newer therapies that incorporate gene therapy and immunologic preconditioning into the regimen.[62]

Hematopoietic stem cells can be harvested from either the bone marrow or the peripheral blood. However, since the introduction of peripheral blood stem cell transplantation (PBSCT) in 1986, blood cells have replaced bone marrow in approximately 100% of autologous and 75% of allogeneic transplantations.[62] For transplantation to be effective, myeloablative doses of chemotherapy have been traditionally administered in order to completely suppress host bone marrow function. However, recent research has demonstrated impaired long-term immune reconstitution in a significant proportion of these people. It appears that a stable mixed chimerism of donor cells in all lineages, including B and myeloid cells, is essential for long-lasting reconstitution. Newer, nonmyeloablative chemotherapeutic conditioning regimens are designed to make room in the bone marrow for donor cells, without completely wiping out bone marrow function, and are associated with better short-term and long-term survival rates.[60–62]

The introduction of gene therapy has radically changed the face of stem cell transplantation. It has allowed the utilization of genetically altered autologous cells to correct preexisting cellular dysfunction. Retroviral vectors carrying the appropriate genetic code are transduced into peripheral blood cells, which are then transplanted back into the host. Depending upon the genetic vector, these genetically altered cells demonstrate sustained engraftment, with multilineage differentiation, increased cell counts, and improvement in both cellular and humoral functioning, without the risk of GVHD and other autoimmune disorders.[47,49,63]

A third potential source of stem cells is umbilical cord blood. Umbilical cord blood is a rich source of primitive hematopoietic blood that can be collected at the time of delivery. Up to 250 mL of umbilical cord blood can be collected without producing detrimental effects to the mother and newborn. Although reliable engraftment of bone marrow can be achieved in children, it is uncertain whether cord blood contains enough stem cells for effective and sustained engraftment in adult transplant recipients.[64]

IN SUMMARY

The immune response is a complex, multidimensional process that requires coordinated activities of both the innate and adaptive immune systems. Because of its complexity, it is not uncommon for one or more normal processes to become disrupted. An immunodeficiency is defined as an absolute or partial loss of the normal immune response that places a person at risk for the development of infection or malignancy. Disorders of the immune system can be classified as primary or secondary disorders. Primary disorders are inherited, as the underlying genetic defect is present as birth, whereas secondary disorders develop sometime later in life in response to another disease entity or condition. The extent to which any or all of these components are compromised dictates the severity of the immunodeficiency.

Immunodeficiency disorders can affect any component of the cellular or humoral immune response. B-lymphocytic or humoral immunodeficiency disorders can affect all circulating Igs, resulting in agammaglobulinemia, or target a single Ig (*e.g.*, IgA immunodeficiency). Defects in humoral immunity increase the risk of recurrent pyogenic infections but have limited impact on the defense against intracellular bacteria (mycobacteria), fungi, protozoa, and most viruses, except those that cause gastrointestinal infection. T-cell immunity is responsible for protection against fungal, protozoan, viral, and intracellular bacterial infections; for control of malignant cell proliferation; and for the coordination of the overall immune response. T-lymphocyte or cell-mediated immune disorders can present as selective T-cell immunodeficiency states or as combined T- and B-cell immunodeficiency disorders. Children born with SCID present with severe opportunistic infections and have a disease course that resembles AIDS. The majority of these children die before the age of 1 unless immune system reconstitution can be achieved through HSCT.

The complement system and phagocytic cells are integral components of innate immunity and can also be targeted in immunodeficiency disorders. The complement system plays a key role in promoting chemotaxis, opsonization, and phagocytosis of invasive pathogens. Deficiencies in complement proteins, control molecules, or receptors can lead to enhanced susceptibility to infectious diseases and autoimmune disorders, particularly SLE. People with phagocytic disorders are exquisitely susceptible to bacterial and fungal infections including *Candida*; however, the exact pathogen varies with the particular disease process. Primary disorders of phagocytosis include LAD disorders, degranulation abnormalities, and defects in microbicidal activity.

HYPERSENSITIVITY DISORDERS

After completing this section of the chapter, the learner will be able to meet the following objectives:

- Describe the adaptive immune responses that protect against microbial agents and hypersensitivity responses.
- Discuss the immune response involved in the development of type I, type II, type III, and type IV hypersensitivity reactions.
- Describe the pathogenesis of common hypersensitivity reactions including allergic rhinitis, food allergy, serum sickness, Arthus reaction, contact dermatitis, and hypersensitivity pneumonitis.

Activation of the immune system normally results in the mobilization and coordination of T-cell and B-cell activity in order to protect the body from invading microorganisms and toxic substances. Unfortunately, this same system is capable of causing serious damage when it does not function as intended. Hypersensitivity is defined as an abnormal and excessive response of the activated immune system that causes injury and damage to host tissues. Disorders caused by immune responses are collectively referred to as *hypersensitivity reactions*. Hypersensitivity reactions are classified as one of four types: type I, IgE-mediated disorders; type II, antibody-mediated disorders; type III, complement-mediated immune disorders; and type IV, T cell–mediated disorders (Table 12.1). They differ with respect to the specific components of the immune response initiated, the onset of symptoms, and the eventual mechanism of injury.

Type I, Immediate Hypersensitivity Disorders

Type I hypersensitivity reactions are IgE-mediated reactions that develop rapidly upon exposure to an antigen. Type I hypersensitivity reactions represent the classic allergic response, and in this context, antigens are referred to as *allergens*. Environmental, medical, and pharmaceutical allergens are all capable of initiating a type I hypersensitivity reaction. Common allergens encountered include pollen proteins, house dust mites, animal dander, foods, household chemicals, and pharmaceutical agents like the antibiotic penicillin. Exposure to the allergen can be through inhalation, ingestion, injection, or skin contact. Depending on the portal of entry, type I reactions may be localized to a discrete area of the body (*e.g.*, contact dermatitis) or systemic causing significant disease (*e.g.*, asthma) and life-threatening anaphylaxis.[65–67]

Two types of cells play a key role in the development of a type I hypersensitivity reactions: type 2 helper T (T_2H) cells and mast cells or basophils. Two distinct subtypes of helper T cells (T_1H or T_2H) develop from activated $CD4^+$ helper T cells based upon the cytokines expressed by the antigen-presenting cells (APCs) at the site of activation. Macrophages and dendritic cells direct the maturation of $CD4^+$ helper T cells toward the T_1H subtype, whereas mast cells and T cells induce differentiation toward the T_2H subtype. The T_1H cells stimulate the differentiation of B cells into IgM- and IgG-producing plasma cells. The T_2H cells direct B lymphocytes to switch class and produce the IgE antibodies necessary for an allergic or hypersensitivity response. In addition, T_2H cytokines are responsible for the mobilization and activation of mast cells, basophils, and eosinophils, inducing inflammatory responses that are distinct from T_1H reactions.[66]

Mast cells, basophils, and eosinophils are essential to the development of type I hypersensitivity reactions. They are members of the *granulocyte* class of leukocytes because they contain granules rich in chemical mediators such as histamine and heparin. These mediators may be preformed or are enzymatically activated in response to T_2H signaling. Once they are released, they are capable of inducing a wide range of cellular responses. Mast cells and basophils are histologically similar and derived from $CD34^+$ progenitor cells.[68] However, basophils are confined to the bloodstream, and mast cells are distributed throughout the connective tissue, especially in areas beneath the skin and mucous membranes of the respiratory, gastrointestinal, and genitourinary tracts and adjacent to blood and lymph vessels.[68] This places the mast cells in close proximity to surfaces with frequent exposure to allergen. Mast cells in different parts of the body and even in a single site can have significant differences in mediator content and sensitivity to agents that produce mast cell degranulation.

Type I hypersensitivity reactions are dependent upon IgE-mediated activation of mast cells and basophils (Fig. 12.2). During the initial exposure to an antigen, allergen-specific IgE

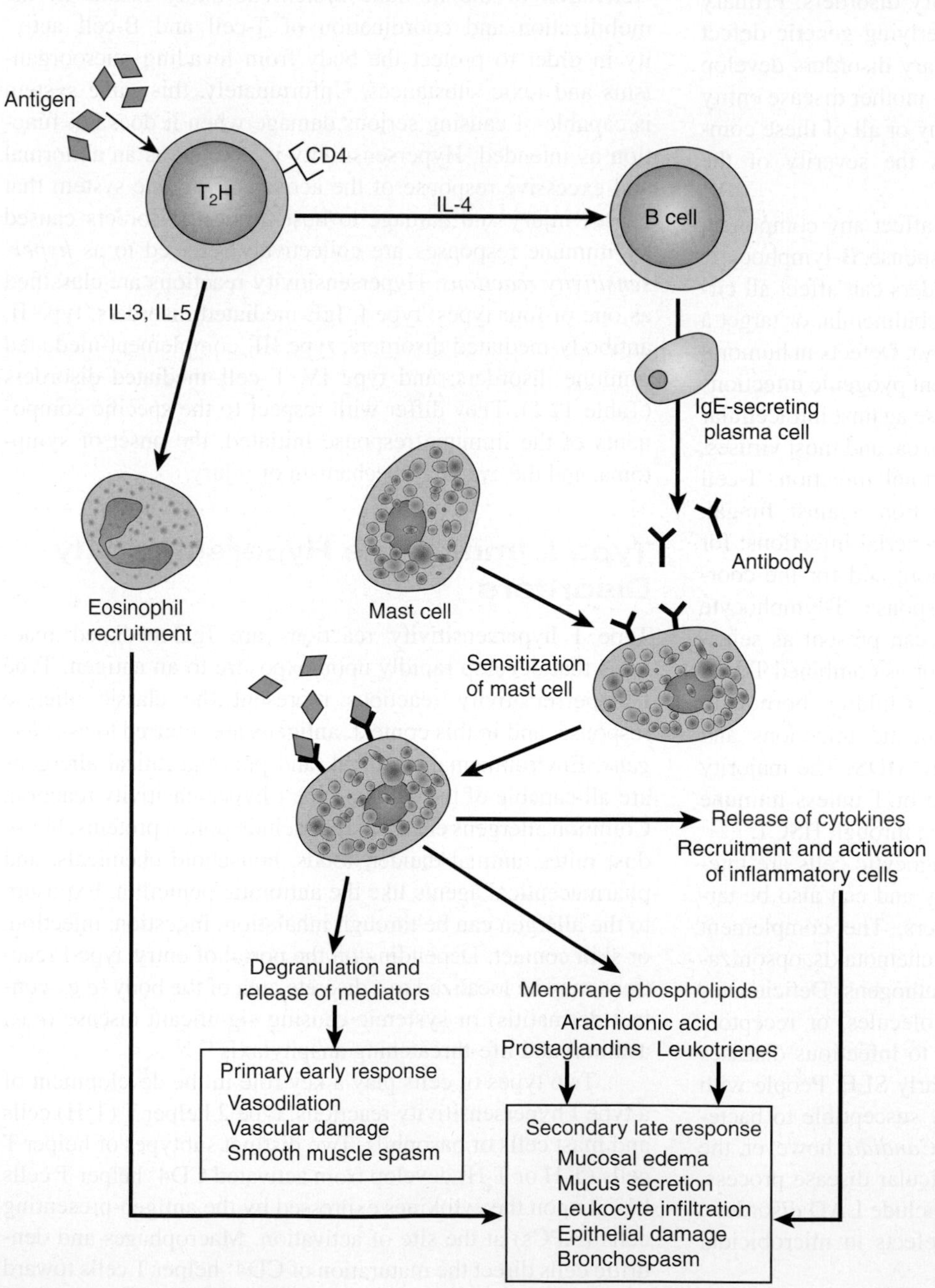

Figure 12.2 • Type I, IgE-mediated hypersensitivity reaction. The stimulation of B-cell differentiation by an antigen-stimulated type 2 helper (T_2H) T cell leads to plasma cell production of IgE and mast cell sensitization. Subsequent binding of the antigen produces degranulation of the sensitized mast cell with release of preformed mediators that leads to a primary or early-phase response. T_2H T-cell recruitment of eosinophils, along with the release of cytokines and membrane phospholipids from the mast cell, leads to a secondary or late-phase response.

is produced as part of the normal humoral response and IgE to the high-affinity IgE receptors known as FcεRI, expressed on the surface of mast cells and basophils.[69,70] In contrast, lymphocytes, eosinophils, and platelets bind IgE via low-affinity FcεRII receptors.[71] On subsequent exposure to an allergen, the multimeric cross-linkages between IgE antibodies are formed creating a bridge between two IgE molecules. When IgE receptors aggregate, they induce a signal transduction that stimulates mast cell degranulation and release of vasoactive chemical mediators, the synthesis and secretion of platelet-activating factor (PAF) and leukotrienes, and the secretion of many growth factors, cytokines, and chemokines.[71]

Most type I hypersensitivity reactions such as bronchial asthma develop in two distinct and well-defined phases: (1) a primary or initial-phase response characterized by vasodilation, vascular leakage, and smooth muscle contraction and (2) a secondary or late-phase response characterized by more intense infiltration of tissues with eosinophils and other acute and chronic inflammatory cells as well as tissue destruction in the form of epithelial cell damage.

The primary or initial-phase response usually begins with 5 to 30 minutes of exposure to an allergen and subsides within 60 minutes. It is mediated by acute mast cell degranulation and the release of preformed and/or enzymatically activated mediators. These mediators include histamine, serotonin, acetylcholine, adenosine, chemotactic mediators, growth factors, and neutral proteases such as chymase and trypsin that lead to generation of kinins. Histamine is the most recognized mediator of type I hypersensitivity reactions. It is a potent vasoactive amine that increases nitric oxide production, relaxes vascular smooth muscle, increases the permeability of capillaries and venules, and causes smooth muscle contraction and bronchial constriction. Acetylcholine mimics many of the actions of histamine and produces bronchial smooth muscle contraction and dilation of small blood vessels via activation of the parasympathetic nervous system. The kinins are a group of potent inflammatory peptides that, once activated through enzymatic modification, produce vasodilation and smooth muscle contraction as well.

The secondary or late phase of the type I hypersensitivity response occurs 2 to 8 hours after resolution of the initial phase and can last for several days. In some cases, the late phase may be significantly prolonged or only partially resolved as in the case of uncontrolled bronchial asthma. It results from the action of lipid mediators and cytokines released from immune cells as part of the normal inflammatory process. The lipid mediators, which are derived from phospholipids found in mast cell membranes, are broken down to form arachidonic acid during the process of mast cell degranulation. Arachidonic acid is then utilized in the synthesis of leukotrienes and prostaglandins, which produce end-organ effects similar to histamine and acetylcholine, except that they have a longer onset and prolonged duration of action. Mast cells also produce cytokines and chemotactic factors that promote migration of eosinophils and leukocytes to the site of allergen exposure, contributing to late-phase response.

It is important to point out that not all IgE-mediated reactions result in hypersensitivity or the development of disease. The IgE-mediated antibody response is a normal part of the immune response to parasitic infection. During the late phase of the response, IgE antibodies are directed against parasite larvae stimulating recruitment of large bodies of inflammatory cells including eosinophils and causing cell-mediated cytotoxicity. This type of type I hypersensitivity reaction is particularly important in developing countries where much of the population is infected with intestinal parasites.

Anaphylactic (Systemic) Reactions

Anaphylaxis is a catastrophic, systemic, life-threatening IgE-mediated hypersensitivity reaction associated with the widespread release of histamine into the systemic circulation that produces massive vasodilation, hypotension, arterial hypoxia, and airway edema.[72] It results from the presence of even minute quantities of allergen that are introduced into the body via the airway, skin, blood, or gastrointestinal mucosa. The level of severity, therefore, depends on the preexisting degree of sensitization and not with the quantity of exposure.

Clinical manifestations occur along a continuum in severity and can be graded on a scale of I to IV.[72] Grade I reactions are usually confined to the cutaneous and mucosal tissues manifesting as erythema and urticaria, with or without angioedema. Grade II reactions progress to include moderate multisystem signs such as hypotension, tachycardia, dyspnea, and gastrointestinal disturbances (*e.g.*, nausea, vomiting, diarrhea, abdominal cramping from mucosal edema). Grade III reactions become life threatening because of the development of bronchospasm, cardiac dysrhythmias, and cardiac collapse. Once a hypersensitivity reaction reaches grade IV, cardiac arrest has occurred, and management is purely resuscitative in nature.

Preventing exposure to potential triggers that cause anaphylaxis is essential because any reaction can be life threatening. All people with potential for anaphylaxis should be advised to wear or carry a medical alert bracelet, necklace, or other identification to inform emergency personnel of the possibility of anaphylaxis. In addition, people with a history of anaphylaxis should be provided with preloaded epinephrine syringes and instructed in their use.

The initial management of anaphylaxis is dependent upon the stage at which a person presents but should always focus on withdrawal of the offending allergen, maintenance of a patent airway, establishment of appropriate intravenous access, volume resuscitation, and administration of epinephrine.[73] It is important to explain to all people with a potential for anaphylaxis that if they have a reaction and self-treat with epinephrine, it is essential for them to seek immediate professional help regardless of their initial response to self-treatment because reactions can reoccur.

Atopic (Local) Reactions

Local hypersensitivity reactions usually occur when the offending allergen is confined to a particular site of exposure.

The term atopy is frequently used to describe these reactions and refers to a genetic predisposition to the development of immediate, type I IgE-mediated hypersensitivity reactions upon exposure to common environmental antigens such as pollens, food, or animal dander. Atopic reactions most commonly manifest as urticarial rash (hives), allergic rhinitis, atopic dermatitis, and bronchial asthma. People prone to atopy frequently develop reactions to more than one environmental allergen with symptoms present at different times throughout the year.

The incidence of immediate hypersensitivity reactions tends to be greater in people with a family history of atopy, yet the genetic basis for these disorders is not completely understood. Because of underlying genetic differences in people with type I hypersensitivity, the exact genome has been difficult to delineate. However, several chromosomal regions have been shown to contain gene sequences linked to the development of asthma and atopy, including the cytokine cluster on chromosome 5q, *interferon-γ* (*IFN-γ*) and STAT6 on 12q, and IL4R on 16p.[74] People with atopic allergic conditions tend to have high total serum and allergen-specific levels of IgE as well as increased numbers of eosinophils, basophils, and mast *cells*. Although the IgE-triggered response is likely a key factor in the pathophysiology of atopic allergic disorders, it is not the only factor and may not be responsible for the development of all forms of atopic dermatitis and asthma.

Allergic Rhinitis. Allergic rhinitis is a common hypersensitivity disorder of the upper respiratory tract that affects between 20% and 40% of the western population. Symptoms include rhinorrhea (runny nose), nasal obstruction, sneezing, nasal itching, and watery eyes (conjunctivitis).[75] The diagnosis of allergic rhinitis is made based upon the person's clinical presentation and a positive skin prick test or the presence of serum-specific IgE antibodies to aeroallergens. People with allergic rhinitis frequently present with other forms of atopy such as allergic asthma and urticaria.[76] Severe attacks may be accompanied by systemic malaise, fatigue, headache, and muscle soreness from sneezing. Fever is absent. The allergens associated with the development of allergic rhinitis are airborne and are therefore deposited directly onto the nasal mucosa. Typical allergens include pollens from ragweed, grasses, trees, and weeds; fungal spores; house dust mites; animal dander; and feathers.

Clinical manifestations are dependent upon the timing and severity of exposure. In people who are chronically exposed to allergens, symptoms can be present throughout the year. This form of atopy is known as *perennial rhinitis*. In contrast, people who present with symptoms only when exposed to high allergen counts, such as in the fall or spring, are said to have *seasonal allergic rhinitis*. Symptoms that become worse at night suggest a household allergen, and symptoms that disappear on weekends suggest occupational exposure.

The allergic response in allergic rhinitis is located specifically in the nasal mucosa. When aeroallergens are inhaled, they are deposited mainly on the nasal mucosa where they are presented to T cells by APCs. In the presence of cellular cytokines, B-cell class switching occurs, resulting in an increase in IgE production.[75,76] Once the allergen–IgE complex is formed, infiltration of the nasal mucosa by T_2H cells, mast cells, basophils, eosinophils, and Langerhans cells takes place, inducing a full cell-mediated immune response.

Treatment of allergic rhinitis focuses on the institution of avoidance measures and control of symptoms. Whenever possible, the offending allergen should be removed from the environment, or exposure should be kept to a minimum. Most symptoms can be controlled with over-the-counter antihistamines and topical nasal decongestants. Tolerance and rebound congestion may occur with chronic administration of topical nasal decongestants, so their use should be limited to less than 1 week. More severe symptoms may require prescription medication including topical nasal corticosteroids (*e.g.*, mometasone or *Nasonex*) and antihistamines (*e.g.*, azelastine HCl). Mast cell stabilizers, such as intranasal cromolyn sodium, that prevent localized mast cell degranulation and release of intracellular mediators may be useful, especially when administered prophylactically. In people whose symptoms cannot be successfully controlled with these measures, a program of desensitization known as immunotherapy ("allergy shots") may be undertaken. Desensitization involves the frequent administration of progressively larger quantities of the offending antigen(s). The antigens stimulate production of high levels of IgG antibodies, which are capable of combining with the antigen and preventing activation of cell-bound IgE antibodies.

Food Allergies. Food allergy is very common in western countries around the world, often manifesting with life-threatening consequences. In fact, food-induced anaphylaxis is the leading cause of emergency room admissions, especially among children.[77] Currently, the prevalence rate of food allergy is between 3% and 6%, and, according to the Centers for Disease Control and Prevention (CDC), this represents an increase of 18% over the past decade.[77,78] The exact etiology of the increase in cases is unknown. Any food is capable of inducing a hypersensitivity reaction in susceptible people, but the most commonly implicated foods include peanuts, tree nuts, and shellfish. In addition, milk is frequently implicated in children.[77,78] People with asthma, adolescents, and those with a personal or family history of food allergy are at increased risk of severe reactions.

The clinical manifestations of food allergy are dependent upon many factors including the amount of food ingested, the presence of an empty stomach, concurrent illness and medication, exercise, and the phase of the menstrual cycle.[77,78] Reactions may differ within a given person during different exposures, but the primary symptoms are seen in the skin, gastrointestinal tract, and respiratory system in approximately 80% of cases. The ability of a specific food to trigger a type I hypersensitivity reaction may be changed during the cooking process because heating can alter (denature) the protein structure of an allergen, so that it is no longer able to trigger the humoral response. Both acute reactions (hives and anaphylaxis) and chronic reactions (asthma, atopic dermatitis, and gastrointestinal disorders) to food allergens can occur.

Anaphylactic reactions to food allergens are common, and the presentation may differ between adults and children. Adults typically present with severe symptoms including cardiovascular collapse, whereas severe abdominal pain, hives, allergic rhinitis, conjunctivitis, and facial flushing are more common in children.[77,78] Within the pediatric population, wheezing and stridor are more common in preschoolers and older children, whereas hives and vomiting are usually seen in infants.[79] The majority of the reactions manifest within 1 hour of exposure, but delayed reactions are possible secondary to delayed absorption of the allergen. A rare form of anaphylaxis associated with food is known as *food-dependent exercise-induced anaphylaxis* (FDEIA). In FDEIA, both exercise and the food allergen are tolerated independently, and symptoms do not occur in the absence of exercise. The pathophysiology is not completely understood but seems to suggest that a pliable state of immunologic tolerance exists in susceptible people. Changes in plasma osmolality and pH, tissue enzyme activity, blood flow distribution, and gastrointestinal permeability may occur during exercise, which result in facilitated allergen recognition and binding.[80,81]

Food allergies can occur at any age but tend to manifest during childhood. The allergic response is activated when a specific food allergen comes in contact with IgE antibody present in the intestinal mucosa and subsequently stimulates local and systemic release of histamine and other cytokines necessary in the allergic response. Carbohydrates, lipids, proteins, or food additives, such as preservatives, colorings, or flavorings, can all serve as potential allergens in the allergic response. Cross-sensitivity to allergens between foods in closely related food groups is common. Therefore, a person can contain common cross-reacting allergens. For example, some people are allergic to all legumes (*i.e.*, beans, peas, and peanuts).

Diagnosis of food allergies is multifaceted and relies upon a careful food history and provocative diet testing. Provocative testing involves the systematic elimination of suspected allergen(s) from the diet for a time to see if the symptoms disappear and then reintroducing the allergens(s) to the diet to determine if the symptoms reappear. Only one food should be tested at a time if definitive diagnosis is sought. Allergen-specific serum IgE levels can also be tested if the risk of provocative food testing is too great.

Treatment of food allergy focuses specifically on the avoidance of the offending allergen. However, this can be difficult, especially in people that are exquisitely sensitive to a particular food protein because foods (processed or fresh) may be contaminated with the protein during handling of the food. Foods that are prepared in the same processing plants that handle tree nuts may be potential allergen sources and, therefore, illicit an allergic response in susceptible people. As a result, warnings are placed on all goods processed in facilities that handle highly allergenic foods. People with severe allergies or a history of anaphylaxis should be educated to carry an EpiPen and to seek emergency care immediately after exposure.

Type II, Antibody-Mediated Disorders

Type II (antibody-mediated) hypersensitivity or *cytotoxic hypersensitivity* reactions are mediated by IgG or IgM antibodies directed against target antigens on specific host cell surfaces or tissues. The antigens may be either intrinsic, inherently part of the host cell, or extrinsic, incorporated into the cell surface upon exposure to a foreign substance or infectious agent. Thus, the tissues that express the target antigens determine the clinical manifestations of type II hypersensitivity reactions. These antigens are known as *tissue-specific antigens*.[82] There are four general mechanisms by which type II hypersensitivity reactions can be propagated, but regardless of the pathway, it is always initiated by the binding of IgG or IgM antibody to tissue-specific antigens. These mechanisms include complement-activated cell destruction, antibody-mediated cell cytotoxicity, complement- and antibody-mediated inflammation, and antibody-dependent modulation of normal cell surface receptors[82] (Fig. 12.3).

Complement-Activated Cell Destruction

The destruction of target cells in type II hypersensitivity reactions can occur as a result of activation of the complement system via the classic pathway. First, formation of the membrane attack complex (MAC) by activation of C5–C9 allows the passage of ions, small molecules, and water into the cell, causing direct lysis of the cell. In addition, IgG and the complement fragment C3b act as opsonins by binding to receptors located on the cell surfaces of macrophages. This process activates the macrophages, which then destroys the target cells by phagocytosis. Thus, activation of the complement system produces a twofold response that culminates in cell destruction.

In people with AIHA, autoantibodies target epitopes located on red blood cells.[83] Erythrocytes coated with these autoantibodies are destroyed by phagocytes in the liver or spleen. Some, but not all, autoantibody types also induce phagocytosis and cell lysis via the complement system. The same process occurs in utero in the development of *erythroblastosis fetalis* or Rh incompatibility. Women who are Rh negative lack RhD antigen on their erythrocytes but produce anti-D antibodies. In the Rh-positive fetus, maternal anti-D antibodies will coat fetal red blood cells containing RhD, allowing them to be removed from the fetal circulation by macrophage- and monocyte-mediated phagocytosis.[84]

Antibody-Dependent Cell Cytotoxicity

Antibody-dependent cell cytotoxicity (ADCC) incorporates components of both the innate and adaptive immune responses in the destruction of target cells but is not dependent upon activation or utilization of complement proteins. Rather, the mechanism relies upon the activity of nonspecific NK cells, but other cells such as macrophages and eosinophils

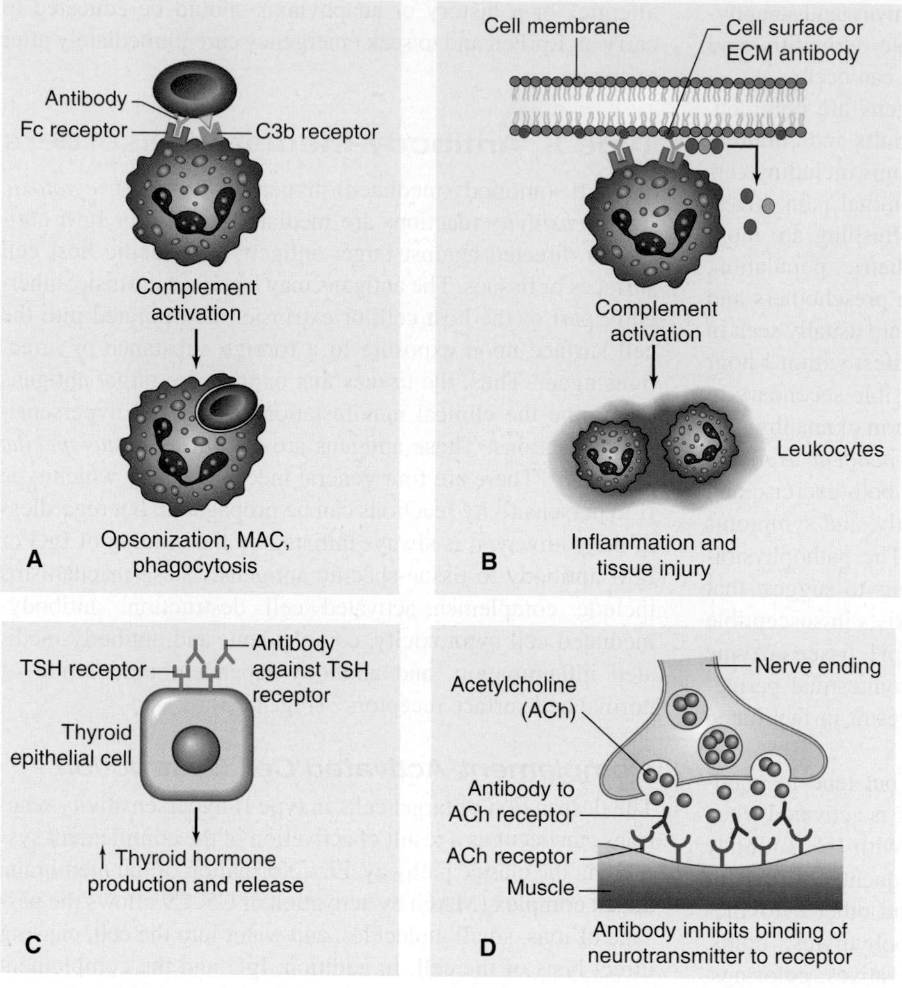

Figure 12.3 • Type II, hypersensitivity reactions result from binding of antibodies to normal or altered surface antigens. **(A)** Opsonization and complement- or antibody receptor–mediated phagocytosis or cell lysis through membrane attack complex (MAC). **(B)** Complement- and antibody receptor–mediated inflammation resulting from recruitment and activation of inflammation-producing leukocytes (neutrophils and monocytes). **(C)** Antibody-mediated cellular dysfunction, in which antibody against the TSH receptor increases thyroid hormone production and **(D)** antibody to acetylcholine receptor inhibits receptor binding of the neurotransmitter in myasthenia gravis.

have been implicated. The Fc fragment of the IgG antibody binds to Fc receptor (FcγR) on the surface of the effector cell, and the variable fragment binds to the epitope on the target cell surface, causing release of chemotactic substances and destruction of the target cell.[85] ADCC is a common antiviral mechanism. It has been implicated in the development of several autoimmune disorders including *pemphigus vulgaris*.

Complement- and Antibody-Mediated Inflammation

When antigens that are normally expressed on vessel walls or that circulate in the plasma are deposited on the surface of endothelial cells or extracellular tissues, the manifestations are the result of localized inflammation as opposed to cell destruction. The presence of antibody in the tissues activates the complement cascade, resulting in the release of the activated complement proteins C3a and C5a, which in turn attracts neutrophils to the area and stimulates the deposition of complement protein C3b. Neutrophils will bind to the Fc antibody fragment or to C3b, but rather than destroying cells via phagocytosis, they undergo degranulation and release chemical mediators (enzyme and oxidases) involved in the inflammatory response. Antibody-mediated inflammation is responsible for the tissue injury seen in Goodpasture disease, which is characterized by the presence of autoantibodies against the α3NC1 domain of collagen IV, an essential protein in the basement membranes of the kidneys and lungs.[86] The antibody-mediated neutrophil activation causes the development of glomerulonephritis, acute renal failure, and hemorrhagic lung disease if immunosuppressive therapy is not initiated.

Antibody-Mediated Cellular Dysfunction

In some type II reactions, the binding of antibody to specific target cell receptors causes the cell to malfunction in some way, rather than initiating the process of cell destruction. The antibody–receptor complex that is formed modulates the function of the receptor by preventing or enhancing interactions with normal ligands, by replacing ligand and directly stimulating receptors, or by destroying the receptor entirely. The symptoms of type II hypersensitivity reactions caused by antibody-mediated cellular dysfunction are dependent upon the specific receptor(s) that are targeted. In Graves disease, autoantibodies, known as *thyrotropin-binding inhibitory Ig*, bind to and activate thyroid-stimulating hormone (TSH) receptors on thyroid cells, stimulating thyroxine production and the development of hyperthyroidism.[87] In contrast, in myasthenia gravis, autoantibodies are directed toward the nicotinic acetylcholine receptors located on the motor end plates within the neuromuscular junction, where they block the action of acetylcholine and stimulate the destruction of the receptors, leading to decreased neuromuscular function.[88]

KEY POINTS

ALLERGIC AND HYPERSENSITIVITY DISORDERS

- Type I hypersensitivity reactions are dependent upon IgE-mediated activation of mast cells and basophils and the subsequent release of chemical mediators of the inflammatory response.
- Type II (antibody-mediated) hypersensitivity or *cytotoxic hypersensitivity* reactions are mediated by IgG or IgM antibodies directed against target antigens on specific host cell surfaces or tissues and result in complement-mediated phagocytosis and cellular injury.
- Type III (immune complex) hypersensitivity is caused by the formation of antigen–antibody immune complexes in the bloodstream, which are subsequently deposited in vascular epithelium or extravascular tissues and which activate the complement system and induce a massive inflammatory response.
- Type IV (cell-mediated) hypersensitivity involves tissue damage in which cell-mediated immune responses with sensitized T lymphocytes cause cell and tissue injury. Although all are T cell mediated, the pathophysiologic mechanisms and sensitized T-cell populations involved differ.

Type III, Immune Complex–Mediated Disorders

Immune complex allergic disorders are caused by the formation of antigen–antibody immune complexes in the bloodstream, which are later deposited in vascular epithelium or extravascular tissues (Fig. 12.4). The deposition of these complexes in the tissues activates the complement system and induces a massive inflammatory response. Like type II hypersensitivity reactions, IgG and IgM antibodies activate immune complex–mediated disorders. However, in type III reactions, the antibody–antigen complexes are formed first in the plasma and then deposited in the tissues. The clinical manifestations may therefore have little to do with the particular antigenic target but rather with the site of immune complex deposition. Immune complexes formed in the circulation can produce damage in any end-organ vessels including those feeding the renal glomerulus, skin, lung, and joint synovium. They can be generalized if the immune complexes are deposited in many organs or localized to a particular organ, such as the kidney, joints, or small blood vessels of the skin. Once deposited, the immune complexes elicit an inflammatory response by activating complement and generating chemotactic factors that recruit neutrophils and other cells of the inflammatory response. The activation of these inflammatory cells by immune complexes and complement, accompanied by the release of potent inflammatory mediators, is directly responsible for the injury. Type III reactions are responsible for the vasculitis seen in many autoimmune diseases including *SLE* and acute glomerulonephritis.

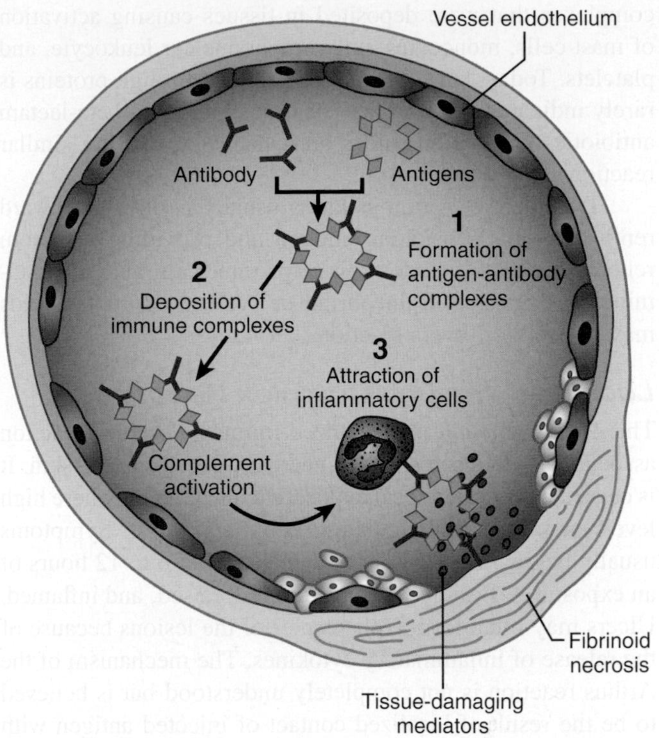

Figure 12.4 • Type III, immune complex reactions involving complement-activating IgG or IgM Igs with (*1*) formation of blood-borne immune complexes that are (*2*) deposited in tissues. Complement activation at the site of immune complex deposition (*3*) leads to attraction of leukocytes that are responsible for vessel and tissue injury.

Systemic Immune Complex Disorders

Serum sickness is a clinical syndrome that results from the formation of insoluble antigen–antibody immune complexes in the presence of antigen excess and subsequent generalized deposition in target tissues such as blood vessels, joints, and the heart and kidneys. The deposited immune complexes activate the complement cascade, increase vascular permeability, and stimulate the recruitment of phagocytic cells. The net result is generalized tissue damage and edema. Clinical manifestations include rash, fever, generalized lymphadenopathy, and arthralgias, which usually begin approximately 1 to 2 weeks after the initial antigen exposure and subside upon withdrawal of the offending agent. In previously sensitized people, severe and life-threatening reactions have been reported. Serum sickness was first described in people receiving foreign serum, such as horse serum, for the treatment of diphtheria and scarlet fever. This antigen load was capable of stimulating the production of large quantities of immune complexes that were deposited in tissues causing activation of mast cells, monocytes, polymorphonuclear leukocyte, and platelets. Today, large volume injection of foreign proteins is rarely indicated, but a variety of drugs including beta-lactam antibiotics and sulfonamides are capable of causing similar reactions.[89]

Treatment of serum sickness usually is directed toward removal of the sensitizing antigen and providing symptom relief. This may include aspirin for joint pain and antihistamines for pruritus. Epinephrine or systemic corticosteroids may be used for severe reactions.

Localized Immune Complex Reactions

The *Arthus reaction* is a localized immune complex reaction associated with discrete tissue necrosis, usually in the skin. It is caused by repeated local exposure to an antigen, where high levels of preformed circulating antibodies exist. Symptoms usually begin within 1 hour and peak within 6 to 12 hours of an exposure.[79] Lesions are typically red, raised, and inflamed. Ulcers may often form at the center of the lesions because of the release of inflammatory cytokines. The mechanism of the Arthus reaction is not completely understood but is believed to be the result of localized contact of injected antigen with circulating IgG antibody. This reaction is the prototypical model for the development of localized vasculitis associated with certain drug reactions in humans.

Type IV, Cell-Mediated Hypersensitivity Disorders

Type IV hypersensitivity reactions differ from type I to III hypersensitivity reactions in that they are cell-mediated and delayed, rather than antibody-mediated and immediate immune responses (Fig. 12.5). The cell-mediated immune response is normally the principal mechanism of defense against a variety of microorganisms, including intracellular pathogens such as *Mycobacterium tuberculosis* and viruses, as well as extracellular agents such as fungi, protozoa, and parasites. However, it can cause cell death and tissue injury in sensitized people in response to topically administered chemical antigens (contact dermatitis) and systemic antigen exposure or as part of the autoimmune process.

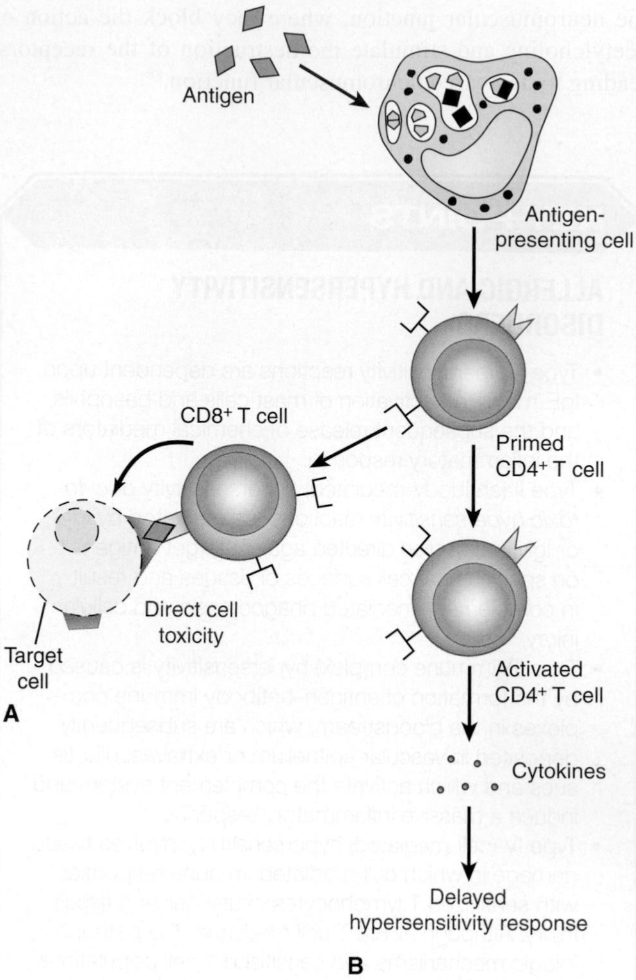

Figure 12.5 • Type IV, cell-mediated hypersensitivity reactions, which include (**A**) direct cell-mediated cytotoxicity in which $CD8^+$ T cells kill the antigen-bearing target cells and (**B**) delayed-type hypersensitivity reactions in which presensitized $CD4^+$ cells release cell-damaging cytokines.

Type IV hypersensitivity reactions are composed of a spectrum of disorders that range from mild to severe in clinical presentation. Although all are T cell mediated, the pathophysiologic mechanisms and sensitized T-cell populations involved differ. Because of the heterogeneity of delayed hypersensitivity reactions, current immunology experts subdivide type IV reactions into four distinct subtypes (IVa, IVb, IVc, and IVd) based upon the immune response, T-cell population, and pathologic characteristics involved.[90] In addition, depending upon the reaction, different T-cell subsets with different cytotoxic and regulatory functions can be activated at different stages of the disease process.

In type IVa hypersensitivity reactions (*e.g.*, eczema), the $CD4^+$-T_1H cells activate monocytes and macrophages through the secretion of large amounts of *IFN-γ*. Activated monocytes stimulate the production of complement-fixing antibodies and activate proinflammatory (*e.g.*, TNF-α and IL-12) and $CD8^+$ responses.[82] Because type IVa responses require the synthesis of effector molecules, they can take up to 24 to 72 hours to develop, which is why they are called "delayed-type" hypersensitivity disorders.

Type IVb and IVd reactions are also considered to be delayed hypersensitivity reactions. Type IVb reactions (*e.g., maculopapular exanthema and bullous exanthema*) are the result of T_2H cell activation and eosinophilic infiltration of the tissues. T_2H cells secrete the cytokines IL-4 and IL-5, which are necessary for activation of mast cell and eosinophilic responses. In addition, these cytokines deactivate macrophages and promote the production of IgE and IgG antibodies by the B lymphocytes. Type IVd reactions are very rare and involve the recruitment and activation of neutrophils by T lymphocytes that specifically secrete IL-8. The only disorder of this subtype is *acute generalized exanthematous pustulosis*

(AGEP), which presents with neutrophil-filled sterile pustules of the skin, fever, and massive leukocytosis.[91]

Type IVc hypersensitivity reactions are cytotoxic responses mediated by $CD4^+$ and $CD8^+$ lymphocytes that secrete perforin and granzyme B.[92] Cytotoxic lymphocytes (CTLs) bind antigen fragments that are displayed on MHC molecules found on the surface of APCs. Peptides derived from cytosolic antigens (*e.g.*, viral) are presented by MHC class I molecules and activate $CD8^+$ T cells, which kill any cell displaying the foreign antigen. Peptides derived from proteins degraded as a result of phagocytic ingestion (*e.g.*, bacteria) are presented on MHC class II molecules, which activate $CD4^+$ T cells. Once activated in this manner, $CD4^+$ T cells can be considered cytotoxic because they can activate other effector cells including cytotoxic $CD8^+$, macrophages, and B lymphocytes.

In viral infections, cell damage is frequently the result of CTL responses rather than cytotoxic effects of the invading organism. While some viruses directly injure infected cells and are said to be cytopathic, other noncytopathic viruses do not. Because CTLs cannot distinguish between cytopathic and noncytopathic viruses, they destroy virtually all cells that are infected regardless of whether or not the virus is dangerous to the cell. In certain forms of hepatitis, for example, the destruction of liver cells is due to the host CTL response and not the virus.

Allergic Contact Dermatitis

Allergic contact dermatitis is a type IV hypersensitivity reaction associated with the activation of T_1H and T-helper lymphocytes. The inflammatory response takes place in two phases, sensitization and elicitation. It is usually confined to sites on the skin that have come in direct contact with a hapten (*e.g.*, cosmetics, hair dyes, metals, topical drugs, plant oils). During the sensitization phase, haptens are captured by dendritic cells, which then migrate to regional lymph nodes and stimulate T-cell production. In addition, local keratinocytes sense haptens and initiate and amplify the local immune response. Reexposure to the specific hapten results in rapid recruitment and activation of memory-specific T cells. The most common form of this condition is the dermatitis that follows an intimate encounter with poison ivy or poison oak antigens, although many other substances can trigger a reaction.

Clinical manifestations of contact dermatitis include an erythematous, papular, and vesicular rash that is associated with intense pruritus and weeping.[93] The affected area often becomes swollen and warm, with exudate formation and crusting. It is not uncommon for a secondary infection to develop. The location of the lesions often provides a clue about the antigen causing the disorder. However, with the same cases of contact dermatitis (*e.g.*, poison ivy), the allergen can be unknowingly spread from one part of the body to another. The severity of the reactions ranges from mild to intense, depending on the person and the allergen. Symptoms usually appear approximately 12 to 24 hours after exposure. Depending on the antigen and the duration of exposure, the reaction may last from days to weeks.

Diagnosis of contact dermatitis is made based upon the characteristics and distribution of the rash as well as the temporal relationship of exposure to the suspected allergen.[93] Patch tests can be performed to confirm the diagnosis. Treatment involves removal of the offending agent followed by application of topical preparations (*e.g.*, ointments, corticosteroid creams) to relieve symptomatic skin lesions and prevent secondary bacterial infections. Severe reactions may require the administration of systemic corticosteroid therapy.

Hypersensitivity Pneumonitis

Hypersensitivity pneumonitis, also known as extrinsic allergic alveolitis, is a form of inflammatory lung disease that results from an exaggerated immune response after exposure to a multitude of inhaled organic particles or related occupational antigens.[94] It was first described by Pepys et al. after exposure to moldy grains and hay and termed "farmer's lung."[95] The offending agent was found to be *Actinomyces*, a bacterium commonly found in moldy foliage. The exact pathophysiologic mechanism of hypersensitivity pneumonitis remains unclear, but evidence supports a role for both type III and type IV immune responses. People demonstrate both high levels of antigen-specific serum IgG levels and combined cellular infiltration and granuloma formation. T_1H cells appear to play a critical role in the development of the disease through the production and release of TNF, IFN-γ, IL-12, and IL-18 in lung tissue.[94] Symptoms, including labored breathing, dry cough, chills and fever, headache, and malaise, usually begin several hours after exposure and subside within hours after the sensitizing antigens are removed. However, long-term sequelae have been reported.

Diagnosis of hypersensitivity pneumonitis is based upon a good history (occupational and otherwise) of exposure to possible antigens. Computed tomography (*CT*) *scan* of the chest demonstrates areas of lobar vascularity and the presence of centrilobular nodules. Removal of the offending agent and administration of oral corticosteroids are the only treatments available.

Latex Allergy

With the institution of universal precautions in the 1980s, the utilization of products containing natural rubber latex increased dramatically. Natural rubber latex is produced from the milky sap of the *Hevea brasiliensis* tree, and at least 13 allergenic proteins have been isolated from it to date, any one of which can illicit an allergic response in susceptible people.[96] In addition, it is a known component of over 40,000 products used in everyday life. As a result, latex allergy has emerged as a significant medical problem in westernized societies. At the peak of latex use in the mid-1990s to late 1990s, 25% to 50% of people with spina bifida or genitourinary anomalies who underwent frequent surgical procedures and 17% of health care workers developed latex allergy as a result of chronic exposure.[96]

Although exposure to natural rubber latex is necessary for sensitization, other factors play a key role in the development of latex allergy. People with a history of atopic reactions, food allergies, and delayed hypersensitivity reactions are more likely to develop an allergic response to latex. The proteins found in latex are found in many naturally occurring substances including tree pollens, avocado, bananas, celery, and pears, so cross-sensitivity is possible. Genetic polymorphisms in over 30 genes located on 15 different chromosomes have been implicated in the development of allergic reaction but have not yet been definitively identified for latex hypersensitivity.[96]

Exposure to latex may occur by a variety of mechanisms including contact with skin and mucous membranes, inhalation, contact with internal tissues, or through intravascular injection. The most severe reactions have resulted from latex proteins coming in contact with the mucous membranes of the mouth, vagina, urethra, or rectum. Children with meningomyelocele and genitourinary anomalies (spina bifida) who undergo frequent examinations and treatments involving the mucosal surface of the bladder or rectum are at particular risk for development of latex allergy.[97] Anaphylactic reactions have been caused by exposure of the internal organs to the surgeon's gloves during surgery.

When natural rubber is processed in the manufacturing of latex-containing products, several accelerants, curing agents, antioxidants, and stabilizers are added to the liquid latex. Because any one of the substances with allergenic potential present in the final latex mixture is capable of triggering an allergic response, it can sometimes makes identification of the offending allergenic agent difficult. To further complicate the picture, when latex gloves are manufactured for use in health care, cornstarch powder is applied to the gloves so they can be more easily put on the hands. Unfortunately, the cornstarch glove powder plays an important role in the allergic response because latex protein particles are readily absorbed by glove powder and can become aerosolized during the application and/or removal of the gloves, causing the development of symptoms in sensitized people. This is especially true in the operating room where high levels of aerosolized latex can be found.

Latex allergy can present as a type I IgE-mediated hypersensitivity reaction, type IV cell-mediated hypersensitivity reaction, or a combination of the two. Frequently, the exact pathophysiologic mechanism is unclear because the activation of the humoral and cell-mediated immune response is so intimately connected.

Type I, IgE-mediated hypersensitivity reactions develop in response to sensitization to one or more of the specific latex proteins. These reactions are immediate and often life threatening, occurring within minutes of exposure. Clinical manifestations range from mild to severe and include urticaria, wheezing, nasal congestion, coryza, rhinoconjunctivitis, bronchospasm, systemic hypotension, anaphylaxis, and cardiovascular collapse.

Type IV hypersensitivity reactions to latex gloves are the most common form of latex allergy seen. In this form of allergy, people usually develop a contact dermatitis to one of the chemical additives rather than the latex proteins within 48 to 96 hours of exposure. The contact dermatitis often affects the dorsum of the hands and is characterized by a vesicular, pruritic rash. When glove contact is continued, the area becomes crusted and thickened. Treatment is with topical corticosteroids during the acute phase and avoidance of all latex-containing products.

Diagnosis of latex allergy is based upon the person's history and the presence of symptoms after exposure to latex-containing products. Because many of the reported reactions to latex gloves are the result of a nonimmunologic, irritant dermatitis, it is important to differentiate between nonallergic and allergic skin reactions.[97] Definitive diagnosis is made through skin prick testing or intradermal injection of allergen and confirmed through latex-specific serum IgE immunoassays. In people with negative immunoassays, a contact test may be performed if the history is compelling as false negatives can occur. Regardless of the technique utilized, all equipment and drugs necessary to treat anaphylaxis must be readily available.[98]

Treatment of latex allergy consists mainly of avoidance measures and requires a great deal of education directed toward the latex-sensitive person and his/her family. People with known latex allergy should avoid contact with any product suspected of containing latex until verified by the manufacturer. All surgical and medical procedures on people with latex allergy should be carried out in a latex-free environment. People with severe type I IgE-mediated hypersensitivity reactions should be instructed to obtain and wear a medic alert bracelet or necklace. Health care workers with severe and life-threatening allergy may be forced to change employment. If type I reactions occur, they are treated with epinephrine, antihistamines (H1 and H2 blockers), and systemic corticosteroids in order to maintain airway patency and restore hemodynamic stability.[97]

IN SUMMARY

Hypersensitivity reactions are exaggerated immunologic responses to environmental, food, or drug antigens that would not affect most of the population. There are four basic categories of hypersensitivity responses: (1) type I responses, which are mediated by the IgE class Igs and include anaphylactic shock, hay fever, and bronchial asthma; (2) type II responses, which involve complement-activated cell destruction (Rh incompatibility), ADCC, complement- and antibody-mediated inflammation (*e.g.*, Goodpasture disease), and antibody-mediated cell dysfunction (*e.g.*, Graves disease and myasthenia gravis); (3) type III, immune complex–mediated hypersensitivity disorders, which involve the formation and deposition of insoluble antigen–antibody complexes in blood vessels causing the development of vasculitis and organ damage as seen in SLE or acute glomerulonephritis, systemic immune complex disease (serum sickness), and local immune complex disease (Arthus reaction); and (4) type

IV cell-mediated hypersensitivity reactions, which are subdivided into four different types based upon the T-cell population involved and the pathophysiologic response.

Latex allergy can involve a type I, IgE-mediated reaction or a type IV, cell-mediated response. The most common type of allergic response to latex is a contact dermatitis caused by a type IV, delayed-type hypersensitivity reaction to rubber additives. The less common, type I IgE-mediated response is caused by sensitization to the latex protein and can precipitate far more serious anaphylactic reactions.

TRANSPLANTATION IMMUNOPATHOLOGY

After completing this section of the chapter, the learner will be able to meet the following objectives:

- Discuss the rationale for matching of HLA or MHC types in organ transplantation.
- Describe the immune mechanisms involved in allogeneic transplant rejection.
- Describe the mechanisms and manifestations of GVHD.

Traditionally, transplantation can be defined as the process of taking cells, tissues, or organs, called a *graft*, from one person and placing them into another person where they take over the normal function of the tissues replaced. Grafts transplanted from another person are known as *allografts*. In certain circumstances, grafts can be taken from one part of the body and transplanted in another part of the body in the same person. These grafts are referred to as *autografts*. The person who provided the graft is referred to as the *donor*, and the person who receives the graft is called either the *recipient* or the *host*. Tissue transplantation has become routine because of improved medical technology, but serious complications still occur. The most important of which is graft rejection mediated by the host's immune system.

In order for transplantation to be successful, it is essential for the host's immune system to recognize the graft as "self" rather than "nonself." It is the function of the T lymphocytes to respond to a limitless number of antigens while at the same time ignoring self-antigens expressed on tissues. The MHC molecules or *HLA*s expressed on the surface of cells enable the lymphocytes to do just this. Circulating B and T lymphocytes destroy cells that express unfamiliar peptide fragments on the MHC. Transplanted tissue can be categorized as an *autologous* graft (autograft) if the donor and recipient are the same person, *syngeneic* graft if the donor and recipient are identical twins, and *allogeneic* (or allograft) if the donor and recipient are unrelated but share similar HLA tissue expression. The HLA molecules that are recognized as foreign on allografts are called *alloantigens*. Donors of solid organ transplants can be living or dead (cadaver) and related or nonrelated (heterologous). The likelihood of rejection varies indirectly with the degree of HLA similarity that exists between the donor and recipient.

Mechanisms Involved in Transplant Rejection

The process of transplant rejection involves a complex but coordinated cell-mediated and antibody-mediated immune response. Although T lymphocytes have received the most attention as mediators of transplant rejection, it is now known that B cells, macrophages, eosinophils, and NK cells have a significant impact on the quality and the quantity of the rejection process. In fact, when T cell–depleting regimens are employed prior to transplantation, the importance of these cells in the rejection process becomes more evident.[99] Three classic forms of rejection exist: cell mediated, antibody mediated, and chronic rejection, although a mixed pattern of rejection can occur as well.

The most common form of acute allograft rejection is T cell mediated and known as *cellular rejection*. It is initiated by the presentation of donor alloantigens to host T lymphocytes by antigen-presenting dendritic cells and macrophages; APCs may come from recipient or donor tissue. When the APCs are donor in origin, T-lymphocyte activation is said to occur via the direct pathway. When the APCs are the recipient's innate cells, T-lymphocyte activation is said to be via the *indirect pathway*, which resembles the pathway normally involved in the recognition of foreign substances. Most of the alloantigen is presented in association with MHC I or II molecules, resulting in destruction of graft cells by $CD8^+$ cytotoxic T cells or the initiation of a delayed hypersensitivity reactions triggered by $CD4^+$ helper T cells.[100]

T cells of the recipient recognize allogeneic MHC molecules on the surface of APCs that have migrated to lymphoid tissue and on the graft itself. $CD8^+$ cells recognize class I MHC molecules and differentiate into mature CTLs, which directly kill the graft tissue as they would any foreign substance. $CD4^+$ helper T cells recognize class II MHC molecules and differentiate into T-helper effector cells, which secrete cytokines that influence almost all other cells of the immune response including B lymphocytes, cytotoxic T cells ($CD8^+$), macrophages, and NK cells. In addition, the cytokines cause increased vascular permeability and local accumulation and activation of macrophages and eventual graft injury. Although it was traditionally believed that T_1H helper cells mediated rejection and T_2H cells promoted tolerance, it is now known that T_2H helper cells alone can be responsible for graft rejection mediated via eosinophil activation.[100]

Antibody-mediated or humoral rejection is caused by B-lymphocyte proliferation and differentiation into plasma cells that produce donor-specific antibodies (DSAs). These antibodies may be preformed if the immune system was exposed pretransplantation, or they may be produced *de novo* following transplantation. B lymphocytes also play an antibody-independent role in graft rejection through the secretion of proinflammatory cytokines and chemokines and the participation in antigen presentation.[99] Antibody-mediated rejection can be hyperacute or acute in origin. *Hyperacute rejection* occurs almost immediately after vascular reperfusion to graft tissue occurs. Preformed antibodies against HLA antigens are deposited in the tissue endothelium and microvasculature where they activate the classic complement pathway causing tissue necrosis and graft injury.[100] Hyperacute rejection is considered a type III hypersensitivity response. *Acute antibody-mediated rejection* occurs within days to weeks after transplantation. The time frame is dependent upon whether or not the recipient received immunosuppressive therapy prior to transplantation. Previous exposure to the relevant HLA antigens is responsible, but unlike in hyperacute rejection, high circulating antibodies are not present at the time of transplantation.[101] Over a period of several days, high titers of complement-fixing antibodies are generated, which cause injury by several mechanisms, including complement-dependent cytotoxicity, inflammation, and antibody-dependent cell-mediated cytotoxicity. Regardless of the mechanism, the initial target of these antibodies in rejection appears to be the graft vasculature.

Chronic rejection involves immune-mediated inflammatory injury to a graft that occurs over a prolonged period. It is most often due to the inability to maintain adequate immunosuppression necessary to control residual circulating antigraft T lymphocytes or antibodies. Chronic rejection manifests itself with a progressive decline in tissue function usually as a result of vascular injury and impaired blood supply.[102] T lymphocytes and macrophages infiltrate the graft and set up a chronic immune response that causes cellular hypertrophy and subendothelial thickening. Antibody-mediated rejection may be responsible for chronic rejection in people with undetected low levels of preexisting or *de novo* DSAs. In renal transplantation, it is characterized by a gradual rise in serum creatinine over a period of 4 to 6 months.

Graft Versus Host Disease

GVHD is a major complication that most frequently occurs after allogeneic stem cell transplantation. There are three fundamental requirements for the development of GVHD:

1. The graft must contain cells that are immunologically competent.
2. The recipient's cells must express antigens that are not present on donor cells.
3. The recipient must be immunologically compromised and incapable of mounting an effective immune response.

Cases of GVHD have also been reported in other settings where tissues containing T lymphocytes, such as blood products, bone marrow, or solid organs (liver), are transplanted into people who are immunocompromised.[103]

GVHD occurs when donor T cells react to HLAs present on host cells. The incidence of acute GVHD directly correlates with the degree of mismatching between recipient and host HLA proteins. Class I HLA (A, B, and C) proteins are expressed on most nucleated cells in the body. Class II HLA proteins (DR, DQ, and DP) are mainly expressed on hemopoietic cells including B lymphocytes, dendritic cells, and monocytes. Class II HLA protein expression can also be stimulated on other cell types during inflammation and tissue injury. Therefore, donors and recipients are matched for class I HLA (A, B, and C) and class II CRB1 antigens in order to decrease the chance of rejection. However, even with tissue matching, 40% of HLA-identical graft recipients develop signs of system GVHD requiring treatment with high-dose steroids. It is believed that GVHD is the result of genetic differences encoded that encode for minor histocompatibility proteins.[103,104]

The development of GVHD involves a three-step process: (1) activation of recipient APCs; (2) activation, proliferation, differentiation, and migration of donor T lymphocytes; and (3) target tissue destruction. Prior to transplantation, host APCs are in a state of heightened activation as a result of the underlying disease process and HSCT preconditioning regimens. As a result, these cells exhibit amplified expression of adhesion molecules, MHC antigens, and costimulatory molecules. Following transplantation, donor T lymphocytes encounter these "heightened" APCs and activate both $CD4^+$ and $CD8^+$ T cells. The result is the stimulation of a complex cascade of cellular mediators and soluble inflammatory agents that amplify tissue injury and promote tissue destruction.

GVHD can be acute or chronic. Acute GVHD usually develops within the first 100 days of transplantation, whereas chronic GVHD occurs sometime after that. However, cases of late-onset acute GVHD have been reported, and in some cases, people present with features of both. Signs and symptoms usually develop first in the skin, coinciding with the engraftment of donor cells. People present with a pruritic, maculopapular rash that starts on the hands and feet but ultimately extends over the entire body. In severe cases, the skin can blister and ulcerations may develop. Gastrointestinal symptoms include nausea, anorexia, diarrhea, and abdominal pain. Gastrointestinal bleeding is an ominous sign as it indicates mucosal ulceration. Liver disease is common but is frequently hard to differentiate from liver involvement normally seen after transplantation. It can progress to the development of veno-occlusive disease, drug toxicity, viral infection, iron overload, extrahepatic biliary obstruction, sepsis, and coma. The severity of acute GVHD is determined based upon the involvement of the three primary target organs affected (skin, GI tract, and liver). Severe GVHD is associated with a poor prognosis and a long-term survival rate of 5%.[103,104]

Chronic GVHD is a major late cause of death after high-dose myeloablative chemoradiotherapy. GVHD can progress to the acute form of the disease, recur sometime after resolution of an acute process, or develop *de novo*. The greatest risk factors for the development of chronic GVHD are advanced recipient age and a previous history of acute GVHD. Signs and symptoms of chronic GVHD are typical of an autoimmune process and can affect all major organ systems within the body.

Prevention of GVHD focuses on regimens that specifically deplete donor T lymphocytes but have been met with mixed long-term success. Regimens including the removal of T cells from donor graft prior to transplantation and the administration of antibodies against T cells in vivo have been studied extensively but are associated with high rates of graft failure. Immunosuppressive or anti-inflammatory drugs such as cyclosporine and tacrolimus or glucocorticoids can be used to block T-cell activation and the action of cytokines.[103,104]

IN SUMMARY

Transplantation can be defined as the process of taking cells, tissues, or organs, called a *graft*, from one person and placing them into another person where they take over the normal function of the tissues replaced. Although advances in medicine had dramatically improved the long-term survival following transplantation, rejection still exists as a major barrier to success. Rejection is the process by which the recipient's immune system recognizes the graft as foreign, mounts an immunologic response, and destroys it. Destruction of the cells or tissues of the graft can be cell mediated, antibody mediated, or a combination of both processes. Hyperacute antibody rejection occurs almost immediately after transplantation and is caused by existing recipient antibodies to graft antigens that initiate an immediate hypersensitivity reaction in the blood vessels of the graft. *Acute antibody-mediated rejection* occurs within days to weeks after transplantation. Previous exposure to the relevant HLA antigens is responsible, but unlike in hyperacute rejection, high circulating antibodies are not present at the time of transplantation. Chronic rejection occurs over a prolonged period and is caused by T cell–generated cytokines that stimulate fibrosis of graft tissue.

GVHD occurs when immunologically competent donor cells are transplanted into recipients who are immunologically compromised. Three basic requirements are necessary for GVHD to develop: (1) the donor cells must be immunologically competent, (2) the recipient tissue must bear antigens foreign to the donor cells, and (3) the recipient must be immunologically compromised so that it cannot destroy the transplanted cells.

AUTOIMMUNE DISEASE

After completing this section of the chapter, the learner will be able to meet the following objectives:

- Discuss the mechanisms of self-tolerance as they relate to the development of autoimmune disease.
- Discuss the possible mechanisms underlying autoimmune disease.
- Describe the criteria for establishing an autoimmune basis for a disease.

Autoimmune diseases are a heterogenous group of disorders that occur when the body's immune system fails to differentiate "self" from "nonself" and mounts an immunologic response against host tissues. Autoimmune diseases can affect almost any cell type, tissue, or organ system. Some autoimmune disorders, such as Hashimoto thyroiditis, are tissue specific. Others, such as SLE, are systemic, affecting multiple organs and systems. Chart 12.2 lists some of the more common autoimmune diseases.

Immunologic Tolerance

A key feature of the immune system is its ability to differentiate between foreign antigens and self-antigens. The capacity of the immune system to differentiate self from nonself is called *self-tolerance*. The development of self-tolerance relies upon two coordinated processes: *central tolerance*, the elimination of autoreactive lymphocytes during maturation in the central lymphoid tissues, and *peripheral tolerance*, the functional suppression of autoreactive lymphocytes in peripheral tissues that have escaped destruction in the thymus.[105] *Autoreactivity* is the process by which an organism acts against its own tissue.

Activation of the immune system requires presentation of foreign antigens to the immunologically active B and T cells. Antigen expression is encoded on the MHC genes, which determine the specific HLA antigens present on cell

CHART 12.2 PROBABLE AUTOIMMUNE DISEASE*

Systemic
Mixed connective tissue disease
Polymyositis–dermatomyositis
Rheumatoid arthritis
Scleroderma
Sjögren syndrome
Systemic lupus erythematosus

Blood
Autoimmune hemolytic anemia
Autoimmune neutropenia and lymphopenia
Idiopathic thrombocytopenic purpura

Other Organs
Acute idiopathic polyneuritis
Atrophic gastritis and pernicious anemia
Autoimmune adrenalitis
Goodpasture syndrome
Hashimoto thyroiditis
Type 1 diabetes mellitus
Myasthenia gravis
Premature gonadal (ovarian) failure
Primary biliary cirrhosis
Sympathetic ophthalmia
Temporal arteritis
Thyrotoxicosis (Graves disease)
Crohn disease, ulcerative colitis

*Examples are not inclusive.

surfaces. During T-cell development in the thymus, T lymphocytes (prothymocytes) undergo random rearrangement of specific gene loci responsible for the coding of antigen receptors. The prothymocytes with TCRs that appropriately bind to MHC are positively selected for, whereas prothymocytes with high affinity for self-antigen or autoreactivity are destroyed.[105] Similar processes take place in the elimination of B lymphocytes that have high affinity for autoantigens. The main objective is to produce a population of B and T lymphocytes that are immunologically unresponsive in the presence of self-antigens prior to their release into the central circulation. Anergy is the complete loss of lymphocyte response to an antigen and can result in a diminished or absent cellular and/or humoral immunologic response.

B-Cell Tolerance

Under normal circumstances, circulating B lymphocytes do not produce antibodies against host tissues. B-cell antibody production is normally kept in check by the help of $CD4^+$ T-helper cells.[106] In addition, autoreactive B lymphocytes can be eliminated by apoptosis in the central lymphoid tissues, spleen, and peripheral lymph nodes, or they can be functionally inactivated in a process known as *anergy*. However, in many autoimmune diseases, the immune system loses its ability to recognize self and produces antibodies, also known as *autoantibodies*, against host tissues. For example, in Graves disease, hyperthyroidism is the result of autoantibody-induced hyperactivity of the TSH receptor (see Fig. 12.3).

T-Cell Tolerance

The primary mechanisms of T-cell tolerance involve a process of positive and negative selection of maturing lymphocytes (Fig. 12.6). When immature lymphocytes migrate into the thymus, the T-cell lineage undergoes TCR gene rearrangement at the α and β loci.[105] At this point, they can mature into either $CD4^+$ or $CD8^+$ cells and are considered to be double positive ($CD4^+/8^+$). After rearrangement, T cells with TCRs that respond appropriately to self-peptide–MHC complexes

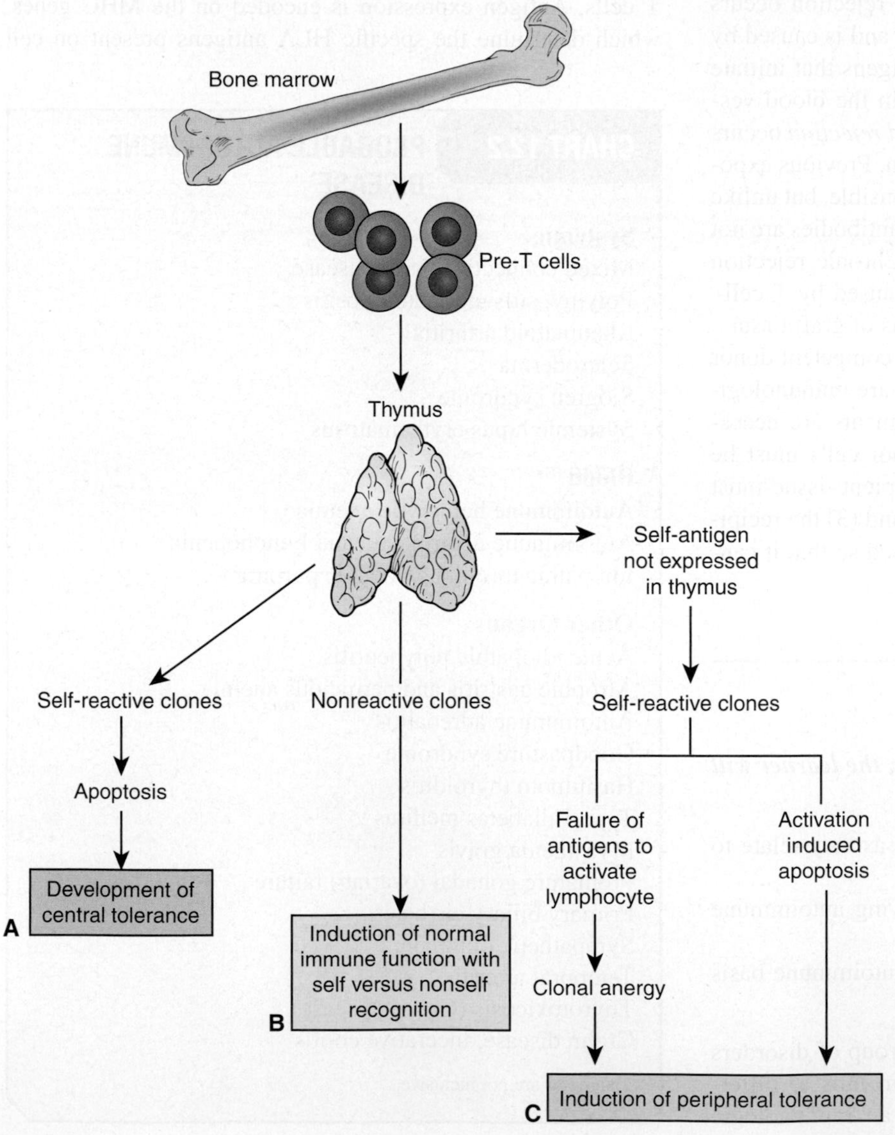

Figure 12.6 • Development of immunologic tolerance. **(A)** Development of central tolerance with deletion of self-reactive T lymphocytes in the thymus. **(B)** Nonreactive lymphocytes with development of normal immune function. **(C)** Induction of peripheral tolerance in self-reactive cells that are not eliminated in the thymus.

and possess little avidity for the antigen are signaled by the release of cytokines and chemokines to migrate into the thymic medulla and mature into $CD4^+/8^-$ and $CD4^-/8^+$ or single-positive lymphocytes. This is known as *positive selection*. In contrast, T cells with TCRs that possess high avidity for the self-peptide–MHC complex are directed to undergo apoptosis or programmed cell death. This is known as clonal deletion or *negative selection* and takes place in the thymic medulla as well. Although the processes governing the selection and maturation of T lymphocytes are extensive, autoreactive T cells can escape into the periphery, where peripheral mechanisms for the development of self-tolerance become important.

Several peripheral mechanisms are available to deal with autoreactive cells that escape central selection. One primary mechanism begins with the development of a specialized subpopulation of T lymphocytes. $CD4^+CD25^+$ regulator T cells are a subset of T lymphocytes produced in the thymus that regulate antigen-specific tolerance. These regulator T cells target and abolish the response of autoreactive T cells that have been released into the peripheral circulation by interrupting the production and release of IL-2. Regulatory T cells are also capable of inducing tolerance to foreign antigens by inhibiting activation and proliferation of naive $CD4^+$ T cells in response to antigen.[105]

The activity of autoreactive T cells can also be inhibited by local anatomic and physiologic factors. Some T cells are located in areas of the body where they fail to come in contact with their corresponding antigens (*e.g.*, blood–brain barrier), so they remain immunologically inactive. In other cases, autoreactive T cells encounter their corresponding antigens, but the costimulatory factors necessary for their activation are missing. The peripheral activation of T cells requires presentation of a peptide antigen in association with MHC molecules on the APCs as well as a set of secondary costimulatory factors. Because costimulatory signals are not strongly expressed on most normal tissues, the encounter of the autoreactive T cells with their specific target antigens fails to initiate an immunologic response resulting in the development of anergy.

Another mechanism essential for the maintenance of functional tolerance involves the apoptotic death of autoreactive T cells when excessive or repeated TCR activation has occurred. This process is referred to as activation-induced cell death (AICD).[107] AICD is necessary in order to prevent activated T cells from inducing an autoimmune response. It is a normal process of the immune system designed to maintain internal homeostasis. AICD is mediated by the interaction between an apoptotic cell surface receptor (called FAS) that is present on the T cell and a soluble membrane messenger molecule known as the FAS ligand (FasL, CD95L). The FAS/FAS ligand bound activates the intracellular processes that result in programmed cell death. The expression of the FAS receptor is markedly increased on the cell surfaces of activated T cells. Therefore, expression of the FAS messenger molecule by the same cohort of activated autoreactive T cells can result in removal of the population from the circulation.

KEY POINTS

IMMUNOLOGIC TOLERANCE

- Immunologic self-tolerance is the ability of the immune system to distinguish between self and nonself antigens. It is mediated through central and peripheral mechanisms that delete autoreactive immune cells or render them unresponsive to autoantigen.
- The development of self-tolerance relies upon two coordinated processes: *central tolerance*, the elimination of autoreactive lymphocytes during maturation in the central lymphoid tissues, and *peripheral tolerance*, the functional suppression of autoreactive lymphocytes in peripheral tissues that have escaped destruction in the thymus.

Mechanisms of Autoimmune Disease

Although it is clear that autoimmune disease results from a loss of self-tolerance, the exact mechanisms are largely unknown. Autoimmune diseases are a heterogeneous group of disorders, so a combination of both genetic and environmental factors plays a significant role. Gender may also be a factor because many autoimmune disorders such as SLE are predominantly seen in women, suggesting that female hormones like estrogens may play a role in the development of certain autoimmune diseases. Estrogen has been shown to have strong immunomodulatory effects including the stimulation of autoreactive B-lymphocyte antibody production, increased leukocyte adhesion to endothelial cells, and increased cytokine production.[108]

Heredity

Although the pathophysiology of autoimmune disease is multifactorial and complex, involving both environmental and genetic influences, it is known that heredity has a significant impact on the prevalence of these disorders. Autoimmune disorders are not inherited in the traditional fashion such as with a single-gene mutation. Rather, people with autoimmune disorders exhibit *susceptibility genes* that act in concert with environmental factors to increase a person's risk of developing the disease process.[109,110] In addition, many of these genes are shared between autoimmune disorders with similar underlying features. For example, type I IFN is a central mediator of the innate immune response stimulating monocyte maturation, plasma cell maturation and Ig class switching, and cytotoxic T-cell activity. People with SLE or systemic sclerosis (SSc) demonstrate defects in the IFN regulatory factor 5 (*IRF5*) gene, resulting in the abnormal transcription of IFN. In other cases, heritable changes occur as a result of changes in gene expression, rather than changes in DNA sequencing. This is termed *epigenetics*. This is the result of the methylation of deoxycytosine (dC) bases in cytosine–guanine DNA base pairs. As a result, the chromatin structure is altered in such a way that it cannot be accessed during the normal processes of DNA transcription and the functions encoded in the DNA sequence cease.

The high concordance rates in first-degree relatives and monozygotic twins provide strong evidence for the role of inheritance in autoimmune disorders. First-degree relatives have a relative risk of rheumatoid arthritis that is two to four times that of the general population. Studies of monozygotic and dizygotic twins indicate that rheumatoid arthritis is approximately 65% heritable with many affected people sharing alleles for the same anticyclic citrullinated peptide (anti-CCP) antibody. It is clear that autoimmunity does not develop in all people with genetic predisposition.[108] Therefore, other factors known as "triggering events" interact to precipitate the altered immune state. In most cases, the event or events that trigger the development of an autoimmune response are unknown, but in many cases, it appears that the "trigger" may be a viral infection, a chemical substance, or a self-antigen from a body tissue that has been hidden from the immune system during development and is suddenly expressed.

Environmental Factors

The role of environment in the development of autoimmune disease is complex. The incidence of some autoimmune diseases, such as type I diabetes mellitus, has increased in recent years faster than would be expected based upon genetic mechanisms alone, suggesting an increased impact of environmental factors in genetically susceptible people.[111] Environmental factors including viral infection, lack of exposure to maternal antibodies through breast-feeding, maternal smoking, and exposure to hazardous chemicals appear to be involved in the pathogenesis of autoimmune disorders, but their precise role in initiating the autoreactive response is largely unknown. Various factors work in concert resulting in the loss of self-tolerance including breakdown of T-cell anergy, release of sequestered antigens, molecular mimicry, and the development of superantigens.

Breakdown in T-Cell Anergy. *Anergy* is a state of reduced function, in which an immunocompetent, antigen-specific T cell is unable to respond to an appropriate stimulus. Anergy can develop if there is loss of normal costimulatory factors in the face of normal T-cell activation or from altered/chronic TCR stimulation. Primary $CD4^+$ and $CD8^+$ T cells' anergy is characterized by defective production of IFN-γ and TNF-α.[112] In addition, regulatory T cells control T-cell activation by failing to express T-cell stimulating inflammatory cytokines. Most normal tissues do not express costimulatory molecules and as a result are protected from circulating autoreactive T cells. However, if normal cells are induced to express costimulatory factors, then normal anergy is inhibited and autoimmunity can develop. This can occur after an infection or in situations where there is tissue necrosis and local inflammation.

Release of Sequestered Antigens. Under normal circumstances, the body does not produce antibodies against self-antigens. If self-antigens have been completely sequestered during T-cell development and reintroduced into the immune system, they are likely to be treated as foreign antigens. This has been documented in cases of autoimmune orchitis and autoimmune uveitis after systemic release of spermatozoa and ocular antigens.[113] Other times, self-antigens may change their structure and, once they come in contact with T cells, are no longer recognized as innate to the host. Once an autoimmune process has been initiated, it tends to become amplified and progress, sometimes with sporadic relapses and remissions. This occurs because the initial inflammatory process releases these altered self-antigens where they encounter the cells of the immune system. The result is continued activation of new lymphocytes that recognize the previously hidden epitopes.

Molecular Mimicry. It is known that viral infections can serve as triggers in many autoimmune processes, but the mechanism by which this occurs is not completely understood. *Molecular mimicry* is one theory that has been postulated to describe the mechanisms by which infectious agents or other foreign substances trigger an immune response against autoantigens. If a susceptible host is exposed to a foreign antigen that is immunologically similar to its own autoantigens (share epitopes), but which differs sufficiently to trigger an immune response, cross-reactivity between the two antigens and damage to host tissues can occur.[114]

Molecular mimicry has been used to explain the cardiac damage associated with acute rheumatic fever after infection with group A beta-hemolytic streptococci and the demyelinating injury in multiple sclerosis.[114] People with rheumatic fever have high levels of circulating antibodies against the type 5 streptococcal M protein, an antigen found in the microbial cell membrane and which demonstrates cross-reactivity with cardiac myosin. Multiple viruses that are destroyed by cytotoxic T cells ($CD8^+$) share common epitopes with the myelin basic proteins targeted in people with multiple sclerosis. However, not everyone exposed to these organisms goes on to develop autoimmunity. This may be due to differences in HLA expression. The HLA type expressed by the cell determines exactly which fragments of a pathogen are displayed on the surface of the APCs for presentation to T cells. Some fragments may be cross-reactive and others may not. In the spondyloarthropathies, B-lymphocyte cross-reactivity exists between gram-negative bacterial membrane peptides, and specific host HLA-B27 antigens have been implicated in the development of the disease.[114]

Superantigens. Superantigens are a family of related substances, including staphylococcal and streptococcal exotoxins, that induce uncontrolled proliferation and activation of T lymphocytes, causing fever, shock, and death. Unlike antigens, superantigens bind as intact molecules to a wide variety of class II MHC molecules on APCs and then to the TCR on the variable region of the β-chain (TCR Vβ). Every superantigen is capable of binding a large subset of TCR Vβ domains and as a result activating up to 20% of all T cells.[115] Superantigens are involved in several diseases, including food poisoning and toxic shock syndrome.

Diagnosis and Treatment of Autoimmune Disease

The diagnosis of autoimmune disorders is not always easy. There are over 80 identified autoimmune disorders, and many have overlapping presentations. In addition, many of the manifestations are nonspecific and are frequently seen in other disease processes that are not of autoimmune etiology. Diagnosis is therefore made based upon evidence of autoimmunity as indicated by history as well as physical and serologic findings. Each autoimmune disease is associated with certain clinical signs and laboratory findings that practitioners screen for during the diagnostic workup. Because the etiology of autoimmunity is multifactorial, it is unlikely that any one specific genetic testing alone will be able to determine a diagnosis with 100% certainty.[116]

The basis for most serologic assays is the demonstration of antibodies directed against tissue antigens or cellular components. The results of serologic testing are correlated with the physical findings during the diagnostic workup. For example, a child who presents with a chronic or acute history of fever, arthritis, and a macular rash and has high levels of antinuclear antibody has a probable diagnosis of SLE. The detection of autoantibodies in the laboratory usually is accomplished by one of three methods: indirect fluorescent antibody (IFA) assays, enzyme-linked immunosorbent assay (ELISA), or particle agglutination of some kind. Each technique relies upon the specificity of antibody for antigen. In the ELISA and IFA, the person's serum is diluted and allowed to react with an antigen-coated surface (*i.e.*, whole, fixed cells for the detection of antinuclear antibodies) so that the antibody present in the sample can bind the antigen. The serum antibody is then linked to an enzyme or secondary antibody producing a visible reaction that allows the amount of antibody present to be quantified. Particle agglutination assays are much simpler because the binding of the person's antibody to antigen-coated particles causes a visible agglutination reaction, and a secondary reaction is not required.[116]

Treatment of autoimmune disorders is dependent upon the magnitude of the presenting manifestations and underlying mechanisms of the disease process. Because in many cases the pathophysiologic mechanisms are not always known, treatment may be purely symptomatic. Corticosteroids and immunosuppressive drugs are the mainstay of therapy directed at arresting or reversing the cellular damage caused by the autoimmune response. Plasmapheresis has been utilized in severe cases to remove autoreactive cells from the circulation.[117]

Recent therapies for the treatment of autoimmune disorders have focused on targeting the specific lymphocytes and cytokines involved in the autoimmune response. For example, type I interferons (IFNα) have been implicated in the development of many autoimmune processes including SLE. Anti-IFN monoclonal antibody therapy has been shown to inhibit the overexpression of IFN genes and suppress the expression of interferon-dependent cytokines (*e.g.*, TNF-α, IL-10, and IL-1). Other recent therapies deplete autoreactive B cells by targeting CD20 (rituximab), modulate B-cell activity without depleting the lymphocyte lineage (epratuzumab), block B-cell growth factors (belimumab), or inhibit the communication between T and B cells by blockade of costimulatory factors (CTLA-4 Ig).[117] Unfortunately, the success of these treatments has been variable.

IN SUMMARY

Autoimmune disorders are caused by a loss of immunologic self-tolerance, which results in damage to body tissues. Autoimmune diseases are a heterogenous group of disorders and depending upon the target of the autoreactive lymphocytes can affect almost any cell or tissue of the body. The ability of the immune system to differentiate self from nonself is called *self-tolerance* and is normally maintained through central mechanisms that delete autoreactive lymphocytes before they come in contact with an autoantigen. Cells that escape deletion by central mechanisms may be suppressed or inactivated in the periphery. Defects in any of these mechanisms can be responsible for the development of autoimmune diseases.

T-cell activity is modulated through the expression of the HLA–MHC complex on cellular surfaces. Antigens are normally presented to TCRs in combination with MHC molecules. This interaction activates a variety of immune processes that culminate in destruction of the "foreign antigen." Disruption of any step in the antigen recognition process can result in the loss of self-tolerance including breakdown of T-cell anergy, release of sequestered antigens, molecular mimicry, and the development of superantigens. Diagnosis of autoimmune disease is made based upon evidence of autoimmunity as indicated by history as well as physical and serologic findings.

ACQUIRED IMMUNODEFICIENCY SYNDROME/HUMAN IMMUNODEFICIENCY VIRUS

The AIDS is a disease caused by infection with the HIV and is characterized by profound immunosuppression with associated opportunistic infections, malignancies, wasting, and CNS degeneration. AIDS is considered a chronic illness today.

THE AIDS EPIDEMIC AND TRANSMISSION OF HIV INFECTION

After completing this section of the chapter, the learner will be able to meet the following objectives:

- State the virus responsible for AIDS and explain how it differs from most other viruses.
- Describe the mechanisms of HIV transmission and relate them to the need for public awareness and concern regarding the spread of AIDS.

According to the latest HIV surveillance report published by CDC, at the end of 2015, an estimated 1.1 million persons aged 13 and older were living with HIV infection in the United States, including an estimated 162,500 (15%) persons whose infections had not been diagnosed.[1,118–122]

Transmission of HIV Infection

HIV is a retrovirus that selectively attacks the $CD4^+$ T lymphocytes, the immune cells responsible for orchestrating and coordinating the immune response to infection. As a consequence, people with HIV infection have a deteriorating immune system and thus are more susceptible to severe infections with ordinarily harmless organisms.[124] The virus responsible for most HIV infection worldwide is called *HIV type 1* (HIV-1). A second type, *HIV type 2* (HIV-2), is endemic in many countries in West Africa but is rarely seen in other parts of the world. The majority of people with HIV-2 (81%) are people who were born in West Africa. People with HIV-2 tend not to develop AIDS.[2,3].

HIV is transmitted from one person to another through sexual contact, through blood-to-blood contact, or perinatally. The CDC transmission categories of HIV for children include perinatal and other. The adult categories include male-to-male sexual contact, intravenous drug use, male-to-male sexual contact and intravenous drug use, heterosexual contact, and other.[3].

Several studies involving more than 1000 uninfected, nonsexual household contacts with persons with HIV infection (including siblings, parents, and children) have shown no evidence of casual transmission. Transmission can occur when infected blood, semen, or vaginal secretions from one person are deposited onto a mucous membrane or into the bloodstream of another person. Sexual contact is the most frequent mode of HIV transmission.[125] HIV is present in semen and vaginal fluids. There is a risk of transmitting HIV when these fluids come in contact with a part of the body that lets them enter the bloodstream. This includes the vaginal and anal mucosa, superficial laceration, wounds, or sores on the skin. Contact with semen occurs during vaginal and anal sexual intercourse, oral sex, and donor insemination. Exposure to vaginal or cervical secretions occurs during vaginal intercourse and oral sex. In most cities in the United States, sexual transmission of HIV is primarily related to vaginal or anal intercourse. However, use of condoms is highly effective in preventing the transmission of HIV.

Because HIV is found in blood, the use of needles, syringes, and other drug injection paraphernalia is a direct route of transmission. Of the reported cases of AIDS in the United States, approximately 25% occurred among people who injected drugs.[125] Transfusions of whole blood, plasma, platelets, or blood cells before 1985 resulted in the transmission of HIV. Seventy to eighty percent of people with hemophilia who were treated with factor VIII supplements before 1985 became infected with HIV.[125] Since 1985, all blood donations in the United States have been screened for HIV, so this is no longer a transmission risk. Other blood products, such as gamma globulin or hepatitis B immune globulin, have not been implicated in the transmission of HIV.

Transmission from mother to infant is the most common way that children become infected with HIV. HIV may be transmitted from infected women to their offspring in utero, during labor and delivery, or through breast-feeding.[6] Ninety percent of infected children acquired the virus from their mother. However, evidence suggests that if mother and infant are treated with one or two additional antiretroviral medications along with zidovudine (standard practice is to administer zidovudine only), a statistically significant decrease in transmission of HIV occurs.[7]

Occupational HIV infection among health care workers is uncommon. Universal Blood and Body Fluid Precautions should be used in encounters with all people in the health care setting because it should be assumed that any person may have a transmissible infection. Occupational risk of infection for health care workers most often is associated with percutaneous inoculation (*i.e.*, needle stick) of blood from a person with HIV infection. Transmission is associated with the size of the needle, amount of blood present, depth of the injury, type of fluid contamination, stage of illness of the person, and viral load of the person.

People with other sexually transmitted diseases (STDs) are at increased risk for HIV infection. The risk of HIV transmission is increased in the presence of genital ulcerative STDs (*i.e.*, syphilis, herpes simplex virus infection, and chancroid) and nonulcerative STDs (*i.e.*, gonorrhea, chlamydial infection, and trichomoniasis). HIV increases the duration and recurrence of STD lesions, treatment failures, and atypical presentation of genital ulcerative diseases because of the suppression of the immune system.

The HIV-infected person is infectious even when no symptoms are present. The point at which an infected person converts from being negative for the presence of HIV antibodies in the blood to being positive is called *seroconversion*. Seroconversion typically occurs within 1 to 3 months after exposure to HIV but can take up to 6 months.[3] The time after infection and before seroconversion is known as the *window period*. During the window period, a person's HIV antibody test result will be negative. Rarely, infection can occur from transfused blood that was screened for HIV antibody and found negative because the donor was recently infected and still in the window period. Consequently, the U.S. FDA requires blood collection centers to screen potential donors through interviews designed to identify behaviors known to present a risk for HIV infection.

KEY POINTS

THE AIDS EPIDEMIC AND TRANSMISSION OF HIV

- AIDS is caused by the HIV.
- HIV is transmitted through blood, semen, vaginal fluids, and breast milk.
- People with HIV infection are infectious even when asymptomatic.

IN SUMMARY

AIDS is an infectious disease of the immune system caused by HIV, a retrovirus that causes profound immunosuppression. The severity of the clinical disease and the absence of a cure or preventive vaccine have increased public awareness and concern. The greatest incidence of HIV in 2010 to 2015 has been in males and people between the age of 25 and 34 years.[1] HIV is transmitted from one person to another through sexual contact, through blood-to-blood contact, or perinatally. Transmission occurs when the infected blood, semen, or vaginal secretions from one person are deposited onto a mucous membrane or into the bloodstream of another person. The primary routes of transmission are through sexual intercourse, through intravenous drug use, and from mother to infant. Blood transfusions and other blood products continue to be routes of transmission in some underdeveloped countries. Occupational exposure in health care settings accounts for only a tiny percentage of HIV transmission. HIV infection is not transmitted through casual contact or by insect vectors. There is growing evidence of an association between HIV infection and other STDs. Infected individuals can transmit the virus to others before their own infections can be detected by antibody tests.

PATHOPHYSIOLOGY AND CLINICAL COURSE

After completing this section of the chapter, the learner will be able to meet the following objectives:

- Describe the structure of HIV and trace its entry and steps in replication within the CD4⁺ T lymphocyte.
- Describe the alterations in immune function that occur in persons with AIDS.
- Relate the altered immune function in persons with HIV infection and AIDS to the development of opportunistic infections, malignant tumors, nervous system manifestations, the wasting syndrome, and metabolic disorders.

Molecular and Biologic Features of HIV

HIV-1 is an enveloped member of the retroviruses specifically the subfamily of lentiviruses.[4]. They can all produce slowly progressive fatal diseases that include wasting syndromes and CNS degeneration. Two genetically different but antigenically related forms of HIV, HIV-1 and HIV-2, have been isolated in people with AIDS. HIV-1 is the type most associated with AIDS in the United States, Europe, and Central Africa, whereas HIV-2 causes a similar disease principally in West Africa. HIV-2 appears to be transmitted in the same manner as HIV-1; it can also cause immunodeficiency as evidenced by a reduction in the number of $CD4^+$ T cells and the development of AIDS. Although the spectrum of disease for HIV-2 is similar to that of HIV-1, it spreads more slowly and causes disease more slowly than HIV-1. Specific tests are now available for HIV-2, and blood collected for transfusion is routinely screened for HIV-2. Because most people with HIV have HIV-1, the discussion focuses on HIV-1.

HIV infects a limited number of cell types in the body, including a subset of lymphocytes called $CD4^+$ T lymphocytes (also known as *T-helper cells* or *$CD4^+$ T cells*), macrophages, and dendritic cells.[11] The $CD4^+$ T cells are necessary for normal immune function. Among other functions, the $CD4^+$ T cell recognizes foreign antigens and helps activate antibody-producing B lymphocytes.[11] The $CD4^+$ T cells also orchestrate cell-mediated immunity, in which cytotoxic $CD8^+$ T cells and natural killer (NK) cells directly destroy virus-infected cells, tubercle bacilli, and foreign antigens. The phagocytic function of monocytes and macrophages is also influenced by $CD4^+$ T cells.

Like other retroviruses, HIV carries its genetic information in ribonucleic acid (RNA) rather than deoxyribonucleic acid (DNA). The HIV virion is spherical and contains an electron-dense core surrounded by a lipid envelope (Fig. 12.7). The virus core contains the major capsid protein p24, two copies of the genomic RNA, and three viral enzymes (protease, reverse transcriptase, and integrase). Because p24 is the most readily detected antigen, it is the target for the antibodies used in screening for HIV infection. The viral core is surrounded by a matrix protein called p17, which lies beneath the viral envelope. The viral envelope is studded with two viral glycoproteins, gp120 and gp41, which are critical for the infection of cells.

Replication of HIV is depicted in Figure 12.8. Each of these steps provides insights into the development of methods used for preventing or treating the infection. The *first step* involves the binding of the virus to the $CD4^+$ T cell. Once HIV has entered the bloodstream, it attaches to the surface of a $CD4^+$ T cell by binding to a CD4 receptor that has a high

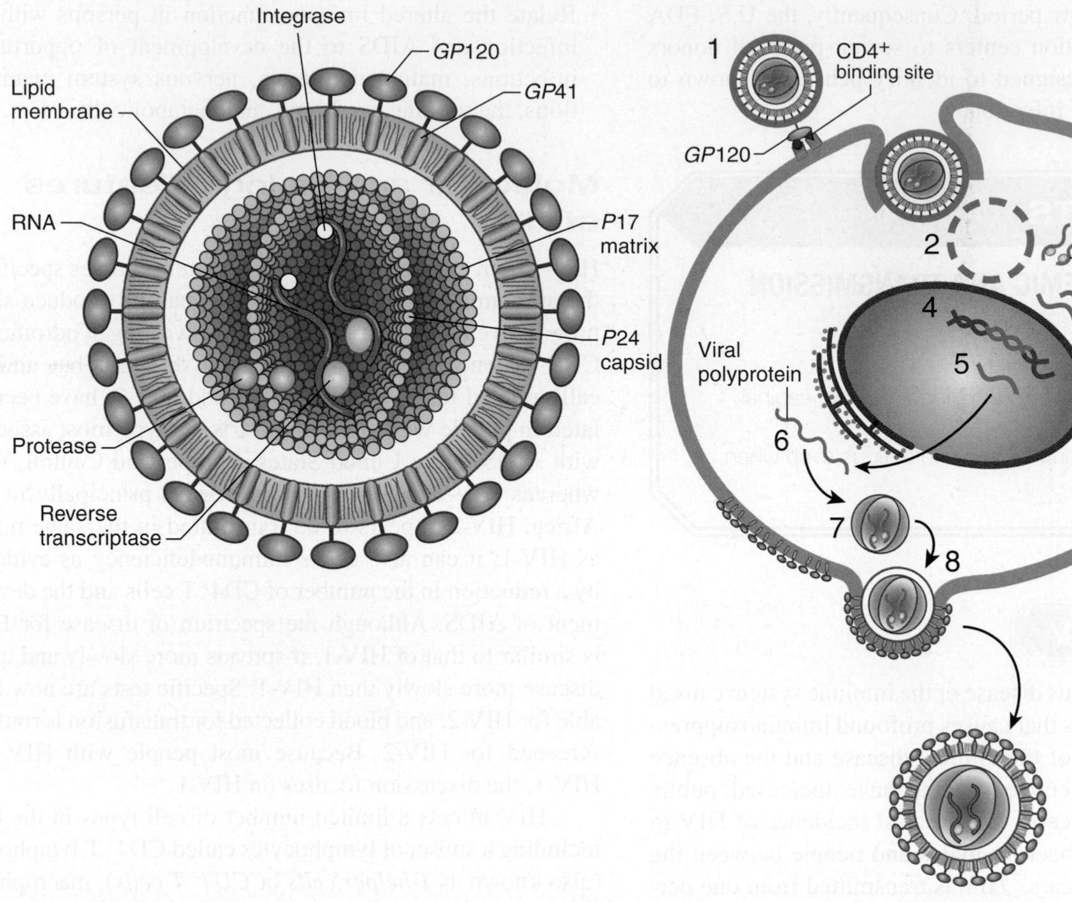

Figure 12.7 • HIV-1 virus. The virus surrounded by a lipid envelope.

affinity for HIV. However, binding to the CD4 receptor is not sufficient for infection; the virus must also bind with other surface molecules (chemokine coreceptors, such as CCR5 and CXCR4) that bind the gp120 and gp41 envelope glycoproteins. This process is known as *attachment*. The *second step* allows for the internalization of the virus. After attachment, the viral envelope peptides fuse to the $CD4^+$ T-cell membrane. Fusion results in an *uncoating* of the virus, allowing the contents of the viral core (the two single strands of viral RNA and the reverse transcriptase, integrase, and protease enzymes) to enter the host cell. The chemokine coreceptors are critical components of the HIV infection process.

The *third step* consists of DNA synthesis. In order for HIV to reproduce, it must change its RNA into DNA. It does this by using the *reverse transcriptase* enzyme. Reverse transcriptase makes a copy of the viral RNA and then in reverse makes another mirror-image copy. The result is double-stranded DNA that carries instructions for viral replication. The *fourth step* is called *integration*. During integration, the new DNA enters the nucleus of the $CD4^+$ T cell and, with the help of the enzyme integrase, is inserted into the cell's original DNA. The *fifth step* involves *transcription* of the double-stranded viral DNA to form a single-stranded messenger RNA (mRNA) with the instructions for building new viruses. Transcription involves activation of the T cell and induction of host cell transcription factors such as nuclear factor-κB (NFκB).[4] To finish, the cycle ribosomal RNA (rRNA) uses the instructions in the mRNA to create a chain of proteins and enzymes called a *polyprotein*. These polyproteins contain the components needed for the next stages in the construction of new viruses. The *seventh step* is called *cleavage*. During cleavage, the protease enzyme cuts the polyprotein chain into the individual proteins that will make up the new viruses. Finally, the proteins and viral RNA are assembled into new HIV viruses and released from the $CD4^+$ T cell.

Treatment of HIV/AIDS relies on the use of agents that interrupt steps of the HIV replication process. Currently, there are multiple drug classes of antiviral agents. The administration of highly active antiretroviral therapy (HAART), also referred to as combined antiretroviral therapy (CAR), typically comprising a combination of three to four antiviral agents, has become the current standard of care.[3].

HIV replication involves the killing of the $CD4^+$ T cell and the release of HIV copies into the bloodstream. These viral particles, or *virions*, invade other $CD4^+$ T cells, allowing the infection to progress (Fig. 12.9). Every day, millions of infected $CD4^+$ T cells are destroyed, releasing billions of viral particles into the bloodstream, but each day, nearly all the $CD4^+$ T cells are replaced and nearly all the viral particles

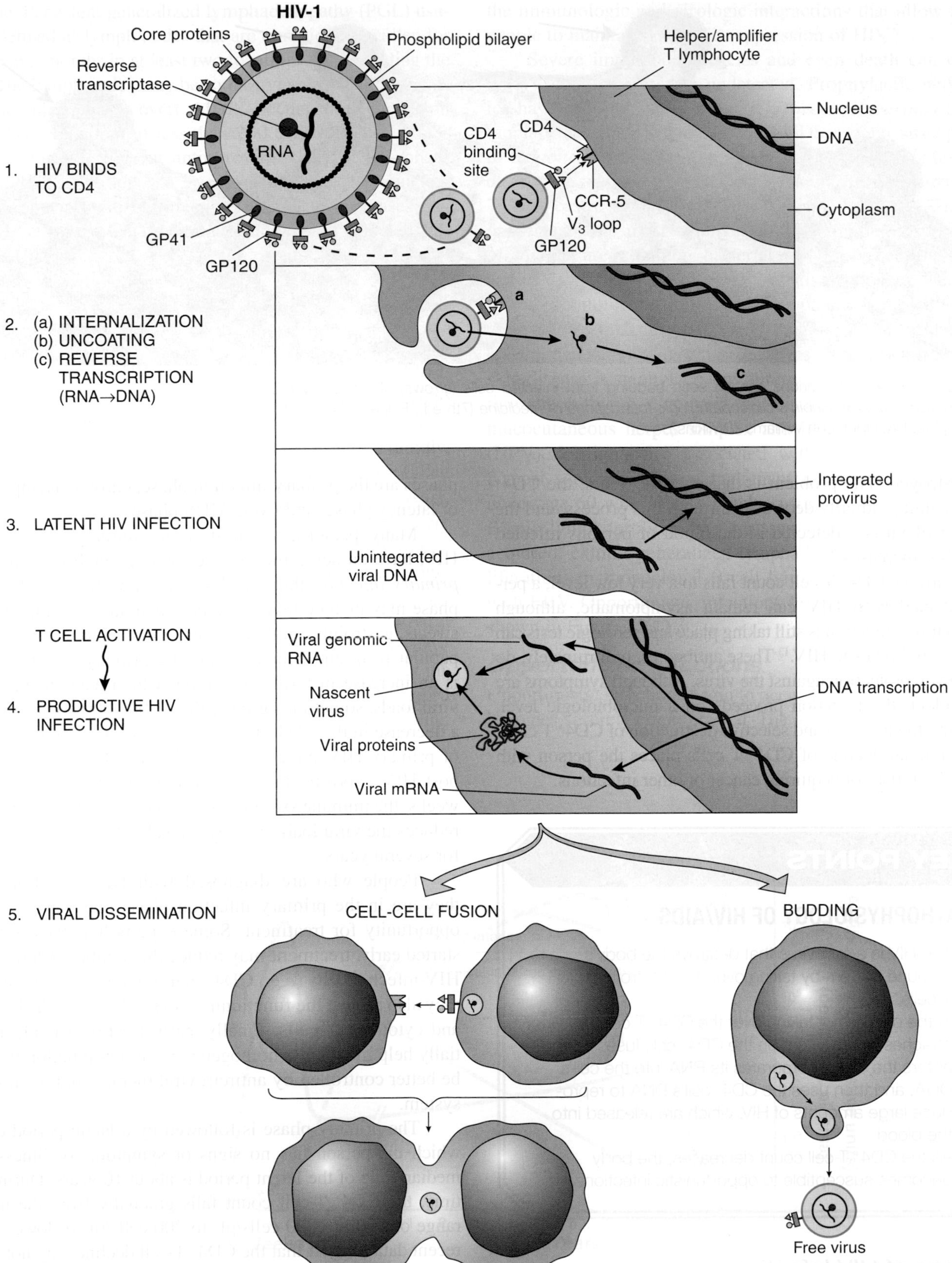

Figure 12.8 • Life cycle of HIV-1 is a multistep process that includes (1) binding CD4 receptor in conjunction with chemokine receptor (*e.g.*, CCR5); (2) internalization, uncoating, and reverse transcription; (3) integration into host DNA as a provisur where it persists in a state of latency; (4) replication in concert with host T-cell activation; and (5) dissemination. (From Strayer D., Rubin R. (Eds.) (2015). *Rubin's clinicopathologic foundations of medicine* (7th ed., Figure 4-23, p. 161). Philadelphia, PA: Lippincott Williams & Wilkins.)

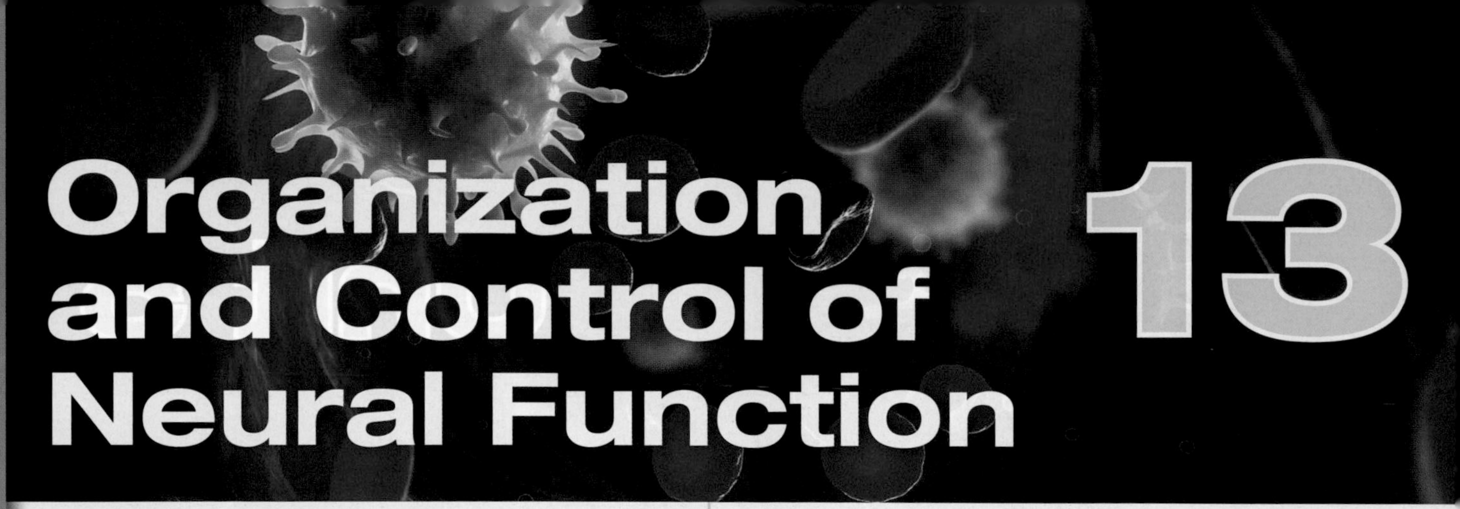

Organization and Control of Neural Function 13

Cynthia Bautista

The major functions of the nervous system include detecting, analyzing, and transmitting information. The sensory system, integrated by the brain, generates signals to motor and autonomic systems to control movement and visceral and endocrine functions. These actions are controlled by neurons, forming a signaling network that includes a motor and sensory system.[1]

The nervous system can be divided into two components—the central nervous system (CNS) and the peripheral nervous system (PNS). The CNS consists of the brain and spinal cord. The PNS consists of cranial nerves (CNs) originating from the brain and spinal nerves originating from the spinal cord. Nerve cells of both the CNS and PNS form incoming (afferent) sensory pathways and outgoing (efferent) motor pathways.

NERVOUS TISSUE CELLS

After completing this section of the chapter, the learner will be able to meet the following objectives:

- Distinguish between the functions of the neurons and neuroglial cells of the nervous system.
- Describe the structure and function of the three parts of a neuron.
- Describe the metabolic requirements of nervous tissue.

Nervous tissue contains two types of cells—neurons and neuroglial cells. The neurons are the functional cells of the nervous system. They exhibit excitability and conduct impulses for the nervous system to function. The neuroglial cells protect the nervous system and provide support for the neurons.

KEY POINTS

THE STRUCTURAL ORGANIZATION OF THE NERVOUS SYSTEM

- The nervous system is divided into two parts—the CNS, consisting of the brain and spinal cord, which are located in the skull and spinal column, and the PNS, which is located outside these structures.
- The nervous system contains two major types of cells: neurons, which are functioning cells of the nervous system, and neuroglial cells, which protect the nervous system and supply metabolic support.

Neurons

Neurons are the functioning cells of the nervous system. Afferent (sensory) neurons transmit information to the CNS, whereas efferent (motor) neurons carry information away from the CNS (Fig. 13.1). Interspersed between the afferent and efferent neurons is a network of interconnecting neurons (also called *interneurons* or *internuncial* neurons) that modulate and control the body's response to sensory input from the internal and external environments.

Neurons have three distinct parts—the cell body, the dendrites, and the axons. These structures form the functional connections, or synapses, with other nerve cells, with receptor cells, or with effector cells. Axonal processes are particularly designed for rapid communication with other neurons and the many body structures innervated by the nervous system.

The cell body (soma) of a neuron contains a large, vesicular nucleus with one or more distinct nucleoli and a well-developed rough endoplasmic reticulum. A neuron's nucleus has the same deoxyribonucleic acid (DNA) and genetic code content present in other cells of the body. Its nucleolus, which is composed of portions of several chromosomes, produces ribonucleic acid (RNA) needed for protein synthesis. The cytoplasm contains large masses of ribosomes that are prominent in most neurons. These acidic RNA masses, which are involved in protein synthesis, stain as dark Nissl bodies with basic histologic stains (see Fig. 13.1).

Dendrites are multiple, short, branched extensions of the nerve cell body. They conduct information toward the cell body and are the main source of information for the neuron. The dendrites and cell body are studded with synaptic terminals that communicate with axons and dendrites of other neurons.

Axons are long efferent processes that project from the cell body. Most neurons have only one axon. However, axons may exhibit multiple branching that results in many axonal terminals. The axon of a neuron conducts nerve impulses from the cell body to its synapse. The axon also provides a physical conduit for the transport of materials between the cell body and the synaptic terminals of the axon. The cell body of the neuron is equipped for a high level of metabolic activity. This is necessary because the cell body must synthesize the cytoplasmic and membrane constituents required to maintain the function of the cell body plus the many proteins and other cytoplasmic

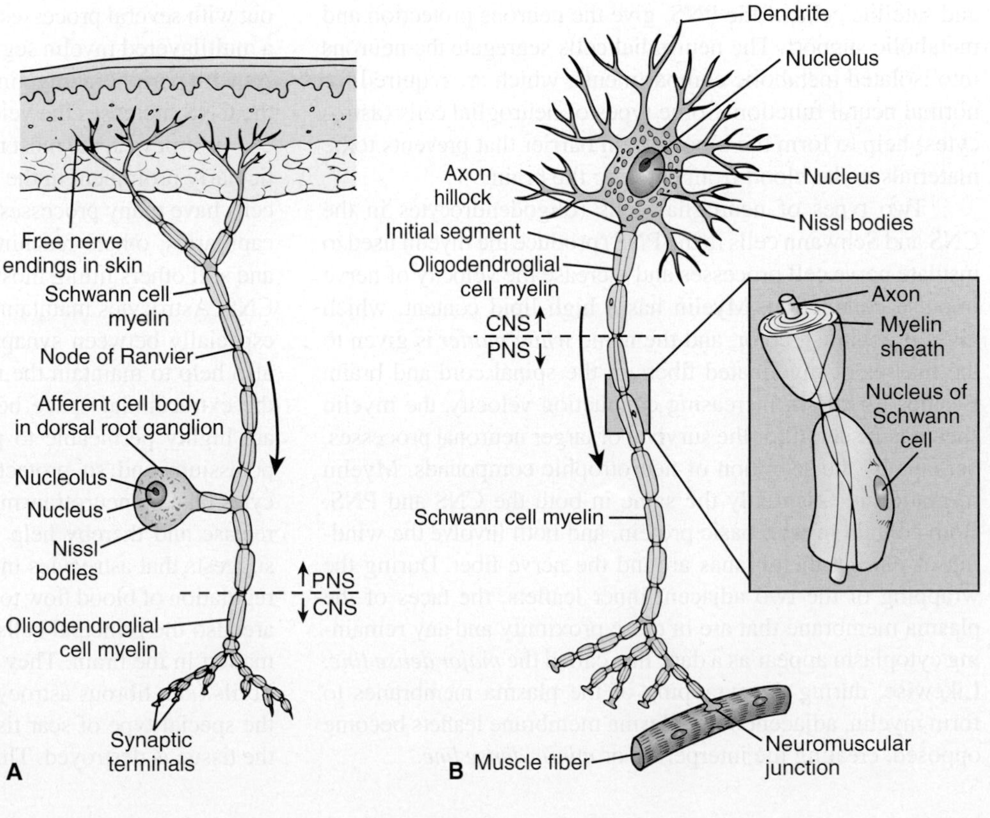

Figure 13.1 • Afferent **(A)** and efferent **(B)** neurons, showing the soma or cell body, dendrites, and axon. *Arrows* indicate the direction for conduction of action potentials.

materials used by the axon and its synaptic terminals. Axons can be very short (0.1 mm) or very long (3.0 m).[2] Axon diameter can vary. Large-diameter axons conduct impulses rapidly, and smaller-diameter axons conduct impulses slowly.

Transportation of materials occurs from the cell body to the axon terminals (anterograde transport) and to a lesser extent in the opposite direction (retrograde transport). The anterograde component consists of fast and slow components. Fast anterograde systems transport molecules such as neurosecretory granules by an energy-dependent system at the rate of 100 to 400 mm/day.[2] Another component of the fast anterograde system transports organelles, including mitochondria. The antidiuretic hormone and oxytocin use the fast anterograde system to travel from hypothalamic neurons through their axons to the posterior pituitary, where the hormones are released into the blood. The slow anterograde component transports materials such as tubulin and cytoplasmic enzymes at a rate of 0.1 to 3.0 mm/day.[2] A fast retrograde component of axonal transport carries materials that are shipped back to the cell body for degradation or reuse. Although much of this material is degraded in lysosomes, retrograde transport is also used to deliver signals to the cell body.

Two motor proteins (kinesin and dynein) are involved in the transport process. Kinesins are generally plus-end–directed motor proteins that transport their cargo anterograde toward the synapse. Cytoplasmic dyneins are minus-end–directed motor proteins that transport their cargo retrograde toward the cell body.

Neuroglial Cells

The neuroglial cells of the nervous system, including the several types of neuroglial cells of the CNS, and the Schwann and satellite cells of the PNS, give the neurons protection and metabolic support. The neuroglial cells segregate the neurons into isolated metabolic compartments, which are required for normal neural function. Some types of neuroglial cells (astrocytes) help to form the blood–brain barrier that prevents toxic materials in the blood from entering the brain.

Two types of neuroglial cells (oligodendrocytes in the CNS and Schwann cells in the PNS) produce the myelin used to insulate nerve cell processes and increase the velocity of nerve impulse conduction. Myelin has a high lipid content, which gives it a whitish color, and the name *white matter* is given to the masses of myelinated fibers in the spinal cord and brain. Besides its role in increasing conduction velocity, the myelin sheath is essential for the survival of larger neuronal processes, perhaps by the secretion of neurotrophic compounds. Myelin formation is essentially the same in both the CNS and PNS. Both contain myelin basic protein, and both involve the winding of plasma membranes around the nerve fiber. During the wrapping of the two adjacent inner leaflets, the faces of the plasma membrane that are in close proximity and any remaining cytoplasm appear as a dark line called the *major dense line*. Likewise, during the wrapping of the plasma membranes to form myelin, adjacent outer plasma membrane leaflets become opposed, creating the interperiod or *minor dense line*.

In some pathologic conditions, the myelin may degenerate or be destroyed. This leaves a section of the axonal process without myelin (demyelinated) while leaving the nearby oligodendroglial or Schwann cells intact. Unless remyelination takes place, the axon eventually dies. The evidence continues to suggest the need for remyelination therapy in multiple sclerosis (a disease characterized by demyelinated lesions [or plaques] in the CNS). Remyelination of lesions that were demyelinated is possible for the person with multiple sclerosis. The use of new imaging technology will need to be established to determine remyelination has occurred in the person with multiple sclerosis.[3]

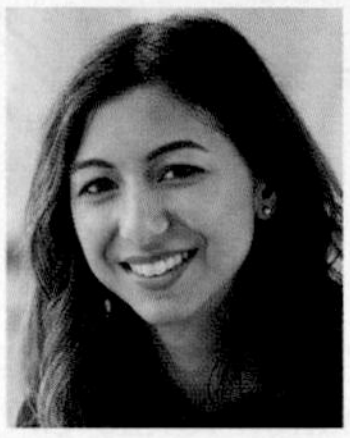

Remember **Ms. Ulrie**, the young woman you met at the beginning of the unit? This young college student has remitting–relapsing multiple sclerosis. She continued to have exacerbations of her disease every few months. She is maintained on a disease-modifying agent and treated with steroids during exacerbations. An MRI is performed every 3 to 6 months to assess for periventricular demyelinated plaques. As her disease progresses, her MRI will show more and more sclerotic plaques.

Neuroglial Cells of the Central Nervous System

Neuroglial cells of the CNS consist of the oligodendrocytes, astrocytes, microglia, and ependymal cells (Fig. 13.2). The *oligodendrocytes* form the myelin in the CNS. Instead of forming a myelin covering for a single axon, these cells reach out with several processes, each wrapping around and forming a multilayered myelin segment around several different axons. As with peripheral myelinated fibers, the covering of axons in the CNS increases the velocity of nerve conduction.

Astrocytes, the most numerous of neuroglial cells, are particularly prominent in the gray matter of the CNS. These large cells have many processes, some reaching to the surface of the capillaries, others reaching to the surface of the nerve cells, and still others filling most of the intercellular space within the CNS. Astrocytes maintain an important link between neurons, especially between synapses, and capillary blood flow. They also help to maintain the right potassium ion concentration in the extracellular space between neurons. Because astrocytes are highly permeable to potassium, they can take up excess potassium and so protect other neurons. In addition, astrocytes take up neurotransmitters from synaptic zones after their release and thereby help regulate synaptic activity. Research suggests that astrocytes may also play an important role in the regulation of blood flow to the cerebral gray matter.[4] Astrocytes are also the principal cells responsible for repair and scar formation in the brain. They can fill their cytoplasm with microfibrils (*i.e.*, fibrous astrocytes), and masses of these cells form the special type of scar tissue that develops in the CNS when the tissue is destroyed. This process is called *gliosis*.

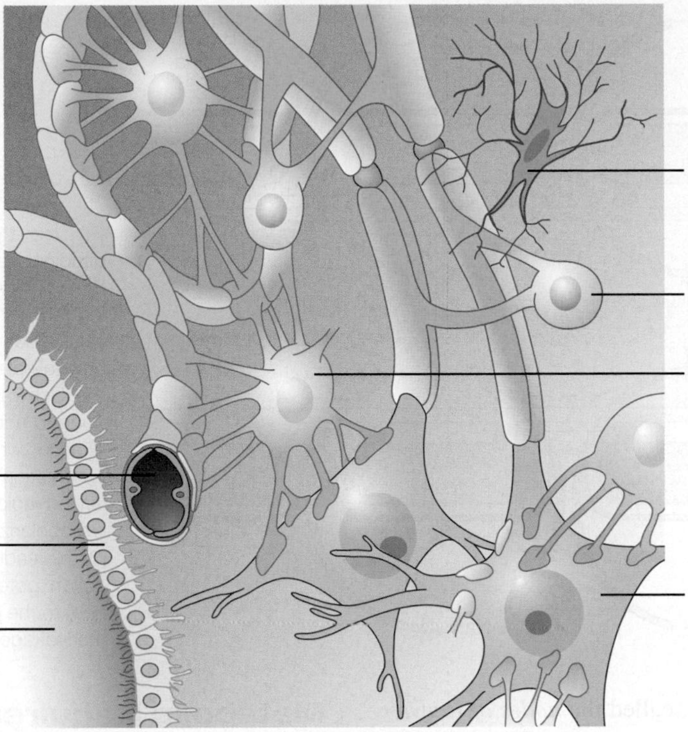

Figure 13.2 • The supporting cells of the CNS. Diagrammatic view of relationships between the glial elements (astrocyte, oligodendrocyte, microglial cell, and ependymal cells), the capillaries, the CSF, and the cell bodies of CNS neurons.

The third type of neuroglial cell, the *microglia*, is a small phagocytic cell that is available for cleaning up debris after cellular damage, infection, or cell death. The fourth type of cell, the *ependymal cell*, forms the lining of the neural tube cavity, the ventricular system. In some areas, these cells combine with a rich vascular network to form the *choroid plexus*, where production of the cerebrospinal fluid (CSF) takes place.

Neuroglial Cells of the Peripheral Nervous System

Satellite and Schwann cells are the two types of neuroglial cells in the PNS. Normally, the nerve cell bodies in the PNS are collected into ganglia, such as the dorsal root and autonomic ganglia. Satellite cells are flattened capsular cells that secrete a basement membrane that protects the cell body from the diffusion of large molecules. A single layer of satellite cells separates each of the cell bodies, and processes of the peripheral nerves are separated from the connective tissue framework of the ganglion.

Schwann cells are close relatives of the satellite cells. The cell membrane and cytoplasm of Schwann cells surround the processes of larger afferent and efferent neurons. During myelination, the Schwann cell wraps around each nerve process several times (Fig. 13.3). Schwann cells line up along the neuronal process, and each of these cells forms its own discrete myelin segment. The end of each myelin segment attaches to the cell membrane of the axon by means of intercellular junctions. Successive Schwann cells are separated

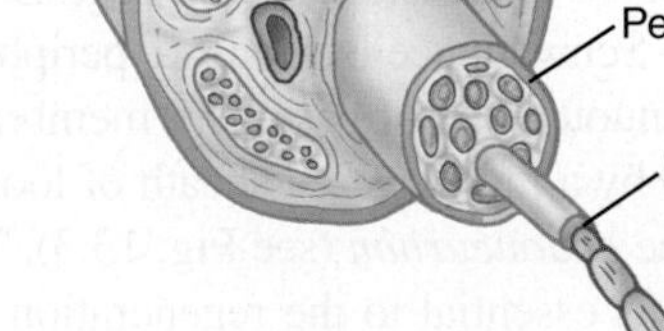

Figure 13.3 • Section of a peripheral nerve containing both afferent (sensory) and efferent (motor) neurons. Schwann cells form a myelin sheath around the larger nerve fibers in the PNS. Successive Schwann cells are separated by short extracellular fluid gaps called the *nodes of Ranvier*, where the myelin is missing and the voltage-gated sodium channels are concentrated.

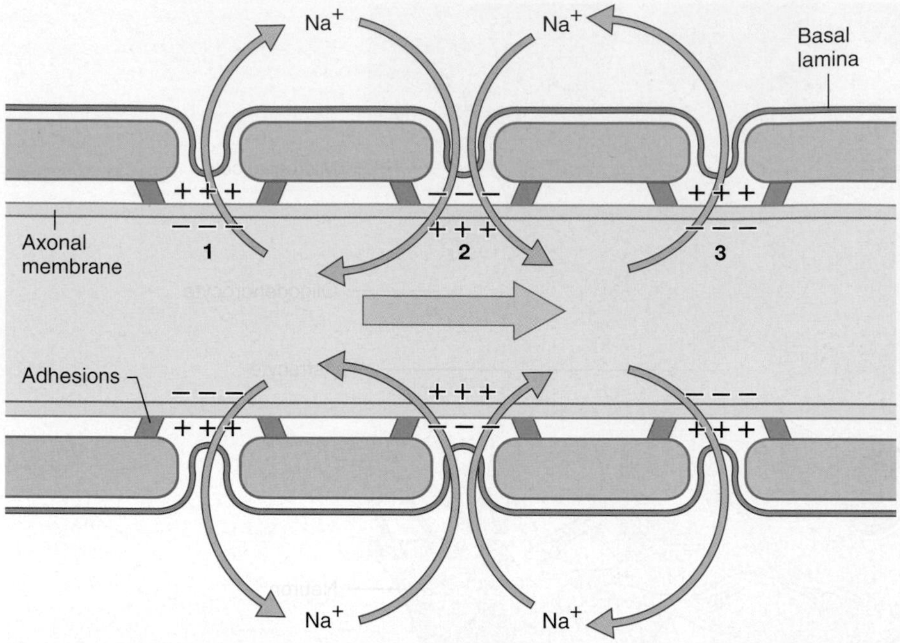

Figure 13.4 • Schematic drawing of a longitudinal section of a myelinated axon in the PNS. Schwann cells insulate the axon, decreasing flow through the membrane. Action potentials occur at the nodes of Ranvier, which are unmyelinated areas of the basal lamina between the Schwann cells. The impulses jump from node to node in a process called *saltatory conduction*, which greatly increases the velocity of conduction. (1) represents the trailing hyperpolarized region behind the action potential, (2) the hypopolarized region at the action potential, and (3) the leading hyperpolarized area ahead of the action potential. The Schwann cell adhesions (*red*) to the plasma membrane of the axon block the leakage of current under the myelin.

by short extracellular fluid gaps, called the *nodes of Ranvier*, where the myelin is missing and voltage-gated sodium channels are concentrated (Fig. 13.4). The nodes of Ranvier increase nerve conduction by allowing the impulse to jump from node to node through the extracellular fluid in a process called *saltatory conduction*. In this way, the impulse can travel more rapidly than it could if it were required to move systematically along the entire nerve process. This increased conduction velocity greatly reduces reaction time or time between the application of a stimulus and the subsequent motor response. The short reaction time is especially important in peripheral nerves with long distances (sometimes 1 to 1.5 m) for conduction between the CNS and distal effector organs.

Each of the Schwann cells along a peripheral nerve is encased in a continuous tube of basement membrane, which in turn is surrounded by a multilayered sheath of loose connective tissue known as the *endoneurium* (see Fig. 13.3). The endoneurial sheath, which is essential to the regeneration of peripheral nerves, provides a collagenous tube through which a regenerating axon can again reach its former target. The endoneurial sheath does not penetrate the CNS. The absence of the endoneurial sheaths is thought to be a major factor in the limited axonal regeneration of CNS nerves compared with those of the PNS.

The endoneurial sheaths are bundled with blood vessels into small bundles or clusters of nerves called *fascicles*. In the nerve, another protective covering called the perineurium surrounds the fascicles. The heavy protective *epineurial sheath* of the peripheral nerve further surrounds the fascicles. The protective layers that surround the peripheral nerve processes are continuous with the connective tissue capsule of the sensory nerve endings and the connective tissue that surrounds the effector structures, such as the skeletal muscle cell. Centrally, the connective tissue layers continue along the dorsal and ventral roots of the nerve and fuse with the meninges that surround the spinal cord and brain.

Metabolic Requirements of Nervous Tissue

Nervous tissue has a high rate of metabolism. The brain receives 15% to 20% (approximately 750 mL/minute) of the total resting cardiac output and consumes 20% of its oxygen.[5] Despite its substantial energy requirements, the brain cannot store oxygen or effectively engage in anaerobic metabolism. An interruption in the blood or oxygen supply to the brain rapidly leads to clinically observable signs and symptoms. Unconsciousness occurs almost simultaneously with cardiac arrest, and the death of brain cells begins within 4 to 6 minutes. Interruption of blood flow also leads to the accumulation of metabolic by-products that are toxic to neural tissue.

Glucose is the major fuel source for the nervous system, but neurons have no provision for storing glucose. Ketones can provide for limited temporary energy requirements. However, these sources are rapidly depleted. Unlike muscle cells, neurons have no glycogen stores and must rely on glucose from the blood or the glycogen stores of supporting neuroglial cells. People receiving insulin for diabetes may experience signs of neural dysfunction and unconsciousness (*i.e.*, insulin reaction or shock) when blood glucose drops because of insulin excess.

IN SUMMARY

Nervous tissue is composed of two types of cells—neurons and neuroglial cells. Neurons are composed of three parts—a cell body, which controls cell activity; the dendrites, which conduct information toward the cell body; and the axon, which carries impulses from the cell body. Axonal transport mechanisms provide the means to convey materials to and from the cell body and axon terminals. The neuroglial cells consist of several types of neuroglial cells in the CNS and Schwann and satellite cells of the PNS. Neuroglial cells protect and provide metabolic support for the neurons, help to regulate blood flow, and aid in segregating them into isolated compartments, which is necessary for normal neuronal function. Nervous system function demands a high proportion of metabolic energy. Glucose is the major fuel for the nervous system. The brain constitutes only 2% of body weight but receives 15% to 20% of the resting cardiac output.

NEUROPHYSIOLOGY

After completing this section of the chapter, the learner will be able to meet the following objectives:

- Describe the three phases of an action potential, and relate the functional importance of ion channels to the different phases.
- Characterize the role of excitatory and inhibitory postsynaptic potentials (IPSPs) as they relate to spatial and temporal summation of membrane potentials.
- Describe how neurotransmitters are synthesized, stored, released, and inactivated.

Neurons are characterized by the ability to communicate with other neurons through electrical impulses or action potentials. Neurons transfer information from one location to another via the frequency and pattern of action potentials.

Action Potentials

Nerve signals are transmitted by action potentials, which are abrupt, pulsatile changes in the membrane potential that last about 5 milliseconds.[2] The cell membranes of excitable tissue, including those of nerve and muscle cells, contain ion channels that are responsible for generating these action potentials. Voltage-dependent gates, which open and close with change in the membrane potential, guard the membrane ion channels. Separate voltage-gated channels exist for the sodium, potassium, and calcium ions. Each type of ion channel has a characteristic membrane potential that opens and closes its channels. Also present are ligand-gated channels that respond to chemical messengers such as neurotransmitters; mechanically, gated channels that respond to physical changes in the cell membrane; and light-gated channels that respond to fluctuations in light levels.

The excitability of neurons can be affected by conditions that alter the resting membrane potential, moving it either closer to or further from the threshold potential. *Hypopolarization* increases the excitability of the postsynaptic neuron by bringing the membrane potential closer to the threshold potential so that a smaller subsequent stimulus is needed to cause the neuron to fire. *Hyperpolarization* brings the membrane potential further from the threshold and has the opposite, inhibitory effect, decreasing the likelihood that an action potential will be generated.

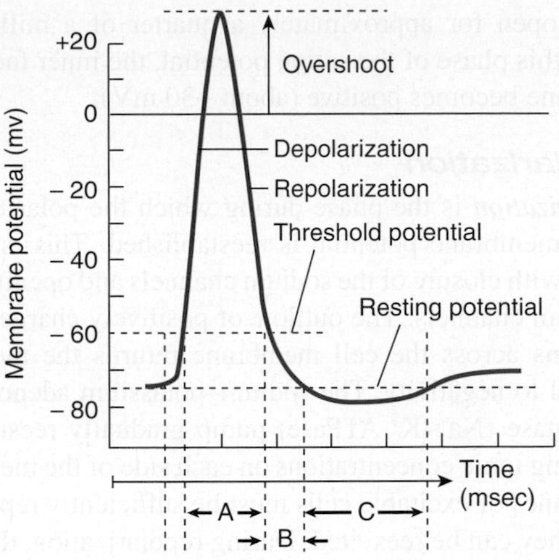

Figure 13.5 • Time course of the action potential recorded at one point of an axon with one electrode inside and one on the outside of the plasma membrane. The rising part of the action potential is called the *spike*. The rising phase plus approximately the first half of the repolarization phase is the absolute refractory period **(A)**. The portion of the repolarization phase that extends from the threshold to the resting membrane potential represents the relative refractory period **(B)**. The remaining portion of the repolarization phase to the resting membrane potential is the negative afterpotential **(C)**. Relative refractory period is the period during which the membrane becomes hyperpolarized as the potential drops below the resting membrane potential.

Action potentials can be divided into three phases—the resting or polarized state, depolarization, and repolarization (Fig. 13.5).

Resting Membrane Potential

The *resting membrane potential* (about −70 mV for large nerve fibers) is the undisturbed period of the action potential during which the nerve is not transmitting impulses. During this period the membrane is said to be *polarized* because of the large separation of charge (*i.e.*, positive on the outside and negative on the inside). The resting phase of the membrane potential continues until some event causes the membrane to increase its permeability to sodium. A *threshold potential* (about −55 mV in large nerve fibers) represents the membrane potential at which neurons or other excitable tissues are stimulated to fire.[6] When the threshold potential is reached, the gate-like structures in the ion channels open. Below the threshold potential, these gates remain tightly closed. The gates function on an all-or-none basis. They are either fully open or fully closed. Under ordinary circumstances, the threshold stimulus is sufficient to open many ion channels, triggering massive depolarization of the membrane (the action potential).

Depolarization

Depolarization is characterized by the flow of electrically charged ions. During the depolarization phase, the membrane suddenly becomes permeable to sodium ions. The rapid inflow of sodium ions produces local currents that travel through the adjacent cell membrane, causing the sodium channels in this part of the membrane to open. In neurons, sodium ion gates remain open for approximately a quarter of a millisecond. During this phase of the action potential, the inner face of the membrane becomes positive (about +30 mV).

Repolarization

Repolarization is the phase during which the polarity of the resting membrane potential is reestablished. This is accomplished with closure of the sodium channels and opening of the potassium channels. The outflow of positively charged potassium ions across the cell membrane returns the membrane potential to negativity. The sodium–potassium adenosine triphosphatase (Na^+–K^+ ATPase) pump gradually reestablishes the resting ionic concentrations on each side of the membrane. Membranes of excitable cells must be sufficiently repolarized before they can be reexcited. During repolarization, the membrane remains refractory until repolarization is approximately one third complete. This period, which lasts 0.4 to 4 ms, is called the *absolute refractory period*. During one portion of the recovery period, the membrane can be excited, although only by a stronger-than-normal stimulus. This period is called the *relative refractory period*.

Synaptic Transmission

Neurons communicate with each other through structures known as *synapses*. Two types of synapses are found in the nervous system—electrical and chemical. *Electrical synapses* permit the passage of current-carrying ions through small openings called *gap junctions* that penetrate the cell junction of adjoining cells and allow current to travel in either direction. The gap junctions allow an action potential to pass directly and quickly from one neuron to another. They may link neurons having close functional relationships into circuits.

The most common type of synapse is the *chemical synapse*. Chemical synapses involve special presynaptic and postsynaptic membrane structures, separated by a synaptic cleft. The presynaptic terminal secretes one and often several chemical transmitter molecules. The secreted neurotransmitters diffuse into the synaptic cleft and bind to receptors on the postsynaptic membrane. In contrast to an electrical synapse, a chemical synapse serves as a rectifier, permitting only one-way communication. Chemical synapses are divided into two types—excitatory and inhibitory. In excitatory synapses, binding of the neurotransmitter to the receptor produces depolarization of the postsynaptic membrane. Binding of the neurotransmitter to the receptor in an inhibitory synapse reduces the postsynaptic neuron's ability to generate an action potential. Most inhibitory neurotransmitters induce hyperpolarization of the postsynaptic membrane by making the membrane more permeable to potassium or chloride, or both.

Chemical synapses are the slowest component in progressive communication through a sequence of neurons, such as in a spinal reflex. In contrast to the conduction of electrical action potentials, each successive event at the chemical synapse—transmitter secretion, diffusion across the synaptic cleft, interaction with postsynaptic receptors, and generation of a subsequent action potential in the postsynaptic neuron—consumes time.

A neuron's cell body and dendrites are covered by thousands of synapses, any or many of which can be active at any moment. Because of the interaction of this rich synaptic input, each neuron resembles a little integrator in which circuits of many neurons interact with one another. It is the complexity of these interactions and the subtle integrations involved in producing behavioral responses that gives the system its intelligence.

Chemical synapses exhibit several relationships. Axons can synapse with dendrites (axodendritic), with the cell body (axosomatic), or with the axon (axoaxonic). Dendrites can synapse with axons (dendroaxonic), other dendrites (dendrodendritic), or the cell body of other neurons (dendrosomatic). Synapses between the nerve cell body and axons (somatoaxonic synapses) also have been observed. Synapses occurring between the cell body of neighboring neurons (somatosomatic) are uncommon, except between some efferent nuclei. The mechanism of communication between the presynaptic and the postsynaptic neuron is similar in all types of synapses. The action potential sweeps into the axonal terminals of the afferent neuron and triggers the rapid release of neurotransmitter molecules from the axonal, or presynaptic, surface.

Excitatory and Inhibitory Postsynaptic Potentials

A neurotransmitter can cause an excitatory or an inhibitory graded potential. When the combination of a neurotransmitter with a receptor site causes partial depolarization of the postsynaptic membrane, it is called an *excitatory postsynaptic potential* (EPSP). In other synapses, the combination of a transmitter with a receptor site is inhibitory in the sense that it causes the local nerve membrane to become hyperpolarized and less excitable. This is called an *inhibitory postsynaptic potential* (IPSP).

Action potentials do not begin in the membrane adjacent to the synapse. They begin in the initial segment of the axon, near the *axon hillock* (see Fig. 13.1), that lies just before the first myelin segment. The initial segment of the axon is more excitable than the rest of the neuron. The local currents resulting from an EPSP (sometimes called a *generator potential*) are usually insufficient to reach threshold and cause depolarization of the axon's initial segment. If several EPSPs occur simultaneously, the area of depolarization can become large enough, and the currents at the initial segment can become strong enough to exceed the threshold potential and initiate an action potential. This summation of depolarized areas is called *spatial summation*. EPSPs also can summate and cause an action potential if they occur in rapid succession. This temporal aspect of the occurrence of two or more EPSPs is called *temporal summation*.

IPSPs also can undergo spatial and temporal summation with each other and with EPSPs, reducing the effectiveness of the latter by a roughly algebraic summation. If the sum of EPSPs and IPSPs keeps the depolarization at the initial segment below threshold levels, no action potential occurs.

Understanding Synaptic Transmission

Neurons communicate with each other through chemical synapses and the use of neurotransmitters. Chemical synapses consist of a presynaptic neuron, a synaptic cleft, and a postsynaptic neuron. The communication process relies on (1) synthesis and release of the neurotransmitter from a presynaptic neuron, (2) binding of the neurotransmitter to receptors in the postsynaptic neuron, and (3) removal of the neurotransmitter from the receptor site.

Neurotransmitter Synthesis and Release

Neurotransmitters are synthesized in the presynaptic neuron and then stored in synaptic vesicles. Communication between the two neurons begins with a nerve impulse that stimulates the presynaptic neuron, followed by movement of the synaptic vesicles to the cell membrane and release of neurotransmitter into the synaptic cleft.

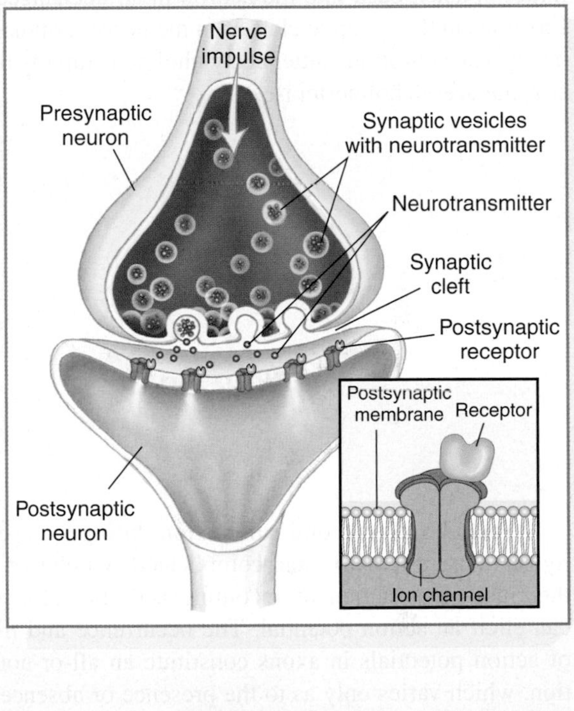

Receptor Binding

Once released from the presynaptic neuron, the neurotransmitter moves across the synaptic cleft and binds to receptors on the postsynaptic neuron. The action of a neurotransmitter is determined by the type of receptor (excitatory or inhibitory) to which it binds. Binding of a neurotransmitter to a receptor with an excitatory function often results in the opening of an ion channel, such as the sodium channel. Many presynaptic neurons also have receptors to which a neurotransmitter binds. The presynaptic receptors function in a negative feedback manner to inhibit further release of the neurotransmitter.

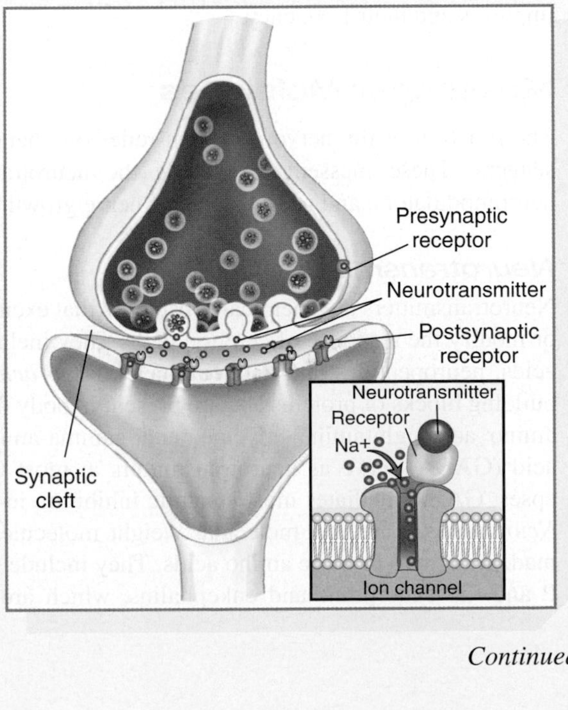

Continued

Understanding Synaptic Transmission *(Continued)*

Neurotransmitter Removal

Precise control of synaptic function relies on the rapid removal of the neurotransmitter from the receptor site. A released neurotransmitter can (1) be taken back up into the neuron in a process called reuptake, (2) diffuse out of the synaptic cleft, or (3) be broken down by enzymes into inactive substances or metabolites. The action of norepinephrine is largely terminated by the reuptake process, in which the neurotransmitter is taken back into the neuron in an unchanged form and reused. Enzymes in the synaptic cleft or in the nerve terminals can also break it down. The neurotransmitter acetylcholine is rapidly broken down by the enzyme acetylcholinesterase.

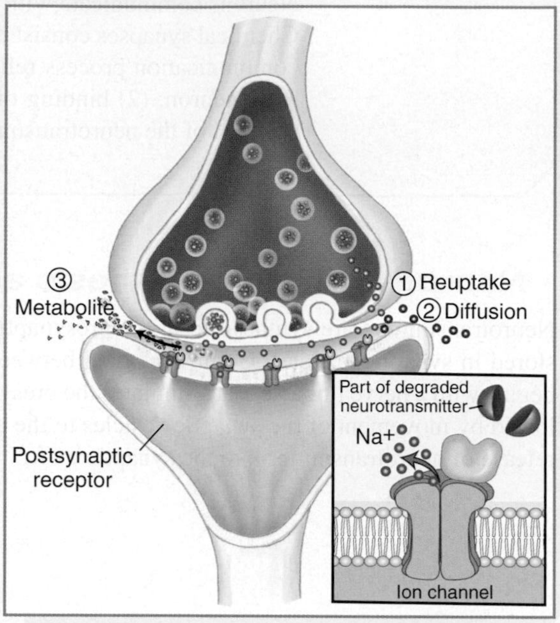

Spatial and temporal summation during synaptic activity serves as a sensitive and complicated switch that requires the right combination of incoming activity before the cell can elicit an action potential. The occurrence and frequency of action potentials in axons constitute an all-or-none situation, which varies only as to the presence or absence of such impulses and their frequency.

Messenger Molecules

The function of the nervous system relies on chemical messengers. These messengers include the neurotransmitters, neuromodulators, and neurotrophic or nerve growth factors.

Neurotransmitters

Neurotransmitters are chemical substances that excite, inhibit, or modify the response of cerebral cells. They include amino acids, neuropeptides, and monoamines. *Amino acids* are the building blocks of proteins and are present in body fluids. The amino acids glutamine, glycine, and gamma-aminobutyric acid (GABA) serve as neurotransmitters at most CNS synapses. GABA mediates most synaptic inhibition in the CNS. *Neuropeptides* are low molecular weight molecules that are made up of two or more amino acids. They include substance P and the endorphins and enkephalins, which are involved in pain sensation and perception. A *monoamine* is an amine molecule containing one amino group (NH_2). Serotonin, dopamine, norepinephrine, and epinephrine are monoamines synthesized from amino acids.

The process of neurotransmission involves the synthesis, storage, and release of a neurotransmitter; the reaction of the neurotransmitter with a receptor; and termination of the receptor action. Neurotransmitters are synthesized in the cytoplasm of the axon terminal. The synthesis of transmitters may require one or more enzyme-catalyzed steps (*e.g.*, one for acetylcholine and three for norepinephrine). Neurons are limited as to the type of transmitter they can synthesize by their enzyme systems. After synthesis, the neurotransmitter molecules are stored in the axon terminal in tiny, membrane-bound sacs called *synaptic vesicles*. These vesicles protect the neurotransmitters from enzyme destruction in the nerve terminal. There may be thousands of vesicles in a single terminal, each containing 10,000 to 100,000 transmitter molecules. The arrival of an impulse at a nerve terminal causes the vesicles to move to the cell membrane and release their transmitter molecules into the synaptic space.

Neurotransmitters exert their actions through specific proteins, called *receptors*, embedded in the postsynaptic membrane. These receptors are tailored precisely to match the size and shape of the transmitter. The interaction between a transmitter and receptor results in a specific physiologic response. The action of a transmitter is determined by the type of receptor (excitatory or inhibitory) to which it binds. Acetylcholine is excitatory when it is released at a myoneural junction, and it is inhibitory when it is released at the sinoatrial node in the heart. Receptors are named according to the type of neurotransmitter with which they interact (*e.g.*, a *cholinergic receptor* is a receptor that binds to acetylcholine).

Rapid removal of a transmitter, once it has exerted its effects on the postsynaptic membrane, is necessary to maintain precise control of neural transmission. A released transmitter can undergo one of these three processes:

1. It can be broken down into inactive substances by enzymes.
2. It can be taken back up into the presynaptic neuron in a process called *reuptake*.
3. It can diffuse into the intercellular fluid until its concentration is too low to influence postsynaptic excitability.

An example of these processes is when acetylcholine is rapidly broken down by acetylcholinesterase into acetic acid and choline, with the choline being taken back into the presynaptic neuron for reuse in acetylcholine synthesis. The catecholamines are largely taken back into the neuron in an unchanged form for reuse. Enzymes in the synaptic space or in the nerve terminals also can degrade catecholamines.

Neuromodulators

Other classes of messenger molecules, known as *neuromodulators*, also may be released from axon terminals. Neuromodulator molecules react with presynaptic or postsynaptic receptors to alter the release of, or response to, neurotransmitters. Neuromodulators may act on postsynaptic receptors to produce slower and longer-lasting changes in membrane excitability. This alters the action of the faster-acting neurotransmitter molecules by enhancing or decreasing their effectiveness. By combining with autoreceptors on its own presynaptic membrane, a transmitter can act as a neuromodulator to augment or inhibit further nerve activity. In some nerves, such as the peripheral sympathetic nerves, a messenger molecule can have both transmitter and modulator functions. For example, norepinephrine can activate α_1-adrenergic postsynaptic receptors to produce vasoconstriction or stimulate α_2-adrenergic presynaptic receptors to inhibit further norepinephrine release.

Neurotrophic Factors

Neurotrophic or nerve growth factors are required to maintain the long-term survival of the postsynaptic cell and are secreted by axon terminals independent of action potentials. Examples include neuron-to-neuron trophic factors in the sequential synapses of CNS sensory neurons. Trophic factors from target cells that enter the axon and are necessary for the long-term survival of presynaptic neurons also have been demonstrated. Target cell-to-neuron trophic factors probably have a great significance in establishing specific neural connections during normal embryonic development.

IN SUMMARY

Neurons are characterized by the ability to communicate with other neurons and body cells through electrical signals called *action potentials*. The cell membranes of neurons contain ion channels that are responsible for generating action potentials. Voltage-dependent gates that open and close with changes in the membrane potential guard these channels. Action potentials are divided into three parts—the resting membrane potential, during which the membrane is polarized, but no electrical activity occurs; the depolarization phase, during which sodium channels open, allowing rapid inflow of the sodium ions that generate the electrical impulse; and the repolarization phase, during which the membrane is permeable to potassium ions, allowing for the efflux of potassium ions and the return to the resting membrane potential.

Synapses are structures that permit communication between neurons. Two types of synapses have been identified—electrical and chemical. Electrical synapses consist of gap junctions between adjacent cells that allow action potentials to move rapidly from one cell to another. Chemical synapses involve special presynaptic and postsynaptic structures, separated by a synaptic cleft. They rely on chemical messengers, released from the presynaptic neuron, that cross the synaptic cleft and then interact with receptors on the postsynaptic neuron.

Neurotransmitters are chemical messengers that control neural function. They selectively cause excitation or inhibition of action potentials. Three major types of neurotransmitters are known—amino acids such as glutamic acid and GABA, neuropeptides such as the endorphins and enkephalins, and monoamines such as epinephrine and norepinephrine. Neurotransmitters interact with cell membrane receptors to produce either excitatory or inhibitory actions. Neuromodulators are chemical messengers that react with membrane receptors to produce slower and longer-acting changes in membrane permeability. Neurotrophic or growth factors, also released from presynaptic terminals, are required to maintain the long-term survival of postsynaptic neurons.

DEVELOPMENTAL ORGANIZATION OF THE NERVOUS SYSTEM

After completing this section of the chapter, the learner will be able to meet the following objectives:

- Define the terms *afferent, efferent, ganglia, association neuron, cell column*, and *tract*.
- Describe the origin and destination of nerve fibers contained in the dorsal and ventral roots.
- Describe the structures innervated by general somatic afferent, special visceral afferent, general visceral afferent, special somatic afferent, general visceral efferent, pharyngeal efferent, and general somatic efferent neurons.

The organization of the nervous system can be described in terms of its development, in which newer functions and greater complexity resulted from the modification and enlargement of more primitive structures. Thus, the rostral or front end of the CNS became specialized, with the more ancient organization being retained in the brain stem and spinal cord. The dominance of the front end of the CNS is reflected in what has been termed a *hierarchy of control*, with the forebrain having control over the brain stem and the brain stem having control over the spinal cord. In the developmental process, newer functions were added to the surface of functionally older systems. As newer functions became concentrated at the rostral end of the nervous system, they also became more vulnerable to injury. Nothing exemplifies this principle better than the persistent vegetative state. This occurs when severe brain injury causes irreversible damage to higher cortical centers, whereas lower stem centers such as those that control breathing remain functional.

Embryonic Development

All body tissues and organs have developed from the three embryonic layers (*i.e.*, ectoderm, mesoderm, and endoderm) that were present during the 3rd week of embryonic life. The body is organized into the soma and viscera. The soma, or body wall, includes all of the structures derived from the embryonic ectoderm, such as the epidermis of the skin and the CNS. Mesodermal connective tissues of the soma include the dermis of the skin, skeletal muscle, bone, and the outer lining of the body cavity (*i.e.*, parietal pleura and peritoneum). The nervous system innervates all somatic structures plus the internal structures making up the viscera. *Viscera* include the great vessels derived from the intermediate mesoderm, the urinary system, and the gonadal structures. It also includes the inner lining of the body cavities, such as the visceral pleura and peritoneum, and the mesodermal tissues that surround the endoderm-lined gut and its derivative organs (*e.g.*, lungs, liver, pancreas).

The nervous system appears very early in embryonic development (week 3). This early development is essential because it influences the development and organization of many other body systems, including the axial skeleton, skeletal muscles, and sensory organs such as the eyes and ears. Throughout life, the organization of the nervous system retains many patterns that were established during embryonic life. It is this early pattern of segmental development in the embryo that is presented as a framework for understanding the nervous system.

During the 2nd week of development, embryonic tissue consists of two layers, the endoderm and the ectoderm. At the beginning of week 3, the ectoderm begins to invaginate and migrates between the two layers, forming a third layer called the mesoderm (Fig. 13.6). Mesoderm along the entire midline of the embryo forms a specialized rod of embryonic tissue

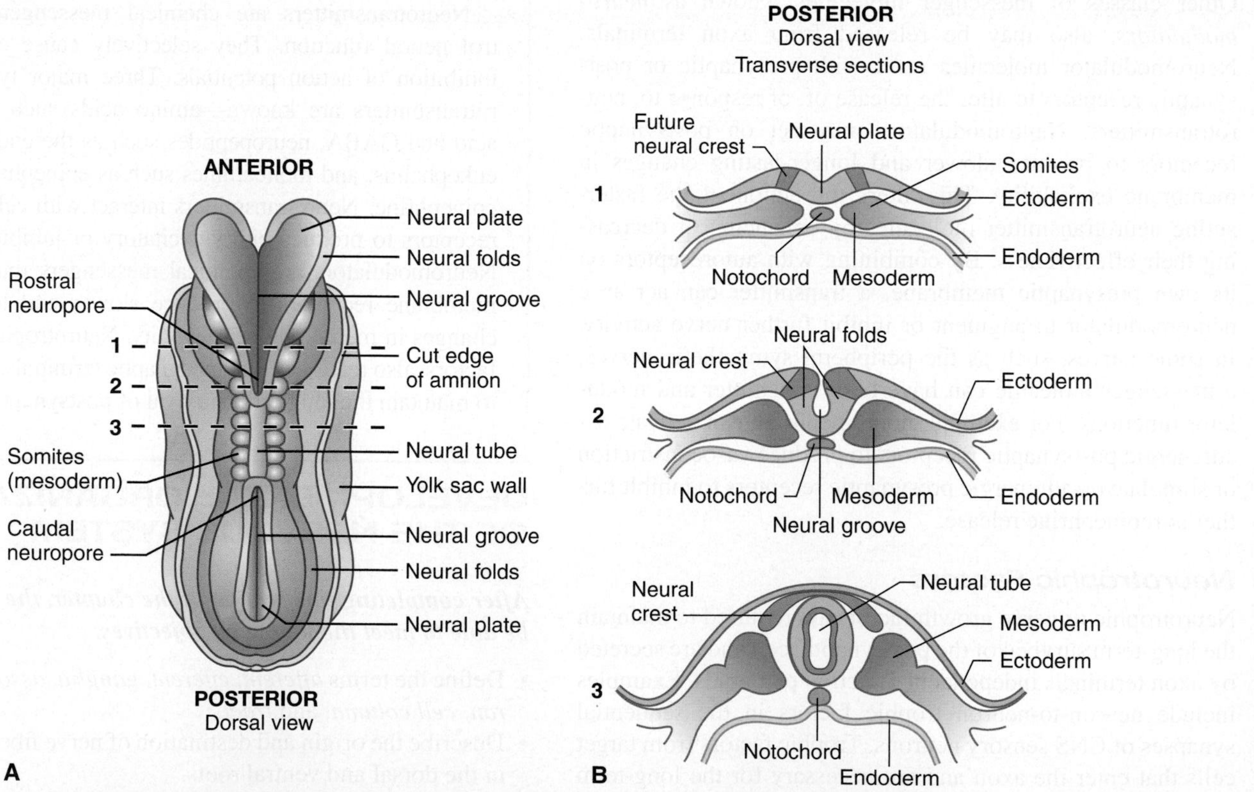

Figure 13.6 • Folding of the neural tube. **(A)** Dorsal view of a six-somite embryo (22 to 23 days) showing the neural folds, neural groove, and fused neural tube. The anterior neuropore closes at about day 25 and the posterior neuropore at about day 27. **(B)** Three cross-sections taken at the levels indicated in **A**. The sections indicate where the neural tube is just beginning to form.

called the *notochord.* The notochord and adjacent mesoderm provide the necessary induction signal for the overlying ectoderm to differentiate and form a thickened structure called the *neural plate*, the primordium of the nervous system. Within the neural plate, an axial groove (*i.e.*, neural groove) develops and sinks into the underlying mesoderm, allowing its walls to fuse across the top and form an ectodermal tube called the *neural tube*. This process, called *closure*, occurs during the later 3rd and 4th weeks of gestation and is vital to the survival of the embryo.

During embryonic development, the neural tube develops into the CNS, whereas the notochord becomes the foundation around which the vertebral column ultimately develops. The surface ectoderm separates from the neural tube and fuses over the top to become the outer layer of the skin. Initial closure of the neural tube begins at the cervical and high thoracic levels and zippers rostrally toward the cephalic end of the embryo and caudally toward the sacrum. Complete closure occurs around day 25 at the rostral-most end of the brain (*i.e.*, anterior neuropore) and around day 27 in the lumbosacral region (*i.e.*, posterior neuropore).

As the neural tube closes, ectodermal cells called *neural crest cells* migrate away from the dorsal surface of the neural tube to become the progenitors of the neurons and supporting cells of the PNS. During this period of embryonic development, neural cell adhesive molecules (N-CAMs) are produced to decrease migration of neural crest cells. In addition, fibronectin molecules are produced to increase the formation of pathways that guide the neural crest cells during their migration. Some of these cells gather into clusters to form the *dorsal root ganglia* at the sides of each spinal cord segment and the *cranial ganglia* that are present in most brain segments. Neurons of these ganglia become the afferent or sensory neurons of the PNS. Other neural crest cells become the pigment cells of the skin or contribute to the formation of the meninges, many structures of the face, and the peripheral ganglion cells of the autonomic nervous system (ANS), including those of the adrenal cortex.

During development, more rostral portions of the embryonic neural tube—approximately 10 segments—undergo extensive modification and enlargement to form the brain (Fig. 13.7). In the early embryo, 3 swellings, or primary vesicles, develop, subdividing these 10 segments into the prosencephalon, or forebrain, containing the first 2 segments; the mesencephalon, or midbrain, which develops from segment 3; and the rhombencephalon, or hindbrain, which develops from segments 4 to 10. The brain stem is formed from modifications of the 10 rostral segments of the wall of the neural tube. In the prosencephalon or forebrain, two pairs of lateral outpouchings develop—the optic cup, which becomes the optic nerve and retina, and the telencephalic vesicles, which become the cerebral hemispheres. Within the prosencephalon, the hollow central canal expands to become enlarged CSF-filled cavities, the first and second (lateral) ventricles. The remaining diencephalic portion of the neural tube develops into the thalamus and hypothalamus. The neurohypophysis (posterior pituitary) grows as a midline ventral outgrowth at the junctions of segments 1 and 2. A dorsal outgrowth, the pineal body, develops between segments 2 and 3.

All brain segments, except segment 2, retain some portion of the basic segmental organization of the nervous system. The evolutionary development of the brain is reflected in the cranial- and upper cervical–paired segmental nerves. This reflects the original pattern of a segmented neural tube, each segment of which has multiple paired branches containing a group of component axons. One segment would have paired branches to body muscles, another set to visceral structures, and so on. The classic pattern of spinal nerve organization, which consists of a pair of dorsal and a pair of ventral roots, is a later evolutionary development that has not occurred in the CNs. Consequently, the CNs, which are arbitrarily numbered 1 through 12, retain the ancient pattern,

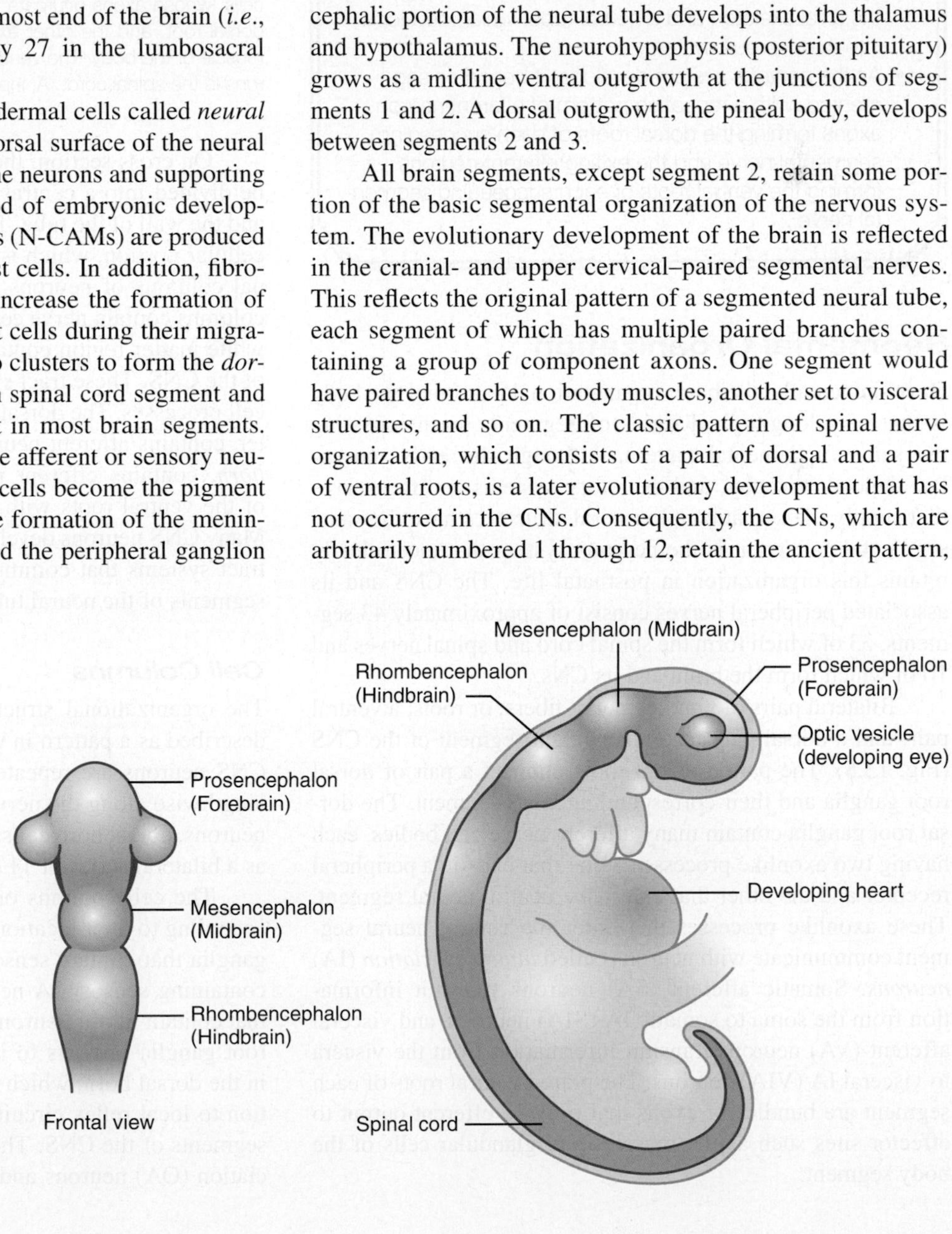

Figure 13.7 • Frontal and lateral views of a 5-week-old embryo showing the brain vesicles and three embryonic divisions of the brain and brain stem.

with more than one CN branching from a single segment. The truly segmental nerve pattern of the CNs is altered because all branches from segment 2 and most of the branches from segment 1 are missing. CN II, also called the *optic nerve*, is not a segmental nerve. It is a brain tract connecting the retina (modified brain) with the first forebrain segment from which it developed.

KEY POINTS

THE DEVELOPMENTAL ORGANIZATION OF THE NERVOUS SYSTEM

- In the process of development, the basic organizational pattern is that of a longitudinal series of segments, each repeating the same basic fundamental organizational pattern: a body wall or soma containing the axial skeleton and a neural tube, which develops into the nervous system.
- As the nervous system develops, it becomes segmented, with a repeating pattern of afferent neuron axons forming the dorsal roots of each succeeding segmental nerve and the exiting efferent neurons forming the ventral roots of each succeeding segmental nerve.

Segmental Organization

Developmentally, the basic organizational pattern of the body is that of a longitudinal series of segments, each repeating the same fundamental pattern. Although the early muscular, skeletal, vascular, and excretory systems and the nerves that supply the somatic and visceral structures have the same segmental pattern, it is the nervous system that most clearly retains this organization in postnatal life. The CNS and its associated peripheral nerves consist of approximately 43 segments, 33 of which form the spinal cord and spinal nerves and 10 of which form the brain and its CNs.

Bilateral pairs of bundled nerve fibers, or roots; a ventral pair; and a dorsal pair accompany each segment of the CNS (Fig. 13.8). The paired dorsal roots connect a pair of dorsal root ganglia and their corresponding CNS segment. The dorsal root ganglia contain many afferent nerve cell bodies, each having two axonlike processes—one that ends in a peripheral receptor and the other that enters the central neural segment. These axonlike processes that enter the central neural segment communicate with neurons called *input association* (IA) *neurons*. Somatic afferent (SA) neurons transmit information from the soma to somatic IA (SIA) neurons, and visceral afferent (VA) neurons transmit information from the viscera to visceral IA (VIA) neurons. The paired ventral roots of each segment are bundles of axons that provide efferent output to effector sites such as the muscles and glandular cells of the body segment.

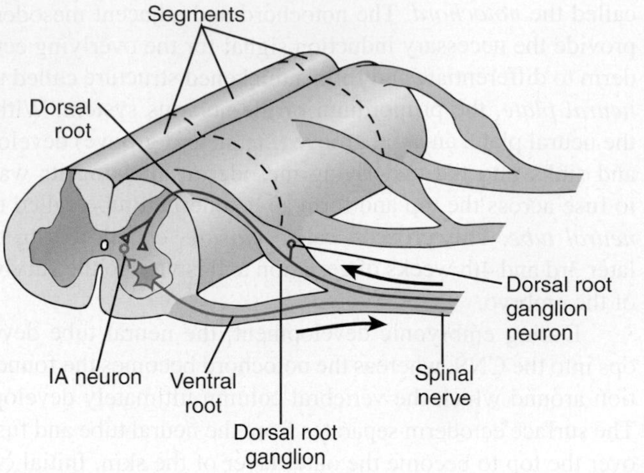

Figure 13.8 • In this diagram of three segments of the spinal cord, three dorsal roots enter the dorsal lateral surface of the cord, and three ventral roots exit. The dorsal root ganglion contains dorsal root ganglion cells, whose axons bifurcate: one process enters the spinal cord in the dorsal root, and the other extends peripherally to supply the skin and muscle of the body. The ventral root is formed by axons from motoneurons in the spinal cord. IA, input association.

On cross section, the hollow embryonic neural tube can be divided into a central canal, or ventricle, containing CSF and the wall of the tube. The latter develops into an inner gray cellular portion, which is functionally divided into longitudinal columns of neurons called the *cell columns*. These cell columns contain nerve cell bodies surrounded by a superficial white matter region containing the longitudinal tract systems of the CNS. These tract systems are composed of many nerve cell processes. The dorsal half, or *dorsal horn* of the gray matter, contains afferent neurons. The ventral portion, or *ventral horn*, contains efferent neurons that communicate by way of the ventral roots with effector cells of the body segment. Many CNS neurons develop axons that grow longitudinally as tract systems that communicate between adjacent and distal segments of the neural tube.

Cell Columns

The organizational structure of the nervous system can be described as a pattern in which functionally specific PNS and CNS neurons are repeated as parallel cell columns running lengthwise along the nervous system. In this pattern, afferent neurons, dorsal horn cells, and ventral horn cells are organized as a bilateral series of 11 cell columns.

The cell columns on each side can be further grouped according to their location in the PNS—four in the dorsal root ganglia that contain sensory neurons, four in the dorsal horn containing sensory IA neurons, and three in the ventral horn that contain motor neurons (Fig. 13.9). Each column of dorsal root ganglia projects to its particular column of IA neurons in the dorsal horn, which then distribute the afferent information to local reflex circuits and to more rostral and elaborate segments of the CNS. The ventral horns contain output association (OA) neurons and lower motor neurons (LMNs). The

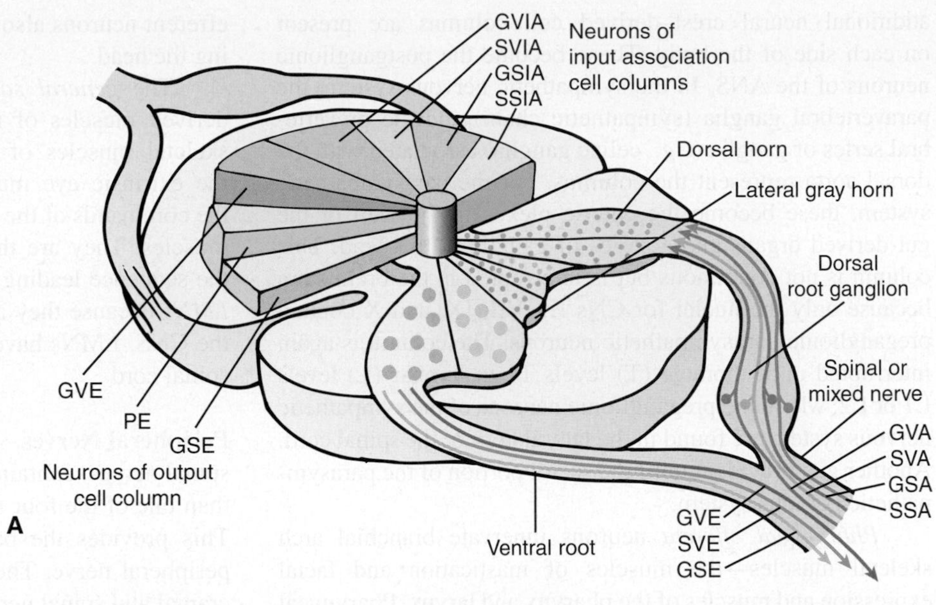

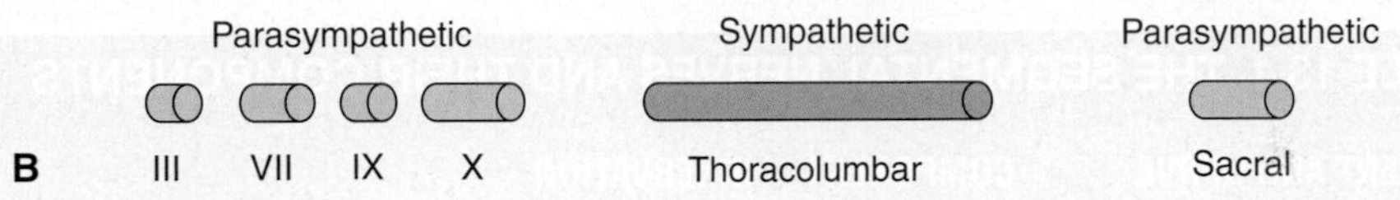

Figure 13.9 • **(A)** Cell columns of the CNS. The cell columns in the dorsal horn contain input association (IA) neurons for the general visceral afferent (GVA), special visceral afferent (SVA), special sensory afferent (SSA), and general somatic afferent (GSA) neurons with cell bodies in the dorsal root ganglion. The cell columns in the ventral horn contain the general visceral efferent (GVE), pharyngeal efferent (PE), and general somite efferent (GSE) neurons and their OA neurons. **(B)** Schematic of the GVE cell column showing both parasympathetic and sympathetic components. The column is not continuous but is interrupted in the brain stem because only the nuclei of CNs III, VII, IX, and X contain preganglionic parasympathetic neurons. The column again is interrupted until levels T1 to L1 or L2, where the preganglionic neurons of the sympathetic portion are found in the lateral horn of the spinal cord. Another gap is evident until the sacral portion of the parasympathetic nervous system.

LMNs provide the final circuitry for organizing efferent nerve activity.

Between the IA neurons and the OA neurons are networks of small internuncial (interneuronal) neurons arranged in complex circuits. Internuncial neurons provide the discreteness, appropriateness, and intelligence of responses to stimuli. Most of the billions of CNS cells in the spinal cord and brain gray matter are internuncial neurons.

Dorsal Horn Cell Columns. Four columns of afferent (sensory) neurons in the dorsal root ganglia directly innervate four corresponding columns of IA neurons in the dorsal horn. These columns are categorized as special and general afferents: special SA, general SA, special VA, and general VA (see Fig. 13.9).

Special somatic afferent fibers are concerned with internal sensory information such as joint and tendon sensation (*i.e.*, proprioception). Neurons in the special SIA column cells relay their information to local reflexes concerned with posture and movement. These neurons also relay information to the cerebellum, contributing to coordination of movement, and to the forebrain, contributing to experience. Afferents innervating the labyrinth and derived auditory end organs of the inner ear also belong to the special SA category.

General somatic afferents innervate the skin and other somatic structures and respond to stimuli such as those that produce pressure or pain. General SIA column cells relay the sensory information to protective and other reflex circuits and project the information to the forebrain, where it is perceived as painful, warm, cold, and the like.

Special visceral afferent cells innervate specialized gut-related receptors, such as the taste buds and receptors of the olfactory mucosa. Their central processes communicate with special VIA column neurons that project to reflex circuits producing salivation, chewing, swallowing, and other responses. Forebrain projection fibers from these association cells provide sensations of taste and smell.

General visceral afferent neurons innervate visceral structures such as the gastrointestinal tract, urinary bladder, and heart and great vessels. They project to the general VIA column, which relays information to vital reflex circuits and sends information to the forebrain regarding visceral sensations such as stomach fullness, bladder pressure, and sexual experience.

Ventral Horn Cell Columns. The ventral horn contains three longitudinal cell columns—general visceral efferent, pharyngeal efferent, and general somatic efferent (see Fig. 13.9). Each of these cell columns contains OA and efferent neurons. The OA neurons coordinate and integrate the function of the efferent motor neurons cells of their column.

General visceral efferent neurons transmit the efferent output of the ANS and are called *preganglionic neurons*. These neurons are structurally and functionally divided into either the sympathetic or the parasympathetic nervous systems. Their axons project through the segmental ventral roots (specifically from a group of neurons originating in the intermediolateral horn of the thoracolumbar cord) to innervate smooth and cardiac muscle and glandular cells of the body, most of which are in the viscera. In the viscera, three additional neural crest–derived cell columns are present on each side of the body. These become the postganglionic neurons of the ANS. In the sympathetic nervous system, the paravertebral ganglia (sympathetic chain) and the prevertebral series of ganglia (*e.g.*, celiac ganglia) associated with the dorsal aorta represent the columns. For the parasympathetic system, these become the enteric plexus in the wall of the gut-derived organs and a series of ganglia in the head. This column is not continuous but is interrupted in the brain stem because only the nuclei for CNs III, VII, IX, and X contain preganglionic parasympathetic neurons. The column is again interrupted until thoracic (T) levels T1 to lumbar (L) levels L1 or L2, where the preganglionic neurons of the sympathetic nervous system are found in the lateral horn of the spinal cord. Another gap is evident until the sacral portion of the parasympathetic nervous system.

Pharyngeal efferent neurons innervate branchial arch skeletal muscles—the muscles of mastication and facial expression and muscles of the pharynx and larynx. Pharyngeal efferent neurons also innervate muscles responsible for moving the head.

The *general somatic efferent* neurons supply somite-derived muscles of the body and head, which include the skeletal muscles of the body and limbs, the tongue, and the extrinsic eye muscles. These efferent neurons transmit the commands of the CNS to peripheral effectors, the skeletal muscles. They are the "final common pathway neurons" in the sequence leading to motor activity. They are often called *LMNs* because they are under the control of higher levels of the CNS. LMNs have their cell bodies in the brain stem and spinal cord.

Peripheral Nerves. Peripheral nerves, including cranial and spinal nerves, contain afferent and efferent processes of more than one of the four afferent and three efferent cell columns. This provides the basis for assessing the function of any peripheral nerve. The functional components of each of the cranial and spinal nerves are presented in Table 13.1.

TABLE 13.1 THE SEGMENTAL NERVES AND THEIR COMPONENTS

SEGMENT AND NERVE	COMPONENT	INNERVATION	FUNCTION
1. Forebrain			
I. Olfactory	SVA	Receptors in olfactory mucosa	Reflexes, olfaction (smell)
2. II. Optic nerve		Optic nerve and retina (part of brain system, not a peripheral nerve)	
3. Midbrain			
V. Trigeminal (V_1) ophthalmic division	SSA	Muscles: upper face: forehead, upper lid	Facial expression, proprioception
	GSA	Skin, subcutaneous tissue; conjunctiva; frontal/ethmoid sinuses	Somesthesia Reflexes (blink)
III. Oculomotor	GVE	Iris sphincter	Pupillary constriction
		Ciliary muscle	Accommodation
	GSE	Extrinsic eye muscles	Eye movement, lid movement
4. Pons			
V. Trigeminal (V_2) maxillary division	SSA	Muscles: facial expression	Proprioception Reflexes (sneeze), somesthesia
	GSA	Skin, oral mucosa, upper teeth, hard palate, maxillary sinus	
V. Trigeminal (V_3) mandibular division	SSA	Lower jaw, muscles: mastication	Proprioception, jaw jerk
	GSA	Skin, mucosa, teeth, anterior two thirds of the tongue	Reflexes, somesthesia
	PE		Mastication: speech
		Muscles: mastication	Protects the ear from loud sounds
		Tensor tympani	Tenses the soft palate
		Tensor veli palatini	
IV. Trochlear	GSE	Extrinsic eye muscle	Moves the eye down and in
5. Caudal Pons			
VIII. Vestibular, cochlear (vestibulocochlear)	SSA	Vestibular end organs	Reflexes, sense of head position
		Organ of Corti	Reflexes, hearing
VII. Facial nerve, intermedius portion	GSA	External auditory meatus	Somesthesia
	GVA	Nasopharynx	Gag reflex: sensation
	SVA	Taste buds of anterior two thirds of the tongue	Reflexes: gustation (taste)
	GVE	Nasopharynx	Mucus secretion, reflexes
		Lacrimal, sublingual, submandibular glands	Lacrimation, salivation
Facial nerve	PE	Muscles: facial expression, stapedius	Facial expression Protects the ear from loud sounds
VI. Abducens	GSE	Extrinsic eye muscle	Lateral eye deviation

TABLE 13.1 THE SEGMENTAL NERVES AND THEIR COMPONENTS *(Continued)*

SEGMENT AND NERVE	COMPONENT	INNERVATION	FUNCTION
6. Middle Medulla			
IX. Glossopharyngeal	SSA	Stylopharyngeus muscle	Proprioception
	GSA	Posterior external ear	Somesthesia
	SVA	Taste buds of posterior one third of the tongue	Gustation (taste)
	GVA	Oral pharynx	Gag reflex: sensation
	GVE	Parotid gland; pharyngeal mucosa	Salivary reflex: mucous secretion
	PE	Stylopharyngeus muscle	Assists swallowing
7–10. Caudal Medulla			
X. Vagus	SSA	Muscles: pharynx, larynx	Proprioception
	GSA	Posterior external ear	Somesthesia
	SVA	Taste buds, pharynx, larynx	Reflexes, gestation
	GVA	Visceral organs (esophagus to midtransverse colon, liver, pancreas, heart, lungs)	Reflexes, sensation
	GVE		Parasympathetic efferent
	PE	Visceral organs as above	Swallowing, phonation, emesis
		Muscles: pharynx, larynx	
XII. Hypoglossal	GSE	Muscles of the tongue	Tongue movement, reflexes
Spinal Segments			
C1–C4 Upper Cervical	PE	Muscles: sternocleidomastoid, trapezius	Head, shoulder movement
XI. Spinal accessory nerve			
Spinal nerves	SSA	Muscles of the neck	Proprioception, DTRs
	GSA	Neck, back of the head	Somesthesia
	GSE	Neck muscles	Head, shoulder movement
C5–C8 Lower Cervical	SSA	Upper limb muscles	Proprioception, DTRs
	GSA	Upper limbs	Reflexes, somesthesia
	GSE	Upper limb muscles	Movement, posture
T1–L2 Thoracic, Upper Lumbar	SSA	Muscles: trunk, abdominal wall	Proprioception
	GSA	Trunk, abdominal wall	Reflexes, somesthesia
	GVA	All of viscera	Reflexes and sensation
	GVE	All of viscera	Sympathetic reflexes, vasomotor control, sweating, piloerection
	GSE	Muscles: trunk, abdominal wall, back	Movement, posture, respiration
L2–S1 Lower Lumbar, Upper Sacral	SSA	Lower limb muscles	Proprioception, DTRs
	GSA	Lower trunk, limbs, back	Reflexes, somesthesia
	GSE	Muscles: trunk, lower limbs, back	Movement, posture
S2–S4 Lower Sacral	SSA	Muscles: pelvis, perineum	Proprioception
	GSA	Pelvis, genitalia	Reflexes, somesthesia
	GVA	Hindgut, bladder, uterus	Reflexes, sensation
	GVE	Hindgut, visceral organs	Visceral reflexes, defecation, urination, erection
S5–Co2 Lower Sacral, Coccygeal	SSA	Perineal muscles	Proprioception
	GSA	Lower sacrum, anus	Reflexes, somesthesia
	GSE	Perineal muscles	Reflexes, posture

Afferent (sensory) components: SSA, special somatic afferent; GSA, general somatic afferent; SVA, special visceral afferent; GVA, general visceral afferent.
Efferent (motor) components: GVE, general visceral efferent (autonomic nervous system); PE, pharyngeal efferent; GSE, general somatic efferent; DTRs, deep tendon reflexes.

Longitudinal Tracts

The gray matter of the cell columns in the CNS is surrounded by bundles of myelinated axons (*i.e.*, white matter) and unmyelinated axons that travel longitudinally along the length of the neural axis. This white matter can be divided into three layers—inner, middle, and outer layer (Fig. 13.10). The inner layer, or *archilayer*, contains short fibers that project for a maximum of approximately five segments before reentering the gray matter. The middle layer, or *paleolayer*, projects to six or more segments. Archilayer and paleolayer fibers have many branches, or collaterals, that enter the gray matter of intervening segments. In the outer layer, or *neolayer*, large-diameter axons that can travel the entire length of the nervous system are found (Table 13.2). *Suprasegmental* is a term that refers to

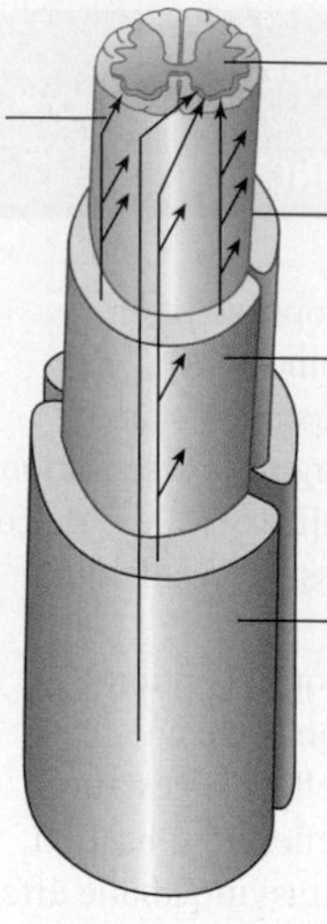

Figure 13.10 • The three concentric subdivisions of the tract systems of the white matter. Migration of neurons into the archilayer converts it into the reticular formation of the white matter.

higher levels of the CNS, such as the brain stem and cerebrum and structures above a given CNS segment. Paleolayer and neolayer fibers have suprasegmental projections.

The longitudinal layers are arranged in bundles, or fiber tracts, that contain axons that have the same destination, origin, and function (Fig. 13.11). These longitudinal tracts are named systematically to reflect their origin and destination; the origin is named first, and the destination is named second. For example, the spinothalamic tract originates in the spinal cord and terminates in the thalamus. The corticospinal tract originates in the cerebral cortex and ends in the spinal cord.

The Inner Layer. Lying deep to the superficial gray matter, the inner layer of white matter contains the axons of neurons that connect neighboring segments of the nervous system. Axons of this layer permit motor neurons of several segments to work together as a functional unit. They also allow the afferent neurons of one segment to trigger reflexes that activate motor units in neighboring segments as well as in the same one. From the standpoint of evolutionary development, this is the oldest of the three layers, and it is sometimes called the *archilayer*. It is the first of the longitudinal layers to become functional, and its circuitry may be limited to reflex types of movements, including reflex movements of the fetus (*i.e.*, quickening) that begin during the 5th month of intrauterine life.

The inner layer of the white matter differs from the other two layers in one important aspect. Many neurons in the embryonic gray matter migrate out into this layer, resulting in a rich mixture of neurons and local fibers called the *reticular formation*. The circuitry of most reflexes is contained in the reticular formation. In the brain stem, the reticular formation becomes quite large and contains major portions of vital reflexes, such as those controlling respiration, cardiovascular function, swallowing, and vomiting. A functional system called the *reticular activating system* operates in the lateral portions of the reticular formation of the medulla, pons, and especially the midbrain. Information derived from all sensory modalities, including those of the somesthetic, auditory, visual, and VA nerves, bombards the neurons of this system.

The reticular activating system has descending and ascending portions. The descending portion communicates with all spinal segmental levels through paleolevel reticulospinal tracts and serves to facilitate many cord-level reflexes. For example, it speeds reaction time and stabilizes postural reflexes. The ascending portion accelerates brain activity, particularly thalamic and cortical activity. This is reflected by the appearance of awake-type patterns of brain wave activity. Sudden stimuli result in protective and attentive postures and increased awareness.

The Middle Layer. The middle layer of the white matter contains most of the major fiber tract systems required for sensation and movement, including the ascending spinoreticular and spinothalamic tracts. This layer consists of larger-diameter and longer suprasegmental fibers, which ascend to the brain stem and are largely functional at birth. These tracts are quite old from an evolutionary standpoint, and, as such, this layer is sometimes called the *paleolayer*. It facilitates many primitive functions, such as the auditory startle reflex, which occurs in response to loud noises. This reflex consists of turning the head and body toward the sound, dilation of the pupils of the eyes, catching of the breath, and quickening of the pulse.

TABLE 13.2 CHARACTERISTICS OF THE CONCENTRIC SUBDIVISIONS OF THE LONGITUDINAL TRACTS IN THE WHITE MATTER OF THE CENTRAL NERVOUS SYSTEM

CHARACTERISTICS	ARCHILAYER TRACTS	PALEOLAYER TRACTS	NEOLAYER TRACTS
Segmental span	Intersegmental (<5 segments)	Suprasegmental (≥5 segments)	Suprasegmental
Number of synapses	Multisynaptic	Multisynaptic but fewer than archilayer tracts	Monosynaptic with target structures
Conduction velocity	Very slow	Fast	Fastest
Examples of functional systems	Flexor withdrawal reflex circuitry	Spinothalamic tracts	Corticospinal tracts

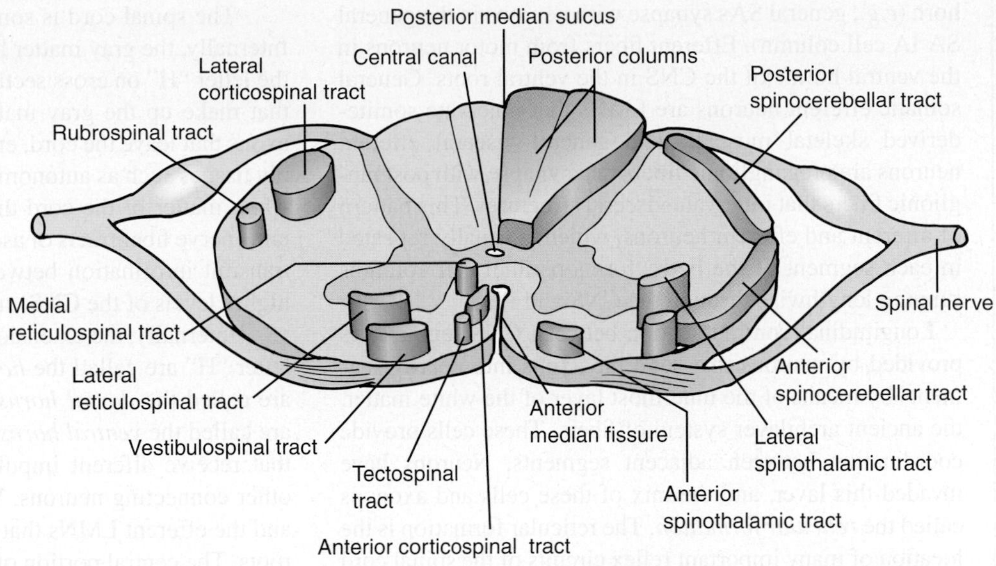

Figure 13.11 • Transverse section of the spinal cord showing selected sensory and motor tracts. The tracts are bilateral but are indicated only on one half of the cord.

The Outer Layer. The outer layer of the tract systems is the newest of the three layers with respect to evolutionary development, and it is sometimes called the *neolayer*. It becomes functional approximately the second year of life, and it includes the pathways needed for bladder training. Myelination of these suprasegmental tracts, which include many pathways required for delicate and highly coordinated skills, is not complete until approximately the fifth year of life. This includes the development of tracts needed for fine manipulative skills, such as the finger–thumb coordination required for using tools and the toe movements needed for acrobatics. Neolayer tracts are the most recently evolved systems and, because they are situated more superficially on the brain and spinal cord, are the most vulnerable to injury. When neolayer tracts are damaged, the paleolayer and archilayer tracts often remain functional, and rehabilitation methods can result in the effective use of the older systems. Delicacy and refinement may be lost, but basic function remains. For example, when the corticospinal system, an important neolayer system that permits the fine manipulative control required for writing, is damaged, the remaining paleolayer systems, if intact, permit the grasping and holding of objects. The hand can still be used to perform basic functions, but the fine manipulative functions of the fingers are lost.

Collateral Communication Pathways. Axons in the archilayer and paleolayer characteristically possess many collateral branches that move into the gray cell columns or synapse with fibers of the reticular formation as the axon passes each succeeding CNS segment. Should a major axon be destroyed at some point along its course, these collaterals provide multisynaptic alternative pathways that bypass the local damage. Neolayer tracts do not possess these collaterals but instead project mainly to the target neurons with which they communicate. Because of this, damage to the neolayer tracts causes permanent loss of function. Damage to the archilayer or paleolayer systems is usually followed by a slow return of function, presumably through the collateral connections.

IN SUMMARY

The CNS develops from the ectoderm of the early embryo by formation of a hollow tube that closes along its longitudinal axis and sinks below the surface. This hollow tube forms the ventricles of the brain and spinal canal, and the sidewall develops to form the brain stem and spinal cord. Development of the CNS requires the coordinated production of many embryonic inductive factors. The brain stem and spinal cord are subdivided into the dorsal horn, which contains neurons that receive and process incoming or afferent sensory information, and the ventral horn, which contains efferent motor neurons that handle the final stages of output processing. The PNS develops from ectodermal cells called *neural crest cells* that migrate away from the dorsal surface of the forming neural tube.

Throughout life, the organization of the nervous system retains many patterns established during early embryonic life. This segmental pattern of early embryonic development is retained in the fully developed nervous system. Each of the 43 or more body segments is connected to the corresponding CNS or neural tube segments by segmental afferent and efferent neurons. Afferent neuronal processes enter the CNS through the dorsal root ganglia and the dorsal roots. Afferent neurons of the dorsal root ganglia are of four types: general SA, special SA, general VA, and special VA. Each of these afferent neurons synapses with its appropriate IA neurons in the cell columns of the dorsal horn (*e.g.*, general SAs synapse with neurons in the general SA IA cell column). Efferent fibers from motor neurons in the ventral horn exit the CNS in the ventral roots. General somatic efferent neurons are LMNs that innervate somite-derived skeletal muscles, and general visceral efferent neurons are preganglionic fibers that synapse with postganglionic fibers that innervate visceral structures. This pattern of afferent and efferent neurons, which is usually repeated in each segment of the body, forms parallel cell columns running lengthwise through the CNS and PNS.

Longitudinal communication between CNS segments is provided by neurons that send the axons into nearby segments by means of the innermost layer of the white matter, the ancient archilayer system of fibers. These cells provide coordination between adjacent segments. Neurons have invaded this layer, and the mix of these cells and axons is called the *reticular formation*. The reticular formation is the location of many important reflex circuits of the spinal cord and brain stem. Paleolayer tracts, located outside the archilayer, provide the longitudinal communication between more distant segments of the nervous system. This layer includes most of the important ascending and descending tracts. The recently evolved neolayer systems, which become functional during infancy and childhood, travel outside the white matter and provide the means for very delicate and discriminative function. The outer position of the neolayer tracts and their lack of collateral and redundant pathways make them the most vulnerable to injury.

STRUCTURE AND FUNCTION OF THE SPINAL CORD AND BRAIN

After completing this section of the chapter, the learner will be able to meet the following objectives:

- Describe the innervation and function of spinal cord reflexes.
- Identify the structures of the hindbrain, midbrain, and forebrain, and describe their functions.
- Identify the cranial nerves, and describe their location and function.

Spinal Cord

In the adult, the spinal cord is found in the upper two thirds of the spinal canal of the vertebral column (Fig. 13.12). It extends from the foramen magnum at the base of the skull to a cone-shaped termination, the conus medullaris, usually at the level of the first or second lumbar vertebra (L1 or L2) in the adult.[2] Consequently, the dorsal and ventral roots of the more caudal portions of the cord elongate during development and angle downward from the cord, forming what is called the *cauda equina* (from the Latin for "horse's tail"). The filum terminale, which is composed of nonneural tissues and the pia mater, continues caudally and attaches to the second sacral vertebra (S2).

The spinal cord is somewhat oval on transverse section. Internally, the gray matter has the appearance of a butterfly or the letter "H" on cross section (see Fig. 13.12). Some neurons that make up the gray matter of the cord have processes or axons that leave the cord, enter the peripheral nerves, and supply tissues such as autonomic ganglia or skeletal muscles. The white matter of the cord that surrounds the gray matter contains nerve fiber tracts of ascending and descending axons that transmit information between segments of the cord or from higher levels of the CNS, such as the brain stem or cerebrum.

Internally, the extensions of the gray matter that form the letter "H" are called the *horns*. Those that extend posteriorly are called the *dorsal horns*, and those that extend anteriorly are called the *ventral horns*. Dorsal horns contain IA neurons that receive afferent impulses through the dorsal roots and other connecting neurons. Ventral horns contain OA neurons and the efferent LMNs that leave the cord through the ventral roots. The central portion of the cord, which connects the dorsal and ventral horns, is called the *intermediate gray matter*. The intermediate gray matter surrounds the central canal. In the thoracic area, the small, slender projections that emerge from the intermediate gray matter are called the *intermediolateral columns* of the horns. These columns contain the visceral OA neurons and the efferent neurons of the sympathetic nervous system.

The amount of gray matter is proportional to how much tissue is innervated by a given segment of the cord (see Fig. 13.12). Larger amounts of gray matter are present in the lower lumbar and upper sacral segments, which supply the lower extremities, and in the fifth cervical segment to the first thoracic segment, which supply the upper limbs. The white matter in the spinal cord also increases progressively toward the brain because ever more ascending fibers are added and the number of descending axons is greater.

The spinal cord and the dorsal and ventral roots are covered by a connective tissue sheath, the pia mater, which also contains the blood vessels that supply the white and gray matter of the cord (Fig. 13.13). On the lateral sides of the spinal cord, extensions of the pia mater, the denticulate ligaments, attach the sides of the spinal cord to the bony walls of the spinal canal. Thus, the cord is suspended by both the denticulate ligaments and the segmental nerves. A fat- and vessel-filled epidural space intervenes between the spinal dura mater and the inner wall of the spinal canal.

The spinal cord and nerves and their supporting structures are protected by the vertebral column. The vertebral body is the anterior, more massive part of the bone that gives strength to the vertebral column and supports body weight. Each vertebral body has two pedicles that extend posteriorly and support the laterally oriented transverse processes of the laminae, which arch medially and fuse to continue as the spinal processes. The vertebral arch and posterior surface of the vertebral body form the wall of the vertebral foramen. The succession of vertebral foramina in the articulated spinal column forms the vertebral canal (spinal canal), which contains the spinal cord, meninges, fat, and spinal nerve roots. The

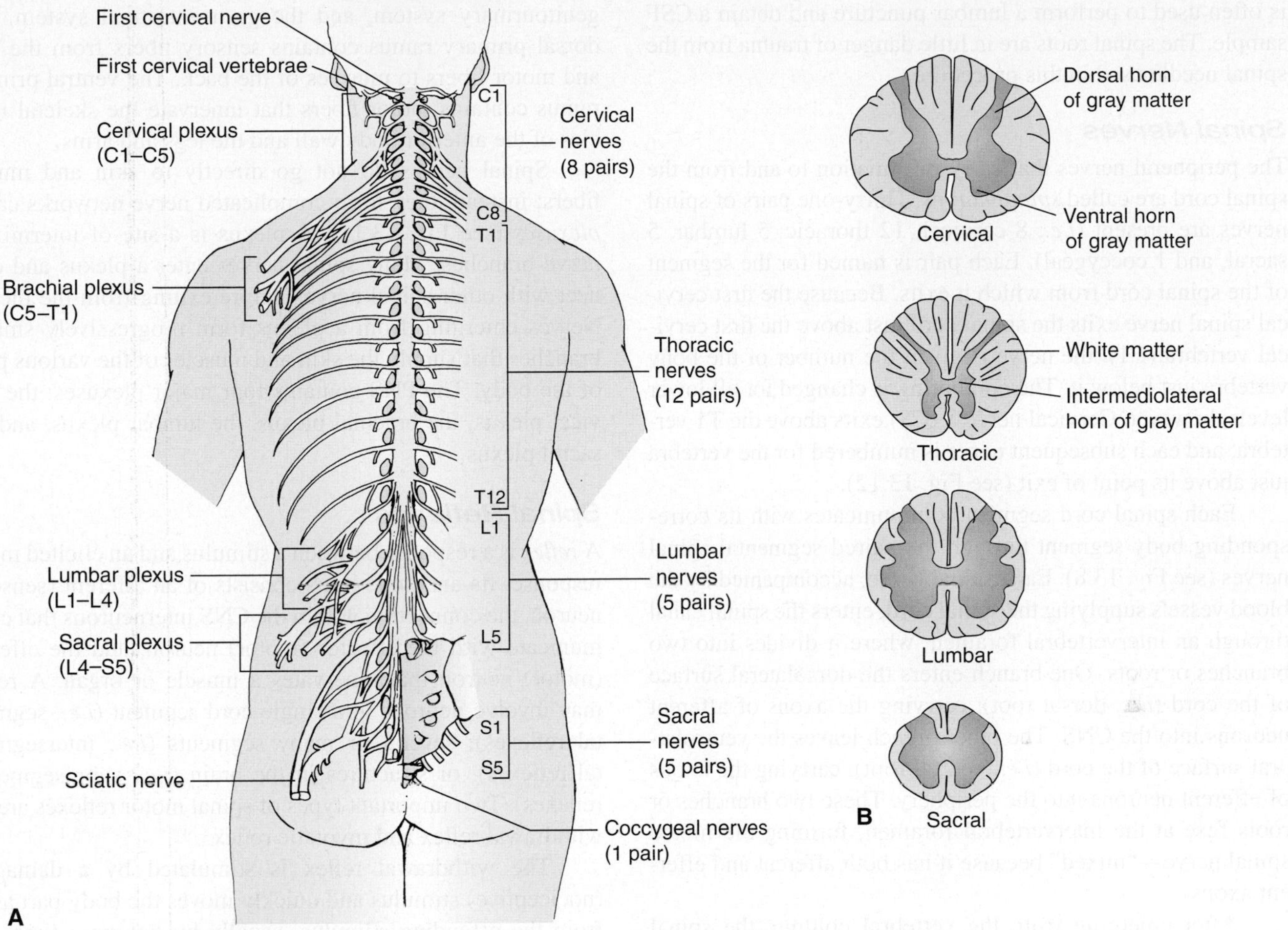

Figure 13.12 • **(A)** Posterior view of the spinal cord, including portions of the major spinal nerves and some of the components of the major nerve plexuses. **(B)** Cross-sectional views of the spinal cord, showing regional variations in gray matter and increasing white matter as the cord ascends.

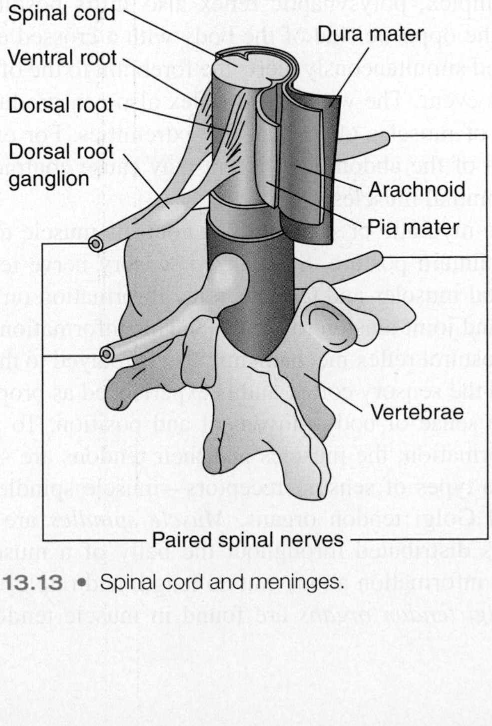

Figure 13.13 • Spinal cord and meninges.

spaces between the vertebral bodies are filled with fibrocartilaginous disks and stabilized with tough ligaments. A gap, the intervertebral foramen, occurs between each two succeeding pedicles, allowing for the exit of the segmental nerves and passage of blood vessels.

Early in fetal life, the spinal cord extends the entire length of the vertebral column, and the spinal nerves exit through the intervertebral foramina (openings) near their level of origin. Because the vertebral column and spinal dura grow faster than the spinal cord, a disparity develops between each succeeding cord segment and the exit of its dorsal and ventral nerve roots through the corresponding intervertebral foramina. In the newborn, the cord terminates at vertebral level L2 or L3, whereas the adult cord usually terminates at the inferior border of L1. In addition, the arachnoid and its enclosed subarachnoid space, which is filled with CSF, do not close down on the filum terminale until they reach the second sacral vertebra. This results in the formation of a pocket of CSF, the *dural cisterna spinalis*, which extends from approximately L2 to S2. Because this area contains an abundant supply of CSF and the spinal cord does not extend this far, the area (L3 or L4) is often used to perform a lumbar puncture and obtain a CSF sample. The spinal roots are in little danger of trauma from the spinal needle used in this procedure.

Spinal Nerves

The peripheral nerves that carry information to and from the spinal cord are called *spinal nerves*. Thirty-one pairs of spinal nerves are present (*i.e.*, 8 cervical, 12 thoracic, 5 lumbar, 5 sacral, and 1 coccygeal). Each pair is named for the segment of the spinal cord from which it exits. Because the first cervical spinal nerve exits the spinal cord just above the first cervical vertebra (C1), the nerve is given the number of the bony vertebra just below it. The numbering is changed for all lower levels, however. Cervical nerve 8 (C8) exits above the T1 vertebra, and each subsequent nerve is numbered for the vertebra just above its point of exit (see Fig. 13.12).

Each spinal cord segment communicates with its corresponding body segment through the paired segmental spinal nerves (see Fig. 13.8). Each spinal nerve, accompanied by the blood vessels supplying the spinal cord, enters the spinal canal through an intervertebral foramen, where it divides into two branches or roots. One branch enters the dorsolateral surface of the cord (*i.e.*, dorsal root), carrying the axons of afferent neurons into the CNS. The other branch leaves the ventrolateral surface of the cord (*i.e.*, ventral root), carrying the axons of efferent neurons into the periphery. These two branches or roots fuse at the intervertebral foramen, forming the mixed spinal nerve—"mixed" because it has both afferent and efferent axons.

After emerging from the vertebral column, the spinal nerve divides into two branches or *rami* (singular, *ramus*)—a small dorsal primary ramus and a larger ventral primary ramus (Fig. 13.14). Thoracic and upper lumbar spinal nerves also produce a third branch, the ramus communicans, which

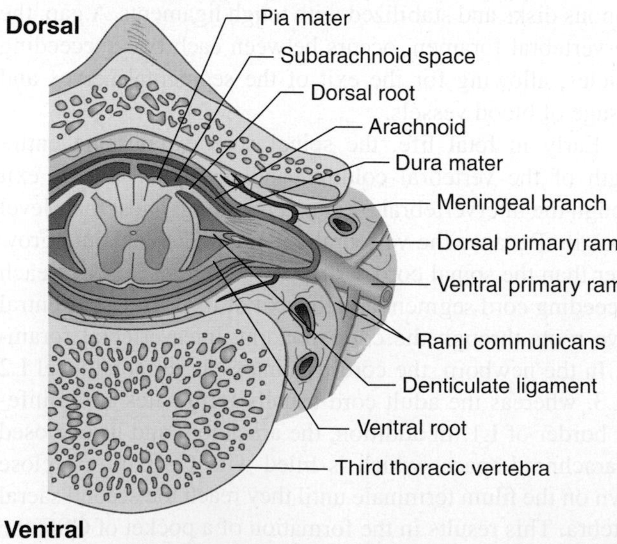

Figure 13.14 • Cross-section of vertebral column at the level of the third thoracic vertebra, showing the meninges, the spinal cord, and the origin of a spinal nerve and its branches or rami.

contains sympathetic axons supplying the blood vessels, the genitourinary system, and the gastrointestinal system. The dorsal primary ramus contains sensory fibers from the skin and motor fibers to muscles of the back. The ventral primary ramus contains motor fibers that innervate the skeletal muscles of the anterior body wall and the legs and arms.

Spinal nerves do not go directly to skin and muscle fibers; instead, they form complicated nerve networks called *plexuses* (see Fig. 13.11). A plexus is a site of intermixing nerve branches. Many spinal nerves enter a plexus and connect with other spinal nerves before exiting from the plexus. Nerves emerging from a plexus form progressively smaller branches that supply the skin and muscles of the various parts of the body. The PNS contains four major plexuses: the cervical plexus, the brachial plexus, the lumbar plexus, and the sacral plexus.

Spinal Reflexes

A *reflex* is a response between a stimulus and an elicited motor response. Its anatomic basis consists of an afferent (sensory) neuron, the connection within the CNS interneurons that communicate with the effector (motor) neuron, and the effector (motor) neuron that innervates a muscle or organ. A reflex may involve neurons in a single cord segment (*i.e.*, segmental reflexes), several or many segments (*i.e.*, intersegmental reflexes), or structures in the brain (*i.e.*, suprasegmental reflexes). Two important types of spinal motor reflexes are the withdrawal reflex and myotatic reflex.

The withdrawal reflex is stimulated by a damaging (nociceptive) stimulus and quickly moves the body part away from the offending stimulus, usually by flexing a limb part (Fig. 13.15). The withdrawal reflex is a powerful reflex, taking precedence over other reflexes associated with locomotion. Any of the major joints may be involved, depending on the site of afferent stimulation. All the joints of an extremity (*e.g.*, finger, wrist, elbow, shoulder) typically are involved. This complex, polysynaptic reflex also shifts postural support to the opposite side of the body with a crossed extensor reflex and simultaneously alerts the forebrain to the offending stimulus event. The withdrawal reflex also can produce contraction of muscles other than the extremities. For example, irritation of the abdominal viscera may cause contraction of the abdominal muscles.

The myotatic or stretch reflex controls muscle tone and helps maintain posture. Specialized sensory nerve terminals in skeletal muscles and tendons relay information on muscle stretch and joint tension to the CNS. This information, which drives postural reflex mechanisms, also is relayed to the thalamus and the sensory cortex and is experienced as proprioception, the sense of body movement and position. To provide this information, the muscles and their tendons are supplied with two types of sensory receptors—muscle spindle receptors and Golgi tendon organs. *Muscle spindles* are stretch receptors distributed throughout the belly of a muscle that transmit information about muscle length and rate of stretch. The *Golgi tendon organs* are found in muscle tendons and

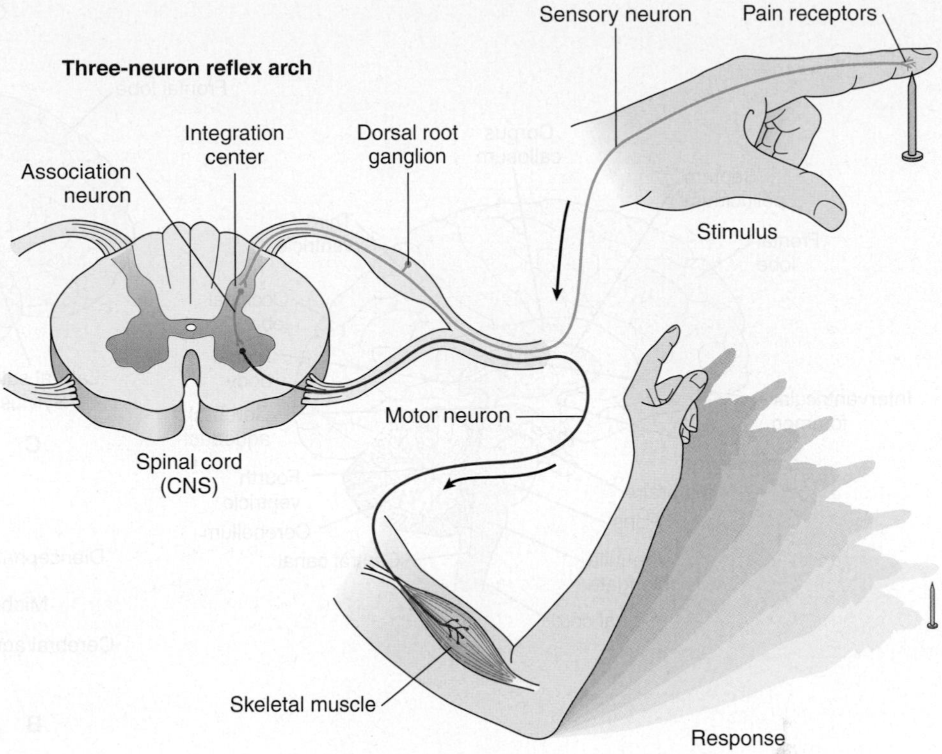

Figure 13.15 • Diagram of withdrawal reflex, showing the essential elements in a spinal reflex arc—a receptor in a sensory neuron, an integration center with an association neuron, and an effector (skeletal muscle).

transmit information about muscle tension or force of contraction at the junction of the muscle and the tendon that attaches to the bone. The likely role of the tendon organs is to equalize the contractile forces of the separate muscle groups, spreading the load over all the fibers to prevent the local muscle damage that might occur when small numbers of fibers are overloaded.

The Brain

Based on its embryonic development, the brain can be divided into three regions—the hindbrain, the midbrain, and the forebrain (see Fig. 13.16A). The hindbrain includes the medulla oblongata, the pons, and its dorsal outgrowth, the cerebellum. Midbrain structures include two pairs of dorsal enlargements, the superior and inferior colliculi. The forebrain, which consists of two hemispheres and is covered by the cerebral cortex, contains central masses of gray matter, the basal ganglia, and the rostral end of the neural tube, the diencephalon, with its adult derivatives—the thalamus and hypothalamus.

The term *brain stem* is often used to include the midbrain, pons, and medulla (Fig. 13.16B). These regions of the neural tube have the organization of spinal cord segments, except that more of the longitudinal cell columns are present, reflecting the increased complexity of the cranial segmental nerves. In the brain stem, the structure and function of the reticular formation have been greatly expanded. In the pons and medulla, the reticular formation contains networks controlling basic breathing, eating, and locomotion functions. Higher-level integration of these functions occurs in the midbrain. The reticular formation is surrounded on the outside by the long tract systems that connect the forebrain with lower parts of the CNS.

Hindbrain

The hindbrain consists of the metencephalon (cerebellum and pons) and the myelencephalon (medulla oblongata). Sleep disorders and stroke are disorders that frequently affect the hindbrain. This area of the brain assists in managing motor activity, posture, and major functions such as respiration and circulation of blood.

Medulla. The medulla oblongata represents the caudal five segments of the brain part of the neural tube. The CN branches entering and leaving it have functions similar to the spinal segmental nerves. Although the ventral horn areas in the medulla are quite small, the dorsal horn areas are enlarged, processing a large amount of the information pouring through the CNs. The segmental peripheral nerve components of the medulla can be divided into those leaving the neural tube ventromedially (*i.e.*, hypoglossal CN) or dorsolaterally (*i.e.*, vagus, spinal accessory, glossopharyngeal, and vestibulocochlear CNs). Because pathologic signs and symptoms reflect the spatial segregation of brain stem components, neurologic syndromes resulting from trauma, tumors, aneurysms, and strokes are often classified as ventral or dorsolateral syndromes.

The general somatic efferent LMNs of the lower segments of the medulla supply the extrinsic and intrinsic muscles of the tongue by means of the *hypoglossal nerve* (CN XII). Damage to the hypoglossal nerve results in weakness or paralysis of tongue muscles. When the tongue is protruded, it deviates toward the damaged and therefore weaker side because of the greater protrusion strength on the normal side. Axons of the hypoglossal nerve exit the medulla adjacent to two long, longitudinal ridges along the medial undersurface of the medulla.

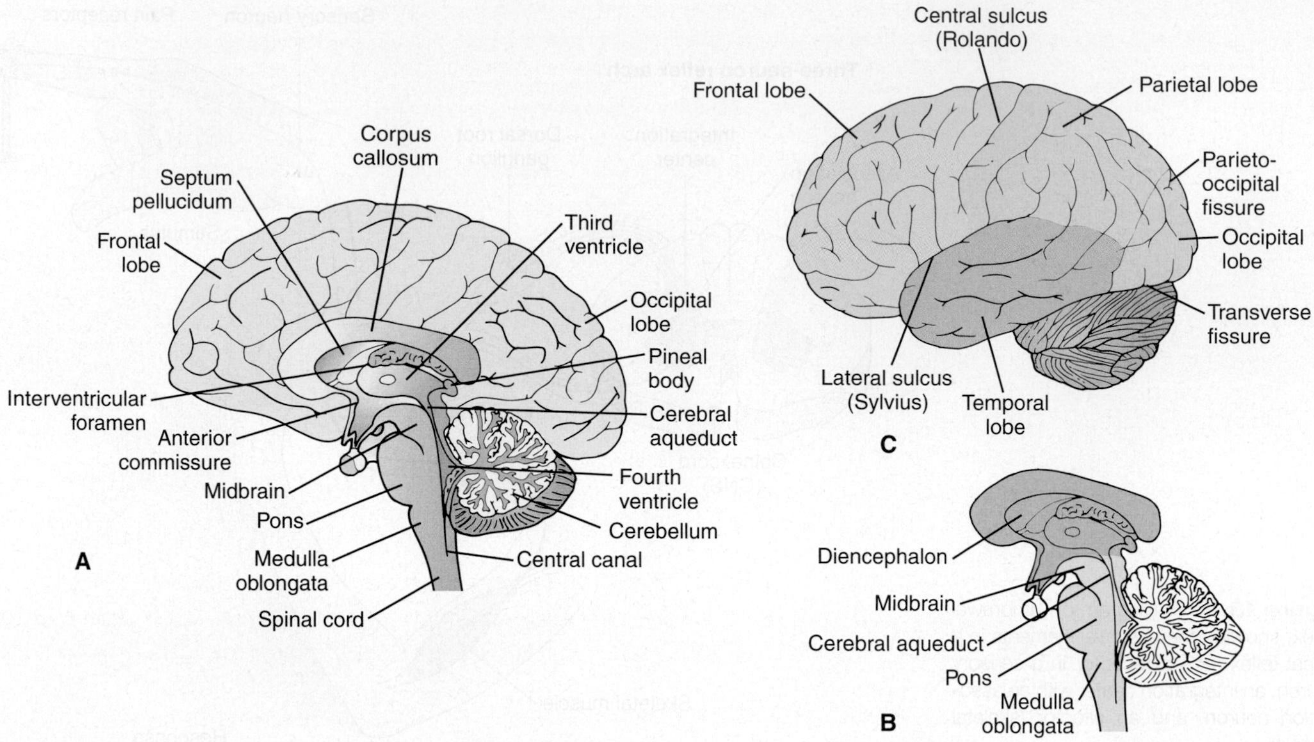

Figure 13.16 • **(A)** Midsagittal section of the brain, showing the structures of the forebrain, midbrain, and hindbrain. **(B)** Diencephalon, brain stem, and the cerebral aqueduct connecting the third and fourth ventricles. **(C)** Lateral view of the cerebral hemispheres.

These ridges, called the *pyramids*, contain the corticospinal fibers, most of which cross to descend in the lateral column to the opposite side of the spinal cord. Lesions of the ventral surface of the caudal medulla result in the syndrome of alternating hypoglossal hemiplegia. These lesions are characterized by signs of ipsilateral (*i.e.*, same side) denervation of the tongue and contralateral (*i.e.*, opposite side) weakness or paralysis of both the upper and lower extremities.

The *vagus nerve* (CN X) has several afferent (sensory) and efferent (motor) components. General SA neurons innervate the external ear, whereas special VA neurons innervate the pharyngeal taste buds. Sensory and motor components of the nerve innervate the pharynx, the gastrointestinal tract (from the laryngeal pharynx to the midtransverse colon), the heart, the spleen, and the lungs.[2] Initiation of many essential reflexes and normal functions depends on intact vagal innervation. The unilateral loss of vagal function can result in slowed gastrointestinal motility, a permanently husky voice, and deviation of the uvula away from the damaged side. Bilateral loss of vagal function can seriously damage reflex maintenance of cardiovascular and respiratory reflexes. Swallowing may become difficult and, occasionally, paralysis of laryngeal structures causes life-threatening airway obstruction.

The sternocleidomastoid, a powerful head-turning muscle, and the trapezius muscle, which elevates the shoulders, are innervated by the *spinal accessory nerve* (CN XI), with LMNs in the upper four cervical spinal segments. Intermediate rootlets from these segmental levels combine and enter the cranial cavity through the foramen magnum and exit the jugular foramen with CNs IX and X. Loss of spinal accessory nerve function results in drooping of the shoulder on the damaged side and weakness when turning the head to the opposite side.

The dorsolateral *glossopharyngeal nerve* (CN IX) contains the same components as the vagus nerve but for a more rostral segment of the gastrointestinal tract and the pharynx. This nerve provides the special visceral sensory innervation of the taste buds of the oral pharynx and the back of the tongue; the afferent innervation of the oral pharynx and the baroreceptors of the carotid sinus; the efferent innervation of the otic ganglion, which controls the salivary function of the parotid gland; and the efferent innervation of the stylopharyngeus muscles of the pharynx. This CN is seldom damaged, but when it is, anesthesia of the ipsilateral oral pharynx develops along with dry mouth resulting from reduced salivation.

The special sensory afferent *vestibulocochlear nerve* (CN VIII), formerly called the *auditory nerve*, is attached laterally at the junction of the medulla oblongata and the pons, often called the *caudal pons*. It consists of two distinct fiber divisions, the cochlear and vestibular divisions, both of which are sensory. Cell bodies in the cochlea of the inner ear produce fibers of the cochlear division. These fibers transmit impulses related to the sense of hearing. The vestibular division arises from two ganglia that innervate cell bodies in the utricle, saccule, and semicircular canals and transmit impulses related to head position and movement of the body through space. Irritation of the cochlear division results in tinnitus (*i.e.*, ringing of the ears); destruction of the nerve results in nerve deafness. Injury to the vestibular division leads to vertigo, nystagmus, and some postural instability.

The *facial nerve* (CN VII) and its intermediate component (the intermedius) is a mixed nerve that has both afferent and efferent components. It emerges from the junction of the pons and medulla. The nervus intermedius, containing the general SA, special VA, general VA, and general visceral efferent neurons, innervates the nasopharynx and taste buds of the palate. It also innervates the anterior two thirds of the tongue, the submandibular and sublingual salivary glands, the lacrimal glands, and the mucous membranes of the nose and roof of the mouth. Loss of this branch of the facial nerve can lead to eye dryness with risk of corneal scarring and blindness. The pharyngeal efferent LMNs of the facial nerve proper innervate muscles that control facial expression, such as wrinkling of the brow and smiling. Unilateral loss of facial nerve function results in flaccid paralysis of the muscles of half the face, a condition called *Bell palsy*.

Pons. The pons (from the Latin for "bridge") develops from the fifth neural tube segment. Internally, the central canal of the spinal cord, which is enlarged in the pons and rostral medulla, forms the fourth ventricle (see Fig. 13.16B). An enlarged area on the ventral surface of the pons contains the pontine nuclei, which receive information from all parts of the cerebral cortex. Axons of these neurons form a massive bundle that swings around the lateral side of the fourth ventricle to enter the cerebellum. In the pons, the reticular formation is large and contains the circuitry for masticating food and manipulating the jaws during speech.

The *abducens nerve* (CN VI), which arises from the caudal pons, sends LMNs out ventrally on either side of the pyramids and then forward into the orbit to innervate the lateral rectus muscle of the eye. As the name suggests, the abducens nerve abducts the eye (lateral or outward rotation); peripheral damage to this nerve results in medial strabismus, which is a weakness or loss of eye abduction.

The *trigeminal nerve* (CN V), which has both sensory and motor subdivisions, exits the brain stem laterally on the forward surface of the pons. The trigeminal is the main sensory nerve conveying the modalities of pain, temperature, touch, and proprioception to the superficial and deep regions of the face. Regions innervated include the skin of the anterior scalp and face, the conjunctiva and orbit, the meninges, the paranasal sinuses, and the mouth, including the teeth and the anterior two thirds of the tongue. LMNs of the trigeminal nerve innervate skeletal muscles involved with mastication and contribute to swallowing and speech, movements of the soft palate, and tension of the tympanic membrane through the tensor tympani muscle. The tensor tympani muscle has a protective reflex function, dampening movement of the middle ear ossicles during high-intensity sound.

Cerebellum. The cerebellum is located in the posterior fossa of the cranium superior to the pons (see Fig. 13.16A). It is separated from the cerebral hemispheres by a fold of dura mater, the tentorium cerebelli. The cerebellum consists of a small, unpaired median portion, called the *vermis*, and two large lateral masses, the *cerebellar hemispheres*.[2] In contrast to the brain stem with its external white matter and internal gray nuclei, the cerebellum, like the cerebrum, has an outer cortex of gray matter overlying the white matter. Next to the fourth ventricle, several masses of gray matter, called the *deep cerebellar nuclei*, border the roof of the fourth ventricle. Cells of the cerebellar cortex and deep nuclei interact, and axons from the latter send information to many regions, particularly to the motor cortex by means of a thalamic relay. Synergistic functions of the cerebellum (*i.e.*, temporal and spatial smoothing) contribute to all movements of the limbs, trunk, head, larynx, and eyes, whether the movement is part of a voluntary movement or of a highly learned semiautomatic or automatic movement. During highly skilled movements, the motor cortex sends signals to the cerebellum, informing it about the movement that is to be performed. The cerebellum makes continuous adjustments, resulting in smoothness of movement, particularly during delicate maneuvers. Highly skillful movement requires extensive motor training, and considerable evidence suggests that many of these learned movement patterns involve cerebellar circuits.

The cerebellum receives proprioceptor input from the vestibular system; feedback from the muscles, tendons, and joints; and indirect signals from the somesthetic, visual, and auditory systems that provide background information for ongoing movement. Sensory and motor information from a given area of the body is sent to the same area in the cerebellum. In this way, the cerebellum can assess continuously the status of each body part—position, rate of movement, and forces such as gravity that are opposing movement. The cerebellum compares what is actually happening with what is intended to happen. It then transmits the appropriate corrective signals back to the motor system, instructing it to increase or decrease the activity of the participating muscle groups so that smooth and accurate movements can be performed.

Another function of the cerebellum is the dampening of muscle movement. All body movements are essentially pendular (*i.e.*, swinging back and forth). As movement begins, momentum develops and must be overcome before the movement can be stopped. This momentum would cause movements to overshoot if they were not dampened. In the intact cerebellum, automatic signals stop movement precisely at the intended point. The cerebellum analyzes proprioceptive information to predict the future position of moving parts, their rapidity of movement, and the projected time course of the movement. This allows the cerebellum to inhibit agonist muscles and excite antagonist muscles when movement approaches the intended target.

Midbrain

The midbrain develops from the fourth segment of the neural tube, and its organization is similar to that of a spinal segment. Internally, the central canal is reestablished as the cerebral aqueduct, connecting the fourth ventricle with the third ventricle (see Fig. 13.16B). Two general somatic efferent CNs, the oculomotor nerve (CN III) and the trochlear nerve (CN IV), exit the midbrain.

Two prominent bundles of nerve fibers, the *cerebral peduncles*, pass along the ventral surface of the midbrain.[2] These fibers include the corticospinal tracts and are the main motor pathways between the forebrain and the pons. On the dorsal surface, four "little hills," the *superior* and *inferior colliculi*, are areas of cortical formation. The inferior colliculi are involved in directional turning and, to some extent, in experiencing the direction of sound sources, whereas the superior colliculi are essential to the reflex mechanisms that control conjugate eye movements when the visual environment is surveyed.

The ventral central gray matter (*i.e.*, ventral horn) of the midbrain contains the LMNs that innervate most of the skeletal muscles that move the optic globe and raise the eyelids. These axons leave the midbrain through the oculomotor nerve (CN III). This nerve also contains the parasympathetic LMNs that control pupillary constriction and ciliary muscle focusing of the lens (see Table 13.1). Damage to the ventrally exiting CN III and to the adjacent cerebral peduncle, which contains the corticospinal axon system on one side, results in paralysis of eye movement combined with contralateral hemiplegia.

A small group of cells in the ventral part of the caudal central gray matter contains the trochlear nerve (CN IV), which innervates the superior oblique eye muscle. This muscle moves the upper part of the eye downward and toward the nose when the eye is adducted or turned inward. The trochlear nerve exits the dorsal surface of the midbrain and decussates (crosses over) before exiting the brain stem. Lesions of the trochlear nerve affect downward gaze on the side opposite the denervated muscle, producing diplopia, or double vision. Walking downstairs becomes particularly difficult. Because the superior oblique muscle has inward rotation of the optic globe as its major function, people with trochlear nerve damage usually carry their heads tilted to the side of damage.

Forebrain

The most rostral part of the brain, the forebrain, consists of the telencephalon, or "end brain," and the diencephalon, or "between brains." The diencephalon forms the core of the forebrain, and the telencephalon forms the cerebral hemispheres.

Diencephalon. Three of the most forward brain segments form an enlarged dorsal horn and ventral horn with a narrow, deep, enlarged central canal—the third ventricle—separating the two sides. This region is called the *diencephalon*. The dorsal horn parts of the diencephalon are the thalamus and subthalamus, and the ventral horn part is the hypothalamus (Fig. 13.17). The optic nerve (CN II) and retina are outgrowths of the diencephalon.

The thalamus consists of two large, egg-shaped masses, one on either side of the third ventricle. It is divided into several major parts, and each part is divided into distinct nuclei, which are the major relay stations for information going to and from the cerebral cortex. All sensory pathways have direct projections to thalamic nuclei, which convey the information to restricted areas of the sensory cortex. Coordination and integration of peripheral sensory stimuli occur in the thalamus, along with some crude interpretation of highly emotion-laden auditory experiences that not only occurs but also can be remembered. For example, a person can recover from a deep coma in which cerebral cortex activity is minimal and remember some of what is said at the bedside.

The thalamus also plays a role in relaying critical information regarding motor activities to and from selected areas

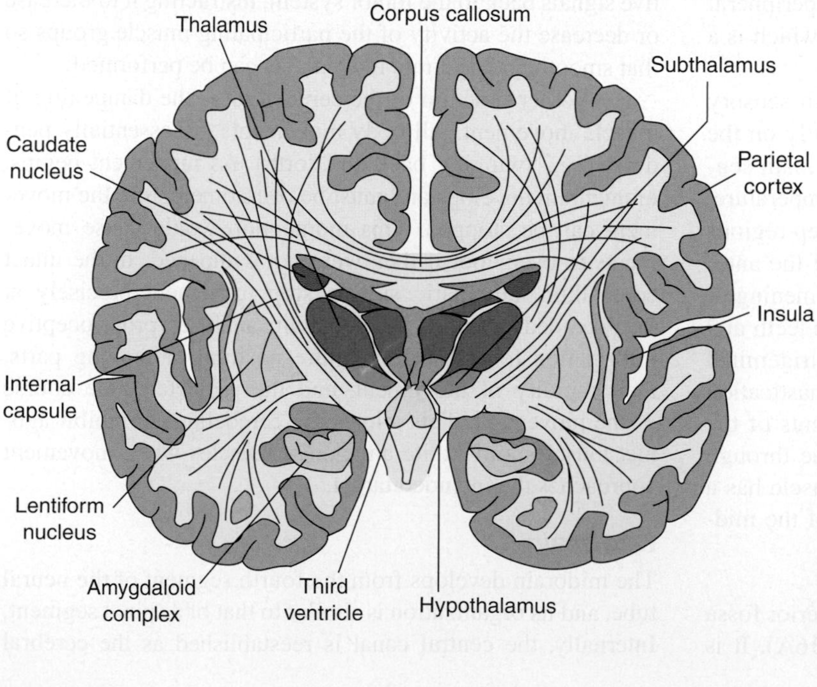

Figure 13.17 • Frontal section of the brain passing through the third ventricle, showing the thalamus, subthalamus, hypothalamus, internal capsule, corpus callosum, basal ganglia (caudate nucleus, lentiform nucleus), amygdaloid complex, insula, and parietal cortex.

of the motor cortex. Two neuronal circuits are significant in this regard. One is the pathway from the cerebral cortex to the pons and cerebellum and then, by way of the thalamus, back to the motor cortex. The second one is the feedback circuit that travels from the cortex to the basal ganglia and then to the thalamus and from the thalamus back to the cortex. The subthalamus also contains movement control systems related to the basal ganglia.

Through its connections with the ascending reticular activating system, the thalamus processes neural influences that are basic to cortical excitatory rhythms (*i.e.*, those recorded on the electroencephalogram), to essential sleep–wakefulness cycles, and to the process of attending to stimuli. Besides their cortical connections, the thalamic nuclei have connections with each other and with neighboring nonthalamic brain structures such as the limbic system. Through their connections with the limbic system, some thalamic nuclei are involved in the relation between stimuli and the emotional responses they evoke.

Inferior to the thalamus and representing the ventral horn portion of the diencephalon is the hypothalamus. It also borders the third ventricle and includes a ventral extension, the neurohypophysis (*i.e.*, posterior pituitary). The hypothalamus is the area of master-level integration of homeostatic control of the body's internal environment. Maintenance of blood gas concentrations, water balance, food consumption, and major aspects of endocrine and ANS control require hypothalamic function.

The internal capsule is a broad band of projection fibers that lies between the thalamus medially and the basal ganglia laterally (see Fig. 13.17). It contains all of the fibers that connect the cerebral cortex with deeper structures, including the basal ganglia, thalamus, midbrain, pons, medulla, and spinal cord.

Cerebral Hemispheres. The two cerebral hemispheres are lateral outgrowths of the diencephalon. Internally, the cerebral hemispheres contain the lateral ventricles, which are connected to the third ventricle of the diencephalon by a small opening called the *interventricular foramen* (see Fig. 13.16A). Axons of the olfactory nerve (CN I) terminate in the most ancient portion of the cerebrum, the olfactory bulb, where initial processing of olfactory information occurs. Projection axons from the olfactory bulb relay information through the olfactory tracts to the thalamus and to other parts of the cerebral cortex (*i.e.*, orbital cortex), where olfactory-related reflexes and olfactory experience occur.

A thick area of myelinated axons called the *corpus callosum* connects the cerebral cortex of the two sides of the brain (see Fig. 13.17). Two smaller commissures, the anterior and posterior commissures, connect the two sides of the more specialized regions of the cerebrum and diencephalon.

The surfaces of the hemispheres are lateral (side), medial (area between the two sides of the brain), and basal (ventral). The cerebral cortex is the recently evolved six-layered neocortex. Many ridges and grooves are present on the surface of the hemispheres. A *gyrus* is the ridge between two grooves, and the groove is called a sulcus or fissure. The cerebral cortex is arbitrarily divided into lobes named after the bones that cover them: the frontal, parietal, temporal, and occipital lobes (see Fig. 13.16C).

Basal Ganglia. A section through the cerebral hemispheres reveals the surface of the cerebral cortex, a subcortical layer of white matter made up of masses of myelinated axons and deep masses of gray matter—the basal ganglia that border the lateral ventricle (see Fig. 13.17). The basal ganglia lie on either side of the internal capsule, just lateral to the thalamus. The basal ganglia consist of the comma-shaped *caudate* (tailed) *nucleus*, the shield-shaped *putamen*, and the *globus pallidus* ("pale globe"). The term *striatum* ("striped body") refers to the caudate plus the putamen. Together, the globus pallidus and putamen make up the *lentiform* (lens-shaped) *nucleus*.[2]

The basal ganglia supply axial and proximal unlearned and learned postures and movements, which enhance and add gracefulness to UMN-controlled manipulative movements. These background movement functions are called *associated movements*. Intact and functional basal ganglia provide arm swinging during walking and running. Basal ganglia also are involved in follow-through movements that accompany throwing a ball or swinging a club. As with the motor cortex, the nuclei on the left side control movement on the right side of the body and vice versa. Circuits connecting the premotor cortex and supplementary motor cortex, the basal ganglia, and parts of the thalamus provide associated movements that accompany highly skilled behaviors. Parkinson disease, Huntington chorea, and some forms of cerebral palsy, among other dysfunctions involving the basal ganglia, result in a frequent or continuous release of abnormal postural or axial and proximal movement patterns. If damage to the basal ganglia is localized to one side, the movements occur on the opposite side of the body. These automatic movement patterns stop only in sleep, but in some conditions, the movements are so violent that falling asleep becomes difficult.

Frontal Lobe. The frontal lobe extends from the frontal pole to the central sulcus (*i.e.*, fissure) and is separated from the temporal lobe by the lateral sulcus. Each frontal lobe can be subdivided rostrally into the frontal pole and laterally into the superior, middle, and inferior gyri, which continue on the undersurface over the eyes as the orbital cortex. These areas are associated with the medial thalamic nuclei, which also are related to the limbic system. Functionally, the prefrontal cortex is thought to be involved in anticipation and prediction of consequences of behavior.

The precentral gyrus (area 4), next to the central sulcus, is the *primary motor cortex* (Fig. 13.18). This area of the cortex provides precise movement control for distal flexor muscles of the hands and feet and of the phonation apparatus required for speech. Just rostral to the precentral gyrus is a region of the frontal cortex called the *premotor* or *motor association*

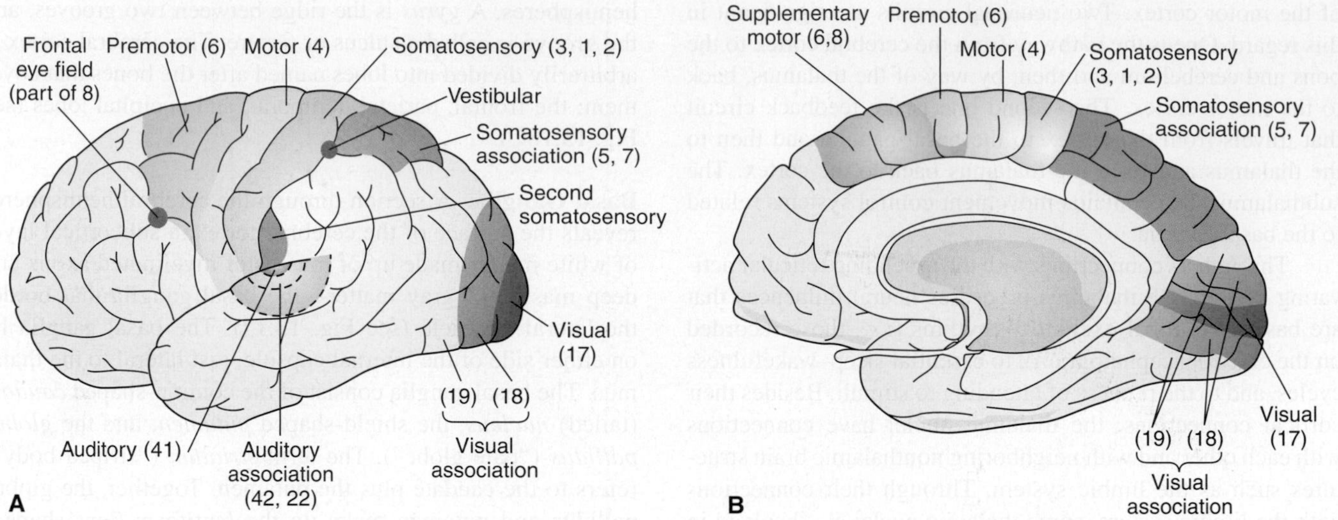

Figure 13.18 • Motor and sensory areas of the cerebral cortex. **(A)** Left lateral view of the cerebral cortex. **(B)** This diagram represents the areas in the brain that has been sectioned in the median plane.

cortex. This region (area 8 and rostral area 6) is involved in the planning of complex learned movement patterns, and damage to these areas results in dyspraxia or apraxia. Such people can manipulate a screwdriver, for instance, but cannot use it to loosen a screw. The primary motor cortex and the association motor cortex are connected with lateral thalamic nuclei, through which they receive feedback information from the basal ganglia and cerebellum. On the medial surface of the hemisphere, the premotor area includes a *supplementary motor cortex* involved in the control of bilateral movement patterns requiring great dexterity.

Parietal Lobe. The parietal lobe of the cerebrum lies behind the central sulcus (*i.e.*, postcentral gyrus) and above the lateral sulcus. A strip of cortex bordering the central sulcus is called the *primary somatosensory cortex* (areas 3, 1, and 2) because it receives very discrete sensory information from the lateral nuclei of the thalamus. Just behind the primary sensory cortex is the *somesthetic association cortex* (areas 5 and 7), which is connected with the thalamic nuclei and with the primary sensory cortex (see Fig. 13.18). This region is necessary for somesthetic perception (*i.e.*, appreciation of the meaningfulness of integrated sensory information from various sensory systems), especially concerning perception of "where" the stimulus is in space and in relation to body parts. Localized lesions of this region can result in the inability to recognize the meaningfulness of an object (a condition called *agnosia*). With the person's eyes closed, a screwdriver can be felt and described as to shape and texture. Nevertheless, the person cannot integrate the sensory information required to identify it as a screwdriver.

Temporal Lobe. The temporal lobe lies below the lateral sulcus and merges with the parietal and occipital lobes. It includes the temporal pole and three primary gyri, the superior, middle, and inferior gyri. The primary auditory cortex (area 41) involves the part of the superior temporal gyrus that extends into the lateral sulcus (see Fig. 13.18). This area is particularly important in discrimination of sounds entering opposite ears. It receives auditory input projections through the inferior colliculus of the midbrain and a ventrolateral thalamic nucleus. The more exposed part of the superior temporal gyrus involves the auditory association or perception area (area 22). The aspects of hearing that attach meaning to certain sound patterns require that this area functions properly. The remaining portions of the temporal cortex are less well defined but apparently are important in long-term memory recall. This is particularly true with respect to perception and memory of complex sensory patterns such as geometric figures and faces (*i.e.*, recognition of "what" or "who" the stimulus is).

Occipital Lobe. The occipital lobe lies posterior to the temporal and parietal lobes and is arbitrarily separated from them (Fig. 13.18). The medial surface of the occipital lobe contains a deep sulcus extending from the limbic lobe to the occipital pole, the *calcarine sulcus*, which is surrounded by the primary visual cortex (area 17).[2] Just superior and inferior and extending onto the lateral side of the occipital pole is the *visual association cortex* (areas 18 and 19). This area is closely connected with the primary visual cortex and with complex nuclei of the thalamus. Integrity of the association cortex is required for gnostic visual function, by which the meaningfulness of visual experience, including experiences of color, motion, depth perception, pattern, form, and location in space, takes place.

The neocortical areas of the parietal lobe, between the somesthetic and the visual cortices, have a function in relating the texture, or "feel," and location of an object with its visual image. Between the auditory and visual association areas, the *parieto-occipital region* is necessary for relating the meaningfulness of a sound and image to an object or person.

Limbic System. The medial aspect of the cerebrum is organized into concentric bands of the cortex, the *limbic system*, which surrounds the connection between the lateral and third ventricles. The innermost band just above and below the cut surface of the corpus callosum is folded out of sight but is an ancient, three-layered cortex ending as the hippocampus in the temporal lobe. Just outside the folded area is a band of transitional cortex, which includes the cingulate and the parahippocampal gyri (Fig. 13.19). The limbic lobe has reciprocal connections with the medial and the intralaminar nuclei of the thalamus, with the deep nuclei of the cerebrum (*e.g.*, amygdaloid nuclei, septal nuclei), and with the hypothalamus. Overall, this region of the brain is involved in emotional experience and in the control of emotion-related behavior. Stimulation of specific areas in this system can lead to feelings of dread, high anxiety, or exquisite pleasure. It also can result in violent behaviors, including attack, defense, or explosive and emotional speech.

Meninges

Inside the skull and vertebral column, the brain and spinal cord are loosely suspended and protected by several connective tissue sheaths called the *meninges* (Fig. 13.20). All surfaces of the spinal cord, brain, and segmental nerves are covered with a delicate connective tissue layer called the *pia mater*. Surface blood vessels and those that penetrate the brain and spinal cord are encased in this protective tissue layer. The second, very delicate, nonvascular, and waterproof layer, called the *arachnoid*, encloses the entire CNS. The CSF is contained in the subarachnoid space. Immediately outside the arachnoid is a continuous sheath of strong connective tissue, the *dura mater*, which provides the major protection for the brain and spinal cord. The cranial dura often splits into two layers, with the outer layer serving as the periosteum of the inner surface of the skull.

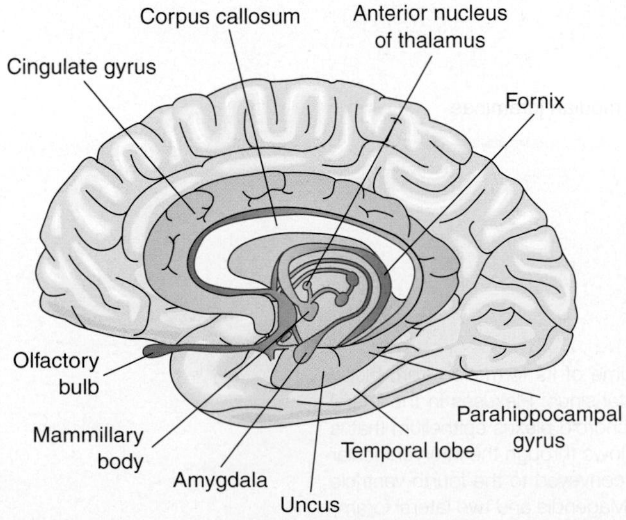

Figure 13.19 • The limbic system includes the limbic cortex (cingulate gyrus, parahippocampal gyrus, uncus) and associated subcortical structures (thalamus, hypothalamus, amygdala).

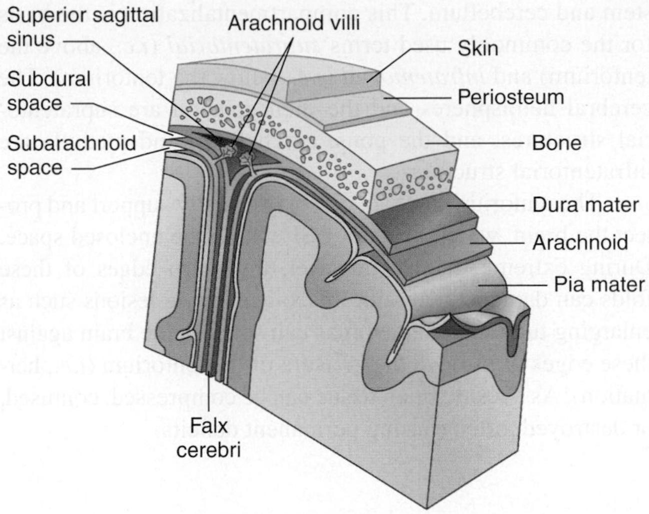

Figure 13.20 • The cranial meninges. Arachnoid villi, shown within the superior sagittal sinus, are one site of CSF absorption into the blood.

The inner layer of the dura forms two major infoldings—a longitudinal infolding called the *falx cerebri* and a transverse infolding called the *tentorium cerebelli* that anchor the brain to the skull (Fig. 13.21). The falx cerebri lies in the longitudinal fissure and separates the two cerebral hemispheres. It attaches to the crista of the ethmoid bone anteriorly and ends by becoming continuous with the tentorium cerebelli. The tentorium cerebelli is a wide crescentic septum that acts as a hammock, supporting the occipital lobes above the cerebellum. The falx cerebri attaches to the tentorium cerebri and holds it up, giving it a tentlike appearance. The tentorium attaches to the petrous portion of the temporal bone and the dorsum sellae of the cranial floor, with a semicircular gap, or incisura, formed at the midline to permit the midbrain to pass forward from the posterior fossa. It also forms a tough septum, separating the anterior and middle cranial fossae, which contain the cerebral hemispheres, from the posterior fossa, found interiorly and containing the brain

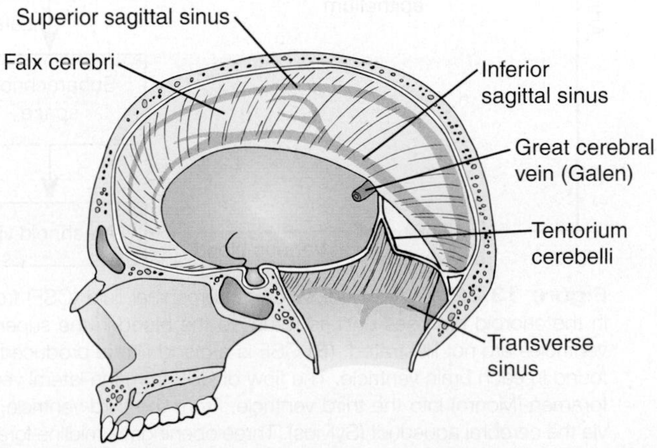

Figure 13.21 • Cranial dura mater. The skull is open to show the falx cerebri and the right and left portions of the tentorium cerebelli, as well as some of the cranial venous sinuses.

stem and cerebellum. This compartmentalization is the basis for the commonly used terms *supratentorial* (*i.e.*, above the tentorium) and *infratentorial* (*i.e.*, below the tentorium). The cerebral hemispheres and the diencephalon are supratentorial structures, and the pons, cerebellum, and medulla are infratentorial structures.

The tentorium and falx cerebri normally support and protect the brain, which floats in CSF within the enclosed space. During extreme trauma, however, the sharp edges of these folds can damage the brain. Space-occupying lesions such as enlarging tumors or hematomas can squeeze the brain against these edges or through the incisura of the tentorium (*i.e.*, herniation). As a result, brain tissue can be compressed, contused, or destroyed, often causing permanent deficits.

Ventricular System and Cerebrospinal Fluid

The ventricular system is a series of CSF-filled cavities in the brain (Fig. 13.22). The CSF provides a supporting and protective fluid for the brain and spinal cord. CSF helps maintain a constant ionic environment that serves as a medium for diffusion of nutrients, electrolytes, and metabolic end products into the extracellular fluid surrounding CNS neurons and neuroglia. Filling the ventricles, the CSF supports the mass of the brain. Because it fills the subarachnoid space surrounding the CNS, a physical force delivered to either the skull or spine is to some extent diffused and cushioned.

A thin layer of neuroglial cells, collectively termed the *ependyma*, lines the ventricles and central canal of the spinal

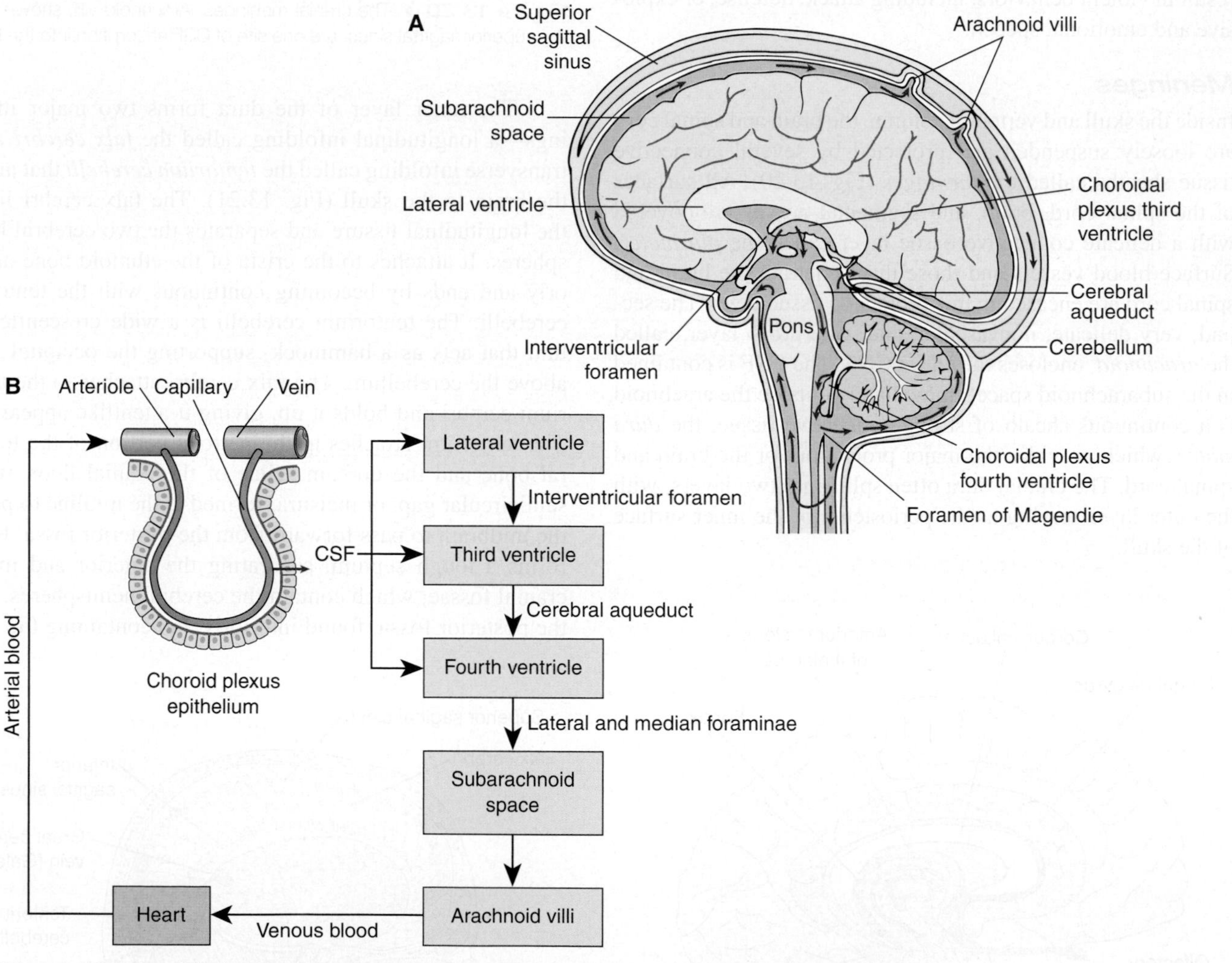

Figure 13.22 • **(A)** The flow of cerebrospinal fluid (CSF) from the time of its formation from blood in the choroid plexuses until its return to the blood in the superior sagittal sinus. Plexuses in the lateral ventricles are not illustrated. **(B)** CSF is a blood filtrate produced by the choroid plexus epithelium that is found in each brain ventricle. The flow of CSF from the lateral ventricles flows through the interventricular foramen (Monro) into the third ventricle. From the third ventricle, CSF is conveyed to the fourth ventricle via the cerebral aqueduct (Sylvius). Three openings, a midline foramen of Magendie and two lateral foramina (Luschka), pass the CSF into the subarachnoid space, where it is returned to the venous circulation through the arachnoid villi.

TABLE 13.3 COMPOSITION OF CEREBROSPINAL FLUID COMPARED WITH PLASMA

SUBSTANCE	PLASMA	CEREBROSPINAL FLUID
Protein (mg/dL)	6000.00	20.00
Na^+ (mEq/L)	135.00	131.00
Cl^- (mEq/L)	101.00	124.00
K^+ (mEq/L)	4.50	2.90
HCO_3^- (mEq/L)	25.00	24.00
pH	7.4	7.32
Glucose (mg/dL)	92.00	61.00

cord. There is a tremendous expansion of the ependyma in the roof of the lateral, third, and fourth ventricles. The CSF is produced by tiny reddish masses of specialized ependymal cells and capillaries, called the *choroid plexus*, which project into the ventricles. CSF is an ultrafiltrate of blood plasma, composed mostly of water with other constituents, making it close to the composition of the brain extracellular fluid (Table 13.3). The amount of CSF produced daily is about 500 mL. The amount of CSF is approximately 125 to 150 mL in the ventricular system at any one time, meaning that the CSF is continuously being absorbed.

The CSF produced in the ventricles must flow through the interventricular foramen, the third ventricle, the cerebral aqueduct, and the fourth ventricle to exit from the ventricular system. Three openings, or foramina, allow the CSF to pass into the subarachnoid space. Two of these, the foramina of Luschka, are located at the lateral corners of the fourth ventricle. The third one, the median foramen of Magendie, is in the midline at the caudal end of the fourth ventricle (see Fig. 13.23). CSF then passes down into the subarachnoid space that surrounds the spinal cord, mainly on its dorsal surface, and moves back up to the cranial cavity along its ventral surface.

Reabsorption of CSF into the vascular system occurs along the sides of the superior sagittal sinus in the anterior and middle fossae. The subarachnoid space has projections, the *arachnoid villi*, which penetrate the inner dura and walls of the superior sagittal sinus. Reabsorption of CSF into the vascular system occurs along a pressure gradient. The normal CSF pressure is in the range of 60 to 180 mm H_2O in the lateral recumbent position.[7] The microstructure of the arachnoid villi are such that if the CSF pressure falls below approximately 50 mm H_2O, the passageways collapse, and reverse flow is blocked. Thus, the arachnoid villi function as one-way valves, permitting CSF outflow into the venous blood of the sagittal sinus but not allowing blood to pass into the arachnoid spaces.

Blood–Brain and Cerebrospinal Fluid–Brain Barriers

Maintenance of a chemically stable environment is essential to the function of the brain. In most regions of the body, extracellular fluid undergoes small fluctuations in pH and concentrations of hormones, amino acids, and potassium ions during routine daily activities such as eating and exercising. When the brain undergoes such fluctuations, the result is uncontrolled neural activity because some substances such as amino acids act as neurotransmitters, and ions such as potassium influence the threshold for neural firing. Two barriers, the blood–brain barrier and the CSF–brain barrier, provide the means for maintaining the stable chemical environment of the brain. Only water, carbon dioxide, and oxygen enter the brain with relative ease. The transport of other substances between the brain and the blood is slower and more controlled.

The blood–brain barrier depends on the unique characteristics of the brain capillaries. Endothelial cells of brain capillaries are joined by continuous tight junctions. In addition, most brain capillaries are surrounded by a basement membrane and by the processes of supporting cells of the brain, called *astrocytes* (Fig. 13.23). The blood–brain barrier permits passage of essential substances while excluding unwanted materials. Reverse transport systems remove materials from the brain. Large molecules, such as proteins and peptides, are largely excluded from crossing the blood–brain barrier. Acute cerebral lesions, such as trauma and infection, increase the permeability of the blood–brain barrier and alter brain concentrations of proteins, water, and electrolytes.

The blood–brain barrier prevents many drugs from entering the brain. Most highly water-soluble compounds are excluded from the brain, especially molecules with high ionic charge such as many of the catecholamines. In contrast, many lipid-soluble molecules cross the lipid layers of the blood–brain barrier with ease. Some drugs, such as the antibiotic chloramphenicol, are highly lipid-soluble and therefore enter

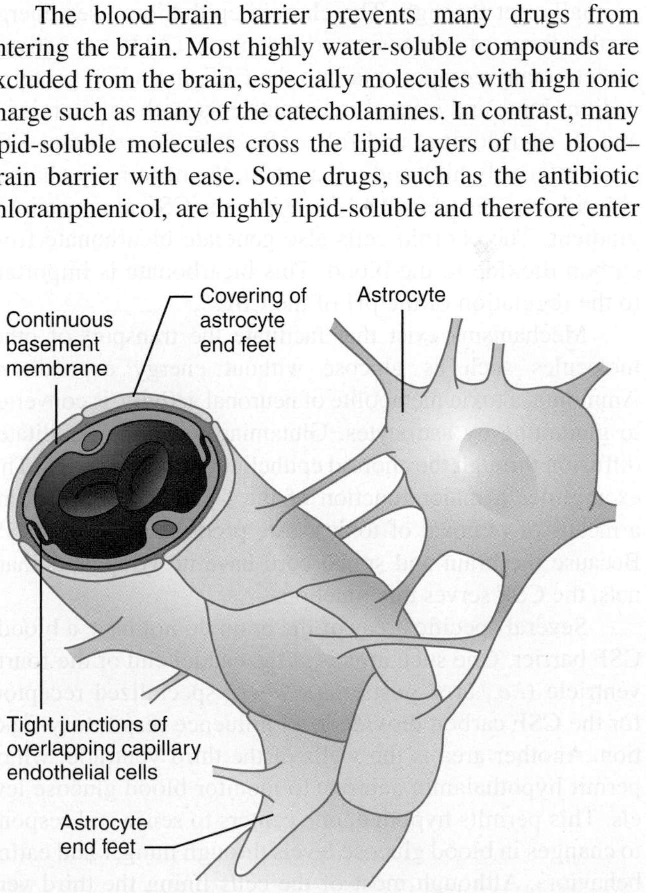

Figure 13.23 • The three components of the blood–brain barrier: the astrocyte and astrocyte end feet that encircle the capillary, the capillary basement membrane, and the tight junctions that join the overlapping capillary endothelial cells.

the brain readily. Other medications have a low solubility in lipids and enter the brain slowly or not at all. Alcohol, nicotine, and heroin are very lipid-soluble and rapidly enter the brain. Some substances that enter the capillary endothelium are converted by metabolic processes to a chemical form incapable of moving into the brain.

The cerebral capillaries are much more permeable at birth than in adulthood, and the blood–brain barrier develops during the early years of life. In severely jaundiced infants, bilirubin can cross the immature blood–brain barrier, producing kernicterus and brain damage. In adults, the mature blood–brain barrier prevents bilirubin from entering the brain, and the nervous system is not affected.

The ependymal cells covering the choroid plexus are linked together by tight junctions, forming a blood–CSF barrier to diffusion of many molecules from the blood plasma of choroid plexus capillaries to the CSF. Water is transported through the choroid epithelial cells by osmosis. Oxygen and carbon dioxide move into the CSF by diffusion, resulting in partial pressures roughly equal to those of plasma. The high sodium and low potassium contents of the CSF are actively regulated and kept relatively constant. Lipids and nonpeptide hormones diffuse through the barrier rather easily, but most large molecules, such as proteins, peptides, many antibiotics, and other medications, do not normally get through. The choroid epithelium uses energy in the form of adenosine triphosphate (ATP) to actively secrete many components into the CSF, including proteins, sodium ions, and several micronutrients such as vitamins C and B_6 (pyridoxine) and folate. Because the resultant CSF has a relatively high sodium content, the negatively charged chloride and bicarbonate diffuse into the CSF along an ionic gradient. The choroid cells also generate bicarbonate from carbon dioxide in the blood. This bicarbonate is important to the regulation of the pH of the CSF.

Mechanisms exist that facilitate the transport of other molecules such as glucose without energy expenditure. Ammonia, a toxic metabolite of neuronal activity, is converted to glutamine by astrocytes. Glutamine moves by facilitated diffusion through the choroid epithelium into the plasma. This exemplifies a major function of the CSF, that of providing a means of removal of toxic waste products from the CNS. Because the brain and spinal cord have no lymphatic channels, the CSF serves this function.

Several specific areas of the brain do not have a blood–CSF barrier. One such area is at the caudal end of the fourth ventricle (*i.e.*, area postrema), where specialized receptors for the CSF carbon dioxide level influence respiratory function. Another area is the walls of the third ventricle, which permit hypothalamic neurons to monitor blood glucose levels. This permits hypothalamic centers to sense and respond to changes in blood glucose levels through hunger and eating behaviors. Although most of the cells lining the third ventricle are ependymal cells, modified ependymal cells called *tanycytes* are also present. Processes of tanycytes extend through the glial lining of the third ventricle to terminate on blood vessels, neurons, or glial cells of the surrounding brain tissue.

IN SUMMARY

In the adult, the spinal cord is in the upper two thirds of the spinal canal of the vertebral column. On transverse section, the spinal cord has an oval shape. Internally, the gray matter has the appearance of a butterfly or letter "H." The dorsal horns contain the IA neurons and receive afferent information from dorsal root and other connecting neurons. The ventral horns contain the OA neurons and efferent LMNs that leave the cord by the ventral roots. Thirty-one pairs of spinal nerves (*i.e.*, 8 cervical, 12 thoracic, 5 lumbar, 5 sacral, and 1 coccygeal) are present. Each pair communicates with its corresponding body segments. The spinal nerves and the blood vessels that supply the spinal cord enter the spinal canal through an intervertebral foramen. After entering the foramen, they divide into two branches, or roots, one of which enters the dorsolateral surface of the cord (*i.e.*, dorsal root), carrying the axons of afferent neurons into the CNS. The other root leaves the ventrolateral surface of the cord (*i.e.*, ventral root), carrying the axons of efferent neurons into the periphery. These two roots fuse at the intervertebral foramen, forming the mixed spinal nerve.

A reflex provides a highly reliable relation between a stimulus and a motor response. Its anatomic basis consists of an afferent (sensory) neuron, the connection with CNS neurons that communicate with the effector (motor) neuron and the effector neuron that innervates a muscle or organ. Reflexes allow the sensory pathway for an involuntary motor response to a stimulus.

The brain can be divided into three parts—the hindbrain, the midbrain, and the forebrain. The hindbrain, consisting of the medulla oblongata, pons, and cerebellum, contains the neuronal circuits for the eating, breathing, and locomotive functions required for survival. CNs III and IV arise from the midbrain, and CNs XII, XI, X, IX, VIII, VII, VI, and V are located in the hindbrain. The forebrain is the most rostral part of the brain. It consists of the diencephalon and the telencephalon. The dorsal horn part of the diencephalon comprises the thalamus and subthalamus, and the ventral horn part is the hypothalamus. The cerebral hemispheres are lateral outgrowths of the diencephalon.

The cerebral hemispheres are divided into lobes—the frontal, parietal, temporal, and occipital lobes—named after the bones of the skull that cover them. Contained in the frontal lobe are the prefrontal premotor area and primary motor cortex; the primary sensory cortex and somesthetic association area are in the parietal cortex; the primary auditory cortex and the auditory association area are in the temporal lobe; and the primary visual cortex and association visual cortex are in the occipital lobe. The limbic system, which is involved in emotional experience and release of emotional behaviors, is located in the medial aspect of the cerebrum. These cortical areas are reciprocally connected with underlying thalamic nuclei through the internal capsule. Thalamic involvement is essential for normal forebrain function.

The brain is enclosed and protected by the dura mater, arachnoid, and pia mater. The protective CSF, in which the brain and spinal cord float, isolates them from minor and moderate trauma. CSF is secreted into the ventricles by the ependymal cells of the choroid plexus, circulates through the ventricular system, and is reabsorbed into the venous system through the arachnoid villi. The CSF–brain barrier and the blood–brain barrier protect the brain from substances in the blood that would disrupt brain function.

THE AUTONOMIC NERVOUS SYSTEM

After completing this section of the chapter, the learner will be able to meet the following objectives:

- Compare the sensory and motor components of the autonomic nervous system with those of the CNS.
- Compare the anatomic location and functions of the sympathetic and parasympathetic nervous systems.
- Describe neurotransmitter synthesis, release, and degradation, and receptor function in the sympathetic and parasympathetic nervous systems.

The ability to maintain homeostasis and perform the activities of daily living in an ever-changing physical environment is largely vested in the ANS. This portion of the nervous system functions at the subconscious level and is involved in regulating, adjusting, and coordinating vital visceral functions such as blood pressure and blood flow, body temperature, respiration, digestion, metabolism, and elimination. The ANS is strongly affected by emotional influences and is involved in many of the expressive aspects of behavior. Blushing, pallor, palpitations of the heart, clammy hands, and dry mouth are several emotional expressions mediated through the ANS. Biofeedback and relaxation exercises have been used for modifying the subconscious functions of the ANS.

As with the somatic nervous system, the ANS is represented in both the CNS and the PNS. The ANS has been defined as a general efferent system innervating visceral organs. The efferent outflow from the ANS has two divisions—the sympathetic nervous system and the parasympathetic nervous system.[8] Afferent inputs to the ANS are provided by VA neurons and are not usually considered a part of the ANS. The two divisions of the ANS are usually viewed as having opposite and antagonistic actions. Exceptions are functions, such as sweating and regulation of arteriolar blood vessel diameter, which are controlled by a single division of the ANS, in this case the sympathetic nervous system.

The functions of the sympathetic nervous system include maintaining body temperature and adjusting blood vessels and blood pressure to meet the changing needs of the body. These adjustments occur in response to changes in routine activities of daily living, such as moving from the supine to the standing position. The sympathoadrenal system also can discharge as a unit when there is a critical threat to the integrity of the individual—the so-called fight-or-flight response. During a stress situation, the heart rate accelerates; blood pressure rises; blood flow shifts from the skin and gastrointestinal tract to the skeletal muscles and brain; blood sugar increases; the bronchioles and pupils dilate; the sphincters of the stomach and intestine and the internal sphincter of the urethra constrict; and the rate of secretion of exocrine glands involved in digestion diminishes. Emergency situations often require vasoconstriction and shunting of blood away from the skin and into the muscles and brain, a mechanism that, should a wound occur, provides for a reduction in blood flow and preservation of vital functions needed for survival. Sympathetic function is often summarized as "catabolic" in that its actions predominate during periods of pronounced energy expenditure, such as when survival is threatened.

In contrast to the sympathetic nervous system, the functions of the parasympathetic nervous system are concerned with conservation of energy, resource replenishment and storage, and maintenance of organ function during periods of minimal activity—the *rest–digest* response. The parasympathetic nervous system slows heart rate, stimulates gastrointestinal function and related glandular secretion, promotes bowel and bladder elimination, and contracts the pupil, protecting the retina from excessive light during periods when visual function is not vital to survival.

The sympathetic and parasympathetic nervous systems are continually active. The effect of this continual activity is referred to as *tone*. The tone of an effector organ or system can be increased or decreased and is usually regulated by a single division of the ANS (*e.g.*, vascular smooth muscle tone is controlled by the sympathetic nervous system). Increased sympathetic activity produces local vasoconstriction from increased vascular smooth muscle tone, and decreased activity results in vasodilation because of decreased tone. In structures such as the sinoatrial node and atrioventricular node of the heart, which are innervated by both divisions of the ANS, one division predominates in controlling tone. In this case, the tonically active parasympathetic nervous system exerts a constraining or braking effect on heart rate, and when parasympathetic outflow is withdrawn, similar to releasing a brake, the heart rate increases. The increase in heart rate that occurs with vagal withdrawal can be further augmented by sympathetic stimulation. Table 13.4 describes the responses of effector organs to sympathetic and parasympathetic impulses.

TABLE 13.4 CHARACTERISTICS OF THE SYMPATHETIC AND PARASYMPATHETIC NERVOUS SYSTEMS

CHARACTERISTIC	SYMPATHETIC OUTFLOW	PARASYMPATHETIC OUTFLOW
Location of preganglionic cell bodies	T1–T12, L1 and L2	CNs: III, VII (intermedius), IX, and X; sacral segments 2, 3, and 4
Relative length of preganglionic fibers	Short—to paravertebral chain of ganglia or to aortic prevertebral ganglia	Long—to ganglion cells near or in the innervated organ
General function	Catabolic—mobilizes resources in anticipation of challenge for survival (preparation for "fight-or-flight" response)	Anabolic—concerned with conservation, renewal, and storage of resources
Nature of peripheral response	Generalized	Localized
Transmitter between preganglionic terminals and postganglionic neurons	ACh	ACh
Transmitter of postganglionic neuron	ACh (sweat glands and skeletal muscle vasodilator fibers), norepinephrine (most synapses), norepinephrine and epinephrine (secreted by adrenal gland)	ACh

ACh, acetylcholine.

KEY POINTS

THE AUTONOMIC NERVOUS SYSTEM

- The ANS functions at the subconscious level and is responsible for maintaining homeostatic functions of the body.
- The ANS has two divisions—the sympathetic and parasympathetic systems. Although the two divisions function together, they are generally viewed as having opposite and antagonistic actions.
- The outflow of both divisions of the ANS consists of a two-neuron pathway: a preganglionic and a postganglionic neuron. Acetylcholine is the neurotransmitter for the preganglionic neurons for both ANS divisions, as well as the postganglionic neurons of the parasympathetic nervous system. Norepinephrine and epinephrine are the neurotransmitters for most sympathetic postganglionic neurons.

Autonomic Efferent Pathways

The outflow of both divisions of the ANS follows a two-neuron pathway. The first motor neuron, called the *preganglionic neuron*, lies in the intermediolateral cell column of the spinal cord or its equivalent location in the brain stem. The second motor neuron, called the *postganglionic neuron*, synapses with a preganglionic neuron in an autonomic ganglion in the PNS. The two divisions of the ANS differ as to location of their preganglionic cell bodies, the relative length of their preganglionic fibers, the nature of their peripheral responses, and their preganglionic and postganglionic neurotransmitters (see Table 13.4). This two-neuron pathway and the interneurons in the autonomic ganglia that add further modulation to ANS function are distinctly different from arrangements in the somatic nervous system.

Most visceral organs are innervated by both sympathetic and parasympathetic fibers (Fig. 13.24). Exceptions include structures such as blood vessels and sweat glands that have input from only one division of the ANS. The fibers of the sympathetic nervous system are distributed to effectors throughout the body, and, as a result, sympathetic actions tend to be more diffuse than those of the parasympathetic nervous system, in which there is a more localized distribution of fibers. The preganglionic fibers of the sympathetic nervous system may traverse a considerable distance and pass through several ganglia before synapsing with postganglionic neurons, and their terminals contact many postganglionic fibers. In some ganglia, the ratio of preganglionic to postganglionic cells may be 1:20; because of this, the effects of sympathetic stimulation are diffuse. Considerable overlap exists, and one ganglion cell may be supplied by several preganglionic fibers. In contrast to the sympathetic nervous system, the parasympathetic nervous system has its postganglionic neurons located very near or in the organ of innervation. Because the ratio of preganglionic to postganglionic communication is often 1:1, the effects of the parasympathetic nervous system are much more circumscribed.

Sympathetic Nervous System

The neurons of the sympathetic nervous system are located primarily in the intermediolateral cell column of the thoracic and upper lumbar segments (T1 to L2) of the spinal cord.[8] Hence, the sympathetic nervous system is often called the *thoracolumbar division* of the ANS. These preganglionic neurons have axons that are largely myelinated and relatively short. Postganglionic neurons of the sympathetic nervous system are located in the paravertebral ganglia of the sympathetic chain of ganglia that lie on either side of the vertebral column or in

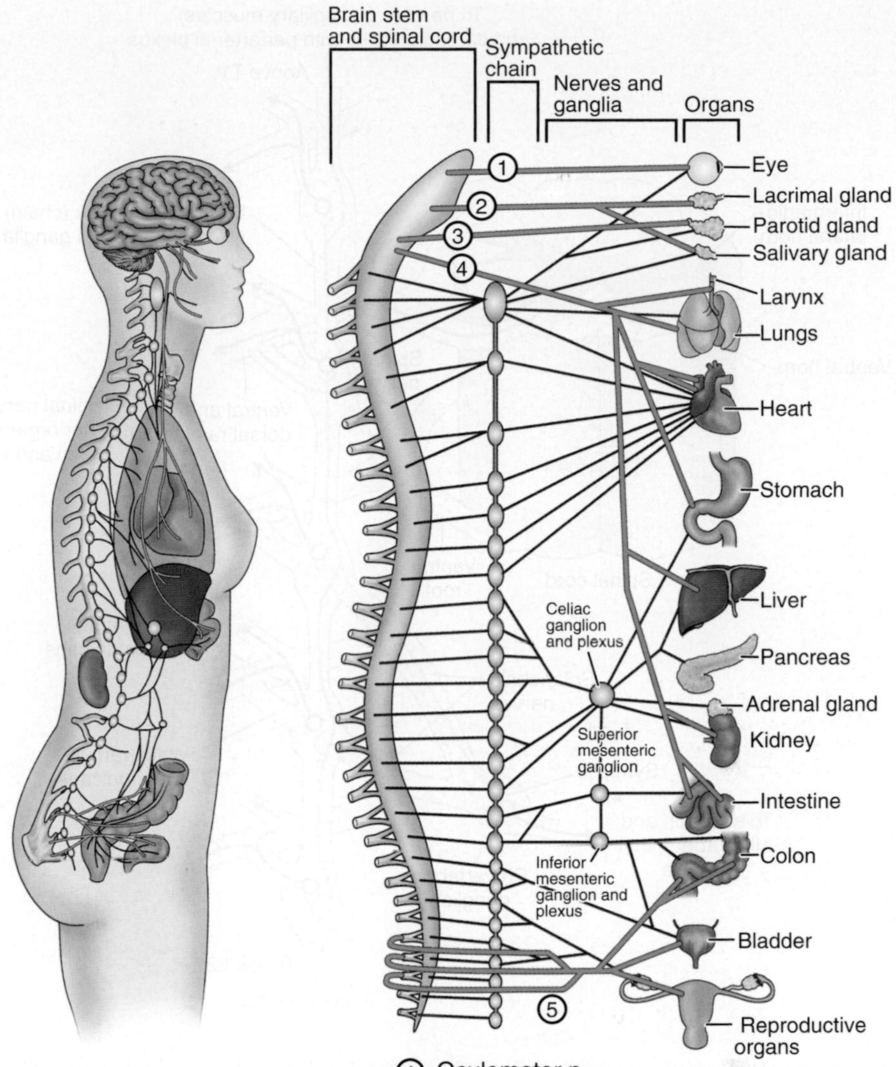

Figure 13.24 • The anatomy of the ANS. (From Hinkle J. L., Cheever, K. H. (2018). *Brunner & Suddarth's textbook of medical-surgical nursing* (4th ed., Fig. 65-10, p. 1954). *Philadelphia*, PA: Lippincott Williams & Wilkins.)

prevertebral sympathetic ganglia such as the celiac ganglia. Besides postganglionic efferent neurons, the sympathetic ganglia contain neurons of the internuncial, short-axon type, similar to those associated with complex circuitry in the brain and spinal cord. Many of these inhibit and others modulate preganglionic to postganglionic transmission.

The axons of the preganglionic neurons leave the spinal cord through the ventral roots of the spinal nerves (T1 to L2), enter the ventral primary rami, and leave the spinal nerve through white rami of the rami communicantes to reach the paravertebral ganglionic chain (Fig. 13.25). In the sympathetic chain of ganglia, preganglionic fibers may synapse with neurons of the ganglion they enter, pass up or down the chain and synapse with one or more ganglia, or pass through the chain and move outward through a splanchnic nerve to terminate in prevertebral ganglia (*i.e.*, celiac, superior mesenteric, or inferior mesenteric) scattered along the dorsal aorta and its branches.

Preganglionic fibers from the thoracic segments of the cord pass upward to form the cervical chain connecting the inferior, middle, and superior cervical sympathetic ganglia with the rest of the sympathetic chain at lower levels. Postganglionic sympathetic axons of the cervical and lower lumbosacral chain ganglia spread further through nerve plexuses along continuations of the great arteries. Cranial structures, particularly blood vessels, are innervated by the spread of postganglionic axons along the external and internal carotid arteries into the face and the cranial cavity. The sympathetic fibers from T1 usually continue up the sympathetic chain into the head; those from T2 pass into the neck; those from T1 to T5 travel to the heart; those from T3, T4, T5, and T6 proceed to the thoracic viscera; those from T7, T8, T9, T10, and T11

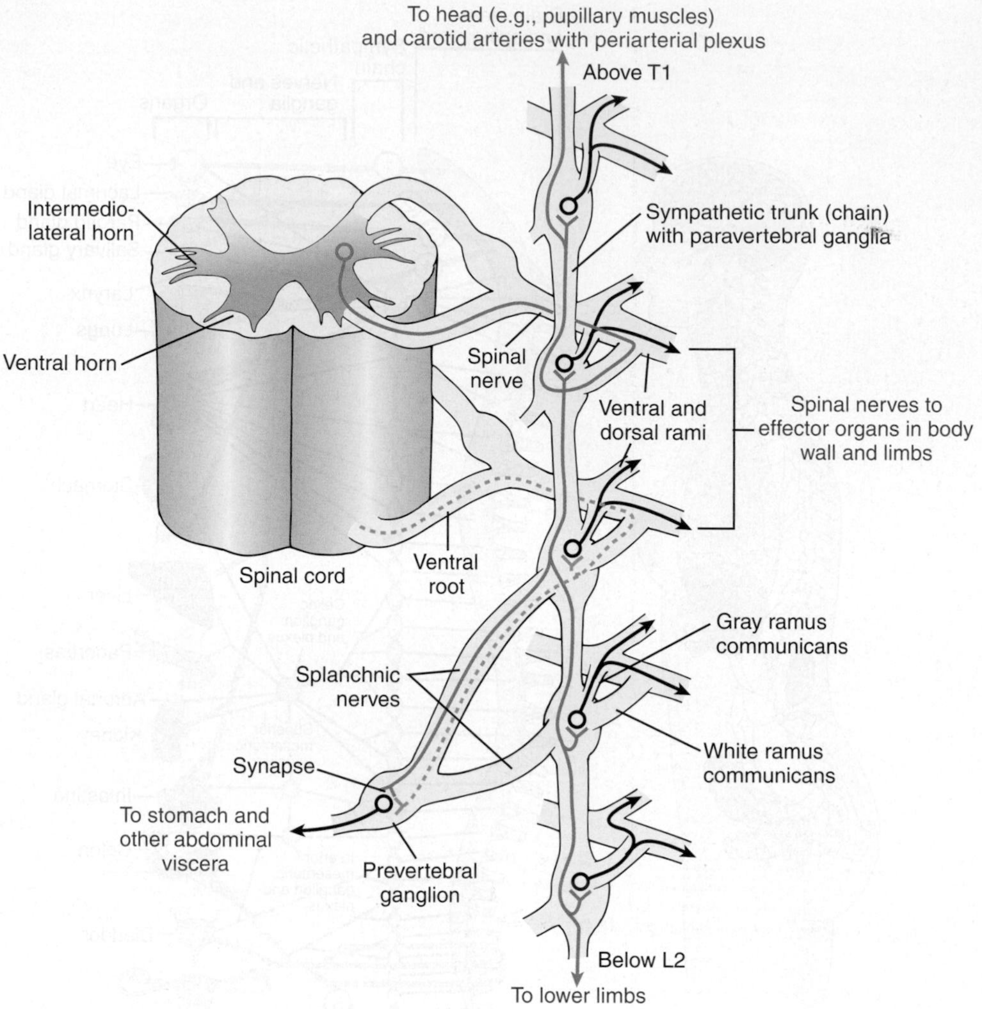

Figure 13.25 • Sympathetic pathways. Sympathetic preganglionic fibers (*blue*) leave the spinal cord by way of the ventral root of the spinal nerves, enter the ventral primary rami, and pass through the white rami to the prevertebral or paravertebral ganglia of the sympathetic chain, where they synapse with postganglionic neurons (*black*). Other preganglionic neurons (*red dotted lines*) travel directly to their destination in the various effector organs.

pass to the abdominal viscera; and those from T12, L1, L2, and L3 pass to the kidneys and pelvic organs. Many preganglionic fibers from the fifth to the last thoracolumbar segments pass through the paravertebral ganglia to continue as the splanchnic nerves. Most of these fibers do not synapse until they reach the celiac or superior mesenteric ganglion; others pass to the adrenal medulla.

The adrenal medulla, which is part of the sympathetic nervous system, contains postganglionic sympathetic neurons that secrete sympathetic neurotransmitters directly into the bloodstream. Some postganglionic fibers, all of which are unmyelinated, exit the paravertebral ganglionic chain and reenter the segmental nerve through unmyelinated branches, called *gray rami*. These segmental nerves are then distributed to all parts of the body wall in the spinal nerve branches. These fibers innervate the sweat glands, piloerector muscles of the hair follicles, all blood vessels of the skin and skeletal muscles, and the CNS itself.

Parasympathetic Nervous System

The preganglionic fibers of the parasympathetic nervous system, also called the *craniosacral division* of the ANS, originate in some segments of the brain stem and sacral segments of the spinal cord.[8] The central regions of origin are the midbrain, pons, medulla oblongata, and sacral spinal cord. The midbrain outflow passes through the oculomotor nerve (CN III) to the ciliary ganglion that lies in the orbit behind the eye; it supplies the pupillary sphincter muscle of each eye and the ciliary muscles that control lens thickness for accommodation. From the caudal pontine, outflow originates the preganglionic fibers of the intermedius component of the facial nerve (CN VII) complex. This outflow synapses in the submandibular ganglion, which sends postganglionic fibers to supply the submandibular and sublingual glands. In addition, preganglionic fibers are distributed to the pterygopalatine ganglia to synapse on postganglionic neurons that supply the lacrimal and nasal glands. Fibers in the glossopharyngeal nerve (CN IX) synapse in the otic ganglia, which supply the parotid salivary glands. The vagus nerve provides parasympathetic innervation for the heart, trachea, lungs, esophagus, stomach, small intestine, proximal half of the colon, liver, gallbladder, pancreas, kidneys, and upper portions of the ureters. The gastrointestinal tract has its own intrinsic network of ganglionic cells located between the smooth muscle layers, called the *enteric nervous system*, which controls local peristaltic and secretory functions. The action of the enteric nervous system can be modified by the activity of the ANS.

Sacral preganglionic axons leave the S2 to S4 segmental nerves by gathering into the pelvic nerves, also called the *nervi erigentes*. The pelvic nerves leave the sacral plexus on each side of the cord and distribute their peripheral fibers to the bladder, uterus, urethra, prostate, distal portion of the transverse colon, descending colon, and rectum. Sacral parasympathetic fibers also supply the venous outflow from the external genitalia to facilitate erectile function.

Except for CNs III, VII, and IX, which synapse in discrete ganglia, the long parasympathetic preganglionic fibers pass uninterrupted to short postganglionic fibers in the organ walls. In the walls of these organs, postganglionic neurons send axons to smooth muscle and glandular cells that modulate their functions.

Central Integrative Pathways

General VA fibers accompany the sympathetic and parasympathetic outflow into the spinal and CNs, bringing chemoreceptor, pressure, organ capsule stretch, and nociceptive information from organs of the viscera to the brain stem, thoracolumbar cord, and sacral cord. Local reflex circuits relating VA and autonomic efferent activity are integrated into a hierarchic control system in the spinal cord and brain stem. Progressively greater complexity in the responses and greater precision in their control occur at each higher level of the nervous system. Most visceral reflexes contain contributions from the LMNs that innervate skeletal muscles as part of their response patterns. The distinction between purely visceral and somatic reflex hierarchies becomes less and less meaningful at the higher levels of hierarchic control and behavioral integration.

The hypothalamus serves as the major control center for most of the autonomically mediated functions. The hypothalamus, with connections to the cerebral cortex, the limbic system, and the pituitary gland, is in a prime position to receive, integrate, and transmit information to other areas of the nervous system. Signals from the hypothalamus can affect almost all the brain stem control centers. For example, stimulation of certain areas, mainly in the posterior hypothalamus, can cause the cardiovascular control centers to increase the arterial blood pressure to more than twice normal. Likewise, other hypothalamic centers control body temperature and increase salivation and gastrointestinal activity.

Reflex adjustments of cardiovascular and respiratory function occur at the level of the brain stem. A prominent example is the carotid sinus baroreflex. Increased blood pressure in the carotid sinus results in increased discharge from afferent fibers that travel by way of CN IX to cardiovascular centers in the brain stem. These centers increase the activity of descending efferent vagal fibers that slow heart rate, while inhibiting sympathetic fibers that increase heart rate and blood vessel tone. Striking features of the ANS are the rapidity and intensity with which it can change visceral function. Within 3 to 5 seconds, it can increase the heart rate to approximately twice its resting level. Bronchial smooth muscle tone is largely controlled by parasympathetic fibers carried in the vagus nerve. These nerves produce mild to moderate constriction of the bronchioles.

Other important ANS reflexes are located at the level of the spinal cord. As with other spinal reflexes, these reflexes are modulated by input from higher centers. When there is a loss of communication between the higher centers and the spinal reflexes, as occurs in spinal cord injury, these reflexes function in an unregulated manner. This results in uncontrolled sweating, vasomotor instability, and reflex bowel and bladder function.

Autonomic Neurotransmission

The generation and transmission of impulses in the ANS occur in the same manner as in other neurons. There are self-propagating action potentials with transmission of impulses across synapses and other tissue junctions by neurohumoral transmitters. However, the somatic motor neurons that innervate skeletal muscles divide into many branches, with each branch innervating a single muscle fiber; in contrast, the distribution of postganglionic fibers of the ANS forms a diffuse neural plexus at the site of innervation. The membranes of the cells of many smooth muscle fibers are connected by conductive protoplasmic bridges, called *gap junctions*, that permit rapid conduction of impulses through whole sheets of smooth muscle, often in repeating waves of contraction. Autonomic neurotransmitters released near a limited portion of these fibers provide a modulating function extending to many effector cells. Smooth muscle layers of the gut and of the bladder wall are examples. Sometimes, isolated smooth muscle cells are individually innervated by the ANS, such as the piloerector cells that elevate the hair on the skin during cold exposure.

The main neurotransmitters of the ANS are acetylcholine and the catecholamines, epinephrine and norepinephrine (Fig. 13.26).[8] Acetylcholine is released at all preganglionic synapses in the autonomic ganglia of both sympathetic and parasympathetic nerve fibers and from postganglionic synapses of all parasympathetic nerve endings. It also is released at sympathetic nerve endings that innervate the sweat glands and cholinergic vasodilator fibers found in skeletal muscle. Norepinephrine is released at most sympathetic nerve endings. The adrenal medulla, which is a modified prevertebral sympathetic ganglion, produces epinephrine along with small amounts of norepinephrine. Dopamine, which is an intermediate compound in the synthesis of norepinephrine, also acts as a neurotransmitter. It is the principal inhibitory transmitter of internuncial neurons in the sympathetic ganglia. It also has vasodilator effects on renal, splanchnic, and coronary blood vessels when given intravenously and is sometimes used in the treatment of shock.

Acetylcholine and Cholinergic Receptors

Acetylcholine is synthesized in the cholinergic neurons from choline and acetyl coenzyme A (acetyl CoA; Fig. 13.27A). After acetylcholine is secreted by the cholinergic nerve endings, it is rapidly broken down by the enzyme acetylcholinesterase. The choline molecule is transported back into the nerve ending, where it is used again in the synthesis of acetylcholine.

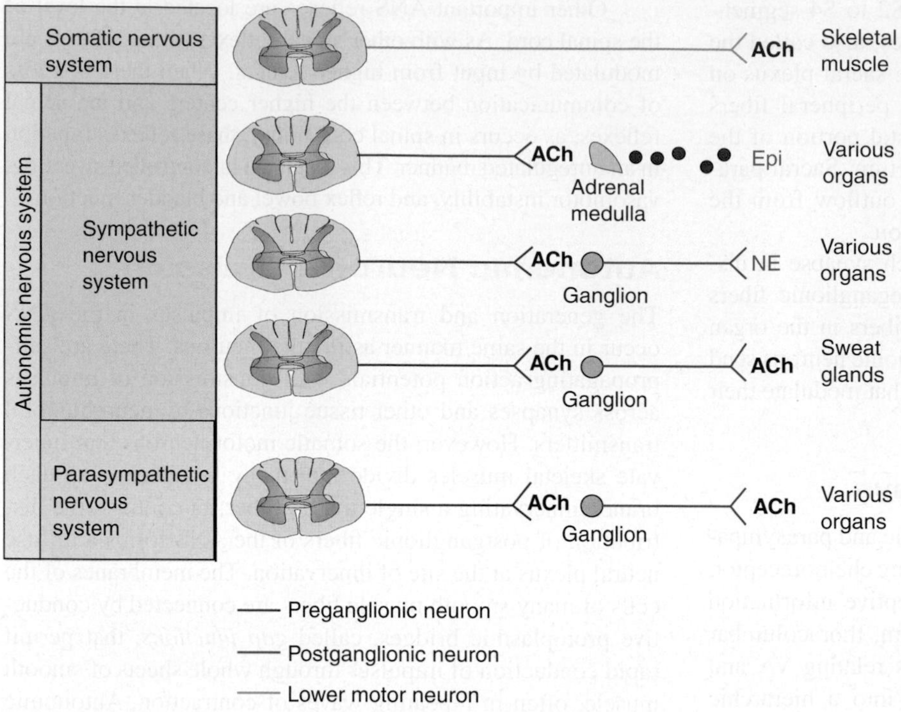

Figure 13.26 • Comparison of neurotransmission in the somatic and autonomic nervous systems. In the somatic nervous system, all LMNs release acetylcholine (ACh) as their neurotransmitter. In the ANS, both sympathetic and parasympathetic preganglionic neurons release ACh as their neurotransmitter. Parasympathetic postganglionic neurons release ACh at the site of organ innervation. Most postganglionic neurons of the sympathetic nervous system release norepinephrine (NE) at the site of organ innervation. The principal neurotransmitter released by the adrenal gland is epinephrine (Epi), which travels to the site of organ innervation through the bloodstream. The postganglionic neurons innervating the sweat gland are sympathetic fibers that use ACh as their neurotransmitter.

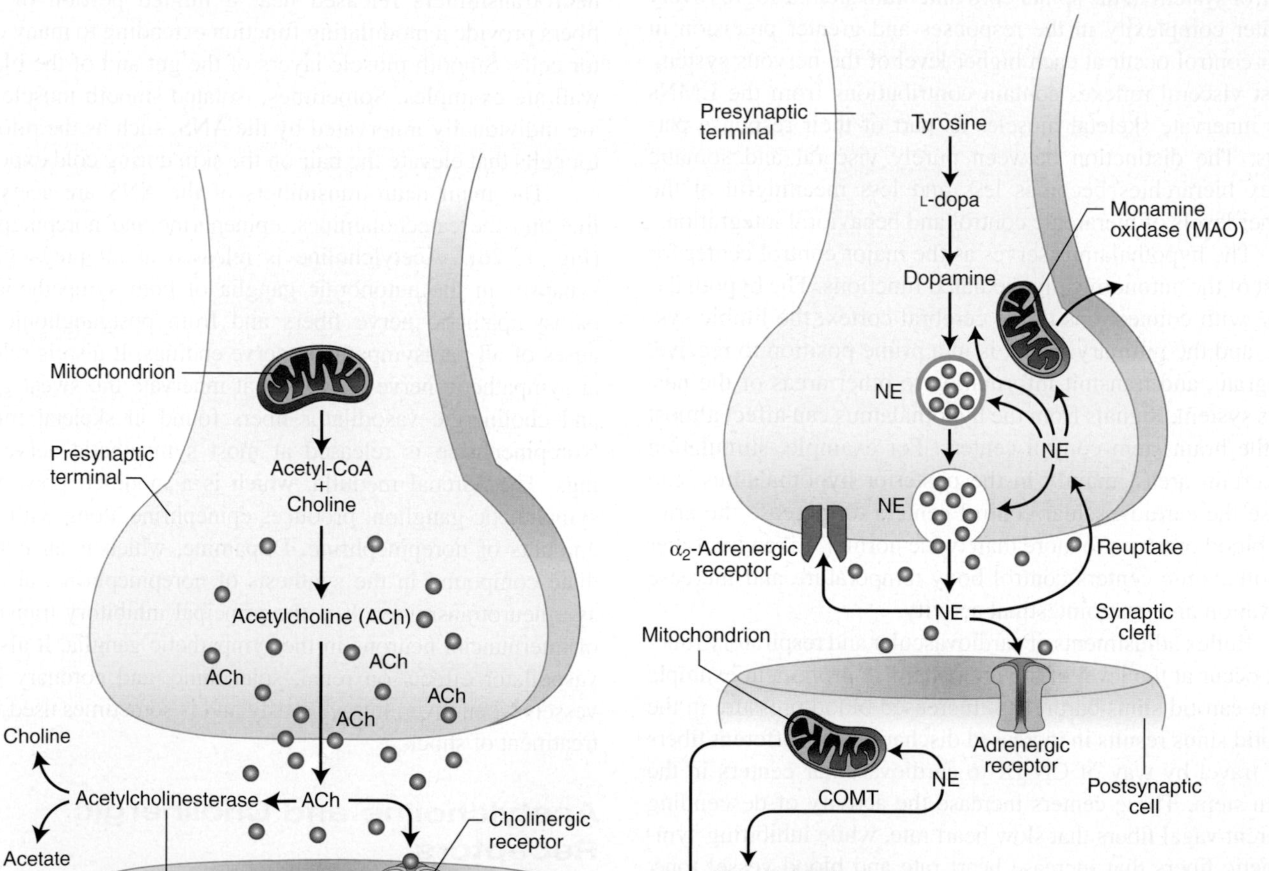

Figure 13.27 • Schematic illustration of cholinergic parasympathetic **(A)** and noradrenergic sympathetic **(B)** neurotransmitter synthesis, release, receptor binding, neurotransmitter degradation, and metabolite transport back into the presynaptic neuron (acetylcholine) and reuptake (norepinephrine). COMT, catechol-*O*-methyltransferase.

Receptors that respond to acetylcholine are called *cholinergic receptors*. Two types of cholinergic receptors are known—muscarinic and nicotinic. Muscarinic receptors are present on the innervational targets of postganglionic fibers of the parasympathetic nervous system and the sweat glands, which are innervated by the sympathetic nervous system. Nicotinic receptors are found in autonomic ganglia and the end plates of skeletal muscle. Acetylcholine is excitatory to most muscarinic and nicotinic receptors, except those in the heart and lower esophagus, where it has an inhibitory effect. The drug atropine is an antimuscarinic or muscarinic cholinergic blocking drug that prevents the action of acetylcholine at excitatory and inhibitory muscarinic receptor sites. Because it is a muscarinic blocking drug, it exerts little effect at nicotinic receptor sites.

Catecholamines and Adrenergic Receptors

The catecholamines, which include norepinephrine, epinephrine, and dopamine, are synthesized in the axoplasm of sympathetic nerve terminal endings from the amino acid tyrosine (see Fig. 13.27B). During catecholamine synthesis, tyrosine is hydroxylated (*i.e.*, has a hydroxyl group added) to form DOPA, and DOPA is decarboxylated (*i.e.*, has a carboxyl group removed) to form dopamine. Dopamine in turn is hydroxylated to form norepinephrine. In the adrenal gland, an additional step occurs during which norepinephrine is methylated (*i.e.*, a methyl group is added) to form epinephrine.

Each step in sympathetic neurotransmitter synthesis requires a different enzyme, and the type of neurotransmitter produced depends on the types of enzymes that are available in a nerve terminal. For example, the postganglionic sympathetic neurons that supply blood vessels synthesize norepinephrine, but postganglionic neurons in the adrenal medulla produce epinephrine or norepinephrine. Epinephrine accounts for approximately 80% of the catecholamines released from the adrenal gland. The synthesis of epinephrine by the adrenal medulla is influenced by glucocorticoid secretion from the adrenal cortex. These hormones are transported through an intra-adrenal vascular network from the adrenal cortex to the adrenal medulla, where they cause the sympathetic neurons to increase their production of epinephrine through increased enzyme activity. Thus, any situation sufficiently stressful to evoke increased levels of glucocorticoids also increases epinephrine levels. As the catecholamines are synthesized, they are stored in vesicles. The final step of norepinephrine synthesis occurs in these vesicles. When an action potential reaches an axon terminal, the neurotransmitter molecules are released from the storage vesicles. The storage vesicles provide a means for concentrated storage of the catecholamines and protect the neurotransmitters from the cytoplasmic enzymes that degrade them.

Besides neuronal synthesis, a second major mechanism exists for the replenishment of norepinephrine in sympathetic nerve terminals. This mechanism consists of the active recapture or reuptake of the released neurotransmitter into the nerve terminal. Between 50% and 80% of the norepinephrine released during an action potential is removed from the synaptic area by an active reuptake process. This process stops the action of the neurotransmitter and allows it to be reused by the neuron. The remainder of the released catecholamines diffuses into the surrounding tissue fluids or is degraded by two special enzymes: catechol-*O*-methyltransferase, which is diffusely present in all tissues, and monoamine oxidase (MAO), which is found in the nerve endings. Some drugs, such as the tricyclic antidepressants, are thought to increase the level of catecholamines at the site of nerve endings in the brain by blocking the reuptake process. Others, such as the MAO inhibitors, increase the levels of neurotransmitters by decreasing their enzymatic degradation.

Catecholamines can cause excitation or inhibition of smooth muscle contraction, depending on the site, dose, and type of receptor present. Norepinephrine has potent excitatory activity and low inhibitory activity. Epinephrine is potent as both an excitatory and an inhibitory agent. The excitatory (α) or inhibitory (β) responses of organs to sympathetic neurotransmitters are mediated by interaction with special structures in the cell membrane called *receptors*.

In vascular smooth muscle, excitation of α receptors causes vasoconstriction, and excitation of β receptors causes vasodilation.[8] Endogenously and exogenously administered norepinephrine produces marked vasoconstriction of the blood vessels in the skin, kidneys, and splanchnic circulation that are supplied with α receptors. The β receptors are most prevalent in the heart, the blood vessels of skeletal muscle, and the bronchioles. Blood vessels in skeletal muscle have α and β receptors. In these vessels, high levels of norepinephrine produce vasoconstriction; low levels produce vasodilation. The low levels are thought to have a diluting effect on norepinephrine levels in the arteries of these blood vessels so that the β effect predominates. With respect to vessels having few receptors, such as those that supply the brain, norepinephrine has little effect.

α-Adrenergic receptors have been further subdivided into α_1 and α_2 receptors and β-adrenergic receptors into β_1 and β_2 receptors. β_1-Adrenergic receptors are found primarily in the heart and can be selectively blocked by β_1 receptor blocking drugs. β_2-Adrenergic receptors are found in the bronchioles and in other sites that have β-mediated functions. α_1-Adrenergic receptors are found primarily in postsynaptic effector sites; they mediate responses in vascular smooth muscle. α_2-Adrenergic receptors are mainly located presynaptically and can inhibit the release of norepinephrine from sympathetic nerve terminals. α_2-Adrenergic receptors are abundant in the CNS and are thought to influence the central control of blood pressure.

The various classes of adrenergic receptors provide a mechanism by which the same adrenergic neurotransmitter can have many selective effects on different effector cells. This mechanism also permits neurotransmitters carried in the bloodstream, whether from neuroendocrine secretion by the adrenal gland or from subcutaneously or intravenously administered drugs, to produce the same effects. The catecholamines produced and released from sympathetic nerve endings are called *endogenous neuromediators*. Sympathetic nerve endings also can be activated by exogenous forms of these neuromediators, which reach the nerve endings through the bloodstream after being injected into the body or administered orally. These drugs mimic the action of the neuromediators and are said to have a *sympathomimetic action.* Other drugs can selectively block the receptor sites on the neurons and temporarily prevent the neurotransmitter from exerting its action.

IN SUMMARY

The ANS regulates, adjusts, and coordinates the visceral functions of the body. The ANS, which is divided into the sympathetic and parasympathetic systems, is an efferent system. It receives its afferent input from VA neurons. The ANS has CNS and PNS components. The outflow of the sympathetic and parasympathetic nervous systems follows a two-neuron pathway, which consists of a preganglionic neuron in the CNS and a postganglionic neuron located outside the CNS. Sympathetic fibers leave the CNS at the thoracolumbar level, and the parasympathetic fibers leave at the cranial and sacral levels. The sympathetic and parasympathetic nervous systems can have opposing effects on visceral function—if one excites, the other inhibits. The hypothalamus serves as the major control center for most ANS functions; local reflex circuits relating VA and autonomic efferent activity are integrated in a hierarchic control system in the spinal cord and brain stem.

The main neurotransmitters for the ANS are acetylcholine and the catecholamines, epinephrine and norepinephrine. Acetylcholine is the transmitter for all preganglionic neurons, for postganglionic parasympathetic neurons, and for selected postganglionic sympathetic neurons. The catecholamines are the neurotransmitters for most postganglionic sympathetic neurons. Neurotransmitters exert their target action through specialized cell surface receptors—cholinergic receptors that bind acetylcholine and adrenergic receptors that bind the catecholamines. The cholinergic receptors are divided into nicotinic and muscarinic receptors, and adrenergic receptors are divided into α and β receptors. Different receptors for the same transmitter at various sites in the same tissue or in other tissues result in differences in tissue responses to the same transmitter. This arrangement also permits the use of pharmacologic agents that act at specific receptor types.

GERIATRIC Considerations

- A decrease in nerve cell mass, overall brain weight, and reduced size of the brain and spinal cord are associated with aging.[9]
- Reaction time slows due to loss of nerve cells; remaining nerve cells have fewer dendrites and demyelination of the cell.[9] Toxicity of the nerve cell may occur due to free radical exposure over the lifetime.[9]
- The ability of the brain to compensate for decreased blood flow decreases with age.[9]

PEDIATRIC Considerations

- Infection, trauma, and congenital malformations can cause neurologic alterations in children.[10]
- During the first 3 to 4 weeks of gestation, the brain and spinal cord are at increased risk for alterations in development when exposed to malnutrition, infection, trauma, and teratogens.[10]
- Because the cranial bones are not fused at birth, the infant is at increased risk for fractures of the skull.[10]
- The more premature the infant, the greater the risk for brain damage because of increased number of fragile capillaries which can result in hemorrhage.[10]
- The increased mobility of the child's spine put them at risk for cervical spine injury.[10]

REVIEW EXERCISES

1. Herpes zoster or shingles is a painful vesicular skin eruption involving the dermatomal distribution of a general SA nerve that is caused by reactivation of the chickenpox virus (varicella–zoster virus) that has remained dormant in the dorsal root ganglion since a childhood infection.
   A. *Explain the reactivation of the varicella–zoster virus.*
2. An event such as cardiac arrest, which produces global ischemia of the brain, can produce a selective loss of recent memory and cognitive skills, while the more vegetative and life-sustaining functions such as breathing are preserved.
   A. *Use principles related to the development of the nervous system and hierarchy of control to explain why.*
3. Usually, spinal cord injury or disease produces both sensory and motor deficits. An exception is infection by the poliomyelitis virus, which produces weakness and paralysis without loss of sensation in the affected extremities.
   A. *Explain, using information on the cell column organization of the spinal cord.*
4. The functions of the sympathetic nervous system are often described in relation to the "fight-or-flight" response. Using this description, explain the physiologic advantage for the following distribution of sympathetic nervous system receptors:
   A. *The presence of β_2 receptors on the blood vessels that provide blood flow to the skeletal muscles during "fight or flight," and the presence of α_1 receptors on the resistance vessels that control blood pressure*

B. The presence of acetylcholine receptors on the sweat glands that allow for evaporative loss of body heat during "fight or flight," and the presence of α_1 receptors that constrict the skin vessels that control blood flow to the skin

C. The presence of β_2 receptors that produce relaxation in the detrusor muscle of the bladder during "fight or flight," and the presence of α_1 receptors that produce contraction of the smooth muscle in the internal sphincter of the bladder

References

1. Hammer G., McPhee S. (2013). *Pathophysiology of disease: An introduction to clinical medicine* (7th ed.). New York: McGraw-Hill.
2. Waxman S. (2017). *Clinical neuroanatomy* (28th ed.). New York, NY: McGraw Hill Education.
3. Harlow D. E., Honce, J. M., Miravalle, A. A. (2013). Remyelination therapy in multiple sclerosis. *Frontiers in Neurology* 6, 1–13.
4. MacVicar B. A., Newman E. A. (2015). Astrocyte regulation of blood flow in the brain. *Cold Spring Harbor Perspectives in Biology* 7, 1–15.
5. Hickey J. (2013). *The clinical practice of neurological and neurosurgical nursing* (7th ed.). Philadelphia, PA: Lippincott Williams & Wilkins.
6. Tortora G., Derrickson B. (2017). *Principles of anatomy and physiology* (15th ed.). Hoboken, NJ: John Wiley & Sons.
7. Rowland, L. P., Pedley, T. A. (2015). *Merritt's Neurology* (13th ed.). Philadelphia, PA: Lippincott Williams & Wilkins.
8. Bader, M. K., Littlejohns, L. R., Olson, D.M. (2016). *AANN Core Curriculum for Neuroscience Nursing*. Chicago, IL: AANN.
9. Eliopoulos, C. Neurologic function. In *Gerontological nursing* (9th ed.). Philadelphia, PA: Wolters Kluwer.
10. Kyle T., Carman S. (Eds.) (2017). Nursing care of the child with an alteration in intracranial regulation/neurologic disorder. In *Essentials of pediatric nursing* (3rd ed.). Philadelphia, PA: Wolters Kluwer.

Somatosensory Function, Pain, Headache, and Temperature Regulation

14

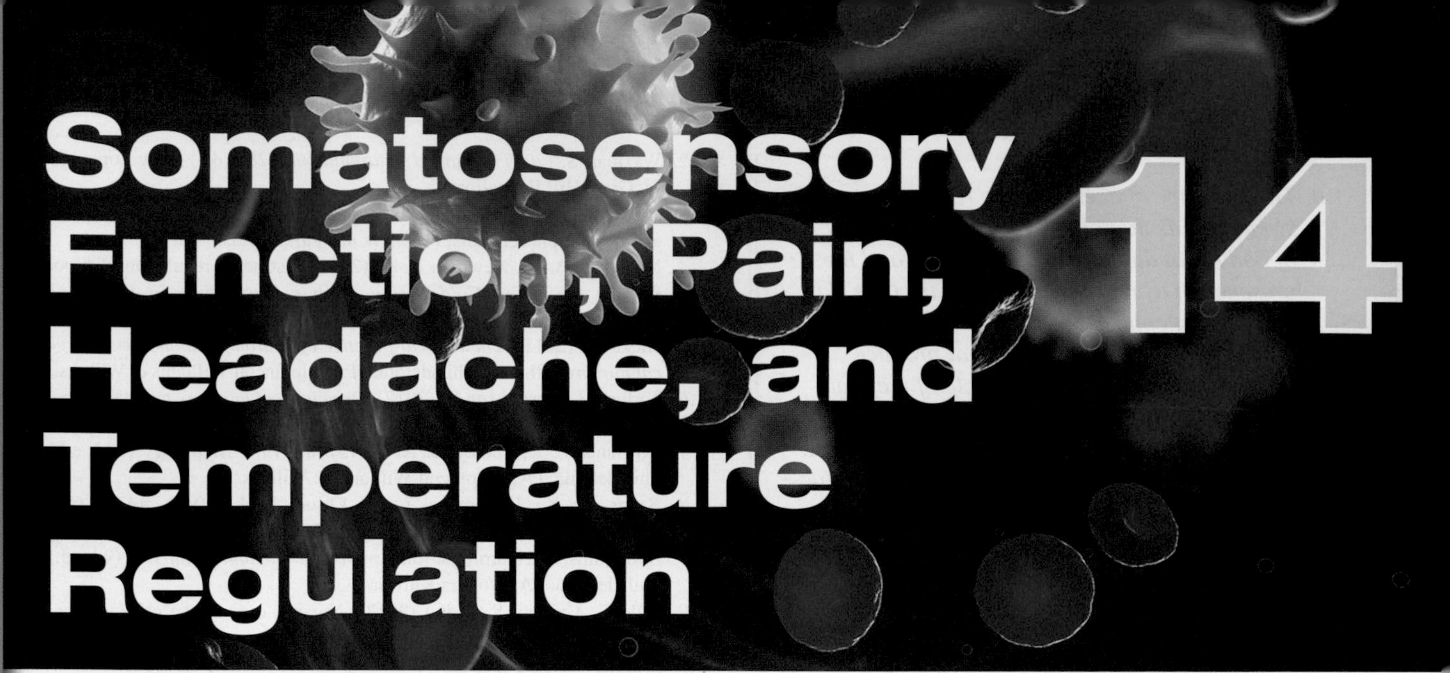

Cynthia Bautista

The somatosensory component of the nervous system provides an awareness of body sensations such as touch, temperature, body position, and pain. The sensory receptors for somatosensory function consist of discrete nerve endings in the skin and other body tissues. Between 2 and 3 million sensory neurons deliver a steady stream of encoded information. Only a small proportion of this information reaches awareness. Most of the information provides input essential for a myriad of reflex and automatic mechanisms.

ORGANIZATION AND CONTROL OF SOMATOSENSORY FUNCTION

After completing this section of the chapter, the learner will be able to meet the following objectives:

- Describe the organization of the somatosensory system in terms of first-, second-, and third-order neurons.
- Summarize the structure and function of the dorsal root ganglion neurons in terms of sensory receptors, conduction velocities, and spinal cord projections.
- Compare the tactile, thermal, and position sense modalities in terms of receptors, adequate stimuli, ascending pathways, and central integrative mechanisms.

The somatosensory system is designed to provide the central nervous system (CNS) with information on touch, temperature, body position, and pain related to deep and superficial body structures. Sensory neurons can be divided into three types that vary in distribution and the type of sensation detected: general somatic, special somatic, and general visceral. *General somatic afferent neurons* have branches with widespread distribution throughout the body and with many distinct types of receptors that result in sensations such as pain, touch, and temperature.[1,2] *Special somatic afferent neurons* have receptors located primarily in muscles, tendons, and joints.[1,2] These receptors sense position and movement of the body. *General visceral afferent neurons* have receptors on various visceral structures that sense fullness and discomfort.[1,2]

Sensory Systems

Sensory systems can be conceptualized as a serial succession of neurons consisting of first-order, second-order, and third-order neurons. *First-order neurons* transmit sensory information from the periphery to the CNS. *Second-order neurons* communicate with various reflex networks and sensory pathways in the spinal cord and travel directly to the thalamus. *Third-order neurons* relay information from the thalamus to the cerebral cortex (Fig. 14.1).

These three primary levels of neural integration provide the organizing framework of the somatosensory system:

- The sensory units, which contain the sensory receptors
- The ascending pathways
- The central processing centers in the thalamus and cerebral cortex

Sensory information usually is relayed and processed in a cephalad (toward the head) direction by the three orders of neurons. Many interneurons process and modify the sensory information at the level of the second- and third-order neurons, and many more participate before coordinated and appropriate learned movement responses occur. The number of participating neurons increases exponentially from the primary through the secondary and the secondary through the tertiary levels.

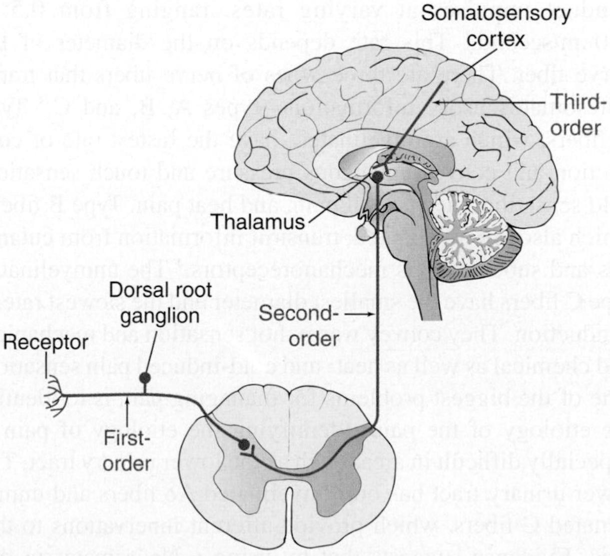

Figure 14.1 • Arrangement of first-order, second-order, and third-order neurons of the somatosensory system.

KEY POINTS

THE SOMATOSENSORY SYSTEM

- The somatosensory system relays information about four major modalities: touch, temperature, body position, and pain.
- Somatosensory information is sequentially transmitted over three types of neurons: first-order neurons, which transmit information from sensory receptors to dorsal horn neurons; second-order CNS association neurons, which communicate with various reflex circuits and transmit information to the thalamus; and third-order neurons, which forward the information from the thalamus to the sensory cortex.

The Sensory Unit

The somatosensory experience arises from information provided by a variety of receptors distributed throughout the body. These receptors monitor four major types or modalities of sensation—stimulus discrimination, tactile sensation, thermal sensation, and position sensation.[1]

Each of the somatosensory modalities is mediated by a distinct system of receptors and pathways to the brain. However, all somatosensory information from the limbs and trunk shares a common class of sensory neurons called *dorsal root ganglion neurons*.[2] Somatosensory information from the face and cranial structures is transmitted by the trigeminal sensory neurons, which function in the same manner as the dorsal root ganglion neurons. The cell body of the dorsal root ganglion neuron, its peripheral branch (which innervates a small area of periphery), and its central axon (which projects to the CNS) form what is called a *sensory unit*.

The fibers of different dorsal root ganglion neurons conduct impulses at varying rates, ranging from 0.5 to 120 m/second.[1] This rate depends on the diameter of the nerve fiber. There are three types of nerve fibers that transmit somatosensory information—types A, B, and C.[3] Type A fibers, which are myelinated, have the fastest rate of conduction and convey cutaneous pressure and touch sensation, cold sensation, mechanical pain, and heat pain. Type B fibers, which also are myelinated, transmit information from cutaneous and subcutaneous mechanoreceptors.[4] The unmyelinated type C fibers have the smallest diameter and the slowest rate of conduction. They convey warm–hot sensation and mechanical and chemical as well as heat- and cold-induced pain sensation. One of the biggest problems for managing pain is to identify the etiology of the pain. Identifying the etiology of pain is especially difficult in areas such as the lower urinary tract. The lower urinary tract has both myelinated Aδ fibers and unmyelinated C fibers, which provide afferent innervations to this area. Evidence suggests that by using a Neurometer in this area, a more comprehensive diagnosis of sensory function can be made. In turn, more effective pharmacologic and nonpharmacologic interventions could be recommended.[5]

Dermatomal Pattern of Dorsal Root Innervation

The somatosensory innervation of the body, including the head, retains a basic segmental organizational pattern that was established during embryonic development. Thirty-three paired spinal nerves provide sensory and motor innervation of the body wall, the limbs, and the viscera. Sensory input to each spinal cord segment is provided by sensory neurons with cell bodies in the dorsal root ganglia.

The region of the body wall that is supplied by a single pair of dorsal root ganglia is called a dermatome. These dorsal root ganglion–innervated strips occur in a regular sequence moving upward from the second coccygeal segment through the cervical segments, reflecting the basic segmental organization of the body and the nervous system (Fig. 14.2). The cranial nerves that innervate the head send their axons to equivalent nuclei in the brain stem. Neighboring dermatomes overlap one another sufficiently so that a loss of one dorsal root or root ganglion results in reduced but not total loss of sensory innervation of a dermatome (Fig. 14.3). Using dermatome maps can help in interpreting the level and extent of sensory deficits that are the result of segmental nerve and spinal cord damage. The information obtained from this exercise can assist in determining the most effective pain management plan.

Spinal Circuitry and Ascending Neural Pathways

On entry into the spinal cord, the central axons of the somatosensory neurons branch extensively and project to neurons in the spinal cord gray matter. Some branches become involved in local spinal cord reflexes and directly initiate motor reflexes (*e.g.*, flexor-withdrawal reflex). Two parallel pathways, the *discriminative pathway* and the *anterolateral pathway*, carry the information from the spinal cord to the thalamic level of sensation, each taking a different route through the CNS. The discriminative pathway crosses at the base of the medulla, and the anterolateral pathway crosses within the first few segments of entering the spinal cord. These pathways relay information to the brain for three purposes—perception, arousal, and motor control. The advantages of having a two-pathway system include the following:

- Sensory information can be handled in two different ways.
- If one pathway is damaged, the other still can provide input.

The Discriminative Pathway. The discriminative pathway, also known as the dorsal column–medial lemniscal pathway, is used for the rapid transmission of sensory information such as discriminative touch.[1] It contains branches of primary afferent axons that travel up the ipsilateral (*i.e.*, same side) dorsal columns of the spinal cord white matter and synapse with highly evolved somatosensory input association neurons in the medulla. The discriminative pathway uses only three neurons to transmit information from a sensory receptor to the somatosensory strip of parietal cerebral cortex of the opposite side of the brain:

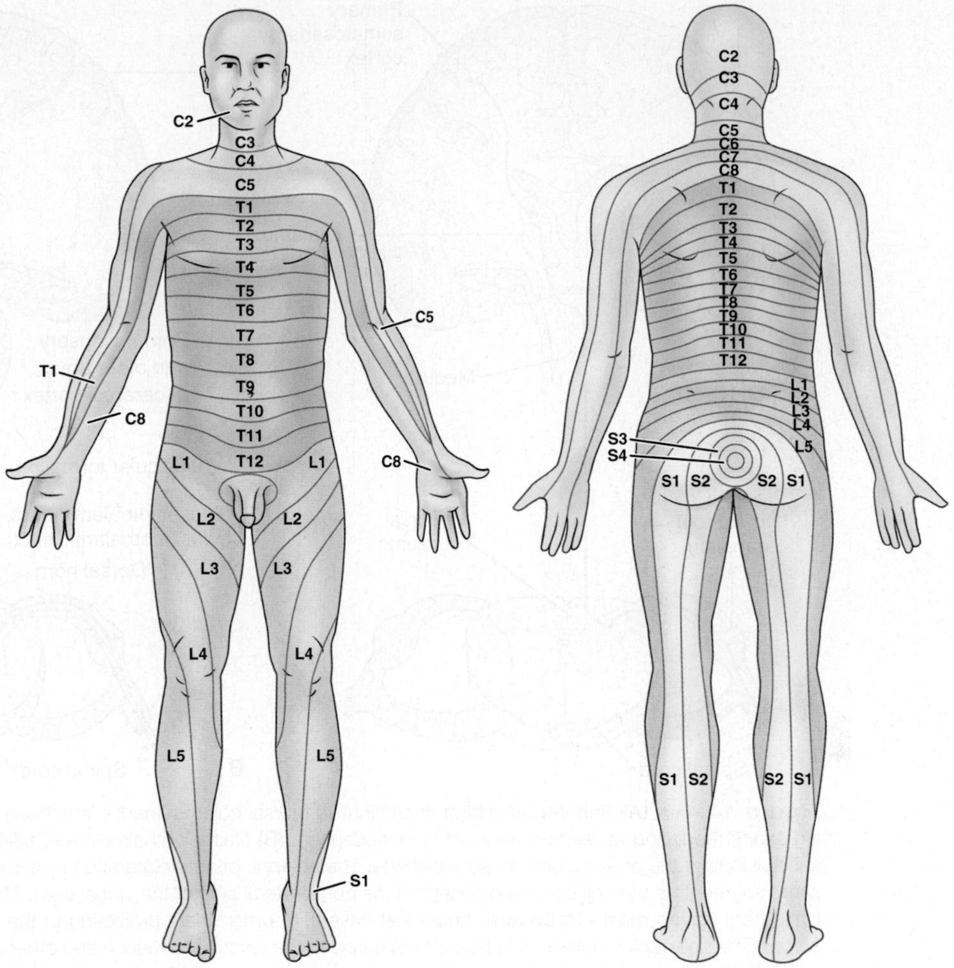

Figure 14.2 • Dermatome distribution. (From Hinkle J. L., Cheever K. H. (2018). *Brunner & Suddarth's textbook of medical-surgical nursing* (14th ed., Figure 65-9, p. 1953). Philadelphia, PA: Lippincott Williams & Wilkins.)

1. The primary dorsal root ganglion neuron, which projects its central axon to the dorsal column nuclei.
2. The dorsal column neuron, which sends its axon through a rapid conducting tract, called the *medial lemniscus*. It then crosses at the base of the medulla and travels to the thalamus on the opposite side of the brain, where basic sensation begins.

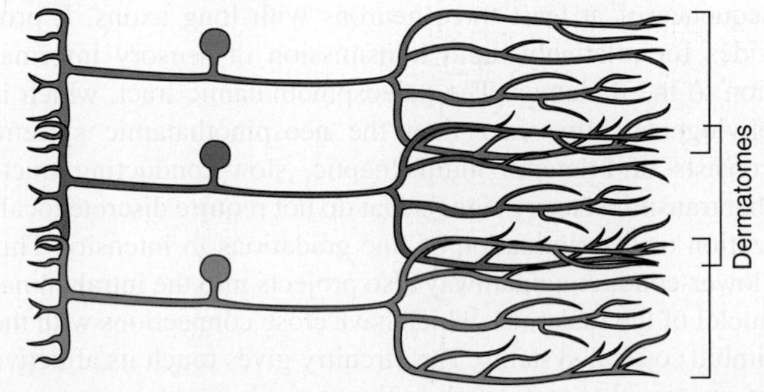

Figure 14.3 • The dermatomes formed by the peripheral processes of adjacent spinal nerves overlap on the body surface. The central processes of these fibers also overlap in their spinal distribution.

3. The thalamic neuron, which projects its axons through the somatosensory radiation to the primary sensory cortex.[1] (Fig. 14.4A)

The medial lemniscus is joined by fibers from the sensory nucleus of the trigeminal nerve (cranial nerve V) that supplies the face. Sensory information arriving at the sensory cortex by this route can be discretely localized and discriminated in terms of intensity.

A distinct feature of the discriminative pathway is that it relays precise information regarding spatial orientation. This is the only pathway taken by the sensations of muscle and joint movement, vibration, and delicate discriminative touch, as is required to differentiate correctly the location of touch on the skin at two neighboring points (*i.e.*, two-point discrimination). An important function of the discriminative pathway is to integrate the input from multiple receptors. The sense of shape and size of an object in the absence of visualization, called *stereognosis*, is based on precise afferent information from muscle, tendon, and joint receptors. For example, a screwdriver is perceived as being different from a knife in terms of its texture (tactile sensibility) and shape based on the relative position of the fingers as they move over the object. This complex interpretive perception requires that both the

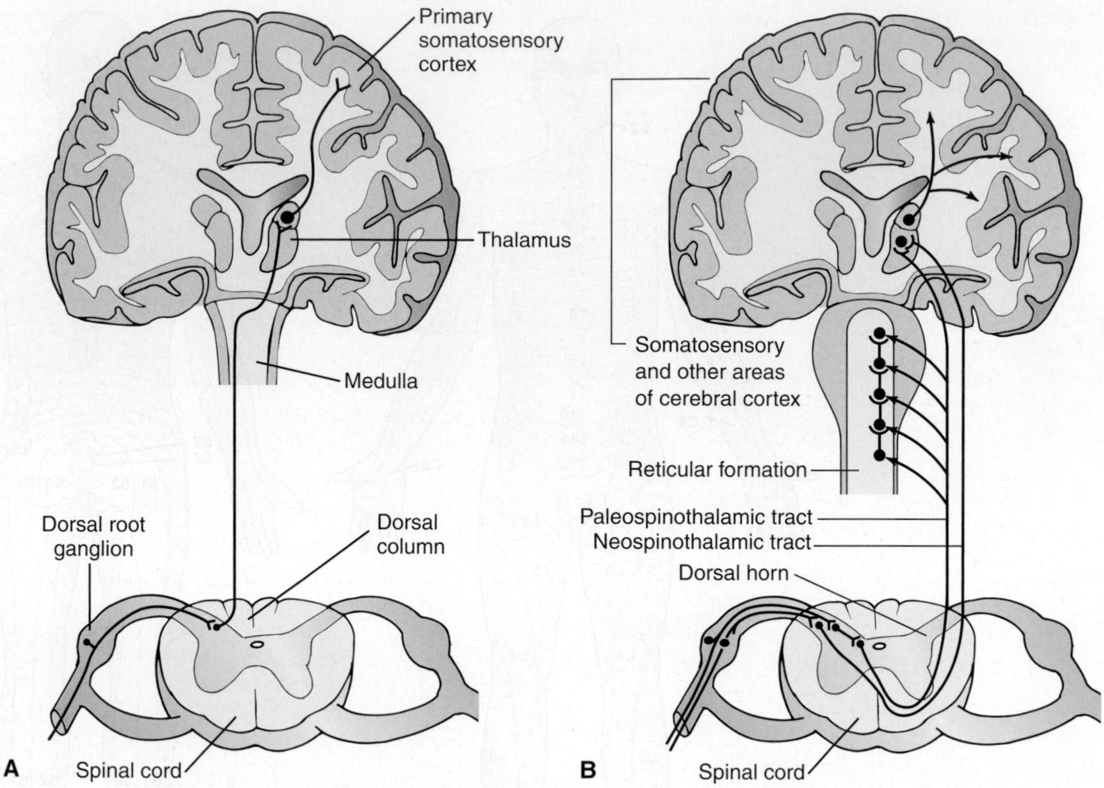

Figure 14.4 • **(A)** Rapid-transmitting discriminative (dorsal column–medial lemniscal) pathway carrying axons mediating tactile sensation and proprioception. **(B)** Neospinothalamic and paleospinothalamic subdivisions of the anterolateral sensory pathway. The neurons of anterolateral pathways cross within the same segment as the cell body and ascend in the contralateral side of the spinal cord. The neospinothalamic tract travels mainly to thalamic nuclei that have third-order fibers projecting to the somatosensory cortex. The paleospinothalamic tract sends collaterals to the reticular formation and other structures, from which further fibers project to the thalamus.

discriminative system and the higher-order parietal association cortex are functioning properly. If the discriminative somatosensory pathway is functional but the parietal association cortex has become discretely damaged, the person can correctly describe the object but does not recognize that it is a screwdriver. This deficit is called astereognosis.

The Anterolateral Pathway. The anterolateral pathways (anterior and lateral spinothalamic pathways) consist of bilateral, multisynaptic, slow-conducting tracts. These pathways provide transmission of sensory information such as pain, thermal sensations, crude touch, and pressure that does not require discrete localization of signal source or fine discrimination of intensity. The fibers of the anterolateral pathway originate in the dorsal horns at the level of the segmental nerve, where the dorsal root neurons enter the spinal cord. They cross in the anterior commissure, within a few segments of origin, to the opposite anterolateral pathway, where they ascend upward toward the brain. The spinothalamic tract fibers synapse with several nuclei in the thalamus, but en route they give off numerous branches that travel to the reticular activating system (RAS) of the brain stem. These projections provide the basis for increased wakefulness or awareness after strong somatosensory stimulation and for the generalized startle reaction that occurs with sudden and intense stimuli. They also stimulate autonomic nervous system responses, such as a rise in heart rate and blood pressure, dilation of the pupils, and the pale, moist skin that results from constriction of the cutaneous blood vessels and activation of the sweat glands.

There are two subdivisions in the anterolateral pathway—the *neospinothalamic tract* and the *paleospinothalamic tract* (Fig. 14.4B).[1] The neospinothalamic tract consists of a sequence of at least three neurons with long axons. It provides for relatively rapid transmission of sensory information to the thalamus. The paleospinothalamic tract, which is phylogenetically older than the neospinothalamic system, consists of bilateral, multisynaptic, slow-conducting tracts that transmit sensory signals that do not require discrete localization or discrimination of fine gradations in intensity. This slower-conducting pathway also projects into the intralaminar nuclei of the thalamus, which have close connections with the limbic cortical systems. The circuitry gives touch its affective or emotional aspects, such as the particular unpleasantness of heavy pressure and the peculiar pleasantness of the tickling and gentle rubbing of the skin.

Central Processing of Somatosensory Information

Perception, or the final processing of somatosensory information, involves awareness of the stimuli, localization and discrimination of their characteristics, and interpretation of their meaning. As sensory information reaches the thalamus, it begins to enter the level of consciousness. In the thalamus, the sensory information is roughly localized and perceived as a crude sense. The full localization, discrimination of the intensity, and interpretation of the meaning of the stimuli require processing by the somatosensory cortex.

The somatosensory cortex is located in the parietal lobe, which lies behind the central sulcus and above the lateral sulcus (Fig. 14.5). The strip of parietal cortex that borders the central sulcus is called the *primary somatosensory cortex* because it receives primary sensory information by direct projections from the thalamus. The *sensory homunculus* reflects the density of cortical neurons devoted to sensory input from afferents in corresponding peripheral areas. Most of the cortical surface is devoted to areas of the body such as the thumb, forefinger, lips, and tongue, where fine touch and pressure discrimination are essential for normal function.

Parallel to and just behind the primary somatosensory cortex (*i.e.*, toward the occipital cortex) lie the somatosensory association areas, which are required to transform the raw material of sensation into meaningful learned perception. Most of the perceptive aspects of body sensation, or somesthesia, require the function of this parietal association cortex. The perceptive aspect, or meaningfulness, of a stimulus pattern involves the integration of present sensation with past learning. For instance, a person's past learning plus present tactile sensation provides the perception of sitting on a soft chair rather than on a hard bicycle seat.

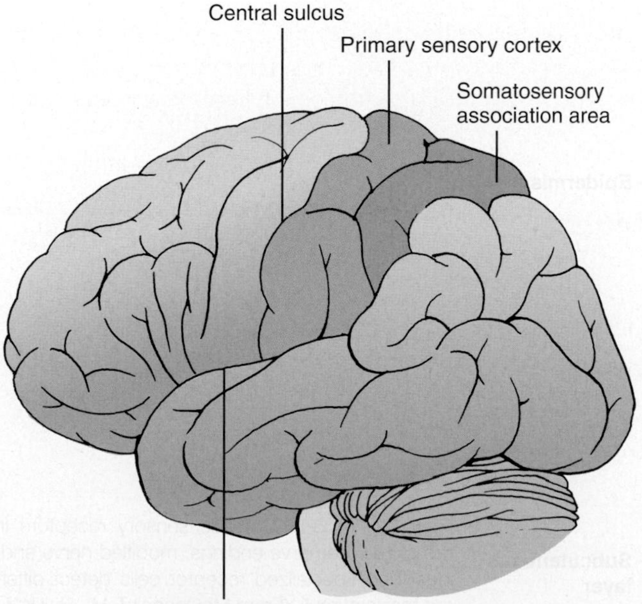

Figure 14.5 • Primary somatosensory cortex and somatosensory association area.

Sensory Modalities

Somatosensory experience can be divided into *modalities*, a term used for qualitative, subjective distinctions between sensations such as touch, heat, and pain. These experiences require the function of sensory receptors and forebrain structures in the thalamus and cerebral cortex. Sensory experience also involves quantitative sensory discrimination or the ability to distinguish between different levels of sensory stimulation.

The receptive endings of different afferent neurons are particularly sensitive to specific forms of physical and chemical energy. They can initiate action potentials to many forms of energy at high energy levels, but they usually are highly tuned to be differentially sensitive to low levels of a particular energy type. For example, a receptive ending may be particularly sensitive to a small increase in local skin temperature. Stimulating the ending with electric current or strong pressure also can result in action potentials. The amount of energy required, however, is much greater than it is for a change in temperature. Other afferent sensory terminals are most sensitive to slight indentations of the skin, and their signals are subjectively interpreted as touch. Cool versus warm, sharp versus dull pain, and delicate touch versus deep pressure are all based on different populations of afferent neurons or on central integration of simultaneous input from several differently tuned afferents.

When information from different primary afferents reaches the forebrain, where subjective experience occurs, the qualitative differences between warmth and touch are called *sensory modalities*. Although the receptor-detected information is relayed to the thalamus and cortex over separate pathways, the experience of a modality, such as cold versus warm, is uniquely subjective.

Stimulus Discrimination

The ability to discriminate the location of a somesthetic stimulus is called acuity and is based on the sensory field in a dermatome innervated by an afferent neuron. High acuity (*i.e.*, the ability to make fine discriminations of location) requires a high density of innervation by afferent neurons. For example, acuity is highest on the lips and cheek but lower on the arm or back. High acuity also requires a projection system through the CNS to the forebrain that preserves distinctions between levels of activity in neighboring sensory fields. Receptors or receptive endings of primary afferent neurons differ as to the intensity at which they begin to fire. For instance, it is possible to assess two-point discrimination by using an open paper clip with its ends bent together to 5 mm apart. When placed on the lips or cheek, the person will readily detect two points of contact. On the back or arm, the ends of the paper clip must be moved progressively farther apart before two points of contact can be detected.

Tactile Sensation

The tactile system, which relays sensory information regarding touch, pressure, and vibration, is considered the basic somatosensory system. Loss of temperature or pain sensitivity leaves the person with no awareness of deficiency. If the tactile system is lost, however, total anesthesia (*i.e.*, numbness) of the involved body part results.

Touch sensation results from stimulation of tactile receptors in the skin and in tissues immediately beneath the skin, pressure from deformation of deeper tissues, and vibration from rapidly repetitive sensory signals. There are at least six types of specialized tactile receptors in the skin and deeper structures—free nerve endings, Meissner corpuscles, Merkel disks, Pacinian corpuscles, hair follicle end organs, and Ruffini end organs (Fig. 14.6).[1]

Free nerve endings are found in skin and many other tissues, including the cornea. They detect touch and pressure. *Meissner corpuscles* are elongated, encapsulated nerve endings present in nonhairy parts of the skin. They are particularly abundant in the fingertips, lips, and other areas where the sense of touch is highly developed. *Merkel disks* are dome-shaped receptors found in nonhairy areas and in hairy parts of the skin. In contrast to Meissner corpuscles, which adapt within a fraction of a second, Merkel disks transmit an initial strong signal that diminishes in strength but is slow in adapting. For this reason, Meissner corpuscles are particularly sensitive to the movement of very light objects over the surface of the skin and to low-frequency vibration. Merkel disks are responsible for giving steady-state signals that allow for continuous determination of touch against the skin.

The *Pacinian corpuscle* is located immediately beneath the skin and deep in the fascial tissues of the body. This type of receptor, which is stimulated by rapid movements of the tissues and adapts within a few hundredths of a second, is important in detecting direct pressure changes and tissue vibration.[2] The *hair follicle end organ* consists of afferent unmyelinated fibers entwined around most of the length of the hair follicle. These receptors, which are rapidly adapting, detect movement on the surface of the body. *Ruffini end organs* are found in the skin and deeper structures, including the joint capsules. These receptors, which have multibranched encapsulated endings, have very little adaptive capacity and are important for signaling continuous states of deformation, such as heavy and continuous touch and pressure because they are sensitive to skin stretch.[2]

Almost all the specialized touch receptors, such as Merkel disks, Meissner corpuscles, hair follicle end organs, Pacinian corpuscles, and Ruffini end organs, transmit their signals in large myelinated nerve fibers (*i.e.*, types Aα, Aβ) that have transmission velocities ranging from 30 to 70 m/second.[1] Most free nerve endings transmit signals by way of small myelinated fibers (*i.e.*, type Aδ) with conduction velocities of 5 to 30 m/second.[1]

The sensory information for tactile sensation enters the spinal cord through the dorsal roots of the spinal nerves. All tactile sensation that requires rapid transmission is transmitted through the discriminative pathway to the thalamus by way of the medial lemniscus. This includes touch sensation requiring a high degree of localization or fine gradations of intensity, vibratory sensation, and sensation that signals movement against the skin. In addition to the ascending discriminative pathway, tactile sensation uses the more primitive and crude anterolateral pathway. The afferent axons that

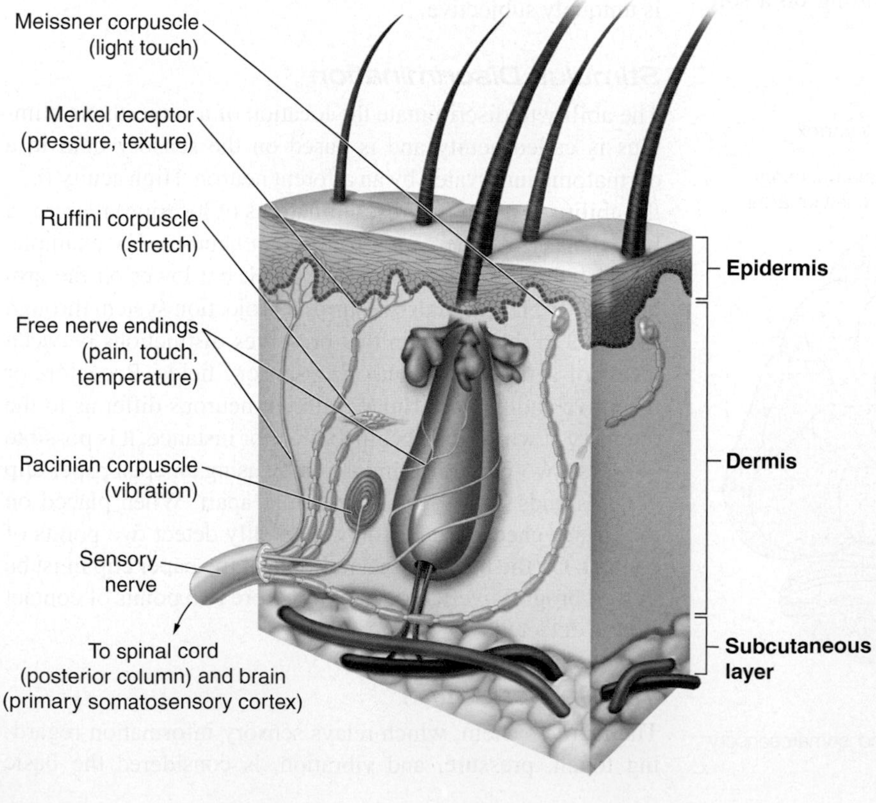

Figure 14.6 • Somatic sensory receptors in the skin. Free nerve endings, modified nerve endings, and specialized receptor cells detect different tactile stimuli. (From McConnell T. H., Hull K. L. (2011). *Human form, human function: essentials of anatomy & physiology*. Philadelphia, PA: Lippincott Williams & Wilkins.)

carry tactile information up the dorsal columns have many branches or collaterals, and some of these synapse in the dorsal horn near the level of dorsal root entry. After several synapses, axons are projected up both sides of the anterolateral aspect of the spinal cord to the thalamus. Few fibers travel all the way to the thalamus. Most synapse on reticular formation neurons that then send their axons on toward the thalamus. The lateral nuclei of the thalamus are capable of contributing a crude, poorly localized sensation from the opposite side of the body. From the thalamus, some projections travel to the somatosensory cortex, especially to the side opposite the stimulus.

Because of multiple routes, total destruction of the anterolateral pathway seldom occurs. The only time this crude alternative system becomes essential is when the discriminative pathway is damaged. Then, despite projection of the anterolateral system information to the somatosensory cortex, only a poorly localized, high-threshold sense of touch remains. These people will lose all sense of joint and muscle movement, body position, and two-point discrimination.

Thermal Sensation

Thermal sensation is discriminated by three types of receptors—cold, warmth, and pain. The cold and warmth receptors are located immediately under the skin at discrete but separate points. In some areas, there are more cold receptors than warmth receptors. For example, the lips have 15 to 25 cold receptors per square centimeter, compared with 3 to 5 in the same-sized area of the finger.[1] Different gradations of heat and cold reception result from the relative degrees of stimulation of the different types of nerve endings. Warmth receptors respond proportionately to increases in skin temperature between 32°C and 48°C and cold receptors to temperatures between 10°C and 40°C.[4] The thermal pain receptors are stimulated only by extremes of temperature such as "freezing cold" (temperatures below 10°C) and "burning hot" (temperatures above 48°C) sensations.[4] Thermal receptors respond rapidly to sudden changes in temperature and then adapt over the next few minutes. They do not adapt completely, however, but continue to respond to steady states of temperature. For example, the sensation of heat one feels on entering a tub of hot water or the extreme degree of cold experienced when going outside on a cold day is the initial response to a change in temperature, followed by an adaptation in which one gets accustomed to the temperature change but still feels the heat or cold because the receptors have not adapted completely.

Thermal afferents, with receptive thermal endings in the skin, send their central axons into the segmental dorsal horn of the spinal cord. On entering the dorsal horn, thermal signals are processed by second-order input association neurons. These association neurons activate projection neurons whose axons then cross to the opposite side of the cord and ascend in the multisynaptic, slow-conducting anterolateral system to the opposite side of the brain. Thalamic and cortical somatosensory regions for temperature are mixed with those for tactile sensibility.

Conduction of thermal information through peripheral nerves is quite slow compared with the rapid tactile afferents that travel through the discriminative system. If a person places a foot in a tub of hot water, the tactile sensation occurs well in advance of the burning sensation. The foot has been removed from the hot water by the local withdrawal reflex well before the excessive heat is perceived by the forebrain. Local anesthetic agents block the small-diameter afferents that carry thermal sensory information before they block the large-diameter axons that carry discriminative touch information.

Position Sensation

Position sense refers to the sense of limb and body movement and position without using vision. It is mediated by input from proprioceptive receptors (muscle spindle receptors and Golgi tendon organs) found primarily in muscles, tendons, and joint capsules. There are two submodalities of proprioception—the stationary or static component (limb position sense) and the dynamic aspects of position sense (kinesthesia). Both of these depend on constant transmission of information to the CNS regarding the degree of angulation of all joints and the rate of change in angulation. In addition, stretch-sensitive receptors in the skin (Ruffini end organs, Pacinian corpuscles, and Merkel cells) also signal postural information. Signals from these receptors are processed through the dorsal column–medial lemniscus pathway. They transmit signals from the periphery to the cerebral cortex, which are then processed in the thalamus before reaching the cerebral cortex. Lesions affecting the posterior column impair position sense. The vestibular system also plays an essential role in position sense.

Clinical Assessment of Somatosensory Function

Performing a neurologic assessment of somatosensory function includes testing the integrity of spinal segmental nerves. A pinpoint pressed against the skin of the sole of the foot that results in a withdrawal reflex, and a complaint of skin pain confirms the functional integrity of the afferent terminals in the skin, the entire pathway through the peripheral nerves of the foot, leg, and thigh to the sacral (S1) dorsal root ganglion and through the dorsal root into the spinal cord segment. It confirms that the somatosensory input association cells receiving this information are functioning and that the reflex circuitry of the cord segments (L5 to S2) is functioning. Also, the lower motor neurons of the L4 to S1 ventral horn can be considered operational, and their axons through the ventral roots, the mixed peripheral nerve, and the motor neuron to the muscles producing the withdrawal response can be considered intact and functional. The communication between the lower motor neuron and the muscle cells is functional, and these muscles have normal responsiveness and strength.

Testing is done at each segmental level, or dermatome, moving upward along the body and neck from coccygeal segments through the high cervical levels to test the functional integrity of all the spinal nerves. Similar dermatomes cover the face and scalp, and these, although innervated by cranial segmental nerves, are tested in the same manner.

Observation of a normal withdrawal reflex rules out peripheral nerve disease, disorders of the dorsal root and ganglion, diseases of the neuromuscular junction, and severe muscle diseases. Normal reflex function also indicates that many major descending CNS tracts are functioning within normal limits. If the person is able to report the pinprick sensation and accurately identify its location, many ascending systems through much of the spinal cord and brain also are functioning normally, as are basic intellect and speech mechanisms.

The integrity of the discriminative dorsal column–medial lemniscus pathway compared with the anterolateral tactile pathways is tested with the person's eyes closed by gently brushing the skin with a wisp of cotton, touching an area with one or two sharp points, touching corresponding parts of the body on each side simultaneously or in random sequence, and passively bending the person's finger one way and then another in random order. If only the anterolateral pathway is functional, the tactile threshold is markedly elevated, two-point discrimination and proprioception are missing, and the person has difficulty discriminating which side of the body received stimulation.

IN SUMMARY

The somatosensory component of the nervous system provides an awareness of body sensations such as touch, temperature, position sense, and pain. There are three primary levels of neural integration in the somatosensory system: the sensory units containing the sensory receptors, the ascending pathways, and the central processing centers in the thalamus and cerebral cortex. A sensory unit consists of a single dorsal root ganglion neuron, its receptors, and its central axon that terminates in the dorsal horn of the spinal cord or medulla. The part of the body innervated by the somatosensory afferent neurons of one set of dorsal root ganglia is called a dermatome. Ascending pathways include the discriminative pathway, which crosses at the base of the medulla, and the anterolateral pathway, which crosses within the first few segments of entering the spinal cord. Perception, or the final processing of somatosensory information, involves centers in the thalamus and somatosensory cortex. In the thalamus, the sensory information is crudely localized and perceived. The full localization, discrimination of the intensity, and interpretation of the meaning of the stimuli require processing by the somatosensory cortex. The *sensory homunculus* reflects the density of cortical neurons devoted to sensory input from afferents in corresponding peripheral areas.

The tactile system relays the sensations of touch, pressure, and vibration. It uses two anatomically separate pathways to relay touch information to the opposite side of the forebrain: the dorsal column discriminative pathway and the anterolateral pathway. Delicate touch, vibration, position, and movement sensations use the discriminative pathway to reach the thalamus, where third-order relay occurs to the primary somatosensory strip of the parietal cortex. Crude tactile sensation is carried by the bilateral slow-conducting anterolateral pathway. Temperature sensations of warm–hot and cool–cold are the result of stimulation to thermal receptors of sensory units projecting to the thalamus and cortex through the anterolateral system on the opposite side of the body. Proprioception is the sense of limb and body movement and position without using vision. Proprioceptive information is processed through the rapid-transmitting dorsal column–medial lemniscus pathway. Testing of the ipsilateral dorsal column (discriminative touch) system or the contralateral temperature projection system permits diagnostic analysis of the level and extent of damage in the somatosensory pathways.

PAIN

After completing this section of the chapter, the learner will be able to meet the following objectives:

- Discuss the differences among the specificity, pattern, gate control, and neuromatrix theories of pain.
- Discuss the difference between the Aδ- and C-fiber neurons in the transmission of pain information.
- Explain the transmission of pain signals with reference to the neospinothalamic, paleospinothalamic, and reticulospinal pathways, including the role of chemical mediators and factors that modulate pain transmission.

The International Association for the Study of Pain defines pain as an "unpleasant sensory and emotional experience associated with actual and potential tissue damage."[6] Pain is when a person reacts to a stimulus by removing the trigger causing the noxious stimulation.[1] It is generally known that the concept of pain perception and reaction to pain can be separated. Distress of pain is more heavily influenced by the reaction to pain than by actual pain intensity. Anxiety, culture, gender, age, past experience, and expectations about pain relief can influence the person's reaction to pain. Pain involves anatomic structures and physiologic behaviors, as well as psychological, social, cultural, and cognitive factors.

Pain is a common symptom that varies widely in intensity and spares no age group. When pain is extremely severe, it disrupts a person's behavior and can consume all of a person's attention. It can be equally devastating for infants and children, young and middle-aged adults, as well as adults over 65 years of age. Both acute pain and chronic pain can be major health problems. Pain is the most common symptom for which people seek medical attention. Acute pain often results from injury, surgery, or invasive medical procedures. It also can be a presenting symptom for some infections (*e.g.*, pharyngitis, appendicitis, otitis media). Chronic pain can be symptomatic of a wide range of health problems (*e.g.*, arthritis, back injury, cancer). Pain of any sort that persists for more than 24 hours has been reported by an estimated 76.5 million Americans.[7]

The experience of pain depends on both sensory perception and stimulation. The perception of pain can be heavily influenced by the endogenous analgesia system that modulates the sensation of pain. This can be illustrated by the phenomenon of soldiers injured in battle or athletes injured during a game who do not perceive major injuries as painful until they leave the battlefield or the game and begin to feel the manifestations of their injuries. Sensory stimulation refers to the processes by which a person experiences pain. An example of this would be nociceptive or neuropathic pain.[8] Pain can be either nociceptive or neuropathic in origin. The receptors for pain (nociceptors) are free nerve endings. When nociceptors are activated in response to actual or impending tissue injury, *nociceptive pain* is the consequence. *Neuropathic pain* arises from direct injury or dysfunction of the sensory axons of peripheral or central nerves.[9] Tissue and nerve injury can result in a wide range of symptoms. These include pain from noninjurious stimuli to the skin (*allodynia*), extreme sensitivity to pain (*hyperalgesia*), and the absence of pain from stimuli that normally would be painful (*analgesia*).[10] The latter, although not painful, can be extremely serious (*e.g.*, in diabetic persons with peripheral neuropathy) because the normally protective early warning system for the presence of tissue injury is absent.

Pain Theories

Traditionally, two theories were offered to explain the physiologic basis for the pain experience—specificity theory and pattern theory. *Specificity theory* regards pain as a separate sensory modality evoked by the activity of specific receptors that transmit information to pain centers or regions in the forebrain where pain is experienced.[11] This theory describes how painful a specific acute injury is predicted to be. However, this theory does not encompass the person's feelings of how the pain feels to him or her, or how the person has handled, or even experienced, pain in the past.[12] *Pattern theory* is comprised of a collective group of theories. It proposes that pain receptors share endings or pathways with other sensory modalities but that different patterns of activity (*i.e.*, spatial or temporal) of the same neurons can be used to signal painful and nonpainful stimuli.[11] For example, light touch applied to the skin would produce the sensation of touch through low-frequency firing of the receptor. On the other hand, intense pressure would produce pain through high-frequency firing of the same receptor. Both specificity and pattern theories focus on the neurophysiologic basis of pain, and both probably apply. Specific nociceptive afferents have been identified. However, almost all afferent stimuli, if driven at a very high frequency, can be experienced as painful.

Gate control theory, a modification of specificity theory, was proposed by Melzack and Wall in 1965 to meet the challenges presented by the pattern theories. This theory postulated the presence of neural gating mechanisms at the segmental spinal cord level to account for interactions between pain and other sensory modalities.[13] The original gate control theory proposed a spinal cord–level network of transmission or projection cells and internuncial neurons, which inhibits the transmission cells, forming a segmental-level gating mechanism that could block projection of pain information to the brain.

According to the gate control theory, the internuncial neurons involved in the gating mechanism are activated by large-diameter, faster-propagating fibers that carry tactile information. The simultaneous firing of the large-diameter touch fibers has the potential for blocking the transmission of impulses from the small-diameter myelinated and unmyelinated pain fibers.[13] Pain therapists have long known that pain intensity can be temporarily reduced during active tactile stimulation. For example, repeated sweeping of a soft-bristled brush on the skin (*i.e.*, brushing) over or near a painful area may result in pain reduction for several minutes to several hours.

Pain modulation is now known to be a much more complex phenomenon than that proposed by the original gate control theory. Tactile information is transmitted by small- and large-diameter fibers. Major interactions between sensory modalities, including the so-called gating phenomenon, occur at several levels of the CNS rostral to the input segment. Perhaps the most puzzling aspect of locally applied stimuli, such as brushing, that can block the experience of pain is the relatively long-lasting effect (minutes to hours) of such treatments. This prolonged effect has been difficult to explain on the basis of specificity theories, including the gate control theory. Other important factors include the effect of endogenous opioids and their receptors at the segmental and brain stem level, descending feedback modulation, altered sensitivity, learning, and culture. Despite this complexity, the Melzack and Wall theory has served a useful purpose. It sparked interest in pain and stimulated research and clinical activity related to the pain-modulating systems.

Melzack developed the *neuromatrix theory* to address further the brain's role in pain as well as the multiple dimensions and determinants of pain.[14] The neuromatrix theory is particularly useful in understanding chronic pain and phantom limb pain, in which there is not a simple one-to-one relationship between tissue injury and pain experience. The neuromatrix theory proposes that the brain contains a widely distributed neural network, called the *body–self neuromatrix*, that contains somatosensory, limbic, and thalamocortical components. Genetic and sensory influences determine the synaptic architecture of an individual's neuromatrix that integrates multiple sources of input and yields the neurosignature pattern that evokes the sensory, affective, and cognitive dimensions of pain experience and behavior. These multiple sources include

- Somatosensory inputs
- Other sensory inputs affecting interpretation of the situation
- Phasic and tonic inputs from the brain addressing such things as attention, expectation, culture, and personality

- Intrinsic neural inhibitory modulation
- Various components of stress regulation systems

The neuromatrix theory may open entire new areas of research, such as an understanding of the role that cortisol plays in chronic pain, the effect estrogen has on pain mediated through the release of peripheral cytokines, and the reported increase in chronic pain that occurs with age.[14]

Pain Mechanisms and Pathways

Pain usually is viewed in the context of tissue injury. The term nociception, which means "pain sense," comes from the Latin word *nocere*, "to injure." Nociceptive stimuli are objectively defined as stimuli of such intensity that they cause, or are close to causing, tissue damage. The withdrawal reflex (*e.g.*, the reflexive withdrawal of a body part from a tissue-damaging stimulus) is used to determine when a stimulus is nociceptive. Stimuli used include pressure from a sharp object, strong electric current to the skin, or application of heat or cold applied to skin. At low levels of intensity, these noxious stimuli do activate nociceptors (pain receptors), but are perceived as painful only when the intensity reaches a level where tissue damage occurs or is imminent.

The mechanisms of pain are many and complex. As with other forms of somatosensation, the pathways are composed of first-, second-, and third-order neurons (Fig. 14.7). The first-order neurons and their receptive endings detect stimuli that threaten the integrity of innervated tissues. Second-order neurons are located in the spinal cord and process nociceptive information. Third-order neurons project pain information to the brain. The thalamus and somatosensory cortex integrate and modulate pain as well as the person's subjective reaction to the pain experience.

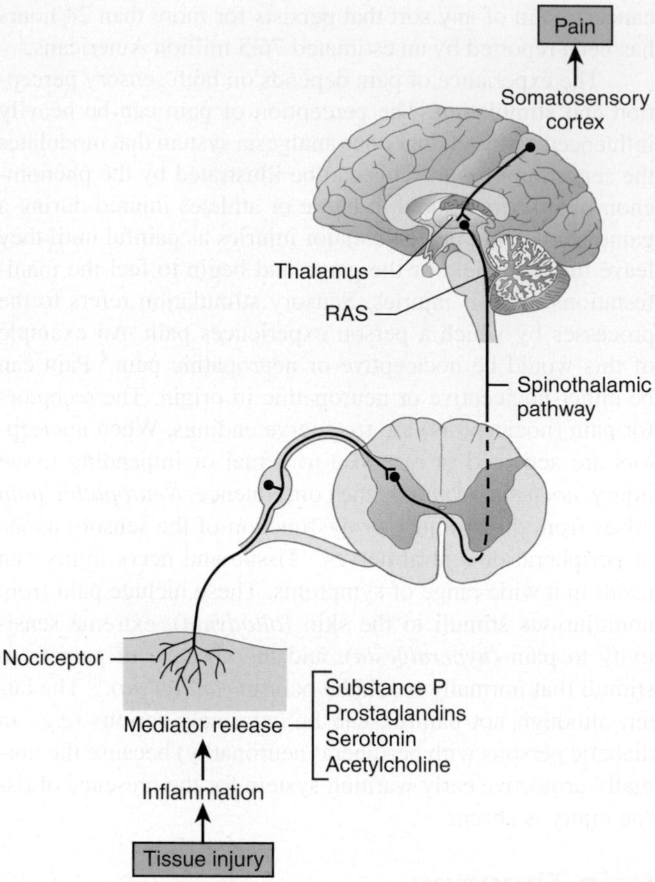

Figure 14.7 • Mechanism of acute pain. Tissue injury leads to release of inflammatory mediators with subsequent nociceptor stimulation. Pain impulses are then transmitted to the dorsal horn of the spinal cord, where they make contract with second-order neurons that cross to the opposite side of the cord and ascend by the spinothalamic tract to the RAS and thalamus. The localization and meaning of pain occur at the level of the somatosensory cortex.

Pain Receptors and Mediators

Nociceptors, or pain receptors, are sensory receptors that are activated by noxious insults to peripheral tissues. Structurally, the receptive endings of the peripheral pain fibers are free nerve endings. These receptive endings, which are widely distributed in the skin, dental pulp, periosteum, meninges, and some internal organs, translate the noxious stimuli into action potentials that are transmitted by a dorsal root ganglion to the dorsal horn of the spinal cord.

Nociceptive action potentials are transmitted through two types of afferent nerve fibers: myelinated Aδ fibers and unmyelinated C fibers. The larger Aδ fibers have considerably greater conduction velocities, transmitting impulses at a rate of 6 to 30 m/second.[1] The C fibers are the smallest of all peripheral nerve fibers; they transmit impulses at the rate of 0.5 to 2.0 m/second.[1] Pain conducted by Aδ fibers traditionally is called *fast pain* and typically is elicited by mechanical or thermal stimuli. C-fiber pain often is described as *slow-wave pain* because it is slower in onset and longer in duration. It is incited by chemical stimuli or by persistent mechanical or thermal stimuli. The slow postexcitatory potentials generated in C fibers are responsible for central sensitization to chronic pain.

Stimulation of Nociceptors

Unlike other sensory receptors, nociceptors respond to several forms of stimulation, including mechanical, thermal, and chemical. Some receptors respond to a single type of stimuli (mechanical or thermal) and others, called *polymodal receptors*, respond to all three types of stimuli (mechanical, thermal, and chemical). Mechanical stimuli can arise from intense pressure applied to skin or from the violent contraction or extreme stretch of a muscle. Both extremes of heat and cold can stimulate nociceptors. Chemical stimuli arise from a number of sources, including tissue trauma, ischemia, and inflammation. A wide range of chemical mediators are released from injured and inflamed tissues, including hydrogen and potassium ions, prostaglandins, leukotrienes, histamine, bradykinin, acetylcholine, and serotonin. These chemical mediators produce their effects by directly stimulating nociceptors or sensitizing them to the effects of nociceptive stimuli, perpetuating the inflammatory responses that lead to the release of chemical agents that act as nociceptive stimuli, or inciting neurogenic reflexes that increase the response to nociceptive stimuli. For example, bradykinin, histamine, serotonin, and potassium activate and also sensitize nociceptors.[1] Adenosine triphosphate (ATP), acetylcholine, and platelets act alone or in concert to sensitize nociceptors through other chemical agents such as prostaglandins. Aspirin and other nonsteroidal anti-inflammatory drugs (NSAIDs) are effective in controlling pain because they block the enzyme needed for prostaglandin synthesis.

Nociceptive stimulation that activates C fibers can cause a response known as *neurogenic inflammation* that produces vasodilation and an increased release of chemical mediators to which nociceptors respond.[1] The C-fiber mechanism is thought to be mediated by a dorsal root neuron reflex that produces retrograde transport and release of chemical mediators, which in turn causes increasing inflammation of peripheral tissues. This reflex can set up a vicious cycle, which has implications for persistent pain and hyperalgesia.[9]

Mediators in the Spinal Cord. In the spinal cord, the transmission of impulses between the nociceptive neurons and the dorsal horn neurons is mediated by chemical neurotransmitters released from central nerve endings of the nociceptive neurons. Some of these neurotransmitters are amino acids (*e.g.*, glutamate), others are amino acid derivatives (*e.g.*, norepinephrine), and still others are low molecular weight peptides composed of two or more amino acids. The amino acid glutamate is a major excitatory neurotransmitter released from the central nerve endings of the nociceptive neurons. Substance P, a neuropeptide, also is released in the dorsal horn by C fibers in response to nociceptive stimulation. Substance P elicits slow excitatory potentials in dorsal horn neurons. Unlike glutamate, which confines its action to the immediate area of the synaptic terminal, some neuropeptides released in the dorsal horn can diffuse some distance because they are not inactivated by reuptake mechanisms. In persistent pain, this may help to explain the excitability and unlocalized nature of many painful conditions. Neuropeptides such as substance P also appear to prolong and enhance the action of glutamate.[1] If these neurotransmitters are released in large quantities or over extended periods, they can lead to secondary hyperalgesia, a condition in which the second-order neurons are overly sensitive to low levels of noxious stimulation.

KEY POINTS

PAIN SENSATION

- The pathway for fast, sharply discriminated pain that moves directly from the receptor to the spinal cord using myelinated Aδ fibers and from the spinal cord to the thalamus using the neospinothalamic tract
- The pathway for slow, continuously conducted pain that is transmitted to the spinal cord using unmyelinated C fibers and from the spinal cord to the thalamus using the more circuitous and slower-conducting paleospinothalamic tract

Spinal Cord Circuitry and Pathways

On entering the spinal cord through the dorsal roots, the pain fibers bifurcate and ascend or descend one or two segments before synapsing with association neurons in the dorsal horn. From the dorsal horn, the axons of association projection neurons cross through the anterior commissure to the opposite side and then ascend upward in the previously described neospinothalamic and paleospinothalamic pathways (Fig. 14.8).

The faster-conducting fibers in the neospinothalamic tract are associated mainly with the transmission of sharp–fast pain information to the thalamus. In the thalamus, synapses are made and the pathway continues to the contralateral parietal somatosensory area to provide the precise location of the pain.

The paleospinothalamic tract is a slower-conducting, multisynaptic tract concerned with the diffuse, dull, aching, and unpleasant sensations that commonly are associated with chronic and visceral pain. This information travels through the small, unmyelinated C fibers. Fibers of this system also project up the contralateral anterolateral pathway to terminate in several thalamic regions, including the intralateral nuclei, which project to the limbic system. It is associated with the emotional or affective–motivational aspects of pain. Spinoreticular fibers from this pathway project bilaterally to the reticular formation of the brain stem. This component of the paleospinothalamic system facilitates avoidance reflexes at all levels. It also contributes to an increase in the electroencephalographic activity associated with alertness and indirectly influences hypothalamic functions associated with sudden alertness, such as increased heart rate and blood pressure. This may explain the tremendous arousal effects of certain pain stimuli.

Dorsal horn (second-order) neurons are divided primarily into two types: wide dynamic range (WDR) neurons that respond to different low-intensity stimuli and nociceptive-specific neurons that respond only to noxious or nociceptive stimuli. When stimuli are increased to a noxious level, the WDR neurons respond more intensely. After more severe damage to peripheral sensory afferents, Aδ and C fibers respond more intensely as they are increasingly stimulated. When C fibers are repetitively stimulated at a rate of once per second, each stimulus produces a progressively increased response from the WDR neurons. This phenomenon of amplification of transmitted signals has been called *windup* and may explain why pain sensation appears to increase with repeated stimulation. Windup and sensitization of dorsal horn neurons have implications for appropriate and early, or even preemptive, pain therapy to avoid the possibility of spinal cord neurons becoming hypersensitive or subject to firing spontaneously.[4]

Brain Centers and Pain Perception

Information from tissue injury is carried from the spinal cord to brain centers in the thalamus where the basic sensation of hurtfulness, or pain, occurs (Fig. 14.9). In the neospinothalamic system, interconnections between the lateral thalamus and the somatosensory cortex are necessary to add precision, discrimination, and meaning to the pain sensation.

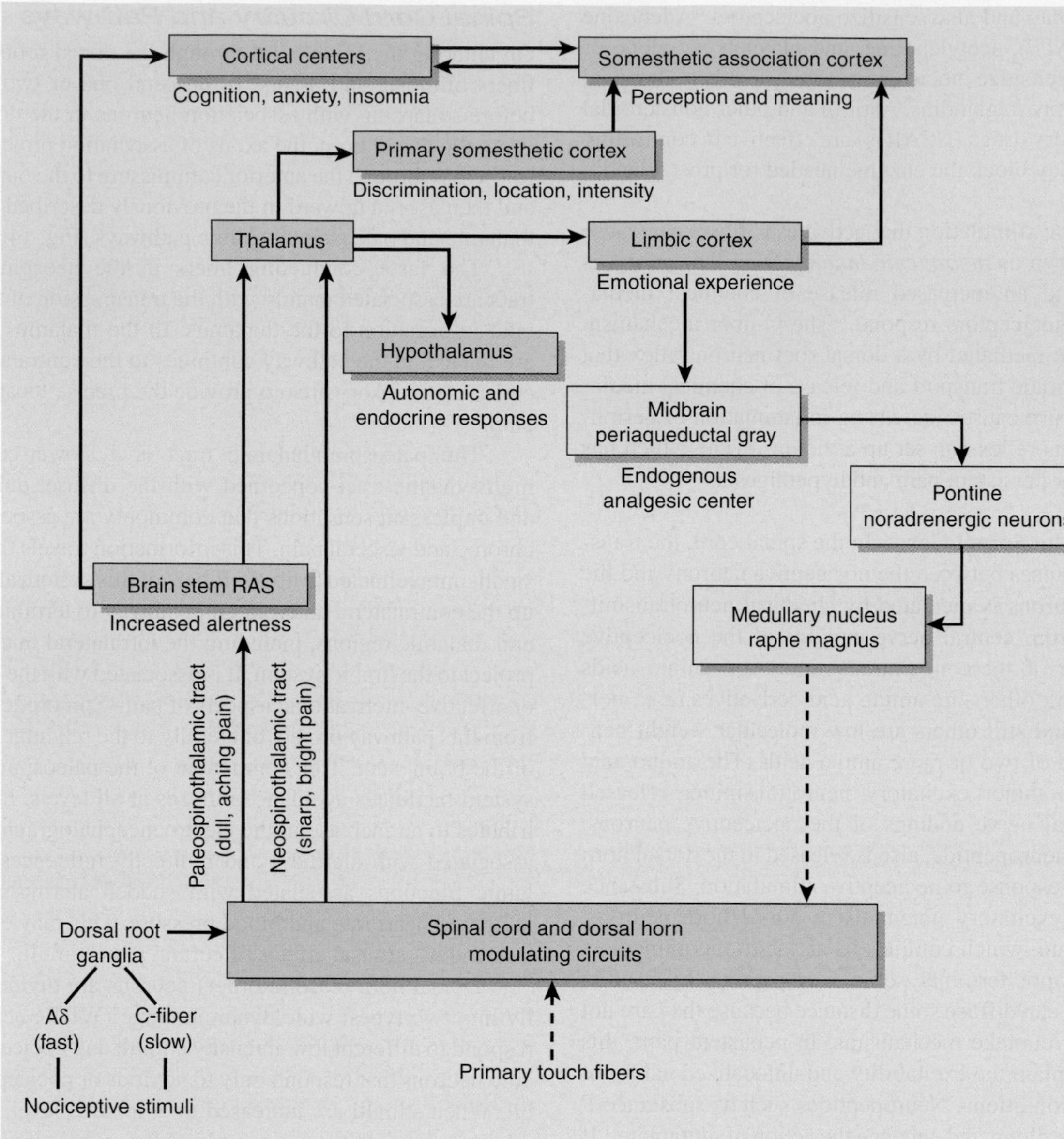

Figure 14.8 • Primary pain pathways. The transmission of incoming nociceptive impulses is modulated by dorsal horn circuitry, which receives input from primary touch receptors and from descending pathways that involve the limbic cortical systems (orbital frontal cortex, amygdala, and hypothalamus), the periaqueductal endogenous analgesic center in the midbrain, pontine noradrenergic neurons, and the NRM in the medulla. *Dashed lines* indicate inhibition or modulation of pain transmission by dorsal horn projection neurons. RAS, reticular activating system.

The paleospinothalamic system projects diffusely from the intralaminar nuclei of the thalamus to large areas of the limbic cortex. These connections probably are associated with the hurtfulness and the mood-altering and attention-narrowing effect of pain.

Research using magnetoencephalography has demonstrated cortical representation of pain sensation in humans and has shown that it is very effective when combined with structural imaging.[15] In healthy adults, nociceptive Aδ afferent stimulation is related to activation in the contralateral primary somatosensory cortex in the parietal lobe, whereas C afferent stimulation is related to activation of the secondary somatosensory cortices and the anterior cingulated cortex, which is part of the limbic system.

Central Pathways for Pain Modulation

A major advance in understanding pain was the discovery of neuroanatomic pathways that arise in the midbrain and brain stem, descend to the spinal cord, and modulate ascending pain impulses. One such pathway begins in an area of the midbrain called the *periaqueductal gray* (PAG) region. Through research it was found that electrical stimulation of the midbrain PAG regions produced a state of analgesia that lasted for many hours. Subsequently, opioid receptors were found to

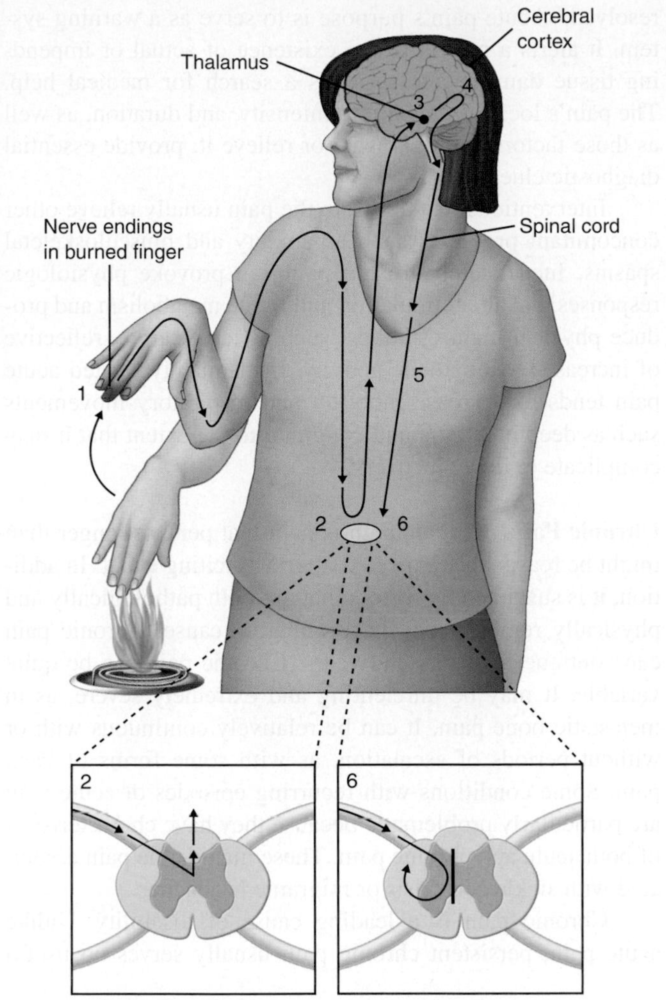

Figure 14.9 • Pain transmission. (*1*) Pain begins as a message received by nerve endings, such as found in a burnt finger. (*2*) The release of substance P, bradykinin, and prostaglandins sensitize the nerve endings, which helps to transmit the pain from the site of injury toward the brain. (*3*) The pain signal then travels as an electrochemical impulse along the length of the nerve to the dorsal horn on the spinal cord, a region that receives signals from all over the body. (*4*) The spinal cord then sends the message to the thalamus, and then to the cortex. (*5*) Pain relief starts with signals from the brain that descend by way of the spinal cord, where (*6*) chemicals such as endorphin S are released in the dorsal horn to diminish the pain message. (From Jensen S. (2015). *Nursing health assessment: a best practice approach* (2nd ed., Figure 6.1, p. 114). Philadelphia, PA: Lippincott Williams & Wilkins.)

be highly concentrated in this and other regions of the CNS where electrical stimulation produced analgesia. Because of these findings, the PAG area of the midbrain often is referred to as the *analgesia system*.[1]

The PAG area receives input from widespread areas of the CNS, including the cerebral cortex, hypothalamus, brain stem reticular formation, and spinal cord by way of the paleospinothalamic and neospinothalamic tracts. This region is intimately connected to the limbic system, which is associated with emotional experience. The neurons of the PAG have axons that descend into an area in the rostral medulla called the *nucleus raphe magnus* (NRM). The axons of these NRM neurons project to the dorsal horn of the spinal cord, where they terminate in the same layers as the entering primary pain fibers (see Fig. 14.8). Serotonin has been identified as a neurotransmitter in the NRM medullary nuclei. It has been shown that tricyclic antidepressant drugs, such as amitriptyline, which enhance the effects of serotonin by blocking its presynaptic uptake, have been found to be effective in the management of certain types of chronic pain.[16] The discovery that norepinephrine can block pain transmission led to studies directed at the combined administration of opioids and clonidine, a central-acting α-adrenergic agonist, for pain relief.

Endogenous Analgesic Mechanisms

There is evidence that opioid receptors and endogenously synthesized opioid peptides, which are morphine-like substances, are found on the peripheral processes of primary afferent neurons and in many regions of the CNS (Fig. 14.9). Three families of endogenous opioid peptides have been identified—the enkephalins, endorphins, and dynorphins. Each family is derived from a distinct precursor polypeptide and has a characteristic anatomic distribution. Although each family usually is located in different groups of neurons, occasionally more than one family is present in the same neuron. For example, proenkephalin peptides are present in areas of the spinal cord and PAG that are related to perception of pain, in the hippocampus and other areas of the brain that modulate emotional behavior, in structures in the basal ganglia that modulate motor control, and in brain stem neurons that regulate autonomic nervous system responses.

Although the endogenous opioid peptides appear to function as neurotransmitters, their full significance in pain control and other physiologic functions is not completely understood. Laboratory studies, although somewhat inconsistent, have found that opioid agonists inhibit calcium channels in dorsal root and trigeminal ganglion neurons as well as on primary afferent neurons. Because it is calcium ions that cause neurotransmitter release at the synapse, such calcium blockage would inhibit synaptic transmission of pain impulses. The characterization of receptors that bind the endogenous opioid peptides is important in understanding the mechanisms of pain control. The identification of these receptors has facilitated a more thorough understanding of the actions of available opioid drugs, such as morphine. It also has facilitated ongoing research into the development of newer preparations, including 24-hour dispensing medications, dermal patches, and intravenous pumps that are self-administered according to perceived need.

Pain Threshold and Tolerance

Pain threshold and tolerance affect a person's response to a painful stimulus. *Pain threshold* is the point at which a stimulus is perceived as painful. *Pain tolerance* is the total pain experience. It is defined as a lesser "response to a drug because of repeated drug administration."[17] Psychological, familial, cultural, and environmental factors significantly influence the amount of pain a person is willing to tolerate. Separation and identification of the role of each of these two aspects of pain continue to pose fundamental problems for the pain management team.

Types of Pain

Pain can be classified according to duration (acute or chronic), location (cutaneous or deep and visceral), and site of referral. Classification based on associated medical diagnosis (*e.g.*, surgery, trauma, cancer, sickle cell disease, fibromyalgia) is also very useful in planning appropriate pain management interventions.

Acute and Chronic Pain

The most widely accepted classification of pain is according to its duration. Pain research emphasizes the importance of differentiating acute pain from chronic pain. The diagnosis and therapy for each is distinctive because they differ in cause, function, mechanisms, and psychological sequelae (Table 14.1)

Traditionally, the distinction between acute and chronic pain has relied on a single continuum of time with some interval (*e.g.*, 6 months). Some conditions such as osteoarthritis exhibit dimensions of both acute and chronic pain.

Acute Pain. Acute pain is pain that is elicited by injury to body tissues and activation of nociceptive stimuli at the site of local tissue damage.[1] It is generally of short duration and tends to resolve when the underlying pathologic process has resolved.[1] Acute pain's purpose is to serve as a warning system. It alerts a person to the existence of actual or impending tissue damage and prompts a search for medical help. The pain's location, radiation, intensity, and duration, as well as those factors that aggravate or relieve it, provide essential diagnostic clues.

Interventions that alleviate the pain usually relieve other concomitant problems such as anxiety and musculoskeletal spasms. Inadequately treated pain can provoke physiologic responses that alter circulation and tissue metabolism and produce physical manifestations, such as tachycardia, reflective of increased sympathetic activity. Inadequately treated acute pain tends to decrease mobility and respiratory movements such as deep breathing and coughing to the extent that it may complicate or delay recovery.

Chronic Pain. Chronic pain is pain that persists longer than might be reasonably expected after an inciting event. In addition, it is sustained by factors that are both pathologically and physically remote from the originating cause. Chronic pain can continue for years and years. Chronic pain can be quite variable. It may be unrelenting and extremely severe, as in metastatic bone pain. It can be relatively continuous with or without periods of escalation, as with some forms of back pain. Some conditions with recurring episodes of acute pain are particularly problematic because they have characteristics of both acute and chronic pain. These include the pain associated with sickle cell crisis or migraine headaches.

Chronic pain is a leading cause of disability. Unlike acute pain, persistent chronic pain usually serves no useful

TABLE 14.1 CHARACTERISTICS OF ACUTE AND CHRONIC PAIN

CHARACTERISTIC	ACUTE PAIN	CHRONIC PAIN
Onset	Recent	Continuous or intermittent
Duration	Short (<6 months)	6 months or more
Autonomic responses	Consistent with sympathetic fight or flight response* Increased heart rate Increased stroke volume Increased blood pressure Increased pupillary dilation Increased muscle tension Decreased gut motility Decreased salivary flow (dry mouth)	Absence of autonomic responses
Psychological component	Associated anxiety	Increased irritability Associated depression Somatic preoccupation Withdrawal from outside interests Decreased strength of relationships
Other types of response		Decreased sleep Decreased libido Appetite changes

*Responses are approximately proportional to intensity of the stimulus.

function. To the contrary, it imposes physiologic, psychological, familial, and economic stresses and may exhaust a person's resources. In contrast to acute pain, psychological and environmental influences may play an important role in the development of behaviors associated with chronic pain.

The biologic factors that influence chronic pain include peripheral mechanisms, peripheral–central mechanisms, and central mechanisms. Peripheral mechanisms result from persistent stimulation of nociceptors and are mostly involved with chronic musculoskeletal, visceral, and vascular disorders. Peripheral–central mechanisms are related to abnormal function of the peripheral and central portions of the somatosensory system, such as those resulting from partial or complete loss of descending inhibitory pathways or spontaneous firing of regenerated nerve fibers. They include conditions such as causalgia, phantom limb pain, and postherpetic neuralgia. Central pain mechanisms are associated with disease or injury of the CNS and characterized by burning, aching, hyperalgesia, dysesthesia, and other abnormal sensations. Central pain is associated with conditions such as thalamic lesions (thalamic pain), spinal cord injury, surgical interruption of pain pathways, and multiple sclerosis.

People with chronic pain may not exhibit the somatic, autonomic, or affective behaviors often associated with acute pain. As painful conditions become prolonged and continuous, autonomic nervous system responses tend to decrease. In addition, loss of appetite, sleep disturbances, and depression often are associated with chronic pain. Amazingly, depression commonly is relieved once the pain is removed. The link between depression and decreased pain tolerance may be explained by the similar manner in which both respond to changes in the biologic pathways of serotonergic and noradrenergic systems. Tricyclic antidepressants and other medications with serotonergic and noradrenergic effects have been shown to relieve a variety of chronic pain syndromes.[17]

Cutaneous and Deep Somatic Pain

Pain can also be classified according to its location. *Cutaneous pain* arises from superficial structures. It is a sharp pain with a burning quality that may be abrupt or slow in onset. It can be localized accurately and may be distributed along the dermatomes. Because of an overlap of nerve fiber distribution between the dermatomes, the boundaries of pain frequently are not as clear-cut as dermatome diagrams indicate.

Deep somatic pain originates in deep body structures (*e.g.*, periosteum, muscles, tendons, joints, and blood vessels). It is more diffuse than cutaneous pain. Various stimuli, such as strong pressure exerted on bone, ischemia to a muscle, and tissue damage, can produce deep somatic pain. An example of this is the pain that a person experiences from a sprained ankle. Radiation of pain from the original site of injury can occur.

Visceral Pain

Visceral pain has its origin in the visceral organs and is one of the most common pains produced by disease. Although similar to somatic pain in many ways, both the neurologic mechanisms and the perception of visceral pain differ from somatic pain. One of the most important differences between surface pain and visceral pain is the type of damage that causes pain. Strong contractions, distention, or ischemia affecting the walls of the viscera can induce severe pain. There is a low density of nociceptors in the viscera compared with the skin. There is functional divergence of visceral input within the CNS, which occurs when many second-order neurons respond to a stimulus from a single visceral afferent.

Visceral nociceptive afferents from the thorax and abdomen travel along the cranial and spinal nerve pathways of the autonomic nervous system. For many years, it was believed that the spinothalamic and spinoreticular tracts carried visceral nociceptive information. Identification of new pathways is sometimes quite important clinically for determining new pain management techniques.

Referred Pain

Referred pain is pain that is perceived at a site different from its point of origin but innervated by the same spinal segment. It is hypothesized that visceral and somatic afferent neurons converge on the same dorsal horn projection neurons (Fig. 14.10). For this reason, it can be difficult for the brain to correctly identify the original source of pain. Pain that originates in the abdominal or thoracic viscera is diffuse and poorly localized and often perceived at a site far removed from the affected area. For example, the pain associated with myocardial infarction commonly is referred to the left arm, neck, and chest, which may delay diagnosis and treatment of a potentially life-threatening condition.

Referred pain may arise alone or concurrent with pain located at the origin of the noxious stimuli. This lack of correspondence between the location of the pain and the location of the painful stimuli can make diagnosis difficult. Although the term *referred* usually is applied to pain that originates in the viscera and is experienced as if originating from the body wall, it also may be applied to pain that arises from somatic structures. For example, pain referred to the chest wall could

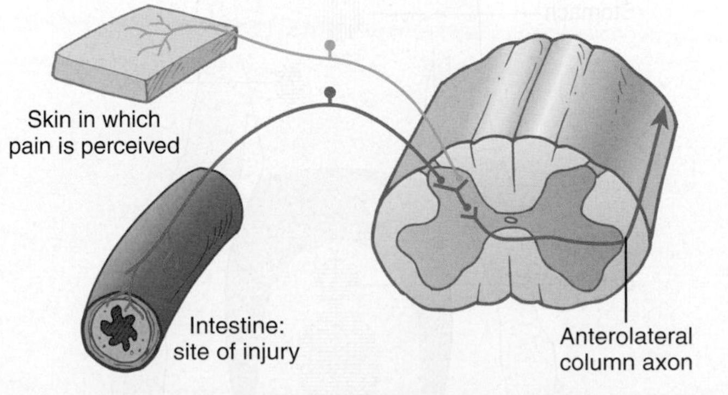

Figure 14.10 • Convergence of cutaneous and visceral inputs onto the same second-order projection neuron in the dorsal horn of the spinal cord. Although virtually all visceral inputs converge with cutaneous inputs, most cutaneous inputs do not converge with other sensory inputs.

be caused by nociceptive stimulation of the peripheral portion of the diaphragm, which receives somatosensory innervation from the intercostal nerves. An understanding of pain referral is of great value in diagnosing illness. The typical pattern of pain referral can be derived from our understanding that the afferent neurons from visceral or deep somatic tissue enter the spinal cord at the same level as the afferent neurons from the cutaneous areas to which the pain is referred (Fig. 14.11).

The sites of referred pain are determined embryologically with the development of visceral and somatic structures that share the same site for entry of sensory information into the CNS and then move to more distant locations. For example, a person with peritonitis may complain of pain in the shoulder. Internally, there is inflammation of the peritoneum that lines the central part of the diaphragm. In the embryo, the diaphragm originates in the neck, and its central portion is innervated by the phrenic nerve, which enters the cord at the level of the third to fifth segments (C3 to C5). As the fetus develops, the diaphragm descends to its adult position between the thoracic and abdominal cavities while maintaining its embryonic pattern of innervation. Thus, fibers that enter the spinal cord at the C3 to C5 levels carry information from both the neck area and the diaphragm, and the diaphragmatic pain is interpreted by the forebrain as originating in the shoulder or neck area.

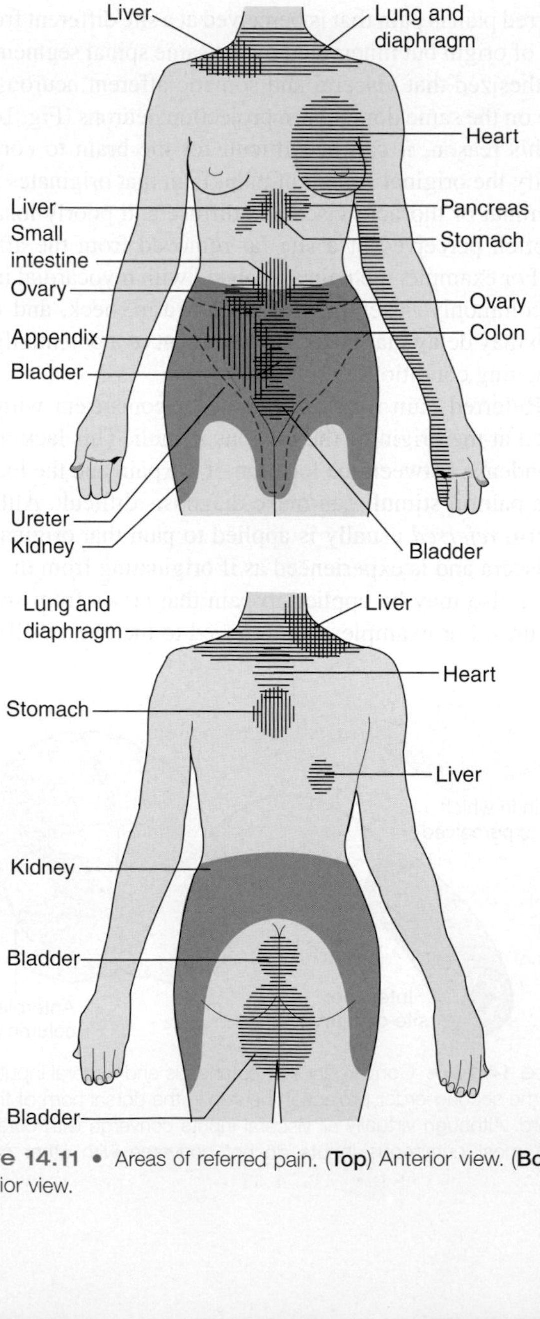

Figure 14.11 • Areas of referred pain. (**Top**) Anterior view. (**Bottom**) Posterior view.

Although the visceral pleura, pericardium, and peritoneum are said to be relatively free of pain fibers, the parietal pleura, pericardium, and peritoneum do react to nociceptive stimuli. Visceral inflammation can involve parietal and somatic structures, and this may give rise to diffuse local or referred pain. For example, when the parietal peritoneum is irritated from appendicitis, it typically gives rise to pain directly over the inflamed area in the lower right quadrant, evoking pain referred to the umbilical area.

Muscle spasm, or *guarding*, occurs when somatic structures are involved. Guarding is a protective reflex rigidity. Its purpose is to protect the affected body parts (*e.g.*, an abscessed appendix or a sprained muscle). This protective guarding may cause blood vessel compression and give rise to the pain of muscle ischemia, causing local and referred pain.

KEY POINTS

TYPES OF PAIN

- Pain can be classified according to duration (acute or chronic), location (cutaneous or deep and visceral), and site of referral.
- Acute pain is a self-limiting pain that lasts less than 6 months.
- Chronic pain is persistent pain that lasts longer than 6 months, lacks the autonomic and somatic responses associated with acute pain, and is accompanied by loss of appetite, sleep disturbances, depression, and other debilitating responses.

Assessment of Pain

Careful assessment of pain assists clinicians in diagnosing, managing, and relieving the person's pain. Assessment includes such things as the nature, severity, location, and radiation of the pain. As with other disease states, eliminating the cause of the pain is preferable to simply treating the symptom of pain. A careful history often provides information about the triggering factors (*i.e.*, injury, infection, or disease) and the site of nociceptive stimuli (*i.e.*, peripheral receptor or visceral organ). A comprehensive pain history should include

- Pain onset
- Description, localization, radiation, intensity, quality, and pattern of the pain
- Anything that relieves or exacerbates it
- The person's personal reaction to the pain

Unlike many other bodily responses, such as temperature and blood pressure, the nature, severity, and distress of pain cannot be measured objectively. To overcome this problem, various methods have been developed for quantifying a person's pain based on the person's report. They include numeric pain intensity, visual analog, and verbal descriptor scales. Most pain questionnaires assess a single aspect of pain such as pain intensity. For example, a *numeric pain intensity* scale asks people to select which number best represents the intensity of their pain, where 0 represents no pain and 10 represents the most intense pain imaginable. A *visual analog* scale also can be used. It is a straight line, often 10 cm in length, with a word description (*e.g.*, "no pain" and "the most intense pain imaginable") at each of the ends of the line representing the continuum of pain intensity. People are asked to choose a point on the continuum that represents the intensity of their pain. The response can be quantified by measuring the line to determine the distance of the mark, measured in millimeters, from the "no pain" end of the line. *Verbal descriptor* scales consist of several numerically ranked choices of words such as none = 0, slight = 1, mild = 2, moderate = 3, and severe = 4. The word chosen is used to determine the numeric representation of pain severity on an ordinal scale.

Management of Pain

The therapeutic approaches to managing acute and chronic pain differ markedly. In acute pain, therapy is directed at providing pain relief by interrupting the nociceptive stimulus. Because the pain is self-limited, in that it resolves as the injured tissues heal, long-term therapy usually is not needed. Chronic pain management is much more complex and is based on multiple considerations, including life expectancy.

Managing Acute Pain

Acute pain should be aggressively managed and pain medication provided before the pain becomes severe. This allows the person to be more comfortable and active and to assume a greater role in directing his or her own care. Part of the reluctance of health care workers to provide adequate relief for acute pain has been fear of addiction. However, addiction to opioid medications is thought to be virtually nonexistent when these drugs are prescribed for acute pain. Usually, less medication is needed when the drug is given before the pain becomes severe and the pain pathways become sensitized.

Managing Chronic Pain

Management of chronic pain requires early attempts to prevent pain and adequate therapy for acute bouts of pain. Specific treatment depends on the cause of the pain, the natural history of the underlying health problem, as well as the life expectancy of the person. If the organic illness causing the pain cannot be cured, then noncurative methods of pain control become the cornerstone of treatment. Treatment methods for chronic pain can include neural blockade, electrical modalities (*e.g.*, transcutaneous electrical nerve stimulation [TENS]), physical therapy, cognitive–behavioral interventions, and nonnarcotic and narcotic medications. Nonnarcotic medications such as tricyclic antidepressants, antiepileptic medications, and NSAIDs serve as useful adjuncts to opioids for the treatment of different types of chronic pain. Chronic pain is best handled by a multidisciplinary team that includes specialists in areas such as anesthesiology, nursing, physical therapy, social services, and surgery.

Cancer is a common cause of chronic pain. The goal of chronic cancer pain management should be pain alleviation and prevention. Pain control remains a significant problem despite the advances in understanding and management of pain. Analgesics, adjuvant drugs, cognitive or behavioral strategies, physical modalities, and nerve blocks are used for many forms of chronic pain. Depending on the form and stage of the cancer, other treatments such as palliative radiation, antineoplastic therapies, and palliative surgery may help to control the pain. The World Health Organization has created an analgesic ladder for cancer pain that assists clinicians in choosing the appropriate analgesic.[18]

Nonpharmacologic Pain Management

A number of nonpharmacologic methods of pain control often are used in pain management. These include cognitive–behavioral interventions, physical agents such as heat and cold, and electroanalgesia. Often these methods are used in addition to analgesics rather than as the only form of pain management.

Cognitive–Behavioral Interventions. Cognitive–behavioral interventions, which often are helpful for people experiencing acute as well as chronic pain, include relaxation, distraction, cognitive reappraisal, imagery, meditation, and biofeedback. If the person is having surgery or a painful procedure, it is ideal to teach these techniques before the pain begins (*e.g.*, before surgery). If the person is already in severe pain, the use of cognitive–behavioral interventions should be based on the person's ability to master the technique as well as his or her response to the intervention. For example, it may be a more appropriate adjunct to analgesics for a terminally ill person in severe pain to use self-selected relaxing music rather than trying to teach that person an intervention requiring more attention (*e.g.*, meditation or cognitive reappraisal).

Relaxation is one of the best-evaluated cognitive–behavioral approaches to pain relief. The relaxation method need not be complex. Relatively simple strategies, such as slow, rhythmic breathing and brief jaw relaxation procedures, have been successful in decreasing self-reported pain and analgesic use.

Distraction (*i.e.*, focusing a person's attention on stimuli other than painful stimuli or negative emotions) does not eliminate pain, but it can make pain more tolerable. It may serve as a type of sensory shielding whereby attention to pain is sacrificed to pay attention to other stimuli that are easily perceived. Examples of distraction include counting, repeating phrases or poems, and engaging in activities that require concentration, such as projects, activities, work, conversation, or describing pictures. Television, adventure movies, music, and humor also can provide distraction. *Cognitive reappraisal* is a form of self-distraction or cognitive control in which people focus their attention on the positive aspects of the experience and away from their pain. Individuals using distraction may not appear to be in severe pain. Nonetheless, it is inappropriate to assume that a person who copes with pain by using distraction does not have pain. Prescribed analgesics should not be denied to people simply because they appear to be coping with their pain without medication. Appropriate assessment is needed to determine the person's level of pain and what other interventions for pain may be needed.

Imagery consists of using one's imagination to develop a mental picture. In pain management, therapeutic guided imagery (*i.e.*, goal-directed imaging) is used. It can be used alone or in conjunction with other cognitive–behavioral interventions (*e.g.*, relaxation or biofeedback) to develop sensory images that may decrease the perceived intensity of pain. It also can be used to lessen anxiety and reduce muscle tension. *Meditation* also can be used, but it requires practice and the ability to concentrate to be effective.

Biofeedback is used to provide feedback to a person concerning the status of some body function (*e.g.*, finger temperature, temporal artery pulsation, blood pressure, or muscle tension). It involves a process of learning designed to make the person aware of certain of his or her own body functions for the purpose of modifying these functions at a conscious level. Interest in biofeedback increased with the possibility of using this treatment modality in the management of migraine and tension headaches or for other pain that has a muscle tension component.

Physical Agents. Heat and cold are physical agents that are used to provide pain relief. The choice of physical agent depends on the type of pain being treated and, in many cases, personal preference.

Heat has long been used to relieve pain. Heat dilates blood vessels and increases local blood flow. It also can influence the transmission of pain impulses and increase collagen extensibility. An increase in local circulation can reduce the level of nociceptive stimulation by reducing local ischemia caused by muscle spasm or tension, increase the removal of metabolites and inflammatory mediators that act as nociceptive stimuli, and help to reduce swelling and relieve pressure on local nociceptive endings. The heat sensation is carried to the posterior horn of the spinal cord and may exert its effect by modulating projection of pain transmission. It also may trigger the release of endogenous opioids. Heat also alters the viscosity of collagen fibers in ligaments, tendons, and joint structures so that they are more easily extended and can be stretched further before the nociceptive endings are stimulated. Thus, heat often is applied before therapy aimed at stretching joint structures and increasing range of motion. Care must be taken not to use excessive heat. When excessive heat is used, the heat itself becomes a noxious stimulus, which results in actual or impending tissue damage and pain. In certain conditions, the use of heat is controversial, and in some conditions (*e.g.*, peripheral vascular disease) where increased blood flow or metabolism would be detrimental, the use of heat is contraindicated.

Like heat, the application of *cold* may produce a dramatic reduction in pain. Cold exerts its effect on pain through circulatory and neural mechanisms. The initial response to local application of cold is sudden local vasoconstriction. This initial vasoconstriction is followed by alternating periods of vasodilation and vasoconstriction during which the body "hunts" for its normal level of blood flow to prevent local tissue damage. The vasoconstriction is caused by local stimulation of sympathetic fibers and direct cooling of blood vessels, and the hyperemia by local autoregulatory mechanisms. In situations of acute injury, cold is used to produce vasoconstriction and prevent extravasation of blood into the tissues. Pain relief results from decreased swelling and decreased stimulation of nociceptive endings. The vasodilation that follows can be useful in removing substances that stimulate nociceptive endings.

Cold also can have a marked and dramatic effect on pain that results from the spasm-induced accumulation of metabolites in muscle. In terms of pain modulation, cold may reduce afferent activity reaching the posterior horn of the spinal cord by modulating sensory input. The application of cold is a noxious stimulus and may influence the release of endogenous opioids from the PAG area. Cold packs should be flexible to conform to body parts easily, adequately wrapped to protect the skin, and applied no more than 15 to 20 minutes at a time.

Stimulus-Induced Analgesia. Stimulus-induced analgesia is one of the oldest known methods of pain relief. Electrical stimulation methods of pain relief include TENS, electrical acupuncture, and neurostimulation. TENS refers to the transmission of electrical energy across the surface of the skin to the peripheral nerve fibers. TENS units have been developed that are convenient, easily transported, and relatively economical to use. Most are approximately the size of a deck of cards. These battery-operated units deliver an electrical current to a target site.

The system usually consists of three parts—a pair of electrodes, lead wires, and a stimulator. The electrical stimulation is delivered in a pulsed waveform that can be varied in terms of pulse amplitude, width, and rate. The type of stimulation used varies with the type of pain being treated. The physiologic pathways and an understanding of the pain mechanisms involved determine electrode placement. They may be placed on either side of a painful area, over an affected dermatome, over an affected peripheral nerve where it is most superficial, or over a nerve trunk. For example, the electrodes commonly are placed medial and lateral to the incision when treating postoperative pain.

There probably is no single explanation for the physiologic effects of TENS. Each specific type of stimulator may have different sites of action and may be explained by more than one theory. The gate control theory was proposed as one possible mechanism. According to this theory, pain information is transmitted by small-diameter Aδ and C fibers. Large-diameter afferent A fibers and small-diameter fibers carry tactile information mediating touch, pressure, and kinesthesia. TENS may function on the basis of differential firing of impulses in the large fibers that carry nonpainful information. Accordingly, increased activity in these larger fibers purportedly modulates transmission of painful information to the forebrain. TENS has the advantage that it is noninvasive, easily regulated by the person or health professional, and effective in some forms of acute and chronic pain. Its use can be taught before surgery, affording a reduction in postoperative analgesic medication and, possibly, preventing the development of persistent pain.

Acupuncture. The practice of acupuncture involves introducing needles into specific points on the surface of the body. Charts are available that describe the points of needle placement that are used to relieve pain at certain anatomic sites. In addition to needles, sometimes palpation is used. Acupuncture is widely available in pain clinics even though large, high-quality, randomized studies on the effects of acupuncture for chronic pain are not plentiful.

Neurostimulation. Neurostimulation delivers low-voltage electrical stimulation to the spinal cord or targeted peripheral nerve to block the sensation of pain. Melzack and Wall (gate theory) proposed that neurostimulation activates the body's pain-inhibiting system. For a totally implantable system, the power source (battery) and lead(s) are surgically implanted.

Pharmacologic Treatment

Analgesics have been used for many years to relieve pain of short duration. An analgesic drug is a medication that acts on the nervous system to decrease or eliminate pain without inducing loss of consciousness. Analgesic drugs do not cure the underlying cause of the pain, but their appropriate use may prevent acute pain from progressing to chronic pain. Another benefit of analgesic drugs is that they enable the person to achieve mobility after surgery, for example, when exercises such as coughing and deep breathing may be required.

The ideal analgesic would be effective, nonaddictive, and inexpensive. In addition, it would produce minimal adverse effects and not affect the person's level of consciousness. Although long-term treatment with opioids can result in opioid tolerance (*i.e.*, more drug being needed to achieve the same effect) and physical dependence, this should not be confused with addiction. Long-term drug-seeking behavior is rare in people who are treated with opioids only during the time that they require pain relief. The unique needs and circumstances presented by each person in pain must be addressed to achieve satisfactory pain management. The use of analgesics is only one aspect of a comprehensive pain management program with acute pain, and even more so with chronic pain.

Nonnarcotic Analgesics. Common nonnarcotic oral analgesic medications include aspirin, other NSAIDs, and acetaminophen. Aspirin, or acetylsalicylic acid, acts centrally and peripherally to block the transmission of pain impulses. It also has antipyretic and anti-inflammatory properties. The action of aspirin and other NSAIDs is through the inhibition of the cyclooxygenase (COX) enzymes, which mediate the biosynthesis of prostaglandins. The NSAIDs also decrease the sensitivity of blood vessels to bradykinin and histamine, affect cytokine production by T lymphocytes, reverse vasodilation, and decrease the release of inflammatory mediators from granulocytes, mast cells, and basophils.[17] Acetaminophen is an alternative to the NSAIDs. Although usually considered equivalent to aspirin as an analgesic and antipyretic agent, it lacks anti-inflammatory properties.

Opioid Analgesics. The term *opioid* or *narcotic* is used to refer to a group of medications, natural or synthetic, which has morphine-like actions.[17] The older term *opiate* was used to designate drugs derived from opium—morphine, codeine, and many other semisynthetic congeners of morphine. Opioids are used for relief of short-term pain and for more long-term use in conditions such as cancer pain. When given for temporary relief of severe pain, such as that occurring after surgery, there is much evidence that opioids given routinely before the pain starts (preemptive analgesia) or becomes extreme are far more effective than those administered in a sporadic manner. People who are treated in this manner seem to require fewer doses and are able to resume regular activities sooner.

Although the analgesic and psychopharmacologic properties of morphine have been known for centuries, the fact that the brain contains its own endogenous opioid-like chemicals, the endorphins (enkephalins, endorphins, and dynorphins), has become known only within the last 40 to 50 years.

The opioid analgesics are characterized by their interaction with three types of opioid receptors, designated mu (μ, for "morphine"), delta (δ), and kappa (κ).[17] Each receptor type has been cloned, and subtypes have been identified using receptor-binding and molecular studies. Morphine and most opioids that are used clinically exert their effects through the mu receptor. Kappa receptor opioids are effective analgesics, but their side effects have proven troublesome, and the clinical impact of delta receptor opioids has been negligible.

It is well documented that the mu receptors modulate both the therapeutic effect of analgesia, as well as the side effects of respiratory depression, miosis, reduced gastrointestinal motility (causing constipation), feelings of well-being or euphoria, and physical dependence. The mu receptors are found at presynaptic and postsynaptic sites in the spinal dorsal horn and in the ascending pathways of the brain stem, thalamus, and cortex as well as the descending inhibitory system that modulates pain at the spinal cord. Their spinal location has been used clinically by direct application of opioid analgesics to the spinal cord by injection, infusion, or implantable intrathecal device (pump), which provides regional anesthesia while minimizing the unwanted respiratory depression, nausea and vomiting, and sedation that occur with systemically administered drugs that act at the brain level. Mu receptors are also found in peripheral sensory neurons after inflammation. This location supports the exploration and eventual clinical use of locally applied opioids (*e.g.*, intraarticular instillation of opioids after knee surgery).

As more information becomes available regarding the opioids and their receptors, it seems likely that pain medications can be developed that act selectively at certain receptor sites, providing more effective pain control while producing fewer adverse effects and affording less danger of addiction.

Adjuvant Analgesics. Adjuvant analgesics include medications such as tricyclic antidepressants, antiepileptic medications, and neuroleptic anxiolytic agents. The fact that the pain suppression system has nonendorphin synapses raises the possibility that potent, centrally acting, nonopiate medications may be useful in relieving pain. Serotonin has been shown to play an important role in producing analgesia. The tricyclic antidepressant medications (*i.e.*, imipramine, amitriptyline, and doxepin) that block the removal of serotonin from the synaptic cleft have been shown to produce pain relief in some people. These medications are particularly useful in some chronic painful conditions, such as postherpetic neuralgia.[16,17]

Certain antiepileptic medications, such as carbamazepine and gabapentin, have analgesic effects in some pain conditions. These medications, which suppress spontaneous neuronal firing, are particularly useful in the management of pain that occurs after nerve injury (neuropathic pain), including diabetic neuropathy and chronic regional pain syndrome. Other agents, such as the corticosteroids, may be used to decrease inflammation and the nociceptive stimuli responsible for pain.[17]

Surgical Intervention

If surgery removes the problem causing the pain, such as a tumor pressing on a nerve or an inflamed appendix, it can be curative. In other instances, surgery is used for symptom management rather than for cure. Surgery for severe, intractable pain of peripheral or central origin has met with some success. It can be used to remove the cause or block the transmission of intractable pain from phantom limb pain, severe neuralgia, inoperable cancer of certain types, and causalgia.

IN SUMMARY

Pain is an elusive and complex phenomenon; it is a symptom common to many illnesses. It is a highly individualized experience that is shaped by a person's culture and previous life experiences, and it is difficult to measure. Scientifically, pain is viewed within the context of nociception. Nociceptors are receptive nerve endings that respond to noxious stimuli. Pain receptors respond to mechanical, thermal, and chemical stimuli. Nociceptive neurons transmit impulses to the dorsal horn neurons using chemical neurotransmitters. The neospinothalamic and the paleospinothalamic pathways are used to transmit pain information to the brain. Several neuroanatomic pathways as well as endogenous opioid peptides modulate pain in the CNS.

Pain can be classified according to duration, location, and referral as well as associated medical diagnoses. Acute pain is self-limiting pain that ends when the injured tissue heals, whereas chronic pain is pain that lasts much longer than the anticipated healing time for the underlying cause of the pain. Pain can arise from cutaneous, deep somatic, or visceral locations. Referred pain is pain perceived at a site different from its origin. Pain threshold, pain tolerance, age, sex, and other factors affect a person's reaction to pain.

Treatment modalities for pain include the use of physiologic, cognitive, and behavioral measures; heat and cold; stimulation-induced analgesic methods; and pharmacologic agents singly or in combination. It is becoming apparent that even with chronic pain, the most effective approach is early treatment or even prevention. After pain is present, the greatest success in pain assessment and management is achieved with the use of an interdisciplinary approach.

After completing this section of the chapter, the learner will be able to meet the following objectives:

- Define allodynia, hypoesthesia, hyperesthesia, paresthesias, hyperpathia, analgesia, and hypoalgesia and hyperalgesia.
- Describe the cause and characteristics and treatment of neuropathic pain, trigeminal neuralgia, postherpetic neuralgia, and complex regional pain syndrome.
- Discuss possible mechanisms of phantom limb pain.

Alterations in Pain Sensitivity

Sensitivity to and perception of pain vary among people and in the same person under different conditions and in different parts of the body. Irritation, mild hypoxia, and mild compression of a peripheral nerve often result in hyperexcitability of the sensory nerve fibers or cell bodies. This is experienced as unpleasant hypersensitivity (*i.e.*, hyperesthesia) or increased painfulness (*i.e.*, *hyperalgesia*). Primary hyperalgesia describes pain sensitivity that occurs directly in damaged tissues. Secondary hyperalgesia occurs in the surrounding uninjured tissue. Possible causes of hyperalgesia include increased sensitivity to noxious stimuli, a decrease in the threshold of nociceptors, an increase in pain produced by suprathreshold stimuli, and the windup phenomenon.[19]

Hyperpathia is a syndrome in which the sensory threshold is raised, but when it is reached, continued stimulation, especially if repetitive, results in a prolonged and unpleasant experience. This pain can be explosive and radiates through a peripheral nerve distribution. It is associated with pathologic changes in peripheral nerves, such as localized ischemia. Spontaneous, unpleasant sensations called *paresthesias* occur with more severe irritation (*e.g.*, the pins and needles sensation that follows temporary compression of a peripheral nerve). The general term *dysesthesia* is given to distortions (usually unpleasant) of somesthetic sensation that typically accompany partial loss of sensory innervation.

More severe pathologic processes can result in reduced or lost tactile (*e.g., hypoesthesia, anesthesia*), temperature (*e.g., hypothermia, athermia*), and pain sensation (*i.e., hypoalgesia*). *Analgesia* is the absence of pain on noxious stimulation or the relief of pain without loss of consciousness. The inability to sense pain may result in trauma, infection, and even loss of a body part or parts. Inherited insensitivity to pain may take the form of congenital indifference or congenital insensitivity to pain. Congenital indifference is when the transmission of nerve impulses appears normal but appreciation of painful stimuli at higher levels appears to be absent. Congenital insensitivity is when a peripheral nerve defect apparently exists such that the transmission of painful nerve impulses does not result in perception of pain. Whatever the cause, people who lack the ability to perceive pain are at constant risk of tissue damage because pain is not serving its protective function.[20]

Allodynia (Greek *allo*, "other," and *odynia*, "painful") is the term used for the puzzling phenomenon of pain that follows a nonnoxious stimulus to apparently normal skin. Nonnoxious stimuli may include wind, touching sheets, and showering. This term is intended to refer to instances in which otherwise normal tissues may be abnormally innervated or may be referral sites for other loci that give rise to pain with nonnoxious stimuli. It can result from increased responsiveness within the spinal cord (central sensitization) or a reduction in the threshold for nociceptor activation (peripheral sensitization). One type of allodynia involves *trigger points*, which are highly localized points on the skin or mucous membrane that can produce immediate intense pain at that site or elsewhere when stimulated by light tactile stimulation. Myofascial trigger points are foci of exquisite tenderness found in many muscles and can be responsible for pain projected to sites remote from the points of tenderness. Trigger points are widely distributed in the back of the head and neck and in the lumbar and thoracic regions. These trigger points cause reproducible myofascial pain syndromes in specific muscles. These pain syndromes are the major source of pain in people at chronic pain treatment centers.

Special Types of Pain

Neuropathic Pain

Neuropathic pain refers to pain that is caused by some problem with the neurologic system. When peripheral nerves are affected by injury or disease, it can lead to unusual and sometimes intractable sensory disturbances. The notable features that point to neuropathic processes as a cause of pain include widespread pain that is not otherwise explainable and evidence of sensory deficit (*e.g.*, numbness, paresthesias). Depending on the cause, few or many axons could be damaged and the condition could be unilateral or bilateral. Neuropathic pain is distinguished from other pain conditions where the pain stimulus begins in nonneuronal tissues.

Causes of neuropathic pain can be categorized according to the extent of peripheral nerve involvement. Conditions that can lead to pain by causing damage to peripheral nerves in a single area include nerve entrapment, nerve compression from a tumor mass, and various neuralgias (*e.g.*, trigeminal, postherpetic, and posttraumatic). Conditions that can lead to pain by causing damage to peripheral nerves in a wide area include diabetes mellitus, long-term alcohol use, and hypothyroidism. Diabetes often causes a length-dependent neuropathy (meaning that the longest axons in a peripheral nerve are most vulnerable). Injury to a nerve also can lead to a multisymptom, multisystem syndrome called *complex regional pain syndrome*. Nerve damage associated with amputation is believed to be a cause of phantom limb pain.

Neuropathic pain can vary with the extent and location of disease or injury. There may be allodynia or pain that is stabbing, jabbing, burning, or shooting. The pain may be persistent or intermittent. The diagnosis depends on the mode of onset, the distribution of abnormal sensations, the quality of the pain, and other relevant medical conditions (*e.g.*, diabetes, hypothyroidism, alcohol use, rash, or trauma). Injury to peripheral nerves sometimes results in pain that persists beyond the time required for the tissues to heal. Peripheral pathologic processes (*e.g.*, neural degeneration, neuroma formation, and generation of abnormal spontaneous neural discharges from the injured sensory neuron) and neural plasticity (*i.e.*, changes in CNS function) are the primary working hypotheses to explain persistent neuropathic pain.

Treatment methods include measures aimed at restoring or preventing further nerve damage (*e.g.*, surgical resection of a tumor causing nerve compression, improving glycemic control for people with diabetes who have painful neuropathies), and interventions for the palliation of pain. Although many adjuvant analgesics are used for neuropathic pain, pain control often is difficult. The initial approach in seeking adequate pain control is to try these drugs in sequence and then in combination and also with nonpharmacologic interventions. The adjuvant analgesics can be divided into two general classes, including neuropathic and bone pain. Often the neuropathic category of pain is treated with tricyclic antidepressants, antiepileptics, local anesthetics, and alpha 2 adrenergic agonists.[16] Most frequently bone pain is treated with glucocorticoids, bisphosphonates, osteoclast inhibitors, and skeletal muscle relaxants.[16]

Poor pain control or unacceptable side effects may lead to a trial with other medications. If there has been a poor response to the adjuvant analgesics, opioids also can be used. However, concerns about side effects and the remote possibility of addiction must be considered. When opioids are used, the use of long-acting opioids with a plan for breakthrough pain is desirable because it addresses the typically continuous nature of neuropathic pain. Nonpharmacologic therapies also are used for neurogenic pain. Electrical stimulation of the peripheral nerve or spinal cord can be used for radiculopathies and neuralgias.

Neuralgia

Neuralgia is characterized by severe, brief, often repetitive attacks of lightning-like or throbbing pain. It occurs along the distribution of a spinal or cranial nerve and usually is precipitated by stimulation of the cutaneous region supplied by that nerve.

Trigeminal Neuralgia. Trigeminal neuralgia, or *tic douloureux*, is one of the most common and severe neuralgias. It is characterized by recurring, sudden onset of sharp, stabbing, pains without numbness in one or more nerve branches of cranial nerve five.[3] Considerable controversy remains regarding the pathophysiology of trigeminal neuralgia. However, most agree it is caused by demyelination of axons in the ganglion, root, and nerve.[16]

Treatment of trigeminal neuralgia includes pharmacologic and surgical modalities. Other interventions include avoidance of precipitating factors (*e.g.*, stimulation of trigger spots) and eye injury because of irritation, provision for adequate nutrition, and avoidance of social isolation. Carbamazepine (Tegretol), an antiepileptic drug, is recognized as a first-line agent for treatment of trigeminal neuralgia.[16] Surgical release of vessels, dural structures, or scar tissue surrounding the semilunar ganglion or root in the middle cranial fossa often eliminates the symptoms.

Postherpetic Neuralgia. Herpes zoster (also called *shingles*) is caused by the same herpes virus (varicella-zoster virus) that causes chickenpox and is thought to represent a localized recurrent infection by the varicella-zoster virus that has remained latent in the dorsal root ganglia since the initial attack of chickenpox.[16] Reactivation of viral replication is associated with a decline in cellular immunity. The probability of developing herpes zoster increases after the age of 60.[16] Increased risk of herpes zoster occurs with impaired cellular immunity.

During the acute attack of herpes zoster, the reactivated virus travels from the affected sensory ganglia and peripheral nerve to the skin of the corresponding dermatomes, causing a unilateral localized vesicular eruption and hyperpathia. In the acute infection, proportionately more of the large nerve fibers are destroyed. Regenerated fibers appear to have smaller diameters. Because there is a relative loss of large fibers with age, older adults are particularly prone to pain because of the shift in the proportion of large- to small-diameter nerve fibers. People with postherpetic neuralgia may experience constant pain ("burning, aching, throbbing"), intermittent pain ("stabbing, shooting"), and stimulus-evoked pain (allodynia).

Early treatment of shingles with antiviral drugs such as acyclovir or valacyclovir that inhibit herpes virus deoxyribonucleic acid (DNA) replication may reduce the severity of herpes zoster. Initially, postherpetic neuralgia can be treated with a topical anesthetic agent, lidocaine–prilocaine cream or 5% lidocaine gel. A tricyclic antidepressant medication, such as amitriptyline or desipramine, may be used for pain relief. Regional nerve blockade has been used with limited success.

A recent trial investigating a new live attenuated herpes zoster vaccine among adults 60 years of age and older, designed to boost their cell-mediated immunity to the varicella-zoster virus, demonstrated dramatic decreases in the incidence of herpes zoster and postherpetic neuralgia.[16] As a result, the vaccine, Zostavax, was approved by the U.S. Food and Drug Administration (FDA) for prevention of herpes zoster in persons 60 years of age and older and offers approximately 60% protection.[16]

Phantom Limb Pain

Phantom limb pain, a type of neurologic pain, follows amputation of a limb or part of a limb. The pain can start out as tingling, squeezing, or heaviness, followed by burning, cramping, or shooting pain.[21] It may disappear spontaneously or persist for many years.

There are multiple theories as to the causes of phantom limb pain. One rationale is that the end of a regenerating nerve becomes trapped in the scar tissue of the amputation site. It is known that when a peripheral nerve is cut, the scar tissue that forms becomes a barrier to regenerating outgrowth of the axon. The growing axon often becomes trapped in the scar tissue, forming a tangled growth (*i.e.*, neuroma) of small-diameter axons, including primary nociceptive afferents and sympathetic efferents. It has been proposed that these afferents show increased sensitivity to innocuous mechanical stimuli and to sympathetic activity and circulating catecholamines. A related theory moves the source of phantom limb pain to the spinal cord, suggesting that the pain is due to the spontaneous firing of spinal cord neurons that have lost their normal sensory input from the body. In this case, a closed self-exciting neuronal loop in the posterior horn of the spinal cord is postulated to send impulses to the brain, resulting in pain. Even the slightest irritation to the amputated limb area can initiate this cycle. Other theories propose that the phantom limb pain may arise in the brain itself. In one hypothesis, the pain is caused by changes in the flow of signals through somatosensory areas of the brain. In other words, there appears to be plasticity even in the adult CNS. Treatment of phantom limb pain has been accomplished using sympathetic blocks, TENS of the large myelinated afferents innervating the area, hypnosis, and relaxation training.

IN SUMMARY

Pain may occur with or without an adequate stimulus, or it may be absent in the presence of an adequate stimulus—either of which describes a pain disorder. There may be analgesia (absence of pain), hyperalgesia (increased sensitivity to pain), hypoalgesia (a decreased sensitivity to painful stimuli), hyperpathia (an unpleasant and prolonged response to pain), hyperesthesia (an abnormal increase in sensitivity to sensation), hypoesthesia (an abnormal decrease in sensitivity to sensations), paresthesia (abnormal touch sensation such as tingling or "pins and needles" in the absence of external stimuli), or allodynia (pain produced by stimuli that do not normally cause pain).

Neuropathic pain may be due to trauma or disease of neurons in a focal area or in a more global distribution (*e.g.*, from endocrine disease or neurotoxic medications). Neuralgia is characterized by severe, brief, often repetitive attacks of lightning-like or throbbing pain that occurs along the distribution of a spinal or cranial nerve and usually is precipitated by stimulation of the cutaneous region supplied by that nerve. Trigeminal neuralgia, or tic douloureux, is one of the most common and severe neuralgias. It is manifested by facial tics or spasms. Postherpetic neuralgia is a chronic pain that can occur after shingles, an infection of the dorsal root ganglia and corresponding areas of innervation by the varicella-zoster virus. Phantom limb pain, a neurologic pain, can occur after amputation of a limb or part of a limb.

HEADACHE AND ASSOCIATED PAIN

After completing this section of the chapter, the learner will be able to meet the following objectives:

- Differentiate between the occurrence and manifestations of migraine headache, cluster headache, tension-type headache, and headache due to temporomandibular joint (TMJ) syndrome.
- Characterize the nonpharmacologic and pharmacologic methods used in treatment of headache.
- Cite the most common cause of TMJ pain.

Headache

Headache is a very common health problem. Over 18 million Americans visit their health care provider because of a headache annually.[16] Although head and facial pain have characteristics that distinguish them from other pain disorders, they also share many of the same features.

Headache is caused by several conditions. Some headaches represent primary disorders and others occur secondary to other disease conditions in which head pain is a symptom. The most common types of primary or chronic headaches are migraine headache, tension-type headache, cluster headache, and chronic daily headache (CDH). Although most causes of secondary headache are benign, some are indications of serious disorders such as meningitis, brain tumor, or cerebral aneurysm. Other times a person may experience a headache post head trauma. Generally the research suggests people with mild traumatic brain injury (TBI) have more problems with headache than those with moderate or severe TBI.[22] The sudden onset of a severe, intractable headache in an otherwise healthy person is more likely related to a serious intracranial disorder, such as subarachnoid hemorrhage or meningitis, than to a chronic headache disorder. Headaches that disturb sleep, exertional headaches (*e.g.*, triggered by physical or sexual activity or a Valsalva maneuver), and headaches accompanied by neurologic symptoms such as drowsiness, visual or limb disturbances, or altered mental status also are suggestive of underlying intracranial lesions or other pathologic processes. Other red flags for secondary headache disorder include a fundamental change or progression in headache pattern or a new headache in people older than 50 years of age, or in people with cancer, immunosuppression, or pregnancy.[23,24] Older adults need a comprehensive assessment of any headache if they have not had headaches before becoming an older adult.[25]

The diagnosis and classification of headaches often is difficult. It requires a comprehensive history and physical examination to exclude secondary causes. The history should include factors that precipitate headache, such as foods and food additives, missed meals, and association with the menstrual period. A careful medication history is essential because many medications can provoke or aggravate headaches. Alcohol also can cause or aggravate headache. A headache diary in which the person records his or her headaches and concurrent or antecedent events may be helpful in identifying factors that contribute to headache onset.

In 2013, the International Headache Society (IHS) published the third edition of *The International Classification of Headache Disorders* (ICHD-3).[24] The classification system is divided into three sections: (1) primary headaches, (2) secondary headaches, and (3) painful cranial neuropathies, other facial pains and other headaches.[24]

Migraine Headache

Migraine headaches affect many people and especially women. Migraine headaches tend to run in families and are thought to be inherited as an autosomal dominant trait with incomplete penetrance.

Etiology and Pathogenesis

The pathophysiologic mechanisms of the pain associated with migraine headaches remain poorly understood. Although many alternative theories exist, it is well established that during a migraine the trigeminal nerve becomes activated.[26] Stimulation of the trigeminal sensory fibers may lead to the release of neuropeptides, causing painful neurogenic inflammation within the meningeal vasculature.[27] Another possible mechanism implicates neurogenic vasodilation of meningeal blood vessels as a key component of the inflammatory processes that occur during migraine. Supporting the neurogenic basis for migraine is the frequent presence of premonitory symptoms before the headache begins: the presence of focal neurologic disturbances, which cannot be explained in terms of cerebral blood flow.[27]

Hormonal variations, particularly in estrogen levels, play a role in the pattern of migraine attacks. For many women, migraine headaches coincide with their menstrual periods. Dietary substances, such as monosodium glutamate, aged cheese, and chocolate, also may precipitate migraine headaches. The actual triggers for migraine are the chemicals in the food, not allergens.

Clinical Manifestations

The ICHD-3 classifies migraine headaches into two major subtypes, migraine without aura and migraine with aura.[24]

Migraine without aura is a pulsatile, throbbing, unilateral headache that typically lasts 1 to 2 days and is aggravated by routine physical activity. The headache is accompanied by nausea and vomiting, which often is disabling, and sensitivity to light and sound. Visual disturbances occur quite commonly and consist of visual hallucinations such as stars, sparks, and flashes of light. Migraine with aura has similar symptoms, but with the addition of reversible visual symptoms, including positive features (*e.g.*, flickering lights, spots, or lines) or negative features (loss of vision); fully reversible sensory symptoms, including positive features (feeling of pins or needles) or negative features (numbness); and fully reversible speech disturbances or neurologic symptoms that precede the headache.[24] The aura usually develops over a period of 5 to 20 minutes and lasts from 5 minutes to an hour. Although only a small percentage of people with migraine experience an aura before an attack, many people without aura have prodromal symptoms, such as fatigue and irritability, that precede the attack by hours or even days.[26]

The other ICHD-3 migraine headache subtypes are chronic migraine, complications of migraine (*e.g.*, status migrainosus, persistent aura without infarction, migrainous infarction, and migraine aura-triggered seizures), probable migraine, and episodic syndromes that may be associated with migraine.[24] Retinal migraines are a rare form of migraine characterized by recurrent attacks of fully reversible scintillations (visual sensation of sparks or flashes of light), scotomata (visual blind spots), or blindness affecting one eye, followed within an hour by migrainous headache. The ICHD-3 classifies chronic migraine when a headache meeting the criteria for migraine is present on 15 or more days per month for 3 months or more, in the absence of medication overuse. Migrainous infarction is an uncommon occurrence in which one or more otherwise typical aura symptoms persist beyond 1 hour and neuroimaging confirms ischemic infarction. Strictly applied, these criteria distinguish this disorder from stroke, which must be excluded.[24]

Migraine headache also can present as a mixed headache, including symptoms typically associated with tension-type headache, sinus headache, or CHD. These are called *transformed migraine* and are difficult to classify. Although nasal symptoms are not one of the diagnostic criteria for migraine, they frequently accompany migraine and are probably because of cranial parasympathetic activation. Sinus pain may indicate either a headache due to sinus inflammation or migraine.

Migraine headaches occur in children as well as adults. Before puberty, migraine headaches are equally distributed between the sexes. The essential diagnostic criterion for migraine in children is the presence of recurrent headaches separated by pain-free periods. Diagnosis is generally based on the child experiencing three of the following—abdominal pain, nausea or vomiting, throbbing headache, unilateral location, associated aura, relief during sleep, and a positive family history. Symptoms vary widely among children, from those that interrupt activities and cause the child to seek relief in a dark environment to those detectable only by direct questioning. A common feature of migraine in children is intense nausea and vomiting. The vomiting may be associated with abdominal pain and fever. Thus, migraine may be confused with other conditions such as appendicitis. Because headaches in children can be a symptom of other, more serious disorders, including intracranial lesions, it is important that other causes of headache be ruled out.

Treatment

The treatment of migraine headaches includes preventive and abortive nonpharmacologic and pharmacologic treatment.

Nonpharmacologic treatment includes the avoidance of migraine triggers, such as foods or smells that precipitate an attack. Many people with migraines benefit from maintaining regular eating and sleeping habits. Measures to control stress, which also can precipitate an attack, also are important. During an attack, many people find it helpful to retire to a quiet, darkened room until symptoms subside.

Pharmacologic treatment involves both abortive therapy for acute attacks and preventive therapy. A wide range of medications is used to treat the acute symptoms of migraine headache. Based on clinical trials, first-line agents include acetylsalicylic acid; combinations of acetaminophen, acetylsalicylic acid, and caffeine; NSAIDs (*e.g.*, naproxen sodium, ibuprofen); serotonin ($5\text{-}HT_1$) receptor agonists (*e.g.*, sumatriptan, naratriptan, rizatriptan, zolmitriptan); ergotamine derivatives (*e.g.*, dihydroergotamine); and antiemetic medications (*e.g.*, ondansetron, metoclopramide).[16,27] Nonoral routes of administration may be preferred in people who develop severe pain rapidly or on awakening, or in those with severe nausea and vomiting. Sumatriptan has been approved for intranasal administration. Frequent use of abortive headache medications may cause rebound headache.

Preventive pharmacologic treatment may be necessary if migraine headaches become disabling, if they occur more than two or three times a month, if abortive treatment is being used more than two times a week, or if the person has hemiplegic migraine, migraine with prolonged aura, or migrainous infarction.[16,27] In most cases, preventive treatment must be taken daily for months to years. First-line agents include β-adrenergic blocking medications (*e.g.*, propranolol, atenolol), antidepressants (amitriptyline), and antiepileptic medications (divalproex sodium, sodium valproate).[16] When a decision to discontinue preventive therapy is made, the medications should be withdrawn gradually.

Other effective medications are available, but they can have serious side effects in some people. For example, because of the risk of coronary vasospasm, the $5\text{-}HT_1$ receptor agonists should not be given to people with coronary artery disease.

Cluster Headache

Cluster headaches are relatively uncommon headaches that occur more frequently in men than women and typically begin in the third decade of life.[28] These headaches tend to occur in clusters over weeks or months, followed by a long, headache-free remission period. Cluster headache is a type of primary neurovascular headache that typically includes severe, unrelenting, unilateral pain.

Etiology and Pathogenesis

The underlying pathophysiologic mechanisms of cluster headaches are not completely known, although recently it has been noted that heredity, through an autosomal dominant gene, plays some role in the pathogenesis of cluster headache. The most likely pathophysiologic mechanisms include the interplay of vascular, neurogenic, metabolic, and humoral factors. Activation of the trigeminovascular system and the cranial autonomic parasympathetic reflexes is thought to explain the pain and autonomic symptoms. The hypothalamus is believed to play a key role. The possible role of the regulating centers in the anterior hypothalamus is implicated from observations of circadian biologic changes and neuroendocrine disturbances (*e.g.*, changes in cortisol, prolactin, and testosterone) that occur in both active periods and during clinical remission. Magnetic resonance imaging has demonstrated dilated intracranial arteries on the painful side. Loss of vascular tone is believed to result from a defect in the sympathetic perivascular innervation.

Clinical Manifestations

The pain associated with cluster headache is of rapid onset and builds to a peak in approximately 10 to 15 minutes, lasting for 15 to 180 minutes. The pain behind the eye radiates to the ipsilateral trigeminal nerve (*e.g.*, temple, cheek, gum). The headache frequently is associated with one or more symptoms such as restlessness or agitation, conjunctival redness, lacrimation specifically on one side, nasal congestion, rhinorrhea, forehead and facial sweating, miosis, ptosis, and eyelid edema.

Treatment

Because of the relatively short duration and self-limited nature of cluster headache, oral preparations typically take too long to reach therapeutic levels. The most effective treatments are those that act quickly. Oxygen inhalation may be indicated for home use. Prophylactic medications for cluster headaches include verapamil, lithium carbonate, corticosteroids, and sodium valproate.[27]

Tension-Type Headache

The most common type of headache is tension-type headache. Unlike migraine and cluster headaches, tension-type headache usually is not sufficiently severe that it interferes with daily activities.

Etiology and Pathogenesis

The exact mechanisms of tension-type headache are not known and the hypotheses of causation are contradictory. One popular theory is that tension-type headache results from sustained tension of the muscles of the scalp and neck; however, some research has found no correlation between muscle contraction and tension-type headache. It is thought that migraine headache may be transformed gradually into chronic tension-type headache. Tension-type headaches also may be caused by oromandibular dysfunction, psychogenic stress, anxiety, depression, and muscular stress. They also may result from overuse of analgesics or caffeine.

Clinical Manifestations

Tension-type headaches frequently are described as dull, aching, diffuse, nondescript headaches, occurring in a hatband distribution around the head, and not associated with nausea or vomiting or worsened by activity. They can be infrequent, episodic, or chronic.

Treatment

Tension-type headaches often are more responsive to nonpharmacologic techniques, such as biofeedback, massage, acupuncture, relaxation, imagery, and physical therapy, than other types of headache. For people with poor posture, a combination of range-of-motion exercises, relaxation, and posture improvement may be helpful.

The medications of choice for acute treatment of tension-type headaches are analgesics, including acetylsalicylic acid; acetaminophen; and NSAIDs.[16,27] People with infrequent tension-type headache usually self-medicate using over-the-counter analgesics to treat the acute pain and do not require prophylactic medication. These agents should be used cautiously because rebound headaches can develop when the medications are taken regularly.

Because the "dividing lines" between tension-type headache, migraine, and CDH often are vague, addition of medications as well as the entire range of migraine medications may be tried in refractory cases. Other medications used concomitantly with analgesics include sedating antihistamines (*e.g.*, promethazine and diphenhydramine), antiemetics (*e.g.*, metoclopramide and prochlorperazine), or sedatives (*e.g.*, butalbital).

Chronic Daily Headache

The term *chronic daily headache* is used to refer to headaches that occur 15 days or more a month, for greater than 3 months.[27] Little is known about the prevalence and incidence of CDH. Diagnostic criteria for CDH are not provided in the IHS classification system.

Etiology and Pathogenesis

The cause of CDH is unknown, although there are several hypotheses. They include transformed migraine headache, evolved tension-type headache, new daily persistent headache, and posttraumatic headache. Although overuse of symptomatic medications has been related to CDH, there is a group of people in whom CDH is unrelated to excessive use of medications.

Clinical Manifestations

In many people, CDH retains certain characteristics of migraine, whereas in others it resembles chronic tension-type headache. CDH may be associated with chronic and episodic tension-type headache. New daily persistent headache may have a rapid onset, with no history of migraine, tension-type headache, trauma, or psychological stress.

Treatment

For people with CDH, a combination of pharmacologic and behavioral interventions may be necessary. As with tension-type headaches, nonpharmacologic techniques, such as biofeedback, massage, acupuncture, relaxation, imagery, and physical therapy, may be helpful. Measures to reduce or eliminate medication, including caffeine, overuse may be helpful.

Temporomandibular Joint Pain

A common cause of head pain is TMJ syndrome. It usually is caused by an imbalance in joint movement because of poor bite, bruxism (*i.e.*, teeth grinding), or joint problems.[27] The pain almost always is referred and commonly presents as facial muscle pain, headache, neck ache, or earache. Referred pain is aggravated by jaw function. Headache associated with this syndrome is common in adults and children and can cause chronic pain problems.

Treatment of TMJ pain is aimed at correcting the problem, and in some cases, this may be difficult. The initial therapy for TMJ should be directed toward relief of pain and improvement in function. Pain relief often can be achieved with use of the NSAIDs. Muscle relaxants may be used when muscle spasm is a problem.

IN SUMMARY

Head pain is a common disorder that is caused by several conditions. Some headaches represent primary disorders and others occur secondary to another disease state in which head pain is a symptom. Primary headache disorders include migraine headache, tension-type headache, cluster headache, and CDH. Although most causes of secondary headache are benign, some are indications of serious disorders such as meningitis, brain tumor, or cerebral aneurysm. TMJ syndrome is one of the major causes of headaches. It usually is caused by an imbalance in joint movement because of poor bite, teeth grinding, or joint problems such as inflammation, trauma, and degenerative changes.

PAIN IN CHILDREN AND OLDER ADULTS

After completing this section of the chapter, the learner will be able to meet the following objectives:

- Differentiate between the pain response in children and older adults.
- Explain how pain assessment may differ in children and older adults.
- Explain how pain treatment may differ in children and older adults.

Pain frequently is underrecognized and undertreated in both children and older adults. In addition to the common obstacles to adequate pain management, such as concern about the effects of analgesia on respiratory status and the potential for addiction to opioids, there are additional deterrents to adequate pain management in children and older adults. In very young children and confused older adults, there are several additional factors. These include the extreme difficulty of assessing the location and intensity of pain in people who are cognitively immature or cognitively impaired and the argument that even if they feel pain, they do not remember it.[19]

Pain in Children

Human responsiveness to painful stimuli begins in the neonatal period and continues through the life span. Although the specific and localized behavioral reactions are less marked in the younger neonate or the more cognitively impaired individual, protective or withdrawal reflexes in response to nociceptive stimuli are clearly demonstrated. Pain pathways, cortical and subcortical centers, and neurochemical responses associated with pain transmission are developed and functional by the last trimester of pregnancy. Neonates clearly perceive pain, as demonstrated by their integrated physiologic response to nociceptive stimuli. Dorsal horn neurons in neonates have a wider receptive field and lower excitatory threshold than those in older children.

As infants and children mature, their responses to pain become more complex and reflective of their maturing cognitive and developmental processes. Children do feel pain and have been shown to reliably and accurately report pain. They also remember pain. This is evidenced in studies of children with cancer, whose distress during painful procedures increases over time without intervention, and in neonates in intensive care units, who demonstrate protective withdrawal responses to a heel stick after repeated episodes.

Pain Assessment

To treat pain adequately, ongoing assessment of the presence of pain and response to treatment is essential.[16] Self-report is usually regarded as the most reliable estimate of pain. With children 8 years of age or older, numeric scales (*i.e.*, 1 to 10) and word graphic scales (*i.e.*, "none," "a little," "most I have ever experienced") can be used. With children 3 to 8 years of age, scales with faces of actual children or cartoon faces can be used to obtain a report of pain. The Wong-Baker FACES Pain Rating Scale (http://wongbakerfaces.org) is useful in children as young as 3 to 4 years of age and contains both pictures and brief description of the pain. The provider explains the pictures using the words under each picture. Another supplementary strategy for assessing a child's pain is to use a body outline and ask the child to indicate where the hurt is located. Care must be taken in assessing children's reports of pain because their reports may be influenced by a variety of factors, including age, anxiety and fear levels, and parental presence. Some physiologic measures, such as heart rate, are convenient to measure and respond rapidly to brief nociceptive stimuli, but they are nonspecific. Relying on indicators of sympathetic nervous system activity and behaviors can also be problematic because they can be caused by things other than pain (*e.g.*, anxiety and activity) and they do not always accompany pain, particularly chronic pain.

Pain Management

The management of children's pain basically falls into two categories—pharmacologic and nonpharmacologic. In terms of pharmacologic interventions, many of the analgesics used in adults can be used safely and effectively in children and adolescents. However, it is critical when using specific medications to determine that the medication has been approved for use with children and that it is dosed appropriately according to the child's weight and level of physiologic development. Age-related differences in physiologic functioning, notably in neonates, will affect drug action. Neonates and infants have decreased levels of the hepatic enzymes needed for metabolism of many analgesics. The levels of these hepatic enzymes quickly increase to adult levels in the first few months of life. The renal excretion of drugs depends on renal blood flow, glomerular filtration rate, and tubular secretion, all of which are decreased in neonates, particularly premature neonates.

The overriding principle in all pediatric pain management is to treat each child's pain on an individual basis and to match the analgesic agent with the cause and the level of pain. A second principle involves maintaining the balance between the level of side effects and pain relief such that pain relief is obtained with as little opioid and sedation as possible. One strategy toward this end is to time the administration of analgesia so that a steady blood level is achieved and, as much as possible, pain is prevented. This requires that the child receive analgesia on a regular dosing schedule, not "as needed." Also, most drugs are packaged primarily for adult use, and dose calculations and serial dilutions may predispose to medication errors.

Nonpharmacologic strategies can be very effective in reducing the overall amount of pain and amount of analgesia used. In addition, some nonpharmacologic strategies can reduce anxiety and increase the child's level of self-control during pain. Children can be taught to use simple distraction and relaxation and other techniques such as application of heat and cold. Other nonpharmacologic techniques can be taught to the child to provide psychological preparation for a painful procedure or surgery. These include positive self-talk, imagery, play therapy, modeling, and rehearsal. The nonpharmacologic interventions must be developmentally appropriate, and if possible, the child and parent should be taught these techniques when the child is not in pain (*e.g.*, before surgery or a painful procedure) so that it is easier to practice the technique.

Pain in Older Adults

Among adults, the prevalence of pain in the general population increases with age. Research is inconsistent about whether there are age-related changes in pain perception. Some apparent age-related differences in pain may be due to differences in willingness to report the pain rather than actual differences in pain. The older adult may be reluctant to report pain so as not to be a burden or out of fear of the diagnoses, tests, medications, or costs that may result from an attempt to diagnose or treat their pain. It is important for the provider to ask very specific questions to older adults regarding their pain in order to elicit the correct information so best management of the pain can be given.[29]

Pain Assessment

The assessment of pain in older adults can range from relatively simple in a well-informed, alert, cognitively intact person with pain from a single source and no comorbidities to extraordinarily difficult in a confused person. When possible, a person's report of pain is the gold standard, but behavioral signs of pain should also be considered. Accurately diagnosing pain when the person has many health problems or some decline in cognitive function can be particularly challenging. In recent years, there has been increased awareness of the need to address issues of pain in people with dementia. The Assessment for Discomfort in Dementia Protocol is one example of the efforts to improve assessment and pain management in these people. It includes behavioral criteria for assessing pain and recommended interventions for pain. Its use has been shown to improve pain management.[30]

Pain Management

When prescribing pharmacologic and nonpharmacologic methods of pain management for the older population, care must be taken to consider the cause of the pain, the person's health status, the concurrent therapies, and the person's mental status. In the older population, where the risk of adverse events is higher, the nonpharmacologic options are usually less costly and cause fewer side effects.

The role of mental focus and anxiety is important, and relaxation techniques, massage, and biofeedback may also be useful nonpharmacologic interventions. Physical therapy and occupational therapy bring a variety of modalities, including the use of braces or splints, changes in biomechanics, and exercise, all of which have been shown to promote pain relief.

Although efficacy is important when considering the use of pharmacologic agents for pain relief in the elderly population, cost and safety must also be considered. Safety issues that must be considered among older adults include changes in drug metabolism, other disease comorbidity, and polypharmacy. Older adults may have physiologic changes that affect the pharmacokinetics of medications prescribed for pain management. These changes include decreased blood flow to organs, delayed gastric motility, reduced kidney function, and decreased albumin related to poor nutrition.[17] Older adults also often have many coexisting health problems, leading to polypharmacy. The addition of analgesics to a complex medication regimen is even more likely to cause drug interactions and complicate compliance in older adults. However, these considerations should not preclude the appropriate use of analgesic drugs to achieve pain relief. Nonopioids are generally the first line of therapy for mild to moderate pain, and acetaminophen is usually the first choice because it is relatively safe for older adults.[16] Opioids are used for more severe pain and for palliative care. As with younger people, adjuvant analgesics are effectively used for treatment of pain in older adults. The use of some assessment tool to evaluate the level of pain and effectiveness of treatment is essential. Monitoring for side effects is also critical.

IN SUMMARY

Children experience and remember pain, and even fairly young children are able to accurately and reliably report their pain. Recognition of this has changed the clinical practice of health professionals involved in the assessment of children's pain. Pharmacologic (including opioids) and nonpharmacologic pain management interventions have been shown to be effective in children. Nonpharmacologic techniques must be based on the developmental level of the child and should be taught to both children and parents.

Pain is a common symptom in older adults. Assessment, diagnosis, and treatment of pain in older adults can be complicated. Older adults may be reluctant or cognitively unable to report their pain. Diagnosis and treatment can be complicated by comorbidities and age-related changes in cognitive and physiologic function.

CONCEPTS IN ACTION BODY TEMPERATURE REGULATION

After completing this section of the chapter, the learner will be able to meet the following objectives:

- Differentiate between body core temperature and skin temperature.
- Identify the differences between methods used for measuring body temperature.
- Define the terms *conduction*, *radiation*, *convection*, and *evaporation*, and relate them to the mechanisms for gain and loss of heat from the body.

Most biochemical processes in the body are affected by changes in temperature. Metabolic processes speed up or slow down depending on whether body temperature is rising or falling. *Core body temperature* (*i.e.*, intracranial, intrathoracic, and intra-abdominal) normally is maintained within a range of 36.0°C to 37.5°C (97.0°F to 99.5°F).[31] Within this range, there are individual differences. For example, core temperature of most females increases approximately 0.5°C to 1.0°C during the postovulation phase of their menstrual cycle.[31] There are also diurnal variations. Internal core temperatures reach their highest point in late afternoon and evening and their lowest point in the early morning hours (Fig. 14.12). In fact, the core body temperature is generally lowest between 3:00 and 6:00 AM and highest during the late afternoon, 3:00 to 6:00 PM.[31]

Body temperature reflects the difference between heat production and heat loss and varies with exercise and extremes of environmental temperature. For instance, exercise can increase metabolic heat production 10-fold.[31] Thankfully, thermoregulatory responses such as sweating simultaneously increase heat loss, and thus keep body temperature from rising dangerously high. Shivering, on the other hand, increases metabolic heat production. This thermoregulatory response can offset the increased heat loss resulting from cold ambient conditions. Properly protected and hydrated, the body can function in environmental conditions that range from −50°C (−58°F) to +50°C (122°F). The failure to adequately manage heat production and/or loss results in devastating consequences. For instance, ice crystals can form in tissues exposed to very cold and damp ambient temperatures. At the other extreme, very high temperatures (+45°C, 113°F) cause proteins to coagulate and/or aggregate. As will be discussed later in this chapter, much smaller, systemic changes in body temperature can be equally devastating, leading to tissue damage, organ failure, coma, and even death.[32]

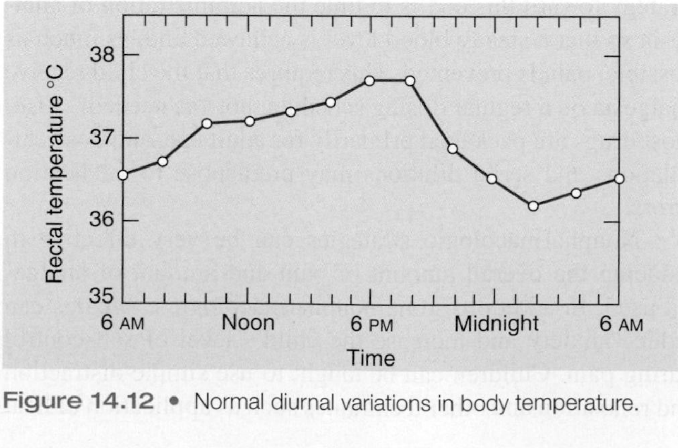

Figure 14.12 • Normal diurnal variations in body temperature.

KEY POINTS

THERMOREGULATION

- Core body temperature is a reflection of the balance between heat gain and heat loss by the body. Metabolic processes produce heat, which must be dissipated.
- The hypothalamus is the thermal control center for the body; it receives information from peripheral and central thermoreceptors and compares that information with its temperature set point.
- An increase in core temperature results from vasoconstriction and shivering, a decrease in temperature results from vasodilation and sweating.

Most of the body's heat is produced by the deeper core tissues (*i.e.*, muscles and viscera), which are insulated from the environment and protected against heat loss by an outer shell of subcutaneous tissues and skin (Fig. 14.13). The thickness of the shell depends on blood flow. In a warm environment, blood flow is increased and the thickness of the outer shell is decreased, allowing for greater dissipation of heat. In a cold environment, the vessels supplying blood flow to the skin and underlying tissues, including those of the limbs and more superficial muscles of the neck and trunk, constrict. This increases the thickness of the shell and helps to minimize the loss of core heat for the body. The subcutaneous fat layer contributes to the insulation value of the outer shell because of its thickness and because it conducts heat only about one third as effectively as other tissues.

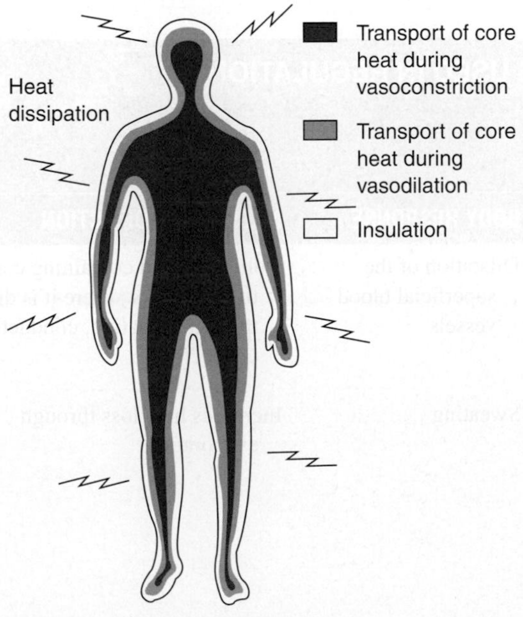

Figure 14.13 • Control of heat loss. Body heat is produced in the deeper core tissues of the body, which is insulated by the subcutaneous tissues and skin to protect against heat loss. During vasodilation, circulating blood transports heat to the skin surface, where it dissipates into the surrounding environment. Vasoconstriction decreases the transport of core heat to the skin surface, and vasodilation increases transport.

Temperatures differ in various parts of the body, with core temperatures being higher than those at the skin surface. The rectal temperature is used as a measure of core temperature and is considered the most accurate parameter.[1] Rectal temperatures usually range from 37.3°C (99.1°F) to 37.6°C (99.6°F). Core temperatures may also be obtained from the esophagus using a flexible thermometer, from a pulmonary artery catheter that is used for thermodilution measurement of cardiac output, or from a urinary catheter with a thermosensor that measures the temperature of urine in the bladder. Because of location, pulmonary artery and esophageal temperatures closely reflect the temperatures of the heart and thoracic organs.

Concept Mastery Alert

The pulmonary artery catheter is the preferred measurement when body temperatures are changing rapidly and need to be followed reliably on an acutely ill person in an intensive care setting.

The oral temperature, taken sublingually, is usually 0.2°C (0.36°F) to 0.51°C (0.9°F) lower than the rectal temperature. However, it usually follows changes in core temperature closely. The axillary temperature also can be used as an estimate of core temperature. However, the parts of the axillary fossa must be pressed closely together for an extended period (5 to 10 minutes for a glass thermometer) because this method requires considerable heat to accumulate before the final temperature is reached.

Ear-based thermometry uses an infrared sensor to measure the blood flow originating from the carotid artery at the tympanic membrane and is considered to directly reflect core temperature.[33] It is popular in all health care settings because of its ease and speed of measurement, acceptability to people, and cost savings in the personnel time that is required to take a temperature. However, there is continuing debate regarding the accuracy of this method.[34]

Core body and skin temperatures are sensed and integrated by thermoregulatory regions in the hypothalamus (particularly, the preoptic–anterior hypothalamic area) and other brain structures (*i.e.*, thalamus and cerebral cortex). Temperature-sensitive ion channels, identified as a subset of the transient receptor potential family (thermoTRPs), present in peripheral and central sensory neurons are activated by innocuous (warm and cool) and noxious (hot and cold) stimuli.[35] Peripheral signals regarding temperature are initiated by changes in local membrane potentials that are transmitted to the brain through dorsal root ganglia.[35] The *set point* of the hypothalamic thermoregulatory center is the ideal core temperature for the individual, helping regulate the temperature of the body core within the normal range of 36.0°C (96.8°F) to 37.5°C (99.5°F). When body temperature begins to rise above the set point, the hypothalamus signals the central and peripheral nervous systems to initiate heat-dissipating behaviors. Likewise, when the temperature falls below the set point, signals from the hypothalamus elicit physiologic behaviors that increase heat conservation and production. Core temperatures above 41°C (105.8°F) or below 34°C (93.2°F) usually mean that the body's ability to thermoregulate has been impaired. Body responses that produce, conserve, and dissipate heat are described in Table 14.2. Spinal cord injuries that transect the cord at T6 or above can seriously impair temperature regulation because the thermoregulatory centers in the hypothalamus can no longer control skin blood flow and sweating.

In addition to reflexive and automatic thermoregulatory mechanisms, humans engage in voluntary behaviors to help regulate body temperature based on their conscious sensation of being too hot or too cold. These behaviors include the selection of proper clothing and regulation of environmental temperature through heating systems and air conditioning. Body positions that hold the extremities close to the body prevent heat loss and are commonly assumed in cold weather.

Mechanisms of Heat Production

Metabolism is the body's main source of heat production or thermogenesis. Many factors impact the metabolic rate, including

- Metabolic rate of each cell
- Any factor that may increase the basal metabolic rate (BMR), such as that caused by muscle activity
- Extra metabolism caused by hormones, such as thyroxine, growth hormone, or testosterone
- Any extra metabolism caused by the sympathetic nervous system stimulation on cells
- Extra metabolism caused by increased cellular chemical activity
- Thermogenic effect of food digestion, absorption, or storage[1]

There is a 0.55°C (1°F) increase in body temperature for every 7% increase in metabolism. The sympathetic neurotransmitters, epinephrine and norepinephrine, which are released when an increase in body temperature is needed, act at the cellular level to shift body metabolism to heat production rather than energy generation. This may be one of the reasons fever tends to produce feelings of weakness and fatigue. Thyroid hormone increases cellular metabolism, but this response usually requires several weeks to reach maximal effectiveness.

Fine involuntary actions such as shivering and chattering of the teeth can produce a three- to fivefold increase in body temperature. *Shivering* is initiated by impulses from the hypothalamus, resulting in an increase in body temperature and increased use of oxygen.[36] Although shivering is an attempt to decrease the body temperature, it actually increases it and increases the use of oxygen.[36]

The first muscle change that occurs with shivering is a general increase in muscle tone, followed by an oscillating rhythmic tremor involving the spinal-level reflex that controls muscle tone. Physical exertion increases body temperature. Muscles convert most of the energy in the fuels they consume into heat rather than mechanical work. With strenuous

TABLE 14.2 HEAT GAIN AND HEAT LOSS RESPONSES USED IN REGULATION OF BODY TEMPERATURE

HEAT GAIN		HEAT LOSS	
BODY RESPONSE	**MECHANISM OF ACTION**	**BODY RESPONSE**	**MECHANISM OF ACTION**
Vasoconstriction of the superficial blood vessels	Confines blood flow to the inner core of the body, with the skin and subcutaneous tissues acting as insulation to prevent loss of core heat	Dilatation of the superficial blood vessels	Delivers blood containing core heat to the periphery where it is dissipated through radiation, conduction, and convection
Contraction of the pilomotor muscles that surround the hairs on the skin	Reduces the heat loss surface of the skin	Sweating	Increases heat loss through evaporation
Assumption of the huddle position with the extremities held close to the body	Reduces the area for heat loss		
Shivering	Increases heat production by the muscles		
Increased production of epinephrine	Increases the heat production associated with metabolism		
Increased production of thyroid hormone	Is a long-term mechanism that increases metabolism and heat production		

exercise, more than three fourths of the increased metabolism resulting from muscle activity appears as heat within the body; the remainder appears as mechanical work.[37]

Mechanisms of Heat Loss

Most of the body's heat losses occur at the skin surface as heat from the blood moves to the skin and from there into the surrounding environment. There are numerous arteriovenous (AV) anastomoses under the skin surface that allow blood to move directly from the arterial to the venous system.[3] These AV anastomoses are much like the radiators in a heating system. When the shunts are open, body heat is freely dissipated to the skin and surrounding environment; when the shunts are closed, heat is retained in the body. The blood flow in the AV anastomoses is controlled almost exclusively by the sympathetic nervous system in response to changes in core temperature and environmental temperature. Contraction of the *pilomotor muscles* of the skin, which raises skin hairs and produces goose bumps, also aids in heat conservation by reducing the surface area available for heat loss.

Heat is lost from the body through radiation, conduction, and convection from the skin surface; through the evaporation of sweat and insensible perspiration; through the exhalation of air that has been warmed and humidified; and through heat lost in urine and feces. Of these mechanisms, only heat losses that occur at the skin surface are directly under hypothalamic control.

Radiation

Radiation is the transfer of heat through air or a vacuum. Heat from the sun is carried by radiation. Heat loss by radiation varies with the temperature of the environment. Environmental temperature must be less than that of the body for heat loss to occur. In a nude person sitting inside a normal temperature room, approximately 60% of body heat typically is dissipated by radiation.[1]

Conduction

Conduction is the direct transfer of heat from one molecule to another. Blood carries, or conducts, heat from the inner core of the body to the skin surface. Normally only a small amount of body heat is lost through conduction to a cooler surface. Cooling blankets or mattresses that are used for reducing fever rely on conduction of heat from the skin to the cool surface of the mattress. Heat also can be conducted in the opposite direction—from the external environment to the body surface. For instance, body temperature may rise slightly after a hot bath.

Water has a specific heat several times greater than air, so water absorbs far greater amounts of heat than air does. The loss of body heat can be excessive and life threatening in situations of cold water immersion or cold exposure in damp or wet clothing.

The conduction of heat to the body's surface is influenced by blood volume. In hot weather, the body compensates by increasing blood volume as a means of dissipating heat. A mild swelling of the ankles during hot weather provides evidence of blood volume expansion. Exposure to cold produces a cold diuresis and a reduction in blood volume as a means of controlling the transfer of heat to the body's surface.[38]

Convection

Convection refers to heat transfer through the circulation of air currents. Normally, a layer of warm air tends to remain near the body's surface. Convection causes continual removal of the warm layer and replacement with air from the surrounding environment. The wind-chill factor that often is included in the weather report combines the effect of convection because of wind with the still-air temperature.

Evaporation

Evaporation involves the use of body heat to convert water on the skin to water vapor. Water that diffuses through the skin independent of sweating is called *insensible perspiration.* Insensible perspiration losses are greatest in a dry environment. Sweating occurs through the sweat glands and is controlled by the sympathetic nervous system. Sweating is mediated by acetylcholine. This is unlike other sympathetically mediated functions in which the catecholamines serve as neuromediators. The impact of this is that anticholinergic drugs, such as atropine, can interfere with heat loss by interrupting sweating.

Evaporative heat losses involve insensible perspiration and sweating, with 0.58 cal being lost for each gram of water that is evaporated.[1] As long as body temperature is greater than the atmospheric temperature, heat is lost through radiation. However, when the temperature of the surrounding environment becomes greater than skin temperature, evaporation is the only way the body can rid itself of heat. Any condition that prevents evaporative heat losses causes the body temperature to rise.

IN SUMMARY

Core body temperature is normally maintained within a range of 36.0°C to 37.5°C (97.0°F to 99.5°F). Core body and skin temperatures are sensed and integrated by thermoregulatory regions in the hypothalamus and other brain structures that function to modify heat production and heat loss as a means of regulating body temperature. Metabolic processes that occur within deeper core structures (*i.e.*, muscles and viscera) of the body produce most of the body's heat. The sympathetic neurotransmitters (epinephrine and norepinephrine) and thyroid hormone act at the cellular level to shift body metabolism to heat production, whereas shivering and chattering of the teeth use the heat liberated from involuntary muscle movements to increase body temperature. Most of the body's heat losses occur at the skin surface as heat from the blood moves through the skin and from there into the surrounding environment. Heat is lost from the skin through radiation, conduction, convection, and evaporation of perspiration and sweat. Contraction of the *pilomotor muscles* of the skin aids in heat conservation by reducing the surface area available for heat loss.

INCREASED BODY TEMPERATURE

After completing this section of the chapter, the learner will be able to meet the following objectives:

- Characterize the physiology of fever.
- Differentiate between the physiologic mechanisms involved in fever and hyperthermia.
- Compare the mechanisms of malignant hyperthermia and neuroleptic malignant syndrome.

Both fever and hyperthermia describe conditions in which body temperature is higher than the normal range. Fever is due to an upward displacement of the thermostatic set point of the thermoregulatory center in the hypothalamus. This is in contrast to hyperthermia, in which the set point is unchanged, but the mechanisms that control body temperature are ineffective in maintaining body temperature within a normal range during situations when heat production outpaces the ability of the body to dissipate that heat.

Fever

Fever, or *pyrexia*, describes an elevation in body temperature that is caused by an upward displacement of the thermostatic set point of the hypothalamic thermoregulatory center. Temperature is one of the most frequent physiologic responses to be monitored during illness.

KEY POINTS

FEVER

- Fever represents an increase in body temperature that results from a cytokine-induced increase in the set point of the thermostatic center in the hypothalamus.
- Fever is a nonspecific response that is mediated by endogenous pyrogens released from host cells in response to infectious or noninfectious disorders.

Mechanisms

Many proteins, breakdown products of proteins, and certain other substances released from bacterial cell membranes can cause the set point to rise. Fever is resolved when the condition that caused the increase in the set point is removed. Fevers that are regulated by the hypothalamus usually do not rise above 41°C (105.8°F), suggesting a built-in thermostatic safety mechanism. Temperatures above that level are usually the result of superimposed activity, such as convulsions, hyperthermic states, or direct impairment of the temperature control center.

Pyrogens are exogenous or endogenous substances that produce fever. *Exogenous pyrogens* are derived from outside the body and include such substances as bacterial products, bacterial toxins, or whole microorganisms. Exogenous pyrogens induce host cells to produce fever-producing mediators called *endogenous pyrogens*. When bacteria or breakdown products of bacteria are present in blood or tissues, phagocytic cells of the immune system engulf them. These phagocytic cells digest the bacterial products and then release pyrogenic cytokines, principally interleukin-1 (IL-1), interleukin-6 (IL-6), and tumor necrosis factor-α (TNF-α), into the bloodstream for transport to the hypothalamus, where they exert their action.[3] These cytokines induce prostaglandin E_2 (PGE_2), which is a metabolite of arachidonic acid (an intramembrane fatty acid). It is hypothesized that when interleukin (IL-1B) interacts with the endothelial cells of the blood–brain barrier in the capillaries of the organum vasculosum laminae terminalis (OVLT), which is in the third ventricle above the optic chiasm, PGE_2 is released into the hypothalamus.[31]

At this point, PGE_2 binds to receptors in the hypothalamus to induce increases in the thermostatic set point through the second messenger cyclic adenosine monophosphate (cAMP). In response to the increase in its thermostatic set point, the hypothalamus initiates shivering and vasoconstriction that raise the body's core temperature to the new set point, and fever is established.

Although the central role of PGE_2 in raising the set point of the hypothalamic thermoregulatory center and producing fever is not questioned, research suggests that the febrile response to invading Gram-negative bacteria and their products (mainly endotoxic lipopolysaccharides) is mediated by PGE_2.[31]

In addition to their fever-producing actions, the endogenous pyrogens mediate a number of other responses. For example, IL-1 and TNF-α are inflammatory mediators that produce other signs of inflammation such as leukocytosis, anorexia, and malaise. Many noninfectious disorders, such as myocardial infarction, pulmonary emboli, and neoplasms, produce fever. In these conditions, the injured or abnormal cells incite the production of endogenous pyrogens. For example, trauma and surgery can be associated with up to 3 days of fever. Some malignant cells, such as those of leukemia and Hodgkin disease, secrete chemical mediators that function as endogenous pyrogens.

A fever that has its origin in the CNS is sometimes referred to as a *neurogenic fever*. It usually is caused by damage to the hypothalamus because of CNS trauma, intracerebral bleeding, or an increase in intracranial pressure. Neurogenic fever is characterized by a high temperature that is resistant to antipyretic therapy and is not associated with sweating.

Purpose

The purpose of fever is not completely understood. However, from a purely practical standpoint, fever is a valuable index to health status. For many, fever signals the presence of an infection and may legitimize the need for medical treatment. There is little research to support the belief that fever below 40°C (104°F) is harmful. In fact, animal studies have demonstrated a clear survival advantage in infected members with fever compared with animals that were unable to produce a fever. It has also been shown that small elevations in temperature such as those that occur with fever enhance immune function by T lymphocyte proliferation.[3] Many of the microbial agents that cause infection grow best at normal body temperatures, and their growth is inhibited by temperatures in the fever range.

Even mild fever, however, is negative in many situations, such as in older adults who have cardiac or pulmonary disease, because it causes more of a demand for oxygen. For every elevated 1°C of temperature, the BMR increases by 7% and causing increased work for the heart. Fever can also produce confusion, tachycardia, and tachypnea. Cell damage can occur when temperatures are elevated greater than 42.2°C (108°F), and this can ultimately cause life-threatening acidosis, hypoxia, and hyperkalemia.[38]

Patterns

The patterns of temperature change in people with fever vary. Additionally, the average diurnal variation in temperature yields a peak rise in the late afternoon or early evening.[32] These patterns can be described as intermittent, remittent, sustained, or relapsing (Fig. 14.14). An *intermittent fever* is one in which temperature returns to normal at least once every 24 hours. In a *remittent fever*, the temperature does not return to normal and varies a few degrees in either direction. In a *sustained* or *continuous fever*, the temperature remains above normal with minimal variations (usually <0.55°C or 1°F). A *recurrent* or *relapsing fever* is one in which there is one or more episodes of fever, each as long as several days, with one or more days of normal temperature between episodes.

Critical to the analysis of a fever pattern is the relation of heart rate to the level of temperature elevation. Most people respond to an increase in temperature with an appropriate increase in heart rate. The observation that a rise in temperature is not accompanied by the anticipated change in heart rate can provide useful information about the cause of the fever. For example, a heart rate that is slower than would be anticipated can occur with Legionnaire disease and drug fever, and a heart rate that is more rapid than anticipated can be symptomatic of hyperthyroidism and pulmonary emboli.

Clinical Manifestations

The physiologic behaviors that occur during the development of fever can be divided into four successive stages (Fig. 14.15):

1. A prodrome
2. A chill, during which the temperature rises
3. A flush
4. Defervescence

During the *first* or *prodromal* period, there are nonspecific complaints such as mild headache and fatigue, general malaise, and fleeting aches and pains. During the *second stage* or *chill*, there is the uncomfortable sensation of being chilled and the onset of generalized shaking (rigors), although the temperature is rising. Vasoconstriction and piloerection usually precede the onset of shivering. At this point, the skin is pale and covered with goose flesh. There is a feeling of being cold and an urge to put on more clothing or covering and to curl up in a position that conserves body heat. When the shivering has caused the body temperature to reach the new set point of the temperature control center, the shivering ceases, and a sensation of warmth develops. At this point, the *third stage* or *flush* begins, during which cutaneous vasodilation occurs and the skin becomes warm and flushed. The *fourth*, or *defervescence*, stage of the febrile response is marked by the initiation of sweating. Not all people proceed through the four stages of fever development. Sweating may be absent, and fever may develop gradually with no indication of a chill or shivering.

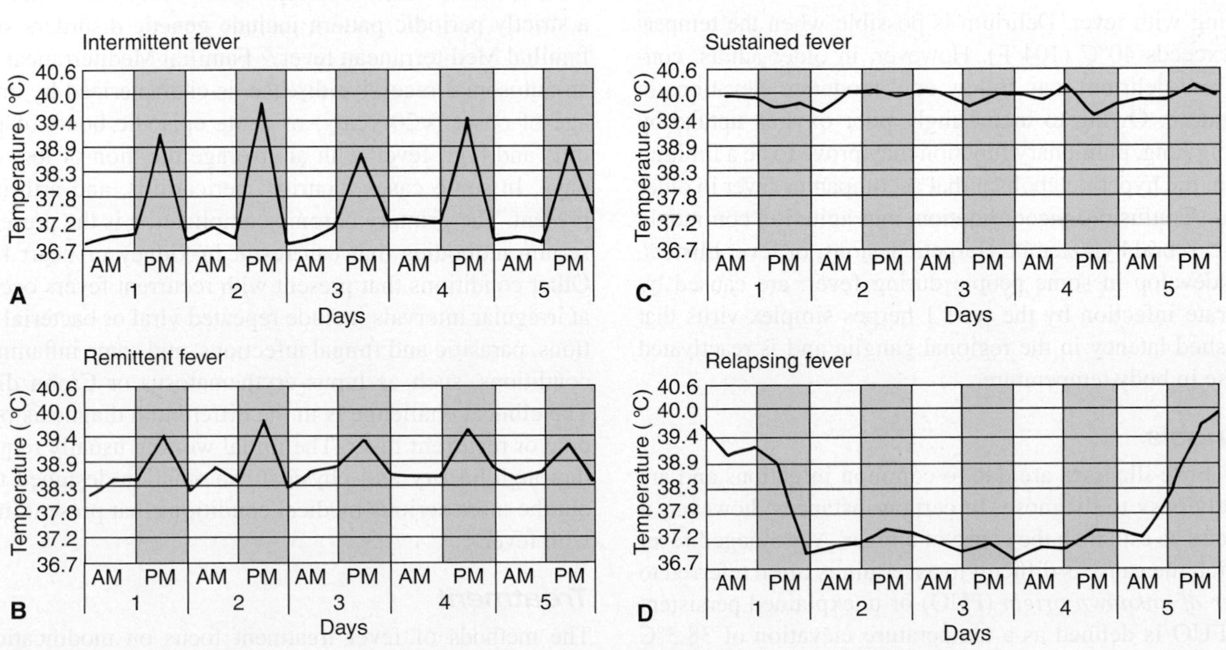

Figure 14.14 • Schematic representation of fever patterns: (A) intermittent, (B) remittent, (C) sustained, and (D) recurrent or relapsing.

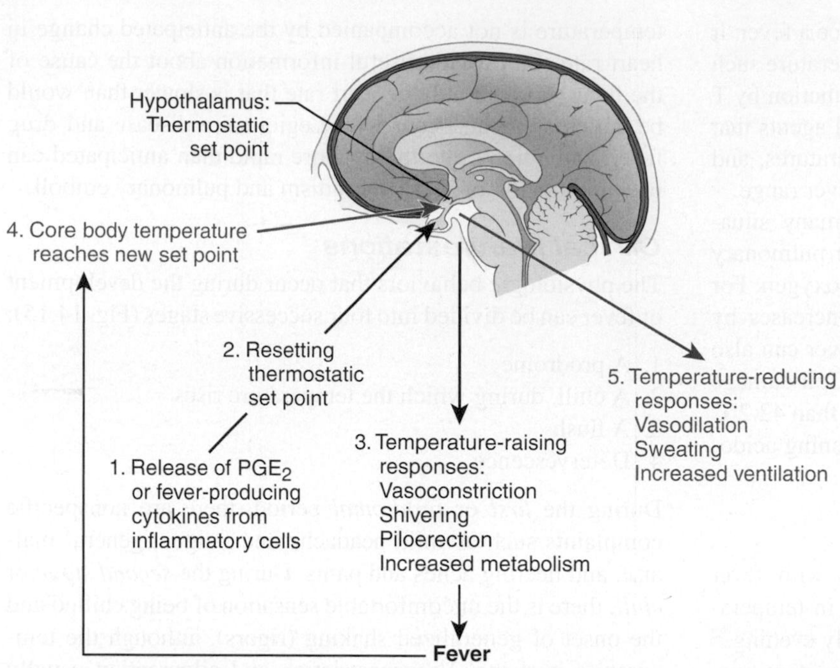

Figure 14.15 • Mechanisms of fever. (*1*) Release of prostaglandin E_2 (PGE_2) or fever-producing cytokines from inflammatory cells; (*2*) resetting of the thermostatic set point in the hypothalamus to a higher level (prodrome); (*3*) generation of hypothalamus-mediated responses that raise body temperature (chill); (*4*) development of fever with elevation of body to new thermostatic set point; and (*5*) production of temperature-lowering responses (flush and defervescence) and return of body temperature to a lower level.

Common clinical manifestations of fever are anorexia, myalgia, arthralgia, and fatigue. These discomforts are worse when the temperature rises rapidly or exceeds 39.5°C (103.1°F). Respiration is increased, and the heart rate usually is elevated. Dehydration occurs because of sweating and the increased vapor losses because of the rapid respiratory rate. Many of the manifestations of fever are related to the increases in the metabolic rate, increases in oxygen demands, and use of body proteins as an energy source. With prolonged fever, there is an increased breakdown of endogenous fat stores. If fat breakdown is rapid, metabolic acidosis may result.

Headache is a common accompaniment of fever and is thought to result from the vasodilation of cerebral vessels occurring with fever. Delirium is possible when the temperature exceeds 40°C (104°F). However, in older adults, confusion and delirium may follow only moderate elevations in temperature. Owing to increasingly poor oxygen uptake by the aging lung, pulmonary function may prove to be a limiting factor in the hypermetabolism that accompanies fever in older persons. Confusion, incoordination, and agitation commonly reflect cerebral hypoxemia. Herpetic lesions, or fever blisters, which develop in some people during fever, are caused by a separate infection by the type 1 herpes simplex virus that established latency in the regional ganglia and is reactivated by a rise in body temperature.

Diagnosis

Most febrile illnesses are due to common infections and are relatively easy to diagnose. In certain instances, however, it is difficult to establish the cause of a fever. A prolonged fever for which the cause is difficult to ascertain is often referred to as *fever of unknown origin* (FUO) or unexplained persistent fever. FUO is defined as a temperature elevation of 38.3°C (101°F) or higher that is present for 3 weeks or longer and includes 1 week of comprehensive diagnostic testing that does not identify a diagnosis.[27] Among the causes of FUO are malignancies (*i.e.*, lymphomas, metastases to the liver and CNS); infections such as human immunodeficiency virus, tuberculosis, or abscessed infections; and drug fever. Malignancies, particularly non-Hodgkin lymphoma, are important causes of FUO in the elderly. Cirrhosis of the liver is another cause of FUO.

Recurrent or periodic fevers may occur in predictable intervals or without any discernible time pattern. They may be associated with no discernible cause, or they can be the presenting symptom of several serious illnesses, often preceding the other symptoms of those diseases by weeks or months. Conditions in which recurrent fevers occur but do not follow a strictly periodic pattern include genetic disorders such as familial Mediterranean fever.[27] Familial Mediterranean fever, an autosomal recessive disease, is characterized by an early age of onset (<20 years) of acute episodic bouts of peritonitis and high fever with an average duration of less than 2 days. In some cases pleuritis, pericarditis, and arthritis are present. The primary chronic complication is the presence of serum antibodies that can result in kidney or heart failure. Other conditions that present with recurrent fevers occurring at irregular intervals include repeated viral or bacterial infections, parasitic and fungal infections, and some inflammatory conditions, such as lupus erythematosus or Crohn disease. The clinical challenge is in the differential diagnosis of periodic or recurrent fever. The initial workup usually requires a thorough history and physical examination designed to rule out the more serious medical conditions that present initially with fever.

Treatment

The methods of fever treatment focus on modifications of the external environment intended to increase heat transfer from the internal to the external environment, support of the hypermetabolic state that accompanies fever, protection of vulnerable body organs and systems, and treatment of the infection or condition causing the fever. Because fever is a disease symptom, its manifestation suggests the need for diagnosis and treatment of the primary cause.

Modification of the environment ensures that the environmental temperature facilitates heat transfer away from the body. Sponge baths with cool water or an alcohol solution can be used to increase evaporative heat losses, but caution is necessary, so the person is not cooled too quickly. It is better to bring the person to a health care practice to obtain advice on whether the person may need intravenous lines for hydration and other medical attention. More profound cooling can be accomplished through the use of forced air blankets or a cooling mattress, which facilitates the conduction of heat from the body into the coolant solution that circulates through the mattress. Care must be taken so that the cooling method does not produce vasoconstriction and shivering that decrease heat loss and increase heat production.

Adequate fluids and sufficient amounts of simple carbohydrates are needed to support the hypermetabolic state and prevent the tissue breakdown that is characteristic of fever. Additional replacement fluids are needed for sweating and to balance the insensible water losses from the lungs that accompany an increase in respiratory rate. Fluids also are needed to maintain an adequate vascular volume for heat transport to the skin surface.

Antipyretic drugs, such as aspirin, ibuprofen, and acetaminophen, often are used to alleviate the discomforts of fever and protect vulnerable organs, such as the brain, from extreme elevations in body temperature. It is thought that these drugs act by resetting the set point of the temperature-regulating center in the hypothalamus to a lower level, presumably by blocking the activity of COX, an enzyme that is required for the conversion of arachidonic acid to PGE_2. However, evidence suggests that the routine administration of antipyretics does not decrease the duration of the fever or illness.[36,39] Because of the risk of Reye syndrome, the Centers for Disease Control and Prevention, FDA, and American Academy of Pediatrics Committee on Infectious Diseases advise against the use of aspirin and other salicylates in children with influenza or chickenpox.

Fever in Children

Fever occurs frequently in infants and young children and is a common reason for visits to the emergency department. Infants and young children have decreased immunologic function and are more commonly infected with virulent organisms. Also, the mechanisms for controlling temperature are not as well developed in infants as they are in older children and adults. Even though infants with fever may not appear ill, this does not imply an absence of bacterial disease. In infants younger than 3 months, a mild elevation in temperature (*i.e.*, rectal temperature of 38°C [100.4°F]) can indicate serious infection.

Although the differential diagnosis of fever is quite broad and includes both infectious and noninfectious causes, the majority of febrile children have an underlying infection. The most common causes are minor or more serious infections of the respiratory system, gastrointestinal tract, urinary tract, or CNS. The epidemiology of serious bacterial disease has changed dramatically with the introduction of the *Haemophilus influenzae* and *Streptococcus pneumoniae* vaccines in developed countries. *H. influenzae* type b has been nearly eliminated, and the incidence of pneumococcal disease caused by vaccine and cross-reactive vaccine serotypes has declined substantially. Fever in infants and children can be classified as low risk or high risk, depending on the probability of the infection progressing to bacteremia or meningitis and signs of toxicity. Infants between the ages of 1 and 28 days with a fever should be considered to have a bacterial infection that can cause bacteremia or meningitis. Signs of toxicity include lethargy, poor feeding, hypoventilation, poor tissue oxygenation, and cyanosis. A white blood cell count with differential and blood cultures usually is taken in high-risk infants and children to determine the cause of fever. A chest radiograph should be obtained in febrile infants younger than 3 months of age with at least one sign of a respiratory illness (*e.g.*, tachypnea, crackles, decreased breath sounds, wheezing, coughing).[27] Febrile children who are younger than 1 year of age and girls between 1 and 2 years of age should be considered at risk for a urinary tract infection.[27]

The approach to treatment of the young child who has a fever without a known source varies depending on the age of the child. High-risk infants and infants who are younger than 28 days are often hospitalized for evaluation of their fever and treatment.[27]

Fever in Older Adults

In the elderly, even slight elevations in temperature may indicate serious infection or disease, most often caused by bacteria. This is because the elderly often have a lower baseline temperature, and although they increase their temperature during an infection, it may fail to reach a level that is equated with significant fever.[27,40] Normal body temperature and the circadian pattern of temperature variation often are altered in the elderly. Fever in the older adult does increase the older adult's immunologic response, but it is generally a much weaker response compared to younger people.[40]

It has been suggested that older adults with serious infections present with an absent or blunted febrile response.[41] The probable mechanisms for the blunted fever response include a disturbance in sensing of temperature by the thermoregulatory center in the hypothalamus, alterations in release of endogenous pyrogens, and the failure to elicit responses such as vasoconstriction of skin vessels, increased heat production, and shivering that increase body temperature during a febrile response.

Absence of fever may delay diagnosis and initiation of antimicrobial treatment. Therefore, it is important to perform a thorough history and physical examination focusing on other signs of infection and sepsis in older adults. Signs of infection in older adults when fever is absent include unexplained changes in functional capacity, worsening of mental status, weakness and fatigue, and weight loss.

Another factor that may delay recognition of fever in older adults is the method of temperature measurement. It has been suggested that rectal and tympanic membrane methods are more effective in detecting fever in the elderly. This is because conditions such as mouth breathing, tongue tremors, and agitation often make it difficult to obtain accurate oral temperatures in older adults.

Hyperthermia

Hyperthermia describes an increase in body temperature that occurs without a change in the set point of the hypothalamic thermoregulatory center. It occurs when the thermoregulatory mechanisms are overwhelmed by heat production, excessive environmental heat, or impaired dissipation of heat.[40] It includes (in order of increasing severity) heat cramps, heat exhaustion, and heatstroke. Malignant hyperthermia describes a rare genetic disorder of anesthetic-related hyperthermia. Hyperthermia also may occur as the result of a drug reaction.

A number of factors predispose individuals to hyperthermia. If muscle exertion is continued for long periods in warm weather, as often happens with athletes, military recruits, and laborers, excessive heat loads are generated. Because adequate circulatory function is essential for heat dissipation, elderly people and those with cardiovascular disease are at increased risk for hyperthermia. Drugs that increase muscle tone and metabolism or reduce heat loss (*e.g.*, diuretics, neuroleptics, drugs with anticholinergic action) can impair thermoregulation. Infants and small children who are left in a closed car for even short periods in hot weather are at risk for hyperthermia.

The best approach to heat-related disorders is prevention, primarily by avoiding activity in hot environments, increasing fluid intake, and wearing climate- and activity-appropriate clothing. The ability to tolerate a hot environment depends on both temperature and humidity. A high relative humidity retards heat loss through sweating and evaporation and decreases the body's cooling ability. The *heat index* is the temperature that the body senses when both the temperature and humidity are combined.

KEY POINTS

HYPERTHERMIA

- Hyperthermia is a pathologic increase in core body temperature without a change in the hypothalamic set point. The thermoregulatory center is overwhelmed by either excess heat production, impaired heat loss, or excessive environmental heat.
- Malignant hyperthermia is an autosomal dominant disorder in which an abnormal release of intracellular stores of calcium causes uncontrolled skeletal muscle contractions, resulting in a rapid increase in core body temperature. This usually is in response to an anesthetic.

Heat Cramps

Heat cramps are slow, painful, skeletal muscle cramps and spasms, usually occurring in the muscles that are most heavily used and lasting for 1 to 3 minutes. Cramping results from salt depletion that occurs when fluid losses from heavy sweating are replaced by water alone. The muscles are tender, and the skin usually is moist. Body temperature may be normal or slightly elevated. There almost always is a history of vigorous activity preceding the onset of symptoms.

Heat Exhaustion

Heat exhaustion is related to a gradual loss of salt and water, usually after prolonged and heavy exertion in a hot environment. The symptoms include thirst, fatigue, nausea, oliguria, giddiness, and finally delirium. Gastrointestinal flulike symptoms are common. Hyperventilation in association with heat exhaustion may contribute to heat cramps and tetany by causing respiratory alkalosis. The skin is moist, the rectal temperature usually is higher than 37.8°C (100°F) but below 40°C (104°F), and the heart rate is elevated. Signs of heat cramps may accompany heat exhaustion.

Heatstroke

Heatstroke is a severe, life-threatening failure of thermoregulatory mechanisms resulting in an excessive increase in body temperature—a core temperature greater than 40°C (104°F); a hot, dry skin; absence of sweating; and possible CNS abnormalities such as delirium, convulsions, and loss of consciousness.[42] On average there are 5946 persons treated annually in hospital emergency departments for exercise-related heatstroke in the United States.[43] The risk of developing heatstroke in response to heat stress is increased in conditions (*i.e.*, alcoholism, obesity, diabetes mellitus, and chronic cardiac, renal, or mental disease) and with drugs (*i.e.*, alcohol, anticholinergics, beta blockers, or tricyclic antidepressants) that impair vasodilation and sweating.[42]

The pathophysiology of heatstroke is thought to result from the direct effect of heat on body cells and the release of cytokines (*e.g.*, interleukins, TNF-α, and interferon) from heat-stressed endothelial cells, leukocytes, and epithelial cells that protect against tissue injury. The net result is a combination of local and systemic inflammatory responses that may result in acute respiratory distress syndrome, acute renal failure, disseminated intravascular coagulation, and multiorgan disorders.

The symptoms of heatstroke include tachycardia, hyperventilation, dizziness, weakness, emotional lability, nausea and vomiting, confusion, delirium, blurred vision, convulsions, collapse, and coma. The skin is hot and usually dry, and the pulse is typically strong initially. The blood pressure may be elevated at first, but hypotension develops as the condition progresses. As vascular collapse occurs, the skin becomes cool. Associated abnormalities include electrocardiographic changes consistent with heart damage, blood coagulation disorders, potassium and sodium depletion, and signs of liver damage.

Treatment consists of measures to support the function of vital organs while instituting cooling procedures aimed at producing a rapid reduction in core temperature. Care must be taken that the cooling methods used do not produce vasoconstriction or shivering and thereby decrease the cooling rate or induce heat production.

Drug Fever

Drug fever has been defined as fever coinciding with the administration of a drug and disappearing after the drug has been discontinued.[32] Drugs can induce fever by several mechanisms. They can interfere with heat dissipation, they can alter temperature regulation by the hypothalamic centers, they can act as direct pyrogens, they can injure tissues directly, or they can induce an immune response.

Exogenous thyroid hormone increases the metabolic rate and can increase heat production and body temperature. Research demonstrates that propylthiouracil (PTU) has several side effects including fever and that use of PTU can induce fever and cause interstitial pneumonia.[44] Peripheral heat dissipation can be impaired by atropine and anticholinergic drugs, antihistamines, phenothiazine antipsychotic drugs, and tricyclic antidepressants, which decrease sweating, or by amphetamines (especially ecstasy), cocaine, and sympathomimetic drugs, which produce peripheral vasoconstriction.[2] Intravenously administered drugs can lead to infusion-related phlebitis with production of cellular pyrogens that produce fever. Treatment with anticancer drugs can cause the release of endogenous pyrogen from the cancer cells that are destroyed. Overdoses of serotonin reuptake inhibitors or use in people taking monoamine oxidase (MOA) inhibitors can cause agitation, hyperactivity, and hyperthermia (serotonin syndrome).[32]

The most common cause of drug fever is a *hypersensitivity reaction*. Hypersensitivity drug fevers develop after several weeks of exposure to the drug, cannot be explained in terms of the drug's pharmacologic action, are not related to drug dose, disappear when the drug is stopped, and reappear when the drug is readministered. The fever pattern is typically spiking in nature and exhibits a normal diurnal rhythm. Persons with drug fevers often experience other signs of hypersensitivity reactions, such as arthralgias, urticaria, myalgias, gastrointestinal discomfort, and rashes.

Temperatures of 38.9°C to 40.0°C (101.8°F to 104.0°F) are common in drug fever. The person may be unaware of the fever and appear to be well for the degree of fever that is present. The absence of an appropriate increase in heart rate for the degree of temperature elevation is an important clue to the diagnosis of drug fever. A fever often precedes other, more serious effects of a drug reaction. For this reason, the early recognition of drug fever is important. Drug fever should be suspected whenever the temperature elevation is unexpected and occurs despite improvement in the condition for which the drug was prescribed.

Malignant Hyperthermia

Malignant hyperthermia is an autosomal dominant metabolic disorder in which heat generated by uncontrolled skeletal muscle contraction can produce severe and potentially fatal hyperthermia.[32] Generally, the mutation involves the RYR1 gene on chromosome 19q13.1.[32] The muscle contraction is caused by an abnormal release of intracellular calcium from the sarcoplasmic reticulum through calcium release channels. The release of calcium at an abnormally high rate also leads to a sustained hypermetabolic rate and a subsequent loss of cellular integrity. The sustained hypermetabolism results in excess lactate production, high ATP consumption, increased oxygen consumption and carbon dioxide production, and elevated heat production.

In affected people, an episode of malignant hyperthermia is triggered by exposure to certain stresses or general anesthetic agents, which can cause an acute or insidious onset of symptoms.[45] The syndrome most frequently is associated with the halogenated anesthetic agents (halothane) and the depolarizing muscle relaxant succinylcholine. There also are various nonoperative precipitating factors, including trauma, exercise, environmental heat stress, and infection. The condition is particularly dangerous in a young person who has a large muscle mass to generate heat.

In addition to a steady rise in end-tidal carbon dioxide levels, an initial sign of the disorder, when the condition occurs during anesthesia, is skeletal muscle rigidity. Cardiac arrhythmias and a hypermetabolic state follow in rapid sequence unless the triggering event is immediately discontinued. In addition to discontinuing the triggering agents, treatment includes measures to cool the body, cardiopulmonary support, and the administration of dantrolene, a muscle relaxant drug that acts by blocking the release of calcium from the sarcoplasmic reticulum.

Neuroleptic Malignant Syndrome

The neuroleptic malignant syndrome is associated with neuroleptic (psychotropic) medications and may occur in as many as 0.02% to 3.23% of people taking such drugs.[32] Most of these drugs block dopamine receptors in the basal ganglia and hypothalamus. Hyperthermia is thought to result from alterations in the function of the hypothalamic thermoregulatory center. Because many of the neuroleptic drugs produce an increase in muscle contraction similar to that of malignant hyperthermia, it has been suggested that the disorder may be caused by a spectrum of inherited defects in genes that are responsible for a variety of calcium regulatory mechanisms in sympathetic neurons (*e.g.*, dopaminergic neurons). The syndrome usually has an explosive onset and is characterized by hyperthermia, muscle rigidity, alterations in consciousness, and autonomic nervous system dysfunction. The hyperthermia is accompanied by tachycardia, cardiac dysrhythmias, labile blood pressure dyspnea, and tachypnea.[32]

Treatment for neuroleptic malignant syndrome includes the immediate discontinuance of the neuroleptic drug, measures to decrease body temperature, and treatment of dysrhythmias and other complications of the disorder. Bromocriptine (a dopamine agonist) and dantrolene (a muscle relaxant) may be used as part of the treatment regimen.

IN SUMMARY

Fever and hyperthermia refer to an increase in body temperature outside the normal range. True fever is a disorder of thermoregulation in which there is an upward displacement of the set point for temperature control. In hyperthermia, the set point is unchanged, but the challenge to temperature regulation exceeds the thermoregulatory center's ability to control body temperature. Fever can be caused by a number of factors, including microorganisms, trauma, and drugs or chemicals, all of which incite the release of endogenous pyrogens. The reactions that occur during fever consist of four stages: a prodrome, a chill, a flush, and a defervescence. A fever can follow an intermittent, remittent, sustained, or recurrent pattern. The manifestations of fever are largely related to dehydration and an increased metabolic rate. Even a low-grade fever in high-risk infants or in older adults can indicate serious infection.

The treatment of fever focuses on modifying the external environment as a means of increasing heat transfer to the external environment, supporting the hypermetabolic state that accompanies fever, protecting vulnerable body tissues, and treating the infection or condition causing the fever.

Hyperthermia, which varies in severity based on the degree of core temperature elevation and the severity of cardiovascular and nervous system involvement, includes heat cramps, heat exhaustion, and heatstroke. Among the factors that contribute to the development of hyperthermia are prolonged muscular exertion in a hot environment, disorders that compromise heat dissipation, and hypersensitivity drug reactions. Malignant hyperthermia is an autosomal dominant disorder that can produce a severe and potentially fatal increase in body temperature. The condition commonly is triggered by general anesthetic agents and muscle relaxants used during surgery. The neuroleptic malignant syndrome is associated with neuroleptic drug therapy and is thought to result from alterations in the function of the thermoregulatory center or from uncontrolled muscle contraction.

DECREASED BODY TEMPERATURE

After completing this section of the chapter, the learner will be able to meet the following objectives:

- Define *hypothermia*.
- Compare the manifestations of mild, moderate, and severe hypothermia and relate them to changes in physiologic functioning that occur with decreased body temperature.
- Describe the causes of heat loss and hypothermia in the newborn infant and in the person undergoing surgery.

Hypothermia

Hypothermia is defined as a core temperature (*i.e.*, rectal, esophageal, or tympanic) less than 35°C (95°F).[46] Accidental hypothermia may be defined as a spontaneous decrease in core temperature, usually in a cold environment and associated with an acute problem but without a primary disorder of the temperature-regulating center. In children, the rapid cooling process, in addition to the diving reflex that triggers apnea and circulatory shunting to establish a heart–brain circulation, may account for the surprisingly high survival rate after cold water submersion. The diving reflex is greatly diminished in adults.

Systemic hypothermia may result from exposure to prolonged cold (atmospheric or submersion). The condition may develop in otherwise healthy people in the course of accidental exposure. Because water conducts heat more readily than air, body temperature drops rapidly when the body is submerged in cold water or when clothing becomes wet. In people with altered homeostasis due to debility or disease, hypothermia may follow exposure to relatively small decreases in atmospheric temperature.

Many underlying conditions can contribute to the development of hypothermia. Malnutrition decreases the fuel available for heat generation, and loss of body fat decreases tissue insulation. Alcohol and sedative drugs dull mental awareness to cold temperatures and impair judgment to seek shelter or put on additional clothing. Alcohol also inhibits shivering. People with cardiovascular disease, cerebrovascular disease, spinal cord injury, and hypothyroidism also are predisposed to hypothermia.

Neonatal Hypothermia

Infants are particularly at risk for hypothermia because of their high ratio of surface area to body mass. Relative to body weight, the body surface area of an infant is three times that of an adult, and in infants with low birth weight, the insulating layer of subcutaneous fat is thinner. The newborn infant is particularly at risk, but the premature newborn is at greatest risk for heat loss and hypothermia.31 Under the usual delivery room conditions (20°C to 25°C [68°F to 77°F]), an infant's skin temperature falls approximately 0.3°C/minute and deep body temperature by approximately 0.1°C/minute. The heat loss occurs by convection to the cooler surrounding air, by conduction to cooler materials on which the infant is resting, by radiation to nearby cooler solid objects, and by evaporation from the moist skin. The unstable body temperature of a preterm infant can drop precipitously after delivery, and this hypothermia is associated with an increase in morbidity and mortality.

The newborn infant does have one important process to fight against hypothermia. This process is called nonshivering thermogenesis, and it occurs primarily in the liver, brown fat tissue, and brain.[1] Brown fat differs from regular adipose tissue because it has a high number of mitochondria. Newborns have this brown fat tissue in their necks and upper back. The brown fat has an uncoupling protein called UCP1 (thermogenin), which allows oxidation of fatty acids to produce heat. The extreme cold temperature stimulates a release of epinephrine and TSH, which causes a release of T_3 and T_4. Epinephrine activates the 5′/3′-monodeiodinase, which assists with the conversion of T_4 to the more rapid-acting T_3. The T_3 acts in the brown fat to release the mitochondrial oxidation from phosphorylation. This, in turn, causes more heat production.[1]

Perioperative Hypothermia

People who undergo surgical procedures are also at risk for hypothermia. It is especially important to prevent hypothermia in thin, debilitated, intoxicated, and older people undergoing surgery by using rewarming therapies and other nursing interventions such as decreased skin exposure and preoperative warming.[47] Perioperative hypothermia is the result of a cold environment and impaired thermoregulatory mechanisms brought about by anesthetics and other drugs. For each one degree temperature loss, there is a 7% decrease in metabolic demands by the body.[48] Both general and regional anesthetic agents disrupt many of the body's thermoregulatory mechanisms. General anesthetic agents lower the metabolic rate and decrease vasoconstriction and shivering thresholds. Postanesthetic shivering is a common complication of modern anesthesia. Apart from discomfort, postanesthesia shivering is associated with a number of potentially dangerous sequelae, including increased oxygen consumption and carbon dioxide production, increased cardiorespiratory effort, and effects of increased catecholamine (epinephrine and norepinephrine) release. These effects can pose a problem to recovery in vulnerable populations such as older adults and people with marginal cardiopulmonary reserves, impaired oxygen-carrying capacity (anemia), and other health problems.

A number of methods are used to prevent heat loss during surgery. Core temperature monitoring, accompanied by passive and active methods to maintain normal body temperature, should be part of routine inoperative monitoring. In many cases, some form of active rewarming is required. Preoperatively, people are assessed carefully for any type of infection, if one is found, surgery will be postponed.

Clinical Manifestations

The signs and symptoms of hypothermia include poor coordination, stumbling, slurred speech, irrationality and poor judgment, amnesia, hallucinations, blueness and puffiness of the skin, dilation of the pupils, decreased respiratory rate, weak and irregular pulse, and stupor. With mild hypothermia, intense shivering generates heat and sympathetic nervous system activity is raised to resist lowering of temperature. Vasoconstriction can be profound, heart rate is accelerated, and stroke volume is increased. Blood pressure increases slightly, and hyperventilation is common. Exposure to cold augments urinary flow (*i.e.*, cold diuresis) before there is any fall in temperature. Dehydration and increased hematocrit may develop within a few hours of even mild hypothermia, augmented by an extracellular to intracellular water shift.

With moderate hypothermia, shivering gradually decreases, and the muscles become rigid. Heart rate and stroke volume are reduced, and blood pressure falls, along with metabolic rate. Associated with this decrease in metabolic rate is a decrease in oxygen consumption and carbon dioxide production. There is roughly a 7% decrease in oxygen consumption for every 1°C (2°F) decrease in temperature. A decrease in carbon dioxide production leads to a decrease in respiratory rate. Respirations decrease as temperatures drop below 32.2°C (90°F). Decreases in mentation, the cough reflex, and respiratory tract secretions may lead to difficulty in clearing secretions and aspiration. In terms of cardiovascular function, a gradual decline in heart rate and cardiac output occurs as hypothermia progresses. Blood pressure initially rises and then gradually falls. There is increased risk of dysrhythmia developing, probably from myocardial hypoxia and autonomic nervous system imbalance. Ventricular fibrillation is a major cause of death in hypothermia.

Carbohydrate metabolism and insulin activity are decreased, resulting in a hyperglycemia that is proportional to the level of cooling. A cold-induced loss of cell membrane integrity allows intravascular fluids to move into the skin, giving the skin a puffy appearance. Acid–base disorders occur with increased frequency at temperatures below 25°C (77°F) unless adequate ventilation is maintained. Extracellular sodium and potassium concentrations decrease, and chloride levels increase. There is a temporary loss of plasma from the circulation along with sludging of red blood cells and increased blood viscosity as the result of trapping in the small vessels and skin.

Diagnosis and Treatment

Oral temperatures are markedly inaccurate during hypothermia because of severe vasoconstriction and sluggish blood flow. Electronic thermometers with flexible probes are available for measuring rectal, bladder, and esophageal temperatures. Most clinical thermometers measure temperature only in the range of 35°C to 42°C (95°F to 107.6°F); a special thermometer that registers as low as 25°C (77°F) or an electrical thermistor probe is needed for monitoring temperatures in people with hypothermia. Treatment of hypothermia consists of rewarming, support of vital functions, and the prevention and treatment of complications.

Therapeutic Hypothermia

Controlled hypothermia may be used after brain injury and during certain types of surgery to decrease inflammation and brain metabolism. This controlled therapeutic hypothermia has been found helpful for people who have had cardiac arrest because of ventricular fibrillation in terms of increasing the person's neurologic outcomes.[47] Intraoperatively, especially with cardiothoracic surgery, people are kept hypothermic between 82.4°F and 89.6°F to decrease metabolic demands and prevent ischemic injury.[48] Myocardial ischemia is prevented by injecting cold cardioplegia solution at 39.2°F into the aortic root under pressure.[48] This solution is heavily composed of potassium, which causes asystole and hypothermia to protect the myocardium during the surgery.[48] Additionally, to maintain myocardial hypothermia, an iced normal saline slush is administered topically. There are, however, some potential complications to cold cardioplegia, such as ventricular dysrhythmias, decreased cerebral blood flow, and postoperative myocardial depression. Therefore, some surgeons use a normothermic blood cardioplegia.[48] After the surgery is complete, warmed blood is perfused to people who were hypothermic during surgery. It takes some time to rewarm the person back to 98.6°F core body temperature, and the rewarming has to be performed slowly. Attempts to prevent shivering and severe vasoconstriction are made.[48] However, if there is a bleeding problem postoperatively, restoration of body temperature needs to be done as quickly and as safely as possible. Currently there is much controversy over using hypothermia for situations such as TBI, cardiac arrest, spinal cord injury, stroke, increased intracranial pressure, hepatic encephalopathy, and spinal cord injury.[49]

IN SUMMARY

Hypothermia is a potentially life-threatening disorder in which the body's core temperature drops below 35°C (95°F). Accidental hypothermia can develop in otherwise healthy people in the course of accidental exposure and in older adults or disabled people with impaired perception of or response to cold. Alcoholism, cardiovascular disease, malnutrition, and hypothyroidism contribute to the risk of hypothermia. Hypothermia is also a common occurrence in newborn infants, particularly those born prematurely, and in people undergoing an operation. The greatest effect of hypothermia is a decrease in the metabolic rate, leading to a decrease in carbon dioxide production and respiratory rate. Clinical manifestations of hypothermia include poor coordination, stumbling, slurred speech, irrationality, poor judgment, amnesia, hallucinations, blueness and puffiness of the skin, dilation of the pupils, decreased respiratory rate, weak and irregular pulse, stupor, and coma. Treatment of hypothermia includes passive or active rewarming, support of vital functions, and the prevention and treatment of complications.

GERIATRIC Considerations

- Persistent pain is commonly widespread in the older adult; fibromyalgia and generalized osteoarthritis are identified as causes.[50]
- Body temperature is lower in older adults (96.9°F to 98.3°F), making it important to record a baseline to determine when fever may be present.[51]
- An undetected elevation in temperature places stress on the heart, increasing the heart rate 10 beats/minute for each 1°F elevation.[51]

PEDIATRIC Considerations

- Children manifest chronic pain the same as acute pain.[52]
- Psychological and environmental factors play a much bigger role in pain perception than for the adult.[52]
- Children of any age, including newborns, experience pain. In the younger infant, facial expression (squeezing eyes shut, mouth open) indicates pain.[52]
- FACES pain rating scale (http://wongbakerfaces.org) can be used in very young children (3 to 4 years) to describe the degree of pain.
- Temperament has been found to predict both distress and pain levels in children.[52]
- Use the least invasive method to assess a child's temperature. Oral temperature is reliable once the child can cooperate, usually about age 5. The rectal method should be avoided in the immunocompromised child.[52]

REVIEW EXERCISES

1. A 25-year-old man is admitted to the emergency department with acute abdominal pain that began in the epigastric area and has now shifted to the lower right quadrant of the abdomen. There is localized tenderness and guarding or spasm of the muscle over the area. His heart rate and blood pressure are elevated, and his skin is moist and cool from perspiring. He is given a tentative diagnosis of appendicitis and referred for surgical consultation.
   A. *Describe the origin of the pain stimuli and the neural pathways involved in the pain that this man is experiencing.*
   B. *Explain the neural mechanisms involved in the spasm of the overlying abdominal muscles.*
   C. *What is the significance of his cool, moist skin and increased heart rate and blood pressure?*
2. A 65-year-old woman with breast cancer is receiving hospice care in her home. She is currently receiving a long-acting opioid analgesic supplemented with a short-acting combination opioid and nonnarcotic medication for breakthrough pain.
   A. *Explain the difference between the mechanisms and treatment of acute and chronic pain.*
   B. *Describe the action of opioid drugs in the treatment of pain.*
   C. *Define the terms tolerance and cross-tolerance as they refer to the use of opioids for treatment of pain.*

D. Describe the common side effects associated with the use of opioid drugs to relieve pain in persons with cancer.

3. A 42-year-old woman presents with sudden, stabbing-type facial pain that arises near the right side of her mouth and then shoots toward the right ear, eye, and nostril. She is holding her hand to protect her face because the pain is "triggered by touch, movement, and drafts." Her initial diagnosis is trigeminal neuralgia.
   A. Explain the distribution and mechanisms of the pain, particularly the triggering of the pain by stimuli applied to the skin.
   B. What are possible treatment methods for this woman?
4. A 21-year-old woman presents to the student health center with complaints of a throbbing pain on the left side of her head, nausea and vomiting, and extreme sensitivity to light, noise, and head movement. She also tells you she had a similar headache 3 months ago that lasted for 2 days and states that she thinks she is developing migraine headaches like her mother. She is concerned because she has been unable to attend classes and has exams next week.
   A. Are this woman's history and symptoms consistent with migraine headaches? Explain.
   B. Use the distribution of the trigeminal nerve and the concept of neurogenic inflammation to explain this woman's symptoms.
5. A 72-year-old man presents to the emergency department after a fall with a complaint of the "worst headache ever experienced." He is able to answer your questions with increasing difficulty.
   A. Differentiate primary headache from secondary headache.
   B. Given the information that you have, what type of headache do you suspect, and why?
6. A 3-year-old child is seen in a pediatric clinic with a temperature of 39°C (102.2°F). Her skin is warm and flushed, her pulse is 120 beats/minute, and her respirations are shallow and rapid at 32 breaths/minute. Her mother states that her daughter has complained of a sore throat and has refused to drink or take medications to bring her temperature down.
   A. Explain the physiologic mechanisms of fever generation.
   B. Are the warm and flushed skin, rapid heart rate, and increased respirations consistent with this level of fever?
   C. After receiving an appropriate dose of acetaminophen, the child begins to sweat, and the temperature drops to 37.2°C (98.9°F). Explain the physiologic mechanisms responsible for the drop in temperature.
7. A 25-year-old man was brought to the emergency department after having been found unconscious in a snow bank. The outdoor temperature at the time he was discovered was −23.3°C (−10°F). His car, which was stalled a short distance away, contained liquor bottles, suggesting that he had been drinking. His temperature on admission was 29.8°C (85.6°F). His heart rate was 40 beats/minute and his respirations were 18 breaths/minute and shallow. His skin was cool, his muscles rigid, and his digits blue.
   A. What factors might have contributed to this man's state of hypothermia?
   B. Is this man able to engage in physiologic behaviors to control loss of body heat?
   C. Given the two methods that are available for taking this man's temperature (oral or rectal), which would be more accurate? Explain.
   D. What precautions should be considered when deciding on a method for rewarming this man?

References

1. Guyton A., Hall J. E. (2016). *Textbook of medical physiology* (13th ed.). Philadelphia, PA: Elsevier Saunders.
2. Ross M. H., Pawlina W. (2016). *Histology: a text and atlas with correlated cell and molecular biology* (7th ed.). Philadelphia, PA: Lippincott Williams & Wilkins.
3. Rowland L., Pedley T. (Eds.) (2015). *Merritt's neurology* (13th ed.). Philadelphia, PA: Lippincott Williams & Wilkins.
4. Tortora G., Derrickson B. (2014). *Principles of anatomy & physiology* (14th ed.). Hoboken, NJ: John Wiley & Sons.
5. Quaghebeur J., Wyndaele J. (2015). A review of techniques used for evaluating lower urinary tract symptoms and the level of quality of life in patients with chronic pelvic pain syndrome. *Itch & Pain* 2, 1–6.
6. International Association for the Study of Pain. (1994). Definition of pain. [Online]. Available: https://www.iasp-pain.org/Taxonomy#Pain. Accessed December 23, 2017
7. The American Academy of Pain Medicine. (2018). Highlights from the National Center for Health Statistics Report: Health, United States, 2006, Special Feature on Pain. [Online]. Available: http://www.painmed.org/PatientCenter/Facts_on_Pain.aspx#incidence Accessed March 16, 2018.
8. Falk S., Dickenson A. (2014). Pain and nociception: Mechanisms of cancer-induced bone pain. *Journal of Clinical Oncology* 32, 1647–1654.
9. Cohan S. P., Mao J.. (2014). Neuropathic pain: mechanisms and their clinical implications. *British Medical Journal* 348, 1–12.
10. Shaygan M., Boger A., Kroner-Herwig B. (2014). Neuropathic sensory symptoms: Association with pain and psychological factors. *Neuropsychiatric Disease and Treatment* 10, 897–906.
11. Moayedi M., Davis K. D. (2013). Theories of pain: From specificity to gate control. *Journal of Neurophysiology* 109, 5–12.
12. Prescott S. A., Ma Q., Koninck Y. (2014). Normal and abnormal coding of painful sensations. *National Neuroscience* 17(2), 183–191.
13. Melzack R., Wall P. D. (1965). Pain mechanisms: A new theory. *Science* 150, 971–979.
14. Melzack R. (1999). From the gate to the neuromatrix. *Pain* 6(Suppl.), S121–S126.
15. Gopalakrishnan R., Burgess R. C., Plow E. B., et al. (2014). A magnetoencephalography study of multi-modal processing of pain anticipation in primary sensory cortices. *Neuroscience* 304, 176–189.

16. Dunphy L. M., Winland-Brown J., Porter B., et al. (2015). *Primary care: the art and science of advanced practice nursing* (4th ed.). Philadelphia, PA: FA Davis.
17. Lehne R. A. (2015). *Pharmacology for nursing care* (9th ed.). St. Louis, MO: Elsevier.
18. Carlson C. L. (2016). Effectiveness of the World Health Organization cancer pain relief guidelines: An integrative review. *Journal of Pain Research* 9, 515–534.
19. Jensen S. (2015). *Nursing health assessment: a best practice approach* (2nd ed.). Philadelphia, PA: Lippincott Williams & Wilkins.
20. Kumaz R., Asci M., Balta O., et al. (2017). Congenital insensitivity to pain syndrome accompanied by neglected orthopedic traumas and complications. *Archive of Clinical Cases* 4(1), 27–33.
21. McCormick Z., Chang-Chien G., Marshall B., et al. (2014). Phantom limb pain: A systematic neuroanatomical-based review of pharmacologic treatment. *Pain Medicine* 15, 292–305.
22. D'Onofrio F., Russo A., Conte F., et al. (2014). Post-traumatic headaches: an epidemiological overview. *Neurological Science* 35(Suppl 1), S203–S206.
23. Chaudhry P., Friedman D. I. (2015). Neuroimaging in secondary headache disorders. *Current Pain and Headache Reports* 19, 1–11.
24. Olesen J., Bendtsen L., Dodick D., et al. (2013). The International Classification of Headache Disorders (3rd ed. beta version). *Cephalalgia* 33(9), 629–808.
25. Hershey L., Bednarczyk E. (2013). Treatment of headache in the elderly. *Current Treatment Options in Neurology* 15, 56–62.
26. Noseda R., Burstein R. (2013). Migraine pathophysiology: Anatomy of the trigeminovascular pathway and associated neurological symptoms, CSD, sensitization and modulation of pain. *Pain* 154(Suppl 1), 1–21.
27. Goroll A. H., Mulley A. G. (2014). *Primary care medicine: office evaluation and management of the adult patient* (7th ed.). Philadelphia, PA: Lippincott Williams & Wilkins.
28. Weaver-Agostoni J. (2013). Cluster headache. *American Family Physician* 88(2), 122–128.
29. Hadjistavropoulos T., Herr K., Prkachim K. M., et al. (2014). Pain assessment in elderly adults with dementia. *The Lancet* 13, 1–13.
30. Achterberg W., Pieper M. J., van Dalen-Kok A. H., et al. (2013). Pain management in patients with dementia. *Clinical Interventions in Aging* 8, 1471–1482.
31. Boron Q. F., Boulpaep E. L. (2016). *Medical physiology* (3rd ed.). Philadelphia, PA: Elsevier.
32. Andreoli T. E., Benjamin I. J., Griggs R. C., et al. (2015). *Andreoli and Carpenter's cecil essentials of medicine* (9th ed.). Philadelphia, PA: Elsevier.
33. Gasim G., Musa I., Abdien M., et al. (2013). Accuracy of tympanic temperature measurement using an infrared tympanic membrane thermometer. *BioMed Central Research Notes* 6, 1–5.
34. Pak S., Lee H., Kwack M., et al. (2014). Systematic review and meta-analysis of the diagnostic accuracy of an infrared tympanic thermometer for use with adults. *International Journal of Nursing* 1(2), 115–134.
35. Auliciems A. (2014). Thermal sensation and cell adaptability. *International Journal of Biometeorology* 58, 325–335.
36. Golembiewski J. (2015). Pharmacological management of perioperative shivering. *Journal of PeriAnesthesia Nursing* 30(4), 357–359.
37. Flouris D., Schlader Z. J. (2015). Human behavioral thermoregulation during exercise in the heat. *Scandinavian Journal of Medical Science of Sports* 25(Suppl 1), 52–64.
38. Rubin R., Strayer D. (Eds.) (2015). *Rubin's pathology: clinicopathologic foundations of medicine* (7th ed.). Philadelphia, PA: Lippincott Williams & Wilkins.
39. Egi M., Makino S., Mizobuchi, S. (2018). Management of fever in critically ill patients with infection. *Journal of Emergency Critical Care Medicine* 2(10), 1–6.
40. Outzen M. (2009). Management of fever in older adults. *Journal of Gerontological Nursing* 35(5), 17–23.
41. Norman D. C. (2016). Clinical features of infection in older adults. *Clinical Geriatric Medicine* 32,433–441.
42. Pryor R., Roth R., Suyama J., et al. (2015). Exertional heat illness: Emerging concepts and advances in prehospital care. *Prehospital Disaster Medicine* 30(3), 297–305.
43. Nichols A. (2014). Heat-related illness in sports and exercise. *Current Review Musculoskeletal Medicine* 7, 355–365.
44. Ferreira C., Costa T., Marques A. V. (2015). Diffuse alveolar haemorrhage secondary to propylthiouracil-induced vasculitis. *British Medical Journal Case Report* published online: DOI: 10.1136/bcr-2014-208289.
45. Rosenberg H., Pollock N., Shiemann A., et al. (2015). Malignant hyperthermia: a review. *Orphanet Journal of Rare Disease* 10, 1–19.
46. Davis C. (2017). *Hypothermia*. Accessed online: https://www.emedicinehealth.com/hypothermia/article_em.htm#what_is_hypothermia.
47. Plitnick K., Biehle K. J., Meinken C. (2015). Shivering suppression in therapeutic hypothermia. *Nursing 2015 Critical Care* 10(5), 22–26.
48. Morton M. G., Fontaine D. K. (2017). *Critical care nursing: a holistic approach* (11th ed.). Philadelphia, PA: Lippincott Williams & Wilkins.
49. Alvis-Miranda H. R., Alcala-Cerra G., Rubiano A. M., et al. (2014). Therapeutic hypothermia in brain trauma injury: controversies. *Romanian Neurosurgery* 3, 259–268.
50. Galicia-Castillo M. C., Weiner D. K. Treatment of persistent pain in older adults. In Crowley M. (Ed.) *UpToDate*. Retrieved March 16, 2018 from https://www.uptodate.com/contents/treatment-of-persistent-pain-in-older-adults.
51. Eliopoulos C. (2018). *Gerontological Nursing* (9th ed.). Philadelphia, PA: Wolters Kluwer.
52. Kyle T., Carman S. (2017). *Essentials of Pediatric Nursing* (3rd ed.). Philadelphia, PA: Wolters Kluwer.

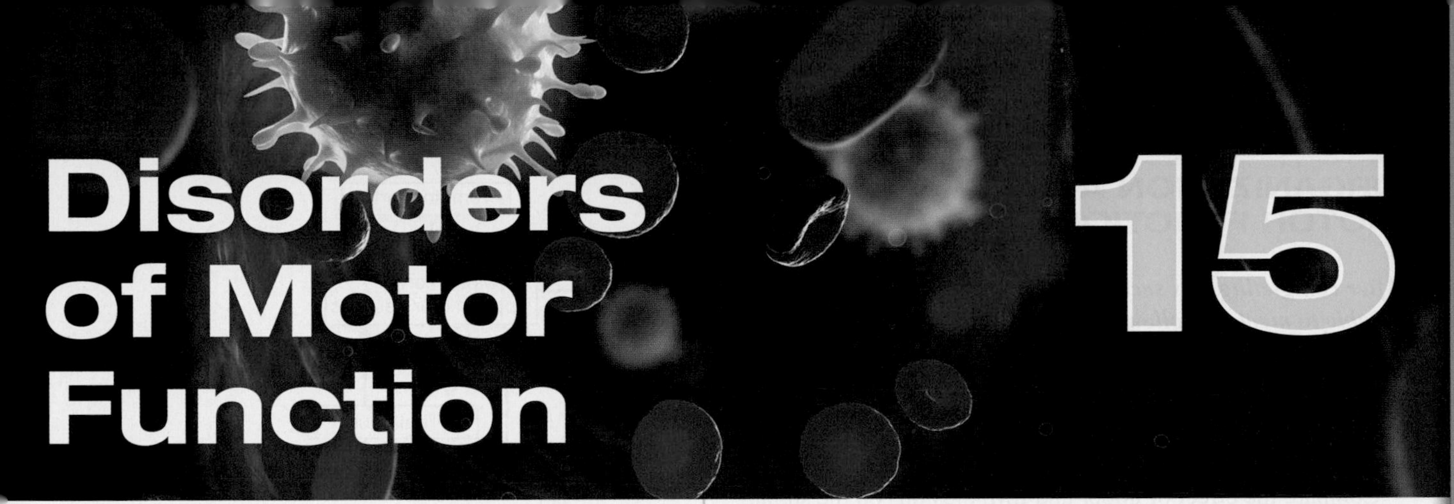

Disorders of Motor Function

15

Cynthia Bautista

Skeletal muscles are required to carry out skilled movements that coordinate and execute these contractions in a manner that provides for smooth, purposeful, and coordinated movement. In some cases, purposeless and disruptive movements can be almost as disabling as absence of movement. This chapter provides an introduction to the organization and control of motor function, followed by a discussion of disorders of motor function, including muscular dystrophy and disorders of the neuromuscular junction, peripheral nerves, basal ganglia and cerebellum, and upper motor neurons (UMNs).

KEY POINTS

MOTOR SYSTEMS

- Motor systems require upper motor neurons that project from the motor cortex to the brain stem or spinal cord, where they directly or indirectly innervate the lower motor neurons (LMNs) of the contracting muscles; sensory feedback from the involved muscles that is continuously relayed to the cerebellum, basal ganglia, and sensory cortex; and a functioning neuromuscular junction that links nervous system activity with muscle contraction.
- The pyramidal motor system originating in the motor cortex provides control of delicate muscle movement, and the extrapyramidal system originating in the basal ganglia provides the background for the more crude, supportive movement patterns.
- The efficiency of the movement by the motor system depends on a background of muscle tone provided by the stretch reflex and vestibular system input to maintain stable postural support.

ORGANIZATION AND CONTROL OF MOTOR FUNCTION

After completing this section of the chapter, the learner will be able to meet the following objectives:

- Define the term *motor unit* and characterize its mechanism of controlling skeletal muscle movement.
- Indicate between the functions of the primary, premotor, and supplemental motor cortices.
- Compare the effect of upper and LMN lesions on the spinal cord stretch reflex function and muscle tone.

Motor function, whether it involves walking, running, or precise finger movements, requires movement and maintenance of posture. This is described as maintaining optimal body position. Structures throughout the neuromuscular system control posture.[1] The neuromuscular system consists of the motor unit (motor neuron and the muscle fibers it innervates); the spinal cord, which contains the basic reflex circuitry for posture and movement; and the descending pathways from brain stem circuits, the cerebellum, basal ganglia, and the motor cortex.

Organization of Movement

The motor systems are organized in a functional hierarchy, each concerned with increased levels of complexity (Fig. 15.1). The lowest level of the hierarchy occurs at the spinal cord, which contains the basic reflex circuitry needed to coordinate the function of the motor units involved in the planned movement. Above the spinal cord is the brain stem. Above the brain stem are the cerebellum and basal ganglia—structures that modify the actions of the brain stem systems. Overseeing these supraspinal structures are the motor centers in the cerebral cortex. The highest level of function, which occurs at the level of the frontal cortex, is concerned with the purpose and planning of the motor movement. The efficiency of movement depends on input from sensory systems that operate in parallel with the motor systems.

The Spinal Cord

The spinal cord contains the neuronal circuits that mediate a variety of reflexes and automatic rhythmic movements. Similar circuits governing reflex movements of the face and mouth are located in the brain stem. The simplest circuits are monosynaptic, containing only a primary motor neuron. However, most reflexes are polysynaptic, involving one or more interposed interneurons. The interneurons and motor neurons also receive input from axons descending from higher centers. These supraspinal signals can modify reflex responses to peripheral stimuli by facilitating or inhibiting different populations of interneurons. They also coordinate movements through these interneurons.

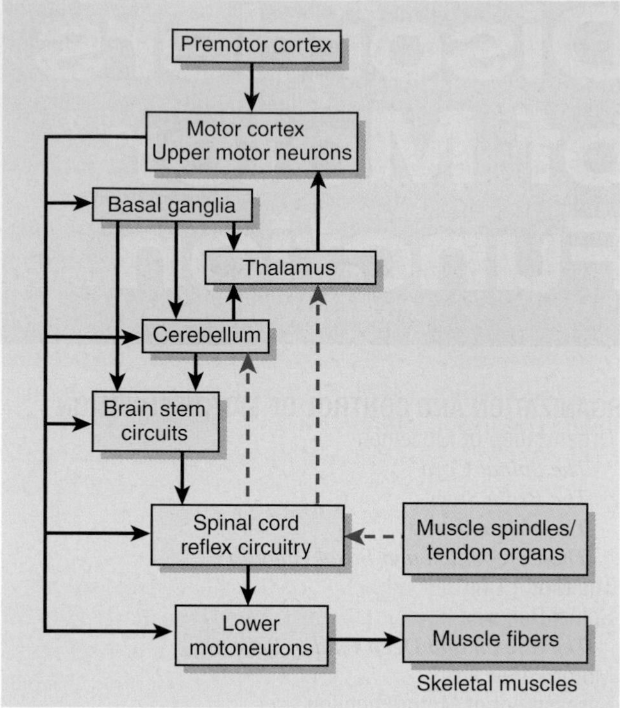

Figure 15.1 • The motor control system. The final common pathway transmits all CNS commands to the skeletal muscles. This path is influenced by sensory input from the muscle spindles and tendon organs (*dashed lines*) and descending signals from the cerebral cortex and brain stem. The cerebellum and basal ganglia influence the motor function indirectly, using brain stem and cortical pathways.

The Brain Stem

The brain stem contains two descending systems—the medial and lateral pathways (Fig. 15.2). The medial pathways provide for the basic postural control systems that the cortical

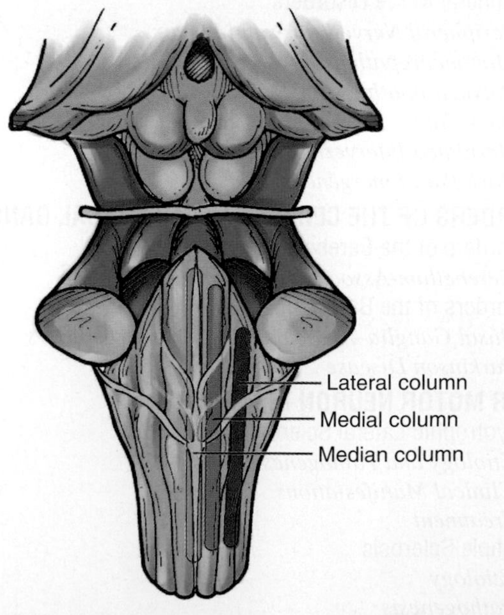

Figure 15.2 • The median, medial, and lateral columns of the reticular formation. (From Hickey J. V. (2014). *The clinical practice of neurological and neurosurgical nursing* (7th ed). Philadelphia, PA: Wolters Kluwer.)

motor areas use to organize highly differentiated movements. The medial pathways consist of tracts that descend in the ipsilateral ventral columns of the spinal cord and terminate in interneurons that influence motor neurons of axial and proximal muscles. These axial and proximal muscles are responsible for postural reflexes, such as those needed for pacing of steps during walking or running and recovery of posture when balance is disrupted.

The lateral brain stem pathways are more concerned with goal-directed movements. They terminate on the interneurons in the dorsolateral part of the spinal gray matter and thus influence the motor neurons that control distal muscles of the limbs. These descending pathways modify the activity of extensor and flexor motor neurons to produce complex motor movements such as walking and running.

The Motor Cortex

The cortex represents the highest level of motor function. The primary, premotor, and supplementary motor cortices located in the posterior part of the frontal lobe initiate and control precise, skillful, and intentional movements of the distal and especially flexor muscles of the limbs and speech apparatus[2] (Fig. 15.3). These motor areas receive information from the thalamus and somatosensory cortex and, indirectly, from the cerebellum and basal ganglia.

The primary motor cortex (area 4 if using Brodmann classification of the brain cortical areas), also called the *motor strip*, is located on the rostral surface and adjacent portions of the central sulcus.[2] The primary motor cortex controls specific muscle movement sequences. It is also the first level of descending control for precise motor movements. The neurons in the primary motor cortex are arranged in a somatotopic array or distorted map of the body called the *motor homunculus*[3] (Fig. 15.4). The areas of the body that require the greatest dexterity have the largest cortical areas devoted to them. More than half of the primary motor cortex is concerned with controlling the muscles of the hands, of facial expression, and of speech.

The premotor cortex (Brodmann areas 6 and 8), which is located just anterior to the primary motor cortex, sends some fibers into the corticospinal tract but mainly innervates the primary motor strip. Nerve signals generated by the premotor cortex produce much more complex *patterns* of movement

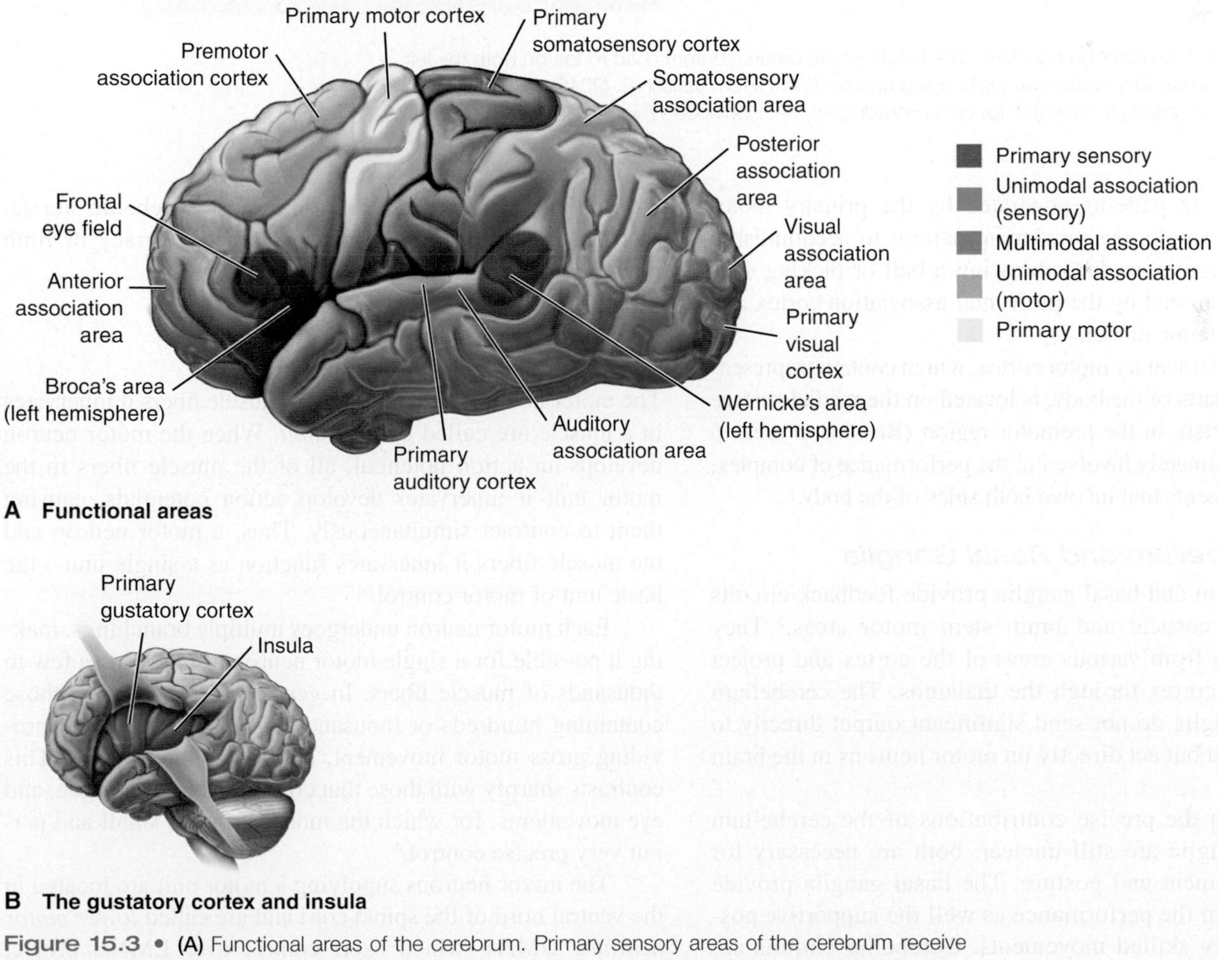

Figure 15.3 • **(A)** Functional areas of the cerebrum. Primary sensory areas of the cerebrum receive sensory information from many sources. The motor association cortex organizes movements, and the primary motor cortex sends commands to individual muscles. **(B)** By pulling back the parietal and temporal lobes, the gustatory cortex and insula are visible. (From McConnell T. H., Hull K. L. (2011). *Human form human function: Essentials of anatomy & physiology* (p. 297). Philadelphia, PA: Lippincott Williams & Wilkins.)

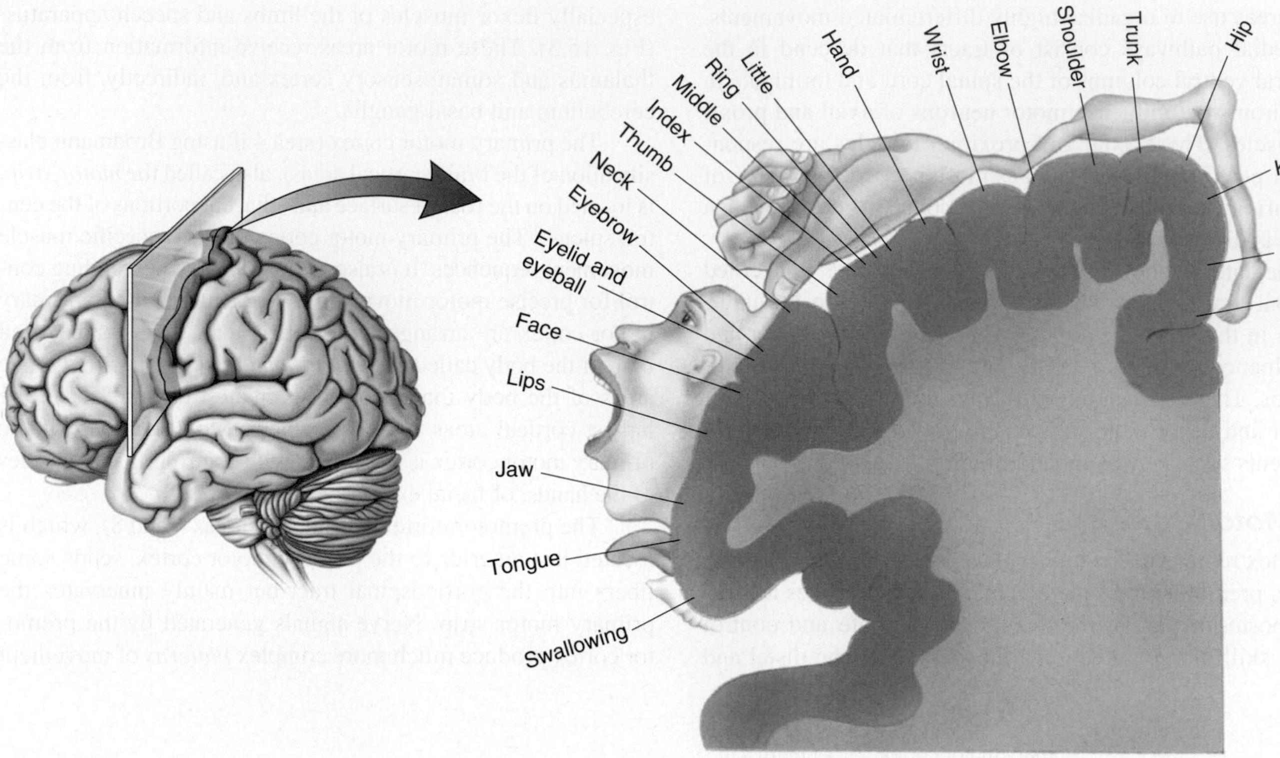

Figure 15.4 • The motor homunculus. The functions are organized from head to toe on both the left and right sides, similar to a person who is hanging upside down. (From Jensen S. (2015). *Nursing health assessment: A best practice approach* (p. 651). Philadelphia, PA: Lippincott Williams & Wilkins.)

than the discrete patterns generated by the primary motor cortex. For example, the movement pattern to accomplish a particular objective, such as throwing a ball or picking up a fork, is programmed by the prefrontal association cortex and associated thalamic nuclei.

The supplementary motor cortex, which contains representations of all parts of the body, is located on the medial surface of the hemisphere in the premotor region (Brodmann areas 6 and 8). It is intimately involved in the performance of complex, skillful movements that involve both sides of the body.

The Cerebellum and Basal Ganglia

The cerebellum and basal ganglia provide feedback circuits that regulate cortical and brain stem motor areas.[2] They receive inputs from various areas of the cortex and project to the motor cortex through the thalamus. The cerebellum and basal ganglia do not send significant output directly to the spinal cord but act directly on motor neurons in the brain stem.

Although the precise contributions of the cerebellum and basal ganglia are still unclear, both are necessary for smooth movement and posture. The basal ganglia provide gracefulness to the performance as well the supportive posture for highly skilled movements. Cerebellar circuits are involved with the timing and coordination of movements that are in progress and with learning of motor skills. Damage to the cerebellum by vascular lesions of certain familial degenerative disorders produces cerebellar ataxia, a characteristic loss of coordination and accuracy of limb movement.

The Motor Unit

The motor neuron and the group of muscle fibers it innervates in a muscle are called a *motor unit*. When the motor neuron develops an action potential, all of the muscle fibers in the motor unit it innervates develop action potentials, causing them to contract simultaneously. Thus, a motor neuron and the muscle fibers it innervates function as a single unit—the basic unit of motor control.

Each motor neuron undergoes multiple branchings, making it possible for a single motor neuron to innervate a few to thousands of muscle fibers. In general, large muscles, those containing hundreds or thousands of muscle fibers and providing gross motor movement, have large motor units. This contrasts sharply with those that control the hand, tongue, and eye movements, for which the motor units are small and permit very precise control.[4]

The motor neurons supplying a motor unit are located in the ventral horn of the spinal cord and are called *lower motor neurons*. UMNs, which exert control over LMNs, project from the motor strip in the cerebral cortex to the ventral horn and are fully contained in the central nervous system (CNS) (Fig. 15.5).

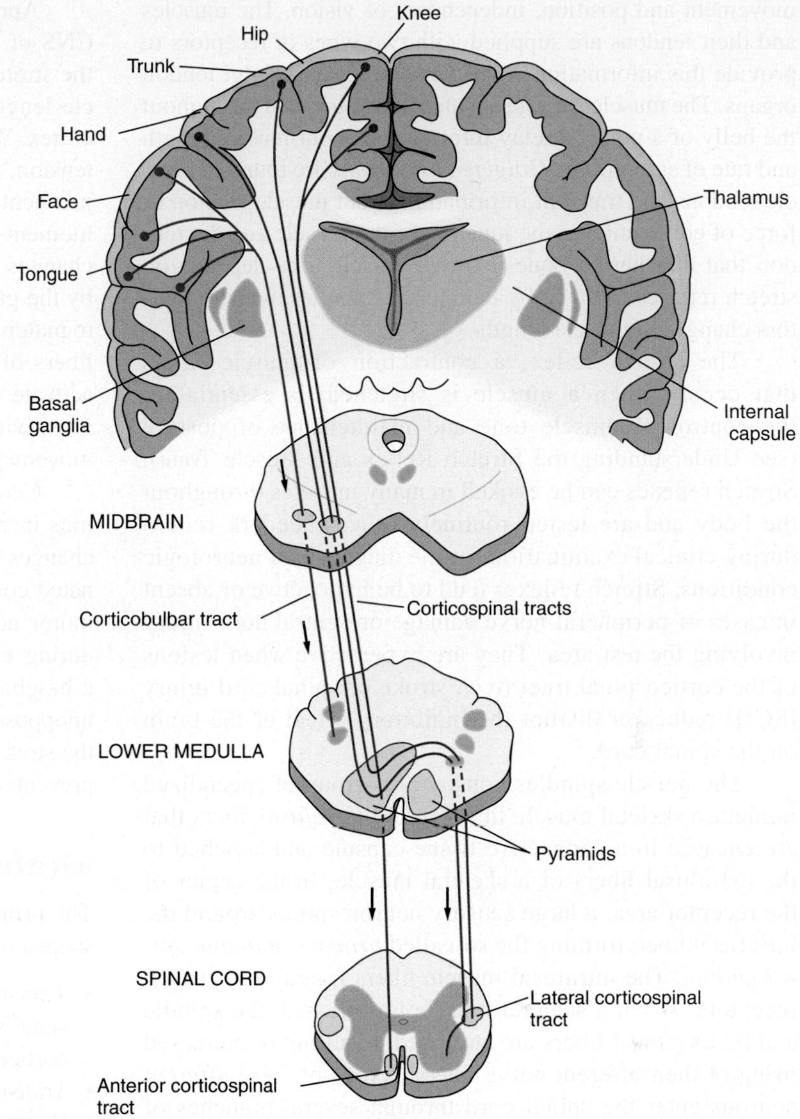

Figure 15.5 • Motor pathways. Descending tracts carry motor and muscle information from the cortex to the cranial and peripheral nerves. (From Jensen S. (2015). *Nursing health assessment: A best practice approach* (p. 651). Philadelphia, PA: Lippincott Williams & Wilkins.)

Spinal Reflexes

Reflexes are coordinated, involuntary motor responses that are initiated by a stimulus applied to peripheral receptors. Some reflexes, such as the flexor withdrawal reflex, initiate movements to avoid hazardous situations. Others, such as the stretch reflex or crossed extensor reflex, serve to integrate motor movements so they function in a coordinated manner. The anatomic basis of a reflex consists of an afferent neuron that synapses either directly with an effector neuron that innervates a muscle or with an interneuron that synapses with an effector neuron. A reflex may involve neurons in a single cord segment (*i.e.*, segmental reflexes), several or many segments (*i.e.*, intersegmental reflexes), or structures in the brain (*i.e.*, suprasegmental reflexes).

There is a significant amount of reflex circuitry in the spinal cord for the coordinated control of movements, particularly stereotyped movements concerned with locomotion. Many of these reflexes work equally well in decerebrate animals (those in which the brain has been destroyed) as long as the spinal cord is intact. Other spinal reflexes require the activity of the brain for their successful completion. In addition, the brain is advised of many types of spinal cord reflex activities and can then inhibit or facilitate them.

The Stretch and Deep Tendon Reflexes

For skeletal muscle to perform normally, the brain must be continually informed of the current state of the muscles, and the muscles must exhibit tone (resistance to active and passive stretch at rest). This will depend on the transmission of information regarding the sense of body position, movement, and muscle tone to the CNS. Information from these sensory afferents is relayed to the cerebellum and cerebral cortex and is experienced as proprioception or the sense of body movement and position, independent of vision. The muscles and their tendons are supplied with two types of receptors to provide this information—muscle spindles and Golgi tendon organs. The muscle spindles, which are distributed throughout the belly of a muscle, relay information about muscle length and rate of stretch. The *Golgi tendon organs* are found in muscle tendons and transmit information about muscle tension or force of contraction at the junction of the muscle and the tendon that attaches to bone. Normal muscle tone depends on stretch reflexes initiated by the muscle spindles, which monitors changes in muscle length.

The stretch reflex, a contraction of muscle fibers that occurs when a muscle is stretched, is essential to the control of muscle tone and maintenance of posture (see Understanding the Stretch Reflex and Muscle Tone). Stretch reflexes can be evoked in many muscles throughout the body and are tested routinely (*e.g.*, knee-jerk reflex) during clinical examination for the diagnosis of neurologic conditions. Stretch reflexes tend to be hypoactive or absent in cases of peripheral nerve damage or ventral horn injury involving the test area. They are hyperactive when lesions of the corticospinal tract (*e.g.*, stroke or spinal cord injury [SCI]) reduce or disrupt the inhibitory effect of the brain on the spinal cord.

The muscle spindles consist of a group of specialized miniature skeletal muscle fibers called *intrafusal fibers* that are encased in a connective tissue capsule and attached to the extrafusal fibers of a skeletal muscle. In the center of the receptor area, a large sensory neuron spirals around the intrafusal fiber, forming the so-called *primary* or *annulospiral ending*. The intrafusal muscle fibers function as stretch receptors. When a skeletal muscle is stretched, the spindle and its intrafusal fibers are stretched, resulting in increased firing of their afferent nerve fibers. Axons of these afferent neurons enter the spinal cord through several branches of the dorsal root. Some branches end in the segment of entry. Others ascend to adjacent segments, influencing intersegmental reflex function. Still, others ascend in the dorsal column of the cord to the medulla of the brain stem. Segmental branches make connections, along with other branches, that pass directly to the anterior gray matter of the spinal cord and establish monosynaptic contact with each of the LMNs that have motor units in the muscle containing the spindle receptor. This produces an opposing muscle contraction. Another segmental branch of the same afferent neuron innervates an internuncial neuron that is inhibitory to motor units of antagonistic muscle groups. This disynaptic inhibitory pathway is the basis for the reciprocal activity of agonist and antagonist muscles (*i.e.*, when an agonist muscle is stretched, the antagonists relax). Reciprocal innervation is useful not only for the stretch reflex but for voluntary movements. Relaxation of the antagonist muscle during movements enhances the speed and efficiency because the muscles that act as prime movers are not working against the contraction of opposing muscle.[2]

Another function of the stretch reflex is to inform the CNS of the status of muscle length. Ascending fibers from the stretch reflex ultimately provide information about muscle length to higher centers in the cerebellum and cerebral cortex. When a skeletal muscle lengthens or shortens against tension, a feedback mechanism needs to be available for readjustment such that the spindle apparatus remains sensitive to moment-to-moment changes in muscle stretch, even while changes in muscle length are occurring. This is accomplished by the gamma motor neurons that adjust spindle fiber length to match the length of the extrafusal muscle fiber. Descending fibers of motor pathways synapse with and simultaneously activate both alpha and gamma motor neurons so that the sensitivity of the spindle fibers is coordinated with muscle movement.

Central control over the gamma motor neurons also permits increases or decreases in muscle tone in anticipation of changes in the muscle force. The CNS, through its coordinated control of the muscle's alpha and the spindle's gamma motor neurons, can suppress the stretch reflex. This occurs during centrally programmed movements, such as pitching a baseball, that require a muscle to produce a full range of unopposed motion. Without this programmed adjustability of the stretch reflex, any movement is immediately opposed and prevented.

Motor Pathways

The primary motor cortex contains many layers of pyramid-shaped output neurons that

- Transmit to the premotor and somatosensory areas on same side of the cortex (*i.e.*, premotor and somatosensory cortices)
- Transmit to the opposite side of the cortex
- Descend to subcortical structures such as the basal ganglia and thalamus

The large pyramidal cells located in the fifth layer transmit to the brain stem and spinal cord. The axons of these UMNs transmit through the subcortical white matter and internal capsule to the deep surface of the brain stem, through the ventral bulge of the pons, and to the ventral surface of the medulla, where they form a ridge or pyramid. About 90% of the corticospinal axons cross the midline at the junction of the medulla and cervical spinal cord to form the lateral corticospinal tract in the lateral white matter of the spinal cord.[4] This tract extends throughout the spinal cord. The remaining 10% of uncrossed fibers travel down the ventral column of the cord, mainly to cervical levels, where they cross and innervate contralateral LMNs.[4]

Motor tracts are classified as belonging to one of two motor pathways—the pyramidal (direct) and extrapyramidal (indirect) pathways. According to this classification system, the pyramidal pathway consists of the motor pathways originating in the motor cortex and terminating in the corticobulbar

Understanding The Stretch Reflex and Muscle Tone

Muscle tone is controlled by the stretch reflex, which monitors changes in muscle length. The activity of the stretch reflex can be divided into three steps: (1) activation of the stretch receptors, (2) integration of the reflex in the spinal cord, and (3) regulation of reflex sensitivity by higher centers in the brain. Testing the knee-jerk reflex provides a means of assessing that reflex.

Stretch Reflex Receptors

Skeletal muscle is composed of two types of muscle fibers—a large number of extrafusal fibers, which control muscle movement, and a smaller number of intrafusal fibers, which control muscle tone. The intrafusal fibers are encapsulated in sheaths, forming a muscle spindle that runs parallel to the extrafusal fibers. Each intrafusal fiber is innervated by a large Ia sensory nerve fiber, which encircles the central noncontractile portion of the fiber to form the so-called *annulospiral ending*. Because the spindles are oriented parallel to the extrafusal muscle fibers, stretching of the extrafusal fibers also stretches the spindle fibers and stimulates the receptive endings of the Ia afferent neuron.

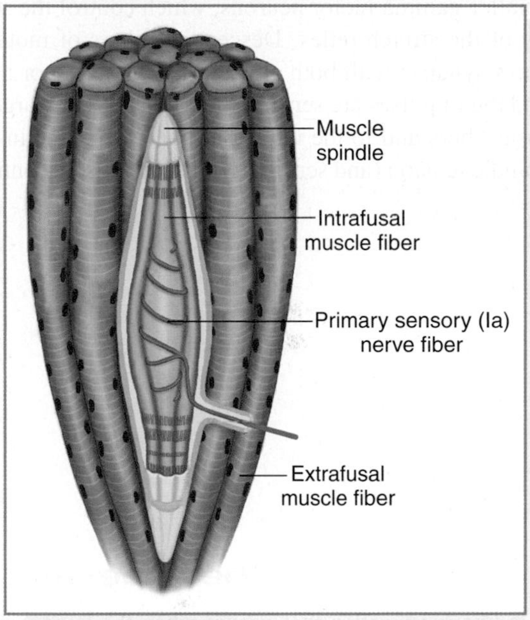

Spinal Reflex Centers

Afferent impulses from the Ia sensory fiber of the muscle spindle are transmitted to the spinal cord, where they synapse with alpha motor neurons of the stretched muscle to form a monosynaptic reflex arc, *monosynaptic* because only one synapse separates the primary sensory input from the motor neuron output. The reflex muscle contraction that follows resists further stretching of the muscle. As this spinal reflex activity is occurring, impulses providing information on muscle length are transmitted to higher centers in the brain. It is the coordinated activity of all the monosynaptic reflexes supplying the extrafusal fibers in a skeletal muscle that provides the muscle tone needed for organized movement.

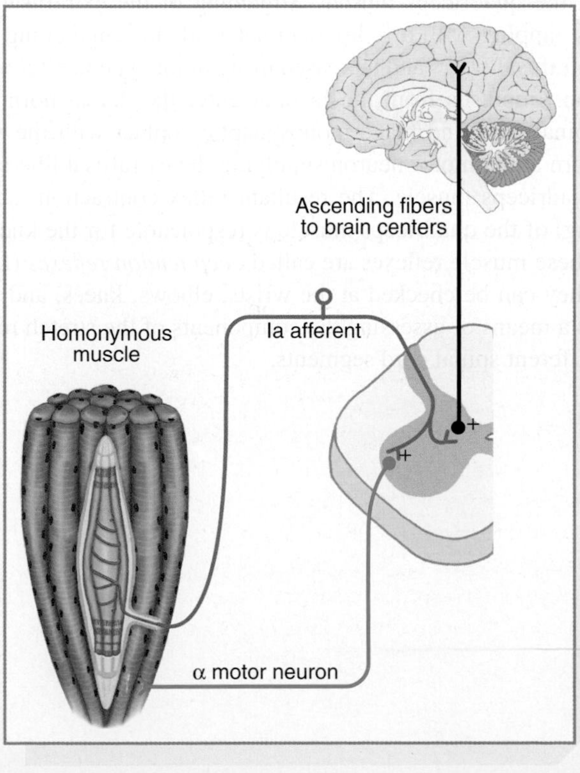

Continued

Understanding The Stretch Reflex and Muscle Tone *(Continued)*

Brain Center Connections

Although a spinal reflex can function independently, its sensitivity is adjusted by higher centers in the brain. Both types of muscle fibers are supplied with motor neurons—the extrafusal fibers with large alpha motor neurons, which produce muscle contraction, and the intrafusal fibers with smaller gamma motor neurons, which control the sensitivity of the stretch reflex. Descending fibers of motor pathways synapse with both alpha and gamma motor neurons, and the impulses are sent simultaneously to the large extrafusal fibers and to the intrafusal fibers to maintain muscle spindle tension (and sensitivity) during muscle contraction.

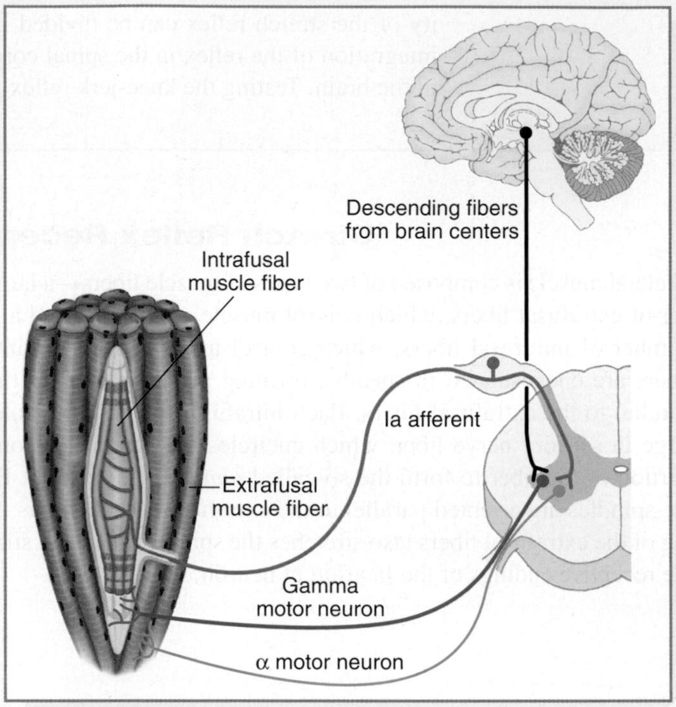

The Knee-Jerk Reflex

The knee-jerk reflex that occurs when the knee is tapped with a reflex hammer tests for the intactness of the stretch reflex arc in the quadriceps muscle. Stretching of the extrafusal fibers by tapping with a reflex hammer leads to lengthening of the intrafusal fibers and increased firing of the type Ia afferent neuron. Impulses from the Ia fiber enter the dorsal horn of the spinal cord and make monosynaptic contact with the ventral horn alpha motor neuron supplying the extrafusal fibers in the quadriceps muscle. The resultant reflex contraction (shortening) of the quadriceps muscle is responsible for the knee jerk. These muscle reflexes are called *deep tendon reflexes* (DTRs). They can be checked at the wrists, elbows, knees, and ankles as a means of assessing the components of the stretch reflex at different spinal cord segments.

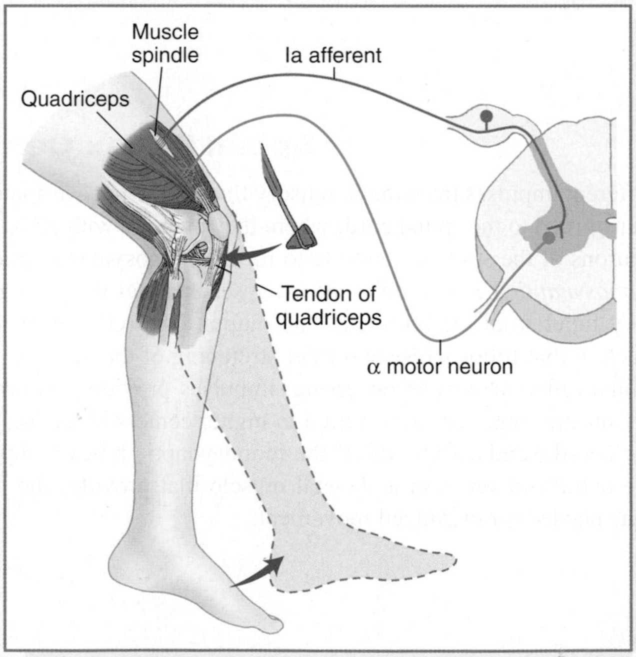

fibers in the brain stem and the corticospinal fibers in the spinal cord. Other fibers from the cortex and basal ganglia project to the brain stem reticular formation and reticulospinal pathways to LMNs of proximal and extensor muscles. These fibers do not decussate in the pyramids, hence the name *extrapyramidal system.* Disorders of the pyramidal tracts (*e.g.*, stroke) are characterized by spasticity and paralysis, whereas those affecting the extrapyramidal tracts (*e.g.*, Parkinson disease) result in involuntary movements, muscle rigidity, and immobility without paralysis.

Assessment of Motor Function

Assessing the motor system should include assessment of

- Body position
- Involuntary movements
- Muscle characteristics (strength, size, and tone)
- Spinal reflexes
- Coordination[5]

Body Position and Involuntary Movements

Observe the body position of the person when moving and at rest. Continually observe for involuntary movements, and note the location, quality, rate, and rhythm of the movements.

Muscle Characteristics

Muscle Strength. Moving each extremity against gravity and resistance tests strength. Abnormalities in any part of the motor pathway can produce impaired strength or muscle weakness. Paralysis refers to loss of movement, and paresis to weakness or incomplete loss of strength. The pattern of weakness may be helpful in the localization of the lesion.

- *Monoparesis* or *monoplegia* results from the destruction of pyramidal UMN innervation of one limb.
- *Hemiparesis* or *hemiplegia results from the destruction of pyramidal UMN innervation of* both limbs on one side.
- *Diparesis* or *diplegia or paraparesis* or *paraplegia results from the destruction of pyramidal UMN innervation of* both upper or lower limbs.
- *Tetraparesis* or *tetraplegia*, also called *quadriparesis* or *quadriplegia, results from the destruction of pyramidal UMN innervation of* all four limbs.

Paresis or paralysis can be further designated as of UMN or LMN origin. UMN lesions of the motor cortex or corticospinal tract typically affect the extensors in the upper extremities more than the flexors, whereas in the lower extremities, the flexors are more affected. In LMN or peripheral nerve disorders, the weakness is predominantly in the distal limb, whereas in muscle disorders, such as muscular dystrophy, proximal limb function may be affected sooner than distal limb function.

Muscle Size. The size of muscle (whether muscles are normal sized, enlarged, or atrophied) also helps localize the lesion and sometimes provides helpful hints to the pathologic process. Muscular atrophy, or loss of muscle bulk, usually results from LMN lesions as well as diseases of the muscles themselves. Hypertrophy refers to an increase in muscle bulk with a proportionate increase in strength. Pseudohypertrophy, as occurs with Duchenne muscular dystrophy (DMD), refers to an increase in bulk without an accompanying increase in strength.

Fasciculations are visible squirming and twitching movements of muscle fibers that can be seen as flickers under the skin. They are caused by spontaneous contractions of all the muscle fibers in a motor unit because of irritation and hyperexcitability of the cell body and its motor neuron and suggest LMN disease.

Muscle Tone. Muscle tone is the normal state of muscle tension. Palpate for muscle tone by palpating the muscle while at rest and during passive stretching. With the person at rest, the joints are put through the normal range of motion (flexion and extension) by the examiner. Disorders of skeletal muscle tone are characteristic of many nervous system lesions. Any interruption of the stretch reflex pathway by peripheral nerve injury, pathologic process of the neuromuscular junction, injury to the spinal cord, or damage to the corticospinal system can result in disturbances of muscle tone.

Abnormalities of muscle tone may be described as hypotonia (less than normal), flaccidity (absent), or hypertonia, rigidity, spasticity, or tetany (all indicating higher-than-normal tone). Typically, UMN lesions produce increased tone, whereas LMN lesions produce decreased tone. Increased resistance that varies and commonly becomes worse at the extremes of the range of motion is called spasticity. Resistance that becomes worse throughout the range and in both directions is called *rigidity*. Decreased resistance suggests disease of the LMNs or the acute stages of SCI. Marked floppiness indicates hypotonic or flaccid muscles.

Spinal Reflex Activity

Testing of DTRs (see Understanding the Stretch Reflex and Muscle Tone) can provide important information about the status of the CNS in controlling muscle function. Hyperactive reflexes are suggestive of a UMN disorder. *Clonus* is the rhythmic contraction and alternate relaxation of a limb that is caused by suddenly stretching a muscle and gently maintaining it in the stretched position. It is seen in the hypertonia of spasticity associated with UMN lesions, such as SCI. *Hyporeflexia* or *areflexia* suggests the presence of an LMN lesion. The distribution of abnormality in the reflexes is also helpful in determining the location of the lesion. For example, hyperreflexia in both lower extremities would suggest a lesion in the spinal cord, whereas hyperreflexia on one side of the body would suggest a lesion in the UMN along the motor pathway (*e.g.*, in the motor cortex or internal capsule).

Coordination of Movement

Coordination of muscle movement requires that four areas of the nervous system function in an integrated manner:

- The motor system for muscle strength
- The cerebellar system for rhythmic movement and steady posture
- The vestibular system for posture and balance
- The sensory system for position sense

In cerebellar disease, one movement cannot be followed quickly by its opposite movement, and movements are slow, irregular, clumsy, unsteady, and inappropriately varying in their speed, force, and direction. *Dysdiadochokinesia* is the failure to accurately perform rapid alternating movements. Ataxia is a term used to describe a wide-based, unsteady gait. *Dysmetria* is a term used to describe inaccuracies of movements leading to a failure to reach a specified target. It is possible to test for dysmetria by having the person touch the examiner's finger and then alternately touch his or her finger. These movements are normally smooth and accurate. Asking the person to touch the examiner's finger with an outstretched arm and finger, first with the eyes open and then closed, provides a test for position sense. Repetitive and consistent deviation to one side (referred to as past pointing), which is worse with the eyes closed, suggests cerebellar or vestibular disease.

Chorea (abnormal writhing movements), *dystonia* (abnormal simultaneous contractions of agonist and antagonist muscles, leading to abnormal postures), tremor (rhythmic movements of a particular body part), *bradykinesia* (slowness of movements), and myoclonus (involuntary jerking movement) indicate abnormalities in the basal ganglia, although the exact localization may be difficult to determine.

IN SUMMARY

Motor function, whether it involves walking, running, or precise finger movements, requires movement and maintenance of posture. The system consists of the LMNs, which are located in the ventral horn of the spinal cord and the group of muscle fibers it innervates in the muscle; spinal cord circuitry and reflexes; and the UMNs that project from the motor cortex to the opposite side of the medulla, where they form a pyramid before crossing the midline to form the lateral corticospinal tract in the spinal cord. The primary, premotor, and supplementary motor cortices provide the voluntary control of motor function which is directed by the motor cortex. The primary motor cortex is responsible for execution of a movement, the premotor cortex for generating a plan of movement, and the supplemental motor cortex for rehearsing the motor sequences of a movement, including those involving both sides of the body. As with other parts of the nervous system, the motor systems are organized in a functional hierarchy of, from bottom to top, the spinal cord, brain stem, and motor cortex, each with circuits that, through their input and output connections, can contribute to the organization and regulation of complex motor responses.

Proper control of muscle function requires the function of reflex circuitry that monitors the functional status of the muscle fibers on a moment-by-moment basis along with the excitation of the muscle by the LMNs located in the spinal cord. The muscle spindles of the stretch reflex function to monitor and correct for changes in muscle length when extrafusal fibers are either shortened (by contraction) or lengthened (by stretch).

Assessments of muscle strength, size, tone, reflexes, patterns of motor movement, and posture provide the means for determining the location of disorders of motor function. Paresis (weakness) and paralysis (loss of muscle movement) reflect a loss of muscle strength. UMN lesions tend to produce spastic paralysis and LMN lesions, flaccid paralysis. Changes in muscle size are characterized by a loss of muscle mass (atrophy) or an increase in muscle mass (hypertrophy). Muscle tone is maintained through the combined function of the spinal cord stretch reflex, and higher centers monitor and buffer UMN innervation of the LMNs. Hypotonia or flaccidity is a condition of less-than-normal muscle tone, and hypertonia or spasticity is a condition of excessive tone. Abnormal and uncoordinated movements and postures are suggestive of a cerebellar or basal ganglia pathologic process.

DISORDERS OF THE MOTOR UNIT

After completing this section of the chapter, the learner will be able to meet the following objectives:

- Define the term *peripheral nervous system* and describe the characteristics of peripheral nerves.
- Compare the cause and manifestations of peripheral mononeuropathies with polyneuropathies.

Most of the diseases of the motor unit cause weakness and atrophy of skeletal muscles. The distinguishing features of these diseases vary depending on which of the components of the motor unit is primarily affected—the cell body of the motor neuron, its axon, the neuromuscular junction, or the muscle fibers.[6,7] Disorders affecting the nerve cell body are often referred to as *lower motor neuron disorders*. Those affecting the nerve axon are referred to as *peripheral neuropathies*. Finally, those affecting the muscle fibers are referred to as *myopathies*.

Skeletal Muscle Disorders

Muscle Atrophy

Maintenance of muscle strength requires relatively frequent movements against resistance. Reduced use results in muscle atrophy, which is characterized by a reduction in the diameter of the muscle fibers because of a loss of protein filaments.[7] When a normally innervated muscle is not used for long periods, the muscle cells shrink in diameter, and although the muscle cells do not die, they lose much of their contractile proteins and become weakened. This is called *disuse atrophy*, and it occurs with conditions such as immobilization and chronic illness. Evidence suggests that all skeletal muscle atrophy is not exactly the same because of different signaling pathways that manage skeletal muscle protein turnover. If this is proven, individualized therapies can be developed for each type of disuse atrophy to allow more targeted prevention.[8]

The most extreme examples of muscle atrophy are found in people with disorders that deprive muscles of their innervation. This is called *denervation atrophy*. During early embryonic development, outgrowing skeletal nerves innervate partially mature muscle cells. If the developing muscle cells are not innervated, they do not mature and eventually die. In the process of innervation, randomly contracting muscle cells become enslaved by the innervating neurons, and from then on, the muscle cell contracts only when stimulated by that particular neuron. If the LMN dies or its axon is destroyed, the skeletal muscle cell is again free of neural domination. When this happens, it begins to have temporary spontaneous contractions, called *fibrillations*. In contrast to previously described fasciculations, fibrillations are not visible clinically and can be detected only by electromyography (EMG). The muscle also begins to lose its contractile proteins, and, after several months, if not reinnervated, it is replaced by fibrous connective tissue, which makes rehabilitation difficult. Atrophy of denervation can often be delayed by electrically stimulating the muscle periodically while waiting to determine if the damaged nerve fiber regenerates.

Muscular Dystrophy

Muscular dystrophy is a term applied to a number of genetic disorders that produce progressive deterioration of skeletal muscles because of mixed muscle cell hypertrophy, atrophy, and necrosis. They are primary diseases of muscle tissue and probably do not involve the nervous system. As the muscle undergoes necrosis, fat and connective tissue replace the muscle fibers, which increases muscle size and results in muscle weakness (Fig. 15.6). The increase in muscle size resulting from connective tissue infiltration is called *pseudohypertrophy*. The muscle weakness is insidious in onset but continually progressive, varying with the type of disorder.

The most common form of the disease is DMD, which occurs once in every 3500 live male births.[9] DMD is inherited as a recessive single-gene defect on the X chromosome and is transmitted from the mother to her male offspring. A spontaneous (mutation) form may occur in girls. Another form of dystrophy, *Becker muscular dystrophy*, is similarly X-linked but manifests later in childhood or adolescence and has a slower course of progression.

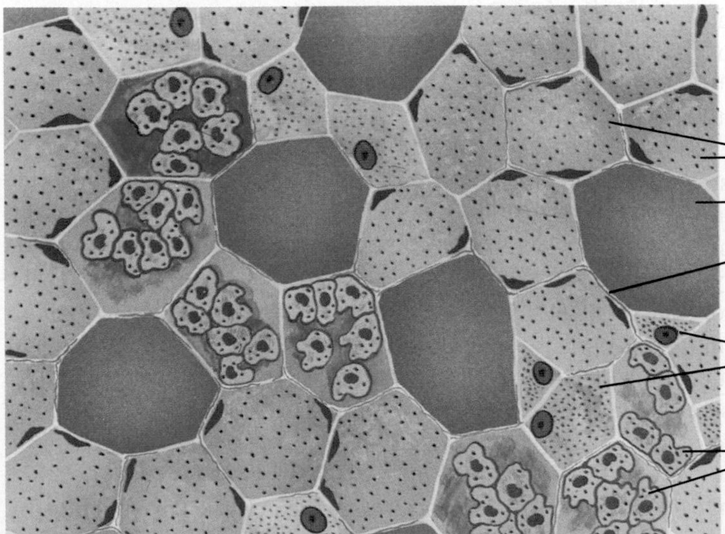

Figure 15.6 • Duchenne muscular dystrophy. The pathologic changes in skeletal muscle. Some fibers are slightly larger and darker than normal. These represent overcontracted segments of sarcoplasm situated between degenerated segments. Other fibers are packed with macrophages that remove degenerated sarcoplasm. Other fibers are smaller than normal and have granular sarcoplasm. These fibers have enlarged, vesicular nuclei with prominent nucleoli and represent regenerating fibers. Developing endomysial fibrosis is represented by the deposition of collagen around individual muscle fibers. The changes are those of a chronic, active noninflammatory myopathy. (From Strayer D. S., Rubin E., Saffitz J. E., et al. (Eds.) (2015). *Rubin's pathology: Clinicopathologic foundations of medicine* (7th ed., Chapter 31). Philadelphia, PA: Lippincott Williams & Wilkins.)

Etiology and Pathogenesis. DMD is caused by mutations in a gene located on the short arm of the X chromosome that codes for a protein called *dystrophin*. Dystrophin is a large cytoplasmic protein located on the inner surface of the sarcolemma or muscle fiber membrane. The dystrophin molecules are concentrated over the Z bands of the muscle, where they form a strong link between the actin filaments of the intracellular contractile apparatus and the extracellular connective tissue matrix.[6,7] It is thought that abnormalities in the dystrophin-associated protein complex compromise sarcolemma integrity, particularly with sustained contractions. This disruption in integrity may be responsible for the observed increased fragility of dystrophic muscle, excessive influx of calcium ions, and release of soluble muscle enzymes such as creatine kinase into the serum. The degenerative process in DMD consists of a relentless necrosis of muscle fibers, accompanied by a continuous process of repair and regeneration, and progressive fibrosis. The degenerative process eventually outpaces the regenerative capacity of the muscle, causing a gradual replacement of muscle fibers by fibrofatty connective tissue. The end stage is characterized by almost complete loss of skeletal muscle fibers, with relative sparing of intrafusal fibers of the muscle spindles.[7]

Clinical Manifestations. Signs of muscle weakness manifested by frequent falling usually become evident beginning when the child is between 2 and 3 years old. The postural muscles of the hips and shoulders are usually the first to be affected. Pseudohypertrophy of the calf muscles eventually develops. Imbalances between agonist and antagonist muscles lead to abnormal postures and the development of contractures and joint immobility. Scoliosis is common. Function of the distal muscles usually is preserved well enough that the child can continue to use eating utensils and a computer keyboard. Function of the extraocular muscles also is well preserved, as is the function of the smooth muscle controlling bladder and bowel activity. Incontinence is an uncommon and late event. Respiratory muscle involvement results in weak and ineffective cough, frequent respiratory infections, and decreasing respiratory reserve. DMD also affects cardiac muscle, and cardiomyopathy is a common feature of the disease. The severity of cardiac involvement, however, does not necessarily correlate with skeletal muscle weakness. Some people die at an early age from severe cardiomyopathy, whereas others maintain adequate cardiac function until the terminal stages of the disease. Death from respiratory and cardiac muscle involvement usually occurs in young adulthood.

Diagnosis. Important diagnostic data for this disease would include observation of the child's voluntary movements and a complete family history. Serum levels of the enzyme creatine kinase, which leaks from damaged muscle fibers, can be used to assist the diagnosis. Muscle biopsy, which shows a mixture of muscle cell degeneration and regeneration and reveals fat and scar tissue replacement, is diagnostic of the disorder. Echocardiography, electrocardiography, and chest radiography are used to assess cardiac function. A specific molecular genetic diagnosis is possible by demonstrating defective dystrophin via immunohistochemical staining of sections of muscle biopsy tissue or by polymerase chain reaction (PCR) analysis of genomic deoxyribonucleic acid (DNA) derived from leukocytes in a blood sample. The same methods of DNA analysis may be used on blood samples to establish carrier status in female relatives at risk, such as sisters and cousins.

Treatment. Management of the disease is directed toward maintaining ambulation and preventing deformities. Passive stretching, correct or counterposturing, and splints help to prevent deformities. Precautions should be taken to avoid respiratory infections. Although there have been exciting advances in identifying the gene and gene product involved in DMD, there is no known cure. Understanding the specific gene modifiers and relevant pathways that alter the course of the disease is necessary to develop targeted treatment options. Genotyping modifiers can identify people with specific phenotypes in order to develop personalized treatment.[10]

Disorders of the Neuromuscular Junction

The neuromuscular junction serves as a synapse between a motor neuron and a skeletal muscle fiber. It consists of the axon terminals of a motor neuron and a specialized region of the muscle membrane called the motor *end plate*. The transmission of impulses at the neuromuscular junction is mediated by the release of the neurotransmitter *acetylcholine* from the axon terminals. Acetylcholine binds to specific receptors in the end-plate region of the muscle fiber surface to cause muscle contraction (Fig. 15.7). Acetylcholine is active in the neuromuscular junction only for the brief period of time that it takes to generate an action potential in the innervated muscle cell. In the synaptic space are large quantities of the enzyme *acetylcholinesterase*, which destroy acetylcholine a few milliseconds after it has been released. The rapid inactivation of acetylcholine allows repeated muscle contractions and gradations of contractile force.

Drug- and Toxin-Induced Disorders

A number of drugs can alter neuromuscular function by changing the release, inactivation, or receptor binding of acetylcholine. A drug that acts on the postjunctional membrane of the motor end plate to prevent the depolarizing effect of the neurotransmitter is curare. To facilitate relaxation of involved musculature during surgical procedures, curare-type drugs are used to block the neuromuscular transmission. Drugs such as physostigmine and neostigmine inhibit the action of acetylcholinesterase and allow acetylcholine released from the motor neuron to accumulate and

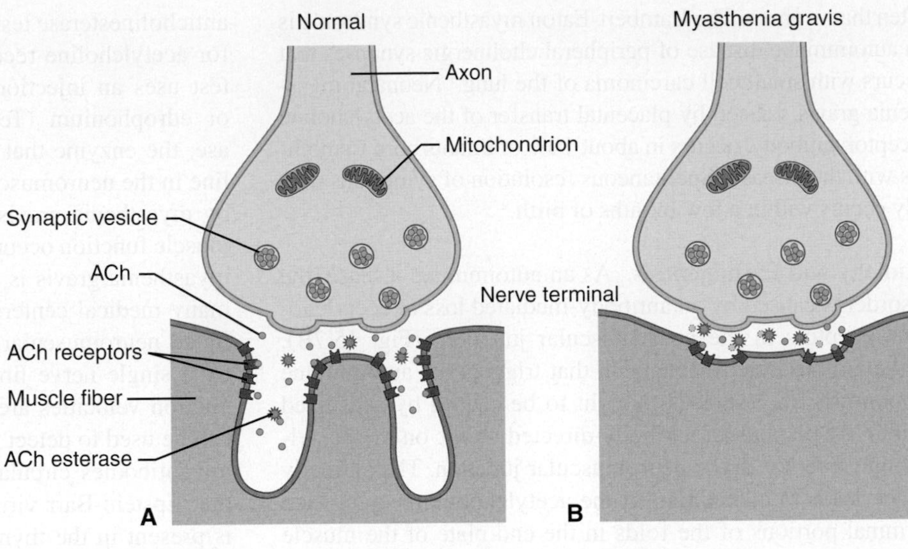

Figure 15.7 • Neuromuscular junction. **(A)** Acetylcholine (ACh) released from the motor neurons in the myoneural junction crosses the synaptic space to reach receptors that are concentrated in the folds of the end plate of the muscle fiber. Once released, ACh is rapidly broken down by the enzyme acetylcholinesterase (ACh esterase). **(B)** Decrease in ACh receptors in myasthenia gravis.

prolong its action.[11] These drugs are used in the treatment of myasthenia gravis.

Neurotoxins from the botulism organism (*Clostridium botulinum*) produce paralysis by blocking acetylcholine release.[7] Clostridia are anaerobic, gram-positive, spore-forming bacilli found worldwide in soils, marine and fresh water sediments, and the intestines of many animals. Classic food-borne botulism occurs through ingestion of soil-grown foods that are not properly cooked or preserved.[7] Spores can be dormant, are resistant to heat, and germinate in low-acidity and low-nitrate environments. Canned vegetables, items preserved in garlic oil, and soups are usually the cause of sporadic outbreaks. Ingestion of the spores leads to toxin synthesis and absorption of the toxins from the intestinal tract. Wound botulism occurs through colonization of wounds with *C. botulinum*.[7] Infant botulism, now the most commonly reported form of the disease, occurs through infant ingestion of *C. botulinum* spores.[12] An infant's immature gastrointestinal tract allows the spores to germinate and elaborate the botulinum toxins. Infants usually develop botulism by ingesting *C. botulinum* spores, which are found in the soil or in honey products.[12]

The classic clinical features of botulism include nausea, vomiting, constipation, cranial nerve abnormalities, hypotonia, hyperreflexia, and respiratory distress. Other common symptoms include difficulty speaking, dysphagia, paralysis, and urinary retention. Constipation may be present in affected infants for a variable time and precede weakness by several weeks. On average, symptoms appear within 18 to 36 hours of ingestion; however, symptoms can occur as soon as 6 hours and as long as 10 days after ingestion.

Pharmacologic preparations of the botulinum toxin (botulinum type A toxin [Botox] and botulinum type B toxin [Myobloc]) have become available for use in treating eyelid and eye movement disorders.[7] It also is used for treatment of spasmodic torticollis, spasmodic dysphonias (laryngeal dystonia), and other dystonias. The drug is injected into the target muscle using the electrical activity recorded from the tip of a special EMG injection needle to guide the injection. The treatment is not permanent and usually needs to be repeated at a specific time.

The aminoglycoside antibiotics (*e.g.*, gentamicin) prevent the release of acetylcholine from nerve endings and may produce a clinical disturbance similar to botulism. Once the drug is eliminated from the body, the symptoms usually subside rapidly. These drugs are particularly dangerous in people with pre-existing disturbances of neuromuscular transmission, such as myasthenia gravis.

The organophosphates that are used in some insecticides bind acetylcholinesterase to prevent the breakdown of acetylcholine. They produce excessive and prolonged acetylcholine action with a depolarization block of cholinergic receptors, including those of the neuromuscular junction.[13] The organophosphates are well absorbed from the skin, lungs, gut, and conjunctiva of the eye, making them particularly effective as insecticides but also potentially dangerous to humans. Certain organophosphates are rapidly metabolized to inactive products in humans and are considered safe for sale to the general public. The sale of other insecticides, such as parathion, which is not effectively metabolized to inactive products, has been banned. Other organophosphate compounds are developed as *nerve gases* with military potential. If absorbed in high enough concentrations, they have lethal effects from depolarization block and loss of respiratory muscle function.

Myasthenia Gravis

Myasthenia gravis is a disorder of transmission at the neuromuscular junction because of antibody-mediated attack on nicotinic AChR or muscle-specific tyrosine kinase (MuSK) that affects communication between the motor neuron and the innervated muscle.[9] This autoimmune disease may occur at any age, but the peak incidence occurs in young adulthood. The disease is approximately three times more common in women than men. A smaller, second peak occurs in later life and affects men more often than women. The Lambert-Eaton myasthenic syndrome is an autoimmune disease of peripheral cholinergic synapses that occurs with small cell carcinoma of the lung.[9] Neonatal myasthenia gravis, caused by placental transfer of the acetylcholine receptor antibody, occurs in about 10% of infants born to mothers with the disease. Spontaneous resolution of symptoms usually occurs within a few months of birth.[9]

Etiology and Pathogenesis. As an autoimmune disease, the disorder is caused by an antibody-mediated loss of acetylcholine receptors in the neuromuscular junction[9] (Fig. 15.7B). Although the exact mechanism that triggers the autoimmune response is unclear, it is thought to be caused by sensitized helper T cells and an antibody-directed attack on the acetylcholine receptor in the neuromuscular junction. The antibody attack leads to a shedding of the acetylcholine receptor–rich terminal portions of the folds in the end plate of the muscle fiber, fewer receptors, and a widened synaptic space that impairs signal transmission. The antibodies do not directly block binding of acetylcholine to prevent neuromuscular transmission. Approximately 70% of people with myasthenia gravis also have thymic abnormalities, such as a thymoma (*i.e.*, thymus tumor) or thymic hyperplasia (*i.e.*, increased thymus weight from an increased number of thymus cells).[9]

Clinical Manifestations. In people with myasthenia gravis who have a reduced postsynaptic membrane area and fewer acetylcholine receptors, each release of acetylcholine from the presynaptic membrane results in a lower-amplitude end-plate potential. This results in both muscle weakness and fatigability with sustained effort. Most commonly affected are the eye and periorbital muscles, with ptosis because of eyelid weakness or diplopia because of weakness of the extraocular muscles as an initial symptom. The disease may progress from ocular muscle weakness to generalized weakness, including respiratory muscle weakness. Chewing and swallowing may be difficult. Weakness in limb movement usually is more pronounced in proximal than in distal parts of the extremity, so that climbing stairs and lifting objects are difficult. As the disease progresses, the muscles of the lower face are affected, causing speech impairment. In most people, symptoms are least evident when arising in the morning, but grow worse with effort and as the day proceeds.

People with myasthenia gravis may experience a sudden exacerbation of symptoms and weakness known as *myasthenic crisis*. Myasthenic crisis occurs when muscle weakness becomes severe enough to compromise ventilation to the extent that ventilatory support and airway protection are needed. Myasthenic crisis usually occurs during a period of stress, such as infection, emotional upset, pregnancy, alcohol ingestion, cold exposure, or surgery. Cholinergic crisis results from inadequate or excessive doses of the anticholinesterase drugs used in treatment of myasthenia gravis.

Diagnosis and Treatment. The diagnosis of myasthenia gravis is based on history and physical examination, the anticholinesterase test, nerve stimulation studies, and an assay for acetylcholine receptor antibodies. The anticholinesterase test uses an injection of neostigmine bromide (Prostigmin) or edrophonium (Tensilon) that inhibits acetylcholinesterase, the enzyme that decreases the breakdown of acetylcholine in the neuromuscular junction. When weakness is caused by myasthenia gravis, a dramatic transitory improvement in muscle function occurs. An advance in diagnostic methods for myasthenia gravis is single-fiber EMG, which is available in many medical centers. Single-fiber EMG detects delayed or failed neuromuscular transmission in muscle fibers supplied by a single nerve fiber. The standard EMG and nerve conduction velocities are usually normal. An immunoassay test can be used to detect the presence of antiacetylcholine receptor antibodies circulating in the blood. Research has found that Epstein-Barr virus, a lymphotropic human herpes virus, is present in the thymuses of many people with myasthenia gravis.[14] Most children diagnosed with myasthenia gravis are found to already have antibodies to acetylcholine receptors, and their degree of disease is influenced by their genetics and environment.[15]

Treatment methods include the use of pharmacologic agents; immunosuppressive therapy, including corticosteroid drugs; management of myasthenic crisis; thymectomy; and plasmapheresis or intravenous immunoglobulin. Medications that may exacerbate myasthenia gravis, such as the aminoglycoside antibiotics, should be avoided. Pharmacologic treatment with reversible anticholinesterase drugs inhibits the breakdown of acetylcholine at the neuromuscular junction by acetylcholinesterase. Pyridostigmine and neostigmine are the drugs of choice. Corticosteroid drugs, which suppress the immune response, are used in cases of a poor response to anticholinesterase drugs and thymectomy. Immunosuppressant drugs (*e.g.*, azathioprine, cyclosporine) also may be used, often in combination with plasmapheresis.

Plasmapheresis removes antibodies from the circulation and provides short-term clinical improvement. It is used primarily to stabilize the condition of people in myasthenic crisis or for short-term treatment in people undergoing thymectomy. Intravenous immunoglobulin also produces improvement in people with myasthenia gravis. Although the effect is temporary, it may last for weeks to months. The indications for its use are similar to those for plasmapheresis. The mechanism of action of intravenous immunoglobulin is unknown. Thymectomy, or surgical removal of the thymus, may be used as a treatment for myasthenia gravis. Because the mechanism whereby surgery exerts its effect is unknown, the treatment is controversial. Removal of the thymus is frequently recommended for young people with myasthenia gravis, and these people generally have less of a progression of myasthenia.

Lower Motor Neuron Disorders

LMN diseases are progressive neurologic illnesses that selectively affect the anterior horn cells of the spinal cord and cranial nerve motor neurons.[7] An example of a disorder that involves purely LMNs is a distinctive group of degenerative disorders that begin in childhood or adolescence called *spinal muscular atrophy* (SMA). Weakness and muscle atrophy are prominent findings in all forms of the disorder. This condition is likely to be inherited, usually in an autosomal recessive fashion, and is caused by the deletion of the survival motor neuron-1 gene (*SMN1*). This disorder is classified as type I (Werdnig-Hoffman disease), type II (intermediate), and type III (Kugelberg-Welander disease).[7] Some forms of SMA result from degeneration of the anterior horn cells but are not caused by deletion of the *SMN1* gene. The most severe form may be symptomatic at birth or in the first months of life. In addition to hypotonia in the infant, people frequently die from respiratory failure.[7]

Peripheral Nerve Disorders

The peripheral nervous system consists of the motor and sensory branches of the cranial and spinal nerves, the peripheral parts of the autonomic nervous system, and the peripheral ganglia. A peripheral neuropathy is any primary disorder of the peripheral nerves. The result usually is muscle weakness, with or without atrophy and sensory changes.

Unlike nerves in the CNS, peripheral nerves are fairly strong and resilient. They contain a series of connective tissue sheaths that enclose their nerve fibers. An outer fibrous sheath called the *epineurium* surrounds the medium-sized to large nerves. Inside, a sheath called the *perineurium* invests each bundle of nerve fibers. In addition, within each bundle, a delicate sheath of connective tissue known as the *endoneurium* surrounds each nerve fiber. Inside the endoneurial sheath are the Schwann cells that produce the myelin sheath that surrounds the peripheral nerves. Each Schwann cell can myelinate only one segment of a single axon—the one that it covers. Therefore, myelination of an entire axon requires the participation of a long line of these cells.

Peripheral Nerve Injury and Repair

There are two main types of peripheral nerve injury based on the target of the insult—segmental demyelination involving the Schwann cell and axonal degeneration involving the neuronal cell body or its axon. The peripheral nerve disorders can affect a spinal nerve or nerve root, a nerve plexus, peripheral nerve trunk (mononeuropathies), or multiple peripheral nerves (polyneuropathies).

Segmental Demyelination. Segmental demyelination occurs when there is a disorder of the Schwann cell (as in Guillain-Barré syndrome) or damage to the myelin sheath (*e.g.*, sensory neuropathies), without a primary abnormality of the axon.[7] It typically affects some Schwann cells while sparing others. The denuded axon provides a stimulus for remyelination, and the population of cells in the endoneurium has the capacity to replace the injured Schwann cells. These cells proliferate and encircle the axon and, in time, remyelinate the denuded portion. However, the new myelin sheath is thin in proportion to the axon, and over time, many chronic demyelinating neuropathies give way to axonal injury.[7]

Axonal Degeneration. Axonal degeneration is caused by primary injury to a neuronal cell body or its axon. Damage to the axon may be due either to a focal event occurring at some point along the length of the nerve (*e.g.*, trauma or ischemia) or to a more generalized abnormality affecting the neuronal cell body (neuropathy).

Damage to a peripheral nerve axon, whether because of injury or neuropathy, results in degenerative changes, followed by breakdown of the myelin sheath and Schwann cells. In distal axonal degeneration, the proximal axon and neuronal cell body, which synthesizes the material required for nourishing and maintaining the axon, remain intact. In neuropathies and crushing injuries in which the endoneurial tube remains intact, the outgrowing fiber will grow down this tube to the structure that is originally innervated by the neuron (Fig. 15.8). However, it can take weeks or months for the regrowing fiber to reach its target organ and for communicative function to be re-established. More time is required for the Schwann cells to form new myelin segments and for the axon to recover its original diameter and conduction velocity.

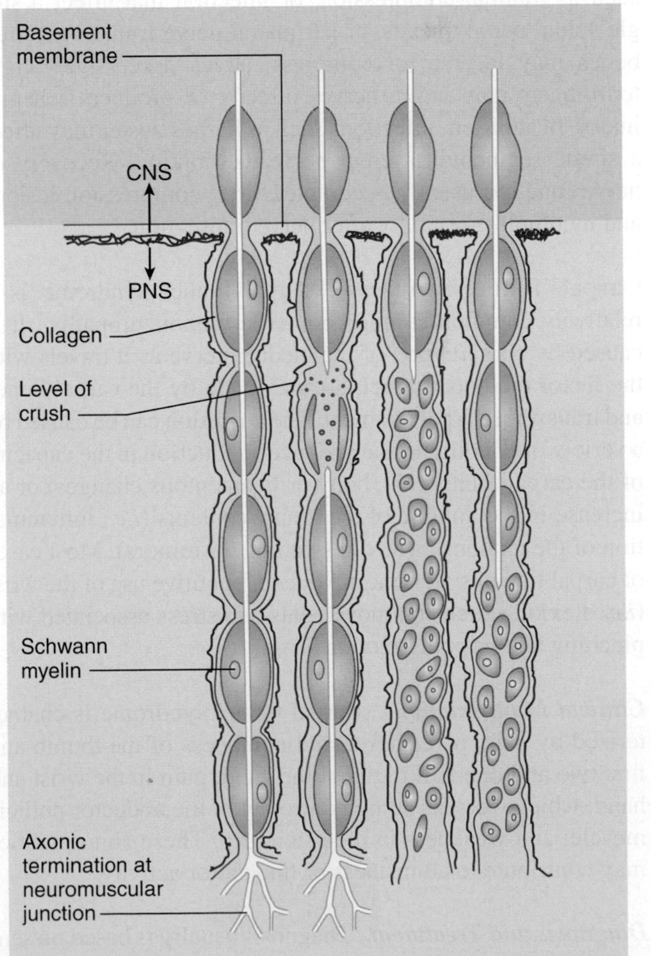

Figure 15.8 • Sequential stages in efferent axon degeneration and regeneration within its endoneurial tube, after peripheral nerve crush injury. PNS, peripheral nervous system.

The successful regeneration of a nerve fiber in the peripheral nervous system depends on many factors. If a nerve fiber is destroyed relatively close to the neuronal cell body, the chances are that the nerve cell will die, and if it does, it will not be replaced. If a crushing type of injury has occurred, partial or often full recovery of function occurs. Cutting-type trauma to a nerve is an entirely different matter. Connective scar tissue forms rapidly at the wound site, and when it does, only the most rapidly regenerating axonal branches are able to get through to the intact distal endoneurial tubes. Many scar-inhibiting agents have been used in an effort to reduce this hazard, but have met with only moderate success. In another attempt to improve nerve regeneration, various types of tubular implants have been placed to fill longer gaps in the endoneurial tube.

Neuropathies involving the neuronal cell body are much less common than those affecting the axons. In these cases, there is little potential for recovery of function because death of the neuronal cells precludes axonal regeneration.

Mononeuropathies

Mononeuropathies usually are caused by localized conditions such as trauma, compression, or infection that affect a single spinal nerve, plexus, or peripheral nerve trunk. Fractured bones may lacerate or compress nerves. Excessively tight tourniquets may injure nerves directly or produce ischemic injury. In addition, infections such as herpes zoster may affect a single segmental afferent nerve distribution. Recovery of nerve function usually is complete after compression lesions and incomplete or faulty after nerve transection.

Carpal Tunnel Syndrome. Carpal tunnel syndrome is a relatively common compression-type mononeuropathy.[7] It is caused by compression of the median nerve as it travels with the flexor tendons through a canal made by the carpal bones and transverse carpal ligament. The condition can be caused by a variety of conditions that produce a reduction in the capacity of the carpal tunnel (*i.e.*, bony or ligamentous changes) or an increase in the volume of the tunnel contents (*i.e.*, inflammation of the tendons, synovial swelling, or tumors). Most cases of carpal tunnel syndrome are due to repetitive use of the wrist (*i.e.*, flexion–extension movements and stress associated with pinching and gripping motions).

Clinical Manifestations. Carpal tunnel syndrome is characterized by pain, paresthesia, and numbness of the thumb and first two and one-half digits of the hand; pain in the wrist and hand, which worsens at night; atrophy of the abductor pollicis muscle; and weakness in precision grip. These abnormalities may contribute to clumsiness of fine motor activity.

Diagnosis and Treatment. Diagnosis usually is based on sensory disturbances confined to median nerve distribution and a positive Tinel or Phalen sign.[16] The *Tinel sign* is the development of a tingling sensation radiating into the palm of the hand that is elicited by light percussion over the median nerve at the wrist. The *Phalen maneuver* is performed by having the person hold the wrist in complete flexion for approximately a minute. If numbness and paresthesia along the median nerve are reproduced or exaggerated, the test result is considered to be positive. EMG and nerve conduction studies often are done to confirm the diagnosis and exclude other causes of the disorder.

Treatment includes avoidance of movements that cause nerve compression, splinting, and anti-inflammatory medications. Measures to decrease the causative repetitive movements should be initiated. Splints may be confined to nighttime use. When splinting is ineffective, corticosteroids may be injected into the carpal tunnel to reduce inflammation and swelling. Surgical intervention consists of operative division of the volar carpal ligaments as a means of relieving pressure on the median nerve.

Polyneuropathies

Polyneuropathies involve demyelination or axonal degeneration of multiple peripheral nerves that leads to symmetric sensory, motor, or mixed sensorimotor deficits. Typically, the longest axons are involved first, with symptoms beginning in the distal part of the extremities. If the autonomic nervous system is involved, there may be postural hypotension, constipation, and impotence. Polyneuropathies can result from immune mechanisms (*e.g.*, Guillain-Barré syndrome), toxic agents (*e.g.*, arsenic polyneuropathy, lead polyneuropathy, alcoholic polyneuropathy), and metabolic diseases (*e.g.*, diabetes mellitus, uremia). Different causes tend to affect axons of different diameters and to affect sensory, motor, or autonomic neurons to different degrees.

Guillain-Barré Syndrome. Guillain-Barré syndrome is an acute immune-mediated polyneuropathy.[17] The syndrome defines a clinical entity that is characterized by rapidly progressive ascending symmetrical limb weakness and loss of tendon reflexes. It has been described as the most common cause of acute, flaccid nontraumatic paralysis. There are several manifestations of the disorder, including pure motor axonal degeneration and axonal degeneration of both motor and sensory nerves.[7] The disorder is manifested by infiltration of mononuclear cells around the capillaries of the peripheral neurons, edema of the endoneurial compartment, and demyelination of ventral spinal roots. The cause of the Guillain-Barré syndrome probably has an immune component. Most people report having had an acute, influenza-like illness before the onset of symptoms. In addition, about one third of people with Guillain-Barré syndrome have antibodies against nerve gangliosides.

Clinical Manifestations. Progressive ascending muscle weakness of the limbs, producing a symmetric flaccid paralysis, characterizes the disorder. Symptoms of paresthesia and numbness often accompany the loss of motor function. Paralysis may progress to involve the respiratory muscles, which will mandate the use of a ventilator for these people. Autonomic nervous system involvement that causes postural hypotension, arrhythmias, facial flushing, abnormalities of sweating, and urinary retention is common. Pain is another common feature of Guillain-Barré syndrome. Guillain-Barré syndrome may have a rapid development of ventilatory failure and autonomic disturbances that threaten circulatory function or it may present as a slow, insidious process. Cranial nerve involvement might transpire resulting in facial, oculomotor, or bulbar weakness. Severity and duration of Guillain-Barré syndrome is diverse and can range from mild weakness with spontaneous recovery, to developing tetraplegic and ventilator dependence with no signs of recovery for several months or longer.[18]

Treatment. Treatment includes support of vital functions and prevention of complications such as skin breakdown and thrombophlebitis. Treatment is most effective if initiated early in the course of the disease.[18] Plasmapheresis and high-dose intravenous immunoglobulin therapy are generally the mainstay of treatment.

Back Pain

Low back pain or low back strain is a common problem that affects almost 70% of people at least once in their lifetime.[16] It affects men and women equally, with onset most often occurring between the ages of 30 and 50 years.[16] Risk factors include heavy lifting, smoking, obesity, and depressive symptoms.[19] However, low back pain is common even in people without these risk factors. Although acute low back pain resolves within 3 to 6 weeks in most people, recurrences are common.[16]

Back pain can result from many interrelated problems involving spinal structures, including facet joints, vertebral periosteum, ligaments, paravertebral musculature and fascia, and spinal nerve roots. People with low back pain frequently experience musculoligamentous injuries and age-related degenerative changes in the intervertebral disks and facet joints. Other causes include disk herniation, which is a herniated nucleus pulposus and spinal stenosis, which is characterized by narrowing of the central canal, typically from hypertrophic degenerative changes.[16]

The diagnostic measures used in the evaluation of back pain include history and physical examination, including a thorough neurologic examination. Other diagnostic methods include radiographs of the back and magnetic resonance imaging (MRI). MRI or radiography is not generally recommended early in the course of low back pain. The diagnostic challenge is to identify those people who require further evaluation for more serious problems.

Treatment of back pain usually is conservative and consists of analgesic medications, muscle relaxants, and instruction in the correct mechanics for lifting and methods of protecting the back.[16] Pain relief is usually provided using nonsteroidal anti-inflammatory drugs, other analgesics, and muscle relaxants. Because of the overwhelming frequency of sleep disorders with low back pain, it is important for the provider to also manage the sleep problem.[20]

Herniated Intervertebral Disk

The intervertebral disk is considered the most critical component of the load-bearing structures of the spinal column. The intervertebral disk consists of a soft, gelatinous center called the *nucleus pulposus*, which is encircled by a strong, ringlike collar of fibrocartilage called the *annulus fibrosus*.[2] The structural components of the disk make it capable of absorbing shock and changing shape while allowing movement. With dysfunction, the nucleus pulposus can be squeezed out of place and herniate through the annulus fibrosus, a condition referred to as a *herniated*, *ruptured*, or *slipped disk* (Fig. 15.9A and B).

Etiology and Pathogenesis. The intervertebral disk can become dysfunctional because of trauma, the effects of aging, or degenerative disorders of the spine. Trauma results from activities such as lifting while in the flexed position, slipping, falling on the buttocks or back, or suppressing a sneeze. With aging, the gelatinous center of the disk dries out and loses much of its elasticity, causing it to fray and tear. Degenerative

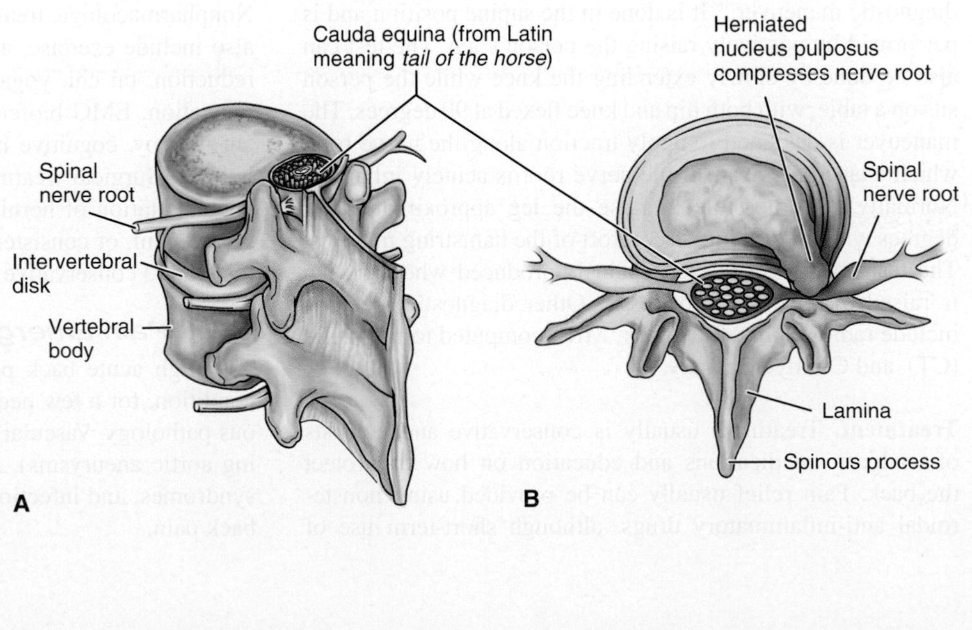

Figure 15.9 • **(A)** Normal lumbar spine vertebrae, intervertebral disks, and spinal nerve root. **(B)** Ruptured vertebral disk. (From Hinkle J. L., Cheever K. H. (2014). *Brunner & Suddarth's textbook of medical-surgical nursing* 13th ed., p. 2074. Philadelphia, PA: Lippincott Williams & Wilkins.)

processes such as osteoarthritis or ankylosing spondylitis predispose to malalignment of the vertebral column.

The cervical and lumbar regions are the most flexible areas of the spine and are most often involved in disk herniations. Usually, herniation occurs at the lower levels of the lumbar spine, where the mass being supported and the bending of the vertebral column are greatest. Most lumbar herniations occur in the L4 or L5 to S1 regions. With herniations of the cervical spine, the most frequently involved levels are C6 to C7 and C5 to C6. Protrusion of the nucleus pulposus usually occurs posteriorly and toward the intervertebral foramen and its contained spinal nerve root (see Fig. 15.9B).

The level at which a herniated disk occurs is important. When the injury occurs in the lumbar area, only the nerve fibers of the cauda equina are involved. Because these elongated dorsal and ventral roots contain endoneurial tubes of connective tissue, regeneration of the nerve fibers is likely. However, several weeks or months are required for full recovery to occur because of the distance to the innervated muscle or skin of the lower limbs.

Clinical Manifestations. The signs and symptoms of a herniated disk are localized to the area of the body innervated by the nerve roots and include both motor and sensory manifestations (Fig. 15.10). Pain is the first and most common symptom of a herniated disk. The nerve roots of L4, L5, S1, S2, and S3 give rise to a syndrome of back pain that spreads down the back of the leg and over the sole of the foot. The pain is usually intensified with coughing, sneezing, straining, stooping, standing, and the jarring motions that occur during walking or riding. Slight motor weakness may occur, although major weakness is rare. The most common sensory deficits from spinal nerve root compression are paresthesias and numbness, particularly of the leg and foot. A herniated disk must be differentiated from other causes of acute back pain.

Diagnosis. Diagnostic measures include history and physical examination. Neurologic assessment includes testing of muscle strength and reflexes. The straight-leg test is an important diagnostic maneuver.[16] It is done in the supine position and is performed by passively raising the person's leg. The test can also be done by slowly extending the knee while the person sits on a table, with both hip and knee flexed at 90 degrees. The maneuver is designed to apply traction along the nerve root, which exacerbates pain if the nerve root is acutely inflamed. Normally, it is possible to raise the leg approximately 90 degrees without causing discomfort of the hamstring muscles. The test result is positive if pain is produced when the leg is raised to 60 degrees or less.[16] Other diagnostic methods include radiographs of the back, MRI, computed tomography (CT), and CT myelography.

Treatment. Treatment usually is conservative and consists of analgesic medications and education on how to protect the back. Pain relief usually can be provided using nonsteroidal anti-inflammatory drugs, although short-term use of opioid pain medications may be required for severe pain. Muscle relaxants may be used on a short-term basis. For the initial treatment of acute or subacute low back pain, guidelines suggest nonpharmacologic treatment including superficial heat, massage, acupuncture, or spinal manipulation. Nonpharmacologic treatment of chronic low back pain should also include exercise, acupuncture, mindfulness-based stress reduction, tai chi, yoga, motor control exercise, progressive relaxation, EMG biofeedback, low-level laser therapy, operant therapy, cognitive behavioral therapy, or spinal manipulation.[21] Surgical treatment may be indicated when there is documentation of herniation by an imaging procedure, consistent pain, or consistent neurologic deficit that has failed to respond to conservative therapy.

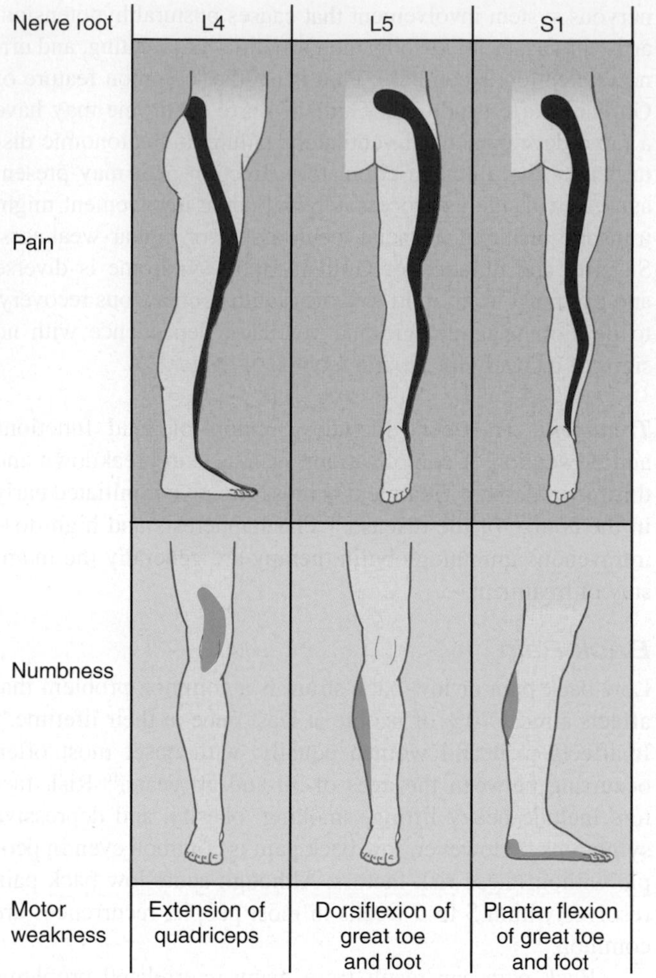

Figure 15.10 • Dermatomes of the leg (L1 through S5) where pain and numbness would be experienced with spinal root irritation.

Back Pain Emergencies

Although acute back pain is usually a non–life-threatening condition, for a few people, it can be a manifestation of serious pathology. Vascular catastrophes (abdominal and dissecting aortic aneurysms), malignancy, spinal cord compression syndromes, and infectious processes may all present as acute back pain.

Clinical findings, commonly referred to as *red flags*, which indicate the possibility of more serious disease include

- Gradual onset of pain
- Age younger than 20 years or older than 50 years
- Thoracic back pain
- History of trauma, fever, chills, night sweats, immunosuppression, or malignancy
- Unintentional weight loss
- Recent procedure known to cause bacteremia
- History of intravenous drug use[16]

The gradual onset of pain may be indicative of malignancy or infection. Back pain that begins before 20 years of age suggests congenital or developmental disorders, and new-onset pain in people 50 years of age or older is more likely to be a manifestation of serious conditions such as an aortic aneurysm, malignancy, or compression fracture. Pain that is aggravated by lying down is a red flag for malignancy or infection; and pain that improves with sitting or slight flexion of the spine suggests the presence of spinal stenosis. Reports of neurologic symptoms such as paresthesia, motor weakness, urinary or fecal incontinence, or gait abnormalities require additional diagnostic tests to rule out spinal cord compression.

IN SUMMARY

The motor unit consists of the LMN, the neuromuscular junction, and the skeletal muscle that the nerve innervates. Disorders of the neuromuscular unit include muscular dystrophy and myasthenia gravis. *Muscular dystrophy* is a term used to describe several disorders that produce progressive deterioration of skeletal muscle because of necrosis followed by fibrofatty tissue replacement. One form, DMD, is inherited as an X-linked trait and transmitted by the mother to her male offspring. Myasthenia gravis is a disorder of the neuromuscular junction resulting from a deficiency of functional acetylcholine receptors, which causes weakness of the skeletal muscles. Because the disease affects the neuromuscular junction, there is no loss of sensory function. The most common manifestations are weakness of the eye muscles, with ptosis and diplopia.

Peripheral nerve disorders involve motor and sensory neurons outside the CNS. There are two main types of peripheral nerve injury based on target of the insult: segmental demyelination involving the Schwann cell and axonal degeneration involving the nerve axon or cell body. Peripheral nerve disorders include mononeuropathies, involving a single spinal nerve, plexus, or peripheral nerve, and polyneuropathies that involve demyelination or axonal degeneration of multiple peripheral nerves that leads to symmetric sensory, motor, or mixed sensorimotor deficits. Carpal tunnel syndrome, a mononeuropathy, is caused by compression of the median nerve that passes through the carpal tunnel in the wrist. Guillain-Barré syndrome is a subacute polyneuropathy, probably because of immune mechanisms, that causes progressive ascending motor, sensory, and autonomic nervous system manifestations. Respiratory involvement may occur and necessitate mechanical ventilation.

Acute back pain is most commonly the result of conditions such as muscle strain; treatment focuses on measures to improve activity tolerance. A herniated intervertebral disk is characterized by protrusion of the nucleus pulposus into the spinal canal with irritation or compression of the nerve root. Usually, herniation occurs at the lower levels of the lumbar and sacral (L4 or L5 to S1) and cervical (C6 to C7 and C5 to C6) regions of the spine. The signs and symptoms of a herniated disk are localized to the area of the body innervated by the affected nerve roots and include pain and both motor and sensory manifestations.

DISORDERS OF THE CEREBELLUM AND BASAL GANGLIA

After completing this section of the chapter, the learner will be able to meet the following objectives:

- Relate the functions of the cerebellum to production of vestibulocerebellar ataxia, decomposition of movement, and cerebellar tremor.
- Describe the functional organization of the basal ganglia and communication pathways with the thalamus and cerebral cortex.

Disorders of the Cerebellum

The cerebellum is a structure located in the posterior fossa and attached to the pons, medulla, and midbrain by the three paired cerebellar peduncles.[2,7] It has sometimes been referred to as the *silent area* of the brain because electrical stimulation does not produce any conscious sensation and rarely causes any motor movements.[7] However, removal or damage to the cerebellum causes movements to become highly abnormal. The cerebellum is especially vital during rapid muscular activities such as running, typing, and even talking. Loss of cerebellar function can result in total incoordination of these functions even though paralysis does not ensue.

The functions of the cerebellum are integrated into many connected afferent and efferent pathways throughout the brain. An extensive and important afferent pathway is the *corticopontocerebellar* pathway, which originates in the cerebral motor and premotor cortices as well as the somatosensory cortex. Other important afferent pathways link the cerebellum to input from the basal ganglia, muscle and joint tension information from the stretch receptors, visual input from the eyes, and balance and equilibrium sensation from the vestibular system in the inner ear. There are three general efferent pathways leading out of the cerebellum:

- *Vestibulocerebellar pathway:* functions in close association with the brain stem vestibular nuclei to maintain equilibrium and posture
- *Spinocerebellar pathway:* provides the circuitry for coordinating the movements of the distal portions of the limbs, especially the hands and fingers
- *Cerebrocerebellar pathway:* transmits output information in the upward direction to the brain, functioning in a feedback manner with the motor and somatosensory systems to coordinate sequential body and limb movements

Cerebellum-Associated Movement Disorders

The signs of cerebellar dysfunction can be grouped into three classes—vestibulocerebellar disorders, cerebellar ataxia or decomposition of movement, and cerebellar tremor. These disorders occur on the side of cerebellar damage and are caused by congenital defect, vascular accident, or growing tumor. Visual monitoring of movement cannot compensate for cerebellar defects, and the movement abnormalities occur whether the eyes are open or closed.

Damage to the part of the cerebellum associated with the vestibular system leads to difficulty or inability to maintain a steady posture of the trunk, which normally requires constant readjusting movements. This is an unsteadiness of the trunk, called *truncal ataxia*, and can be so severe that standing is not possible. The ability to fix the eyes on a target also can be affected. Constant conjugate readjustment of eye position, called nystagmus, results and makes reading extremely difficult, especially when the eyes are deviated toward the side of cerebellar damage.

Cerebellar ataxia and tremor are different aspects of defects in the smooth, continuously correcting functions. Cerebellar dystaxia or, if severe, ataxia is characterized by a decomposition of movement, with each succeeding component of a complex movement occurring separately instead of being blended into a smoothly proceeding action. Because ethanol specifically affects cerebellar function, people who are inebriated often walk with a staggering and unsteady gait. Rapid alternating movements such as supination–pronation–supination of the hands are jerky and performed slowly. Reaching to touch a target breaks down into small sequential components, each going too far, followed by overcorrection. The finger moves jerkily toward the target, misses, corrects in the other direction, and misses again, until the target is finally reached. This is called *over- and underreaching* or *dysmetria*. Multiple sclerosis (MS) is the most common cause of cerebellar ataxia.[22] In up to 26% of preschool children, acute postinfectious cerebellar ataxia can occur with a prior history of varicella.[23]

Cerebellar tremor is a rhythmic back-and-forth movement of a finger or toe that worsens as the target is approached. The tremor results from the inability of the damaged cerebellar system to maintain ongoing fixation of a body part and to make smooth, continuous corrections in the trajectory of the movement; overcorrection occurs, first in one direction and then the other. Often, the tremor of an arm or leg can be detected during the beginning of an intended movement. The common term for cerebellar tremor is *intention tremor*. It is possible to assess cerebellar function as it relates to tremor by asking a person to touch one heel to the opposite knee, to gently move the toes along the back of the opposite shin, or to touch the nose with a finger.

Cerebellar function also can affect the motor skills of chewing and swallowing (dysphagia) and of speech (dysarthria). Normal speech requires smooth control of respiratory muscles and highly coordinated control of the laryngeal, lip, and tongue muscles. Cerebellar dysarthria is characterized by slow, slurred speech of continuously varying loudness. Speech therapy can provide rehabilitative efforts, including learning to slow the rate of speech and to compensate as much as possible using less-affected muscles.

Disorders of the Basal Ganglia

The basal ganglia are a group of deep, interrelated subcortical nuclei that provide an essential role in control of movement. They function in the organization of inherited and highly learned and rather automatic movement programs, especially those affecting the trunk and proximal limbs. The basal ganglia are thought to be particularly important in starting, stopping, and monitoring movements ordered and executed by the cortex, especially those that are relatively slow and sustained, or stereotyped, such as arm-swinging during walking. They also help to regulate the intensity of these movements, and they act to inhibit antagonistic or unnecessary movements. The function of the basal ganglia is not limited to motor functions. They also are involved in cognitive and perceptual functions.

The structural components of the basal ganglia include the caudate nucleus, putamen, and the globus pallidus.[2] They are located lateral and caudal to the thalamus, occupying a large portion of the interior of both cerebral hemispheres. The caudate and putamen are collectively referred to as the *striatum*, and the putamen and the globus pallidus form a wedge-shaped region called the *lentiform nucleus*. Two other structures, the *substantia nigra* of the midbrain *and subthalamic nucleus* of the diencephalon, are considered part of the basal ganglia[2] (Fig. 15.11). The dorsal part of the substantia nigra contains cells that use dopamine as a neurotransmitter and are rich in a black pigment called *melanin*. The high concentration of melanin gives the structure a black color, hence the name *substantia nigra*. The axons of the substantia nigra form the *nigrostriatal pathway*, which supplies dopamine to the striatum. The subthalamic nucleus lies just below the thalamus and above the anterior portion of the substantia nigra. The glutaminergic cells of this nucleus are the only excitatory projections to the basal ganglia.

Associated with the basal ganglia are several thalamic nuclei. For the motor and premotor cortices, these nuclei are

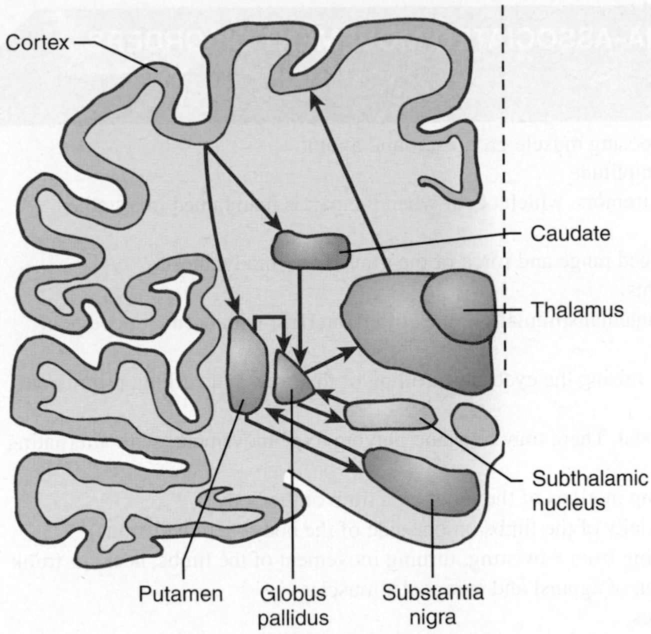

Figure 15.11 • Structures and basal neural circuitry of the basal ganglia.

the ventral lateral (VL) and the ventral anterior (VA) nuclei. Each region of the cerebral cortex is interconnected with a corresponding region of the ventral row of thalamic nuclei. The cortex-to-thalamus and thalamus-to-cortex feedback circuitries are excitatory and, if unmodulated, would produce hyperactivity of the cortical area, causing stiffness and rigidity of the face, body, and limbs, and, if alternating, a continuous tremor (*i.e.*, tremor at rest). For many semiautomatic stereotyped movements, thalamic excitability is modulated through inhibition by the basal ganglia. The basal ganglia form a major component of an inhibitory loop from each specific cortical region. Discrete inhibitory cortex-to-basal ganglia and thalamus-to-cortex loops modulate the function of all cerebral cortex regions.

The basal ganglia have input structures that receive afferent information from outside structures, internal circuits that connect the various structures of the basal ganglia, and output structures that deliver information to other brain centers. The striatum represents the major input structure for the basal ganglia. Virtually, all principal pathways for executing learned patterns of movement pass through the striatum. Other basal ganglia structures such as the substantia nigra and subthalamic nuclei are interconnected to one another or with the input and output nuclei and are components of the internal structures.

The output functions of the basal ganglia are mainly inhibitory. Looping circuits from specific cortical centers pass through the basal ganglia to modulate the excitability of certain thalamic nuclei and thus influence the cortical control of highly learned, automatic, and stereotyped motor functions. The two output nuclei of the basal ganglia, the globus pallidus and the substantia nigra, tonically inhibit their target nuclei in the thalamus. The basal ganglia also have a cognitive function. This function is closely connected with the cerebral cortex in that the basal ganglia monitor sensory information coming into the brain and apply it to information stored in memory. The cognitive control of motor activities determines, subconsciously and within seconds, which patterns of movement will be needed to achieve a goal. The caudate nucleus, which receives large amounts of input from the association areas of the brain, plays a major role in the cognitive control of motor activity.

Multiple pathways provide excitatory signals that balance the large number of inhibitory signals transmitted by GABA (γ-aminobutyric acid) ergic and dopaminergic neurons. One of these circuits involves a *neostriatal inhibitory projection* on the substantia nigra. The substantia nigra projects dopaminergic axons back on the striatum. Parkinsonism is a deficiency in the dopaminergic projection of this modulating circuit. The function of the striatum also involves local cholinergic interneurons. The destruction of these interneurons is thought to be related to the choreiform movements of Huntington disease, another basal ganglia–related syndrome.

Basal Ganglia–Associated Movement Disorders

Disorders of the basal ganglia comprise a complex group of motor disturbances characterized by tremor and other involuntary movements, changes in posture and muscle tone, and poverty and slowness of movement. They include tremors and tics, hypokinetic disorders, and hyperkinetic disorders[1] (Table 15.1).

Lesions of the basal ganglia disrupt movement. The various types of involuntary movements often occur in combination and appear to have a common underlying cause. There are hypokinetic and hyperkinetic disorders, which can be explained as having pathology in the indirect or direct pathways linking the basal ganglia with the thalamocortical motor circuit. Overactivity of the indirect pathway relative to the direct pathway would result in hypokinetic disorders such as Parkinson disease. Underactivity of the indirect pathway would result in hyperkinetic disorders such as chorea and ballismus.

Parkinson Disease

Parkinson disease is a degenerative disorder of basal ganglia function that results in variable combinations of tremor, rigidity, akinesia/bradykinesia, and postural changes. The disorder is characterized by progressive destruction of the nigrostriatal pathway, with subsequent reduction in striatal concentrations of dopamine. The prevalence of Parkinson disease in the United States is estimated at 1.0% of the population over 65 years of age.[16] The mean onset of Parkinson disease is 57 years of age, with approximately 60,000 new cases being diagnosed annually.

The clinical syndrome arising from the degenerative changes in basal ganglia function often is referred to as *parkinsonism.* In Parkinson disease, also known as *idiopathic*

TABLE 15.1 CHARACTERISTICS OF BASAL GANGLIA–ASSOCIATED MOVEMENT DISORDERS

MOVEMENT DISORDER	CHARACTERISTICS
Tremor	Involuntary, oscillating contractions of opposing muscle groups around a joint Usually fairly uniform in frequency and amplitude Can occur as resting tremors and postural tremors, which occur when the part is maintained in a stable position
Hypokinetic disorders	Slowness in initiating movement and reduced range and force of the movement (bradykinesia)
Chorea	Irregular wriggling and writhing movements Accentuated by movement and by environmental stimulation; they often interfere with normal movement patterns May be grimacing movements of the face, raising the eyebrows, rolling of the eyes, and curling, protrusion, withdrawal of the tongue In the limbs, the movements largely are distal. There may be piano playing–type movements with alternating extension and flexion of the fingers
Athetosis	Continuous, wormlike, twisting, and turning motions of the joints of a limb or the body
Ballismus	Violent, sweeping, flinging motions, especially of the limbs on one side of the body (hemiballismus)
Dystonia	Abnormal maintenance of a posture resulting from a twisting, turning movement of the limbs, neck, or trunk Often the result of simultaneous contraction of agonist and antagonist muscles Can result in grotesque and twisted postures
Dyskinesias	Bizarre wriggling and writhing movements Frequently involve the face, mouth, jaw, and tongue, causing grimacing, pursing of the lips, or protrusion of the tongue Limbs affected less often Tardive dyskinesia is an untoward reaction that can develop with long-term use of some antipsychotic medications

parkinsonism, dopamine depletion results from degeneration of the dopamine nigrostriatal system. Parkinsonism can also develop as a postencephalitic syndrome, as a side effect of therapy with antipsychotic drugs that block dopamine receptors, as a toxic reaction to a chemical agent, or as an outcome of severe carbon monoxide poisoning. In addition, symptoms of parkinsonism can occur when damage to the nigrostriatal pathway occurs in such conditions as cerebral vascular disease, brain tumors, repeated head trauma, or a degenerative neurologic disease.

The primary brain abnormality found in all people with Parkinson disease is degeneration of the nigrostriatal dopamine neurons.[16] On microscopic examination, there is loss of pigmented substantia nigra neurons (Fig. 15.12). Some residual nerve cells are atrophic, and few contain *Lewy bodies*, which are visualized as spherical, eosinophilic cytoplasmic inclusions. Lewy bodies are produced inside degenerated neurons in many people with Parkinson disease or parkinsonism.[16]

Etiology and Pathogenesis. Although the cause of Parkinson disease is still unknown, it is widely believed that most cases are caused by an interaction of environmental and genetic factors. Over the past several decades, several pathologic processes (*e.g.*, oxidative stress and mitochondrial disorders) that might lead to degeneration have been identified as causes of Parkinson disease. Some environmental factors have been identified that increase the risk of Parkinson disease. Occupational contact with specific agricultural pesticides has been related to the development of Parkinson disease. Rural living with private wells has been noted as a risk factor for Parkinson disease, especially if the area has been sprayed with herbicides and pesticides. Interestingly, smoking cigarettes and drinking coffee have a lower risk of Parkinson disease.[24] Multiple genes have been identified that illustrate there are different types of Parkinson disease depending on whether the person inherits a dominant or recessive gene.[25] In fact, it has been found that the recessive form causes a milder set of symptoms than the dominant form, which resembles the more complex and severe form of Parkinson disease with Lewy bodies.[25] Although rare, the autosomal dominant form of the disease has received considerable attention because α-synuclein is one of the major components of the Lewy bodies that are found in brain tissue of people with Parkinson disease.[7,25] Mutations in a second gene coding the protein *parkin* is associated with an autosomal recessive, early-onset form of Parkinson disease. The parkin protein acts as an enzyme (*i.e.*, ubiquitin ligase) in the ubiquitin-conjugating system that targets defective and abnormally folded proteins for destruction. Loss of normal parkin function is postulated to cause abnormal proteins to aggregate and cause neurodegenerative changes.[7] The relationship of genetics to Parkinson disease is beginning to provide more information that helps explain the etiology of parkinsonism, similar to the epidemiologic studies, which have identified multiple environmental risks. Also there

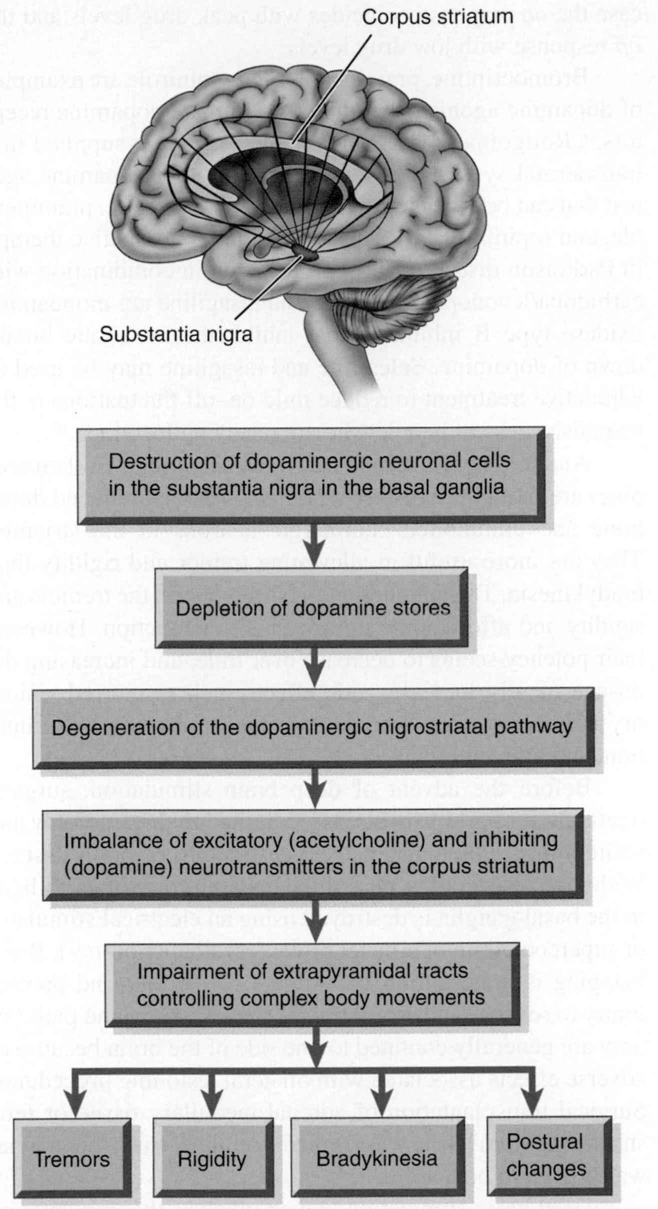

Figure 15.12 • Pathophysiology of Parkinson disease. The nuclei in the substantia nigra project fibers to the corpus striatum. The nerve fibers carry dopamine to the corpus striatum. The loss of dopamine nerve cells from the brain's substantia nigra is thought to be responsible for the symptoms of parkinsonism. (From Hinkle J. L., Cheever K. H. (2014). *Brunner & Suddarth's textbook of medical-surgical nursing* 13th ed., p. 2063. Philadelphia, PA: Lippincott Williams & Wilkins.)

are several new diagnostic tools available regarding genomic, proteomic, transcriptomic, lipidomic, and metabolomic molecules and signaling pathways that determine the diagnosis of Parkinson disease.[25] There are also syndromes that can cause parkinsonism and not the actual idiopathic Parkinson disease such as 1-methyl-4phenyl-1,2,3,6–tetrahydropyridine (MPTP)-induced parkinsonism, postinfectious parkinsonism, striatonigral degeneration, and progressive supranuclear palsy where the common finding is loss of pigmented dopaminergic neurons in the substantia nigra.[7]

Clinical Manifestations. The cardinal manifestations of Parkinson disease are tremor, rigidity, and bradykinesia or slowness of movement.[16] Tremor is the most visible manifestation of the disorder. The tremor affects the distal segments of the limbs, mainly the hands and feet; head, neck, face, lips, and tongue; or jaw. It is characterized by rhythmic, alternating flexion and contraction movements (4 to 6 beats/minute) that resemble the motion of rolling a pill between the thumb and forefinger. The tremor usually is unilateral, occurs when the limb is supported and at rest, and disappears with movement and sleep. The tremor eventually progresses to involve both sides of the body.

Rigidity is defined as resistance to movement of both flexors and extensors throughout the full range of motion. It is most evident during passive joint movement and involves jerky, cogwheel-type or ratchet-like movements that require considerable energy to perform. Flexion contractions may develop due to the rigidity. As with tremor, rigidity usually begins unilaterally but progresses to involve both sides of the body.

Bradykinesia is characterized by slowness in initiating and performing movements and difficulty with sudden, unexpected stopping of voluntary movements. Unconscious associative movements occur in a series of disconnected steps rather than in a smooth, coordinated manner. This is the most disabling of the symptoms of Parkinson disease. People with the disease have difficulty initiating walking and difficulty turning. While walking, they may freeze in place and feel as if their feet are glued to the floor, especially when moving through a doorway or preparing to turn. When they walk, they lean forward to maintain their center of gravity and take small, shuffling steps without swinging their arms, and they have difficulty changing their stride. Manifestations of advanced-stage parkinsonism include falls, fluctuations in motor function, neuropsychiatric disorders, and sleep disorders. Loss of postural reflexes predisposes to falling, often backward. Emotional and voluntary facial movements become limited and slow as the disease progresses, and facial expression becomes stiff and masklike. There is loss of the blinking reflex and a failure to express emotion. The tongue, palate, and throat muscles become rigid. The person may drool because of difficulty in moving the saliva to the back of the mouth and swallowing it. The speech becomes slow and monotonous, without modulation, and poorly articulated.

Because the basal ganglia also influence the autonomic nervous system, people with Parkinson disease often have excessive and uncontrolled sweating, sebaceous gland secretion, and salivation. Autonomic symptoms, such as lacrimation, dysphagia, orthostatic hypotension, thermal regulation, constipation, impotence, and urinary incontinence, may be present, especially late in the disease.

Cognitive dysfunction may also be an important feature associated with Parkinson disease. The most severe form of dementia is seen in about 20% of people with Parkinson disease. Deficits in visuospatial discrimination, frontal lobe executive function, and memory retrieval (compared with formation of new memories, as seen in Alzheimer disease) are more typical of the cognitive dysfunction seen in people with Parkinson disease than in other forms of dementia. Deficits in executive functioning may be among the earliest signs of cognitive decline, as evidenced by difficulty in planning, starting, and carrying out tasks. Dementia, when it does occur, is usually a late manifestation of the disease, and the rate of decline is slow compared with Alzheimer disease.

Treatment. The approach to treatment of Parkinson disease must be highly individualized. It is significant to realize that there is no treatment that will totally prevent the disease progression. Treatment only manages the symptoms.[16] Nonpharmacologic interventions offer group support, education, daily exercise, and adequate nutrition. Botulinum toxin injections may be used in the treatment of dystonias such as eyelid spasm and limb dystonias that frequently are associated with Parkinson disease. People with parkinsonism other than idiopathic Parkinson disease usually do not respond significantly to medications developed for Parkinson disease.

Pharmacologic treatment usually is determined by the severity of symptoms. Antiparkinson drugs act by increasing the functional ability of the underactive dopaminergic system or by reducing the excessive influence of excitatory cholinergic neurons. Drugs that improve the function of the dopaminergic system include those that increase dopamine levels (levodopa), stimulate dopamine receptors (dopamine receptor agonists), or retard the breakdown of dopamine (monoamine oxidase inhibitors). Because dopamine transmission is disrupted in Parkinson disease, there is a preponderance of cholinergic activity, which may be treated with anticholinergic drugs.[26]

Dopamine does not cross the blood–brain barrier. Administration of levodopa, a precursor of dopamine that does cross the blood–brain barrier, has yielded significant improvement in clinical symptoms of Parkinson disease and remains the most effective drug for treatment. The evidence of decreased dopamine levels in the striatum in Parkinson disease led to the administration of large doses of the synthetic compound levodopa, which is absorbed from the intestinal tract, crosses the blood–brain barrier, and is converted to dopamine by centrally acting dopa decarboxylase. When levodopa (a decarboxylase inhibitor) is given in combination with carbidopa, the peripheral metabolism of levodopa is reduced, plasma levels of levodopa are increased and its half-life is longer, more levodopa is available for entry into the brain, and a smaller dose is needed.[26] A later adverse effect of levodopa treatment is the so-called *on–off phenomenon*, in which frequent, abrupt, and unpredictable fluctuations in motor performance occur during the day. These fluctuations include *on* periods without dyskinesia, *on* periods with dyskinesia, and periods of bradykinesia (the *off* response). Some fluctuations reflect the timing of drug administration, in which case the *on* response coincides with peak drug levels and the *off* response with low drug levels.

Bromocriptine, pramipexole, and ropinirole are examples of dopamine agonists that directly stimulate dopamine receptors.[26] Rotigotine is a dopamine agonist that is supplied in a transdermal system. Apomorphine is another dopamine agonist that can be given intravenously. Bromocriptine, pramipexole, and ropinirole can be used as initial or adjunctive therapy in Parkinson disease. They can be given in combination with carbidopa/levodopa. Selegiline and rasagiline are monoamine oxidase type B inhibitors that inhibit the metabolic breakdown of dopamine. Selegiline and rasagiline may be used as adjunctive treatment to reduce mild on–off fluctuations in the responsiveness of people who are receiving levodopa.[16]

Anticholinergic drugs (*e.g.*, trihexyphenidyl, benztropine) are thought to restore a *balance* between reduced dopamine and uninhibited cholinergic neurons in the striatum. They are more useful in alleviating tremor and rigidity than bradykinesia. The anticholinergic drugs lessen the tremors and rigidity and afford some improvement of function. However, their potency seems to decrease over time, and increasing the dosage merely increases side effects such as blurred vision, dry mouth, bowel and bladder problems, cognitive dysfunction, and hallucinations.[16]

Before the advent of deep brain stimulation, surgical treatment for Parkinson disease is limited to thalamotomy and pallidotomy, which also caused destruction of brain tissue.[16] With these procedures, part of the thalamus or globus pallidus in the basal ganglia is destroyed using an electrical stimulator or supercooled tip of a metal probe (cryothalamotomy). Brain mapping is done during the surgery to identify and prevent injury to sensory and motor tracts. Thalamotomy and pallidotomy are generally confined to one side of the brain because of adverse effects associated with bilateral lesioning procedures. Surgical transplantation of adrenal medullary tissue or fetal substantia nigra tissue was studied in clinical trials, but neither was proven to be helpful.

Deep brain stimulation, which involves the implantation of electrodes into the subthalamic nuclei or the pars interna of the globus pallidus, is performed more frequently for treatment of Parkinson disease in the United States because it is considered to be nondestructive and reversible.[16] The electrodes are connected to a surgically implanted impulse generator that delivers electrical simulation to block the abnormal nerve activity that causes tremor and abnormal motor activity in Parkinson disease. The deep brain stimulation system allows the stimulation to be programmed to control the person's symptoms, and the stimulation parameters can be changed over time as the disease progresses. Deep brain stimulation is used for people with Parkinson disease who respond to levodopa but experience side effects associated with it (*e.g.*, motor fluctuation or dyskinesia). It is not a cure but serves to increase the duration of the *on* periods, allows for a reduction in medication dosages (in subthalamic nuclei stimulation), and improves function.

IN SUMMARY

Alterations in coordination of muscle movements and abnormal muscle movements result from disorders of the cerebellum and basal ganglia. The functions of the cerebellum, which are especially vital during rapid muscular movements, use afferent input from various sources, including the stretch receptors, proprioceptors, tactile receptors in the skin, visual input, and vestibular system. Cerebellar disorders include vestibulocerebellar dysfunction, cerebellar ataxia, and cerebellar tremor.

The basal ganglia organize basic movement patterns into more complex patterns and release them when commanded by the motor cortex, contributing gracefulness to cortically initiated and controlled skilled movements. Disorders of the basal ganglia are characterized by involuntary movements, alterations in muscle tone, and disturbances in posture. These disorders include tremor, tics, hemiballismus, chorea, athetosis, dystonias, and dyskinesias.

Parkinsonism, a disorder of the basal ganglia, is characterized by destruction of the nigrostriatal pathway, with a subsequent reduction in striatal concentrations of dopamine. This results in an imbalance between the inhibitory effects of dopaminergic basal ganglia functions and an increase in the excitatory cholinergic functions. The disorder is manifested by resting tremor, increased muscle tonus and rigidity, slowness of movement (*i.e.*, bradykinesia), gait disturbances, and impaired autonomic postural responses. The disease usually is slowly progressive over several decades. The tremor often begins in one or both hands and then becomes generalized. Postural changes and gait disturbances continue to become more pronounced, resulting in significant disability.

UPPER MOTOR NEURON DISORDERS

After completing this section of the chapter, the learner will be able to meet the following objectives:

- Relate the pathologic UMN and LMN changes that occur in amyotrophic lateral sclerosis (ALS) to the manifestations of the disease.
- Explain the significance of demyelination and plaque formation in MS.
- State the effects of SCI on ventilation and communication, the autonomic nervous system, cardiovascular function, sensorimotor function, and bowel, bladder, and sexual functions.

UMN disorders involve neurons that are fully contained within the CNS. They include the motor neurons arising in the motor areas of the cortex and their fibers as they project through the brain and descend in the spinal cord. ALS is a mixed UMN and LMN disorder. Disorders that affect UMNs include MS and SCI.

Amyotrophic Lateral Sclerosis

ALS, also known as *Lou Gehrig disease* after the famous New York Yankees baseball player, is a devastating neurologic disorder that selectively affects motor function. ALS has an annual incidence of 1 per 100,000 population.[7] ALS is primarily a disorder of middle to late adulthood, affecting people most frequently in their fifties, with men developing the disease nearly twice as often as women.

ALS affects motor neurons in three locations—the anterior horn cells (LMNs) of the spinal cord; the motor nuclei of the brain stem, particularly the hypoglossal nuclei; and the UMNs of the cerebral cortex.[7] The fact that the disease is more extensive in the distal parts of the affected tracts in the lower spinal cord rather than the proximal parts suggests that affected neurons first undergo degeneration at their distal terminals and that the disease proceeds until ultimately the parent nerve cell dies. A remarkable feature of the disease is that the entire sensory system, the regulatory mechanisms of control and coordination of movement, and the intellect remain intact. The neurons for ocular motility and the parasympathetic neurons in the sacral spinal cord also are spared.

The death of LMNs leads to denervation, with subsequent shrinkage of musculature and muscle fiber atrophy. It is this fiber atrophy, called *amyotrophy*, which appears in the name of the disease. The loss of nerve fibers in lateral columns of the white matter of the spinal cord, along with fibrillary gliosis, imparts a firmness or sclerosis to this CNS tissue. The term *lateral sclerosis* designates these changes.

Etiology and Pathogenesis

The cause of LMN and UMN destruction in ALS is uncertain. Five percent of cases are familial. The others are believed to be sporadic, with no family history of the disease.[7] The gene for a subset of familial ALS has been mapped to superoxide dismutase 1 (*SOD1*) on chromosome 21.[7] The neurofilament proteins, which function in the axonal transport of molecules, are destroyed with ALS. Other genetic loci for ALS have been mapped but not yet cloned. Another suggested mechanism of pathogenesis in ALS is exotoxic injury through activation of glutamate-gated ion channels, which are distinguished by their sensitivity to *N*-methyl-D-aspartic acid. Although autoimmunity has been suggested as a cause of ALS, the disease does not respond to the immunosuppressant agents that normally are used in treatment of autoimmune disorders.

Clinical Manifestations

The symptoms of ALS may be referable to UMN or LMN involvement. Manifestations of UMN lesions include weakness, spasticity or stiffness, and impaired fine motor control.[7] Dysphagia (difficulty swallowing), dysarthria (impaired articulation of speech), and dysphonia (difficulty making the sounds of speech) may result from brain stem LMN involvement or from dysfunction of UMNs descending to the brain stem. Manifestations of LMN destruction include fasciculations, weakness, muscle atrophy, and hyporeflexia.[7] Muscle cramps involving the distal legs often are an early symptom. The most common clinical presentation is slowly progressive weakness and atrophy in distal muscles of one upper extremity. This is followed by regional spread of clinical weakness, reflecting involvement of neighboring areas of the spinal cord. Eventually, UMNs and LMNs involving multiple limbs and the head are affected. In the more advanced stages, muscles of the palate, pharynx, tongue, neck, and shoulders become involved, causing impairment of chewing, swallowing, and speech. Dysphagia with recurrent aspiration and weakness of the respiratory muscles produces the most significant acute complications of the disease. Death usually results from involvement of cranial nerves and respiratory musculature.

Treatment

Currently, there is no cure for ALS. Management of people with ALS is challenging and requires a multidisciplinary team. Measures to assist people with the disorder to manage their symptoms (*e.g.*, weakness and muscle spasms, dysphagia, communication difficulty, excessive watery saliva, and emotional lability), nutritional status, and respiratory muscle weakness allow people with the disorder to survive longer than would otherwise have been the case. Riluzole, an antiglutamate drug, has been proven to prolong survival in ALS.[27] The drug is designed to decrease glutamate accumulation and slow the progression of the disease. Clinical trials are focused on exercise programs, nutritional interventions, transplanted stem cells, and antisense therapy.[27]

Multiple Sclerosis

As with other demyelinating disorders, MS is characterized by inflammation and destruction of mostly the white matter of the CNS myelin.[16,28] The peripheral nervous system is spared, and there is usually no evidence of an associated systemic disease. MS is estimated to affect 400,000 people in the United States.[29] The age of onset is typically between 20 and 30 years, with women being affected twice as frequently as men.[16] MS results in significant functional and often work-related disability in people who are in the prime of their productivity.

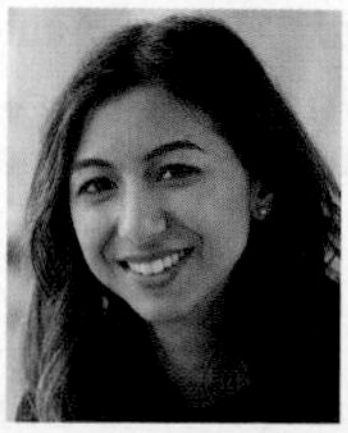

Remember **Ms. Ulrie,** whom you were introduced to in the Unit V case study opening scenario? Ms. Ulrie is a 22-year-old college student who is diagnosed with remitting–relapsing MS. Ms. Ulrie fits the age of onset of MS, which is typically between 20 and 30 years of age. She also has a family member with MS (her grandmother), and her female gender puts her at higher risk for MS compared to males. It will be challenging for Ms. Ulrie to be successful with her college studies during exacerbations of MS.

Etiology

MS occurs more commonly in people of Northern European ancestry and is uncommon in Asians.[29] It has been observed that the disease is more common in northern latitudes, perhaps related to the selective migration of people with a susceptible genetic background to these regions.[29] The prevalence is low in Asia, Africa, and northern South America.

The person with MS has a 10% to 20% chance of having a family member with MS.[29] The risk without having any family history is 1/1000.[7] People with the human leukocyte antigen HLA-DR2 haplotype are particularly at risk for MS.[30]

Pathogenesis

MS is believed to be an immune-mediated disorder that occurs in people who are genetically susceptible. Although the target antigen has not been identified, the data suggest an immune response to a protein in the CNS.

The lesions of MS consist of hard, sharp-edged, demyelinated patches that are visible throughout the white matter as well as sometimes the gray matter of the CNS[7] (Fig. 15.13). These lesions, which represent the result of acute myelin breakdown, are called *plaques*. The lesions have a predilection for the optic nerves, periventricular white matter, brain stem, cerebellum, and spinal cord white matter.[7] In an active plaque, there is evidence of ongoing myelin breakdown. The sequence of myelin breakdown is not well understood, although it is known that the lesions contain small amounts of myelin basic proteins and increased amounts of proteolytic enzymes, macrophages, lymphocytes, and plasma cells.

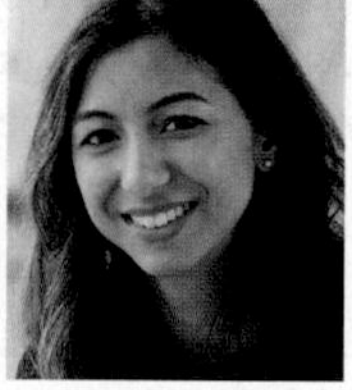

Ms. Ulrie had an MRI, which illustrated she already had one or two periventricular plaques. This would explain some of her symptoms of blurry vision, upper extremity weakness, tingling, and numbness of both hands. On neurologic examination, she had blurry vision in the right eye, motor weakness, and a feeling of pins and needles in both hands. She also complained of being very fatigued.

Oligodendrocytes are decreased in number and may be absent, especially in older lesions. Acute, subacute, and chronic lesions often are seen at multiple sites throughout the CNS.

MRI has shown that the lesions of MS may occur in two stages:

1. A first stage that involves the sequential development of small inflammatory lesions
2. A second stage during which the lesions extend and consolidate and when demyelination and gliosis (scar formation) occur

It is not known whether the inflammatory process, present during the first stage, is directed against myelin or against the oligodendrocytes that produce myelin.

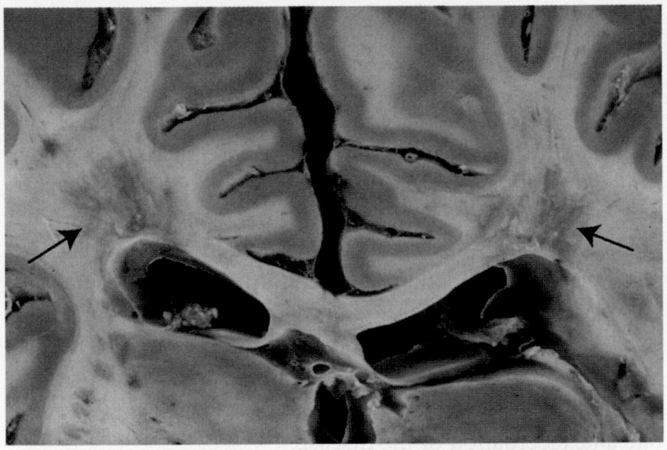

Figure 15.13 • Multiple sclerosis. This fresh coronal section shows darker hues of the somewhat irregular periventricular plaques (*arrows*) reflecting the loss of myelin, which imparts the normal glistening white appearance of white matter. (From Strayer D. S., Rubin E., Saffitz J. E., et al. (Eds.) (2015). *Rubin's pathology: Clinicopathologic foundations of medicine* (7th ed., Chapter 32). Philadelphia, PA: Lippincott Williams & Wilkins.)

Clinical Manifestations and Course

The pathophysiology of MS involves the demyelination of nerve fibers in the white matter of the brain, spinal cord, and optic nerve. In the CNS, myelin is formed by the oligodendrocytes, chiefly those lying among the nerve fibers in the white matter. This function of the oligodendrocytes is equivalent to that of the Schwann cells in the peripheral nervous system. The properties of the myelin sheath—high electrical resistance and low capacitance—permit it to function as an electrical insulator. Demyelinated nerve fibers display a variety of conduction abnormalities, ranging from decreased conduction velocity to conduction blocks. The interruption of neural conduction in the demyelinated nerves is manifested by a variety of symptoms, depending on the location and extent of the lesion. Areas commonly affected by MS are the optic nerve (visual field), corticobulbar tracts (speech and swallowing), corticospinal tracts (muscle strength), cerebellar tracts (gait and coordination), spinocerebellar tracts (balance), medial longitudinal fasciculus (conjugate gaze function of the extraocular eye muscles), and posterior cell columns of the spinal cord (position and vibratory sensation). Typically, an otherwise healthy person presents with an acute or subacute episode of paresthesias, optic neuritis (*i.e.*, visual clouding or loss of vision in part of the visual field with pain on movement of the globe), diplopia, or specific types of gaze paralysis.

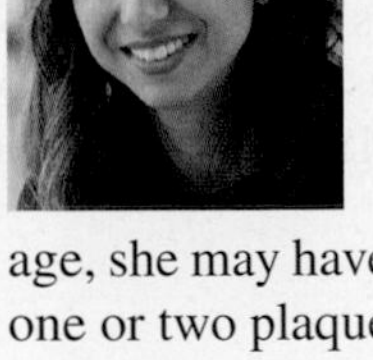

Ms. Ulrie presented with blurry vision in the right eye, which is indicative of optic neuritis. She had been feeling fine until a week ago when she experienced this acute episode of symptoms. The symptoms persisted, so she went to the emergency department. At 22 years of age, she may have had the MS for a while given that she had one or two plaques already as illustrated in her MRI.

Paresthesias are evidenced as numbness, tingling, burning sensations, or pressure on the face or involved extremities, with symptoms ranging from annoying to severe. Pain from spasticity also may be a factor that can be alleviated by appropriate stretching exercises. Other common symptoms are abnormal gait, bladder and sexual dysfunction, vertigo, nystagmus, fatigue, and speech disturbance. These symptoms usually last for several days to weeks and then completely or partially resolve. After a period of normal or relatively normal function, new symptoms appear. Psychological manifestations, such as mood swings, may represent an emotional reaction to the nature of the disease or, more likely, involvement of the white matter of the cerebral cortex. Depression, euphoria, inattentiveness, apathy, forgetfulness, and loss of memory may occur. Fatigue is one of the most common problems for people with MS. Fatigue often is described as a generalized low-energy feeling not related to depression and different from weakness. Fatigue has a harmful impact on activities of daily living and sustained physical activity. Interventions such as spacing activities and setting priorities often are helpful.

The course of the disease may fall into one of four categories:

1. Relapsing–remitting
2. Secondary progressive
3. Primary progressive
4. Progressive relapsing[7,16]

The *relapsing–remitting* form of the disease is characterized by episodes of acute worsening with recovery and a stable course between relapses.

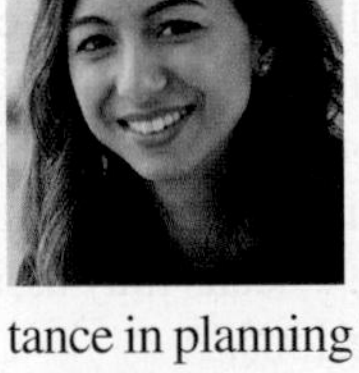

It will be difficult for **Ms. Ulrie** if she progresses to having speech disturbances; mood swings, which would indicate white matter involvement; forgetfulness; and loss of memory as a college student. She is very fatigued, which is another frequent symptom, and she will need to have some assistance in planning her hectic course schedule so she can manage it. Ms. Ulrie is diagnosed with the relapsing–remitting form of MS so she should have some stable times in between exacerbations if she is able to organize herself and get adequate rest. This will indeed be difficult as a college student.

Secondary progressive disease involves a gradual neurologic deterioration with or without superimposed acute relapses in a person with previous relapsing–remitting disease. *Primary progressive disease* is characterized by nearly continuous neurologic deterioration from onset of symptoms. The *progressive relapsing* category of disease involves gradual neurologic deterioration from the onset of symptoms but with subsequent superimposed relapses.[7,16]

Diagnosis

The diagnosis of MS is based on established clinical and, when necessary, laboratory criteria. There is no one definitive diagnostic test. Advances in cerebrospinal fluid (CSF) analysis and

MRI have greatly simplified the procedure. A definite diagnosis of MS requires evidence of one of the following patterns:

- Two or more episodes of exacerbation separated by 1 month or more and lasting more than 24 hours, with subsequent recovery
- A clinical history of clearly defined exacerbations and remissions, with or without complete recovery, followed by progression of symptoms over a period of at least 6 months
- Slow and stepwise progression of signs and symptoms over a period of at least 6 months[16]

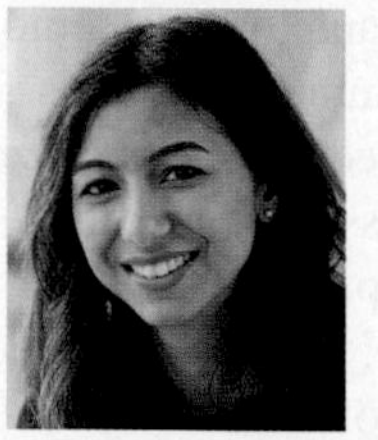

With a more detailed history taking session, the neurologist can determine that Ms. Ulrie had similar symptoms, but especially visual blurriness about 6 months prior to this event. She says she just took it easy and rested because it is summertime and all the symptoms went away. She had not seen a physician for this previous episode because she felt it was due to stress of the previous academic year. She also did not have the fatigue that she has now nor is the blurriness as bad in her eye.

Primary progressive MS may be suggested by a progressive course that lasts longer than 6 months. A person who has not had a relapse or progression of symptoms is described as having stable MS.

MRI can be used as an adjunct to clinical diagnosis. MRI studies can detect lesions even when CT scans appear normal. A computer-assisted method of MRI can measure lesion size. Many new areas of myelin abnormality are asymptomatic. Serial MRI studies can be done to detect asymptomatic lesions, monitor the progress of existing lesions, and evaluate the effectiveness of treatment. Although MRI can be used to provide evidence of disseminated lesions in people with the disease, normal findings do not exclude the diagnosis. Electrophysiologic evaluations (*e.g.*, evoked potential studies) and CT scans may assist in the identification and documentation of lesions.

Although no laboratory test can be used to diagnose MS, examination of the CSF is helpful. A large percentage of people with MS have elevated immunoglobulin G (IgG) levels, and some have oligoclonal patterns (*i.e.*, discrete electrophoretic bands) even with normal IgG levels. Total protein or lymphocyte levels may be mildly elevated in the CSF. These test results can be altered in a variety of inflammatory neurologic disorders and are not specific for MS.

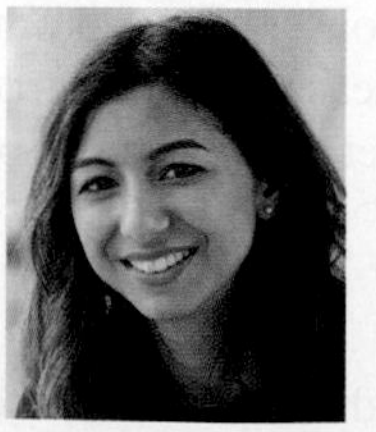

The CSF from the lumbar puncture results are protein 0.40/L, lymphocytes 3×10^6/L, and oligoclonal bands present. Oligoclonal bands are not found in normal CSF, but are found in 90% of people with MS. These results added to the confirmation of the diagnosis for Ms. Ulrie.

Treatment

Most treatment measures for MS are directed at modifying the course and managing the primary symptoms of the disease. The variability in symptoms, unpredictable course, and lack of specific diagnostic methods have made the evaluation and treatment of MS difficult. People who are minimally affected by the disorder require no specific treatment. The person should be encouraged to maintain as healthy a lifestyle as possible, including good nutrition and adequate rest and relaxation. Physical therapy may help maintain muscle tone. Every effort should be made to avoid excessive fatigue, physical deterioration, emotional stress, viral infections, and extremes of environmental temperature, which may precipitate an exacerbation of the disease.

The pharmacologic agents used in the management of MS fall into three categories:

1. Those used to treat acute attacks or initial demyelinating episodes
2. Those used to modify the course of the disease
3. Those used to treat symptoms of the disorder

Corticosteroids are the mainstay of treatment for acute attacks of MS. These agents are thought to reduce the inflammation, improve nerve conduction, and have important immunologic effects. Long-term administration does not, however, appear to alter the course of the disease and can have harmful side effects. Plasmapheresis and intravenous immunoglobulin have also proven beneficial in some cases.

The agents used to modify the course of the disease include interferon beta, glatiramer acetate, and mitoxantrone.[16] These agents have shown some benefit in reducing exacerbations in people with relapsing–remitting MS. Interferon beta is a cytokine that acts as an immune enhancer. Interferon is administered by injection and is usually well tolerated. The most common side effects are flulike symptoms for 24 to 48 hours after each injection, and these usually subside after 2 to 3 months of treatment. Glatiramer acetate is a synthetic polypeptide that simulates parts of the myelin basic protein. Although the exact mechanism of action is unknown, the drug seems to block myelin-damaging T cells by acting as a myelin decoy. The drug is given daily by subcutaneous injection.[16]

Mitoxantrone is an antineoplastic agent that prevents the ligation of DNA strands and thus delays the cell cycle progression and has immunomodulatory properties. Acute drug side effects include nausea and alopecia. Recently, a humanized monoclonal antibody, natalizumab, has also been approved for relapsing–remitting MS. Its action is suppression of leukocyte entry into the CNS.[26]

Among the medications used to manage the chronic problems associated with MS are dantrolene, baclofen, or diazepam for spasticity; cholinergic drugs for bladder problems; and antidepressant drugs for depression. A high-fiber diet is recommended for people with MS who experience constipation.

Vertebral and Spinal Cord Injury

SCI represents damage to the neural elements of the spinal cord. SCI is primarily a disorder of young people, with most injuries occurring in the 29- to 42-year age group.[31] In the United States, there are 282,000 people with spinal cord injuries.[31] The most common cause of SCI is motor vehicle crash, followed by falls, violence (primarily gunshot wounds), and recreational sporting activities.[31] Life expectancy for people with SCI continues to increase, but is somewhat below life expectancy for those without SCI. Mortality rates are significantly higher during the first year after injury than during subsequent years, particularly for people who are severely injured.[31]

Most SCIs involve damage to the vertebral column or supporting ligaments as well as the spinal cord. Because of extensive tract systems that connect sensory afferent neurons and LMNs with high brain centers, SCIs commonly involve both sensory and motor function. Although the discussion in this section of the chapter focuses on traumatic SCI, much of the content is applicable to SCI caused by other disorders, such as congenital deformities (*e.g.*, spina bifida), tumors, ischemia and infarction, and bone disease with pathologic fractures of the vertebrae.

Injury to the Vertebral Column

Injuries to the vertebral column include fractures, dislocations, and subluxations. A fracture can occur at any part of the bony vertebrae, causing fragmentation of the bone. It most often involves the pedicle, lamina, or processes (*e.g.*, facets). Dislocation or subluxation (partial dislocation) injury causes the vertebral bodies to become displaced, with one overriding another and preventing correct alignment of the vertebral column. Damage to the ligaments or bony vertebrae may make the spine unstable. In an unstable spine, further unguarded movement of the spinal column can impinge on the spinal canal, causing compression or overstretching of neural tissue.

Most SCI injuries occur due to a combination of writhing movements and a compressive force. Flexion injuries (*i.e.*, hyperflexion) occur when forward bending of the spinal column exceeds the limits of normal movement. Typical flexion injuries result, for example, when the head is struck from behind, as in a fall with the back of the head as the point of impact. Extension injuries occur with excessive forced bending (*i.e.*, hyperextension) of the spine backward. A typical extension injury involves a fall in which the chin or face is the point of impact, causing hyperextension of the neck.

Concept Mastery Alert

Injuries of flexion and extension occur more commonly in the cervical spine (C4 to C6) than in any other area. Limitations imposed by the ribs, spinous processes, and joint capsules in the thoracic and lumbar spine make this area less flexible and less susceptible to flexion and extension injuries than the cervical spine.

A compression injury, causing the vertebral bones to shatter, squash, or even burst, occurs when there is spinal loading (*i.e.*, axial load) from a high-velocity blow to the top of the head, such as a diving injury (Fig. 15.14A). Compression injuries may occur when the vertebrae are weakened by conditions such as osteoporosis and cancer with bone metastasis. Axial rotation injuries can produce highly unstable injuries. Maximal axial rotation occurs in the cervical region, especially between C1 and C2, and at the lumbosacral joint (Fig. 15.14B). Coupling of vertebral motions is common in injury when two or more individual motions occur (*e.g.*, lateral bending and axial rotation).

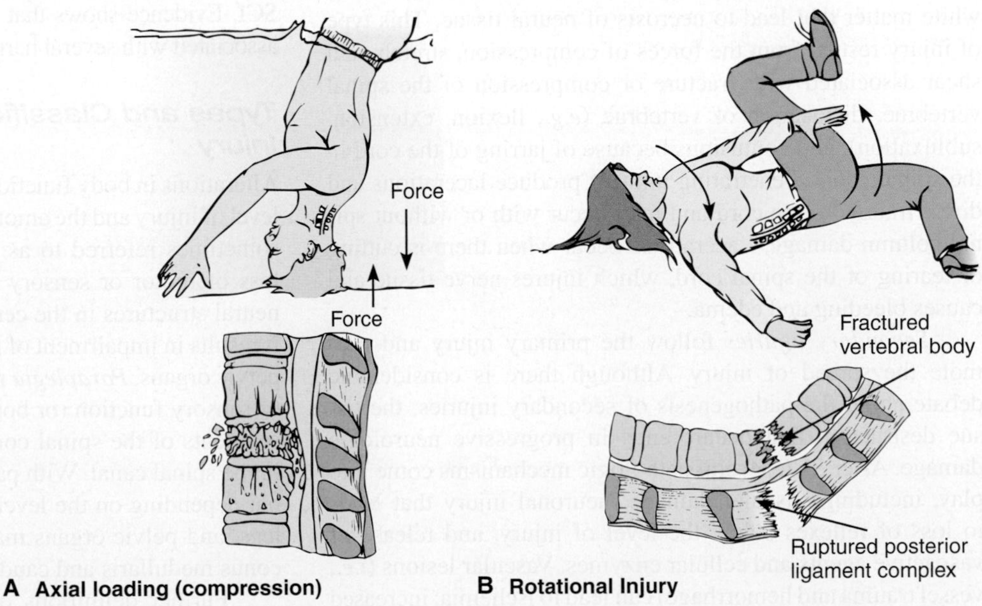

Figure 15.14 • (A) Compression vertebral fracture secondary to axial loading as occurs when a person falls from a height and lands on the buttocks. **(B)** Rotational injury, in which there is concurrent fracture and tearing of the posterior ligamentous complex, is caused by extreme lateral flexion or twisting of the head or neck. (From Morton P. G., Fontaine D. K. (2018). *Critical care nursing: A holistic approach* (11th ed., p. 941). Philadelphia, PA: Lippincott Williams & Wilkins.)

Acute Spinal Cord Injury

SCI involves damage to the neural elements of the spinal cord. The damage may result from direct trauma to the cord from penetrating wounds or indirect injury resulting from vertebral fractures, fracture–dislocations, or subluxations of the spine. The spinal cord may be contused, not only at the site of injury but above and below the trauma site causing it to swell. Traumatic injury may be complicated by the loss of blood flow to the cord, with resulting infarction.

Sudden, complete transection of the spinal cord results in complete loss of motor, sensory, reflex, and autonomic function below the level of injury. The immediate response to SCI is often referred to as *spinal shock*. It is characterized by flaccid paralysis with loss of tendon reflexes below the level of injury, absence of somatic and visceral sensations below the level of injury, and loss of bowel and bladder function. Loss of systemic sympathetic vasomotor tone may result in vasodilation, increased venous capacity, and hypotension. These manifestations occur regardless of whether the level of the lesion eventually will produce spastic (UMN) or flaccid (LMN) paralysis. The basic mechanisms accounting for transient spinal shock are unknown. Spinal shock may last for hours, days, or weeks. Usually, if reflex function returns by the time the person reaches the hospital, the neuromuscular changes are reversible. This type of reversible spinal shock may occur in football-type injuries, in which jarring of the spinal cord produces a concussion-like syndrome with loss of movement and reflexes, followed by full recovery within days. In people in whom the loss of reflexes persists, hypotension and bradycardia may become critical but manageable problems. In general, the higher the level of injury (*i.e.*, T6 and above), the greater is the effect.

Pathophysiology. The pathophysiology of acute SCI can be divided into two types—primary and secondary.[2] The *primary neurologic injury* occurs at the time of mechanical injury and is irreversible. It is characterized by small hemorrhages in the gray matter of the cord, followed by edematous changes in the white matter that lead to necrosis of neural tissue. This type of injury results from the forces of compression, stretch, and shear associated with fracture or compression of the spinal vertebrae, dislocation of vertebrae (*e.g.*, flexion, extension, subluxation), and contusions because of jarring of the cord in the spinal canal. Penetrating injuries produce lacerations and direct trauma to the cord and may occur with or without spinal column damage. Lacerations occur when there is cutting or tearing of the spinal cord, which injures nerve tissue and causes bleeding and edema.

Secondary injuries follow the primary injury and promote the spread of injury. Although there is considerable debate about the pathogenesis of secondary injuries, the tissue destruction that occurs ends in progressive neurologic damage. After SCI, several pathologic mechanisms come into play, including vascular damage, neuronal injury that leads to loss of reflexes below the level of injury, and release of vasoactive agents and cellular enzymes. Vascular lesions (*i.e.*, vessel trauma and hemorrhage) can lead to ischemia, increased vascular permeability, and edema. Blood flow to the spinal cord may be further compromised by spinal shock that results from a loss of vasomotor tone and neural reflexes below the level of injury. The release of vasoactive substances (*i.e.*, norepinephrine, serotonin, dopamine, and histamine) from the wound tissue causes vasospasm and impedes blood flow in the microcirculation, producing further necrosis of blood vessels and neurons. The release of proteolytic and lipolytic enzymes from injured cells causes delayed swelling, demyelination, and necrosis in the neural tissue in the spinal cord.

Treatment. The goal of management of acute SCI is to reduce the neurologic deficit and prevent any additional loss of neurologic function. Most traumatic injuries to the spinal column render it unstable, mandating measures such as immobilization with collars and backboards and limiting the movement of people at risk for, or with known, SCI. Every person with multiple trauma or head injury is automatically treated as though he or she has a cervical cord injury until this is ruled out with imaging.

The nature of the injury determines further methods of stabilization and treatment. In unstable injuries of the cervical spine, cervical traction improves or restores spinal alignment, decompresses neural structures, and facilitates recovery. Fractures and dislocations of the thoracic and lumbar vertebrae may be initially stabilized by restricting the person to bed rest and turning him or her in a logrolling manner to keep the spine rigid. Gunshot or stab wounds of the spinal column may not produce structural instability and may not require immobilization.

The goal of early surgical intervention for an unstable spine is to provide internal skeletal stabilization so that early mobilization and rehabilitation can occur. One of the more important aspects of early SCI care is the prevention and treatment of spinal or systemic shock and the hypoxia associated with compromised respiration. The cord must be perfused to prevent hypoxia. The clinical benefit of methylprednisolone in the treatment of SCI has no supporting evidence, and it is therefore not recommended to administer methylprednisolone for the treatment of SCI. Evidence shows that the use of high-dose steroids can be associated with several harmful side effects.[32]

Types and Classification of Spinal Cord Injury

Alterations in body function that result from SCI depend on the level of injury and the amount of cord involvement. *Tetraplegia*, sometimes referred to as *quadriplegia*, is the impairment or loss of motor or sensory function (or both) after damage to neural structures in the cervical segments of the spinal cord.[32] It results in impairment of function in the arms, trunk, legs, and pelvic organs. *Paraplegia* refers to impairment or loss of motor or sensory function (or both) in the thoracic, lumbar, or sacral segments of the spinal cord from damage of neural elements in the spinal canal. With paraplegia, arm functioning is spared, but depending on the level of injury, functioning of the trunk, legs, and pelvic organs may be impaired. Paraplegia includes conus medullaris and cauda equina injuries.

Further definitions of SCI describe the extent of neurologic damage as *complete* or *incomplete*.[32] Complete cord injuries can result from severance of the cord, disruption of nerve fibers although they remain intact, or interruption of blood supply to that segment, resulting in complete destruction of neural tissue and UMN or LMN paralysis. With complete injuries, no motor or sensory function is preserved in sacral segments S4 to S6. Incomplete SCI implies there is some residual motor or sensory function below the level of injury. The prognosis for return of function is better in an incomplete injury because of preservation of axonal function. Incomplete injuries may manifest in a variety of patterns, but can be organized into certain patterns or *syndromes* that occur more frequently and reflect the predominant area of the cord that is involved. Types of incomplete lesions include the central cord syndrome, Brown-Séquard syndrome, anterior cord syndrome, and conus medullaris syndrome.

Central Cord Syndrome. A condition called *central cord syndrome* occurs when injury is predominantly in the central gray or white matter of the cord[33] (Fig. 15.15). Because the corticospinal tract fibers are organized with those controlling the arms located more centrally and those controlling the legs located more laterally, some external axonal transmission may remain intact. Motor function of the upper extremities is affected, but the lower extremities may not be affected or may be affected to a lesser degree, with some sparing of sacral sensation. Bowel, bladder, and sexual functions usually are affected to various degrees, and this may parallel the degree of lower extremity involvement. This syndrome occurs almost exclusively in the cervical cord, rendering the lesion a UMN lesion with spastic paralysis. Central cord damage is more frequent in older adults with narrowing or stenotic changes in the spinal canal that are related to arthritis. Damage also may occur in people with congenital stenosis.

Brown-Séquard Syndrome. A condition called *Brown-Séquard syndrome* results from damage to a hemisection of the anterior and posterior cord[34] (Fig. 15.16). The effect is an ipsilateral loss of voluntary motor function from the corticospinal tract and proprioception loss with a contralateral loss of pain and temperature sensation from the lateral spinothalamic tracts for all levels below the lesion.

Anterior Cord Syndrome. Anterior cord syndrome usually is caused by damage from infarction of the anterior spinal artery, resulting in damage to the anterior two thirds of the cord[1] (Fig. 15.17). The deficits include loss of motor function provided by the corticospinal tracts and loss of pain and temperature sensation from damage to the lateral spinothalamic tracts. The posterior one third of the cord is relatively unaffected, preserving the dorsal column axons that convey position, vibration, and touch sensation.

Conus Medullaris and Cauda Equina Syndromes. The conus medullaris syndrome involves damage to the conus medullaris or the sacral cord (*i.e.*, T12 to L1, lower end of spinal cord) and lumbar nerve roots in the neural canal. Functional deficits resulting from this type of injury usually result in flaccid bowel and bladder and altered sexual function. Sacral segments occasion-

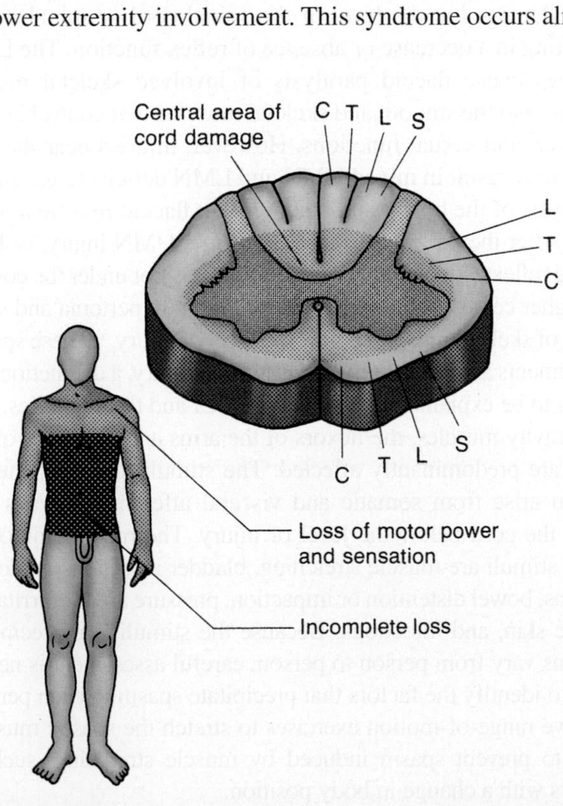

Figure 15.15 • Central cord syndrome. A cross-section of the cord shows central damage and the associated motor and sensory loss (*C*, cervical; *L*, lumbar; *S*, sacral; *T*, thoracic.) (From Hickey J. V. (2014). *The clinical practice of neurological and neurosurgical nursing* (7th ed., first figure in Chart 17–2, p. 398). Philadelphia, PA: Lippincott Williams & Wilkins.)

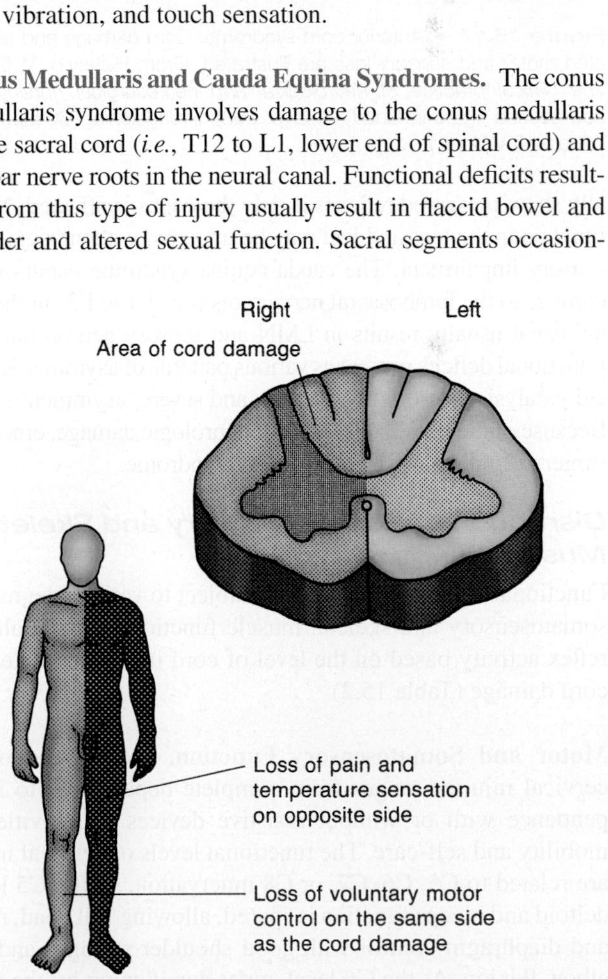

Figure 15.16 • Brown-Séquard syndrome. Cord damage and associated motor and sensory loss are illustrated. (From Hickey J. V. (2014). *The clinical practice of neurological and neurosurgical nursing* (7th ed., third figure in Chart 17–2, p. 399). Philadelphia, PA: Lippincott Williams & Wilkins.)

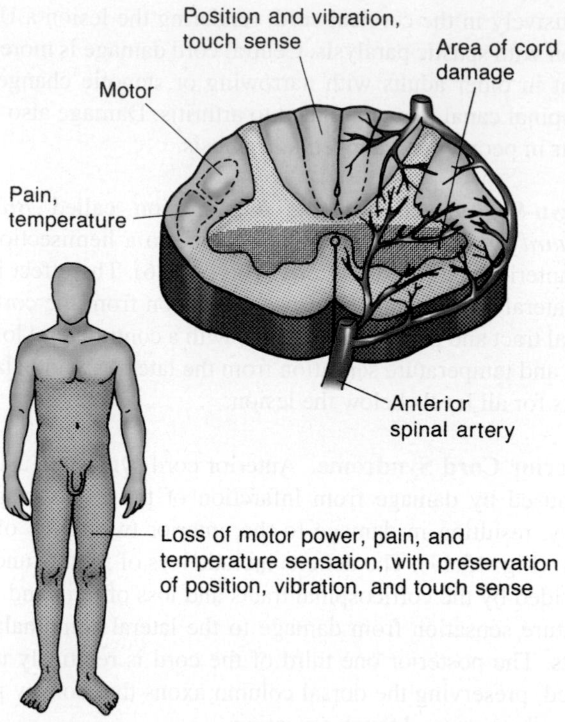

Figure 15.17 • Anterior cord syndrome. Cord damage and associated motor and sensory loss are illustrated. (From Hickey J. V. (2014). *The clinical practice of neurological and neurosurgical nursing* (7th ed., second figure in Chart 17–2, p. 398). Philadelphia, PA: Lippincott Williams & Wilkins.)

ally show preserved reflexes if only the conus is affected. Motor function in the legs and feet may be impaired without significant sensory impairment. The cauda equina syndrome occurs when damage to the lumbosacral nerve roots (*i.e.*, L1 to L2) in the spinal canal usually results in LMN and sensory neuron damage. Functional deficits present as various patterns of asymmetric flaccid paralysis, sensory impairment, and severe, asymmetric pain. Because of the possible permanent neurologic damage, emergent surgery is indicated for cauda equina syndrome.

Disruption of Somatosensory and Skeletal Muscle Function

Functional abilities after SCI are subject to various degrees of somatosensory and skeletal muscle function loss and altered reflex activity based on the level of cord injury and extent of cord damage (Table 15.2).

Motor and Somatosensory Function. Motor function in cervical injuries ranges from complete dependence to independence with or without assistive devices in activities of mobility and self-care. The functional levels of cervical injury are related to C5, C6, C7, or C8 innervation. At the C5 level, deltoid and biceps function is spared, allowing full head, neck, and diaphragm control with good shoulder strength and full elbow flexion. At the C6 level, wrist dorsiflexion by the wrist extensors is functional, allowing tenodesis, which is the natural bending inward and flexion of the fingers when the wrist is extended and bent backward. Tenodesis is a key movement because it can be used to pick up objects when finger movement is absent. A functional C7 injury allows full elbow flexion and extension, wrist plantar flexion, and some finger control. At the C8 level, finger flexion is added.

Thoracic cord injuries (T1 to T12) allow full upper extremity control with limited to full control of intercostal and trunk muscles and balance. Injury at the T1 level allows full fine motor control of the fingers. Because of the lack of specific functional indicators at the thoracic levels, the level of injury usually is determined by sensory level testing.

Functional capacity in the L1 through L5 nerve innervations allows hip flexion, hip abduction (L1 to L3), movement of the knees (L2 to L5), and ankle dorsiflexion (L4 to L5). Sacral (S1 to S5) innervation allows for full leg, foot, and ankle control and innervation of perineal musculature for bowel, bladder, and sexual functions.

Reflex Activity. Spinal cord reflexes are fully integrated in the spinal cord and can function independent of input from higher centers. Altered spinal reflex activity after SCI is essentially determined by the level of injury and whether UMNs or LMNs are affected. With UMN injuries at T12 and above, the cord reflexes remain intact, whereas communication pathways with higher centers have been interrupted. This results in spasticity of involved skeletal muscle groups and of smooth and skeletal muscles that control bowel, bladder, and sexual functions. In LMN injuries at T12 or below, the reflex circuitry itself has been damaged at the level of the spinal cord or spinal nerve, resulting in a decrease or absence of reflex function. The LMN injuries cause flaccid paralysis of involved skeletal muscle groups and the smooth and skeletal muscles that control bowel, bladder, and sexual functions. However, injuries near the T12 level may result in mixed UMN and LMN deficits (*e.g.*, spastic paralysis of the bowel and bladder with flaccid muscle tone).

After the period of spinal shock in a UMN injury, isolated spinal reflex activity and muscle tone that is not under the control of higher centers return. This may result in hypertonia and spasticity of skeletal muscles below the level of injury.[34] These spastic movements are involuntary instead of voluntary, a distinction that needs to be explained to people with SCI and their families. The antigravity muscles, the flexors of the arms and extensors of the legs, are predominantly affected. The stimuli for reflex muscle spasm arise from somatic and visceral afferent pathways that enter the cord below the level of injury. The most common of these stimuli are muscle stretching, bladder infections or stones, fistulas, bowel distention or impaction, pressure areas or irritation of the skin, and infections. Because the stimuli that precipitate spasms vary from person to person, careful assessment is necessary to identify the factors that precipitate spasm in each person. Passive range-of-motion exercises to stretch the spastic muscles help to prevent spasm induced by muscle stretching, such as occurs with a change in body position.

Spasticity is not detrimental and may even facilitate maintenance of muscle tone to prevent muscle wasting, improve venous return, and aid in mobility. Spasms become detrimental when they impair safety. They also reduce the

TABLE 15.2 FUNCTIONAL ABILITIES BY LEVEL OF CORD INJURY

INJURY LEVEL	SEGMENTAL SENSORIMOTOR FUNCTION	DRESSING, EATING	ELIMINATION	MOBILITY*
C1	Little or no sensation or control of head and neck; no diaphragm control; requires continuous ventilation	Dependent	Dependent	Limited. Voice-controlled or sip-n-puff electric wheelchair
C2–C3	Head and neck sensation; some neck control; independent of mechanical ventilation for short periods	Dependent	Dependent	Same as for C1
C4	Good head and neck sensation and motor control; some shoulder elevation; diaphragm movement	Dependent; may be able to eat with adaptive sling	Dependent	Limited to voice-, mouth-, head-, chin-, or shoulder-controlled electric wheelchair
C5	Full head and neck control; shoulder strength; elbow flexion	Independent with assistance	Maximal assistance	Electric or modified manual wheelchair; needs transfer assistance
C6	Fully innervated shoulder; wrist extension or dorsiflexion	Independent or with minimal assistance	Independent or with minimal assistance	Independent in transfers and wheelchair
C7–C8	Full elbow extension; wrist plantar flexion; some finger control	Independent	Independent	Independent; manual wheelchair
T1–T5	Full hand and finger control; use of intercostal and thoracic muscles	Independent	Independent	Independent; manual wheelchair
T6–T10	Abdominal muscle control; partial to good balance with trunk muscles	Independent	Independent	Independent; manual wheelchair
T11–L5	Hip flexors, hip abductors (L1–L3), knee extension (L2–L4), knee flexion, and ankle dorsiflexion (L4–L5)	Independent	Independent	Short distance to full ambulation with assistance
S1–S5	Full leg, foot, and ankle control; innervation of perineal muscles for bowel, bladder, and sexual functions (S2–S4)	Independent	Normal to impaired bowel and bladder function	Ambulate independently with or without assistance

*Assistance refers to adaptive.

ability to make functional gains in mobility and activities of daily living. Spasms also may cause trauma to bones and tissues, leading to joint contractures and skin breakdown.

Respiratory Muscle Function. In order for ventilation to occur, the expiratory and inspiratory muscles need to be innervated by the spinal cord. Segments C3 to C5 through the phrenic nerves innervate the main muscle of ventilation, the diaphragm. Spinal segments T1 through T7 innervate the intercostal muscles, which function in elevating the rib cage and are needed for coughing and deep breathing. The major muscles of expiration are the abdominal muscles, which receive their innervation from levels T6 to T12.

Although the ability to inhale and exhale may be preserved at various levels of SCI, functional deficits in ventilation are most apparent in the quality of the breathing cycle and the ability to oxygenate tissues, eliminate carbon dioxide, and mobilize secretions. Cord injuries involving C1 to C3 result in a lack of respiratory effort, and people who are affected require assisted ventilation. Although a C3 to C5 injury allows partial or full diaphragmatic function, ventilation is diminished because of the loss of intercostal muscle function, resulting in shallow breaths and a weak cough. Below the C5 level, as less intercostal and abdominal musculature is affected, the ability to take a deep breath and cough is less impaired. Maintenance therapy consists of muscle training to strengthen existing muscles for endurance and mobilization of secretions. The ability to speak is compromised with assisted ventilation, whether continuous or intermittent. Thus, ensuring adequate communication of needs is also essential.

Disruption of Autonomic Nervous System Function

If there is an SCI, all autonomic nerve function below the injury site will be stopped. This includes sympathetic outflow from the thoracic and lumbar cord and parasympathetic outflow from the sacral cord. Because of their sites of exit from the CNS, the cranial nerves, such as the vagus, are unaffected. Depending on the level of injury, the spinal reflexes that control autonomic nervous system function are largely isolated from the rest of the CNS. Afferent sensory input that enters the spinal cord is unaffected, as is the efferent motor output from the cord. Lacking are the regulation and integration of reflex function by centers in the brain and brain stem. This results in a situation in which the autonomic reflexes below the level of injury are uncontrolled, whereas those above the level of injury function in a relatively controlled manner.

Sympathetic nervous system regulation of circulatory function and body temperature (*i.e.*, thermoregulation) presents some of the most severe problems in SCI. The higher the level of injury and the greater the surface area affected, the more profound are the effects on circulation and thermoregulation. People with injury at the T6 level or above experience problems in regulating vasomotor tone. Those with injuries below the T6 level usually have sufficient sympathetic function to maintain adequate vasomotor function. The level of injury and its corresponding problems may vary among people, and some dysfunctional effects may be seen at levels below T6. With lower lumbar and sacral injuries, sympathetic function remains essentially unaltered.

Vasovagal Response. The vagus nerve (cranial nerve X), which is unaffected in SCI, normally exerts a continuous inhibitory effect on heart rate. Vagal stimulation that causes a marked bradycardia is called the *vasovagal response*. Visceral afferent input to the vagal centers in the brain stem of people with tetraplegia or high-level paraplegia can produce marked bradycardia when unchecked by a dysfunctional sympathetic nervous system. Severe bradycardia and even asystole can result when deep endotracheal suctioning or rapid position change elicits the vasovagal response. Preventive measures, such as hyperoxygenation before, during, and after suctioning, are advised. Rapid position changes should be avoided or anticipated, and anticholinergic drugs should be immediately available to counteract severe episodes of bradycardia.

Autonomic Dysreflexia. Autonomic dysreflexia, also known as *autonomic hyperreflexia*, represents an acute episode of exaggerated sympathetic reflex responses that occur in people with injuries at T6 and above, in which CNS control of spinal reflexes is lost (Fig. 15.18). It does not occur until spinal

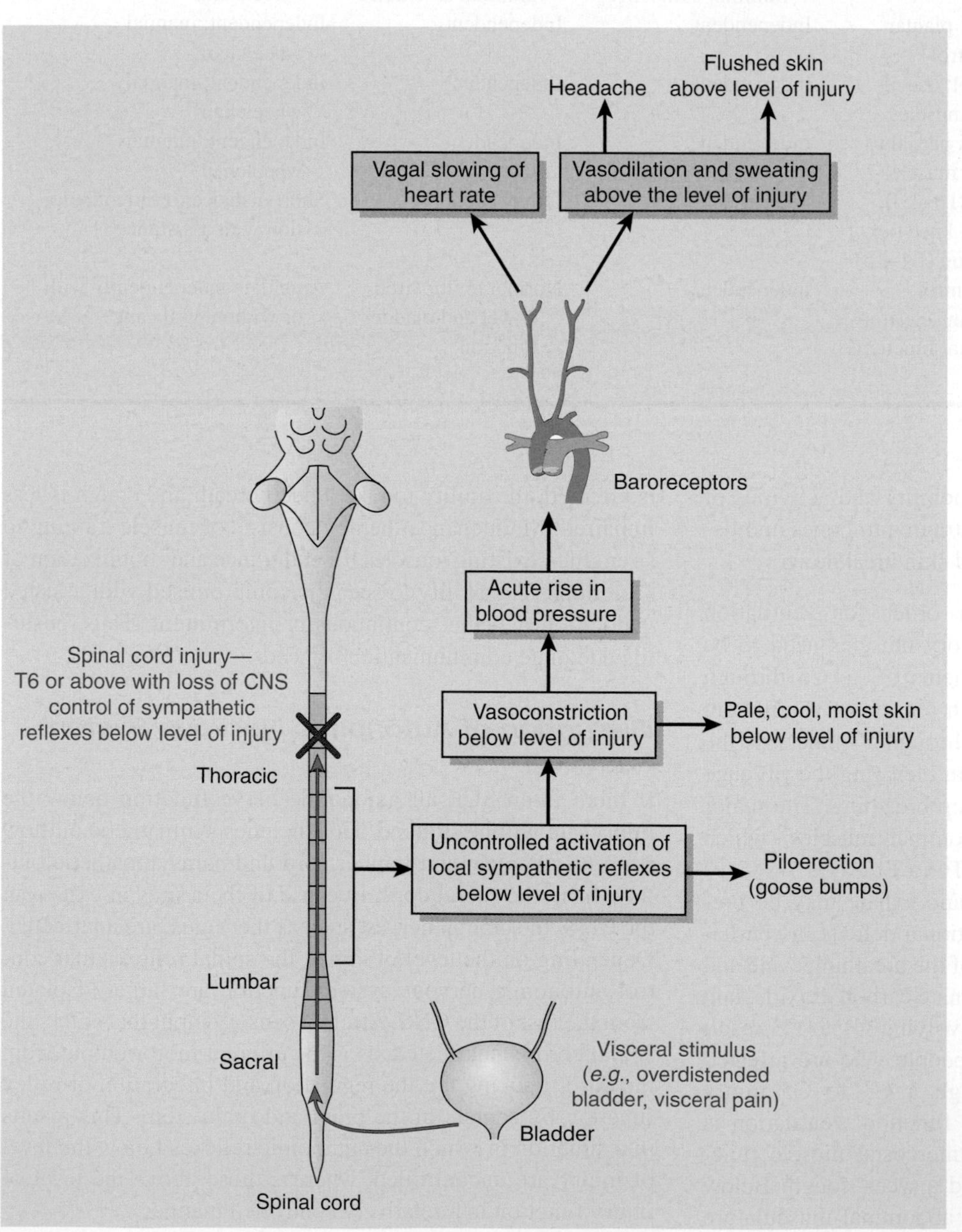

Figure 15.18 • Mechanisms of autonomic dysreflexia.

shock has resolved and autonomic reflexes return, most often within the first 6 months after injury. It is most unpredictable during the first year after injury, but can occur throughout the person's lifetime.

Autonomic dysreflexia is characterized by mild to severe hypertension, skin pallor, and gooseflesh associated with the piloerector response. Because baroreceptor function and parasympathetic control of heart rate travel by way of the cranial nerves, these responses remain intact. Continued hypertension produces a baroreflex-mediated vagal slowing of the heart rate to bradycardic levels. There is an accompanying baroreflex-mediated vasodilation, with flushed skin and profuse sweating above the level of injury, headache ranging from dull to severe and pounding, nasal stuffiness, and feelings of anxiety. A person may experience one, several, or all of the symptoms with each episode.

The stimuli initiating the dysreflexic response include visceral distention, such as a full bladder or rectum; stimulation of pain receptors, as occurs with pressure ulcers, ingrown toenails, dressing changes, and diagnostic or operative procedures; and visceral contractions, such as ejaculation, bladder spasms, or uterine contractions. In many cases, the dysreflexic response results from a full bladder.

Autonomic dysreflexia is a clinical emergency, and without prompt and adequate treatment, convulsions, loss of consciousness, and even death can occur. The major components of treatment include monitoring blood pressure while removing or correcting the initiating cause or stimulus. The person should be placed in an upright position, and all support hose or binders should be removed to promote venous pooling of blood and reduce venous return, thereby decreasing blood pressure. If the stimuli have been removed or the stimuli cannot be identified and the upright position is established, but the blood pressure remains elevated, drugs that block autonomic function are administered. Prevention of the type of stimuli that trigger the dysreflexic event is advocated.

Postural Hypotension. Postural, or orthostatic, hypotension can occur with injuries at T4 to T6 and above and is due to the interruption of sympathetic outflow to blood vessels in the extremities and abdomen. Pooling of blood, along with gravitational forces, impairs venous return to the heart, and there is a subsequent decrease in cardiac output when the person is placed in an upright position. The signs of orthostatic hypotension include dizziness, pallor, excessive sweating above the level of the lesion, complaints of blurred vision, and possibly fainting. Postural hypotension usually is prevented by slow changes in position and measures to promote venous return.

Disruption of Bladder, Bowel, and Sexual Functions

Loss of bladder function results from disruption of neural pathways between the bladder and the reflex voiding center at the S2 to S4 level (*i.e.*, an LMN lesion) or between the reflex voiding center and higher brain centers for communication and coordinated sphincter control (*i.e.*, a UMN lesion). People with UMN lesions or spastic bladders lack awareness of bladder filling (*i.e.*, storage) and voluntary control of voiding (*i.e.*, evacuation). In LMN lesions or flaccid bladder dysfunction, lack of awareness of bladder filling and lack of bladder tone render the person unable to void voluntarily or involuntarily.

Bowel elimination is a coordinated function involving the enteric nervous system, the autonomic nervous system, and the CNS. People with SCI above S2 to S4 develop spastic functioning of the defecation reflex and loss of voluntary control of the external anal sphincter. Damage to the cord at the S2 to S4 level causes flaccid functioning of the defecation reflex and loss of anal sphincter tone. Even though the enteric nervous system innervation of the bowel remains intact, without the defecation reflex, peristaltic movements are ineffective in evacuating stool.

Sexual function, like bladder and bowel control, is mediated by the S2 to S4 segments of the spinal cord. The genital sexual response in SCI, which is manifested by an erection in men and vaginal lubrication in women, may be initiated by mental or touch stimuli, depending on the level of injury. The T11 to L2 cord segments have been identified as the mental stimulus, or psychogenic, sexual response area, where autonomic nerve pathways in communication with the forebrain leave the cord and innervate the genitalia. The S2 to S4 cord segments have been identified as the sexual-touch reflex center. In T10 or higher injuries, reflex sexual response to genital touch may occur freely. However, a sexual response to mental stimuli (T11 to L2) does not occur because of the spinal lesion blocking the communication pathway. In an injury at T12 or below, the sexual reflex center may be damaged, and there may be no response to touch.

In men, the lack of erectile ability or inability to experience penile sensations or orgasm is not a reliable indicator of fertility, which should be evaluated by an expert. In women, fertility is parallel to menses. Usually, it is delayed 3 to 5 months after injury.

Disruption of Other Functions

Temperature Regulation. The central mechanisms for thermoregulation are in the hypothalamus. In response to cold, the hypothalamus stimulates vasoconstrictor responses in peripheral blood vessels, particularly those of the skin. This results in decreased loss of body heat. Heat production results from increased metabolism, voluntary activity, or shivering. To reduce heat, hypothalamus-stimulated mechanisms produce vasodilation of skin blood vessels to dissipate heat, and sweating to increase evaporative heat losses.

After SCI, the communication between the thermoregulatory centers in the hypothalamus and the sympathetic effector responses below the level of injury is disrupted. The ability to control blood vessel responses that conserve or dissipate heat is lost, as are the abilities to sweat and shiver. Higher levels of injury tend to produce greater disturbances in thermoregulation. In tetraplegia and high paraplegia, there are few defenses against changes in the environmental temperature, and body temperature tends to assume the temperature of the external environment, a condition known as *poikilothermy*.

People with lower-level injuries have various degrees of thermoregulation. Disturbances in thermoregulation are chronic and may cause continual loss of body heat. Treatment consists of education in the adjustment of clothing and awareness of how environmental temperatures affect the person's ability to accommodate to these changes.

Deep Vein Thrombosis and Edema. People with SCI are at high risk for development of deep vein thrombosis (DVT) and pulmonary embolism. The high risk for DVT in people with acute SCI is due to immobility, decreased vasomotor tone below the level of injury, and hypercoagulability and stasis of blood flow. Electrical stimulation applied to the lower limbs has been reported to provide some benefit by achieving muscular contraction and improving venous flow. Local pain, a common symptom of DVT, is often absent because of sensory deficits. Thus, a regular schedule of visual inspection for local signs of DVT (*e.g.*, swelling) is important. Testing of people at high risk for DVT includes plethysmography and duplex ultrasonography.

Dependent edema is also a common problem in people with SCI. The development of edema is related to decreased peripheral vascular resistance, decreased muscle tone in the paralyzed limbs, and immobility that causes increased venous pressure and abnormal pooling of blood in the abdomen, lower limbs, and upper extremities. Positioning to minimize gravitational forces or by using compression devices (*e.g.*, support stockings, binders) that encourage venous return usually relieves edema in the dependent body parts.

Skin Integrity. The entire surface of the skin is innervated by cranial or spinal nerves organized into dermatomes that show cutaneous distribution. The CNS and autonomic nervous system also play a vital role in skin function. The sympathetic nervous system, through control of vasomotor and sweat gland activity, influences the health of the skin by providing adequate circulation, excretion of body fluids, and temperature regulation. The lack of sensory warning mechanisms and voluntary motor ability below the level of injury, coupled with circulatory changes, places the person with spinal cord injury at major risk for disruption of skin integrity. Significant factors associated with disruption of skin integrity are pressure, shearing forces, and localized trauma and irritation. Relieving pressure, allowing adequate circulation to the skin, and skin inspection are primary ways of maintaining skin integrity. Of all the complications after SCI, skin breakdown is the most preventable.

Future Directions in Repair of the Injured Spinal Cord

Currently, strategies for repairing the injured spinal cord focus on promoting the regrowth of interrupted nerve fiber tracts, using nerve growth–stimulating factors or molecules that suppress inhibitors of neuronal extension; bridging spinal cord lesions with scaffolds that are impregnated with nerve growth factors, which promote axon growth and reduce the barriers caused by scar tissue; repairing damaged myelin and restoring nerve fiber conductivity in the lesion area; and enhancing CNS plasticity by promoting compensatory growth of spared, intact nerve fibers above and below the level of injury. Although these strategies may not allow for complete repair of the spinal cord so as to recreate what was present before the injury, even small successes may be useful for someone with SCI.

IN SUMMARY

UMN lesions are those involving neurons completely contained in the CNS. ALS is a progressive and devastating neurologic disorder that selectively affects motor function. It affects LMNs in the spinal cord as well as UMNs in the brain stem and cerebral cortex. MS is a slowly progressive demyelinating disease of the CNS. The most common symptoms are paresthesias, optic neuritis, and motor weakness. The disease is usually characterized by exacerbations and remissions. Initially, near-normal function returns between exacerbations.

SCI is a disabling neurologic condition most commonly caused by motor vehicle accidents, falls, and sports injuries. Dysfunctions of the nervous system after SCI comprise various degrees of sensorimotor loss and altered reflex activity based on the level of injury and extent of cord damage. Depending on the level of injury, the physical problems of SCI include spinal shock; ventilation and communication problems; autonomic nervous system dysfunction that predisposes to the vasovagal response, autonomic hyperreflexia, impaired body temperature regulation, and postural hypotension; impaired muscle pump and venous innervation leading to edema of dependent areas of the body and risk for DVT; altered sensorimotor integrity that contributes to uncontrolled muscle spasms, altered pain responses, and threats to skin integrity; alterations in bowel and bladder elimination; and impaired sexual function.

GERIATRIC Considerations

- Research has led to development of single-photon emission computed tomography (SPECT), which detects changes in neurotransmitters such as dopamine. This finding will allow providers to recognize disorders such as Parkinson disease earlier to improve treatment outcomes.[35]
- Decreases in strength and agility are normal findings with aging; however, localized weakness is associated with disease.[36]
- Decreased nerve input into muscles that occurs with aging contributes to atrophy in the hands.[36]
- Falls in the elderly are attributed to degeneration of nerve cells in the inner ear.[37]
- Neurofibrillary tangles used to diagnose Alzheimer disease can also be present in the elderly with normal cognitive function.[37]

PEDIATRIC Considerations

- Inability to perform finger-to-nose movement and a positive Romberg sign may indicate an alteration in cerebellar function.[38]
- Absence or asymmetry of reflexes indicates cerebral dysfunction.[38]

REVIEW EXERCISES

1. A 32-year-old woman presents with complaints of drooping eyelids, difficulty chewing and swallowing, and weakness of her arms and legs that is less severe in the morning but becomes worse as the day progresses. She complains that climbing stairs and lifting objects are becoming increasingly difficult. Clinical examination confirms weakness of the eyelid and jaw muscles. She is told that she may have myasthenia gravis and is scheduled for a blood test to assess for antibodies.
   A. *Explain the pathogenesis of this woman's symptoms as it relates to myasthenia gravis.*
   B. *Explain how information from the antibody blood test can be used to assist in the diagnosis of the disorder.*
   C. *Explain the rationale for avoiding the use of aminoglycoside antibiotics for treatment of infections in this woman.*
2. A 66-year-old man complains of right-hand tremor at rest that interferes with his various graphic design creations. He also complains of dragging his left leg when walking, being unsteady when turning, and a stooped over posture. Upon examination, he is found to also have mild rigidity in all limbs, flat facies, hypophonia, and impaired rapid alternating movements. Based on his clinical presentation, he is diagnosed with Parkinson disease.
   A. *How would you go about helping him to outline the role of the cerebellum and basal ganglia in performing the motor movements associated with these maneuvers?*
3. A 20-year-old man suffered an SCI at the C2 to C3 level as the result of a motorcycle accident.
   A. *Explain the effects of this man's injury on ventilation and communication; sensorimotor function; autonomic nervous system function; bowel, bladder, and sexual functions; and temperature regulation.*
   B. *Autonomic dysreflexia, which is a threat to people with SCI at T6 or above, is manifested by hypertension, often to extreme levels, and bradycardia; constriction of skin vessels below the level of injury; and severe headache and nasal stuffiness. Explain the origin of the elevated blood pressure and bradycardia. The condition does not occur until after shock has resolved and usually occurs only in people with injuries at T6 and above. Explain.*

References

1. Patton K., Thibodeau G. (2016). *Anatomy & physiology* (9th ed., p. 333). Philadelphia, PA: Elsevier.
2. Hall J. E. (2016). *Guyten and Hall textbook of medical physiology* (13th ed.). Philadelphia, PA: Elsevier.
3. Penfield W., Rasmussen T. (1950). *The cerebral cortex of man*. New York, NY: Macmillan.
4. Tortora G., Derrickson B. (2017). *Principles of anatomy & physiology* (15th ed.). New York, NY: John Wiley.
5. Bickley L. S., Szilagyi P. G. (2013). *Bates' guide to physical examination and history taking* (11th ed., pp. 708–718). Philadelphia, PA: Lippincott Williams & Wilkins.
6. Anthony D. P., Anthony D. C. (2015). Peripheral nerve and skeletal muscle. In Kumar V., Abbas A. K., Fausto N. (Eds.), *Robbins and Cotran pathologic basis of disease* (9th ed., pp. 1227–1250). Philadelphia, PA: Elsevier.
7. Strayer D. S., Rubin E., Saffitz J. E., et al. (Eds.) (2015). *Rubin's pathology: Clinicopathologic foundations of medicine* (7th ed.). Philadelphia, PA: Lippincott Williams & Wilkins.
8. Malavaki C. J., Sakkas G. K., Mitrou G. I., et al. (2015). Skeletal muscle atrophy: disease-induced mechanisms may mask disuse atrophy. *Journal of Muscle Research and Cell Motility* 36(6), 405–421.
9. Louis E., Mayer S. A., Rowland L. P. (Eds.) (2015). *Merritt's neurology*. Philadelphia, PA: Wolters Kluwer.
10. Vo A. H., McNally E. (2015). Modifier genes and their effect on Duchenne muscular dystrophy. *Current Opinion in Neurology* 28(5), 528–534.
11. Katzung B., Trevor A. (2015). *Basic and clinical pharmacology* (13th ed.). New York, NY: Lange Medical Books/McGraw-Hill.
12. Rosow L. K., Strober J. B. (2015). Infantile botulism: Review and clinical update. *Pediatric Neurology* 52(5), 487–492.
13. King A. M., Aaron C. K. (2015). Organophosphate and carbamate poisoning. *Emergency Medicine Clinics of North America* 33, 133–151.
14. Cavalcante P., Galbardi B., Franzi S., et al. (2016). Increased expression of toll-like receptors 7 and 9 in myasthenia gravis thymus characterized by active Epstein-Barr virus infection. *Immunobiology* 221(4), 516–527.
15. Della Marina A., Trippe H., Lutz S., et al. (2014). Juvenile myasthenia gravis: Recommendations for diagnostic approaches and treatment. *Neuropediatrics* 45(2), 75–83.
16. Dunphy L. M., Windland-Brown J. E., Porter B. O., et al. (2015). *Primary care: The art and science of advanced practice nursing* (4th ed.). Philadelphia, PA: FA Davis.
17. Ansar V., Valadi N. (2015). Guillain-Barre syndrome. *Primary Care; Clinics in Office Practice* 42(2), 189–193.
18. Willison H. J., Jacobs B. C., van Doorn P. A. (2016). Guillain–Barre syndrome. *Lancet* 388, 717–727.
19. Maher C., Underwood M., Buchbinder R. (2017). Non-specific low back pain. *Lancet* 389, 736–747.
20. Bahouq H., Allali F., Rkain H., et al. (2013). Prevalence and severity of insomnia in chronic low back pain patients. *Rheumatology International* 33, 1277–1281.
21. Oaseem A., Wilt T. J., McLean R. M., et al. (2017). Noninvasive treatments for acute, subacute, and chronic low back pain: A clinical practice

guideline from the American College of Physicians. *Annals of Internal Medicine* 166, 514–530.
22. Wilkins A. (2017). Cerebellar dysfunction in multiple sclerosis. *Frontiers in Neurology* 8, 1–6.
23. Sivaswamy L. (2014). Approach to acute ataxia in childhood: Diagnosis and evaluation. *Pediatric Annals* 43(4), 153–159.
24. Derkinderen P., Shannon K., Brundin P. (2014). Gut feelings about smoking and coffee in Parkinson's disease. *Movement Disorders* 29(18), 976–979.
25. Miller D. B., O'Callaghan J. P. (2015). Biomarkers of Parkinson's disease: present and future. *Metabolism* 64(301), S40–S46.
26. Lehne R. A. (2013). *Pharmacology for nursing care* (8th ed.). Philadelphia, PA: Elsevier.
27. Gordon P. H. (2013). Amyotrophic lateral sclerosis: An update for 2013 clinical features, pathophysiology, management and therapeutic trials. *Aging and Disease* 4(5), 295–310.
28. Hickey J. V. (2014). *The clinical practice of neurological and neurosurgical nursing* (7th edition). Philadelphia, PA: Wolters Kluwer.
29. Bader M. K., Littlejohns L. R., Olson D.M. (2016). *AANN core curriculum for neuroscience nursing*. Chicago, IL: AANN
30. Sawcer S., Franklin R. J., Ban M. (2014). Multiple sclerosis genetics. *Lancet Neurology* 13, 700–709.
31. National Spinal Cord Injury Statistical Center. (2016). *Facts and figures at a glance*. Birmingham, AL: University of Alabama at Birmingham.
32. Hurlbert R. J., Hadley M.N., Walters B. C., et al. (2013). Pharmacological therapy for acute spinal cord injury. *Neurosurgery* 72(3), 93–105.
33. Bonner S., Smith C. (2013). Initial management of acute spinal cord injury. *Continuing Education in Anesthesia, Critical Care, & Pain* 13(6), 224–231.
34. Morton P. G., Fontaine D. K. (2018). *Critical care nursing: A holistic approach* (11th ed.). Philadelphia, PA: Lippincott Williams & Wilkins.
35. Fischbach F. T., Dunning M. B. (2015). *Nurse's quick reference to common laboratory and diagnostic tests*. (6th ed.) Philadelphia, PA: Lippincott Williams & Wilkins.
36. Hinkle J. L., Cheever K. H. (2018). *Brunner & Suddarth's textbook of medical-surgical nursing*. Philadelphia, PA: Wolters Kluwer.
37. Eliopoulos C. (2018). *Gerontological nursing*. (9th Ed). Philadelphia, PA: Wolters Kluwer.
38. Bowden V. R., Greenberg C. S. (2014). *Children and their families: The continuum of nursing care*. (3rd Ed). Philadelphia, PA: Wolters Kluwer.

16 Disorders of Brain Function

Cynthia Bautista

The brain is susceptible to injury by trauma, ischemia, tumors, degenerative processes, and metabolic derangements. Brain injuries can be categorized as traumatic (*i.e.*, epidural hematoma, subdural hematoma, concussion, contusion, or diffuse axonal injury) or nontraumatic (*i.e.*, stroke, infection, tumor, or seizure). Brain injuries can cause a change in level of consciousness and alterations in cognition, motor, and sensory function. Brain damage can result from the effects of ischemia, excitatory amino acids, edema, and increased intracranial pressure (ICP).

MANIFESTATIONS AND MECHANISMS OF BRAIN INJURY

After completing this section of the chapter, the learner will be able to meet the following objectives:

- Identify the levels of consciousness and their characteristics.
- Describe the determinants of intracranial pressure and compensatory mechanisms used to prevent ICP.
- Discuss cytotoxic, vasogenic, and interstitial cerebral edema.

The brain is protected from external forces by the rigid confines of the skull and the cushioning afforded by the cerebrospinal fluid (CSF). The metabolic stability required by its electrically active cells is maintained by a number of regulatory mechanisms, including the blood–brain barrier and autoregulatory mechanisms that ensure its blood supply. Nonetheless, the brain remains remarkably vulnerable to injury by trauma, ischemia, tumors, degenerative processes, and metabolic derangements.

Manifestations of Brain Injury

Brain injury, whether because of trauma, stroke, or other pathologic processes, is manifested by changes in the level of consciousness and alterations in cognitive, motor, and sensory function. Focal brain injury causes focal neurologic deficits that may, or may not, alter consciousness. Global brain injury nearly always results in altered levels of consciousness, ranging from inattention to stupor or coma.

The cerebral hemispheres are the most susceptible to damage, and the most frequent sign of brain dysfunction is an altered level of consciousness and change in behavior. As the brain structures in the diencephalon, midbrain, pons, and medulla are sequentially affected, additional signs related to pupillary and eye movement reflexes, motor function, and respiration become evident (Table 16.1). Hemodynamic and respiratory instability are the last signs to occur because their regulatory centers are located low in the medulla.

With progressive neurologic deterioration, the person's neurologic capabilities appear to deteriorate in a stepwise fashion. Similarly, as neurologic function returns, there appears to be a stepwise progress to higher levels of consciousness. Deterioration of brain function from supratentorial lesions tends to follow a rostral-to-caudal stepwise progression, which is observed as the brain initially compensates for injury and subsequently decompensates with loss of autoregulation and cerebral perfusion. Infratentorial (brain stem) lesions may lead to an early, sometimes abrupt disturbance in consciousness without any orderly rostrocaudal progression of neurologic signs.

Altered Levels of Consciousness

All forms of brain injury and disease can lead to altered levels of consciousness. Consciousness is the state of awareness of self and the environment and of being able to orient to new stimuli.[1] It is divided into two components:

1. Arousal and wakefulness
2. Content and cognition[2]

Arousal and wakefulness require the concurrent functioning of both cerebral hemispheres and an intact reticular activating system (RAS) in the brain stem. The content and cognition aspects of consciousness are determined by a functioning cerebral cortex.

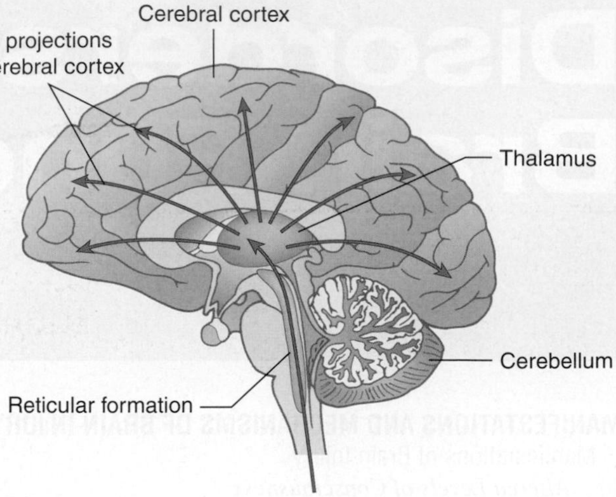

Figure 16.1 • The brain stem reticular formation and RAS. Ascending sensory tracts send axon collateral fibers to the reticular formation. These give rise to fibers synapsing in the nonspecific nuclei of the thalamus. From there, the nonspecific thalamic projections influence widespread areas of the cerebral cortex and limbic system.

Anatomic and Physiologic Basis of Consciousness. The reticular formation is a diffuse, primitive system of interlacing nerve cells and fibers in the brain stem that receive input from multiple sensory pathways (Fig. 16.1). Anatomically, the reticular formation constitutes the central core of the brain stem, extending from the medulla through the pons to the midbrain, that is continuous caudally with the spinal cord and rostrally with the subthalamus, the hypothalamus, and the thalamus.[2] Fibers from the RAS also project to the autonomic nervous system and motor systems. The hypothalamus plays a predominant role in maintaining homeostasis through integration of somatic, visceral, and endocrine functions. Inputs

TABLE 16.1 KEY SIGNS IN ROSTRAL-TO-CAUDAL PROGRESSION OF BRAIN LESIONS

LEVEL OF BRAIN INJURY	KEY CLINICAL SIGNS
Diencephalon	Impaired consciousness; small, reactive pupils; intact oculocephalic response; abnormal flexion posturing; Cheyne-Stokes respirations
Midbrain	Coma; fixed, midsize pupils; impaired oculocephalic response; central neurogenic hyperventilation; extension posturing
Pons	Coma; fixed, miotic (small) pupils; dysconjugate gaze; impaired oculovestibular response; loss of corneal reflex; hemiparesis/quadriparesis; extension posturing; apneustic respirations
Medulla	Coma, fixed pupils, flaccidity, loss of gag and cough reflexes, ataxic/apneic respirations

TABLE 16.2 DESCENDING LEVELS OF CONSCIOUSNESS AND THEIR CHARACTERISTICS

LEVEL OF CONSCIOUSNESS	CHARACTERISTICS
Full consciousness	Awake, alert, and oriented to time, place, and person; comprehends spoken and written word and is able to express ideas
Confusion	Disoriented to time, place, or person; memory difficulty; difficulty following commands
Lethargy	Oriented to time, place, and person; very slow in mental processes, motor activity, and speech; responds to pain appropriately
Obtundation	Responds verbally with a word; arousable with stimulation; responds appropriately to painful stimuli; follows simple commands; appears very drowsy
Stupor	Unresponsive except to vigorous and repeated stimuli; responds appropriately to painful stimuli; lies quiet with minimal spontaneous movement; may have incomprehensible sounds and/or eye opening
Coma	Does not respond appropriately to stimuli; sleeplike state with eyes closed; does not make any verbal sounds

Data from Hickey J. V. (2014). *The clinical practice of neurological and neurosurgical nursing* (7th ed.). Philadelphia, PA: Lippincott Williams & Wilkins.

from the reticular formation, vestibulospinal projections, and other motor systems are integrated to provide a continuously adapting background of muscle tone and posture to facilitate voluntary motor actions. Reticular formation neurons that function in regulation of cardiovascular, respiratory, and other visceral functions are intermingled with those that maintain other reticular formation functions.

Ascending fibers of the reticular formation, known as the ascending RAS, transmit activating information to all parts of the cerebral cortex. The flow of information in the ascending RAS activates the hypothalamic and limbic structures that regulate emotional and behavioral responses such as those that occur in response to pain and loud noises, and they exert facilitatory effects on cortical neurons. Without cortical activation, a person is less reactive to environmental stimuli, and the level of consciousness is reduced.

The pathways for the ascending RAS travel from the medulla through the midbrain, such that lesions of the brain stem can interrupt RAS activity, leading to altered levels of consciousness and coma. Any deficit in level of consciousness, from mild confusion to stupor or coma, indicates direct injury either to the RAS or to both cerebral hemispheres concurrently. For example, consciousness may decline because of severe systemic metabolic derangements that affect both hemispheres or from head trauma causing shear injuries to white matter of both the RAS and the cerebral hemispheres. Brain injuries that affect a hemisphere unilaterally and spare the RAS, such as cerebral infarction, usually do not cause impaired consciousness.

Levels of Consciousness. Levels of consciousness reflect awareness and response to the environment. A person who is fully conscious is totally aware of her or his surroundings and able to react to stimuli in the environment.[1] Levels of consciousness exist on a continuum that includes consciousness, confusion, lethargy, obtundation, stupor, and coma (Table 16.2).

The earliest signs of diminution in level of consciousness are inattention, mild confusion, disorientation, and blunted responsiveness. With further deterioration, the person who is experiencing delirium becomes markedly inattentive and variably lethargic or agitated. The person may progress to become obtunded and may respond only to vigorous or noxious stimuli.

The Glasgow Coma Scale provides an organized method to assess level of consciousness. This scale is for easy use as a bedside assessment for impaired consciousness in people with brain injury[3,4] (Table 16.3). Numbered scores are given to responses of eye opening and verbal and motor responses. The total score is the sum of the best response in each category.

KEY POINTS

BRAIN INJURY AND LEVELS OF CONSCIOUSNESS

- Consciousness is a global function that depends on a diffuse neural network that includes both cerebral hemispheres and activity of the RAS.
- Impaired consciousness implies diffuse brain injury to both cerebral hemispheres simultaneously or the RAS at any level (medulla through thalamus).
- In contrast, local brain injury causes focal neurologic deficit but does not disrupt consciousness.

TABLE 16.3 THE GLASGOW COMA SCALE

TEST	SCORE*
Eye Opening (E)	
Spontaneous	4
To speech	3
To painful stimuli	2
No response	1
Motor Response (M)	
Obeys commands	6
Localizes pain	5
Normal flexion (withdrawal)	4
Abnormal flexion (decorticate)	3
Extension (decerebrate)	2
No response	1
Verbal Response (V)	
Oriented	5
Confused conversation	4
Inappropriate words	3
Incomprehensible sounds	2
No response	1

*GCS score = E + M + V. Best possible score = 15; worst possible score = 3.
From Teasdale, G., Jennett, B. (1974). Assessment of coma and impaired consciousness. A practical scale. *Lancet* 304(7872), 81–84. Copyright © 1974 Elsevier. With permission.

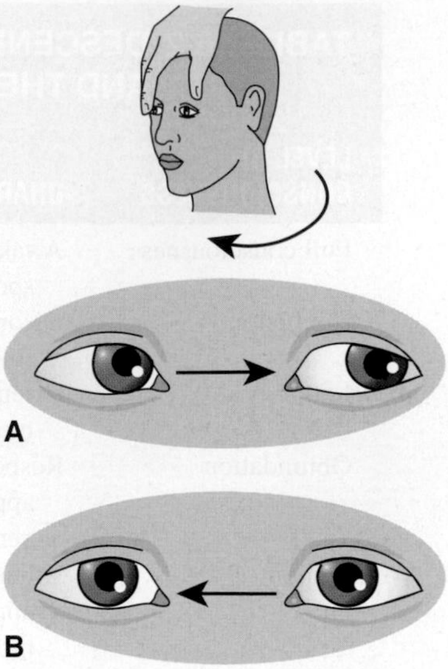

Figure 16.2 • Doll's-head response. The *doll's-head eye response* demonstrates the always-present vestibular static reflexes without forebrain interference or suppression. Severe damage to the forebrain or to the brain stem rostral to the pons often results in loss of rostral control of these static vestibular reflexes. If the person's head is moved from side to side or up and down, the eyes will move in conjugate gaze to the opposite side **(A)**, much like those of a doll with counterweighted eyes. If the doll's-head phenomenon is observed, brain stem function at the level of the pons is considered intact (in a person who is comatose). In the person who is unconscious without intact brain stem function and vestibular static reflexes, the eyes stay in midposition (fixed) or turn in the same direction **(B)** as the head is turned.

Other Manifestations of Deteriorating Brain Function

Additional elements in the initial neurologic evaluation of a person with brain injury include checking for abnormalities in the size of the pupils and their reaction to light, evidence of abnormal flexion or extension posturing, and altered patterns of respiration.

Pupillary Reflexes and Eye Movements. Although the pupils may initially respond briskly to light, they become nonreactive and dilated as brain function deteriorates. A bilateral loss of the pupillary light response is indicative of lesions of the brain stem. A unilateral loss of the pupillary light response may be due to a lesion of the optic or oculomotor pathways. The oculocephalic reflex (doll's-head eye movement) can be used to determine whether the brain stem centers for eye movement are intact (Fig. 16.2).

If the oculocephalic reflex is inconclusive, and if there are no contraindications, the oculovestibular reflex (*i.e.*, cold caloric test, in which cold water is instilled into the ear canal) may be used to elicit nystagmus.

Abnormal Flexion and Extension Posturing. With the early onset of unconsciousness, there is some combative and purposeful movement in response to pain. As coma progresses, noxious stimuli can initiate rigidity and abnormal postures if the motor tracts are interrupted at specific levels. These abnormal postures are classified as decorticate and decerebrate.[2] Decerebrate (extensor) posturing results from increased muscle excitability (see Fig. 16.6A). It is characterized by rigidity of the arms with palms of the hands turned away from the body and with stiffly extended legs and plantar flexion of the feet. This response occurs with rostral-to-caudal deterioration, when lesions of the diencephalon extend to involve the midbrain and upper brain stem. Decorticate posturing is characterized by flexion of the arms, wrists, and fingers, with adduction of the upper extremities, internal rotation, and plantar flexion of the lower extremities (see Fig. 16.6B). Decorticate posturing results from lesions of the cerebral hemisphere or internal capsule. Both decerebrate and decorticate posturing are poor prognostic signs.

Respiratory Responses. Early respiratory changes include yawning and sighing, with progression to Cheyne-Stokes breathing. With progression of injury continuing to the midbrain, respirations change to central neurogenic hyperventilation, in which the frequency of respirations may exceed 40 breaths per minute because of uninhibited stimulation of inspiratory and expiratory centers. With medullary involvement, respirations become ataxic (*i.e.*, totally uncoordinated and irregular). Apnea may occur because of a lack of responsiveness to carbon dioxide stimulation. Complete ventilatory assistance is often required at this point.

Brain Death

Brain death is defined as the irreversible loss of function of the brain, including the brain stem.[5] Irreversibility implies that brain death cannot be reversed. Some conditions such as drug and metabolic intoxication can cause cessation of brain functions that is completely reversible, even when they produce clinical cessation of brain functions and electroencephalographic (EEG) silence. This needs to be excluded before declaring a person brain dead.

With advances in scientific knowledge and technology that have provided the means for artificially maintaining ventilatory and circulatory function, the definition of death has had to be continually reexamined. In 2010, the Quality of Standards Subcommittee of the American Academy of Neurology published the evidence-based guideline update for clinical parameters for determining brain death and procedures for testing people older than 18 years of age.[5] According to these parameters, "brain death is the absence of clinical brain function when the proximate cause is known and demonstrably irreversible."[5] This update found that complex–spontaneous motor movements and false-positive triggering of the ventilator may occur in people who are brain dead. They also found insufficient evidence to determine the minimally acceptable observation period to ensure that neurologic functions have ceased irreversibly. It is safe to determine apnea with the apneic oxygenation diffusion, but there is insufficient evidence to determine the comparative safety of techniques used for apnea testing. The newer ancillary tests also had insufficient evidence to determine cessation of brain function.[5] Longer periods of observation of absent brain activity are required if the person is a child and in cases of drug overdose (*e.g.*, barbiturates, other central nervous system [CNS] depressants), drug toxicity (*e.g.*, neuromuscular blocking drugs, aminoglycoside antibiotics), and neuromuscular diseases such as myasthenia gravis, hypothermia, and shock. Medical circumstances may require the use of confirmatory tests.

Medical documentation should include cause and irreversibility of the condition, absence of brain stem reflexes and motor responses to pain, absence of respiration with a pressure of carbon dioxide (PCO_2) of 60 mm Hg or more, and the justification for use of confirmatory tests and their results. Apnea is confirmed after ventilation with pure oxygen 10 minutes before withdrawal from the ventilator, followed by passive flow of oxygen. This method allows the PCO_2 to rise to 60 mm Hg after a 10-minute period of apnea, without hazardously lowering the oxygen content of the blood. If respiratory reflexes are intact, the hypercarbia that develops should stimulate ventilatory effort within 30 seconds. Spontaneous breathing efforts indicate that the brain stem is functioning. Confirmatory tests of brain death include conventional angiography (*i.e.*, no intracerebral filling at the level of the carotid bifurcation or circle of Willis), transcranial Doppler ultrasonography, technetium-99 m hexamethylpropyleneamine oxime brain scan (*i.e.*, no uptake of isotope in brain parenchyma), somatosensory-evoked potentials, and EEG.

Persistent Vegetative State

Advances in the care of people with brain injury during the past several decades have resulted in survival of many people who previously would have died. Unfortunately, most people in prolonged coma who survive evolve to what often is called the *persistent vegetative state*. The vegetative state is characterized by loss of all cognitive functions and the unawareness of self and surroundings. Reflex and vegetative functions remain, including sleep–wake cycles.[6] These people have spontaneous eye opening without concurrent awareness, often confusing hopeful families. People in the vegetative state require nonoral feeding and full nursing care.

The criteria for diagnosis of vegetative state include the absence of awareness of self and environment and an inability to interact with others; the absence of sustained or reproducible voluntary behavioral responses; lack of language comprehension; sufficiently preserved hypothalamic and brain stem function to maintain life; bowel and bladder incontinence; and variably preserved cranial nerve (*e.g.*, pupillary, gag) and spinal cord reflexes.[6] The diagnosis of persistent vegetative state requires that the condition has continued for at least 1 month. The minimally conscious state has been defined as a state of arousal similar to persistent vegetative state, but with the distinction of the objective presence of some awareness on the part of the person.[7]

Mechanisms of Brain Injury

Injury to brain tissue can result from a number of conditions, including trauma, tumors, stroke, metabolic derangements, and degenerative disorders. Brain damage resulting from these disorders involves several common pathways, including the effects of ischemia, excitatory amino acid injury, cerebral edema, and injury because of ICP. In many cases, the mechanisms of injury are interrelated.

Hypoxic and Ischemic Injury

The energy requirements of the brain are provided mainly by adenosine triphosphate (ATP). The ability of the cerebral circulation to deliver oxygen in sufficiently high concentrations to facilitate metabolism of glucose and generate ATP is essential to brain function. Although the brain makes up only 2% of the body's weight, it receives 15% of the resting cardiac output and accounts for 20% of the oxygen consumption.[8,9] Thus, deprivation of oxygen or blood flow can have a deleterious effect on brain structures.

By definition, hypoxia denotes a deprivation of oxygen with maintained blood flow (perfusion), whereas ischemia is a situation of greatly reduced or interrupted blood flow. The brain tends to have different sensitivities to the two conditions. Whereas hypoxia interferes with the delivery of oxygen, ischemia interferes with delivery of oxygen and glucose as well as the removal of metabolic wastes. Hypoxia usually is seen in conditions such as exposure to reduced atmospheric pressure, carbon monoxide poisoning, severe anemia, and failure to oxygenate the blood. Because hypoxia indicates decreased oxygen levels in all brain tissue, it produces a generalized depressant effect on the brain. Neurons are capable of substantial anaerobic metabolism and are fairly tolerant of pure hypoxia. It commonly produces euphoria, listlessness, drowsiness, and impaired problem solving. Unconsciousness and seizures may occur when hypoxia is sudden and severe. However, the effects of severe hypoxia (*i.e.*, anoxia) on brain function seldom are seen because the condition rapidly leads to cardiac arrest and ischemia.

Cerebral ischemia can be focal, as in stroke, or global, as in cardiac arrest. In global ischemia, the blood flow to the entire brain is compromised. In contrast, during focal ischemia, only a region of the brain is underperfused, as in ischemic stroke. Collateral circulation provides blood flow to uninvolved brain areas during focal ischemia. The collateral perfusion may even provide sufficient substrates to the borders of the focal ischemic region to maintain a low level of metabolic activity, thereby preserving membrane integrity. At the same time, interruption in delivery of glucose under these anaerobic conditions may result in additional lactic acid production and depletion of ATP stores.[8]

Global Ischemia. Global ischemia occurs when blood flow is inadequate to meet the metabolic needs of the entire brain. The result is a spectrum of neurologic disorders reflecting global brain dysfunction. Unconsciousness occurs within seconds of severe global ischemia, such as that resulting from complete cessation of blood flow, as in cardiac arrest, or with marked decrease in blood flow, as in serious cardiac arrhythmias. If cerebral circulation is restored immediately, consciousness is regained quickly. However, if blood flow is not promptly restored, severe pathologic changes take place. Energy sources, glucose and glycogen, are exhausted in 2 to 4 minutes, and cellular ATP stores are depleted in 4 to 5 minutes. Approximately 50% to 75% of the total energy requirement of neuronal tissue is spent on mechanisms for maintenance of ionic gradients across the cell membrane (*e.g.*, sodium–potassium pump), resulting in fluxes of sodium, potassium, and calcium ions.[10] Excessive influx of sodium results in neuronal and interstitial edema. The influx of calcium initiates a cascade of events, including release of intracellular and nuclear enzymes that cause cell destruction. When ischemia is sufficiently severe or prolonged, infarction or death of all the cellular elements of the brain occurs. Even if blood flow is restored, if ischemic thresholds for injury are exceeded, then permanent cell death ensues. Furthermore, reperfusion of injured tissues can lead to secondary brain injury through the delivery of inflammatory cells and toxic by-products, including excitatory amino acids. Such reperfusion injury compounds the initial ischemic damage.

The pattern of global ischemia reflects the anatomic arrangement of the cerebral vessels and the sensitivity of various brain tissues to oxygen deprivation[11] (Fig. 16.3). Selective neuronal sensitivity to a lack of oxygen is most apparent in the Purkinje cells of the cerebellum and neurons in the Sommer sector of the hippocampus, where cell death occurs earliest after global ischemia. The anatomic arrangement of the cerebral blood vessels predisposes to two types of injury: watershed infarcts and laminar necrosis.

Watershed infarcts are concentrated in anatomically vulnerable border zones between the overlapping territories

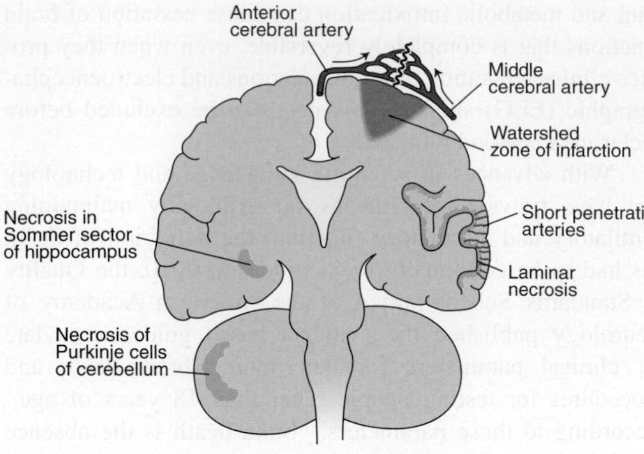

Figure 16.3 • Consequences of global ischemia. A global insult induces lesions that reflect the vascular architecture (watershed infarcts, laminar necrosis) and the sensitivity of individual neuronal systems (pyramidal cells of the Sommer section, Purkinje cells). (Courtesy of Dimitri Karetnikov, artist.) (From Strayer D. S., Rubin E. (Eds.) (2015). *Rubin's pathology: Clinicopathologic foundations of medicine* (Fig. 32-23, p. 1427). Philadelphia, PA: Lippincott Williams & Wilkins.)

supplied by the major cerebral arteries, notably the middle, anterior, and posterior cerebral arteries. The overlapping territory at the distal ends of these vessels forms extremely vulnerable areas in terms of global ischemia, called *watershed zones*. During events such as severe hypotension, these distal territories undergo a profound lowering of blood flow, predisposing to focal ischemia and infarction of brain tissues. Therefore, global ischemia can result in focal infarcts that occur in the border zones between major vascular territories. This is in contrast to primarily focal ischemia in which the pattern of infarction is within a vascular territory. Laminar necrosis refers to short, serpiginous segments of necrosis that occur within and parallel to the cerebral cortex, in areas supplied by the penetrating arteries. The gray matter of the cerebral cortex receives its major blood supply through short penetrating arteries that emerge at right angles from larger vessels in the pia mater and then form a cascade as they repeatedly branch, forming a rich capillary network. An abrupt loss of arterial blood pressure markedly diminishes flow through these capillary channels. Because the third cortical layer is most sensitive to ischemia, the necrosis that develops is laminar and is most severe in this deep layer of the cortex.

The neurologic deficits that result from global ischemic injury vary widely. If the period of nonflow or low flow is minimal, the neurologic damage usually is minimal to nonexistent. When the period is extensive or resuscitation is lengthy, the early neurologic clinical picture is that of coma; fixed, dilated pupils; and abnormal motor posturing. If the person survives, there may be gradual improvement in neurologic status, although permanent cognitive and focal deficits usually persist and can prevent a return to preischemic levels of functioning.

An exception to this time frame is the circumstance of cold-water drowning in which the person, especially a child, is submerged in cold water for longer than 30 minutes.[12] Hypothermia develops and reduces the cerebral metabolic requirements for oxygen, minimizes intracellular acidosis, and lessens the effects of excitotoxic by-products. In this case, recovery can be rapid and remarkable, and resuscitation efforts should not be discontinued precipitously.

Treatment of global cerebral ischemia varies with the underlying cause (*e.g.*, cardiac arrest, hanging, asthma attack). General goals common to all causes are aimed at providing oxygen to the injured brain and decreasing the metabolic needs of brain tissue during the nonflow state. Hemodynamic support aimed at restoring systemic and cerebral perfusion is required. Respiratory support including mechanical ventilation and supplemental oxygen may be indicated. Methods that decrease brain temperature as a means of decreasing brain metabolism are effective in certain people after cardiac arrest.[13] Normovolemic hemodilution may be used to overcome sludging of cerebral blood flow during reperfusion. Because both hypoglycemia and hyperglycemia adversely affect the outcome in people with global ischemia, control of blood glucose around the level of 140 mg/dL is appropriate.[14]

Excitotoxic Brain Injury

In many neurologic disorders, injury to neurons may be caused by various mediators, including excitatory amino acids, catecholamines, nitric oxide, free radicals, inflammatory cells, apoptosis, and intracellular proteases.[15] The final common pathway for neuronal cell injury and death triggered by excessive activity of the excitatory neurotransmitters and their receptor-mediated effects is termed excitotoxicity supratentorial. The neurologic conditions involved in excitotoxic injury range from acute insults such as stroke, hypoglycemic injury, and trauma to chronic degenerative disorders such as Huntington disease and possibly Alzheimer dementia.

Glutamate is the principal excitatory neurotransmitter in the brain, and its interaction with specific receptors is responsible for many higher-order functions, including memory, cognition, movement, and sensation.[15] Many of the actions of glutamate are coupled with receptor-operated ion channels. One subtype in particular, the glutamate *N*-methyl-D-aspartate (NMDA) receptor, has been implicated in causing CNS injury.[15] This subtype of glutamate receptor opens a large-diameter calcium channel that permits calcium and sodium ions to enter the cell and allows potassium ions to exit, resulting in prolonged (seconds) action potentials. Extracellular concentrations of glutamate are tightly regulated, with excess amounts removed and actively transported into astrocytes and neurons.

During prolonged ischemia, the glutamate transport mechanisms become immobilized, causing extracellular glutamate to accumulate. In addition, intracellular glutamate is released from the damaged cells. This glutamate excess then drives the uncontrolled opening of NMDA receptor-operated channels, producing an increase in intracellular calcium. Excess intracellular calcium leads to a series of calcium-mediated processes called the *calcium cascade* (Fig. 16.4),

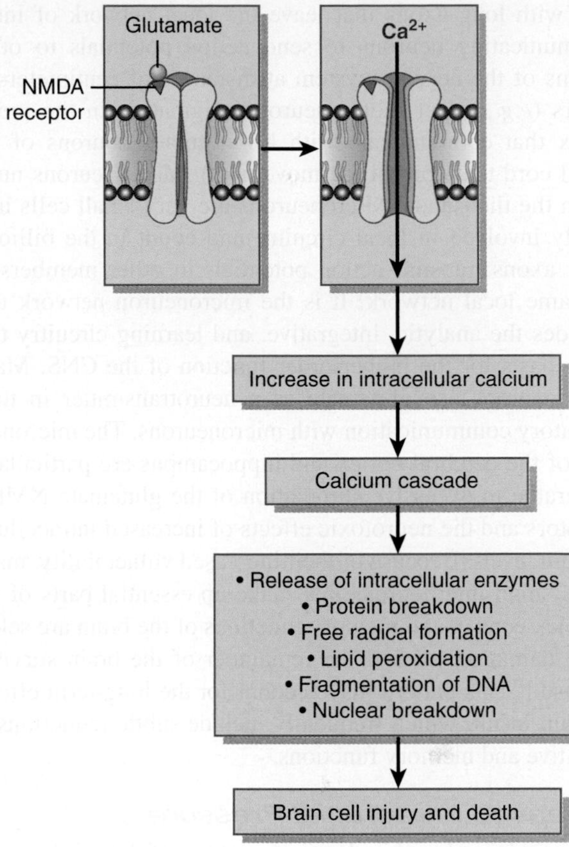

Figure 16.4 • The role of the glutamate NMDA receptor in brain cell injury.

including the release of intracellular enzymes that cause protein breakdown, free radical formation, lipid peroxidation, fragmentation of deoxyribonucleic acid (DNA), mitochondrial injury, nuclear breakdown, and eventually cell death.

The effects of acute glutamate toxicity may be reversible if the excess glutamate can be removed or if its effects can be blocked before the full cascade of events progresses. Drugs called *neuroprotectants* are being developed to interfere with the calcium cascade and thus reduce brain cell injury. These pharmacologic strategies may protect viable brain cells from irreversible damage in the setting of excitotoxicity. Pharmacologic strategies being explored include those that inhibit the synthesis or release of excitatory amino acid transmitters; block the NMDA receptors; stabilize the membrane potential to prevent initiation of the calcium cascade using lidocaine and certain barbiturates; and specifically block certain intracellular proteases, endonucleases, and lipases that are known to be cytotoxic.[15] The drug riluzole, which acts presynaptically to inhibit glutamate release, currently is being used in the treatment of amyotrophic lateral sclerosis (see Chapter 16). In the setting of ischemic stroke, multiple mechanisms of pharmacologic action, including NMDA receptor blockade, nitric oxide manipulation, inflammatory suppression, and potassium channel opening, are being studied.[15]

CNS neurons can be divided into two major categories: macroneurons and microneurons. Macroneurons are large cells with long axons that leave the local network of intercommunicating neurons to send action potentials to other regions of the nervous system at distances of centimeters to meters (*e.g.*, upper motor neurons originating in the motor cortex that communicate with lower motor neurons of the spinal cord that control leg movement). Macroneurons number in the thousands. Microneurons are very small cells intimately involved in local circuitry and count in the billions. Their axons transmit action potentials to other members of the same local network. It is the microneuron network that provides the analytic, integrative, and learning circuitry that is the basis for the higher-order function of the CNS. Many macroneurons use glutamate as a neurotransmitter in their excitatory communication with microneurons. The microneurons of the cerebral cortex and hippocampus are particularly vulnerable to excessive stimulation of the glutamate NMDA receptors and the neurotoxic effects of increased intracellular calcium levels. Because of their increased vulnerability, many of the small interneurons that make up essential parts of the complex control and memory functions of the brain are selectively damaged, even if the remainder of the brain survives the insult. This pattern may account for the long-term effects of brain insult, which frequently include subtle reductions in cognitive and memory functions.

Increased Intracranial Pressure

The brain is enclosed in the rigid confines of the skull, or cranium, making it particularly susceptible to increases in ICP. Increased ICP is a common pathway for brain injury from different types of insults and agents. Excessive ICP can obstruct cerebral blood flow, destroy brain cells, displace brain tissue (as in herniation), and otherwise damage delicate brain structures (Table 16.4).

The cranial cavity contains blood (approximately 10%), brain tissue (approximately 80%), and CSF (approximately 10%) in the rigid confines of a nonexpandable skull.[2] Each of these three volumes contributes to the ICP, which normally is maintained within a range of 0 to 15 mm Hg when measured in the lateral ventricles. The volumes of each of these components can vary slightly without causing marked changes in ICP. This is because small increases in the volume of one component can be compensated for by a decrease in the volume of one or both of the other two components. This dynamic equilibrium is called the *Monro-Kellie hypothesis*.[2] Abnormal variation in intracranial volume with subsequent changes in ICP can be caused by a volume change in any of the three intracranial components. For example, an increase in tissue volume can result from a brain tumor, brain edema, or bleeding into brain tissue. An increase in blood volume develops when there is vasodilation of cerebral vessels or obstruction of venous outflow. Excess production, decreased absorption, or obstructed circulation of CSF affords the potential for an increase in the CSF component. The Monro-Kellie hypothesis explains the reciprocal compensation that occurs among the three intracranial compartments (blood, brain tissue, and CSF).[2]

Of the three intracranial volumes, tissue volume is relatively restricted in its ability to undergo change. CSF and blood volume are best able to compensate for changes in ICP. Initial increases in ICP are buffered by a translocation of CSF to the spinal subarachnoid space and increased reabsorption of CSF. The compensatory ability of the blood compartment is limited by the small amount of blood that is in the cerebral circulation. The cerebral blood vessels contain less than 10% of the intracranial volume, most of which is contained in the low-pressure venous system. As the volume-buffering capacity of this compartment become exhausted, venous pressure increases, and cerebral blood volume and ICP rise. Also, cerebral blood flow is highly controlled by autoregulatory mechanisms, which affect its compensatory capacity. Conditions such as ischemia and an elevated partial PCO_2 in the blood produce a compensatory vasodilation of the cerebral blood vessels. A decrease in PCO_2 has the opposite effect. For this reason, hyperventilation, which results in a decrease in PCO_2 levels, is sometimes used in the treatment of ICP.

The impact of increases in blood, brain tissue, or CSF volumes on ICP varies among people and depends on the amount of increase, effectiveness of compensatory mechanisms, and compliance of brain tissue. Compliance represents the ratio of change in volume to the resulting change in pressure (compliance = change in volume/change in pressure).[2] In the case of intracranial volumes and pressure, an increase in intracranial volume will have little, or no, effect on ICP as long as compliance is high. Factors that influence compliance include the amount of volume increase, the time frame for accommodation, and the size of the intracranial compartments. For example, small volume increments over long periods of time

TABLE 16.4 EARLY AND LATE SIGNS OF INCREASED ICP

SIGNS	EARLY SIGN	LATE SIGN
Level of consciousness	Decreased alertness to drowsy	Stupor or coma
Pupil size and reaction to light	Small and sluggish reaction	Large and nonreactive
Motor function	Hemiparesis	Hemiplegia
Vital signs	No change	Hypertension, widened pulse pressure, bradycardia, abnormal respiratory patterns
Other signs	Headache, slurred speech	Vomiting

can be accommodated more easily than a comparable amount introduced over a short time.

The cerebral perfusion pressure (CPP), which represents the difference between the mean arterial pressure (MAP) and the ICP (CPP = MAP − ICP), is the pressure gradient driving blood flow to the brain.[9,16] Normal CPP ranges from 70 to 100 mm Hg. Brain ischemia develops at levels below 40 mm Hg.[2] When the pressure in the cranial cavity approaches or exceeds the MAP, tissue perfusion becomes inadequate, cellular hypoxia results, and neuronal death may occur. The highly specialized cortical neurons are the most sensitive to oxygen deficit. A decrease in the level of consciousness is one of the earliest and most reliable signs of increased ICP. The continued cellular hypoxia leads to general neurologic deterioration. The level of consciousness may deteriorate from alertness through confusion, lethargy, obtundation, stupor, and coma.

One of the late signs seen with a marked increase in ICP is the Cushing triad (reflex), which is triggered by ischemia of the vasomotor center in the brain stem. Neurons in the vasomotor center respond directly to ischemia by producing a marked increase in MAP in an attempt to increase CPP, accompanied by a widening of the pulse pressure and reflex slowing of the heart rate. These three signs (*i.e.*, hypertension, bradycardia, and widened pulse pressure), called the *Cushing reflex,* are important but late indicators of increased ICP.[17]

Brain Herniation

The brain is protected by the nonexpandable skull and supporting septa, the falx cerebri and the tentorium cerebelli, that divide the intracranial cavity into fossae or compartments that normally protect against excessive movement. The falx cerebri is a sickle-shaped septum that separates the two hemispheres. The tentorium cerebelli divides the cranial cavity into anterior and posterior fossae. This inflexible dural sheath extends posteriorly from the bony petrous ridges and anterior to the clinoid process, sloping downward and outward from its medial edge to attach laterally to the occipital bone. Extending posteriorly into the center of the tentorium is a large semicircular opening called the *incisura* or *tentorial notch.* The temporal lobe rests on the tentorial incisura, and the midbrain occupies

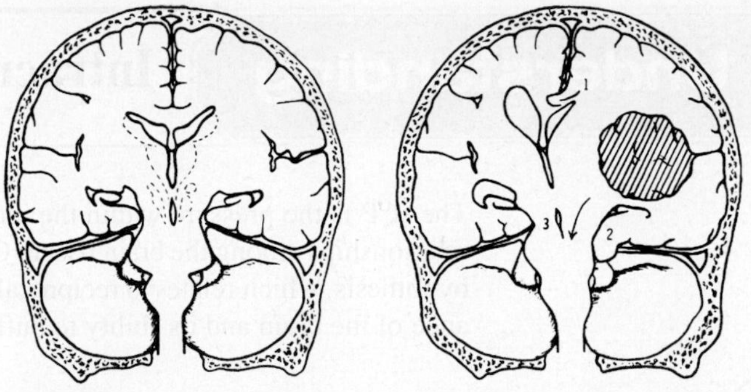

Figure 16.5 • Patterns of herniation. Normal brain **(left)**, supratentorial herniations **(right)**. (*1*) Herniation of cingulated gyrus under the falx cerebri. (*2*) Herniation of the temporal lobe into the tentorial notch. (*3*) Downward displacement of the brain stem through the notch. (From Hickey J. V. (2014). *The clinical practice of neurological and neurosurgical nursing* (7th ed., p. 1427). Philadelphia, PA: Lippincott Williams & Wilkins.)

the anterior portion of the tentorial notch. The cerebellum is closely opposed to the dorsum of the midbrain and fills the posterior part of the notch. Other important anatomic associations exist among the anterior cerebral, internal carotid, posterior communicating, and posterior and superior cerebellar arteries and the incisura. The oculomotor nerve (cranial nerve III) emerges from the mediolateral surface of each peduncle just caudal to the tentorium.

Brain herniation represents a displacement of brain tissue under the falx cerebri or through the tentorial notch or incisura of the tentorium cerebelli (see Fig. 16.5). It occurs when an elevated ICP in one brain compartment causes displacement of the cerebral tissue toward an area of lower ICP. The different types of herniation syndromes are based on the area of the brain that has herniated and the structure under which it has been pushed. They commonly are divided into two broad categories, supratentorial and infratentorial, based on whether they are located above or below the tentorium.

Supratentorial Herniations. There are three major patterns of supratentorial herniation: cingulate, central transtentorial, and uncal transtentorial. Table 16.5 describes the key structures

TABLE 16.5 KEY STRUCTURES AND CLINICAL SIGNS OF CINGULATE, CENTRAL, AND UNCAL HERNIATIONS

HERNIATION SYNDROME	KEY STRUCTURES INVOLVED	KEY CLINICAL SIGNS
Cingulate	Anterior cerebral artery	Leg weakness
Central transtentorial	RAS	Altered level of consciousness
	Corticospinal tract	Decorticate posturing
		Rostral–caudal deterioration
Uncal	Cerebral peduncle	Hemiparesis
	Oculomotor nerve	Ipsilateral pupil dilation
	Posterior cerebral artery	Visual field loss
	Cerebellar tonsil	Respiratory arrest
	Respiratory center	

Understanding Intracranial Pressure

The ICP is the pressure within the intracranial cavity. It is determined by (1) the pressure–volume relationships among the brain tissue, CSF, and blood in the intracranial cavity; (2) the Monro-Kellie hypothesis, which relates to reciprocal changes among the intracranial volumes; and (3) the compliance of the brain and its ability to buffer changes in intracranial volume.

Intracranial Volumes and Pressure

The ICP represents the pressure exerted by the essentially incompressible tissue and fluid volumes of the three compartments contained within the rigid confines of the skull—the brain tissue and interstitial fluid (80%), the blood (10%), and the CSF (10%).

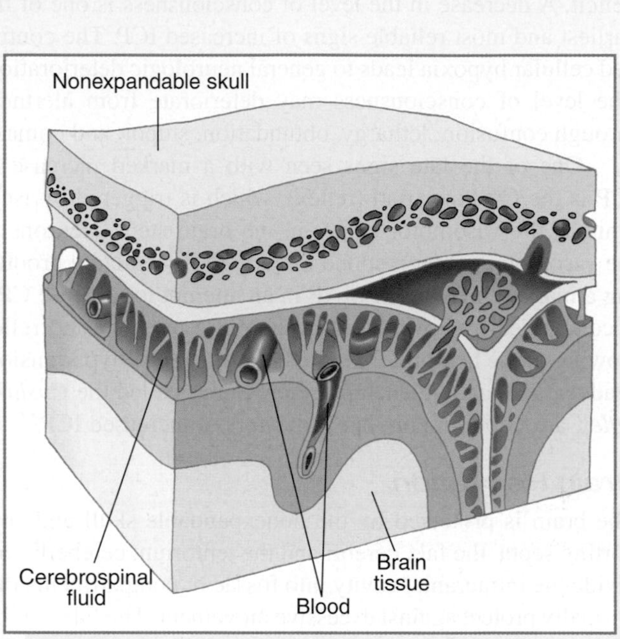

Monro-Kellie Hypothesis

Normally, a reciprocal relationship exists among the three intracranial volumes such that the ICP is maintained within normal limits. Because these volumes are practically incompressible, a change in one component must be balanced by an almost equal and opposite effect in one or both of the remaining components. This is known as the *Monro-Kellie hypothesis*.

Of the three intracranial volumes, the fluid in the CSF compartment is the most easily displaced. The CSF **(A)** can be displaced from the ventricles and cerebral subarachnoid space to the spinal subarachnoid space, and it can also undergo increased absorption or decreased production. Because most of the blood in the cranial cavity is contained in the low-pressure venous system, venous compression **(B)** serves as a means of displacing blood volume.

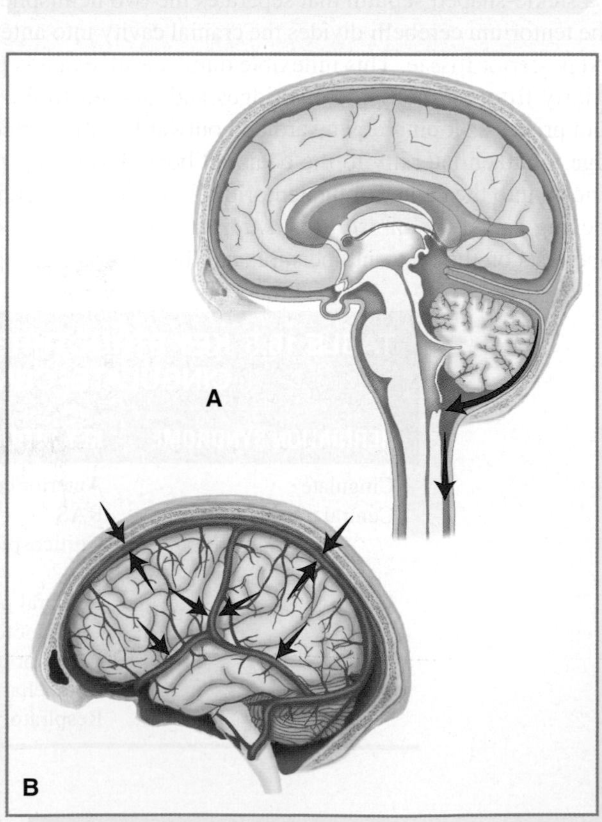

Understanding Intracranial Pressure *(Continued)*

Compliance and the Volume–Pressure Curve

Compliance, which refers to the ease with which a substance can be compressed or deformed, is a measure of the brain's ability to maintain its ICP during changes in intracranial volume. Compliance (C) represents the ratio of change (Δ) in volume (V) to change in pressure (P): $C = \Delta V/\Delta P$.

The dynamic effects of changes in intracranial volume and compliance on ICP can be illustrated on a graph with the volume represented on the horizontal axis and ICP on the vertical axis. The shape of the curve demonstrates the effect on ICP of adding volume to the intracranial cavity. From points A to B, the compensatory mechanisms are adequate, compliance is high, and the ICP remains relatively constant as volume is added to the intracranial cavity. At point B, the ICP is relatively normal, but the compensatory mechanisms have reached their limits, compliance is decreased, and ICP begins to rise with each change in volume. From points C to D, the compensatory mechanisms have been exceeded, and ICP rises significantly with each increase in volume as compliance is lost.

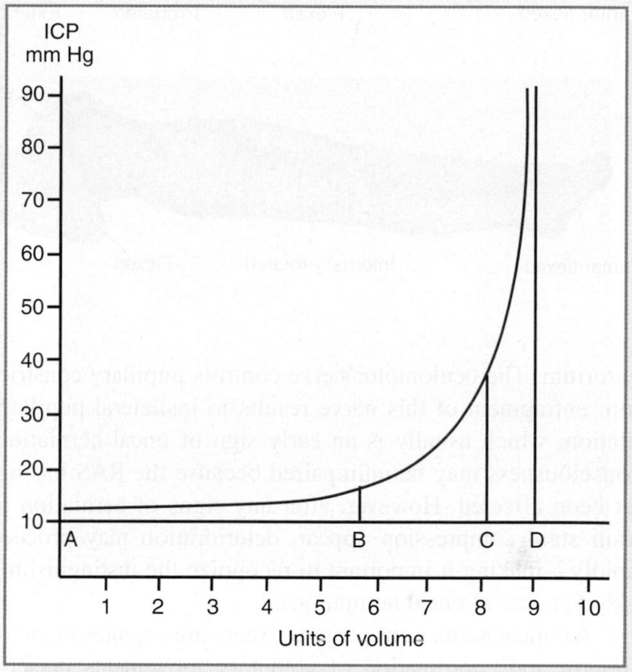

and clinical signs of these three types of herniations. Of the three, cingulate herniation poses the less serious threat in terms of clinical outcomes.[2] Transtentorial herniations result in two distinct syndromes: an uncal syndrome and a central syndrome. Clinically, they display distinct patterns early in their course, but both merge in a similar pattern once they begin to involve the midbrain level and below (brain stem structures).

Cingulate herniation involves displacement of the cingulate gyrus and hemisphere beneath the sharp edges of the falx cerebri to the opposite side of the brain. Displacement of the falx can compress the local brain tissue and blood supply from the anterior cerebral artery, causing ischemia and edema, which further increase ICP levels. Unilateral or bilateral leg weakness is an early sign of impending cingulate herniation.

Central transtentorial herniations involve the downward displacement of the cerebral hemispheres, basal ganglia, diencephalon, and midbrain through the tentorial incisura. The diencephalon may be compressed tightly against the midbrain with such force that edema and hemorrhage result. It may or may not be associated with uncal or lateral herniation. In the early diencephalic stage, there is clouding of consciousness, bilaterally small pupils (approximately 2 mm in diameter) with a full range of constriction, and motor responses to pain that are purposeful or semipurposeful (localizing) and often asymmetric. The clouding of consciousness, which is often a first sign of central herniations, is caused by pressure on the RAS in the upper midbrain, which is responsible for wakefulness. As the herniation progresses to the late diencephalic stage, painful stimulation results in decorticate posturing, which may be asymmetric (see Fig. 16.6B), and there is waxing and waning of respirations with periods of apnea (Cheyne-Stokes respirations). With midbrain involvement, the pupils are fixed and midsize (approximately 5 mm in diameter), and reflex adduction of the eyes is impaired; pain elicits decerebrate posturing (Fig. 16.6B); and respirations change from Cheyne-Stokes to neurogenic hyperventilation, in which the frequency may exceed 40 breaths per minute because of uninhibited stimulation of the inspiratory and expiratory centers. Progression to involve the lower pons and upper medulla produces fixed, midpoint (3- to 5-mm) pupils with loss of reflex abduction and adduction of the eyes, and absence of motor responses or only leg flexion on painful stimuli. Once the area of herniation has progressed beyond the diencephalon and into the midbrain and brain stem, the process is generally irreversible and the prognosis poor.[2]

Uncal herniation occurs when a lateral mass pushes the brain tissue centrally and forces the medial aspect of the temporal lobe, which contains the uncus and hippocampal gyrus, under the edge of the tentorial incisura, into the posterior fossa. As a result, the diencephalon and midbrain are compressed and displaced laterally to the opposite side of the tentorium. Cranial nerve III (oculomotor nerve) and the posterior cerebral artery frequently are caught between the uncus and the

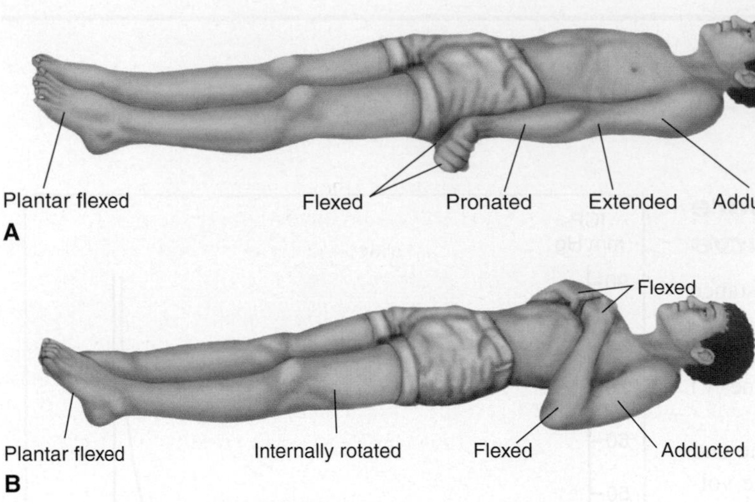

Figure 16.6 • Abnormal posturing. **(A)** Decerebrate posturing. In decerebrate rigidity, the upper arms are held at the sides with elbows, wrists, and fingers flexed. The legs are extended and internally rotated. The feet are plantar flexed. **(B)** Decorticate posturing. In decorticate rigidity, the jaws are clenched and neck extended. The arms are adducted and stiffly extended at the elbows with the forearms pronated and the wrists and fingers flexed.(From Hickey J. V. (2014). *The clinical practice of neurological and neurosurgical nursing* (7th ed., p. 173). Philadelphia, PA: Lippincott Williams & Wilkins.)

tentorium. The oculomotor nerve controls pupillary constriction; entrapment of this nerve results in ipsilateral pupillary dilation, which usually is an early sign of uncal herniation. Consciousness may be unimpaired because the RAS has not yet been affected. However, after any signs of herniation or brain stem compression appear, deterioration may proceed rapidly—making it important to recognize the distinguishing early features of uncal herniations.

As uncal herniations progress, there are changes in motor strength and coordination of voluntary movements because of compression of the descending motor pathways. It is not unusual for initial changes in motor function to occur ipsilateral to the side of the brain damage because of compression of the contralateral cerebral peduncles. This may result in a false localizing sign of hemiparesis on the same side as cranial nerve III, rather than on the opposite side, which would be the case if a singular lesion in the midbrain is the cause. As the condition progresses, bilateral positive Babinski responses and respiratory changes (*e.g.*, Cheyne-Stokes respirations, ataxic patterns) occur. Decorticate and decerebrate posturing may develop, followed by dilated, fixed pupils, flaccidity, and respiratory arrest.

Infratentorial Herniation. Infratentorial herniation results from increased pressure in the infratentorial compartment. It often progress rapidly and can cause death because it is likely to involve the lower brain stem centers that control vital cardiopulmonary functions. Herniation may occur superiorly (upward) through the tentorial incisura or inferiorly (downward) through the foramen magnum.

Upward displacement of brain tissue can cause blockage of the aqueduct of Sylvius and lead to hydrocephalus and coma. Downward displacement of the midbrain through the tentorial notch or the cerebellar tonsils through the foramen magnum can interfere with medullary functioning and cause cardiac or respiratory arrest. In cases of pre-existing ICP elevations, herniation may occur when the pressure is released from below, such as in a lumbar puncture. If the CSF pathway is blocked and fluid cannot leave the ventricles, the volume expands, and fluid is displaced downward through the tentorial notch. The expanding volume causes all function at a given level to cease as destruction progresses in a rostral-to-caudal direction. The result of this displacement is brain stem ischemia and hemorrhage extending from the diencephalon to the pons. If the lesion expands rapidly, displacement and obstruction occur quickly, leading to irreversible infarction and hemorrhage.

Cerebral Edema

Cerebral edema, or brain swelling, occurs with an increase in water and sodium content causing an increase in brain volume.[18] There are two types of brain edema: vasogenic and cytotoxic.[8,18] Vasogenic edema occurs when integrity of the blood–brain barrier is disrupted, allowing fluid to escape into the extracellular fluid that surrounds brain cells. Cytotoxic edema involves the actual swelling of brain cells themselves. The impact of brain edema depends on the brain's compensatory mechanisms and the extent of the swelling.

Vasogenic Edema. Vasogenic edema occurs with conditions that impair the function of the blood–brain barrier and allow transfer of water and protein from the vascular into the interstitial space. It occurs in conditions such as tumors, prolonged ischemia, hemorrhage, brain injury, and infectious processes (*e.g.*, meningitis). Vasogenic edema occurs primarily in the white matter of the brain, possibly because the white matter is more compliant than the gray matter. Vasogenic edema can displace a cerebral hemisphere and can be responsible for various types of herniation. The functional manifestations of vasogenic edema include focal neurologic deficits, disturbances in consciousness, and severe intracranial hypertension.

Cytotoxic Edema. Cytotoxic edema involves an increase in intracellular fluid. It can result from hypoosmotic states such as water intoxication or severe ischemia that impair the function of the sodium–potassium membrane pump. Ischemia also results in the inadequate removal of anaerobic metabolic end products such as lactic acid, producing extracellular acidosis. If blood flow is reduced to low levels for extended periods or to extremely low levels for a few minutes, cellular edema can cause the cell membrane to rupture, allowing the escape of intracellular contents into the surrounding extracellular fluid. This leads to damage of neighboring cells. The altered osmotic conditions result in water entry and cell swelling. Major changes in cerebral function, such as stupor and coma, occur with cytotoxic edema. The edema associated with ischemia may be severe enough to produce cerebral infarction with necrosis of brain tissue.

Treatment. Although cerebral edema is viewed as a pathologic process, it does not necessarily disrupt brain function unless it increases the ICP. The localized edema surrounding a brain tumor or abscess rapidly begins to reduce signs of brain edema with glucocorticoid therapy, but use of these drugs is not effective for cerebral infarction, intracranial hemorrhage (ICH), subarachnoid hemorrhage (SAH), or traumatic brain injury (TBI) edema. The mechanism of action of the glucocorticoid therapy in the treatment of cerebral edema is a direct normalizing effect on endothelial cell function. Osmotherapy (*e.g.*, 20% mannitol (0.5 to 1.5 g/kg) or 3%, 7%, 10%, or 23% hypertonic saline in repeated boluses) may be useful in the acute phase of vasogenic and cytotoxic edema.

Hydrocephalus

Enlargement of the CSF compartment occurs with hydrocephalus, which is defined as an abnormal increase in CSF volume in any part or all of the ventricular system. The two causes of hydrocephalus are decreased absorption of CSF and obstruction of CSF flow. There are two types of hydrocephalus: noncommunicating and communicating.

Noncommunicating or obstructive hydrocephalus occurs when obstruction in the ventricular system prevents the CSF from reaching the arachnoid villi. CSF flow can be obstructed by congenital malformations, from tumors encroaching on the ventricular system, and by inflammation or hemorrhage. The ependyma (*i.e.*, lining of ventricles and CSF-filled spaces) is especially sensitive to viral infections, particularly during embryonic development; ependymitis is believed to be the cause of congenital aqueductal stenosis.[11]

Communicating hydrocephalus is caused by impaired reabsorption of CSF from the arachnoid villi into the venous system. Decreased absorption can result from a block in the CSF pathway to the arachnoid villi or a failure of the villi to transfer the CSF to the venous system. It can occur if too few villi are formed, if postinfective (meningitis) scarring occludes them, or if the villi become obstructed with fragments of blood or infectious debris. Adenomas of the choroid plexus can cause an overproduction of CSF. This form of hydrocephalus is much less common than that resulting from decreased absorption of CSF.

Similar pathologic patterns occur with noncommunicating and communicating types of hydrocephalus. The cerebral hemispheres become enlarged, and the ventricular system beyond the point of obstruction is dilated. The sulci on the surface of the brain become effaced and shallow, and the white matter is reduced in volume. The presence and extent of the ICP are determined by fluid accumulation and the type of hydrocephalus, the age at onset, and the rapidity and extent of pressure rise. Computed tomographic (CT) and magnetic resonance imaging (MRI) scans are used to diagnose all types of hydrocephalus. The usual treatment is a shunting procedure, which provides an alternative route for return of CSF to the circulation.

Signs and symptoms of hydrocephalus vary greatly, depending on the rapidity of onset. When hydrocephalus develops in utero or before the cranial sutures have fused in infancy, the ventricles expand beyond the point of obstruction, the cranial sutures separate, the head expands, and there is bulging of the fontanels. Because the skull is able to expand, signs of increased ICP may be absent and intelligence spared. However, seizures are not uncommon, and in severe cases, optic nerve atrophy leads to blindness. Weakness and uncoordinated movement are common. Surgical placement of a shunt allows for diversion of excess CSF fluid, preventing extreme enlargement of the head and neurologic deficits.

In adults, head enlargement does not occur because the cranial sutures are fully fused. Thus, signs and symptoms are likely. Slowly developing hydrocephalus is unlikely to produce an increase in ICP, but it may still produce deficits such as progressive dementia and gait changes, as in normal-pressure hydrocephalus (*pseudotumor cerebri*) in the elderly. In contrast, acute-onset hydrocephalus in adults usually is marked by symptoms of increased ICP, including headache, vomiting, and papilledema or lateral rectus palsy from pressure effects on the cranial nerves. If the obstruction is not relieved, progression to herniation ensues (see previous discussion of herniation). Treatment includes surgical decompression and shunting.

IN SUMMARY

Brain injury is manifested by changes in the level of consciousness and alterations in motor, sensory, and cognitive function. Consciousness is a state of awareness of self and environment. It exists on a continuum from normal wakefulness and sleep to the pathologic states of stupor and coma. In progressive brain injury, the onset of coma may follow a rostral-to-caudal progression with characteristic changes in levels of consciousness, respiratory activity, pupillary and oculovestibular reflexes, and muscle tone occurring as the diencephalon through the medulla are affected.

Brain death is defined as the irreversible loss of function of the brain, including that of the brain stem. Clinical examination must disclose at least the absence of responsiveness, brain stem reflexes, and respiratory effort. The vegetative state is characterized by loss of all cognitive functions and the unawareness of self and surroundings, whereas reflex and vegetative functions remain intact.

Many of the agents that cause brain damage do so through common pathways, including hypoxia or ischemia, accumulation of excitatory neurotransmitters, increased ICP, and cerebral edema. Deprivation of oxygen (*i.e.*, hypoxia) or blood flow (*i.e.*, ischemia) can have deleterious effects on the brain structures. Focal ischemia causes localized brain injury, as in stroke. Global ischemia, as in cardiac arrest, occurs when blood flow to the entire brain is inadequate, causing global deficits such as altered mental status.

TRAUMATIC BRAIN INJURY

After completing this section of the chapter, the learner will be able to meet the following objectives:

- Describe the effects of primary and secondary brain injuries.
- Summarize the different types of hematomas that can occur in the brain.
- Identify focal versus diffuse brain injuries.

The brain is enclosed in the protective confines of the rigid bony skull. Although the skull generally affords protection to the soft tissues of the CNS from external forces, it also imposes risks as a source of injury from internal forces. The bony structures of the internal surface of the skull can induce traumatic and ischemic brain injuries when intracranial tissues increase in volume (swelling or bleeding) or shift (swelling or mechanical trauma). Furthermore, fractures of the skull can compress sections of the nervous system and cause penetrating wounds.

TBI is the leading cause of death and disability among people younger than 24 years of age. The main causes of TBI are motor vehicle crashes, falls, and assaults, with the most common cause of fatal head injuries being motor vehicle crashes involving vehicles and pedestrians.[16]

Traumatic brain injuries can involve the scalp, skull, meninges, or brain. Skull fractures can be classified as linear, comminuted, depressed, and basilar. A linear skull fracture is a break in the continuity of bone. A comminuted skull fracture refers to a splintered or multiple fracture line. When bone fragments are embedded into the brain tissue, the fracture is said to be depressed. A fracture of the bones that form the base of the skull is called a basilar skull fracture.

Radiologic examination usually is needed to confirm the presence and extent of a skull fracture. This evaluation is important because of the possible damage to the underlying tissues. The ethmoid cribriform plate, through which the olfactory fibers enter the skull, represents the most fragile portion of the neurocranium and is shattered in basal skull fractures. A frequent complication of basilar skull fractures is leakage of CSF from the nose (rhinorrhea) or ear (otorrhea); this occurs because of the proximity of the base of the skull to the nose and ears. This break in protection of the brain becomes a probable source of infection of the meninges or of brain substance. There may be subconjunctival hemorrhage of the eye or periorbital ecchymosis. Skull fractures can damage the cranial nerves (I, II, III, VII, and VIII) as they exit the cranial vault.

Primary and Secondary Brain Injuries

The effects of traumatic head injuries can be divided into two categories:

1. Primary injuries, in which damage is caused by impact
2. Secondary injuries, in which damage results from the subsequent brain swelling, infection, or cerebral hypoxia

The primary brain injuries include focal (*e.g.*, contusion, laceration, hemorrhage) and diffuse (*e.g.*, concussion, diffuse axonal injury) injuries. Secondary brain injuries are often diffuse or multifocal, including edema, infection, and hypoxic brain damage. Although the skull and CSF provide protection for the brain, they also can contribute to trauma. When the mechanical forces inducing brain injury cause bouncing of the brain in the closed confines of the rigid skull, a contusion, coup–contrecoup injury can occur. Because the brain floats freely in the CSF, blunt force to the head accelerates the brain within the skull, and then the brain decelerates abruptly on hitting the inner skull surfaces (Fig. 16.7). The direct contusion of the brain at the site of external force is referred to as a *coup* injury, whereas the rebound injury on the opposite side of the brain is the *contrecoup* injury. As the brain strikes the rough surface of the cranial vault, brain tissue, blood vessels, nerve tracts, and other structures are bruised and torn, resulting in contusions and hematomas.

The most common cause of secondary brain injury is ischemia. It can result from the hypoxia and hypotension that occur during the resuscitation process or from the impairment of regulatory mechanisms by which cerebrovascular responses maintain an adequate blood flow and oxygen supply.[19]

The significance of secondary injuries depends on the extent of damage caused by the primary injury. In mild brain injury, there may be momentary loss of consciousness without noticeable neurologic symptoms or residual damage, except for possible residual amnesia. Microscopic changes usually can be detected in the neurons and glia within hours of injury, but brain imaging is negative. Concussion is a transient neurogenic dysfunction caused by some mechanical force to the brain.[16] Although recovery usually takes place within 24 hours, mild symptoms, such as headache, irritability, insomnia, and poor concentration and memory, may persist for months. This is known as the *postconcussion syndrome*. The memory loss usually includes an interval of time preceding the accident (retrograde amnesia) and after the injury (anterograde amnesia). The duration of retrograde amnesia correlates with the severity of the brain injury. Because these cognitive complaints are vague and subjective, they sometimes are regarded as being of psychological origin. Postconcussion syndrome can have a significant effect on activities of daily living and return to employment. People with postconcussion syndrome may need cognitive retraining, medications, or psychological support.

In moderate brain injury, many small hemorrhages and some swelling of brain tissue occur. These contusions often are distributed along the rough, irregular inner surface of the brain and are more likely to occur in the frontal or temporal lobes, resulting in cognitive and motor deficits. Moderate brain injury is characterized by a period of unconsciousness and may be associated with focal manifestations such as hemiparesis, aphasia, and cranial nerve palsy. In this type of injury, the contusions often can be visualized on CT scan.

Severe brain injury involves extensive primary and secondary injury to brain structures. In severe head injury, the

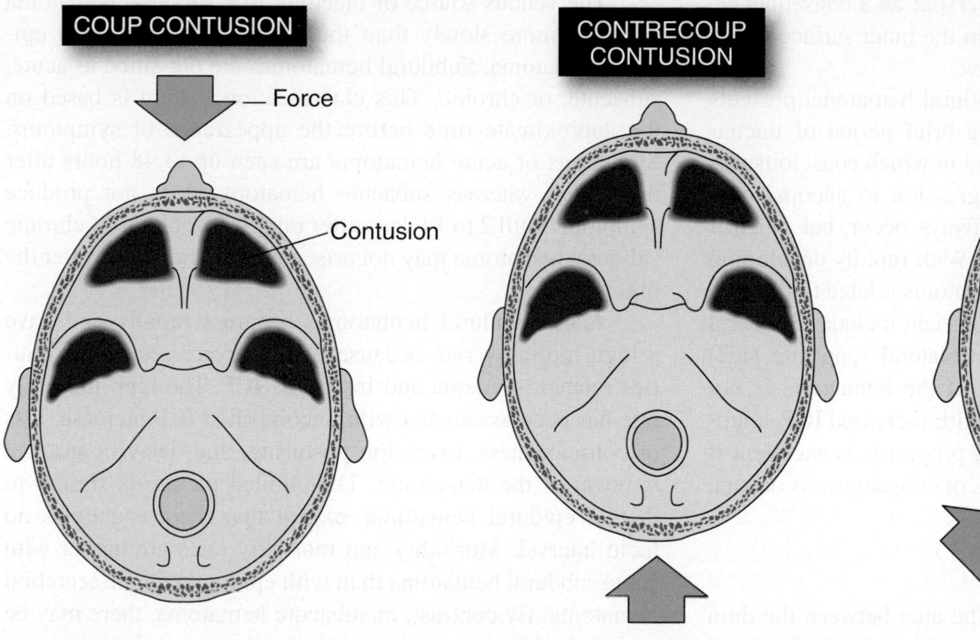

Figure 16.7 • Biomechanics of cerebral contusion. The cerebral hemispheres float in the cerebrospinal fluid. Rapid deceleration or acceleration of the skull causes the cortex to impact forcefully into the anterior and middle fossa. The position of a contusion is determined by the direction of the force and the intracranial anatomy. (From Strayer D. S., Rubin E. (Eds.) (2015). *Rubin's Pathology: Clinicopathologic foundations of medicine* (7th ed., Fig. 32-18, p. 1423). Philadelphia, PA: Wolters Kluwer.)

primary injury is instantaneous and irreversible, resulting from shearing and pressure forces that cause diffuse axonal injury, disruption of blood vessels, and tissue damage. Contusions and intracerebral, subdural, epidural, and SAHs are often evident on CT scan. It often is accompanied by severe neurologic deficits such as coma, hemiplegia, and elevated ICP. Severe brain injuries often occur with injury to other parts of the body such as the neck, extremities, chest, and abdomen.

Hematomas

Hematomas result from vascular injury and bleeding. Depending on the anatomic position of the ruptured vessel, bleeding can occur in any of several compartments, including the epidural, subdural, intracerebral, and subarachnoid spaces.

Epidural Hematoma

Epidural hematomas usually are caused by head injury in which the temporal area of the skull is fractured. An epidural hematoma is one that develops between the inner table of the bones of the skull and the dura (Fig. 16.8). It usually results from a tear in an artery, most often the middle meningeal, usually in association with a skull fracture.[8] Because bleeding is arterial in origin, rapid expansion of the hematoma compresses the brain. Epidural hematoma is more common in a young person because the dura is less firmly attached to

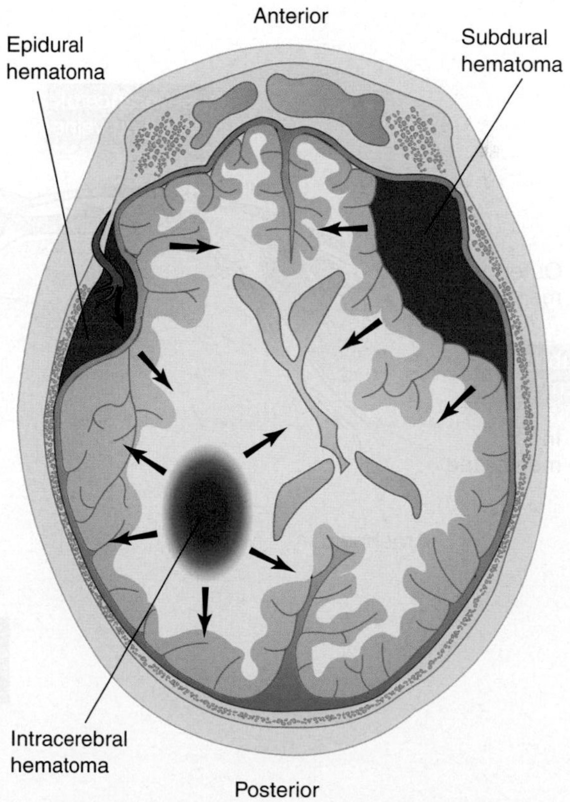

Figure 16.8 • Location of epidural, subdural, and intracerebral hematomas.

the skull surface than in an older person; as a consequence, the dura can be easily separated from the inner surface of the skull, allowing the hematoma to grow.

Typically, a person with an epidural hematoma presents with a history of head injury and a brief period of unconsciousness followed by a lucid period in which consciousness is regained, followed by rapid progression to unconsciousness. The lucid interval does not always occur, but when it does, it is of great diagnostic value. With rapidly developing unconsciousness, there are focal symptoms related to the area of the brain involved. These symptoms can include ipsilateral (same side) pupil dilation and contralateral (opposite side) hemiparesis from uncal herniation. If the hematoma is not removed, the condition progresses, with increased ICP, tentorial herniation, and death. However, prognosis is excellent if the hematoma is removed before loss of consciousness occurs.

Subdural Hematoma

A subdural hematoma develops in the area between the dura and the arachnoid (subdural space) and usually is the result of a tear in the small bridging veins that connect veins on the surface of the cortex to dural sinuses. The bridging veins pass from the pial vessels through the CSF-filled subarachnoid space, penetrate the arachnoid and the dura, and empty into the intradural sinuses.[11] These veins are readily snapped in head injury when the brain moves suddenly in relation to the skull (Fig. 16.9).

The venous source of bleeding in a subdural hematoma develops more slowly than the arterial bleeding in an epidural hematoma. Subdural hematomas are classified as acute, subacute, or chronic. This classification system is based on the approximate time before the appearance of symptoms. Symptoms of acute hematoma are seen up to 48 hours after the injury, whereas subacute hematoma does not produce symptoms until 2 to 14 days after injury. Symptoms of chronic subdural hematoma may not arise until several weeks after the injury.

Acute subdural hematomas progress rapidly and have a high mortality rate because of the severe secondary injuries related to edema and increased ICP. The high mortality rate has been associated with uncontrolled ICP increase, loss of consciousness, extension posturing, and delay in surgical removal of the hematoma. The clinical picture is similar to that of epidural hematoma, except that there usually is no lucid interval. Morbidity and mortality rates are higher with acute subdural hematoma than with epidural and intracerebral hematoma. By contrast, in subacute hematoma, there may be a period of improvement in the level of consciousness and neurologic symptoms, only to be followed by deterioration if the hematoma is not removed.

Symptoms of chronic subdural hematoma develop weeks after a head injury, so much later that the person may not remember having had a head injury. Chronic subdural hematoma is more common in alcoholics and older adults because brain atrophy causes the brain to shrink away from the dura

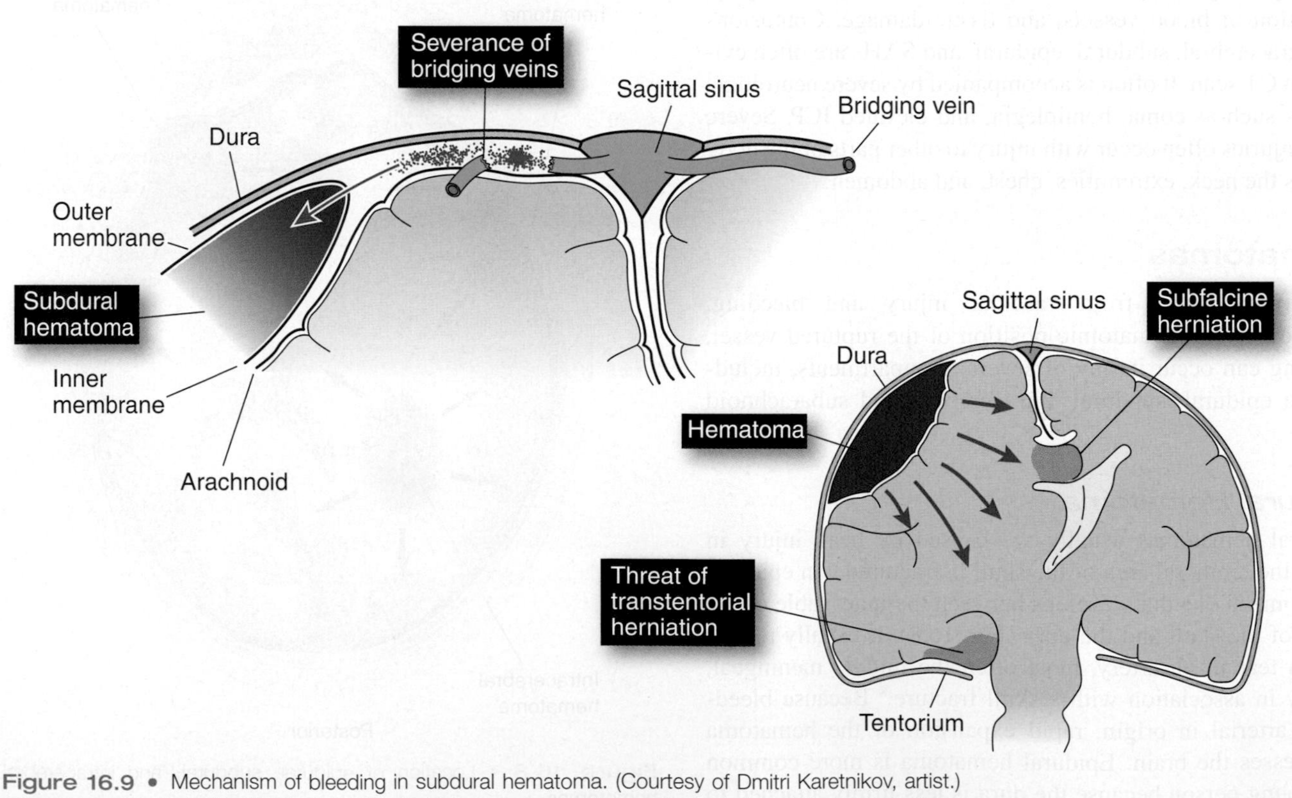

Figure 16.9 • Mechanism of bleeding in subdural hematoma. (Courtesy of Dmitri Karetnikov, artist.) (From Strayer D. S., Rubin E. (Eds.) (2015). *Rubin's pathology: Clinicopathologic foundations of medicine* (7th ed., p. 1463). Philadelphia, PA: Wolters Kluwer.)

and stretch fragile bridging veins. These veins rupture, causing slow seepage of blood into the subdural space. Fibroblastic activity causes the hematoma to become encapsulated. The sanguineous fluid in this encapsulated area has high osmotic pressure and draws in fluid from the surrounding subarachnoid space; the mass expands, exerting pressure on the cranial contents. In some instances, the clinical picture is less defined, with the most prominent symptom being a decreasing level of consciousness indicated by drowsiness, confusion, headache, and apathy.

Traumatic Intracerebral Hematomas

Traumatic intracerebral hematomas may be single or multiple. They can occur in any lobe of the brain but are most common in the frontal or temporal lobes, related to the bony prominences on the inner skull surface (Fig. 16.10). They may occur in association with the severe motion that the brain undergoes during head injury, or a contusion can coalesce into a hematoma. Intracerebral hematomas occur more frequently in older adults and alcoholics, whose cerebral vessels are more friable.

The signs and symptoms produced by an intracerebral hematoma depend on its size and location in the brain. Signs of increased ICP can be manifested if the hematoma is large and encroaching on vital structures. A hematoma in the temporal lobe can be dangerous because of the potential for lateral herniation.

Treatment of an intracerebral hematoma can be medical or surgical. For a large hematoma with a rapidly deteriorating neurologic condition, surgery to evacuate the clot usually is indicated. Surgery may not be needed in someone who is neurologically stable despite neurologic deficits; in this case, the hematoma may resolve much like a contusion.

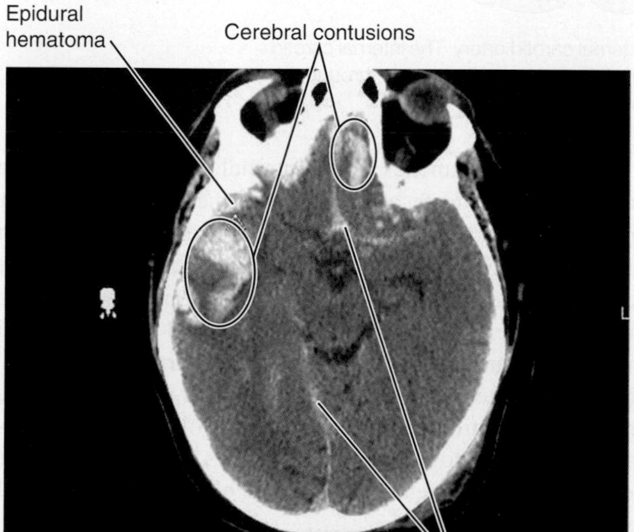

Figure 16.10 • CT scan of the brain in TBI, showing hemorrhagic cerebral contusions in right temporal and bifrontal lobes, SAH, and epidural hematoma.

IN SUMMARY

The effects of traumatic brain injuries can be divided into two categories: primary and secondary injuries. Primary injuries result from direct impact, resulting in skull fracture, concussion, or contusion. In secondary injuries, damage results from the subsequent brain swelling; epidural, subdural, or intracerebral hematoma formation; infection; cerebral hypoxia; and ischemia. Even if there is no break in the skull, a blow to the head can cause severe and diffuse brain damage. Such closed injuries vary in severity and can be classified as focal or diffuse. Diffuse injuries include concussion and diffuse axonal injury. Focal injuries include contusion, laceration, and hemorrhage.

CEREBROVASCULAR DISEASE

After completing this section of the chapter, the learner will be able to meet the following objectives:

- Identify the major vessels in the cerebral circulation.
- Describe the autoregulation of cerebral blood flow.
- Summarize the pathologies of ischemic and hemorrhagic stroke.

Cerebrovascular disease encompasses a number of disorders involving vessels in the cerebral circulation. These disorders include transient ischemic attacks (TIAs) and stroke result in disruption of the cerebral circulation.

Cerebral Circulation

Cerebral Blood Vessels

The blood flow to the brain is supplied by the two internal carotid arteries anteriorly and the vertebral arteries posteriorly (Fig. 16.11A). The internal carotid artery, a terminal branch of the common carotid artery, branches into several arteries: ophthalmic, posterior communicating, anterior choroidal, anterior cerebral, and middle cerebral (see Fig. 16.11B). Most of the arterial blood in the internal carotid arteries is distributed through the anterior and middle cerebral arteries. The anterior cerebral arteries supply the medial surface of the frontal and parietal lobes and the anterior half of the thalamus, the corpus striatum, part of the corpus callosum, and the anterior limb of the internal capsule. The genu and posterior limb of the internal capsule and medial globus pallidus are fed by the anterior choroidal branch of the internal carotid artery. The middle cerebral artery passes laterally, supplying the lateral basal ganglia and the insula, and then emerges on the lateral cortical surface, supplying the inferior frontal gyrus, the motor and premotor frontal cortex concerned with delicate face and hand control. It is the major vascular source for the language cortices (frontal and superior temporal), the primary and association auditory cortex (superior temporal gyrus), and the primary and association somatosensory cortex for the face and hand (postcentral gyrus,

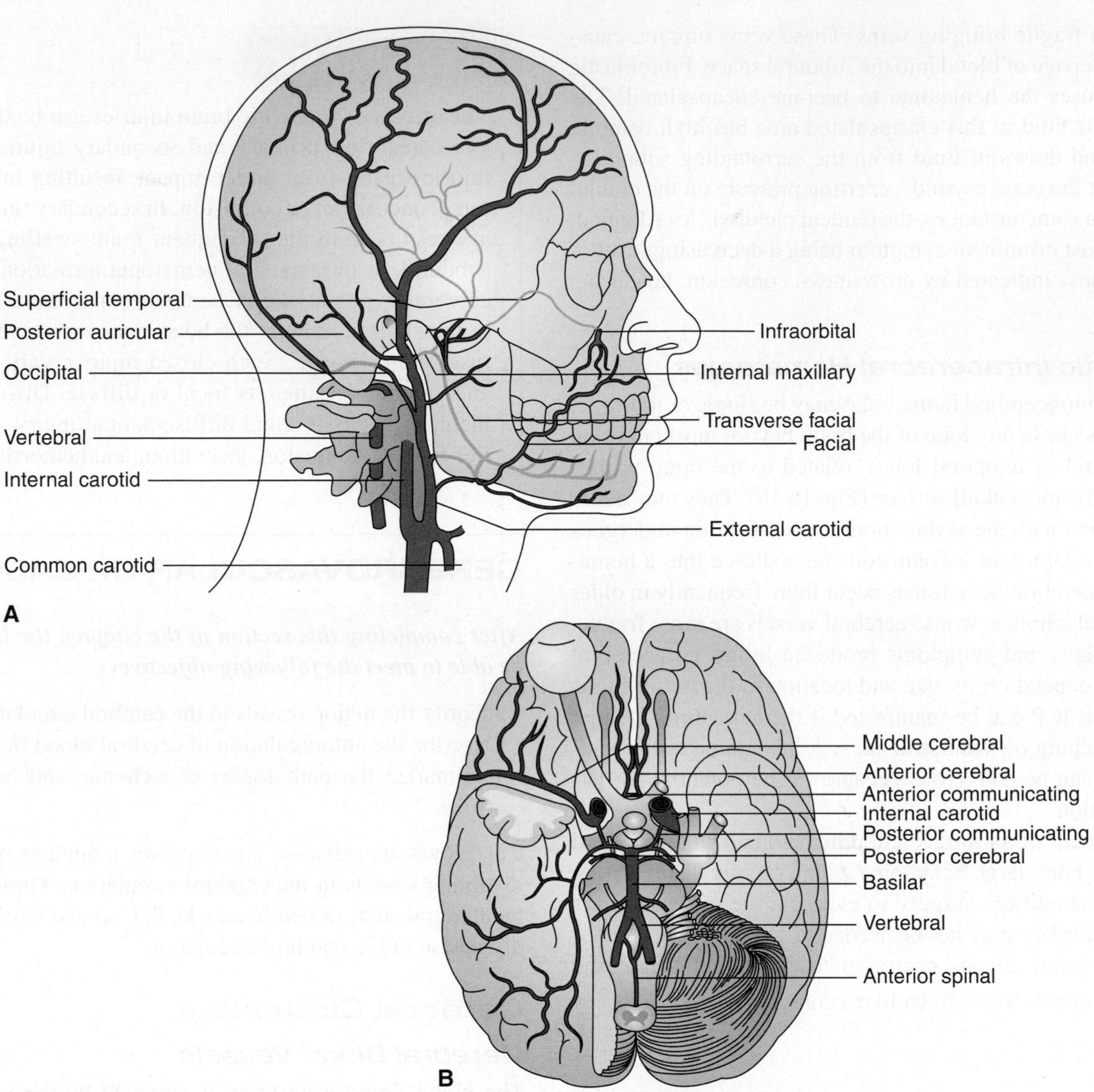

Figure 16.11 • Cerebral circulation. **(A)** Branches of the right external carotid artery. The internal carotid artery ascends to the base of the brain. The right vertebral artery is also shown as it ascends through the transverse foramen of the cervical vertebrae. **(B)** The cerebral arterial circle (circle of Willis).

parietal). The middle cerebral artery is functionally a continuation of the internal carotid; emboli of the internal carotid most frequently become lodged in branches of the middle cerebral artery. The consequences of ischemia of these areas may be the most devastating, resulting in damage to the fine manipulative skills of the face and upper limbs and to receptive and expressive communication functions (*e.g.*, aphasia).

The two vertebral arteries arise from the subclavian artery and enter the foramina in the transverse spinal processes at the level of the sixth cervical vertebra and continue upward through the foramina of the upper six vertebrae; they wind behind the atlas and enter the skull through the foramen magnum and unite to form the basilar artery, which then diverges to terminate in the posterior cerebral arteries. Branches of the basilar and vertebral arteries supply the medulla, pons, cerebellum, midbrain, and caudal part of the diencephalon. The posterior cerebral arteries supply the remaining occipital and inferior regions of the temporal lobes and the thalamus.

The distal branches of the internal carotid and vertebral arteries communicate at the base of the brain through the circle of Willis; this anastomosis of arteries can provide continued circulation if blood flow through one of the main vessels is disrupted (see Fig. 16.11B). For instance, occlusion of one middle cerebral artery may have limited consequences if the anterior and posterior communicating arteries are patent, allowing collateral flow from the ipsilateral posterior cerebral and opposite carotid arteries. Without collateral input, cessation of blood flow in cerebral arteries results in ischemic neural damage as metabolic needs of electrically active cells exceed nutrient supply.

The cerebral circulation is drained by two sets of veins that empty into the dural venous sinuses: the deep (great) cerebral venous system and the superficial venous system. In contrast to the superficial cerebral veins that travel through the pia mater on the surface of the cerebral cortex, the deep system is well protected. These vessels connect directly to the sagittal sinuses in the falx cerebri by bridging veins. They travel through the CSF-filled subarachnoid space and penetrate the arachnoid and then the dura to reach the dural venous sinuses. This system of sinuses returns blood to the heart primarily through the internal jugular veins. Alternate routes for venous flow also exist; for example, venous blood may exit through the emissary veins that pass through the skull and through veins that traverse various foramina to empty into extracranial veins.

The intracranial venous system has no valves. The direction of flow depends on gravity or the relative pressure in the venous sinuses compared with that of the extracranial veins. Increases in intrathoracic pressure, as can occur with coughing or performance of the Valsalva maneuver (*i.e.*, exhaling against a closed glottis), produce a rise in central venous pressure that is reflected back into the internal jugular veins and to the dural sinuses.

Regulation of Cerebral Blood Flow

The blood flow to the brain is maintained at approximately 750 mL/minute or one sixth of the resting cardiac output.[17] The regulation of blood flow to the brain is controlled largely by autoregulatory or local mechanisms that respond to the metabolic needs of the brain. Cerebral autoregulation has been classically defined as the ability of the brain to maintain constant cerebral blood flow despite changes in systemic arterial pressure. This allows the cerebral cortex to adjust cerebral blood flow locally to satisfy its metabolic needs. The autoregulation of cerebral blood flow is efficient within an MAP range of approximately 60 to 140 mm Hg.[17] Although total cerebral blood flow remains relatively stable throughout marked changes in cardiac output and arterial blood pressure, regional blood flow may vary markedly in response to local changes in metabolism. If blood pressure falls below 60 mm Hg, cerebral blood flow becomes severely compromised, and if it rises above the upper limit of autoregulation, blood flow increases rapidly and overstretches the cerebral vessels. In people with hypertension, this autoregulatory range shifts to higher MAP levels.

At least three metabolic factors affect cerebral blood flow: carbon dioxide, hydrogen ion, and oxygen concentration. Increased carbon dioxide provides a potent stimulus for vasodilation—a doubling of the PCO_2 in the blood results in a doubling of cerebral blood flow. Increased hydrogen ion concentrations also increase cerebral blood flow, serving to wash away the neurally depressive acidic materials.[17] Profound extracellular acidosis induces vasomotor paralysis, in which case cerebral blood flow may depend entirely on the systemic arterial blood pressure. Decreased oxygen concentration also increases cerebral blood flow.

Concept Mastery Alert

Decreased oxygen saturation increases cerebral blood flow, as does an increased carbon dioxide level. Both of these factors result in less oxygen for the cells of the brain. The body attempts to compensate by increasing blood flow to the area.

The deep cerebral blood vessels appear to be completely controlled by autoregulation. However, the superficial and major cerebral blood vessels are innervated by the sympathetic nervous system. Under normal physiologic conditions, local regulatory and autoregulatory mechanisms override the effects of sympathetic stimulation. However, when local mechanisms fail, sympathetic control of cerebral blood pressure becomes important.[17] For example, when the arterial pressure rises to very high levels during strenuous exercise or in other conditions, the sympathetic nervous system constricts the large and intermediate-sized superficial blood vessels as a means of protecting the smaller, more easily damaged vessels. Sympathetic reflexes are believed to cause vasospasm in the intermediate and large arteries in some types of brain damage, such as that caused by rupture of a cerebral aneurysm.

Stroke

Stroke is the syndrome of acute focal neurologic deficit from a vascular disorder that injures brain tissue. Stroke remains one of the leading causes of mortality and morbidity in the United States. Each year, 795,000 Americans are afflicted with stroke; many survivors are left with at least some degree of neurologic impairment.[20] There are two main types of strokes: ischemic and hemorrhagic. Ischemic strokes are caused by an interruption of blood flow in a cerebral vessel and are the most common type of stroke, accounting for 87% of all strokes.[20] Hemorrhagic strokes account for 13% of all strokes, 10% intracerebral hemorrhage, and 3% SAH.[20] A hemorrhagic stroke usually is from a blood vessel rupture caused by hypertension, aneurysm, or arteriovenous malformation and has a much higher fatality rate than ischemic strokes.

Etiology

The risk factors for stroke are age, sex, race, prior stroke, family history, hypertension, smoking, diabetes mellitus, cardiac disease, hypercholesteremia, and hypercoagulopathy.[21] The incidence of stroke increases with age, with men's stroke incidence rates being greater than female rates at younger ages, but not at older ages. Because females live longer than men, more females die of stroke each year. Blacks and some Hispanic/Latino Americans have a higher incidence of all stroke types and higher mortality rates compared with Whites.[21] Blood pressure is a powerful determinant of stroke risk. The higher the blood pressure, the greater the risk of stroke.[21] Heart disease, particularly atrial fibrillation and other conditions that predispose to clot formation on the wall of the heart or valve leaflets or to paradoxical embolism through right-to-left shunting, predisposes to cardioembolic stroke. Polycythemia, sickle cell disease (during sickle cell crisis), and blood disorders predispose to clot formation in the cerebral vessels.

Other, modifiable behavioral risk factors include obesity, physical inactivity, alcohol, illicit drug use, hypercoagulability disorders, hormone replacement therapy, and oral contraceptive use.[21] An increased risk of stroke is associated with hormone replacement therapy.[21] Light to moderate consumption of alcohol is associated with reduced risk of stroke, but heavier consumption of alcohol increases risk of stroke.[21] Several drugs of abuse, cocaine, amphetamines, and heroin, are associated with stroke.[21,22]

Elimination or control of risk factors for stroke (*e.g.*, use of tobacco, control of blood lipids and blood sugar, reduction of hypertension) offers the best opportunity to prevent cerebral ischemia from cerebral atherosclerosis. Primary prevention of stroke by early detection and treatment of modifiable risk factors offers significant advantages over waiting until a serious event has occurred.

Ischemic Stroke

Ischemic strokes are caused by cerebrovascular obstruction by thrombosis or emboli (Fig. 16.12). Ischemic stroke can be classified into five main mechanisms of stroke subtypes and their frequency: 20% large artery thrombosis (atherosclerotic disease), 25% small penetrating artery thrombosis disease (lacunar stroke), 20% cardiogenic embolism, 30% cryptogenic stroke (undetermined cause), and 5% other.[2]

Ischemic Penumbra in Evolving Stroke. During the evolution of a stroke, there usually is a central core of dead or dying cells, surrounded by an ischemic band or area of minimally perfused cells called the *penumbra* (border zone). Brain cells of the penumbra receive marginal blood flow, their metabolic activities are impaired, but the structural integrity of the brain cells is maintained.[15] Whether the cells of the penumbra continue to survive depends on the successful timely return of adequate circulation, the volume of toxic products released by the neighboring dying cells, the degree of cerebral edema, and alterations in local blood flow. If the toxic products result in additional death of cells in the penumbra, the border zone of dead or dying tissue enlarges, and the volume of surrounding ischemic tissue increases.

Transient Ischemic Attacks. TIAs are a transient episode of neurologic dysfunction caused by focal brain, spinal cord, or retinal ischemia, without acute infarction.[23] A TIA reflects a temporary disturbance in focal cerebral blood flow, which reverses before infarction occurs. The causes of TIAs are the same as those of ischemic stroke and include atherosclerotic disease of cerebral vessels and emboli. TIAs are important because they may provide warning of impending stroke. There is a higher risk of early stroke after TIA, 10% to 15% have a stroke within 3 months, with 50% occurring in 48 hours.[23] Diagnosis of TIA before a stroke may permit surgical or medical intervention that prevents an eventual stroke and the associated neurologic deficits.

Thrombotic Stroke. Thrombi are the most common cause of ischemic strokes, usually occurring in atherosclerotic blood vessels. In the cerebral circulation, atherosclerotic plaques are found most commonly at arterial bifurcations. Common sites of plaque formation include larger vessels of the brain, notably the origins of the internal carotid and vertebral arteries, and junctions of the basilar and vertebral arteries. Cerebral infarction can result from an acute local thrombosis and occlusion at the site of chronic atherosclerosis, with or without embolization of the plaque material distally, or from critical perfusion

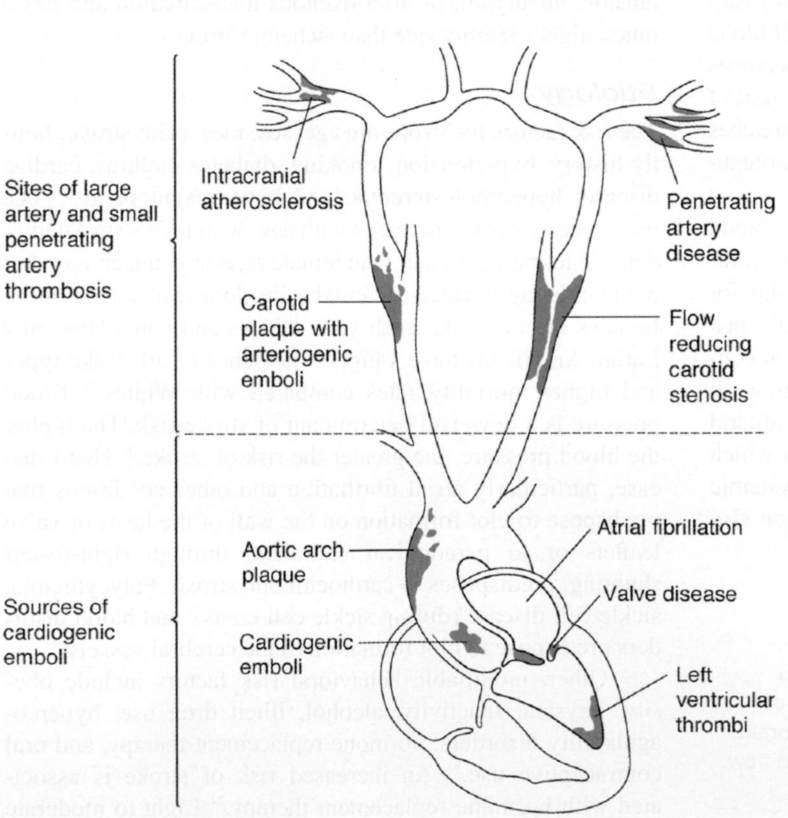

Figure 16.12 • The most frequent sites of arterial and cardiac abnormalities causing ischemic stroke. (From Hickey J. V. (2014). *The clinical practice of neurological and neurosurgical nursing* (7th ed., p. 531). Philadelphia, PA: Lippincott Williams & Wilkins.)

failure distal to a stenosis (watershed). These infarcts often affect the cortex, causing aphasia or neglect, visual field defects, or transient monocular blindness (amaurosis fugax). In most cases of stroke, a single cerebral artery and its territories are affected. Usually, thrombotic strokes are seen in older people and frequently are accompanied by evidence of atherosclerotic heart or peripheral arterial disease.

Lacunar Stroke. Lacunar infarcts are small (1.5- to 2-cm) to very small (3- to 4-mm) infarcts located in the deeper, noncortical parts of the brain or in the brain stem. They are found in the territory of single deep penetrating arteries supplying the internal capsule, basal ganglia, or brain stem. They result from occlusion of the smaller penetrating branches of large cerebral arteries, commonly the middle cerebral and posterior cerebral arteries. In the process of healing, lacunar infarcts leave behind small cavities, or *lacunae* (*lakes*). They are thought to result from arteriolar lipohyalinosis or microatheroma, commonly in the settings of chronic hypertension or diabetes. Six basic causes of lacunar infarcts have been proposed: embolism, hypertension, small-vessel occlusive disease, hematologic abnormalities, small intracerebral hemorrhages, and vasospasm. Because of their size and location, lacunar infarcts usually do not cause cortical deficits like aphasia or apraxia. Instead, they produce classic recognizable *lacunar syndromes* such as pure motor hemiplegia, pure sensory hemiplegia, and dysarthria with the clumsy hand syndrome. CT or MRI may show several lacunae as well as diffuse white matter changes associated with dementia.

Embolic Stroke. An embolic stroke is caused by a moving blood clot that travels from its origin to the brain. It usually affects the larger proximal cerebral vessels, often lodging at bifurcations. The most frequent site of embolic strokes is the middle cerebral artery, reflecting the large territory of this vessel and its position as the terminus of the carotid artery. Although most cerebral emboli originate from a thrombus in the left heart, they also may originate in an atherosclerotic plaque in the carotid arteries. The embolus travels quickly to the brain and becomes lodged in a smaller artery through which it cannot pass. Embolic stroke usually has a sudden onset with immediate maximum deficit.

Various cardiac conditions predispose to formation of emboli that produce embolic stroke, including rheumatic heart disease, atrial fibrillation, recent myocardial infarction, ventricular aneurysm, mobile aortic arch atheroma, and bacterial endocarditis. The use of transesophageal echocardiography has implicated a patent foramen ovale as a source for paradoxical venous emboli to the arterial system.

Hemorrhagic Stroke

The most frequently fatal stroke results from the spontaneous rupture of a cerebral blood vessel.[24–26] The resulting intracerebral hemorrhage can cause a focal hematoma, edema, compression of the brain contents, or spasm of the adjacent blood vessels. The most common predisposing factors are advancing age and hypertension. Aneurysms and arteriovenous malformations are structural abnormalities that can also cause sudden hemorrhage. A cerebral hemorrhage occurs suddenly, usually when the person is active. Vomiting commonly occurs at the onset, and headache often occurs. Focal symptoms depend on which vessel is involved. In the most common situation, hemorrhage into the basal ganglia results in contralateral hemiplegia, with initial flaccidity progressing to spasticity. The hemorrhage and resultant edema exert great pressure on the brain substance, and the clinical course progresses rapidly to coma and frequently to death.

Aneurysmal Subarachnoid Hemorrhage. Aneurysmal SAH is a type of hemorrhagic stroke caused by the rupture of a cerebral aneurysm, and the resulting bleeding into the subarachnoid space can extend well beyond the site of origin, flooding the basal cistern, ventricles, and spinal subarachnoid space.[8,11,27] An aneurysm is a bulge at the site of a localized weakness in the muscular wall of an arterial vessel. Most cerebral aneurysms are small saccular aneurysms called *berry aneurysms.* They usually occur in the anterior circulation and are found at bifurcations and other junctions of vessels such as those in the circle of Willis (Fig. 16.13). They are thought to arise from a congenital defect in the media of the involved vessels. Their incidence is higher in people with certain disorders, including polycystic kidney disease, fibromuscular dysplasia, coarctation of the aorta, and arteriovenous malformations of the brain.[8,11] Other causes of cerebral aneurysms are atherosclerosis, hypertension, and bacterial infections.

Rupture of a cerebral aneurysm results in SAH. The probability of rupture increases with the size of the aneurysm, more likely in those bigger than 3 to 5 mm.[27] Of the various environmental factors that may predispose to aneurysmal SAH, cigarette smoking, hypertension, and excessive alcohol intake appear to constitute the greatest threat.[27,28] Intracranial aneurysms are rare in children, and the mean age for SAH is approximately 50 years. The mortality and morbidity rates

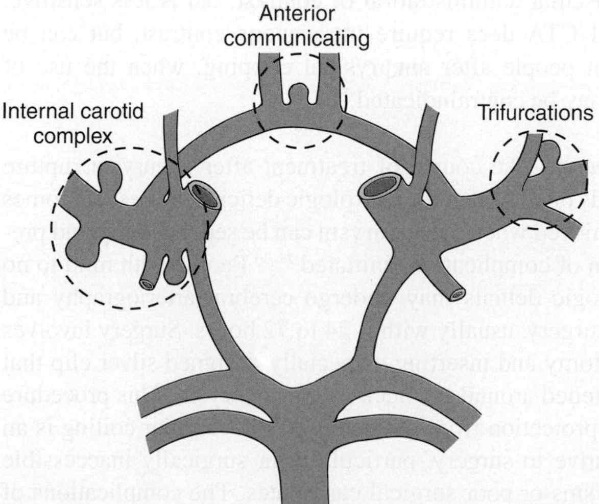

Figure 16.13 • Common sites of berry aneurysms.

with aneurysmal SAH are high, with only one third of people recovering without major disability.[28]

Clinical Manifestations. The signs and symptoms of cerebral aneurysms can be divided into two phases: those presenting before rupture and bleeding and those presenting after rupture and bleeding. Most small aneurysms are asymptomatic. Intact aneurysms frequently are found at autopsy as an incidental finding.[8] Approximately 10% to 20% of people with SAH have a history of atypical headaches occurring days to weeks before the onset of hemorrhage, suggesting the presence of a small leak.[27,28] These headaches are characterized by sudden onset and often are accompanied by nausea, vomiting, and dizziness. The onset of subarachnoid aneurysmal rupture often is heralded by a sudden and severe headache, described as *the worst headache of my life*.[27,28] If the bleeding is severe, the headache may be accompanied by collapse and loss of consciousness. Vomiting may accompany the presenting symptoms. Other manifestations include signs of meningeal irritation such as nuchal rigidity (neck stiffness) and photophobia (light intolerance); cranial nerve deficits, especially cranial nerve II, and sometimes III and IV (diplopia and blurred vision); stroke syndromes (focal motor and sensory deficits); cerebral edema and increased ICP; and pituitary dysfunction (diabetes insipidus and hyponatremia). Hypertension, a frequent finding, and cardiac arrhythmias result from massive release of catecholamines triggered by the SAH.

Diagnosis. The diagnosis of SAH and intracranial aneurysms is made by clinical presentation, noncontrast CT scan, lumbar puncture if CT is normal and suspicion of SAH is strong, and angiography.[27,28] To identify the aneurysm at the source of bleeding, conventional angiography, magnetic resonance angiography (MRA), and helical (spiral) computed tomography angiography (CTA) are used. Conventional catheter angiography is the definitive diagnostic tool for detecting the aneurysm. MRA is noninvasive and does not require the intravascular administration of contrast, but is less sensitive. Helical CTA does require intravenous contrast, but can be used in people after aneurysmal clipping, when the use of MRI may be contraindicated.

Treatment. The course of treatment after aneurysm rupture depends on the extent of neurologic deficit. The best outcomes are achieved when the aneurysm can be secured early and prevention of complications initiated.[28–30] People with mild to no neurologic deficits may undergo cerebral arteriography and early surgery, usually within 24 to 72 hours. Surgery involves craniotomy and inserting a specially designed silver clip that is tightened around the neck of the aneurysm. This procedure offers protection from rebleeding. Endovascular coiling is an alternative to surgery, particularly in surgically inaccessible aneurysms or poor surgical candidates. The complications of aneurysmal rupture include rebleeding, vasospasm with cerebral ischemia, hydrocephalus, hypothalamic dysfunction, and seizure activity. Rebleeding and vasospasm are the most serious and most difficult to treat. Rebleeding, which has its highest incidence on the first day after the initial rupture, results in further and usually catastrophic neurologic deficits.

Vasospasm is a dreaded complication of aneurysmal rupture. The condition is difficult to treat and is associated with a high incidence of morbidity and mortality. Although the description of aneurysm-associated vasospasm is relatively uniform, its proposed mechanisms are controversial. Usually, the condition develops within 3 to 10 days (peak, 7 days) after aneurysm rupture and involves a focal narrowing of the cerebral artery or arteries that can be visualized on arteriography or by transcranial Doppler. The neurologic status gradually deteriorates as blood supply to the brain in the region of the spasm is decreased; this usually can be differentiated from the rapid deterioration seen in rebleeding. Vasospasm is treated by attempting to improve CPP through the use of vasoactive drugs or administration of intravenous fluids to achieve euvolemia. Endovascular techniques include intra-arterial vasodilators and mechanical dilation of vessels with balloon angioplasty. Nimodipine, a drug that blocks calcium channels and selectively acts on cerebral blood vessels, may be used to reduce the incidence and severity of delayed ischemic deficits from vasospasm following aneurysmal rupture.

Another complication of aneurysm rupture is the development of hydrocephalus. It is caused by plugging of the arachnoid villi with products from lysis of blood in the subarachnoid space. Hydrocephalus is diagnosed by serial CT scans showing increasing size of the ventricles and by the clinical signs of increased ICP. Ventriculostomy, lumbar drain, or ventricular-peritoneal shunt may be used to treat hydrocephalus to decrease the increased ICP.

Arteriovenous Malformations. Arteriovenous malformations are a complex tangle of abnormal arteries and veins linked by one or more fistulas.[2] These vascular networks lack a capillary bed, and the small arteries have a deficient muscularis layer. Arteriovenous malformations are thought to arise from failure in development of the capillary network in the embryonic brain. As the child's brain grows, the malformation acquires additional arterial contributions that enlarge to form a tangled collection of thin-walled vessels that shunt blood directly from the arterial to the venous circulation. Arteriovenous malformations typically present before 40 years of age and affect men and women equally. Rupture of vessels in the malformation causing hemorrhagic stroke accounts for approximately 1% of all strokes.[2]

Pathophysiology. The hemodynamic effects of arteriovenous malformations are twofold. First, blood is shunted from the high-pressure arterial system to the low-pressure venous system without the buffering advantage of the capillary network. The draining venous channels are exposed to high levels of pressure, predisposing them to rupture and hemorrhage. Second, the elevated arterial and venous pressures divert blood away from the surrounding tissue, impairing tissue perfusion.

Clinical Manifestations. Clinically, this is evidenced by slowly progressive neurologic deficits. The major clinical manifestations of arteriovenous malformations are intracerebral and SAH, seizures, headache, and progressive neurologic deficits. Headaches often are severe, and people with the disorder may describe them as throbbing and synchronous with their heartbeat. Other, focal symptoms depend on the location of the lesion and include visual symptoms (*i.e.*, diplopia and hemianopia), hemiparesis, mental deterioration, and speech deficits.

Diagnosis and Treatment. Definitive diagnosis often is obtained through cerebral angiography. Treatment methods include surgical excision, endovascular occlusion, radiosurgery, and conservative treatment.[2] Because of the nature of the malformation, each of these methods is accompanied by some risk for complications. If the arteriovenous malformation is accessible, surgical excision usually is the treatment of choice. Endovascular treatment involves the insertion of microcatheters into the cerebral circulation for delivery of embolic materials (*e.g.*, microballoons, sclerosing agents, microcoils, or quick drying glue) into the arteriovenous malformation vessels.[2] Radiosurgery may involve the use of a Gamma Knife, proton beam, or linear accelerator.

Clinical Manifestations of Stroke

The specific manifestations of stroke or TIA are determined by the cerebral artery that is affected, by the area of brain tissue that is supplied by that vessel, and by the adequacy of the collateral circulation. Symptoms of stroke/TIA always are sudden in onset and focal and usually are one sided. The most common symptoms are a facial droop, arm weakness, and slurred speech. Other frequent stroke symptoms are unilateral numbness, vision loss in one eye (amaurosis fugax) or to one side (hemianopia), language disturbance (aphasia), and sudden, unexplained imbalance or ataxia. In the event of TIA, symptoms rapidly resolve spontaneously, usually within minutes, although the underlying mechanisms are the same as for stroke. The specific stroke signs depend on the specific vascular territory compromised (Table 16.6). As a generalization, carotid ischemia causes monocular visual loss or aphasia (dominant hemisphere) or hemineglect (nondominant hemisphere), contralateral sensory or motor loss, or other discrete cortical signs such as apraxia and agnosia. Vertebrobasilar ischemia induces ataxia, diplopia, hemianopia, vertigo, cranial nerve deficits, contralateral hemiplegia, sensory deficits (either contralateral or crossed, *i.e.*, contralateral body and ipsilateral face), and arousal defects. Discrete subsets of these vascular syndromes usually occur, depending on which branches of the involved artery are blocked.

Stroke-Related Motor Deficits. Motor deficits are most common, followed by deficits of language, sensation, and cognition. After a stroke affecting the corticospinal tract such as the motor cortex, posterior limb of the internal capsule, basis pontis, or medullary pyramids, there is profound weakness on the contralateral side. Involvement at the level of the motor cortex is most often in the territory of the middle

TABLE 16.6 SIGNS AND SYMPTOMS OF STROKE BY INVOLVED CEREBRAL ARTERY

CEREBRAL ARTERY	BRAIN AREA INVOLVED	SIGNS AND SYMPTOMS*
Anterior cerebral	Infarction of the medial aspect of one frontal lobe if lesion is distal to communicating artery; bilateral frontal infarction if flow in other anterior cerebral artery is inadequate	Paralysis of contralateral foot or leg; impaired gait; paresis of contralateral arm; contralateral sensory loss over toes, foot, and leg; problems making decisions or performing acts voluntarily; lack of spontaneity, easily distracted; slowness of thought; aphasia depends on the hemisphere involved; urinary incontinence; cognitive and affective disorders
Middle cerebral	Massive infarction of most of lateral hemisphere and deeper structures of the frontal, parietal, and temporal lobes; internal capsule; basal ganglia	Contralateral hemiplegia (face and arm); contralateral sensory impairment; aphasia; homonymous hemianopia; altered consciousness (confusion to coma); inability to turn eyes toward paralyzed side; denial of paralyzed side or limb (hemiattention); possible acalculia, alexia, finger agnosia, and left–right confusion; vasomotor paresis and instability
Posterior cerebral	Occipital lobe; anterior and medial portion of temporal lobe	Homonymous hemianopia and other visual defects such as color blindness, loss of central vision, and visual hallucinations; memory deficits, perseveration (repeated performance of same verbal or motor response)
	Thalamus involvement	Loss of all sensory modalities; spontaneous pain; intentional tremor; mild hemiparesis; aphasia
	Cerebral peduncle involvement	Oculomotor nerve palsy with contralateral hemiplegia
Basilar and vertebral	Cerebellum and brain stem	Visual disturbance such as diplopia, dystaxia, vertigo, dysphagia, dysphonia

*Depend on the hemisphere involved and adequacy of collaterals.

cerebral artery, usually with a sparing of the leg, which is supplied by the anterior cerebral artery. Subcortical lesions of the corticospinal tracts cause equal weakness of the face, arm, and leg. Within 6 to 8 weeks, the initial weakness and flaccidity is replaced by hyperreflexia and spasticity. Spasticity involves an increase in the tone of affected muscles and usually an element of weakness. The flexor muscles usually are more strongly affected in the upper extremities and the extensor muscles more strongly affected in the lower extremities. There is a tendency toward foot drop; outward rotation and circumduction of the leg with gait; flexion at the wrist, elbow, and fingers; lower facial paresis; slurred speech; an upgoing toe to plantar stimulation (Babinski sign); and dependent edema in the affected extremities. A slight corticospinal lesion may be indicated only by clumsiness in carrying out fine coordinated movements rather than obvious weakness. Passive range-of-motion exercises help to maintain joint function and to prevent edema, shoulder subluxation (*i.e.*, incomplete dislocation), and muscle atrophy and may help to re-establish motor patterns. If no voluntary movement or movement on command appears within a few months, significant function usually will not return to that extremity.

Stroke-Related Dysarthria and Aphasia. Dysarthria is a disorder of speech, manifest as the imperfect articulation of speech sounds or changes in voice pitch or quality. It results from a stroke affecting the muscles of the pharynx, palate, tongue, lips, or mouth and does not relate to the content of speech. A person with dysarthria may demonstrate slurred speech while still retaining language ability or may have a concurrent language problem as well. *Aphasia* is a general term that encompasses varying degrees of inability to comprehend, integrate, and express language. Aphasia may be localized to the dominant cerebral cortex or thalamus, usually the left side in 95% of people who are right handed and 70% of people who are left handed. In children, language dominance can readily shift to the unaffected hemisphere, resulting in more transient language deficits after stroke. A stroke in the territory of the middle cerebral artery is the most common aphasia-producing stroke.

Aphasia can be categorized as receptive or expressive, or as fluent or nonfluent. Fluency relates to the ease and spontaneity of conversational speech and is more strictly defined by the rate of speech, with *fluent* denoting many words and *nonfluent* few words. Expressive or nonfluent aphasia is characterized by an inability to easily communicate spontaneously or translate thoughts or ideas into meaningful speech or writing. Speech production is limited, effortful, and halting and often may be poorly articulated because of a concurrent dysarthria. The person may be able, with difficulty, to utter or write two or three words, especially those with an emotional overlay. Comprehension is normal, and the person seems to be fully aware of his or her deficits but is unable to correct them. This often leads to frustration, anger, and depression. Expressive, nonfluent aphasia is associated with lesions of the Broca area at the dominant inferior frontal lobe cortex (areas 44 and 45).

Fluent speech requires little or no effort, is articulate, and is of increased quantity. The term *fluent* refers only to the ease and rate of verbal output and does not relate to the content of speech or the ability of the person to comprehend what is being said. Verbal utterances are often paraphasic, meaning that letters, syllables, or whole words are substituted for the target words. There are three categories of fluent aphasia: Wernicke, anomic, and conductive aphasia. Wernicke aphasia is characterized by an inability to comprehend the speech of others or to comprehend written material. Lesions of the posterior superior temporal or lower parietal lobe (areas 22 and 39) are associated with receptive, fluent aphasia. Anomic aphasia is speech that is nearly normal except for a difficulty with finding singular words. Conductive aphasia is manifest as impaired repetition and speech riddled with letter substitutions, despite good comprehension and fluency. Conductive aphasia (*i.e.*, disconnection syndrome) results from destruction of the fiber system under the insula that connects the Wernicke and Broca areas.

Stroke-Related Cognitive and Other Deficits. Stroke can also cause cognitive, sensory, visual, and behavioral deficits. One distinct cognitive syndrome is that of hemineglect or hemi-inattention. Usually caused by strokes affecting the nondominant (right) hemisphere, hemineglect is the inability to attend to and react to stimuli coming from the contralateral (left) side of space. People may not visually track, orient, or reach to the neglected side. They may neglect to use the limbs on that side, despite normal motor function, and may not shave, wash, or comb that side. Such people are unaware of this deficit, which is another form of their neglect (*anosognosia*). Other cognitive deficits include apraxia (impaired ability to carry out previously learned motor activities despite normal sensory and motor function), agnosia (impaired recognition with normal sensory function), memory loss, behavioral syndromes, and depression. Sensory deficits affect the body contralateral to the lesion and can manifest as numbness, tingling paresthesias, or distorted sensations such as dysesthesia and neuropathic pain. Visual disturbances from stroke are diverse, but most common are hemianopia from a lesion of the optic radiations between the lateral geniculate body and the temporal or occipital lobes, or monocular blindness from occlusion of the ipsilateral central retinal artery, a branch of the internal carotid.

Diagnosis and Treatment of Stroke

Diagnosis. Accurate diagnosis of acute stroke is based on a complete history and neurologic examination. A careful history, including documentation of previous TIAs, the time of onset, the specific focal symptoms (to determine the likely vascular territory), and any coexisting diseases, can help to determine the type of stroke that is involved. The diagnostic evaluation should aim to determine the presence of ischemia or hemorrhage, identify the stroke or TIA mechanism (*i.e.*, large-vessel or small-vessel atherothrombotic, cardioembolic, hemorrhagic, other or cryptogenic), characterize the severity of clinical deficits, and unmask the presence of risk factors.

Brain imaging studies document the brain infarction, whereas vascular imaging reveals the anatomy and pathologic processes of the related blood vessels. CT scans and MRI have become essential brain imaging tools in diagnosing stroke, differentiating cerebral hemorrhage from ischemia, and excluding intracranial lesions that mimic stroke clinically. CT scans are a necessary screening tool in the acute setting for rapid identification of hemorrhage, but are insensitive to ischemia within 24 hours and to any brain stem or small infarcts. MRI is superior for imaging ischemic lesions in all territories and differentiating other nonstroke pathologic processes (*e.g.*, tumors, contusion, infection). MRI techniques such as perfusion- and diffusion-weighted imaging (DWI) can reveal cerebral ischemia immediately after onset and identify areas of potentially reversible damage (*i.e.*, penumbra). MR DWI is used in settings of emergency stroke evaluation to rapidly identify the area and volume of ischemia, identifying candidates for emergency treatments.

Vascular imaging is accomplished with CTA, MRA, catheter-based *conventional* arteriography, and ultrasonography. All except ultrasonography can demonstrate the site of vascular abnormality (intracranial and extracranial) and afford visualization of most intracranial vascular areas. However, each modality has relative strengths and weaknesses. MRA is noninvasive and most widely available, but less sensitive and specific than CTA or catheter angiography. CTA is exquisitely detailed for a noninvasive technique, but is limited in availability and requires iodinated contrast, which is nephrotoxic. Catheter angiography remains the gold standard in sensitivity and allows visualization of dynamic patterns of collateral flow, but is invasive and requires significant contrast doses. CTA and MRA have largely replaced angiography as a screening tool for vascular lesions. Ultrasonographic techniques allow quick bedside assessment of the carotid bifurcation (duplex ultrasonography) or of flow velocities in the cerebral circulation (transcranial Doppler).

Treatment. Salvaging brain tissue, preventing secondary stroke, and minimizing long-term disability are the treatment goals for an acute ischemic stroke. The care of people with stroke has shifted away from the *nearest hospital* to certified *stroke centers*. These are hospitals that have been certified by some external agency, most commonly the state or Joint Commission on Accreditation of Healthcare Organizations, the federal agency overseeing all facilities that care for people with Medicare.[31] Certification establishes that a hospital can manage people who have had stroke with appropriate care throughout the continuum, from emergency treatments, through the inpatient stay, and into the rehabilitation phase. With this advancement, the medical and lay communities together acknowledge that care of the person with stroke requires specialized personnel and resources to minimize the devastating costs to society from stroke, the leading cause of adult disability in the United States.

Stroke care begins with emergency treatments aimed at reversing the evolving ischemic brain injury. The realization that there is a window of opportunity during which ischemic but viable brain tissue can be salvaged has led to the use of reperfusion techniques and neuroprotective strategies in the early treatment of ischemic stroke. Although the results of emergent treatment of hemorrhagic stroke have been less dramatic, continued efforts to reduce disability have been promising. Reperfusion techniques include thrombolytic drugs (administered either intravenously or intra-arterially), catheter-directed mechanical clot disruption, and augmentation of CPP during acute stroke. The use of thrombolytic agents for treatment of stroke was first investigated in the late 1960s, but it was quickly abandoned because of hemorrhagic complications resulting from treatment many hours beyond the time window of penumbral cell viability and because exclusion of people with hemorrhagic stroke was difficult before CT scanning was available. The interest in thrombolytic therapy has increased because of thrombolytic agents and the availability of rapid diagnostic scanning methods that are able to differentiate between ischemic and hemorrhagic stroke.

The first and only agent approved by the U.S. Food and Drug Administration (FDA) for treatment of acute ischemic stroke is tissue plasminogen activator (tPA), which was approved in 1996. A subcommittee of the Stroke Council of the American Heart Association has developed guidelines for the use of tPA for acute stroke.[14] These guidelines recommend that in people with suspected stroke, the diagnosis of hemorrhagic stroke be excluded through the use of CT scanning before administration of thrombolytic therapy, which must be administered within 3 hours of onset of symptoms. The major risk of treatment with thrombolytic agents is ICH. A number of conditions, including therapeutic levels of oral anticoagulant medications, a history of gastrointestinal or urinary tract bleeding in the previous 21 days, prior stroke or head injury within 3 months, major surgery within the past 14 days, and a blood pressure greater than 185/110 mm Hg, are considered contraindications to intravenous thrombolytic therapy.[14] A longer time window for treatment with tPA has been tested formally and should be administered to eligible people who can be treated in the time period of 3 to 4.5 hours after stroke.[32]

Emerging treatments for ischemic stroke are being increasingly used as alternative methods of reperfusion beyond intravenous thrombolysis. Catheter-based methods allow recanalization of a directly visualized cerebral clot with intra-arterial techniques. The interventional specialist might mechanically disrupt the clot, deliver thrombolytic drug intra-arterially at the clot surface, or urgently stent intracranial vessels to restore flow. Generally, although person selection is more stringent for these invasive methods, people can be treated past the 3-hour time window for intravenous tPA. However, these methods require an experienced interventional angiography team and extensive institutional infrastructure and thus remain limited to tertiary care centers. Other experimental treatments include neuroprotection with drugs that limit the calcium cascade (see Fig. 16.4), and treatments like hypothermia that decrease brain metabolic demands in the setting of ischemia are being actively investigated in clinical trials.

Poststroke treatment is aimed at preventing recurrent stroke and medical complications while promoting the fullest possible recovery of function. The risk of stroke recurrence is highest in the first week after stroke or TIA, so the early implementation of antiplatelet agents in most cases, or warfarin (an anticoagulant) in cardioembolic stroke, is imperative. Long-term stroke recurrence is most effectively prevented with aggressive reduction of risk factors, primarily hypertension, diabetes, smoking, and hyperlipidemia. In cases of carotid territory stroke with carotid stenosis, revascularization with surgery or stenting should be considered. Early hospital care also requires careful prevention of aspiration, deep vein thrombosis, and falls. Recovery is maximized with early and aggressive rehabilitation efforts that include all members of the rehabilitation team—physician, nurse, speech therapist, physical therapist, and occupational therapist—and the family. The successful treatment of stroke depends on education of the public, paramedics, and health care professionals about the need for both early diagnosis and treatment and for risk factor reduction and prevention. The message should be that prevention is the key and to treat stroke symptoms as an emergency. Effective medical and surgical procedures may preserve brain function and prevent disability.

IN SUMMARY

A stroke is an acute focal neurologic deficit caused by a vascular disorder that injures brain tissue. It is the fifth leading cause of death in the United States and a major cause of disability. There are two main types of stroke: ischemic and hemorrhagic. Ischemic stroke, which is the most common type, is caused by cerebrovascular obstruction by a thrombus or emboli. Hemorrhagic stroke, which is associated with greater morbidity and mortality, is caused by the rupture of a blood vessel and bleeding into the brain.

One form of hemorrhagic stroke, known as aneurysmal SAH, results from a ruptured cerebral aneurysm. Presenting symptoms include worst headache of life, nuchal rigidity, photophobia, and nausea. Complications include rebleeding, vasospasm, and hydrocephalus.

Arteriovenous malformations are congenital abnormal communications between arterial and venous channels that result from failure in development of the capillary network in the embryonic brain. The vessels in the arteriovenous malformations may enlarge to form a space-occupying lesion, become weak and predisposed to bleeding, and divert blood away from other parts of the brain; they can cause brain hemorrhage, seizures, headache, and other neurologic deficits.

The acute manifestations of stroke depend on the location of the blood vessel that is involved and can include motor, sensory, language, speech, and cognitive disorders. Early diagnosis and treatment with thrombolytic agents can prevent disabling brain injury from ischemic stroke. Treatment of long-term neurologic deficits from stroke is primarily symptomatic, involving the combined efforts of the health care team, the person who has had stroke, and the family.

INFECTIONS AND NEOPLASMS

After completing this section of the chapter, the learner will be able to meet the following objectives:

- Discuss the assessment and management of meningitis.
- Describe the symptoms of encephalitis.
- Identify the classification of major brain tumors.
- Describe the general clinical manifestations of brain tumors.

Infections

Infections of the CNS may be classified according to the structure involved, including:

- Meninges—meningitis
- Brain parenchyma—encephalitis
- Spinal cord—myelitis
- Brain and spinal cord—encephalomyelitis

They also may be classified by the type of invading organism, including bacterial, viral, fungal, or other. In general, pathogens enter the CNS through the bloodstream by crossing the blood–brain barrier or by direct invasion through skull fracture or a bullet hole or, rarely, by contamination during surgery or lumbar puncture.

Meningitis

Meningitis is an inflammation of the pia mater, the arachnoid, and the CSF-filled subarachnoid space. Inflammation spreads rapidly because of CSF circulation around the brain and spinal cord. The inflammation usually is caused by an infection, but chemical meningitis can occur. There are two types of acute infectious meningitis: acute purulent meningitis (usually bacterial) and acute lymphocytic (usually viral) meningitis.[8] Factors responsible for the severity of meningitis include virulence factors of the pathogen, host factors, brain edema, and the presence of permanent neurologic sequelae.

Bacterial Meningitis. Most cases of bacterial meningitis are caused by *Streptococcus pneumoniae* (the pneumococcus) or *Neisseria meningitidis* (the meningococcus), except in neonates (infected most by group B streptococci).[33] Other pathogens that cause infection in adults are gram-negative bacilli and *Listeria monocytogenes. Haemophilus influenzae* was a leading cause of meningitis in decades. However, incidence of infection caused by this organism has declined dramatically during recent years because of vaccination against *H. influenzae*.

Epidemics of meningococcal meningitis occur in settings such as the military, where the recruits must reside in close contact. The very young and the very old are at highest risk for pneumococcal meningitis. Risk factors associated with contracting meningitis include head trauma with basilar skull fractures, otitis media, sinusitis or mastoiditis, neurosurgery, dermal sinus tracts, systemic sepsis, or immunocompromise.

Pathophysiology. In the pathophysiologic process of bacterial meningitis, the bacterial organisms replicate and undergo lysis in the CSF, releasing endotoxins or cell wall fragments. These substances initiate the release of inflammatory mediators, which set off a complex sequence of events permitting pathogens, neutrophils, and albumin to move across the capillary wall into the CSF. As the pathogens enter the subarachnoid space, they cause inflammation, characterized by a cloudy, purulent exudate. Thrombophlebitis of the bridging veins and dural sinuses or obliteration of arterioles by inflammation may develop, causing vascular congestion and infarction in the surrounding tissues. Ultimately, the meninges thicken and adhesions form. These adhesions may impinge on the cranial nerves, giving rise to cranial nerve palsies, or may impair the outflow of CSF, causing hydrocephalus.

Clinical Manifestations. The most common symptoms of acute bacterial meningitis are fever and chills; headache; stiff neck; back, abdominal, and extremity pains; and nausea and vomiting.[9] Other signs include seizures, cranial nerve palsies, and focal cerebral signs. Meningococcal meningitis causes a petechial rash with palpable purpura in most people. These petechiae vary in size from pinhead to large ecchymoses or even areas of skin gangrene that slough if the person survives. Other types of meningitis also may produce a petechial rash. People infected with *H. influenzae* or *S. pneumoniae* may present with difficulty in arousal and seizures, whereas those with *N. meningitidis* infection may present with delirium or coma.[34] The development of brain edema, hydrocephalus, or increased cerebral blood flow can increase ICP.

Meningeal signs (*e.g.*, photophobia and nuchal rigidity), such as those seen in SAH, also may be present. Two assessment techniques can help determine whether meningeal irritation is present. The Kernig sign is resistance to extension of the knee while the person is lying with the hip flexed at a right angle. The Brudzinski sign is elicited when flexion of the neck induces flexion of the hip and knee. These postures reflect resistance to the painful stretching of the inflamed meninges from the lumbar level to the head. Cranial nerve damage (especially the eighth nerve, with resulting deafness) and hydrocephalus may occur as complications of pyogenic meningitis.

Diagnosis. Diagnosis of bacterial meningitis is based on the history and physical examination, along with laboratory data. Lumbar puncture findings, which are necessary for accurate diagnosis, include a cloudy and purulent CSF under increased pressure. The CSF typically contains large numbers of polymorphonuclear neutrophils (up to $90,000/mm^3$), increased protein content, and reduced sugar content. Bacteria can be seen on smears and can easily be cultured with appropriate media. Occasionally, previous antibiotic use limits culture sensitivities, in which case latex agglutination can be used, or polymerase chain reaction (PCR) testing for *N. meningitidis*, *H. influenzae*, and *Listeria* species. Because complications associated with lumbar puncture include life-threatening cerebral herniation, people who are at risk (*i.e.*, those who are immunocompromised, had a seizure within a week, have papilledema, or have specific neurologic abnormalities) should have a CT scan before undergoing the procedure.

Treatment. Treatment includes urgent antibiotics while diagnostic testing ensues.[2,9,18,34] Delay in initiation of antimicrobial therapy, most frequently because of performance of medical imaging before performance of lumbar puncture or transfer to another medical facility, can result in poor outcomes.[3,34] Initial choice of antibiotics includes broad-spectrum coverage with a third-generation cephalosporin, vancomycin, and sometimes ampicillin. Further adjustment of antibiotics is driven by results of CSF cultures. Effective antibiotics produce rapid lysis of the pathogen, which produces inflammatory mediators that have the potential for exacerbating the abnormalities of the blood–brain barrier. To suppress this pathologic inflammation, adjunctive corticosteroid therapy is increasingly administered with or just before the first dose of antibiotics in people of all ages.[2,9,18,33]

People who have been exposed to someone with meningococcal meningitis should be treated prophylactically with antibiotics.[33] Effective polysaccharide vaccines are available to protect against meningococcal groups A, C, Y, and W-135. These vaccines are recommended for military recruits and college students, who are at increased risk for invasive meningococcal disease.

Viral Meningitis. Viral meningitis manifests in much the same way as bacterial meningitis, but the course is less severe and the CSF findings are markedly different. There are lymphocytes in the fluid rather than polymorphonuclear cells, the protein content is only moderately elevated, and the sugar content usually is normal. The acute viral meningitides are self-limited and usually require only symptomatic treatment, except for herpes simplex virus (HSV) type 2, which responds to intravenous acyclovir. Viral meningitis can be caused by many different viruses, most often enteroviruses, including coxsackievirus, poliovirus, and echovirus. Others include Epstein-Barr virus, mumps virus, HSV, and West Nile virus. Although often the virus cannot be identified, newer assays are emerging that allow in some circumstances for rapid identification of viral ribonucleic acid (RNA) in CSF.

Encephalitis

Encephalitis represents a generalized infection of the parenchyma of the brain or spinal cord. A virus usually causes it, but it also may be caused by bacteria, fungi, and other organisms. The nervous system is subject to invasion by many viruses, such as arbovirus, poliovirus, and rabies virus. The mode of transmission may be the bite of a mosquito (arbovirus), a rabid animal (rabies virus), or ingestion (poliovirus). Common causes of encephalitis in the United States are HSV and West Nile virus. Less frequent causes of encephalitis are toxic substances such as ingested lead and vaccines for measles and mumps.

The pathologic picture of encephalitis includes local necrotizing hemorrhage, which ultimately becomes generalized, with prominent edema. There is progressive degeneration of nerve cell bodies. The histologic picture, although rather general, may demonstrate some specific characteristics. For example, the poliovirus selectively destroys the cells of the anterior horn of the spinal cord.

Like meningitis, encephalitis is characterized by fever, headache, and nuchal rigidity. However, more often, people also experience neurologic disturbances, such as lethargy, disorientation, seizures, focal paralysis, delirium, and coma. Diagnosis of encephalitis is made by clinical history and presenting symptoms, in addition to traditional CSF studies.

Brain Tumors

Primary brain tumors account for 2% of all cancer deaths. The American Cancer Society estimates that there were 22,850 new cases and more than 15,320 deaths from brain and other nervous system cancers in 2015.[35] Metastases to the brain develops in 10% to 15% of people with cancer.[9] In children, primary brain tumors are second only to leukemia.[35] The mortality rate among this age group approaches 30%.[36]

Types of Tumors

For most neoplasms, the term *malignant* is used to describe the tumor's lack of cell differentiation, its invasive nature, and its ability to metastasize. However, the terms *benign* and *malignant* do not apply to brain tumors in the same sense as they do to tumors in other parts of the body. In the brain, even a well-differentiated and histologically benign tumor may grow and cause death because of its location. Most histologically benign tumors infiltrate the normal brain tissue, preventing total resection and allowing for tumor recurrence. Classification of brain tumors is based on histopathologic characteristics. The World Health Organization (WHO) system is the most widely used classification system for brain tumors.[2,9]

Brain tumors can be divided into three basic types:

- Primary intracranial tumors of neuroepithelial tissue (*e.g.*, neurons, neuroglia)
- Primary intracranial tumors that originate in the skull cavity but are not derived from the brain tissue itself (*e.g.*, meninges, pituitary gland, pineal gland, primary CNS lymphoma)
- Metastatic tumors[11]

Collectively, neoplasms of astrocytic origin are the most common type of primary brain tumor in adults, followed by primary CNS lymphoma.

Glial Tumors. Glial tumors are divided into two main categories: astrocytic and oligodendroglial. For purposes of classification, astrocytic tumors can be subdivided into fibrillary (infiltrating) astrocytic tumors and pilocytic astrocytomas.

Fibrillary or diffuse astrocytomas account for 80% of adult primary brain tumors. They are most common in middle age, with the anaplastic astrocytomas having a peak incidence in the sixth decade. Although they usually are found in the cerebral hemispheres, they also can occur in the cerebellum, brain stem, or spinal cord. Astrocytomas of the cerebral hemispheres commonly are divided into three grades of increasing pathologic anaplasia and rapidity of progression: well-differentiated lesions, designated *astrocytomas*; intermediate-grade tumors, termed *anaplastic astrocytomas*; and the least differentiated and most aggressive, designated *glioblastoma multiforme*. Clinically, infiltrating astrocytic tumors present with symptoms of increased ICP (*e.g.*, headache) or focal abnormalities related to their position (*e.g.*, seizures).

Pilocytic astrocytomas are distinguished from other astrocytomas by their cellular appearance and their benign behavior. Typically, they occur in children and young adults and usually are located in the cerebellum, but they also can be found in the floor and walls of the third ventricle, in the optic chiasm and nerves, and occasionally in the cerebral hemispheres. The prognosis of people with pilocytic astrocytomas is influenced primarily by their location. The prognosis is usually better for people with surgically resectable tumors, such as those located in the cerebellar cortex, than for people with less accessible tumors, such as those involving the hypothalamus or brain stem.

Oligodendrogliomas are tumors of the oligodendrocytes or their precursors, or with histologic features representing both oligodendrocytes and astrocytes. They represent approximately 5% to 20% of glial tumors and are most common in middle life.[37] The prognosis of people with oligodendrogliomas is less predictable than for people with infiltrating astrocytomas. It depends on the histologic grade of the tumor, its location, and recognition of molecular features that can be linked to chemosensitivity.[37] The oligodendroglial tumors are prone to spontaneous hemorrhage owing to their delicate vasculature.

Ependymomas. Ependymomas are derived from the single layer of epithelium that lines the ventricles and spinal canal. Although they can occur at any age, they are more common in children and affect the lining of ventricle; they constitute 12% of all adult CNS tumors.[37] The spinal cord is the most common site for ependymomas occurring in middle age. The clinical features depend on the location of the neoplasm. Intracranial tumors are often associated with hydrocephalus and evidence of increased ICP.

Meningiomas. Meningiomas develop from the meningothelial cells of the arachnoid and are outside the brain. They usually have their onset in the middle or later years of life and constitute approximately 35% of primary brain tumors in this age group.[37] Meningiomas are slow-growing, well-circumscribed, and often highly vascular tumors. They usually are benign, and complete removal is possible if the tumor does not involve vital structures.

Primary Central Nervous System Lymphomas. Primary CNS lymphoma is a rare tumor that accounts for 4% of all CNS tumors. These deep, periventricular, and diffuse tumors are especially common in people who are immunocompromised and are associated with the Epstein-Barr virus and derived from large B cells. Most are malignant, and recurrence is common despite treatment. Behavioral and cognitive changes, hemiparesis, and aphasia are common presenting symptoms. Visual field deficits occur in about 20% of people.[37] Biopsy is usually performed, and then the lymphoma is treated with chemotherapy.

Etiology

A few environmental risk factors can contribute to the risk of developing a brain tumor.[18] High-dose irradiation increases the risk of gliomas, meningiomas, and nerve sheath tumors. Acquired immune suppression also increases the risk for primary CNS lymphoma. Other environmental risk factors and occupational exposures have not been convincingly demonstrated to increase the risk of brain tumors (*e.g.*, head trauma, industrial exposure to polyvinyl chloride, dietary exposure to N-nitrosourea compounds).[18] Several genetic syndromes increase the risk of brain tumors like neurofibromatosis type 1 and 2, Li-Fraumeni syndrome, tuberous sclerosis, von Hippel-Lindau syndrome, and Burkitt syndrome.[18]

Clinical Manifestations

Intracranial tumors give rise to focal disturbances in brain function and increased ICP. Focal disturbances occur because of brain compression, tumor infiltration, disturbances in blood flow, and brain edema.

Tumors may be located intra-axially (*i.e.*, within brain tissue) or extra-axially (*i.e.*, outside brain tissue, but within the cranium). Disturbances in brain function usually are greatest with fast-growing, infiltrative, intra-axial tumors because of compression, infiltration, and necrosis of brain tissue. Extra-axial tumors, such as meningiomas, may reach a large size without producing signs and symptoms. Cysts may form in tumors and contribute to brain compression. The clinical manifestations of brain tumors depend on the size and location of the tumor. General signs and symptoms include headache, nausea, vomiting, mental changes, papilledema, visual disturbances (*e.g.*, diplopia), alterations in sensory and motor function, and seizures. Because the volume of the intracranial cavity is fixed, brain tumors cause a generalized increase in ICP when they reach sufficient size or produce edema. Cerebral edema usually is of the vasogenic type, which develops around the tumors and is characterized by increased brain water and expanded extracellular fluid. The edema is thought to result from increased permeability of tumor capillary endothelial cells. Tumors can also obstruct the flow of CSF in the ventricular cavities and produce hydrocephalic dilation of the proximal ventricles and atrophy of the cerebral hemispheres. With very slow-growing tumors, complete compensation of ventricular volumes can occur, but with rapidly growing tumors, increased ICP is an early sign. Depending on the location of the tumor, brain displacement and herniation of the uncus or cerebellum may occur.

Headache that accompanies brain tumors results from compression or distortion of pain-sensitive dural or vascular structures. It may be felt on the same side of the head as the tumor, but more commonly is diffuse. In the early stages, the headache is mild and occurs in the morning on awakening and improves with head elevation. The headache becomes more constant as the tumor enlarges and often is worsened by coughing, bending, or sudden movements of the head.

Vomiting occurs with or without nausea, may be projectile, and is a common symptom of increased ICP and brain stem compression. Direct stimulation of the vomiting center, which is located in the medulla, may contribute to the vomiting that occurs with brain tumors. The vomiting is often associated with headache. Papilledema (edema of the optic disk) results from increased ICP and obstruction of the CSF pathways. It is associated with decreased visual acuity, diplopia, and deficits in the visual fields. Visual defects associated with papilledema often are the reason that people with brain tumor seek medical care.

Personality and mental changes are common with brain tumors. People with brain tumors often are irritable initially and later become quiet and apathetic. They may become forgetful, seem preoccupied, and appear to be psychologically depressed. Because of the mental changes, a psychiatric consultation may be sought before a diagnosis of brain tumor is made.

Focal signs and symptoms are determined by the location of the tumor. Tumors arising in the frontal lobe may grow to large size, increase the ICP, and cause signs of generalized brain dysfunction before focal signs are recognized. Tumors that impinge on the visual system cause visual loss or visual field defects long before generalized signs develop. Certain areas of the brain have a relatively low threshold for seizure activity. Temporal lobe tumors often produce seizures as their first symptom. Hallucinations of smell or hearing and déjà vu phenomena are common focal manifestations of temporal lobe tumors. Brain stem tumors commonly produce upper and lower motor neuron signs, such as weakness of facial muscles and ocular palsies that occur with or without involvement of sensory or long motor tracts. Cerebellar tumors often cause ataxia of gait.

Diagnosis and Treatment

The diagnosis of brain tumors is mainly done with an MRI. Gadolinium-enhanced MRI is the test of choice for identifying and localizing the presence and extent of tumor involvement. CT scans may fail to reveal certain mass lesions such as low-grade tumors or posterior fossa masses. Diagnostic maneuvers that suggest a possible tumor and indicate the need for MRI include physical and neurologic examinations and visual field and funduscopic examination. Cerebral angiography can be used to visualize the tumor's vascular supply, information that is important when planning surgery. MRI may be supplemented with positron emission tomography to better characterize the metabolic properties of the tumor, useful in planning treatment.[18] MRA and CTA can be used to distinguish vascular masses from tumors.

The three general methods for treatment of brain tumors are surgery, irradiation, and chemotherapy. Surgery is part of the initial management of virtually all brain tumors; it establishes the diagnosis and achieves tumor removal in many cases. The development of microsurgical neuroanatomy, the operating microscope, and advanced stereotactic and ultrasonographic technology; the fusion of imaging systems with resection techniques; and the intraoperative monitoring of evoked potentials or the EEG have improved the effectiveness of surgical resection. The degree of removal may be limited by the location of the tumor and its invasiveness. Stereotactic surgery uses three-dimensional coordinates and CT and MRI to localize a brain lesion precisely. Ultrasonographic technology has been used for localizing and removing tumors. The ultrasonic aspirator, which combines a vibrating head with suction, permits atraumatic removal of tumors from cranial nerves and important cortical areas. Intraoperative monitoring of evoked potentials is an important adjunct to some types of surgery. For example, evoked potentials can be used to monitor auditory, visual, speech, or motor responses during surgery done under local anesthesia.

Most malignant brain tumors respond to external irradiation. Irradiation can increase longevity and sometimes can allay symptoms when tumors recur. The treatment dose depends on the tumor's histologic type, radioresponsiveness, and anatomic site and on the level of tolerance of the surrounding tissue. *Gamma Knife* combines stereotactic localization of tumor with radiosurgery, allowing delivery of high-dose radiation to deep tumors while sparing surrounding brain. Radiation therapy is avoided in children younger than 2 years of age because of the long-term effects, which include developmental delay, panhypopituitarism, and secondary tumors.

The use of chemotherapy for brain tumors is somewhat limited by the blood–brain barrier. Chemotherapy can be used as an adjunct to surgery and radiation therapy. Chemotherapeutic agents can be administered intravenously, intra-arterially, intrathecally (*i.e.*, into the spinal canal), or intraventricularly. Chemotherapy is standard of care for high-grade gliomas.[9]

IN SUMMARY

Infections of the CNS may be classified according to the structures involved (*e.g.*, meningitis, encephalitis) or the type of organism causing the infection. The damage caused by infection may predispose to hydrocephalus, seizures, or other neurologic defects.

Brain tumors account for 2% of all cancer deaths and are the second most common type of cancer in children. Brain tumors can arise primarily from intracranial structures, and tumors from other parts of the body often metastasize to the brain. Primary brain tumors can arise from any structure in the cranial cavity. Most begin in brain tissue, but the pituitary, the pineal region, and the meninges also are sites of tumor development. Brain tumors cause focal disturbances in brain function and increased ICP. Focal disturbances result from brain compression, tumor infiltration, disturbances in blood flow, and cerebral edema. The clinical manifestations of brain tumor depend on the size and location of the tumor. General signs and symptoms include headache, nausea, vomiting, mental changes, papilledema, visual disturbances, alterations in motor and sensory function, and seizures. Diagnostic tests include physical examination, visual field testing and funduscopic examination, CT scans, MRI studies, brain scans, and cerebral angiography. Treatment includes surgery, radiation therapy, and chemotherapy.

SEIZURE DISORDERS

After completing this section of the chapter, the learner will be able to meet the following objectives:

- Discuss the causes of seizures.
- Describe the origin of seizure activity in focal and generalized seizures and compare the manifestations of a focal seizure and generalized seizures.

A seizure represents the abnormal behavior caused by an electrical discharge from neurons in the cerebral cortex. A seizure is a discrete clinical event with associated signs and symptoms that vary according to the site of neuronal discharge in the brain. Manifestations of seizure generally include sensory, motor, autonomic, or psychic phenomena. Americans have a 10% chance of experiencing a single seizure in their lifetime.[9] Seizure activity is the most common disorder encountered in pediatric neurology, and among adults its, incidence is exceeded only by cerebrovascular disorders. In most people, the first seizure episode occurs before 20 years of age. After 20 years of age, a seizure is caused most often by a structural change, trauma, tumor, or stroke.

Seizures may occur during almost all serious illnesses or injuries affecting the brain, including metabolic derangements, infections, tumors, drug abuse, vascular lesions, congenital deformities, and brain injury. A seizure is a single event of abnormal discharge that results in an abrupt, altered state of cerebral function.[2] Epilepsy is a chronic disorder of recurrent discharges from neurons.[2] The current classification system endorsed by the International League Against Epilepsy classifies seizures into two categories: as occurring in and rapidly engaging bilaterally distributed networks (generalized) and within networks limited to one hemisphere and either discretely localized or more widely distributed (focal).[38]

KEY POINTS

SEIZURES

- Focal seizures begin in a specific area of the cerebral hemisphere. There are two major groups for focal seizures: without impairment of consciousness (aware) and with impaired consciousness (impaired awareness).
- Generalized seizures begin simultaneously in both cerebral hemispheres. They include unconsciousness and involve varying bilateral degrees of symmetric motor responses without evidence of localization to one hemisphere. These seizures are divided into two groups: motor and nonmotor.

Etiology

Many theories have been proposed to explain the cause of the abnormal brain electrical activity that occurs with seizures. Seizures may be caused by alterations in cell membrane permeability or distribution of ions across the neuronal cell membranes. Another cause may be decreased inhibition of cortical or thalamic neuronal activity or structural changes that alter the excitability of neurons. Neurotransmitter imbalances such as an acetylcholine excess or γ-aminobutyric acid (GABA, an inhibitory neurotransmitter) deficiency have been proposed as causes. Certain epilepsy syndromes have been linked to specific genetic mutations causing ion channel defects.[39]

Classification

The International Classification of Epileptic Seizures determines seizure type by clinical symptoms and EEG activity. It divides seizures into two broad categories:

- Focal onset, in which the seizure begins in a specific or focal area of one cerebral hemisphere
- Generalized onset, which begin simultaneously in both cerebral hemispheres[38] (Chart 20.1)

The system also has a category for seizures of unknown onset, such as epileptic spasms.

Focal Seizures

Focal seizures are the most common type of seizure among newly diagnosed cases. For focal seizures, the original distinctions of simple partial, complex partial, and so on have been eliminated. Instead, these seizures must be differentiated into two major groups—without impairment of consciousness or awareness and with impairment of consciousness or awareness.[38]

Although descriptors of focal seizures may be used based on the earlier classification of seizures, the following revised descriptors of degree of impairment developed by the International League Against Epilepsy Commission on Classification and Terminology, 2017, can help differentiate in the evaluation of each person who is experiencing focal seizures:

CHART 16.1 CLASSIFICATION OF SEIZURES

Focal Onset
- Without impairment of consciousness or awareness (aware)
- With impairment of consciousness or awareness (impaired awareness)

Motor Onset
- Automatisms
- Atonic
- Clonic
- Epileptic spasms
- Hyperkinetic
- Myoclonic
- Tonic

Nonmotor Onset
- Autonomic
- Behavior arrest
- Cognitive
- Emotional
- Sensory

Generalized Onset

Motor
- Tonic–clonic
- Clonic
- Tonic
- Myoclonic
- Myoclonic–tonic–clonic
- Myoclonic–tonic
- Atonic
- Epileptic spasms

Nonmotor (absence)
- Typical
- Atypical
- Myoclonic
- Eyelid myoclonia

Unknown Onset

Motor
- Tonic–clonic
- Epileptic spasm

Nonmotor
- Behavior arrest

From Fisher R. S., Cross J. H., French J. A., et al. (2017). Operational classification of seizure types by the International League Against Epilepsy. *Epilepsia* 58(4), 522–530. Copyright © 2017 International League Against Epilepsy. Reprinted by permission of John Wiley & Sons, Inc.

- **Focal onset without impairment of consciousness or awareness**
  - Focal seizures with observable motor or autonomic components. (This roughly corresponds to the concept of *simple partial seizure*. 'Focal motor and

autonomic are terms that may adequately convey this concept depending on the seizure manifestations.)
  - Focal seizures involving subjective sensory or psychic phenomena only (This corresponds to the concept of an aura.)
- **Focal onset with impairment of consciousness or awareness** (This roughly corresponds to the concept of complex partial seizure.)
  - Focal seizures evolving to a bilateral, convulsive seizure (involving tonic, clonic, or tonic and clonic components) (This expression replaces the term *secondarily generalized seizure.*)[38]

Seizures Without Impairment of Consciousness or Awareness. These types of seizures usually involve only one hemisphere and are not accompanied by loss of consciousness or responsiveness. These seizures have been referred to as simple partial seizures, elementary partial seizures, partial seizures with elementary symptoms.

The observed clinical signs and symptoms depend on the area of the brain where the abnormal neuronal discharge is taking place. If the motor area of the brain is involved, the earliest symptom is motor movement corresponding to the location of onset on the contralateral side of the body. The motor movement may remain localized or may spread to other cortical areas. If the sensory portion of the brain is involved, there may be no observable clinical manifestations. Sensory symptoms correlating with the location of seizure activity on the contralateral side of the brain may involve somatic sensory disturbance (*e.g.*, tingling and crawling sensations) or special sensory disturbance (*i.e.*, visual, auditory, gustatory, or olfactory phenomena). When abnormal cortical discharge stimulates the autonomic nervous system, flushing, tachycardia, diaphoresis, hypotension or hypertension, or pupillary changes may be evident.

The term prodrome or *aura* traditionally has meant a stereotyped warning sign of impending seizure activity described by the person who is affected. The aura actually represents a simple partial seizure, reflecting only a small area of abnormal electrical activity in the brain. Simple partial seizures may progress to complex partial seizures or generalized tonic–clonic seizures that result in unconsciousness. Most people perceive the aura as a warning sign of impending complex partial seizures or other generalized seizures.

Seizures with Impairment of Consciousness or Awareness. These types of seizures involve impairment of consciousness and often arise from the temporal lobe. The seizure begins in a localized area of the brain but may progress rapidly to involve both hemispheres. These seizures are sometimes referred to as *psychomotor seizures,* reflecting their typical manifestations.

These types of seizures often are accompanied by automatisms. Automatisms are repetitive, nonpurposeful activities such as lip smacking, grimacing, patting, or rubbing clothing. Confusion during the postictal state (after a seizure) is common. Hallucinations and illusional experiences such as déjà vu (familiarity with unfamiliar events or environments) or jamais vu (unfamiliarity with a known environment) have been reported. There may be overwhelming fear, uncontrolled forced thinking or a flood of ideas, and feelings of detachment and depersonalization. A person with this type of seizure disorder sometimes is misdiagnosed as having a psychiatric disorder.

These seizures are focal at onset but then become generalized as the ictal neuronal discharge spreads, involving deeper structures of the brain, such as the thalamus or the reticular formation. Discharges spread to both hemispheres, resulting in progression to tonic–clonic seizure activity. These seizures may start as seizures with or without consciousness or awareness and may be preceded by subjective sensory or psychic phenomena. These subjective sensory or psychic phenomena, often a stereotyped peculiar sensation that precedes the seizure, are the result of partial seizure activity. A history of subjective sensory or psychic phenomena is clinically useful to identify the seizure as partial and not generalized in onset. However, absence of subjective sensory or psychic phenomena does not reliably exclude a focal onset because many bilateral, convulsive seizures generalize too rapidly to generate subjective sensory or psychic phenomena.

Generalized Seizures

Generalized seizures are the most common type of seizure. These seizures are classified as generalized when clinical signs, symptoms, and supporting EEG changes indicate involvement of both hemispheres at onset. The clinical symptoms include unconsciousness and involve varying bilateral degrees of symmetric motor responses without evidence of localization to one hemisphere. These seizures are divided into two categories: motor and nonmotor.[38]

Motor

Tonic–Clonic Seizures. Tonic–clonic seizures, formerly called grand mal seizures, are the most common major motor seizure. Frequently, a person has a vague warning (probably a focal seizure) and experiences a sharp tonic contraction of the muscles with extension of the extremities and immediate loss of consciousness. Incontinence of bladder and bowel is common. Cyanosis may occur from contraction of airway and respiratory muscles. The tonic phase is followed by the clonic phase, which involves rhythmic bilateral contraction and relaxation of the extremities. At the end of the clonic phase, the person remains unconscious until the RAS begins to function again. This is called the postictal phase. The tonic–clonic phases last approximately 60 to 90 seconds.

Myoclonic Seizures. Myoclonic seizures involve brief involuntary muscle contractions induced by stimuli of cerebral origin. A myoclonic seizure involves bilateral jerking of muscles, generalized or confined to the face, trunk, or one or more extremities.

Clonic Seizures. Clonic seizures begin with a loss of consciousness and sudden hypotonia. This is followed by limb jerking that may or not be symmetrical.

Tonic Seizures. In a tonic seizure, there is a sudden onset of increased tone, which is maintained in the extensor muscles. It is often associated with falling.

Atonic Seizures. In atonic seizures, there is a sudden, split-second loss of muscle tone leading to slackening of the jaw, drooping of the limbs, or falling to the ground. These seizures also are known as drop attacks.

Nonmotor

Absence Seizures. Absence seizures are generalized, nonconvulsive epileptic events and are expressed mainly as disturbances in consciousness. Formerly referred to as petit mal seizures, absence seizures typically occur only in children and cease in adulthood or evolve to generalized motor seizures. Children may present with a history of school failure that predates the first evidence of seizure episodes. Although typical absence seizures have been characterized as a blank stare, motionlessness, and unresponsiveness, motion occurs in many cases of absence seizures. This motion takes the form of automatisms such as lip smacking, mild clonic motion (usually in the eyelids), increased or decreased postural tone, and autonomic phenomena. There often is a brief loss of contact with the environment. The seizure usually lasts only a few seconds, and then the person is able to resume normal activity immediately. The manifestations often are so subtle that they may pass unnoticed. Because automatisms and unresponsiveness are common to complex partial seizures, the latter often are mistakenly labeled as *petit mal* seizures.

Atypical absence seizures are similar to typical absence seizures except for greater alterations in muscle tone and less abrupt onset and cessation. In practice, it is difficult to distinguish typical from atypical absence seizures without the benefit of supporting EEG findings. However, it is important to distinguish between focal seizures with impairment of consciousness or awareness and absence seizures because the drugs of choice for treatment are different. Medications that are effective for focal seizures may increase the frequency of absence seizures.

Diagnosis and Treatment

The diagnosis of seizure disorders is based on a thorough history and neurologic examination, including a full description of the seizure. The physical examination and laboratory studies help exclude any metabolic disease (*e.g.*, hyponatremia) that could precipitate seizures. MRI scans are used to identify structural defects such as temporal lobe sclerosis or underlying congenital malformations causing the seizure. One of the most useful diagnostic tests is the EEG, which is used to record changes in the brain's electrical activity. It is used to support the clinical diagnosis of epilepsy, to provide a guide for prognosis, and to assist in classifying the seizure disorder.

The first rules of treatment are to protect the person from injury during a seizure, preserve brain function by aborting or preventing seizure activity, and treat any underlying disease. People with epilepsy should be advised to avoid situations that could be dangerous or life threatening if seizures occur. Treatment of the underlying disorder may reduce the frequency of seizures. After the underlying disease is treated, the aim of treatment is to bring the seizures under control with the least possible disruption in lifestyle and minimum side effects from medication.

Anticonvulsant Medications

The categories and causes of epilepsy are extremely diverse, so a single antiepileptic drug for treatment is unlikely to be etiologically specific. Instead, antiepileptic drug treatment can be specified according to seizure type. Adequate seizure control is achieved in about two thirds of people with appropriate antiepileptic drug treatment.[40]

Choice of drugs used as first-line therapy for seizure disorders has changed since the newer drugs were introduced because they have much better side effect profiles.[2] Carbamazepine, gabapentin, lamotrigine, levetiracetam, oxcarbazepine, topiramate, valproic acid, and zonisamide are the drugs of choice in treating focal seizures or tonic–clonic seizures resulting from focal seizures. Ethosuximide or valproic acid is the drug of choice for absence seizures. Valproic acid, carbamazepine, oxcarbazepine, and lamotrigine are helpful for people with many of the minor motor seizures and tonic–clonic seizures. Myoclonic seizures can be treated with valproic acid. Atonic seizures are highly resistant to therapy. Each of the new drugs—gabapentin, lamotrigine, topiramate, and oxcarbazepine— is approved for use as monotherapy in adults who have focal seizures alone or with secondarily generalized (grand mal) seizures. The other agents are approved as add-on therapy when the first-line agent is not fully effective. In all cases, side effect profiles and person-specific factors affect choice of antiepileptic medications.

Women of childbearing age require special consideration concerning fertility, contraception, and pregnancy. Many of the drugs interact with oral contraceptives; some affect hormone function or decrease fertility. All such women should be advised to take folic acid supplementation. For women with epilepsy who become pregnant, antiseizure drugs increase the risk for congenital abnormalities and other perinatal complications. Carbamazepine, phenytoin, phenobarbital, primidone, and valproic acid can interfere with vitamin D metabolism and predispose to osteoporosis.

Whenever possible, a single drug should be used in epilepsy therapy. Monotherapy eliminates drug interactions and additive side effects. Determining the proper dose of the anticonvulsant drug is often a long and tedious process, which can be very frustrating for the person with epilepsy. Consistency in taking the medication is essential. Anticonvulsant drugs never should be discontinued abruptly. The dose should be decreased slowly to prevent seizure recurrence. The most frequent cause of recurrent seizures is a person not complying with drug regimens. Ongoing education and support are extremely important in the management of seizures. The psychosocial implications of a diagnosis of epilepsy continue to have a large impact on those affected with the disorder.

The neurologist and primary care physician must work together when a person on anticonvulsant medication becomes ill and must take additional medications. Some drugs act synergistically, and others interfere with the actions of anticonvulsant medications. This situation needs to be carefully monitored to avoid overmedication or interference with successful seizure control.

Surgical Therapy

Surgical treatment may be an option for people with epilepsy that is refractory to drug treatment.[41] With the use of modern neuroimaging and surgical techniques, a single epileptogenic lesion can be identified and removed without leaving a neurologic deficit. The most common surgery consists of removal of the amygdala and an anterior part of the hippocampus and entorhinal cortex, as well as a small part of the temporal pole, leaving the lateral temporal neocortex intact. Another surgical procedure involves partial removal of the corpus callosum to prevent spread of a unilateral seizure to a generalized seizure. Some people who are refractory to treatment benefit from an implantable electrical stimulator of the vagus nerve. Modern epilepsy surgery requires a multidisciplinary team of highly skilled surgeons and specialists working together in an epilepsy center. Most procedures require only a few hours in the operating room and a few days' stay in the hospital after surgery. Epilepsy surgery is increasingly considered a treatment modality for people with medically intractable epilepsy.

Psychogenic Nonepileptic Seizures

Psychogenic nonepileptic seizures (PNES) have no epileptiform activity on EEG but exhibit paroxysmal events that look like epileptic seizures. The major cause is usually psychologically based. The person could have experienced any of the following historical factors: antiepileptic drugs that do not relieve seizures, episodes that are consistently associated with emotional/environmental triggers, presence of a witness, or history of chronic pain, psychiatric illness, or trauma. The health care provider should be familiar with the following common factors associated with PNES: gradual onset, side-to-side head shaking, closed eyelids during event, partial responsiveness during seizure, and rapid postictal reorientation. People are diagnosed using video-assisted EEG to record events along with psychological testing. Treatment for PNES consists of attending to the underlying psychological stressors and conflicts, comorbidities, and maladaptive emotional/cognitive functioning. On average, about 50% of these people will continue to experience PNES.[42]

Status Epilepticus

Seizures that do not stop spontaneously or occur in succession without recovery are called *status epilepticus*. Status epilepticus is a medical emergency and, if not promptly treated, may lead to respiratory failure and death.

The disorder occurs most frequently in the young and old. Morbidity and mortality rates are highest in older adults and people with acute symptomatic seizures, such as those related to anoxia or cerebral infarction.[43] Approximately one third of people have no history of a seizure disorder, and in another one third, status epilepticus occurs as an initial manifestation of epilepsy.[43] If status epilepticus is caused by neurologic or systemic disease, the cause needs to be identified and treated immediately because the seizures probably will not respond until the underlying cause has been corrected.

Treatment consists of appropriate life support measures. Medications are given to control seizure activity. Intravenously administered diazepam or lorazepam is considered first-line therapy for the condition. The prognosis is related to the underlying cause as well as the duration of the seizures themselves.

Nonconvulsive Seizures

Nonconvulsive seizures (NCS) are common in the person in intensive care unit (ICU). At least 20% of people who are comatose in a general ICU have NCS. The prevalence of NCS is about 48% of people who remain comatose after a generalized seizure. It occurs in at least 20% of people with acute structural brain lesions (*e.g.*, traumatic injury). It is important to identify people at risk for NCS. People with a past medical history of tumor, epilepsy, meningitis, and/or encephalitis may be at risk for NCS. Specific clinical features that the health care provider can assess for are twitching of oral or ocular muscles along with eye deviation. NCS cannot be detected without continuous EEG monitoring. People who are comatose require 48 hours of continuous EEG recording to detect seizure activity. MRI findings have shown encephalomalacia. Seizure duration is strongly associated with outcome.[44]

IN SUMMARY

Seizures are caused by spontaneous, uncontrolled, paroxysmal, transitory discharges from cortical centers in the brain. Seizures may occur as a reversible symptom of another disease condition or as a recurrent condition called *epilepsy*. Epileptic seizures are classified as focal or generalized seizures. Focal seizures have evidence of local onset, beginning in one hemisphere. Generalized seizures involve both hemispheres from the start and include unconsciousness and rapidly occurring, widespread, bilateral symmetric motor responses. They include minor motor seizures such as absence and akinetic seizures, and major motor or grand mal seizures. Control of seizures is the primary goal of treatment and is accomplished with anticonvulsant medications. Anticonvulsant medications interact with each other and need to be monitored closely when more than one drug is used. Status epilepticus is a medical emergency and, if not promptly treated, may lead to respiratory failure and death. NCS are common in the person in ICU and cannot be detected without continuous EEG monitoring.

GERIATRIC Considerations

- As the brain ages, loss of neurons contributes to reduced cerebral blood flow and nerve conduction.[45]
- A change in mental status should never be considered a normal part of aging; mental processing declines with age but memory, language, and judgment remain unimpaired.[45]
- Changes in the nervous system function are nonspecific and slow to evolve, which can result in a decline in status that is overlooked.[46]

PEDIATRIC Considerations

- Parents are integral to assessing neurologic function in infants and children. They are usually the first to notice changes in level of consciousness.[47]
- Primitive reflexes (Moro, tonic neck, and withdrawal reflexes) are important in assessing neurologic health in infants because they can't perform tasks on command.[47]
- When positioning an infant for lumbar puncture, place upright with head flexed forward. For the child, position on the side with head flexed forward and knees flexed to the abdomen.[47]
- The majority of seizures start in childhood and begin external to the brain with an infection, high fever, or toxin.[47]
- Neural tube defects are the most common congenital anomaly of the CNS.[47]
- A dramatic decrease in positional plagiocephaly (asymmetry in head shape without fused sutures) has resulted from the *back to sleep* program, which teaches parents to place infants supine to sleep to prevent sudden infant death syndrome.[47]
- To decease head injury in children, Healthy People 2020 supports legislation to require bicycle helmets.[48]

REVIEW EXERCISES

1. A 20-year-old man is an unbelted driver involved in a motor vehicle crash and presents in a coma.
   A. *What are the clinical signs of coma?*
   B. *Where does the source of coma localize in the brain?*
   C. *Which complications of traumatic brain injury might lead to coma?*
   D. *What are the key treatment options to manage increased intracranial pressure?*
2. A 65-year-old woman presents with a 1-hour history of right-sided facial droop, arm weakness, and dysarthria. An immediate CT scan of the brain is negative.
   A. *Where in the brain is the pathologic process?*
   B. *What are the indications to administer intravenous tissue plasminogen activator?*
   C. *What are the possible causes of this stroke, and what diagnostic tests would reveal the cause?*
3. A child is taken to the emergency department with lethargy, fever, and a stiff neck on examination.
   A. *What findings on initial lumbar puncture indicate bacterial versus viral meningitis?*
   B. *In the case of bacterial meningitis, what are the most likely organisms?*
4. A 60-year-old man develops involuntary shaking of his right arm, which spreads to the face; then he collapses with whole-body shaking and loss of consciousness. After 1 minute, the shaking stops, and he is confused and disoriented.
   A. *What type of seizure is suggested by the clinical manifestations?*
   B. *Assuming this is his first seizure, what diagnostic tests should be performed to identify a cause for the seizure?*
   C. *If he has a long history of similar recurrent seizures, what treatments should be instituted? What treatments should be considered if he has failed multiple adequate trials of anticonvulsant medications?*

References

1. Posner J. B., Saper, C. B., Schiff, N. Plum, F. (2007). *The diagnosis of stupor and coma* (4th ed.). London, UK: Oxford University Press.
2. Hickey J. V. (2014). *The clinical practice of neurological and neurosurgical nursing* (7th ed.). Philadelphia, PA: Lippincott Williams & Wilkins.
3. Reith, F. C. M., Van den Brande, R., Synnot, A., et al. (2016). The reliability of the Glasgow: A systematic review. *Intensive Care Medicine* 42, 3–15.
4. Teasdale, G., Maas, A., Lecky, F., et al. (2014). The Glasgow coma scale at 40 years: Standing the test of time. *Lancet Neurology* 13, 844–854.
5. Spinello, I. M. (2015). Brain death determination. *Journal of Intensive Care Medicine* 30(6), 326–337.
6. Bender, A., Jox, R. J., Grill, E., et al. (2015). Persistent vegetative state and minimally conscious state. *Deutsches Arzteblatt International* 112, 235–242.
7. Ragazzoni, A., Pirulli, C., Veniero, D., et al. (2013). Vegetative versus minimally conscious sates: A study using TMS-EEG, sensory and event-related potentials. *PLoS One* 8(2), 1–11.
8. Frosch M. P., Anthony D., DeGirofami U. (2015). The central nervous system. In Kumar V., Abbas A. K., Aster J. (Eds.), *Robbins and Cotran pathologic basis of disease* (9th ed., pp. 1251–1318). Philadelphia, PA: Elsevier Saunders.
9. Bader M., Littlejohns L., Olson, D. (2016). *AANN core curriculum for neuroscience nursing*. Glenview, IL: American Association of Neuroscience Nurses.
10. Richmond T. S. (1997). Cerebral resuscitation after global brain ischemia: Linking research to practice. *AACN Clinical Issues* 8, 171–181.
11. Strayer D. S., Rubin E. (Eds.) (2015). *Rubin's Pathology: Clinicopathologic foundations of medicine* (7th ed.). Philadelphia, PA: Lippincott Williams & Wilkins.

12. Kleboom, J. K., Verkade, H. J., Burgrhof, J. G., et al. (2015). Outcome after resuscitation beyond 30 minutes in drowned children with cardiac arrest and hypothermia: Dutch nationwide retrospective cohort study. *British Medical Journal* 350, h418.
13. Callaway, C., Donnino, M. W., Fink, E. L., et al. (2015). Part 8: Post-cardiac arrest care: 2015 American Heart Association Guidelines Update for cardiopulmonary resuscitation and emergency cardiovascular care. *Circulation* 2015, s465–s482.
14. Jauch, E. C., Saver, J. L., Adams, H. P., et al. (2013). Guidelines for the early management of patients with acute ischemic stroke patient. *Stroke* 40, 870–947.
15. Aminoff M. J., Greenberg, D. A., Simon, R. P. (2015). *Clinical neurology* (9th ed.). New York, NY: McGraw-Hill.
16. Vos, P. E., Diaz-Arrastia, R. (2015). *Traumatic brain injury*. Oxford, UK: John Wiley & Sons.
17. Guyton A. C., Hall J. E. (2016). *Textbook of medical physiology* (13th ed.). Philadelphia, PA: Elsevier Saunders.
18. Louis E. D., Mayer S. A., Rowland L. P. (2016). *Merritt's neurology* (13th ed.). Philadelphia, PA: Lippincott Williams & Wilkins.
19. Tran, L. V. (2014). Understanding the pathophysiology of traumatic brain injury and the mechanisms of action of neuroprotective interventions. *Journal of Trauma Nursing* 121(1), 1–58.
20. Benjamin, E., Blaha,N., Chluve, S. E., et al. (2017). Heart disease and stroke statistics—2011 update: A report from the American Heart Association. *Circulation* 136, e10–e209.
21. Meschia, J. F., Bushnell, C., Boden-Albala, B., et al. (2014). Guidelines for the primary prevention of stroke: A statement for healthcare professionals from the American Heart Association/American Stroke Association. *Stroke* 45, 3754–3832.
22. Fonseca, A. C., Ferro, J. M. (2013). Drug abuse and stroke. *Current Neurology and Neuroscience Reports* 13, 1–9.
23. Sacco, R. L., Kasner, S. E., Broderick, J. P., et al. (2013). An updated definition of stroke for the 21st century. *Stroke* 44, 2064–2089.
24. Brouwers, H., Chang, Y., Falcone, G. J., et al. (2014). Predicting hematoma expansion after primary intracerebral hemorrhage. *The Journal of the American Medical Association* 71(2), 158–164.
25. Godoy, D. A., Pinero, G. R., Koller, P., et al. (2015). Steps to consider in the approach and management of critically ill patient with spontaneous intracerebral hemorrhage. *World Journal of Critical Care Medicine* 4(3), 213–229.
26. Hemphill, J. C., Greenberg, A. M., Anderson, C. S., et al. (2015). Guidelines for the management of spontaneous intracerebral hemorrhage. *Stroke* 46, 2032–2060.
27. D'Souza S. (2015). Aneurysmal subarachnoid hemorrhage. *Journal of Neurosurgical Anesthesiology* 27(3), 222–240.
28. Connolly E., Rabinstein, A. A., Carhuapoma, J. R., et al. (2012) Guidelines for the management of aneurysmal subarachnoid hemorrhage. *Stroke* 43, 1711–1737.
29. van Donkelaar, C. E., Bakker, N. A., Veeger, N. J., et al. (2015). Predictive factors for rebleeding after aneurysmal subarachnoid hemorrhage. *Stroke* 46(2), 2100–2106.
30. Gathier, C. S., Dankbaar, J. W., van der Jagt, M., et al. (2015). Effects of induced hypertension of cerebral perfusion in delayed cerebral ischemic after aneurysmal subarachnoid hemorrhage. *Stroke* 46, 3277–3281.
31. Man, S., Cox, M., Patel, P., et al. (2017). Differences in acute ischemic stroke quality of care and outcomes by primary stroke center certification organization. *Stroke* 48, 412–419.
32. del Zoppo G., Saver J., Jauch E., et al. (2009). Expansion of the time window for treatment of acute ischemic stroke with intravenous tissue plasminogen activator. *Stroke* 40, 2945–2948.
33. van de Beek D., Brouwer, M., Hasbum, R., et al. (2016). Community-acquired bacterial meningitis. *Nature Reviews Disease Primers* 2, 1–20.
34. van de Beek D., Cabellos, C., Dzupova, O., et al. (2016). European society of clinical microbiology and infectious disease guideline: diagnosis and treatment of acute bacterial meningitis. *Clinical Microbiology and Infection* 32, S37–S62.
35. Siegel, R. L., Miller, K. D., Jemal, A. (2015). Cancer statistics, 2015. *CA: A Cancer Journal for Clinicians* 65, 5–29.
36. Ater, J. L., Kuttesch, J. F. (2016). Brain tumors in childhood. In Kliegman, R., Stanton, B, St. Germe, J., et al. (Eds.). *Nelson textbook of pediatrics* (20th ed., Chapter 497). Philadelphia, PA: Elsevier Saunders.
37. Henke Yarbo, C., Wujcik, D., Holmes Gobel, B. (Eds.) (2016). *Central nervous system cancer. Cancer nursing* (Chapter 49) Burlington, MA: Jones and Bartlett Learning.
38. Fisher, R. S., Cross, J. H., French, J. A., et al. (2017). Operational classification of seizure types by the International League Against Epilepsy. *Epilepsia* 58(4), 522–530.
39. Husain, A. M. (Ed.) (2016). *Practical epilepsy*. New York, NY: Demos Medical.
40. Katzung, B., Trevor, A. (2015). *Basic and clinical pharmacology* (13th ed.). New York, NY: McGraw-Hill Medical.
41. Jette, N., Wiebe, S. (2013). Update on the surgical treatment of epilepsy. *Current Opinion in Neurology* 26, 201–207.
42. Doss, R. C., LaFrance, W. C. (2015). Psychogenic non-epileptic seizures. *Seminar in Epileptology* 18(4), 337–343.
43. Betjemann, J. P., Lowenstein, D. H. (2015). Status epilepticus in adults. *Lancet Neurology* 14, 615–624.
44. Laccheo, I., Sonmezturk, H., Bhatt, A. B., et al. (2015). Non-convulsive status epilepticus and non-convulsive seizures in neurological ICU patients. *Neurocritical Care* 22, 202–211.
45. Hinkle, J. L., Cheever, K. H. (2018). *Brunner & Suddarth's textbook of medical-surgical nursing* (14th ed.). Philadelphia, PA: Wolters Kluwer.
46. Eliopoulos, C. (2018). *Gerontological nursing* (9th ed.). Philadelphia, PA: Wolters Kluwer.
47. Kyle, T., Carman, S. (2017). *Essentials of pediatric nursing* (3rd ed.). Philadelphia, PA: Wolters Kluwer.
48. Healthy People.gov 2020. Bicycle helmet safety institute. http://www.healthypeople.gov

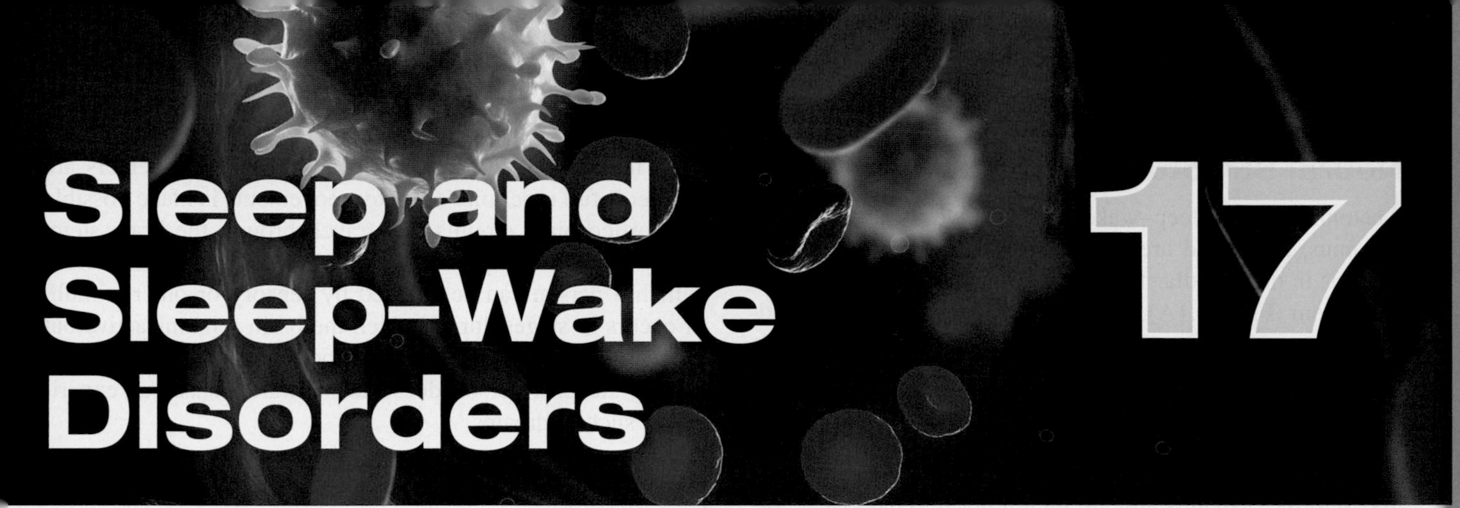

Sleep and Sleep–Wake Disorders

17

Christine Paquin Kurtz

As humans, we spend approximately a third of our lives asleep. We all know what sleep feels like. Yet defining sleep, describing what happens when we sleep, and explaining why we sleep is more difficult. Of equal concern is an understanding of factors that interfere with sleep. For many people, the inability to engage in appropriate periods of normal, restful sleep seriously impairs their functioning. The content in this chapter is divided into three parts:

1. The neurobiology of sleep
2. Sleep–wake disorders
3. Sleep and sleep disorders in children and older adults

NEUROBIOLOGY OF SLEEP

After completing this section of the chapter, the learner will be able to meet the following objectives:

- Identify the major brain structures that are involved in sleep.
- Describe the different stages of sleep in terms of the electroencephalogram tracing, eye movements, motor movements, heart rate, blood pressure, and cerebral activity.

Sleep is part of what is called the *sleep–wake cycle*. In contrast to wakefulness, which is a time of mental activity and energy expenditure, sleep is a period of inactivity and restoration of mental and physical function. It has been suggested that sleep provides time for entering information that has been acquired during periods of wakefulness into memory and for reestablishing communication between various parts of the brain. Sleep also is a time when other body systems restore energy and repair tissues. Muscle activity and digestion decrease, and sympathetic nervous system activity is diminished. Many hormones, such as growth hormone, are produced in a cyclic manner correlating with the sleep–wake cycle, suggesting that growth and tissue repair may occur during sleep.

Neural Structures and Pathways

Anatomically, the sleep–wake cycle involves structures in the thalamus, associated areas of the cerebral cortex, and interneurons in the reticular formation of the midbrain, pons, and brain stem (Fig. 17.1A). The reticular formation of the midbrain, pons, and brain stem monitors and modulates the activity of various circuits controlling wakefulness. The thalamus and the cerebral cortex function in tandem, with all sensory information being relayed to the thalamus and from there to the cerebral cortex. For example, visual impulses from the retina go to the thalamus and are then relayed to the visual cortex. The pathways between each sensory area of the thalamus and the cortex form two-way communication loops called the *thalamocortical system*.[1,2] Communication between each sensory area of the thalamus and its companion area in the cortex is kept orderly by several neuronal control systems, including the midbrain reticular formation, which controls the level of background activity so that external stimuli can be processed.

The Sleep–Wake Cycle

The sleep–wake cycle normally consists of a synchronous pattern of wakefulness and sleep. Wakefulness is a state of being aware of the environment—of receiving and responding to information arriving from all the senses, placing that information into memory, and recalling and integrating present experiences with previously stored memories. During wakefulness, both the thalamocortical system and brain stem centers are active. A full repertoire of motor movements is made possible by corticospinal circuits that travel through the brain stem. Sleep represents a period of diminished consciousness from which a person can be aroused by sensory or other stimuli. It occurs in stages during which the brain remains active but does not effectively process sensory information. However, during sleep, a person does have inward conscious experiences such as dreams.[3]

Brain Waves

Many of the advances in understanding the sleep–wake cycle have come about because of the ability to record brain waves through the use of the electroencephalogram (EEG). The source of the brain waves is the alternating excitatory and inhibitory nerve activity in postsynaptic potentials in cortical neurons.[3] During the recording of an EEG, the postsynaptic potentials are averaged and filtered to improve the quality of the signal. As such, the EEG does not measure the activity of a single neuron but rather the combined activity and "cross talk" among many hundreds of neurons responding to a given stimulus.

The normal EEG consists of brain waves of various frequencies (measured in cycles per second, or hertz [Hz]) and amplitude (measured in microvolts [μV]) (Fig. 17.2). Four types of EEG waves are used to describe brain activity during the sleep–wake cycle: alpha, beta, delta, and theta.[1–3] The

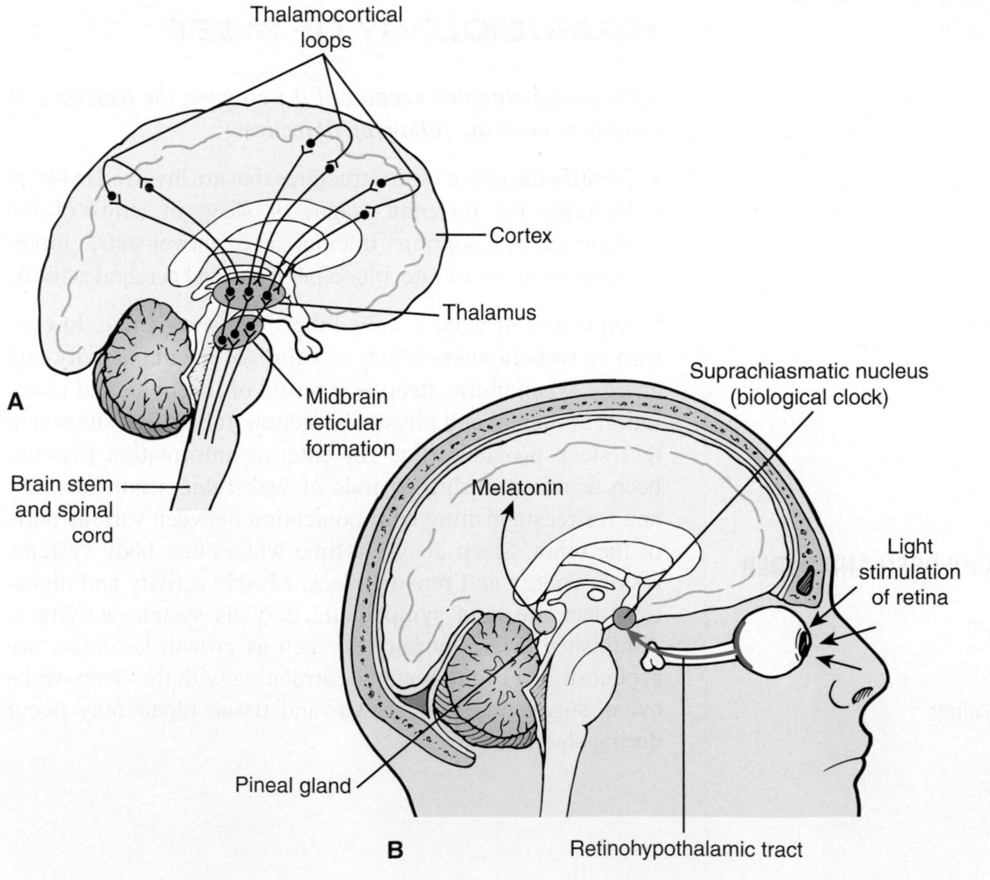

Figure 17.1 • **(A)** Brain structures involved in sleep. **(B)** Location of the SCN (biologic clock) with input from the retina and its association with the pineal gland and melatonin production.

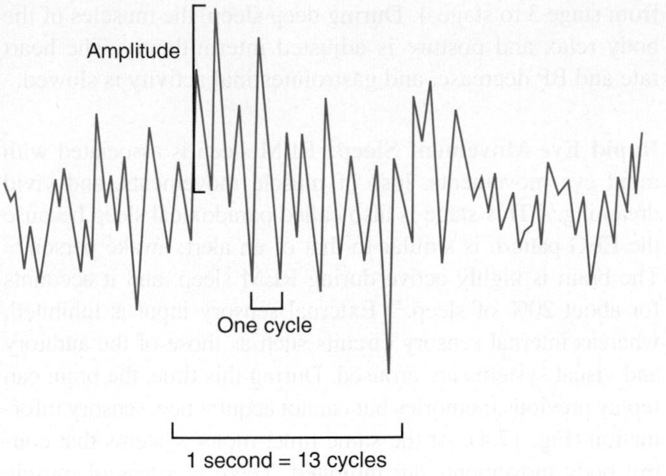

Figure 17.2 • The amplitude and frequency characteristics of an EEG tracing.

alpha wave, which has a frequency of 8 to 13 Hz, occurs when a person is awake with eyes closed. When the eyes are open, the EEG becomes desynchronized and the dominant frequency changes to the low-amplitude beta waves with a frequency greater than 13 to 30 Hz. The increased frequency of the beta waves is thought to reflect a higher level of brain activity produced by firing of a large number of neurons, and the low amplitude a lack of synchronization resulting from nerve activity occurring in many different brain sites at the same time. The theta (4 to 7 Hz) and delta (0.5 to 4 Hz) waves are observed during sleep.[2] The low-frequency, higher-amplitude waves that occur during sleep indicate that fewer neurons are firing and that those that are active are more highly synchronized and less affected by sensory stimulation. During REM sleep, beta waves are present.

Sleep Stages

There are two types of sleep: rapid eye movement (REM) and non–rapid eye movement (NREM) sleep.[2,4] These two types of sleep alternate with each other and are characterized by differences in eye movements, muscle tone and body movements, heart rate and blood pressure (BP), breathing patterns, brain wave activity, and dreaming (Table 17.1). A complete sleep cycle takes about 90 to 110 minutes.

Non–Rapid Eye Movement Sleep. NREM sleep, or slow-wave sleep, is a quiet type of sleep characterized by a relatively inactive, yet fully regulating brain and a fully movable body.[4] It accounts for about 80% of sleep.[2,4] The brain stem coordinates activity between the spinal cord and various reflexes such as swallowing and chewing. NREM sleep normally is encountered when the person first becomes drowsy. Falling asleep does not occur all at once. It is divided into four stages that reflect an increasing depth of sleep (Fig. 17.3):

- Stage 1
- Stage 2
- Stage 3
- Stage 4

Stage 1 consists of low-voltage, mixed-frequency, alpha wave EEG activity. It occurs at sleep onset and is a brief (1 to 7 minutes) transitional stage between wakefulness and true sleep. During this stage, people can be easily aroused simply by touching them, calling their name, or quietly closing a door. People may experience sudden muscle contractions called hypnic jerks, similar to a "jump" we may experience when we are startled.[5] Oftentimes these contractions are preceded by a sensation of falling. In addition to its role at sleep onset, stage 1 serves as a transitional stage for repeated sleep cycles throughout the night. Stage 1 is usually shorter during the first third of sleeping, and the longest during the last third of sleeping.[4] A common sign of severely disrupted sleep is an increase or decrease in stage 1 sleep.

Stage 2 is deeper than stage 1, lasting approximately 10 to 25 minutes. During stage 2 sleep, EEG activity includes predominantly theta waves that are interrupted by sleep spindles consisting of bursts of high-frequency (12 to 14 Hz) waves.

TABLE 17.1 ELECTROENCEPHALOGRAM, EYE AND MOTOR MOVEMENTS, VITAL FUNCTIONS, AND CEREBRAL ACTIVITY DURING SLEEP

SLEEP STAGE	ELECTROENCEPHALOGRAM	EYE MOVEMENTS	MOTOR MOVEMENTS	HEART RATE, BLOOD PRESSURE, RESPIRATIONS	CEREBRAL ACTIVITY
Stage 1	Low-voltage, mixed-frequency alpha waves	Slow, rolling movements	Moderate activity	Slows	Decreases
Stage 2	Low-voltage 4- to 7-Hz and 12- to 14-Hz sleep spindles, theta waves with spindles	Slow, rolling movements	Moderate activity	Slows	Decreases
Stages 3 and 4	High-voltage delta, 0.5- to 4-Hz waves	Slow, rolling movements	Moderate activity	Slows	Decreases
REM sleep	Low-voltage, mixed-frequency, 13- to 80-Hz beta waves	Clusters of rapid eye movements	Suppressed with loss of muscle tone	Increases, variable	Increases

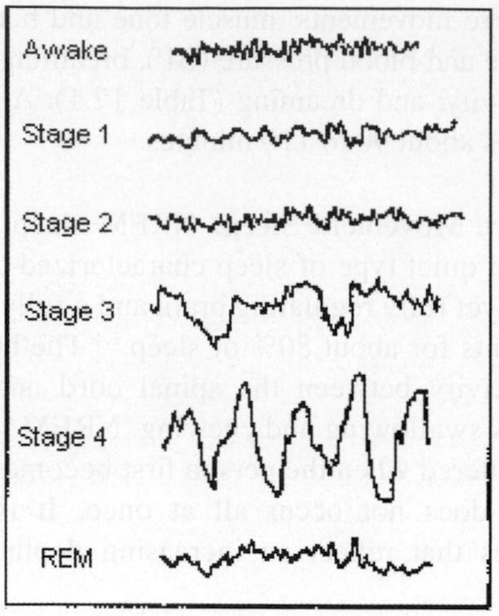

Figure 17.3 • Brain waves during wakefulness. NREM sleep stages 1, 2, 3, and 4 and REM sleep.

Spindle activity appears to be important in the overnight integration of new memories and existing neocortical knowledge.[6] A more intense stimulus is required for arousal in this stage.

Stages 3 and 4 represent deep sleep and are dominated by high-voltage, low-frequency (0.5 to 4 Hz) delta waves. Stage 3 usually lasts only a few minutes and is transitional to stage 4, which lasts for approximately 20 to 40 minutes in the first cycle. An increasingly larger stimulus is required for arousal from stage 3 to stage 4. During deep sleep, the muscles of the body relax and posture is adjusted intermittently. The heart rate and BP decrease, and gastrointestinal activity is slowed.

Rapid Eye Movement Sleep. REM sleep is associated with rapid eye movements, loss of muscle movements, and vivid dreaming.[2,4] This stage is also called paradoxical sleep because the EEG pattern is similar to that of an alert, awake person.[1,2] The brain is highly active during REM sleep, and it accounts for about 20% of sleep.[2,4] External sensory input is inhibited, whereas internal sensory circuits such as those of the auditory and visual systems are aroused. During this time, the brain can replay previous memories but cannot acquire new sensory information (Fig. 17.4). At the same time, motor systems that control body movements are inhibited. There is a loss of muscle movement and muscle tone. The result is an extraordinary set of paradoxes, in which people see things in their dreams but cannot move. They imagine being engaged in activities such as running, flying, or dancing but are paralyzed.

There also are changes in autonomic nervous system–controlled functions during REM sleep—BP, heart rate, and respirations increase and fluctuate and temperature regulation is lost. Cerebral blood flow and metabolic rate decrease. The brain is highly active and brain metabolism may increase as much as 20%.[1] Sleep-related penile erection occurs during this stage of sleep.

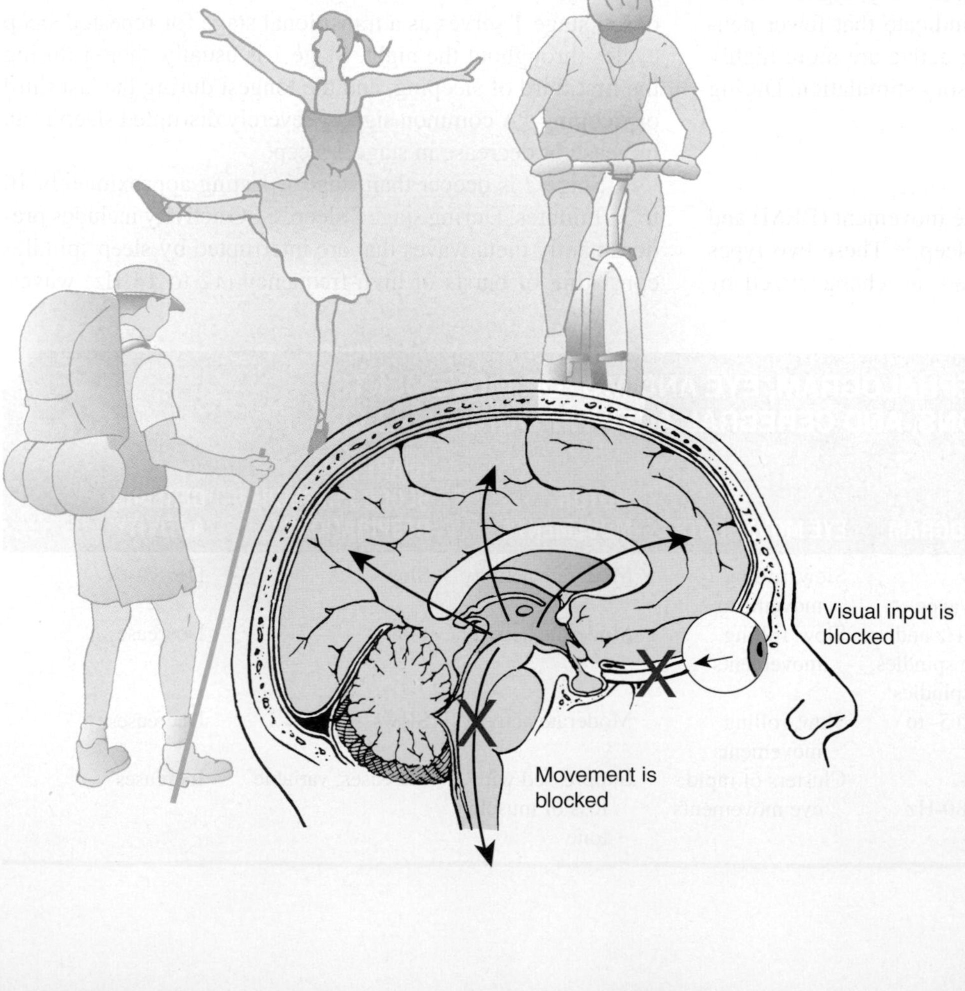

Figure 17.4 • Dreaming during REM sleep when sensory and motor activity are blocked.

It has been shown that adequate amounts of REM sleep are necessary for normal daytime functioning. Deprivation of REM sleep is associated with anxiety, irritability, inability to concentrate, and, if deprivation is severe enough, disturbed behavior.

Moving between Sleep Stages. There is a rather predictable pattern of shifting between one NREM stage and another during a typical night's sleep.[1,2] At sleep onset, there is a stepwise descent from lighter stage 1 sleep to deeper stage 4 sleep, followed by an abrupt ascent back toward stage 1. However, in place of stage 1, the first REM episode usually occurs. REM sleep is comparatively short (1 to 5 minutes) during the first sleep cycle but gradually becomes longer across the night. Stages 3 and 4 occupy less time in the second and subsequent sleep cycles and disappear altogether in later cycles as stage 2 expands to occupy the NREM sleep cycle. By morning, nearly all of the sleep cycle is spent in stages 1 and 2 and REM.[1,3]

Breathing during Sleep

Breathing normally changes during sleep. Stages 1 and 2 of NREM sleep are characterized by a cyclic waning and waxing of the tidal volume and respiratory rate, which may include brief periods (5 to 15 seconds) of apnea. After sleep has stabilized during stages 3 and 4 of NREM sleep, breathing becomes more regular. Ventilation usually is 1 to 2 L/minute less than during quiet wakefulness, the arterial carbon dioxide partial pressure (PCO_2) is 2 to 4 mm Hg greater, and the arterial oxygen partial pressure (PO_2) is 3 to 9 mm Hg less.[7] Involuntary respiratory control mechanisms, such as responses to hypercapnia, hypoxia, and lung inflation, are intact during NREM sleep and critically important to maintaining ventilation.

During REM sleep, respirations become irregular, but not periodic, and may include short periods of apnea. Breathing during REM sleep has many features of the voluntary control that integrates breathing with acts such as walking, talking, and swallowing. However, their influence on breathing is diminished.

Dreaming

Dreams are recollections of mental activity that occurred during sleep. They occur during all stages of sleep, but the majority of dreams occur during REM and sleep onset (stages 1 and 2). Dreams that occur during REM sleep tend to be bizarre and colorful. Dreams that occur during stages 1 and 2 of sleep tend to be shorter, have fewer associations, and lack the color and emotion of those that occur during REM sleep.[2]

The purpose of dreaming is unclear. Evidence suggests that dreaming, like other physiologic functions, is important to learning and memory processing. It has been suggested that dreaming may be the result of reprogramming of the central nervous system (CNS; *i.e.*, rearranging previous experiences) in preparation for the next day's conscious experiences.

KEY POINTS

SLEEP–WAKE CYCLE

- The sleep–wake cycle normally consists of a synchronous pattern of wakefulness and sleep. Wakefulness is a state of being aware of the environment, receiving and responding to sensory input, recalling and integrating experiences into memory, and purposeful body movements.
- Sleep, which is a period of inactivity and restoration of mental and physical function, is characterized by alternations between NREM (slow-wave sleep) and REM (paradoxical) sleep.[2]

Circadian Rhythms

Normally, sleep and wakefulness occur in a cyclic manner, integrated into the 24-hour light–dark solar day. The term **circadian**, from the Latin *circa* ("about") and *dies* ("day"), is used to describe these 24-hour diurnal rhythms. The function of the circadian time system is to provide a temporal organization for physiologic processes and behaviors as a means of promoting effective adaptation to the environment. At the behavioral level, this is expressed in regular cycles of sleep and waking and body functions such as temperature regulation and hormone secretion based on changes in the 24-hour light–dark solar day.

The daily rhythm of the sleep–wake cycle is part of a timekeeping system created by an internal pacemaker or clock.[2,8] The light/dark environment that accounts for the circadian rhythm involves a widely distributed network in the brain and the periphery.[8] Because the intrinsic sleep–wake cycle tends to be longer than 24 hours, a daily resetting of the circadian clock is necessary to synchronize with the environmental day. This process is called *entrainment* and normally is accomplished by exposure to the light–dark changes of the solar day.

The circadian clock appears to be controlled by a small group of hypothalamic cells, called the *suprachiasmatic nucleus* (SCN), located just above the optic chiasm and lateral to the third ventricle[2,3,8] (see Fig. 17.1). The SCN, which receives light–dark input from the retina, exhibits a rhythm of neuronal firing that is high during the day and low during the night. Although light serves as the primary stimulus for resetting the circadian clock via the SCN, other stimuli such as locomotion and activity, food availability, glucocorticoid level, and temperature are able to reset the peripheral clock.[8] The major projections from the SCN are to the anterior pituitary, with lesser ones to the basal forebrain and midline thalamus. Projections to the anterior pituitary provide for diurnal regulation of growth hormone and cortisol secretion; those to hypothalamic centers, for changes in metabolism and body temperature; and those to the brain stem reticular formation, for changes in autonomic nervous system–regulated functions such as heart rate and BP (Fig. 17.5).

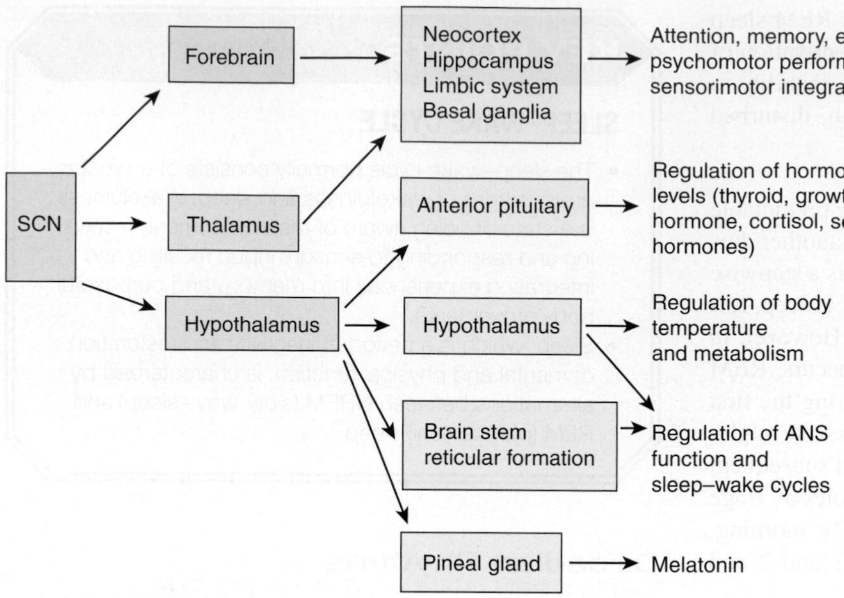

Figure 17.5 • Projections from the suprachiasmatic nucleus (SCN) to the forebrain, thalamus, and hypothalamus. ANS, autonomic nervous system.

Melatonin

Melatonin, a hormone produced by the pineal gland, is thought to help regulate the sleep–wake cycle and, possibly, circadian rhythm.[2,3,9] The pineal gland synthesizes and releases melatonin at night, a rhythm that is under direct control of the SCN (see Fig. 17.1). Large numbers of melatonin receptors are present in the SCN, suggesting a feedback loop between the SCN and the pineal gland. Administration of melatonin produces phase-shifting changes in the circadian rhythm, similar to those caused by light. There has been recent interest in the use of melatonin in treatment of various sleep disorders, particularly those related to a shift in the circadian rhythm. Although synthetic preparations are available without prescription in health food stores and pharmacies, their potency, purity, safety, and effectiveness cannot be ensured. Melatonin is not regulated by the Food and Drug Administration.[2,10] There also is a lack of clinical trial evidence about appropriate dosage, adverse effects, drug interactions, and the effects of melatonin on various disease states.[10] A pharmacologic melatonin receptor agonist, ramelteon (Rozerem), is available also as a prescription drug (to be discussed).

IN SUMMARY

Sleep is part of what is called the *sleep–wake cycle*. In contrast to wakefulness, which is a time of mental activity and energy expenditure, sleep is a period of inactivity and restoration of mental and physical function. There are two types of sleep: REM and NREM. REM sleep is associated with rapid eye movements, loss of muscle movements, and vivid dreaming. External sensory input is inhibited, whereas internal sensory circuits such as those of the auditory and visual systems are aroused. NREM sleep is a quiet type of sleep characterized by a relatively inactive, yet fully regulating brain, and a fully movable body. It is divided into four stages that reflect an increasing depth of sleep. Stage 1 is a brief transitional stage that occurs at the onset of sleep, during which a person is easily aroused. Stage 2 is a deeper sleep, lasting approximately 10 to 25 minutes, during which EEG activity is interrupted by sleep spindles consisting of bursts of high-frequency waves. Stages 3 and 4 represent deep sleep, during which the muscles of the body relax, the heart rate and BP decrease, and gastrointestinal activity is slowed.

Normally, sleep and wakefulness occur in a cyclic manner, called the *circadian rhythm*, and are integrated into the 24-hour light–dark solar day. The circadian clock is thought to be controlled by the SCN in the hypothalamus. The SCN, which receives light–dark input from the retina, exhibits a rhythm of neuronal firing that is high during the day and low during the night. Melatonin, a hormone produced by the pineal gland, is thought to help regulate the sleep–wake cycle.

SLEEP DISORDERS

After completing this section of the chapter, the learner will be able to meet the following objectives:

- Characterize non–24-hour sleep–wake rhythm disorder experienced by visually impaired people, sleep disorders associated with acute shifts in the sleep–wake cycle due to intercontinental travel and shift work, and advanced sleep–wake phase and delayed sleep–wake phase disorders.
- Explain the physiologic mechanisms, contributing factors, and manifestations of obstructive sleep apnea and describe the methods used in diagnosis and treatment of the disorder.
- Describe the diagnosis and treatment of short-term and chronic insomnia and narcolepsy.

Sleep disorders cover a broad spectrum of symptoms including the inability to fall asleep and stay asleep, circadian rhythm and sleep–wake transition disorders, sleep-related breathing and movement disorders, and excessive sleepiness. Although sleep disorders have existed for centuries, it is only within the past three to four decades that attention has focused on their diagnosis and classification. The development of the *Diagnostic Classification of Sleep and Arousal Disorders* by the Association of Sleep Disorders in 1979 heralded the emergence of the discipline of sleep medicine. This was followed by the *International Classification of Sleep Disorders* (ICSD), which was produced by the American Academy of Sleep Medicine, in association with the European Sleep Research Society, the Japanese Society of Sleep Research, and the Latin American Sleep Society. First produced in 1990, the ICSD was revised in 1997, 2005, and again in 2014 as ICSD-3.[5] ICSD-3 classifies sleep disorders into six major categories (Chart 17.1).

Diagnostic Methods

The diagnosis of sleep disorders usually is based on an adequate sleep history and physical examination. A sleep diary or sleep log often is helpful in describing sleep problems and arriving at a diagnosis.[11] In some cases, sleep laboratory studies may be needed to arrive at an accurate diagnosis.

Sleep History

A sleep history is fundamental to the process of identifying the nature of a sleep disorder.[11] The history should include the person's perception of the sleep problem, sleep schedule (*e.g.*, times of retiring and arising), problems with falling asleep and maintaining sleep, quality of sleep, daytime sleepiness and impact of the sleep disorder on daytime functioning, general emotional and physical problems, sleep hygiene (*e.g.*, eating and drinking before retiring), and sleep environment (*e.g.*, bed comfort, room temperature, noise, light). Because drugs such as over-the-counter medications, herbal preparations, and prescription medications can influence sleep, a careful drug history is important. It also is important to obtain information about the use of alcohol, caffeine, tobacco, and illegal substances.

CHART 17.1 INTERNATIONAL CLASSIFICATION OF SLEEP–WAKE DISORDERS

- Insomnia
- Sleep-related breathing disorders
- Central disorders of hypersomnolence
- Circadian rhythm sleep–wake disorders
- Parasomnias
- Sleep-related movement disorders
- Isolated symptoms, apparently related to normal variants and unresolved issues
- Other sleep disorders

Adapted from American Academy of Sleep Medicine. (2014). *International classification of sleep disorders* (3rd ed.). Darien, IL: American Academy of Sleep Medicine, with permission.

Sleep Log/Diary

A sleep log/diary is a person's written account of his or her sleep experience. It usually is recommended that the diary be kept for at least 2 weeks. The diary should record the person's account of his or her bedtime, wake-up time, total sleep time, time of sleep onset, time needed to prepare for bed and to fall asleep, use of sleep medications, number of awakenings, subjective assessment of sleep quality, time out of bed in the morning, and daytime naps and symptoms. A number of sample forms are available to health care professionals for distribution to their clients.

Actigraphy and Polysomnography

Actigraphy. Actigraphy measures muscle motion and is the most appropriate method for obtaining objective measurements of sleep duration and efficiency outside the sleep laboratory.[12,13] The actigraph is a compact device that is worn on the wrist or ankle to measure body movement, which is an indirect indicator of wakefulness and sleep. Depending on the unit that is used, it can collect information for up to several weeks.

Polysomnography. A typical sleep study, or *polysomnography* (PSG), involves the use of the EEG, electrooculogram (EOG), electromyogram (EMG), electrocardiogram (ECG), breathing movements, and pulse oximetry.[12] The EOG records eye movements. Because the eye is like a small battery with the retina negative to the cornea, an electrode placed on the skin near the eye records changes in voltage as the eye rotates in its socket. The EMG records the electrical activity from muscle movement. It is recorded from the surface of the skin. It typically is recorded from under the chin because muscles in this area of the body show very dramatic changes associated with the sleep cycle. The ECG is used to measure the heart rate and detect cardiac arrhythmias. The pulse oximeter (ear or finger) measures arterial oxygen saturation.

The multiple sleep latency test (MSLT) is used to evaluate daytime sleepiness. The American Academy of Sleep Medicine recommends this test be done after sleeping as much as possible for a week prior to the test, and especially the night before. MSLT values of less than 5 minutes indicate sleepiness, whereas values over 10 minutes are considered normal alertness. An MSLT result of less than 8 minutes is considered abnormal when diagnosing sleep disorders, such as narcolepsy.[5] Polysomnographic recordings are made during three to five naps spaced 2 hours apart during the day. Special attention is paid to how much time elapses from when the lights go out to the first evidence of sleep. This interval is called *sleep latency*.

Circadian Rhythm Sleep–Wake Disorders

Circadian rhythm sleep disorders occur when there is an incompatibility between circadian rhythms and sleep patterns. Sleep problems due to alternations in circadian rhythms are related to intrinsic factors (non–24-hour sleep–wake rhythm disorder [N24SWD], irregular sleep–wake rhythm disorder [ISWR], advanced sleep phase disorder, and delayed sleep phase disorder) and acute shifts in the sleep–wake cycle (jet lag and shift work).[5]

Non–24-Hour Sleep–Wake Rhythm Disorder

Non–24-hour sleep–wake rhythm disorder, also referred to as free-running disorder, consists of a lack of synchronization between the internal sleep–wake rhythm and the external 24-hour day. This results in symptoms of insomnia or excessive sleepiness.[5] Most people with the disorder are blind or have brain lesions that affect the SCN. Studies have shown that one half to two thirds of blind people have N24SWD.[14]

Strengthening the light–dark cycle is a treatment option for both blind and sighted people with N24SWD as the circadian visual pathway remains intact in some blind people.[15] Treatment for blind people also includes melatonin and the melatonin receptor agonist tasimelteon (Hetlioz). Bright light exposure and melatonin administration have been shown to be effective treatments for N24SWD in sighted people.[14]

Irregular Sleep–Wake Rhythm

ISWR is characterized by a lack of consistent pattern to the sleep–wake cycle. Total sleep time may be relatively normal but sleep periods are shortened and dispersed throughout the day and night. The causes of this disorder are unknown. It is most common in people with neurodevelopmental and neurodegenerative disorders.[16] Contributing factors include poor sleep hygiene behaviors and decreased environmental synchronizing factors such as daytime activity and light exposure.[5] Treatment includes bright light exposure during the day hours. The disorder usually is unresponsive to sedative and stimulant medications.

Delayed and Advanced Sleep–Wake Phase Disorder

Change in sleep phase disorders include delayed sleep–wake phase disorder (DSWPD) and advanced sleep–wake phase disorder (ASWPD). The disorders may arise because of developmental changes in the sleep–wake cycle or because of poor sleep habits.

The main symptoms of *delayed sleep phase syndrome (DSWPD)* are extreme difficulty in falling asleep at a conventional hour of the night and awakening on time in the morning for school, work, or other responsibilities. In adults, there is evidence of association between some mental illnesses, such as mood disorders, and DSWPD.[5] DSWPD is most common in adolescents whose frustrated parents cannot wake them up in time for school and have trouble getting them to go to bed at night. Staying up late is fairly common among teenagers, who are strongly influenced by peer pressure, defiance of parental rules, and other pressures. It has been suggested that social pressure may contribute to, but may not be the only reason for, changes in a teenager's sleep pattern. Rather, puberty may be accompanied by a lengthening of the intrinsic circadian rhythm, with a corresponding increase in evening wakefulness, which in turn leads to later sleep onset and arising.

Diagnosis of DSWPD is usually made from information in a sleep history, confirmed with a 2-week sleep log or diary. The presence of concurrent psychopathologic disorders or chronic sedative or alcohol use should be considered. There are no quick remedies for DSWPD. In adolescents, commonsense remedies such as setting earlier bedtimes and using multiple alarm clocks for waking up have been used, but with minimal success. The use of bright light may be helpful in maintaining morning wakefulness.[15,17] Supplementation with melatonin may be effective but the exact dosage has not been determined.[17]

ASWPD is essentially the mirror image of DSWPD—early sleep onset and early arising. People with ASWPD have trouble staying awake in the evening and have to curtail evening activities to avoid falling asleep.[16] The pathophysiologic basis of ASWPD is presumed to be a partial defect in phase delay capability, with the possibility that people with the disorder have an inherently fast circadian timing system. This disorder often occurs in older adults. Diagnosis of ASWPD is based on history and information from a sleep diary. Other pathologic causes, such as sleep apnea or depressive and bipolar disorders, should be ruled out. The need for treatment depends on how disruptive a person perceives the problem to be. Current treatment methods, which focus largely on sleep schedule changes, are somewhat limited.[16]

Acute Shifts in the Sleep–Wake Cycle

The normal diurnal clock is set for a 24-hour day and resists changes in its pattern by as little as 1 to 2 hours/day. This means that there is a limited range of day lengths to which humans can synchronize. Imposed sleep–wake schedules of less than 23 hours or more than approximately 26 hours, such as those that occur with intercontinental jet travel and switches in the work shift, produce increasing sleep difficulties.

Jet Lag Disorder. *Jet lag*, a popular term for symptoms of sleep disturbance that occur with air travel that crosses several time zones, is caused by the sudden loss of synchrony between a traveler's intrinsic circadian clock and the local time of the flight's destination. The severity and duration of symptoms vary depending on the number of time zones crossed, direction of travel (eastward versus westward), take-off and arrival times, and age. Most people who cross three or four time zones experience some sleep disturbance, usually lasting two to four nights.

Circadian rhythms take longer to resynchronize to local time after eastward flights than westward flights. There is a natural tendency for the circadian clock to move later each day, making it more difficult to phase advance than to phase delay.[5] Eastward travel requires a phase advance, wherein bedtime occurs sooner than the person's internal clock is ready for sleep. Because the human time system seems to be less flexible in adjusting to sudden time changes after 35 years of age, age also affects adjustment to time zone changes.

Manifestations of jet lag syndrome include insomnia, daytime sleepiness, decreased alertness and performance, general malaise, and gastrointestinal symptoms.[5] Other symptoms, such as eye and nasal irritation, headache, abdominal distention, dependent edema, and intermittent dizziness, result from cabin conditions and usually remit sooner than symptoms of jet lag. Frequent travelers, such as airline personnel and business travelers, may develop chronic sleep disturbances accompanied by malaise, irritability, and performance impairment. Jet lag usually is milder in infrequent travelers but may reduce the enjoyment of a vacation or effectiveness of business transactions. People with preexisting sleep disorders such as sleep apnea often experience a worsening of symptoms with jet travel.

Management of jet lag focuses on efforts either to maintain the home time schedule or to adapt to the new time zone schedule. For people crossing four or fewer time zones for only a few days, trying to maintain a schedule that is nearer to the home time schedule may be helpful, especially with westward travel. For trips of only 1 to 2 days, short-acting hypnotics may be helpful.[10] For longer stays, adapting to the new time schedule as quickly as possible is probably a better strategy. For stays of all length, good sleep hygiene, including keeping a regular sleep–wake schedule and avoiding excessive alcohol and caffeine, is recommended to improve sleep and adjust to a new sleep schedule. Staying well-hydrated and eating regular meals appropriate to the new time zone are also helpful. Alertness may be improved with short naps and caffeine but should be avoided close to bedtime.[10]

Shift Work Disorder. Shift work disorder includes excessive sleepiness and insomnia due to a work schedule that requires wakefulness during the worker's intrinsic sleep time.[5] Shift work usually creates an environment in which some circadian clock–setting cues (*e.g.*, artificial light and rest–activity) are shifted, whereas others (*e.g.*, natural light–dark schedule, family and social routines) are not. This situation almost never allows for a complete shift of the circadian system. To complicate the situation, most night shift workers revert to a nighttime sleeping schedule on days off. The effect of abruptly attempting to sleep at normal hours after working nights and sleeping days is biologically equivalent to a 6- to 10-hour eastbound jet flight.

Manifestations of sleep disorders of night shift workers include shortened and interrupted daytime sleep after the night shift, somnolence and napping at work, sleepiness while commuting home, and insomnia on the nights off from work. The abrupt transitions required of workers and interruptions that occur from sleeping during the day hours naturally result in a degree of sleep deprivation.[18] Arriving at a sleep schedule that is most supportive of the worker's intrinsic circadian rhythm often is difficult for night shift workers. Beginning sleep at noon rather than earlier in the morning may produce a more normal sleep period in relation to shift onset but may exacerbate insomnia on nights off. Sleeping in absolute darkness during daytime by using blackout shades or eye masks may benefit the night worker's sleep.

Insomnia

Insomnia is the most common sleep disorder that affects the general population.[19] Criteria for the diagnosis of insomnia include

- Difficulty initiating and/or maintaining sleep
- Adequate opportunity and circumstances for sleep
- Daytime consequences such as fatigue, daytime sleepiness, irritability, and impaired attention or memory[5]

Estimates of the prevalence of insomnia vary depending on the method used in the diagnosis and monitoring of the condition. According to the fifth edition of the *Diagnostic and Statistical Manual of Mental Disorders*, approximately one third of adults report insomnia symptoms.[5,19] An estimated 10% of adults have chronic insomnia.[5] Risk factors of insomnia include female gender, advancing age, and anxious temperament or worry-prone personality. While it is most often associated with other disorders that are psychiatric, medical, or substance related, it usually has an independent course and requires separate treatment.[5] The *International Classification of Sleep Disorders*, third edition, includes three categories of insomnia: chronic insomnia disorder, short-term insomnia disorder, and other insomnia disorder.

Chronic Insomnia Disorder

Diagnosis of chronic insomnia includes the symptoms of difficulty in initiating or maintaining sleep despite adequate opportunity for sleep and daytime impairment that has occurred at least three times a week for at least 3 months' duration.[5,19]

Chronic insomnia often is related to medical or psychiatric disorders. Factors such as pain, immobility, and hormonal changes associated with pregnancy or menopause also can cause insomnia. Interrupted sleep can accompany other sleep disorders such as restless leg syndrome (RLS) and sleep apnea. Many health problems worsen during the night. Heart failure, respiratory disease, and gastroesophageal reflux can cause frequent awakening during the night.[5] Mood and anxiety disorders are the most frequent cause of insomnia in people with psychiatric diagnoses.[19]

A number of drugs can lead to poor-quality sleep. Drugs commonly related to insomnia are caffeine, nicotine, stimulating antidepressants, alcohol, and recreational drugs. Although alcohol initially may induce sleep, it often causes disrupted and fragmented sleep. Sleep also is disrupted in people undergoing alcohol or sleep medication withdrawal.

Short-Term Insomnia Disorder

The diagnosis of short-term insomnia disorder, also referred to as adjustment or acute insomnia, is made when the criteria for insomnia are present for less than 3 months.[5] Short-term insomnia often is caused by an identifiable emotional and physical stressor. Some common examples include loss of a loved one by death or divorce, major illness, and sleep schedule problems. A common cause of short-term insomnia is an unfamiliar sleep environment, such as that encountered when traveling.

Factors that contribute to a nonconducive sleep environment include excessive noise, extremes of temperature, an uncomfortable sleep surface, or being forced to sleep in an uncomfortable position. Hospital intensive care units with their noise, intensive lighting, and frequent interruptions for monitoring vital signs and providing treatments are excellent examples of nonconducive sleep environments. Common stress-related causes of insomnia are expected occurrences such as being "on call" for work or stressful life events. Sleep schedule changes include jet lag and sleep disruption due to shift work.

Diagnosis

The diagnosis of insomnia is aided by a sleep history. Questions should address both sleep and daytime functioning. If the person has a bed partner, it is important to ask the partner if the person with insomnia snores, has unusual movement during sleep, or is excessively drowsy during the day. Because sleep needs vary from person to person, a 1- to 2-week sleep diary can be useful in diagnosing the sleep problem and in serving as a baseline for treatment of effects.[11] Other factors that need to be explored are the use of drugs such as caffeine, tobacco, and alcohol as well as prescription and over-the-counter drugs that affect the sleep–wake cycle. Identification of physical and psychological factors that interfere with sleep also is important. Actigraphy or PSG may be used as diagnostic tools. PSG is the most sensitive tool to evaluate sleep and wakefulness. However, it is expensive and, because of the numerous monitoring electrodes, can actually disrupt sleep. Its use as a diagnostic tool for insomnia is usually limited to cases in which other sleep disorders, such as sleep apnea, are suspected.[12]

Treatment

Treatment of insomnia includes education and counseling regarding better sleep habits (sleep hygiene), behavioral therapy aimed at changing maladaptive sleep habits, and the judicious use of pharmacologic interventions. The cause and duration of insomnia are particularly important in deciding on a treatment strategy. With short-term insomnia, treatment stresses the development of good sleep hygiene and judicious short-term use of sedatives or hypnotics. Careful assessment is required to determine the cause of insomnia. Depending on the findings, treatment options include behavioral strategies, such as relaxation therapy, sleep restriction therapy, stimulus control therapy, and cognitive therapy. Sedatives and hypnotics, which tend to become less effective with time and may cause dependence, are used with caution.

Sleep hygiene refers to a set of rules and information about personal and environmental activities that affect sleep. These rules include establishing a regular wake-up time to help set the circadian clock and regularity of sleep onset, maintaining a practice of sleeping only as long as needed to feel refreshed, providing a quiet sleep environment that is neither too hot nor too cold, and avoiding the use of alcohol and caffeine (coffee, colas, tea, chocolate) before retiring for sleep.

Cognitive–behavioral therapy is first-line treatment for adults with insomnia disorder. It includes cognitive therapy and behavioral interventions such as sleep restriction therapy, stimulus control therapy, and sleep hygiene education.[20] Cognitive therapy involves identifying dysfunctional beliefs and attitudes about sleep and replacing them with more adaptive substitutes. Sleep restriction therapy consists of curtailing the amount of time spent in bed in an effort to increase the sleep efficiency (time asleep/time in bed). People with insomnia often increase their time in bed in the misguided belief that it will provide more opportunity to sleep. Stimulus control therapy focuses on reassociating the bed and bedroom with sleep rather than sleeplessness. It is important that the bed and bedroom be identified with sleep and not with reading, watching television, or working. People who cannot fall asleep should be instructed to turn on the light and do something else outside the bed, preferably in another room.

Pharmacologic treatment usually is reserved for short-term (4 to 5 weeks) management of insomnia—either as the sole treatment or as adjunctive therapy until the underlying problem can be addressed.[20] The most common type of agents used to promote sleep are the benzodiazepine receptor agonists (BZRAs) such as zolpidem (Ambien), zaleplon (Sonata), and eszopiclone (Lunesta). Ramelteon is the first and only nonscheduled drug approved by the U.S. Food and Drug Administration for treatment of insomnia. It was approved in 2005 for sleep-onset insomnia and can be prescribed for long-term use. Ramelteon is a melatonin receptor agonist with high selectivity for melatonin (MT)-1 and MT-2 receptors in the SCN of the hypothalamus, receptors that are believed to be involved in sleep promotion and maintenance of the circadian rhythm.[21] Ramelteon has no appreciable binding to gamma-aminobutyric acid (GABA) receptors and hence no anxiolytic or abuse potential. However, recent studies demonstrate no statistically significant difference between ramelteon and placebo on sleep outcomes.[20]

Sedating antidepressants also may be prescribed, particularly when insomnia is due to depression. Antihistamines have sedative effects and may be used to induce sleep. The most commonly used agents are diphenhydramine and doxylamine. Most over-the-counter sleep medications include an antihistamine. Adverse effects of antihistamines include daytime sleepiness, cognitive impairments, and anticholinergic effects. Falls and fractures are more frequent in people using hypnotic or other psychotherapeutic agents. Melatonin, available in both natural and synthetic forms, is one of the most popular over-the-counter sleep aids.

KEY POINTS

SLEEP DISORDERS

- Primary sleep disorders include insomnia (repeated difficulty with sleep initiation and duration, and impaired daytime function), narcolepsy (characterized by excessive daytime sleepiness), breathing-related sleep disorder (disordered respirations during sleep), and circadian rhythm sleep disorder (misalignment between sleep pattern and societal norms).
- The parasomnias, which are undesirable physical phenomena that occur almost exclusively during sleep or are exaggerated by sleep, include nightmares, sleepwalking, and sleep terrors.

Narcolepsy

Narcolepsy is a disorder of central hypersomnolence characterized by "daily periods of irrepressible need to sleep or daytime lapses into sleep occurring for at least 3 months" (p. 146).[5] Daytime sleepiness is the most common initial symptom of narcolepsy. It is most apparent in boring, sedentary situations and often is relieved by movement. Although the sleepiness that occurs with narcolepsy is similar to that experienced after sleep deprivation, it is different in that no amount of nighttime sleep produces full alertness. The periods of daytime sleep usually are brief, lasting 30 minutes or less, and often are accompanied by brief interruptions of speech or irrelevant words, lapses in memory, and nonsensical activities. The ICSD third edition defines two types of narcolepsy, type 1 and type 2. Type 1 includes the presence of cataplexy.[5] Cataplexy is characterized by brief periods of muscle weakness brought about by emotional reactions such as laughter, anger, or fear. Associated features of narcolepsy include sleep paralysis, hypnagogic hallucinations, and automatic behaviors. Sleep paralysis is a terrifying experience that occurs on falling asleep or on awakening, during which people find themselves unable to move, speak, or even breathe deeply.

Hypnagogic hallucinations are vivid hallucinations that occur at the onset of sleep. Similar hallucinations may occur on awakening (*i.e.*, hypnopompic hallucinations). These hallucinations are usually visual or auditory, although tactile components may occur.[22] The exact boundary between hypnagogic hallucinations and dreams is not a clear one.

Generally beginning in puberty, narcolepsy has a peak incidence between ages 15 and 30.[12] The mechanisms underlying the manifestations of narcolepsy appear to be linked to an abnormality in REM sleep regulation. The occurrence of REM sleep at sleep onset or within 10 to 15 minutes of sleep onset is the most characteristic and striking manifestation of the disorder. Periods of sleep-onset REM are thought to indicate impaired sleep–wake regulation rather than increased need for REM sleep. The sleep paralysis, dreamlike hallucinations, and loss of muscle tone that occur during cataplexy are similar to behaviors that occur during REM sleep.

Etiology

Although the cause of narcolepsy is unknown, there are indications that the disorder may have a genetic component. People with narcolepsy have been shown to have an unusually high rate of a specific human leukocyte antigen (HLA) subtype (HLA DQB1-0602).[5,19] This association is seen in approximately 85% of cases with cateplexy.[23] Importantly, this association is substantially lower in people who have received the diagnosis of narcolepsy but do not have cataplexy.[23] The strong association between HLA type and cataplexy raises the possibility that narcolepsy is an autoimmune disease.

Research has suggested a link between an identified group of neurotransmitters called *hypocretins* and narcolepsy. The hypocretins (hypocretin 1 and hypocretin 2) are secreted by cells in the area of the hypothalamus that is related to wakefulness. Studies suggest that narcolepsy with cataplexy is caused by hypocretin deficiency. Although the cause of this deficiency is not completely known, it is believed to be due to an autoimmune response leading to deterioration of hypocretin neurons in people with the HLA DQB 1-0602 allele.[24] Narcolepsy may also be caused by neurologic insults that affect levels of hypocretin, such as hypothalamic lesions, and vascular, or inflammatory, brain trauma.[25]

Diagnosis and Treatment

Sleep laboratory studies are usually required for accurate diagnosis of narcolepsy. Both daytime and nighttime studies usually are done.[26] Nighttime PSG is usually performed to determine the presence and severity of sleep apnea, limb movement disorders, and nocturnal sleep disturbance. A daytime MSLT usually is done the next day. People with narcolepsy are observed to have a short period of sleep latency (<8 minutes, often <5 minutes) during daytime studies, along with a rapid onset of REM sleep (usually within 10 minutes). A mean sleep latency of less than 8 minutes and two or more periods of sleep-onset REM during the repeated nap opportunities are considered diagnostic of narcolepsy.[5,22]

There is no known cure for narcolepsy. Therefore, the goal of treatment is symptom management.[22] Patient education about good sleep hygiene, maintaining regular sleep patterns, and avoiding sleep deprivation should be included in the treatment plan for narcolepsy. People should also be warned about the risks of driving when excessively sleepy. Several short (15- to 20-minute) naps per day may decrease excessive daytime sleepiness. Unfortunately, such lifestyle changes are usually insufficient to adequately control the symptoms of narcolepsy.

Pharmacologic treatment of narcolepsy focuses on the use of stimulant medications such as methylphenidate (Ritalin), amphetamines (*e.g.*, Adderall, Desoxyn), modafinil (Provigil), and armodafinil (Nuvigil), which are FDA approved for the treatment of narcolepsy. Sodium oxybate (Xyrem), a CNS depressant, is FDA approved for the treatment of cataplexy and excessive daytime sleepiness.[22] It is believed to help by consolidating and improving the quality of nighttime sleep. Tricyclic antidepressants and the selective serotonin reuptake inhibitors (SSRIs) have been used successfully to treat the cataleptic attacks.[22]

Sleep-Related Movement Disorders

A variety of spontaneous limb movements occur during normal sleep. Many of these movements demonstrate characteristic rates and patterns during certain stages of sleep. Many movement disorders occur during stage 2 NREM sleep. Some occur during normal sleep in all people at some time or another. Others are not part of normal sleep patterns and can be disruptive of sleep. Among the abnormal motor disorders are periodic limb movement disorder (PLMD) and RLS.

Periodic Limb Movement Disorder

PLMD is characterized by episodes of repetitive movement of the large toe with flexion of the ankle, knee, and hip during sleep.[5,27,28] It can occur simultaneously in both legs, alternate between legs, or occur unilaterally. The disorder results in disrupted sleep quality and daytime functioning. The condition occurs most frequently during light (stages 1 and 2 NREM) sleep compared with deep (stages 3 and 4 NREM) sleep and REM sleep. The incidence of the disorder, which occurs equally in men and women, increases with age. The disorder frequently accompanies RLS.[27] People with PLMD are often unaware of periodic limb movements, but their bed partners may report the symptoms.

The cause of PLMD is largely unknown. It has been observed that the movements mimic the Babinski reflex, suggesting removal of an excitatory influence over a subcortical inhibitory system allowing for facilitation of abnormal movements during sleep. There is also an autonomic response that accompanies the periodic leg movements. A rapid rise in heart rate and arterial BP is followed by bradycardia and return of BP to normal.[28] The disorder is considered a diagnosis of exclusion, and diagnosis is facilitated with use of EMG recordings from both tibialis anterior muscles. A person must experience both the periodic leg movements in sleep and a disruption in daytime functioning to receive the diagnosis of PLMD.[5,27]

Restless Legs Syndrome

RLS is a sleep disorder characterized by the following:

1. An urge to move the limbs with or without sensations
2. Worsening at rest or inactivity
3. Improving with activity or movement
4. Worsening in the evening or night[5]

The prevalence of the condition is estimated at 5% to 10% of the general population in Europe and North America.[5] Although the prevalence increases with age, it has a variable age of onset and can even occur in children. Approximately 7 out of 10 people may experience the disorder sometime in their lifetime.[27]

The disorder, which is thought to have its origin in the CNS, can occur as a primary or secondary disorder. There is a high familial incidence of primary RLS, suggesting a genetic disorder. Secondary causes of RLS include iron deficiency, neurologic disorders such as spinal cord and peripheral nerve lesions, pregnancy, uremia, and medications. Although the neurologic basis of RLS has not been determined, recent research suggests that it may involve homeostatic mechanisms that regulate the influx and efflux of iron from cells of the CNS that regulate motor movements.[29] Cerebrospinal fluid ferritin (the main iron storage molecules in the CNS) levels are lower in people with RLS. Of interest is the role of iron in dopaminergic transmission in the CNS. Iron is an important cofactor for tyrosine hydroxylase, the rate-limiting enzyme in dopamine synthesis, and also plays a major role in the functioning of postsynaptic dopamine receptors.[29]

Diagnosis of RLS is based on a history of

1. A compelling urge to move the legs, usually associated with unpleasant sensations
2. Motor restlessness, as seen by activities such as pacing, tossing and turning in bed, or rubbing the legs
3. Symptoms that become worse at rest and are relieved by activity
4. Symptoms that are worse in the evening or at night[29,30]

Laboratory tests to determine secondary causes of RLS usually are done. Because RLS may be a symptom of iron deficiency, serum ferritin and iron saturation should be assessed. This is important because iron deficiency is frequently present in the absence of anemia. Sleep studies usually are not required because the condition can be diagnosed on the basis of history and clinical findings.

Treatment of RLS varies depending on the severity of symptoms. Dopaminergic agents are the first-line drugs for most people with RLS.[27,30] These include ropinirole (Requip), pramipexole (Mirapex), levodopa, and carbidopa (Sinemet). Antiseizure agents (gabapentin), BZDs (*e.g.*, clonazepam, temazepam), and opioids (*e.g.*, codeine, propoxyphene, or oxycodone) are second-line agents.[30] Although pharmacologic treatment is helpful for many people with RLS, those with mild symptoms may not require medications. For many people, deliberate manipulation of the muscles through ambulation, kicking movements, stretching, or massage may provide relief. Good sleep habits are important. Because a high prevalence of iron deficiency has been found among people with RLS, treatment of the deficiency may improve or resolve symptoms.

Sleep-Related Breathing Disorders

Sleep-disordered breathing (SDB) is associated with several conditions that result in altered respirations. Each condition has specific clinical presentations along with methods of diagnosis, treatment, and follow-up. These breathing disorders result in sleep deprivation and interfere with work, driving, and social activities. The most common SDB is sleep apnea.

Sleep Apnea

Sleep apnea is an SDB, accompanied by daytime symptoms, most often excessive sleepiness. There are two types of sleep apnea: central and obstructive.[31] *Central sleep apnea* is not common, and the etiology is unknown.[32] However, it is associated with underlying pathologic conditions such as Cheyne-Stokes breathing or environmental causes such as high-altitude periodic breathing.[31,33] It is characterized by a cessation or decrease in ventilatory effort during sleep and is usually associated with oxygen desaturation. *Obstructive sleep apnea (OSA)* syndrome, which is caused by upper airway obstruction and characterized by snoring, disrupted sleep, and excessive daytime sleepiness, is the much more common type. Although airflow ceases, respiratory muscles continue to function. This is one of the features that distinguishes central sleep apnea from OSA. The majority of people with central sleep apnea also have some obstructive events.[33]

Obstructive Sleep Apnea

Apnea is defined as cessation of airflow through the nose and mouth for 10 seconds or longer.[5,32,33] The apneic periods typically last for 10 to 30 seconds,[5] and some people may have as many as 300 to 500 apneic periods per night.[1] An accompanying reduction in tidal volume due to a decrease in the depth and rate of respiration (called *hypopnea*) is associated with a decrease in arterial oxygen saturation. An adult may experience up to five events an hour without symptoms. As the number of hypopnea events increases, so does the severity of symptoms. Five or greater events per hour in combination with reports of excessive daytime sleepiness are indicative of OSA.[5]

Pathogenesis. A critical pathophysiologic feature of OSA is sleep-related partial or full collapse of the upper airway at the level of the pharynx.[1,34] All skeletal muscles except the diaphragm undergo a decrease in tone during sleep. This loss of muscle tone is most pronounced during REM sleep. The loss of muscle tone in the upper airways predisposes to airway obstruction as the negative airway pressure produced by contraction of the diaphragm brings the vocal cords together, collapses the pharyngeal wall, and sucks the tongue back into the throat (Fig. 17.6). Airway collapse is accentuated in people with conditions that cause narrowing of the upper airway or weakness of the throat muscles.

Etiology. Conditions that predispose to OSA include male gender, increasing age, a positive family history, and obesity. Alcohol and other drugs that depress the CNS tend to increase the severity of obstructive episodes. Most people who develop sleep apnea are obese. Large neck girth in both male and female snorers is highly predictive of sleep apnea. Neck circumferences greater than 40 cm are correlated with OSA, even more so than body mass index (BMI).[34] Men have a higher risk for OSA than women. The reason for this is not entirely clear, but gonadal hormones may play a role.[34] Postmenopausal women are at higher risk than premenopausal women. People with specific endocrine disorders, namely, acromegaly, Cushing syndrome, hypothyroidism, and type 2 diabetes mellitus, are

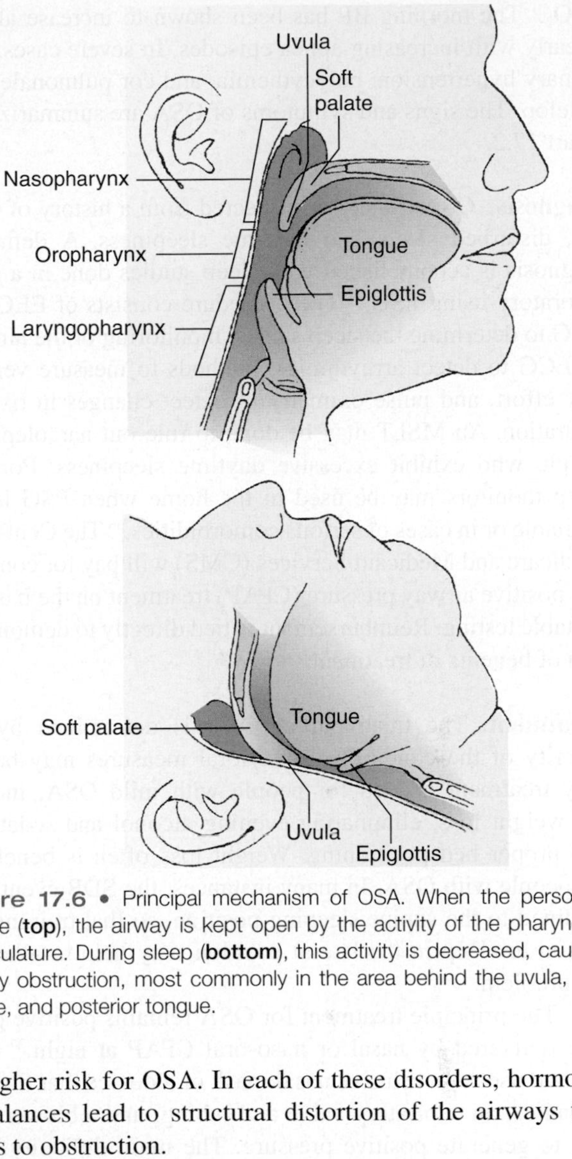

Figure 17.6 • Principal mechanism of OSA. When the person is awake (**top**), the airway is kept open by the activity of the pharyngeal musculature. During sleep (**bottom**), this activity is decreased, causing airway obstruction, most commonly in the area behind the uvula, soft palate, and posterior tongue.

at higher risk for OSA. In each of these disorders, hormonal imbalances lead to structural distortion of the airways that leads to obstruction.

Clinical Manifestations. OSA is characterized by loud snoring and labored breathing interrupted by periods of silence soon followed by apnea.[1,34] Abnormal gross motor movements during sleep are common. In many cases, the snoring precedes by many years the onset of other signs of sleep apnea. The most common presenting symptoms are persistent and excessive daytime sleepiness and a history of snoring. Other symptoms include morning headache, memory and judgment problems, irritability, difficulty concentrating, and depression. People with OSA are more likely to fall asleep at inappropriate times and have higher rates of automobile and work-related accidents. Men may complain of impotence. In children, a decline in school performance may be the only indication of the problem.

Increased sympathetic activity can lead to an increased risk of cardiovascular disease.[1] OSA is associated with sleep-related cardiac arrhythmias, hypertension, and heart failure. Frequent apneic periods may result in increased systemic and pulmonary BPs and significant decreases in PO_2 and increased

PCO_2.[1] The morning BP has been shown to increase almost linearly with increasing apnea episodes. In severe cases, pulmonary hypertension, polycythemia, and cor pulmonale may develop. The signs and symptoms of OSA are summarized in Chart 17.2.

Diagnosis. OSA usually is suspected from a history of snoring, disturbed sleep, and daytime sleepiness. A definitive diagnosis is accomplished with sleep studies done in a sleep laboratory using PSG.[33] The procedure consists of EEG and EOG to determine the sleep stages, monitoring of the airflow, an ECG to detect arrhythmias, methods to measure ventilatory effort, and pulse oximetry to detect changes in oxygen saturation. An MSLT may be done to rule out narcolepsy in people who exhibit excessive daytime sleepiness. Portable sleep monitors may be used in the home when PSG is not available or in cases of serious comorbidities.[35] The Center for Medicare and Medicaid Services (CMS) will pay for continuous positive airway pressure (CPAP) treatment on the basis of portable testing. Reimbursement is tied directly to demonstration of benefits of treatment.[36]

Treatment. The treatment of OSA is determined by the severity of the condition. Behavioral measures may be the only treatment needed for people with mild OSA, including weight loss, eliminating evening alcohol and sedatives, and proper bed positioning. Weight loss often is beneficial for people with OSA. In many instances, the SDB events are confined to the supine sleeping position, so that training the person to sleep in the lateral position may help to alleviate the problem.

The principle treatment for OSA remains positive pressure delivered by nasal or naso-oral CPAP at night.[37] This method uses an occlusive nasal mask or a device that fits into the nares, an expiratory valve and tubing, and a blower system to generate positive pressure. The main difficulty with CPAP is that many people find it unacceptable. Common complaints include dryness of the mouth, claustrophobia, and noise.

CHART 17.2 SIGNS AND SYMPTOMS OF OBSTRUCTIVE SLEEP APNEA

- Excessive daytime sleepiness
- Noisy snoring
- Observed apnea
- Insomnia
- Heartburn
- Nocturia
- Morning headaches
- Dry mouth
- Erectile dysfunction
- Hypertension

Oral or dental appliances that displace the tongue forward and move the mandible to a more anterior and forward position may be an option for persons with mild to moderate OSA and those who don't tolerate CPAP treatment.[37] People who snore but do not have sleep apnea also may use these devices. They should be fitted by a dentist or orthodontist experienced in their use. Side effects of the devices include excessive salivation and temporomandibular joint discomfort.

Several surgical procedures have been used to correct airway obstruction, including nasal septoplasty (*i.e.*, repair of the nasal septum) and uvulopalatopharyngoplasty (*i.e.*, excision of excess soft tissue on the palate, uvula, and posterior pharyngeal wall). Both of these procedures have met with limited success. Severe cases of sleep apnea may require a tracheostomy (*i.e.*, surgical placement of a tube into the trachea for the purpose of maintaining an open airway). The tracheostomy tube remains occluded during the day and is opened during the night.

Obesity Hypoventilation Disorder. Obesity hypoventilation disorder (OHD) is also known as the pickwickian syndrome, named after the fat boy in Charles Dickens' *The Posthumous Papers of the Pickwick Club*, published in 1837, is characterized by obesity, hypersomnolence, periodic breathing, hypoxemia, and right-sided heart failure. The American Academy of Sleep Medicine advises against referring to this disorder as pickwickian syndrome.[5] This condition is now called obesity hypoventilation syndrome (OHS). OHS is defined as follows:

1. A BMI ≥ 30 kg/m^2
2. Chronic hypoventilation leading to hypoxia and hypercapnia when awake
3. Hypoventilation that is not due to lung parenchymal or airway disease

Parasomnias

Parasomnias are undesirable episodes or behaviors that occur during sleep.[5] They include nightmares, sleepwalking (somnambulism), and sleep terrors. Sleepwalking, sleep terrors, and bed-wetting often are seen in children and may be considered normal to some degree at a certain age. They are less common in adults and may be indicative of other pathologic processes. For example, sleepwalking and sleep terrors may occur in people with poorly controlled cardiac insufficiency after myocardial infarction. In rare cases, sleepwalking and sleep terrors may be the first sign of a slowly evolving brain tumor. Finally, sleepwalking and sleep terrors may be triggered by disorders interacting with the sleep–wake cycle. Particularly in older adults, health problems such as a febrile illness may enhance NREM sleep nightmares, sleep terrors, and sleepwalking.

Nightmare Disorder

Nightmares are vivid and terrifying nocturnal episodes in which the dreamer is abruptly awakened from sleep. Usually there is difficulty returning to sleep. Nightmares significantly affect 10% to 50% of children between 3 and 5 years of age to the degree that parents are disturbed.[5] About half of adults admit to an occasional nightmare; 1% of adults report having a nightmare at least once a week.[26] Most nightmares occur during REM sleep. Most REM-altering disorders and medications that affect REM sleep affect dreaming.

Nightmares are a defining symptom of posttraumatic stress disorder (PTSD).[19] These nightmares occur after intensely frightening or highly emotional experiences and are associated with disturbed sleep and daytime hyperarousability. People with PTSD report awakening from dreams that involve reliving the trauma. The frequency of PTSD nightmares increases with the severity of trauma, and they can persist for long periods after the traumatic experience.

Sleepwalking and Sleep Terrors

Sleepwalking and sleep terrors usually occur during stages 3 and 4 of NREM sleep. Because stages 3 and 4 are more prolonged during the first third of the night, sleepwalking and sleep terrors usually occur during this time.[38] Sleep terrors are characterized by sudden, loud, terrified screaming and prominent autonomic nervous system activation (tachycardia, tachypnea, diaphoresis, and mydriasis). Sleepwalking is characterized by complex automatic behaviors, such as aimless wandering, furniture rearranging, urinating in closets, and going outdoors. During a typical episode, the sleepwalker appears dazed and relatively unresponsive to the communication efforts of others. On awakening, there may be a brief period of confusion or disorientation. The sleepwalker usually has no memory or only a vague awareness of what has happened. Lifetime prevalence of sleepwalking is 6.9% most commonly occurring in childhood. In a recent study, the current prevalence (over a 12-month period) of sleepwalking was 5% in children and 1.5% in adults suggesting very few people begin sleepwalking in adulthood.[39] Sleep deprivation, use of sedatives, alternations in sleep schedule, and stress are associated with sleep terrors and sleepwalking in adults.[5]

Diagnosis and treatment of sleepwalking and sleep terrors depends on age. Because most children eventually outgrow the disorders, parents may simply need to be reassured and instructed in safety measures. Insufficient sleep may precipitate episodes of sleepwalking. Therefore, parents should make certain that the child goes to bed on time and gets enough sleep. In adults, a through medical, psychiatric, and sleep history should be done to eliminate other causes of the disorder, such as Parkinson disease, hyperthyroidism, and migraine.[40] Because sleepwalking can be dangerous, it is important that the environment be safe. Dangerous objects should be removed, and bolts should be placed on doors and windows. No attempt should be made to interrupt the sleepwalking event because such efforts may be frightening.

Pharmacologic treatment of sleepwalking includes the selective use of the BZDs (particularly diazepam and clonazepam)[41,42] or the tricyclic antidepressant imipramine.[43] In older adults, treatment focuses on reversing the underlying causes of delirium. Because medications are a frequent cause of delirium in older adults, a complete drug history should be done with the intent of eliminating medications that might be causing the disorder.

IN SUMMARY

Sleep disorders include the circadian rhythm sleep disorders, insomnias, narcolepsy, sleep-related movement disorders, sleep apnea, and the parasomnias. Sleep problems due to *alterations in circadian rhythm* are related to intrinsic factors (N24SWRD, ISWR, ASPD, and DSPD) and acute shifts in the sleep–wake cycle (jet lag and shift work). *Insomnia* represents a subjective problem of insufficient sleep and impairment in daytime functioning despite an adequate opportunity to sleep. It includes acute and chronic problems in falling asleep and maintaining sleep, or waking up too early with consequences such as fatigue, decreased concentration, attention, and memory, and impaired performance in social or work situations.

Narcolepsy is a disorder of daytime sleep attacks, hallucinations occurring at the onset of sleep, and sleep paralysis. Narcolepsy may occur with or without cataplexy. Among the *movement disorders* that occur during sleep are PLMD and RLS. PLMD is characterized by episodes of repetitive movement of the large toe with flexion of the ankle, knee, and hip during sleep, usually involving both legs. RLS is a neurologic disorder characterized by an irresistible urge to move the legs, usually owing to a "creeping," "crawling," or uncomfortable sensation. It usually is worse during periods of inactivity and often interferes with sleep.

Obstructive sleep apnea (OSA) is a serious, potentially life-threatening disorder characterized by brief periods of apnea or breathing cessation during sleep, loud snoring interrupted by periods of silence, and abnormal gross motor movements. It is accompanied by complaints of persistent daytime sleepiness, morning headache, memory and judgment problems, irritability, difficulty concentrating, and depression. OSA also is associated with sleep-related cardiac arrhythmias, hypertension, and heart failure. The parasomnias are undesirable physical phenomena that occur almost exclusively during sleep or are exaggerated by sleep. They include nightmares, sleepwalking, and sleep terrors.

SLEEP AND SLEEP DISORDERS IN CHILDREN AND OLDER ADULTS

After completing this section of the chapter, the learner will be able to meet the following objectives:

- Characterize normal sleep patterns of infants and small children and relate them to the development of sleep disorders.
- Describe the normal changes in sleep stages that occur with aging and relate them to sleep problems in the older adults.

Sleep patterns change as the brain develops in the fetus and neonate, matures during adolescence and early adulthood, and begins to decline with aging.

Sleep and Sleep Disorders in Children

Sleep Patterns in Children

A child's circadian rhythms and sleep patterns are established early in life. The first behavioral manifestations of sleep patterns occur between 28 and 30 weeks of gestation, when movement of the fetus is interrupted by periods of quiet.[44] At 32 weeks, periods of quiescence begin to occur at regular intervals, suggesting the beginnings of a sleep–wake cycle.

Newborns (0 to 2 months) usually sleep approximately 16 to 20 hours/day. Equally distributed over night- and daytime, sleep periods generally last 1 to 4 hours interspersed with 1- to 2-hour periods of wakefulness.[45] Initially, sleep–wake patterns are based on hunger. Around 2 to 4 months of age, circadian rhythms are developed. The sleep states of infants are slightly different than older children and adults. Infants have three basic sleep states: "active (REM-like; 50% of sleep), quiet (NREM-like), and intermediate (with features of both)."[45] Although infants have some capacity to concentrate sleep in one part of the day, this capacity must be developed in the weeks after birth. As development progresses, the infant is able to concentrate sleep during the night and remain awake for longer periods during the day. As the cyclic structure of the sleep–wake cycle progresses, the amount of time spent in REM sleep decreases. By the time the child is 6 months of age, three distinct stages of NREM sleep occur.

Sleep Disorders in Children

Although sleep complaints are common among adults, children usually do not complain about sleep problems, although their parents might. The usual concerns of parents include irregular sleep habits, insufficient or too much sleep, nightmares, sleep terrors, sleepwalking, and bed-wetting. Complaints of excessive daytime sleepiness or sleep attacks not accounted for by an inadequate amount of sleep may be due to a more serious health or sleep problem (*e.g.*, narcolepsy). In these cases, a careful sleep history, physical examination, and other diagnostic tests may be needed. Three of the more common sleep problems of children are discussed in this section of the chapter, including sleep terrors, confusional arousals, and sleepwalking.

Sleep Terrors. Sleep terrors are marked by repeated episodes of awakening from slow-wave (stage 3) sleep. They usually occur during the first third of the night; most are brief, but they may last for up to 40 minutes.[5] Sleep terrors are most common in early childhood. In one study, the prevalence was 34.4% at 1½ years, decreased to 13.4% at 5 years, and was 5.3% at 13 years.[46] The disorder gradually resolves in children and usually disappears during adolescence. The course is variable, usually occurring at intervals of days or weeks. In a typical episode, the child sits up abruptly in bed, appears frightened, and demonstrates signs of extreme anxiety, including dilated pupils, excessive perspiration, rapid breathing, and tachycardia. Until the agitation and confusion subsides, efforts to comfort or help the child are futile. There usually is no memory of the episode. Occasionally, the child recounts a sense of terror on being aroused during a night terror, but there is only fragmentary recall of dreamlike images. Treatment consists primarily of educating and reassuring the family. The child should be assisted in settling down without awakening. The child must be protected if he or she gets up and walks about during the episodes.

Confusional Arousals. Confusional arousals are common affecting 17.3% of children aged 3 to 13 years.[5] They usually occur during the first third of the night when the brain is partially asleep while remaining partially awake. During these events, children present with marked confusion, slow and inappropriate responses to questions, and nonpurposeful activities. They do not express fear, terror, or panic. Children spontaneously return to sleep and have no recollection of the event in the morning. Recovery from sleep deprivation tends to increase the incidence of confusional arousals.

Sleepwalking. Sleepwalking, common in children between the ages of 5 and 12 years, involves repeated episodes of complex motor movements that lead to leaving the bed and walking without the child being conscious of the episode or remembering that it occurred.[12] As with sleep terrors, it normally occurs in NREM sleep stages 3 and 4 during the first third of the sleep period.

A sleepwalking episode typically lasts for a few minutes to half an hour, during which time the child sits up; makes purposeful movements such as picking at the bed coverings; and then proceeds to semipurposeful movements such as getting out of bed, walking around, opening doors, dressing, or going to the bathroom. Often they end up in the parent's bedroom. Commonly, they are unresponsive to the efforts of others to communicate with them. Confusion and disorientation are typical of the events, and on awakening, there is no memory of the event. There may be manifestations of extreme autonomic nervous system activity such as tachycardia, rapid breathing, perspiration, and urination.

Sleepwalking is reported in approximately 5% of children.[39] Frequent sleepwalking events, defined as one to four times a week, occur in 1% to 6% of children.[47] It occurs more frequently in children in whom there is a family history of sleepwalking. Sleepwalking can begin as soon as the child is able to walk and may start at any age. Children who sleepwalk usually stop doing so by the time they reach puberty. The primary concern is injury during an episode. Children may bump into things, fall down stairs, or even leave their home during an episode. Therefore, gates should be placed across stairs and windows and doors should be locked so the child cannot leave the house.

Sleep and Sleep Disorders in Older Adults

Complaints of difficulty sleeping occur in over 50% of adults aged 65 years and older, and 30% of older adults experience chronic insominia.[9] However, this increased prevalence should not be expected as a phenomenon of aging. Instead, the difficulties with sleeping are often the result of medical and psychosocial comorbidities.[19] The consequences of chronic sleep problems in older adults can be considerable. Left uncorrected, a sleep disorder affects the quality of life. Loss of sleep and use of sedating medications may lead to falls and accidents. Sleep-related disorders of breathing may have serious cardiovascular, pulmonary, and CNS effects.

There are a number of changes that occur in the sleep–wake cycle as a person ages. Older adults have repeated and frequent interruptions of sleep with longer periods of wakefulness along with a shorter duration of stages 3 and 4 and REM sleep.[2] Additionally, the deepest stages of NREM sleep frequently are reduced.[2,9] Compared with younger people, adults in their 70s need 30 to 60 minutes less sleep than adults in their 20s.[9] They often take longer to fall asleep, they awaken earlier, and they have more nighttime arousals. Environmental influences, particularly auditory stimuli, often are more disruptive in older adults. With an increase in nighttime wakefulness, there is an increase in daytime fatigue and daytime napping. An often-overlooked cause of nocturnal awakenings in the older adult population is nocturia or need to urinate during the night.

The causes of sleep disorders in older adults include age-related changes in sleep architecture, secondary sleep disturbances, primary sleep disorders, lack of exercise, and poor sleep habits. Factors that predispose to secondary sleep disturbances include physical and mental illness, medication effects, and emotional stress. A variety of medical illnesses contribute to sleep disorders in older adults, including arthritic pain, respiratory problems, cardiac disease, and neurologic disorders. Nightmares and nighttime fears are common in older adults with Parkinson disease, particularly those who are receiving levodopa. Psychiatric illness, such as depression, is a common cause of disturbed sleep in this age group. Primary sleep disorders such as sleep apnea, RLS, and PLMD also increase in old age. Many medications used to treat chronic medical and psychiatric conditions have stimulating effects and interfere with sleep. These include some of the antidepressants, decongestants, bronchodilators, corticosteroids, and antihypertensives. Alcohol use also may serve as a deterrent to sleep in older adults. Sleep–wake problems may be compounded further by inappropriate interventions initiated by the older adult, his or her family, or health care providers.

Sleep also is disturbed in disorders characterized by dementia. Episodes of nocturnal wandering, confusion, and delirium can occur despite normal daytime functioning. People with Alzheimer disease often have increased periods of nighttime awakening and daytime napping.

Diagnosis of sleep disorders in older adults requires a comprehensive sleep history, inquiries about pain and anxiety or depression, review of current sleep hygiene practices, drug use history, spousal or bed partner reports, a comprehensive physical examination, and appropriate laboratory tests.[9] Interventions to assist the older adult include education about good sleep habits. The development of a sleep ritual is essential.[9] Treatment of a medical disorder and changes in medication regimes and timing of medication doses can often improve sleep. Avoidance of alcohol and stimulants before bedtime and improving sleep hygiene are other measures that can be used to improve sleep. Although hypnotics can be used to treat transient insomnia, they often fail to provide long-term relief of chronic sleep disturbances.

IN SUMMARY

Circadian rhythms and sleep patterns are established early in life. In the newborn, REM sleep occurs at sleep onset, and periods of sleep and awakening are distributed throughout the day. As the cyclic structure of the sleep–wake cycle progresses, the amount of time spent in REM sleep decreases. By the time the child is 6 months of age, three distinct stages of NREM sleep occur. At 9 months, about 70% to 80% of infants sleep through the night and may nap at predictable times during the day. Although sleep complaints are common among adults, children usually do not complain about sleep problems, although their parents might. The usual concerns of parents include irregular sleep habits, insufficient or too much sleep, nightmares, sleep terrors, and sleepwalking.

Complaints of sleep disorders are common in older adults. The sleep–wake cycle changes that occur with aging are evidenced by more fragmented sleep and shorter duration of stage 3 and stage 4 sleep. Older adults also have more health problems that interrupt sleep, they are apt to be on medications that interfere with sleep, and they are more likely to have sleep disorders such as insomnia, RLS, and sleep-disturbed breathing. Left uncorrected, sleep disorders in older adults affect the quality of life. Loss of sleep and use of sedating medications may lead to falls and accidents.

GERIATRIC Considerations

- Older adults frequently have sleep problems, such as sleep apnea and insomnia. These problems are often unrecognized and undertreated. Older adults usually experience insomnia symptoms for several years before receiving a formal diagnosis.[48]
- Negative consequences of insomnia in late life include decreased quality of life, risk for falls, psychological and physical difficulties, economic and social costs, risk for nursing home placement, and mortality.[48]
- Significant changes occur in sleep with advancing age, with a reduction in total sleep time from an average of 8.9 hours (young adults) to 7.4 (older adults), and an increase in nocturnal awake time.[49]
- Are changes in sleep quality part of the normal aging process or due to comorbidities that accompany aging?[50] Geriatric people often experience insomnia because of physiologic and neurologic changes that occur during the aging process.[51]

PEDIATRIC Considerations

- The irregular sleep schedule of newborns is due to the immature circadian rhythm regulated by light and dark.[52]
- Nighttime fears and nightmares are common among toddlers and preschoolers.[52]
- School-age children still need 9 to 11 hours of sleep; because of their interest in technology and caffeine, sleep issues are common.[52]
- Active sleep of the neonate and term infant mimics the adult rapid eye movement sleep cycle, which may take on characteristics such as smiling and sucking. Quiet sleep of the neonate and term infant correlates with the non–rapid eye movement sleep of adults with regular heart rate and respirations.[53]

REVIEW EXERCISES

1. A frustrated mother complains that her teenage son stays up at night and then has trouble waking up and getting to school on time.
   A. *Is there a developmental explanation for these behaviors?*
   B. *What suggestions would you make to this mother?*
2. A 30-year-old woman presents with complaints of fatigue, irritability, and difficulty concentrating. She relates that for the past 3 months or more, she has had difficulty falling asleep and staying asleep despite remaining in bed and focusing on measures to help her sleep. She laughingly tells you she has even tried counting sheep.
   A. *What type of diagnostic measure would prove useful in determining whether this woman's problem is related to insomnia?*
   B. *If the woman is diagnosed with insomnia, what type of treatment would be indicated?*

References

1. Hall J. E. (2016). *Guyton and Hall Textbook of medical physiology* (13th ed., pp. 738, 763–767). Philadelphia, PA: Elsevier.
2. Barrett K. E., Barman S. M., Boitano S., et al. (2016). *Ganong's review of medical physiology* (25th ed., pp. 272–275). New York, NY: McGraw Hill Education.
3. Sherwood L. (2016). *Human physiology: From cells to systems* (9th ed., pp. 168–172). Boston, MA: Cengage Learning.
4. Carskadon M. A., Dement W. C. (2016). Normal human sleep: An overview. In Kryger M. H., Roth T., Dement W. C. (Eds.), *Principles and practice of sleep medicine* (6th ed.). St. Louis, MO: Elsevier Saunders.
5. American Academy of Sleep Medicine. (2014). *International classification of sleep disorders: Diagnostic and coding manual* (3rd ed.). Darien, IL: Author.
6. Lambon Ralph M., Tamminen J., Tamminen J., et al. (n.d). The role of sleep spindles and slow-wave activity in integrating new information in semantic memory. *Journal of Neuroscience* 33(39), 15376–15381.
7. Heinzer R. C., Sériés F. (2016). Physiology of the upper and lower airways. In Kryger M. H., Roth T., Dement W. C. (Eds.), *Principles and practice of sleep medicine* (6th ed., pp. 174–185). St. Louis, MO: Elsevier Saunders.
8. Potter G. D. M., Skene D. J., Arendt J., et al. (2016). Circadian Rhythm and Sleep Disruption: Causes, Metabolic Consequences, and Countermeasures. *Endocrine Reviews* 37(6), 584–608. Available: http://doi.org.ezproxy.uthsc.edu/10.1210/er.2016-1083.
9. Delgado D., Canham L., Cotterill N., et al. (2017). Protocol for a randomized, double blind, placebo controlled, crossover trial of Melatonin for treatment of Nocturia in adults with Multiple Sclerosis (MeNiMS). *BMC Neurology* 17(1), 63. doi:10.1186/s12883-017-0845-y.
10. Reid K. J., Abbott S. M. (2015). Jet lag and shift work disorder. *Sleep Medicine Clinics* 10(4), 523–535. doi:http://dx.doi.org/10.1016/j.jsmc.2015.08.006.
11. Sateia M. J., Buysse D. J., Krystal A. D., et al. 2017. Clinical practice guideline for the pharmacologic treatment of chronic insomnia in adults: An American Academy of Sleep Medicine clinical practice guideline. *Journal of Clinical Sleep Medicine* 13(2):307–349.
12. Marino M., Li Y., Rueschman M. N., et al. (2013). Measuring sleep: Accuracy, sensitivity, and specificity of wrist actigraphy compared to polysomnography. *Sleep* 36(11), 1747–1755. Available: http://doi.org/10.5665/sleep.3142.
13. Meltzer L. J., Walsh C. M., Peightal A. A. (2015). Comparison of actigraphy immobility rules with polysomnographic sleep onset latency in children and adolescents. *Sleep & Breathing = Schlaf & Atmung* 19(4), 1415–1423. Available: http://doi.org/10.1007/s11325-015-1138-6.
14. Uchiyama M., Lockley S. (2015). Non-24-Hour Sleep-Wake Rhythm Disorder in sighted and blind patients. *Sleep Medicine Clinics of North America* 10, 495–516. doi:http://dx.doi.org/10.1016/j.jsmc2015.07.006.
15. Lack L., Wright H. (2012). Circadian rhythm disorders I: Phase-advanced & phase-delayed syndromes. In Morin C. M., Espie C. A. (Eds.), *The Oxford Handbook of Sleep and Sleep Disorders*. Oxford University Press. Retrieved October 15, 2017, from http://www.oxfordhandbooks.com/view/10.1093/oxfordhb/9780195376203.001.0001/oxfordhb-9780195376203-e-028.
16. Auger R. R., Burgess H. J., Emens J. S., et al. (2015). Clinical Practice Guideline for the Treatment of Intrinsic Circadian Rhythm Sleep-Wake Disorders: Advanced Sleep-Wake Phase Disorder (ASWPD), Delayed Sleep-Wake Phase Disorder (DSWPD), Non-24-Hour Sleep-Wake Rhythm Disorder (N24SWD), and Irregular Sleep-Wake Rhythm Disorder (ISWRD). An Update for 2015. *Journal of Sleep Medicine* 11(10), 1199–1236. doi:http://dx.doi.org/10.5664/jcsm.5100.
17. Auger R., Burgess H., Emens J., et al. (2015). Clinical Practice Guideline for the Treatment of Intrinsic Circadian Rhythm Sleep-Wake Disorders: Advanced Sleep-Wake Phase Disorder (ASWPD), Delayed Sleep-Wake Phase Disorder (DSWPD), Non-24-Hour Sleep-Wake Rhythm Disorder (N24SWD), and Irregular Sleep-Wake Rhythm Disorder (ISWRD). An Update for 2015. *Journal of Clinical Sleep Medicine* 11(10), 1199–1236. doi:10.5664/jcsm.5100.
18. Costa G. (2016). Sleep deprivation due to shift work. *Handbook of Clinical Neurology* 131, 437–446.
19. American Psychiatric Association. (2013). *Diagnostic and statistical manual of mental disorders. Text revision* (45th ed.). Washington, DC: Author.
20. National Guideline Clearinghouse. (2016). *Guideline Summary: Management of Chronic Insomnia Disorder in Adults: A Clinical Practice Guideline from the American College of Physicians*. Agency for Research and Healthcare Quality. Retrieved from: http://www.guideline.gov.
21. Mor M., Bedini A., Spadoni G., et al. (n.d). Pharmacokinetic and pharmacodynamic evaluation of ramelteon: An insomnia therapy. *Expert Opinion on Drug Metabolism and Toxicology* 11(7), 1145–1156.
22. Ahmed I., Thorpy M. (2010). Clinical features, diagnosis, and treatment of narcolepsy. *Clinics in Chest Medicine* 31, 371–381. doi:10.1016/j.ccm.2010.02.014.

23. Bidaki R., Zarei M., Toosi A., et al. (2012). A review on genetics of sleep disorders. *Iranian Journal of Psychiatry and Behavioral Sciences* 6(1), 12–19.
24. Liblau R. S., Vassalli A., Seifinejad A., et al. (2015). Hypocretin (orexin) biology and the pathophysiology of narcolepsy with cataplexy. *Lancet* 14, 318–328.
25. Leschziner G. (2014). Narcolepsy: A clinical review. *Practical Neurology* 14, 323–331.
26. Zak R. S., Mallea J. M., Aurora R. N. (2011). Management of parasomnias. In Avidan A. Y., Zee P. C. (Eds.), *Handbook of sleep medicine* (2nd ed., pp. 177–190). Philadelphia, PA: Lippincott Williams & Wilkins.
27. Malhotra R. K., Avidan A. Y. (2012). Parasomnias and their mimics. *Neurologic Clinics* 304, 1067–1094.
28. Lanfranchi P. A., Somers V. K. (2016). Cardiovascular physiology: Autonomic control in health and in sleep disorders. In Kryger M. H., Roth T., Dement W. C. (Eds.), *Principles and practice of sleep medicine* (6th ed., pp. 226–236). St. Louis, MO: Elsevier Saunders.
29. Allen R. P., Montplaisir J., Walters A., et al. (2016). Restless legs syndrome and periodic limb movements during sleep. In Kryger M. H., Roth T., Dement W. C. (Eds.), *Principles and practice of sleep medicine* (6th ed., pp. 923–934). St. Louis, MO: Elsevier Saunders.
30. National Institute of Neurological Disorders and Stroke. (2017). Restless legs syndrome fact sheet. [Online]. Available: https://www.ninds.nih.gov/Disorders/Patient-Caregiver-Education/Fact-Sheets/Restless-Legs-Syndrome-Fact-Sheet.
31. Sateia M. J., Thorpy M. J. (2016). Classification of sleep disorders. In Kryger M. H., Roth T., Dement W. C. (Eds.), *Principles and practice of sleep medicine* (6th ed., pp. 618–625). St. Louis, MO: Elsevier Saunders.
32. Philips B. (2011). Sleep-disordered breathing. In Avidan A. Y., Zee P. C. (Eds.), *Handbook of sleep medicine* (2nd ed., pp. 13–29). Philadelphia, PA: Lippincott Williams & Wilkins.
33. Zinchuk A. V., Thomas R. J. (2016). Central sleep apnea: Diagnosis and management. In Kryger M. H., Roth T., Dement W. C. (Eds.), *Principles and practice of sleep medicine* (6th ed., pp. 1059–1075). St. Louis, MO: Elsevier Saunders.
34. Guilleminault C., Takaoka S. (2016). Signs and symptoms of obstructive sleep apnea and upper airway resistance syndrome. In Kryger M. H., Roth T., Dement W. C. (Eds.), *Principles and practice of sleep medicine* (6th ed., pp. 3–10). St. Louis, MO: Elsevier Saunders.
35. National Guideline Clearinghouse. (2013). *Diagnosis of obstructive sleep apnea in adults: A clinical practice guideline from the American Colleges of Physicians*. Retrieved from: http://www.guideline.gov.
36. Centers for Medicare and Medicaid Services. (2015). Decision memo for continuous positive airway pressure (CPAP) therapy for obstructive sleep apnea (OSA) (CAG-00093R2). [Online]. Available: https://www.cms.gov/Medicare/Coverage/Coverage-with-Evidence-Development/Continuous-Positive-Airway-Pressure-CPAP-Therapy-For-Obstructive-Sleep-Apnea-OSA-2404.html.
37. National Guideline Clearinghouse. (2013). *Management of obstructive sleep apnea in adults: A clinical practice guideline from the American Colleges of Physicians*. Retrieved from: http://www.guideline.gov.
38. Fleetham J. A., Fleming J. A. E. (2014). Parasomnias. *Canadian Medical Association Journal* 186(8), E273–E280. Available: http://doi.org/10.1503/cmaj.120808.
39. Stallman H. M., Kohler M. (2016). Prevalence of sleepwalking: A systematic review and meta-analysis. *PLoS One* 11(11), e0164769. doi:10.1371/journal.pone.0164769.
40. American Academy of Sleep Medicine (2017). *Sleep walking-overview and facts*. Available: http://www.sleepeducation.org/sleep-disorders-by-category/parasomnias/sleepwalking/symptoms-risk-factors.
41. Hodoba D., Schmidt D. (2012). Biperiden for treatment of somnambulism in adolescents and adults with or without epilepsy: Clinical observations. *Epilepsy & Behavior* 25, 517–528.
42. Cochen De Cock V. (2016). Sleepwalking. *Current Treatment Options in Neurology* 18(6), 1–9. doi:10.1007/s11940-015-0388-8.
43. Reiter J., Rosen D. (2014). The diagnosis and management of common sleep disorders in adolescents. *Current Opinion in Pediatrics* 26, 407–412. doi:10.1097/MOP.0000000000000113.
44. Bathory E., Tomopoulos S. (2017). Sleep regulation, physiology and development, sleep duration and patterns, and sleep hygiene in infants, toddlers, and pre-school age children. *Current Problems in Pediatric and Adolescent Health Care* 47(2), 29–42.
45. Davis K. F., Owens J. A. (2011). Sleep disorders in children. In Avidan A. Y., Zee P. C. (Eds.), *Handbook of sleep medicine* (2nd ed., pp. 239–260). Philadelphia, PA: Lippincott Williams & Wilkins.
46. Petit D., Pennestri M., Paquet J., et al. (2015). Childhood sleepwalking and sleep terrors: A longitudinal study of prevalence and familial aggregation. *JAMA Pediatrics* 169(7), 653–658. doi:10.1001/jamapediatrics.2015.127.
47. Carter K. A., Hathaway N. E., Lettieri C. F. (2014). Common sleep disorders in children. *American Family Physician* 89(5), 368–377.
48. Rodriguez J. C., Dzierzewski J. M., Alessi C. A. (2015). Sleep problems in the elderly. *Medical Clinics North America* 99(2), 431–439. Available: https://www.ncbi.nlm.nih.gov/pmc/articles/PMC4406253.
49. Gooneratne N. S., Vitiello M. V. (2014). Sleep in older adults: Normative changes, sleep disorders, and treatment options. *Clinics in Geriatric Medicine* 30(3), 591–627.
50. Jordan A., Edwards B., Edwards B. A., et al. (n.d.). Aging and sleep: Physiology and pathophysiology. *Seminars in Respiratory and Critical Care Medicine* 31(5), 618–633.
51. Edmonds C., Swanoski M. A review of suvorexant, doxepin, ramelteon, and tasimelteon for the treatment of insomnia in geriatric patients. *Consultant Pharmacist* 2017 32(3):156–160. doi:10.4140/TCP.n.2017.156.
52. National Sleep Foundation. (2017). Children and sleep. Available: https://sleepfoundation.org/sleep-topics/children-and-sleep.
53. Scraggs T. L. (2012). EEG maturation: Viability through adolescence. *Neurodiagnostic Journal* 52, 176–203.

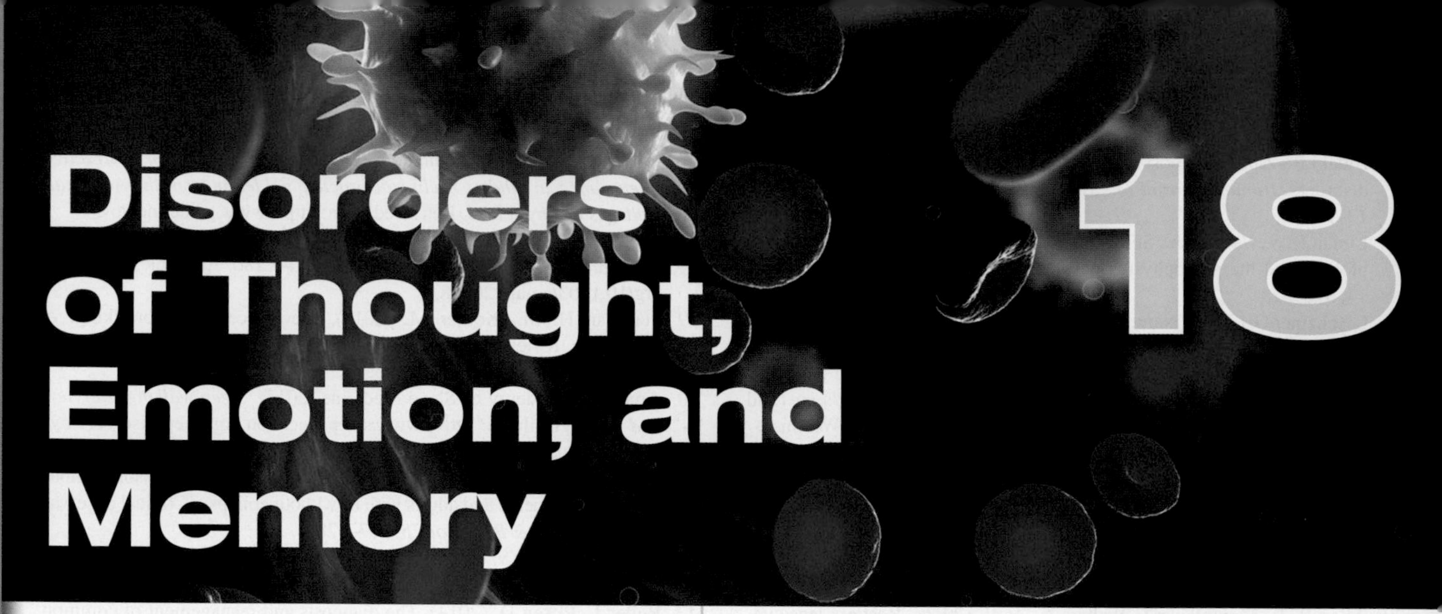

Disorders of Thought, Emotion, and Memory

18

Elizabeth M. Long

The purpose of this chapter is to present both the pathophysiology of common psychiatric disorders, also referred to as mental illness, and orders of memory and cognition. These disorders are characterized by imbalances of thought, mood, and/or behaviors, which interfere with people's ability to function. The Diagnostic and Statistical Manual of Mental Disorders (*DSM-5*) is an evidence-based manual recognizing 297 different diagnoses of mental illness.[1] Please consult that source for specific criteria for each disorder discussed in this chapter. There is a 17.9% prevalence of mental illness among US adults,[2] highlighting the need for a clear understanding of these disorders and appropriate evidence-based treatments.

PSYCHIATRIC DISORDERS

After completing this section of the chapter, the learner will be able to meet the following objectives:

- Identify the prevalence of mental illness across the life span.
- Discuss the role of biologic, psychological, and environmental factors in the disorders of thought and emotion.
- Identify the effect of specific neurochemicals in the development of disorders of thought and emotion.

Incidence and Prevalence

Mental health affects how well our brain and body function, how we handle stress, and how we relate to others, and also, it affects our ability to work and enjoy life. Mental illness is common among Americans with one in five experiencing the consequences of a psychiatric disorder in any given year. One in 25 adults lives with serious mental illness, such as schizophrenia, bipolar disorder, or major depression. Children are not exempt. Fifty percent of all chronic mental illness begins before age 14, and 75% begins by age 24.[3] Importantly, 30% of people with a physical disorder have a coexisting psychiatric disorder.[4] Fifty percent of people with a substance use disorder have a coexisting psychiatric disorder.[2,3]

The Diagnosis of Psychiatric Disorders

Psychiatric diagnoses are made using the *Diagnostic and Statistical Manual of Mental Disorders (DSM-5)*.[1] These disorders consist of symptom categories or syndromes of observable traits often occurring together. A different international coding system developed by the World Health Organization, the *International Statistical Classification of Diseases and Related Health Problems (ICD-10)*, corresponds with some of the *DSM-5* codes.[5] Psychopathology is determined by symptoms relying on subjective judgments, based on social norms. Neuroimaging and other diagnostic tests are generally performed to rule out neurologic or medical conditions, which may be causing symptoms but are generally not diagnostic of the psychiatric disorder.

Understanding Psychiatric Disorders

There is increasing evidence psychiatric disorders can be caused by multiple causes: biologic, psychological, and environmental conditions or a combination of these factors. Biologic factors consist of genetics, infections, brain defects or injury, poor nutrition, exposure to toxins, or abnormalities in fetal development. Psychological factors include stress, early loss of a parent, or neglect. Environmental factors may involve dysfunctional family dynamics, cultural expectations, and substance use.

The Role of Genetics

Epigenetics, the study of heritable changes in gene expression not involving changes to the underlying DNA sequence, involves a change in phenotype without a change in genotype, which affects how cells read genes without changing the DNA. Endophenotypes is a term used to describe specific phenotypes with a clear genetic connection to psychiatric illness. Research using endophenotypes suggests that multiple pathways contribute to psychiatric diagnosis.[6–11]

The Stress–Diathesis Theory

The stress–diathesis model of psychiatric disorders evolved from a recognition that genetics (diathesis) and environment (stress) both contribute to the development of psychiatric disorders.[10] Large-scale epidemiologic and case-controlled studies suggest trauma because of a variety of reasons underlies a wide range of psychiatric disorders as well as medical illness.[12] The body's response and the long-term consequences of a disturbing event depend on a multitude of factors, such as age, developmental stage, coping skills, support system, cognitive deficits, preexisting neural physiology, and the nature of the trauma.[13]

The incidence of mental health problems such as obesity, sexually transmitted diseases, alcoholism, severe and persistent mental illness, psychosis, substance abuse, eating disorders, anxiety, and depression has been significantly and positively correlated with what is termed adverse childhood experiences (ACE). Prospective studies involving ACE confirm those with episodes of maternal neglect, and physical and sexual abuse were almost three times as likely to experience major depression by their early 30s. These study participants were at risk for high inflammation levels (high-sensitivity C-reactive protein level >3 mg/L) and clustering of metabolic risk biomarkers (obesity, high blood pressure, high total cholesterol, low high-density lipoprotein cholesterol, high glycated hemoglobin, and low maximum oxygen consumption levels). These physiologic changes predisposed a person to develop cardiovascular disease, doubling the risk for heart disease.[14] Long-term emotional, immune, and metabolic changes result from exposure to adverse psychosocial experiences in childhood.

Researchers have found the key pathway for these physiologic changes is the complex bodily reactions to the stress response. Trauma is different from stress. Trauma refers to events leaving a person helpless. Stress refers to a state of burdened response to outside stressors, resulting in deterioration and dysfunction. Stress responses are beneficial in mobilizing the body for action, but prolonged activation of the stress response particularly in early childhood leads to profound long-term physical changes. Early adversity has been found to alter the DNA in the brain through a process called methylation. Methyl groups affix genes that govern the production of stress hormone receptors in the brain, preventing the brain from regulating its response to stress. Research evidence suggests exposure to stress can induce long-lasting changes in DNA methylation and its relationship to the pathogenesis of some psychiatric disorders.[6,15]

Parental nurturing can mediate this epigenetic response. In the absence of nurturing, children have difficulties with attention and following directions. As teenagers, they are more likely to engage in high-risk behavior and, as adults, show increased aggression, impulsive behavior, weakened cognition, and an inability to discriminate between real and imagined threats. Traumatic events and prolonged stress are thought to underlie or contribute to wide range of psychiatric disorders and medical problems.[16]

Information Processing

Information processing systems are distributed throughout the brain and display synchronized oscillations. This synchronization allows for the creation of neural temporal maps so perception, memory, cognition, emotion, language, and sensations result from the interactions between these systems of neural networks.

Neuroplasticity is the capacity of the nervous system to change its structure and function in response to biologic, psychological, and environmental events. Psychopathology is thought to result when there is a dysregulation disrupting the integration of neural networks and plasticity. The more intense the arousal of the amygdala, the stronger the memory imprint, and the less likely the experience is processed. Neuronal circuits connect the amygdala to the prefrontal lobe in the cortex serving as the translator of the emotion so amygdala activation can be modulated.[17–19]

Perception is the final stage of information processing. Perception consists of the input of sensory information from the outside world and the processing of this information into meaning. All sensory information from the external world is transmitted to the thalamus and then projected to the somatosensory cortex and prefrontal association area. The prefrontal association area keeps track of where information has been put in long-term memory and is responsible for retrieving and then integrating memories with sensory input for decision-making. For example, visual stimuli from the retina are transmitted to centers in the thalamus through the optic nerve; from there, it is relayed to the primary visual cortex in the occipital lobe and then to the visual association cortex, where meaning is understood. It is the conscious awareness of sensory stimuli that results in behavioral responses to the sensation. For people with trauma, brain injury, or degenerative changes, information processing and cognitive function may be impaired.[18,19]

Neurochemicals

Neurochemicals and neurohormones play key roles in mediating endocrine and behavioral responses to stress. These messenger substances are made of amino acids and include hormones in the endocrine system, neurotransmitters in the autonomic nervous system (ANS), immune cells, and neuropeptides. Genes are turned off and on by these messenger molecules with more than 300 messenger molecules identified. These molecules typically are stored in vesicles in the presynaptic axonal terminal and released by the process of exocytosis. Neurotransmitters transmit signals across the synapse and activate the receptors of the postsynaptic cell and include small-molecule and neuroactive peptides. Neurotransmitters, important in the development and treatment of psychiatric disorders, are acetylcholine (ACh), dopamine (DA), glutamate, gamma-aminobutyric acid (GABA), norepinephrine (NE), epinephrine, and serotonin (5-HT). Neurotransmission involves several discrete steps including synthesis, storage and release, binding to receptors on the postsynaptic membrane, and removal of the transmitter from the synaptic cleft.[19,20]

Neurotransmitters are excitatory and/or inhibitory. Excitatory neurotransmitters such as glutamate increase the probability the target cell will fire an action potential by mediating the depolarization of the target cell. Excitatory transmitters serve as the body's stimulants promoting wakefulness, energy, and activity through regulating many of the body's most basic functions, including thought processes, higher thinking, and sympathetic (neuroexcitatory) activity. Inhibitory neurotransmitters such as GABA serve as the body's natural tranquilizers, generally serving to induce sleep, promote calmness, and decrease aggression. Acetylcholine and norepinephrine have both excitatory and inhibitory receptors and can mediate sympathetic arousal and/or agitation, as well as parasympathetic calming.[20]

An outline of selected neurochemical response patterns in stress and potential psychiatric disorders is included in Table 18.1.[18–20]

Neurohormonal factors mediate behavioral responses to stress. There is considerable evidence that the regulation of corticotropin-releasing hormone (CRH) and the hypothalamic–pituitary–adrenal (HPA) axis are essential for adaptation to stress, and traumatic experiences early in life are particularly disruptive to these systems. Elevation of CRH because of trauma early in life may cause long-term pathophysiologic changes.[21] Cortisol is released during the stress response and is an important hormone contributing to increased arousal, vigilance, inhibition of growth and reproduction, and containment of the immune response. Excessive cortisol can have serious deleterious effects on all systems of the body and plays an important role in the formation, processing, and retrieval of memories. Dehydroepiandosterone (DHEA) is another adrenal steroid released under stress along with cortisol. It is thought DHEA facilitates learning and memory and appears to enhance cognition and performance under stress.[22,23]

Memory

Memory can be classified as immediate, recent, or remote.[19] Immediate memory is typically confined to remembering information for a period of several seconds to minutes (*e.g.*, 7 to 10 digits of a telephone number). It is thought memories involve implicit information with respect to the ability to pay attention. Recent memory encompasses remembering something from minutes to days, whereas long-term memory, which lasts for years, is generally thought to result from actual structural changes in the synapses. Brain structures critical to the formation of memories include the amygdala, the hippocampus, the prefrontal cortex, and the cerebellum.[19]

Memory is stored in neural networks across the brain, and these connections are linked together and organized around associated emotions, thoughts, images, and sensations. These interconnected biochemical and neuronal networks serve as templates for future experiences depending on how the memory was perceived and stored in the brain. Pathways of neurons are shaped by experience and continually revised by new and ongoing experiences depending on plasticity of the specific brain structure.

Behavior is altered by environmental cues processed through learning and memory. Learning changes the pattern of receptors in the information network. There are two forms of memory: implicit memory, which is largely unconscious

TABLE 18.1 NEUROCHEMICALS AND POSSIBLE DISORDERS OF THOUGHT, EMOTION, AND MEMORY

NEUROCHEMICALS	PROPOSED ACTION	BRAIN REGION	PSYCHIATRIC DISORDER
Acetylcholine (Ach)	Excitatory or inhibitory Learning and memory	Basal ganglia Motor cortex	Neurocognitive disorders (NCDs)
Dopamine (DA)	Involuntary motor movement Mood states Reward systems Judgment	Substantia nigra Ventral segmental area of midbrain	Schizophrenia Mood disorders Anxiety disorders Substance use disorders NCDs
Norepinephrine (NE) and epinephrine (E)	Learning and memory Reward systems	Sympathetic nervous system	Mood disorders Anxiety disorder
Serotonin (5-HT)	Appetite, sleep, and mood Hallucinations Pain perception	Raphe nucleus in the brain stem	Schizophrenia Mood disorders Anxiety disorders NCDs
Amino acids γ-Aminobutyric acid (GABA), glutamate, aspartate, and glycine	Inhibits excitability of neurons	Throughout brain	Schizophrenia Mood disorders Anxiety disorders Substance use disorders NCDs
Corticotropin-releasing hormone	Activates fear behaviors Increases motor activity	Hypothalamic–pituitary–adrenal axis	Mood disorders
Cortisol	Mobilizes energy Increases arousal	Hypothalamus	Mood disorders
DHEA	Neuroprotective Positive mood effect	Hypothalamus	Mood disorders
Enkephalins	Nociception	Central nervous system	Substance use disorders

and includes somatic, motor, emotional, and procedural memories, and explicit memory, which is involved with processing the factual knowledge of people, places, and things and its meaning. People with psychiatric disorders not only experience specific cortical dysfunctions but may have trouble in the proposed pathways for learning and memory.

Thought processes involve a pattern of stimuli from many parts of the nervous system at the same time and in a definite sequence. Each thought requires simultaneous input from portions of the cerebral cortex, the thalamus, the limbic system, and the reticular formation in the brain stem. The prefrontal association cortex processes information from many areas of the brain, is necessary to achieve thinking, and can keep track of bits of information and recall them simultaneously from working memory. This allows planning, goal setting, and problem solving. Thoughts are expressed in the form of language through the functions of the left hemisphere, the Broca area in the frontal lobe for word formation, and the Wernicke area in the temporal lobe for language comprehension.[19] Figure 18.1 illustrates the four lobes of the cerebral cortex.

One of the most important structures in the brain processing memory is the hippocampus. This structure of the brain is not fully developed until between 16 and 18 months of age. It is here, deep in the limbic brain, where information from the neocortex is processed, transmitted, and integrated.[23] The hippocampus is important for explicit memory, reality testing, and inhibition of the amygdala. Research has found the size of the amygdala and hippocampus is significantly reduced for those who have been significantly traumatized.[17] The excessive stimulation of the amygdala interferes with hippocampal functioning, so the ability to accurately describe the traumatic experience is impaired. This inability to integrate the traumatic memory into a coherent narrative may leave a person with images and sensations without the words, and/or there may only be a somatic memory of the experience. The decreased functioning and size of the hippocampus is thought to result in behavioral disinhibition and an inability to learn from experience.

Another important structure with respect to memory is the cerebellum, the largest structure in the brain. The cerebellum is activated when information processing and semantic memory occurs. The cerebellum is important in memory because it allows for attention to be shifted rapidly, accurately, smoothly, and efficiently.[24] Figure 18.2 illustrates brain structures important for memory and information processing.

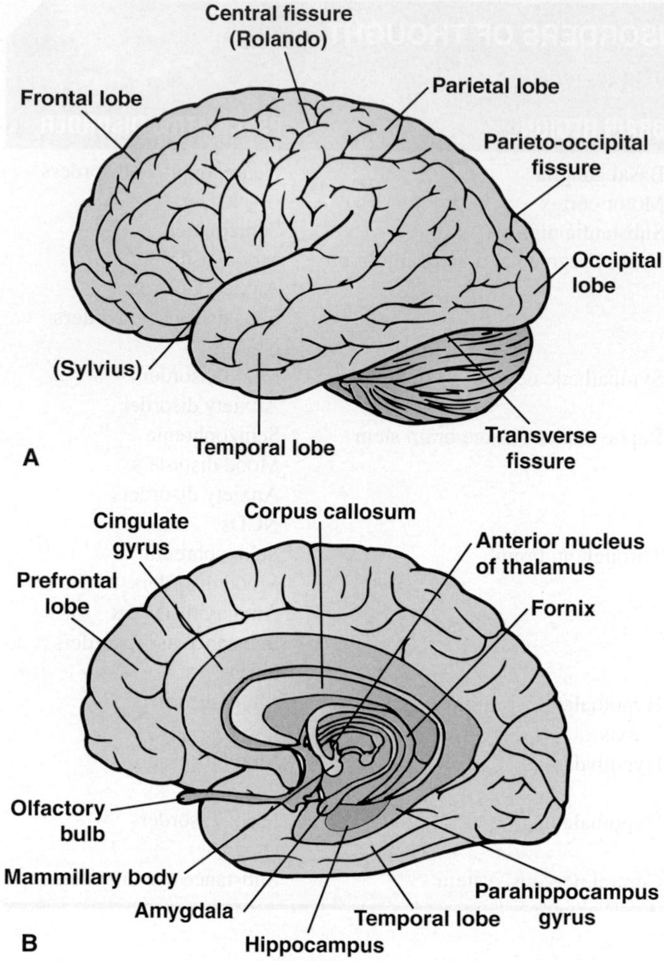

Figure 18.1 • **(A)** Lateral aspects of the cerebral hemispheres, including the frontal, temporal, parietal, and occipital lobes. **(B)** The structure of the limbic cortex, which includes the limbic cortex (cingulate gyrus, parahippocampal gyrus, hippocampus) and associated subcortical structures (thalamus, hypothalamus, amygdala).

IN SUMMARY

Because the brain integrates the processes of learning, memory, and emotions, symptoms may be somatic, cognitive, and/or emotional impairment or a combination of all these dimensions. People with psychiatric disorders and brain injuries often experience difficulty in the proposed pathways for learning and memory. These difficulties are likely to influence behavior and can result in significant problems in daily living and functioning in relationships and work. An increased understanding of the complex interactions among the different parts of the brain will assist in the development of more effective psychotherapies and more efficacious use of psychotropic drugs.

TYPES OF PSYCHIATRIC DISORDERS

After completing this section of the chapter, the learner will be able to meet the following objectives:

- Discuss underlying neuropathophysiology of schizophrenia.
- Describe the manifestations and diagnostic criteria for depressive disorders.
- Describe the manifestations of panic disorder, generalized anxiety disorder, phobias, and obsessive–compulsive disorder and the underlying pathophysiology of each.

Schizophrenia

Schizophrenia is a chronic debilitating psychotic disorder affecting 1% of the population and results in marked impairment in functioning.[3,25] Schizophrenia affects a person's thoughts, feelings, perceptions, and overall behavior while

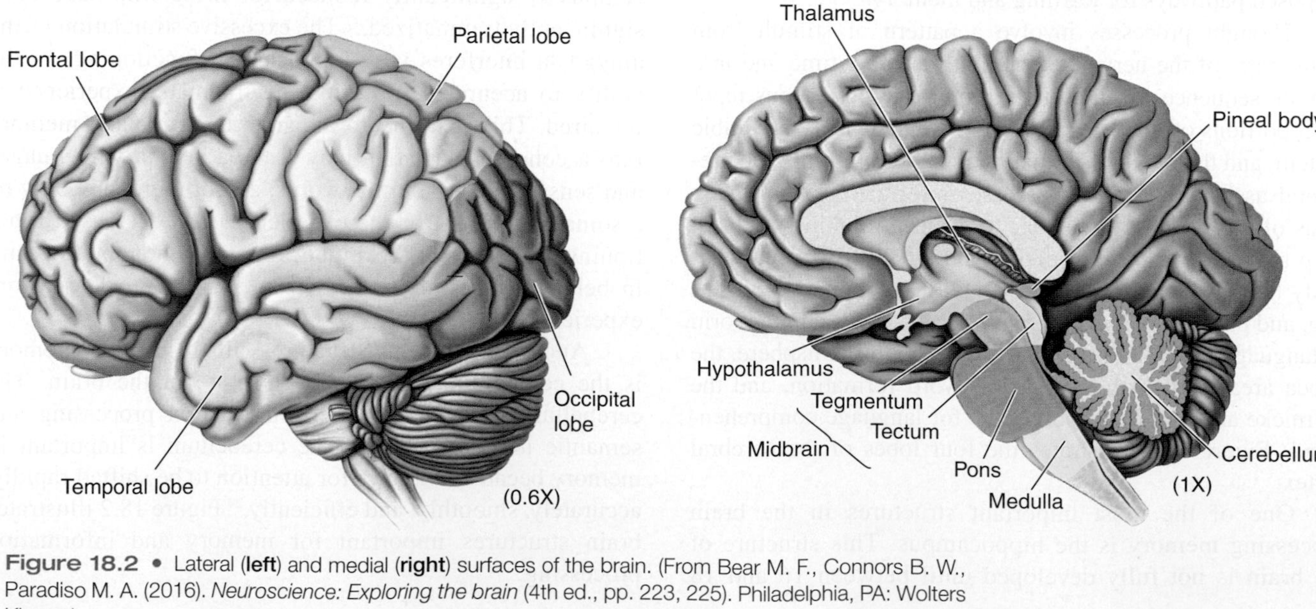

Figure 18.2 • Lateral (**left**) and medial (**right**) surfaces of the brain. (From Bear M. F., Connors B. W., Paradiso M. A. (2016). *Neuroscience: Exploring the brain* (4th ed., pp. 223, 225). Philadelphia, PA: Wolters Kluwer.)

TABLE 18.2 POSITIVE SYMPTOMS OF SCHIZOPHRENIA REFLECTING ALTERED SPEECH PATTERNS IN SCHIZOPHRENIA

SPEECH PATTERN	DESCRIPTION
Neologisms	Using invented words
Derailment	Loose associations
Tangentiality	Inability to stick to the original point
Incoherence	Loss of logical connections
Word salad	Groups of disconnected words

interfering with filtering of stimuli from the environment. The onset of the disorder typically occurs between the ages of 16 and 30. The prevalence of schizophrenia is greater in men throughout most of adulthood but is equal to women by the age of 50 or 60. Proposed risk factors for schizophrenia include childhood trauma, malnutrition, long-term cannabis use, Vitamin D deficiency, migrant status, older fathers, prenatal famine, retroviruses, chronic amphetamine use, obstetrical complications, poverty, and other psychosocial disorders.[26] Another risk factor is having a close relative with schizophrenia. In fact, first-degree relatives of a person with schizophrenia have a 10-fold greater prevalence of the illness than the population at large.[26,27]

Schizophrenia spectrum and psychotic disorders are characterized by symptoms such as delusions, hallucinations or false perceptions, psychosis resulting in a break with reality, disjointed behaviors and speech, limited emotions, and impaired ability to reason and problem solve, along with social dysfunction. The criteria for schizophrenia require two or more psychotic manifestations that last 6 months before diagnosis is made.[28]

Clinical Manifestations

Characteristics of schizophrenia include *positive* and *negative symptoms* reflecting the presence of abnormal behaviors. *Positive* or *psychotic symptoms* include:

- Incomprehensible speech
- Hallucinations
- Delusions
- Grossly disorganized or catatonic behavior

Frequently, people with schizophrenia lose the ability to sort and interpret incoming stimuli, which impairs the ability to respond appropriately to the environment. An enhancement or a blunting of the senses is very common in the early stages of schizophrenia. Sounds may be experienced as louder and more intrusive; colors may be brighter and sharper. Sensory overload owing to a loss of the ability to screen external sensory stimuli occurs. Some people with schizophrenia have a blunted response to pain. Examples of altered speech patterns reflecting positive schizophrenia symptoms are included in Table 18.2.[18,19]

Hallucinations and *delusions* are *hallmarks of schizophrenia* and may be related to the inability to filter, interpret, and respond appropriately to stimuli. Auditory hallucinations are especially common. Auditory hallucinations range from simple repetitive sounds to many voices speaking at once. Sometimes, the voices are pleasant, but often, they accuse and curse. When visual hallucinations occur, they are usually in conjunction with auditory hallucinations.[18,29]

Delusions are false ideas that cannot be corrected by reason. They range from simply believing people are watching them (ideas of reference) to beliefs they are being punished and/or manipulated by others (delusions of paranoia). Delusions of being a historical figure (*e.g.*, Jesus Christ or the President) also are common and are called grandiose delusions. Sometimes, the delusions include a belief the affected person can control others with his or her thoughts.[18]

The *negative symptoms* of schizophrenia reflect the absence of normal social and interpersonal behaviors. Examples of these negative behaviors are included in Table 18.3.[18,19] *Negative symptoms* are the most difficult to treat and often

TABLE 18.3 NEGATIVE SYMPTOMS OF SCHIZOPHRENIA REFLECTING ABSENCE OF NORMAL SOCIAL AND INTERPERSONAL BEHAVIORS

BEHAVIOR	DESCRIPTION
Alogia	Tendency to speak very little
Avolition	Lack of motivation for goal-oriented activity
Apathy	Lack of interest or concern
Affective flattening	Lack of emotional expression
Inappropriate affect	Affect does not match the situation
Anhedonia	Inability to experience pleasure in things ordinarily pleasurable

TABLE 18.4 NEGATIVE SYMPTOMS OF SCHIZOPHRENIA REFLECTING DISORGANIZED BEHAVIOR

BEHAVIOR	DESCRIPTION
Catatonic excitement	Hyperactive, purposeless activity with abnormal movements such as grimacing or posturing
Echopraxia	Imitation of another person's movement
Regressed behavior	Go back to behavior of another time
Stereotypy	Repetitive, idiosyncratic movements
Hypervigilance	Enhanced state of sensory stimulation
Waxy flexibility	Posture held in odd fixed position for extended periods of time

are severe and persistent between acute episodes of illness.[9] Another component of the negative symptoms of schizophrenia is referred to as *disorganized behavior*. In addition to agitation or aggression, other specific disorganized behavior may occur and is included in Table 18.4.[18,19]

Neurophysiology of Symptoms

The complete set of pathogenic mechanisms underlying schizophrenia is not clear. Research suggests that changes in the dysregulation of the dopamine and serotonergic system[23,29] and other neurotransmitter changes such as decreased glutamate activity through dysfunction of its *N*-methyl-D-aspartate receptor play a role.[30] Many of the symptoms of impaired cognition seen in schizophrenia are thought to be tied to deficits in GABA. Lower production of this amino acid has been found in the dorsolateral prefrontal cortex and may be a consequence of mRNA dysfunction.[30] Neuroimaging suggests several functional abnormalities occur in schizophrenia. These include excessive loss of cortical gray matter, abnormal cortical thinning, reduced numbers of synaptic structures on neurons, reduced dendritic spine density of pyramidal neurons in the prefrontal cortex, and arrested migration of hippocampal neurons. Enlargement of the lateral and third ventricles; a reduction in frontal lobe, temporal lobe, and amygdala; and diminished neuronal content in the thalamus have also been noted.[29,31–33] Interestingly, genetically identical twins are only 50% concordant for developing schizophrenia, suggesting 50% of the variance is attributed to environmental or other nongenetic contributions.[6]

Treatment

Schizophrenia is considered a chronic illness with remissions and exacerbations. Goals of treatment for schizophrenia are to induce a remission, prevent a recurrence, and improve behavioral, cognitive, and psychosocial functions. Early intervention programs are associated with a better treatment response.[33] The goal is *recovery*. According to the Substance Abuse and Mental Health Services Administration (SAMHSA), four dimensions supporting mental health recovery include health, home, purpose, and community.[34] Treatment in the community is preferred. However, hospitalization may be indicated if a person is a danger to self or others, is unable to provide basic care for self, or refuses to eat or drink.

Pharmacologic treatment with antipsychotics is often helpful with the positive symptoms of schizophrenia. Both typical and atypical antipsychotic drugs address these positive symptoms. The negative symptoms of schizophrenia respond more favorably to the atypical antipsychotic drugs. Often antipsychotics are combined with benzodiazepines or antiparkinson agents during the acute phase of treatment to reduce the risk of extrapyramidal effects from large doses of antipsychotic agents. Both categories of drugs exert their effect by blocking dopamine receptors, although the atypical antipsychotics have a more refined blockade action. The atypical antipsychotics also exert some of their effects through blockade of serotonin (5-hydroxytryptamine [HT]) receptors. Treatment with atypical or second-generation antipsychotics has been implicated in the development of metabolic syndrome. Often there is a rapid weight gain upon initiation of treatment during the first year, and obesity, insulin resistance, hypertension, high triglyceride level, and low HDL cholesterol levels develop. Long-acting antipsychotics are a potential treatment option that may improve compliance and decrease hospital readmissions.[35] Maintenance of pharmacotherapy is difficult because of the cost of the medications, the side effect profile, and the disease process.

Evidence supports psychosocial interventions—which include patient and family education, housing support, vocational rehabilitation, social skills training, family interventions, cognitive–behavioral therapy, and cognitive training—are effective for many people with schizophrenia.[18,36] Psychosocial interventions are important to help people learn about and live successfully with their illness. Family members may need assistance in learning about the illness and the best ways to support each other and their family member with schizophrenia.

Mood Disorders

Mood disorders are relatively common, but only half of those who need treatment are diagnosed and treated. The *DSM-5* section on mood disorders includes depression and bipolar disorders.[1] The 12-month prevalence of mood disorders in the United States is 9.5%, with 45% of these cases classified as severe. Mood disorder rates are higher among people living in or near poverty.[37,38]

Depressive Disorders

The *DSM-5* recognizes eight types of depressive disorders.[1] Prevalence of depression is higher in people from families with a history of mood disorders than in the population at large. The prevalence of major depression among women is double that in men.[37] Data suggest that major depressive episodes (MDE) occur in 6.7% of adults yearly and 12.8% of adolescents.[2,3] In all age groups, MDE has increased. Depression can vary in intensity and often is recurrent. The average onset of depression is the in the mid-30s. The age of onset of depression has been decreasing, with increasing MDE in ages 18 to 25 years of age.[39] The earlier and more frequent the onset of symptoms, the more likely it is medications will be required for symptom relief. Depression in older adults often appears with an element of confusion and often is left untreated. A first episode of depression occurring after 65 years of age can be a precursor to neurocognitive disorder and should precipitate both assessment and treatment of the depression, as well as a complete evaluation for neurocognitive disorders. Early intervention often greatly slows progression, allowing the older adult to maintain independence and quality of life.[39]

Major Depressive Disorder. People with major depressive disorder (MDD) experience loss of interest in previously enjoyed activities and resist attempts to engage them in such activities. Recurring thoughts of suicide, lack of appetite, inability to concentrate, difficulty or complete inability to make decisions, and feelings of worthlessness are common. Lack of energy, decreased motor skills, substance abuse, and a range of sleep disturbances from insomnia to oversleep can be characteristic. The criteria for diagnosis include the presence of symptoms most of the day nearly every day for a minimum of 2 weeks that interfere with activities such as work or functioning. Depression has various subclassifications distinguished by symptom patterns.[40]

Persistent Depressive Disorders (Dysthymia). Dysthymia is a chronic but mild state of depression lasting at least 2 years. There is a roller-coaster presentation in which the person may move from major to less severe depression,[41] often feeling sad. At least two of the following must also be present: altered sleep pattern (too much or not enough), fatigue, altered eating patterns (lack of appetite or overeating), inability to concentrate, poor self-esteem, and feelings of hopelessness. Stress is thought to play a role in dysthymia, and although the cause is idiopathic, there is a pattern of familiar expression, environmental, psychological, and biochemical contributing factors.[42]

Premenstrual Dysphoric Disorder. Premenstrual dysphoric disorder (PMDD) is related to the menstrual cycle and must not merely represent an exacerbation of the symptoms of another psychiatric disorder. The exact cause of this disorder is not clear but relates to the hormonal fluctuation a few days to 2 weeks before menstruation. Many women experience premenstrual syndrome, in which breast tenderness, abdominal pain, water retention, acne, back pain, and disturbances of sleep are present. In contrast, those with PMDD experience exhaustion, anger, a feeling of insecurity or loss of control, and a lack of desire for relationships. In 3% to 8% of women experiencing PMDD, these psychological issues prevent them from participating in their everyday lives. PMDD stops with menopause.[43]

Disruptive Mood Dysregulation Disorder. Disruptive mood dysregulation disorder (DMDD) is a relatively new diagnosis occuring in children and adolescents. DMDD is characterized by extreme moodiness in which the child (between 6 and 18 years of age) experiences anger, temper outburst, and irritability. Every day for most of the day, the child will exhibit anger and irritability. Temper outburst may average 3 or more times weekly along with difficulty functioning because of irritability when interacting with others. Criteria for diagnosis includes the presence of these symptoms gradually over 12 or more months.[44]

Depressive Disorder Due to Another Medical Conditions and Substances. Depressive disorders must be differentiated from medication side effects and medical illnesses. Depression often co-occurs with physical illnesses, notably myocardial infarction. Depression negatively impairs prognosis, affecting both behavioral and physiologic aspects of recovery, and increases the risk of death.[4,21] Medical conditions associated with depression include endocrine disorders, cardiovascular disease, neurologic disorders, autoimmune conditions, infectious diseases, certain cancers, and nutritional deficiencies.[45]

Neurophysiology of Symptoms. Epidemiologic and neurobiologic studies suggest interactions between biologic and psychosocial factors over time explain the risk of developing MDD. Multiple possible biologic theories have been identified in the development of depressive disorder including inflammation, HPA axis hyperactivity, low levels of neurotrophic growth factor, and low levels of vitamin D. Growing evidence supports some forms of depression may be linked to ongoing inflammation in the body. Higher inflammatory markers (C-reactive protein) have been noted in people with depression.[46] Disturbances in the function of the HPA axis also may play a critical role in depression. Early life stressors such as neglect or trauma can produce chronically elevated levels of cortisol.[47] Low levels of neurotrophic growth factor have been found in the hippocampus in postmortem tissue. Neuroimaging indicates smaller hippocampal volumes and hippocampal hypertrophy in people who have depression and have experienced early abuse.[21] Several mechanisms of action have been proposed to explain the association between vitamin D and depression. Vitamin D receptors have been found in the amygdala. Vitamin D may exert a neuroprotective function.[48,49] Circadian rhythms also are an area of serious research interest.[50]

Neurologic disorders of the limbic system and basal ganglia are also involved in the development of mood disorders. Neurotransmitter dysfunction is linked to depression. Research points to an imbalance of serotonin and/or epinephrine leading to depressive disorders. Current research also points to the role of dopamine in depressive disorders.[29] The monoaminergic hypothesis of depression attributes decreased levels of these neurotransmitters in the synaptic cleft, due either to decreased presynaptic release or decreased postsynaptic sensitivity, as the underlying pathologic process in depression.[50,51] Many studies have found reduced plasma, cerebrospinal fluid, and brain GABA levels in depression. Animal studies have also found that chronic stress can reduce or deplete GABA levels. Several studies suggest GABA and cholinergic receptors play an important role in the development of depression. Cortisol and DHEA are being studied as possible contributors to depression.[51]

Treatment. Antidepressants alleviate depressive symptoms by increasing the activity of norepinephrine and serotonin at postsynaptic membrane receptors. The most widely used mechanism of action of antidepressants is to inhibit the reuptake of serotonin at the presynaptic space. Formulations vary and target different neurotransmitters. Examples are selective serotonin reuptake inhibitors (SSRIs), serotonin antagonist and reuptake inhibitors (SARIs), and the serotonin and norepinephrine reuptake inhibitors (SNRIs).[52]

Tricyclic antidepressants block the reuptake of serotonin and NE by the presynaptic membrane. The monoamine oxidase (MAO) inhibitors increase the concentration of serotonin and NE by reducing the degradation of these neurotransmitters by MAO but are used less often because of their side effect profile and required dietary restrictions.[18,19,52]

Electroconvulsive therapy, a procedure that electrically stimulates a generalized seizure, can be an effective treatment for severe depression.[52] Phototherapy, or light therapy, uses artificial light to influence the production of melatonin and the function of the catecholamine systems. It is often a first-line treatment for depression associated that is with seasonal changes.[52] Evidence points to a combination of antidepressants, interpersonal therapy, cognitive–behavioral therapy, and problem-solving therapy for improved outcomes.[18,19,52]

Bipolar Disorder

Bipolar disorder is mood disorder with depressive components. The components discussed in major depression must be met in addition to the *cardinal symptom of bipolar disorder mania.* There is a lifetime prevalence of nearly 2.5% for bipolar disorders worldwide. The median age of onset is 25 years of age, with women having a higher frequency of occurrence. However, the disorder often presents in adolescence.[2,3,53] People with bipolar disturbances experience high (euphoria) to low (depression) mood swings. Often, people go undiagnosed for 10 years after onset of symptoms.[40]

Clinical Manifestations

There are four types of bipolar disorder, which are based on the severity and deviation from the euthymic or normal mood state[40]:

- Bipolar I disorder: The person has one or more manic episodes in which the mood is elevated, expansive, or even irritable alternating with major depressive episodes. Mood swings are common along with transferred rage. Manic episodes may interfere with work or school because of distraction and flight of ideas. Episodes begin suddenly and last from a few days to a few months. The depressive symptoms are more severe and are less responsive to conventional therapies than the manic symptoms.
- Bipolar II disorders: The person has a major depressive episode and at least one hypomanic or less severe manic episode. The hypomanic symptoms are present for at least 4 days.
- Cyclothymia: This disorder is similar to Type I but has less severe symptoms. Symptoms of hypomania and nonpsychotic depression are present for at least 2 years, or 1 year for children and adolescents. This disorder is one of exclusion—that is, the person with cyclothymia does not meet the criteria for a major depressive or manic episode.
- Rapid cycling: This term characterizes the person who has four or more manic episodes for at least 2 weeks in a year. Remission (either partial or complete) is replaced with clinical manifestations of the opposite type. Depressive symptoms are pronounced.

Neurophysiology of Symptoms. Studies on bipolar disorders suggest causation is multifold with impaired neuroplasticity as a key feature.[54] Biologically, bipolar disorders are thought to be a result of genetic, neuroendocrine, autonomic, and immune dysregulation.[6,50] There is a strong genetic basis for development. Recent studies suggest pathologic mechanisms in bipolar disorder may be linked to the same mechanisms as schizophrenia.[55–57] Some data suggest bipolar endophenotypes and/or resilience factors may play a role in development.[58]

Neuroimaging studies consistently show abnormalities in the subgenual prefrontal cortex in people with familial bipolar disorder, a region related to responses to emotional experiences. In some cases, a reduction in the volume of gray matter in the prefrontal cortex, with an associated decrease in activity in the region, was seen.[59] Clinical studies have suggested this area of the brain is important for mood states and has extensive connections with the limbic system.

Treatment. Treatment involves both psychosocial interventions used to treat depression and pharmacologic agents. Agents aimed at neurotransmitter and neurohormonal dysregulation are antipsychotics, and some anticonvulsants can block dopamine receptors and are potent antimanics. Some antidepressants and mood regulators modulate glutamate transmission and provide rapid alleviation of depressive symptoms with ketamine infusion. The gold standard in the treatment of bipolar depression is lithium. It is thought to reduce intracellular myoinositol concentration and increase neuronal growth cone spreading at therapeutic concentrations. It is known to inhibit the accumulation of cyclic adenosine monophosphate (cAMP) and may down-regulate second-messenger systems associated with cAMP-linked receptors.[52]

Antipsychotics, lithium, and some anticonvulsants can stabilize mood by regulation of sleep and circadian rhythm. When social and circadian rhythms are regulated, recurrences may be delayed. Unfortunately, many people with bipolar disorder do not believe they need treatment, particularly during the manic phase of the illness, and tend to self-medicate with alcohol or recreational drugs.[60] It is not unusual for people with bipolar depression to be diagnosed with substance use disorders.[2,3,12]

Anxiety Disorders

Anxiety disorders are characterized by intense fearfulness occurring without a precipitating potentially dangerous event and are accompanied by subjective and objective manifestations. Anxiety disorders are the most prevalent of the psychiatric disorders, affecting approximately 18.1% of all people.[3] Women are 60% more likely than men to experience an anxiety disorder over their lifetime. The *DSM-5* classifies phobias, panic disorder and selective mutism as anxiety disorders.[1]

Generalized Anxiety Disorder

Generalized anxiety disorder (GAD) is characterized by excessive anxiety and worry about several events or activities. A person with GAD finds it difficult to control the worry. The most frequent age GAD is diagnosed in ages 45 to 59.[56] Criteria for diagnosis of GAD is chronic and excessive worry and anxiety that interferes with daily activities and relationships for the majority of days for at least 6 months. Apprehension, anxiety, tension, and autonomic hyperactivity are exhibited. Fatigue, inability to concentrate, and sleep disturbances may result. About half of all people with GAD experience depression.[40]

Separation Anxiety Disorder

In separation anxiety, both adults and children become distressed when separating from home or an attachment figure. Although separation anxiety is normal in infants up to age 2, when the distress continues beyond the developmental level, separation anxiety disorder is present. Sadness, lack of concentration, fear of monsters or dangerous situations, and withdrawing from others are common characteristics of SAD. Headaches and nausea, sleep disturbances, nightmares, fear of being alone, and even anger may be experienced with separation.[40]

Selective Mutism

Selective mutism is an anxiety disorder in which a person is too afraid to speak in social or select settings. It is most commonly found in children who have a phobia of speaking or a fear of people. Although the cause is unknown, genetic factors are thought to have an influence. To be characterized with the disorder, a person must experience its symptoms for more than 1 month.[61]

Phobias

A phobia is a strong irrational fear of something posing little or no real threat. There are various types of phobias including animal, situational (traveling), and bodily.[40] Agoraphobia, a phobia closely associated with panic disorder, is a marked fear or anxiety about actual or anticipated inability to leave a public space.[62] Social Anxiety Disorder (Social Phobia) affects 7% of both children and adults. The median age of onset is 13 years of age.[40]

Panic Disorder

People with Panic disorder experience recurrent unexpected surges of recurrent fear or intense discomfort accompanied by physical or behavioral symptoms.[40] The prevalence of panic disorder is between 2% and 3% for adolescents and adults.[1,3] People with panic attack also have feelings of being out of control; fear of death; physical manifestations such as palpitations, sweats, chills, tingling or numbness; chest or stomach pain; dyspnea; and nausea.[63,64]

The diagnosis of panic disorder may be made more difficult by the presence of symptoms such as chest pain and shortness of breath that also are associated with potentially serious medical conditions. Often those with panic attacks initially are seen in emergency room settings with a person convinced they are experiencing a heart attack.

Panic attacks usually last 15 to 30 minutes, but sometimes continue for an hour.[18,19,62] Environmental and stressful life events appear to be involved in the causation of panic attacks. Children with separation anxiety often develop panic disorder as adults. In addition, early traumas such as socioeconomic disadvantages and a history of physical or sexual abuse are associated with the development of panic disorder.[64]

Anxiety Disorder Due to Substance/ Medication or Medical Conditions

Anxiety can be due to substance intoxication or withdrawal and/or to a medication treatment. In addition, anxiety symptoms can be the physiologic mechanism of another medical condition. Common conditions include endocrine, cardiovascular, respiratory, metabolic, and neurologic disorders.[65]

Neurophysiology of Symptoms

Anxiety disorders are thought to be caused by an interaction of multiple biologic and psychosocial factors. The major mediators of anxiety appear to be GABA, NE, serotonin, and dopamine. Underaction of the serotonergic system and overactivation of adrenergic system occur. The autonomic system—specifically the sympathetic nervous system—is involved in the stress response. Corticosteroid activation may increase or decrease activity of neural pathways, inducing anxiety.[6,65] Specifically, the anxiety disorder of panic is thought to be related to hyperactive amygdala, limbic, and cortical prefrontal cortex involvement. Genetic risk variants such as altered neuroplasticity have been proposed to stimulate the fear network.[62] Glutamate is the primary excitatory neurotransmitter in the central nervous system and is involved in virtually every neuronal pathway, including those underlying normal and pathologic anxiety states.

Treatment

Treatment includes the use of behavioral, psychological, and drug therapies. Cognitive behavioral therapy is an important component in the treatment of anxiety disorders. First-line, evidence-based pharmacologic treatment for anxiety disorders include specific SSRIs, SNRIs, and 5-HT_{1a} agonists.[66,67] There is growing evidence of the greater effectiveness of SSRIs in the treatment of panic, but full response to medication can take 12 or more weeks.[60] These agents result in limbic, paralimbic, and frontal hyperactivity normalization and serotonergic suppression. Second-line treatments include benzodiazepines. These drugs increase the activity of the $GABA_A$ receptor, which increases the flow of chloride ions across the cell membrane, hyperpolarizing the membrane and thus inhibiting firing of target cells. Because of the high level of physiologic and psychological dependence, benzodiazepines are no longer considered first-line agents in the treatment of anxiety disorders and are indicated for short-term use only.[67] Several drugs have proved effective for the treatment of social phobia, including SSRIs, benzodiazepines, and MAO inhibitors. Social phobia also has been particularly responsive to behavioral and cognitive therapies.[66,67]

Obsessive–Compulsive and Related Disorders

The *DSM-5* separates obsessive–compulsive disorder (OCD) from the anxiety disorders. Obsessive–compulsive and related disorders (OCRDs) include obsessive–compulsive disorder (OCD), body dysmorphic disorder, hoarding disorder, and trichotillomania and excoriation.[1]

Obsessive–Compulsive Disorder

Obsessive–compulsive disorders are characterized by the need to repeat distressful, uncontrollable thoughts (obsessions) and behaviors (compulsions).[68] Obsessive–compulsive disorder (OCD) among adults in the United States has an estimated lifetime prevalence of 2.3%.[2,3] This disorder is often underdiagnosed in children because it may appear as a behavior problem with impulsive angry outbursts and thus may be confused with attention deficit disorders or poor school performance.[69–71]

Body Dysmorphic Disorder

Body dysmorphic disorder (BDD) is a body-image disorder causing severe emotional distress and difficulties in daily functioning. It is characterized by persistent preoccupations with an imagined or slight imperfection in one's appearance. Research shows it affects men and women almost equally.[71]

Hoarding Disorder

Hoarding disorder is characterized by a persistent difficulty discarding or parting with possessions, despite the actual value. There is a perceived need to save the items and distress associated with discarding them. The accumulation of possessions congests and clutters active living areas and substantially compromises their intended use. The accumulation of the items causes distress or impairment in social, occupational, or other important areas of functioning (including maintaining an environment safe for oneself or others).[71]

Trichotillomania and Excoriation Disorders

A new *DSM-5* classification of OCRDs, excoriation disorder (dermatillomania), is characterized by recurrent and excessive picking, scratching, or rubbing of normal skin.[71] The lifetime prevalence of trichotillomania disorder is estimated to be 1%.[1]

Neurophysiology of Symptoms

The exact neurobiology of OCRDs is not clear. Environmental and genetic factors are thought to contribute to the development of OCD such as perinatal events, psychosocial stressors, trauma, and inflammatory processes.[72] Neuroimaging studies repeatedly demonstrate disruption in the orbitofrontal cortex, cingulated cortex, basal ganglia, and more recently regions within the parietal lobe, in the pathophysiology of obsessions and compulsions. In addition, smaller white matter volume in dorsolateral prefrontal and cingulate cortices has been shown.[73] Excessive activation of anterior cingulate cortex is thought to be present in people presenting with OCRDs. Recent research points to the role of glutamate signaling in the development of OCRDs.[69,74,75]

Treatment

Treatment of OCRDs includes psychotherapy, pharmacotherapy, electroconvulsive therapy, transcranial magnetic simulation, and in extreme cases deep brain stimulation surgery.[76] Psychotherapy includes exposure and response prevention. Certain SSRIs are the preferred pharmacotherapy.[76]

Substance Use Disorders

The terms substance abuse and substance dependence have been grouped into the single category *Substance Use Disorders* (SUD) by providers since 2013. Several substances in the *DSM-5* are recognized as playing a role in SUD including alcohol, caffeine, cannabis, hallucinogens, inhalants, opioids, sedatives, stimulants, and/or tobacco.[1] The annual prevalence rate of SUD in people aged 12 and older is 8.1%.[2,3] One out of eight people who have a SUD also experience an alcohol or additional SUD. Approximately 40% of adults with a SUD have a co-occurring mental illness. Abuse of substances such as drugs or alcohol before the age of 20 can change the development of the brain and increase the chance of addiction later in life.[77] Preoccupation with use is the overarching assessment and includes giving up important activities, more time spent using or procuring substance, and continued use with worsening of problems (physical, mental, emotional) caused by SUD.[78]

Neurophysiology of Symptoms

Current and ongoing research has pointed to a complex, multifactorial etiology, including psychosocial, biologic, and environmental factors. Genetics and environmental factors are proposed to be equally important in the development of SUD. Addiction may be up to 50% inheritable.[77] Activation of the brain's reward system is central to the development of substance use disorders.[79] Neurobiologic theories suggest neuronal plasticity and metaplasticity in the mesolimbic system can promote reward-based learning and the development of addiction.[80] Neuroimaging of brain functioning suggests dopamine is associated with substance use. Substances facilitating dopamine transmission acquire incentive and reinforcing properties and facilitate drug-seeking behavior. The pathophysiologic mechanisms of each substance class are different, but the activation of the reward system in all is similar.

The substance alcohol's effects on dopamine release are likely mediated through interactions with other neurotransmitter systems, such as glutamate, GABA, corticotropin-releasing factor, and 5-HT, as well as through interactions with the endorphins and enkephalins. The up-regulation of NMDA receptors and changes in glutamate signaling pathways may be increased with chronic exposure to alcohol. Plasticity at glutamatergic synapses on dopamine neurons may regulate how vulnerable a person is to developing addiction.[80]

Cocaine and amphetamines raise the level of dopamine in the nucleus accumbens by blocking the dopamine transporter, prolonging the time dopamine remains in the synaptic cleft. Nicotine enhances the release of dopamine by acting on presynaptic cholinergic receptors.[81,82] There is a reported increase in GABA levels in opiate use. Opioids bind to opiate receptors, which are the binding sites for enkephalins, dynorphins, and endorphins.[83]

Treatment

Treatment of SUD requires an understanding of physiologic alterations in brain function causing relapse, even years after abstinence. Precipitants for relapse include stress, environmental cues, and exposure to the substance. Relapses are not uncommon and should not be considered as failures in treatment but rather a reflection of the nature of the illness. Because there is a high comorbidity between depression and SUD, professional treatment of preexisting psychiatric problems often decreases the use of illicit substances and helps prevent relapse. Treatments are varied and include biologic, behavioral, and psychosocial interventions. Targeting the reward pathways of the brain can be part of ongoing treatment for SUD. Currently, three medications, which act as alcohol antagonists or deterrents, are approved by the U.S. Food and Drug Administration (FDA) for the treatment of alcohol SUD in adults.[84,85] Other medications are used to block opiate receptors and euphoric effects. None of the approved agents eliminate cravings[85,86] and work best with other therapies, such as behavioral therapies, cognitive–behavioral therapies, and psychodynamic, interpersonal, group, and family therapies.

IN SUMMARY

The development of a psychiatric disorder depends on a multitude of factors including cumulative and developmental trauma, social supports, attachment, and a person's neurobiologic and psychological profile. These factors create changes in the brain and in neural functioning. Recent research has deepened our understanding of how this complex interplay and genetics contributes to psychopathology. Through identifying those who are vulnerable and at risk for developing psychopathology, clinicians can begin to frame interventions strengthening resilience and maintaining psychological well-being.[87–89] The growing body of knowledge of the pathophysiology of psychiatric disorders continues to lead to evidence-based therapies for enhancing resilience and the prevention of psychiatric disorders.

DISORDERS OF MEMORY AND COGNITION

After completing this section of the chapter, the learner will be able to meet the following objectives:

- Compare the presentations of Neurocognitive Disorders because of Alzheimer disease, vascular disorders, frontotemporal degeneration, Lewy body, and substance use.
- Describe the changes in brain tissue occurring with Alzheimer disease.

Cognition refers to all the processes by which the sensory input is transformed, reduced, elaborated, stored, recovered, and used. It involves the perception of sensory input and the ability to learn and manipulate new information, recognize familiar objects and recollect past experiences, solve problems, think abstractly, and make judgments. The cognitive domains involved with neurocognitive disorders include memory, language, perceptual motor, social cognition and executive function, and complex attention.[1,80,90]

Normal Cognitive Aging

Memory shows a slow, progressive decline over the life span, and it is important to differentiate what can be termed "normal cognitive aging" from disorders of memory and cognition. Many older adults, of course, remain intellectually intact and make outstanding contributions later in life. Learning new information is slowed, but remote memory remains intact. Executive functioning diminishes minimally with aging. Vocabulary and most cognitive abilities remain resilient during normal aging. Conceptual reasoning, memory, and processing speed decline gradually over time. However, in normal aging, this slowing does not affect functional abilities.[91,92]

Neurocognitive Disorders

The *DSM-5* has replaced the terminology of dementia with neurocognitive disorders (NCD), the preferred scientific term. Neurocognitive disorders is an overall term for a decline in mental function severe enough to interfere with a person's ability to perform usual daily activities and is not a normal part of the aging process. Symptoms of NCD can vary but include memory loss, communication and language issues (word finding), difficulty performing complex tasks (bill paying), and judgment issues.[93,94] These are directly related to the cognitive domains of memory, language, perceptual motor, social cognition, executive function, and complex attention. Specific etiologic subtypes of neurocognitive dysfunction are classified by the *DSM-5*. Each subtype must also meet the criteria for mild or moderate NCD.[1] It is estimated 13.8% of people aged 72 and older have some form of neurocognitive disorder.[95]

The individual NCDs affect cognitive domains of memory, language, executive function, perceptual motor, social cognition, and complex attention. Each NCD has unique presentations and features. Research into the pathogenesis of these disorders is ongoing, and there is a growing body of evidence to guide treatment.

Neurocognitive Disorders Due to Delirium

Delirium is an acute fluctuating confusional state, which develops over a short period of time.[18] Prevalence is estimated to be 1% to 2% in those 65 and older and 10% among those 85 and older.[96] Extremes of age, neurocognitive disorders, functional impairments, a history of SUD, and sensory impairments increase the risk for development of delirium. Medical conditions, medications, uncontrolled pain, drug withdrawal, urinary retention, and fecal impaction are also common precipitating factors. Studies suggest inflammation and impaired oxidative metabolism are part of the pathogenesis of delirium. In addition, impaired neurotransmitter transmission of acetylcholine, serotonin, gamma-aminobutyric acid (GABA), and dopamine play a role in the development of delirium.[96]

In delirium cognition is unsystematic, portrayed by decreased consciousness, alteration in sleep, and abnormal psychomotor actions.[40] Treatment of delirium is supportive with efforts to eliminate the underlying cause.[52]

Neurocognitive Disorders Due to Alzheimer Disease

Neurocognitive disorders because of Alzheimer disease (AD) occur in middle or late life and account for 60% to 80% of all cases of NCD. The disorder affects more than 5.2 million in the United States and may be the sixth leading cause of death in the United States. The risk for development of AD increases with age. It is estimated almost 50% of people 85 years of age and older live with NCD because of AD, with two thirds being women. Projections estimate 7.1 million Americans will develop NCD because of AD by the year 2050.[95]

Clinical Manifestations. Neurocognitive disorders because of AD follow an insidious and progressive course, with an average survival of 8 to 10 years after diagnosis.[95] The *hallmark symptoms are loss of short-term memory, difficulty with language, and changes in behavior*. Various stages of the disease have been recognized, ranging from four to seven stages identified by the Alzheimer's Association. All are characterized by progressive degenerative changes.[95] Table 18.5 illustrates the stages, manifestations and cognitive domains

TABLE 18.5 COGNITIVE DOMAINS AFFECTED WITH PROGRESSION OF AD

STAGE	MANIFESTATIONS	COGNITIVE DOMAIN AFFECTED
Stage 1 No impairment	Forgetfulness	Memory
Stage 2 Very mild decline	Occasional short-term memory Occasional aphasia	Memory Language
Stage 3 Mild decline	Short term memory (STM), name recall Occasional aphasia Concentration issues	Memory Language Complex attention
Stage 4 Moderate decline	STM recall Episodic long-term memory recall (LTM) Aphasia issues Difficulty completing multitask steps	Memory Language Complex attention Executive function
Stage 5 Moderately severe decline	Disoriented to time and place More LTM deficits Difficulty dressing appropriately	Memory Language Attention Executive function Perceptual motor
Stage 6 Severe decline	Disoriented to person, time, place More profound episodic LTM deficits Reversed sleep pattern Loss of bladder and bowel control Enhancement of previously suppressed personality characteristics Paranoid delusions	Memory Language Attention Executive function Perceptual motor Social cognition
Stage 7 Very severe decline	Unresponsive Loss of motor control Abnormal reflexes Difficulty swallowing Death	Memory Language Attention Executive function Perceptual motor Social cognition

Source: Smits L., et al. (2015). Trajectories of cognitive decline in different types of dementia. *Psychological Medicine* 45(5), 1051–1059. doi:10.1017/S0033291714002153; Alzheimer's Association. (2016). 2016 Alzheimer's disease facts and figures. *Alzheimer's and Dementia* 12(4), 1–80. Available: https://www.alz.org/documents_custom/2016-facts-and-figures.pdf; Sadock B., Sadock V. (2014). *Synopsis of psychiatry* (11th ed.). Philadelphia, PA: Lippincott Williams & Wilkins.

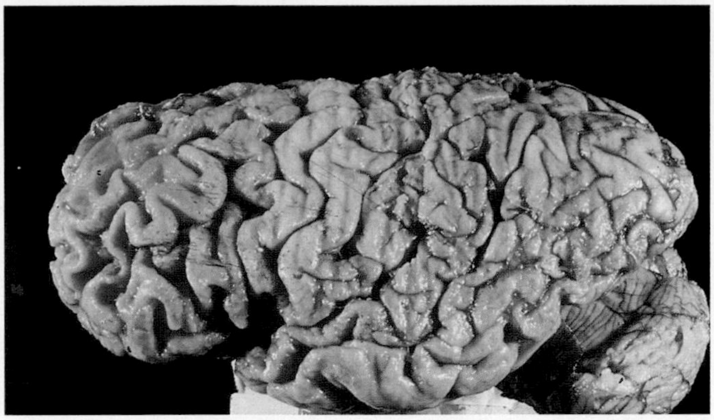

Figure 18.3 • Severe cortical brain atrophy. There is severe frontotemporal atrophy that may indicate Alzheimer or Pick disease. The frontal atrophy indicates changes in executive function and impaired judgment. (From Rubin R., Strayer D. (Eds.) (2012). *Rubin's pathology: Clinicopathologic foundations of medicine* (6th ed., p. 1349). Philadelphia, PA: Lippincott Williams & Wilkins.)

affected with the progression of AD. Depression, agitation, and sleep disorders are common in this disorder.

Neurophysiology of Symptoms. Alzheimer disease is characterized by cortical atrophy and loss of neurons, particularly in the parietal and temporal lobes. Severe cortical atrophy found in AD is illustrated in Figure 18.3. Pathogenic aspects of AD are not completely understood but are thought to be a combination of neurotransmission disruption, oxidative stress, neuroinflammation, and other factors.

Neurotransmitters with a significant role in AD pathogenesis include Ach, GABA, NMDA, and L-arginine,[97,98,99] Arginine metabolism is thought to be altered in the hippocampus. Other neurotransmitters may play a role in oxidative stress, which is known to be involved in AD.[91,100] Studies suggest decreased cholinergic transmission in the brain is associated with cognitive impairments. Additional studies have shown interaction of beta-amyloid (Aβ) with cholinergic receptors. Disrupted signaling in the cholinergic and glutamatergic systems at the cortex causes hippocampus, amygdala, frontal cortex, and parietal defects.[100]

The classic neuropathologic findings in AD are neurofibrillary tangles and amyloid (neuritic) plaques. The major microscopic features of AD are related to widespread cellular degeneration and diffuse synaptic and neuronal loss, and neurofibrillary tangles. The neuritic plaques are dense aggregates of amyloid beta (Aβ). Current genetic, pathologic, and biochemical and cellular studies support an imbalance between the production and removal of Aβ, causing accumulation as a key factor in the pathogenesis of AD. Neuritic plaques are illustrated in Figure 18.4.[101,102]

Familial AD is caused by mutations in amyloid precursor protein (APP), presenilin 1 (PS-1), presenilin 2 (PS-2), and Apolipoprotein E-e4 (APOE4). These mutations lead to changes in Aβ.[103] The dominant component of the amyloid core is Aβ, a peptide derived from the proteolysis of a larger membrane-spanning amyloid precursor

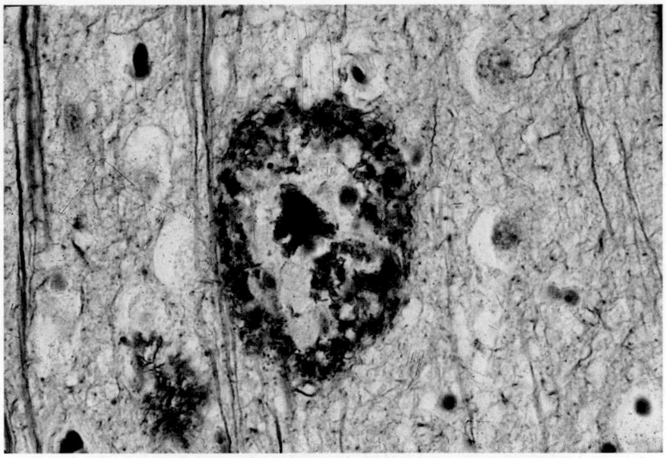

Figure 18.4 • Neuritic plaques with Alzheimer disease. The plaques are accumulations of polymerized *B*-amyloid with a ring of neuritic processes. (From Rubin R., Strayer D. (Eds.) (2012). *Rubin's pathology: Clinicopathologic foundations of medicine* (6th ed., p. 1345). Philadelphia, PA: Lippincott Williams & Wilkins.)

protein (APP). There is increasing evidence that Aβ is the critical molecule in the pathogenesis of AD.[103] Research is now looking at relationships between oxygen species, neuronal apoptosis, and calcium. Oxygen species may augment Aβ production and aggregation as well facilitate tau phosphorylation. Studies also suggest Aβ may impair calcium homeostasis and contribute to oxygen species disrupting the membrane.[104,105]

The neurofibrillary tangles, found in the cytoplasm of abnormal neurons, consist of fibrous proteins wound around each other in a helical fashion (Fig. 18.5). These tangles are resistant to chemical or enzymatic breakdown and persist in brain tissue long after the neuron in which they arose has died and disappeared. A major component of the paired helical filaments is an abnormally hyperphosphorylated form of the protein tau, an axonal microtubule-associated protein enhancing microtubule assembly.[106]

Inherited early-onset AD symptoms appear before the age of 65 and represent 1% to 2% of AD cases. Studies suggest genetic factors contributing to AD are like those in Down syndrome.[106,107]

Concept Mastery Alert

One of the genetic changes associated with AD occurs on chromosome 21, which is the same chromosome affected in Down syndrome. Virtually all people with Down syndrome exhibit pathologic features of AD as they age.

Diagnosis and Treatment. A diagnosis of AD can only be confirmed by microscopic examination of tissue obtained from a cerebral biopsy or at autopsy. The diagnosis is based on clinical findings. Neuroimaging and metabolic screening are important steps in excluding other conditions when diagnosing NCD because of AD.

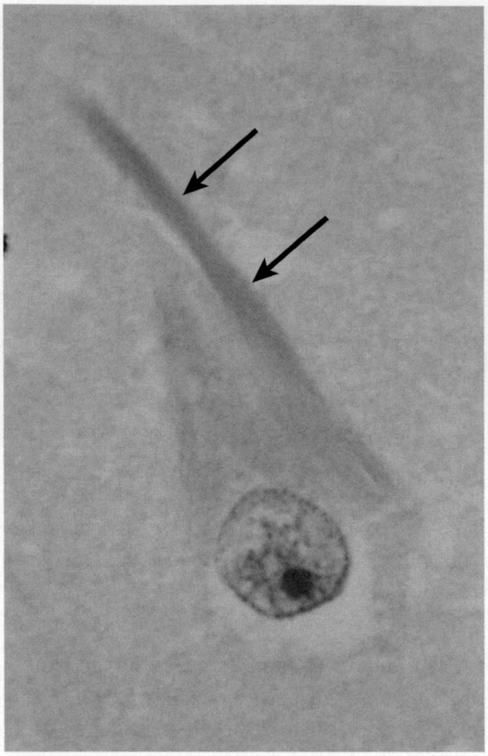

Figure 18.5 • Neurofibrillary tangles. These tangles are made up of intraneuronal accumulations of tau protein. The sites and complexity of tangles do correlate with clinical symptoms. (From Rubin R., Strayer D. (Eds.) (2012). *Rubin's pathology: Clinicopathologic foundations of medicine* (6th ed., p. 1346). Philadelphia, PA: Lippincott Williams & Wilkins.)

There is no curative treatment for AD. Medications may slow progression and improve depression, agitation, or sleep disorders. Cholinesterase inhibitors have been shown to be effective in slowing the progression of the disease by potentiating the action of available Ach and inhibiting acetylcholinesterase. *N*-methyl-D-aspartate antagonists act by interfering with the glutamatergic excitotoxicity caused by the ischemia and amyloid deposits associated with the disease, or they may provide symptomatic improvement through effects on the function of hippocampal neurons.[108] Antipsychotics are not approved for use in treating agitation with AD. Appropriate interventions include environmental adjustments, redirection, and finding the underlying cause of the behavior. Personalized music playlists are an evidence-based practice showing great success in decreasing agitated behaviors in people with AD.[109,110]

Two major goals of care are maintaining socialization and providing support for caregivers. Groups such as the Alzheimer's Association are effective in providing support. Daycare and respite centers are available in many areas to provide relief for caregivers and appropriate stimulation for the people.

Neurocognitive Disorders Due to Vascular Disease

Neurocognitive disorders because of vascular disease, formerly known as multi-infarct dementia, account for approximately 10% of all NCD types[97] and are caused by injury resulting from ischemic or hemorrhagic damage to the brain. Damage to large vessels may cause sudden symptoms, with small vessel damage leading to a slower onset of symptoms.[1] Research suggests cerebral vessel pathology might be an underrecognized risk factor for AD.[86] Early cognitive domains affected are perceptual motor, complex attention, and executive function. Symptoms of depression are often present. The *incidence is closely associated with stroke*, as well as hypertension, arrhythmias, myocardial infarction, peripheral vascular disease, lipid abnormalities, diabetes mellitus, autoimmune and infectious vasculitis, and smoking.[111]

Neurocognitive Disorders Due to Traumatic Brain Injury (TBI)

Neurocognitive disorders because of traumatic brain injury (TBI) are caused by long-term consequences of a brain injury. The prevalence of NCD due to TBI is increasing.[112]

Neurocognitive Disorder Due to Parkinson Disease

Approximately 10% of people with Parkinson disease (PD) develop the symptoms of an NCD. Neurocognitive symptoms generally occur after age 70 and *after development of the classic clinical manifestations of PD* such as bradykinesia, tremor, rigidity, and postural instability.[108,113] In NCD because of PD, aggregates of α-Synuclein protein (Lewy bodies) accumulate in the substantia nigra. The aggregates are thought to cause degeneration of the nerve cells that produce dopamine.[102,108] Cognitive impairment slowly but gradually worsens within all cognitive domains. Dementia is more common in PD, and clinical manifestations include unintentional muscle movements or twitching, visual hallucinations, memory disorders, visual–spatial deficits, slowness of movement and thought, REM sleep behavior disorder, mood disturbances (depression, agitation, and anxiety), and rigidity in posture. Cerebral changes in PD are similar to those of AD.[94,108]

Treatment includes supportive care and pharmacologic agent including cholinesterase inhibitors, N-methyl-D-aspartic acid, and dopaminergics.[51,108]

Neurocognitive Disorders Due to Lewy Body Disease

In Lewy body disease (LBD), aggregates of α-Synuclein protein (Lewy bodies) accumulate in the nuclei of cortical neurons controlling memory and motor control cortical. These proteins replace nerve cell structures. Clinical manifestations early in the disease are fluctuations in alertness and attention and recurrent visual hallucinations.[113] Lewy body disease is often confused for Alzheimer disease but has earlier onset and includes parkinsonian features and behaviors that include delusions, aggression, and depression.[40] Treatment includes cholinesterase inhibitors, N-methyl-D-aspartic acid, and dopaminergics. Important to avoid in LBD are neuroleptics and first-generation antipsychotics.[108]

Neurocognitive Disorders Due to Frontotemporal Degeneration (FTD)

Frontotemporal degeneration (FTD), originally known as Pick disease and frontotemporal dementia, is a progressive deterioration of the frontal and anterior lobes of the brain. Mutations in five genes have been identified in FTD. The encoding of the tau protein, growth factor precursor gene granulin are the most common gene markers. A histopathologic state underlies the clinical symptoms, and structural imaging shows anterior temporal and frontal lobe atrophy.[19] The disorder has a strong familial component, with 30% to 50% of people diagnosed with FTD reporting at least one relative with the disorder. *Disease onset is before 65 years of age.*[95]

There are two distinct clinical presentations indicating the symptoms of FTD:

- Behavior (more common)
  - Disinhibited and impulsive actions.
  - Apathy.
  - Inappropriate social behavior.
  - Behavioral abnormalities can be quite extreme and can be misdiagnosed as schizophrenia or psychotic depression.
- Language (less common)
  - Disturbances in understanding.
  - Disturbances in expression.[114]

Research reveals genetic and pathologic changes associated with FTD are the same genes involved in amyotrophic lateral sclerosis.[114,115] *Neuroimaging can be helpful in distinguishing FTD from other types of cognitive disorders.* Typically, structural imaging shows anterior temporal and frontal lobe atrophy. The course of the disease is relentless, with death ensuing within 2 to 10 years.

Neurocognitive Disorders Due to Huntington Disease

Huntington disease (HD) is caused by a genetic mutation of the HTT gene. There is a 50% chance of developing HD if one parent has disorder.[116] The first and most severely affected neurons are of the caudate nucleus and putamen of the basal ganglia. The neurochemical changes occurring with the disease are complex (Fig. 18.6). A decrease in GABA in the basal ganglia causes less inhibition of the thalamus, which results in increased release of the excitatory neurotransmitter glutamate to the frontal cortex.[116] Dysfunction of both the indirect and direct motor pathways within the basal ganglia in HD causes a wide range of motor symptoms called dyskinesias. Studies suggest alterations in dopamine balance, related to glutamate receptor function, may also have a significant role in behavioral and cognitive alterations in HD.[117] As the disease progresses, increasing numbers of neurons are affected, leading to brain atrophy.

Most adults show clinical manifestations in middle life; however, cognitive and psychological abnormalities begin in

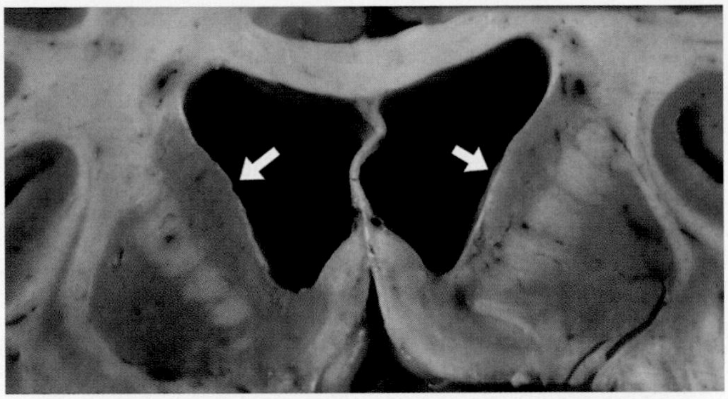

Figure 18.6 • Huntington disease. The caudal nuclei (*arrows*) are atrophied and lead into enlarged lateral ventricles. A small degree of cortical atrophy is also seen. (From Rubin R., Strayer D. (Eds.) (2012). *Rubin's pathology: Clinicopathologic foundations of medicine* (6th ed., p. 1351). Philadelphia, PA: Lippincott Williams & Wilkins.)

early adulthood. Appearance may be disheveled, and mood swings may progress to aggressive behavior. Suicidal tendencies increase as disease progresses because there is no cure. Chorea (jerky involuntary movements) increases with stress and peaks after 10 years of onset. Some memory deficits and slowing of cognitive function may accompany impulsiveness, frustration, and hostility as the frontal lobe deteriorates.[40] The immediate cause of death is usually infection.[1] There is no cure for HD. Treatment is supportive and aimed at symptom relief.[117]

Neurocognitive Disorders Due to HIV Infection

Neurocognitive disorders can develop because of HIV infection. Recent studies suggest the brain may act as a reservoir for HIV infection, causing persistent inflammation. Excessive glutamate is released upon HIV infection and is associated with neurotoxicity.[118] Treatment is supportive.

Neurocognitive Disorders Due to Prion Disease

Prion diseases (spongiform encephalopathies) are rare and fatal disorders caused by misfolding of endogenous protein into an infectious pathologic prion protein. Creutzfeldt-Jakob disease (CKD), a prion disease, affects only one person per million each year worldwide and has been linked to eating beef infected with bovine spongiform encephalopathy. The condition may be hereditary, idiopathic, or acquired through contaminated tissue or surgical instruments.[89,119,120] Degeneration of the pyramidal and extrapyramidal systems occurs, causing cognition changes within 6 months of onset. Death often occurs within months, although a few people may survive for several years.[99] Early symptoms consist of abnormalities in personality and perceptual motor coordination and impaired memory and judgment. Extreme cognitive decline, insomnia, blindness, and ataxia follow as the disease progresses.[119,120] There is no effective treatment for CJD.

Neurocognitive Disorders Due to Substances/Medications

Substance/medication induced NCD is characterized by neurocognitive impairments persisting beyond acute withdrawal of the substance. Risk factors for substance/medication-induced NCDs include defective coping mechanisms and long history of substance abuse.[121] Symptoms of alcohol-related mild or major NCD include impairments in memory, executive function, social cognition, complex attention, and perceptual motor skills. In some instances, suspending alcohol use leads to improvements in cognitive functioning; often, however, the damage is permanent and irreversible.[122]

Wernicke-Korsakoff syndrome can result from chronic alcohol use. Figure 18.7 illustrates the areas of the brain impacted by chronic ethanol (alcohol) use including cortical atrophy. Clinical manifestations include discrete memory impairment and confabulation, acute weakness and paralysis of the extraocular muscles, nystagmus, ataxia, and confusion. Peripheral neuropathy may be evident. Other symptoms are an unsteady gait and complaints of diplopia. There may be signs attributable to alcohol withdrawal such as delirium, confusion, and hallucinations. This disorder is caused by a deficiency of thiamine (vitamin B_1), which directly interferes with production of glucose, the brain's main nutrient.[122]

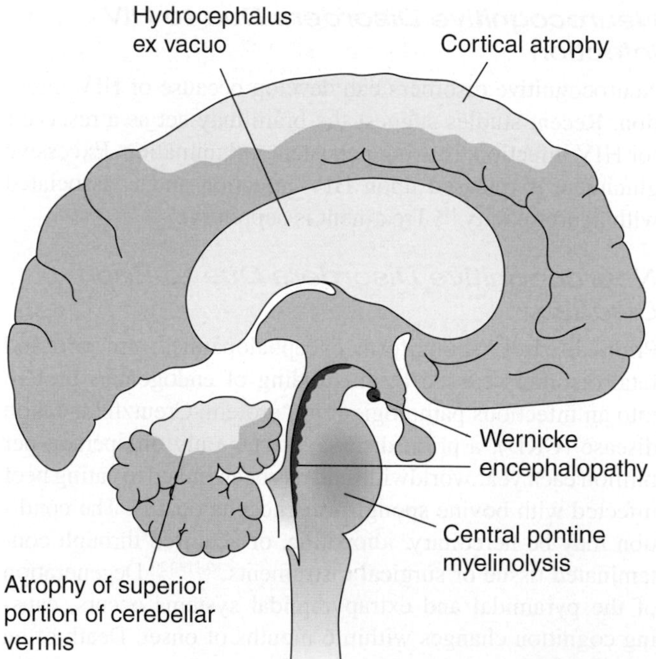

Figure 18.7 • Region of brain with lesions associated with chronic ethanol abuse. This illustrates what the Wernicke-Korsakoff syndrome involves. (From Rubin R., Strayer D. (Eds.) (2012). *Rubin's pathology: Clinicopathologic foundations of medicine* (6th ed., p. 1342). Philadelphia, PA: Lippincott Williams & Wilkins.)

IN SUMMARY

Cognition refers to all the processes by which sensory input is transformed, reduced, elaborated, stored, recovered, and used. It is important to differentiate what can be termed "normal cognitive aging" from disorders of memory and cognition. Memory problems that are associated with normal aging tend to reflect a generalized decrease in the efficiency with which information is processed and retrieved. Memory of a past event can be based on retrieval that is accompanied by recollection of specific details or on the feeling that the event is old or new based on its familiarity. There is evidence that recollection is more dependent on the hippocampus, whereas familiarity is more dependent on the entorhinal cortex and that healthy aging has greater effects on recollection than familiarity.

Dementia represents a syndrome of deterioration in cognitive function severe enough to interfere with occupational or social performance. The diagnosis of dementia is based on history; complete physical and neurologic examination; evaluation of cognitive, behavioral, and functional status; and laboratory (particularly thyroid hormone and vitamin B_{12}) and neuroimaging studies. There are several potentially reversible causes of dementia that can be remembered by the mnemonic DEMENTIA: *d*rug (any drug with anticholinergic activity), *e*motional (depression), *m*etabolic (thyroid function), *e*yes and ears declining, *n*ormal pressure hydrocephalus, *t*umor or other space-occupying lesion, *i*nfection (HIV or syphilis), and *a*nemia (vitamin B_{12} or folate deficiency).

The major syndromes of progressive dementia include Alzheimer disease, vascular dementia, FTD, CJD, Wernicke-Korsakoff syndrome, HD, PD, and dementia with Lewy bodies. By far the most common cause of dementia (60% to 80%) is Alzheimer disease. The condition is a major health problem among the elderly. It is characterized by cortical atrophy and loss of neurons, and the presence of neuritic plaques, granulovacuolar degeneration, and cerebrovascular deposits of amyloid. The disease follows an insidious and progressive course that begins with memory impairment and terminates in an inability to recognize family or friends and the loss of control over bodily functions. Ischemic or hemorrhagic damage is associated with vascular dementia and FTD with atrophy of the frontotemporal lobes. CJD is a rare, rapidly progressive form of dementia. Wernicke-Korsakoff syndrome most often results from chronic alcoholism. HD is a hereditary disorder characterized by chronic and progressive chorea, psychological changes, and dementia. There is controversy as to whether dementia with Lewy bodies is connected to Alzheimer and PA. Currently, dementia with Lewy bodies is categorized as an alpha-synucleinopathy.

GERIATRIC Considerations

- Depression and cardiovascular diseases have similar pathologic mechanisms and together negatively impact the prognosis of elderly people.[123]
- Although not a normal part of the aging process, depression most often occurs when other physical health conditions or comorbidities are present.[123]
- Older adults seldom report depressed moods as their primary complaint; instead, physical or somatic take priority.[123]
- With aging, body cells may lose their ability to repair damage from gene mutations, resulting in an accumulation of genetic changes that result in diseases such Alzheimer disease.[124]
- Alzheimer disease is the sixth leading cause of death for older adults, and the prevalence of AD increases with age; it is estimated that as many as half of those 85 years and older are affected by AD.[124]
- Baby boomers have a higher rate of alcohol and drug abuse than previous generations, placing them at a higher risk for falls, memory problems, liver disease, and sleep problems.[125]

PEDIATRIC Considerations

- Children often reveal anxiety and depression through somatic complaints such as stomach aches or nausea. Recurring complaints would warrant investigating the presence of anxiety, depression, or another mental health issue.[126]
- An example of separation anxiety disorder is children refusing to go to school.[126]
- Obsessive–compulsive disorder is a familial brain disorder that develops or worsens following a streptococcal infection.[126]
- In adolescence, mood disorders such as depression carry a high risk for suicide.[126]

REVIEW EXERCISES

1. A 45-year-old woman was brought to the emergency department after being picked up by the police. She was wandering in and out of traffic saying someone was after her and was recognized as a homeless person. Her appearance is dirty and disheveled, and she is wearing several layers of clothing, although it is summer. She smacks her lips and at times does not seem to understand questions. Periodically, she laughs for no apparent reason and often repeats the words of her questioner. She has a 20-year history of schizophrenia with multiple admissions.
   A. *List the positive and negative signs she exhibits.*
   B. *What are the brain areas and transmitters responsible for these signs?*
   C. *What are the clinical manifestations and criteria leading to her diagnosis?*
2. A 35-year-old woman was recently admitted with suicidal tendencies shortly after a diagnosis of major depression. She had lost 40 pounds in the last 6 months. She appears tired and supplies only short answers to questions. She complains of dizziness and informs the health care giver that it is not her business to discuss her suicidal thoughts. Her husband says she relies heavily on alcohol, is not able to sleep, and has missed work the last 5 days.
   A. *Describe some of her manifestations.*
   B. *Provide an explanation for her tiredness.*
   C. *What areas of the brain and neurotransmitters are involved in depression?*
   D. *What other physical conditions can mimic the signs of depression?*
3. A 40-year-old woman is seen in the emergency department in a state of severe panic. She has had panic attacks for several months and had not sought treatment until her husband came home and found her sitting in the bedroom unable to move. She had been there all day and had soiled her clothing. In the emergency department, she appeared frightened and paced in one area. She had difficulty understanding questions and cooperated only if she could pace. The husband relates his wife had been under a lot of stress in her job and had recently lost some important clients.
   A. *What are some manifestations of her panic?*
   B. *What is the biologic cause of anxiety disorders (include the brain structures and neurotransmitters involved)?*
   C. *Describe the physiologic manifestations of a panic attack.*
4. A 70-year-old man presents to the clinic with forgetfulness that seems to be getting worse. He has been having trouble remembering names and is not participating in community activities because he is afraid he will get lost. He states he is afraid he has Alzheimer disease. His wife states, "this is just part of getting old."
   A. *What are the normal signs of aging?*
   B. *What are the stages, symptoms, and cognitive domains affected with Alzheimer disease?*
   C. *What are the hallmark pathologic signs of Alzheimer disease?*
   D. *What are other neurocognitive disorders that could present with memory loss?*

References

1. American Psychiatric Association. (2013). *Diagnostic and statistical manual of mental disorders, DSM-5*. Washington, DC: American Psychiatric Association.
2. Substance Abuse and Mental Health Services. (2016). Key substance use and mental health indicators in the United States: Results from the 2016 national survey on drug use and health. Available: https://www.samhsa.gov/data/sites/default/files/NSDUH-FFR1-2016/NSDUH-FFR1-2016.pdf
3. National Institute of Health. (2017). *Mental health by the numbers*. Available: https://www.nami.org/Learn-More/Mental-Health-By-the-Numbers
4. Walker E., Druss B. (2016). A public health perspective on mental and medical comorbidity. *JAMA Psychiatry* 316(10), 1104–1105. doi:10.1001/jama.2016.10486
5. World Health Organization. (2016). *Classifications of diseases: ICD 11*. Available: http://www.who.int/classifications/icd/en/
6. Smoller J. (2016). The genetics of stress-related disorders: PTSD, depression, and anxiety disorders. *Neuropsychopharmacology Reviews* 41, 297–319. doi:10.1038/npp.2015.266
7. Greenwood T., et al. (2016). Genetic assessment of additional endophenotypes from the Consortium on the Genetics of Schizophrenia Family Study. *Schizophrenia Research* 170(1), 30–40. doi:10.1016/j.schres.2015.11.008.
8. Braff D. (2017). The importance of endophenotypes in schizophrenia research. *Schizophrenia Research* 163(1), 1–8. doi:10.1016/j.schres.2015.02.007
9. Light G., et al. (2014). Comparison of the heritability of schizophrenia and endophenotypes in the COGS-1 Family Study. *Schizophrenia Bulletin* 40(6), 1404–1411. doi:10.1093/schbul/sbu064
10. Klengel T., Binder E. (2015). Epigenetics of stress-related psychiatric disorders and gene × environment interactions. *Neuron* 86(6), 1343–1357. doi:10.1016/j.neuron.2015.05.036
11. Adams R., Ritter C., Bonfine N. (2015). Epidemiology of trauma: Childhood adversities, neighborhood problems, discrimination, chronic strains, life events, and daily hassles among people with a severe mental illness. *Psychiatry Research* 230(2), 609–615. doi:10.1016/j.psychres.2015.10.012
12. Hasin D., Grant B. (2015). The national epidemiologic survey on alcohol and related conditions (NESARC) waves 1 and 2: Review and summary of findings. *Social Psychiatry and Psychiatric Epidemiology* 50(11), 1609–1640. doi:10.1007/s00127-015-1088-0
13. Substance Abuse and Mental Health Services Administration. (2014). Understanding the impact of trauma. In *Trauma-Informed Care in Behavioral Health Services: Treatment Improvement Protocol (TIP) Series, No. 57*. Available: https://www.ncbi.nlm.nih.gov/books/NBK207191/
14. Center for Disease Control. (2016). Violence prevention. Adverse childhood experiences. Available: https://www.cdc.gov/violenceprevention/acestudy/index.html
15. Guitivano S., Kaminsky A. (2016). Role of epigenetic factors in the development of mental illness throughout life. *Neuroscience Research* 102, 56–66. doi:10.1016/j.neures.2014.08.003
16. Institute of Medicine and National Research Council. (2014). *New directions in child abuse and neglect research*. Washington, DC: The National Academies Press.
17. Cacciaglia R., et al. (2017). Trauma exposure relates to heightened stress, altered amygdala morphology and deficient extinction learning: Implications for psychopathology. *Psychoneuroendocrinology* 76, 19–28. doi:10.1016/j.psyneuen.2016.11.012
18. Boyd M. (2018). *Psychiatric nursing, contemporary practice* (5th ed.). Philadelphia, PA: Lippincott Williams & Wilkins.
19. Sadock B., Sadock V. (2014). *Synopsis of psychiatry* (11th ed.). Philadelphia, PA: Lippincott Williams & Wilkins.
20. Charney D., Sklar P., Buxbaum N. E. (Eds.) (2014). *Neurobiology of mental illness* (4th ed.). New York, NY: Oxford Press.
21. De Bellis M., Zisk A. (2014). The biological effects of childhood trauma. *Child and Adolescent Psychiatric Clinics of North America* 23(2), 185–222. doi:10.1016/j.chc.2014.01.002
22. Kamina H., Kertes D. (2017). Cortisol and DHEA in development and psychopathology. *Hormones & Behavior* 89, 69–85. doi:10.1016/j.yhbeh.2016.11.018
23. Herman J., et al. (2016). Regulation of the hypothalamic-pituitary-adrenocortical stress response. *Comprehensive Physiology* 6(2), 603–621. doi:10.1002/cphy.c150015
24. Koziol L., et al. (2014). Consensus paper: The cerebellum's role in movement and cognition. *Cerebellum* 13(1), 151–177. doi:10.1007/s12311-013-0511-x
25. U.S. National Institutes of Mental Health. (2016). *Schizophrenia*. Available: https://www.nimh.nih.gov/health/topics/schizophrenia/index.shtml
26. Davis J., et al. (2016). A review of vulnerability and risks for schizophrenia: Beyond the two hit hypothesis. *Neuroscience and Biobehavioral Reviews* 65, 185–194. doi:10.1016/j.neubiorev.2016.03.017
27. Chou I.-J., et al. (2017). Familial aggregation and heritability of schizophrenia and co-aggregation of psychiatric illnesses in affected families. *Schizophrenia Bulletin* 43(5), 1070–1078. doi:10.1093/schbul/sbw1
28. Schulz S. C. (2018). Schizophrenia. *Merck manual professional version*. Available: http://www.merckmanuals.com/professional/psychiatric-disorders/schizophrenia-and-related-disorders/schizophrenia#v1029197. Accessed February 14, 2018
29. Grace A. (2016). Dysregulation of the dopamine system in the pathophysiology of schizophrenia and depression. *Nature Reviews. Neuroscience* 17(8), 524–532. doi:10.1038/nrn.2016.57
30. Howes O., McCutcheon R., Stone J. (2015). Glutamate and dopamine in schizophrenia: An update for the 21st century. *Journal of Psychopharmacology* 29(2), 97–115. doi:10.1177/0269881114563634
31. Sekar A., et al. (2016). Schizophrenia risk from complex variation of complement component 4. *Nature* 530(7589), 177–183. doi:10.1038/nature16549
32. Caitlin E., et al. (2015). Dendritic spine alterations in schizophrenia. *Neuroscience Letters* 601(5), 46–53. doi:10.1016/j.neulet.2014.11.042
33. Matosin N., et al. (2016). Molecular evidence of synaptic pathology in the CA1 region in schizophrenia. *NPJ Schizophrenia* 2, 16022. doi:10.1038/npjschz.2016.22
34. Substance Abuse and Mental Health Services Administration. (2017). *Recovery and recovery support*. Available: https://www.samhsa.gov/recovery
35. Marcus S., et al. (2015). Antipsychotic adherence and rehospitalization in schizophrenia patients receiving oral versus long acting injectable antipsychotics following hospital discharge. *Journal of Managed Care & Specialty Pharmacy* 21(9), 754–769. doi:10.18553/jmcp.2015.21.9.754
36. Agency for Healthcare Research and Quality. (2016). *Effective health care program: Treatments for adults with schizophrenia*. Available: https://effectivehealthcare.ahrq.gov/topics/schizophrenia-adult/research-protocol/
37. National Institute of Mental Health. (2017). *Any mood disorder among adults*. Available: https://www.nimh.nih.gov/health/statistics/prevalence/any-mood-disorder-among-adults.shtml
38. Center for Disease Control. (2015). *Depression in the U.S. household population, 2009–2012*. Available: https://www.cdc.gov/nchs/data/databriefs/db172.htm
39. Harris M. (2017). Cognitive issues: Decline, delirium, depression, dementia. *Nursing Clinics of North America* 52(3), 363–374. doi:10.1016/j.cnur.2017.05.001
40. Mohr W. K. (2013). *Psychiatric-mental health nursing evidenced-based concepts, skills, and practices*. Philadelphia, PA: Wolters Kluwer.
41. National Institute of Mental Health. (2016). *Depression*. Available: https://www.nimh.nih.gov/health/topics/depression/index.shtml. Accessed February 14, 2018.
42. Chand S. P., Whitten R. A. (2017). *Depression [updated 2017 November 25]. StatPearls [Internet]*. Treasure Island (FL): StatPearls Publishing. Available from: https://www-ncbi-nlm-nih-gov.ezproxy.uthsc.edu/books/NBK430847/
43. PubMed Health. (2017). *Premenstrual syndrome: Overview*. Available: https://www.ncbi.nlm.nih.gov/pubmedhealth/PMH0072449/?report=printable. Accessed February 14, 2018.
44. National Institute for Mental Health. *Disruptive mood dysregulation disorder overview*. Available: https://www.nimh.nih.gov/health/topics/disruptive-mood-dysregulation-disorder-dmdd/disruptive-mood-dysregulation-disorder.shtml. Accessed February 14, 2018.

45. Lichtman J., et al. (2014). Depression as a risk factor for poor prognosis among patients with acute coronary syndrome: Systematic review and recommendations. *Circulation* 129, 1350–1369. doi:10.1161/CIR.0000000000000019
46. Wium-Andersen M., et al. (2013). Elevated C-reactive protein levels, psychological distress, and depression in 73,131 individuals. *JAMA Psychiatry* 70(2), 176–184. doi:10.1001/2013.jamapsychiatry.102
47. Fakhoury M. (2016). Revisiting the serotonin hypothesis: Implications for major depressive disorders. *Molecular Neurobiology* 53(5), 2778–2786. doi:10.1007/s12035-015-9152-z
48. Milaneschi Y., et al. (2014). The association between low vitamin D and depressive disorders. *Molecular Psychiatry* 19(4), 444–451. doi:10.1038/mp.2013.36
49. Verduijn J., et al. (2015). Pathophysiology of major depressive disorder: Mechanisms involved in etiology are not associated with clinical progression. *Translational Psychiatry* 5(9), e649. doi:10.1038/tp.2015.137
50. Jagannath A., Peirson S., Foster R. (2013). Sleep and circadian rhythm disruption in neuropsychiatric illness. *Current Opinion in Neurobiology* 23(5), 888–894. doi:10.1016/j.conb.2013.03.008
51. Pytkaa K., et al. (2016). The role of glutamatergic, GABA-ergic, and cholinergic receptors in depression and antidepressant-like effect. *Pharmacological Reports* 68(2), 443–450. doi:10.1016/j.pharep.2015.10.006
52. American Psychological Association. (2016). *Practice guidelines for the psychiatric evaluation of adults* (3rd ed.). Arlington, VA: American Psychological Association.
53. GBD 2016 Disease and Injury Incidence and Prevalence Collaborators. (2017). Global, regional, and national incidence, prevalence, and years lived with disability for 328 diseases and injuries for 195 countries, 1990–2016: A systematic analysis for the global burden of disease study 2016. *Lancet* 390, 1211–1259. doi:10.1016/S0140-6736(17)32154-2
54. Machado-Vieira R., et al. (2014). Multiple levels of impaired neural plasticity and cellular resilience in bipolar disorder: Developing treatments using an integrated translational approach. *World Journal of Biological Psychiatry* 15(2), 84–95. doi:10.3109/15622975.2013.830775
55. Altamura A. C., Buoli M., Pozzoli S. (2014). Role of immunological factors in the pathophysiology and diagnosis of bipolar disorder: Comparison with schizophrenia. *Psychiatry & Clinical Neurosciences* 68(1), 21–36. doi:10.1111/pcn.12089
56. Schubert K. O., Föcking M., Cotter D. R. (2015). Proteomic pathway analysis of the hippocampus in schizophrenia and bipolar affective disorder implicates 14-3-3 signaling, aryl hydrocarbon receptor signaling, and glucose metabolism: Potential roles in GABAergic interneuron pathology. *Schizophrenia Research* 167, 64–72. doi:10.1016/j.schres.2015.02.002
57. Steen N., et al. (2014). Altered systemic cortisol metabolism in bipolar disorder and schizophrenia spectrum disorders. *Journal of Psychiatric Research* 52, 57–62. doi:10.1016/j.jpsychires.2014.01.017
58. McNamara R., Strawn J. (2015). Nonheritable risk factors for bipolar disorder. In Strakowski S. M., DelBello M. P., Adler C. M., et al. (Eds.) *Bipolar disorder in youth: Presentation, treatment, and neurobiology* (pp. 109-130). New York, NY: Oxford University Press.
59. Wise T., et al (2014). Diagnostic and therapeutic utility of neuroimaging in depression: An overview. *Neuropsychiatric Disease and Treatment* 10, 1509–1522. doi:10.2147/NDT.S50156
60. Levin J., et al. (2016). Medication adherence in patients with bipolar disorder: A comprehensive review. *CNS Drugs* 30(9), 819. doi:10.1007/s40263-016-0368-x
61. Selective Mutism Foundation. (2018). *What is selective mutism?* Available: http://www.selectivemutismfoundation.org/info-on-selective-mutism/what-is-selective-mutism. Accessed February 14, 2018.
62. Asmundson G., Taylor S., Smits J. (2014). Panic disorder and agoraphobia: An overview and commentary on DSM-5 changes. *Depression and Anxiety* 31(6), 480–486. doi:10.1002/da.22277
63. National Institute of Mental Health. (2017). *Panic disorder: When fear overwhelms*. Available https://www.nimh.nih.gov/health/publications/panic-disorder-when-fear-overwhelms/index.shtml. Accessed February 22, 2018
64. Wolf M. R., Nochajski T. H., Farrell H. G. (2015). The effects of childhood sexual abuse and other trauma on drug court participants. *Journal of Social Work Practice in The Addictions* 15(1), 44. doi:10.1080/1533256X.2014.996228
65. Craske, M. G., et al. (2016). Anxiety. *Lancet* 388(10063); 3048–3059. doi:10.1016/S0140-6736(16)30381-6
66. Jakubovski E., Bloch M. H. (2016). Anxiety disorder-specific predictors of treatment outcome in the coordinated anxiety learning and management (CALM) trial. *Psychiatric Quarterly* 87(3), 445–464. doi:10.1007/s11126-015-9399-6
67. Anxiety and Depression Association of America. (2015). *Clinical practice review for GAD*. Available: https://adaa.org/resources-professionals/practice-guidelines-gad
68. Freed P. E. (2018). Obsessive compulsive and related disorders management of obsessions and compulsions. In Boyd M. (Eds.) *Psychiatric nursing contemporary practice* (6th ed., pp. 453–469). Philadelphia, PA: Wolters Kluwer.
69. Anxiety and Depression Association of America. (2015). *Clinical practice review for OCD*. Available: https://adaa.org/resources-professionals/practice-guidelines-ocd
70. Abramovitch A., et al. (2015). Comorbidity between attention deficit/hyperactivity disorder and obsessive-compulsive disorder across the lifespan: A systematic and critical review. *Harvard Review of Psychiatry* 23(4), 245–262. doi:10.1097/HRP.0000000000000050
71. Van Ameringen M., Patterson B., Simpson W. (2014). DSM-5 obsessive-compulsive and related disorders: Clinical implications of new criteria. *Depression and Anxiety* 31(6), 487–493. doi:10.1002/da.22259
72. Pauls D., et al. (2014). Obsessive-compulsive disorder: An integrative genetic and neurobiological perspective. *Nature Reviews. Neuroscience* 15(6), 410–424. doi:10.1038/nrn3746
73. Bargallo N. (2014). White matter structural alterations in pediatric obsessive–compulsive disorder: Relation to symptom dimensions. *Progress in Neuropsychopharmacology & Biological Psychiatry* 54, 249–258. doi:10.1016/j.pnpbp.2014.06.009
74. Monzani B., et al. (2014). The structure of genetic and environmental risk factors for dimensional representations of DSM-5 obsessive-compulsive spectrum disorders. *JAMA Psychiatry* 71(2), 182–189. doi:10.1001/jamapsychiatry.2013.3524
75. Zhu Y., et al. (2015). Decreased thalamic glutamate level in unmedicated adult obsessive-compulsive disorder patients detected by proton magnetic resonance spectroscopy. *Journal of Affective Disorders* 178, 193–200. doi:10.1016/j.jad.2015.03.008
76. Bokor G., Anderson P. D. (2014). Obsessive–compulsive disorder. *Journal of Pharmacy Practice* 27(2), 116–130. doi:10.1177/0897190014521996
77. National Council on Alcoholism and Drug Dependence. (2015). *Family history and genetics*. Available: https://www.ncadd.org/about-addiction/family-history-and-genetics
78. Dugosh K. L., Cacciola J. S. (2017). Clinical assessment of substance use disorders. In Hermann R. (Ed.) *UpToDate*. Available: https://www.uptodate.com/contents/clinicalassessment of substanceabusedisorders
79. Freeman T., et al. (2015). Dopamine, urges to smoke, and the relative salience of drug versus non-drug reward. *Social Cognitive and Affective Neuroscience* 10(1), 85–92. doi:10.1093/scan/nsu026
80. Leamy T., et al. (2016). Alcohol misuse in emerging adulthood: Association of dopamine and serotonin receptor genes with impulsivity-related cognition. *Addictive Behaviors* 63, 29–36. doi:10.1016/j.addbdh.2016.05.008
81. National Institute on Drug Abuse. (2017). *Impacts of drugs on neurotransmission*. Available: https://www.drugabuse.gov/news-events/nida-notes/2017/03/impacts-drugs-neurotransmission
82. Wingo T., et al. (2016). Novelty seeking and drug addiction in humans and animals: From behavior to molecules. *Journal of Neuroimmune Pharmacology* 11(3), 456. doi:10.1007/s11481-015-9636-7
83. Bodnar R. (2016). Endogenous opiates and behavior. *Peptides* 75, 18–70. doi:10.1016/j.peptides.2015.10.009
84. Wackernah R., Minnick M., Clapp P. (2014). Alcohol use disorder: Pathophysiology, effects, and pharmacologic options for treatment. *Substance Abuse and Rehabilitation* 5, 1–12. doi:10.2147/SAR.S37907

85. U.S. Department of Health and Human Services. (2016). *Facing addiction in America: The surgeon general's report on alcohol, drugs, and health*. Washington, DC: HHS.
86. Amstadter A., et al. (2016). The relationship between genetic and environmental influences on resilience and on common internalizing and externalizing psychiatric disorders. *Social Psychiatry and Psychiatric Epidemiology* 51(5), 669–678. doi:10.1007/s00127-015-1163-6
87. Teicher M., Samson J. (2016). Annual research review: Enduring neurobiological effects of childhood abuse and neglect. *Journal of Child Psychology & Psychiatry* 57(3), 241–266. doi:10/1111/jcpp.12507
88. Shrivastava A., Desousa A. (2016). Resilience: A psychobiological construct for psychiatric disorders. *Indian Journal of Psychiatry* 58(1), 38. doi:10.4103/0019-5545.174365
89. Smits L., et al. (2015). Trajectories of cognitive decline in different types of dementia. *Psychological Medicine* 45(5), 1051–1059. doi:10.1017/S0033291714002153
90. Harada C., et al. (2013). Normal cognitive aging. *Clinics in Geriatric Medicine* 29(4), 737–752. doi:10.1016/j.cger.2013.07.002
91. Smith C., Cotter V. (2016). Age related changes. In Boltz M., Capezuti E., Fulmer T., et al. (Eds.) *Evidence based geriatric protocols for best practice* (pp. 23–41). New York: Springer.
92. Alzheimer's Association. (2017). *What is dementia?* Available: http://www.alz.org/what-is-dementia.asp
93. Alzheimer's Association. (2011). In brief for healthcare professionals: New Diagnostic Criteria and guidelines for Alzheimer's disease. Available: https://www.alz.org/health-care-professionals/documents/InBrief_Issue7_Final.pdf
94. Alzheimer's Association. (n.d.). In brief for healthcare professionals: Differentiating dementias. Available: https://www.alz.org/health-care-professionals/documents/InBrief_Issue7_Final.pdf
95. Alzheimer's Association. (2016). 2016 Alzheimer's disease facts and figures. *Alzheimer's and Dementia* 12(4), 1–80. Available: https://www.alz.org/documents_custom/2016-facts-and-figures.pdf
96. Adamis D., et al. (2015). A comparison of delirium diagnosis in elderly medical inpatients using the CAM, DRS-R98, DSM-IV and DSM-5 criteria. *International Psychogeriatrics* 27(6), 883–889. doi:10.1017/S1041610214002853
97. Arvanitakis Z., et al. (2016). Articles: Relation of cerebral vessel disease to Alzheimer's disease dementia and cognitive function in elderly people: A cross-sectional study. *Lancet Neurology* 15(9), 934–943. doi:10.1016/S1474-4422(16)30029-1
98. Ramesh K., Hemachandra R. (2016). Therapeutics of neurotransmitters in Alzheimer's disease. *Journal of Alzheimer's Disease* 57(4), 1049–1069. doi:10.3233/JAD-161118
99. Liu P., et al. (2014). Altered arginine metabolism in Alzheimer's disease brains. *Neurobiology of Aging* 35(9), 1992–2003. doi:10.1016/j.neurobiolaging.2014.03.013
100. Sanabria-Castro A., Alvarado-Echeverría I., Monge-Bonilla C. (2017). Molecular pathogenesis of Alzheimer's disease: An update. *Annals of Neurosciences* 24(1), 46–54. doi:10.1159/000464422
101. Villemagne V., et al. (2017). Aβ-amyloid and Tau imaging in dementia. *Seminars in Nuclear Medicine* 47, 75–88. doi:10.1053/j.semnuclmed.2016.09.006
102. Alzheimer's Association. (2017). What we know today about Alzheimer's: *The search for Alzheimer's causes and risk factors*. Alzheimer's Research Center. Available: http://www.alz.org/research/science/alzheimers_disease_causes.asp
103. Cai Y., An S., Kim S. (2015). Mutations in presenilin 2 and its implications in Alzheimer's disease and other dementia-associated disorders. *Clinical Interventions in Aging* 10, 1163–1172. doi:10.2147/CIAS85808
104. Fonseca A., Cardoso S., Pereira C. (2015). Calcium and redox homeostasis in Alzheimer's disease: a focus on the endoplasmic reticulum. *Therapeutic Targets for Neurological Diseases* 1, 1–13. doi:10.14800/ttnd.428
105. Makhaeva G., et al. (2015). Conjugates of γ-carbolines and phenothiazine as new selective inhibitors of butyrylcholinesterase and blockers of NMDA receptors for Alzheimer disease. *Scientific Reports* 18(5);13164. doi:10.1038/srep13164
106. Lee J., et al. (2017). Candidate gene analysis for Alzheimer's disease in adults with Down syndrome. *Neurobiology of Aging* 56, 150–158. doi:10.1016/j.neurobiolaging.2017.04.018
107. Hamlett E., et al. (2017). Neuronal exosomes reveal Alzheimer's disease biomarkers in Down syndrome. *Alzheimer's & Dementia: Journal of The Alzheimer's Association* 13(5); 541–549. doi:10.1016/j.jalz.2016.08.012
108. Walter C., et al. (2014). Differentiating Alzheimer's disease, Lewy body, and Parkinson dementia using DSM-5. *Journal for Nurse Practitioners* 10(4), 262–270. doi:10/1016/jnurpra.2014.01.002
109. Thomas K. et al. (2017). Individualized music program is associated with improved outcomes for U.S. nursing home residents with dementia. *American Journal of Geriatric Psychiatry* 25(9), 931–938. doi:10.1016/jagp2017.04.008
110. Long E. (2017). Innovative approach to managing behavioral and psychological dementia. *Journal for Nurse Practitioners* 13(7), 475–481. doi:10.1016.j/nurpra.2017.05.003
111. Alzheimer's Association. (2017). Health care professionals and Alzheimer's: Differential diagnosis of vascular dementia. Available: http://www.alz.org/health-care-professionals/differential-diagnosis-vascular-dementia.asp
112. Centers for Disease Control and Prevention. (2015). *Report to congress on traumatic brain injury in the United States: Epidemiology and rehabilitation*. Atlanta, GA: National Center for Injury Prevention and Control; Division of Unintentional Injury Prevention.
113. Aarsland D. (2015). Epidemiology of dementia associated with Parkinson's disease. In Emre M. (Ed.) *Cognitive impairment and dementia in Parkinson's disease* (pp. 5–16).Oxford, UK: Oxford University Press.
114. Alzheimer's Association. (2017). *Frontotemporal dementia*. Available: http://www.alz.org/dementia/fronto-temporal-dementia-ftd-symptoms.asp#types
115. Scaber J., Talbot K. (2016). What is the role of TDP-43 in C9orf72-related amyotrophic lateral sclerosis and frontotemporal dementia? *Brain: A Journal of Neurology* 139(12), 3057–3059. doi:10.1093/brain/aww264
116. World Health Organization. (2017). *Genomic resource centre: Genes and human disease*. Available: http://www.who.int/genomics/public/geneticdiseases/en/index2.html
117. Cepeda C., et al. (2014). The role of dopamine in Huntington's disease. *Progress in Brain Research* 211, 235–254. doi:10.1016/B978-0-444-63425-2.00010-6
118. Saylor D., et al. (2016). HIV-associated neurocognitive disorder—Pathogenesis and prospects for treatment. *Neurology* 12(4), 234–248. doi:10.1038/nrneurol.2016.27
119. Hugo J., Ganguli M. (2014). Dementia and cognitive impairment: Epidemiology, diagnosis, and treatment. *Clinics in Geriatric Medicine* 30(3), 421–442. doi:10.1016/j.cger.2014.04.001
120. Leitão M., et al. (2016). CSF Tau proteins reduce misdiagnosis of sporadic Creutzfeldt-Jakob disease suspected cases with inconclusive 14-3-3 result. *Journal of Neurology* 263(9), 1847. doi:10.1007/s00415-016-8209-x
121. Hartney E. (2017). What is mild neurocognitive disorder due to substance/medication use? Available: https://www.verywellmind.com/medication-or-substance-induced-neurocognitive-disorder-4144778. Accessed February 22, 2018
122. Rawat P., et al. (2016).Neuropathology in neuropsychiatric disorders secondary to alcohol misuse. In Preedy V. (Ed.) *Neuropathology of drug addictions and substance misuse* (pp. 627-636). London, UK: Elsevier.
123. Jiang W. (2018). Depression & cardiovascular disorders in the elderly. *Psychiatric Clinics of North America* (1), 29–37. doi:10.1016/j.psc.2017.10.003.
124. Hinkle J. L., Cheever K. H. (2018). *Brunner & Suddarth's textbook of medical-surgical nursing* (14th ed.). Philadelphia, PA: Wolters Kluwer.
125. Kettaneh A. A. (2015). Substance abuse among the elderly population: Overview and management. *Journal of Applied Rehabilitation Counseling* 46(4), 11–17.
126. Bowden V., Greenberg C. S. (2014). *Children and their families: The continuum of nursing care*. (3rd ed.). Philadelphia, PA: Wolters Kluwer.

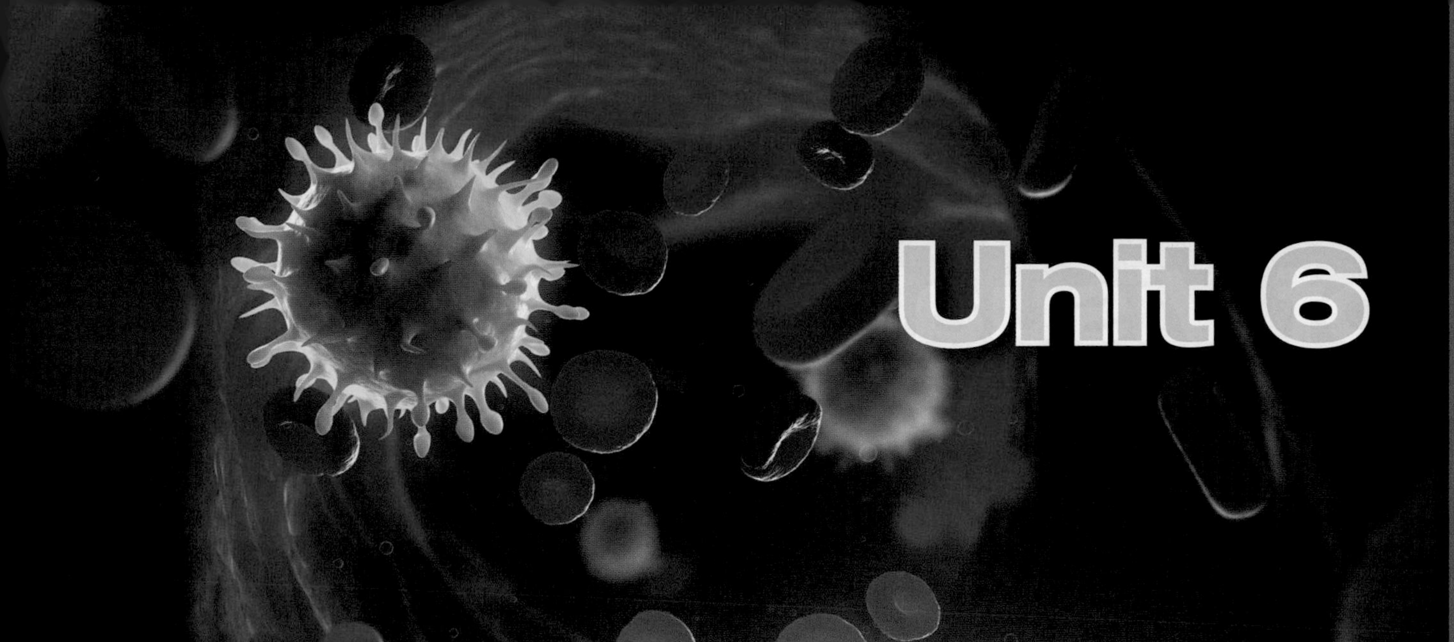

Unit 6

Disorders of Special Sensory Function

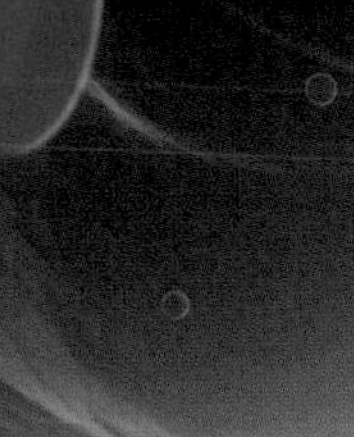

Mr. Pall, a 20-year-old college student, presents to his primary care provider complaining of a 2-day history of "almost painless" left red eye. He attended a friend's gig at a local club 48 hours ago. He stayed out late at the club, which was full of cigarette smoke. However, he states that smoke has never bothered his eyes before.

He denies any trauma to his eye but reports a head cold of several days' duration. He has a history of 5 years of contact lens use (daily wear). His medical history is positive for allergic rhinoconjunctivitis, fracture of the right wrist at age 9 from skateboarding, and an appendectomy last summer. He says that he may have fallen asleep without removing his contacts, which happens about twice a month. He denies blurry vision, any change in vision since the redness began, or pain in eyeball with or without eye movement. He reports that his "left eye is glued shut" upon waking. Upon examination, the primary care provider notes an extremely red, injected, and swollen left conjunctiva with slight yellow drainage. Right eye shows similar findings, but to a lesser extent.

Vision can be corrected to within normal limits (WNL), and no foreign bodies are noted upon fluorescein stain. The primary care provider diagnoses Mr. Pall with left and right bacterial conjunctivitis and prescribes antibiotic drops. Mr. Pall is taught how to administer the drops as well as hygienic practices to prevent reinfection.

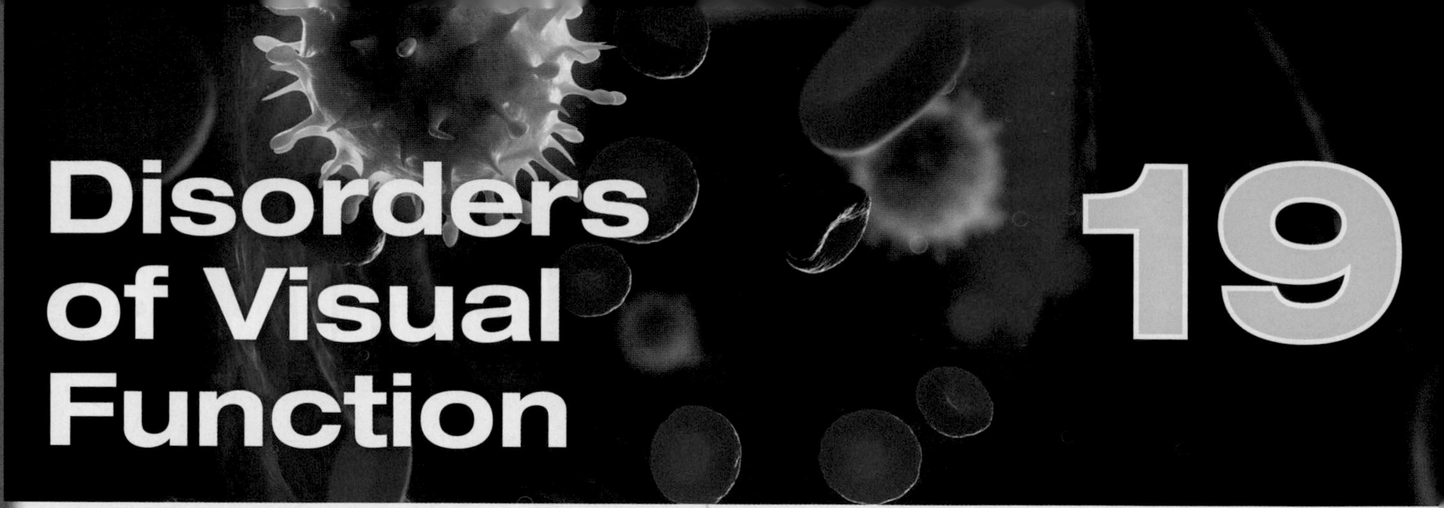

Disorders of Visual Function

19

Diane Smith

The World Health Organization (WHO) reports that 161 million people worldwide are visually impaired: 124 million have low vision, and 37 million are blind.[1] An additional 153 million have visual impairment due to uncorrected refractive errors (nearsightedness, farsightedness, or astigmatism).[1] In 2017, the World Health Assembly stated that more than 90% of the world's visually impaired people live in low- and middle-income countries.[1] The WHO is a founding partner of Vision 2020 and is working to eliminate the main causes of avoidable blindness by the year 2020.[1]

Alterations in vision can result from disorders of the eyelids and optic globe (conjunctiva, cornea, and uvea), intraocular pressure (glaucoma), lens (cataract), vitreous humor and retina (retinopathy and macular degeneration), optic pathways and visual cortex, and extraocular muscles and eye movement. The optic globe, commonly called the *eyeball*, is a remarkably mobile, nearly spherical structure contained in a pyramid-shaped cavity of the skull called the *orbit*. The eyeball occupies only the anterior one fifth of the orbit. The remainder is filled with muscles, nerves, the lacrimal gland, and adipose tissue that support the normal position of the optic globe. Exposed surfaces of the eyes are protected by the eyelids, which are mucous membrane–lined skin flaps that provide a means for shutting out most light. Tears bathe

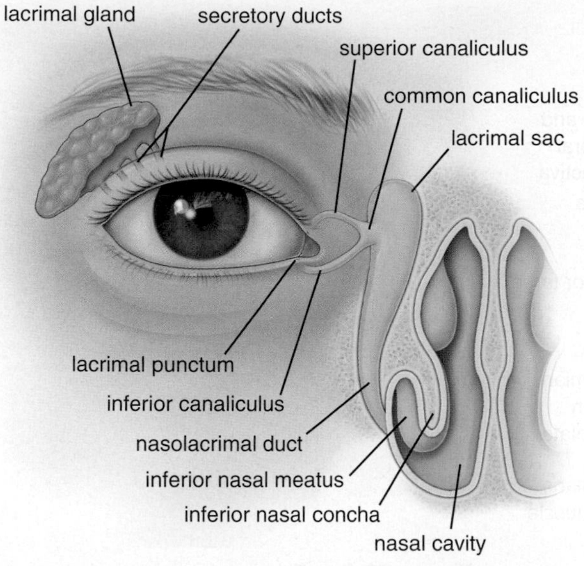

Figure 19.1 • Schematic diagram of the eye and lacrimal apparatus. (From Pawlina W. (2016). *Histology: A text and atlas: With correlated cell and molecular biology* (7th ed., p. 923, Fig. 24.18). Philadelphia, PA: Wolters Kluwer.)

the anterior surface of the eye. They prevent friction between it and the lid, maintain hydration of the cornea, and protect the eye from infection and irritation by foreign objects. Figure 19.1 illustrates the eyelid and lacrimal apparatus.

Three distinct layers form the wall of the eyeball—the sclera or outer supporting layer, the uvea or middle vascular layer, and the retina, which is composed of the neuronal retinal layer and the outer pigmented layer (see Fig. 19.2). The outer layer of the eyeball consists of a tough, opaque, white, fibrous layer called the *sclera*. It is strong yet elastic and maintains the shape of the globe. The sclera is continuous with the cornea anteriorly and with the cranial dural sheath that surrounds and protects the optic nerve posteriorly. The choroid (uvea) predominantly provides vascular support of the retina, whereas the retina is the neurosensory tissue that provides the sensory input for sight.

KEY POINTS

VISION

- Vision is a special sensory function that incorporates the visual receptor functions of the eyeball, the optic nerve, and optic pathways that carry and distribute sensory information from the optic globe to the central nervous system (CNS) via photoreceptors in the retina and the primary and visual association cortices that translate the sensory signals into visual images.
- Binocular vision depends on the coordination of three pairs of extraocular nerves that provide for the conjugate eye movements, with optical axes of the two eyes maintained parallel with one another as the eyes rotate in their sockets.

DISORDERS OF THE ACCESSORY STRUCTURES OF THE EYE

After completing this section of the chapter, the learner will be able to meet the following objectives:

- Describe the cause of eyelid weakness.
- Compare and contrast *entropion* and *ectropion*.
- Compare and contrast marginal blepharitis, a hordeolum, and a chalazion regarding causes and manifestations.

Disorders of the Eyelids

The upper and lower eyelids, the *palpebrae*, are modified folds of skin with associated muscle and cartilaginous plates that protect the eyeball. The palpebral fissure is the oval opening between the upper and lower eyelids. At the corners of the eye, where the upper and lower lids meet, is an angle called the *canthus*. The lateral canthus is the outer, or temporal,

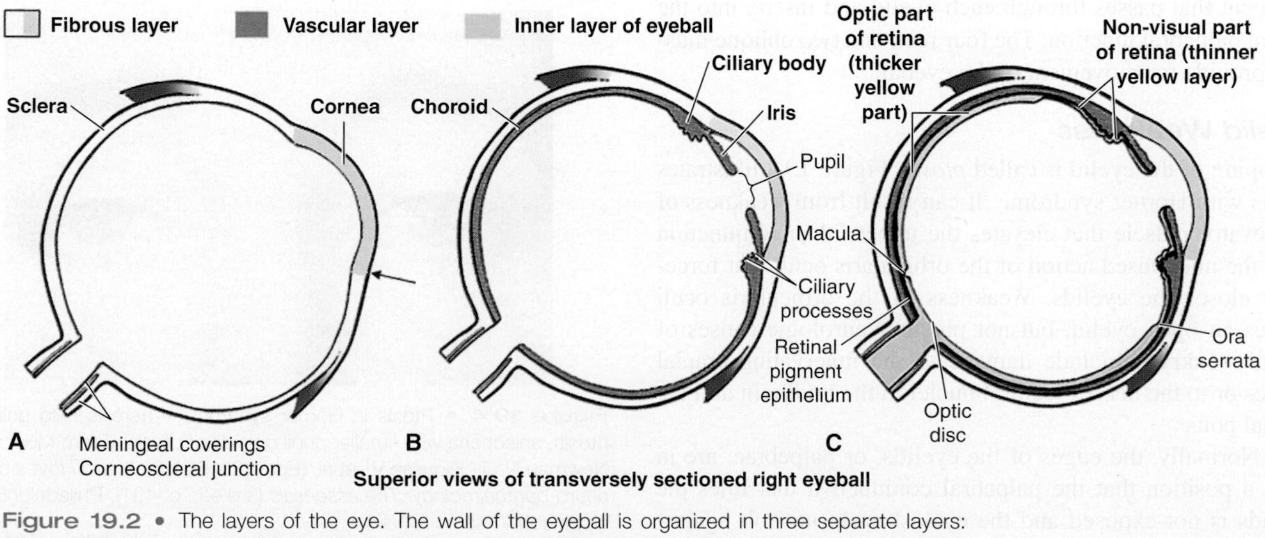

Figure 19.2 • The layers of the eye. The wall of the eyeball is organized in three separate layers: **(A)** an outer fibrous layer, **(B)** a middle vascular layer, and **(C)** an inner photosensitive layer, the retina. (From Moore K. L., Agur A. M., Dalley A. F. (2015). *Essential clinical anatomy* (5th ed., p. 522, Fig. 7.26). Philadelphia, PA: Wolters Kluwer/Lippincott Williams & Wilkins.)

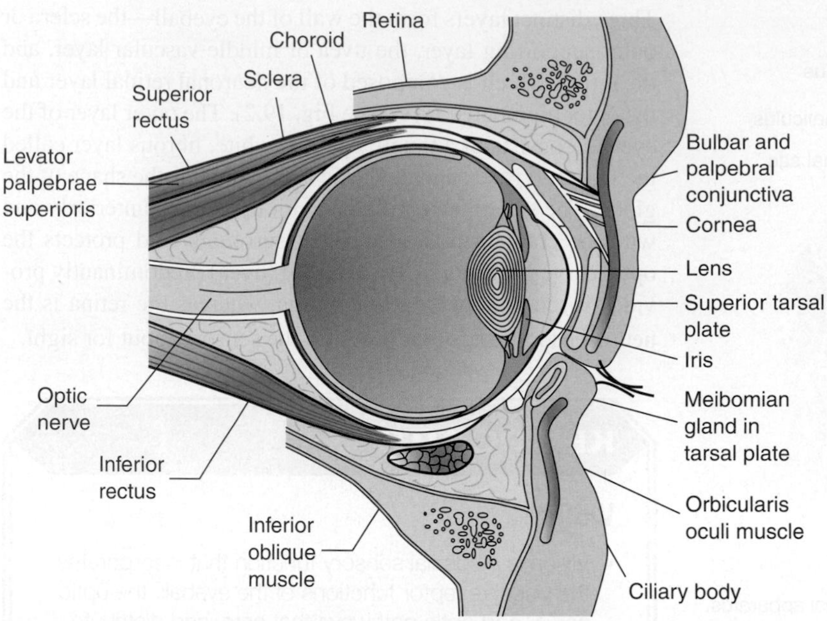

Figure 19.3 • The eye and its appendages: anterior view.

angle, and the medial canthus is the inner, or nasal, angle. In each lid, a tarsus, or plate of dense connective tissue, gives the lid its shape (Fig. 19.3). Each tarsus contains modified sebaceous glands, called *meibomian glands*, the ducts of which open onto the eyelid margins. Sebaceous secretions of the meibomian glands enable airtight closure of the lids and prevent rapid evaporation of tears.

Two striated muscles, the levator palpebrae superioris and the orbicularis oculi, provide for movement of the eyelids. The levator palpebrae superioris, innervated by the oculomotor nerve (cranial nerve [CN] III), serves to raise the upper lid. Encircling the eye is the orbicularis oculi muscle, which is supplied by the facial nerve (CN VII). When this muscle contracts, it closes the eyelids. Between the nose and medial angle of the eye is the medial palpebral ligament, which connects to the medial margin of the orbit (see Fig. 19.3). A similar palpebral ligament attaches to the lateral margin of the orbit. The orbicularis oculi nerve inserts into the medial palpebral ligament that passes through each eyelid and inserts into the lateral palpebral junction. The four recti and two oblique muscles provide for movement of the eyeball.

Eyelid Weakness

Drooping of the eyelid is called *ptosis*. Figure 19.4 illustrates ptosis with Horner syndrome. It can result from weakness of the levator muscle that elevates the upper lid in conjunction with the unopposed action of the orbicularis oculi that forcefully closes the eyelids. Weakness of the orbicularis oculi causes an open eyelid, but not ptosis. Neurologic causes of eyelid weakness include damage to the innervating cranial nerves or to the nerves' central nuclei in the midbrain and the caudal pons.

Normally, the edges of the eyelids, or palpebrae, are in such a position that the palpebral conjunctiva that lines the eyelids is not exposed and the eyelashes do not rub against the cornea. Turning in of the lid margin is called *entropion*. It is usually caused by scarring of the palpebral conjunctiva or degeneration of the fascial attachments to the lower lid that occurs with aging. Corneal irritation may occur as the eyelashes turn inward. *Ectropion* refers to eversion of the lower lid margin and is the most frequent bilateral lid condition. It is caused by relaxation of the orbicularis oculi muscle because of CN VII weakness or the aging process.[2] Ectropion causes tearing and ocular irritation and may lead to inflammation of the cornea.

Entropion and ectropion can be treated surgically. Contraction of the resulting scar tissue usually draws the lid up to its normal position.

Eyelid Inflammation

Blepharitis is a common chronic bilateral inflammation involving the lashes and lid margins (Fig. 19.5). Two main

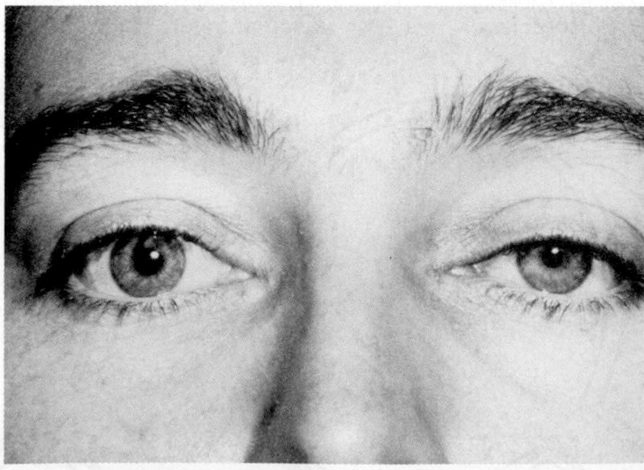

Figure 19.4 • Ptosis in Horner syndrome—there is mild unilateral ptosis, anisocoria with smaller pupil on side of ptosis. (From Miller N. R., Newman N. J., Biousse V., et al. (Eds.) (2016). *Walsh and Hoyt's clinical neuro-ophthalmology: The essentials* (3rd ed., p. 431). Philadelphia, PA: Lippincott Williams & Wilkins.)

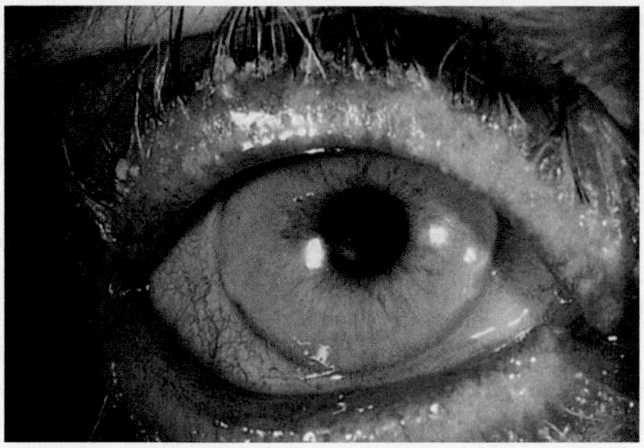

Figure 19.5 • Blepharitis—inflammation of margin of eyelid. (From Jensen S. (2015). *Nursing health assessment: A best practice approach* (2nd ed., p. 341). Philadelphia, PA: Lippincott Williams & Wilkins.)

types of anterior blepharitis occur—inflammatory and infectious. The inflammatory form is usually associated with seborrhea (*i.e.*, dandruff) of the scalp or brows. Infectious blepharitis may be caused by *Staphylococcus epidermidis* or *Staphylococcus aureus*, in which case the lesions are often ulcerative. The main symptoms of anterior blepharitis are irritation, burning, redness, and itching of the eyelid margins. Treatment includes careful cleaning with a damp applicator to remove the scales. When the disorder is associated with a microbial infection, an antibiotic (ointment or drops) is prescribed.[3]

Posterior blepharitis is inflammation of the eyelids that involves the meibomian glands. It may result from a bacterial infection, particularly with staphylococci, or dysfunction of the meibomian glands, in which there is a strong association with acne rosacea.[3] The meibomian glands and their orifices are inflamed, with dilation of the glands, plugging of the orifices, and abnormal secretions. The tears may be frothy and abnormally greasy from the meibomian secretions. Treatment of posterior blepharitis is determined by associated conjunctival and corneal changes. Initial therapies can include warm compresses and lid massage. Systemic antibiotic therapy can be prescribed, guided by results of bacterial cultures.[3]

A *hordeolum*, or *stye*, is usually caused by an infection of the meibomian gland or other structures of the eyelid margin. The infection is usually caused by *S. aureus*. Symptoms include pain, redness, and swelling. Applying warm, moist compresses to the site assists in treatment. A referral to an ophthalmologist may be required if the infection does not resolve after 2 to 3 days. Topical antibiotics or medications with corticosteroids are no longer recommended.[3]

A *chalazion* is a focal chronic inflammation developing when the meibomian gland becomes obstructed. A small, painless nodule develops on the tarsus. Treatment consists of warm, moist compresses. Referral to an ophthalmologist may be necessary if the nodule does not resolve. Antibiotics are not given because this is not an infectious process.[3]

Disorders of the Lacrimal System

The lacrimal system includes the major lacrimal gland, which produces the tears; the puncta, canaliculi, and tear sac, which collect the tears; and the nasolacrimal duct, which empties the tears into the nasal cavity. The lacrimal gland lies in the orbit, superior and lateral to the eyeball (see Fig. 19.1). Approximately 12 small ducts connect the lacrimal gland to the superior conjunctival fornix. Tears contain approximately 98% water, 1.5% sodium chloride, and small amounts of potassium, albumin, and glucose. The function of tears is to provide a smooth optical surface by abolishing minute surface irregularities. Tears also wet and protect the delicate surface of the cornea and conjunctiva. They flush and remove irritating substances and microorganisms and provide the cornea with necessary nutrient substances. Tears also contain lysozymes and immunoglobulin A (IgA), IgG, and IgE, which synergistically act to protect against infection. Although IgA predominates, IgE concentrations are increased in some allergic conditions.

Dry Eyes

Dry eye is a multifactorial disease characterized by unstable tear film causing a variety of symptoms and/or visual impairment, potentially accompanied by ocular surface damage.[4]

The thin film of tears that covers the cornea is essential in preventing drying and damage of the outer layer of the cornea as well as providing immune protection. This tear film is composed of three layers:

1. An outer lipid layer, which is derived from the meibomian glands and which limits evaporative loss
2. An intermediate aqueous layer, secreted by the lacrimal glands
3. An inner mucin layer, which overlies the cornea and epithelial cells[5]

Dry eye symptoms are common and can be divided into two categories: aqueous-deficient and evaporative.[5] The aqueous-deficient category is associated with autoimmune diseases and disorders. The evaporative category has a variety of causes, but the most common are related to an obstruction of meibomian gland openings. Other causes include poor eyelid closure, infrequent blinking, and contact lens wear.[5] People may complain that the eyes feel gritty. There may be pain or burning, light sensitivity, redness, or itching. Occasionally, vision may be blurred.[5] Artificial tears are commonly used for relief of symptoms. Persistent discomfort requires an evaluation by a health care provider.[5]

Dacryocystitis

Dacryocystitis is an inflammation and infection of the lacrimal sac and occurs secondary to an anatomical obstruction (dacryostenosis) of the tear duct (nasolacrimal duct). The symptoms include tearing and discharge, pain, swelling, and tenderness. The treatment includes application of warm compresses and topical and oral antibiotic therapy.

In infants, dacryostenosis is usually caused by failure of the nasolacrimal ducts to open spontaneously before birth. Definitive treatment requires surgery.[6]

IN SUMMARY

The eyelids serve to protect the eye. Ptosis refers to drooping of the upper lid, which is caused by injury to CN III. Entropion, which refers to turning in the upper eyelid and eyelashes, is discomforting and causes corneal irritation. Ectropion, or eversion of the lower eyelid, causes tearing and may lead to corneal inflammation. Marginal blepharitis is the most common disorder of the eyelids. It commonly is caused by a staphylococcal infection or seborrhea (*i.e.*, dandruff).

The lacrimal system includes the major lacrimal gland, which produces the tears; the puncta and tear sac, which collect the tears; and the nasolacrimal duct, which empties the tears into the nasal cavity. Tears protect the cornea from drying and irritation. Impaired tear production or conditions that prevent blinking and the spread of tears produce drying of the eyes and predispose them to corneal irritation and injury. Dacryocystitis is an inflammation caused by an infection of the lacrimal sac.

DISORDERS OF THE CONJUNCTIVA, CORNEA, AND UVEAL TRACT

After completing this section of the chapter, the learner will be able to meet the following objectives:

- Compare symptoms associated with red eye caused by conjunctivitis, corneal irritation, and acute glaucoma.
- Characterize the manifestations, treatment, and possible complications of bacterial, *Acanthamoeba*, and herpes keratitis.
- Describe tests used in assessing the pupillary reflex and cite the possible causes of abnormal pupillary reflexes.

Disorders of the Conjunctiva

The conjunctiva is a delicate mucous membrane that lines the anterior surface of both eyelids as the *palpebral conjunctiva* and folds back over the anterior surface of the optic globe as the *ocular* or *bulbar conjunctiva.*[7] The ocular conjunctiva covers only the sclera or white portion of the optic globe, not the cornea. When both eyes are closed, the conjunctiva lines the closed conjunctival sac. Although the conjunctiva protects the eye, its main function is the production of a lubricating mucus that bathes the eye and keeps it moist.

Conjunctivitis, or inflammation of the conjunctiva (*i.e.*, red or pink eye), is one of the most common forms of eye disease. It may result from bacterial or viral infection, allergens, chemical agents, physical irritants, or radiant energy. Depending on the cause, conjunctivitis can vary in severity from a mild hyperemia (redness) with tearing to severe conjunctivitis with purulent drainage. The conjunctiva is extremely sensitive to irritation and inflammation.

Clinical manifestations of conjunctivitis include a foreign body sensation, a scratching or burning sensation, itching, and photophobia. Severe pain suggests corneal rather than conjunctival disease. A discharge, or exudate, may be present. It is usually watery when the conjunctivitis is caused by allergy, a foreign body, or viral infection and mucopurulent in the presence of bacterial or fungal infection. A characteristic of many forms of conjunctivitis is papillary hypertrophy. This occurs because the palpebral conjunctiva is bound to the tarsus by fine fibrils. As a result, inflammation that develops between the fibrils causes the conjunctiva to be elevated in mounds called **papillae**. When the papillae are small, the conjunctiva has a smooth, velvety appearance. Red papillary conjunctivitis suggests bacterial or chlamydial conjunctivitis. In allergic conjunctivitis, the papillae often become flat-topped, polygonal, and milky in color and have a cobblestone appearance.

The diagnosis of conjunctivitis is based on history, physical examination, and microscopic and culture studies to identify the cause. Because a red eye may be the sign of several eye conditions, it is important to differentiate between redness caused by conjunctivitis and that caused by more serious eye disorders, such as corneal lesions and acute glaucoma. In contrast to corneal lesions and acute glaucoma, conjunctivitis produces infection (*i.e.*, enlargement and redness) of the peripheral conjunctival blood vessels rather than those radiating around the corneal limbus. Conjunctivitis also produces only mild discomfort compared with the moderate to severe discomfort associated with corneal lesions or the severe and deep pain associated with acute glaucoma. Infectious forms of conjunctivitis are usually bilateral and may involve other family members and associates. Unilateral disease suggests sources of irritation such as foreign bodies or chemical irritation.

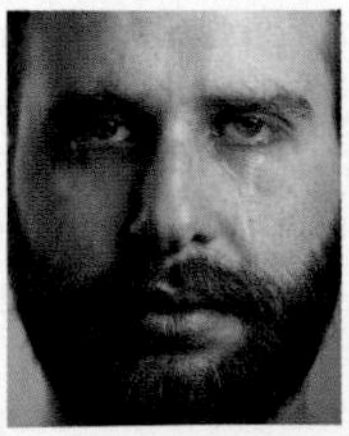

Remember Mr. Pall from the unit opener case study. His primary care provider diagnosed him with bacterial conjunctivitis based on the history and physical examination findings. He complains of his left eye being stuck together like glue because of the huge amounts of yellow drainage upon awakening, and Mr. Pall has no other concerns besides the conjunctivitis, except that he has an upper respiratory infection. On physical examination, injected and swollen conjunctiva, red eye, and large amounts of drainage were found. He has some slight discomfort but no pain.

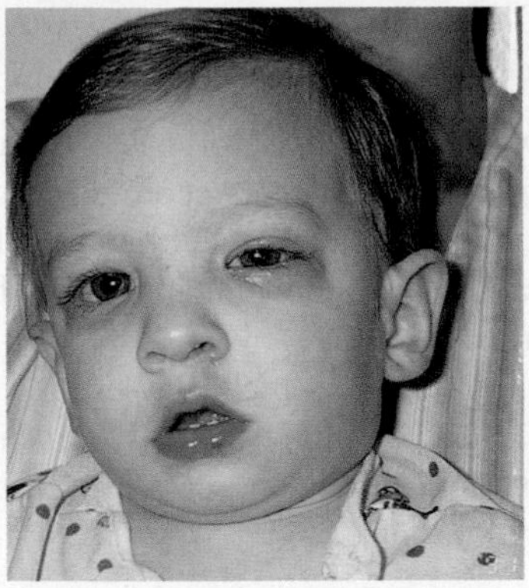

Figure 19.6 • Allergic conjunctivitis—usually bilateral and common in people with allergic conditions. (From Jensen S. (2015). *Nursing health assessment: A best practice approach* (2nd ed., p. 341). Philadelphia, PA: Lippincott Williams & Wilkins.)

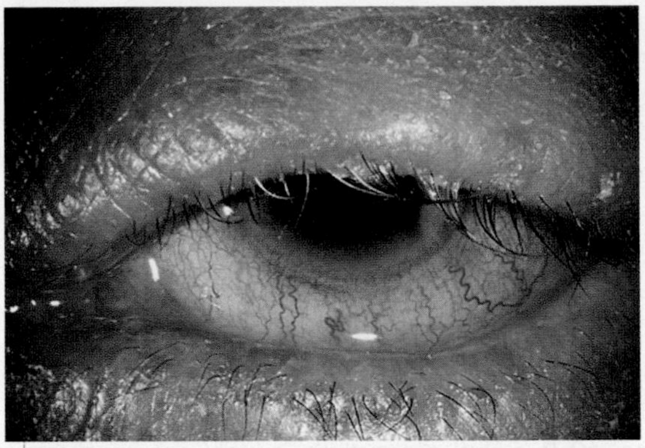

Figure 19.7 • Bacterial conjunctivitis—usually purulent discharge and infected conjunctiva. (From Jensen S. (2015). *Nursing health assessment: A best practice approach* (2nd ed., p. 341). Philadelphia, PA: Lippincott Williams & Wilkins.)

Allergic Conjunctivitis

Allergic conjunctivitis encompasses a spectrum of conjunctival conditions usually characterized by itching. The most common of these is seasonal allergic rhinoconjunctivitis, or hay fever. Seasonal allergic conjunctivitis is an IgE-mediated hypersensitivity reaction precipitated by small airborne allergens such as pollens.[3] It typically causes bilateral tearing, itching, and redness of the eyes (Fig. 19.6).

The treatment of seasonal allergic rhinoconjunctivitis includes allergen avoidance and the use of cold compresses and eye washes with tear substitute. Allergic conjunctivitis also has been successfully treated with oral second-generation, nonsedating antihistamines.[3]

Infectious Conjunctivitis

Causes of infectious conjunctivitis include bacteria, viruses, gonorrhea, herpes, and chlamydia. Infections may spread from areas adjacent to the conjunctiva or may be blood-borne, such as in measles or chickenpox. Newborns can contract conjunctivitis during the birth process.

Bacterial Conjunctivitis. Bacterial conjunctivitis may present as a hyperacute, acute, or chronic infection. *Hyperacute conjunctivitis* is a severe, sight-threatening ocular infection most commonly caused by *Neisseria gonorrhoeae* and less commonly caused by *Neisseria meningitidis*. In newborns, *N. gonorrhoeae is the cause of the most serious type of conjunctivitis*.[3] In adults and adolescents, infection occurs through autoinoculation from infected genitalia. The infection has an abrupt onset and is characterized by a copious amount of yellow-green drainage. The symptoms, which typically are progressive, include conjunctival redness; chemosis (swelling around the cornea); lid swelling; and tender, swollen preauricular lymph nodes (Fig. 19.7). Gonococcal ocular infections left untreated result in corneal ulceration with ultimate perforation and sometimes permanent loss of vision. Diagnostic methods include immediate Gram staining of ocular specimens and special cultures for *Neisseria* species. Treatment includes systemic antibiotics supplemented with ocular antibiotics.[3]

Acute bacterial conjunctivitis typically presents with burning, tearing, and mucopurulent or purulent discharge. Common agents of bacterial conjunctivitis are *Streptococcus pneumoniae*, *S. aureus*, and *Haemophilus influenzae* in adults. In children, *Moraxella catarrhalis* is also common.[3] Infection normally begins in one eye and within 24 to 48 hours spreads to the unaffected eye. Drainage may be green, white, or yellow. Treatment may include local application of antibiotic drops or ointment.

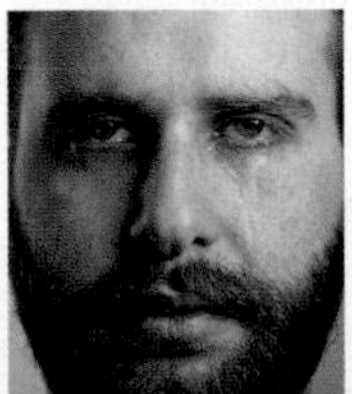

Mr. Pall had not had conjunctivitis previously, but living in a college dormitory would increase his risk of picking it up easily. He also mentioned that he had a head cold (upper respiratory infection) for several days duration and could have infected his eye himself from cross contact with the nasal drainage from his upper respiratory infection. Most likely, of the three common bacteria (*S. pneumoniae*, *S. aureus*, and *H. influenzae*) that cause conjunctivitis, Mr. Pall has *S. pneumoniae*. Because of the irritation from the contacts and cigarette smoke at the party the evening before, Mr. Pall may have touched his eyes frequently, therefore infecting the conjunctiva.

Viral Conjunctivitis. Etiologic agents of viral conjunctivitis include adenoviruses, herpesviruses, and enteroviruses. One of the most common causes of viral conjunctivitis is adenovirus type.[3] The infection, which causes generalized conjunctival hyperemia, copious tearing, and minimal exudate, is usually associated with an upper respiratory tract infection (Fig. 19.8). Children are affected more often than are adults.

Swimming pools contaminated because of inadequate chlorination are common sources of infection.[3] Symptoms

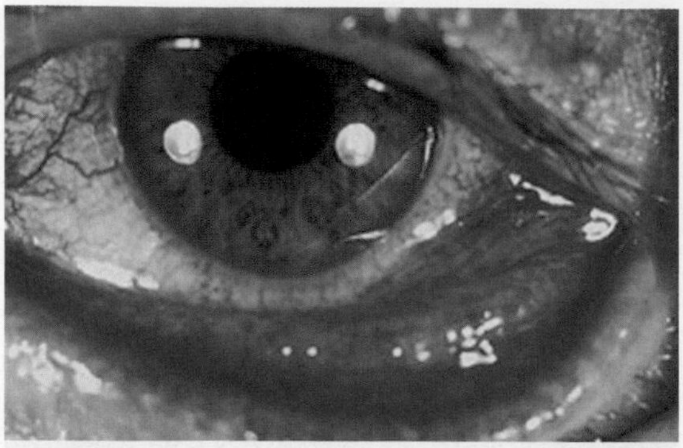

Figure 19.8 • Viral conjunctivitis—usually clear discharge, which may be accompanied by sinus congestion and rhinorrhea. (From Jensen S. (2015). *Nursing health assessment: A best practice approach* (2nd ed., p. 341). Philadelphia, PA: Lippincott Williams & Wilkins.)

will resolve over time with the use of cool compresses and artificial tears. Topical antibiotics may be given if a secondary infection is present. Topical antivirals are not recommended.[3]

Chlamydial Conjunctivitis. There are two types of chlamydial eye infections:

- Trachoma, which includes serotypes A through C, causing chronic keratoconjunctivitis. According to the WHO, it is the leading cause of preventable blindness. It is rare in the United States and Europe while commonly found in developing countries.[3,8]
- Inclusion conjunctivitis, which is associated with serotypes D through K. It is a common, sexually transmitted infection in adolescents and adults and can be transmitted to vaginally delivered infants.[3]

Sexually transmitted eye infections should be evaluated and treated promptly by a health care provider.

Disorders of the Cornea

At the anterior part of the eyeball, the outer covering of the eye is modified to form the transparent cornea, which bulges anteriorly from its junction with the sclera (Fig. 19.9).

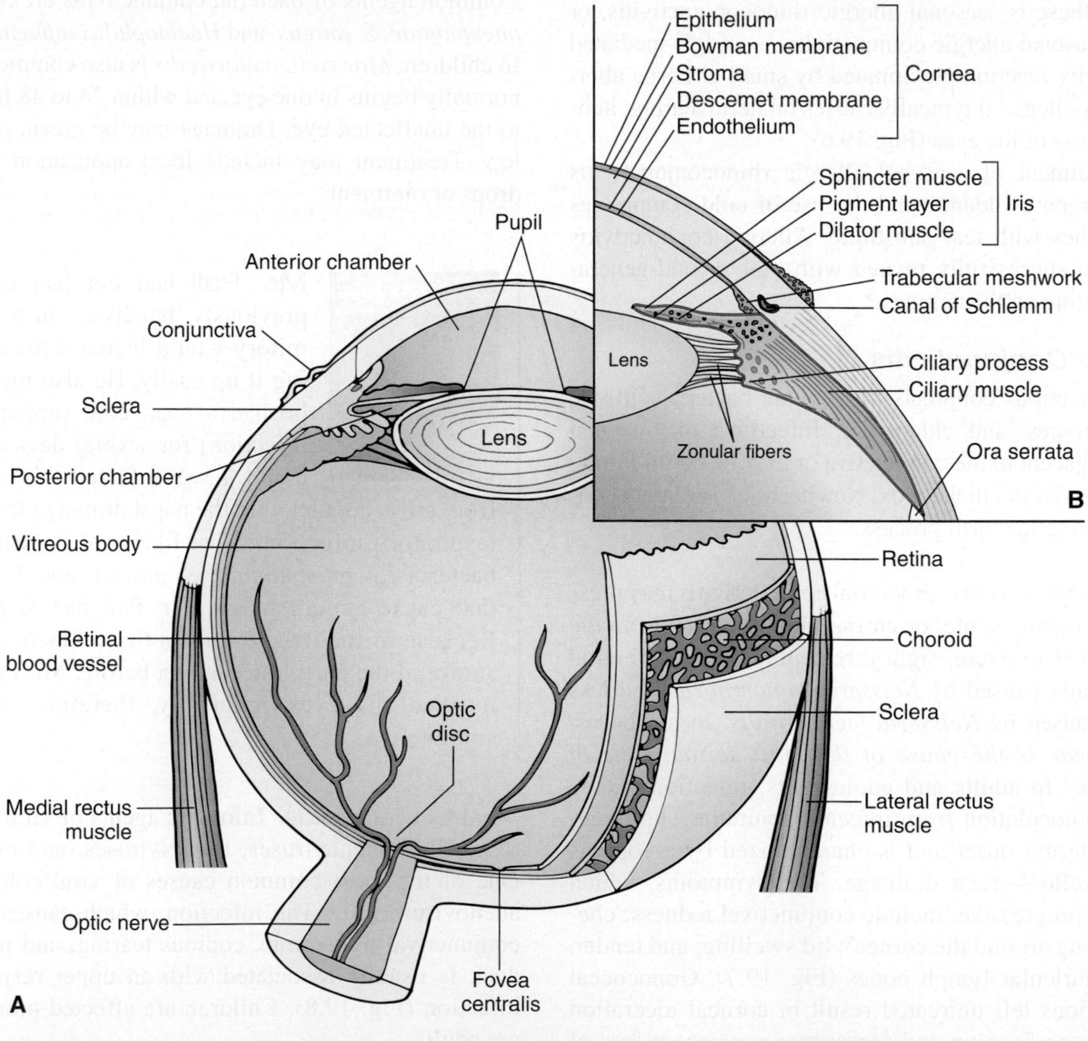

Figure 19.9 • (A) Transverse section of the eyeball. (B) Enlargement of the anterior and posterior chambers of the eye, showing the layers of the cornea, the structures of the iris, aqueous drainage system (trabecular meshwork, canal of Schlemm), and the ciliary process and ciliary muscle.

A major part of the refraction (*i.e.*, bending) of light rays and focusing of vision occurs in the cornea. Three layers of tissue form the cornea:

1. An extremely thin outer epithelial layer, which is continuous with the bulbar conjunctiva
2. A middle layer called the *substantia propria* or *stroma*
3. An inner endothelial layer, which lies next to the aqueous humor of the anterior chamber.[9]

The substantia propria is composed of regularly arranged collagen bundles embedded in a mucopolysaccharide matrix. This organization of the collagen fibers, which makes the substantia propria transparent, is necessary for light transmission. Hydration within a limited range is necessary to maintain the spacing of the collagen fibers and transparency. The three layers of the cornea are separated by two important basement membranes: the Bowman and Descemet membranes. The *Bowman membrane*, which lies between the corneal epithelium and stoma, acts as a barrier to infection. It does not regenerate. If damaged, an opaque scar forms that can impair vision. The *Descemet membrane*, which lies between the corneal endothelium and stroma, has a feltlike appearance and consists of interwoven fibers and pores. Unlike the Bowman membrane, it regenerates readily after injury.

The cornea is avascular and obtains its nutrient and oxygen supply by diffusion from blood vessels of the adjacent sclera, from the aqueous humor at its deep surface, and from tears. The corneal epithelium is heavily innervated by sensory neurons (trigeminal nerve [CN V], ophthalmic division [CN V_1]). Epithelial damage causes discomfort that ranges from a foreign body sensation and burning of the eyes to severe, incapacitating pain. Reflex lacrimation is common.

Disorders of the cornea include trauma, inflammation and infection, abnormal corneal deposits, and degenerative processes such as arcus senilis. Diagnosis of corneal disorders is based on history of trauma, medication use, and signs and symptoms associated with corneal irritation and disease.[9] Because of the discomfort involved, examination of the eye is often eased by instillation of a local anesthetic agent. Fluorescein staining can be used to outline an ulcerated area. The biomicroscope (slit lamp) is used for proper examination of the cornea. In cases of an infectious etiology, scrapings from the ulcer are obtained for staining and culture studies.

Corneal Trauma

The integrity of the epithelium and the endothelium is necessary to maintain hydration of the cornea within a limited range. Damage to either structure leads to edema and loss of transparency. Among the causes of corneal edema is the prolonged wearing of contact lenses, which can deprive the epithelium of oxygen, disrupting its integrity. Corneal edema also occurs after a sudden rise in intraocular pressure. With corneal edema, the cornea appears dull, uneven, and hazy. In addition, visual acuity decreases and iridescent vision (*i.e.*, rainbows around lights) occurs.

Trauma that causes abrasions of the cornea can be extremely painful, but if minor, the abrasions usually heal in a few days. The epithelial layer can regenerate, and small defects heal without scarring. If the stroma is damaged, healing occurs more slowly, and the danger of infection is increased. Injuries to the Bowman membrane and the stromal layer heal with scar formation that impairs the transmission of light.

Keratitis

Keratitis refers to inflammation of the cornea, which can result in partial or total loss of vision caused by infectious or noninfectious sources. Infectious sources include bacteria, viruses, fungi, and amebae. Noninfectious causes include eye trauma, chemical exposure, and ultraviolet exposure. Contact lens wear is a major risk factor for infectious keratitis.[10] Symptoms of keratitis can include pain, photophobia, conjunctival hyperemia (redness), and corneal cloudiness with stromal involvement.[11] Immediate evaluation and treatment by a health care provider should be sought.

Herpes Simplex Keratitis. Herpes simplex virus (HSV) keratitis is the leading cause of corneal scarring and opacity causing blindness worldwide.[12] Most cases are caused by HSV type 1, the cause of labial or lip infections. However, in neonatal infections acquired during passage through the birth canal, approximately 80% are caused by HSV type 2 (the cause of genital herpes). The disease can occur as a primary or recurrent infection.[13] Primary epithelial infections are the optical counterpart of labial herpes with similar immunologic and pathologic features as well as a similar time course. During childhood, mild primary HSV infection may go unnoticed. After the initial primary infection, the virus may persist in a quiescent or latent state in the trigeminal ganglion and possibly in the cornea without causing signs of infection.

Recurrent infection may be precipitated by various poorly understood, stress-related factors that reactivate the virus. Involvement is usually unilateral. The first symptoms are irritation, photophobia, and tearing. Some reduction in vision may occur when the lesion affects the central part of the cornea. Because corneal anesthesia occurs early in the disease, the symptoms may be minimal, and the person may delay seeking medical care. A history of fever blisters or other herpetic infection is often noted, but corneal lesions may be the only sign of recurrent herpes infection. Most typically, the corneal lesion involves the epithelium and has a typical branching pattern. These epithelial lesions heal without scarring. Herpetic lesions that involve the stromal layer of the cornea produce increasingly severe corneal opacities. Although previously thought to be a purely immunologic response to viral particles or virally induced cellular changes, there is increasing evidence that infection due to active viral particles can occur in stromal and possibly endothelial cells, as well as other tissues in the anterior segment such as the iris and trabecular endothelium.

The treatment of HSV keratitis focuses on eliminating viral replication in the cornea while minimizing the damaging effects of the inflammatory process. Topical antiviral agents such as trifluridine drops, vidarabine or acyclovir ointment, or ganciclovir gel are used to promote healing.[14,15] Oral antiviral agents (*e.g.*, acyclovir) can be used but have not been studied in comparative trials for efficacy, and resistance to these drugs has been increasing. The use of topical corticosteroids is contraindicated.[14,15]

Varicella–Zoster Ophthalmicus. Herpes zoster or shingles is a relatively common infection caused by herpesvirus type 3, the same virus that causes varicella (chickenpox). It occurs when the varicella virus, which has remained dormant in the neurosensory ganglia since the primary infection, is reactivated. Herpes zoster ophthalmicus, which represents 10% to 25% of all cases of herpes zoster, occurs when reactivation of the latent virus occurs in the ganglia of the ophthalmic division of the trigeminal nerve.[9,13] Immunocompromised people, particularly those with human immunodeficiency virus (HIV) infection, are at higher risk for developing herpes zoster ophthalmicus than are those with a normally functioning immune system.

Herpes zoster ophthalmicus usually presents with malaise, fever, headache, and burning and itching of the periorbital area. These symptoms commonly precede the ocular eruption by a day or two. The rash, which is initially vesicular, becomes pustular and then crusting. Involvement of the tip of the nose and lid margins indicates a high likelihood of ocular involvement. Ocular signs include conjunctivitis, keratitis, and anterior uveitis, often with elevated intraocular pressure. People with corneal disease present with varying degrees of decreased vision, pain, and sensitivity to light.

Treatment includes the use of high-dose oral antiviral drugs (*i.e.*, acyclovir, valacyclovir, famciclovir). Initiation of treatment within the first 72 hours after the appearance of the rash reduces the incidence of ocular complications but not the postherpetic neuralgia.

***Acanthamoeba* Keratitis.** *Acanthamoeba* is a free-living protozoan in contaminated water frequented by travelers. *Acanthamoeba* keratitis is a rare but serious and sight-threatening complication of exposure from continuous wearing of soft contact lenses, either extended wear or those worn overnight beyond doctor-recommended periods, or when poor disinfection techniques are used. It also may occur in non–contact lens wearers after exposure to contaminated water or soil. It is characterized by pain that is disproportionate to the clinical manifestations, redness of the eye, and photophobia. The disorder commonly is misdiagnosed as herpes keratitis or fungal keratitis. Diagnosis is confirmed by fluorescein staining of the eye.[16] Corneal biopsies with cultures may be indicated. To preserve vision, an immediate referral to a health care provider is required.[17–19]

Abnormal Corneal Deposits

The cornea frequently is the site for deposition of abnormal metabolic products. In hypercalcemia, calcium salts can precipitate in the cornea, producing a cloudy band keratopathy. Cystine crystals are deposited in cystinosis, cholesterol esters in hypercholesterolemia, and a golden ring of copper (*i.e.*, Kayser-Fleischer ring) in hepatolenticular degeneration due to Wilson disease. Pharmacologic agents, such as chloroquine, can result in crystal deposits in the cornea.

Arcus senilis is an extremely common, bilateral, benign corneal degeneration that may occur at any age but is more common in the elderly. It consists of a grayish-white infiltrate, approximately 2 mm wide, that occurs at the periphery of the cornea. It may represent an extracellular lipid infiltration and commonly is associated with hyperlipidemia, so lipid studies should be done if it is found in people under the age of 50. Arcus senilis does not produce visual symptoms, and there is no treatment necessary for this finding in older adults.

Corneal Transplantation

Over 40,000 corneal transplants are performed in the United States yearly.[20] Unlike kidney or heart transplantation procedures, which are associated with considerable risk of rejection of the transplanted organ, corneal transplants entail minimal danger of rejection. However, corneas that have been subjected to burns or that are unhealthy lose their "immune-privileged" status and become susceptible to graft rejection. The risk for immune rejection lasts a lifetime. Any use of human corneas for transplantation has the risk for immune rejection.[8]

Disorders of the Uveal Tract

The middle vascular layer, or uveal tract, is an incomplete ball with gaps at the pupil and the optic nerve. The pigmented uveal tract has three distinct regions: the choroid, ciliary body, and the iris. The *choroid* is a highly vascular, dark brown membrane that forms the posterior five sixths of the uveal tract. Its blood vessels provide nourishment for the other layers of the eyeball. Its brown pigment, produced by melanocytes, absorbs light within the eyeball and light that penetrates the retina. The light-absorptive function prevents the scattering of light and is important for visual acuity, particularly with high background illumination levels. The *ciliary body* is a thickened ring of tissue that encircles the lens. It has smooth muscle and secretory functions. Its smooth muscle function contributes to changes in lens shape and its secretory function to the production of aqueous humor.

The iris is an adjustable diaphragm that permits changes in pupil size and in the light entering the eye. The posterior surface of the iris is formed by a two-layer epithelium continuous with those layers covering the ciliary body. The anterior layer contains the dilator or radial muscles of the iris. Just anterior to these muscles is a layer of highly vascular connective tissue. Embedded in this layer are concentric rings of smooth muscle that compose the sphincter muscle of the pupil. The anterior layer of the iris forms an irregular anterior surface, containing many fibroblasts and melanocytes. Eye color differences result from the density of the pigment. The amount of pigment decreases from that found in dark brown eyes through shades of brown and green to that found in blue eyes.

Several mutations affect the pigment of the uveal tract, including albinism. *Albinism* is a genetic (autosomal recessive trait) deficiency of tyrosinase, the enzyme needed for the synthesis of melanin by the melanocytes. Tyrosinase-negative albinism, also called *classic albinism*, is characterized by an absence of tyrosinase. Affected people have white hair, pink skin, and light blue eyes. In these people, excessive light penetrates the unpigmented iris and choroid and, to some extent, the anterior sclera. Their photoreceptors are flooded with excess light, and visual acuity is markedly reduced. Excess stimulation of the photoreceptors at normal or high illumination levels is experienced as painful photophobia, a symptom of many disease processes.

Uveitis

Inflammation of the entire uveal tract, which supports the lens and neural components of the eye, is called uveitis. Uveitis is caused by infectious (virus, bacteria, fungi, or parasite) or noninfectious (autoimmune, malignant, or idiopathic) agents. One type of noninfectious etiology, autoimmune, results from an inflammatory disorder of ocular tissue with clinical features in common and an immunologically based cause. A serious consequence of uveitis can be the involvement of the underlying retina. Parasitic invasion of the choroid can result in local atrophic changes that usually involve the retina; examples include toxoplasmosis and histoplasmosis. Metastatic uveal tumors from malignancies such as breast, lung, and colon cancers have been documented. Primary uveal lymphoma is not common but occurs and requires radiation treatment.[9,21]

The Pupil and Pupillary Reflexes

Contraction or relaxation of the sphincter and radial muscles of the iris controls changes in pupil size. The pupillary reflex, which controls the size of the pupillary opening, is controlled by the autonomic nervous system, with the parasympathetic nervous system producing pupillary constriction or miosis and the sympathetic nervous system producing pupillary dilation or mydriasis. The sphincter muscle that produces pupillary constriction is innervated by postganglionic parasympathetic neurons of the ciliary ganglion and other scattered ganglion cells between the scleral and choroid layers. Part of the oculomotor (CN III) nucleus is called the *Edinger-Westphal nucleus*.[22] This autonomic nucleus, found in the midbrain, provides the preganglionic innervation for these parasympathetic axons. Pupillary dilation by the radial muscles is provided by sympathetic innervation under excitatory descending control from the hypothalamus. Innervation is derived from preganglionic neurons in the upper thoracic cord, which send axons along the sympathetic chain to synapse with postganglionic neurons in the superior ciliary ganglion. Postganglionic fibers travel along the surfaces of the carotid and smaller arteries to reach the eye.

A region in the midbrain called the pretectum controls the pupillary reflex. Pretectal areas on each side of the brain are connected, explaining the binocular aspect of the light reflex. The afferent stimuli for pupillary constriction arise in the ganglionic cells of the retina and are transmitted to the *pretectal nuclei* at the junction of the thalamus and the midbrain and from there to preganglionic neurons in the oculomotor (CN III) nuclei (Fig. 19.10).

Shining a penlight into one eye of the person tests normal function of the pupillary reflex mechanism. To avoid a change in pupil size due to accommodation, ask the person to stare into the distance. A rapid constriction of the pupil exposed to light should occur; this is called the *direct pupillary light reflex*. Because the reflex is normally bilateral, the contralateral

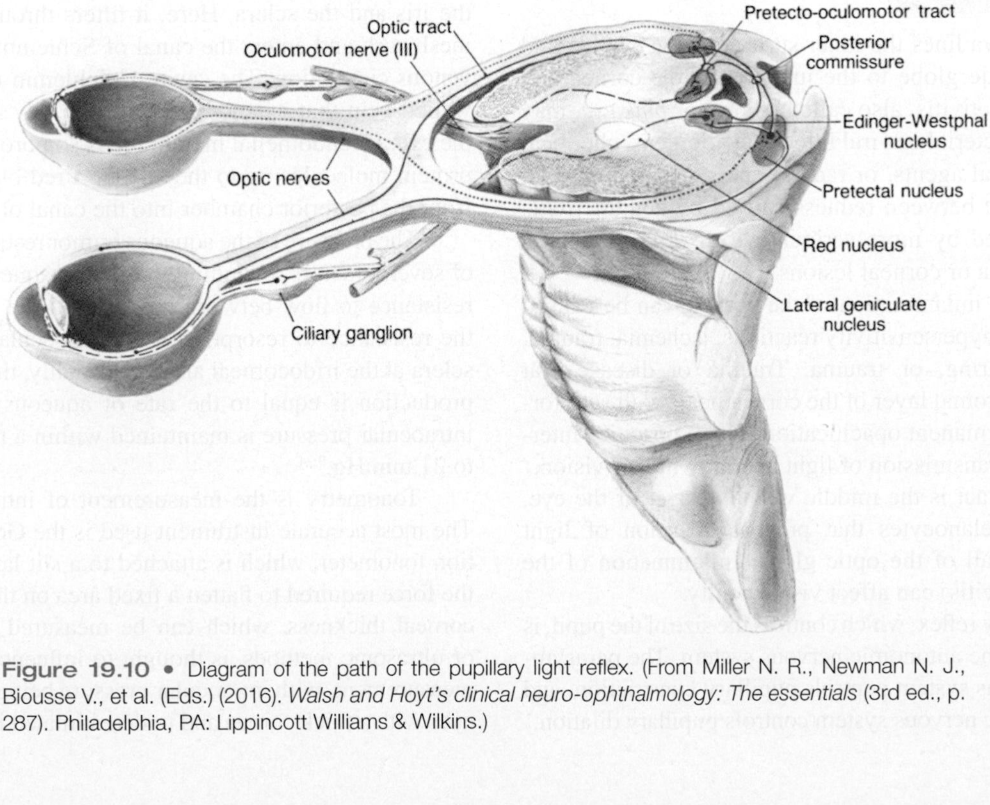

Figure 19.10 • Diagram of the path of the pupillary light reflex. (From Miller N. R., Newman N. J., Biousse V., et al. (Eds.) (2016). *Walsh and Hoyt's clinical neuro-ophthalmology: The essentials* (3rd ed., p. 287). Philadelphia, PA: Lippincott Williams & Wilkins.)

pupil also should constrict, a reaction called the *consensual pupillary light reflex*. The circuitry of the light reflex is partially separated from the main optic pathway. This is illustrated by the fact that the pupillary reflex remains unaffected when lesions to the optic radiations or the visual cortex occur.

Integrity of the dual autonomic control of pupillary diameter is vulnerable to trauma, tumor enlargement, or vascular disease. With diffuse damage to the forebrain involving the thalamus and hypothalamus, the pupils are typically small but respond to light. Damage to the CN III nucleus results in permanent pupillary dilation in the affected eye. Lesions affecting the cervical spinal cord or the ascending sympathetic ganglionic chain in the neck or internal carotid artery (*e.g.*, Horner syndrome) can interrupt the sympathetic control of the iris dilator muscle, resulting in permanent pupillary constriction. Tumors of the orbit that compress structures behind the eye can eliminate all pupillary reflexes, usually before destroying the optic nerve.

Pharmacologic agents can also differentially affect pupillary size. Bilateral pupillary constriction is characteristic of opiate usage. Pupillary dilation results when topical parasympathetic blocking agents, such as atropine, are applied and sympathetic pupillodilatory function is left unopposed. Sympathomimetic agents can enhance dilation. Ophthalmologists and optometrists use these medications to facilitate the examination of the transparent media and fundus of the eye. Miotic drugs (*e.g.*, pilocarpine), which are used in the treatment of angle-closure glaucoma (to be discussed), produce pupil constriction and in that manner facilitate aqueous humor circulation.

IN SUMMARY

The conjunctiva lines the inner surface of the eyelids and covers the optic globe to the junction of the cornea and sclera. Conjunctivitis, also called *red eye* or *pink eye*, may result from bacterial or viral infection, allergens, chemical agents, physical agents, or radiant energy. It is important to differentiate between redness caused by conjunctivitis and that caused by more serious eye disorders, such as acute glaucoma or corneal lesions.

Keratitis, or inflammation of the cornea, can be caused by infections, hypersensitivity reactions, ischemia, trauma, defects in tearing, or trauma. Trauma or disease that involves the stromal layer of the cornea heals with scar formation and permanent opacification. These opacities interfere with the transmission of light and may impair vision.

The uveal tract is the middle vascular layer of the eye. It contains melanocytes that prevent diffusion of light through the wall of the optic globe. Inflammation of the uveal tract (uveitis) can affect visual acuity.

The pupillary reflex, which controls the size of the pupil, is controlled by the autonomic nervous system. The parasympathetic nervous system controls pupillary constriction, and the sympathetic nervous system controls pupillary dilation.

INTRAOCULAR PRESSURE AND GLAUCOMA

After completing this section of the chapter, the learner will be able to meet the following objectives:

- Describe the formation and outflow of aqueous humor from the eye and relate to the development of glaucoma.
- Compare open-angle and angle-closure glaucoma in terms of pathology, symptomatology, diagnosis, and treatment.
- Explain why glaucoma leads to blindness.

Glaucoma is now described as optic neuropathy rather than a disease of elevated pressure in the eye. It is considered the leading cause of irreversible blindness worldwide. Projections suggest that over 100 million people will be affected by 2040, many of whom live in Asia and Africa.[23] There are two types of glaucoma: primary open-angle and primary angle-closure. Primary open-angle can occur when intraocular pressure is within a normal range (10 to 21 mm Hg); however, an increase in pressure is considered a risk factor. Primary angle-closure is somewhat rare but more prevalent in the Asian population.[3] Both types of glaucoma will be discussed in this section.

Control of Intraocular Pressure

The intraocular pressure is largely regulated by the aqueous humor, which fills the anterior and posterior chambers of the eye. The aqueous humor is produced by the ciliary body and passes from the posterior chamber through the pupil into the anterior chamber (Fig. 19.11A).[24] Aqueous humor leaves through the iridocorneal angle between the anterior surface of the iris and the sclera. Here, it filters through the trabecular meshwork and enters the canal of Schlemm for return to the venous circulation. The canal of Schlemm is actually a thin-walled vein that extends circumferentially around the iris of the eye. Its endothelial membrane is so porous that even large protein molecules up to the size of a red blood cell can pass from the posterior chamber into the canal of Schlemm.

The pressure of the aqueous humor results from a balance of several factors, including the rate of aqueous secretion, the resistance to flow between the iris and the ciliary body, and the resistance to resorption at the trabeculated region of the sclera at the iridocorneal angle. Normally, the rate of aqueous production is equal to the rate of aqueous outflow, and the intraocular pressure is maintained within a normal range of 9 to 21 mm Hg.[9,24]

Tonometry is the measurement of intraocular pressure. The most accurate instrument used is the Goldmann applanation tonometer, which is attached to a slit lamp and measures the force required to flatten a fixed area on the cornea. Central corneal thickness, which can be measured by either optical or ultrasonic methods, is thought to influence the accuracy of measurement, with intraocular pressure being overestimated in eyes with a thick cornea and underestimated in eyes with a thin

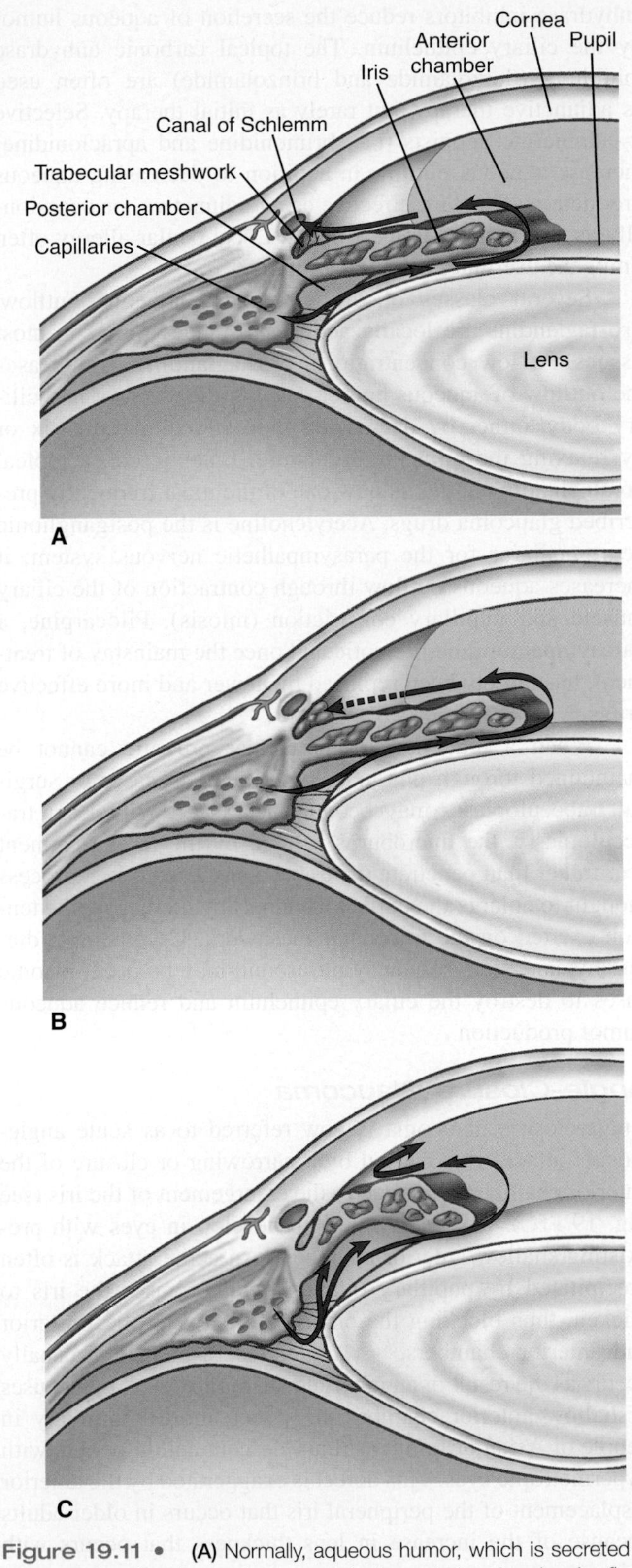

Figure 19.11 • **(A)** Normally, aqueous humor, which is secreted in the posterior chamber, gains access to the anterior chamber by flowing through the pupil. In the angle of the anterior chamber, it passes through the canal of Schlemm into the venous system. **(B)** In open-angle glaucoma, the outflow of aqueous humor is obstructed at the trabecular meshwork. **(C)** In angle-closure glaucoma, the aqueous humor encounters resistance to flow through the pupil. Increased pressure in the posterior chamber produces a forward bowing of the peripheral iris, so that the iris blocks the trabecular meshwork.

cornea. Another type of tonometer, the noncontact ("air-puff") tonometer, which uses the rebound force of a small puff of air blown against the cornea to estimate the intraocular pressure, is not as accurate as the applanation tonometer. However, this method does not require anesthetic drops because no instrument touches the eye. It is therefore more easily used by technicians and is useful in screening programs.[25]

Glaucoma

Glaucoma usually results from congenital or acquired lesions of the anterior segment of the eye that mechanically obstruct aqueous outflow. Glaucoma is commonly classified as open-angle (*i.e.*, wide-angle) or angle-closure (*i.e.*, narrow-angle) glaucoma, depending on the location of the compromised outflow and may occur as a primary or secondary disorder. Primary glaucoma can occur without evidence of preexisting ocular or systemic disease. Secondary glaucoma can result from inflammatory processes that affect the eye, from tumors, or from blood cells of trauma-produced hemorrhage that obstruct the outflow of aqueous humor.

In people with glaucoma, temporary or permanent impairment of vision results from degenerative changes in the retina and optic nerve and from corneal edema and opacification. Damage to optic nerve axons in the region of the optic nerve can be recognized on ophthalmoscopic examination. The normal optic disc has a central depression called the *optic cup*. With progressive atrophy of axons caused by increased intraocular pressure, pallor of the optic disc develops, and the size and depth of the optic cup increase. Because changes in the optic cup precede visual field loss, regular ophthalmoscopic examinations are important for detecting eye changes that occur with increased intraocular pressure. Many attempts have been made to quantify the optic disc changes in people with glaucoma using various photographic techniques and, more recently, scanning laser imaging systems.

Advances in computer technology allow detection and quantification of visual changes due to glaucoma. These tests of vision include white-on-white and blue-on-yellow visual field testing, testing of contrast sensitivity, and dark adaptation. Scanning laser technology and optical coherence tomography tests can detect damage to retinal ganglion axons before visual field loss occurs.

Primary Open-Angle Glaucoma

Primary open-angle glaucoma is the most common form of glaucoma.[24,26] The condition is characterized by an abnormal increase in intraocular pressure that occurs without obstruction at the iridocorneal angle, hence the name *open-angle glaucoma*. Instead, it usually occurs because of an abnormality of the trabecular meshwork that controls the flow of aqueous humor into the canal of Schlemm[24,26] (see Fig. 19.11B). Secondary open-angle glaucoma occurs as a result of other conditions, including the formation of red cell fragments after trauma and iris pigment epithelial granules that may clog the trabecular meshwork.

The condition is usually asymptomatic and chronic, causing progressive damage to the optic nerve and visual field loss unless it is appropriately treated. Elevated intraocular pressure is a risk factor for open-angle glaucoma, but it is not the only diagnostic factor. Some people maintain a higher intraocular pressure without evidence of optic nerve damage or visual field loss.[3]

Etiology. The etiology of primary open-angle glaucoma remains unclear. Major risk factors for this disorder include an age of 40 years and older, black race, a positive first-degree family history, myopia, and increased intraocular pressure.[26] Other risk factors with moderate to fair epidemiologic evidence include hypertension, type 2 diabetes, hyperthyroidism, migraine headaches, and sleep apnea.[26] In some people, the use of moderate amounts of topical or inhaled corticosteroid medications can cause an increase in intraocular pressure. Sensitive people also may sustain an increase in intraocular pressure with the use of systemic corticosteroid drugs. There is emerging evidence that central corneal thickness is also an important predictor for the development of primary open-angle glaucoma, and it may be a relevant predictor of both glaucoma progression and response to intraocular pressure–lowering drugs.[26]

Diagnosis. Diagnostic methods include applanation tonometry, ophthalmoscopic visualization of the optic nerve, and central visual field testing. Measurement of intraocular pressures provides a means of assessing glaucoma risk. Because the condition is usually asymptomatic, people at risk for open-angle glaucoma should have regular direct ophthalmoscopic examinations, on both eyes, concentrating on the optic disc. Optic disc changes frequently are noted before visual field defects become apparent. Periodic stereoscopic assessment of the optic disc by an eye care provider trained in the detection of glaucoma is strongly recommended for at-risk people.

Treatment. The elevation in intraocular pressure in people with open-angle glaucoma is usually treated pharmacologically or, in cases where pharmacologic treatment fails, by increasing aqueous outflow through a surgically created pathway. Drugs used in the long-term management of glaucoma fall into five classes: β-adrenergic antagonists, prostaglandin analogs, adrenergic agonists, carbonic anhydrase inhibitors, and cholinergic agonists.[26] Most glaucoma drugs are applied topically. However, systemic side effects may occur. When treatment with one drug does not reduce the intraocular pressure to the target level, a drug from a different class may be used or a second medication may be added as adjunctive therapy.

Topical β-adrenergic antagonists are usually the drugs of first choice for lowering intraocular pressure. The β-adrenergic antagonists are thought to lower intraocular pressure by decreasing aqueous humor production in the ciliary body. Systemic adsorption of these eye drops can cause bradycardia and bronchospasm in people with asthma. Carbonic anhydrase inhibitors reduce the secretion of aqueous humor by the ciliary epithelium. The topical carbonic anhydrase inhibitors (dorzolamide and brinzolamide) are often used as adjunctive therapy, but rarely as initial therapy. Selective α_2-adrenergic agonists (*i.e.*, brimonidine and apraclonidine) increase aqueous outflow in addition to decreasing aqueous production. They are effective as an adjunctive, or occasionally as a primary, treatment agent. Local ocular allergy often limits the usefulness of apraclonidine.[26]

Several classes of drugs increase aqueous outflow. Prostaglandins are locally acting substances found in most tissues. At low concentrations, prostaglandin $F_{2\alpha}$ increases the outflow of aqueous humor through the iris root and ciliary body, either by decreasing the extracellular matrix or by relaxing the ciliary musculature. Latanoprost, a topical prostaglandin analog, is now one of the most frequently prescribed glaucoma drugs. Acetylcholine is the postganglionic neuromediator for the parasympathetic nervous system; it increases aqueous outflow through contraction of the ciliary muscle and pupillary constriction (miosis). Pilocarpine, a parasympathomimetic miotic and once the mainstay of treatment, has largely been replaced by newer and more effective drugs.[26]

When a reduction in intraocular pressure cannot be maintained through pharmacologic methods, laser or surgical trabeculoplasty may become necessary. With laser trabeculoplasty, the microburns created by the laser treatment scar rather than penetrate the trabecular meshwork, a process thought to enlarge the outflow channels by increasing the tension exerted on the trabecular meshwork. Cryotherapy, diathermy, and high-frequency ultrasound may be used in some cases to destroy the ciliary epithelium and reduce aqueous humor production.

Angle-Closure Glaucoma

Angle-closure glaucoma is now referred to as acute angle-closure attack. It is caused by a narrowing or closure of the anterior chamber angle due to the enlargement of the iris (see Fig. 19.11C). It is most likely to develop in eyes with preexisting shallow anterior chambers. An acute attack is often precipitated by pupillary dilation, which causes the iris to thicken, thus blocking the circulation between the posterior and anterior chambers.[26–28] Angle-closure glaucoma usually occurs as the result of an inherited anatomic defect that causes a shallow anterior chamber. It is seen more commonly in people of Asian or Inuit (Eskimo) descent and in people with hypermetropic eyes. This defect is exaggerated by the anterior displacement of the peripheral iris that occurs in older adults because of the increase in lens thickness that occurs with aging.

Clinical Manifestations. Symptoms of acute angle-closure glaucoma are related to sudden, intermittent increases in intraocular pressure. Administration of topical pharmacologic agents such as atropine drops that cause pupillary dilation (mydriasis) also can precipitate an acute episode of increased intraocular pressure in people with the potential for angle-closure glaucoma. Some systemic (oral) medications have been reported to precipitate an acute attack as well. Attacks of increased intraocular pressure are manifested by ocular pain and blurred or iridescent vision caused by corneal edema.[24,27,28] The pupil may be enlarged and fixed. Symptoms are often spontaneously relieved by sleep and conditions that promote pupillary constriction. With repeated or prolonged attacks, the eye becomes reddened, and edema of the cornea may develop, giving the cornea a hazy appearance. A unilateral, often excruciating, headache is common. Nausea and vomiting may occur, causing the headache to be confused with migraine.

Some people with congenitally narrow anterior chambers never develop symptoms, and others develop symptoms only in older age. Because of the dangers of vision loss, those with narrow anterior chambers should be warned about the significance of blurred vision, halos, and ocular pain. Sometimes, decreased visual acuity and an unreactive pupil may be the only clues to angle-closure glaucoma in older adults.

Diagnosis and Treatment. The depth of the anterior chamber can be evaluated by side/shadow illumination or by a technique called *gonioscopy*. Gonioscopy uses a special contact lens and mirrors or prisms to view and measure the angle of the anterior chamber. The side/shadow illumination method uses only a penlight. The light source is held at the temporal side of the eye and directed horizontally across the iris. In people with a normal-sized anterior chamber, the light passes through the chamber to illuminate both halves of the iris. In people with a narrow anterior chamber, only the half of the iris adjacent to the light source is illuminated, whereas a shadow is cast on the half of the iris opposite the light source.

Acute angle-closure glaucoma is an ophthalmic emergency. Treatment is initially directed at reducing the intraocular pressure, usually with pharmacologic agents. Once the intraocular pressure is under control, a laser peripheral iridotomy is performed to create a permanent opening between the anterior and posterior chambers, allowing the aqueous humor to bypass the pupillary block. The anatomic abnormalities responsible for angle-closure glaucoma are usually bilateral, and prophylactic surgery is often performed on the other eye.

Congenital and Infantile Glaucoma

There are several types of childhood glaucoma, including congenital glaucoma that is present at birth and infantile glaucoma that develops during the first 2 to 3 years of life. As with glaucoma in adults, childhood glaucoma can occur as a primary or secondary disorder.

Etiology and Pathophysiology. Congenital glaucoma is caused by a disorder in which the anterior chamber retains its fetal configuration, with aberrant trabecular meshwork extending to the root of the iris, or is covered by a membrane. In general, it has a much poorer prognosis than infantile glaucoma. Primary infantile glaucoma occurs in approximately 1 in 10,000 live births but accounts for 2% to 15% of people in institutions for the blind.[27,29] It is bilateral in 65% to 80% of cases and occurs more commonly in boys than girls. About 10% of cases have a familial origin, and the rest are either sporadic or possibly multifactorial with reduced penetrance.[27,29] The familial cases are usually transmitted as an autosomal dominant trait with potentially high penetrance. Recent studies suggest a mutation in chromosome 2 (2p21 region). This gene is expressed in the tissues of the anterior chamber of the eye, and its protein product plays an important role in the metabolism of molecules that are used in signaling pathways during the terminal stages of anterior chamber development.[29]

Clinical Manifestations and Treatment. The earliest symptoms of congenital or infantile glaucoma are excessive tearing and photophobia. Affected infants tend to be fussy, have poor eating habits, and rub their eyes frequently. Diffuse edema of the cornea usually occurs, giving the eye a grayish-white appearance. Chronic elevation of the intraocular pressure before the age of 3 years causes enlargement of the entire optic globe. Early surgical treatment is necessary to prevent blindness.[29]

IN SUMMARY

Glaucoma (optic neuropathy) is a leading cause of blindness worldwide. It is characterized by conditions that cause an increase in intraocular pressure and that, if untreated, can lead to atrophy of the optic disc and progressive blindness. The aqueous humor is formed by the ciliary epithelium in the posterior chamber and flows through the pupil to the angle formed by the cornea and the iris. Here, it filters through the trabecular meshwork and enters the canal of Schlemm for return to the venous circulation. Glaucoma results from overproduction or impeded outflow of aqueous humor from the anterior chamber of the eye.

There are two types of glaucoma: open-angle and angle-closure. Open-angle glaucoma is caused by microscopic obstruction of the trabecular meshwork. Open-angle glaucoma is usually asymptomatic, and considerable loss of the visual field often occurs before medical treatment is sought. Routine screening by applanation tonometry provides one of the best means for early detection of glaucoma before vision loss has occurred. Angle-closure glaucoma is caused by a narrow anterior chamber and blockage of the outflow channels at the angle formed by the iris and the cornea. This occurs when the iris becomes thickened during pupillary dilation. Congenital glaucoma is caused by a disorder in which the anterior chamber retains its fetal configuration, with aberrant trabecular meshwork extending to the root of the iris, or is covered by a membrane. Early surgical treatment is necessary to prevent blindness.

DISORDERS OF THE LENS AND LENS FUNCTION

After completing this section of the chapter, the learner will be able to meet the following objectives:

- Describe changes in eye structure that occur with nearsighted and farsighted vision.
- Describe changes in lens structure that occur with cataract.
- Cite risk factors and visual changes associated with cataract.

The function of the eye is to transform light energy into nerve signals that can be transmitted to the cerebral cortex for interpretation. Optically, the eye is similar to a camera. It contains a lens system that focuses an inverted image, an aperture (*i.e.*, the pupil) for controlling light exposure, and a retina that corresponds to the film and records the image.

Disorders of Refraction and Accommodation

The lens is an avascular, transparent, biconvex body, the posterior side of which is more convex than the anterior side. A thin, highly elastic lens capsule is attached to the surrounding ciliary body by delicate suspensory radial ligaments called *zonules*, which hold the lens in place (see Fig. 19.9). The tough elastic sclera, in providing for a change in lens shape, acts as a bow, and the zonule and the lens capsule act as the bowstring. The suspensory ligaments and lens capsule are normally under tension, causing the lens to have a flattened shape for distant vision. Contraction of the muscle fibers of the ciliary body narrows the diameter of the ciliary body, relaxes the fibers of the suspensory ligaments, and allows the lens to relax to a more convex shape for near vision.

When light passes from one medium to another, its velocity is decreased or increased, and the direction of light transmission is changed. This change in direction of light rays is called *refraction*. When light rays pass through the center of a lens, their direction is not changed. However, other rays passing peripherally through a lens are bent (Fig. 19.12A). The refractive power of a lens is usually described as the distance (in meters) from its surface to the point at which the rays come into focus (*i.e.*, focal length). Usually, this is reported as the reciprocal of this distance (*i.e.*, diopters).[23] For example, a lens that brings an object into focus at 0.5 m has a refractive power of 2 diopters ($1/0.5 = 2$). With a fixed-power lens, the closer an object is to the lens, the further behind the lens is its focus point. The closer the object, the stronger and more precise the focusing system must be.

In the eye, the major refraction of light begins at the convex corneal surface. Further refraction occurs as light moves from the posterior corneal surface to the aqueous humor, from the aqueous humor to the anterior lens surface, from the anterior lens surface to the posterior lens surface, and from the posterior lens surface to the vitreous humor.

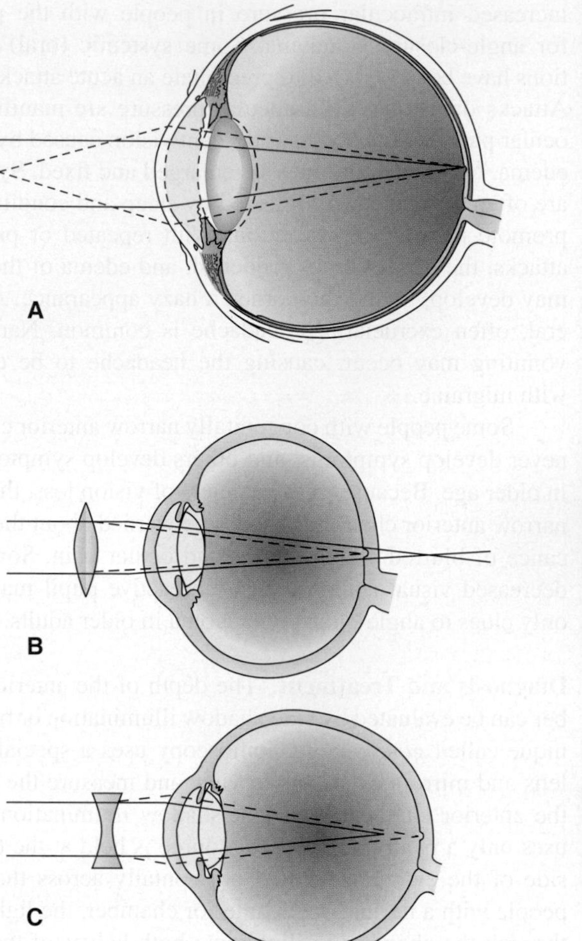

Figure 19.12 • **(A)** Accommodation. The *solid lines* represent rays of light from a distant object, and the *dotted lines* represent rays from a near object. The lens is flatter for the former and more convex for the latter. In each case, the rays of light are brought to a focus on the retina. **(B)** Hyperopia corrected by a biconvex lens, shown by the *dashed lines*. **(C)** Myopia corrected by a biconcave lens, shown by the *dashed lines*.

Disorders of Refraction

A perfectly shaped optic globe and cornea result in optimal visual acuity, producing a sharp image in focus at all points on the retinal surface in the posterior part, or fundus, of the eye. Unfortunately, individual differences in formation and growth of the eyeball and cornea frequently result in inappropriate focal image formation. If the anteroposterior dimension of the eyeball is too short, the image is theoretically focused posterior to (behind) the retina. This is called *hyperopia* or *farsightedness*. In such cases, the accommodative changes of the lens can bring distant images into focus, but near images become blurred. Hyperopia (Fig. 19.12B) is corrected by appropriate convex-surface lenses. If the anteroposterior dimension of the eyeball is too long, the focus point for an infinitely distant target is anterior to the retina. This condition is called *myopia* or *nearsightedness* (Fig. 19.12C). People with myopia can see close objects without problems because accommodative changes in their lens bring near objects into focus, but distant objects are blurred. Myopia can be corrected with an appropriate concave-surface lens. Refractive corneal surgeries such as laser in situ keratomileusis (LASIK), photorefractive keratectomy, and radial keratotomy can be performed to correct the corneal curvature to create accurate optical focus.[30,31]

Refractive defects of the corneal surface do not permit the formation of a sharp image. Nonuniform curvature of the refractive medium with regard to the horizontal and vertical planes is called *astigmatism*. Astigmatism is usually the result of an asymmetric bowing of the cornea, but it can result from defects in the cornea, lens, or the retina. Lens correction is available to sharpen focus in case of such refractive error.

Disorders of Accommodation

Because the retina is at a fixed distance from the lens, adjustability in the refractive power of the lens is needed so that a clear image is maintained as gaze is shifted from a far to a near object. The process by which the refractive power of the lens is increased, and the diverging light rays are bent more sharply, is called accommodation. Accommodation is neurologically associated with convergence of the eyes and pupillary constriction and results from thickening of the lens through contraction of the ciliary muscle. Contraction of the ciliary muscles is controlled mainly by the parasympathetic fibers of the oculomotor CN III. In near vision, pupillary constriction (*i.e.*, miosis) improves the clarity of the retinal image. This must be balanced against the resultant decrease in light intensity reaching the retina. During changes from near to far vision, pupillary dilation partially compensates for the reduced size of the retinal image by increasing the light entering the pupil. A third component of accommodation involves the reflex narrowing of the palpebral opening during near vision and widening during far vision.

Paralysis of the ciliary muscle, with loss of accommodation, is called *cycloplegia*.[32,33] Pharmacologic cycloplegia is sometimes necessary to aid refractive examination of the eye, especially in small children who are unable to hold a steady degree of accommodation during the examination. Lens shape is totally controlled by the pretectal region and the parasympathetic pathways through the oculomotor nerve to the ciliary muscle. Accommodation is lost with destruction of this pathway.

The term presbyopia refers to a decrease in accommodation that occurs because of aging. The lens consists of transparent fibers arranged in concentric layers, of which the external layers are the newest and softest. No loss of lens fibers occurs with aging; instead, additional fibers are added to the outermost portion of the lens. As the lens ages, it thickens, and its fibers become less elastic, so that the range of focus or accommodation is diminished to the point where reading glasses become necessary for near vision.

Cataracts

A cataract is a lens opacity that interferes with the transmission of light to the retina. It has been estimated that 18 million people in the world are visually disabled because of cataracts.[32,34] Cataracts are the most common cause of age-related visual loss in the world. They are found in approximately 50% of those between 65 and 74 years of age and in 70% of those older than 75 years.[1] Cataract surgery is the most common surgical procedure covered by Medicare, with more than 1 million procedures performed annually. More than 95% of people undergoing cataract surgery experience visual improvement if there is no ocular comorbidity.[32,34,35]

Causes and Types of Cataracts

The cause of cataract development is thought to be multifactorial, with different factors being associated with different types of opacities. The pathogenesis of cataracts is not completely understood. Several risk factors have been proposed, including the effects of aging, genetic influences, environmental and metabolic influences, drugs, and injury.[36,37] Metabolically induced cataracts are caused by disorders of carbohydrate metabolism (diabetes) or inborn errors of metabolism. Long-term exposure to sunlight (ultraviolet B radiation) and heavy smoking have been associated with increased risk of cataract formation.[36] Occasionally, cataracts occur as a developmental defect (*i.e.*, congenital cataracts) or secondary to trauma or diseases.[33,36]

Cataracts can result from several drugs. Corticosteroid drugs have been implicated as causative agents in cataract formation. Both systemic and inhaled corticosteroids have been cited as risk factors.[35] Other drugs associated with cataracts include the phenothiazines, amiodarone, and strong miotic ophthalmic drugs such as phospholine iodide.[37] Frequent examination of lens transparency should accompany the use of these and any other medications with potential cataract-forming effects.

Traumatic Cataract. Traumatic cataracts are usually caused by foreign body injury to the lens or blunt trauma to the eye. Foreign body injury that interrupts the lens capsule allows aqueous and vitreous humor to enter the lens and initiate cataract formation. Other causes of traumatic cataract are overexposure to heat (*e.g.*, glassblower cataract) or to ionizing radiation. The radiation dose necessary to cause a cataract varies with the amount and type of energy; younger lenses are most vulnerable.

Congenital Cataract. A congenital cataract is one that is present at birth. Among the causes of congenital cataracts are genetic defects, toxic environmental agents, and viruses such as rubella. Cataracts and other developmental defects of the ocular apparatus depend on the total dose of the agent and the embryonic stage at the time of exposure. During the last trimester of fetal life, genetically or environmentally influenced malformation of the superficial lens fibers can occur. Congenital lens opacities may occur in children of mothers with diabetes.[36] Most congenital cataracts are not progressive and are not dense enough to cause significant visual impairment. However, if the cataracts are bilateral and the opacity is significant, lens extraction should be done on one eye by the age of 2 months to permit the development of vision (see later section on amblyopia). If the surgery is successful, the contralateral lens should be removed soon after.

Senile Cataract. Cataracts are the most common cause of age-related vision loss in the world.[36] With normal aging, the nucleus and the cortex of the lens enlarge as new fibers are formed in the cortical zones of the lens. In the nucleus, the old fibers become more compressed and dehydrated. Metabolic changes occur and lens proteins become more insoluble, and concentrations of calcium, sodium, potassium, and phosphate increase. During the early stages of cataract formation, a yellow pigment and vacuoles accumulate in the lens fibers. The unfolding of protein molecules, cross-linking of sulfhydryl groups, and conversion of soluble to insoluble proteins lead to the loss of lens transparency. The onset is gradual, and the only symptoms are increasingly blurred vision and visual distortion.

Clinical Manifestations

The manifestations of cataract depend on the extent of opacity and whether the defect is bilateral or unilateral. With the exception of traumatic or congenital cataract, most cataracts are bilateral. Age-related cataracts, which are the most common type, are characterized by increasingly blurred vision and visual distortion. Visual acuity for far and near objects decreases. Dilation of the pupil in dim light improves vision. With nuclear cataracts (those involving the lens nucleus), the refractive power of the anterior segment often increases to produce an acquired myopia. People with hyperopia may experience a "second sight" or improved reading acuity until increasing opacity reduces acuity. Central lens opacities may divide the visual axis and cause an optical defect in which two or more blurred images are seen. Posterior subcapsular cataracts are located in the posterior cortical layer and usually involve the central visual axis. In addition to decreased visual acuity, cataracts tend to cause light entering the eye to be scattered, thereby producing glare or the abnormal presence of light in the visual field.

Diagnosis and Treatment

Diagnosis of cataract is based on ophthalmoscopic examination and the degree of visual impairment on the Snellen vision test. On ophthalmoscopic examination, cataracts may appear as a gross opacity filling the pupillary aperture or as an opacity silhouetted against the red background of the fundus. A Snellen test acuity of 20/50 is a common requirement for drivers of motor vehicles, so tests of potential vision (*i.e.*, the ability to see well after surgery) may be done to ensure that the visual loss can be corrected to necessary functional levels if the cataract were removed.

There is no effective medical treatment for cataract. Strong bifocals, magnification, appropriate lighting, and visual aids may be used as the cataract progresses. Surgery is the only treatment for correcting cataract-related vision loss. Surgery usually involves lens extraction and intraocular lens implantation. It is commonly performed on an outpatient basis with the use of local anesthesia. The use of extracapsular surgery, which leaves the posterior capsule of the lens intact, has significantly improved the outcomes of cataract surgery. The cataract lens is usually removed using phacoemulsification techniques.[37] Phacoemulsification involves ultrasonic fragmentation of the lens into fine pieces, which then are aspirated from the eye.

One of the greatest advances in cataract surgery has been the development of reliable intraocular implants. Monofocal intraocular lenses that correct for distance vision are available, and eyeglasses may be needed for near vision, although this has been addressed by the recent introduction of multifocal intraocular lenses.

IN SUMMARY

The lens is a biconvex, avascular, colorless, and almost transparent structure suspended behind the iris. The shape of the lens is controlled by the ciliary muscle, which contracts and relaxes the zonule fibers, thus changing the tension on the lens capsule and altering the focus of the lens. Refraction, which refers to the ability to focus an object on the retina, depends on the size and shape of the eyeball and the cornea and on the focusing ability of the lens. Errors in refraction occur when the visual image is not focused on the retina because of individual differences in the size or shape of the eyeball or cornea. In hyperopia, or farsightedness, the image theoretically falls behind the retina. In myopia, or nearsightedness, the image falls in front of the retina. Accommodation is the process by which a clear image is maintained as the gaze is shifted from a far to a near object. It is associated with convergence of the eyes and pupillary constriction, and thickening of the lens results from contraction of the ciliary muscle. Presbyopia is a change in the lens that occurs because of aging such that the lens becomes thicker and less able to change shape and accommodate for near vision.

A cataract is a lens opacity. It can occur as the result of congenital influences, metabolic disturbances, infection, injury, and aging. The most common type of cataract is the senile cataract that occurs with aging. The treatment for a totally opaque or mature cataract is surgical extraction. An intraocular lens implant may be inserted during the surgical procedure to replace the removed lens; otherwise, thick convex lenses or contact lenses are used to compensate for the loss of lens function.

DISORDERS OF THE VITREOUS AND RETINA

After completing this section of the chapter, the learner will be able to meet the following objectives:

- Cite the manifestations and long-term visual effects of papilledema.
- Describe the pathogenesis of background and proliferative diabetic retinopathies and their mechanisms of visual impairment.
- Explain the pathology and visual changes associated with macular degeneration.

The posterior segment, comprising five sixths of the eyeball, contains the transparent vitreous humor and the neural retina. The innermost layer of the eyeball, the fundus, is visualized through the pupil with an ophthalmoscope.

Disorders of the Vitreous

Vitreous humor (*i.e.*, vitreous body) is a colorless, amorphous biologic gel that fills the posterior cavity of the eye (see Fig. 19.2). It consists of approximately 99% water, some salts, glycoproteins, proteoglycans, and dispersed collagen fibrils. The vitreous is attached to the ciliary body and the peripheral retina in the region of the ora serrata and to the periphery of the optic disc.

Disease, aging, and injury can disturb the factors that maintain the water of the vitreous humor in suspension, causing liquefaction of the gel to occur. With the loss of gel structure, fine fibers, membranes, and cellular debris develop. When this occurs, floaters (images) can often be noticed as these substances move within the vitreous cavity during head movement. In disease, blood vessels may grow from the surface of the retina or optic disc onto the posterior surface of the vitreous, and blood may fill the vitreous cavity.

In a procedure called a *vitrectomy*, the removal and replacement of the vitreous with a balanced saline solution can restore sight in some people with vitreous opacities resulting from hemorrhage or vitreoretinal membrane formations that cause legal blindness. Using this procedure, a small probe with a cutting tip is used to remove the opaque vitreous and membranes. The procedure is difficult and requires complex instrumentation. It is of no value if the retina is not functional.

Disorders of the Retina

The function of the retina is to receive visual images, partially analyze them, and transmit this modified information to the brain.[38] It is composed of two layers: the inner neural retina that contains the photoreceptors and an outer melanin-containing layer that rests on, and is firmly attached to, the choriocapillaris, the capillary layer of the choroid. A non–light-sensitive portion of the retina, along with the retinal pigment epithelium, continues anteriorly to form the posterior surface of the iris. A wavy border called the *ora serrata* exists at the junction between the light-sensitive and the non–light-sensitive retinas. Separating the vascular portion of the choroid from pigmented cells of the retina is a thin layer of elastic tissue, the *Bruch membrane*, which contains collagen fibrils in its superficial and deep portions. Cells of the pigmented layer receive their nourishment by diffusion from the choriocapillaris.

Disorders of the retina and its function include derangements of the pigment epithelium (*e.g.*, retinitis pigmentosa), ischemic conditions caused by disorders of the retinal blood supply, disorders of the retinal vessels such as retinopathies that cause hemorrhage and the development of opacities, separation of the pigment and sensory layers of the retina (*i.e.*, retinal detachment), abnormalities of the Bruch membrane and choroid (*e.g.*, macular degeneration), and malignant tumors of the nuclear layer of the retina (*i.e.*, retinoblastoma). Because the retina has no pain fibers, most diseases of the retina are painless and do not cause redness of the eye.

The Neural Retina

The neural retina is composed of three layers of neurons: a posterior layer of photoreceptors, a middle layer of bipolar cells, and an inner layer of ganglion cells that communicate with the photoreceptors (Fig. 19.13). A pattern of light on the retina falls on a massive array of photoreceptors. These photoreceptors synapse with bipolar and other interneurons before action potentials in ganglion cells relay the message to specific regions of the brain and the brain stem associated with vision. For rods, this microcircuitry involves the convergence of signals from many rods on a single ganglion

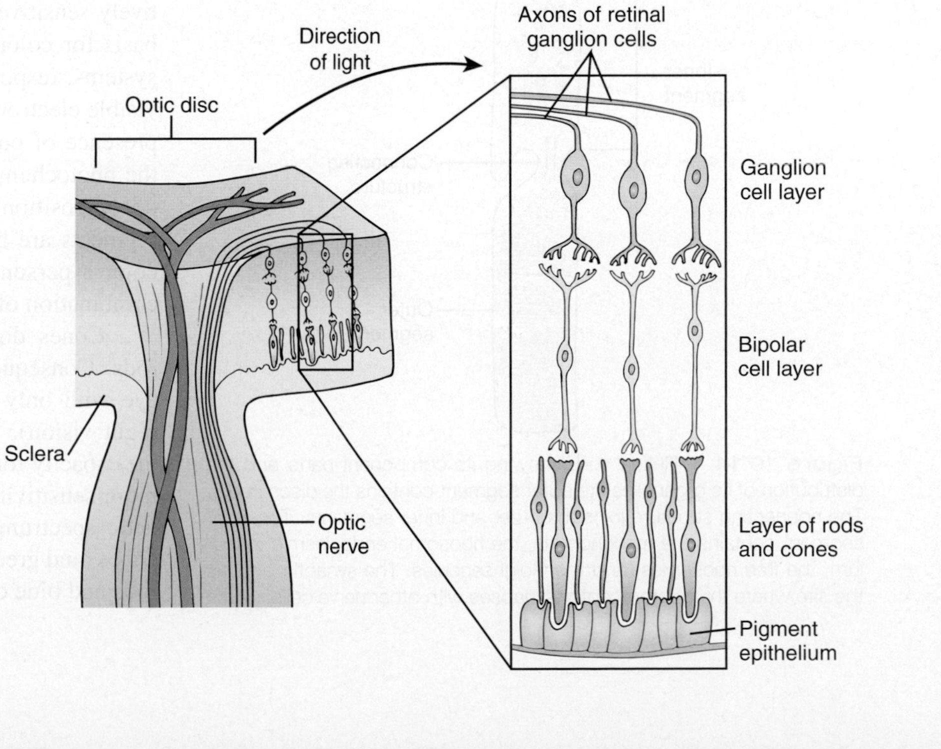

Figure 19.13 • Organization of the human retina. The optic pathway begins with photoreceptors (rods and cones) in the retina. The responses of the photoreceptors are transmitted by the bipolar cells to the ganglion cell layer of the retina.

cell. This arrangement maximizes spatial summation and the detection of stimulated (light versus dark) receptors. The interneurons, composed of horizontal and amacrine cells, have cell bodies in the bipolar layer, and they play an important role in modulating retinal function. A superficial marginal layer contains the axons of the ganglion cells as they collect and leave the eye through the optic nerve. These fibers lie beside the vitreous humor. Light must pass through the transparent inner layers of the sensory retina before it reaches the photoreceptors.

Photoreceptors

Two types of photoreceptors are present in the retina: rods, capable of black–white discrimination, and cones, capable of color discrimination. Both types of photoreceptors are thin, elongated, mitochondria-filled cells with a single, highly modified cilium (Fig. 19.14). The cilium has a short base, or inner segment, and a highly modified outer segment. The plasma membrane of the outer segment is tightly folded to form membranous discs (rods) or conical shapes (cones) containing visual pigment. These discs are continuously synthesized at the base of the outer segment and shed at the distal end. Discarded membranes are phagocytized by the retinal pigment cells. If this phagocytosis is disrupted, as in retinitis pigmentosa, the sensory retina degenerates.

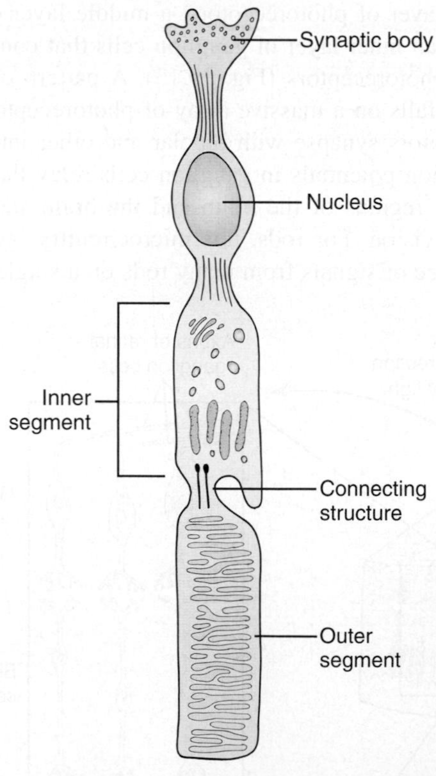

Figure 19.14 • Retinal rod, showing its component parts and the distribution of its organelles. Its outer segment contains the discs (rods). The connecting structure joins the outer and inner segments. The inner segment contains the mitochondria, the ribosomal endoplasmic reticulum, the free ribosomes, and the Golgi saccules. The synaptic body is the site where the photoreceptor synapses with other nerve cells.

Rods. Photoreception involves the transduction of light energy into an altered ionic membrane potential of the rod cell. Light passing through the eye penetrates the nearly transparent neural elements to produce decomposition of the photochemical substance (visual pigment) called *rhodopsin* in the outer segment of the rod. Light that is not trapped by a rhodopsin molecule is absorbed by the retinal pigment melanin or deeper choroid melanin. Rhodopsin consists of a protein called *opsin* and a vitamin A–derived pigment called *retinal*. During light stimulation, rhodopsin is broken down into its component parts, opsin and retinal; retinal subsequently is converted into vitamin A. The reconstitution of rhodopsin occurs during total darkness; vitamin A is transformed into retinal, and then opsin and retinal combine to form rhodopsin. Considerable stores of vitamin A are present in the retinal pigment cells and in the liver; therefore, a vitamin A deficiency must be present for weeks or months to affect the photoreceptive process. Reduced sensitivity to light, a symptom of vitamin A deficiency, initially affects night vision; however, this is quickly reversed by injection or ingestion of the vitamin.

Rod-based vision is particularly sensitive to detecting light, especially moving light stimuli, at the expense of clear pattern discrimination. Rod vision is particularly adapted for night and low-level illumination. Dark adaptation is the process by which rod sensitivity increases to the optimum level. This requires approximately 4 hours in total or near-total darkness and is referred to as scotopic vision (night vision). During daylight or high-intensity bombardment, the concentration of vitamin A increases, whereas the concentration of the photopigment retinal decreases. During dark adaptation, an increase in synthesis of retinal from vitamin A results in a higher concentration of rhodopsin available to capture light energy.

Cones and Color Sensitivity. Cone receptors that are selectively sensitive to different wavelengths of light provide the basis for color vision. Three types of cones, or cone–color systems, respond to the blue, green, and red portions of the visible electromagnetic spectrum. This selectivity reflects the presence of one of three color-sensitive molecules to which the photochemical substance (visual pigment) is bound. The decomposition and reconstitution processes of the cone visual pigments are believed to be similar to that of the rods. The color a person perceives depends on which set of cones or combination of sets of cones is stimulated in a given image.

Cones do not have the dark adaptation capability of rods. Consequently, the dark-adapted eye is a rod receptor eye with only black-gray-white discrimination (scotopic or night vision). The light-adapted eye (*photopic vision*) adds the capacity for color discrimination. Rhodopsin has its maximum sensitivity in the blue-green region of the electromagnetic spectrum. If red lenses are worn in daylight, the red cones (and green cones to some extent) are in use, whereas the rods and blue cones are essentially in the dark, and therefore, dark adaptation proceeds. This method is used by military and night-duty airport control tower personnel to allow adaptation to take place before they go on duty in the dark.

Macula and Fovea. An area approximately 1.5 mm in diameter near the center of the retina, called the *macula lutea* (*i.e.*, "yellow spot"), is especially adapted for acute and detailed vision.[38] This area is composed entirely of cones. In the central portion of the macula, the *fovea centralis* (foveola), the blood vessels and innermost layers are displaced to one side instead of resting on top of the cones (Fig. 19.15). This allows light to pass unimpeded to the cones without passing through several layers of the retina. Of the approximately 6.4 million cones in the retina, 200,000 are located in the fovea. The density of cones drops off rapidly away from the fovea. Rods are not present in the fovea, but their numbers increase as the cones decrease in density toward the periphery of the retina.

Color Blindness. "Color blindness" is a misnomer for a condition in which people appear to confuse or mismatch colors or experience reduced acuity for color discrimination. These people are often unaware of their defect until they attempt to discriminate between red and green traffic lights or show difficulty matching colors. Color blindness is inherited as an X-linked deficiency of a specific type of retinal photoreceptor. The most common abnormality is red-green color blindness. The deficiency is usually partial but can be complete. Rarely are two of the color mechanisms missing; when this occurs, usually red and green are missing. Complete lack of color discrimination is rare. For such people, the world is experienced entirely as black, gray, and white.

The genetically color-blind person has never experienced the full range of normal color vision and is unaware of what he or she is missing. Color discrimination is necessary for everyday living, and color-blind people, knowingly or unknowingly, make color discriminations based on other criteria, such as brightness or position. For example, the red light of a traffic signal is always the upper light, and the green is the lower light. Color-blind people experience difficulties when brightness differences are small, and discrimination must be based on hue and saturation qualities.

Retinitis Pigmentosa. Retinitis pigmentosa represents a group of hereditary diseases that cause slow degenerative changes in the retinal photoreceptors. The disease can be inherited as an autosomal dominant (20% to 30%) and autosomal

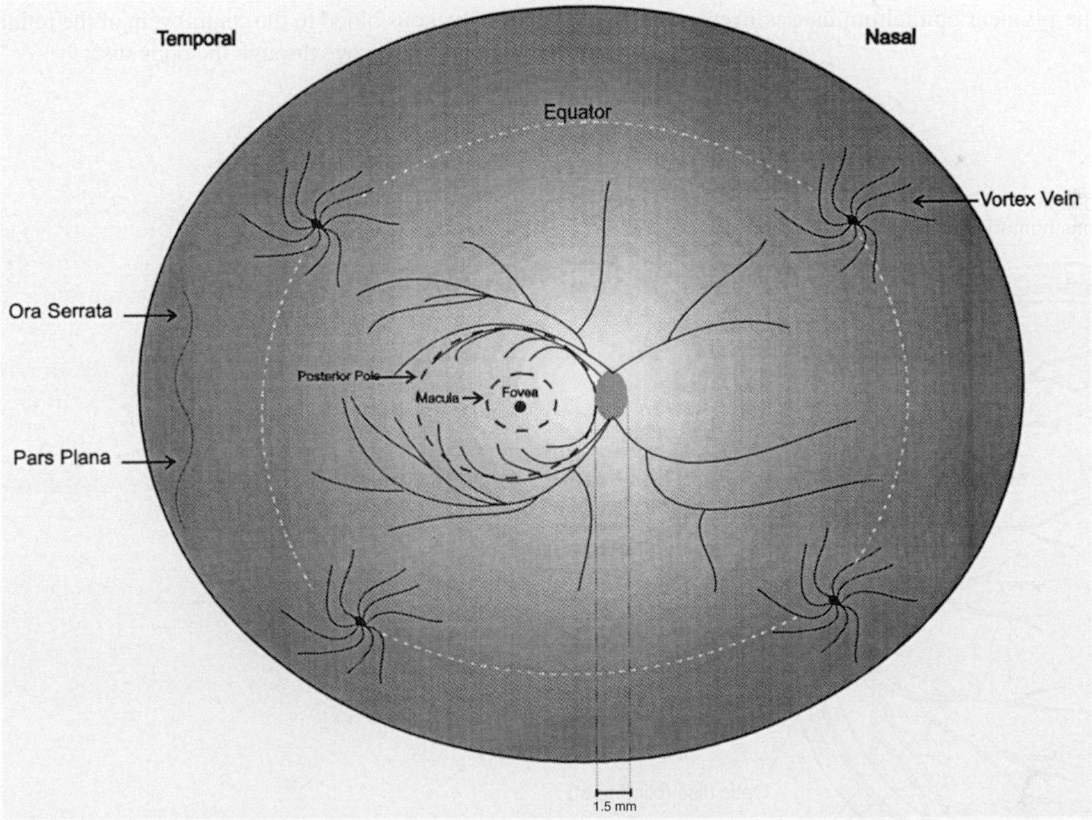

Figure 19.15 • Anatomy of retina as viewed by funduscopic examination. (From Miller N. R., Newman N. J., Biousse V., et al. (Eds.) (2008). *Walsh and Hoyt's clinical neuro-ophthalmology: The essentials* (2nd ed., p. 43). Philadelphia, PA: Lippincott Williams & Wilkins.)

recessive (10% to 15%). The remaining percent is X-link associated. There are over 100 gene mutations associated with retinitis pigmentosa.[39] Nonocular diseases can be associated with retinitis pigmentosa such as Usher syndrome, Refsum disease, and Bardet-Biedl syndrome.[39]

In cases known as rod–cone dystrophy (formally called *rod–cone retinitis pigmentosa*), the rods are the predominantly affected photoreceptor cells. This generally produces a number of characteristic clinical symptoms, including night blindness, which is usually an early symptom, and bilateral symmetric loss of midperipheral fields. Although there is relative preservation of macular vision, the visual field defects gradually increase both centrally and peripherally. With progression, cone photoreceptor cells are also affected and day vision and central visual acuity are compromised. The rate of visual failure is variable.[39]

Disorders of Retinal Blood Supply

The blood supply for the retina is derived from two sources: the choriocapillaris (*i.e.*, the capillary layer of the choroid) and branches of the central retinal artery (Fig. 19.16). Oxygen and other nutritional substances needed by the retina and its component parts (pigment cells, rods, and cones) are supplied by diffusion from blood vessels in the choroid. Because the choriocapillaris provides the only blood supply for the fovea centralis (*i.e.*, foveola), detachment of this part of the sensory retina from the pigment epithelium causes irreparable visual loss.

> **KEY POINTS**
>
> **DISORDERS OF THE RETINAL BLOOD SUPPLY**
>
> - The blood supply for the retina is derived from the central retinal artery, which supplies blood flow for the entire inside of the retina, and from vessels in the choroid, which supply the rods and cones.
> - The retinopathies, which are disorders of the retinal vessels, interrupt blood flow to the visual receptors, leading to visual impairment.
> - Retinal detachment separates the visual receptors from the choroid, which provides their major blood supply.

The bipolar, horizontal, amacrine, and ganglion cells, and the ganglion cell axons that gather at the optic disc, are supplied by branches of the retinal artery.[38] The central artery of the retina is a branch of the ophthalmic artery. It enters the globe through the optic disc. Branches of this artery radiate over the entire retina, except the central fovea, which is surrounded by, but is not crossed by, arterial branches. The central artery of the retina is an end artery, meaning that it does not anastomose with other arteries. This is critical because an infarct in this artery will totally deprive distal structures of their vascular supply. Retinal veins follow a distribution parallel to the arterial branches and carry venous blood to the central vein of the retina, which exits the back of the eye through the optic disc.

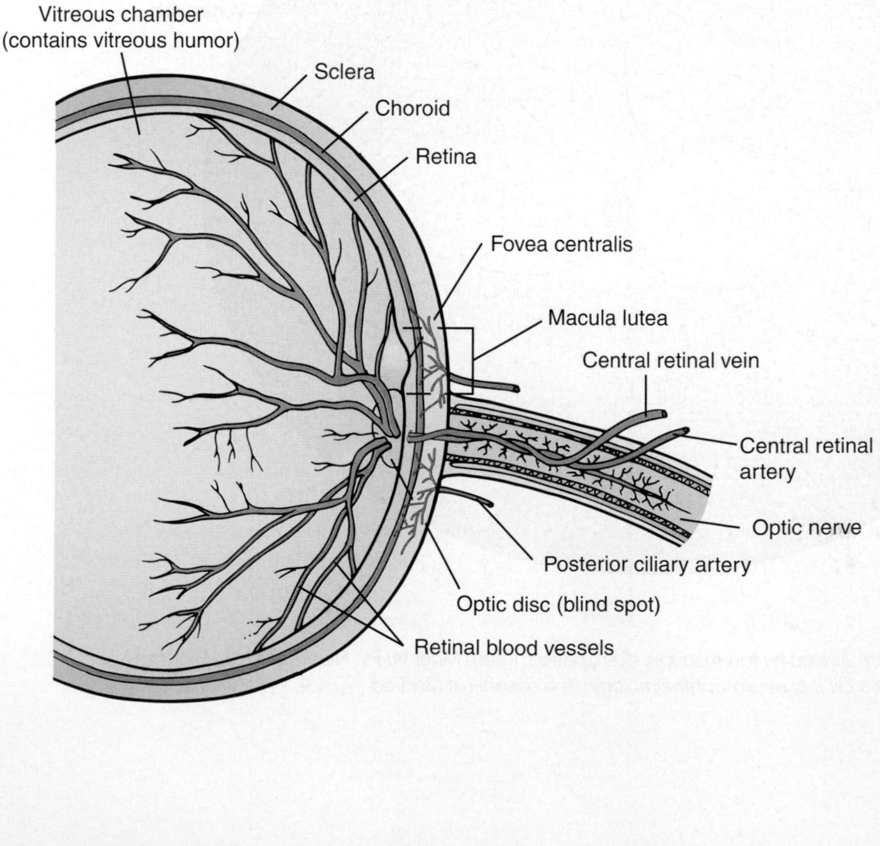

Figure 19.16 • Retinal circulation.

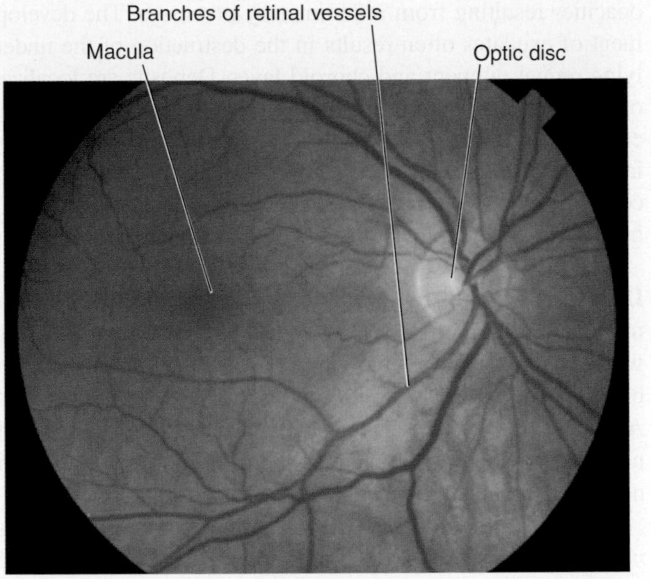

Figure 19.17 • Funduscopic image of normal retina. (From Moore K. L., Dalley A. F., Agur A. M. R. (2018). *Clinically oriented anatomy* (8th ed., p. 905, Fig. 8.52). Philadelphia, PA: Wolters Kluwer.)

Funduscopic examination of the eye with an ophthalmoscope provides an opportunity to examine the retinal blood vessels and other aspects of the retina (Fig. 19.17). Because the retina is an embryonic outgrowth of the brain and the blood vessels are to a considerable extent representative of brain blood vessels, the ophthalmoscopic examination of the fundus of the eye permits the study and diagnosis of metabolic and vascular diseases of the brain as well as pathologic processes that are specific to the retina.

Functioning of the retina, like that of other cellular portions of the CNS, depends on an oxygen supply from the vascular system. One of the earliest signs of decreased perfusion pressure in the head region is a graying-out or blackout of vision, which usually precedes loss of consciousness. This can occur during large increases in intrathoracic pressure, which interfere with the return of venous blood to the heart, as occurs with the Valsalva maneuver, with systemic hypotension, and during sudden postural changes (*e.g.*, postural hypotension).

Ischemia of the retina occurs during general circulatory collapse. If a person survives cardiopulmonary arrest, for instance, permanently decreased visual acuity can occur as a result of edema and the ischemic death of retinal neurons. This is followed by primary optic nerve atrophy proportional to the extent of ganglionic cell death. The ophthalmic artery, the source of the central artery of the retina, takes its origin from the internal carotid artery.[38] Intermittent retinal ischemia can accompany internal carotid or common carotid stenosis. *Amaurosis fugax* is characterized by transient episodes of monocular visual loss lasting 5 to 10 minutes.[40] People with the disorder often describe a curtain coming down from above or across their vision, usually with complete return of vision within seconds or minutes. Besides the vision loss, contralateral hemiplegia or sensory deficits may accompany the episodes. The condition, commonly due to emboli, is most often the result of carotid artery disease.[40]

Papilledema. The central retinal artery enters the eye through the optic papilla in the center of the optic nerve. An accompanying vein exits alongside the same path. The entrance and exit of the central retinal artery and vein running through the tough scleral tissue at the optic papilla can be compromised by any condition causing persistent increased intracranial pressure. The most common of these conditions are cerebral tumors, subdural hematomas, hydrocephalus, and malignant hypertension.

Usually, the thin-walled, low-pressure veins are the first to collapse, with the consequent backup and slowing of arterial blood flow. Under these conditions, capillary permeability increases and leakage of fluid results in edema of the optic papilla, called *papilledema*. The interior surface of the papilla is normally cup-shaped and can be evaluated for cupping with an ophthalmoscope. With papilledema, sometimes called *choked disc*, the optic cup is distorted by protrusion into the interior of the eye (Fig. 19.18). Because this sign does not occur until the intracranial pressure is significantly elevated, compression damage to the optic nerve fibers passing through the lamina cribrosa may have begun. As a warning sign, papilledema occurs quite late. Unresolved papilledema results in the destruction of the optic nerve axons and blindness. Pseudopapilledema can result from benign intracranial hypertension or optic disc drusen (calcified deposits in the optic papilla).

Retinopathies

Disorders of the retinal vessels can result in microaneurysms, neovascularization, hemorrhage, and formation of retinal opacities. *Microaneurysms* are outpouchings of the retinal vasculature. On ophthalmoscopic examination, they appear as minute, unchanging red dots associated with blood vessels. These microaneurysms tend to leak plasma, resulting in localized edema that gives the retina a hazy appearance. Microaneurysms can be identified with certainty using fluorescein angiography; the fluorescein dye is injected intravenously, and the retinal vessels subsequently are photographed

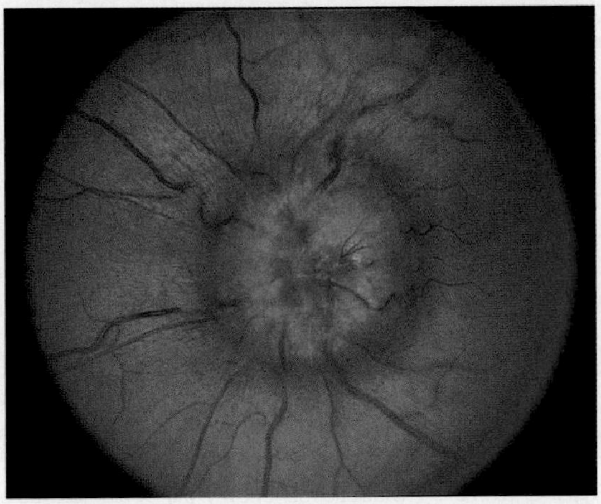

Figure 19.18 • Chronic papilledema. The optic nerve head is congested and protrudes anteriorly toward the interior of the eye. It has blurred margins, and vessels within it are poorly seen. (From Klintworth G. K. (2015). The eye. In Rubin R., Strayer D. E. (Eds.) *Rubin's pathology: Clinicopathologic foundations of medicine* (7th ed., p. 1518, Fig. 33-15). Philadelphia, PA: Lippincott Williams & Wilkins.)

using a special ophthalmoscope and fundus camera. The microaneurysms may bleed, but areas of hemorrhage and edema tend to clear spontaneously. However, they reduce visual acuity if they encroach on the macula and cause degeneration before they are absorbed.

Neovascularization involves the formation of new blood vessels. They can develop from the choriocapillaris, extending between the pigment layer and the sensory layer, or from the retinal veins, extending between the sensory retina and the vitreous cavity and sometimes into the vitreous. These new blood vessels are fragile, leak protein, and are likely to bleed. Neovascularization occurs in many conditions that impair retinal blood flow, including stasis because of hyperviscosity of blood or decreased flow, vascular occlusion, sickle cell disease, sarcoidosis, diabetes mellitus, and retinopathy of prematurity.[40–42]

Hemorrhage can be preretinal, intraretinal, or subretinal. *Preretinal hemorrhages* occur between the retina and the vitreous. These hemorrhages are usually large because the blood vessels are only loosely restricted; they may be associated with a subarachnoid or subdural hemorrhage and are usually regarded as a serious manifestation of the disorder. They usually reabsorb without complications unless they penetrate into the vitreous. *Intraretinal hemorrhages* occur because of abnormalities of the retinal vessels, diseases of the blood, increased pressure in the retinal vessels, or vitreous traction on the vessels. Systemic causes include diabetes mellitus, hypertension, and blood dyscrasias. *Subretinal hemorrhages* are those that develop between the choroid and pigment layer of the retina. A common cause of subretinal hemorrhage is neovascularization. Photocoagulation may be used to treat microaneurysms and neovascularization.

Light normally passes through the transparent inner portions of the sensory retina before reaching the photoreceptors. *Opacities* such as hemorrhages, exudate, cotton-wool spots, edema, and tissue proliferation can produce a localized loss of transparency observable with an ophthalmoscope. Exudates are opacities resulting from inflammatory processes. The development of exudates often results in the destruction of the underlying retinal pigment and choroid layer. Deposits are localized opacities consisting of lipid-laden macrophages or accumulated cellular debris. Cotton-wool spots are retinal opacities with hazy, irregular outlines. They occur in the nerve fiber layer and contain cell organelles. Cotton-wool patches are associated with retinal trauma, severe anemia, papilledema, and diabetic retinopathy.

Diabetic Retinopathy. Diabetic retinopathy is the most common cause of blindness in the industrialized countries of the world. It ranks first as the cause of newly reported cases of blindness in people between the ages of 20 and 74 years.[40,43] Advances in treatment have greatly reduced the risk of blindness from diabetes, but because diabetes is so common, retinopathy remains an important cause of visual impairment.

Diabetic retinopathy can be divided into two types: *nonproliferative* (*i.e.*, background) and *proliferative*.[41–43] Background or nonproliferative retinopathy is confined to the retina. It involves engorgement of the retinal veins, thickening of the capillary endothelial basement membrane, and development of capillary microaneurysms (Fig. 19.19A). Small intraretinal hemorrhages may develop and microinfarcts may cause cotton-wool spots and leakage of exudates. A sensation of glare (because of the scattering of light) is a common complaint. The most common cause of decreased vision in people with background retinopathy is macular edema. The edema is caused primarily by the breakdown of the inner blood–retina barrier at the level of the capillary endothelium, allowing leakage of fluid and plasma constituents into the surrounding retina.

Proliferative diabetic retinopathy represents a more severe retinal change than background retinopathy (Fig. 19.19B). It is characterized by formation of new, fragile blood vessels (*i.e.*, neovascularization) at the disc and elsewhere in the retina. These vessels grow in front of the retina along the posterior surface of the vitreous or into the vitreous. They

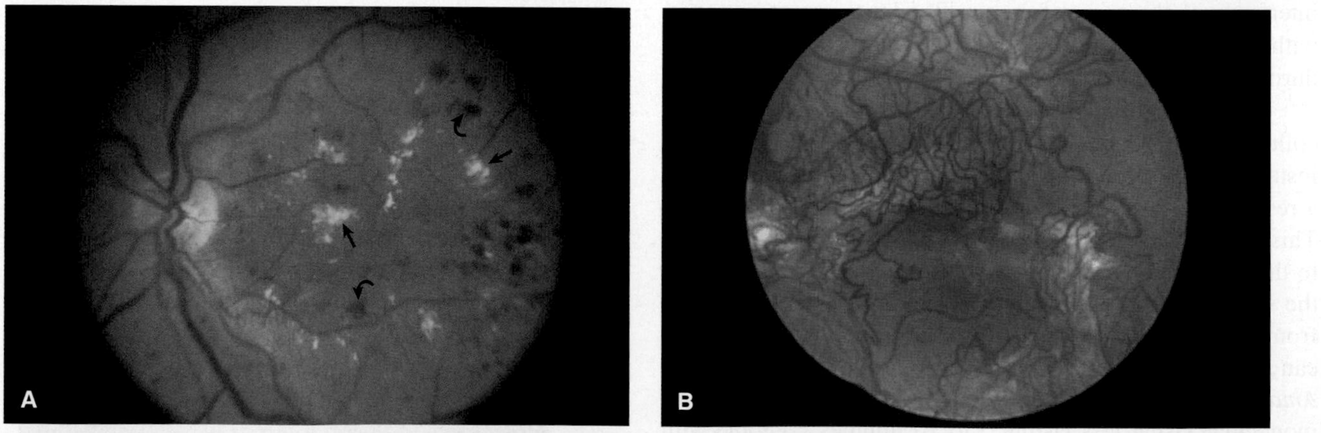

Figure 19.19 • Diabetic retinopathy. **(A)** Ocular fundus of a person with background diabetic retinopathy. Several yellowish "hard" exudates (*straight arrows*) and several relatively small retinal hemorrhages (*curved arrows*) are present. **(B)** A vascular frond (top half) has extended anteriorly to the retina in the eye with proliferative diabetic retinopathy. (From Klintworth G. K. (2015). The eye. In Rubin R., Strayer D. E. (Eds.) *Rubin's pathology: Clinicopathologic foundations of medicine* (7th ed., p. 1514, Fig. 33-10A and B). Philadelphia, PA: Lippincott Williams & Wilkins.)

threaten vision in two ways. First, because they are abnormal, they often bleed easily, leaking blood into the vitreous cavity and decreasing visual acuity. Second, the blood vessels attach firmly to the retinal surface and posterior surface of the vitreous, such that normal movement of the vitreous may exert a pull on the retina, causing retinal detachment and progressive blindness. Because early proliferative diabetic retinopathy is likely to be asymptomatic, it must be identified early, before bleeding occurs and obscures the view of the fundus or leads to fibrosis and retinal detachment.

The cause of diabetic retinopathy is uncertain. Several biochemical mechanisms have been proposed as explanations for the development and progression of diabetic retinopathy and have led to exploration of possible treatments.[41,44] However, except for the demonstration that chronically elevated levels of blood glucose contribute to the development and progression of retinopathy and other complications of diabetes, no mechanism can be regarded as established. Hypertension is also thought to increase the risk for the development and progression of diabetic retinopathy. Recent evidence suggests that the renin–angiotensin system is activated by chronically elevated levels of blood glucose. Angiotensin II increases vascular permeability and promotes angiogenesis, and it has been suggested that a relationship may exist between angiotensin II and vascular endothelial growth factor (VEGF) in ocular tissues.[44,45] Accordingly, angiotensin-converting enzyme inhibitors or receptor blockers may be useful agents for preventing the progression of diabetic retinopathy. In addition to chronic hyperglycemia and hypertension, several studies have indicated the association of diabetic exudative retinopathy with hypercholesteremia and combined inflammatory mediators on the retinal microvasculature.[45]

Preventing diabetic retinopathy from developing or progressing is considered the best approach to preserving vision. Growing evidence suggests that careful control of blood glucose levels in people with diabetes mellitus may retard the onset and progression of retinopathy. The ACCORD Eye Study Group demonstrated that intensive management of people with type 1 diabetes to maintain blood glucose at near-normal levels limited the risk of developing retinopathy. There also is a need for intensive management of hypertension and hyperlipidemia, both of which have been shown to increase the risk of diabetic retinopathy in people with diabetes.[43]

Regular dilated eye examinations are an effective approach to detecting and treating vision-threatening diabetic retinopathy. Current guidelines recommend that people with diabetes have yearly eye examinations, although deviations from this guideline are appropriate in certain low-risk groups. For people with moderate to severe nonproliferative retinopathy, more frequent examinations are often necessary to determine when to initiate treatment. People with any levels of macular edema, severe nonproliferative diabetic retinopathy, or any proliferative retinopathy require the prompt care of an ophthalmologist who is knowledgeable and experienced in the management and treatment of diabetic retinopathy. Women with preexisting diabetes who plan to become pregnant should have a comprehensive eye examination and be counseled about the risk for initiation or progression of diabetic retinopathy. Women with diabetes who become pregnant should have a comprehensive eye examination in the first trimester and close follow-up throughout pregnancy.

Photocoagulation using an argon laser provides the major direct treatment modality for diabetic retinopathy.[41,42] Treatment strategies include laser photocoagulation applied directly to leaking microaneurysms and grid photocoagulation with a checkerboard pattern of laser burns applied to diffuse areas of leakage and thickening.[41] Because laser photocoagulation destroys the proliferating vessels and the ischemic retina, it reduces the stimulus for further neovascularization. However, photocoagulation of neovascularization near the disc is not recommended.[41] Vitrectomy has proved effective in removing vitreous hemorrhage and severing vitreoretinal membranes that develop.

Because of the limitations of current treatment measures, new pharmacologic therapies that target the underlying biochemical mechanisms that cause diabetic retinopathy are being investigated. Recent interest has focused on intravitreal corticosteroid injections.[42,44]

Hypertensive Retinopathy. As with other blood vessels in the body, the retinal vessels undergo changes in response to chronically elevated blood pressure. In the initial, vasoconstrictor stage, there is vasospasm and an increase in retinal arterial tone because of local autoregulatory mechanisms. On ophthalmoscopy, this stage is represented by a general narrowing of the retinal arterioles. Persistently elevated blood pressure results in the compensatory thickening of arteriolar walls, which effectively reduces capillary perfusion pressure. With severe, uncontrolled hypertension, there is disruption of the blood–retina barrier, necrosis of smooth muscle and endothelial cells, exudation of blood and lipids, and retinal ischemia. These changes are manifested in the retina by microaneurysms, intraretinal hemorrhages, hard exudates, and cotton-wool spots. Swelling of the optic disc may occur at this stage and usually indicates severely elevated blood pressure (malignant hypertension). Older adults often have more rigid vessels that are unable to respond to the same degree as those in younger people.

Studies have shown that signs of hypertensive retinopathy regress with control of blood pressure.[45] There is also evidence that advanced signs of hypertensive retinopathy (*e.g.*, retinal hemorrhages, microaneurysms, and cotton-wool spots) predict stroke and death from stroke independent of elevated blood pressure and other risk factors.[45] People with these signs may benefit from close monitoring of cerebrovascular risk and intensive measures to reduce the risk.

Retinal Detachment

Retinal detachment involves the separation of the neurosensory retina from the pigment epithelium (Fig. 19.20). It occurs when traction on the inner sensory layer or a tear in this layer allows fluid, usually vitreous, to accumulate between the two layers.[38,46] There are four types of retinal detachments:

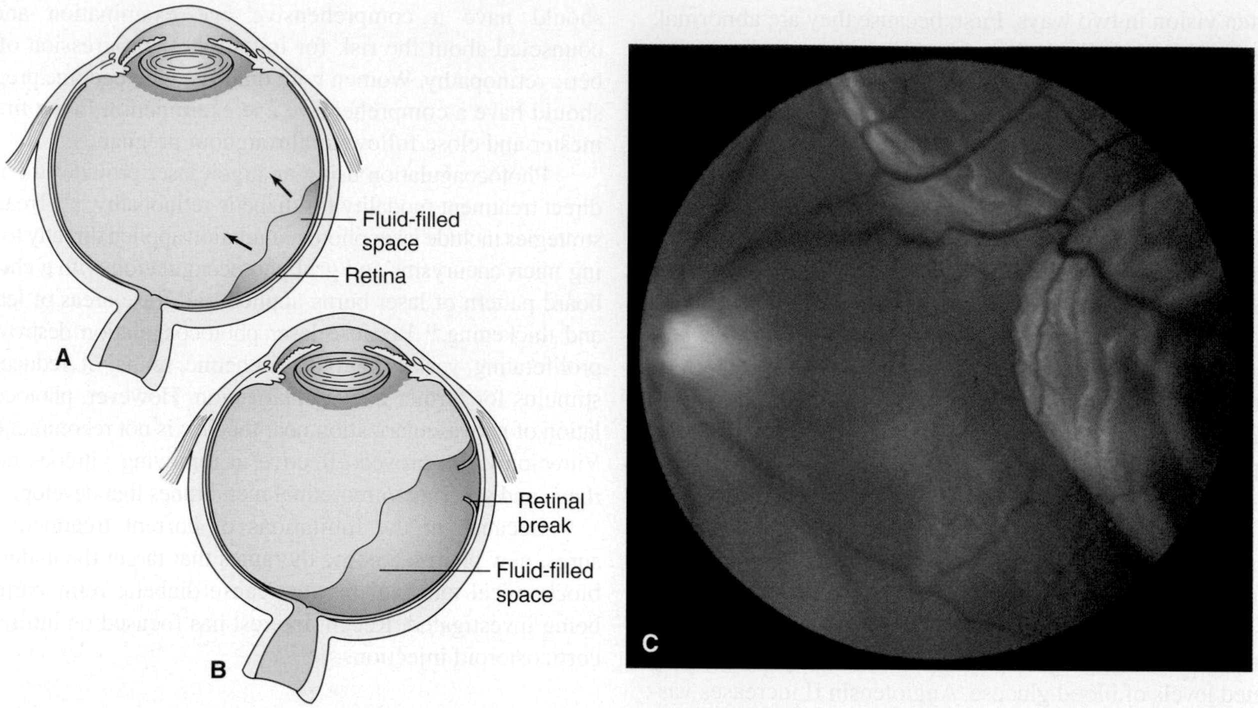

Figure 19.20 • Retinal detachment. **(A)** Changes in the vitreous structure cause it to shrink and separate from the retina, causing posterior vitreous detachment; **(B)** sustained fluid collection and tractional forces cause the retina to tear (rhegmatogenous retinal detachment). **(C)** Ophthalmoscopic photograph of retinal detachment. (From Moore K. L., Dalley A. F., Agur A. M. R. (2018). *Clinically oriented anatomy* (8th ed., p. 918, Figure B8.25). Philadelphia, PA: Lippincott Williams & Wilkins.)

exudative, traction, rhegmatogenous, and combined traction/rhegmatogenous.[46–48]

Exudative (or serous) *retinal detachment* results from the accumulation of serous or hemorrhagic fluid in the subretinal space due to severe hypertension, inflammation, or neoplastic effusions. It usually resolves with successful treatment of the underlying disease and without visual impairment. *Traction retinal attachment* occurs with mechanical forces on the retina, usually mediated by fibrotic tissue, resulting from previous hemorrhage (*e.g.*, from diabetic retinopathy), injury, infection, or inflammation. Intraocular surgery such as cataract extraction may produce traction on the peripheral retina that causes eventual detachment months or even years after surgery. Correction of traction retinal detachment requires disengaging scar tissue from the retinal surface, and vision outcomes are often poor.

Rhegmatogenous detachment (*rhegma* is the Greek for "rent" or "hole") is the most common type of retinal detachment. The vitreous is a hydrated gel whose structure is maintained by a collagenous and mucopolysaccharide matrix. As people age, this macromolecular network begins to liquefy and collapse. As this occurs, the vitreous shrinks and partly separates from the retinal surface, a condition known as *posterior vitreous detachment* (see Fig. 19.20). Rhegmatogenous detachment occurs when the liquid vitreous enters the subretinal space through the retinal tear. Detachment of the neural retina from the retinal pigment layer separates the receptors from their major blood supply, the choroid. If retinal detachment continues for some time, permanent destruction and blindness of that part of the retina occur.

Etiology and Pathophysiology. Risk factors for retinal detachment can include but are not limited to advancing age, myopia, previous eye surgeries, intraocular tumors, and diabetes. Approximately one in four people between the ages of 61 and 70 years develops a posterior vitreous detachment. In about 10% to 15% of these people, a retinal tear or hole forms as the vitreous pulls away from the retina, especially in the periphery where the retina is thinner.[38,46] People with high grades of myopia may have abnormalities in the peripheral retina that predispose to sudden detachment. In moderate to severe myopia or nearsightedness, the axial (anteroposterior) length of the eye is increased, resulting in an egg-shaped globe. As a result, there is greater vitreoretinal traction, and posterior vitreous detachment may occur at a younger age than in people without myopia. Also, the retina tends to be thinner and more prone to formation of a hole or tear. Other, less common risk factors include a family history of retinal detachment, a history of congenital eye disease (glaucoma, cataracts), and hereditary vitreopathies with abnormal vitreous gel.

Clinical Manifestations and Diagnosis. The primary symptom of retinal detachment consists of painless changes in vision. Commonly, flashing lights or sparks, followed by small floaters or spots in the field of vision, occur as the vitreous pulls away from the posterior pole of the eye. As detachment progresses, the person perceives a shadow or dark curtain progressing across the visual field. Because the process begins in the periphery and spreads circumferentially and posteriorly, initial visual disturbances may involve only one quadrant of the visual field. Large peripheral detachments may occur without involvement of the macula, so that visual acuity remains unaffected.

Diagnosis is based on a history of visual disturbances (*e.g.*, presence of floaters, luminous rays, or light flashes) and the ophthalmoscopic appearance of the retina. The direct (handheld) ophthalmoscope is useful in detecting an altered red reflex sometimes associated with retinal detachment. However, because the view is narrow, a negative examination with direct ophthalmoscopy cannot exclude the diagnosis of retinal detachment. Ophthalmologists and optometrists use indirect examination techniques that greatly enhance visualization of the peripheral retina.[46]

Treatment. Because there is a variable interval between a retinal break and retinal detachment, treatment methods focus on early detection and prevention of further vitreous detachment and retinal tear formation. Symptomatic retinal breaks are usually treated with laser or cryotherapy to seal the retinal tears so that the vitreous can no longer leak into the subretinal space. The treatment is more than 95% effective in preventing progression of a retinal tear and preventing retinal detachment.[38] The primary treatment of traction retinal detachment is vitreoretinal surgery and may involve vitrectomy, membrane removal, scleral buckling, or pneumatic retinopexy. Scleral buckling is the primary surgical procedure performed to reattach the retina.[46–48] With scleral buckling, a piece of silicone (*i.e.*, the buckle) is sutured and infolded into the sclera, physically indenting the sclera so it contacts the separated pigment and retinal layers. A less invasive procedure, pneumatic retinopexy, involves the intraocular injection of an expandable gas instead of a piece of silicone to form the indentation.[46–48]

Macular Degeneration

Macular degeneration is characterized by degenerative changes in the central portion of the retina (the macula) that result primarily in loss of central vision (see Fig. 19.1B). Age-related macular degeneration (AMD) is the most common cause of reduced vision and legal blindness worldwide.[49,50] Risk factors include age over age 50 years, female sex, white race, cigarette smoking, nutritional factors, cardiovascular diseases, and genes that are implicated in the regulation of lipid pathways.[49–53]

There are two types of AMD: an atrophic nonexudative or "dry" form and an exudative or "wet" form. Although both types are progressive, they differ in terms of manifestations, prognosis, and management. Although most people with AMD manifest nonproliferative changes only, those who experience severe vision loss do so from the development of the exudative form of the disease.

Clinical Manifestations and Diagnosis. Nonexudative AMD is characterized by various degrees of atrophy and degeneration of the outer retina, Bruch membrane, and the choriocapillaris. It does not involve leakage of blood or serum. Therefore, it is called *dry age-related macular degeneration* (Fig. 19.21). On ophthalmoscopic examination, there

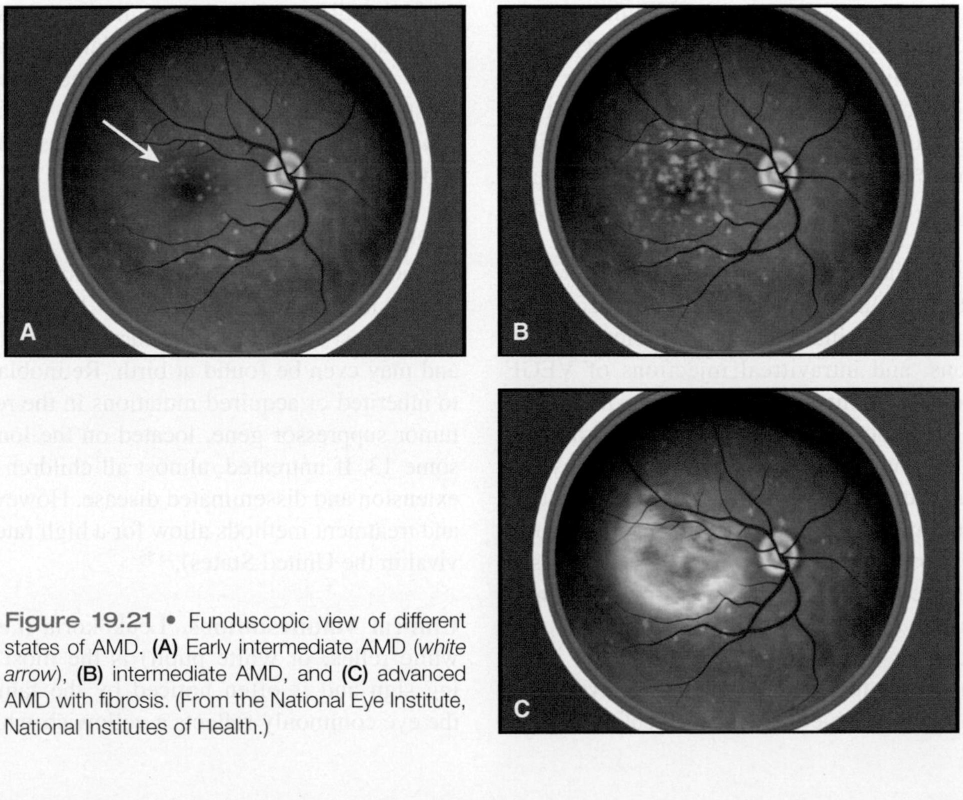

Figure 19.21 • Funduscopic view of different states of AMD. **(A)** Early intermediate AMD (*white arrow*), **(B)** intermediate AMD, and **(C)** advanced AMD with fibrosis. (From the National Eye Institute, National Institutes of Health.)

are visible changes in the retinal pigmentary epithelium and pale yellow spots, called *drusen*, which may occur individually or in groups throughout the macula. Histopathologically, most drusen contain remnants of materials representative of focal detachment of the pigment epithelium. With time, the drusen enlarge, coalesce, and increase in number. The level of associated visual impairment is variable and may be minimal. Most people with macular drusen do not experience significant loss of central vision, and the atrophic changes may stabilize or progress slowly. However, people with the nonexudative form of AMD need to be followed closely because the exudative stage may develop suddenly, at any time. Careful monitoring for metamorphopsia, or distorted vision of straight lines, can aid in the early detection of retinal damage.

The exudative or "wet form" of macular degeneration is characterized by the formation of a choroidal neovascular membrane that separates the pigmented epithelium from the neuroretina. These new blood vessels have weaker walls than normal and are prone to leakage. The leakage of serous or hemorrhagic fluid into the subretinal space causes separation of the pigmented epithelium from the neurosensory retina. Over time, the subretinal hemorrhages organize to form scar tissue, causing death of the underlying retinal tissue and loss of all visual function in the corresponding macular area (see Fig. 19.21). The early stages of subretinal neovascularization may be difficult to detect with an ophthalmoscope. Therefore, there is a need to be alert for recent or sudden changes in central vision, blurred vision, or scotomata in people with evidence of AMD.

Although some subretinal neovascular membranes may regress spontaneously, the natural course of exudative macular degeneration is toward irreversible loss of central vision. People with late-stage disease often find it difficult to see at long distances (*e.g.*, in driving), do close work (*e.g.*, reading), see faces clearly, or distinguish colors. However, they may not be severely incapacitated because the peripheral retinal function usually remains intact. With the use of low-vision aids, many of them are able to continue many of their normal activities.

Treatment. Effective therapies for exudative or wet-type macular degeneration include thermal laser photocoagulation, photodynamic therapy, intravitreal and periocular corticosteroid injections, and intravitreal injections of VEGF inhibitors. The decision about specific therapies must take into account the likelihood of visual recovery, which is greater with smaller, more recent lesions, as well as the risks of the various therapies. Currently, there is no established effective treatment for the dry form of macular degeneration, and most current therapies and new investigational treatments are directed at choroidal (or subretinal) neovascularization.[53,54]

Photodynamic laser therapy, which involves the intravenous injection of a dye that is subsequently activated by retinal laser irradiation to produce selective vascular damage, is indicated when the neovascular membrane is well defined. Conventional photocoagulation of subfoveal neovascular membranes is associated with an inevitable immediate reduction in vision because of associated retinal damage and thus is indicated only for extrafoveal membranes. Various surgical procedures to excise subfoveal neovascular membranes or position the macula away from them continue to be investigated.

The VEGF inhibitors that are administered by intravitreal injection include pegaptanib, ranibizumab, and bevacizumab. Pegaptanib is a VEGF inhibitor for the treatment of slow vision loss in eyes affected by all subtypes of AMD. Ranibizumab is a recombinant humanized monoclonal antibody with specificity for VEGF for the treatment of the wet form of AMD. Bevacizumab is approved in the United States as an intravenous infusion for treatment of colorectal cancer. Although bevacizumab has not been approved for ophthalmologic neovascular use, it can be used on an off-label basis. The corticosteroids have an angiostatic activity that appears to be independent of their hormone activity. The intravitreal injection of these agents bypasses the blood–ocular barrier, achieving therapeutic levels in the eye while avoiding systemic side effects.[53,54]

In addition to currently used and forthcoming treatments, there is interest in the so-called preventative category of treatments. Tobacco smoking is consistently identified as a preventable AMD risk. Therefore, elimination of tobacco smoking should be one of the first therapeutic recommendations. Preventative recommendations also include dietary supplementation with antioxidants and minerals such as vitamin E (α-tocopherol), vitamin C (ascorbic acid), zinc, and β-carotene for people at risk for developing macular degeneration and for slowing the progression of AMD in people with the disease.[53,54] Although dietary supplements seems reasonable, more experimental data and randomized clinical trials are needed to support their therapeutic value and their most effective composition in terms of single- or multiple-supplement combinations, as well as dosing of particular supplements.

Retinoblastoma

Retinoblastoma is the most common intraocular malignant neoplasm of children, affecting 1 in 20,000.[55] The tumor occurs most frequently in children younger than 2 years of age and may even be found at birth. Retinoblastomas are related to inherited or acquired mutations in the retinoblastoma (*Rb*) tumor suppressor gene, located on the long arm of chromosome 13. If untreated, almost all children die of intracranial extension and disseminated disease. However, new diagnostic and treatment methods allow for a high rate of cure (93% survival in the United States).[55,56]

Clinical Manifestations. Leukokoria (*i.e.*, cat's-eye reflex, white reflex, or white pupil) is the most common presenting sign and is often noticed by the family; light entering the eye commonly reflects a yellowish-white color similar to

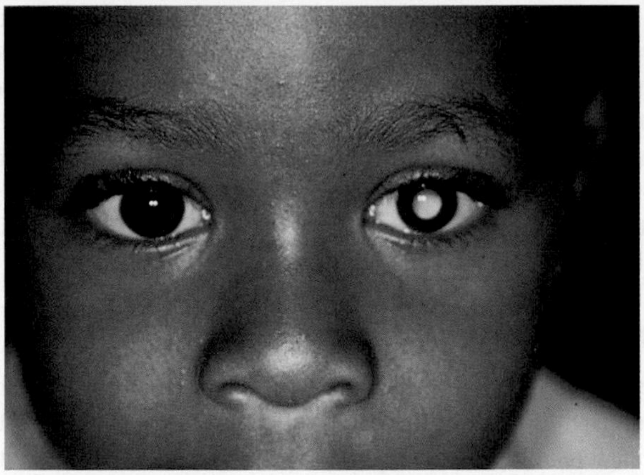

Figure 19.22 • The white pupil reflex (leukokoria) in the left eye of a child with intraocular retinoblastoma. (From Klintworth G. K. (2015). The eye. In Rubin R., Strayer D. E. (Eds.) *Rubin's pathology: Clinicopathologic foundations of medicine* (7th ed., p. 1523, Fig. 33-22A). Philadelphia, PA: Lippincott Williams & Wilkins.)

that of the membranous covering of a cat's eye (Fig. 19.22). Strabismus (squint) is the second most common sign.[57] Red, tearing, and painful eyes are a late sign of the disorder. Limited or poor vision is also a late sign. Most retinoblastomas occur sporadically and are unilateral. Up to 25% of sporadic retinoblastomas and most inherited forms of the disorder are bilateral.

Diagnosis and Treatment. Diagnostic measures for detection of retinoblastoma are usually prompted by abnormal results of an eye examination in the hospital nursery or health care provider's office. All children with a family history of retinoblastoma should be screened soon after birth. Screening should be repeated every 4 to 6 weeks until 1 year of age and then every 2 to 3 months until 3 years of age.[56,57] Congenital cataracts are an important cause of childhood leukokoria and should be ruled out. A definitive diagnosis usually requires ophthalmoscopic examination under general anesthesia by an ophthalmologist to obtain complete visualization of both eyes, which facilitates photographing and mapping of the tumors. CT or MRI scans are used to evaluate the extent of intraocular disease and extraocular spread.

The goals of treatment are primarily to save the child's life and secondarily to save the eye. Treatment options include laser thermotherapy, cryotherapy, chemotherapy, and enucleation (removal of the eye). Advances in genetics have enabled emerging therapies such as intravitreal chemotherapy and tumor hypoxia; the goal of both is preserving the globe (eyeball).[58–60] The choice of treatment is determined by the size of the tumor and its location and extension, as well as the visual potential and age of the child. Up to 45% of children treated with eye-preserving therapy may need subsequent therapy for recurrence of tumor, and up to 10% of children with unilateral tumors will develop a tumor in the contralateral eye.[57]

IN SUMMARY

The neural retina covers the inner aspect of the posterior two thirds of the eyeball and is continuous with the optic nerve. It contains the neural receptors for vision, and it is here that light energy of different frequencies and intensities is converted to graded local potentials, which then are converted to action potentials and transmitted to visual centers in the brain. The photoreceptors normally shed portions of their outer segments. Cells in the pigment epithelium phagocytize these segments. Failure of phagocytosis, as occurs in one form of retinitis pigmentosa, results in degeneration of the pigment layer and blindness.

The retina receives its blood from two sources: the choriocapillaris, which supplies the pigment layer and the outer portion of the sensory retina adjacent to the choroid, and the branches of the retinal artery, which supply the inner half of the retina. Retinal blood vessels are normally apparent through the ophthalmoscope. Neovascularization involves the formation of new, fragile blood vessels that leak protein and are likely to bleed. Although the cause of neovascularization is uncertain, research links the process with a VEGF produced by the lining of blood vessels. Hypoxia is a key regulator of VEGF-induced retinal neovascularization.

Disorders of retinal vessels can result from many local and systemic disorders, including diabetes mellitus and hypertension. They cause vision loss through changes that result in hemorrhage, production of opacities, and separation of the pigment epithelium and sensory retina. Retinal detachment involves separation of the sensory receptors from their blood supply; it causes blindness unless reattachment is accomplished promptly. Macular degeneration is characterized by loss of central vision due to destructive changes of the macula of the retina. There are two types of AMD: a nonexudative "dry form" that causes atrophy and degeneration of the outer retina and an exudative "wet form" that results in formation of a choroidal neovascular membrane with vessels that leak blood and serum and predispose to separation of the pigmented epithelium from the neuroretina. Although there are currently no effective therapies for the dry form of AMD, effective forms of treatment for the wet form include photodynamic therapy, laser photocoagulation, and intravitreal injection of corticosteroids and VEGF inhibitors.

Retinoblastoma is an intraocular malignant neoplasm of children (most often those younger than 2 years of age) that is caused by inherited or acquired mutations in the retinoblastoma (*Rb*) tumor suppressor gene. The most common presenting sign is leukokoria (white reflex or white pupil), with strabismus being the second most common sign. With new diagnostic and treatment methods, nearly 95% of retinoblastomas are cured in the United States.

DISORDERS OF NEURAL PATHWAYS AND CORTICAL CENTERS

After completing this section of the chapter, the learner will be able to meet the following objectives:

- Characterize what is meant by a *visual field defect*.
- Define the terms *hemianopia, quadrantanopia, heteronymous hemianopia,* and *homonymous hemianopia* and relate them to disorders of the optic pathways.
- Describe visual defects associated with disorders of the visual cortex and visual association areas.

Full visual function requires the normally developed brain-related functions of photoreception and the pupillary reflex. These functions depend on the integrity of all optic pathways, including retinal circuitry and the pathway from the optic nerve to the visual cortex and other visual regions of the brain and brain stem.

Optic Pathways

Visual information is carried to the brain by axons of the retinal ganglion cells, which form the optic nerve. Surrounded by pia mater, cerebrospinal fluid, arachnoid, and the dura mater, the optic nerve represents an outgrowth of the brain rather than a peripheral nerve. The optic nerve extends from the back of the optic globe through the orbit and the optic foramen, into the middle cranial fossa, and onto the optic chiasm at the base of the brain[55] (Fig. 19.23). Axons from the nasal portion of the retina remain medial, and those from the temporal retina remain lateral in the optic nerve.

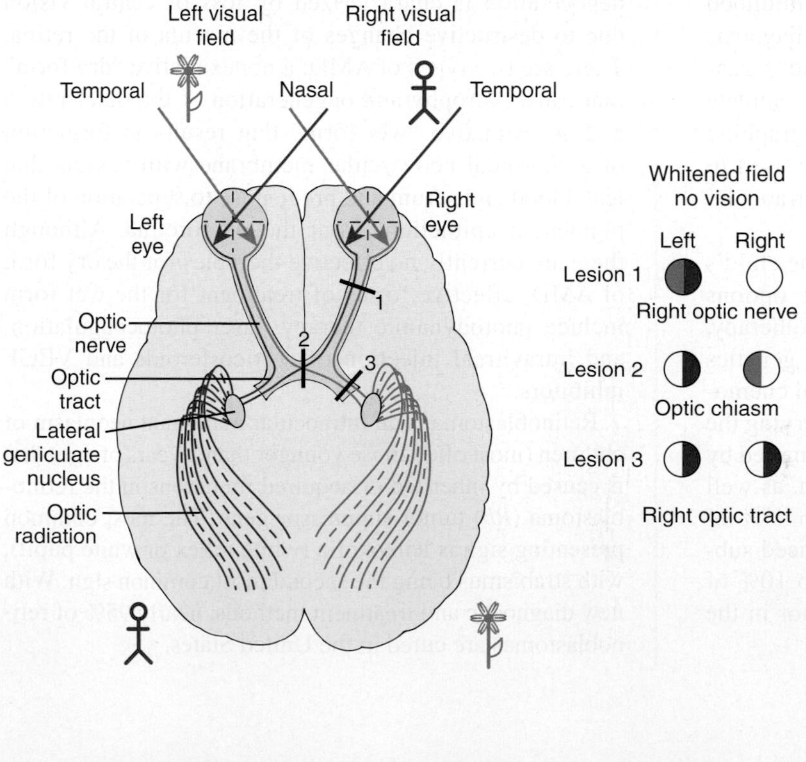

Figure 19.23 • Diagram of optic pathways. The *red lines* indicate the right visual field and the *blue lines* the left visual field. Note the crossing of fibers from the medial half of each retina at the optic chiasm. Lesion 1 (right optic nerve) produces unilateral blindness. Lesion 2 (optic chiasm) may involve only those fibers that originate in the nasal half of each retina and cross to the opposite side in the optic chiasm; visual loss involves the temporal half of each field (bitemporal hemianopia). Lesion 3 (right optic tract) interrupts fibers (and vision) originating on the same side of both eyes (homonymous) with loss of vision from half of each field (hemianopia).

The two optic nerves meet and fuse in the optic chiasm, beyond which they are continued as the optic tracts. In the optic chiasm, axons from the nasal retina of each eye cross to the opposite side and join with the axons of the temporal retina of the contralateral eye to form the optic tracts. Thus, one optic tract contains fibers from both eyes that transmit information from the same visual hemifield (half-field).

Visual Cortex

The primary visual cortex (area 17) surrounds the calcarine fissure, which lies in the occipital lobe. It is at this level that visual sensation is first experienced (Fig. 19.24). Immediately surrounding area 17 are the visual association cortices (areas 18 and 19) and several other association cortices. These association cortices, with their thalamic nuclei, must be functional to add meaningfulness to visual perception.

Circuitry in the primary visual cortex and the visual association areas is extremely discrete with respect to the location of retinal stimulation. For example, specific neurons respond to the particular orientation of a moving edge, specific colors, or familiar shapes. This elaborate organization of the visual cortex, with its functionally separate and multiple representations of the same visual field, provides the major basis for visual sensation and perception. Because of this discrete circuitry, lesions of the visual cortex must be large to be detected clinically.

Visual Fields

The *visual field* refers to the area that is visible during fixation of vision in one direction. Because visual system deficits are often expressed as visual field deficits rather than as direct

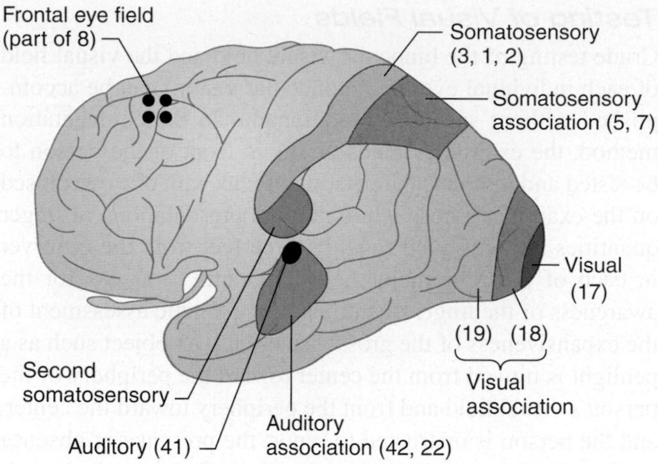

Figure 19.24 • Lateral view of the cortex illustrating the location of the visual, visual association, auditory, and auditory association areas.

measures of neural function, the terminology for normal and abnormal visual characteristics usually is based on visual field orientation.

Most of the visual field is *binocular* or seen by both eyes. This binocular field is subdivided into central and peripheral portions. Central portions of the retina provide high visual acuity and correspond to the field focused on the central fovea; the peripheral and surrounding portion provides the capacity to detect objects, particularly moving objects. Beyond the visual field shared by both eyes, the left lateral periphery of the visual field is seen exclusively by the left nasal retina, and the right peripheral field is seen by the right nasal retina.

As with a camera, the simple lens system of the eye inverts the image of the external world on each retina. In addition, the right and left sides of the visual field also are reversed. The right binocular visual field is seen by the left retinal halves of each eye—the nasal half of the right eye and the temporal half of the left eye.

Once the level of the retina is reached, the nervous system plays a consistent role. The upper half of the visual field is received by the lower half of the retinas of both eyes. Representations of this upper half of the field are carried in the lower half of each optic nerve: They synapse in the lower half of the lateral geniculate nucleus (LGN) of each side of the brain (see Fig. 19.19). Neurons in this part of the LGN send their axons through the inferior half of the optic radiation, looping into the temporal lobe to terminate in the lower half of the primary visual cortex on each side of the brain.

Because of the lateral separation of the two eyes, each eye contributes a different image of the world to the visual field. This is called *binocular disparity*. Disparity between the laterally displaced images seen by the two eyes provides a powerful source of three-dimensional depth perception for objects within a distance of 30 m. Beyond that distance, binocular disparity becomes insignificant: Depth perception is based on other cues (*e.g.*, the superimposition of the image of near objects over that of far objects and the faster movement of near objects than of far objects).

Visual Field Defects

Visual field defects result from damage to the retina, optic pathways, or the visual cortex. Perimetry or visual field testing, in which the limits of the visual field of each eye are measured and plotted in an arc, is used to identify defects and determine the location of lesions.

Retinal Defects. All of us possess a hole, or *scotoma*, in our visual field, of which we are unaware. Because the optic disc, where the optic nerve fibers exit the retina, does not contain photoreceptors, the corresponding location in the visual field constitutes a blind spot approximately 15 degrees temporal to fixation of each eye. Local retinal damage caused by small vascular lesions and other localized pathologic processes can produce additional blind spots. As with the normal blind spot, people are usually not aware of the existence of scotomata in their visual field unless they encounter problems seeing objects in certain restricted parts of the visual field.

Absences near or in the center of the bilateral visual field can be annoying and even disastrous. Although the hole is not recognized as such, the person finds that a part of a printed page appears or disappears, depending on where the fixation point is held. Most people learn to position their eyes to use the remaining central foveal vision for high-acuity tasks. Defects in the peripheral visual field, including the monocular peripheral fields, are less annoying but potentially more dangerous. People who are unaware of the defect, when walking or driving an automobile, do not see cars or bicyclists until their image reaches the functional visual field. This is sometimes too late to avert an accident. Once these people become aware of the defect, they can learn to shift their gaze constantly to obtain visual coverage of important parts of the visual field. If the damage is at the retinal or optic nerve level, only the monocular field of the damaged eye becomes a problem. A lesion affecting the central foveal vision of one eye can result in complaints of eye strain during reading and other close work because only one eye is being used.

Disorders of the Optic Pathways

Localized damage to the optic tracts, LGN, optic radiation, or primary visual cortex affects corresponding parts of the visual fields of both eyes (see Fig. 19.19). Examination of visual system function is of particular importance because lesions at various points along the pathway have characteristic symptoms that assist in the localization of the lesion.

Among the disorders that can interrupt the optic pathway are vascular lesions, trauma, and tumors. For example, normal visual system function depends on adequate perfusion of the ophthalmic artery and its branches; the central artery of the retina; the anterior and middle cerebral arteries, which supply the intracranial optic nerve, chiasm, and optic tracts; and the posterior cerebral artery, which supplies the LGN, optic radiation, and visual cortex. The adequacy of posterior cerebral artery function depends on that of the vertebral and basilar arteries that supply the brain stem. Vascular insufficiency in any one of these arterial systems can seriously affect vision.

Visual field defects of each eye and of the two eyes together are useful in localizing lesions affecting the system. Blindness in one eye is called *anopia*. If half of the visual field for one eye is lost, the defect is called hemianopia, and if a quarter of the field is lost, it is called *quadrantanopia*. Enlarging pituitary tumors can produce longitudinal damage through the optic chiasm with loss of the medial fibers of the optic nerve representing both nasal retinas and both temporal visual half-fields. The loss of different half-fields in the two eyes is called a *heteronymous loss*, and the abnormality is called *heteronymous hemianopia*. Destruction of one or both lateral halves of the chiasm is common with multiple aneurysms of the circle of Willis. In this condition, the function of one or both temporal retinas is lost, and the nasal fields of one or both eyes are lost. The loss of the temporal fields (nasal retina) of both eyes is called *bitemporal heteronymous anopia*. With both eyes open, the person with bilateral defects still has the full binocular visual field.

Loss of the optic tract, LGN, full optic radiation, or complete visual cortex on one side results in loss of the corresponding visual half-fields in each eye. *Homonymous* means "the same" for both eyes. In left-side lesions, the right visual field is lost for each eye and is called *complete right homonymous hemianopia*. Partial injury to the left optic tract, LGN, or optic radiation can result in the loss of a quarter of the visual field in both eyes. This is called *homonymous quadrantanopia*, and depending on the lesion, it can involve the upper (superior) or lower (inferior) fields. Because the optic radiation fibers for the superior quarter of the visual field traverse the temporal lobe, superior quadrantanopia is more common.

Disorders of the Visual Cortex

Discrete damage to the binocular portion of the primary visual cortex also can result in scotomata in the corresponding visual fields. The central high-acuity portion of the visual field is located at the occipital pole. If the visual loss is in the central high-acuity part of the field, severe loss of visual acuity and pattern discrimination occurs. Mechanical trauma to the cortex results in firing of neurons, experienced as flashes of light or "seeing stars." Destruction of the polar visual cortex causes severe loss of visual acuity and pattern discrimination. Such damage is permanent and cannot be corrected with lenses.

The bilateral loss of the entire primary visual cortex, called *cortical blindness*, eliminates all visual experience. Crude analysis of visual stimulation at reflex levels, such as eye-orienting and head-orienting responses to bright moving lights, pupillary reflexes, and blinking at sudden bright lights, may be retained even though vision has been lost. Extensive damage to the visual association cortex (areas 18 and 19) that surrounds an intact primary visual cortex results in a loss of the learned meaningfulness of visual images (*i.e.*, visual agnosia). The person can see the patterns of color, shapes, and movement, but no longer can recognize formerly meaningful stimuli. Familiar objects can be described but not named or reacted to meaningfully. However, if other sensory modalities, such as hearing and touch, can be applied, full recognition occurs. This disorder represents a problem of recognition rather than intellect.

Testing of Visual Fields

Crude testing of the binocular visual field and the visual field of each individual eye (*i.e.*, monocular vision) can be accomplished without specialized equipment. In the confrontation method, the examiner stands or sits in front of the person to be tested and instructs the person to focus with one eye closed on the examiner's nose while random presentations of finger quantities are presented roughly three feet from the observer in each of the four major field quadrants to assess for the awareness of the finger quantities.[61] In a kinetic assessment of the expansiveness of the gross visual field, an object such as a penlight is moved from the center toward the periphery of the person's visual field and from the periphery toward the center, and the person is instructed to report the presence or absence of the object. By moving the object through the vertical, horizontal, and oblique aspects of the visual field, a crude estimate can be made of the visual field. Large field defects can be estimated by the confrontation method, and it may be the only way for testing young children and uncooperative adults.

Accurate determination of the presence, size, and shape of smaller holes, or scotomata, in the visual field of a particular eye can be demonstrated only by perimetry. This is done by having the person look with one eye toward a central spot directly in front of the eye while the head is stabilized by a chin rest or bite board. A small dot of light or a colored object is moved back and forth in all areas of the visual field. The person reports whether the stimulus is visible and, if a colored stimulus is used, what the perceived color is. A hemispheric support is used to control and standardize the movement of the test object, and a plot of radial coordinates of the visual field is made. Automated perimetry uses static dots of varying intensity and color, as well as flicker frequency stimuli, to assess higher levels of retinal cell function. Perimetry provides a means of determining alterations from normal and, with repeated testing, a way of following the progress of the condition causing the visual field defect or its treatment.

IN SUMMARY

Visual information is carried to the brain by axons of the retinal ganglion cells that form the optic nerve. The two optic nerves meet and fuse in the optic chiasm. The axons of each nasal retina cross in the chiasm and join the uncrossed fibers of the temporal retina of the opposite eye in the optic tract to form the optic tracts. The fibers of each optic tract then synapse in the LGN and, from there, travel by way of the optic radiations to the primary visual cortex in the calcarine area of the occipital lobe. Damage to the visual association cortex can result in the phenomenon of seeing an object without the ability to recognize it (*i.e.*, visual agnosia). Optic pathway or visual cortex damage leads to visual field defects that can be identified through visual field testing. Perimetry, which maps the sensitivity contours of the visual field, can be used to determine the presence, size, and shape of smaller holes, or scotomata, in the visual field of an eye.

DISORDERS OF EYE MOVEMENT

After completing this section of the chapter, the learner will be able to meet the following objectives:

- Describe the function and innervation of the extraocular muscles.
- Explain the difference between paralytic and nonparalytic strabismus.
- Define *amblyopia* and explain its pathogenesis.

For complete visual function, it is necessary that the two eyes focus on the same fixation point, that the image of the object falls simultaneously on the fovea of each eye, and that the retinal and CNS visual mechanisms are functional. It is through these mechanisms that an object is simultaneously imaged on the fovea of both eyes and perceived as a single image. Strabismus and amblyopia are two disorders that affect this highly integrated system.

Extraocular Eye Muscles and Their Innervation

Each eyeball can rotate around its vertical axis (lateral or medial rotation in which the pupil moves away from or toward the nose), its horizontal left-to-right axis (vertical elevation or depression, in which the pupil moves up or down), and longitudinal horizontal axis in which the top of the pupil moves toward or away from the nose.

Three pairs of extraocular muscles—the superior and inferior recti, the medial and lateral recti, and the superior and inferior obliques—control the movement of each eye (Fig. 19.25). The four rectus muscles are named according to where they insert into the sclera on the medial, lateral, inferior, and superior surfaces of each eye. The two oblique muscles insert on the lateral posterior quadrant of the eyeball—the superior oblique on the upper surface and the inferior oblique on the lower. Each of the three sets of muscles in each eye is reciprocally innervated so that one muscle relaxes when the other contracts. Reciprocal contraction of the medial and lateral recti moves the eye from side to side (adduction and abduction); the superior and inferior recti move the eye up and down (elevation and depression). The oblique muscles rotate (intorsion and extorsion) the eye around its optic axis. A seventh muscle, the levator palpebrae superioris, elevates the upper lid.

The extraocular muscles are innervated by three cranial nerves. The abducens nerve (CN VI) innervates the lateral rectus, the trochlear nerve (CN IV) innervates the superior oblique, and the oculomotor nerve (CN III) innervates the remaining four muscles (Table 19.1). The CN VI (abducens) nucleus, in the caudal pons, innervates the lateral rectus muscle, which rotates the ipsilateral (same side) eye laterally (abduction). Partial or complete damage to this nerve results in weakness or complete paralysis of the muscle. Medial gaze is normal, but the affected eye fails to rotate laterally with an attempted gaze toward the affected side, a condition called *medial strabismus*. The CN IV (trochlear) nucleus, at the junction of the pons and midbrain, innervates the contralateral or opposite-side superior oblique muscle, which rotates the top of the globe inward toward the nose, a movement called *intorsion*. In combination with other muscles, it also contributes strength to movement of the innervated eye downward and inward.

The CN III (oculomotor) nucleus, which extends through a considerable part of the midbrain, contains clusters of lower motor neurons for each of the five eye muscles it innervates: inferior rectus, superior rectus, inferior oblique, medial rectus, and levator palpebrae superioris. The medial rectus, superior rectus, and inferior rectus rotate the eye in the directions shown in Table 19.1. The action of the inferior rectus is antagonistic to the superior rectus. Because of its plane of attachment to the globe, the inferior oblique rotates the eye in the frontal plane (*i.e., torsion*), pulling the top of the eye laterally (*i.e., extorsion*). CN III also innervates the levator palpebrae superioris muscle that elevates the upper eyelid and is involved

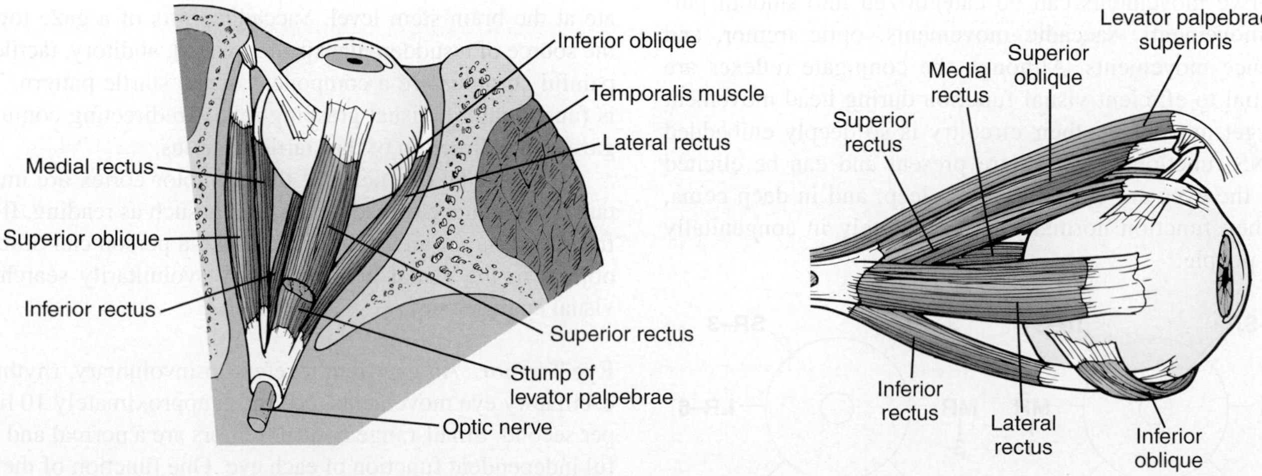

Figure 19.25 • Extraocular muscles of the right eye.

TABLE 19.1 EYE IN PRIMARY POSITION: EXTRINSIC OCULAR MUSCLE ACTIONS

MUSCLE*	INNERVATION	PRIMARY	SECONDARY	TERTIARY
MR: medial rectus	III	Adduction		
LR: lateral rectus	VI	Abduction		
SR: superior rectus	III	Elevation	Intorsion	Adduction
IR: inferior rectus	III	Depression	Extorsion	Adduction
SO: superior oblique	IV	Intorsion	Depression	Abduction
IO: inferior oblique	III	Extorsion	Elevation	Abduction

*In the schema of the functional roles of the six extraocular muscles, the major directional force applied by each muscle is indicated on the top. These muscles are arranged in functionally opposing pairs per eye and in parallel opposing pairs for conjugate movements of the two eyes. The numbers associated with each muscle indicate the cranial nerve innervation: 3, oculomotor (III) cranial nerve; 4, trochlear (IV) cranial nerve; 6, abducens (VI) cranial nerve.

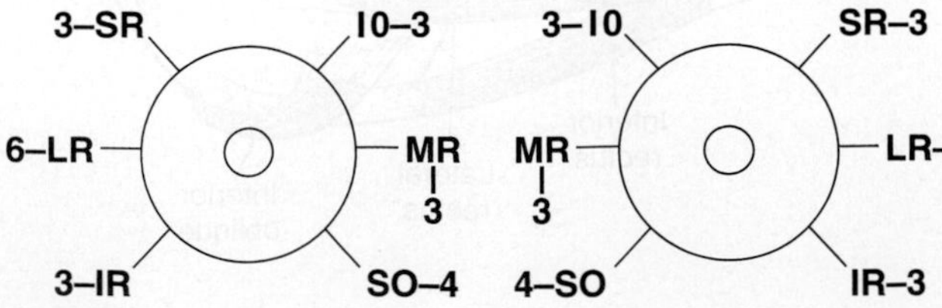

in vertical gaze eye movements. As the eyes rotate upward, the upper eyelid is reflexively retracted, and in the downward gaze, it is lowered, restricting exposure of the conjunctiva to air and reducing the effects of drying.

Communication between the eye muscle nuclei of each side of the brain occurs primarily through the posterior commissure at the rostral end of the midbrain. Longitudinal communication among the three nuclei occurs along a fiber tract called the *medial longitudinal fasciculus* (MLF), which extends from the midbrain to the upper part of the spinal cord. Each pair of eye muscles is reciprocally innervated, by the MLF or other associated pathways, so that as one muscle contracts, the other relaxes. These MLF-linked communication paths are vulnerable to damage in the caudal midbrain and pons. Damage to the pontine MLF on one side of the brain results in loss of this linkage, such that lateral deviation of the ipsilateral eye is no longer linked to adduction on the contralateral side. If the MLF is damaged bilaterally, the linkage is lost for lateral gaze in either direction.

Eye Movements and Gaze

Conjugate movements are those in which the optical axes of the two eyes are kept parallel, sharing the same visual field. *Gaze* refers to the act of looking steadily in one direction. Eye movements can be categorized into smooth pursuit movements, saccadic movements, optic tremor, and vergence movements. Although the conjugate reflexes are essential to efficient visual function during head movement or target movement, their circuitry is so deeply embedded in CNS function that they are present and can be elicited when the eyes are closed, during sleep, and in deep coma, and they function normally and accurately in congenitally blind people.

Smooth Pursuit Movements. Smooth pursuit movements are tracking movements that serve to maintain an object at a fixed point in the center of the visual fields of both eyes. The object may be moving with the eyes following, or the object may be stationary with the head moving. Normal eye posture is a conjugate gaze directed straight forward with the head held in a forward-looking posture. Smooth pursuit movements normally begin from this position. In fact, holding a strongly deviated gaze becomes tiring after about 30 seconds, and most people will make head and body rotation adjustments to bring the eyes to a central position within that time.

Asking the person to follow a finger or another object as it is moved slowly through the visual field tests voluntary pursuit movements. Successful conjugate following requires a functional optic system communicating to the superior colliculus and to the primary visual cortex.

Saccadic Eye Movements. Saccadic eye movements are sudden, jerky conjugate movements that quickly change the fixation point. During reading, the fixation pattern involves a focus on a word or short series of words and then a sudden jump of the eyes to a new fixation point on the next word or phrase. During the saccade, a person does not experience the blur of the rapidly moving visual field. Saccadic movements are automatic reflex movements that, in most situations, operate at the brain stem level. Saccadic shifts of a gaze toward the source of a sudden, unexpected visual, auditory, tactile, or painful stimulus are a component of the startle pattern. This is functionally a visual grasping reflex, redirecting conjugate gaze in the direction of the startle stimulus.

The frontal eye fields of the premotor cortex are important for voluntary saccadic movements such as reading. If this frontal premotor area is not functional, a person can describe objects in the visual field but cannot voluntarily search the visual environment.

Eye Tremor. An eye tremor refers to involuntary, rhythmic, oscillatory eye movements, occurring approximately 10 times per second. Small-range optical tremors are a normal and useful independent function of each eye. One function of the fine optic tremor is to constantly move a bright image onto a new bank of cones, permitting previously stimulated receptors quickly to recover from adaptation.

Vergence Eye Movements. Vergence eye movements are those that move the eyes in opposite directions to keep the image of an object precisely positioned on the fovea of each eye. Convergence and divergence, which assist in maintaining a binocularly fixed image in near vision, have a major role in accurate depth perception. The vergence system is driven by retinal disparity (*i.e.*, differential placement of an object's image on each retina). A nearby target (<30 ft) moving in the same dimension as the optical axis elicits a reflex mechanism that provides redirection of the optical axes of each eye away from parallel (*i.e.*, in opposite directions) in the horizontal plane. This process permits a continued binocular focus on the near target. Perception of depth is a higher-order function of the cortical visual system and is based on one or more of several classes of stimuli, such as superimposition and relative movement.

Strabismus

Strabismus, or squint, refers to any abnormality of eye coordination or alignment that results in loss of binocular vision. When images from the same spots in visual space do not fall on corresponding points of the two retinas, diplopia, or double vision, occurs. Strabismus affects approximately 4% of children younger than 6 years of age.[62,63] Because 30% to 50% of these children sustain permanent secondary loss of vision, or amblyopia, if the condition is left untreated, early diagnosis and treatment are essential.

In standard terminology, the disorders of eye movement are described according to the direction of movement. *Esotropia* refers to medial (inward) deviation, *exotropia* to lateral (outward) deviation, *hypertropia* to upward deviation, *hypotropia* to downward deviation, and *cyclotropia* to torsional deviation. The term *concomitance* refers to equal deviation in all directions of gaze. A nonconcomitant strabismus is one that varies with the direction of gaze. Strabismus may be divided into nonparalytic (concomitant) forms, in which there is no primary muscle impairment, and paralytic (nonconcomitant) forms, in which there is weakness or paralysis of one or more of the extraocular muscles. Strabismus is called *intermittent,* or *periodic,* when there are periods in which the eyes are parallel. It is monocular when the same eye always deviates and the opposite eye fixates. Figure 19.26 illustrates abnormalities in eye movement associated with esotropia and exotropia.

Nonparalytic Strabismus

Nonparalytic esotropia is the most common type of strabismus. The individual ocular muscles have no obvious defect, and the amount of deviation is constant or relatively constant

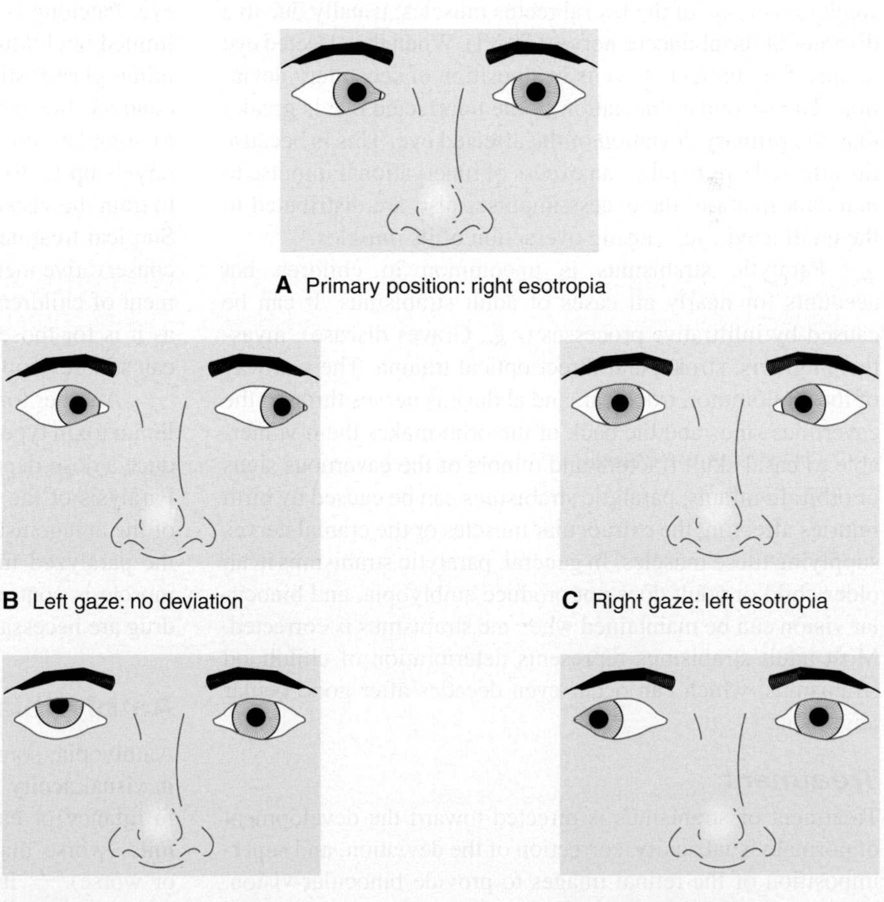

Figure 19.26 • **(A–C)** Paralytic strabismus associated with paralysis of the right lateral rectus muscle: **(A)** primary position of the eyes (looking straight ahead), **(B)** left gaze with no deviation, and **(C)** right gaze with left esotropia. **(D)** Primary position of the eyes with weakness of the right inferior rectus and right hypertropia. **(E)** Primary position of the eyes with weakness of the right medial rectus and right exotropia.

in the various directions of gaze. With persistent deviation, secondary abnormalities may develop because of overactivity or underactivity of the extraocular muscles in some fields of gaze.

The disorder may be nonaccommodative, accommodative, or a combination of the two. Infantile esotropia is the most common cause of nonaccommodative strabismus. It occurs in the first 6 months of life, with large-angle deviations, in an otherwise developmentally and neurologically normal infant. Eye movements are full, and the child often uses each eye independently to alter fixation (cross-fixation). The cause of the disorder is unclear. Research suggests that idiopathic strabismus may have a genetic basis; siblings often present with similar disorders.

Accommodative strabismus is caused by disorders such as uncorrected hyperopia of a significant degree, in which the esotropia occurs with accommodation that is undertaken to focus clearly. Onset of this type of esotropia characteristically occurs between 18 months and 4 years of age because accommodation is not well developed until that time. The disorder most often is monocular but may be alternating.

Paralytic Strabismus

Paralytic strabismus results from paresis (*i.e.*, weakness) or plegia (*i.e.*, paralysis) of one or more of the extraocular muscles. When the normal eye fixates, the affected eye is in the position of primary deviation. In the case of esotropia, there is weakness of one of the lateral rectus muscles, usually due to a disorder of the abducens nerve (CN VI). When the affected eye fixates, the unaffected eye is in a position of secondary deviation. The secondary deviation of the unaffected eye is greater than the primary deviation of the affected eye. This is because the affected eye requires an excess of innervational impulse to maintain fixation; the excess impulses also are distributed to the unaffected eye, causing overaction of its muscles.[63,64]

Paralytic strabismus is uncommon in children but accounts for nearly all cases of adult strabismus. It can be caused by infiltrative processes (*e.g.*, Graves disease), myasthenia gravis, stroke, and direct optical trauma. The pathway of the oculomotor, trochlear, and abducens nerves through the cavernous sinus and the back of the orbit makes them vulnerable to basal skull fracture and tumors of the cavernous sinus or orbit. In infants, paralytic strabismus can be caused by birth injuries affecting the extraocular muscles or the cranial nerves supplying these muscles. In general, paralytic strabismus in an older child or adult does not produce amblyopia, and binocular vision can be maintained when the strabismus is corrected. Most adult strabismus represents deterioration of childhood strabismus, which can occur even decades after good ocular alignment.

Treatment

Treatment of strabismus is directed toward the development of normal visual acuity, correction of the deviation, and superimposition of the retinal images to provide binocular vision. Early and adequate treatment is crucial because a delay in or lack of treatment can lead to amblyopia and permanent loss of vision. In addition to its effects on visual function, strabismus can have an adverse impact on interpersonal relationships, self-image, schoolwork, and participation in extracurricular activities. Children begin to develop negative attitudes toward classmates with strabismus.

Treatment includes both surgical and nonsurgical methods. Infantile esotropia is usually treated surgically by weakening the medial rectus muscle on each eye while the infant is under general anesthesia. Surgery in children with esotropia should be done as early as possible to preserve stereoscopic acuity. Early surgical treatment also appears to result in better outcomes than later intervention. Recurrent strabismus is common with infantile esotropia, and multiple surgeries are often required.[64,65]

Nonsurgical treatment includes glasses, occlusive patching, and eye exercises (*i.e.*, pleoptics). Glasses are often used in the treatment of accommodative esotropia that occurs with hypermetropia (farsightedness). Because accommodation is linked with convergence, focusing drives the eyes inward, producing esotropia. Intermittent exotropia is commonly treated with patching, use of overminus glasses, and eye exercises. Although no appreciable deviation is present when the child with intermittent strabismus sees near objects, the deviation becomes obvious when the child views distant objects or is fatigued. Patching for 1 to 2 hours daily for several months works by preventing, rather than treating, suppression of an eye. Patching is most effective in infants, and the efficacy is limited in children older than 3 years of age. The use of overminus glasses stimulates accommodative convergences, which contracts the exotropic drift. Vision therapy involves exercises to stimulate convergence (*e.g.*, focusing on reading-distance targets up to 30 minutes several times a day) and techniques to train the visual system to recognize the suppressed images. Surgical treatment of intermittent exotropia is indicted when conservative methods fail to correct the deviation. Early treatment of children with intermittent exotropia is not as crucial as it is for those with constant deviations because stereopsis can still develop.

Another form of treatment involves the injection of botulinum toxin type A (Botox) into the extraocular muscle to produce a dose-dependent paralysis of that extraocular muscle.[66] Paralysis of the muscle shifts the eye into the field of action of the antagonist muscle. During the time the eye is deviated, the paralyzed muscle is stretched, whereas the antagonistic muscle is contracted. Usually, two or more injections of the drug are necessary to obtain a lasting effect.

Amblyopia

Amblyopia, sometimes called *lazy eye*, describes a decrease in visual acuity resulting from abnormal visual development in infancy or early childhood. The vision loss ranges from mild (worse than 20/25) to severe (legal blindness, 20/200 or worse).[62,63] It is the leading cause of visual impairment, affecting 1% to 4% of the population. With early detection and treatment, most cases of amblyopia are reversible and the most severe forms of the condition can be prevented.

Etiology and Pathophysiology

Normal development of the thalamic and cortical circuitry necessary for binocular visual perception requires simultaneous binocular use of each fovea during a critical period early in life (0 to 5 years). Amblyopia can result from visual deprivation (*e.g.*, cataracts, ptosis) or abnormal binocular interactions (*e.g.*, strabismus, anisometropia) during visual immaturity. In infants with unilateral cataracts that are dense, central, and larger than 2 mm in diameter, this time is before 2 months of age.[67] In conditions causing abnormal binocular interactions, one image is suppressed to provide clearer vision. In esotropia, vision of the deviated eye is suppressed to prevent diplopia. A similar situation exists in anisometropia, in which the refractive indexes of the two eyes are different. Although the eyes are correctly aligned, they are unable to focus together, and the image of one eye is suppressed.

Treatment

The reversibility of amblyopia depends on the maturity of the visual system at the time of onset and the duration of the abnormal experience. Occasionally in strabismus, some people alternate eye fixation and do not experience deep amblyopia or diplopia. With late adolescent or adult onset, this habit pattern must be unlearned after correction. Amblyopia is remarkably responsive to treatment if the treatment is initiated early in life. Thus, all infants and young children should be evaluated for visual conditions that could lead to amblyopia.

The treatment of children with the potential for development of amblyopia must be instituted well before the age of 6 years to avoid the suppression phenomenon. Surgery for congenital cataracts and ptosis should be done early. Severe refractive errors should be corrected. In children with strabismus, the alternate blocking of the vision in one eye and then the other forces the child to use both eyes for form discrimination. The duration of occlusion of vision in the good eye must be short (2 to 5 hours/day) and closely monitored, or deprivation amblyopia can develop in the good eye as well. Although amblyopia is not likely to occur after 8 or 9 years of age, some plasticity in central circuitry is evident even in adulthood. For example, after refractive correction for long-standing astigmatism in adults, visual acuity improves slowly, requiring several months to reach normal levels.

Eye Examination in Infants and Children

Early detection and prompt treatment of ocular disorders in children are important to prevent amblyopia and lifelong visual impairment. The American Academy of Pediatrics in association with the American Association of Certified Orthoptists, American Association of Pediatric Ophthalmology and Strabismus, and American Academy of Ophthalmology recommends that all newborn infants be examined in the nursery for structural abnormalities and have a red reflex test performed to check for abnormalities in the back of the eye (posterior segment) and opacities in the visual axis, such as cataracts or corneal opacity.[64,65] An infant with an abnormal red reflex requires immediate referral to an eye care specialist. Visual examinations should then be performed on all well-child visits. These should include age-appropriate evaluation of visual acuity, ocular alignment, and ocular media clarity (cataracts, tumors).

Visual assessment of infants and children younger than 3 years of age is accomplished by determining whether each eye can fixate on an object, maintain fixation, and then follow the object in various gaze positions. Failure to perform these maneuvers indicates significant visual impairment. The assessment should be done binocularly and monocularly. If poor fixation is noted binocularly after 3 months of age, a significant bilateral eye or brain abnormality should be suspected and the child should be referred for further evaluation. Emphasis should be placed on screening for visual acuity as soon as the child is cooperative enough to complete the examination and at least at 6 months, 2 years, and 4 years old. Decreased vision in one eye requires evaluation for ocular deviation or other ocular abnormalities, which may be difficult to discern on screening examination.[67] Strabismus deviations of only a few degrees, too small to be detected by gross inspection, can lead to amblyopia and vision loss.

Every effort should be made to ensure that eye examinations are performed by properly prepared examiners, using appropriate testing conditions, instruments, and techniques. The results of vision assessments and visual acuity measurements, along with instructions for follow-up care, should be clearly communicated to the parents. Parents' observations are also important. Questions about whether the child's eyes seem straight or seem to cross or drift, or appear lazy; whether the child's eyelids droop or one eyelid tends to close; and, in older children, whether the child seems to see well or tends to hold objects close to his or her face when trying to focus can provide helpful information.[62–67]

IN SUMMARY

Binocular vision depends on the extraocular muscles and their innervating cranial nerves to move the eye up and down and rotate it around its optical axis. For full visual function, it is necessary that the two eyes point toward the same fixation point and the two images become fused. Binocular fusion is controlled by ocular reflex mechanisms that adjust the orientation of each eye to produce a single image. The term *conjugate gaze* refers to the use of both eyes to look steadily in one direction. During conjugate eye movements, the optical axes of the two eyes are maintained parallel with each other as the eyes rotate upward, downward, or from side to side in their sockets.

Strabismus refers to abnormalities in the coordination of eye movements, with loss of binocular eye alignment. This inability to focus a visual image on corresponding parts of the two retinas results in diplopia. Esotropia refers to medial deviation, exotropia to lateral deviation, hypertropia to upward deviation, hypotropia to downward deviation, and cyclotropia to torsional deviation. Paralytic strabismus is caused by weakness or paralysis of the extraocular muscles, whereas nonparalytic strabismus results from the inappropriate length or insertion of the extraocular muscles or from accommodation disorders.

Amblyopia (*i.e.*, lazy eye) is a decrease in visual acuity resulting from abnormal visual development in infancy and early childhood. It results from inadequately developed CNS circuitry because of visual deprivation (*e.g.*, cataracts) or abnormal binocular interactions (*e.g.*, strabismus) during visual immaturity.

GERIATRIC Considerations

- Cornea shows infiltration of degenerative lipid material around the limbus (arcus senilis), and pupil size decreases.[68]
- Lens loses elasticity and may become hard and glass-like. The lens's inability to change shape results in near vision or presbyopia.[1]
- The transparent fiber of the lens begins to thicken and yellow, which is the beginning of the senile cataract.[68]
- The aging person needs more light to see because of decreased adaptation to darkness (which contributes to trouble driving at night.[68]
- Visual disturbances that begin in the fourth decade of life increase the risk for falls because of changes in depth perception distortion.[69]

PEDIATRIC Considerations

- At birth, eye function is limited but rapidly matures during the first 6 months and then fully matures by age 4 or 5 years.[70]
- At birth, infants are very sensitive to bright light, and their pupils are small to limit light entering the eye. Peripheral vision is intact, but central vision is still developing.[71]
- Retinopathy of prematurity, if untreated, can result in blindness. Strabismus may occur even if ROP is resolved.[72]

REVIEW EXERCISES

1. The mother of a 3-year-old boy notices that his left eye is red and watering when she picks him up from day care. He keeps rubbing his eye as if it itches. The next morning, however, she notices that both eyes are red, swollen, and watering. Being concerned, she takes him to the pediatrician in the morning and is told that he has "pink eye." She is told that the infection should go away by itself.
   A. *What part of the eye is involved?*
   B. *What type of conjunctivitis do you think this child has: bacterial, viral, or allergic?*
   C. *Why didn't the pediatrician order an antibiotic?*
   D. *Is the condition contagious? What measures should she take to prevent its spread?*
2. During a routine eye examination to get new glasses because she had been having difficulty with her distant vision, a 75-year-old woman is told that she is developing cataracts.
   A. *What type of visual changes occurs as the result of a cataract?*
   B. *What can the woman do to prevent the cataracts from getting worse?*
   C. *What treatment may she eventually need?*
3. A 50-year-old woman is told by her "eye doctor" that her intraocular pressure is slightly elevated and that although there is no evidence of damage to her eyes now, she is at risk for developing glaucoma and should have regular eye examinations.
   A. *Describe the physiologic mechanisms involved in the regulation of intraocular pressure.*
   B. *What are the risk factors for developing glaucoma?*
   C. *Explain how an increase in intraocular pressure produces its damaging effects.*
4. The parents of a newborn infant have been told that their son has congenital cataracts in both eyes and will require cataract surgery to prevent loss of sight.
   A. *Explain why the infant is at risk for losing his sight if the cataracts are not removed.*
   B. *When should this procedure be done to prevent loss of vision?*

References

1. World Health Organization. (2017). Blindness and visual impairment. [Online]. Available: www.WHO.int. Accessed July 1, 2017.
2. Michels K. S., Czyz C. N., Cahill K. V., et al. (2014). Age-matched, case-controlled comparison of clinical indicators for development of entropion and ectropion. *Journal of Ophthalmology* 2014, 231487. Available: http://doi.org/10.1155/2014/
3. Uphold C. R., Graham M. V. (2013). *Clinical guidelines in family practice* (pp. 301–302, 304–307). North Miami Beach, FL: Barmarrae Books, Inc.

4. Tsubota K., Yokoi N., Shimazaki J., et al. (2016). New perspectives on dry eye definition and diagnosis: A consensus report by the Asia Dry Eye Society. *The Ocular Surface* 15(1), 65–67.
5. Goldberg R., Banta J. (2013). Dry eye syndrome. In Buttarom T., Trybulski J., Baily P., et al. (Eds.) *Primary care a collaborative practice* (pp. 333–335). St. Louis, MO: Elsevier Mosby.
6. Kossler A., Banta, J. (2013). Nasolacrimal duct obstruction and dacryocystitis. In Buttarom T., Trybulski J., Baily P., et al. (Eds.) *Primary care a collaborative practice* (pp. 335–336). St. Louis, MO: Elsevier Mosby.
7. Gilbard J. P. (2009). Dry eye and blepharitis: Approaching the patient with chronic eye irritation. *Geriatrics* 64(6), 22–26.
8. World Health Organization. (2017). Trachoma. [Online]. Available: www.WHO.int. Accessed July 4, 2017.
9. Riordan-Eva P. (2011). Anatomy and embryology of the eye. In Riordan-Eva P., Cunningham E. T. (Eds.) *Vaughan & Asbury's general ophthalmology* (18th ed., pp. 1-26). New York: McGraw-Hill.
10. Collier S., Gronostaj M., et al. (2014). Estimated burden of keratitis. [Online]. Available: www.cdc.gov. Accessed July 5, 2017.
11. Weiss M., Banta J. (2013). Evaluation and management of eye disorders. In Buttarom T., Trybulski J., Baily P., et al. (Eds.) *Primary care a collaborative practice* (p. 320). St. Louis, MO: Elsevier Mosby.
12. Farooq A. V., Shukla D. (2012). Herpes simplex epithelial and stromal keratitis: An epidemiologic update. *Survey of Ophthalmology* 57(5), 448–462. Available: http://doi.org/10.1016/j.survophthal.2012.01.005
13. Biswell R. (2011). Cornea. In Riodan-Eva P., Cunningham E. T. (Eds.) *Vaughan & asbury's general ophthalmology* (18th ed., pp. 120–144). New York: McGraw-Hill.
14. Guess S., Stone D., Chodosh J. (2007). Evidence-based treatment of herpes simplex virus keratitis: A systematic review. *The Ocular Surface Journal* 15(3), 240–250.
15. Piret J., Boivin G. (2016). Antiviral resistance in herpes simplex virus and varicella-zoster virus infections: Diagnosis and management. *Current Opinion Infectious Disease* 29(6), 654–662.
16. Kumar R., Cruzat A., Hamrah P. (2010). Current state of in vivo confocal microscopy in management of microbial keratitis. *Seminars in Ophthalmology* 25(5-6), 166–170.
17. Ikeda Y., Miyazaki D., et al. (2012). Assessment of real-time polymerase chain reaction detection of acanthamoeba and prognosis determinants of acanthamoeba keratitis. *Ophthalmology* 119(6), 1111–1119.
18. Seal D. (2003). Acanthamoeba keratitis update-incidence, molecular epidemiology and new drugs for treatment. *Eye Journal* 17(8), 893–905.
19. Iovieno A., Gore D., Carnt N., et al. (2014). Acanthamoeba sclerokeratitis: Epidemiology, clinical features and treatment outcomes. *Ophthalmology* 121(12), 2340–2347.
20. National Eye Institute. (2017). Corneal Transplantation. [On-line]. Available: https://www.nei.nih.gov. Accessed July 8, 2017.
21. Caspi R. (2010). A look at autoimmunity and inflammation in the eye. *Journal of Clinical Investigation* 120(9), 3073–3083.
22. Miller N., Newman N., Biousse V., et al. (Eds.) (2008). *Walsch and Hoyt's clinical neuro-ophthalmology: The essentials* (2nd ed). Philadelphia, PA: Lippincott Williams & Wilkins.
23. Tham Y., Li X., Wong T., et al. (2014). Global prevalence of glaucoma and projections of glaucoma burden through 2040: A systematic review and meta-analysis. *Ophthalmology* 121(11), 2081–2090.
24. Salmon J. (2011). Glaucoma. In Riordan-Eva P., Cunningham E. T. (Eds.) *Vaughan & Asbury's general ophthalmology* (18th ed., pp. 22–237). New York: McGraw-Hill.
25. Fernandez-Bahamonde J., Roman-Rodriguez C., Fernandez-Ruiz M. (2011). Central corneal thickness as a predictor of visual field loss in primary open angle glaucoma for a Hispanic population. *Seminars in Ophthalmology* 26(1), 28–32.
26. Prum B., Rosenberg L., et al. (2016). Primary open-angle glaucoma preferred practice pattern guidelines. *Ophthalmology* 123(1), 41–111.
27. Tarongoy P, Ho C., Walton D. (2009). Angle closure glaucoma: The role of the lens in the pathogenesis prevention and treatment. *Survey of Ophthalmology* 54(2), 211–225.
28. Lai J., Gangwani R. (2012). Medication induced acute angle closure attack. *Hong Kong Medical Journal* 18(2), 139–145.
29. Mandal A., Chakrabarti D. (2011). Update on congenital glaucoma. *Indian Journal of Ophthalmology* 59(Suppl), 148–157.
30. Riorodan-Eva P. (2011). Optics and refractions. In Riordan-Eva P., Cunningham E. T. (Eds.) *Vaughan & Ashbury's general ophthalmology*. (18th ed., pp. 396–411). New York: McGraw-Hill.
31. Messmer J. (2010). LASIK: A primer for family physicians. *American Family Physician* 81(1), 42–47.
32. Krantz E., Cruickshanks K., Klein B., et al. (2010). Measuring refraction in adults in epidemiological studies. *Archives of Ophthalmology* 128(1), 88–92.
33. Harper R., Shock J. (2011). Lens. In Riordan-Eva P,. Cunningham E. (Eds.) *Vaughan & Ashbury's general ophthalmology* (18th ed., pp. 174–181).
34. Townsend J., Banta J. (2013). Cataracts. In Buttaro T., Trybulski J., Bailey P., et al. (Eds.) *Primary care: A collaborative practice* (4th ed. pp. 322–324). St. Louis, MO: Elsevier Mosby.
35. Vizzeri G., Weinreb R. (2010). Cataract surgery and glaucoma. *Current Opinion in Ophthalmology* 21(1), 20–24.
36. Pringle E., Graham E. (2011). Ocular disorders associated with systemic disease. In Riordan-Eva P., Cunningham E. T. (Eds.) *Vaughn & Ashbury's general ophthalmology* (18th ed., pp. 314–346). New York: McGraw-Hill.
37. Riordan-Eva P. (2011). Disorders of the eyes and lids. In McPhee S., Papadakis M. (Eds.) *Current medical diagnosis and treatment* (50th ed., pp. 166–197). New York: McGraw-Hill.
38. Fletcher E., Chong N., Augsburger J. et al. (2011). Retina. In Riordan-Eva P., Cunningham E. T. (Eds.) *Vaughn & Ashbury's general ophthalmology* (18th ed., pp. 190–221). New York: McGraw-Hill.
39. Genetics Home Reference. (2017). Retinitis Pigmentosa. [Online]. Available: https://ghr.nlm.nih.gov. Accessed July 12, 2017.
40. Beran D., Murphy-Lavoie H. (2009). Acute, painless vision loss. *Journal of the Louisiana State Medical Society* 161(4), 214–216, 218–223.
41. Fante R., Durairaj V., Oliver S. (2010). Diabetic retinopathy: An update on treatment. *The American Journal of Medicine* 123(3), 213–216.
42. Zhang X., Saaddine J., Chou C., et al. (2010). Prevalence of diabetic retinopathy in the United States, 2005-2008. *Journal of the American Medical Association* 304(6), 649–656.
43. The ACCORD Study Group and ACCORD Eye Study Group. (2010). Effects of medical therapies on retinopathy progression in type 2 diabetes. *New England Journal of Medicine* 363, 233–244.
44. Heng L., Comyn O., Peto C., et al. (2013). Diabetic retinopathy: Pathogenesis, clinical grading, management and future developments. *Diabetic Medicine* 30(6), 640–650.
45. Cuspidi C., Negri F., Giudici V., et al. (2009). Retinal changes and cardiac remodeling in systemic hypertension. *Therapeutic Advances in Cardiovascular Disease* 3(3), 205–214.
46. D'Amico D. (2008). Primary retinal detachment. *New England Journal of Medicine*.359(22), 2346–2354.
47. Sun Q., Sun T., Xu Y., et al. (2012). Primary vitrectomy verses scleral buckling for the treatment of rhegmatogenous retinal detachment: A meta-analysis of randomized controlled clinical trials. *Current Eye Research* 37(6), 492–499.
48. Hatef E., Sena D., Fallano K., et al. (2015). Pneumatic retinopexy verses scleral buckle for repairing simple rhegmatogenous retinal detachments. *Cochrane Database of Systematic Review [Online]* (5), CD008350. Available: www.cochranelibrary.com. Accessed July 14, 2017.
49. Kokotas H., Grigoriadou M., Petersen M. (2011). Age-related macular degeneration: Genetic and clinical findings. *Clinical Chemistry and Laboratory Medicine* 49(4), 601–616.
50. Klein R., Myers C., Klein B. (2014). Vasodilator, blood pressure-lowering medications, and age-related macular degeneration: The Beaver Dam Eye Study. *Ophthalmology* 121(8), 1604–1611.
51. Chiang A., Regillo C. (2011). Preferred therapies for neovascular age-related macular degereration. *Current Opinion in Ophthalmology* 22(3), 199–204.

52. Jonasson F., Fisher D., Eiriksdottir G., et al. (2014). Five-year incidence, progression, and risk factors for age-related macular degeneration: the age, gene/environment susceptibility study. *Ophthalmology* 121(9), 1766–1772.
53. Lim L., Mitchell P., Seddon J. et al. (2012). Age-related macular degeneration. *Lancet* 379(9827), 1728–1738.
54. Yehoshua Z., Rosenfeld P., Albini T. (2011). Current clinical trials in dry AMD and the definition of appropriate clinical outcome measures. *Seminars in Ophthalmology* 26(3), 167–180.
55. Klintworth G. (2008). The eye. In Rubin R., Strayer D. (Eds.) *Rubin's pahology: clinicopathologic foundations of medicine* (5th ed., pp. 1265–1266). Philadelphia, PA: Lippincott Williams & Wilkins.
56. Li J., Coats D., Fung D., et al. (2010). The detection of simulated retinoblastoma by using red-reflex testing. *Pediatrics* 126(1), 292–207.
57. Kembhavi S., Sable N., Vora T., et al. (2011). Leukocoria: All that's white is not retinoblastoma. *Journal of Clinical Oncology* 29(19), 586–587.
58. Nale P. (2011). Early recognition of recurrence key to successfully treating retinoblastoma. *Ocular Surgery News* 29(10), 18.
59. Smith S., Smith B. (2013). Evaluating the risk of extraocular tumor spread following intravitreal injection therapy for retinoblastoma: a systematic review. *British Journal of Ophthalmology* 97(10), 1231–1236.
60. Villegas V., Hess D., Wildner A., et al. (2013). Retinoblastoma. *Current Opinions in Ophthalmology* 24(6), 581–588.
61. Kerr N., Chew S., Eady E., et al. (2010). Diagnostic accuracy of confrontation visual field test. *Neurology* 74(15), 1184–1190.
62. Motley W., Asbury T. (2004). Strabismus. In Riordan-Eva P., Cunningham E. T. (Eds.) *Vaughan & Ashbury general ophthalmology* (18th ed., pp. 238–258). New York: McGraw-Hill.
63. Granet D., Khayali S. (2011). Amblyopia and strabismus. *Pediatric Annals* 40(2), 89–94.
64. Minnal V., Rosenberg J. (2011). Refractive surgery: A treatment for and a cause of strabismus. *Current Opinion in Ophthalmology* 22(4), 222–225.
65. Wang L., Nelson L. (2010). One muscle strabismus surgery. *Current Opinion in Ophthalmology* 21(5), 335–340.
66. Rowe F., Noonan C. (2017). Botulinum toxin for the treatment of strabismus. *Cochrane Database of Systematic Reviews* 3. [Online]. Available: onlinelibrary.wiley.com. Accessed July 29, 2017.
67. Hered R. (2011). Effective vision screening of young children in the pediatric office. *Pediatric Annals* 40(2), 76–82.
68. Jansen S. (2015). *Nursing health assessment: A best practice approach* (2nd ed). Philadelphia, PA: Wolters Kluwer.
69. Epiopoulos C. (2018). Vision and hearing. In *Gerontological nursing* (9th ed., pp. 364–377).
70. Boyd K. (2017). *Baby's vision development: What to expect the first year*. American Academy of Opthalmology. Available: https://www.aao.org/eye-health/tips-prevention/baby-vision-development-first-year
71. Kyle T. (2017). *Essentials of pediatric nursing* (3rd ed). Philadelphia, PA: Wolters Kluwer Health.
72. Griffith M., Alarcon E. I., Brunette I. (2016). Regenerative approaches for the cornea. *Journal of Internal Medicine* 280(3), 276–286. doi:10.1111/joim.12502.

Disorders of Hearing and Vestibular Function

20

Maeghan Arnold, Deena Garner, and Sharon Stevenson

The ear is a sensory organ of hearing and vestibular equilibrium consisting of three parts: the external, middle, and inner ear. The external and middle ears are designed to capture and transmit sound waves to the inner ear while amplifying sound. The inner ear, which is fluid-filled, contains structures necessary for hearing and balance. The fluid in the inner ear conducts and transmits sound waves and vibrations. Acute otitis media, or inflammation of the middle ear, is a leading cause of primary care visits and the number one reason for antimicrobial prescriptions for children. Hearing loss is one of the most common disabilities experienced by people in the United States, particularly among older adults. It is also a cause of impaired language development in children. Vertigo, a disorder of vestibular function, is also a common cause of disability among older adults. This chapter is divided into two parts: the first focuses on disorders of the ear and auditory function and the second on disorders of the inner ear and vestibular function.

DISORDERS OF THE AUDITORY SYSTEM

After completing this section of the chapter, the learner will be able to meet the following objectives:

- Relate the functions of the eustachian tube to the development of middle ear problems, including acute otitis media and otitis media with effusion.
- Describe the disease process associated with otosclerosis and relate it to progressive conductive hearing loss.
- Differentiate between conductive, sensorineural, and mixed hearing loss and name the common causes of each.

Disorders of the External Ear

The external ear consists of the auricle and the external acoustic meatus (Fig. 20.1). The auricle, or pinna, which collects sound, is composed of cartilage that is covered by a thin skin

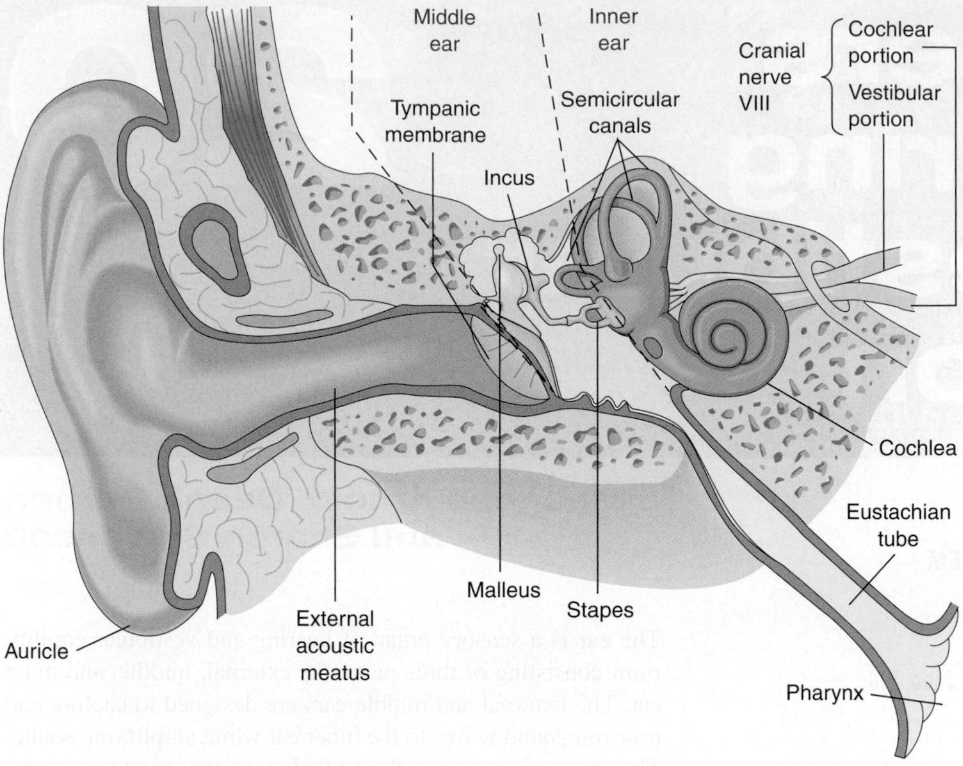

Figure 20.1 • External, middle, and internal subdivisions of the ear.

and very fine hair.[1] The rim, or helix, is somewhat thicker, and the fleshy earlobe lacks surrounding cartilage. The funnel shape of the auricle concentrates high-frequency sound into the ear canal.

The external acoustic meatus, or ear canal, is approximately 2.5-cm long in adults.[1] In infants and young children, the canal is relatively shorter so extra care must be taken when inspecting it with an otoscope. A thin layer of skin containing fine hairs, sebaceous glands, and ceruminous glands lines the ear canal. These glands produce cerumen, or earwax, which has certain antimicrobial properties and is thought to serve a protective function.

Branches of the trigeminal nerve (cranial nerve [CN] V) innervate the anterior portion of the auricle and external part of the ear canal. The posterior portions of the auricle and the wall of the ear canal are innervated by auricular branches of the facial (CN VII), glossopharyngeal (CN IX), and vagus (CN X) nerves. Because of the vagal innervation, the insertion of a speculum or an otoscope into the external ear canal can stimulate coughing or vomiting reflexes.

The tympanic membrane, approximately 1 cm in diameter, is a thin, semitransparent membrane that separates the external ear from the middle ear.[1] The tympanic membrane is covered with thin skin externally and the mucous membrane of the middle ear internally. The tympanic membrane vibrates when audible sound waves enter the external auditory canal. Movements of the membrane are transmitted through the middle ear to the inner ear.

When viewed through an otoscope, the tympanic membrane appears as a shallow, oval cone pointing inward toward its apex, the umbo (Fig. 20.2). Landmarks include the lightened stripe over the handle of the malleus; the umbo at the end of the handle; the *pars tensa* (tense part), which constitutes most of the drum; a thinner membrane, the *pars flaccida* (flaccid part); and the small area above the malleus attachment. A bright light reflected from an otoscope's illuminator, called the *cone of light*, radiates from the umbo. The tympanic membrane is semitransparent. The *chorda tympani*, a small, whitish cord, crosses the middle ear from back to front and can be seen just under its upper edge. The *chorda tympani* is a branch of the facial nerve (CN VII).

The function of the external ear is disturbed when sound transmission is obstructed by impacted cerumen, inflammation (*i.e.*, otitis externa), or drainage from the external ear (otorrhea).

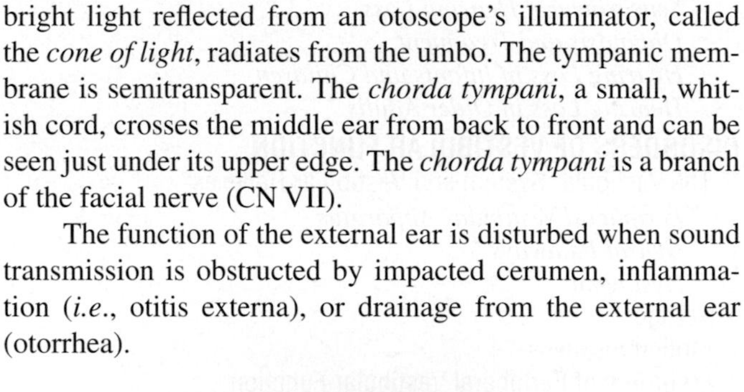

Figure 20.2 • Bony landmarks of the tympanic membrane. (From Bickley L. S. (2017). *Bates' guide to physical examination and history taking* (12th ed., Figure 7-40). Philadelphia, PA: Wolters Kluwer.)

Impacted Cerumen

Cerumen, or earwax, is a protective secretion produced by the sebaceous and ceruminous glands of the skin that lines the ear canal. Although cerumen is beneficial in cleaning, protecting, and lubricating the ear, the cerumen can accumulate and narrow the canal causing reversible conductive hearing loss.[2]

Impacted cerumen usually produces no symptoms unless it hardens and touches the tympanic membrane or the canal becomes irritated by a buildup of hardened cerumen. Clinical manifestations may include pain, itching, and a sensation of fullness. As the canal becomes completely occluded, a person may experience a feeling of fullness, a conductive hearing loss, vertigo, and tinnitus (*i.e.*, ringing in the ears). Because the external auditory canal is innervated by the auricular branch of the vagus nerve, coughing or even cardiac deceleration can result from stimulation of the canal by cerumen impaction or removal attempts.[2]

Removal of cerumen is only indicated when visualization of the ear canal and tympanic membrane is necessary. In most cases, cerumen can be removed by manual extraction using a curette or gentle irrigation using a bulb syringe and warm tap water. Manual extraction is performed using a plastic curette or hook while visualizing the ear canal. Ear irrigation is performed using warm water to avoid inducing a feeling of disequilibrium. The ear canal should be dried thoroughly after irrigation to avoid introducing an infection. Irrigation should be avoided in an only-hearing ear or one that is postsurgical, prone to infection, or questionable for perforation of the tympanic membrane. Consideration must be given to conditions such as an immunocompromised state, diabetes mellitus, and radiation to the head and neck.[2]

Cerumen that has become hardened or impacted can be softened by instillation of a few drops of a ceruminolytic agent, a compound that disintegrates earwax. Typically, these agents are instilled in the affected ear one or two times daily for up to 4 days before irrigation. Instilling ceruminolytic agents can result in discomfort, transient hearing loss, dizziness, and skin irritation. Overuse should be avoided because this may make impaction worse. Ceruminolytic agents should not be used in ears that may have a perforated tympanic membrane or that have an active infection of the ear canal.[2]

Otitis Externa

Otitis externa (OE), also called swimmer's ear, involves inflammation of the external ear that can vary in severity. It can be caused by infectious agents, irritation (*e.g.*, wearing glasses, hearing aids, or earphones), or allergic reactions. OE is a common disease that affects all age groups.[3] OE is more prevalent in hot and humid conditions, and peak incidence occurs in children aged 7 to 12 years.

Etiology. Predisposing factors include swimming, trauma to the canal caused by cleaning or scratching, cerumen buildup, hearing aid use, and allergies or skin conditions such as eczema and seborrhea. Bacterial infections are the cause of 91% of acute OE cases. The most common bacterial pathogens are gram-negative rods (*Pseudomonas aeruginosa*, *Proteus* species) and fungi (*Aspergillus*) that grow in the presence of excess moisture.[3]

Clinical Manifestations and Treatment. Otitis externa commonly occurs in the summer and is manifested by itching, redness, tenderness, discharge, impaired hearing, and narrowing of the ear canal because of swelling. Inflammation of the pinna or canal makes movement of the ear painful. There may be watery or purulent drainage and intermittent hearing loss.[4]

Treatment usually includes the use of eardrops containing an appropriate antimicrobial or antifungal agent. For bacterial infections, a corticosteroid solution may be combined with an antimicrobial to reduce inflammation. Systemic oral agents are not indicated. Over-the-counter treatment with white vinegar may be used for mild cases only if the tympanic membrane is not perforated. Protection of the ear from additional moisture (*i.e.*, use of earplugs) and avoidance of trauma from scratching with cotton-tipped applicators and other devices are important. Preventing recurrences is important, particularly in people who swim frequently.[4]

Disorders of the Middle Ear and Eustachian Tube

The middle ear is an air-filled space inside the temporal bone, which contains three tiny bones called *ossicles*. These bones are the *malleus (hammer)*, *incus*, *(anvil)*, and *stapes (stirrup)*[1] (Fig. 20.1). The middle ear begins as a thin, translucent membrane called the *tympanic membrane*. The tympanic membrane appears pearly gray to light pink with peripheral blood vessels. The tympanic membrane can be divided into the *pars flaccida* and the *pars tensa*. The pars flaccida is the smaller, upper, triangular section above the *short process of malleus*, and the pars tensa consists of the remaining portion of the tympanic membrane. The tympanic membrane is attached to the temporal bone by a fibrous border called the *annulus*. The malleus holds the tympanic membrane slightly inward, which causes the oval membrane to be slightly concave. The concave shape creates a "cone of light" when light is reflected on the tympanic membrane.

The translucency of the membrane allows visualization of the middle ear, which includes the malleus: The *umbo* is the tip of the malleus that meets the membrane, the *manubrium (handle of malleus)* is attached to the membrane, and the short process of the malleus is another landmark of the tympanic membrane.[1] The middle ear is connected to the nasopharynx by the *eustachian tube*. The walls of the eustachian tube are typically collapsed and valvelike, opening only during swallowing, chewing, and yawning or when expansion is forced.[1] The eustachian tube has three main functions: to protect the middle ear from sound and pressure, to drain secretions from the middle ear, and to equalize pressure on both sides of the tympanic membrane.[1]

The malleus (hammer), incus, (anvil), and stapes (stirrup) are connected by synovial joints and are covered with the epithelial lining of the cavity.[1] The ossicles move when sound waves reach the tympanic membrane, transmitting sound from the external ear canal to the inner ear.[1] The head of the malleus communicates with the incus, which communicates with the stapes. The stapes attaches to the *oval window*, which vibrates from sound, separates the inner and middle ear, and is in contact with the inner ear fluid. Lying inferior to the oval window, the *round window* communicates with the inner ear and acts as a valve by bulging outward when fluid pressure increases in the inner ear.[1]

KEY POINTS

DISORDERS OF THE MIDDLE EAR

- The middle ear is a small, air-filled compartment in the temporal bone. It is separated from the outer ear by the tympanic membrane; communication between the nasopharynx and the middle ear occurs through the eustachian tube; and tiny bony ossicles that span the middle ear transmit sound to the sensory receptors in the inner ear.
- Otitis media (OM) refers to inflammation of the middle ear. It can represent an acute otitis media (AOM), which has an abrupt onset and is usually related to bacterial infection, or otitis media with effusion (OME), which is associated with fluid in the middle ear without the manifestations of infection and does not usually require treatment with antimicrobial agents.

Eustachian Tube Dysfunction

The eustachian tube extends from the middle ear to the nasopharynx and allows air or secretions to enter or leave the middle ear cavity (Fig. 20.1). The eustachian tube serves three basic functions:

1. Equalization of pressure on both sides of the tympanic membrane
2. Protection of the middle ear from excessively loud sound, abrupt changes in pressure, and nasopharyngeal secretions
3. Drainage of middle ear secretions into the nasopharynx

The nasopharyngeal entrance to the eustachian tube, which usually is closed, is opened by the action of the trigeminal (CN V)-innervated *tensor veli palatini muscle*. Opening of the eustachian tube, which normally occurs with swallowing and yawning reflexes, allows for equalization of pressure in the middle ear with that of the atmosphere. This equalization of pressure ensures that sound transmission is not reduced and rupture does not result from sudden changes in external pressure, as occurs during plane travel.[5]

The eustachian tube is lined with a mucous membrane that continues into the pharynx. Infections from the nasopharynx can travel to the middle ear, causing acute otitis media (AOM) (discussed later in this chapter). Toward the nasopharynx, the eustachian tube is lined by columnar epithelium with mucus-secreting cells. Expansion of mucus-secreting cells is thought to contribute to the mucoid secretions that develop during certain types of OM.[5]

Abnormalities in eustachian tube function are important factors in the development of middle ear infections. There are two important types of eustachian tube dysfunction: abnormal patency and obstruction. The *abnormally patent tube* does not close or does not close completely. In infants and children with an abnormally patent tube, air and secretions often are pushed into the eustachian tube during crying and nose blowing. The eustachian tubes of children are short and positioned nearly horizontal, allowing air and secretions from the pharynx to move to the middle ear.[5]

Obstruction of the eustachian tube can be functional or mechanical. *Functional obstruction* results from the persistent collapse of the eustachian tube because of a lack of tubal stiffness or poor function of the tensor veli palatini muscle that controls the opening of the eustachian tube. It is common in young children because the amount and rigidity of the cartilage supporting the eustachian tube are less than in older children and adults. Changes in the craniofacial base also reduce the efficiency of the tensor muscle. In addition, craniofacial disorders, such as a cleft palate, alter the attachment of the tensor muscle, producing functional obstruction of the eustachian tube.

Mechanical obstruction results from internal obstruction or external compression of the eustachian tube. Ethnic differences in the structure of the palate may increase the likelihood of obstruction. The most common internal obstruction is caused by swelling and secretions resulting from allergy and viral respiratory infections. External compression by prominent or enlarged adenoidal tissue surrounding the opening of the eustachian tube may make drainage less effective. Tumors also may obstruct drainage. With obstruction, air in the middle ear is absorbed, causing a negative pressure and the passage of watery capillary fluid into the middle ear.

Barotrauma

Barotrauma is ear pain or damage resulting from rapid changes in air pressure or imbalances between the middle ear and the atmosphere. It occurs most often when there is a sudden change in atmospheric pressure, such as during rapid airplane or sea-level descent, when the air must move through the eustachian tube to equalize pressure in the middle ear. If the eustachian tube is completely or even partially blocked by infection, swelling, or inflammation from a common cold or allergy, air is prevented from moving in and out of the middle ear. Pain, hearing loss, bruising to the tympanic membrane, or even rupture of the tympanic membrane (Fig. 20.3) can result from the differing pressures.[6]

Barotrauma most often occurs in people who travel while suffering from an upper respiratory tract infection.

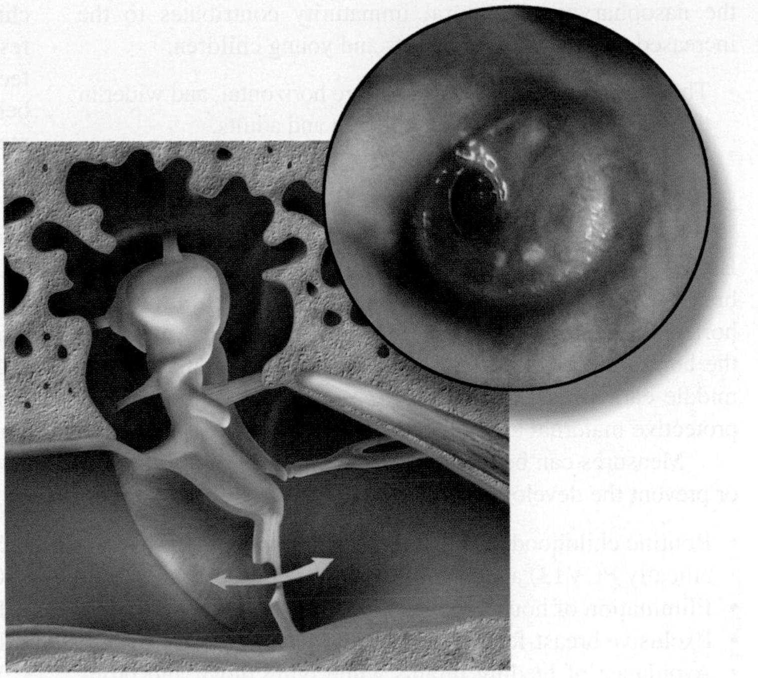

Figure 20.3 • Perforation of the tympanic membrane. (From Anatomical Chart Company, Middle Ear Conditions chart.)

Decongestants, such as nose drops or nasal sprays, may be used 30 to 60 minutes prior to ascent or descent to reduce congestion and open the eustachian tubes.[6] Acute negative middle ear pressure that persists on the ground is treated with decongestants and attempts at autoinflation with yawning, swallowing, or chewing gum. More severe hearing loss or discomfort may require that the person consult an otolaryngologist.

Barotrauma often results in the perforation of the tympanic membrane if exposed to concussive forces such as a direct blow or an explosion (Fig. 20.3). Traumatic perforations must be assessed for signs of injury to other structures on the middle or inner ear. Symptoms such as hearing loss, vertigo, nystagmus, or possible leakage of cerebrospinal fluid warrant urgent consultation by an otolaryngologist.

Otitis Media

Otitis media (OM) refers to inflammation of the middle ear without reference to etiology or pathogenesis. The term OM is broad and includes conditions caused by bacterial and viral processes.

Acute otitis media (AOM) is an acute bacterial or viral infection in the middle ear[6] (Fig. 20.4). It usually has an abrupt onset of signs and symptoms related to middle ear inflammation, such as otalgia and fever, and an accompanying upper respiratory infection. *Otitis media with effusion* (OME), or serous otitis media, refers to the presence of fluid in the middle ear without signs and symptoms of acute ear infection. OME can develop spontaneously because of poor eustachian tube function, accompany a viral upper respiratory tract infection, or occur as a prelude or a sequela to AOM.[6] Because OME does not require treatment with antimicrobial agents, it is important to differentiate OME from AOM to avoid unnecessary use of antimicrobial agents.

Risk Factors. Although AOM may occur in any age group, it is most frequently diagnosed in children between the ages of 3 months and 3 years. Smoking in the household is a significant risk factor for AOM. Other risk factors include prematurity, daycare attendance, having an unimmunized status, bottle-feeding, feeding in the supine position, being overweight or obese, a family history of OM, being of the male gender, and sharing a bedroom. AOM is more frequent in children with craniofacial anomalies or congenital syndromes associated with craniofacial anomalies.[6]

The most important factor that contributes to AOM is believed to be a dysfunction of the eustachian tube that allows reflux of fluid and bacteria into the middle ear space from

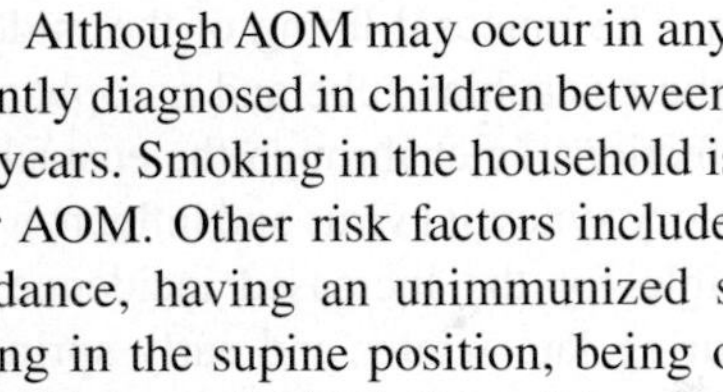

Figure 20.4 • Acute otitis media of the right ear. (From Jensen S. (2015). *Nursing health assessment: A best practice approach* (2nd ed., p. 370). Philadelphia, PA: Lippincott Williams & Wilkins.)

the nasopharynx. Structural immaturity contributes to the increased risk of AOM in infants and young children:

- The eustachian tube is shorter, more horizontal, and wider in this age group than in older children and adults.
- Infection can spread more easily through the eustachian canal of infants who spend most of their day in the supine position.

Bottle-fed infants have a higher incidence of AOM than breast-fed infants, probably because they are held in a more horizontal position during feeding, and swallowing while in the horizontal position facilitates the reflux of milk into the middle ear.[7] Breast-feeding also provides for the transfer of protective maternal antibodies to the infant.

Measures can be taken to reduce the risk of contracting, or prevent the development of, AOM[6,7]:

- Routine childhood vaccinations against pneumococci (specifically PCV13) and an annual influenza vaccine
- Elimination of household smoking
- Exclusive breast-feeding until at least 6 months of age
- Avoidance of feeding infants while lying down and propping bottles
- Use of xylitol (liquid or chewing gum)
- Selecting daycare facilities with a small staff-to-child ratio

Etiology. The etiology of AOM may be of either bacterial or viral origin. The mucosal lining of the middle ear is continuous with the eustachian tube and nasopharynx, and most middle ear infections enter through the eustachian tube (Fig. 20.1). Respiratory syncytial virus and influenza are the viruses most responsible for the increased incidence rate of AOM in children during late winter and early spring. Respiratory viruses may infect the middle ear mucosa, either alone or in combination with bacteria. Although a virus is usually the initial causative agent in the development of AOM, bacteria may proliferate in the fluid of the middle ear. Most cases of AOM follow an uncomplicated upper respiratory tract infection that has been present for several days. *Streptococcus pneumoniae*, *Haemophilus influenza*, *Moraxella catarrhalis*, and *Streptococcus pyogenes* (group A streptococci) are the most common infecting bacterial organisms responsible for the development of AOM.

Clinical Manifestations. AOM is characterized by the following key criteria:

- Acute onset of otalgia (or pulling of the ears in an infant) that may interfere with sleep and/or activity
- Fever (>39°C)
- Irritability
- Otorrhea
- Hearing loss
- Evidence of middle ear inflammation
- Middle ear effusion (decreases mobility of the tympanic membrane)

Children older than 3 years of age may have rhinorrhea, or runny nose, vomiting, and diarrhea. In contrast, younger children often have nonspecific signs and symptoms that manifest as ear tugging, irritability, nighttime awakening, and poor feeding. Ear pain usually increases as the effusion accumulates behind the tympanic membrane. Perforation of the tympanic membrane may occur acutely, allowing purulent material from the eustachian tube to drain into the external auditory canal. This may prevent spread of the infection into the temporal bone or intracranial cavity. Healing of the tympanic membrane usually follows resolution of the middle ear infection.

As mentioned earlier in this chapter, OME is a condition in which the tympanic membrane is intact and there is an accumulation of fluid in the middle ear without signs or symptoms of infection. The duration of the effusion may range from less than 3 weeks to more than 3 months. Although often asymptomatic and afebrile, clinical findings of OME include[7]:

- Complaint of intermittent ear pain
- Sensation of fullness in the ear
- Complaint of hearing loss
- Dizziness
- Decreased tympanic membrane mobility
- Visible air–fluid level with or without bubble

Many cases of OME resolve spontaneously, but some experience recurrent OME. Persistent middle ear fluid from OME results in decreased motility of the tympanic membrane and serves as a barrier to sound conduction.

Diagnosis. Distinguishing between AOM and OME is often straightforward, but each condition may evolve into the other without any clearly differentiating physical findings. Because of the increasing antimicrobial resistance, distinguishing between AOM and OME has become increasingly important.

Both AOM without otorrhea (drainage from the ear) and OME are accompanied by otoscopic signs of MME, namely, the presence of at least two or three abnormalities:

- White- or yellow-appearing tympanic membrane (may be seen in either AOM or OME)
- Tympanic membrane that appears amber (usually seen in OME)
- Opacification of tympanic membrane other than scarring (may be seen in either)
- Decreased or absent motility of tympanic membrane (may be seen in either)

With OME, the tympanic membrane is often cloudy with distinct impairment of mobility, and an air–fluid level or bubble may be visible in the middle ear.

A definitive diagnosis of AOM requires the following[7]:

- History of acute onset of signs and symptoms
- The presence of MME confirmed by bulging of tympanic membrane, limited or absent mobility by pneumatic otoscopy, air–fluid level behind tympanic membrane, and or otorrhea
- Signs and symptoms of middle ear inflammation confirmed by erythema of tympanic membrane or onset of pain.

Unless intense, erythema alone is insufficient to support a diagnosis of AOM because erythema without other abnormalities may result from crying or vascular flushing. Pneumatic otoscopy is the most efficient way to make the diagnosis and should be used to either make or confirm the diagnosis. The use of the pneumatic otoscope allows the introduction of air into the ear canal for the purpose of determining tympanic membrane mobility. The movement of the tympanic membrane is decreased in some cases of AOM and absent in chronic middle ear infection. The diagnosis of AOM can also be confirmed using tympanometry. *Tympanometry* is helpful in detecting effusion in the middle ear or high negative middle ear pressure. Portable tympanometers (resembling an otoscope) and desktop instruments are available.

Tympanocentesis (puncture of the tympanic membrane with a needle) may be done to relieve pain from an effusion or to obtain a specimen of middle ear fluid for culture and sensitivity testing. The procedure involves the insertion of a needle through the inferior part of the tympanic membrane. This procedure is rarely attempted and is only useful in a situation involving a toxic or immunocompromised person or in the presence of a resistant infection. If tympanocentesis is warranted, a referral to an otolaryngologist should be made. If the person has undergone surgery for the placement of tympanostomy tubes, also known as pressure equalization tubes (PETs), the collection of ear drainage from the external ear canal can be cultured to determine the causative agent of the infection.

Treatment. The treatment of OM focuses on symptom control and management of the underlying pathologic process. A number of options for pain management are available, including the local application of heat or cold, distraction, and use of weight- and age-appropriate analgesic medications such as acetaminophen, ibuprofen, and naproxen. Myringotomy (incision of the tympanic membrane), performed by an otolaryngologist, can be used for relief of pressure in the person who is in severe pain.

The extensive use of antimicrobial agents contributes to the development of bacterial resistance, and evidence exists for the efficacy and safety of two alternative approaches to routine antibiotic prescription: observation or "watchful waiting" and follow-up. Observation for 48 to 72 hours without antimicrobial agents is an option with uncomplicated AOM. These approaches involve waiting to see if symptoms improve before beginning antibiotic therapy. Factors to consider when deciding whether to defer treatment include the person's age (healthy children 6 months to 2 years), severity of illness, and certainty of the diagnosis. If observation is recommended, it is essential that the person have ready access to communication, follow-up, and a mechanism for obtaining medication if needed. A follow-up visit is recommended if the person has not shown signs of symptom improvement after 48 to 72 hours to confirm or exclude AOM. If the person was initially given antimicrobial agents but shows no sign of improvement, the antimicrobial agent should be changed.

Most cases of OME resolve spontaneously within a 3-week to 3-month period. The management options for this duration include observation, detailed charting to include location (unilateral or bilateral), the description of fluid, and any associated symptoms. Other management options include conducting hearing tests and identifying persons at risk for speech, language, or learning delays. There is no evidence that decongestants, antibiotics, and nasal steroids are of any benefit in the management of OME.[6]

Referral to an otolaryngologist is indicated if the effusion persists for 4 months or longer. Because there is concern over hearing loss and its effect on learning and speech, a hearing evaluation is recommended when OME persists for 3 months or longer or at any time that language delay, learning problems, or a significant hearing loss is suspected.

Children with recurrent OM should be evaluated to rule out any anatomic variations (*e.g.*, enlarged adenoids), allergies, and immunologic abnormalities. Surgical treatment (*e.g.*, tympanostomy tubes, adenoidectomy) may be indicated if the effusion has persisted for 4 months or longer and is accompanied by persistent hearing loss and other manifestations.

Tympanostomy tube insertion is the preferred initial procedure and does not typically include the removal of adenoids unless the child has additional indications, such as postnasal obstruction from enlarged adenoids. The tubes usually are inserted under general anesthesia. The ears of children with tubes must be kept out of water. The adverse effects of tube placement include the following:

- Recurrent otorrhea
- Persistent perforation
- Scarring
- Atrophy of the tympanic membrane
- Cholesteatoma

Adenoidectomy plus myringotomy (without tube insertion) has been effective in older children. Recent research indicates that prompt insertion of tympanostomy tubes for persistent OME in otherwise healthy children who were younger than 3 years of age did not improve developmental outcomes (*e.g.*, literacy, attention, social skills, and academic achievement) as compared with delayed insertion in children in whom effusion continued unremittingly.[6]

Complications of Otitis Media. The complications of OM include hearing loss, adhesive OM, cholesteatoma, mastoiditis, and intracranial complications such as otologic meningitis.

Hearing loss, which is a common complication of OM, usually is conductive and temporary based on the duration of the effusion. Hearing loss that is associated with fluid collection usually resolves when the effusion clears. Permanent hearing loss may occur as the result of damage to the tympanic membrane or other middle ear structures. Cases of sensorineural hearing loss are rare. Children younger than 3 years of age with recurrent OME are at increased risk of impaired language development. Persistent and episodic conductive hearing loss in children may impair their cognitive, linguistic, and emotional development.[6]

Cholesteatoma is usually the result of a chronic ear infection and involves the formation of an epidermal cyst of the middle ear or mastoid.[6] The cyst, which can be small (approximately 2 mm in diameter) or large (approximately 4 cm in diameter), consists of desquamated debris from the keratinizing, squamous epithelial lining of the middle ear.[7] Surrounding structures can be destroyed by the growth of the cholesteatoma. The cysts can be congenital, primary acquired, or secondary acquired. Research indicates the formation may be related to the inflammatory process, TM perforation, or the collection of desquamated tissue in the middle ear.[7] Cholesteatomas commonly appear whitish or pearllike in color. Symptoms commonly include painless drainage from the ear and hearing loss. Treatment involves surgery to remove the cholesteatomatous material.

Mastoiditis is a suppurative infection of the mastoid cells.[7] Mastoiditis can develop as the result of chronic middle ear infection. The mucoperiosteal lining of the mastoid air cells becomes inflamed, resulting in swelling and obstruction from mastoid drainage.[6] Treatment of AOM with antimicrobial medication does not eliminate the occurrence of mastoiditis. The incidence of mastoiditis isn't known, but its prevalence has decreased since the introduction of modern antibiotics.[7] Although uncommon, mastoiditis can be life threatening. It is most common during childhood, specifically between the ages of 6 and 13 months.[7] Clinical manifestations include[6]:

- Chronic or concurrent AOM
- Fever
- Otalgia
- Persistent OM
- Swelling in the supra-auricular or postauricular area

Mastoiditis, suspected or confirmed, warrants immediate referral to the closest surgical hospital.

Intracranial complications are uncommon since the advent of antimicrobial therapy. Although rare, these complications can develop when the infection spreads through vascular channels or by direct extension. These complications are seen more often with chronic suppurative OM and mastoiditis. They include otogenic meningitis, brain abscess, lateral sinus thrombophlebitis or thrombosis, labyrinthitis, and facial nerve paralysis. Any child who develops persistent headache, tinnitus, stiff neck, or visual or other neurologic symptoms should be investigated for possible intracranial complications.

Otosclerosis

Otosclerosis is a disease of the bone of the otic capsule that causes the formation of new spongy bone around the stapes and oval window.[6] The newly formed bone causes the stapes to become fixed or immobile, resulting in conductive hearing loss. In most cases, the condition is hereditary and follows an autosomal dominant pattern of inheritance. It most commonly affects Caucasian females. Although otosclerosis may begin at any time in life, it typically appears during adolescence and progresses during early adulthood. Pregnancy seems to accelerate the disease. Generally, both ears are affected, but the rate of hearing loss is not symmetric.[1]

During active bone resorption, the bone structure appears spongy and softer than normal (*i.e.*, osteospongiosis). The resorbed bone is replaced by an overgrowth of new, hard, sclerotic bone. The process is slowly progressive, involving more areas of the temporal bone, especially in front of and behind the stapes footplate. As the disease invades the footplate, the pathologic bone increasingly restricts the stapes, reducing the transmission of sound. Pressure of otosclerotic bone on middle ear structures or the vestibulocochlear nerve (CN VIII) may contribute to the development of tinnitus, sensorineural hearing loss, and vertigo.[6]

The symptoms of otosclerosis involve an insidious hearing loss. Initially, the affected person is unable to hear a whisper or someone speaking at a distance. In the earliest stages, the bone conduction by which the person's own voice is heard remains relatively unaffected. At this point, the person's own voice sounds unusually loud, and the sound of chewing becomes intensified. Because bone conduction is maintained, persons with otosclerosis may be able to use the telephone but have difficulty in carrying on face-to-face conversations. Many are able to hear better in a noisy environment, probably because the masking effect of background noise causes other persons to speak louder.[1]

The treatment of otosclerosis can be medical or surgical. A hearing aid may allow a person with conductive hearing loss to hear and interact with others. To slow bone resorption and overgrowth, sodium fluoride may be recommended. Surgical treatment involves a stapedectomy and reconstruction of the middle ear (stapedotomy). During a stapedectomy, the diseased stapes is removed using a microsurgical technique. A prosthesis is inserted, with one end connecting to the incus and the other inserted into the oval window. During a stapedotomy, a small hole is created in the footplate of the stapes and a wire or ribbon is inserted. Surgical intervention is usually successful at restoring hearing.[6]

Disorders of the Inner Ear

The inner ear is composed of intricate channels that facilitate hearing and position sense. Structurally, it consists of an outer bony labyrinth located in the otic capsule of the petrous part of the temporal bone and an inner membranous labyrinth. The membranous labyrinth lies in the bony labyrinth and consists of a complex system of sacs and ducts (*i.e.*, semicircular

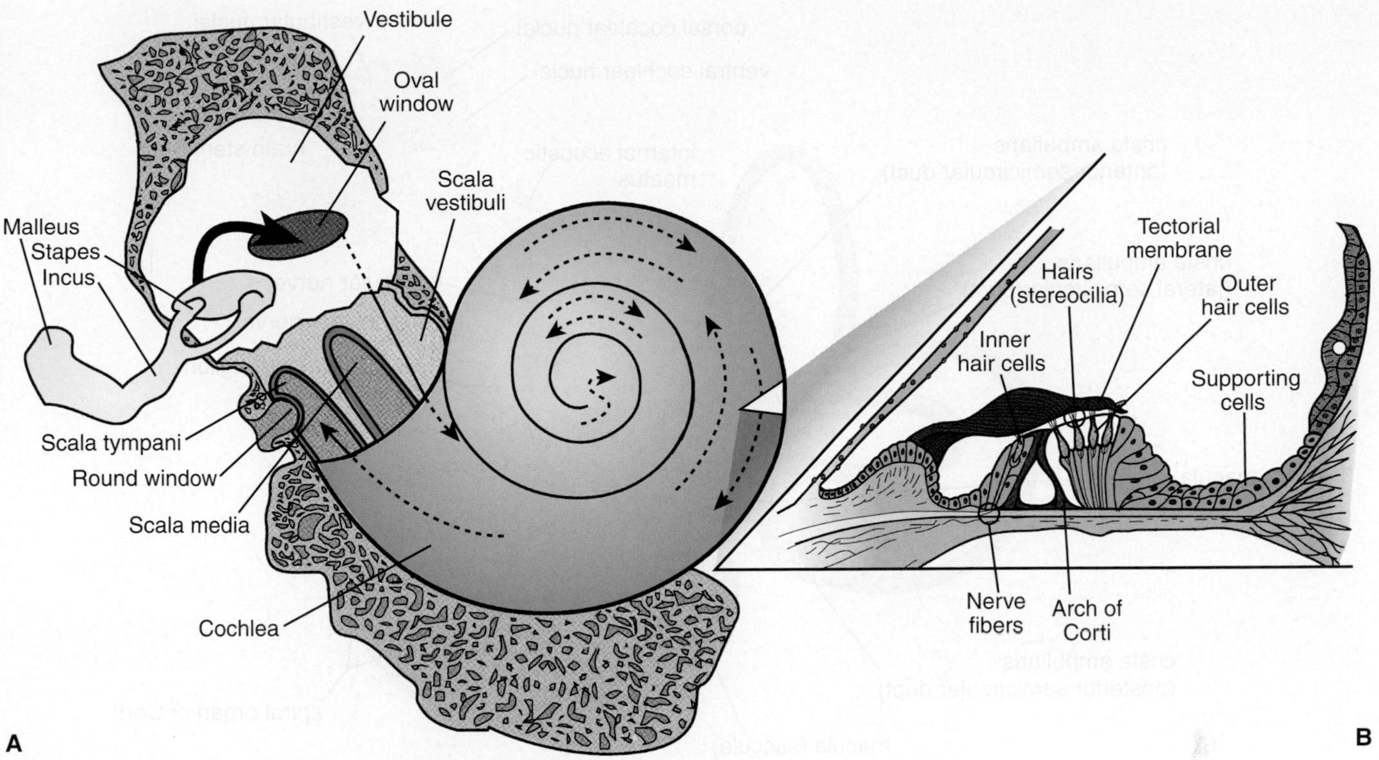

Figure 20.5 • The cochlea and the organ of Corti. **A.** The pea-sized, snail shaped cochlea is a coiled system and the the hearing portion of the inner ear. **B.** An enlargement of a cross-section of the organ of Corti, showing the relationships among the hair cells and the membranes. Hair cells in the organ of Corti transduce fluid movement into neural signals. (From Rhoades, R. A., Bell, D. A. (2018). *Medical physiology* (5th ed., Figure 4.18, p. 72). Philadelphia, PA: Wolters Kluwer).

ducts). The bony labyrinth, which occupies a space with a diameter less than 1.5 cm, is a series of cavities (the cochlea, vestibule, and semicircular canals)[8] (Fig. 20.5). The receptors for hearing are contained in the cochlea, and those for head position sense are contained in the semicircular ducts, the utricle, and the saccule. The vestibule is the central egg-shaped cavity of the bony labyrinth that lies posterior to the cochlea and anterior to the semicircular canals. It contains the utricle and saccule and parts of the balancing apparatus (vestibular labyrinth). The vestibule features the oval window on its lateral wall, occupied by the base of the stapes.

The cochlea is the shell-shaped part of the bony labyrinth that contains the inner membranous cochlear duct, the part of the inner ear concerned with hearing. The spiral canal of the cochlea, which is shaped like a snail shell, begins at the vestibule and winds around a central core of spongy bone called the *modiolus*. The modiolus contains canals for blood vessels and for distribution of the cochlear nerve. The cochlea consists of three tubes coiled side by side:

1. The *scala vestibuli*
2. The *scala media*
3. The *scala tympani*

The vestibular membrane, also known as *Reissner membrane*, separates the scala vestibuli and scala media from each other. The basilar membrane separates the scala tympani from the scala media. On the surface of the basilar membrane lies the spiral organ of Corti, which contains a series of electromechanically sensitive cells, the *hair cells*. They are the receptive organs that generate nerve impulses in response to sound vibrations.

The endolymph and perilymph are the two types of fluids in the inner ear. The scala vestibuli and scala tympani communicate directly with the subarachnoid space around the brain, so the perilymph is similar to cerebrospinal fluid.[8] The endolymph that fills the scala media is an entirely different fluid; it is secreted by the stria vascularis on the outer wall of the scala media (Fig. 20.6). The perilymph that fills the scala vestibuli and scala tympani has a high sodium (Na^+) concentration, whereas the endolymph that fills the scala media has a high potassium (K^+) content. This is significant because there is a direct current resting membrane potential of about +80 mV that exists between the endolymph and perilymph, with positivity inside the scala media and negativity outside the scala media. This difference in polarity causes a current, called the *endolymphatic potential*, and is generated

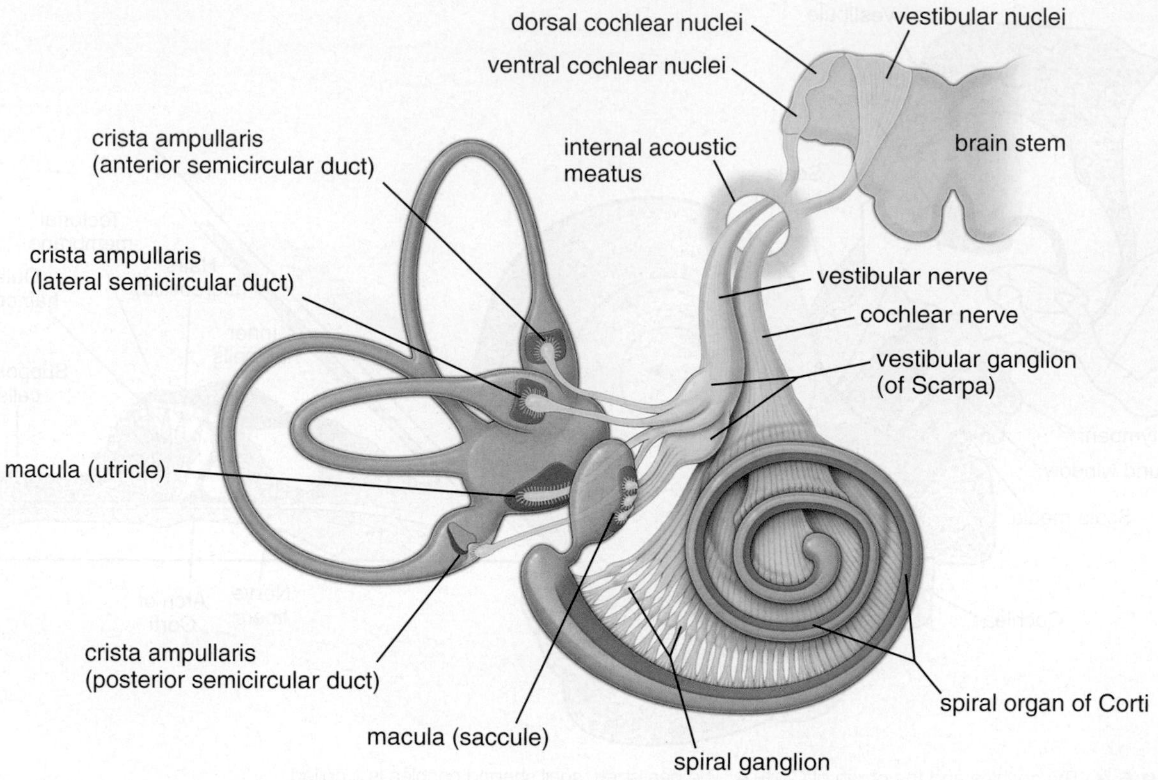

Figure 20.6 • Spiral organ of Corti has been removed from the cochlear duct and greatly enlarged to show the inner and outer hair cells, the basilar membrane, and the cochlear nerve fibers. (From Pawlina W., Ross M. H. (2016). *Histology: A text and atlas with correlated cell and molecular biology* (7th ed., Figure 25.24, p. 954). Philadelphia, PA: Wolters Kluwer.)

by a continual exchange of K^+ ions into the scala media by Na^+/K^+ adenosine triphosphatase (ATPase) pumps in the stria vascularis. This current is believed to sensitize the hair cells of the organ of Corti, increasing their ability to respond to the slightest sound.

Unlike light, which can be transmitted through a vacuum (*e.g.*, outer space), sound is a pressure disturbance that originates from a vibrating object and then spreads via the molecules of an elastic medium. Sound waves, which are delivered by the stapes footplate to the perilymph, travel throughout the fluid of the inner ear, including up the scala vestibuli, to the apex of the cochlea (Fig. 20.6). The vestibular membrane is thin, so the sound vibrations from the scala vestibuli are readily transmitted into the scala media. Therefore, as far as sound conduction is concerned, the scala media and scala vestibuli function as a single chamber.

As the pressure wave descends through the endolymph of the scala media, it sets the entire basilar membrane vibrating. The basilar membrane, which becomes progressively larger from its base to its distal apex, resonates at higher frequencies near the base and at lower frequencies toward its apex as the fluid pressure wave travels up the cochlear spiral. This provides the major basis for recognition of sound, known as pitch.

On top of the basilar membrane and extending along its entire length is an elaborate arrangement of columnar epithelium called the *spiral organ of Corti* (Fig. 20.5). Continuous rows of hair cells separated into inner and outer rows can be found in the columnar arrangement of the spiral organ. The cells have hairlike cilia that protrude through openings and support the reticular membrane into the endolymph of the cochlear duct. A gelatinous mass, the tectorial membrane, extends from the medial side of the duct to enclose the cilia of the outer hair cells. The hair cells in the organ of Corti are programmed to respond to distortion of the cochlear duct induced by compression waves moving through the perilymph, which move up and down in the surrounding scala vestibuli and scala tympani. If enough hair cells are destroyed in a particular segment of the cochlea, hearing loss of particular tones can occur.

Neural Pathways

Information flows from the hair cells in the organ of Corti to neurons that have their cell bodies in the cochlear ganglion and follows a spiral course in the bony modiolus of the cochlear spiral. Afferent fibers from the spiral ganglion (*i.e.*, vestibulocochlear or auditory nerve [CN VIII]) travel to the cochlear nuclei in the caudal pons. Consequently, impulses from either ear are transmitted through the auditory pathways to both sides of the brain stem.

From the inferior colliculus (located in the midbrain), the auditory pathway passes to the medial geniculate nucleus of the thalamus, where all the fibers synapse. From the medial geniculate nuclei, the auditory tract spreads through the auditory radiation to the primary auditory cortex (area 41), located mainly in the superior temporal gyrus and insula. This area and its corresponding higher-order thalamic nuclei are required for high-acuity loudness discrimination and precise discrimination of pitch. The auditory association cortex (areas 42 and 22) borders the primary cortex on the superior temporal gyrus. This area and its associated higher-order thalamic nuclei are necessary for auditory gnosis, or the meaningfulness of sound, to occur. Experience and the precise analysis of momentary auditory information are integrated during this process.

Tinnitus

Tinnitus (from the Latin word *tinniere*, meaning "to ring") is the perception of abnormal ear or head noises that are not produced by an external stimulus.[8] Although it often is described as "ringing of the ears," tinnitus may also assume a hissing, roaring, buzzing, or humming sound. Tinnitus may be constant or intermittent and unilateral or bilateral. Tinnitus affects 10% to 15% of the population; however, it is primarily associated with the elderly or those who work in loud areas.[8]

For clinical purposes, tinnitus is subdivided into objective and subjective tinnitus.[8] *Objective tinnitus* refers to those rare cases in which the sound is detected or potentially detectable by another observer. Typical causes of objective tinnitus include vascular abnormalities or neuromuscular disorders. In some vascular disorders, for example, sounds generated by turbulent blood flow (*e.g.*, arterial bruits or venous hums) are conducted to the auditory system. Vascular disorders typically produce a pulsatile form of tinnitus.

Subjective tinnitus refers to noise perception when there is no noise stimulation of the cochlea. A number of causes and conditions have been associated with subjective tinnitus. Intermittent periods of mild, high-pitched tinnitus lasting for several minutes are common in people who have normal hearing.

Etiology. Impacted cerumen is a benign cause of tinnitus, which resolves after the earwax is removed. Conditions associated with more persistent tinnitus include noise-induced hearing loss, presbycusis (sensorineural hearing loss that occurs with aging), hypertension, atherosclerosis, head injury, and cochlear or labyrinthine infection or inflammation.

The physiologic cause of subjective tinnitus is largely unknown. It is likely due to several mechanisms, including abnormal firing of auditory receptors, cochlear dysfunction, auditory nerve damage, or alterations in processing of the signal.

Diagnosis and Treatment. Because tinnitus is a symptom, the diagnosis relies heavily on the person's ability to describe the symptoms that have been impacting the person's hearing and other aspects of life. A history of medication or stimulant use and dietary factors that may cause tinnitus should be obtained. Tinnitus often accompanies hearing disorders, and tests of auditory function are usually done. Causes of objective tinnitus, such as serious vascular abnormalities, should be ruled out.

Treatment measures include elimination of drugs or other substances that are suspected of causing tinnitus, such as caffeine, some cheeses, red wine, and foods containing monosodium glutamate (MSG). The use of an externally produced sound (*i.e.*, noise generators or tinnitus-masking devices) may be used to mask or inhibit the tinnitus. Medications (including antihistamines, anticonvulsant drugs, calcium channel blockers, benzodiazepines, and antidepressants) have been used for tinnitus alleviation, but most are not effective, and many produce undesirable side effects. For persistent tinnitus, psychological interventions may be needed to help the person deal with the stress and distraction associated with the condition. Tinnitus retraining therapy, which includes directive counseling and extended use of low-noise generators to facilitate auditory adaptation to the tinnitus, has met with considerable success. Surgical intervention (*i.e.*, cochlear nerve section, vascular decompression) is a last resort for people in whom all other interventions have failed and in whom the disorder is disabling.

Disorders of the Central Auditory Pathways

The auditory pathways in the brain involve communication between the two sides of the brain at many levels. As a result, strokes, tumors, abscesses, and other focal abnormalities seldom produce more than a mild reduction in auditory acuity on the side opposite the lesion. For intelligibility of auditory language, lateral dominance becomes important. On the dominant side, usually the left side, the more medial and dorsal portion of the auditory association cortex is of crucial importance. This area is called the *Wernicke area.* People with damage to this area of the brain can speak intelligibly and read normally but are unable to understand the meaning of major aspects of audible speech. This condition is called auditory receptive aphasia.

Tumors or other irritative foci that affect the way sounds are perceived in the primary auditory cortex can produce roaring or clicking sounds, which can manifest as auditory hallucinations. Focal seizures that originate in or near the auditory cortex often are immediately preceded by a prodrome (*i.e.*, an aura) and then the perception of ringing or other sounds. Damage to the auditory association cortex, especially if bilateral, results in an inability to recognize or remember sounds (*i.e.*, auditory agnosia). If the damage is in the dominant hemisphere, speech recognition can be affected (*i.e.*, sensory or receptive aphasia).

Hearing Loss

Hearing is a specialized sense that provides the ability to perceive vibration of sound waves. Functions of the ear include receiving sound waves, distinguishing their frequency, translating this information into nerve impulses, and transmitting these impulses to the central nervous system (CNS). The compression waves that produce sound have frequency and intensity. *Frequency* indicates the number of waves per unit time (reported in cycles per second [cps] or hertz [Hz]). The human ear is most sensitive to waves in the frequency range of 1000 to 3000 Hz. Most people cannot hear compression waves that have a frequency higher than 20,000 Hz. Waves of higher frequency are called *ultrasonic waves*, meaning that they are above the audible range. In the audible frequency range, the subjective experience correlated with sonic frequency is the pitch of a sound. Waves below 20 to 30 Hz are experienced as a rattle or drumbeat rather than a tone.

Wave intensity is represented by amplitude or units of sound pressure. Generally, the intensity (in power units or ergs per square centimeter) of a sound is expressed as the ratio of intensities between the sound and a reference value. A 10-fold increase in sound pressure is called a *bel*, after Alexander Graham Bell. Because this representation is too crude to be of use, the decibel (dB), or 1/10 of a bel, is used.

Nearly 36 million Americans (17%) have hearing loss. Hearing loss in general is classified as:

- Mild (the most quiet sounds heard by people with their better ear are 26 to 40 dB)
- Moderate (the most quiet sounds heard by people with their better ear are 41 to 55 dB)
- Moderately severe (the most quiet sounds heard by people with their better ear are 56 to 70 dB)
- Severe (the most quiet sounds heard by people with their better ear are 71 to 90 dB)
- Profound (the most quiet sounds heard by people with their better ear are 91 dB or greater in adults and 70 dB or greater in children)[8]

The term "hard of hearing" is sometimes used for people who have difficulty hearing and is defined as hearing loss greater than 20 to 25 dB in adults and greater than 15 dB in children.

There are many causes of hearing loss or deafness. Age and suddenness of onset provide important clues as to the cause of hearing loss. Most hearing loss fits into the categories of conductive, sensorineural, or mixed deficiencies.[8] Hearing loss may be hereditary or acquired, sudden or progressive, unilateral or bilateral, partial or complete, and reversible or irreversible. Chart 20.1 summarizes common causes of conductive and sensorineural hearing loss.

KEY POINTS

HEARING LOSS

- Hearing is a sensory function that incorporates the sound-transmitting properties of the external ear canal, the eardrum that separates the external and middle ear, the bony ossicles of the middle ear, the sensory receptors of the cochlea in the inner ear, the neural pathways of the vestibulocochlear or auditory nerve, and the primary auditory and auditory association cortices.
- Hearing loss can be caused by conductive disorders; this means that auditory stimuli are not transmitted properly through the structures of the ear to the sensory receptors in the inner ear. Hearing loss can also be caused by sensorineural disorders that affect the inner ear, auditory nerve, or auditory pathways. Hearing loss can also be a combination of conductive and sensorineural disorders (mixed hearing loss).

CHART 20.1 COMMON CAUSES OF CONDUCTIVE AND SENSORINEURAL HEARING LOSS

Conductive Hearing Loss
- External ear conditions
  - Impacted earwax or foreign body
  - Otitis externa
- Middle ear conditions
  - Trauma
  - Otitis media (acute and with effusion)
  - Otosclerosis
  - Tumors

Sensorineural Hearing Loss
- Trauma
  - Head injury
  - Noise
- CNS infections (*e.g.*, meningitis)
- Degenerative conditions
  - Presbycusis
- Vascular
  - Atherosclerosis
  - Sudden deafness
- Ototoxic drugs (*e.g.*, aminoglycosides, salicylates, loop diuretics)
- Tumors
  - Vestibular schwannoma (acoustic neuroma)
  - Meningioma
  - Metastatic tumors
- Idiopathic
  - Ménière disease

Mixed Conductive and Sensorineural Hearing Loss
- Middle ear conditions
  - Barotrauma
  - Cholesteatoma
  - Otosclerosis
- Temporal bone fracture

Conductive Hearing Loss

Conductive hearing loss occurs when auditory stimuli are not adequately transmitted through the auditory canal, tympanic membrane, middle ear, or ossicle chain to the inner ear.[9] Temporary hearing loss can occur as the result of impacted cerumen in the outer ear or fluid in the middle ear. Foreign bodies, including pieces of cotton and insects, may impair hearing. More permanent causes of hearing loss are thickening or damage of the tympanic membrane or involvement of the bony structures (ossicles and oval window) of the middle ear because of otosclerosis or Paget disease.

Sensorineural Hearing Loss

Sensorineural, or perceptive, hearing loss occurs with disorders that affect the inner ear, auditory nerve, or auditory pathways of the brain.[9] With this type of deafness, sound waves are conducted to the inner ear, but abnormalities of the cochlear apparatus or auditory nerve decrease or distort the transfer of information to the brain. Tinnitus often accompanies cochlear nerve irritation. Abnormal function resulting from damage or malformation of the central auditory pathways and circuitry is included in this category.

Etiology. Sensorineural hearing loss is usually irreversible and occurs most commonly in the higher frequencies. Sensorineural hearing loss may have a genetic cause or may result from intrauterine infections such as maternal rubella or developmental malformations of the inner ear. Genetic hearing loss may result from mutation in a single gene (monogenetic) or from a combination of mutations in different genes and environmental factors (multifactorial). Hearing loss may begin before development of speech (prelingual) or after speech development (postlingual). Most prelingual forms are present at birth. Hereditary forms of hearing loss also can be classified as being part of a syndrome in which other abnormalities are present or, as nonsyndromic, in which deafness is the only abnormality.

Sensorineural hearing loss also can result from trauma to the inner ear, tumors that encroach on the inner ear or sensory neurons, vascular disorders with hemorrhage, or thrombosis of vessels that supply the inner ear. Other causes of sensorineural deafness are infections and drugs. Sudden sensorineural hearing loss represents an abrupt loss of hearing that occurs instantaneously or on awakening. It most commonly is caused by viral infections, circulatory disorders, or rupture of the labyrinth membrane that can occur during tympanotomy.

Environmentally induced deafness can occur through direct exposure to an excessively intense sound, as in the workplace or at a concert. This is a particular problem in older adults who were working in noisy environments before the mid-1960s, when there were no laws mandating the use of devices for protective hearing. Sustained or repeated exposure to noise pollution at sound intensities greater than 100 to 120 dB can cause corresponding mechanical damage to the organ of Corti. If the damage is severe, permanent sensorineural deafness to the corresponding sound frequencies occurs. Wearing earplugs or ear protection is important under many industrial conditions and for musicians and music listeners exposed to high sound amplification.

A number of infections can cause hearing loss. Deafness or some degree of hearing impairment is the most common serious complication of bacterial meningitis in infants and children. The mechanism causing hearing impairment seems to be a suppurative labyrinthitis or neuritis resulting in the loss of hair cells and damage to the auditory nerve. Untreated suppurative OM also can extend into the inner ear and cause sensorineural hearing loss through the same mechanisms.

Among the neoplasms that impair hearing are *acoustic neuromas*, which are benign Schwann cell tumors affecting CN VIII. These tumors usually are unilateral and cause hearing loss by compressing the cochlear nerve or interfering with blood supply to the nerve and cochlea. Other neoplasms that can affect hearing include meningiomas and metastatic brain tumors. The temporal bone is a common site of metastases in people with cancer.

Drugs that damage inner ear structures are labeled *ototoxic*. Vestibular symptoms of ototoxicity include light-headedness and dizziness. If toxicity is severe, cochlear symptoms consisting of tinnitus or hearing loss occur. This type of hearing loss is sensorineural; it can occur in one or both ears and may be temporary or permanent. Several classes of drugs have been identified as having ototoxic potential, including aminoglycosides, antimalarials, some chemotherapeutic drugs, loop diuretics (*e.g.*, *furosemide [Lasix]*), and salicylates (*e.g.*, aspirin).[8] The symptoms of drug-induced hearing loss may be transient, as is often the case with salicylates and diuretics, or they may be permanent. The risk of ototoxicity depends on the total dose of the drug and its concentration in the bloodstream. This risk is increased in people with impaired kidney function because they are unable to excrete medications effectively, as well as those who have previously received another potentially ototoxic drug.

Diagnosis and Treatment

Diagnosis. Diagnosis of hearing loss is aided by obtaining a comprehensive history of associated otologic factors such as otalgia, otorrhea, tinnitus, and self-described hearing difficulties. Additionally, a thorough physical examination is needed to assess for otorrhea, impacted cerumen, or injury to the tympanic membrane. Hearing tests including conventional audiometry and high-frequency audiometry are most frequently used to diagnose ototoxicity.[8] A history of occupational and noise exposure is important, as is the use of medications with ototoxic potential. Testing for hearing loss includes a number of methods, including a person's reported ability to hear an observer's voice, use of a tuning fork to test air and bone conduction, audioscopes, and auditory brain stem evoked responses (ABRs).

Tuning forks are used to differentiate conductive and sensorineural hearing loss. A 512-Hz or higher-frequency tuning fork is used because frequencies below this level elicit a vibratory response.[9] The Weber test evaluates conductive hearing loss by lateralization of sound. The test is done by placing the lightly vibrating tuning fork on the forehead or top of the head. In people with conductive losses, the sound is louder on the side with the hearing loss, but in persons with sensorineural loss, it radiates to the side with the better hearing.[9] The Rinne test compares air and bone conduction.[9] The test is done by alternately placing the tuning fork on the mastoid bone and in front of the ear canal. In conductive losses, bone conduction exceeds air conduction. In sensorineural losses, the opposite occurs.[9]

An audioscope is a rechargeable battery–powered, handheld instrument that combines a pure-tone screening audiometer and otoscope into a single unit. It produces pure sounds at 500, 1000, 2000, and 4000 Hz, at loudness levels of 20, 25, and 40 dB. If a person cannot hear pure tones at 1000 to 2000 Hz (usual speech frequencies), referral for a full audiogram is indicated. The audiogram is an important method of analyzing a person's hearing and is generally considered the gold standard for diagnosis of hearing loss. It is done by an audiologist and requires highly specialized sound production and control equipment. Pure tones of controlled intensity are delivered, usually to one ear at a time, and the minimum intensity needed for hearing to be experienced is plotted as a function of frequency.

The ABR is a noninvasive method that permits functional evaluation of certain parts of the central auditory pathways. Electroencephalographic (EEG) electrodes and high-gain amplifiers produce a record of the electrical wave activity elicited during repeated tests of either or both ears. ABR recording involves subjecting the ear to loud clicks and using a computer to pick up nerve impulses as they are processed in the midbrain. With this method, certain early waves that come from discrete portions of the pons and midbrain auditory pathways can be correlated with specific sensorineural abnormalities. Also, magnetic resonance imaging (MRI) and computed tomography (CT) are used to identify tumors in the brain.

Treatment. Hearing loss can have many consequences. Social isolation and depressive disorders are common in hearing-impaired elderly. Safety issues, both in and out of the home, may become significant.

Treatment of hearing loss can range from simple removal of impacted cerumen in the external auditory canal to surgical procedures such as those used to reconstruct the tympanic membrane. For other people, hearing aids and cochlear implants are an option. Although many assistive devices are available to people with hearing loss, understanding on the part of family and friends is perhaps the most important. It is important that those speaking to people with hearing impairment face the person and articulate so that lipreading cues can be used.

Hearing aids remain the mainstay of treatment for many people with conductive and sensorineural hearing loss. With microcircuitry, hearing aids are designed with computer chips that allow multiple programs to be placed in a single hearing aid. The various programs allow the user to select a specific setting for different listening situations. The development of microcircuitry has also made it possible for hearing aids to be miniaturized to the point that, in many cases, they can be placed deep in the ear, where they take advantage of the normal shape of the external ear and ear canal. Although modern hearing aids have improved greatly, they cannot replicate the hearing person's ability to hear both soft and loud noises. They also fail to consistently filter out distorted or background noise. Other aids for the hearing impaired include alert and signal devices, assistive listening devices from telephone companies, and dogs trained to respond to various sounds.

Cochlear implants for profound hearing loss have been very effective, and over 200,000 people worldwide have received one.[8] These prostheses are inserted into the scala tympani of the cochlea and work by providing direct stimulation to the auditory nerve, bypassing the area that is absent or nonfunctional in a deaf cochlea. For the implant to work, the auditory nerve must be functional. Although early implants used a single electrode, current implants use multielectrode placement, enhancing speech perception. Most people who become deaf after learning speech derive substantial benefit when cochlear implants are used in conjunction with lipreading. Some are able to understand some speech without lipreading, and some are able to communicate by telephone.

Hearing Loss in Infants and Children

Even slight or unilateral hearing loss can negatively impact the young child's language development. Although estimates vary depending on the group surveyed and testing methods used, 1 to 3 babies out of 1000 will be born with a permanent hearing loss. When considering less severe or transient conductive hearing loss that is commonly associated with middle ear disease in young children, the numbers are even greater.

The cause of hearing impairment in children may be conductive or sensorineural. Most conductive hearing loss is caused by middle ear infections. Causes of sensorineural hearing impairment include genetic, infectious, traumatic, and ototoxic factors. Genetic causes are probably responsible for as much as 50% of sensorineural hearing loss in children. Hearing loss affects 1 to 3 of 1000 newborns; this number increases if the newborn is in an intensive care setting.[10] Congenital cytomegalovirus is the most common cause of sensorineural hearing loss in newborns.[11]

Postnatal causes of sensorineural hearing loss include beta-hemolytic streptococcal sepsis in the newborn and bacterial meningitis. *Streptococcus pneumoniae* is the most common cause of bacterial meningitis that results in sensorineural hearing loss after the neonatal period. This cause may become less frequent with the routine administration of the conjugate pneumococcal vaccine. Other causes of sensorineural hearing loss are toxins and trauma. Early in pregnancy, the embryo is particularly sensitive to toxic substances, including ototoxic drugs such as the aminoglycosides and loop diuretics. Trauma, particularly head trauma, may cause sensorineural hearing loss.

Hearing impairment can have a major impact on the development of a child. Therefore, early identification through screening programs is strongly advocated. The American Academy of Pediatrics (AAP) and the Joint Commission on Infant Hearing (JCIH) published a position paper calling for universal screening of all infants by physiologic measurements before 1 month of age, with proper intervention no later than 6 months of age.[12] The currently recommended screening techniques are either the transient evoked otoacoustic emissions (TEOAEs) or the ABR. Both methodologies are noninvasive, relatively quick (<5 minutes), and easy to perform. The TEOAE measures sound waves generated in the inner ear (cochlea) in response to clicks or tone bursts emitted and recorded by a minute microphone placed in the external ear canals of the infant. The ABR uses three electrodes pasted to the infant's scalp to measure the EEG waves generated by clicks. Because many children become hearing impaired after the neonatal period and are not identified by neonatal screening programs, the AAP and JCIH recommend that all infants with risk factors for delayed onset of progressive hearing loss receive ongoing audiologic and medical monitoring and at appropriate intervals thereafter.[12]

Once hearing loss has been identified, a full developmental and speech and language evaluation is needed.

Hearing Loss in Older Adults

The term *presbycusis* is used to describe degenerative hearing loss that occurs with advancing age.[13] Approximately 45% of the population aged 65 years and older is hearing impaired.[13] Because of its high prevalence, presbycusis is a common social and health problem.

The hearing loss associated with presbycusis is typically gradual, bilateral, and characterized by high-frequency hearing loss.[13] It is further characterized by reduced hearing sensitivity and speech understanding in noisy environments, slowed central processing of acoustic information, and impaired localization of sound sources. The disorder first reduces the ability to understand speech and, later, the ability to detect, identify, and localize sounds. The most common complaint of people with presbycusis is not that they cannot hear but rather that they cannot understand with clarity what is being said.[13] For example, they often confuse words like *mash* with *math*, *map* with *mat*, and *Sunday* with *some day*. High-frequency warning sounds, such as beepers, turn signals, and escaping steam, are not heard and localized, with potentially dangerous results. Because the age at which problems occur varies widely, it seems likely that the disorder results from a mixture of acquired auditory stresses, trauma, and otologic diseases in addition to the aging process.

Given the high prevalence of presbycusis in people of retirement age and the adverse effects of hearing loss on well-being, screening for hearing loss should be performed at annual health care visits. The single question "do you have a hearing problem?" is usually an effective method of screening. Screening audiometry administered by someone trained in its use is a practical and cost-effective method for detecting significant hearing loss. The equipment needed for screening audiometry is lightweight, low cost, and well accepted by persons being tested. (Clinical measures for hearing loss such as whispered voice tests and finger friction tests are reportedly imprecise and are not reliable methods for screening.)

Several otologic abnormalities can be identified and treated. Cerumen impaction may cause conductive hearing loss.[14] Many older adults are on multiple medications, some of which may possess ototoxic potential.

The majority of hearing loss in older adults is sensorineural. In mild to severe hearing loss, the most effective treatment is hearing amplification with hearing aids, lipreading, and assistive listening devices (*e.g.*, hearing aids with the telephone, captioning on televised programs, flashing alarms). Cochlear implants are indicated at any age for people with bilateral hearing losses not materially helped by hearing aids.

IN SUMMARY

Hearing is a specialized sense whose external stimulus is the vibration of sound waves. Our ears receive sound waves, distinguish their frequencies, translate this information into nerve impulses, and transmit them to the CNS. Anatomically, the auditory system consists of the outer ear, middle ear, and inner ear, the auditory pathways, and the auditory cortex. The middle ear is a tiny, air-filled cavity in the temporal bone. A connection exists between the middle ear and the nasopharynx. This connection, called the *eustachian tube*, allows equalization of pressure between the middle ear and the atmosphere. The inner ear contains the receptors for hearing.

Disorders of the auditory system include infections of the external and middle ear, otosclerosis, and conduction and sensorineural deafness. OE is an inflammatory process of the external ear. OM is an inflammation of the middle ear without reference to etiology or pathogenesis. AOM, which refers to an acute middle ear infection, is one of the most common illnesses in children. It usually follows an upper respiratory tract infection, has an abrupt onset, and is characterized by otalgia, fever, and hearing loss. OME refers to the presence of fluid in the inner ear without signs and symptoms of acute ear infection. The effusion that accompanies OM can persist for weeks or months, interfering with hearing and impairing speech development. It is important to differentiate OME from AOM to avoid unnecessary antimicrobial use. Otosclerosis is a familial disorder of the otic capsule. It causes bone resorption followed by excessive replacement with sclerotic bone. The disorder eventually causes immobilization of the stapes and conduction deafness.

Deafness, or hearing loss, can develop as the result of a number of auditory disorders. It can be conductive, sensorineural, or mixed. Conduction deafness occurs when transmission of sound waves from the external ear to the inner ear is impaired. Sensorineural deafness can involve cochlear structures of the inner ear or the neural pathways that transmit auditory stimuli. Sensorineural hearing loss can result from genetic or congenital disorders, trauma, infections, vascular disorders, tumors, or ototoxic drugs. Hearing loss in infants and young children impairs language and speech development. In the elderly, hearing loss is a common condition resulting in significant loss of social well-being. Treatment of hearing loss includes the use of hearing aids and, in some cases of profound deafness, implantation of cochlear prosthesis.

DISORDERS OF VESTIBULAR FUNCTION

After completing this section of the chapter, the learner will be able to meet the following objectives:

- Explain the function of the vestibular system with respect to postural reflexes and maintaining a stable visual field despite marked changes in head position.
- Compare the manifestations and pathologic processes associated with benign paroxysmal positional vertigo and Ménière disease.
- Distinguish the characteristics of peripheral and central vestibular disorders.

The Vestibular System and Vestibular Reflexes

By about 24 weeks of gestational age, the vestibular system has reached adult form and size.[15] Located in the inner ear, the vestibular system is primarily responsible for balance. The vestibular system includes the vestibular apparatus, and CNS connections contribute to the reflex activity needed for detecting and maintaining postural orientation and perception of motion. Beyond maintaining posture and balance, the vestibular system also integrates visual input from the eyes and proprioceptive input from the peripheral nerves through the spinal cord.[16]

Disorders of the vestibular system are characterized by vertigo, nystagmus, tinnitus, nausea and vomiting, and autonomic nervous system manifestations. Despite the discomfort of these symptoms, few cases are life-threatening conditions.[16] There are many types of vestibular disorders (Table 20.1).

TABLE 20.1 COMMON DISORDERS AFFECTING THE VESTIBULAR SYSTEM

TYPE OF DISORDER	PATHOLOGY
Acoustic neuroma	A noncancerous growth or tumor on the vestibulocochlear nerve
Benign paroxysmal positional vertigo (BPPV)	Disorder of otoliths
Ménière disease	Dislodgement of otoliths that participate in the receptor function of the vestibular system
Motion sickness	Repeated stimulation of the vestibular system such as during car, air, and boat travel
Labyrinthitis	Acute viral or bacterial infection of the vestibular pathways
Vestibular migraine	Dizziness or vertigo occurs with or without headache; related to the neurotransmitter serotonin

These disorders can be a major cause for the sensation of dizziness, vision changes, or unsteadiness.

Peripheral Vestibular Apparatus

The peripheral vestibular apparatus is contained in the bony labyrinth of the inner ear. It has two chambers: The *outer bony labyrinth* is filled with perilymph fluid, and the *inner membranous labyrinth* is filled with endolymph fluid. The membranous labyrinth has three semicircular canals and two otolithic organs (the utricle and saccule). Each ear contains these five structures, which supply sensory information to coordinate eye and head movement.[17] The semicircular canals are located perpendicular to each other and detect rotational movement, whereas the utricle and saccule detect linear movement. The smaller saccule extends into the cochlea through the ductus reuniens, and the utricle lies between the cochlea and semicircular ducts (Fig. 20.7). Small patches of hair cells are located in a membranous ampulla of the three semicircular ducts and the maculae of the saccule and utricle.[5]

The cavities of the three semicircular canals, the lateral, anterior, and posterior canals, are oriented in one of three planes of space. The lateral (horizontal) canals are in the same plane, whereas the anterior (superior) canal of one side is parallel with the posterior (inferior) canal on the other side, and the two function as a pair. Located in each semicircular canal is a corresponding semicircular duct, which communicates with the utricle. Each of these ducts has an enlarged swelling at one end called an ampulla. The ampulla contains a ridge that is covered by a sensory epithelium with hair cells that are raised into a crest, called the *crista ampullaris* (Fig. 20.6). These hair cells are innervated by the primary afferents of the vestibular nerve, which is a subdivision of the eighth CN. The hair cells of the crista ampullaris extend into a flexible gelatinous mass, called the *cupula*, which essentially closes off fluid flow through the semicircular ducts (Fig. 20.7). When the head begins to move, gravity produces a change in the endolymph, which causes the hair cells to bend, generating impulses carried by the vestibular branch of the eighth CN. Because all the hair cells in each semicircular canal share a common orientation, angular acceleration in one direction increases afferent nerve activity, whereas acceleration in the opposite direction diminishes nerve activity. Impulses from the semicircular ducts are particularly important in reflex movement of the eyes and keep images steady on the retina when the head moves. Vestibular nystagmus is a complex phenomenon that occurs during and immediately after rotational motion.[18] As you rotate your head, your eyes slowly drift in the opposite direction and then jump rapidly back toward the direction of rotation to establish a new fixation point.

Both the saccule and utricle have an equilibrium receptor, called a macula, that relates to changes in head position. Each macula is a small, flat epithelial patch with supporting cells and sensory hair cells. The sides and bases synapse with sensory endings of the vestibular nerve (Fig. 20.8). Each group of hair cells has multiple small cilia called *stereocilia*, plus one large cilium, the *kinocilium*. The kinocilium is located at

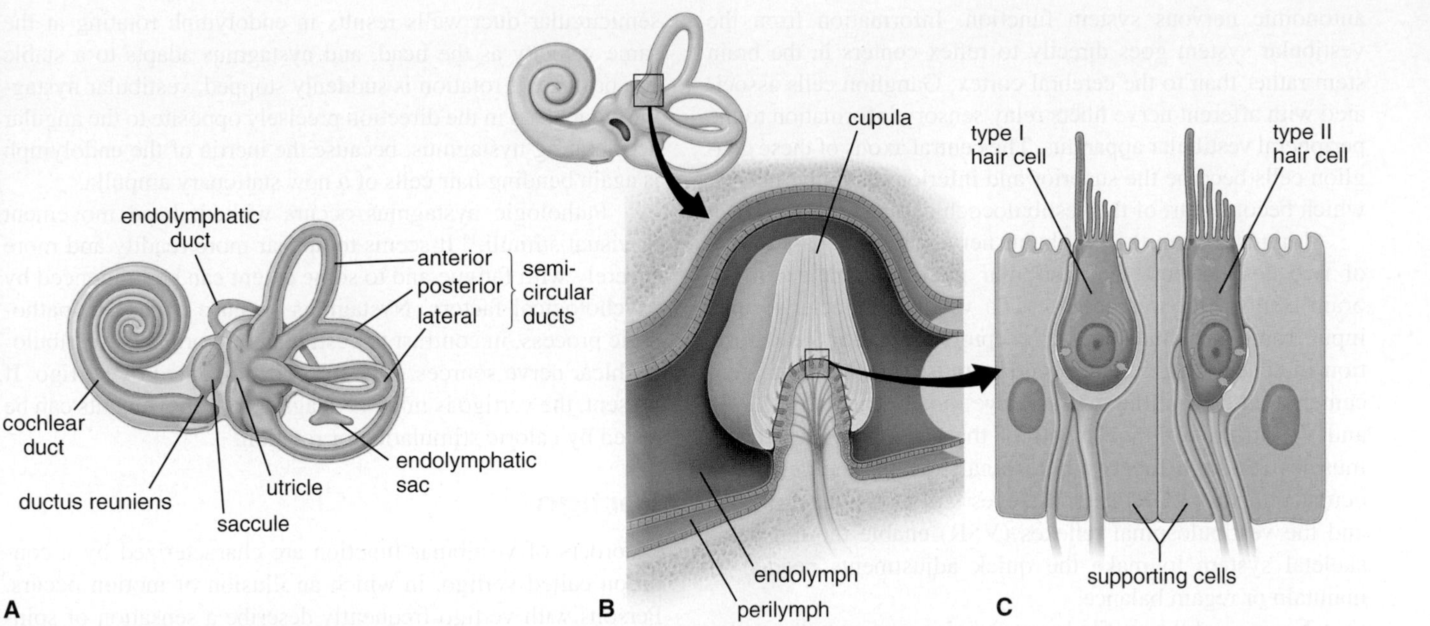

Figure 20.7 • **(A)** The osseous and membranous labyrinth of the left ear showing the utricle and saccule with their maculae and three semicircular canals and their ampullae. **(B)** Location of the crista ampullaris and its connection to the vestibular branch of CN VIII. **(C)** The location of the cupula and movement of hair cells of the crista ampullaris with head movement. (From Pawlina W., Ross M. H. (2016). *Histology: A text and atlas with correlated cell and molecular biology* (7th ed., Figures 25.8C (p. 942), 25.12B and C (p. 946)). Philadelphia, PA: Wolters Kluwer.)

one side of the cell, and the stereocilia become progressively shorter toward the other side of the cell. Tiny short hairs connect the tip of each stereocilium to the next longer stereocilium and finally to the kinocilium. Movement of the head in one direction causes movement of the adjoined stereocilia and kinocilium and depolarization or activation of the receptor. Movement of the head in the other direction causes hyperpolarization or inactivation of the receptor.

The hair cells in both the utricular and saccular maculae are embedded in a flattened gelatinous mass, the *otolithic membrane*, which is studded with tiny stones (calcium carbonate crystals) called *otoliths*. Although they are small, the density of the otoliths increases the membrane's weight and its resistance to change in motion. When the head is tilted, the gelatinous mass shifts its position because of the pull of the gravitational field, bending the stereocilia of the macular hair cells. The otoliths are sensitive to static or changing head movements, depending on the direction that the cilia are bending. In a condition called *benign paroxysmal positional vertigo* (BPPV), changes in head position cause a sensation of whirling or spinning. With this condition, the otoliths become dislodged from their gelatinous base and drift into the semicircular canals, causing vertigo.

Neural Pathways

The response to body imbalance, such as stumbling, must be fast and reflexive. The vestibular system has extensive links with neural pathways controlling vision, hearing, and

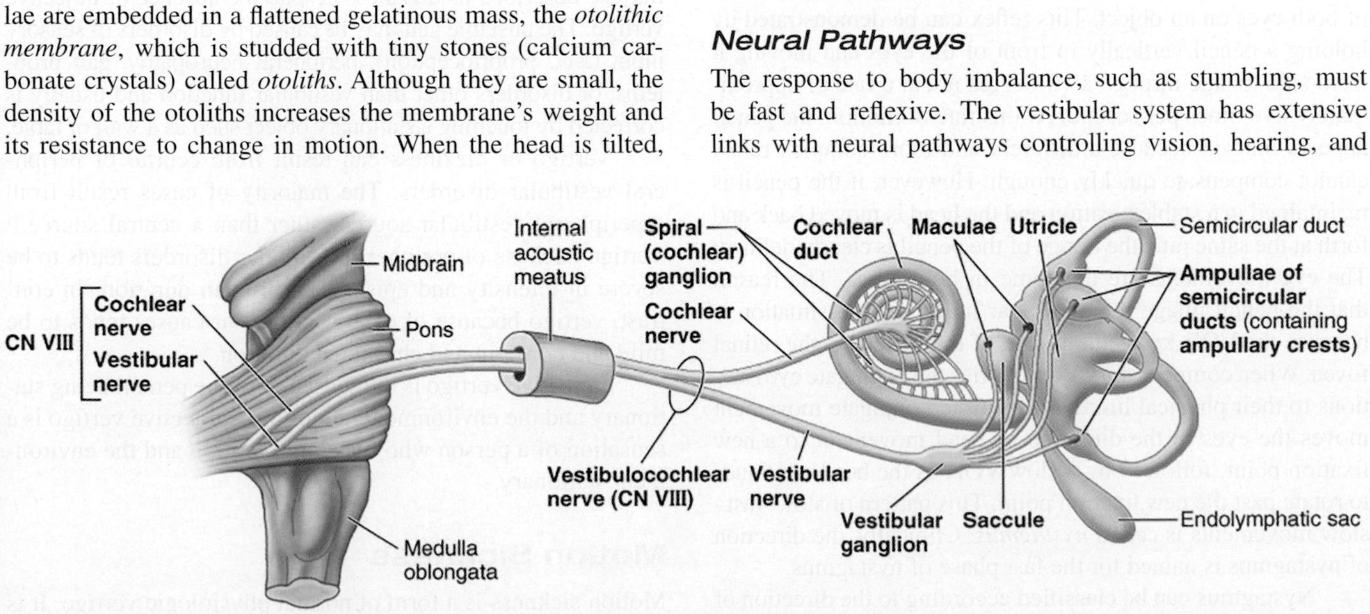

Figure 20.8 • Vestibulocochlear nerve (CN VIII). (From Moore K. L., Anne M. R., Dalley A. F. *Essential clinical anatomy* (5th ed., Figure 7.78, p. 573). Philadelphia, PA: Lippincott Williams & Wilkins.)

autonomic nervous system function. Information from the vestibular system goes directly to reflex centers in the brain stem rather than to the cerebral cortex. Ganglion cells associated with afferent nerve fibers relay sensory information to the peripheral vestibular apparatus. The central axons of these ganglion cells become the superior and inferior vestibular nerves, which become part of the vestibulocochlear nerve (CN VIII).

Impulses from the vestibular nerves initially pass to one of two destinations: the vestibular nuclear complex in the brain stem or the cerebellum. The vestibular nuclei receive input from visual and somatic receptors that report head position in space. These nuclei send impulses to the brain stem centers that control the extrinsic eye movements (CN III, IV, and VI) and reflex movements of the neck, limb, and trunk muscles (through the vestibulospinal tracts). The vestibulo-ocular reflexes (VOR) keep the eyes still as the head moves, and the vestibulospinal reflexes (VSR) enable the musculoskeletal system to make the quick adjustments needed to maintain or regain balance.

Neurons of the vestibular nuclei also project to the thalamus, the temporal cortex, the somatosensory area of the parietal cortex, and the chemoreceptor trigger zone. The thalamic and cortical projections provide the basis for the subjective experiences of position in space and of rotation. Connections with the chemoreceptor trigger zone stimulate the vomiting center in the brain. This is thought to account for the nausea and vomiting that accompany vestibular disorders.

Nystagmus

Nystagmus can be either physiologic or pathologic. Physiologically, nystagmus refers to the involuntary rhythmic and oscillatory eye movements caused by altered input from the vestibular nuclei during head movement.[19] The VOR produces slow compensatory conjugate eye rotations that occur in the opposite direction of head movement and stabilize fixation of both eyes on an object. This reflex can be demonstrated by holding a pencil vertically in front of the eyes and moving it from side to side through a 10-degree arc at a rate of approximately five times per second. At this rate of motion, the pencil appears blurred because a different and more complex reflex cannot compensate quickly enough. However, if the pencil is maintained in a stable position and the head is moved back and forth at the same rate, the image of the pencil is clearly defined. The eye movements are the same in both cases. The reason that the pencil image remains clear in the second situation is because the VOR keeps the image of the pencil on the retinal fovea. When compensatory VOR carries the conjugate eye rotations to their physical limit, a very rapid conjugate movement moves the eyes in the direction of head movement to a new fixation point, followed by a slow VOR as the head continues to rotate past the new fixation point. This pattern of slow–fast–slow movements is called *nystagmus*. Clinically, the direction of nystagmus is named for the fast phase of nystagmus.

Nystagmus can be classified according to the direction of eye movement: horizontal, vertical, rotary (torsional), or mixed. If head rotation is continued, friction between endolymph and semicircular duct walls results in endolymph rotating at the same velocity as the head, and nystagmus adapts to a stable eye posture. If rotation is suddenly stopped, vestibular nystagmus reappears in the direction precisely opposite to the angular accelerating nystagmus, because the inertia of the endolymph is again bending hair cells of a now stationary ampulla.

Pathologic nystagmus occurs without head movement or visual stimuli.[19] It seems to appear more readily and more severely with fatigue and to some extent can be influenced by psychological factors. Nystagmus because of a CNS pathologic process, in contrast to vestibular end organ or vestibulocochlear nerve sources, seldom is accompanied by vertigo. If present, the vertigo is mild. Nystagmus eye movements can be tested by caloric stimulation or rotation.

Vertigo

Disorders of vestibular function are characterized by a condition called vertigo, in which an illusion of motion occurs. Persons with vertigo frequently describe a sensation of spinning, "to-and-fro" motion, or falling.

Concept Mastery Alert

With vertigo, the person may be stationary and the environment in motion (*i.e.*, objective vertigo), or the person may be in motion and the environment stationary (*i.e.*, subjective vertigo).

Vertigo is different than light-headedness, faintness, or syncope. It is considered more of a spinning of oneself or the surroundings. Presyncope, which is characterized by a feeling of light-headedness or "blacking out," is commonly caused by postural hypotension or a global impairment of cerebral circulation that limits blood flow.[20] An inability to maintain normal gait may be described as dizziness despite the absence of objective vertigo. The unstable gait may be caused by disorders of sensory input (*e.g.*, proprioception), peripheral neuropathy, gait problems, or disorders other than vestibular function and usually is corrected by touching a stationary object such as a wall or table.

Vertigo or dizziness can result from central or peripheral vestibular disorders. The majority of cases result from a peripheral vestibular source rather than a central source.[21] Vertigo because of peripheral vestibular disorders tends to be severe in intensity and episodic or brief in duration. In contrast, vertigo because of central vestibular causes tends to be mild and constant and chronic in duration.

Objective vertigo is the sensation of the person being stationary and the environment in motion. Subjective vertigo is a sensation of a person who may be in motion and the environment stationary.

Motion Sickness

Motion sickness is a form of normal physiologic vertigo. It is caused by repeated rhythmic stimulation of the vestibular system, such as that encountered in car, air, or boat travel. Vertigo, malaise, nausea, and vomiting are the principal symptoms. Autonomic signs, including lowered blood pressure, tachycardia, and excessive sweating, may occur. Hyperventilation, which commonly accompanies motion sickness, produces changes in blood volume and pooling of blood in the lower extremities, leading to postural hypotension and sometimes to syncope. Some persons experience a variant of motion sickness, complaining of sensing the rocking motion of the boat after returning to ground. This usually resolves after the vestibular system becomes accustomed to the stationary influence of being back on land.

Motion sickness can usually be suppressed by supplying visual signals that more closely match the motion signals being supplied to the vestibular system. For example, looking out the window and watching the environment move when experiencing motion sickness associated with car travel provides the vestibular system with the visual sensation of motion. However, reading a book provides the vestibular system with a misinterpretation that the environment is stable. Motion sickness usually decreases in severity with repeated exposure. Anti–motion sickness drugs also may be used to reduce or relieve the symptoms. These drugs work by suppressing the activity of the vestibular system.

Disorders of Peripheral Vestibular Function

Disease or damage to the vestibular system can result in dysfunction of this system. Disorders of peripheral vestibular function occur when otolith debris enters the semicircular canals, causing gravitational sensitivity, as in BPPV, or is unbalanced by unilateral involvement of one of the vestibular organs, as in Ménière disease.[22] The inner ear is vulnerable to injury caused by fracture of the petrous portion of the temporal bones; by infection of nearby structures, including the middle ear and meninges; and by blood-borne toxins and infections. Damage to the vestibular system can occur as an adverse effect of certain drugs or from allergic reactions to foods. The aminoglycosides (*e.g.*, streptomycin, gentamicin) have a specific toxic affinity for the vestibular portion of the inner ear. Alcohol can cause transient episodes of vertigo. The cause of peripheral vertigo remains unknown in approximately half of the cases.

Severe irritation or damage of the vestibular end organs or nerves results in severe balance disorders reflected by instability of posture, ataxia, and falling accompanied by vertigo. With irritation, falling is away from the affected side. With destruction, it is toward the affected side. Adaptation to asymmetric stimulation occurs within a few days, after which the signs and symptoms diminish and eventually are lost. After recovery, there usually is a slightly reduced acuity for tilt, and the person walks with a somewhat broadened base to improve postural stability. The neurologic basis for this adaptation to unilateral loss of vestibular input is not understood. After adaptation to the loss of vestibular input from one side, the loss of function of the opposite vestibular apparatus produces signs and symptoms identical to those resulting from unilateral rather than bilateral loss. Within weeks, adaptation is again sufficient for movement and even for driving a car. Such a person relies heavily on visual and proprioceptive input from muscle and joint sensors and has severe orientation difficulty in the dark, particularly when moving over uneven areas.

Benign Paroxysmal Positional Vertigo

Benign paroxysmal positional vertigo (BPPV) is the most common cause of pathologic vertigo and usually develops after the fourth decade of life. It is characterized by brief periods of vertigo, usually lasting less than 1 minute, that are precipitated by a change in head position. The most prominent symptom of BPPV is vertigo that occurs in bed when the person rolls into a lateral position.[22] It also commonly occurs when the person is getting in and out of bed, bending over and straightening up, or extending the head to look up. It also can be triggered by amusement rides that feature turns and twists.

BPPV is thought to result from damage to the delicate sensory organs of the inner ear, the semicircular ducts, and the otoliths. BPPV is a common recurrence with people who have Ménière disease or have experienced head trauma.[22] People experiencing BPPV have a movement of the otoliths from the utricle into the endolymph of the semicircular canal, which continue to move even when the head is stationary.[21] Movement of the otoliths or free-floating debris causes this portion of the vestibular system to become more sensitive, such that any movement of the head in the plane parallel to the posterior duct may cause vertigo and nystagmus. There usually is a several second delay between head movement and onset of vertigo, representing the time it takes to generate the exaggerated endolymph activity. Symptoms usually subside with continued movement, probably because the movement causes the debris to be redistributed throughout the endolymph system and away from the posterior semicircular canal.

Diagnosis is based on tests that involve the use of a change in head position to elicit vertigo and nystagmus, such as the Dix-Hallpike maneuver.[23] BPPV often is successfully treated with drug therapy to control vertigo-induced nausea. Nondrug therapies using the rolling over maneuver and canalith repositioning are successful for many people.[21] Canalith repositioning involves a series of maneuvers in which the head is moved to different positions in an effort to reposition the free-floating debris in the endolymph of the semicircular canals.

Acute Vestibular Neuronitis

Acute vestibular neuronitis, or labyrinthitis, represents an inflammation of the vestibular nerve and is characterized by an acute onset generally within a couple of hours. Manifestations include vertigo, nausea, and vomiting lasting several days and not associated with auditory or other neurologic presentations. Generally these symptoms resolve in about 10 to 14 days. A large percentage of people report an upper respiratory tract illness 1 to 2 weeks before onset of symptoms, suggesting a viral origin. The condition also can occur in people with herpes zoster oticus. In some people, attacks of acute vestibulopathy recur over months or years. There is no way to determine whether a person who experiences a first attack will have repeated attacks.

Ménière Disease

Ménière disease is a disorder of the inner ear because of distention of the endolymphatic compartment of the inner ear. The classic triad of symptoms includes hearing loss, vertigo, and tinnitus.[24] The primary lesion appears to be in the endolymphatic sac, which is thought to be responsible for endolymph filtration and excretion. A number of pathogenetic mechanisms have been postulated, including an increased production of endolymph, decreased production of perilymph accompanied by a compensatory increase in volume of the endolymphatic sac, and decreased absorption of endolymph caused by malfunction of the endolymphatic sac or blockage of endolymphatic pathways.

Etiology. The cause of Ménière disease is unknown, but it is known that this syndrome is of peripheral origin with vertigo. A number of conditions—such as trauma, infection, specific drugs (certain antibiotics), and toxins—have been identified as possible etiologies of Ménière disease. The most common form of the disease is classified as idiopathic and is thought to be caused by a single viral injury to the fluid transport system of the inner ear.[24]

Clinical Manifestations. Ménière disease is characterized by fluctuating episodes of tinnitus, feelings of ear fullness, and violent rotary vertigo that often render the person unable to sit or walk. There is a need to lie quietly with the head fixed in a comfortable position, avoiding all head movements that aggravate the vertigo. Symptoms referable to the autonomic nervous system, including pallor, sweating, nausea, and vomiting, usually are present. The more severe the attack, the more prominent are the autonomic manifestations. A fluctuating hearing loss occurs, which returns to normal after the episode subsides. Initially, the symptoms tend to be unilateral, resulting in rotary nystagmus caused by an imbalance in vestibular control of eye movements. Because initial involvement usually is unilateral and because the sense of hearing is bilateral, many persons with the disorder are not aware of the full extent of their hearing loss. However, as the disease progresses, the person will experience worsening of hearing. The episodes of vertigo diminish and then disappear, although the person may be unsteady, especially in the dark.

Diagnosis and Treatment. Methods used in the diagnosis of Ménière disease include audiograms, vestibular testing by electronystagmography (ENG), and petrous pyramid radiographs. The administration of hyperosmolar substances, such as glycerin and urea, often produces acute temporary hearing improvement in persons with Ménière disease. This method sometimes is used as a diagnostic measure of endolymphatic hydrops. The diuretic furosemide also may be used for this purpose.

The management of Ménière disease focuses on attempts to reduce the distention of the endolymphatic space and can be medical or surgical. Pharmacologic management consists of suppressant drugs (*e.g.*, prochlorperazine, promethazine, diazepam), which act centrally to decrease the activity of the vestibular system. Diuretics are used to reduce endolymph fluid volume. A low-sodium diet is recommended in addition to these medications. The steroid hormone, prednisone, may be used to maintain satisfactory hearing and resolve dizziness.

Surgical methods include the creation of an endolymphatic shunt in which excess endolymph from the inner ear is diverted into the subarachnoid space or the mastoid (endolymphatic sac surgery) and vestibular nerve section or chemical ablation.[25] Advances in vestibular nerve section have facilitated the monitoring of CN VII and CN VIII potentials.

Disorders of Central Vestibular Function

Abnormal nystagmus and vertigo can occur as a result of CNS lesions involving the cerebellum and lower brain stem. Central causes of vertigo include brain stem ischemia, tumors, and multiple sclerosis. When brain stem ischemia is the cause of vertigo, it usually is associated with other brain stem signs such as diplopia, ataxia, dysarthria, or facial weakness. Compression of the vestibular nuclei by cerebellar tumors invading the fourth ventricle results in progressively severe signs and symptoms. In addition to abnormal nystagmus and vertigo, vomiting and a broad-based and dystaxic gait become progressively more evident.

Centrally derived nystagmus usually has equal excursion in both directions (*i.e.*, pendular). In contrast to peripherally generated nystagmus, CNS-derived nystagmus is relatively constant rather than episodic. It can occur in any direction (rather than primarily in the horizontal or torsional [rotatory] dimensions), often changes direction through time, and cannot be suppressed by visual fixation. Repeated induction of nystagmus results in rapid diminution or "fatigue" of the reflex with peripheral abnormalities, but fatigue is not characteristic of central lesions. Abnormal nystagmus can make reading and other tasks that require precise eye positional control difficult.

Diagnosis and Treatment of Vestibular Disorders

Diagnostic Tests

Diagnosis of vestibular disorders is based on a description of the symptoms, a history of trauma or exposure to agents that are destructive to vestibular structures, and physical examination. Physical and neurologic examinations—including gait assessment, oculomotor assessment, and positional testing—are used to help make the diagnosis. Other tests performed when vestibular dysfunction is suspected are discussed next.

Romberg Test. The Romberg test is one of the oldest sensory tests used to demonstrate disorders of static vestibular function. The person being tested is requested to stand with feet together and arms extended forward so that the degree of sway and arm stability can be observed. The person then is asked to close his or her eyes. When visual clues are removed, postural stability is based on proprioceptive sensation from the joints, muscles, and tendons and from static vestibular reception. Deficiency in vestibular static input is indicated by greatly increased sway and a tendency for the arms to drift toward the side of deficiency.

If vestibular input is severely deficient, the subject falls toward the deficient side. Care must be taken because defects of proprioceptive projection to the forebrain also result in some arm drift and postural instability toward the deficient side. Only if two-point discrimination and vibratory sensation from the lower and upper limbs are bilaterally normal can the deficiency be attributed to the vestibular system.

Electronystagmography and Videonystagmography. ENG is an examination that records eye movements in response to vestibular, visual, cervical (vertigo triggered by somatosensory input from head and neck movements), rotational, and positional stimulation. Electrodes are placed lateral to the outer canthus of each eye and above and below each eye. A ground electrode is placed on the forehead. With ENG, the velocity, frequency, and amplitude of spontaneous or induced nystagmus and the changes in these measurements brought by a loss of fixation, with the eyes open or closed, can be quantified. The advantages of ENG are that it is easily administered, is noninvasive, does not interfere with vision, and does not require head restraint.

The VNG, which has replaced the ENG in clinical practice, uses infrared goggles to record and measure eye movements on camera. The test captures ocular mobility using different eye maneuvers, eye tracking, head positioning, and caloric stimulation. Caloric testing has historically used water irrigation, but air has become the medium of choice. This test involves stimulating the inner ear, one ear at a time, with warm air followed by cold air and comparing measured responses.[23]

Other Tests. The rotational chair test rotates a person in the dark to stimulate nystagmus, and horizontal movements can be measured. A head MRI with contrast should also be considered when assessing vestibular dysfunction.[23]

In peripheral lesions, nystagmus is usually horizontal and with a rotary component; the fast beat usually beats away from the disease side. Several types of maneuvers can be used to provoke vertigo and observe for nystagmus. Usually, the examiner has the person sitting upright on an examining table with the head turned toward the examiner, with the person's eyes focused on the examiner's finger. The person is then properly supported and lowered rapidly to the supine position with the head extending over the upper end of the examining table and placed about 30 degrees lower than the body. The person is observed for nystagmus for about 30 seconds while in that position. The test can be performed with the head turned to either side or with the person looking straight ahead.

Vertigo arising from central lesions tends to develop gradually, and nystagmus is not always present, can occur in any direction, and can be dissociated in the two eyes. ENG is often useful in documenting the characteristics of the nystagmus. Further evaluation of central vertigo usually requires MRI.

Treatment

Pharmacologic Methods. Depending on the cause, vertigo may be treated pharmacologically. Medications used for symptomatic relief include antihistamines, anticholinergic agents, antiemetics, and benzodiazepines. Antihistamines and anticholinergic drugs suppress vestibular symptoms. Benzodiazepines and antiemetics can be sedating and are reserved for severe symptoms not responsive to other medications.[24] Although the antihistamines have long been used in treating vertigo, little is known about their mechanism of action.

Vestibular Rehabilitation Exercises. Vestibular rehabilitation has been shown to be helpful as a treatment for peripheral vestibular disorders. Physical therapists are usually involved in developing a program including habituation exercises, balance retraining exercises, and a general conditioning program for people to use at home.[25] The habituation exercises take advantage of physiologic fatigue of the neurovegetative response to repetitive movement or positional stimulation and are done to decrease motion-provoked vertigo, light-headedness, and unsteadiness. The exercises are selected to provoke the vestibular symptoms. The person moves quickly into the position that causes symptoms, holds the position until the symptoms subside (*i.e.*, fatigue of the neurovegetative response), relaxes, and then repeats the exercise for a prescribed number of times. The exercises usually are repeated twice daily.

Balance retraining exercises consist of activities directed toward improving individual components of balance that may be abnormal. General conditioning exercises, a vital part of the rehabilitation process, are individualized to the person's preferences and lifestyle. It is recommended that the person practice these exercises about five times per week.

IN SUMMARY

The vestibular system plays an essential role in the equilibrium sense, which is closely integrated with the visual and proprioceptive (position) senses. Receptors in the semicircular canals, utricle, and saccule of the vestibular system, located in the inner ear, respond to changes in linear and angular acceleration of the head. The vestibular nerve fibers travel in CN VIII to the vestibular nuclei at the junction of the medulla and pons; some fibers pass through the nuclei to the cerebellum. Cerebellar connections are necessary for temporally smooth, coordinated movements during ongoing head movements, tilt, and angular acceleration. The vestibular nuclei also connect with nuclei of the oculomotor (CN III), trochlear (CN IV), and abducens (CN VI) nerves that control eye movement. *Nystagmus* is a term used to describe vestibular-controlled eye movements that occur in response to angular and rotational movements of the head. The vestibulospinal tract, which provides for the control of muscle tone in the axial muscles, including those of the back, provides the support for maintaining balance. Neurons of the vestibular nuclei also project to the thalamus, to the temporal cortex, and to the somatosensory area of the parietal cortex. The thalamic and cortical projections provide the basis for the subjective experiences of position in space and of rotation and vertigo.

Vertigo, an illusory sensation of motion of either oneself or one's surroundings, tinnitus, and hearing loss are common manifestations of vestibular dysfunction, as are autonomic manifestations such as perspiration, nausea, and vomiting. Common disorders of the vestibular system include motion sickness, BPPV, and Ménière disease.

BPPV is a condition believed to be caused by free-floating particles in the posterior semicircular canal. It presents as a sudden onset of dizziness or vertigo that is provoked by certain changes in head position. Ménière disease, which is caused by an overaccumulation of endolymph, is characterized by severe, disabling episodes of tinnitus, feelings of ear fullness, and violent rotary vertigo. The diagnosis of vestibular disorders is based on a description of the symptoms, a history of trauma or exposure to agents destructive to vestibular structures, and tests of eye movements (*i.e.*, nystagmus) and muscle control of balance and equilibrium. Among the methods used in treatment of the vertigo that accompanies vestibular disorders are habituation exercises and antivertigo drugs. These drugs act by diminishing the excitability of neurons in the vestibular nucleus.

GERIATRIC Considerations

- Older people with impaired hearing may be shunned by others and may avoid situations in which they must interact.[26]
- 10% of older adults describe having difficulty hearing telephone conversations.
- Acute otitis externa increases in the elderly population because of comorbid conditions and use of hearing aids.[3]
- Ear irrigation is a simple method to remove cerumen accumulations in the older person's ear canal but can result in dizziness and increased risk of falls.[26]
- Tinnitus (ringing of the ears) is often found with age-related hearing loss, ear injury, medications, and cardiovascular disease in the older person.[26]
- Although hearing aids can help older people with hearing impairment improve their hearing, if they are uncomfortable with or need help in caring for the device, they may need support.[26]

PEDIATRIC Considerations

- Hearing is fully developed at birth, as evidenced by the newborn's ability to distinguish parents' voices and be soothed by familiar music.[27]
- For neonates with acute otitis media, feeding difficulties may be the only indication that sepsis is present.[3]
- Infants (9 to 12 months) who are unable to repeat syllables such as "ma-ma" should be referred for hearing assessment.[27]
- A decline in school performance is an indication that hearing evaluation is needed.[27]

REVIEW EXERCISES

1. A mother notices that her 13-month-old child is fussy and tugging at his ear and he refuses to eat his breakfast. When she takes his temperature, it is 37.8°C (100°F). Although the child attends daycare, the mother has kept him home and made an appointment with the child's health care provider. In the provider's office, his temperature is 37.9°C (100.2°F), he is somewhat irritable, and he has a clear nasal drainage. His left tympanic membrane shows normal landmarks and mobility on pneumatic otoscopy. His right tympanic membrane is erythematous, and there is decreased mobility on pneumatic otoscopy.
   A. *What risk factors are present that predispose this child to the development of AOM?*
   B. *Are his signs and symptoms typical of OM in a child of this age?*
   C. *What are the most likely pathogens? What treatment would be indicated?*
   D. *Later in the week, the mother notices that the child does not seem to hear as well as he did before developing the infection. Is this a common occurrence, and should the mother be concerned about transient hearing loss in a child of this age?*
2. A granddaughter is worried that her grandfather is "losing his hearing." Lately, he has been staying away from social gatherings that he always enjoyed, saying everybody mumbles. He is defiant in maintaining that there is nothing wrong with his hearing. However, he does complain that his ears have been ringing a lot lately.

A. What are common manifestations of hearing loss in older adults?
B. What type of evaluation would be appropriate for determining if this man has a hearing loss and the extent of his hearing loss?
C. What are some things that the granddaughter might do so that her grandfather could hear her better when she is talking to him?

3. A 70-year-old man complains that he gets this terrible feeling "like the room is moving around" and becomes nauseated when he rolls over in bed or bends over suddenly. It usually goes away once he has been up for a while. He has been told that his symptoms are consistent with BPPV.
A. What is the pathophysiology associated with this man's vertigo?
B. Why do the symptoms subside once he has been up for a while?
C. What methods are available for treatment of the disorder?

References

1. Lemone P., Burke K. M., Bauldoff G., et al. (2015). *Medical-Surgical nursing: Clinical reasoning in patient care* (6th ed.). Boston, MA: Pearson Education.
2. Schwartz S. R., Magit A.M., Rosenfeld R.M., et al. (2017). *Clinical practice guideline (update): Earwax (cerumen impaction)*. Sage Publications. doi: 10.1177/0194599816671491.
3. Waitzman A. A. (2017). *Otitis externa*. Available: https://emedicine.medscape.com/article/994550-overview#a1. Accessed November 9, 2017.
4. Rosenfeld R. M., Schwartz S. P., Cannon C. R., et al. Clinical practice guideline: Acute otitis externa. *Otolaryngology–Head and Neck Surgery* 2014;150(1 Suppl):S1–S24.
5. Scanlon V. C., Sanders T. (2015). *Essentials of anatomy and physiology* (7th ed.). Philadelphia, PA: F.A. Davis.
6. Porter R. S., Kaplan J. L. (2016). *Merck manual: Professional version*. Whitehouse Station, NJ: Merck Sharp & Dohme Corporation.
7. Burns C. E., Dunn A. M., Brady M. A., et al. (2017). *Pediatric primary care* (6th ed.). St. Louis, MO: Saunders Elsevier.
8. Pensak M. L., Choo D. I. (2015). *Clinical otology* (4th ed.). New York, NY: Thieme Medical Publishers, Inc.
9. Bickley L. S. (2017). *Bates' guide to physical examination and history taking* (12th ed.). Philadelphia, PA: Wolters Kluwer.
10. Simpson K. R., Creehan P. A. (2014). *Perinatal nursing* (4th ed.). Philadelphia, PA: Wolters Kluwer.
11. Youngkin E. Q., Davis M.S., Schadewald D. M., et al. (2013). *Women's health: A primary care clinical guide* (4th ed.). Upper Saddle River, NJ: Pearson Education Inc.
12. American Academy of Pediatrics. (2017). *Pediatric clinical practice guidelines & policies: A compendium of evidence-based research for pediatric practice* (17th ed.). Elk Grove Village, IL: American Academy of Pediatrics.
13. Cook R. L., Nelson K. C. (2018). Presbycusis. In *The 5-minute clinical consult* (26th ed.). Philadelphia, PA: Wolters Kluwer.
14. Venes D. (2017). *Taber's cyclopedic medical dictionary* (23rd ed.). Philadelphia, PA: F.A. Davis Company.
15. Hill M. (2017). Hearing development: Embryology of the ear. In A. M. Tharpe, R. Seewald (Eds.) *Comprehensive handbook of pediatric audiology*. Kenilworth, NJ: Plural Publishing, Inc.
16. Kaplan J. L., Porter R. S. (2016). *Merck manual professional version*. Whitehouse Station, NJ: Merck Sharp & Dohme Corp., A Subsidiary of Merck & Co., Inc.
17. Cacace A. T., Kleine E., Holt A. G., et al. (2016). *Scientific foundations of audiology: Perspectives from physics, biology, modeling, and medicine*. San Diego, CA: Plural Publishing, Inc.
18. Lambert S. R., Lyons C. J. (2017). *Taylor and Hoyt's pediatric ophthalmology and strabismus* (5th ed.). Edinburgh, New York: Elsevier.
19. Bowling B. (2016). *Kanski's clinical ophthalmology* (8th ed.). Edinburgh: Elsevier.
20. Goldman L., Schafer A. (2016). *Goldman-Cecil medicine* (25th ed.). Philadelphia, PA: Elsevier.
21. Adams J. (2013). *Emergency medicine: Clinical essentials* (2nd ed.). Philadelphia, PA: Elsevier/Saunders.
22. Netter F. H., Jones H. R., Srinivasan J., et al. (2013). *Netter's neurology* (2nd ed.). Philadelphia, PA: Elsevier/Saunders.
23. Louis E. D., Mayer S. A., Rowland, L. P. (2016). *Merritt's neurology* (13th ed.). Philadelphia, PA: Wolters Kluwer.
24. Samuels M. A. (2017). *Scientific American Neurology*. Hamilton, ON: Decker Intellectual Properties, Inc.
25. O'Sullivan S. B., Schmitz T. J., Fulk G. D. (2014). *Physical rehabilitation* (6th ed.). Philadelphia, PA: F.A. Davis Company.
26. Elipoulos C. (2018). Vision and hearing. In *Gerontological nursing* (9th ed., pp. 364–377). Philadelphia, PA: Wolters Kluwer.
27. Bowden V. R., Greenberg C. S. (2014). The child with altered sensory status. In *Children and their families the continuum of nursing care* (3rd ed., pp. 1462–1519). Philadelphia, PA: Wolters Kluwer.

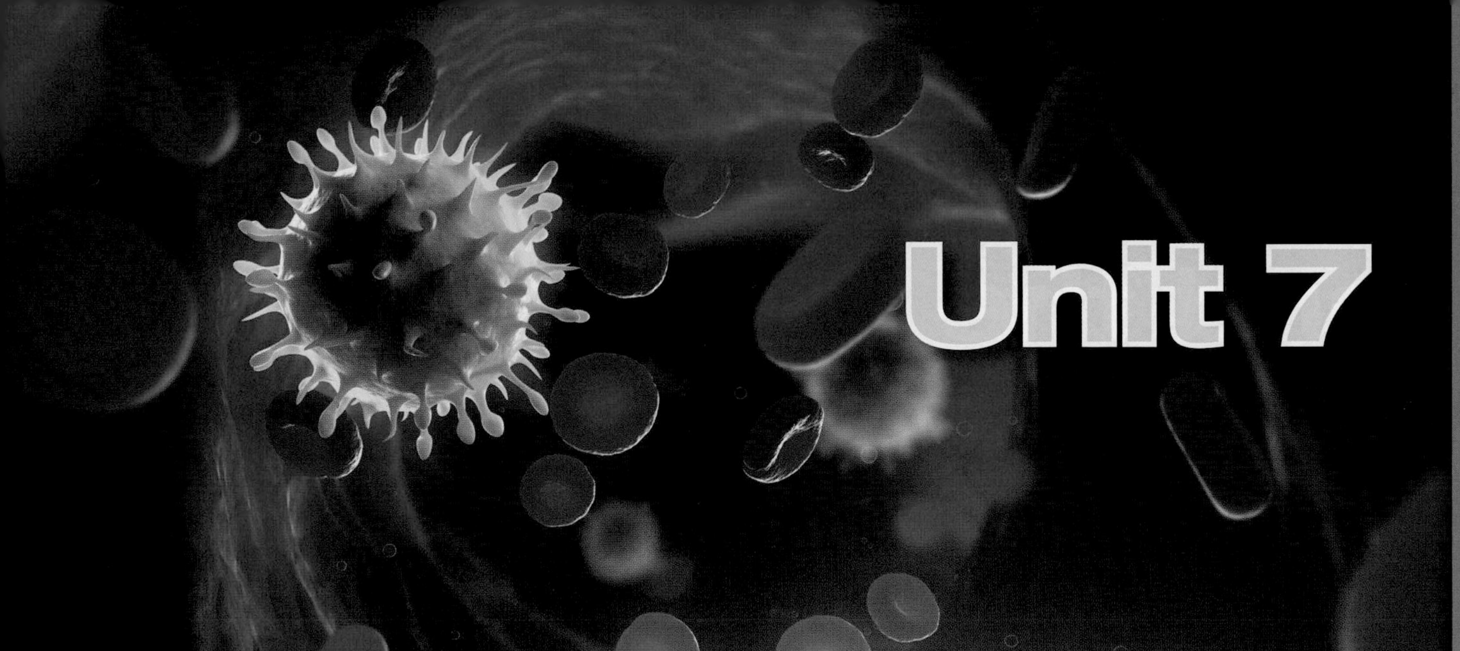

Unit 7

Disorders of the Hematopoietic System

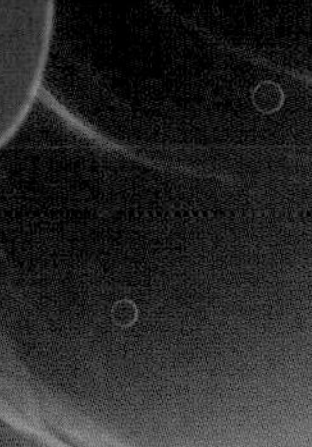

Mrs. Cretena, a 48-year-old woman, presents for her annual physical examination. She complains of fatigue and heavy menses over the last 6 months. She has four children and works full time, so she had not really thought much of the fatigue until she talked to a friend who recommended that she should have her hemoglobin level tested. Her laboratory data reflected the following: RBC = $4.2 \times 10^6/mm^3$ (normal range for females: 4.0 to $5.5 \times 10^6/mm^3$), hematocrit = 35% (normal range for females: 36% to 48%), and hemoglobin = 10 g/dL (normal range for females: 12.0 to 16.0 g/dL). Her red blood cell indices indicated a microcytic hypochromic anemia caused by iron deficiency. She was told to take ferrous sulfate three times a day (TID) and return for a follow-up in 2 weeks.

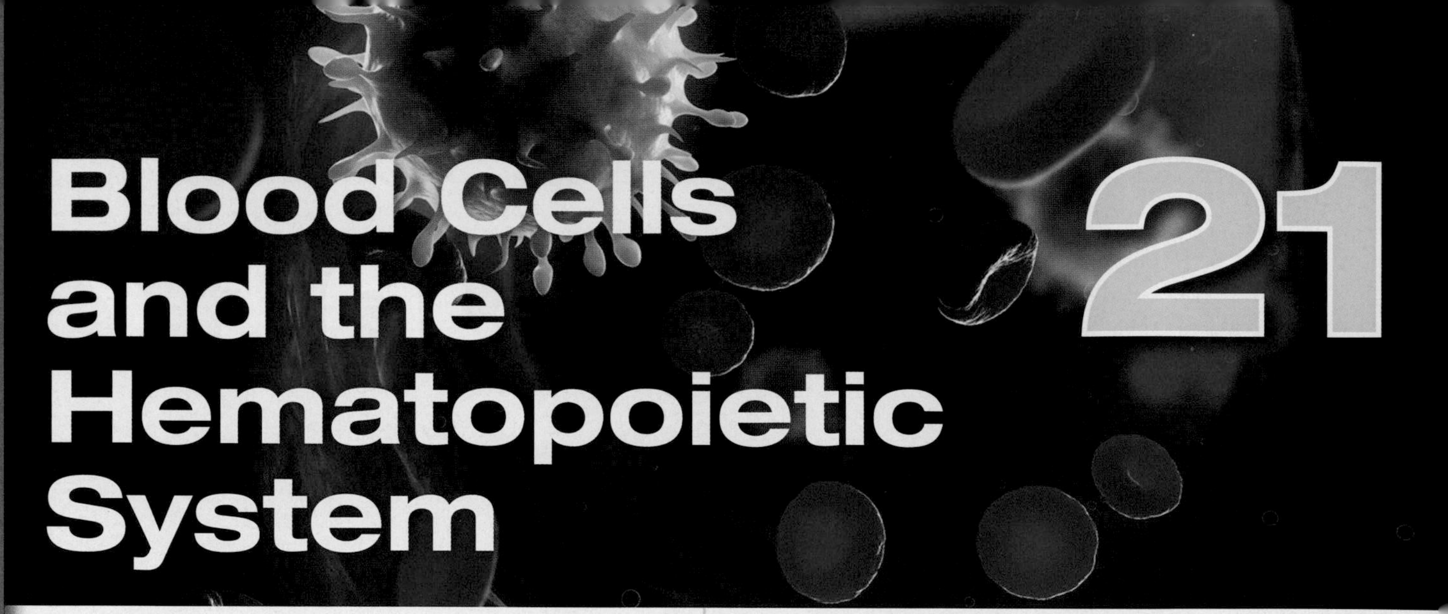

Blood Cells and the Hematopoietic System

21

Jacqueline Rosenjack Burchum

Blood is a specialized connective tissue that consists of blood cells (erythrocytes, leukocytes, and thrombocytes) suspended in an extracellular fluid, known as *plasma*. Blood accounts for about 7% to 8% of total body weight.[1] The total volume of blood in the average adult is about 5 to 6 L, and it circulates throughout the body within the confines of the circulatory system. Because blood circulates throughout the body, it is an ideal vehicle for transport of materials to and from the many cells of the body.

COMPOSITION OF BLOOD AND FORMATION OF BLOOD CELLS

After completing this section of the chapter, the learner will be able to meet the following objectives:

- Describe the composition and functions of plasma.
- Understand the function and life span of blood cells.
- Trace the process of hematopoiesis from stem cell to mature blood cell.

Blood components are easily identified in the laboratory. When a blood specimen is spun in a centrifuge, it separates into distinct layers (Fig. 21.1).

The bottom layer (approximately 42% to 47% of the whole blood volume) contains the erythrocytes or red blood cells (RBCs). The intermediate fluffy-looking layer (approximately 1%) containing the leukocytes, or white blood cells (WBCs), is white or gray. This layer is called the buffy coat.[2] Above the WBCs is a thin layer of thrombocytes that is not discernible to the naked eye. The translucent, yellowish fluid that forms above the RBCs, WBCs, and thrombocytes is the plasma, which comprises approximately 55% of the blood total volume.

KEY POINTS

COMPOSITION OF THE BLOOD

- The most abundant type of blood cells, the RBC, functions in oxygen and carbon dioxide transport.
- The WBCs serve various roles in immunity and inflammation.
- Thrombocytes are small cell fragments that are involved in blood clotting.

TABLE 21.1 PLASMA COMPONENTS

PLASMA	PERCENTAGE OF PLASMA VOLUME	DESCRIPTION
Water	90–91	
Proteins	6.5–8	
Albumin		54% Plasma proteins
Globulins		38% Plasma proteins
Fibrinogen		7% Plasma proteins
Other substances	1–2	Hormones, enzymes, carbohydrates, fats, amino acids, gases, electrolytes, excretory products

Plasma

By weight, plasma is 90% to 91% water, 6.5% to 8% proteins, and 2% other small molecular substances (Table 21.1). Plasma serves a number of vital functions. It operates as a transport vehicle for nutrients, chemical messengers, metabolites, and other materials.[3] For example, plasma carries hormones from their site of secretion to the target organ. It transports blood urea nitrogen, a waste product of metabolism, to the kidneys for excretion. It transports the RBCs that pick up oxygen at the pulmonary alveoli for distribution to the tissues. Plasma also participates in electrolyte and acid–base balance, and it contains the plasma proteins that contribute to the osmotic regulation of body fluids. In addition, because water has a high capacity to hold heat, plasma can absorb and distribute much of the heat that is generated in the body.

Plasma Proteins

The plasma proteins are the most abundant solutes in plasma. It is the presence of these proteins that distinguish the composition of plasma from that of interstitial fluid. The major types of plasma proteins are albumin, globulins, and fibrinogen. Except for the blood-borne hormones and gamma globulins, most plasma proteins are produced by the liver, which secretes them into the blood. Albumin is the most abundant plasma protein, making up approximately 54% of all plasma proteins. It is too large to pass through the pores in the capillary wall; therefore, it remains in the circulation, where it contributes to the plasma osmotic pressure and maintenance of blood volume. (See Chapter 14.) Albumin also serves as a carrier for certain substances and acts as a blood buffer.

The globulins comprise approximately 38% of all plasma proteins. There are three types of globulins—the *alpha globulins* that transport bilirubin and steroids, the *beta globulins* that transport iron and copper, and the *gamma globulins* that constitute the antibodies of the immune system.

Fibrinogen makes up approximately 7% of the plasma proteins. Fibrinogen is a soluble protein that polymerizes to form the insoluble protein fibrin during blood clotting. The presence of fibrinogen and clotting factors differentiates plasma from serum. When these are removed from plasma, as occurs when a blood specimen is allowed to clot, the liquid that remains is the serum.[2]

A variety of proteins comprise the remaining 1% of the plasma proteins. These include hormones, enzymes, complement, and carriers for lipids.

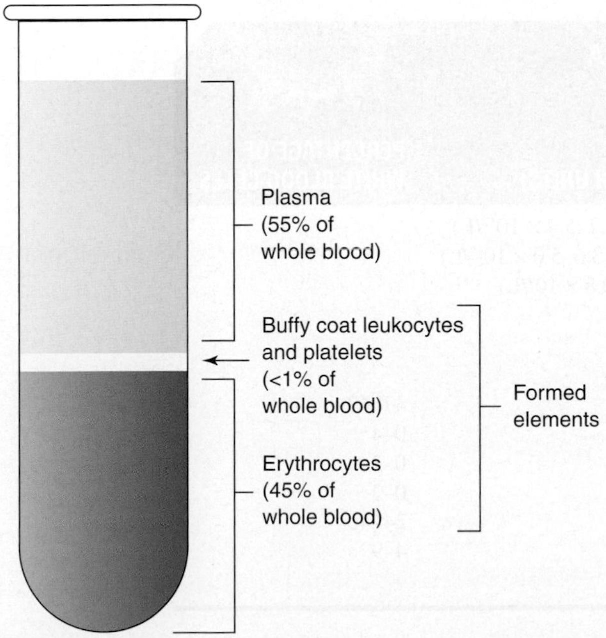

Figure 21.1 • Layering of blood components in an anticoagulated and centrifuged blood sample.

Blood Cells

The formed elements in the blood—the RBCs, WBCs, and thrombocytes—originate in the bone marrow.[2] Figure 21.2 illustrates a blood smear. Although they are called blood cells, only the WBCs are true cells. RBCs have no nuclei or organelles, and thrombocytes are just cell fragments.

Most blood cells do not divide. Therefore, division of cells in the bone marrow must continually renew them. Table 21.2 lists the normal values for the blood cells.

Erythrocytes

The erythrocytes, or RBCs, are the most numerous of the formed elements. They are small, biconcave disks having an average diameter of 6 to 8 μm.[4] They have a thickness at the edge of approximately 2.6 μm, but at the center, thickness is only 0.8 μm.[2] This gives them a large surface area that, combined with

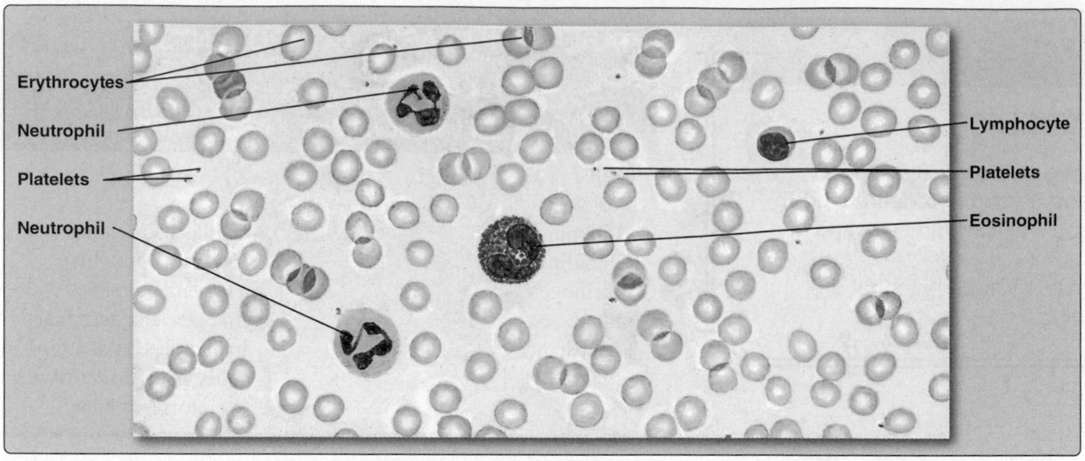

Figure 21.2 • Human blood smear showing erythrocytes, neutrophils, eosinophils, lymphocytes, and platelets. (From Leeper-Woodford S. A., Adkinson L. R. (2016). *Lippincott illustrated reviews: Integrated systems* (Fig. 4.46). Philadelphia, PA: Wolters Kluwer.)

their high elasticity, allows them to easily deform into just about any shape needed in order to move through the small capillaries of the circulatory system.[4]

The primary function of RBCs is to carry oxygen to the body's tissues. This is accomplished by the oxygen-carrying protein, *hemoglobin*, which is contained within each RBC.[1] It is the hemoglobin that imparts the red color to these cells. In addition to transport of oxygen, RBCs contribute to carbon dioxide transport for excretion and to regulate acid–base balance.[1]

The life span of an RBC is approximately 120 days. Ninety percent of the aged RBCs are phagocytosed in the bone marrow, spleen, and liver.[2] The other 10% of RBCs break down within the blood vessels, where they release small, insignificant amounts of hemoglobin into the circulatory system.[2] In order to maintain sufficient numbers of RBCs, the bone marrow continually releases new RBCs as old or damaged RBCs are removed from the circulation.

Leukocytes

The leukocytes, or WBCs, are 10 to 12 μm in diameter and thus much larger than RBCs.[2] However, they constitute only 1% of the total blood volume. They originate in the bone marrow and circulate throughout the lymphoid tissues of the body.

WBCs are crucial to our defense against disease in the following ways:

- They are responsible for the immune response that protects against disease-causing microorganisms.
- They identify and destroy cancer cells.
- They participate in the inflammatory response and wound healing.

TABLE 21.2 BLOOD CELL COUNT OF A TYPICAL ADULT*

BLOOD CELLS	NUMBER OF CELLS/mL (SI UNITS)	PERCENTAGE OF WHITE BLOOD CELLS
Red blood cell count	Male: 4.2–5.4 × 10^6/μL (4.2–5.4 × 10^{12}/L) Female: 3.6–5.0 × 10^6/μL (3.6–5.0 × 10^{12}/L)	
White blood cell count	4.8–10.8 × 10^3/μL (4.8–10.8 × 10^9/L)	
Differential count		
Granulocytes		
Neutrophils		
Segs		47–63
Bands		0–4
Eosinophils		0–3
Basophils		0–2
Lymphocytes		24–40
Monocytes		4–9
Platelet count	150–400 × 10^3	

RBC indices:
MCV (mean corpuscular volume) 80–100 fL.
MCH (mean cell hemoglobin) 27–34 pg/cell.
MCHC (mean corpuscular hemoglobin concentration) 31–35 g/dL.
*Values for infants and children vary significantly according to age.

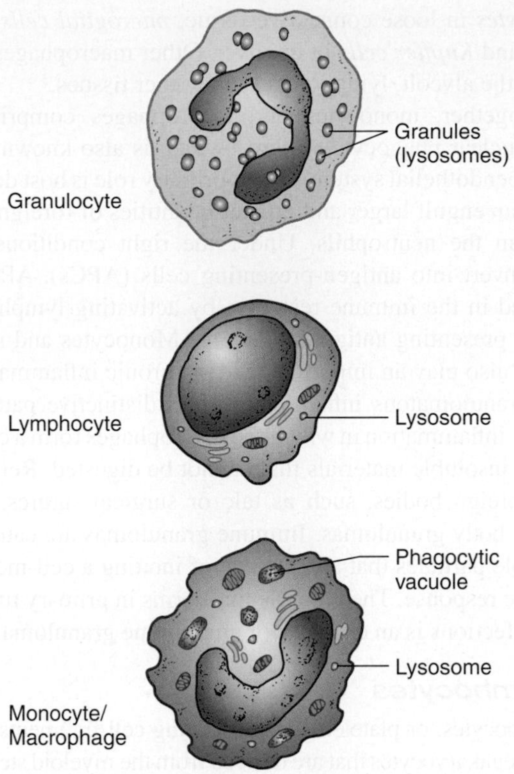

Figure 21.3 • White blood cells.

WBCs are commonly classified into two groups based on the presence or absence of specific cytoplasmic granules that can take up certain stains (Fig. 21.3). WBCs visibly containing these granules are classified as *granulocytes.* WBCs that lack these specific granules are classified as *agranulocytes*.[2]

Granulocytes. Granulocytes are spherical with distinctive multilobar nuclei. All are phagocytes, which have the ability to engulf microbes and other substances. The granules within the granulocyte's cytoplasm contain chemicals and enzymes that break down the engulfed microbes.[5]

Granulocytes are divided into three types—neutrophils, eosinophils, and basophils—according to the staining properties of their specific granules. Eosinophils derive their name from the staining of granules by an acid dye called eosin. Basophils are so named because their granules readily take up a basic dye.[2] Neutrophils derived their name from a former belief that neutrophils were stained by "neutral dyes" that combine acidic and basic dyes; however, the exact mechanism of neutrophils' staining is unknown.[2]

Neutrophils. The neutrophils constitute 55% to 65% of the total WBCs.[2] Because these WBCs have nuclei that are divided into three to five lobes, they are often called *polymorphonuclear leukocytes* or *PMNs*.[2] The stained neutrophil is a pale lilac[6] or tan color.[5]

The neutrophils are primarily responsible for maintaining normal host defenses against invading bacteria and fungi, cell debris, and a variety of foreign substances. (See Chapter 13.) Therefore, they increase in number during bacterial and systemic fungal infections and other instances that call them into action. Neutrophils have a short life span that varies from 5 hours[6] to approximately 4 to 5 days.[1] The pool of circulating neutrophils (*i.e.*, those that are measured in the blood count) is in a closely maintained equilibrium with a similar-sized pool of cells marginating along the walls of small blood vessels. In response to chemotactic factors, the marginating neutrophils deform in order to squeeze through capillary pores to exit the circulation at sites of inflammation.[1]

The bone marrow releases large numbers of neutrophils in response to an acute systemic bacterial infection. Immature neutrophils, called *band cells*, are often released as part of this response. As the stores of mature neutrophils are depleted, band cells make up an increasing component of circulating WBCs. Figure 21.4 illustrates the development stages of the neutrophil.

Eosinophils. Eosinophils are similar in size to neutrophils, but they contain bilobed (two-lobed) nuclei,[2] and their cytoplasmic granules stain a red color.[6] Eosinophils reside primarily in the tissues rather than within the circulation.[7] In the blood, they constitute 1% to 3% of the total WBCs.

Eosinophils have important host defense roles in allergic reactions, parasitic infections, and chronic immune responses associated with conditions such as asthma.[6] Therefore, eosinophils increase in number in response to allergic responses, worm infestations, and asthma.[2] In response to allergies, eosinophils release enzymes such as histaminase to inactivate histamine and other inflammatory substances, thereby decreasing the severity of inflammatory reactions.[2] Although they are phagocytes, the eosinophils in parasitic worm infections

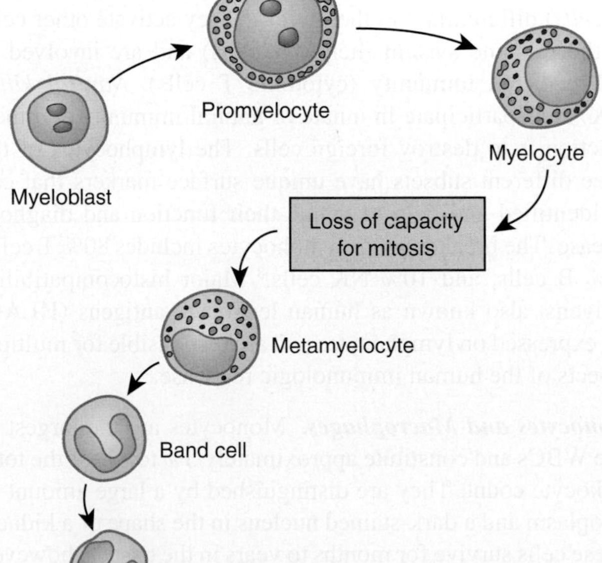

Figure 21.4 • Developmental stages of the neutrophil, which begins its development in the bone marrow as a myeloblast.

are too small to phagocytize the parasite. In these instances, eosinophils use surface markers to attach themselves to the parasite and then kill the parasite through the release of hydrolytic enzymes and toxic proteins.[1]

Basophils. The basophils, also of similar size to neutrophils, are the least numerous of the WBCs, accounting for only 0.3% to 0.5% of the total WBCs. The stained basophil has dark-blue granules that are so large and abundant that they sometimes conceal the appearance of the nucleus.[6] These granules contain heparin, an anticoagulant; histamine, a vasodilator; and other mediators of inflammation such as bradykinin and leukotrienes.[2] In this way, basophils are similar to mast cells. (See Chapter 34.) Like the mast cells and the eosinophils, the basophils are involved in allergic and hypersensitivity reactions.[1]

Agranulocytes. Agranulocytes, also known as *mononuclear leukocytes*, are distinguished from granulocytes by their finer granules and their single-lobed nucleus. The granulocytes are divided into two types—lymphocytes and monocytes.

Lymphocytes. Lymphocytes account for 20% to 30% of the total blood WBCs.[2] They are the main functional cells of the immune system. They move between blood and lymph tissue, where they may be stored for hours or years. Their function in the lymph nodes or spleen is to defend against microorganisms through the immune response.

There are three types of lymphocytes—B lymphocytes, T lymphocytes, and natural killer cells. The *B lymphocytes (B cells)* are so named because they were first recognized as a separate population in the bursa of Fabricius in birds and bursa-equivalent organs (*e.g.*, bone marrow) in mammals. They differentiate to form antibody-producing plasma cells and are involved in humoral-mediated immunity. The *T lymphocytes (T cells)* differentiate in the thymus. They activate other cells of the immune system (helper T cells) and are involved in cell-mediated immunity (cytotoxic T cells). *Natural killer (NK) cells* participate in innate or natural immunity and their function is to destroy foreign cells. The lymphocytes of the three different subsets have unique surface markers that can be identified and help to define their function and diagnose disease. The breakdown of lymphocytes includes 80% T cells, 10% B cells, and 10% NK cells.[8] Major histocompatibility antigens, also known as human leukocyte antigens (HLAs), are expressed on lymphocytes and are responsible for multiple aspects of the human immunologic response.[8]

Monocytes and Macrophages. Monocytes are the largest in size WBCs and constitute approximately 3% to 8% of the total leukocyte count. They are distinguished by a large amount of cytoplasm and a dark-stained nucleus in the shape of a kidney. These cells survive for months to years in the tissues; however, the life span of the circulating monocyte is approximately 1 to 3 days, three to four times longer than that of the granulocytes.[1]

Monocytes are produced in the bone marrow. After leaving the vascular system and entering the tissues, they transform into macrophages. The specific activity of macrophages depends on their location. The macrophages are known as *histiocytes* in loose connective tissue, *microglial cells* in the brain, and *Kupffer cells* in the liver. Other macrophages function in the alveoli, lymph nodes, and other tissues.[3]

Together, monocytes and macrophages comprise the mononuclear phagocyte system,[3] which is also known as the reticuloendothelial system.[5] Their primary role is host defense. They can engulf larger and greater quantities of foreign material than the neutrophils. Under the right conditions, they can convert into antigen-presenting cells (APCs). APCs are involved in the immune response by activating lymphocytes and by presenting antigen to T cells. Monocytes and macrophages also play an important role in chronic inflammation.

Granulomatous inflammation is a distinctive pattern of chronic inflammation in which the macrophages form a capsule around insoluble materials that cannot be digested. Relatively inert foreign bodies, such as talc or surgical sutures, incite foreign body granulomas. Immune granulomas are caused by insoluble particles that are capable of inciting a cell-mediated immune response. The tubercle that forms in primary tuberculosis infections is an example of an immune granuloma.

Thrombocytes

Thrombocytes, or platelets, are circulating cell fragments of the large megakaryocytes that are derived from the myeloid stem cell. They contribute to formation of the platelet plug to help control bleeding after injury to a vessel wall (Fig. 21.5). Their cytoplasmic granules release mediators required for the blood coagulation process. Thrombocytes have a membrane but no nucleus, cannot replicate, and, if not used, last approximately 10 days in the circulation before the phagocytic cells of the spleen remove them.[2]

Formation of Blood Cells (Hematopoiesis)

Hematopoiesis (from the Greek *haima*, "blood," and *poiesis*, "making") is the production of blood cells. It begins in the yolk sac during the second week of embryonic development[2] and then transitions to the liver and spleen around the second month of gestation. At approximately 7 months of gestation, this function is gradually taken over by the bone marrow.[4] The bone marrow continues to serve as the primary site of blood cell production throughout life. In children, this occurs primarily in the distal long bones. In adults, hematopoiesis is largely restricted to the flat bones of the axial skeleton.[4]

Medullary and Extramedullary Hematopoiesis

Medullary hematopoiesis refers to blood cell production that occurs within the bone marrow. The blood-forming population of bone marrow is made up of three types of cells—self-renewing stem cells, differentiated progenitor (parent) cells, and functional mature blood cells. At sites where the marrow is hematopoietically active, it produces so many RBCs that are red, hence the name *red bone marrow*. Fat cells are also present in bone marrow, but they are inactive in terms of blood cell generation. The fat cell can be visualized in the bone marrow in Figure 21.6. Marrow that is made up predominantly of fat

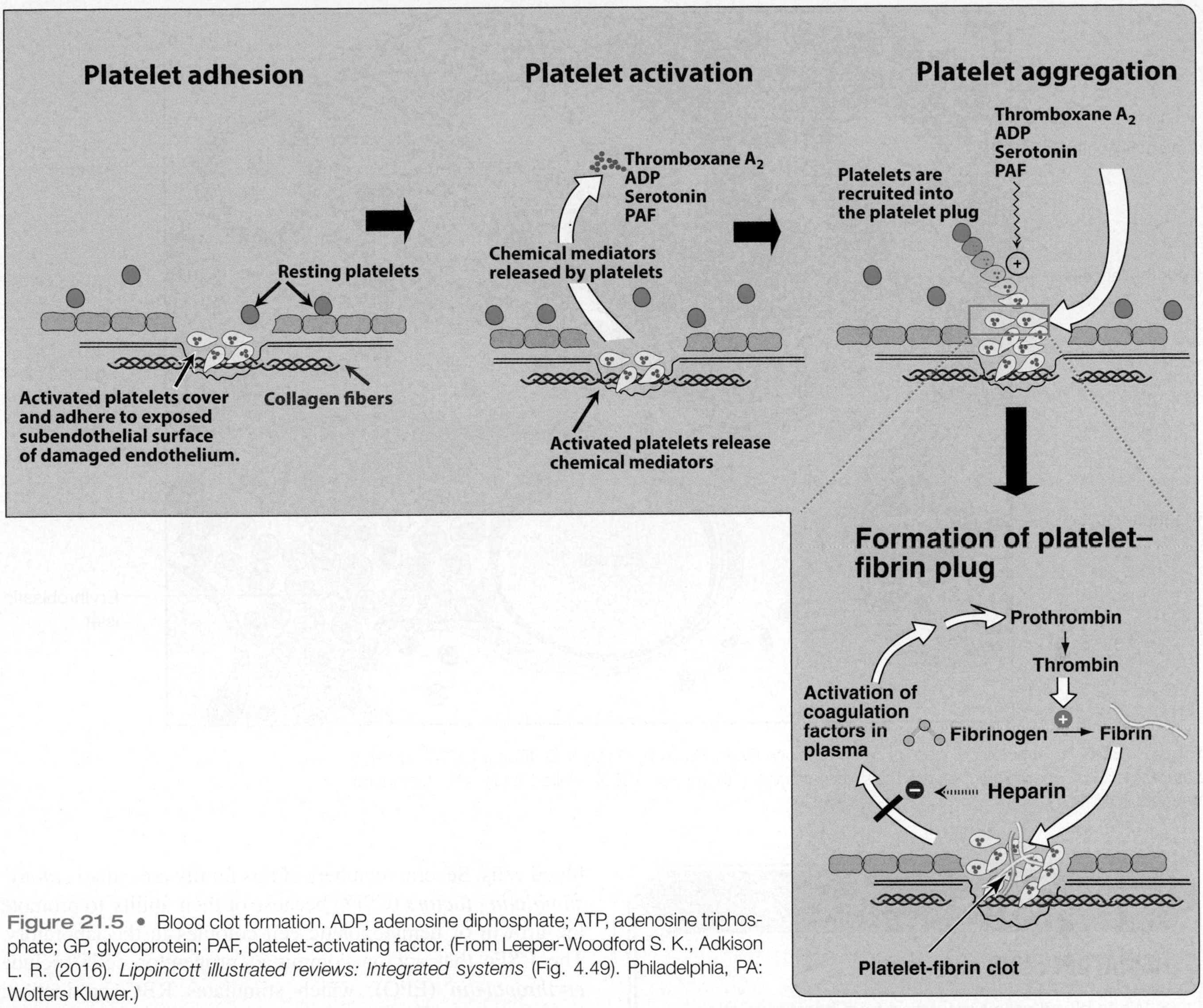

Figure 21.5 • Blood clot formation. ADP, adenosine diphosphate; ATP, adenosine triphosphate; GP, glycoprotein; PAF, platelet-activating factor. (From Leeper-Woodford S. K., Adkison L. R. (2016). *Lippincott illustrated reviews: Integrated systems* (Fig. 4.49). Philadelphia, PA: Wolters Kluwer.)

cells is called *yellow bone marrow*. During active skeletal growth, red marrow in long bones is gradually replaced by yellow marrow. This occurs with the transition from long bone hematopoiesis to axial skeletal hematopoiesis. In adults, red marrow is largely restricted to the flat bones of the pelvis, ribs, and sternum. However, when the demand for red cell replacement increases, as in hemolytic anemia, there can be resubstitution of red marrow for yellow marrow.

Extramedullary hematopoiesis is blood cell production that occurs in places other than within the bone marrow. Although the liver and spleen cease hematopoiesis during fetal development, they retain hematopoietic ability. If the bone marrow becomes incapable of producing sufficient numbers of blood cells, as occurs during some pathologic conditions, the liver and spleen will resume hematopoiesis.[3]

Blood Cell Precursors

All blood cells are derived from *pluripotent stem cells* (Fig. 21.7). As its name implies, pluripotent (from *pluri*, "several," and *potent*, "capable of") cells are capable of producing several types of cells. All of the blood cell precursors of the erythrocyte (*i.e.*, red cell), myelocyte (*i.e.*, granulocyte or monocyte), lymphocyte (*i.e.*, T lymphocyte and B lymphocyte), and megakaryocyte (*i.e.*, thrombocyte) series are derived from these special cells. Pluripotent stem cells have a lifelong potential for proliferation and self-renewal, which makes them an indispensable and lifesaving source of reserve cells for the entire hematopoietic system.

Pluripotent stem cells develop into functionally mature cells through a process of differentiation. Several levels of differentiation lead to the development of committed, unipotential cells, which are the progenitors for each of the blood cell types. These progenitor cells are referred to as *colony-forming units* (CFUs). These progenitor cells have only limited capacity for self-renewal but retain the potential to differentiate into lineage-specific precursor cells. Precursor cells have morphologic characteristics that permit them to be recognized as the first cell of a particular cell line. They have lost their ability for self-renewal but undergo cell division and differentiation, eventually giving rise to mature lymphocytes, myelocytes, megakaryocytes, or erythrocytes.[1]

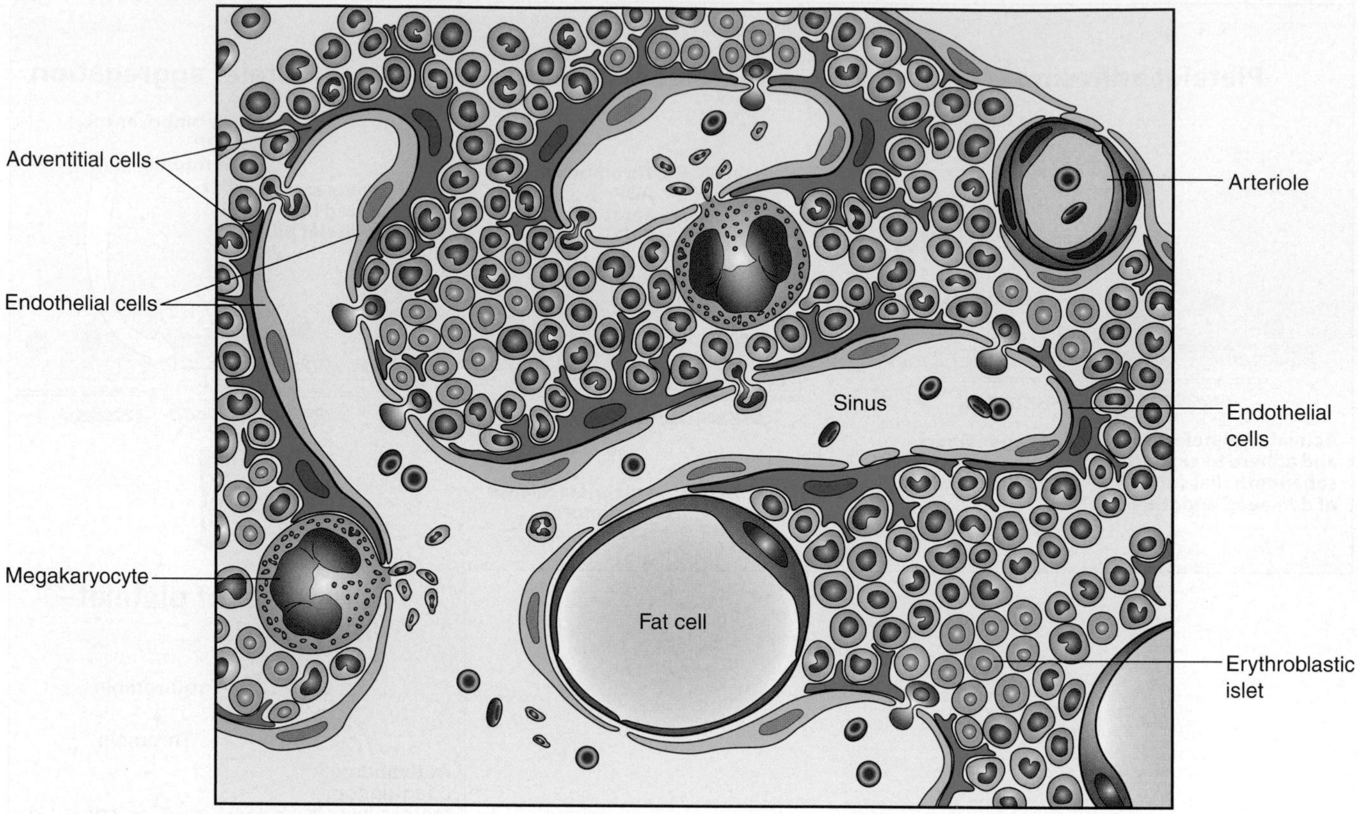

Figure 21.6 • Structure of normal bone marrow. (From Rubin R., Strayer D. (Eds.). (2015). *Rubin's pathology: Clinicopathologic foundations of medicine* (7th ed., p. 1080). Philadelphia, PA: Lippincott Williams & Wilkins.)

KEY POINTS

HEMATOPOIESIS

- White blood cells are formed from hematopoietic stem cells that differentiate into committed progenitor cells, which in turn develop into the myelogenous and lymphocytic lineages needed for the formation of the different blood cell types.
- The growth and reproduction of the different stem cells are controlled by colony-stimulating factors (CSFs) and other cytokines and chemical mediators.

Regulation of Hematopoiesis

Under normal conditions, the numbers and total mass for each type of circulating blood cell remain relatively constant. The blood cells are produced in different numbers according to needs and regulatory factors. This regulation of blood cells is thought to be at least partially controlled by hormone-like growth factors called cytokines. The cytokines are a family of short-lived mediators that stimulate the proliferation, differentiation, and functional activation of the various blood cells.

Many cytokines derived from lymphocytes or bone marrow stromal cells stimulate the growth and production of new blood cells. Several members of this family are called *colony-stimulating factors* (CSFs) because of their ability to promote the growth of hematopoietic cell colonies in the laboratory. The CSFs that act on committed progenitor cells include *erythropoietin* (EPO), which stimulates RBC production; *granulocyte–monocyte colony-stimulating factor* (GM-CSF), which stimulates progenitors for granulocytes, monocytes, erythrocytes, and megakaryocytes; *granulocyte colony–stimulating factor* (G-CSF), which promotes the proliferation of neutrophils; *macrophage colony–stimulating factor* (M-CSF), which induces macrophage colonies; and *thrombopoietin* (TPO), which stimulates the differentiation of thrombocytes. Other cytokines, such as the interleukins, interferons, and tumor necrosis factor, support the proliferation of stem cells and the development of lymphocytes and act synergistically to aid the multiple functions of the CSFs.

The genes for most hematopoietic growth factors have been cloned, and their recombinant proteins have been generated for management of a wide range of clinical conditions. Some examples of the clinically useful factors include EPO, TPO, G-CSF, and GM-CSF. They are used to treat bone marrow failure caused by chemotherapy or aplastic anemia, the anemia of kidney failure and cancer, hematopoietic neoplasms, infectious diseases such as acquired immunodeficiency syndrome (AIDS), and congenital and myeloproliferative disorders. Growth factors are used to

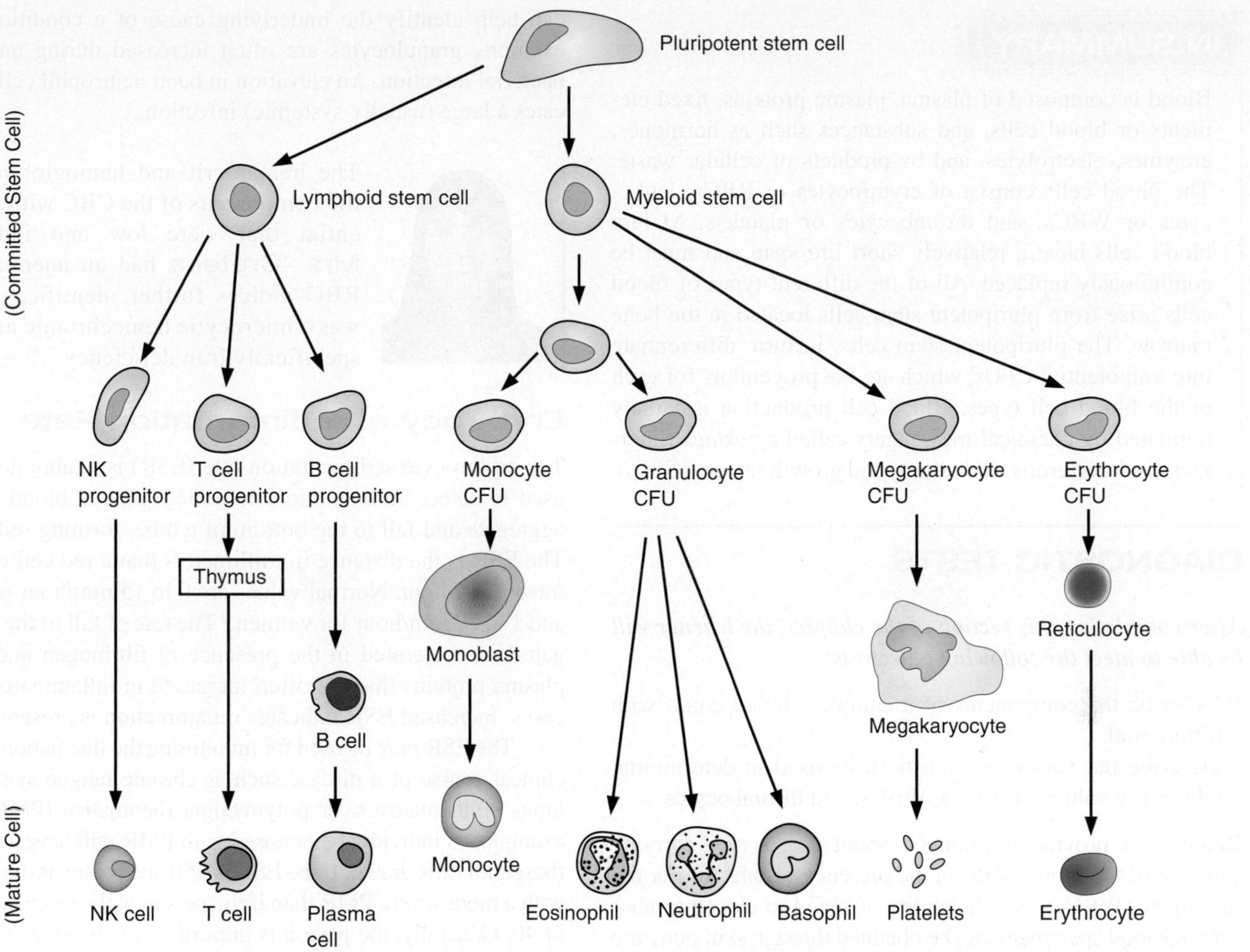

Figure 21.7 • Major maturational stages of blood cells. CFU, colony-forming unit; NK, natural killer cell.

increase peripheral stem cells for transplantation and to accelerate cell proliferation after bone marrow engraftment. Many of these uses are still investigational and new factors are being created.

Disorders of Hematopoietic Stem Cells

Underproliferation of the stem cell population may result in failure to produce one or several cell types. For example, aplastic anemia develops when the multipotent stem cells fail to grow and provide cells for differentiation. *Pancytopenia* (from *pan*, "all"; *cyto*, "cell"; and *penia*, "lacking") is a reduction in the number of all blood cell types. Persons with pancytopenia have concomitant anemia (low RBC levels), thrombocytopenia (low thrombocyte levels), and granulocytopenia (low granulocyte levels).

Myeloproliferative diseases are characterized by a hypercellular bone marrow and elevated blood cell counts. Unregulated overproduction of the red cell mass is termed polycythemia. Thrombocytosis occurs when the bone marrow produces too many thrombocytes. Leukemias represent a spectrum of diseases characterized by an abnormal proliferation of WBCs.

Management of these and many other disorders uses hematopoietic stem cells as part of the treatment. Many people with leukemia obtain stem cell transplants that greatly impact their ability to have a remission from the disease. Stem cell transplants focus on correcting bone marrow failure, immunodeficiencies, hematologic defects and malignancies, and inherited errors of metabolism. Sources of the stem cells include bone marrow and umbilical cord blood, which replenish the recipient with a normal population of pluripotent stem cells. Stem cell transplants may be derived from the recipient (autologous) or from a histocompatible donor (allogeneic). Autologous transplants are often used to replenish stem cells after high-dose chemotherapy or irradiation. Umbilical cord blood from HLA-matched donors is a transplant option for children and carries less risk of graft-versus-host disease. See Chapters 22, 23, and 24 for a more detailed description of the pathogenesis, clinical manifestations, and treatment of these stem cell disorders.

IN SUMMARY

Blood is composed of plasma, plasma proteins, fixed elements or blood cells, and substances such as hormones, enzymes, electrolytes, and by-products of cellular waste. The blood cells consist of erythrocytes or RBCs, leukocytes or WBCs, and thrombocytes or platelets. Mature blood cells have a relatively short life span and must be continuously replaced. All of the different types of blood cells arise from pluripotent stem cells located in the bone marrow. The pluripotent stem cells, in turn, differentiate into unipotential CFUs, which are the progenitors for each of the blood cell types. Blood cell production is largely regulated by chemical messengers called *cytokines* (interleukins, interferons, and others) and growth factors (CSFs).

DIAGNOSTIC TESTS

After completing this section of the chapter, the learner will be able to meet the following objectives:

- Describe the components of a complete blood count with differential.
- Describe the various diagnostic tests used in determining laboratory values for RBCs, WBCs, and thrombocytes.

Blood tests provide information about the oxygen-carrying capacity of the blood (RBCs), the presence of infection or tissue injury (WBCs), and the ability of blood to clot (thrombocytes). Blood specimens can be obtained through skin puncture (capillary blood), venipuncture, arterial puncture, or bone marrow aspiration. Each specimen has a specific procedure that correlates to what collection tube to use; whether the specimen should be gently agitated after collection; whether the specimen needs to be refrigerated, iced, or not; and other specific details that must be followed in order to generate accurate findings.

Blood Count

The blood count provides information regarding the number of blood cells and their structural and functional characteristics. A complete blood count (CBC) is a commonly performed laboratory test that determines the number of RBCs, WBCs, and thrombocytes per unit of blood. Measurements of hemoglobin, hematocrit, mean corpuscular volume (MCV), mean corpuscular hemoglobin concentration (MCHC), and mean cell hemoglobin (MCH) are usually included in the CBC.

The MCV, MCHC, and MCH, which are called the RBC indices, reflect the size, shape, or color of cells. These indices are often used to determine what type of anemia a person has. For example, a low MCV indicates a small cell, and a low MCHC and MCH indicate a pale cell. These findings are commonly seen in iron deficiency anemia.

The white cell differential count is the determination of the relative proportions (percentages) of individual white cell types. Knowing which type of WBC is increased or decreased can help identify the underlying cause of a condition. For example, granulocytes are often increased during an acute bacterial infection. An elevation in band neutrophil cells indicates a large (usually systemic) infection.

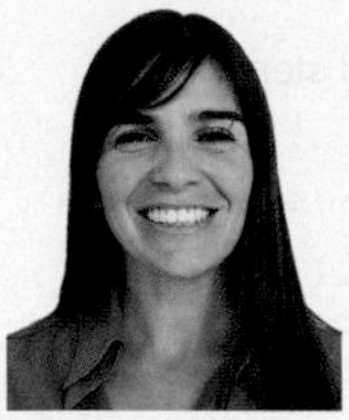

The hematocrit and hemoglobin were the components of the CBC with differential that were low and indicated Mrs. Cretena had an anemia. The RBC indices further identified that it was a microcytic hemochromic anemia, specifically iron deficiency.

Erythrocyte Sedimentation Rate

The erythrocyte sedimentation rate (ESR) is a laboratory test used to detect inflammation. In anticoagulated blood, RBCs aggregate and fall to the bottom of a tube, forming sediment. The ESR is the distance in millimeters that a red cell column travels in 1 hour. Normal values are 0 to 15 mm/hour for men and 1 to 20 mm/hour for women.[9] The rate of fall of the aggregates is accelerated in the presence of fibrinogen and other plasma proteins that are often increased in inflammatory diseases. Increased ESR indicates inflammation is present.

The ESR may be used for monitoring the fluctuations in the clinical course of a disease such as chronic fatigue syndrome, lupus erythematosus, or polymyalgia rheumatica (PMR). For example, an individual diagnosed with PMR will have an initial (baseline) ESR drawn. If the ESR is >60, the person is diagnosed with a more severe PMR than if the person had an elevated ESR of 40. Generally, the person is prescribed prednisone, and then at follow-up visits, the dose of prednisone will be gradually decreased depending on the ESR and the person's symptoms.

Bone Marrow Aspiration and Biopsy

Tests of bone marrow function are done on samples obtained using bone marrow aspiration or bone marrow biopsy. Bone marrow aspiration is performed with a special needle inserted into the bone marrow cavity, through which a sample of marrow is withdrawn. Usually, the posterior iliac crest is used in all people older than 12 to 18 months of age. Other sites include the anterior iliac crest, sternum, and spinous processes T10 through L4. The sternum is not commonly used in children because the cavity is too shallow and there is danger of mediastinal and cardiac perforation. Because aspiration disturbs the marrow architecture, this technique is used primarily to determine the type of cells present and their relative numbers for diagnostic purposes. Stained smears of bone marrow aspirates are usually subjected to several studies, including determination of the erythroid to myeloid cell count (*i.e.*, normal ratio is 1:3), differential cell count, search for abnormal cells, evaluation of iron stores in reticulum cells, and special stains and immunochemical studies.[9]

Bone marrow biopsy is done with a special biopsy needle inserted into the posterior iliac crest. It is likely a bone marrow biopsy (instead of a bone marrow aspiration) will be needed to diagnose an acute leukemia; the aspirate procedure may not obtain a specimen, given that there are so many WBCs in the marrow. This would also be true with someone who was pancytopenic, and there is little to no hematopoietic activity.[9] Biopsy removes an actual sample of bone marrow tissue and allows study of the architecture of the tissue. It is used to determine the marrow-to-fat ratio and the presence of fibrosis, plasma cells, granulomas, and cancer cells. The major hazard of these procedures is the slight risk of hemorrhage. This risk is increased in people with a reduced platelet count or any type of bleeding tendency.

IN SUMMARY

Diagnostic tests of the blood include the CBC, the ESR, and bone marrow aspiration and biopsy. The CBC is used to describe the number and characteristics of the RBCs, WBCs, and thrombocytes. The ESR is used to detect inflammation. Bone marrow aspiration is removal of the fluid portion of marrow from within the bone marrow cavity. Bone marrow aspirate analysis focuses on cellular morphology and determination of a differential cell count. A bone marrow biopsy removes a sample of solid bone marrow, which permits study of the marrow's overall cellularity and detection of focal lesions and the extent of the marrow by pathologic processes.

GERIATRIC Considerations

- Active bone marrow is replaced with fat as people age, limiting the body's response to needs for blood cells.[10]
- Leukopenia (decreased white blood cell count) and anemia (decreased red blood cell count) are more common in older adults because of limited bone marrow function.[10]
- Limited growth factor in the aging person causes a decrease in erythropoiesis.[10]
- Myeloid malignancies are more common in older adults because of stem cell damage in the DNA.[10]

PEDIATRIC Considerations

- The bone marrow is the site for hematopoiesis beginning the 20th week of gestation and into young adulthood.[11]
- Infants and adolescents are more susceptible to iron deficiency anemia because of growth spurts and nutritional deficits.[11]
- Ethnicity, white or East Asian children, contributes to a lower hemoglobin value.[11]
- Newborns' red blood cells demonstrate anisocytosis (a variation in size) and poikilocytosis (a variation in shape).[11]
- Stem cells formed in the liver commit to a unique lineage: myeloid, monocytic, lymphoid, or platelets.[11]

REVIEW EXERCISES

1. A 14-year-old boy is admitted to the emergency department with severe abdominal pain and a tentative diagnosis of appendicitis. His white blood cell count shows an elevated number of white blood cells with an increased percentage of "band cells."
   A. *Explain the significance of this finding.*
2. Many of the primary immunodeficiency disorders, in which there is a defect in the development of immune cells of T- or B-lymphocyte origin, can be cured with allogeneic stem cell transplantation from an unaffected donor.
   A. *Explain why stem cells are used rather than mature lymphocytes. You might want to refer to Figure 21.7.*
   B. *Describe how the stem cells would go about the process of repopulating the bone marrow.*

References

1. Hall J. E. (2015). *Guyton and Hall textbook of medical physiology* (13th ed., pp. 445–464, 483–495). Philadelphia, PA: Elsevier Saunders.
2. Pawlina W. (2016). *Histology: A text and atlas with correlated cell and molecular biology* (7th ed., pp. 270–312). Philadelphia, PA: Wolters-Kluwer.
3. McKenzie S. (2014). *Clinical laboratory hematology* (3rd ed., pp. 2–5, 26–34). Boston, MA: Pearson.
4. Ciesla B. (2012). *Hematology in practice* (2nd ed., pp. 32–58). Philadelphia, PA: F. A. Davis.
5. Hutson, P. R. (2017). Hematology: Red and white blood cell tests. In Lee M. (Ed.), *Basic skills in interpreting laboratory data* (6th ed.). Bethesda, MD: American Society of Health-System Pharmacists.
6. Aster J. C., Bunn H. F. (2017). *Pathophysiology of blood disorders* (2nd ed.). New York, NY: McGraw-Hill.
7. Weller P. F., Klion A. D. (2017). Approach to the patient with unexplained eosinophilia. In Mahoney D. H., Bochner B. S. (Eds.), *UpToDate*. Waltham, MA: UpToDate Inc. Available: http://www.uptodate.com
8. Warren J. S., Strayer D. S. (2015). Immunopathology. In Rubin R., Strayer D. (Eds.), *Rubin's pathology: Clinicopathologic foundations of medicine* (7th ed., pp. 131–168). Philadelphia, PA: Lippincott Williams & Wilkins.
9. Fischbach F., Dunning M. (2009). *A manual of laboratory and diagnostic tests* (8th ed.). Philadelphia, PA: Lippincott Williams & Wilkins.
10. Hinkle J. L., Cheever K. H. (2018). Assessment of hematologic function and treatment modalities. In *Brunner & Suddarth's textbook of medical-surgical nursing* (14th ed., p. 908). Philadelphia, PA: Wolters Kluwer.
11. Bowden V. R., Greenberg C. S. (2014). The child with altered hematologic status. In *Children and their families the continuum of nursing care* (3rd ed., pp. 1172–1226). Philadelphia, PA: Wolters Kluwer.

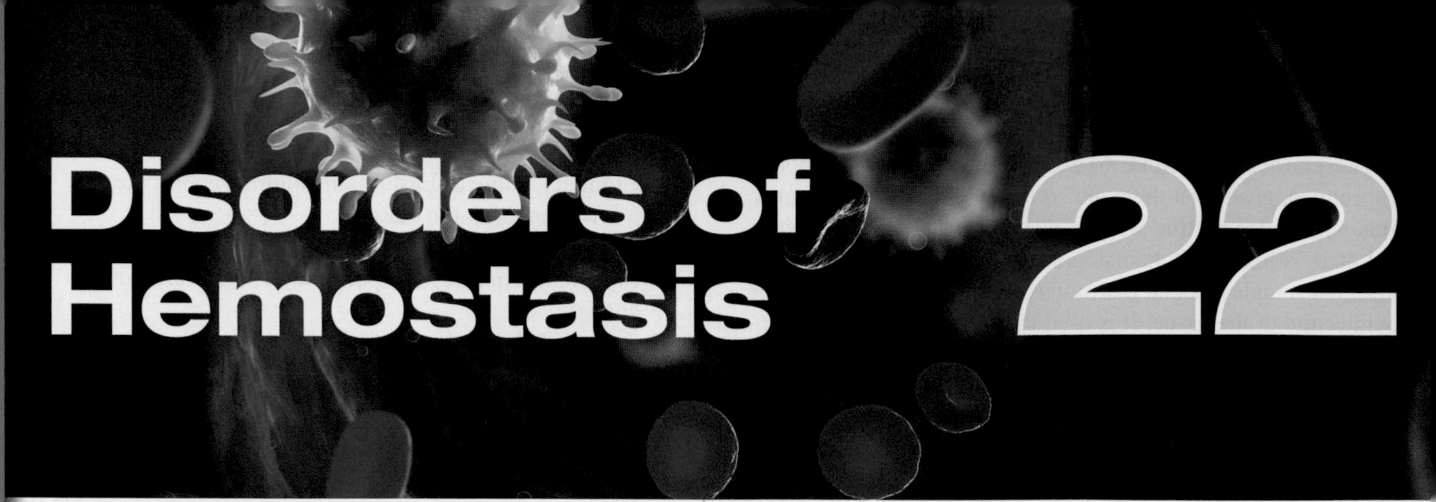

Disorders of Hemostasis 22

Paige Wimberley

Hemostasis refers to the stoppage of blood flow. The normal process of hemostasis is regulated by a complex array of activators and inhibitors that maintain blood fluidity and prevent blood from leaving the vascular compartment. Hemostasis is normal when it seals a blood vessel to prevent blood loss and hemorrhage. It is abnormal when it causes inappropriate blood clotting or when clotting is insufficient to stop the flow of blood from the vascular compartment. Disorders of hemostasis fall into two main categories—the inappropriate formation of clots within the vascular system (thrombosis) and the failure of blood to clot in response to an appropriate stimulus (bleeding).

MECHANISMS OF HEMOSTASIS

After completing this section of the chapter, the learner will be able to meet the following objectives:

- Describe the three stages of hemostasis.
- Describe the purpose of blood coagulation.
- Explain the functions of clot retraction and clot dissolution.

Hemostasis is divided into three stages:

1. Vascular constriction
2. Formation of the platelet plug
3. Blood coagulation[1]

During the process of hemostasis, hairlike fibrin strands glue the aggregated platelets together to form the structural basis of the blood clot. In the presence of fibrin, plasma becomes gel-like and traps red blood cells and other formed elements in the blood. Hemostasis is complete when fibrous tissue grows into the clot and seals the hole in the vessel.

Vascular Constriction

Vessel spasm constricts the vessel and reduces blood flow. It is a transient event that usually lasts minutes or hours.[2] Vessel spasm is initiated by endothelial injury and caused by local and humoral mechanisms. Neural reflexes and thromboxane A_2 (TXA_2), a prostaglandin released from platelets, and other mediators such as serotonin, contribute to vasoconstriction.[2] The most powerful vasoconstrictor is endothelin 1.[1] Prostacyclin, another prostaglandin released from the vessel endothelium, produces vasodilation and inhibits platelet aggregation in the surrounding uninjured endothelium.[2]

Formation of the Platelet Plug

Small breaks in the vessel wall are often sealed with a platelet plug rather than a blood clot. Platelets, or *thrombocytes*, arise from *megakaryocytes*.[1] The platelet has a half-life of approximately 8 to 12 days, and then, it is broken down and eliminated by macrophages.[1] The normal serum concentration is about 150,000 to 400,000 platelets per microliter (μL) of blood.[3] Platelet production is controlled by a protein called *thrombopoietin* that causes proliferation and maturation of megakaryocytes.[1] The sources of thrombopoietin include the liver, kidney, smooth muscle, and bone marrow.

Platelets are anuclear cell fragments but have many characteristics of cells. Platelets are spherically shaped, with an asymmetrical plasma membrane that is covered with a coat of glycoproteins, glycosaminoglycans, and coagulation proteins (Fig. 22.1). One of the important glycoproteins is GPIIb/IIIa, which binds fibrinogen and bridges platelets to one another.[1] The platelet shape is maintained by microtubules and actin and myosin filaments that support the cell membrane. Platelets have mitochondria and enzyme systems capable of producing adenosine triphosphate (ATP) and adenosine diphosphate (ADP). They also have the enzymes needed for synthesis of the prostaglandin, TXA_2, required for their function in hemostasis.

Platelets contain two specific types of granules (α- and δ-granules) that release mediators for hemostasis.[2] The α-granules express the P-selectin, an adhesive protein, on their surface and contain fibrinogen, von Willebrand factor (vWF), fibronectin, factors V and VIII, platelet factor 4 (a heparin-binding chemokine), platelet-derived growth factor (PDGF), transforming growth factor-alpha (TGF-α), and thrombospondin.[3] The release of growth factors results in the proliferation and growth of vascular endothelial cells, smooth muscle cells, and fibroblasts and is important in vessel repair. The δ-granules, or dense granules, contain ADP and ATP, ionized calcium, histamine, serotonin, and epinephrine, which contribute to vasoconstriction.[3]

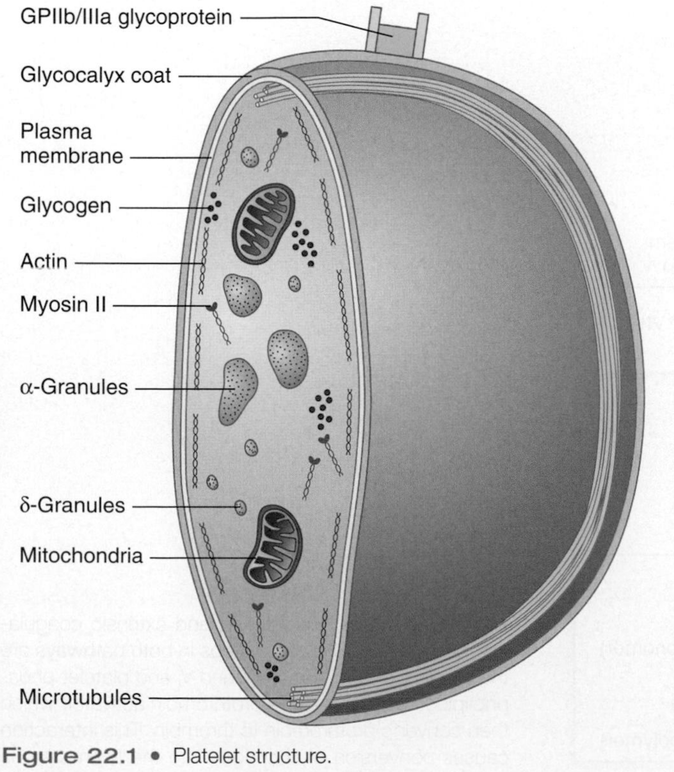

Figure 22.1 • Platelet structure.

Platelet plug formation involves activation, adhesion, and aggregation of platelets. Platelets are attracted to a damaged vessel wall, become activated, and change from smooth disks to spiny spheres, exposing glycoprotein receptors on their surfaces. Platelet adhesion requires a protein molecule called *von Willebrand factor*, which leaks into the injured tissue from the plasma.[1] This factor is produced by the endothelial cells of blood vessels and circulates in the blood as a carrier protein for coagulation factor VIII. Adhesion to the vessel subendothelial layer occurs when the platelet receptor binds to vWF at the injury site, linking the platelet to exposed collagen fibers.[3]

Platelet aggregation occurs soon after adhesion. The secretion of the contents of the platelet granules mediates it. The release of the dense body contents is particularly important because calcium is required for the coagulation component of hemostasis, and ADP is a mediator of platelet aggregation. ADP release also facilitates the release of ADP from other platelets, leading to amplification of the aggregation process. Besides ADP, platelets secrete the prostaglandin TXA_2, which is an important stimulus for platelet aggregation. The combined actions of ADP and TXA_2 lead to the expansion of the enlarging platelet aggregate, which becomes the primary hemostatic plug. Stabilization of the platelet plug occurs as the coagulation pathway is activated on the platelet surface, and fibrinogen is converted to fibrin. This creates a fibrin meshwork that cements the platelets and other blood components together.[1] P-selectin is also part of the platelet aggregation process because it binds leukocytes, which, with platelet substances such as PDGF, participate in healing of the vessel wall.[2]

The platelet membrane plays an important role in platelet adhesion and the coagulation process. The coat of glycoproteins on its surface controls interactions with the vessel endothelium. Platelets normally avoid adherence to the endothelium but interact with injured areas of the vessel wall and the deeper exposed collagen.[1] Glycoprotein (GPIIb/IIIa) receptors on the platelet membrane bind fibrinogen and link platelets together. Defective platelet plug formation causes bleeding in people who are deficient in platelets or vWF. In addition to sealing vascular breaks, platelets play an almost continuous role in maintaining normal vascular integrity. They may supply growth factors for endothelial and arterial smooth muscle cells.[1] Most platelet defects result in bleeding, which is usually superficial and localized.[4]

Platelet inhibitors are important pharmacologic agents that work at different points in the adhesion–activation–aggregation progression.[5] Cyclooxygenase-1 (COX-1) inhibitors (such as aspirin) clot formation in people who are at risk for myocardial infarction, stroke, or peripheral artery disease. Low-dose aspirin therapy inhibits prostaglandin synthesis, including TXA_2.

Clopidogrel and ticlopidine achieve their antiplatelet effects by inhibiting the ADP pathway in platelets. Unlike aspirin, these drugs have an effect on prostaglandin synthesis. Both clopidogrel and ticlopidine prolong the bleeding time. However, the most serious side effects of ticlopidine have been neutropenia and thrombotic thrombocytopenic purpura (TTP).[5]

Drugs that act as GPIIb/IIIa receptor inhibitors (tirofiban, eptifibatide, abciximab) have been developed for use in the treatment of acute coronary syndromes.[5] However, acute and delayed thrombocytopenia has been reported after use of these agents, suggesting that further investigation is needed to understand the mechanisms leading to the thrombocytopenia and improve methods for detection of this complication.[5]

KEY POINTS

HEMOSTASIS

- Hemostasis is the orderly, stepwise process for stopping bleeding that involves vasospasm, formation of a platelet plug, and the development of a fibrin clot.
- The blood clotting process requires the presence of platelets produced in the bone marrow, vWF generated by the vessel endothelium, and clotting factors synthesized in the liver, using vitamin K.

Blood Coagulation

The coagulation cascade is part of the hemostatic process. It is a stepwise process resulting in the conversion of the soluble plasma protein, fibrinogen, into fibrin. The insoluble fibrin strands create a meshwork that cements platelets and other blood components together to form the clot.

Many substances that promote clotting (procoagulation factors) or inhibit it (anticoagulation factors) control the coagulation process. Each of the procoagulation or coagulation factors, identified by Roman numerals, performs a specific step in the coagulation process. The activation of one procoagulation factor or proenzyme is designed to activate the next factor in the sequence (cascade effect). Because most of the inactive procoagulation factors are present in the blood at all times, the multistep process ensures that a massive episode of intravascular clotting does not occur. It also means that abnormalities of the clotting process occur when one or more of the factors are deficient or when conditions lead to inappropriate activation of any of the steps.

Most of the coagulation factors are proteins synthesized in the liver. Vitamin K is necessary for the synthesis of factors II, VII, IX, and X, prothrombin, and protein C. If there is a deficiency of vitamin K or liver failure so that not enough prothrombin is created, a bleeding tendency will develop.[1] Calcium (factor IV) is required in all but the first two steps of the clotting process.[1] The body usually has sufficient amounts of calcium for these reactions. Inactivation of the calcium ion prevents blood from clotting when it is removed from the body. The addition of citrate to blood stored for transfusion purposes prevents clotting by chelating ionic calcium. Ethylenediaminetetraacetic acid (EDTA), another chelator, is often added to blood samples used for analysis in the clinical laboratory.

The coagulation process results from the activation of what have traditionally been designated the *intrinsic* and the *extrinsic* pathways, both of which form prothrombin activator[1,3,4] (Fig. 22.2). The intrinsic pathway, which is a

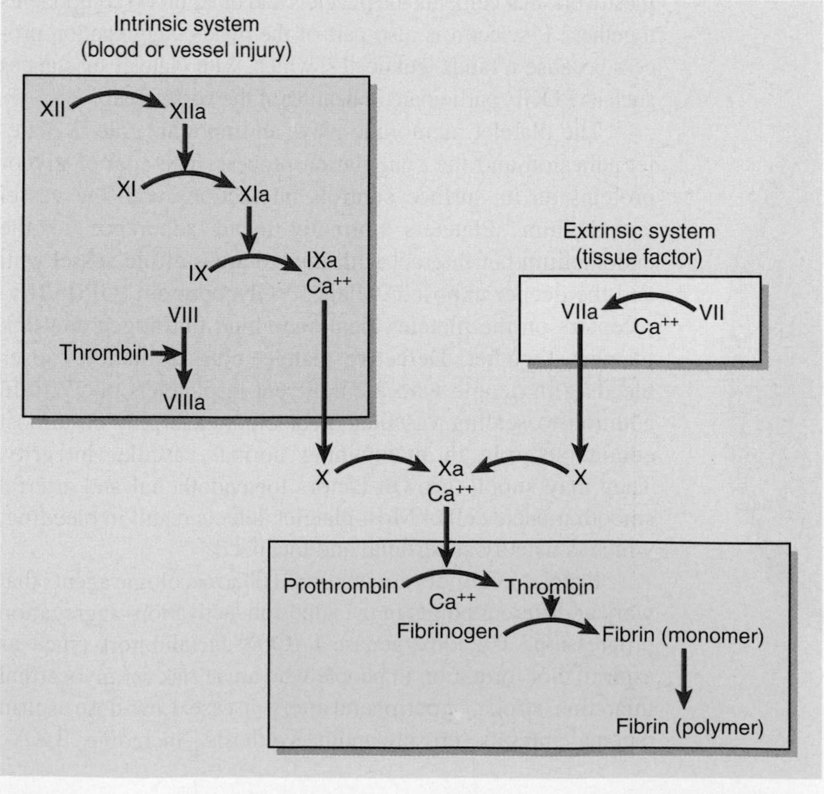

Figure 22.2 • The intrinsic and extrinsic coagulation pathways. The terminal steps in both pathways are the same. Calcium, factors X and V, and platelet phospholipids combine to form prothrombin activator, which then converts prothrombin to thrombin. This interaction causes conversion of fibrinogen into the fibrin strands that create the insoluble blood clot.

relatively slow process (can cause clotting in 1 to 6 minutes), begins in the circulation with the activation of factor XII.[1] The extrinsic pathway, which is a much faster process (can cause clotting in 15 seconds), begins with trauma to the blood vessel or surrounding tissues and the release of tissue factor or tissue thromboplastin, an adhesive lipoprotein, from the subendothelial cells.[1,3] It is composed of phospholipids from the membranes along with a lipoprotein complex that acts as a proteolytic enzyme.[1] The terminal steps in both pathways are the same—the activation of factor X and the conversion of prothrombin to thrombin. Thrombin then acts as an enzyme to convert fibrinogen to fibrin, the material that stabilizes a clot. Both pathways are needed for normal hemostasis, and many interrelations exist between them. Each system is activated when blood passes out of the vascular system. The intrinsic system is activated as blood comes in contact with collagen in the injured vessel wall. The extrinsic system is activated when blood is exposed to tissue extracts. However, bleeding that occurs because of defects in the extrinsic system usually is not as severe as that resulting from defects in the intrinsic pathway.[1,3]

Blood coagulation is regulated by several natural anticoagulants. Antithrombin III inactivates coagulation factors and neutralizes thrombin, the last enzyme in the pathway for the conversion of fibrinogen to fibrin. When antithrombin III is complexed with naturally occurring heparin, its action is accelerated to inactivate thrombin, factor Xa, and other coagulation factors. This complex activation provides protection against uncontrolled thrombus formation on the endothelial surface.[1,5]

Protein C, a plasma protein, acts as an anticoagulant by inactivating factors V and VIII. Protein C or PC antigen (factor V Leiden) is produced in the liver and prevents thrombosis. Protein C deficiency is 35% to 58% congenital but can also be acquired if one has severe liver failure, vitamin K deficiency, or malignancy.[8] This disorder is an inherited defect in factor V and causes increased risk for clotting. It is able to be measured by a protein C resistance test, and the normal range should be between 0.60 and 1.25 of normal PC antigen.[8] Women with factor V Leiden combined with the prothrombotic influence of pregnancy are at high risk for adverse pregnancy outcomes such as venous thromboembolism (VTE) disorders, preeclampsia, fetal loss, and placental abruption.[6]

Protein S, another plasma protein, accelerates the action of protein C. A deficiency of either protein C or S puts one at risk for thrombosis. A protein S test is performed to determine if the deficiency is inherited or acquired because often people with autoimmune disorders are at risk for protein S deficiency.[4] The normal range for females is 0.50 to 1.20 of normal activity, and for males, the range is 0.60 to 1.30.[7]

Plasmin breaks down fibrin into fibrin degradation products that act as anticoagulants. It has been suggested that some of these natural anticoagulants may play a role in the bleeding that occurs with disseminated intravascular coagulation (DIC).

Anticoagulant drugs, such as warfarin and heparin, are used to prevent thromboembolic disorder (i.e., deep vein thrombosis and pulmonary embolism). Warfarin acts by decreasing prothrombin and other procoagulation factors. It alters vitamin K in a manner that reduces its ability to participate in synthesis of the vitamin K–dependent coagulation factors in the liver. Warfarin is readily absorbed after oral administration. Its maximum effect takes 36 to 72 hours because of the varying half-lives of preformed clotting factors that remain in the circulation. Heparin is naturally formed and released in small amounts by mast cells in connective tissue surrounding capillaries. Pharmacologic preparations of heparin are extracted from animal tissues. Heparin binds to antithrombin III, causing a conformational change that increases the ability of antithrombin III to inactivate thrombin, factor Xa, and other clotting factors. By promoting the inactivation of clotting factors, heparin ultimately suppresses the formation of fibrin. Heparin is unable to cross the membranes of the gastrointestinal tract and must be given by injection, usually by intravenous infusion. Low molecular weight heparins have been developed that inhibit activation of factor X but have little effect on thrombin and other coagulation factors. The low molecular weight heparins are given by subcutaneous injection and require less frequent administration and monitoring compared with the standard (unfractionated) heparin.

Warfarin has a narrow therapeutic window, leading to many potential complications. In addition, the person needs to have frequent laboratory testing of their anticoagulant time with an International Normalized Ratio (INR) test.[8] Therefore, new oral anticoagulants (NOAC) have been developed. The mechanism of action of NOACs is more specific than vitamin K antagonists (VKA); NOACs inhibit coagulation factor IIa or activated factor Xa. Advantages of NOAC include the rapidity of onset, fewer interactions with food and other drugs, and a more predictable anticoagulant effect.[9]

Clot Retraction

Clot retraction normally occurs within 20 to 60 minutes after a clot has formed, contributing to hemostasis by squeezing serum from the clot and joining the edges of the broken vessel.[1] Platelets, through the action of their actin and myosin filaments, also contribute to clot retraction and hemostasis. Clot retraction requires large numbers of platelets, and failure of clot retraction is indicative of a low platelet count.

Clot Dissolution

The dissolution of a blood clot begins shortly after its formation. This allows blood flow to be reestablished and permanent tissue repair to take place. The process by which a blood clot dissolves is called *fibrinolysis*. As with clot formation, clot dissolution requires a sequence of steps controlled by activators and inhibitors. Plasminogen, the proenzyme for the fibrinolytic process, normally is present in the blood in its inactive form. It is converted into its active form, plasmin, by plasminogen activators formed in the vascular endothelium, liver, and kidneys. The plasmin formed from plasminogen digests the fibrin strands of the clot and certain clotting factors, such as fibrinogen, factor V, factor VIII, prothrombin, and factor XII. Circulating plasmin is rapidly inactivated by α_2-plasmin inhibitor, which limits the fibrinolytic process to the local clot and prevents it from occurring in the entire circulation.[10]

Two naturally occurring plasminogen activators are tissue-type plasminogen activator and urokinase-type plasminogen activator. The liver, plasma, and vascular endothelium are the major sources of physiologic activators. These activators are released in response to a number of stimuli, including vasoactive drugs, venous occlusion, elevated body temperature, and exercise. The activators are unstable and rapidly inactivated by inhibitors synthesized by the endothelium and the liver. For this reason, chronic liver disease may cause altered fibrinolytic activity. A major inhibitor, plasminogen activator inhibitor-1, in high concentrations has been associated with deep vein thrombosis, coronary artery disease, and myocardial infarction.[1] Several tissue plasminogen activators (alteplase, reteplase, tenecteplase), produced by recombinant DNA technology, are available for use in treatment of acute myocardial infarction, acute ischemic stroke, and pulmonary embolism.

Understanding Hemostasis

Hemostasis, which refers to the stoppage of blood flow, is divided into three stages:

1. Vessel vasoconstriction
2. Formation of the platelet plug
3. Development of a blood clot as a result of the coagulation process

Clot retraction and clot dissolution are also significant to hemostasis. The process involves the interaction of substrates, enzymes, protein cofactors, and calcium ions that circulate in the blood or are released from platelets and cells in the vessel wall.

Vessel Vasoconstriction

Injury to a blood vessel causes vascular smooth muscle in the vessel wall to contract. This instantaneously reduces the flow of blood from the vessel rupture. Both local nervous reflexes and local humoral factors such as TXA_2, which is released from platelets, contribute to the vasoconstriction.

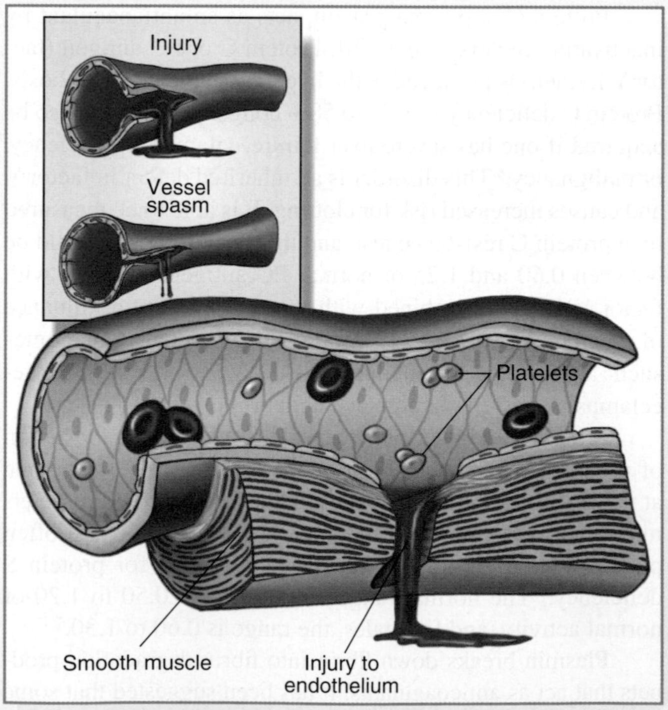

Understanding Hemostasis *(Continued)*

Formation of the Platelet Plug

Seconds after vessel injury, vWF, released from the endothelium, binds to platelet receptors, causing adhesion of the platelets to the exposed collagen fibers **(inset)**. As the platelets adhere to the collagen fibers on the damaged vessel wall, they become activated and release ADP and TXA_2. The ADP and TXA_2 attract additional platelets, leading to platelet aggregation.

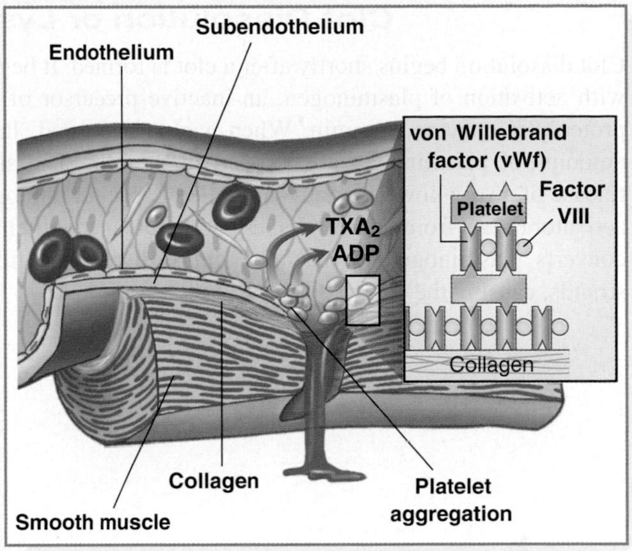

Blood Coagulation

Blood coagulation is a complex process involving the sequential activation of various factors in the blood. There are two coagulation pathways: (1) the intrinsic pathway begins in the circulation and is initiated by activation of circulating factor XII and (2) the extrinsic pathway, which is activated by a cellular lipoprotein called *tissue factor* that becomes exposed when tissues are injured. Both pathways lead to the activation of factor X, the conversion of prothrombin to thrombin, and conversion of fibrinogen to the insoluble fibrin threads that hold the clot together.

Additionally, the two following processes occur which allow for dissolution of the newly formed clot.

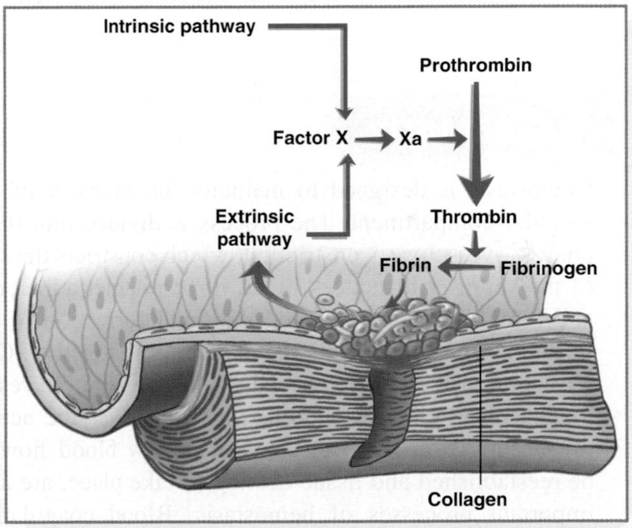

Clot Retraction

Within a few minutes after a clot is formed, the actin and myosin in the platelets that are trapped in the clot begin to contract in a manner similar to that in muscles. As a result, the fibrin strands of the clot are pulled toward the platelets, thereby squeezing serum (plasma without fibrinogen) from the clot and causing it to shrink.

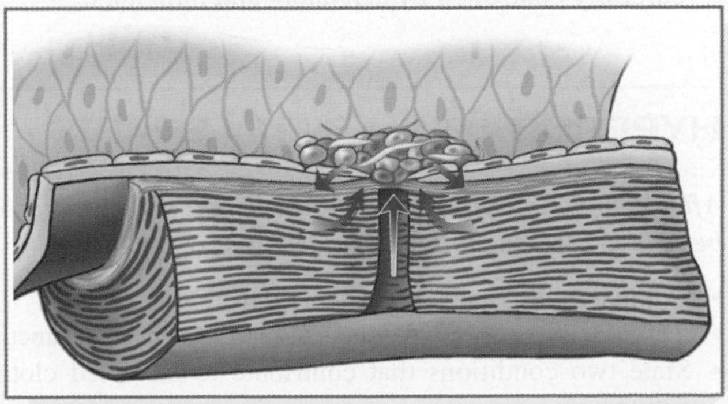

Continued

Understanding Hemostasis *(Continued)*

Clot Dissolution or Lysis

Clot dissolution begins shortly after a clot is formed. It begins with activation of plasminogen, an inactive precursor of the proteolytic enzyme, plasmin. When a clot is formed, large amounts of plasminogen are trapped in the clot. The slow release of a very powerful activator called tissue plasminogen activator (t-PA) from injured tissues and vascular endothelium converts plasminogen to plasmin, which digests the fibrin strands, causing the clot to dissolve.

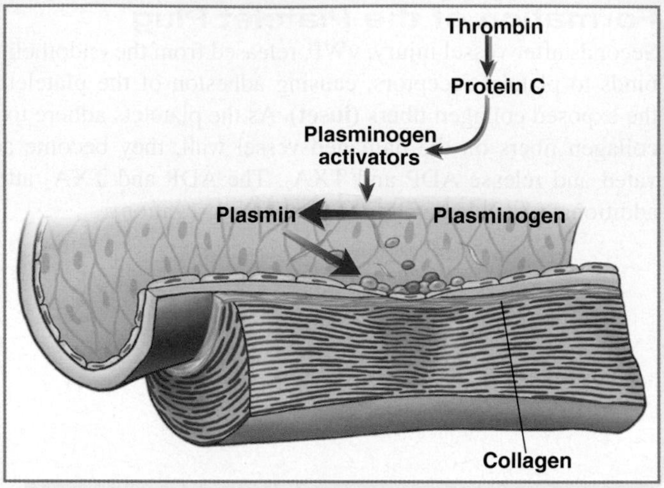

IN SUMMARY

Hemostasis is designed to maintain the integrity of the vascular compartment. The process is divided into three phases—vessel vasoconstriction, which constricts the size of the vessel and reduces blood flow; platelet adherence and formation of the platelet plug; and formation of the fibrin clot, which cements the platelet plug together. Clot retraction, which pulls the edges of the injured vessel together, and clot dissolution, which involves the action of plasmin to dissolve the clot and allow blood flow to be reestablished and tissue healing to take place, are also important processes of hemostasis. Blood coagulation requires the stepwise activation of coagulation factors, carefully controlled by activators and inhibitors.

HYPERCOAGULABILITY STATES

After completing this section of the chapter, the learner will be able to meet the following objectives:

- Compare normal and abnormal clotting.
- Describe the causes and effects of increased platelet function.
- State two conditions that contribute to increased clotting activity.

Hypercoagulability represents an exaggerated form of hemostasis that predisposes to thrombosis and blood vessel occlusion. There are two general forms of hypercoagulability states—conditions that create increased platelet function and conditions that cause accelerated activity of the coagulation system. Chart 22.1 summarizes conditions commonly

CHART 22.1 CONDITIONS ASSOCIATED WITH HYPERCOAGULABILITY STATES

Increased Platelet Function
Atherosclerosis
Diabetes mellitus
Smoking
Elevated blood lipid and cholesterol levels
Increased platelet levels

Accelerated Activity of the Clotting System
Pregnancy and the puerperium
Use of oral contraceptives
Postsurgical state
Immobility
Congestive heart failure
Malignant diseases

associated with hypercoagulability states. Arterial thrombi are usually due to turbulence and composed largely of platelet aggregates. On the other hand, venous thrombi are usually due to stasis of flow and composed largely of platelet aggregates and fibrin complexes that result from activation of the coagulation cascade.

Hypercoagulability Associated with Increased Platelet Function

Hypercoagulability because of increased platelet function results in platelet adhesion, formation of platelet clots, and disruption of blood flow. The causes of increased platelet function are disturbances in flow, endothelial damage, and increased sensitivity of platelets to factors that cause adhesiveness and aggregation. Atherosclerotic plaques disturb blood flow, causing endothelial damage and promoting platelet adherence. Platelets that adhere to the vessel wall release growth factors, which cause proliferation of smooth muscle and thereby contribute to the development of atherosclerosis. Smoking, elevated levels of blood lipids and cholesterol, hemodynamic stress, and diabetes mellitus predispose to vessel damage, platelet adherence, and eventual thrombosis.

Thrombocytosis

The term *thrombocytosis* is used to describe elevations in the platelet count above 1,000,000/μL. Thrombocytosis can occur as a reactive process (secondary thrombocytosis) or as an essential process (primary thrombocytosis).[11,12]

Etiology and Pathogenesis. Thrombopoietin is the key hormone in the regulation of megakaryocyte differentiation and platelet formation, although various cytokines (*e.g.*, interleukin-6 and interleukin-11) may also play a role.[2] Megakaryocytes and their platelet progeny have receptors for thrombopoietin. Thrombopoietin is carried in the plasma attached to receptors on the surface of circulating platelets and in an unbound form that is free to promote megakaryocyte proliferation. When the platelet count falls, more unbound thrombopoietin is available to stimulate megakaryocyte proliferation, and when the platelet count rises, less thrombopoietin is available to stimulate proliferation. Thus, megakaryocyte proliferation and platelet production are normally controlled in a negative feedback mechanism by the platelet count.[2]

The most common cause of secondary thrombocytosis is a disease state that stimulates thrombopoietin production. The result is increased megakaryocyte proliferation and platelet production. However, the platelet count seldom exceeds 1,000,000/μL. The common underlying causes of secondary thrombocytosis include tissue damage because of surgery, infection, cancer, and chronic inflammatory conditions such as rheumatoid arthritis and Crohn disease.[12] Usually, the only clinically apparent signs are those of the underlying disease. Thrombocytosis may also occur in other myeloproliferative disorders such as polycythemia vera and myelogenous leukemia.

Primary or essential thrombocytosis represents a myeloproliferative (bone marrow) disorder of the hematopoietic stem cells.[11] Although thrombopoietin levels are often normal in essential thrombocytosis, abnormalities in the thrombopoietin receptor and platelet binding cause higher-than-expected levels of free thrombopoietin. This leads to increased megakaryocyte proliferation and platelet production. Dysfunction of the platelets produced contributes to the major clinical features of bleeding and thrombosis.

Clinical Manifestations and Treatment. The common clinical manifestations of essential thrombocytosis are thrombosis and hemorrhage. Thrombotic events include deep vein thrombosis and pulmonary embolism and portal and hepatic vein thrombosis. Some people experience erythromelalgia, a painful throbbing and burning of the fingers caused by occlusion of the arterioles by platelet aggregates. Typically, the disorder is characterized by long asymptomatic periods punctuated by occasional thrombotic episodes and hemorrhagic crises, both of which occur in people with very high platelet counts. Treatment includes the use of platelet-lowering drugs (*e.g.*, hydroxyurea) in high-risk cases.[12] Aspirin may be a highly effective adjunctive therapy in people with recurrent thrombotic complications.

KEY POINTS

HYPERCOAGULABILITY STATES

- Arterial thrombi are associated with conditions that produce turbulent blood flow and platelet adherence.
- Venous thrombi are associated with conditions that cause stasis of blood flow with increased concentrations of coagulation factors.

Hypercoagulability Associated with Increased Clotting Activity

Thrombus formation because of activation of the coagulation system can result from primary (genetic) or secondary (acquired) disorders affecting the coagulation components of the blood clotting process (*i.e.*, an increase in procoagulation factors or a decrease in anticoagulation factors).

Inherited Disorders

A common hereditary thrombophilia, Factor V Leiden, causes activated protein C resistance.[13] Activated protein C resistance accounts for approximately 20% of initial episodes of thrombosis, 50% of familial thrombosis, and 60% of thrombotic events in those with normal levels of protein C, protein S, antithrombin, and antiphospholipid antibodies.[13]

Hypercoagulability is associated with increased risk of VTE. High morbidity and mortality are associated with

VTE.[14,16] VTE, which includes pulmonary embolism and deep vein thrombosis, can be divided into genetic and acquired. The incidence of genetic VTE is relatively low.[15]

Acquired Disorders

Among the acquired or secondary factors that lead to increased coagulation and thrombosis are venous stasis because of prolonged bed rest and immobility, myocardial infarction, cancer, hyperestrogenic states, smoking, obesity, and oral contraceptives.[17] People with a malignancy develop VTE more often than those without a malignancy. Approximately 20% to 25% of those presenting with primary VTE will be found to have an occult malignancy.[15]

Stasis of blood flow causes accumulation of activated clotting factors and platelets and prevents their interactions with inhibitors. Slow and disturbed flow is a common cause of venous thrombosis in the immobilized or postsurgical person. Inflammation is believed to contribute to stasis. Heart failure also contributes to venous congestion and thrombosis. Hyperviscosity syndromes (polycythemia) and deformed red blood cells in sickle cell disease increase the resistance to flow and cause small-vessel stasis.

The incidence of stroke, thromboemboli, and myocardial infarction is greater in women who use oral contraceptives, particularly those older than 35 years of age and those who are heavy smokers. Clotting factors are also increased during normal pregnancy. These changes, along with limited activity during the puerperium (immediate postpartum period), predispose to venous thrombosis.

Hypercoagulability also is common in cancer and sepsis. Many tumor cells are thought to release tissue factor molecules, which, along with the increased immobility and sepsis seen in people with malignant disease, contribute to thrombosis in these people.

As a result of these varied avenues for VTE to develop, prophylaxis has become a quality indicator of health care. The American College of Chest Physicians has developed and published standards for prevention of VTE, which include low molecular weight heparin, unfractionated heparin, and compression stockings and/or intermittent pneumatic stockings. These guidelines are to be implemented based on assessing the person's risk factors and current condition using the Caprini risk score. This score stratifies person into four risk categories. Interventions are then selected to prevent VTE.[16]

Antiphospholipid Syndrome

Another cause of increased venous and arterial thrombosis is the *antiphospholipid syndrome*. This condition is associated with autoantibodies (primarily immunoglobulin G [IgG]) directed against protein-binding phospholipids, which results in increased coagulation activity.[15] The common features of antiphospholipid syndrome are venous and arterial thrombi, recurrent fetal loss, and thrombocytopenia. The disorder can be a primary condition occurring in isolation with signs of hypercoagulability or a secondary condition sometimes associated with systemic lupus erythematosus.[4]

Etiology and Pathogenesis. Although the mechanisms for this syndrome are unknown, several potential pathways have been identified:

- The antibodies may interfere with the coagulation cascade, leading to a hypercoagulability state.
- The antibodies may directly bind to the endothelial cell surface, causing secretion of cytokines that result in activation and aggregation of platelets.
- The antibodies may target a serum phospholipid-binding protein that functions as an anticoagulant.

In addition to the action of the antibodies, it seems likely that other factors play a role in determining whether a person develops clinical manifestations of the disorder. Although speculative, these factors may include vascular trauma or the presence of infection that leads to cytokine production and endothelial cell activation.[4]

Clinical Manifestations. People with the disorder present with a variety of clinical manifestations, typically those characterized by recurrent venous and arterial thrombi. Cardiac valvular vegetations associated with adherence of thrombi and thrombocytopenia because of excessive platelet consumption may also occur. Venous thrombosis, especially in the deep leg veins, occurs in up to 50% of people with the syndrome, half of whom develop pulmonary emboli. Arterial thrombosis involves the brain in up to 50% of cases, causing transient ischemic attacks or strokes.[15] Other sites for arterial thrombosis are the coronary arteries of the heart and the retinal, renal, and peripheral arteries. Women with the disorder commonly have a history of recurrent pregnancy losses because of ischemia and thrombosis of the placental vessels. These women also have increased risk of giving birth to a premature infant owing to pregnancy-associated hypertension and uteroplacental insufficiency.

In most people with antiphospholipid syndrome, the thrombotic events occur as a single episode at one anatomic site. In some people, recurrences may occur months or years later and mimic the initial event. Occasionally, someone may present with multiple vascular occlusions involving many organ systems. This rapid onset condition is termed *catastrophic antiphospholipid syndrome* and is associated with a high mortality rate.[18]

Treatment. Treatment of the syndrome focuses on removal or reduction in factors that predispose to thrombosis, including advice to stop smoking and counseling against use of estrogen-containing oral contraceptives by women. The acute thrombotic event is treated with anticoagulants (heparin and warfarin) and immune suppression in refractory cases. Aspirin and anticoagulant drugs, as well as newer, non–vitamin K anticoagulants, may be used to prevent future thrombosis.[18]

IN SUMMARY

Hypercoagulability causes excessive clotting and contributes to thrombus formation. It results from conditions that foster an increase in platelet numbers or function or accelerated activity of the coagulation system. Thrombocytosis, an elevation in the platelet count, can occur as a reactive process (secondary thrombocytosis) or an essential process (primary thrombocytosis). Increased platelet function usually results from disorders such as atherosclerosis that damage the vascular endothelium and disturb blood flow or from conditions such as smoking that increase sensitivity of platelets to factors that promote adhesiveness and aggregation.

Factors that cause accelerated activity of the coagulation system include blood flow stasis, resulting in an accumulation of coagulation factors, and alterations in the components of the coagulation system (*i.e.*, an increase in procoagulation factors or a decrease in anticoagulation factors). The antiphospholipid syndrome, an acquired venous and arterial clotting disorder, manifests as a primary disorder or can be a secondary disorder associated with systemic lupus erythematosus. It is associated with antiphospholipid antibodies, which promote thrombosis that can affect many organs.

BLEEDING DISORDERS

After completing this section of the chapter, the learner will be able to meet the following objectives:

- Differentiate the mechanisms of drug-induced thrombocytopenia and idiopathic thrombocytopenia.
- Describe the manifestations of thrombocytopenia.
- State three common defects of coagulation factors and their etiologies.
- Differentiate between the mechanisms of bleeding in hemophilia A and von Willebrand disease.
- Describe the effect of vascular disorders on hemostasis.
- Explain the physiologic basis of acute disseminated intravascular coagulation.

Bleeding disorders or impairment of blood coagulation can result from defects in any of the factors that contribute to hemostasis. Bleeding can occur as a result of disorders associated with platelet number or function, coagulation factors, and blood vessel integrity.

Bleeding Associated with Platelet Disorders

Bleeding because of platelet disorders reflects a decrease in platelet number because of decreased production, increased destruction, or impaired function of platelets. Spontaneous bleeding from platelet disorders most often involves small vessels of the mucous membranes and skin. Common sites of bleeding are the mucous membranes of the nose, mouth, gastrointestinal tract, and uterine cavity. Cutaneous bleeding is seen as pinpoint hemorrhages (petechiae) and purple areas of bruising (purpura) in dependent areas where the capillary pressure is higher (Fig. 22.3). Petechiae are seen almost exclusively in conditions of platelet deficiency and not platelet dysfunction. Bleeding of the intracranial vessels is a rare danger with severe platelet depletion.

Thrombocytopenia

A reduction in platelet number, also referred to as *thrombocytopenia,* is an important cause of generalized bleeding. Thrombocytopenia usually refers to a decrease in the number of circulating platelets to a level less than 150,000/μL.[19] The greater the decrease in the platelet count, the greater the risk of bleeding. Thrombocytopenia can result from a decrease in platelet production, increased sequestration of platelets in the spleen, or decreased platelet survival.

Decreased platelet production because of loss of bone marrow function occurs in aplastic anemia. Replacement of bone marrow by malignant cells, such as that occurring in leukemia, also results in decreased production of platelets. Radiation therapy and drugs such as those used in the treatment of cancer may depress bone marrow function and reduce platelet production. Infection with human immunodeficiency virus (HIV) or cytomegalovirus may suppress the production of megakaryocytes, the platelet precursors.

Production of platelets may be normal, but excessive pooling of platelets in the spleen may occur. Although the spleen normally sequesters 30% to 40% of the platelets before release into the circulation, the proportion can be as great as 90% when the spleen is enlarged in splenomegaly.[1] When necessary, hypersplenic thrombocytopenia may be treated with splenectomy.

Reduced platelet survival is caused by a variety of immune and nonimmune mechanisms. Platelet destruction

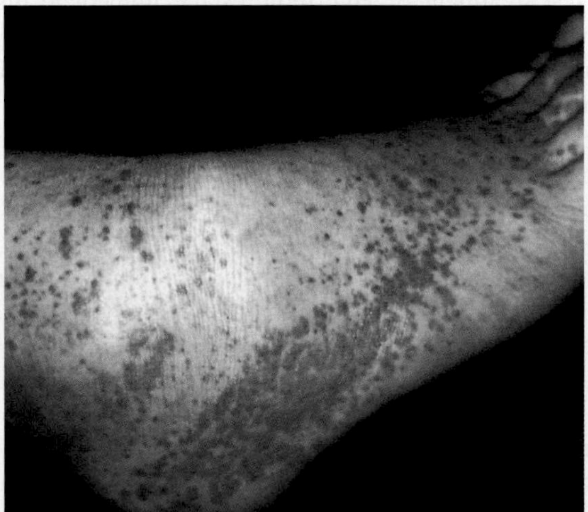

Figure 22.3 • Clinically mild cutaneous vasculitis with palpable purpura and petechiae. (From Hall J. C., Hall B. J. (2017). *Sauer's manual of skin diseases* (11th ed., p. 176). Philadelphia, PA: Lippincott Williams & Wilkins.)

may be caused by antiplatelet antibodies. The antibodies may be directed against platelet self-antigens or against antigens on the platelets from blood transfusions or pregnancy. The antibodies target the platelet membrane glycoproteins GPIIb/IIIa and GPIb/IX. Nonimmune destruction of platelets results from mechanical injury because of prosthetic heart valves or malignant hypertension, which results in small-vessel narrowing. In acute DIC or TTP, excessive platelet consumption leads to a deficiency.[4]

Drug-Induced Thrombocytopenia. Some drugs, such as aspirin, atorvastatin, and some antibiotics, may cause drug-induced immune thrombocytopenia (DITP).[19] These drugs induce an antigen–antibody response and formation of immune complexes that cause platelet destruction by complement-mediated lysis. In people with drug-associated thrombocytopenia, there is a rapid fall in the platelet count within 2 to 3 days of resuming a drug or 7 or more days (*i.e.*, the time needed to mount an immune response) after starting a drug for the first time. The platelet count rises rapidly after the drug is discontinued.

Heparin-Induced Thrombocytopenia. Heparin-induced thrombocytopenia (HIT) is associated with the anticoagulant drug heparin. Ten percent of people treated with heparin develop a mild, transient thrombocytopenia within 2 to 5 days of starting the drug.[19] However, approximately 1% to 5% of people treated with heparin experience life-threatening thromboembolic events 1 to 2 weeks after the start of therapy.[4] HIT is caused by an immune reaction directed against a complex of heparin and platelet factor 4, a normal component of platelet granules that binds tightly to heparin. The binding of antibody to platelet factor 4 produces immune complexes that activate the remaining platelets, leading to thrombosis. In addition, prothrombotic platelet particles and induction of tissue factor continue to promote coagulation.[19]

The treatment of HIT requires the immediate discontinuation of heparin therapy and the use of alternative anticoagulants to prevent thrombosis recurrence. The newer low molecular weight heparin has been shown to be effective in reducing the incidence of heparin-induced complications compared with the older, high molecular weight form of the drug.

Immune Thrombocytopenic Purpura. Immune thrombocytopenic purpura (ITP) results in platelet antibody formation and excess destruction of platelets. Primary ITP is an autoimmune disease in which platelets are directly destroyed or their formation inhibited by the immune system. Primary ITP occurs in both genders and affects children and adults, though the incidence is highest in females aged 30 to 59 and in persons older than 60.[20] Primary ITP is classified as "newly diagnosed" (from diagnosis until 3 months), "persistent," (from diagnosis until 3 to 12 months) or "chronic" (from diagnosis until >12 months).[20] Immune thrombocytopenia purpura is also referred to as idiopathic or having unknown cause.

Autoimmune disorders and chronic infections such as *Helicobacter pylori*, hepatitis C virus, and HIV contribute to secondary forms of ITP. When these related diseases are present, expected hemorrhagic symptoms may be absent.[20]

Etiology and Pathogenesis. The thrombocytopenia that occurs in ITP is thought to result from multiple mechanisms, including antiplatelet antibodies against glycoproteins (IIb/IIIa and Ib/IX) in the platelet membrane. The platelets, which are made more susceptible to phagocytosis because of the antibody, are destroyed in the spleen. Plasma levels of thrombopoietin, the major factor that stimulates growth and development of megakaryocytes, are not elevated in people with ITP.[21] Evidence suggests that ITP is caused by T-cell dysfunction, specifically CD4 and T regulatory cells, which trigger the autoimmune response and proceed to thrombocytopenia.[21]

Clinical Manifestations. Manifestations of ITP include a history of bruising, bleeding from gums, epistaxis (*i.e.*, nosebleed), melena, and abnormal menstrual bleeding in those with moderately reduced platelet counts. Because the spleen is the site of platelet destruction, splenic enlargement may occur. The condition may be discovered incidentally or as a result of signs of bleeding, often into the skin (*i.e.*, purpura and petechiae) or oral mucosa.

Diagnosis and Treatment. Diagnosis of ITP usually is based on severe thrombocytopenia (platelet counts <20,000 to 30,000/μL) and exclusion of other causes. Tests for the platelet-bound antibodies are available but lack specificity (*e.g.*, they react with platelet antibodies from other sources). The secondary form of ITP sometimes mimics the idiopathic form of the disorder; therefore, the diagnosis is made only after excluding other known causes of thrombocytopenia.

The decision to treat ITP is based on the platelet count and the degree of bleeding. Many persons with ITP do well without treatment. Corticosteroids are usually used as initial therapy. Other effective initial treatments include intravenous immune globulin. However, this treatment is expensive, and the beneficial effect lasts only 1 to 2 weeks.

Thrombotic Thrombocytopenic Purpura. Thrombotic thrombocytopenic purpura (TTP) is a combination of thrombocytopenia, hemolytic anemia, renal failure, fever, and neurologic abnormalities. It is a rare disorder that likely results from introduction of platelet-aggregating substances into the circulation.[4]

Etiology and Pathogenesis. Thrombotic thrombocytopenic purpura (TTP) is caused by a deficiency of ADAMTS13, which is responsible for severing large vWF multimers. The unchecked platelet aggregation results in microvascular occlusions leading to end organ failure. Approximately 1% of all TTP is hereditary, whereas the remaining 99% is acquired. The following are known to decrease ADAMTS13 activity: hemolytic uremic syndrome, cancer, infections, pregnancy, several drugs, and autoimmune diseases affecting connective tissues.[22]

The onset of TTP is abrupt, and the outcome may be fatal. Widespread vascular occlusions result from thrombi in the arterioles and capillaries of many organs, including the heart, brain, and kidneys. Erythrocytes become fragmented as they circulate through the partly occluded vessels, causing hemolytic anemia and jaundice.

Clinical Manifestations and Treatment. The clinical manifestations include purpura, petechiae, vaginal bleeding, and neurologic symptoms ranging from headache to seizures and altered consciousness. Emergency treatment for TTP includes *plasmapheresis,* a procedure that involves removal of plasma from withdrawn blood and replacement with fresh-frozen plasma. Plasma infusion provides the deficient enzyme. With plasmapheresis and plasma infusion treatment, there is a complete recovery in 80% of cases.[22]

Impaired Platelet Function

Impaired platelet function (also called *thrombocytopathia*) may result from inherited disorders of adhesion (*e.g.,* von Willebrand disease) or acquired defects resulting from drugs, disease, or surgery. Defective platelet function is also common in uremia, presumably because of unexcreted waste products. Chart 22.2 lists drugs that impair platelet function.

CHART 22.2 DRUGS THAT MAY PREDISPOSE TO BLEEDING*

Interference with Platelet Production or Function
Acetazolamide
Antimetabolite and anticancer drugs
Antibiotics such as penicillin and the cephalosporins
Aspirin and salicylates
Carbamazepine
Clofibrate
Colchicine
Dipyridamole
Thiazide diuretics
Gold salts
Heparin
NSAIDs
Quinine derivatives (quinidine and hydroxychloroquine)
Sulfonamides

Interference with Coagulation Factors
Amiodarone
Anabolic steroids
Warfarin
Heparin

Decrease in Vitamin K Levels
Antibiotics
Clofibrate

*This list is not intended to be inclusive.

Concept Mastery Alert

The action of aspirin is irreversible acetylation of platelet cyclooxygenase activity. In contrast, ITP results in platelet antibody formation and excess destruction of platelets and can result from use of heparin or quinidine.

KEY POINTS

BLEEDING DISORDERS

- Disorders of platelet plug formation include a decrease in platelet numbers because of inadequate platelet production (bone marrow dysfunction), excess platelet destruction (thrombocytopenia), abnormal platelet function (thrombocytopathia), or defects in vWF.
- Impairment of the coagulation stage of hemostasis is caused by a deficiency in one or more of the clotting factors.
- Disorders of blood vessel integrity result from structurally weak vessels or vessel damage because of inflammation and immune mechanisms.

Bleeding Associated with Coagulation Factor Deficiencies

Blood coagulation defects can result from deficiencies or impaired function of one or more of the clotting factors, including vWF. Deficiencies can arise because of inherited disease or defective synthesis or increased consumption of the clotting factors. Bleeding resulting from clotting factor deficiencies typically occurs after injury or trauma. Large bruises, hematomas, and prolonged bleeding into the gastrointestinal or urinary tracts or joints are common.

Inherited Disorders

Von Willebrand disease and hemophilia (A and B) are two of the most common inherited disorders of bleeding. Von Willebrand disease is considered the most frequent inherited coagulopathy and affects approximately 1% to 2% of the population.[4] Hemophilia A (factor VIII deficiency) affects 1 in 5000 male live births. Hemophilia B (factor IX deficiency) occurs in approximately 1 in 20,000 people, accounting for 15% of people with hemophilia.[4] It is genetically and clinically similar to hemophilia A. Von Willebrand disease and hemophilia A are caused by defects involving the factor VIII–vWF complex. vWF, which is synthesized by the endothelium and megakaryocytes, is required for platelet adhesion to the subendothelial matrix of the blood vessel. It also serves as the carrier for factor VIII and is important for the stability of factor VIII in the circulation by preventing its proteolysis. Factor VIII coagulant protein, the functional portion, is produced by the liver and endothelial cells. Thus, factor VIII and vWF, synthesized separately, come together and circulate in the plasma as a unit that serves to promote clotting and adhesion of platelets to the vessel wall.[4]

Von Willebrand Disease. Von Willebrand disease is a relatively common hereditary bleeding disorder characterized by a deficiency or defect in vWF. As many as 20 variants of von Willebrand disease have been described.[4] These variants can be grouped into two categories—types 1 and 3, which are associated with reduced levels of vWF, and type 2, which is characterized by defects in vWF.

Classification. Type 1, an *autosomal dominant disorder*, accounts for approximately 70% of cases and is relatively mild. Type 2, also an autosomal dominant disorder, accounts for about 25% of cases and is associated with mild to moderate bleeding. Type 3, which is a relatively rare *autosomal recessive disorder*, is associated with extremely low levels of functional vWF and correspondingly severe clinical manifestations.[4] People with von Willebrand disease have a compound defect involving platelet function and the coagulation pathway.

Clinical Manifestations. Clinical manifestations include spontaneous bleeding from the nose, mouth, and gastrointestinal tract, excessive menstrual flow, and a prolonged bleeding time in the presence of a normal platelet count. Most cases (*i.e.*, types 1 and 2) are mild and require no treatment, and many people with the disorder are diagnosed when surgery or dental extraction results in prolonged bleeding. In severe cases (*i.e.*, type 3), life-threatening gastrointestinal bleeding and joint hemorrhage may be similar to that seen in hemophilia.[4] The bleeding associated with von Willebrand disease is usually mild, and no treatment is routinely administered other than avoidance of aspirin.

Hemophilia A. Hemophilia A is an X-linked recessive disorder that primarily affects males. Although it is a hereditary disorder, there is no family history of the disorder in approximately 30% of newly diagnosed cases, suggesting that it has arisen as a new mutation in the factor VIII gene.[4] Approximately 90% of people with hemophilia produce insufficient quantities of the factor, and 10% produce a defective form. The percentage of normal factor VIII activity in the circulation depends on the genetic defect and determines the severity of hemophilia (*i.e.*, 6% to 30% in mild hemophilia, 2% to 5% in moderate hemophilia, and 1% or less in severe forms of hemophilia). In mild or moderate forms of the disease, bleeding usually does not occur unless there is a local lesion or trauma such as surgery or a dental procedure. The mild disorder may not be detected in childhood. In severe hemophilia, bleeding usually occurs in childhood (*e.g.*, it may be noticed at the time of circumcision) and is spontaneous and severe, often occurring several times a month.

Clinical Manifestations. Characteristically, bleeding occurs in soft tissues, the gastrointestinal tract, and the hip, knee, elbow, and ankle joints. Spontaneous joint bleeding usually begins when a child begins to walk. Often, a target joint is prone to repeated bleeding. The bleeding causes inflammation of the synovium, with acute pain and swelling. Without proper treatment, chronic bleeding and inflammation cause joint fibrosis and contractures, resulting in major disability.

Treatment. The prevention of trauma is important in people with hemophilia. Aspirin and other NSAIDs that affect platelet function should be avoided. Factor VIII replacement therapy administered at home has reduced the typical musculoskeletal damage. It is initiated when bleeding occurs or as prophylaxis with repeated bleeding episodes. The recombinant products and continuous infusion pumps may allow prevention rather than therapy for hemorrhage. The development of inhibitory antibodies to recombinant factor VIII is still a major complication of treatment.

The cloning of the factor VIII gene and progress in gene delivery systems have led to the hope that hemophilia A may be cured by gene replacement therapy. Carrier detection and prenatal diagnosis can now be done by analysis of direct gene mutation or DNA linkage studies. Prenatal amniocentesis or chorionic villus sampling is used to predict complications and determine therapy. It may eventually be used to select people for gene addition.

Acquired Disorders

Coagulation factors V, VII, IX, X, XI, and XII, prothrombin, and fibrinogen are synthesized in the liver. In liver disease, synthesis of these clotting factors is reduced, and bleeding may result. Of the coagulation factors synthesized in the liver, factors II, VII, IX, and X and prothrombin require the presence of vitamin K for normal activity. In vitamin K deficiency, the liver produces the clotting factor but in an inactive form. Vitamin K is a fat-soluble vitamin that is continuously being synthesized by intestinal bacteria. This means that a deficiency in vitamin K is not likely to occur unless intestinal synthesis is interrupted or absorption of the vitamin is impaired. Vitamin K deficiency can occur in the newborn infant before the establishment of the intestinal flora. It can also occur as a result of treatment with broad-spectrum antibiotics that destroy intestinal flora. Because vitamin K is a fat-soluble vitamin, its absorption requires bile salts. Vitamin K deficiency may result from impaired fat absorption caused by liver or gallbladder disease.

Bleeding Associated with Vascular Disorders

Bleeding resulting from vascular disorders is sometimes referred to as *nonthrombocytopenic purpura*. These disorders may occur because of structurally weak vessel walls or because of damage to vessels by inflammation or immune responses. Most often, they are characterized by easy bruising and the spontaneous appearance of petechiae and purpura of the skin and mucous membranes. In people with bleeding disorders caused by vascular defects, the platelet count and results of other tests for coagulation factors are normal.

Among the vascular disorders that cause bleeding are hemorrhagic telangiectasia, an uncommon autosomal dominant disorder characterized by thin-walled, dilated capillaries and arterioles; vitamin C deficiency (*i.e.*, scurvy), resulting in poor collagen synthesis and failure of the endothelial cells to be cemented together properly, which causes a fragile vascular wall; Cushing disease, causing protein wasting and loss of vessel tissue support because of excess cortisol; and senile purpura (*i.e.*, bruising in elderly persons), caused by impaired collagen synthesis in the aging process. Vascular defects also occur in the course of DIC or as a result of microthrombi and corticosteroid therapy.

Disseminated Intravascular Coagulation

DIC is a paradox in the hemostatic sequence and is characterized by widespread coagulation and bleeding in the vascular compartment. It is not a primary disease but occurs as a complication of a wide variety of conditions. DIC begins with massive activation of the coagulation sequence as a result of unregulated generation of thrombin, resulting in systemic formation of fibrin. In addition, levels of all the major anticoagulants are reduced (Fig. 22.4). The microthrombi that result cause vessel occlusion and tissue ischemia. Multiple organ failure may ensue. Clot formation consumes all available coagulation proteins and platelets, and severe hemorrhage results.

Etiology and Pathogenesis

The disorder can be initiated by activation of the intrinsic or extrinsic pathway or both. Activation through the extrinsic pathway occurs with liberation of tissue factors and is associated with obstetric complications, trauma, bacterial sepsis, and cancers.

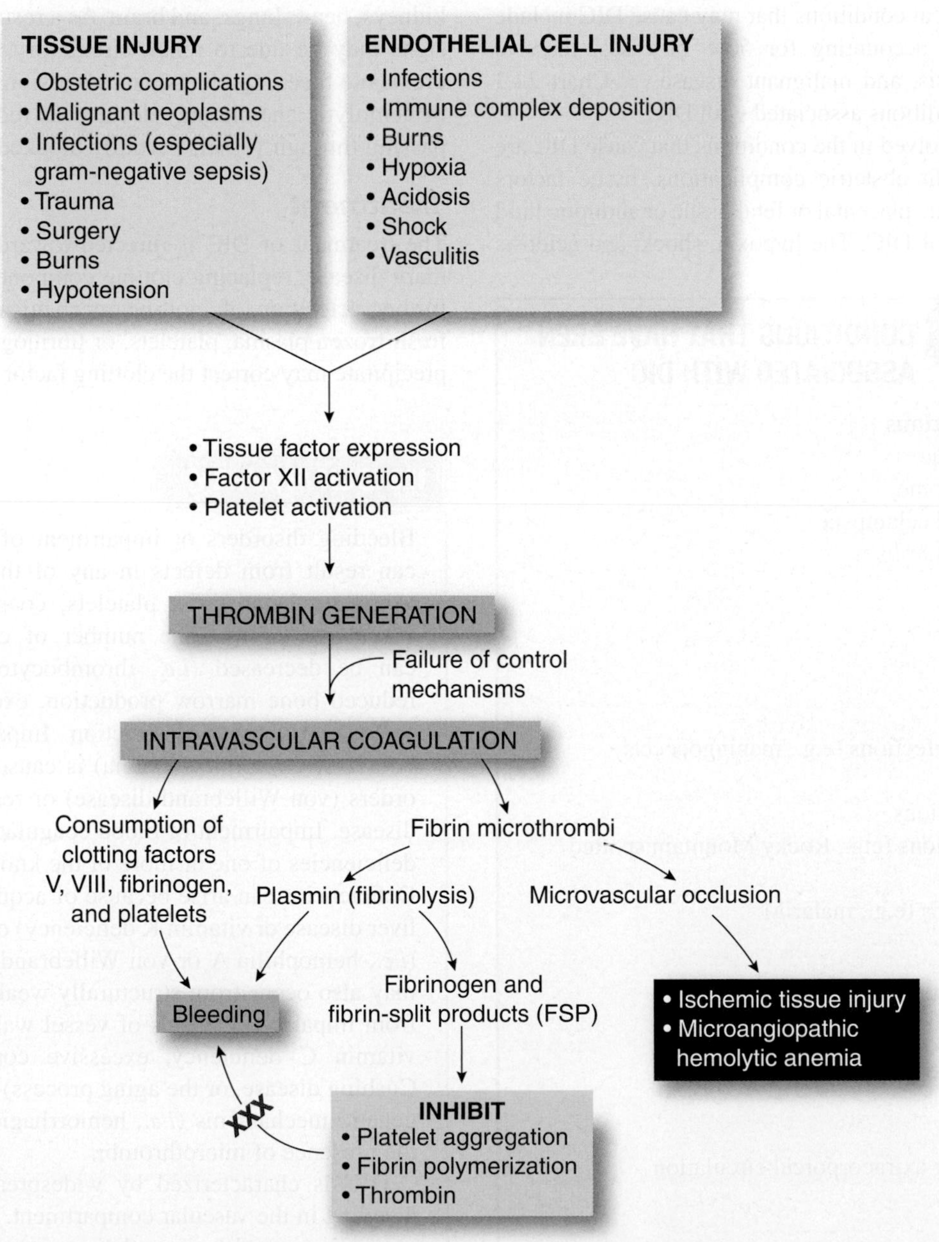

Figure 22.4 • Pathophysiology of DIC. The DIC syndrome is triggered by tissue injury, endothelial cell injury, or a combination of both of these processes. Due to the failure of the normal mechanisms controlling hemostasis, intravascular coagulation occurs. (From Valdez R., Zutter M., Florea A. D., et al. (2015). Hematopathology. In Rubin R., Strayer D. (Eds.), *Rubin's pathology: Clinicopathologic foundations of medicine* (7th ed., p. 1113). Philadelphia, PA: Lippincott Williams & Wilkins.)

The intrinsic pathway may be activated through extensive endothelial damage, with activation of factor XII. Endothelial damage may be caused by viruses, infections, immune mechanisms, stasis of blood, or temperature extremes. Impaired anticoagulation pathways are also associated with reduced levels of antithrombin and the protein C anticoagulant system in DIC. There is evidence that the underlying cause of DIC is infection or inflammation and the cytokines (tumor necrosis factor, interleukin-1, and others) liberated in the process are the pivotal mediators.[23,24] These cytokines not only mediate inflammation but also can increase the expression of tissue factor on endothelial cells and simultaneously decrease the expression of thrombomodulin. Thrombomodulin, a glycoprotein that is present on the cell membrane of endothelial cells, binds thrombin and acts as an additional regulatory mechanism in coagulation. Common clinical conditions that may cause DIC include obstetric disorders, accounting for 50% of cases, massive trauma, shock, sepsis, and malignant disease.[23,24] Chart 22.3 summarizes the conditions associated with DIC.

The factors involved in the conditions that cause DIC are often interrelated. In obstetric complications, tissue factors released from necrotic placental or fetal tissue or amniotic fluid may be the trigger of DIC. The hypoxia, shock, and acidosis that may coexist also contribute by causing endothelial injury. Gram-negative bacterial infections result in the release of endotoxins, which activate both the extrinsic pathway by release of tissue factor and the intrinsic pathway through endothelial damage. Endotoxins also inhibit the activity of protein C.[23,24]

CHART 22.3 CONDITIONS THAT HAVE BEEN ASSOCIATED WITH DIC

Obstetric Conditions
Abruptio placentae
Dead fetus syndrome
Preeclampsia and eclampsia
Amniotic fluid embolism

Cancers
Metastatic cancer
Leukemia

Infections
Acute bacterial infections (e.g., meningococcal meningitis)
Acute viral infections
Rickettsial infections (e.g., Rocky Mountain spotted fever)
Parasitic infections (e.g., malaria)

Shock
Septic shock
Severe hypovolemic shock

Trauma or Surgery
Burns
Massive trauma
Surgery involving extracorporeal circulation
Snake bite
Heat stroke

Hematologic Conditions
Blood transfusion reactions

Clinical Manifestations

Although coagulation and formation of microemboli characterize DIC, its acute manifestations usually are more directly related to the bleeding problems that occur. The bleeding may be present as petechiae, purpura, oozing from puncture sites, or severe hemorrhage.

Uncontrolled postpartum bleeding may indicate DIC. Microemboli may obstruct blood vessels and cause tissue hypoxia and necrotic damage to organ structures, such as the kidneys, heart, lungs, and brain. As a result, common clinical signs may be due to renal, circulatory, or respiratory failure, acute bleeding ulcers, or convulsions and coma. A form of hemolytic anemia may develop as red cells are damaged passing through vessels partially blocked by thrombus.[23,24]

Treatment

The treatment of DIC is directed toward managing the primary disease, replacing clotting components, and preventing further activation of clotting mechanisms. Transfusions of fresh-frozen plasma, platelets, or fibrinogen-containing cryoprecipitate may correct the clotting factor deficiency.

IN SUMMARY

Bleeding disorders or impairment of blood coagulation can result from defects in any of the factors that contribute to hemostasis: platelets, coagulation factors, or vascular integrity. The number of circulating platelets can be decreased (*i.e.*, thrombocytopenia) because of reduced bone marrow production, excess pooling in the spleen, or immune destruction. Impaired platelet function (*i.e.*, thrombocytopathia) is caused by inherited disorders (von Willebrand disease) or results from drugs or disease. Impairment of blood coagulation can result from deficiencies of one or more of the known clotting factors. Deficiencies can arise because of acquired disorders (*i.e.*, liver disease or vitamin K deficiency) or inherited diseases (*i.e.*, hemophilia A or von Willebrand disease). Bleeding may also occur from structurally weak vessels that result from impaired synthesis of vessel wall components (*i.e.*, vitamin C deficiency, excessive cortisol levels as in Cushing disease, or the aging process) or from damage by genetic mechanisms (*i.e.*, hemorrhagic telangiectasia) or the presence of microthrombi.

DIC is characterized by widespread coagulation and bleeding in the vascular compartment. It begins with massive activation of the coagulation cascade and generation of microthrombi that cause vessel occlusion and tissue ischemia. Clot formation consumes all available coagulation proteins and platelets, and severe hemorrhage results.

GERIATRIC Considerations

- Prolonged INR without obvious cause or anticoagulation therapy occurs frequently among elderly persons. This prolonged INR is used to predict 30-day mortality.[25]
- Older adults with hemophilia were likely managed with blood component transfusion when younger, placing them at risk for hepatitis B and C infections.[26]
- Arthropathy is a major cause of morbidity in older persons with hemophilia, complicated by the increased risk of bleed with the use of NSAIDs for pain control.[26]
- Cardiac disease is common in the elderly population and complicated with the challenge that management using surgical interventions and antiplatelet therapy places people with hemophilia or other hematologic conditions at higher risk.[26]

PEDIATRIC Considerations

- ITP is the most common thrombocytopenic disorder among children.[27]
- ITP often follows an upper respiratory infection; however, varicella, mononucleosis, and vaccination for smallpox and measles have triggered the immune system.[27]
- In children with hemophilia, target joints are susceptible to chronic hemophilic arthropathy if bleeding is not treated effectively when it occurs.[28]
- Cerebrospinal meningitis is at epidemic levels in children; the endotoxins released trigger the inflammatory response, and consumption of platelets may result in disseminated intravascular disease.[28]
- Acquired coagulation disorders in children who are ill occur more frequently than congenital coagulation disorders.[25]

REVIEW EXERCISES

1. A 55-year-old man has begun taking one 81-mg aspirin tablet daily on the recommendation of his physician. The physician had told him that this would help to prevent heart attack and stroke.
   A. *What is the desired action of aspirin in terms of heart attack and stroke prevention?*
   B. *The drug clopidogrel (Plavix) is often prescribed along with aspirin to prevent thrombosis in persons with severe atherosclerotic disease who are at risk for myocardial infarction or stroke. Explain the rationale for using the two drugs together.*
2. The drug desmopressin acetate (DDAVP), which is a synthetic analog of arginine vasopressin, increases the half-life of factor VIII and is sometimes used to treat bleeding in males with mild hemophilia.
   A. *Explain.*
3. A 29-year-old new mother, who delivered her infant 3 days ago, is admitted to the hospital with chest pain and is diagnosed as having venous thrombosis with pulmonary emboli.
   A. *What factors would contribute to this woman's risk of developing thromboemboli?*
4. The new mother is admitted to the intensive care unit and started on low molecular weight heparin and warfarin. She is told that she will be discharged in a day or two and will remain on the heparin for 5 days and the warfarin for at least 3 months.
   A. *Explain the action of heparin and warfarin. Why is heparin administered for 5 days during the initiation of warfarin treatment?*
   B. *Anticoagulation with heparin and warfarin is not a definitive treatment for clot removal in pulmonary embolism but a form of secondary prevention. Explain.*

References

1. Hall J. E. (2016). *Guyton and Hall textbook of medical physiology* (13th ed., pp. 483–494). Philadelphia, PA: Elsevier.
2. Smith S. A., Travers R. J., Morrissey J. H. (2015). How it all starts: Initiation of the clotting cascade. *Critical Reviews in Biochemistry and Molecular Biology* 50(4), 326–336. doi: 10.3109/10409238.2015.1050550.
3. Xu X. R., Zhang D., Oswald B. E., et al. (2016). Platelets are versatile cells: New discoveries in hemostasis, thrombosis, immune responses, tumor metastasis and beyond. *Critical Reviews in Clinical Laboratory Sciences* 53(6), 409–430. doi: 10.1080/10408363.2016.1200008.
4. Aster J. C., Bunn H. F. (2017). *Pathophysiology of blood disorders* (2nd ed., pp. 156–213). New York, NY: McGraw Hill Education.
5. Shifrin M. M., Widmar, S. B. (2016). Platelet inhibitors. *Nursing Clinics of North America* 51, 29–43.
6. Franchi F., Biguzzi E., Martinelli I., et al. (2013). Normal reference ranges of antithrombin, protein C and protein S: Effect of sex, age, and hormonal status. *Thrombosis Research* 132, e152–e157. doi: 10.1016/j.thromres.2013.07.003.
7. Minuk L., Lazo-Langner A., Kovacs J., et al. (2010). Levels of protein C and protein S tested in the acute phase of a venous thrombolic event are not falsely elevated. *Thrombosis Journal* 8, 10. https://doi.org/10.1186/1477-9560-8-10
8. Pengo V., Banzato A., Bison E., et al. (2016). Efficacy and safety rivaroxaban vs. warfarin in high-risk patients with antiphospholipid syndrome: Rationale and design of the Trial on Rivaroxaban in AntiPhospholipid Syndrome (TRAPS) Trial. *Lupus* 25, 301–306.
9. Loffredo L., Perri L., Violi F. (2015). Impact of new oral anticoagulants on gastrointestinal bleeding in atrial fibrillation: A meta-analysis of interventional trials. *Digestive and Liver Disease* 47, 429–431.
10. Randi A. M., Laffan M. A. (2016). Von Willebrand factor and angiogenesis: Basic and applied issues. *Journal of Thrombosis and Haemostasis* 15, 13–20.

11. Chapin J. C., Hajjar K. A. (2015). Fibrinolysis and the control of blood coagulation. *Blood Reviews* 29, 17–24.
12. Nelson N. D., Marcogliese A., Bergstrom K., et al. (2016). Thrombopoietin measurement as a key component in the evaluation of pediatric thrombocytosis. *Pediatric Blood Cancer* 63, 1484–1487.
13. Sharma D., Singh G. (2017). Thrombocytosis in gynecological cancers. *Journal of Cancer Research and Therapeutics* 13(2), 193–197.
14. Cott M. V., Khor B., Zehnder J. L. (2016). Factor V Leiden. *American Journal of Hematology* 91, 46–49.
15. Tinholt M., Sandset P. M., Iversen N. (2016). Polymorphism of the coagulation system and risk of cancer. *Thrombosis Research* 140S1, S49–S54.
16. Wen S., Duan Q., Yang F., et al. (2017). Early diagnosis of venous thromboembolism as a clinical primary symptom of occult cancer: Core proteins of a venous thrombus (review). *Oncology Letters* 14, 491–496.
17. Pollak A. W., McDane R. D. (2014). Succinct review of the new VTE prevention and management guidelines. *Mayo Clinic Proceedings* 89(3), 394–408.
18. Rosendaal F. R. (2016). Causes of venous thrombosis. *Thrombosis Journal* 14(Suppl 1), 24. doi: 10.1186/s12959-016-0108-y.
19. Pengo V., Banzato A., Bison E., et al. (2016). Efficacy and safety of rivaroxaban vs warfarin in high-risk patients with antiphospholipid syndrome: Rationale and design of Trial on Rivaroxaban in AntiPHospholipid Syndrome (TRAPS) trial. *Lupus* 2016;25(3):301–306.
20. Ali N., Auerbach H. E. (2017). New-onset acute thrombocytopenia in hospitalized patients: pathophysiology and diagnostic approach. *Journal of Community Hospital Internal Medicine Perspectives* 7, 157–167.
21. Bădulescu O., Bădescu M., Ciocoiu M., et al. (2017). Immune thrombocytopenic purpura: Correlations between thrombocytopenia severity and its clinical symptoms. *Archives of the Balkan Medical Union*, 52(1), 9–14.
22. Perer M., Garrido T. (2017). Advances in the pathophysiology of primary immune thrombocytopenia. *Hematology* 22, 42–53.
23. Kessler C. S., Khan B. A., Lai-Miller K. (2012). Thrombotic thrombocytopenic purpura: A hematological emergency. *Journal of Emergency Medicine* 43, 538–544.
24. Singh B. (2014). *Disseminated intravascular coagulation (DIC): Clinical manifestations, diagnosis, and treatment options*. New York, NY: Nova Science Publishers.
25. Van Ommen C., Peters M. (2012). Clinical practice: The bleeding child. Part I: Primary hemostatic disorders. *European Journal of Pediatrics* 171(1), 1–10. doi: 10.1007/s00431-011-1532-4.
26. van Herrewegen F., Meijers J., Peters M., et al. (2012). Clinical practice: The bleeding child. Part II: Disorders of secondary hemostasis and fibrinolysis. *European Journal of Pediatrics* 171(2), 207–214. doi: 10.1007/s00431-011-1571-x.
27. Hinkle J. L., Cheever K. H. (2018). Hematologic function. In *Brunner & Sudarth's textbook of medical-surgical nursing* (14th ed.). Philadelphia, PA: Wolters Kluwer.
28. Bowden V. R., Greenberg C. S. (2014). The child with altered hematologic status. In *Children and their families the continuum of nursing care* (3rd ed.). Philadelphia, PA: Wolters Kluwer.

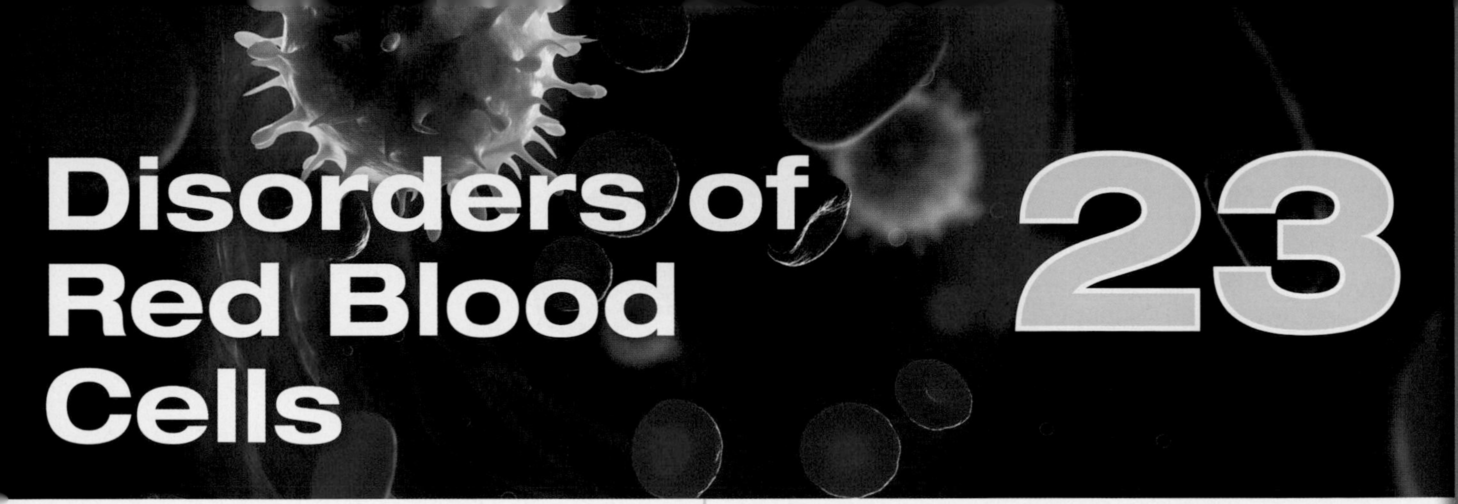

Disorders of Red Blood Cells 23

Jacqueline Rosenjack Burchum

Although the lungs provide the means for gas exchange between the external and internal environments, it is the hemoglobin in the red blood cells that transports oxygen to the tissues. The red blood cells also function as carriers of carbon dioxide and participate in acid–base balance. This chapter focuses on the red blood cell, blood types and transfusion therapy, anemia, polycythemia, and age-related changes in the red blood cells.

THE RED BLOOD CELL

After completing this section of the chapter, the learner will be able to meet the following objectives:

- Discuss the function of iron in the formation of hemoglobin.
- Describe the formation, transport, and elimination of bilirubin.
- Describe red blood cell count, percentage of reticulocytes, hemoglobin, hematocrit, mean corpuscular volume, and mean corpuscular hemoglobin concentration as it relates to the diagnosis of anemia.

The erythrocytes are 500 to 1000 times more numerous than other blood cells and are the most common type of blood cell.[1] The mature erythrocyte (also called a red blood cell or red cell) is a nonnucleated, biconcave disk (Fig. 23.1A). This unique shape contributes in two ways to the oxygen transport function of the erythrocyte. The biconcave shape provides a larger surface area for oxygen diffusion than would a spherical cell of the same volume, and the thinness of the cell membrane enables oxygen to diffuse rapidly between the exterior and the innermost regions of the cell (Fig. 23.1).

Another structural feature that facilitates the transport function of the red blood cell is the flexibility of its membrane. It can squeeze through capillaries easily and therefore has the ability to reach peripheral body tissue.[2] A complex network of fibrous proteins, especially one called *spectrin*, maintains the biconcave shape and flexibility of the red cell membrane

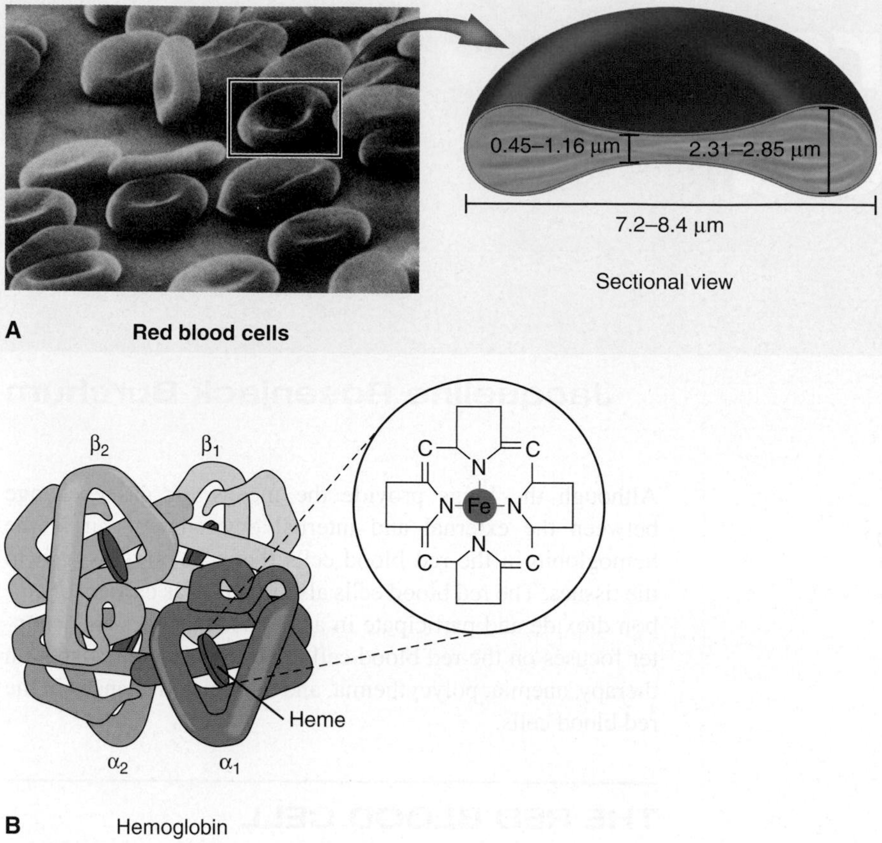

Figure 23.1 • Physical characteristics of RBCs. **(A)** RBCs are biconcave disks without nuclei. **(B)** Hemoglobin molecule, showing the four iron (Fe)-containing heme subunits and their structure. (From Pawline W. (2016). *Histology: A text and atlas: With correlated cell and molecular biology* (pp. 273, 276). Philadelphia, PA: Wolters Kluwer.)

(Fig. 23.2). Spectrin forms an attachment with another protein, called *ankyrin*, which resides on the inner surface of the membrane and is anchored to an integral protein that spans the membrane. This unique arrangement of proteins imparts elasticity and stability to the membrane and allows it to deform easily.[3]

The primary function of the red blood cell, facilitated by the hemoglobin molecule, is to transport oxygen to the tissues. Because oxygen is poorly soluble in plasma, about 95% to 98% is carried bound to hemoglobin. The hemoglobin molecule is composed of two pairs of structurally different alpha (α) and beta (β) polypeptide chains (see Fig. 23.1B). Each of the four polypeptide chains consists of a globin (protein) portion and a heme unit.[1] Thus, each molecule of hemoglobin can carry four molecules of oxygen. Hemoglobin is a natural pigment. Because of its iron content, it appears red when oxygen is attached and has a bluish cast when deoxygenated.[2] The production of each type of globin chain is controlled by individual structural genes with five different gene loci. Mutations, which can occur anywhere in these five loci, have resulted in over 550 types of abnormal hemoglobin molecules.[4]

The two major types of normal hemoglobin are adult hemoglobin (HbA) and fetal hemoglobin (HbF). HbA consists of a pair of α chains and a pair of β chains. HbF is the predominant hemoglobin in the fetus from the 3rd through the 9th months of gestation. It has a pair of gamma (γ) chains substituted for the α chains. Because of this chain substitution, HbF has a higher affinity for oxygen than HbA.[4] This affinity facilitates the transfer of oxygen across the placenta from the HbA in the mother's blood to the HbF in the fetus's blood. HbF is generally replaced within 6 months of birth with HbA.

KEY POINTS

RED BLOOD CELLS

- The function of red blood cells, facilitated by the iron-containing hemoglobin molecule, is to transport oxygen from the lungs to the tissues.
- The red blood cell, which has a life span of approximately 120 days, is broken down in the spleen; the degradation products such as iron and amino acids are recycled.

Hemoglobin Synthesis

The rate at which hemoglobin is synthesized depends on the availability of iron for heme synthesis. A lack of iron results in relatively small amounts of hemoglobin in the red blood cells. The amount of iron in the body is approximately 2 g in women and up to 6 g in men.[2] Body iron is found in several compartments. Most iron (approximately 80%) is complexed to heme in hemoglobin, with small amounts found in the myoglobin of muscle, the cytochromes, and the iron-containing enzymes. The other 20% is stored in the bone marrow, liver,

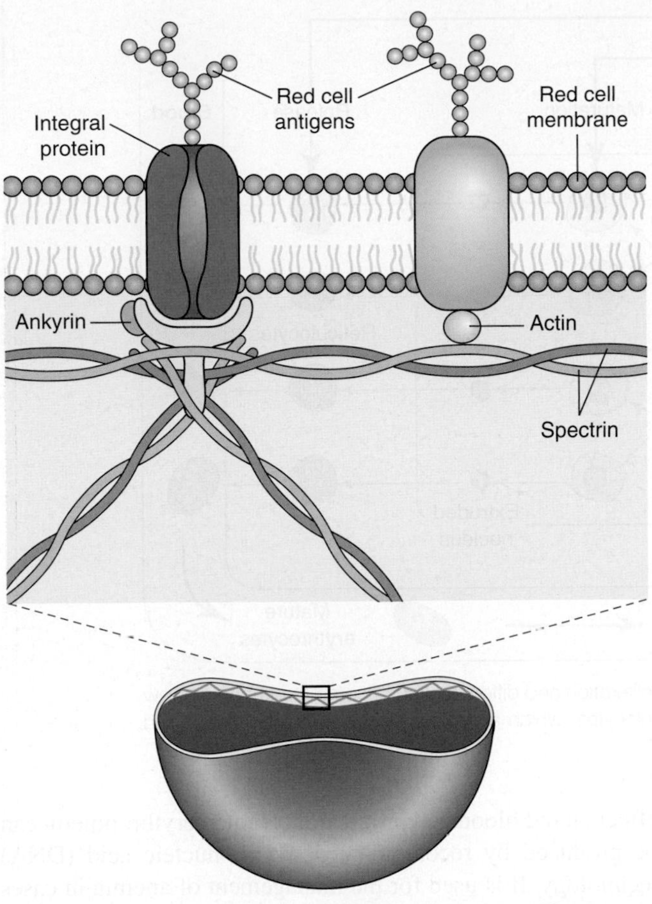

Figure 23.2 • Cross-sectional side view of the biconcave structure of the red blood cell and diagram showing the cytoskeleton and flexible network of spectrin proteins that attach to the ankyrin protein, a transmembrane protein that resides on the inner surface of the membrane and is anchored to an integral protein that spans the membrane.

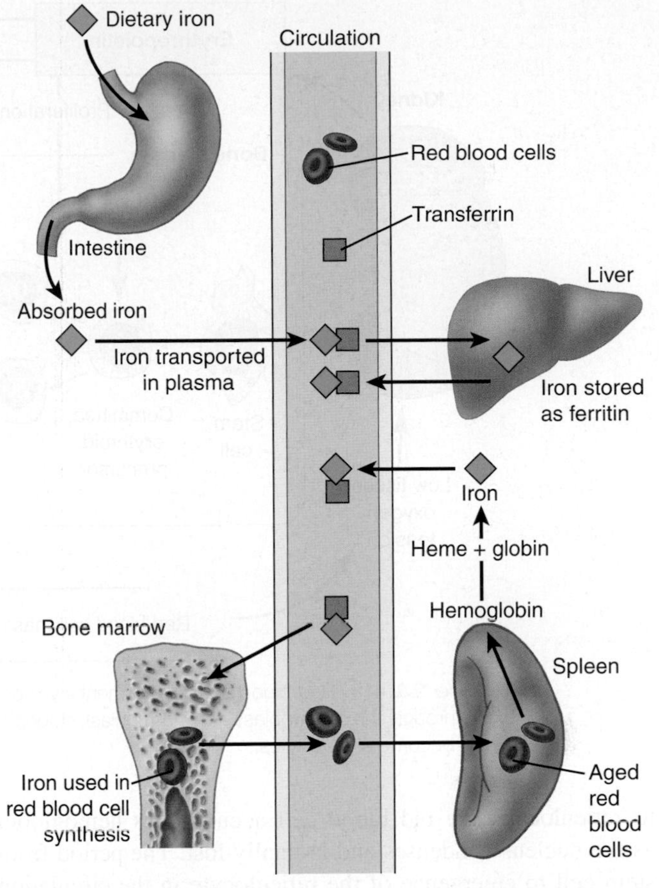

Figure 23.3 • Diagrammatic representation of the iron cycle, including its absorption from the gastrointestinal tract, transport in the circulation, storage in the liver, recycling from aged red cells destroyed in the spleen, and use in the bone marrow synthesis of red blood cells.

spleen, and other organs. Normally, some iron is sequestered in the intestinal epithelial cells and is lost in the feces as these cells slough off.

When red blood cells age and are destroyed in the spleen, the iron from their hemoglobin is released into the circulation and returned to the bone marrow for incorporation into new red blood cells. This recycled iron from old erythrocytes is the primary source of iron used in the production of new erythrocytes.[5]

Dietary iron also helps to maintain body stores. Iron, principally derived from meat, is absorbed in the small intestine, especially the duodenum (Fig. 23.3). When body stores of iron are diminished or erythropoiesis is stimulated, absorption is increased. (Conversely, in iron overload, excretion of iron is accelerated.) The iron that is absorbed enters the circulation, where it immediately combines with a β-globulin, *apotransferrin*, to form *transferrin*, which is then transported in the plasma.[1] From the plasma, iron can be deposited in tissues such as the liver, where it is stored as *ferritin*, a protein–iron complex, which can easily return to the circulation. Serum ferritin levels, which can be measured in the laboratory, provide an index of body iron stores. Clinically, decreased ferritin levels usually indicate the need for prescription of iron supplements such as ferrous sulfate. Transferrin can also deliver iron to the developing red cell in bone marrow by binding to membrane receptors. This iron is taken up by the developing red cell, where it is used in heme synthesis.[5]

Red Cell Production

Erythropoiesis refers to the production of red blood cells. After birth, red cells are produced in the red bone marrow. Until 5 years of age, almost all bones produce red cells to meet the growth needs of a child, after which bone marrow activity in long bones gradually declines. In adults, red cell production takes place mainly in the membranous bones of the vertebrae, sternum, ribs, and pelvis.[3] With this reduction in activity, the red bone marrow is replaced with fatty yellow bone marrow.

The red blood cells are derived from precursor cells called *erythroblasts*, which are formed continuously from the pluripotent stem cells in the bone marrow (Fig. 23.4). The red cell precursors move through a series of divisions, each producing a smaller cell as they continue to develop into mature red blood cells. Hemoglobin synthesis begins at the early erythroblast stage and continues until the cell becomes a mature erythrocyte. During its transformation from normoblast

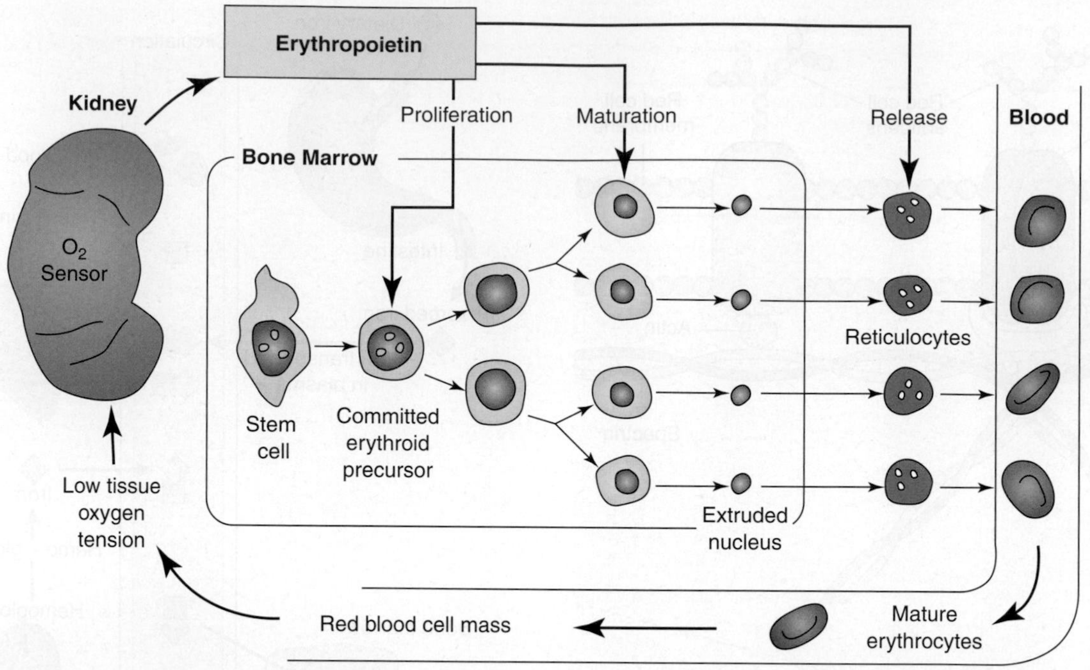

Figure 23.4 • Red blood cell development involves the proliferation and differentiation of committed bone marrow cells through the erythroblast and normoblast stages to reticulocytes, which are released into the bloodstream and finally become erythrocytes.

to reticulocyte, the red blood cell accumulates hemoglobin as the nucleus condenses and is finally lost. The period from stem cell to emergence of the reticulocyte in the circulation normally takes approximately 1 week. Maturation of reticulocyte to erythrocyte takes approximately 24 to 48 hours. During this process, the red cell loses its mitochondria and ribosomes, along with its ability to produce hemoglobin and engage in oxidative metabolism. Most maturing red cells enter the blood as reticulocytes. Approximately 1% of the body's total complement of red blood cells is generated from bone marrow each day, and the reticulocyte count therefore serves as an index of the erythropoietic activity of the bone marrow.[2]

Erythropoiesis is governed for the most part by tissue oxygen needs. Any condition that causes a decrease in the amount of oxygen that is transported in the blood produces an increase in red cell production. The oxygen content of the blood does not act directly on the bone marrow to stimulate red blood cell production. Instead, the decreased oxygen content is sensed by the peritubular cells in the kidneys, which then produce a hormone called *erythropoietin*. Normally, about 90% of all erythropoietin is produced by the kidneys, with the remaining 10% formed in the liver. Although erythropoietin is the key regulator of erythropoiesis, a number of growth factors, including granulocyte colony–stimulating factor (G-CSF), granulocyte–macrophage (GM)-CSF, and insulin-like growth factor-1 (IGF-1), are involved in the early stages of erythropoiesis.[2] Erythropoietin acts primarily in later stages of erythropoiesis to induce the erythrocyte colony–forming units to proliferate and mature through the normoblast stage into reticulocytes and mature erythrocytes. In the absence of erythropoietin, as in kidney failure, hypoxia has little or no effect on red blood cell production. Human erythropoietin can be produced by recombinant deoxyribonucleic acid (DNA) technology. It is used for the management of anemia in cases of chronic renal failure, for anemias induced by chemotherapy in persons with malignancies, and in the treatment of anemia in human immunodeficiency virus (HIV)–infected persons.[2]

Because red blood cells are released into the blood as reticulocytes, the percentage of these cells is higher when there is a marked increase in red blood cell production. In some severe forms of anemia, the reticulocytes (normally about 1%) may account for as much as 30% of the total red cell count. In some situations, red cell production is so accelerated that numerous erythroblasts appear in the blood.[2]

Red Cell Destruction

Mature red blood cells have a life span of approximately 4 months, or 120 days. As the red blood cell ages, a number of changes occur—metabolic activity in the cell decreases, enzyme activity declines, and adenosine triphosphate (ATP) decreases. Membrane lipids become reduced and the cell membrane becomes more fragile, causing the red cell to self-destruct as it passes through narrow places in the circulation and in the small trabecular spaces in the spleen.[2] The rate of red cell destruction (1% per day) normally is equal to the rate of red cell production, but in conditions such as hemolytic anemia, the cell's life span may be shorter.

The destruction of red blood cells is facilitated by a group of large phagocytic cells found in the spleen, liver, bone marrow, and lymph nodes. These phagocytic cells recognize old and defective red cells and then ingest and destroy them in a series of enzymatic reactions. During these reactions, the amino acids from the globulin chains and iron from the heme units are salvaged and reused (Fig. 23.5). The bulk of the heme unit is converted to bilirubin, the pigment of bile, which is insoluble in plasma and attaches to plasma proteins for transport. Bilirubin is removed from the blood by the liver and conjugated with glucuronide to render it water soluble so that it can be excreted in the bile. Excess elimination of bilirubin in the bile because of increased red cell destruction can lead to the development of bilirubin gallstones. The plasma-insoluble form of bilirubin is referred to as *unconjugated bilirubin* and the water-soluble form as *conjugated bilirubin*. Serum levels of conjugated and unconjugated bilirubin can be measured in the laboratory and are reported as direct and indirect, respectively. If red cell destruction and consequent bilirubin production are excessive, unconjugated bilirubin accumulates in the blood. This results in a yellow discoloration of the skin, called *jaundice*.[2]

When red blood cell destruction takes place in the circulation, as in hemolytic anemia, the hemoglobin remains in the plasma. The plasma contains a hemoglobin-binding protein called *haptoglobin*.[4] Other plasma proteins, such as albumin, can also bind hemoglobin. With extensive intravascular destruction of red blood cells, hemoglobin levels may exceed the hemoglobin-binding capacity of haptoglobin and other plasma proteins. When this happens, free hemoglobin appears in the blood (*i.e.*, hemoglobinemia) and is excreted in the urine (*i.e.*, hemoglobinuria).[4] Because excessive red blood cell destruction can occur in hemolytic transfusion reactions, urine samples are tested for free hemoglobin after a transfusion reaction.

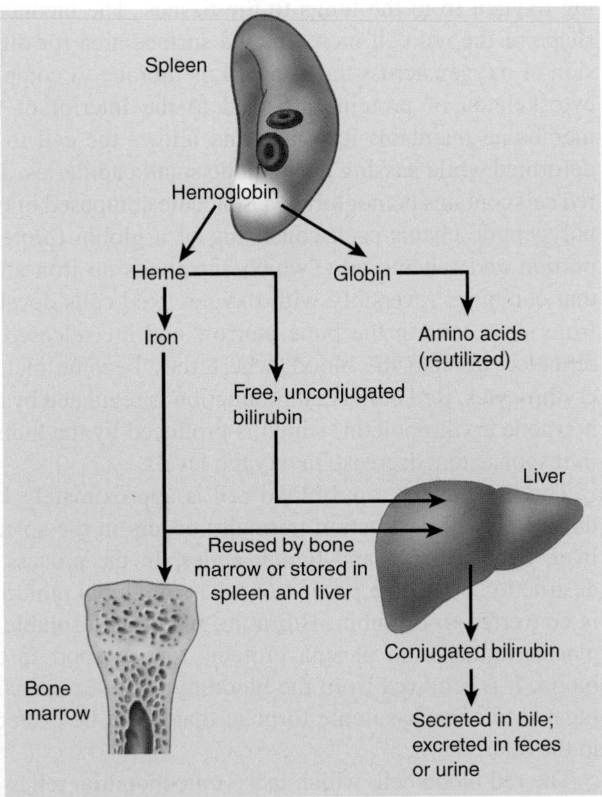

Figure 23.5 • Destruction of red blood cells and fate of hemoglobin.

Red Cell Metabolism and Hemoglobin Oxidation

The red blood cell, which lacks mitochondria, relies on glucose and the glycolytic pathway for its metabolic needs. The enzyme-mediated anaerobic metabolism of glucose generates the ATP needed for normal membrane function and ion transport. The depletion of glucose or the functional deficiency of one of the glycolytic enzymes leads to the premature death of the red blood cell. An offshoot of the glycolytic pathway is the production of 2,3-diphosphoglycerate (2,3-DPG), which binds to the hemoglobin molecule and reduces the affinity of hemoglobin for oxygen. This facilitates the release of oxygen at the tissue level. An increase in the concentration of 2,3-DPG occurs in conditions of chronic hypoxia such as chronic lung disease, anemia, and residence at high altitudes.[1]

Certain chemicals (*e.g.*, nitrates and sulfates) and drugs that oxidize hemoglobin to an inactive form interrupt the oxidation of hemoglobin (the combining of hemoglobin with oxygen). The nitrite ion reacts with hemoglobin to produce methemoglobin, which has a low affinity for oxygen. Large doses of nitrites can result in high levels of methemoglobin, causing pseudocyanosis and tissue hypoxia. For example, sodium nitrate, which is used in curing meats, can produce methemoglobin when taken in large amounts. In nursing infants, the intestinal flora is capable of converting significant amounts of inorganic nitrate (*e.g.*, from well water) to nitrite.

A hereditary deficiency of glucose-6-phosphate dehydrogenase (G6PD) predisposes to oxidative denaturation of hemoglobin, with resultant red cell injury and lysis. Deficiency of G6PD is an anemia that is most frequently seen in black men. Hemolysis usually occurs as the result of oxidative stress generated by either an infection or exposure to certain drugs or foods.

Laboratory Tests

Red blood cells can be studied by means of a sample of blood (Table 23.1). In the laboratory, automated blood cell counters rapidly provide accurate measurements of red cell content and cell indices. The *red blood cell count* measures the total number of red blood cells in a microliter (μL) of blood. The *percentage of reticulocytes* (normally approximately 1%) provides an index of the rate of red cell production. The *hemoglobin* (grams per deciliter [dL] or 100 milliliters [mL] of blood) measures the hemoglobin content of the blood. The major components of blood are the red cell mass and plasma volume. The *hematocrit* measures the red cell mass in a 100-mL plasma volume. To determine the hematocrit, a sample of blood is placed in a glass tube, which is then centrifuged to separate the cells and the plasma. The hematocrit may be deceptive because it varies with the quantity of extracellular fluid, rising with dehydration and falling with overexpansion of extracellular fluid volume (Fig. 23.6).

TABLE 23.1 STANDARD LABORATORY VALUES FOR RED BLOOD CELLS

TEST	NORMAL VALUES	SIGNIFICANCE
Red Blood Cell Count (RBC)		
Men	4.2–5.4 × 10^6/μL	Number of red cells in the blood
Women	3.6–5.0 × 10^6/μL	
Reticulocytes	1.0%–1.5% of total RBC	Rate of red cell production
Hemoglobin		
Men	14–16.5 g/dL	Hemoglobin content of the blood
Women	12–15 g/dL	
Hematocrit		
Men	40%–50%	Volume of cells in 100 mL of blood
Women	37%–47%	
Mean corpuscular volume	85–100 fL	Size of the red cell
Mean corpuscular hemoglobin concentration	31–35 g/dL	Concentration of hemoglobin in the red cell
Mean cell hemoglobin	27–34 pg/cell	Red cell mass

Red cell indices are used to differentiate types of anemias by size or color of red cells. The *mean corpuscular volume* (*MCV*) reflects the volume or size of the red cells. The MCV falls in microcytic (small cell) anemia and rises in macrocytic (large cell) anemia. Some anemias are normocytic (*i.e.*, cells are of normal size or MCV). The *mean corpuscular hemoglobin concentration* (*MCHC*) is the concentration of hemoglobin in each cell. Hemoglobin accounts for the color of red blood cells. Anemias are described as *normochromic* (normal color or MCHC) or *hypochromic* (decreased color or MCHC). Mean *cell hemoglobin* (MCH) refers to the mass of the red cell and is less useful in classifying anemias.[1]

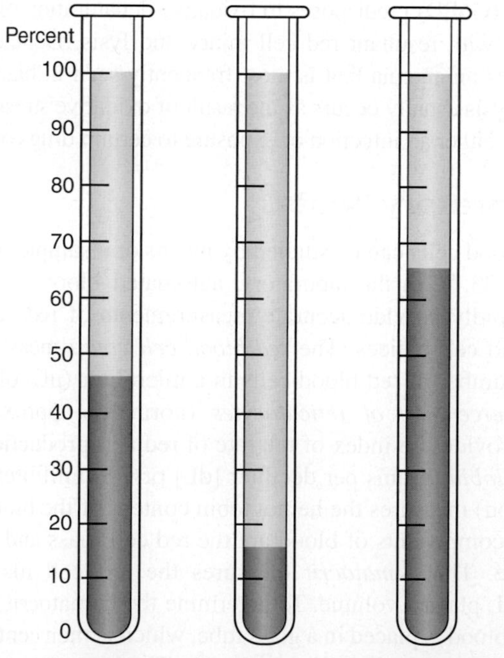

Figure 23.6 • Hematocrit. The hematocrit measures the percentage of cells in 100 mL of plasma: **(A)** normal, **(B)** decreased in anemia, and **(C)** increased in polycythemia.

A stained blood smear provides information about the size, color, and shape of red cells and the presence of immature or abnormal cells. If blood smear results are abnormal, examination of the bone marrow may be indicated. Bone marrow commonly is aspirated with a needle from the posterior iliac crest or the sternum. The aspirate is stained and observed for number and maturity of cells and abnormal types.

IN SUMMARY

The red blood cell provides the means for transporting oxygen from the lungs to the tissues. The biconcave shape of the red cell increases the surface area for diffusion of oxygen across the thin cell membrane. A complex cytoskeleton of proteins attached to the interior of the membrane maintains its shape and allows the cell to be deformed while passing through the small capillaries. The red cell contains hemoglobin, a molecule composed of two polypeptide chains each consisting of a globin (protein) portion and a heme unit, which surrounds an iron atom that combines reversibly with oxygen. Red cells develop from stem cells in the bone marrow and are released as reticulocytes into the blood, where they become mature erythrocytes. Red blood cell production is regulated by the hormone erythropoietin, which is produced by the kidney in response to a decrease in oxygen levels.

The life span of a red blood cell is approximately 120 days. Red cell destruction normally occurs in the spleen, liver, bone marrow, and lymph nodes. In the process of destruction, the heme portion of the hemoglobin molecule is converted to bilirubin. Bilirubin, which is insoluble in plasma, attaches to plasma proteins for transport in the blood. It is removed from the blood by the liver and conjugated to a water-soluble form so that it can be excreted in the bile.[1]

The red blood cell, which lacks mitochondria, relies on glucose and the glycolytic pathway for its metabolic needs.

The end product of the glycolytic pathway, 2,3-DPG, increases the release of oxygen to the tissues during conditions of hypoxia by reducing hemoglobin's affinity for oxygen.[1]

In the laboratory, automated blood cell counters rapidly provide accurate measurements of red blood cell count and cell indices. A stained blood smear provides information about the size, color, and shape of red cells and the presence of immature or abnormal cells. If blood smear results are abnormal, examination of the bone marrow may be indicated.

BLOOD TYPES AND TRANSFUSION THERAPY

After completing this section of the chapter, the learner will be able to meet the following objectives:

- Differentiate red cell antigens from antibodies in people with type A, B, AB, or O blood.
- Explain the determination of the Rh factor.
- List the signs and symptoms of a blood transfusion reaction.

Anemias of various causes are treated with transfusions of whole blood or red blood cells only when oxygen delivery to the tissues is compromised, as evidenced by measures of oxygen transport and use, hemoglobin, and hematocrit. Current recommendations suggest transfusion for people with hemoglobin levels less than 7 g/dL, depending on age, illness, risk factors, and surgical procedures.[6] Acute massive blood loss usually is replaced with whole blood transfusion. Most anemias, however, are treated with transfusions of red cell concentrates, which supply only the blood component that is deficient.

Several blood components that are used for transfusion are prepared and stored under specific conditions and have unique uses, as described in Table 23.2. These red cell components are derived principally from voluntary blood donors. However, before a red cell or whole blood transfusion from a volunteer donor source can occur, a series of procedures is required to ensure a successful transfusion. Donor and recipient samples are typed to determine ABO and Rh groups and screened for unexpected red cell antibodies. The crossmatch is performed by incubating the donor cells with the recipient's serum and observing for agglutination. If none appears, the donor and recipient blood types are compatible.

The use of autologous donation and transfusion has been advocated since the early 1980s. Autologous transfusion refers to the procedure of receiving one's own blood—usually to replenish a surgical loss—thereby eliminating the risk of blood-borne disease or transfusion reaction.[7] Autologous blood can be provided by several means—predeposit, normovolemic hemodilution, and intraoperative salvage. A person who is anticipating elective orthopedic, vascular, or open heart surgery may predeposit blood (*i.e.*, have the blood collected up to 6 weeks in advance and stored) for later transfusion during the surgery. Hemodilution involves the removal of one or two units of blood immediately before surgery followed by the infusion of intravenous crystalloids or colloids to maintain circulatory volume. The collected blood is transfused during or at the completion of surgery, if needed. Intraoperative blood salvage is the collection of bloodshed from the operative site for reinfusion into the person. Semiautomated devices are used to collect, anticoagulate, wash, and resuspend red cells for reinfusion during many procedures, including vascular, cardiac, and orthopedic surgery.[7]

ABO Blood Groups

ABO compatibility is essential for effective transfusion therapy and requires knowledge of ABO antigens and antibodies. There are four major ABO blood groups determined by the presence or absence of two red cell antigens (A and B). People who have neither A nor B antigens are classified as having type O blood. Those with A antigens are classified as having type A blood; those with B antigens, as having type B blood; and those with A and B antigens, as having type AB blood (Table 23.3). The ABO blood groups are genetically determined. The type O gene is apparently functionless in production of a red cell antigen. Each of the other genes is expressed by the presence of a strong antigen on the surface of the red cell. Six genotypes, or gene combinations, result in four phenotypes, or blood type expressions. In the United States, types O and A are the most common.

ABO antibodies predictably develop in the serum of people whose red cells lack the corresponding antigen. Persons with type A antigens on their red cells develop type B antibodies; persons with type B antigens develop type A antibodies in their serum; people with type O blood develop type A and type B antibodies; and people with type AB blood develop neither A nor B antibodies. The ABO antibodies usually are not present at birth but begin to develop at 3 to 6 months of age and reach maximum levels between the ages of 5 and 10 years.[7]

Rh Types

The D antigen of the Rh system is also important in transfusion compatibility and is routinely tested. The Rh type is coded by three gene pairs—C, c; D, d; and E, e. Each allele, with the exception of d, codes for a specific antigen. The D antigen is the most immunogenic. People who express the D antigen are designated Rh-positive, and those who do not express the D antigen are Rh-negative. Unlike serum antibodies for the ABO blood types, which develop spontaneously after birth, Rh antibodies develop after exposure to one or more of the Rh antigens, usually through pregnancy or transfusions, and persist for many years.[2] Because it takes several weeks to produce antibodies, a reaction may be delayed and usually is mild. If subsequent transfusions of Rh-positive blood are given to a person who has become sensitized, the person may have a severe, immediate reaction.

TABLE 23.2 BLOOD AND BLOOD COMPONENTS COMMONLY USED IN TRANSFUSION THERAPY*

COMPONENT	COMPOSITION	INDICATIONS AND CONSIDERATIONS
Whole blood	Cells and plasma, hematocrit about 40%	Volume replacement and oxygen-carrying capacity; usually used only in significant bleeding (>25% blood volume lost)
PRBCs	RBCs with little plasma (hematocrit about 75%); some platelets and WBCs remain	↑ RBC mass; symptomatic anemia: • Platelets within the unit are not functional • WBCs within the unit may cause reaction and are not functional
Platelets—random	Platelets (5.5×10^{10} platelets/unit), plasma; some RBCs, WBCs	Bleeding because of severe ↓ platelets Prevent bleeding when platelets <5000–10,000/mm^3 Survival ↓ in presence of fever, chills, infection Repeated treatment leads to ↓ survival because of alloimmunization.
Platelets—single donor	Platelets (3×10^{11} platelets/unit) 1 unit is equivalent to 6–8 units of random platelets.	Used for repeated treatment: • ↓ alloimmunization risk by limiting exposure to multiple donors
Plasma	Plasma; all coagulation factors Complement	Bleeding in people with coagulation factor deficiencies; plasmapheresis
Granulocytes	Neutrophils (>1×10^{10}/unit); some lymphocytes, RBCs, and platelets will remain within the unit.	Severe neutropenia in selected people; controversial
Lymphocytes	Lymphocytes (number varies)	Stimulate graft-versus-host disease effect
Cryoprecipitate	Fibrinogen ≥150 mg/bag, AHF (VIII:C) 80–110 units/bag, von Willebrand factor; fibronectin	von Willebrand disease Hypofibrinogenemia Hemophilia A
AHF	Factor VIII	Hemophilia A
Factor IX concentrate	Factor IX	Hemophilia B (Christmas disease)
Factor IX complex	Factors II, VII, IX, X	Hereditary factor VII, IX, X deficiency; hemophilia A with factor VII inhibitors
Albumin	Albumin 5%, 25%	Hypoproteinemia; burns; volume expansion by 5% to ↑ blood volume; 25% leads to ↓ hematocrit
IV gamma-globulin	Immunoglobulin G antibodies	Hypogammaglobulinemia (in CLL, recurrent infections); ITP; primary immunodeficiency states
Antithrombin III concentrate (AT III)	AT III (trace amounts of other plasma proteins)	AT III deficiency with or at risk for thrombosis

*The composition of each type of blood component is described as well as the most common indications for using a given blood component. RBCs, platelets, and fresh-frozen plasma are the blood products most commonly used. When transfusing these blood products, it is important to realize that the individual product is always "contaminated" with very small amounts of other blood products (*e.g.,* WBCs mixed in a unit of platelets). This contamination can cause some difficulties, particularly isosensitization, in certain people.

↑, increased; ↓, decreased; AHF, antihemophilic factor; CLL, chronic lymphocytic leukemia; ITP, idiopathic thrombocytopenic purpura; IV, intravenous; PRBCs, packed red blood cells; RBCs, red blood cells; WBCs, white blood cells.

Reprinted from Hinkle J. L., Cheever K. H. (2018). *Brunner & Suddarth's textbook of medical-surgical nursing* (14th ed., Table 32-4, p. 915). Philadelphia, PA: Wolters Kluwer; adapted from American Red Cross. (2015a). Blood components. Retrieved on September 14, 2015 at: www.redcrossblood.org/learn-about-blood/blood components; Dzieczkowski J. S., Anderson K. C. (2015). Transfusion biology and therapy. In Kasper D., Fauci A., Hauser S., et al. (Eds.), *Harrison's principles of internal medicine* (19th ed.). Retrieved on May 25, 2016 at: accessmedicine.mhmedical.com.laneproxy.stanford.edu/content.aspx?bookid=1130&Sectionid=79732248.

Blood Transfusion Reactions

The seriousness of blood transfusion reactions prompts the need for extreme caution when blood is administered. Because most transfusion reactions result from administrative errors or misidentification, care should be taken to identify correctly the recipient and the transfusion source. The recipient's vital signs should be monitored before and during the transfusion, and careful observation for signs of transfusion reaction is imperative.

In the event of a blood transfusion reaction, the transfusion should be stopped immediately. Venous access should be maintained because it may be necessary to infuse intravenous solutions to ensure diuresis, administer medications,

TABLE 23.3 ABO BLOOD GROUP SYSTEM

GENOTYPE	RED CELL ANTIGENS	BLOOD TYPE	SERUM ANTIBODIES
OO	None	O	AB
AO	A	A	B
AA	A	A	B
BO	B	B	A
BB	B	B	A
AB	AB	AB	None

and take blood samples. Additionally, the donated blood will need to be tested to determine factors that contributed to the reaction.

The Centers for Disease Control and Prevention (CDC) has identified 11 types of transfusion reactions.[8] The reactions and classification criteria are provided in Table 23.4. The most common or concerning reactions are addressed in the discussion that follows.

Acute Hemolytic Transfusion Reactions

Acute hemolytic transfusion reactions (AHTF) occurs when there is destruction of donor red cells by reaction with antibody in the recipient's serum.[7] It can be life-threatening, but fortunately, it is rare: It occurs in 1 out of 76,000 transfusions. The majority of these (1 out of 40,000 transfusions) is caused by ABO incompatibility. Typical signs and symptoms may occur following as little as 10 mL of blood transfusion.[7]

Hemoglobin that is released from the hemolyzed donor cells is filtered in the glomeruli of the kidneys. Because of the adverse effects of the filtered hemoglobin on renal tubular flow, two possible complications of an AHTF are oliguria and renal failure.[9] In addition to other testing, a urine specimen should be examined for the presence of hemoglobin, urobilinogen, and red blood cells.

TABLE 23.4 CLASSIFICATION OF BLOOD TRANSFUSION REACTIONS

BLOOD TRANSFUSION REACTION	CASE DEFINITION*
Allergic reaction	**Definitive:** Two or more of the following occurring during or within 4 hours of cessation of transfusion: • Conjunctival edema • Edema of the lips, tongue, and uvula • Erythema and edema of the periorbital area • Generalized flushing • Hypotension • Localized angioedema • Maculopapular rash • Pruritus (itching) • Respiratory distress; bronchospasm • Urticaria (hives) **Probable:** ANY 1 of the following occurring during or within 4 hours of cessation of transfusion: • Conjunctival edema • Edema of the lips, tongue, and uvula • Erythema and edema of the periorbital area • Localized angioedema • Maculopapular rash • Pruritus (itching) • Urticaria (hives) (CDC, 2017, p. 12)
Acute hemolytic transfusion reaction	**Definitive:** Occurs during or within 24 hours of cessation of transfusion with new onset of ANY of the following signs/symptoms: • Back/flank pain • Chills/rigors • Disseminated intravascular coagulation (DIC) • Epistaxis • Fever • Hematuria (gross visual hemolysis) • Hypotension • Oliguria/anuria • Pain and/or oozing at IV site • Renal failure

(Continued)

TABLE 23.4 CLASSIFICATION OF BLOOD TRANSFUSION REACTIONS *(Continued)*

BLOOD TRANSFUSION REACTION	CASE DEFINITION*
Acute hemolytic transfusion reaction (*Continued*)	*AND* Two or more of the following: • Decreased fibrinogen • Decreased haptoglobin • Elevated bilirubin • Elevated LDH • Hemoglobinemia • Hemoglobinuria • Plasma discoloration c/w hemolysis • Spherocytes on blood film *AND EITHER* • (IMMUNE MEDIATED) Positive direct antiglobulin test (DAT) for anti-IgG or anti-C3 *AND* Positive elution test with alloantibody present on the transfused red blood cells *OR* • (NON–IMMUNE MEDIATED) Serologic testing is negative, and physical cause (*e.g.*, thermal, osmotic, mechanical, chemical) is confirmed. **Probable:** Meets signs and symptoms criteria for acute hemolysis *AND EITHER* • (IMMUNE MEDIATED) Physical cause is excluded but serologic evidence is not sufficient to meet definitive criteria *OR* • (NON–IMMUNE MEDIATED) Physical cause is suspected and serologic testing is negative (CDC, 2017, p. 15).
Delayed hemolytic transfusion reaction	**Definitive:** Positive direct antiglobulin test (DAT) for antibodies developed between 24 hours and 28 days after cessation of transfusion *AND EITHER* • Positive elution test with alloantibody present on the transfused red blood cells *OR* • Newly identified red blood cell alloantibody in recipient serum *AND EITHER* • Inadequate rise of posttransfusion hemoglobin level or rapid fall in hemoglobin back to pretransfusion levels *OR* • Otherwise unexplained appearance of spherocytes **Probable:** Newly identified red blood cell alloantibody demonstrated between 24 hours and 28 days after cessation of transfusion *BUT* Incomplete laboratory evidence to meet definitive case definition criteria *NOTE:* Person may be asymptomatic or have symptoms that are similar to but milder than AHTR; symptoms are not required to meet case definition criteria (CDC, 2017, p. 16).
Delayed serologic transfusion reaction	Absence of clinical signs of hemolysis *AND* Demonstration of new, clinically significant antibodies against red blood cells *BY EITHER* • Positive direct antiglobulin test (DAT) *OR* • Positive antibody screen with newly identified RBC alloantibody (CDC, 2017, p. 17)

TABLE 23.4 CLASSIFICATION OF BLOOD TRANSFUSION REACTIONS *(Continued)*

BLOOD TRANSFUSION REACTION	CASE DEFINITION*
Febrile non-hemolytic transfusion reaction	Occurs during or within 4 hours of cessation of transfusion *AND EITHER* • Fever (greater than or equal to 38°C/100.4°F oral and a change of at least 1°C/1.8°F) from pretransfusion value *OR* • Chills/rigors are present (CDC, 2017, p. 14).
Hypotensive transfusion reaction	All other adverse reactions presenting with hypotension are excluded *AND* Hypotension occurs during or within 1 hour after cessation of transfusion. • Adults (18 years and older): Drop in systolic BP of greater than or equal to 30 mm Hg and systolic BP less than or equal to 80 mm Hg • Infants, children, and adolescents (1 year to less than 18 years old): Greater than 25% drop in systolic BP from baseline (*e.g.*, drop in systolic BP of 120 mm Hg to below 90 mm Hg) • Neonates and small infants (less than 1 year old OR any age and less than 12 kg body weight): Greater than 25% drop in basline value using whichever measurement is being recorded (*e.g.*, mean BP) (CDC, 2017, p. 13)
Transfusion-associated circulatory overload (TACO)	New onset or exacerbation of three or more of the following within 6 hours of cessation of transfusion: • Acute respiratory distress (dyspnea, orthopnea, cough) • Elevated brain natriuretic peptide (BNP) • Elevated central venous pressure (CVP) • Evidence of left heart failure • Evidence of positive fluid balance • Radiographic evidence of pulmonary edema (CDC, 2017, p. 9)
Transfusion-related acute lung injury (TRALI)	*NO* evidence of acute lung injury (ALI) prior to transfusion *AND* ALI onset during or within 6 hours of cessation of transfusion *AND* Hypoxemia defined by any of these methods: • PaO_2/FiO_2 less than or equal to 300 mm Hg • Oxygen saturation less than 90% on room air • Other clinical evidence *AND* Radiographic evidence of bilateral infiltrates *AND* No evidence of left atrial hypertension (*i.e.*, circulatory overload) (CDC, 2017, p. 10)
Transfusion-associated dyspnea (TAD)	Acute respiratory distress occurring within 24 hours of cessation of transfusion *AND* Allergic reaction, TACO, and TRALI definitions are not applicable (CDC, 2017, p. 11).
Transfusion-associated graft-versus-host disease	**Definitive:** A clinical syndrome occurring from 2 days to 6 weeks after cessation of transfusion characterized by: Characteristic rash: erythematous, maculopapular eruption centrally that spreads to extremities and may, in severe cases, progress to generalized erythroderma and hemorrhagic bullous formation • Diarrhea • Fever • Hepatomegaly • Liver dysfunction (*i.e.*, elevated ALT, AST, alkaline phosphatase, and bilirubin) • Marrow aplasia • Pancytopenia *AND* • Characteristic histological appearance of skin or liver biopsy **Probable:** Meets definitive criteria *EXCEPT* Biopsy negative or not done (CDC, 2017, p. 18)

(Continued)

TABLE 23.4 CLASSIFICATION OF BLOOD TRANSFUSION REACTIONS *(Continued)*

BLOOD TRANSFUSION REACTION	CASE DEFINITION*
Transfusion-transmitted infection	Laboratory evidence of a pathogen in the transfusion recipient (CDC, 2017, p. 20)
Post transfusion purpura	**Definitive:** Alloantibodies in the person directed against HPA or other platelet-specific antigen detected at or after development of thrombocytopenia *AND* Thrombocytopenia (*i.e.*, decrease in platelets to less than 20% of pretransfusion count) **Probable:** Alloantibodies in the person directed against HPA or other platelet-specific antigen detected at or after development of thrombocytopenia *AND* Decrease in platelets to levels between 20% and 80% of pretransfusion count (CDC, 2017, p. 19)

*CDC case definitions are reported verbatim to avoid misinterpretation.

Adapted from Centers for Disease Control and Prevention (CDC). (2017). *National healthcare safety network biovigilance component hemovigilance module surveillance protocol* (pp. 9–30). Available: https://www.cdc.gov/nhsn/PDFs/Biovigilance/BV-HV-protocol-current.pdf.

Delayed Hemolytic Transfusion Reactions

Delayed hemolytic transfusion reactions (DHTR) may occur 1 to 2 weeks after transfusion and are caused by undetected antibodies in the recipient's serum. The estimated incidence of DHTR is about 1:1500 transfusions, and the reaction is accompanied by a fall in hemoglobin and jaundice.[9] However, recipients may be asymptomatic.

Febrile Reactions

The estimated incidence of febrile reactions ranges from 0.1% to 1% of those receiving transfusions. Recipient antibodies directed against the donor's white cells cause an increase in temperature approximately 2 hours after the transfusion begins.[9] Antipyretics are used to treat this reaction. Future febrile reactions may be avoided by the use of leukocyte-reduced blood.

Allergic Reactions

Allergic reactions occur in 1% to 3% of people receiving blood transfusions and are the most common reactions. They are caused by antibodies against donor proteins. Allergic reactions may range from a mild rash with itching to life-threatening anaphylactic reactions.[8] Mild reactions can be relieved with antihistamines.[9]

Anaphylactic reactions are uncommon, occurring in 1 out of every 20,000 to 50,000 transfusions. Like allergic reactions, they are caused by antibodies to donor proteins, specifically IgA, C4, and haptoglobin. The reaction is severe and life-threatening. Signs and symptoms include cardiovascular collapse with hypotension and tachycardia, bronchospasm, hypoxemia, angioedema, and urticaria. Treatment includes epinephrine, antihistamines, and glucocorticoids.[9]

Transfusion-Related Acute Lung Injury

The underlying cause of transfusion-related acute lung injury (TRALI) is human leukocyte antigen (HLA) in the donor blood. Occurrence, although not common (1 in 10,000 cases), is fatal in 10% to 20% of those affected. Within 6 hours of receiving a transfusion, the recipient develops pulmonary edema with hypotension and hypoxemia. Treatment is supportive.[9]

Transfusion-Associated Circulatory Overload

Transfusion-associated circulatory overload (TACO) most commonly strikes people already at high risk for overload. These are primarily people with heart or renal problems and people who are older than 60 years. TACO occurs in approximately 1% of transfusions and has a mortality rate of 1.4% to 8.3%. The main symptom is acute respiratory distress. Treatment involves diuretics to reduce overload and supplemental oxygen to meet oxygen demand.[9] Maintaining an upright position can help manage orthopnea and prevent worsening pulmonary edema related to gravity-related fluid shifts.

IN SUMMARY

Transfusion therapy provides the means for replacement of red blood cells and other blood components. Red blood cells contain surface antigens, and reciprocal antibodies are found in the serum. Four major ABO blood types are determined by the presence or absence of two red cell antigens—A and B. The D antigen determines the Rh-positive type; absence of the D antigen determines the Rh-negative type. ABO and Rh types must be determined in recipient and donor blood before transfusion to ensure compatibility.

ANEMIA

After completing this section of the chapter, the learner will be able to meet the following objectives:

- Describe the manifestations of anemia and their mechanisms.
- Describe the relation between vitamin B_{12} deficiency and megaloblastic anemia.
- Compare characteristics of the red blood cells in acute blood loss, hereditary spherocytosis, sickle cell disease, iron deficiency anemia, and aplastic anemia.

Anemia is defined as an abnormally low number of circulating red blood cells or level of hemoglobin, or both, resulting in diminished oxygen-carrying capacity. There are four primary causes of anemia: (1) excessive loss of red blood cells from bleeding, (2) destruction (hemolysis) of red blood cells, (3) defective red blood cell production, or (4) inadequate red blood cell production because of bone marrow failure.

Anemia is not a disease, but an indication of some disease process or alteration in body function. The effects of anemia can be grouped into three categories:

1. Manifestations of impaired oxygen transport and the resulting compensatory mechanisms
2. Reduction in red cell indices and hemoglobin levels
3. Signs and symptoms associated with the pathologic process that is causing the anemia

The manifestations of anemia depend on its severity, the rapidity of its development, and the person's age and health status.

In anemia, the oxygen-carrying capacity of hemoglobin is reduced, causing tissue hypoxia. Tissue hypoxia can give rise to fatigue, weakness, dyspnea, and sometimes angina. Hypoxia of brain tissue results in headache, faintness, and dim vision. The redistribution of the blood from cutaneous tissues or a lack of hemoglobin causes pallor of the skin, mucous membranes, conjunctiva, and nail beds. Tachycardia and palpitations may occur as the body tries to compensate with an increase in cardiac output. A flow-type systolic heart murmur may result from changes in blood viscosity. Ventricular hypertrophy and high-output heart failure may develop in people with severe anemia, particularly those with preexisting heart disease. Erythropoiesis is accelerated and may be recognized by diffuse bone pain and sternal tenderness. In addition to the common anemic manifestations, hemolytic anemias are accompanied by jaundice caused by increased blood levels of bilirubin. In aplastic anemia, petechiae and purpura (*i.e.*, minute hemorrhagic spots and purplish areas on the skin caused by small-vessel bleeding) are the result of reduced platelet function.[10]

Laboratory tests are useful in determining the severity and cause of the anemia. The red cell count and hemoglobin levels provide information about the severity of the anemia, whereas red cell characteristics such as size (normocytic, microcytic, macrocytic), color (normochromic, hypochromic), and shape often provide information about the cause of anemia (Fig. 23.7).[11]

KEY POINTS

ANEMIA

- Anemia, which is a deficiency of red cells or hemoglobin, results from excessive bleeding, increased destruction (hemolysis) of red blood cells, production of defective red blood cells, or production of insufficient numbers of red blood cells.
- Blood loss anemia is characterized by loss of iron-containing red blood cells from the body; hemolytic anemia involves destruction of red blood cells in the body with iron being retained in the body.

Blood Loss Anemia

The clinical and red cell manifestations associated with blood loss anemia depend on the rate of hemorrhage and whether the bleeding loss is internal or external. With rapid blood loss, circulatory shock and circulatory collapse may occur. With more slowly developing anemia, the amount of red cell mass lost may reach 50% without the occurrence of signs and symptoms.[1]

The effects of *acute* blood loss are mainly because of loss of intravascular volume, which can lead to cardiovascular collapse and shock. A fall in the red blood cell count, hematocrit, and hemoglobin is caused by hemodilution resulting from movement of fluid into the vascular compartment. Initially, the red cells are normal in size and color (normocytic, normochromic). The hypoxia that results from blood loss stimulates proliferation of committed erythroid stem cells in the bone marrow. It takes about 5 days for the progeny of stem cells to differentiate fully, an event that is marked by increased reticulocytes in the blood. If the bleeding is controlled and sufficient iron stores are available, the red cell concentration returns to normal within 3 to 4 weeks. External bleeding leads to iron loss and possible iron deficiency, which can hamper restoration of red cell counts.

Chronic blood loss does not affect blood volume but instead leads to iron deficiency anemia when iron stores are depleted. Gastrointestinal bleeding and menstrual disorders commonly cause it. Because of compensatory mechanisms, people are commonly asymptomatic until the hemoglobin level is less than 8 g/dL. The red cells that are produced have too little hemoglobin, so they are small and pale, giving rise to microcytic hypochromic anemia (see Fig. 23.7).[5]

Hemolytic Anemias

Hemolytic anemia is characterized by

- The premature destruction of red cells
- The retention in the body of iron and the other products of hemoglobin destruction
- An increase in erythropoiesis

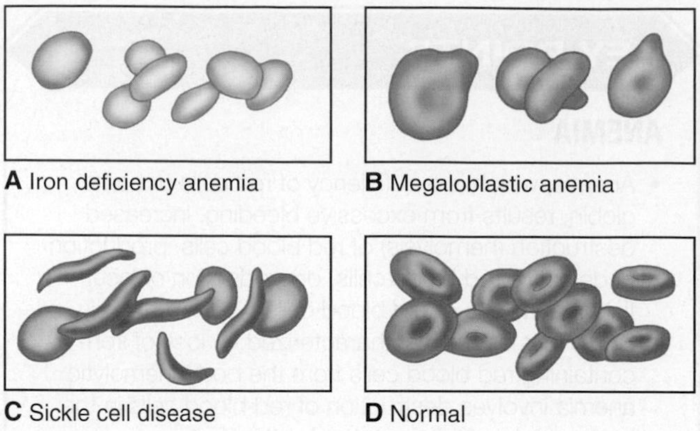

Figure 23.7 • Red cell characteristics seen in different types of anemia: **(A)** microcytic and hypochromic red cells, characteristic of iron deficiency anemia; **(B)** macrocytic and misshaped red blood cells, characteristic of megaloblastic anemia; **(C)** abnormally shaped red blood cells seen in sickle cell disease; and **(D)** normocytic and normochromic red blood cells, as a comparison.

Almost all types of hemolytic anemia are distinguished by normocytic and normochromic red cells. Because of the red blood cell's shortened life span, the bone marrow usually is hyperactive, resulting in an increased number of reticulocytes in the circulating blood. As with other types of anemias, the person experiences easy fatigability, dyspnea, and other signs and symptoms of impaired oxygen transport.

In hemolytic anemia, red cell breakdown can occur within or outside the vascular compartment.[5] *Intravascular hemolysis* is less common and occurs as a result of complement fixation in transfusion reactions, mechanical injury, or toxic factors. It is characterized by hemoglobinemia, hemoglobinuria, jaundice, and hemosiderinuria. *Extravascular hemolysis* occurs when red cells become less deformable, making it difficult for them to traverse the splenic sinusoids. The abnormal red cells are sequestered and phagocytized by macrophages.[11] The manifestations of extravascular hemolysis include anemia and jaundice.

Another classification of hemolytic anemia is based on whether the cause is intrinsic or extrinsic. *Intrinsic* causes include defects of the red cell membrane, the various hemoglobinopathies, and inherited enzyme defects.[5] Two main types of hemoglobinopathies can cause red cell hemolysis: the abnormal substitution of an amino acid in the hemoglobin molecule, as in sickle cell disease, and the defective synthesis of one of the polypeptide chains that form the globin portion of hemoglobin, as in the thalassemias.

Extrinsic or acquired forms of hemolytic anemia are caused by agents external to the red blood cell, such as drugs, bacterial and other toxins, antibodies, and physical trauma.[5] Although all these factors can cause premature and accelerated destruction of red cells, they cannot all be treated in the same way. Some respond to splenectomy, others to treatment with corticosteroid hormones, and still others do not resolve until the primary disorder is corrected.

Inherited Hemolytic Anemias

There are also a group of inherited hemolytic anemias such as sickle cell anemia, thalassemia, and hereditary spherocytosis. People who inherit one of these anemias can have very different clinical manifestations, depending on the genotype they have. In fact, a person could be acutely ill or may have little to no clinical manifestations.

Hereditary Spherocytosis. Hereditary spherocytosis is mostly transmitted as an autosomal dominant trait and is the most common inherited disorder of the red cell membrane.[1] The disorder is caused by abnormalities of the spectrin, ankyrin, protein 4.2, or band 3 membrane proteins that lead to a gradual loss of the membrane surface. The loss of membrane relative to cytoplasm causes the cell to lose its lipid bilayer from the red blood cell cytoskeleton. The red cell forms a spherical shape and cannot easily traverse the spleen.[1] Gradually, most of these cells lose more of their surface membrane and die.

Clinical signs are variable but typically include mild hemolytic anemia, jaundice, splenomegaly, and bilirubin gallstones. A life-threatening aplastic crisis may occur when a sudden disruption of red cell production (often from a parvovirus B19) causes a rapid drop in hematocrit and the hemoglobin level.[1] The disorder usually is treated with splenectomy to reduce red cell destruction. Blood transfusions may be required in a crisis.[1]

Sickle Cell Disease. Sickle cell disease is an inherited disorder in which an abnormal hemoglobin (hemoglobin S [HbS]) leads to chronic hemolytic anemia, pain, and organ failure. The HbS gene is transmitted by recessive inheritance and can manifest as sickle cell trait (*i.e.*, heterozygote with one HbS gene) or sickle cell disease (*i.e.*, homozygote with two HbS genes). Sickle cell disease affects approximately 100,000 Americans.[12]

Etiology and Pathogenesis. The abnormal structure of HbS results from a point mutation in the β chain of the hemoglobin molecule, with an abnormal substitution of a single amino acid, valine, for glutamic acid (Fig. 23.8). Variations in proportions exist, and the concentration of HbS correlates with the risk of sickling. In the homozygote with sickle cell disease, the HbS becomes sickled when deoxygenated or at a low oxygen tension. The deoxygenated hemoglobin aggregates and polymerizes in the cytoplasm, creating a semisolid gel that changes the shape and deformability of the cell. The sickled cell may return to normal shape with oxygenation in the lungs. However, after repeated episodes of deoxygenation, the cells remain permanently sickled. The person with sickle cell trait who has less HbS has little tendency to sickle and is virtually asymptomatic. HbF inhibits the polymerization of HbS. Therefore, most infants with sickle cell disease do not begin to experience the effects of the sickling until after 8 to 10 weeks of age, when the HbF has been replaced by HbS.[1]

There are two major consequences of red blood cell sickling—chronic hemolytic anemia and blood vessel occlusion. Premature destruction of the cells because of the rigid,

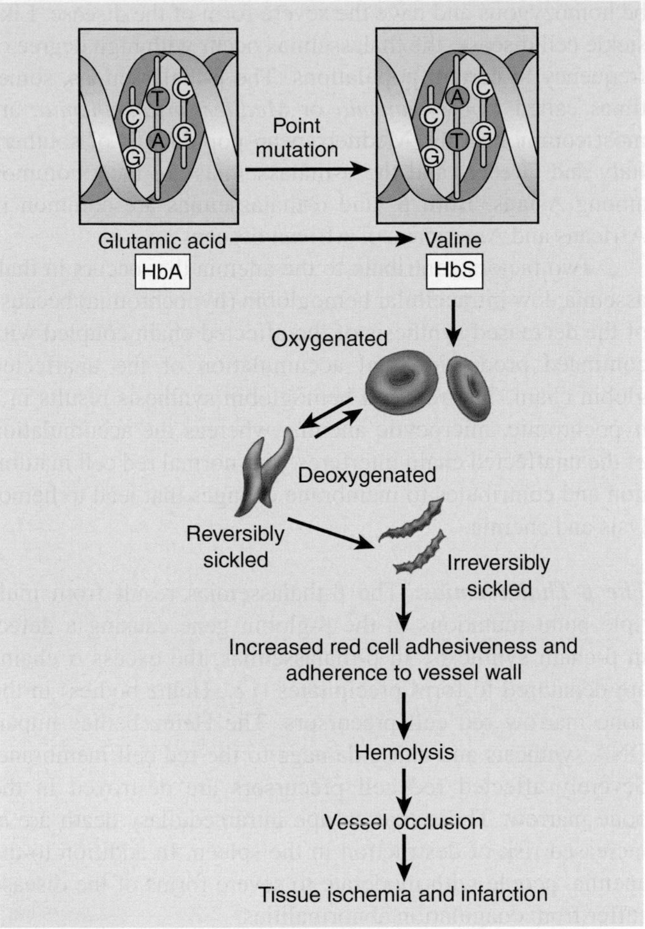

Figure 23.8 • Mechanism of sickling and its consequences in sickle cell disease.

nondeformable membrane occurs in the spleen, causing hemolysis and anemia from a decrease in red cell numbers. Vessel occlusion is a complex process involving an interaction among the sickled cells, endothelial cells, leukocytes, platelets, and other plasma proteins. Factors associated with sickling and vessel occlusion include cold, stress, physical exertion, infection, and illnesses that cause hypoxia, dehydration, or acidosis. The rate of HbS polymerization is affected by the concentration of hemoglobin in the cell. Dehydration increases the hemoglobin concentration and contributes to the polymerization and resulting sickling. Acidosis reduces the affinity of hemoglobin for oxygen, resulting in more deoxygenated hemoglobin and increased sickling.

Clinical Manifestations. People who are homozygous for the HbS gene experience severe hemolytic anemia, chronic hyperbilirubinemia, and vaso-occlusive crises. The hyperbilirubinemia that results from the breakdown products of hemoglobin often leads to jaundice and the production of pigment stones in the gallbladder.

Blood vessel occlusion causes most of the severe complications. An acute pain episode results from vessel occlusion and hypoxia and can occur suddenly in almost any part of the body.[5] Commonly, obstruction by sickled cells occurs in the abdomen, chest, bones, and joints. Many areas may be affected simultaneously. Infarctions caused by sluggish blood flow may cause chronic damage to the liver, spleen, heart, kidneys, retina, and other organs (Fig. 23.9). *Acute chest syndrome* occurs with vessel occlusion in the lungs and is a leading cause of death in people with sickle cell disease.[13] Acute chest syndrome is characterized by sudden chest pain. Cough develops due to pulmonary infiltrates. Respiratory insufficiency results in dyspnea.[5] Painful bone crises may be caused by marrow infarcts. Children have an increased susceptibility to osteomyelitis and may experience growth retardation. Transient ischemic attack or cerebral hemorrhage may precede a stroke, and approximately one quarter of people with sickle cell disease develop neurologic complications.[5]

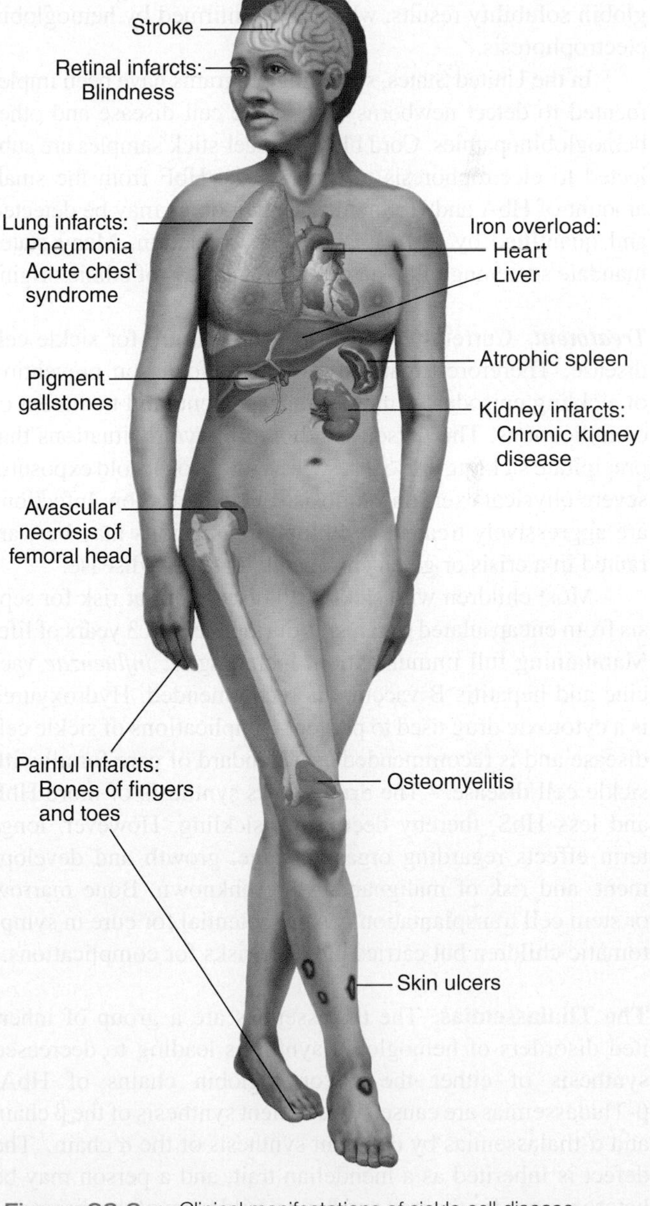

Figure 23.9 • Clinical manifestations of sickle cell disease.

The spleen is especially susceptible to damage by HbS. Because of the spleen's sluggish blood flow and low oxygen tension, hemoglobin in red cells traversing the spleen becomes deoxygenated, causing ischemia. Splenic injury begins in early childhood, characterized by intense congestion, and is usually asymptomatic. The congestion causes functional asplenia and predisposes the person to life-threatening infections by encapsulated organisms, including *Streptococcus pneumoniae*, *Haemophilus influenzae* type b, and *Klebsiella* species. Neonates and small children have not had time to create antibodies to these organisms and rely on the spleen for their removal. In the absence of specific antibody to the polysaccharide capsular antigens of these organisms, splenic activity is essential for removing these organisms when they enter the blood.

Diagnosis and Screening. Neonatal diagnosis of sickle cell disease is made on the basis of clinical findings and hemoglobin solubility results, which are confirmed by hemoglobin electrophoresis.

In the United States, screening programs have been implemented to detect newborns with sickle cell disease and other hemoglobinopathies. Cord blood or heel-stick samples are subjected to electrophoresis to separate the HbF from the small amount of HbA and HbS. Other hemoglobins may be detected and quantified by further laboratory evaluation. Many states mandate screening of all newborns, regardless of ethnic origin.

Treatment. Currently, there is no known cure for sickle cell disease. Therefore, treatment strategies focus on prevention of sickling episodes, symptom management, and treatment of complications. The person is advised to avoid situations that precipitate sickling episodes, such as infections, cold exposure, severe physical exertion, acidosis, and dehydration. Infections are aggressively treated, and blood transfusions may be warranted in a crisis or given chronically in severe disease.

Most children with sickle cell disease are at risk for sepsis from encapsulated organisms during the first 3 years of life. Maintaining full immunization, including *H. influenzae* vaccine and hepatitis B vaccine, is recommended. Hydroxyurea is a cytotoxic drug used to prevent complications of sickle cell disease and is recommended as a standard of care for all with sickle cell disease.[13] The drug allows synthesis of more HbF and less HbS, thereby decreasing sickling. However, long-term effects regarding organ damage, growth and development, and risk of malignancies are unknown. Bone marrow or stem cell transplantation has the potential for cure in symptomatic children but carries multiple risks for complications.

The Thalassemias. The thalassemias are a group of inherited disorders of hemoglobin synthesis leading to decreased synthesis of either the α- or β-globin chains of HbA. β-Thalassemias are caused by deficient synthesis of the β chain and α-thalassemias by deficient synthesis of the α chain.[1] The defect is inherited as a mendelian trait, and a person may be heterozygous for the trait and have a mild form of the disease or be homozygous and have the severe form of the disease. Like sickle cell disease, the thalassemias occur with high degree of frequency in certain populations. The β-thalassemias, sometimes called *Cooley anemia* or *Mediterranean anemia*, are most common in the Mediterranean populations of southern Italy and Greece, and the α-thalassemias are most common among Asians. Both β- and α-thalassemias are common in Africans and Americans of African descent.

Two factors contribute to the anemia that occurs in thalassemia: low intracellular hemoglobin (hypochromia) because of the decreased synthesis of the affected chain coupled with continued production and accumulation of the unaffected globin chain. The reduced hemoglobin synthesis results in a hypochromic, microcytic anemia, whereas the accumulation of the unaffected chain interferes with normal red cell maturation and contributes to membrane changes that lead to hemolysis and anemia.

The β-Thalassemias. The β-thalassemias result from multiple point mutations in the β-globin gene causing a defect in β-chain synthesis. In β-thalassemias, the excess α chains are denatured to form precipitates (*i.e.*, Heinz bodies) in the bone marrow red cell precursors. The Heinz bodies impair DNA synthesis and cause damage to the red cell membrane. Severely affected red cell precursors are destroyed in the bone marrow. Those that escape intramedullary death are at increased risk of destruction in the spleen. In addition to the anemia, people with moderate to severe forms of the disease suffer from coagulation abnormalities.

The clinical manifestations of the β-thalassemias are based on the severity of the anemia. The presence of one normal gene in heterozygous persons (thalassemia minor) usually results in sufficient normal hemoglobin synthesis to prevent severe anemia. People who are homozygous for the trait (thalassemia major) have severe, blood transfusion–dependent anemia that is evident at 6 to 9 months of age when the hemoglobin switches from HbF to HbA. If transfusion therapy is not started early in life, severe growth retardation occurs in children with the disorder.

In severe β-thalassemia, marked anemia produced by ineffective hematopoiesis and hemolysis leads to increased erythropoietin secretion and hyperplasia in the bone marrow and sites of extramedullary hematopoiesis. The expanding mass of erythropoietic marrow invades the bony cortex, impairs bone growth, and produces other bone abnormalities. There is thinning of the cortical bone, with new bone formation evident on the maxilla and frontal bones of the face (*i.e.*, chipmunk facies). The long bones, ribs, and vertebrae may become vulnerable to fracture because of osteoporosis or osteopenia, which contributes to increased morbidity in older people. Enlargement of the spleen (splenomegaly) and liver (hepatomegaly) results from extramedullary hematopoiesis and increased red cell destruction.

Iron overload is a major complication of β-thalassemia. Excess iron stores, which accumulate from increased dietary absorption and repeated transfusions, are deposited in the myocardium, liver, and endocrine organs and induce organ damage. Cardiac, hepatic, and endocrine diseases are common causes of morbidity and mortality from iron overload.

Regular blood transfusions to maintain hemoglobin levels at 9 to 10 g/dL improve growth and development and prevent most of the complications, and iron chelation therapy can reduce the iron overload and extend life expectancy.[14] Stem cell transplantation is a potential cure for low-risk people, particularly in younger people with no complications of the disease or its treatment, and has excellent results.[14] In the future, stem cell gene replacement may provide a cure for many with the disease.

The α-Thalassemias. The α-thalassemias are caused by a gene deletion that results in defective α-chain synthesis.[14] Synthesis of the α-globin chains of hemoglobin is controlled by two pairs or four genes. Hence, α-thalassemia shows great variation in severity related to the number of gene deletions. Silent carriers who have a deletion of a single α-globin gene are asymptomatic, and those with deletion of two genes have the α-thalassemia trait and exhibit mild hemolytic anemia. Deletion of three of the four α-chain genes leads to unstable aggregates of α chains called *hemoglobin H* (HbH). This disorder is the most important clinical form and is common in Asians. The β chains are more soluble than the α chains, and their accumulation is less toxic to the red cells, so that senescent rather than precursor red cells are affected. Most people with HbH have chronic moderate hemolytic anemia and may require blood transfusions in time of fever or illness or with certain medications.[14] The most severe form of α-thalassemia occurs in infants in whom all four α-globin genes are deleted and is called hydrops fetalis syndrome. Such a defect results in a hemoglobin molecule (Hb Bart) that is formed exclusively from the chains of HbF. Hb Bart, which has an extremely high oxygen affinity, cannot release oxygen in the tissues.[14] Hydrops fetalis syndrome usually results in death in utero or shortly after birth.

Inherited Enzyme Defects. The most common inherited enzyme defect that results in hemolytic anemia is a deficiency of G6PD.[14] The gene that determines this enzyme is located on the X chromosome, and the defect is expressed only in males and homozygous females. There are multiple genetic variants of this disorder found in all populations but particularly in African and Mediterranean groups.[14] The disorder makes red cells more vulnerable to oxidants and causes direct oxidation of hemoglobin to methemoglobin, which cannot transport oxygen, and denaturing of the hemoglobin molecule to form Heinz bodies, which are precipitated in the red blood cell. Hemolysis usually occurs as the damaged red blood cells move through the narrow vessels of the spleen, causing hemoglobinemia, hemoglobinuria, and jaundice. The hemolysis is short-lived, occurring 2 to 3 days after the trigger event. In black people, the defect is mildly expressed and is not associated with chronic hemolytic anemia unless triggered by oxidant drugs, acidosis, or infection.

The antimalarial drug primaquine, the sulfonamides, nitrofurantoin, aspirin, phenacetin, some chemotherapeutics, and other drugs cause hemolysis.[14] Free radicals generated by phagocytes during infections also are possible triggers. The disorder can be diagnosed through the use of a G6PD assay or screening test.

Acquired Hemolytic Anemias

Several acquired factors exogenous to the red blood cell produce hemolysis by direct membrane destruction or by antibody-mediated lysis.[1] Various drugs, chemicals, toxins, venoms, and infections such as malaria destroy red cell membranes. Hemolysis can also be caused by mechanical factors such as prosthetic heart valves, vasculitis, and severe burns. Obstructions in the microcirculation, as in disseminated intravascular coagulation, thrombotic thrombocytopenic purpura, and renal disease, may traumatize the red cells by producing turbulence and changing pressure gradients.

Many hemolytic anemias are immune mediated, caused by antibodies that destroy the red cell. Autoantibodies may be produced in response to drugs and disease. Alloantibodies come from an exogenous source and are responsible for transfusion reactions and hemolytic disease of the newborn.[1]

The autoantibodies that cause red cell destruction are of two types: warm-reacting antibodies of the immunoglobulin G (IgG) type, which are maximally active at 37°C, and cold-reacting antibodies of the IgM type, which are optimally active at or near 4°C.[1]

The *warm-reacting antibodies* cause no morphologic or metabolic alteration in the red cell. Instead, they react with antigens on the red cell membrane, causing destructive changes that lead to spherocytosis, with subsequent phagocytic destruction in the spleen or reticuloendothelial system (RES). They lack specificity for the ABO antigens but may react with the Rh antigens. The reactions have a rapid onset and may be severe and life-threatening. Fatigue is a common complaint and jaundice and moderate splenomegaly are present. Angina or congestive heart failure may also occur. There are varied causes for this anemia. Approximately 50% are idiopathic, and 50% are drug induced (*e.g.*, penicillin) or related to some other disorder. The drug-induced hemolysis is commonly benign.[15]

The *cold-reacting antibodies* activate complement. Chronic hemolytic anemia caused by cold-reacting antibodies occurs with lymphoproliferative disorders and as an idiopathic disorder of unknown cause.[1] The hemolytic process occurs in distal body parts, where the temperature may fall below 30°C. Vascular obstruction by red cells results in pallor, cyanosis of the body parts exposed to cold temperatures, and Raynaud phenomenon. Hemolytic anemia caused by cold-reacting antibodies develops in only a few people and is rarely severe.[15]

The direct antiglobulin test (DAT), also known as the direct Coombs test, is used to diagnose immune hemolytic anemias.[16] It detects the presence of antibody or complement on the surface of the red cell. In this test, red cells that have been washed free of serum are mixed with antihuman globulin reagent. The red cells agglutinate if the reagent binds to and bridges the antibody or complement on adjacent red cells. The DAT result is positive in cases of autoimmune hemolytic anemia, erythroblastosis fetalis (Rh disease of the newborn), transfusion reactions, and drug-induced hemolysis. The indirect antiglobulin test detects antibody in the serum, and the result is positive for specific antibodies.[16] It is used for antibody detection and cross-matching before transfusion.[7]

Anemias of Deficient Red Cell Production

Anemia may result from the decreased production of erythrocytes by the bone marrow. A deficiency of nutrients for hemoglobin synthesis (iron) or DNA synthesis (cobalamin or folic acid) may reduce red cell production by the bone marrow. A deficiency of red cells also results when the marrow itself fails or is replaced by nonfunctional tissue.

Iron Deficiency Anemia

Iron deficiency is a common worldwide cause of anemia affecting people of all ages. The anemia results from dietary deficiency, loss of iron through bleeding, or increased demands.[5] Because iron is a component of heme, a deficiency leads to decreased hemoglobin synthesis and consequent impairment of oxygen delivery.

Etiology and Pathogenesis. Body iron is used for multiple mechanisms every day. When red cells become senescent and are broken down, their iron is released and reused in the production of new red cells. Despite this efficiency, small amounts of iron are lost in the feces and need to be replaced by dietary uptake. Iron balance is maintained by the absorption of 1 to 2 mg daily to replace the iron lost in the feces.[1] The average western diet supplies about 20 mg.[1] The absorbed iron is more than sufficient to supply the needs of most people but may be barely adequate in toddlers, adolescents, and women of child-bearing age. Dietary deficiency of iron is not common in developed countries except in certain populations. Most iron is derived from meat, and when meat is not available, as for impoverished populations, or is not a dietary constituent, as for vegetarians, iron deficiency may occur.

The usual reason for iron deficiency in adults in the western world is chronic blood loss because there is inadequate iron available for recycling. In men and postmenopausal women, blood loss may occur from gastrointestinal bleeding because of peptic ulcer, vascular lesions, intestinal polyps, hemorrhoids, or cancer.[5] In women of child-bearing age, iron demand is increased because of losses from menstruation. Additionally, in pregnant women, fetal development increases iron requirements for erythropoiesis.[5]

A child's growth places extra demands on the body. Blood volume increases, with a greater need for iron. Iron requirements are proportionally higher in infancy (3 to 24 months) than at any other age, although they are also increased in childhood and adolescence. In infancy, the two main causes of iron deficiency anemia are low iron levels at birth because of maternal deficiency and a diet consisting mainly of cow's milk, which is low in absorbable iron.

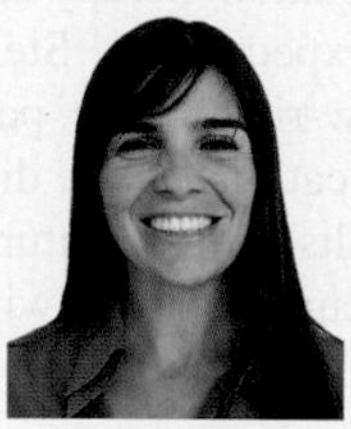

Remember Mrs. Cretena from the unit opener case study who was diagnosed with a microcytic hypochromic anemia that turned out to be iron deficiency anemia? Her PCP referred her to a nutritionist last week. At this visit, she explained that she was a vegetarian and did not eat any red meat. Her dietary history also revealed that she did not have sufficient amounts of protein and iron in her daily diet. Mrs. Cretena came in today for a follow-up visit with her PCP. She volunteered more information regarding her heavy menses at this second visit. She said that she was saturating approximately 16 large pads/day, which was up from her "normal" amount of about 10 large pads/day. When asked when she last visited her gynecologist, she replied that it had been about 10 years ago (after her last child was born). A gynecologist visit was made for her immediately following this primary care visit.

Given this extra information, it becomes easy to understand why Mrs. Cretena has developed iron deficiency anemia. Her hematocrit, hemoglobin, and ferritin were low. With a hemoglobin of 10 g/dL and a MCHC = 29 g/dL (31 to 35 g/dL) and a MCV = 76 fL (80 to 100 fL), the color of her hemoglobin was pale and the size of her cells was small. A second blood sample will be obtained at this visit to assess if taking the ferrous sulfate is helping. It most likely will show larger cell size for the new erythrocytes. Therefore, she will have anisocytosis given she already has small cells still present. As she improves her diet, continues taking ferrous sulfate, and has less loss of blood with her menses, her hemoglobin will increase and cells will become normocytic and normochromic as the anemia resolves.

Clinical Manifestations. The manifestations of iron deficiency anemia are related to impaired oxygen transport and lack of hemoglobin. Depending on the severity of the anemia, fatigability, palpitations, dyspnea, angina, and tachycardia may occur. Pica, a craving for substances lacking nutritional value such as clay or ice, may develop. Other clinical manifestations can include a spoon-shaped deformity of the fingernails called koilonychia, smooth tongue, sores in the corners of the mouth, and sometimes dysphagia.[5]

Diagnosis and Treatment. Low hemoglobin and hematocrit, decreased iron stores, and low serum iron and ferritin characterize iron deficiency anemia. The red cells are decreased in number and are microcytic and hypochromic (see Fig. 23.7). Poikilocytosis (irregular shape) and anisocytosis (irregular size) are also present. Laboratory values indicate reduced MCHC and MCV.

Prevention of iron deficiency is a primary concern in infants and children. Avoidance of cow's milk, iron supplementation at 4 to 6 months of age in breast-fed infants, and use of iron-fortified formulas and cereals are recommended for infants younger than 1 year of age.[17] In the 2nd year, a diet rich in iron-containing foods and use of iron-fortified vitamins will help prevent iron deficiency.

The treatment of iron deficiency anemia in children and adults is directed toward controlling chronic blood loss, increasing dietary intake of iron, and administering supplemental iron. Ferrous sulfate, which is the usual oral replacement therapy, replenishes iron stores in several months.

Megaloblastic Anemias

Megaloblastic anemias are caused by impaired DNA synthesis that results in enlarged red cells (MCV > 100 fL) because of impaired maturation and division.[1] Vitamin B_{12} and folic acid deficiencies are the most common conditions associated with megaloblastic anemias. Because megaloblastic anemias develop slowly, there are often few symptoms until the anemia is far advanced.[1]

Vitamin B_{12}–Deficiency Anemia. Vitamin B_{12}, also known as *cobalamin*, serves as a cofactor for two important reactions in humans. It is essential for DNA synthesis and nuclear maturation, which in turn leads to normal red cell maturation and division.[1] Vitamin B_{12} is also involved in a reaction that prevents abnormal fatty acids from being incorporated into neuronal lipids. This abnormality may predispose to myelin breakdown and produce some of the neurologic complications of vitamin B_{12} deficiency.[1] Currently, approximately 5% to 20% of older adults have B_{12} deficiency because of malabsorption. Risk factors for this deficiency include long-term use of drugs such as proton pump inhibitors, gastrointestinal diseases such as sprue or ileitis, surgeries such as a gastrectomy or gastric bypass, and parasites.[5]

Etiology and Pathogenesis. Vitamin B_{12} is found in all foods of animal origin. Dietary deficiency is rare and usually found only in strict vegetarians who avoid all dairy products as well as meat and fish. Normal body stores of 1000 to 5000 micrograms (μg) provide the daily requirement of 1 μg for a number of years.[10] Therefore, deficiency of vitamin B_{12} develops slowly. Vitamin B_{12} is absorbed by a unique process. After release from the animal protein, it is bound to intrinsic factor, a protein secreted by the gastric parietal cells (Fig. 23.10). The vitamin B_{12}–intrinsic factor complex protects vitamin B_{12} from digestion by intestinal enzymes. The complex travels to the ileum, where it binds to membrane receptors on the epithelial cells. Vitamin B_{12} is then separated from intrinsic factor and transported across the membrane into the circulation. There, it is bound to its carrier protein, transcobalamin II, which transports vitamin B_{12} to its storage and tissue sites. Any defects in this pathway may cause a deficiency.

Pernicious anemia is a specific form of megaloblastic anemia caused by atrophic gastritis and failure to produce

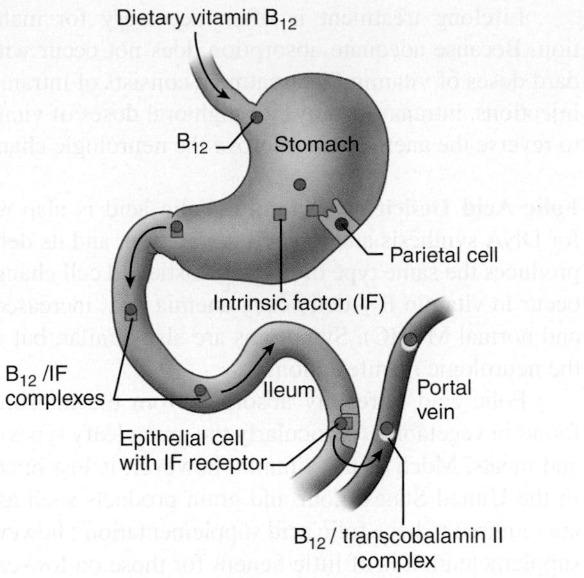

Figure 23.10 • Absorption of vitamin B_{12}.

intrinsic factor that leads to failure to absorb vitamin B_{12}. Pernicious anemia is believed to result from immunologically mediated, possibly autoimmune, destruction of the gastric mucosa. The resultant chronic atrophic gastritis is marked by loss of parietal cells and production of antibodies that interfere with binding of vitamin B_{12} to intrinsic factor. Other causes of vitamin B_{12}–deficiency anemia include gastrectomy, ileal resection, inflammation or neoplasms in the terminal ileum, and malabsorption syndromes. The hallmark of vitamin B_{12} deficiency is megaloblastic anemia. When vitamin B_{12} is deficient, the red cells that are produced are abnormally large because of excess cytoplasmic growth and structural proteins (see Fig. 23.7). The cells have immature nuclei and show evidence of cellular destruction. They have flimsy membranes and are oval rather than biconcave. These oddly shaped cells have a short life span that can be measured in weeks rather than months.

Clinical Manifestations. The loss of red cells results in a moderate to severe anemia and mild jaundice. The MCV is elevated because the cells are larger than normal, and the MCHC is normal. Neurologic changes that accompany the disorder are caused by deranged methylation of myelin protein. Demyelination of the dorsal and lateral columns of the spinal cord causes symmetric paresthesias of the feet and fingers, loss of vibratory and position sense, and eventual spastic ataxia. In more advanced cases, cerebral function may be altered. In some cases, confusion and dementia and other neuropsychiatric changes may precede hematologic changes.

Diagnosis and Treatment. Diagnosis of vitamin B_{12} deficiency is made by finding an abnormally low vitamin B_{12} serum level. The diagnosis of pernicious anemia, as the cause of the deficiency, is usually made by the detection of parietal cell and intrinsic factor antibodies.[5]

Lifelong treatment is often necessary for malabsorption. Because adequate absorption does not occur with standard doses of vitamin B_{12}, treatment consists of intramuscular injections, intranasal sprays, or high oral doses of vitamin B_{12} to reverse the anemia and improve the neurologic changes.[5]

Folic Acid Deficiency Anemia. Folic acid is also required for DNA synthesis and red cell maturation, and its deficiency produces the same type of megaloblastic red cell changes that occur in vitamin B_{12}–deficiency anemia (*i.e.*, increased MCV and normal MCHC). Symptoms are also similar, but without the neurologic manifestations.[5]

Folic acid is readily absorbed from the intestine. It is found in vegetables (particularly the green leafy types), fruits, and meats. Much of the vitamin, however, is lost in cooking. In the United States, flour and grain products such as cereal are required to have folic acid supplementation[5]; however, this supplementation is of little benefit for those on low-carbohydrate diets in which these foods are restricted.

A dietary deficiency may result in anemia in a few months. The most common causes of folic acid deficiency are malnutrition or dietary lack of folic acid, especially in older adults. Alcohol suppresses folate absorption and impairs enterohepatic recirculation, so people with chronic alcohol intake are at greater risk.[5] Malabsorption of folic acid also may be due to syndromes such as celiac disease or other intestinal disorders. In neoplastic disease, tumor cells compete for folate, and deficiency is common. Methotrexate, a folic acid analog used in the treatment of cancer, can also impair the action of folic acid by blocking its conversion to the active form.[5]

Because pregnancy increases the need for folic acid 5- to 10-fold, a deficiency commonly occurs. Poor dietary habits, anorexia, and nausea are other reasons for folic acid deficiency during pregnancy. It is well known there is an association between folate deficiency and neural tube defects (*e.g.*, spina bifida, anencephaly) in the growing fetus. Accordingly, all women of child-bearing age with male sexual partners are advised to ensure an intake of 0.4 mg of folic acid to maintain serum levels adequate to prevent neural tube deficits in their offspring.[18]

Aplastic Anemia

Aplastic anemia describes a disorder of pluripotential bone marrow stem cells that results in a reduction of all three hematopoietic cell lines—red blood cells, white blood cells, and platelets.[5] Pure red cell aplasia, in which only the red cells are affected, rarely occurs.[5] Anemia results from the failure of the marrow to replace senescent red cells that are destroyed and leave the circulation, although the cells that remain are of normal size and color. At the same time, because the leukocytes, particularly the neutrophils, and the thrombocytes have a short life span, a deficiency of these cells usually is apparent before the anemia becomes severe.[1]

Etiology and Pathogenesis. Among the causes of aplastic anemia are exposure to high doses of radiation, chemicals, and toxins that suppress hematopoiesis directly or through immune mechanisms. Chemotherapy and irradiation commonly result in bone marrow depression, which causes pancytopenia (anemia, thrombocytopenia, and neutropenia). Identified toxic agents include benzene, the antibiotic chloramphenicol, and the alkylating agents and antimetabolites used in the treatment of cancer. Aplastic anemia caused by exposure to chemical agents may be an idiosyncratic reaction because it affects only certain susceptible people. It typically occurs weeks after a drug is initiated but can occur earlier. Such reactions often are severe and sometimes irreversible and fatal.

Aplastic anemia can develop in the course of many infections. It has been reported most often as a complication of viral hepatitis, mononucleosis, and other viral illnesses, including acquired immunodeficiency syndrome (AIDS).

Rarely, aplastic anemia can occur in the absence of toxic substances or infections. These cases are called *idiopathic aplastic anemia*. Because idiopathic aplastic anemia sometimes responds to immunosuppressive drugs, the mechanism underlying the pathogenesis is believed to be an autoimmune response targeting the hematopoietic cells.[5]

Clinical Manifestations. The onset of aplastic anemia may be insidious, or it may strike with suddenness and great severity. It can occur at any age. The initial presenting symptoms include weakness, fatigability, and pallor caused by anemia. Petechiae (*i.e.*, small, punctate skin hemorrhages) and ecchymoses (*i.e.*, bruises) often occur on the skin, and bleeding from the nose, gums, vagina, or gastrointestinal tract may occur because of decreased platelet levels. The decrease in the number of neutrophils increases susceptibility to infection.

Diagnosis and Treatment. With aplastic anemia, there is a gradual onset with some fatigue or possibly some bleeding from the gums or the person may complain that he is having difficulty clotting. Once the person presents to the physician, the aplastic anemia may be life-threatening. There are no specific physical findings such as hepatosplenomegaly or lymphadenopathy. The complete blood count (CBC) shows pancytopenia, which means decreased red and white blood cells and platelets. The red blood cell indices indicate normochromic and normocytic anemia.[10]

Perhaps, one of the most helpful findings to determine the etiology of the pancytopenia is determined in the patient's history. Most likely, the person has taken a drug or acquired a virus, which has caused the aplastic anemia.

Therapy for aplastic anemia includes discontinuing any drugs or chemicals that precipitated the condition. Hematopoietic stem cell replacement or immunosuppressive therapy can reverse the condition in most people.[5]

Chronic Disease Anemias

Anemia often occurs as a complication of chronic infections, inflammation, and cancer. Of the anemias that occur secondary to chronic conditions, anemia because of chronic renal failure is especially common and frequently severe. The kidneys are the primary site for the synthesis of erythropoietin, the colony-stimulating factor that stimulates stem cells to differentiate into erythrocytes. The damaged kidney secretes inadequate amounts of erythropoietin; therefore, fewer red blood cells are produced.[5]

Chronic renal failure almost always results in anemia, primarily because of a deficiency of erythropoietin. Unidentified uremic toxins and retained nitrogen associated with chronic renal failure also interfere with the actions of erythropoietin and with red cell production and survival.[1] Hemolysis and blood loss associated with hemodialysis and bleeding tendencies also contribute to the anemia of renal failure. Therapy for these anemias includes treatment for the underlying disease, erythropoietin therapy, iron supplementation, and blood transfusions. In order to avoid the adverse effect of thrombosis associated with erythropoietin therapy, the hemoglobin should be maintained at 12 g/dL or below.[5]

"Anemia of critical illness" is common in the intensive care unit, with more than 90% of people having low hemoglobin levels secondary to their comorbidities. In critically ill people, low erythropoietin concentrations and anemia also appear to be caused by inflammatory cytokines. In this population, it is suggested that red blood cell transfusions be restricted to reduce the risk of transmission of infectious agents and immune modulation.

IN SUMMARY

Anemia is a condition of an abnormally low number of circulating red blood cells or hemoglobin level, or both. It is not a disease, but a manifestation of a disease process or alteration in body function. The manifestations of anemia are those associated with impaired oxygen transport; alterations in red blood cell number, hemoglobin content, and cell structure; and the signs and symptoms of the underlying process causing the anemia.

Anemia can result from excessive blood loss, red cell destruction because of hemolysis, or deficient hemoglobin or red cell production. Blood loss anemia can be acute or chronic. With bleeding, iron and other components of the erythrocyte are lost from the body. Hemolytic anemia is characterized by the premature destruction of red cells, with retention in the body of iron and the other products of red cell destruction. Hemolytic anemia can be caused by defects in the red cell membrane, hemoglobinopathies (sickle cell disease or thalassemia), or inherited enzyme defects (G6PD deficiency). Acquired forms of hemolytic anemia are caused by agents extrinsic to the red blood cell, such as drugs, bacterial and other toxins, antibodies, and physical trauma. Iron deficiency anemia, which is characterized by decreased hemoglobin synthesis, can result from dietary deficiency, loss of iron through bleeding, or increased demands for red cell production. Vitamin B_{12} and folic acid deficiencies impair red cell production by interfering with DNA synthesis. Aplastic anemia is caused by bone marrow suppression and usually results in a reduction of white blood cells and platelets, as well as red blood cells. Chronic diseases such as inflammatory disorders (rheumatoid arthritis), cancers, and chronic kidney disease cause anemia through the production of inflammatory cytokines that interfere with erythropoietin production or response.

POLYCYTHEMIA

After completing this section of the chapter, the learner will be able to meet the following objectives:

- Define the term *polycythemia.*
- Compare causes of polycythemia vera and secondary polycythemia.
- Describe the manifestations of polycythemia.

Polycythemia is an abnormally high total red blood cell mass with a hematocrit greater than 54% in men and greater than 47% in women.[1] A hematocrit greater than 50% can cause cardiac dysfunction and vascular obstruction, whereas a hematocrit greater than 60% can lead to hypoxia.[1] Polycythemia is categorized as *relative* or *absolute*. In *relative* polycythemia, also called Gaisböck syndrome, the hematocrit rises because of a loss of plasma volume without a corresponding decrease in red cells.[1] This may occur with water deprivation, excessive diuretic usage, or gastrointestinal losses. Relative polycythemia is corrected by increasing the vascular fluid volume. *Absolute* polycythemia is a rise in hematocrit because of an increase in total red cell mass and is classified as primary or secondary.

Absolute Polycythemia: Primary

Primary polycythemia, or *polycythemia vera*, is a neoplastic disease of the pluripotent cells of the bone marrow characterized by an absolute increase in total red blood cell mass accompanied by elevated white cell and platelet counts. In polycythemia vera, the clinical manifestations are variable and are related to an increase in the red cell count, hemoglobin level, and hematocrit with increased blood volume and viscosity. Viscosity rises exponentially with the hematocrit and can interfere with cardiac output and blood flow. Hypertension is common, and there may be complaints of headache, dizziness, inability to concentrate, and some difficulty with hearing and vision because of decreased cerebral blood flow.[2] Venous stasis gives rise to a plethoric appearance or dusky redness, even cyanosis, particularly of the lips, fingernails, and mucous membranes. Because of the increased concentration of blood cells, the person may experience itching and pain in the fingers or toes, and the hypermetabolism may induce night sweats and weight loss. Thromboembolism and hemorrhage, because of platelet abnormalities, are common complications that can be prevented by phlebotomy. The goal of treatment in primary polycythemia is to reduce blood viscosity. Withdrawing blood by periodic phlebotomy to reduce red cell volume can do this.

Concept Mastery Alert

Symptoms associated with polycythemia vera include headache, hearing difficulty, dusky red appearance, and cyanosis of the lips, fingernails, and mucous membranes. Possible complications associated with the increased number of RBCs include blood clots because of increased blood thickness, enlarged spleen associated with work to removed extra RBCs, hypertension because of increased viscosity and increased oxygen consumption, and chest pain because of oxygen-rich blood not reaching organs especially the heart.

Absolute Polycythemia: Secondary

Secondary polycythemia results from a physiologic increase in the level of erythropoietin, commonly as a compensatory response to hypoxia. Conditions causing hypoxia include living at high altitudes, chronic heart and lung disease, and smoking. Native people who live at high altitudes of 14,000 to 17,000 feet develop secondary polycythemia or physiologic polycythemia where their RBC count is generally 6 to 7 million/mm^3. This allows them to perform all types of heavy labor at high altitude.[2] The resultant release of erythropoietin by the kidney causes the increased formation of red blood cells in the bone marrow. Neoplasms that secrete erythropoietin may also cause a secondary polycythemia. Kidney disease such as hydronephrosis or renal cysts may obstruct blood flow, cause hypoxia, and lead to an increase in erythropoietin. Treatment of secondary polycythemia focuses on relieving hypoxia. For example, continuous low-flow oxygen therapy can be used to correct the severe hypoxia that occurs in some people with chronic obstructive pulmonary disease. This form of treatment is thought to relieve the pulmonary hypertension and polycythemia and to delay the onset of cor pulmonale.

IN SUMMARY

Polycythemia describes a condition in which the red blood cell mass is increased. It can present as a relative or absolute. Relative polycythemia results from a loss of vascular fluid and is corrected by replacing the fluid. Absolute polycythemia is further classified as a primary or secondary disorder. Absolute primary polycythemia, or polycythemia vera, is a proliferative disease of the bone marrow with an absolute increase in total red blood cell mass accompanied by elevated white cell and platelet counts. Absolute secondary polycythemia results from increased erythropoietin levels caused by hypoxic conditions such as chronic heart and lung disease. Many of the manifestations of polycythemia are related to increased blood volume and viscosity that lead to hypertension and stagnation of blood flow.

AGE-RELATED CHANGES IN RED BLOOD CELLS

After completing this section of the chapter, the learner will be able to meet the following objectives:

- Describe the function of hemoglobin F in the neonate, and describe the red blood cell changes that occur during the early neonatal period.
- Cite the factors that predispose to hyperbilirubinemia in the infant.
- Describe the pathogenesis of hemolytic disease of the newborn.
- Compare conjugated and unconjugated bilirubin in terms of production of encephalopathy in the neonate.
- Explain the action of phototherapy in the treatment of hyperbilirubinemia in the neonate.
- State the changes in the red blood cells that occur with aging.

Red Cell Changes in the Neonate

At birth, changes in the red blood cell reflect the transition to extrauterine life and the need to transport oxygen from the lungs (Table 23.5). Hemoglobin concentrations at birth are high, reflecting the high synthetic activity in utero to provide adequate oxygen delivery. Toward the end of the first postnatal week, hemoglobin concentration begins to decline, gradually falling to a minimum value at approximately age 2 months. The red cell count and hematocrit likewise fall. The factors responsible for the decline include reduced red cell production and plasma dilution caused by increased blood volume with growth. Neonatal red cells also have a shorter life span of 50 to 70 days and are thought to be more fragile than those of older adults. During the early neonatal period, there is also a switch from HbF to HbA. The switch to HbA provides greater unloading of oxygen to the tissues because HbA has a lower affinity for oxygen compared with HbF. Infants who are small for gestational age or born to diabetic or smoking mothers or who experienced hypoxia in utero have higher total hemoglobin levels, higher HbF levels, and a delayed switch to HbA.

A physiologic anemia of the newborn develops at approximately 2 months of age. It seldom produces symptoms and cannot be altered by nutritional supplements. Anemia of prematurity, an exaggerated physiologic response in infants with low birth weight, is thought to result from a poor erythropoietin response. A contributing factor is the frequent blood sampling often required in these infants. The hemoglobin level rapidly declines after birth to a low of 7 to 10 g/dL at approximately 6 weeks of age. Signs and symptoms include apnea, poor weight gain, pallor, decreased activity, and tachycardia. In infants born before 33 weeks' gestation or those with hematocrits below 33%, the clinical features are more evident.

Anemia at birth, characterized by pallor, congestive heart failure, or shock, usually is caused by hemolytic disease of

TABLE 23.5 RED CELL VALUES FOR CHILDREN

TEST	SPECIMEN	REFERENCE RANGE
Erythrocyte count (RBC)	Cord blood	3.9–5.5 millions of cells/mm^3
	1–3 days (capillary)	4.0–6.6 millions of cells/mm^3
	1 week	3.9–6.3 millions of cells/mm^3
	2 weeks	3.6–6.2 millions of cells/mm^3
	1 month	3.0–5.4 millions of cells/mm^3
	2 months	2.7–4.9 millions of cells/mm^3
	3–6 months	3.1–4.5 millions of cells/mm^3
	0.5–2 years	3.7–5.3 millions of cells/mm^3
	2–6 years	3.9–5.3 millions of cells/mm^3
	6–12 years	4.0–5.2 millions of cells/mm^3
	12–18 years (male)	4.3–5.2 millions of cells/mm^3
	12–18 years (female)	4.1–5.1 millions of cells/mm^3
Hematocrit	1 day (capillary)	48%–69% PRC*
	2 days	48%–75% PRC
	3 days	44%–72% PRC
	2 months	28%–42% PRC
	6–12 years	35%–45% PRC
	12–18 years (male)	37%–49%
	12–18 years (female)	36%–46% PRC
Hemoglobin	1–3 days (capillary)	14.5–22.2 g/dL
	2 months	9.0–14.0 g/dL
	6–12 years	11.5–15.5 g/dL
	12–18 years (male)	13.0–16.0 g/dL
	12–18 years (female)	12.0–16.0 g/dL

*PRC, percent packed red blood cells (volume red cells/volume whole blood cells × 100).
Adapted from Bowden V. R., Greenberg C. S. (2014). *Children and their families: The continuum of care* (3rd ed., pp. 1656, 1658–1659). Philadelphia, PA: Lippincott Williams & Wilkins, Appendix D Reference Ranges for Laboratory Tests, with permission.

the newborn. Bleeding from the umbilical cord, internal hemorrhage, congenital hemolytic disease, and frequent blood sampling are other possible causes of anemia. The severity of symptoms and presence of coexisting disease may warrant red cell transfusion.

Hyperbilirubinemia in the Neonate

Hyperbilirubinemia, an increased level of serum bilirubin, is a common cause of jaundice in the neonate. A benign, self-limited condition, it most often is related to the developmental state of the neonate. Rarely, cases of hyperbilirubinemia are pathologic and may lead to kernicterus and serious brain damage.

Physiologic jaundice appears in term infants on the 2nd or 3rd day of life. Ordinarily, the indirect bilirubin in umbilical cord blood is 1 to 3 mg/dL and increases by no more than 5 mg/dL in 24 hours, giving rise to jaundice. The increase in bilirubin is related to the increased red cell breakdown and the inability of the immature liver to conjugate bilirubin. Premature infants exhibit a slower rise and longer duration of serum bilirubin levels, perhaps because of poor hepatic uptake and reduced albumin binding of bilirubin. Peak bilirubin levels of 8 to 12 mg/dL appear on days 5 to 7. Most neonatal jaundice resolves spontaneously within 1 week and is untreated.

The cause of jaundice is made on the basis of history and clinical and laboratory findings. Many factors cause elevated bilirubin levels in the neonate, including breast-feeding, hemolytic disease of the newborn, hypoxia, infections, and acidosis. Bowel or biliary obstruction and liver disease are less common causes. Associated risk factors include prematurity, Asian ancestry, and maternal diabetes. These neonates accumulate significant levels of unconjugated bilirubin 7 days after birth, with maximum levels of 10 to 30 mg/dL reached in the third week of life. It is thought that the breast milk contains fatty acids that inhibit bilirubin conjugation in the neonatal liver. A factor in breast milk is also thought to increase the absorption of bilirubin in the duodenum. This type of jaundice disappears if breast-feeding is discontinued. Nursing can be resumed in 3 to 4 days without any hyperbilirubinemia ensuing.

Hyperbilirubinemia places the neonate at risk for the development of a neurologic syndrome called *kernicterus*. This condition is caused by the accumulation of unconjugated bilirubin in brain cells. Unconjugated bilirubin is lipid-soluble, crosses the permeable blood–brain barrier of the neonate, and is deposited in cells of the basal ganglia, causing brain damage. Asphyxia and hyperosmolality may also contribute by damaging the blood–brain barrier and allowing bilirubin to cross and enter the cells. The level of unconjugated bilirubin and the duration of exposure that will be toxic to the infant are unknown. Symptoms may appear 2 to 5 days after birth in term infants or by day 7 in premature infants. Lethargy, poor feeding, and short-term behavioral changes may be evident in mildly affected infants. Severe manifestations include rigidity, tremors, ataxia, and hearing loss. Extreme cases cause seizures and death. Most survivors are seriously damaged and by 3 years of age exhibit involuntary muscle spasm, seizures, mental retardation, and deafness.

Hyperbilirubinemia in the neonate is treated with phototherapy or exchange transfusion. Phototherapy is more commonly used to treat jaundiced infants and reduce the risk of kernicterus. Exposure to fluorescent light in the blue range of the visible spectrum (420- to 470-nm wavelength) reduces bilirubin levels. Bilirubin in the skin absorbs the light energy and is converted to a structural isomer that is more water soluble and can be excreted in the stool and urine. Effective treatment depends on the area of skin exposed and the infant's ability to metabolize and excrete bilirubin. Frequent monitoring of bilirubin levels, body temperature, and hydration is critical to the infant's care. Exchange transfusion is considered when signs of kernicterus are evident or hyperbilirubinemia is sustained or rising and unresponsive to phototherapy.

Hemolytic Disease of the Newborn

Erythroblastosis fetalis, or hemolytic disease of the newborn, occurs in Rh-positive infants of Rh-negative mothers who have been sensitized.[1] The mother can produce anti-Rh antibodies from pregnancies in which the infants are Rh-positive or by blood transfusions of Rh-positive blood. The Rh-negative mother usually becomes sensitized during the first few days after delivery, when fetal Rh-positive red cells from the placental site are released into the maternal circulation. Because the antibodies take several weeks to develop, the first Rh-positive infant of an Rh-negative mother usually is not affected. Infants with Rh-negative blood have no antigens on their red cells to react with the maternal antibodies and are not affected.

After an Rh-negative mother has been sensitized, the Rh antibodies from her blood are transferred to subsequent infants through the placental circulation. These antibodies react with the red cell antigens of the Rh-positive infant, causing agglutination and hemolysis. This leads to severe anemia with compensatory hyperplasia and enlargement of the blood-forming organs, including the spleen and liver, in the fetus. Liver function may be impaired, with decreased production of albumin causing massive edema, called *hydrops fetalis*. If blood levels of unconjugated bilirubin are abnormally high because of red cell hemolysis, there is a danger of kernicterus developing in the infant, resulting in severe brain damage or death.

Several advances have served significantly to decrease the threat to infants born to Rh-negative mothers—prevention of sensitization, antenatal identification of the at-risk fetus, and intrauterine transfusion to the affected fetus. The injection of Rh immune globulin (*i.e.*, gamma globulin–containing Rh antibody) prevents sensitization in Rh-negative mothers who have given birth to Rh-positive infants if administered at 28 weeks' gestation and within 72 hours of delivery, abortion, genetic amniocentesis, or fetal–maternal bleeding. After sensitization has developed, the immune globulin is of no value. Since 1968, the year Rh immune globulin was introduced, the incidence of sensitization of Rh-negative women has dropped dramatically. Early prenatal care and screening of maternal blood continue to be important in reducing immunization. Efforts to improve therapy are aimed at production of monoclonal anti-D, the Rh antibody.

Exchange transfusions are administered after birth by removing and replacing the infant's blood volume with type O Rh-negative blood. The exchange transfusion removes most of the hemolyzed red cells and some of the total bilirubin, treating the anemia and hyperbilirubinemia.

Red Cell Changes with Aging

Anemia is an increasingly common health problem in people of advanced age.[5] The highest prevalence is in men aged 85 years and older. Undiagnosed and untreated anemia can have severe complications and is associated with increased risk of mortality.

Hemoglobin levels decline after middle age. In studies of men older than 60 years of age, mean hemoglobin levels ranged from 15.3 to 12.4 g/dL, with the lowest levels found in the oldest adults. The decline is less in women. In most asymptomatic older adults, lower hemoglobin levels result from iron deficiency and anemia of chronic disease caused by inflammatory disease, malignancy, or chronic kidney disease (CKD).[5]

As with other body systems, the capacity for red cell production changes with aging. The location of bone cells involved in red cell production shifts toward the axial skeleton, and the number of progenitor cells declines. Although many older adults are able to maintain hemoglobin and hematocrit levels within a range similar to that of younger adults, during a stress situation such as bleeding, the red blood cells of older adults are not replaced as promptly as those of their younger counterparts. This inability to replace red blood cells closely correlates with the increased prevalence of anemia in older adults. Inflammatory cytokines, which have been found to increase with age, may mediate this reduced sensitivity to erythropoietin.

The diagnosis of anemia in older adults requires a complete physical examination, a CBC, and studies to rule out comorbid conditions such as malignancy, gastrointestinal conditions that cause bleeding, and pernicious anemia. The CBC should include a peripheral blood smear and a reticulocyte count and index. The treatment of anemia in older adults should focus on the underlying cause and correction of the red cell deficit. Although erythropoietin remains the treatment of choice for anemias associated with cancer and renal disease, its potential complications especially regarding cardiovascular disease remain to be established.

IN SUMMARY

Hemoglobin concentrations at birth are high, reflecting the in utero need for oxygen delivery. Toward the end of the first postnatal week, these levels begin to decline, gradually falling to a minimum value at approximately 2 months of age. During the early neonatal period, there is a shift from HbF to HbA. Many infants have physiologic jaundice because of hyperbilirubinemia during the first week of life, probably related to increased red cell breakdown and the inability of the infant's liver to conjugate bilirubin. The term *kernicterus* describes elevated levels of lipid-soluble, unconjugated bilirubin, which can be toxic to brain cells. Depending on severity, kernicterus is treated with phototherapy or exchange transfusions (or both). Hemolytic disease of the newborn occurs in Rh-positive infants of Rh-negative mothers who have been sensitized. It involves hemolysis of infant red cells in response to maternal Rh antibodies that have crossed the placenta. Administration of Rh immune globulin to the mother within 72 hours of delivery of an Rh-positive infant, abortion, or amniocentesis prevents sensitization.

Anemia is an increasingly common health problem in older adults. With the increasing numbers of older adults, this will become more of a health care challenge. As with many other tissue cells, the capacity for red cell replacement decreases with aging. Although most older adults are able to maintain their hemoglobin and hematocrit levels within a normal range, they are unable to replace their red cells as promptly as their younger counterparts during a stress situation such as bleeding. This inability to replace red blood cells closely correlates with the increased prevalence of anemia in older adults, which is usually the result of bleeding, infection, malignancy, or chronic disease.

GERIATRIC Considerations

- Hematocrit levels in both men and women are lower after age 60 because of a decreased production of RBCs by the bone marrow, leading to fatigue.[19]
- The most common hematologic system disorder in aging is anemia, which can be attributed to decreased production of RBCs and chronic illnesses or infections.[20]
- Anemia in the elderly should be investigated; it is never normal.[20]
- Nutrient deficiencies lead to alteration in RBCs. Folate, vitamin B_{12} (pernicious anemia), and vitamin C deficiencies are more common in older adults because of altered absorption, interference by medications, and malabsorption.[20]

PEDIATRIC Considerations

- Fetal hemoglobin has a shorter life span, putting the infant at risk for anemia.[21]
- Preterm infants lack transplacental iron transfer, leading to anemia. In term infants, physiologic anemia occurs around 4 to 6 months because of increased blood volume and growth.[21]
- The normal value for hematocrit is higher in infants because of the many macrocytic (large-size RBCs) present.[19]
- Thalassemia, a congenital anemia caused by deficient globin chain synthesis in thalassemic erythrocytes, is most common in infants and children from the Mediterranean region, where malaria has been epidemic.[22]
- Two common tests are used to evaluate red blood cells. The complete blood count (CBC) with differential is used to evaluate cellular components, and a bone marrow examination evaluates blood cell development.[22]

REVIEW EXERCISES

1. Forty students in a hematology class conducted a laboratory exercise that involved determining their blood type. In a subsequent laboratory discussion, they discovered that 16 students had type A blood, 20 had type O blood, 3 had type B blood, and only 1 had type AB blood.
   A. *What types of blood antigens and antibodies would students with type A, type O, and type AB blood have?*
   B. *What could be the possible blood types of the parents of students with type B blood, type O blood, and type AB blood?*
   C. *If these students required a blood transfusion, what type of blood could those with type A, type O, and type AB receive? (Assume the blood is of the same Rh type.)*
2. A 29-year-old woman presents with generalized fatigue. Her physical examination reveals a heart rate of 115 beats/minute, blood pressure of 115/75 mm Hg, and respiratory rate of 28 breaths/minute. Her skin and nail beds are pale. Her laboratory results include red blood cell count $3.0 \times 10^6/\mu L$, hematocrit 30%, hemoglobin 9 g/dL, and a decrease in serum ferritin levels.
   A. *What disorder do you suspect this woman has?*
   B. *What additional data would be helpful in determining the etiology of her condition?*

C. Which of her signs reflect the body's attempt to compensate for the hypoxemia associated with this disorder?

D. What is the significance of the low ferritin level, and how could it be used to make decisions related to her treatment?

3. A 65-year-old woman presents to the clinic for evaluation and treatment of numbness in her lower extremities. She has no other complaints. She takes medication for hypertension, two calcium supplements, and a multivitamin daily. Her laboratory results include red blood cell count 3.0 × $10^6/\mu L$, hematocrit 20%, hemoglobin 9 g/dL, and a markedly elevated MVC.

   A. What type of anemia does she have?

   B. What is the reason for her neurologic symptoms?

   C. What type of treatment would be appropriate?

4. A 12-year-old boy with sickle cell disease presents in the emergency department with severe chest pain. His mother reports that he was doing well until he came down with a respiratory tract infection. She also states he insisted on playing basketball with the other boys in the neighborhood even though he wasn't feeling well.

   A. What is the most likely cause of pain in this boy?

   B. Infections and aerobic-type exercise that increase the levels of deoxygenated hemoglobin produce sickling in people who are homozygous for the sickle cell gene and have sickle cell disease, but not in people who are heterozygous and have sickle cell trait. Explain.

   C. People with sickle disease experience anemia but not iron deficiency. Explain.

References

1. Valdez R., Zutter M., Li S., et al. (2015). Hematopathology. In Rubin E., Gorstein F., Rubin R., et al. (Eds.), *Rubin's pathology: Clinicopathologic foundations of medicine* (7th ed., pp. 1079–1171). Philadelphia, PA: Lippincott Williams & Wilkins.
2. Hall J. E. (2015). *Guyton and Hall textbook of medical physiology* (13th ed., pp. 445–464, 483–495). Philadelphia, PA: Elsevier Saunders.
3. Ciesla B. (2012). *Hematology in practice* (2nd ed., pp. 32–58). Philadelphia, PA: F. A. Davis.
4. Ross M., Pawlina W. (2016). *Histology: A text and atlas with correlated cell and molecular biology* (7th ed., pp. 270–312). Philadelphia, PA: Wolters-Kluwer.
5. Aster J. C., Bunn H. F. (2017). *Pathophysiology of blood disorders* (2nd ed.). New York, NY: McGraw-Hill.
6. Carson J. L., Guyatt G., Heddle N. M., et al. (2016). Clinical practice guidelines from the AABB: Red blood cell transfusion thresholds and storage. *Journal of the American Medical Association* 316(19), 2025–2035.
7. Howard P. R. (2017). *Basic and applied concepts of blood banking and transfusion practices* (4th ed., pp. 94–118, 313–314). St. Louis, MO: Elsevier.
8. United States Centers for Disease Control and Prevention. *The National Healthcare Safety Network (NHSN) Manual: Biovigilance Component v2.4*. Atlanta, GA: Division of Healthcare Quality Promotion, National Center for Emerging and Zoonotic Infectious Diseases. Available: http://www.cdc.gov/nhsn/PDFs/Biovigilance/BV-HV-protocol-current.pdf
9. Weinstein R. (2016). *Red cell transfusion: A pocket guide for the clinician. American Society of Hematology*. Available: http://www.hematology.org/Clinicians/Guidelines-Quality/Quick-Ref/6976.aspx
10. Goroll A. H., Mulley A. G. (2014). *Primary care medicine: Office evaluation and management of the adult patient* (7th ed., pp. 629–663). Philadelphia, PA: Lippincott Williams & Wilkins.
11. McKenzie S. (2015). *Clinical laboratory hematology* (3rd ed., pp. 178–194). Boston, MA: Pearson.
12. United States Centers for Disease Control and Prevention (CDC). (2016). *Sickle cell disease: Data and statistics*. Available: https://www.cdc.gov/ncbddd/sicklecell/data.html
13. National Heart, Lung, and Blood Institute. (2014). *Evidence based management of sickle cell disease: Expert panel report*. Available: https://www.nhlbi.nih.gov/sites/www.nhlbi.nih.gov/files/sickle-cell-disease-report%20020816.pdf
14. Nussbaum R. L., McInnes R. R., Willard H. F. (2016). *Thompson & Thompson genetics in medicine* (8th ed., pp. 198–214). Philadelphia, PA: Elsevier.
15. Schrier S. L., Brugnara C. (2017). *Pathogenesis of autoimmune hemolytic anemia: Warm agglutinins and drugs*. In Mentzer W. C. (Ed.), *UpToDate*. Available: http://www.uptodate.com/contents/pathogenesis-of-autoimmune-hemolytic-anemia-warm-agglutinins-and-drugs
16. Schrier S. L., Brugnara C. (2017). Pathogenesis of autoimmune hemolytic anemia: Cold agglutinin disease. In Mentzer W. C. (Ed.), *UpToDate*. Available: http://www.uptodate.com/contents/pathogenesis-of-autoimmune-hemolytic-anemia-cold-agglutinin-disease
17. American Academy of Pediatrics. (2015). *Vitamin D and iron supplements for babies: AAP recommendations*. Available: https://www.healthychildren.org/English/ages-stages/baby/feeding-nutrition/Pages/Vitamin-Iron-Supplements.aspx
18. United States Centers for Disease Control and Prevention (CDC). (2016). *Folic acid recommendations*. Available: https://www.cdc.gov/ncbddd/folicacid/recommendations.html
19. Fischbach F. T., Dunning M. B. (2015). *A manual of laboratory and diagnostic tests* (9th ed.). Philadelphia, PA: Wolters Kluwer Health.
20. Miller C. A. (2015). *Nursing for wellness in older adults* (7th ed.). Philadelphia, PA: Wolters Kluwer.
21. Kyle T., Carman S. (2017). Nursing care of the child with an alteration in perfusion. In Kyle T., & Carman S. (Eds.), *Essentials of pediatric nursing* (3rd ed., p. 907). Philadelphia, PA: Wolters Kluwer.
22. Bowden V. R., Greenberg C. S. (2014). The child with altered hematologic status. In Bowden, V. R., & Greenberg C. S. (Eds.), *Children and their families the continuum of nursing care* (3rd ed., pp. 1172–1183). Philadelphia, PA: Wolters Kluwer Health/Lippincott Williams & Wilkins

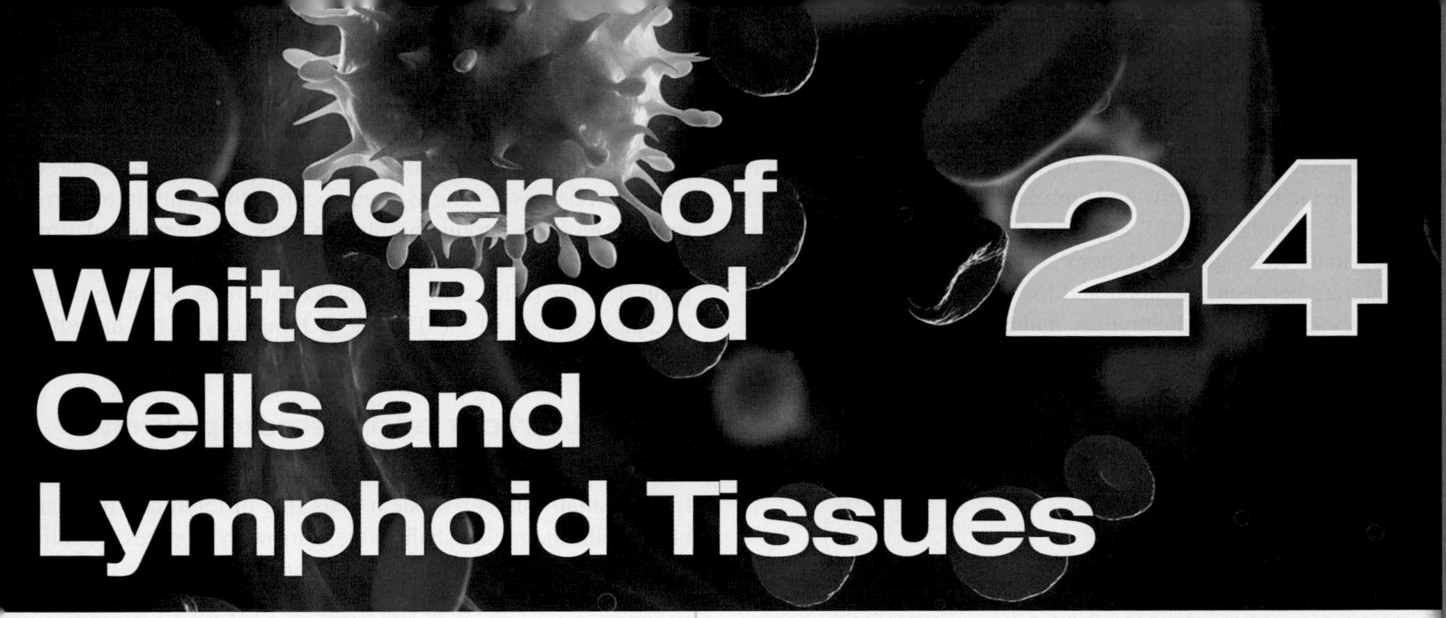

Disorders of White Blood Cells and Lymphoid Tissues

24

Paige Wimberley

The white blood cells and lymphoid tissues where these cells originate and mature function to protect the body against invasion by foreign agents. Disorders of the white blood cells include leukopenia, in which there is a deficiency in leukocytes, and proliferative disorders, in which there is an expansion of leukocytes. The proliferative disorders may be reactive, as occurs with infection, or neoplastic, as occurs with malignant lymphomas and leukemia. This chapter focuses on leukopenia, infectious mononucleosis, malignant lymphomas, leukemias, and plasma cell dyscrasias (multiple myeloma).

HEMATOPOIETIC AND LYMPHOID TISSUES

After completing this section of the chapter, the learner will be able to meet the following objectives:

- Describe the different types of white blood cells and structures of the lymphoid system where they circulate and mature.
- Trace the development of the different white blood cells from their origin in the pluripotent bone marrow stem cell to their circulation in the bloodstream.

The hematopoietic system encompasses all the blood cells and their precursors. It includes the myeloid or bone marrow tissue, in which the blood cells are formed, and the lymphoid tissues of the lymph nodes, thymus, and spleen, in which the white blood cells circulate, mature, and function. The development of the different blood cells involves interactions among precursor bone marrow cells and a variety of growth factors, cytokines (chemical messengers), and gene products such as transcription factors.

Leukocytes (White Blood Cells)

The white blood cells include the granulocytes (*i.e.*, neutrophils, eosinophils, and basophils), monocytes/macrophages, and lymphocytes. The granulocytes and the agranular monocytes/macrophages are derived from the myeloid stem cell in the bone marrow and circulate in the blood (Fig. 24.1). The T lymphocytes (T cells) and B lymphocytes (B cells) originate from lymphoid stem cells in the bone marrow and migrate between the blood and the lymphatic system. T lymphocytes mature in the thymus, and B lymphocytes in the bone marrow. The T lymphocytes differentiate to form CD4+ helper T cells, which serve to orchestrate the immune response, and CD8+ cytotoxic T cells, which provide for cell-mediated immune responses. The B lymphocytes differentiate to form immunoglobulin-producing plasma cells. Another population of lymphocytes includes the large granular lymphocytes, or natural killer (NK) cells, which do not share the specificity or characteristics of the T or the B lymphocytes but have the ability to lyse target cells.[1]

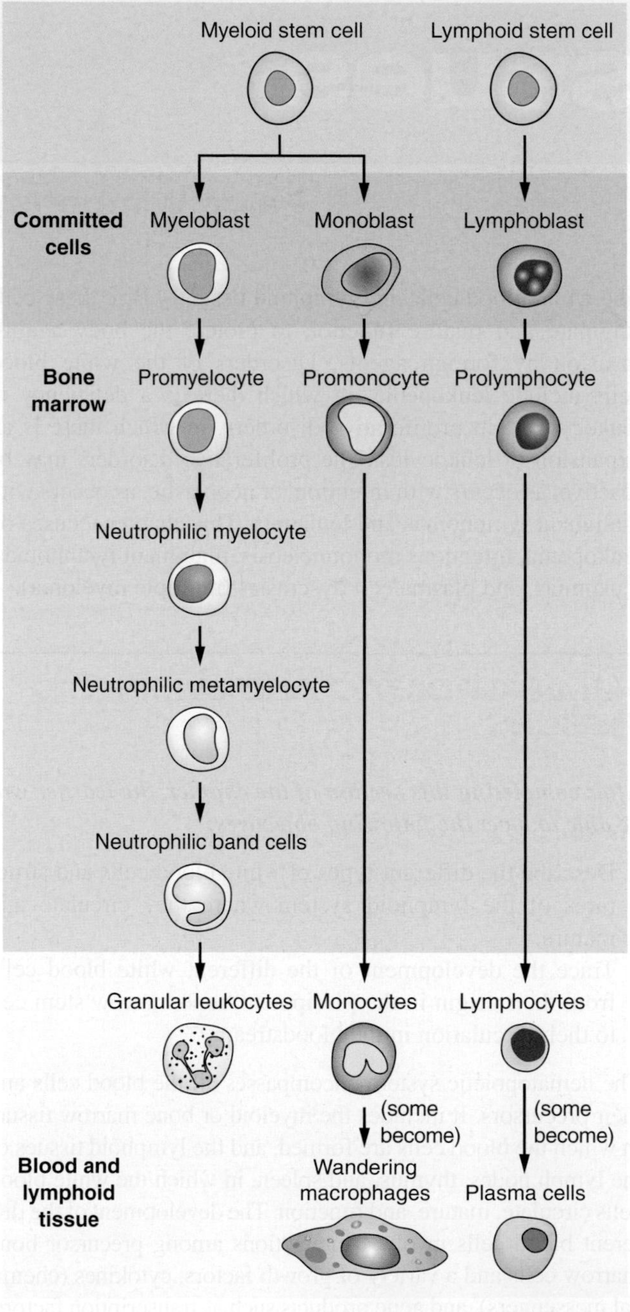

Figure 24.1 • Leukocytes originate from multipotential stem cells in the bone marrow. Granular leukocytes (neutrophils, eosinophils, basophils) have their origin in the myeloid stem cells and develop through a sequence involving myeloblasts. Monocytes, like granulocytes, are progeny of the myeloid stem cell line but develop along a pathway involving monoblasts. Only lymphocytes originate from the lymphoid stem cell line. They develop through a sequence involving lymphoblasts and are released from the bone marrow as prolymphocytes, which undergo further differentiation in the lymphoid organs.

Bone Marrow and Hematopoiesis

The entire hematopoietic system, with all its complexity, arises from a small number of stem cells that differentiate to form blood cells and replenish the bone marrow by a process of self-renewal. All the hematopoietic precursors, including the erythroid (red blood cell), myelocyte (granulocyte and monocyte), lymphocyte (T cell and B cell), and megakaryocyte (platelet) series, are derived from a small population of cells called *pluripotent stem cells* (Fig. 24.2). These cells are capable of providing *progenitor cells* (*i.e.*, parent cells) for myelopoiesis and lymphopoiesis, processes by which myeloid and lymphoid blood cells are made. Several levels of differentiation lead to the development of committed *unipotent cells*, which are the progenitors for each of the different blood cell types.

Hematopoietic Growth Factors

Like erythropoiesis, leukopoiesis, or production of white blood cells, is controlled by hematopoietic growth factors. The *hematopoietic growth factors* are a family of glycoproteins that support hematopoietic colony formation. These growth factors can be categorized into three groups: the growth factors that are involved in the development of a specific cell lineage; those that affect the early multipotential progenitor cells; and those that induce the expression of growth factor genes in other cells.[2] Cytokines or chemical messengers, such as interleukin (IL)-1, IL-4, IL-6, and interferon, act synergistically to support the functions of the growth factors.

There are several lineage-specific growth factors: erythropoietin, granulocyte–macrophage colony-stimulating factor (GM-CSF), and monocyte–macrophage colony-stimulating factor (M-CSF). Although the hematopoietic growth factors act at different points in the proliferation and differentiation pathway, their functions overlap. For example, GM-CSF stimulates the growth and function of granulocyte, macrophage, and eosinophil progenitor cells and induces IL-1 gene expression in neutrophils and peripheral mononuclear leukocytes. Cytokines, such as IL-3, act on the most immature bone marrow progenitor cells, thereby promoting the development of cells that can differentiate into a number of cell types. The identification and characterization of the various growth factors and cytokines have led to their use in treating a wide range of diseases, including bone marrow failure, hematopoietic neoplasms, infectious diseases, and congenital and myeloproliferative disorders.

Leukocyte Developmental Stages

Leukocyte development begins with the myeloid and lymphoid stem cells in the bone marrow. The granulocyte and monocyte cell lines derive from the myeloid stem cells and the lymphocytes from the lymphoid stem cells (see Fig. 24.1). The

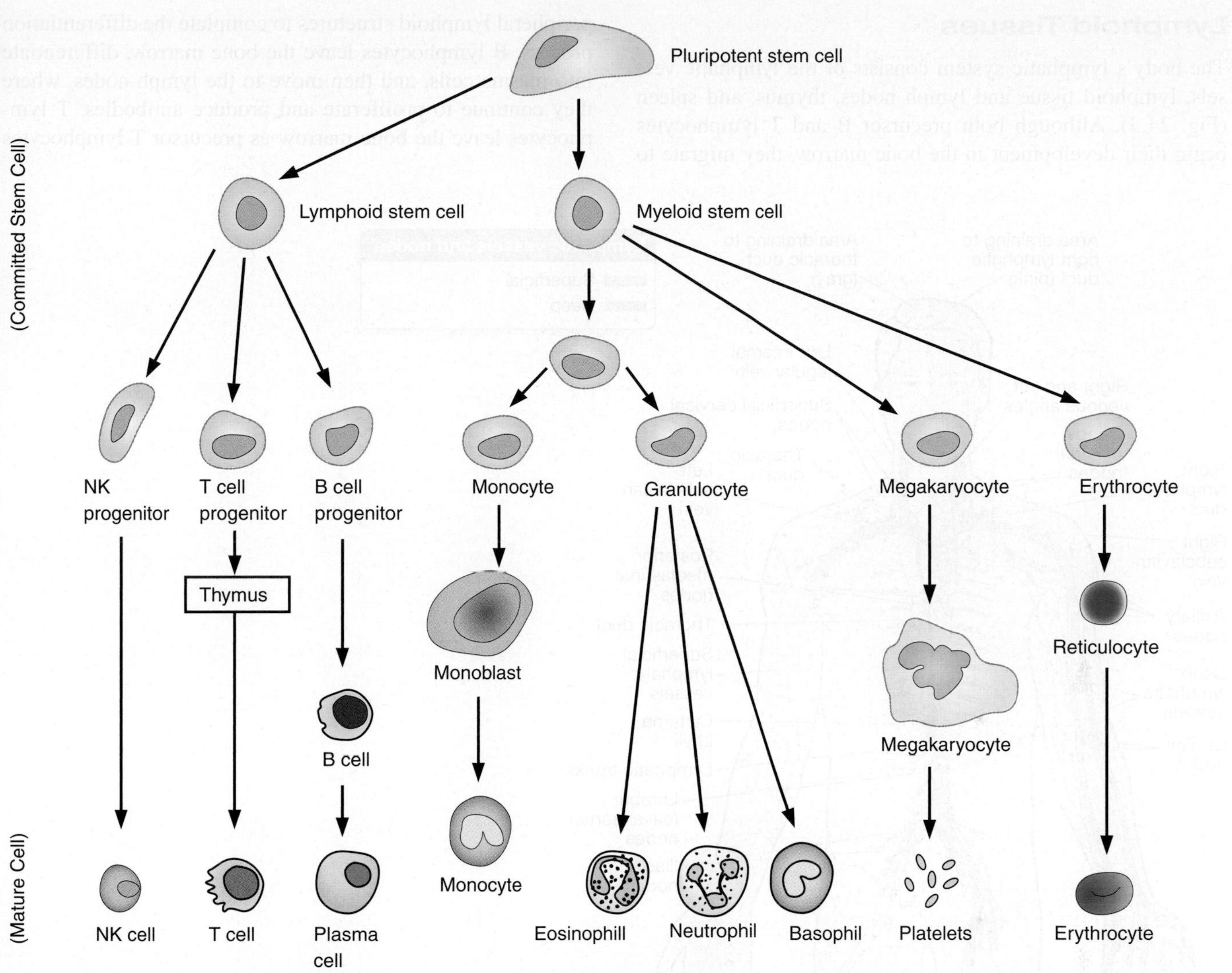

Figure 24.2 • Major developmental stages of blood cells. NK, natural killer cell. (From Porth C. M. (2015). *Essentials of pathophysiology* (4th ed., Fig. 11-1, p. 242). Philadelphia, PA: Lippincott Williams & Wilkins.)

immature precursor cells for each of the cell lines are called *blast cells. Myeloblasts*, which are the granulocytic precursor cells, have round to oval nuclei, with delicate chromatin and a blue to gray cytoplasm. During the next stage of development, the myeloblasts are transformed into *promyelocytes* with similar nuclei, but with a cytoplasm containing many primary granules. In the subsequent *metamyelocyte* stage, the nuclei distort and become arclike, producing the band developmental stage. Maturation from metamyelocyte to mature neutrophil involves progressive condensation of nuclear chromatin, increasing nuclear lobulation, and the appearance of secondary (specific) granules. Eosinophils and basophils undergo similar developmental stages but develop different secondary granules. Like granulocytes, monocytes develop from the granulocyte–monocyte progenitor cell and progress through a monoblast and promonocyte stage. By contrast, lymphocytes derive from lymphoid stem cells and progress through the lymphoblast and prolymphocyte stages. The prolymphocytes leave the bone marrow and travel to the lymphoid tissues, where further differentiation into T and B lymphocytes occurs. The names of the various leukocyte developmental stages are often used in describing blood cell changes that occur in hematopoietic disorders (*e.g.*, acute lymphoblastic leukemia [ALL] and acute promyelocytic leukemia).

KEY POINTS

HEMATOPOIESIS

- The white blood cells are formed from hematopoietic stem cells that differentiate into committed progenitor cells that in turn develop into the myelocytic and lymphocytic lineages needed for the formation of the different types of white blood cell.
- The life span of white blood cells is relatively short so that constant renewal is necessary to maintain normal blood levels. Any conditions that decrease the availability of stem cells or hematopoietic growth factors produce a decrease in white blood cells.

Lymphoid Tissues

The body's lymphatic system consists of the lymphatic vessels, lymphoid tissue and lymph nodes, thymus, and spleen (Fig. 24.3). Although both precursor B and T lymphocytes begin their development in the bone marrow, they migrate to peripheral lymphoid structures to complete the differentiation process. B lymphocytes leave the bone marrow, differentiate into plasma cells, and then move to the lymph nodes, where they continue to proliferate and produce antibodies. T lymphocytes leave the bone marrow as precursor T lymphocytes

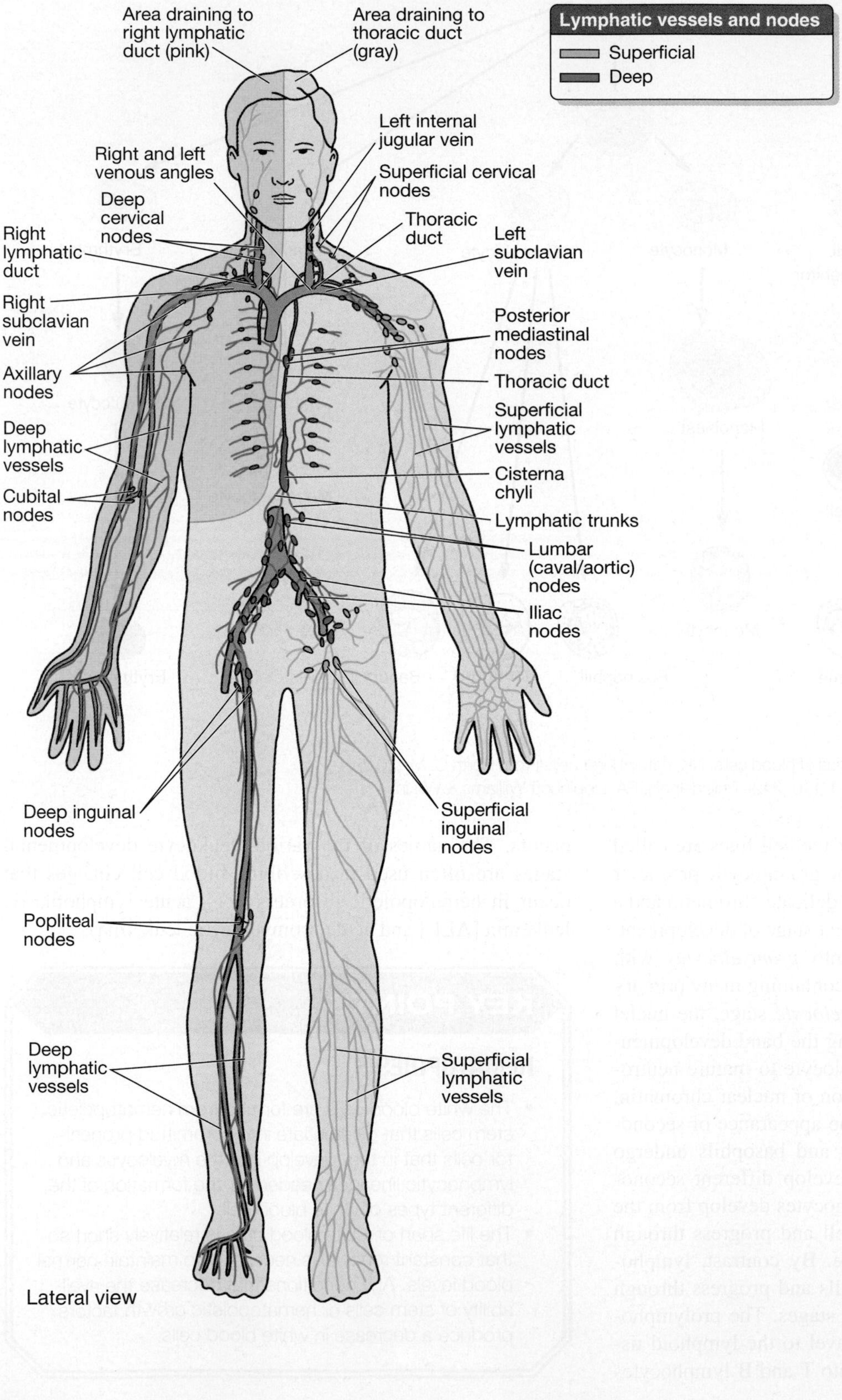

Figure 24.3 • Lymphatic system. **(A)** The right lymphatic duct drains lymph from the right side of the head and neck and the right upper limbs (shaded). The thoracic duct drains the remainder of the body. Deep lymphatic vessels are shown on the right, and superficial lymphatic vessels are shown on the left. **(B)** Lymph flow from extracellular spaces through a lymph node. Small black arrows indicate the flow of interstitial fluid out of blood capillaries into the lymphatic capillaries. (From Moore K. L., Agur A. M., Dalley A. F. (2015). *Essential clinical anatomy* (5th ed., Fig. 1-18, p. 26). Philadelphia, PA: Wolters Kluwer/Lippincott Williams & Wilkins.)

travel to the thymus, where they differentiate into CD4+ helper T cells and CD8+ cytotoxic T cells, after which many of them move to lymph nodes, where they undergo further proliferation.

Lymph nodes consist of organized collections of lymphoid tissue located along the lymphatic vessels.[3] Typically grayish-white and ovoid or bean-shaped, they range in size from 1 mm to about 1 to 2 cm in diameter. A fibrous capsule and radiating trabeculae provide a supporting structure, and a delicate reticular network contributes to internal support (Fig. 24.4). The parenchyma of the lymph node is divided into an outer or superficial cortex and an inner medulla. The superficial cortex contains well-defined B-cell and T-cell domains. The B-cell–dependent cortex consists of two types of follicles: immunologically inactive follicles, called *primary follicles*, and active follicles that contain germinal centers, called *secondary follicles*. Germinal centers contain large lymphocytes (centroblasts) and small lymphocytes with cleaved nuclei (centrocytes). The mantle zone is the small layer of B cells surrounding the germinal centers. The portion of the cortex between the medullary and superficial cortex is called the *paracortex*. This region contains most of the T cells in the lymph nodes.

Although some lymphocytes enter the lymph nodes through the afferent lymphatic channels, most enter through the wall of postcapillary venules located in the deep cortex. These vessels, which are lined with specialized endothelial cells that possess receptors for antigen-primed lymphocytes, signal lymphocytes to leave the circulation and migrate through the lymph nodes. Both B and T cells leave the bloodstream through these channels.[1,4,5] The T cells remain in the paracortex and the B cells migrate to the follicular area of the cortex. Most lymphocytes leave the lymph node by entering the lymphatic sinuses, from which they enter the efferent lymphatic vessel.

The alimentary canal, respiratory passages, and genitourinary systems are guarded by accumulations of lymphoid tissue that are not enclosed in a capsule. This form of lymphoid tissue is called *diffuse lymphoid tissue* or *mucosa-associated lymphoid tissue* (MALT) because of its association with mucous membranes (Fig. 24.5).[3] Lymphocytes are found in the subepithelium of these tissues. Lymphomas can arise from MALT as well as lymph node tissue.

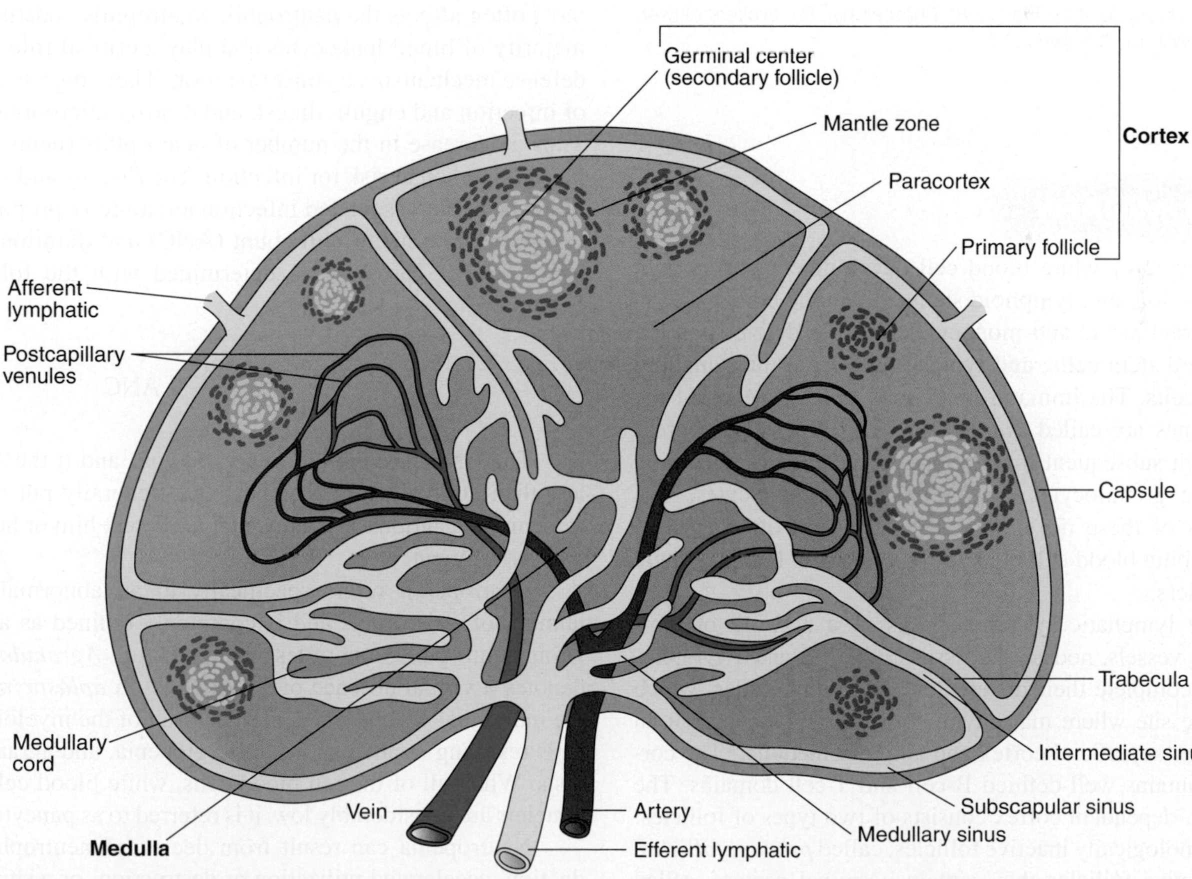

Figure 24.4 • Structures of normal lymph node. (From Rubin R., Strayer D. E. (Eds.) (2015). *Rubin's pathology: Clinicopathologic foundations of medicine* (7th ed., Fig. 26-46, p. 1131). Philadelphia, PA: Lippincott Williams & Wilkins.)

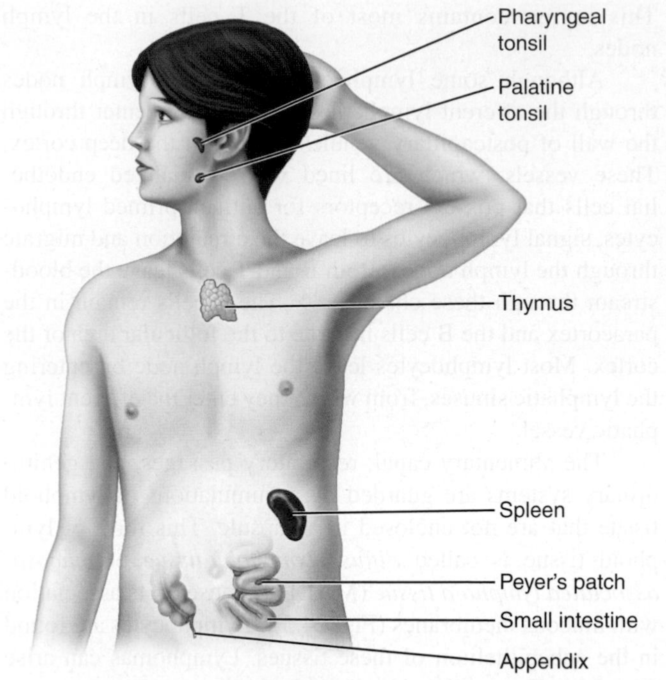

Figure 24.5 • Mucosa-associated lymphoid tissue (MALT). This type of lymphoid tissue protects the body's entry points. (From McConnell T. H., Hull K. L. (2011). *Human form human function: Essentials of anatomy & physiology* (p. 473, Fig. 12-8). Philadelphia, PA: Wolters Kluwer/Lippincott Williams & Wilkins.)

IN SUMMARY

Leukocyte or white blood cell development begins with the myeloid and lymphoid stem cells in the bone marrow. The granulocyte and monocyte cell lines derive from the myeloid stem cells, and lymphocytes from the lymphoid stem cells. The immature precursor cells for each of the cell lines are called *blast cells*. The blast cells progress through subsequent maturational stages before becoming mature granulocytes, monocytes, or lymphocytes. The names of these developmental stages are often used in describing blood cell changes that occur in hematopoietic disorders.

The lymphatic system consists of a network of lymphatic vessels, nodes, and tissues where B and T lymphocytes complete their differentiation. Lymph nodes, which are the site where many lymphomas originate, exhibit an outer or superficial cortex and an inner medulla.[4] The cortex contains well-defined B-cell and T-cell domains. The B-cell–dependent cortex consists of two types of follicles: immunologically inactive follicles, called *primary follicles*, and active follicles that contain germinal centers, called *secondary follicles*. Most of the T cells are contained in the paracortex, the area between the medullary and superficial cortices.

NONNEOPLASTIC DISORDERS OF WHITE BLOOD CELLS

After completing this section of the chapter, the learner will be able to meet the following objectives:

- Define the terms *leukopenia, neutropenia, granulocytopenia*, and *aplastic anemia*.
- Describe the mechanism of symptom production in neutropenia.

The number of leukocytes, or white blood cells, in the peripheral circulation normally ranges from 5000 to 10,000 cells/μL (also expressed as 5 to 10 × 10^3 cells/μL, or 5000 to 10,000 cells/mm^3 of blood).[1] The nonneoplastic disorders of white blood cells include a deficiency of leukocytes (leukopenia) and proliferative disorders in which there are increased numbers of leukocytes.

Neutropenia (Agranulocytosis)

The term *leukopenia* describes a decrease in the absolute number of leukocytes in the blood. Although leukopenia may affect any of the specific types of white blood cells, it most often affects the neutrophil. Neutrophils constitute the majority of blood leukocytes and play a critical role in host defense mechanisms against infection. They migrate to sites of infection and engulf, digest, and destroy microorganisms. Thus a decrease in the number of neutrophils (neutropenia) places a person at risk for infection. The risk for and severity of neutropenia-associated infection are directly proportional to the absolute neutrophil count (ANC) and duration of the neutropenia.[3] The ANC is determined with the following formula[5]:

$$\frac{\text{segs} + \text{bands} \times \text{WBC}}{100} = \text{ANC}$$

The ANC is supposed to be 1000/μL, and if the ANC is less than 500 cells/mm^3, the person is generally put on neutropenic precautions in the hospital to protect him or her from the environment.[6]

Neutropenia refers specifically to an abnormally low number of neutrophils and is commonly defined as a circulating neutrophil count of less than 1000/μL. *Agranulocytosis* denotes a virtual absence of neutrophils. In *aplastic anemia*, the individual will have a depletion of all of the myeloid stem cells resulting in anemia, thrombocytopenia, and agranulocytosis. When all of the red blood cells, white blood cells, and platelets are considerably low, it is referred to as pancytopenia.

Neutropenia can result from decreased neutrophil production, accelerated utilization or destruction, or a shift from the blood to the tissue compartments. It can be present at birth (congenital) or arise from a number of factors that occur later in life and do not have a hereditary component (acquired).

Congenital Neutropenia

Inherited disorders of proliferation and maturation of myeloid stem cell lines are relatively rare and have a high degree of variability in severity and symptomatology. Approximately one half are due to neutrophil elastase (ELANE) mutations. ELANE mutations are not associated with extra hemopoietic presentations.[7]

Congenital neutropenias can be divided into two subtypes: congenital (permanent) severe neutropenia and cyclic neutropenia, which has variable expression. Severe congenital neutropenia is usually diagnosed in infants under 6 months of age, and counts are usually less than 2 g/L.[7] Severe bacterial and/or fungal infections are associated with its discovery. The risk of severe infection is inversely related to the neutrophil count—that is, the lower the neutrophil count, the higher the risk of infection.

Cyclic (intermittent) neutropenia is often discovered in children under 2 years of age and is usually associated with acute stomatologic disorders. Cyclic neutropenia occurs with periodic oscillations between normal and abnormal neutrophils. In some instances, the bone marrow may function normally for a period of time. As a result the risk for severe life-threatening infections exists but frequency is reduced. The cycles may become less noticeable in older adults and then the disorder begins to resemble chronic neutropenia.

Severe congenital neutropenia, or *Kostmann syndrome*, is characterized by an arrest in myeloid maturation at the promyelocyte stage of development that can be inherited as either an autosomal dominant or autosomal recessive trait.[8] The autosomal dominant disease is usually associated with mutations in the neutrophil elastase gene, which in turn leads to apoptosis of bone marrow myeloid cells. The autosomal recessive severe congenital neutropenia or Kostmann syndrome is due to mutations in the HAX-1 gene, which causes a loss of mitochondrial potential. The disorder is characterized by severe bacterial infections. Before the GM-CSFs became available for clinical use, two thirds of children died of fatal infections before reaching adolescence. Approximately 20% of people with the disorder develop acute myelogenous leukemia (AML).[8]

Acquired Neutropenia

Acquired neutropenia encompasses a broad spectrum of causative processes and includes primary and secondary autoimmune neutropenia, infection-related neutropenia, and drug-induced neutropenia (Chart 24.1). A number of bone marrow disorders, hematopoietic malignancies, and radiation therapy may induce neutropenia.

Autoimmune Neutropenia. Autoimmune neutropenia results from antibodies directed against neutrophil cell membrane antigens or bone marrow progenitors. The autoimmune forms of neutropenia may be classified as primary (*i.e.*, those not associated with other detectable pathologic processes) or secondary (*i.e.*, those associated with another disease condition).[9]

CHART 24.1 PRINCIPAL CAUSES OF NEUTROPENIA

Congenital
- Alloimmune neonatal neutropenia (transfer of maternal antibodies)
- Cyclic neutropenia
- Kostmann syndrome (severe congenital neutropenia)

Acquired
Autoimmune
- Primary (rare, usually occurs in children and runs a benign course)
- Secondary
  - Systemic lupus erythematous
  - Felty syndrome in people with RA
- Infection related
- Many types of infections agents, but most commonly viruses
- Mechanisms include increased consumption of neutrophils, production of autoantibodies, direct infiltration of hematopoietic cells, and bone marrow suppression

Drug related
- Immune-mediated reactions in which drugs act as haptens (*e.g.*, penicillin, propylthiouracil, aminopyrine)
- Accelerated apoptosis (clozapine [antipsychotic agent])
- Cancer chemotherapeutic drugs (bone marrow depression)

Radiation therapy to bone marrow
Hematologic malignancies

Primary autoimmune neutropenia is a rare disorder of early childhood, during which a moderate to severe neutropenia is observed. The condition is usually benign, with mild to moderate infections for children. The disorder is rare in adults. Because primary autoimmune neutropenia is self-limiting, treatment is usually restricted to the use of antimicrobial agents for people who experience recurrent infections.

Secondary immune-associated neutropenia is often associated with systemic autoimmune disorders, mainly rheumatoid arthritis (RA) and systemic lupus erythematosus (SLE).[9] Felty syndrome, a variant of RA, is a triad of splenomegaly, recurrent pulmonary infections, and neutropenia.[9] The neutropenia is the result of antineutrophil antibodies and high levels of circulating immune complexes, which induce neutrophil apoptosis. Coupled with the end-organ manifestations of RA, the majority of people with Felty syndrome are susceptible to serious bacterial infection that sometimes leads to sepsis and poor clinical outcome.

Several antibody-mediated mechanisms are believed to be responsible for the neutropenia seen in people with SLE. These include the development of antineutrophil antibodies, along with increased neutrophil apoptosis and decreased neutrophil production by the bone marrow. Similar to Felty syndrome, continued treatment of SLE to control symptoms is the preferred method of treatment.

Infection-Related Neutropenia. Many different types of infectious diseases, including viral, bacterial, rickettsial, and parasitic, may cause neutropenia, the most common being viral. Infections may produce neutropenia in multiple ways such as decreased neutrophil production, loss of neutrophils by toxins, or problems resulting in neutrophil sequestration in the spleen. Neutropenia is also a common manifestation of acquired immunodeficiency syndrome (AIDS), in which a virus-induced suppression of marrow cell proliferation is often aggravated by infectious consumption of neutrophils and by antiviral drugs.[4]

Drug-Related Neutropenia. Drug-induced neutropenia is attributed to a number of drugs, especially those used in the treatment of cancer.[10,11] The risk for development of chemotherapy-induced neutropenia is influenced by patient- and treatment-related disease, oncologic disease, and other comorbidities. One of the most important patient-related factors is age. Older adults are at greater risk than younger people because of age-related cellular changes in neutrophils.[12] Patient-related factors include disease burden, nutritional and hydration status, and previous history of anemia or neutropenia. Treatment-related factors include radiation therapy to the bone marrow, extensive prior chemotherapy, and treatment regimen.

The term *idiosyncratic* is used to describe drug reactions that are different from the effect obtained in most people and that cannot be explained in terms of allergy. Idiosyncratic reactions occur as an immune-mediated or direct damage to myeloid precursors and cell lineage.[10] The reaction is reversible on discontinuation of the drug.

Febrile neutropenia is often related to chemotherapy-induced neutropenia and is associated with significant mortality and morbidity.[11] Febrile neutropenia (FN)—defined as oral temperature greater than 38.3°C and an ANC less than 0.5×10^9/L[12]—is a key factor limiting the dose of many cytotoxic drugs.[11] Most cases are associated with bacterial infections, but FN may develop as a result of fungal or viral infections. Primary prophylaxis with G-CSF is useful against the development of FN.[12]

Neutrophils provide the first line of defense against organisms that inhabit the skin and gastrointestinal tract. Thus, early signs of infection due to neutropenia, particularly those associated with a mild to moderate decrease in neutrophils, include mild skin lesions, stomatitis, pharyngitis, and diarrhea. Signs and symptoms of more severe neutropenia include malaise, chills, and fever, followed in sequence by marked weakness and fatigability. Untreated infections can be rapidly fatal, particularly if the ANC drops below 250/μL. With severe neutropenia, the usual signs of infection may not be present because of a lack of a sufficient number of neutrophils to produce an inflammatory response.

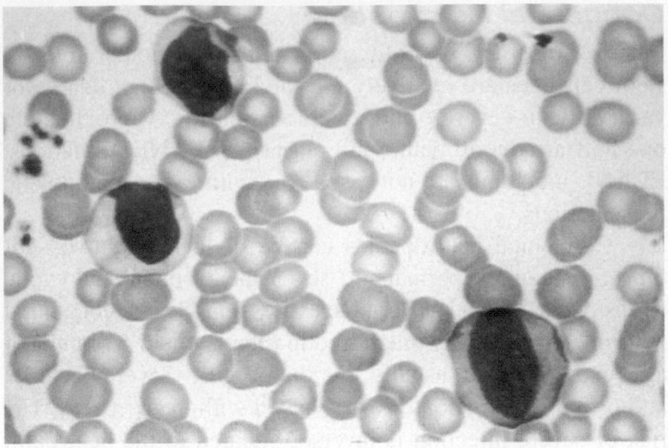

Figure 24.6 • Infectious mononucleosis. An absolute lymphocytosis caused by a heterogeneous population of small and larger lymphoid cells, including atypical lymphocytes, is characteristic of the Epstein-Barr virus–driven disorder. (From Rubin R., Strayer D. E. (Eds.) (2015). *Rubin's pathology: Clinicopathologic foundations of medicine* (7th ed., Fig. 26-50, p. 1134). Philadelphia, PA: Lippincott Williams & Wilkins.)

Infectious Mononucleosis

Infectious mononucleosis is a self-limiting lymphoproliferative disorder. Eighty-five percent of the time it is caused by the Epstein-Barr virus (EBV), a member of the herpesvirus family (Fig. 24.6).[13] Epstein-Barr virus is responsible for approximately 90% of all cases of infectious mononucleosis, with cytomegalovirus (CMV) accounting for the remainder.[14] Approximately 35% to 50% of infections with EBV result in infectious mononucleosis, most often in adolescents and young adults.[13] Once an individual is infected, the virus will remain present in the B lymphocytes for a lifetime.[13]

Clinical Course

The onset of infectious mononucleosis usually is insidious. The incubation period lasts 4 to 6 weeks.[14] A prodromal period, which lasts for several days, follows and is characterized by malaise, anorexia, and chills. The prodromal period precedes the onset of fever, pharyngitis, and lymphadenopathy. Occasionally, the disorder comes on abruptly with a high fever. Most people seek medical attention for severe pharyngitis, which usually is most severe on days 5 to 7 and persists for 7 to 14 days. The lymph nodes are typically enlarged throughout the body, particularly in the cervical, axillary, and groin areas. Palatal petechiae may be present in those with sore throat and lymphadenopathy.[15]

A maculopapular generalized rash has been reported in 3% to 15% of people. The rash often follows treatment with beta-lactam antibiotics.[16]

Complications

Splenomegaly occurs in approximately 50% to 60% of cases.[14] The spleen may be enlarged two to three times its normal size, and rupture of the spleen occurs in less than

0.5% of cases.[15] Hepatitis may also occur. These are thought to be immune mediated. Hepatitis is characterized by hepatomegaly, nausea, anorexia, and jaundice. Although discomforting, it usually is a benign condition that resolves without causing permanent liver damage. Other potential complications include myocarditis, upper airway obstruction, encephalitis, and hemolytic anemia.[15] Those who have X-linked lymphoproliferative syndrome have a greater risk of complications and are more likely to die from the infection.[15]

Blood testing includes the monospot and serologic testing. The monospot tests for heterophile antibodies, which are considered the hallmark of an EBV infection.[14] The development of the heterophile antibodies take time to develop, resulting in false negatives early in the disease. An increase in IgM and IgG antibodies early in the disease are indicative of an EBV infection.

Most people with infectious mononucleosis recover without incident. The acute phase of the illness usually lasts for 2 to 3 weeks, after which recovery occurs rapidly. Some degree of debility and lethargy may persist for 2 to 3 months. Treatment is primarily symptomatic and supportive.

IN SUMMARY

Neutropenia, which represents a marked reduction in the absolute number of neutrophils, is one of the major disorders of the white blood cells. It can occur as a congenital or acquired disorder. Congenital neutropenia consists primarily of cyclic neutropenia, which is characterized by cyclic (18- to 24-day) oscillations of peripheral neutrophils, and severe congenital neutropenia or Kostmann syndrome, which is associated with severe bacterial infections. The acquired neutropenias encompass a wide spectrum of causative processes, including immunologically mediated bone marrow suppression or neutrophil injury and destruction; infection-mediated mechanisms, including increased peripheral utilization; and drug-mediated mechanisms, particularly those related to the use of cancer chemotherapeutic agents. Neutropenia may also be caused by a number of bone marrow conditions, hematopoietic malignancies, and radiation therapy. Because the neutrophil is essential to host defenses against bacterial and fungal infections, severe and often life-threatening infections are common in people with neutropenia.

Infectious mononucleosis is a self-limited lymphoproliferative disorder caused by the B-lymphotropic EBV, a member of the herpesvirus family. The highest incidence of infectious mononucleosis is found in adolescents and young adults, and it is seen more frequently in the upper socioeconomic classes of developed countries. The virus is usually transmitted in the saliva. The disease is characterized by fever, generalized lymphadenopathy, sore throat, and the appearance in the blood of atypical lymphocytes and several antibodies, including the well-known heterophil antibodies that are used in the diagnosis of infectious mononucleosis. Most people with infectious mononucleosis recover without incident. Treatment is largely symptomatic and supportive.

NEOPLASTIC DISORDERS OF LYMPHOID AND HEMATOPOIETIC ORIGIN

After completing this section of the chapter, the learner will be able to meet the following objectives:

- Use the concepts regarding the central and peripheral lymphoid tissues to describe the site of origin of the malignant lymphomas and leukemias.
- Explain how changes in chromosomal structure and gene function can contribute to the development of malignant lymphomas and leukemias.

The neoplastic disorders of lymphoid origin represent the most important of the white blood cell disorders. The neoplasia of lymphoid origin can arise from both B and T cells as well as tumors representing various stages of lymphocyte development.[17,18] The major categories include non-Hodgkin lymphomas (NHLs), Hodgkin lymphoma (HL), lymphoid leukemias, and plasma cell dyscrasias. The clinical features of these neoplasms are largely determined by their cell of origin, the progenitor cell from which they originated, and the molecular events involved in their transformation into a malignant neoplasm. Because blood cells circulate throughout the body, these neoplasms are often disseminated from the onset.

Malignant Lymphomas

The lymphomas are a diverse group of solid tumors composed of neoplastic lymphoid cells that vary with respect to molecular features, genetics, clinical presentation, and treatment. Approximately 8260 new cases of HLs were diagnosed in the United States in 2017, of which about 1070 will eventually die.[19] The incidence of new NHL cases in the United States in 2017 was 72,240, and there were 20,140 deaths in 2017 from NHL.[19] Incidence rates for both NHL and HL remained stable from 2004 until 2013, whereas death rates declined from 2005 to 2014.[19]

Approximately 5% of cancers in children under 14 years of age are NHLs including Burkitt lymphoma. Hodgkin lymphoma accounts for 3%, occurring most often during adolescence.[19]

Non-Hodgkin Lymphomas

The NHLs represent a clinically diverse group of B-cell, T-cell, or NK-cell origin. They represent about 4% of all new cases of cancer diagnosed in the United States.[19]

Non-Hodgkin lymphomas arise from the lymphocytes, and the site of their origination varies according to their common lymphoid progenitor.[21] Alterations in the developmental process of these cells can lead to any of the subtypes of lymphoid neoplasm with varying characteristics.[21] The exact cause of the alterations is unknown; however, pathogens such as EBV, Human T-lymphotropic virus 1, and Helicobacter pylori have been linked to specific subtypes.[18]

Characterization of NHLs include cellular morphology, immunophenotype, clinical symptoms, and level of aggression.[18–22] Incidence of the disease has increased since the 1970s, and subtypes vary widely worldwide.[20] These variations are believed to occur because of environmental, genetic, and other unidentified factors.[20,23] Differential diagnosis is important in treatment planning, as is disease staging, disease location, the person's general health and history, including any previous treatments for cancers.[18,22] Staging is accomplished using the Ann Arbor system.

Mature B-Cell Lymphomas. B-cell lymphomas are the most common NHL subtype and originate either from the germinal center B or activated B cells that have exited the germinal centers.[18,20] More commonly diagnosed B-cell subtypes include follicular lymphoma, immunoblastic large cell lymphoma, and mantle cell lymphoma.[24]

Follicular lymphomas are derived from germinal center B cells and consist of a mixture of centroblasts and centrocytes (Fig. 24.7). Follicular lymphoma tumors resemble primary lymphoid follicles, secrete cytokines, induce T-cell exhaustion and apoptosis, and interact with resident T helper cells to promote their survival and proliferation.[25] Follicular lymphomas are usually indolent, and prognosis for long-term survival is good.[26] However, there is an increased risk for second cancers for those over 65 years, males, and those treated with radiation.[26] The lymphoma predominantly affects lymph nodes. Other sites of involvement include the spleen, bone marrow, peripheral blood, head and neck region, gastrointestinal tract, and skin. Over time, approximately one of three follicular lymphomas transforms into a fast-growing diffuse large B-cell lymphoma.[17]

Diffuse large B-cell lymphomas are a heterogeneous group of aggressive germinal or postgerminal center neoplasms. The disease occurs in all age groups but is most prevalent between 60 and 70 years of age. The cause of diffuse large B-cell lymphoma is unknown but may involve EBV or HIV infections. It is a rapidly evolving, multifocal, nodal and extranodal tumor. Manifestations are typically seen at the time

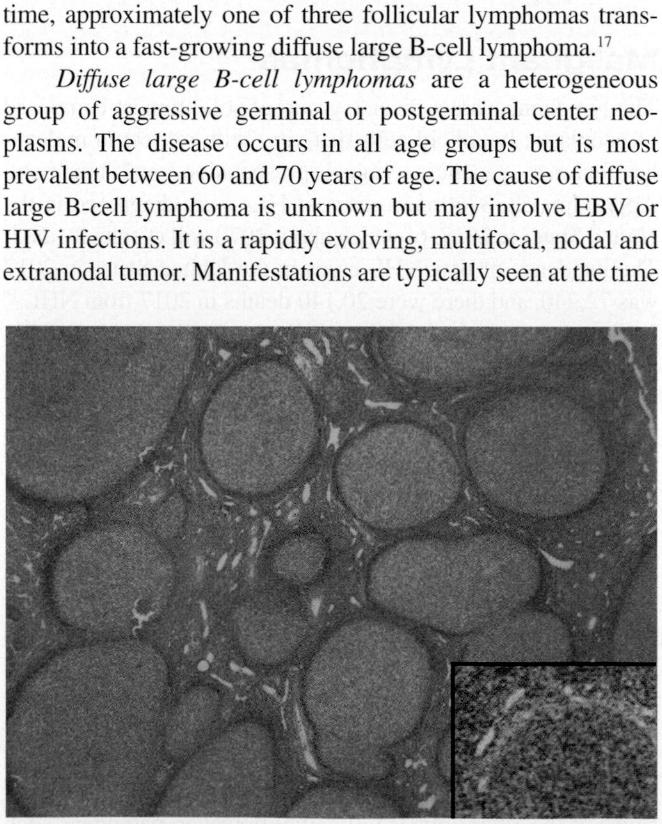

Figure 24.7 • Follicular lymphoma. The normal lymph node architecture is replaced by malignant lymphoid follicles in a back-to-back pattern. The *inset* illustrates malignant lymphoid follicle germinal centers. (From Rubin R., Strayer D. E. (Eds.) (2015). *Rubin's pathology: Clinicopathologic foundations of medicine* (7th ed., Fig. 26-58, p. 1144). Philadelphia, PA: Lippincott Williams & Wilkins.)

of presentation. As a group, diffuse large B-cell lymphomas are rapidly fatal if untreated.

Burkitt lymphoma, one of the most aggressive and rapidly growing tumors of the NHLs, is a disorder of germinal center B cells.[17] It is endemic in regions of Africa where both EBV and malarial infection are common.[23] Virtually 100% of people with African Burkitt lymphoma have evidence of previous EBV infection (Fig. 24.8).

Mantle cell lymphomas constitute less than 10% of NHLs and have their origin in the naive B cell. After the precursor stage, B cells undergo immunoglobulin (Ig) gene rearrangements and develop into surface IgM- and IgD-positive naive B cells. These cells give rise to mantle cell lymphoma. Mantle cell lymphomas do not occur in children, but affect older people (median age, 60 years). They have a rapid rate of progression, and half of people do not tend to survive 3 years.

Marginal zone lymphomas (MZL) refers to related forms of NHL that affect B cells including mucosal-associated lymphoid tissue (MALT), nodal-marginal zone lymphoma, and splenic marginal zone lymphoma. MALT involve late-stage memory B cells that reside in the marginal zone or outermost compartment of the lymph node follicle. MALT lymphomas tend to remain localized for prolonged periods and to follow an indolent course. MALT develop in epithelial tissues of the gastrointestinal and respiratory tracts and remain localized. Prolonged inflammation promotes continued mutations. These additional mutations allow the tumor to become antigen independent and metastasize.[27]

Clinical Manifestations. The manifestations of NHL depend on lymphoma type (*i.e.*, indolent or aggressive) and the stage of the disease. People with indolent or slow-growing lymphomas usually present with painless lymphadenopathy, which may be isolated or widespread. Involved lymph nodes may be present in the retroperitoneum, mesentery, and pelvis. The indolent lymphomas are usually disseminated at the time of diagnosis, and bone marrow involvement is frequent. With or without treatment, the natural course of the disease may fluctuate over 5 to 10 or more years. Many low-grade lymphomas eventually transform into more aggressive forms of lymphoma/leukemia.

People with intermediate or more aggressive forms of lymphoma usually present with accompanying constitutional symptoms such as fever, drenching night sweats, or weight loss. Frequently, there is increased susceptibility to bacterial, viral, and fungal infections associated with hypogammaglobulinemia and a poor humoral antibody response, rather than the impaired cellular immunity seen with HL. Because of their high growth fraction, these lymphomas tend to be sensitive to radiation and chemotherapy.

Diagnosis and Treatment. A lymph node biopsy is used to confirm the diagnosis of NHL and immunophenotyping to determine the lineage and clonality. Staging of the disease is important in selecting a treatment for people with NHL.

Treatment of NHL depends on the histologic type, stage of the disease, and clinical status of the person. For early-stage disease involving a single or limited node involvement,

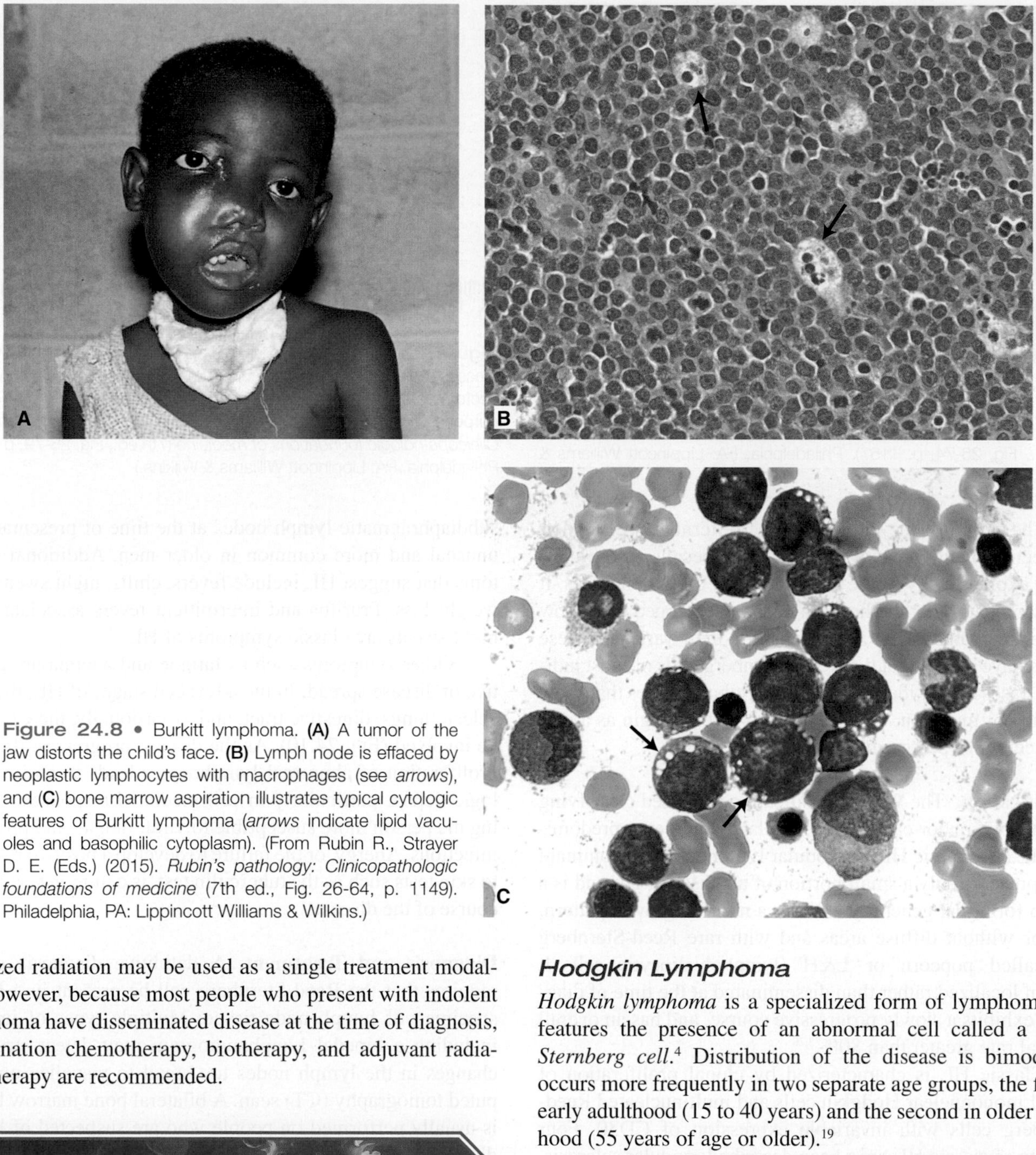

Figure 24.8 • Burkitt lymphoma. **(A)** A tumor of the jaw distorts the child's face. **(B)** Lymph node is effaced by neoplastic lymphocytes with macrophages (see *arrows*), and **(C)** bone marrow aspiration illustrates typical cytologic features of Burkitt lymphoma (*arrows* indicate lipid vacuoles and basophilic cytoplasm). (From Rubin R., Strayer D. E. (Eds.) (2015). *Rubin's pathology: Clinicopathologic foundations of medicine* (7th ed., Fig. 26-64, p. 1149). Philadelphia, PA: Lippincott Williams & Wilkins.)

localized radiation may be used as a single treatment modality. However, because most people who present with indolent lymphoma have disseminated disease at the time of diagnosis, combination chemotherapy, biotherapy, and adjuvant radiation therapy are recommended.

KEY POINTS

MALIGNANT LYMPHOMAS

- The lymphomas represent malignancies that arise in the peripheral lymphoid tissues.
- NHLs represent a group of heterogeneous lymphocytic cancers that are multicentric in origin and spread to various tissues throughout the body, including the bone marrow.
- HL is a group of cancers characterized by Reed-Sternberg cells that begins as a malignancy in a single lymph node and then spreads to contiguous lymph nodes.

Hodgkin Lymphoma

Hodgkin lymphoma is a specialized form of lymphoma that features the presence of an abnormal cell called a *Reed-Sternberg cell*.[4] Distribution of the disease is bimodal. It occurs more frequently in two separate age groups, the first in early adulthood (15 to 40 years) and the second in older adulthood (55 years of age or older).[19]

HL differs from NHL in several respects. First, it usually arises in a single node or chain of nodes, whereas NHL frequently originates at extranodal sites and spreads to anatomically contiguous nodes.[5] Second, HL is characterized by the presence of large, atypical, mononuclear tumor cells, called *Reed-Sternberg cells* (Fig. 24.9). These cells, which frequently constitute less than 1% of the total cell population, are a diagnostic hallmark of the disease.

Etiology and Pathogenesis. As with NHLs, the cause of HL is largely unknown. Although exposure to carcinogens and viruses as well as genetic and immune mechanisms have been proposed as causes, none has been proved to be involved in the pathogenesis of the disease.

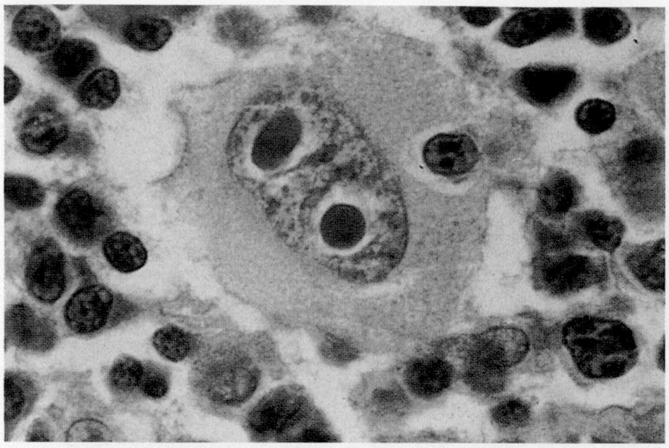

Figure 24.9 • Classic Reed-Sternberg cell. Mirror-image nuclei contain large eosinophilic nucleoli. (From Rubin R., Strayer D. E. (Eds.) (2015). *Rubin's pathology: Clinicopathologic foundations of medicine* (7th ed., Fig. 26-74, p. 1157). Philadelphia, PA: Lippincott Williams & Wilkins.)

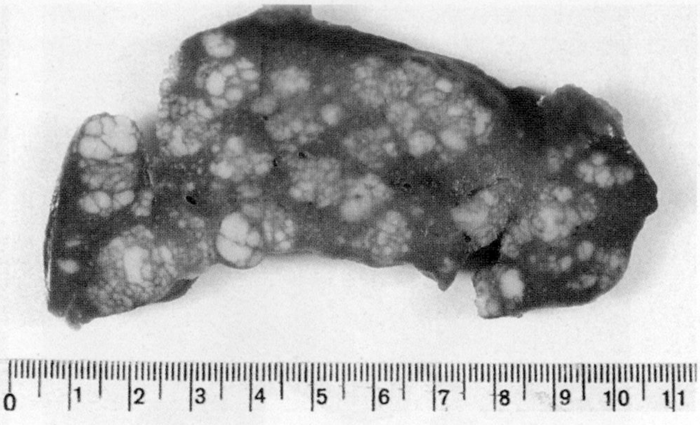

Figure 24.10 • Hodgkin lymphoma involving the spleen. Multiple masses replace the normal splenic parenchyma. Laparotomy and splenectomy are no longer routinely performed for diagnostic and staging purposes. (From Rubin R., Strayer D. E. (Eds.) (2015). *Rubin's pathology: Clinicopathologic foundations of medicine* (7th ed., Fig. 26-79, p. 1160). Philadelphia, PA: Lippincott Williams & Wilkins.)

The origin of the neoplastic Reed-Sternberg cell of HL has been difficult to study, in large part because these cells do not express many of the markers found on lymphocytes. It is only recently that methods have been developed that allow for the microanalysis of these cells and their variants. These studies have shown that the Reed-Sternberg cells of most individual cases harbor identical immunoglobulin genes that show evidence of mutation, establishing the cell of origin as a germinal center or postgerminal center B cell.

Classification. The WHO classification proposed classifying HL into two major categories: nodular lymphocyte-predominant HL and classic HL.[4,28] Nodular lymphocyte-predominant HL represents only a small portion of all cases of HL and is a unique form that generally exhibits a nodular growth pattern, with or without diffuse areas and with rare Reed-Sternberg cells called "popcorn" or "L&H" (lymphohistiocytic) cells. It is often localized rather than disseminated at the time of diagnosis, exhibits a slowly progressive course, and has an overall survival rate greater than 80%.[5,28]

Classic HL is characterized by clonal proliferation of typical mononuclear Hodgkin cells and multinucleated Reed-Sternberg cells with invariable expression of CD30. Four variants of classic HL have been described: nodular sclerosis, mixed cellularity, lymphocyte rich, and lymphocyte depleted. The nodular sclerotic type is the most common and is often found in adolescent and young adult women, 15 to 35 years of age.[5] Lymphocyte-rich HL is a newly defined entity, and lymphocyte-depleted HL is rarely diagnosed.

Clinical Manifestations. Most people with HL present with painless enlargement of a single node or group of nodes. The initial lymph node involvement typically is above the level of the diaphragm (*i.e.*, in the neck, supraclavicular area, or axilla). Mediastinal masses are frequent and are sometimes discovered on routine chest radiography. There may be complaints of chest discomfort with cough or dyspnea. Involvement of subdiaphragmatic lymph nodes at the time of presentation is unusual and more common in older men. Additional symptoms that suggest HL include fevers, chills, night sweats, and weight loss. Pruritus and intermittent fevers associated with night sweats are classic symptoms of HL.

Other symptoms such as fatigue and anemia are indicative of disease spread. In the advanced stages of HL, the liver, spleen, lungs, digestive tract, and, occasionally, the CNS may be involved (Fig. 24.10). As the disease progresses, the rapid proliferation of abnormal lymphocytes leads to an immunologic defect, particularly in cell-mediated responses, rendering the person more susceptible to viral, fungal, and protozoal infections. Anergy, or the failure to develop a positive response to skin tests such as the tuberculin test, is common early in the course of the disease.

Diagnosis and Treatment. A definitive diagnosis of HL requires that the Reed-Sternberg cell be present in a biopsy specimen of lymph node tissue. Multiple types of imaging including a bipedal lymphangiogram may detect structural changes in the lymph nodes too small to visualize on computed tomography (CT) scan. A bilateral bone marrow biopsy is usually performed on people who are suspected of having disseminated disease.

People with HL are staged according to the number of lymph nodes involved, whether the lymph nodes are on one or both sides of the diaphragm, and whether there is disseminated disease involving the bone marrow, liver, lung, or skin. The staging of HL is of great clinical importance because the choice of treatment and the prognosis ultimately are related to the distribution of the disease.

Irradiation and chemotherapy are used in treating the disease. Most people with localized disease are treated with radiation therapy. A combined approach using radiation, biotherapy, and chemotherapy is used in people with advanced disease. The accuracy of staging techniques, delivery of radiation, and curative efficacy of combination chemotherapy regimens have improved the survival rate of people with HL. Five year survival rates for early stage HL ranges from 94% to 96%.[29]

Leukemias

The leukemias are malignant neoplasms of cells originally derived from hematopoietic precursor cells. They are characterized by diffuse replacement of bone marrow with unregulated, proliferating, immature neoplastic cells. In most cases, the leukemic cells spill out into the blood, where they are seen in large numbers. The term *leukemia* (*i.e.*, "white blood") was first used by Virchow to describe a reversal of the usual ratio of red blood cells to white blood cells. The leukemic cells may also infiltrate the liver, spleen, lymph nodes, and other tissues throughout the body, causing enlargement of these organs.

In the United States in 2017, approximately 62,130 new cases of leukemia were diagnosed , and approximately 24,500 people were expected to die of the disease.[19] Leukemia is the most common cause of cancer in children and adolescents. It accounts for about 29%[19] of cancers in children. Although it commonly is thought of as a childhood disease, leukemia is diagnosed 10 times more frequently in adults than children.

Classification

The leukemias commonly are classified according to their predominant cell type (*i.e.*, lymphocytic or myelocytic) and whether the condition is acute or chronic. Biphenotypic leukemias demonstrate characteristics of both lymphoid and myeloid lineages. A rudimentary classification system, the French-American-British (FAB) Cooperative Group classification, is still being used and divides leukemia into four types: acute lymphocytic (lymphoblastic) leukemia (ALL), chronic lymphocytic leukemia (CLL), acute myelogenous (myeloblastic) leukemia (AML), and chronic myelogenous leukemia (CML). However, new classification systems with multiple subtypes that differentiate many characteristics and employ gene expression profiling are being used clinically for diagnosis and treatment.[30] The *lymphocytic leukemias* involve immature lymphocytes and their progenitors that originate in the bone marrow but infiltrate the spleen, lymph nodes, CNS, and other tissues. The *myelogenous leukemias* involve the pluripotent myeloid stem cells in bone marrow and interfere with the maturation of all blood cells, including the granulocytes, erythrocytes, and thrombocytes.

Etiology and Molecular Biology

The causes of leukemia are largely unknown. The incidence of leukemia among people who have been exposed to high levels of radiation is unusually high. An increased incidence of leukemia also is associated with exposure to benzene, many unknown toxins, drugs, chemicals, and gases. Leukemia may occur as a second cancer after aggressive chemotherapy for other cancers, such as HL. The existence of a genetic predisposition to development of acute leukemia is suggested by the increased leukemia incidence among a number of congenital disorders, including Down syndrome, neurofibromatosis, and Fanconi anemia. There also are numerous reports of multiple cases of acute leukemia occurring within the same family.

The molecular biology of leukemia suggests that the event or events causing the disorders exert their effects through dysregulation of genes that normally regulate blood cell development and homeostasis.[5] Cytogenetic studies have shown that recurrent chromosomal changes occur in over one half of all cases of leukemia. Most commonly, these are structural changes classified as translocations, written t(8;21), in which a part of one (*e.g.*, 8) chromosome becomes located on another chromosome (*e.g.*, 21) and vice versa; inversions, written inv(16), in which part of a chromosome (*e.g.*, 16) is upside down and now in reverse order, but still attached to the original chromosome; and deletions, written del(7) or −7, in which part of a chromosome (*e.g.*, 7) has been lost. It is the disruption or dysregulation of specific genes and gene products occurring at the site of these chromosome aberrations that contributes to the development of leukemia.[29] In many instances, these genes and their products have been shown to be directly or indirectly involved in the normal development or maintenance of the hematopoietic system. Thus, it would appear that leukemia results, at least in part, from disruption in the activity of genes that normally regulate blood cell development. Figure 24.11 compares a normal blood smear to one with leukemia. Advances in molecular biology regarding leukemia are beginning to provide a more complete understanding of the molecular complexity of leukemia for the purposes of diagnosis, classification, treatment, and monitoring of clinical outcomes.

One of the more studied translocations is the Philadelphia chromosome, which was the first chromosomal abnormality identified in cancer. The Philadelphia chromosome translocation, t(9;22), represents a reciprocal translocation between the long arm of chromosome 22 and the long arm of chromosome 9.[4] During the translocation, a large portion of 22q is translocated to 9q, and a smaller piece of 9q is moved to 22q (Fig. 24.12). The portion of 9q that is translocated contains *ABL*, a proto-oncogene that is the cellular homolog of the Abelson murine leukemic virus. The *ABL* gene is received at a specific site on 22q called the *breakpoint cluster region* (BCR). The resulting *BCR-ABL* fusion gene codes for a novel protein that differs from that of the normal *ABL* gene in that it possesses tyrosine kinase activity (a characteristic activity of transforming genes).[4] The presence of the tyrosine kinase generated by the fusion gene allows affected cells to bypass the regulated signals that control normal cell growth and differentiation and instead undergo malignant transformation to become leukemic cells. The Philadelphia chromosome translocation is found in more than 90% of people with CML and in some people with acute leukemia. The development of tyrosine kinase inhibitors has contributed to the targeted approach for treatment of leukemias that display the Philadelphia chromosome translocation.[31]

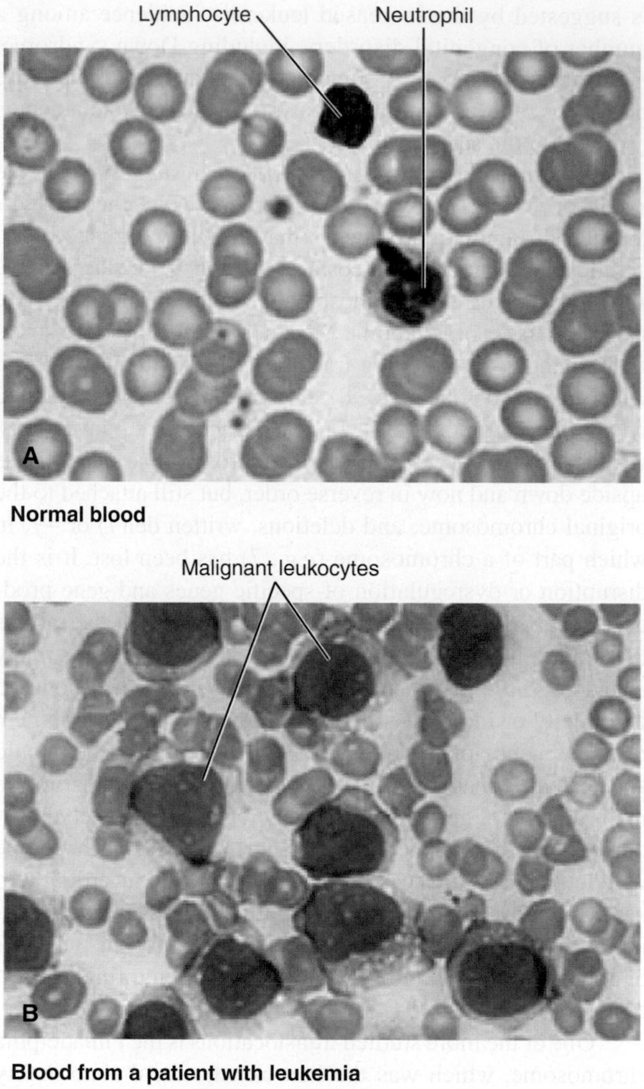

Figure 24.11 • Leukemia. **(A)** Normal blood with normal neutrophil and lymphocyte. **(B)** Blood from a person with leukemia illustrating numerous abnormal leukocytes. (From McConnell T. H., Hull K. L. (2011). *Human form, human function: Essentials of anatomy & physiology* (p. 386). Philadelphia, PA: Lippincott Williams & Wilkins.)

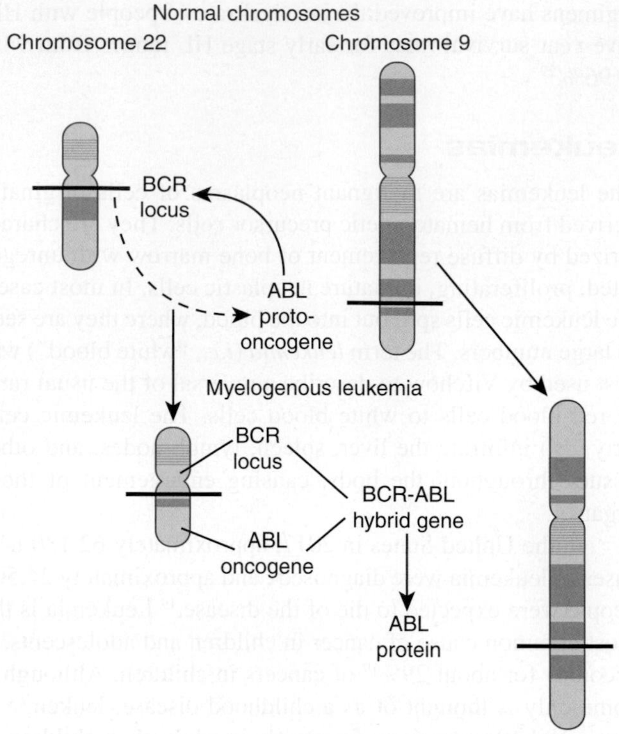

Figure 24.12 • The Philadelphia (Ph) chromosome is formed by breaks at the ends of the long arms of chromosomes 9 and 22, allowing the *ABL* proto-oncogene on chromosome 9 to be translocated to the breakpoint cluster region (*BCR*) on chromosome 22. The result is a new fusion gene coding for the BCR-ABL protein, which is presumably involved in the pathogenesis of CML.

Acute Leukemias

The acute leukemias are cancers of the hematopoietic progenitor cells.[4] They usually have a sudden onset with signs and symptoms related to depressed bone marrow function (Table 24.1). There are two types of acute leukemia: ALL and AML. ALL occurs most frequently in children, accounting for three out of four cases of childhood leukemia cases. However, about one third of cases of ALL occur in adults, and most of the deaths from the disease occur in adults (about four out of five). In the United States, over 5970 new cases of ALL adults are predicted in 2017.[19] In addition, over 1400 cases of ALL will result in death.[19] AML is mainly a disease of older adults, but it is also seen in children and young adults.[19] In children and adolescents, AML accounts for one in four cases of leukemia. The American Cancer Society predicts there will be 21,380 new cases of AML with approximately 10,590 deaths in 2017.[19]

ALL encompasses a group of neoplasms composed of precursor B (pre-B) or T (pre-T) lymphocytes referred to as *lymphoblasts* (see Fig. 24.13). Approximately 90% of people with ALL have numeric and structural changes in the chromosomes of their leukemic cells. They include hyperploidy (*i.e.*, more than 50 chromosomes), polyploidy (*i.e.*, three or more sets of chromosomes), and chromosomal translocations and deletions. Many of these chromosomal aberrations serve to dysregulate the expression and function of transcription factors required for normal hematopoietic cell development.

The AMLs are a diverse group of neoplasms affecting myeloid precursor cells in the bone marrow.[4] Most are associated with acquired genetic alterations that inhibit terminal myeloid differentiation. As a result, normal marrow elements are replaced by an accumulation of relatively undifferentiated blast cells with a resultant suppression of the remaining progenitor cells that leads to anemia, neutropenia, and thrombocytopenia. Specific chromosomal abnormalities, including translocations, are seen in a large number of AMLs. One subtype of AML, acute promyelocytic leukemia, which represents 10% of adult cases of AML, is associated with a t(15;17) chromosomal translocation.[32] This translocation produces a fusion gene that encodes a portion of the transcription factor, retinoic acid receptor-a (RARa), fused to a portion of another

TABLE 24.1 CLINICAL MANIFESTATIONS OF LEUKEMIA AND THEIR PATHOLOGIC BASIS*

CLINICAL MANIFESTATIONS	PATHOLOGIC BASIS
Bone marrow depression	
Malaise, easy fatigability	Anemia
Fever	Infection or increased metabolism by neoplastic cells
Bleeding	Decreased thrombocytes
Petechiae	
Ecchymosis	
Gingival bleeding	
Epistaxis	
Bone pain and tenderness upon palpation	Subperiosteal bone infiltration, bone marrow expansion, and bone resorption
Headache, nausea, vomiting, papilledema, cranial nerve palsies, seizures, coma	Leukemic infiltration of the CNS
Abdominal discomfort	Generalized lymphadenopathy, hepatomegaly, splenomegaly due to leukemic cell infiltration
Increased vulnerability to infections	Immaturity of the white cells and ineffective immune function
Hematologic abnormalities	Physical and metabolic encroachment of leukemia cells on red blood cells and thrombocyte precursors
Anemia	
Thrombocytopenia	
Hyperuricemia and other metabolic disorders	Abnormal proliferation and metabolism of leukemia cells

*Manifestations vary with the type of leukemia.

protein, PML. This change in the retinoic acid receptor produces a block in differentiation that can be overcome with pharmacologic doses of retinoic acid.

Clinical Manifestations. Although ALL and AML are distinct disorders, they typically present with similar clinical features. Both are characterized by an abrupt onset of symptoms, including fatigue resulting from anemia; low-grade fever, night sweats, and weight loss due to the rapid proliferation and hypermetabolism of the leukemic cells; bleeding due to a decreased platelet count; and bone pain and tenderness due to bone marrow expansion.[32–34] Infection results from neutropenia, with the risk of infection rising steeply as the neutrophil count falls below 500 cells/μL. Generalized lymphadenopathy, splenomegaly, and hepatomegaly caused by infiltration of leukemic cells occur in all acute leukemias but are more common in ALL.

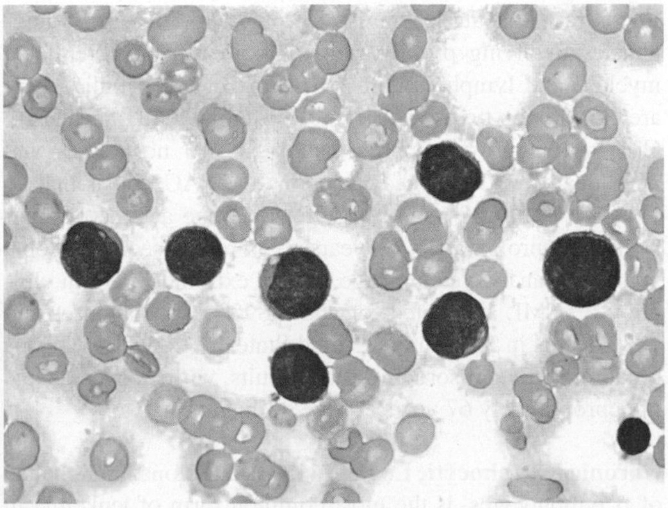

Figure 24.13 • Acute lymphoblastic leukemia. The lymphoblasts in peripheral blood have irregular and indented nuclei with fine nuclear chromatin, visible nucleoli, and variable amounts of agranuolar cytoplasm. (From Rubin R., Strayer D. E. (Eds.) (2015). *Rubin's pathology: Clinicopathologic foundations of medicine* (7th ed., Fig. 26-56, p. 1138). Philadelphia, PA: Lippincott Williams & Wilkins.)

In addition to the common manifestations of acute leukemia (*i.e.*, fatigue, weight loss, fever, easy bruising), infiltration of malignant cells in the skin, gums, and other soft tissues is particularly common in the monocytic form of AML. The leukemic cells may also cross the blood–brain barrier and establish sanctuary in the CNS. CNS involvement is more common in ALL than AML, and is more common in children than adults. Signs and symptoms of CNS involvement include cranial nerve palsies, headache, nausea, vomiting, papilledema, and occasionally seizures and coma.

Leukostasis is a condition in which the circulating blast count is markedly elevated (usually 100,000 cells/μL). The high number of circulating leukemic blasts increases blood viscosity and predisposes to the development of leukoblastic emboli with obstruction of small blood vessels in the pulmonary and cerebral circulations. Occlusion of the pulmonary vessels leads to vessel rupture and infiltration of lung tissue, resulting in sudden shortness of breath and progressive dyspnea. Cerebral leukostasis leads to diffuse headache and lethargy, which can progress to confusion and coma.

Once identified, leukostasis requires immediate and effective treatment to lower the blast count rapidly. Initial treatment uses apheresis to remove excess blast cells, followed by chemotherapy to stop leukemic cell production in the bone marrow.[33,34]

Hyperuricemia occurs as the result of increased proliferation or increased breakdown of purine nucleotides (*i.e.*, one of the components of nucleic acids) secondary to the leukemic cell death that results from chemotherapy. It may increase before and during treatment. Prophylactic therapy with rasburicase (Elitek), a recombinant version of a urate oxidase enzyme, is generally administered to prevent renal complications secondary to uric acid crystallization in the urine filtrate.[34]

Diagnosis. A definitive diagnosis of acute leukemia is based on blood and bone marrow studies. It requires the demonstration of leukemic cells in the peripheral blood, bone marrow, or extramedullary tissue. Laboratory findings reveal the presence of immature white blood cells (blasts) in the circulation and bone marrow, where they may constitute 60% to 100% of the cells. As these cells proliferate and begin to crowd the bone marrow, the development of other blood cell lines in the marrow is suppressed. Consequently, there is a loss of mature myeloid cells, such as erythrocytes, granulocytes, and platelets. Anemia is almost always present, and the platelet count is decreased. Immunophenotyping is performed to determine the lineage subtype of the leukemia.[30]

Bone marrow biopsy may be used to determine the molecular characteristics of the leukemia, the degree of bone marrow involvement, and the morphology and histology of the disease. Cytogenetic studies, which are used to determine chromosomal abnormalities, are one of the most powerful prognostic indicators in acute leukemia. Certain chromosomal abnormalities respond more favorably to certain types of treatment and have a better prognosis than other abnormalities.

In ALL, the staging includes a lumbar puncture to assess CNS involvement. Imaging studies that include CT scans of the chest, abdomen, and pelvis may also be obtained to identify additional sites of disease.

Treatment. Treatment of ALL and AML consists of several phases and includes *induction therapy*, which is designed to elicit a remission; *intensification therapy*, which is used to produce a further reduction in leukemic cells after a remission is achieved; and *maintenance therapy*, which serves to maintain the remission. The goal of induction therapy is the production of a severe bone marrow response with destruction of leukemic progenitor cells followed by normal bone marrow recovery. The likelihood of achieving a remission depends on a number of factors, including age, type of leukemia, and stage of the disease at time of presentation. Of these factors, age is probably the most significant prognostic variable.

Massive necrosis of malignant cells can occur during the initial phase of chemotherapy treatment. This phenomenon, known as *tumor lysis syndrome*, can lead to life-threatening metabolic disorders, including hyperkalemia, hyperphosphatemia, hyperuricemia, hypomagnesemia, hypocalcemia, and acidosis, with the potential for causing acute renal failure. Aggressive prophylactic hydration with alkaline solutions and administration of rasburicase (Elitek) to reduce uric acid levels are used to counteract these effects.

As with ALL, treatment of AML consists of a number of phases. Treatment usually consists of induction therapy followed by intensive consolidation therapy. Induction therapy consists of intensive chemotherapy to effect aplasia of the bone marrow. During this period, supportive transfusion and treatment with antimicrobial agents often are needed.

Bone marrow or stem cell transplantation may be considered for people with ALL and AML who have failed to respond to other forms of therapy.[33,34] Because of the risk of complications, bone marrow transplantation is not usually recommended for people older than 50 to 55 years of age.[34,35]

KEY POINTS

LEUKEMIAS

- Leukemias are malignant neoplasms arising from the transformation of a single blood cell line derived from hematopoietic stem cells.
- Because leukemic cells are immature and poorly differentiated, they proliferate rapidly and have a long life span, they do not function normally, they interfere with the maturation of normal blood cells, and they circulate in the bloodstream, cross the blood–brain barrier, and infiltrate many body organs.

Chronic Leukemias

In contrast to acute leukemias, chronic leukemias are malignancies involving proliferation of more fully differentiated myeloid and lymphoid cells. As with acute leukemia, there are two major types of chronic leukemia: CLL and CML. CLL accounted for approximately 20,110 new cases and 4600 deaths in the United States in 2017.(ACA) It is mainly a disorder of older people. The average age at time of diagnosis is approximately 72 years. It is rarely seen in people younger than 40 years of age, and is extremely rare in children.[19,35] CML accounted for about 8950 new diagnoses and 1080 deaths in 2011 in the United States.[19] As with CLL, it is predominantly a disorder of older adults, with an average age of approximately 67 years at time of diagnosis.[19]

Chronic Lymphocytic Leukemia. CLL, a clonal malignancy of B lymphocytes, is the most common form of leukemia in adults in the Western world. In the past, CLL was viewed as a homogeneous disease of immature, immune-incompetent, minimally self-renewing B cells, which accumulated because of faulty apoptotic mechanisms. Some people with CLL survive for many years without therapy and eventually succumb to unrelated diseases, whereas others have a rapidly fatal disease despite aggressive therapy. Immunophenotyping confirms CLL diagnosis. A number of B-cell markers are evaluated to make the differential diagnosis, along with CLL-specific genomic aberrations. The number of genomic alterations increases over the course of the disease.[33]

The clinical signs and symptoms of CLL are largely related to the progressive infiltration of the bone marrow and lymphoid tissues by neoplastic lymphocytes and to secondary immunologic defects. People with the indolent form of CLL are often asymptomatic at the time of diagnosis, and lymphocytosis is noted on a complete blood count obtained for another, unrelated disorder. As the disease progresses, lymph nodes gradually increase in size and new nodes are involved, sometimes in unusual areas such as the scalp, orbit, pharynx, pleura, gastrointestinal tract, liver, prostate, and gonads. People with the aggressive form of CLL experience a more rapid sequence of clinical deterioration characterized by increasing lymphadenopathy, hepatosplenomegaly, fever, abdominal pain, weight loss, progressive anemia, and thrombocytopenia, with a rapid rise in lymphocyte count.

Hypogammaglobulinemia is common in CLL, especially in people with advanced disease. An increased susceptibility to infection reflects an inability to produce specific antibodies and abnormal activation of complement. The most common infectious organisms are those that require opsonization for bacterial killing, such as *Streptococcus pneumoniae*, *Staphylococcus aureus*, and *Haemophilus influenzae*.

The diagnostic hallmark of CLL is isolated lymphocytosis. The white blood cell count is usually greater than 20,000/μL and may be elevated to several hundred thousand. Usually, 75% to 98% are lymphocytes. The hematocrit and platelet counts are usually normal at presentation. Cytogenetic studies may provide prognostic information.[33,34] The finding of deletion of chromosome 17p or 11q is a poor prognostic indicator.[33]

Treatment of CLL usually depends on the presence of prognostic indicators.[33] People with the low-risk or indolent form of CLL usually do not require specific treatment for many years after diagnosis and eventually die of apparently unrelated causes. Reassurance that people with the disorder can live a normal life for many years is important. Many people with intermediate-risk disease may remain stable for many years as well, whereas others may develop complications and need treatment within a few months. Most people with high-risk CLL require treatment at diagnosis. Complications such as autoimmune hemolytic anemia or thrombocytopenia may require treatment with corticosteroids or splenectomy.

In younger people with aggressive disease, an allogeneic ablative (destruction of bone marrow cells by irradiation or chemotherapy) or nonmyeloablative stem cell transplant is a treatment option. In a nonmyeloablative type of transplant, the goal is marrow suppression, destruction of leukemia cells by the donor's lymphocytes, known as "graft-versus-leukemia" effect, and marrow recovery with donor cells.

Chronic Myelogenous Leukemia. CML is a disorder of the pluripotent hematopoietic progenitor cell. It is characterized by excessive proliferation of marrow granulocytes, erythroid precursors, and megakaryocytes. The CML cells harbor a distinctive cytogenic abnormality, the previously described *Philadelphia chromosome*.[4] It is generally believed that CML develops when a single, pluripotent hematopoietic stem cell acquires a Philadelphia chromosome. Although CML originates in the pluripotent stem cells, granulocyte precursors remain the dominant leukemic cell type.

The clinical course of CML is commonly divided into three phases:

1. A chronic phase of variable length
2. A short accelerated phase
3. A terminal blast crisis phase

The onset of the chronic phase is usually slow, with nonspecific symptoms such as weakness and weight loss. The most characteristic laboratory finding at the time of presentation is leukocytosis with immature granulocyte cell types in the peripheral blood. Anemia and, eventually, thrombocytopenia develop. Anemia causes weakness, easy fatigability, and exertional dyspnea. Splenomegaly is often present at the time of diagnosis; hepatomegaly is less common; and lymphadenopathy is relatively uncommon.

The accelerated phase of CML is characterized by enlargement of the spleen and progressive symptoms. Splenomegaly often causes a feeling of abdominal fullness and discomfort. An increase in basophil count and more immature cells in the blood or bone marrow confirm transformation to the accelerated phase. During this phase, constitutional symptoms such as low-grade fever, night sweats, bone pain, and weight loss develop because of rapid proliferation and hypermetabolism of the leukemic cells. Bleeding and easy bruising may arise from dysfunctional platelets. Generally, the accelerated phase is short (6 to 12 months).

The terminal blast crisis phase of CML represents evolution to acute leukemia and is characterized by an increasing number of myeloid precursors, especially blast cells, in the blood. Constitutional symptoms become more pronounced during this period, and splenomegaly may increase significantly. Isolated infiltrates of leukemic cells can involve the skin, lymph nodes, bones, and CNS. With very high blast counts (>100,000 cells/μL), symptoms of leukostasis may occur.

A diagnostic feature of CML is an elevated white blood count, with a median count of 150,000/μL at the time of diagnosis, although in some cases, it is only modestly increased. The hallmark of the disease is the presence of the BCR-ABL gene product, which can be detected in the peripheral blood. This is best done using the polymerase chain reaction (PCR), which has supplanted cytogenetics in identifying the Philadelphia chromosome. Bone marrow examination is not usually necessary for diagnosis but is useful for prognosis and detecting additional chromosomal abnormalities.

The goals of treatment for CML include a hematologic response characterized by normalized blood counts; a cytogenetic response demonstrated by the reduction or elimination of the Philadelphia chromosome from the bone marrow; and a molecular response confirmed by the elimination of the BCR-ABL fusion protein.[40] The only available curative treatment for CML is allogeneic bone marrow or stem cell transplantation. In most transplantation centers, full myoablative transplants are available to children and adults younger than 60 years of age who have an HLA-matched sibling donor or an unrelated molecular-matched donor. Nonmyeloablative or "mini-transplants" are available to people younger than 70 years of age who have sibling HLA-matched or unrelated HLA-matched donors.

Plasma Cell Dyscrasias

Plasma cell dyscrasias are characterized by expansion of a single clone of immunoglobulin-producing plasma cells and a resultant increase in serum levels of a single monoclonal immunoglobulin or its fragments. The plasma cell dyscrasias include multiple myeloma; localized plasmacytoma (solitary myeloma); lymphoplasmacytic lymphoma; primary or immunocyte amyloidosis due to excessive production of light chains; and monoclonal gammopathy of undetermined significance (MGUS).

Monoclonal gammopathy of undetermined significance is characterized by the presence of the monoclonal immunoglobulin in the serum without other findings of multiple myeloma. MGUS is considered a premalignant condition.[38] Approximately 2% per year of people with MGUS will go on to develop a plasma cell dyscrasia (multiple myeloma, lymphoplasmacytic lymphoma, or amyloidosis). The strong link between MGUS and multiple myeloma suggests that a first oncogenic event produces MGUS and a second event results in multiple myeloma.[4]

Multiple Myeloma

Multiple myeloma is a B-cell malignancy of terminally differentiated plasma cells. The high morbidity and mortality rates of this disorder are associated with its end-organ destruction.[37] It occurs most frequently in people older than 60 years of age, with the median age of people with multiple myeloma being 71 years.

The cause of multiple myeloma is unknown. Risk factors are thought to include chronic immune stimulation, autoimmune disorders, exposure to ionizing radiation, and occupational exposure to pesticides or herbicides (*e.g.*, dioxin).[36] Myeloma has been associated with exposure to Agent Orange during the Vietnam War. A number of viruses have been associated with the pathogenesis of myeloma.

Pathogenesis. Multiple myeloma is characterized by proliferation of malignant plasma cells in the bone marrow and osteolytic bone lesions throughout the skeletal system (Fig. 24.14). As with other hematopoietic malignancies, it

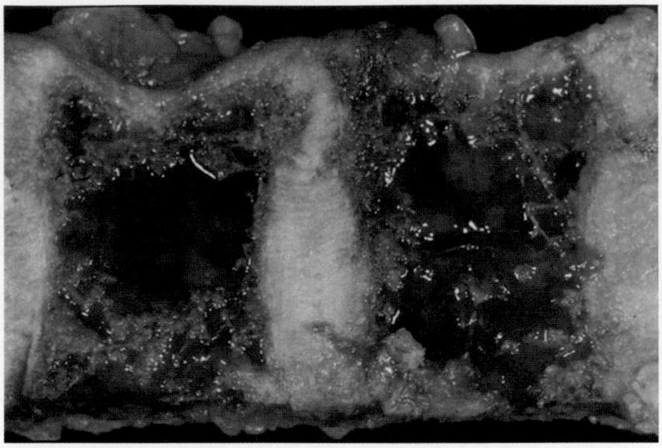

Figure 24.14 • Plasma cell myeloma. Multiple lytic bone lesions are present in the vertebra. Bones such as this are prone to pathologic fracture. (From Rubin R., Strayer D. E. (Eds.) (2015). *Rubin's pathology: Clinicopathologic foundations of medicine* (7th ed., Fig. 26-65, p. 1151). Philadelphia, PA: Lippincott Williams & Wilkins.)

is now recognized that multiple myeloma is associated with chromosomal abnormalities, including deletions of 13q and translocations involving the IgG locus on chromosome 14.[32,37] One fusion partner is a fibroblast growth factor receptor gene on chromosome 4, which is truncated to produce a constitutively active receptor. Changes also occur in the bone marrow microenvironment, including the induction of angiogenesis, the suppression of cell-mediated immunity, and the development of paracrine signaling loops involving cytokines such as IL-6 and vascular endothelial growth factor. Other growth factors that are implicated in multiple myeloma include granulocyte CSF, interferon-α, and IL-10. The development of bone lesions in multiple myeloma is thought to be related to an increase in expression by osteoblasts of the receptor activator of the nuclear factor-κB (NF-κB) ligand (RANKL).[36]

One of the characteristic features resulting from the proliferating osteoclasts in multiple myeloma is the unregulated production of a monoclonal antibody referred to as the *M protein* because it is detected as an M spike on protein electrophoresis. In most cases the M protein is either IgG (60%) or IgA (20% to 25%).[37] In the remaining 15% to 20% of cases, the plasma cells produce only abnormal proteins, termed *Bence Jones proteins*, that consist of light chains of the immunoglobulin molecule. Because of their low molecular weight, the Bence Jones proteins are readily excreted in the urine. People with this form of the disease (light-chain disease) have Bence Jones proteins in their serum, but lack the M component. However, up to 80% of myeloma cells produce both complete immunoglobulins as well as excess light chains. Therefore, both M proteins and Bence Jones proteins are present. Many of the light-chain proteins are directly toxic to renal tubular structures, which may lead to tubular destruction and, eventually, to renal failure.

Clinical Manifestations. The main sites involved in multiple myeloma are the bones and bone marrow. In addition to the

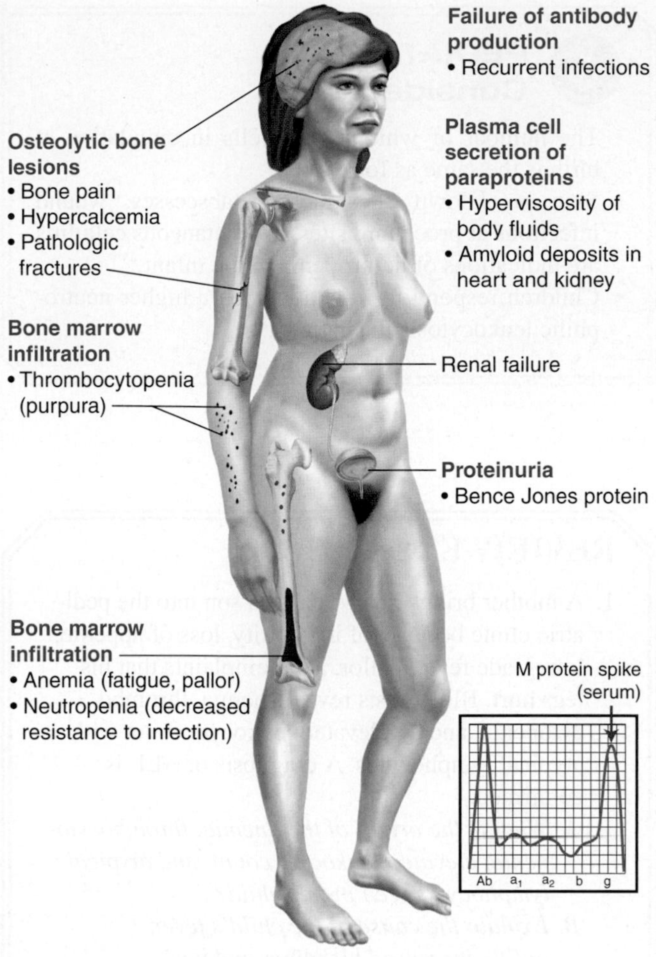

Figure 24.15 • Clinical features of multiple myeloma.

abnormal proliferation of marrow plasma cells, there is proliferation and activation of osteoclasts, which leads to bone resorption and destruction (Fig. 24.15). This increased bone resorption predisposes the person to pathologic fractures and hypercalcemia. Paraproteins secreted by the plasma cells may cause a hyperviscosity of body fluids and may break down into amyloid, a proteinaceous substance deposited between cells, causing heart failure and nephropathy. Although multiple myeloma is characterized by excessive production of monoclonal immunoglobulin, levels of normal immunoglobulins are usually depressed. This contributes to a general susceptibility to recurrent bacterial infections.

The malignant plasma cells also can form plasmacytomas (plasma cell tumors) in bone and soft tissue sites. The most common site of soft tissue plasmacytomas is the gastrointestinal tract. The development of plasmacytomas in bone tissue is associated with bone destruction and localized pain. Osteolytic lesions and compression fractures may be seen in the axial skeleton and proximal long bones. Occasionally, the lesions may affect the spinal column, causing vertebral collapse and spinal cord compression.

Bone pain is one of the first symptoms to occur in approximately three fourths of all people diagnosed with multiple myeloma. Bone destruction also impairs the production of erythrocytes and leukocytes and predisposes the person to anemia and recurrent infections. Many people experience weight loss and weakness. Renal insufficiency occurs in approximately half of all people with multiple myeloma. Neurologic manifestations caused by neuropathy or spinal cord compression also may be present.

Diagnosis and Treatment. Diagnosis of multiple myeloma is based on clinical manifestations, blood tests, and bone marrow examination.[38,39] The classic triad of bone marrow plasmacytosis (more than 10% plasma cells), lytic bone lesions, and either the serum M-protein spike or the presence of Bence Jones proteins in the urine is definitive for a diagnosis of multiple myeloma. Bone radiographs are important in establishing the presence of bone lesions. Anemia is almost universal. Other laboratory features include hypercalcemia, an elevated erythrocyte sedimentation rate, and signs of kidney failure.

The treatment of multiple myeloma is changing rapidly.[39,40] For several decades, melphalan (an alkylating agent) and prednisone have remained the cornerstone for treatment of multiple myeloma. Cumulative exposure to melphalan, however, is associated with increased risk of marrow toxicity, including myelodysplasia, acute leukemia, and impaired stem cell production. This is an important consideration in people who are candidates for autologous stem cell transplants. The addition of anthracyclines, alternative alkylating agents and interferon has yielded minimal improvement in treatment outcomes. Although the incorporation of new classes of medications in the treatment of multiple myeloma has seen a shift in the older treatment regimens, the conventional approaches have not been excluded.

High-dose chemotherapy with autologous stem cell transplantation is considered appropriate front-line therapy for people younger than 70 years of age newly diagnosed with multiple myeloma. Allogeneic transplantation offers prolonged disease-free outcomes and potential cure, but at a high cost of treatment-related mortality. Because of this, "mini-transplants" using non–marrow-ablative chemotherapy may be used to provide sufficient immune suppression to allow donor engraftment and subsequent graft-versus-tumor effect.

IN SUMMARY

The lymphomas (NHL and HL) represent malignant neoplasms of cells native to lymphoid tissue that have their origin in the secondary lymphoid structures such as the lymph nodes and MALTs. The NHLs are a group of neoplastic disorders that originate in the lymphoid tissues, usually the lymph nodes. The NHLs are multicentric in origin and spread early to various lymphoid tissues throughout the body, especially the liver, spleen, and bone marrow. HL is characterized by painless and progressive enlargement of a single node or group of nodes. It is believed to originate in one area of the lymphatic system and, if unchecked, spreads throughout the lymphatic network.

The leukemias are malignant neoplasms of the hematopoietic precursor cells that originate in the bone marrow. They are classified according to cell type (*i.e.*, lymphocytic or myelocytic) and whether the disease is acute or chronic. The lymphocytic leukemias involve immature lymphocytes and their progenitors that originate in the bone marrow but infiltrate the spleen, lymph nodes, CNS, and other tissues. The myelogenous leukemias involve the pluripotent myeloid stem cells in bone marrow and interfere with the maturation of all blood cells, including the granulocytes, erythrocytes, and thrombocytes.

The acute leukemias (*i.e.*, ALL, which primarily affects children, and AML, which primarily affects adults) have a sudden onset with symptoms of depressed bone marrow function (anemia, fatigue, bleeding, and infections); bone pain; and generalized lymphadenopathy, splenomegaly, and hepatomegaly. The chronic leukemias, which largely affect adults, have a more insidious onset. CLL often has the most favorable clinical course, with many persons living long enough to die of other, unrelated causes. The course of CML is slow and progressive, with transformation to a course resembling that of AML.

Multiple myeloma is a plasma cell dyscrasia characterized by expansion of a single clone of immunoglobulin-producing plasma cells and a resultant increase in serum levels of a single monoclonal immunoglobulin or its fragments. The main sites involved in multiple myeloma are the bones and bone marrow. In addition to the abnormal proliferation of marrow plasma cells, there is proliferation and activation of osteoclasts that leads to bone resorption and destruction, and predisposes to increased risk for pathologic fractures and development of hypercalcemia. Paraproteins secreted by the plasma cells may cause hyperviscosity of body fluids and may break down into amyloid, a proteinaceous substance deposited between cells that can cause heart failure and neuropathy. Bone marrow involvement leads to increased risk of infection due to suppressed humoral and cell-mediated immunity and anemia due to impaired red cell production.

GERIATRIC Considerations

- If the WBC response to infections is inadequate,[41] an overwhelming infection such as sepsis can result.
- Leukopenia, a decrease in WBCs in the elderly individual, is due to a decreased production of the growth factors needed for hematopoiesis by stromal cells located in the marrow or a decreased response to the growth factors.[42]
- In the aging adult, the DNA of stem cells is damaged, increasing the risk of myeloid malignancies, such as acute myeloid leukemia (AML).[42]
- Myelosuppression of the bone marrow in the aging individual results from medications that prevent the bone marrow from producing sufficient WBCs.[42]

PEDIATRIC Considerations

- The number of white blood cells in circulation at birth is the same as for adults.[43]
- Skin breakdown at skinfolds, abscesses, wound infections at procedure sites, and cutaneous cellulitis are indications of neutropenia in the infant.[43]
- Children respond to infection with a higher neutrophilic leukocytosis than adults.[41]

REVIEW EXERCISES

1. A mother brings her 4-year-old son into the pediatric clinic because of irritability, loss of appetite, low-grade fever, pallor, and complaints that his legs hurt. Blood tests reveal anemia, thrombocytopenia, and an elevated leukocyte count with atypical lymphocytes. A diagnosis of ALL is confirmed.
   A. *What is the origin of the anemia, thrombocytopenia, elevated leukocyte count, and atypical lymphocytes seen in this child?*
   B. *Explain the cause of the child's fever, pallor, increased bleeding, and bone pain.*
   C. *The parents are informed that the preferred treatment for ALL consists of aggressive chemotherapy with the purpose of achieving a remission. Explain the rationale for using chemotherapy to treat leukemia.*
   D. *The parents are told that the child will need intrathecal chemotherapy administered by a lumbar puncture. Why is this treatment necessary?*
2. A 36-year-old man presents to his health care clinic with fever, night sweats, weight loss, and a feeling of fullness in his abdomen. Subsequent lymph node biopsy reveals a diagnosis of NHL.
   A. *Although lymphomas can originate in any of the lymphoid tissues of the body, most originate in the lymph nodes, and most (80% to 85%) are of B-cell origin. Hypothesize as to why B cells are more commonly affected than T cells.*
   B. *Monoclonal antibodies are being used in the treatment of NHL. Explain how these agents exert its effect and why they are specific for B-cell lymphomas.*

References

1. Hall J. E. (2016). *Guyton and Hall textbook of medical physiology* (13th ed.). Philadelphia, PA: Elsevier.
2. Sarker J. M., Pearce S. M., Nelson R. P., et al. (2017). An integrative multi-lineage model of variation in leukopoiesis and acute myelogenous leukemia. *BMC Systems Biology* 11, 78. doi:10.1186/s12918-017-0469-2.
3. Ross M. H., Pawline W. (2017). *Histology: A text and atlas* (6th ed.). Philadelphia, PA: Lippincott Williams & Wilkins.
4. Hsu M. C., Itkin M. (2016). Lymphatic anatomy. *Techniques in Vascular and Interventional Radiology* 19, 247–254.
5. Aster J. C., Bunn H. F. (2017). *Pathophysiology of blood disorders* (2nd ed.). New York: MacGraw Hill.
6. Carman C. V., Martinelli R. (2015). T lymphocyte-endothelial interactions: Emerging understanding of trafficking and antigen-specific immunity. *Frontiers in Immunology* 6, 603. doi:10.3389/fimmu.2015.00603.
7. Nayak R., Trump L. R., Aronow B. J., et al. (2015). Pathogenesis of ELANE-mutant severe neutropenia revealed by induced pluripotent stem cells. *Journal of Clinical Investigation* 125, 3103–3116.
8. Klimiankou M., Mellor-Heineke S., Zeidler C., et al. (2016). Role of CSF3R mutations in the pathomechanism of congential neutropenia and secondary acute myeloid leukemia. *Annals of the New York Academy of Sciences* 1370, 119–125.
9. Afzal W., Owlia M. B., Hasni S., et al. (2017). Autoimmune neutropenia updates: Etiology, pathology, and treatment. *Southern Medical Journal* 110(4), 300–307. doi:10.14423/SMJ.0000000000000637.
10. Moore D. C. (2016). Drug-induced neutropenia: A focus on rituximab-induced late-onset neutropenia. *Pharmacy and Therapeutics* 41(12), 765–768.
11. Saeed A. N., Al-Atiyyat N. (2015). Management of chemotherapy-induced febrile neutropenia among adult oncology patients: A review. *Canadian Oncology Nursing Journal* 25, 281–284.
12. Klastersky J., de Naurois J., Rolston K., et al. (2016). Management of febrile neutropaenia: ESMO clinical practice guidelines. *Annals of Oncology* 27(suppl 5), v111–v118.
13. Zhong Y. (2012). Epstein-Barr Virus infection and lymphoproliferative disorder after hmatopoietic cell transplantation. *Clinical Journal of Oncology Nursing* 16, 211–214.
14. Kessenich C. R., Flanagan M. (2015). Diagnosis of infectious mononucleosis. *Nurse Practitioner* 40(8), 13–16.
15. Womack H., Jimenez M. (2015). Common questions about infectious mononucleosis. *American Family Physician* 91, 372–376.
16. Thompson D. F., Ramos C. L. (2017). Antibiotic-induced rash in patients with infectious mononucleosis. *Annals of Pharmacotherapy* 51, 154–162.
17. Zhang X. M., Aguilera N. (2014). New immunohistochemistry for B-Cell lymphoma and Hodgkin lymphoma. *Archives of Pathology & Laboratory Medicine* 138, 1666–1672.
18. Armitage J. O., Gascoyne R. D., Lunning M. A., et al. (2017). Non-Hodgkin lymphoma. *Lancet* 390, 298–310.
19. American Cancer Association. (2017). *Cancer facts & figures:2017*. Atlanta, GA: American Cancer Society.
20. Skrabek P., Turner D., Seftel M. (2013). Epidemiology of non-Hodgkin lymphoma. *Transfusion and Apheresis Science* 49, 133–138.
21. Ninkovic S., Lambert J. (2017). Non-Hodgkin lymphoma. *Medicine* 45, 297–304.
22. King H., Myatt R. (2014). An overview of non-Hodkin's lymphoma. *Cancer Nursing Practice* 13(1), 31–38.
23. 't Mannetje A., DeRoos A. J., Boffetta P., et al. (2016). Occupation and risk of non-hodgkin lymphoma and its subtypes: a pooled analysis from the interlymph consortium. *Environmental Health Perspectives* 124, 396–405.
24. Howlader N., Noone A. M., Krapcho M., et al. (Eds). (April 2017). *SEER cancer statistics review, 1975–2014*. Bethesda, MD: National Cancer Institute. Available: http://seer.cancer.gov/csr/1975_2014/, based on November 2016 SEER data submission, posted to the SEER web site.
25. Czerwinski D. K., Long S. R., Khodadoust M., et al. (2016). Examining the heterogeneity of follicular lymphoma by multi-parameter flow cytometry in previously untreated patients. *Blood* 128(22), 2947. Available: http://www.bloodjournal.org/content/128/22/2947
26. Giri S., Bhatt V. R., Verma V., et al. (2017). Original study: Risk of second primary malignancies in patients with follicular lymphoma: A United States population-based study. *Clinical Lymphoma Myeloma & Leukemia* 17, 569–574. doi:10.1016/j.clml.2017.06.028.
27. Park Y. K., Choi J. E., Jung W. Y., et al. (2016). Mucosa-associated lymphoma tissue (MALT) lymphoma as an unusual cause of malignant hilar biliary stricture: A case report with literature review. *World Journal of Surgical Oncology* 14, 167. doi:10.1186/s1 2957-016-0928-z.
28. National Cancer Institute. (2017). *Surveillance, epidemiology, and end results program*. Available: https://seer.cancer.gov/statfacts/html/hodg.html
29. Herst J., Crump M., Baldassare F. G., et al. (2017). Management of early–stage Hodgkin Lymphoma: A practice guideline. *Clinical Oncology* 29, e5–e12.
30. Arber D. A., Orazi A., Hasserjian R., et al. (2016). The 2016 revision to the World Health Organization classification of myeloid neoplasms and acute leukemia. *Blood* 20, 2391–2405.
31. Bernt K. M., Hunger S. P. (2015). Current concepts in pediatric Philadelphia chromosome-positive acute lymphoblastic leukemia. *Frontiers in Oncology* 4(54), 1–24. doi:10.3389/fonc.2014.00054.
32. Mwirigi A., Dillion R., Raj K. (2017). Acute leukaemia. *Medicine* 45, 280–286.
33. Scarfo L., Ferrari A. J. M., Ghia P. (2016). Chronic lymphocyte leukaemai. *Critical Reviews in Oncology/Hematology* 104, 170–182.
34. Widick P., Winer E. S. (2016). Leukocytosis and leukemia. *Primary Care; Clinics in Office Practice* 43, 575–587.
35. Rowswell-Turner R. B., Barr P. M. (2017). Treatment of chronic lymphocytic leukemia in older adults. *Journal of Geriatric Oncology* 8, 315–319.
36. Holt S. (2014). *Multiple myeloma: Risk factors, diagnosis, and treatments*. New York: Nova Science Publishers.
37. Blancas-Mejia L. M., Martin E. B., Williams A., et al. (2017). Kinetic stability and sequence/structure studies of urine-derived Bence-Jones proteins from multiple myeloma and light chain amyloidosis patients. *Biophysical Chemistry* 230, 89–98.
38. Ahn I. E., Mailankody S., Korde N., et al. (2015). Dilemmas in treating smoldering multiple myeloma. *Journal of Clinical Oncology* 33, 115–123.
39. Kazandjian D. (2016). Multiple myeloma epidemiology and survival: A unique malignancy. *Seminars in Oncology* 43, 676–681.
40. Palumbo A., et al. (2015). Revised International Staging System for multiple myeloma: A report from International Myeloma Working Group. *Journal of Clinical Oncology* 33, 2863–2869.
41. Fischbach F. T., Dunning M. B. (2015). *A manual of laboratory and diagnostic tests* (9th ed.). Philadelphia, PA: Wolters Kluwer.
42. Thomas M. L. (2018). Assessment of hematologic function and treatment modalities. In Hinkle J. L., Cheever, K. H. (Ed.), *Brunner & Suddarth's textbook of medical-surgical nursing* (14th ed., pp. 902–924). Philadelphia, PA: Wolters Kluwer.
43. Soistmann H. C. (2014). The child with altered hematologic status. In Bowden V. R., Greenberg C. S. (Ed.), *Children and their families the continuum of care* (3rd ed., pp. 1172–1227). Philadelphia, PA: Wolters Kluwer.

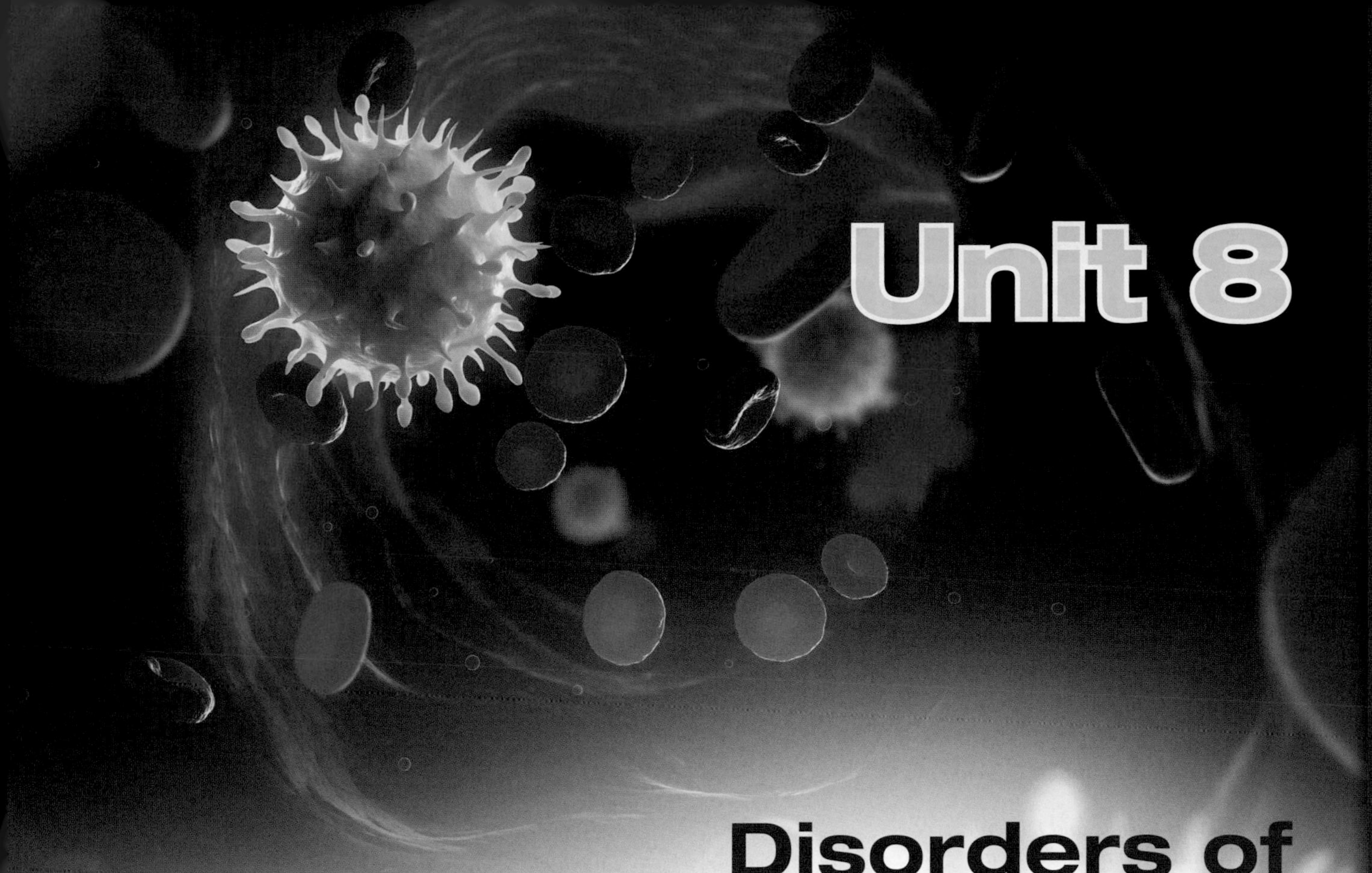

Unit 8

Disorders of Cardiovascular Function

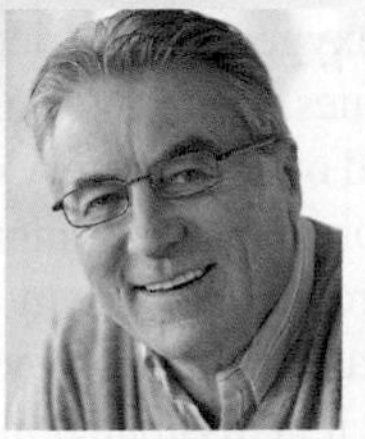

Mr. Brown, a 65-year-old male, presents with concerns about high blood pressure. He recently checked his blood pressure at a retail store, and the readout suggested that he consult a health care provider. Approximately 8 years ago, he was prescribed an angiotensin-converting enzyme (ACE) inhibitor to lower his blood pressure, which was then "borderline hypertensive." At that time, he refused a diuretic because he feared the side effect of frequent urination. He completed the 30-day prescription, thought that he was cured, and never refilled his prescription or followed up with his health care provider.

His father died at 70 of a "heart attack" and had been diagnosed with hypertension and an aortic abdominal aneurysm in his 50s. Mr. Brown quit smoking in his 20s and has an occasional glass of wine. He reports shortness of breath with exertion and denies chest pain. His vital signs are as follows: blood pressure, 160/90 mm Hg; pulse, 90 bpm/minute; respiration rate, 16/minute; temperature, 98.5°F; height, 5′8″; weight, 190 lb; and body mass index (BMI), 28.9 (classified as overweight). Physical examination reveals jugular vein distention (JVD); a loud, systolic ejection murmur without audible thrill (abbreviated as III/VI SEM); and mild bilateral edema in his lower limbs. An electrocardiogram (ECG) reveals multiple incidences of premature atrial contractions (PACs). The ECG shows left ventricular hypertrophy and atrial enlargement and an ejection fraction (EF) of 40%. His fasting lipoprotein profile is as follows: total cholesterol, 260; LDL cholesterol, 150; HDL cholesterol, 35; and triglycerides, 150 (all in mg/dL). Mr. Brown is diagnosed with hypertension, hypercholesteremia, and heart failure. According to the New York Heart Association system of classification, his heart failure is categorized as class II (NYHA II), meaning that his symptoms are mild. He is prescribed a statin, a beta-adrenergic receptor blocker, a diuretic, and an ACE inhibitor and scheduled to have a cardiac catheterization. Mr. Brown is also educated about the importance of follow-up care and provided with a low-sodium, low-cholesterol diet plan and an exercise regimen (for after his cardiac catheterization).

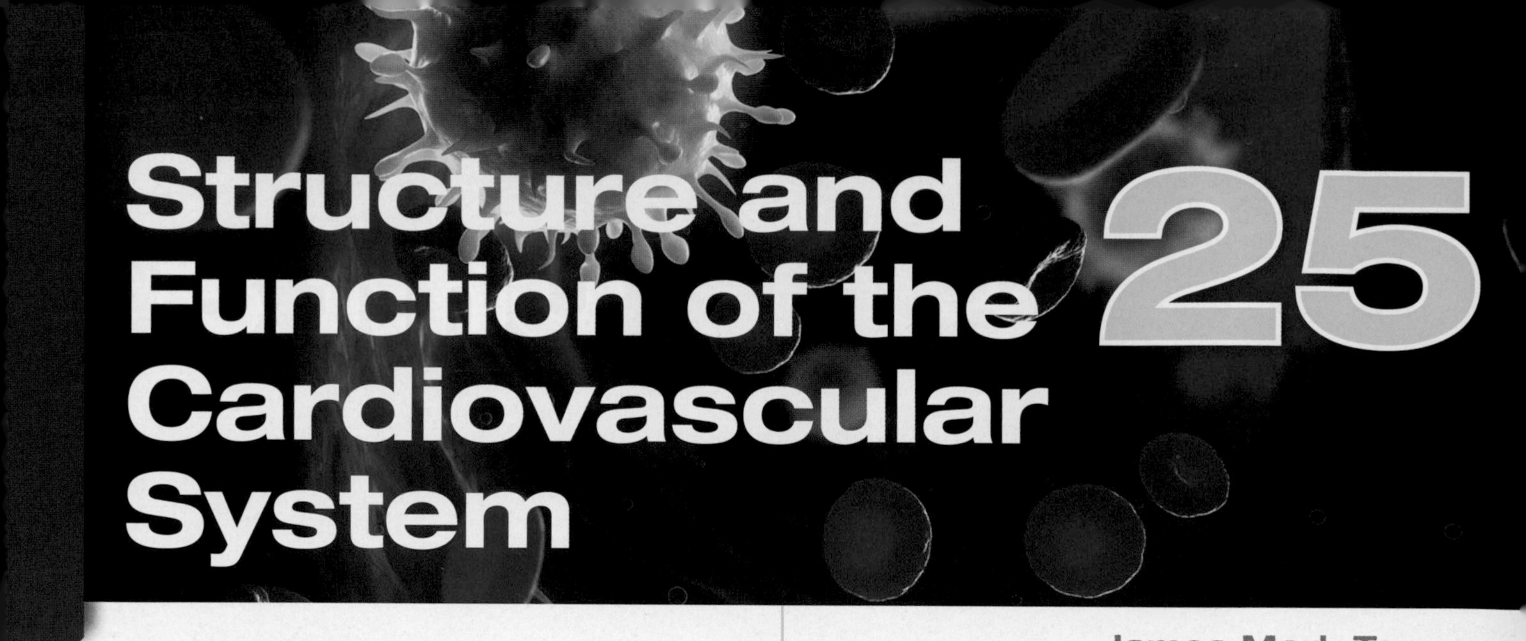

Structure and Function of the Cardiovascular System

25

James Mark Tanner

The main function of the circulatory system, which consists of the heart and blood vessels, is transportation. The circulatory system delivers oxygen and nutrients needed for metabolic processes to the tissues. It carries waste products from the tissues to the kidneys and other excretory organs for elimination. It also circulates electrolytes and hormones needed to regulate body function. The circulatory system also plays an important role in body temperature regulation by transporting core heat to the periphery, where it is dissipated into the external environment.

THE HEART AS A PUMP

After completing this section of the chapter, the learner will be able to meet the following objectives:

- Describe the structural components and function of the pericardium, myocardium, endocardium, and the heart valves and fibrous skeleton.
- Define the terms *preload* and *afterload*.
- State the formula for calculating the cardiac output and explain the effects that venous return, cardiac contractility, and heart rate have on cardiac output.

The heart is a four-chambered muscular pump approximately the size of a fist. It beats an average of 70 times each minute, 24 hours each day, and 365 days each year for a lifetime. In 1 day, this pump moves more than 1800 gallons of blood throughout the body.

Functional Anatomy of the Heart

The heart is located between the lungs in the mediastinal space of the intrathoracic cavity in a loose-fitting sac called the *pericardium*. Its broader side (*i.e.*, base) faces upward, and its tip (*i.e.*, apex) points downward, forward, and to the left. The heart is positioned obliquely, so that the right side of the heart is almost fully in front of the left side of the heart, with only a small portion of the lateral left ventricle on the frontal plane of the heart (Fig. 25.1). When the hand is placed on the thorax, the main impact of the heart's contraction, or *point of maximum impulse (PMI)*, is felt against the chest wall at a point between the fifth and sixth ribs, a little below the nipple and approximately 3 inches to the left of the midline.

The wall of the heart is composed three layers: the epicardium, which lines the pericardial cavity; the myocardium or muscle layer; and the smooth endocardium, which lines the chambers of the heart (Fig. 25.2). A fibrous skeleton supports the valvular structures of the heart. The interatrial and interventricular septa divide the heart into a right and a left pump, each composed of two muscular chambers, including a thin-walled atrium, which serves as a reservoir for blood coming into the heart, and a thick-walled ventricle, which pumps blood out of

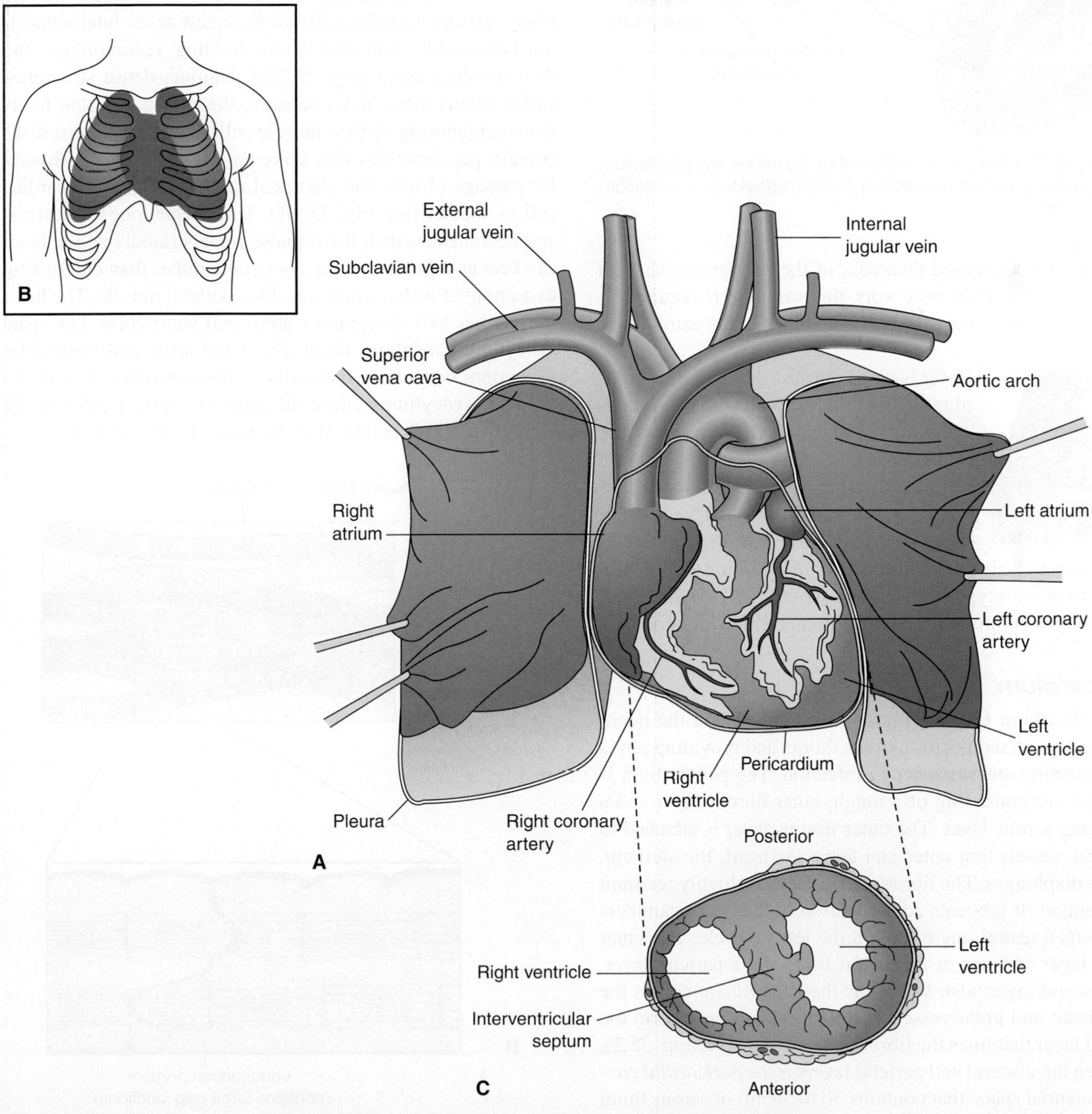

Figure 25.1 • (A) Anterior view of the heart, lungs, and great vessels (note that the lungs, which normally fold over part of the heart's anterior, have been pulled back). **(B)** The heart in relation to the sternum, ribs, and lungs. **(C)** Cross-section of the heart showing the increased thickness of the left ventricle compared with the right.

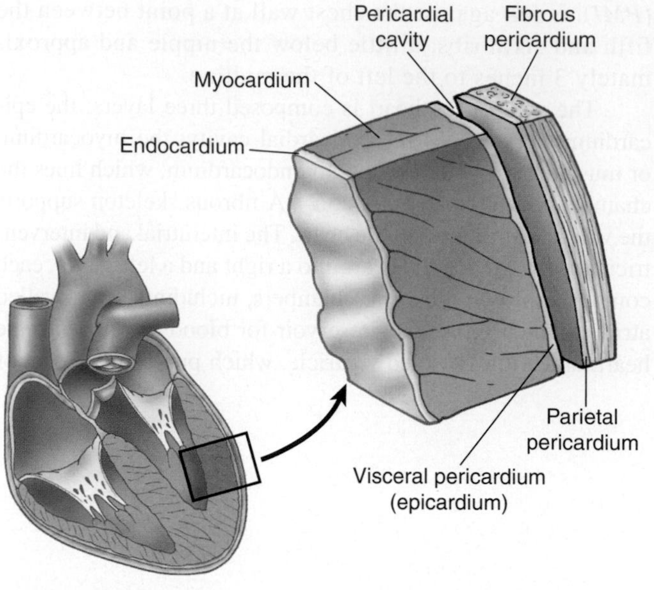

Figure 25.2 • Layers of the heart showing the visceral pericardium, pericardial cavity, parietal pericardium, fibrous pericardium, myocardium, and endocardium.

the heart. The increased thickness of the left ventricular wall results from the additional work this ventricle is required to perform in order to move oxygenated blood to the extremities.

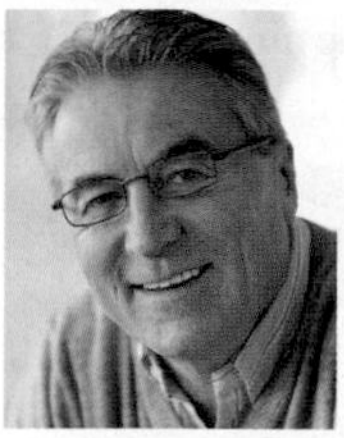

Refer back to the case study at the beginning of the unit. **Mr. Brown** has longstanding, untreated high blood pressure (hypertension). His echocardiogram revealed thickening of the left ventricular wall, a change known as left ventricular hypertrophy (LVH). Mr. Brown's LVH indicates that his left ventricle has been working abnormally hard to move oxygenated blood out of the heart to the rest of his body, a common finding in patients with hypertension.

Pericardium

The pericardium forms a fibrous covering around the heart, holding it in a fixed position in the thorax and providing physical protection and a barrier to infection. The pericardium is a trilayer sac consisting of a tough, outer fibrous layer and a thin, inner serous layer. The outer fibrous layer is attached to the great vessels that enter and leave the heart, the sternum, and the diaphragm. The fibrous pericardium is highly resistant to distention. It prevents acute dilation of the heart chambers and exerts a restraining effect on the left ventricle. The inner serous layer consists of a visceral layer and a parietal layer. The visceral layer, also known as the *epicardium*, covers the entire heart and great vessels and then folds over to form the parietal layer that lines the fibrous pericardium (see Fig. 25.2). Between the visceral and parietal layers is the *pericardial cavity*, a potential space that contains 30 to 50 mL of serous fluid. This fluid acts as a lubricant to minimize friction as the heart contracts and relaxes against surrounding structures.

CONCEPTS IN ACTION *Myocardium*

The myocardium, or muscular portion of the heart, forms the wall of the atria and ventricles. Cardiac muscle cells, like skeletal muscle, are striated and composed of *sarcomeres* that contain actin and myosin filaments. They are smaller and more compact than skeletal muscle cells and contain many large mitochondria, which provides them with the energy needed to pump continuously.

The contractile properties of cardiac muscle are similar to those of skeletal muscle, except the contractions are involuntary and the duration of contraction is much longer. Unlike the orderly longitudinal arrangement of skeletal muscle fibers, cardiac muscle cells are arranged as an interconnecting latticework, with their fibers dividing, recombining, and then dividing again (Fig. 25.3A). Unique, dense structures, called *intercalated disks*, separate the cardiac muscle fibers from neighboring cardiac muscle cells. The intercalated disks contain gap junctions that serve as low-resistance pathways for passage of ions and electrical impulses from one cardiac cell to another (see Fig. 25.3B). Thus, when one myocardial cell becomes excited, the impulse travels rapidly so the heart can beat as a single unit, or *syncytium*, rather than contracting as a group of isolated units, as does skeletal muscle. The heart muscle has two syncytium—atrial and ventricular. The atrial syncytium constitutes the walls of the atria, and ventricular syncytium constitutes the walls of the ventricles. These two types of syncytiums allow the atria to contract prior to the ventricles, which is important to proper heart function.

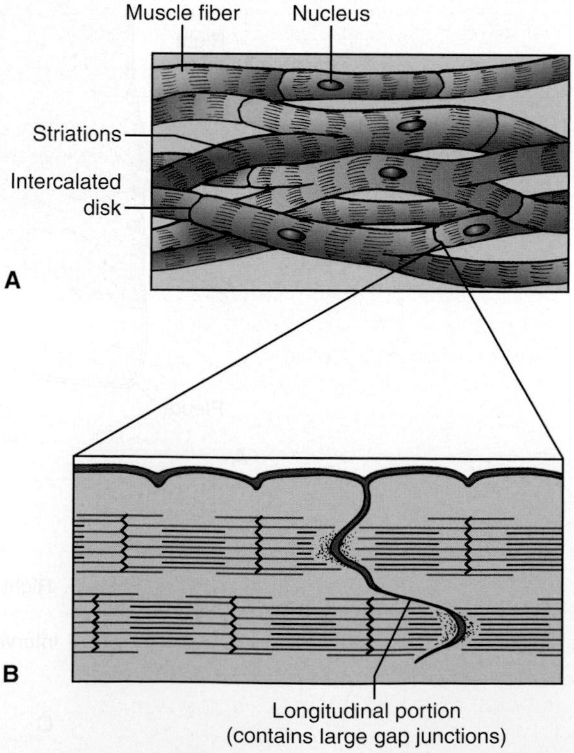

Figure 25.3 • **(A)** Cardiac muscle fibers showing their branching structure. **(B)** Area indicated where cell junctions lie in the intercalated disks.

As in skeletal muscle, cardiac muscle contraction involves actin and myosin filaments, which interact and slide along one another during muscle contraction. A number of important proteins regulate actin–myosin binding. These include tropomyosin and the troponin complex. The troponin complex consists of three subunits (troponin T, troponin I, and troponin C) that regulate calcium-mediated contraction in striated muscle. In clinical practice, the measurement of serum levels of the cardiac forms of troponin T and troponin I is used in the diagnosis of myocardial infarction.

Although cardiac muscle cells require calcium for contraction, they have a less well-defined sarcoplasmic reticulum for storing calcium than skeletal muscle cells. Thus, cardiac muscle relies more heavily than skeletal muscle on an influx of extracellular calcium ions for contraction. The cardiac glycosides (*e.g.*, digoxin) are inotropic drugs that increase cardiac contractility by increasing the free calcium concentration in the vicinity of the actin and myosin filaments.

Endocardium

The endocardium is a thin, three-layered membrane that lines the heart. The innermost layer consists of smooth endothelial cells supported by a thin layer of connective tissue. The endothelial lining of the endocardium is continuous with the lining of the blood vessels that enter and leave the heart. The middle layer consists of dense connective tissue with elastic fibers. The outer layer, composed of irregularly arranged connective tissue cells, contains blood vessels and branches of the conduction system and is continuous with the myocardium.

Heart Valves and Fibrous Skeleton

An important structural feature of the heart is its fibrous skeleton, which consists of four interconnecting valve rings and surrounding connective tissue. It separates the atria and ventricles and forms a rigid support for attachment of the valves and insertion of the cardiac muscle (Fig. 25.4). The tops of the valve rings are attached to the muscle tissue of the atria, pulmonary trunks, and aorta. The bottoms are attached to the ventricular walls. For the heart to function effectively, blood flow must occur in a one-way direction, moving in a forward (antegrade) manner through the chambers of the right heart to the lungs and then through the chambers of the left heart to the systemic circulation (Fig. 25.5). The heart's two atrioventricular (AV) (*i.e.*, tricuspid and mitral) valves and two semilunar (*i.e.*, pulmonary and aortic) valves provide this unidirectional flow.

When closed, the AV valves prevent backflow of blood from the ventricles to the atria during systole. The thin edges of the AV valves form cusps, two on the left side of the heart (*i.e.*, *bicuspid valve*), and three on the right side (*i.e.*, *tricuspid valve*). The bicuspid valve is also known as the *mitral valve*. The AV valves are supported by the *papillary muscles*, which project from the wall of the ventricles, and the *chordae tendineae*, which attach to the valve (Fig. 25.6). Contraction of the papillary muscles at the onset of systole ensures closure by producing tension on the leaflets of the AV valves before the full force of ventricular contraction pushes against them. The chordae tendineae are cordlike structures that support the AV valves and prevent them from everting into the atria during systole.

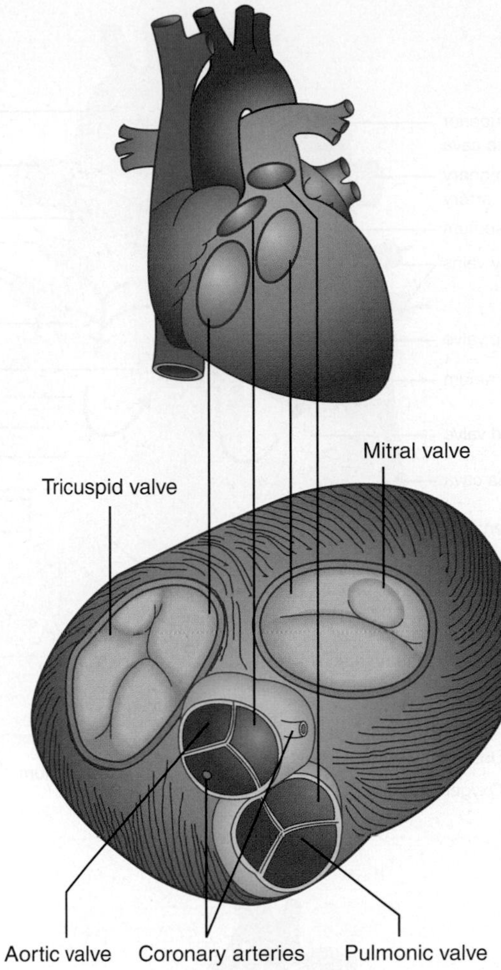

Figure 25.4 • Fibrous skeleton of the heart, which forms the four interconnecting valve rings and support for attachment of the valves and insertion of cardiac muscle.

The *aortic* and *pulmonic valves* prevent backflow from the aorta and the pulmonary arteries into the ventricles during diastole. The pulmonic valve, which is located between the right ventricle and the pulmonary artery, controls the flow of blood into the pulmonary circulation, and the aortic valve, located between the left ventricle and the aorta, controls the flow of blood into the systemic circulation. Because their flaps are shaped like half-moons, they are often referred to as the *semilunar valves*. The semilunar valves have three cuplike cusps that are attached to the valve rings (Fig. 25.7B). These cuplike structures collect the *retrograde*, or backward, flow of blood that occurs toward the end of systole, enhancing closure. For the development of a perfect seal along the free edges of the semilunar valves, each valve cusp must have a triangular shape, which is facilitated by a nodular thickening at the apex of each leaflet (see Fig. 25.7A). Behind the semilunar valves are the *sinuses of Valsalva*. In these sinuses, eddy currents develop that tend to keep the valve cusps away from the vessel walls. The openings for the coronary arteries are located behind the right

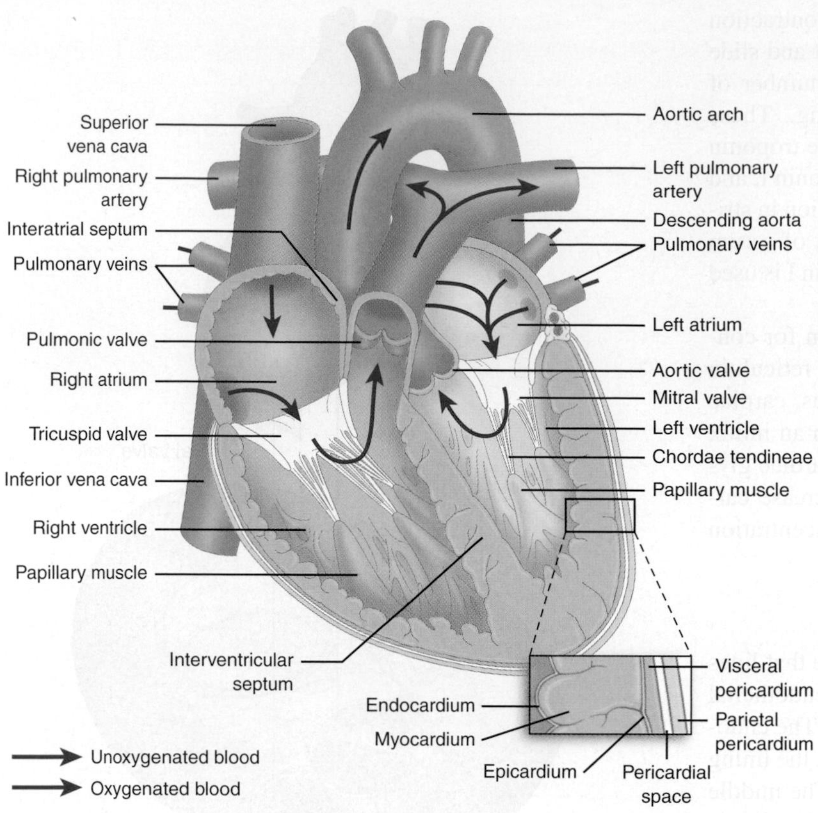

Figure 25.5 • Structures of the heart. *Arrows* show the course of blood flow through the heart chambers. (From Hinkle J., Cheever K. (2018). *Brunner and Suddarth's textbook of medical-surgical nursing* (14th ed., p. 685, Fig. 25-1). Philadelphia, PA: Wolters Kluwer.)

and left cusps, respectively, of the aortic valve. Were it not for the presence of the sinuses of Valsalva and the eddy currents, the valve cusps would block the coronary artery openings.

There are no valves at the atrial sites (*i.e.*, venae cavae and pulmonary veins) where blood enters the heart. This means that excess blood is pushed back into the veins when the atria become distended. For example, the jugular veins typically become prominent in severe right-sided heart failure when they normally should be flat or collapsed. Likewise, the pulmonary venous system becomes congested when outflow from the left side of the heart is impeded.

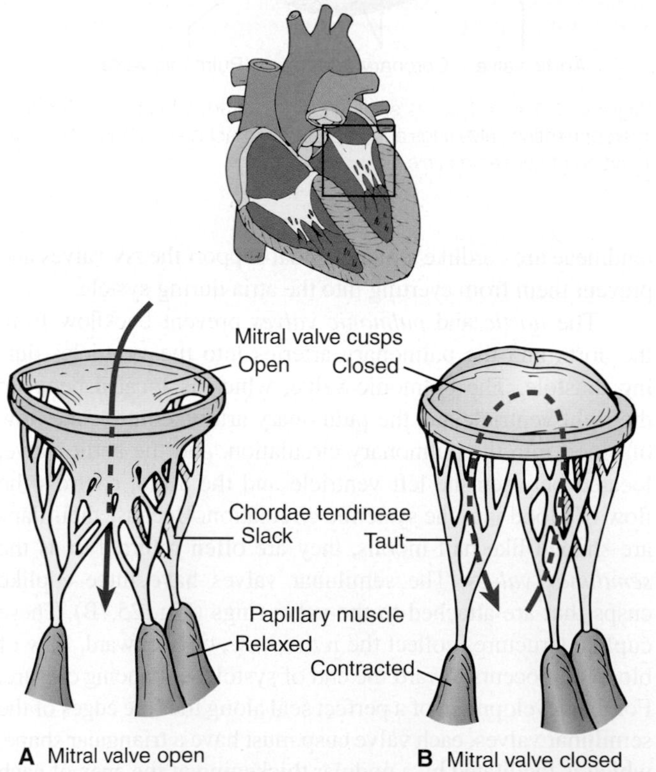

Figure 25.6 • The mitral (AV) valve showing the papillary muscles and chordae tendineae. **(A)** The open mitral valve with relaxed papillary muscles and slack chordae tendineae. **(B)** The closed mitral valve with contracted papillary muscles and taut chordae tendineae that prevent the valve cusps from everting into the atria.

KEY POINTS

THE HEART

- The heart is a four-chambered pump consisting of two atria (the right atrium, which receives blood returning to the heart from the systemic circulation, and the left atrium, which receives oxygenated blood from the lungs) and two ventricles (a right ventricle, which pumps blood to the lungs, and a left ventricle, which pumps blood into the systemic circulation). The heart valves control the direction of blood flow from the atria to the ventricles (the AV valves), from the right side of the heart to the lungs (pulmonic valve), and from the left side of the heart to the systemic circulation (aortic valve).

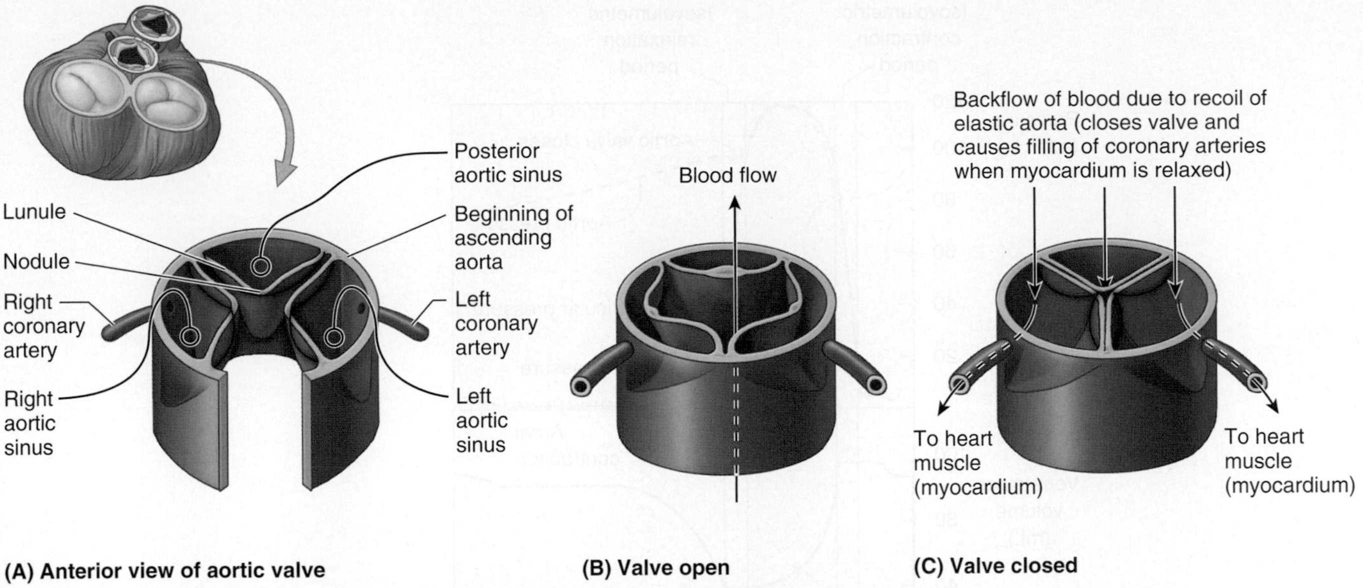

Figure 25.7 • Diagram of the aortic valve. **(A)** The position of the aortic valve at the base of the ascending aorta is indicated. **(B)** The appearance of the three leaflets of the aortic valve when the aorta is cut open and spread out, flat. (From Moore K. L., Dalley A. F., Agur A. M. R. (2018). *Clinically oriented anatomy* (8th ed., p. 366). Philadelphia, PA: Wolters Kluwer.)

Cardiac Cycle

The term *cardiac cycle* is used to describe the rhythmic pumping action of the heart. The cardiac cycle is divided into two parts:

- *Systole*, the period during which the ventricles are contracting
- *Diastole*, the period during which the ventricles relax and fill with blood

Simultaneous changes occur in the left atrial pressure, left ventricular pressure, aortic pressure, ventricular volume, ECG, and heart sounds during the cardiac cycle (Fig. 25.8).

The electrical activity, recorded on the ECG, precedes the mechanical events of the cardiac cycle. The small, rounded P wave of the ECG represents depolarization of the sinoatrial (SA) node (*i.e.*, pacemaker of the heart), the atrial conduction tissue, and the atrial muscle mass. The QRS complex registers the depolarization of the ventricular conduction system and the ventricular muscle mass. The T-wave on the ECG occurs during the last half of systole and represents repolarization of the ventricles.

Ventricular Systole and Diastole

Ventricular systole is divided into two periods—the isovolumetric contraction period and the ejection period. The *isovolumetric contraction period*, which begins with closure of the AV valves and occurrence of the first heart sound, or S1, heralds the onset of systole. Immediately after closure of the AV valves, there is an additional 0.02 to 0.03 second during which the semilunar (pulmonary and aortic) valves remain closed. During this period (see Fig. 25.8), the ventricular pressures rise abruptly because both the AV and semilunar valves are closed and no blood is leaving the ventricles. The ventricles continue to contract until left ventricular pressure is slightly higher than aortic pressure and right ventricular pressure is higher than pulmonary artery pressure. At this point, the semilunar valves open, signaling the onset of the *ejection period.* Approximately 60% of the stroke volume is ejected during the first quarter of systole. The remaining 40% is ejected during the next two quarters of systole. Little blood is ejected from the heart during the last quarter of systole, although the ventricle remains contracted. At the end of systole, the ventricles relax, causing a precipitous fall in intraventricular pressures. As this occurs, blood from the large arteries flows back toward the ventricles, causing the aortic and pulmonic valves to snap shut. This event is marked by the second heart sound or S2.

The aortic pressure reflects changes in the ejection of blood from the left ventricle. There is a rise in pressure and stretching of the elastic fibers in the aorta as blood is ejected into the aorta at the onset of systole. The aortic pressure continues to rise and then begins to fall during the last quarter of systole as blood flows out of the aorta into the peripheral vessels. The *incisura*, or notch, in the aortic pressure tracing represents closure of the aortic valve. This is caused by a short period of backflow of blood immediately before closure of the valve. The aorta is highly elastic and as such stretches during systole to accommodate the blood that is being ejected from the left heart. During diastole, recoil of the elastic fibers in the aorta serves to maintain the aortic pressure.

Diastole is marked by ventricular relaxation and filling. After closure of the semilunar valves, the ventricles continue to relax for another 0.03 to 0.06 second (referred to as the *isovolumetric relaxation period*). During this time, both the semilunar and AV valves remain closed, and the ventricular volume remains the same, as the ventricular pressure drops

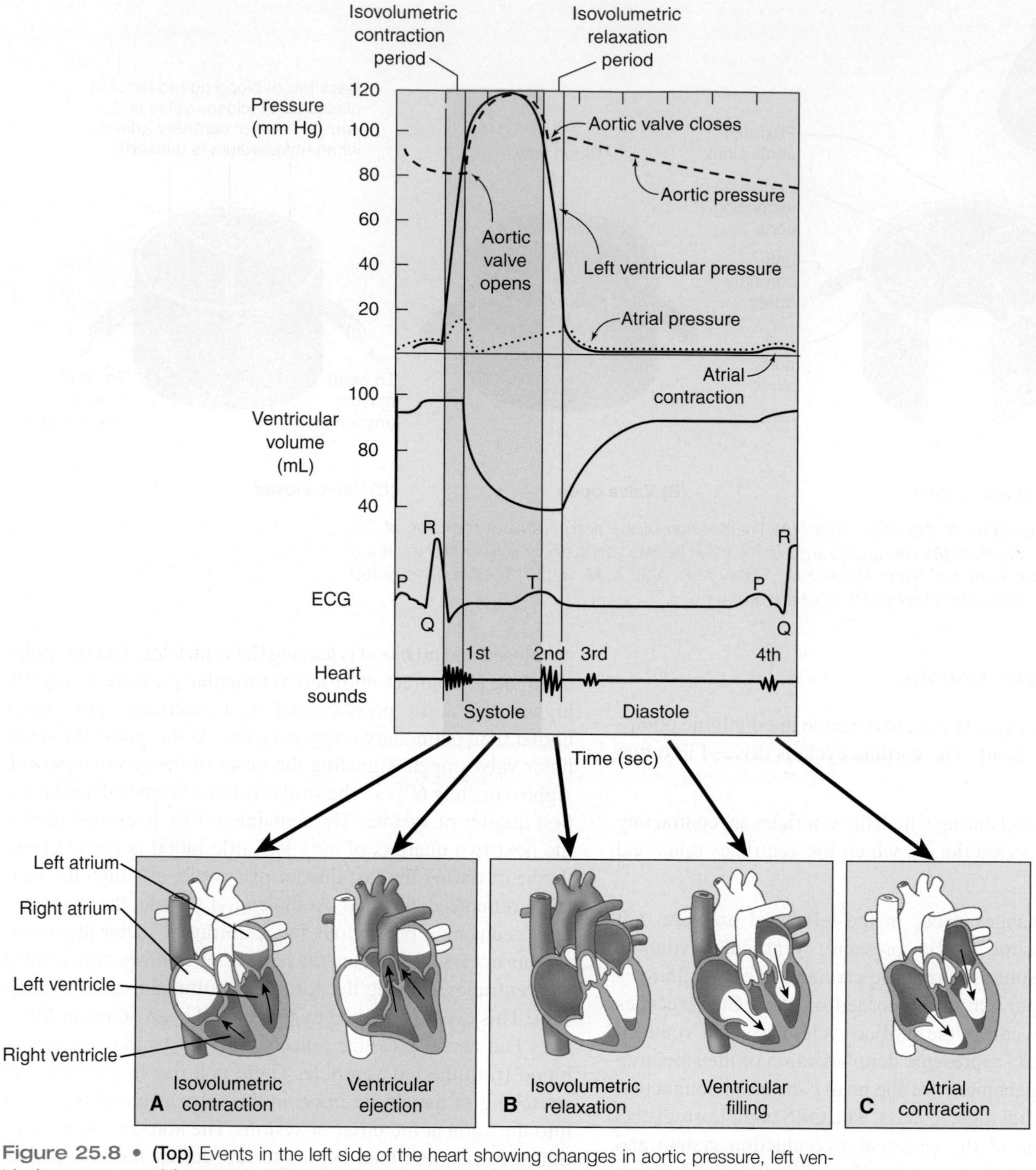

Figure 25.8 • **(Top)** Events in the left side of the heart showing changes in aortic pressure, left ventricular pressure, atrial pressure, left ventricular volume, the electrocardiogram (ECG), and heart sounds during the cardiac cycle. **(Bottom)** Position of the AV and semilunar valves during (*A*) isovolumetric contraction and ventricular ejection, (*B*) isovolumetric relaxation and ventricular filling, and (*C*) atrial contraction.

until it becomes less than the atrial pressure (see Fig. 25.8). As this occurs, the AV valves open and blood that has been accumulating in the atria during systole moves into the ventricles. Most of ventricular filling occurs during the first third of diastole, which is called the *rapid filling period*. During the middle third of diastole, inflow of blood into the ventricles constitutes a minimal amount. The last third of diastole is marked by atrial contraction, which gives an additional thrust to ventricular filling, which accounts for approximately 20% of the filling of the ventricles.[1] When audible, the third heart sound is heard during the rapid filling period of diastole as blood flows into a distended or noncompliant ventricle. The fourth heart sound occurs during the last third of diastole as the atria contract.

During diastole, the ventricles increase their volume to approximately 120 mL (*i.e.*, the *end-diastolic volume*). At the end of systole, approximately 40 to 50 mL of blood (*i.e.*, the *end-systolic volume*) remains in the ventricles (see Fig. 25.8). The difference between the end-diastolic and end-systolic volumes (approximately 70 mL) is called the *stroke volume*. The *ejection fraction*, which is the stroke volume divided by the end-diastolic volume, represents the fraction or percentage of the end-diastolic volume that is ejected from the heart during systole. The left ventricular ejection fraction (normally about 55% to 75% when determined by echocardiography or angiocardiography) is frequently used to evaluate the prognosis of people with a variety of heart diseases.

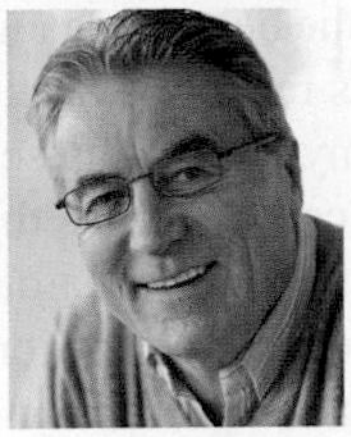

Refer back to Mr. Brown, whose ejection fraction is measured at 40%. This is below normal (normal is about 55% to 75%) and indicates a poor prognosis. In fact, his low ejection fraction is a result of the complications of long-standing hypertension, and he has already been diagnosed with New York Heart Association stage II heart failure.

Atrial Filling and Contraction

There are three main atrial pressure waves that occur during the cardiac cycle—the a, c, and v waves. The *a wave* occurs during the last part of diastole and is caused by atrial contraction. The *c wave* occurs as the ventricles begin to contract, and their increased pressure causes the AV valves to bulge into the atria. The *v wave* occurs toward the end of systole when the AV valves are still closed and results from a slow buildup of blood in the atria. The right atrial pressure waves are transmitted to the internal jugular veins as pulsations. These pulsations can be observed visually and may be used to assess cardiac function. For example, exaggerated a waves occur when the volume of the right atrium is increased because of impaired emptying into the right ventricle.

Because there are no valves between the junctions of the central veins (*i.e.*, venae cavae and pulmonary veins) and the atria, atrial filling occurs during both systole and diastole. During normal quiet breathing, right atrial pressure usually varies between −2 and +2 mm Hg. It is this low atrial pressure that maintains the movement of blood from the systemic circulation into the right atrium and from the pulmonary veins into the left atrium.

Right atrial pressure is regulated by a balance between the ability of the heart to move blood out of the right heart and through the left heart into the systemic circulation and the tendency of blood to flow from the peripheral circulation into the right atrium. When the heart pumps strongly, right atrial pressure is decreased and atrial filling is enhanced. Right atrial pressure is also affected by changes in intrathoracic pressure. It is decreased during inspiration when intrathoracic pressure becomes more negative, and it is increased during coughing or forced expiration when intrathoracic pressure becomes more positive. Venous return is a reflection of the amount of blood in the systemic circulation that is available for return to the right heart and the force that moves blood back to the right side of the heart. Venous return is increased when the blood volume is expanded or when right atrial pressure falls, and it is decreased in hypovolemic shock or when right atrial pressure rises.

Although the main function of the atria is to store blood as it enters the heart, these chambers also act as pumps that aid in ventricular filling. This function becomes more important during periods of increased activity when the diastolic filling time is decreased because of an increase in heart rate or when heart disease impairs ventricular filling. In these two situations, the cardiac output would fall drastically were it not for the action of the atria. It has been estimated that atrial contraction can contribute as much as 20% to cardiac reserve during periods of increased need, while having little or no effect on cardiac output during rest.

Regulation of Cardiac Performance

The efficiency of the heart as a pump often is measured in terms of *cardiac output* or the amount of blood the heart pumps each minute. The cardiac output (CO) is the product of the *stroke volume* (SV) and the *heart rate* (HR) and can be expressed by the equation $CO = SV \times HR$. The cardiac output varies with body size and the metabolic needs of the tissues. It increases with physical activity and decreases during rest and sleep. The average cardiac output in resting normal adults ranges from 4 to 6.0 L/minute. If a highly trained athlete is performing at an extreme exercise level, the heart may be required to pump four to six times this amount.

The *cardiac reserve* refers to the maximum percentage of increase in cardiac output that can be achieved above the normal resting level. The normal young adult has a cardiac reserve of approximately 300% to 400%. Cardiac performance is influenced by the work demands of the heart and the ability of the coronary circulation to meet its metabolic needs.

The heart's ability to increase its output according to body needs mainly depends on four factors:

- *Preload* or ventricular filling
- *Afterload* or resistance to ejection of blood from the heart
- *Cardiac contractility*
- *Heart rate*

Heart rate and cardiac contractility are strictly cardiac factors, meaning they originate in the heart, although they are controlled by various neural and humoral mechanisms. Preload and afterload, on the other hand, are mutually dependent on the behavior of the heart and the vasculature. Not only do they determine the cardiac output, they are themselves determined by the cardiac output and certain vascular characteristics.

Preload

The preload represents the volume work of the heart. It is usually considered the end-diastolic pressure when the ventricle has been filled.[2] It is called the *preload* because it is the work or load imposed on the heart before the contraction begins. Preload represents the amount of blood that the heart must pump with each beat. It is largely determined by the venous return to the heart and the accompanying stretch of the cardiac muscle fibers.

The increased force of contraction that accompanies an increase in ventricular end-diastolic volume is referred to as the *Frank-Starling mechanism* or Starling law of the heart (Fig. 25.9).[3] The anatomic arrangement of the actin and myosin filaments in the myocardial muscle fibers is such that the tension or force of contraction depends on the degree to which the muscle fibers are stretched just before the ventricles begin

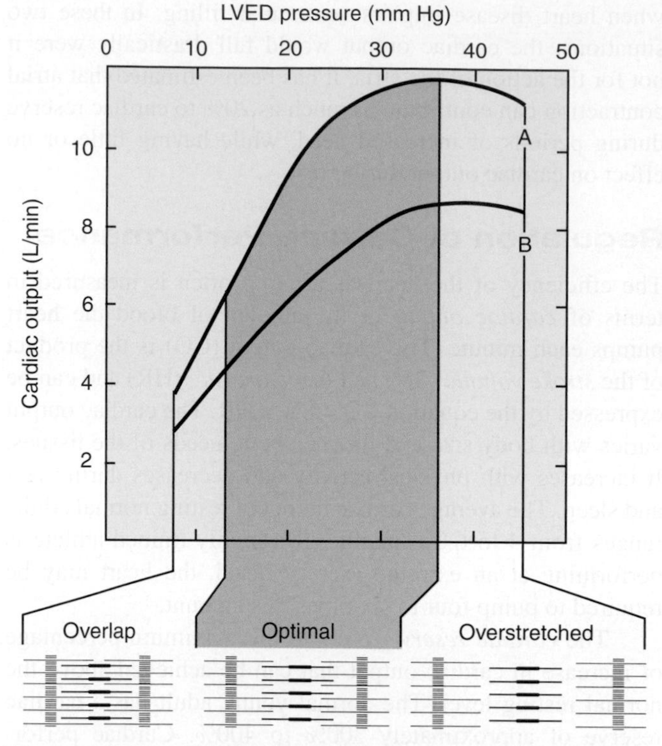

Figure 25.9 • The Frank-Starling ventricular function curve in a normal heart. **(Top)** An increase in left ventricular end-diastolic (LVED) pressure produces an increase in cardiac output (*curve B*) by means of the Frank-Starling mechanism. The maximum force of contraction and increased stroke volume are achieved when diastolic filling causes the muscle fibers to be stretched about two and one half times their resting length. In *curve A*, an increase in cardiac contractility produces an increase in cardiac output without a change in LVED volume and pressure. **(Bottom)** Stretching of the actin and myosin filaments at the different LVED filling pressures.

to contract. The maximum force of contraction and cardiac output is achieved when venous return produces an increase in left ventricular end-diastolic filling (*i.e.*, preload) such that the muscle fibers are stretched about two and one half times their normal resting length. When the muscle fibers are stretched to this degree, there is optimal overlap of the actin and myosin filaments needed for maximal contraction.

The Frank-Starling mechanism allows the heart to adjust its pumping ability to accommodate various levels of venous return. When a greater amount of blood flows into the ventricles, the cardiac muscle is stretched to a greater length. Cardiac output is less when decreased filling causes excessive overlap of the actin and myosin filaments or when excessive filling causes the filaments to be pulled too far apart.

Afterload

The afterload is the pressure in which the muscle exerts its contractile force in order to move blood into the aorta. It is called the *afterload* because it is the work presented to the heart after the contraction. The systemic arterial blood pressure is the main source of afterload work on the left heart, and the pulmonary arterial pressure is the main source of afterload work on the right heart. The afterload work of the left ventricle is also increased with narrowing (*i.e.*, stenosis) of the aortic valve. For example, in the late stages of aortic stenosis, the left ventricle may need to generate systolic pressures up to 300 mm Hg to move blood through the diseased and narrow valve.[2,4]

Cardiac Contractility

Cardiac contractility refers to the ability of the heart to change its force of contraction without changing its resting (*i.e.*, diastolic) length. The contractile state of the myocardial muscle is determined by biochemical and biophysical properties that govern the actin and myosin interactions in the myocardial cells. It is strongly influenced by the number of calcium ions that are available to participate in the contractile process.

An *inotropic* influence is one that modifies the contractile state of the myocardium independent of the Frank-Starling mechanism (see Fig. 25.9, top curve). For example, sympathetic stimulation produces a positive inotropic effect by increasing the calcium that is available for interaction between the actin and myosin filaments. Hypoxia exerts a negative inotropic effect by interfering with the generation of adenosine triphosphate (ATP), which is needed for muscle contraction.

Heart Rate

The heart rate determines the frequency with which blood is ejected from the heart. Therefore, as the heart rate increases, cardiac output tends to increase. As the heart rate increases, the time spent in diastole is reduced, and there is less time for the ventricles to fill. At a heart rate of 75 beats/minute, one cardiac cycle lasts 0.8 second, of which approximately 0.3 second is spent in systole and approximately 0.5 second in diastole. As the heart rate increases, the time spent in systole remains approximately the same, whereas that spent in diastole decreases. This leads to a decrease in stroke volume and, at high heart rates, a decrease in cardiac output. One of the dangers of ventricular tachycardia is a reduction in cardiac output because the heart does not have time to fill adequately.

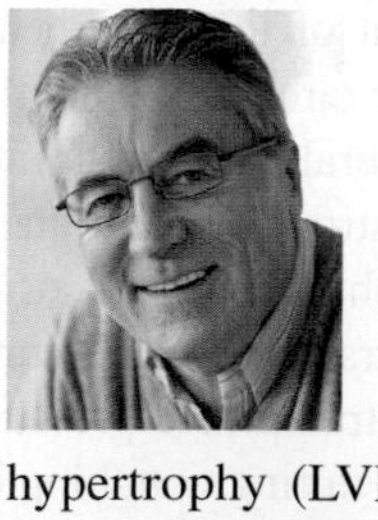

Refer back to Mr. Brown, who has a high afterload due to high blood pressure. His left ventricle has been working harder than normal to overcome the increased resistance and eject blood into the aorta. This increased workload has stimulated muscle growth, leading to left ventricular hypertrophy (LVH). The thickened ventricular wall does not stretch easily during diastolic filling, so blood pools in the left atrium, leading to left atrial enlargement (LAE). LAE puts Mr. Brown at increased risk for arrhythmias.

IN SUMMARY

The heart is a four-chambered muscular pump that lies in the pericardial sac within the mediastinal space of the intrathoracic cavity. The wall of the heart is composed of an outer epicardium, which lines the pericardial cavity; a fibrous skeleton; the myocardium, or muscle layer; and the smooth endocardium, which lines the chambers of the heart. The four heart valves control the direction of blood flow.

The cardiac cycle describes the pumping action of the heart. It is divided into two parts: systole, during which the ventricles contract and blood is ejected from the heart, and diastole, during which the ventricles are relaxed and blood is filling the heart. The stroke volume (approximately 70 mL) represents the difference between the end-diastolic volume (approximately 120 mL) and the end-systolic volume (approximately 40 to 50 mL). The electrical activity of the heart, as represented on the ECG, precedes the mechanical events of the cardiac cycle. The heart sounds signal the closing of the heart valves during the cardiac cycle. Atrial contraction occurs during the last third of diastole. Although the main function of the atria is to store blood as it enters the heart, atrial contraction acts to increase cardiac output during periods of increased activity when the filling time is reduced or in disease conditions in which ventricular filling is impaired.

The heart's ability to increase its output according to body needs depends on the preload, or filling of the ventricles (*i.e.*, end-diastolic volume); the afterload, or resistance to ejection of blood from the heart; cardiac contractility, which determines the force of contraction; and the heart rate, which determines the frequency with which blood is ejected from the heart. The maximum force of cardiac contraction occurs when an increase in preload stretches muscle fibers of the heart to approximately two and one half times their resting length (*i.e.,* Frank-Starling mechanism).

ORGANIZATION OF THE CIRCULATORY SYSTEM

After completing this section of the chapter, the learner will be able to meet the following objectives:

- Compare the function and distribution of blood flow and blood pressure in the systemic and pulmonary circulations.
- State the relation between blood volume and blood pressure in arteries, veins, and capillaries of the circulatory system.

Pulmonary and Systemic Circulations

The circulatory system can be divided into two parts:

- The *pulmonary circulation*, which moves blood through the lungs and creates a link with the gas exchange function of the respiratory system
- The *systemic circulation*, which supplies all the other tissues of the body (Fig. 25.10)

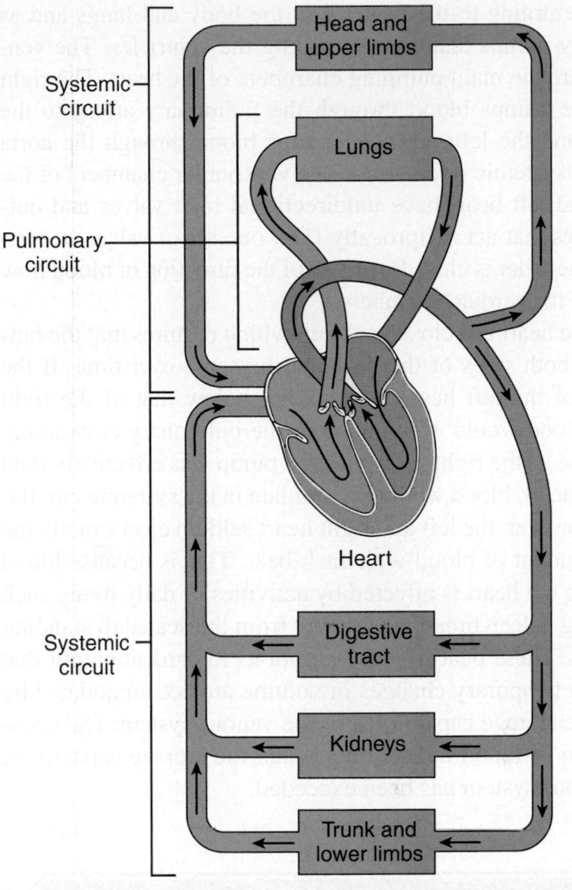

Figure 25.10 • Systemic and pulmonary circulations. The right side of the heart pumps blood to the lungs, and the left side of the heart pumps blood to the systemic circulation.

The pulmonary circulation consists of the right heart, the pulmonary artery, the pulmonary capillaries, and the pulmonary veins. The pulmonary vessels are unique in that the pulmonary artery is the only artery that carries venous blood, and the pulmonary veins are the only veins that carry arterial blood. Pulmonary circulation is considered low pressure and low resistance because it is a short system only involving blood to and from the lungs. The low pressure of the pulmonary circulation allows blood to move through the lungs more slowly, which is important for gas exchange. The systemic circulation consists of the left heart, the aorta and its branches, the capillaries that supply the brain and peripheral tissues, and the systemic venous system and the vena cava. The veins from the lower portion of the body merge to form the inferior vena cava, and those from the head and upper extremities merge to form the superior vena cava, both of which empty into the right heart. This circulation is more complex with higher pressures because it involves a complex vascular tree that provides substantial resistance to blood flow due to the effects of gravity.

The heart functions as a pump for the body. The right heart sends blood to the pulmonary circulatory system, and the left heart sends blood to the peripheral circulatory system. Both sides of the heart are further divided into two chambers—an *atrium* and a *ventricle*. The atria function as reservoirs for blood returning to the heart from the body and lungs and as auxiliary pumps that assist in filling the ventricles. The ventricles are the main pumping chambers of the heart. The right ventricle pumps blood through the pulmonary artery to the lungs, and the left ventricle pumps blood through the aorta into the systemic circulation. The ventricular chambers of the right and left heart have unidirectional inlet valves and outlet valves that act reciprocally (*i.e.*, one set of valves is open while the other is closed) to control the direction of blood flow through the cardiac chambers.

The heart is a closed system, which requires that the outputs of both sides of the heart be the same over time. If the output of the left heart were to fall below that of the right heart, blood would accumulate in the pulmonary circulation. Likewise, if the right heart were to pump less effectively than the left heart, blood would accumulate in the systemic circulation. However, the left and right heart seldom eject exactly the same amount of blood with each beat. This is because blood return to the heart is affected by activities of daily living such as taking a deep breath or moving from the seated to standing position. These beat-by-beat variations in cardiac output that result in temporary changes in volume are accommodated by the large storage capabilities of the venous system. The accumulation of blood occurs only when the storage capacity of the venous system has been exceeded.

KEY POINTS

FUNCTIONAL ORGANIZATION OF THE CIRCULATORY SYSTEM

- The circulatory system consists of the heart, which pumps blood; the arterial system, which distributes oxygenated blood to the tissues; the venous system, which collects deoxygenated blood from the tissues and returns it to the heart; and the capillaries, where exchange of gases, nutrients, and wastes takes place.
- The circulatory system is a closed system that is divided into two parts: the low-pressure pulmonary circulation, linking circulation and gas exchange in the lungs, and the high-pressure systemic circulation, providing oxygen and nutrients to the tissues.

Volume and Pressure Distribution

Effective blood flow in the circulatory system depends on sufficient blood volume to fill the blood vessels as well as a pressure difference across the system that provides the force to move blood forward. The total blood volume is a function of age and body weight, ranging from 85 to 90 mL/kg in the neonate and from 70 to 75 mL/kg in the adult. Approximately 4% of the blood at any given time is in the left heart, 16% is in the arteries and arterioles, 4% is in the capillaries, 64% is in the venules and veins, and 4% is in the right heart. The arteries and arterioles have thick, elastic walls and function as a distribution system to carry blood away from the heart and have the highest pressure. Arterioles, sometimes referred to as resistance vessels, provide the bulk of resistance to the circulatory flow. They provide resistance because of the layer of smooth muscle that encapsulates their vessel walls. Capillaries are small, thin-walled vessels that link the arterial and venous sides of the circulation and allow the exchange of oxygen and metabolites generated by the various tissues. Because of their small size and large surface area, the capillaries contain the smallest amount of blood. The venules and veins, which contain the largest amount of blood, are thin-walled, high compliance vessels that function as a reservoir to collect blood from the capillaries and return it to the right heart.

Blood moves from the arterial to the venous side of the circulation along a pressure gradient, moving from an area of higher pressure to one of lower pressure. The pressure distribution in the different parts of the circulation is almost an inverse of the volume distribution (see Fig. 25.11). The pressure in the arterial side of the systemic circulation, which contains approximately one sixth of the blood volume, is much greater than the pressure on the venous side of the circulation, which contains approximately two thirds of the blood. It is the pressure difference between the arterial and venous sides of the circulation (approximately 84 mm Hg) that provides the driving force for flow of blood in the systemic circulation. The pulmonary circulation has a similar arterial–venous pressure difference but of a lesser magnitude. Because the pulmonary and systemic circulations are connected and function as a closed system, blood can be shifted from one circuit to the other. Shifts in intrathoracic pressure and body position can cause shifts in blood volume. A shift of blood from one system to the other has a much greater effect in the pulmonary circulation because it contains less blood volume than the systemic circulation. The blood volume of the pulmonary circulation, which is approximately 4.7 to 5 L in the average-size adult, can vary from as low as 50% of normal to as high as 200% of normal. An increase in intrathoracic pressure, which impedes venous return to the right heart, can produce a transient shift from the pulmonary to the systemic circulation of as much as 250 mL. Body position also affects the distribution of blood volume. In the recumbent position, approximately 25% to 30% of the total blood volume is in the central circulation. On standing, this blood is displaced to the lower part of the body due to the force of gravity.

IN SUMMARY

The circulatory system functions as a transport system that circulates nutrients and other materials to the tissues and removes waste products. The circulatory system can be divided into two parts—the pulmonary circulation and the systemic circulation. The heart pumps blood throughout the system, and the blood vessels serve as tubes through

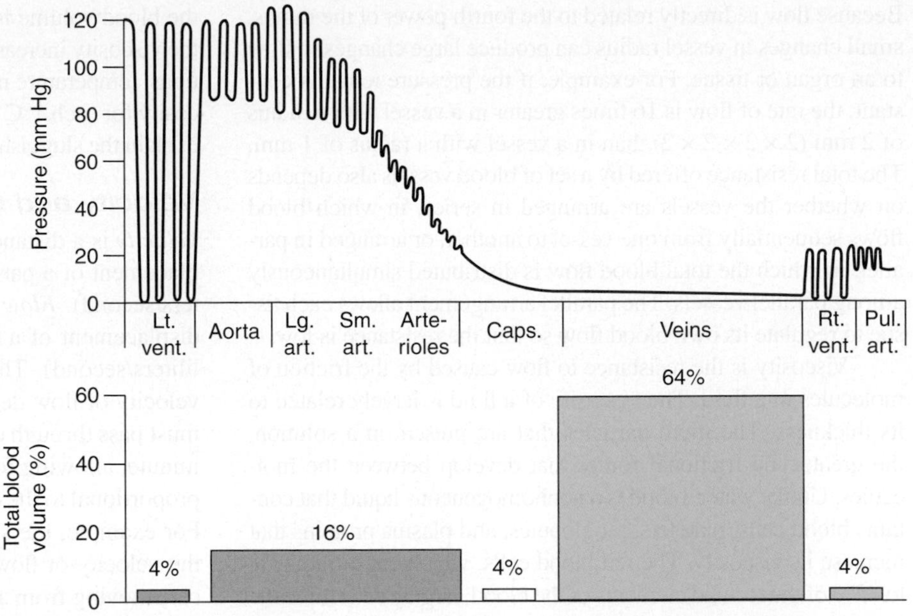

Figure 25.11 • Pressure and volume distribution in the systemic circulation. The graphs show the inverse relation between internal pressure and volume in different portions of the circulatory system. (From Klabunde R. E. (2012). *Cardiovascular physiology concepts* (2nd ed., p. 96). Philadelphia, PA: Lippincott Williams & Wilkins.)

which blood flows. The arterial system carries blood from the heart to the tissues, and the veins carry it back to the heart. The cardiovascular system is a closed system, with a right and left heart connected in series. The systemic circulation (which involves the left heart) provides blood flow for all the tissues. The right heart provides blood flow for the pulmonary circulation. Blood moves throughout the circulation along a pressure gradient, moving from the high-pressure arterial system to the low-pressure venous system. In the circulatory system, pressure is inversely related to volume. The pressure on the arterial side of the circulation, which contains only approximately one sixth of the blood volume, is much greater than the pressure on the venous side of the circulation, which contains approximately two thirds of the blood.

PRINCIPLES OF BLOOD FLOW

After completing this section of the chapter, the learner will be able to meet the following objectives:

- Define the term *hemodynamics* and describe the effects of blood pressure, vessel radius, vessel length, vessel cross-sectional area, and blood viscosity on blood flow.
- Use the law of Laplace to explain the effect of radius size on the pressure and wall tension in a vessel.
- Use the term *compliance* to describe the characteristics of arterial and venous blood vessels.

The term *hemodynamics* refers to the basic principles of physics, specifically Ohm law, that govern blood flow in the circulatory system and fluid movement in general. The concepts of flow, pressure, resistance, and capacitance as applied to blood flow in the cardiovascular system will be used in subsequent chapters to describe the hemodynamic changes that occur with disorders of the cardiovascular system.

Relationships between Blood Flow, Pressure, and Resistance

The most important factors governing the flow of blood in the cardiovascular system are *pressure*, *resistance*, and *flow*. Ohm law states that current (I) equals the voltage difference (ΔV) divided by the resistance (R). When relating this to blood flow, the voltage difference is the pressure difference or pressure gradient (ΔP), the resistance is the resistance to flow (R), and the current is the blood flow (F).[3] Blood flow (F) through a vessel or series of blood vessels is determined by the pressure difference (P1 – P2) between the two ends of the vessel and the resistance (R) that blood must overcome as it moves through the vessel ($F = \Delta P/R$). In the cardiovascular system, blood flow is represented by the cardiac output. Resistance is the opposition to flow caused by friction between the moving blood and the stationary vessel wall. In the peripheral circulation, the collective resistance of all the vessels in that part of the circulation is referred to as the *peripheral vascular resistance* (PVR) or, sometimes, as the *systemic vascular resistance* (SVR). The flow, pressure, and resistance relationships also can be applied on a smaller scale to determine the blood flow and resistance to flow of a single organ such as the kidney. Renal artery pressure, renal vein pressure, and renal vascular resistance determine blood flow to the kidney.

Resistance to Flow

The blood vessels and the blood itself constitute resistance to flow. The French physician Poiseuille derived a helpful equation for understanding the relationship between resistance, blood vessel diameter (radius), and blood viscosity factors that affect blood flow. The equation $F = \Delta P \text{ (pressure)} \times \pi \times r \text{ (radius)}^4/8 \times L$ (length) $\times\ \eta$ (viscosity) expands on the previous equation, $F = \Delta P/R$, by relating flow to two determinants of resistance: vessel radius and blood viscosity. The length of vessels does not usually change, and 8 is a constant that does not change.

Because flow is directly related to the fourth power of the radius, small changes in vessel radius can produce large changes in flow to an organ or tissue. For example, if the pressure remains constant, the rate of flow is 16 times greater in a vessel with a radius of 2 mm (2 × 2 × 2 × 2) than in a vessel with a radius of 1 mm. The total resistance offered by a set of blood vessels also depends on whether the vessels are arranged in series, in which blood flows sequentially from one vessel to another, or arranged in parallel, in which the total blood flow is distributed simultaneously among parallel vessels. The parallel arrangement allows each tissue to regulate its own blood flow so that the resistance is low.

Viscosity is the resistance to flow caused by the friction of molecules in a fluid. The viscosity of a fluid is largely related to its thickness. The more particles that are present in a solution, the greater the frictional forces that develop between the molecules. Unlike water, blood is a nonhomogeneous liquid that contains blood cells, platelets, fat globules, and plasma proteins that increase its viscosity. The red blood cells, which constitute 40% to 45% of the formed elements of the blood, largely determine the viscosity of the blood. A hematocrit measurement is performed in order to measure the proportion of red blood cells in blood. For example, if a person has a hematocrit of 38, then 38% of the blood volume is red blood cells. If the hematocrit increases, the viscosity increases, and vice versa. Also, under special conditions, temperature may affect viscosity. There is a 2% rise in viscosity for each 1°C decrease in body temperature. This fact helps explain the sluggish blood flow seen in people with hypothermia.

Velocity and Cross-Sectional Area

Velocity is a distance measurement. It refers to the rate of displacement of a particle of fluid with respect to time (centimeters/second). *Flow* is a volume measurement. It refers to the displacement of a volume of fluid with respect to time (milliliters/second). The cross-sectional area of a vessel and the velocity of flow determine it. The same volume of blood flow must pass through each segment of the circulatory system each minute, allowing for continuous flow; the velocity is inversely proportional to the cross-sectional area of the vessel (v = F/A).[2] For example, the smaller the cross-sectional area, the greater the velocity of flow. This phenomenon can be compared with cars moving from a two-lane to a single-lane section of a highway. To keep traffic moving at its original pace, cars would have to double their speed in the single-lane section of the highway. So it is with blood flow in the circulatory system.

Understanding The Hemodynamics of Blood Flow

The term *hemodynamics* is used to describe factors such as (1) pressure and resistance, (2) vessel radius, (3) cross-sectional area and velocity of flow, and (4) laminar versus turbulent flow that affect blood flow through the blood vessels in the body.

Pressure, Resistance, and Flow

The flow (F) of fluid through a tube, such as blood through a blood vessel, is directly related to a pressure difference ($P_1 - P_2$) between the two ends of the tube and inversely proportional to the resistance (R) that the fluid encounters as it moves through the tube.

The resistance to flow, in peripheral resistance units (PRUs), is determined by the blood viscosity, vessel radius, and whether the vessels are aligned in series or in parallel. In vessels aligned in series, blood travels sequentially from one vessel to another such that the resistance becomes additive (*e.g.*, 2 + 2 + 2 = 6 PRU). In vessels aligned in parallel, such as capillaries, the blood is not confined to a single channel but can travel through each of several parallel channels such that the resistance becomes the reciprocal of the total resistance (*i.e.*, 1/R). As a result, there is no loss of pressure, and the total resistance (*e.g.*, 1/2 + 1/2 + 1/2 = 3/2 PRU) is less than the resistance of any of the channels (*i.e.*, 2) taken separately.

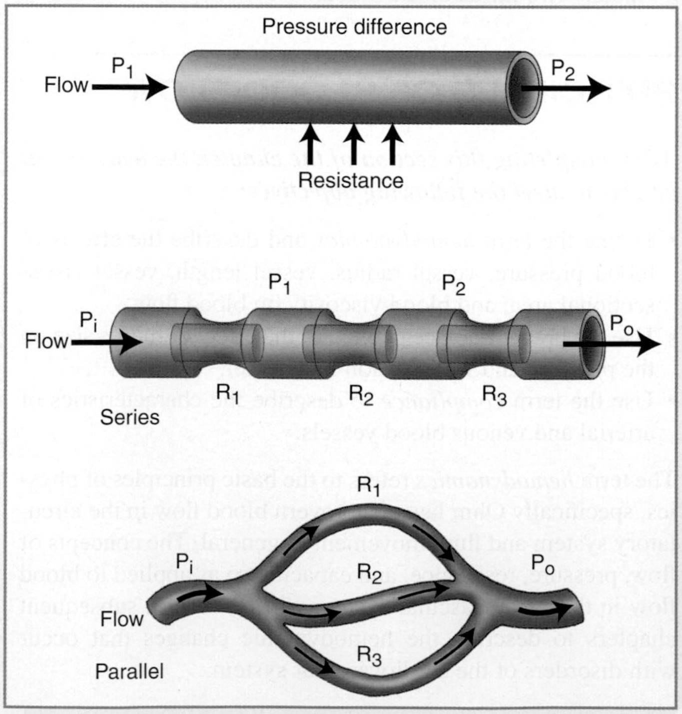

Understanding The Hemodynamics of Blood Flow *(Continued)*

Vessel Radius

In addition to pressure and resistance, the rate of blood flow through a vessel is affected by the fourth power of its radius (the radius multiplied by itself four times). Thus, blood flow in vessel B with a radius of 2 mm will be 16 times greater than in vessel A with a radius of 1 mm.

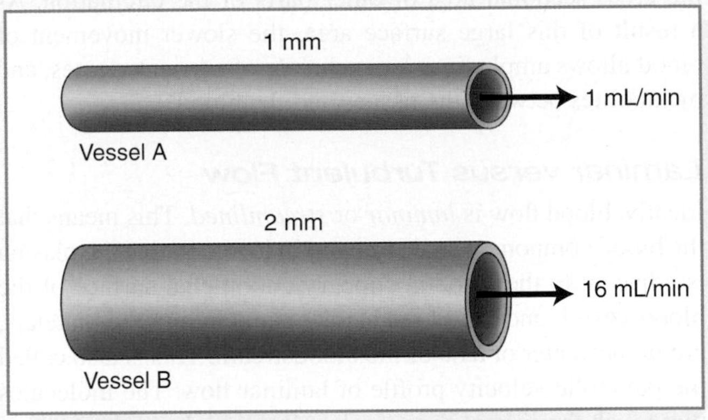

Cross-Sectional Area and Velocity of Flow

The velocity or rate of forward movement of the blood is affected by the cross-sectional area of a blood vessel. As the cross-sectional area of a vessel increases (sections 1 and 3), blood must flow laterally as well as forward to fill the increased area. As a result, the mean forward velocity decreases. In contrast, when the cross-sectional area is decreased (section 2), the lateral flow decreases and the mean forward velocity is increased.

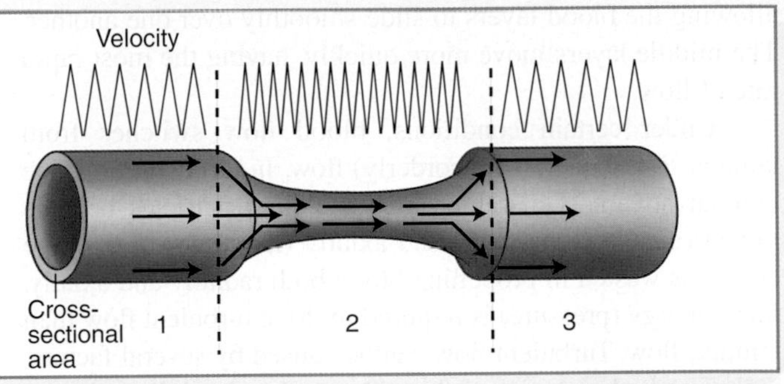

Laminar and Turbulent Flow

Blood flow is normally laminar, with platelets and blood cells remaining in the center or axis of the bloodstream. Laminar blood flow can be described as layered flow in which a thin layer of plasma adheres to the vessel wall, while the inner layers of blood cells and platelets shear against this motionless layer. This allows each layer to move at a slightly faster velocity, with the greatest velocity occurring in the central part of the bloodstream.

Turbulent blood flow is flow in which the blood elements do not remain confined to a definite lamina or layer, but develop vortices (*i.e.*, a whirlpool effect) that push blood cells and platelets against the wall of the vessel. More pressure is required to force a given flow of blood through the same vessel (or heart valve) when the flow is turbulent rather than laminar. Turbulence can result from an increase in velocity of flow, a decrease in vessel diameter, or low blood viscosity. Turbulence is usually accompanied by vibrations of the fluid and surrounding structures. Some of these vibrations in the cardiovascular system are in the audible frequency range and may be detected as murmurs or bruits.

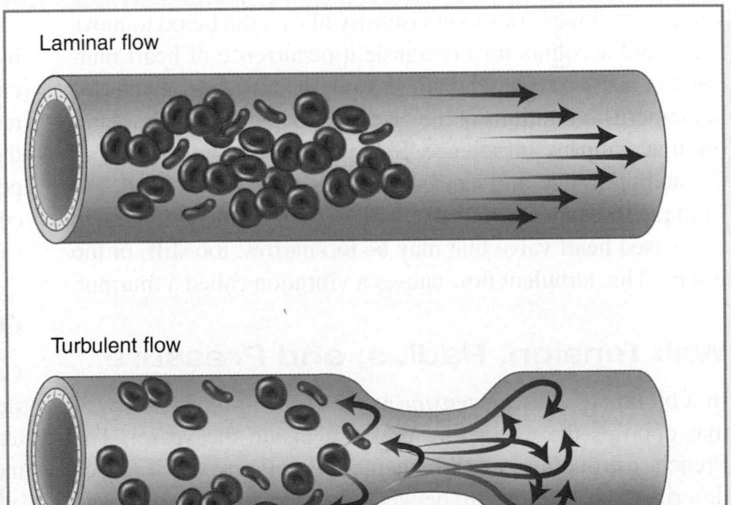

The linear velocity of blood flow in the circulatory system varies widely from 30 to 35 cm/second in the aorta to 0.2 to 0.3 mm/second in the capillaries. This is because even though each individual capillary is very small, the total cross-sectional area of all the systemic capillaries greatly exceeds the cross-sectional area of other parts of the circulation. As a result of this large surface area, the slower movement of blood allows ample time for exchange of nutrients, gases, and metabolites between the tissues and the blood.

Laminar versus Turbulent Flow

Ideally, blood flow is *laminar* or *streamlined*. This means that the blood components are arranged in layers so that the plasma is adjacent to the smooth, slippery endothelial surface of the blood vessel, and the blood elements, including the platelets, are in the center or *axis* of the bloodstream. This is also called the parabolic velocity profile of laminar flow. The molecules that touch the side of the vessel wall move slower because of adherence to the wall.[1] This arrangement reduces friction by allowing the blood layers to slide smoothly over one another. The middle layers move more quickly, having the most rapid rate of flow.

Under certain conditions, blood flow switches from laminar to turbulent (or disorderly) flow. In turbulent flow, the laminar stream is disrupted, and the fluid particles become mixed radially (crosswise) and axially (lengthwise). Because energy is wasted in propelling blood both radially and axially, more energy (pressure) is required to drive turbulent flow than laminar flow. Turbulent flow can be caused by several factors, including high velocity of flow, change in vessel diameter, an obstruction in a vessel, and low blood viscosity. The tendency for turbulence to occur is increased in direct proportion to the velocity of flow. Low blood viscosity allows the blood to move faster and accounts for the transient occurrence of heart murmurs in some people who are severely anemic (*i.e.*, decreased hematocrit). Vibrations of the blood and surrounding structures often accompany turbulence. Some of these vibrations are in the audible range and can be heard using a stethoscope. For example, a heart murmur results from turbulent flow through a diseased heart valve that may be too narrow, too stiff, or too floppy. This turbulent flow causes a vibration called a murmur.

Wall Tension, Radius, and Pressure

In a blood vessel, *wall tension* is the force in the vessel wall that opposes the distending pressure inside the vessel. The French astronomer and mathematician Pierre de Laplace described the relationship between wall tension, pressure, and the radius of a vessel or sphere. This relationship, which has come to be known as the *law of Laplace*, can be expressed by the equation $P = T/r$, in which T is wall tension, P is the intraluminal pressure, and r is vessel radius.[3] Accordingly, the internal pressure expands the vessel until it is exactly balanced by the tension in the vessel wall. The smaller the radius, the greater the pressure needed to balance the wall tension. The law of Laplace can also be used to express the effect of the radius on wall tension ($T = P \times r$). This correlation can be compared with a partially inflated balloon. Because the pressure in the balloon is equal throughout, the tension in the section with the smaller radius is less than the tension in the section with the larger radius. The same principle holds true for an arterial aneurysm, in which the tension and risk of rupture increase as the aneurysm grows.

The law of Laplace was later expanded to include wall thickness ($T = P \times r$/wall thickness). Thus, wall tension is inversely related to wall thickness—the thicker the vessel wall, the lower the tension, and vice versa. In hypertension, arterial vessel walls hypertrophy and become thicker, thereby reducing the tension and minimizing wall stress.

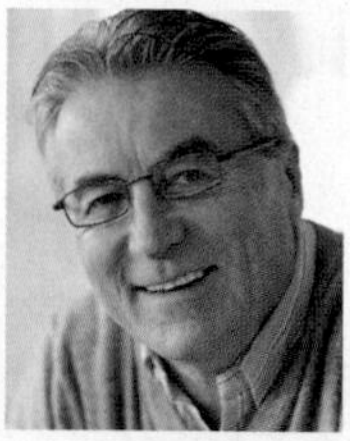

Remember **Mr. Brown** from the case study. His father had hypertension and an abdominal aortic aneurysm. Aneurysms occur when wall tension exceeds the structural capacity of the arterial wall. The arterial wall thickening induced by hypertension helps protect against aneurysms by keeping the wall tension low. However, as discussed in Chapter 26, hypertension is also associated with atherosclerosis, an arterial disease that weakens the structural capacity of the arterial wall. Overall, Mr. Brown will be less vulnerable to aneurysms if he corrects his hypertension.

The law of Laplace can also be applied to the pressure required to maintain the patency of small blood vessels. Provided that the thickness of a vessel wall remains constant, it takes more pressure to overcome wall tension and keep a vessel open as its radius decreases in size. The *critical closing pressure* refers to the point at which blood vessels collapse so that blood can no longer flow through them. For example, in circulatory shock, there is a decrease in blood volume and vessel radii, along with a drop in blood pressure. As a result, many of the small blood vessels collapse as blood pressure drops to the point where it can no longer overcome the wall tension. The collapse of peripheral veins often makes it difficult to insert venous lines that are needed for fluid and blood replacement.

Distention and Compliance

Compliance refers to the total quantity of blood that can be stored in a given portion of the circulation for each millimeter of mercury (mm Hg) rise in pressure. Compliance is the increase in volume divided by the increase in pressure. In other words, the ability of a vessel to distend and increase volume with increasing pressure is quantified as compliance. The most distensible of all vessels are the veins, which can increase their volume with only slight changes in pressure. This allows the veins to function as a reservoir for storing large quantities of blood that can be returned to the circulation when it is needed. The compliance of a vein is approximately 24 times that of its corresponding artery because it is 8 times as distensible and has a volume 3 times as great.

IN SUMMARY

Blood flow is influenced by the pressure difference between the two ends of the vessel, the vessel length, its radius and cross-sectional area, the viscosity of the blood, and tension of the vessel wall. The rate of flow is directly related to the pressure difference between the two ends of the vessel and the vessel radius and inversely related to vessel length and blood viscosity. The cross-sectional area of a vessel influences the velocity of flow. As the cross-sectional area decreases, the velocity is increased and vice versa. Laminar blood flow is a flow in which there is layering of blood components in the center of the bloodstream, which reduces friction. In contrast to laminar flow, turbulent flow is disordered flow, in which the blood moves crosswise and lengthwise in blood vessels. The law of Laplace describes the relationship between wall tension, transmural pressure, and radius. This law states that the pressure needed to overcome wall tension becomes greater as the radius decreases. Wall thickness also affects wall tension. It increases as the wall becomes thinner and decreases as the wall becomes thicker. Compliance of blood vessels refers to the total quantity of blood that can be stored in a given part of the circulatory system for each mm Hg rise in pressure.

THE SYSTEMIC CIRCULATION AND CONTROL OF BLOOD FLOW

After completing this section of the chapter, the learner will be able to meet the following objectives:

- Compare the structure and function of arteries and veins.
- Use the equation blood pressure = cardiac output × peripheral vascular resistance to explain the regulation of arterial blood pressure.
- Define autoregulation and characterize mechanisms responsible for short-term and long-term regulation of blood flow.

The vascular system functions in the delivery of oxygen and nutrients and removal of waste products from the tissues. It consists of the arteries and arterioles, the capillaries, and the venules and veins. Although blood vessels of the vascular system are often compared with a system of rigid pipes and tubes, this analogy serves only as a starting point. Blood vessels are dynamic structures that constrict and relax to adjust blood pressure and flow to meet the varying needs of the many different tissue types and organ systems. Structures such as the heart, brain, liver, and kidneys require a large and continuous flow to carry out their vital functions. In other tissues such as the skin and skeletal muscle, the need for blood flow varies with the level of function. For example, there is a need for increased blood flow to the skin during fever and for increased skeletal muscle blood flow during exercise.

Blood Vessels

All blood vessels, except the capillaries, have walls composed of three layers, or coats, called *tunicae* (Fig. 25.12). The outermost layer of a vessel, called the *tunica externa* or *tunica adventitia*, is composed primarily of loosely woven collagen fibers that protect the blood vessel and anchor it to the surrounding structures. The middle layer, the *tunica media*, is largely a smooth muscle layer that constricts to regulate and control the diameter of the vessel. Larger arteries have an external elastic lamina that separates the tunica media from the tunica externa. The innermost layer, the *tunica intima*, consists of a single layer of flattened endothelial cells with minimal underlying subendothelial connective tissue. The endothelial layer provides a smooth and slippery inner surface for the vessel. This smooth inner lining, as long as it remains intact, prevents platelet adherence and blood clotting.

The layers of the different types of blood vessels vary with vessel function. The walls of the arterioles, which control blood pressure, have large amounts of smooth muscle. Veins are thin-walled, distensible, and collapsible vessels. Capillaries are single-cell–thick vessels designed for the exchange of gases, nutrients, and waste materials.

Vascular Smooth Muscle

Vascular smooth muscle cells, which form the predominant cellular layer in the tunica media, produce vasoconstriction or dilation of blood vessels. Smooth muscle contracts slowly and generates high forces for long periods with low energy requirements. It uses only 1/10 to 1/300 the energy of skeletal muscle. These characteristics are important in structures, such as blood vessels, that must maintain their tone day in and day out.

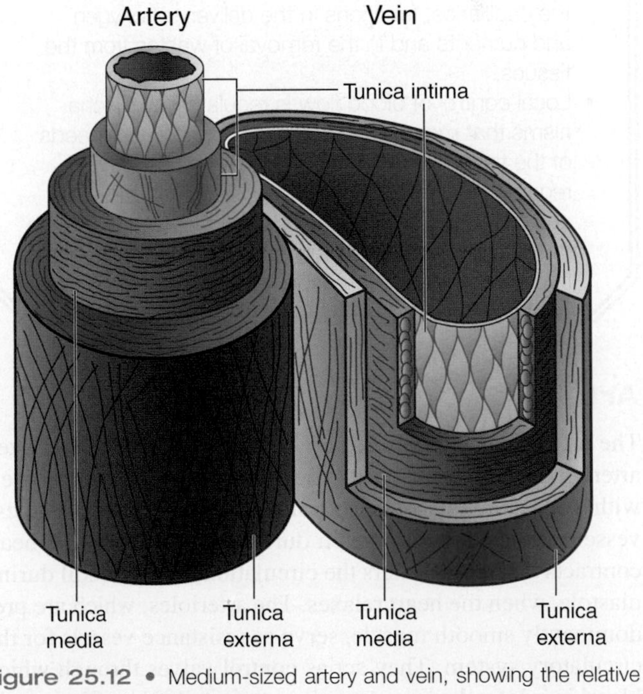

Figure 25.12 • Medium-sized artery and vein, showing the relative thicknesses of the three layers.

Compared with skeletal and cardiac muscles, smooth muscle has less well-developed sarcoplasmic reticulum for storing intracellular calcium, and it has very few fast sodium channels. Depolarization of smooth muscle instead relies largely on extracellular calcium, which enters through calcium channels in the muscle membrane. Sympathetic nervous system control of vascular smooth muscle tone occurs through receptor-activated opening and closing of the calcium channels. In general, α-adrenergic receptors are excitatory in that they cause the channels to open and produce vasoconstriction. β-Adrenergic receptors are inhibitory in that they cause the channels to close and produce vasodilation. Calcium channel–blocking drugs cause vasodilation by blocking calcium entry through the calcium channels.

Smooth muscle contraction and relaxation also occur in response to local tissue factors such as lack of oxygen, increased hydrogen ion concentrations, and excess carbon dioxide. Nitric oxide (formerly known as the *endothelium-derived relaxing factor*) acts locally to produce smooth muscle relaxation and regulate blood flow. These factors are discussed more fully in the section "Local and Humoral Control of Blood Flow."

KEY POINTS

THE VASCULAR SYSTEM AND CONTROL OF BLOOD FLOW

- The vascular system, which consists of the arterial system (a high-pressure system delivering blood to the tissues), the venous system (a low-pressure system that collects blood from the capillaries), and the capillaries, functions in the delivery of oxygen and nutrients and in the removal of wastes from the tissues.
- Local control of blood flow is regulated by mechanisms that match blood flow to the metabolic needs of the tissue. Over the short term, the tissues autoregulate flow through the synthesis of vasodilators and vasoconstrictors derived from the tissue, smooth muscle, or endothelial cells; over the long term, blood flow is regulated by creation of a collateral circulation.

Arterial System

The arterial system consists of the large- and medium-sized arteries and the arterioles. Arteries are thick-walled vessels with large amounts of elastic fibers. The elasticity of these vessels allows them to stretch during systole, when the heart contracts and blood enters the circulation, and to recoil during diastole, when the heart relaxes. The arterioles, which are predominantly smooth muscle, serve as resistance vessels for the circulatory system. They act as control valves through which blood is released as it moves into the capillaries. Changes in the activity of sympathetic fibers that innervate these vessels cause them to constrict or to relax as needed to maintain blood pressure.

Arterial Pressure Pulsations

The delivery of blood to the tissues of the body depends on pressure pulsations or waves of pressure that are generated by the intermittent ejection of blood from the left ventricle into the distensible aorta and large arteries of the arterial system. The arterial pressure pulse represents the energy that is transmitted from molecule to molecule along the length of the vessel (Fig. 25.13). In the aorta, this pressure pulse is transmitted at a velocity of 4 to 6 m/second, which is approximately 20 times faster than the flow of blood. Therefore, the pressure pulse has no direct relation to blood flow and could occur if there was no flow at all. When taking a pulse, it is the pressure pulses that are felt, and it is the pressure pulses that produce the Korotkoff sounds heard during blood pressure measurement. The tip or maximum deflection of the pressure pulsation coincides with the systolic blood pressure, and the minimum point of deflection coincides with the diastolic pressure. The pulse pressure is the difference between systolic and diastolic pressure. If all other factors are equal, the magnitude of the pulse pressure reflects the volume of blood ejected from the left ventricle in a single beat.

Both the pressure values and the conformation of the pressure wave change as it moves though the peripheral arteries, such that pulsations in the large arteries are even greater than those in the aorta (see Fig. 25.13). In other words, systolic pressure and pulse pressure are higher in large arteries than in

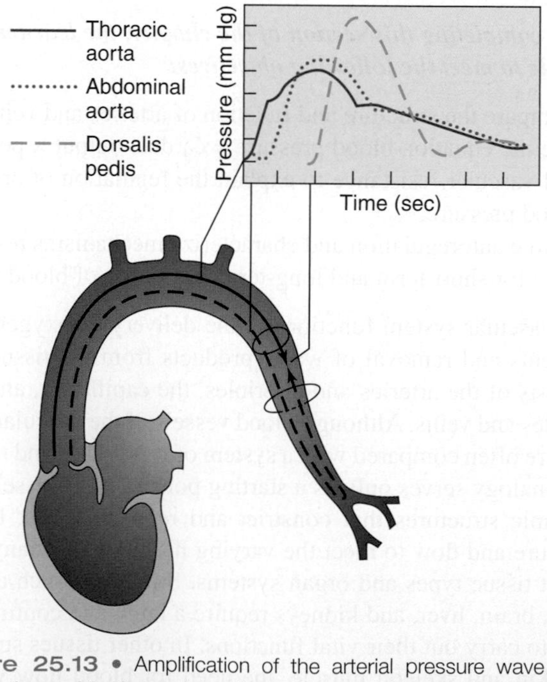

Figure 25.13 • Amplification of the arterial pressure wave as it moves forward in the peripheral arteries. This amplification occurs as a forward-moving pressure wave merges with a backward-moving reflected pressure wave. **(Inset)** The amplitude of the pressure pulse increases in the thoracic aorta, abdominal aorta, and dorsalis pedis.

the aorta. The increase in pulse pressure in the "downstream" arteries is due to the fact that immediately after ejection from the left ventricle, the pressure wave travels at a higher velocity than the blood itself, augmenting the downhill pressure. Furthermore, at branch points of arteries, pressure points are reflected backward, which also tends to augment pressure at those sites. With peripheral arterial disease, there is a delay in the transmission of the reflected wave so that the pulse decreases rather than increases in amplitude.

After its initial amplification, the pressure pulse becomes smaller and smaller as it moves through the smaller arteries and arterioles, until it disappears almost entirely in the capillaries. This damping of the pressure pulse is caused by the resistance and ability to distend characteristics of these vessels. The increased resistance of these small vessels impedes the transmission of the pressure waves. However, their ability to distend is great enough that any small change in flow does not cause a pressure change. Although the pressure pulses usually are not transmitted to the capillaries, there are situations in which this does occur. For example, injury to a finger or other area of the body often results in a throbbing sensation. In this case, extreme dilation of the small vessels in the injured area produces a reduction in the dampening of the pressure pulse. Capillary pulsations also occur in conditions that cause exaggeration of aortic pressure pulses, such as aortic regurgitation or patent ductus arteriosus.

Venous System

The venous system is a low-pressure system that returns blood to the heart. The venules collect blood from the capillaries, and the veins transport blood back to the right heart. Because blood from the systemic veins flows into the right atrium of the heart, the pressure in the right atrium is called the *central venous pressure*. Right atrial pressure is regulated by the ability of the right ventricle to pump blood into the lungs and the tendency of blood to flow from the peripheral veins into the right atrium. The normal right atrial pressure is about 0 mm Hg, which is equal to atmospheric pressure. It can increase to 20 to 30 mm Hg in conditions such as right heart failure and the rapid transfusion of blood at a rate that greatly increases total blood volume and causes excessive quantities of blood to attempt to flow into the heart from the systemic veins.

The veins and venules are thin-walled, distensible, and collapsible vessels. The veins are capable of enlarging and storing large quantities of blood, which can be made available to the circulation as needed. Even though the veins are thin walled, they are muscular. This allows them to contract or expand to accommodate varying amounts of blood. Veins are innervated by the sympathetic nervous system. When blood is lost from the circulation, the veins constrict as a means of maintaining intravascular volume.

Valves in the veins of extremities prevent retrograde flow (Fig. 25.14). Thus, with the help of skeletal muscles that surround and intermittently compress the leg veins in a milking manner, blood is moved forward to the heart through these one-way valves. This pumping action is known as the

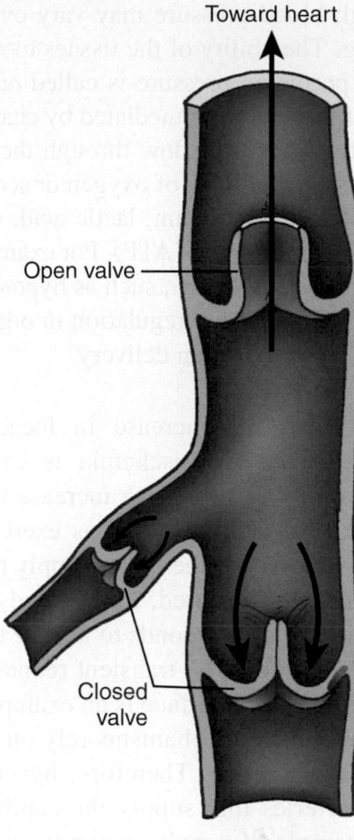

Figure 25.14 • Portion of a femoral vein opened, to show the valves. The direction of flow is upward. Backward flow closes the valve.

venous or *muscle pump*. It facilitates blood flow return at low pressure back to the heart against gravity. There are no valves in the abdominal or thoracic veins. Therefore, pressure changes in the abdominal and thoracic cavities, respectively, cause the venous blood flow in these veins.

Because the venous system is a low-pressure system, blood flow must oppose the effects of gravity. In a person in the standing position, the weight of the blood in the vascular column causes an increase of 1 mm Hg in pressure for every 13.6 mm of distance below the level of the heart. Were it not for the valves in the veins and the action of the skeletal muscles, the venous pressure in the feet would be about +90 mm Hg in the standing adult. Gravity has no effect on the venous pressure in a person in the recumbent position because the blood in the veins is then at the level of the heart.

Local and Humoral Control of Blood Flow

Tissue blood flow is regulated on a minute-to-minute basis in relation to tissue needs and on a longer-term basis through the development of collateral circulation. Neural mechanisms regulate the cardiac output and blood pressure needed to support these local mechanisms.

Short-Term Autoregulation

Local control of blood flow is governed largely by the nutritional needs of the tissue. For example, blood flow to organs such as the heart, brain, and kidneys remains relatively constant, although blood pressure may vary over a range of 60 to 180 mm Hg. The ability of the tissues to maintain constant changes in perfusion pressure is called *autoregulation*. Autoregulation of blood flow is mediated by changes in blood vessel tone due to changes in flow through the vessel or by local tissue factors, such as lack of oxygen or accumulation of tissue metabolites (*i.e.*, potassium, lactic acid, or adenosine, which is a breakdown product of ATP). For example, a change in systemic arterial pressure (*e.g.*, such as hypotension during circulatory shock) leads to autoregulation in organs to ensure adequate blood flow and oxygen delivery.

Reactive Hyperemia. An increase in local blood flow following a brief period of ischemia is called *reactive hyperemia*. The ability of tissues to increase blood flow in situations of increased activity, such as exercise, is called *functional hyperemia*. When the blood supply to an area has been occluded and then restored, local blood flow through the tissues increases within seconds to restore the metabolic equilibrium of the tissues. The transient redness seen on an arm after leaning on a hard surface is an example of reactive hyperemia. Local control mechanisms rely on a continuous flow from the main arteries. Therefore, hyperemia cannot occur when the arteries that supply the capillary beds are narrowed. For example, if a major coronary artery becomes occluded, the opening of channels supplied by that vessel cannot restore blood flow.

Endothelial Control of Vascular Function. One of the important functions of the endothelial cells lining the arterioles and small arteries is the synthesis and release of factors that control vessel dilation. Intact endothelium produces a factor that causes relaxation of vascular smooth muscle. Originally, this factor was called *endothelium-derived relaxing factor*; it is now known as *nitric oxide*. The normal endothelium maintains a continuous release of nitric oxide, which is formed from L-arginine and oxygen through the action of an enzyme called *nitric oxide synthase* (Fig. 25.15). The production of nitric oxide can be stimulated by a variety of endothelial *agonists*, including acetylcholine, bradykinin, histamine, and thrombin. *Shear stress* on the endothelium resulting from an increase in blood flow or blood pressure also stimulates nitric oxide production and vessel relaxation. Nitric oxide also inhibits platelet aggregation and secretion of platelet contents, many of which cause vasoconstriction. Nitric oxide is released into the vessel lumen (to inactivate platelets) and away from the lumen (to relax smooth muscle) and protects against both thrombosis and vasoconstriction. Nitroglycerin, which is used in the treatment of angina, produces its effects by causing the release of nitric oxide in vascular smooth muscle of the target tissues.

The endothelium also produces a number of vasoconstrictor substances, including *angiotensin II*, vasoconstrictor prostaglandins, and *endothelin-1*. The endothelin-1, a 21 amino acid peptide, is present in all endothelial cells and requires very small amounts to cause vasoconstriction. For example, after a blood vessel is damaged, local endothelin is released to vasoconstrict the vessel and prevent extensive bleeding.[2]

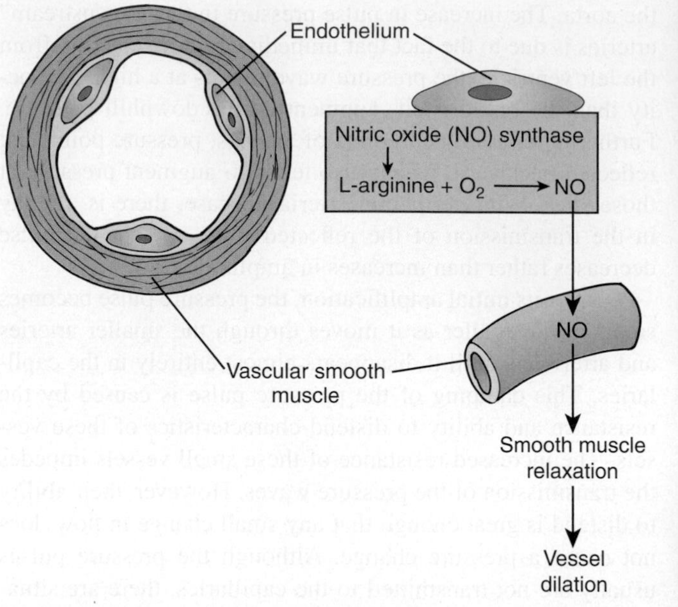

Figure 25.15 • Function of nitric oxide in smooth muscle relaxation.

Long-Term Regulation of Blood Flow

Long-term regulation allows a more complete control of blood flow compared to short-term regulation. One way to regulate blood flow is to change the amount of vascularity over a prolonged period. This process is called *angiogenesis*. If the metabolism in the tissue is increased for a long period of time, vascularity increases and vice versa. There is actual physical reconstruction of the tissue vasculature to meet the metabolic need of the tissue. This regeneration occurs much better in younger tissue compared to older tissue. In addition, *vascular endothelial growth factor*, *fibroblast growth factor*, *and angiotensin* have been isolated in tissues that have insufficient blood supply. These growth factors cause new vessels to spring new growth. Blood vessels can also disappear due to certain other substances, such as *angiostatin* and *endostatin*, in which the exact physiologic mechanism is unknown. Oxygen also plays a role in the long-term regulation of blood flow.[2,3] For example, if the atmospheric oxygen is low, then the vascularity increases to compensate for the low oxygen. This is seen in animals that live in higher altitude where oxygen levels are low.

Furthermore, collateral circulation is a mechanism for the long-term regulation of local blood flow. In the heart and other vital structures, anastomotic channels exist between some of the smaller arteries. These channels permit perfusion of an area by more than one artery. When one artery becomes occluded, these anastomotic channels increase in size, allowing blood from a patent artery to perfuse the area supplied by the occluded vessel. For example, people with extensive obstruction of a coronary blood vessel may rely on collateral circulation to meet the oxygen needs of the myocardial tissue normally supplied by that vessel. As with other long-term compensatory mechanisms, the recruitment of collateral circulation is most efficient when obstruction to flow is gradual rather than sudden.

Humoral Control of Vascular Function

Humoral control of blood flow involves the effect of vasodilator and vasoconstrictor substances in the blood. Some of these substances are formed by special glands and transported in the blood throughout the entire circulation. Others are formed in local tissues and aid in the local control of blood flow. Among the most important of the humoral factors are norepinephrine and epinephrine, angiotensin II, histamine, serotonin, bradykinin, and the prostaglandins.

Norepinephrine and Epinephrine. Norepinephrine is an especially powerful vasoconstrictor hormone. Epinephrine is less so and in some tissues (*e.g.*, skeletal muscle) even causes mild vasodilation. Stimulation of the sympathetic nervous system during stress or exercise causes local constriction of veins and arterioles because of the release of norepinephrine from sympathetic nerve endings. In addition, sympathetic stimulation causes the adrenal medullae to secrete both norepinephrine and epinephrine into the blood. These hormones then circulate in the blood, causing direct sympathetic stimulation of blood vessels in all parts of the body.

Angiotensin II. Angiotensin II is another powerful vasoconstrictor substance. Angiotensin II is produced as a part of the renin–angiotensin–aldosterone system and normally acts on many arterioles simultaneously to increase the PVR, thereby increasing the arterial blood pressure.

Histamine. Histamine has a powerful vasodilator effect on arterioles and has the ability to increase capillary permeability, allowing leakage of both fluid and plasma proteins into the tissues. Histamine is largely derived from mast cells in injured tissues and basophils in the blood. In certain tissues, such as skeletal muscle, the activity of the mast cells is mediated by the sympathetic nervous system. When sympathetic control is withdrawn, the mast cells release histamine.

Serotonin. Serotonin is liberated from aggregating platelets during the clotting process. It causes vasoconstriction and plays a major role in control of bleeding. Serotonin is found in the brain and lung tissues, and there is some speculation that it may be involved in the vascular spasm associated with some allergic pulmonary reactions and migraine headaches.

Bradykinin. The kinins (*i.e.*, kallidins and bradykinin) are liberated from the globulin kininogen, which is present in body fluids. Bradykinin causes intense dilation of arterioles, increased capillary permeability, and constriction of venules. It is thought that the kinins play special roles in regulating blood flow and capillary leakage in inflamed tissues. It is also believed that bradykinin helps to regulate blood flow in the skin as well in the salivary and gastrointestinal glands.

Prostaglandins. Prostaglandins are synthesized from constituents of the cell membrane (*i.e.*, the long-chain fatty acid *arachidonic acid*). Tissue injury incites the release of arachidonic acid from the cell membrane, which initiates prostaglandin synthesis. There are several prostaglandins (*e.g.*, E_2, F_2, D_2), which are subgrouped according to their solubility; some produce vasoconstriction and some produce vasodilation. As a rule of thumb, those in the E group are vasodilators, and those in the F group are vasoconstrictors. The corticosteroid hormones produce an anti-inflammatory response by blocking the release of arachidonic acid, preventing prostaglandin synthesis.

IN SUMMARY

The walls of all blood vessels, except the capillaries, are composed of three layers: the tunica externa, tunica media, and tunica intima. The layers of the vessel vary with its function. Arteries are thick-walled vessels with large amounts of elastic fibers. The walls of the arterioles, which control blood pressure, have large amounts of smooth muscle. Veins are thin-walled, distensible, and collapsible vessels. Venous flow is designed to return blood to the heart. It is a low-pressure system and relies on venous valves and the action of muscle pumps to offset the effects of gravity.

The delivery of blood to the tissues of the body depends on pressure pulses that are generated by the intermittent ejection of blood from the left ventricle into the distensible aorta and large arteries of the arterial system. The combination of the arteries' ability to distend and their resistance to flow reduces the pressure pulsations so that constant blood flow occurs by the time blood reaches the capillaries.

The mechanisms that control local blood flow are designed to ensure adequate delivery of blood to the capillaries in the microcirculation, where the exchange of cellular nutrients and wastes occurs. Local control is governed largely by the needs of the tissues and is regulated by local tissue factors such as lack of oxygen and the accumulation of metabolites. Reactive hyperemia is a local increase in blood flow that occurs after a temporary occlusion of blood flow. It is a compensatory mechanism that decreases the oxygen debt of the deprived tissues. Long-term regulation of blood flow includes angiogenesis, vascular endothelial growth factor, fibroblast growth factor, and angiotensin, which increase tissue vascularity, while angiostatin and endostatin have been found to dissolve blood vessels. Collateral circulation improves local blood flow by the development of collateral vessels.[2,3] The endothelium-derived relaxing factor (mainly nitric oxide) and humoral factors, such as norepinephrine and epinephrine, angiotensin II, histamine, serotonin, bradykinin, and the prostaglandins, contribute to the regulation of blood flow.

THE MICROCIRCULATION AND LYMPHATIC SYSTEM

After completing this section of the chapter, the learner will be able to meet the following objectives:

- Define the term *microcirculation*.
- Describe the structure and function of the capillaries.
- Explain the forces that control the fluid exchange between the capillaries and the interstitial spaces.

The term *microcirculation* refers to the functions of the smallest blood vessels, the capillaries and the neighboring lymphatic vessels, which transport nutrients to tissues and remove excreta from the cells.

Structure and Function of the Microcirculation

The structures of the microcirculation include the arterioles, capillaries, and venules. Blood enters the microcirculation through an arteriole, passes through the capillaries, and leaves through a small venule. The metarterioles serve as thoroughfare channels that link arterioles and capillaries (Fig. 25.16). Small cuffs of smooth muscle, the precapillary sphincters, are positioned at the arterial end of the capillary. The smooth muscle tone of the arterioles, venules, and precapillary sphincters serves to control blood flow through the capillary bed. Depending on venous pressure, blood flows through the capillary channels when the precapillary sphincters are open.

Capillary Structure and Function

Capillaries are microscopic vessels that connect the arterial and venous segments of the circulation. In each person, there are approximately 10 billion capillaries, with a total surface area of 500 to 700 m.[2] Capillary walls are composed of a single layer of endothelial cells and their basement membrane (Fig. 25.17). The endothelial cells form a tube just large enough to allow the passage of red blood cells, one at a time.

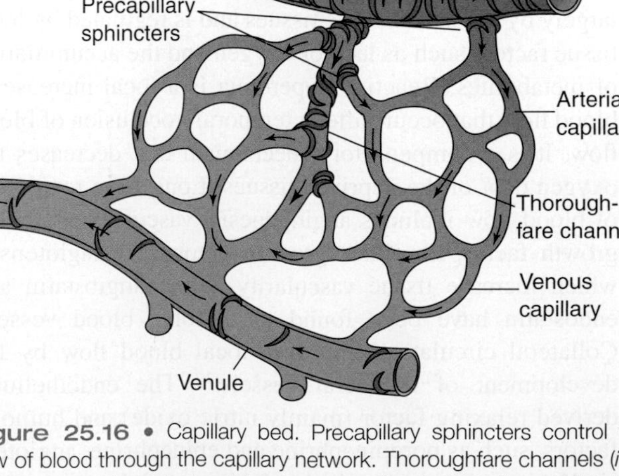

Figure 25.16 • Capillary bed. Precapillary sphincters control the flow of blood through the capillary network. Thoroughfare channels (*i.e.*, arteriovenous shunts) allow blood to move directly from the arteriole into the venule without moving through nutrient channels of the capillary.

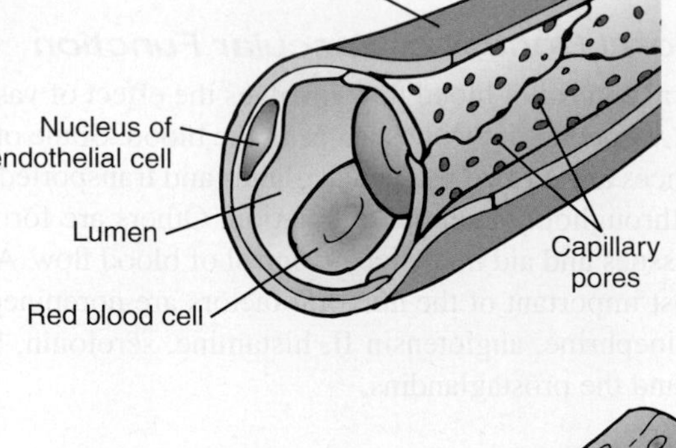

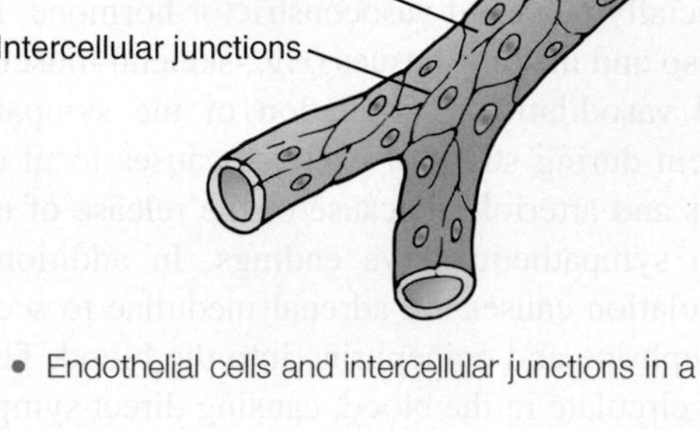

Figure 25.17 • Endothelial cells and intercellular junctions in a section of capillary.

Water-filled junctions, called the *capillary pores*, join the capillary endothelial cells and provide a pathway for passage of substances through the capillary wall. The size of the capillary pores varies with capillary function. In the brain, the endothelial cells are joined by tight junctions that form the blood–brain barrier. This prevents substances that would alter neural excitability from leaving the capillary. In organs that process blood contents, such as the liver, capillaries have large pores so that substances can pass easily through the capillary wall. The glomerular capillaries in the kidney have small openings called *fenestrations* that pass directly through the middle of the endothelial cells. This allows large amounts of small molecular and ionic substances to filter through the glomeruli without having to pass through the clefts between the endothelial cells.

Because of their thin walls and close proximity to the cells of metabolically active tissues, capillaries are particularly well suited for the exchange of gases and metabolites between cells and the bloodstream. This exchange of substances occurs through spaces between tissue cells called the *interstitium*. The interstitium is supported by *collagen* and *elastin* fibers and filled with *proteoglycan* (sugar–protein) molecules that combine with water to form a tissue gel. The tissue gel acts like a sponge to entrap the interstitial fluid and provide for distribution of the fluid, even to those cells that are most distant from the capillary.

Fluids, electrolytes, gases, and substances of small and large molecular weights move across the capillary endothelium by diffusion, filtration, and pinocytosis. The exchange of gases and fluids across the capillary wall occurs by simple diffusion. Lipid-soluble substances such as oxygen and carbon dioxide readily exchange across the endothelial cells by diffusion. Water flows through the capillary endothelial cell membranes through water-selective channels called *aquaporins*. Water and water-soluble substances such as electrolytes, glucose, and amino acids also diffuse between the endothelial cells in the capillary pores. Pinocytosis is responsible for the movement of white blood cells and large protein molecules.

Control of Blood Flow in the Microcirculation

Blood flow through capillary channels, designed for exchange of nutrients and metabolites, is called *nutrient flow*. In some parts of the microcirculation, blood flow bypasses the capillary bed, moving through a connection called an *arteriovenous shunt*, which directly connects an arteriole and a venule. This type of blood flow is called *nonnutrient flow* because it does not allow for nutrient exchange. Nonnutrient channels are common in the skin and are important in terms of heat exchange and temperature regulation.

Capillary–Interstitial Fluid Exchange

The hydrostatic and osmotic pressures of the capillary and interstitial fluids, as well as the permeability of the capillary wall, largely control the direction and magnitude of fluid movement across the capillary wall. The direction of fluid movement can either be into or out of the capillary. When net fluid movement is out of the capillary into the interstitial spaces, it is called *filtration*. When net movement is from the interstitium into the capillary, it is called *absorption* (Fig. 25.18).

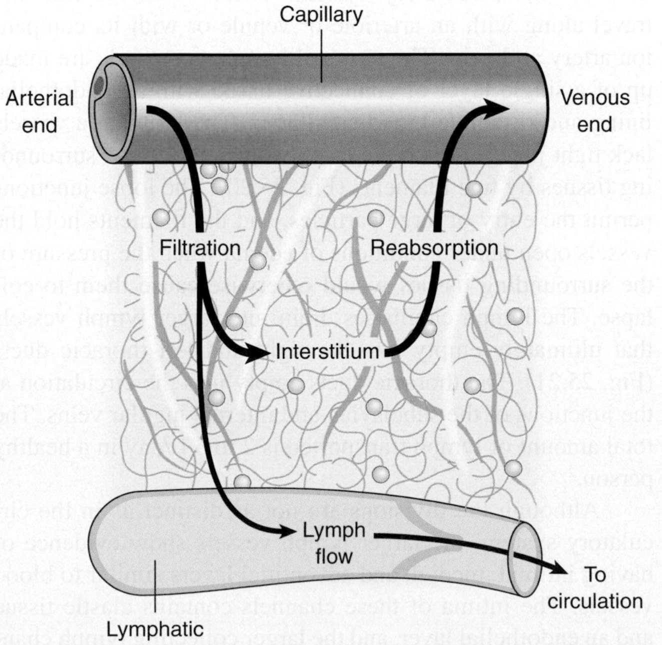

Figure 25.18 • Capillary filtration and lymph flow. Fluid is filtered out of the capillary and into the interstitium at the arterial end of the capillary. Most of the fluid is reabsorbed at the venous end of the capillary, with the rest of the fluid entering the terminal lymphatics for return to the circulation.

The capillary hydrostatic pressure represents the fluid pressure that tends to push water and its dissolved substances through the capillary pores into the interstitium. The osmotic pressure caused by the plasma proteins in the blood tends to pull fluid from the interstitial spaces back into the capillary. This pressure is termed *colloidal osmotic pressure* to differentiate the osmotic effects of the plasma proteins, which are suspended colloids, from the osmotic effects of substances such as sodium and glucose, which are dissolved crystalloids. Capillary permeability controls the movement of water and substances, such as the plasma proteins that influence osmotic pressure, into the interstitial spaces. Also important to this exchange mechanism is the lymphatic system, which removes excess fluid and osmotically active proteins and large particles from the interstitial spaces and returns them to the circulation.

Hydrostatic Forces

The capillary hydrostatic pressure is the principal force in capillary filtration. Both the arterial and venous pressures (the capillaries being interspersed between the arteries and veins) determine the hydrostatic pressure (blood pressure) within the capillaries. An increase in small artery and arterial pressure elevates capillary hydrostatic pressure. However, a reduction in each of these pressures has the opposite effect. A change in venous pressure has a greater effect on the capillary hydrostatic pressure than does the same change in arterial pressure. About 80% of increased venous pressure, such as that caused by venous thrombosis or congestive heart failure, is transmitted back to the capillary. The previously discussed effects on gravity on venous pressure also affect capillary hydrostatic pressure. When a person stands, the hydrostatic pressure is greater in the legs and lower in the head.

The interstitial hydrostatic pressure is the pressure exerted by the interstitial fluids outside the capillary. It can be positive or negative. A positive interstitial fluid pressure opposes capillary filtration, and a negative interstitial fluid pressure increases the movement of fluid out of the capillary into the interstitium. In the normal nonedematous state, the interstitial hydrostatic pressure is close to zero or slightly negative (−1 to −4 mm Hg) and has very little effect on capillary filtration or outward movement of fluid.

Osmotic Forces

The key factor that restrains fluid loss from the capillaries is the colloidal osmotic pressure (approximately 28 mm Hg) generated by the plasma proteins. The plasma proteins are large molecules that disperse in the blood and occasionally escape into the tissue spaces. Because the capillary membrane is almost impermeable to the plasma proteins, these particles exert an osmotic force that pulls fluid into the capillary and offsets the pushing force of the capillary filtration pressure. The plasma contains a mixture of plasma proteins, including albumin, globulins, and fibrinogen. Albumin, which is the smallest and most abundant of the plasma proteins, accounts for approximately 70% of the total osmotic pressure. It is the number, not the size, of the particles in solution that controls the osmotic pressure.

Although the size of the capillary pores prevents most plasma proteins from leaving the capillary, small amounts escape into the interstitial spaces and exert an osmotic force that tends to pull fluid from the capillary into the interstitium. This amount is increased in conditions such as inflammation in which an increase in capillary permeability allows plasma proteins to escape into the interstitium. The lymphatic system is responsible for removing proteins from the interstitium. In the absence of a functioning lymphatic system, interstitial colloidal osmotic pressure increases, causing fluid to accumulate. Normally, a few white blood cells, plasma proteins, and other large molecules enter the interstitial spaces. These cells and molecules, which are too large to reenter the capillary, rely on the loosely structured wall of the lymphatic vessels for return to the vascular compartment.

Balance of Hydrostatic and Osmotic Forces

Normally, the movement of fluid between the capillary bed and the interstitial spaces is continuous. As Ernest H. Starling pointed out, a state of equilibrium exists as long as equal amounts of fluid enter and leave the interstitial spaces. This is referred to as "Starling forces" and is illustrated in Figure 25.19. In the diagram, the hydrostatic pressure at the arterial end of the capillary is higher than at the venous end.[5,6] The pushing force of the capillary hydrostatic pressure on the arterial end of the capillary, along with the pulling effects of the interstitial colloidal osmotic pressure, contributes to the net outward movement of fluid. The capillary colloidal osmotic pressure and opposing interstitial osmotic pressure determine the reabsorption of fluid at the venous end of the capillary. A slight imbalance in forces causes slightly more filtration of fluid into interstitial spaces than absorption back into the capillary. It is this fluid that is returned to the circulation by the lymphatic system.

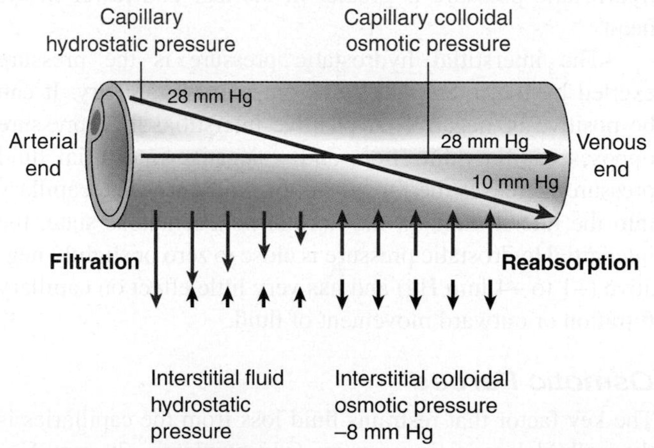

Figure 25.19 • Capillary–interstitial fluid exchange equilibrium. Normally, the forces (capillary hydrostatic pressure, interstitial colloidal osmotic pressure, and the opposing interstitial fluid pressure) that control the outward movement of fluid from the capillary (filtration) are almost balanced by the forces (capillary colloidal osmotic pressure and interstitial colloidal osmotic pressure) that pull fluid back into the capillary (reabsorption).

The Lymphatic System

The lymphatic system represents an accessory route through which fluid can flow into the blood from interstitial spaces.[3] This system, commonly called the *lymphatics*, serves almost all body tissues, except cartilage, bone, epithelial tissue, and tissues of the central nervous system (CNS). However, even most of these tissues have prelymphatic channels that eventually flow into areas supplied by the lymphatics. Lymph is derived from interstitial fluids that flow through the lymph channels. It contains plasma proteins and other osmotically active particles that rely on the lymphatics for movement back into the circulatory system. The lymphatic system is also the main route for absorption of nutrients, particularly fats, from the gastrointestinal tract. The lymphatic system also filters the fluid at the lymph nodes and removes foreign particles such as bacteria. When lymph flow is obstructed, a condition called *lymphedema* occurs. Involvement of lymphatic structures by malignant tumors and removal of lymph nodes at the time of cancer surgery are common causes of lymphedema.

The lymphatic system is made up of vessels similar to those of the circulatory system. These vessels commonly travel along with an arteriole or venule or with its companion artery and vein. The terminal lymphatic vessels are made up of a single layer of connective tissue with an endothelial lining and resemble blood capillaries. The lymphatic vessels lack tight junctions and are loosely anchored to the surrounding tissues by fine filaments (Fig. 25.20). The loose junctions permit the entry of large particles, and the filaments hold the vessels open under conditions of edema when the pressure of the surrounding tissues would otherwise cause them to collapse. The lymph capillaries drain into larger lymph vessels that ultimately empty into the right and left thoracic ducts (Fig. 25.21). The thoracic ducts empty into the circulation at the junctions of the subclavian and internal jugular veins. The total amount of lymph transported is 2 to 3 L/day in a healthy person.[2]

Although the divisions are not as distinct as in the circulatory system, the larger lymph vessels show evidence of having intimal, medial, and adventitial layers similar to blood vessels. The intima of these channels contains elastic tissue and an endothelial layer, and the larger collecting lymph channels contain smooth muscle in their medial layer. Contraction

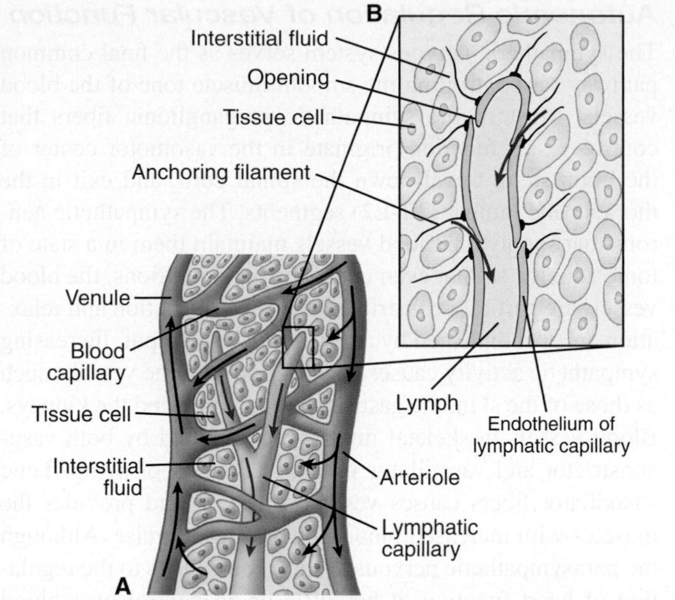

Figure 25.20 • **(A)** Location of the lymphatic capillary. Fluid from the arterial side of the capillary bed moves into the interstitial spaces and is reabsorbed in the venous side of the capillary bed. **(B)** Details of the lymphatic capillary with its anchoring filaments and overlapping edges that serve as valves and can be pushed open, allowing the inflow of interstitial fluid and its suspended particles.

of this smooth muscle assists in propelling lymph toward the thorax. External compression of the lymph channels by pulsating blood vessels in the vicinity and active and passive movements of body parts also aid in forward propulsion of lymph. The interstitial fluid pressure and the activity of lymph pumps determine the rate of flow (approximately 120 mL/hour) through the lymphatic system via all of the various lymph channels.

IN SUMMARY

Exchange of fluids between the vascular compartment and the interstitial spaces occurs at the capillary level. The capillary hydrostatic pressure pushes fluids out of the capillaries, and the colloidal osmotic pressure exerted by the plasma proteins pulls fluids back into the capillaries. Albumin, which is the smallest and most abundant of the plasma proteins, provides the major osmotic force for return of fluid to the vascular compartment. Normally, slightly more fluid leaves the capillary bed than can be reabsorbed. This excess fluid is returned to the circulation by way of the lymphatic channels.

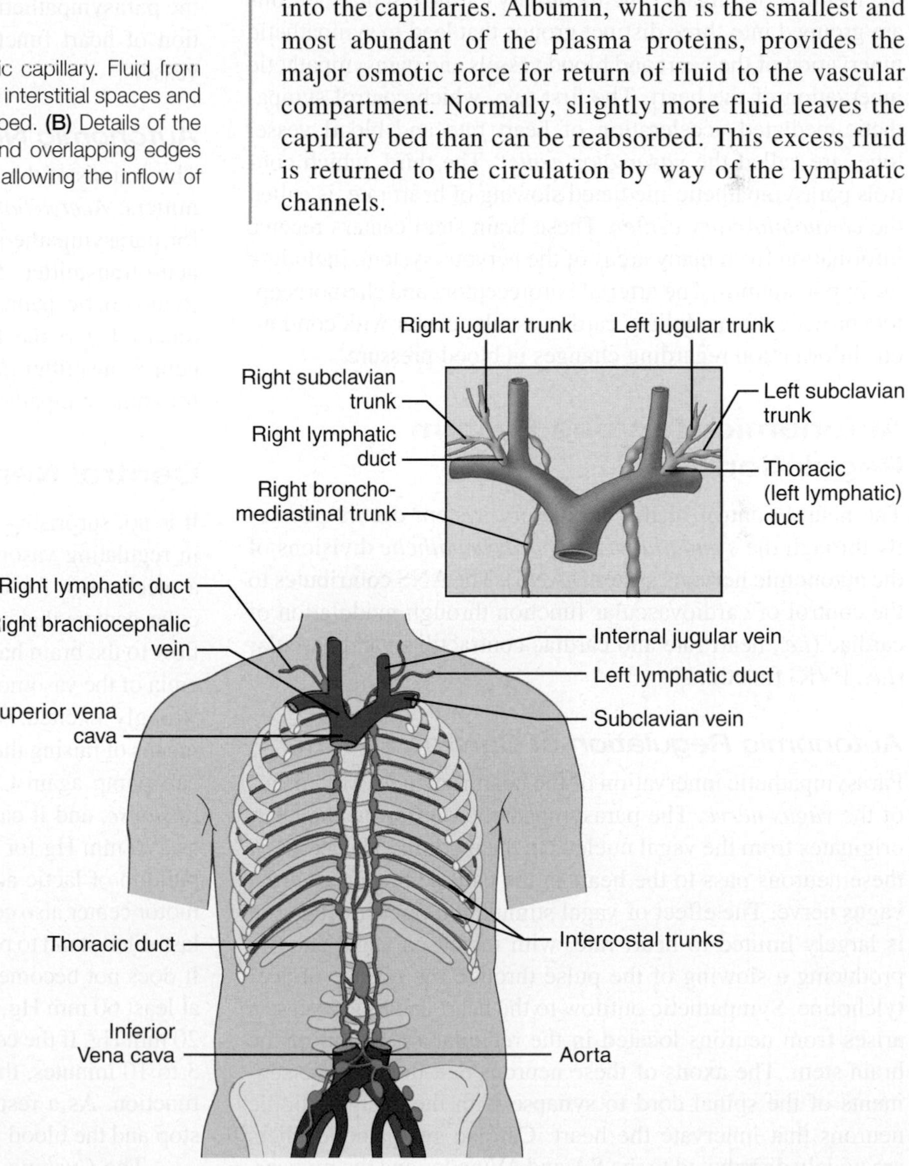

Figure 25.21 • Lymphatic system, showing the thoracic duct and position of the left and right lymphatic ducts **(inset)**.

NEURAL CONTROL OF CIRCULATORY FUNCTION

After completing this section of the chapter, the learner will be able to meet the following objectives:

- Relate the performance of baroreceptors and chemoreceptors in the control of cardiovascular function.
- Describe the distribution of the sympathetic and parasympathetic nervous systems in the innervation of the circulatory system and their effects on heart rate and cardiac contractility.
- Relate the role of the CNS in terms of regulating circulatory function.

The neural control centers for the integration and modulation of cardiac function and blood pressure are located bilaterally in the medulla oblongata. The medullary cardiovascular neurons are grouped into three distinct groups that lead to sympathetic innervation of the heart and blood vessels and parasympathetic innervation of the heart. The first two, which control sympathetic-mediated acceleration of heart rate and blood vessel tone, are called the *vasomotor center*. The third, which controls parasympathetic-mediated slowing of heart rate, is called the *cardioinhibitory center*. These brain stem centers receive information from many areas of the nervous system, including the hypothalamus. The arterial baroreceptors and chemoreceptors provide the medullary cardiovascular center with continuous information regarding changes in blood pressure.

Autonomic Nervous System Regulation

The neural control of the circulatory system occurs primarily through the *sympathetic* and *parasympathetic* divisions of the autonomic nervous system (ANS). The ANS contributes to the control of cardiovascular function through modulation of cardiac (*i.e.*, heart rate and cardiac contractility) and vascular (*i.e.*, PVR) functions.

Autonomic Regulation of Cardiac Function

Parasympathetic innervation of the heart is achieved by means of the *vagus nerve*. The parasympathetic outflow to the heart originates from the vagal nucleus in the medulla. The axons of these neurons pass to the heart in the cardiac branches of the vagus nerve. The effect of vagal stimulation on heart function is largely limited to heart rate, with increased vagal activity producing a slowing of the pulse through the release of acetylcholine. Sympathetic outflow to the heart and blood vessels arises from neurons located in the reticular formation of the brain stem. The axons of these neurons exit the thoracic segments of the spinal cord to synapse with the postganglionic neurons that innervate the heart. Cardiac sympathetic fibers are widely distributed to the SA and AV nodes and the myocardium. Increased sympathetic activity produces an increase in the heart rate and the velocity and force of cardiac contraction.

Autonomic Regulation of Vascular Function

The sympathetic nervous system serves as the final common pathway for controlling the smooth muscle tone of the blood vessels. Most of the sympathetic preganglionic fibers that control vessel function originate in the vasomotor center of the brain stem, travel down the spinal cord, and exit in the thoracic and lumbar (T1-L2) segments. The sympathetic neurons that supply the blood vessels maintain them in a state of tonic activity, so that even under resting conditions, the blood vessels are partially constricted. Vessel constriction and relaxation are accomplished by altering this basal input. Increasing sympathetic activity causes constriction of some vessels, such as those of the skin, the gastrointestinal tract, and the kidneys. Blood vessels in skeletal muscle are supplied by both vasoconstrictor and vasodilator fibers. Activation of sympathetic vasodilator fibers causes vessel relaxation and provides the muscles with increased blood flow during exercise. Although the parasympathetic nervous system contributes to the regulation of heart function, it has little or no control over blood vessels.

Autonomic Neurotransmitters

The actions of the ANS are mediated by chemical neurotransmitters. *Acetylcholine* is the postganglionic neurotransmitter for parasympathetic neurons, and *norepinephrine* is the main neurotransmitter for postganglionic sympathetic neurons. Sympathetic neurons also respond to epinephrine, which is released into the bloodstream by the adrenal medulla. The neurotransmitter *dopamine* can also act as a neurotransmitter for some sympathetic neurons.

Central Nervous System Responses

It is not surprising that the CNS, which plays an essential role in regulating vasomotor tone and blood pressure, would have a mechanism for controlling the blood flow to the cardiovascular centers that control circulatory function. When the blood flow to the brain has been sufficiently interrupted to cause ischemia of the vasomotor center, these vasomotor neurons become strongly excited. This causes massive vasoconstriction as a means of raising the blood pressure to levels as high as the heart can pump against. This response is called the *CNS ischemic response*, and it can raise the blood pressure to levels as high as 270 mm Hg for as long as 10 minutes. It is thought that the buildup of lactic acid and other acidic substances in the vasomotor center also contributes to the CNS ischemic response as a last-ditch stand to preserve the blood flow to vital brain centers.[1] It does not become activated until blood pressure has fallen to at least 60 mm Hg, and it is most effective in the range of 15 to 20 mm Hg. If the cerebral circulation is not reestablished within 3 to 10 minutes, the neurons of the vasomotor center cease to function. As a result, the tonic impulses to the blood vessels stop and the blood pressure falls precipitously.

The *Cushing reaction* is a special type of CNS response resulting from an increase in intracranial pressure.[1,3] When the intracranial pressure rises to levels that equal intra-arterial pressure, blood vessels to the vasomotor center become compressed, initiating the CNS ischemic response. The purpose of this reflex is to produce a rise in arterial pressure to levels above intracranial pressure so that the blood flow to the vasomotor center can be reestablished. Should the intracranial pressure rise to the point that the blood supply to the vasomotor center becomes inadequate, vasoconstrictor tone is lost, and the blood pressure begins to fall. The elevation in blood pressure associated with the Cushing reflex is usually of short duration and should be considered a protective homeostatic mechanism. It helps protect the vital centers of the brain from nutrition loss if the CNS fluid rises high enough to compress the cerebral arteries.[3] The brain and other cerebral structures are located within the rigid confines of the skull, with no room for expansion. Therefore, any increase in intracranial pressure tends to compress the blood vessels that supply the brain.

IN SUMMARY

The neural control centers for the regulation of cardiac function and blood pressure are located in the reticular formation of the lower pons and medulla of the brain stem, where the integration and modulation of ANS responses occur. These brain stem centers receive information from many areas of the nervous system, including the hypothalamus. Both the parasympathetic and sympathetic nervous systems innervate the heart. The parasympathetic nervous system functions in regulating heart rate through the vagus nerve, with increased vagal activity producing a slowing of heart rate. The sympathetic nervous system has an excitatory influence on heart rate and contractility, and it serves as the final common pathway for controlling the smooth muscle tone of the blood vessels.

GERIATRIC Considerations

- With age, the conduction system slows, producing a slower heart rate due to a loss of function of the cells throughout the conduction system.[6]
- With age, the size of the heart increases due to hypertrophy and thickening of the heart wall, leading to a decreased cardiac output as a result of decreased contractility and volume.[6]
- Aging leads to the stiffening of valves, preventing them from closing properly. Murmurs and backflow occur due to the malfunctioning of the stiff valves.[6]
- Stress or a decline in health status due to illness puts an increased demand on the aging heart; the heart is unable to respond as quickly, and the elderly person often experiences fatigue, irregular and pounding heartbeat, and shortness of breath. This can also occur during exercise.[6]

PEDIATRIC Considerations

- Cardiovascular disorders in children are divided into two major categories: congenital heart disease and acquired heart disease.[7] Congenital heart disease (CHD) accounts for the majority of birth defects, with 32,000 babies born annually with CHD defects.[8]
- The etiology of CHD is idiopathic; however, it is believed that there are multifactorial causes such as genetics and maternal exposure to environmental factors.[7]
- When assessing the heart of a child younger than age 7, keep in mind that the heart lies more horizontally with the apex below the fourth intercostal space.[7]
- Harmless murmurs and physiologic splitting of heart sound may be heard in infancy or childhood.[7]
- Many chromosome defects are associated with CHD such as Down syndrome, trisomy 13/18, and cri-du-chat.[7]

REVIEW EXERCISES

1. In people with atherosclerosis of the coronary arteries, symptoms of myocardial ischemia do not usually occur until the vessel has been 75% occluded.
   A. *Use the Poiseuille law to explain.*
2. Once an arterial aneurysm has begun to form, it continues to enlarge as the result of the increased tension in its wall.
   A. *Explain the continued increase in size using the law of Laplace.*
   B. *Using information related to cross-sectional area and velocity of flow, explain why there is stasis of blood flow with the tendency to form clots in aneurysms with a large cross-sectional area.*
3. Use events in the cardiac cycle depicted in Figure 25.10 to explain.
   A. *The effect of hypertension on the isovolumetric contraction period*
   B. *The effect of an increase in heart rate on the time spent in diastole*
   C. *The effect of an increase in the isovolumetric relaxation period on the diastolic filling of the ventricle*

(Continued)

4. Use the Frank-Starling ventricular function curve depicted in Figure 25.11 to explain the changes in cardiac output that occur with changes in respiratory effort.
   A. *What happens to cardiac output during increased inspiratory effort in which a marked decrease in intrathoracic pressure produces an increase in venous return to the right heart?*
   B. *What happens to cardiac output during increased expiratory effort in which a marked increase in intrathoracic pressure produces a decrease in venous return to the right heart?*
   C. *Given these changes in cardiac output that occur during increased respiratory effort, what would you propose as one of the functions of the Frank-Starling curve?*

References

1. St. John S., Cerkvenic J., Borlaug B., et al. (2015). Effects of cardiac resynchronization therapy on cardiac remodeling and contractile function: results from resynchronization reverses remodeling in systolic left ventricular dysfunction (REVERSE). *Journal of the American Heart Association* 4(9), 1–9.
2. Mohrman D., Heller L. (2010). *Cardiovascular physiology* (7th ed.). New York: McGraw-Hill.
3. Guyton A., Hall J. E. (2011). *Textbook of medical physiology* (12th ed., pp. 157–189, 191–211). Philadelphia, PA: Saunders.
4. Freeman W., Kobayashi Y. (2016). Invasive assessment of the coronary microcirculation. *JACC: Cardiovascular Interventions* 25(9), 802–804.
5. Yolmaz-Erol A., Atasever B., Mathura K., et al. (2007). Cardiac resynchronization improves microcirculation. *Journal of Cardiac Failure* 13(2), 95–99.
6. Brunner, L. S., Suddarth, D. S., Smeltzer, S. O., et al. (2018). *Brunner and Suddarth's textbook of medical-surgical nursing* (14th ed., p. 678). Philadelphia, PA: Lippincott.
7. Kyle T., Carman S. (2017). *Essentials of pediatric nursing* (3rd ed., pp. 652–700). Philadelphia, PA: Wolters Kluwer.
8. American Heart Association. (2015). *Understand your risk for congenital heart defects*. Available: http://www.heart.org/HEARTORG/Conditions/CongenitalHeartDefects/UnderstandYourRiskforCongenitalHeartDefects/Understand-Your-Risk-for-Congenital-Heart-Defects_UCM_001219_Article.jsp#.WfDsRohryUk.

Disorders of Blood Flow and Blood Pressure Regulation

26

Linda C. Mefford

Blood flow through the systemic circulatory system depends on a system of patent blood vessels and adequate perfusion pressure. Structural disorders of the arteries and arterioles decrease blood flow to the tissues, causing impaired delivery of oxygen and nutrients and leading to the accumulation of waste products from cellular metabolism. Venous structural disorders interfere with the outflow of blood from capillary beds, causing both fluid and cellular waste products to be trapped in the tissues. Disturbances in blood flow can result from pathologic changes in the vessel wall, vascular obstruction, vasospasm, or vasodilation.

Blood pressure is highly variable and must be carefully regulated to ensure adequate perfusion to all cells of the body.

Assuring a constant flow of blood to vital organs such as the heart, brain, and kidneys is essential to life. Although a critical decrease in blood flow (hypotension) can produce an immediate threat to life, a continuous elevation of blood pressure (hypertension) contributes to premature death and disability because of the damaging effects of elevated pressure on blood vessels.

BLOOD VESSEL STRUCTURE AND FUNCTION

After completing this section of the chapter, the learner will be able to meet the following objectives:

- Describe the functions of the endothelial cells and define the term *endothelial dysfunction.*
- Describe the function of vascular smooth muscle and its role in vascular repair.

The walls of all blood vessels except the capillaries are composed of three distinct layers: (1) an outer layer of loosely woven connective collagen tissue (the *tunica externa*); (2) a middle layer of circumferentially arranged layers of smooth muscle cells, or SMCs (the *tunica media*); and (3) an inner layer consisting of a single layer of endothelial cells and underlying subendothelial connective tissue (the *tunica intima*). The thin capillaries consist of a single layer of endothelial cells surrounded intermittently by cells called *pericytes.* These pericytes share some characteristics that are similar to SMCs.[1] Figure 26.1 illustrates the layers of the arterial walls, including differences among the three layers of tunica. Figure 26.2

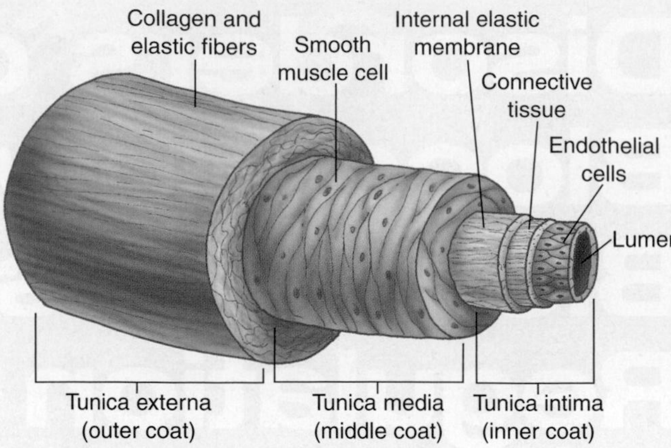

Figure 26.1 • Diagram of a typical artery showing the tunica externa, tunica media, and tunica intima.

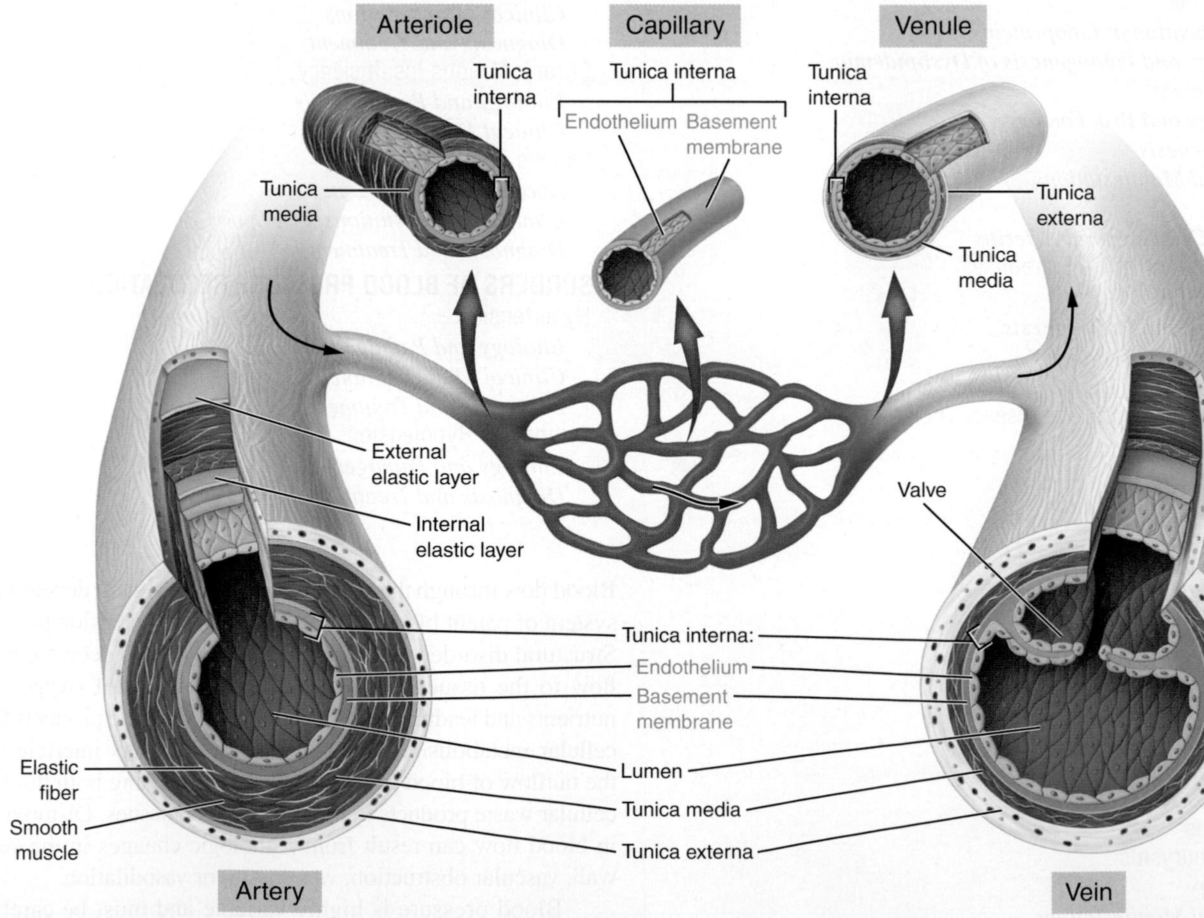

Figure 26.2 • Blood vessels—microanatomy of the artery, vein, and capillary beds. (From McConnell T. H., Hull K. L. (2011). *Human form, human function: Essentials of anatomy & physiology*. (Figure 11-12, p. 433). Philadelphia, PA: Wolters Kluwer/Lippincott Williams & Wilkins.)

TABLE 26.1 THE STRUCTURE AND FUNCTION OF THE BLOOD VESSELS

VESSEL	STRUCTURE	FUNCTION
Artery	Three-layered wall with thick tunica media, which gives it the properties of contractility and elasticity	Transport of blood away from the heart, maintenance of blood pressure
Arteriole	Three-layered wall, with much thinner layers and smaller lumen than in arteries	Transport of blood away from the heart, help control blood pressure by regulation of peripheral resistance through vasoconstriction and vasodilation
Capillary	Microscopic size with single-layered wall of endothelium	Thin walls permit the exchange of materials between the blood and interstitial fluid
Venule	Three-layered wall with very thin layers, which gradually enlarge as they near the heart	Transport of blood from capillary beds toward the heart
Vein	Three-layered wall, with thinner tunica media and larger lumen than in arteries. Include internal valves to aid in the unidirectional flow of blood toward the heart	Transport of blood from venules toward the heart

From Wingerd B. (2014). *The human body: Concepts of anatomy and physiology*. Philadelphia, PA: Lippincott Williams & Wilkins.

illustrates the comparative microanatomy of veins, arteries, and capillaries. Table 26.1 describes the structure and function of the blood vessels.

Endothelium

Approximately 60,000 miles of specialized squamous epithelial cells form a continuous lining for the entire vascular system called the *endothelium*.[2] Endothelium is a versatile, multifunctional tissue that plays an active role in controlling vascular function. This semipermeable membrane plays essential roles in homeostatic functions such as transfer of molecules across the vascular wall, platelet adhesion and blood clotting, modulation of blood flow and vascular resistance, metabolism of hormones, regulation of immune and inflammatory reactions, and elaboration of factors that influence the growth of other cell types (particularly vascular SMCs).[3]

Endothelial cells respond to various stimuli by structural and functional alterations, collectively described by the term *endothelial dysfunction*. Endothelial dysfunction can be caused by factors such as inflammation, hemodynamic stress, certain lipid molecules, and hypoxia. Dysfunctional endothelial cells secrete cytokines, growth factors, procoagulant or anticoagulant factors, and a variety of other biologically active products. They also influence the reactivity of the underlying SMCs through production of both relaxing factors (*e.g.*, nitric oxide) and contracting factors (*e.g.*, endothelins).[1,2]

Vascular Smooth Muscle Cells

Vascular SMCs in the tunica media constrict and dilate blood vessels in response to hormonal and neural stimulation (particularly in response to the sympathetic branch of the autonomic nervous system [ANS]). Nerves do not enter the tunica media to directly synapse with vascular SMCs; instead, the neurotransmitter norepinephrine diffuses into the tunica media. The resulting action potentials are propagated along the SMCs through gap junctions, causing contraction of the entire muscle layer and thus reducing the radius of the vessel lumen. This decreased radius then increases the resistance to flow through the vessel.[2]

Vascular SMCs also synthesize biologic molecules such as collagen, elastin, growth factors, and cytokines. When injured, SMCs migrate into the tunica intima, where they proliferate.[1] Thus, SMCs are important in both normal vascular repair and pathologic processes such as atherosclerosis. Growth promoters and inhibitors stimulate the migratory and proliferative activities of vascular SMCs. Growth promoters include platelet-derived growth factor, thrombin, fibroblast growth factor, and cytokines such as interferon gamma and interleukin-1. Growth inhibitors include nitric oxide.[3,4]

IN SUMMARY

With the exception of capillaries, the walls of blood vessels are composed of three layers—an outer layer of loosely woven connective tissue, a middle layer of vascular smooth muscle, and an inner layer of endothelial cells. Capillaries are composed only of a single layer of endothelial cells. Vascular endothelial cells control the transfer of molecules across capillary walls and are also actively involved in modulating the processes of platelet adhesion and coagulation, as well as in regulating blood flow and vascular resistance. Endothelial cells also play a role in regulating immune and inflammatory reactions and elaborating factors that serve as hormones and growth factors (particularly growth factors that influence the SMCs). Many of the factors produced by vascular SMCs are important in both normal vascular repair and pathologic processes such as atherosclerosis. The term *endothelial dysfunction* describes several types of potentially reversible changes in endothelial function that occurs in response to environmental stimuli.

REGULATION OF SYSTEMIC ARTERIAL BLOOD PRESSURE

After completing this section of the chapter, the learner will be able to meet the following objectives:

- Define the terms *systolic blood pressure, diastolic blood pressure, pulse pressure*, and *mean arterial blood pressure.*
- Explain how cardiac output (CO) and peripheral vascular resistance (PVR) interact in determining systolic and diastolic blood pressure.

In a person with a healthy heart, blood is continually being rhythmically ejected into the systemic circulation from the left ventricle into the aorta. Blood pressure rises during systole (as the left ventricle contracts) and falls as the heart relaxes during diastole. The contour of the arterial pressure tracing shown in Figure 26.3 illustrates the pressure changes that typically occur within the large arteries of the systemic circulation. A rapid upstroke in the pulse contour occurs during left ventricular contraction, followed by a slower rise to the peak blood pressure. Approximately 70% of the blood that leaves the left ventricle is ejected during the first one third of systole, accounting for the rapid rise in the pressure contour. The end of systole is marked by a brief downward deflection and formation of the *dicrotic notch*, reflecting the point at which ventricular pressure falls below aortic pressure. That pressure change triggers the sudden closure of the aortic valve, which then leads to a small rise in intra-aortic pressure resulting from the continued contraction of the aorta and other large vessels against the closed aortic valve. As the ventricles relax and blood flows into the peripheral vessels during diastole, the arterial pressure falls rapidly at first, then continues to decline more slowly as the driving force decreases.[3]

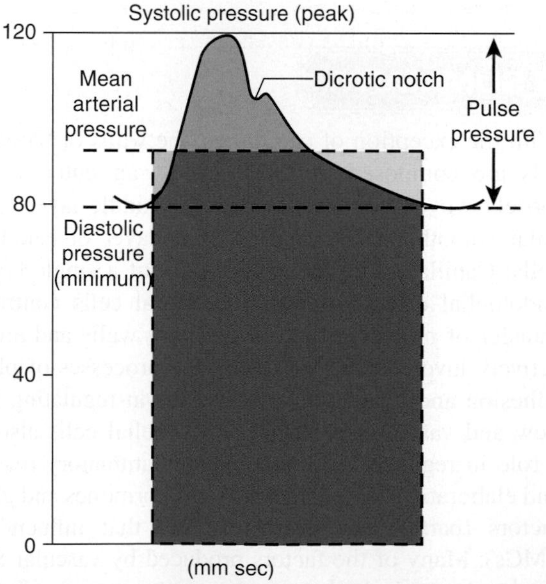

Figure 26.3 • Intra-arterial pressure tracing made from the brachial artery. Pulse pressure is the difference between systolic and diastolic pressures. The darker area represents the MAP, which can be calculated by using the formula of mean arterial pressure = diastolic pressure + pulse pressure/3.

The pressure at the height of the pressure pulse (the *systolic pressure*) ideally is less than 120 mm Hg in adults, with the lowest pressure (the *diastolic pressure*) less than 80 mm Hg (Fig. 26.3). The difference between systolic and diastolic pressures (approximately 40 mm Hg in healthy adults) is called the *pulse pressure.* Two major factors affect the magnitude of the pulse pressure—the volume of blood ejected from the left ventricle during a single beat (the *stroke volume*) and the degree of total distensibility within the arterial tree (reflecting the ability of the arterial vasculature to accept the blood ejected from the heart). Arterial distensibility is determined by the combination of (1) the elastic properties of the aorta and large arteries and (2) the degree of resistance to flow into the smaller vessels. The *mean arterial pressure (MAP)*, which is approximately 90 to 100 mm Hg in adults, is a measure of the average pressure in the arterial system during ventricular contraction and relaxation. MAP serves as a good indicator of tissue perfusion and is determined by 60% of the diastolic pressure and 40% of the systolic pressure. Notice that MAP is not a simple mathematical average of systolic and diastolic pressures because a greater fraction of each cardiac cycle is spent in diastole (relaxation) than in systole (contraction).[3]

MAP is a function of CO and PVR. The components of CO are stroke volume (SV) and heart rate (HR), expressed mathematically by the equation: CO = SV × HR. Therefore, MAP can be expressed mathematically as follows: MAP = CO × PVR. The PVR reflects both changes in the radius of the arterioles and the viscosity (thickness) of the blood. The arterioles often are referred to as the *resistance vessels* because they can selectively constrict or relax to control the resistance to outflow of blood into the capillaries. The body maintains its blood pressure by (a) adjusting CO to compensate for changes in PVR and (b) adjusting PVR to compensate for changes in CO.[3]

Mechanisms of Blood Pressure Regulation

Although different tissues in the body have some capability to autoregulate their own blood flow, it is necessary for the arterial pressure to remain relatively constant to ensure adequate tissue perfusion. The mechanisms used to regulate arterial pressure depend on whether acute control or long-term control is needed.[3] (See Fig. 26.4.)

Acute Regulation

Acute regulation of blood pressure (over seconds to minutes) is necessary to correct temporary imbalances, such as during physical exercise or changes in body position. These acute regulatory mechanisms also maintain blood pressure at survival levels during life-threatening situations. The acute control of blood pressure relies mainly on neural and humoral mechanisms, with neural mechanisms producing the most rapid response.[3]

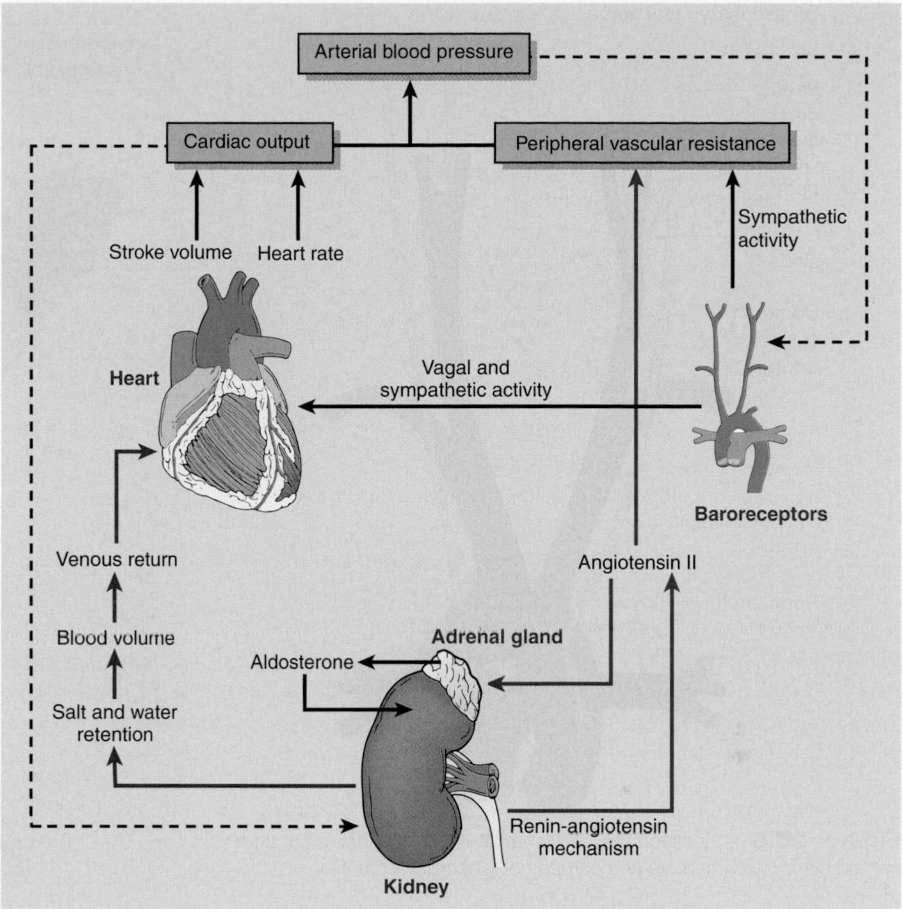

Figure 26.4 • Mechanisms of blood pressure regulation. The *solid lines* represent the mechanisms for renal and baroreceptor control of blood pressure through changes in CO and PVR. The *dashed lines* represent the stimulus for regulation of blood pressure by the baroreceptors and the kidneys.

Neural Mechanisms. The neural control centers for blood pressure regulation are located in the reticular formation of the medulla and the lower third of the pons, where integration and modulation of ANS responses occur. This area of the brain contains the vasomotor and cardiac control centers, often collectively referred to as the *cardiovascular center.* The cardiovascular center transmits parasympathetic impulses to the heart through the vagus nerve and sympathetic impulses to the heart and blood vessels through the spinal cord and peripheral sympathetic nerves. Vagal stimulation of the heart produces a slowing of HR, whereas sympathetic stimulation produces increases in both HR and cardiac contractility. Blood vessels are selectively innervated by the sympathetic nervous system (SNS). Increased sympathetic activity produces constriction of the small arteries and arterioles with a resultant increase in PVR.[3]

The ANS control of blood pressure is mediated through intrinsic circulatory reflexes, extrinsic reflexes, and higher neural control centers. The circulatory *intrinsic reflexes*, including the *baroreceptor* and *chemoreceptor reflexes*, are controlled within the circulatory system and are essential for rapid and short-term regulation of blood pressure. The sensors for *extrinsic reflexes* are found outside the circulation. These extrinsic reflexes include blood pressure responses associated with factors such as pain and cold. The neural pathways for these reactions are more diffuse, and their responses are less consistent than those of the intrinsic reflexes. Many of these responses are channeled through the hypothalamus, which plays an essential role in the control of SNS responses. Examples of higher neural control include blood pressure responses caused by variations in mood and emotion.[3]

The *baroreceptors or pressoreceptors* are pressure-sensitive receptors located in the walls of blood vessels and the heart. The carotid and aortic baroreceptors are located in strategic positions between the heart and the brain (Fig. 26.5). They respond to changes in the stretch of the vessel wall by sending impulses to the cardiovascular centers in the brain stem to effect appropriate changes in HR, strength of cardiac contraction, and vascular smooth muscle tone. For example, the fall in blood pressure that occurs on moving from the lying to the standing position produces a decrease in the stretch of the baroreceptors. This triggers a resultant increase in HR and a sympathetically induced vasoconstriction that produces an increase in PVR.[3]

The *arterial chemoreceptors* are chemosensitive cells that monitor blood levels of oxygen, carbon dioxide, and hydrogen ions. These chemoreceptors are located in the carotid bodies (which lie in the bifurcation of the two common carotid arteries) and in the aortic bodies of the aorta (see Fig. 26.5). Because of their locations, these chemoreceptors are always in close contact with arterial blood. Although the

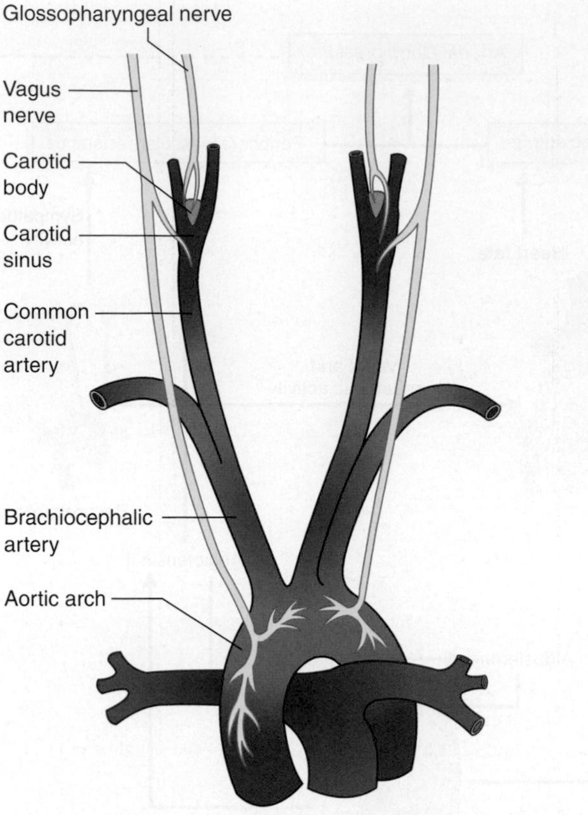

Figure 26.5 • Location and innervation of the aortic arch and carotid sinus baroreceptors and carotid body chemoreceptors.

main function of the chemoreceptors is to regulate ventilation, they also communicate with cardiovascular centers in the brain stem and can induce widespread vasoconstriction. Whenever the arterial blood pressure drops below a critical level, the chemoreceptors are stimulated because of diminished oxygen supply and a buildup of carbon dioxide and hydrogen ions.[3] In people with chronic lung disease, systemic and pulmonary hypertension may develop in response to hypoxemia. People with sleep apnea may also experience an increase in blood pressure because of the hypoxemia that occurs during the apneic periods.[1,4–6]

Humoral Mechanisms. A number of humoral mechanisms contribute to blood pressure regulation, including the *renin–angiotensin–aldosterone system*, *vasopressin* (also called *Antidiuretic Hormone*), and *epinephrine/norepinephrine.* These substances acutely regulate blood pressure by altering vascular tone. Norepinephrine/epinephrine also modifies blood pressure by increasing HR and cardiac contractility.[3]

The *renin–angiotensin–aldosterone system* plays a central role in blood pressure regulation. Renin is an enzyme that is synthesized, stored, and released by the juxtaglomerular cells of the kidneys. Renin release occurs in response to increased SNS activity or decreased blood pressure, extracellular fluid volume, or extracellular sodium concentration. Most of the renin leaves the kidney and enters the bloodstream, where it acts enzymatically to convert an inactive circulating plasma protein called *angiotensinogen* to angiotensin I (Fig. 26.6). Angiotensin I is then converted to angiotensin II. This conversion occurs almost entirely while blood is flowing through the lungs, catalyzed by an enzyme called the *angiotensin-converting enzyme* (ACE) produced in the endothelium of the blood vessels of the lung. Although angiotensin II has a half-life of only several minutes, renin persists in the circulation for 30 minutes to 1 hour, leading to

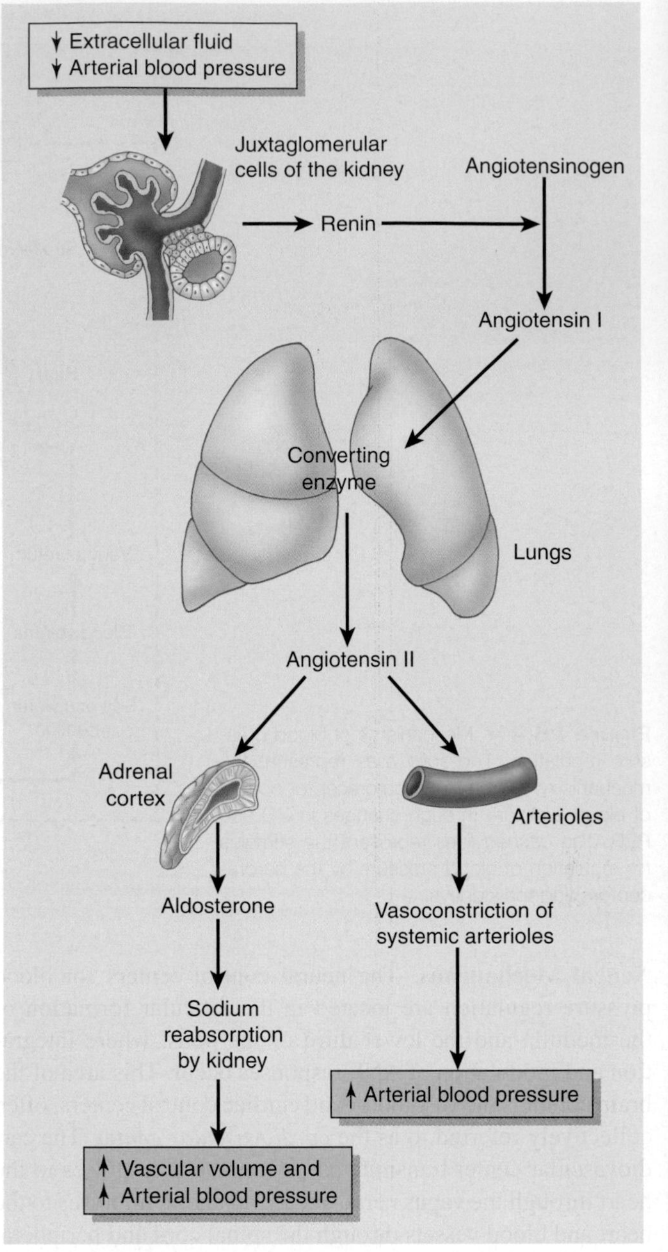

Figure 26.6 • Control of blood pressure by the renin–angiotensin–aldosterone system. Renin enzymatically converts the plasma protein angiotensinogen to angiotensin I; ACE in the lung converts angiotensin I to angiotensin II; and angiotensin II produces vasoconstriction and increases salt and water retention through direct action on the kidney and through increased aldosterone secretion by the adrenal cortex.

Understanding Determinants of Blood Pressure

The arterial blood pressure is the force that moves blood through the arterial system, reflecting the intermittent contraction and relaxation of the left ventricle. It is determined by factors including the blood volume, elastic properties of the blood vessels, CO, and PVR.

Arterial Blood Pressure

The arterial blood pressure represents the force that distributes blood to the capillaries throughout the body. The highest arterial pressure is the systolic pressure (coinciding with ventricular contraction), and the lowest is the diastolic pressure (coinciding with ventricular relaxation). The aorta and its major branches conduct blood between the heart and the arterioles. The arterioles, which are the terminal components of the arterial system, serve as resistance vessels that regulate the distribution of blood to the capillary beds. Because the arteries are fairly compliant and the arterioles provide high resistance to blood flow, the arterial system acts as a filter that converts the pulsatile flow generated by the heart into a more steady, nonpulsating flow through the capillaries. As blood exits the capillary beds, the low-pressure venous system collects blood and then returns it to the heart, thus maintaining the diastolic filling pressure needed to produce an adequate CO to repeat the process of filling the arterial tree with blood.

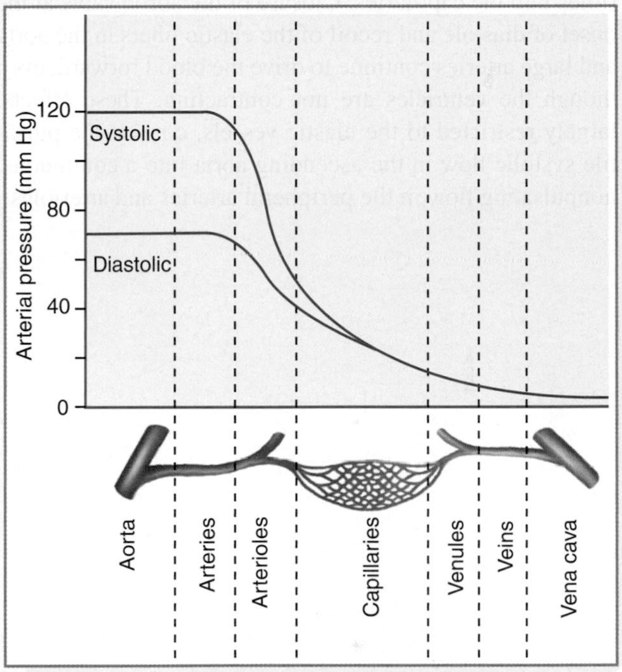

Systolic Pressure

The systolic blood pressure reflects the combined factors of (a) the volume of blood (SV) ejected from the ventricles with each beat; (b) the rate and force with which the blood is ejected; and (c) the elasticity, or compliance, of the aorta and large arteries. The blood ejected from the heart during systole does not move directly through the entire circulation. Instead, a substantial fraction of the SV is stored in large arteries. Because the walls of these vessels are elastic, they can be stretched to accommodate a large volume of blood without an appreciable change in pressure. The systolic pressure often increases with aging as the aorta and large arteries lose their elasticity and become more rigid.

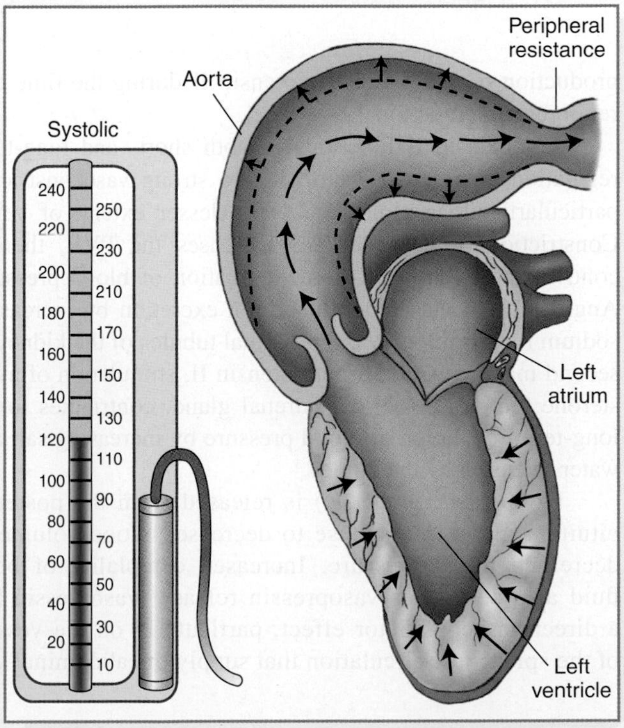

Continued

Understanding Determinants of Blood Pressure *(Continued)*

Diastolic Pressure

The diastolic blood pressure reflects the combined factors of (a) the closure of the aortic valve, (b) the energy that has been stored in the elastic fibers of the large arteries during systole, and (c) the resistance to flow through arterioles into the capillaries. Closure of the aortic valve at the onset of diastole and recoil of the elastic fibers in the aorta and large arteries continue to drive the blood forward, even though the ventricles are not contracting. These effects, largely restricted to the elastic vessels, convert the pulsatile systolic flow in the ascending aorta into a continuous, nonpulsating flow in the peripheral arteries and arterioles.

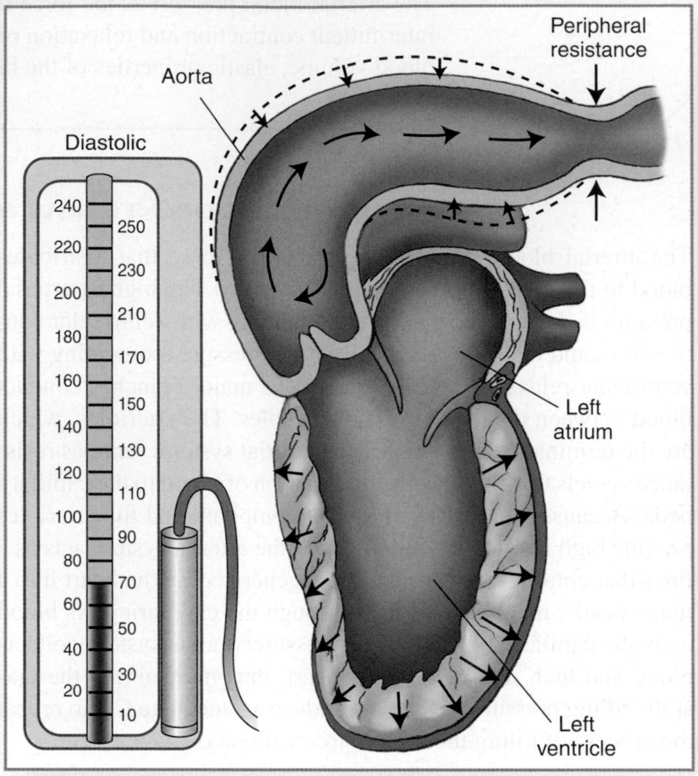

production of additional angiotensin II during the time that renin remains functional.[3]

Angiotensin II functions in both short- and long-term regulation of blood pressure. It is a strong vasoconstrictor, particularly of arterioles and, to a lesser extent, of veins. Constriction of the arterioles increases the PVR, thereby contributing to the short-term regulation of blood pressure. Angiotensin II also reduces sodium excretion by increasing sodium reabsorption by the proximal tubules of the kidney. A second major function of angiotensin II, stimulation of aldosterone secretion from the adrenal gland, contributes to the long-term regulation of blood pressure by increasing salt and water retention by the kidney.[3]

Vasopressin (or ADH) is released from the posterior pituitary gland in response to decreased blood volume or decreased blood pressure. Increased osmolality of body fluid also stimulates vasopressin release. Vasopressin has a direct vasoconstrictor effect, particularly on the vessels of the splanchnic circulation that supply the abdominal viscera. However, long-term increases in vasopressin cannot maintain an increase in blood pressure. Vasopressin does not contribute to the hypertension produced by sodium-retaining hormones or other vasoconstricting substances. It has been suggested that vasopressin plays a permissive role in hypertension through its water-retaining properties or as a neurotransmitter that serves to modify ANS function.[3] The antidiuretic actions of vasopressin are discussed in Chapter 32.

The catecholamines epinephrine and, to a lesser extent, norepinephrine are released from the adrenal gland into the bloodstream when the SNS is activated. These catecholamine molecules increase blood pressure by inducing vasoconstriction and by increasing HR and cardiac contractility.[3]

Long-Term Regulation

Long-term mechanisms control the daily, weekly, and monthly regulation of blood pressure. Although the neural and hormonal mechanisms involved in the short-term regulation of blood pressure act rapidly, they are unable to maintain their effectiveness over time. Instead, the long-term regulation of blood pressure is largely vested in the kidneys and their role in the regulation of the extracellular fluid volume.[3]

Extracellular fluid volume and arterial blood pressure are regulated around an equilibrium point, representing the normal pressure for a given person.[3] When the body contains excess extracellular fluid because of increased water and salt intake, the arterial pressure rises. This rise in arterial pressure results in increases in the rate at which the kidneys excrete both water (*i.e., pressure diuresis*) and salt (*i.e., pressure natriuresis*). According to this model of kidney function, arterial pressure can be increased by two mechanisms: (a) shifting the elimination of salt and water to a higher pressure level and (b) changing the extracellular fluid level at which diuresis and natriuresis occur. A number of factors can influence the function of the kidneys in the long-term regulation of blood pressure. For example, excess sympathetic nerve activity or the release of vasoconstrictor substances can alter the transmission of arterial pressure to the kidney. Similarly, changes in neural and humoral control of kidney function can shift the diuresis–natriuresis process to a higher fluid or pressure level, thereby initiating an increase in arterial pressur.[3]

An increase in fluid volume can elevate blood pressure by two general mechanisms: (a) through a direct effect on the preload component of CO and (b) through an indirect effect on PVR through the mechanisms that autoregulate blood flow. Autoregulatory mechanisms distribute blood flow to the various tissues of the body according to their metabolic needs. When the blood flow to a specific tissue bed is excessive, local blood vessels constrict, and when the flow is deficient, the local vessels dilate. This is what is meant by autoregulation of blood flow. In situations of increased extracellular fluid volume with a resultant increase in CO, all of the tissues of the body are exposed to the same increase in flow. This results in a generalized constriction of arterioles and an increase in the PVR (and blood pressure).[3]

Circadian Variations in Blood Pressure

These acute and chronic mechanisms attempt to regulate blood pressure around a particular set point. However, this set point varies in a characteristic circadian pattern, with nocturnal blood pressure tending to decline by 10% to 20%. A decrease in nocturnal dipping of blood pressure has been shown to be a useful predictor of the likelihood of adverse cardiovascular events (with a decline in nocturnal blood pressure dipping serving as a stronger predictor of adverse cardiac effects than daytime blood pressure levels). The degree of nocturnal blood pressure dipping has been noted to decrease in people who repetitively experience shortened sleep periods, reflecting an increased risk for cardiovascular problems in people who do not get adequate sleep.[7]

IN SUMMARY

The alternating contraction and relaxation of ventricular muscle produce a pressure pulse that moves blood through the circulatory system. The elastic walls of the aorta stretch during systole and relax during diastole to maintain the diastolic pressure. The *systolic blood pressure* denotes the highest point of the pressure pulse and the *diastolic blood pressure* the lowest point. The *pulse pressure* (which reflects the pulsatile nature of arterial blood flow) is the difference between the systolic and diastolic pressures. The *MAP* is the average blood pressure in the systemic circulation. Systolic pressure is determined primarily by the characteristics of the *SV*, whereas diastolic pressure is determined largely by the *PVR*, reflecting the condition of the arteries and arterioles and their abilities to accept the runoff of blood from the aorta.

The regulation of blood pressure involves both acute and long-term mechanisms. The acute mechanisms are responsible for regulating blood pressure on a minute-by-minute or hour-by-hour basis during activities such as physical exercise and changes in body position. The acute regulation of blood pressure relies mainly on neural and humoral mechanisms, the most rapid of which are the neural mechanisms. The long-term mechanisms, those maintaining blood pressure over days, weeks, and even years, are largely vested in the kidney and the regulation of extracellular fluid volume.

DISORDERS OF SYSTEMIC ARTERIAL BLOOD FLOW

After completing this section of the chapter, the learner will be able to meet the following objectives:

- Describe possible mechanisms involved in the development of atherosclerosis.
- Describe the pathology associated with the vasculitides and relate it to disease conditions associated with vasculitis.
- Distinguish between the pathology and manifestations of aortic aneurysms and dissection of the aorta.

The arterial system distributes blood to all the tissues in the body. There are three types of arteries: large elastic arteries, including the aorta and its distal branches; medium-sized arteries, such as the coronary and renal arteries; and small arteries and arterioles that pass through the tissues. The large arteries function mainly in transport of blood. The medium-sized arteries are composed predominantly of circular and spirally arranged SMCs. Distribution of blood flow to the various organs and tissues of the body is controlled by contraction and relaxation of the smooth muscle of these vessels. The small arteries and arterioles regulate capillary blood flow. Each of these different types of arteries tends to be affected by different disease processes.[1,3,4]

Disease of the arterial system affects body function by impairing blood flow. The effect of impaired blood flow on the body depends on the structures involved and the extent of altered flow. The term *ischemia* denotes a reduction in arterial flow to a level that is insufficient to meet the oxygen demands of the tissues. *Infarction* refers to an area of ischemic necrosis in an organ produced by occlusion of its arterial blood supply or its venous drainage. The discussion in this section focuses on blood lipids and dyslipidemia, atherosclerosis, vasculitis, arterial disease of the extremities, and arterial aneurysms.

KEY POINTS

DISORDERS OF SYSTEMIC ARTERIAL BLOOD FLOW

- Atherosclerosis is a progressive disease characterized by the formation of fibrofatty plaques in the intima of large- and medium-sized vessels, including the aorta, coronary arteries, and cerebral vessels. The major risk factors for atherosclerosis are hypercholesterolemia and inflammation.
- Vasculitis is an inflammation of the blood vessel wall resulting in vascular tissue injury and necrosis. Arteries, capillaries, and veins may be affected. The inflammatory process may be initiated by direct injury, infectious agents, or immune processes.
- Aneurysms represent an abnormal localized dilatation of an artery because of a weakness in the vessel wall. As the aneurysm increases in size, the tension in the wall of the vessel increases, and it may rupture. The increased size of the vessel may also exert pressure on adjacent structures.

Dyslipidemia

Dyslipidemia refers to a condition of imbalance of the lipid components of the blood. Hyperlipidemia is an excess of lipids in the blood. Lipids are classified as triglycerides, phospholipids, and cholesterol. They are a diverse group of compounds that have many key biologic functions. Triglycerides, which are used in energy metabolism, are combinations of three fatty acids and a single glycerol molecule. Phospholipids, which contain a phosphate group, are important structural constituents of lipoproteins, blood-clotting components, the myelin sheath, and cell membranes. Although cholesterol is not composed of fatty acids, its steroid nucleus is synthesized from fatty acids, and thus, its chemical and physical activity is similar to that of other lipid substances.[3]

Classification of Lipoproteins

Because cholesterol and triglyceride are hydrophobic molecules that are insoluble in plasma, they combine with specific water-soluble proteins called *apoproteins*. This binding with apoproteins allows the creation of a water-soluble molecule that can travel through the plasma. The hydrophobic fat-based molecules (i.e., cholesterol and triglycerides) and the apoproteins combine to form a transport molecule called a *lipoprotein*. The structure of the lipoprotein is a hydrophobic core encapsulated by a stabilizing coat composed of the water-soluble apoproteins and the hydrophilic heads of phospholipids. These lipoproteins transport cholesterol and triglycerides to various tissues for energy utilization, lipid deposition, steroid hormone production, and bile acid formation.[3] The molecular structure of these lipoprotein particles is illustrated in Figure 26.7.

Lipoproteins are classified into five types according to their densities as measured by ultracentrifugation: chylomicrons, very-low-density lipoprotein (VLDL), intermediate-density lipoprotein (IDL), low-density lipoprotein (LDL), and high-density lipoprotein (HDL). VLDL carries large amounts of triglycerides that have a lower density than cholesterol. LDL is the main carrier of cholesterol, whereas HDL is actually 50% protein (Fig. 26.8).[3]

It is the apoproteins within the lipoprotein particle that seem to control the interactions and ultimate metabolic fate of the lipoproteins. Various classes and subtypes of apoproteins have been identified. In particular, elevated levels of the subtype lipoprotein(a) are increasingly linked through research to a variety of pathophysiologic conditions, including atherosclerosis, atherosclerotic coronary vascular disease, calcific aortic valve stenosis, and autoimmune disorders.[8–10] Apolipoprotein (aproprotein B) combines with the lipids to carry them throughout the vascular system. Its involvement in the metabolism of lipids (fats) and role as the primary protein of VLDL and LDL contributes to plaque formation and atherosclerosis.

Two sites of lipoprotein synthesis have been identified—the small intestine and the liver. The chylomicrons, which are the largest of the lipoprotein molecules, are synthesized in the wall of the small intestine. They are involved in the

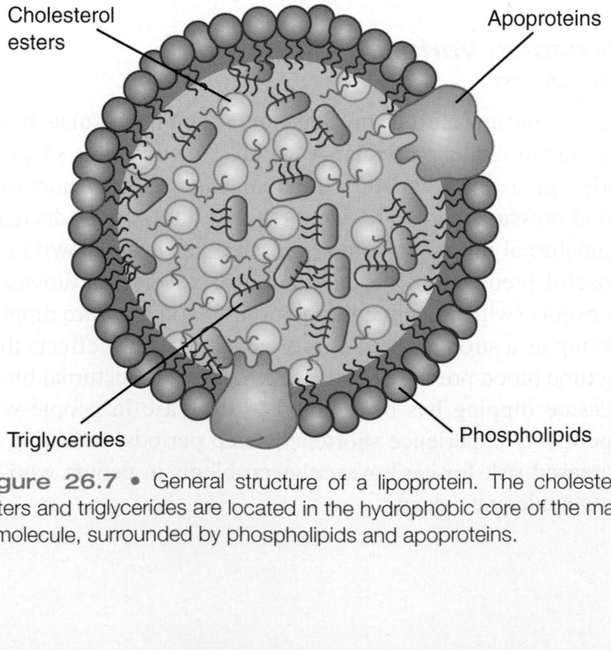

Figure 26.7 • General structure of a lipoprotein. The cholesterol esters and triglycerides are located in the hydrophobic core of the macromolecule, surrounded by phospholipids and apoproteins.

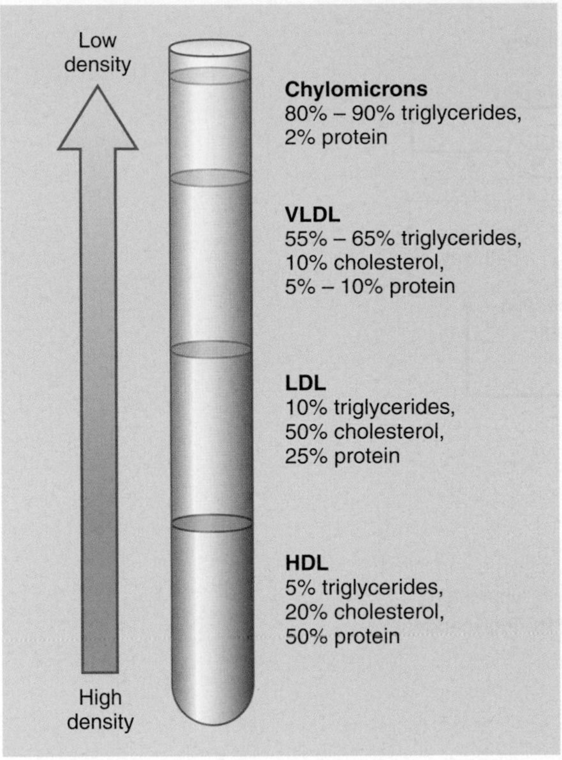

Figure 26.8 • Lipoproteins are named based on their protein content, which is measured in density. Because fats are less dense than proteins, as the proportion of triglycerides decreases, the density increases.

transport of dietary (exogenous pathway) triglycerides and cholesterol that have been absorbed from the gastrointestinal tract. Chylomicrons transfer their triglycerides to the cells of adipose and skeletal muscle tissue. Cholesterol remains in the remnant chylomicron particles after the triglycerides are removed. Ultimately, the residual cholesterol is then taken up by the liver, which synthesizes it for the development of VLDL and/or excretes it in the bile.[3]

The liver synthesizes and releases VLDL and HDL. The VLDLs contain large amounts of triglycerides and lesser amounts of cholesterol esters and provide the primary pathway for transport of the endogenous triglycerides produced in the liver.[1] VLDLs also serve as the body's main source of energy during prolonged fasting. Like chylomicrons, VLDLs carry their triglycerides to fat and muscle cells, where the triglycerides are removed. The resulting IDL fragments (which are reduced in triglyceride content and enriched in cholesterol) travel to the liver where they are recycled to reform VLDL, or these IDLs are also converted to LDL in the vascular compartment. IDLs are the main source of LDL.[3] This pathway of lipoprotein synthesis and transport is depicted in Figure 26.9.

LDL, sometimes called the *bad cholesterol*, serves as the primary transport molecule for cholesterol. LDL is removed from the circulation either by LDL receptors or by scavenger cells such as monocytes or macrophages. Approximately 70% of LDL is removed through the LDL receptor–mediated pathway, with the remainder removed by the scavenger pathway.[1] Although LDL receptors are widely distributed, approximately 75% are located on hepatocytes. Thus, the liver plays an extremely important role in LDL metabolism. LDL receptor–mediated removal involves binding of LDL to cell surface receptors, followed by *endocytosis* (a phagocytic process in which LDL is engulfed and moved into the cell in the form of a membrane-covered endocytic vesicle). Within the cell, the endocytic vesicles fuse with lysosomes and the LDL molecule is enzymatically degraded, causing free cholesterol to be released into the cellular cytoplasm. Other nonhepatic tissues (*i.e.*, adrenal glands, SMCs, endothelial cells, and lymphoid cells) also use the LDL receptor–mediated pathway to obtain cholesterol needed for membrane and hormone synthesis. These tissues can control their cholesterol intake by adding or removing LDL receptors.[1,3,4]

The scavenger pathway of LDL removal involves ingestion by phagocytic monocytes and macrophages. These scavenger cells have receptors that bind LDL that has been oxidized or chemically modified. The amount of LDL removed by the scavenger pathway is directly related to the plasma cholesterol level. When the quantity of LDL receptors is decreased or when LDL levels exceed receptor availability, the amount of LDL removed by scavenger cells is greatly increased. The uptake of LDL by macrophages in the arterial wall can lead to the development of atherosclerosis.[1,3,4]

HDL is often referred to as the *good cholesterol* because HDL facilitates the reverse transport of cholesterol (carrying cholesterol from the peripheral tissues back to the liver, where it can be secreted into the bile and eliminated from the body through the bowel as part of feces).[5] Although clear mechanisms of action have not yet been identified, it is thought that HDL may also be protective against atherosclerosis through roles in reducing oxidative stress and reducing inflammation.[3] It has been observed that regular exercise, moderate alcohol consumption, and certain lipid medications increase HDL levels, whereas smoking, the metabolic syndrome, and excess alcohol consumption are associated with decreased levels of HDL.[1,4,11]

Etiology and Pathogenesis of Dyslipidemia

Serum cholesterol levels may be elevated as a result of an increase in any of the lipoproteins—the chylomicrons, VLDL, IDL, LDL, or HDL. The commonly used classification system for dyslipidemia is based on the type of lipoprotein involved. Factors that can raise blood lipid levels include nutrition, genetics, medications, comorbid conditions, and metabolic diseases. Most cases of elevated levels of cholesterol are probably multifactorial. Some people may have increased sensitivity to dietary cholesterol, others may have a lack of LDL receptors, and still others may have an altered synthesis of the apoproteins involved with lipid transport.[4]

Dyslipidemia may be classified as either primary or secondary. Primary dyslipidemia refers to abnormalities in blood lipid and cholesterol levels that develop independent of other health problems or lifestyle behaviors, whereas secondary dyslipidemia is associated with other health problems and behaviors. Dyslipidemia is characterized by combinations of

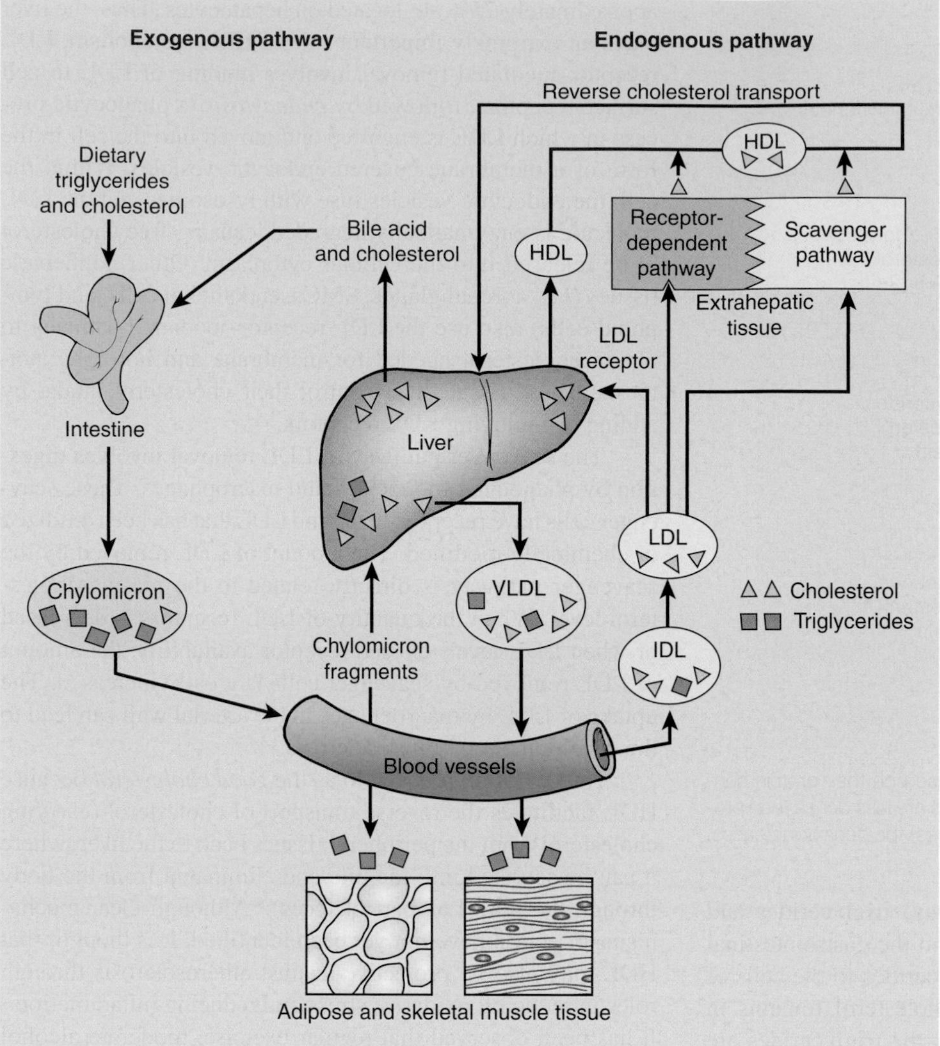

Figure 26.9 • Schematic representation of the exogenous and endogenous pathways for triglyceride and cholesterol transport.

the following patterns of blood lipids: increased triglycerides, increased total blood cholesterol, increased LDL cholesterol, and decreased HDL cholesterol.[12]

Primary Dyslipidemia. Many types of primary dyslipidemia have a genetic basis. There may be a defective synthesis of certain apoproteins, a lack of receptors for lipids, defective lipid receptors, or genetically determined defects in the handling of cholesterol by cells.[4] For example, the LDL receptor is deficient or defective in the genetic disorder known as *familial hypercholesterolemia.*

Familial Hypercholesterolemia. Familial hypercholesterolemia is an autosomal dominant disorder of lipid metabolism resulting from a mutation in a gene located on the short arm of chromosome 19 that codes for a receptor for LDL.[4] Because most of the circulating cholesterol is removed through receptor-dependent mechanisms, blood cholesterol levels are markedly elevated in people with this disorder. The disorder is a common inherited disorder in the United States, with the heterozygous form occurring in 1 in 500 adults. The recessive homozygous form is more rare, with an incidence of 1 case per million.[4] In the heterozygous form of the disease, blood LDL levels typically have a mean value of approximately 350 mg/dL. Although people with the heterozygous form of the disease commonly have an elevated cholesterol level from birth, they do not develop symptoms until adult life, when they often develop *xanthomas* (*i.e.*, cholesterol deposits) along the tendons (Fig. 26.10) and atherosclerosis appears. In contrast, people with the homozygous form of the disease may experience blood levels of LDL as high as 1,000 mg/dL. This population with homozygous disease will also typically develop tendon xanthomas and atherosclerotic vascular lesions during childhood, and they are at greater risk for death from myocardial ischemic disease during the young adult years. Therefore, it is particularly important for people with the homozygous form to receive early pharmacologic treatment with medications such as statins to lower blood levels of LDL.[4]

Secondary Dyslipidemia. Causes of secondary dyslipidemia include dietary factors, obesity, and the metabolic changes associated with Type 2 diabetes mellitus. To promote optimal

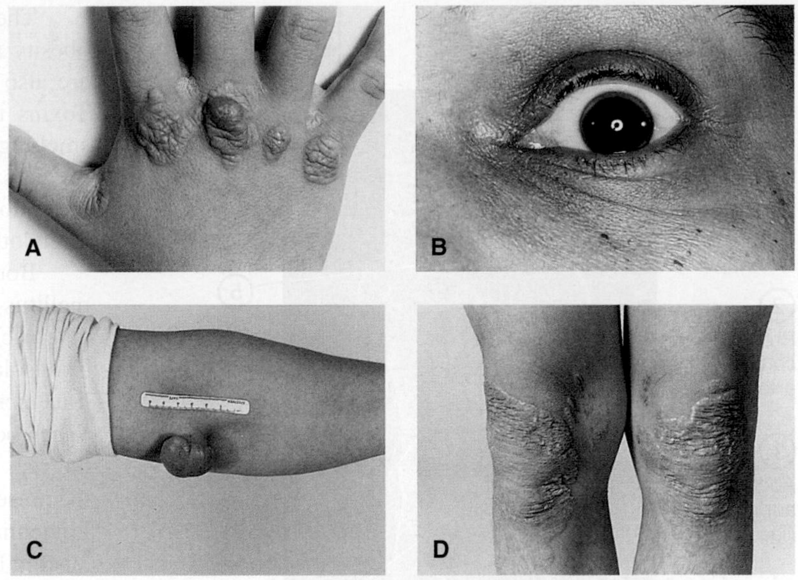

Figure 26.10 • Xanthomas in the skin and tendons **(A, C, D)**. Arcus lipoides represents the deposition of lipids in the peripheral cornea **(B)**. (From Strayer D., Rubin R., Saffitz J. E., et al. (Eds.) (2015). *Rubin's pathology: Clinicopathologic foundations of medicine* (7th ed., Fig. 26-24, p. 600). Philadelphia, PA: Wolters Kluwer.)

blood levels of lipid and cholesterol, recommendations are to adopt a dietary pattern that emphasizes fruits, vegetables, and whole grains, along with low-fat dairy products, chicken, fish, legumes, and nuts. Dietary oils should be nontropical vegetable oils. Intake of sweets (including sugary beverages) and red meat should be minimized. These dietary recommendations are consistent with the DASH diet (***D***ietary ***A***pproaches to ***S***top ***H***ypertension) or a Mediterranean dietary approach.[13]

Ongoing research into the metabolic changes associated with obesity continues to reveal connections between adiposity and dyslipidemia. The dyslipidemia pattern associated with obesity typically consists of elevated triglycerides, elevated LDL cholesterol, and decreased HDL cholesterol. The mechanisms of obesity-associated dyslipidemia appear to be related to the chemical activity of adipose tissue. Adipocytes secrete proinflammatory chemicals called adipokines. Additionally, some people also have many macrophages embedded within the areas of adipose tissue deposition. The combination of the adipokine secretion and macrophage activity leads to a chronic low grade state of systemic inflammation in some people with obesity. Additionally, free fatty acids are continually secreted into the blood as a result of hydrolytic activity within the adipocytes. This combination of elevated free fatty acids and systemic inflammation is thought to disrupt the glucose homeostatic mechanisms, contributing to the development of insulin resistance by body cells. The insulin resistance results in use of nonglucose energy sources, leading to further increases in levels of blood lipids. The development of insulin resistance is more strongly associated with an intra-abdominal location of adipose tissue.[14]

The typical presentation of dyslipidemia that occurs in people with Type 2 diabetes mellitus includes elevation of triglycerides and low HDL cholesterol. Type 2 diabetes mellitus is characterized by the development of a state of insulin resistance along with a collection of metabolic alterations, including dyslipidemia, called the *metabolic syndrome*. Since the metabolic syndrome was first described in 1988, multiple diagnostic criteria have been suggested. In 2009, a consensus definition was proposed collaboratively by several key international organizations.[15] In this consensus statement, the metabolic syndrome was defined as the presence of three or more of the following:

- Elevated fasting blood glucose (or current treatment for diabetes)
- Elevated blood pressure (or current treatment for hypertension)
- Elevated waist circumference (by country-specific norms), reflecting increased abdominal fat deposits
- Dyslipidemia reflected by increased blood triglycerides and/or decreased HDL cholesterol in the blood (or receiving current treatment for dyslipidemia).[16]

Because abdominal obesity is one of the definitional characteristics of the metabolic syndrome, it is uncertain whether the metabolic changes originate from the previously described chemical and immune changes associated with the excess adipose tissue or whether the insulin resistance of type 2 diabetes mellitus develops first and the obesity is a consequence of the changes in glucose regulation.[16]

Other systemic disorders that can elevate lipids include hypothyroidism, nephrotic syndrome, and obstructive liver disease.[1,4] Medications such as beta-blockers, estrogens, and protease inhibitors (used in the treatment of human immunodeficiency virus [HIV] infection) can also increase lipid levels.[17]

Atherosclerosis

Atherosclerosis is a type of arteriosclerosis or hardening of the arteries. The term *atherosclerosis*, which comes from the Greek words *atheros* ("gruel" or "paste") and *sclerosis* ("hardness"), denotes the formation of fibrofatty lesions in the intimal lining

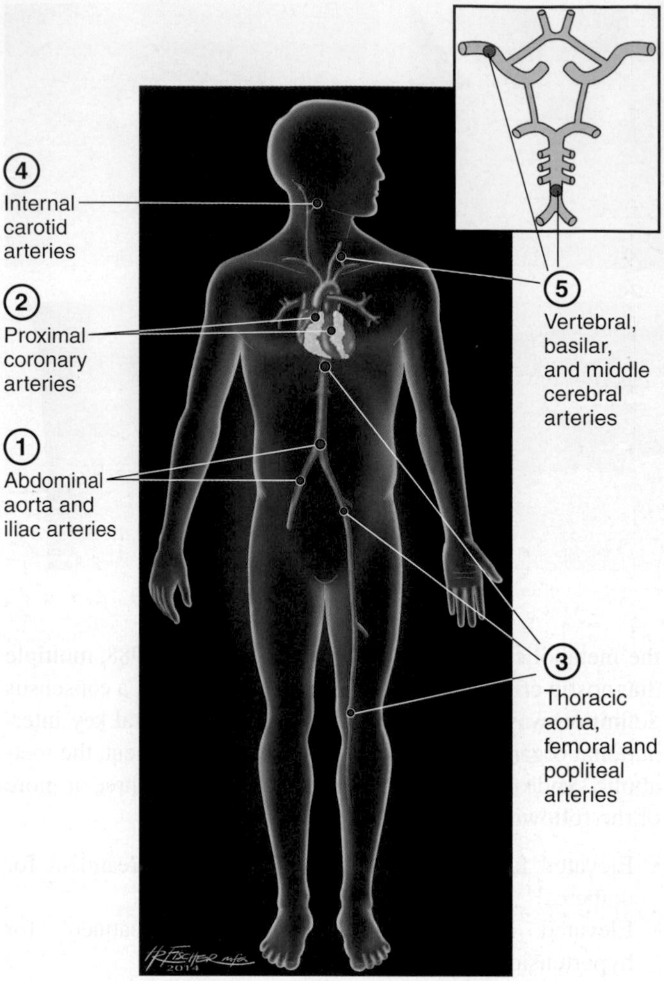

Figure 26.11 • Sites of severe atherosclerosis in order of frequency. (From Strayer D., Rubin R., Saffitz J. E., et al. (Eds.) (2015). *Rubin's pathology: Clinicopathologic foundations of medicine* (6th ed., Fig. 16-17, p. 594). Philadelphia, PA: Wolters Kluwer.)

of the large- and medium-sized arteries such as the aorta and its branches, the coronary arteries, and the large vessels that supply the brain. The common sites at which severe atherosclerotic lesions tend to form are shown in Figure 26.11.

Etiology and Risk Factors

The major risk factor for atherosclerosis is hypercholesterolemia and especially elevations in LDL cholesterol levels. Hypercholesterolemia is one of several risk factors for atherosclerosis that can be modified by dietary and life style changes and by medications. Additional nonmodifiable risk factors include increasing age, family history of heart disease, and male sex. Several genetically determined alterations in lipoprotein and cholesterol metabolism have also been identified.[4] Other factors being equal, men are at greater risk for development of atherosclerotic coronary vascular disease (CVD) than are premenopausal women, probably because of the protective effects of natural estrogens. After menopause, the incidence of atherosclerosis-related diseases in women increases, and the frequency of myocardial infarction in men and women tends to equalize.[1,3,4]

The traditional cardiac risk factors of cigarette smoking, obesity and visceral fat, hypertension, and diabetes mellitus are also risk factors for the development of atherosclerosis. Toxins that enter the bloodstream as a result of cigarette smoking can damage endothelial tissue. Prolonged smoking of years of one pack or more per day doubles the damage to the endothelium. However, stopping smoking reduces the risk of endothelial damage significantly.[1]

Both hypertension (high blood pressure) and diabetes mellitus are independent risk factors for the development of atherosclerosis, but they also have additive, synergistic effects. The isolated presence of either hypertension or diabetes mellitus increases the risk for atherosclerosis by at least twofold. When both hypertension and diabetes mellitus exist together, the risk for atherosclerosis increases to an eightfold risk. In the presence of the triad of hypertension, diabetes, and hyperlipidemia, the risk for atherosclerosis increases to almost a 20-fold likelihood.[3]

Other factors associated with an increased risk for development of atherosclerosis include physical inactivity, stressful life patterns, blood levels of C-reactive protein (CRP), and serum homocysteine levels.[4] Considerable interest in the role of systemic inflammation in the etiology of atherosclerosis has emerged. CRP is an acute phase reactant protein of the inflammatory process. Blood levels of CRP have been demonstrated to be a useful but nonspecific biologic marker of the presence of systemic inflammation. CRP molecules have also been noted to be present within some atherosclerotic plaque, further implicating the role of inflammation in plaque formation. Therefore, blood levels of CRP serve as an effective clinical marker of risk for atherosclerotic vascular disease (see Chapter 9).[4] The high-sensitivity CRP test is recommended as a screening test for cardiovascular risk.[18] This high-sensitivity test differs from the standard CRP test that is used for assessing the degree of inflammation present when a bacterial infection is suspected (in which case, a large rise in CRP would be expected as the immune system mounts an inflammatory response against the invading bacteria). The high-sensitivity CRP test can detect the presence of smaller quantities levels of CRP, making it a useful test to monitor for small rises in CRP levels as a screening test for cardiovascular risk in apparently healthy people.[19]

Homocysteine is derived from the metabolism of dietary methionine, an amino acid that is abundant in animal protein. The normal metabolism of homocysteine requires adequate levels of folate, vitamin B_6, vitamin B_{12}, and riboflavin. Homocysteine inhibits elements of the anticoagulant cascade and is associated with endothelial damage, which is thought to be an important first step in the development of atherosclerosis.[1,4] A rare autosomal recessive disorder called homocystinuria is caused by an inherited defect in the production of an enzyme to metabolize homocysteine, resulting in high serum levels of homocysteine. People with homocystinuria are at risk for early development of severe atherosclerosis because of the high blood levels of homocysteine.[4] Although research into the use of homocysteine levels as a risk factor for cardiovascular disease is being done, current recommendations for screening do not include routine assessment of blood homocysteine levels.[18]

Pathogenesis

The lesions associated with atherosclerosis are of three types: the fatty streak, the fibrous atheromatous plaque, and the complicated lesion. The latter two are responsible for the clinically significant manifestations of the disease. Figure 26.12 shows the general structure of atherosclerotic plaque.

Fatty streaks are thin, flat, yellow intimal discolorations that progressively enlarge by becoming thicker and slightly elevated as they grow in length. Histologically, they consist of macrophages and SMCs that have become distended with lipid to form foam cells. Fatty streaks are present in children, often in the first year of life.[1,2] This occurs regardless of geographic setting, sex, or race. They increase in number until about 20 years of age, and then they remain static or regress. Damage to the endothelium is an early marker that can later become atherosclerotic. Once the endothelium is damaged circulating monocytes and lipids begin to adhere to the area. This *fibrous atheromatous plaque* is characterized by the gray to pearly white appearance because of the macrophages that ingest and oxidize accumulated lipoproteins and form a visible fatty steak. Over time, the fatty steaks grow larger and proliferate into the smooth muscle. As the lesions increase in size, they encroach on the lumen of the artery. The macrophages release substances that cause inflammation and eventually may occlude the vessel or predispose to thrombus formation, causing a reduction of blood flow.[3] Because blood flow is inversely related to the fourth power of the vessel radius, the reduction in blood flow becomes increasingly greater as the atherosclerotic disease progresses.[3]

The more advanced complicated lesions contain hemorrhage, ulceration, and scar tissue deposits. Thrombosis is the most important complication of atherosclerosis. Slowing and turbulence of blood flow in the region of the plaque and ulceration of the plaque cause it. The thrombus may cause occlusion of small vessels in the heart and brain. In addition, aneurysms may develop in arteries weakened by extensive plaque formation.[4]

Although risk factors associated with atherosclerosis have been identified through epidemiologic studies, many unanswered questions remain regarding the mechanisms by which these risk factors contribute to the development of atherosclerosis. The vascular endothelial layer, which consists of a single layer of cells with cell-to-cell attachments, normally serves as a selective barrier that protects the subendothelial layers by interacting with blood cells and other blood components. One hypothesis of plaque formation suggests that injury to the endothelial vessel layer is the initiating factor in the development of atherosclerosis.[1,4] The fact that atherosclerotic lesions tend to form where vessels branch or where there is turbulent flow suggests that hemodynamic factors also play a role.

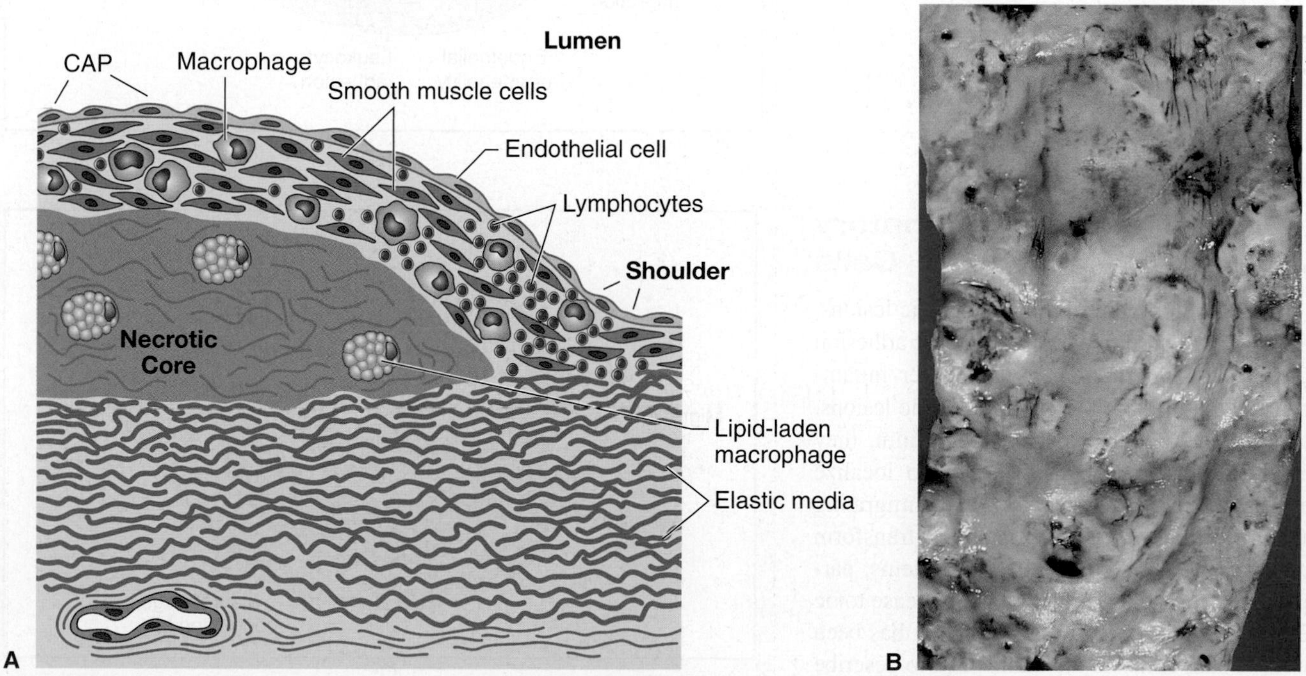

Figure 26.12 • Fibrofatty plaque of atherosclerosis. **(A)** In this fully developed fibrous plaque, the core contains lipid-filled macrophages and necrotic SMC debris. The "fibrous" cap is composed largely of SMCs, which produce collagen, small amounts of elastin, and glycosaminoglycans. Also shown are infiltrating macrophages and lymphocytes. Note that the endothelium over the surface of the fibrous cap frequently appears intact. **(B)** The aorta shows discrete raised, tan plaques. Focal plaque ulcerations are also evident. (From Rubin R., Strayer D. S., Saffitz J. E., et al. (Eds.) (2015). *Rubin's pathology: Clinicopathologic foundations of medicine.* (7th ed., Fig. 16-12A and D, p. 589). Philadelphia, PA: Wolters Kluwer.)

Understanding The Development of Atherosclerosis

Atherosclerosis is characterized by the development of atheromatous lesions within the intimal lining of the large- and medium-sized arteries that protrude into and can eventually obstruct blood flow. The development of atherosclerotic lesions is a progressive process involving (a) endothelial cell injury, (b) migration of inflammatory cells, (c) SMC proliferation and lipid deposition, and (d) gradual development of the atheromatous plaque with a lipid core.

Endothelial Cell Injury

The vascular endothelium consists of a single layer of cells with cell-to-cell attachments, which normally protects the subendothelial layers from interacting with blood cells and other blood components. Agents such as smoking, elevated LDL levels, immune mechanisms, and mechanical stress associated with hypertension share the potential for causing endothelial injury with adhesion of monocytes and platelets.

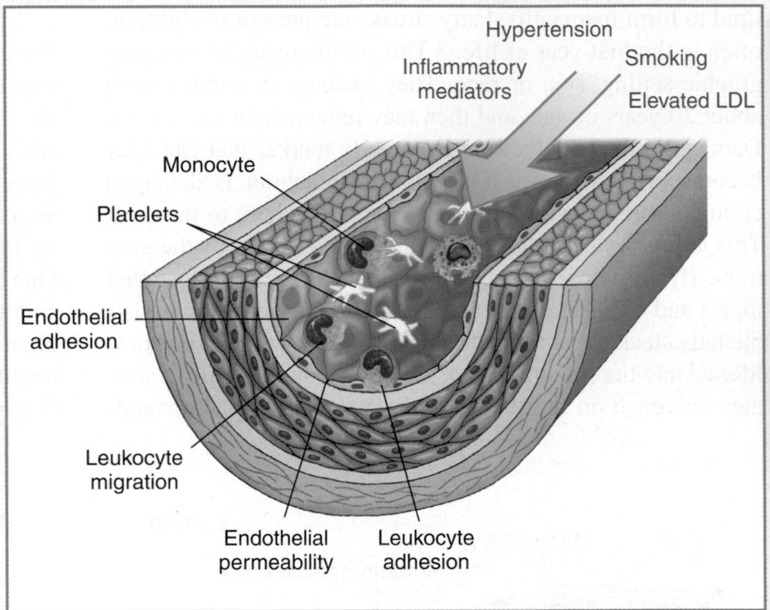

Migration of Inflammatory Cells

Early in the development of atherosclerotic lesions, endothelial cells begin to express selective adhesion molecules that bind monocytes and other inflammatory cells that initiate the atherosclerotic lesions. After monocytes adhere to the endothelium, they migrate between the endothelial cells to localize in the intima of the vascular wall. After migrating into the vascular wall, the monocytes transform into macrophages, which engulf lipoproteins, particularly LDL. Activated macrophages release toxic oxygen species that oxidize the LDL that has been engulfed. "Foam cells" is the name used to describe macrophages which have engulfed and oxidized LDL.

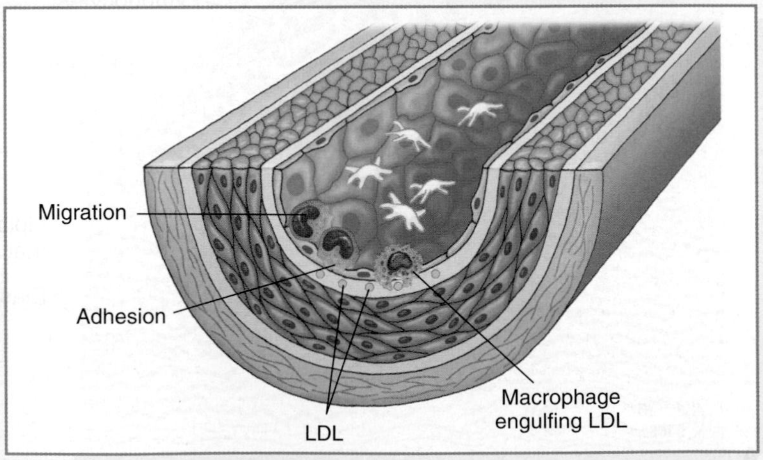

Understanding The Development of Atherosclerosis *(Continued)*

Lipid Accumulation and Smooth Muscle Cell Proliferation

The recruitment of monocytes, their differentiation into macrophages, the subsequent ingestion and oxidation of lipids by macrophages, and their transformation into foam cells is protective because this process removes excess lipids from the circulation. However, progressive accumulation of foam cells within the vessel wall eventually leads to lesion progression. The macrophages also produce growth factors that contribute to the migration and proliferation of SMCs and the elaboration of ECM within the vascular wall. Ultimately, the foam cell macrophages die, producing deposits of necrotic cellular debris and lipids within the vascular wall.

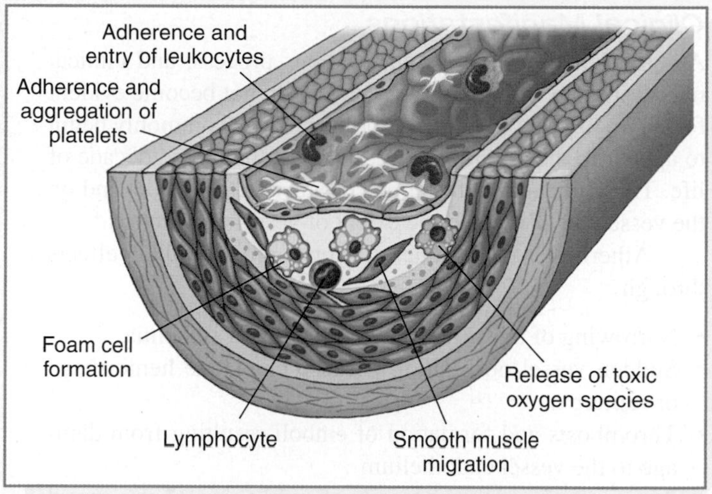

Plaque Structure

Atherosclerotic plaques consist of an aggregation of SMCs, macrophages, and other leukocytes; ECM, including collagen and elastic fibers; and intracellular and extracellular lipids. Typically, the superficial fibrous cap is composed of SMCs and dense ECM. Immediately beneath and to the side of the fibrous cap is a cellular area (the shoulder) consisting of macrophages, SMCs, and lymphocytes. Below the fibrous cap is a central core of lipid-laden foam cells and fatty debris. Rupture, ulceration, or erosion of an unstable or vulnerable fibrous cap may lead to hemorrhage into the plaque or thrombotic occlusion of the vessel lumen.

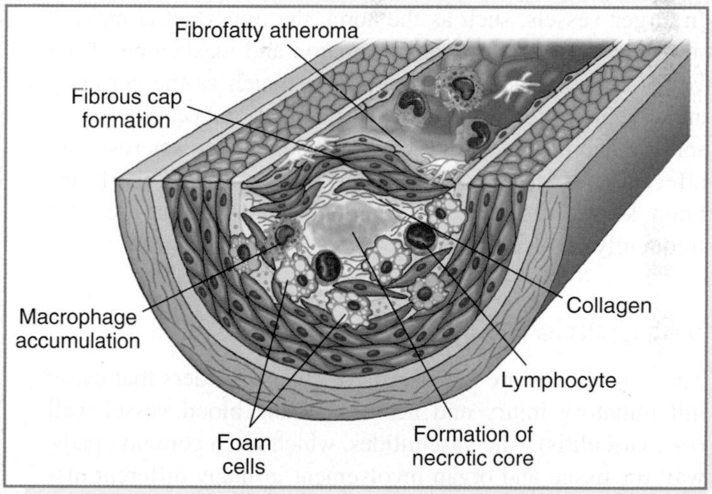

Hyperlipidemia is also believed to play an active role in the pathogenesis of the atherosclerotic lesion, with special concern related to increased blood levels of LDL because of its higher cholesterol content. Interactions between the endothelial layer of the vessel wall and white blood cells, particularly the monocytes, normally occur throughout life; these interactions increase when blood cholesterol levels are elevated. One of the earliest responses to elevated cholesterol levels is the attachment of monocytes to the endothelium. The monocytes have been observed to emigrate through the cell-to-cell attachments of the endothelial layer into the subendothelial spaces, where they transform into macrophages.[4]

Activated macrophages release free radicals that oxidize LDL. Oxidized LDL is toxic to the endothelium, causing endothelial loss and exposure of the subendothelial tissue to blood components. This leads to platelet adhesion, platelet aggregation, and fibrin deposition. Platelets and activated macrophages release various factors that are thought to promote growth factors that modulate the proliferation of SMCs and deposition of extracellular matrix (ECM) in the lesions.[1,4] Activated macrophages also ingest oxidized LDL (by uptake through the scavenger receptor) to become foam cells. These foam cells have been noted to be present in all stages of atherosclerotic plaque formation. Lipids released from necrotic foam cells accumulate to form the lipid core of unstable plaques. Histologically, a large central lipid core, inflammatory infiltrate, and a thin fibrous cap typically characterized these unstable atherosclerotic plaques.[1,4] (See Fig. 26.12.)

These unstable plaques, or "vulnerable plaques," are at risk of rupture. This plaque rupture often occurs at the shoulder of the plaque where the fibrous cap is thinnest (because of the presence of local inflammatory cells and mediators that degrade the cap) and the mechanical stresses highest.[1,4]

Clinical Manifestations

Atherosclerosis begins as an insidious process, and clinical manifestations of the disease typically do not become evident for 20 to 40 years or longer. Fibrous plaques commonly begin to appear in the arteries of Americans in their third decade of life. The clinical manifestations of atherosclerosis depend on the vessels involved and the extent of vessel obstruction.[4]

Atherosclerotic plaques (lesions) produce their effects through

- Narrowing of the vessel and production of ischemia
- Sudden vessel obstruction because of plaque hemorrhage or rupture
- Thrombosis and formation of emboli resulting from damage to the vessel endothelium
- Aneurysm formation because of weakening of the vessel wall.[1,4]

In larger vessels, such as the aorta, the important complications are those of thrombus formation and weakening of the vessel wall. In medium-sized arteries, such as the coronary and cerebral arteries, ischemia and infarction because of vessel occlusion are more common. Although atherosclerosis can affect any organ or tissue, the arteries supplying the heart, brain, kidneys, lower extremities, and small intestine are most frequently involved.[4]

Vasculitis

The vasculitides are a group of vascular disorders that cause inflammatory injury and necrosis of the blood vessel wall (*i.e.*, vasculitis). The vasculitides, which are a common pathway for tissue and organ involvement in many different disease conditions, involve the endothelial cells and SMCs of the vessel wall.[2] Vessels of any type (arteries, veins, and capillaries) in virtually any organ can be affected. Because they may affect veins and capillaries, the terms *vasculitis*, *angiitis*, and *arteritis* often are used interchangeably. Clinical manifestations often include fever, myalgia, arthralgia, and malaise. Vasculitis may result from direct injury to the vessel, infectious agents, or immune processes, or they may be secondary to other disease states such as systemic lupus erythematosus. Physical agents such as cold (*i.e.*, frostbite), irradiation (*i.e.*, sunburn), mechanical injury, immune mechanisms, and toxins may secondarily cause vessel damage, often leading to necrosis of the vessels. Small vessel vasculitides are sometimes associated with *antineutrophil cytoplasmic antibodies* (ANCAs). ANCAs are antibodies directed against certain proteins in the cytoplasm of neutrophils. These autoantibodies may cause endothelial damage.[1] Serum ANCA titers, which can correlate with disease activity, may serve as a useful quantitative diagnostic marker for these disorders.

The vasculitides are commonly classified based on etiology, pathologic findings, and prognosis. One classification system divides the conditions into three groups: (a) small vessel, (b) medium-sized vessel, and (b) large vessel vasculitides[1,4] (Table 26.2). Small vessel refers to small arteries (ANCA-associated disease only), arterioles, venules, and capillaries; medium vessels refer to medium- and small-sized arteries and arterioles; and large vessel refers to the aorta and its major tributaries. The small vessel vasculitides are involved in a number of different diseases, most of which are mediated by type III immune complex hypersensitivity reaction. They commonly involve the skin and are often a complication of an underlying disease (*i.e.*, vasculitis associated with neoplasms or connective tissue disease) and exposure to environmental agents (*i.e.*, serum sickness and urticarial vasculitis). ANCA-positive small vessel vasculitis includes microscopic polyangiitis, Wegener granulomatosis, and the Churg-Strauss syndrome.[20]

Medium-sized vessel vasculitides produce necrotizing damage to medium-sized muscular arteries of major organ systems. This group includes polyarteritis nodosa, Kawasaki disease, and thromboangiitis obliterans. Large vessel vasculitides involve large elastic arteries. They include giant cell (temporal) arteritis, polymyalgia rheumatica, and Takayasu arteritis. Giant cell (temporal) arteritis will be considered as a case model.

Giant Cell Temporal Arteritis

Temporal arteritis (*i.e.*, giant cell arteritis), the most common of the vasculitides, is a focal inflammatory condition of medium-sized and large arteries. It predominantly affects branches of arteries originating from the aortic arch, including the superficial temporal, vertebral, ophthalmic, and posterior ciliary arteries. The disorder progresses to involve the entire artery wall with focal necrosis and granulomatous inflammation involving multinucleated giant cells. It is more common in older adults, with a 2:1 female-to-male ratio. The cause is unknown. However, an autoimmune origin, such as an initial T cell–mediated immune response, has been suggested.[1] The disorder often is insidious in onset and may be heralded by the sudden onset of headache, tenderness over the artery, swelling and redness of the overlying skin, blurred vision or diplopia, and facial pain. Almost one half of affected people have systemic involvement in the form of polymyalgia rheumatica. Up to 10% of people with giant cell arteritis go on to develop aortic aneurysm (especially thoracic).

Arterial Disease of the Extremities

Disorders of the circulation in the extremities often are referred to as *peripheral vascular disorders.* In many respects, the disorders that affect arteries in the extremities are the same as those affecting the coronary and cerebral arteries because all of these vascular disorders produce ischemia, pain, impaired function, and in some cases infarction and tissue necrosis. Not only are the effects similar, but also the pathologic conditions that impair circulation in the extremities are identical. This section focuses on acute arterial occlusion of the extremities, atherosclerotic occlusive disease, thromboangiitis obliterans, and Raynaud disease and phenomenon.

TABLE 26.2 CLASSIFICATION OF THE VASCULITIDES

GROUP	EXAMPLES	CHARACTERISTICS
Small vessel vasculitis	Microscopic polyangiitis	Necrotizing vasculitis with few or no immune deposits affecting medium and small blood vessels, including capillaries, venules, and arterioles; necrotizing glomerulonephritis and involvement of the pulmonary capillaries are common
	Wegener granulomatosis	Granulomatous inflammation involving the respiratory tract and necrotizing vasculitis affecting capillaries, venules, arterioles, and arteries; necrotizing glomerulonephritis is common
Medium-sized vessel vasculitis	Polyarteritis nodosa	Necrotizing inflammation of medium-sized or small arteries without vasculitis in arteries, capillaries, or venules; usually associated with underlying disease or environmental agents
	Kawasaki disease	Involves large, medium-sized, and small arteries (frequently the coronaries) and is associated with mucocutaneous lymph node syndrome; usually occurs in small children
	Thromboangiitis obliterans	Segmental, thrombosing, acute and chronic inflammation of the medium-sized and small arteries, principally the tibial and radial arteries but sometimes extending to the veins and nerves of the extremities; occurs almost exclusively in men who are heavy smokers
Large vessel vasculitis	Giant cell (temporal) arteritis	Granulomatous inflammation of the aorta and its major branches with predilection for extracranial vessels of the carotid artery; infiltration of vessel wall with giant cells and mononuclear cells; usually occurs in people older than 50 years of age and is often associated with polymyalgia rheumatic
	Takayasu arteritis	Granulomatous inflammation of the aorta and its branches; usually occurs in people younger than 50 years of age

Acute Arterial Occlusion

Acute arterial occlusion is a sudden event that interrupts arterial flow to the affected tissues or organ. Most acute arterial occlusions are the result of an embolus or a thrombus. Although much less common than emboli and thrombus, trauma or arterial spasm caused by arterial cannulation can be another cause of acute arterial occlusion.

Etiology and Pathogenesis

An embolus is a freely moving particle such as a blood clot that breaks loose and travels in the larger vessels of the circulation until lodging in a smaller vessel and occluding blood flow. Most emboli arise in the heart and are caused by conditions that cause blood clots to develop on the wall of a heart chamber or valve surface. Emboli usually are a complication of heart disease: ischemic heart disease with or without infarction, atrial fibrillation, or rheumatic heart disease. Prosthetic heart valves can be another source of emboli. Other types of emboli are fat emboli that originate from bone marrow of fractured bones, air emboli from the lung, and amniotic fluid emboli that develop during childbirth.

A thrombus is a blood clot that forms on the wall of a vessel and continues to grow until reaching a size that obstructs blood flow. Thrombi often arise as the result of erosion or rupture of the fibrous cap of an arteriosclerotic plaque.

Clinical Manifestations

The signs and symptoms of acute arterial occlusion depend on the artery involved and the adequacy of the collateral circulation. Emboli tend to lodge in bifurcations of the major arteries, including the aorta and iliac, femoral, and popliteal arteries.[4] The presentation of acute arterial embolism is often described as that of the seven "Ps":

- Pistol shot (acute onset)
- Pallor
- Polar (cold)
- Pulselessness
- Pain
- Paresthesia
- Paralysis

Occlusion in an extremity causes sudden onset of acute pain with numbness, tingling, weakness, pallor, and coldness. There often is a sharp line of demarcation between the oxygenated tissue above the line of obstruction and the ischemic tissue below the line of obstruction. Pulses are absent below the level of the occlusion. These changes are followed rapidly by cyanosis, mottling, and loss of sensory, reflex, and motor function. Tissue death occurs unless blood flow is restored.[1,4]

Diagnosis and Treatment

Diagnosis of acute arterial occlusion is based on signs of impaired blood flow. It uses visual assessment, palpation of pulses, and methods to assess blood flow. Treatment of acute arterial occlusion is aimed at restoring blood flow. An embolectomy, surgical removal of the embolus, is the optimal therapy when a large artery is occluded.[1,4]

Thrombolytic therapy (*i.e.*, streptokinase or tissue plasminogen activator) may be used in an attempt to dissolve the clot. Anticoagulant therapy (*i.e.*, heparin) usually is given to prevent extension of the embolus and to prevent progression of the original thrombus. Application of cold should be avoided, and the extremity should be protected from injury resulting from hard surfaces and overlying bedclothes.[1,4,17]

Atherosclerotic Occlusive Disease (Peripheral Artery Disease)

Atherosclerosis is an important cause of peripheral artery disease (PAD) and is seen most commonly in the vessels of the lower extremities. The condition is sometimes referred to as *arteriosclerosis obliterans.* The superficial femoral and popliteal arteries are the most commonly affected vessels. When lesions develop in the lower leg and foot, the tibial, common peroneal, or pedal vessels are the arteries most commonly affected. The disease is seen most commonly in people as they advance in age.[1,4]

Etiology

The risk factors for this disorder are similar to those for atherosclerosis. Cigarette smoking contributes to the progress of the atherosclerosis of the lower extremities and to the development of symptoms of ischemia. People with diabetes mellitus develop more extensive and rapidly progressive vascular disease than do people who do not have diabetes.[1,4]

Clinical Manifestations

As with atherosclerosis in other locations, the signs and symptoms of vessel occlusion are gradual. Usually, there is at least a 50% narrowing of the vessel before symptoms of ischemia arise. The primary symptom of chronic obstructive arterial disease is *intermittent claudication* or pain with walking.[1,4] Typically, people with the disorder complain of calf pain because the gastrocnemius muscle has the highest oxygen consumption of any muscle group in the leg during walking. Some people may complain of a vague aching feeling or numbness, rather than pain. Other activities such as swimming, bicycling, and climbing stairs use other muscle groups and may not incite the same degree of discomfort as walking.[1,4]

Other signs of ischemia include atrophic changes and thinning of the skin and subcutaneous tissues of the lower leg and diminution in the size of the leg muscles. The foot often is cool, and the popliteal and pedal pulses are weak or absent. Limb color blanches with elevation of the leg because of the effects of gravity on perfusion pressure and becomes deep red when the leg is in the dependent position because of an autoregulatory increase in blood flow and a gravitational increase in perfusion pressure.[1,4]

When blood flow is reduced to the extent that it no longer meets the minimal needs of resting muscle and nerves, ischemic pain at rest, ulceration, and gangrene develop. As tissue necrosis develops, there typically is severe pain in the region of skin breakdown, which is worse at night with limb elevation and is improved with standing.[1,4]

Diagnosis

Diagnostic methods include inspection of the limbs for signs of chronic low-grade ischemia such as subcutaneous atrophy, brittle toenails, hair loss, pallor, coolness, or dependent rubor. Palpation of the femoral, popliteal, posterior tibial, and dorsalis pedis pulses allows for an estimation of the level and degree of obstruction. Blood pressures may be taken at various levels on the leg to determine the level of obstruction. A Doppler ultrasound device may also be used for detecting pulses. Ultrasound imaging, magnetic resonance imaging (MRI) arteriography, spiral computed tomographic (CT) arteriography, and invasive contrast angiography may also be used as diagnostic methods.[1,4]

Treatment

The two goals of treatment in people with PAD are (1) to decrease their considerable cardiovascular risk and (2) to reduce symptoms. People with PAD should be evaluated for coexisting coronary and cerebrovascular atherosclerosis. It is also important to address other cardiovascular risk factors, including smoking, hypertension, high lipid levels, and diabetes. Smoking cessation should be encouraged, and the coexisting health conditions should be treated appropriately. Medications that may be useful include antiplatelet agents to minimize thrombosis and statins to lower cholesterol. The tissues of extremities affected by atherosclerosis are easily injured and slow to heal. Treatment includes measures directed at protection of the affected tissues and preservation of functional capacity. Walking (slowly) to the point of claudication may be encouraged to increase collateral circulation. Percutaneous or surgical vascular intervention is typically reserved for the person with disabling claudication or limb-threatening ischemia.[1,4,17]

Thromboangiitis Obliterans

Thromboangiitis obliterans, or Buerger disease, is an inflammatory (*i.e.*, vasculitis) arterial disorder that causes thrombus formation. The disorder affects the medium-sized arteries, usually the plantar and digital vessels in the foot and lower leg. Arteries in the arm and hand also may be affected. It is characterized by segmental, thrombosing, and acute and chronic inflammation. Although primarily an arterial disorder, the inflammatory process often extends to involve adjacent veins and nerves. Usually, the disease is seen in people less than 35 years of age who are heavy cigarette smokers.[1,4]

Etiology and Pathogenesis

The pathogenesis of Buerger disease remains speculative. However, cigarette smoking and in some instances tobacco chewing seem to be involved. It has been suggested that the nicotine has a direct effect on the endothelial cell toxicity and may trigger an immune response.[1] Genetic influences are suggested because it is more prevalent in certain ethnic groups.

Clinical Manifestations

Pain is the predominant symptom of the disorder. It is usually related to distal arterial ischemia. During the early stages of the disease, there is intermittent claudication in the arch of the foot and the digits. In severe cases, pain is present even when the person is at rest. The impaired circulation increases sensitivity to cold. The peripheral pulses are diminished or absent, and there are changes in the color of the extremity. In moderately advanced cases, the extremity becomes cyanotic when the person assumes a dependent position, and the digits may turn reddish blue even when in a nondependent position. With lack of blood flow, the skin assumes a thin, shiny look and hair growth and skin nutrition suffer. Chronic ischemia causes thick, malformed nails. If the disease continues to progress, tissues eventually ulcerate and gangrenous changes arise that may necessitate amputation.[1,4]

Diagnosis and Treatment

Diagnostic methods are similar to those for atherosclerotic disease of the lower extremities. As part of the treatment program for thromboangiitis obliterans, it is mandatory that the person stop smoking cigarettes or using tobacco. Even passive smoking and nicotine replacement therapy should be eliminated. Other treatment measures are of secondary importance and focus on methods for producing vasodilation and preventing tissue injury.[1,4]

Raynaud Disease and Phenomenon

Raynaud disease or phenomenon is a functional disorder caused by intense vasospasm of the arteries and arterioles in the fingers and, less often, the toes. This is a common disorder affecting 3% to 5% of the population and is more common in women than men. The disorder is divided into two types—the primary type, called *Raynaud disease*, occurs without demonstrable cause, and the secondary type, called *Raynaud phenomenon*, is associated with other disease states or known causes of vasospasm.[1,4]

Etiology and Pathogenesis

Vasospasm implies an excessive vasoconstrictor response to stimuli that normally produce only moderate vasoconstriction. In contrast to other regional circulations that are supplied by vasodilator and vasoconstrictor fibers, the cutaneous vessels of the fingers and toes are innervated only by sympathetic vasoconstrictor fibers. In these vessels, vasodilation occurs by withdrawal of sympathetic stimulation. Cooling of specific body parts such as the head, neck, and trunk produces a sympathetic-mediated reduction in digital blood flow, as does emotional stress.[1,4]

Raynaud disease is precipitated by exposure to cold or by strong emotions and usually is limited to the fingers. It also follows a more benign course than Raynaud phenomenon, seldom causing tissue necrosis. The cause of vasospasm in primary Raynaud disease is unknown. Raynaud phenomenon is associated with previous vessel injury, such as frostbite, occupational trauma associated with the use of heavy vibrating tools, collagen diseases, neurologic disorders, and chronic arterial occlusive disorders. Another occupation-related cause is the exposure to alternating hot and cold temperatures such as that experienced by butchers and food preparers. Raynaud phenomenon is often the first symptom of collagen diseases, such as scleroderma and systemic lupus erythematosus.[1,4]

Clinical Manifestations

In Raynaud disease and Raynaud phenomenon, ischemia because of vasospasm causes changes in skin color that progress from pallor to cyanosis, a sensation of cold, and changes in sensory perception, such as numbness and tingling. The color changes usually are first noticed in the tips of the fingers, later moving into one or more of the distal phalanges (Fig. 26.13). After the ischemic episode, there is a period of hyperemia with intense redness, throbbing, and paresthesias. The period of hyperemia is followed by a return to normal color. Although all of the fingers usually are affected symmetrically, in some cases only one or two digits are involved, or only a portion of the digit is affected.[1,4]

In severe, progressive cases usually associated with Raynaud phenomenon, trophic changes may develop. The nails may become brittle, and the skin over the tips of the affected fingers may thicken. Nutritional impairment of these structures may give rise to arthritis. Ulceration and superficial gangrene of the fingers, although infrequent, may occur.[1,4]

Diagnosis and Treatment

The initial diagnosis is typically based on history of vasospastic attacks supported by other evidence of the disorder. Treatment measures are directed toward eliminating factors that cause

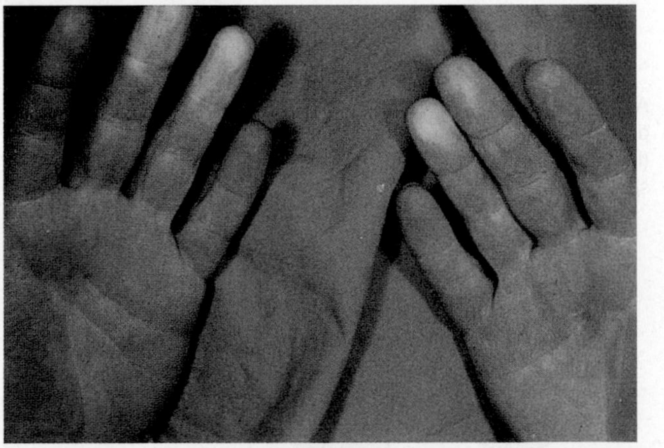

Figure 26.13 • Raynaud phenomenon. The tips of the fingers show marked pallor. (From Rubin R., Strayer D. S., Saffitz J. E., et al. (Eds.) (2015). *Rubin's pathology: Clinicopathologic foundations of medicine* (7th ed., Fig. 16-29, p. 604). Philadelphia, PA: Wolters Kluwer.)

vasospasm and protecting the digits from trauma during an ischemic episode. Abstinence from smoking, protection from cold, and controlling emotional stress are priorities.[1,4]

Aneurysms

An *aneurysm* is an abnormal localized dilation of a blood vessel. Aneurysms can occur in arteries and veins, but they are most common in the aorta. Aneurysms can assume several forms and may be classified according to their cause, location, and anatomic features. Figure 26.14 shows the common locations and forms of aneurysms.

There are two structural types of aneurysms: true aneurysms and false aneurysms. A *true aneurysm* is one in which the aneurysm is bounded by a complete vessel wall. The blood in a true aneurysm remains within the vascular compartment. *False aneurysm* or *pseudoaneurysm* represents a localized *dissection* or tear in the inner wall of the artery with formation of an extravascular hematoma that causes vessel enlargement. Unlike true aneurysms, only by the outer layers of the vessel wall or supporting tissues bound false aneurysms.[1,4]

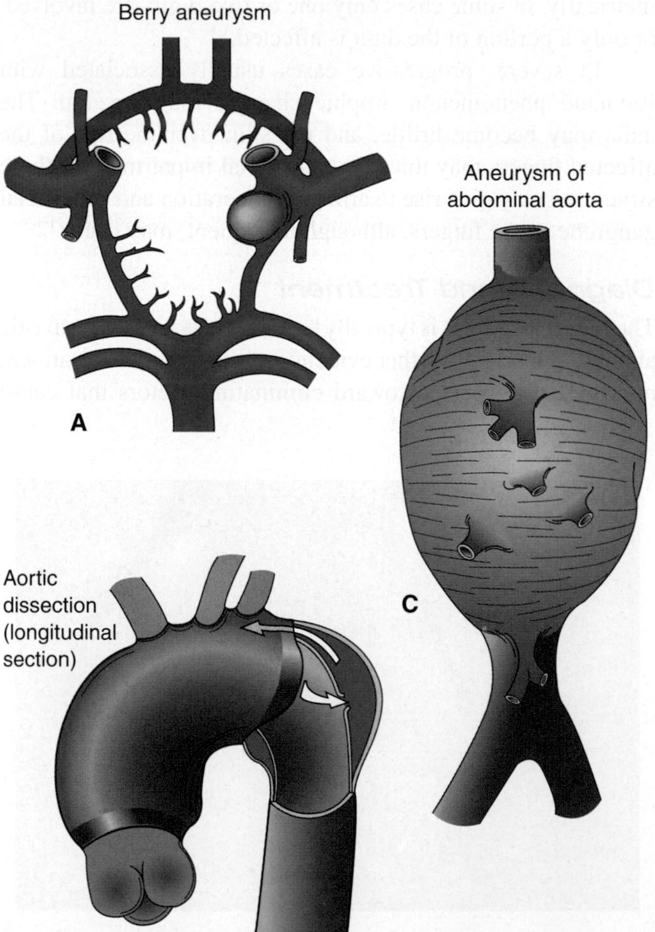

Figure 26.14 • Three forms of aneurysms: **(A)** berry aneurysm in the circle of Willis, **(B)** aortic dissection, and **(C)** fusiform-type aneurysm of the abdominal aorta.

A *berry aneurysm* (Fig. 26.14A) is a true aneurysm that consists of a small, spherical dilation of the vessel at a bifurcation.[1,4] This type of aneurysm usually is found in the circle of Willis in the cerebral circulation. A *fusiform aneurysm* (Fig. 26.14C) is a true aneurysm that involves the entire circumference of the vessel and is characterized by a gradual and progressive dilation of the vessel. These aneurysms, which vary in diameter (up to 20 cm) and length, may involve the entire ascending and transverse portions of the thoracic aorta or may extend over large segments of the abdominal aorta. A *saccular aneurysm* is a true aneurysm that extends over part of the circumference of the vessel and appears saclike.[4] A *dissecting aneurysm* (Fig. 26.14B) is a false aneurysm resulting from a tear in the intimal layer of the vessel that allows blood to enter the vessel wall, dissecting its layers to create a blood-filled cavity. If dissection occurs in the aorta, it is a life-threatening condition (see discussion in the next section).

The weakness that leads to aneurysm formation may be caused by several factors, including congenital defects, trauma, infections, and atherosclerosis. Once initiated, the aneurysm grows larger as the tension in the vessel increases. This is because the tension in the wall of a vessel is equal to the pressure multiplied by the radius (*i.e.*, tension pressure × radius). In this case, the pressure in the segment of the vessel affected by the aneurysm does not change but remains the same as that of adjacent portions of the vessel. As an aneurysm increases in diameter, the tension in the wall of the vessel increases in direct proportion to its increased size. If untreated, the aneurysm may rupture because of the increased tension. Even an unruptured aneurysm can cause damage by exerting pressure on adjacent structures and interrupting blood flow.

Aortic Aneurysms

Aortic aneurysms may involve any part of the aorta—the ascending aorta, aortic arch, descending aorta, thoracoabdominal aorta, or abdominal aorta. Multiple aneurysms may be present. Fig. 26.15 shows a large abdominal aortic aneurysm. Note that the aneurysm in Figure 26.15 is showing a true aneurysm, with all layers of the vessel weakened and thrombus formation inside the lumen of the aorta. Compare this with the contrasting image of a false dissecting aortic aneurysm that is shown in Figure 26.14B.

Etiology

The two most common causes of aortic aneurysms are atherosclerosis and degeneration of the vessel media. Half of the people with aortic aneurysms have hypertension. Aortic aneurysms usually develop more frequently in men after the age of 50 years who smoke cigarettes.[4]

Clinical Manifestations

The signs and symptoms of aortic aneurysms depend on the size and location. An aneurysm also may be asymptomatic, with the first evidence of its presence being associated with vessel rupture. Aneurysms of the thoracic aorta are less

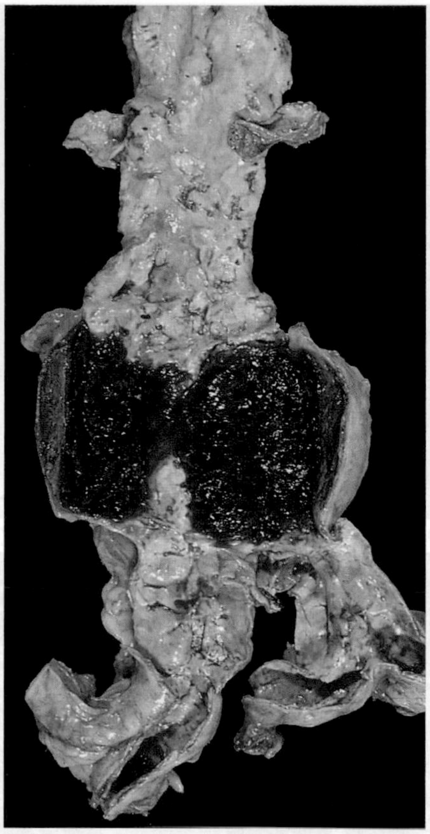

Figure 26.15 • Atherosclerotic aneurysm of the abdominal aorta. The aneurysm has been opened longitudinally to reveal a large thrombus in the lumen. The aorta and common iliac arteries display complicated lesions of atherosclerosis. (From Rubin R., Strayer D. S., Saffitz J. E., et al. (Eds.) (2015). *Rubin's pathology: Clinicopathologic foundations of medicine* (7th ed., Fig. 16-38, p. 611). Philadelphia, PA: Wolters Kluwer.)

common than abdominal aortic aneurysms and may present with substernal, back, and neck pain. There also may be dyspnea, stridor, or brassy cough caused by pressure on the trachea. Hoarseness may result from pressure on the recurrent laryngeal nerve, and there may be difficulty swallowing because of pressure on the esophagus. The aneurysm also may compress the superior vena cava, causing distention of neck veins and edema of the face and neck.[1,4]

Abdominal aortic aneurysms are located most commonly below the level of the renal artery and involve the bifurcation of the aorta and proximal end of the common iliac arteries.[1,4] The infrarenal aorta is normally 2 cm in diameter; an aneurysm is defined as an aortic diameter greater than 3 cm. They can involve any part of the vessel circumference (saccular) or extend to involve the entire circumference (fusiform). Most abdominal aneurysms are asymptomatic. Because an aneurysm is of arterial origin, a pulsating mass may provide the first evidence of the disorder. Typically, aneurysms larger than 4 cm are palpable. The mass may be discovered during a routine physical examination, or the affected person may complain of its presence. Calcification, which frequently exists on the wall of the aneurysm, may be detected during abdominal radiologic examination. Pain may be present and varies from mild mid-abdominal or lumbar discomfort to severe abdominal and back pain. As the aneurysm expands, it may compress the lumbar nerve roots, causing lower back pain that radiates to the posterior aspects of the legs. The aneurysm may extend to and impinge on the renal, iliac, or mesenteric arteries or to the vertebral arteries that supply the spinal cord. An abdominal aneurysm also may cause erosion of vertebrae. Stasis of blood favors thrombus formation along the wall of the vessel (Fig. 26.15), and peripheral emboli may develop, causing symptomatic arterial insufficiency.[1,4]

With thoracic and abdominal aneurysms, the most dreaded complication is rupture. The likelihood of rupture correlates with increasing aneurysm size. The risk of rupture rises from less than 2% for small abdominal aneurysms (<4 cm in diameter) to 5% to 10% per year for aneurysms larger than 5 cm in diameter.[4]

Diagnosis and Treatment

Diagnostic methods include use of ultrasonography, echocardiography, CT scans, and MRI. Surgical repair frequently is the treatment of choice.[1,4]

Aortic Dissection

Aortic dissection (dissecting aneurysm) is an acute, life-threatening condition. It involves hemorrhage into the vessel wall with longitudinal tearing of the vessel wall to form a blood-filled channel (Fig. 26.16). Unlike atherosclerotic aneurysms, aortic dissection often occurs without evidence of previous vessel dilation. More than 95% of the cases of dissecting aneurysm show transverse tear in the intima and internal media. The dissection can originate anywhere along the length of the aorta. The majority of the dissections involve the ascending aorta.[4] The second most common site is the thoracic aorta just distal to the origin of the subclavian artery.

Etiology and Pathogenesis

Aortic dissection is caused by conditions that weaken or cause degenerative changes in the elastic and smooth muscle of the layers of the aorta. It is most common in the 40- to 60-year-old age group and more prevalent in men than in women.[1] Two risk factors predispose to aortic dissection—hypertension and degeneration of the medial layer of the vessel wall. There is a history of hypertension in most cases.[1] Aortic dissection is also associated with connective tissue diseases, such as Marfan syndrome. It may also occur during pregnancy because of changes in the aorta that occur during this time. Other factors that predispose to dissection are congenital defects of the aortic valve (*i.e.*, bicuspid or unicuspid valve structures) and aortic coarctation. Aortic dissection is a potential complication of cardiac surgery or catheterization. Surgically related dissection may occur at the points where the aorta has been incised or cross-clamped. It also has been reported at the site where the saphenous vein was sutured to the aorta during coronary artery bypass surgery.

Aortic dissections are commonly classified into two types, type A and type B, as determined by the level of

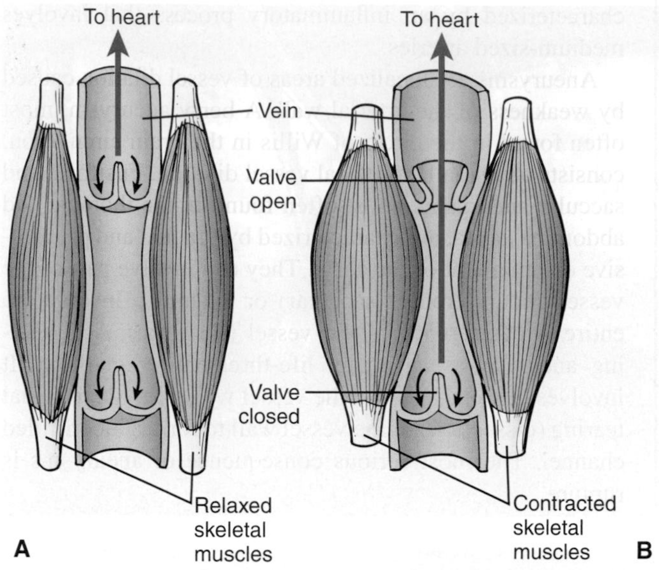

Figure 26.17 • The skeletal muscle pumps and their function in promoting blood flow in the deep and superficial calf vessels of the leg.

person walks, the action of the leg muscles serves to increase flow in the deep venous channels and return venous blood to the heart (Fig. 26.17). This function of the leg muscles (the gastrocnemius and soleus muscles of the lower extremities) can be compared with the pumping action of the heart and is therefore referred to as the *skeletal muscle pump*.[4] During muscle contraction, which is similar to systole, valves in the communicating channels close to prevent backward flow of blood into the superficial system, as blood in the deep veins is moved forward by the action of the contracting muscles. During muscle relaxation, which is similar to diastole, the communicating valves open, allowing blood from the superficial veins to move into the deep veins.

Although its structure enables the venous system to serve as a storage area for blood, it also renders the system susceptible to problems related to stasis and venous insufficiency. This section focuses on three common problems of the venous system—varicose veins, venous insufficiency, and venous thrombosis.

KEY POINTS

DISORDERS OF THE VENOUS CIRCULATION

- Veins are thin-walled, distensible vessels that collect blood from the tissues and return it to the heart. The venous system is a low-pressure system that relies on the pumping action of the skeletal muscles to move blood forward and the presence of venous valves to prevent retrograde flow.
- Disorders of the venous system produce congestion of the affected tissues and predispose to clot formation because of stagnation of flow and activation of the clotting system.

Varicose Veins

Varicose, or dilated, tortuous veins of the lower extremities are common and often lead to secondary problems of venous insufficiency (Fig. 26.18). Varicose veins are described as being primary or secondary. Primary varicose veins originate in the superficial saphenous veins, and secondary varicose veins result from impaired flow in the deep venous channels. Approximately 80% to 90% of venous blood from the lower extremities is transported through the deep channels. The development of secondary varicose veins becomes inevitable when flow in these deep channels is impaired or blocked. The most common cause of secondary varicose veins is deep vein thrombosis (DVT). Other causes include congenital or acquired arteriovenous (AV) fistulas, congenital venous malformations, and pressure on the abdominal veins caused by pregnancy or a tumor.[1,3,4]

The incidence of varicose veins rises with age. The prevalence of varicose veins is 50% in people older than 50 years. The condition is more common in females between 30 and 50 years of age, especially if there is a strong familial predisposition.[4] There is also a higher incidence in obese people, because of the increase in intra-abdominal pressure, and among people who stand for the majority of their day because of an occupation (*e.g.*, nurses).

Etiology and Pathogenesis

Prolonged standing and increased intra-abdominal pressure are important contributing factors in the development of primary

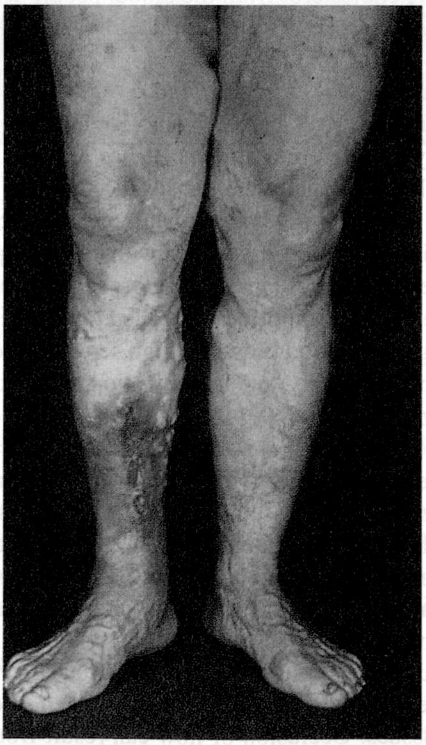

Figure 26.18 • Varicose veins of the legs. Severe varicosities of the superficial leg veins have led to stasis dermatitis and secondary ulcerations. (From Strayer D., Rubin R., Saffitz J. E., et al. (Eds.) (2015). *Rubin's pathology: Clinicopathologic foundations of medicine* (7th ed., Fig. 16-41, p. 614). Philadelphia, PA: Wolters Kluwer.)

varicose veins. Prolonged standing increases venous pressure and causes dilation and stretching of the vessel wall. One of the most important factors in the elevation of venous pressure is the hydrostatic effect associated with the standing position. When a person is in the erect position, the full weight of the venous columns of blood is transmitted to the leg veins. The effects of gravity are compounded in people who stand for long periods without using their leg muscles to assist in pumping blood back to the heart.[1,3,4]

Because there are no valves in the inferior vena cava or common iliac veins, blood in the abdominal veins must be supported by the valves located in the external iliac or femoral veins. When intra-abdominal pressure increases, as it does during pregnancy, or when the valves in these two veins are absent or defective, the stress on the saphenofemoral junction is increased. The high incidence of varicose veins in women who have been pregnant also suggests a hormonal effect on venous smooth muscle contributing to venous dilation and valvular incompetence. Lifting also increases intra-abdominal pressure and decreases flow of blood through the abdominal veins. Occupations that require repeated heavy lifting also predispose to development of varicose veins.[1,3,4]

Prolonged exposure to increased pressure causes the venous valves to become incompetent so they no longer close properly. When this happens, the reflux of blood causes further venous enlargement, pulling the valve leaflet apart and causing more valvular incompetence in sections of adjacent distal veins. Another consideration in the development of varicose veins is the fact that the superficial veins have only subcutaneous fat and superficial fascia for support, but the deep venous channels are supported by muscle, bone, and connective tissue. Obesity reduces the support provided by the superficial fascia and tissues, increasing the risk for development of varicose veins.[1,3,4]

Clinical Manifestations

The signs and symptoms associated with primary varicose veins vary. Many women with superficial varicose veins complain of their unsightly appearance. In many cases, aching in the lower extremities and edema, especially after long periods of standing, may occur. The edema usually subsides at night when the legs are elevated. When the communicating veins are incompetent, symptoms are more common.[22]

Diagnosis and Treatment

The diagnosis of varicose veins can often be made after a thorough history and physical examination, especially inspection of the extremities involved. The Doppler ultrasonic flow probe may also be used to assess flow in the large vessels. Angiographic studies using a radiopaque contrast medium may be used to assess venous function.[22]

After the venous channels have been repeatedly stretched and the valves rendered incompetent, little can be done to restore normal venous tone and function. Ideally, measures should be taken to prevent the development and progression of varicose veins. This would include weight loss and measures to avoid activities, such as continued standing, that produce prolonged elevation of venous pressure. Treatment measures for varicose veins focus on improving venous flow and preventing tissue injury. When correctly fitted, elastic support stockings or leggings compress the superficial veins and prevent distention. Prescription stockings measured to fit properly afford the most precise control. These stockings should be applied before the standing position is assumed, when the leg veins are empty.[22]

Sclerotherapy, which often is used in the treatment of small residual varicosities, involves the injection of a sclerosing agent into the collapsed superficial veins to produce fibrosis of the vessel lumen. Surgical treatment consists of removing the varicosities and the incompetent perforating veins; however, this is limited to people with patent deep venous channels.[22]

Chronic Venous Insufficiency

The term *venous insufficiency* refers to the pathophysiologic of persistent venous hypertension on the structure and function of the venous system of the lower extremities.

Etiology and Pathogenesis

The causation is multifactorial, including factors such as increased venous hydrostatic pressure (as with prolonged standing), incompetent valves in the veins, deep vein obstructions (as with DVT), decreased function of the skeletal muscle pumps, inflammatory processes, and endothelial dysfunction.[1,4,23]

With venous insufficiency, effective unidirectional flow of blood and emptying of the deep veins cannot occur. If the muscle pumps are ineffective, blood may be driven in a retrograde direction. Secondary failure of the communicating and superficial veins subjects the subcutaneous tissues to high pressures.[1,4,23]

Clinical Manifestations

Clinical manifestations are associated with impaired blood flow. In contrast to the ischemia caused by arterial insufficiency, venous insufficiency leads to tissue congestion, edema, and eventual impairment of tissue nutrition. The edema is exacerbated by long periods of standing. Necrosis of subcutaneous fat deposits can occur, followed by skin atrophy. Brown pigmentation of the skin caused by hemosiderin deposits resulting from the breakdown of red blood cells is common. Secondary lymphatic insufficiency may occur, with progressive sclerosis of the lymph channels because of increased demand for clearance of interstitial fluid. People with longstanding venous insufficiency may also experience stiffening of the ankle joint and loss of muscle mass and strength.[1,4,23]

In advanced venous insufficiency, impaired tissue nutrition causes stasis dermatitis and the development of stasis or venous ulcers (Fig. 26.18). Stasis dermatitis is characterized by the presence of thin, shiny, bluish brown, irregularly

Renal Hypertension. With the dominant role that the kidney assumes in blood pressure regulation, it is not surprising that the largest single cause of secondary hypertension is renal disease. Decreased urine formation, retention of salt and water, and hypertension are common complications of acute kidney disorders such as acute glomerulonephritis, acute renal failure, and acute urinary tract obstruction. Hypertension also commonly occurs with chronic pyelonephritis, polycystic kidney disease, diabetic nephropathy, and end-stage renal disease. In older adults, a sudden onset of secondary hypertension often is associated with atherosclerotic disease of the renal blood vessels.[1,3,4]

Renovascular hypertension refers to hypertension caused by reduced renal blood flow and activation of the renin–angiotensin–aldosterone mechanism. It is the most common cause of secondary hypertension, accounting for 1% to 2% of all cases of hypertension.[40] The reduced renal blood flow that occurs with renovascular disease causes the affected kidney to release excessive amounts of renin, increasing circulating levels of angiotensin II. Angiotensin II, in turn, acts as a vasoconstrictor to increase PVR and as a stimulus for increased aldosterone levels and sodium retention by the kidney. One or both of the kidneys may be affected. When the renal artery of only one kidney is involved, the unaffected kidney is subjected to the detrimental effects of the elevated blood pressure.[1,3,4]

Two major types of renovascular disease have been described—atherosclerosis of the proximal renal artery and fibromuscular dysplasia, a noninflammatory vascular disease that affects the renal arteries and branch vessels. Atherosclerotic stenosis of the renal artery is seen most often in older adults, particularly those with comorbidities for atherosclerosis. Fibromuscular dysplasia is more common in women and tends to occur in younger age groups, often people in the 30 to 50 years age range. Pathogenic mechanisms are uncertain; however, the incidence tends to increase with environmental factors such as smoking.[40]

Disorders of Adrenocortical Hormones. Increased levels of adrenocortical hormones can also give rise to hypertension because of hormonally induced renal retention of salt and water. Primary hyperaldosteronism (excess production of aldosterone because of adrenocortical hyperplasia or adenoma) and excess levels of glucocorticoid (Cushing disease or syndrome) tend to raise the blood pressure.[42]

Pheochromocytoma. A pheochromocytoma is a tumor of chromaffin tissue, which contains sympathetic nerve cells that stain with chromium salts and release catecholamine. The tumor is most commonly located in the adrenal medulla but can arise in other sites, such as the sympathetic ganglia, where there is chromaffin tissue. Although rare, the presence of a pheochromocytoma can cause serious hypertensive crises.[41]

Coarctation of the Aorta. Coarctation of the aorta is a congenital condition in which there is a narrowing in the area of the arch of the aorta. The aortic narrowing increases the resistance to blood flow, causing the left ventricle to increase pressure in the attempt to overcome the resistance. Because the subclavian arteries typically arise above the location of the narrowing, the result is hypertension in the upper extremities and normal or low blood pressures in the lower extremities. Coarctation can be surgically repaired to remove the restriction to flow through the aorta and normalize blood pressure.[43]

Oral Contraceptive Drugs. The use of oral contraceptives is a common cause of secondary hypertension in young women. The cause of the increased blood pressure is largely unknown, although it has been suggested that the probable cause is volume expansion because both estrogens and synthetic progesterones used in oral contraceptive pills cause sodium retention. Fortunately, the hypertension associated with oral contraceptives usually disappears after the drug has been discontinued, although it may take as long as 3 months for this to happen.[4,17]

Clinical Manifestations of Hypertension

Primary hypertension is typically an asymptomatic disorder. When symptoms do occur, they are often related to the long-term effects of hypertension on other *target organ* systems such as the kidneys, heart, eyes, and blood vessels. The morbidity and mortality related to hypertension are progressive over the whole range of systolic and diastolic pressures, with *target-organ damage* varying markedly among people with similar levels of hypertension. People with secondary hypertension are also at risk for these target organ effects; however, those people may also demonstrate clinical manifestations related to the primary disease process that is causing the secondary hypertension. Chart 26.1 presents a listing of clinical indicators that indicate the presence of target organ damage.

CHART 26.1 CONSEQUENCES OF TARGET ORGAN DAMAGE IN HYPERTENSION

- Heart
  - Angina (because of myocardial ischemia)
  - Myocardial Infarction
  - Heart failure
- Brain
  - Stroke or transient ischemic attack
- Chronic kidney disease or kidney failure
- Peripheral artery disease
- Retinopathy
- Sexual Dysfunction

Source: American Heart Association (2018). Health Threats from High Blood Pressure. Downloaded from: http://www.heart.org/HEARTORG/Conditions/HighBloodPressure/LearnHowHBPHarmsYourHealth/Health-Threats-From-High-Blood-Pressure_UCM_002051_Article.jsp.

Target Organ Damage. The increased perfusion pressure of hypertension can cause directly damage to target organs. In addition, the increased intravascular pressure can damage vascular endothelial cells, which increases the risk of the development of atherosclerotic vascular disease (which further impairs organ perfusion). Target-organ damage particularly affects organs that are highly vascular in structure or strongly dependent upon adequate blood supply for appropriate function, including the heart, brain, kidneys, and the retina of the eyes. Therefore, hypertension is a leading cause of ischemic heart and brain disease, end-stage renal disease, and visual impairment or blindness from retinopathy.[4,26]

Hypertension is a major risk factor for atherosclerosis because it promotes and/or accelerates plaque formation and possible rupture. It predisposes to all major atherosclerotic cardiovascular disorders, including coronary heart disease, heart failure, stroke, and PAD. The risk for coronary artery disease and stroke depends to a great extent on other risk factors, such as obesity, smoking, and dyslipidemia as well as genetic predisposition.[1,4]

An elevation in blood pressure increases the workload of the left ventricle by increasing the pressure against which the heart must pump as it ejects blood into the systemic circulation. The pressure over time increases the workload of the heart. Over time, the left ventricular wall remodels and hypertrophies to compensate for the increased pressure work. This left ventricular hypertrophy is a major risk factor for coronary heart disease, cardiac dysrhythmias, sudden death, and congestive heart failure because it cannot pump efficiently.[1,4]

Chronic hypertension leads to nephrosclerosis, a common cause of chronic kidney disease. The damage to the kidneys is caused by multiple mechanisms. One of the major ways hypertension causes damage to the kidneys is through glomerular hypoperfusion. This hypoperfusion then causes glomerulosclerosis and tubulointerstitial fibrosis. Other ways that have been studied include endothelial dysfunction from high glomerular pressures. Hypertensive kidney disease is more common in blacks than whites. Hypertension also plays an important role in accelerating the course of other types of kidney disease, particularly diabetic nephropathy.[1,4]

Dementia and cognitive impairment occur more commonly in people with hypertension. Hypertension, particularly systolic hypertension, is a major risk factor for ischemic stroke and intracerebral hemorrhage.[1,4] Narrowing and sclerosis of small penetrating arteries in the subcortical regions of the brain are common findings on autopsy in people with chronic hypertension.[1,4] These changes are thought to contribute to hypoperfusion, loss of autoregulation of blood flow, and impairment of the blood–brain barrier, ultimately leading to subcortical white matter demyelination. Effective antihypertensive therapy strongly reduces the risk of development of significant white matter changes. However, existing white matter changes, once established, do not appear to be reversible.[1,4]

Hypertension also affects the eye in sometimes devastating ways. Hypertensive retinopathy affects the retina through a series of microvascular changes.[1,4] The eye of a person with hypertension will initially have increased vasomotor tone, which causes generalized arteriolar narrowing. As hypertension persists, arteriosclerotic changes become worse and include media wall hyperplasia, intimal thickening, and hyaline degeneration. These long-term changes can cause more severe AV nicking and may cause blindness (Fig. 26.20). Acute increases in blood pressure can lead to hemorrhages, microaneurysms, and hard exudates. A strong association exists between retinopathy and hypertension. This is a target organ that would need to be evaluated regularly in a person with hypertension to prevent extensive damage to the eyes.[1,4]

Hypertensive Emergency. A small number of people with hypertension develop an accelerated and potentially fatal form hypertension called a *hypertensive emergency*, which is characterized by sudden, marked elevations in blood pressure (>180/120 mm Hg) complicated by evidence of acute or worsening target organ damage. It is critical that emergent interventions be implemented to return blood pressure to safe levels to prevent permanent organ dysfunction or death. Acute organ damage from hypertensive emergency can include ischemic stroke, hypertensive encephalopathy, cardiac ischemia, and retinal hemorrhage.[26,44,45]

Diagnosis and Treatment

Hypertension is diagnosed by sequential blood pressure measurements that indicate a consistent elevation of the pressure

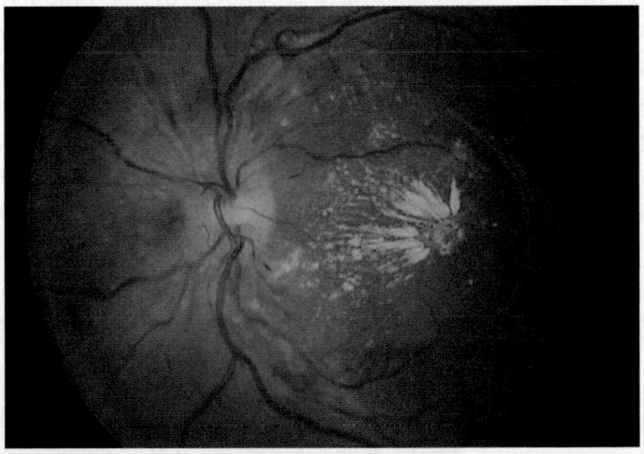

Figure 26.20 • Hypertensive retinopathy. Various abnormalities develop within the retina in hypertension. The commonly associated arteriolosclerosis affects the appearance of the retinal microvasculature. Light reflected from the thickened arteriolar walls mimics silver or copper wire. Blood flow through the retinal venules is not well visualized at the sites of arteriolar–venular crossings. This effect is due to a thickening of the venular wall rather than to an impediment to blood flow caused by compression; the column of blood proximal to the compression is not wider than the part distal to the crossing. Impaired axoplasmic flow within the nerve fiber layer, caused by ischemia, results in swollen axons with cytoplasmic bodies. Such structures resemble cotton on funduscopy ("cotton-wool spots"). Hemorrhages are common in the retina, and exudates frequently form a star around the macula. (From Strayer D., Rubin R., Saffitz J. E., et al. (Eds.) (2015). *Rubin's pathology: Clinicopathologic foundations of medicine* (7th ed., Fig. 33-8, p. 1512). Philadelphia, PA: Wolters Kluwer.)

within the systemic arterial circuit. Threshold criteria for the diagnosis and management of hypertension continue to shift as new scientific evidence emerges. The most recent clinical management guidelines for adults in the United States were issued in November 2017 as a joint publication of the American College of Cardiology (ACC) and the American Heart Association (AHA).[26] The 2017 ACC/AHA diagnostic guidelines and recommendations for clinical management are included as Table 26.3.

These revised 2017 guidelines reflect a significantly lower diagnostic threshold for hypertension than in previous guidelines, with the lower threshold for diagnosis of stage 1 hypertension recommended at systolic blood pressure levels of 130 to 139 mm Hg or diastolic blood pressure levels at 80 to 89 mm Hg.[26] These revised diagnostic levels are in comparison to the previous diagnostic thresholds established by the Joint National Committee 7 guidelines from 2003,[46] which were systolic blood pressure of 140 to 159 mm Hg or diastolic blood pressure of 90 to 99 mm Hg. The clinical management of primary hypertension is focused toward reducing the effects of modifiable factors through lifestyle and behavior changes and with medication therapy. Clinical management of secondary hypertension is directed at the primary disease.

High Blood Pressure in Pregnancy. Hypertensive disorders of pregnancy complicate up to 10% of pregnancies and are a major cause of mortality and morbidity for both mothers and babies in the United States and worldwide. Most adverse events are attributable directly to the preeclampsia syndrome. Pregnant women can also have an underlying chronic hypertension, which also manifests adverse effects during the pregnancy.[47,48] The decreased placental blood flow that occurs with hypertensive disorders of pregnancy also affects the fetus, frequently disrupting fetal growth and leading to preterm delivery. In women with preeclampsia, delivery of the fetus is curative. The timing of delivery becomes a difficult decision in preterm pregnancies because the welfare of both the mother and the infant must be taken into account.

In 2013, the American College of Obstetricians and Gynecologists (ACOG) published a new classification system for high blood pressure in pregnancy. The ACOG guidelines include the following four classifications: preeclampsia–eclampsia, chronic hypertension, chronic hypertension with superimposed preeclampsia, and gestational hypertension.[47] As the prevalence of chronic hypertension increases in the population, more women are entering pregnancy with an underlying comorbidity of chronic hypertension. The pathophysiology of chronic hypertension has been previously discussed; therefore, the focus of this section will be on preeclampsia–eclampsia and gestational hypertension.

Preeclampsia–Eclampsia. According to the 2013 ACOG report,[47] preeclampsia is a multisystem disorder of pregnancy that includes the following characteristics:

- Hypertension, with systolic blood pressure ≥140 mm Hg and/or diastolic blood pressure ≥90 mm Hg.
- Thrombocytopenia, with platelet counts ≤100,000/μL
- Impaired liver function, reflected by elevation of liver transaminases (to levels twice the normal)
- Renal insufficiency of new onset, evidenced by elevated creatinine levels to ≥1.1 mg/dL or twice the normal levels
- Pulmonary edema
- Disturbances of vision or cerebral disturbances (both new in onset).

Edema and proteinuria are also often associated with preeclampsia; however, these findings are no longer requirements for the diagnosis of preeclampsia.[47]

The specific cause of preeclampsia is unknown; however, considerable evidence suggests that placental dysfunction is the key factor. A decrease in placental blood flow may lead to the release of toxic mediators that contribute to endothelial

TABLE 26.3 CLASSIFICATION OF BLOOD PRESSURE IN ADULTS (BY THE 2017 GUIDELINES OF THE AMERICAN COLLEGE OF CARDIOLOGY AND AMERICAN HEART ASSOCIATION)

BLOOD PRESSURE CLASSIFICATION	SYSTOLIC BLOOD PRESSURE (MM HG)	DIASTOLIC BLOOD PRESSURE (MM HG)
Normal	<120	***and*** <80
Elevated	120–129	***and*** <80
Stage 1 hypertension	130–139	***or*** 80–89
Stage 2 hypertension	>140	***or*** ≥90

Modified with permission from Whelton P. K., Carey R. M., Aronow W. S., et al. (2017). ACC/AHA/AAPA/ABC/ACPM/AGS/APhA/ASH/ASPC/NMA/PCNA guideline for the prevention, detection, evaluation, and management of high blood pressure in adults: a report of the American College of Cardiology/American Heart Association Task Force on Clinical Practice Guidelines. *Hypertension* 71(6), 1269–1324.

dysfunction in blood vessels throughout the body, particularly in the kidney, brain, liver, and heart. Additional factors that are being investigated as contributors to the pathophysiology include genetics, disruptions in the renin–angiotensin system, and possible antiangiogenic factors. In severe cases, complications include hypoperfusion of vital organs, disseminated intravascular coagulation (DIC), cerebral hemorrhage, hepatic failure, and acute renal failure.[47,48]

The "eclampsia" phase of the syndrome is heralded by the onset of seizures because of the neurologic involvement. Another serious complication is HELLP syndrome, a life-threatening phenomenon characterized by the combination of **H**emolysis, **E**levated **L**iver enzymes, and **L**ow **P**latelet count.[47]

Gestational Hypertension. Gestational hypertension is characterized by elevation of blood pressure of new onset occurring after the pregnancy has reached 20 weeks gestation, without evidence of proteinuria or the other clinical manifestations that are diagnostic of preeclampsia. Blood pressure often normalizes after delivery; however, the occurrence of gestational hypertension may be a risk factor for the later development of chronic hypertension.[47]

High Blood Pressure in Children and Adolescents. Although the incidence of hypertension among children and adolescents has historically been low, recent data indicate increasing prevalence. This may be due in part to increasing prevalence of obesity and other lifestyle factors, such as decreased physical activity and increased intake of high-calorie, high-salt foods. Secondary hypertension also remains a common form of high blood pressure in infants and children.[4,48]

Blood pressure norms for children are based on age-, height-, and sex-specific percentile norms. According to 2017 updated recommendations of the American Academy of Pediatrics, normal blood pressure for children less than 13 years of age is defined as a blood pressure greater than 90th percentile norms. For adolescents 13 years and older, a normal blood pressure is defined as a blood pressure below 120/80 mm Hg.[48]

High Blood Pressure in Older Adults. Among the aging processes that contribute to an increase in blood pressure are a stiffening of the large arteries, particularly the aorta; decreased baroreceptor sensitivity; increased PVR; and decreased renal blood flow. With aging, the elastin fibers in the walls of the arteries are gradually replaced by collagen fibers that render the vessels stiffer and less compliant. Because of increased wall stiffness, the aorta and large arteries are less able to buffer the increase in systolic pressure that occurs as blood is ejected from the left heart, and they are less able to store the energy needed to maintain the diastolic pressure. As a result, the systolic pressure increases, the diastolic pressure remains unchanged or decreases, and the pulse pressure, or difference between the systolic pressure and diastolic pressure, widens.[1,3,4]

KEY POINTS

HYPERTENSION

- Hypertension represents an elevation in systolic and/or diastolic blood pressure.
- Primary (essential) hypertension is characterized by a chronic elevation in blood pressure that occurs without evidence of other disease. Secondary hypertension is characterized by an elevation of blood pressure that results from some other disorder, such as kidney disease.

Orthostatic Hypotension

Orthostatic or postural hypotension is an abnormal drop in blood pressure on assumption of the standing position. A 2011 consensus definition for orthostatic hypotension is "a sustained reduction in systolic pressure of at least 20 mm Hg or more or diastolic blood pressure of 10 mm Hg within 3 minutes of standing or head-up tilt on a tilt table to at least 60 degrees" (Freeman et al., 2011, p. 46). This consensus definition was endorsed by multiple international neurologic professional groups, who also recognize that this numeric change in blood pressure values may be accompanied by clinical symptoms or may be asymptomatic. This expert consensus document also recognizes that supine hypertension is also present at times. For those people with supine hypertension, the document advises that a blood pressure reduction of 30 mm Hg would be a more appropriate metric.[49] Clinicians also recognize that it is equally important to also assess for the presence of orthostatic symptoms (*e.g.*, dizziness, syncope), which are perhaps more relevant than the numeric decrease in blood pressure, and that blood pressure decreases may also occur after 3 minutes in an upright position.[50]

Etiology and Pathogenesis

After the assumption of the upright posture from the supine position, approximately 500 to 700 mL of blood is rapidly shifted to the lower part of the body, with an accompanying decrease in central blood volume and arterial pressure. Maintenance of blood pressure during position change is quite complex, involving the rapid initiation of cardiovascular, neurohumoral, and muscular responses. When the standing position is assumed in the absence of circulatory reflexes or blood volume, blood pools in the lower part of the body, CO falls, blood pressure drops, and blood flow to the brain is inadequate. As a result, symptoms of decreased blood flow to the CNS may occur, including feelings of weakness, nausea, light-headedness, dizziness, blurred vision, palpitations, and syncope (*i.e.*, fainting).[1,4]

The decrease in blood pressure that occurs on standing is usually transient, lasting through several cardiac cycles. Normally, the baroreceptors located in the thorax and carotid sinus area sense the decreased pressure and initiate reflex constriction of the veins and arterioles and an increase in HR, which brings blood pressure back to normal. The initial adjustment to orthostatic stress is mediated exclusively by the ANS. Within a few minutes of standing, blood levels of ADH and sympathetic neuromediators increase as a secondary means of ensuring maintenance of normal blood pressure in the standing position. Under normal conditions, the renin–angiotensin–aldosterone system is also activated when the standing position is assumed, and even more so in situations of hypotensive orthostatic stress.[1,3,4]

Muscle movement in the lower extremities also aids venous return to the heart by pumping blood out of the legs. The unconscious slight body and leg movement during standing (postural sway) is recognized as an important factor in moving venous blood back to the heart.[51] Crossing the legs, which involves contraction of the agonist and antagonist muscles, has been shown to be a simple and effective way of increasing CO and, therefore, blood pressure.

A wide variety of conditions, acute and chronic, are associated with orthostatic hypotension. Although orthostatic hypotension can occur in all age groups, it is seen more frequently in older adults, especially in those who are sick and frail. Any disease condition that reduces blood volume, impairs mobility, results in prolonged inactivity, or impairs ANS function may also predispose to orthostatic hypotension. Adverse effects of medications are also commonly encountered causes of orthostatic hypotension, such as diuretics.[1,3,4]

Effects of Aging. Weakness and dizziness on standing are common complaints of older adults, with episodes of orthostatic hypotension presenting an increased risk for falls in this population. Although orthostatic tolerance is well maintained in healthy older people, with advancing age there is an increasing tendency toward arterial pressure instability and postural hypotension. Although orthostatic hypotension may be either systolic or diastolic, that associated with aging seems more often to be systolic. Several deficiencies in the circulatory response may predispose to this problem in older adults, including diminished ability to produce an adequate increase in the HR, ventricular SV, or PVR; decreased function of the skeletal muscle pumps; and decreased blood volume. Because cerebral blood flow primarily depends on systolic pressure, people with impaired cerebral circulation may experience symptoms of weakness, ataxia, dizziness, and syncope when their arterial pressure falls even slightly. This may happen in older adults who are immobilized for even brief periods or whose blood volume is decreased owing to inadequate fluid intake or overzealous use of diuretics.[1,3,4,51]

Reduced Blood Volume. Orthostatic hypotension often is an early sign of reduced blood volume or fluid deficit. When blood volume is decreased, the vascular compartment is only partially filled. Although CO may be adequate when a person is in the recumbent position, it often decreases to the point of causing weakness and fainting when the person assumes the standing position. Common causes of orthostatic hypotension related to hypovolemia are excessive use of diuretics, excessive diaphoresis, loss of gastrointestinal fluids through vomiting and diarrhea, and loss of fluid volume associated with prolonged bed rest.[1,3,4]

Bed Rest and Impaired Mobility. Prolonged bed rest promotes a reduction in plasma volume, a decrease in venous tone, failure of peripheral vasoconstriction, and weakness of the skeletal muscles that support the veins and assist in returning blood to the heart. Physical deconditioning follows even short periods of bed rest. After 3 to 4 days, the blood volume is decreased. Loss of vascular and skeletal muscle tone is less predictable but probably becomes maximal after approximately 2 weeks of bed rest.[1,3,4]

Drug-Induced Hypotension. Antihypertensive drugs and psychotropic drugs are the most common cause of chronic orthostatic hypotension. In most cases, the orthostatic hypotension is well tolerated. However, if the hypotension causes light-headedness or syncope, the dosage of the drug is usually reduced or a different drug substituted.[17]

Disorders of the Autonomic Nervous System. The SNS plays an essential role in adjustment to the upright position. Sympathetic stimulation increases HR and cardiac contractility and causes constriction of peripheral veins and arterioles. Orthostatic hypotension caused by altered ANS function is common in peripheral neuropathies associated with diabetes mellitus, after injury or disease of the spinal cord, or as the result of a cerebral vascular accident in which sympathetic outflow from the brain stem is disrupted.[1,3,4]

KEY POINTS

ORTHOSTATIC HYPOTENSION

- Orthostatic or postural hypotension represents an abnormal drop in blood pressure on assumption of the upright position because of pooling of blood in the lower part of the body.
- Orthostatic hypotension may be accompanied by a decrease in cerebral perfusion that causes a feeling of light-headedness, dizziness, and, in some cases, fainting. It poses a particular threat for falls in the elderly.

Diagnosis and Treatment

Orthostatic hypotension can be assessed with the auscultatory method of blood pressure measurement. It is strongly recommended that a second person be available when blood pressure is measured in the standing position to prevent injury should the person become faint. The seated position may be used in people who are unable to stand; however, the postural blood pressure changes may be missed. A thorough physical should be done to determine the cause and seriousness of the condition. A careful history should be taken to elicit information about symptoms, particularly dizziness and history of syncope and falls; medical conditions, particularly those such as diabetes mellitus that predispose to orthostatic hypotension; use of prescription and over-the-counter drugs; and symptoms of ANS dysfunction, such as erectile or bladder dysfunction. A physical examination should document blood pressure in both arms and the HR while in the supine, sitting, and standing positions and should note the occurrence of symptoms. Noninvasive, 24-hour ambulatory blood pressure monitoring may be used to determine blood pressure responses to other stimuli of daily life, such as food ingestion and exertion.[49–52]

Treatment of orthostatic hypotension is primarily directed toward alleviating the cause and helping people learn ways to cope with the disorder and prevent falls and injuries. Medications that predispose to postural hypotension should be avoided. Correcting the fluid deficit and trying a different antihypertensive medication are examples of measures designed to correct the cause. Measures designed to help people prevent symptomatic orthostatic drops in blood pressure include gradual ambulation to allow the circulatory system to adjust (*i.e.*, sitting on the edge of the bed for several minutes and moving the legs to initiate skeletal muscle pump function before standing); avoidance of situations that encourage excessive vasodilation (*e.g.*, drinking alcohol, exercising vigorously in a warm environment); and avoidance of excess diuresis (*e.g.*, use of diuretics), diaphoresis, or loss of body fluids. Tight-fitting elastic support hose or an abdominal support garment may help prevent pooling of blood in the lower extremities and abdomen.[49–52]

IN SUMMARY

Hypertension is one of the most common cardiovascular disorders. It may occur as a primary disorder (*i.e.*, essential hypertension) or as a symptom of some other disease (*i.e.*, secondary hypertension). The incidence of essential hypertension increases with age; the condition is seen more frequently among blacks, and it may be associated with a family history of high blood pressure, metabolic syndrome, obesity, and increased sodium intake. Causes of secondary hypertension include kidney disease and adrenal cortical disorders (hyperaldosteronism and Cushing disease), which increase sodium and water retention; pheochromocytomas, which increase catecholamine levels; and coarctation of the aorta, which produces an increase in blood flow and systolic blood pressure in the arms and a decrease in blood flow and systolic pressure in the legs. Uncontrolled hypertension increases the risk of heart disease, renal complications, retinopathy, and stroke.

Hypertension that occurs during pregnancy can be divided into four categories: preeclampsia–eclampsia, chronic hypertension, chronic hypertension with superimposed preeclampsia, and gestational hypertension. Preeclampsia–eclampsia is a life-threatening complication of pregnancy that is thought to be related to the placenta and widespread endothelial dysfunction. Gestational hypertension is a new onset finding of increased blood pressure after 20 weeks gestation, without signs of preeclampsia.

The prevalence of hypertension in children and adolescents appears to be increasing, partly as a result of an increase in childhood obesity, and lifestyle factors such as physical inactivity and increased intake of high-calorie and high-salt foods. Hypertension is a common pathophysiologic condition in older adults. A frequent finding in this population is an isolated systolic hypertension thought to be related to the loss of elastin fibers in the aorta and the inability of the aorta to stretch during systole.

Orthostatic hypotension refers to an abnormal decrease in systolic and diastolic blood pressures that occur on assumption of the upright position. An important consideration in orthostatic hypotension is the occurrence of dizziness and syncope. Among the factors that contribute to its occurrence are decreased fluid volume, medications, aging, defective function of the ANS, and the effects of immobility. Diagnosis of orthostatic hypotension relies on blood pressure measurements in the supine and upright positions, and a history of symptomatology, medication use, and disease conditions that contribute to a postural drop in blood pressure. Treatment includes correcting the reversible causes and assisting the person to compensate for the disorder and prevent falls and injuries.

GERIATRIC Considerations

- Because the coronary arteries of females are narrower than in males, atherosclerosis makes diagnostic procedures such as cardiac catheterization and treatments such as angioplasty challenging.[53]
- Because of the protective benefit of estrogen, women usually develop coronary artery disease 10 years later than men.[53]
- The sensitivity to baroreceptor regulation of blood pressure decreases with age.[54]
- The incidence of decreased tissue perfusion increases with age because of varicose veins, atherosclerosis, hypertension, and congestive heart failure.[54]
- Hypertension associated with aging is primarily caused from vasoconstriction and increased afterload.[54]
- The risk for hyperlipidemia increases with age because of comorbidities such as diabetes, hypothyroidism, and use of some medications such as corticosteroids and thiazide diuretics.[54]

PEDIATRIC Considerations

- Heart failure usually occurs in infants because of congenital heart defects, which are often repaired during the first year of life. Well children who present later with heart failure usually have acquired cardiac disease such as viral disease affecting the heart muscle, bacterial infection of the endocarditis, or rheumatic fever.[55]
- Congenital heart disease is the primary reason for children to develop heart failure.[55]
- Hyperlipidemia in children is the beginning of atherosclerosis manifested in later life.[55]
- Auscultation is the preferred assessment methods to measure blood pressure in children because of lack of reference standards needed in automatic devices.[55]

REVIEW EXERCISES

1. A 55-year-old male executive presents at the clinic for his regular checkup. He was diagnosed with hypertension 5 years ago and has been taking a diuretic and a β-adrenergic blocker to control his blood pressure. His blood pressure is currently being maintained at about 135/70 mm Hg. His total cholesterol level is 180 mg/dL, and his HDL cholesterol is 30 mg/dL. He is otherwise well. He is a nonsmoker. He has recently read in the media about "inflammation" and the heart and expresses concern about his risk of CHD.
   A. *Identify risk factors for atherosclerosis present in this history.*
   B. *Explain the role of HDL in the prevention of atherosclerosis.*
2. A 62-year-old man presents at the emergency department of his local hospital with complaints of excruciating, "ripping" pain in his upper back. He has a history of poorly controlled hypertension. His radial pulse and blood pressure, which on admission were 92 and 140/80 mm Hg, respectively, become unobtainable in both arms. A transesophageal echocardiogram reveals a dissection of the descending aorta. Aggressive blood pressure control is initiated with the goal of reducing the systolic pressure and pulsatile blood flow (pulse pressure).
   A. *Explain how aortic dissection differs from a thoracic aorta aneurysm.*
   B. *Explain the role of poorly controlled hypertension as an etiologic factor in dissecting aneurysms.*
   C. *Why did his radial pulse and blood pressure become unobtainable?*
   D. *Explain the need for aggressive control of aortic pressure and pulsatile blood flow.*
3. A 34-year-old, otherwise healthy woman complains of episodes lasting several hours in which her fingers become pale and numb. This is followed by a period during which the fingers become red, throbbing, and painful. She lives in the Northeast and notices it more in the fall and winter months.
   A. *What do you think is causing this woman's problem?*
   B. *She relates that the episodes often occur when her fingers become cold or when she becomes upset. Explain the possible underlying mechanisms.*
   C. *What types of measures could be used to treat this woman?*
4. A 47-year-old African American man who is an executive in a law firm has his blood pressure taken at a screening program and is told that his pressure is 142/90 mm Hg. His father and older brother have hypertension, and his paternal grandparents had a history of stroke and myocardial infarction. The patient enjoys salty foods and routinely uses a saltshaker to add salt to meals his wife prepares, drinks about four beers while watching television in the evening, and gained 15 lb in the past year. Although his family has encouraged him to engage in physical activities with them, he states he is either too busy or too tired.
   A. *According to the 2017 ACC/AHA guidelines, into what category does the patient's blood pressure fall? What are his risk factors for hypertension?*
   B. *Explain how an increased salt intake might contribute to his increase in blood pressure.*
   C. *What lifestyle changes would you suggest to the patient? Explain the rationale for your suggestions.*
5. A 36-year-old woman enters the clinic complaining of headache and not feeling well. Her blood pressure is 175/90 mm Hg. Her renal test results are abnormal, and follow-up tests confirm that she has a stricture of the left renal artery.
   A. *Would this woman's hypertension be classified as primary or secondary?*
   B. *Explain the physiologic mechanisms underlying her blood pressure elevation.*
6. A 75-year-old woman residing in an extended care facility has multiple health problems, including diabetes, hypertension, and heart failure. Lately, she has been feeling dizzy when she stands up, and she has almost fallen on several occasions.

Her family is concerned and wants to know why this is happening and what they can do to prevent her from falling and breaking her hip.

A. *How would you go about assessing this woman for orthostatic hypotension?*

B. *What are some causes of orthostatic hypotension in elderly people?*

C. *How might this woman's medical conditions and their treatment contribute to her orthostatic hypotension?*

References

1. Kumar V., Abbas A. K., Aster J. C. (2015). *Robbins & Cotran Pathologic Basis of Disease* (9th ed.). Philadelphia, PA: Elsevier Saunders.
2. Ross M., Pawlina W. (2015). *Histology: A Text and Atlas* (7th ed.). Philadelphia, PA: Lippincott Williams & Wilkins.
3. Hall J. E. (2015). *Guyton and Hall Textbook of Medical Physiology* (13th ed.). Philadelphia, PA: Elsevier.
4. Rubin R., Strayer D. S., Saffitz J. E., et al. (Eds.) (2015). *Rubin's pathology: Clinicopathologic Foundations of Medicine* (7th ed.). Philadelphia, PA: Wolters Kluwer.
5. Hopps E., Caimi G. (2015). Obstructive sleep apnea syndrome: Links between pathophysiology and cardiovascular complications. *Clinical and Investigative Medicine* 38(6), E362–E370.
6. Wang L., Li N., Yao X., et al. (2017). Detection of secondary causes and coexisting diseases in hypertensive patients: OSA and PA are the common causes associated with hypertension. *BioMed Research International* Article ID 8295010, 8 pages https://doi.org/10.1155/2017/8295010
7. Yang H., Haack M., Gautam S., et al. (2017). Repetitive exposure to shortened sleep leads to blunted sleep-associated blood pressure dipping. *Journal of Hypertension* 35(6), 1187–1194.
8. Missala I., Kassner U., Steinhagen-Thiessen E. (2012). A systematic literature review of the association of lipoprotein(a) and autoimmune diseases and atherosclerosis. *International Journal of Rheumatology.* Article ID 480784, 10 pages. DOI: 10.1155/2012/480784
9. Schmitz G., Orso E. (2015). Lipoprotein(a) hyperlipidemia as cardiovascular risk factor: Pathophysiological aspects. *Clinical Research in Cardiology Supplement* 10:21–25.
10. Tsimikas S. (2016). The re-emergence of lipoprotein(a) in a broader clinical arena. *Progress in Cardiovascular Diseases* 59(2016) 135–144.
11. Wakabayashi I. (2016). A U-shaped relationship between alcohol consumption and cardiometabolic index in middle-aged men. *Lipids in Health and Disease* 15(50), 1–7. DOI: 10.1186/s12944-016-0217-4
12. Kennedy M. J., Jellerson K. D., Snow M. Z., et al. (2013). Challenges in the pharmacologic management of obesity in children and adolescents. *Pediatric Drugs* 15, 335–342. DOI: 10.1007/s40272-013-0028-2
13. Eckel R. H., Jakicic J. M., Ard J. D., et al. (2013). AHA/ACC guideline on lifestyle management to reduce cardiovascular risk: A report of the American College of Cardiology American/Heart Association Task Force on Practice Guidelines. *Circulation* 2013;129(25 Suppl 2):S76–S99.
14. Heymsfield S. B., Wadden T. A. (2017). Mechanisms, pathophysiology, and management of obesity. *New England Journal of Medicine* 376, 254–266. DOI: 10.1056/NEJMra1514009
15. Alberti KG, Eckel RH, Grundy SM, et al. (2009). Harmonizing the metabolic syndrome: A joint interim statement of the International Diabetes Federation Task Force on Epidemiology and Prevention; National Heart, Lung, and Blood Institute; American Heart Association; World Heart Federation; International Atherosclerosis Society; and International Association for the Study of Obesity. *Circulation* 120, 1640–1645.
16. McCracken E., Monagahan M., Sreenivasan S. (2018). Pathophysiology of the metabolic syndrome. *Clinics in Dermatology* 36, 14–20. DOI: https://doi.org/10.1016/j.clindermatol.2017.09.004
17. Lehne R. A. (2016). *Pharmacology for Nursing Care* (9th ed.). St. Louis, MO: Elsevier.
18. Goff D. C. Jr, Lloyd-Jones D. M., Bennett G., et al. (2013). 2013 ACC/AHA guideline on the assessment of cardiovascular : a report of the American College of Cardiology/American Heart Association Task Force on Practice Guidelines. *Circulation* 29(25 Suppl 2), :S49–S73. DOI: 10.1161/01.cir.0000437741.48606.98
19. American Association of Clinical Chemistry Lab Tests Online. (2018). *High-sensitivity C-reactive protein.* Downloaded from: https://labtestsonline.org/tests/high-sensitivity-c-reactive-protein-hs-crp
20. Jennette J. C. (2013). Overview of the 2012 revised international Chapel Hill Consensus Conference nomenclature of vasculotides. *Clinical and Experimental Nephrology* 17(5), 603–606.
21. Steuer J., Bjorck M., Mayer D., et al. (2013) Distinction between acute and chronic type B aortic dissection: Is there a sub-acute phase? *European Journal of Vascular and Endovascular Surgery* 45(6), 627–631.
22. Chen J. C. (2017) Current therapy for primary varicose veins. *British Columbia Medical Journal* 59(8), 418–423.
23. Mazuchova J., Pec M., Halasova E., et al. (2016). News in pathogenesis of chronic venous insufficiency. *Acta Medica Martiniana* 16(2), 5–8. DOI: 10.1515/acm-2016-0006
24. Nasr H., Scriven J. M. (2015). Superficial thrombophlebitis (superficial venous thrombosis). *The British Medical Journal* 350, h2039. DOI: 10.1136/bmj.h2039
25. Douketis J. D. (2016). Deep venous thrombosis (DVT). *Merck Manual Professional Edition.* Downloaded from: http://www.merckmanuals.com/professional/cardiovascular-disorders/peripheral-venous-disorders/deep-venous-thrombosis-dvt
26. Whelton P. K., Carey R. M., Aronow W. S., et al. (2017). ACC/AHA/AAPA/ABC/ACPM/AGS/APhA/ASH/ASPC/NMA/PCNA guideline for the prevention, detection, evaluation, and management of high blood pressure in adults: A report of the American College of Cardiology/American Heart Association Task Force on Clinical Practice Guidelines. *Hypertension* 71(6), 1269–1324.
27. U.S. Department of Health and Human Services Centers for Disease Control. (2016). *Health, United States, 2016 with Chartbook on Long-Term Trends in Health.* Downloaded from: https://www.cdc.gov/nchs/data/hus/hus16.pdf
28. World Health Organization (2017). *Global Health Observatory Data on Raised Blood Pressure.* Downloaded from: http://www.who.int/gho/ncd/risk_factors/blood_pressure_text/en/
29. Flynn J. T., Kaelber D. C., Baker-Smith C. M., et al. (2017). Clinical practice guidelines for screening and management of high blood pressure in children and adolescents. *Pediatrics* 140(3):e20171904
30. Garfinkle M. A. (2017). Salt and essential hypertension: Pathophysiology and implications for treatment. *Journal of the American Society of Hypertension* 11(6), 385–391. DOI: http://dx.doi.org/10.1016/j.jash.2017.04.006
31. American Heart Association. (2016). *High Blood Pressure and African Americans.* Downloaded from: http://www.heart.org/HEARTORG/Conditions/HighBloodPressure/UnderstandSymptomsRisks/High-Blood-Pressure-and-African-Americans_UCM_301832_Article.jsp
32. Willey J. Z., Moon Y. P., Kahn E., et al. (2014). Population attributable risks of hypertension and diabetes for cardiovascular disease and stroke in the northern Manhattan study. *Journal of the American Heart Association* 3, e001106. DOI: 10.1161/JAHA.114.001106
33. Everett B., Zajacova A. (2015). Gender differences in hypertension and hypertension awareness among young adults. *Biodemography and Social Biology* 61(1), 1–17. DOI: 10.1080/19485565.2014.929488.
34. Han L., Liu Y., Duan S., et al. (2016). DNA methylation and hypertension: Emerging evidence and challenges. *Briefings in Functional Genomics* 15(6), 460–469. DOI: 10.1093/bfgp/elw014
35. Fanning E., O'Shea D.. (2018). Genetics and the metabolic syndrome. *Clinics in Dermatology* 36, 9–13. https://doi.org/10.1016/j.clindermatol.2017.09.003
36. Elijovich F., Weinberger M. H., Anderson C. A. M.; on behalf of the American Heart Association Professional and Public Education Committee of the Council on Hypertension; Council on Functional

Genomics and Translational Biology; and Stroke Council. (2016). Salt sensitivity of blood pressure: A scientific statement from the American Heart Association. *Hypertension* 68, e7–e46. DOI: 10.1161/HYP.0000000000000047.

37. McEvoy J. W., Blaha M. J., DeFilippis A. P., et al. (2015). Cigarette smoking and cardiovascular events: Role of inflammation and subclinical atherosclerosis. *Arteriosclerosis, Thrombosis, and Vascular Biology* 35(3), 700–709.
38. Ahmad M., Makati D., Akbar S. (2017). Review of and updates on hypertension in obstructive sleep apnea. *International Journal of Hypertension* Article ID 1848375, 13 pages. DOI: https://doi.org/10.1155/2017/1848375
39. Foster C. A., Church K. S., Poddar M. (2017). Licorice-induced hypertension: A case of pseudohyperaldosteronism due to jelly bean ingestion. *Postgraduate Medicine* 129(3), 329–331.
40. Samadian F., Dalli N., Jamalian A. (2017). New insights into pathophysiology, diagnosis, and treatment of renovascular hypertension. *Iranian Journal of Kidney Diseases* 11(2), 79–89.
41. Lenders J. W. M., Duo Q. Y., Eisenhofer G., et al. (2014). Pheochromocytoma and paraganglioma: An endocrine society clinical practice guideline. *Journal of Clinical Endocrinology and Metabolism* 99(6), 1915–1942.
42. Funder J. W., Carey R. M., Mantero F., et al. (2016). The management of primary aldosteronism: Case detection, diagnosis, and treatment: An endocrine society clinical practice guideline. *Journal of Clinical Endocrinology and Metabolism* 101(5), 1889–1916.
43. American Heart Association. (2017). *Coarctation of the Aorta.* Downloaded at: http://www.heart.org/HEARTORG/Conditions/CongenitalHeartDefects/AboutCongenitalHeartDefects/Coarctation-of-the-Aorta-CoA_UCM_307022_Article.jsp
44. Golshani C., Lieberman R. M., Fischer R. M., et al. (2017). Hypertensive crisis with massive retinal and choroidal infarction. *American Journal of Ophthalmology Case Reports* 6, 58–60.
45. American Heart Association. (2017). *Hypertensive Crisis: When You Should Call 9-1-1 for Blood Pressure.* Downloaded from: http://www.heart.org/HEARTORG/Conditions/HighBloodPressure/GettheFactsAboutHighBloodPressure/Hypertensive-Crisis-When-You-Should-Call-9-1-1-for-High-Blood-Pressure_UCM_301782_Article.jsp
46. U.S. Department of Health and Human Services. (2003). *The seventh report of the Joint National Committee on Detection, Evaluation, and Treatment of High Blood Pressure.* (NIH publication 03-5233). [Online.] Available: www.nhlbi.nih.gov/guidelines/hypertension/jnc7full.pdf
47. American College of Obstetricians and Gynecologists Task Force on Hypertension in Pregnancy. (2013). *Hypertension in Pregnancy.* Downloaded at: https://www.acog.org/Resources-And-Publications/Task-Force-and-Work-Group-Reports/Hypertension-in-Pregnancy
48. Jena M., Mishra S., Jena S., et al. (2016). Pregnancy induced hypertension & pre-eclampsia: Pathophysiology & recent management trends: A review. *International Journal of Pharmaceutical Research and Allied Sciences* 5(3), 326–334
49. Freeman R., Wieling W., Axelrod F. B., et al. (2011). Consensus statement on the definition 47(4), orthostatic hypotension, neutrally mediated syncope and the postural tachycardia syndrome. *Autonomic Neuroscience: Basic and Clinical* 161, 46–48. DOI: 10.1016/j.autneu.2011.02.004
50. Chisolm P. Anpalahan M. (2017). Orthostatic hypotension: Pathophysiology, assessment, treatment and the paradox of supine hypotension. *Internal Medicine Journal* 47(4), 370–379. DOI: 10.1111/imj.13171
51. Wieling W., vanDijk N., Thijs R. D., et al. (2014). Physical countermeasures to increase orthostatic tolerance. *Journal of Internal Medicine* 277(1), 69–82. DOI: 10.1111/joim.12249
52. Shaw B. H., Claydon V. E. (2014). The relationship between orthostatic hypotension and falling in older adults. *Clinical Autonomic Research* 24, 3–13. DOI: 10.1007/s10286-013-0219-5
53. Hinkle J. L., Cheever K. H. (2018). *Brunner & Suddarth's Textbook of Medical-surgical Nursing* (14th ed.). Philadelphia, PA: Wolter Kluwers.
54. Eliopoulos C. (2018). *Gerontological Nursing* (9th ed.). Philadelphia, PA: Wolters Kluwer.
55. Critchfield D. (2014). The Child with altered cardiovascular status. In Bowden V., Greenberg C. S. (Ed.), *Children and Their Families: The Continuum of Nursing Care*. (3rd ed.). Philadelphia, PA: Wolters Kluwer.

Disorders of Cardiac Function, and Heart Failure and Circulatory Shock

27

Herodotos Ellinas

This chapter focuses on common heart problems that affect persons in all age groups. It is organized into two parts: "Disorders of Cardiac Function" and "Heart Failure and Circulatory Shock." The "Disorders of Cardiac Function" part of this chapter includes disorders of the pericardium, coronary artery disease (CAD), cardiomyopathies, infectious and immunologic disorders of the heart, and valvular heart disease. The "Heart Failure and Circulatory Shock" part of this chapter includes heart disease (in infants and children), heart failure (in children, adults, and older adults) and circulatory shock. Although cardiovascular disease (CVD) and heart failure are often thought to be the same, CVD typically refers to conditions with narrow or blocked vessels that place the person at risk for such events as a stroke or myocardial infarction, whereas heart failure refers to failure of the heart as a pump.

DISORDERS OF CARDIAC FUNCTION

CVD is the leading cause of death in males and females in the United States. Because of economic advances, social structures, and demographics, low- and middle-income countries are seeing an accelerated increase in CVD, surpassing infectious diseases.[1] It is estimated that the direct and indirect costs of CVD in the United States alone were $316.12 billion in 2012 to 2013 with projections that direct costs will triple by 2030.[2] To reduce this increase in morbidity, mortality, and cost, strategies such as population-based public health measures, preventative programs for high-risk subgroups, and the allocation of resources for treatments for CVD can be useful.[1]

DISORDERS OF THE PERICARDIUM

After completing this section of the chapter, the learner will be able to meet the following objectives:

- Characterize the function of the pericardium.
- Compare the clinical manifestations of acute pericarditis and chronic pericarditis.
- Describe the physiologic impact of pleural effusion on cardiac function and relate it to cardiac tamponade.

The pericardium, sometimes referred to as the *pericardial sac*, is a double-layered serous membrane that isolates the heart from other thoracic structures, maintains its position in the thorax, prevents it from overfilling, and serves as a barrier to infection. The pericardium consists of two layers: a thin inner layer, called the *visceral pericardium*, that adheres to the epicardium; and an outer fibrous layer, called the *parietal pericardium*, that is attached to the great vessels that enter and leave the heart, the sternum, and the diaphragm. These two layers of the pericardium are separated by a potential space, the *pericardial cavity*, which contains about 50 mL of serous fluid. This fluid acts as a lubricant that prevents frictional forces from developing as the heart contracts and relaxes. Although there is little blood supply to the pericardium, it is well innervated and inflammation can cause severe pain.[3]

The pericardium is subject to many of the same pathologic processes (*e.g.*, congenital disorders, infections, trauma, immune mechanisms, and neoplastic disease) that affect other structures of the body. Pericardial disorders frequently are associated with or result from another disease in the heart or the surrounding structures (Chart 27.1).

CHART 27.1 CLASSIFICATION OF DISORDERS OF THE PERICARDIUM

Inflammation

Acute inflammatory pericarditis

- Infectious
- Viral (echovirus, coxsackievirus, and others)
- Bacterial (*e.g.*, tuberculosis, *Staphylococcus*, *Streptococcus*)
- Fungal
- Immune and collagen disorders
- Rheumatic fever
- Rheumatoid arthritis
- Systemic lupus erythematosus
- Metabolic disorders
- Uremia
- Electrolyte imbalance secondary to end-stage renal disease
- Myxedema
- Ischemia and tissue injury
- Myocardial infarction
- Cardiac surgery
- Chest trauma
- Physical and chemical agents
- Radiation therapy
- Untoward reactions to medications, such as hydralazine, procainamide, and anticoagulants
- Chronic inflammatory pericarditis

Neoplastic Disease

- Primary
- Secondary (*e.g.*, carcinoma of the lung or breast, lymphoma)

Congenital Disorders

- Complete or partial absence of the pericardium
- Congenital pericardial cysts

KEY POINTS

DISORDERS OF THE PERICARDIUM

- The pericardium isolates the heart from other thoracic structures, maintains its position in the thorax, and prevents it from overfilling.
- The two layers of the pericardium are separated by a thin layer of serous fluid, which prevents frictional forces from developing between the visceral and parietal layers of the pericardium.
- Disorders that produce inflammation of the pericardium interfere with the friction-reducing properties of the pericardial fluid and produce pain.
- Disorders that increase the fluid volume of the pericardial sac interfere with cardiac filling and produce a subsequent reduction in cardiac output.

Acute Pericarditis

Pericarditis represents an inflammatory process of the pericardium. *Acute pericarditis*, defined as signs and symptoms resulting from a pericardial inflammation of less than 2 weeks, may occur as an isolated disease or as the result of systemic disease. Viral infections (especially infections with coxsackieviruses and echoviruses) are the most common cause of pericarditis and probably are responsible for many cases classified as idiopathic. Other causes of acute pericarditis include bacterial or mycobacterial infections, connective tissue diseases (*e.g.*, systemic lupus erythematosus, rheumatoid arthritis), uremia, postcardiac surgery, neoplastic invasion of the pericardium, radiation, trauma, drug toxicity, and contiguous inflammatory processes of the myocardium or lung.[3,4]

Like other inflammatory conditions, acute pericarditis often is associated with increased capillary permeability. The capillaries that supply the serous pericardium become permeable, allowing plasma proteins, including fibrinogen, to leave the capillaries and enter the pericardial space. This results in an exudate that varies in type and amount according to the causative agent. Acute pericarditis frequently is associated with a fibrinous (fibrin-containing) exudate (Fig. 27.1), which heals by resolution or progresses to deposition of scar tissue and formation of adhesions between the layers of the serous pericardium. Inflammation also may involve the superficial myocardium and the adjacent pleura.

Clinical Manifestations

The manifestations of acute pericarditis include a triad of chest pain, pericardial friction rub, and electrocardiographic (ECG) changes. The clinical findings may vary according to the causative agent. Nearly all people with acute pericarditis have chest pain. The pain usually is abrupt in onset and sharp, occurring in the precordial area, and may radiate to the neck,

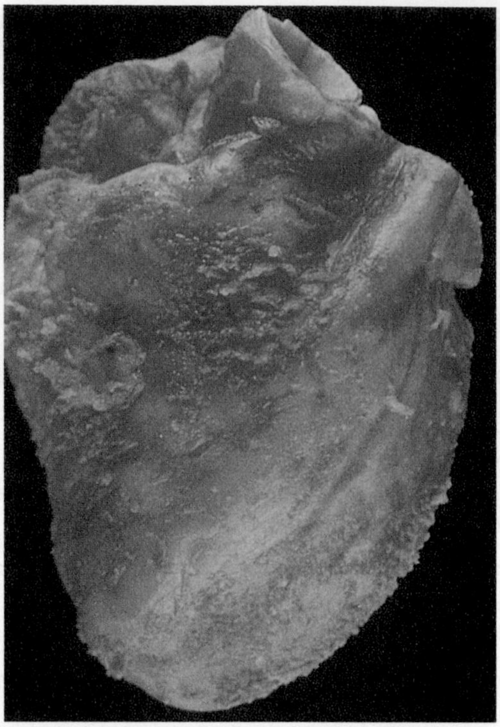

Figure 27.1 • Fibrinous pericarditis. The heart of a patient who died of untreated uremia displays a shaggy, fibrinous exudate covering the visceral pericardium. (From Strayer D. E., Rubin R. (Eds.) (2015). *Rubin's pathology: Clinicopathologic foundations of medicine* (7th ed., Fig. 17-52, p. 675) Philadelphia, PA: Lippincott Williams & Wilkins.)

back, abdomen, or side. Pain in the scapular ridge may be due to irritation of the phrenic nerve. The pain typically is worse with deep breathing, coughing, swallowing, and positional changes because of changes in venous return and cardiac filling. The person often finds relief by sitting up and leaning forward. It is important to differentiate the chest pain from pericarditis from acute myocardial infarction or pulmonary embolism (PE).

Diagnosis

Diagnosis of acute pericarditis is based on clinical manifestations, ECG, chest radiography, and echocardiography. A pericardial friction rub, often described as high pitched or scratchy, results from the rubbing and friction between the inflamed pericardial surfaces. The friction rub is typically described as having three components, which correspond to atrial systole, ventricular systole, and rapid filling of the ventricle. Because it results from the rubbing together of the inflamed pericardial surfaces, large effusions are unlikely to produce a friction rub. Except in uremic pericarditis, the ECG changes in pericarditis typically evolve through four progressive stages: diffuse ST-segment elevations and PR-segment depression, normalization of the ST and PR segments, widespread T-wave inversions, and normalization of T waves. Laboratory markers of systemic inflammation may also be present, including an elevated white blood cell count, elevated erythrocyte sedimentation rate (ESR), and increased C-reactive protein (CRP).[4] Although increased CRP is not present in all cases, it can be used to monitor disease activity and length of treatment needed.[5]

Treatment

Acute idiopathic pericarditis is frequently self-limiting and presumed to be viral. Symptoms are usually successfully treated with nonsteroidal anti-inflammatory drugs (NSAIDs).[3,4] Colchicine can be added to the treatment regimen and has also been shown to be of benefit in people who have a slow response to NSAIDs. Colchicine produces its anti-inflammatory effects by preventing the polymerization of microtubules, which leads to the inhibition of leukocyte migration and phagocytosis. When infection is present, antibiotics specific for the causative agent usually are prescribed. Corticosteroids may be used for treatment of persons with connective tissue disease or severely symptomatic pericarditis that is not responsive to NSAIDs and colchicine. Corticosteroids should be avoided if possible because of an increased number of side effects, recurrences, and hospitalizations.

Relapsing pericarditis can occur in up to 30% of people with acute pericarditis who respond satisfactorily to treatment.[3] A minority of these people develop recurrent bouts of pericardial pain, which can sometimes be chronic and debilitating. The process commonly is associated with autoimmune disorders, such as lupus erythematosus, rheumatoid arthritis, scleroderma, and myxedema, but may also occur following viral pericarditis. Treatment includes the use of anti-inflammatory medications such as NSAIDs initially and then treatment with colchicine. If reoccurrence continues, colchicine prophylaxis is warranted. If colchicine is not tolerated, then low-dose corticosteroids can be initiated.[3]

Pericardial Effusion and Cardiac Tamponade

Pericardial effusion refers to the accumulation of fluid in the pericardial cavity, usually as a result of an inflammatory or infectious process. It may also develop as the result of neoplasms, cardiac surgery, trauma, cardiac rupture due to myocardial infarction, and dissecting aortic aneurysm. The pericardial cavity has little reserve volume. The pressure–volume relationship between the normal pericardial and cardiac volumes can be dramatically affected by only small amounts of fluid once critical levels of effusion are present. Because right heart filling pressures are lower than that of the left heart, increases in pressure are usually reflected in signs and symptoms of right-sided heart failure before equalization is achieved.

Pathogenesis

The amount of fluid, the rapidity with which it accumulates, and the elasticity of the pericardium determine the effect the effusion has on cardiac function. Small pericardial effusions may produce no symptoms or abnormal clinical findings. Even a large effusion that develops slowly may cause few or no symptoms, provided the pericardium is able to stretch and avoid compressing the heart. However, a sudden accumulation of even 200 mL of fluid may raise intracardiac pressure to levels that seriously limit the venous return to the heart.[4] Symptoms of cardiac compression also may occur with relatively small accumulations of fluid if the pericardium has become thickened by scar tissue or neoplastic infiltrations.

Pericardial effusion can lead to a condition called *cardiac tamponade*, in which there is compression of the heart due to the accumulation of fluid, pus, or blood in the pericardial sac. This life-threatening condition can be caused by infections, neoplasms, and bleeding.[3,4] Cardiac tamponade results in increased intracardiac pressure, progressive limitation of ventricular diastolic filling, and reductions in stroke volume and cardiac output. The severity of the condition depends on the amount of fluid present and the rate at which it accumulates.

A significant accumulation of fluid in the pericardium results in increased adrenergic stimulation, which leads to tachycardia and increased cardiac contractility. There is elevation of central venous pressure (CVP), jugular venous distention, a fall in systolic blood pressure, narrowed pulse pressure, muffled heart sounds, and signs of circulatory shock. People with slowly developing cardiac tamponade usually appear acutely ill, but not to the extreme seen in those with rapidly developing tamponade.

Diagnosis

A key diagnostic finding is *pulsus paradoxus*, or an exaggeration of the normal variation in the systemic arterial pulse volume with respiration.[3,4] Normally, the decrease in intrathoracic pressure that occurs during inspiration accelerates venous flow, increasing right atrial and right ventricular filling. This causes the interventricular septum to bulge to the left, producing a slight decrease in left ventricular filling, stroke volume output, and systolic blood pressure. In cardiac tamponade, the left ventricle (LV) is compressed from within by movement of the interventricular septum and from without by fluid in the pericardium (Fig. 27.2). This produces a marked decrease in left ventricular filling and left ventricular stroke volume output. Pulsus paradoxus can be determined by palpation, cuff sphygmomanometry, or arterial pressure monitoring. With pulsus paradoxus, the arterial pulse as palpated at the carotid or femoral artery becomes weakened or absent during inspiration and becomes stronger during expiration. Palpation provides only a gross estimate of the degree of pulsus paradoxus. It is more sensitively estimated when the blood pressure cuff is used to compare the Korotkoff sounds during inspiration and expiration—a decline in systolic pressure greater than 10 mm Hg during inspiration is suggestive of tamponade. Arterial pressure monitoring allows visualization of the arterial pressure waveform and measurement of the blood pressure drop during inspiration.

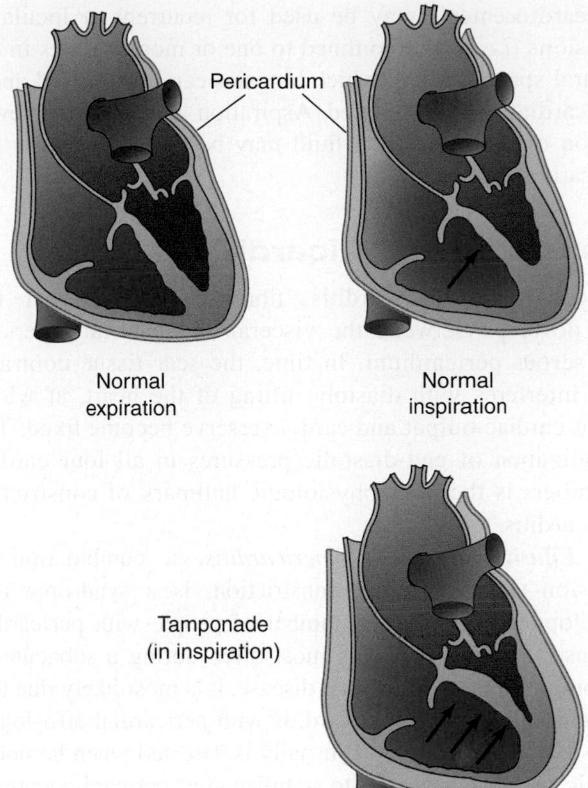

Figure 27.2 • Effects of respiration and cardiac tamponade on ventricular filling and cardiac output. During inspiration, venous flow into the right heart increases, causing the interventricular septum to bulge into the LV. This produces a decrease in left ventricular volume, with a subsequent decrease in stroke volume output. In cardiac tamponade, the fluid in the pericardial sac produces further compression of the LV, causing an exaggeration of the normal inspiratory decrease in stroke volume and systolic blood pressure.

The echocardiogram is a rapid, accurate, and widely used method of evaluating pericardial effusion. The ECG often reveals nonspecific T-wave changes and low QRS voltage. Usually, only moderate to large effusions can be detected by chest radiography.

Treatment

Treatment of pericardial effusions depends on the progression to cardiac tamponade. In small pericardial effusions or mild cardiac tamponade, NSAIDs, colchicine, or corticosteroids may minimize fluid accumulation. Pericardiocentesis, or removal of fluid from the pericardial sac, often with the aid of echocardiography, is the initial treatment of choice. Closed pericardiocentesis, which is performed with a needle inserted through the chest wall, may be an emergency lifesaving measure in severe cardiac tamponade. Open pericardiocentesis may be used for recurrent or loculated effusions (*i.e.*, those confined to one or more pockets in the pleural space), during which biopsies can be obtained and a pericardial window created. Aspiration and laboratory evaluation of the pericardial fluid may be used to identify the causative agent.

Constrictive Pericarditis

In constrictive pericarditis, fibrous, calcified scar tissue develops between the visceral and parietal layers of the serous pericardium. In time, the scar tissue contracts and interferes with diastolic filling of the heart, at which point cardiac output and cardiac reserve become fixed. The equalization of end-diastolic pressures in all four cardiac chambers is the pathophysiologic hallmark of constrictive pericarditis.[5]

Effusive–constrictive pericarditis, a combination of effusion–tamponade and constriction, is a syndrome that develops in a significant number of people with pericardial disease. Because it occurs most often during a subacute or chronic course of pericardial disease, it is most likely due to a transition from acute pericarditis with pericardial effusion to constrictive pericarditis. It usually is detected when hemodynamic measurements fail to stabilize after pericardiocentesis. There are many causes, but the most common is idiopathic with the exception of being possibly caused by malignant disease, radiation, and tuberculosis. People with the disorder usually require pericardiectomy.[3,5]

Etiology and Clinical Manifestations

Long-standing inflammation from mediastinal radiation, cardiac surgery, or infection is usually the cause of constrictive pericarditis. Ascites is a prominent early finding and may be accompanied by pedal edema, dyspnea on exertion, and fatigue. The jugular veins also are distended. The Kussmaul sign is an inspiratory distention of the jugular veins caused by the inability of the right atrium, encased in its rigid pericardium, to accommodate the increase in venous return that occurs with inspiration. Exercise intolerance, muscle wasting, and weight loss develop in end-stage constrictive pericarditis.

Diagnosis

Chest radiography and Doppler and transesophageal echocardiography are helpful in the diagnosis of constrictive pericarditis. Doppler echocardiogram and cardiac catheterization are especially useful in the differentiation of constrictive pericarditis from restrictive cardiomyopathy, as are computed tomography (CT) and magnetic resonance imaging (MRI). In chronic constrictive pericarditis, surgical removal or resection of the pericardium (*i.e.*, pericardiectomy) is often the treatment of choice.[3]

IN SUMMARY

The pericardium is a two-layered membranous sac that isolates the heart from other thoracic structures, maintains its position in the thorax, and prevents it from overfilling; it also may help prevent infection. Disorders of the pericardium include acute and chronic pericarditis, pericardial effusion and cardiac tamponade, and constrictive and effusive–constrictive pericarditis. The major threat of pericardial disease is compression of the heart chambers.

Acute pericarditis may be infectious in origin, or it may be due to systemic diseases. It is characterized by chest pain, ECG changes, and pericardial friction rub. Recurrent pericarditis is usually associated with autoimmune disorders, and symptoms may be minimal. Pericardial effusion, either acute or chronic, refers to the presence of an exudate in the pericardial cavity. It can increase intracardiac pressure, compress the heart, and interfere with venous return to the heart. The amount of exudate, the rapidity with which it accumulates, and the elasticity of the pericardium determine the effect the effusion has on cardiac function. Cardiac tamponade represents a life-threatening compression of the heart resulting from excess fluid in the pericardial sac. In constrictive pericarditis, scar tissue develops between the visceral and parietal layers of the serous pericardium. In time, the scar tissue contracts and interferes with cardiac filling.

CORONARY ARTERY DISEASE

After completing this section of the chapter, the learner will be able to meet the following objectives:

- Describe blood flow in the coronary circulation and relate it to the determinants of myocardial oxygen supply and demand.
- Define the term *acute coronary syndrome* (ACS) and distinguish among chronic stable angina, unstable angina (UA), non–ST-segment elevation myocardial infarction (NSTEMI), and ST-segment elevation myocardial infarction (STEMI) in terms of pathology, symptomatology, ECG changes, and serum cardiac markers.
- Define the treatment goal for ACS.

The term *coronary artery disease* (CAD) describes heart disease caused by impaired coronary blood flow. In most cases, CAD is caused by atherosclerosis, which affects not only the coronary arteries but arteries in other areas of the body. Diseases of the coronary arteries can cause myocardial ischemia and angina, myocardial infarction or heart attack, cardiac arrhythmias, conduction defects, heart failure, and

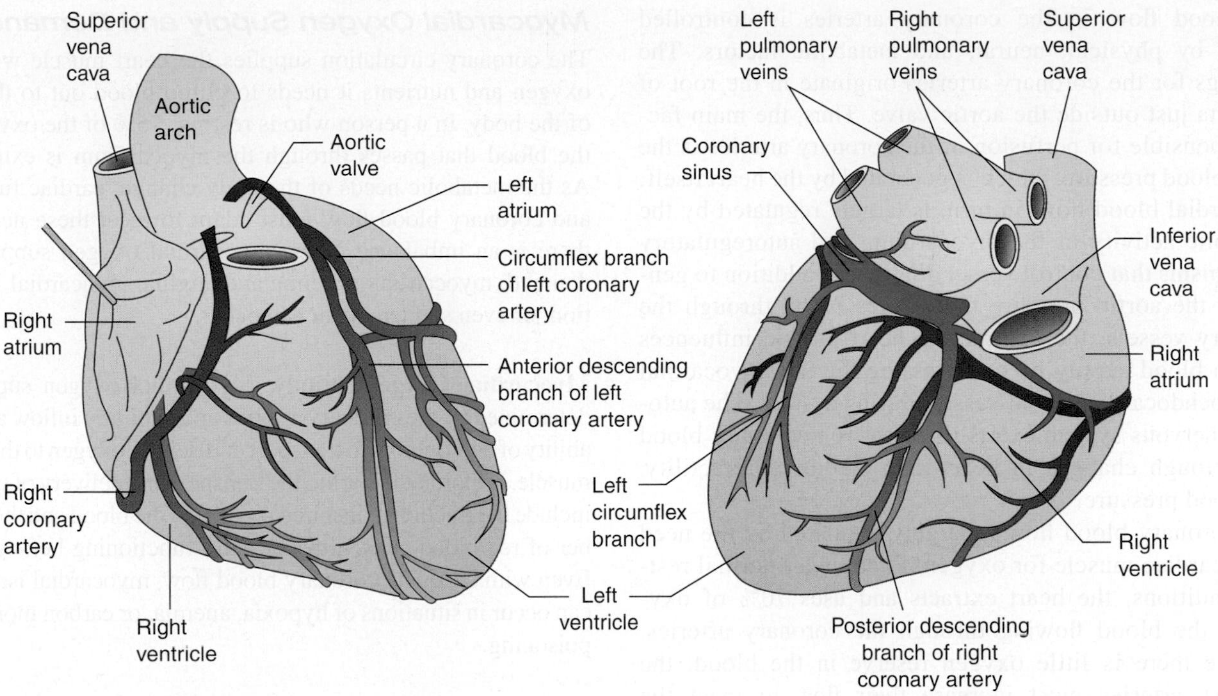

Figure 27.3 • Coronary arteries and some of the coronary sinus veins.

sudden death. Each year, more than 790,000 Americans have new or recurrent myocardial infarctions.[6]

Major risk factors for CAD include cigarette smoking, elevated blood pressure, elevated serum total and low-density lipoprotein (LDL) cholesterol, low serum high-density lipoprotein (HDL) cholesterol, diabetes, advancing age, abdominal obesity, and physical inactivity.[2] Individuals with diabetes and metabolic syndrome are at particularly increased risk for development of CVD and have significant morbidity from the disease.[2]

Coronary Circulation

The Coronary Arteries

The two main coronary arteries, the left and the right, arise from the coronary sinus just above the aortic valve (Fig. 27.3). The left coronary artery supplies blood flow to the anterior and left lateral portions of the LV. The *left main coronary artery* then divides into the left anterior descending and circumflex branches. The *left anterior descending artery* passes down through the groove between the two ventricles, giving off diagonal branches, which supply the LV, and perforating branches, which supply the anterior portion of the interventricular septum and the anterior papillary muscle of the LV. The *circumflex branch* of the left coronary artery passes to the left and moves posteriorly in the groove that separates the left atrium and ventricle, giving off branches that supply the left lateral wall of the LV. The *right coronary artery* lies in the right atrioventricular (AV) groove, and its branches supply most of the right ventricle and the posterior part of the LV in 80% to 90% of people. The right coronary artery usually moves to the back of the heart, where it forms the *posterior descending artery*, which normally supplies the posterior portion of the heart, interventricular septum, sinoatrial (SA) and AV nodes, and posterior papillary muscle. By convention, the coronary artery that supplies the posterior third of the septum (either the right coronary artery or the left circumflex) is called *dominant*. In a right dominant circulation, present in approximately four fifths of people, the left circumflex perfuses the lateral wall of the LV, and the right coronary artery supplies the entire right ventricular free wall and the posterior third of the septum. Thus, occlusion of the right as well as the left coronary artery can cause left ventricular damage.

The large epicardial coronary arteries lie on the surface of the heart, with smaller intramyocardial arteries branching and penetrating the myocardium before merging with a network or plexus of subendocardial vessels. Although there are no connections between the large coronary arteries, there are anastomotic channels that join the small arteries. With gradual occlusion of the larger vessels, the smaller collateral vessels increase in size and provide alternative channels for blood flow. One of the reasons CAD does not produce symptoms until it is far advanced is that the collateral channels develop at the same time the atherosclerotic changes are occurring.

Blood flow in the coronary arteries is controlled largely by physical, neural, and metabolic factors. The openings for the coronary arteries originate in the root of the aorta just outside the aortic valve. Thus, the main factor responsible for perfusion of the coronary arteries is the aortic blood pressure, which is generated by the heart itself. Myocardial blood flow, in turn, is largely regulated by the metabolic activity of the myocardium and autoregulatory mechanisms that control vessel dilation. In addition to generating the aortic pressure that moves blood through the coronary vessels, the contracting heart muscle influences its own blood supply by compressing the intramyocardial and subendocardial blood vessels during systole. The autonomic nervous system exerts its effects on coronary blood flow through changes in heart rate, cardiac contractility, and blood pressure.

Coronary blood flow is largely regulated by the need of the cardiac muscle for oxygen. Even under normal resting conditions, the heart extracts and uses 70% of oxygen in the blood flowing through the coronary arteries. Because there is little oxygen reserve in the blood, the coronary arteries must increase their flow to meet the metabolic needs of the myocardium during periods of increased activity. The normal resting blood flow through the coronary arteries averages approximately 225 mL/minute or about 4% to 5% of the total cardiac output.[7] During strenuous exercise, coronary flow may increase four- to fivefold to meet the energy requirements of the heart.

One of the major determinants of coronary blood flow is the metabolic activity of the heart. Numerous agents, referred to as *metabolites*, are thought to act as mediators for the vasodilation that accompanies increased cardiac work. These substances, which include potassium ions, lactic acid, carbon dioxide, and adenosine, are released from working myocardial cells. Of these substances, adenosine appears to have the greatest vasodilator effect and is perhaps the critical mediator of local blood flow.[7]

The endothelial cells that line the blood vessels, including the coronaries, normally form a barrier between the blood and the arterial wall. They also synthesize several substances that, when released, can affect relaxation or constriction of the smooth muscle in the arterial wall. Potent vasodilators produced by the endothelium include nitric oxide, prostacyclin, and endothelium-derived hyperpolarizing factor (EDHF). The most important of these is nitric oxide. Most vasodilators and vasodilating stimuli exert their effects through nitric oxide. Products from aggregating platelets, thrombin, the products of mast cells, and increased shear force, which is responsible for so-called flow-mediated vasodilation, stimulate the synthesis and release of nitric oxide.[7] The endothelium also is the source of vasoconstricting factors, the best known of which are the endothelins.

Myocardial Oxygen Supply and Demand

The coronary circulation supplies the heart muscle with the oxygen and nutrients it needs to pump blood out to the rest of the body. In a person who is resting, 75% of the oxygen in the blood that passes through the myocardium is extracted. As the metabolic needs of the body change, cardiac function and coronary blood flow must adapt to meet these needs. If there is an imbalance in the myocardial oxygen supply and demand, myocardial ischemia and angina, myocardial infarction, or even sudden death can occur.

Myocardial Oxygen Supply. Myocardial oxygen supply is determined by the coronary arteries and capillary inflow and the ability of hemoglobin to transport and deliver oxygen to the heart muscle. Important factors in the transport and delivery of oxygen include the fraction of inspired oxygen in the blood and the number of red blood cells with normally functioning hemoglobin. Even with adequate coronary blood flow, myocardial ischemia can occur in situations of hypoxia, anemia, or carbon monoxide poisoning.

Myocardial Oxygen Demand. There are three major determinants of myocardial oxygen demand (MVO_2): the heart rate, left ventricular contractility, and systolic pressure or myocardial wall stress or tension (Fig. 27.4). The heart rate is the most important factor in myocardial oxygen demand for two reasons:

As the heart rate increases, myocardial oxygen consumption or demand also increases.

Subendocardial coronary blood flow is reduced because of the decreased diastolic filling time with increased heart rates.[7]

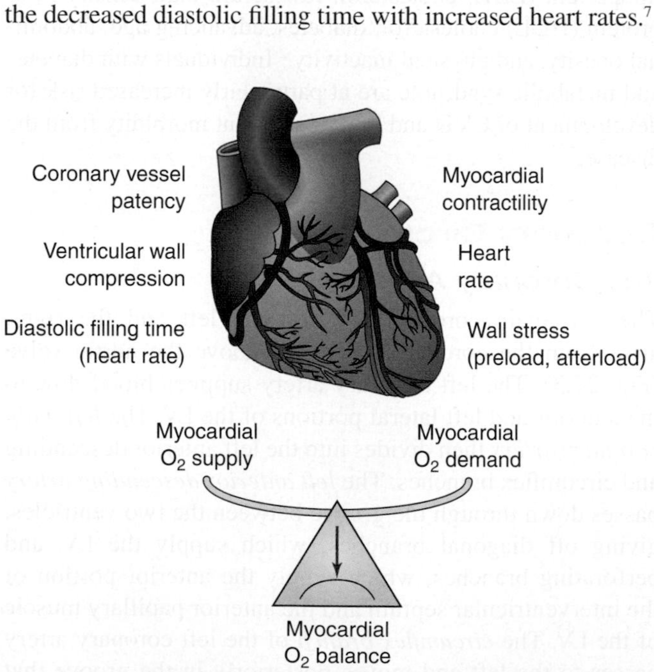

Figure 27.4 • Myocardial oxygen (O_2) balance is determined by factors that affect myocardial O_2 supply and myocardial O_2 demand (MVO_2).

Understanding Myocardial Blood Flow

Blood flow in the coronary vessels that supply the myocardium is influenced by (1) the aortic pressure, (2) autoregulatory mechanisms, and (3) compression of the intramyocardial vessels by the contracting heart muscle.

Aortic Pressure

The two main coronary arteries that supply blood flow to the myocardium arise in the sinuses behind the two cusps of the aortic valve. Because of their location, the pressure and flow of blood in the coronary arteries reflects that of the aorta. During systole, when the aortic valve is open, the velocity of blood flow and position of the valve cusps cause the blood to move rapidly past the coronary artery inlets, and during diastole, when the aortic valve is closed, blood flow and the aortic pressure are transmitted directly into the coronary arteries.

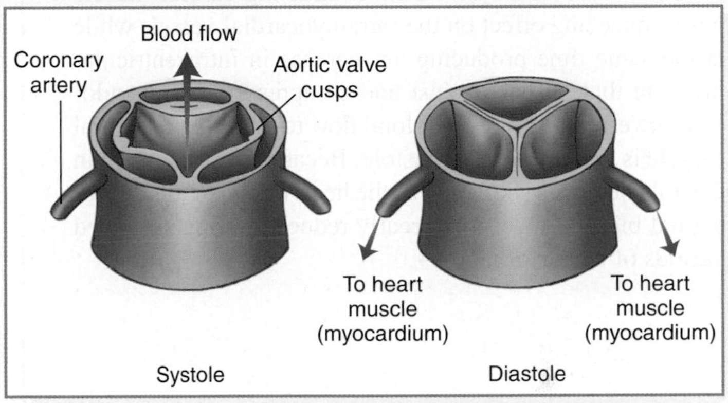

Autoregulatory Mechanisms

The heart normally extracts 60% to 80% of the oxygen in the blood delivered to it, leaving little in reserve. Accordingly, oxygen delivery during periods of increased metabolic demand depends on autoregulatory mechanisms that regulate blood flow through a change in vessel tone and diameter. During increased metabolic demand, vasodilation produces an increase in blood flow; during decreased demand, vasoconstriction or return of vessel tone to normal produces a reduction in flow. The mechanisms that link the metabolic activity of the heart to changes in vessel tone result from vasoactive mediators released from myocardial cells and the vascular endothelium.

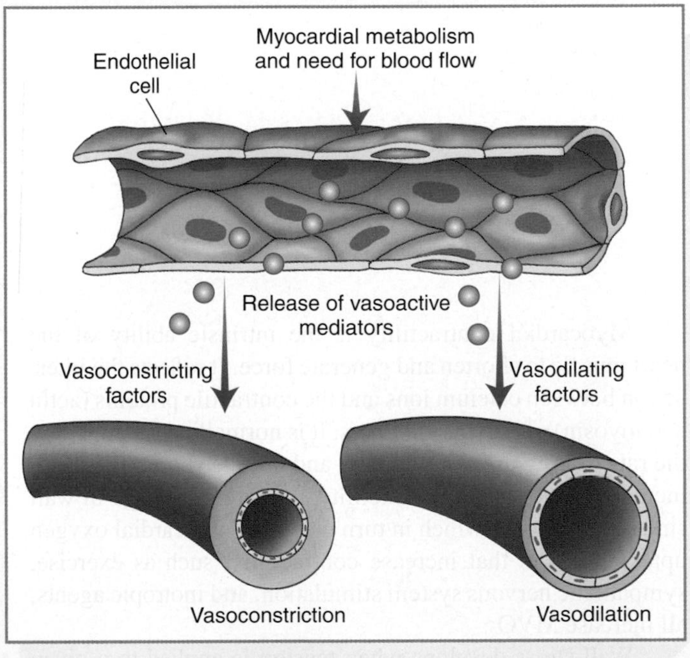

Continued

Understanding Myocardial Blood Flow (Continued)

Vessel Compression

The large coronary arteries lie on the epicardial surface of the heart, with smaller intramyocardial vessels branching off and moving through the myocardium before merging with a plexus of vessels that supply the subendocardial muscle with blood. During systole, the contracting cardiac muscle has a squeezing effect on the intramyocardial vessels while at the same time producing an increase in intraventricular pressure that pushes against and compresses the subendocardial vessels. As a result, blood flow to the subendocardial muscle is greatest during diastole. Because the time spent in diastole becomes shortened as the heart rate increases, myocardial blood flow can be greatly reduced during sustained periods of tachycardia.

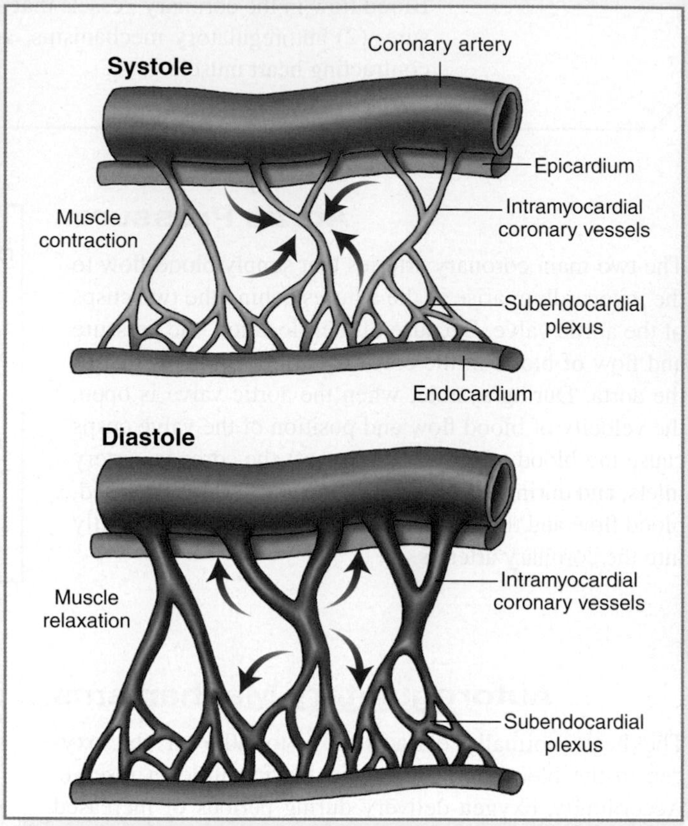

Myocardial contractility is the intrinsic ability of the heart muscle to shorten and generate force. It reflects the interaction between calcium ions and the contractile proteins (actin and myosin) of the muscle fibers. It is normally determined by the rate of pressure development and muscle shortening. With increased myocardial contractility, the rate of change in wall stress is increased, which in turn increases myocardial oxygen uptake. Factors that increase contractility, such as exercise, sympathetic nervous system stimulation, and inotropic agents, all increase MVO_2.

Wall stress develops when tension is applied to a given area. Left ventricular wall stress can be thought of as the average tension that individual muscle fibers must generate to shorten against a developed intraventricular pressure. It is proportional to the product of the intraventricular pressure and ventricle radius divided by the thickness of the ventricle wall. Thus, at a given pressure, wall stress is increased by an increase in radius (ventricular dilation) and by a decrease in wall thickness. The term *preload* is used to describe the distending force of the ventricular wall as it fills prior to contraction.[7] Changes in preload are assessed by using the left ventricular end-diastolic (LVED) pressure. This can be measured indirectly by using the pulmonary artery occlusive (or wedge) pressure, obtained through a pulmonary artery catheter. *Afterload* is the "load" against which the heart must contract to eject blood. A major component of the left ventricular afterload is the aortic pressure, or pressure that the ventricle must generate to eject blood into the aorta.[7] An increase in wall stress, whether caused by an increase in preload or afterload, increases MVO_2 because as cardiac muscle fibers develop more tension, they require a greater rate of adenosine triphosphate (ATP) use. Because wall stress is inversely related to wall thickness, ventricular hypertrophy serves as an adaptive mechanism by which the ventricle is able to offset the increase in wall stress that accompanies increased aortic pressure or aortic valve stenosis.

Assessment of Coronary Blood Flow and Myocardial Perfusion

Among the methods used in the evaluation of coronary blood flow and myocardial perfusion are ECG, exercise stress testing, echocardiography, and Doppler ultrasonographic imaging; cardiac MRI and CT; and cardiac catheterization and angiography. These assessment modalities vary widely and are undergoing constant technologic advances.[8]

Electrocardiography. The 12-lead ECG is the most frequently used cardiovascular diagnostic procedure. It can be used not only for the diagnosis and treatment of CAD but also for the identification of ventricular conduction defects, arrhythmias, electrolyte imbalances, drug effects, and genetically mediated electrical or structural abnormalities. The standard 12-lead ECG uses electrodes to record electrical potential differences, generated by ion currents (action potentials) during the cardiac cycle, between prescribed sites on the body. Proper electrode placement and patient position are important because they can change the recorded amplitudes and axes of the ECG, which can effect interpretation.

Ambulatory ECG monitoring often is done to detect transient ST-segment and T-wave changes that occur and are not accompanied by symptoms (*i.e.*, silent ischemia). Continuous ambulatory ECG monitoring can be done using a Holter monitor and/or event monitor. Another method, called *signal-averaged* or *high-resolution ECG*, accentuates the QRS complex so that low-amplitude afterpotentials can be identified. These low-amplitude afterpotentials can sometimes be correlated with high risk of ventricular arrhythmias, and sudden death may be detected.

Exercise Stress Testing. Exercise stress testing is a means of observing cardiac function under stress and is typically performed in adults with symptoms of known or suspected ischemic heart disease. It is also used to check for physiologic response post MI or revascularization, functional capacity for an exercise program and/or cardiac rehabilitation, efficacy of medication or surgical treatments, and the severity of arrhythmias and preoperatively to assess functional status.[8]

Treadmill exercise, which is the most commonly used method of cardiovascular stress testing, requires higher levels of myocardial performance than other forms of exercise. The goal is to achieve maximum level of exertion based on patient age if possible. While trying to do this, blood pressure is monitored during exercise testing, and the ECG pattern is recorded for the purposes of determining heart rate and detecting myocardial ischemic changes. Chest pain, severe shortness of breath, arrhythmias, ST-segment changes on the ECG, or a decrease in blood pressure suggests CAD. If one or more of these signs or symptoms are present, the test is usually terminated.

Pharmacologic stress testing may be used to simulate the stress of exercise in persons who cannot participate in active forms of exercise because of orthopedic, neurologic, or peripheral vascular disorders or other conditions. The intravenous infusion of dipyridamole, adenosine, or dobutamine can be used. Dipyridamole blocks the cellular reabsorption of adenosine, an endogenous vasodilator, and increases coronary blood flow three to five times above baseline levels. In people with significant CAD, the resistance vessels distal to the stenosis already are maximally dilated to maintain normal resting flow. In these people, further vasodilation does not produce an increase in blood flow. Intravenous injection of adenosine has comparable effects. Dobutamine, a sympathomimetic agent, increases myocardial contractility and stroke volume. During stress echocardiography, low-dose dobutamine identifies myocardial viability, and high-dose dobutamine identifies myocardial ischemia.[8]

Exercise stress testing in certain populations can pose a challenge. Women who engage in an exercise stress test are less sensitive to exercise-induced ST-segment depression. To increase accuracy of test results in women, radionuclide testing has been suggested but is not in the American College of Cardiology/American Heart Association (ACC/AHA) guidelines. Testing in older adults is also challenging because of their decrease in exercise capacity. They usually have lightheadedness and fatigue due to deconditioning and muscle fatigue. This may require a modified protocol but is not a contradiction to exercise stress testing.[8]

Echocardiography. Echocardiography is still the most widely used diagnostic test to check for structure and function of the heart. It uses ultrasound signals that are inaudible to the human ear.[9] The ultrasound signal is reflected (*i.e.*, echoes) whenever there is a change in the resistance to transmission of the sound beam. Thus, it is possible to create a moving image of the internal structures of the heart because the chest wall, blood, and different heart structures all reflect ultrasound differently. The echocardiogram is useful for determining ventricular dimensions and valve movements, obtaining data on the movement of the left ventricular wall and septum, estimating diastolic and systolic volumes, and viewing the motion of individual segments of the left ventricular wall during systole and diastole.

There are several different forms of echocardiography, including two-dimensional (2-D), M-mode, three-dimensional (3-D), Doppler, and contrast echocardiography. M-mode echocardiography, which was the earliest form of cardiac ultrasonography, uses a stationary ultrasound beam to produce a one-dimensional or "ice-pick" view of the heart. *Two-dimensional echocardiography* uses a moving ultrasound beam to produce an integrated view of the heart comprising multiple pie-shaped images. *Doppler echocardiography* uses ultrasound to record blood flow within the heart. Contrast use has improved the delineation of structures on the left side of the heart. Three-dimensional images of the heart can be obtained via newer transducers from a full volume 3-D echocardiographic image.

Transesophageal echocardiography uses a 2-D echocardiography transducer placed at the end of a flexible endoscope to obtain echocardiographic images from the esophagus. This placement allows echocardiographic images of cardiac structures to be obtained from different viewpoints, rather than only from the surface of the chest. Transesophageal echocardiography is particularly useful in assessing valve function. Stress echocardiography, with or without the use of pharmacologic agents, is used in conjunction with dynamic exercise. Rest and stress images are recorded, stored, and then analyzed for global and regional left ventricular size, shape, and function. Reduced systolic wall thickening seen on stress echocardiography identifies myocardial ischemia.

Nuclear Cardiac Imaging. Nuclear cardiac imaging techniques involve the use of radionuclides (*i.e.*, radioactive substances) and are essentially noninvasive. Three types of nuclear cardiology tests are commonly used: myocardial perfusion imaging, positron emission tomography (PET), and radionuclide angiocardiography. With all three of these tests, a scintillation (gamma) camera is used to record the radiation emitted from the radionuclide. Single-photon emission computed tomography (SPECT), which uses a multiple-head camera to obtain a series of planar images over a 180- to 360-degree arc around the thorax, is the most widely used imaging technique at present.[10]

Myocardial perfusion imaging is used to visualize the regional distribution of blood flow. *Myocardial perfusion scintigraphy* uses thallium-201 or one of the newer technetium-based agents that are extracted from the blood and taken up by functioning myocardial cells. Thallium-201, an analog of potassium, is distributed to the myocardium in proportion to the magnitude of blood flow. After injection, an external detection device registers the distribution of the radioactive material. An ischemic area appears as a "cold spot" that lacks radioactive uptake. The most important application of this technique has been its use during stress testing for evaluation of ischemic heart disease.

Positron emission tomography (PET) uses positron-emitting agents to demonstrate either the perfusion or metabolic status of the myocardium. The radioisotopes used as positron emitters are the naturally occurring, small atomic weight atoms (*e.g.*, carbon, nitrogen, oxygen) that are the predominant constituents of organic compounds such as glucose. During ischemia, cardiac muscle shifts from fatty acid to glucose metabolism. Thus, a radioactive tracer such as fluorodeoxyglucose can be used to distinguish a transiently dysfunctional ("stunned") myocardium from scar tissue by showing persistent glucose metabolism in areas of reduced blood flow.

Radionuclide angiocardiography provides actual visualization of the ventricular structures during systole and diastole and a means for evaluating ventricular function during rest and exercise stress testing. A radioisotope such as technetium-labeled albumin, which does not leave the capillaries but remains in the blood and is not bound to the myocardium, is used for this type of imaging. This type of nuclear imaging can be used to determine right and left ventricular volumes, ejection fractions, regional wall motion, and cardiac contractility. This method also is useful in the diagnosis of intracardiac shunts.

Cardiac Magnetic Resonance Imaging and Computed Tomography. The cardiac MRI creates a spatially resolved map of radio signals and, compared with x-ray–based techniques, is much safer. Cardiac MRI uses gadolinium as a contrast agent and ECG gating to prevent artifacts and blurring from periodic cardiac cycles.[11] In nearly all current scanners, this is achieved by gating (triggering) the acquisition of MRI data to the R wave of the ECG. Cardiac MRI is used for quantifying the volume, mass, and function of the ventricles. MRI cannot be used in people with certain implanted devices such as pacemakers and defibrillators, unless approved by the FDA and after special programming adjustments.[11]

CT is an x-ray–based technique that obtains cross-sectional views of the body through rotation of the x-ray scanner around the person. Several generations of CT technology have been developed, including conventional CT, contrast-enhanced CT, and electron beam CT. CT cardiac imaging can be performed with or without injection of a contrast agent. Noncontrast CT studies are used primarily to assess coronary artery calcification. Contrast-enhanced studies can be used to assess cardiac chambers, great cardiac vessels, and sometimes the coronary artery lumen.[12] The electron beam CT, developed specifically for cardiac imaging, is a useful technique for identifying persons with or at risk for CAD. Unlike conventional CT, in which the scanner moves around the person, in electron beam CT, only the electron beam moves.

Cardiac Catheterization and Arteriography. Cardiac catheterization is one of the most widely used invasive procedures in the assessment of CAD. Cardiac catheterization involves the passage of flexible catheters into the great vessels and chambers of the heart. In right heart catheterization, the catheter is inserted into a peripheral vein (usually the femoral) and then advanced into the right heart. The left heart catheter is inserted retrograde through a peripheral artery (usually the brachial or femoral) into the aorta and left heart. The cardiac catheterization laboratory, where the procedure is done, is equipped for viewing and recording fluoroscopic images of the heart and vessels in the chest and for measuring pressures in the heart and great vessels. It also has equipment for cardiac output studies and for obtaining samples of blood for blood gas analysis. Angiographic studies are done by injecting a radiographic contrast medium into the heart so that an outline of the moving structures can be visualized and filmed.

Coronary arteriography involves the injection of a radiographic contrast medium into the coronary arteries, permitting visualization of lesions in these vessels. It is used to identify and establish the extent of coronary artery narrowing, perform percutaneous coronary intervention (PCI) and placement of coronary artery stents, and determine appropriateness for coronary artery bypass graft surgery.[13] Intracoronary physiologic measurements (Doppler ultrasonography, fractional flow reserve) can also be obtained with new sensor guidewire technology.

Coronary Atherosclerosis and the Pathogenesis of Coronary Artery Disease

Atherosclerosis is the most common cause of CAD, is slow and progressive, and can begin at a very young age in the United States and other developed countries of the world.

Atherosclerosis can affect one or all three of the major epicardial coronary arteries and their branches. Clinically significant lesions may be located anywhere in these vessels but tend to predominate in the first several centimeters of the left anterior descending and left circumflex or the entire length of the right coronary artery.[14] Sometimes the major secondary branches also are involved.

CAD is commonly divided into two types of disorders: the ACS and chronic ischemic heart disease. The *acute coronary syndrome* represents a spectrum of acute ischemic heart diseases ranging from UA to myocardial infarction resulting from disruption of an atherosclerotic plaque. *Chronic ischemic heart disease* is characterized by recurrent and transient episodes of myocardial ischemia and stable angina that result from narrowing of a coronary artery lumen because of atherosclerosis and/or vasospasm.

Stable Versus Unstable Plaque. There are two types of atherosclerotic lesions:

1. Fixed or stable plaque, which obstructs blood flow
2. Unstable/vulnerable plaque or high-risk plaque, which can rupture and cause platelet adhesion and thrombus formation

The fixed or stable plaque is commonly implicated in stable angina and the unstable plaque in UA and myocardial infarction. In most cases, the myocardial ischemia underlying UA, acute myocardial infarction, stroke, and, in many cases, sudden cardiac death (SCD) is precipitated by abrupt plaque changes, followed by thrombosis. The major determinants of plaque vulnerability to disruption include the size of the lipid-rich core, the stability and thickness of its fibrous cap, the presence of inflammation, and the lack of smooth muscle cells (Fig. 27.5). Plaques with a thin fibrous cap overlaying a large lipid core are at high risk for rupture.

Although plaque disruption may occur spontaneously, it is often triggered by hemodynamic factors such as blood flow characteristics and vessel tension. For example, a sudden surge of sympathetic activity with an increase in blood pressure, heart rate, force of cardiac contraction, and coronary blood flow is thought to increase the risk of plaque disruption. Indeed, many people with myocardial infarction report a trigger event, most often emotional stress or physical activity. Plaque disruption also has a diurnal variation, occurring most frequently during the first hour upon awakening, suggesting that physiologic factors such as surges in coronary artery tone and blood pressure may promote atherosclerotic plaque disruption and subsequent platelet deposition. It has been suggested that the sympathetic nervous system is activated upon awakening, resulting in changes in platelet aggregation and fibrinolytic activity that tend to favor thrombosis.

Thrombosis and Vessel Occlusion. Local thrombosis occurring after plaque disruption results from a complex interaction among its lipid core, smooth muscle cells, macrophages, and collagen. The lipid core provides a stimulus for platelet aggregation and thrombus formation. Both smooth muscle and foam cells in the lipid core contribute to the expression of tissue factor in unstable plaques. Once exposed to blood, tissue factor initiates the extrinsic coagulation pathway, resulting in the local generation of thrombin and deposition of fibrin.[14,15]

Platelets play an important role in linking plaque disruption to acute CAD. As a part of the response to plaque disruption, platelets adhere to the endothelium and release

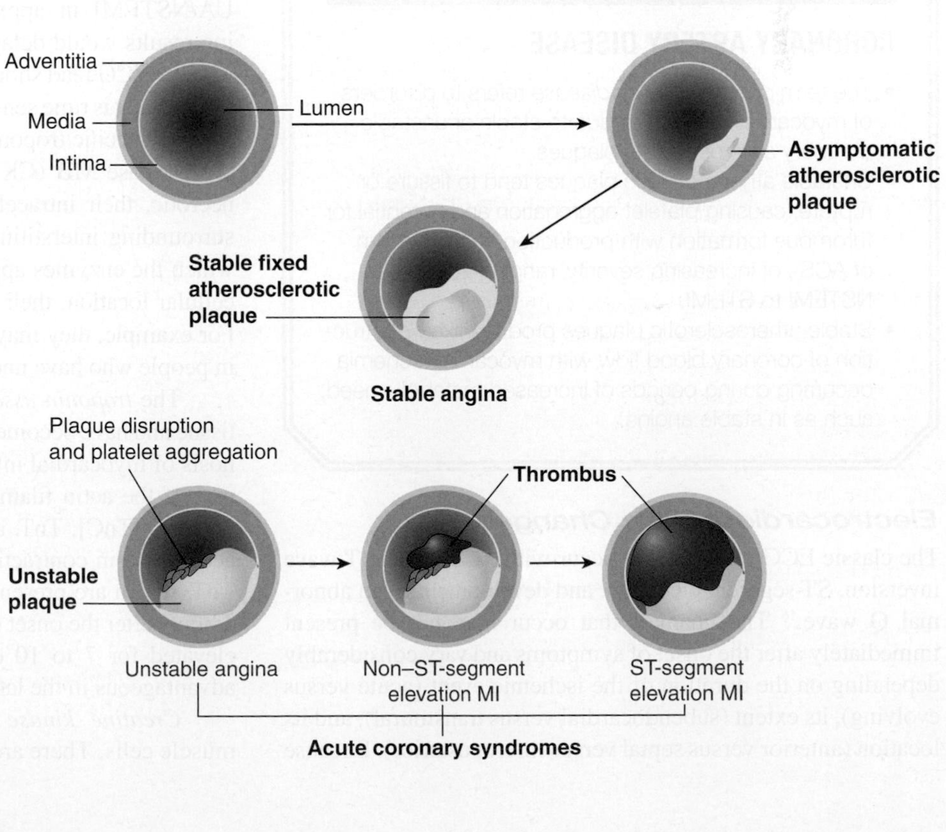

Figure 27.5 • Atherosclerotic plaque: stable fixed atherosclerotic plaque in stable angina and unstable plaque with plaque disruption and platelet aggregation in the ACSs.

substances (*i.e.*, adenosine diphosphate [ADP], thromboxane A_2, and thrombin) that promote further aggregation of platelets and thrombus formation. The platelet membrane, which contains glycoprotein receptors that bind fibrinogen and link platelets together, contributes to thrombus formation. Platelet adhesion and aggregation occurs in several steps. First, release of ADP, thromboxane A_2, and thrombin initiates the aggregation process. Second, glycoprotein IIb/IIIa receptors on the platelet surface are activated. Third, fibrinogen binds to the activated glycoprotein receptors, forming bridges between adjacent platelets.

There are two types of thrombi formed as a result of plaque disruption—white platelet-containing thrombi and red fibrin-containing thrombi. The thrombi in UA have been characterized as grayish-white and presumably platelet rich. Red thrombi, which develop with vessel occlusion in myocardial infarction, are rich in fibrin and red blood cells superimposed on the platelet component and completely obstruct blood flow.[15]

Acute Coronary Syndrome

ACS includes UA, non–ST-segment elevation (non–Q-wave) myocardial infarction, and ST-segment elevation (Q-wave) myocardial infarction. People without ST-segment elevation on ECG are those in whom thrombotic coronary occlusion is subtotal or intermittent, whereas those with ST-segment elevation are usually found to have complete coronary occlusion on angiography, and many ultimately have Q-wave myocardial infarction.

KEY POINTS

CORONARY ARTERY DISEASE

- The term *coronary artery disease* refers to disorders of myocardial blood flow due to stable or unstable coronary atherosclerotic plaques.
- Unstable atherosclerotic plaques tend to fissure or rupture, causing platelet aggregation and potential for thrombus formation with production of a spectrum of ACSs of increasing severity, ranging from UA to NSTEMI to STEMI.
- Stable atherosclerotic plaques produce fixed obstruction of coronary blood flow with myocardial ischemia occurring during periods of increased metabolic need, such as in stable angina.

Electrocardiographic Changes

The classic ECG changes that occur with ACS involve T-wave inversion, ST-segment elevation, and development of an abnormal Q wave.[16] The changes that occur may not be present immediately after the onset of symptoms and vary considerably depending on the duration of the ischemic event (acute versus evolving), its extent (subendocardial versus transmural), and its location (anterior versus septal versus inferoposterior). Because these changes usually occur over time and are seen on the ECG leads that view the involved area of the myocardium, provision for continuous and serial 12-lead ECG monitoring is indicated. The repolarization phase of the action potential (T-wave and ST segment on the ECG) is usually the first to be involved during myocardial ischemia and injury. As the involved area becomes ischemic, myocardial repolarization is altered, causing changes in the T wave. This is usually represented by T-wave inversion, although a hyperacute T-wave elevation may occur as the earliest sign of infarction. ST-segment changes occur with ischemic myocardial injury and, depending on what leads are involved, can indicate the lesion of interest. Normally, the ST segment of the ECG is nearly isoelectric (*e.g.*, flat along the baseline) because all healthy myocardial cells attain the same potential during early repolarization. Acute severe ischemia reduces the resting membrane potential and shortens the duration of the action potential in the ischemic area. These changes create a voltage difference between the normal and ischemic areas of the myocardium that leads to a so-called current of injury between these regions. It is these currents of injury that are represented on the surface ECG as a deviation of the ST segment. When the acute injury is transmural, the overall ST vector is shifted in the direction of the outer epicardium, resulting in ST-segment elevation.[16] With Q-wave infarction, abnormal Q waves and R wave loss develop because there is no depolarizing current conduction from the necrotic tissue. When the injury is confined primarily to the subendocardium, the overall ST segment is shifted toward the inner ventricular layer, resulting in an overall depression and not elevation of the ST segment.

Serum Biomarkers

Even though cardiac biomarkers aid clinicians in diagnosing UA/NSTEMI in approximately one third of people, awaiting results would delay reperfusion treatment for STEMI. The 12-lead ECG read should initiate reperfusion treatment because this therapy is time sensitive. Serum biomarkers for ACS include cardiac-specific troponin I (TnI) and troponin T (TnT) and creatine kinase MB (CK-MB). As the myocardial cells become necrotic, their intracellular contents begin to diffuse into the surrounding interstitium and then into the blood. The rate at which the enzymes appear in the blood depends on their intracellular location, their molecular weight, and local blood flow. For example, they may appear at an earlier than predicted time in people who have undergone successful reperfusion therapy.[17]

The *troponin assays* have high specificity for myocardial tissue and have become the primary biomarker tests for the diagnosis of myocardial infarction. The troponin complex, which is part of the actin filament, consists of three subunits (*i.e.*, troponin C [TnC], TnT, and TnI) that regulate calcium-mediated actin–myosin contractile process in a striated muscle. TnI and TnT, which are present in cardiac muscle, begin to rise within 3 hours after the onset of myocardial infarction and may remain elevated for 7 to 10 days after the event. This is especially advantageous in the late diagnosis of myocardial infarction.[17]

Creatine kinase is an intracellular enzyme found in muscle cells. There are three isoenzymes of CK, with the MB isoenzyme being highly specific for injury to myocardial tissue. Serum levels of CK-MB exceed normal ranges within 4 to 8 hours of myocardial injury and decline to normal within 2 to 3 days.[17]

When comparing troponin and CK-MB, the troponin level identifies necrosis in cardiac muscles earlier than CK-MB. Clinicians examining cardiac biomarkers should focus on troponin levels, rather than CK-MB levels, for diagnosis and for establishing the success of reperfusion.[17]

Unstable Angina/Non–ST-Segment Elevation Myocardial Infarction

UA/NSTEMI is considered to be a clinical syndrome of myocardial ischemia ranging from stable angina to myocardial infarction.[18] Typically, UA and NSTEMI differ in whether the ischemia is severe enough to cause sufficient myocardial damage to release detectable quantities of serum cardiac markers. People who have no evidence of serum markers for myocardial damage are considered to have UA, whereas a diagnosis of NSTEMI is indicated if a serum marker of myocardial injury is present.

The pathophysiology of UA/NSTEMI can be divided into five phases:

1. The development of the unstable plaque that ruptures or plaque erosion with superimposed nonocclusive thrombosis
2. An obstruction such as spasm, constriction, dysfunction, or adrenergic stimuli
3. Severe narrowing of the coronary lumen
4. Inflammation
5. Any physiologic state causing ischemia related to decreased oxygen supply such as fever or hypotension

Inflammation can play a prominent role in plaque instability, with inflammatory cells releasing cytokines that cause the fibrous cap to become thinner and more vulnerable to rupture or erosion. The pain associated with UA/NSTEMI has a persistent and severe course and is characterized by at least one of three features:

1. It occurs at rest (or with minimal exertion), usually lasting more than 20 minutes (if not interrupted by nitroglycerin).
2. It is severe and described as frank pain and of new onset (*i.e.*, within 1 month).
3. It is more severe, prolonged, or frequent than previously experienced.

Risk stratification of people presenting with UA/NSTEMI is important because the outcome can range from excellent, with little change in treatment, to NSTEMI or death, requiring aggressive treatment. UA/NSTEMI is classified by severity based on clinical history, ECG pattern, and serum biomarkers. UA/NSTEMI is classified as:

1. Class I (new-onset severe angina)
2. Class II (angina at rest within the past month, but not within the last 48 hours)
3. Class III (angina at rest within 48 hours)

The ECG pattern in UA/NSTEMI demonstrates ST-segment depression (or transient ST-segment elevation) and T-wave changes. The degree of ST-segment deviation has been shown to be an important measure of ischemia and prognosis.

ST-Segment Elevation Myocardial Infarction

Acute STEMI, also known as *heart attack*, is characterized by the ischemic death of myocardial tissue associated with atherosclerotic disease of the coronary arteries. The area of infarction is determined by the coronary artery that is affected and by its distribution of blood flow (Fig. 27.6). Approximately 30% to 40% of infarcts affect the right coronary artery, 40% to 50% affect the left anterior descending artery, and the remaining 15% to 20% affect the left circumflex artery.[17]

Pathophysiology. The extent of the infarct depends on the location and extent of occlusion, amount of heart tissue supplied by the vessel, duration of the occlusion, metabolic needs of the affected tissue, extent of collateral circulation, and other factors such as heart rate, blood pressure, and cardiac rhythm. An infarct may involve the endocardium, myocardium, epicardium, or a combination of these. Transmural infarcts involve the full thickness of the ventricular wall and most commonly occur when there is obstruction of a single artery (Fig. 27.7). Subendocardial infarcts involve the inner one third to one half of the ventricular wall and occur more frequently in the presence of severely narrowed but still patent arteries. Most infarcts are transmural, involving the free wall of the LV and the interventricular septum.

The principal biochemical consequence of myocardial infarction is the conversion from aerobic to anaerobic metabolism with inadequate production of energy to sustain normal myocardial function. As a result, a striking loss of contractile function occurs within 60 seconds of onset.[17] Changes in cell structure (*i.e.*, glycogen depletion and mitochondrial swelling) develop within several minutes. These early changes are reversible if blood flow is restored. Although gross tissue changes are not apparent for hours after onset of myocardial infarction, the ischemic area ceases to function within a matter of minutes, and irreversible damage to cells occurs in approximately 40 minutes. Irreversible myocardial cell death (necrosis) occurs after 20 to 40 minutes of severe ischemia.[17] Microvascular injury occurs in approximately 1 hour and follows irreversible cell injury. If the infarct is large enough, it depresses overall left ventricular function and pump failure ensues.

Multiple dynamic structural changes maintain cardiac function in persons with STEMI. Both the infarcted and noninfarcted areas of the ventricle undergo progressive changes in size, shape, and thickness, comprising early wall thinning, healing, hypertrophy, and dilation, collectively termed *ventricular remodeling*. As the nonfunctioning muscle in the infarcted area becomes thin and dilated, the muscle in the surrounding, noninfarcted area becomes thicker as it undergoes adaptive hypertrophy, so it can take over the work of the muscle in the infarcted zone. However, the adaptive effect of

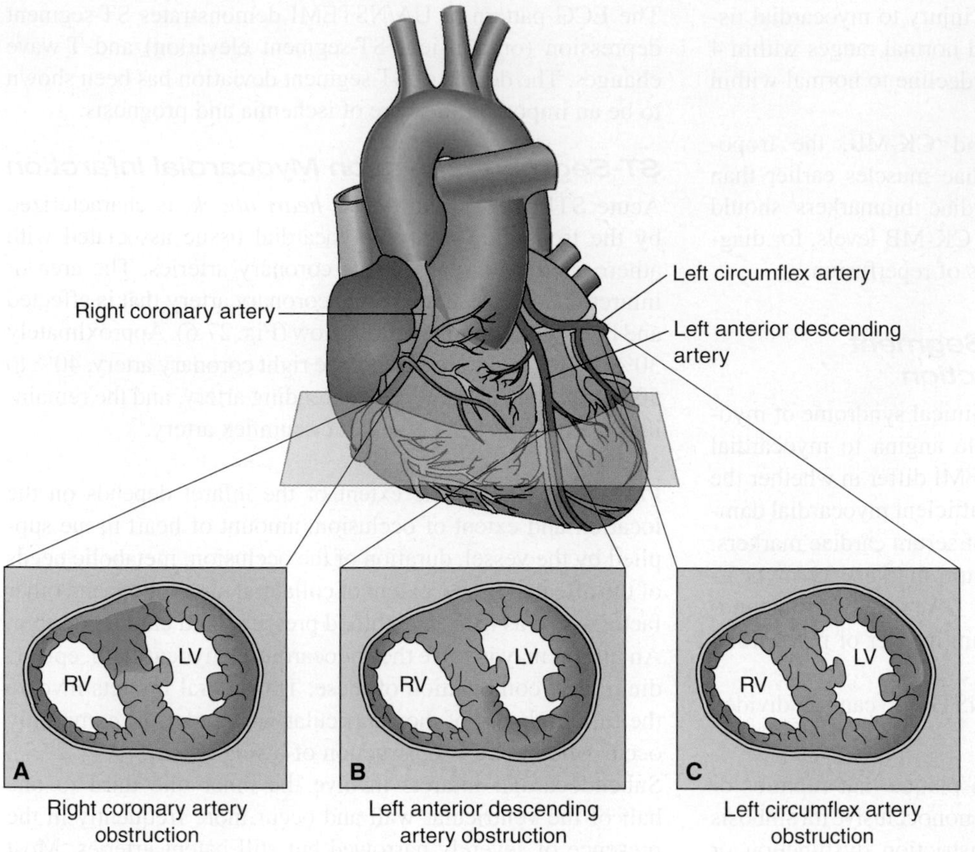

Figure 27.6 • Areas of the heart affected by occlusion of the **(A)** right coronary artery, **(B)** left anterior descending coronary artery, and **(C)** left circumflex coronary artery. RV, right ventricle; LV, left ventricle.

remodeling may be overwhelmed by aneurysm formation or depression of myocardial function, causing further impairment of ventricular function.[17]

Clinical Manifestations. STEMI may occur as an abrupt-onset event or as a progression from UA/NSTEMI. The onset of STEMI usually is abrupt, with pain as the significant symptom. The pain typically is severe and crushing, often described as being constricting, suffocating, or like "something sitting on my chest." It usually is substernal, radiating to the left arm, neck, or jaw, although it may be experienced in other areas of the chest. Unlike that of angina, the pain associated with STEMI is more prolonged and not relieved by rest or nitroglycerin, and narcotics frequently are required. Some persons may not describe it as "pain" but as "discomfort." Women often experience atypical ischemic-type chest discomfort, whereas the elderly may complain of shortness of breath more frequently than chest pain.[19]

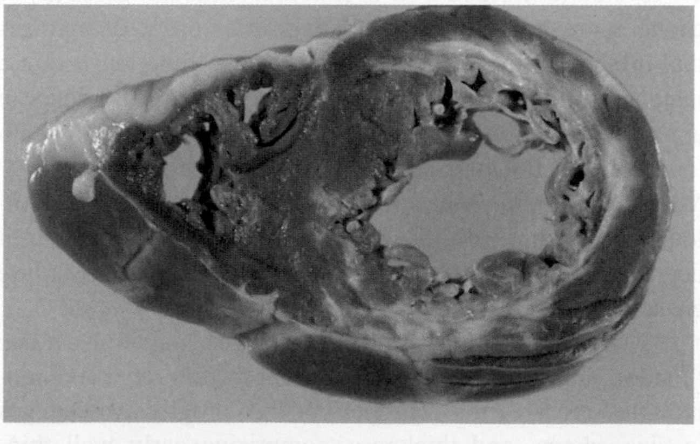

Figure 27.7 • Acute myocardial infarct. A transverse section of the heart of a person who died a few days after the onset of severe chest pain shows a transmural infarct in the anteroseptal region of the LV (left anterior descending [LAD] coronary artery territory). The necrotic myocardium is soft, yellowish, and sharply demarcated (*arrows*). (From Strayer D. E., Rubin R. (Eds.) (2015). *Rubin's pathology: Clinicopathologic foundations of medicine* (7th ed., Fig. 17-15, p. 643) Philadelphia, PA: Lippincott Williams & Wilkins.)

Gastrointestinal complaints are common with STEMI. There may be a sensation of epigastric distress; nausea and vomiting may occur. These symptoms are thought to be related to the severity of the pain and vagal stimulation. The epigastric distress may be mistaken for indigestion, and the person may seek relief with antacids or other home remedies, which only delays getting medical attention. Complaints of fatigue and weakness, especially of the arms and legs, are common. Pain and sympathetic stimulation combine to give rise to tachycardia, anxiety, restlessness, and feelings of impending doom. A productive cough may be present with frothy, pink sputum. The skin often is pale, cool, and moist. Impairment of myocardial function may lead to hypotension and shock.

Sudden death from STEMI is death that occurs within 1 hour of symptom onset.[17] It usually is attributed to fatal arrhythmias, which may occur without evidence of infarction. Early hospitalization after onset of symptoms greatly improves the chances of averting sudden death because appropriate resuscitation facilities are immediately available when the ventricular arrhythmia occurs.

Management of Acute Coronary Syndrome

Because the specific diagnosis of STEMI often is difficult to make at the time of entry into the health care system, the immediate management of UA/NSTEMI and STEMI is generally the same. The prognosis in STEMI is largely related to the occurrences of two general complications—arrhythmias and mechanical complications (pump failure). The majority of deaths from STEMI are due to the sudden development of ventricular arrhythmias. Therefore, the major elements in management of people with STEMI include

- Recognition of symptoms and prompt seeking of medical care
- Prompt deployment of an emergency medical team capable of resuscitation procedures, including defibrillation
- Expeditious transport to a hospital equipped for managing arrhythmias and providing advanced cardiac life support
- Expeditious implementation of reperfusion therapy within 60 to 90 minutes[17,18]

People who experience signs and symptoms of STEMI often delay seeking treatment, despite current public information regarding the benefits of early treatment. People who delay seeking treatment in the hospital include older adults, women, African Americans, people of low socioeconomic status, people with a history of angina and/or diabetes, and people who consult a relative.

Emergency department goals for management of ACS include identification of people who are candidates for reperfusion therapy. The history and physical examination should be conducted thoroughly, but efficiently, so as not to delay reperfusion therapy. Prior episodes of CVD, including ACS, coronary bypass surgery, or PCI, should be ascertained. Evaluation of the person's chief complaint, typically chest pain, along with other associated symptoms is essential in differentiating ACS from other diagnoses.

For any person presenting to the emergency department with symptoms of ACS, expeditious workup (within 10 minutes) should be performed including a 12-lead ECG. The typical ECG changes may not be present immediately after the onset of symptoms, except as arrhythmias. Diagnostic ECG tracings (*i.e.*, ST-segment elevation, prolongation of the Q wave, and inversion of the T wave) may be difficult to identify in people with STEMI who present with chest pain. Therefore, serial ECG tracings should be obtained. Some added difficulties include premature ventricular contractions, which are common arrhythmias after myocardial infarction. The occurrence of other arrhythmias and conduction defects depends on the areas of the heart and conduction pathways that are included in the infarct. A new bundle branch block, particularly left bundle branch block, also serves as a criterion for STEMI and indicates a need for rapid reperfusion.

Commonly indicated treatment regimens include administration of oxygen, aspirin, nitrates, pain medications, antiplatelet and anticoagulant therapy, and β-adrenergic blocking agents (beta-blockers). People with ECG evidence of infarction should receive immediate reperfusion therapy with a thrombolytic agent or PCI within 60 to 90 minutes.[20] The importance of intensive insulin control to maintain normal blood glucose (80 to 110 mg/dL) in people who are critically ill has been supported by multiple studies. Current ACC/AHA guidelines recommend the maintenance of strict glucose control during STEMI.[19]

Pain relief is a major objective in the treatment of STEMI. It is accomplished through a combination of oxygen, nitrates, analgesics (*e.g.*, morphine), and β-adrenergic blocking agents. The administration of oxygen augments the oxygen content of inspired air and increases the oxygen saturation of hemoglobin. Arterial oxygen levels may fall precipitously after STEMI, and oxygen administration helps to maintain the oxygen content of the blood perfusing the coronary circulation. In people with severe heart failure from STEMI, continuous positive-pressure ventilation or endotracheal intubation and support with mechanical ventilation may be necessary.

Nitroglycerin is given because of its vasodilating effect and ability to relieve coronary pain. The vasodilating effects of the drug decrease venous return (*i.e.*, reduce preload) and arterial blood pressure (*i.e.*, reduce afterload), thereby reducing oxygen consumption. Nitroglycerin may also limit infarction size and is most effective if given within 4 hours of symptom onset. Nitroglycerin usually is administered sublingually initially, after which the need for intravenous infusion is assessed. The use of intravenous nitroglycerin may be indicated for treatment of ongoing ischemic pain, control of hypertension, or management of pulmonary congestion. Nitroglycerin should not be administered to people with severe hypotension or to people who have received a phosphodiesterase inhibitor for erectile dysfunction within the previous 24 hours.

Although a number of analgesic agents have been used to treat the pain of STEMI, morphine is usually the drug of choice.[17] It is indicated if chest pain is unrelieved with oxygen and nitrates. The reduction in anxiety that accompanies the administration of morphine contributes to a decrease in restlessness and autonomic nervous system activity, with a subsequent decrease in the metabolic demands of the heart. It is commonly given intravenously because of the rapid onset of action. The intravenous route also bypasses the variable rate of absorption of subcutaneous or intramuscular sites, which often are underperfused because of the decrease in cardiac output that occurs after infarction.

β-Adrenergic blocking drugs act as antagonists that block β-receptor–mediated functions of the sympathetic nervous system and thus decrease myocardial oxygen demand by reducing heart rate and cardiac contractility and systemic arterial blood pressure. The lengthening of diastole caused by the slower heart rate may enhance myocardial perfusion, especially to the subendocardium. Beta-blockers also alter resting myocardial membrane potentials and may decrease life-threatening ventricular arrhythmias. Because sympathetic nervous system activity increases the metabolic demands of the myocardium, oral or intravenous beta-blockers are usually administered within the first few hours after the onset of STEMI. They should not be given in STEMI caused by cocaine use because it may accentuate coronary spasm, though there is controversy regarding the use of β-adrenergic agents in the setting of ACS. Other relative contraindications to beta-blockers include symptomatic bradycardia, hypotension, moderate to severe left ventricular failure, shock, and second- or third-degree heart block.

Platelets play a major role in the thrombotic response to atherosclerotic plaque disruption; therefore, inhibition of platelet aggregation is an important aspect in the early treatment of both UA/NSTEMI and STEMI. Aspirin (*i.e.*, acetylsalicylic acid) is the preferred antiplatelet agent for preventing platelet aggregation in people with ACS. Aspirin, which acts by inhibiting synthesis of the prostaglandin thromboxane A_2, is thought to promote reperfusion and reduce the likelihood of rethrombosis. The actions of aspirin are related to the presence of the acetyl group, which irreversibly acetylates the critical platelet enzyme, cyclooxygenase, which is required for thromboxane A_2 synthesis. Because the action is irreversible, the effect of aspirin on platelet function lasts for the lifetime of the platelet—approximately 8 to 10 days. For people who are unable to take aspirin because of hypersensitivity or gastrointestinal intolerance, clopidogrel may be prescribed. Clopidogrel is a thienopyridine derivative that reduces platelet aggregation by inhibiting the ADP pathway in platelets. Unlike aspirin, it has no effect on prostaglandin synthesis. Results of several studies have resulted in recommendations by the AHA for the use of clopidogrel along with aspirin for people with UA/NSTEMI and for preprocedural loading and long-term therapy for people undergoing PCI. Antithrombin agents are also used in the treatment of people with ACS. Anticoagulation therapy, which targets the coagulation pathway and formation of the fibrin clot, involves the use of unfractionated and low–molecular-weight heparin. The rationale for the use of antithrombin therapy in people with STEMI is the prevention of deep vein thrombosis (DVT), pulmonary emboli, and cerebral embolization.

Angiotensin-converting enzyme (ACE) inhibitors are often used during the early and convalescent phases of STEMI, demonstrating a benefit in terms of decreased mortality rate. ACE inhibitors increase cardiac output and stroke volume and reduce systemic vascular resistance as well as pulmonary capillary wedge pressure (PCWP). This, in turn, reduces LV dysfunction and decreases SCD. The greatest benefit is in those people with previous infarctions, heart failure, and tachycardia. ACE inhibitors usually are started within the first 24 hours, after fibrinolytic therapy has been completed. Therapy with ACE inhibitors is usually begun with low-dose oral administration and is increased steadily to full dose.[19] Although the use of ACE inhibitors as short-term therapy for people with UA/NSTEMI does not appear to have benefits, long-term use is helpful in preventing recurrent ischemic episodes.[17]

Reperfusion Strategies. The term *reperfusion* refers to reestablishment of blood flow through use of pharmacologic agents (fibrinolytic therapy), PCI, or coronary artery bypass grafting (CABG). All people presenting with STEMI should be assessed for reperfusion therapy as soon as possible on entry into the health care system. Time since onset of symptoms, risk of STEMI, possible risks associated with fibrinolytic therapy, and time required for transport to a skilled PCI laboratory should all be considered.

Early reperfusion (within 15 to 20 minutes) after onset of occlusion can prevent necrosis and improve myocardial perfusion in the infarct zone. Reperfusion after a longer interval can salvage some of the myocardial cells that would have died owing to longer periods of ischemia. It also may prevent the microvascular injury that occurs over a longer period. Even though much of the viable myocardium existing at the time of reflow, or reperfusion, ultimately recovers, critical abnormalities in biochemical function may persist, causing impaired ventricular function. The recovering area of the heart is often referred to as a hibernating myocardium. Because myocardial function is lost before cell death occurs, a hibernating myocardium may not be capable of sustaining life, and persons with large areas of dysfunctional myocardium may require life support until the stunned regions regain their function.[20]

Fibrinolytic Therapy. Fibrinolytic drugs dissolve blood and platelet clots and are used to reduce mortality, limit infarct size, encourage infarct healing and myocardial remodeling, and reduce the potential for life-threatening arrhythmias. These agents interact with plasminogen to generate plasmin, which lyses fibrin clots and digests clotting factors V and VIII, prothrombin, and fibrinogen. The fibrinolytic agents include streptokinase, alteplase, reteplase, and tenecteplase-tPA. The best results occur if treatment is initiated within 30 minutes of symptom onset. The magnitude of the benefit declines after this period, but it is possible that some benefit can be achieved for up to 12 hours after the onset of pain. The person must be a low-risk candidate for complications caused by bleeding, with no intracranial hemorrhage or significant trauma within the last 3 months. The primary complication of fibrinolytic therapy is intracranial hemorrhage, which usually occurs within the first 24 hours of treatment.[17]

Percutaneous Coronary Intervention. PCI is indicated as an early invasive procedure for people with UA/NSTEMI who have no serious comorbidity and who have lesions amenable to PCI.[20] PCI includes percutaneous transluminal coronary angioplasty (PTCA), stent implantation, atherectomy, and thrombectomy. The goal in PCI is to perform the procedure within 90 minutes of the person's first medical contact (the "door-to-balloon interval").[20]

Balloon PTCA involves dilation of a stenotic atherosclerotic plaque with an inflatable balloon (Fig. 27.8). The procedure is similar to cardiac catheterization for coronary angiography, in that the double-lumen balloon dilation catheter is introduced percutaneously into the femoral or brachial

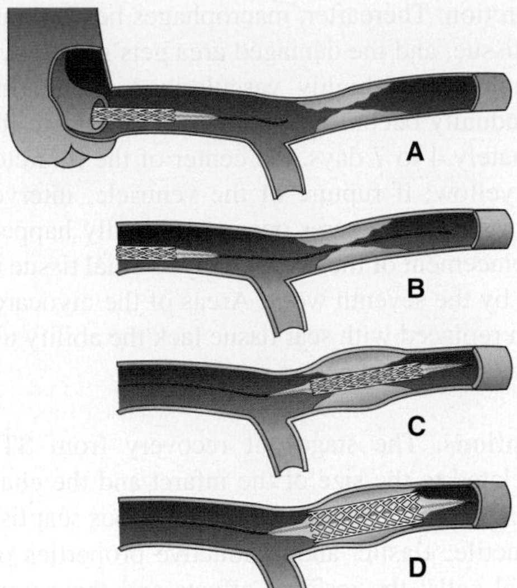

Figure 27.8 • Balloon-expandable stent insertion. **(A)** Insertion of a guide catheter with a collapsed balloon-expandable stent mounted over a guidewire into a coronary artery. **(B)** Advancement of guidewire across the coronary lesion. **(C)** Positioning of the balloon-expandable stent across the lesion. **(D)** Balloon inflation with expansion of the stent. Once the stent is expanded, the balloon system is removed.

artery and advanced under fluoroscopic view into the stenotic area of the affected coronary vessel. There, it is used to expand the coronary arterial lumen by stretching and tearing the atherosclerotic plaque and, to a lesser extent, by distributing the plaque along its longitudinal axis. This procedure is frequently used in conjunction with the placement of stents. Acute complications of PTCA include thrombosis and vessel dissection; longer-term complications involve restenosis of the dilated vessel.

The use of *coronary stenting* has been shown to improve short- and long-term outcomes compared with PTCA alone. People undergoing stent procedures are treated with antiplatelet and anticoagulant medications to prevent thrombosis, which is a major risk of the procedure.[20] The bare metal self-expanding wire mesh stents that were used initially had high thrombosis rates and have largely been replaced by balloon-expandable stents. Radiation brachytherapy was used to improve restenosis of the stents and involved the use of localized intracoronary artery radiation for reduction of in-stent restenosis. The procedure is credited with inhibiting cell proliferation and vascular lesion formation and preventing constrictive arterial remodeling. This procedure has limitations including the need for radiation therapy and has been shown to be inferior to drug-eluting stents.[20] Bare metal stents are being used in 20% to 30% of the people who require PCI.

Drug-eluting stents (with sirolimus, paclitaxel, zotarolimus, and everolimus) are also being used to suppress local neointimal proliferation that causes restenosis of the coronary artery.[20] Recent clinical trials found that long-term use up to 1 year of aspirin and clopidogrel is recommended to prevent restenosis. *Atherectomy* (*i.e.*, cutting of the atherosclerotic plaque with a high-speed circular blade from within the vessel) is a mechanical technique to remove atherosclerotic tissue during angioplasty. Laser, angioplasty devices are also used. However, with the availability of stents, these procedures are used less frequently than in the past. Thrombectomy (removal of the thrombus) involves the use of a special catheter device to fracture the thrombus into small pieces and then pull the fracture fragments into the catheter tip, so they can be propelled proximally and removed.

Coronary Artery Bypass Grafting. CABG is one of the most common surgeries performed in the world, providing relief of angina, improvement in exercise tolerance, and prolongation of life. The procedure involves revascularization of the affected myocardium by placing a saphenous vein graft between the aorta and the affected coronary artery distal to the site of occlusion or by using the internal mammary artery as a means of revascularizing the left anterior descending artery or its branches (Fig. 27.9). One to five distal anastomoses commonly are done.

Emergent or urgent CABG, as a reperfusion strategy, is indicated in situations such as failed PCI with persistent pain or hemodynamic instability or for people who are not candidates for PCI or fibrinolytic therapy.[19,21] In considering CABG as a treatment option, the risk for hospital mortality and other

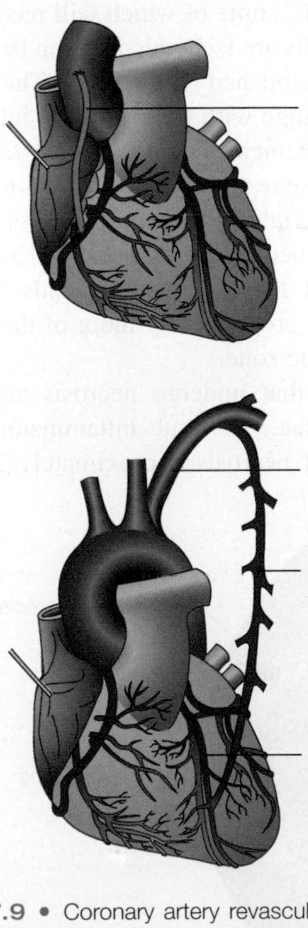

Figure 27.9 • Coronary artery revascularization. **(Top)** Saphenous vein bypass graft. The vein segment is sutured to the ascending aorta and the right coronary artery at a point distal to the occluding lesion. **(Bottom)** Mammary artery bypass graft. The mammary artery is anastomosed to the anterior descending left coronary artery, bypassing the obstructing lesion.

complications must be taken into account. Advanced age, poor left ventricular function, and the urgency with which surgery is performed increase the risk of early mortality. Serious complications, such as stroke, mediastinitis, and renal dysfunction, also increase the mortality and morbidity associated with CABG. The use of preoperative antibiotics and perioperative administration of beta-blockers help in reducing the incidence of postoperative infection and atrial fibrillation.

CABG does not alter the progress of the CAD, and although the rate of return of angina is low for the first 5 years, about 50% of vein grafts are closed 10 years after CABG. The use of internal mammary artery grafts, however, has shown excellent late patency. Aspirin is the drug of choice for prophylaxis against early saphenous vein graft closure and is continued indefinitely.[2] New surgical techniques in the treatment of CAD continue to evolve in an effort to reduce adverse effects of the midline sternotomy incision, cardiopulmonary bypass, and global cardioplegic arrest. Some of these include "off-pump" CABG, the development of robotic coronary bypass, and transmyocardial laser revascularization.[2]

Postinfarction Recovery Period

After a myocardial infarction, there usually are three zones of tissue damage: a zone of myocardial tissue that becomes necrotic because of an absolute lack of blood flow; a surrounding zone of injured cells, some of which will recover; and an outer zone in which cells are ischemic and can be salvaged if blood flow can be reestablished (Fig. 27.10). The boundaries of these zones may change with time after the infarction and with the success of treatment measures to reestablish blood flow. If blood flow can be restored within the 20- to 40-minute time frame, loss of cell viability does not occur or is minimal. The progression of ischemic necrosis usually begins in the subendocardial area of the heart and extends through the myocardium to involve progressively more of the transmural thickness of the ischemic zone.

Myocardial cells that undergo necrosis are gradually replaced with scar tissue. An acute inflammatory response develops in the area of necrosis approximately 2 to 3 days after infarction. Thereafter, macrophages begin removing the necrotic tissue, and the damaged area gets gradually replaced by an ingrowth of highly vascularized granulation tissue, which gradually becomes less vascular and more fibrous. At approximately 4 to 7 days, the center of the infarcted area is soft and yellow; if rupture of the ventricle, interventricular septum, or valve structures occurs, it usually happens at this time. Replacement of the necrotic myocardial tissue usually is complete by the seventh week. Areas of the myocardium that have been replaced with scar tissue lack the ability to contract and initiate or conduct action potentials.

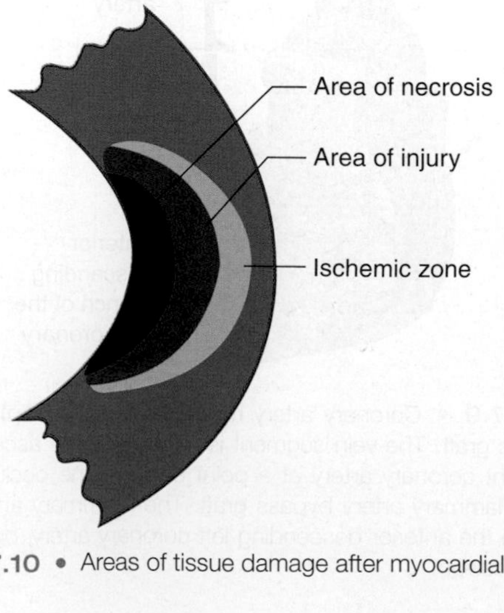

Figure 27.10 • Areas of tissue damage after myocardial infarction.

Complications. The stages of recovery from STEMI are closely related to the size of the infarct and the changes that have taken place in the infarcted area. Fibrous scar tissue lacks the contractile, elastic, and conductive properties of normal myocardial cells; the residual effects and the complications are determined essentially by the extent and location of the injury. Among the complications of STEMI are sudden death, pericarditis, stroke, thromboemboli, and mechanical defects (*e.g.*, mitral valve regurgitation, ventricular septal rupture, left ventricular wall rupture, and left ventricular aneurysm). Depending on its severity, myocardial infarction has the potential for compromising the pumping action of the heart. Heart failure and cardiogenic shock are dreaded complications of STEMI.

Life-threatening arrhythmias can be the first symptom of an ACS, differing in mechanism from chronic stable angina. With ACS, mechanisms may be related to reentry, abnormal automaticity, and electrolyte imbalances, particularly potassium and magnesium. Symptomatic bradycardia and heart block are also complications of ACS and are treated according to the guidelines for implantation of cardiac pacemakers and antiarrhythmic devices.[2]

Pericarditis tends to occur in people with large infarcts and a lower ejection fraction. It may appear as early as the second or third day postinfarction or up to several weeks later. This late complication, called *Dressler syndrome*, occurs weeks to months after STEMI and is thought to be an autoimmune response. In contrast to the pain associated with STEMI, the pain with pericarditis is sharp and stabbing and aggravated by deep inspiration and positional changes. Because of reperfusion therapy, this complication has been greatly reduced.

Acute stroke is another complication of STEMI. Risk factors for stroke after a STEMI include hypertension, older age, history of previous stroke, decreased ejection fraction, and atrial fibrillation. Thromboemboli, presenting as DVT or pulmonary emboli, do not present as frequently as in the past because of the use of anticoagulant therapy.

Mechanical defects result from changes that occur in the necrotic and subsequently inflamed myocardium and include rupture of the ventricular septum, papillary muscle, or free ventricular wall[17] (Fig. 27.11). Partial or complete rupture of a papillary muscle is a rare but often fatal complication of transmural myocardial infarction.[17] It is detected by the presence of a new systolic murmur and clinical deterioration,

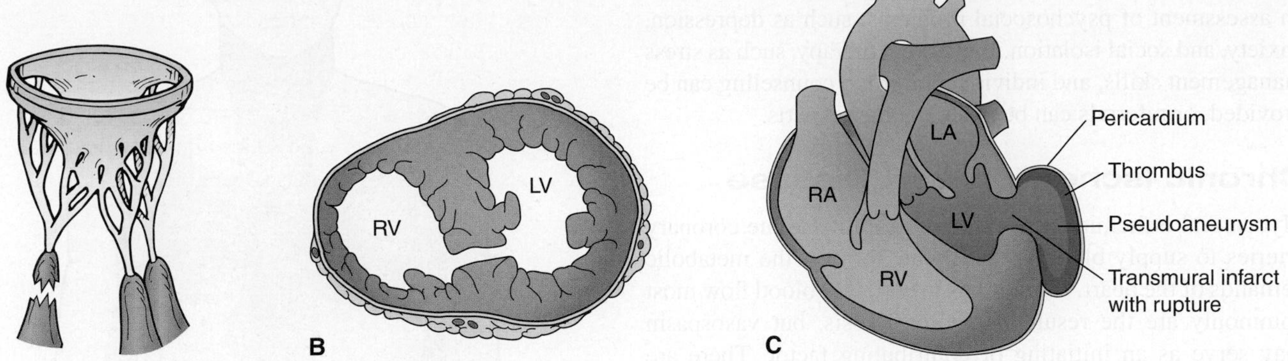

Figure 27.11 • Acute mechanical complications of myocardial infarction. **(A)** Papillary muscle rupture. **(B)** Interventricular septum rupture. **(C)** Rupture of the free wall of the LV with pseudoaneurysm formation. RA, right atrium; LA, left atrium; RV, right ventricle; LV, left ventricle.

often with pulmonary edema. More frequently, postinfarction mitral valve regurgitation results from early ischemic dysfunction of the papillary muscle and underlying myocardium. Ventricular septal rupture occurs less frequently than in the past because of the use of reperfusion therapy. Previously thought to require surgical intervention only in symptomatic people, surgical repair is now recommended for all people with ventricular septal rupture. Complete rupture of the free wall of the infarcted ventricle occurs in 1% to 6% of people and usually results in immediate death.[17] It usually occurs 3 to 7 days postinfarction, usually involves the anterior wall, and is more frequent in older women. Incomplete or gradual rupture may be sealed off by the pericardium, creating a pseudoaneurysm that requires early surgical intervention because delayed complete rupture is common.

A left ventricular aneurysm, a sharply delineated area of scar tissue that bulges paradoxically during systole (Fig. 27.12),

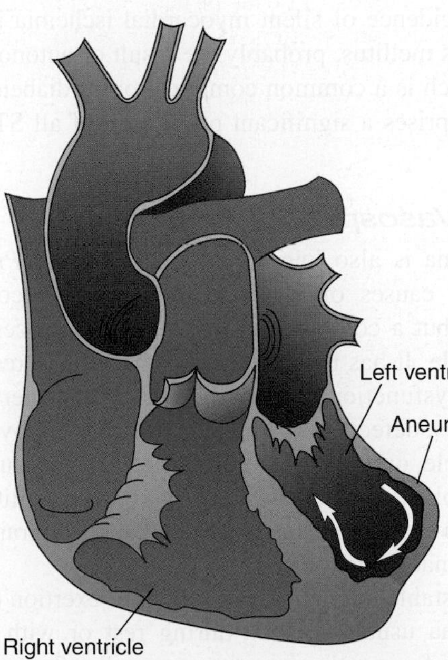

Figure 27.12 • Paradoxical movement of a left ventricular aneurysm during systole.

develops in 10% of people dying in the hospital of STEMI.[17] They usually present on the anterior portion of the LV after occlusion of the left anterior descending coronary artery and become evident 4 to 8 weeks after infarct. They rarely rupture but may be associated with arterial emboli, ventricular arrhythmias, and heart failure. Surgical resection may be performed for these indications when other treatment measures fail.[17]

Cardiac Rehabilitation

Cardiac rehabilitation programs are recommended for people after ACS and incorporate strategies to improve adherence to medical therapies and lifestyle changes. Components of cardiac rehabilitation include exercise, nutrition, smoking cessation, psychosocial management, and education. Education is an essential component of cardiac rehabilitation programs and is often incorporated with other aspects of the program. This includes education related to exercise, nutrition, smoking cessation, and medications. Adherence to a cardiac rehabilitation program, or to any of its components, can be extremely difficult. Among the factors that influence participation and adherence are physician referral, reimbursement issues, distance and transportation, and social support.[22]

An exercise program is an integral part of a cardiac rehabilitation program. It includes activities such as walking, swimming, and bicycling. These exercises involve changes in muscle length and rhythmic contractions of muscle groups. Most exercise programs are individually designed to meet each person's physical and psychological needs. The goal of the exercise program is to increase the maximal oxygen consumption by the muscle tissues, so that these persons are able to perform more work at a lower heart rate and blood pressure.[22]

In addition to exercise, cardiac risk factor modification incorporates strategies for smoking cessation, weight loss, stress reduction, and control of hypertension and diabetes (when present). Nutrition counseling has direct effects on weight, serum lipids, blood pressure, diabetes, and other factors. The choice of diet is based on beneficial effect, as well as the social and cultural needs of the person. Dietary patterns are assessed and specific goals determined and communicated with the person.[22] Cardiac rehabilitation programs should include an assessment of psychosocial problems, such as depression, anxiety, and social isolation. Behavioral therapy, such as stress management skills, and individual or group counseling can be provided, or referrals can be made to other experts.

Chronic Ischemic Heart Disease

Myocardial ischemia occurs when the ability of the coronary arteries to supply blood is inadequate to meet the metabolic demands of the heart. Limitations in coronary blood flow most commonly are the result of atherosclerosis, but vasospasm may serve as an initiating or contributing factor. There are several major types of chronic ischemic CAD: chronic stable angina, silent myocardial ischemia, variant or vasospastic angina, chest pain with normal coronary angiography, and ischemic cardiomyopathy.

Stable Angina

Chronic stable angina is associated with a fixed coronary obstruction that produces a disparity between coronary blood flow and metabolic demands of the myocardium. Stable angina is the initial manifestation of ischemic heart disease in approximately half of persons with CAD.[23] Although most people with stable angina have atherosclerotic heart disease, angina does not develop in a considerable number of people with advanced coronary atherosclerosis. This probably is because of their sedentary lifestyle, the development of adequate collateral circulation, or the inability of these people to perceive pain. In many instances, myocardial infarction occurs without a history of angina.

Angina pectoris usually is precipitated by situations that increase the work demands of the heart, such as physical exertion, exposure to cold, and emotional stress. The pain typically is described as a constricting, squeezing, or suffocating sensation. It usually is steady, increasing in intensity only at the onset and end of the attack. The pain of angina commonly is located in the precordial or substernal area of the chest; it is similar to myocardial infarction in that it may radiate to the left shoulder, jaw, arm, or other areas of the chest (Fig. 27.13). In some people, the arm or shoulder pain may be confused with arthritis; in others, epigastric pain is confused with indigestion. Angina commonly is categorized according to whether it occurs with exercise, occurs during rest, is of new onset, or is of increasing severity.

Typically, chronic stable angina is provoked by exertion or emotional stress and relieved within minutes by rest or the use of nitroglycerin. A delay of more than 5 to 10 minutes before relief is obtained suggests that the symptoms are not due to ischemia or that they are due to severe ischemia. Angina that occurs at rest, is of new onset, or is increasing in intensity or duration denotes an increased risk for myocardial infarction and should be evaluated immediately using the criteria for ACS.

Silent Myocardial Ischemia

Silent myocardial ischemia occurs in the absence of anginal pain. The factors that cause silent myocardial ischemia appear

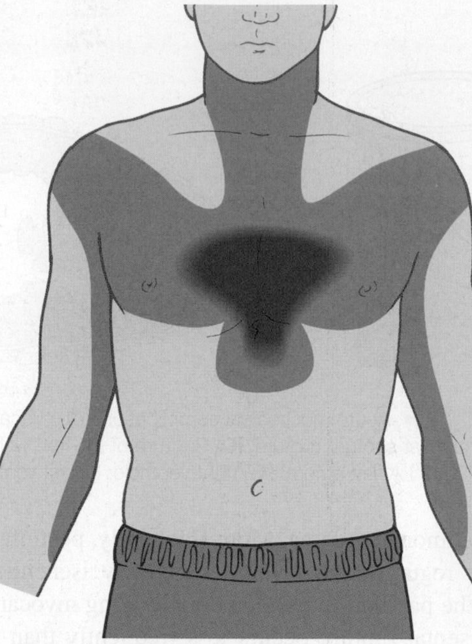

Figure 27.13 • Areas of pain due to angina.

to be the same as those responsible for angina: impaired blood flow from the effects of coronary atherosclerosis or vasospasm. Silent myocardial ischemia affects three populations—people who are asymptomatic without other evidence of CAD, people who have had a myocardial infarct and continue to have episodes of silent ischemia, and people with angina who also have episodes of silent ischemia.[23] The reason for the painless episodes of ischemia is unclear. The episodes may be shorter and involve less myocardial tissue than those producing pain. Another explanation is that persons with silent angina have defects in pain threshold or pain transmission, or autonomic neuropathy with sensory denervation. There is evidence of an increased incidence of silent myocardial ischemia in people with diabetes mellitus, probably the result of autonomic neuropathy, which is a common complication of diabetes. Silent STEMI comprises a significant proportion of all STEMIs in older adults.

Variant (Vasospastic) Angina

Variant angina is also known as *vasospastic* or *Prinzmetal angina*. The causes of variant angina are not completely understood, but a combination of pathologic processes may be responsible. It has been suggested that it may result from endothelial dysfunction, hyperactive sympathetic nervous system responses, defects in the handling of calcium by vascular smooth muscle, or an alteration in nitric oxide production.[18,23] In some people, it is associated with hypercontractility of vascular smooth muscle and is associated with migraine headaches or Raynaud phenomenon.

Unlike stable angina that occurs with exertion or stress, variant angina usually occurs during rest or with minimal exercise and frequently occurs nocturnally (between midnight and 8 AM). Arrhythmias often occur when the pain is severe, and most people are aware of their presence during an attack. ECG changes are significant if recorded during an attack. These abnormalities include ST-segment elevation or depression, T-wave peaking, U-wave inversion, and rhythm disturbances. People with variant angina who have serious arrhythmias during spontaneous episodes of pain are at a higher risk of sudden death.

Chest Pain with Normal Coronary Angiography

Exercise-induced chest pain with normal coronary angiography is frequently described as *cardiac syndrome X*. This disorder should not be confused with metabolic syndrome, which was formerly described as *syndrome X*. The cause of the chest pain has not been established but is thought to reflect a problem with the microvasculature and/or increased cardiac pain perception. The alternate name *microvascular angina* has been suggested for this disorder.

Ischemic Cardiomyopathy

Ischemic cardiomyopathy describes CAD that results in myocardial dysfunction. This can present with symptoms of cardiomyopathy without a known history of CAD in people who have had multiple MIs or have occluded arteries. It is important to recognize the difference between ischemic and dilated cardiomyopathy (DCM) because ischemic cardiomyopathy may be reversed upon presentation. Ischemic cardiomyopathy caused by multiple MIs has a poor prognosis because there is greater damage compared to those who have occluded lesions that can be reversed.

Diagnosis

The diagnosis of angina is based on a detailed pain history, the presence of risk factors, invasive and noninvasive studies, and laboratory data. Noncoronary causes of chest pain, such as esophageal reflux or musculoskeletal disorders, are ruled out.

Noninvasive testing for chronic stable angina includes ECG, echocardiography, exercise stress testing, nuclear imaging studies, CT, and possibly cardiac MRI. Because the resting ECG is often normal, exercise testing is often used in evaluating people with angina. Ischemia that is asymptomatic at rest is detected by precipitation of typical chest pain or ST-segment changes on the ECG. Although noninvasive testing is valuable in the diagnosis of chronic stable angina, cardiac catheterization and coronary arteriography are needed for definitive diagnosis.[13,17] Serum biochemical markers for myocardial infarction are normal in people with chronic stable angina. Metabolic abnormalities are frequently detected, such as hypercholesterolemia and other dyslipidemias, carbohydrate intolerance, and insulin resistance.

Treatment

Comprehensive and individualized assessment, lifestyle changes, and treatments are needed for people with chronic stable angina. The treatment goals for stable angina are directed toward symptom reduction and prevention of myocardial infarction through nonpharmacologic strategies, pharmacologic therapy, and coronary interventions. PCI relieves symptoms for people with chronic stable angina but does not extend the life span. CABG is usually indicated in people with double- or triple-vessel disease.[21]

Nonpharmacologic methods are aimed at symptom control and lifestyle modifications to reduce risk factors for coronary disease. They include smoking cessation, stress reduction, a regular exercise program, limiting dietary intake of cholesterol and saturated fats, weight reduction if obesity is present, and avoidance of cold that produces vasoconstriction. The goal of pharmacologic treatment of angina is to relieve ischemia and alleviate symptoms, prevent myocardial infarction and death, and improve the quality of life. Pharmacologic agents used in chronic stable angina include aspirin or clopidogrel, beta-blockers in people without contraindications or calcium antagonists when beta-blockers are contraindicated, and ACE inhibitors in people who also have diabetes or left ventricular systolic dysfunction (see previous discussion in section on Acute Coronary Syndrome). In people with established CAD, including chronic stable angina, the use of lipid-lowering agents or statins is recommended, even in the presence of mild to moderate elevations of LDL cholesterol.

Nitrates, both short acting and long acting, are vasodilators used in the treatment of chronic stable angina and in silent myocardial ischemia.[23] Nitrates exert their effect mainly through a decrease in venous return to the heart with a resultant decrease in intraventricular volume. Arterial pressure also decreases. Decreased intraventricular pressure and volume are associated with decreased wall tension and myocardial oxygen requirement. Although they are not vasodilators, beta-blocking drugs are extremely useful in management of angina associated with effort. The benefits of beta-blocking agents are due primarily to their hemodynamic effects—decreased heart rate, blood pressure, and myocardial contractility—which decrease myocardial oxygen requirements at rest and during exercise. The calcium channel–blocking drugs, also called *calcium antagonists*, block activated and inactivated L-type calcium channels in cardiac and smooth muscle. The therapeutic effects of the calcium channel–blocking agents result from coronary and peripheral artery dilation and from decreased myocardial metabolism associated with the decrease in myocardial contractility. Persons with variant angina usually respond to treatment with calcium antagonists.

IN SUMMARY

CAD is a disorder of impaired coronary blood flow, usually caused by atherosclerosis. Myocardial ischemia occurs when there is a disparity between myocardial oxygen supply and demand and can present as chronic ischemic heart disease or ACS. Diagnostic methods for CAD include ECG, exercise stress testing, nuclear imaging studies, CT, MRI, and angiographic studies in the cardiac catheterization laboratory.

The ACS, which includes UA/NSTEMI and STEMI, results from multiple pathophysiologic processes, including unstable atherosclerotic plaques, platelet aggregation, and thrombus formation. UA is an accelerated form of angina in which the pain occurs more frequently, is more severe, and lasts longer than in chronic stable angina. Myocardial infarction refers to the ischemic death of myocardial tissue associated with obstructed blood flow in the coronary arteries due to plaque disruption and occlusion of blood flow. NSTEMI and STEMI differ in terms of extent of myocardial damage. The complications of STEMI include potentially fatal arrhythmias, heart failure and cardiogenic shock, pericarditis, thromboemboli, rupture of cardiac structures, and ventricular aneurysms. Diagnostic methods include the use of ECG monitoring and serum biomarkers. Treatment goals focus on reestablishment of myocardial blood flow through rapid reperfusion of the occluded coronary artery, prevention of clot extension through use of aspirin and other antiplatelet and antithrombotic agents, alleviation of pain, administration of oxygen, and the use of vasodilators (nitroglycerin) and β-adrenergic blocking agents to reduce the work demands on the heart.

The chronic ischemic heart diseases include chronic stable angina, silent myocardial ischemia, variant (vasospastic) angina, chest pain with normal angiography, and ischemic cardiomyopathy. Chronic stable angina is associated with a fixed atherosclerotic obstruction and pain that is precipitated by increased work demands on the heart and relieved by rest. Variant angina can result from spasms of the coronary arteries or other dysfunctions. Silent myocardial ischemia and ischemic cardiomyopathy occur without CAD symptoms.

CARDIOMYOPATHIES

After completing this section of the chapter, the learner will be able to meet the following objectives:

- Define the term *cardiomyopathy* as it relates to both the mechanical and electrical function of the myocardium.
- Differentiate among the pathophysiologic changes that occur with hypertrophic cardiomyopathy (HCM), arrhythmogenic right ventricular cardiomyopathy (ARVC), dilated cardiomyopathies, and myocarditis.
- Describe the treatment strategies of both primary and secondary cardiomyopathy.

The definition and classification of the cardiomyopathies have evolved tremendously with the advance of molecular genetics. The definition and classification of cardiomyopathies were updated in an AHA scientific statement incorporating not only the advances of cardiac molecular genetics but other newly diagnosed diseases, as well as ion channelopathies.[24] This scientific statement defines cardiomyopathies as:

> A heterogeneous group of diseases of the myocardium associated with mechanical and/or electrical dysfunction that usually (but not invariably) exhibit inappropriate ventricular hypertrophy or dilatation and are due to a variety of causes that frequently are genetic
>
> Cardiomyopathies either are confined to the heart or are part of generalized systemic disorders, often leading to cardiovascular death or progressive heart failure–related disability.[24]

Based on this definition, the classification of cardiomyopathies is divided into two major groups: *primary* and *secondary*. The primary cardiomyopathies represent heart disorders that are confined to the myocardium, whereas the secondary cardiomyopathies represent myocardial changes that occur with a variety of systemic (multiorgan) disorders. Cardiomyopathies are usually associated with disorders related to mechanical (*e.g.*, heart failure) or electrical (*e.g.*, life-threatening arrhythmias) mechanisms.

Primary Cardiomyopathies

The primary cardiomyopathies are classified as genetic, mixed, or acquired, based on their etiology.[24] The genetic cardiomyopathies include HCM, ARVC, left ventricular noncompaction cardiomyopathy, inherited conduction system disorders, and ion channelopathies. The mixed cardiomyopathies, which include DCM, are of both genetic and nongenetic origin. Acquired cardiomyopathies include those that have their origin in the inflammatory process (*e.g.*, myocarditis), stress ("Takotsubo" pericarditis), or pregnancy (peripartum cardiomyopathy). In many cases, the cause is unknown, in which case it is referred to as an *idiopathic cardiomyopathy*.

Genetic Cardiomyopathies

Hypertrophic Cardiomyopathy. HCM is characterized by unexplained left ventricular hypertrophy with disproportionate thickening of the interventricular septum, abnormal diastolic filling, cardiac arrhythmias, and, in some cases, intermittent left ventricular outflow obstruction[25] (Fig. 27.14). It is one of the most common types of cardiomyopathy, occurring in approximately 1 person in 500 of the general population.[25] HCM is the most common cause of SCD in young athletes. The propensity to sudden death seems to be genetic, and implantable cardioverter defibrillators (ICDs) have been proved to be lifesaving.[25] Other complications that occur include atrial fibrillation, stroke, and heart failure.

HCM is an autosomal dominant heart disease caused by mutations in the genes encoding proteins of the cardiac sarcomere contractile proteins. Histologically, HCM appears as myocyte hypertrophy with myofibril disarray and increased cardiac fibrosis. Currently, nine genes can be identified in genetic tests that are associated with HCM, with the β-myosin heavy chain and the myosin-binding protein C genes being the most common. More than 400 individual mutations have been identified and are unique from family to family. Some phenotypic correlates can be made from specific mutations; however, there are many exceptions, indicating that genetic modifiers and environmental factors are also important.[25] Although HCM is inherited, it may present anywhere from

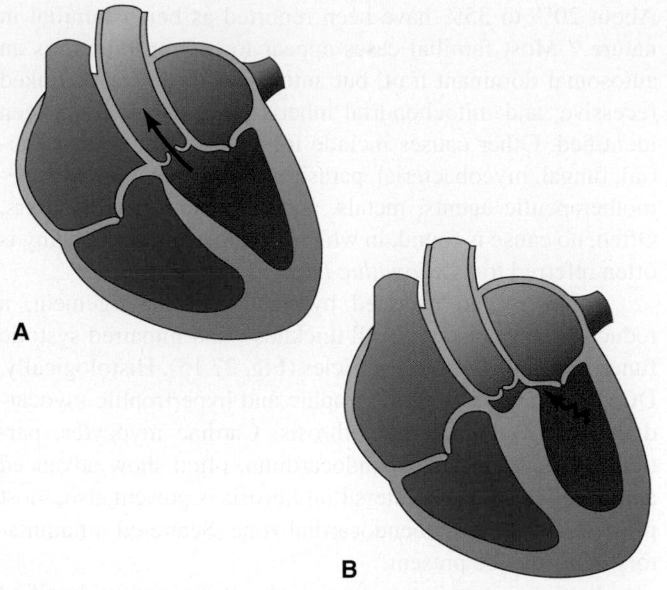

Figure 27.14 • Vertical section of the heart showing **(A)** a normal heart and **(B)** a heart with HCM in which disproportionate thickening of interventricular septum causes intermittent left ventricular outflow obstruction.

early childhood to late adulthood with a broad category of manifestations and variable clinical course. The basic physiologic abnormalities in HCM are reduced left ventricular chamber size, poor compliance with reduced stroke volume that results from impaired diastolic filling, mitral regurgitation, and, in about 25% of cases, dynamic obstruction of left ventricular outflow.[25] Clinical manifestations in the majority of the cases are asymptomatic but may include dyspnea, chest pain during exertion, exercise intolerance, syncope, and arrhythmias. Owing to massive hypertrophy, high left ventricular chamber pressure, and potentially abnormal intramural arteries, focal myocardial ischemia often develops even in the absence of CAD; thus, anginal pain is common. HCM is frequently associated with the development of left ventricular outflow obstruction during rest or exertion that is caused by systolic anterior motion (SAM) of the mitral valve and contact of the mitral valve with the ventricular septum. Clinical manifestations are highly variable and may progress to end-stage heart failure with left ventricular remodeling and systolic dysfunction.

Diagnosis of HCM is frequently established with 2-D echocardiography, demonstrating nondilated left ventricular hypertrophy, in the absence of other cardiac or systemic diseases. ECG is abnormal in 95% of the cases showing left ventricular hypertrophy. Continuous ambulatory monitoring is useful in detection of arrhythmias. Cardiac MRI can also be helpful in determining the site and extent of hypertrophy. The value of electrophysiologic testing remains controversial. Genetic testing, through bidirectional deoxyribonucleic acid (DNA) sequence analysis, provides accurate diagnosis and precise identification of gene mutations, if the gene involved is one of the few that can be identified through testing.[25]

Medical management of HCM is primarily focused on people with obstructive HCM who are symptomatic. The first-line approach to relief of symptoms is pharmacologic therapy designed to block the effects of catecholamines that exacerbate outflow obstruction and to slow the heart rate to enhance diastolic filling. β-Adrenergic blockers are generally the initial choice for persons with symptomatic HCM. The calcium channel blocker verapamil can also be used. It can, however, exacerbate left ventricular outflow obstruction and is not recommended for people with severe outflow obstruction and pronounced symptoms. Disopyramide may also be added to beta-blocker or verapamil because it tends to decrease the gradient and improves symptoms in some people.[25]

In obstructive HCM that is refractory to drug therapy, septal myectomy, alcohol ablation of the interventricular septum, and dual-chamber and biventricular pacing are alternative treatment options. Atrial fibrillation is treated with pharmacologic rate control, cardioversion, and coagulation. An ICD should be used for people with HCM who are at risk for SCD. People at risk for SCD would include those who have had a prior cardiac arrest or have sustained ventricular tachycardia or ventricular fibrillation, a first-degree relative with premature SCD related to HCM, repetitive ventricular tachycardia, ventricular wall thickness greater than 30 mm, hypotensive response to exercise, and recent unexplained syncope.[26] About 5% of people develop end-stage HCM and require standard therapy for advanced heart failure, including consideration for heart transplantation.

Arrhythmogenic Right Ventricular Cardiomyopathy/Dysplasia. ARVC/arrhythmogenic right ventricular dysplasia (ARVD) is a heart muscle disease where fibrofatty infiltration of the right ventricular myocardium causes right-sided heart failure and various rhythm disturbances, particularly ventricular tachycardia.[27] It ranks second, after HCM, as the leading cause of SCD in young athletes. The incidence of ARVC/D varies from about 1 in 2000 to 1 in 5000, affecting men more frequently than women. It is inherited as an autosomal dominant trait in 30% to 50% of cases with eight genes identified, although some recessive forms have been identified that present somewhat differently than ARVC/D.[27]

The disorder is characterized by progressive loss of myocytes, with partial or complete replacement of the right ventricular muscle with fatty or fibrofatty tissue. The disorder is associated with reentrant ventricular tachyarrhythmias of right ventricular origin that are often precipitated by exercise-induced discharge of catecholamines. Clinical manifestations are thought to present in three phases. In the early "concealed phase," individuals are generally asymptomatic but are at risk for SCD especially during exertion. In the "electrical phase," people often present with palpitations and/or syncope. It is during this phase that right ventricular changes are identified using echocardiography. Then later in the "diffuse phase," people can have biventricular heart failure. Other symptoms may include abdominal pain and mental confusion.

Diagnosis of ARVC/D is based on clinical, ECG, echocardiographic, Holter monitor, cardiac MRI, signal-averaged electrocardiography (SAECG), and histologic findings. Personal and family history, including first- and second-degree relatives, is important. Characteristic findings on 12-lead ECG include ventricular tachycardia with left bundle branch block pattern, T-wave inversion in the right precordial leads, and epsilon waves (small deflections just beyond the QRS complex). Right ventricular bundle branch block may also be present. Cardiac MRI and right ventricular angiography can be used in the assessment of ARVC/D.

Treatment for ARVC/D is aimed at prevention of SCD. Although ARVC/D cannot be cured, the goal of treatment is to control the arrhythmias with combinations of various antiarrhythmic agents.[27] Radiofrequency ablation is used in drug-refractory cases, although it is completely successful in only 30% to 65% of cases, with multiple ablations sometimes needed. ICD placement is also indicated for drug-refractory cases and for those who have survived an SCD episode. ICD placement for others is debatable because no risk stratification system exists. Final options for treatment include ventriculotomy and heart transplantation.

Ion Channelopathies. Ion channels are pore-forming proteins that provide pathways for movement of ions across cell membranes. Diseases caused by mutations in genes encoding ion channel subunits or proteins are called *ion channelopathies*.[28] In the heart, these ion channel disorders include the long QT syndrome (LQTS), short QT syndrome (SQTS), Brugada syndrome, and catecholaminergic polymorphic ventricular tachycardia.

LQTS and SQTS are caused by sodium or potassium ion channel gene mutations. LQTS, which is probably the most common of the ion channelopathies, is identified on 12-lead ECG by a prolonged QT interval. It causes a polymorphic ventricular tachycardia known as *torsade de pointes*. First described in 2000, the SQTS is characterized by short QT interval (<330 ms) on the ECG, which can lead to ventricular tachycardia or fibrillation and SCD.[28]

Brugada syndrome was described originally in 1992 as a clinical entity related to a sodium channel gene mutation. It is associated with SCD in young people, particularly young Southeast Asian men who experience SCD during sleep. The disorder is characterized on ECG by right bundle branch block and ST-segment elevation in the anterior leads (V3–V4).[28] Catecholaminergic polymorphic ventricular tachycardia is caused by an abnormal receptor that regulates calcium release from the sarcoplasmic reticulum. It is triggered by vigorous physical activity or acute emotion and leads to syncope, polymorphic ventricular tachycardia, and SCD. The ECG of a person with Brugada syndrome is characteristic consisting of right bundle branch pattern and ST-segment elevation in V1 to V3.[27]

Mixed (Genetic and Nongenetic) Cardiomyopathies

Dilated Cardiomyopathy. DCM is a common cause of heart failure and the leading indication for heart transplantation. About 20% to 35% have been reported as being familial in nature.[29] Most familial cases appear to be transmitted as an autosomal dominant trait, but autosomal recessive, X-linked recessive, and mitochondrial inheritance patterns have been identified. Other causes include infections (*i.e.*, viral, bacterial, fungal, mycobacterial, parasitic), toxins, alcoholism, chemotherapeutic agents, metals, and multiple other disorders. Often, no cause is found, in which case the cardiomyopathy is often referred to as *idiopathic DCM*.

DCM is characterized by ventricular enlargement, a reduction in ventricular wall thickness, and impaired systolic function of one or both ventricles (Fig. 27.15). Histologically, DCM is characterized by atrophic and hypertrophic myocardial fibers and interstitial fibrosis. Cardiac myocytes, particularly those in the subendocardium, often show advanced degenerative changes. Interstitial fibrosis is present also, most prominently in the subendocardial zone. Scattered inflammatory cells may be present.

It can present in nearly any age. It is usually identified when clinical manifestations of DCM appear, such as dyspnea, orthopnea, and reduced exercise capacity. In the end stages, people with DCM often have ejection fractions of less than 25% (normal is approximately 50% to 60%).[29] As the disease progresses, stasis of blood in the walls of the heart chambers can lead to thrombus formation and systemic emboli. Secondary mitral valve regurgitation and abnormal cardiac rhythms are common. Death is usually due to heart failure or arrhythmias and can occur suddenly.

The treatment of DCM is directed toward relieving the symptoms of heart failure and reducing the work of the heart. Pharmacologic agents include diuretics to reduce preload, beta-blockers to reduce heart rate and myocardial oxygen demand, afterload-reducing agents to improve contractility and decrease left ventricular filling pressures, and ACE inhibitors to promote vasodilation. Anticoagulants to prevent thrombus formation and antiarrhythmics may also be used. Other

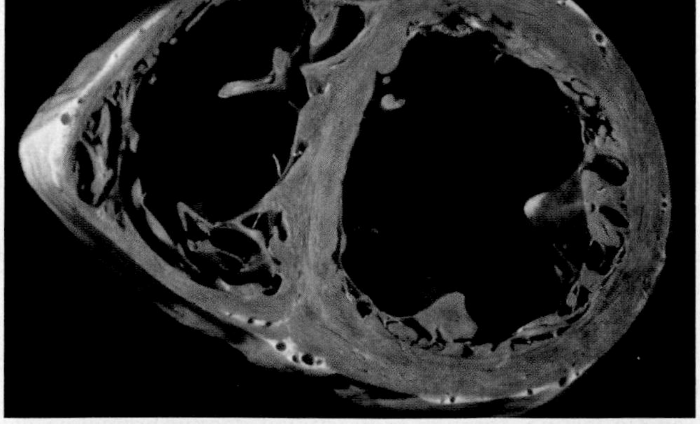

Figure 27.15 • Idiopathic DCM. A transverse section of the enlarged heart reveals conspicuous dilation of both ventricles. Although the ventricular wall appears thinned, the increased mass of the heart indicates considerable hypertrophy. (From Strayer D. E., Rubin R. (Eds.) (2015). *Rubin's pathology: Clinicopathologic foundations of medicine* (7th ed., Fig. 17-42, p. 665) Philadelphia, PA: Lippincott Williams & Wilkins.)

treatments may include a biventricular pacemaker, a biventricular ICD, and, in cases that are refractory to treatment, cardiac transplantation. Removing or avoiding causative agents (if identified); avoiding myocardial depressants, including alcohol; and encouraging activity as tolerated are also important.

Primary Restrictive Cardiomyopathy. Restrictive cardiomyopathy is a rare form of heart muscle disease in which ventricular filling is restricted because of excessive rigidity of the ventricular walls.[27] Restrictive cardiomyopathy can be idiopathic or associated with distinct diseases that affect the myocardium, principally radiation fibrosis, amyloidosis, sarcoidosis, or metastatic tumors. Genetics may also play a role because familial forms of restrictive cardiomyopathy have been reported.[27]

Symptoms of restrictive cardiomyopathy include dyspnea, paroxysmal nocturnal dyspnea, orthopnea, hepatomegaly, peripheral edema, ascites, fatigue, and weakness. The manifestations of restrictive cardiomyopathy resemble those of constrictive pericarditis. In the advanced form of the disease, all the signs of heart failure are present except cardiomegaly.

Acquired Cardiomyopathies

Myocarditis (Inflammatory Cardiomyopathy). Myocarditis is the inflammation of the myocardium, but its classification, diagnosis, and treatment are complex. Clinical findings can vary greatly, from nonspecific symptoms, such as fever, myalgias, or exertional dyspnea, to hemodynamic collapse and sudden death. The incidence and prevalence of myocarditis have been difficult to ascertain because of the wide variation in clinical presentation.

Although there are a number of etiologies associated with myocarditis, it is usually caused by a viral infection, most commonly an enterovirus (coxsackievirus group B).[30] Adenovirus and parvovirus in young children have also been identified as causative agents. Other etiologies include bacterial or fungal infections, hypersensitivity to certain drugs, and autoimmune diseases, such as systemic lupus erythematosus. Myocarditis is a frequent pathologic cardiac finding in persons with acquired immunodeficiency syndrome (AIDS), although it is unclear whether it is due to the human immunodeficiency virus infection itself or to a secondary infection.

Acute viral myocarditis appears to progress through three phases, the acute viral infection, autoimmune activation, and ongoing myocardial injury, resulting in DCM.[30] The three phases present with varying clinical manifestations and varying indications for treatment. Phases 1 and 2 produce inflammatory responses to the initial viral infection. However, activation of the immune system in response to virus-specific antigens can also elicit inflammatory responses by the host, independent of the initial viral infection, which can lead to tissue damage in the host organism. As leukocytes, lymphocytes, and macrophages penetrate the myocardium, interstitial edema and focal myocyte necrosis lead to replacement fibrosis.[30] It has been suggested that autoreactive T cells and host-generated cytokines, including tumor necrosis factor [TNF]-α, interleukin-1, and interleukin-6, may play prominent roles in the myocardial changes that occur with mycocarditis.[30] Some cases of myocarditis progress to phase 3, which is characterized by ongoing myocardial injury that ultimately results in acute or chronic DCM, severe left ventricular failure, or life-threatening arrhythmias.

The signs and symptoms of myocarditis vary from asymptomatic to cardiogenic shock. Some persons may present with a viral syndrome such as fever, chills, nausea, vomiting, arthralgia, and myalgia, occurring up to 6 weeks before the diagnosis of myocarditis. Other persons may present with heart failure without antecedent symptoms. The onset of heart failure may be gradual or abrupt and fulminant. Emboli may occur because of the procoagulant effect of cytokines combined with decreased myocardial contractility. At times, the presentation may mimic ACS, with ST-segment and T-wave changes, positive cardiac markers, and regional wall motion abnormalities despite normal coronary arteries. People may also present with AV block or complete heart block. Viral myocarditis in children or young adults is often nonspecific, with symptoms such as fever and poor eating.

No clinical practice guidelines exist, and although standardized diagnostic guidelines have been proposed (*i.e.*, Dallas criteria), these criteria separate initial biopsies into no myocarditis, borderline myocarditis, and myocarditis. There have been several factors suggesting they are no longer adequate.

Endomyocardial biopsy findings, obtained through cardiac catheterization, remain the gold standard for establishing the diagnosis of acute myocarditis, despite limited accuracy.[30,31] Other diagnostic methods include the use of serum cardiac biomarkers (*i.e.*, CK, TnI, TnT) and immunohistochemical staining. Echocardiography is usually performed in the initial evaluation of suspected myocarditis, although the findings can be nonspecific. Other myocardial imaging techniques that are being evaluated include nuclear imaging with gallium- or indium-labeled antimyosin antibodies and cardiac MRI.

Many cases of myocarditis can be mild and self-limiting, so first-line treatment remains largely supportive.[30,31] Initial treatments include supplemental oxygen, bed rest, and antibiotics, if needed. In persons with more severe myocarditis, hemodynamic support with vasopressors and positive inotropic agents may be needed. ACE inhibitors, beta-blockers, and spironolactone (an aldosterone antagonist) may be used to prevent further clinical deterioration in people with DCM due to myocarditis.[31] An ICD should be considered for those with documented life-threatening arrhythmias. Biventricular involvement usually indicates poorer prognosis. Immunosuppressive therapy continues to be investigated as a treatment for myocarditis, but routine use is not supported.

Peripartum Cardiomyopathy. Peripartum cardiomyopathy is a rare heart muscle disorder that occurs during the last trimester of pregnancy or the first 5 to 6 months after delivery. The disorder is relatively rare in the United States, but in some regions of Africa, it is encountered in as much as 1% of pregnant women. The incidence is greater in African American, multiparous, or older women and in women with twin fetuses, with preeclampsia, or who use tocolytic therapy to prevent premature labor and delivery.[32]

Although the etiology of peripartum cardiomyopathy is unknown, several causes have been proposed, including infectious, immunologic, nutritional, drug-induced, and genetic factors. Some women exhibit inflammatory cells in heart biopsies taken during the symptomatic phase of the disorder, suggesting a disordered immune response. It presents just as LV systolic dysfunction such as shortness of breath at rest and/or exertional, palpitations, edema, and orthopnea.

Diagnosis of peripartum cardiomyopathy can be challenging because symptoms that can occur normally in late pregnancy are similar to the early signs of heart failure. A joint workshop of the National Heart, Lung, and Blood Institute and the Office of Rare Diseases of the National Institutes of Health, in 1997, identified four criteria for the definition of peripartum cardiomyopathy:

1. Heart failure in the last month of pregnancy or within 5 months after delivery.
2. No identifiable cause of heart failure.
3. No identifiable cause of heart failure before the last month of pregnancy.
4. Evidence of systolic dysfunction.[32]
5. Management of peripartum cardiomyopathy includes standard therapy for heart failure.

However, potential teratogenic effects and excretion of drugs during breast-feeding need to be considered. The aim of therapy is to reduce fluid and salt intake, reduce preload and afterload, increase myocardial contractility, and try to prevent complications such as mortality. Prognosis depends on resolution of the heart failure. About half of women with peripartum cardiomyopathy spontaneously recover normal cardiac function; the other half are left with persistent left ventricular dysfunction or progress to overt heart failure and early death.[32]

Stress or Takotsubo ("Broken Heart Syndrome") Cardiomyopathy. Stress cardiomyopathy was first described in Japan, where most cases have occurred, although cases have increased in the United States.[33] In Japan, it was called *takotsubo* after the fishing pot with a narrow neck and wide base used to trap octopus. The term *transient left ventricular apical ballooning* has also been used to describe this syndrome.

Stress or takotsubo cardiomyopathy has been identified in the clinical setting as a transient, reversible left ventricular dysfunction in response to profound psychological or emotional stress. The syndrome occurs primarily in middle-aged women who present with acute STEMI but who, on cardiac catheterization, have no evidence of CAD. There is, however, impaired myocardial contractility characterized by apical ballooning of the LV with hypercontractility of the basal LV.[33]

The mechanism for myocardial stunning in stress cardiomyopathy is unclear, although some theories suggest ischemia from coronary artery spasm, microvascular spasm, hormonal predisposition, or direct myocyte injury. When catecholamine levels return to normal, the interventricular gradient resolves and left ventricular function recovers.[33] Treatment is the same as that for heart failure, including short-term use of anticoagulants; most people demonstrate rapid improvement and an excellent prognosis.

Secondary Cardiomyopathies

Secondary cardiomyopathy is a heart muscle disease in the presence of a multisystem disorder (Chart 27.2). There are numerous conditions reported to involve the myocardium. Some of these disorders produce accumulation of abnormal substances between myocytes (extracellular), whereas others produce accumulation of abnormal substances within myocytes (intracellular).

CHART 27.2 CONDITIONS ASSOCIATED WITH SECONDARY CARDIOMYOPATHIES*

Autoimmune Disorders
Systemic lupus erythematosus
Rheumatoid arthritis
Scleroderma
Polyarteritis nodosa

Endocrine Disorders
Acromegaly
Diabetes mellitus
Hypothyroidism and hyperthyroidism
Hyperparathyroidism

Familial Storage Diseases
Glycogen storage disease
Mucopolysaccharidoses
Hemochromatosis

Infiltrative Disorders
Amyloidosis
Sarcoidosis
Radiation-induced fibrosis

Neuromuscular/Neurologic Disorders
Friedreich ataxia
Muscular dystrophy
Neurofibromatosis

Nutritional Deficiencies
Thiamine (beriberi)
Protein (kwashiorkor)

Toxins
Alcohol and its metabolites
Arsenic
Cancer chemotherapeutic agents (anthracyclines [doxorubicin, daunorubicin], cyclophosphamide)
Catecholamines
Hydrocarbons

*Not intended to be inclusive.

Almost 100 distinct myocardial diseases can result in the clinical features of DCM. They include cardiomyopathies associated with drugs, diabetes mellitus, muscular dystrophy, autoimmune disorders, and cancer treatment agents (radiation and cancer drugs). Alcoholic cardiomyopathy is the single most common identifiable cause of DCM in the United States and Europe. Doxorubicin (Adriamycin) and other anthracycline drugs, used in the treatment of cancer, are potent agents whose usefulness is limited by cumulative dose-dependent cardiac toxicity. Another cancer chemotherapeutic agent with cardiotoxic potential is cyclophosphamide (Cytoxan). Unlike the primary myocyte injury that occurs with doxorubicin, the principal insult with cyclophosphamide appears to be vascular, leading to myocardial hemorrhage.

IN SUMMARY

The cardiomyopathies involve both mechanical and electrical etiologies of myocardial dysfunction. They are currently identified as either primary or secondary cardiomyopathies, based on genetic or other organ system involvement. Symptoms related to most cardiomyopathies, whether primary or secondary, are those associated with heart failure and SCD. Treatments are related to symptom management and prevention of lethal arrhythmias.

The primary cardiomyopathies include genetic, mixed, or acquired types. The genetic cardiomyopathies include HCM, ARVC, left ventricular noncompaction cardiomyopathy, inherited conduction system disorders, and ion channelopathies. The mixed cardiomyopathies, which include DCM, are of both genetic and acquired origin. Acquired cardiomyopathies include those that have their origin in the inflammatory process (*e.g.*, myocarditis), stress (takotsubo), or pregnancy (peripartum cardiomyopathy). In many cases, the cause is unknown, in which case the cardiomyopathy is referred to as *idiopathic*.

The secondary cardiomyopathies are heart diseases in which myocardial involvement occurs as part of a generalized systemic (multiorgan) disorder. They include cardiomyopathies associated with drugs, diabetes mellitus, muscular dystrophy, autoimmune disorders, and cancer treatment agents (radiation and chemotherapeutic drugs).

INFECTIOUS AND IMMUNOLOGIC DISORDERS

After completing this section of the chapter, the learner will be able to meet the following objectives:

- Distinguish between the roles of infectious organisms in infective endocarditis (IE) and rheumatic fever (RF).
- Describe the relation between the infective vegetations associated with IE and the extracardiac manifestations of the disease.
- Describe the long-term effects of RF and outline primary and secondary prevention strategies for RF and rheumatic heart disease.

Infective Endocarditis

IE is a serious and potentially life-threatening infection of the inner surface of the heart. It is characterized by colonization or invasion of the heart valves and the mural endocardium by a microbial agent, leading to the formation of bulky, friable vegetations and destruction of underlying cardiac tissues.[34]

The incidence, demographics, and characteristics of IE have changed over the past decade. The classic picture of a person with preexisting RHD and community-associated bacteremia no longer represents the majority of cases of IE. More common causes now are mitral valve prolapse, congenital heart disease, prosthetic heart valves, and implantable devices such as pacemakers and defibrillators.[34,35] Host factors such as neutropenia, immunodeficiency, malignancy, therapeutic immunosuppression, diabetes, and alcohol or intravenous drug use are predisposing factors. Infections of these intracardiac, arterial, and venous devices are nosocomially acquired in medical centers throughout the developed world.[34]

Traditionally, IE has been classified on clinical grounds into acute or subacute–chronic forms, depending on the onset, etiology, and severity of the disease. Usually, the onset of acute cases is rapid and involves people with normal cardiac valves who are either healthy and perhaps have a history of intravenous drug use or are debilitated. Subacute–chronic cases evolve over months; these people usually have valve abnormalities. The development of drug-resistant strains of microorganisms due to the indiscriminate use of antibiotics and an increase in the number of immunocompromised persons has made classification of acute and subacute–chronic cases more difficult.[35]

Etiology and Pathogenesis

Staphylococcal infections have now emerged as the leading cause of IE, with streptococci and enterococci as the other two most common causes. Other causative agents include the so-called HACEK group (*Haemophilus* species, *Actinobacillus actinomycetemcomitans*, *Cardiobacterium hominis*, *Eikenella corrodens*, and *Kingella kingae*), gram-negative bacilli, and fungi.[35] The causative agents differ somewhat in the major high-risk groups. For example, *Staphylococcus aureus* is the major offender in intravenous drug abusers, whereas prosthetic heart valve IE tends to be caused by coagulase-negative staphylococci (*e.g.*, *Staphylococcus epidermidis*). Also, *S. epidermidis* has been associated with implantable devices and health care–associated infections.[35] Foremost among the factors leading to the development of IE is seeding of the blood with microbes. The portal of entry into the bloodstream may be an obvious infection, a dental or surgical procedure that causes transient bacteremia, injection of a contaminated substance directly into the blood by intravenous drug users, or an occult source in the oral cavity or gut. Endothelial injury, bacteremia, and altered hemodynamics can all incite the formation of a fibrin–platelet thrombus along the endothelial lining. The thrombus is susceptible to bacterial seeding from transient bacteremia, causing continued monocyte activation and cytokine and tissue factor production. This results in progressive enlargement of infected valvular vegetations.

In both acute and subacute–chronic forms of IE, friable, bulky, and potentially destructive vegetative lesions form on the heart valves (Fig. 27.16). The aortic and mitral valves are the most common sites of infection, although the right heart may also be involved, particularly in intravenous drug abusers. These vegetative lesions consist of a collection of infectious organisms and cellular debris enmeshed in the fibrin strands of clotted blood. The lesions may be singular or multiple, may grow as large as several centimeters, and usually are found loosely attached to the free edges of the valve surface.[35] The infectious loci continuously release bacteria into the bloodstream and are a source of persistent bacteremia. As the lesions grow, they cause valve destruction, leading to valvular regurgitation, ring abscesses with heart block, pericarditis, aneurysm, and valve perforation.

The intracardiac vegetative lesions also have local and distant systemic effects.[35] The loose organization of these lesions permits the organisms and fragments of the lesions to form emboli and travel in the bloodstream, causing cerebral, systemic, or pulmonary emboli. The fragments may lodge in small blood vessels, causing small hemorrhages, abscesses, and infarction of tissue. The bacteremia also can initiate immune responses thought to be responsible for skin manifestations, polyarthritis, glomerulonephritis, and other immune disorders.

Clinical Manifestations

The incubation period for onset of symptoms is approximately 2 weeks or less in greater than 80% of people. However, if the infection is *Candida* related, the incubation period can be up to 5 months. Initial symptoms of IE can include fever

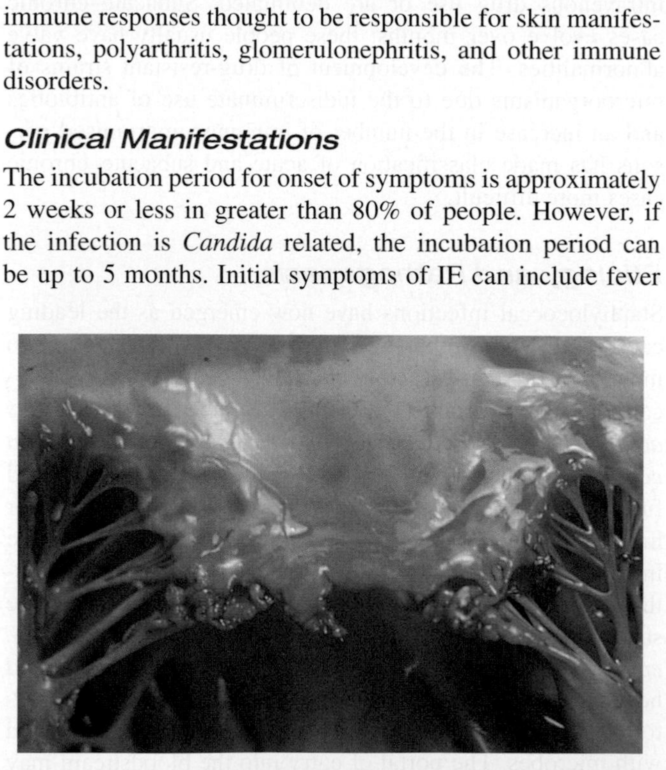

Figure 27.16 • Bacterial endocarditis. The mitral valve shows destructive vegetations, which have eroded through the free margin of the valve leaflet. (From Strayer D. E., Rubin R. (Eds.) (2015). *Rubin's pathology: Clinicopathologic foundations of medicine* (7th ed., Fig. 17-34, p. 657) Philadelphia, PA: Lippincott Williams & Wilkins.)

and signs of systemic infection, change in the character of an existing heart murmur, and evidence of embolic distribution of the vegetative lesions.[35] In the acute form, the fever usually is spiking and accompanied by chills. In the subacute form, the fever usually is low grade, of gradual onset, and frequently accompanied by other systemic signs of inflammation, such as spleen enlargement, anorexia, malaise, and lethargy. Small petechial hemorrhages frequently result when emboli lodge in the small vessels of the skin, nail beds, and mucous membranes. Splinter hemorrhages (*i.e.*, dark red lines) under the nails of the fingers and toes are common.[35] Cough, dyspnea, arthralgia or arthritis, diarrhea, and abdominal or flank pain may occur as the result of systemic emboli. Congestive heart failure can develop from valve destruction, coronary artery embolism, or myocarditis. Renal insufficiency can also develop from destruction or antimicrobial toxicities.

Diagnosis

IE continues to pose major challenges in diagnosis and treatment, despite advances in its epidemiology and microbiology. The diagnosis of IE cannot be made through any single test but rather includes the use of clinical, laboratory, and echocardiographic features.[35] The Duke criteria, which were modified by a committee of the AHA in 2005, provide health care professionals with a standardized assessment of persons with suspected IE that integrates blood culture evidence of infection, echocardiographic findings, clinical symptoms and signs, and laboratory information.[35] The modified Duke criteria are classified into major criteria (positive blood culture for IE, evidence of endocardial involvement) and minor criteria (predisposition to IE, predisposing heart condition, or intravenous drug use; fever with a temperature greater than 38 °C; vascular phenomenon such as evidence of arterial emboli; immunologic phenomenon such as glomerulonephritis; microbiologic evidence such as blood culture that does not meet major criteria). Cases are classified as "definite" if they fulfill two major criteria, one major criterion plus two minor criteria, or five minor criteria. Cases are defined as "possible" if they fulfill one major criterion and one minor criterion or three minor criteria. Diagnosis of IE is rejected if an alternative diagnosis is made, the infection resolves with antibiotic treatment for 4 days or less, or there is no histologic evidence of infection.[34]

The blood culture remains the most definitive diagnostic procedure and is essential to guide treatment. Three separate sets of blood cultures from three separate venipuncture sites should be obtained within 24 hours. However, the indiscriminate use of antibiotics has made identifying the causative organism much more difficult. The modified Duke criteria recommend the inclusion of *S. aureus* as a major criterion, whether it is a nosocomial or a community-acquired infection as well as *viridans streptococci*, *Streptococci bovis*, and HACEK groups. A single positive blood culture for *Coxiella burnetii* and an anti–phase I IgG antibody titer greater than 1:800 are also considered major criteria. Negative blood cultures can delay diagnosis and treatment and have a profound effect on outcome.[35] This can occur because of prior antibiotic administration or because the causative organisms are slow growing, require special culture media, or are not readily cultured.

Echocardiography is the primary technique for detection of vegetations and cardiac complications resulting from IE and is an important tool in the diagnosis and management of disease. The ACC/AHA recommends echocardiography in all people who are suspected of having IE. Echocardiographic evidence of endocardial involvement is now the major criterion in the modified Duke criteria. It is recommended that transthoracic echocardiography be used in low initial risk or low clinical suspicion and transesophageal echocardiography be used in moderate to high clinical suspicion. High-suspicion individuals include prosthetic valves, prior IE, complex congenital disease, heart failure, or new-onset heart murmur.[34]

Treatment

Treatment of IE focuses on identifying and eliminating the causative microorganism, minimizing the residual cardiac effects, and treating the pathologic effect of emboli. The choice of antimicrobial therapy depends on the organism cultured and whether it occurs in a native or prosthetic valve. *S. aureus*, the most common cause of IE, is primarily the result of nosocomial infections from intravascular catheters, surgical wounds, and indwelling prosthetic devices. Guidelines for the prevention and management of nonvalvular cardiovascular device–related infections are presented in the literature.[34,35] The widespread emergence of multidrug-resistant organisms, including *S. aureus*, poses a serious challenge in the treatment of IE. In addition to antibiotic therapy, surgery may be needed for unresolved infection, severe heart failure, and significant emboli.

The majority of people with IE are cured with medical or surgical treatment. People who have had infectious endocarditis should be educated about its signs and symptoms and informed of the possibility of relapse or recurrence. Immediate medical attention should be sought if signs or symptoms recur. Prevention of IE through the use of prophylactic antibiotics is controversial. The current recommendations conclude that only a very small number of IE cases might be prevented by antibiotic prophylaxis for dental procedures. Therefore, prophylaxis is recommended only for people with previous IE, congenital heart disease (such as unrepaired cyanotic coronary heart disease repaired with prosthetic material or with residual defects), prosthetic cardiac valve, and cardiac transplantation who develop cardiac valvulopathy. It is not recommended based solely on an increased lifetime risk of acquiring IE.[34,35]

Rheumatic Heart Disease

RF and rheumatic heart disease (RHD) are complications of the immune-mediated response to group A (beta-hemolytic) streptococcal (GAS) throat infection.[36] The most serious aspect of RF is the development of chronic valvular disorders that produce permanent cardiac dysfunction and sometimes cause fatal heart failure years later. Although RF and RHD are rare in developed countries, they continue to be major health problems in underdeveloped countries, where inadequate health care, poor nutrition, and crowded living conditions still prevail.[36,37]

Pathogenesis

Beta-hemolytic streptococci are divided into several serologic groups based on their cell wall polysaccharide antigen. Group A is further subdivided into more than 130 distinct M types, which are responsible for the vast majority of infections. The M protein best defines the virulence of the bacterium and has been studied most intensively with regard to cross-reactivity with heart tissue.[37] Although GAS causes both pharyngitis and skin (impetigo) infections, only the pharyngitis has been linked with RF and RHD.

The pathogenesis of RF still remains unclear. The time frame for development of symptoms in relation to the sore throat and the presence of antibodies to GAS strongly suggests an immunologic origin.[36,37] It is thought that antibodies directed against the M protein of certain strains of streptococci cross-react with glycoprotein antigens in the heart, joints, and other tissues to produce an autoimmune response through a phenomenon called *molecular mimicry*. The onset of symptoms 2 to 3 weeks after infection and the absence of streptococci in the lesion support this belief. Although only a small percentage of persons with untreated GAS pharyngitis develop RF, the incidence of recurrence with a subsequent untreated infection is substantially greater. These observations and more recent studies suggest a genetic predisposition to the development of the disease. Also, environmental elements can affect the development of RF. It has been found that people who live in overcrowded areas, such as military barracks, have a higher incidence of RF due to the high virulence with rapid transmission.[37]

Clinical Manifestations

RF can manifest as an acute, recurrent, or chronic disorder. The *acute stage* of RF includes a history of an initiating streptococcal infection and subsequent involvement of the connective tissue elements of the heart, blood vessels, joints, and subcutaneous tissues. Common to all is a lesion called the *Aschoff body*,[36,37] which is a localized area of tissue necrosis surrounded by immune cells. The *recurrent phase* usually involves extension of the cardiac effects of the disease. The *chronic phase* of RF is characterized by permanent deformity of the heart valves and is a common cause of mitral valve stenosis. Chronic RHD usually does not appear until at least 10 years after the initial attack, sometimes decades later.

Most people with RF have a history of sore throat, headache, fever (101°F to 104°F), abdominal pain, nausea, vomiting, swollen glands (usually at the angle of the jaw), and other signs and symptoms of streptococcal infection. Other clinical manifestations associated with an acute episode of RF are related to the acute inflammatory process and the structures involved in the disease process. The course of the disease is characterized by a constellation of findings that includes migratory polyarthritis of the large joints, carditis, erythema marginatum, subcutaneous nodules, and Sydenham chorea.[36,37] Laboratory markers of acute inflammation include an elevated white blood cell count, ESR, and CRP. These elevated levels of acute-phase reactants are not specific for RF but provide evidence of an acute inflammatory response.

Polyarthritis. Polyarthritis is the most common and frequently the first manifestation of RF in 75% of cases. It may be the only major criterion in adolescents and adults. The arthritis, which may range from arthralgia to disabling arthritis, most often involves the larger joints, particularly the knees and ankles, and occurs less frequently in the wrists, elbows, shoulders, and hips. It is almost always migratory, affecting one joint and then moving to another. Untreated, the arthritis lasts approximately 4 weeks. A striking feature of rheumatic arthritis is the dramatic response (usually within 48 hours) to salicylates. Arthritis usually heals completely and leaves no functional residua.

Carditis. Acute rheumatic carditis, which complicates the acute phase of RF, can affect the endocardium, myocardium, or pericardium. The involvement of the endocardium and valvular structures produces the permanent and disabling effects of RF. Carditis mostly manifests itself as mitral regurgitation and less commonly aortic regurgitation although all four valves can be involved. During the acute inflammatory stage of the disease, the valvular structures become red and swollen, and small vegetative lesions develop on the valve leaflets. The acute inflammatory changes gradually proceed to development of fibrous scar tissue, which tends to contract and cause deformity of the valve leaflets and shortening of the chordae tendineae. In some cases, the edges or commissures of the valve leaflets fuse together as healing occurs.

Clinical features of endocarditis/valvulitis, without a history of RHD, include the presence of an apical holosystolic murmur of mitral regurgitation or a basal early diastolic murmur of aortic regurgitation. In someone with a history of RHD, a change in the character of these murmurs or a new murmur would indicate acute rheumatic carditis.

Subcutaneous Nodules, Erythema Marginatum, and Sydenham Chorea. *Subcutaneous nodules* are hard, painless, and freely movable and usually occur over the extensor muscles of the wrist, elbow, ankle, and knee joints, ranging in size from 0.5 to 2 cm. Subcutaneous nodules rarely occur alone in RF and occur most often in association with moderate to severe carditis.

Erythema marginatum lesions are maplike, macular areas most commonly seen on the trunk or inner aspects of the upper arm and thigh but never on the face. They occur early in the course of a rheumatic attack and tend to occur with subcutaneous nodules as well as carditis. They are transitory and disappear during the course of the disease.

Sydenham chorea is the major central nervous system manifestation of RF. It is seen most frequently in young girls and rarely occurs after 20 years of age. There typically is an insidious onset of irritability and other behavior problems. The child often is fidgety, cries easily, begins to walk clumsily, and drops things. The choreiform movements are spontaneous, rapid, purposeless jerking movements that interfere with voluntary activities. Facial grimaces are common, and even speech may be affected. The chorea is self-limited, usually running its course within a matter of weeks or months, but recurrences are not uncommon. A previous streptococcal infection can be detected only in about two thirds of cases, making differential diagnosis more difficult.

Diagnosis

There are no specific laboratory tests that can establish a diagnosis of RF. Because of the variety of signs and symptoms, the Jones criteria for the diagnosis of RF, which were first proposed in 1944 and have undergone multiple reviews by the AHA and the World Health Organization (WHO), are designed to assist in standardizing the diagnosis of RF.[36,37] The Jones criteria divide the clinical features of RF into major and minor categories, based on prevalence and specificity. The presence of two major signs (*i.e.*, carditis, polyarthritis, chorea, erythema marginatum, and subcutaneous nodules) or one major and two minor signs (*i.e.*, arthralgia, fever, and elevated ESR, CRP, or leukocyte count), accompanied by evidence of a preceding GAS infection, indicates a high probability of RF.

The use of echocardiography has enhanced the understanding of both acute and chronic RHD. It is useful in assessing the severity of valvular stenosis and regurgitation, the chamber size and ventricular function, and the presence and size of pleural effusions. Doppler ultrasonography may be useful in identifying cardiac lesions in persons who do not show typical signs of cardiac involvement during an attack of RF but is not considered either a major or minor Jones criterion at this time.

Treatment and Prevention

It is important that streptococcal infections be promptly diagnosed and treated to prevent RF. The gold standard for detecting a streptococcal infection is throat culture. However, it takes 24 to 48 hours to produce a result, delaying treatment. The development of rapid tests for direct detection of GAS antigens has provided at least a partial solution for this problem. Both the throat culture and the rapid antigen tests are highly specific for GAS infection but are limited in terms of their sensitivity (*e.g.*, the person may have a negative test result but have a streptococcal infection). A negative antigen test result should be confirmed with a throat culture when a streptococcal infection is suspected.[36] The presence of GAS in the upper respiratory tract can indicate either a carrier or infectious state, the latter of which can be defined by a rising antibody response. Serologic examinations for streptococcal antibodies (antistreptolysin O and antideoxyribonuclease B) are measured for retrospective confirmation of recent streptococcal infections in persons thought to have acute RF. There is, however, no single specific laboratory test result that is pathognomonic for acute or recurrent RF.

Treatment of acute RF is designed to control the acute inflammatory response and prevent cardiac complications and recurrence of the disease. During the acute phase, antibiotics, anti-inflammatory drugs, and selective restriction of activities are prescribed. No clinical isolate of GAS is resistant to penicillin; therefore, penicillin, or erythromycin (or a newer macrolide antibiotic) in penicillin-allergic people, is the treatment of choice for GAS infection.[36] Narrow-spectrum cephalosporins have also been given successfully but should be avoided in people who have a history of anaphylaxis to penicillin. Salicylates and corticosteroids can be used to suppress the inflammatory response but should not be given until the diagnosis of RF is confirmed. Surgery is indicated for chronic rheumatic valve disease and is determined by the severity of the symptom or the evidence that cardiac function is significantly impaired. Procedures used include closed mitral commissurotomy, valve repair, and valve replacement.

The person who has had an attack of RF is at high risk for recurrence after subsequent GAS throat infections. Penicillin is still the treatment of choice for secondary prophylaxis, with erythromycin used in penicillin-allergic individuals. The duration of prophylaxis depends on whether residual valvular disease is present or absent. Compliance with a plan for prophylactic administration of penicillin requires that the person and his or her family understand the morbidity associated with such recurrent infections. People are also urged to promptly report streptococcal infections to their physicians for adequate treatment and to their dentists for adequate protection during dental procedures that may traumatize the oral mucosa.

IN SUMMARY

IE involves the invasion of the endocardium by pathogens that produce vegetative lesions on the endocardial surface. The loose organization of these lesions permits the organisms and fragments of the lesions to be disseminated throughout the systemic circulation. Although several organisms can cause the condition, staphylococci have now become the leading cause of IE. Treatment of IE focuses on identifying and eliminating the causative microorganism, minimizing the residual cardiac effects, and treating the pathologic effect of emboli.

RF, which is associated with an antecedent GAS throat infection, is an important cause of heart disease. Its most serious and disabling effects result from involvement of the heart valves. Because there is no single laboratory test result, sign, or symptom that is pathognomonic for acute RF, the Jones criteria are used to establish the diagnosis during the acute stage of the disease. Primary and secondary prevention strategies focus on appropriate antibiotic therapy.

VALVULAR HEART DISEASE

After completing this section of the chapter, the learner will be able to meet the following objectives:

- State the function of the heart valves and relate alterations in hemodynamic function of the heart that occur with valvular disease.
- Compare the effects of stenotic and regurgitant mitral and aortic valvular heart disease on cardiovascular function.

The past several decades have brought remarkable advances in the treatment and outlook for people with valvular heart disease. This is undoubtedly due to improved methods for noninvasive monitoring of ventricular function, improvement in prosthetic valves, advances in valve reconstruction procedures, and the development of useful guidelines to improve the timing of surgical interventions.[26] However, valvular heart disease continues to produce considerable morbidity and mortality.

Hemodynamic Derangements

The function of the heart valves is to promote unidirectional flow of blood through the chambers of the heart. Dysfunction of the heart valves can result from a number of disorders, including congenital defects, trauma, ischemic damage, degenerative changes, and inflammation. Although any of the four heart valves can become diseased, the most commonly affected are the mitral and aortic valves. Disorders of the pulmonary and tricuspid valves are not as common, because of the low pressure in the right side of the heart.

The heart valves consist of thin leaflets of tough, flexible, endothelium-covered fibrous tissue firmly attached at the base to the fibrous valve rings. Capillaries and smooth muscle are present at the base of the leaflet but do not extend up into the valve. The leaflets of the heart valves may be injured or become the site of an inflammatory process that can deform their line of closure. Healing of the valve leaflets often is associated with increased collagen content and scarring, causing the leaflets to shorten and become stiffer. The edges of the healing valve leaflets can fuse together so that the valve does not open or close properly.

Two types of mechanical disruptions occur with valvular heart disease: narrowing of the valve opening so it does not open properly and distortion of the valve so it does not close properly (Fig. 27.17). *Stenosis* refers to a narrowing of the valve orifice and failure of the valve leaflets to open normally. Blood flow through a normal valve can increase by five to seven times the resting volume; consequently, valvular stenosis must be severe before it causes problems. Significant narrowing of the valve orifice increases the resistance to blood flow through the valve, converting the normally smooth laminar flow to a less efficient turbulent flow.

This increases the volume and work of the chamber emptying through the narrowed valve—the left atrium in the case

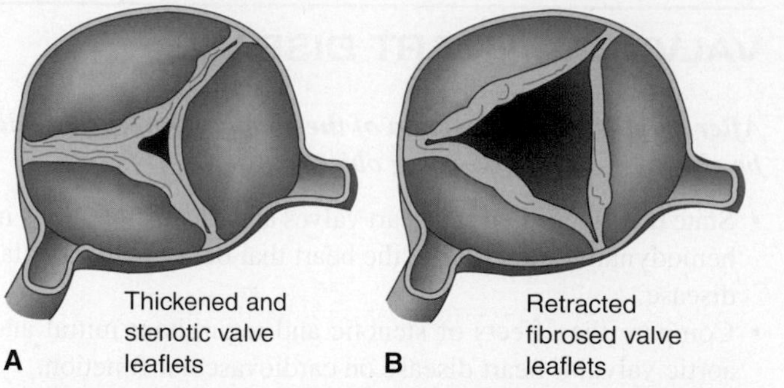

Figure 27.17 • Disease of the aortic valve as viewed from the aorta. **(A)** Stenosis of the valve opening. **(B)** An incompetent or regurgitant valve that is unable to close completely.

of mitral stenosis and the LV in aortic stenosis. Symptoms usually are noticed first during situations of increased flow, such as exercise. An incompetent or regurgitant valve permits backward flow to occur when the valve should be closed—flowing back into the LV during diastole when the aortic valve is affected and back into the left atrium during systole when the mitral valve is diseased.

The effects of valvular heart disease on cardiac function are related to alterations in blood flow across the valve and to the resultant increase in work demands on the hearts. Many valvular heart defects are characterized by heart murmurs resulting from turbulent blood flow through a diseased valve.

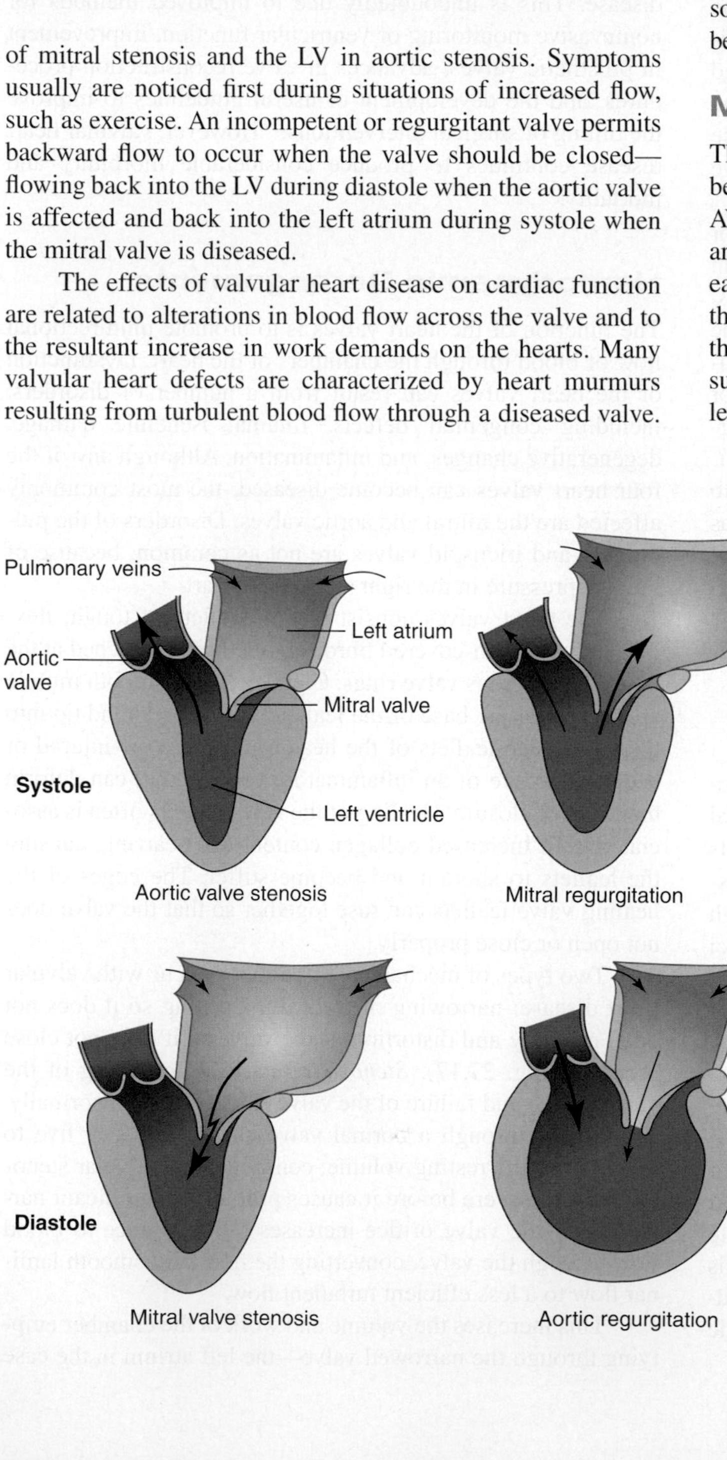

Figure 27.18 • Alterations in hemodynamic function that accompany aortic valve stenosis, mitral valve regurgitation, mitral valve stenosis, and aortic valve regurgitation. The *thin arrows* indicate direction of normal flow and *thick arrows* the direction of abnormal flow.

Disorders in valve flow and heart chamber size for mitral and aortic valve disorders are illustrated in Figure 27.18.

Echocardiography, described earlier in the chapter, provides a means of visualizing valvular motion and valvular closing patterns as well as blood flow. Pulsed Doppler ultrasonography provides a semiquantitative or qualitative estimation of the severity of transvalvular gradients, right ventricular systolic pressure, and valvular regurgitation. Color flow Doppler provides a visual pattern of flow velocities over the anatomic 2-D or 3-D echocardiographic image. This allows for demonstration of turbulence from stenotic and regurgitant valves.

Transesophageal echocardiography with Doppler ultrasonography is used to obtain echocardiographic data when surface sound transmission is poor. It provides clearer images and allows better visualization of the AV valves and prosthetic heart valves.

Mitral Valve Disorders

The mitral valve controls the directional flow of blood between the left atrium and the LV. The edges or cusps of the AV valves are thinner than those of the semilunar valves; they are anchored to the papillary muscles by the chordae tendineae. During much of systole, the mitral valve is subjected to the high pressure generated by the LV as it pumps blood into the systemic circulation. During this period of increased pressure, the chordae tendineae prevent the eversion of the valve leaflets into the left atrium.

KEY POINTS

VALVULAR HEART DISEASE

- The heart valves determine the direction of blood flow through the heart chambers.
- Valvular heart defects exert their effects by obstructing flow of blood (stenotic valve disorders) or allowing backward flow of blood (regurgitant valve disorders).

Mitral Valve Stenosis

Mitral valve stenosis represents the incomplete opening of the mitral valve during diastole, with left atrial distention and impaired filling of the LV. Mitral valve stenosis most commonly is the result of RF.[26,38] Less frequently, the defect is congenital and manifests during infancy or early childhood or in older adults related to annular calcification. Mitral valve stenosis is a continuous, progressive, lifelong disorder consisting of a slow, stable course in the early years and progressive acceleration in later years.

Pathogenesis. Mitral valve stenosis is characterized by fibrous replacement of valvular tissue, along with stiffness and fusion of the valve apparatus (Fig. 27.18). Typically, the mitral cusps fuse at the edges and involvement of the chordae tendineae causes shortening, which pulls the valvular structures more deeply into the ventricles. As the resistance to flow through the valve increases, the left atrium becomes dilated and left atrial pressure rises.[38] The increased left atrial pressure eventually is transmitted to the pulmonary venous system, causing pulmonary congestion.

The rate of flow across the valve depends on the size of the valve orifice, the driving pressure (*i.e.*, atrial minus ventricular pressure), and the time available for flow during diastole. The normal mitral valve area is 4 to 5 cm^2. Symptoms develop as the gradient across the valve becomes worse so that the left atrial pressure is greater than the left ventricular pressure. As the condition progresses, symptoms of decreased cardiac output occur during extreme exertion or other situations that cause tachycardia and thereby reduce diastolic filling time. In the late stages of the disease, pulmonary vascular resistance increases with the development of pulmonary hypertension; this increases the pressure against which the right heart must pump and eventually leads to right-sided heart failure.

Clinical Manifestations. The signs and symptoms of mitral valve stenosis depend on the severity of the obstruction and are related to the elevation in left atrial pressure and pulmonary congestion, decreased cardiac output owing to impaired left ventricular filling, and left atrial enlargement with development of atrial arrhythmias and mural thrombi. The symptoms are those of heart failure development including pulmonary congestion, nocturnal paroxysmal dyspnea, and orthopnea. Palpitations, chest pain, weakness, and fatigue are common complaints.

Premature atrial beats, paroxysmal atrial tachycardia, and atrial fibrillation may occur as a result of distention of the left atrium. Fibrosis of the internodal and interatrial tracts, along with damage to the SA node, may occur from the rheumatic process itself. Atrial fibrillation develops in 30% to 40% of people with symptomatic mitral stenosis.[38] Together, the fibrillation and distention predispose to mural thrombus formation. The risk of arterial embolization, particularly stroke, is significantly increased in people with atrial fibrillation.

Diagnosis. The murmur of mitral valve stenosis is heard during diastole when blood is flowing through the constricted valve orifice; it is characteristically a low-pitched, rumbling murmur, best heard at the apex of the heart. The first heart sound often is accentuated and delayed because of the increased left atrial pressure; an opening snap may precede the diastolic murmur as a result of the elevation in left atrial pressure. The 2-D and Doppler echocardiograms are most commonly used to diagnose mitral stenosis. These echocardiograms confirm the diagnosis of mitral stenosis, evaluate mitral valve morphology and hemodynamics, and measure pulmonary artery pressures. They also rule out other causes of mitral stenosis and assist in identifying the most appropriate treatment.

Treatment. Medical treatment of mitral valve stenosis is aimed at relieving signs of decreased cardiac output and pulmonary congestion. Loop diuretics are initiated to relieve some of the congestion. In atrial fibrillation, the goals are to control ventricular rate and prevent systemic embolization with anticoagulation therapy. Antibiotic prophylaxis against recurrent RF is recommended. Surgical interventions, including balloon valvotomy, commissurotomy, and valve repair or replacement, may be used to treat degenerative and functional mitral valve disease.[38,39] Balloon mitral valvotomy has been shown to be superior to closed and open commissurotomy. Although some countries continue to practice closed commissurotomy, most centers choose to perform MVR if balloon mitral valvotomy fails. The type of valve replaced depends somewhat on person's preferences. If a mechanical prosthesis is used, lifetime anticoagulation is indicated.

Mitral Valve Regurgitation

Mitral valve regurgitation is characterized by incomplete closure of the mitral valve, with the left ventricular stroke volume being divided between the forward stroke volume that moves into the aorta and the regurgitant stroke volume that moves back into the left atrium during systole (Fig. 27.19).

Etiology and Pathogenesis. Mitral valve regurgitation can result from many processes. RHD is associated with a rigid and thickened valve that does not open or close completely. In addition to RHD, mitral regurgitation can result from rupture of the chordae tendineae or papillary muscles, papillary muscle dysfunction, or stretching of the valve structures due to dilation of the LV or valve orifice. Mitral valve prolapse is a common cause of mitral valve regurgitation.

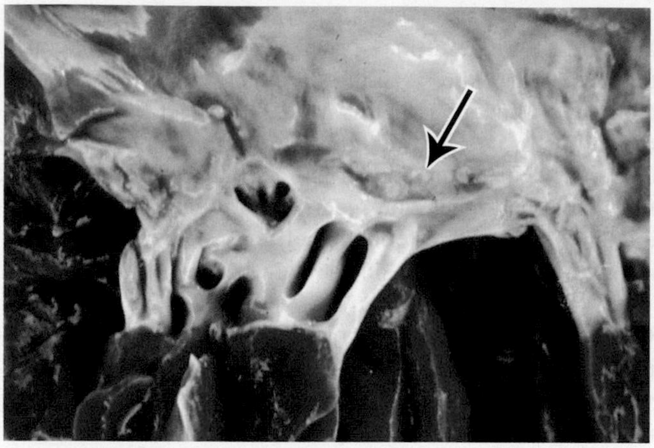

Figure 27.19 • Chronic rheumatic valvulitis. A view of the mitral valve from the left atrium shows rigid, thickened, and fused leaflets with a narrow orifice, creating the characteristic "fish-mouth" (*arrow*) appearance of rheumatic mitral stenosis. (From Strayer D. E., Rubin R. (Eds.) (2015). *Rubin's pathology: Clinicopathologic foundations of medicine* (7th ed., Fig. 17-30, p. 654) Philadelphia, PA: Lippincott Williams & Wilkins.)

Acute mitral valve regurgitation may occur abruptly, such as with papillary muscle dysfunction after myocardial infarction, valve perforation in IE, or ruptured chordae tendineae in mitral valve prolapse. In acute severe mitral regurgitation, acute volume overload increases left ventricular preload, allowing a modest increase in left ventricular stroke volume. However, the forward stroke volume (that moves through the aorta into the systemic circulation) is reduced, and the regurgitant stroke volume leads to a rapid rise in left atrial pressure and pulmonary edema and decrease in cardiac output. Acute mitral valve regurgitation almost always is symptomatic. If severe, mitral valve replacement often is indicated.

The hemodynamic changes associated with chronic mitral valve regurgitation occur more slowly, allowing for recruitment of compensatory mechanisms. An increase in LVED volume permits an increase in total stroke volume, with restoration of forward flow into the aorta. Augmented preload and reduced or normal afterload (provided by unloading the LV into the left atrium) facilitate left ventricular ejection. At the same time, a gradual increase in left atrial size allows for accommodation of the regurgitant volume at a lower filling pressure.

Clinical Manifestations. The increased volume work associated with mitral regurgitation is relatively well tolerated, and many people with the disorder remain asymptomatic for many years, developing symptoms between 6 and 10 years after diagnosis. The degree of left ventricular enlargement reflects the severity of regurgitation.[40] As the disorder progresses, left ventricular function becomes impaired, the forward (aortic) stroke volume decreases, and the left atrial pressure increases, with the subsequent development of pulmonary congestion. Typical symptoms are those of LV failure such as dyspnea on exertion, paroxysmal nocturnal dyspnea, and orthopnea. Surgery should be performed before the onset of these symptoms.

A characteristic feature of mitral valve regurgitation is an enlarged LV, a hyperdynamic left ventricular impulse, and a pansystolic (throughout systole) murmur. Mitral regurgitation, like mitral stenosis, predisposes to atrial fibrillation.

Diagnosis and Treatment. The 2-D Doppler echocardiogram is useful in mitral regurgitation to evaluate left ventricular and atrial size, measure the ejection fraction, and assist in decision-making regarding surgery through assessment of the severity of the regurgitation. In some people with mitral regurgitation, preload reduction can be beneficial and may be treated with ACE inhibitors and biventricular pacing. Surgeries used in the treatment of mitral regurgitation include mitral valve repair and valve replacement with or without removal of the mitral apparatus. Mitral valve surgery is recommended in severe mitral regurgitation or symptomatic people where mitral valve regurgitation is possibly underestimated. Mitral valve repair avoids the use of anticoagulation needed with artificial valves.[39,40]

Mitral Valve Prolapse

Sometimes referred to as the *floppy mitral valve syndrome*, mitral valve prolapse occurs in 1% to 2.5% of the general population. The disorder is seen more frequently in women than in men and may have a familial basis. Familial mitral valve prolapse is transmitted as an autosomal trait, and several chromosomal loci have been identified. Although the exact cause of the disorder usually is unknown, it has been associated with Marfan syndrome, osteogenesis imperfecta, and other connective tissue disorders and with cardiac, hematologic, neuroendocrine, metabolic, and psychological disorders.

Pathogenesis. Pathologic findings in people with mitral valve prolapse include a myxedematous (mucinous) degeneration of mitral valve leaflets that causes them to become enlarged and floppy so that they prolapse or balloon back into the left atrium during systole (Fig. 27.20).

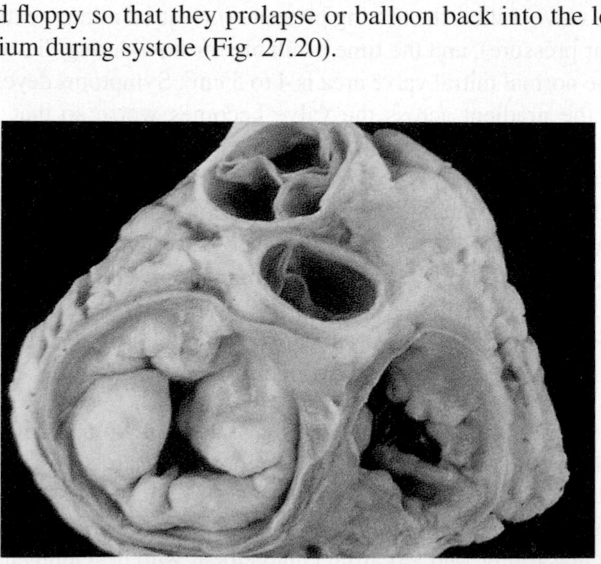

Figure 27.20 • Mitral valve prolapse. A view of the mitral valve from the left atrium shows redundant and deformed leaflets that billow into the left atrial cavity. (From Strayer D. E., Rubin R. (Eds.) (2015). *Rubin's pathology: Clinicopathologic foundations of medicine* (7th ed., Fig. 17-38A, p. 659) Philadelphia, PA: Lippincott Williams & Wilkins.)

Secondary fibrotic changes reflect the stresses and injury that the ballooning movements impose on the valve. Certain forms of mitral valve prolapse may arise from disorders of the myocardium that place undue stress on the mitral valve because of abnormal movement of the ventricular wall or papillary muscle. Mitral valve prolapse may or may not cause mitral regurgitation.

Clinical Manifestations and Diagnosis. Most people with mitral valve prolapse are asymptomatic, and the disorder is discovered during a routine physical examination. A minority of people have chest pain mimicking angina, dyspnea, fatigue, anxiety, palpitations, and lightheadedness. Unlike angina, the chest pain often is prolonged, ill defined, and not associated with exercise or exertion. The pain has been attributed to ischemia resulting from traction of the prolapsing valve leaflets. The anxiety, palpitations, and arrhythmias may result from abnormal autonomic nervous system function that commonly accompanies the disorder. The disorder is characterized by a spectrum of auscultatory findings, ranging from a silent form to one or more midsystolic clicks followed by a late systolic or holosystolic murmur. The clicks are caused by the sudden tensing of the mitral valve apparatus as the leaflets prolapse. Two-dimensional and Doppler echocardiographies are valuable noninvasive studies used to diagnose mitral valve prolapse.

Treatment. The treatment of mitral valve prolapse focuses on the relief of symptoms and the prevention of complications.[39] People with palpitations and mild tachyarrhythmias or increased adrenergic symptoms and those with chest discomfort, anxiety, and fatigue often respond to therapy with the β-adrenergic blocking drugs. In many cases, the cessation of stimulants such as caffeine, alcohol, and cigarettes may be sufficient to control symptoms. Transient ischemic attacks occur more frequently in persons with mitral valve prolapse. Therefore, in people with documented events who are in sinus rhythm with no atrial thrombi, daily aspirin therapy is recommended. Most people with mitral valve prolapse are encouraged to participate in regular exercise and lead a normal life. People who develop severe valve dysfunction may require valve surgery.

Aortic Valve Disorders

The aortic valve is located between the LV and the aorta. The aortic valve has three cusps and sometimes is referred to as the *aortic semilunar valve* because its leaflets are crescent or moon shaped (Fig. 27.17). The aortic valve has no chordae tendineae. Although their structures are similar, the cusps of the aortic valve are thicker than those of the mitral valve. The middle layer of the aortic valve is thickened near the middle, where the three leaflets meet, ensuring a tight seal. Between the thickened tissue and their free margins, the leaflets are thinner and flimsy.

An important aspect of the aortic valve is the location of the orifices for the two main coronary arteries, which are located behind the valve and at right angles to the direction of blood flow. It is the lateral pressure in the aorta that propels blood into the coronary arteries. During the ejection phase of the cardiac cycle, the lateral pressure is diminished by conversion of potential energy to kinetic energy as blood moves forward into the aorta. This process is grossly exaggerated in aortic valve stenosis because of the high flow velocities.

Aortic Valve Stenosis

Aortic valve stenosis, often referred to simply as *aortic stenosis*, is characterized by increased resistance to ejection of blood from the LV into the aorta (Fig. 27.18). The most common causes of aortic valve stenosis are congenital valve malformations and acquired calcification of a normal tricuspid valve. Congenital malformations may result in unicuspid, bicuspid, or misshaped valve leaflets. Acquired aortic stenosis is usually the consequence of calcification associated with the normal "wear and tear" of either a previously normal aortic valve or congenitally bicuspid valves (with which approximately 1% of the population is born).[41] The incidence of acquired aortic valve stenosis is 2% to 4% in adults older than 65 years of age.[41]

Pathogenesis. The progression of calcific aortic stenosis is usually slow and varies widely among individuals. Valve changes range from mild thickening without obstruction to severe calcification with impaired leaflet motion and obstructed left ventricular outflow.[41] Processes in the development of calcific aortic valve disease have been shown to be similar to those in CAD. Both conditions are more common in men, older persons, and persons with hypercholesterolemia derived in part from an active inflammatory process.[41] Early lesions of aortic sclerosis show focal subendothelial plaque-like lesions, similar to the initial phases of an atherosclerotic lesion. Aortic sclerosis is distinguished from aortic stenosis by the degree of valve impairment. In aortic sclerosis, the valve leaflets are abnormally thickened, but the obstruction to outflow is minimal, whereas in aortic stenosis the functional area of the valve has decreased enough to cause measurable obstruction to outflow. Calcification of the aortic valve progresses from the base of the cusps to the leaflets. This reduces leaflet motion and effective valve area but without commissural fusion. As calcification progresses, the leaflets become more rigid, there is worsening obstruction to left ventricular outflow, and fusion of the commissures leads to aortic stenosis.

Because aortic stenosis develops gradually, the LV has time to adapt. With increased systolic pressure from obstruction, the left ventricular wall becomes thicker, or hypertrophies, but a normal chamber volume is maintained. This increase in wall thickness can maintain a normal ejection fraction. Little hemodynamic disturbance occurs as the valve area is reduced by half its normal area (from a normal 3 to 4 cm^2 to 1.5 to 2 cm^2). However, an additional reduction in valve area from one half to one fourth of its normal size produces severe obstruction to flow and a progressive pressure overload on the LV. At this point, the increased work of the heart begins to exceed the coronary blood flow reserve, causing both systolic and diastolic dysfunction and signs of heart failure.[39,41]

Diagnosis. Aortic stenosis is usually first diagnosed with auscultation of a loud systolic ejection murmur or a single or paradoxically split second heart sound. Eventually, the classic symptoms of angina, syncope, and heart failure develop, although more subtle signs of a decrease in exercise tolerance or exertional dyspnea should be monitored closely. Angina occurs in approximately two thirds of people with advanced aortic stenosis and is similar to that observed in CAD. Dyspnea, marked fatigability, peripheral cyanosis, and other signs of low-output heart failure usually are not prominent until late in the course of the disease. Syncope (fainting) is most commonly due to the reduced cerebral circulation that occurs during exertion when the arterial pressure declines consequent to vasodilation in the presence of a fixed cardiac output.

Echocardiography can be used to evaluate the severity of calcified aortic lesions, left ventricular size and function, degree of ventricular hypertrophy, and presence of associated valve disorders and plays a major part in decision-making for aortic valve replacement. Evaluation with echocardiography is recommended as follows:

- Yearly in people with severe aortic stenosis
- Every 1 to 2 years with moderate stenosis
- Every 3 to 5 years with mild stenosis

Treatment. There is no effective medical therapy for severe aortic stenosis, although aggressive risk factor modification is indicated such as lipid-lowering and hypertensive management.[39,41] In children with congenital aortic stenosis, the valve leaflets are merely fused and balloon valvotomy may provide substantial benefit; valve replacement is the most effective treatment. Medical interventions are prescribed to relieve symptoms of heart failure for those people who are ineligible for surgical intervention. For people with symptomatic aortic stenosis, valve replacement almost always improves symptoms.

Aortic Valve Regurgitation

Aortic valve regurgitation (or aortic regurgitation) is the result of an incompetent aortic valve that allows blood to flow back to the LV during diastole (Fig. 27.18). As a result, the LV must increase its stroke volume to include blood entering from the lungs as well as that leaking back through the regurgitant valve.

Etiology and Pathogenesis. This defect may result from conditions that cause scarring of the valve leaflets or from enlargement of the valve orifice to the extent that the valve leaflets no longer meet. There are various causes of aortic regurgitation, including RF, idiopathic dilation of the aorta, congenital abnormalities, IE, and Marfan syndrome. Other causes include hypertension, trauma, and failure of a prosthetic valve.

Acute aortic regurgitation is characterized by the presentation of a sudden, large regurgitant volume to an LV of normal size that has not had time to adapt to the volume overload. It is caused most commonly by disorders such as IE, trauma, or aortic dissection. Although the heart responds with use of the Frank-Starling mechanisms and an increase in heart rate, these compensatory mechanisms fail to maintain the cardiac output. As a result, there is severe elevation in LVED pressure, which is transmitted to the left atrium and pulmonary veins, culminating in pulmonary edema. A decrease in cardiac output leads to sympathetic stimulation and a resultant increase in heart rate and peripheral vascular resistance that cause the regurgitation to worsen. Death from pulmonary edema, ventricular arrhythmias, or circulatory collapse is common in severe acute aortic regurgitation.

Chronic aortic regurgitation, which usually has a gradual onset, represents a condition of combined left ventricular volume and pressure overload. As the valve deformity increases, regurgitant flow into the LV increases, diastolic blood pressure falls, and the LV progressively enlarges. Hemodynamically, the increase in left ventricular volume results in the ejection of a large stroke volume that usually is adequate to maintain the forward cardiac output until late in the course of the disease. Most persons remain asymptomatic during this compensated phase, which may last for decades. The only sign for many years may be a soft systolic aortic murmur.

Clinical Manifestations and Diagnosis. As the disease progresses, signs and symptoms of left ventricular failure begin to appear. These include exertional dyspnea, orthopnea, and paroxysmal nocturnal dyspnea. In aortic regurgitation, failure of aortic valve closure during diastole causes an abnormal drop in diastolic pressure. Because coronary blood flow is greatest during diastole, the drop in diastolic pressure produces a decrease in coronary perfusion. Although angina is rare, it may occur when the heart rate and diastolic pressure fall to low levels. People with severe aortic regurgitation often complain of an uncomfortable awareness of heartbeat, particularly when lying down, and chest discomfort due to pounding of the heart against the chest wall. Tachycardia, occurring with emotional stress or exertion, may produce palpitations, head pounding, and premature ventricular contractions.

The major physical findings relate to the widening of the arterial pulse pressure. Korotkoff sounds may persist to zero, even though intra-arterial pressure rarely falls below 30 mm Hg.[39,41] The large stroke volume and wide pulse pressure may result in prominent carotid pulsations in the neck (Corrigan pulse), head bobbing (de Musset sign), systolic pulsations in the fingernail bed on gentle pressure (Quincke pulse), throbbing peripheral pulses, and a left ventricular impulse that causes the chest to move with each beat. The hyperkinetic pulse of more severe aortic regurgitation, called a *water-hammer pulse*, is characterized by distention and quick collapse of the artery. The turbulence of flow across the aortic valve produces a holodiastolic decrescendo murmur heard best at the left sternal border. In severe aortic regurgitation, a middiastolic rumble at the apex can be heard, called the *Austin Flint* murmur.

Treatment. The treatment for acute or severe chronic aortic regurgitation is aortic valve replacement. Surgery is recommended whenever people are symptomatic, regardless of left ventricular function. In asymptomatic people, valve replacement remains controversial. However, in people with left ventricular systolic dysfunction or with severe left ventricular dilation, valve replacement is also recommended, even if these people are asymptomatic.[39,41]

Medication therapy in aortic regurgitation has been studied in clinical trials. The goal of medical therapy is to improve forward stroke volume and reduce regurgitant volume, usually through the use of afterload reducers. There is no strong indication for medical therapy based on the clinical trials. There is only a weak recommendation for afterload reduction. The first-line agent that is recommended in people with asymptomatic severe aortic regurgitation, especially in hypertensive people, is ACE inhibitors. Surgery remains the primary therapy for symptomatic severe aortic regurgitation.[41]

IN SUMMARY

Dysfunction of the heart valves can result from a number of disorders, including congenital defects, trauma, ischemic heart disease, degenerative changes, and inflammation. Rheumatic endocarditis is a common cause. Valvular heart disease produces its effects through disturbances of blood flow. A stenotic valvular defect is one that causes a decrease in blood flow through a valve, resulting in impaired emptying and increased work demands on the heart chamber that empties blood across the diseased valve. A regurgitant valvular defect permits the blood flow to continue when the valve is closed. Valvular heart disorders produce blood flow turbulence and often are detected through cardiac auscultation.

HEART FAILURE AND CIRCULATORY SHOCK

Adequate perfusion of body tissues depends on the pumping ability of the heart, a vascular system that transports blood to the cells and back to the heart, sufficient blood to fill the circulatory system, and tissues that are able to extract and use oxygen and nutrients from the blood. Heart failure and circulatory shock are separate conditions that reflect failure of the circulatory system. Both conditions exhibit common compensatory mechanisms even though they differ in terms of pathogenesis and causes.

HEART FAILURE IN ADULTS

After completing this section of the chapter, the learner will be able to meet the following objectives:

- Explain how the Frank-Starling mechanism, sympathetic nervous system, renin–angiotensin–aldosterone mechanism, natriuretic peptides (NPs), endothelins, and myocardial hypertrophy and remodeling function as adaptive and maladaptive mechanisms in heart failure.
- Differentiate high-output versus low-output heart failure, systolic versus diastolic heart failure, and right-sided versus left-sided heart failure in terms of causes, impact on cardiac function, and major manifestations.
- Differentiate chronic heart failure from acute heart failure syndromes (AHFS) and methods of diagnosis, assessment, and management.

Heart failure has been defined as a complex syndrome resulting from any functional or structural disorder of the heart that results in or increases the risk of developing manifestations of low cardiac output and/or pulmonary or systemic congestion.[42] In the United States, heart failure costs the nation more than $30 billion per year, and in 2009, it affected more than 5 million people. Heart failure can occur in any age group but primarily affects older adults. Although morbidity and mortality rates from other CVDs have decreased over the past several decades, the incidence of heart failure is increasing at an alarming rate. Approximately 400,000 to 700,000 people are diagnosed with heart failure each year in the United States.

The syndrome of heart failure can be produced by any heart condition that reduces the pumping ability of the heart. Among the most common causes of heart failure are CAD, hypertension, DCM, and valvular heart disease.[42] Because many of the processes leading to heart failure are long-standing and progress gradually, heart failure can often be prevented or its progression slowed by early detection and intervention. The importance of these approaches is emphasized by the ACC/AHA guidelines that have incorporated a classification system of heart failure that includes four stages:

1. Stage A—High risk for developing heart failure, but no identified structural abnormalities and no signs of heart failure
2. Stage B—The presence of structural heart disease, but no history of signs and symptoms of heart failure
3. Stage C—Current or prior symptoms of heart failure with structural heart disease
4. Stage D—Advanced structural heart disease and symptoms of heart failure at rest on maximum medical therapy[42,43]

This staging system recognizes that there are established risk factors and structural abnormalities that are characteristic of the four stages of heart failure. People normally progress from one stage to another unless disease progression is slowed or stopped by treatment.

KEY POINTS

HEART FAILURE

- The function of the heart is to move deoxygenated blood from the venous system through the right heart into the pulmonary circulation and oxygenated blood from the pulmonary circulation through the left heart and into the arterial circulation.
- Systolic dysfunction represents a decrease in cardiac myocardial contractility and an impaired ability to eject blood from the LV, whereas diastolic dysfunction represents an abnormality in ventricular relaxation and filling.

Pathophysiology of Heart Failure

Cardiac output is the amount of blood that the ventricles eject each minute. The heart has the amazing capacity to adjust its cardiac output to meet the varying needs of the body. During sleep, the cardiac output declines, and during exercise, it increases markedly. The ability to increase cardiac output during increased activity is called the *cardiac reserve*. For example, competitive swimmers and long-distance runners have large cardiac reserves. During exercise, the cardiac output of these athletes rapidly increases to as much as five to six times their resting level.[44] In sharp contrast with healthy athletes, people with heart failure often use their cardiac reserve at rest. For them, just climbing a flight of stairs may cause shortness of breath because they have exceeded their cardiac reserve.

Control of Cardiac Performance and Output

Cardiac output, which is the major determinant of cardiac performance, reflects how often the heart beats each minute (heart rate) and how much blood it pumps with each beat (stroke volume) and can be expressed as the product of the heart rate and stroke volume (*i.e.*, cardiac output = heart rate × stroke volume). The heart rate is regulated by a balance between the activity of the sympathetic nervous system, which produces an increase in heart rate, and the parasympathetic nervous system, which slows it down, whereas the stroke volume is a function of preload, afterload, and myocardial contractility.[44,45]

Preload and Afterload. The work that the heart performs consists mainly of ejecting blood that has returned to the ventricles during diastole into the pulmonary or systemic circulation. It is determined largely by *preload* and *afterload*.

Preload reflects the volume or loading conditions of the ventricle at the end of diastole, just before the onset of systole. It is the volume of blood stretching the heart muscle at the end of diastole and is normally determined by the venous return to the heart. During any given cardiac cycle, the maximum volume of blood filling the ventricle is present at the end of diastole. Known as the *end-diastolic volume*, this volume causes an increase in the length of the myocardial muscle fibers. Within limits, as end-diastolic volume or preload increases, the stroke volume increases in accord with the Frank-Starling mechanism.

Afterload represents the force that the contracting heart muscle must generate to eject blood from the filled heart. The main components of afterload are the systemic (peripheral) vascular resistance and ventricular wall tension. When the systemic vascular resistance is elevated, as with arterial hypertension, an increased left intraventricular pressure must be generated to first open the aortic valve and then move blood out of the ventricle and into the systemic circulation. This increased pressure equates to an increase in ventricular wall stress or tension. As a result, excessive afterload may impair ventricular ejection and increase wall tension.

Myocardial Contractility. Myocardial contractility, also known as *inotropy*, refers to the contractile performance of the heart. It represents the ability of the contractile elements (actin and myosin filaments) of the heart muscle to interact and shorten against a load. Contractility increases cardiac output independent of preload and afterload.

The interaction between the actin and myosin filaments during cardiac muscle contraction and relaxation (*i.e.*, cross-bridge attachment and detachment) requires the use of energy supplied by the breakdown of ATP and the presence of calcium ions (Ca^{++}).

As with skeletal muscle, when an action potential passes over the cardiac muscle fiber, the impulse spreads to the interior of the muscle fiber along the membranes of the transverse (T) tubules. The T tubule action potentials in turn act to cause release of Ca^{++} from the sarcoplasmic reticulum (Fig. 27.21). These Ca^{++} ions diffuse into the myofibrils and catalyze the chemical reactions that promote sliding of the actin and myosin filaments along one another to produce muscle shortening. In addition to the Ca^{++} ions released from the sarcoplasmic reticulum, a large quantity of extracellular Ca^{++} also diffuses into the sarcoplasm through voltage-dependent L-type Ca^{++} channels in T tubules at the time of the action potential. Without the extra Ca^{++} that enters through the L-type Ca^{++} channels, the strength of the cardiac contraction would be considerably weaker. Opening of the L-type Ca^{++} channels is facilitated by the second messenger cyclic adenosine monophosphate (cAMP), the formation of which is coupled to β-adrenergic receptors. The catecholamines (norepinephrine and epinephrine) exert their inotropic effects by binding to these receptors. The L-type calcium channel also contains several other types of drug receptors. The dihydropyridine Ca^{++} channel–blocking drugs (*e.g.*, nifedipine) exert their effects by binding to one site, whereas diltiazem and verapamil appear to bind to closely related but not identical receptors in another region. Blockade of the Ca^{++} channels in cardiac muscle by these drugs results in a reduction in contractility throughout the heart and a decrease in sinus node pacemaker rate and in AV node conduction velocity.

Another mechanism that can modulate inotropy is the sodium ion (Na^+)/Ca^{++} exchange pump and the ATPase-dependent Ca^{++} pump on the myocardial cell membrane (Fig. 27.21). These pumps transport Ca^{++} out of the cell, thereby preventing the cell from becoming overloaded with Ca^{++}. If Ca^{++} extrusion is inhibited, the rise in intracellular Ca^{++} can increase inotropy. Digitalis and related cardiac glycosides are inotropic agents that exert their effects by inhibiting the Na^+/potassium ion (K^+)–ATPase pump, which increases intracellular Na^+; this in turn leads to an increase in intracellular Ca^{++} through the Na^+/Ca^{++} exchange pump.

Systolic Versus Diastolic Dysfunction

Classification separates the pathophysiology of heart failure into systolic and diastolic failure or dysfunction based on the ventricular ejection fraction.[46,47] *Ejection fraction* is the percentage of blood pumped out of the ventricles with each contraction. A normal ejection fraction is about 55% to 70%. In systolic ventricular dysfunction, myocardial contractility is impaired, leading to a decrease in the ejection fraction and cardiac output. Diastolic ventricular dysfunction is characterized by a normal ejection

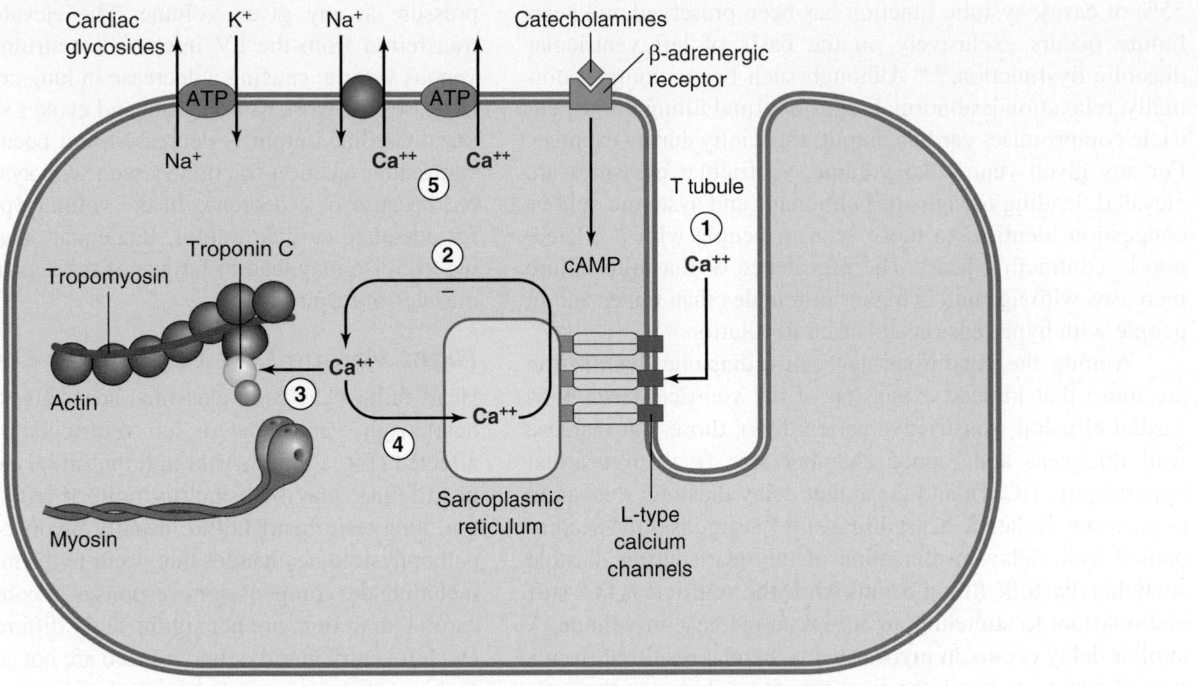

Figure 27.21 • Schematic representation of the role of calcium ions (Ca^{++}) in cardiac excitation–contraction coupling. The influx (site 1) of extracellular Ca^{++} through the L-type Ca^{++} channels in the T tubules during excitation triggers (site 2) release of Ca^{++} by the sarcoplasmic reticulum. This Ca^{++} binds to TnC (site 3). The Ca^{++}–troponin complex interacts with tropomyosin to unblock active sites on the actin and myosin filaments, allowing cross-bridge attachment and contraction of the myofibrils (systole). Relaxation (diastole) occurs as a result of calcium reuptake by the sarcoplasmic reticulum (site 4) and extrusion of intracellular Ca^{++} by the sodium Na^+/Ca^{++} exchange transporter or, to a lesser extent, by the Ca^{++} ATPase pump (site 5). Mechanisms that raise systolic Ca^{++} increase the level of developed force (inotropy). Binding of catecholamines to β-adrenergic receptors increases Ca^{++} entry by phosphorylation of the Ca^{++} channels through a cAMP-dependent second messenger mechanism. The cardiac glycosides increase intracellular Ca^{++} by inhibiting the Na^+/K^+–ATPase pump. The elevated intracellular Na^+ reverses the Na^+/Ca^{++} exchange transporter (site 5), so less Ca^{++} is removed from the cell. (Modified from Klabunde R. E. (2005). *Cardiovascular Physiology Concepts* (p. 46). Philadelphia, PA: Lippincott Williams & Wilkins.)

fraction but impaired diastolic ventricular relaxation, leading to a decrease in ventricular filling that ultimately causes a decrease in preload, stroke volume, and cardiac output. Many people with heart failure have combined elements of both systolic and diastolic ventricular dysfunction, and the division between systolic and diastolic dysfunction may be somewhat artificial, particularly as it relates to manifestations and treatment.[47] It is important to note that ventricular dysfunction is not synonymous with heart failure. It can, however, lead to heart failure. With both systolic and diastolic ventricular dysfunction, compensatory mechanisms are usually able to maintain adequate resting cardiac function until the later stages of heart failure.

Systolic Dysfunction. Systolic dysfunction is primarily defined as a decrease in myocardial contractility, characterized by an ejection fraction of less than 40%. A normal heart ejects approximately 65% of the blood that is present in the ventricle at the end of diastole. In systolic heart failure, the ejection fraction declines progressively with increasing degrees of myocardial dysfunction. In very severe forms of heart failure, the ejection fraction may drop to a single-digit percentage. With a decrease in ejection fraction, there is a resultant increase in end-diastolic volume (preload), ventricular dilation, and ventricular wall tension and a rise in ventricular end-diastolic pressure.[5] The increased volume, added to the normal venous return, leads to an increase in ventricular preload. The rise in preload is thought to be a compensatory mechanism to help maintain stroke volume through the Frank-Starling mechanism despite a drop-in ejection fraction. Although it serves as a compensatory mechanism, increased preload can also lead to one of the most deleterious consequences of systolic ventricular dysfunction—accumulation of blood in the atria and the venous system (which empties into the atria), causing pulmonary or peripheral edema.

Systolic dysfunction commonly results from conditions that impair the contractile performance of the heart (*e.g.*, ischemic heart disease and cardiomyopathy), produce a volume overload (*e.g.*, valvular insufficiency and anemia), or generate a pressure overload (*e.g.*, hypertension and valvular stenosis) on the heart. The extent of systolic ventricular dysfunction can be estimated by measuring the cardiac output and ejection fraction and by assessment for manifestations of left-sided heart failure, particularly pulmonary congestion.

Diastolic Dysfunction. Although heart failure is commonly associated with impaired systolic function, in approximately

55% of cases, systolic function has been preserved and heart failure occurs exclusively on the basis of left ventricular diastolic dysfunction.[48,49] Although such hearts contract normally, relaxation is abnormal. The abnormal filling of the ventricle compromises cardiac output, especially during exercise. For any given ventricular volume, ventricular pressures are elevated, leading to signs of pulmonary and systemic venous congestion identical to those seen in people with a dilated, poorly contracting heart. The prevalence of diastolic failure increases with age and is higher in females than males and in people with hypertension and atrial fibrillation.[48,49]

Among the conditions that cause diastolic dysfunction are those that impede expansion of the ventricle (*e.g.*, pericardial effusion, constrictive pericarditis), those that increase wall thickness and reduce chamber size (*e.g.*, myocardial hypertrophy, HCM), and those that delay diastolic relaxation (*e.g.*, aging, ischemic heart disease).[48,49] Aging is often accompanied by a delay in relaxation of the heart during diastole such that diastolic filling begins while the ventricle is still stiff and resistant to stretching to accept an increase in volume. A similar delay occurs in myocardial ischemia, resulting from a lack of energy to break the rigor that forms between the actin and myosin filaments and to move Ca^{++} out of the cytosol and back into the sarcoplasmic reticulum.[48,49]

Diastolic function is further influenced by the heart rate, which determines how much time is available for ventricular filling. An increase in heart rate shortens the diastolic filling time.[7] Thus, diastolic dysfunction can be aggravated by tachycardia or an arrhythmia and improved by a reduction in heart rate, which allows the heart to fill over a longer period.

With diastolic dysfunction, blood is unable to move freely into the LV, causing an increase in intraventricular pressure at any given volume. The elevated pressures are transferred from the LV into the left atrium and pulmonary venous system, causing a decrease in lung compliance, which increases the work of breathing and evokes symptoms of dyspnea. Cardiac output is decreased, not because of a reduced ventricular ejection fraction as seen with systolic dysfunction but because of a decrease in the volume (preload) available for adequate cardiac output. Inadequate cardiac output during exercise may lead to fatigue of the legs and the accessory muscles of respiration.

Right Versus Left Ventricular Dysfunction

Heart failure has been classified according to the side of the heart (right ventricular or left ventricular) that is primarily affected (Fig. 27.22). Although the initial event that leads to heart failure may be primarily right or left ventricular in origin, long-term heart failure usually involves both sides. The pathophysiologic changes that occur in the myocardium itself, including the compensatory responses in conditions like myocardial infarction, are not significantly different between right and left ventricular dysfunction and are not addressed in detail in this section.

Right Ventricular Dysfunction. Right-sided heart failure impairs the ability to move deoxygenated blood from the systemic circulation into the pulmonary circulation. Consequently, when the right ventricle fails, there is a reduction in the amount of blood moved forward into the pulmonary circulation and then into the left side of the heart, ultimately causing a reduction of left ventricular cardiac output. Also, if the right ventricle does not move the blood forward, there is accumulation or congestion of blood into the systemic venous

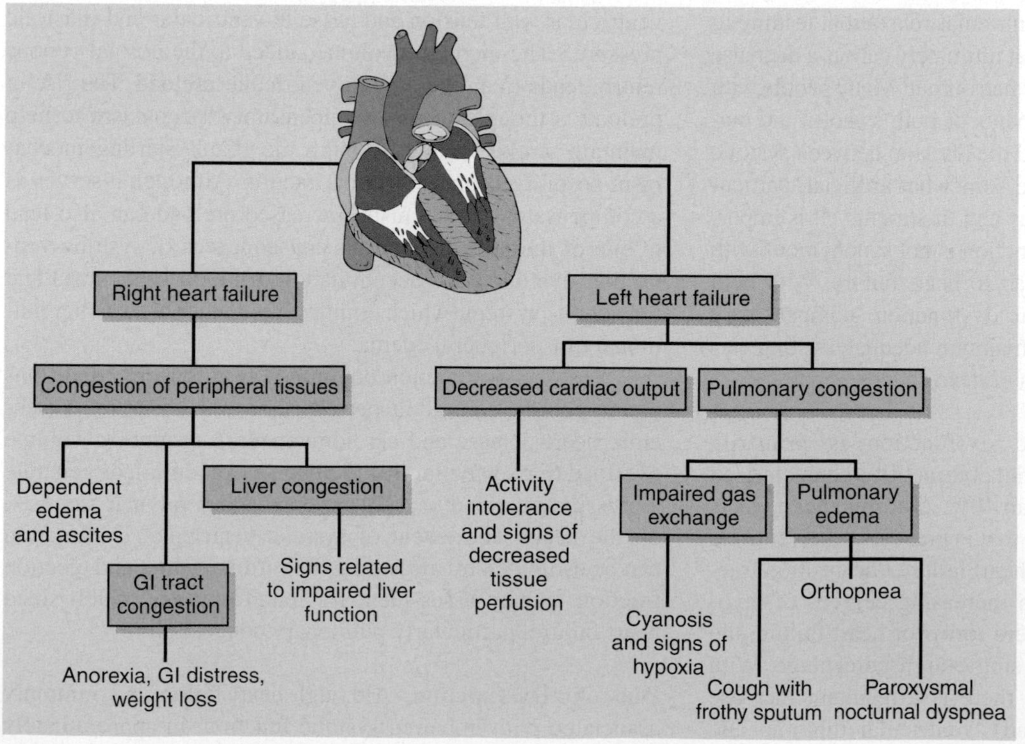

Figure 27.22 • Manifestations of left- and right-sided heart failure. GI, gastrointestinal.

system. This causes an increase in right ventricular end-diastolic, right atrial, and systemic venous pressures. A major effect of right-sided heart failure is the development of peripheral edema (Fig. 27.22). Because of the effects of gravity, the edema is most pronounced in the dependent parts of the body. When the person is in the upright position, edema is seen in the lower extremities; when the person is supine, the edema is seen in the area over the sacrum. The accumulation of edema fluid is evidenced by a gain in weight (*i.e.*, 1 pint [568 mL] of accumulated fluid results in a 1 lb [0.45 kg] weight gain). Daily measurement of weight can be used as a means of assessing fluid accumulation in a person with chronic heart failure. As a rule, a weight gain of more than 2 lb (0.90 kg) in 24 hours or 5 lb (2.27 kg) in 1 week is considered a sign of worsening failure.[48]

Right-sided heart failure also produces congestion of the viscera. As venous distention progresses, blood backs up in the hepatic veins that drain into the inferior vena cava, and the liver becomes engorged. This may cause hepatomegaly and right upper quadrant pain. In severe and prolonged right-sided heart failure, liver function is impaired and hepatic cells may die. Congestion of the portal circulation also may lead to engorgement of the spleen and the development of ascites. Congestion of the gastrointestinal tract may interfere with digestion and absorption of nutrients, causing anorexia and abdominal discomfort. The jugular veins, which are above the level of the heart, are normally not visible in the standing position or when sitting with the head at higher than a 30-degree angle. In severe right-sided heart failure, the external jugular veins become distended and can be visualized when the person is sitting up or standing.

The causes of right ventricular dysfunction include conditions that impede blood flow into the lungs or compromise the pumping effectiveness of the right ventricle. Left ventricular failure is the most common cause of right ventricular failure. Sustained pulmonary hypertension also causes right ventricular dysfunction and failure. Pulmonary hypertension occurs in people with chronic pulmonary disease, severe pneumonia, pulmonary embolus, or aortic or mitral stenosis. When the right-sided heart failure occurs in response to chronic pulmonary disease, it is referred to as *cor pulmonale*.[48] Other common causes include stenosis or regurgitation of the tricuspid or pulmonic valves, right ventricular infarction, and cardiomyopathy. Right ventricular dysfunction with heart failure is also caused by congenital heart defects such as tetralogy of Fallot and ventricular septal defect.

Left Ventricular Dysfunction. Left-sided heart failure impairs the movement of blood from the low-pressure pulmonary circulation into the high-pressure arterial side of the systemic circulation. With impairment of left heart function, there is a decrease in cardiac output to the systemic circulation. Blood accumulates in the LV, left atrium, and pulmonary circulation, which causes an elevation in pulmonary venous pressure (Fig. 27.22). When the pressure in the pulmonary capillaries (normally approximately 10 mm Hg) exceeds the capillary osmotic pressure (normally approximately 25 mm Hg), there is a shift of intravascular fluid into the interstitium of the lung resulting in pulmonary edema (Fig. 27.23). An episode of pulmonary edema often occurs at night, after the person has been reclining for some time and the gravitational forces have been removed from the circulatory system. It is then that the edema fluid that had been sequestered in the lower extremities during the day is returned to the vascular compartment and redistributed to the pulmonary circulation.

The most common causes of left ventricular dysfunction are hypertension and acute myocardial infarction. Left ventricular heart failure and pulmonary congestion can develop very rapidly in people with acute myocardial infarction. Even when the infarcted area is small, there may be a surrounding area of ischemic tissue. This may result in large areas of ventricular wall hypokinesis or akinesis and rapid onset of pulmonary congestion and edema. Stenosis or regurgitation of the aortic or mitral valve also creates the level of left-sided backflow that results in pulmonary congestion. As pulmonary

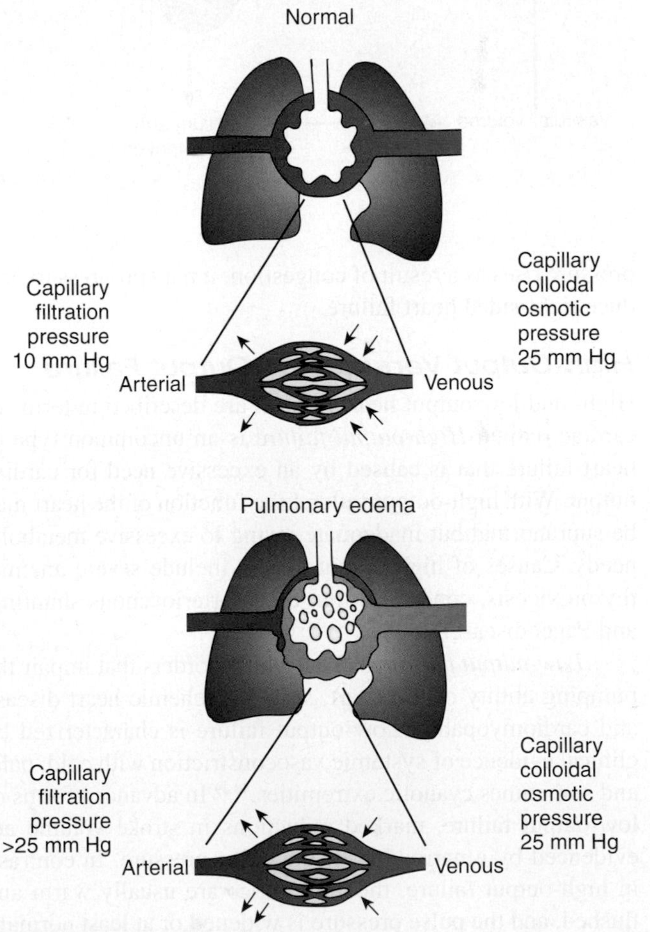

Figure 27.23 • Mechanism of respiratory symptoms in left-sided heart failure. In the normal exchange of fluid in the pulmonary capillaries **(top)**, the capillary filtration pressure that moves fluid out of the capillary into the lung is less than the capillary colloidal osmotic pressure that pulls fluid back into the capillary. Development of pulmonary edema **(bottom)** occurs when the capillary filtration pressure exceeds the capillary colloidal osmotic pressure that pulls fluid back into the capillary.

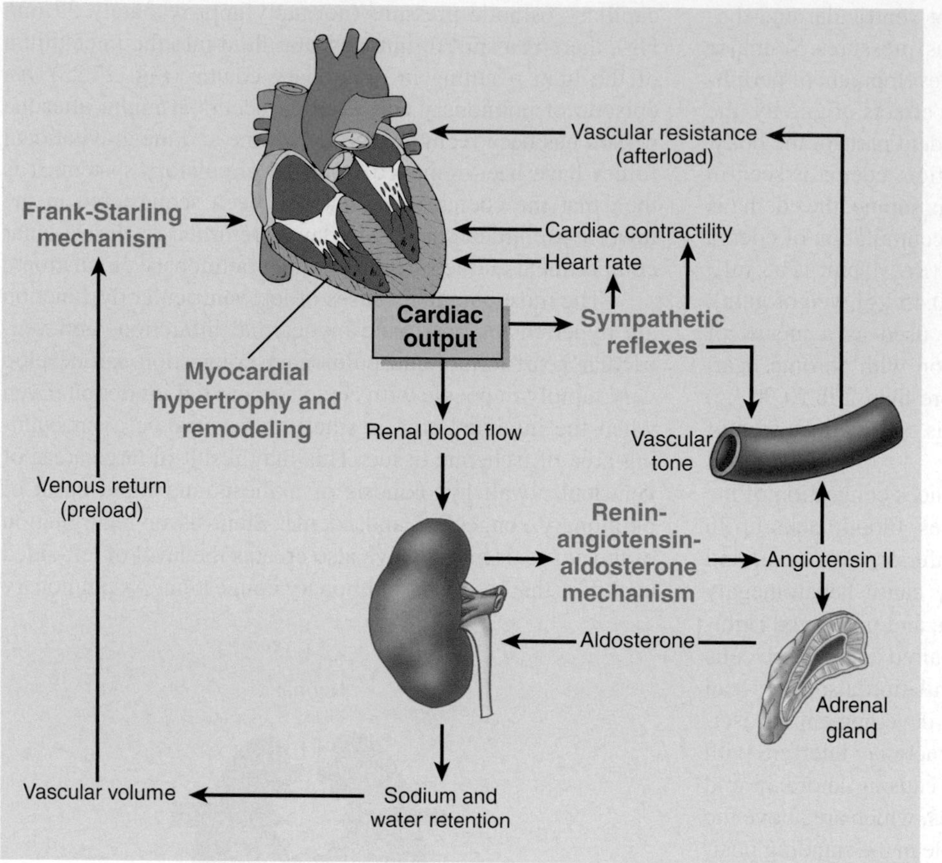

Figure 27.24 • Compensatory mechanisms in heart failure. The Frank-Starling mechanism, sympathetic reflexes, renin–angiotensin–aldosterone mechanism, and myocardial hypertrophy function in maintaining cardiac output for the failing heart.

pressure rises as a result of congestion, it may progress to produce right-sided heart failure.

High-Output Versus Low-Output Failure

High- and low-output heart failures are described in terms of cardiac output. *High-output failure* is an uncommon type of heart failure that is caused by an excessive need for cardiac output. With high-output failure, the function of the heart may be supranormal but inadequate owing to excessive metabolic needs. Causes of high-output failure include severe anemia, thyrotoxicosis, conditions that cause arteriovenous shunting, and Paget disease.

Low-output failure is caused by disorders that impair the pumping ability of the heart, such as ischemic heart disease and cardiomyopathy. Low-output failure is characterized by clinical evidence of systemic vasoconstriction with cold, pale, and sometimes cyanotic extremities.[48,49] In advanced forms of low-output failure, marked reductions in stroke volume are evidenced by a narrowing of the pulse pressure. In contrast, in high-output failure, the extremities are usually warm and flushed, and the pulse pressure is widened or at least normal.

Compensatory Mechanisms

In heart failure, the cardiac reserve is largely maintained through compensatory or adaptive responses such as the Frank-Starling mechanism, activation of neurohumoral influences such as the sympathetic nervous system reflexes, the renin–angiotensin–aldosterone mechanism, cardiac NPs, locally produced vasoactive substances, and myocardial hypertrophy and remodeling[49] (Fig. 27.24).

The first of these adaptations occurs rapidly over minutes to hours of myocardial dysfunction and may be adequate to maintain the overall pumping performance of the heart at relatively normal levels. Myocardial hypertrophy and remodeling occur slowly over months to years and play an important role in the long-term adaptation to hemodynamic overload. In the failing heart, early decreases in cardiac function may go unnoticed because these compensatory mechanisms maintain the cardiac output. However, these mechanisms contribute not only to the adaptation of the failing heart but also to the pathophysiology of heart failure.[49]

Frank-Starling Mechanism. The Frank-Starling mechanism operates through an increase in preload (Fig. 27.25). With increased diastolic filling, there is increased stretching of the myocardial fibers and more optimal approximation of the heads on the thick myosin filaments to the troponin binding sites on the thin actin filaments, with a resultant increase in the force of the next contraction. In the normally functioning heart, the Frank-Starling mechanism serves to match the outputs of the two ventricles. As illustrated in Figure 27.25, there is no one single Frank-Starling curve. An increase in contractility, or inotropy, will increase cardiac output at any end-diastolic volume, causing the curve to move up and to

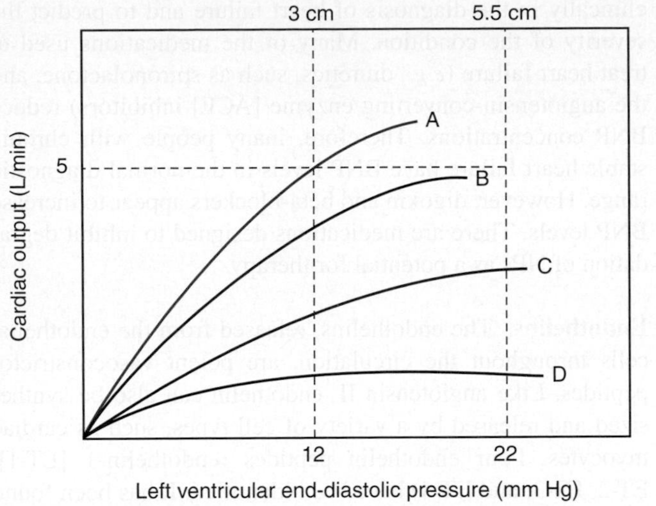

Figure 27.25 • Left ventricular function curves. *Curve A:* Normal function curve, with a normal cardiac output and optimal LVED filling pressure. *Curve B:* Compensated heart failure with normal cardiac output at higher LVED pressures. *Curve C:* Decompensated heart failure with a decrease in cardiac output and elevated LVED, with eventual elevation of pulmonary capillary pressure and development of pulmonary congestion. *Curve D:* Cardiogenic shock, with an extreme decrease in cardiac output and marked increase in LVED pressures.

the left, whereas a decrease in inotropy will cause the curve to move down and to the right. In heart failure, inotropy is decreased compared with normal. Thus, the stroke volume will not be as high as with normal inotropy, regardless of the increase in preload.

In heart failure, a decrease in cardiac output and renal blood flow leads to increased sodium and water retention, a resultant increase in vascular volume and venous return to the heart, and an increase in ventricular end-diastolic volume. Within limits, as preload and ventricular end-diastolic volume increase, there is a resultant increase in cardiac output. Although this may preserve the resting cardiac output, the resulting chronic elevation of LVED pressure is transmitted to the atria and the pulmonary circulation, causing pulmonary congestion.

An increase in muscle stretch, as occurs with the Frank-Starling mechanism, also causes an increase in ventricular wall tension with a resultant increase in myocardial oxygen consumption. Because increased wall tension increases myocardial oxygen requirements, it can produce ischemia and contribute to further impairment of inotropy, moving the Frank-Starling curve farther down and to the right (Fig. 27.25). In this situation, the increase in preload is no longer contributing to compensation but rather causing heart failure to worsen. The use of diuretics in people with heart failure helps to reduce vascular volume and ventricular filling, thereby unloading the heart and reducing ventricular wall tension.

Sympathetic Nervous System Activity. Stimulation of the sympathetic nervous system plays an important role in the compensatory response to decreased cardiac output and stroke volume. Both cardiac sympathetic tone and catecholamine (epinephrine and norepinephrine) levels are elevated during the late stages of most forms of heart failure. By direct stimulation of heart rate and cardiac contractility, regulation of vascular tone, and enhancement of renal sodium and water retention, the sympathetic nervous system initially helps to maintain perfusion of the various body organs. In people who progress to more severe heart failure, blood is diverted to the more critical cerebral and coronary circulations.

Although the sympathetic nervous system response is meant to augment blood pressure and cardiac output and is the most immediate compensatory mechanism, it can become maladaptive. An increase in sympathetic activity by stimulation of the β-adrenergic receptors of the heart leads to tachycardia, vasoconstriction, and cardiac arrhythmias. Acutely, tachycardia significantly increases the workload of the heart, thus increasing myocardial oxygen demand, and cardiac ischemia and cardiomyopathy both contribute to worsening of heart failure. By promoting arrhythmias, the catecholamines released with sympathetic nervous system stimulation also may contribute to the high rate of sudden death seen with heart failure.

There is evidence that prolonged sympathetic stimulation may also lead to desensitization of β-adrenergic receptors without affecting α-adrenergic receptors. Even though circulating norepinephrine levels are increased in people with heart failure, the lack of functioning β-adrenergic receptors in relation to α-adrenergic receptors may lead to vasoconstriction and an increase in systemic vascular resistance. An increase in systemic vascular resistance causes an increase in cardiac afterload and ventricular wall stress, thus increasing myocardial oxygen consumption. Other effects include decreased renal perfusion and additional augmentation of the renin–angiotensin–aldosterone system, as well as decreased blood flow to skin, muscle, and abdominal organs.

Renin–Angiotensin–Aldosterone Mechanism. One of the most important effects of lowered cardiac output in heart failure is a reduction in renal blood flow and glomerular filtration rate, which leads to sodium and water retention. With decreased renal blood flow, there is a progressive increase in renin secretion by the kidneys with parallel increases in circulating levels of angiotensin II. The increased concentration of angiotensin II contributes directly to a generalized and excessive vasoconstriction, as well as facilitates norepinephrine release and inhibits reuptake of norepinephrine by the sympathetic nervous system.

Angiotensin II also provides a powerful stimulus for aldosterone production by the adrenal cortex. Aldosterone increases tubular reabsorption of sodium, with an accompanied increase in water retention. Because aldosterone is metabolized in the liver, its levels are further increased when heart failure causes liver congestion. Angiotensin II also increases the level of antidiuretic hormone (ADH), which serves as a vasoconstrictor and inhibitor of water excretion. In heart failure, the progressive accumulation of fluid leads to ventricular dilation and increased wall tension. The increased oxygen demand that accompanies increased wall tension eventually outweighs the compensatory Frank-Starling mechanism, reducing inotropy and progressing heart failure.

In addition to their individual effects on sodium and water balance, angiotensin II and aldosterone are also involved in regulating the inflammatory and reparative processes that follow tissue injury. In this capacity, they stimulate inflammatory cytokine production (*e.g.*, TNF and interleukin-6), attract inflammatory cells (*e.g.*, neutrophils and macrophages), activate macrophages at sites of injury and repair, and stimulate the growth of fibroblasts and synthesis of collagen fibers. Fibroblast and collagen deposition results in ventricular hypertrophy and myocardial wall fibrosis, which decreases compliance (*i.e.*, increases stiffness), ultimately causing inappropriate remodeling of the heart and progression of both systolic and diastolic ventricular dysfunction.[49] Thus, the progression of heart failure may be augmented by aldosterone-mediated effects on both the vasculature and myocardium.

Natriuretic Peptides. The heart muscle produces and secretes a family of related peptide hormones (NPs) that have potent diuretic, natriuretic, and vascular smooth muscle effects and also interact with other neurohumoral mechanisms that affect cardiovascular function. Two of the four known NPs most commonly associated with heart failure are atrial natriuretic peptide (ANP) and brain natriuretic peptide (BNP).

As the name indicates, ANP is released from atrial cells in response to atrial stretch, pressure, or fluid overload. BNP is primarily secreted by the ventricles as a response to increased ventricular pressure or fluid overload. In early heart failure, NT-proBNP can be detected as a precursor for BNP in the blood. Although the NPs are not secreted from the same chambers in the heart, they have very similar functions. In response to increased chamber stretch and pressure, they promote rapid and transient natriuresis and diuresis through an increase in the glomerular filtration rate and an inhibition of tubular sodium and water reabsorption.

The NPs also facilitate complex interactions with the neurohormonal system, inhibiting the sympathetic nervous system, the renin–angiotensin–aldosterone system, endothelin inflammatory cytokines, and vasopressin. Suppression of the sympathetic nervous system causes both venous and arterial dilation with consequent reduction in venous return to the heart (decreased preload) and cardiac filling pressures and a decrease in afterload (arterial vasodilation). Inhibition of angiotensin II and vasopressin by the NPs reduces renal fluid retention. In addition, the NPs directly affect the central nervous system and the brain, inhibiting the secretion of vasopressin and the function of the salt appetite and thirst center.

Circulating levels of both ANP and BNP are reportedly elevated in people with heart failure. BNP and NT-proBNP levels can be detected through blood work and commercial assays. The concentrations are well correlated with the extent of ventricular dysfunction, increasing up to 30-fold in people with advanced heart disease. Assays of BNP are used clinically in the diagnosis of heart failure and to predict the severity of the condition. Many of the medications used to treat heart failure (*e.g.*, diuretics, such as spironolactone, and the angiotensin-converting enzyme [ACE] inhibitors) reduce BNP concentrations. Therefore, many people with chronic stable heart failure have BNP levels in the normal diagnostic range. However, digoxin and beta-blockers appear to increase BNP levels. There are medications designed to inhibit degradation of NPs as a potential for therapy.

Endothelins. The endothelins, released from the endothelial cells throughout the circulation, are potent vasoconstrictor peptides. Like angiotensin II, endothelin can also be synthesized and released by a variety of cell types, such as cardiac myocytes. Four endothelin peptides (endothelin-1 [ET-1], ET-2, ET-3, and ET-4) have been identified. It has been found that the endothelins induce vascular smooth muscle cell proliferation and cardiac myocyte hypertrophy; increase the release of ANP, aldosterone, and catecholamines; and exert antinatriuretic effects on the kidneys. Production of ET-1 is regulated by many factors that are significant for cardiovascular function and have implications for heart failure. Plasma ET-1 levels also correlate directly with pulmonary vascular resistance, and it is thought that the peptide may play a role in mediating pulmonary hypertension in people with heart failure. There are at least two types of endothelin receptors—type A and type B. Type A receptor is associated with smooth muscle constriction and hypertrophy, whereas type B receptor is associated with vasodilation. Because ET-1 can act on the heart to cause hypertrophy and sodium and water retention, an endothelin receptor antagonist is now available for use in people with pulmonary arterial hypertension due to severe heart failure.

Inflammatory Mediators. There is ongoing research examining the relationship between inflammatory markers, especially CRP, and heart failure. Elevated CRP levels have been associated with adverse consequences in people with heart failure. They have also been shown to be predictive of the development of heart failure in high-risk groups. Of particular interest are the interactions between CRP and mediators, such as angiotensin II and norepinephrine. This inflammatory relationship continues to be examined. However, it is difficult to test because it is not understood how to decrease the inflammatory effect in heart failure.

Myocardial Hypertrophy and Remodeling. The development of myocardial hypertrophy constitutes one of the principal mechanisms by which the heart compensates for an increase in workload.[48,49] Although ventricular hypertrophy improves the work performance of the heart, it is also an important risk factor for subsequent cardiac morbidity and mortality. Inappropriate hypertrophy and remodeling can result in changes in structure (*i.e.*, muscle mass, chamber dilation) and function (*i.e.*, impaired systolic or diastolic function) that often lead to further pump dysfunction and hemodynamic overload.

Myocardial hypertrophy and remodeling involve a series of complex events at both the molecular and cellular levels. The myocardium is composed of myocytes, or muscle cells, and nonmyocytes. The myocytes are the functional units of cardiac muscle. Their growth is limited by an increment in cell size, as opposed to an increase in cell number. The nonmyocytes include cardiac macrophages, fibroblasts, vascular smooth muscle, and endothelial cells. These cells, which are present in the interstitial space, remain capable of an increase in cell number and provide support for the myocytes. The nonmyocytes also determine many of the inappropriate changes that occur during myocardial hypertrophy. For example, uncontrolled cardiac fibroblast growth is associated with increased synthesis of collagen fibers, myocardial fibrosis, and ventricular wall stiffness. Not only does ventricular wall stiffness increase the workload of the heart, but the fibrosis and remodeling that occur may lead to electrical conduction abnormalities in which the heart contracts in an uncoordinated manner, known as *cardiac dyssynchrony*, causing reduced systolic heart function.[47]

Recent research has focused on the type of hypertrophy that develops in people with heart failure. At the cellular level, cardiac muscle cells respond to stimuli from stress placed on the ventricular wall by pressure and volume overload by initiating several different processes that lead to hypertrophy. These include stimuli that produce the following:

- *Symmetric hypertrophy* with a proportionate increase in muscle length and width, as occurs in athletes
- *Concentric hypertrophy* with an increase in wall thickness, as occurs in hypertension
- *Eccentric hypertrophy* with a disproportionate increase in muscle length, as occurs in DCM (Fig. 27.26)

When the primary stimulus for hypertrophy is *pressure overload*, the increase in wall stress leads to parallel replication of myofibrils, thickening of the individual myocytes, and concentric hypertrophy. Concentric hypertrophy may preserve systolic function for a time, but eventually the work performed by the ventricle exceeds the vascular reserve, predisposing to ischemia. When the primary stimulus is *ventricular volume overload*, the increase in wall stress leads to replication of myofibrils in series, elongation of the cardiac muscle cells, and eccentric hypertrophy. Eccentric hypertrophy leads to a decrease in ventricular wall thickness with an increase in diastolic volume and wall tension.

Acute Heart Failure Syndromes

The AHFS are "defined as gradual or rapid changes in heart failure signs and symptoms resulting in a need for urgent therapy."[50] These symptoms are primarily the result of severe pulmonary edema due to elevated left ventricular filling pressures, with or without a low cardiac output.[50] The syndromes are among the most common disorders seen in emergency departments, and chronic heart failure, often complicated by episodes of acute worsening, is the most common cause of the syndrome.

AHFS are thought to encompass three different types of conditions:

1. Worsening of chronic systolic or diastolic dysfunction that appears to respond to treatment, approximately 80%
2. New-onset acute heart failure that occurs secondary to a precipitating event such as a large myocardial infarction or a sudden increase in blood pressure superimposed on a noncompliant LV
3. Worsening of end-stage/advanced heart failure that is refractory to treatment, with predominantly left ventricular systolic dysfunction associated with a low-output state[50,51]

The difference between new-onset AHFS and AHFS caused by chronic heart failure is in the degree of physiologic response, which is more pronounced in the new-onset AHFS and subtler in chronic heart failure because of the compensatory pathophysiology. For example, with new-onset AHFS, the person will have a stronger sympathetic response with enhanced pulmonary vascular permeability causing rapid and dramatic symptoms of pulmonary edema. Because many compensatory mechanisms operate in people with chronic heart failure, they tolerate higher pulmonary vascular pressures. Chronic changes in neurohormonal regulation lead to stronger activation of the angiotensin–aldosterone system with a resultant volume overload, and venous congestion becomes more prominent in both the systemic and pulmonary circulations.

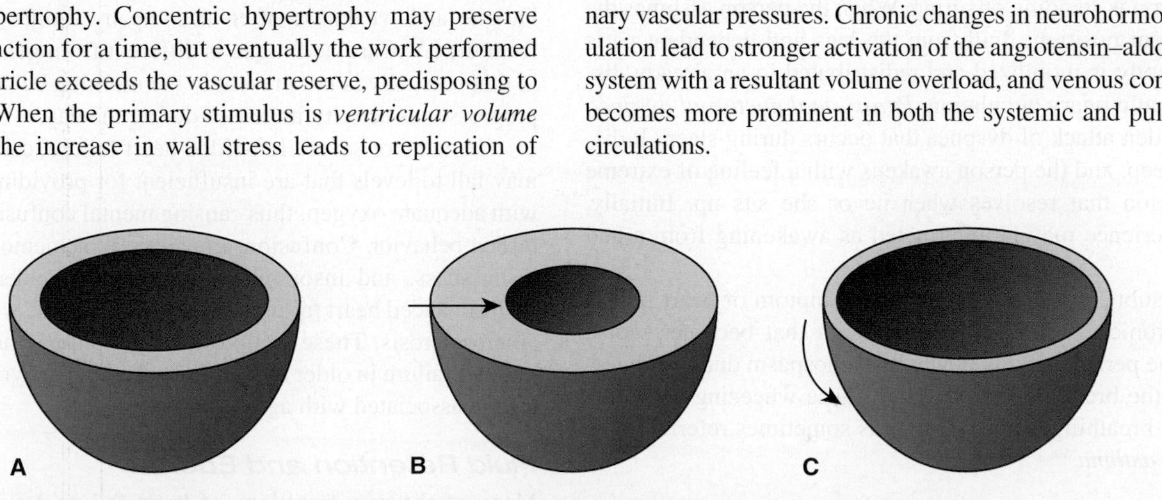

Figure 27.26 • Different types of myocardial hypertrophy. **(A)** Normal symmetric hypertrophy with proportionate increases in myocardial wall thickness and length. **(B)** Concentric hypertrophy with a disproportionate increase in wall thickness. **(C)** Eccentric hypertrophy with a disproportionate decrease in wall thickness and ventricular dilation.

Clinical Manifestations of Heart Failure

The manifestations of heart failure depend on the extent and type of cardiac dysfunction that is present and the rapidity with which it develops. A person with previously stable compensated heart failure may develop signs of heart failure for the first time when the condition has advanced to a critical point, such as with a progressive increase in pulmonary hypertension in a person with mitral valve regurgitation. Overt heart failure also may be precipitated by conditions such as infection, emotional stress, uncontrolled hypertension, or fluid overload.[50] Many people with serious underlying heart disease, regardless of whether they have previously experienced heart failure, may be relatively asymptomatic as long they carefully adhere to their treatment regimen. A dietary excess of sodium is a frequent cause of sudden cardiac decompensation.

The manifestations of heart failure reflect the physiologic effects of the impaired pumping ability of the heart, decreased renal blood flow, and activation of the sympathetic compensatory mechanisms. The severity and progression of symptoms depend on the extent and type of dysfunction that is present (systolic versus diastolic, right- versus left-sided). The signs and symptoms include shortness of breath and other respiratory manifestations, fatigue and limited exercise tolerance, fluid retention and edema, cachexia and malnutrition, and cyanosis. People with severe heart failure may exhibit diaphoresis and tachycardia.

Respiratory Manifestations

Shortness of breath due to congestion of the pulmonary circulation is one of the major manifestations of left-sided heart failure. Perceived shortness of breath (*i.e.*, breathlessness) is called *dyspnea*. Dyspnea related to an increase in activity is called *exertional dyspnea*. *Orthopnea* is shortness of breath that occurs when a person is supine. Gravitational forces cause fluid to become sequestered in the lower legs and feet when the person is standing or sitting. When the person assumes the recumbent position, fluid from the legs and dependent parts of the body is mobilized and redistributed to an already distended pulmonary circulation. *Paroxysmal nocturnal dyspnea* is a sudden attack of dyspnea that occurs during sleep. It disrupts sleep, and the person awakens with a feeling of extreme suffocation that resolves when he or she sits up. Initially, the experience may be interpreted as awakening from a bad dream.

A subtle and often overlooked symptom of heart failure is a chronic dry, nonproductive cough that becomes worse when the person is lying down. Bronchospasm due to congestion of the bronchial mucosa may cause wheezing and difficulty in breathing. This condition is sometimes referred to as *cardiac asthma*.[50]

Cheyne-Stokes Respiration. Cheyne-Stokes respiration is a pattern of periodic breathing characterized by gradual increase in depth (and sometimes rate) of breathing to a maximum, followed by a decrease resulting in apnea. Although no longer associated solely with heart failure, it is recognized as an independent risk factor for worsening of heart failure. It has been suggested that Cheyne-Stokes respirations may not be just a marker for increasing severity of heart failure but may also aggravate it.[50] During sleep, Cheyne-Stokes breathing causes recurrent awakening and thereby reduces slow-wave and rapid eye movement (REM) sleep. The recurrent cycling of hypoventilation/apnea and hyperventilation may also increase sympathetic activity and predispose to arrhythmias. Nocturnal oxygen has been seen to improve sleep, exercise tolerance, and cognitive function.

Acute Pulmonary Edema. Acute pulmonary edema is the most dramatic symptom of AHFS. It is a life-threatening condition in which capillary fluid moves into the alveoli.[50,52] The accumulated fluid in the alveoli and airways causes lung stiffness, makes lung expansion more difficult, and impairs the gas exchange function of the lung. With the decreased ability of the lungs to oxygenate the blood, the hemoglobin leaves the pulmonary circulation without being fully oxygenated, resulting in shortness of breath and cyanosis.

The person with severe pulmonary edema is usually seen sitting and gasping for air. The pulse is rapid, the skin is moist and cool, and the lips and nail beds are cyanotic. As the pulmonary edema worsens and oxygen supply to the brain drops, confusion and stupor appear. Dyspnea and air hunger are accompanied by a productive cough with frothy (resembling beaten egg whites) and often blood-tinged sputum—the effect of air mixing with the serum albumin and red blood cells that have moved into the alveoli. The movement of air through the alveolar fluid produces fine crepitant sounds called *crackles*, which can be heard with chest auscultation. As fluid moves into the larger airways, the crackles become louder and coarser.

Fatigue, Weakness, and Mental Confusion

Fatigue and weakness often accompany diminished output from the LV. Cardiac fatigue is different from general fatigue in that it usually is not present in the morning but appears and progresses as activity increases during the day.

In acute or severe left-sided heart failure, cardiac output may fall to levels that are insufficient for providing the brain with adequate oxygen, thus causing mental confusion and disturbed behavior. Confusion, impairment of memory, anxiety, restlessness, and insomnia are common in elderly persons with advanced heart failure, particularly in those with cerebral atherosclerosis. These symptoms may confuse the diagnosis of heart failure in older adults because of their myriad of other causes associated with aging.

Fluid Retention and Edema

Many of the manifestations of heart failure result from the increased capillary pressures (increased hydrostatic pressures) that develop in the peripheral circulation in people with right-sided heart failure and in the pulmonary circulation in people with left-sided heart failure. The increased capillary pressure reflects an overfilling of the vascular system because of increased sodium and water retention and venous congestion, referred to earlier as *backward* failure, resulting from impaired cardiac output.[50,52]

Nocturia is a nightly increase in urine output that occurs relatively early in the course of heart failure. It occurs because of the increased cardiac output, renal blood flow, and glomerular filtration rate that follow the increased blood return to the heart when the person is in a supine position. *Oliguria*, which is a decrease in urine output, is a late sign related to a severely reduced cardiac output and resultant renal failure.

Transudation of fluid into the pleural cavity (hydrothorax) or the peritoneal cavity (ascites) may occur in people with advanced heart failure. Because the pleural veins drain into both the systemic and pulmonary venous beds, hydrothorax is observed more commonly in people with hypertension involving both venous systems.[50] Pleural effusion occurs as the excess fluid in the lung interstitial spaces crosses the visceral pleura, which in turn overwhelms the capacity of the pulmonary lymphatic system. Ascites occurs in people with increased pressure in the hepatic veins and veins draining the peritoneum. It usually reflects right ventricular failure and long-standing elevation of systemic venous pressure in chronic heart failure.[50,51]

Cachexia and Malnutrition

Cardiac cachexia is a condition of malnutrition and tissue wasting that occurs in people with end-stage heart failure. A number of factors probably contribute to its development, including the fatigue and depression that interfere with food intake, congestion of the liver and gastrointestinal structures that impairs digestion and absorption and produces feelings of fullness, and the circulating toxins and mediators released from poorly perfused tissues that impair appetite and contribute to tissue wasting.

Cyanosis

Cyanosis is the bluish discoloration of the skin and mucous membranes caused by excess desaturated hemoglobin in the blood; it often is a late sign of heart failure. Cyanosis may be central, caused by arterial desaturation resulting from impaired pulmonary gas exchange, or peripheral, caused by venous desaturation resulting from extensive extraction of oxygen at the capillary level. Central cyanosis is caused by conditions that impair oxygenation of the arterial blood, such as pulmonary edema, left heart failure, or right-to-left cardiac shunting. Peripheral cyanosis is caused by conditions such as low-output heart failure that result in delivery of poorly oxygenated blood to the peripheral tissues or by conditions such as peripheral vasoconstriction that cause excessive removal of oxygen from the blood. Central cyanosis is best monitored in the lips and mucous membranes because these areas are not subject to conditions, such as a cold environment, that cause peripheral cyanosis. People with right-sided or left-sided heart failure may develop cyanosis especially around the lips and in the peripheral parts of the extremities.

Arrhythmias and Sudden Cardiac Death

Both atrial and ventricular arrhythmias occur in people with heart failure. Atrial fibrillation is the most common arrhythmia. Clinical manifestations associated with atrial fibrillation are related to loss of atrial contraction, tachycardia, irregular heart rate, and a drop in blood pressure.[50–52] There is also strong evidence that people with heart failure are at increased risk for sudden cardiac arrest, that is, unwitnessed death or death that occurs within 1 hour of the symptom onset.[50–52] In people with ventricular dysfunction, sudden death is caused most commonly by ventricular tachycardia or ventricular fibrillation.

Diagnosis and Treatment

Diagnosis. Diagnostic methods in heart failure are directed toward establishing the cause of the disorder and determining the extent of the dysfunction. Medical guidelines for diagnosis and treatment are clearly described in the AHA guidelines for heart failure management.[53] Because heart failure represents the failure of the heart as a pump and can occur in the course of a number of heart diseases or other systemic disorders, the diagnosis of heart failure often is based on signs and symptoms related to the failing heart itself, such as shortness of breath and fatigue. The functional classification of the New York Heart Association (NYHA) is one guide to classifying the extent of dysfunction.

The NYHA functional classification classifies dysfunction into four classes[50]:

1. Class I—People who have known heart disease without symptoms during ordinary activity
2. Class II—People who have heart disease who have slight limitations but not extreme fatigue, palpitations, dyspnea, or angina pain during regular activity
3. Class III—People with heart disease who are comfortable at rest but ordinary activity does result in fatigue, palpitations, dyspnea, and angina pain
4. Class IV—People who have marked progressive cardiac disease and are not comfortable at rest or minimal activity

The methods used in the diagnosis of heart failure include risk factor assessment, history and physical examination, laboratory studies, ECG, chest radiography, and echocardiography. The history should include information related to dyspnea, cough, nocturia, generalized fatigue, and other signs and symptoms of heart failure. A complete physical examination includes assessment of heart rate, heart sounds, blood pressure, jugular veins for venous congestion, lungs for signs of pulmonary congestion, and lower extremities for edema. Laboratory tests are used in the diagnosis of anemia and electrolyte imbalances and to detect signs of chronic liver congestion. Measurements of BNP and NT-proBNP can be useful if the diagnosis of heart failure is uncertain and as risk stratification. The use of serial BNP or NT-proBNP levels has not yet been well established.

Echocardiography plays a key role in assessing right and left ventricular wall motion (normal, akinesis, or hypokinesis), wall thickness, ventricular chamber size, valve function, heart defects, ejection fraction, and pericardial disease. ECG findings may indicate atrial or ventricular hypertrophy, underlying disorders of cardiac rhythm, or conduction abnormalities such as right or left bundle branch block. Radionuclide ventriculography and cardiac angiography are recommended if there is reason to suspect CAD as the underlying cause for heart failure. Chest x-rays provide information about the size and shape of the heart and pulmonary vasculature. The cardiac silhouette can be used to detect cardiac hypertrophy and dilation. Chest x-rays can indicate the relative severity of the failure by revealing if pulmonary edema is predominantly vascular or interstitial or has advanced to the alveolar and bronchial stages. Cardiac magnetic resonance imaging (CMRI) and cardiac computed tomography (CCT) are used to document ejection fraction, ventricular preload, and regional wall motion.

Invasive hemodynamic monitoring may be used for assessment in acute, life-threatening episodes of heart failure. These monitoring methods include CVP, pulmonary artery pressure monitoring, thermodilution measurements of cardiac output, and intra-arterial measurements of blood pressure. CVP reflects the amount of blood returning to the heart. Measurements of CVP are best obtained by a catheter inserted into the superior vena cava–right atrial junction through a peripheral vein or by the right atrial port (opening) in a pulmonary artery catheter. This pressure is decreased in hypovolemia and increased in right-sided heart failure. The changes that occur in CVP over time usually are more significant than the absolute numeric values obtained during a single reading.

Ventricular volume pressures are obtained by means of a flow-directed, balloon-tipped pulmonary artery catheter. This catheter is introduced through a peripheral or central vein and then advanced into the right atrium. The balloon is then inflated with air, enabling the catheter to float through the right ventricle into the pulmonary artery until it becomes wedged in a small pulmonary vessel (Fig. 27.27). With the balloon inflated, the catheter monitors pulmonary capillary pressures (also called *pulmonary capillary wedge pressure* [PCWP]), which is in direct communication with pressures from the left heart. The pulmonary capillary pressures provide a means of assessing the pumping ability of the left heart.

Intra-arterial blood pressure monitoring provides a means for continuous monitoring of blood pressure. It is used in people with acute heart failure when aggressive intravenous medication therapy or a mechanical assist device is required. Measurements are obtained through a small catheter inserted into a peripheral artery, usually the radial artery. The catheter is connected to a pressure transducer, and beat-by-beat measurements of blood pressure are recorded. The monitoring system displays the contour of the pressure waveform and the systolic, diastolic, and mean arterial pressures, along with the heart rate and rhythm.

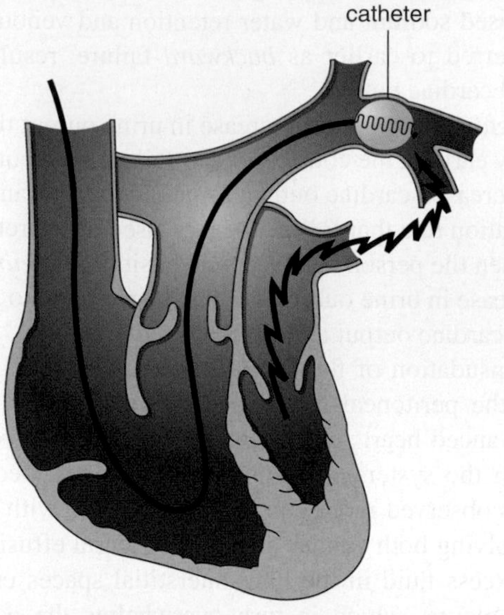

Figure 27.27 • Balloon-tipped pulmonary artery catheter positioned in a small pulmonary vessel. The PCWP, which reflects the left ventricular diastolic pressure, is measured with the balloon inflated.

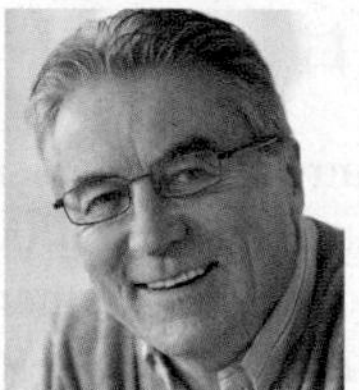

Remember Mr. Brown from the unit opener case study? He was diagnosed with high blood pressure and hypercholesterolemia. His subsequent cardiac catheterization revealed mild ischemic occlusion that did not meet the criteria for a cardiac stent or angioplasty. This result, along with his low ejection fraction of 40%, indicated that the supply of oxygen to his heart muscle was moderately impaired, reducing the force developed by the LV. Therefore, he was diagnosed with ischemic cardiomyopathy and was classified as having Stage B (American Heart Association) and class II (NYHA) heart failure.

Treatment. The goals of treatment are determined by the rapidity of onset and severity of the heart failure. People with AHFS require urgent therapy directed at stabilizing and correcting the cause of the cardiac dysfunction. For people with chronic heart failure, the goals of treatment are directed toward relieving the symptoms, improving the quality of life, and reducing or eliminating risk factors (*e.g.*, hypertension, diabetes, obesity) with a long-term goal of slowing, halting, or reversing the cardiac dysfunction.[50–53]

Treatment measures for both acute and chronic heart failure include nonpharmacologic and pharmacologic approaches. Mechanical support devices, including the intra-aortic balloon pump (for acute failure) and the ventricular assist device (VAD), sustain life in people with severe heart failure. Heart transplantation remains the treatment of choice for many people with end-stage heart failure.

Nonpharmacologic Methods. Exercise intolerance is typical in people with chronic heart failure.[51] Consequently, individualized exercise training is important to maximize muscle conditioning. People who are not accustomed to exercise and those with more severe heart failure are started at a lower intensity and shorter sessions than those who are mostly asymptomatic. Sodium and fluid restriction and weight management are important for all people with heart failure individualized to the severity of heart failure. Counseling, health teaching, and ongoing evaluation programs help people with heart failure to manage and cope with their treatment regimen.

Pharmacologic Treatment. Once heart failure is moderate to severe, pharmacologic in conjunction with nonpharmacologic management is important to prevent and treat acute heart failure and manage chronic heart failure. Evidence-based agents recommended for treatment and management include diuretics, ACE inhibitors or angiotensin II receptor blockers, β-adrenergic blockers, and digoxin.[50–53] The choice of pharmacologic agents is based on symptomatology of the person.

Diuretics are among the most frequently prescribed medications for moderate to severe heart failure.[50–53] They promote the excretion of fluid and help to sustain cardiac output and tissue perfusion by reducing preload and allowing the heart to operate at a more optimal part of the Frank-Starling curve. Thiazide and loop diuretics are both used. In emergencies, such as acute pulmonary edema, loop diuretics such as furosemide can be administered intravenously. When given as a bolus infusion, intravenous furosemide acts within minutes to increase venous capacitance so that right ventricular output and pulmonary capillary pressures are decreased.

The *ACE inhibitors*, which prevent the conversion of angiotensin I to angiotensin II, have been used effectively in the treatment of chronic heart failure. The renin–angiotensin–aldosterone system is activated early in the course of heart failure and plays an important role in its progression. It results in an increase in angiotensin II, which causes vasoconstriction, unregulated ventricular remodeling, and increased aldosterone production with a subsequent increase in sodium and water retention by the kidneys. ACE inhibitors have been shown to limit these harmful complications. The *angiotensin II receptor blockers* appear to have similar but more limited beneficial effects. They have the advantage of not causing a cough, which is a troublesome side effect of the ACE inhibitors for many people. Aldosterone has a number of deleterious effects in people with heart failure. *Aldosterone receptor antagonists* may be used in combination with other agents for people with moderately severe to severe heart failure.

β-Adrenergic receptor blocking drugs are used to decrease left ventricular dysfunction associated with activation of the sympathetic nervous system. Large clinical trials have shown that long-term therapy with β-adrenergic receptor blocking agents reduces morbidity and mortality in people with chronic heart failure. The mechanism of this benefit remains unclear, but it is likely that chronic elevations of catecholamines and sympathetic nervous system activity cause progressive myocardial damage, leading to a worsening of left ventricular function and a poorer prognosis in people with heart failure. Large, landmark clinical trials of people with stable NYHA class II and III heart failure have demonstrated significant reductions in the overall mortality rate with treatment with various β-adrenergic receptor blocking agents.[52,53]

Digitalis has been a recognized treatment for heart failure for over 200 years. The various forms of digitalis are called *cardiac glycosides*. They improve cardiac function by increasing the force and strength of ventricular contractions. By decreasing SA node activity and decreasing conduction through the AV node, they also slow the heart rate and increase diastolic filling time. Although not a diuretic, digitalis promotes urine output by improving cardiac output and renal blood flow. The role of digitalis in the treatment of heart failure has been studied in clinical trials over the past several decades. The results of these studies remain controversial and mixed; there seems to be a growing consensus that although it does not necessarily reduce mortality rates, digitalis can possibly prevent clinical deterioration and hospitalization.

Vasodilator drugs have not been extensively studied as a lone treatment for the management of heart failure but can be effective in symptom management. Agents such as isosorbide dinitrate and hydralazine may be added to other standard medications for people with chronic heart failure. Vasodilators such as nitroglycerin, nitroprusside, and nesiritide (B-type NP) are used in AHFS to improve left heart performance by decreasing the preload (through vasodilation) or reducing the afterload (through arteriolar dilation), or both.[52,53]

Oxygen Therapy. Oxygen therapy increases the oxygen content of the blood and is most often used in people with acute episodes of heart failure. Continuous positive airway pressure (CPAP) is recommended to reduce the need for endotracheal intubation in people with AHFS. Because CPAP increases intrathoracic pressure, it also has the potential for decreasing venous return and left ventricular preload, thereby improving the cardiac ejection fraction and stabilizing the hemodynamic status in persons with severe heart failure. Bilevel positive airway pressure (BiPAP), which is like CPAP but also delivers higher pressures during inspiration, is argued by some to be superior to CPAP in that it decreases the respiratory rate and heart rate and improves oxygenation more quickly or more substantially than CPAP.[53]

Cardiac Resynchronization and Implantable Cardioverter–Defibrillators. Some people with heart failure have abnormal intraventricular conduction that results in dyssynchronous and ineffective contractions. Cardiac resynchronization therapy involves the placement of pacing leads into the right ventricle and LVs as a means of resynchronizing the contraction of the two ventricles. Cardiac resynchronization has been shown to improve ventricular function and blood pressure, improve quality of life, and reduce the risk of death.[54]

People with heart failure are at significant risk of SCD from ventricular fibrillation or ventricular tachycardia.

Implantation of a cardioverter–defibrillator is indicated in selected people with heart failure to prevent SCD.[54] A cardioverter–defibrillator is a programmable implanted device that monitors the cardiac rhythm. It has the capacity to pace the heart and deliver electrical shocks to terminate lethal arrhythmias when needed.

Mechanical Support and Heart Transplantation. Refractory heart failure reflects deterioration in cardiac function that is unresponsive to medical or surgical interventions. With improved methods of treatment, more people are reaching a point where a cure is unachievable and death is imminent without mechanical support or heart transplantation.

Since the early 1960s, significant progress has been made in improving the efficacy of *VADs*, which are mechanical pumps used to support ventricular function. VADs are used to decrease the workload of the myocardium while maintaining cardiac output and systemic arterial pressure. This decreases the workload of the ventricle and allows it to rest and recover. They may be used in people who fail or have difficulty being weaned from cardiopulmonary bypass after cardiac surgery, those who develop cardiogenic shock after myocardial infarction, those with end-stage cardiomyopathy, and those who are awaiting cardiac transplantation. Earlier and more aggressive use of VADs as a bridge to transplantation and destination therapy (permanent support) has been shown to increase survival.[55] VADs that allow the person to be mobile and managed at home are sometimes used for long-term or permanent support for treatment of end-stage heart failure, rather than simply as a bridge to transplantation. VADs can be used to support the function of the LV, right ventricle, or both.[55]

Heart transplantation is the preferred treatment for people with end-stage cardiac failure and otherwise good life expectancy.[55] Despite the overall success of heart transplantation, donor availability remains a key problem, and only about 5000 procedures are completed each year with thousands being denied transplantation each year.

Other novel surgical therapies that are being explored include left ventricular remodeling. Left ventricular remodeling is a surgical procedure designed to restore the size and shape of the ventricle and is thought to be a viable surgical alternative to cardiac transplantation for people with severe left ventricular dysfunction.[55]

IN SUMMARY

Heart failure occurs when the heart fails to pump sufficient blood to meet the metabolic needs of body tissues. The physiology of heart failure reflects the interplay between a decrease in cardiac output that accompanies impaired function of the failing heart and the compensatory mechanisms that preserve the cardiac reserve. Compensatory mechanisms include the Frank-Starling mechanism, sympathetic nervous system activation, the renin–angiotensin–aldosterone mechanism, NPs, the endothelins, and myocardial hypertrophy and remodeling. In the failing heart, early decreases in cardiac function may go unnoticed because these compensatory mechanisms maintain the cardiac output. In severe and prolonged heart failure, the compensatory mechanisms no longer are effective and instead contribute to the progression of heart failure.

Heart failure may be described in terms of systolic versus diastolic dysfunction and right ventricular versus left ventricular dysfunction. With systolic dysfunction, there is impaired ejection of blood from the heart during systole; with diastolic dysfunction, there is impaired filling of the heart during diastole. Right ventricular dysfunction is characterized by congestion in the peripheral circulation and left ventricular dysfunction by congestion in the pulmonary circulation. Heart failure can present as a chronic condition characterized by decreased cardiac function or as an AHFS. The AHFS represents a gradual or rapid change in heart failure signs and symptoms, indicating need for urgent therapy. These symptoms are primarily the result of pulmonary congestion due to elevated left ventricular filling pressures with or without a low cardiac output.

The manifestations of heart failure include edema, nocturia, fatigue and impaired exercise tolerance, cyanosis, signs of increased sympathetic nervous system activity, and impaired gastrointestinal function and malnutrition. In right-sided heart failure, there is dependent edema of the lower parts of the body, engorgement of the liver, and ascites. In left-sided heart failure, pulmonary congestion with shortness of breath and chronic, nonproductive cough are common.

The diagnostic methods in heart failure are directed toward establishing the cause and extent of the disorder. Treatment is directed toward correcting the cause whenever possible, improving cardiac function, maintaining the fluid volume within a compensatory range, and developing an activity pattern consistent with individual limitations in cardiac reserve. Among the medications used in the treatment of heart failure are diuretics, ACE inhibitors and angiotensin receptor blocking agents, β-adrenergic receptor blockers, digoxin, and vasodilators. Mechanical support devices, including the VADs, sustain life in people with severe heart failure. Heart transplantation remains the treatment of choice for many people with end-stage heart failure.

HEART DISEASE IN INFANTS AND CHILDREN

After completing this section of the chapter, the learner will be able to meet the following objectives:

- Describe the flow of blood in the fetal circulation, state the function of the foramen ovale and ductus arteriosus, and describe the changes in circulatory function that occur at birth.
- Describe the anatomic defects and altered patterns of blood flow in children with atrial septal defects, ventricular septal defects, endocardial cushion defects, pulmonary stenosis, tetralogy of Fallot, patent ductus arteriosus, transposition of

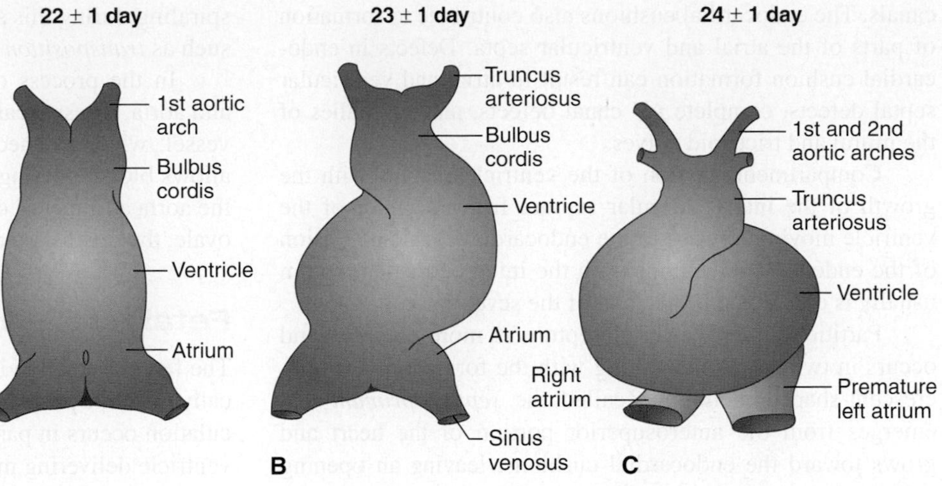

Figure 27.28 • Ventral view of the developing heart. **(A)** Fusion of the heart tubes to form a single tube; it is at this stage that the heart begins to beat. **(B)** Cardiac looping, in which the heart begins to bend ventrally and to the right, bringing the primitive ventricle leftward and in continuity with the sinus venosus (future left and right atria), with the future right ventricle being shifted rightward and in continuity with the bulbus cordis (future aorta and pulmonary artery), and **(C)** folding is complete.

the great vessels, coarctation of the aorta, and single-ventricle anatomy.
- Describe the manifestations related to the acute, subacute, and convalescent phases of Kawasaki disease.

Approximately 1 of every 115 to 125 infants born has a congenital heart defect, making this the most common form of structural birth defect.[1] Advances in diagnostic methods and surgical treatment have greatly increased the long-term survival and outcomes for children born with congenital heart defects. Surgical correction of most defects is now possible, often within the first weeks of life, and the majority of affected children are expected to survive into adulthood.

Although thousands of infants born each year will have a congenital heart disease, other children will develop an acquired heart disease, including Kawasaki disease.

Embryonic Development of the Heart

The heart is the first functioning organ in the embryo. Its first pulsatile movements begin during the third week after conception. This early development of the heart is essential to the rapidly growing embryo as a means of circulating nutrients and removing waste products. Most of the development of the heart and blood vessels occurs between the third and eighth weeks of embryonic life.[56]

The developing heart begins as two endothelial tubes that fuse into a single tubular structure.[56] The early heart structures develop as the tubular heart elongates and forms alternating dilations and constrictions. A single atrium and ventricle along with the bulbus cordis develop first (Fig. 27.28). This is followed by formation of the truncus arteriosus and the sinus venosus, a large venous sinus that receives blood from the embryo and developing placenta. The early pulsatile movements of the heart begin in the sinus venosus and move blood out of the heart by way of the bulbus cordis, truncus arteriosus, and aortic arches.

A differential growth rate in the early cardiac structures, along with fixation of the heart at the venous and arterial ends, causes the tubular heart to bend over on itself. As the heart bends, the atrium and the sinus venosus come to lie behind the bulbus cordis, truncus arteriosus, and ventricle. This looping of the primitive heart results in the heart's alignment in the left side of the chest with the atrium located behind the ventricle. Malrotation during formation of the ventricular loop can cause various malpositions, such as dextroposition of the heart.

The embryonic heart undergoes further development as partitioning of the chambers occurs. Partitioning of the AV canal, atrium, and ventricle begins in the fourth week and essentially is complete by the fifth week. Septation of the heart begins as tissue bundles called the *endocardial cushions* form in the midportion of the dorsal and ventral walls of the heart in the region of the AV canal and begin to grow inward. Until septation begins, a single AV canal exists between the atria and the ventricles. As the endocardial cushions enlarge, they meet and fuse to form separate right and left AV canals (Fig. 27.29). The mitral and tricuspid valves develop in these

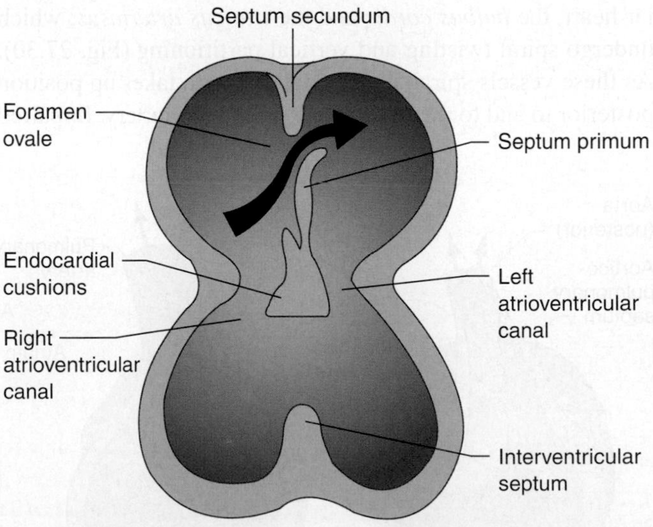

Figure 27.29 • Development of the endocardial cushions, right and left AV canals, interventricular septum, and septum primum and septum secundum of the foramen ovale. Note that blood from the right atrium flows through the foramen ovale to the left atrium.

canals. The endocardial cushions also contribute to formation of parts of the atrial and ventricular septa. Defects in endocardial cushion formation can result in atrial and ventricular septal defects, complete AV canal defects, and anomalies of the mitral and tricuspid valves.

Compartmentalization of the ventricles begins with the growth of the interventricular septum from the floor of the ventricle moving upward to the endocardial cushions. Fusion of the endocardial cushions with the interventricular septum usually is completed by the end of the seventh week.

Partitioning of the atrial septum is more complex and occurs in two stages, beginning with the formation of a thin, crescent-shaped membrane called the *septum primum* that emerges from the anterosuperior portion of the heart and grows toward the endocardial cushions, leaving an opening called the *foramen primum* between its lower edge and the endocardial cushions. A second membrane, called *septum secundum*, also begins to grow from the upper wall of the atrium on the right side of the septum primum. As this membrane grows toward the endocardial cushions, it gradually overlaps an opening in the upper part of the septum primum, forming an oval opening with a flap-type valve called the *foramen ovale* (Fig. 27.22). The upper part of the septum primum gradually disappears, with the remaining part becoming the valve of the foramen ovale. The foramen ovale forms a communicating channel between the two upper chambers of the heart. This opening, which typically closes shortly after birth, allows blood from the umbilical vein to pass directly into the left heart, bypassing the lungs.

To complete the transformation into a four-chambered heart, provision must be made for separating the blood pumped from the right side of the heart, which is to be diverted into the pulmonary circulation, from the blood pumped from the left side of the heart, which is to be pumped to the systemic circulation. This separation of blood flow is accomplished by developmental changes in the outflow channels of the tubular heart, the *bulbus cordis* and the *truncus arteriosus*, which undergo spiral twisting and vertical partitioning (Fig. 27.30). As these vessels spiral and divide, the aorta takes up position posterior to and to the right of the pulmonary artery. Impaired spiraling during this stage of development can lead to defects such as *transposition of the great vessels*.

In the process of forming a separate pulmonary trunk and aorta, a vessel called the *ductus arteriosus* develops. This vessel, which connects the pulmonary artery and the aorta, allows blood entering the pulmonary trunk to be shunted into the aorta as a means of bypassing the lungs. Like the foramen ovale, the ductus arteriosus usually closes shortly after birth.[56]

Fetal and Perinatal Circulation

The fetal circulation is different anatomically and physiologically from the postnatal circulation. Blood flow in the fetal circulation occurs in parallel rather than in series, with the right ventricle delivering most of its output to the placenta for oxygen uptake and the LV pumping blood to the heart, brain, and primarily upper body of the fetus.[57] Before birth, oxygenation of blood occurs through the placenta, and after birth, it occurs through the lungs. The fetus is maintained in a low-oxygen state (PO_2 30 to 35 mm Hg; hemoglobin O_2 saturation 60% to 70%). To compensate, fetal cardiac output is higher than at any other time in life (400 to 500 mL/kg/minute), and fetal hemoglobin has a higher affinity for oxygen.[57] Also, the pulmonary vessels in the fetus are markedly constricted because of the fluid-filled lungs and the heightened hypoxic stimulus for vasoconstriction that is present in the fetus. As a result, blood flow through the lungs is less than at any other time in life.

In the fetus, blood enters the circulation through the umbilical vein and returns to the placenta through the two umbilical arteries (Fig. 27.31). A vessel called the *ductus venosus* allows the majority of the blood from the umbilical vein to bypass the hepatic circulation and pass directly into the inferior vena cava. From the inferior vena cava, blood flows into the right atrium, where approximately 40% of the blood volume moves through the foramen ovale into the left atrium. It then passes into the LV and is ejected into the ascending aorta to perfuse the head and upper extremities. In this way, the best-oxygenated blood from the placenta is used to perfuse the brain. At the same time, venous blood from the head and upper extremities returns to the right side of the heart through

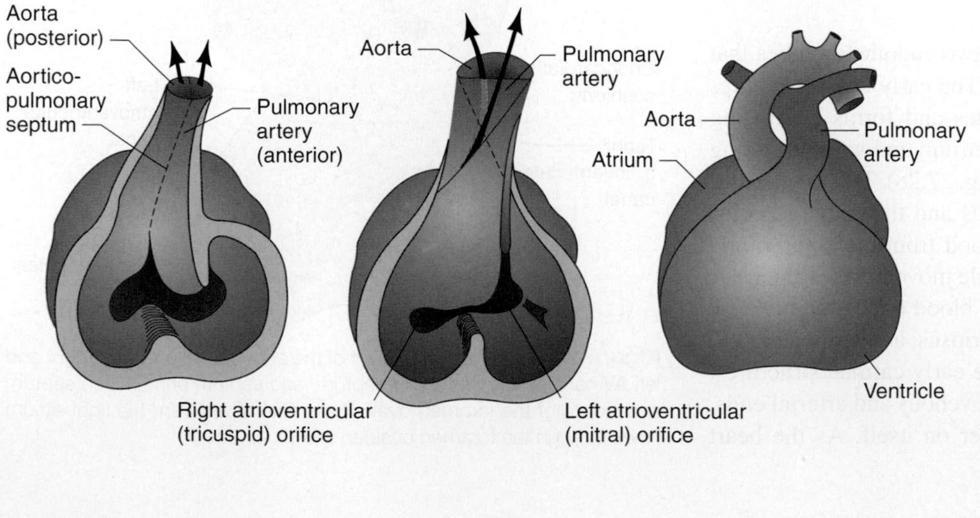

Figure 27.30 • Separation and twisting of the truncus arteriosus to form the pulmonary artery and aorta.

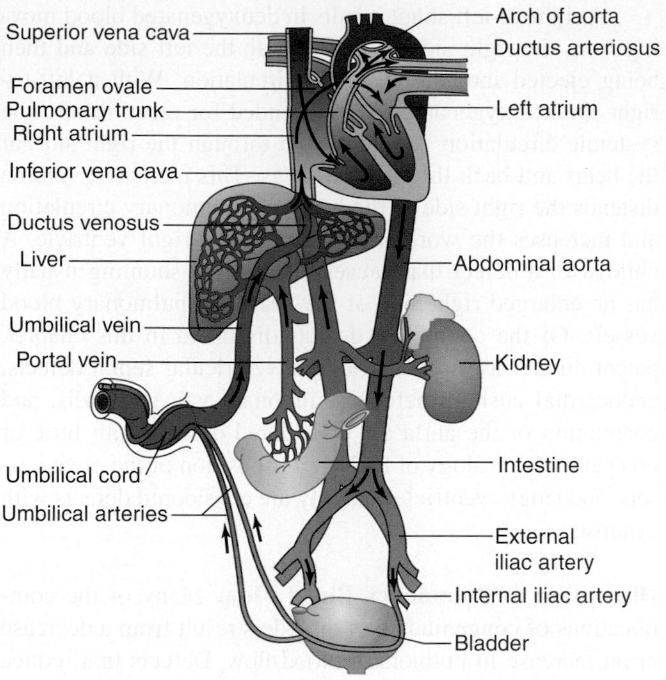

Figure 27.31 • Fetal circulation.

the superior vena cava, moves into the right ventricle, and is ejected into the pulmonary artery. Because of the very high pulmonary vascular resistance that is present, almost 90% of blood ejected into the pulmonary artery gets diverted through the ductus arteriosus into the descending aorta. This blood perfuses the lower extremities and is returned to the placenta by the umbilical arteries.

At birth, the infant takes its first breath and switches from placental to pulmonary oxygenation of the blood. The most dramatic alterations in the circulation after birth are the elimination of the low-resistance placental vascular bed and the marked pulmonary vasodilation that is produced by initiation of ventilation. Within minutes of birth, pulmonary blood flow increases from 35 mL/kg/minute to 160 to 200 mL/kg/minute.[57] The pressure in the pulmonary circulation and the right side of the heart falls as fetal lung fluid is replaced by air and as lung expansion decreases the pressure transmitted to the pulmonary blood vessels. With lung inflation, the alveolar oxygen tension increases, causing reversal of the hypoxemia-induced pulmonary vasoconstriction of the fetal circulation. Cord clamping and removal of the low-resistance placental circulation produce an increase in systemic vascular resistance and a resultant increase in left ventricular pressure. The resultant decrease in right atrial pressure and increase in left atrial pressure produce closure of the foramen ovale flap valve. Reversal of the fetal hypoxemic state also produces constriction of ductal smooth muscle, contributing to closure of the ductus arteriosus by 72 hours post birth. After the initial precipitous fall in pulmonary vascular resistance, a more gradual decrease in pulmonary vascular resistance is related to regression of the medial smooth muscle layer in the pulmonary arteries. During the first 2 to 9 weeks of life, gradual thinning of the smooth muscle layer results in further decreases in pulmonary vascular resistance. By the time a healthy, term infant is several weeks old, the pulmonary vascular resistance has fallen to adult levels.

Several factors, including alveolar hypoxia, prematurity, lung disease, and congenital heart defects, may affect postnatal pulmonary vascular development. Alveolar hypoxia is one of the most potent stimuli of pulmonary vasoconstriction and pulmonary hypertension in the neonate. During this period, the pulmonary arteries remain highly reactive and can constrict in response to hypoxia, acidosis, hyperinflation of the alveoli, and hypothermia. Thus, hypoxia during the first days of life may delay or prevent the normal decrease in pulmonary vascular resistance.

Much of the development of the smooth muscle layer in the pulmonary arterioles occurs during late gestation; as a result, infants born prematurely have less medial smooth muscle. These infants follow the same pattern of smooth muscle regression, but because less muscle exists, the muscle layer may regress in a shorter time. The pulmonary vascular smooth muscle in premature infants also may be less responsive to hypoxia. For these reasons, a premature infant may demonstrate a larger decrease in pulmonary vascular resistance and a resultant shunting of blood from the aorta through the ductus arteriosus to the pulmonary artery within hours of birth.

Congenital Heart Defects

The major development of the fetal heart occurs between the fourth and seventh weeks of gestation, and most congenital heart defects arise during this time. Most congenital heart defects are thought to be multifactorial in origin, resulting from an interaction between a genetic predisposition toward development of a heart defect and environmental influences.

Knowledge about the genetic basis of congenital heart defects has grown dramatically in recent years. This area of research is particularly important as more individuals with congenital heart disease survive into adulthood and consider having children of their own. Recent knowledge suggests that the genetic contribution to congenital heart disease has been underestimated in the past. Some heart defects, such as aortic stenosis, atrial septal defect of the secundum type, pulmonary valve stenosis, tetralogy of Fallot, and certain ventricular septal defects, have a stronger familial predisposition than others.

Chromosomal abnormalities are also associated with congenital heart defects, and as much as 30% of children with congenital heart disease have an associated chromosomal abnormality. Heart disease is found in nearly 100% of children with trisomy 18, 50% of those with trisomy 21, and 35% of those with Turner syndrome. Another syndrome with cardiac malformations is Williams syndrome (7q11.23 microdeletion), which is associated with supravalvar aortic and pulmonary stenoses.

As much as 30% of congenital cardiac defects may be attributable to identifiable and potentially modifiable risk factors, including teratogenic influences, and adverse maternal conditions such as febrile illnesses, systemic lupus erythematosus, diabetes mellitus, maternal alcohol ingestion, and treatment with anticonvulsant medications, retinoids, lithium, and other prescription or nonprescription drugs. Proper prenatal care, especially periconceptive multivitamin intake with folic acid, may reduce the risk of cardiac disease in the fetus.

Pathophysiology

Congenital heart defects produce their effects mainly through abnormal shunting of blood, production of cyanosis, and disruption of pulmonary blood flow.

Abnormal Shunting of Blood. Shunting of blood refers to the diversion of blood flow from one system to the other—from the arterial to the venous system (*i.e.*, left-to-right shunt) or from the venous to the arterial system (*i.e.*, right-to-left shunt). The shunting of blood in congenital heart defects is determined by the presence, position, and size of an abnormal opening between the right and left circulations and the degree of resistance to flow through the opening.

The vascular resistance of the systemic and pulmonary circulations influences the direction of shunting. Because of the high pulmonary vascular resistance in the neonate, atrial and ventricular septal defects usually do not produce significant shunt or symptoms during the first weeks of life.

As the pulmonary vascular smooth muscle regresses in the neonate, the resistance in the pulmonary circulation falls below that of the systemic circulation; in uncomplicated atrial or ventricular septal defects, blood shunts from the left side of the heart to the right. In more complicated ventricular septal defects, increased resistance to outflow may affect the pattern of shunting. For example, defects that increase resistance to aortic outflow (*e.g.*, aortic valve stenosis, coarctation of the aorta, hypoplastic left heart syndrome) increase left-to-right shunting, and defects that obstruct pulmonary outflow (*e.g.*, pulmonary valve stenosis, tetralogy of Fallot) increase right-to-left shunting.[58] Crying, defecating, or even the stress of feeding may increase pulmonary vascular resistance and cause an increase in right-to-left shunting and cyanosis in infants with septal defects.

Cyanotic Versus Acyanotic Disorders. Congenital heart diseases are commonly divided into two categories: acyanotic and cyanotic. Defects that result in a left-to-right shunt are usually categorized as acyanotic disorders because shunted systemic circulation blood mixing with pulmonary circulation blood is not enough to significantly change normal levels of oxygen saturation.

Defects that produce shunting of blood from the right to the left side of the heart or result in obstruction of pulmonary blood flow are categorized as cyanotic disorders.[58] Cyanosis, a bluish color of the skin, most notable in the nail beds and mucous membranes, develops when sufficient deoxygenated blood from the right side of the heart mixes with oxygenated blood in the left side of the heart. Abnormal color becomes obvious when the oxygen saturation falls below 80% in the capillaries (equal to 5 g of deoxygenated hemoglobin).

A right-to-left shunt results in deoxygenated blood moving from the right side of the heart to the left side and then being ejected into the systemic circulation. With a left-to-right shunt, oxygenated blood intended for ejection into the systemic circulation is recirculated through the right side of the heart and back through the lungs. This increased volume distends the right side of the heart and pulmonary circulation and increases the workload placed on the right ventricle. A child with a defect that causes left-to-right shunting usually has an enlarged right side of the heart and pulmonary blood vessels. Of the congenital defects discussed in this chapter, patent ductus arteriosus, atrial and ventricular septal defects, endocardial cushion defects, pulmonary valve stenosis, and coarctation of the aorta are considered defects with little or no cyanosis; tetralogy of Fallot, transposition of the great vessels, and single-ventricle anatomy are considered defects with cyanosis.

Disruption of Pulmonary Blood Flow. Many of the complications of congenital heart disorders result from a decrease or an increase in pulmonary blood flow. Defects that reduce pulmonary blood flow (*e.g.*, pulmonary stenosis) typically cause symptoms of fatigue, dyspnea, and failure to thrive. In contrast to the arterioles in the systemic circulation, the arterioles in the pulmonary circulation are normally thin-walled vessels that can accommodate the various levels of stroke volume that are ejected from the right heart. The thinning of the pulmonary vessels occurs during the first weeks after birth, during which the vessel media thin and pulmonary vascular resistance decreases. In a term infant who has a congenital heart defect that produces markedly increased pulmonary blood flow (*e.g.*, ventricular septal defect), the increased flow stimulates pulmonary vasoconstriction and delays or reduces the normal involutional thinning of the small pulmonary arterioles. In most cases during early infancy, pulmonary vascular resistance is only slightly elevated, and the major contribution to pulmonary hypertension is the increased blood flow. However, in some infants with a large right-to-left shunt, the pulmonary vascular resistance never decreases.

Congenital heart defects that persistently increase pulmonary blood flow or pulmonary vascular resistance have the potential of causing pulmonary hypertension and producing irreversible pathologic changes in the pulmonary vasculature. When shunting of systemic blood flow into the pulmonary circulation threatens permanent injury to the pulmonary vessels, a surgical procedure should be done to reduce the flow temporarily or permanently. Pulmonary artery banding consists of placing a constrictive band around the main pulmonary artery, thereby increasing resistance to outflow from the right ventricle. The banding technique is a temporary measure to alleviate symptoms and protect the pulmonary vasculature in anticipation of later surgical repair of the defect.

Manifestations and Treatment

It is increasingly common for heart defects to be diagnosed prenatally.[59] Infants can be evaluated shortly after birth to confirm the diagnosis and develop a treatment plan. Reliable diagnostic images of the fetal heart can be obtained as early as 12 weeks of gestation. Among the disorders that can be diagnosed with certainty by fetal echocardiography are AV septal defects, hypoplastic left heart syndrome, aortic valve stenosis, HCM, pulmonic valve stenosis, and transposition of the great arteries. Disorders that result in an abnormal four-chamber view, an image typically obtained during routine prenatal ultrasonography, are the most likely to be detected.[59]

In the postnatal period, congenital heart defects may present with numerous signs and symptoms. Over 40 different types of congenital heart defects have been described with variable severity and therefore unpredictable presentation for infants and children with congenital heart disease. Some defects, such as patent ductus arteriosus and small ventricular septal defects, close spontaneously. In other, less severe defects, there may be no obvious signs and symptoms, and the disorder may be discovered during a routine health examination. Cyanosis, pulmonary congestion, cardiac failure, and decreased peripheral perfusion are the chief concerns in children with more severe defects. Such defects often cause problems immediately after birth or early in infancy. The child may exhibit cyanosis, respiratory difficulty, and fatigability and is likely to have difficulty with feeding and failure to thrive. A generalized cyanosis that persists longer than 3 hours after birth suggests congenital heart disease.[60]

An oxygen challenge (administration of 100% oxygen for 10 minutes) can help to determine whether congenital heart disease is present in a cyanotic newborn. An arterial blood sample is taken during this time. If the partial pressure of oxygen (PO_2) is greater than 250 mm Hg, cyanotic heart disease can be ruled out; if the PO_2 is 160 to 250 mm Hg, heart disease is unlikely; failure of the PO_2 to rise to these levels is strongly suggestive of cyanotic heart disease.[58] Because infant cyanosis may appear as duskiness, it is important to assess the color of the mucous membranes, fingernails, toenails, tongue, and lips. Pulmonary congestion in the infant causes an increase in respiratory rate, orthopnea, grunting, wheezing, coughing, and crackles. A chest radiograph can quickly differentiate infants who have reduced pulmonary vascular markings (densities) from those who have normal or increased markings. The infant whose peripheral perfusion is markedly decreased may be in a shocklike state.

Heart failure manifests itself as tachypnea or dyspnea at rest or on exertion. For the infant, this most commonly occurs during feeding. Recurrent respiratory infections and excessive sweating may also be reported. Also, syncope or near syncope can occur. Growth failure results from unresolved heart failure.[60] The treatment plan usually includes supportive therapy (*e.g.*, digoxin, diuretics, and feeding supplementation) designed to help the infant compensate for the limitations in cardiac reserve and to prevent complications. Surgical intervention often is required for severe defects. It may be done in the early weeks of life or, conditions permitting, delayed until the child is older. Children with structural congenital heart disease and those who have had corrective surgery may have a higher-than-expected risk for development of IE.

Prophylactic antibiotic therapy before dental procedures or other periods of increased risk for bacteremia is suggested for children with

- Unrepaired cyanotic heart disease, including those with palliative shunts and conduits or repaired congenital heart disease with residual defects at the site or adjacent to the site of a prosthetic patch or prosthetic device (which inhibit endothelialization)
- Prior IE
- Prosthetic cardiac valves
- Prosthetic material used for cardiac valve repair
- Cardiac transplant with valve regurgitation[61,62]

Types of Defects

Congenital heart defects can affect almost any of the cardiac structures or central blood vessels. Defects include communication between heart chambers, interrupted development of the heart chambers or valve structures, malposition of heart chambers and great vessels, and altered closure of fetal communication channels. The particular defect reflects the embryo's stage of development at the time it occurred. It is common for multiple defects to be present in one child and for some congenital heart disorders, such as tetralogy of Fallot, to involve several defects.

The development of the heart is simultaneous and sequential; a heart defect may reflect the multiple developmental events that were occurring simultaneously or sequentially. Most infants who have a congenital heart defect usually do not have a major problem during infancy. Only about one third of infants who are born with anomalies have a disease state that is critical. Over 40 types of defects have been identified, the most common being ventricular septal defects, which are responsible for 28% to 42% of all congenital heart disorders.[60]

Patent Ductus Arteriosus. The ductus arteriosus plays a vital role in diverting blood from the right side of the heart and away from the lungs to the systemic circulation during fetal life (Fig. 27.32G). With the onset of spontaneous respiration after birth, muscular constriction of the ductal tissue typically closes this vessel. The initiating step of ductal closure in the healthy infant is believed to be the sharp increase in arterial oxygen saturation and subsequent fall in pulmonary vascular resistance after birth. Additional factors that are thought to contribute to ductal closure are a fall in endogenous levels of prostaglandins and adenosine and the release of vasoactive substances. After constriction, the lumen of the ductus becomes permanently sealed with fibrous tissue within 2 to 3 weeks.

For 90% of full-term infants, the ductus is functionally closed by 48 hours of age.[63] Full-term infants with abnormalities of circulation or ventilation and premature infants are those most likely to exhibit persistent patency of the ductus arteriosus. Arterial oxygenation, circulating prostaglandins, genetic predetermination, and other, unknown factors interact to determine the mechanism of ductal closure.[63] Circulating

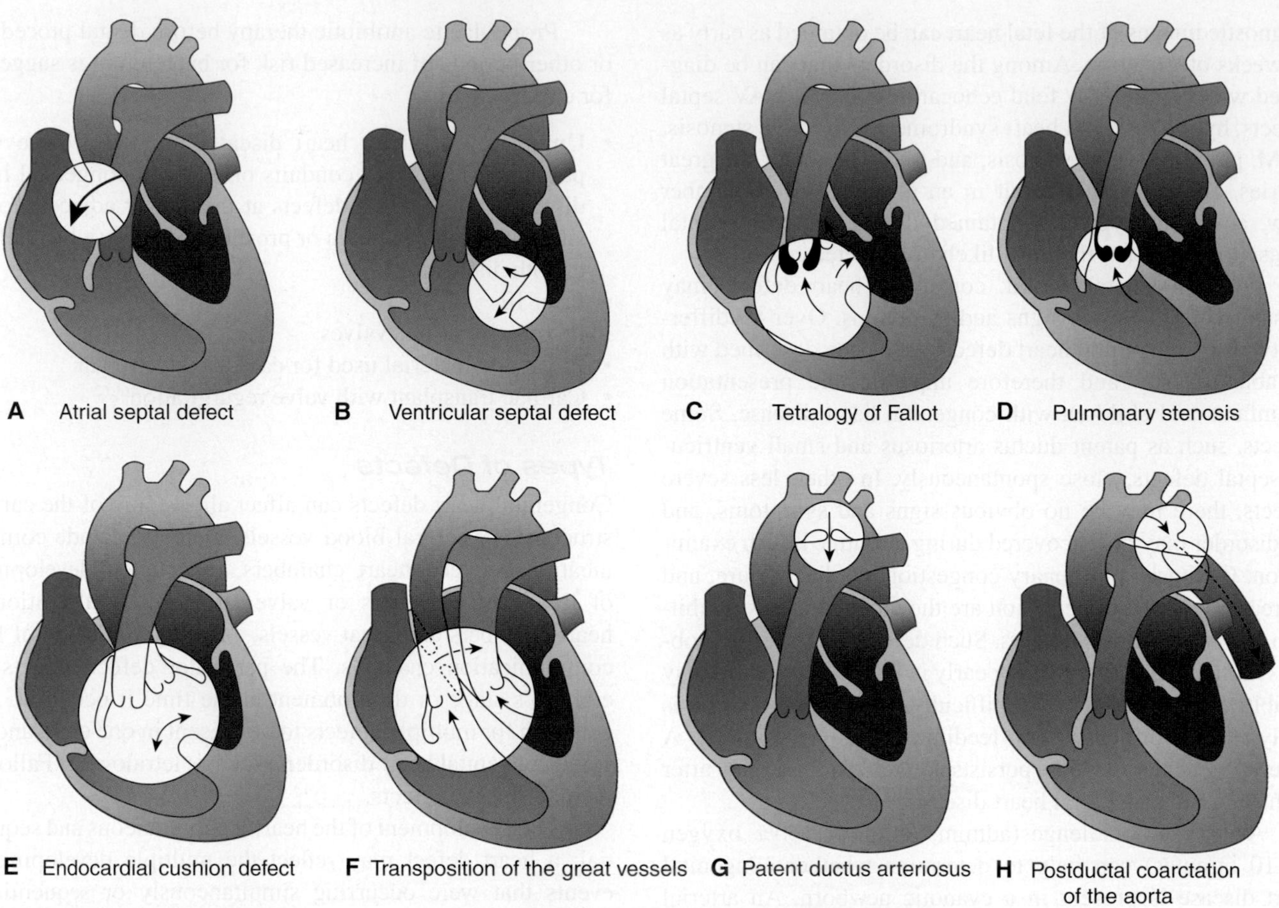

Figure 27.32 • Congenital heart defects. **(A)** Atrial septal defect. Blood is shunted from left to right. **(B)** Ventricular septal defect. Blood is usually shunted from left to right. **(C)** Tetralogy of Fallot. This involves a ventricular septal defect, dextroposition of the aorta, right ventricular outflow obstruction, and right ventricular hypertrophy. Blood is shunted from right to left. **(D)** Pulmonary stenosis, with decreased pulmonary blood flow and right ventricular hypertrophy. **(E)** Endocardial cushion defects. Blood flows between the chambers of the heart. **(F)** Transposition of the great vessels. The pulmonary artery is attached to the left side of the heart and the aorta to the right side. **(G)** Patent ductus arteriosus. The high-pressure blood of the aorta is shunted back to the pulmonary artery. **(H)** Postductal coarctation of the aorta.

prostaglandin levels are directly related to gestational age, and the incidence of patent ductus arteriosus in infants with birth weights less than 1000 g may be as high as 50%.[63]

Persistent patency of the ductus arteriosus is defined as a duct that remains open beyond 3 months in the full-term infant. The size of the persistent ductus and the difference between the systemic and pulmonary vascular resistance determine its clinical manifestations. Blood typically shunts across the ductus from the higher-pressure left side (systemic circulation) to the lower-pressure right side (pulmonary circulation). A murmur is typically detected within days or weeks of birth. The murmur is loudest at the second left intercostal space, is continuous through systole and diastole, and has a characteristic "machinery" sound.[60,63] A widened pulse pressure is common because of the continuous runoff of aortic blood into the pulmonary artery. Diagnostic methods include chest radiography and echocardiography. There are increased pulmonary markings on chest radiography and enlargement of the left heart from the increased pulmonary venous return if it is a larger shunt. Chest x-rays are normal in small shunts.[60] Echocardiography is used to determine the presence, size, direction (*i.e.*, left to right or right to left), and physical consequences of the shunt.

An untreated patent ductus can result in important long-term complications that may include congestive heart failure, IE, pulmonary vascular disease, aneurysm formation, thromboembolism, and calcification.[60] The potential risk of complications and the extremely low procedural morbidity and mortality justify closure of a patent ductus even when the shunt is small. In the premature infant, a patent ductus can produce respiratory distress and impede weaning from mechanical ventilation. Indomethacin, an inhibitor of prostaglandin synthesis and an NSAID, has proven effective in the treatment of patent ductus in premature infants.[60] There has been some success with the use of ibuprofen, which is also an inhibitor of prostaglandin synthesis and an NSAID; however, the long-term effects on chronic lung disease and pulmonary hypertension are still unknown. Together, NSAIDs result in the functional closure of patent ductus in about 80% of people.

When this medical management fails, surgical intervention is recommended. In the full-term infant or older child, closure can be achieved with either surgical ligation or device occlusion. Surgery typically involves a small left thoracotomy or thoracoscopic approach that allows ligation of the vessel. Implantable devices, most commonly coils, have allowed successful ductus closure to be done in the catheterization laboratory on an outpatient basis. The anatomy of the ductus and the size of the person are key determinants of the applicability of this technique.

Although closure of a patent ductus is uniformly recommended when it is present as an isolated lesion, deliberate maintenance of ductal patency can be a lifesaving therapy for children with complex forms of congenital heart disease who have ductal-dependent pulmonary or systemic blood flow or those with obligatory mixing of the arterial and venous circulations (*i.e.*, transposition of the great arteries). Intravenous infusion of prostaglandin E_1 has proven to be extremely effective in maintaining ductal patency or reopening the ductus in newborns. Today, this therapy is routinely administered to newborns with suspected congenital heart defects until they can be transported to a specialized center where a diagnosis can be confirmed.[60]

Atrial Septal Defects. Any persistent opening that allows shunting of blood across the atrial septum is considered an atrial septal defect. The defect may be single or multiple and vary from a small, asymptomatic opening to a large, symptomatic opening. The typology of the defect is determined by its position and may include a secundum atrial defect (the most common form), an ostium primum defect, a sinus venosus defect, or a patent foramen ovale (Fig. 27.32A). The defect occurs more frequently in girls than boys, as much as 2:1.[60] As much as 50% of children with congenital heart disorders have an atrial septal defect as a part of their diagnosis.

Many atrial septal defects are asymptomatic and discovered incidentally during a routine physical examination at a few years of age.[63] Intracardiac shunting is usually from left to right and may increase with age as the right ventricle becomes more compliant. In most cases, there is a moderate shunt resulting in dilation of the right heart chambers and overperfusion of the pulmonary circulation. The increased volume of blood that must be ejected from the right heart prolongs closure of the pulmonary valve and produces a separation (fixed splitting) of the aortic and pulmonary components of the second heart sound. Children with undiagnosed atrial defects are at risk for pulmonary vascular disease, although this is a rare occurrence before 20 years of age. Rarely, infants with a large shunt may develop congestive heart failure and failure to thrive, prompting early closure of the defect.[60,63]

Atrial septal defects that measure 8 mm or more are unlikely to undergo spontaneous closure. Smaller defects may be observed for spontaneous closure in the young child. However, surgical or transcatheter closure is recommended in children with persistent defects to reduce the long-term risk of pulmonary vascular disease and atrial arrhythmias.[63] Both transcatheter device and surgical closures are effective and of low risk. Use of the transcatheter approach is determined by the position and size of the defect. Transcatheter device closure has been particularly effective for small to medium-sized secundum septal defects and patent foramen ovale. Sinus venosus defects, which are frequently associated with partial anomalous pulmonary venous return and ostium primum defects, require surgical closure. Surgery requires the use of cardiopulmonary bypass and mild hypothermia. Most defects are effectively closed using the person's native septal tissue or a pericardial or synthetic patch. There is a very low incidence of residual sequelae or need for reintervention if closure occurred during the first two decades of life.

Ventricular Septal Defects. A ventricular septal defect is an opening in the ventricular septum that results from an incomplete separation of the ventricles during early fetal development (Fig. 27.32B). These defects may be single or multiple and may occur in any position along the ventricular septum. Ventricular septal defects are the most common form of congenital heart defect, accounting for 28% to 42% of congenital heart disorders.[64] Distribution between males and females is relatively even. Ventricular septal defect may be the only cardiac defect, or it may occur in association with multiple cardiac anomalies.

The ventricular septum originates from two sources: the interventricular groove of the folded tubular heart that gives rise to the muscular part of the septum and the endocardial cushions that extend to form the membranous portion of the septum. The upper membranous portion of the septum is the last area to close, typically by the seventh week of gestation, and it is here that most defects occur. Depending on the size of the opening and the pulmonary vascular resistance, the signs and symptoms of a ventricular septal defect may range from an asymptomatic murmur to congestive heart failure.[60]

The physical size of the ventricular septal defect is a major, but not the only, determinant of left-to-right shunt. The pulmonary vascular resistance in relation to systemic vascular resistance also determines the shunt's magnitude. In a small communicating defect (<0.5 cm^2), the higher pressure in the LV drives the shunt to the left, and the size of the defect limits the magnitude of the shunt. Most children with such defects are asymptomatic and have a low risk for development of pulmonary vascular disease.

In a larger, nonrestrictive shunt (usually >1 cm^2), right and left ventricular pressure is equalized, and the degree of shunting is determined by the ratio of pulmonary to systemic vascular resistance. After birth in infants with large ventricular septal defects, pulmonary vascular resistance may remain higher than normal, and the size of the left-to-right shunt may initially be limited. As the pulmonary vascular resistance continues to fall in the first few weeks after birth because of normal involution of the media of the small pulmonary arterioles, the magnitude of the left-to-right shunt increases. Eventually, a large left-to-right shunt develops, and clinical symptoms (*e.g.*, tachypnea; diaphoresis, especially with feeding; and failure to thrive) become apparent. In most cases during infancy, pulmonary vascular pressure is only slightly elevated, and the major contributor to pulmonary hypertension is an increase in pulmonary blood flow. In some infants with a large septal defect, pulmonary arteriolar thickness never decreases. With continued exposure to high pulmonary blood flow, pulmonary vascular obstructive disease develops. In untreated people, the pulmonary vascular resistance can eventually exceed the systemic resistance. In this case, a reversal of shunt flow occurs, and the child demonstrates progressive cyanosis as deoxygenated blood moves from the right to the left side of the heart. These symptoms, coupled with irreversible changes in the pulmonary vasculature, represent an end-stage form of congenital heart disease called *Eisenmenger complex*. People who develop this have a life expectancy of about 43 years, and the cause of death is progressive heart failure.[60]

The treatment of a ventricular septal defect depends on the size of the defect, accompanying hemodynamic derangements, and symptomatology. Children with small or medium-sized defects may be followed without intervention if they remain free from signs of congestive heart failure or pulmonary hypertension. Ventricular defects do not increase in size, and some spontaneously close over time.[63] Detailed 2-D echocardiography is usually adequate to diagnosis the size and position of a defect as well as to estimate pulmonary pressures. Cardiac catheterization is usually reserved for cases where it is necessary to confirm the degree and reversibility of pulmonary vascular resistance.

Congestive heart failure is treated medically. Symptomatic infants may require feeding supplements or tube feeding to promote growth and development. In the symptomatic infant in whom complete repair cannot be achieved because of size or other complicating lesions, a palliative procedure may be performed to reduce symptoms. Placement of a synthetic band around the main pulmonary artery (pulmonary artery banding) can reduce pulmonary blood flow until complete repair can be accomplished. Surgical closure of the defect is completed by placement of a synthetic or autologous patch effectively to close the shunt across the ventricular septum. These procedures are typically done electively in the infant or young child and are associated with low morbidity and mortality rates. Transcatheter device closure of ventricular septal defects is another option for defect closure with improved complication risk in the recent years.

Endocardial Cushion Defects. The AV canal connects the atria to the ventricles during early cardiac development. The endocardial cushions surround this canal and contribute tissue to the lower part of the atrial septum, the upper part of the ventricular septum, the septal leaflet of the tricuspid valve, and the anterior leaflet of the mitral valve.[64] Any flaw in the development of these tissues results in an endocardial cushion defect. Approximately 3% of all congenital heart defects are endocardial cushion defects, with a nearly equal incidence in boys and girls. Endocardial cushion defects have a strong association with trisomy 21 and are seen in as much as 50% of children with this genetic disorder.[64]

Several variations of endocardial cushion defects are possible. The defect may be described as *partial* or *complete*. The anatomy of the AV valve determines its classification. In partial AV canal defects, the two AV valve rings are complete and separate. The most common type of partial AV canal defect is an ostium primum defect, often associated with a cleft in the mitral valve. In a complete canal defect, there is a common AV valve orifice along with defects in both the atrial and ventricular septal tissue (Fig. 27.32E). Other cardiac defects may be associated with endocardial cushion defects and most commonly include cardiac malposition defects and tetralogy of Fallot.[65,66]

Physiologically, endocardial cushion defects result in abnormalities similar to those described for atrial or ventricular septal defects. The direction and magnitude of a shunt in a child with an endocardial cushion defect are determined by the combination of defects and the child's pulmonary and systemic vascular resistances. The hemodynamic effects of an isolated ostium primum defect are those of the previously described atrial septal defect. These children are largely asymptomatic during childhood. With a complete AV canal defect, pulmonary blood flow is increased after pulmonary vascular resistance falls because of left-to-right shunting across both the ventricular and atrial septal defects. Children with complete defects often have effort intolerance, easy fatigability, failure to thrive, recurrent infections, and other signs of congestive heart failure, particularly when the shunt is large. Pulmonary hypertension and increased pulmonary vascular resistance result if the lesion is left untreated.

The timing of treatment for endocardial cushion defects is determined by the severity of the defect and symptoms. With an ostium primum defect, surgical repair usually is planned on an elective basis before the child reaches school age. The defect in the atrial septum is closed with a patch, and mitral valvuloplasty is performed if the valve is regurgitant. Corrective surgery is required for all complete AV canal defects. This is typically performed early in the infant's life and requires patching of both the atrial and ventricular septal defects and separation of the AV valve apparatus to create competent mitral and tricuspid valves. Infants with severe symptoms may require a palliative procedure where the main pulmonary artery is banded to reduce pulmonary blood flow. This typically improves the infant's ability to grow and develop until a complete repair can be performed. Total surgical repair of complete AV canal defects can be accomplished with low operative risk. Reoperation may be required in approximately 11.7% of children.

Pulmonary Stenosis. Obstruction of blood flow from the right ventricle to the pulmonary circulation is termed *pulmonary stenosis*. The obstruction can occur as an isolated valvular lesion, within the right ventricular chamber, in the pulmonary arteries, or as a combination of stenoses in multiple areas. It is a relatively common defect, estimated to account for approximately 10% of all congenital cardiac disease, and is often associated with other abnormalities.[63]

Pulmonary valvular defects, the most common type of obstruction, usually produce some impairment of pulmonary blood flow and increase the workload imposed on the right side of the heart (Fig. 27.32D). Most children with pulmonary valve stenosis have mild stenosis that does not increase in severity. These children are largely asymptomatic and are diagnosed by the presence of a systolic murmur. Moderate or greater stenosis has been shown to progress over time, particularly before 12 years of age, so these children require careful follow-up. Critical pulmonary stenosis in the neonate is evidenced by cyanosis due to right-to-left atrial-level shunting and right ventricular hypertension. These infants require prostaglandin E_1 to maintain circulation to the lungs through the ductus arteriosus.[33]

Pulmonary valvotomy is the treatment of choice for all valvular defects with pressure gradients from the right ventricle to the pulmonary circulation greater than 30 mm Hg. Transcatheter balloon valvuloplasty has been quite successful in this lesion. Stenosis in the peripheral pulmonary arteries can also be effectively treated with balloon angioplasty.[63] Recently, stents have been used with success. Stents are used for children with pulmonary artery stenosis to keep the vessels open. This is used when balloon dilation has failed.[60]

Tetralogy of Fallot. Tetralogy of Fallot is the most common cyanotic congenital heart defect.[60] As the name implies, tetralogy of Fallot consists of four associated defects:

1. A ventricular septal defect involving the membranous septum and the anterior portion of the muscular septum
2. Dextroposition or shifting to the right of the aorta, so that it overrides the right ventricle and is in communication with the septal defect
3. Obstruction or narrowing of the pulmonary outflow channel, including pulmonary valve stenosis, a decrease in the size of the pulmonary trunk, or both
4. Hypertrophy of the right ventricle because of the increased work required to pump blood through the obstructed pulmonary channels[66] (Fig. 27.32C)

Variations of the defect can be a right aortic arch and a persistent left superior vena cava. When this is seen, it is called *pentalogy of Fallot*.[60]

Cyanosis is caused by a right-to-left shunt across the ventricular septal defect. The degree of cyanosis is determined by the restriction of blood flow into the pulmonary bed. Right ventricular outflow obstruction causes deoxygenated blood from the right ventricle to shunt across the ventricular septal defect and be ejected into the systemic circulation. The degree of obstruction may be dynamic and can increase during periods of stress, causing hypercyanotic attacks ("tet spells"). These spells typically occur in the morning during crying, feeding, or defecating. These activities increase the infant's oxygen requirements. Crying and defecation may further increase pulmonary vascular resistance, thereby increasing right-to-left shunting and decreasing pulmonary blood flow. With the hypercyanotic spell, the infant becomes acutely cyanotic, hyperpneic, irritable, and diaphoretic. Later in the spell, the infant becomes limp and may lose consciousness. Placing the infant in the knee–chest position increases systemic vascular resistance, thus decreasing right-to-left shunting and increasing pulmonary blood flow. During a hypercyanotic spell, toddlers and older children may spontaneously assume the squatting position, which functions like the knee–chest position to relieve the spell. Turbulent flow across the narrow right ventricular outflow track produces a characteristic harsh systolic ejection murmur. Auscultation during a hypercyanotic spell reveals a diminished or absent murmur due to the dramatic reduction in pulmonary blood flow.[66]

Total surgical correction is required for all children with tetralogy of Fallot. However, before surgery, iron deficiency anemia should be addressed in order to prevent stroke. Dehydration is monitored closely to prevent thrombotic complications, propranolol can be administered to prevent hypoxic spells, and sodium bicarbonate and alpha-adrenergic agonists are administered if acidosis is present.

Early definitive repair in infancy is currently advocated in most centers experienced in intracardiac surgery in infants. When extreme cyanosis is present in a small infant or when there is associated marked hypoplasia of the pulmonary arteries, a palliative procedure to facilitate pulmonary blood flow may be necessary. This is accomplished by placing a prosthetic shunt between a systemic artery and the pulmonary artery (modified Blalock-Taussig shunt). Balloon dilation of the pulmonary valve may also afford palliation in some infants. Total correction is then carried out later in infancy or early childhood. Complete repair includes patch closure of the ventricular septal defect and relief of any right ventricular outflow tract obstruction. Repair is associated with a mortality rate of less than 3%; however, people need long-term follow-up to monitor for residual lesions, right ventricular dilation or dysfunction, and arrhythmias.[66] They also need to be monitored because they continue to be at risk for IE.

Transposition of the Great Arteries. In complete transposition of the great arteries, the aorta arises from the right ventricle, and the pulmonary artery arises from the LV (Fig. 27.32F). Complete transposition occurs in 1 per 4000 live births and is the most common reason for pediatric cardiology referral in the first 2 weeks of life.

Cyanosis is the most common presenting symptom resulting from an anomaly that allows the systemic venous return to be circulated through the right heart and ejected into the aorta and the pulmonary venous return to be recirculated to the lungs through the LV and main pulmonary artery.[60] In infants born with this defect, survival depends on communication between the right and left sides of the heart in the form of a patent ductus arteriosus or septal defect. Ventricular septal defects are present in 50% of infants, of which 10% have a small VSD, with transposition of the great arteries at birth and may allow effective mixing of blood. Prostaglandin E_1 should be administered to neonates when this lesion is suspected in an effort to maintain the patency of the ductus arteriosus. Balloon atrial septostomy may be done to increase the blood flow between the two sides of the heart. In this procedure, a balloon-tipped catheter is inserted into the heart through the vena cava and then passed through the foramen ovale into the left atrium. The balloon is then inflated and pulled back through the foramen ovale, enlarging the opening as it goes.

Corrective surgery is essential for long-term survival. An arterial switch procedure, the current operation of choice, has survival rates greater than 90%.[60] This procedure, which corrects the relation of the systemic and pulmonary blood flows, is preferably performed in the first 2 to 3 weeks of life, before the postnatal reduction in pulmonary vascular resistance occurs. The coronary arteries are moved to the left-sided great artery, and any ventricular septal defects are closed during the same operation. Complications of the arterial switch procedure may include coronary insufficiency, supravalvar pulmonary stenosis, neoaortic regurgitation, and rhythm abnormalities.[65]

Coarctation of the Aorta. Coarctation of the aorta is a localized narrowing of the aorta, proximal to (preductal), distal to (postductal), or opposite the entry of the ductus arteriosus (juxtaductal; see Fig. 27.32H). Approximately 98% of coarctations are juxtaductal. Constriction of aberrant ductal tissue extending into the aortic wall is believed to be the cause of obstruction.[63] The anomaly occurs more often in males than females, as much as 3:1. It is frequently associated with other congenital cardiac lesions, most commonly bicuspid aortic valve (46%), and occurs in approximately 10% of subjects with Turner syndrome, suggesting a genetic linkage.[60,63]

The classic sign of coarctation of the aorta is a disparity in pulsations and blood pressures in the arms and legs. The femoral, popliteal, and dorsalis pedis pulsations are weak or delayed compared with the bounding pulses of the arms and carotid vessels. Normally, the systolic blood pressure in the legs obtained by the cuff method is 10 to 20 mm Hg higher than in the arms. In coarctation, the pressure in the legs is lower and may be difficult to obtain. People with coarctation are often identified during a diagnostic workup for hypertension. Most people with moderate coarctation remain otherwise asymptomatic owing to collateral vessels that form around the area of narrowing. Left untreated, however, coarctation will result in left ventricular hypertension and hypertrophy and significant systemic hypertension. Infants with severe coarctation demonstrate early symptoms of heart failure and may present in critical condition upon ductal closure. Reopening of the duct with prostaglandin E_1, if possible, and emergent surgery are needed in this subgroup.[63]

Children with coarctation causing a blood pressure gradient between the arms and legs of 20 mm Hg or greater should be treated ideally by 2 years of age to reduce the likelihood of persistent hypertension.[63] A surgical approach typically involves resection of the narrowed segment of the aorta and end-to-end anastomosis of healthy tissue. This can usually be accomplished without cardiopulmonary bypass, with a mortality rate near zero. Balloon angioplasty with or without stent placement has also been used, although the presence of residual gradients and the reliability of the surgical approach have limited this technique.[60,63] The most common complications after repair of coarctation are persistent hypertension and recoarctation. Operative mortality rates increase if an associated defect is present.

Functional Single-Ventricle Anatomy. Several forms of complex congenital heart disease result in only one functional ventricle. There may be a single right or a single LV or a ventricle of indeterminate morphology. Hypoplastic left heart syndrome is the most common form of single right ventricular anatomy. Tricuspid valve atresia is the most common cause of a single LV. Several other forms of double-inlet ventricle have been described; however, all forms of this disease result in similar pathologic effects and follow a common pathway of intervention.[60]

All forms of single-ventricle anatomy result in a common mixing chamber of pulmonary and systemic venous return and cause varying degrees of cyanosis. The single ventricle must supply both the pulmonary and systemic circulations.[60] The amount of blood flow to each circulation is determined by the resistance in each system. As pulmonary vascular resistance falls, flow to the pulmonary circulation will be preferential, and systemic circulation will be compromised. In some defects, such as hypoplastic left heart syndrome, systemic flow depends on a patent ductus arteriosus. Neonates with this lesion typically present with extreme cyanosis and symptoms of heart failure as the ductus begins to close.[63]

Although functional single-ventricle anatomy cannot be completely repaired, the surgical palliation of these defects has been one of the most innovative accomplishments in intervention for congenital heart disease. The goal of surgical palliation is to redirect systemic venous return directly to the pulmonary arteries and allow the single ventricle to deliver oxygenated blood to the systemic circulation. This is accomplished in a series of two- to three-staged surgical procedures during the child's first years of life. Currently, a modified Fontan approach is done surgically. Cardiac transplantation is also used as an intervention for the most complex forms of single-ventricle congenital heart disease (Fig. 27.33).

Survival rates for children with complex forms of single-ventricle heart disease have improved markedly, but long-term outcomes remain uncertain. Ventricular dysfunction, arrhythmias, and thromboses plague this population. Defining the optimal medical and surgical management strategies for these people remains an active area of research in pediatric cardiology and cardiac surgery.[60]

Adults with Congenital Heart Disease

Successful treatment of congenital heart disease in the pediatric population has resulted in a growing number of adult survivors with a variety of repaired, unrepaired, and palliated congenital cardiac lesions. An epidemiologic study on the prevalence and age distribution of congenital heart disease identified a prevalence of 6 per 1000 adults.[60,67]

Although the majority of adults with congenital heart disease will have undergone treatment and perhaps surgery as children, most congenital heart defects must be considered

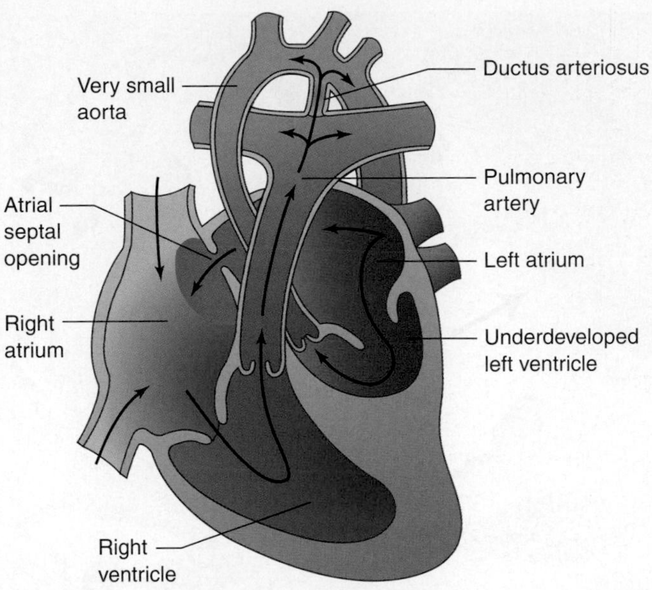

Figure 27.33 • Functional single-ventricle anatomy with an underdeveloped LV and small ascending aorta. Because of the markedly decreased left ventricular compliance, most of the pulmonary venous blood returning to the left atrium shunts left to right at the atrial level. Pulmonary arterial blood flows into the pulmonary arteries as well as right to left across a patent ductus arteriosus into the aorta.

chronic conditions requiring long-term surveillance and care. Only the simplest isolated lesions can be considered completely repaired.[67] Chronic physiologic concerns include arrhythmias, hemodynamic problems, complications of prolonged cyanosis, endocarditis, residual lesions, and the need for reoperation. The underlying heart defect can also have significant implications for other aspects of health, such as exercise tolerance, noncardiac surgery, and pregnancy. Several important psychosocial issues also require consideration, including neurocognitive achievement, employment, insurability, family planning, treatment adherence, and understanding of the underlying condition and risks. Life expectancy for some of the most complex lesions (*e.g.*, hypoplastic left heart syndrome) is unknown because the oldest survivors to date were born in the 1980s. A growing medical specialty has emerged designed specifically to provide adults with congenital heart disease the specialized services they need from practitioners who understand both the complexities of their cardiac problems and other issues of adult health care.

Kawasaki Disease

Kawasaki disease, also known as *mucocutaneous lymph node syndrome*, is an acute febrile disease of young children. First described in Japan in 1967 by Dr. Tomisaku Kawasaki, the disease affects the skin, brain, eyes, joints, liver, lymph nodes, and heart. The disease is the most common cause of acquired heart disease in young children, with 15% to 25% of cases resulting in coronary artery aneurysms or ectasias that may lead to myocardial infarction, sudden death, or chronic coronary insufficiency.[37,68] More than 4000 children with Kawasaki disease are hospitalized annually in the United States.[68] Over 80% of people with Kawasaki disease are 4 years of age or younger, with a male-to-female ratio of 1.5:1. Although it is most common in Japan, the disease affects children of many races, occurs worldwide, and is increasing in frequency.

Pathogenesis

The disease is characterized by a vasculitis (*i.e.*, inflammation of the blood vessels) that begins in the small vessels (*i.e.*, arterioles, venules, and capillaries) and progresses to involve some of the larger arteries, such as the coronaries. The exact etiology and pathogenesis of the disease remain unknown, but it is thought to be of immunologic origin. Immunologic abnormalities, including increased activation of helper T cells and increased levels of immune mediators and antibodies that destroy endothelial cells, have been detected during the acute phase of the disease. It has been hypothesized that some unknown antigen, possibly a common infectious agent, triggers the immune response in a genetically predisposed child.

Clinical Manifestations

The clinical course of the disease has been described in three phases: the acute, subacute, and convalescent phases.[37,68] The *acute phase* begins with an abrupt onset of fever, followed by conjunctivitis, rash, involvement of the oral mucosa, redness and swelling of the hands and feet, and enlarged cervical lymph nodes (Fig. 27.34). The fever typically is high, reaching 40°C (104°F) or more, has an erratic spiking pattern, is unresponsive to antibiotics, and persists for 5 or more days. The conjunctivitis, which is bilateral, begins shortly after the onset of fever, persists throughout the febrile course of the disease, and may last as long as 4 to 8 weeks. There is no exudate, discharge, or conjunctival ulceration, differentiating it from many other types of conjunctivitis. The rash usually is deeply erythematous and may take several forms, the most common of which is a nonpruritic urticarial rash with large erythematous plaques or a measles-type rash. Although the rash usually is generalized, it may be accentuated centrally or peripherally. Some children have a perianal rash with a diaper-like distribution. Oropharyngeal manifestations include fissuring of the lips, diffuse erythema of the oropharynx, and hypertrophic papillae of the tongue, creating a "strawberry" appearance. The hands and feet become swollen and painful and have reddened palms and soles. The rash, oropharyngeal manifestations, and changes in hands and feet appear within 1 to 3 days of fever onset and usually disappear as the fever subsides. Lymph node involvement is the least constant feature of the disease. It is cervical and unilateral, with a single, firm, enlarged lymph node mass that usually is larger than 1.5 cm in diameter.

The *subacute phase* begins with defervescence and lasts until all signs of the disease have disappeared. During the subacute phase, desquamation (*i.e.*, peeling) of the skin of the fingers and toe tips begins and progresses to involve the entire surface of the palms and soles. Patchy peeling of skin areas other than the hands and feet may occur in some children. The convalescent stage persists from the complete resolution of symptoms until all signs of inflammation have disappeared.

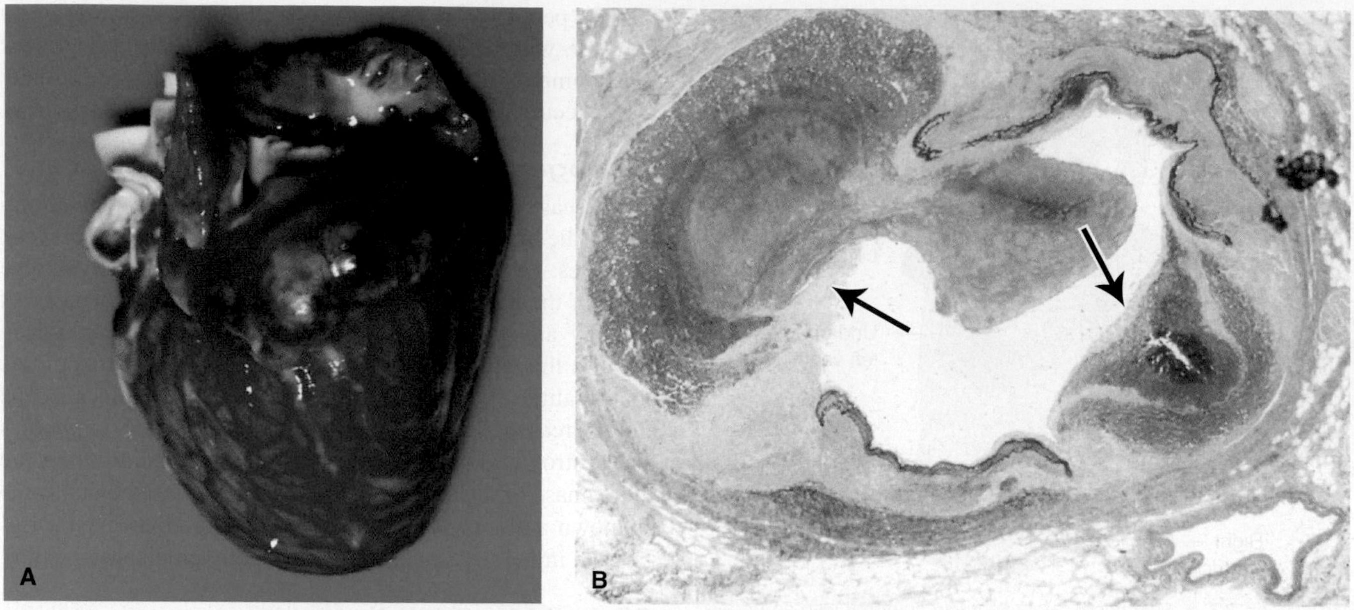

Figure 27.34 • Kawasaki disease. **(A)** The heart of a child who died from Kawasaki disease shows conspicuous coronary artery aneurysms. **(B)** A microscopic section of a coronary artery from the same person details with arrows small aneurysms filled with thrombus. (From Strayer D. E., Rubin R. (Eds.) (2015). *Rubin's pathology: Clinicopathologic foundations of medicine* (7th ed., Fig. 16-35, p. 609) Philadelphia, PA: Lippincott Williams & Wilkins.)

This usually takes approximately 8 weeks, although inflammatory changes in the coronary arteries may persist as long as 4 years.

In addition to the major manifestations that occur during the acute stage of the illness, there are several associated, less specific characteristics of the disease, including arthritis, urethritis and pyuria, gastrointestinal manifestations (*e.g.*, diarrhea, abdominal pain), hepatitis, and hydrops of the gallbladder. Arthritis or arthralgia occurs in approximately 30% of children with the disease, characterized by symmetric joint swelling involving large and small joints. Central nervous system involvement occurs in almost all children and is characterized by pronounced irritability and lability of mood.

Cardiac involvement is the most important manifestation of Kawasaki disease. Coronary artery abnormalities develop in approximately 15% to 25% of children, manifested by coronary artery dilation and aneurysm formation as seen on 2-D echocardiography. The manifestations of coronary artery involvement include signs and symptoms of myocardial ischemia or, rarely, overt myocardial infarction or rupture of the aneurysm. Pericarditis, mitral regurgitation, pericardial effusions, myocarditis, endocarditis, aortic regurgitation, heart failure, and arrhythmias also may develop. Death from Kawasaki disease is estimated to occur in 2% of people and is almost always cardiac in nature, most often occurring during the convalescent phase of the illness, usually from thromboses or coronary arterial aneurysms.[37]

Diagnosis and Treatment

No specific diagnostic test for Kawasaki disease is available; therefore, the diagnosis is made on clinical grounds following published guidelines.[37,68] The guidelines specify fever persisting at least 5 days or more without another source in association with at least four principal features, including oral changes that may include erythema or cracking of the lips, strawberry tongue, and erythema of the oral mucosa; bilateral, nonexudative conjunctivitis; polymorphous rash, generally with truncal involvement, nonvesicular; changes of extremities that may include erythema and edema of the hands or feet and desquamation of fingers and toes 1 to 3 weeks after onset of illness; and cervical lymphadenopathy, often unilateral, with at least one node that is 1.5 cm in size.[37] Chest radiographs, ECG tests, and 2-D echocardiography are used to detect coronary artery involvement and follow its progress. Coronary angiography may be used to determine the extent of coronary artery involvement.

Intravenous gamma globulin (2 g/kg single infusion) and aspirin are considered the best therapies for prevention of coronary artery abnormalities in children with Kawasaki disease. During the acute phase of the illness, aspirin usually is given in larger doses (80 to 100 mg/kg/day divided in four doses) for its anti-inflammatory and antipyretic effects. After the fever is controlled, the aspirin dose is lowered (3 to 5 mg/kg/day, single dose), and the drug is given for its anti–platelet-aggregating effects for up to 8 weeks.[37]

Recommendations for cardiac follow-up evaluation (*i.e.*, stress testing and sometimes coronary angiography) are based on the level of coronary artery changes. Anticoagulant therapy may be recommended for children with multiple or large coronary aneurysms. Some restrictions in activities such as participation in competitive sports may be advised for children with significant coronary artery abnormalities.[37,68]

IN SUMMARY

Congenital heart defects arise during fetal heart development, which occurs during weeks 3 through 8 after conception, and reflect the stage of development at the time the causative event occurred. Several factors contribute to the development of congenital heart defects, including genetic and chromosomal influences, viruses, and environmental agents such as drugs and radiation. The exact cause of the defect often is unknown. These defects are relatively common and are the most common cause of death related to a birth defect.

Congenital heart defects may produce no effects, or they may markedly affect cardiac function. The defects may produce shunting of blood from the right to the left side of the heart or from the left to the right side of the heart. Left-to-right shunts typically increase the volume of the right side of the heart and pulmonary circulation, and right-to-left shunts transfer deoxygenated blood from the right side of the heart to the left side, diluting the oxygen content of blood that is being ejected into the systemic circulation and causing cyanosis. The direction and degree of shunt depend on the size and position of the defect that connects the two sides of the heart and the difference in resistance between the two sides of the circulation. Congenital heart defects often are classified as defects that produce cyanosis and those that produce little or no cyanosis. Depending on the severity of the defect, congenital heart defects may be treated medically or surgically. Medical and surgical treatment often is indicated in children with severe defects.

Kawasaki disease is an acute febrile disease of young children that affects the skin, brain, eyes, joints, liver, lymph nodes, and heart. The disease can produce aneurysmal disease of the coronary arteries and is the most common cause of acquired heart disease in young children.

HEART FAILURE IN CHILDREN AND OLDER ADULTS

After completing this section of the chapter, the learner will be able to meet the following objectives:

- Describe the causes of heart failure in infants and children.
- Explain how the aging process affects cardiac function and predisposes to ventricular dysfunction.
- Identify how the signs and symptoms of heart failure may differ between younger and older adults.

Heart Failure in Infants and Children

As in adults, heart failure in infants and children results from the inability of the heart to maintain the cardiac output required to sustain metabolic demands.[69] The etiology of heart failure, however, is very different between children and adults. Structural (congenital) heart defects are the most common cause of heart failure in children. Surgical correction of congenital heart defects may cause heart failure as a result of intraoperative manipulation of the heart and resection of heart tissue, with subsequent alterations in pressure, flow, and resistance relations. Usually, the heart failure that results is acute and resolves after the effects of the surgical procedure have subsided. Another cause of heart failure in children is cardiomyopathy related to a genetic or inherited disorder, infectious disease, drugs, toxins, and Kawasaki disease.[68] Chart 27.3 lists some of the more common causes of heart failure in children, which include the following:

- Inflammatory heart disorders (*e.g.*, myocarditis, RF, bacterial endocarditis, Kawasaki disease)
- Cardiomyopathy
- Congenital heart disorders

CHART 27.3 CAUSES OF HEART FAILURE IN CHILDREN

Newborn Period
Congenital heart defects
Severe left ventricular outflow disorders
Hypoplastic left heart
Critical aortic stenosis or coarctation of the aorta
Large arteriovenous shunts
Ventricular septal defects
Patent ductus arteriosus
Transposition of the great vessels
Heart muscle dysfunction (secondary)
Asphyxia
Sepsis
Hypoglycemia
Hematologic disorders (*e.g.*, anemia)

Infants 1 to 6 Months
Congenital heart disease
Large arteriovenous shunts (ventricular septal defect)
Heart muscle dysfunction
Myocarditis
Cardiomyopathy
Pulmonary abnormalities
Bronchopulmonary dysplasia
Persistent pulmonary hypertension

Toddlers, Children, and Adolescents
Acquired heart disease
Cardiomyopathy
Viral myocarditis
Rheumatic fever
Endocarditis
Systemic disease
Sepsis
Kawasaki disease
Renal disease
Sickle cell disease
Congenital heart defects
Nonsurgically treated disorders
Surgically treated disorders

Clinical Manifestations

Many of the signs and symptoms of heart failure in infants and children are similar to those in adults. In children, overt symptoms of heart failure occur late in the disease process.[69] Breathlessness, tachypnea, and tachycardia felt as palpitations are the most common symptoms.[69] Other symptoms include fatigue, effort intolerance, cough, anorexia, and abdominal pain. A subtle sign of cardiorespiratory distress in infants and children is a change in disposition or responsiveness, including irritability or lethargy. Sympathetic stimulation produces peripheral vasoconstriction and diaphoresis. Decreased renal blood flow often results in a decrease in urine output despite adequate fluid intake.

When right ventricular function is impaired, systemic venous congestion develops. Hepatomegaly due to liver congestion often is one of the first signs of systemic venous congestion in infants and children. However, dependent edema or ascites rarely is seen unless the CVP is extremely high. Because of their short, fat necks, jugular venous distention is difficult to detect in infants. It is not a reliable sign until the child is of school age or older. A third heart sound, or gallop rhythm, is a common finding in infants and children with heart failure. It results from rapid filling of a noncompliant ventricle. However, it is difficult to distinguish at high heart rates.

Most commonly, children develop interstitial pulmonary edema rather than alveolar pulmonary edema. This reduces lung compliance and increases the work of breathing, causing tachypnea and increased respiratory effort. Older children display use of accessory muscles (*i.e.*, scapular and sternocleidomastoid). Head bobbing and nasal flaring may be observed in infants. Signs of respiratory distress often are the first and most noticeable indication of heart failure in infants and young children. Pulmonary congestion may be mistaken for bronchiolitis or lower respiratory tract infection. The infant or young child with respiratory distress often grunts with expiration. This grunting effort (essentially, exhaling against a closed glottis) is an instinctive effort to increase end-expiratory pressures and prevent collapse of small airways and the development of atelectasis. Respiratory crackles are uncommon in infants and usually suggest development of a respiratory tract infection. Wheezes may be heard, particularly if there is a large left-to-right shunt.

Infants with heart failure often show increased tachypnea, fatigue, and diaphoresis during feeding.[69] Weight gain is slow owing to high energy requirements and low calorie intake. Diaphoresis occurs (because of increased sympathetic tone) particularly over the head and neck. They may have repeated lower respiratory tract infections. Peripheral perfusion usually is poor, with cool extremities; tachycardia is common (resting heart rate >150 beats/minute); and the respiratory rate is increased (resting rate >50 breaths/minute).[69]

Diagnosis and Treatment

Diagnosis of heart failure in infants and children is based on symptomatology, chest radiographic films, ECG findings, and echocardiographic techniques to assess cardiac structures and ventricular function (*i.e.*, end-systolic and end-diastolic diameters), arterial blood gases to determine intracardiac shunting and ventilation–perfusion inequalities, and other laboratory studies to determine anemia and electrolyte imbalances.

Treatment of heart failure in infants and children includes measures aimed at improving cardiac function and eliminating excess intravascular fluid. Oxygen delivery must be supported and oxygen demands controlled or minimized. Whenever possible, the cause of the disorder is corrected (*e.g.*, medical treatment of sepsis and anemia, surgical correction of congenital heart defects). With congenital anomalies that are amenable to surgery, medical treatment often is needed for a time before surgery and usually is continued in the immediate postoperative period. For some children, only medical management can be provided.

Medical management of heart failure in infants and children is similar to that in the adult, although it is tailored to the special developmental needs of the child. Inotropic agents such as digitalis often are used to increase cardiac contractility. Diuretics may be given to reduce preload and vasodilating medications used to manipulate the afterload. Medication doses must be carefully tailored to control for the child's weight and conditions such as reduced renal function. Daily weighing and accurate measurement of intake and output are imperative during acute episodes of failure. Most children feel better in the semiupright position. An infant seat is useful for infants with chronic heart failure. Activity restrictions usually are designed to allow children to be as active as possible within the limitations of their heart disease. Infants with heart failure often have problems feeding. Small, frequent feedings usually are more successful than larger, less frequent feedings. Severely ill infants may lack sufficient strength to suck and may need to be tube-fed.

The treatment of heart failure in children should be designed to allow optimal physical and psychosocial development. It requires the full involvement of the parents, who often are the primary care providers. Therefore, parent education and support are essential.

Heart Failure in Older Adults

Heart failure is largely a disease of aging. It is one of the most common causes of disability in older adults and is the most frequent hospital admission and discharge diagnosis for older adults (those older than 65 years) in the United States and Canada.[70] Among the factors that have contributed to the increased numbers of older adults with heart failure are the improved therapies for ischemic and hypertensive heart disease.[71] Thus, people who would have died from acute myocardial disease 20 years ago are now surviving but with residual left ventricular dysfunction. Advances in treatment of other diseases have also contributed indirectly to the rising prevalence of heart failure in the older population.

Coronary heart disease, hypertension, arrhythmias, and valvular heart disease (particularly aortic stenosis and mitral regurgitation) are common causes of heart failure in older adults.[72] In contrast to the etiology in middle-aged people with heart failure, factors other than systolic failure contribute to heart failure in older adults. Preserved left ventricular function may be seen in 40% to 80% of older adults with heart failure. Aging is associated with impaired left ventricular filling due to changes in myocardial relaxation and compliance. These alterations lead to a shift in the left ventricular pressure–volume relationship, such that small increases in left ventricular volume lead to greater increases in left ventricular diastolic pressure. This increase in diastolic pressure further compromises left ventricular filling and leads to increases in left atrial, pulmonary venous, and pulmonary capillary pressures and thus predisposes to pulmonary congestion and heart failure.[71,72] Although diastolic heart failure accounts for less than 10% of heart failure cases in people younger than 60 years of age, it accounts for greater than 50% of cases after age 75 years.[71,72]

There are a number of changes associated with aging that contribute to the development of heart failure in older adults.[71,72] First, reduced responsiveness to β-adrenergic stimulation limits the heart's capacity to maximally increase heart rate and contractility. A second major effect of aging is increased vascular stiffness, which leads to a progressive increase in systolic blood pressure with advancing age, which in turn contributes to the development of left ventricular hypertrophy and altered diastolic filling. Third, in addition to increased vascular stiffness, the heart itself becomes stiffer and less compliant with age. The changes in diastolic stiffness result in important alterations in diastolic filling and atrial function. A reduction in ventricular filling not only affects cardiac output but produces an elevation in diastolic pressure that is transmitted back to the left atrium, where it stretches the muscle wall and predisposes to atrial ectopic beats and atrial fibrillation. The fourth major effect of cardiovascular aging is altered myocardial metabolism at the level of the mitochondria. Although older mitochondria may be able to generate sufficient ATP to meet the normal energy needs of the heart, they may not be able to respond under stress.

Clinical Manifestations

The manifestations of heart failure in older adults often are masked by other disease conditions.[53] Nocturia and nocturnal incontinence are early symptoms but may be caused by other conditions such as prostatic hypertrophy. Lower extremity edema may reflect venous insufficiency. Impaired perfusion of the gastrointestinal tract is a common cause of anorexia and profound loss of lean body mass. Loss of lean body mass may be masked by edema. Exertional dyspnea, orthopnea, and impaired exercise tolerance are cardinal symptoms of heart failure in both younger and older adults with heart failure. However, with increasing age, which is often accompanied by a more sedentary lifestyle, exertional dyspnea becomes less prominent. Instead of dyspnea, the prominent sign may be restlessness. Chart 27.4 summarizes the clinical manifestations of heart failure in older adults.

CHART 27.4 MANIFESTATIONS OF HEART FAILURE IN OLDER ADULTS

Symptoms

Nocturia or nocturnal incontinence
Fatigue
Cognitive impairment (*e.g.*, problem solving, decision-making)
Depression
Restlessness/acute delirium
Sleep disturbance
History of falls
Loss of appetite

Signs

Dependent edema (ankle edema when sitting up and sacral edema when supine)
Pulmonary crackles (usually late sign)

Physical signs of heart failure, such as elevated jugular venous pressure, hepatic congestion, S_3 gallop, and pulmonary crackles, occur less commonly in older adults, in part because of the increased incidence of diastolic failure, in which signs of right-sided heart failure are late manifestations and a third heart sound is typically absent.[71]

Instead, behavioral changes and altered cognition such as short-term memory loss and impaired problem-solving are more common. Depression is common in older adults with heart failure and shares the symptoms of sleep disturbances, cognitive changes, and fatigue.[53]

Older adults also maintain a precarious balance between the managed symptom state and acute symptom exacerbation. During the managed symptom state, they are relatively symptom-free while adhering to their treatment regimen. Acute symptom exacerbation, often requiring emergency medical treatment, can be precipitated by seemingly minor conditions such as poor adherence to sodium restriction, infection, or stress. Failure to promptly seek medical care is a common cause of progressive acceleration of symptoms.

Diagnosis and Treatment

The diagnosis of heart failure in older adults is based on the history, physical examination, chest radiograph, and ECG findings.[17,71,72] However, the presenting symptoms of heart failure often are difficult to evaluate. Symptoms of dyspnea on exertion are often interpreted as a sign of "getting older" or attributed to deconditioning from other diseases. Ankle edema is not unusual in older adults because of decreased skin turgor and the tendency of older adults to be more sedentary with the legs in a dependent position.

Treatment of heart failure in older adults involves many of the same methods as in younger people, with medication dose adaptations to reduce age-related adverse and toxic events.[53] ACE inhibitors may be particularly beneficial to preserve cognitive and functional capacities.[53] Activities may be restricted to a level that is commensurate with the cardiac reserve. Seldom is bed rest recommended or advised. Bed rest causes rapid deconditioning of skeletal muscles and increases the risk of complications such as orthostatic hypotension and thromboemboli. Instead, carefully prescribed exercise programs can help to maintain activity tolerance. Even walking around a room usually is preferable to continuous bed rest. Sodium restriction usually is indicated. Because older adults have the highest hospital readmission rates, education is extremely important, and it is imperative to involve the family members and caregivers in their management and treatment. It is also important to have a multidisciplinary approach to their care with frequent contact because they will have other comorbid conditions and can deteriorate rapidly.

IN SUMMARY

The mechanisms of heart failure in children and older adults are similar to those in adults. However, the causes and manifestations may differ because of age. In children, heart failure is seen most commonly during infancy and immediately after heart surgery. It can be caused by congenital and acquired heart defects and is characterized by fatigue, effort intolerance, cough, anorexia, abdominal pain, and impaired growth. Treatment of heart failure in children includes correction of the underlying cause whenever possible. For congenital anomalies that are amenable to surgery, medical treatment often is needed for a time before surgery and usually is continued in the immediate postoperative period. For many children, only medical management can be provided.

In older adults, age-related changes in cardiovascular function contribute to heart failure but are not in themselves sufficient to cause heart failure.[71] The clinical manifestations of heart failure often are different and superimposed on other disease conditions. Therefore, heart failure often is more difficult to diagnose in older adults than in younger people. Because older adults are more susceptible to adverse and toxic medication reactions, medication doses need to be adapted and more closely monitored.

CIRCULATORY FAILURE (SHOCK)

After completing this section of the chapter, you should be able to meet the following objectives:

- Compare the causes, pathophysiology, and chief characteristics of cardiogenic, hypovolemic, obstructive, and distributive shock.
- Describe the complications of shock as they relate to the lungs, kidneys, gastrointestinal tract, and blood clotting.
- State the rationale for treatment measures to correct and reverse shock.

Circulatory shock can be described as an acute failure of the circulatory system to supply the peripheral tissues and organs of the body with an adequate blood supply, resulting in cellular hypoxia.[73] Hypoperfusion of systemic tissue results from deficient cardiac output.[74] Most often, hypotension and hypoperfusion are present, but shock may occur in the presence of normal vital signs. Shock is not a specific disease but a syndrome that can occur in the course of many life-threatening traumatic conditions or disease states. It can be caused by an alteration in cardiac function (cardiogenic shock), a decrease in blood volume (hypovolemic shock), excessive vasodilation with maldistribution of blood flow (distributive shock), or obstruction of blood flow through the circulatory system (obstructive shock). The main types of shock are summarized in Chart 27.5 and depicted in Figure 27.35.

Pathophysiology of Circulatory Shock

Circulatory failure results in hypoperfusion of organs and tissues, which in turn results in insufficient supply of oxygen and nutrients for cellular function. There are compensatory physiologic responses that eventually decompensate into various shock states if the condition is not properly treated in a timely manner. The most immediate of the compensatory

CHART 27.5 CLASSIFICATION OF CIRCULATORY SHOCK

Cardiogenic
Myocardial damage (myocardial infarction, contusion)
Sustained arrhythmias
Acute valve damage, ventricular septal defect
Cardiac surgery

Hypovolemic
Loss of whole blood
Loss of plasma
Loss of extracellular fluid

Obstructive
Inability of the heart to fill properly (cardiac tamponade)
Obstruction to outflow from the heart (pulmonary embolus, cardiac myxoma, pneumothorax, or dissecting aneurysm)

Distributive
Loss of sympathetic vasomotor tone (neurogenic shock)
Presence of vasodilating substances in the blood (anaphylactic shock)
Presence of inflammatory mediators (septic shock)

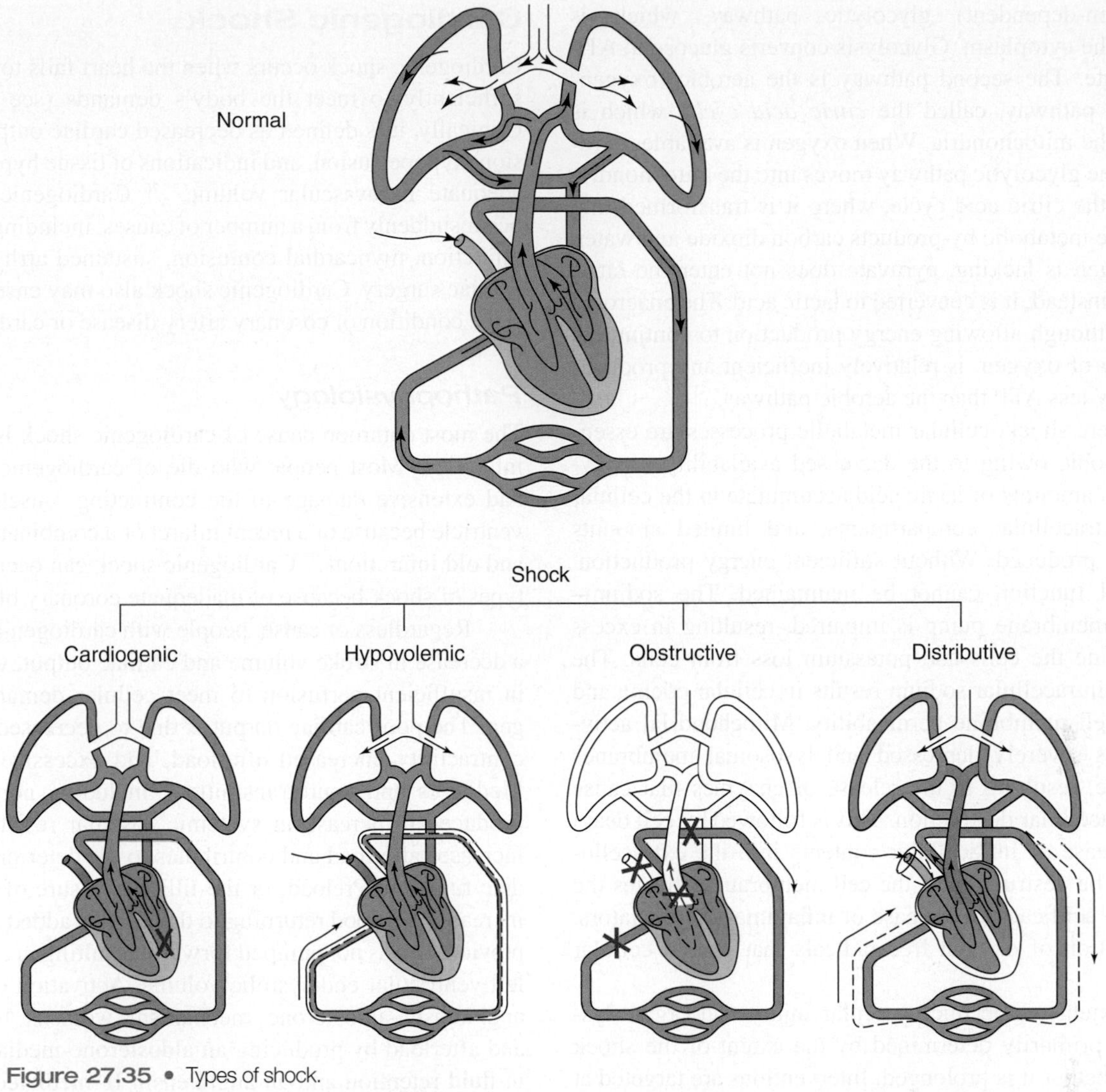

Figure 27.35 • Types of shock.

mechanisms are the sympathetic and renin systems, which are designed to maintain cardiac output and blood pressure.

There are two types of adrenergic receptors for the sympathetic nervous system: α and β. The β-receptors are further subdivided into β_1 and β_2 receptors. Stimulation of the α-receptors causes vasoconstriction, stimulation of β_1 receptors an increase in heart rate and force of myocardial contraction, and of β_2 receptors vasodilation of the skeletal muscle beds and relaxation of the bronchioles. In shock, there is an increase in sympathetic outflow that results in increased epinephrine and norepinephrine release and activation of both α- and β-receptors. Thus, increases in heart rate and vasoconstriction occur in most types of shock. There also is an increase in renin release, leading to an increase in angiotensin II, which augments vasoconstriction and leads to an aldosterone-mediated increase in sodium and water retention by the kidneys. In addition, there is local release of vasoconstrictors, including norepinephrine, angiotensin II, vasopressin, and endothelin, which contribute to arterial and venous vasoconstriction.

The compensatory mechanisms that the body recruits are not effective over the long term and become detrimental when the shock state is prolonged. The intense vasoconstriction causes a decrease in tissue perfusion and insufficient supply of oxygen. Cellular metabolism is impaired, vasoactive inflammatory mediators such as histamine are released, production of oxygen free radicals is increased, and excessive lactic acid and hydrogen ions result in intracellular acidity.[74] Each of these factors promotes cellular dysfunction or death. If circulatory function is re-established, whether the shock is irreversible or the person will survive is determined largely at the cellular level.

Shock ultimately exerts its effect at the cellular level, with failure of the circulation to supply the cell with the oxygen and nutrients needed for production of ATP. The cell uses ATP for a number of purposes, including operation of the sodium–potassium membrane pump that moves sodium out of the cell and potassium back into the cell. The cell uses two pathways to convert nutrients to energy. The first is the anaerobic (non–oxygen-dependent) glycolytic pathway, which is located in the cytoplasm. Glycolysis converts glucose to ATP and pyruvate. The second pathway is the aerobic (oxygen-dependent) pathway, called the *citric acid cycle*, which is located in the mitochondria. When oxygen is available, pyruvate from the glycolytic pathway moves into the mitochondria and enters the citric acid cycle, where it is transformed into ATP and the metabolic by-products carbon dioxide and water. When oxygen is lacking, pyruvate does not enter the citric acid cycle; instead, it is converted to lactic acid. The anaerobic pathway, although allowing energy production to continue in the absence of oxygen, is relatively inefficient and produces significantly less ATP than the aerobic pathway.

In severe shock, cellular metabolic processes are essentially anaerobic owing to the decreased availability of oxygen. Excess amounts of lactic acid accumulate in the cellular and the extracellular compartments, and limited amounts of ATP are produced. Without sufficient energy production, normal cell function cannot be maintained. The sodium–potassium membrane pump is impaired, resulting in excess sodium inside the cells and potassium loss from cells. The increase in intracellular sodium results in cellular edema and increased cell membrane permeability. Mitochondrial activity becomes severely depressed and lysosomal membranes may rupture, resulting in the release of enzymes that cause further intracellular destruction. This is followed by cell death and the release of intracellular contents into the extracellular space. The destruction of the cell membrane activates the arachidonic acid cascade, release of inflammatory mediators, and production of oxygen free radicals that extend cellular damage.

The extent of the microvascular injury and organ dysfunction is primarily determined by the extent of the shock state and whether it is prolonged. Interventions are targeted at both prevention and early intervention, when possible.

KEY POINTS

CIRCULATORY SHOCK

- Circulatory shock can result from failure of the heart as a pump, a loss of fluid from the vascular compartment (hypovolemic shock), obstruction of flow through the vascular compartment (obstructive shock), or an increase in the size of the vascular compartment that interferes with the distribution of blood (distributive shock).
- The manifestations of shock reflect both the impaired perfusion of body tissues and the body's attempt to maintain tissue perfusion through conservation of water by the kidney, translocation of fluid from the extracellular to the intravascular compartment, and activation of sympathetic nervous system mechanisms that increase heart rate and divert blood from less to more essential body tissues.

Cardiogenic Shock

Cardiogenic shock occurs when the heart fails to pump blood sufficiently to meet the body's demands (see Fig. 27.35). Clinically, it is defined as decreased cardiac output, hypotension, hypoperfusion, and indications of tissue hypoxia, despite adequate intravascular volume.[75,76] Cardiogenic shock may occur suddenly from a number of causes, including myocardial infarction, myocardial contusion, sustained arrhythmias, and cardiac surgery. Cardiogenic shock also may ensue as an end-stage condition of coronary artery disease or cardiomyopathy.

Pathophysiology

The most common cause of cardiogenic shock is myocardial infarction. Most people who die of cardiogenic shock have had extensive damage to the contracting muscle of the left ventricle because of a recent infarct or a combination of recent and old infarctions.[77] Cardiogenic shock can occur with other types of shock because of inadequate coronary blood flow.

Regardless of cause, people with cardiogenic shock have a decrease in stroke volume and cardiac output, which results in insufficient perfusion to meet cellular demands for oxygen. The poor cardiac output is due to decreased myocardial contractility, increased afterload, and excessive preload.[75,76] Mediators and neurotransmitters, including norepinephrine, produce an increase in systemic vascular resistance, which increases afterload and contributes to the deterioration of cardiac function. Preload, or the filling pressure of the heart, is increased as blood returning to the heart is added to blood that previously was not pumped forward, resulting in an increase in left ventricular end-systolic volume. Activation of the renin–angiotensin–aldosterone mechanism worsens both preload and afterload by producing an aldosterone-mediated increase in fluid retention and an angiotensin II–mediated increase in vasoconstriction. The increased resistance (*i.e.*, afterload) to ejection of blood from the left ventricle, in combination with a decrease in myocardial contractility, results in an increase in end-systolic ventricular volume and preload, which further impairs the heart's ability to pump effectively.

Eventually, coronary artery perfusion is impaired because of the increased preload and afterload, and cardiac function decreases because of poor myocardial oxygen supply. There is an increase in intracardiac pressures due to volume overload and ventricular wall tension in both diastole and systole. Excessive pressures decrease coronary artery perfusion during diastole, and increased wall tension decreases coronary artery perfusion during systole. If treatment is unsuccessful, cardiogenic shock may result in a systemic inflammatory response syndrome. This is evidenced by increased white blood cell count, increased temperature, and release of inflammatory markers such as CRP.[75,76]

Clinical Manifestations

Signs and symptoms of cardiogenic shock include indications of hypoperfusion with hypotension, although a preshock state of hypoperfusion may occur with a normal blood pressure. The lips, nail beds, and skin may become cyanotic because of stagnation of blood flow and increased extraction of oxygen from the hemoglobin as it passes through the capillary bed. Mean arterial and systolic blood pressures decrease because of poor stroke volume, and there is a narrow pulse pressure and near-normal diastolic blood pressure because of arterial vasoconstriction.[77] Urine output decreases because of lower renal perfusion pressures and the increased release of aldosterone. Elevated preload is reflected in a rise in CVP and PCWP. Neurologic changes, such as alterations in cognition or consciousness, may occur because of low cardiac output and poor cerebral perfusion.

Treatment

Treatment of cardiogenic shock requires striking a precarious balance between improving cardiac output, reducing the workload and oxygen needs of the myocardium, and increasing coronary perfusion. Fluid volume must be tightly regulated to maintain the filling pressure and optimize stroke volume in people who are fluid overloaded. Pulmonary edema and arrhythmias should be monitored, corrected, or prevented to increase stroke volume and decrease the oxygen demands of the heart. Coronary artery perfusion is increased by promoting coronary artery vasodilation, increasing blood pressure, decreasing ventricular wall tension, and decreasing intracardiac pressures.

Pharmacologic treatment includes the use of vasodilators such as nitroprusside and nitroglycerin. Both nitroprusside and nitroglycerin cause coronary artery dilation, which increases myocardial oxygen delivery. Nitroprusside causes arterial and venous dilation, producing a decrease in venous return to the heart and a reduction in arterial resistance against which the left heart must pump.[75,76] At lower doses, the main effects of nitroglycerin are on the venous vascular beds and coronary arteries. At high doses, it also dilates the arterial beds. Both medications may result in a decrease in diastolic arterial pressure that results in a lower systemic vascular resistance (afterload). The systolic arterial pressure is maintained by an increase in ventricular stroke volume, which is ejected against the lowered systemic vascular resistance. The improvement in heart function increases stroke volume and enables blood to be redistributed from the pulmonary vascular bed to the systemic circulation.

Positive inotropic agents are used to improve cardiac contractility. Both dobutamine and milrinone are effective medications in that they result in increased contractility and arterial vasodilation. Dobutamine is a synthetic agent consisting of two isomers, one of which is a potent β_1-adrenergic receptor agonist and α_1-adrenergic receptor antagonist and the other is a mild β_2-adrenergic receptor agonist and α_1-adrenergic receptor agonist. The combination tends to produce vasodilation and a positive inotropic action. Milrinone increases myocardial contractility by increasing the movement of Ca^{++} into myocardial cells during an action potential (see Fig. 27.21). The increase in stroke volume results in a decrease in end-systolic volume and a reduction in preload. With a decrease in preload pressures, coronary artery perfusion is improved during diastole. Thus, stroke volume and myocardial oxygen supply are improved with a minimal increase in myocardial oxygen demand. Catecholamines increase cardiac contractility but must be used with extreme caution because they also result in arterial constriction and increased heart rates, which worsen the imbalance between myocardial oxygen supply and demand.

The intra-aortic balloon pump, also referred to as *counterpulsation*, enhances coronary and systemic perfusion yet decreases afterload and myocardial oxygen demands.[74] The device, which pumps in synchrony with the heart, consists of a 10-inch-long balloon that is inserted through a catheter into the descending aorta (Fig. 27.36). The balloon is timed to inflate during ventricular diastole and deflate just before

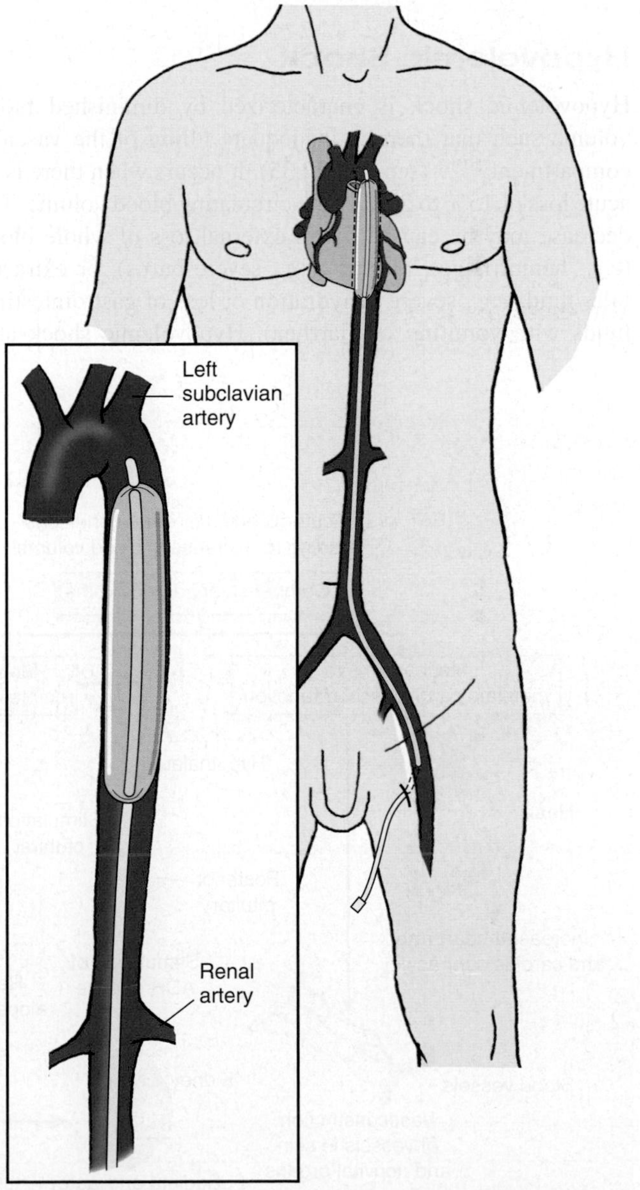

Figure 27.36 • Proper position of the balloon catheter, illustrating percutaneous insertion. (From Morton P. G., Fontaine D. K. (2018). *Critical Care Nursing: A Holistic Approach* (11th ed., Fig. 18-18, p. 293). Philadelphia, PA: JB Lippincott.)

ventricular systole. Diastolic inflation creates a pressure wave in the ascending aorta that increases coronary artery blood flow and a less intense wave in the lower aorta that enhances organ perfusion. The abrupt balloon deflation at the onset of systole results in a displacement of blood volume that lowers the resistance to ejection of blood from the left ventricle. Thus, the heart's pumping efficiency is increased, myocardial oxygen supply is increased, and myocardial oxygen consumption is decreased.

When cardiogenic shock is caused by myocardial infarction, several aggressive interventions can be used successfully. Fibrinolytic therapy, percutaneous coronary intervention, or CABG may be used to prevent or treat cardiogenic shock.[77] Reperfusion of the coronary arteries is expected to improve myocardial function.

Hypovolemic Shock

Hypovolemic shock is characterized by diminished blood volume such that there is inadequate filling of the vascular compartment[73,75,76] (see Fig. 27.35). It occurs when there is an acute loss of 15% to 20% of the circulating blood volume. The decrease may be caused by an external loss of whole blood (*e.g.*, hemorrhage), plasma (*e.g.*, severe burns), or extracellular fluid (*e.g.*, severe dehydration or loss of gastrointestinal fluids with vomiting or diarrhea). Hypovolemic shock also can result from an internal hemorrhage or from third-space losses, when extracellular fluid is shifted from the vascular compartment to the interstitial space or compartment.

Pathophysiology

Hypovolemic shock, which has been the most widely studied type of shock, is often used as a prototype in discussions of the manifestations of shock. Figure 27.37 shows the effect of removing blood from the circulatory system during approximately 30 minutes.[73] Approximately 10% of the total blood volume can be removed without changing cardiac output or arterial pressure. The average blood donor loses approximately 500 mL or 10% of their blood without experiencing adverse effects. As increasing amounts of blood (10% to 25%) are removed, the stroke volume falls, but arterial pressure is maintained because of sympathetic-mediated increases in heart rate and vasoconstriction. Vasoconstriction results in an increased diastolic pressure and narrow pulse pressure. Blood pressure is the product of cardiac output and systemic vascular resistance (blood pressure = cardiac output × systemic vascular resistance). An increase in systemic vascular resistance maintains mean arterial pressure for a short time despite decreased cardiac output. Cardiac output and tissue perfusion decrease before signs of hypotension appear. Cardiac output and arterial pressure fall to zero when approximately 30% to 40% of the total blood volume has been removed.[73,75,76]

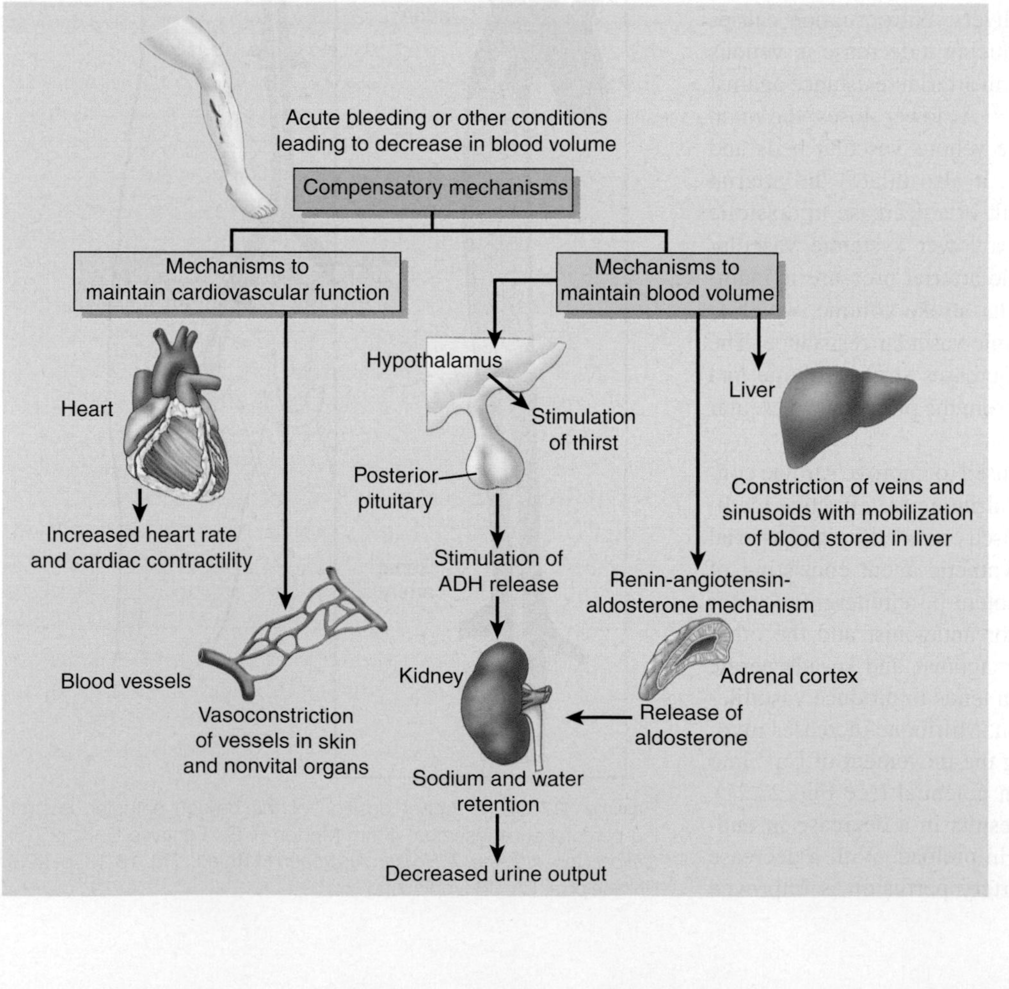

Figure 27.37 • Compensatory mechanisms used to maintain circulatory function and blood volume in hypovolemic shock. ADH, antidiuretic hormone.

Compensatory Mechanisms. Without compensatory mechanisms to maintain cardiac output and blood pressure, the loss of vascular volume would result in a rapid progression from the initial to the progressive and irreversible stages of shock. The most immediate of the compensatory mechanisms are the sympathetic-mediated responses designed to maintain cardiac output and blood pressure (Fig. 27.37). Within seconds after the onset of hemorrhage or the loss of blood volume, tachycardia, increased cardiac contractility, vasoconstriction, and other signs of sympathetic and adrenal medullary activity appear. The sympathetic vasoconstrictor response also mobilizes blood that has been stored in the venous side of the circulation as a means of increasing venous return to the heart. There is considerable capacity for blood storage in the large veins of the abdomen, and approximately 350 mL of blood that can be mobilized in shock is stored in the liver.[73] Sympathetic stimulation does not initially cause constriction of the cerebral and coronary vessels, and blood flow to the heart and brain is maintained at essentially normal levels as long as the mean arterial pressure remains above 70 mm Hg.[73]

Compensatory mechanisms designed to restore blood volume include absorption of fluid from the interstitial spaces, conservation of sodium and water by the kidneys, and thirst. Extracellular fluid is distributed between the interstitial spaces and the vascular compartment. When there is a loss of vascular volume, capillary pressures decrease, and water is drawn into the vascular compartment from the interstitial spaces. The maintenance of vascular volume is further enhanced by renal mechanisms that conserve fluid. A decrease in renal blood flow and glomerular filtration rate results in activation of the renin–angiotensin–aldosterone mechanism, which produces an increase in sodium reabsorption by the kidneys. The decrease in blood volume also stimulates centers in the hypothalamus that regulate ADH release and thirst. ADH, also known as *vasopressin*, constricts the peripheral arteries and veins and greatly increases water retention by the kidneys. Although the mechanism of ADH is more sensitive to changes in serum osmolality, a decrease of 10% to 15% in blood volume serves as a strong stimulus for thirst[73,75,76]

During the early stages of hypovolemic shock, vasoconstriction decreases the size of the vascular compartment and increases systemic vascular resistance. This response usually is all that is needed when the injury is slight and blood loss is minimal. As hypovolemic shock progresses, vasoconstriction of the blood vessels that supply the skin, skeletal muscles, kidneys, and abdominal organs becomes more severe, with a further decrease in blood flow and conversion to anaerobic metabolism resulting in cellular injury.

Clinical Manifestations

The signs and symptoms of hypovolemic shock depend on its severity and are closely related to low peripheral blood flow and excessive sympathetic stimulation. They include thirst, increased heart rate, cool and clammy skin, decreased arterial blood pressure, decreased urine output, and changes in mentation. Laboratory tests of hemoglobin and hematocrit provide information regarding the severity of blood loss or hemoconcentration due to dehydration. Serum lactate and arterial pH provide information about the severity of acidosis due to anaerobic metabolism. Metabolic acidosis revealed by arterial blood gas measurement is the gold standard diagnostic test.[75,76] Acute, fatal hemorrhagic shock is characterized by metabolic acidosis, coagulopathy, and hypothermia, followed by circulatory failure.[75,76]

An increase in heart rate is an early sign of hypovolemic shock, as the body tries to maintain cardiac output despite the decrease in stroke volume. As shock progresses, the pulse becomes weak and thready, indicating vasoconstriction and reduced filling of the vascular compartment. Thirst is an early symptom in hypovolemic shock. Although the underlying cause is not fully understood, it probably is related to decreased blood volume and increased serum osmolality.

Arterial blood pressure is decreased in moderate to severe shock. However, controversy exists over the value of blood pressure measurements in the early diagnosis and management of shock. This is because compensatory mechanisms tend to preserve blood pressure until shock is relatively far advanced. Furthermore, a normal arterial pressure does not ensure adequate perfusion and oxygenation of vital organs at the cellular level. This does not imply that blood pressure should not be closely monitored in people at risk for development of shock, but it does indicate the need for other assessment measures.

As shock progresses, the respirations become rapid and deep, to compensate for the increased production of acid and decreased availability of oxygen. Decreased intravascular volume results in decreased venous return to the heart and a decreased CVP. When shock becomes severe, the peripheral veins may collapse. Sympathetic stimulation leads to intense vasoconstriction of the skin vessels, which results in cool and mottled skin. In hemorrhagic shock, the loss of red blood cells results in pallor of the skin and mucous membranes.

Urine output decreases very quickly in hypovolemic shock. Compensatory mechanisms decrease renal blood flow as a means of diverting blood flow to the heart and brain. Oliguria of 20 mL/hour or less indicates inadequate renal perfusion. Continuous measurement of urine output is essential for assessing the circulatory and volume status of the person in shock.

Restlessness, agitation, and apprehension are common in early shock because of increased sympathetic outflow and increased levels of epinephrine. As the shock progresses and blood flow to the brain decreases, restlessness is replaced by altered arousal and mentation. Loss of consciousness and coma may occur if the person does not receive or respond to treatment.

Treatment

The duration and amount of fluid loss are directly related to mortality. Therefore, the treatment of hypovolemic shock is directed toward correcting or controlling the underlying cause and improving tissue perfusion. Ongoing loss of blood must be corrected. Oxygen is administered to increase oxygen delivery to the tissues. Medications usually are administered intravenously. Frequent measurements of heart rate and cardiac rhythm, blood pressure, and urine output are used to assess the severity of circulatory compromise and to monitor treatment.

In hypovolemic shock, the goal of treatment is to restore vascular volume.[75,76] This can be accomplished through intravenous administration of fluids and blood. The crystalloids (*e.g.*, isotonic saline and Ringer lactate) are readily available and effective, at least temporarily. Plasma volume expanders (*e.g.*, pentastarch and colloidal albumin) have a high molecular weight, do not necessitate blood typing, and remain in the vascular space for longer periods than crystalloids such as dextrose and saline. The use of crystalloids versus colloids has not been studied in large clinical trials. Therefore, the use of one versus the other to decrease morbidity has not been established. Blood or blood products (packed or frozen red cells) are administered based on hematocrit and hemodynamic findings. Fluids and blood are best administered based on volume indicators such as CVP and urine output.

Vasoactive medications are agents capable of constricting or dilating blood vessels. Considerable controversy exists about the advantages or disadvantages related to the use of these drugs. As a general rule, vasoconstrictor agents are not used as a primary form of therapy in hypovolemic shock and may be detrimental. These agents are given only when volume deficits have been corrected yet hypotension persists.

Distributive Shock

Distributive or vasodilatory shock is characterized by loss of blood vessel tone, enlargement of the vascular compartment, and displacement of the vascular volume away from the heart and central circulation.[75,76,78] In distributive shock, the capacity of the vascular compartment expands to the extent that a normal volume of blood does not fill the circulatory system (see Fig. 27.35). Therefore, this type of shock is also referred to as *normovolemic shock*. Two main causes result in the loss of vascular tone: a decrease in the sympathetic control of vasomotor tone and the release of excessive vasodilator substances. It can also occur as a complication of vessel damage resulting from prolonged and severe hypotension due to hemorrhage, known as *irreversible* or *late-phase hemorrhagic shock*.[78] There are three shock states that share the basic circulatory pattern of distributive shock: neurogenic shock, anaphylactic shock, and septic shock.[75,76]

Neurogenic Shock

Neurogenic shock is caused by decreased sympathetic control of blood vessel tone due to a defect in the vasomotor center in the brain stem or the sympathetic outflow to the blood vessels.[73] The term *spinal shock* describes the neurogenic shock that occurs in people with spinal cord injury. Output from the vasomotor center can be interrupted by brain injury, the depressant action of drugs, general anesthesia, hypoxia, or lack of glucose (*e.g.*, insulin reaction). Fainting due to emotional causes is a transient form of impaired sympathetic outflow. Many general anesthetic agents can cause a neurogenic shock–like reaction, especially during induction, because of interference with sympathetic nervous system function. Spinal anesthesia or spinal cord injury above the midthoracic region can interrupt the transmission of outflow from the vasomotor center. In contrast to other shock states due to the loss of blood volume or impaired cardiac function, the heart rate in neurogenic shock often is slower than normal, and the skin is dry and warm. This type of distributive shock is rare and usually transitory.

Anaphylactic Shock

Anaphylaxis is a clinical syndrome that represents the most severe systemic allergic reaction.[8] Anaphylactic shock results from an immunologically mediated reaction in which vasodilator substances such as histamine are released into the blood. These substances cause vasodilation of arterioles and venules along with a marked increase in capillary permeability. The vascular response in anaphylaxis is often accompanied by life-threatening laryngeal edema and bronchospasm, circulatory collapse, contraction of gastrointestinal and uterine smooth muscle, and urticaria (hives) or angioedema.

Etiology. Among the most frequent causes of anaphylactic shock are reactions to medications, such as penicillin; foods, such as nuts and shellfish; and insect venoms. The most common cause is stings from insects of the order Hymenoptera (*i.e.*, bees, wasps, and fire ants). Latex allergy causes life-threatening anaphylaxis in a growing segment of the population. Health care workers and others who are exposed to latex are developing latex sensitivities that range from mild urticaria, contact dermatitis, and mild respiratory distress to anaphylactic shock.[75,76,79] The onset and severity of anaphylaxis depend on the sensitivity of the person and the rate and quantity of antigen exposure.

Clinical Manifestations. Signs and symptoms associated with impending anaphylactic shock include the following:

- Abdominal cramps
- Apprehension
- Warm or burning sensation of the skin
- Itching
- Urticaria (*i.e.*, hives)
- Coughing
- Choking
- Wheezing
- Chest tightness
- Difficulty in breathing

After blood begins to pool peripherally, there is a precipitous drop in blood pressure, and the pulse becomes so weak that it is difficult to detect. Life-threatening airway obstruction may ensue as a result of laryngeal angioedema or bronchial spasm. Anaphylactic shock often develops suddenly; death can occur within minutes unless appropriate medical intervention is promptly instituted.

Treatment. Treatment includes immediate discontinuation of the inciting agent or institution of measures to decrease its absorption (*e.g.*, application of ice to the site of an insect bite), close monitoring of cardiovascular and respiratory function, and maintenance of respiratory gas exchange, cardiac output, and tissue perfusion. Epinephrine is given in an anaphylactic reaction because it constricts blood vessels and relaxes the smooth muscle in the bronchioles, thus restoring cardiac and respiratory function.[79,80] Other treatment measures include the administration of oxygen, antihistamine drugs, and corticosteroids. The person should be placed in a supine position. This is extremely important because venous return can be severely compromised in the sitting position. This in turn produces a pulseless mechanical contraction of the heart and predisposes to arrhythmias. In several cases, death has occurred immediately after assuming the sitting position.[79,80]

Prevention. The prevention of anaphylactic shock is preferable to treatment. Once a person has been sensitized to an antigen, the risk of repeated anaphylactic reactions with subsequent exposure is high. All health care providers should question people regarding previous drug reactions and inform people as to the name of the medication they are to receive before it is administered or prescribed. People with known hypersensitivities should wear MedicAlert jewelry and carry an identification card to alert medical personnel if they become unconscious or unable to relate this information. People who are at risk for anaphylaxis should be provided with emergency medications (*e.g.*, epinephrine autoinjector) and instructed in procedures to follow in case they are inadvertently exposed to the offending antigen.[79,80]

Sepsis and Septic Shock

Septic shock, which is the most common type of vasodilatory shock, is associated with severe infection and the systemic response to infection (Fig. 27.38).[81,82] *Sepsis* is currently defined as suspected or proven infection, plus a systemic inflammatory response syndrome (*e.g.*, fever, tachycardia, tachypnea, elevated white blood cell count, altered mental state, and hyperglycemia in the absence of diabetes).[81,82] *Septic shock* is defined as severe sepsis with hypotension, despite fluid resuscitation, with a high risk for mortality.[81]

It is estimated that sepsis occurs in 1.5 million people each year in the United States, and about 250,000 die.[83] The growing incidence has been attributed to enhanced awareness of the diagnosis, increased number of resistant organisms, growing number of immunocompromised and older adults, and greater use of invasive procedures. With early intervention and advances in treatment methods, the mortality rate has decreased.[81–83]

Pathophysiology. The pathogenesis of sepsis involves a complex process of cellular activation resulting in the release of proinflammatory mediators such as cytokines, recruitment of neutrophils and monocytes, involvement of neuroendocrine reflexes, and activation of complement, coagulation, and

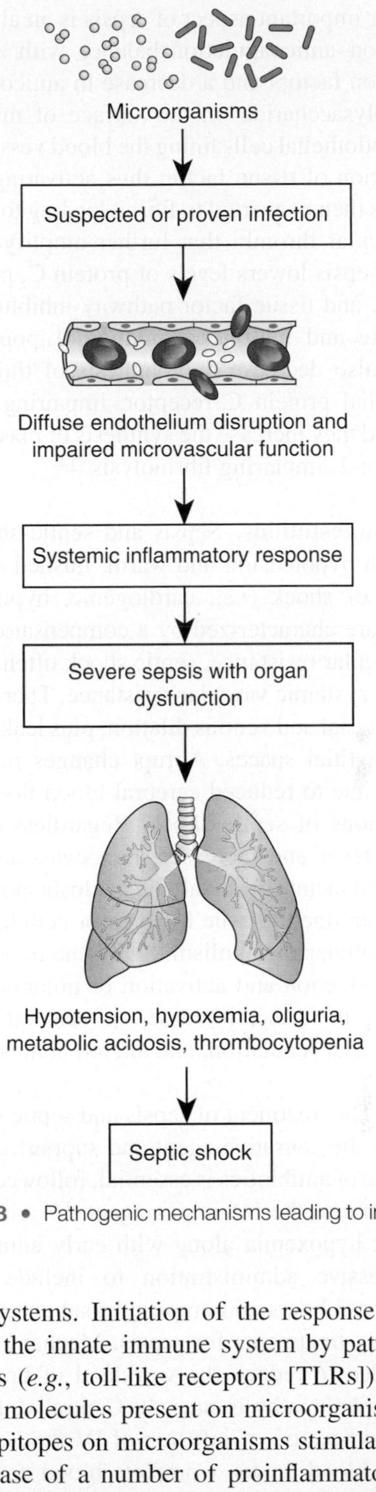

Figure 27.38 • Pathogenic mechanisms leading to infection to septic shock.

fibrinolytic systems. Initiation of the response begins with activation of the innate immune system by pattern recognition receptors (*e.g.*, toll-like receptors [TLRs]) that interact with specific molecules present on microorganisms. Binding of TLRs to epitopes on microorganisms stimulates transcription and release of a number of proinflammatory and anti-inflammatory mediators. Two of these mediators, TNF-α and interleukin-1, are involved in leukocyte adhesion, local inflammation, neutrophil activation, suppression of erythropoiesis, generation of fever, tachycardia, lactic acidosis, ventilation–perfusion abnormalities, and other signs of sepsis as discussed earlier. Although activated neutrophils kill microorganisms, they also injure the endothelium by releasing mediators that increase vascular permeability. In addition, activated endothelial cells release nitric oxide, a potent vasodilator that acts as a key mediator of septic shock.

Another important aspect of sepsis is an alteration of the procoagulation–anticoagulation balance with an increase in procoagulation factors and a decrease in anticoagulation factors. Lipopolysaccharide on the surface of microorganisms stimulates endothelial cells lining the blood vessels to increase their production of tissue factor, thus activating coagulation. Fibrinogen is then converted to fibrin, leading to the formation of microvascular thrombi that further amplify tissue injury. In addition, sepsis lowers levels of protein C, protein S, antithrombin III, and tissue factor pathway inhibitor, substances that modulate and inhibit coagulation. Lipopolysaccharide and TNF-α also decrease the synthesis of thrombomodulin and endothelial protein C receptor, impairing activation of protein C, and they increase the synthesis of plasminogen activator inhibitor-1, impairing fibrinolysis.[81,83]

Clinical Manifestations. Sepsis and septic shock typically manifest with hypotension and warm, flushed skin. Whereas other forms of shock (*i.e.*, cardiogenic, hypovolemic, and obstructive) are characterized by a compensatory increase in systemic vascular resistance, septic shock often presents with a decrease in systemic vascular resistance. There is hypovolemia due to arterial and venous dilation, plus leakage of plasma into the interstitial spaces. Abrupt changes in cognition or behavior are due to reduced cerebral blood flow and may be early indications of septic shock. Regardless of the underlying cause, fever and increased leukocytes are present. An elevated serum lactate or metabolic acidosis indicates anaerobic metabolism due to tissue hypoxia or cellular dysfunction and altered cellular metabolism.[81,82] Tissue hypoxia produces continued production and activation of inflammatory mediators, resulting in further increases in vascular permeability, impaired vascular regulation, and altered hemostasis.

Treatment. The treatment of sepsis and septic shock focuses on control of the causative agent and support of the circulation. Early use of antibiotics is essential, followed by antibiotic therapy specific to the infectious agent.[81,82] Airway management to treat hypoxemia along with early administration of fluids (aggressive administration to include crystalloids) within the first 3 hours and empiric broad-spectrum antibiotics are priority treatments for sepsis. Mechanical ventilation may be needed to reduce the workload of breathing, especially if encephalopathy is present. Central venous access is recommended because of infusion of IV fluids, medications, and frequent blood draws. Complete blood counts with differential, coagulation studies including D-dimer levels, serum lactate, and liver function tests are diagnostic and indicate the severity. Blood cultures from at least two different sites are obtained prior to antibiotic therapy.[82]

Obstructive Shock

The term *obstructive shock* describes circulatory shock that results from mechanical obstruction of the flow of blood through the central circulation (great veins, heart, or lungs; see Fig. 27.35). Obstructive shock may be caused by a number of conditions, including dissecting aortic aneurysm, cardiac tamponade, pneumothorax, atrial myxoma, and evisceration of abdominal contents into the thoracic cavity because of a ruptured hemidiaphragm. The most frequent cause of obstructive shock is PE.

The primary physiologic result of obstructive shock is elevated right heart pressure due to impaired right ventricular function. Pressures are increased despite impaired venous return to the heart. Signs of right-sided heart failure occur, including elevation of CVP and jugular venous distention. Treatment modalities focus on correcting the cause of the disorder, frequently with surgical interventions such as pulmonary embolectomy, pericardiocentesis (*i.e.*, removal of fluid from the pericardial sac) for cardiac tamponade, or the insertion of a chest tube for correction of a tension pneumothorax or hemothorax. In severe or massive pulmonary embolus, fibrinolytic drugs may be used to break down the clots causing the obstruction.

Complications of Shock

Many body systems are destroyed by shock. Five major complications of severe shock are the following:

1. Pulmonary injury
2. Acute renal failure
3. Gastrointestinal ulceration
4. Disseminated intravascular coagulation (DIC)
5. Multiple organ dysfunction syndrome (MODS)

These complications of shock are serious and often fatal.

Acute Lung Injury/Acute Respiratory Distress Syndrome

Acute lung injury/acute respiratory distress syndrome (ALI/ARDS) is a potentially lethal form of pulmonary injury that may be either the cause or result of shock. ARDS is a more severe aspect of ALI and is differentiated primarily for early intervention, prevention, and research purposes.

ALI/ARDS is marked by the rapid onset of profound dyspnea that usually occurs 12 to 48 hours after the initiating event. The respiratory rate and effort of breathing increase. Arterial blood gas analysis establishes the presence of profound hypoxemia that is refractory to supplemental oxygen. The hypoxemia results from impaired matching of ventilation and perfusion and from the greatly reduced diffusion of blood gases across the thickened alveolar membranes.

The Berlin definition of ARDS requires that the following criteria be present:

- Respiratory symptoms are present within 1 week of known clinical insult or new/worsening symptoms during the week.
- Chest x-ray or computed tomography shows bilateral opacities found with pulmonary edema not caused by pleural effusion, atelectasis, or pulmonary nodules.

- Cardiac failure or hypervolemia must not be the only cause for respiratory failure.
- Impairment of oxygenation must be present; severity of the hypoxemia determines the severity of the ARDS.[84]

Interventions for ALI/ARDS focus on increasing the oxygen concentration in the inspired air and supporting ventilation mechanically to optimize gas exchange while avoiding oxygen toxicity and preventing further lung injury. Although the delivery of high levels of oxygen using high-pressure mechanical ventilatory support and positive end-expiratory pressure may correct the hypoxemia, the mortality rate, which was previously greater than 50%, has declined (the exact rate of change is uncertain but attributed to improved mechanical ventilation and supportive care).[85] The use of sedation and analgesic agents increases tolerance to mechanical ventilation while also decreasing energy consumption. Evidence surrounding the use and effectiveness of muscle relaxants to improve oxygenation lacks scientific proof. Nutritional support can decrease catabolic losses and improve the immune response. Nosocomial pneumonia is a complication of ARDS leading to prolonged mechanical ventilation and increased rate of mortality. Even with prophylactic treatment, the risk of DVT and PE is high and contributes to immobility, trauma, and activation of the coagulation pathway. To prevent gastrointestinal complications such as risk for GI bleed, prophylaxis against stress ulcers is recommended.[85]

Acute Renal Failure

The renal tubules are particularly vulnerable to ischemia, and acute renal failure is an important factor in mortality because of severe shock. Most cases of acute renal failure are due to impaired renal perfusion or direct injury to the kidneys. The degree of renal damage is related to the severity and duration of shock. The normal kidney is able to tolerate severe ischemia for 15 to 20 minutes. The renal dysfunction most frequently seen after severe shock is acute tubular necrosis. Acute tubular necrosis usually is reversible, although return to normal renal function may require weeks or months. Continuous monitoring of urinary output during shock provides a means of assessing renal blood flow. Frequent monitoring of serum creatinine and blood urea nitrogen levels also provides valuable information regarding renal status.

Mediators implicated in septic shock are powerful vasoconstrictors capable of activating the sympathetic nervous system and causing intravascular clotting. They have been shown to trigger all the separate physiologic mechanisms that contribute to the onset of acute renal failure.

Gastrointestinal Complications

The most important risk factors for gastrointestinal complications are shock and administration of drugs used to treat shock. Splanchnic perfusion and intolerance to enteral nutrition may lead to hypoperfusion of the gut. The gastrointestinal tract is particularly vulnerable to ischemia because of the changes in distribution of blood flow to its mucosal surface. In shock, there is widespread constriction of blood vessels that supply the gastrointestinal tract, causing a redistribution of blood flow and a severe decrease in mucosal perfusion. People may experience loss of appetite, nausea, or vomiting. Superficial mucosal lesions of the stomach and duodenum can develop within hours of severe trauma, sepsis, or burns. Bowel obstruction or bleeding may occur after the decrease in perfusion in shock. Hemorrhage usually has its onset within 2 to 10 days after the original insult and often begins without warning. Poor perfusion in the gastrointestinal tract has been credited with allowing intestinal bacteria to enter the bloodstream, thereby contributing to the development of sepsis and shock.[75,76] Shock can result in intestinal and gastric mucosa tissue damage due to decreased supply of ATP during shock states. When ischemia is present, the gastrointestinal tract is at risk for reperfusion injury, where oxygen supply that is restored produces free radicals, leading to tissue damage. The glycoprotein mucous layer that forms a protective physical barrier in the gut is decreased during shock states.

Histamine type 2 receptor antagonists, proton pump inhibitors, or sucralfate may be given prophylactically to prevent gastrointestinal ulcerations caused by shock. Nasogastric tubes, when attached to intermittent suction, also help to diminish the accumulation of hydrogen ions in the stomach. Enteral nutrition may also reduce the risk of GI bleed. Intravenous proton pump inhibitors are used to treat severe upper gastrointestinal bleeding.[75,86]

Disseminated Intravascular Coagulation

DIC is characterized by widespread activation of the coagulation system with resultant formation of fibrin clots and thrombotic occlusion of small and midsized vessels. The systemic formation of fibrin results from increased generation of thrombin, the simultaneous suppression of physiologic anticoagulation mechanisms, and the delayed removal of fibrin as a consequence of impaired fibrinolysis. Clinically overt DIC is reported to occur in as much as 1% of hospitalized people and in 30% to 50% of people with sepsis.[86] As with other systemic inflammatory responses, the derangement of coagulation and fibrinolysis is thought to be mediated by inflammatory mediators and cytokines.

The contribution of DIC to morbidity and mortality in sepsis depends on the underlying clinical condition and the intensity of the coagulation disorder. Depletion of the platelets and coagulation factors increases the risk of bleeding. Deposition of fibrin in the vasculature of organs contributes to ischemic damage and organ failure. However, it remains uncertain whether DIC was a predictor of unfavorable outcome or merely a marker of the seriousness of the underlying condition causing the DIC.

The management of sepsis-induced DIC focuses on treatment of the underlying disorder and measures to interrupt the coagulation process. Platelet and factor replacement to correct bleeding and heparin for people with excessive fibrin deposits is recommended.[87,88]

Multiple Organ Dysfunction Syndrome

MODS represents the presence of altered organ function in an acutely ill person such that homeostasis cannot be maintained without intervention. As the name implies, MODS commonly affects multiple organ systems, including the kidneys, lungs, liver, brain, and heart. MODS is a particularly life-threatening complication of shock, especially septic shock. It has been reported as the most frequent cause of death in the noncoronary intensive care unit. Mortality rates vary but range from 40% to 75% in people with MODS due to sepsis.[89] Mortality rates increase with an increased number of organs failing. A high mortality rate is associated with failure of the brain, liver, kidneys, and lungs. The pathogenesis of MODS is not clearly understood, and current management therefore is primarily supportive. Elevated levels of endotoxins consistent with septic shock are also found in multiple organ dysfunction. Apoptosis is also delayed during sepsis, contributing to multiple organ failure. Major risk factors for the development of MODS are severe trauma, sepsis, prolonged periods of hypotension, hepatic dysfunction, infarcted bowel, advanced age, and alcohol abuse. Interventions for multiple organ failure are focused on support of the affected organs.[89,90]

IN SUMMARY

Circulatory shock is an acute emergency in which body tissues are deprived of oxygen and cellular nutrients or are unable to use these materials in their metabolic processes. Circulatory shock may develop because the heart is unable to adequately pump blood through the circulatory system (cardiogenic shock), there is insufficient blood in the circulatory system (*i.e.*, hypovolemic shock), there is a maldistribution of blood due to abnormalities in the vascular resistance (*i.e.*, distributive shock), or blood flow or venous return is obstructed (*i.e.*, obstructive shock). Three types of shock share the basic circulatory pattern of distributive shock: neurogenic shock, anaphylactic shock, and septic shock. Septic shock, which is the most common of the three types, is associated with a severe, overwhelming inflammatory response and has a high mortality rate.

The manifestations of hypovolemic shock, which serves as a prototype for circulatory shock, are related to low peripheral blood flow and excessive sympathetic stimulation. The low peripheral blood flow produces thirst, changes in skin temperature, decreased blood pressure, increased heart rate, decreased venous pressure, decreased urine output, and changes in the sensorium. The intense vasoconstriction that serves to maintain blood flow to the heart and brain causes a decrease in tissue perfusion, impaired cellular metabolism, liberation of lactic acid, and, eventually, cell death. Whether the shock is irreversible or the person will survive is determined largely by changes that occur at the cellular level.

The complications of shock result from the deprivation of blood flow to vital organs or systems, such as the lungs, kidneys, gastrointestinal tract, and blood coagulation system. Shock can cause or be accompanied by ALI/ARDS, which is characterized by changes in the permeability of the alveolar–capillary membrane with development of interstitial edema and severe hypoxemia that does not respond to oxygen therapy. The renal tubules are particularly vulnerable to ischemia, and acute renal failure is an important complication of shock. Gastrointestinal ischemia may lead to gastrointestinal bleeding and increased vascular permeability to intestinal bacteria, which can cause further sepsis and shock. DIC is characterized by formation of small clots in the circulation. It is thought to be caused by inappropriate activation of the coagulation cascade because of toxins or other products released as a result of the shock state. Multiple organ failure, perhaps the most ominous complication of shock, rapidly depletes the body's ability to compensate and recover from a shock state.

GERIATRIC Considerations

- The heart's very limited ability to regenerate is due to a very slow rate of replacement of the cardiac stem cells and myocytes.[91]
- The ventricles become stiffer with age resulting in increased filling (diastolic) pressure leading to greater risk for diastolic heart failure.[91]
- Thirty-five percent of older adults are obese, which is a risk factor for coronary heart disease and atherosclerosis; black women aged 65 and older are at the greatest risk.[92]
- Symptoms associated with peptic ulcer disease in older adults are more severe than in younger adults, leading to dehydration, hemorrhage, infection, and risk of shock.[93]
- The decreased ability of the older adult to quickly respond to shock makes it imperative to observe for symptoms such as restlessness, which is the primary symptom of hypoxia; administer prophylactic oxygen; and carefully monitor intake and output.[93]

PEDIATRIC Considerations

- Levels of brain (b-type) natriuretic protein (BNP) are a biomarker to indicate severity of heart failure in infants.[91]
- Cardiac hypertrophy in infants rereleases atrial natriuretic factor usually restricted to the atrium after birth along with contractile proteins to compensate for decreased cardiac output.[91]
- Evidence of maternal rubella infection during the first 4 weeks of gestation is the greatest risk for congenital cardiac defects. Persistent patent ductus arteriosus is the most common congenital cardiac defect in mothers infected with rubella during the early weeks of gestation.[91]
- Acute renal failure in children is most often the result of hypovolemic or septic shock.[94]
- A line of demarcation of skin temperature is a sign that the child may be developing shock with accompanying cardiovascular compromise.[94]
- Neonates exhibit a paradoxical phenomenon of exhibiting bradycardia rather than tachycardia seen in infants and children in shock.[94]

REVIEW EXERCISES

1. A 45-year-old man presents in the emergency department complaining of substernal chest pain that is also felt in his left shoulder. He is short of breath and nauseated. His blood pressure is 160/90 mm Hg, and his heart rate is 100 beats/minute. His ECG shows an ST-segment elevation in leads II, III, and AVF. He is given oxygen, aspirin, and nitroglycerin. Blood tests reveal elevated CK-MB and TnI.
   A. *What is the probable cause of the man's symptoms?*
   B. *What is the significance of the ST-segment changes?*
   C. *What is the significance of elevated CK-MB and TnI?*
   D. *Relate the actions of aspirin, nitroglycerin, and oxygen to the treatment of this man's condition.*
2. A 50-year-old woman presents with complaints of paroxysmal nocturnal dyspnea and orthopnea, palpitations, and fatigue. An echocardiogram demonstrates a thickened, immobile mitral valve with anterior and posterior leaflets moving together, slow early diastolic filling of the ventricle, and left atrial enlargement.
   A. *What is the probable cause of this woman's symptoms?*
   B. *Explain the pathologic significance of the slow early diastolic filling, distended left atrium, and palpitations.*
   C. *Given the echocardiographic data, what type of cardiac murmur would you expect to find in this woman?*
   D. *Which circulation (systemic or pulmonary) would you expect to be affected as this woman's mitral valve disorder progresses?*
3. A 75-year-old male with long-standing hypertension and angina due to coronary heart disease presents with ankle edema, nocturia, increased shortness of breath with activity, and a chronic nonproductive cough. He has a past history of smoking two packs per day and drinking, but he says he now does not smoke and is now sober. His blood pressure is 170/80 and his heart rate is 100. ECG and chest radiography indicate the presence of left ventricular hypertrophy.
   A. *Relate the presence of uncontrolled hypertension and CAD to the development of heart failure in this man.*
   B. *Explain the significance of left ventricular hypertrophy in terms of both a compensatory mechanism and a pathologic mechanism in the progression of heart failure.*
   C. *Explain the management and treatment for this diagnosis.*
4. A 4-month-old male infant is brought into the pediatric clinic by his mother. She reports that she noted over the past several weeks that her baby's lips and mouth and his fingernails and toenails have become a bluish-gray color. She also states that he seems to tire easily and that even nursing seems to wear him out. Lately, he has had several spells where he has suddenly turned blue, has had difficulty breathing, and has been very irritable. During one of these spells, he turned limp and seemed to have passed out for a short time. An echocardiogram reveals a thickening of the right ventricular wall with overriding of the aorta, a large subaortic ventricular septal defect, and narrowing of the pulmonary outflow with stenosis of the pulmonary valve.
   A. *What is this infant's probable diagnosis?*
   B. *Describe the shunting of blood that occurs with this disorder and its relationship to the development of cyanosis.*
   C. *The surgical creation of a shunt between the aorta and pulmonary artery may be performed as a palliative procedure for infants with marked hypoplasia of the pulmonary artery, with corrective surgery performed*

later in childhood. Explain how this procedure increases blood flow to the lungs.

5. A 21-year-old man is admitted to the emergency department with excessive blood loss after an automobile injury. He is alert and anxious, his skin is cool and moist, his heart rate is 135, and his blood pressure is 100/85. He is receiving intravenous fluids, which were started at the scene of the accident by an emergency medical technician. He has been typed and cross-matched for blood transfusions, and a urinary catheter has been inserted to monitor his urinary output. His urinary output has been less than 10 mL since admission, and his blood pressure has dropped to 85/70. Efforts to control his bleeding have been unsuccessful, and he is being prepared for emergency surgery.
   A. *Use information regarding the compensatory mechanisms in circulatory shock to explain this man's presenting symptoms, including urinary output.*
   B. *The treatment of hypovolemic shock is usually directed at maintaining the circulatory volume through fluid resuscitation rather than maintaining the blood pressure through the use of vasoactive medications. Explain.*

References

1. Gaziano T. A., Prabhakaran D., Gaziano J. M. (2015). Global burden of cardiovascular disease. In Mann D. L., Zipes D. P., Libby P., et al. (Eds.) *Braunwald's heart disease: A textbook of cardiovascular medicine* (10th ed., pp. 1–20). Philadelphia, PA: Elsevier Saunders.
2. Roger V. L., Go A. S., Lloyd-Jones D., et al. (2012). Heart disease and stroke statistics—2012 update. A report from the American Heart Association Statistics Committee and Stroke Statistics Subcommittee. *Circulation* 125, e2–e220.
3. LeWinter M. M., Tischler M. D. (2015). Pericardial diseases. In Mann D. L., Zipes D. P., Libby P. (Eds.) *Braunwald's heart disease: A textbook of cardiovascular medicine* (10th ed., pp. 1636–1657). Philadelphia, PA: Elsevier Saunders.
4. O'Gara P. T., Kushner F. G., Ascheim D. D., et al. (2013). ACC/AHA guidelines for the management of patients with ST-elevation myocardial infarction. *Circulation* 110, e362–e425.
5. Guyton A., Hall J. E. (2016). *Textbook of medical physiology* (13th ed., pp. 259–270). Philadelphia, PA: Elsevier Saunders.
6. Center for Disease Control. (2017). *Heart attack.* Available: https://www.cdc.gov/heartdisease/heart_attack.htm. Accessed February 28, 2018.
7. Opie L. H., Bers D. M. (2015). Mechanisms of cardiac contraction and relaxation. In Mann D. L., Zipes D. P., Libby P., et al. (Eds.) *Braunwald's heart disease: A textbook of cardiovascular medicine* (10th ed., pp. 429–453). Philadelphia, PA: Elsevier Saunders.
8. Myers J. (2011). Exercise testing. In Woods S. L., Froelicher E. S., Motzer S. U., et al. (Eds.) *Cardiac nursing* (6th ed., pp. 420–435). Philadelphia, PA: Lippincott Williams & Wilkins.
9. Solomon S. D., Wu Justina, Gillam L. D. (2015). Echocardiography. In Mann D. L., Zipes D. P., Libby P., et al. (Eds.) *Braunwald's heart disease: A textbook of cardiovascular medicine* (10th ed., pp. 179–260). Philadelphia, PA: Elsevier Saunders.
10. Udelson J. E., Dilsizian V., Bonow R. O. (2015). Nuclear cardiology. In Mann D. L., Zipes D. P., Libby P., et al. (Eds.) *Braunwald's heart disease: A textbook of cardiovascular medicine* (10th ed., pp. 271–319). Philadelphia, PA: Elsevier Saunders.
11. Kwong R. Y. (2015). Cardiovascular magnetic resonance. In Mann D. L., Zipes D. P., Libby P., et al. (Eds.) *Braunwald's heart disease: A textbook of cardiovascular medicine* (10th ed., pp. 320–340). Philadelphia, PA: Elsevier Saunders.
12. Taylor A. J. (2015). Cardiac computed tomography. In Mann D. L., Zipes D. P., Libby P., et al. (Eds.) *Braunwald's heart disease: A textbook of cardiovascular medicine* (10th ed., pp. 341–363). Philadelphia, PA: Elsevier Saunders.
13. Davidson C. J., Bonow R. O. (2015). Cardiac catheterization. In Mann D. L., Zipes D. P., Libby P., et al. (Eds.) *Braunwald's heart disease: A textbook of cardiovascular medicine* (10th ed., pp. 364–391). Philadelphia, PA: Elsevier Saunders.
14. Falk E., Fuster V. (2017). Atherothrombosis: Disease burden, activity, and vulnerability. In Fuster V., Walsh R. A., Harrington R. A., et al. (Eds.) *Hurst's the heart* (14th ed., chapter 32). New York, NY: McGraw-Hill.
15. Badimon J. J., Ibanez B., Fuster V., et al. (2017). Coronary thrombosis: Local and systemic factors. In Fuster V., Walsh R. A., Harrington R. A., et al. (Eds.) *Hurst's the heart* (14th ed., chapter 33). New York, NY: McGraw-Hill.
16. Mirvis D. M., Goldberger A. L. (2015). Electrocardiography. In Mann D. L., Zipes D. P., Libby P., et al. (Eds.) *Braunwald's heart disease: A textbook of cardiovascular medicine* (10th ed., pp. 114–154). Philadelphia, PA: Elsevier Saunders.
17. Scirica B. M., Morrow D. A. (2015). ST-elevation myocardial infarction: Pathology, pathophysiology, and clinical features; and ST-elevation myocardial infarction: Management. In Bonow R. O., Mann D. L., Zipes D., et al. (Eds.) *Braunwald's heart disease: A textbook of cardiovascular medicine* (10th ed., pp. 1068–1094). Philadelphia, PA: Elsevier Saunders.
18. Giugliano R. P., Cannon C. P., Braunwald E. (2015). Non-ST elevation acute coronary syndromes. In Mann D. L., Zipes D. P., et al. (Eds.) *Braunwald's heart disease: A textbook of cardiovascular medicine* (10th ed., pp.1155–1181). Philadelphia, PA: Elsevier Saunders.
19. Canty J. M., Duncker D. J. (2015). Coronary blood flow and myocardial ischemia. In Mann D. L., Zipes D. P., et al. (Eds.) *Braunwald's heart disease: A textbook of cardiovascular medicine* (10th ed., pp. 1029–1056). Philadelphia, PA: Elsevier Saunders.
20. Mauri L., Bhatt D. (2015). Percutaneous coronary interventions. In Mann D. L., Zipes D. P., Libby P., et al. (Eds.) *Braunwald's heart disease: A textbook of cardiovascular medicine* (10th ed., pp. 1245–1268). Philadelphia, PA: Elsevier Saunders.
21. Hills L. D., Smith P. K., Anderson J. L., et al. (2011). 2011 ACC/AHA Guideline for coronary artery bypass graft surgery. *Circulation* 124, e652–e735.
22. Thompson P. D. (2015). Exercise-based, comprehensive rehabilitation. In Mann D. L., Zipes D. P., Libby P., et al. (Eds.) *Braunwald's heart disease: A textbook of cardiovascular medicine* (10th ed., pp. 1015–1020). Philadelphia, PA: Elsevier Saunders.
23. Morrow D. A., Boden W. B. (2015). Stable ischemic heart disease. In Mann D. L., Zipes D. P., Libby P., et al. (Eds.) *Braunwald's heart disease: A textbook of cardiovascular medicine* (10th ed., pp. 1182–1244). Philadelphia, PA: Elsevier Saunders.
24. Maron B. J., Towbin J. A., Thiene G., et al. (2006). Contemporary definitions and classification of the cardiomyopathies. *Circulation* 113, 1807–1816.
25. Chowdhry S., Jacoby D., Moon J. C., et al. (2016). Update on hypertrophic cardiomyopathy and a guide to the guidelines. *Nature Reviews Cardiology* 13, 651–675.
26. Otto C. M., Bonow R. O. (2015). Valvular heart disease. In Mann D. L., Zipes D. P., Libby P., et al. (Eds.) *Braunwald's heart disease: A textbook of cardiovascular medicine* (10th ed., pp. 1446–1523). Philadelphia, PA: Elsevier Saunders.

27. Arbustini E., Favalli B., Narula N., et al. (2017). Genetic basis of cardiovascular disease. In Fuster V., Walsh R. A., Harrington R. A., et al. (Eds.) *Hurst's the heart* (14th ed., chapter 9). New York, NY: McGraw-Hill.
28. Priori S., Napolitano C. (2017). Genetics of channelopathies and clinical implications. In Fuster V., Walsh R. A., Harrington R. A., et al. (Eds.) *Hurst's the heart* (14th ed., chapter 80). New York, NY: McGraw-Hill.
29. Arbustini E., Serrio A., Favalli V., et al. (2017). Dilated cardiomyopathies. In Fuster V., Walsh R. A., Harrington R. A., et al. (Eds.) *Hurst's the heart* (14th ed., chapter 58). New York, NY: McGraw-Hill.
30. Arbustini E., Agozzino M., Favalli V., et al. (2017). Myocarditis. In Fuster V., Walsh R. A., Harrington R. A., et al. (Eds.) *Hurst's the heart* (14th ed., chapter 63). New York, NY: McGraw-Hill.
31. Maisch B., Pankuweit S. (2013). Standard and etiology-directed evidence-based therapies in myocarditis: State of the art and future perspectives. *Heart Failure Reviews* 18, 761–795.
32. Johnson-Coyle L., Jensen L., Sobey A. (2012). Peripartum cardiomyopathy: Review and practice guidelines. *American Journal of Critical Care* 21, 89–98.
33. Tarkin J. M., Khetyar M., Kaski J. C. (2008). Management of Takotsubo syndrome. *Cardiovascular Drugs and Therapy* 22, 71–77.
34. Baddour L. M., Freeman W. K., Suri R. M., et al. (2015). Cardiovascular infections. In Mann D. L., Zipes D. P., Libby P., et al. (Eds.) *Braunwald's heart disease: A textbook of cardiovascular medicine* (10th ed., pp. 1524–1550). Philadelphia, PA: Elsevier Saunders.
35. Badour L., Wilson W., Bayer A. (2015). Infective endocarditis: diagnosis, antimicrobial therapy, and management of complications. *Circulation* 132, 1435–1486.
36. Mayosi B. M. (2015). Rheumatic fever. In Bonow R. O., Mann D. L., Zipes D. P., et al. (Eds.) *Braunwald's heart disease: A textbook of cardiovascular medicine* (10th ed., pp. 1834–1842). Philadelphia, PA: Elsevier Saunders.
37. Mason J. C. (2015). Rheumatic diseases and the cardiovascular system. In Bonow R. O., Mann D. L., Zipes D. P., et al. (Eds.) *Braunwald's heart disease: A textbook of cardiovascular medicine* (10th ed., pp. 1876–1892). Philadelphia, PA: Elsevier Saunders.
38. Bahl V. K., Math R. S., Carabello B. A. (2017). Mitral stenosis. In Fuster V., Walsh R. A., Harrington R. A., et al. (Eds.) *Hurst's the heart* (14th ed., chapter 50). New York, NY: McGraw-Hill.
39. Nishimura R. A., Otto C. M., Bonow R. O., et al. (2014). ACC/AHA 2014 guideline for the management of patients with valvular heart disease. *Circulation* 129, e521–e643
40. Groarke J. D., Carabello B. A., O'Gara P. T. (2017). Ischemic mitral regurgitation. In Fuster V., Walsh R. A., Harrington R. A., et al. (Eds.) *Hurst's the heart* (14th ed., chapter 49). New York, NY: McGraw-Hill.
41. Carabello B. A., Hahn R. T.. (2017). Aortic valve disease. In Fuster V., Walsh R. A., Harrington R. A., et al. (Eds.) *Hurst's the heart* (14th ed., chapter 47). New York, NY: McGraw-Hill.
42. Yancy C. W., Jessup M., Bozkurt B., et al. (2013). 2013 ACC/AHA 2013 guidelines for the management of heart failure. *Circulation* 128, e240–e327.
43. Yancy C. W., Jessup M., Bozkurt B., et al. (2016). 2016 ACCF/AHA/HFSA Focused update on new pharmacological therapy for heart failure. *Circulation* 134, 1977–2016.
44. Guyton A. C., Hall J. E. (2016). *Textbook of medical physiology* (13th ed., pp. 245–258). Philadelphia, PA: Elsevier Saunders.
45. Opie L. H., Bers D. M. (2015). Mechanisms of cardiac contraction and relaxation. In Bonow R. O., Mann D. L., Zipes D. P., et al., (Eds.) *Braunwald's heart disease: A textbook of cardiovascular medicine* (10th ed., pp. 429–453). Philadelphia, PA: Elsevier Saunders.
46. Januzzi J. L., Mann D. L. (2015). Clinical assessment of heart failure. In Bonow R. O., Mann D. L., Zipes D. P., et al. (Eds.) *Braunwald's heart disease: A textbook of cardiovascular medicine* (10th ed., pp. 473–483). Philadelphia, PA: Elsevier Saunders.
47. Mann D. (2015). Management of heart failure with reduced ejection fraction. In Bonow R. O., Mann D. L., Zipes D. P., et al. (Eds.) *Braunwald's heart disease: A textbook of cardiovascular medicine* (10th ed., pp. 512–546). Philadelphia, PA: Elsevier Saunders.
48. Hasenfuss G., Mann D. (2015). Pathophysiology of heart failure. In Bonow R. O., Mann D. L., Zipes D. P., et al. (Eds.) *Braunwald's heart disease: A textbook of cardiovascular medicine* (10th ed., pp. 454–472). Philadelphia, PA: Elsevier Saunders.
49. Gaggin H. K., Dec G. W. (2017). Pathophysiology of heart failure. In Fuster V., Walsh R. A., Harrington R. A., et al. (Eds.) *Hurst's the heart* (14th ed., chapter 68). New York, NY: McGraw-Hill.
50. Felker G. M., Teerlink J. R. (2015). Diagnosis and management of acute heart failure. In Bonow R. O., Mann D. L., Zipes D. P., et al. (Eds.) *Braunwald's heart disease: A textbook of cardiovascular medicine* (10th ed., pp. 484–511). Philadelphia, PA: Elsevier Saunders.
51. Ahmad T., Butler J., Borlaug B. (2017). The diagnosis and management of chronic heart failure. In Fuster V., Walsh R. A., Harrington R. A., et al. (Eds.) *Hurst's the heart* (14th ed., chapter 70). New York, NY: McGraw-Hill.
52. Bloom M. W., Cole R. T., Butler J. (2017). Evaluation and management of acute heart failure. In Fuster V., Walsh R. A., Harrington R. A., et al. (Eds.) *Hurst's the heart* (14th ed., chapter 71). New York, NY: McGraw-Hill.
53. Yancy C. W., Jessup M. (2017). 2017 ACC/AHA/HFSA Focused Update of the 2013 ACCF/AHA Guideline for the Management of Heart Failure. *Circulation* 136, e137–e161.
54. Upadhyay G. A., Singh J. P. (2017). Pacemakers and defibrillators. In Fuster V., Walsh R. A., Harrington R. A., et al. (Eds.) *Hurst's the heart* (14th ed., chapter 89). New York, NY: McGraw-Hill.
55. Jessup M., Acker M. A. (2015). Surgical management of heart failure. In Bonow R. O., Mann D. L., Zipes D. P., et al. (Eds.) *Braunwald's heart disease: A textbook of cardiovascular medicine* (10th ed., pp. 575–589). Philadelphia, PA: Elsevier Saunders.
56. Van Praagh R. (2006). Embryology. In Keane J. F., Lock J. E., Fyler D. C. (Eds.) *Nadas' Pediatric Cardiology* (2nd ed., pp. 13–25). Philadelphia, PA: Elsevier Saunders.
57. Freed M. D. (2006). Fetal and transitional circulation. In Keane J. F., Lock J. E., Fyler D. C. (Eds.) *Nadas' Pediatric Cardiology* (2nd ed., pp. 75–79). Philadelphia, PA: Elsevier Saunders.
58. Nadas A. S., Fyler D. C. (2006). Hypoxemia. In Keane J. F., Lock J. E., Fyler D. C. (Eds.) *Nadas' Pediatric Cardiology* (2nd ed., pp. 97–101). Philadelphia, PA: Elsevier Saunders.
59. Webb G. D., Smallhorn J. F., Therrien J., et al. (2015). Congenital heart disease. In Mann D. L., Zipes D. P., et al. (Eds.) *Braunwald's heart disease: A textbook of cardiovascular medicine* (10th ed., pp. 1391–1445). Philadelphia, PA: Elsevier Saunders.
60. Lin J. P., Child J. S. (2017). Congenital heart disease in adolescents and adults. In Fuster V., Walsh R. A., Harrington R. A., et al. (Eds.) *Hurst's the heart* (14th ed., chapter 56). New York, NY: McGraw-Hill.
61. Colan S. D. (2006). Cardiomyopathies. In Keane J. F., Lock J. E., Fyler D. C. (Eds.) *Nadas' Pediatric Cardiology* (2nd ed., pp. 415–445). Philadelphia, PA: Elsevier Saunders.
62. Nishimura R. A., Otto C. M., Bonow R. O., et al. (2017). 2017 ACC/AHA focused update of the 2014 guideline for the management of patients with valvular heart disease. *Circulation* 135(25), e1159–e1195.
63. Keane J. F., Geva T., Fyler D. C. (2006). Atrial septal defect, ventricular septal defect, coarctation of the aorta, single ventricle, pulmonary stenosis. In Keane J. F., Lock J. E., Fyler D. C. (Eds.) *Nadas' Pediatric Cardiology* (2nd ed., pp. 527–558, 603–616, 627–644, 743–752). Philadelphia, PA: Elsevier Saunders.
64. Marx G. R., Fyler D. C. (2006). Endocardial cushion defects. In Keane J. F., Lock J. E., Fyler D. C. (Eds.) *Nadas' Pediatric Cardiology* (2nd ed., pp. 663–674). Philadelphia, PA: Elsevier Saunders.

65. Fulton D. R., Fyler D. C. (2006). D-Transposition of the great arteries. In Keane J. F., Lock J. E., Fyler D. C. (Eds.) *Nadas' Pediatric Cardiology* (2nd ed., pp. 645–662). Philadelphia, PA: Elsevier Saunders.
66. LoBreitbart R. E., Fyler D. C. (2006). Tetralogy of Fallot. In Keane J. F., Lock J. E., Fyler D. C. (Eds.) *Nadas' Pediatric Cardiology* (2nd ed., pp. 559–580). Philadelphia, PA: Elsevier Saunders.
67. Landzberg M. (2006). Adult congenital heart disease. In Keane J. F., Lock J. E., Fyler D. C. (Eds.) *Nadas' Pediatric Cardiology* (2nd ed., pp. 833–841). Philadelphia, PA: Elsevier Saunders.
68. Fulton D. R., Newburger J. W. (2006). Kawasaki disease. In Keane J. F., Lock J. E., Fyler D. C. (Eds.) *Nadas' Pediatric Cardiology* (2nd ed., pp. 401–413). Philadelphia, PA: Elsevier Saunders.
69. Bernstein D. (2016). Heart failure. In Kliegman R. M., Stanton B. F., et al. (Eds.) *Nelson Textbook of Pediatrics* (20th ed., pp. 2282–2288). Philadelphia, PA: Elsevier Saunders.
70. American Heart Association. (2017). Heart disease and stroke statistics: 2017 update at a glance. [Online]. Available: www.americanheart.org/downloadable/heart/.pdf. Accessed October 12, 2017.
71. Rich M. W. (2011). Heart failure in older adults. *Medical Clinics of North America* 95(3), 439–461.
72. Schwartz J. B., Zipes D. P. (2015). Cardiovascular disease in the elderly. In Bonow R. O., Mann D. L., Zipes D. P., et al. (Eds.) *Braunwald's heart disease: A textbook of cardiovascular medicine* (10th ed., pp. 1711–1743). Philadelphia, PA: Elsevier Saunders.
73. Guyton A. C., Hall J. E. (2016). *Textbook of medical physiology* (13th ed., pp. 169–291). Philadelphia, PA: Elsevier.
74. Bloom M. M., Cole R. T., Butler J.. Evaluation and management of acute heart failure. In: Fuster V., Harrington R. A., Narula J., Eapen Z. J. (Eds.) *Hurst's the heart* (14th ed.) New York, NY: McGraw-Hill. http://accessmedicine.mhmedical.com/content.aspx?bookid=2046&sectionid=176562062. Accessed May 22, 2018
75. Gaieski D. F., Mikkelsen M. (2018). Evaluation of and initial approach to the adult patient with undifferentiated hypotension and shock. In Finley G. (Ed.) *UpToDate*. Retrieved May 15, 2015 from https://www-uptodate-comcontents/evaluation-of-and-initial-approach-to-the-adult-patient-with-undifferentiated-hypotension-and-shock?search=evaluation%20and%20management%20of%20shock%20states:%20hypovolemic,%20distributive,%20and%20cardiogenic%20shock&source=search_result&selectedTitle=3~150&usage_type=default&display_rank=3
76. Gaieski D. F., Mikkelsen M. E. (2018). Definition, classification, etiology, and pathophysiology of shock in adults. In Finlay G. (Ed.) *UpToDate.* Retrieved May 15, 2018 from https://www-uptodate-com/contents/definition-classification-etiology-and-pathophysiology-of-shock-in-adults?search=evaluation%20and%20management%20of%20shock%20states:%20hypovolemic,%20distributive,%20and%20cardiogenic%20shock&source=search_result&selectedTitle=4~150&usage_type=default&display_rank=4f
77. Hochman J. S., Reyentovich A.. In Saperia G. M. (Ed.) *UpToDate*. Prognosis and treatment of cardiogenic shock complicating acute myocardial infarction. Retrieved May 15, 2018 from https://www-uptodate-com/contents/prognosis-and-treatment-of-cardiogenic-shock-complicating-acute-myocardial-infarction?search=cardiogenic%20shock:%20complicating%20myocardial%20infarction:%20an%20overview&source=search_result&selectedTitle=1~150&usage_type=default&display_rank=1
78. Smith N, Silberman M. *Shock, Distributive. Updated 2017 October 31. In: StatPearls [Internet]*. Treasure Island (FL): StatPearls Publishing; 2018 Jan. Available: https://www-ncbi-nlm-nih-gov.ezproxy.uthsc.edu/books/NBK470316/. Retrieved May 15, 2018.
79. Kelso J. M. (2018). Anaphylaxis: Confirming the diagnosis and determining the cause(s). In Feldweg A. M. (Ed.) *UpToDate.* Retrieved May 15, 2018 from https://www-uptodate-com/contents/anaphylaxis-confirming-the-diagnosis-and-determining-the-causes?search=anaphylaxis:%20confirming%20the%20diagnosis%20and%20determing%20the%20cause&source=search_result&selectedTitle=1~150&usage_type=default&display_rank=1
80. Campbell R. L., Kelso J. M. (2017). Anaphylaxis: Emergency treatment. In Feldweg A. M. (Ed.) *UpToDate*. Retrieved May 15, 2018 from https://www-uptodate-com/contents/anaphylaxis-emergency-treatment?search=anaphylaxis%20treatment&source=search_result&selectedTitle=1~150&usage_type=default&display_rank=1
81. Neviere R. (2018). Sepsis syndromes in adults: Epidemiology, definitions, clinical presentation, diagnosis, and prognosis. In Finlay G. (Ed.) *UpToDate.* Retrieved May 15, 2018 from https://www-uptodate-com/contents/sepsis-syndromes-in-adults-epidemiology-definitions-clinical-presentation-diagnosis-and-prognosis?search=sepsis%20syndromes%20in%20adults:%20epidemiology,%20definitions,&source=search_result&selectedTitle=1~150&usage_type=default&display_rank=1
82. Schmidt G. A., Mandel J. (2018). Evaluation and management of suspected sepsis and septic shock in Adults. In Finlay G. (Ed.) *UpToDate.* Retrieved May 15, 2018 from https://www-uptodate-com / contents/evaluation-and-management-of-suspected-sepsis-and-septic-shock-in-adults?search=evaluation%20and%20managment%20of%20suspected%20sepsis%20and%20septic%20shock%20in%20adults&source=search_result&selectedTitle=1~150&usage_type=default&display_rank=1
83. Center for Disease Control and Prevention. (2017). *Sepsis.* Available: https://www-uptodate-com.ezproxy.uthsc.edu/contents/clinical-features-diagnosis-and-treatment-of-disseminated-intravascular-coagulation-in-adults?search=recombinant%20human%20activated%20protein%20C%20and%20septic%20shock&source=search_result&selectedTitle=4~150&usage_type=default&display_rank=4. Retrieved May 15, 2018
84. Siegel M. D. (2017). Acute respiratory distress syndrome: Clinical features and diagnosis in adults. In Finlay G. (Ed.) *UpToDate.* Retrieved May 15, 2018 from https://www-uptodate-com/contents/acute-respiratory-distress-syndrome-clinical-features-and-diagnosis-in-adults?search=acute%20lung%20injury%20and%20shock&source=search_result&selectedTitle=2~150&usage_type=default&display_rank=2
85. Siegel M. D. (2018). Acute respiratory distress syndrome: Supportive care and oxygenation in adults. In Finlay G. (Ed.) *UpToDate.* Retrieved May 15, 2018 from https://www-uptodate-com. /contents/acute-respiratory-distress-syndrome-supportive-care-and-oxygenation-in-adults?search=acute%20lung%20injury%20and%20shock&source=search_result&selectedTitle=5~150&usage_type=default&display_rank=5
86. Weinhouse G. L. (2018). Stress ulcer prophylaxis in the intensive care unit. In Finlay G. (Ed.) *UpToDate.* Retrieved May 15, 2018 from https://www-uptodate-com. /contents/stress-ulcer-prophylaxis-in-the-intensive-care-unit/print?search=use%20of%20histamine%20type%202%20receptor%20antagonist%20to%20prevent%20gastrointestinal%20ulcers&source=search_result&selectedTitle=4~150&usage_type=default&display_rank=4
87. Levi M. M. (2017). *Disseminated intravascular coagulation clinical presentation*. Available: https://emedicine.medscape.com/article/199627-clinical#b3. Accessed May 15, 2018
88. Leung L. L. K. (2017). Clinical features, diagnosis, and treatment of disseminated intravascular coagulation in adults. In Timjauer J. S. (Ed.) *UpToDate.* Retrieved May 15, 2018 from https://www-uptodate-co / contents/clinical-features-diagnosis-and-treatment-of-disseminated-intravascular-coagulation-in-adults?search=recombinant%20human%20activated%20protein%20C%20and%20septic%20shock&source=search_result&selectedTitle=4~150&usage_type=default&display_rank=4
89. La-Khafaji A. H. (2018). *Multiple organ dysfunction syndrome in sepsis.* Available: https://emedicine.medscape.com/article/169640-overview. Retrieved May 15, 2018
90. Neviere R. (2018). Pathophysiology of sepsis. In Finlay G. (Ed.) *UptoDate.* Retrieved May 15, 2018 from https://www-uptodate-com/contents/pathophysiology-of-sepsis/print?search=pathogenesis%20

and%20management%20of%20multiple%20organ%20dysfunction%20or%20failure%20in%20acute%20sepsis%20and%20septic%20shock&source=search_result&selectedTitle=6~150&usage_type=default&display_rank=6
91. Strayer D. S., Rubin E. (2015). *Rubin's Pathology Clinicopathologic Foundations* (7th ed.). Philadelphia, PA: Wolters Kluwer.
92. Miller C. A. (2015). *Nursing for Wellness in Older Adults* (7th ed). Philadelphia, PA: Wolter Kluwers.
93. Eliopoulos C. (2018). *Gerontological Nursing* (9th ed.). Philadelphia, PA: Wolters Kluwer.
94. Kyle T., Carman S. (2017). *Essentials of Pediatric Nursing* (3rd ed.). Philadelphia, PA: Wolters Kluwer.

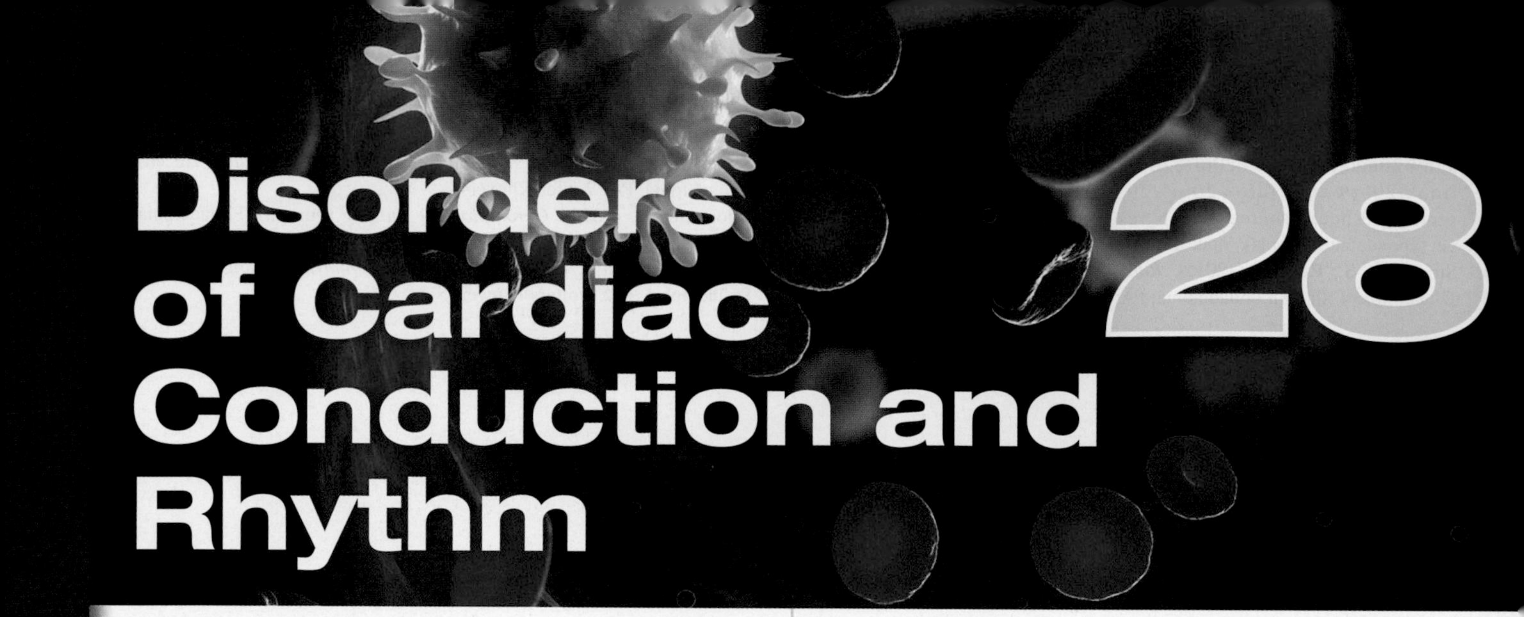

Disorders of Cardiac Conduction and Rhythm

28

Jaclyn Conelius

Heart muscle is unique in that it is capable of generating and rapidly conducting its own electrical impulses or action potentials. These action potentials result in excitation of muscle fibers throughout the myocardium. Impulse formation and conduction result in weak electrical currents that spread through the entire body. It is these impulses that are recorded on an electrocardiogram. Disorders of cardiac impulse generation and conduction range from benign arrhythmias to those causing serious disruption of heart function and sudden cardiac death.

CARDIAC CONDUCTION SYSTEM

After completing this section of the chapter, the learner will be able to meet the following objectives:

- Describe the cardiac conduction system, including the five phases of cardiac action potential.
- Illustrate an ECG tracing labeling the electrical signals of the conduction system of the heart.

In certain areas of the heart, the myocardial cells have been modified to form the specialized cells of the conduction system. These specialized cells have the ability to self-excitation, which is the capability of initiating and conducting impulses.[1] It is the conduction system that maintains the pumping efficiency of the heart. Specialized pacemaker cells generate impulses at a faster rate than other types of heart tissue, and the conduction tissue transmits these impulses more rapidly than other cardiac cell types. Because of these properties, a normal conduction system controls the rhythm of the heart.

The specialized excitatory and conduction system of the heart consists of the sinoatrial (SA) node, in which the normal rhythmic impulse is generated; the internodal pathways between the atria and the ventricles; the atrioventricular (AV) node and bundle of His, which conduct the impulse from the atria to the ventricles; and the Purkinje fibers, which conduct

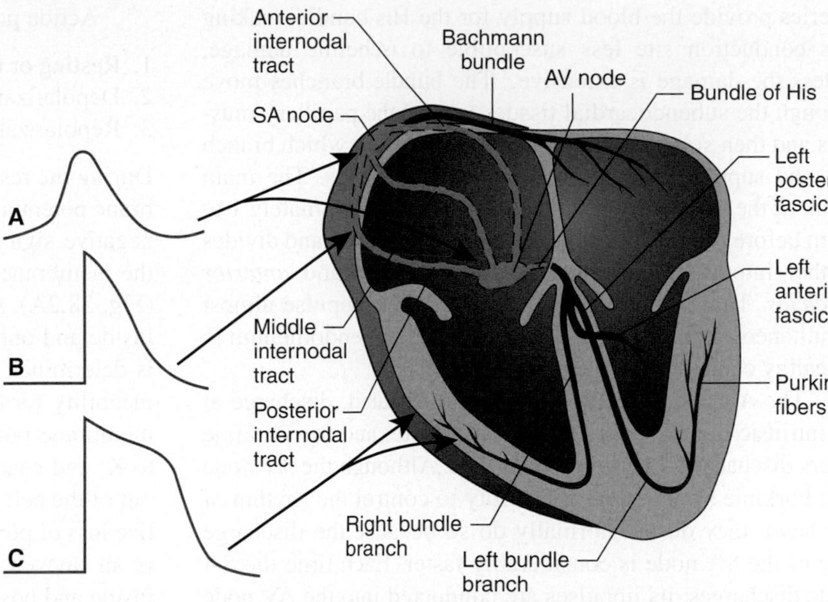

Figure 28.1 • Conduction system of the heart and action potentials. *A*, Action potential of sinoatrial (SA) and atrioventricular (AV) nodes; *B*, atrial muscle action potential; *C*, action potential of ventricular muscle and Purkinje fibers.

the impulses through the entire tissue of the right and left ventricles (Fig. 28.1).

The heart essentially has two conduction systems: one that controls atrial activity and one that controls ventricular activity. The atrial conduction begins with the SA node, which has the fastest intrinsic rate of firing (60 to 100 beats/minute), normally serving as the pacemaker of the heart. It is a spindle-shaped strip of specialized muscle tissue, about 10 to 20 mm in length and 2 to 3 mm wide, located in the posterior wall of the right atrium just below the opening of the superior vena cava and less than 1 mm from the epicardial surface.[2] Impulses originating in the SA node travel through the atria to the AV node. Because of the anatomic location of the SA node, the progression of atrial depolarization occurs in an inferior, leftward, and somewhat posterior direction, and the right atrium is depolarized slightly before the left atrium.[1,3] There are three internodal pathways between the SA node and the AV node, including the anterior (Bachmann), middle (Wenckebach), and posterior (Thorel) internodal tracts. These three tracts **anastomose** with each other proximally to the AV node. This large muscle bundle originates along the anterior border of the SA node and travels posteriorly around the aorta to the left atrium.[1,4]

The AV junction connects the two conduction systems and provides for one-way conduction between the atria and ventricles. The AV node is a compact, ovoid structure measuring approximately 1 × 3 × 5 mm and located on the posterior wall slightly beneath the right atrial endocardium, anterior to the opening of the coronary sinus, and immediately above the insertion of the septal leaflet of the tricuspid valve.[1,4] It is important to note that everywhere except for the AV node in a healthy heart, the atrial muscle is separated from the ventricular muscle in order to prevent cardiac impulses firing inappropriately.

The AV node is divided into three functional regions:

- The AN or transitional region, located between the atria and the rest of the node
- The N or middle region (*i.e.*, the node proper)
- The NH region, in which nodal fibers merge with the bundle of His, which is the upper portion of the specialized conduction system[1,5]

In the AN portion of the node, atrial fibers connect with very small junctional fibers of the node itself. The velocity of conduction through the AN and N fibers is very slow (approximately one half that of normal cardiac muscle), which greatly delays transmission of the impulse.[1,4] A further delay occurs as the impulse travels through the N region into the NH region, which connects with the *bundle of His* (also called the *AV bundle*). This delay provides a mechanical advantage whereby the atria complete their ejection of blood before ventricular contraction begins. Under normal circumstances, the AV node provides the only connection between the atrial and ventricular conduction systems. Its main job is to coordinate atrial and ventricular conduction. The atria and ventricles would beat independently of each other if the transmission of impulses through the AV node were blocked.

The *Purkinje system*, which initiates ventricular conduction, has large fibers that allow for rapid conduction. Once the impulse enters the Purkinje system, it spreads almost immediately to the whole ventricle (0.03 second).[1] This rapid rate of conduction throughout the Purkinje system is necessary for the swift and efficient ejection of blood from the heart. The fibers of the Purkinje system originate in the AV node and proceed to form the bundle of His, which extends through the fibrous tissue between the valves of the heart and into the ventricular system. Because of its proximity to the aortic valve and the mitral valve ring, the bundle of His is predisposed to inflammation and deposits of calcified debris that can interfere with impulse conduction.[1] The bundle of His penetrates into the ventricles and almost immediately divides into *right* and *left bundle branches* that straddle the interventricular septum. Branches from the anterior and posterior descending coronary arteries provide the blood supply for the His bundle, making this conduction site less susceptible to ischemic damage, unless the damage is extensive.[2] The bundle branches move through the subendocardial tissues toward the papillary muscles and then subdivide into the Purkinje fibers, which branch out and supply the outer walls of the ventricles. The main trunk of the left bundle branch extends for approximately 1 to 2 cm before fanning out as it enters the septal area and divides further into two segments: the *left posterior* and *anterior fascicles*. These Purkinje fibers transmit the impulse almost simultaneously to the right and left ventricular endothelium in a healthy conduction system.

The AV nodal fibers, when not stimulated, discharge at an intrinsic rate of 40 to 60 times a minute, and the Purkinje fibers discharge 15 to 40 times/minute. Although the AV node and Purkinje system have the ability to control the rhythm of the heart, they do not normally do so because the discharge rate of the SA node is considerably faster. Each time the SA node discharges, its impulses are conducted into the AV node and Purkinje fibers, causing them to fire. The AV node can assume the pacemaker function of the heart, should the SA node fail to discharge, and the Purkinje system can assume the pacemaker function of the ventricles, should the AV node fail to conduct impulses from the atria to the ventricles. Under these circumstances, the heart rate reflects the intrinsic firing rate of the prevailing structures.

KEY POINTS

CARDIAC CONDUCTION SYSTEM

- Normally, impulses are generated in the SA node, which has the fastest rate of firing and travel through the AV node to the Purkinje system in the ventricles.
- Cardiac action potentials are divided into five phases: phase 0, or the rapid upstroke of the action potential; phase 1, or early repolarization; phase 2, or the plateau; phase 3, or final repolarization period; and phase 4, or diastolic repolarization period.

Action Potentials

An action potential represents the sequential change in electrical potential that occurs across a cell membrane when excitation occurs and causes the heart to conduct this electrical impulse across the atrium and ventricle. These potential or voltage differences, often referred to as membrane potentials, represent the flow of current associated with the passage of ions through ion channels in the cell membrane. The sodium (Na^+), potassium (K^+), and calcium (Ca^{++}) ions are the major charge carriers in cardiac muscle cells. Disorders of the ion channels along with disruption in the flow of these current-carrying ions are increasingly being linked to the generation of cardiac arrhythmias and conduction disorders.

Action potentials can be divided into three phases:

1. Resting or unexcited state
2. Depolarization
3. Repolarization

During the resting phase, cardiac cells exhibit a resting membrane potential that typically ranges from −60 to −90 mV. The negative sign before the voltage indicates that the inside of the membrane is negatively charged in relation to the outside (Fig. 28.2A). Although different kinds of ions are found both inside and outside of the membrane, the membrane potential is determined largely by Na^+ and K^+ and the membrane permeability for these two ions. During the resting phase of the membrane potential, the membrane is selectively permeable to K^+ and nearly impermeable to Na^+. As a result, K^+ diffuses out of the cell along its concentration gradient, causing a relative loss of positive ions from inside the membrane. The result is an uneven distribution of charge with negativity on the inside and positivity on the outside.

Depolarization represents the period of time (measured in milliseconds [ms]) during which the polarity of the membrane potential is reversed. It occurs when the cell membrane suddenly becomes selectively permeable to a current-carrying ion such as Na^+, allowing it to move into a cell and change the membrane potential so it becomes positive on the inside and negative on the outside (Fig. 28.2B).

Repolarization involves reestablishment of the resting membrane potential. It has a somewhat slower process, involving the outward flow of electrical charges and the return of the membrane potential to its resting state.[6] During repolarization, membrane permeability for K^+ again increases, allowing the positively charged K^+ to move outward across the membrane. This outward movement removes positive charges from inside the cell; thus, the voltage across the membrane again becomes negative on the inside and positive on the outside (Fig. 28.2C). The adenosine triphosphatase (ATPase)-dependent sodium–potassium pump assists in repolarization by pumping positively charged Na^+ out across the cell membrane and returning K^+ to the inside of the membrane.[7]

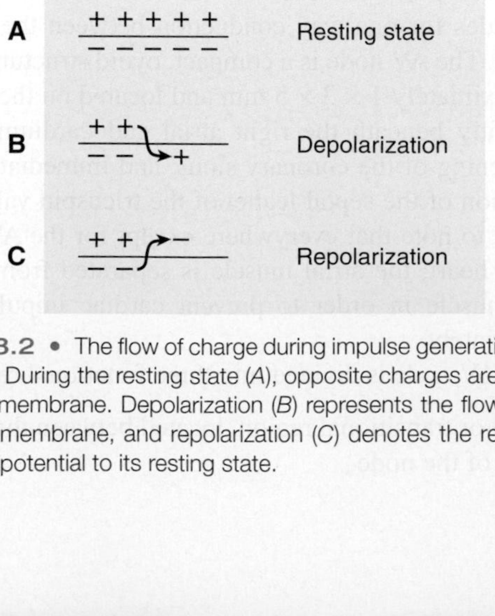

Figure 28.2 • The flow of charge during impulse generation in excitable tissue. During the resting state (*A*), opposite charges are separated by the cell membrane. Depolarization (*B*) represents the flow of charge across the membrane, and repolarization (*C*) denotes the return of the membrane potential to its resting state.

Action Potential Phases

The action potentials in cardiac muscle are typically divided into five phases:

1. *Phase 0*—upstroke or rapid depolarization
2. *Phase 1*—rapid repolarization period
3. *Phase 2*—plateau
4. *Phase 3*—final, rapid repolarization period
5. *Phase 4*—diastolic depolarization (Fig. 28.3B)

Cardiac muscle has three types of membrane ion channels that contribute to the voltage changes that occur during the different phases of the cardiac action potential. They are the fast Na^+ channels, slow calcium (Ca^{++}) channels, and K^+ channels.

During *phase 0*, in atrial and ventricular muscle and in the Purkinje system, the fast Na^+ channels in the cell membrane are stimulated to open, resulting in the rapid influx of Na^+. The point at which the Na^+ channels open is called the *depolarization threshold*. When the cell has reached this threshold, a rapid influx of Na^+ occurs. The exterior of the cell now is negatively charged in relation to the highly positive interior of the cell. This influx of Na^+ produces a rapid, positively directed change in the membrane potential, resulting in the electrical spike during phase 0 of the action potential.[2,6] The membrane potential shifts from a resting membrane potential of approximately −90 to +20 mV. The rapid depolarization that

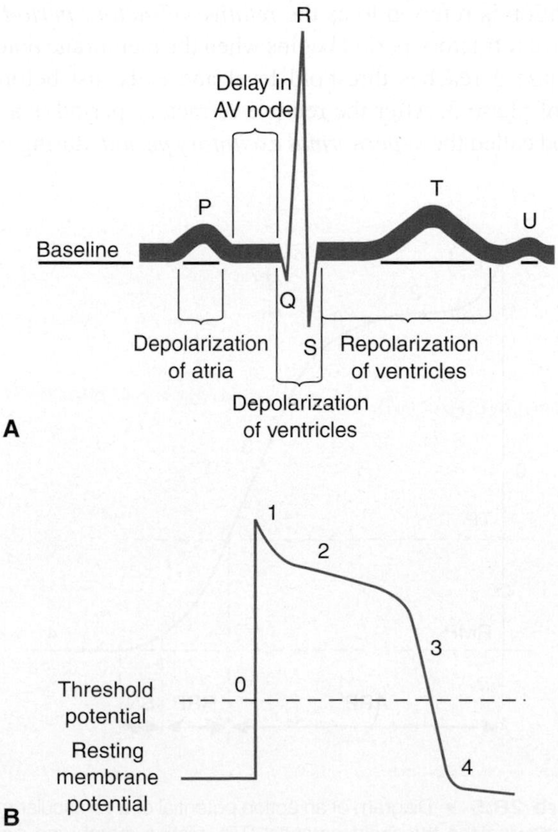

Figure 28.3 • Relation between **(A)** the electrocardiogram and **(B)** phases of the ventricular action potential.

comprises phase 0 is responsible for the QRS complex on the electrocardiogram (ECG) (Fig. 28.3A). Depolarization of a cardiac cell tends to cause adjacent cells to depolarize because the voltage spike of the cell's depolarization stimulates the Na^+ channels in nearby cells to open. Therefore, when a cardiac cell is stimulated to depolarize, a wave of depolarization is propagated across the heart, cell by cell.

Phase 1 occurs at the peak of the action potential and signifies inactivation of the fast Na^+ channels with an abrupt decrease in sodium permeability. The slight downward slope is thought to be caused by the influx of a small amount of negatively charged chloride ions and efflux of potassium.[2] The decrease in intracellular positivity reduces the membrane potential to a level near 0 mV, from which the plateau, or phase 2, arises.

Phase 2 represents the plateau of the action potential. If K^+ permeability increased to its resting level at this time, as it does in nerve fibers or skeletal muscle, the cell would repolarize rapidly. Instead, K^+ permeability is low, allowing the membrane to remain depolarized throughout the phase 2 plateau. A concomitant influx of Ca^{++} into the cell through the slow Ca^{++} channels contributes to the phase 2 plateau.[2,7] Calcium ions entering the muscle during this phase also play a key role in the contractile process. These unique features of the phase 2 plateau cause the action potential of cardiac muscle (several hundred milliseconds) to last 3 to 15 times longer than that of skeletal muscle and produce a corresponding increased period of contraction.[1] The phase 2 plateau coincides with the ST segment of the ECG.

Phase 3 reflects rapid repolarization and begins with the downslope of the action potential. During the phase 3 repolarization period, the slow Ca^{++} channels close and the influx of Ca^{++} and Na^+ ceases. There is a sharp rise in K^+ permeability, contributing to the rapid outward movement of K^+ and reestablishment of the resting membrane potential (−90 mV). At the conclusion of phase 3, the distribution of K^+ and Na^+ returns the membrane to the normal resting state. The T wave on the ECG corresponds with phase 3 of the action potential.

Phase 4 represents the resting membrane potential. During phase 4, the activity of the Na^+/K^+-ATPase pump contributes to maintaining the resting membrane potential by transporting Na^+ out of the cell and moving K^+ back in. Phase 4 corresponds to diastole.[2]

Fast and Slow Responses

There are two main types of action potentials in the heart—the fast response and the slow response. The *fast response* occurs in the normal myocardial cells of the atria, the ventricles, and the Purkinje fibers (Fig. 28.4A). It is characterized by the opening of voltage-dependent Na^+ channels called the *fast sodium channels*. The fast response cardiac cells do not normally initiate cardiac action potentials. The fast response cells have a constant resting potential, rapid depolarization, and then a longer period of sustained depolarization before repolarization. This allows impulse conduction to be rapid to adjacent cells. Myocardial fibers with a fast response are capable of conducting electrical activity at relatively rapid rates (0.5 to 5.0 m/second), thereby providing a high safety factor for conduction.[8]

The *slow response* occurs in the SA node, which is the natural pacemaker of the heart, and the conduction fibers of the AV node (Fig. 28.4B). The hallmark of these pacemaker cells is a spontaneous phase 4 depolarization. The membrane permeability of these cells allows a slow inward leak of current to occur through the slow channels during phase 4. This leak continues until the threshold for firing is reached, at which point the cell spontaneously depolarizes. Under normal conditions, the slow response, sometimes referred to as the *calcium current*, does not contribute significantly to depolarization of the atria and ventricles. Its primary role in normal atrial and ventricular cells is to provide for the entrance of calcium for the excitation–contraction mechanism that couples the electrical activity with muscle contraction.

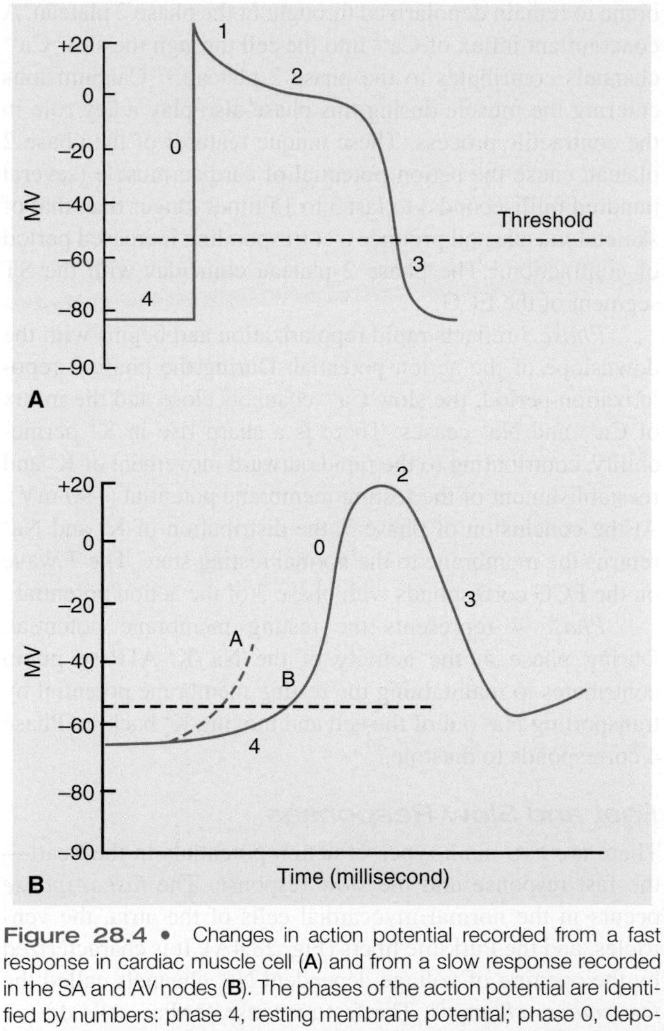

Figure 28.4 • Changes in action potential recorded from a fast response in cardiac muscle cell (A) and from a slow response recorded in the SA and AV nodes (B). The phases of the action potential are identified by numbers: phase 4, resting membrane potential; phase 0, depolarization; phase 1, brief period of repolarization; phase 2, plateau; and phase 3, repolarization. The slow response is characterized by a slow, spontaneous rise in the phase 4 membrane potential to threshold levels; it has a lesser amplitude and shorter duration than the fast response. Increased automaticity (*A*) occurs when the rate of phase 4 depolarization is increased.

The rate of pacemaker cell discharge varies with the resting membrane potential and the slope of phase 4 depolarization (Fig. 28.3). Catecholamines (*i.e.*, epinephrine and norepinephrine) increase heart rate by increasing the slope or rate of phase 4 depolarization. Acetylcholine, a parasympathetic mediator, slows the heart rate by decreasing the slope of phase 4.

The fast response of atrial and ventricular muscle can be converted to a slow pacemaker response under certain conditions. For example, such conversions may occur spontaneously in people with severe coronary artery disease and in areas of the heart where blood supply has been markedly compromised. Impulses generated by these cells can lead to ectopic beats and serious arrhythmias.

Absolute and Relative Refractory Periods

The pumping action of the heart requires alternating contraction and relaxation. There is a period in the action potential during which the membrane cannot be stimulated to generate another action potential (Fig. 28.5). This period, known as the *absolute or effective refractory period*, includes phases 0, 1, and 2 and part of phase 3. During this time, the cell cannot depolarize again under any circumstances. This acts as a safety margin for the heart in order to prevent any stimulation or generate any extra beats. When repolarization has returned the membrane potential to below threshold, although not yet at the resting membrane potential (−90 mV), the cell is capable of responding to a greater-than-normal stimulus. This condition is referred to as the *relative refractory period*. The relative refractory period begins when the membrane potential in phase 3 reaches threshold level and ends just before the end of phase 3. After the relative refractory period is a short period called the *supernormal excitatory period*, during which

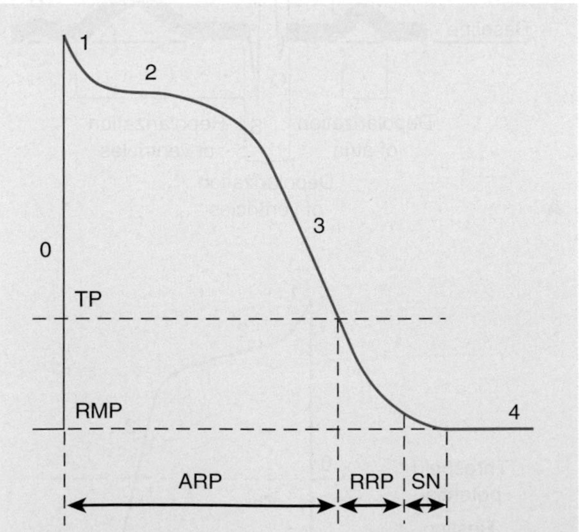

Figure 28.5 • Diagram of an action potential of a ventricular muscle cell, showing the threshold potential (TP), resting membrane potential (RMP), absolute refractory period (ARP), relative refractory period (RRP), and supernormal (SN) period.

a weak stimulus can evoke a response. The supernormal excitatory period extends from the terminal portion of phase 3 until the beginning of phase 4. It is during this period that cardiac arrhythmias develop.[8]

Electrocardiography

The ECG is a graphic recording of the electrical activity of the heart or a picture of the heart as it contracts. The electrical currents generated by the heart spread through the body to the skin, where they can be sensed by appropriately placed electrodes, amplified, and viewed on an oscilloscope or chart recorder.

The deflection points of an ECG are designated by the letters P, Q, R, S, and T. The P wave represents the SA node and atrial depolarization; the QRS complex (*i.e.*, beginning of the Q wave to the end of the S wave) depicts ventricular depolarization; and the T wave portrays ventricular repolarization. The isoelectric line between the P wave and the Q wave represents depolarization of the AV node, bundle branches, and Purkinje system. Atrial repolarization occurs during ventricular depolarization and is hidden in the QRS complex. Figure 28.6 depicts the electrical activity of the conduction system on an ECG tracing.

The ECG records the potential difference in charge between two electrodes as the depolarization and repolarization waves move through the heart and are conducted to the skin surface. The shape of the recorder tracing is determined by the direction in which the impulse spreads through the heart muscle in relation to electrode placement. A depolarization wave that moves toward the recording electrode registers as a positive, or upward, deflection. Conversely, if the impulse moves away from the recording electrode, the deflection is downward, or negative. When there is no flow of charge between electrodes, the potential is zero, and a straight line is recorded at the baseline of the chart.

Conventionally, 12 leads (6 limb leads and 6 chest leads) are recorded for a diagnostic ECG, each providing a unique view of the electrical forces of the heart from a different position on the body's surface. The six limb leads view the electrical forces as they pass through the heart on the frontal or vertical plane. The electrodes are attached to the four extremities or representative areas on the body near the shoulders and lower chest or abdomen. The electrical potential recorded from any one extremity should be the same no matter where the electrode is placed on the extremity. The six chest leads provide a view of the electrical forces as they pass through the heart on the horizontal plane. They are moved to different positions on the chest, including the right and left sternal borders and the left anterior surface (Fig. 28.7). The right lower extremity lead is used as a ground electrode.[8] When indicated, additional electrodes may be applied to other areas of the body, such as the back or right anterior chest to record from other areas of the heart. However, this is not done routinely.

Although accurate ECG placement and lead selection are important aspects of ECG monitoring, there have been many studies that identified two common errors: misplaced electrode placement and inappropriate lead selection for individual clinical situations.[9] Improper lead placement can significantly change QRS morphology, resulting in misdiagnosis of cardiac arrhythmias or failure to detect existing conduction defects.

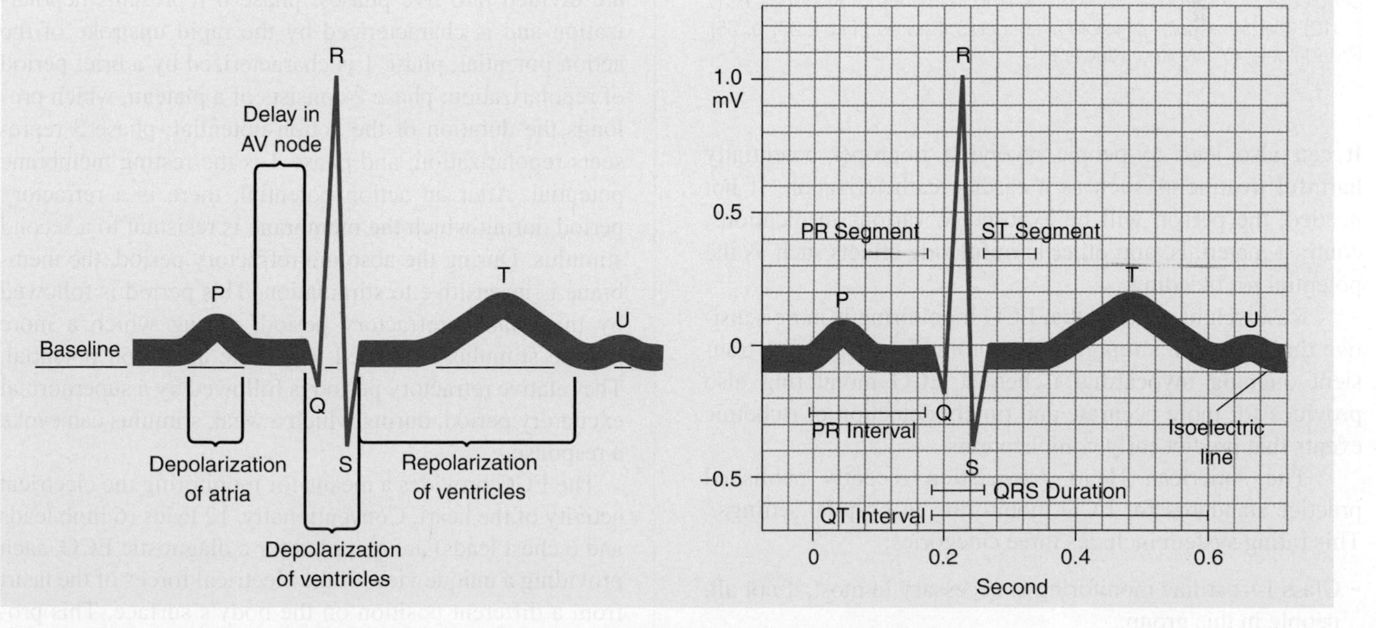

Figure 28.6 • Diagram of the ECG (lead II) and representative depolarization and repolarization of the atria and ventricles. The P wave represents atrial depolarization, the QRS complex ventricular depolarization, and the T-wave ventricular repolarization. Atrial repolarization occurs during ventricular depolarization and is hidden under the QRS complex.

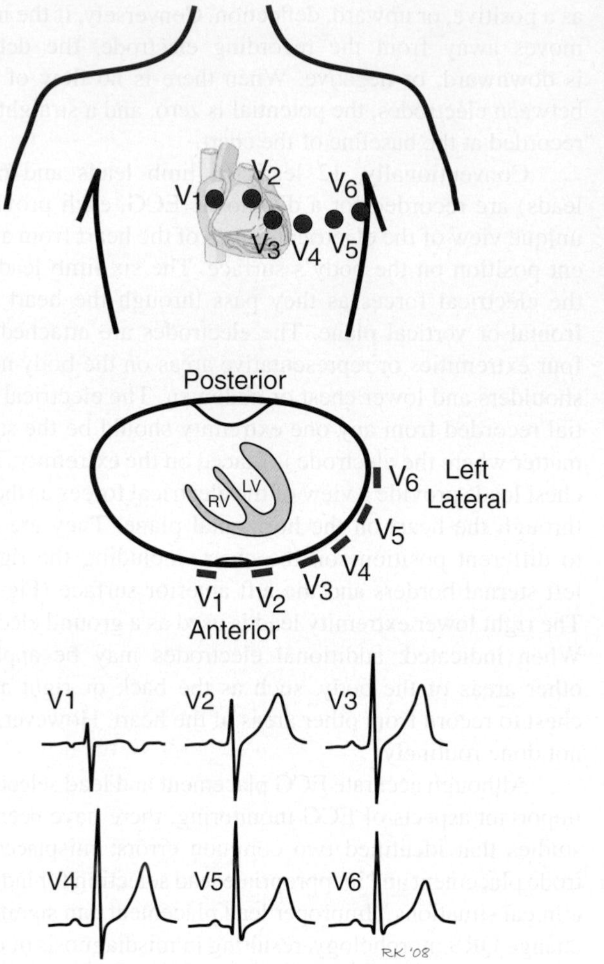

Figure 28.7 • Placement of the six precordial chest leads and the normal appearance of the ECG recording for leads V_1–V_6. These electrodes record electrical activity in the horizontal plane, which is perpendicular to the frontal plane of the limb leads. (From Klabunde R. E. (2012). *Cardiovascular physiology concepts* (2nd ed., Fig. 2.20, p. 35). Philadelphia, PA: Wolters Kluwer.)

It can also lead to people receiving improper potentially harmful treatments such as a cardiac catheterization. If not needed, the person will be exposed to various medications, contrast materials, and other harmful side effects such as the potential for bleeding.

Research has shown that ECG monitoring is more sensitive than a person's report of symptoms for identifying transient ongoing myocardial ischemia. ECG monitoring also provides for more accurate and timely detection of ischemic events that predict early complications.

The American Heart Association recently published practice standards for ECG monitoring in hospital settings.[8] This rating system includes three categories:

- Class I—cardiac monitoring is necessary in most, if not all, people in this group.
- Class II—cardiac monitoring may be beneficial in some people, but it is not an essential component of care for these people.
- Class III—cardiac monitoring is not indicated because the risk of a serious event for these people is so low that monitoring is not viewed as therapeutic.

Examples of people categorized as class I are those who have been resuscitated from a cardiac arrest, are in the early phase of ACS, have unstable coronary syndromes or newly diagnosed high-risk coronary lesions, or have undergone cardiac surgery within the past 48 to 72 hours. In addition, recommendations for staffing, training, documentation, and approaches for improving quality of ECG monitoring were presented. It is recommended that these practice standards be adhered to when making determinations about ECG monitoring.

IN SUMMARY

The rhythmic contraction and relaxation of the heart rely on the specialized cells of the heart's conduction system. Specialized cells in the SA node have the fastest inherent rate of impulse generation known as automaticity and act as the pacemaker of the heart. Impulses from the SA node travel through the atria to the AV node and then to the AV bundle and the ventricular Purkinje system. The AV node provides the only connection between the atrial and ventricular conduction systems. The atria and the ventricles function independently of each other when AV node conduction is blocked.

Action potentials represent the sequential changes in electrical potentials that are associated with the movement of current-carrying ions through ion channels in the cell membrane. The action potentials of cardiac muscle are divided into five phases: phase 0 represents depolarization and is characterized by the rapid upstroke of the action potential; phase 1 is characterized by a brief period of repolarization; phase 2 consists of a plateau, which prolongs the duration of the action potential; phase 3 represents repolarization; and phase 4 is the resting membrane potential. After an action potential, there is a refractory period during which the membrane is resistant to a second stimulus. During the absolute refractory period, the membrane is insensitive to stimulation. This period is followed by the relative refractory period, during which a more intense stimulus is needed to initiate an action potential. The relative refractory period is followed by a supernormal excitatory period, during which a weak stimulus can evoke a response.

The ECG provides a means for monitoring the electrical activity of the heart. Conventionally, 12 leads (6 limb leads and 6 chest leads) are recorded for a diagnostic ECG, each providing a unique view of the electrical forces of the heart from a different position on the body's surface. This procedure allows for advanced arrhythmia detection and early identification of ischemia- and infarction-related changes in people with ACS.

DISORDERS OF CARDIAC RHYTHM AND CONDUCTION

After completing this section of the chapter, the learner will be able to meet the following objectives:

- Characterize the effects of atrial arrhythmias including atrial flutter and atrial fibrillation (AF) on heart rhythm.
- Describe the characteristics of first-, second-, and third-degree heart block, ventricular tachycardia, and ventricular fibrillation.

There are two types of disorders of the cardiac conduction system: disorders of rhythm and disorders of impulse conduction. There are many causes of cardiac arrhythmias and conduction disorders, including congenital defects or degenerative changes in the conduction system, myocardial ischemia and infarction, fluid and electrolyte imbalances, and the effects of pharmacologic agents. Arrhythmias are not necessarily pathologic; they can occur in both healthy and diseased hearts. Disturbances in cardiac rhythms exert their harmful effects by interfering with the heart's pumping ability. Excessively rapid heart rates (tachyarrhythmias) reduce the diastolic filling time, causing a subsequent decrease in the stroke volume output and in coronary perfusion while increasing the myocardial oxygen needs. Abnormally slow heart rates (bradyarrhythmias) may impair blood flow to vital organs such as the brain.

KEY POINTS

PHYSIOLOGIC BASIS OF ARRHYTHMIA GENERATION

- Cardiac arrhythmias represent disorders of cardiac rhythm related to alterations in automaticity, excitability, conductivity, or refractoriness of specialized cells in the conduction system of the heart.

Mechanisms of Arrhythmias and Conduction Disorders

The specialized cells in the conduction system manifest four inherent properties that contribute to the genesis of all cardiac rhythms, both normal and abnormal. They are automaticity, excitability, conductivity, and refractoriness. An alteration in any of these four properties may produce arrhythmias or conduction defects.

The ability of certain cells in the conduction system spontaneously to initiate an impulse or action potential is referred to as *automaticity*. The SA node has an inherent discharge rate of 60 to 100 times/minute. It normally acts as the pacemaker of the heart because it reaches the threshold for excitation before other parts of the conduction system have recovered sufficiently to be depolarized. If the SA node fires more slowly or SA node conduction is blocked, another site that is capable of automaticity takes over as pacemaker.[1,3] Other regions that are capable of automaticity include the atrial fibers that have plateau-type action potentials, the AV node, the bundle of His, and the bundle branch Purkinje fibers. These pacemakers have a slower rate of discharge than the SA node. The AV node has an inherent firing rate of 40 to 60 times/minute, and the Purkinje system fires at a rate of 15 to 40 times/minute. The SA node may be functioning properly, but because of additional precipitating factors, other cardiac cells can assume accelerated properties of automaticity and begin to initiate impulses. These additional factors might include injury, hypoxia, electrolyte disturbances, enlargement or hypertrophy of the atria or ventricles, and exposure to certain chemicals or drugs.

An *ectopic pacemaker* is an excitable focus outside the normally functioning SA node. These pacemakers can reside in other parts of the conduction system or in muscle cells of the atria or ventricles. A premature contraction occurs when an ectopic pacemaker initiates a beat. Premature contractions do not follow the normal conduction pathways, they are not coupled with normal mechanical events, and they often render the heart refractory or incapable of responding to the next normal impulse arising in the SA node. They occur without incident in persons with healthy hearts in response to sympathetic nervous system stimulation or other stimulants, such as caffeine. In the diseased heart, premature contractions may lead to more serious arrhythmias.

Excitability describes the ability of a cell to respond to an impulse and generate an action potential. Myocardial cells that have been injured or replaced by scar tissue do not possess normal excitability. For example, during the acute phase of an ischemic event, involved cells become depolarized. These ischemic cells remain electrically coupled to the adjacent nonischemic area; current from the ischemic zone can induce reexcitation of cells in the nonischemic zone.

Conductivity is the ability to conduct impulses, and *refractoriness* refers to the extent to which the cell is able to respond to an incoming stimulus. The refractory period of cardiac muscle is the interval in the repolarization period during which an excitable cell has not recovered sufficiently to be excited again. Disturbances in conductivity or refractoriness predispose to arrhythmias.

The phenomenon, known as reentry, is the cause of many tachyarrhythmias.[1,5] Under normal conditions, an electrical impulse is conducted through the heart in an orderly, sequential manner. The electrical impulse then dies out and does not reenter adjacent tissue because that tissue has already been depolarized and is refractory to immediate stimulation. However, fibers that were not activated during the initial wave of depolarization can recover excitability before the initial impulse dies out, and they may serve as a link to reexcite areas of the heart that were just discharged and have recovered from the initial depolarization.[2] This activity disrupts the normal conduction sequence. For reentry to occur,

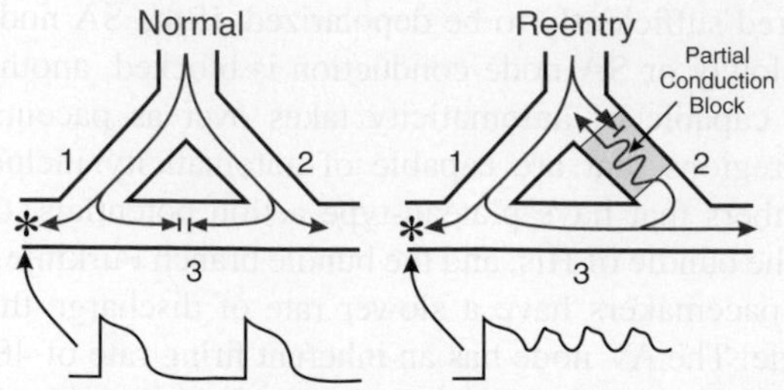

Figure 28.8 • Mechanism of reentry. With normal conduction of action potentials, impulses traveling down branches 1 and 2 cancel out each other in branch 3. Reentry can occur if branch 2 has impaired conduction and blocks orthograde impulses but slowly conducts retrograde impulses. If a retrograde impulse emerging from branch 2 reaches excitable tissue (after the ERP, but before the next normal impulse), a premature action potential can be conducted down branch 1. If this occurs with successive action potentials, tachycardia occurs. (From Klabunde R. E. (2012). *Cardiovascular physiology concepts* (2nd ed., Fig. 2.11, p. 24). Philadelphia, PA: Wolters Kluwer.)

there must be areas of slow conduction and a unidirectional conduction block (Fig. 28.8). For previously depolarized areas to repolarize adequately to conduct an impulse again, slow conduction is necessary. Unidirectional block is necessary to provide a one-way route for the original impulse to reenter, thereby blocking other impulses entering from the opposite direction from extinguishing the reentrant circuit.[2] Reentry requires a triggering stimulus such as an extrasystole to start the circuit.

Reentry may occur anywhere in the conduction system. The functional components of a reentry circuit can be large and include an entire specialized conduction system, or the circuit can be microscopic. It can include myocardial tissue, AV nodal cells, junctional tissue, or the ventricles. Factors contributing to the development of a reentrant circuit include ischemia, infarction, and elevated serum potassium levels. Scar tissue interrupts the normally low-resistance paths between viable myocardial cells, slowing conduction, promoting asynchronous myocardial activation, and predisposing to unidirectional conduction block. There are several forms of reentry. The first is anatomic reentry. It involves an anatomic obstacle around which the circulating current must pass and results in an excitation wave that travels in a set pathway.[2] Arrhythmias that arise as a result of anatomic reentry are paroxysmal supraventricular tachycardias, as seen in Wolff-Parkinson-White syndrome, AF, atrial flutter, AV nodal reentry, and some ventricular tachycardias. Functional reentry does not rely on an anatomic structure to circle but instead depends on the local differences in conduction velocity and refractoriness among neighboring fibers that allow an impulse to circulate repeatedly around an area.[2] The last type of reentry is spiral reentry. It is initiated by a current that does not proceed down a regular pathway; rather, it breaks away, then curls and rotates. These impulses become erratic and irregular in the atrium. This is what is seen in AF.

Types of Arrhythmias and Conduction Disorders

Sinus Node Arrhythmias

In a healthy heart driven by sinus node discharge, the rate ranges between 60 and 100 beats/minute. On the ECG, a P wave may be observed to precede every QRS complex. Normal sinus rhythm has been considered the "normal" rhythm of a healthy heart. In normal sinus rhythm, a P wave precedes each QRS complex, and the R-R intervals remain relatively constant over time (Fig. 28.9). Alterations in the function of the SA node lead to changes in rate or rhythm of the heartbeat.

For example, respiratory sinus arrhythmia is a cardiac rhythm characterized by gradual lengthening and shortening of R-R intervals (see Fig. 28.9). This variation in cardiac cycles is related to intrathoracic pressure changes that occur with respiration and resultant alterations in autonomic control of the SA node. Inspiration causes acceleration of the heart rate, and expiration causes slowing and does not require any treatment. Respiratory sinus arrhythmia accounts for most heart rate variability in healthy people. Heart rate variability is the beat-to-beat variation of the cardiac signal and is considered to be an index of autonomic nervous system balance.

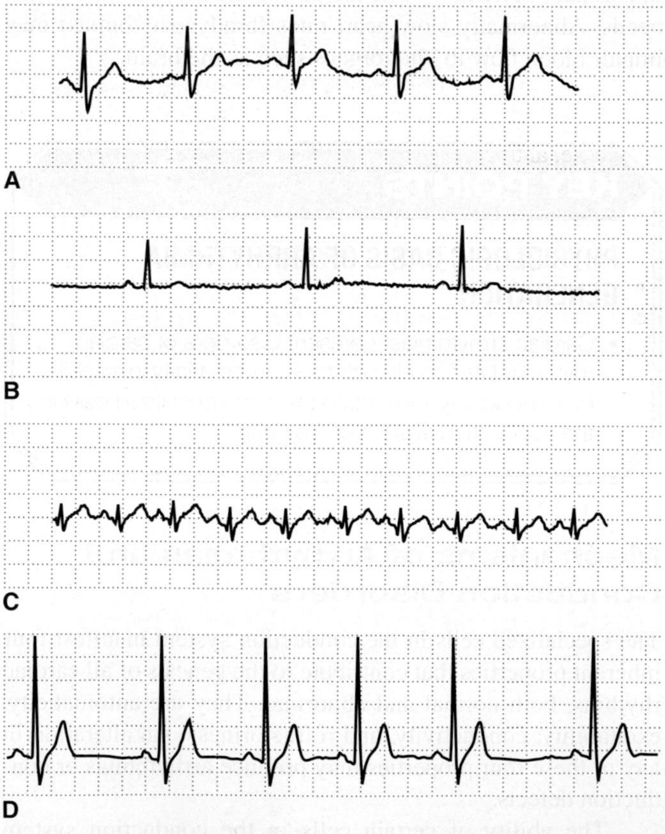

Figure 28.9 • Electrocardiographic tracings of rhythms originating in the sinus node. **(A)** Normal sinus rhythm (60 to 100 beats/minute). **(B)** Sinus bradycardia (<60 beats/minute). **(C)** Sinus tachycardia (>100 beats/minute). **(D)** Respiratory sinus arrhythmia, characterized by gradual lengthening and shortening of R-R intervals.

Therefore, a decreased heart rate variability has been associated with altered health states, including MI, congestive heart failure, hypertension, stable angina, diabetes mellitus, and chronic obstructive pulmonary disease (COPD).[9]

Sinus Bradycardia. Sinus bradycardia describes a slow (<60 beats/minute) heart rate (see Fig. 28.9). In sinus bradycardia, a P wave precedes each QRS. A normal P wave and PR interval (0.12 to 0.20 second) indicates that the impulse originated in the SA node rather than in another area of the conduction system that has a slower inherent rate. Vagal stimulation as well as some medications decreases the firing rate of the SA node and conduction through the AV node to cause a decrease in heart rate. This rhythm may be normal in trained athletes, who maintain a large stroke volume, and during sleep. In most cases, sinus bradycardia is benign unless it is associated with hemodynamic decompensation, such as dizziness and fatigue. It may also be an indicator of poor prognosis when it occurs in conjunction with acute MI and after resuscitation from cardiac arrest.[10]

Sinus Pause or Arrest. Sinus arrest refers to failure of the SA node to discharge and results in an irregular pulse. The impulse fails to proceed through the AV node. An escape rhythm develops as another pacemaker takes over. Sinus arrest may result in prolonged periods of asystole and often predisposes to other arrhythmias. Causes of sinus arrest include disease of the SA node, digitalis toxicity, stroke, MI, acute myocarditis, excessive vagal tone, sleep apnea, quinidine, lidocaine, and hyperkalemia or hypokalemia.[10,11]

Sinus Tachycardia. Sinus tachycardia refers to a rapid heart rate (>100 beats/minute) that has its origin in the SA node (see Fig. 28.9). A normal P wave and PR interval should precede each QRS complex. The mechanism of sinus tachycardia is enhanced automaticity related to sympathetic stimulation or withdrawal of vagal tone. Sinus tachycardia is a normal response during fever, blood loss, anxiety, pain, and exercise, and in situations that incite sympathetic stimulation. It may be associated with congestive heart failure, MI, and hyperthyroidism. Pharmacologic agents such as atropine, isoproterenol, epinephrine, and quinidine also can cause sinus tachycardia.[11,12]

Sick Sinus Syndrome. Sick sinus syndrome (SSS) is a term that describes a number of forms of cardiac impulse formation and intra-atrial and AV conduction abnormalities.[11–14] The syndrome most frequently is the result of total or subtotal destruction of the SA node, areas of nodal–atrial discontinuity, inflammatory or degenerative changes of the nerves and ganglia surrounding the node, or pathologic changes in the atrial wall.[10] In addition, occlusion of the sinus node artery may be a significant contributing factor. SSS is most often idiopathic but can be seen in people with coronary artery disease, fibrosis infective processes, certain drugs, and collagen vascular diseases.[12,13] In children, the syndrome is most commonly associated with congenital heart defects, particularly after corrective cardiac surgery.[14]

The arrhythmias associated with SSS include spontaneous persistent sinus bradycardia that is not appropriate for the physiologic circumstances, prolonged sinus arrest or exit block, combinations of SA and AV node conduction disturbances, or alternating paroxysms of rapid regular or irregular atrial tachyarrhythmias and periods of slow atrial and ventricular rates (bradycardia–tachycardia syndrome).[10,12,14] Most commonly, the term *sick sinus syndrome* is used to refer to the bradycardia–tachycardia syndrome. The bradycardia is caused by disease of the sinus node (or other intra-atrial conduction pathways), and the tachycardia is caused by paroxysmal atrial or junctional arrhythmias. People with this syndrome often are asymptomatic. The most common manifestations of SSS are light-headedness, dizziness, and syncope, and these symptoms are related to the bradyarrhythmias.[14] When persons with SSS experience palpitations, they are generally the result of tachyarrhythmias and are suggestive of the presence of bradycardia–tachycardia syndrome.

Treatment depends on the rhythm problem and frequently involves the implantation of a permanent pacemaker. Pacing for the bradycardia, combined with drug therapy to treat the tachycardia, often is required in the bradycardia–tachycardia syndrome.[10,11] Medications that affect SA node discharge must be used cautiously if no pacemaker is implanted.

KEY POINTS

SUPRAVENTRICULAR AND VENTRICULAR ARRHYTHMIAS

- Supraventricular arrhythmias represent disorders of atrial rhythm or conduction above the ventricles.
- Ventricular arrhythmias represent disorders of ventricular rhythm or conduction and can be life threatening.

Arrhythmias of Atrial Origin

Impulses from the SA node pass through the conductive pathways in the atria to the AV node. Arrhythmias of atrial origin include premature atrial contractions (PAC), multifocal and focal atrial tachycardia, atrial flutter, and AF (Fig. 28.10).

Premature Atrial Contractions. PACs are contractions that originate in the atrial conduction pathways or atrial muscle cells and occur before the next expected SA node impulse. This impulse to contract usually is transmitted to the ventricle and back to the SA node. The location of the ectopic focus determines the configuration of the P wave. In general, the closer the ectopic focus is to the SA node, the more the ectopic complex resembles a normal sinus complex. The retrograde transmission to the SA node often interrupts the timing of the next sinus beat, such that a pause occurs between the

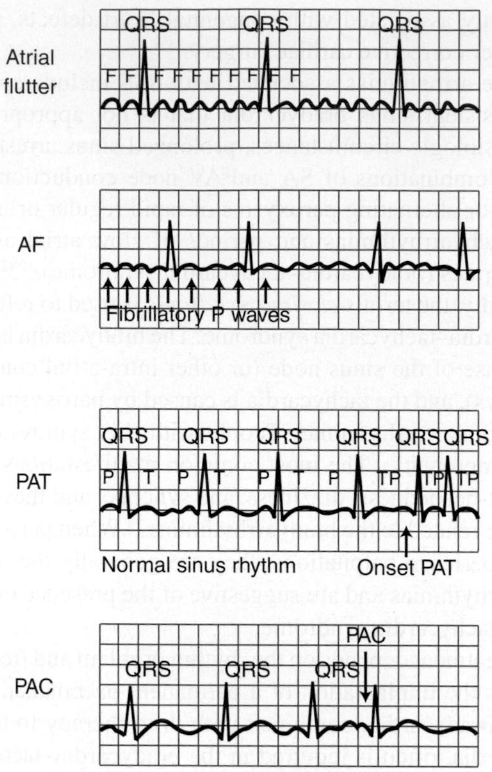

Figure 28.10 • Electrocardiographic tracings of atrial arrhythmias. Atrial flutter (*first tracing*) is characterized by the atrial flutter (*F*) waves occurring at a rate of 240 to 450 beats/minute. The ventricular rate remains regular because of the conduction of every sixth atrial contraction. Atrial fibrillation (AF) (*second tracing*) has grossly disorganized atrial electrical activity that is irregular with respect to rate and rhythm. The ventricular response is irregular, and no distinct *P* waves are visible. The *third tracing* illustrates paroxysmal atrial tachycardia (PAT), preceded by a normal sinus rhythm. The *fourth tracing* illustrates premature atrial contractions (PACs).

two normally conducted beats. In healthy people, PACs may be the result of stress, alcohol, tobacco, or caffeine. They also have been associated with MI, digitalis toxicity, low serum potassium or magnesium levels, and hypoxia.

Atrial Tachycardia. Atrial tachycardia can be multifocal (coming from several ectopic areas in the atrium) or focal (coming from one area in the atrium). In multifocal atrial tachycardia, the P waves look different based on where they originate in the atrium and become irregular with rates greater than 100 beats/minute. Focal atrial tachycardia is regular, with rates around 100 to 250 beats/minute. Depending on what type of atrial tachycardia is present, there may be different organic causes. Multifocal atrial tachycardia is usually seen in older adults with COPDs, hypoxia, and electrolyte disorders. Focal atrial tachycardia is usually associated with caffeine, alcohol intake, mitral valve disease, rheumatic heart disease, acute MI, COPD, hypokalemia, and digitalis toxicity. Multifocal atrial tachycardia is treated by addressing the underlying disease. Focal can be treated by identifying the underlying cause, the use of antiarrhythmics, or (if those fail) a radiofrequency (RF) catheter ablation of the ectopic focus causing the atrial tachycardia.[15]

Atrial Flutter. Atrial flutter is a rapid atrial ectopic tachycardia, with a rate that ranges from 240 to 450 beats/minute. There are two types of atrial flutter: typical and atypical flutter.[10,15] The most common, typical atrial flutter (sometimes called type I), is a result of a reentry rhythm in the right atrium, which can be entrained and interrupted with atrial pacing techniques. The atrial rate in typical type I flutter usually is in the vicinity of 300 beats/minute, but it can range from 240 to 340 beats/minute.

In typical atrial flutter, the ECG reveals a defined sawtooth pattern in leads AVF, V_1, and V_5.[16] The ventricular response rate and regularity are variable and depend on the AV conduction sequence. When regular, the ventricular response rate usually is a defined fraction of the atrial rate (*i.e.*, when conduction from the atria to the ventricles is 2:1, an atrial flutter rate of 300 would result in a ventricular response rate of 150 beats/minute). The QRS complex may be normal or abnormal, depending on the presence or absence of preexisting intraventricular conduction defects or aberrant ventricular conduction.

Atrial flutter rarely is seen in normal, healthy people. It may be seen in people of any age in the presence of underlying atrial abnormalities. Subgroups that are at particularly high risk for development of atrial flutter include children, adolescents, and young adults who have undergone corrective surgery for complex congenital heart diseases.[15]

Atrial Fibrillation. Atrial fibrillation (AF) is characterized as rapid disorganized atrial activation and uncoordinated contraction by the atria.[17] In most cases, multiple, small reentrant circuits are constantly arising in the atria, colliding, being extinguished, and arising again. Fibrillation occurs when the atrial cells cannot repolarize in time for the next incoming stimulus. AF is characterized on the ECG by a grossly disorganized pattern of atrial electrical activity that is irregular with respect to rate and rhythm and the absence of discernible P waves. Atrial activity is depicted by fibrillatory (f) waves of varying amplitude, duration, and morphology. These f waves appear as random oscillation of the baseline. Because of the random conduction through the AV node, QRS complexes appear in an irregular pattern.

AF is classified into three categories—paroxysmal, persistent, and permanent.[17] Paroxysmal AF self-terminates and lasts no longer than 7 days, while persistent lasts greater than 7 days and usually requires intervention such as a cardioversion. AF is classified as permanent when attempts to terminate are failed and the person remains in AF. During AF, the atrial rate typically ranges from 400 to 600 beats/minute, with many impulses blocked at the AV node. The ventricular response is completely irregular ranging from 80 to 180 beats/minute in the untreated state. Because of changes in stroke volumes resulting from varying periods of diastolic filling, not all ventricular beats produce a palpable pulse. The difference between the apical rate and the palpable peripheral pulses is called the *pulse deficit*. The pulse deficit increases when the ventricular rate is high.

AF can be seen in people without any apparent disease, or it may occur in people with coronary artery disease, mitral valve disease, ischemic heart disease, hypertension, MI, pericarditis, congestive heart failure, digitalis toxicity, and hyperthyroidism. Spontaneous conversion to sinus rhythm within 24 hours of AF is common, occurring in up to two thirds of people with the disorder.[17]

AF is the most common chronic arrhythmia, with an incidence and prevalence that increase with age. The incidence of AF increases with age. For example, it occurs in less than 0.5% of the population aged less than 50 years and increases by 2% at ages 60 to 69 years old. The prevalence is also greater in men than in women.[17]

The symptoms of chronic AF vary. Some people have minimal symptoms, and others have severe symptoms, particularly at the onset of the arrhythmia. The symptoms may range from palpitations to acute pulmonary edema. Fatigue and other nonspecific symptoms are common in the elderly. The condition predisposes people to thrombus formation in the atria, with subsequent risk of embolic stroke.

The treatment of AF depends on its cause, regency of onset, and persistence. It can be treated with antiarrhythmic medications to control rate or medically convert to sinus rhythm. Also, anticoagulant medications may be used to prevent embolic stroke depending on their risk for stroke.[18] Cardioversion may be considered in some persons, particularly when pulmonary edema or unstable cardiac status is present.

Paroxysmal Supraventricular Tachycardia. Paroxysmal supraventricular tachycardia refers to tachyarrhythmias that originate above the bifurcation of the bundle of His and have a sudden onset and termination. The heart rate may be 140 to 240 beats/minute and be perfectly regular despite exercise or change in position. Most people remain asymptomatic except for an awareness of the rapid heartbeat, but some may experience shortness of breath, especially if the episodes are prolonged. The most common mechanism for paroxysmal supraventricular tachycardia is reentry. It may be the result of AV nodal reentry, Wolff-Parkinson-White syndrome (caused by an accessory conduction pathway between the atria and ventricles), or intra-atrial or sinus node reentry.

Junctional Arrhythmias

The AV node can act as a pacemaker in the event the SA node fails to initiate an impulse. Junctional rhythms can be transient or permanent, and they usually have a rate of 40 to 60 beats/minute. Junctional fibers in the AV node or bundle of His also can serve as ectopic pacemakers, producing premature junctional complexes. Another rhythm originating in the junctional tissues is nonparoxysmal junctional tachycardia. This rhythm usually is of gradual onset and termination. However, it may occur abruptly if the dominant pacemaker slows sufficiently. The rate associated with junctional tachycardia ranges from 70 to 130 beats/minute, but it may be faster.[2] The P waves may precede, be buried in, or follow the QRS complexes, depending on the site of the originating impulses. The clinical significance of nonparoxysmal junctional tachycardia is the same as for atrial tachycardias. Catheter ablation therapy has been used successfully to treat some people with recurrent or intractable junctional tachycardia. Nonparoxysmal junctional tachycardia is observed most frequently in people with underlying heart disease, such as inferior wall MI or myocarditis, or after open heart surgery. It also may be present in persons with digitalis toxicity.

Disorders of Ventricular Conduction and Rhythm

The junctional fibers in the AV node join with the bundle of His, which divides to form the right and left bundle branches. The bundle branches continue to divide and form the Purkinje fibers, which supply the walls of the ventricles (see Fig. 28.1). As the cardiac impulse leaves the junctional fibers, it travels through the AV bundle. Next, the impulse moves down the right and left bundle branches that lie beneath the endocardium on either side of the septum. It then spreads out through the walls of the ventricles. Interruption of impulse conduction through the bundle branches is called *bundle-branch block*. These blocks usually do not cause alterations in the rhythm of the heartbeat. Instead, a bundle-branch block interrupts the normal progression of depolarization, causing the ventricles to depolarize one after the other because the impulses must travel through muscle tissue rather than through the specialized conduction tissue. This prolonged conduction causes the QRS complex to be wider than the normal 0.08 to 0.12 second. The left bundle branch bifurcates into the left anterior and posterior fascicles.

Long QT Syndrome and Torsade de Pointes

The *long QT syndrome* (LQTS) is characterized by a prolongation of the QT interval that may result in a characteristic type of polymorphic ventricular tachycardia called *torsade de pointes* and sudden cardiac death.[10,12] *Torsade de pointes* (*i.e.*, "twisting or rotating around a point") is a specific type of ventricular tachycardia (Fig. 28.11). The term refers to the polarity of the QRS complex, which swings from positive to negative and vice versa. The QRS abnormality is characterized by large, bizarre, polymorphic QRS complexes that vary, often from beat to beat, in amplitude and direction, as well as in rotation of the complexes around the isoelectric line. The rate of tachycardia is 100 to 180, but it can be as fast as 200 to 300 per minute. The rhythm is highly unstable and may terminate in ventricular fibrillation or revert to sinus rhythm.

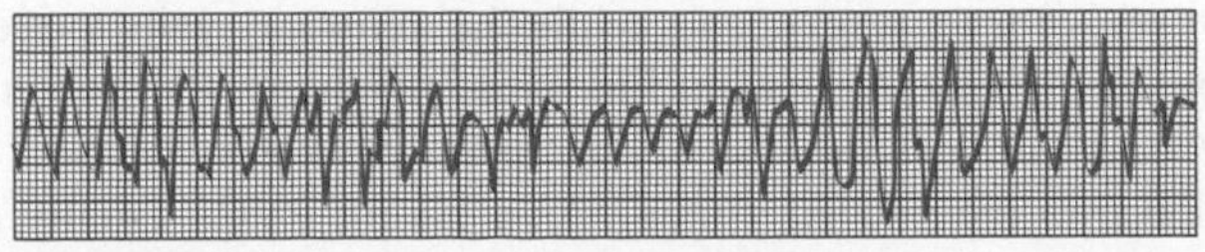

Figure 28.11 • Torsade de pointes. (From Morton P. G., Fontaine D. K. (2018). *Critical care nursing: A holistic approach* (11th ed., Fig. 17-27B, p. 227). Philadelphia, PA: Wolters Kluwer.)

Various agents and conditions that reduce the magnitude of outward repolarizing potassium currents enhance the magnitude of the inward depolarizing sodium and calcium currents, or both can cause LQTS. Thus, there is delayed repolarization of the ventricles with development of early depolarizing afterpotentials that initiate the arrhythmia. Typically, the QT interval is measured in a lead in which the T wave is prominent, and its end is easily distinguished, such as V_2 or V_3. Because the QT interval shortens with tachycardia and lengthens with bradycardia, it is typically corrected for heart rate and is noted as QT_c.[19] Nonetheless, a QT_c greater than 440 milliseconds in men and greater than 460 milliseconds in women has been linked with episodes of sudden arrhythmia death syndromes.

LQTSs have been classified into inherited and acquired forms, both of which are associated with the development of torsade de pointes and sudden cardiac death. The hereditary forms of LQTS are caused by disorders of membrane ion channel proteins, with either potassium channel defects or sodium channel defects.[20,21]

Acquired LQTS has been linked to a variety of conditions, including cocaine use, exposure to organophosphorus compounds, electrolyte imbalances, marked bradycardia, MI, subarachnoid hemorrhage, autonomic neuropathy, human immunodeficiency virus infection, and protein-sparing fasting.[21] Medications linked to LQTS include digitalis, antiarrhythmic agents (*e.g.*, amiodarone, procainamide, and quinidine), verapamil (calcium channel blocker), haloperidol (antipsychotic agent), and erythromycin (antibiotic).[19] The acquired forms of LQTS often are classified as pause dependent because the torsade de pointes associated with them generally occurs at slow heart rates or in response to short–long–short R-R interval sequences. Treatment of acquired forms of LQTS is directed primarily at identifying and withdrawing the offending agent, although emergency measures that modulate the function of transmembrane ion currents can be lifesaving.

Ventricular Arrhythmias

Arrhythmias that arise in the ventricles generally are considered more serious than those that arise in the atria because they afford the potential for interfering with the pumping action of the heart.

Premature Ventricular Contractions. A premature ventricular contraction (PVC) is caused by a ventricular ectopic pacemaker. After a PVC occurs, the ventricle usually is unable to repolarize sufficiently to respond to the next impulse that arises in the SA node. This delay, commonly referred to as a *compensatory pause*, occurs while the ventricle waits to reestablish its previous rhythm (Fig. 28.12). When a PVC occurs, the diastolic volume usually is insufficient for ejection of blood into the arterial system. As a result, PVCs usually do not produce a palpable pulse, or the pulse amplitude is significantly diminished. In the absence of heart disease, PVCs typically are not clinically significant. The incidence of PVCs

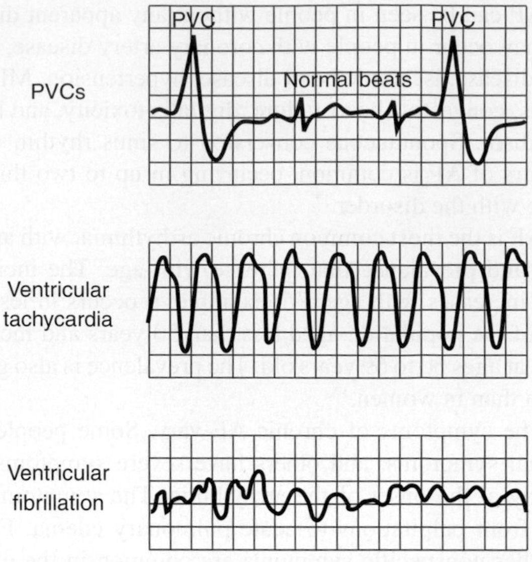

Figure 28.12 • Electrocardiographic (ECG) tracings of ventricular arrhythmias. Premature ventricular contractions (PVCs) (*top tracing*) originate from an ectopic focus in the ventricles, causing a distortion of the QRS complex. Because the ventricle usually cannot repolarize sufficiently to respond to the next impulse that arises in the SA node, a PVC frequently is followed by a compensatory pause. Ventricular tachycardia (*middle tracing*) is characterized by a rapid ventricular rate of 70 to 250 beats/minute and the absence of P waves. In ventricular fibrillation (*bottom tracing*), there are no regular or effective ventricular contractions, and the ECG tracing is totally disorganized.

is greatest with ischemia, acute MI, history of MI, ventricular hypertrophy, infection, increased sympathetic nervous system activity, or increased heart rate.[22] PVCs also can be the result of electrolyte disturbances or medications.

A special pattern of PVC called *ventricular bigeminy* is a condition in which each normal beat is followed by or paired with a PVC. This pattern often is an indication of digitalis toxicity or heart disease. The occurrence of frequent PVCs in the diseased heart predisposes to the development of other, more serious arrhythmias, including ventricular tachycardia and ventricular fibrillation.

Ventricular Tachycardia. Ventricular tachycardia describes a cardiac rhythm originating distal to the bifurcation of the bundle of His, in the specialized conduction system in ventricular muscle, or both.[2] It is characterized by a ventricular rate of 70 to 250 beats/minute, and the onset can be sudden or insidious. Usually, ventricular tachycardia is exhibited electrocardiographically by wide, tall, bizarre-looking QRS complexes that persist longer than 0.12 second (see Fig. 28.12). QRS complexes can be uniform in appearance, *monomorphic*, or they can vary randomly, in a repetitive manner (*e.g.*, torsade de pointes), in an alternating pattern (*e.g.*, bidirectional), or in a stable but changing fashion, polymorphic.[12] Ventricular tachycardia can be sustained, lasting more than 30 seconds and requiring intervention, or it can be nonsustained and stop spontaneously. This rhythm is dangerous because it eliminates atrial kick and can cause a reduction in diastolic filling time to the point at which cardiac output is severely diminished or nonexistent.

Ventricular Flutter and Fibrillation. These arrhythmias represent severe derangements of cardiac rhythm that terminate fatally within minutes unless corrective measures are taken promptly. The ECG pattern in ventricular flutter has a sine-wave appearance with large oscillations occurring at a rate of 150 to 300 per minute.[10] In ventricular fibrillation, the ventricle quivers but does not contract. The classic ECG pattern of ventricular fibrillation is that of gross disorganization without identifiable waveforms or intervals (see Fig. 28.12). When the ventricles do not contract, there is no cardiac output, and there are no palpable or audible pulses. Immediate defibrillation using a nonsynchronized, direct-current electrical shock is mandatory for ventricular fibrillation and for ventricular flutter that has caused loss of consciousness.[10]

Disorders of Atrioventricular Conduction

Under normal conditions, the AV junction, which consists of the AV node with its connections to the entering atrial internodal pathways, the AV bundle, and the nonbranching portion of the bundle of His, provides the only connection for transmission of impulses between the atrial and ventricular conduction systems. Junctional fibers in the AV node have high-resistance characteristics that cause a delay in the transmission of impulses from the atria to the ventricles. This delay provides optimal timing for the atrial contribution to ventricular filling and protects the ventricles from abnormally rapid rates that arise in the atria. Conduction defects of the AV node are most commonly associated with fibrosis or scar tissue in fibers of the conduction system. Conduction defects also may result from medications, including digoxin, β-adrenergic blocking agents, calcium channel–blocking agents, and class 1A antiarrhythmic agents.[23] Additional contributing factors include electrolyte imbalances, acute MI, idiopathic fibrosis of the conduction system, inflammatory disease, or cardiac surgery. Some other less common causes include infections, autoimmune, oncologic, and iatrogenic disorders.

Heart block refers to abnormalities of impulse conduction. It may be normal, physiologic (*e.g.*, vagal tone), or pathologic. It may occur from a conduction block in the atrium, AV nodal fibers, or in the AV bundle (*i.e.*, bundle of His), which is continuous with the Purkinje conduction system that supplies the ventricles. The PR interval on the ECG corresponds with the time it takes for the cardiac impulse to travel from the SA node to the ventricular pathways. Normally, the PR interval ranges from 0.12 to 0.20 second.

First-Degree AV Block. First-degree AV block is characterized by a prolonged PR interval (>0.20 second; Fig. 28.13). The prolonged PR interval indicates delayed AV conduction, but all atrial impulses are conducted to the ventricles. This condition usually produces a regular atrial and ventricular rhythm. Clinically significant PR interval prolongation can result from conduction delays in the AV node itself, the

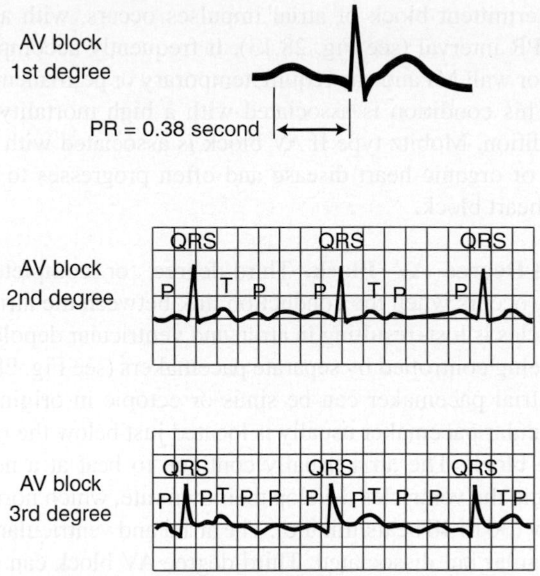

Figure 28.13 • Electrocardiographic changes that occur with alterations in AV node conduction. The *top tracing* shows the prolongation of the PR interval, which is characteristic of first-degree AV block. The *middle tracing* illustrates Mobitz type II second-degree AV block, in which the conduction of one or more P waves is blocked. In third-degree AV block (*bottom tracing*), impulses conducted through the AV node are completely blocked, and the atria and ventricles develop their own rates of impulse generation.

His–Purkinje system, or both.[18] When the QRS complex is normal in contour and duration, the AV delay almost always occurs in the AV node and rarely in the bundle of His. In contrast, when the QRS complex is prolonged, showing a bundle branch block pattern, conduction delays may be in the AV node or the His–Purkinje system. First-degree block may be the result of disease in the AV node, such as ischemia or infarction, or of infections such as rheumatic fever or myocarditis.[21,23] Isolated first-degree heart block usually is not symptomatic, and temporary or permanent cardiac pacing is not indicated but should be monitored.

Second-Degree AV Block. Second-degree AV block is characterized by intermittent failure of conduction of one or more impulses from the atria to the ventricles. The nonconducted P wave can appear intermittently or frequently. A distinguishing feature of second-degree AV block is that conducted P waves relate to QRS complexes with recurring PR intervals; that is, the association of P waves with QRS complexes is not random.[18] Second-degree AV block has been divided into two types: type I (*i.e.*, Mobitz type I or Wenckebach phenomenon) and type II (*i.e.*, Mobitz type II). A *Mobitz type I* AV block is characterized by progressive lengthening of the PR interval until an impulse is blocked and the sequence begins again. It frequently occurs in persons with inferior wall MI, particularly with concomitant right ventricular infarction. The condition usually is associated with an adequate ventricular rate and rarely is symptomatic. It usually is transient and does not require temporary pacing.[18] In the *Mobitz type II* AV block, an intermittent block of atrial impulses occurs, with a constant PR interval (see Fig. 28.13). It frequently accompanies anterior wall MI and can require temporary or permanent pacing. This condition is associated with a high mortality rate. In addition, Mobitz type II AV block is associated with other types of organic heart disease and often progresses to complete heart block.

Third-Degree AV Block. Third-degree, or complete AV block, occurs when the conduction link between the atria and ventricles is lost, resulting in atrial and ventricular depolarization being controlled by separate pacemakers (see Fig. 28.13). The atrial pacemaker can be sinus or ectopic in origin. The ventricular pacemaker usually is located just below the region of the block. The atria usually continue to beat at a normal rate, and the ventricles develop their own rate, which normally is slow (30 to 40 beats/minute). The atrial and ventricular rates are regular but dissociated. Third-degree AV block can result from an interruption at the level of the AV node, in the bundle of His, or in the Purkinje system. Third-degree blocks at the level of the AV node usually are congenital, whereas blocks in the Purkinje system usually are acquired. Normal QRS complexes, with rates ranging from 40 to 60 complexes per minute, usually are displayed on the ECG when the block occurs proximal to the bundle of His.

Complete heart block causes a decrease in cardiac output with possible periods of syncope (fainting), known as a *Stokes-Adams attack*.[18] Other symptoms include dizziness, fatigue, exercise intolerance, or episodes of acute heart failure.[1] Most people with complete heart block require a permanent cardiac pacemaker.

Inherited Types of Arrhythmias

Cardiac arrhythmias most commonly occur in the presence of cardiac disease, electrolyte disorders, or other demonstrable abnormalities. Ischemic heart disease is the primary cause for the development of ventricular fibrillation, and structural heart defects such as hypertrophic and dilated cardiomyopathies account for most of the remaining cases. For many years, people who had died suddenly were referred to as having *idiopathic ventricular fibrillation* when in fact ion channel abnormalities or channelopathies were the underlying cause.[24] Over the past several decades, considerable evidence has been collected indicating that these cases are genetically determined abnormalities of proteins in the ion channels that control the electrical activity of the heart. Many genes have been associated with inherited arrhythmogenic channelopathies, and it is expected that more will be identified and linked to sudden death in people with apparently healthy hearts.[24,25] Among the inherited arrhythmogenic disorders are congenital LQTS, SQTS, Brugada syndrome, and catecholaminergic polymorphic ventricular tachycardia.

Congenital Long QT Syndrome. Congenital LQTS is an inherited arrhythmogenic disease characterized by life-threatening ventricular arrhythmias. Hundreds of gene mutations have been identified on the three major and nine minor LQTS susceptible genes.[20] The ECG marker for LQTS consists of a prolonged QT interval, abnormal morphology of the T wave, and a characteristic polymorphic ventricular tachycardia (torsade de pointes). The severity of the clinical manifestations in LQTS varies, ranging from full-blown disease with marked prolongation of the QT interval and recurrent syncope to subclinical forms with borderline QT-interval prolongation and no arrhythmias or syncopal episodes.

Depending on which gene is affected, long-term treatment with β-adrenergic receptor blockers, permanent pacing, or left cardiac sympathetic denervation is frequently effective.[25] Placement of an implantable cardioverter–defibrillator is recommended for people in whom recurrent syncope, sustained ventricular arrhythmias, or sudden cardiac arrest occurs despite drug treatment.

Short QT Syndrome. Short QT syndrome (SQTS) was first described in 2000 and is associated with a QT interval less than 330 milliseconds. There are still limited data on the syndrome. However, of the research that has been performed, most people with this disorder are asymptomatic, and some have history of syncope. The treatment of choice remains an implantable cardioverter–defibrillator to prevent sudden cardiac death.[16,26]

Brugada Syndrome. First described in 1992, Brugada syndrome is an autosomal dominant disorder characterized by ST-segment elevation in precordial leads V_1 to V_3, right bundle-branch block, and susceptibility to ventricular tachycardia.[25] Symptoms associated with this ECG include syncope, palpitations, chest discomfort, cardiac arrest, and nocturnal agonal respiration. It has so far been associated with a single gene encoding for the cardiac sodium channel. The disorder typically manifests in adulthood with very incomplete penetrance, and a high percentage of mutation carriers are asymptomatic.[26] Even though the disorder is inherited as an autosomal trait, a male-to-female ratio of 8:1 is observed in clinical manifestations.[24]

Catecholaminergic Polymorphic Ventricular Tachycardia. Catecholaminergic polymorphic ventricular tachycardia (CPVT) is a disorder characterized by ventricular tachycardia, syncope, and sudden death occurring in familial or sporadic cases in the absence of cardiac disease or ECG abnormalities.

The ECG of people with CPVT is usually remarkably normal, and they do not have structural heart disease. Physical activity and acute emotions are the specific triggers for arrhythmias in people with CPVT. The complexity of the arrhythmias progressively increases with an increase in workload, from isolated premature beats to bigeminy to runs of ventricular tachycardia. It is particularly important to perform genetic analyses to identify mutations. If left untreated, the disorder is highly malignant, but the prognosis improves considerably once the disorder is correctly identified and treatment is implemented.[27] Antiadrenergic treatment with beta-blockers is the cornerstone of therapy for CPVT. The use of an implantable cardioverter–defibrillator may be necessary when exercise stress testing. Holter monitoring indicates that beta-blockers do not provide complete arrhythmia protection, but they also do not increase the risk of cardiac arrest.[24]

Diagnostic Methods. The diagnosis of cardiac rhythm and conduction disorders usually is made on the basis of the surface ECG, Holter ECG monitoring, or implantable loop ECG recording. Further clarification of conduction defects and cardiac arrhythmias can be obtained using exercise stress testing and electrophysiologic studies.

Surface ECG

A resting surface ECG records the impulses originating in the heart as they are recorded at the body surface. These impulses are recorded for a limited time and during periods of inactivity. Although there are no complications related to the procedure, errors related to misdiagnosis may result in iatrogenic heart disease.[5,6] The resting ECG is the first approach to the clinical diagnosis of disorders of cardiac rhythm and conduction, but it is limited to events that occur during the period the ECG is being monitored.

Holter ECG Monitoring

Holter monitoring is one form of long-term monitoring during which a person wears a device that digitally records two or three ECG leads for up to 48 hours. During this time, the person keeps a diary of his or her activities or symptoms, which later are correlated with the ECG recording. Most recording devices also have an event marker button that can be pressed when the individual experiences symptoms, which assists the technician or physician in correlating the diary, symptoms, and ECG changes during analysis. Newer Holter recorders are capable of providing a derived 12-lead ECG. Holter monitoring is useful for documenting arrhythmias, conduction abnormalities, and ST-segment changes. The interpretative accuracy of long-term Holter recordings varies with the system used and clinician expertise. Most computer software packages used to scan Holter recordings are sufficiently accurate to meet clinical demand. The majority of people who have ischemic heart disease exhibit PVCs, particularly those who have recently experienced MI.[28] The frequency of PVCs increases progressively over the first several weeks and decreases approximately 6 months postinfarction. Holter recordings also are used to determine antiarrhythmic drug efficacy, episodes of myocardial ischemia, QT prolongation, and heart rate variability.

Intermittent ECG recorders, event recorders, also are used in the diagnosis of arrhythmias and conduction defects. There are two basic types of recorders that perform this type of monitoring.[28] The first continuously monitors rhythm and is programmed to recognize abnormalities. In the second variety, the unit does not continuously monitor the ECG and therefore cannot automatically recognize abnormalities. The latter form relies on the person to activate the unit when he or she is symptomatic. The data are stored in memory or transmitted telephonically to an ECG receiver, where they are recorded. These types of ECG recordings are useful in people who have transient symptoms.

Implantable Loop ECG Recorder

If Holter and event monitors do not produce any diagnostic information and a person continues to have symptoms, a loop recorder can be implanted. This device is implanted under the skin in the left upper chest area. It continuously monitors the person's ECG and can be programmed to store patient-activated events when they are symptomatic. The loop recorder can be in place for as long as 3 years. It is useful for documenting arrhythmias, antiarrhythmic drug efficacy, episodes of myocardial ischemia, QT prolongation, pauses, and heart rate variability.

Exercise Stress Testing

The exercise stress test elicits the body's response to measured increases in acute exercise. This technique provides information about changes in heart rate, blood pressure, respiration, and perceived level of exercise. It is useful in determining exercise-induced alterations in hemodynamic response and ECG ischemic-type ST-segment changes and can detect and classify disturbances in cardiac rhythm and conduction associated with exercise.[29] These changes are indicative of a poorer prognosis in people with known coronary disease and recent MI. If a person cannot walk on a treadmill, there are pharmacologic alternatives. The stress echocardiogram can visualize the motion and pumping to see if there is lack of blood flow to a certain area of the heart. This entails the person walking on a treadmill as if they were doing a regular stress test, then lying on a table immediately afterward for the echocardiogram images.

Electrophysiologic Studies

Electrophysiologic testing is used for the diagnosis and management of complex arrhythmias. It involves the passage of two or more electrode catheters into the right side of the heart. These catheters are inserted into the femoral, subclavian, internal jugular, or antecubital veins and positioned with fluoroscopy into the high right atrium near the sinus node, the area of the His bundle, the coronary sinus that lies in the posterior AV groove, and into the right ventricle.[3] The electrode catheters are used to stimulate the heart and record intracardiac ECGs. During the study, overdrive pacing, cardioversion, or defibrillation may be necessary to terminate tachycardia induced during the stimulation procedures.

The primary indications for electrophysiologic testing are:

- To determine a person's potential for arrhythmia formation
- To evaluate recurrent syncope of cardiac origin, when ambulatory ECG has not provided the diagnosis

- To differentiate supraventricular from ventricular arrhythmias
- To locate arrhythmogenic foci for therapeutic interventions such as catheter ablation procedures or antitachycardia devices[11]

Testing can also define reproducible arrhythmia induction characteristics and hence can be used to evaluate the therapeutic efficacy of a particular treatment modality.

Electrophysiologic methods can also be used as interventions. These interventions may include pacing a person out of tachycardia or ablation therapy. Ablation therapy involves the destruction of myocardial tissue by delivering electrical energy over electrodes on a catheter placed next to an area related to the onset or maintenance of arrhythmias.

Risks associated with electrophysiologic testing are small. Most electrophysiologic studies do not involve left-sided heart access, and therefore, the risk of MI, stroke, or systemic embolism is less than observed with coronary arteriography. The addition of therapeutic maneuvers, such as ablation therapy, to the procedure increases the risk of complications, which include venous thrombosis and pulmonary emboli.[30]

Treatment

The treatment of cardiac rhythm or conduction disorders is directed toward controlling the arrhythmia, correcting the cause, and preventing more serious or fatal arrhythmias. Correction may involve simply adjusting an electrolyte disturbance or withholding a medication such as digitalis. Preventing more serious arrhythmias often involves drug therapy, electrical stimulation, or surgical intervention.

Pharmacologic Treatment

Antiarrhythmic drugs act by modifying the disordered formation and conduction of impulses that induce cardiac muscle contraction. These drugs are classified into four major groups (class I through class IV) according to the drug's effect on the action potential of the cardiac cells.[11] Although drugs in one category have similar effects on conduction, they may vary significantly in their hemodynamic effects. Two other types of antiarrhythmic drugs, the cardiac glycosides and adenosine, are not included in this classification schema. The cardiac glycosides (*i.e.*, digitalis drugs) slow the heart rate and are used in the management of arrhythmias such as atrial tachycardia, atrial flutter, and AF. Adenosine, an endogenous nucleoside that is present in every cell, is used for emergency intravenous treatment of paroxysmal supraventricular tachycardia involving the AV node. It interrupts AV node conduction and slows SA node firing.[31,32]

Class I Drugs. Class I drugs act by blocking the fast sodium channels. These drugs affect impulse conduction, excitability, and automaticity to various degrees and therefore have been divided further into three groups: IA, IB, and IC. Class IA drugs (*e.g.*, quinidine, procainamide, disopyramide) decrease automaticity by depressing phase 4 of the action potential, decrease conductivity by moderately prolonging phase 0, and prolong repolarization by extending phase 3 of the action potential.[31,32] Because these drugs are effective in suppressing ectopic foci and treating reentrant arrhythmias, they are used for supraventricular and ventricular arrhythmias. Class IB drugs (*e.g.*, lidocaine, mexiletine) decrease automaticity by depressing phase 4 of the action potential, have little effect on conductivity, decrease refractoriness by decreasing phase 2, and shorten repolarization by decreasing phase 3. These drugs have little or no effect on sodium channels in resting cells. However, they shorten the action potential and are powerful inhibitors of sodium-dependent conduction in depolarized cells, making them effective in depressing conduction in ischemic areas of the heart.[24] Drugs in this group are used for treating ventricular arrhythmias only and have little or no effect on myocardial contractility. Class IC drugs (*e.g.*, propafenone, moricizine, flecainide) decrease conductivity by markedly depressing phase 0 of the action potential but have little effect on refractoriness or repolarization. Their primary action is inhibition of sodium channel opening. Drugs in this class are used for life-threatening ventricular arrhythmias and supraventricular tachycardias.

Class II Drugs. Class II drugs (*e.g.*, propranolol, metoprolol, atenolol, timolol, sotalol) are β-adrenergic blocking drugs that act by blunting the effect of sympathetic nervous system stimulation on the heart, thereby inhibiting calcium channel opening. These drugs decrease automaticity by depressing phase 4 of the action potential. They also decrease heart rate and cardiac contractility. These medications are effective for treatment of supraventricular arrhythmias and tachyarrhythmias by counteracting action on arrhythmogenesis of catecholamines.[24]

Class III Drugs. Class III drugs (*e.g.*, amiodarone, bretylium, ibutilide, dofetilide, sotalol) act by inhibiting the potassium current and repolarization, thereby extending the action potential and refractoriness. They have little inhibiting effect on depolarizing currents. Sotalol has both β-adrenergic receptor blocking (class II) and action potential prolonging (class III) actions. It may cause QT prolongation and should be discontinued if there is a greater than 15% increase from baseline.[32] Sotalol is used to treat AF and ventricular tachycardia related to old MI. Amiodarone not only can cause QT prolongation, but it has additional extracardiac side effects such as thyroid, hepatic, and pulmonary toxicities. These toxicities need to be monitored on a regular basis and taken into account when deciding to initiate treatment for AF and ventricular arrhythmias. Dofetilide is used for the treatment of AF and flutter as well as to prevent recurrences and control rate. Unlike amiodarone, it does not have associated toxicities, but it does prolong the QT interval.[24] Ibutilide may also cause QT prolongation, but this prolongation returns to normal in 3 to 4 hours after the infusion is discontinued. These agents are used in the treatment of serious ventricular arrhythmias.

Class IV Drugs. Class IV drugs (*e.g.*, verapamil, diltiazem, mibefradil) act by blocking the slow calcium channels, thereby depressing phase 4 and lengthening phases 1 and 2 of the action potential. By blocking the release of intracellular calcium ions, these agents reduce the force of myocardial contractility, thereby decreasing myocardial oxygen demand. These drugs are used to slow the SA node pacemaker and inhibit conduction in the AV node, slowing the ventricular response in atrial tachycardias, and to terminate reentrant paroxysmal supraventricular tachycardias when the AV node functions as a reentrant pathway.[24]

Electrical Interventions. The correction of conduction defects, bradycardias, and tachycardias can involve the use of a pacemaker, cardioversion, or defibrillation. Electrical interventions can be used in emergency and elective situations. Efforts directed at cardiac electrostimulation date back more than a century. During this time, tremendous strides have been made in the effectiveness of cardiac pacing.

Cardiac Pacemaker. A cardiac pacemaker is an electronic device that delivers an electrical stimulus to the heart. It is used to initiate heartbeats in situations when the normal pacemaker of the heart is defective. These situations include certain types of AV heart block, symptomatic bradycardia in which the rate of cardiac contraction and consequent cardiac output are inadequate to perfuse vital tissues, as well as other cardiac arrhythmias. A pacemaker may be used as a temporary or a permanent measure. Pacemaker leads can pace the atria, the ventricles, or the atria and ventricles sequentially, or overdrive pacing can be used. Overdrive pacing may be used to try to treat recurrent ventricular tachycardia and reentrant atrial or ventricular tachyarrhythmias and to terminate atrial flutter.

Temporary pacemakers are useful for treatment of symptomatic bradycardias and to perform overdrive pacing. They can be placed transcutaneously, transvenously, or epicardially. External temporary pacing, also known as *transcutaneous pacing*, involves the placement of large patch electrodes on the anterior and posterior chest wall, which then are connected by a cable to an external pulse generator.

Internal temporary pacing, also known as *transvenous pacing*, involves the passage of a venous catheter with electrodes on its tip into the right atrium or ventricle, where it is wedged against the endocardium. The electrode then is attached to an external pulse generator. This procedure is performed under fluoroscopic or electrocardiographic direction. During open thoracotomy procedures, epicardial pacing wires sometimes are placed. These wires are brought out directly through the chest wall and also can be attached to an external pulse generator, if necessary.

Permanent cardiac pacemakers may become necessary for a variety of reasons. Permanent pacemakers require a pulse generator and implantation of pacing wires into the epicardium that deliver the electrical stimuli.[33] Ongoing evaluation of the pacemaker's sensing, firing, and battery life is necessary on a regular basis.[22]

Synchronized Cardioversion and Defibrillation. Synchronized cardioversion and defibrillation are two reliable methods for treating ventricular tachycardia, and cardioversion is the definitive treatment for AF. The discharge of electrical energy that is synchronized with the R wave of the ECG is referred to as *synchronized cardioversion*, and unsynchronized discharge is known as *defibrillation*. The goal of both of these techniques is to provide an electrical pulse to the heart in such a way as to depolarize the heart completely during passage of the current. This electrical current interrupts the disorganized impulses, allowing the SA node to regain control of the heart. Defibrillation and synchronized cardioversion can be delivered externally through large patch electrodes on the chest or internally through small paddle electrodes placed directly on the myocardium, patch electrodes sewn into the epicardium, or transvenous wires placed in the right ventricle. There are pacemakers and implantable cardioverter–defibrillators that can perform antitachycardia pacing, cardioversion, and defibrillation when programmed by a specialized health care provider.[33]

Concept Mastery Alert

The electricity in nonsynchronized defibrillation depolarizes the entire heart, interrupting the chaotic rhythm and allowing the SA node to take control.

Automatic implantable cardioverter–defibrillators (AICDs) are being used successfully to treat people with life-threatening ventricular tachyarrhythmias by the use of intrathoracic electrical countershock.[33] Reliable sensing and detection of ventricular tachyarrhythmias are essential for proper functioning of the AICD. Sensing and detection are accomplished through endocardial leads. The AICD can also be programmed to provide antitachycardia pacing, which will pace faster than the ventricular rate to try to terminate the arrhythmia. All AICDs respond to ventricular tachyarrhythmia at fast rates by delivering an electrical shock between intrathoracic electrodes within 10 to 20 seconds of its onset. This time frame provides nearly a 100% likelihood of reversal of the arrhythmia, supporting the utility of this device as a reliable and effective means of preventing sudden cardiac death in survivors of out-of-hospital cardiac arrest. There are three types of AICDS: single-chamber, dual-chamber, and biventricular defibrillators. These devices are monitored regularly in person and remotely, and there are specific guidelines established on how often they need to be evaluated by a health care provider.[22]

Ablation and Surgical Interventions

Ablation therapy is used for treating recurrent, life-threatening supraventricular and ventricular tachyarrhythmias. Ablative therapy may be performed by catheter or surgical techniques. It involves localized destruction, isolation, or excision of cardiac tissue that is considered to be arrhythmogenic.[3,28]

The first catheter ablation procedures were performed using direct-current shocks, but this energy source has largely been replaced by RF energy, which is delivered by an external generator and destroys tissue by heat production.[28] RF ablation uses RF waves to destroy defective or aberrant electrical conduction pathways. RF ablation remains the most common method for ablating cardiac arrhythmias. An additional kind of energy that was developed was cryoenergy, or freezing. Cryoablation involves the direct application of an extremely cold probe to arrhythmogenic cardiac tissue. Catheter-delivered cryoablation causes damage by freezing cellular structures of defective or aberrant electrical conduction pathways.[3,28] When comparing RF ablation and cryoablation, there are no significant differences in efficacy and complications. The type of energy used is based on the physician preference and type of arrhythmia.[23]

Additional surgical interventions such as coronary artery bypass surgery, ventriculotomy, and endocardial resection may be used to improve myocardial oxygenation, remove arrhythmogenic foci, or alter electrical conduction pathways.[34] Coronary artery bypass surgery improves myocardial oxygenation by increasing blood supply to the myocardium. Ventriculotomy involves the removal of aneurysm tissue and the resuturing of the myocardial walls to eliminate the paradoxical ventricular movement and the foci of arrhythmias. In endocardial resection, endocardial tissue that has been identified as arrhythmogenic through the use of electrophysiologic testing or intraoperative mapping is surgically removed. Ventriculotomy and endocardial resection have been performed with cryoablation or laser ablation as an adjunctive therapy.

IN SUMMARY

Disorders of cardiac rhythm arise as the result of disturbances in impulse generation or conduction in the heart. Normal sinus rhythm and respiratory sinus arrhythmia (*i.e.*, heart rate speeds up and slows down in concert with respiratory cycle) are considered normal cardiac rhythms. Cardiac arrhythmias are not necessarily pathologic; they occur in healthy and diseased hearts. Sinus arrhythmias originate in the SA node. They include sinus bradycardia (heart rate <60 beats/minute); sinus tachycardia (heart rate >100 beats/minute); sinus arrest, in which there are prolonged periods of asystole; and SSS, a condition characterized by periods of bradycardia alternating with tachycardia.

Atrial arrhythmias arise from alterations in impulse generation that occur in the conduction pathways or muscle of the atria. They include PACs, atrial flutter (*i.e.*, atrial depolarization rate of 240 to 450 beats/minute), and AF (*i.e.*, grossly disorganized atrial depolarization that is irregular with regard to rate and rhythm). Atrial arrhythmias often go unnoticed unless they are transmitted to the ventricles.

Arrhythmias that arise in the ventricles commonly are considered more serious than those that arise in the atria because they afford the potential for interfering with the pumping action of the heart. The LQTS represents a prolongation of the QT interval that may result in torsade de pointes and sudden cardiac death. A PVC is caused by a ventricular ectopic pacemaker. Ventricular tachycardia is characterized by a ventricular rate of 70 to 250 beats/minute. Ventricular fibrillation (*e.g.*, ventricular rate >350 beats/minute) is a fatal arrhythmia unless it is successfully treated with defibrillation. Arrhythmogenic cardiomyopathies are inherited disorders of the ion channels that control the electrical activity of the heart. Among the inherited arrhythmogenic disorders are congenital LQTS, SQTS, Brugada syndrome, and CPVT.

Alterations in the conduction of impulses through the AV node lead to disturbances in the transmission of impulses from the atria to the ventricles. There can be a delay in transmission (*i.e.*, first-degree heart block), failure to conduct one or more impulses (*i.e.*, second-degree heart block), or complete failure to conduct impulses between the atria and the ventricles (*i.e.*, third-degree heart block). Conduction disorders of the bundle of His and Purkinje system, called *bundle-branch blocks*, cause a widening of and changes in the configuration of the QRS complex of the ECG.

The diagnosis of disorders of cardiac rhythm and conduction typically is accomplished using surface ECG recordings or electrophysiologic studies. Surface electrodes can be used to obtain a 12-lead ECG; signal-averaged electrocardiographic studies in which multiple samples of QRS waves are averaged to detect ventricular late action potentials; and Holter monitoring, which provides continuous ECG recordings for up to 48 hours and loop recording, which provides continuous recording up to 3 years. Electrophysiologic studies use electrode catheters inserted into the right heart through a peripheral vein as a means of directly stimulating the heart while obtaining an intracardiac ECG recording.

Both medications and electrical devices are used in the treatment of arrhythmias and conduction disorders. Antiarrhythmic drugs act by modifying disordered formation and conduction of impulses that induce cardiac muscle contraction. They include drugs that act by blocking the fast sodium channels, β-adrenergic blocking drugs that decrease sympathetic outflow to the heart, drugs that act by inhibiting the potassium current and repolarization, calcium channel–blocking agents, cardiac glycosides (*i.e.*, digitalis drugs), and adenosine, which is used for emergency intravenous treatment of paroxysmal supraventricular tachycardia involving the AV mode. Electrical devices include temporary and permanent cardiac pacemakers that are used to treat symptomatic bradycardias or to provide overdrive pacing procedures; defibrillators that are used to treat atrial and ventricular fibrillation; external or internally implanted cardioversion devices, which can be used to treat ventricular tachycardia; and RF ablation and cryoablation therapy, which are used to destroy specific irritable foci in the heart. Surgical procedures can be performed to excise irritable or dysfunctional tissue, to replace cardiac valves, or to provide better blood supply to the myocardial muscle wall.

GERIATRIC Considerations

- Digitalis toxicity is the leading cause of arrhythmias associated with aging.[34]
  - Other factors associated with arrhythmias and aging include hypokalemia, angina pectoris, decreased coronary artery blood flow, and acute blood loss.
- Because older adults have a higher rate of mortality from cardiac arrest, monitoring of digoxin levels and assessing for weakness, confusion, low heart rate, fainting, and irregular heart rate can prevent complications.[34]
- Atrial fibrillation, the most common chronic cardiac arrhythmia, is associated with comorbidities; 80% have hypertension, and the majority have heart failure, ischemia, or high levels of fat or lipid in the blood.[34]

PEDIATRIC Considerations

- Sinus tachycardia is common in children following cardiac surgery. Anesthesia, incisions, and manipulations during surgery can lead to arrhythmias in the immediate postoperative period.[27]
- Sinus bradycardia is associated with an immature newborn conduction system.[27]
- Fever, dehydration, pain, anxiety, acidosis, anemia, and sepsis can lead to sinus tachycardia in children.[27]
- Wolff-Parkinson-White syndrome is the most common symptomatic arrhythmia in the newborn with heart rates reaching 220 beats per minute (bpm) in infants and 180 bpm in children.[27]
- Short QT syndrome, a rare autosomal dominant arrhythmia, most often results from alterations in potassium channels and places child at risk for malignant arrhythmias.[26]
- Congenital alterations in conduction are often the result of maternal autoantibodies such as in systemic lupus erythematosus.[35]

REVIEW EXERCISES

1. A 75-year-old woman with a history of congestive heart failure presents to the clinic complaining of feeling tired. Her heart rate is 121 beats/minute, and the rhythm is irregular.
   A. *What type of arrhythmia do you think she might be having? What would it look like if you were to obtain an ECG?*
   B. *What causes this irregularity?*
   C. *Why do you think she is feeling tired?*
   D. *What are some of the concerns with this type of arrhythmia?*
2. A 45-year-old man appears at the urgent care center with complaints of chest discomfort, shortness of breath, and generally not feeling well. You assess vital signs and find that his temperature is 99.2°F, blood pressure 180/90, pulse 90 and slightly irregular, and respiratory rate 26. You do an ECG, and the readings from the anterior leads indicate that he is experiencing an ischemic episode.
   A. *You attach him to a cardiac monitor and see that his underlying rhythm is normal sinus rhythm, but he is having frequent premature contractions that are more than 0.10 second in duration. What type of premature contractions do you suspect?*
   B. *What would you expect his pulse to feel like?*
   C. *What do you think the etiology of this arrhythmia might be? How might it be treated?*

References

1. Guyton A. C., Hall J. E. (2016). *Textbook of medical physiology* (131th ed., pp. 109–123, 155–165, 1115–1127, 1157). Philadelphia, PA: Elsevier Saunders.
2. Rubart M., Zipes D. P. (2012). Genesis of cardiac arrhythmias: Electrophysiologic considerations. In Bonow R. O., Mann D. L., Zipes D. P., et al. (Eds.), *Braunwald's heart disease: A textbook of cardiovascular medicine* (9th ed., pp. 653–687). Philadelphia, PA: Elsevier Saunders.
3. Fogoros R. N. (2012). *Electrophysiologic testing* (5th ed., pp. 4–12, 210–256). Hoboken, NJ: Wiley-Blackwell.
4. Klabunde R. (2012). *Cardiovascular physiology concepts* (2nd ed., pp. 1–67). Philadelphia, PA: Lippincott Williams & Wilkins.
5. Rao B. N. V. R. (2017). *Clinical examination in cardiology* (2nd ed., p. 48). Philadelphia, PA: Elsevier Saunders.
6. Garcia T. (2015). Acquiring the 12 lead electrocardiogram doing it right every time. *Journal of Emergency Nursing* 41(6), 474–478.
7. Morton P. G., Fontaine D. K. (2018). Anatomy and physiology of the cardiovascular system. In *Critical care nursing: A holistic approach* (11th ed., pp. 173–183). Philadelphia, PA: Wolters Kluwer.
8. Drew B., Califf R., Funk M., et al. (2004). Practice standards for electrocardiographic monitoring in hospital settings. *Circulation* 110, 2721–2746.
9. Jones T., Goldberger Z. (2016). Errors in electrocardiography monitoring, computerized EGC, other sites of ECG recording. In Stroobandt R. X., Serge Barold S., Sinnaeve A. F. (Eds.), *ECG from basics to essentials: Step by step*. Chichester, UK: John Wiley & Sons, Ltd.
10. Olgin J. L., Zipes D. P. (2012). Specific arrhythmias: Diagnosis and treatment. In Bonow R. O., Mann D. L., Zipes D. P., et al. (Eds.), *Braunwald's heart disease: A textbook of cardiovascular medicine* (13th ed., pp. 771–823). Philadelphia, PA: Elsevier Saunders.
11. Bashore T. M., Granger C. B. Jackson K., et al. (2017). The heart. In Papadakis M. A., McPhee S. J., Rabow, M.W. (Eds.), *Current medical diagnosis and treatment* (56th ed., pp. 322–438). New York: McGraw-Hill.
12. Morton P. G., Reck K., Headley, J. M. (2018). Patient assessment: Cardiovascular system. In *Critical care nursing: A holistic approach* (11th ed., pp. 184–261). Philadelphia, PA: Wolters Kluwer.
13. Ewy G. (2014). Sick sinus syndrome. *Journal of the American College of Cardiology* 64(6), 539–540.
14. Semelka M., Gera J., Usman S.(2013). Sick sinus syndrome: A review. *American Academy of Family Physicians* 87(10), 691–696.
15. Page R. L., Joglar J. A., Caldwell M. A., et al. (2016). 2015 ACC/AHA/HRS guideline for the management of adult patients with supraventricular tachycardia. *Journal of the American College of Cardiology* 67(13), e27–e115, doi: 10.1016/j.jacc.2015.08.856.

16. Mazzanti A., Kanthan A., Montefore N., et al. (2014). Novel insight into the natural history of short QT syndrome. *Journal of the American College of Cardiology* 63(13), 1300–1308.
17. Members W. C., January C. T., Wann L. S., et al. (2014). 2014 AHA/ACC/HRS guideline for the management of patients with atrial fibrillation: A report of the American College of Cardiology/American Heart Association Task Force on Practice Guidelines and the Heart Rhythm Society. *Circulation* 130(23), e199.
18. Curtis A. (2013). Practice implication of the atrial fibrillation guidelines. *American Journal of Cardiolology* 111, 1660–1670.
19. Earl G., Hankins S. (2016). Drug-induced long QT syndrome. *Nursing2017 Critical Care* 11(5), 5–10.
20. Nakano Y., Shimizu W. (2015). Genetics of long QT syndrome. *Journal of Human Genetics* 61, 51–55.
21. Abrams D., MacRae C. (2014). Long QT syndrome. *Circulation* 129, 1524–1529.
22. Knight B. P. (2017 Up to Date). Patient education: Implantable cardioverter-defibrillators (Beyond the Basics). Available: https://www.uptodate.com/contents/implantable-cardioverter-defibrillators-beyond-the-basics?
23. Garg J., Chaudhary R., Palaniswamy C., et al. (2016). Cryoballoon versus radiofrequency ablation for atrial fibrillation: A meta-analysis of 16 clinical trials. *Journal of Atrial Fibrillation* 9(3), 1429.
24. Steinberg J., Mittal S. (2017). *Electrophysiology: The basics* (2nd ed., pp. 301–322, 271–298). Philadelphia, PA: Wolters Kluwer.
25. Tester D. J., Ackerman M. J. (2012). *Genetics of cardiac arrhythmias*. In Bonow R. O., Mann D. L., Zipes D. P., et al. (Eds.), *Braunwald's heart disease: A textbook of cardiovascular medicine* (9th ed., pp. 81–90). Philadelphia, PA: Elsevier Saunders.
26. Khera S., Jacobson J. T. (2016). Short QT syndrome in current clinical practice. *Cardiology in Review* 24(4), 190–193.
27. Bowden V. R., Greenberg C. S. (2014). The child with altered cardiovascular status. In *Children and their families the continuum of nursing care* (3rd ed., pp. 646–647). Philadelphia, PA: Wolters Kluwer.
28. Miller J. M., Zipes D. P. (2012). Diagnosis of cardiac arrhythmias. In Bonow R. O., Mann D. L., Zipes D. P., et al. (Eds.), *Braunwald's heart disease: A textbook of cardiovascular medicine* (9th ed., pp. 702–709). Philadelphia, PA: Elsevier Saunders.
29. Garner K. K., Pomeroy W., Arnold J. J. (2017). Exercise stress testing: Indications and common questions. *American Family Physician* 96(5), 293–299.
30. Synder M. L., Coombs V. J., Barquist K. C., et al. (2018). Patient management: Cardiovascular system. In *Critical care nursing: A holistic approach* (11th ed., pp. 261–336). Philadelphia, PA: Wolters Kluwer.
31. Kumar K., Zimetbaum P. J. (2013). Antiarrhythmic drugs 2013: State of the art. *Invasive Electrophysiology and Pacing* 14, 409–416.
32. Parker M., Sanoski C. (2016). Clinical Pearls in using antiarrhythmic drugs in the outpatient setting. *Journal of Pharmacy Practice* 29(1), 77–86.
33. Fisher J. D. et al. (1992) Antitachycardia pacing, cardioversion, and defibrillation: From the past to the future. In Alt E., Klein H., Griffin J. C. (Eds.), *The implantable cardioverter/defibrillator*. Berlin, Heidelberg: Springer.
34. Eliopoulos C. (2018). Circulation. In *Gerontological nursing* (9th ed., pp. 268–291). Philadelphia, PA: Wolters Kluwer.
35. Strayer D. S., Rubin E. (Eds). (2015). *Rubin's pathology clinicopathologic foundations of medicine*. (7th ed.). Philadelphia, PA: Wolters Kluwer.

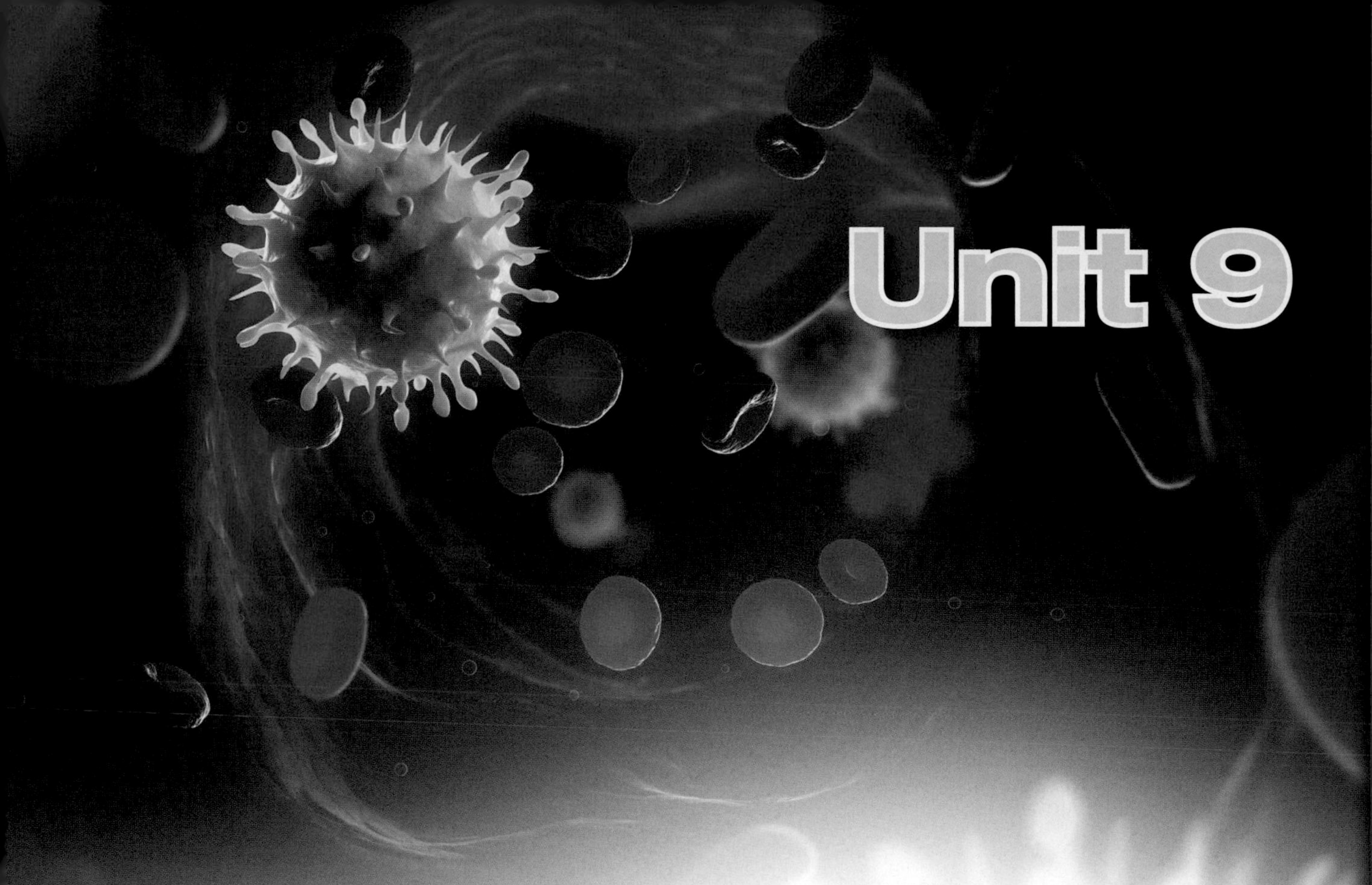

Unit 9

Disorders of Respiratory Function

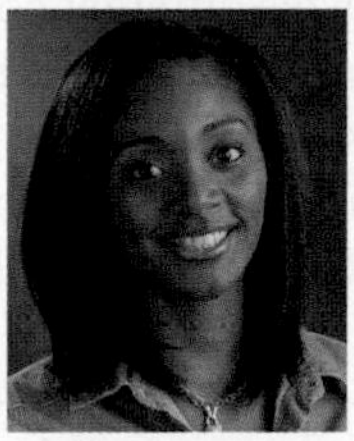

Ms. French, who is 24 years old, presents to the emergency department with shortness of breath (SOB) and a nonproductive cough. Her vital signs are as follows: temperature, 99.3°F; heart rate, 132 beats/minute; respiratory rate, 20 breaths/minute; blood pressure, 110/64 mm Hg; and pulse oximetry, 93% on room air. Physical examination reveals decreased breath sounds on the right side, sharp chest pain with inspiration, and soreness in her right calf. Ms. French has taken oral contraceptives daily for 6 years but takes no other medications. She smokes 1 pack of cigarettes per day. There is no significant family history for heart disease. An electrocardiogram (ECG) shows sinus tachycardia. Chest x-ray is not significant. A computed tomography (CT) scan reveals a small thrombus in the right main pulmonary artery. Arterial blood gases (ABGs) at time of presentation are as follows: pH, 7.47; $PaCO_2$, 31 mm Hg; PaO_2, 86 mm Hg; SaO_2, 93%; and HCO_3^-, 24 mEq/L. These values indicate she is in respiratory alkalosis. Serum levels are within normal limits, except D-dimer, 0.7 mg/L (normal: <0.5 mg/L) and troponin I, 0.2 ng/mL (normal: 0.0 to 0.4 ng/mL). Ms. French is diagnosed with a pulmonary embolism, and immediate treatment with heparin is instituted.

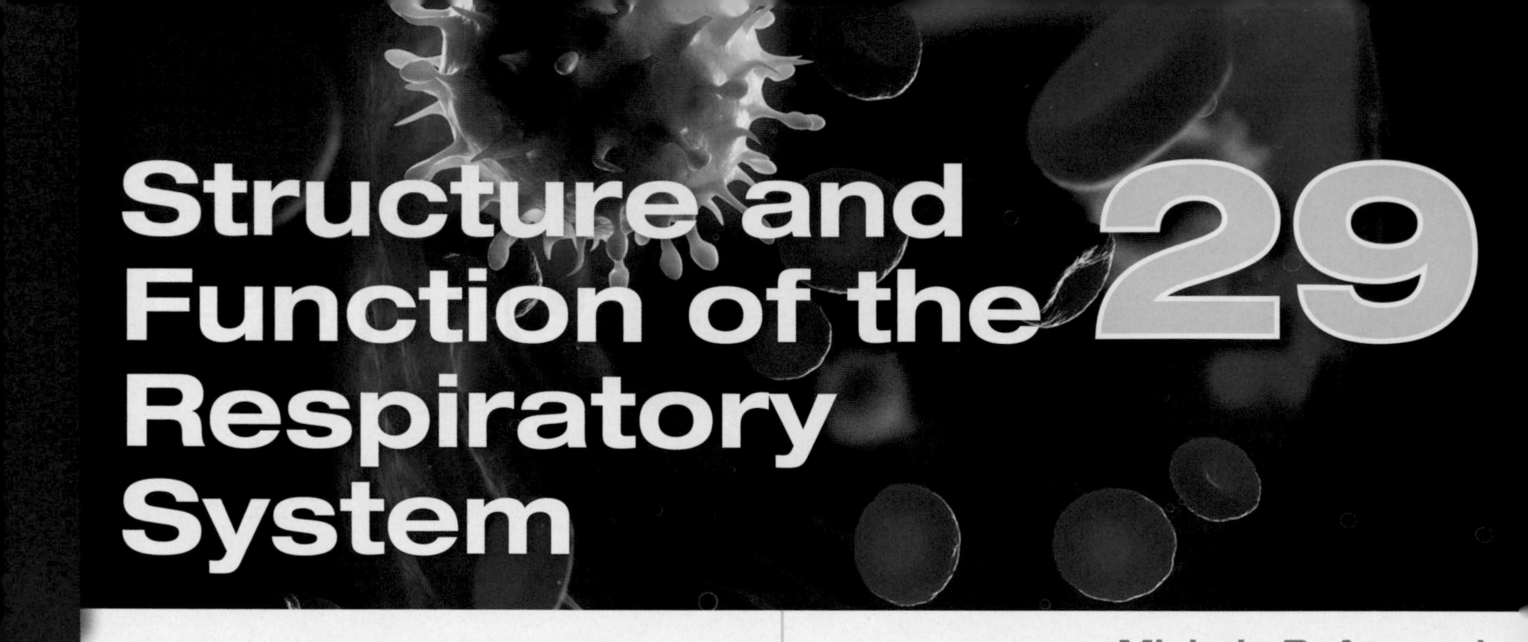

Structure and Function of the Respiratory System 29

Michele R. Arwood

CHAPTER OUTLINE

The primary function of the respiratory system, which consists of the airways and lungs, is gas exchange. Oxygen from the air is transferred to the blood, and carbon dioxide from the blood is eliminated into the atmosphere. In addition to gas exchange, the lungs serve as a host defense by providing a barrier between the external environment and the inside of the body. Finally, the lung is also a metabolic organ that synthesizes and metabolizes different compounds.

This chapter focuses on the structural organization of the respiratory system, exchange of gases between the atmosphere and the lungs, exchange of gases in the lungs and its transport in the blood, and control of breathing.

STRUCTURAL ORGANIZATION OF THE RESPIRATORY SYSTEM

After completing this section of the chapter, the learner will be able to meet the following objectives:

- State the difference between the conducting and the respiratory airways.

- Trace the movement of air through the airways, beginning in the nose and oropharynx and moving into the respiratory tissues of the lung.
- Differentiate the function of the bronchial and pulmonary circulations that supply the lungs.

The respiratory system consists of the air passages (two lungs) and the blood vessels that supply them. It also consists of the structures that provide a ventilator mechanism, that is, the rib cage and the respiratory muscles, which include the diaphragm—the principal respiratory muscle.

The lungs are soft, spongy, cone-shaped organs located side by side in the chest cavity (Fig. 29.1). They are separated from each other by the *mediastinum* (*i.e.*, the space between the lungs) and its contents—the heart, blood vessels, lymph nodes, nerve fibers, thymus gland, and esophagus. The upper part of the lung, which lies against the top of the thoracic cavity, is called the *apex*, and the lower part, which lies against the diaphragm, is called the *base*. The lungs are divided into lobes, three in the right lung and two in the left.

Functionally, the respiratory system can be divided into two parts: the *conducting airways*, through which air moves as it passes between the atmosphere and the lungs, and the *respiratory tissues* of the lungs, where gas exchange takes place.

KEY POINTS

CONDUCTING AND RESPIRATORY AIRWAYS

- Respiration requires ventilation, or movement of gases into and out of the lungs; perfusion, or movement of blood through the lungs; and diffusion of gases between the lungs and the blood.
- Ventilation depends on the conducting airways, including the nasopharynx and oropharynx, larynx, and tracheobronchial tree, which move air into and out of the lungs but do not participate in gas exchange.
- Gas exchange takes place in the respiratory airways of the lungs, where gases diffuse across the alveolar–capillary membrane as they are exchanged between the air in the lungs and the blood that flows through the pulmonary capillaries.

Conducting Airways

The conducting airways consist of the nasal passages, mouth and pharynx, larynx, trachea, bronchi, and bronchioles (see Fig. 29.1). Besides functioning as a conduit for airflow, the

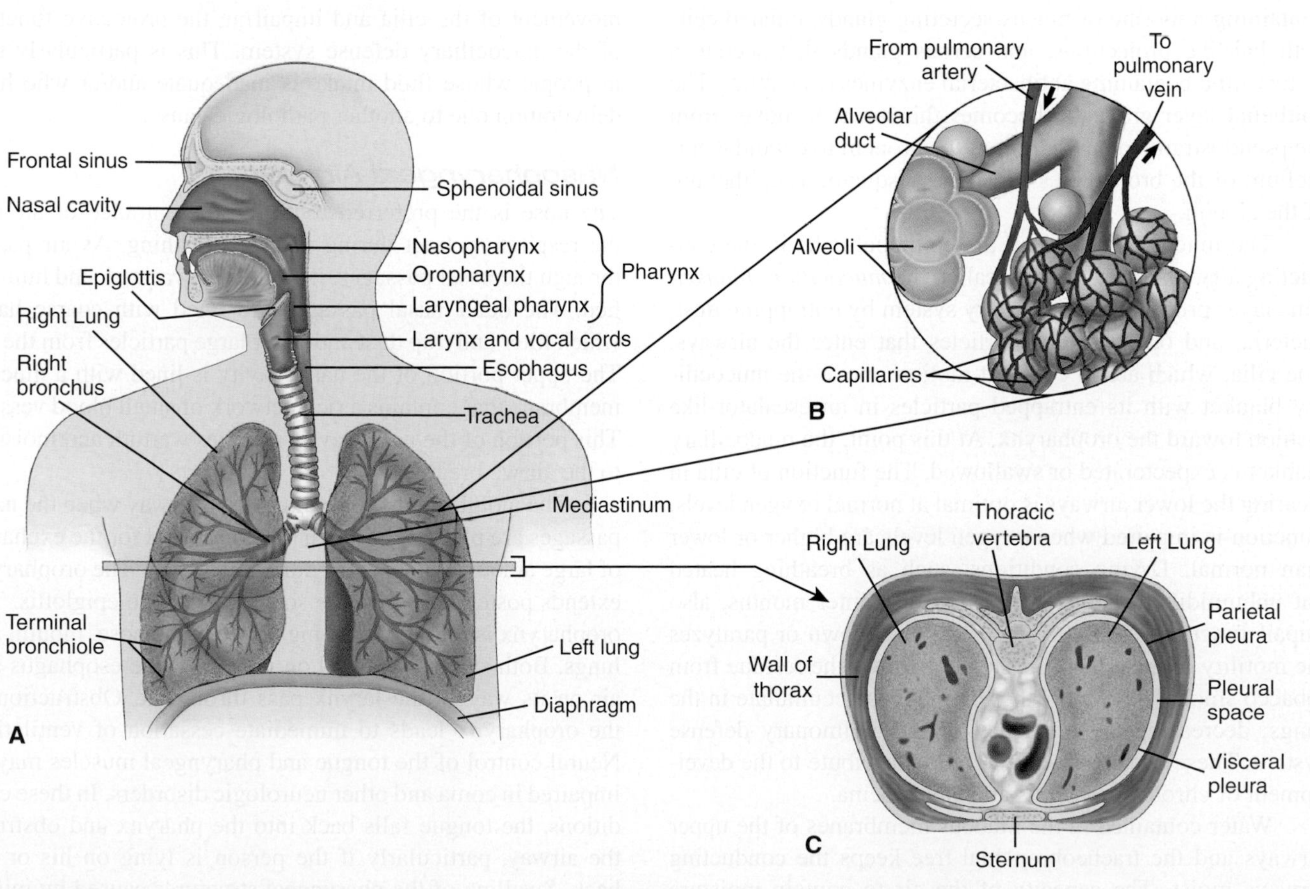

Figure 29.1 • The respiratory system. **(A)** Upper respiratory structures and the structures of the thorax. **(B)** Alveoli. **(C)** A horizontal cross-section of the lungs. (From Hinkle J. L., Cheever K. H. (2018). *Brunner & Suddarth's textbook of medical-surgical nursing* (14th ed., Figure 20-3, p. 482). Philadelphia, PA: Wolters Kluwer.)

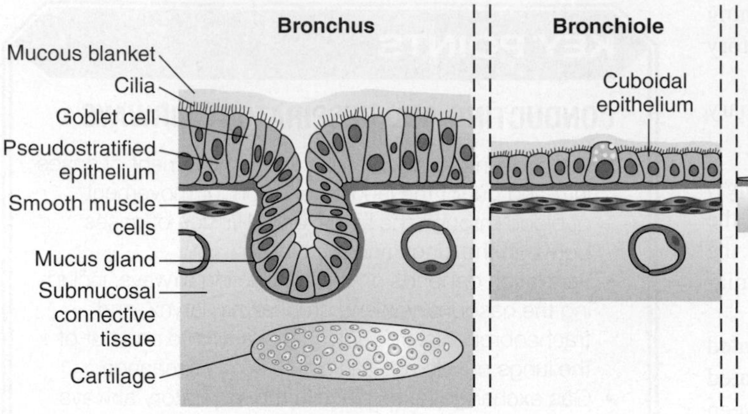

Figure 29.2 • Airway wall structure: bronchus, bronchiole, and alveolus. The bronchial wall contains pseudostratified epithelium, smooth muscle cells, mucus glands, connective tissue, and cartilage. In smaller bronchioles, a simple epithelium is found, cartilage is absent, and the wall is thinner. The alveolar wall is designed for gas exchange, rather than structural support. (From Porth C. M. (2015). *Essentials of pathophysiology* (4th ed., Fig. 21-6, p. 517). Philadelphia, PA: Lippincott Williams & Wilkins.)

conducting airways serve to "condition" the inspired air. The air we breathe is warmed, filtered, and moistened as it moves through these structures. Heat is transferred to the air from the blood flowing through the walls of the respiratory passages. The mucociliary blanket removes foreign materials, and water from the mucous membranes is used to moisten the air.

A combination of cartilage, elastic and collagen fibers, and smooth muscle provides the airways with the rigidity and flexibility needed to maintain airway patency and ensure an uninterrupted supply of air. Most of the conducting airways are lined with ciliated pseudostratified columnar epithelium, containing a mosaic of mucus-secreting glands, ciliated cells with hairlike projections, and serous glands that secrete a watery fluid containing antibacterial enzymes (Fig. 29.2). The epithelial layer gradually becomes thinner as it moves from the pseudostratified epithelium of the bronchi to cuboidal epithelium of the bronchioles and then to squamous epithelium of the alveoli.

The mucus produced by the epithelial cells in the conducting airways forms a layer, called the *mucociliary blanket*. This layer protects the respiratory system by entrapping dust, bacteria, and other foreign particles that enter the airways. The cilia, which are in constant motion, move the mucociliary blanket with its entrapped particles in an escalator-like fashion toward the oropharynx. At this point, the mucociliary blanket is expectorated or swallowed. The function of cilia in clearing the lower airways is optimal at normal oxygen levels. Function is impaired when oxygen levels are higher or lower than normal. Drying conditions, such as breathing heated but unhumidified indoor air during the winter months, also impair function. Cigarette smoking slows down or paralyzes the motility of the cilia. This slowing allows the residue from tobacco smoke, dust, and other particles to accumulate in the lungs, decreasing the efficiency of this pulmonary defense system. These changes are thought to contribute to the development of chronic bronchitis and emphysema.

Water contained in the mucous membranes of the upper airways and the tracheobronchial tree keeps the conducting airways moist. The capacity of the air to contain moisture without condensation increases as the temperature rises. Thus, the air in the alveoli, which is maintained at body temperature, usually contains considerably more moisture than does the atmosphere-temperature air that we breathe. The difference between the moisture contained in the air we breathe and that found in the alveoli is drawn from the moist surface of the mucous membranes that line the conducting airways. This is a source of insensible water loss. When a person has a fever, the water vapor in the lungs increases, causing more water to be lost from the respiratory mucosa. Also, fever usually is accompanied by an increase in respiratory rate so that more air needing to be moisturized passes through the airways. As a result, respiratory secretions thicken, preventing free movement of the cilia and impairing the protective function of the mucociliary defense system. This is particularly true in people whose fluid intake is inadequate and/or who have dehydration due to another pathologic cause.

Nasopharyngeal Airways

The nose is the preferred route for the entrance of air into the respiratory tract during normal breathing. As air passes through the nasal passages, it is filtered, warmed, and humidified. The outer nasal passages are lined with coarse hairs, which filter and trap dust and other large particles from the air. The upper portion of the nasal cavity is lined with a mucous membrane that contains a rich network of small blood vessels. This portion of the nasal cavity supplies warmth and moisture to the air we breathe.

The mouth serves as an alternative airway when the nasal passages are plugged or when there is a need for the exchange of large amounts of air (*e.g.*, during exercise). The oropharynx extends posteriorly from the soft palate to the epiglottis. The oropharynx is the only opening between the nose, mouth, and lungs. Both swallowed food on its way to the esophagus and air on its way to the larynx pass through it. Obstruction of the oropharynx leads to immediate cessation of ventilation. Neural control of the tongue and pharyngeal muscles may be impaired in coma and other neurologic disorders. In these conditions, the tongue falls back into the pharynx and obstructs the airway, particularly if the person is lying on his or her back. Swelling of the pharyngeal structures caused by injury, infection, or severe allergic reaction or the presence of a foreign body also predisposes a person to airway obstruction.

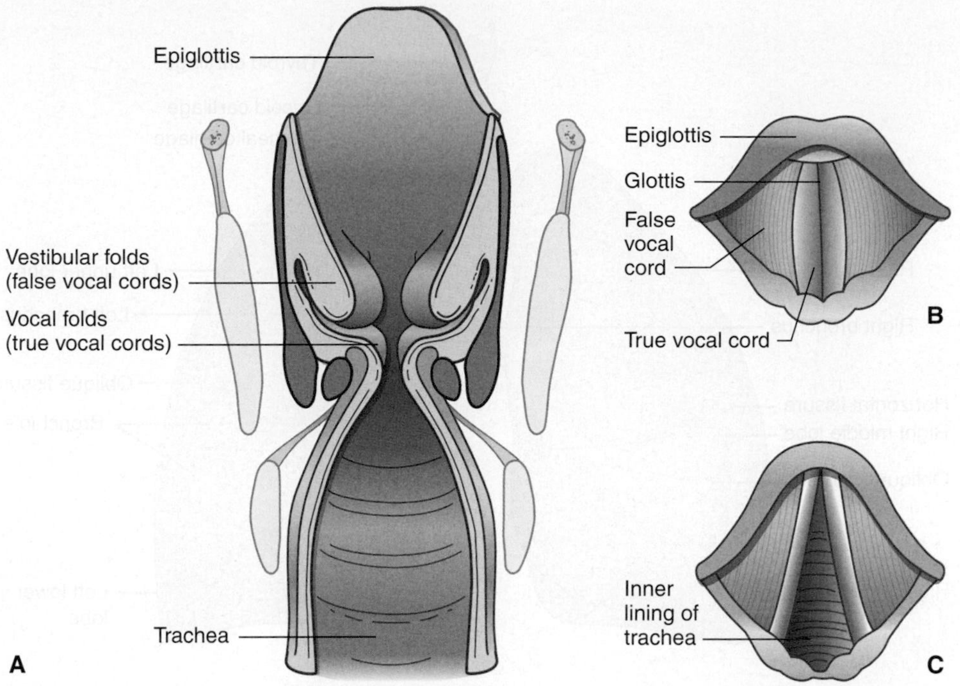

Figure 29.3 • **(A)** Coronal section showing the position of the epiglottis, the vestibular folds (true vocal cords), vocal folds (false vocal cords), and glottis. **(B)** Vocal cords viewed from above with glottis closed and **(C)** with glottis open.

Larynx

The larynx connects the oropharynx with the trachea. It is located between the upper airways and the lungs. The walls of the larynx are supported by firm cartilaginous structures that prevent collapse during inspiration. The functions of the larynx can be divided into two categories: those associated with speech and those associated with protecting the lungs from substances other than air.

The cavity of the larynx is divided into two pairs of shelflike folds stretching from front to back with an opening in the midline (Fig. 29.3). The upper pair of folds, called the *vestibular folds*, has a protective function. The lower pair of folds, called the *vocal folds*, produces the vibrations required for making vocal sounds. The vocal folds and the elongated opening between them are called the *glottis*. A complex set of muscles controls the opening and closing of the glottis. The *epiglottis*, which is located above the larynx, is a large, leaf-shaped piece of cartilage that is covered with epithelium. When only air is flowing through the larynx, the inlet of the larynx is open and the free edges of the epiglottis point upward. During swallowing, the larynx is pulled superiorly and the free edges of the epiglottis move downward to cover the larynx, thus routing liquids and foods into the esophagus.

In addition to opening and closing the glottis for speech, the vocal folds of the larynx can perform a sphincter function, closing off the airways. When confronted with substances other than air, the laryngeal muscles contract and close off the airway. At the same time, the cough reflex is initiated as a means of removing a foreign substance from the airway. If the swallowing mechanism is partially or totally paralyzed, food and fluids can enter the airways instead of the esophagus when a person attempts to swallow. These substances are not easily removed. When they are pulled into the lungs, they can cause a serious inflammatory condition called *aspiration pneumonia*.

Tracheobronchial Tree

The tracheobronchial tree, which consists of the trachea, bronchi, and bronchioles, can be viewed as a system of branching tubes flowing through the lobes of the lungs. There are approximately 23 levels of branching, beginning with the conducting airways and ending with the respiratory airways, where gas exchange takes place (see Fig. 29.4).

The trachea, or windpipe, is a continuous tube that connects the larynx and the major bronchi of the lungs. The walls of the trachea are supported by horseshoe- or C-shaped rings of hyaline cartilage, which prevent it from collapsing when the pressure in the thorax becomes negative (Fig. 29.5). The open part of the C ring, which abuts the esophagus, is connected by smooth muscle. Because this portion of the trachea is not rigid, the esophagus can expand anteriorly as swallowed food passes through it.

The trachea extends to the superior border of the fifth thoracic vertebra, where it divides to form the right and left main or primary bronchi. Between the main bronchi is a keellike ridge, called the *carina* (Fig. 29.6). The mucosa of the carina is highly sensitive. For example, violent coughing is initiated when a foreign object (*e.g.*, whole grape or large piece of hot dog or even the tip of the suction catheter) makes contact with it. The structure of the primary bronchi is similar to the trachea in that these airways are lined with a mucosal surface and supported by cartilaginous rings. Each primary bronchus, accompanied by the pulmonary arteries, veins, and lymph vessels, enters the lung through a slit called the *hilum*.

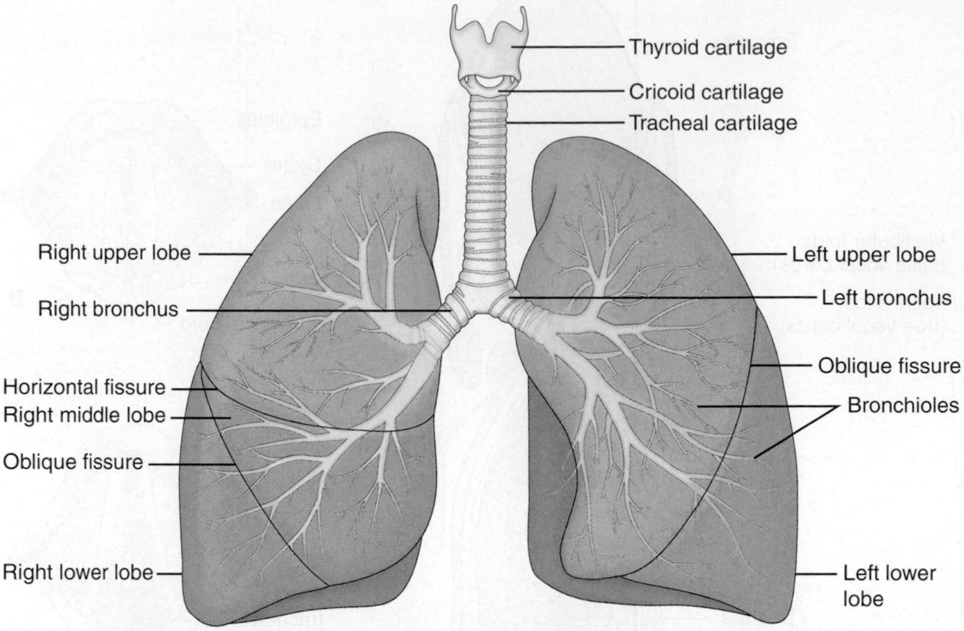

Figure 29.4 • Anterior view of the lungs. The lungs consist of five lobes. The right lung has three lobes (upper, middle, and lower); the left has two lobes (upper and lower). The lobes are further subdivided into fissures. The bronchial tree, another lung structure, inflates with air to fill the lobes. (From Hinkle J. L., Cheever K. H. (2018). *Brunner & Suddarth's textbook of medical-surgical nursing* (14th ed., Figure 20-4, p. 483). Philadelphia, PA: Wolters Kluwer.)

On entering the lungs, each primary bronchus divides into secondary or lobular bronchi that supply each of the lobes of the lung—three in the right lung and two in the left (see Fig. 29.6). The right middle lobe bronchus is of relatively small diameter and length and sometimes bends sharply near its bifurcation. It is surrounded by a collar of lymph nodes that drain the middle and the lower lobe and is particularly subject to obstruction. The secondary bronchi, in turn, divide to form the segmental bronchi, which supply the bronchopulmonary segments of the lung. The trachea is the zero generation, the two mainstem bronchi are the first generation, and as the airways get smaller and smaller, their generation number is identified (Fig. 29.7).

There are 10 segments on the right lung and 9 on the left. These segments are identified according to their location in the lung (*e.g.*, the apical segment of the right upper lobe) and are the smallest named units in the lung. Lung disorders such as atelectasis and pneumonia often are localized to a particular bronchopulmonary segment. The structure of the secondary and segmental bronchi is similar, for the most part, to that of the primary bronchi. However, irregular plates of hyaline cartilage that completely surround the lumina of the bronchi replace the C-shaped cartilage rings. In addition, there are two layers of smooth muscle spiraling in opposite directions (Fig. 29.8).

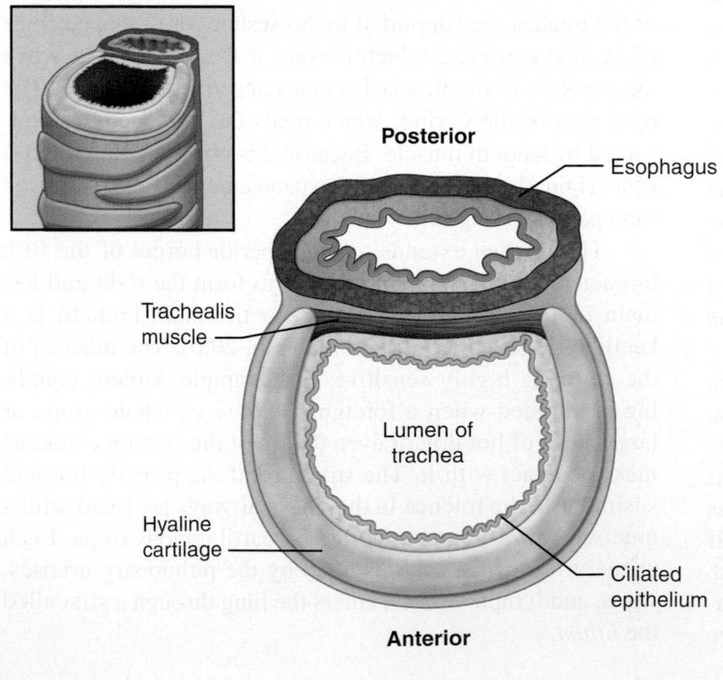

Figure 29.5 • Cross-section of the trachea, illustrating its relationship to the esophagus, the position of the supporting hyaline cartilage rings in its wall, and the trachealis muscle connecting the free ends of the cartilage rings.

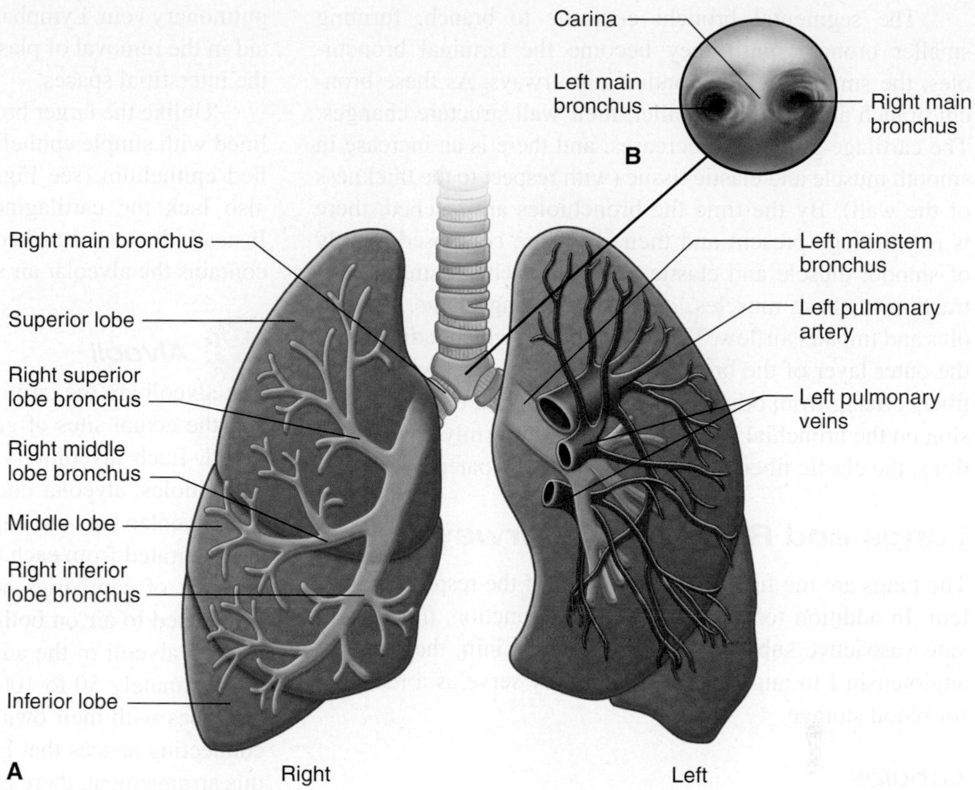

Figure 29.6 • **(A)** Anterior view of respiratory structures, including the lobes of the lung, the larynx, trachea, and the main bronchi on the left and the main pulmonary artery and vein on the right. **(B)** The carina is located at the bifurcation of the right and left mainstem bronchi.

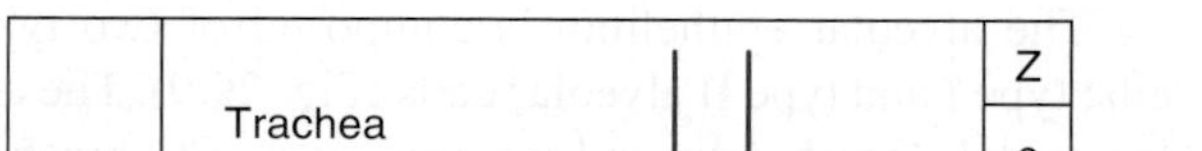

Figure 29.7 • Idealization of the human airways according to Weibel. Note that the first 16 generations (Z) make up the conducting airways, and the last 7 make up the respiratory zone (or the transitional and respiratory zones). (From West J. B. (2016). *Respiratory physiology: The essentials* (10th ed., Figure 1.4, p. 6). Philadelphia, PA: Lippincott Williams & Wilkins.)

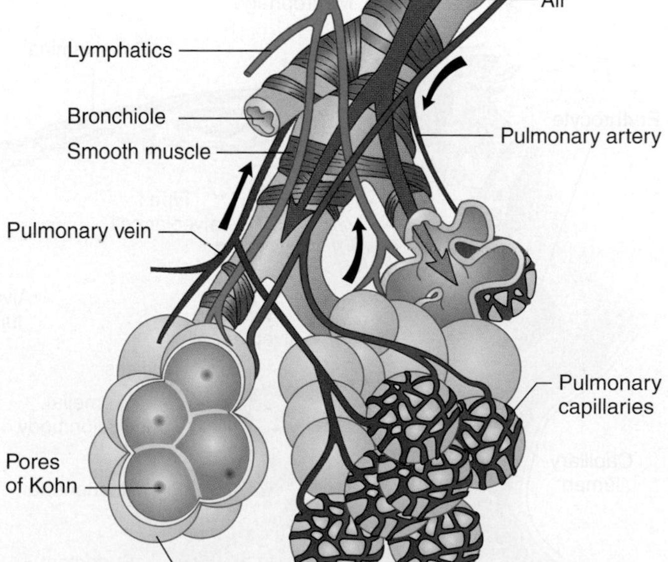

Figure 29.8 • Lobule of the lung, showing the bronchial smooth muscle fibers, pulmonary blood vessels, and lymphatics.

The segmental bronchi continue to branch, forming smaller bronchi, until they become the terminal bronchioles, the smallest of the conducting airways. As these bronchi branch and become smaller, their wall structure changes. The cartilage gradually decreases, and there is an increase in smooth muscle and elastic tissue (with respect to the thickness of the wall). By the time the bronchioles are reached, there is no cartilage present and their walls are composed mainly of smooth muscle and elastic fibers. Bronchospasm, or contraction of these muscles, causes narrowing of the bronchioles and impairs airflow. The elastic fibers, which radiate from the outer layer of the bronchial wall and connect with elastic fibers arising from other parts of the bronchial tree, exert tension on the bronchial walls. By pulling uniformly in all directions, the elastic fibers help maintain airway patency.

Lungs and Respiratory Airways

The lungs are the functional structures of the respiratory system. In addition to their gas exchange function, they inactivate vasoactive substances such as bradykinin, they convert angiotensin I to angiotensin II, and they serve as a reservoir for blood storage.

Lobules

The gas exchange function of the lung takes place in the lobules of the lungs, which are the smallest functional units of the lungs. A branch of a terminal bronchiole, an arteriole, the pulmonary capillaries, and a venule supply each lobule (see Fig. 29.8).

Gas exchange takes place in the terminal respiratory bronchioles and the alveolar ducts and sacs. Blood enters the lobules through a pulmonary artery and exits through a pulmonary vein. Lymphatic structures surround the lobule and aid in the removal of plasma proteins and other particles from the interstitial spaces.

Unlike the larger bronchi, the respiratory bronchioles are lined with simple epithelium rather than ciliated pseudostratified epithelium (see Fig. 29.2). The respiratory bronchioles also lack the cartilaginous support of the larger airways. Instead, they are attached to the elastic spongelike tissue that contains the alveolar air spaces.

Alveoli

The alveoli are the terminal air spaces of the respiratory tract and the actual sites of gas exchange between the air and the blood. Each alveolus is a small outpouching of respiratory bronchioles, alveolar ducts, and alveolar sacs (see Fig. 29.8). The alveolar sacs are cup-shaped, thin-walled structures that are separated from each other by thin alveolar septa. A single network of capillaries occupies most of the septa, so blood is exposed to air on both sides. There are approximately 300 million alveoli in the adult lung, with a total surface area of approximately 50 to 100 m^2.[1] Unlike the bronchioles, which are tubes with their own separate walls, the alveoli are interconnecting spaces that have no separate walls. As a result of this arrangement, there is a continual mixing of air in the alveolar structures. Small holes in the alveolar walls, the pores of Kohn, also contribute to the mixing of air.

The alveolar epithelium is composed of two types of cells: type I and type II alveolar cells (Fig. 29.9). The alveoli also contain brush cells and macrophages. The brush cells, which are few in number, are thought to act as receptors that monitor the air quality of the lungs. The macrophages, which

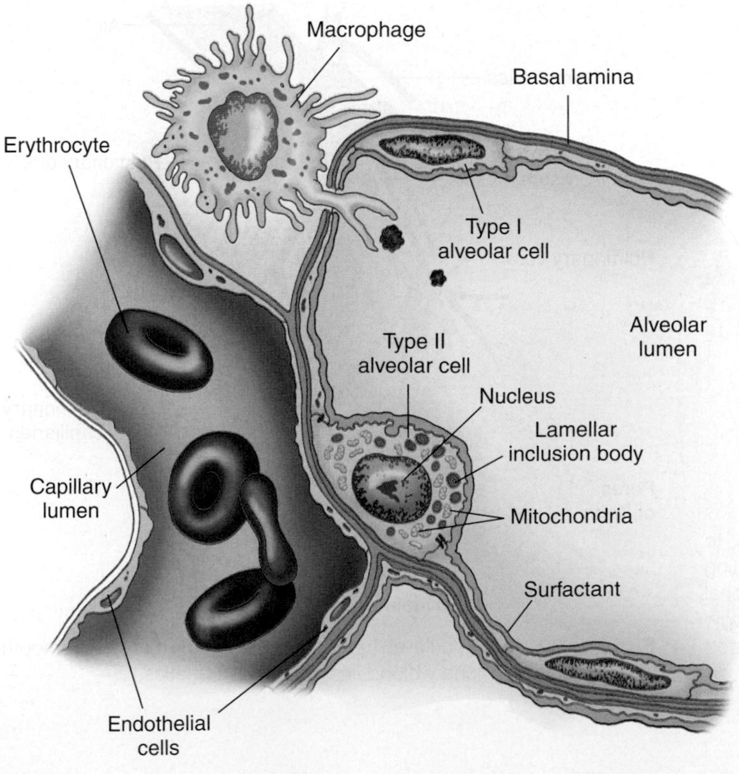

Figure 29.9 • Schematic illustration of type I and type II alveolar cells and their relationship to the alveoli and pulmonary capillaries. Type I alveolar cells constitute most of the alveolar surface. Type II alveolar cells, which produce surfactant, are located at the corners between adjacent alveoli. Also shown are the endothelial cells, which line the pulmonary capillaries, and an alveolar macrophage.

are present in both the alveolar lumen and the septum of the alveoli, function to remove offending material from the lung.

Type I Alveolar Cells. The type I alveolar cells, also known as *type I pneumocytes*, are extremely thin squamous cells with a thin cytoplasm and flattened nucleus that occupy about 95% of the surface area of the alveoli. They are joined to one another and to other cells by occluding junctions. These junctions form an effective barrier between the air and the components of the alveolar wall. Type I alveolar cells are not capable of cell division.

Type II Alveolar Cells. The type II alveolar cells, also called *type II pneumocytes*, are small cuboidal cells located at the corners of the alveoli. Type II cells are as numerous as type I cells, but because of their different shape, they cover only about 5% of the alveolar surface area. The type II cells synthesize pulmonary surfactant, a substance that decreases the surface tension in the alveoli and allows for greater ease of lung inflation. They are also the progenitor cells for type I cells. After lung injury, they proliferate and restore both type I and type II alveolar cells.

Pulmonary surfactant is a complex mixture of phospholipids, neutral lipids, and proteins that is synthesized in the type II alveolar cells. Type II alveolar cells are rich in mitochondria and are metabolically active. Their apical cytoplasm contains stacks of parallel membrane sheets or lamellae, called the lamellar bodies. All of the components of surfactant are synthesized by the alveolar type II cells and stored as preformed units in the lamellar bodies. Secretion of surfactant occurs by exocytosis. The major route of clearance of surfactant within the lung is through reuptake by the type II cells. After reuptake, the phospholipids are either recycled or degraded and reused in the synthesis of new phospholipids.

The surfactant molecules produced by the type II alveolar cells reduce the surface tension at the air–epithelium interface and modulate the immune functions of the lung. There are four types of surfactant, each with a different molecular structure: surfactant apoproteins A (SP-A), B (SP-B), C (SP-C), and D (SP-D). SP-B and SP-C reduce the surface tension at the air–epithelium interface and increase lung compliance and ease of lung inflation. SP-B is particularly important to the generation of the surface-reducing film that makes lung expansion possible. For example, SP-B–deficiency disorders are often a result of single-gene disorders that cause acute and chronic respiratory dysfunction. SP-C is necessary for decreasing surface tension and stopping end-expiratory alveolar collapse.[2] SP-A and SP-D do not reduce surface tension but contribute to host defenses that protect against pathogens that have entered the lung. They are members of the collectin protein family that function as a part of the innate immune system. Collectively, they opsonize pathogens, including bacteria and viruses, to facilitate phagocytosis by macrophages. They also regulate the production of inflammatory mediators. SP-A and SP-D are directly bactericidal, meaning they can kill bacteria in the absence of immune system effector cells. SP-D can be used to predict problems with acute lung injury (ALI) and acute respiratory distress syndrome (ARDS). Both of these conditions can best be predicted by using a combination of biomarkers (SP-D, neutrophil chemotactic factor, and interleukin-8) and clinical predictors (Acute Physiology and Chronic Health Evaluation III [APACHE III]). Therefore, it is most significant to measure SP-D in people experiencing chest trauma.[3]

Alveolar Macrophages. The macrophages are present in both the connective tissue of the septum and in the air spaces of the alveolus. They are responsible for the removal of offending substances from the alveoli. In the air spaces, they scavenge the surface to remove inhaled particulate matter, such as dust and pollen. Some macrophages pass up the bronchial tree in the mucus and are disposed of by swallowing or coughing when they reach the pharynx. Others enter the septal connective tissue, where, filled with phagocytosed materials, they remain for life. Thus, at autopsy, urban dwellers, as well as smokers, usually show many alveolar macrophages filled with carbon and other polluting particles from the environment. The alveolar macrophages also phagocytose insoluble infectious agents such as *Mycobacterium tuberculosis*. The activated macrophages then aggregate to form a fibrin-encapsulated granuloma, called a *tubercle*, to contain the infection. The tubercle bacillus can remain dormant in this stage or be reactivated years later, when the person's immunologic tolerance wanes as the result of old age or immunosuppressive disease or therapy.

Pulmonary Vasculature and Lymphatic Supply

Pulmonary and Bronchial Circulations

The lungs are provided with a dual blood supply, the pulmonary and bronchial circulations. The pulmonary circulation arises from the pulmonary artery and provides for the gas exchange function of the lungs (see Fig. 29.8). Deoxygenated blood leaves the right heart through the pulmonary artery. The pulmonary artery divides into a left pulmonary artery that enters the left lung and a right pulmonary artery that enters the right lung. Return of oxygenated blood to the heart occurs by way of the pulmonary veins, which empty into the left atrium. This is the only part of the circulation where arteries carry deoxygenated blood and veins carry oxygenated blood.

The bronchial circulation distributes blood to the conducting airways and the supporting structures of the lung. The bronchial circulation also has a secondary function of warming and humidifying incoming air as it moves through the conducting airways. The bronchial arteries arise from the thoracic aorta and enter the lungs with the major bronchi. They divide and subdivide along with the bronchi as they move out into the lung, supplying them and other lung structures with oxygen. The blood from the capillaries in the bronchial circulation drains into the bronchial veins, with the blood from the larger bronchial veins emptying into the vena cava. Blood from the smaller bronchial veins empties into the pulmonary veins. Because the bronchial circulation does not participate in gas exchange, this blood is deoxygenated. As a result, it dilutes the oxygenated blood returning to the left side of the heart through the pulmonary veins.

The bronchial blood vessels are the only ones that can undergo angiogenesis (formation of new vessels) and develop collateral circulation when vessels in the pulmonary circulation are obstructed, as in pulmonary embolism. The development of new blood vessels helps to keep lung tissue alive until the pulmonary circulation can be restored.

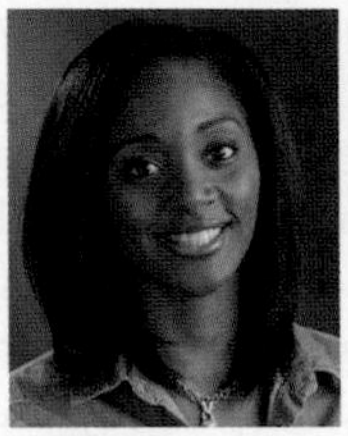

Remember Ms. French, the person with pulmonary embolism you met at the beginning of the unit? In pulmonary embolism, an area of the pulmonary vasculature becomes obstructed by an embolus, impairing blood flow to the alveoli and interfering with gas exchange.

Lymphatic Circulation

The lungs are also supplied with lymphatic drainage that parallels their dual blood supply. One set of lymph vessels, the superficial vessels, drains the surface of the lung and travels in the connective tissue of the visceral pleura. A second set of the vessels, the deep lymphatic vessels, follows the pulmonary arteries, pulmonary veins, and bronchial tree down to the level of the respiratory bronchioles (see Fig. 29.8). Both of these systems have numerous interconnections, and both form networks that drain into the hilar lymph nodes at the base of each lung. Particulate matter entering the lung is partly removed through these channels, as are the plasma proteins that have escaped from the pulmonary capillaries. The latter function is particularly important in keeping the lungs dry and in preventing the accumulation of fluid in the pleural cavity.

Innervation

The sympathetic and parasympathetic divisions of the autonomic nervous system innervate the lung. It is parasympathetic stimulation, through the vagus nerve, that is responsible for the slightly constricted smooth muscle tone in the normal resting lung. There is no voluntary motor innervation of the lung, nor are there pain fibers. Pain fibers are found only in the pleura.

Stimulation of the parasympathetic nervous system leads to airway constriction and increased glandular secretion. Parasympathetic innervation of the lung arises from the vagal nuclei in the medulla. Preganglionic fibers from the vagal nuclei descend in the vagus nerve to ganglia adjacent to the airways and blood vessels of the lung. Postganglionic fibers from the ganglia then complete the network that innervates smooth muscle, blood vessels, and epithelial cells, including the goblet and submucosal glands. Both the preganglionic and postganglionic fibers contain excitatory (cholinergic) motor neurons that respond to acetylcholine. Parasympathetic innervation is greater in the large airways and diminishes toward the smaller airways.

Stimulation of the sympathetic nervous system causes airway relaxation, blood vessel constriction, and inhibition of glandular secretion. Sympathetic innervation arises from the cell bodies in paravertebral sympathetic ganglia. Neurotransmitters of the sympathetic nervous system include the catecholamines norepinephrine and epinephrine.

Pleura

A thin, transparent, double-layered serous membrane, called the *pleura*, lines the thoracic cavity and encases the lungs (see Fig. 29.10). The outer parietal layer lines the pulmonary cavities and adheres to the thoracic wall, the mediastinum, and the diaphragm. The inner visceral pleura closely covers the lung and is adherent to all its surfaces. It is continuous with the parietal pleura at the hilum of the lung, where the major bronchus and pulmonary vessels enter and leave the lung. A thin film of serous fluid separates the two pleural layers, allowing the two layers to glide over each other and yet hold together. In this way, there is no separation between the lungs and the chest wall, which would potentially allow for infectious processes to build up and negatively impact chest wall expansion. The pleural cavity is a potential space in which serous fluid or inflammatory exudate can accumulate. The term *pleural effusion* is used to describe an abnormal collection of fluid or exudate in the pleural cavity.

IN SUMMARY

The respiratory system consists of the air passages and the lungs, where gas exchange takes place. Functionally, the air passages of the respiratory system can be divided into two parts: the conducting airways, through which air moves as it passes into and out of the lungs, and the respiratory tissues, where gas exchange actually takes place. The conducting airways include the nasal passages, mouth and nasopharynx, larynx, and tracheobronchial tree. Air is warmed, filtered, and humidified as it passes through these structures.

The lungs are the functional structures of the respiratory system. In addition to their gas exchange function, they inactivate vasoactive substances such as bradykinin; they convert angiotensin I to angiotensin II; and they serve as a reservoir for blood. The lobules, which are the functional units of the lung, consist of the respiratory bronchioles, alveoli, and pulmonary capillaries. It is here that gas exchange takes place. Oxygen from the alveoli diffuses across the alveolar–capillary membrane into the blood, and carbon dioxide from the blood diffuses into the alveoli. There are two types of alveolar cells: type I and type II. Type I cells, which provide the gas exchange function of the lung, are extremely thin squamous cells lining most of the surface of the alveoli. Type II cells, which produce surfactant and serve as progenitor cells for type I cells, are small cuboidal cells. There are four types of pulmonary surfactant protein (SP): SP-A, SP-B, SP-C, and SP-D. SP-B and SP-C provide the critical surface tension–lowering properties necessary for ease of lung inflation. SP-A

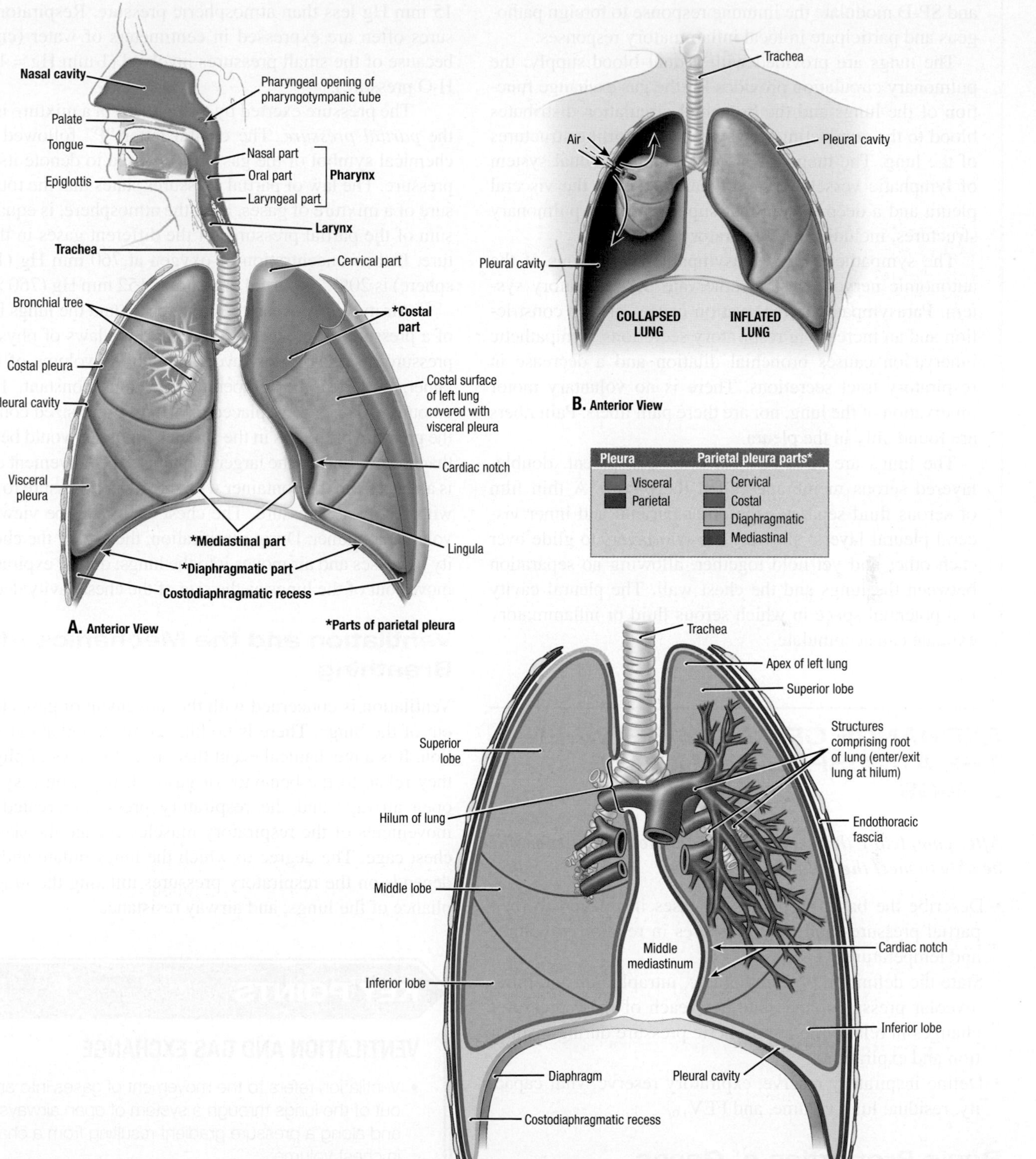

Figure 29.10 • Respiratory system and pleura. **(A)** Overview. **(B)** Pleural cavity and pleura. **(C)** Diagrammatic section through heart and lungs with pulmonary vessels and tracheobronchial tree. The lungs invaginate a continuous membranous pleural sac; the visceral (pulmonary) pleura covers the lungs, and the parietal pleura lines the thoracic cavity; the visceral and parietal pleurae are continuous around the root of the lung. The parietal pleura can be divided regionally into the costal, diaphragmatic, mediastinal and cervical parts; note the costodiaphragmatic recess. The pleural cavity is potential space between the visceral and parietal pleurae that contains a thin layer of fluid. If a sufficient amount of air enters the pleural cavity, the surface tension adhering visceral to parietal pleura (lung to thoracic wall) is broken, and the lung collapses (atelectasis) because of its inherent elasticity (elastic recoil). When a lung collapses, the pleural cavity—normally a potential space—becomes a real space **(B)** and may contain air (pneumothorax), blood (hemothorax), etc. (From Agur A. M. R., Dalley, A. F. (2017). *Grant's atlas of anatomy* (14th ed., Figure 3.27, p. 220). Philadelphia, PA: Lippincott Williams & Wilkins.)

and SP-D modulate the immune response to foreign pathogens and participate in local inflammatory responses.

The lungs are provided with a dual blood supply: the pulmonary circulation provides for the gas exchange function of the lungs and the bronchial circulation distributes blood to the conducting airways and supporting structures of the lung. The lungs are also supplied by a dual system of lymphatic vessels: a superficial system in the visceral pleura and a deep system that supplies deeper pulmonary structures, including the respiratory bronchioles.

The sympathetic and parasympathetic divisions of the autonomic nervous system innervate the respiratory system. Parasympathetic innervation causes airway constriction and an increase in respiratory secretions. Sympathetic innervation causes bronchial dilation and a decrease in respiratory tract secretions. There is no voluntary motor innervation of the lung, nor are there pain fibers. Pain fibers are found only in the pleura.

The lungs are encased in a thin, transparent, double-layered serous membrane called the *pleura*. A thin film of serous fluid separates the outer parietal and inner visceral pleural layers, allowing the two layers to glide over each other and yet hold together, allowing no separation between the lungs and the chest wall. The pleural cavity is a potential space in which serous fluid or inflammatory exudate can accumulate.

EXCHANGE OF GASES BETWEEN THE ATMOSPHERE AND THE LUNGS

After completing this section of the chapter, the learner will be able to meet the following objectives:

- Describe the basic properties of gases in relation to their partial pressures and their pressures in relation to volume and temperature.
- State the definition of intrathoracic, intrapleural, and intra-alveolar pressures, and state how each of these pressures changes in relation to atmospheric pressure during inspiration and expiration.
- Define inspiratory reserve, expiratory reserve, vital capacity, residual lung volume, and $FEV_{1.0}$.

Basic Properties of Gases

The air we breathe is made up of a mixture of gases, mainly nitrogen and oxygen. These gases exert a combined pressure called the *atmospheric* or *barometric pressure*. The pressure at sea level, which is defined as 1 atmosphere, is 760 millimeters of mercury (mm Hg, or torr) or 14.7 pounds per square inch (PSI). When measuring respiratory pressures, atmospheric pressure is assigned a value of zero. A respiratory pressure of +15 mm Hg means that the pressure is 15 mm Hg above atmospheric pressure, and a respiratory pressure of −15 mm Hg is 15 mm Hg less than atmospheric pressure. Respiratory pressures often are expressed in centimeters of water (cm H_2O) because of the small pressures involved (1 mm Hg = 1.35 cm H_2O pressure).

The pressure exerted by a single gas in a mixture is called the *partial pressure*. The capital letter "P" followed by the chemical symbol of the gas (PO_2) is used to denote its partial pressure. The law of partial pressures states that the total pressure of a mixture of gases, as in the atmosphere, is equal to the sum of the partial pressures of the different gases in the mixture. If the concentration of oxygen at 760 mm Hg (1 atmosphere) is 20%, its partial pressure is 152 mm Hg (760 × 0.20).

Air moves between the atmosphere and the lungs because of a pressure difference. According to the laws of physics, the pressure of a gas varies inversely with the volume of its container, provided the temperature remains constant. If equal amounts of a gas were placed in two different-sized containers, the pressure of the gas in the smaller container would be greater than the pressure in the larger container. The movement of gases is always from the container with the greater pressure to the one with the lesser pressure. The chest cavity can be viewed as a volume container. During inspiration, the size of the chest cavity increases and air moves into the lungs; during expiration, air moves out of the lungs as the size of the chest cavity decreases.

Ventilation and the Mechanics of Breathing

Ventilation is concerned with the movement of gases into and out of the lungs. There is nothing complicated about ventilation. It is a mechanical event that obeys the laws of physics as they relate to the behavior of gases. It relies on a system of open airways and the respiratory pressures created as the movements of the respiratory muscles change the size of the chest cage. The degree to which the lungs inflate and deflate depends on the respiratory pressures inflating the lung, compliance of the lungs, and airway resistance.

KEY POINTS

VENTILATION AND GAS EXCHANGE

- Ventilation refers to the movement of gases into and out of the lungs through a system of open airways and along a pressure gradient resulting from a change in chest volume.
- During inspiration, air is drawn into the lungs as the respiratory muscles expand the chest cavity; during expiration, air moves out of the lungs as the chest muscles recoil and the chest cavity becomes smaller.
- The ease with which air is moved into and out of the lung depends on the resistance of the airways, which is inversely related to the fourth power of the airway radius, and lung compliance, or the ease with which the lungs can be inflated.

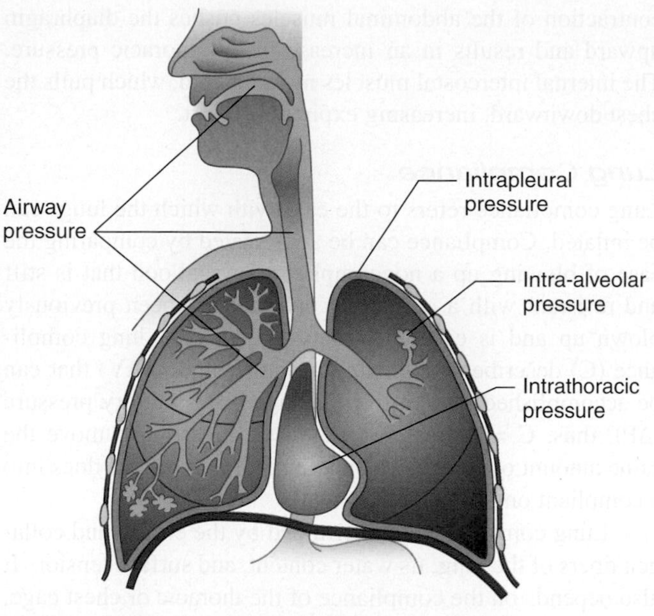

Figure 29.11 • Partitioning of respiratory pressures.

Respiratory Pressures

The pressure inside the airways and alveoli of the lungs is called the *intrapulmonary pressure* or *alveolar pressure*. The gases in this area of the lungs are in communication with atmospheric pressure (Fig. 29.11). When the glottis is open and air is not moving into or out of the lungs, as occurs just before inspiration or expiration, the intrapulmonary pressure is zero or equal to atmospheric pressure.

The pressure in the pleural cavity is called the *intrapleural pressure*. The intrapleural pressure of a normal inflated lung is always negative in relation to alveolar pressure, approximately –4 mm Hg between breaths when the glottis is open and the alveolar spaces are open to the atmosphere. The lungs and the chest wall have elastic properties, each pulling in the opposite direction. If removed from the chest, the lungs would contract to a smaller size, and the chest wall, if freed from the lungs, would expand. The opposing forces of the chest wall and lungs create a pull against the visceral and parietal layers of the pleura, causing the pressure in the pleural cavity to become negative. During inspiration, the elastic recoil of the lungs increases, causing intrapleural pressure to become more negative than during expiration. Without the negative intrapleural pressure holding the lungs against the chest wall, their elastic recoil properties would cause them to collapse. Although intrapleural pressure is negative in relation to alveolar pressure, it may become positive in relation to atmospheric pressure (*e.g.*, during forced expiration and coughing). The *transpulmonary* (*trans* = "across") *pressure* is the difference between the alveolar and intrapleural pressures and is used in determining pulmonary compliance.

The *intrathoracic pressure* is the pressure in the thoracic cavity. It is equal to the intrapleural pressure and is the pressure to which the lungs, heart, and great vessels are exposed. Forced expiration against a closed glottis, such as occurs during defecation and the Valsalva maneuver, produces marked increases in intrathoracic pressure and impedes venous return to the right atrium.

Chest Cage and Respiratory Muscles

The lungs and major airways share the chest cavity with the heart, great vessels, and esophagus. The chest cavity is a closed compartment bounded on the top by the neck muscles and at the bottom by the diaphragm. The outer walls of the chest cavity are formed by 12 pairs of ribs, the sternum, the thoracic vertebrae, and the intercostal muscles that lie between the ribs. Mechanically, the act of breathing depends on the fact that the chest cavity is a closed compartment whose only opening to the external atmosphere is through the trachea.

Ventilation consists of inspiration and expiration. During *inspiration*, the size of the chest cavity increases, the intrathoracic pressure becomes more negative, and air is drawn into the lungs. *Expiration* occurs as the elastic components of the chest wall and lung structures that were stretched during inspiration recoil, causing the size of the chest cavity to decrease and the pressure in the chest cavity to increase.

The diaphragm is the principal muscle of inspiration. When the diaphragm contracts, the abdominal contents are forced downward and the chest expands from top to bottom (Fig. 29.12). During normal levels of inspiration,

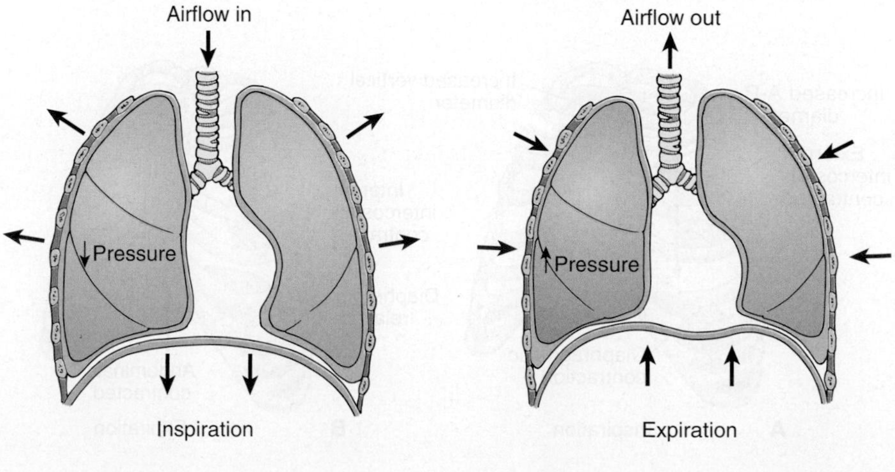

Figure 29.12 • Movement of the diaphragm and changes in chest volume and pressure during inspiration and expiration. During inspiration, contraction of the diaphragm and expansion of the chest cavity produce a decrease in intrathoracic pressure, causing air to move into the lungs. During expiration, relaxation of the diaphragm and chest cavity produces an increase in intrathoracic pressure, causing air to move out of the lungs.

the diaphragm moves approximately 1 cm, but this can be increased to 10 cm on forced inspiration. The diaphragm is innervated by the phrenic nerve roots, which arise from the cervical level of the spinal cord, mainly from C4 but also from C3 and C5. People who sustain spinal cord injury above C3 lose the function of the diaphragm and require mechanical ventilation. Paralysis of one side of the diaphragm causes the chest to move up on that side rather than down during inspiration because of the negative pressure in the chest. This is called *paradoxical movement*.

The external intercostal muscles, which also aid in inspiration, connect to the adjacent ribs and slope downward and forward (Fig. 29.13). When they contract, they raise the ribs and rotate them slightly so that the sternum is pushed forward. This enlarges the chest from side to side and from front to back. The intercostal muscles receive their innervation from nerves that exit the central nervous system at the thoracic level of the spinal cord. Paralysis of these muscles usually does not have a serious effect on respiration because of the effectiveness of the diaphragm.

The accessory muscles of inspiration include the scalene muscles and the sternocleidomastoid muscles. The scalene muscles elevate the first two ribs, and the sternocleidomastoid muscles raise the sternum to increase the size of the chest cavity. These muscles contribute little to quiet breathing but contract vigorously during exercise. For the accessory muscles to assist in ventilation, they must be stabilized in some way. For example, people with bronchial asthma often brace their arms against a firm object during an attack as a means of stabilizing their shoulders so that the attached accessory muscles can exert their full effect on ventilation. The head commonly is bent backward so that the scalene and sternocleidomastoid muscles can elevate the ribs more effectively.

Expiration is largely passive. It occurs as the elastic components of the chest wall and lung structures that were stretched during inspiration recoil, causing air to leave the lungs as the intrathoracic pressure increases. When needed, the abdominal and the internal intercostal muscles can be used to increase expiratory effort (see Fig. 29.13B). The increase in intra-abdominal pressure that accompanies the forceful contraction of the abdominal muscles pushes the diaphragm upward and results in an increase in intrathoracic pressure. The internal intercostal muscles move inward, which pulls the chest downward, increasing expiratory effort.

Lung Compliance

Lung compliance refers to the ease with which the lungs can be inflated. Compliance can be appreciated by comparing the ease of blowing up a noncompliant new balloon that is stiff and resistant with a compliant one that has been previously blown up and is easy to inflate. Specifically, lung compliance (C) describes the change in lung volume (ΔV) that can be accomplished with a given change in respiratory pressure (ΔP); thus, $C = \Delta V/\Delta P$. It takes more pressure to move the same amount of air into a noncompliant lung than it does into a compliant one.

Lung compliance is determined by the elastin and collagen fibers of the lung, its water content, and surface tension. It also depends on the compliance of the thoracic or chest cage. It is diminished by conditions that reduce the natural elasticity of the lung, block the bronchi or smaller airways, increase the surface tension in the alveoli, or impair the flexibility of the thoracic cage.

Elastin and Collagen Fibers. Lung tissue is made up of elastin and collagen fibers. The elastin fibers are easily stretched and increase the ease of lung inflation, whereas the collagen fibers resist stretching and make lung inflation more difficult. In lung diseases such as interstitial lung disease and pulmonary fibrosis, the lungs become stiff and noncompliant as the elastin fibers are replaced with scar tissue. Pulmonary congestion and edema produce a reversible decrease in pulmonary compliance.

Elastic recoil describes the ability of the elastic components of the lung to recoil to their original position after having been stretched. Overstretching lung tissues, as occurs with emphysema, causes the elastic components of the lung to lose their recoil, making the lung easier to inflate but more difficult to deflate because of its inability to recoil.

Surface Tension. An important factor in lung compliance is the *surface tension* or attraction forces of the surface

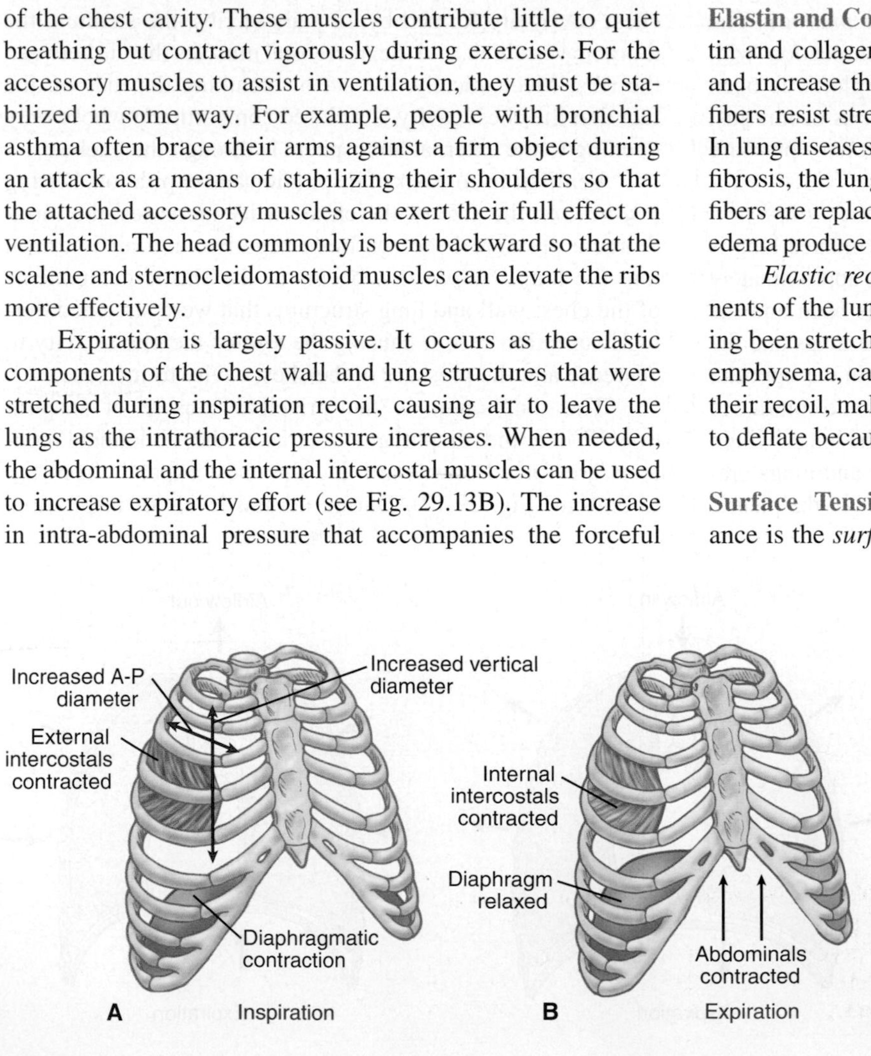

Figure 29.13 • Expansion and contraction of the chest cage during expiration and inspiration, demonstrating especially diaphragmatic contraction, elevation of the rib cage, and function of the (A) external and (B) internal intercostals.

molecules in the alveoli. The alveoli are lined with a thin film of liquid, and it is at the interface between this liquid film and the alveolar air that surface tension develops. This is because the forces that hold the water molecules of the liquid film together are stronger than those that hold the air molecules in the alveoli together. In the alveoli, excess surface tension causes water molecules in the liquid film to contract, making lung inflation difficult.

The units of surface tension are those of force per unit length. The relationship between the pressure within a sphere such as an alveolus and the tension in the wall can be described using the law of Laplace (pressure = 2 × surface tension/radius).[4] If the surface tension were equal throughout the lungs, the alveoli with the smallest radii would have the greatest pressure, and this would cause them to empty into the larger alveoli (Fig. 29.14A). The reason this does not occur is because of surface tension–lowering molecules, called *surfactant*, that line the inner surface of the alveoli.

Pulmonary surfactant is a complex mixture of phospholipids, neutral lipids, and proteins that is synthesized in the type II alveolar cells. Substances that are termed surfactants consist of two parts with opposing properties that are irreversibly bound to each other. One part is polar and seeks aqueous fluid or hydrophilic (water-attracting) surfaces; the other is nonpolar and seeks oil, air, or hydrophobic (water-repelling) surfaces (see Fig. 29.14B). Pulmonary surfactant forms a monolayer, with its hydrophilic surface binding to liquid film on the surface of the alveoli and its hydrophobic surface facing outward toward the gases in the alveolar air. It is this monolayer that interrupts the surface tension that develops at the air–liquid interface in the alveoli.

Pulmonary surfactant protein (SP), particularly SP-B, exerts several important effects on lung inflation. It lowers the surface tension and it increases lung compliance and ease of lung inflation.[2] Without surfactant, lung inflation would be extremely difficult. In addition, it helps to keep the alveoli dry and prevent pulmonary edema. This is because water is pulled out of the pulmonary capillaries into the alveoli when increased surface tension causes the alveoli to contract. Surfactant also provides for stability and more even inflation of the alveoli. Alveoli, except those at the pleural surface, are surrounded by other alveoli. Thus, the tendency of one alveolus to collapse is opposed by the traction exerted by the surrounding alveolus. The surfactant molecules are also more densely packed in small alveoli than in large alveoli (see Fig. 29.14C). In postoperative and bedridden people, shallow and quiet breathing often impairs the spreading of surfactant. Encouraging these people to cough and deep breathe enhances the spreading of surfactant. This allows for a more even distribution of ventilation and prevention of atelectasis.

The type II alveolar cells that produce surfactant do not begin to mature until the 26th to 27th week of gestation; consequently, many premature infants have difficulty producing sufficient amounts of surfactant. This can lead to alveolar collapse and severe respiratory distress. This condition,

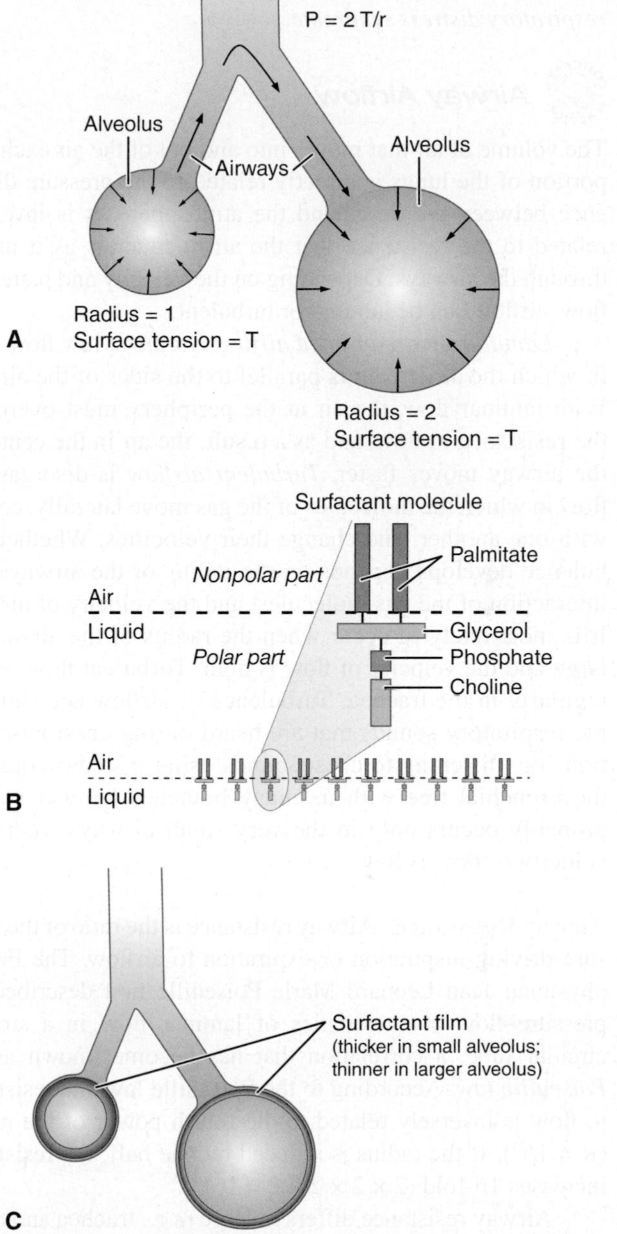

Figure 29.14 • **(A)** The effect of the surface tension (forces generated at the fluid–air interface) and radius on the pressure and movement of gases in the alveolar structures. According to the law of Laplace (P = 2T/r, P = pressure, T = tension, r = radius), the pressure generated within the sphere is inversely proportional to the radius. Air moves from the alveolus with a small radius and higher pressure to the alveolus with the larger radius and lower pressure. **(B)** Surfactant molecules, showing their hydrophilic heads attached to the fluid lining of the alveolus and their hydrophobic tails oriented toward the air interface. **(C)** The surfactant molecules form a monolayer (*shaded in blue*) that disrupts the intermolecular forces and lowers the surface tension more in the smaller alveolus with its higher concentration of surfactant than in the larger alveolus with the lower concentration.

called *infant respiratory distress syndrome*, is the single most common cause of respiratory disease in premature infants. Surfactant dysfunction also is possible in the adult. This usually occurs as the result of severe injury or infection and can contribute to the development of a condition called *acute respiratory distress syndrome*.

Airway Airflow

The volume of air that moves into and out of the air exchange portion of the lungs is directly related to the pressure difference between the lungs and the atmosphere. It is inversely related to the resistance that the air encounters as it moves through the airways. Depending on the velocity and pattern of flow, airflow can be laminar or turbulent.

Laminar or *streamlined airflow* occurs at low flow rates in which the air stream is parallel to the sides of the airway. With laminar flow, the air at the periphery must overcome the resistance to flow, and as a result, the air in the center of the airway moves faster. *Turbulent airflow* is disorganized flow in which the molecules of the gas move laterally, collide with one another, and change their velocities. Whether turbulence develops depends on the radius of the airways, the interaction of the gas molecules, and the velocity of airflow. It is most likely to occur when the radius of the airways is large and the velocity of flow is high. Turbulent flow occurs regularly in the trachea. Turbulence of airflow accounts for the respiratory sounds that are heard during chest auscultation (*i.e.*, listening to chest sounds using a stethoscope). In the bronchial tree with its many branches laminar airflow probably occurs only in the very small airways where the velocity of flow is low.

Airway Resistance. Airway resistance is the ratio of the pressure driving inspiration or expiration to airflow. The French physician Jean Léonard Marie Poiseuille first described the pressure–flow characteristics of laminar flow in a straight circular tube, a correlation that has become known as the *Poiseuille law*. According to the Poiseuille law, the resistance to flow is inversely related to the fourth power of the radius ($R = 1/r^4$). If the radius is reduced by one half, the resistance increases 16-fold ($2 \times 2 \times 2 \times 2 = 16$).

Airway resistance differs in large (*e.g.*, trachea and bronchi), medium-sized (*e.g.*, segmental), and small (*e.g.*, bronchioles) airways. Therefore, the total airway resistance is equal to the sum of the resistances in these three types of airways. The site of most of the resistance along the bronchial tree is the medium size bronchi, with the smallest airways contributing very little to the total airway resistance.[5] This is because most of these airways are arranged in parallel and their resistances are added as reciprocals (*i.e.*, total combined resistance = 1/R + 1/R, etc.). Although the resistance of each individual bronchiole may be relatively high, their great number results in a large total cross-sectional area, causing their total resistance to be low. Many airway diseases, such as emphysema and chronic bronchitis, begin in the small airways. Early detection of these diseases is often difficult because a considerable amount of damage must be present before the usual measurements of airway resistance can be detected.

Airway resistance is greatly affected by lung volumes. Resistance is less during inspiration than expiration. This is because elastic fibers connect the outside of the airways to the surrounding lung tissues. As a result, these airways are pulled open as the lungs expand during inspiration, and they become narrower as the lungs deflate during expiration (Fig. 29.15). This is one of the reasons why people with conditions that increase airway resistance, such as asthma (reactive airway), usually have less difficulty breathing during inspiration than during expiration.

Airway resistance is also affected by the bronchial smooth muscle tone that controls airway diameter. The smooth muscles in the airway, from the trachea down to the terminal bronchioles, are under autonomic nervous system control. Stimulation of the parasympathetic nervous system causes bronchial constriction as well as increased mucus secretion. Sympathetic stimulation has the opposite effect.

Airway Compression during Forced Expiration. Airway resistance does not change much during normal quiet breathing. However, it is significantly increased during forced expiration, such as in vigorous exercise. Airflow through the collapsible airways in the lungs depends on the distending airway (intrapulmonary) pressures that hold the airways open

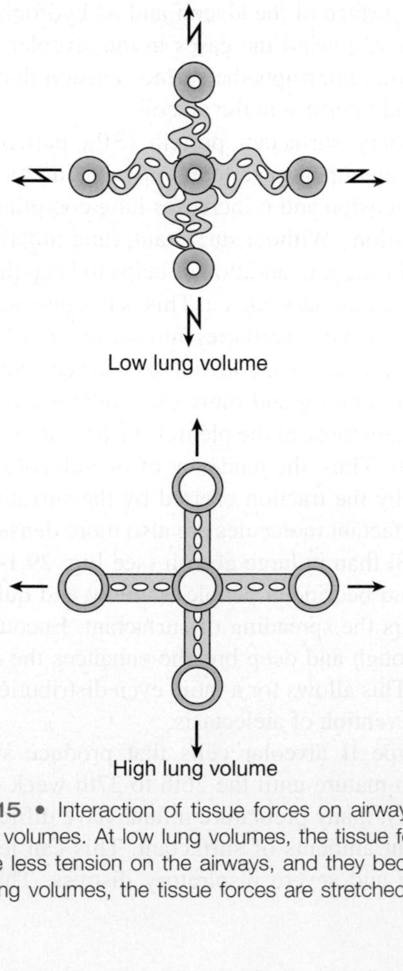

Figure 29.15 • Interaction of tissue forces on airways during low and high lung volumes. At low lung volumes, the tissue forces tend to fold and place less tension on the airways, and they become smaller; during high lung volumes, the tissue forces are stretched and pull the airways open.

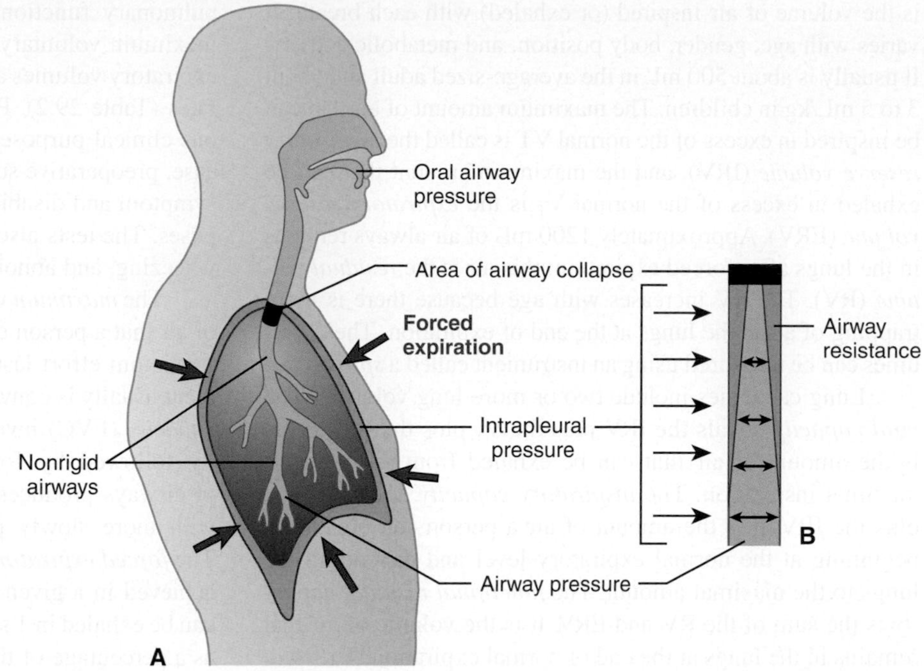

Figure 29.16 • Mechanism that limits maximal expiratory flow rate. **(A)** Airway patency and airflow in the nonrigid airways of the lungs rely on a transpulmonary pressure gradient in which airway pressure is greater than intrapleural pressure. **(B)** Airway resistance normally produces a drop in airway pressure as air moves out of the lungs. The increased intrapleural pressure that occurs with forced expiration produces airway collapse in the nonrigid airways at the point where intrapleural pressure exceeds airway pressure.

and the external (intrapleural or intrathoracic) pressures that surround and compress the airways. The difference between these two pressures (intrathoracic pressure minus airway pressure) is called the *transpulmonary pressure*. For airflow to occur, the distending pressure inside the airways must be greater than the compressing pressure outside the airways.

During forced expiration, the transpulmonary pressure is decreased because of a disproportionate increase in the intrathoracic pressure compared with airway pressure. The resistance that air encounters as it moves out of the lungs causes a further drop in airway pressure. If this drop in airway pressure is sufficiently great, the surrounding intrathoracic pressure will compress the collapsible airways (*i.e.*, those that lack cartilaginous support), causing airflow to be interrupted and air to be trapped in the terminal airways (Fig. 29.16).

This type of airway compression usually is seen only during forced expiration in people with normal respiratory function. However, it may occur during normal breathing in people with lung diseases. For example, in conditions that increase airway resistance, such as emphysema, the pressure drop along the smaller airways is magnified, and an increase in intra-airway pressure is needed to maintain airway patency. Measures such as pursed-lip breathing increase airway pressure and improve expiratory flow rates in people with chronic obstructive pulmonary disease (COPD). This is also the basis for using positive end-expiratory pressure in people who are being mechanically ventilated. Infants who are having trouble breathing often grunt to increase their expiratory airway pressures and keep their airways open.

Lung Volumes

Lung volumes, or the amount of air exchanged during ventilation, can be subdivided into three components: (1) the tidal volume, (2) the inspiratory reserve volume, and (3) the expiratory reserve volume (Fig. 29.17). The *tidal volume* (V_T)

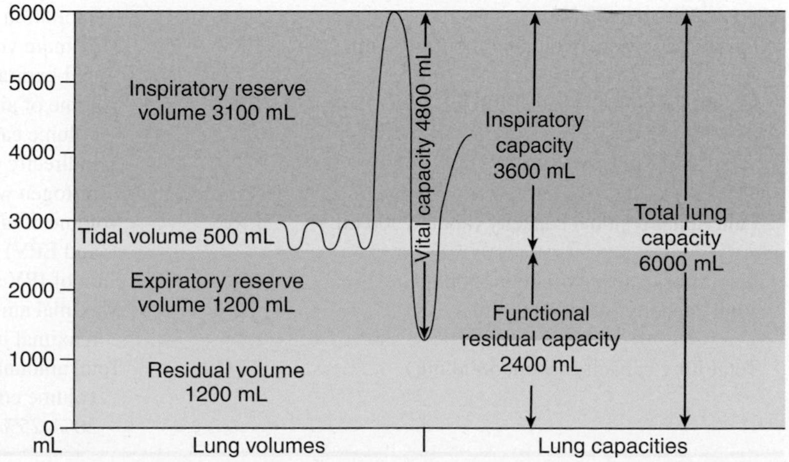

Figure 29.17 • Tracings of respiratory volumes **(left)** and lung capacities **(right)** as they would appear if made using a spirometer. The tidal volume (*yellow*) represents the amount of air inhaled and exhaled during normal breathing; the inspiratory reserve volume (*pink*), the maximal amount of air in excess of the tidal volume that can be forcefully inhaled; the maximal expiratory reserve (*blue*), the maximal amount of air that can be exhaled in excess of the tidal volume; and the residual volume (*green*), the air that continues to remain in the lung after maximal expiratory effort. The inspiratory capacity represents the sum of the inspiratory reserve volume and the tidal volume; the functional residual capacity, the sum of the maximal expiratory reserve and residual volumes; and the total lung capacity, the sum of all the volumes.

is the volume of air inspired (or exhaled) with each breath. It varies with age, gender, body position, and metabolic activity. It usually is about 500 mL in the average-sized adult and about 3 to 5 mL/kg in children. The maximum amount of air that can be inspired in excess of the normal VT is called the *inspiratory reserve volume* (IRV), and the maximum amount that can be exhaled in excess of the normal V_T is the *expiratory reserve volume* (ERV). Approximately 1200 mL of air always remains in the lungs after forced expiration; this air is the *residual volume* (RV). The RV increases with age because there is more trapping of air in the lungs at the end of expiration. These volumes can be measured using an instrument called a *spirometer*.

Lung capacities include two or more lung volumes. The *vital capacity* equals the IRV plus the V_T plus the ERV. This is the amount of air that can be exhaled from the point of maximal inspiration. The *inspiratory capacity* equals the V_T plus the IRV. It is the amount of air a person can breathe in beginning at the normal expiratory level and distending the lungs to the maximal amount. The *functional residual capacity* is the sum of the RV and ERV. It is the volume of air that remains in the lungs at the end of normal expiration. The *total lung capacity* is the sum of all the volumes in the lungs. The RV cannot be measured with the spirometer because this air cannot be expressed from the lungs. It is measured by indirect methods, such as the helium dilution method, nitrogen washout method, or body plethysmography.[4] Lung volumes and capacities are summarized in Table 29.1.

Pulmonary Function Studies

The previously described lung volumes and capacities are anatomic or static measures determined by lung volumes and measured without relation to time. The spirometer also is used to measure dynamic lung function (*i.e.*, ventilation with respect to time). These tests often are used in assessing pulmonary function. Pulmonary function measures include maximum voluntary ventilation, forced vital capacity, forced expiratory volumes and flow rates, and forced inspiratory flow rates (Table 29.2). Pulmonary function is measured for various clinical purposes, including diagnosis of respiratory disease, preoperative surgical and anesthetic risk evaluation, and symptom and disability evaluation for legal or insurance purposes. The tests also are used for evaluating dyspnea, cough, wheezing, and abnormal radiologic or laboratory findings.

The *maximum voluntary ventilation* measures the volume of air that a person can move into and out of the lungs during maximum effort lasting for 12 to 15 seconds. This measurement usually is converted to liters per minute. The *forced vital capacity* (FVC) involves full inspiration to total lung capacity followed by forceful maximal expiration. Obstruction of airways produces a FVC that is lower than that observed with more slowly performed vital capacity measurements. The *forced expiratory volume* (FEV) is the expiratory volume achieved in a given time period. The $FEV_{1.0}$ is the FEV that can be exhaled in 1 second. The $FEV_{1.0}$ frequently is expressed as a percentage of the FVC. The $FEV_{1.0}$ and FVC are used in the diagnosis of obstructive lung disorders.

The *forced inspiratory vital flow* (FIF) measures the respiratory response during rapid maximal inspiration. Calculation of airflow during the middle half of inspiration ($FIF_{25\%-75\%}$) relative to the forced midexpiratory flow rate ($FEF_{25\%-75\%}$) is used as a measure of respiratory muscle dysfunction because inspiratory flow depends more on effort than does expiration.[1,4]

Efficiency and the Work of Breathing

The *minute volume*, or total ventilation, is the amount of air that is exchanged in 1 minute. It is determined by the metabolic needs of the body. The minute volume is equal to the V_T multiplied by the respiratory rate, which is normally about

TABLE 29.1 LUNG VOLUMES AND CAPACITIES

VOLUME	SYMBOL	MEASUREMENT
Tidal volume (about 500 mL at rest)	V_T	Amount of air that moves into and out of the lungs with each breath
Inspiratory reserve volume (about 3000 mL)	IRV	Maximum amount of air that can be inhaled from the point of maximal expiration
Expiratory reserve volume (about 1100 mL)	ERV	Maximum volume of air that can be exhaled from the resting end-expiratory level
Residual volume (about 1200 mL)	RV	Volume of air remaining in the lungs after maximal expiration. This volume cannot be measured with the spirometer. It is measured indirectly using methods such as the helium dilution method, the nitrogen washout technique, or body plethysmography.
Functional residual capacity (about 2300 mL)	FRC	Volume of air remaining in the lungs at end-expiration (sum of RV and ERV)
Inspiratory capacity (about 3500 mL)	IC	Sum of IRV and TV
Vital capacity (about 4600 mL)	VC	Maximal amount of air that can be forcibly exhaled from the point of maximal inspiration
Total lung capacity (about 5800 mL)	TLC	Total amount of air that the lungs can hold. It is the sum of all the volume components after maximal inspiration. This value is about 20%–25% less in females than in males.

TABLE 29.2 PULMONARY FUNCTION TESTS

TEST	SYMBOL	MEASUREMENT*
Maximal voluntary ventilation	MVV	Maximum amount of air that can be breathed in a given time
Forced vital capacity	FVC	Maximum amount of air that can be rapidly and forcefully exhaled from the lungs after full inspiration. The expired volume is plotted against time.
Forced expiratory volume achieved in 1 second	$FEV_{1.0}$	Volume of air expired in the first second of FVC
Percentage of FVC	$FEV_{1.0}/FVC\%$	Volume of air expired in the first second, expressed as a percentage of FVC
Forced midexpiratory flow rate	$FEF_{25\%–75\%}$	The forced midexpiratory flow rate determined by locating the points on the volume–time curve recording obtained during FVC corresponding to 25% and 75% of FVC and drawing a straight line through these points. The slope of this line represents the average midexpiratory flow rate.
Forced inspiratory flow rate	$FIF_{25\%–75\%}$	FIF is the volume inspired from RV at the point of measurement. $FIF_{25\%–75\%}$ is the slope of a line between the points on the volume pressure tracing corresponding to 25% and 75% of the inspired volume.

*By convention, all the lung volumes and rates of flow are expressed in terms of body temperature and pressure and saturated with water vapor (BTPS), which allows for a comparison of the pulmonary function data from laboratories with different ambient temperatures and altitudes.

6000 mL (500 mL V_T × respiratory rate of 12 breaths/minute) in the average-sized adult during normal activity. The efficiency of breathing is determined by matching the V_T and respiratory rate in a manner that provides an optimal minute volume while minimizing the work of breathing.

The work of breathing is determined by the amount of effort required to move air through the conducting airways and by the ease of lung expansion, or compliance. Expansion of the lungs is difficult for people with stiff and noncompliant lungs. They usually find it easier to breathe if they keep their V_T low and breathe at a more rapid rate (*e.g.*, 300 × 20 = 6000 mL) to achieve their minute volume and meet their oxygen needs. In contrast, people with obstructive airway disease usually find it less difficult to inflate their lungs but expend more energy in moving air through the airways. As a result, these people take deeper breaths and breathe at a slower rate (*e.g.*, 600 × 10 = 6000 mL) to achieve their oxygen needs.

IN SUMMARY

The movement of air between the atmosphere and the lungs follows the laws of physics as they relate to gases. The air in the alveoli contains a mixture of gases, including nitrogen, oxygen, carbon dioxide, and water vapor. With the exception of water vapor, each gas exerts a pressure that is determined by the atmospheric pressure and the concentration of the gas in the mixture. Water vapor pressure is affected by temperature but not atmospheric pressure. Air moves into the lungs along a pressure gradient. The pressure inside the airways and alveoli of the lungs is called *intrapulmonary* (or *alveolar*) *pressure*; the pressure in the pleural cavity is called *pleural pressure*; and the pressure in the thoracic cavity is called *intrathoracic pressure*.

Breathing is the movement of gases between the atmosphere and the lungs. It requires a system of open airways and pressure changes resulting from the action of the respiratory muscles in changing the volume of the chest cage. The diaphragm is the principal muscle of inspiration, assisted by the external intercostal muscles. The scalene and sternocleidomastoid muscles elevate the ribs and act as accessory muscles for inspiration. Expiration is largely passive, aided by the elastic recoil of the respiratory muscles that were stretched during inspiration. When needed, the abdominal and internal intercostal muscles can be used to increase expiratory effort.

Lung compliance describes the ease with which the lungs can be inflated. The elastic and collagen fibers of the lung, the water content, the surface tension of the alveoli, and the compliance of the chest wall determine lung compliance. It also reflects the surface tension at the air–epithelium interface of the alveoli. Surfactant molecules, produced by type II alveolar cells, reduce the surface tension in the lungs and thereby increase lung compliance.

The volume of air that moves into and out of the air exchange portion of the lungs is directly related to the pressure difference between the lungs and the atmosphere and inversely related to the resistance that the air encounters as it moves through the airways. Depending on the velocity and pattern of flow, airflow can be laminar or turbulent. Airway resistance refers to the impediment to flow that the air encounters as it moves through the airways. It differs with airway size, being greatest in the medium-sized bronchi and lowest in the smaller bronchioles.

Lung volumes and lung capacities reflect the amount of air that is exchanged during normal and forced breathing. The tidal volume (V_T) is the amount of air that moves into and out of the lungs during normal breathing. The inspiratory reserve volume (IRV) is the maximum amount of air that can be inspired in excess of the normal V_T. The expiratory reserve volume (ERV) is the maximum amount that can be exhaled in excess of the normal V_T. The residual volume (RV) is the amount of air that remains in the lungs after forced expiration. Lung capacities include two or more lung volumes. The vital capacity equals the IRV plus the V_T plus the ERV and is the amount of air that can be exhaled from the point of maximal inspiration. The minute volume, which is determined by the metabolic needs of the body, is the amount of air that is exchanged in 1 minute (*i.e.*, respiratory rate and V_T).

EXCHANGE AND TRANSPORT OF GASES

After completing this section of the chapter, the learner will be able to meet the following objectives:

- Differentiate between pulmonary and alveolar ventilation.
- Explain why ventilation and perfusion must be matched.
- Cite the difference between dead air space and shunt.
- Explain the significance of a shift to the right and a shift to the left in the oxygen–hemoglobin dissociation curve.

The primary functions of the lungs are oxygenation of the blood and removal of carbon dioxide. Pulmonary gas exchange is conventionally divided into three processes:

- Ventilation—the flow of gases into and out of the alveoli of the lungs
- Perfusion—the flow of blood in the adjacent pulmonary capillaries
- Diffusion—the transfer of gases between the alveoli and the pulmonary capillaries

The efficiency of gas exchange requires that alveolar ventilation occur adjacent to perfused pulmonary capillaries.

Ventilation

Ventilation refers to the exchange of gases in the respiratory system. There are two types of ventilation: pulmonary and alveolar. *Pulmonary ventilation* refers to the total exchange of gases between the atmosphere and the lungs. *Alveolar ventilation* is the exchange of gases within the gas exchange portion of the lungs. Ventilation requires a system of open airways and a pressure difference that moves air into and out of the lungs. It is affected by body position and lung volume as well as by disease conditions that affect the heart and respiratory system.

Distribution of Ventilation

The distribution of ventilation between the apex and base of the lung varies with body position and the effects of gravity on intrapleural pressure (Fig. 29.18). In the seated or standing position, gravity exerts a downward pull on the lung, causing intrapleural pressure at the apex of the lung to become more negative than that at the base of the lung. As a result, the

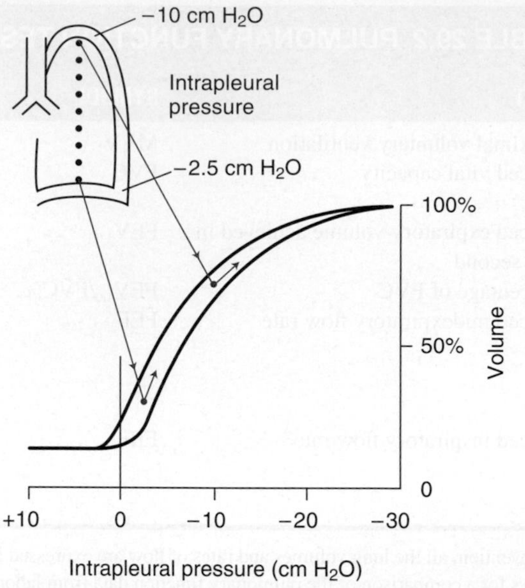

Figure 29.18 • Explanation of the regional differences in ventilation down the lung. Because of the weight of the lung, the **intrapleural pressure** is less negative at the base than at the apex. As a consequence, the basal lung is relatively compressed in its resting state but expands more on inspiration than does the apex. (From West J. B. (2016). *Respiratory physiology: The essentials* (10th ed., Figure 7.8, p. 118). Philadelphia, PA: Lippincott Williams & Wilkins.)

alveoli at the apex of the lung are more fully expanded than those at the base of the lung. The same holds true for dependent portions of the lung in the supine or lateral position. In the supine position, ventilation in the lowermost (posterior) parts of the lung exceeds that in the uppermost (anterior) parts. In the lateral position (*i.e.*, lying on the side), the dependent lung is better ventilated.

Lung volumes also affect the distribution of ventilation. Compliance reflects the change in volume that occurs with a change in pressure. It is less in fully expanded alveoli, which have difficulty accommodating more air, and greater in alveoli that are less inflated. During full inspiration in the seated or standing position, the airways are pulled open and air moves into the more compliant portions of the lower lung. At low lung volumes, the opposite occurs. In this case, the pleural pressure at the base of the lung exceeds airway pressure compressing the airways so that ventilation is greatly reduced. In addition, the airways in the upper part of the lung remain open so that the top of the lung is better ventilated than the bottom.

Even at low lung volumes, some air remains in the alveoli of the lower portion of the lungs, preventing their collapse. According to the law of Laplace, the pressure needed to overcome the tension in the wall of a sphere or an elastic tube is inversely related to its radius. Therefore, the small airways close first, trapping some gas in the alveoli. There may be increased trapping of air in the alveoli of the lower part of the lungs in older people and in those with lung disease (*e.g.*, emphysema). This condition is thought to result from a loss in the elastic recoil properties of the lungs, so that the intrapleural pressure, created by the elastic recoil of the lung and chest wall, becomes less negative. In these people, airway closure occurs at the end of normal instead of low lung volumes, trapping larger amounts of air with a resultant increase in the residual lung volume.

Dead Air Space

Dead space refers to the air that must be moved with each breath but does not participate in gas exchange. The movement of air through dead space contributes to the work of breathing but not to gas exchange. There are two types of dead space:

- Anatomic dead space: that contained in the conducting airways
- Alveolar dead space: that contained in the respiratory portion of the lung

The volume of anatomic airway dead space is fixed at approximately 150 to 200 mL, depending on body size. It constitutes air contained in the nose, pharynx, trachea, and bronchi. The creation of a tracheostomy (surgical opening in the trachea) decreases anatomic dead space ventilation because air does not have to move through the nasal and oral airways. Alveolar dead space, normally about 5 to 10 mL, constitutes alveolar air that does not participate in gas exchange. When alveoli are ventilated but deprived of blood flow, they do not contribute to gas exchange and thereby constitute alveolar dead space.

The *physiologic dead space* includes the anatomic dead space plus alveolar dead space. In people with normal respiratory function, physiologic dead space is about the same as anatomic dead space. Only in lung disease does physiologic dead space increase. Alveolar ventilation is equal to the minute ventilation minus the physiologic dead space ventilation.

KEY POINTS

MATCHING OF VENTILATION AND PERFUSION

- Exchange of gases between the air in the alveoli and the blood in pulmonary capillaries requires a matching of ventilation and perfusion.
- Dead air space refers to the volume of air that is moved with each breath but does not participate in gas exchange. Anatomic dead space is that contained in the conducting airways that normally do not participate in gas exchange. Alveolar dead space results from alveoli that are ventilated but not perfused.
- Shunt refers to blood that moves from the right to the left side of the circulation without being oxygenated. With an anatomic shunt, blood moves from the venous to the arterial side of the circulation without going through the lungs. Physiologic shunting results from blood moving through unventilated parts of the lung.

Perfusion

The primary functions of the pulmonary circulation are to perfuse or provide blood flow to the gas exchange portion of the lung and to facilitate gas exchange. The pulmonary circulation serves several important functions in addition to gas exchange. It filters all the blood that moves from the right to the left side of the circulation; it removes most of the thromboemboli that might form; and it serves as a reservoir of blood for the left side of the heart.

The gas exchange function of the lungs requires a continuous flow of blood through the respiratory portion of the lungs. Deoxygenated blood enters the lung through the pulmonary artery, which has its origin in the right side of the heart and enters the lung at each hilum, along with the right and left main bronchi. The pulmonary arteries branch in a manner similar to that of the airways. The small pulmonary arteries accompany the bronchi as they move down the lobules and branch to supply the capillary network that surrounds the alveoli (see Fig. 29.8). The oxygenated capillary blood is collected in the small pulmonary veins of the lobules. It then moves to the larger veins to be collected in the four large pulmonary veins that empty into the left atrium.

The pulmonary blood vessels are thinner, more compliant, and offer less resistance to flow than those in the systemic circulation. In addition, the pressures in the pulmonary system are much lower (*e.g.*, 22/8 mm Hg versus 120/70 mm Hg pressure in systemic circulation). The low pressure and low resistance of the pulmonary circulation accommodate the delivery of varying amounts of blood from the systemic circulation without producing signs and symptoms of congestion. The volume in the pulmonary circulation is approximately 500 mL, with approximately 100 mL of this volume located in the pulmonary capillary bed. When the input of blood from the right heart and output of blood to the left heart are equal, pulmonary blood flow remains constant. Small differences between input and output can result in large changes in pulmonary volume if the differences continue for many heartbeats. The movement of blood through the pulmonary capillary bed requires that the mean pulmonary arterial pressure be greater than the mean pulmonary venous pressure. Pulmonary venous pressure increases in left-sided heart failure, allowing blood to accumulate in the pulmonary capillary bed and cause pulmonary edema.

Distribution of Blood Flow

As with ventilation, the distribution of pulmonary blood flow is affected by body position and gravity. In the upright position, the distance of the upper apices of the lung above the level of the heart may exceed the perfusion capabilities of the mean pulmonary arterial pressure (approximately 12 mm Hg). Therefore, blood flow in the upper part of the lungs is less than that in the base or bottom part of the lungs (Fig. 29.19). In the supine position, the lungs and the heart are at the same level, and blood flow to the apices and base of the lungs becomes

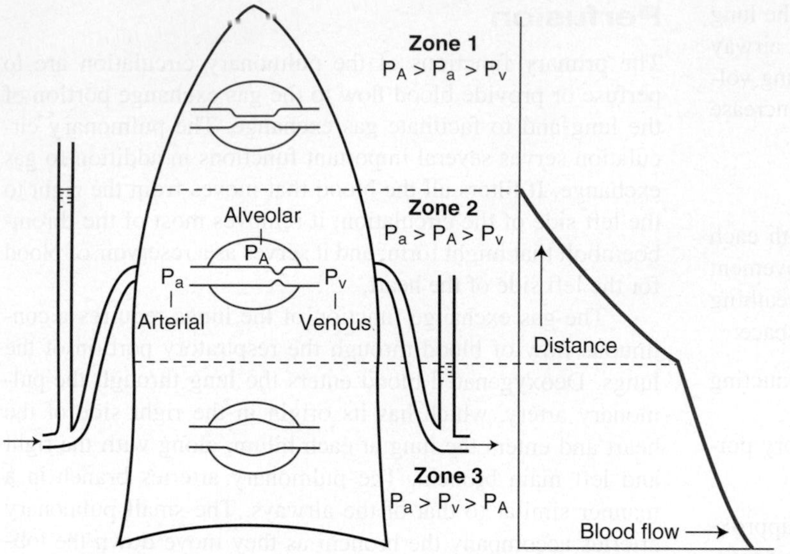

Figure 29.19 • Explanation of uneven distribution of blood flow in the lung, based on the pressures affecting the capillaries. (From West J. B. (2016). *Respiratory physiology: The essentials* (10th ed., Figure 4.8, p. 50). Philadelphia, PA: Lippincott Williams & Wilkins.)

more uniform. In this position, blood flow to the posterior or dependent portions (*e.g.*, bottom of the lung when lying on the side) exceeds flow in the anterior or nondependent portions of the lungs.

Hypoxia-Induced Vasoconstriction

The blood vessels in the pulmonary circulation are highly sensitive to alveolar oxygen levels and undergo marked vasoconstriction when exposed to hypoxia. The precise mechanism for this response is unclear. When alveolar oxygen levels drop below 60 mm Hg, marked vasoconstriction may occur. At very low oxygen levels, the local flow may be almost abolished. In regional hypoxia, which occurs with atelectasis, vasoconstriction is localized to a specific region of the lung. In this case, vasoconstriction has the effect of directing blood flow away from the hypoxic regions of the lungs. When alveolar hypoxia no longer exists, blood flow is restored.

Generalized hypoxia, which occurs at high altitudes and in people with chronic hypoxia due to lung disease, causes vasoconstriction throughout the lung. Prolonged hypoxia can lead to pulmonary hypertension and increased workload on the right heart, causing cor pulmonale. A low blood pH produces a similar effect, particularly when alveolar hypoxia is present (*e.g.*, during circulatory shock).

Shunt

Shunt refers to blood that moves from the right to the left side of the circulation without being oxygenated. As with dead air space, there are two types of shunts: physiologic and anatomic. In an *anatomic shunt*, blood moves from the venous to the arterial side of the circulation without moving through the lungs. Anatomic intracardiac shunting of blood occurs with congenital heart defects. In a *physiologic shunt*, there is mismatching of ventilation and perfusion within the lung. This results in insufficient ventilation to provide the oxygen needed to oxygenate the blood flowing through the alveolar capillaries. Physiologic shunting of blood usually results from destructive lung disease that impairs ventilation or from heart failure that interferes with movement of blood through sections of the lungs.

Mismatching of Ventilation and Perfusion

The gas exchange properties of the lung depend on matching ventilation and perfusion, ensuring that equal amounts of air and blood are entering the respiratory portion of the lungs. Both dead air space and shunt produce a mismatching of ventilation and perfusion, as depicted in Figure 29.20. With shunt (depicted on the left), there is perfusion without ventilation, resulting in a low ventilation–perfusion ratio. It occurs in conditions such as atelectasis in which there is airway obstruction.

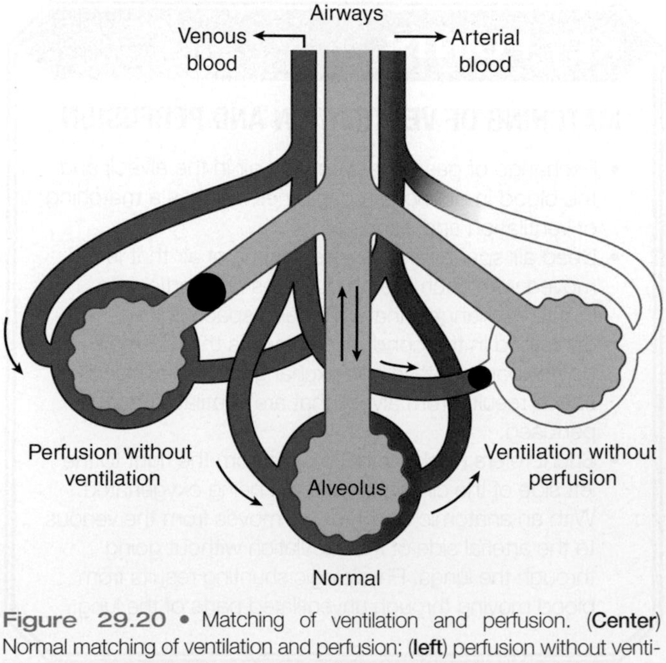

Figure 29.20 • Matching of ventilation and perfusion. (**Center**) Normal matching of ventilation and perfusion; (**left**) perfusion without ventilation (*i.e.*, shunt); (**right**) ventilation without perfusion (*i.e.*, dead air space).

With dead air space (depicted on the right), there is ventilation without perfusion, resulting in a high ventilation–perfusion ratio. It occurs in conditions such as pulmonary embolism, which impairs blood flow to a part of the lung. The arterial blood leaving the pulmonary circulation reflects mixing of blood from normally ventilated and perfused areas of the lung as well as areas that are not ventilated (dead air space) or perfused (shunt). Many of the conditions that cause mismatching of ventilation and perfusion involve both dead air space and shunt. In chronic obstructive lung disease, for example, there may be impaired ventilation in one area of the lung and impaired perfusion in another area.

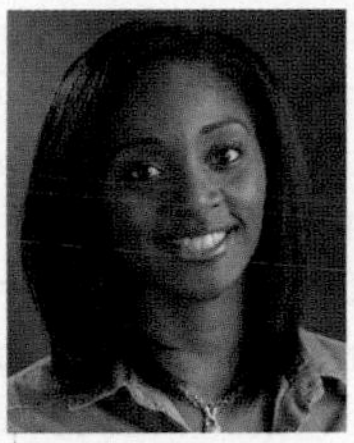

In a person with pulmonary embolism like Ms. French, ventilation/perfusion mismatch occurs because blood flow to part of the lung is impaired. Ms. French's increased respiratory rate is a clinical manifestation of her impaired gas exchange from the ventilation/perfusion mismatch.

Diffusion

Diffusion occurs in the respiratory portions of the lung and refers to the movement of gases across the alveolar–capillary membrane. The *Fick law of diffusion* can describe gas diffusion in the lung. The Fick law states the volume of a gas ($\dot{V}_{gas}$) diffusing across the membrane per unit time is directly proportional to the partial pressure difference of the gas ($P_1 - P_2$), the surface area (SA) of the membrane, and the diffusion coefficient (D) and is inversely proportional to the thickness (T) of the membrane (Fig. 29.21).[1]

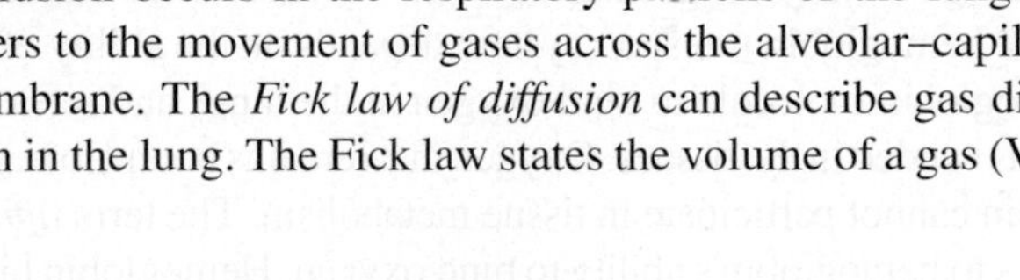

Figure 29.21 • The Fick law of diffusion states that the diffusion of a gas (V_{gas}) across a sheet of tissue is related to the surface area (SA) of the tissue, the diffusion constant (D) for the gas, and the partial pressure difference ($P_1 - P_2$) on either side of the tissue and is inversely proportional to the thickness (T) of the tissue.

Several factors influence the diffusion of gases in the lung. The administration of high concentrations of oxygen increases the difference in partial pressure between the two sides of the membrane and increases the diffusion of the gas. Diseases that destroy lung tissue (*i.e.*, surface area for diffusion) or increase the thickness of the alveolar–capillary membrane adversely influence the diffusing capacity of the lungs.

The removal of one lung, for example, reduces the diffusing capacity by one half. The thickness of the alveolar–capillary membrane and the distance for diffusion are increased in people with pulmonary edema or pneumonia. The characteristics of the gas and its molecular weight and solubility constitute the diffusion coefficient and determine how rapidly a gas diffuses through the respiratory membranes. For example, carbon dioxide diffuses 20 times more rapidly than oxygen because of its greater solubility in the respiratory membranes.

The diffusing capacity provides a measure of the rate of gas transfer in the lungs per partial pressure gradient. Because the initial alveolar–capillary difference for oxygen cannot be measured, carbon monoxide (CO) is used to determine the diffusing capacity. Measuring CO has several advantages:

- Its uptake is not limited by diffusion or blood flow.
- There is essentially no CO in venous blood.
- Its affinity for hemoglobin is 210 times that of oxygen, ensuring that its partial pressure will remain essentially zero in the pulmonary capillary.

The most common technique for making this measurement is the *single-breath test*. This test involves the inhalation of a single breath of dilute CO, followed by a breath-hold of 10 seconds. The diffusing capacity can be calculated using the lung volume and the percentage of CO in the alveoli at the beginning and end of the 10-second breath-hold.

Oxygen and Carbon Dioxide Transport

Although the lungs are responsible for the exchange of gases with the external environment, it is the blood that transports these gases between the lungs and body tissues. The blood carries oxygen and carbon dioxide in the physically dissolved state and in combination with hemoglobin. Carbon dioxide also is converted to bicarbonate and transported in that form.

Dissolved oxygen and carbon dioxide exert a partial pressure that is designated in the same manner as the partial pressures in the gas state. In the clinical setting, blood gas measurements are used to determine the partial pressure of oxygen (PO_2) and carbon dioxide (PCO_2) in the blood.

TABLE 29.3 ARTERIAL BLOOD GAS RANGES

PARAMETER	RANGE
1. pH = acid or base	7.35–7.45
2. PCO_2 = partial pressure of carbon dioxide	35–45 mm Hg
3. HCO_3^-= bicarbonate	22–26 mEq/L
4. PO_2 = partial pressure of oxygen	80–100 mm Hg

Concept Mastery Alert

Arterial blood commonly is used for measuring blood gases. Venous blood is not used because venous levels of oxygen and carbon dioxide reflect the metabolic demands of the tissues rather than the gas exchange function of the lungs.

The PO_2 of arterial blood normally is above 80 mm Hg, and the PCO_2 is in the range of 35 to 45 mm Hg (Table 29.3). Normally, the ABGs are the same or nearly the same as the partial pressure of the gases in the alveoli. The arterial PO_2 often is written PaO_2, and the alveolar PO_2 as PAO_2, with the same types of designations being used for PCO_2. This text uses PO_2 and PCO_2 to designate both arterial and alveolar levels of the gases.

Oxygen Transport

Oxygen is transported in two forms:

- In chemical combination with hemoglobin
- In the dissolved state

Hemoglobin carries about 98% to 99% of oxygen in the blood and is the main transporter of oxygen. The remaining 1% to 2% of the oxygen is carried in the dissolved state. Only the dissolved form of oxygen passes through the capillary wall, diffuses through the cell membrane, and makes itself available for use in cell metabolism. The oxygen content (measured in mL/100 mL) of the blood includes the oxygen carried by hemoglobin and in the dissolved state.

Hemoglobin Transport. Hemoglobin is a highly efficient carrier of oxygen. Hemoglobin with bound oxygen is called *oxyhemoglobin*. When oxygen is removed, it is called *deoxygenated* or *reduced hemoglobin*. Each gram of hemoglobin carries approximately 1.34 mL of oxygen when it is fully saturated. This means that a person with a hemoglobin level of 14 g/100 mL carries 18.8 mL of oxygen per 100 mL of blood.

In the lungs, oxygen moves across the alveolar–capillary membrane, through the plasma, and into the red blood cell, where it forms a loose and reversible bond with the hemoglobin molecule. In normal lungs, this process is rapid. Therefore, even with a fast heart rate, the hemoglobin is almost completely saturated with oxygen during the short time it spends in the pulmonary capillaries. As the oxygen moves out of the capillaries in response to the needs of the tissues, the hemoglobin saturation drops. It is approximately 95% to 97% saturated as the blood leaves the left side of the heart. It then drops to approximately 75% saturation as the mixed venous blood returns to the right side of the heart.

Dissolved Oxygen. The partial pressure of oxygen represents the level of dissolved oxygen in plasma. The amount of dissolved oxygen depends on its partial pressure and its solubility in the plasma. In the normal lung at 760 mm Hg atmospheric pressure, the PO_2 of arterial blood is approximately 100 mm Hg. The solubility of oxygen in plasma is fixed and very small. For every 1 mm Hg of PO_2 present, 0.003 mL of oxygen becomes dissolved in 100 mL of plasma. This means that at a normal arterial PO_2 of 100 mm Hg, the blood carries only 0.3 mL of dissolved oxygen in each 100 mL of plasma. This amount (approximately 1%) is very small compared with the amount that can be carried in an equal amount of blood when oxygen is attached to hemoglobin.

However, this small amount can become a lifesaving mode of transport in cases of CO poisoning, when most of the hemoglobin sites are occupied by CO and are unavailable for transport of oxygen. The use of a hyperbaric chamber, in which 100% oxygen can be administered at high atmospheric pressures, increases the amount of oxygen that can be carried in the dissolved state and is used for people with severe burns, especially those impacting the respiratory system, and in people with multiple types of wounds such as the immunosuppressed or those with diabetes who have trouble healing.

Binding Affinity of Hemoglobin for Oxygen. The efficiency of the hemoglobin transport system depends on the ability of the hemoglobin molecule to bind oxygen in the lungs and release it as it is needed in the tissues. Oxygen that remains bound to hemoglobin cannot participate in tissue metabolism. The term *affinity* refers to hemoglobin's ability to bind oxygen. Hemoglobin binds oxygen more readily when its affinity is increased and releases it more readily when its affinity is decreased.

The hemoglobin molecule is composed of four polypeptide chains with an iron-containing heme group. Because oxygen binds to the iron atom, each hemoglobin molecule can bind four molecules of oxygen when it is fully saturated. Oxygen binds cooperatively with the heme groups on the hemoglobin molecule. After the first molecule of oxygen binds to hemoglobin, the molecule undergoes a change in shape. As a result, the second and third molecules bind more readily, and binding of the fourth molecule is even easier. In a like manner, the unloading of the first molecule of oxygen enhances the unloading of the next molecule and so on. Thus, the affinity of hemoglobin for oxygen changes with hemoglobin saturation.

Hemoglobin's affinity for oxygen is also influenced by pH, carbon dioxide concentration, and body temperature. It binds oxygen more readily under conditions of increased pH (alkalosis), decreased carbon dioxide concentration, and decreased body temperature, and it releases it more readily under conditions of decreased pH (acidosis), increased carbon dioxide concentration, and fever. For example, increased tissue metabolism generates carbon dioxide and metabolic acids and thereby decreases the affinity of hemoglobin for oxygen. Heat also is a by-product of tissue metabolism, explaining the effect of fever on oxygen binding.

Red blood cells contain a metabolic intermediate called *2,3-diphosphoglycerate (2,3-DPG)* that also affects the affinity of hemoglobin for oxygen. An increase in 2,3-DPG enhances unloading of oxygen from hemoglobin at the tissue level. Conditions that increase 2,3-DPG include exercise, hypoxia that occurs at high altitude, and chronic lung disease.[1]

The Oxygen Dissociation Curve. The relation between the oxygen carried in combination with hemoglobin and the PO_2 of the blood is described by the *oxygen–hemoglobin dissociation curve*, which is shown in Figure 29.22. The *x*-axis of the graph depicts the PO_2 or dissolved oxygen. It reflects the partial pressure of the oxygen in the lungs (*i.e.*, the PO_2 is approximately 100 mm Hg when room air is being breathed, but can rise to 200 mm Hg or higher when oxygen-enriched air is breathed). The left *y*-axis depicts hemoglobin saturation or the amount of oxygen that is carried by the hemoglobin. The right *y*-axis depicts oxygen content or total amount of the oxygen content being carried in the blood.

The S-shaped oxygen dissociation curve has a flat top portion representing binding of oxygen to hemoglobin in the lungs and a steep portion representing its release into the tissue capillaries (see Fig. 29.22A). The S shape of the curve reflects the effect that oxygen saturation has on the conformation of the hemoglobin molecule and its affinity for oxygen. At approximately 100 mm Hg PO_2, a plateau occurs. At this point, the hemoglobin is approximately 98% saturated. Increasing the alveolar PO_2 above this level does not increase the hemoglobin saturation. Even at high altitudes, when the partial pressure of oxygen is considerably decreased, the hemoglobin remains relatively well saturated. At 60 mm Hg PO_2, for example, the hemoglobin is still approximately 89% saturated.

The steep portion of the dissociation curve—between 60 and 40 mm Hg—represents the removal of oxygen from the hemoglobin as it moves through the tissue capillaries. This portion of the curve reflects a considerable transfer of oxygen from hemoglobin to the tissues with only a small drop in PO_2. This ensures a gradient for oxygen to move into body cells. The tissues normally remove approximately 5 mL of oxygen per 100 mL of blood, and the hemoglobin of mixed venous blood is approximately 75% saturated as it returns to the right side of the heart. In this portion of the dissociation curve (saturation < 75%), the rate at which oxygen is released from hemoglobin is determined largely by tissue uptake. During strenuous exercise, for example, the muscle cells may remove as much as 15 mL of oxygen per 100 mL of blood from hemoglobin.

Hemoglobin can be regarded as a buffer system that regulates the delivery of oxygen to the tissues. In order to function as a buffer system, the affinity of hemoglobin for oxygen must change with the metabolic needs of the tissues. This change is represented by a shift to the right or left in the dissociation curve (see Fig. 29.22B). A shift to the right indicates that the tissue PO_2 is greater for any given level of hemoglobin saturation and represents reduced affinity of the hemoglobin for oxygen at any given PO_2. It usually is caused by conditions that reflect increased tissue metabolism, such as fever or acidosis, or by an increase in PCO_2. High altitude and conditions such as pulmonary insufficiency, heart failure,

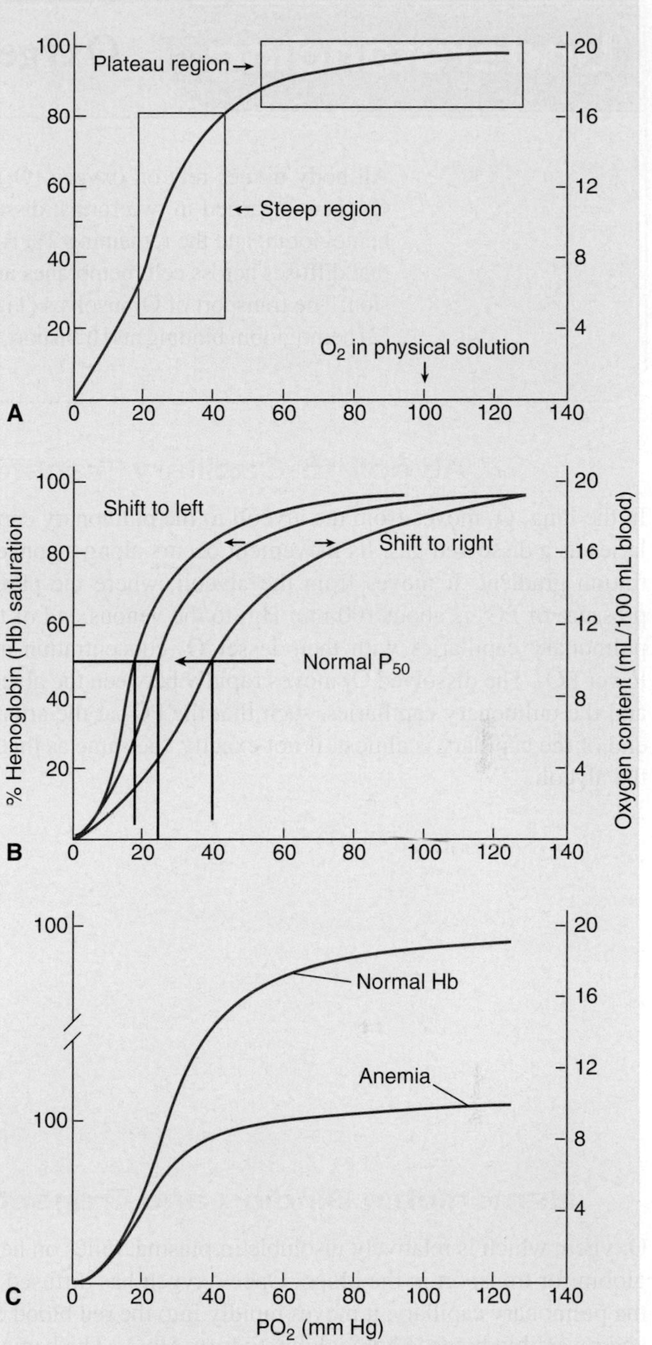

Figure 29.22 • Oxygen–hemoglobin dissociation curve. **(A)** Left boxed area represents the steep portion of the curve where oxygen is released from hemoglobin (Hb) to the tissues and the top boxed area the plateau of the curve where oxygen is loaded onto hemoglobin in the lung. **(B)** The effect of body temperature, arterial PCO_2, and pH on hemoglobin affinity for oxygen as indicated by a shift in the curve and position of the P_{50}. A shift of the curve to the right because of an increase in temperature or PCO_2 or decreased pH favors release of oxygen to the tissues. A decrease in temperature or PCO_2 or increase in pH shifts the curve to the left and has the opposite effect. The P_{50} is the partial pressure of oxygen required to saturate 50% of hemoglobin with oxygen. **(C)** Effect of anemia on the oxygen-carrying capacity of blood. The hemoglobin can be completely saturated, but the oxygen content of the blood is reduced.

Understanding Oxygen Transport

All body tissues rely on oxygen (O_2) that is transported in the blood to meet their metabolic needs. Oxygen is carried in two forms: dissolved and bound to hemoglobin. About 98% of O_2 is carried by hemoglobin, and the remaining 2% is carried in the dissolved state. Dissolved oxygen is the only form that diffuses across cell membranes and produces a partial pressure (PO_2), which, in turn, drives diffusion. The transport of O_2 involves (1) transfer from the alveoli to the pulmonary capillaries in the lung, (2) hemoglobin binding and transport, and (3) the dissociation from hemoglobin in the tissue capillaries.

Alveoli-to-Capillary Transfer

In the lung, O_2 moves from the alveoli to the pulmonary capillaries as a dissolved gas. Its movement occurs along a concentration gradient. It moves from the alveoli, where the partial pressure of PO_2 is about 100 mm Hg, to the venous end of the pulmonary capillaries with their lesser O_2 concentration and lower PO_2. The dissolved O_2 moves rapidly between the alveoli and the pulmonary capillaries, such that the PO_2 at the arterial end of the capillary is almost, if not exactly, the same as that in the alveoli.

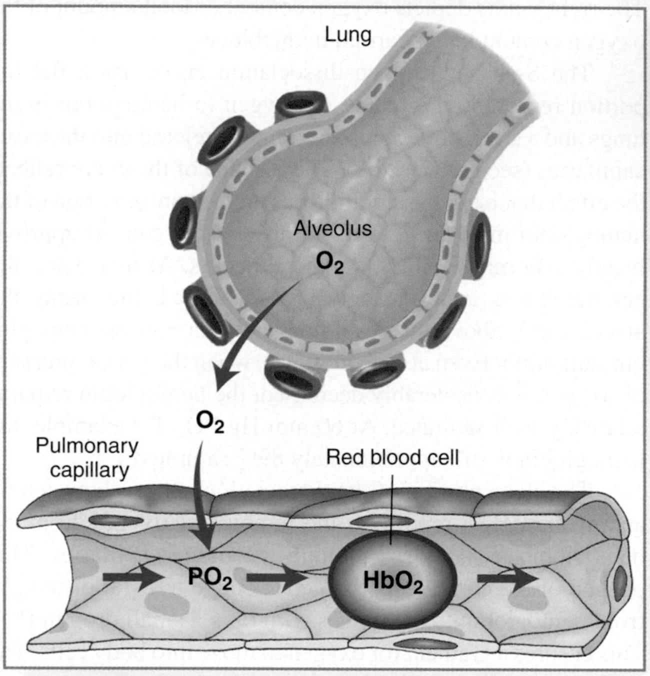

Hemoglobin Binding and Transport

Oxygen, which is relatively insoluble in plasma, relies on hemoglobin for transport in the blood. Once oxygen has diffused into the pulmonary capillary, it moves rapidly into the red blood cells and reversibly binds to hemoglobin to form HbO_2. The hemoglobin molecule contains four heme units, each capable of attaching an oxygen molecule. Hemoglobin is 100% saturated when all four units are occupied and is usually about 97% saturated in the systemic arterial blood. The capacity of the blood to carry O_2 is dependent both on hemoglobin levels and the ability of the lungs to oxygenate the hemoglobin.

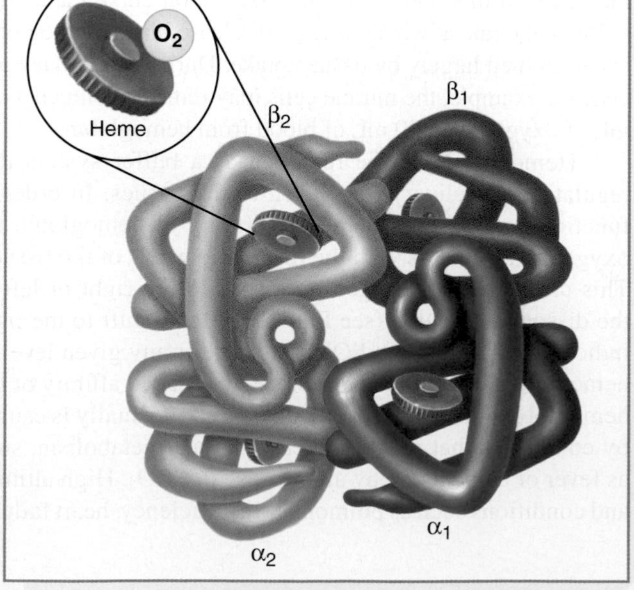

Understanding Oxygen Transport *(Continued)*

Oxygen Dissociation in the Tissues

The dissociation or release of O_2 from hemoglobin occurs in the tissue capillaries where the PO_2 is less than that of the arterial blood. As oxygen dissociates from hemoglobin, it dissolves in the plasma and then moves into the tissues where the PO_2 is less than that in the capillaries. The affinity of hemoglobin for O_2 is influenced by the carbon dioxide (PCO_2) content of the blood and its pH temperature and 2,3-diphosphoglycerate (2,3-DPG), a by-product of glycolysis in red blood cells. Under conditions of high metabolic demand, in which the PCO_2 is increased and the pH is decreased, the binding affinity of hemoglobin is decreased. During decreased metabolic demand, when the PCO_2 is decreased and the pH is increased, the affinity is increased.

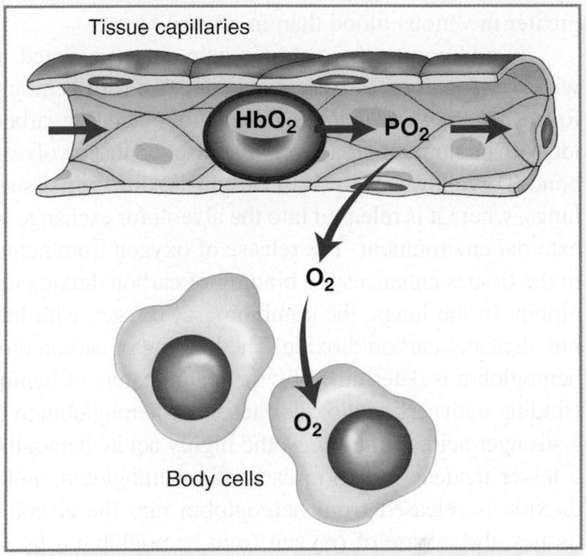

and severe anemia also cause the oxygen dissociation curve to shift to the right. A shift to the left in the oxygen dissociation curve represents an increased affinity of hemoglobin for oxygen. It occurs in situations associated with a decrease in tissue metabolism, such as alkalosis, decreased body temperature, and decreased PCO_2 levels. The degree of shift can be determined by the P_{50}, or the partial pressure of oxygen that is needed to achieve a 50% saturation of hemoglobin. Returning to Figure 29.22B, the dissociation curve on the left has a P_{50} of approximately 20 mm Hg; the normal curve, a P_{50} of 26 mm Hg; and the curve on the right, a P_{50} of 39 mm Hg.

The oxygen content (measured in mL/dL blood) represents the total amount of oxygen carried in the blood, including the dissolved oxygen and that carried by the hemoglobin (see Fig. 29.22C). The amount of hemoglobin-bound oxygen is determined by the concentration of hemoglobin (in g/dL), the oxygen-binding capacity of hemoglobin (1.34 mL O_2/g hemoglobin), and the percentage saturation of the hemoglobin. The dissolved oxygen content is the product of the oxygen solubility (0.0003 mL O_2/dL) times the PO_2. Thus, an anemic person may have a normal PO_2 and hemoglobin saturation level but decreased oxygen content because of the lower amount of hemoglobin for binding oxygen.

Carbon Dioxide Transport

Carbon dioxide is transported in the blood in three forms:

- As dissolved carbon dioxide (10%)
- Attached to hemoglobin (30%)
- As bicarbonate (60%)

Acid–base balance is influenced by the amount of dissolved carbon dioxide and the bicarbonate level in the blood.

As carbon dioxide is formed during the metabolic process, it diffuses out of cells into the tissue spaces and then into the capillaries. The partial pressure of the gas and its solubility coefficient (0.03 mL/100 mL/1 mm Hg PCO_2) determine the amount of dissolved carbon dioxide that can be carried in plasma. Carbon dioxide is 20 times more soluble in plasma than is oxygen. Thus, the dissolved state plays a greater role in transport of carbon dioxide compared with oxygen.

Most of the carbon dioxide diffuses into the red blood cells, where it either forms carbonic acid or combines with hemoglobin. *Carbonic acid* (H_2CO_3) is formed when carbon dioxide combines with water. The process is catalyzed by an enzyme called *carbonic anhydrase*, which is present in large quantities in red blood cells. Carbonic anhydrase increases the rate of the reaction between carbon dioxide and water approximately 5000-fold. Carbonic acid readily ionizes to form bicarbonate (HCO_3^-) and hydrogen (H^+) ions. The hydrogen ion combines with the hemoglobin, which is a powerful acid–base buffer, and the bicarbonate ion diffuses into plasma in exchange for a chloride ion. This exchange is made possible by a special bicarbonate–chloride carrier protein in the red blood cell membrane. As a result of the bicarbonate–chloride shift, the chloride and water content of the red blood cell is greater in venous blood than in arterial blood.

In addition to the carbonic anhydrase–mediated reaction with water, carbon dioxide reacts directly with hemoglobin to form *carbaminohemoglobin*. The combination of carbon dioxide with hemoglobin is a reversible reaction that involves a loose bond. This allows transport of carbon dioxide from tissues to the lungs, where it is released into the alveoli for exchange with the external environment. The release of oxygen from hemoglobin in the tissues enhances the binding of carbon dioxide to hemoglobin. In the lungs, the combining of oxygen with hemoglobin displaces carbon dioxide. The binding of carbon dioxide to hemoglobin is determined by the acidic nature of hemoglobin. Binding with carbon dioxide causes the hemoglobin to become a stronger acid. In the lungs, the highly acidic hemoglobin has a lesser tendency to form carbaminohemoglobin, and carbon dioxide is released from hemoglobin into the alveoli. In the tissues, the release of oxygen from hemoglobin causes hemoglobin to become less acid, thereby increasing its ability to combine with carbon dioxide and form carbaminohemoglobin.

IN SUMMARY

The primary functions of the lungs are oxygenation of the blood and removal of carbon dioxide. Pulmonary gas exchange is conventionally divided into three processes: ventilation, or the flow of gases into the alveoli of the lungs; perfusion, or movement of blood through the adjacent pulmonary capillaries; and diffusion, or transfer of gases between the alveoli and the pulmonary capillaries.

Ventilation is the movement of air between the atmosphere and the lungs and perfusion is the flow of blood into and out of the gas exchange portions of the lung. Pulmonary ventilation refers to the total exchange of gases between the atmosphere and the lungs, and alveolar ventilation to ventilation in the gas exchange portion of the lungs. The distribution of alveolar ventilation and pulmonary capillary blood flow varies with lung volume and body position. In the upright position and at high lung volumes, ventilation is greatest in the lower parts of the lungs. The upright position also produces a decrease in blood flow to the upper parts of the lung, resulting from the distance above the level of the heart and the low mean arterial pressure in the pulmonary circulation. The efficiency of gas exchange requires matching of ventilation and perfusion, so that equal amounts of air and blood enter the respiratory portion of the lungs. Two conditions interfere with matching of ventilation and perfusion: dead air space, in which areas of the lungs are ventilated but not perfused, and shunt, in which areas of the lungs are perfused but not ventilated.

The diffusion of gases in the lungs is influenced by four factors: the surface area available for diffusion; the thickness of the alveolar–capillary membrane, through which the gases diffuse; the differences in the partial pressure of the gas on either side of the membrane; and the diffusion characteristics of the gas.

The blood transports oxygen to the cells and returns carbon dioxide to the lungs. Oxygen is transported in two forms: in chemical combination with hemoglobin and physically dissolved in plasma (PO_2). Hemoglobin is an efficient carrier of oxygen. Approximately 98% to 99% of oxygen is transported in this manner. The relationship between the oxygen carried in combination with hemoglobin and the oxygen–hemoglobin dissociation curve describes the PO_2 of the blood. Carbon dioxide is carried in three forms: attached to hemoglobin (30%), dissolved carbon dioxide (10%), and bicarbonate (60%).

CONTROL OF BREATHING

After completing this section of the chapter, the learner will be able to meet the following objectives:

- Compare the neural control of the respiratory muscles, which control breathing, with that of cardiac muscle, which controls the pumping action of the heart.
- Trace the integration of the cough reflex from stimulus to explosive expulsion of air that constitutes the cough.
- Define dyspnea and list three types of conditions in which dyspnea occurs.

Unlike the heart, which has inherent rhythmic properties and can beat independently of the nervous system, the muscles that control respiration require continuous input from the nervous system. Movement of the diaphragm, intercostal muscles, sternocleidomastoid, and other accessory muscles that control ventilation is integrated by neurons located in the pons and medulla. These neurons are collectively referred to as the *respiratory center* (Fig. 29.23).

Respiratory Center

The respiratory center consists of two dense, bilateral aggregates of respiratory neurons. These neurons are involved in initiating inspiration and expiration and incorporating afferent impulses into motor responses of the respiratory muscles. The first, or dorsal, group of neurons in the respiratory center is concerned primarily with inspiration. These neurons control the activity of the phrenic nerves that innervate the diaphragm and drive the second, or ventral, group of respiratory neurons. They are thought to integrate sensory input from the lungs and airways into the ventilatory response. The second group of neurons, which contains inspiratory and expiratory neurons, controls the spinal motor neurons of the intercostal and abdominal muscles.

The pacemaker properties of the respiratory center result from the cycling of the two groups of respiratory neurons:

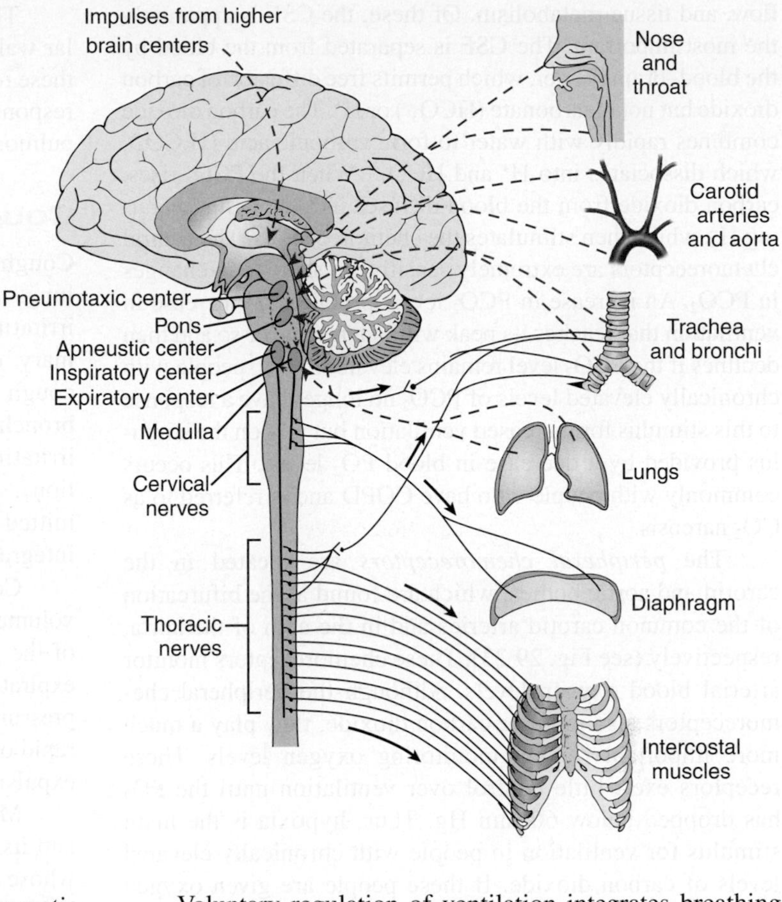

Figure 29.23 • Schematic representation of activity in the respiratory center. Impulses traveling over afferent neurons (*dashed lines*) communicate with central neurons, which activate efferent neurons that supply the muscles of respiration. Respiratory movements can be altered by a variety of stimuli.

the *pneumotaxic center* in the upper pons and the *apneustic center* in the lower pons (see Fig. 29.23). These two groups of neurons contribute to the function of the respiratory center in the medulla. The apneustic center has an excitatory effect on inspiration, tending to prolong inspiration. The pneumotaxic center switches inspiration off, assisting in the control of respiratory rate and inspiratory volume. Brain injuries that damage the connection between the pneumotaxic and apneustic centers result in an irregular breathing pattern that consists of prolonged inspiratory gasps interrupted by expiratory efforts.

Axons from the neurons in the respiratory center cross in the midline and descend in the ventrolateral columns of the spinal cord. The tracts that control expiration and inspiration are spatially separated in the cord, as are the tracts that transmit specialized reflexes (*i.e.*, coughing and hiccupping) and voluntary control of ventilation. Only at the level of the spinal cord are the respiratory impulses integrated to produce a reflex response.

Regulation of Breathing

The control of breathing has automatic and voluntary components. The automatic regulation of ventilation is controlled by input from two types of sensors or receptors: chemoreceptors and lung receptors. Chemoreceptors monitor blood levels of oxygen, carbon dioxide, and pH and adjust ventilation to meet the changing metabolic needs of the body. Lung receptors monitor breathing patterns and lung function.

Voluntary regulation of ventilation integrates breathing with voluntary acts such as speaking, blowing, and singing. These acts, which are initiated by the motor and premotor cortex, cause a temporary suspension of automatic breathing. The automatic and voluntary components of respiration are regulated by afferent impulses transmitted to the respiratory center from a number of sources. Afferent input from higher brain centers is evidenced by the fact that a person can consciously alter the depth and rate of respiration. Fever, pain, and emotion exert their influence through lower brain centers. Vagal afferents from sensory receptors in the lungs and airways are integrated in the dorsal area of the respiratory center.

Chemoreceptors

Tissue needs for oxygen and the removal of carbon dioxide are regulated by chemoreceptors that monitor blood levels of these gases. Input from these sensors is transmitted to the respiratory center, and ventilation is adjusted to maintain the ABGs within a normal range.

There are two types of chemoreceptors: central and peripheral. The most important chemoreceptors for sensing changes in the PCO_2 of the blood are the *central chemoreceptors*, which are located in chemosensitive regions near the respiratory center in the medulla. The central chemoreceptors are surrounded by brain extracellular fluid and respond to changes in its hydrogen ion (H^+) concentration. The composition of the extracellular fluid surrounding the chemoreceptors is governed by the cerebral spinal fluid (CSF), local blood flow, and tissue metabolism. Of these, the CSF is apparently the most important. The CSF is separated from the blood by the blood–brain barrier, which permits free diffusion of carbon dioxide but not bicarbonate (HCO_3^-) or H^+. The carbon dioxide combines rapidly with water to form carbonic acid (H_2CO_3), which dissociates into H^+ and HCO_3^-. When the PCO_2 rises, carbon dioxide from the blood diffuses into the CSF, liberating H^+, which then stimulates the chemoreceptors. The central chemoreceptors are extremely sensitive to short-term changes in PCO_2. An increase in PCO_2 levels produces an increase in ventilation that reaches its peak within a minute or so and then declines if the PCO_2 level remains elevated. Thus, people with chronically elevated levels of PCO_2 no longer have a response to this stimulus for increased ventilation but rely on the stimulus provided by a decrease in blood PO_2 levels. This occurs commonly with people who have COPD and is referred to as CO_2 narcosis.

The *peripheral chemoreceptors* are located in the carotid and aortic bodies, which are found at the bifurcation of the common carotid arteries and in the arch of the aorta, respectively (see Fig. 29.23). These chemoreceptors monitor arterial blood oxygen levels. Although the peripheral chemoreceptors also monitor carbon dioxide, they play a much more important role in monitoring oxygen levels. These receptors exert little control over ventilation until the PO_2 has dropped below 60 mm Hg. Thus, hypoxia is the main stimulus for ventilation in people with chronically elevated levels of carbon dioxide. If these people are given oxygen therapy at a level sufficient to increase the PO_2 above that needed to stimulate the peripheral chemoreceptors, their ventilation may be seriously depressed.

Lung Receptors

Lung and chest wall receptors monitor the status of breathing in terms of airway resistance and lung expansion. There are three types of lung receptors: stretch, irritant, and juxtacapillary receptors.

Stretch receptors are located in the smooth muscle layers of the conducting airways. They respond to changes in pressure in the walls of the airways. When the lungs are inflated, these receptors inhibit inspiration and promote expiration. They are important in establishing breathing patterns and minimizing the work of breathing by adjusting respiratory rate and V_T to accommodate changes in lung compliance and airway resistance.

The *irritant receptors* are located between the airway epithelial cells. They are stimulated by noxious gases, cigarette smoke, inhaled dust, and cold air. Stimulation of the irritant receptors leads to airway constriction and a pattern of rapid, shallow breathing. This pattern of breathing probably protects respiratory tissues from the damaging effects of toxic inhalants. It also is thought that the mechanical stimulation of these receptors may ensure more uniform lung expansion by initiating periodic sighing and yawning. It is also possible that these receptors are involved in the bronchoconstriction response that occurs in some people with bronchial asthma.

The *juxtacapillary* or *J receptors* are located in the alveolar wall, close to the pulmonary capillaries. It is thought that these receptors sense lung congestion. These receptors may be responsible for the rapid, shallow breathing that occurs with pulmonary edema, pulmonary embolism, and pneumonia.[5]

Cough Reflex

Coughing is a neurally mediated reflex that protects the lungs from accumulation of secretions and from entry of irritating and destructive substances. It is one of the primary defense mechanisms of the respiratory tract. The cough reflex is initiated by receptors located in the tracheobronchial wall. These receptors are extremely sensitive to irritating substances and to the presence of excess secretions. Afferent impulses from these receptors are transmitted through the vagus to the medullary center, which integrates the cough response.

Coughing itself requires the rapid inspiration of a large volume of air (usually about 2.5 L), followed by rapid closure of the glottis and forceful contraction of the abdominal and expiratory muscles. As these muscles contract, intrathoracic pressures are elevated to levels of 100 mm Hg or more. The rapid opening of the glottis at this point leads to an explosive expulsion of air.

Many conditions can interfere with the cough reflex and its protective function. The reflex is impaired in people whose abdominal or respiratory muscles are weak. This problem can be caused by disease conditions that lead to muscle weakness or paralysis, by prolonged inactivity, or as an outcome of surgery involving these muscles. Bed rest interferes with expansion of the chest and limits the amount of air that can be taken into the lungs in preparation for coughing, making the cough weak and ineffective. Disease conditions that prevent effective closure of the glottis and laryngeal muscles interfere with production of the marked increase in intrathoracic pressure that is needed for effective coughing. The presence of a nasogastric tube, for example, may prevent closure of the upper airway structures and may fatigue the receptors for the cough reflex that are located in the area. The cough reflex also is impaired when there is depressed function of the medullary centers in the brain that integrate the cough reflex. Interruption of the central integration aspect of the cough reflex can arise as the result of disease of this part of the brain or the action of drugs that depress the cough center.

Dyspnea

Dyspnea is a subjective sensation or a person's perception of difficulty in breathing that includes the perception of labored breathing and the reaction to that sensation. The terms *dyspnea*, *breathlessness*, and *shortness of breath (SOB)* often are used interchangeably. Dyspnea is observed in at least three major cardiopulmonary disease states:

- Primary lung diseases, such as pneumonia, asthma, and emphysema
- Heart disease that is characterized by pulmonary congestion

- Neuromuscular disorders, such as myasthenia gravis and muscular dystrophy, that affect the respiratory muscles

Although dyspnea commonly is associated with respiratory disease, it also occurs for some people only during exercise and is referred to as exercise-induced reactive airway disorder or exercise-induced asthma.

The cause of dyspnea is unknown. Four types of mechanisms have been proposed to explain the sensation:

- Stimulation of lung receptors
- Increased sensitivity to changes in ventilation perceived through central nervous system mechanisms
- Reduced ventilatory capacity or breathing reserve
- Stimulation of neural receptors in the muscle fibers of the intercostals and diaphragm and of receptors in the skeletal joints

The first of the suggested mechanisms is stimulation of lung receptors. These receptors are stimulated by the contraction of bronchial smooth muscle, the stretch of the bronchial wall, pulmonary congestion, and conditions that decrease lung compliance. The second category of proposed mechanisms focuses on central nervous system mechanisms that transmit information to the cortex regarding respiratory muscle weakness or a discrepancy between the increased effort of breathing and inadequate respiratory muscle contraction. The third type of mechanism focuses on a reduction in ventilatory capacity or breathing reserve. A reduction in breathing reserve (*i.e.*, maximum voluntary ventilation not being used during a given activity) to less than 65% to 75% usually correlates well with dyspnea. The fourth possible mechanism is stimulation of muscle and joint receptors in the respiratory musculature because of a discrepancy in the tension generated by these muscles and the V_T that results. These receptors, once stimulated, transmit signals that bring about an awareness of the breathing discrepancy. Like other subjective symptoms, such as fatigue and pain, dyspnea is difficult to quantify because it relies on a person's perception of the problem.

The most common method for measuring dyspnea is a retrospective self-perceived determination of the level of daily activity at which a person experiences dyspnea. Several scales are available for this use. One of these uses four grades of dyspnea to evaluate disability. The visual analog scale may be used to assess breathing difficulty that occurs with a given activity, such as walking a certain distance. The visual analog scale consists of a continuum line (often 10 cm in length) with descriptors such as "easy to breathe" on one end and "very difficult to breathe" on the other. The person being assessed selects a point on the scale that describes his or her perceived dyspnea.

The treatment of dyspnea depends on the cause. For example, people with impaired respiratory function may require oxygen therapy, and those with pulmonary edema may require measures to improve heart function. Methods to decrease anxiety, breathing retraining, and energy conservation measures may be used to decrease the subjective sensation of dyspnea.

IN SUMMARY

The respiratory system requires continuous input from the nervous system. Movement of the diaphragm, intercostal muscles, and other respiratory muscles is controlled by neurons of the respiratory center located in the pons and medulla. The control of breathing has automatic and voluntary components. The automatic regulation of ventilation is controlled by two types of receptors: lung receptors, which protect respiratory structures, and chemoreceptors, which monitor the gas exchange function of the lungs by sensing changes in blood levels of carbon dioxide, oxygen, and pH. There are three types of lung receptors: stretch receptors, which monitor lung inflation; irritant receptors, which protect against the damaging effects of toxic inhalants; and J receptors, which are thought to sense lung congestion. There are two groups of chemoreceptors: central and peripheral. The central chemoreceptors are the most important in sensing changes in carbon dioxide levels, and the peripheral chemoreceptors function in sensing arterial blood oxygen levels.

Voluntary respiratory control is needed for integrating breathing and actions such as speaking, blowing, and singing. These acts, which are initiated by the motor and premotor cortex, cause temporary suspension of automatic breathing. The cough reflex protects the lungs from the accumulation of secretions and from the entry of irritating and destructive substances; it is one of the primary defense mechanisms of the respiratory tract. Dyspnea is a subjective sensation of difficulty in breathing that is seen in cardiac, pulmonary, and neuromuscular disorders that affect the respiratory muscles.

GERIATRIC Considerations

- A decrease in surface area and elasticity of the alveoli in older adults causes less effective exchange of oxygen and carbon dioxide and chest wall expansion.[6]
- Respiratory dead space, the area where oxygen and carbon dioxide are not exchanged, increases with age,[6] resulting in a ventilation/perfusion inequality.
- Older adults lack the ability to quickly increase respirations[6] resulting in decreased compensation to correct acid base imbalances.

PEDIATRIC Considerations

- Children have an increased risk for respiratory distress because of narrow airways and immature chemoreceptors that respond to oxygen and carbon dioxide levels in the blood.[7]
- Hypoxia, a decreased oxygen concentration in arterial blood, results from an increased need for oxygen.[7]
- Barrel chest is often present in infants and toddlers.[7]
- A decreased lung capacity and immature intercostal muscles result in less pulmonary reserve, placing children at risk for hypoxemia.[7]
- Chest retraction associated with respiratory distress is due to a compliant and flexible bony chest of a child.[7]
- Normal newborns have lower normal oxygen saturation taking at least an hour to reach the desired normal saturation levels of 88%.[8]

REVIEW EXERCISES

1. Calculate the *partial pressure* of oxygen (PO_2) in the alveoli at an atmospheric pressure at sea level (760 mm Hg); Denver, Colorado, at 5431 feet (621 mm Hg); and Berthoud Pass, Colorado at 12,490 feet (477 mm Hg). Consider that the oxygen concentration is 21% and the water vapor pressure in the lungs is 47 mm Hg.
2. Use the solubility coefficient for oxygen and the oxygen dissociation curve depicted in Figure 29.22 to answer the following questions:
   A. *What is the hemoglobin saturation at a high altitude in which the barometric pressure is 500 mm Hg (consider oxygen to represent 21% of the total gases)?*
   B. *It is usually recommended that the hemoglobin saturation of people with chronic lung disease be maintained at about 89% to 90% when they are receiving supplemental low-flow oxygen. What would their PO_2 be at this level of hemoglobin saturation and what is the rationale for keeping the PO_2 at this level?*
   C. *What is the oxygen content of a person with a hemoglobin level of 6 g/dL who is breathing room air?*
   D. *What is the oxygen content of a person with CO poisoning who is receiving 100% oxygen at 3 atmospheres' pressure in a hyperbaric chamber? Consider that most of the person's hemoglobin is saturated with CO.*

References

1. Boron W. F., Boulpaep E. L. (2017). *Medical physiology* (3rd ed.). Philadelphia, PA: WB Saunders.
2. Coleman W. B., Songalis T. (2018). *Molecular pathology: The molecular basis of human disease* (2nd ed.). San Diego, CA: Elsevier.
3. Gaunsbaek M. Q., Rasmussen K. J., Beers M. F., (2013). Lung surfactant protein D (SP-D) response and regulation during acute and chronic lung injury. *Lung* 191(3), 295–303.
4. Andreoli T., Benjamin I., Griggs R., et al. (Eds.) (2016). *Andreoli and Carpenter's Cecil essentials of medicine* (9th ed.). St. Louis, MO: Elsevier.
5. West J. B. (2012). *Respiratory physiology: The essentials* (9th ed.). Philadelphia, PA: Lippincott Williams & Wilkins.
6. Hinkle J. L., Cheever K. H. (2018). *Brunner & Suddarth's textbook of medical-surgical nursing* (14th ed.). Philadelphia, PA: Wolters Kluwer.
7. Kline-Tilford A. M. (2014). The child with altered respiratory status. In Bowden V., Greenberg C. S. (Eds.) *Children and their families the continuum of nursing care* (3rd ed.). Philadelphia, PA: Wolters Kluwer.
8. World Health Organization. (2016). *Oxygen therapy for children.* Geneva, Switzerland: WHO Document Production Services.

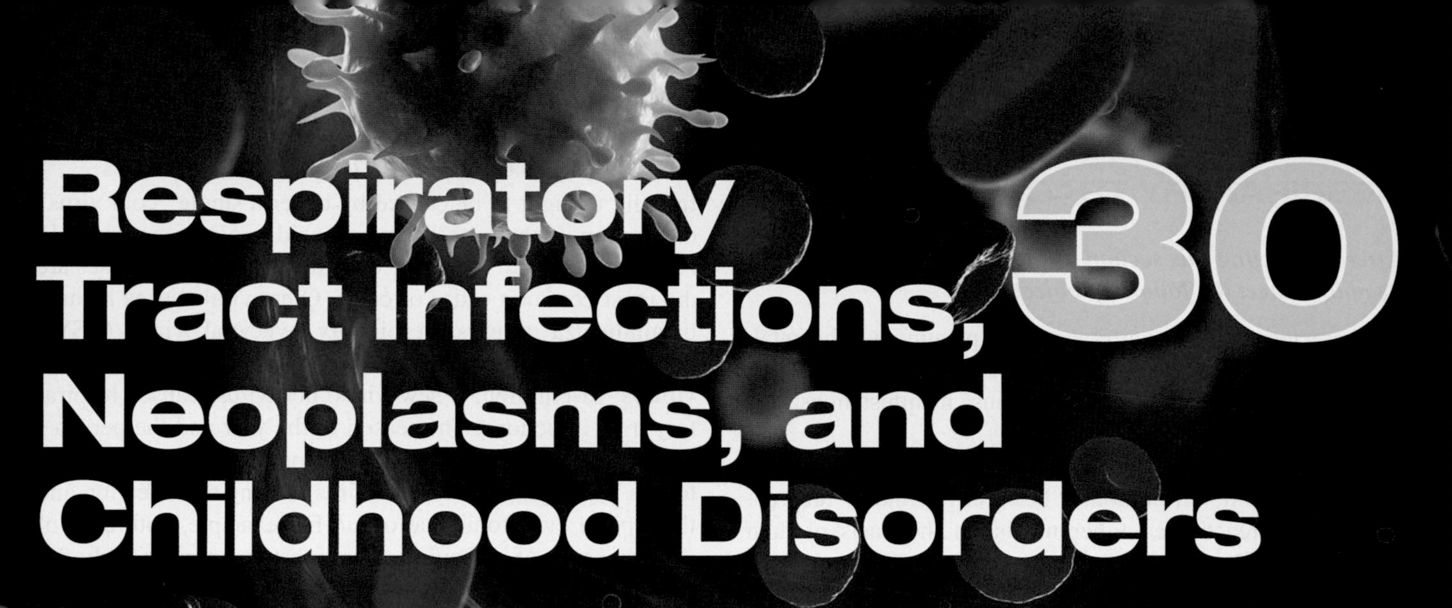

Respiratory Tract Infections, Neoplasms, and Childhood Disorders

30

Tracy McClinton, Emma Murray, and Stephanie Nikbakht

Respiratory illnesses represent one of the more common reasons for visits to the physician, admission to the hospital, and forced inactivity among all age groups. The common cold, although not usually serious, is a frequent cause of missed work and school days. Pneumonia is the eighth leading cause of death in the United States, particularly among the elderly and those with compromised immune function.[1] In addition, it is the largest infectious cause of death among children in the world.[2] Tuberculosis remains one of the deadliest diseases in the world and affects one third of the world population.[3] A large number of people have multidrug-resistant TB, and many are immunocompromised. Immunocompromised people experience all types of bacterial, viral, and fungal infections. The most frequently seen fungal infections include histoplasmosis, coccidioidomycosis, and blastomycosis. Lung cancer remains the leading cause of cancer death worldwide.[4] Children with upper and lower airway infections represent a large number of visits to primary care providers. Premature infants, especially those who experience respiratory distress syndrome (RDS), are at high risk for chronic respiratory infections and other complications such as bronchopulmonary dysplasia (BPD).

RESPIRATORY TRACT INFECTIONS

After completing this section of the chapter, the learner will be able to meet the following objectives:

- Characterize community-acquired pneumonia, hospital-acquired pneumonia, and pneumonia in immunocompromised people in terms of pathogens, manifestations, and prognosis.
- Describe the immunologic properties of the tubercle bacillus, and differentiate between primary tuberculosis and reactivated tuberculosis on the basis of their pathophysiology.

The respiratory tract is susceptible to infectious processes caused by multiple types of microorganisms. Infections can involve the upper respiratory tract (*i.e.*, nose, oropharynx, and larynx), the lower respiratory tract (*i.e.*, lower airways and lungs), or the upper and lower airways. For the most part, the signs and symptoms of respiratory tract infections depend on the function of the structure involved, the severity of the infectious process, and the person's age and general health status. The discussion in this section of the chapter focuses on the common cold, rhinosinusitis, influenza, pneumonia, tuberculosis, and fungal infections of the lung. Acute respiratory infections in children are discussed in the last section of the chapter.

Viruses are the most frequent cause of respiratory tract infections. They can cause infections ranging from a self-limited cold to life-threatening pneumonia. Moreover, viral infections can damage bronchial epithelium, obstruct airways, and lead to secondary bacterial infections. Each viral species has its own pattern of respiratory tract involvement. For example, the rhinoviruses grow best at 33°C and often exacerbate asthma attacks, acute wheezing, or pneumonia.[5] Viruses are able to move from the nasal cavity to the upper airways by binding to the intercellular adhesion molecule (ICAM-1). People with compromised immunologic response are most susceptible to having a virus cause serious gas exchange or ventilation problems.[6]

Other microorganisms, such as bacteria (*e.g.*, pneumococci, staphylococci), mycobacteria (*e.g.*, *Mycobacterium tuberculosis*), fungi (*e.g.*, *Histoplasma capsulatum* [histoplasmosis], *Coccidioides immitis* [coccidioidomycosis], and *Blastomyces dermatitidis* [blastomycosis]), and opportunistic organisms (*e.g.*, *Pneumocystis jirovecii*), also produce infections of the lung. In turn, many of these infections produce significant morbidity and mortality.

The Common Cold

The common cold is a viral infection of the upper respiratory tract. It occurs more frequently than any other respiratory tract infection. Most adults have three to four colds per year, whereas the average school child may have up to 6 to 8 per year.[6]

Etiology and Pathogenesis

Initially thought to be caused by either a single "cold virus" or a group of them, the common cold is now recognized to be associated with a number of viruses.[6] The rhinoviruses are the most common cause of colds. Other viral causes include parainfluenza viruses, respiratory syncytial virus (RSV), human metapneumovirus (hMPV), coronaviruses, and adenoviruses. In children, a new virus, bocavirus, causes respiratory tract infections. The season of the year and the person's age, immunologic state, and prior exposure are important factors in identifying the type of virus causing the infection and the type of symptoms that occur. For example, outbreaks of colds because of rhinoviruses are most common in early fall and late spring. Colds because of RSV peak in the winter and spring months, and infections because of the adenoviruses and coronaviruses are more frequent during the winter and spring months. Infections resulting from the RSV and parainfluenza viruses are most common and severe in infants and children younger than 6 years of age. Infections occur less frequently and with milder symptoms with increasing age until after 65 years of age. Parainfluenza viruses often produce lower respiratory symptoms with first infections, but less severe upper respiratory symptoms with reinfections.

The "cold viruses" are spread rapidly from person to person. Children are the major reservoir of cold viruses, often acquiring a new virus from another child in school or day care. The fingers are the greatest source of spread, and the nasal mucosa and conjunctival surface of the eyes are the most common portals for entry of the virus. The illness lasts on average about 7 days with an incubation period of about 2 days.[7] Aerosol spread of colds through coughing and sneezing is much less important than the spread through direct mucous membrane contact by fingers picking up the virus from contaminated surfaces and carrying it to the nasal membranes and eyes.[7]

Clinical Manifestations

The condition usually begins with a feeling of dryness and stuffiness affecting mainly the nasopharynx. This is followed by excessive production of nasal secretions and tearing of the eyes, which is often referred to as rhinitis. Usually, the secretions remain clear and watery. The mucous membranes of the upper respiratory tract become reddened and swollen. Often there is postnasal dripping (PND), which irritates the pharynx and larynx, causing sore throat and hoarseness. The affected person may experience headache and generalized malaise. In severe cases, there may be chills, fever, and exhaustion. Viral shedding may begin shortly before symptoms.[7]

Treatment

The common cold is an acute and self-limited illness in people who are otherwise healthy. Therefore, symptomatic treatment with rest and antipyretic drugs is usually all that is needed. Antibiotics are ineffective against viral infections and are not recommended. Many over-the-counter (OTC) remedies are available for treating the common cold. Antihistamines are popular OTC drugs because of their action in drying nasal secretions. However, they may dry up bronchial secretions and worsen the cough, and they may cause dizziness, drowsiness, and impaired judgment. If these drugs are used too frequently over too many days, they can cause rebound symptoms. In addition, there is no evidence that they shorten the duration of the cold. Decongestant drugs (*i.e.*, sympathomimetic agents) are available in OTC nasal sprays, drops, and oral cold medications. These drugs constrict the blood vessels in the swollen nasal mucosa and reduce nasal swelling. Rebound nasal swelling can occur with indiscriminate use of nasal drops and sprays. Oral preparations containing decongestants may cause systemic vasoconstriction and elevation of blood pressure when given in doses large enough to relieve nasal congestion. Thus, people with hypertension, heart disease, hyperthyroidism, diabetes mellitus, or other health problems should avoid taking these drugs.[8]

There is controversy regarding the use of vitamin C to reduce the incidence and severity of colds and influenza. Vitamin C intake has been found to be beneficial in shortening the duration of the cold if taken before the onset of the cold, but it has shown no true effect on incidence with the general population. Others have found Vitamin C intake to be of questionable value in decreasing the severity of a common cold.[8]

Rhinosinusitis

Rhinosinusitis refers to inflammation involving the nasal sinuses.

The paranasal sinuses are air sacs that develop during embryogenesis from a series of ridges and furrows within the cartilaginous capsule surrounding the developing nasal cavity. As development progresses, outpouchings from these furrows become lined with ciliated respiratory epithelium and invade the surrounding facial bones to become the major sinuses. Each sinus remains in constant communication with the nasal cavity through narrow openings or *ostia*. The sinuses are named for the bone in which they are located—frontal, ethmoid, maxillary, and sphenoidal (Fig. 30.1A). The *frontal sinuses* open into the middle meatus of the nasal cavity. The *ethmoid sinuses* consist of 3 to 15 air cells on each side of the ethmoid, with each maintaining a separate path to the nasal chamber. The anterior ethmoid, frontal, and maxillary sinuses all drain into the nasal cavity through a narrow passage called the *ostiomeatal complex* (see Fig. 30.1B). Defects in the anterior ethmoid sinus can obstruct the ostiomeatal complex and cause secondary disease of the frontal or maxillary sinuses. The *maxillary sinuses* are located inferior to the bony orbit and superior to the hard palate, and their openings are located superiorly and medially in the sinus, a location that impedes drainage. The *sphenoidal sinuses* are located just anterior to the pituitary fossa behind the posterior ethmoid sinuses, with their openings draining into the sphenoethmoid recess at the top of the nasal cavity (see Fig. 30.1C).

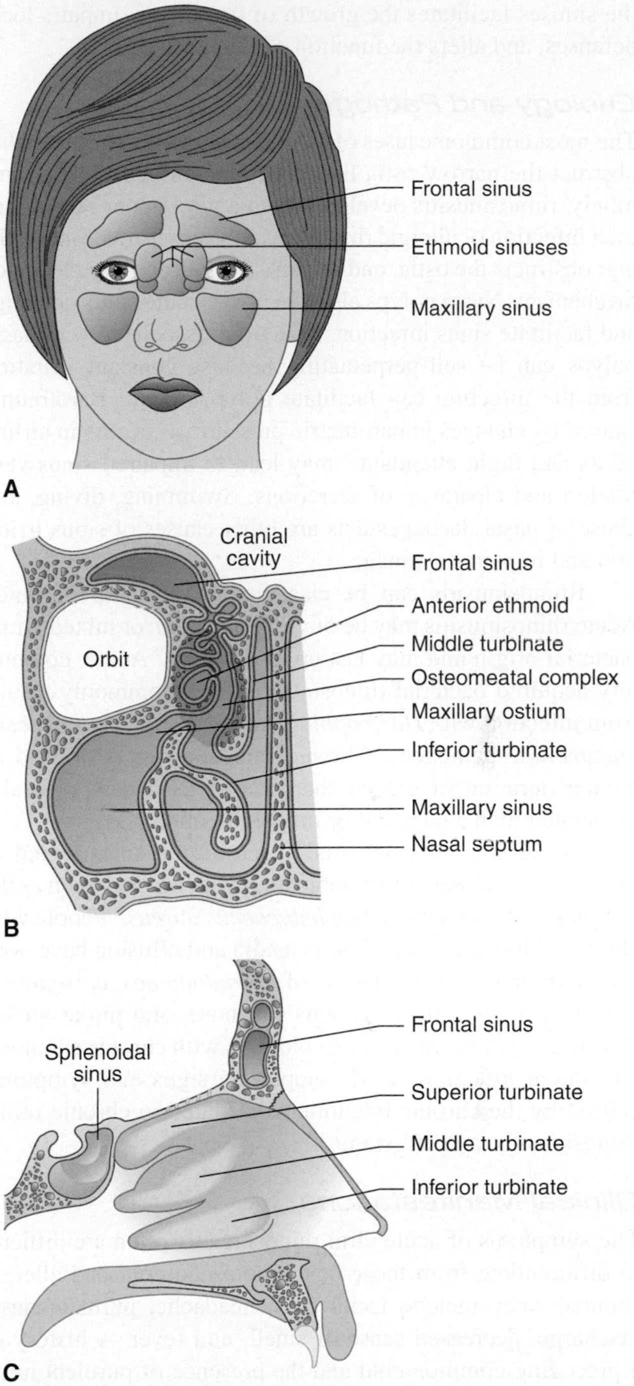

Figure 30.1 • Paranasal sinuses. **(A)** Frontal view showing the frontal, ethmoid, and maxillary sinuses. **(B)** Cross-section of nasal cavity (anterior view). The shaded area is the osteomeatal complex, which is the final common pathway for drainage of the anterior ethmoid, frontal, and maxillary sinuses. **(C)** Lateral wall, left nasal cavity showing the frontal sphenoidal sinuses and the superior, middle, and inferior turbinates.

Each sinus is lined with a mucosal surface that is continuous with that of the nasal passages. An active mucociliary clearance mechanism helps move fluid and microorganisms out of the sinuses and into the nasal cavity. Mucociliary clearance, along with innate and adaptive immune mechanisms, helps to keep the sinuses sterile. The lower oxygen content in the sinuses facilitates the growth of organisms, impairs local defenses, and alters the function of immune cells.

Etiology and Pathogenesis

The most common causes of rhinosinusitis are conditions that obstruct the narrow ostia that drain the sinuses.[9] Most commonly, rhinosinusitis develops when a viral upper respiratory tract infection or allergic rhinitis, which causes mucosal swelling, obstructs the ostia, and impairs the mucociliary clearance mechanism. Nasal polyps also can obstruct the sinus openings and facilitate sinus infection. Infections associated with nasal polyps can be self-perpetuating because constant irritation from the infection can facilitate polyp growth. Barotrauma caused by changes in barometric pressure, as occurs in airline pilots and flight attendants, may lead to impaired sinus ventilation and clearance of secretions. Swimming, diving, and abuse of nasal decongestants are other causes of sinus irritation and impaired drainage.

Rhinosinusitis can be classified as acute or chronic.[9] Acute rhinosinusitis may be of viral, bacterial, or mixed viral–bacterial origin and may last up to 4 weeks.[9] Acute, community-acquired bacterial rhinosinusitis most commonly results from infection with *Haemophilus influenzae* or *Streptococcus pneumoniae* pathogens. Chronic rhinosinusitis is defined as having duration of greater than 12 weeks and is generally associated with a bacterial or fungal infection.[9]

In chronic rhinosinusitis, anaerobic organisms tend to predominate, alone or in combination with aerobes such as the *Streptococcus* species or *Staphylococcus aureus*.[9] People with chronic rhinosinusitis and otitis media and effusion have been found to have accumulation of *Pseudomonas aeruginosa*, which forms biofilm in various ear, nose, and throat areas.[9] This finding of the presence of biofilms with chronic ear, nose, and throat infections lends support to signs and symptoms caused by the chronic inflammation related to chronic otitis, rhinosinusitis, and effusion.[9]

Clinical Manifestations

The symptoms of acute viral rhinosinusitis often are difficult to differentiate from those of the common cold and allergic rhinitis. They include facial pain, headache, purulent nasal discharge, decreased sense of smell, and fever. A history of a preceding common cold and the presence of purulent nasal drainage, pain on bending, unilateral maxillary pain, and pain in the teeth are common with involvement of the maxillary sinuses. The symptoms of acute viral rhinosinusitis usually resolve within 5 to 7 days without medical treatment.[6] Acute bacterial rhinosinusitis is suggested by symptoms that worsen after 5 to 7 days or persist beyond 10 days, or symptoms that are out of proportion to those usually associated with a viral upper respiratory tract infection.[9] People who are immunocompromised, such as those with leukemia, aplastic anemia, a bone marrow transplant, or HIV infection, often present with fever of unknown origin, rhinorrhea, or facial edema. Often, other signs of inflammation such as purulent drainage are absent.

In people with chronic rhinosinusitis, symptoms may consist of sinus pressure with nasal congestion. The symptoms may persist for years with periods of greater severity than others.[9] The person may complain of a headache that is dull and constant. People with chronic rhinosinusitis may have superimposed bouts of acute rhinosinusitis. The epithelial changes that occur during acute rhinosinusitis usually are reversible, but the mucosal changes that occur with chronic rhinosinusitis often are irreversible.

Diagnosis and Treatment

The diagnosis of rhinosinusitis usually is based on symptom history and a physical examination that includes inspection of the nose and throat.[9] Headache because of sinusitis needs to be differentiated from other types of headache. Bending forward, coughing, or sneezing usually exaggerates sinusitis headache. Physical examination findings in acute bacterial sinusitis and viral sinusitis are often times difficult to differentiate with regard to diagnosis.[9]Sinus radiographs and computed tomography (CT) scans may be used. CT scans usually are reserved for diagnosis of chronic rhinosinusitis or to exclude complications.[9] Treatment of rhinosinusitis depends on the cause and includes appropriate use of antibiotics, mucolytic agents, and symptom relief measures. About two thirds of people with acute bacterial rhinosinusitis improve without antibiotic treatment. Most people with viral upper respiratory infections improve within 7 days. Treatment of bacterial infections consists of repeated courses of antibiotics that are culture-guided. Some antibiotic courses may be 3 to 4 weeks or longer. Treatment may also consist of mechanical nasal irrigation and intranasal glucocorticoids.[9] In addition to antibiotic therapy, the treatment of acute rhinosinusitis includes measures to promote adequate drainage by reducing nasal congestion. Oral and topical decongestants may be used for this purpose. The use of intranasal decongestants should be limited to 3 to 5 days to prevent rebound vasodilation. Antihistamines tend to dry up secretions and are not recommended as adjunctive treatment in acute viral or bacterial rhinosinusitis. Mucolytic agents such as guaifenesin may be used to thin secretions. Topical corticosteroids may be used to decrease inflammation in people with allergic rhinitis or rhinosinusitis. Nonpharmacologic measures include saline nasal sprays, nasal irrigation, and mist humidification. However, although no studies have been conducted, most providers feel these nasal sprays and irrigations are not effective.

Surgical intervention directed at correcting obstruction of the ostiomeatal openings may be indicated in people with chronic rhinosinusitis that is resistant to other forms of therapy. Indications for surgical intervention include obstructive nasal polyps and obstructive nasal deformities.

Complications

Because of the sinuses' proximity to the brain and orbital wall, sinusitis can lead to intracranial and orbital wall complications. Intracranial complications are seen most commonly with infection of the frontal and ethmoid sinuses because of their proximity to the dura and drainage of the veins from the frontal sinus into the dural sinus. Orbital complications can range from edema of the eyelids to orbital cellulitis and subperiosteal abscess formation. Facial swelling over the involved sinus, abnormal extraocular movements, protrusion of the eyeball, periorbital edema, or changes in mental status may indicate intracranial complications and require immediate medical attention.[10]

Influenza

Influenza is one of the most important causes of acute upper respiratory tract infection in humans. Influenza, combined with pneumonia, is the eighth leading cause of death in the United States.[1] Rates of infection are highest among children and older adults, but rates of serious illness and death are highest among people 65 years of age or older.[11]

The viruses that cause influenza belong to the Orthomyxoviridae family, whose members are characterized by a segmented, single-stranded ribonucleic acid (RNA) genome.[12] There are three types of influenza viruses that cause epidemics in humans: types A, B, and C. Influenza A differs in its ability to infect multiple species, including avian and mammalian species. The influenza A virus is further divided into subtypes based on two surface glycoproteins: hemagglutinin (HA) and neuraminidase (NA).[12] HA is an attachment protein that allows the virus to enter epithelial cells in the respiratory tract, and NA facilitates viral replication from the cell.[12] Contagion results from the ability of the influenza A virus to develop new HA and NA subtypes against which the population is not protected. An antigenic shift, which involves a major genetic rearrangement in either antigen, may lead to epidemic or pandemic infection. Lesser changes, called *antigenic drift*, find the population partially protected by cross-reacting antibodies. Influenza B and C undergo less frequent antigenic shifts than influenza A, probably because few related viruses exist in mammalian or avian species.[12]

As with many viral respiratory tract infections, influenza is more contagious than bacterial respiratory tract infections. In contrast to the rhinoviruses, transmission occurs by inhalation of droplet nuclei rather than touching contaminated objects. Most infected people develop symptoms of the disease, increasing the likelihood of contagion through spread of infectious droplets. Young children are most likely to become infected and also to spread the infection. The incubation period for influenza is 1 to 4 days, with 2 days being the average. People become infectious starting 1 day before their symptoms begin and remain infectious through approximately 1 week after illness onset.[12] Viral shedding can continue for approximately 3 weeks.

Pathogenesis

The influenza viruses can cause three types of infections: an uncomplicated upper respiratory infection (rhinotracheitis), viral pneumonia, and a respiratory viral infection followed by a bacterial infection. Influenza initially establishes upper airway infection. In doing this, the virus first targets and kills mucous-secreting, ciliated, and other epithelial cells, leaving gaping holes between the underlying basal cells and allowing extracellular fluid to escape. This is the reason for the "runny nose" that is characteristic of this phase of the infection. If the virus spreads to the lower respiratory tract, the infection can cause severe shedding of bronchial and alveolar cells down to a single-cell–thick basal layer. Additionally, compromising the natural defenses of the respiratory tract, influenza infection promotes bacterial adhesion to epithelial cells. Pneumonia may result from a viral pathogenesis or from a secondary bacterial infection.

Clinical Manifestations

In the early stages, the symptoms of influenza often are indistinguishable from other viral infections. There is an abrupt onset of fever and chills, rigors, malaise, muscle aching, headache, profuse, watery nasal discharge, nonproductive cough, and sore throat.[12] One distinguishing feature of an influenza viral infection is the rapid onset, sometimes in as little as 1 to 2 minutes, of profound malaise. The symptoms of uncomplicated rhinotracheitis usually peak by days 3 to 5 and disappear by days 7 to 10. The aforementioned symptoms can be caused by any of the influenza A or B viruses. Influenza C virus infection causes symptoms similar to the common cold.

Viral pneumonia occurs as a complication of influenza, most frequently in older adults or in people with cardiopulmonary disease. However, it has been reported in pregnant women and in healthy, immunocompetent people. It typically develops within 1 day after onset of influenza and is characterized by rapid progression of symptoms. Adults with underlying comorbidities (e.g., heart failure, COPD) have exacerbations when hospitalized with influenza.[12] The clinical course of influenza pneumonia progresses rapidly. It can cause hypoxemia and death within a few days of onset. Survivors often develop diffuse pulmonary fibrosis.

Secondary complications typically include sinusitis, otitis media, bronchitis, bacterial pneumonia, and, in young children, croup; secondary complications may rarely include parotitis or bacterial tracheitis.[12] People in whom secondary bacterial pneumonia develops usually report that they were beginning to feel better when they experienced a return of fever, shaking chills, pleuritic chest pain, and productive cough. The most common causes of secondary bacterial pneumonia are *S. pneumoniae*, *S. aureus*, *H. influenzae*, and *Moraxella catarrhalis*. This form of pneumonia commonly produces less tachypnea and is usually milder than primary influenza pneumonia. Influenza-related deaths can result from pneumonia as well as exacerbations of cardiopulmonary conditions and other disease. Reye syndrome (fatty liver with encephalitis) is a rare complication of influenza, particularly in young children who have been given aspirin as an antipyretic agent.

Diagnosis and Treatment

The appropriate treatment of people with influenza depends on accurate and timely diagnosis. Early diagnosis can reduce the inappropriate use of antibiotics and provide the opportunity for use of an antiviral drug. Rapid diagnostic tests, which are available for use in outpatient settings, allow health care providers to diagnose influenza more accurately, consider treatment options more carefully, and monitor the influenza type and its prevalence in their community.[13]

The goals of treatment for influenza are designed to limit the infection to the upper respiratory tract. The symptomatic approach for treatment of uncomplicated influenza rhinotracheitis focuses on rest, keeping warm, managing the fever, and keeping well hydrated. Analgesics and cough medications can also be used. Rest decreases the oxygen requirements of the body and reduces the respiratory rate and the chance of spreading the virus from the upper to lower respiratory tract. Keeping warm helps maintain the respiratory epithelium at a core body temperature of 37°C (or higher if fever is present), thereby inhibiting viral replication, which is optimal at 35°C. Drinking large amounts of liquids ensures that the function of the epithelial lining of the respiratory tract is not further compromised by dehydration. Antiviral medications may be indicated in some people. Antibacterial antibiotics should be reserved for bacterial complications.

Four antiviral drugs are available for treatment of influenza: amantadine (Symmetrel), rimantadine (Flumadine), zanamivir (Relenza), peramivir (Rapivab), and oseltamivir (Tamiflu).[12] The first-generation antiviral drugs amantadine and rimantadine are similarly effective against influenza A but not influenza B. These agents inhibit the uncoating of viral RNA in the host cells and prevent its replication. Both drugs are effective in prevention of influenza A in high-risk groups and in treatment of people who acquire the disease. Unfortunately, resistance to the drugs develops rapidly, and strains that are resistant to amantadine also are resistant to rimantadine. Amantadine stimulates release of catecholamines, which can produce central nervous system side effects such as anxiety, depression, and insomnia.

The second-generation antiviral drugs zanamivir and oseltamivir are inhibitors of NA, a viral glycoprotein that is necessary for viral replication and release. These drugs, which have been approved for treatment of acute uncomplicated influenza infection, are effective against both influenza A and B viruses. Zanamivir and oseltamivir result in less resistance than amantadine and rimantadine. Zanamivir is administered intranasally, and oseltamivir is administered orally. Zanamivir can cause bronchospasm and is not recommended for people with asthma or chronic obstructive lung disease. To be effective, the antiviral drugs should be initiated within 48 hours after onset of symptoms.[12]

Influenza Immunization

Because influenza is so highly contagious, prevention relies primarily on vaccination. All people 6 months of age and older in the United States are recommended to receive the annual influenza vaccine. The formulation of the vaccines must be changed yearly in response to antigenic changes in the influenza virus. The Centers for Disease Control and Prevention (CDC) Advisory Committee on Immunization Practices (ACIP) annually updates its recommendations for the composition of the vaccine. Influenza vaccines are contraindicated in people with anaphylactic hypersensitivity to eggs or to other components of the vaccine, people with a history Guillain-Barré syndrome, and people with acute febrile illness. Although the inactivated vaccines do not cause asthma exacerbations, they are associated with rare incidents of Guillain-Barré syndrome.[12,13]

The effectiveness of the influenza vaccine in preventing and lessening the effects of influenza infection depends primarily on the age and immunocompetence of the recipient and the match between the virus strains included in the vaccine and those that circulate during the influenza season.[12] When there is a good match, the inactivated vaccine given via intramuscular injection is effective in preventing the illness in approximately 50% to 70% of healthy people younger than 65 years of age.[12] A higher dose of inactivated influenza vaccine is given to seniors older than 65 years.[12]

Avian Influenza (Bird Flu)

Avian influenza, or zoonotic influenza, is an infection caused by avian influenza viruses. The normal hosts for avian influenza viruses are birds and occasionally pigs. These influenza viruses occur naturally among birds.[12] Avian strains of the influenza virus do not usually cause outbreaks of disease in humans unless a reassortment of the virus genome has occurred within an intermediate mammalian host such as a pig. Zoonotic infections that cause a threat are subtypes H_5, H_7, and H_9.[12] In this setting, a virus is produced that contains mammalian characteristics as well as avian characteristics to which humans may not be immune. It is noteworthy that many of the pandemics of the past were thought to arise in Asia, where large human populations live in close proximity to ducks, chickens, and pigs, thus facilitating the phenomenon of viral reassortment. In 2013, an outbreak of avian H_7N_9 was associated with approximately 30% fatality rate of hospitalized people in eastern China.[12]

In past years, a highly pathogenic influenza A subtype, H5N1, was found in poultry in East and Southeast Asian countries.[12] Although the H5N1 strain is highly contagious from one bird to another, its transmission from human to human is relatively inefficient and not sustained. The result is only rare cases in person-to-person transmission. Most cases occur after exposure to infected poultry or surfaces contaminated with poultry droppings. Because infection in humans is associated with a high mortality rate, there is considerable concern that the H5N1 strain might mutate and initiate a pandemic. People who contract avian flu generally complain about typical influenza symptoms along with eye infections, pneumonia, and acute RDS.[12]

There currently is no commercially available vaccine to protect humans against the bird flu. Current commercial rapid diagnostic tests are not optimally sensitive or specific for detection of the virus. Most Asian H5N1 influenza strains are resistant to amantadine and rimantadine. The NA inhibitors, oseltamivir and zanamivir, would probably be effective if administered within 48 hours, but additional studies are needed to demonstrate their effectiveness.

Swine Flu (H1N1)

In June 2009, the World Health Organization identified a world influenza pandemic. This pandemic was caused by an influenza A flu known as the swine-origin influenza A flu (H1N1). H1N1 caused extremely high fevers and was especially serious in young adults less than 25 years of age. Interestingly, older adults were not at higher risk for H1N1 as they tend to be for most infections such as seasonal influenza. This virus is spread from human to human and is generally referred to as the swine flu. The majority of people affected by the virus did not experience severe illness although there were some who needed hospitalization and who even died. The CDC does recommend that most people be vaccinated against H1N1.

Pneumonias

The term *pneumonia* describes inflammation of parenchymal structures of the lung in the lower respiratory tract, such as the alveoli and the bronchioles. It causes more than 1.25 million hospitalizations annually.[13] Pneumonia is the eighth leading cause of death in the United States and the most common cause of death from infectious disease.[2] Etiologic agents include infectious and noninfectious agents. Inhalation of irritating fumes or aspiration of gastric contents, although much less common than infectious causes, can result in severe pneumonia.

Although antibiotics have significantly reduced the mortality rate from pneumonias, these diseases remain an important immediate cause of death among older adults and in people with debilitating diseases.[13] There have been subtle changes in the spectrum of microorganisms that cause infectious pneumonias, including a decrease in pneumonias caused by *S. pneumoniae* and an increase in pneumonias caused by other microorganisms such as *Pseudomonas*, *Candida* and other fungi, and nonspecific viruses. Many of these pneumonias occur in people with impaired immune defenses, including those on immunosuppressant drugs to prevent organ transplant of bone marrow rejection, or in people who frequently take anti-inflammatory drugs.

Because of the overlap in symptomatology and changing spectrum of infectious organisms involved, pneumonias are increasingly being classified according to the setting (community or hospital in which it occurs). Using this classification, pneumonias can be community-acquired and hospital-acquired (nosocomial) pneumonias.[13] People with compromised immune function constitute a special concern in both categories.

Pneumonias can also be classified according to the type of agent (typical or atypical) causing the infection, and distribution of the infection (lobar pneumonia or bronchopneumonia). *Typical pneumonias* result from infection by bacteria that multiply extracellularly in the alveoli and cause inflammation and exudation of fluid into the air-filled spaces of the alveoli (Fig. 30.2). *Atypical pneumonias* are caused by viral and mycoplasma infections that involve the alveolar septum and the interstitium of the lung. They produce less striking symptoms and physical findings than bacterial pneumonia. For example, there is a lack of alveolar infiltration and purulent sputum, leukocytosis, and lobar consolidation on the chest imaging.

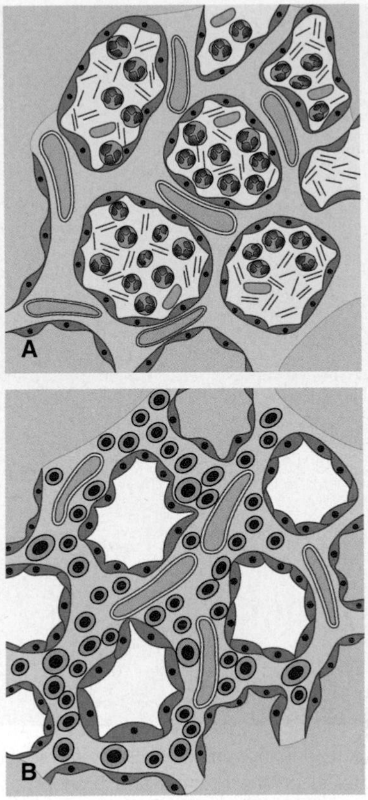

Figure 30.2 • Location of inflammatory processes in (**A**) typical and (**B**) atypical forms of pneumonia.

Acute bacterial pneumonias can be classified as lobar pneumonia or bronchopneumonia, based on their anatomic pattern of distribution (Fig. 30.3). In general, *lobar pneumonia* refers to consolidation of a part or all of a lung lobe, and *bronchopneumonia* signifies a patchy consolidation involving more than one lobe (see Fig. 30.4).

KEY POINTS

PNEUMONIAS

- Pneumonias are respiratory disorders involving inflammation of the lung structures, such as the alveoli and bronchioles.
- Pneumonias due to infectious agents commonly are classified according to the source of infection (community- versus hospital-acquired) and according to the immune status of the host (pneumonia in the immunocompromised person).

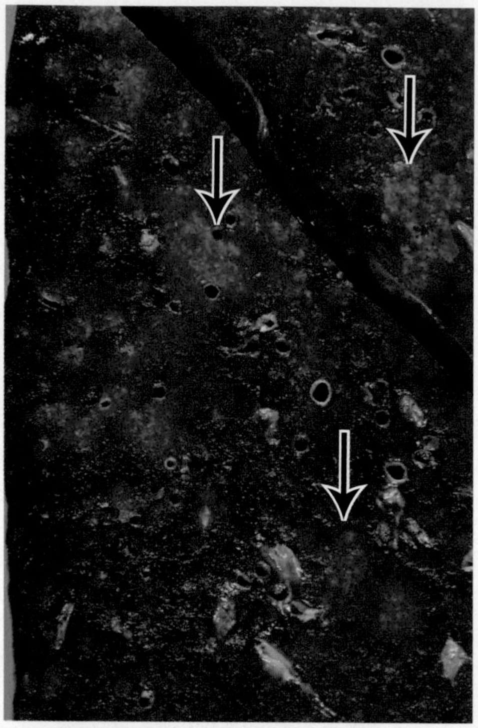

Figure 30.3 • Bronchopneumonia. Scattered foci of consolidation (*arrows*) are centered on the bronchi and bronchioles. (From Strayer D.S., Rubin R. (Eds.) (2015). *Rubin's pathology: Clinicopathologic foundations of medicine* (7th ed., Fig. 18-12, p. 687). Philadelphia, PA: Lippincott Williams & Wilkins.)

Community-Acquired Pneumonia

The term *community-acquired pneumonia* is used to describe infections from organisms found in the community rather than in the hospital or nursing home. It is defined as an infection that begins outside the hospital or is diagnosed within 48 hours after admission to the hospital in a person who has not resided in a long-term care facility for 14 days or more before admission.[14] Community-acquired pneumonia may be further categorized according to risk of mortality and need for hospitalization based on age, presence of coexisting disease, and severity of illness, using physical examination, laboratory, and radiologic findings.[13]

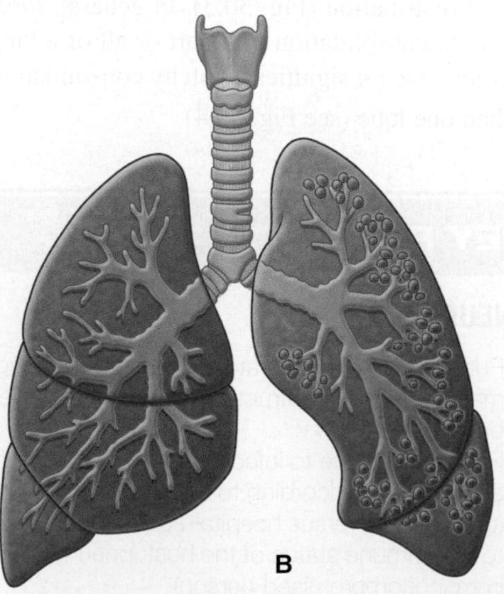

Figure 30.4 • Distribution of lung involvement in (**A**) lobar pneumonia and (**B**) bronchopneumonia.

Community-acquired pneumonia may be either bacterial or viral. The most common cause of infection in all categories is *S. pneumoniae*.[13] Other common pathogens include *H. influenzae*, *S. aureus*, and gram-negative bacilli. Less common agents, although they are becoming more common, are *Mycoplasma pneumoniae*, *Legionella*,[13] *Chlamydia* species, and viruses, sometimes called *atypical agents*. Common viral causes of community-acquired pneumonia include the influenza virus, RSV, adenovirus, and parainfluenza virus.

The methods used in the diagnosis of community-acquired pneumonia depend on age, coexisting health problems, and the severity of illness. In people younger than 65 years of age and without coexisting disease, diagnosis is usually based on history and physical examination, chest radiographs, and knowledge of the microorganisms currently causing infections in the community. Sputum specimens may be obtained for staining procedures and culture. Blood cultures may be done for people requiring hospitalization.

Treatment involves the use of appropriate antibiotic therapy.[13] Empiric antibiotic therapy, based on knowledge regarding an antibiotic's spectrum of action and ability to penetrate bronchopulmonary secretions, often is used for people with community-acquired pneumonia who do not require hospitalization. Hospitalization and more intensive care may be required depending on the person's age, preexisting health status, and severity of the infection.

Hospital-Acquired Pneumonia

Hospital-acquired pneumonia is defined as a lower respiratory tract infection that was not present or incubating on admission to the hospital. Usually, infections occurring 48 hours or more after admission are considered hospital acquired.[13] Hospital-acquired pneumonia is the second most common cause of hospital-acquired infection and has a mortality rate of 30% to 50%.[13] People requiring intubation and mechanical ventilation are particularly at risk. Others at risk include those with compromised immune function, chronic lung disease, and airway instrumentation, such as endotracheal intubation or tracheotomy.

Most hospital-acquired infections are bacterial. The organisms are those present in the hospital environment and include *P. aeruginosa*, *S. aureus*, *Enterobacter* species, *Klebsiella* species, *Escherichia coli*, and *Serratia* species. The organisms that are responsible for hospital-acquired pneumonias are different from those responsible for community-acquired pneumonias, and many of them have acquired antibiotic resistance and are more difficult to treat.

Pneumonia in Immunocompromised People

Pneumonia in immunocompromised people remains a major source of morbidity and mortality. The term *immunocompromised host* usually is applied to people with a variety of underlying defects in host defenses.[15] It includes people with primary and acquired immunodeficiency states, those who have undergone bone marrow or organ transplantation, people with solid organ or hematologic cancers, and those on corticosteroid and other immunosuppressant drugs.

Although almost all types of microorganisms can cause pulmonary infection in immunocompromised people, certain types of immunologic defects tend to favor certain types of infections.[15] Defects in humoral immunity predispose to bacterial infections against which antibodies play an important role, whereas defects in cellular immunity predispose to infections caused by viruses, fungi, mycobacteria, and protozoa. Neutropenia and impaired granulocyte function, as occur in people with leukemia, chemotherapy, and bone marrow depression, predispose to infections caused by *S. aureus*, *Aspergillus*, gram-negative bacilli, and *Candida*. The time course of infection often provides a hint to the type of agent involved. A fulminant pneumonia usually is caused by bacterial infection, whereas an insidious onset usually is indicative of a viral, fungal, protozoal, or mycobacterial infection.

Acute Bacterial (Typical) Pneumonias

Bacterial pneumonias remain an important cause of mortality among older adults and people with debilitating illnesses. The lung below the main bronchi is normally sterile despite frequent entry of microorganisms into the air passages by inhalation during ventilation or aspiration of nasopharyngeal secretions. Most people unknowingly aspirate small amounts of organisms that have colonized their upper airways, particularly during sleep. These organisms do not normally cause infection because of the small numbers that are aspirated and because of the respiratory tract's defense mechanisms that prevent them from entering the distal air passages[13] (Table 30.1). Loss of the cough reflex, damage to the ciliated endothelium that lines the respiratory tract, or impaired immune defenses predispose to colonization and infection of the lower respiratory system. Bacterial adherence also plays a role in colonization of the lower airways. The epithelial cells of critically and chronically ill people are more receptive to binding microorganisms that cause pneumonia. Other clinical risk factors favoring colonization of the tracheobronchial tree include antibiotic therapy that alters the normal bacterial flora, diabetes, smoking, chronic bronchitis, and viral infection.

Bacterial pneumonias are commonly classified according to etiologic agent. This is because the clinical and morphologic features, and thus the therapeutic implications, often vary with the causative agent. The discussion in this section focuses on two types of bacterial pneumonia: pneumococcal pneumonia and Legionnaire disease.

Pneumococcal Pneumonia. *Streptococcus pneumoniae* (pneumococcus) remains the most common cause of bacterial pneumonia.[13] *S. pneumoniae* is a gram-positive diplococcus, possessing a capsule of polysaccharide. The virulence of the pneumococcus is a function of its capsule, which prevents or delays digestion by phagocytes. The polysaccharide is an antigen that primarily elicits a B cell response with antibody production. In the absence of antibody, clearance of the pneumococci from the body relies on the reticuloendothelial system, with the macrophages in the spleen playing a major role in elimination of the organism.[13] This, along with the spleen's role in antibody production, increases the risk for pneumococcal bacteremia in people who are anatomically or functionally asplenic, such as children with sickle cell disease. The initial step in the pathogenesis of pneumococcal infection is the attachment and colonization of the organism to the mucus and cells of the nasopharynx. Colonization does not equate with signs of infection. Perfectly healthy people can be colonized and carry the organism without evidence of infection. Healthy colonized people largely spread particular strains of pneumococci, particularly antibiotic-resistant strains.

The pathologic process of pneumococcal pneumonia can be divided into the four stages—edema, red hepatization, gray hepatization, and resolution[15] (see Fig. 30.5).

During the first stage of pneumococcal pneumonia, the alveoli become filled with a protein-rich edema fluid

TABLE 30.1 RESPIRATORY DEFENSE MECHANISMS AND CONDITIONS THAT IMPAIR THEIR EFFECTIVENESS

DEFENSE MECHANISM	FUNCTION	FACTORS THAT IMPAIR EFFECTIVENESS
Glottic and cough reflexes	Protect against aspiration into tracheobronchial tree	Loss of cough reflex because of stroke or neural lesion, neuromuscular disease, abdominal or chest surgery, depression of the cough reflex because of sedation or anesthesia, presence of a nasogastric tube (tends to cause adaptation of afferent receptors)
Mucociliary blanket	Removes secretions, microorganisms, and particles from the respiratory tract	Smoking, viral diseases, chilling, inhalation of irritating gases
Phagocytic and bactericidal action of alveolar macrophages	Removes microorganisms and foreign particles from the lung	Tobacco smoke, chilling, alcohol, oxygen intoxication
Immune defenses (IgA and IgG and cell-mediated immunity)	Destroy microorganisms	Congenital and acquired immunodeficiency states

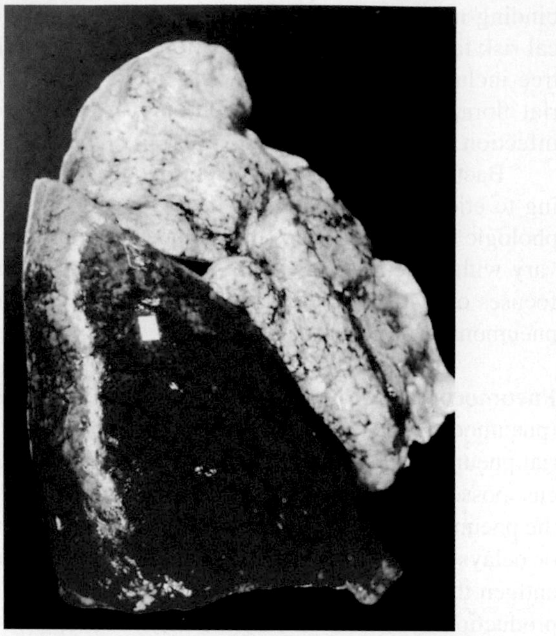

Figure 30.5 • Lobar pneumonia. The entire left lower lobe is consolidated and in the stage of *red* hepatization. The upper lobe is normally expanded. (From Strayer D. S., Rubin R. (Eds.) (2015). *Rubin's pathology: Clinicopathologic foundations of medicine* (7th ed., Fig. 18-11, p. 687). Philadelphia, PA: Lippincott Williams & Wilkins.)

containing numerous organisms (Fig. 30.6). Marked capillary congestion follows, leading to massive outpouring of polymorphonuclear leukocytes and red blood cells. Because the first consistency of the affected lung resembles that of the liver, this stage is referred to as the *red hepatization* stage. The next stage, occurring after 2 or more days, depending on the success of treatment, involves the arrival of macrophages that phagocytose the fragmented polymorphonuclear cells, red blood cells, and other cellular debris. During this stage, which is termed the *gray hepatization* stage, the congestion has diminished but the lung is still firm. The alveolar exudate is then removed and the lung gradually returns to normal.

The signs and symptoms of pneumococcal pneumonia vary widely, depending on the age and health status of the infected person.[15] In previously healthy people, the onset usually is sudden and is characterized by malaise, severe, shaking chills, and fever. During the initial or congestive stage, coughing brings up watery sputum and breath sounds are limited, with fine crackles. As the disease progresses, the character of the sputum changes; it may be blood tinged or rust colored to purulent. Pleuritic pain, a sharp pain that is more severe with respiratory movements, is common. With antibiotic therapy, fever usually subsides in approximately 48 to 72 hours, and recovery is uneventful. Older adults are less likely to experience marked elevations in temperature. In fact, the only sign of pneumonia may be a loss of appetite and deterioration in mental status in older adults.

Treatment includes the use of antibiotics that are effective against *S. pneumoniae*. Multidrug-resistant strains of *S. pneumoniae* are emerging in the United States and other countries, which is why it is vital that the strain of *S. pneumoniae* is susceptible to the antibiotic.

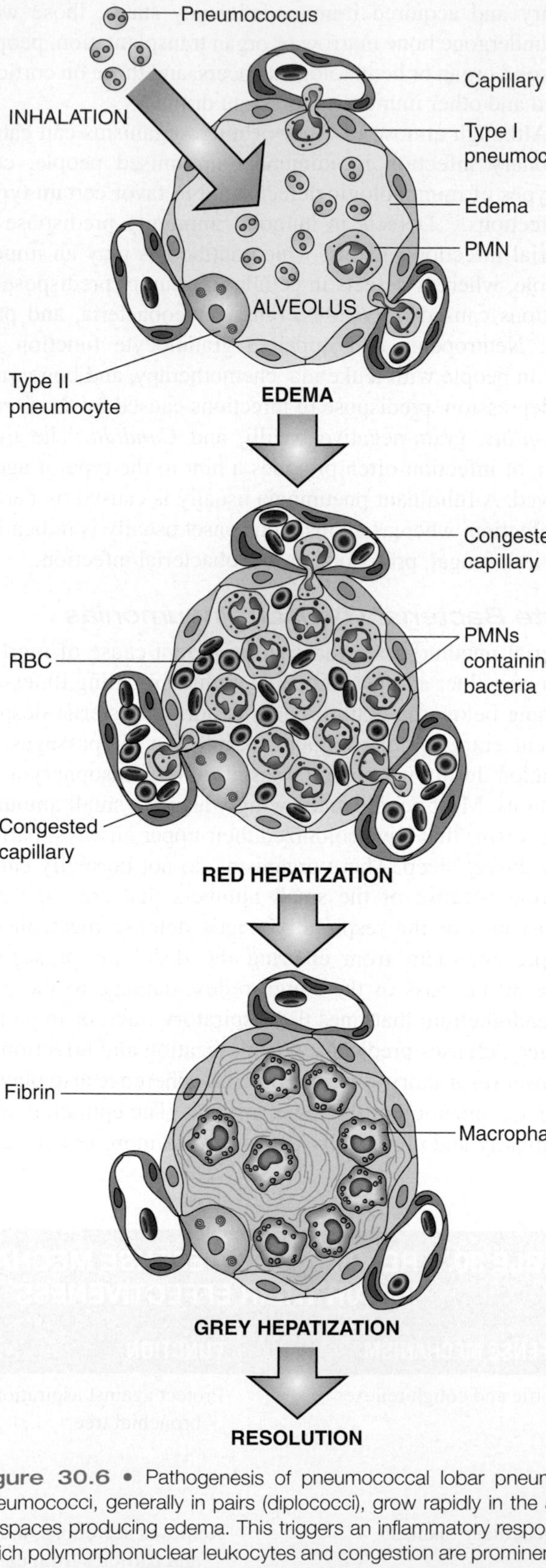

Figure 30.6 • Pathogenesis of pneumococcal lobar pneumonia. Pneumococci, generally in pairs (diplococci), grow rapidly in the alveolar spaces producing edema. This triggers an inflammatory response in which polymorphonuclear leukocytes and congestion are prominent (*red* hepatization). As the inflammation progresses, macrophages replace the polymorphonuclear leukocytes and ingest the debris (*gray* hepatization). The process generally resolves with correct medical management, but complications may occur. (PMN, polymorphonuclear leukocytes; RBC, red blood cell.) (From Rubin R., Strayer D. S. (Eds.) (2012). *Rubin's pathology: Clinicopathologic foundations of medicine* (6th ed.). Philadelphia, PA: Lippincott Williams & Wilkins.)

Pneumococcal pneumonia can be prevented through immunization. The capsular polysaccharides induce antibodies primarily by T-cell–independent mechanisms. The vaccine is recommended for people 65 years of age or older and people aged 2 to 65 years with chronic illnesses, particularly cardiovascular and pulmonary diseases, diabetes mellitus, and alcoholism, who sustain increased morbidity with respiratory infections. Immunization is also recommended for immunocompromised people 2 years of age or older, including those with congenital or acquired immunodeficiency, generalized malignancy, sickle cell disease, splenectomy, multiple myeloma, renal failure, nephrotic syndrome, organ transplantation, and HIV infection.[13,15] Immunization is also recommended for residents in special environments or social settings in which the risk for invasive pneumococcal disease is increased (*e.g.*, Alaskan Natives, certain Native American populations) and for residents of nursing homes and long-term care facilities.

Because their immune system is immature, the antibody response to most pneumococcal capsular polysaccharides usually is poor or inconsistent in children younger than 2 years of age. With the success of *H. influenzae* type B vaccine, *S. pneumoniae* has become the leading cause of bacterial meningitis in the United States. *S. pneumoniae* also contributes substantially to noninvasive respiratory infections and is the most common cause of community-acquired pneumonia, acute otitis media, and sinusitis among young children.[15]

Legionnaire Disease. Legionnaire disease is a form of bronchopneumonia caused by a gram-negative rod, *Legionella pneumophila*.[16] Transmission from person to person has not been documented, and infection normally occurs by acquiring the organism from the environment. Infection typically occurs when water that contains the pathogen is aerosolized into appropriately sized droplets and is inhaled or aspirated by a susceptible host.[16] The disease was first recognized and received its name after an epidemic of severe and, for some, fatal pneumonia that developed among delegates to the 1976 American Legion convention held in a Philadelphia hotel. The spread of infection was traced to a water-cooled air-conditioning system. Although healthy people can contract the infection, the risk is greatest among smokers, people with chronic diseases, and those with impaired cell-mediated immunity.[16]

Symptoms of the disease typically begin approximately 2 to 10 days after infection. Onset is usually abrupt, with malaise, weakness, lethargy, fever, and dry cough. Other manifestations include disturbances of central nervous system function, gastrointestinal tract involvement, arthralgias, and elevation in body temperature.[16] The presence of pneumonia along with diarrhea, hyponatremia, and confusion is characteristic of *Legionella* pneumonia. The disease causes consolidation of lung tissues and impairs gas exchange.

Diagnosis is based on clinical manifestations, radiologic studies, and specialized laboratory tests to detect the presence of the organism. Of these, the *Legionella* urinary antigen test is a relatively inexpensive, rapid test that detects antigens of *L. pneumophila* in the urine.[16] The urine test usually is easier to obtain because people with legionellosis often have a nonproductive cough, and the test results remain positive for weeks despite antibiotic therapy. The test is available as both a radioimmunoassay and an enzyme immunoassay.

Treatment consists of administration of antibiotics that are known to be effective against *L. pneumophila*. Delay in instituting antibiotic therapy significantly increases mortality rates; therefore, antibiotics known to be effective against *L. pneumophila* should be included in the treatment regimen for severe community-acquired pneumonia.[16]

Primary Atypical Pneumonia

The primary atypical pneumonias are caused by a variety of agents, the most common being *M. pneumoniae*. Mycoplasma infections are particularly common among children and young adults.[15] Other etiologic agents include viruses (*e.g.*, influenza virus, RSVs, adenoviruses, rhinoviruses, rubeola [measles], and varicella [chickenpox] viruses) and *Chlamydia cae*.[17] In some cases, the cause is unknown.

The atypical pneumonias are characterized by patchy involvement of the lung, largely confined to the alveolar septum and pulmonary interstitium. The term *atypical* denotes a lack of lung consolidation, production of moderate amounts of sputum, moderate elevation of white blood cell count, and lack of alveolar exudate.[15] The agents that cause atypical pneumonias damage the respiratory tract epithelium and impair respiratory tract defenses, thereby predisposing to secondary bacterial infections. The sporadic form of atypical pneumonia is usually mild with a low mortality rate. It may, however, assume epidemic proportions with intensified severity and greater mortality, as in the influenza pandemics of 1915 and 1918.

The clinical course among people with mycoplasmal and viral pneumonias varies widely from a mild infection (*e.g.*, influenza types A and B, adenovirus) that masquerades as a chest cold to a more serious and even fatal outcome. The symptoms may remain confined to fever, headache, and muscle aches and pains. Cough, when present, is characteristically dry, hacking, and nonproductive. The diagnosis is usually made based on history, physical findings, and chest x-rays. There are a few assessment tools to assist in determining treatment for people with pneumonia that also predict mortality such as the CURB 65.[18]

Tuberculosis

Tuberculosis is the world's foremost cause of death from a single infectious agent. Approximately 10.4 million people are infected globally.[19] This does not include the millions of people who are thought to be latently infected with *M. tuberculosis*. The World Health Organization estimates over 9 million new TB cases occur annually, worldwide.[20] With the introduction of antibiotics in the 1950s, the United States and other Western countries enjoyed a long decline in the number of infections until the mid-1980s. Since that time, the rate of infection has increased, particularly among people infected with HIV. Tuberculosis is more common among foreign-born people from countries with a high incidence of tuberculosis and among residents of high-risk congregate settings such as correctional facilities, drug treatment facilities, and homeless shelters. Outbreaks of a drug-resistant form of tuberculosis have emerged, complicating the selection of drugs and affecting the duration of treatment.

Tuberculosis is an infectious disease caused by the mycobacterium, *M. tuberculosis*. The mycobacteria are slender, rod-shaped aerobic bacteria that do not form spores. They are similar to other bacterial organisms except for an outer waxy capsule that makes them more resistant to destruction; the organism can persist in old necrotic and calcified lesions and remain capable of reinitiating growth. The waxy coat also causes the organism to retain red dye when treated with acid in acid-fast staining.[20] Thus, the mycobacteria are often referred to as *acid-fast bacilli*. Although *M. tuberculosis* can infect practically any organ of the body, the lungs are most frequently involved. The tubercle bacilli are strict aerobes that thrive in an oxygen-rich environment. This explains their tendency to cause disease in the upper lobe or upper parts of the lower lobe of the lung, where the ventilation and oxygen content are greatest.

Mycobacterium tuberculosis hominis is the most frequent form of tuberculosis that threatens humans. Other mycobacteria, including *Mycobacterium avium–intracellulare* (MAI) complex, are much less virulent than *M. tuberculosis hominis*. These mycobacteria rarely cause disease except in severely immunosuppressed people, such as those with HIV infection. Generally, MAI complex is transmitted from eating contaminated food or water.

Mycobacterium tuberculosis hominis is an airborne infection spread by minute, invisible particles, called *droplet nuclei* that are harbored in the respiratory secretions of people with active tuberculosis. Coughing, sneezing, and talking all create respiratory droplets. These droplets evaporate and leave organisms (droplet nuclei), which remain suspended in the air and are circulated by air currents. Thus, living under crowded and confined conditions increases the risk for spread of the disease.

KEY POINTS

TUBERCULOSIS

- Tuberculosis is an infectious disease caused by *M. tuberculosis*, a rod-shaped, aerobic bacterium that is resistant to destruction and can persist in necrotic and calcified lesions for prolonged periods and remain capable of reinstating growth.
- A positive tuberculin skin test results from a cell-mediated immune response and implies that a person has been infected with *M. tuberculosis* and has mounted a cell-mediated immune response. It does not mean that the person has active tuberculosis.

Pathogenesis

The pathogenesis of tuberculosis in a previously unexposed immunocompetent person is centered on the development of a cell-mediated immune response that confers resistance to the organism and development of tissue hypersensitivity to the tubercular antigens.[20] The destructive features of the disease, such as caseating necrosis and cavitation, result from the hypersensitivity immune response rather than the destructive capabilities of the tubercle bacillus.

Macrophages are the primary cell infected with *M. tuberculosis*. Inhaled droplet nuclei pass down the bronchial tree without settling on the epithelium and are deposited in the alveoli. Soon after entering the lung, the bacilli are phagocytosed by alveolar macrophages but resist killing, apparently because cell wall lipids of *M. tuberculosis* block fusion of phagosomes and lysosomes. Although the macrophages that first ingest *M. tuberculosis* cannot kill the organisms, they initiate a cell-mediated immune response that eventually contains the infection. As the tubercle bacilli multiply, the infected macrophages degrade the mycobacteria and present their antigens to T lymphocytes. The sensitized T lymphocytes, in turn, stimulate the macrophages to increase their concentration of lytic enzymes and ability to kill the mycobacteria. When released, these lytic enzymes also damage lung tissue. The development of a population of activated T lymphocytes and related development of activated macrophages capable of ingesting and destroying the bacilli constitutes the cell-mediated immune response, a process that takes about 3 to 6 weeks to become effective.

In people with intact cell-mediated immunity, the cell-mediated immune response results in the development of a gray-white, circumscribed granulomatous lesion, called a *Ghon focus*, that contains the tubercle bacilli, modified macrophages, and other immune cells.[20] It is usually located in the subpleural area of the upper segments of the lower lobes or in the lower segments of the upper lobe. When the number of organisms is high, the hypersensitivity reaction produces significant tissue necrosis, causing the central portion of the Ghon focus to undergo soft, caseous (cheeselike) necrosis. During this same period, tubercle bacilli, free or inside macrophages, drain along the lymph channels to the tracheobronchial lymph nodes of the affected lung, and there evoke the formation of caseous granulomas. The combination of the primary lung lesion and lymph node granulomas is called a *Ghon complex* (Fig. 30.7). The Ghon complex eventually heals, undergoing shrinkage, fibrous scarring, and calcification, the latter visible radiographically. However, small numbers of organisms may remain viable for years. Later, if immune mechanisms decline or fail, latent tuberculosis infection has the potential to develop into secondary tuberculosis.

Clinical Manifestations

Primary Tuberculosis. Primary tuberculosis is a form of the disease that develops in previously unexposed and therefore unsensitized people. It typically is initiated as a result of

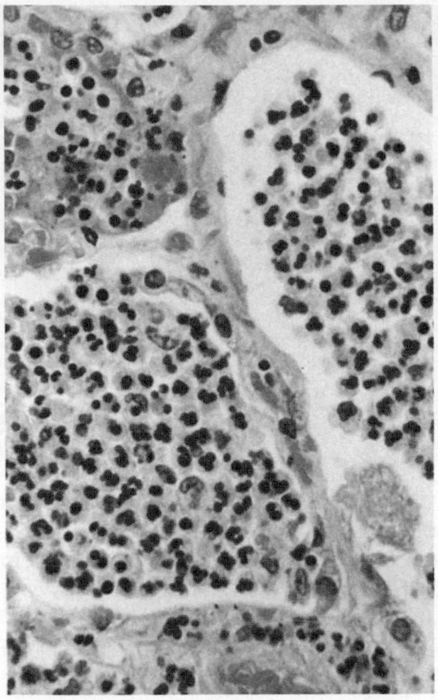

Figure 30.7 • Pneumococcal pneumonia. Alveoli are packed with an exudate composed of polymorphonuclear leukocytes and occasional macrophages. (From Beasley M. B., Travis W. D., Rubin E. (2008). *The respiratory system*; Strayer D. S., Rubin R. (Eds.) (2015). *Rubin's pathology: Clinicopathologic foundations of medicine* (7th ed., Fig. 18-14, p. 689). Philadelphia, PA: Lippincott Williams & Wilkins.)

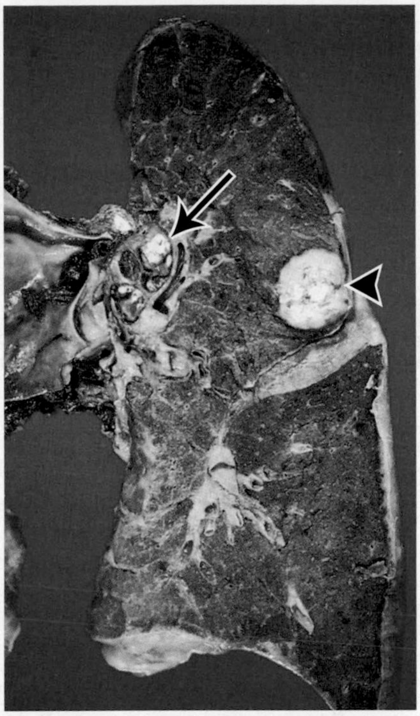

Figure 30.8 • Primary tuberculosis. A healed Ghon complex is represented by a subpleural nodule (*arrowhead*) and involved hilar lymph nodes (*arrow*). (From Strayer D. S., Rubin R. (Eds.) (2015). *Rubin's pathology: Clinicopathologic foundations of medicine* (7th ed., Fig. 18-14, Fig. 18-16, p. 691). Philadelphia, PA: Lippincott Williams & Wilkins.)

inhaling droplet nuclei that contain the tubercle bacillus (Fig. 30.8). Most people with primary tuberculosis go on to develop *latent infection* in which T lymphocytes and macrophages surround the organism in granulomas that limit their spread.[20] People with latent tuberculosis do not have active disease and cannot transmit the organism to others.

In small percentage of newly infected people, the immune response is inadequate. These people go on to develop progressive primary tuberculosis with continued destruction of lung tissue and spread to multiple sites within the lung.[20] People with HIV infection and others with disorders of cell-mediated immunity are more likely to develop progressive tuberculosis if they become infected. In those who develop progressive disease, the symptoms are usually insidious and nonspecific, with fever, weight loss, fatigue, and night sweats.[20] Sometimes the onset of symptoms is abrupt, with high fever, pleuritis, and lymphadenitis. As the disease spreads, the organism gains access to the sputum, allowing the person to infect others.

In rare instances, tuberculosis may erode into a blood vessel, giving rise to hematogenic dissemination. *Miliary tuberculosis* describes minute lesions, resembling millet seeds, resulting from this type of dissemination that can involve almost any organ, particularly the brain, meninges, liver, kidney, and bone marrow.

Primary Progressive Tuberculosis. Primary progressive tuberculosis represents either reinfection from inhaled droplet nuclei or reactivation of a previously healed primary lesion[20] (see Fig. 30.8). It often occurs in situations of impaired body defense mechanisms. The partial immunity that follows primary tuberculosis affords protection against reinfection and to some extent aids in localizing the disease should reactivation occur. In primary progressive tuberculosis, the cell-mediated hypersensitivity reaction can be an aggravating factor, as evidenced by the frequency of cavitation and bronchial dissemination. In severe cases, the cavities may rapidly coalesce and become enlarged in diameter[20] (Fig. 30.9). Pleural effusion and tuberculous empyema are common as the disease progresses.

People with early primary progressive tuberculosis commonly present with low-grade fevers, fatigue, and weight loss.[20] A cough initially is dry but later becomes productive with purulent and sometimes blood-tinged sputum. Dyspnea and orthopnea develop as the disease advances to late primary progressive tuberculosis. Also night sweats, anemia, and rales on lung auscultation are evident as the disease progresses.[20]

Diagnosis

Diagnosing TB has many challenges and is often missed, especially with people who present with less than classic symptoms of TB and who do not fit the most impacted TB population groups.[20] The most frequently used screening methods for pulmonary tuberculosis are tuberculin skin tests and chest x-ray. The tuberculin skin test measures the delayed hypersensitivity (*i.e.*, cell-mediated, type IV) that follows exposure to the tubercle bacillus. People who become tuberculin positive usually remain so for the remainder of their lives. A positive

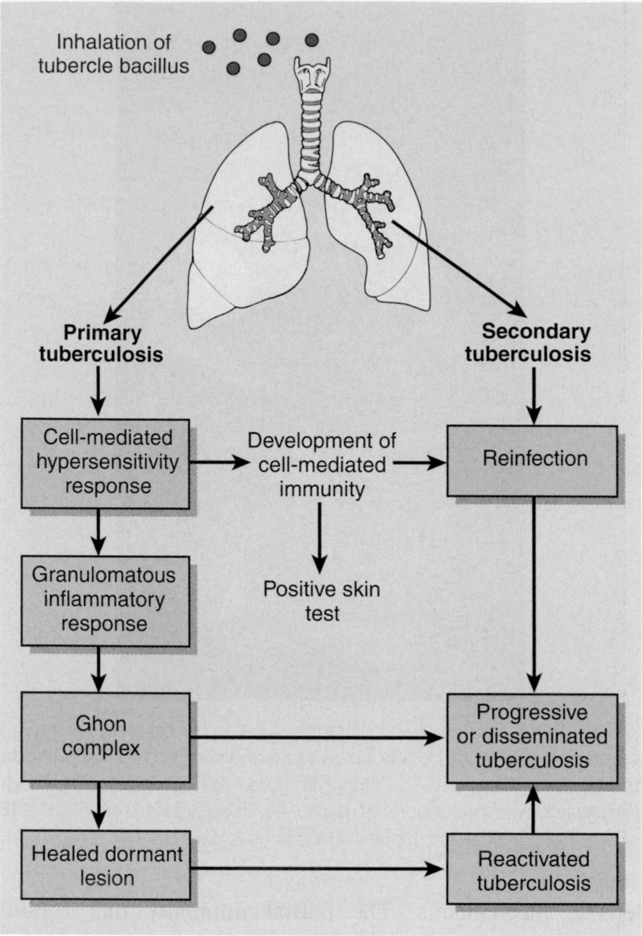

Figure 30.9 • Pathogenesis of tuberculosis infection.

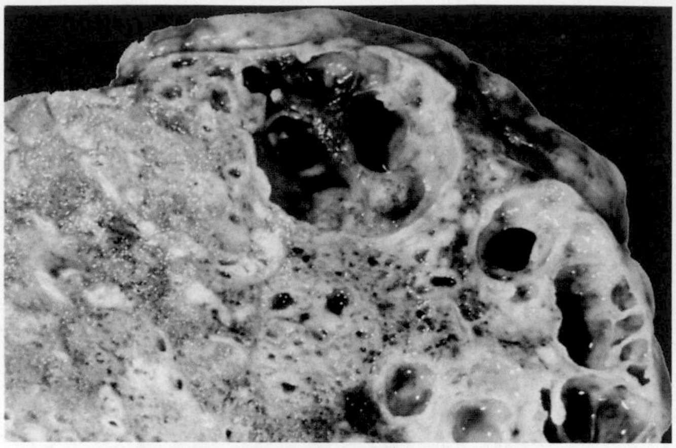

Figure 30.10 • Cavitary tuberculosis. The apex of the left upper lobe shows tuberculous cavities surrounded by consolidated and fibrotic pulmonary parenchyma that contains small tubercles. (From Beasley M. B., Travis W. D., Rubin E. (2008). *The respiratory system*; Strayer D. S., Rubin R. (Eds.) (2015). *Rubin's pathology: Clinicopathologic foundations of medicine* (7th ed., Fig. 18-18, p. 692). Philadelphia, PA: Lippincott Williams & Wilkins.)

reaction to the skin test does not mean that a person has active tuberculosis. It only means that there has been exposure to the bacillus and that cell-mediated immunity to the organism has developed. False-positive and false-negative skin test reactions can occur. False-positive reactions can result from cross-reactions with nontuberculosis mycobacteria, such as *M. avium-intracellulare* complex (see Fig. 30.10). Because the hypersensitivity response to the tuberculin test depends on cell-mediated immunity, a false-negative test result can occur because of immunodeficiency states that result from HIV infection, immunosuppressive therapy, lymphoreticular malignancies, or aging. This is called *anergy*. In the immunocompromised person, a negative tuberculin test result can mean that the person has a true lack of exposure to tuberculosis or is unable to mount an immune response to the test. The QuantiFERON-TB Gold test (QFT-TB Gold) is used to detect active and latent TB by measuring interferon-y (IFN-y), which is part of the cell-mediated immune activity to TB response.[20] It has a 24-hour test results turnaround, but it is expensive and is not available at all health care settings.

Definitive diagnosis of active pulmonary tuberculosis requires identification of the organism from cultures or identification of the organism from deoxyribonucleic acid (DNA) or RNA amplification techniques.[20] Bacteriologic studies (*i.e.*, acid-fast stain and cultures) of early sputum specimens, gastric aspirations, or bronchial washings obtained during fiberoptic bronchoscopy may be used.

Treatment

The goals of treatment are to eliminate all tubercle bacilli from an infected person while avoiding emergence of significant drug resistance. Treatment of active tuberculosis requires the use of multiple drugs.[20] Tuberculosis is an unusual disease in that chemotherapy is required for a relatively long period. The tubercle bacillus is an aerobic organism that multiplies slowly and remains relatively dormant in oxygen-poor caseous material. It undergoes a high rate of mutation and tends to acquire resistance to any one drug. For this reason, multidrug regimens are used for treating people with active tuberculosis.[20] Drug susceptibility tests are used to guide treatment in drug-resistant forms of the disease.

Two groups meet the criteria established for the use of antimycobacterial therapy for tuberculosis: people with active tuberculosis and people who have had contact with cases of active tuberculosis and who are at risk for development of an active form of the disease. Prophylactic treatment is used for people who are infected with *M. tuberculosis* but do not have active disease.[21] This group includes the following:

- People with a positive skin test result who have had close contact with active cases of tuberculosis.
- People who have converted from a negative to positive skin test result within 2 years.
- People who have a history of untreated or inadequately treated tuberculosis.
- People who have chest radiographs with evidence of tuberculosis but no bacteriologic evidence of the active disease.

- People who have special risk factors such as silicosis, diabetes mellitus, prolonged corticosteroid therapy, immunosuppression therapy, end-stage renal disease, chronic malnutrition from any cause, or hematologic or reticuloendothelial cancers.
- People who have a positive HIV test result or have AIDS.
- People who are 35 years of age or younger with a positive reaction of unknown duration (these people are considered to harbor a small number of microorganisms and usually are treated with isoniazid [INH]).

The primary drugs used in the treatment of tuberculosis are INH, rifampin, pyrazinamide (PZA), ethambutol, and streptomycin.[20] INH is remarkably potent against the tubercle bacillus and probably is the most widely used drug for tuberculosis. Although its exact mechanism of action is unknown, it apparently combines with an enzyme that is needed by the INH-susceptible strains of the tubercle bacillus. Resistance to the drug develops rapidly, and combination with other effective drugs delays the development of resistance. Rifampin inhibits RNA synthesis in the bacillus. Although ethambutol and PZA are known to inhibit the growth of the tubercle bacillus, their mechanisms of action are largely unknown. Streptomycin, the first drug found to be effective against tuberculosis, must be given by injection, which limits its usefulness, particularly in long-term therapy. However, it remains an important drug in tuberculosis therapy and is used primarily in people with severe, possibly life-threatening forms of tuberculosis.

Outbreaks of multidrug-resistant tuberculosis have posed a problem for the prophylactic treatment of exposed people, including health care workers.[20] Various treatment protocols are recommended, depending on the type of resistant strain that is identified. Success of chemotherapy for prophylaxis and treatment of tuberculosis depends on strict adherence to a lengthy drug regimen. This often is a problem, particularly for people with asymptomatic tuberculosis infections.

First administered to humans in 1921, the bacillus Calmette-Guérin (BCG) vaccine is used to prevent the development of tuberculosis in people who are at high risk for infection. BCG is an attenuated strain of *M. tuberculosis bovis*.[20] It is administered only to people who have a negative tuberculin skin test result. The vaccine, which is given intradermally, produces a local reaction that can last as long as 3 months and may result in scarring at the injection site. People who have been vaccinated with BCG usually have a positive tuberculin skin test result.

Today, more than 70 years after its development, BCG remains the only tuberculosis vaccine available. Currently, several candidate vaccines are being prepared or are already in the early stages of human testing. Worldwide, BCG is currently used as a major method of prevention for tuberculosis. However, it is not generally recommended in the United States because of the low prevalence of tuberculosis infection, the vaccine's interference with the ability to determine latent tuberculosis with skin tests, and variable effectiveness against pulmonary tuberculosis.[21] Vaccination of health care workers may be considered on an individual basis in settings where people in the hospital are infected with drug-resistant strains of tuberculosis.

Fungal Infections

Fungi are classified as yeasts and molds. Yeasts are round and grow by budding. Molds form tubular structures called *hyphae* and grow by branching and forming spores. Some fungi are *dimorphic*, meaning that they grow as yeasts at body temperatures and as molds at room temperatures. A simple classification of mycoses or diseases caused by fungi divides them into superficial, cutaneous, subcutaneous, or deep (systemic) mycoses. The superficial, cutaneous, or subcutaneous mycoses cause disease of the skin, hair, and nails. Deep fungal infections may produce pulmonary and systemic infections and are sometimes fatal. Virulent fungi that live free in nature, in soil, or in decaying organic matter cause these infections. They are frequently limited to certain geographic regions.

The most common of these are the dimorphic fungi, which include *H. capsulatum* (histoplasmosis), *C. immitis* (coccidioidomycosis), and *B. dermatitidis* (blastomycosis). These fungi form infectious spores, which enter the body through the respiratory system. Most people who become infected with these fungi develop only minor symptoms or none at all. Only a small minority develops serious disease.

The host's cell-mediated immune response is paramount in controlling such infections. Pathologic fungi generally produce no toxins. In the host, they induce a delayed cell-mediated hypersensitivity response to their chemical constituents. Cellular immunity is mediated by antigen-specific T lymphocytes and cytokine-activated macrophages that assume fungicidal properties. The primary pulmonary lesions consist of aggregates of macrophages stuffed with organisms, with similar lesions developing in the lymph nodes that drain the area. These lesions develop into granulomas complete with giant cells and may develop central necrosis and calcification resembling that of primary tuberculosis.

Although most fungal infections are asymptomatic, they can be severe or even fatal in people who have experienced a heavy exposure, have underlying immune deficiencies, or develop progressive disease that is not recognized or treated. Immunocompromised people, particularly those with HIV infection, are especially prone to development of disseminated infection.

Histoplasmosis

Histoplasmosis is caused by the dimorphic fungus *H. capsulatum*. Most cases in the United States occur along the major river valleys of the Midwest—the Ohio and the Mississippi.[22] The organism grows in soil and other areas that have been enriched with bird excreta and bat droppings.[22]

Etiology and Pathogenesis. The infection is acquired by inhaling the fungal spores that are released when the dirt or dust from the infected areas is disturbed. The spores convert to the parasitic yeast phase when exposed to body temperature in the alveoli. They are then carried to the regional lymphatics and from there are disseminated throughout the body in the bloodstream. Dissemination occurs during the first several weeks of infection before specific immunity has developed. After 2 to 3 weeks, cellular immunity develops as long as the host is immunocompetent, establishing the body's ability to control the infection.

Clinical Manifestations. Depending on the host's resistance and immunocompetence, the disease usually causes no symptoms and resolves spontaneously.[22] The average incubation period for the infection to cause symptoms is approximately 1 to 4 weeks after exposure.[22] Most people with *H. capsulatum* infection remain asymptomatic or have mild respiratory illness that is not diagnosed as histoplasmosis. Latent asymptomatic histoplasmosis is characterized by evidence of healed lesions in the lungs or hilar lymph nodes. Primary pulmonary histoplasmosis occurs in otherwise healthy people as a mild, self-limited, febrile respiratory infection. Its symptoms include muscle and joint pains and a nonproductive, dry cough. Erythema nodosum (*i.e.*, subcutaneous nodules) or erythema multiforme (*i.e.*, hivelike lesions) sometimes appears. During this stage of the disease, chest radiographs usually show single or multiple infiltrates.

Chronic histoplasmosis can resemble reactivation tuberculosis. Infiltration of the upper lobes of one or both lungs occurs with cavitation. This form of the disease is more common in middle-aged men who smoke and in people with chronic lung disease. The most common manifestations are a productive cough, chest pain, fever, night sweats, and weight loss. In many people, the disease is self-limited. In others, there is progressive destruction of lung tissue and dissemination of the disease.

Disseminated histoplasmosis can follow primary or chronic histoplasmosis. However, it most often develops as an acute and fulminating infection in the very old or the very young or in people who are immunocompromised, including people who have undergone transplantations, those with hematologic malignancies, and people with AIDS. Although the macrophages of the reticuloendothelial system can remove the fungi from the bloodstream, they are unable to destroy them. Characteristically, this form of the disease produces high fever, generalized lymph node enlargement, hepatosplenomegaly, muscle wasting, anemia, leukopenia, and thrombocytopenia. There may be hoarseness, ulcerations of the mouth and tongue, nausea, vomiting, diarrhea, and abdominal pain. Often, meningitis becomes a dominant feature of the disease.

Diagnosis and Treatment. A number of laboratory tests, including cultures, fungal stain, antigen detection, and serologic tests for antibodies, are used in the diagnosis of histoplasmosis. The type of test that is used depends on the type of involvement that is present. In pulmonary disease, sputum culture is rarely positive, whereas blood or bone marrow cultures from immunocompromised people with acute disseminated disease are positive in approximately 75% of cases. Some people may need a surgical biopsy on their suspicious lung nodule to rule out malignancy.[23] Antigen tests can be performed on blood, urine, cerebrospinal fluid, or bronchoalveolar lavage fluid. A Histoplasma urine antigen assay is particularly useful in detecting disseminated histoplasmosis. The sensitivity for this technique is greater than 95%.[22]

An antifungal drug, such as itraconazole (Sporanox), usually is the drug of choice for treatment of people with disease severe enough to require treatment or those with compromised immune function who are at risk for the development of disseminated disease. For those with immunocompetency, no drug is generally needed because the histoplasmosis tends to resolve spontaneously. People with HIV-related histoplasmosis usually require lifelong suppression therapy with itraconazole.

Coccidioidomycosis

Coccidioidomycosis, "valley fever," is a common fungal infection caused by inhaling the spores of *C. immitis* or *C. posadasii*.[24]

Etiology and Pathogenesis. The disease resembles tuberculosis, and its mechanisms of infection are similar to those of histoplasmosis. It is most prevalent in the deserts in the southwestern United States, principally in parts of California, Arizona, Nevada, New Mexico, and Texas. The *C. immitis* and *C. posadasii* organism lives in soil and can establish new sites in the soil. Events such as dust storms and digging for construction have been associated with increased incidence of the disease.

Clinical Manifestations. The disease most commonly occurs as an acute, primary, self-limited pulmonary infection with or without systemic involvement. However, in some cases it progresses to a disseminated disease. The incubation period is 1 to 4 weeks.[24] About 60% to 80% of infected people are asymptomatic or develop mild respiratory symptoms of primary coccidioidomycosis. The symptoms are usually those of a respiratory tract infection with fever, cough, and pleuritic pain. Dermatologic manifestations may occur in the form of erythyema nodosum days after onset of symptoms.[24,25] The skin lesions usually are accompanied by arthralgias or arthritis without effusion. The terms *desert bumps* and *desert arthritis* are used to describe these manifestations. The presence of skin and joint manifestations indicates strong host defenses because people who have had such manifestations seldom acquire disseminated disease.

Commonly affected structures in disseminated disease are the lymph nodes, meninges, spleen, liver, kidney, skin, and adrenal glands. Meningitis is the most common cause of death. People with diabetes, lung disease, or compromised immune function, infants, smokers, pregnant women, and members of dark-skinned races tend to localize the disease poorly and are at higher risk for disseminated disease.[24,25] In HIV-infected people in endemic areas, coccidioidomycosis is now a common opportunistic infection.

Diagnosis and Treatment. Radiologic studies, including chest radiographic studies and bone scans, are useful in determining disease but cannot distinguish coccidioidomycosis from other pulmonary diseases. A definitive diagnosis requires microscopic or serologic evidence that *C. immitis* or *C. posadasii* is present in body tissues or fluids. Spherules can be visualized in specially stained biopsy specimens. Serologic tests can be done for immunoglobulin M (IgM) and IgG antibody detection.[24]

Treatment depends on the severity of infection. People without associated risk factors such as HIV infection or without specific evidence of progressive disease usually can be managed without antifungal therapy. The oral antifungal drugs itraconazole and fluconazole are used for treatment of less severe forms of infection.[24]

Blastomycosis

Blastomycosis is a fungal infection caused by inhaling the spores of *B. dermatitidis*. The disease is most commonly found in the southeastern and north central United States, especially in areas bordering the Mississippi and Ohio River valleys and states bordering the Great Lakes.[26] *B. dermatitidis* is most commonly found in soil containing decayed vegetation or decomposed wood.

Local suppurative (pus-forming) and granulomatous lesions of the lungs and skin characterize blastomycosis. The symptoms of acute infection, which are similar to those of acute histoplasmosis, include fever, cough, aching joints and muscles, and, uncommonly, pleuritic pain. In contrast to histoplasmosis, the cough in blastomycosis often is productive, and the sputum is purulent. Acute pulmonary infections may be self-limited or progressive. In people with overwhelming pulmonary disease, diffuse interalveolar infiltrates and evidence of acute RDS may develop. Extrapulmonary spread most commonly involves the skin, bones, or prostate. These lesions may provide the first evidence of the disease.

The definitive diagnostic test for *B. dermatitidis* infection is growth of the organism from sputum, tissue biopsy, or body fluid. It generally takes several weeks to grow in mold phase at room temperature. Once growth has occurred, laboratories that use the highly specific and sensitive DNA probe for *B. dermatitidis* can rapidly identify the organism. New diagnostics are being used in clinical trials.[27]

Treatment of the progressive or disseminated form of the disease includes the use of itraconazole. Amphotericin B is recommended for people who are immunosuppressed. In recent clinical trials, medications such as Posaconazole and Voriconazole have shown to be effective against *B. dermatitidis*.[27] Most people with blastomycosis are identified and treated before the development of overwhelming or fatal disease.

IN SUMMARY

Respiratory infections are the most common cause of respiratory illness. They include the common cold, influenza, pneumonias, tuberculosis, and fungal infections. The common cold occurs more frequently than any other respiratory infection. The fingers are the usual source of transmission, and the most common portals of entry are the nasal mucosa and the conjunctiva of the eye. The influenza virus causes three syndromes: an uncomplicated rhinotracheitis, a respiratory viral infection followed by a bacterial infection, and viral pneumonia. The contagiousness of influenza results from the ability of the virus to mutate and form subtypes against which the population is unprotected.

Pneumonia describes an infection of the parenchymal tissues of the lung. Loss of the cough reflex, damage to the ciliated endothelium that lines the respiratory tract, or impaired immune defenses predispose people to pneumonia. Pneumonia can be classified according to the setting in which it occurs (community- or hospital-acquired), type of organism causing the infection (typical or atypical), and location of the infection (lobar pneumonia or bronchopneumonia). People with compromised immune function constitute a special concern in both categories. Community-acquired pneumonia involves infections from organisms that are present more often in the community than in the hospital or nursing home. The most common cause of community-acquired pneumonia is *S. pneumoniae*. Hospital-acquired (nosocomial) pneumonia is defined as a lower respiratory tract infection occurring 48 hours or more after admission. Hospital-acquired pneumonia is the second most common cause of hospital-acquired infection. Acute typical pneumonias, including *S. pneumoniae* and *L. pneumophila* pneumonia, are caused by organisms that multiply extracellularly in the alveoli and cause inflammation and transudation of fluid into the air-filled spaces of the alveoli. Atypical pneumonias are caused by a variety of agents, including *M. pneumoniae* and viruses that invade the alveolar septum and interstitium of the lung.

Tuberculosis is a chronic respiratory infection caused by *M. tuberculosis*, which is spread by minute, invisible particles called *droplet nuclei*. Tuberculosis is a particular threat among HIV-infected people, foreign-born people from countries with a high incidence of tuberculosis, and residents of high-risk congregate settings such as correctional facilities, drug treatment facilities, and homeless shelters. The tubercle bacillus incites a distinctive chronic inflammatory response referred to as *granulomatous inflammation*. The destructiveness of the disease results from the cell-mediated hypersensitivity response that the bacillus evokes rather than its inherent destructive capabilities. Cell-mediated immunity and hypersensitivity reactions contribute to the evolution of the disease. The treatment of tuberculosis has been complicated by outbreaks of drug-resistant forms of the disease.

Infections caused by the fungi *H. capsulatum* (histoplasmosis), *C. immitis* (coccidioidomycosis), and *B. dermatitidis* (blastomycosis) produce pulmonary manifestations that resemble tuberculosis. These infections are common but seldom serious unless they produce progressive destruction of lung tissue or the infection disseminates to organs and tissues outside the lungs.

CANCER OF THE LUNG

After completing this section of the chapter, the learner will be able to meet the following objectives:

- Compare small cell lung cancer (SCLC) and non–small cell lung cancer (NSCLC) in terms of histopathology, prognosis, and treatment methods.
- Define the term *paraneoplastic* and cite three paraneoplastic manifestations of lung cancer.

Because of a general decrease in smoking over the past 30 years, along with early detection and treatment,[28] the number of Americans who develop lung cancer is decreasing. Yet, lung cancer remains the leading cause of cancer death among men and women in the United States with the average age of diagnosis being 70 years.[28] Smoking among teens has increased in recent years, raising the potential for increased rates of lung cancer in the future. In addition, there has been an increase in smoking and lung cancer rates among Native American and Alaskan Natives.[28] Currently, the 5-year survival rate for men diagnosed with lung cancer is between 7% and 12%. For women diagnosed with cancer, the 5-year survival rate is between 8% and 14%. Relative survival for a diagnosis of lung cancer is 18.1% in the United States..[23,29]

Cigarette smoking causes more than 80% of cases of lung cancer. The risk for lung cancer among cigarette smokers increases with duration of smoking and the number of cigarettes smoked per day. Cigarette smokers can benefit at any age from smoking cessation.[30] Industrial hazards also contribute to the incidence of lung cancer. A commonly recognized hazard is exposure to asbestos. The mean risk for lung cancer is significantly greater in asbestos workers compared to the general population. In addition, tobacco smoke contributes heavily to the development of lung cancer in people exposed to asbestos.[4] In addition to cigarette smoking and industrial hazards, there is also evidence to suggest a familial predisposition to lung cancer. This occurrence may be due to a genetic predisposition, with the trait being expressed only in the presence of its major predisposing factor—cigarette smoking.[4] Finally, there is an increased incidence in lung cancer in people who have never smoked, including those exposed to smoking and even in those not exposed to smoking.[4]

Histologic Subtypes and Pathogenesis

Most (about 95%) primary lung tumors are carcinomas that arise from the lung tissue.[4] The remaining 5% are a miscellaneous group that includes bronchial carcinoid tumors (neuroendocrine tumors), bronchial gland tumors, fibrosarcomas, and lymphomas. The lung is also a frequent site of metastasis from cancers in other parts of the body.

Lung cancers are being identified recently as aggressive or nonaggressive, locally invasive, and widely metastatic tumors that arise from the epithelial lining of major bronchi.[31] These tumors begin as small mucosal lesions that may follow one of several patterns of growth. They may form intraluminal masses that invade the bronchial mucosa and infiltrate the peribronchial connective tissue, or they may form large, bulky masses that extend into the adjacent lung tissue. Some large tumors undergo central necrosis and acquire local areas of hemorrhage, and some invade the pleural cavity and chest wall and spread to adjacent intrathoracic structures.[9] All types of lung cancer, especially small cell lung carcinoma, have the capacity to synthesize bioactive products and produce paraneoplastic syndromes. These syndromes are a result of hormonal production of ectopic peptide by the tumor or from autoantibodies released in response to the tumor.[9] Generally, the paraneoplastic syndromes are of endocrine, neurologic, and/or immunologic etiology.

Lung cancer is commonly subdivided into four major categories with percentages of occurrence in each category. These include squamous cell lung carcinoma (25% to 40%), adenocarcinoma (20% to 40%), small cell carcinoma (20% to 25%), and large cell carcinoma (10% to 15%).[9] However, new diagnostic techniques allow more lung cancers to be detected at an earlier stage. This has led to changes being made in the percentages of occurrence in the major categories of lung cancer. For example, in 2011, the adenocarcinomas are estimated to account for 35% to 50% of all lung cancers.[31] For purposes of staging and treatment, lung cancers have been commonly identified as SCLC or NSCLC.[9] The key reason for this classification was that most SCLCs have metastasized by the time of diagnosis and were therefore not amenable to surgery. However, new protocols are being used today in many of the large oncology centers that involve lung cancer biomarkers and new molecular targeted therapies for different types of lung cancer.[31] In fact, a whole new classification system of lung cancers is evolving where non–small cell carcinoma is being used less frequently and large cell carcinoma is being replaced by large cell neuroendocrine carcinoma.[31]

Small Cell Lung Cancers

The SCLCs are characterized by a distinctive cell type—small round to oval cells that are approximately the size of a lymphocyte.[32] The cells grow in clusters that exhibit neither glandular nor squamous organization. Electron microscopic studies demonstrate the presence of neurosecretory granules in some of the tumor cells similar to those found in the bronchial epithelium of the fetus or neonate.[32] The presence of these granules suggests the ability of some of these tumors to secrete polypeptide hormones. The presence of neuroendocrine markers such as neuron-specific enolase and parathormone-like and other hormonally active products suggests that these tumors may arise from the neuroendocrine cells of the bronchial epithelium. This cell type has the strongest association with cigarette smoking and is rarely observed in someone who has not smoked.[32]

The SCLCs are highly malignant, tend to infiltrate widely, disseminate early in their course, and rarely are resectable. Brain metastases are particularly common with SCLC and may provide the first evidence of the tumor. This type of lung cancer is associated with several types of paraneoplastic syndrome, including the syndrome of inappropriate antidiuretic hormone secretion, Cushing syndrome associated with ectopic production of adrenocorticotropic hormone, and the Eaton-Lambert syndrome of neuromuscular disorder.

Non–Small Cell Lung Cancers

The NSCLCs include squamous cell carcinomas, adenocarcinomas, and large cell carcinomas (see Fig. 30.11). Like the SCLCs, these cancers have the capacity to synthesize bioactive products and produce paraneoplastic syndromes.

Squamous Cell Carcinoma. Squamous cell carcinoma is found most commonly in men and is closely correlated with a smoking history. Squamous cell carcinoma tends to originate in the central bronchi as an intraluminal growth and is thus more amenable to early detection through cytologic examination of the sputum than other forms of lung cancer. It tends to spread centrally into major bronchi and hilar lymph nodes and disseminates outside the thorax later than other types of bronchogenic cancers. Squamous cell carcinoma is associated with the paraneoplastic syndromes that produce hypercalcemia.

Adenocarcinoma. Currently, adenocarcinoma is the most common type of lung cancer in North America. Its association with cigarette smoking is weaker than for squamous cell carcinoma. It is the most common type of lung cancer in women and nonsmokers. Adenocarcinomas can have their origin in either the bronchiolar or alveolar tissues of the lung. These tumors tend to be located more peripherally than squamous cell sarcomas and sometimes are associated with areas of scarring (Fig. 30.12). The scars may be due to old infarcts, metallic foreign bodies, wounds, and granulomatous infections such as tuberculosis. In general, adenocarcinomas have a poorer stage-for-stage prognosis than squamous cell carcinomas.

Large Cell Carcinoma. Large cell carcinomas have large, polygonal cells. They constitute a group of neoplasms that are highly anaplastic and difficult to categorize as squamous cell carcinoma or adenocarcinoma. They tend to occur in the periphery of the lung, invading subsegmental bronchi and larger airways. They have a poor prognosis because of their tendency to spread to distant sites early in their course.

Clinical Manifestations

The manifestations of lung cancer can be divided into three categories:

1. Those due to involvement of the lung and adjacent structures.
2. The effects of local spread and metastasis.
3. Nonmetastatic paraneoplastic manifestations involving endocrine, neurologic, and connective tissue function.

As with other cancers, lung cancer also causes nonspecific symptoms such as anorexia and weight loss. Because its symptoms are similar to those associated with smoking and chronic bronchitis, they often are disregarded. Metastases already exist in many people presenting with evidence of

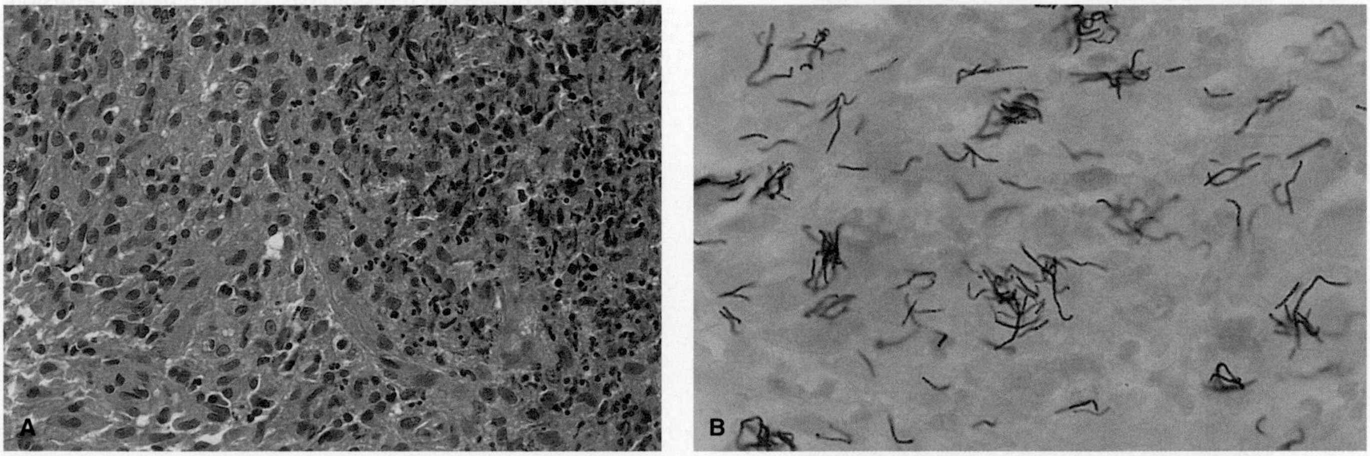

Figure 30.11 • *Mycobacterium avium–intracellulare (MAI)* pneumonia in acquired immunodeficiency syndrome (AIDS). **(A)** The pneumonia is characterized by an extensive infiltrate of macrophages. **(B)** The Ziehl-Neelsen stain shows numerous acid-fast organisms. (From Rubin R., Strayer D. S. (Eds.) (2015). *Rubin's pathology: Clinicopathologic foundations of medicine* (7th ed., Fig. 18-20, p. 693). Philadelphia, PA: Lippincott Williams & Wilkins.)

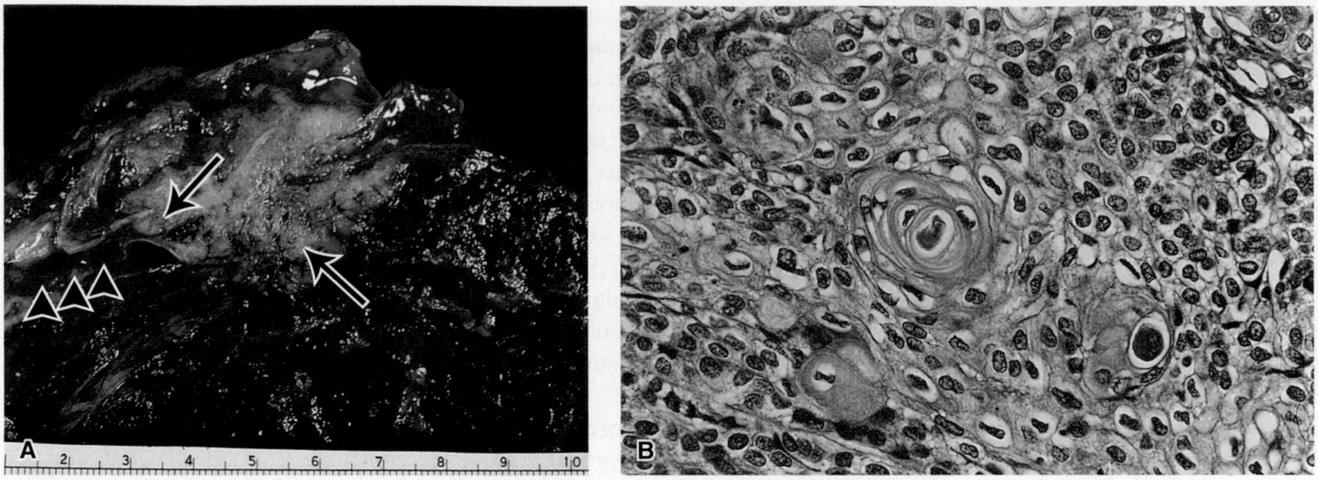

Figure 30.12 • Squamous cell carcinoma of the lung. **(A)** The tumor (*large arrow*) grows within the lumen of a bronchus (*arrowheads* highlight the course of the bronchus) and invades the adjacent intrapulmonary lymph node (*small arrow*). **(B)** A photomicrograph shows well-differentiated squamous cell carcinoma with a keratin pearl composed of cells with brightly eosinophilic cytoplasm. (From Strayer D. S., Rubin R. (Eds.) (2015). *Rubin's pathology: Clinicopathologic foundations of medicine* (7th ed., Fig. 18-79, p. 737). Philadelphia, PA: Lippincott Williams & Wilkins.)

lung cancer (see Fig. 30.13). The most common sites of these metastases are the brain, bone, and liver.

Many of the manifestations of lung cancers result from local irritation and obstruction of the airways and from invasion of the mediastinum and pleural space. The earliest symptoms usually are chronic cough, shortness of breath, and wheezing because of airway irritation and obstruction. Hemoptysis (*i.e.*, blood in the sputum) occurs when the lesion erodes blood vessels. Pain receptors in the chest are limited to the parietal pleura, mediastinum, larger blood vessels, and peribronchial afferent vagal fibers. Dull, intermittent, poorly

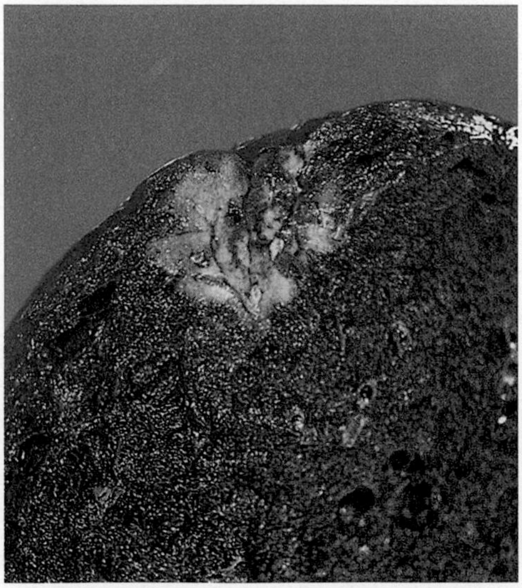

Figure 30.13 • Invasive adenocarcinoma of the lung. A peripheral tumor of the upper right lobe has an irregular border and a tan or gray cut surface and causes puckering of the overlying pleura. (From Strayer D. S., Rubin R. (Eds.) (2015). *Rubin's pathology: Clinicopathologic foundations of medicine* (7th ed., Fig. 18-80, p. 738). Philadelphia, PA: Lippincott Williams & Wilkins.)

localized retrosternal pain is common in tumors that involve the mediastinum. Pain becomes persistent, localized, and more severe when the disease invades the pleura.

Tumors that invade the mediastinum may cause hoarseness because of the involvement of the recurrent laryngeal nerve and cause difficulty in swallowing because of compression of the esophagus. An uncommon complication called the *superior vena cava syndrome* occurs in some people with mediastinal involvement. Interruption of blood flow in this vessel usually results from compression by the tumor or involved lymph nodes. The disorder can interfere with venous drainage from the head, neck, and chest wall. The outcome is determined by the speed with which the disorder develops and the adequacy of the collateral circulation. Tumors adjacent to the visceral pleura often insidiously produce pleural effusion. This effusion can compress the lung and cause atelectasis and dyspnea. It is less likely to cause fever, pleural friction rub, or pain than pleural effusion resulting from other causes.

Diagnosis and Treatment

The diagnosis of lung cancer is based on a careful history and physical examination and on other tests such as chest radiography, bronchoscopy, cytologic studies of the sputum or bronchial washings, percutaneous needle biopsy of lung tissue, and scalene lymph node biopsy.[32] CT scans, MRI studies, and ultrasonography are used to locate lesions and evaluate the extent of the disease. Positron emission tomography (PET) is a noninvasive alternative for identifying metastatic lesions in the mediastinum or distant sites. People with SCLC should also have a CT scan or MRI of the brain for detection of metastasis.

Like other cancers, lung cancer is classified according to extent of disease. NSCLCs are usually classified according to cell type (*i.e.*, squamous cell carcinoma, adenocarcinoma, and large cell carcinoma) and staged according to the TNM international staging system.[32] SCLCs are not staged using the TNM system because micrometastases are assumed to be present at the time of diagnosis. Instead, they are usually classified as limited disease when the tumor is limited to the unilateral hemithorax, or extensive disease when it extends beyond these boundaries.[32]

Treatment methods for NSCLC include surgery, radiation therapy, and chemotherapy.[32] These treatments may be used singly or in combination. Surgery is used for the removal of small, localized NSCLC tumors. It can involve a lobectomy, pneumonectomy, or segmental resection of the lung. Radiation therapy can be used as a definitive or main treatment modality, as part of a combined treatment plan, or for palliation of symptoms. Because of the frequency of metastases, chemotherapy often is used in treating lung cancer. Combination chemotherapy, which uses a regimen of several drugs, usually is used. New targeted treatments are under development with the goal of increasing survival and ultimately providing a cure for this type of cancer.

Therapy for SCLC is based on the stage and currently includes chemotherapy and radiation therapy; however, this is changing as new therapies are developed.[32] Advances in the use of combination chemotherapy, along with thoracic irradiation, have improved the outlook for people with SCLC. Because SCLC may metastasize to the brain, prophylactic cranial irradiation is often indicated. In most people who achieve a complete remission from SCLC, the brain is the most frequent site of relapse. About half of these people develop clinical metastasis within 3 years. Newer combination chemotherapy regimens and targeted therapies are being developed in hopes of providing treatment alternatives that increase survival and produce fewer treatment liabilities.

Management of Lung Cancer in Older Adults

Given the fact that most people are older than 65 years of age when diagnosed with lung cancer, it is important to understand management of lung cancer in older adults. Knowledge about the optimal treatment for older adults is limited because of underrepresentation in clinical trials and failure to evaluate younger versus older people in randomized clinical trials. At present, it is recommended that older adults should be treated based on their general physiologic rather than chronologic age. This includes an evaluation of functional status (ability to be independent in daily tasks at home and in the community), coexisting medical conditions, nutritional status, cognition, psychological functioning, social support, and medication review. Those with good performance status and normal renal and hematologic parameters may be treated surgically or receive standard chemotherapy and radiation for limited-stage disease and combination chemotherapy for extensive-stage disease.

Surgery remains the mainstay for older adults with stages I to III NSCLC. Curative resection is feasible in older adults. The challenge for surgical treatment for older adults is age-related physiologic changes in cardiovascular and respiratory systems that may affect tolerance of surgery.

Radiation can be given with curative intent for older adults who are not surgical candidates. It may also be used for palliation of cancer-related symptoms. Evidence suggests that treatment tolerance and efficacy of thoracic radiation are similar in younger and older people. Age is reported to have no effect on acute or late radiation toxicity, including nausea, dyspnea, esophagitis, or weakness. Chemotherapy is the mainstay of treatment of SCLC. Older adults with good performance status may receive standard chemotherapy for limited disease and combination chemotherapy for extensive-stage disease. Some older adults may require dose reductions or be unable to complete the full chemotherapy course.

IN SUMMARY

Cancer of the lung is a leading cause of death worldwide. Cigarette smoking is implicated in the majority of cases of lung cancer. The risk for lung cancer among cigarette smokers increases with duration of smoking and the number of cigarettes smoked per day. Industrial hazards, such as exposure to asbestos, increase the risk for development of lung cancer. Because lung cancer develops insidiously, it often is far advanced before it is diagnosed. This fact explains the poor 5-year survival rate. Carcinoma, which accounts for 95% of all primary lung cancers, can be subdivided currently into four major categories: squamous cell carcinoma, adenocarcinoma, large cell carcinoma, and small cell carcinoma. For purposes of staging and treatment, lung cancer is divided into SCLC and NSCLC. The main reason for this is that almost all SCLCs have metastasized at the time of diagnosis.

The manifestations of lung cancer can be attributed to the involvement of the lung and adjacent structures, the effects of local spread and metastasis, and paraneoplastic syndromes involving endocrine, neurologic, and hematologic dysfunction. As with other cancers, lung cancer causes nonspecific symptoms such as anorexia and weight loss. Treatment methods for lung cancer include surgery, irradiation, and chemotherapy. The current increase in lung cancer among older adults (those 65 years of age and older) has required a rethinking of the treatment strategies for this age group, with the trend being to base treatment on physiologic rather than chronologic age.

RESPIRATORY DISORDERS IN CHILDREN

After completing this section of the chapter, the learner will be able to meet the following objectives:

- Describe the role of surfactant in lung function in the neonate.
- Describe the possible cause and manifestations of RDS and BPD.

- List the signs of impending respiratory failure in small children.

Acute respiratory diseases are the most common cause of illness in infancy and childhood. This section focuses on

- Lung development, with an emphasis on the developmental basis for lung disorders in children
- Respiratory disorders in the neonate
- Respiratory infections in children

Lung Development

Although other body systems are physiologically ready for extrauterine life as early as 25 weeks of gestation, the lungs require much longer. Immaturity of the respiratory system is a major cause of morbidity and mortality in infants born prematurely. Even at birth, the lungs are not fully mature, and additional growth and maturation continue well into childhood.

Lung development may be divided into five stages: embryonic period, pseudoglandular period, canalicular period, saccular period, and alveolar period.[33,34] The development of the respiratory system begins with the *embryonic period* (weeks 4 to 6 of gestation). During this period, a rudimentary bronchial bud branches from the esophagus to begin formation of the airways and alveolar spaces. The bronchial bud divides into two lung buds that grow laterally. The right bud gives rise to two secondary bronchial buds and the left bud to one secondary bronchial bud. Consequently, at maturity, there are three main (primary) bronchi and three lung lobes on the right and only two main bronchi and two lung lobes on the left. Each secondary bronchial bud subsequently undergoes continuous branching. The tertiary (segmental) bronchi (10 in the right lung and 8 or 9 in the left lung) begin to form during the seventh week. The pulmonary vasculature is a mesenchymal derivative. Soon after their appearance, the bronchial buds are surrounded by a vascular plexus, which originates from the aorta and drains into the major somatic veins. This vascular plexus connects with the pulmonary artery and veins at the seventh week of gestation.

During the *pseudoglandular period* (weeks 5 to 16), the lungs resemble a gland. During this period, the conducting airways are formed. At 17 weeks, all of the major elements of the lung have formed except the gas exchange structures. Respiration is not possible because the airways end in blind tubes. The *canalicular period* (weeks 17 to 27) marks the formation of the primitive alveoli. The lumina of the bronchi and bronchioles become much larger, and the lung tissue becomes more highly vascularized. By the 24th week, each bronchiole has given rise to two or more respiratory bronchioles. Respiration is possible at this time because some primitive alveoli have developed at the ends of the bronchioles.[33,34]

The *saccular period* (weeks 27 to 35) is devoted to the development of the terminal alveolar sacs, which facilitate gas exchange. During this period, the terminal sacs thin out, and capillaries begin to bulge into the terminal sacs. These thin cells are known as type I alveolar cells. By the 25th to 28th weeks, sufficient terminal sacs are present to permit survival. Before this time, the premature lungs are incapable of adequate gas exchange. It is not so much the presence of the thin alveolar epithelium as it is the adequate matching of pulmonary vasculature to it that is critical to survival.[33,34] Type II alveolar cells begin to develop at approximately 24 weeks. These cells produce surfactant, a substance capable of lowering the surface tension of the air–alveoli interface. By the 28th to 30th weeks, sufficient amounts of surfactant are available to prevent alveolar collapse when breathing begins.

The *alveolar period* (late fetal to early childhood) marks the maturation and expansion of the alveoli. Starting as early as 30 weeks and usually by 36 weeks of gestation, the saccular structures become alveoli.[33,34] Alveolar development is characterized by thinning of the pulmonary interstitium and the appearance of a single-capillary network, in which one capillary bulges into each terminal alveolar sac. By the late fetal period, the lungs are capable of respiration because the alveolar–capillary membrane is sufficiently thin to allow for gas exchange.

Although transformation of the lungs from glandlike structures to highly vascular, alveoli-like organs occurs during the late fetal period, mature alveoli do not form for some time after birth. The growth of the lung during infancy and early childhood involves an increase in the number rather than the size of the alveoli. Only one eighth to one sixth of the adult number of alveoli is present at birth. There is a relative slowing of alveolar growth during the first 3 months after birth, and this is followed by a rapid increase in alveolar number during the rest of the first year of life.

Development of Breathing in the Fetus and Neonate

The fetal lung is a secretory organ, and fluids and electrolytes are secreted into the potential air spaces. This fluid appears to be important in stimulating alveolar development. For the fetus to complete the transition from intrauterine to extrauterine life, this fluid must be cleared from the lung soon after birth. Presumably with the onset of labor, the secretion of fluid ceases. During the birth process, pressure on the fetal thorax causes the fluid to be expelled from the mouth and nose. When the lungs expand after birth, the fluid moves into the tissues surrounding the alveoli and is then absorbed into the pulmonary capillaries or removed by the lymphatic system.

Fetal breathing movements occur in utero. These movements are irregular in rate and amplitude, ranging from 30 to 70 breaths/minute, and become more rapid as gestation advances. Because they are rapid and shallow, these movements do not result in movement of fluid into or out of the fetal lung. Instead, they are thought to condition the respiratory muscles and stimulate lung development. The breathing movements in the fetus become more rapid in response to an increase in carbon dioxide levels and become slower in response to hypoxia.

The major difference between respiration in the fetus and the neonate is that there is complete separation between gas exchange and breathing movements in the fetus. The gas supply and exchange depend entirely on maternal mechanisms controlling placental circulation. At birth, dependence on the placental circulation is terminated, and the infant must integrate the two previously separate functions of gas exchange and respiratory movements. Within seconds of clamping the umbilical cord, the infant takes its first breath, and rhythmic breathing begins and persists for life.

Effective ventilation requires coordinated interaction between the muscles of the upper airways, including those of the pharynx and larynx, the diaphragm, and the intercostal muscles of the chest wall. In infants, a specific sequence of upper airway nerve and muscle activity occurs before and early in inspiration. The tongue moves forward to prevent airway obstruction, and the vocal cord abducts, reducing laryngeal resistance. By moving downward, the action of the diaphragm increases chest volume in both the longitudinal and transverse directions. In the infant, the diaphragm inserts more horizontally than in the adult. As a result, contraction of the diaphragm tends to draw the lower ribs inward, especially if the infant is placed in the horizontal position. The function of the intercostal muscles is to lift the ribs during inspiration. In the infant, however, the intercostal muscles are not fully developed, so they function largely to stabilize the chest rather than lift the chest wall.

The chest wall of the neonate is highly compliant. Although this is advantageous during the birth process in that it allows for marked distortion to occur without damaging chest structures, it has implications for ventilation during the postnatal period. A striking characteristic of neonatal breathing is the paradoxical inward movement of the upper chest during inspiration, especially during active sleep. This occurs because of decreased activity of the intercostal muscles during active sleep, which allows the contracting diaphragm to pull the highly compliant chest wall inward. Under circumstances such as crying, the intercostal muscles of the neonate function together with the diaphragm to splint the chest wall and prevent its collapse.

Normally, the infant's lungs also are compliant. This is advantageous to the infant with a compliant chest cage because it takes only small changes in inspiratory pressure to inflate a compliant lung. When respiratory disease develops, lung compliance is reduced, and it takes more effort to inflate the lungs. The diaphragm must generate more negative pressure, causing the compliant chest wall structures to be sucked inward. *Retractions* are abnormal inward movements of the chest wall during inspiration. They may occur intercostally (between the ribs), in the substernal or epigastric area, and in the supraclavicular spaces. Because the chest wall of the infant is compliant, substernal retractions become more obvious with small changes in lung function. Retractions can indicate airway obstruction or atelectasis.

Airway Resistance

Normal lung inflation requires uninterrupted movement of air through the extrathoracic airways (*i.e.*, nose, pharynx, larynx, and upper trachea) and intrathoracic airways (*i.e.*, bronchi and bronchioles). The neonate (0 to 4 weeks of age) breathes predominantly through the nose and does not adapt well to mouth breathing. Any obstruction of the nose or nasopharynx may increase upper airway resistance and increase the work of breathing.

The airways of the infant and small child are much smaller than those of the adult.[33] Because the resistance to airflow is inversely related to the fourth power of the radius (resistance = $1/r^4$), relatively small amounts of mucus secretion, edema, or airway constriction can produce marked changes in airway resistance and airflow. Nasal flaring is a method that infants use to take in more air. This method of breathing increases the size of the nares and decreases the resistance of the small airways.

Normally, the extrathoracic airways in the infant narrow during inspiration and widen during expiration, and the intrathoracic airways widen during inspiration and narrow during expiration.[33] This occurs because the pressure inside the extrathoracic airways reflects the intrapleural pressures that are generated during breathing, whereas the pressure outside the airways is similar to atmospheric pressure. Thus, during inspiration, the pressure inside becomes more negative, causing the airways to narrow, and during expiration it becomes more positive, causing them to widen. In contrast to the extrathoracic airways, the pressure outside the intrathoracic airways is equal to the intrapleural pressure. These airways widen during inspiration as the surrounding intrapleural pressure becomes more negative and pulls them open, and they narrow during expiration as the surrounding pressure becomes more positive.

Lung Volumes and Gas Exchange

The functional residual capacity, which is the air left in the lungs at the end of normal expiration, plays an important role in the infant's gas exchange. In the infant, the functional residual capacity occurs at a higher lung volume than in the older child or adult.[33] This higher end-expiratory volume results from a more rapid respiratory rate, which leaves less time for expiration. However, the increased residual volume is important to the neonate for several reasons: (1) it holds the airways open throughout all phases of respiration, (2) it favors the reabsorption of intrapulmonary fluids, and (3) it maintains more uniform lung expansion and enhances gas exchange. During active sleep, the tone of the upper airway muscles is reduced. Therefore, the time spent in expiration is shorter, and the intercostal activity that stabilizes the chest wall is less. This results in a lower end-expiratory volume and less optimal gas exchange.

Control of Ventilation

Fetal arterial oxygen pressures (PO_2) normally range from 25 to 30 mm Hg, and carbon dioxide pressures (PCO_2) range from 45 to 50 mm Hg, independent of any respiratory movements. Any decrease in oxygen levels induces quiet sleep in the fetus with subsequent cessation of breathing movements, both of which lead to a decrease in oxygen consumption. Switching to oxygen derived from the aerated lung at birth causes an immediate increase in arterial PO_2 to approximately 50 mm Hg; within a few hours, it increases to approximately 70 mm Hg.[35] These levels, which greatly exceed fetal levels, cause the chemoreceptors that sense arterial PO_2 levels to become silent for several days. Although the infant's arterial PO_2 may fluctuate during this critical time, the chemoreceptors do not respond appropriately. It is not until several days after birth that the chemoreceptors "reset" their PO_2 threshold. Only then do they become the major controller of breathing. However, the response seems to be biphasic, with an initial hyperventilation followed by a decreased respiratory rate and even apnea. Periodic breathing and apnea are characteristic of premature infants and reflect patterns of fetal breathing.

Manifestations of Respiratory Disorders or Infection in the Infant or Small Child

Most respiratory disorders in the infant or small child produce a decrease in lung compliance or an increase in airway resistance manifested by changes in breathing patterns, rib cage distortion (retractions), audible sounds, and use of accessory muscles.[33]

Children with restrictive lung disorders, such as pulmonary edema or RDS, breathe at faster rates, and their respiratory excursions are shallow. *Grunting* is an audible noise emitted during expiration. An expiratory grunt is common as the child tries to raise the end-expiratory pressure and thus prolong the period of oxygen and carbon dioxide exchange across the alveolar–capillary membrane.

Increased airway resistance can occur in either the extrathoracic or intrathoracic airways. When the obstruction is in the extrathoracic airways, inspiration is more prolonged than expiration. *Nasal flaring* (enlargement of the nares) helps reduce the nasal resistance and maintain airway patency. It can be a sign of increased work of breathing and is a significant finding in an infant. *Inspiratory retractions*, or pulling in of the soft tissue surrounding the cartilaginous and bony thorax, are often observed with airway obstruction in infants and small children (Fig. 30.14). In conditions such as croup, the pressures distal to the point of obstruction must become more negative to overcome the resistance; this causes collapse of the distal airways, and the increased turbulence of air moving through the obstructed airways produces an audible crowing sound called a *stridor* during inspiration.

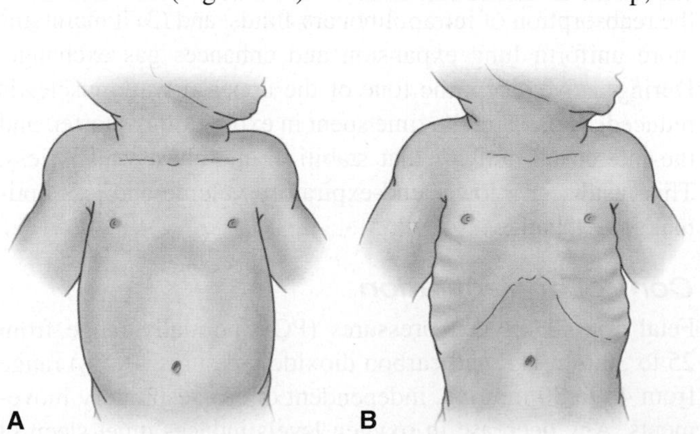

Figure 30.14 • **(A)** Normal inspiratory appearance of the chest during unobstructed breathing in the neonate. **(B)** Sternal and intercostal retractions during obstructed breathing in the neonate.

When the obstruction is in the intrathoracic airways, as occurs with bronchiolitis and bronchial asthma, expiration is prolonged and the child makes use of the accessory expiratory muscles (abdominals). Rib cage retractions may also be present. Intrapleural pressure becomes more positive during expiration because of air trapping. This causes collapse of intrathoracic airways and produces an audible wheezing or whistling sound during expiration.

Respiratory Disorders in the Neonate

The neonatal period is one of transition from placental dependency to air breathing. This transition requires functioning of the surfactant system, conditioning of the respiratory muscles, and establishment of parallel pulmonary and systemic circulations. Respiratory disorders develop in infants who are born prematurely or who have other problems that impair this transition. Among the respiratory disorders of the neonate are the RDS and BPD.

Respiratory Distress Syndrome

RDS, previously known as *hyaline membrane disease*, is one of the most common causes of respiratory disease in premature infants.[36] In these infants, pulmonary immaturity, together with surfactant deficiency, leads to alveolar collapse (Fig. 30.15).

The incidence of RDS is higher among preterm male infants, white infants, infants of diabetic mothers, and those subjected to asphyxia, cold stress, precipitous deliveries, and delivery by cesarean section (when performed before the 38th week of gestation).

Etiology and Pathogenesis. The type II alveolar cells that produce surfactant do not begin to mature until approximately the 25th to 28th weeks of gestation. Consequently, many premature infants are born with poorly functioning type II alveolar cells and have difficulty producing sufficient amounts of surfactant.

Surfactant synthesis is influenced by several hormones, including insulin and cortisol. Insulin tends to inhibit surfactant production; this explains why infants of insulin-dependent diabetic mothers are at increased risk for development of RDS. Cortisol can accelerate maturation of type II cells and formation of surfactant. The reason that premature infants born by cesarean section presumably are at greater risk for development of RDS is that they are not subjected to the stress of vaginal delivery, which is thought to increase the infants' cortisol levels. Surfactant reduces the surface tension in the alveoli, thereby equalizing the retractive forces in the large and small alveoli and reducing the amount of pressure needed to inflate and hold the alveoli open. Without surfactant, the large alveoli remain inflated, whereas the small alveoli become

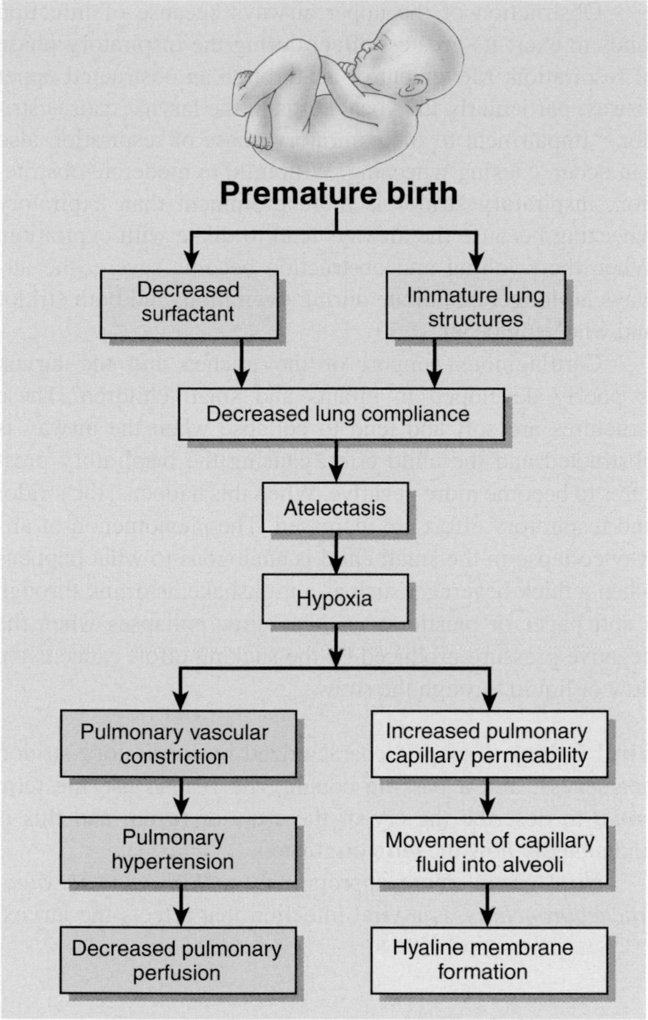

Figure 30.15 • Pathogenesis of RDS in the infant.

difficult to inflate. At birth, the first breath requires high inspiratory pressures to expand the lungs. With normal levels of surfactant, the lungs retain up to 40% of the residual volume after the first breath, and subsequent breaths require far lower inspiratory pressures. With a surfactant deficiency, the lungs collapse between breaths, making the infant work as hard with each successive breath as with the first breath. The airless portions of the lungs become stiff and noncompliant. A hyaline membrane forms inside the alveoli as protein- and fibrin-rich fluids are pulled into the alveolar spaces. The fibrin–hyaline membrane constitutes a barrier to gas exchange, leading to hypoxemia and carbon dioxide retention, a condition that further impairs surfactant production.

Clinical Manifestations. Infants with RDS present with multiple signs of respiratory distress, usually within the first 24 hours of birth. Central cyanosis is a prominent sign. Breathing becomes more difficult, and retractions occur as the infant's soft chest wall is pulled in as the diaphragm descends. Grunting sounds accompany expiration. As the tidal volume drops because of atelectasis, the respiration rate increases (usually to 60 to 120 breaths/minute) in an effort to maintain normal minute ventilation. Fatigue may develop rapidly because of the increased work of breathing. The stiff lungs of infants with RDS also increase the resistance to blood flow in the pulmonary circulation. As a result, a hemodynamically significant patent ductus arteriosus may develop in infants with RDS.

Treatment The basic principles of treatment for infants with suspected RDS focus on the provision of supportive care, including gentle handling and minimal disturbance.[33] An incubator or radiant warmer is used to prevent hypothermia and increased oxygen consumption. Continuous cardiorespiratory monitoring is needed. Monitoring of blood glucose and prevention of hypoglycemia are also recommended. Oxygen levels can be assessed through an arterial (umbilical) line or by a transcutaneous oxygen sensor. Treatment includes administration of supplemental oxygen, continuous positive airway pressure through nasal prongs, and often assisted mechanical ventilation.

Exogenous surfactant therapy is used to prevent and treat RDS.[36] There are two types of surfactants: natural surfactants prepared from animal sources and synthetic surfactants. The surfactants are suspended in saline and administered into the airways, usually through an endotracheal tube. The treatment often is initiated soon after birth in infants who are at high risk for RDS.

Bronchopulmonary Dysplasia

BPD is a chronic lung disease that develops in premature infants who were treated with long-term mechanical ventilation, mainly for RDS.[37] The condition is considered to be present if the neonate is oxygen dependent at 36 weeks after gestation.

Etiology. The disorder is thought to be a response of the premature lung to early injury. High-inspired oxygen concentration and injury from positive-pressure ventilation (*i.e.*, barotrauma) have been implicated.

Clinical Manifestations. BPD is characterized by chronic respiratory distress, persistent hypoxemia when breathing room air, reduced lung compliance, increased airway resistance, and severe expiratory flow limitation. There is a mismatching of ventilation and perfusion with development of hypoxemia and hypercapnia. Pulmonary vascular resistance may be increased and pulmonary hypertension and cor pulmonale (*i.e.*, right heart failure associated with lung disease) may develop. The infant with BPD often demonstrates a barrel chest, tachycardia, rapid and shallow breathing, chest retractions, cough, and poor weight gain.[33] Clubbing of the fingers occurs in children with severe disease. Hepatomegaly and periorbital edema may develop in infants with right heart failure.

The treatment of BPD includes mechanical ventilation and administration of supplemental oxygen. Weaning from ventilation is accomplished gradually, and some infants may require ventilation at home. Rapid lung growth occurs during the first year of life, and lung function usually improves. Most adolescents and young adults who had severe BPD during infancy have some degree of pulmonary dysfunction, consisting of airway obstruction, airway hyperreactivity, or hyperinflation.

Respiratory Infections in Children

In children, respiratory tract infections are common, and although they are troublesome, they usually are not serious. Frequent infections occur because the immune system of infants and small children has not been exposed to many common pathogens. Consequently, they tend to contract infections with each new exposure. Although most of these infections are not serious, the small size of an infant's or child's airways tends to foster impaired airflow and obstruction. For example, an infection that causes only sore throat and hoarseness in an adult may result in serious airway obstruction in a small child.

Upper Airway Infections

Significant acute upper airway infections in infants and small children include viral croup, bacterial tracheitis, and epiglottitis.[33] Croup is the more common and usually is benign and self-limited. Bacterial tracheitis is rare but can occur in children experiencing multiple viral respiratory infections. Epiglottitis is a rapidly progressive and life-threatening condition. The characteristics of croup and epiglottitis infections are described in Table 30.2.

Obstruction of the upper airways because of infection tends to exert its greatest effect during the inspiratory phase of respiration. Movement of air through an obstructed upper airway, particularly the vocal cords in the larynx, causes stridor.[33] Impairment of the expiratory phase of respiration also can occur, causing wheezing. With mild to moderate obstruction, inspiratory stridor is more prominent than expiratory wheezing because the airways tend to dilate with expiration. When the swelling and obstruction become severe, the airways no longer can dilate during expiration, and both stridor and wheezing occur.

Cartilaginous support of the trachea and the larynx is poorly developed in infants and small children. These structures are soft and tend to collapse when the airway is obstructed and the child cries, causing the inspiratory pressures to become more negative. When this happens, the stridor and inspiratory effort are increased. The phenomenon of airway collapse in the small child is analogous to what happens when a thick beverage, such as a milkshake, is drunk through a soft paper or plastic straw. The straw collapses when the negative pressure produced by the sucking effort exceeds the flow of liquid through the straw.

Viral Croup. Croup is characterized by inspiratory stridor, hoarseness, and a barking cough. The British use the term *croup* to describe the cry of the crow or raven, and this is undoubtedly how the term originated.

Viral croup, more appropriately called *acute laryngotracheobronchitis*, is a viral infection that affects the larynx,

TABLE 30.2 CHARACTERISTICS OF EPIGLOTTITIS, CROUP, AND BRONCHIOLITIS IN SMALL CHILDREN

CHARACTERISTICS	EPIGLOTTITIS	CROUP	BRONCHIOLITIS
Common causative agent	*Haemophilus influenzae* type B bacterium	Mainly parainfluenza virus	Respiratory syncytial virus
Most commonly affected age group	2–7 years (peak 3–5 years)	3 months to 5 years	<2 years (most severe in infants younger than 6 months)
Onset and preceding history	Sudden onset	Usually follows symptoms of a cold	Preceded by stuffy nose and other signs
Prominent features	Child appears very sick and toxic Sits with mouth open and chin thrust forward Low-pitched stridor, difficulty swallowing, fever, drooling, anxiety Danger of airway obstruction and asphyxia	Stridor and a wet, barking cough Usually occurs at night Relieved by exposure to cold or moist air	Breathlessness, rapid, shallow breathing, wheezing, cough, and retractions of lower ribs and sternum during inspiration
Usual treatment	Hospitalization Intubation or tracheotomy Treatment with appropriate antibiotic	Mist tent or nebulization if not relieved by exposure to air or moist air Oxygen	Supportive treatment, possibly nebulization therapy or intubation depending on situation

trachea, and bronchi. The parainfluenza viruses account for the majority of cases. Other causes include adenoviruses, rhinovirus, RSV, and influenza A and B viruses.[38] Viral croup usually is seen in children 3 months to 5 years of age. The condition may affect the entire laryngotracheal tree. However, because the subglottic area is the narrowest part of the respiratory tree in this age group, the obstruction usually is greatest in this area. Although the respiratory manifestations of croup often appear suddenly, they usually are preceded by upper respiratory infections that cause rhinorrhea (*i.e.*, runny nose), coryza (*i.e.*, common cold), hoarseness, and low-grade fever. In most children, the manifestation of croup advances only to stridor and slight dyspnea before they begin to recover. The symptoms usually subside when the child is exposed to moist air. For example, letting the bathroom shower run and then taking the child into the bathroom often brings prompt and dramatic relief of symptoms. Exposure to cold air also seems to relieve the airway spasm. Often, severe symptoms are relieved simply because the child is exposed to cold air on the way to the hospital emergency department. Viral croup does not respond to antibiotics, and expectorants, bronchodilating agents, and antihistamines are not helpful. The child should be disturbed as little as possible and carefully monitored for signs of respiratory distress.

Airway obstruction may progress in some children. As obstruction increases, the stridor becomes continuous and is associated with nasal flaring with substernal and intercostal retractions. Agitation and crying aggravate the signs and symptoms, and the child prefers to sit up or be held upright. In the cyanotic, pale, or obstructed child, any manipulation of the pharynx, including use of a tongue depressor, can cause cardiorespiratory arrest and should be done only in a medical setting that has the facilities for emergency airway management. Establishment of an artificial airway may become necessary in severe airway obstruction.

Spasmodic Croup. Spasmodic croup manifests with symptoms similar to those of acute viral croup. Because the child is afebrile and lacks other manifestations of the viral prodrome, it is thought to have an allergic origin. Spasmodic croup characteristically occurs at night and tends to recur with respiratory tract infections. The episode usually lasts several hours and may recur several nights in a row.

Most children with spasmodic croup can be managed effectively at home. An environment of high humidification (*i.e.*, cold-water room humidifier or taking the child into a bathroom with a warm, running shower) lessens irritation and prevents drying of secretions. Or, if there is no success with opening the airway, the child should be brought outside into the cold air, which, in some cases, can assist the child's breathing.

Bacterial Tracheitis. This disorder is also called laryngotracheobronchitis and bacterial croup. It is a rare infection of the trachea secondary to a bacterium, most often *S. aureus*. If seen, it generally follows a viral respiratory infection. The manifestations are similar to viral croup except the child will need an antibiotic because a bacterium causes the infection. These children will need to be diagnosed and treated quickly; otherwise, acute respiratory failure can occur.

Epiglottitis. Acute epiglottitis is a dramatic, potentially fatal condition characterized by inflammatory edema of the supraglottic area, including the epiglottis and pharyngeal structures (see Fig. 30.14). It comes on suddenly, bringing danger of airway obstruction and asphyxia.[33] In the past, the *H. influenzae* type B bacterium was the most commonly identified etiologic agent. It is seen less commonly because the widespread use of immunization against *H. influenzae* type B. Therefore, other agents such as *Streptococcus pyogenes*, *S. pneumoniae*, and *S. aureus* now represent the larger cause of pediatric epiglottitis.

The child appears pale, toxic, and lethargic and assumes a distinctive position—sitting up with the mouth open and the chin thrust forward. The child has difficulty swallowing, a muffled voice, drooling, fever, and extreme anxiety. Moderate to severe respiratory distress is evident. There is inspiratory and sometimes expiratory stridor, flaring of the nares, and inspiratory retractions of the suprasternal notch and supraclavicular and intercostal spaces. Within a matter of hours, epiglottitis may progress to complete obstruction of the airway and death unless adequate treatment is instituted. Epiglottitis is a medical emergency and immediate establishment of an airway by endotracheal tube or tracheotomy usually is needed.

Concept Mastery Alert

If epiglottitis is suspected, the caregiver should keep the child calm and decrease anxiety. The child should never be forced to lie down because this causes the epiglottis to fall backward and may lead to complete airway obstruction. Examination of the throat with a tongue blade or other instrument may cause cardiopulmonary arrest and should be done only by medical personnel experienced in intubation of small children. It also is unwise to attempt any procedure, such as drawing blood, which would heighten the child's anxiety, because this also could precipitate airway spasm and cause death. Recovery from epiglottitis usually is rapid and uneventful after an adequate airway has been established and appropriate antibiotic therapy initiated.

Lower Airway Infections

Lower airway infections produce air trapping with prolonged expiration. Wheezing results from bronchospasm, mucosal inflammation, and edema. The child presents with increased expiratory effort, increased respiratory rate, and wheezing. If the infection is severe, there also are marked intercostal retractions and signs of impending respiratory failure.

Acute Bronchiolitis/Respiratory Syncytial Virus. Acute bronchiolitis is a viral infection of the lower airways, most commonly caused by the RSV.[39] Other viruses, such as parainfluenza-3 virus and some adenoviruses, as well as mycoplasmas, also are causative. The infection produces inflammatory obstruction of the small airways and necrosis of the cells lining the lower airways. It usually occurs during the first 2 years of life, with a peak incidence between 3 and 6 months of age. The source of infection usually is a family member with a minor respiratory illness.

Older children and adults tolerate bronchiolar edema much better than infants and do not manifest the clinical picture of bronchiolitis. Most affected infants in whom bronchiolitis develops have a history of a mild upper respiratory tract infection. These symptoms usually last several days and may be accompanied by fever and diminished appetite. There is then a gradual development of respiratory distress, characterized by a wheezy cough, dyspnea, and irritability. The infant usually is able to take in sufficient air but has trouble exhaling it. Air becomes trapped in the lung distal to the site of obstruction and interferes with gas exchange. Hypoxemia and, in severe cases, hypercapnia may develop. Airway obstruction may produce air trapping and hyperinflation of the lungs or collapse of the alveoli. Infants with acute bronchiolitis have a typical appearance, marked by breathlessness with rapid respirations, a distressing cough, and retractions of the lower ribs and sternum. Crying and feeding exaggerate these signs. Wheezing and crackles may or may not be present, depending on the degree of airway obstruction. In infants with severe airway obstruction, wheezing decreases as the airflow diminishes. Usually, the most critical phase of the disease is the first 48 to 72 hours. Cyanosis, pallor, listlessness, and sudden diminution or absence of breath sounds indicate impending respiratory failure. The characteristics of bronchiolitis are described in Table 30.2.

The latest evidence does not recommend that clinicians administer albuterol or corticosteroids to children with a diagnosis of bronchiolitis. However, nebulized hypertonic saline may be given to hospitalized children.[40]

Infants with respiratory distress usually are hospitalized. Treatment is supportive and includes administration of supplemental oxygen if the oxygen saturation consistently falls below 90%.[33] Evidence suggests that children with respiratory distress needing oxygen should first be given high-flow oxygen via a nasal cannula because it tends to increase oxygen saturation, increase comfort, and increase the overall respiratory condition.[40] Often with young children, a nebulizer is used to administer the steam or bronchodilator. Elevation of the head facilitates respiratory movements and avoids airway compression. Handling is kept at a minimum to avoid tiring. Because the infection is viral, antibiotics are not effective and are given only for a secondary bacterial infection. Dehydration may occur as the result of increased insensible water losses because of the rapid respiratory rate and feeding difficulties, and measures to ensure adequate hydration are needed. If the child is in respiratory distress and adequate hydration cannot be achieved, the child should receive intravenous fluids. Recovery usually begins after the first 48 to 72 hours and usually is rapid and complete. Adequate hand washing is essential to prevent the nosocomial spread of RSV.

Signs of Impending Respiratory Failure

Respiratory problems of infants and small children often originate suddenly, and recovery usually is rapid and complete. Children are at risk for the development of airway obstruction and respiratory failure resulting from obstructive disorders or lung infection. The child with epiglottitis is at risk for airway obstruction. The child with bronchiolitis is at risk for respiratory failure resulting from impaired gas exchange. Children with impending respiratory failure because of airway or lung disease have rapid breathing; exaggerated use of the accessory muscles; retractions, which are more pronounced in the child than in the adult because of more compliant chest; nasal flaring; and grunting during expiration. The signs and symptoms of impending respiratory failure are listed in Chart 30.1.

CHART 30.1 SIGNS OF RESPIRATORY DISTRESS AND IMPENDING RESPIRATORY FAILURE IN THE INFANT AND SMALL CHILD

- Severe increase in respiratory effort, including severe retractions or grunting, decreased chest movement
- Cyanosis that is not relieved by administration of oxygen (40%)
- Heart rate of 150 per minute or greater and increasing bradycardia
- Very rapid breathing (rate 60 per minute in the newborn to 6 months or above 30 per minute in children 6 months to 2 years)
- Very depressed breathing (rate 20 per minute or below)
- Retractions of the supraclavicular area, sternum, epigastrium, and intercostal spaces
- Extreme anxiety and agitation
- Fatigue

IN SUMMARY

Although other body systems are physiologically ready for extrauterine life as early as 25 weeks of gestation, the lungs take longer. Immaturity of the respiratory system is a major cause of morbidity and mortality in premature infants.

Lung development may be divided into five stages: embryonic period, pseudoglandular period, canalicular period, saccular period, and alveolar period. The first three phases are devoted to development of the conducting airways, and the last two phases are devoted to development of the gas exchange portion of the lung. By the 25th to 28th weeks of gestation, sufficient terminal air sacs are present to permit survival. It is also during this period that type II alveolar cells, which produce surfactant, begin to function.

Lung development is incomplete at birth; an infant is born with only one eighth to one sixth the adult number of alveoli. Alveoli continue to be formed during early childhood, reaching the adult number of 300 million alveoli by 8 years of age.

Children with restrictive lung disease breathe at faster rates, and their respiratory excursions are shallow. An expiratory grunt is common as the child tries to raise the functional residual capacity by closing the glottis at the end of expiration. Obstruction of the extrathoracic airways often produces turbulence of airflow and an audible inspiratory crowing sound called *stridor*, and obstruction of the intrathoracic airways produces an audible expiratory wheezing or whistling sound. RDS is one of the most common causes of respiratory disease in premature infants. In these infants, pulmonary immaturity, together with surfactant deficiency, leads to alveolar collapse. BPD is a chronic pulmonary disease that frequently develops in premature infants who were treated with long-term mechanical ventilation.

Acute respiratory disease is the most common cause of illness in infancy and childhood. It accounts for 50% of illnesses in children younger than 5 years of age and 30% of illnesses in children between 5 and 12 years of age. Because of the small size of the airway of infants and children, respiratory tract infections in these groups often are more serious. Infections that may cause only a sore throat and hoarseness in the adult may produce serious obstruction in the child. Among the respiratory tract infections that affect small children are croup, bacterial tracheitis, epiglottitis, and bronchiolitis. Epiglottitis is a life-threatening supraglottic infection that may cause airway obstruction and asphyxia.

GERIATRIC Considerations

- Physiologic changes associated with aging that include fewer cilia and less mucus, ineffective cough and gag reflex, and inconsistent ventilation and blood flow reduce the antibody's effectiveness against antigens and foreign particles.[41]
- Because many older smokers have used tobacco for most of their lifetimes, inflammation of the mucosa, reduced lung capacity, and reduced ciliary performance lead to an increased risk for infection of the respiratory system.[35]
- Older adults should avoid OTC treatment for respiratory issues because of interaction with medications and masking of serious problems. Colds lasting more than 1 week may represent a serious respiratory alteration requiring medical attention.[35]
- Because of age-related changes in the respiratory tract, the common symptoms of pneumonia (cough with phlegm, hyperthermia, and chest discomfort) may not be present, delaying a diagnosis and treatment.[35]

PEDIATRIC Considerations

- Airway infections are caused by diverse organisms that are more serious in malnourished infants and children and those not normally exposed.[42]
- RSV most often occurs as epidemics in nurseries resulting in nosocomial infections.[42]
- Streptococcal pneumonia in the newborn is typically caused by group B streptococci passed from mother to infant through normal flora found in the female genital tract.[42]

REVIEW EXERCISES

1. It is flu season, and although you had a flu shot last year, you have not had one this year. Imagine yourself experiencing an abrupt onset of fever, chills, malaise, muscle aching, and nasal stuffiness.
   A. *Which of these symptoms would lead you to believe you are coming down with the flu?*
   B. *Because you hate to miss classes, you decide to go to the student health center to get an antibiotic. After being seen by a health professional, you are told that antibiotics are ineffective against the flu virus, and you are instructed not to attend classes but instead to go home, take acetaminophen for your fever, go to bed and stay warm, and drink a lot of fluids. Explain the rationale for each of these recommendations.*
   C. *Explain why last year's flu shot did not protect you during this year's flu season.*
2. Bacterial (*e.g., S. pneumoniae*) pneumonia is commonly manifested by a cough productive of sputum, whereas with atypical (*e.g., M. pneumoniae*) pneumonia, the cough is usually nonproductive or absent.
   A. *Explain.*
3. A 4-month-old infant is admitted to the pediatric intensive care unit with a diagnosis of bronchiolitis. The infant is tachypneic, with wheezing, nasal flaring, and retractions of the lower sternum and intercostal spaces during inspiration.
   A. *What is the usual pathogen in bronchiolitis? Would this infection be treated with an antibiotic?*
   B. *Explain the physiologic mechanism involved in the retraction of the lower sternum and intercostal spaces during inspiration.*
   C. *What would be the signs of impending respiratory failure in this infant?*

References

1. Centers for Disease Control. (2016). Leading causes of death. Available: https://www.cdc.gov/nchs/fastats/leading-caues-of-death.htm. Accessed December 12, 2017
2. World Health Organization. (2016). Pneumonia. [Online]. Available: https://www.who.int/mediacentre/factsheets/fs331/en/. Accessed December 12, 2017
3. Centers for Disease Control. (2016). *Tuberculosis.* [Online]. Available: https://www.cdc.gov/tb/statistics/default.htm. Accessed December 12, 2017
4. World Health Organization. (2016). *Cancer.* [Online]. Available: https://www.who.int/mediacentre/factsheets/fs297/en/. Accessed December 12, 2017
5. Tapparel C., Sobo K., Constant S., et al. (2013). Growth and characterization of different human rhinovirus C types in three-dimensional human airway epithelia reconstituted in vitro. *Virology* 446(1–2), 1–8. Available: www.sciencedirect.com/science/article/pii/S0042682213004017. Accessed December 12, 2017
6. Othumpangat S., Noti J., McMillen C., et al. (2016). ICAM-1 regulates the survival of influenza virus in lung epithelial cells during the early stages of infection. *Virology* 487, 85–94. Available: www.sciencedirect.com/science/article/pii/S0042682215004328. Accessed: December 13, 2017
7. Dolin R. Common viral respiratory infections. In Kasper D., Fauci A., Hauser S., et al. (Eds), *Harrison's principles of internal medicine* (19th ed.). New York, NY: McGraw-Hill. Available: http://accessmedicine.mhmedical.com/content.aspx?bookid=1130&sectionid=79738549. Accessed: December 13, 2017.
8. Truven Health Analytics. (2017). *Micromedex Solutions.* Available: http://www.micromedexsolutions.com.ezproxy.uthsc.edu/micromedex2/librarian/CS/C8DF59/ND_PR/evidencexpert/ND_P/evidencexpert/DUPLICATIONSHIELDSYNC/78BD86/ND_PG/evidencexpert/ND_B/evidencexpert/ND_AppProduct/evidencexpert/ND_T/evidencexpert/PFActionId/evidencexpert.IntermediateToDocumentLink?docId=333&contentSetId=7&title=ANTIHISTAMINE%2FDECONGESTANT&servicesTitle=ANTIHISTAMINE%2FDECONGESTANT. Accessed December 13, 2017
9. Rubin M. A., Ford L. C., Gonzales R., et al. (2014). Sore throat, earache, and upper respiratory symptoms. *Harrison's principles of internal medicine* (19th ed.). Kasper D., Hauser S. L., Jameson J. L., et al. New York, NY: McGraw-Hill. Available: http://accessmedicine.mhmedical.com/content.aspx?bookid=1130&sectionid=79725618
10. Kliegman R. M., Stanton B. F. (2016). Sinusitis. In Kliegman R. M., Stanton B. F., Geme J. W. St., et al. (Eds.), *Nelson textbook of pediatrics* (20th ed., pp. 2014–2017). St. Louis: Elsevier, Inc.
11. Centers for Disease Control and Prevention. (2017). *Estimated influenza illnesses, medical visits, hospitalizations, and deaths averted by vaccination in the United States.* Available: https://www.cdc.gov/flu/about/disease/2015-16.htm
12. Hayden F. G. (2016). Influenza. In Goldman L., Schafer A. I. (Eds.), *Goldman-Cecil medicine* (25th ed., pp. 2191–2197). Philadelphia, PA: Saunders, an imprint of Elsevier Inc.
13. Musher D. M. (2016). Overview of pneumonia. In Goldman L., Schafer A. I. (Eds.), *Goldman-Cecil medicine* (25th ed., pp. 610–620). Philadelphia, PA: Saunders, an imprint of Elsevier Inc.
14. Elsevier Point of Care. (2017). *Community-acquired pneumonia in adults.* Available: https://www.clinicalkey.com/#!/content/67-s2.0-77188ebd-e5b9-49a1-88a0-0211995a4b85. Accessed: December 13, 2017
15. Kumar V., Abbas A. K. (2015). The lung. In Kumar V., Abbas A. K., (Eds.), *Robbins and Cotran pathologic basis of disease* (9th ed., pp. 669–726). Philadelphia, PA: Saunders, an imprint of Elsevier Inc.
16. Yu V. L., Pedro-Botet L., Lin Y. E. (2014). Legionella infections. In Kasper D., Fauci A., Hauser S., et al. (Eds), *Harrison's principles of internal medicine* (19th ed.) New York, NY: McGraw-Hill. Available: http://accessmedicine.mhmedical.com/content.aspx?bookid=1130&sectionid=79735876. Accessed: December 13, 2017
17. Gaydos C. A., Quinn T. C. (2014). Chlamydial infections. In Kasper D., Fauci A., Hauser S., et al. (Eds), *Harrison's principles of internal medicine* (19th ed.). New York, NY: McGraw-Hill. Available: http://accessmedicine.mhmedical.com/content.aspx?bookid=1130&sectionid=79737875. Accessed: December 13, 2017
18. Liu J.-L., Xu F., Zhou H., et al. (2016). Expanded CURB-65: A new score system predicts severity of community-acquired pneumonia with superior efficiency. *Scientific Reports* 6, 22911. *PMC*. Web. 12 Dec. 2017.
19. World Health Organization Regional Office for South East Asia. (2017). Tuberculosis/human immunodeficiency virus proteins. Available: http://apps.who.int/iris/handle/10665/254762. Accessed: December 13, 2017
20. Raviglione M. C. (2014). Tuberculosis. In Kasper D., Fauci A., Hauser S., et al. (Eds), *Harrison's principles of internal medicine* (19th ed.). New York, NY: McGraw-Hill. Available: http://accessmedicine.mhmedical.com.ezproxy.uthsc.edu/content.aspx?bookid=1130&sectionid=79737003. Accessed: December 14, 2017
21. Pai M., Rodrigues C. (2015). Management of latent tuberculosis infection: An evidence-based approach. *Lung India: Official Organ of Indian Chest Society* 32(2), 205–207. DOI: 10.4103/0970-2113.156210. Available: https://www.ncbi.nlm.nih.gov/pmc/articles/PMC4429378/. Accessed December 14, 2017
22. Hage C. A., Wheat L. (2014). Histoplasmosis. In Kasper D., Fauci A., Hauser S., et al. (Eds), *Harrison's principles of internal medicine* (19th ed.). New York, NY: McGraw-Hill. Available: http://accessmedicine.mhmedical.com.ezproxy.uthsc.edu/content.aspx?bookid=1130&sectionid=79739792. Accessed: December 14, 2017
23. Jemal A., Ward E. M., Johnson C. J., et al. (2017). Annual report to the nation on the status of cancer, 1975–2014, featuring survival. *JNCI: Journal of the National Cancer Institute* 109(9), https://doi.org/10.1093/jnci/djx030
24. Nosanchuk J. D. (2016). Endemic mycoses. In Nadel J. A., Murray J. F., Gotway M. B., et al. (Eds.), *Murray and Nadel's textbook of respiratory medicine* (6th ed., pp. 646–660). Philadelphia, PA: Elsevier Saunders. Available: https://www-clinicalkey-com.ezproxy.uthsc.edu/#!/content/book/3-s2.0-B9781455733835000373?scrollTo=%23top. Accessed: December 14, 2017
25. Galgiani J. N. (2016). Coccidioidomycosis. In Goldman L., Schafer A. I. (Eds.), *Goldman-Cecil medicine* (25th ed., pp. 2072–2073.e2). Philadelphia, PA: Elsevier Saunders.
26. Jackson M. A., Long S. S. (2015). Red Book 2015: Report of the Committee on Infectious Diseases (30th ed.). Elk Grove Village, IL: American Academy of Pediatrics. Available: EBSCOhost, ezproxy.uthsc.edu/login?url=http://search.ebscohost.com/login.aspx?direct=true&db=nlebk&AN=1076143&site=ehost-live. Accessed November 30, 2017
27. Smith J. A., Gauthier G. (2015). New developments in blastomycosis. *Seminars in Respiratory and Critical Care Medicine* 36(5), 715–728.
28. DeSantis C. E., Lin C. C., Marlotto A. B., et al. (2014). Cancer treatment and survivorship statistics, 2014. *CA: A Cancer Journal for Clinicians* 64, 252–271.
29. National Cancer Institute. (2014). *SEER Cancer Stat Facts: Lung and Bronchus Cancer. Bethesda, MD.* Available: http://seer.cancer.gov/statfacts/html/lungb.html. Accessed December 10, 2017
30. Ridge C. A., McErlean A. M., Ginsberg M. S. (2013). Epidemiology of lung cancer. *Seminars in Interventional Radiology* 30(2), 93–98. DOI: 10.1055/s-0033-1342949
31. Reid P. T., Innes J. A. (2014). Respiratory disease. In Walker B. R., Colledge N. R., Ralston S. H., et al. (Eds), *Davidson's Principles and Practice of Medicine* (22nd ed., pp. 643–732). Philadelphia, PA: Elsevier Churchill Livingstone.
32. Horn L., Lovly C. M., Johnson D. H. (2014). Neoplasms of the lung. In Kasper D., Fauci A., Hauser S., et al. (Eds), *Harrison's principles of internal medicine* (19th ed.). New York, NY: McGraw-Hill. Available: http://accessmedicine.mhmedical.com/content.aspx?bookid=1130&sectionid=79725618
33. Hockenberry M. J., Wilson D. (2015). *Wong's Nursing Care of Infants and Children.* St Louis, MO: Elsevier.
34. Kallapur S. G., Jobe A. H. (2015). Lung development and maturation. In Martin R. J., Faranoff A. A., Walsh M. C. (Eds), *Faranoff and Martin's Neonatal-Perinatal Medicine* (10th ed., pp. 1042–1059). Philadelphia, PA: Elsevier.

35. Eliopoulos C. (2018). Respiration. In *Gerontological Nursing*. Philadelphia, PA: Wolters Kluwer.
36. Wambach J. A., Hamvas A. (2015). Respiratory distress syndrome in the neonate. In Martin R. J., Faranoff A. A., Walsh M. C. (Eds), *Faranoff and Martin's Neonatal-Perinatal Medicine* (10th ed., pp. 1042–1059). Philadelphia, PA: Elsevier.
37. Kair L. R., Leonard D. T., Anderson J. M. (2012). Bronchopulmonary dysplasia. *Pediatrics in Review* 33(6), 255–262.
38. Szentpetery S., Weiner D. J., Finder J. D. (2018). Pulmonary disorders. In Zitelli B. J., McIntire S. C., Nowalk A. J. (Eds), *Zitelli and Davis' Atlas of Pediatric Physical Diagnosis* (7th ed., pp. 593–615). Philadelphia, PA: Elsevier.
39. Bower J., McBride J. T. (2015). Bronchiolitis. In Bennett J. E., Dolin R., Blaser M. J. (Eds), *Mandell, Douglas, and Bennett's Principles of Infectious Diseases* Updated edition (8th ed., pp. 818–822). Philadelphia, PA: Elsevier Saunders.
40. Ralston S. L., Lieberthal A. S., Meissner H. C., et al. (2014). Clinical practice guideline: The diagnosis, management and prevention of bronchiolitis. *Pediatrics* 134, e1474–e1502.
41. Overbaugh K. (2018). Assessment of respiratory function. In Hinkle J. L., Cleever K. H. (Eds.), *Brunner & Suddarth's textbook of medical-surgical nursing* (14th ed., pp. 480–509). Philadelphia: PA: Wolters Kluwer.
42. Strayer D. S., Rubin E. (2015). *Rubin's Pathology Clinicopathologic Foundations of Medicine* (7th ed.). Philadelphia, PA: Wolters Kluwer.

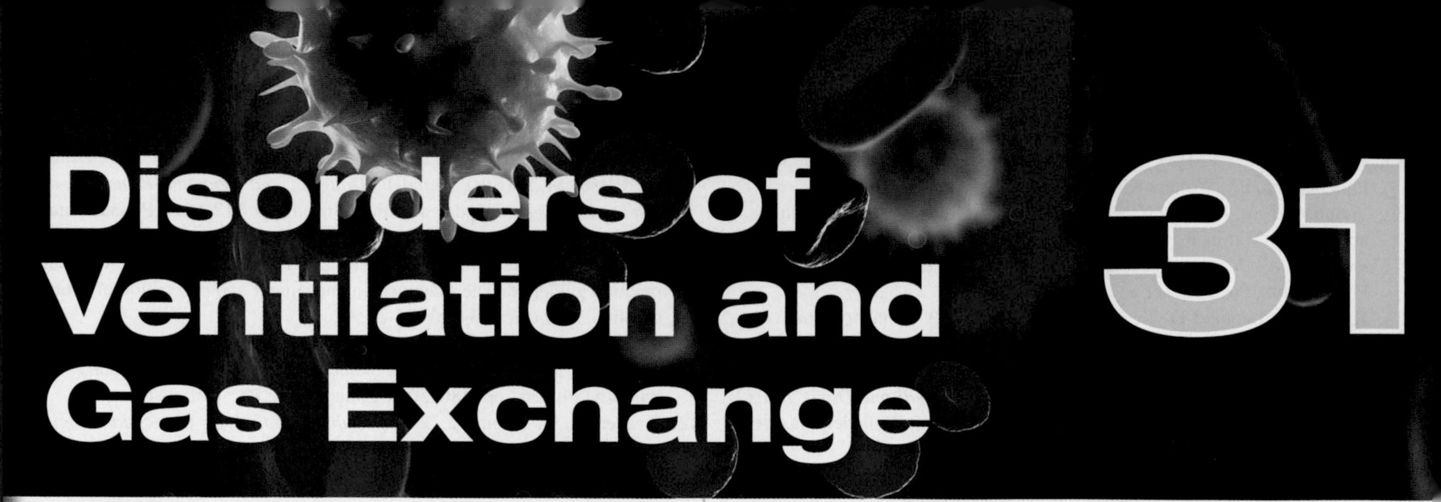

Disorders of Ventilation and Gas Exchange

31

Tracy McClinton and Emma Murray

The major function of the lungs is to exchange oxygen (O_2) and carbon dioxide (CO_2) to support the metabolic functions of the body's tissues. The gas exchange function of the lungs depends on a system of open airways, expansion of the lungs, an adequate surface area for gas diffusion, and adequate blood flow through the pulmonary capillary bed.

Many types of disease are capable of disrupting the normal gas-exchanging function of the lungs. In some cases, the disruption is temporary, and in other cases, it is marked and disabling. In some people, it is due to a system-wide deterioration most probably from an acute trauma or injury. Frequently seen respiratory disorders that disrupt ventilation and pulmonary gas exchange are discussed in the following six sections:

- Physiologic effects of altered ventilation and gas exchange
- Disorders of lung inflation
- Obstructive airway disorders
- Interstitial lung disorders
- Disorders of the pulmonary circulation
- Acute respiratory disorders

It is important to realize that people with an underlying comorbidity such as chronic obstructive pulmonary disease (COPD) who then experience an acute event such as a blunt trauma of the thorax or lupus erythematosus will require more ventilatory assistance and cardiovascular support than those who have "normal" lung function and no autoimmune dysfunction. Also, any person with inflammation from sarcoidosis or an infection such as tuberculosis, or excessive bronchoconstriction from reactive airway disease, will be challenged if he or she acquires a condition causing acute respiratory failure.

PHYSIOLOGIC EFFECTS OF VENTILATION AND DIFFUSION DISORDERS

After completing this section of the chapter, the learner will be able to meet the following objectives:

- Define the terms *hypoxemia* and *hypercapnia*.
- Differentiate between the mechanisms causing disorders of ventilation and diffusion.
- Compare the manifestations of hypoxemia and hypercapnia.

The primary function of the respiratory system is to remove appropriate amounts of CO_2 from the blood entering the pulmonary circulation and to add adequate amounts of O_2 to the blood leaving the pulmonary circulation.[1,2] This section of the chapter provides a brief overview of the causes and manifestations of the hypoxemia and hypercapnia that develop as the result of the impaired ventilation and gas exchange occurring with many of the disorders discussed in the chapter.

Ventilation involves the movement of atmospheric air to the alveoli for provision of O_2 and removal of CO_2. Minute ventilation is the volume of air exchanged per minute and is determined by both the amount of air exchanged with each breath (tidal volume) and the respiratory rate (breaths per minute). *Gas exchange* takes place within the lungs and involves the exchange of O_2 and CO_2 between air in the alveoli and the blood in the pulmonary capillaries. The process involves the diffusion or movement of O_2 from the air in the alveoli (which is rich in O_2 and low in CO_2) to the blood in the pulmonary capillaries. It also involves the transfer of CO_2 from the blood in the pulmonary capillaries (which has low amounts of O_2 and high amounts of CO_2) to the alveoli. Adequate oxygenation of the blood and removal of CO_2 also depend on adequate circulation of blood through the pulmonary blood vessels (perfusion) and appropriate contact between ventilated alveoli and perfused capillaries of the pulmonary circulation (ventilation and perfusion matching) (Fig. 31.1).

As a general rule, oxygenation of the blood depends primarily on factors that promote diffusion of O_2 from the alveoli into the pulmonary capillaries. Removal of CO_2 depends primarily on the minute ventilation (respiratory rate × tidal volume) and elimination of CO_2 from the alveoli (Fig. 31.2).

Hypoxemia

Hypoxemia refers to a reduction in arterial blood O_2 levels, which is considered a PaO_2 less than 95 mm Hg.

Etiology and Pathogenesis

Hypoxemia can result from an inadequate amount of O_2 in the air, a disorder of the respiratory system, dysfunction of the neurologic system, or alterations in circulatory function. The mechanisms whereby respiratory disorders lead to a significant reduction in PO_2 are hypoventilation, impaired diffusion of gases, inadequate circulation of blood through the pulmonary capillaries, and mismatching of ventilation and perfusion.[1,2] Often, more than one mechanism contributes to hypoxemia in a person with respiratory or cardiac disease.

Clinical Manifestations

Hypoxemia produces its effects through tissue hypoxia and the compensatory mechanisms that the body uses to adapt to the lowered oxygen level. Body tissues vary considerably in their vulnerability to hypoxia. Tissues with the greatest need are the brain, lungs, and heart. If the PO_2 of the tissues falls below a critical level, aerobic metabolism ceases and anaerobic metabolism takes over, with formation and release of lactic acid. This results in increased serum lactate levels and metabolic acidosis. The normal range of serum lactate levels is 1 to 0.5 mmol/L in nonacutely ill people.

Mild hypoxemia produces few manifestations. Recruitment of sympathetic nervous system compensatory mechanisms produces an increase in heart rate, peripheral vasoconstriction, diaphoresis, and a mild increase in blood pressure. There may be slight impairment of mental performance and visual acuity and sometimes hyperventilation. This is because hemoglobin saturation still is approximately 90% when the PO_2 is only 60 mm Hg. More pronounced hypoxemia may produce confusion, personality changes, restlessness, agitated or combative behavior, uncoordinated muscle movements, euphoria, impaired judgment, delirium, and, eventually, stupor and coma.

The manifestations of chronic hypoxemia may be insidious in onset and attributed to other causes, particularly in people with chronic lung disease. The body compensates for chronic hypoxemia by increased ventilation, pulmonary vasoconstriction, and increased production of red blood cells. Pulmonary vasoconstriction occurs as a local response to alveolar hypoxia. It increases pulmonary arterial pressure and improves the matching of ventilation and blood flow. Increased production of

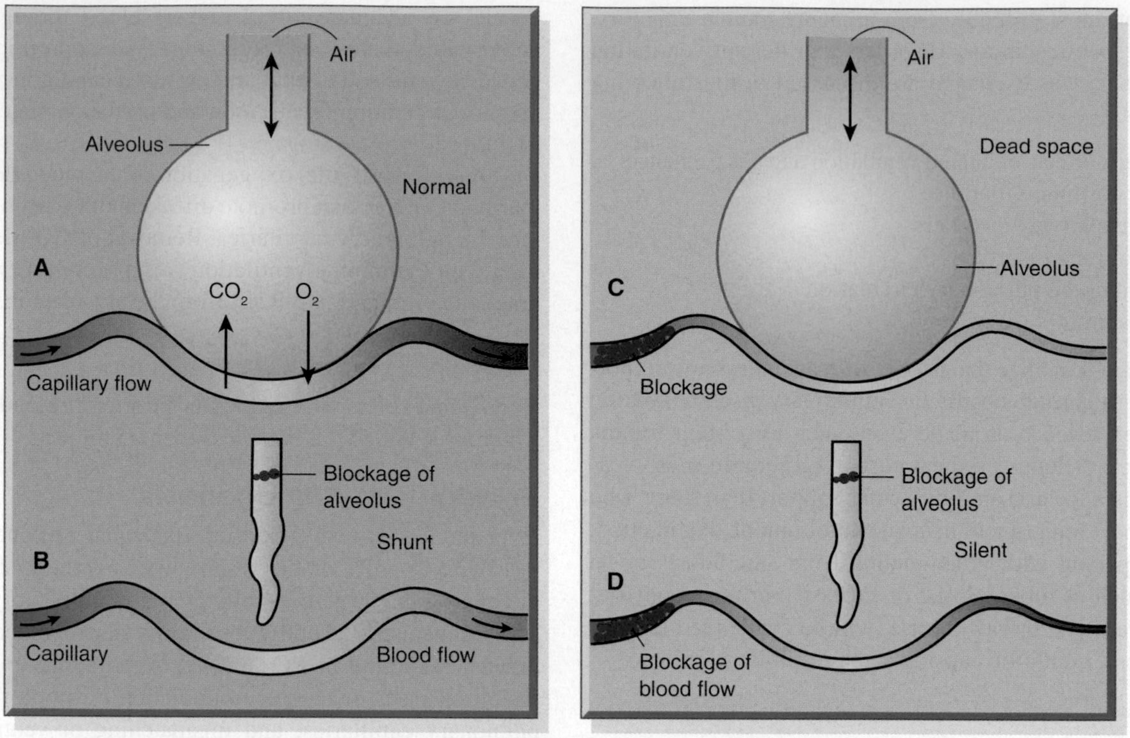

Figure 31.1 • Ventilation–perfusion ratios. Normal ratio **(A)**. In the healthy lung, a given amount of blood passes an alveolus and is matched with an equal amount of gas. The ratio is 1:1 (ventilation matches perfusion). Low ventilation–perfusion ratios: shunts **(B)**. Low ventilation–perfusion states may be called shunt-producing disorders. When perfusion exceeds ventilation, a shunt exists. Blood bypasses the alveoli without gas exchange occurring. This is seen with obstruction of the distal airways, such as with pneumonia, atelectasis, tumor, or a mucous plug. High ventilation–perfusion ratios: dead space **(C)**. When ventilation exceeds perfusion, dead space results. The alveoli do not have an adequate blood supply for gas exchange to occur. This is characteristic of a variety of disorders, including pulmonary emboli, pulmonary infarction, and cardiogenic shock. Silent unit **(D)**. In the absence of both ventilation and perfusion or with limited ventilation and perfusion, a condition known as a silent unit occurs. This is seen with pneumothorax and severe ARDS. (From Hinkle J. L., Cheever K. H. (2018). *Brunner & Suddarth's textbook of medicalsurgical nursing* (14th ed., figures in Chart 20-2, p. 486). Philadelphia, PA: Lippincott Williams & Wilkins.)

red blood cells results from the release of erythropoietin from the kidneys in response to hypoxia. Polycythemia increases the red blood cell concentration and the oxygen-carrying capacity of the blood. Other adaptive mechanisms include a shift to the right in the oxygen dissociation curve, which increases O_2 release to the tissues (see Fig. 29.22).

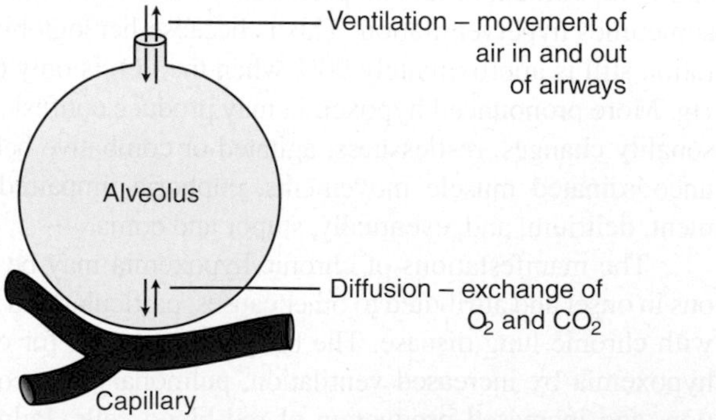

Figure 31.2 • Primary lung functions: ventilation and diffusion. From Morton P. G., Fontaine D. K. (2018). *Critical care nursing: A holistic approach* (11th ed., Fig. 25-1, p. 449). Philadelphia, PA: Lippincott Williams & Wilkins.)

Cyanosis refers to the bluish discoloration of the skin and mucous membranes that result from an excessive concentration of reduced or deoxygenated hemoglobin in the small blood vessels. It usually is most marked in the lips, nail beds, ears, and cheeks. The degree of cyanosis is modified by the amount of cutaneous pigment, skin thickness, and the state of the cutaneous capillaries. Cyanosis is more difficult to distinguish in people with dark skin and in areas of the body with increased skin thickness. Inspect the buccal tissue of the oral mucosa of dark-skinned people because this is the most accurate location to assess for cyanosis. Although cyanosis may be evident in people with respiratory failure, it often is a late sign. A concentration of approximately 5 g/dL of deoxygenated hemoglobin is required in the circulating blood for cyanosis to occur.[1] The absolute quantity of reduced hemoglobin, rather than the relative quantity, is important in producing cyanosis.

People with anemia and low hemoglobin levels are less likely than people with high hemoglobin concentrations to exhibit cyanosis (because they have less hemoglobin to deoxygenate), even though they may be relatively hypoxic because of their decreased ability to transport oxygen. A person with a high hemoglobin level due to polycythemia may be cyanotic without being hypoxic.

Cyanosis can be divided into two types: central and peripheral. *Central cyanosis* is evident in the tongue and lips. It is caused by an increased amount of deoxygenated hemoglobin or an abnormal hemoglobin derivative in the arterial blood. Abnormal hemoglobin derivatives include *methemoglobin*, in which the nitrite ion reacts with hemoglobin. Because methemoglobin has a low affinity for O_2, large doses of nitrites can result in cyanosis and tissue hypoxia. Although nitrites are used in treating angina, the therapeutic dose is too small to cause cyanosis. *Peripheral cyanosis* occurs in the extremities and on the tip of the nose or ears. It is caused by slowing of blood flow to an area of the body, with increased extraction of oxygen from the blood. It results from vasoconstriction and diminished peripheral blood flow, as occurs with cold exposure, shock, heart failure, or peripheral vascular disease. Clubbing may also be evident in people with COPD since there is long-term hypoxia. This is readily seen during a peripheral cardiovascular inspection when the provider assesses peripheral oxygenation/perfusion since the angle of the nail is 180 degrees or greater (Fig. 31.3).

Diagnosis

Diagnosis of hypoxemia is based on clinical observation and diagnostic measures of PO_2 levels. The analysis of arterial blood gases provides a direct measure of the O_2 content of the blood and is the best indicator of the ability of the lungs to oxygenate the blood. Venous oxygen saturation (SvO_2) reflects the body's extraction and utilization of O_2 at the tissue levels. Venous blood samples can be obtained through either a pulmonary artery catheter or a central line. The latter is less invasive but slightly less accurate because the blood has not yet been mixed in the right ventricle.

Noninvasive measurements of arterial O_2 saturation of hemoglobin can be obtained using an instrument called the *pulse oximeter* (Fig. 31.4). The pulse oximeter uses light-emitting diodes and combines plethysmography (*i.e.*, changes in light absorbance and vasodilation) with spectrophotometry (Sp) to measure oxygen saturation.[3] The normal SpO_2 ranges from 90 to 100. Spectrophotometry uses a red-wavelength light that passes through oxygenated hemoglobin and is absorbed by deoxygenated hemoglobin and an infrared wavelength light that is absorbed by oxygenated hemoglobin and passes through deoxygenated hemoglobin. Sensors that can be placed on the ear, finger, toe, or forehead are available. Sensors can be placed on the palm, penis, foot, and arm of infants. The pulse oximeter cannot distinguish between oxygen-carrying hemoglobin and carbon monoxide–carrying hemoglobin. In addition, the pulse oximeter cannot detect elevated levels of methemoglobin. Although pulse oximetry is not as accurate as arterial blood gas measurements, it provides the means for noninvasive and continuous monitoring of O_2 saturation. This is a useful trend indicator of respiratory and circulatory status. However, its reliability is questionable when used with people who are acutely ill. Using a formula that identifies arterial values of pH, PCO_2, and PO_2 from the person's venous values and pulse oximetry has also been effective.[4] Using blood from a central venous line with pulse oximetry may offer more information than arterial specimens in people acutely ill with respiratory disorders.[5]

The ratio between the arterial PaO_2 and the fraction of inspired oxygen (FiO_2), termed the *PF ratio*, is an additional indicator of alterations in diffusion of O_2 at the lung level. In determining this ratio, the PO_2 is divided by the FiO_2. For example, the FiO_2 of a person breathing room air is 0.21 because 21% of atmospheric air is O_2, whereas for the person receiving 40% O_2, the FiO_2 is 0.40. The normal value of the PF ratio is greater than 300.[6] The PF ratio is useful for evaluating improvements or deteriorations in oxygen diffusion regardless of the percentage of supplemental oxygen that is being administered. In addition, the PF ratio is a diagnostic indicator of acute lung injury and acute respiratory distress syndrome (ARDS).

Treatment

Treatment of hypoxemia is directed toward correcting the cause of the disorder and increasing the gradient for diffusion through the administration of supplemental oxygen. Oxygen may be delivered by nasal cannula, mask, or administered directly via an endotracheal or tracheostomy tube in people who are mechanically ventilated. A high-flow administration system is one in which the flow rate and reserve capacity are sufficient to provide all the inspired air.[7] A low-flow administration system delivers less than the total inspired air.[7] The concentration of O_2 being administered (usually determined

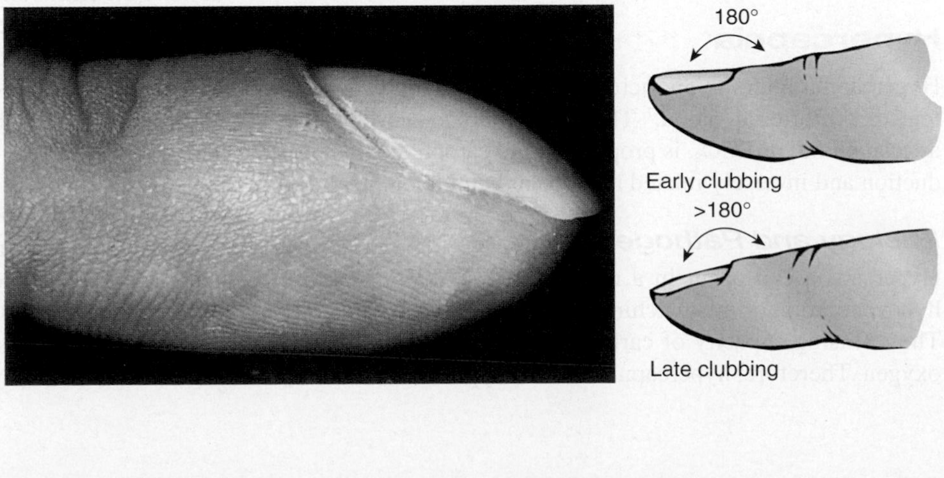

Figure 31.3 • Clubbing. The angle between the nail plate and the proximal nail fold increases to 180 degrees or greater. (From Morton P. G., Fontaine D. K. (2018). *Critical care nursing: A holistic approach* (11th ed., Fig. 24.2, p. 434). Philadelphia, PA: Lippincott Williams & Wilkins.)

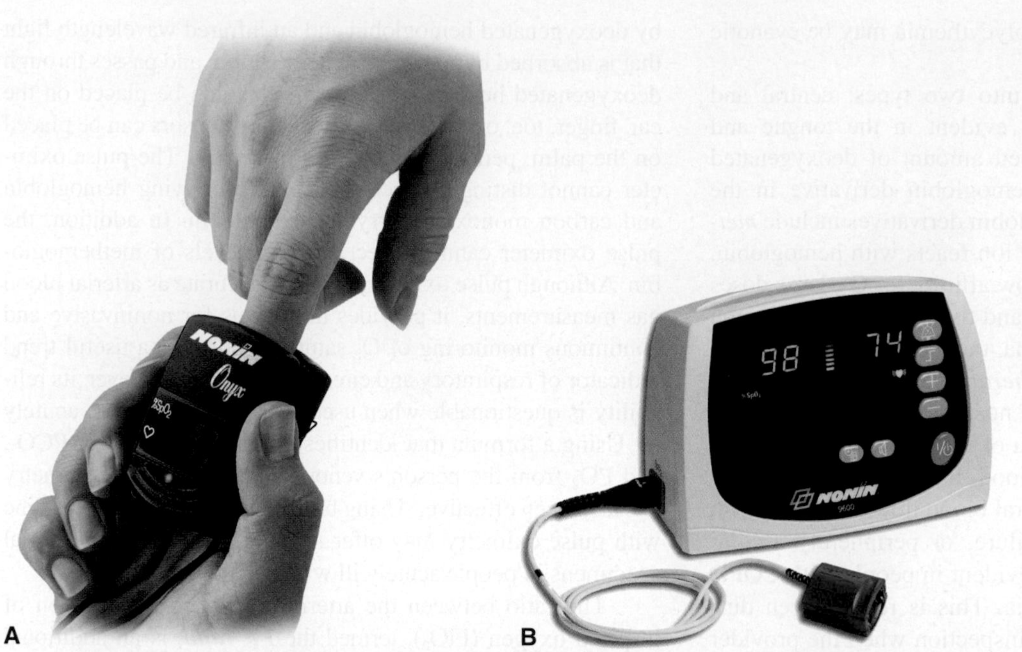

Figure 31.4 • Measuring blood oxygenation with pulse oximetry reduces the need for invasive procedures, such as drawing blood for analysis of oxygen levels. **(A)** Self-contained digital fingertip pulse oximeter, which incorporates the sensor and the display into one unit. **(B)** Tabletop model with sensor attached. Memory permits tracking heart rate and oxygen saturation over time. (From Hinkle J. L., Cheever K. H. (2018). *Brunner & Suddarth's textbook of medicalsurgical nursing* (14th ed., Fig. 20-12, p. 503). Philadelphia, PA: Lippincott Williams & Wilkins.)

by the flow rate) is based on the PO_2. A high-flow rate must be carefully monitored in people with chronic lung disease because increases in PO_2 above 60 mm Hg may depress the ventilatory drive. There also is the danger of oxygen toxicity with high concentrations of oxygen. Continuous breathing of oxygen at high concentrations can lead to diffuse parenchymal lung injury. People with healthy lungs begin to experience respiratory symptoms such as cough, sore throat, substernal tightness, nasal congestion, and painful inspiration after breathing pure oxygen for 24 hours.[2]

KEY POINTS

VENTILATION AND GAS EXCHANGE

- Ventilation is the movement of air volume from the atmosphere to the alveoli.
- Gas exchange is the delivery of oxygen and removal of carbon dioxide from the capillary membrane.

Hypercapnia

Hypercapnia refers to an increase in the carbon dioxide content of the arterial blood.[7] The carbon dioxide level in the arterial blood, or PCO_2, is proportional to carbon dioxide production and inversely related to alveolar ventilation.

Etiology and Pathogenesis

Hypercapnia can occur in a number of disorders that cause hypoventilation or mismatching of ventilation and perfusion.[7] The diffusing capacity of carbon dioxide is 20 times that of oxygen. Therefore, hypercapnia without hypoxemia is usually observed only in situations of hypoventilation.[2] In cases of ventilation–perfusion mismatching, hypercapnia is usually accompanied by a decrease in arterial PO_2 levels.

Conditions that increase carbon dioxide production, such as an increase in metabolic rate or a high-carbohydrate diet, can contribute to the degree of hypercapnia that occurs in people with impaired respiratory function. Changes in the metabolic rate resulting from an increase in activity, fever, or disease can have profound effects on carbon dioxide production. Alveolar ventilation usually rises proportionally with these changes, and hypercapnia occurs only when this increase is inappropriate.

The respiratory quotient (RQ), which is the ratio of carbon dioxide production to oxygen consumption ($RQ = CO_2$ production/O_2 consumption), varies with the type of food metabolized.[1] A characteristic of carbohydrate metabolism is an RQ of 1.0, with equal amounts of carbon dioxide being produced and oxygen being consumed. Because fats contain less oxygen than carbohydrates, their oxidation produces less carbon dioxide (RQ = 0.7). The metabolism of pure proteins (RQ = 0.81) results in the production of more carbon dioxide than the metabolism of fat, but less than the metabolism of carbohydrates. The type of food that is eaten or the types of nutrients that are delivered through enteral feedings (*i.e.*, through a tube placed in the small intestine) or parenteral nutrition (*i.e.*, through a central venous catheter) may influence PCO_2 levels.

Clinical Manifestations and Diagnosis

Hypercapnia affects a number of body functions, including acid–base balance and renal, neurologic, and cardiovascular function. Elevated levels of PCO_2 produce a decrease in pH and respiratory acidosis. The body normally compensates for an increase in PCO_2 by increasing renal bicarbonate (HCO_3^-)

CHART 31.1 SYMPTOMS OF WORK OF BREATHING

Shortness of breath
Diaphoresis
Pursed-lip breathing
Tachypnea or bradypnea/irregular breathing rhythm
Use of accessory muscles
Tachycardia
Abdominal breathing
Cyanosis

retention, which results in an increase in serum HCO_3^- and pH levels. As long as the pH is within normal range, the main complications of hypercapnia are those resulting from the accompanying hypoxia. Because the body adapts to chronic increases in blood levels of carbon dioxide, people with chronic hypercapnia may not have symptoms until the PCO_2 becomes markedly elevated. At this point, they will display symptoms of increased work of breathing (WOB) since they will also be experiencing hypoxemia (Chart 31.1).

The diagnosis of hypercapnia is based on physiologic manifestations, arterial pH, and arterial blood gas levels. $PACO_2$ can also be measured on individuals receiving mechanical ventilation via end-tidal carbon dioxide ($ETCO_2$) measuring at the end of exhalation.[7] Samples of the carbon dioxide at the end of the exhaled breath can be used to identify an estimated $PACO_2$.[7]

Treatment

The treatment of hypercapnia is directed at decreasing the WOB and improving the ventilation–perfusion balance. The use of intermittent rest therapy, such as nocturnal negative pressure ventilation or continuous positive airway pressure, in people with chronic obstructive disease or chest wall disease may be effective in increasing the strength and endurance of the respiratory muscles and improving the PCO_2. Respiratory muscle retraining aimed at improving respiratory muscle strength and their endurance, or both, has been used to improve exercise tolerance and diminish the likelihood of respiratory fatigue. Use of a ventilator may become necessary in situations of acute hypercapnia.

IN SUMMARY

The primary function of the respiratory system is to remove appropriate amounts of CO_2 from the blood entering the pulmonary circulation and provide adequate O_2 to blood leaving the pulmonary circulation. This is accomplished through the process of ventilation, in which air moves into and out of the lungs, and diffusion, in which gases move between the alveoli and the pulmonary capillaries. Although both diffusion and ventilation affect gas exchange, oxygenation of the blood largely depends on diffusion and removal of carbon dioxide on ventilation.

Hypoxemia refers to a decrease in arterial blood oxygen levels that results in a decrease in tissue oxygenation. Hypoxemia can occur as the result of hypoventilation, diffusion impairment, shunt, and ventilation–perfusion impairment. Acute hypoxemia is manifested by increased respiratory effort (increased respiratory and heart rates, use of accessory muscles, pursed-lip breathing, and diaphoresis), cyanosis, and impaired sensory and neurologic function, which is also referred to as WOB. The body compensates for chronic hypoxemia by increased ventilation, pulmonary vasoconstriction, and increased production of red blood cells.

Hypercapnia refers to an increase in carbon dioxide levels. In the clinical setting, four factors contribute to hypercapnia: alterations in carbon dioxide production, disturbance in the gas exchange function of the lungs, abnormalities in function of the chest wall and respiratory muscles, and changes in neural control of respiration. Alterations in respiratory function or the rate decrease minute volume, which is the most common cause of hypercapnia. The manifestations of hypercapnia consist of those associated with a decreased pH (respiratory acidosis); vasodilation of blood vessels, including those in the brain; and depression of central nervous system (CNS) function.

DISORDERS OF LUNG INFLATION

After completing this section of the chapter, the learner will be able to meet the following objectives:

- Characterize the pathogenesis and manifestations of transudative and exudative pleural effusion, chylothorax, and hemothorax.
- Differentiate among the causes and manifestations of spontaneous pneumothorax, secondary pneumothorax, and tension pneumothorax.
- Describe the causes of pleurisy (pleuritis) and differentiate the characteristics of pleural pain from other types of chest pain.

Air entering through the airways inflates the lung, and the negative pressure in the pleural cavity keeps the lung from collapsing. Disorders of lung inflation are caused by conditions that obstruct the airways, cause lung compression, or produce lung collapse. There can be compression of the lung by an accumulation of fluid in the intrapleural space; complete collapse of an entire lung, as in pneumothorax; or collapse of a segment of the lung due to airway obstruction, as in atelectasis.

Disorders of the Pleura

The pleura is a thin, double-layered serous membrane that encases the lungs (Fig. 31.5). The outer *parietal layer* lines

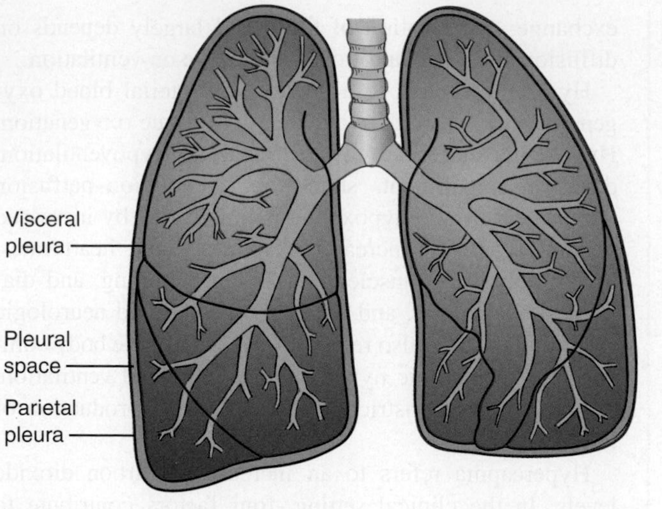

Figure 31.5 • The relationship between the parietal and visceral pleurae and the pleural space, which is the site of fluid accumulation in pleural effusions.

the thoracic wall and superior aspect of the diaphragm. It continues around the heart and between the lungs, forming the lateral walls of the mediastinum. The inner *visceral layer* covers the lung and is adherent to all its surfaces. The pleural cavity or space between the two layers contains a thin layer of serous fluid that lubricates the pleural surfaces and allows the parietal and visceral pleurae to slide smoothly over each other during breathing movements. The pressure in the pleural cavity, which is negative in relation to atmospheric pressure, holds the lungs against the chest wall and keeps them from collapsing. Disorders of the pleura include pleural effusion, hemothorax, pneumothorax, and pleural inflammation.

Pleural Effusion

Pleural effusion refers to an abnormal collection of fluid in the pleural cavity.[8] Like fluid developing in other transcellular spaces in the body, pleural effusion occurs when the rate of fluid formation exceeds the rate of its removal.

Etiology and Pathogenesis. Normally, fluid enters the pleural space from capillaries in the parietal pleura and is removed by the lymphatics situated in the parietal pleura. Fluid can also enter from the interstitial spaces of the lung through the visceral pleura or from small holes in the diaphragm. Accordingly, fluid may accumulate when there is excess fluid formation (from the interstitium of the lung, the parietal pleura, or peritoneal cavity) or when there is decreased removal by the lymphatics.

The fluid that accumulates in a pleural effusion may be a transudate or exudate, purulent (containing pus), chyle, or sanguineous (bloody). The accumulation of a serous transudate (clear fluid) in the pleural cavity often is referred to as *hydrothorax*. The condition may be unilateral or bilateral. The most common cause of hydrothorax is congestive heart failure. Other causes are renal failure, nephrosis, liver failure, and malignancy. An *exudate* is a pleural fluid that has a specific gravity greater than 1.020 and often contains inflammatory cells.

Transudative and exudative pleural effusions are distinguished by measuring the lactate dehydrogenase (LDH) and protein levels in the pleural fluid.[8] LDH is an enzyme that is released from inflamed and injured pleural tissue. Because measurements of LDH are easily obtained from a sample of pleural fluid, it is a useful marker for diagnosis of exudative pleural disorders. Exudative pleural effusion meets at least one of the following criteria:

1. A pleural fluid protein/serum protein ratio greater than 0.5
2. A pleural fluid LDH/serum LDH ratio greater than 0.6
3. A pleural fluid LDH greater than two thirds the upper limit of normal serum LDH[8]

Conditions that produce exudative pleural effusions are bacterial pneumonia, viral infection, pulmonary infarction, and malignancies. These conditions make up approximately 70% of all pleural effusions.[9]

Parapneumonic effusions are a common type of pleural effusion and are largely caused by bacterial infections such as pneumonia. A common type of parapneumonic effusion is *empyema*, an infection in the pleural cavity that results in exudate containing glucose, proteins, leukocytes, and debris from dead cells and tissue.[9] It is caused by an adjacent bacterial pneumonia, rupture of a lung abscess into the pleural space, invasion from a subdiaphragmatic infection, or infection associated with trauma.

Chylothorax is the effusion of lymph in the thoracic cavity. Chyle, a milky fluid containing chylomicrons, is found in the lymph fluid originating in the gastrointestinal tract. The thoracic duct transports chyle to the central circulation. Chylothorax also results from trauma, inflammation, or malignant infiltration obstructing chyle transport from the thoracic duct into the central circulation. It is the most common cause of pleural effusion in the fetus and neonate, resulting from congenital malformation of the thoracic duct or lymph channels. Chylothorax also can occur as a complication of intrathoracic surgical procedures and use of the great veins for total parenteral nutrition and hemodynamic monitoring.[8]

Clinical Manifestations. The manifestations of parapneumonic effusions vary with the cause. Empyemas may be accompanied by fever, increased white blood cell count, and other signs of inflammation. Fluid in the pleural cavity acts as a space-occupying mass; it causes a decrease in lung expansion on the affected side that is proportional to the amount of fluid collected. Characteristic signs of pleural effusion are dullness or flatness to percussion and diminished breath sounds. Hypoxemia may occur due to the decreased surface area and usually is corrected with supplemental oxygen. Dyspnea, the most common symptom, occurs when fluid compresses the lung, resulting in increased effort or rate of breathing. Pleuritic pain usually occurs only when inflammation is present. However, constant discomfort may be felt with large effusions.

Diagnosis and Treatment. Diagnosis of pleural effusion is based on chest radiographs, chest ultrasonography, and computed tomography (CT). Thoracentesis (aspiration of fluid from the pleural space) can be used to obtain a sample of pleural fluid for diagnosis. The treatment of pleural effusion is directed at the cause of the disorder. With large effusions, thoracentesis may be used to remove fluid from the intrapleural space and allow for reexpansion of the lung. A palliative method used for treatment of pleural effusions caused by a malignancy is the injection of a sclerosing agent into the pleural cavity. This method of treatment causes obliteration of the pleural space and prevents the reaccumulation of fluid. Chest tube drainage may be necessary in cases of continued effusion.

Hemothorax

Hemothorax is a specific type of pleural effusion in which there is blood in the pleural cavity.

Etiology and Pathogenesis. Bleeding may be the result of chest injury, a complication of chest surgery, malignancies, or rupture of a great vessel such as an aortic aneurysm. Hemothorax may be classified as minimal, moderate, or large.[9] A minimal hemothorax involves the presence of at least 250 mL of blood in the pleural space.[8] Small amounts of blood usually are absorbed from the pleural space, and the hemothorax usually clears in 10 to 14 days without complication. A moderate hemothorax fills approximately one third of the pleural space and may produce signs of lung compression and loss of intravascular volume. It requires immediate drainage and replacement of intravascular fluids. A large hemothorax fills one half or more of one side of the chest and is usually caused by bleeding from a high-pressure vessel such as an intercostal or mammary artery. It requires immediate drainage and, if the bleeding continues, surgery to control the bleeding.

Clinical Manifestations. In addition to alterations in oxygenation, ventilation, respiration effort, and breath sounds, signs of blood loss, including increased heart rate, may accompany hemothorax. Because hemothorax is abrupt in onset, the manifestations are usually sudden and distressing. One of the complications of untreated moderate or large hemothorax is fibrothorax—the fusion of the pleural surfaces by fibrin, hyaline, and connective tissue—and, in some cases, calcification of the fibrous tissue, which restricts lung expansion.

Diagnosis and Treatment. Diagnosis of hemothorax is based on chest radiographs and decreased arterial saturation, which is indicative of decreased oxygen exchange. If the person is symptomatic or oxygen exchange is compromised, chest tube drainage is indicated.

Pneumothorax

Pneumothorax refers to the presence of air in the pleural space. Pneumothorax causes partial or complete collapse of the affected lung.

Etiology and Pathogenesis. Pneumothorax can occur without an obvious cause or injury (*i.e.*, spontaneous pneumothorax) or as a result of direct injury to the chest or major airways (*i.e.*, traumatic pneumothorax). Tension pneumothorax describes a life-threatening condition in which increased pressure within the pleural cavity impairs both respiratory and cardiac function.

Spontaneous Pneumothorax. Spontaneous pneumothorax is hypothesized to occur due to the rupture of an air-filled bleb, or blister, on the surface of the lung. Rupture of these blebs allows atmospheric air from the airways to enter the pleural cavity (Fig. 31.6). Because alveolar pressure normally is greater than pleural pressure, air flows from the alveoli into the pleural space, causing the involved portion of the lung to collapse as a result of its own recoil. Air continues to flow into the pleural space until a pressure gradient no longer exists or until the decline in lung size causes the leak to seal. Spontaneous pneumothoraces can be divided into primary and secondary pneumothoraces. Primary pneumothorax occurs in otherwise healthy people, whereas secondary pneumothorax occurs in persons with underlying lung disease.

In primary spontaneous pneumothorax, the blebs usually are located at the top of the lungs. The condition is seen most often in tall boys and young men between 10 and 30 years of age. It has been suggested that the difference in pleural pressure from the top to the bottom of the lung is greater in tall people and that this difference in pressure may contribute to the development of blebs. Smoking and family history are factors associated with primary spontaneous pneumothorax.[2] Inflammation of the small airways related to smoking probably contributes to the condition, and cessation of smoking may reduce the recurrence.

Secondary spontaneous pneumothoraces usually are more serious because they occur in people with lung disease. They are associated with many different types of lung conditions that cause trapping of gases and destruction of lung

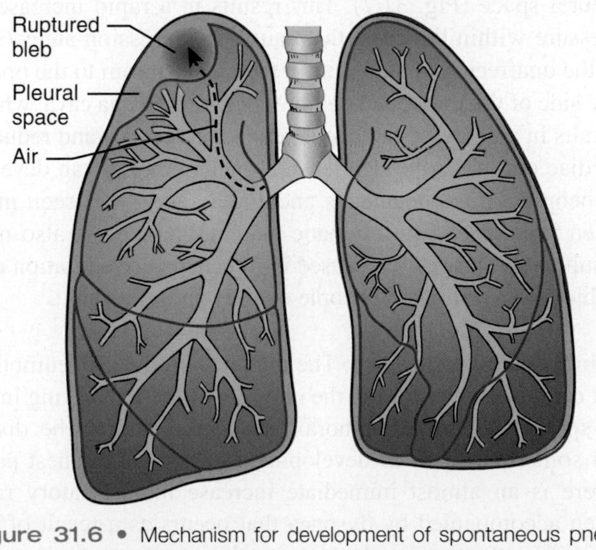

Figure 31.6 • Mechanism for development of spontaneous pneumothorax, in which an air-filled bleb on the surface of the lung ruptures, allowing atmospheric air from the airways to enter the pleural space.

tissue, including asthma, tuberculosis, cystic fibrosis (CF), sarcoidosis, bronchogenic carcinoma, and metastatic pleural diseases. A common cause of secondary spontaneous pneumothorax is emphysema. Secondary spontaneous pneumothorax may be life threatening because of the underlying lung injury and poor compensatory reserves.

Catamenial pneumothorax occurs in relation to the menstrual cycle and usually is recurrent.[10] It typically occurs in women between 30 and 40 years of age who have a history of endometriosis. About one third of all spontaneous pneumothoraces in women who undergo surgery are caused by catamenial pneumothorax.[10] It usually affects the right lung and develops within 72 hours of onset of menses. Although the cause of catamenial pneumothorax is unknown, it has been suggested that air may gain access to the peritoneal cavity during menstruation and then enter the pleural cavity through a diaphragmatic defect.[10] Pleural and diaphragmatic endometrioses also have been implicated as causes of the condition.

Traumatic Pneumothorax. Traumatic pneumothorax may be caused by penetrating or nonpenetrating injuries. Fractured or dislocated ribs that penetrate the pleura are the most common cause of pneumothorax from nonpenetrating chest injuries. Hemothorax may accompany these injuries. Pneumothorax also may accompany fracture of the trachea or major bronchus or rupture of the esophagus. People with pneumothorax due to chest trauma frequently have other complications and may require chest surgery. Medical procedures such as transthoracic needle aspirations, central line insertion, intubation, and positive-pressure ventilation occasionally may cause pneumothorax. Traumatic pneumothorax also can occur as a complication of cardiopulmonary resuscitation.

Tension Pneumothorax. Tension pneumothorax occurs when the intrapleural pressure exceeds atmospheric pressure. It is a life-threatening condition and occurs when injury to the chest or respiratory structures permits air to enter but not leave the pleural space (Fig. 31.7). This results in a rapid increase in pressure within the chest that causes compression atelectasis of the unaffected lung, a shift in the mediastinum to the opposite side of the chest, and compression of the vena cava, which results in a decrease in venous return to the heart and reduced cardiac output.[9] Although tension pneumothorax can develop in people with spontaneous pneumothoraces, it is seen most often in people with traumatic pneumothoraces. It also may result from barotrauma caused by mechanical ventilation due to high tidal volume on people on the ventilator.[11]

Clinical Manifestations. The manifestations of pneumothorax depend on its size and the integrity of the underlying lung. In spontaneous pneumothorax, manifestations of the disorder sometimes include development of ipsilateral chest pain. There is an almost immediate increase in respiratory rate, often accompanied by dyspnea that occurs as a result of the activation of receptors that monitor lung volume. Asymmetry of the chest may occur because of the air being trapped in the pleural cavity on the affected side. This asymmetry may be evidenced during inspiration as a lag in the movement of the affected side, with inspiration delayed until the unaffected lung reaches the same level of pressure as the lung with the air trapped in the pleural space. Percussion of the chest produces a more hyperresonant sound, and breath sounds are decreased or absent over the area of the pneumothorax.

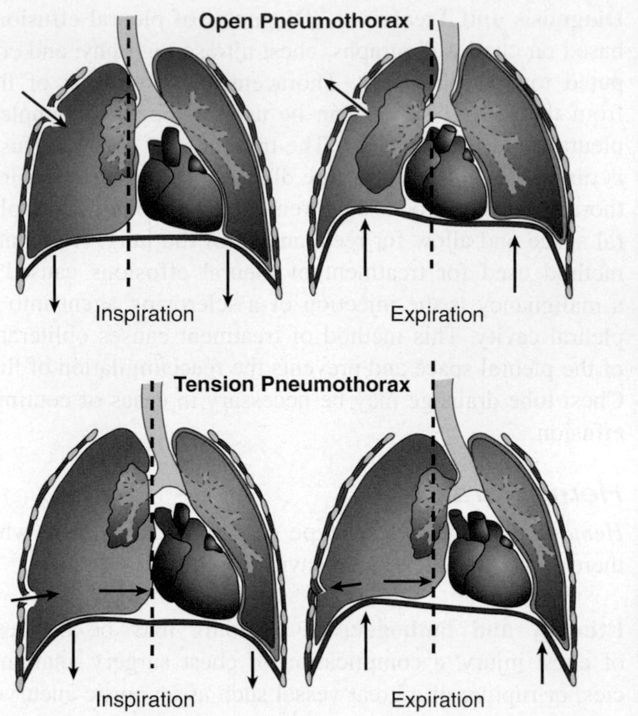

Figure 31.7 • Open or communicating pneumothorax **(top)** and tension pneumothorax **(bottom)**. In an open pneumothorax, air enters the chest during inspiration and exits during expiration. There may be slight inflation of the affected lung because of a decrease in pressure as air moves out of the chest. In tension pneumothorax, air can enter but not leave the chest. As the pressure in the chest increases, the heart and great vessels are compressed and the mediastinal structures are shifted toward the opposite side of the chest. The trachea is pushed from its normal midline position toward the opposite side of the chest, and the unaffected lung is compressed.

With tension pneumothorax, the structures in the mediastinal space shift toward the opposite side of the chest (see Fig. 31.7). When this occurs, the position of the trachea, normally located in the midline of the neck, deviates with the mediastinum. The position of the trachea can be used as a means of assessing for a mediastinal shift. Because of the increase in intrathoracic pressure, stroke volume is impaired to such an extent that cardiac output is decreased despite an increase in heart rate. There may be jugular neck vein distention, subcutaneous emphysema (*i.e.,* presence of air in the subcutaneous tissues of the chest and neck), and clinical signs of shock due to impaired cardiac function.

Hypoxemia usually develops immediately after a large pneumothorax, followed by vasoconstriction of the blood vessels in the affected lung, causing the blood flow to shift to the unaffected lung. In people with primary spontaneous pneumothorax, this mechanism usually returns oxygen saturation to normal within 24 hours. Hypoxemia usually is more serious in persons with underlying lung disease in whom secondary spontaneous pneumothorax develops or in people with underlying heart disease who are unable to compensate with an increase in heart rate and stroke volumes. Regardless of etiology, the hypoxemia caused by the partial or total loss of lung function can be life threatening. Without immediate intervention, the increased thoracic pressure will further impair both cardiac and pulmonary function, resulting in severe hypoxemia and hypotension, which often leads to respiratory and cardiac arrest.

Diagnosis and Treatment. Chest radiograph or CT scan confirms diagnosis of pneumothorax. Perform pulse oximetry and blood gas analysis to determine the effect on blood oxygen levels. Treatment of pneumothorax varies with the cause and extent of the disorder. In small spontaneous pneumothoraces, the air usually reabsorbs spontaneously. Therefore, only observation and follow-up chest radiographs are required. Supplemental oxygen may be used to correct the hypoxemia until the air is reabsorbed. In larger pneumothoraces, the air is removed by needle aspiration or a closed drainage system used with or without suction. This type of drainage system uses a one-way valve or a water-seal chamber to allow air to exit the pleural space and prevent it from reentering the chest.

Emergency treatment of tension pneumothorax involves the prompt insertion of a large-bore needle or chest tube into the affected side of the chest along with one-way valve drainage or continuous chest suction to aid in reinflating the affected lung. Sucking chest wounds, which allow air to pass in and out of the chest cavity, should be treated by promptly covering the area with an airtight bandage (*e.g.,* Vaseline gauze, firm piece of plastic). Chest tubes are inserted as soon as possible to reexpand the lung. Because of the risk for recurrence, people with primary spontaneous pneumothorax should be advised against cigarette smoking, exposure to high altitudes, flying in nonpressurized aircraft, and scuba diving.

KEY POINTS

DISORDERS OF LUNG INFLATION

- The pleura encases the lungs and is made up of two layers, which create the pleural cavity where pathology is often caused by air getting into the space, which is called a pneumothorax, or blood in the pleural space, which would cause a hemothorax.
- Atelectasis is a partial expansion of the lung, which is caused by obstruction or compression of lung tissue.

Pleuritis

Pleuritis (also called *pleurisy*) refers to inflammation of the pleura. Pleuritis is common in infectious processes such as respiratory infections that extend to involve the pleura. Pain is a frequent symptom and most commonly is unilateral and abrupt in onset. When the central part of the diaphragm is irritated, the pain may be referred to the shoulder. Chest movements such as deep breathing and coughing that exaggerate pressure changes in the pleural cavity and increase movement of the inflamed or injured pleural surfaces usually make the pain worse. Because deep breathing is painful, tidal volumes usually are kept small, and breathing becomes more rapid to maintain minute volume. Reflex splinting of the chest muscles may occur, causing a lesser respiratory expansion on the affected side.

It is important to differentiate pleural pain from pain produced by other conditions, such as musculoskeletal strain of chest muscles, bronchial irritation, and myocardial disease. Musculoskeletal pain may occur as the result of frequent, forceful coughing. This type of pain usually is bilateral and located in the inferior portions of the rib cage, where the abdominal muscles insert into the anterior rib cage. Movements associated with contraction of the abdominal muscles make it worse. The pain associated with irritation of the bronchi usually is substernal and dull in character rather than sharp; it is often described as tightening. This type of pain is made worse with coughing but is not affected by deep breathing. Myocardial discomfort or pain usually is located in the substernal area and is not affected by respiratory movements.

Treatment of pleuritis consists of treating the underlying disease and inflammation. Analgesics and nonsteroidal anti-inflammatory drugs (NSAIDs; *e.g.,* ibuprofen, indomethacin) may be used for pleural pain. Although these agents reduce inflammation, they may not entirely relieve the discomfort associated with deep breathing and coughing.

Atelectasis

Atelectasis refers to an incomplete expansion of a lung or portion of a lung. It can be caused by airway obstruction, lung compression such as occurs in pneumothorax or pleural effusion, or increased recoil of the lung due to loss of pulmonary surfactant. The disorder may be present at birth (*i.e.,* primary atelectasis) or develop during the neonatal period or later in life (*i.e.,* acquired or secondary atelectasis).

Etiology and Pathogenesis

Primary atelectasis of the newborn implies that the lung has never been inflated. It is seen most frequently in premature and high-risk infants. A secondary form of atelectasis can occur in infants who established respiration and subsequently experienced impairment of lung expansion. Among the causes of secondary atelectasis in the newborn is respiratory distress syndrome associated with lack of surfactant, airway obstruction due to aspiration of amniotic fluid or blood, and bronchopulmonary dysplasia.

Acquired atelectasis occurs mainly in adults. It is caused most commonly by airway obstruction and lung compression (Fig. 31.8). A mucus plug in the airway or external compression by fluid, tumor mass, exudate, or other matter in the area surrounding the airway can cause obstruction. Portions of alveoli, a small segment of lung, or an entire lung lobe may be involved

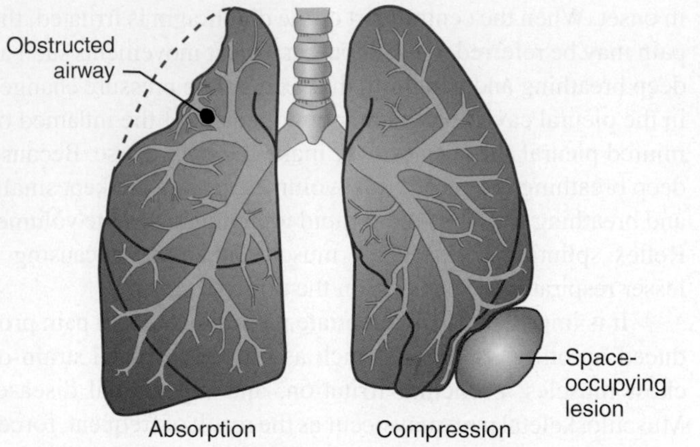

Figure 31.8 • Atelectasis caused by airway obstruction and absorption of air from the involved lung area **(left)** and by compression of lung tissue **(right)**.

in obstructive atelectasis. Complete obstruction of an airway is followed by the absorption of air from the dependent alveoli and collapse of that portion of the lung. Breathing high concentrations of oxygen increases the rate at which gases are absorbed from the alveoli and predisposes to atelectasis. The danger of obstructive atelectasis increases after surgery. Administration of narcotics or anesthesia, pain, and immobility tend to promote retention of viscid bronchial secretions and can cause airway obstruction. The encouragement of coughing and deep breathing, frequent change of position, adequate hydration, and early ambulation decrease the likelihood of atelectasis developing.

Another cause of atelectasis is compression of lung tissue. It occurs when the pleural cavity is partially or completely filled with fluid, exudate, blood, a tumor mass, or air. It is observed most commonly in people with pleural effusion from congestive heart failure or cancer.

Clinical Manifestations

The clinical manifestations of atelectasis include tachypnea, tachycardia, dyspnea, cyanosis, signs of hypoxemia, diminished chest expansion, decreased breath sounds, and intercostal retractions. There may be intercostal retraction (pulling in of the intercostal spaces) over the involved area during inspiration. Signs of respiratory distress are proportional to the extent of lung collapse. If the collapsed area is large, the mediastinum and trachea shift to the affected side. In compression atelectasis, the mediastinum shifts away from the affected lung.

Diagnosis and Treatment

The diagnosis of atelectasis is based on signs and symptoms. Chest radiographs are used to confirm the diagnosis. CT scans may be used to show the exact location of the obstruction.

Treatment depends on the cause and extent of lung involvement. It is directed at reducing the airway obstruction or lung compression and at reinflating the collapsed area of the lung. Ambulation, deep breathing, and body positions that favor increased lung expansion are used when appropriate. Administration of oxygen may be needed to correct the hypoxemia. There are new minimally invasive bronchoscopic procedures that may be used as both a diagnostic and treatment method.

IN SUMMARY

Disorders of the pleura include pleural effusion, hemothorax, pneumothorax, and pleuritis. Pleural effusion refers to the abnormal accumulation of fluid in the pleural cavity. The fluid may be a transudate (*i.e.,* hydrothorax), exudate (*i.e.,* parapneumonic effusion, empyema), or chyle (*i.e.,* chylothorax). Hemothorax refers to the presence of blood in the pleural cavity. Pain is a common symptom of conditions that produce pleuritis or inflammation of the pleura. Characteristically, the pain is unilateral, abrupt in onset, and exaggerated by respiratory movements. Pneumothorax refers to an accumulation of air in the pleural cavity that causes partial or complete collapse of the lung. Pneumothorax can result from rupture of an air-filled bleb on the lung surface or from penetrating or nonpenetrating injuries. A tension pneumothorax is a life-threatening event in which air progressively accumulates in the thorax, collapsing the lung on the injured side and progressively shifting the mediastinum to the opposite side of the thorax, producing severe cardiac and respiratory impairment.

Atelectasis refers to an incomplete expansion of the lung. Primary atelectasis occurs most often in premature and high-risk infants. Acquired atelectasis occurs mainly in adults and is caused most commonly by a mucus plug in the airway or by external compression by fluid, tumor mass, exudate, or other matter in the area surrounding the airway.

OBSTRUCTIVE AIRWAY DISORDERS

After completing this section of the chapter, the learner will be able to meet the following objectives:

- Describe the interaction between one's genetics, alteration of immune response, and environmental agents in the pathogenesis of asthma or reactive airway disease.
- Differentiate between chronic bronchitis and emphysema in terms of pathology and clinical manifestations.
- Describe the genetic abnormality responsible for the manifestations of CF.

Obstructive airway disorders are caused by disorders that limit expiratory airflow. Asthma represents an acute and reversible form of airway disease caused by narrowing of airways due to bronchospasm, inflammation, and increased airway secretions. Chronic obstructive disorders include a variety of airway diseases, such as chronic bronchitis, emphysema, bronchiectasis, and CF.

Physiology of Airway Disease

Air moves through the upper airways (*i.e.,* trachea and major bronchi) into the lower or pulmonary airways (*i.e.,* bronchi and alveoli). In the pulmonary airways, the cartilaginous layer that provides support for the trachea and major bronchi gradually disappears and is replaced with crisscrossing strips of smooth muscle. The contraction and relaxation of the smooth muscle layer, which is innervated by the autonomic nervous system, controls the diameter of the bronchial airways and consequent resistance to airflow. Parasympathetic stimulation, through the vagus nerve and cholinergic receptors, produces bronchial constriction, whereas sympathetic stimulation, through β_2-adrenergic receptors, increases bronchial dilation. At rest, a slight vagal-mediated bronchoconstrictor tone predominates. When there is need for increased airflow, as during exercise, the bronchodilator effects of the sympathetic nervous system are stimulated and the bronchoconstrictor effects of the parasympathetic nervous system are inhibited. Bronchial smooth muscle also responds to inflammatory mediators, such as histamine, that act directly on bronchial smooth muscle cells to produce constriction.

KEY POINTS

AIRWAY DISORDERS

- Changes in airway patency involve changes in airway diameter due to bronchial smooth muscle hyperreactivity or changes in bronchial wall structure, injury to the mucosal lining of the airways, or excess respiratory tract secretions.
- Bronchial asthma is a chronic disorder of the airways that causes episodes of airway obstruction due to bronchial smooth muscle hyperreactivity and airway inflammation. The episodes usually are reversible.
- COPD represents a group of disorders that cause chronic and recurrent obstruction of the pulmonary airways. These disorders can affect patency of the bronchial structures (chronic bronchitis), the gas-diffusing airspaces distal to the terminal bronchioles (emphysema), or a combination of both.

Asthma

Asthma is a chronic disorder of the airways that causes episodes of airway obstruction, bronchial hyperresponsiveness, airway inflammation, and, in some, airway remodeling.[12] More than 25 million people have asthma in the United States. An estimated 7.1 million children have asthma.[13] As adults are living longer, the prevalence of asthma in older adults is increasing.

The strongest risk factor for developing asthma is a genetic predisposition for the development of an immunoglobulin E (IgE)-mediated response to common allergens.[14] IgE is the antibody involved in causing allergic reactions and inflammation.[14] Other risk factors for childhood asthma include family history of asthma, allergies, antenatal exposure to tobacco smoke and pollution, and multiple potentially overlapping genetic predispositions.[15] Asthma severity is impacted by several factors including genetics, age of onset, pollution exposure, atopy, degree of exposure to triggers, environmental triggers such as tobacco smoke and dust mites, and the presence of gastroesophageal reflux disease or respiratory infections[13,14] (see "Severe or Refractory Asthma").

Etiology and Pathogenesis

The common denominator underlying asthma is an exaggerated hyperresponsiveness to a variety of stimuli. Airway inflammation manifested by the presence of inflammatory cells (particularly eosinophils, lymphocytes, and mast cells) and by damage to the bronchial epithelium contributes to the pathogenesis of the disease. There are two subsets of T-helper cells (T_1H and T_2H) that develop from the same precursor $CD4^+$ T lymphocyte.[14,16–18] T_1H cells differentiate in response to microbes and stimulate the differentiation of B cells into immunoglobulin M (IgM)– and IgG-producing plasma cells. T_2H cells, on the other hand, respond to allergens and helminths (intestinal parasites) by stimulating B cells to differentiate into IgE-producing plasma cells, produce growth factors for mast cells, and recruit and activate eosinophils. In people with allergic asthma, T-cell differentiation appears to be skewed toward a proinflammatory T_2H response. Although the molecular basis for this preferential differentiation is unclear, it seems likely that both genetic and environmental factors play a role.[14,16–19]

Cytokines also have an apparent role in the chronic inflammatory response and complications of asthma. Tumor necrosis factor (TNF)-α and interleukins 4 and 5 (IL-4, IL-5) participate in the pathogenesis of bronchial asthma through their effects on the bronchial epithelial and smooth muscle cells.[20–22] Studies suggest that TNF-α, an inflammatory cytokine that is stored and released from mast cells, plays a critical role in the initiation and amplification of airway inflammation in persons with asthma. TNF-α is credited with increasing the migration and activation of inflammatory cells (*i.e.,* eosinophils and neutrophils) and contributing to all aspects of airway remodeling, including proliferation and activation of fibroblasts, increased production of extracellular matrix glycoproteins, and mucous cell hyperplasia.[22]

It has been determined that frequent viral respiratory infections predispose people with asthma to experience an exacerbation of their disease. In fact, frequent viral respiratory infections may also cause the development of asthma in some people.[17] When these respiratory infections are frequent at an early age, there is evidence that the T-helper 2 (T_2H) response is exaggerated. When the CD4 T_2H cytokines IL-4, IL-5, and IL-13 are released, the airways are predisposed for an allergic response, which favors the production of IgE.[16–18]

The National Heart, Lung, and Blood Institute's Expert Panel Report 3 (NHLBI EPR 3): Guidelines for the Diagnosis and Management of Asthma defined asthma as a chronic inflammatory disorder of the airways. The immunologic aspects of asthma including the cascade of neutrophils, eosinophils, lymphocytes, and mast cells cause epithelial injury. This causes airway inflammation, which further increases hyperresponsiveness and decreased airflow.[14] There are multiple mediators and cell types that cause the inflammation and airway bronchoconstriction in asthma. When mast cells are activated, the release of histamine; prostaglandin D_2; cytokines such as IL-1 to IL-5, interferon, TNF, and granulocyte–macrophage colony-stimulating factor; and leukotrienes causes massive bronchoconstriction and inflammation of pulmonary vasculature endothelium. Mast cells can trigger multiple cytokine release, which causes major inflammation of the airway. The contraction of the airways and subsequent swelling leads to further airway obstruction.

The mast cell release may be linked to exercise-induced asthma (EIA), which is when individuals only experience wheezing and bronchospasm during exercise.[19,20] The cause of EIA is unclear but the following two theories are possible explanations. One theory explaining the cause of EIA is based on the loss of heat and water from the tracheobronchial tree because of the need for warming and humidifying large volumes of air.[21] The response commonly is exaggerated when the person exercises in a cold environment. The second theory supporting EIA is the airway rewarming hypothesis, which states that airways cool and then warm during any exercise.[21] This causes congestion in the bronchiolar vessels that surround the bronchial tree and allows fluid exudates to move into the mucosa of the airway, which triggers the inflammatory cascade. It is important to assess the type of air (polluted, cold, or warm), level of exercise, presence/absence of respiratory infectious process, and individual's asthma stability when identifying if a person has EIA.[19]

Eosinophils tend to be present in airways of people with asthma and generate inflammatory enzymes and release leukotrienes and many proinflammatory enzymes.[14,22] It is common to have increased neutrophils in sputum and airways of people experiencing asthma exacerbations.[22] The release of leukotrienes causes more mucus secretion, which often obstructs the airway further and causes more histamine release from the mast cells.[21]

This inflammatory process produces recurrent episodes of airway obstruction, characterized by wheezing, breathlessness, chest tightness, and a cough that often is worse at night and in the early morning. These episodes, which usually are reversible either spontaneously or with treatment, also cause an associated increase in bronchial responsiveness to a variety of stimuli.[17] Chronic inflammation can lead to airway remodeling, in which case airflow limitations may be only partially reversible.[14] This may be due to the long-term effects of the inflammation on the airway structures.[14]

There is a small group of people with the clinical triad of asthma, chronic rhinosinusitis with nasal polyps, and precipitation of asthma and rhinitis attacks in response to aspirin and other NSAIDs.[22] The mechanism of the hypersensitivity reaction is complex and not fully understood, but most evidence points toward an abnormality in arachidonic acid (AA) metabolism. Cyclooxygenase (COX), the rate-limiting enzyme in AA metabolism, exists in two main forms: COX-1 and COX-2. COX-1 is responsible for the synthesis of protective prostaglandins and COX-2 for the synthesis of mediators of inflammation and bronchoconstriction. It has been hypothesized that in people with aspirin-induced asthma, the inhibition of COX-1 shunts the metabolism of AA away from the production of protective prostaglandins and toward the generation of COX-2 and other mediators of inflammation and bronchoconstriction.[22] Avoidance of aspirin and all NSAIDs is a necessary part of the treatment program.

In addition, both emotional factors and changes in hormone levels are thought to contribute to an increase in asthma symptoms. Emotional factors produce bronchospasm by way of vagal pathways. They can act as a bronchospastic trigger, or they can increase airway responsiveness to other triggers through noninflammatory mechanisms. The role of sex hormones in asthma is unclear, although there is much circumstantial evidence to suggest that they may be important. In fact, research shows girls with an early menarche (<11.5 years) had twice the chance of developing asthma in their twenties than girls with average menarche.[23] Up to 40% of women with asthma report a premenstrual increase in asthma symptoms.[24] Female sex hormones have a regulatory role on β_2-adrenergic function, and it has been suggested that abnormal regulation may be a possible mechanism for premenstrual asthma.[24] A study comparing premenopausal women with asthma, menopausal women with asthma, and a control group found that menopausal women with asthma had decreased estradiol concentrations, had high sputum neutrophils, and exhaled IL-6, which is indicative of a neutrophilic inflammation. Women with premenopausal asthma had an eosinophilic inflammatory phenotype.[24]

Clinical Manifestations

Asthma attacks may occur spontaneously or in response to various triggers, respiratory infections, emotional stress, or weather changes. Asthma is often worse at night, referred to as *nocturnal asthma*. Studies of nocturnal asthma suggest that there is a circadian and sleep-related variation in hormones and respiratory function.[25,26] The greatest decrease in respiratory function occurs at about 4:00 AM, at which time cortisol levels are low, melatonin levels high, and eosinophil activity increased.

People with asthma exhibit a wide range of signs and symptoms, from episodic wheezing and feelings of chest tightness to an acute, immobilizing attack. The attacks differ from person to person, and between attacks, many people are symptom-free. A mild attack may produce a feeling of chest tightness, a slight increase in respiratory rate with prolonged expiration, and mild wheezing. A cough may accompany the wheezing. More severe attacks are accompanied by use of the accessory muscles, distant breath sounds due to air trapping, and loud wheezing. As the condition progresses, fatigue develops, the skin becomes moist, and anxiety and apprehension are obvious. Sensations of shortness of breath may be severe, and often the person is able to speak only one or two words before taking a breath. At the point at which airflow is markedly decreased, breath sounds become inaudible with diminished wheezing, and the cough becomes ineffective despite being repetitive and hacking.[17] This point often marks the onset of respiratory failure.

During an asthmatic attack, the airways narrow because of bronchospasm, edema of the bronchial mucosa, and mucus plugging. Expiration becomes prolonged because of progressive airway obstruction. The amount of air that can be forcibly expired in 1 second (forced expiratory volume in 1 second [$FEV_{1.0}$]) and the peak expiratory flow (PEF) rate, measured in liters per second, are decreased. A fall in the PEF to levels below 50% of the predicted value during an acute asthmatic attack indicates a severe exacerbation and the need for emergency department treatment.[17]

During a prolonged attack, air becomes trapped behind the occluded and narrowed airways, causing hyperinflation of the lungs. This produces an increase in the residual volume (RV) along with a decrease in the inspiratory reserve capacity (tidal volume + inspiratory reserve volume [IRC]) and forced vital capacity (FVC), such that the person breathes close to his or her functional residual capacity (residual volume + expiratory reserve volume). As a result, more energy is needed to overcome the tension already present in the lungs, and the accessory muscles (*e.g.,* sternocleidomastoid muscles) are required to maintain ventilation and gas exchange. This increased WOB further increases oxygen demands and causes dyspnea and fatigue. Because air is trapped in the alveoli and inspiration is occurring at higher residual lung volumes, the cough becomes less effective. As the condition progresses, the effectiveness of alveolar ventilation declines, and mismatching of ventilation and perfusion occurs, causing hypoxemia and hypercapnia. Pulmonary vascular resistance may increase as a result of the hypoxemia and hyperinflation, leading to a rise in pulmonary arterial pressure and increased work demands on the right heart.

Diagnosis

The diagnosis of asthma is based on a careful history and physical examination, laboratory findings, and pulmonary function studies. Spirometry provides a means for measuring FVC, $FEV_{1.0}$, PEF, tidal volume, expiratory reserve capacity, and inspiratory reserve capacity. The $FEV_{1.0}/FVC$ ratio can then be calculated. The level of airway responsiveness can be measured by inhalation challenge tests using methacholine (a cholinergic agonist), histamine, or exposure to a nonpharmacologic agent such as cold air.

Small, inexpensive, portable meters that measure PEF are available. Although not intended for use in the diagnosis of asthma, they can be used in clinics and primary care providers' offices and in the home to provide frequent measures of flow rates. Day–night (circadian) variations in asthma symptoms and PEF variability can be used to indicate the severity of bronchial hyperresponsiveness. The person's best performance is established from readings taken over several weeks. This often is referred to as the individual's *personal best* and is used as a reference to indicate changes in respiratory function.[14]

Treatment

The NHLBI EPR 3 classifies four stages of asthma for children greater than 12 years and adults, including intermittent, mild persistent, moderate persistent, and severe persistent.[17] The Expert Panel developed these classification systems in order to direct asthma treatment and to assist in identifying people at high risk for development of life-threatening asthma attacks[14,15] (Table 31.1). Asthma treatment consists of prevention measures, nonpharmacologic measures, desensitization, and pharmacologic management.

Prevention measures to control factors contributing to asthma severity are aimed at limiting exposure to irritants and factors that increase asthma symptoms and precipitate asthma exacerbations. They include education of the person and family regarding measures used in avoiding exposure to irritants and allergens that are known to induce or trigger an attack. A careful history often is needed to identify all the contributory factors. Factors such as nasal polyps, a history of aspirin sensitivity, and gastroesophageal reflux should be considered. Annual influenza vaccination is recommended for people with persistent asthma.

Nonpharmacologic management includes relaxation techniques and controlled breathing, which often help to allay the panic and anxiety that aggravate breathing difficulties. The hyperventilation that often accompanies anxiety and panic is known to act as an asthmatic trigger. In a child, measures to encourage independence as it relates to symptom control, along with those directed at helping to develop a positive self-concept, are essential.

A *program of desensitization* may be undertaken in people with persistent asthma who react to allergens, such as house dust mites, that cannot be avoided. This involves the injection of selected antigens (based on skin tests) to stimulate the production of IgG antibodies that block the IgE response. A course of allergen immunotherapy is typically of 3 to 5 years' duration.[14]

The Expert Panel recommends a stepwise approach to *pharmacologic therapy* based on the classification systems discussed previously.[14] The first line of treatment with any of the persistent forms of asthma includes an inflammatory controller drug that would include inhaled corticosteroids (ICS), mast cell stabilizers, and leukotriene modifiers. ICS are considered the most effective in preventing airway inflammation and generally the drug used.

The *quick-relief medications* such as the short-acting β_2-adrenergic agonists (SABA) (*e.g.,* albuterol, levalbuterol, pirbuterol) relax bronchial smooth muscle and provide prompt relief of symptoms, usually within 30 minutes. They are administered by inhalation (*i.e.,* metered-dose inhaler [MDI] or nebulizer), and their recommended use is in alleviating acute attacks of asthma because regular use does

TABLE 31.1 CLASSIFICATION OF ASTHMA SEVERITY (YOUTHS ≥12 YEARS OF AGE AND ADULTS)*

	SYMPTOMS	DURATION	LUNG FUNCTION
Intermittent	Symptoms ≤2 times a week Asymptomatic and normal PEF between exacerbations Exacerbations brief (from a few hours to a few days); intensity may vary	≤2 days/week; nighttime awakening ≤2 times/month, no interference with normal activity	$FEV_{1.0}$ or EEF ≥80% predicted PEV/FVC normal
Mild	Symptoms >2 times a week but <1 time a day; exacerbations may affect activity	>2 days/week but not daily; times a month; nighttime awakening = 3–4 times/month; minor interference with normal activity	$FEV_{1.0}$ ≥ 80% predicted$FEV_{1.0}$/FVC normal
Moderate	Daily symptoms Daily use of inhaled short-acting β2-adrenergic agonist Exacerbations affect activity Exacerbations ≥2 times a week; may last days	Daily; nighttime awakening ≥1 time/week but less than nightly; some limitations to normal activity	$FEV_{1.0}$ > 60%– < 80% predicted-$FEV_{1.0}$/FVC reduced 5%
Severe	Continual symptoms Limited physical activity Frequent exacerbations	Consistently through the day; nighttime awakenings ≥ 7 times/weekly; severe limitations to normal activity	$FEV_{1.0}$ ≤ 60% predicted $FEV_{1.0}$/FVC reduced > 5%

*Age-specific classification criteria for children provided on website.
$FEV_{1.0}$, forced expiratory volume in 1 second; PEF, peak expiratory flow rate.
Adapted from National Asthma Education and Prevention Program, Third Expert Panel on the Diagnosis and Management of Asthma. Expert Panel Report 3: Guidelines for the Diagnosis and Management of Asthma. Bethesda (MD): National Heart, Lung, and Blood Institute (US); 2007 Aug. Section 3, Component 1: Measures of Asthma Assessment and Monitoring. Available from: https://www.ncbi.nlm.nih.gov/books/NBK7230.

not produce beneficial effects.[14] The anticholinergic medications (*e.g.*, ipratropium) block the postganglionic efferent vagal pathways that cause bronchoconstriction. These medications, which are administered by inhalation, produce bronchodilation by direct action on the large airways and do not change the composition or viscosity of the bronchial mucus. It is thought that they may provide some additive benefit for treatment of asthma exacerbations when administered with inhaled β_2-adrenergic agonists.[14] A short course of systemic corticosteroids, administered orally or parenterally, may be used for treating an acute flare. Although their onset of action is slow (>4 hours), systemic corticosteroids may be used in the treatment of moderate to severe exacerbations because of their action in preventing the progression of the exacerbation, speeding recovery, and preventing early relapses.[14]

The anti-inflammatory agents sodium cromolyn and nedocromil are also used to prevent an asthmatic attack. These agents act by stabilizing mast cells, thereby preventing release of the inflammatory mediators that cause an asthmatic attack. They are used prophylactically to prevent early and late responses but are of no benefit when taken during an attack. Due to the immunomodulatory properties of vitamin D and its abilities to modify proinflammatory and anti-inflammatory responses in the immunologic system, there have been studies suggesting a correlation of vitamin D and more effective management of childhood and asthma exacerbations as well as with steroid-resistant asthma.[27]

Severe or Refractory Asthma

Severe or refractory asthma represents a subgroup of approximately 5% of people with asthma who have more troublesome disease as evidenced by high medication requirements to maintain good symptom control or those who continue to have persistent symptoms despite high medication use.[28] These people are at increased risk for fatal or near-fatal asthma.

Little is known about the causes of severe asthma. Among the proposed risk factors are genetic predisposition, continued allergen or tobacco exposure, infection, intercurrent sinusitis or gastroesophageal reflux disease, and lack of compliance or adherence with treatment measures.[28] It has been proposed that because asthma is a disease involving multiple genes, mutations in genes regulating cytokines, growth factors, or receptors for medications used in treatment of asthma (β_2-adrenergic agonist or glucocorticoid) could be involved. Environmental factors include both allergen and tobacco exposure, with the strongest response occurring in response to house dust, cockroach allergen, and *Alternaria* exposure. Infections may also play a role. Respiratory syncytial virus infections are implicated in children, and pathogens such as mycoplasma and chlamydiae may play a role in adults. Gastroesophageal reflux and chronic sinusitis may also play a role. Although the cause of death during an acute asthmatic attack is largely unknown, both cardiac arrhythmias and asphyxia due to severe airway obstruction have been implicated. It has been suggested that an underestimation of the severity of the attack may be a contributing factor. Deterioration often occurs rapidly during an acute attack, and underestimation of its severity may lead to a life-threatening delay in seeking medical attention. Frequent and repetitive use of β_2-adrenergic agonist inhalers far in excess of the recommended doses may temporarily blunt symptoms and mask the severity of the condition. It has been suggested that people who have a fatal or near-fatal asthmatic attack may not perceive its severity.[28,29] That is, they may not perceive the severity of their condition and consequently not take appropriate measures in terms of seeking medical or emergency treatment.

The long-acting β_2-agonists (LABA) such as salmeterol and formoterol are used to treat severe refractory asthma only if no other treatment is effective. The long-acting β_2-adrenergic agonists have durations of action of at least 12 hours and should not be used to treat acute symptoms or exacerbations. These drugs have a black box warning from the U.S. Food and Drug Administration due to their possibility of causing asthma death, especially if they are used as a monotherapy. Research is also focusing on the use of allergen immunotherapy treatment aimed at T_2H cytokines in specific groups of people with severe asthma. However, only one is currently available.[28,30,31] The only licensed anti-IgE therapy for severe asthma is omalizumab, which has severe potential systemic side effects.[31]

Asthma in Older Adults

For older adults with asthma, who already have a decreased immunologic function due to aging, it is important to be aware of how this lowered immunity impacts their airway inflammation. Studies demonstrate these changes in immune function can seriously affect their conditions.[32]

Asthma in Children

Asthma is a leading cause of chronic illness in children and is responsible for approximately 13.8 million number of lost school days/year. It is the most frequent admitting diagnosis in children's hospitals. Based on information collected by the Centers for Disease Control and Prevention, asthma may have its onset at any age. In addition, asthma is more prevalent in black than white children and results in more frequent disability and more frequent hospitalizations in black children.[33]

As with adults, asthma in children commonly is associated with an IgE-related reaction. It has been suggested that IgE directed against respiratory viruses in particular may be important in the pathogenesis of wheezing illnesses in infants (*i.e.,* bronchiolitis), which often precede the onset of asthma. Other contributing factors include exposure to environmental allergens such as pet dander, dust mite antigens, and cockroach allergens. Exposure to environmental tobacco smoke also contributes to asthma in children.

The signs and symptoms of asthma in infants and small children vary with the stage and severity of an attack. Because airway patency decreases at night, many children have acute signs of asthma at this time. Infants with undiagnosed asthma may have a prolonged cough without cold symptoms, independent of wheezing.[34] Often, previously well infants and children develop what may seem to be a cold with rhinorrhea, rapidly followed by irritability, a tight and nonproductive cough, wheezing, tachypnea, dyspnea with prolonged expiration, and use of accessory muscles of respiration. Cyanosis, hyperinflation of the chest, and tachycardia indicate increasing severity of the attack. Wheezing may be absent in children with extreme respiratory distress. The symptoms may progress rapidly and require a trip to the emergency department or hospitalization.

The expert panel of the Global Initiative for Asthma (GINA) has developed a global strategy with guidelines for management and prevention of asthma in infants and children from 0 to 5 years, 6 to 11 years, and for adults and children 12 years of age and older. As with adults and older children, GINA recommends a stepwise approach to diagnosing and managing asthma in infants and children.[34]

Chronic Obstructive Pulmonary Disease

COPD is characterized by chronic and recurrent obstruction of airflow in the pulmonary airways. Airflow obstruction usually is progressive and is accompanied by inflammatory responses to noxious particles or gases. COPD is a leading cause of morbidity and mortality worldwide. It has been estimated that approximately 30 million Americans[35] have some degree of COPD; 16 million are diagnosed with COPD. Of those diagnosed, 56% are women. In the United States COPD is the fourth leading cause of death following heart disease, cancer, and unintentional injuries.[36] According to the COPD National Action Plan, more than $32 billion was spent on direct costs related to COPD care and $20.4 billion was spent on indirect costs related to COPD in 2010. The projected cost in 2020 is approximately $49 billion.[36,37]

The most common cause of COPD is smoking, and approximately 80% of deaths related to COPD are associated with a history of smoking.[37] A second, less common factor is a hereditary deficiency in α_1-antitrypsin (AAT). Other predisposing factors are asthma and airway hyperresponsiveness. Although clinical findings may be absent during the early stages of COPD, any person with a chronic cough, sputum production, dyspnea and a history to exposures of risk factors such as smoking or indoor/outdoor pollutions should be considered for the diagnosis of COPD.[28,36,37] By the time symptoms appear or are recognized, the disease is usually far advanced. For smokers with early signs of airway disease, there is hope that early recognition, combined with appropriate treatment and smoking cessation, may prevent or delay the usually relentless progression of the disease.

Etiology and Pathogenesis

The mechanisms involved in the pathogenesis of COPD usually are multiple and include inflammation and fibrosis of the bronchial wall, hypertrophy of the submucosal glands and hypersecretion of mucus, and loss of elastic lung fibers and alveolar tissue.[28,37] Inflammation and fibrosis of the bronchial wall, along with excess mucus secretion, obstruct airflow and cause mismatching of ventilation and perfusion. Destruction of alveolar tissue decreases the surface area for gas exchange, and loss of elastic fibers impairs the expiratory flow rate, increases air trapping, and predisposes to airway collapse.

The term *chronic obstructive pulmonary disease* encompasses two types of obstructive airway disease: *emphysema*, with enlargement of airspaces and destruction of lung tissue, and *chronic obstructive bronchitis*, with increased mucus production, obstruction of small airways, and a chronic productive cough. People with COPD often have overlapping features of both disorders.[28,37]

Emphysema. Emphysema is characterized by a loss of lung elasticity and abnormal enlargement of the airspaces distal to the terminal bronchioles, with destruction of the alveolar walls and capillary beds (Fig. 31.9). Enlargement of the airspaces leads to hyperinflation of the lungs and produces an increase in total lung capacity (TLC). Two of the recognized causes of emphysema are smoking, which incites lung injury, and an inherited deficiency of AAT, an antiprotease enzyme that protects the lung from injury. AAT deficiency (AATD) is a genetic risk factor for COPD.[28,38] Mutations in the SERPINA1 gene can cause AATD. Isoelectric focusing is considered to be the gold standard in diagnosis of ATTD. 38)

Emphysema is thought to result from the breakdown of elastin and other alveolar wall components by enzymes, called *proteases*, which digest proteins. Normally, antiprotease enzymes, including AAT, protect the lung. Cigarette smoke and other irritants stimulate the movement of inflammatory cells into the lungs, resulting in increased release of elastase and other proteases. In smokers in whom COPD develops, antiprotease production and release may be inadequate to neutralize the excess protease production such that the process of elastic tissue destruction goes unchecked (Fig. 31.10).

The type and amount of AAT that a person has is determined by a pair of codominant genes referred to as *PI* (protein inhibitor) genes. An AATD is inherited as an autosomal recessive disorder. Most people with clinically diagnosed emphysema before the age of 40 years have an AATD. Smoking and repeated respiratory tract infections, which also decrease AAT levels, contribute to the risk for emphysema in persons with AATD. Laboratory methods are available for measuring AAT levels. Human AAT is available for replacement therapy in people with a hereditary deficiency of the enzyme.

There are two commonly recognized types of emphysema: centriacinar or centrilobular, and panacinar (Fig. 31.11). Centriacinar emphysema is mostly associated with cigarette smoking and affects the respiratory bronchioles predominantly in the upper lobes and in the superior lower lobes.[28] It is the most common type of emphysema and is seen predominantly in male smokers. The panacinar type produces initial involvement of the peripheral alveoli and later extends to involve the more central bronchioles. This type of emphysema is more common in people with AATD. It also is found in

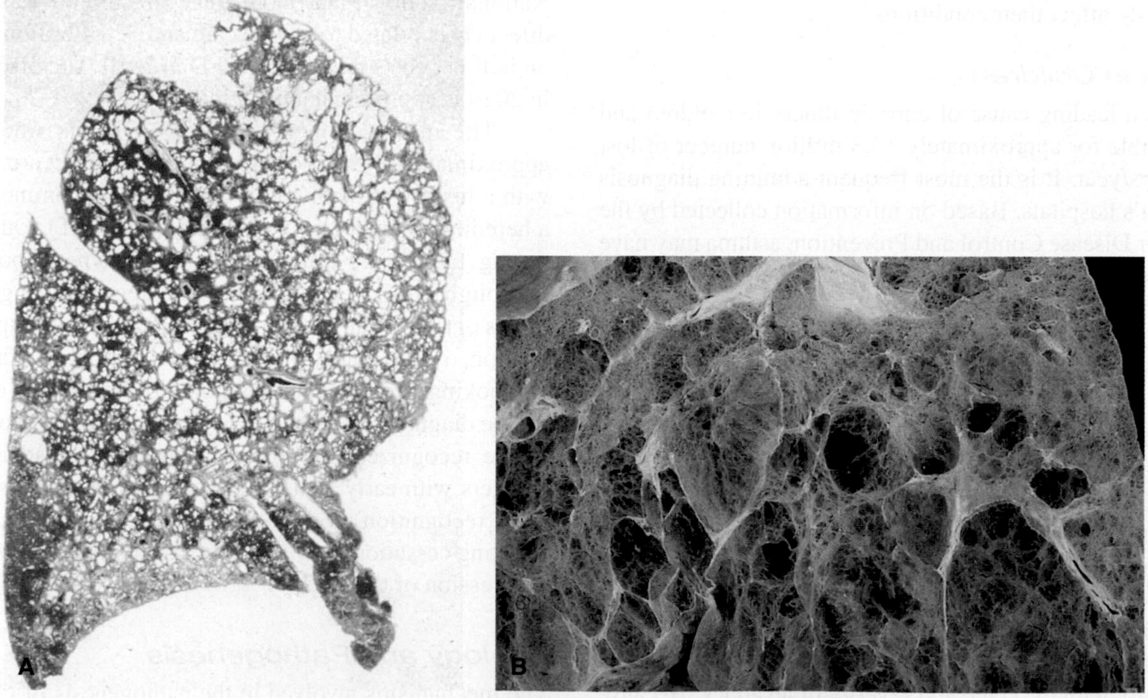

Figure 31.9 • Panacinar emphysema. **(A)** A whole mount of the left lung from a people with severe emphysema reveals widespread destruction of pulmonary parenchyma that in some areas leaves behind a lacy network of supporting tissue. **(B)** The lung from a person with AATD shows a panacinar pattern of emphysema. The loss of alveolar walls has resulted in markedly enlarged airspaces. (From Strayer D., Rubin R. (Eds.) (2015). *Rubin's pathology: Clinicopathologic foundations of medicine* (7th ed., Fig. 18-45, p. 710). Philadelphia, PA: Lippincott Williams & Wilkins.)

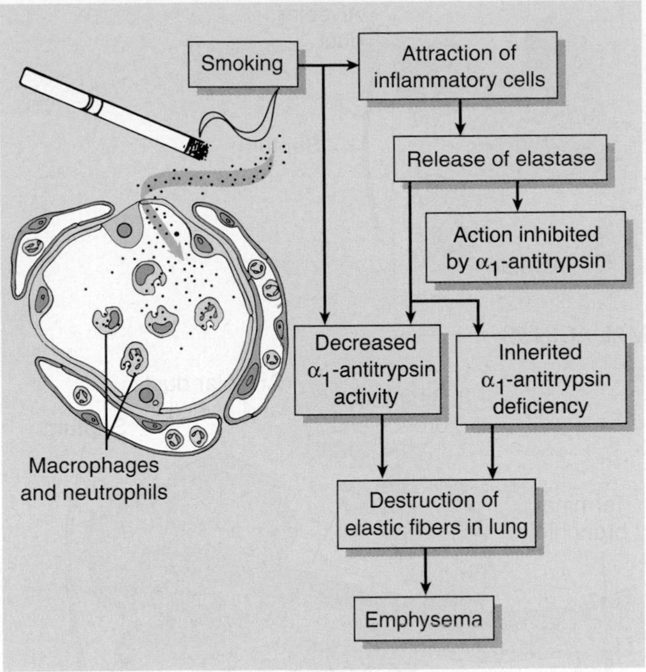

Figure 31.10 • The proteolysis–antiproteolysis theory of the pathogenesis of emphysema. Cigarette (tobacco) smoking is closely related to the development of emphysema. Some products in tobacco smoke induce an inflammatory reaction. The serine elastase in polymorphonuclear leukocytes, a particularly potent elastolytic agent, injures the elastic tissue of the lung. Normally, this enzyme activity is inhibited by a_1-antitrypsin, but tobacco smoke, directly or through the generation of free radicals, inactivates AAT (protease inhibitor). (From Strayer D., Rubin R. (Eds.) (2015). *Rubin's pathology: Clinicopathologic foundations of medicine* (7th ed., Fig. 18-42, p. 708). Philadelphia, PA: Lippincott Williams & Wilkins.)

smokers in association with centriacinar emphysema. In such cases, the panacinar pattern tends to occur in the lower parts of the lung and centriacinar emphysema is seen in the upper parts of the lung.

Chronic Bronchitis. Chronic bronchitis represents airway obstruction of the major and small airways.[28,39] The condition is seen most commonly in middle-aged men and is associated with chronic irritation from smoking and recurrent infections. A clinical diagnosis of chronic bronchitis requires the history of a chronic productive cough for at least 3 consecutive months in at least 2 consecutive years.[39] Typically, the cough has been present for many years, with a gradual increase in acute exacerbations that produce frankly purulent sputum.

The earliest feature of chronic bronchitis is hypersecretion of mucus in the large airways, associated with hypertrophy of the submucosal glands in the trachea and bronchi.[28] Although mucus hypersecretion in the large airways is the cause of sputum overproduction, it is now thought that accompanying changes in the small airways (small bronchi and bronchioles) are physiologically important in the airway obstruction that develops in chronic bronchitis.[28] Histologically, these changes include a marked increase in goblet cells and excess mucus production with plugging of the airway lumen, inflammatory infiltration, and fibrosis of the bronchiolar wall. It is thought that both the submucosal hypertrophy in the larger airways and the increase in goblet cells in the smaller airways are a protective reaction against tobacco smoke and other pollutants. Viral and bacterial infections are common in people with chronic bronchitis and are thought to be a result rather than a cause of the problem.

Clinical Manifestations

The clinical manifestations of COPD usually have an insidious onset. People characteristically seek medical attention in the fifth or sixth decade of life, with manifestations such as fatigue, exercise intolerance, cough, sputum production, or shortness of breath. The productive cough usually occurs in the morning and the dyspnea becomes more severe as the disease progresses. Frequent exacerbations of infection and respiratory insufficiency are common, causing absence from work and eventual disability. The late stages of COPD are characterized by recurrent respiratory infections and chronic respiratory failure. Death usually occurs during an exacerbation of illness associated with infection and respiratory failure.

The mnemonics "pink puffer" and "blue bloater" have been used to differentiate the clinical manifestations of emphysema and chronic obstructive bronchitis. People with predominant emphysema are classically referred to as *pink puffers*, a reference to the lack of cyanosis, the use of accessory muscles, and pursed-lip ("puffer") breathing. With loss of lung elasticity and hyperinflation of the lungs, the airways often collapse during expiration because pressure in surrounding lung tissues exceeds airway pressure. Air becomes trapped in the alveoli and lungs, producing an increase in the anteroposterior dimensions of the chest, the so-called *barrel chest* that is typical of people with emphysema (Fig. 31.12). Such people have a dramatic decrease in breath sounds throughout the chest. Because the diaphragm may be functioning near its maximum ability, the person is vulnerable to diaphragmatic fatigue and acute respiratory failure.

People with a clinical syndrome of chronic bronchitis are classically labeled *blue bloaters*, a reference to cyanosis and fluid retention associated with right-sided heart failure. In practice, differentiation between the two types of COPD is often difficult. This is because people with COPD often have some degree of both emphysema and chronic bronchitis.

The manifestations of COPD represent a progressive change in respiratory function. There is moderate to severe respiratory impairment due to obstruction of airflow, which is greater on expiration than inspiration, resulting in increased WOB but decreased effectiveness. The development of exertional dyspnea, often described as increased effort to breathe, heaviness, air hunger, or gasping, can be insidious and is often reported in the sixth decade. Activities involving significant arm work, particularly above the shoulders, are particularly difficult for persons with COPD. Activities that allow the person to brace the arms and use the accessory muscles are better tolerated. As the disease progresses, breathing becomes increasingly more labored, even at rest. The expiratory phase

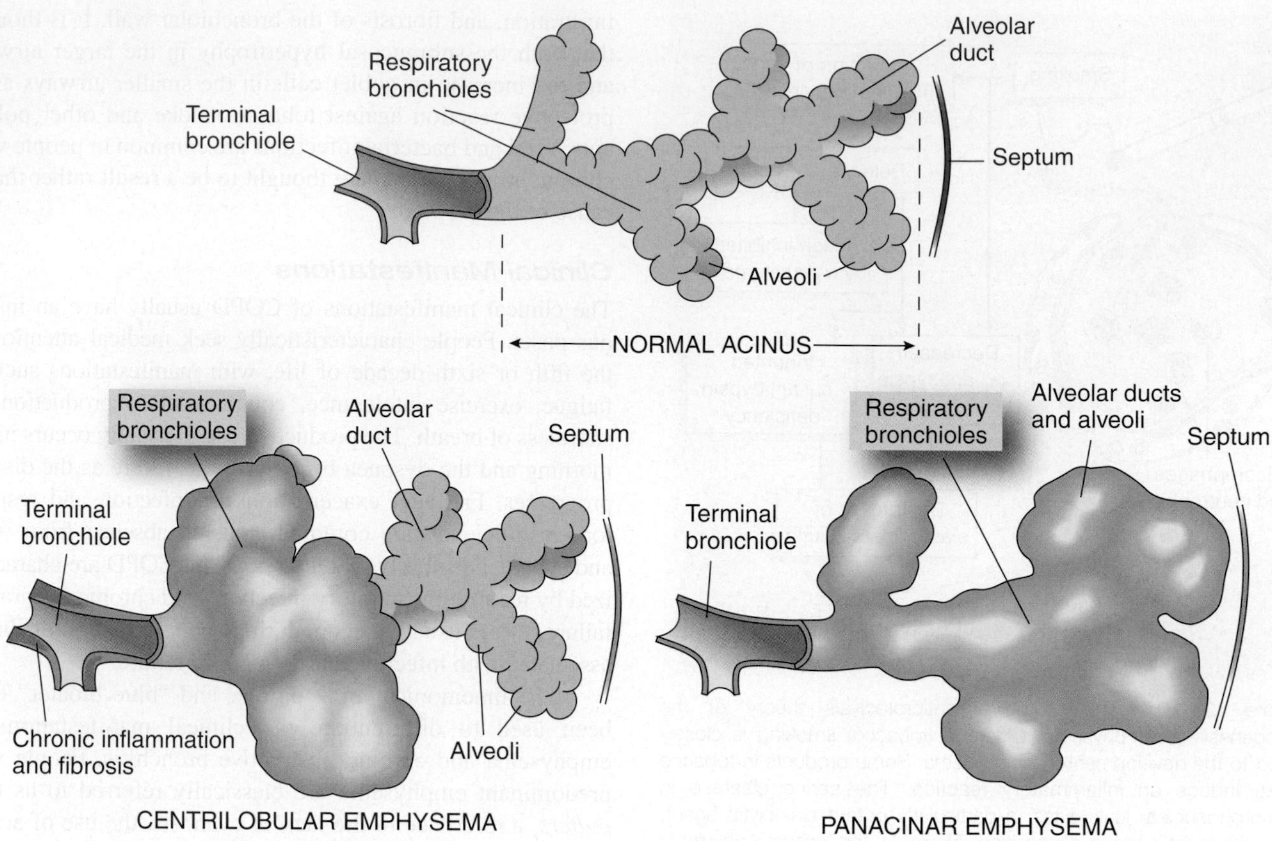

Figure 31.11 • Types of emphysema. The acinus is the gas-exchanging structural unit of the lung distal to the terminal bronchiole. It consists of (from proximal to distal) respiratory bronchioles, alveolar ductus, alveolar sacs, and alveoli. In centrilobular (proximal acinar) emphysema, the respiratory bronchioles are predominantly involved. In paraseptal (distal acinar) emphysema, the alveolar ducts are particularly affected. In panacinar (panlobular) emphysema, the acinus is uniformy damaged. (From Strayer D., Rubin R. (Eds.) (2015). *Rubin's pathology: Clinicopathologic foundations of medicine* (7th ed., Fig. 18-43, p. 709). Philadelphia, PA: Lippincott Williams & Wilkins.)

of respiration is prolonged, and expiratory wheezes and crackles can be heard on auscultation. People with severe airflow obstruction may also exhibit use of the accessory muscles, sitting in the characteristic "tripod" position to facilitate use of the sternocleidomastoid, scalene, and intercostal muscles.[28] Pursed-lip breathing enhances airflow because it increases the resistance to the outflow of air and helps to prevent airway collapse by increasing airway pressure. Eventually, people with COPD are unable to maintain normal blood gases by increasing their breathing effort. Hypoxemia, hypercapnia, and cyanosis develop, reflecting an imbalance between ventilation and perfusion.

Severe hypoxemia, in which arterial PO_2 levels fall below 55 mm Hg, causes reflex vasoconstriction of the pulmonary vessels and further impairment of gas exchange in the lung. It is more common in people with the chronic bronchitis form of COPD. Hypoxemia also stimulates red blood cell production, causing polycythemia. The increase in pulmonary vasoconstriction and subsequent elevation in pulmonary artery pressure further increase the work of the right ventricle. As a result, people with COPD may develop right-sided heart failure with peripheral edema (*i.e.,* cor pulmonale). However, signs of overt right-sided heart failure are seen less frequently since the advent of supplemental oxygen therapy.

Diagnosis

The diagnosis of COPD is based on a careful history and physical examination, pulmonary function studies, chest radiographs, and laboratory tests. Airway obstruction prolongs the expiratory phase of respiration and affords the potential for impaired gas exchange because of mismatching of ventilation and perfusion. The FVC is the amount of air that can be forcibly exhaled after maximal inspiration. In an adult with normal respiratory function, this should be achieved in 4 to 6 seconds. In people with chronic lung disease, the time required for FVC is increased, the $FEV_{1.0}$ is decreased, and the ratio of $FEV_{1.0}$ to FVC is decreased. In severe disease, the FVC is markedly reduced. Lung volume measurements reveal a marked increase in RV, an increase in TLC, and elevation of the RV-to-TLC ratio. These and other measurements of expiratory flow are determined by spirometry and are used in the diagnosis of COPD. Spirometry measurements can be used in staging disease severity. For example, an $FEV_{1.0}$-to-FVC ratio of less than 70% with an $FEV_{1.0}$ of 80% or more, with

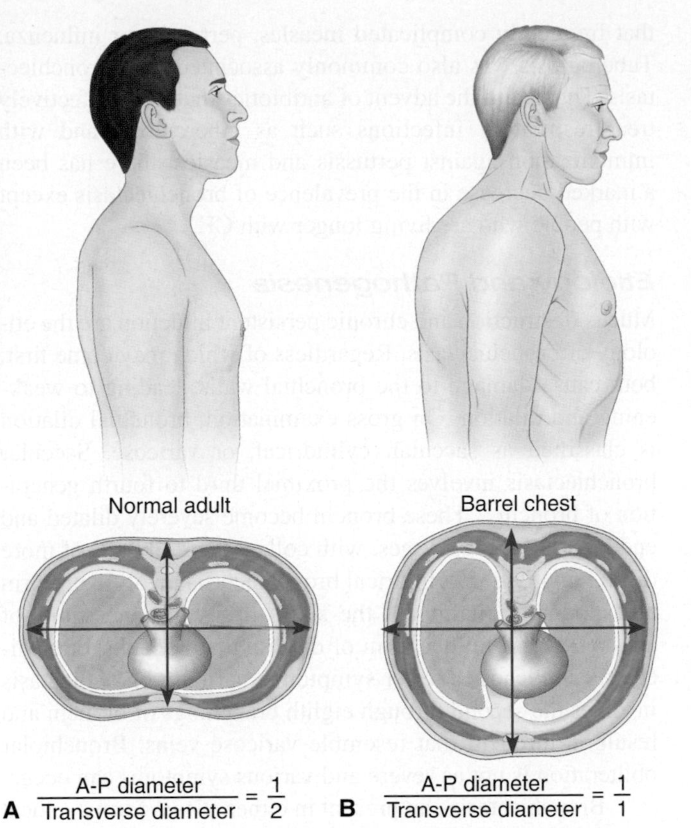

Figure 31.12 • Characteristics of normal chest wall and chest wall in emphysema. **(A)** The normal chest wall and its cross-section. **(B)** The barrel-shaped chest of emphysema and its cross-section. (From Hinkle J. L., Cheever K. H. (2018). *Brunner & Suddarth's textbook of medical-surgical nursing* (14th ed., Fig. 24-3, p. 637). Philadelphia, PA: Lippincott Williams & Wilkins.)

or without symptoms, indicates mild disease, and an $FEV_{1.0}$-to-FVC ratio of less than 70% with an $FEV_{1.0}$ of less than or equal to 50%, with or without symptoms, indicates moderate disease. Severe disease is indicated by an $FEV_{1.0}$ range of 30-50%, and very severe COPD is indicated with an $FEV_{1.0}$ of less than 30%; both with $FEV_{1.0}$-to-FVC ratios less than 70%.[35] Other diagnostic measures become important as the disease advances. Measures of exercise tolerance, nutritional status, hemoglobin saturation, and arterial blood gases can be used to assess the overall impact of COPD on health status and to direct treatment.

Treatment

The treatment of COPD depends on the stage of the disease and often requires an interdisciplinary approach. Smoking cessation is the only measure that slows the progression of the disease. Education of people with COPD and their families is a key to successful management of the disease. Psychosocial rehabilitation must be individualized to meet the specific needs of people with COPD and their families. These needs vary with age, occupation, financial resources, social and recreational interests, and interpersonal and family relationships.

People in more advanced stages of the disease often require measures to maintain and improve physical and psychosocial functioning, pharmacologic interventions, and oxygen therapy. Avoidance of cigarette smoke and other environmental airway irritants is imperative. Wearing a cold-weather mask often prevents dyspnea and bronchospasm due to cold air and wind exposure.

Respiratory tract infections can prove life threatening to people with severe COPD. A person with COPD should avoid exposure to others with known respiratory tract infections and should avoid attending large gatherings during periods of the year when influenza or respiratory tract infections are prevalent. Immunization for influenza and pneumococcal infections decreases the likelihood of their occurrence.

Maintaining and improving physical and psychosocial functioning is an important part of the treatment program for people with COPD. A long-term pulmonary rehabilitation program can significantly reduce episodes of hospitalization and add measurably to a person's ability to manage and cope with his or her impairment in a positive way. This program includes breathing exercises that focus on restoring the function of the diaphragm, reducing the WOB, and improving gas exchange. Physical conditioning with appropriate exercise training increases maximal oxygen consumption and reduces ventilatory effort and heart rate for a given workload. Work simplification and energy conservation strategies may be needed when impairment is severe.

The pharmacologic treatment of COPD includes the use of bronchodilators, including inhaled adrenergic and anticholinergic agents. Inhaled β_2-adrenergic agonists have been the mainstay of treatment of COPD. It has been suggested that long-acting inhaled β_2-adrenergic agonists may be even more effective than the short-acting forms of the drug. The anticholinergic drugs (*e.g.*, ipratropium bromide, tiotropium bromide), which are administered by inhalation, produce bronchodilation by blocking parasympathetic cholinergic receptors that produce contraction of bronchial smooth muscle. These medications, which are administered by inhalation, produce bronchodilation by direct action on the large airways and do not change the composition or viscosity of the bronchial mucus. They also reduce the volume of sputum without altering its viscosity. Because these drugs have a slower onset and longer duration of action, they usually are used on a regular basis rather than on an as-needed basis. Inhalers that combine an anticholinergic drug with a β_2-adrenergic agonist are available.

ICSs often are used in treatment of COPD; there is controversy regarding their usefulness. An explanation for this lack of effect may be related to the fact that corticosteroids prolong the action of neutrophils and hence do not suppress the neutrophilic inflammation seen in COPD. Because corticosteroids are useful in relieving asthma symptoms, they may benefit people with asthma concomitant with COPD. ICSs also may be beneficial in treating acute exacerbations of COPD, minimizing the undesirable effects that often accompany systemic use.

Oxygen therapy is prescribed for selected people with significant hypoxemia (arterial $PO_2 < 55$ mm Hg). Administration of continuous low-flow (1 to 2 L/minute) oxygen to maintain arterial PO_2 levels between 55 and 65 mm Hg decreases dyspnea and pulmonary hypertension and improves neuropsychologic function and activity tolerance. The overall goal of oxygen therapy is to maintain a hemoglobin oxygen saturation of 88% to 92%.[35] Because the ventilatory drive associated with hypoxic stimulation of the peripheral chemoreceptors does not occur until the arterial PO_2 has been reduced to about 60 mm Hg or less, increasing the arterial PO_2 above 60 mm Hg tends to depress the hypoxic stimulus for ventilation and often leads to hypoventilation and carbon dioxide retention. Therefore, clinicians should use caution and not over oxygenate COPD people to seek a higher spirometry goal, as this may depress the drive to breathe.

Bronchiectasis

Bronchiectasis is an uncommon type of COPD characterized by a permanent dilation of the bronchi and bronchioles caused by destruction of the muscle and elastic supporting tissue as the result of a continuous cycle of infection and inflammation (Fig. 31.13). It is not a primary disease but is considered secondary to acquiring frequent infections. In the past, bronchiectasis often followed a necrotizing bacterial pneumonia that frequently complicated measles, pertussis, or influenza. Tuberculosis was also commonly associated with bronchiectasis. Thus, with the advent of antibiotics that more effectively treat respiratory infections such as tuberculosis and with immunization against pertussis and measles, there has been a marked decrease in the prevalence of bronchiectasis except with people who are living longer with CF.

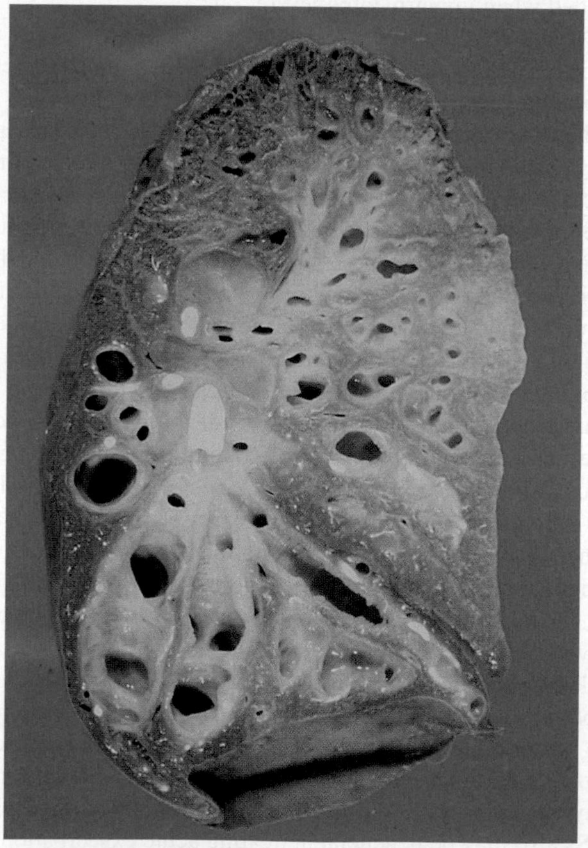

Figure 31.13 • Bronchiectasis. The resected upper lobe shows widely dilated bronchi, with thickening of the bronchial walls and collapse and fibrosis of the pulmonary parenchyma. (From Strayer D., Rubin R. (Eds.) (2015). *Rubin's pathology: Clinicopathologic foundations of medicine* (7th ed., Fig. 18-10, p. 686). Philadelphia, PA: Lippincott Williams & Wilkins.)

Etiology and Pathogenesis

Mucus obstruction and chronic persistent infection are the etiology of bronchiectasis. Regardless of which may come first, both cause damage to the bronchial walls, leading to weakening and dilation. On gross examination, bronchial dilation is classified as saccular, cylindrical, or varicose. Saccular bronchiectasis involves the proximal third to fourth generation of bronchi.[37] These bronchi become severely dilated and end blindly in dilated sacs, with collapse and fibrosis of more distal lung tissue. Cylindrical bronchiectasis involves uniform and moderate dilation of the sixth to eighth generations of airways. It is a milder form of disease than saccular bronchiectasis and leads to fewer symptoms. Varicose bronchiectasis involves the second through eighth branchings of bronchi and results in bronchi that resemble varicose veins. Bronchiolar obliteration is not as severe and various symptoms can occur.

Bronchiectasis can present in either of two forms: a local obstructive process involving a lobe or segment of a lung or a diffuse process involving much of both lungs. *Localized or focal bronchiectasis* is most commonly caused by conditions such as tumors, foreign bodies, and mucus plugs that produce atelectasis and infection due to obstructed drainage of bronchial secretions. It can affect any area of the lung, the area being determined by the site of obstruction or infection. *Generalized or diffuse bronchiectasis* usually is bilateral and most commonly affects the lower lobes.[28] It is due largely to inherited impairments of host mechanisms or acquired disorders that permit introduction of infectious organisms into the airways. They include inherited conditions such as CF, in which airway obstruction is caused by impairment of normal mucociliary function; congenital and acquired immunodeficiency states, which predispose to respiratory tract infections; lung infection (*e.g.*, tuberculosis, fungal infections, lung abscess); and exposure to toxic gases that cause airway obstruction.

Clinical Manifestations

Bronchiectasis is associated with a number of abnormalities that profoundly affect respiratory function, including atelectasis, obstruction of the smaller airways, and diffuse bronchitis. People with bronchiectasis have recurrent bronchopulmonary infection; coughing; production of copious amounts of foul-smelling, purulent sputum; and hemoptysis. Weight loss and anemia are common.

In addition, the manifestations of bronchiectasis are similar to those seen in chronic bronchitis and emphysema. As in the latter two conditions, chronic bronchial obstruction leads to marked dyspnea and cyanosis. Clubbing of the fingers, which is not usually seen in other types of obstructive lung diseases, is more common in moderate to advanced bronchiectasis.

Diagnosis and Treatment

Diagnosis is based on history and imaging studies. The condition often is evident on chest radiographs. High-resolution CT scanning of the chest allows for definitive diagnosis. Accuracy of diagnosis is important because interventional bronchoscopy or surgery may be palliative or curative in some types of obstructive disease.

Treatment consists of early recognition and treatment of infection along with regular postural drainage and chest physical therapy. Persons with this disorder benefit from many of the rehabilitation and treatment measures used for chronic bronchitis and emphysema.

Cystic Fibrosis

CF, which is the major cause of severe chronic respiratory disease in children, is an autosomal recessive disorder involving the exocrine glands in the epithelial lining of the respiratory, gastrointestinal, and reproductive tracts.[40] CF affects about 30,000 children and adults in the United States and more than 10 million persons are asymptomatic carriers of the defective gene.[40] The defective gene, cystic fibrosis transmembrane regulator (CFTR), and its protein product cause excessive thick mucus that obstructs lungs and the pancreas. In addition to chronic respiratory disease, CF is manifested by pancreatic exocrine deficiency and elevation of sodium chloride in the sweat. Nasal polyps, sinus infections, pancreatitis, and cholelithiasis also are seen with CF. Most boys with CF have congenital bilateral absence of the vas deferens with azoospermia.

Etiology and Pathogenesis

CF is caused by mutations in a single gene on the long arm of chromosome 7 that encodes for the CFTR, which functions as a chloride (Cl^-) channel in epithelial cell membranes. Mutations in the CFTR gene render the epithelial membrane relatively impermeable to the chloride ion (Fig. 31.14). There are greater than 1000 possible CFTR changes that can occur. However, the most common CFTR gene mutation is called the delta F508, in which the deletion of the amino acid phenylalanine at the 508 position results in a severe phenotype. Due to the deletion of this amino acid, chloride channels are misfolded and are not inserted into the cell membrane.[41] Others have a partial loss or mutation of the CFTR gene so their phenotype is less severe and often goes unnoticed until they have an acute injury such as pneumonia and may need intubation and mechanical ventilation.

The impact on impaired Cl^- transport due to the CFTR gene mutation ultimately affects the reabsorption of NaCl, which results in high concentrations of NaCl in the sweat of individuals with CF.[42] The impaired transport of Cl^- ultimately leads to a series of secondary events, including increased absorption of Na^+ and water from the airways into the blood.

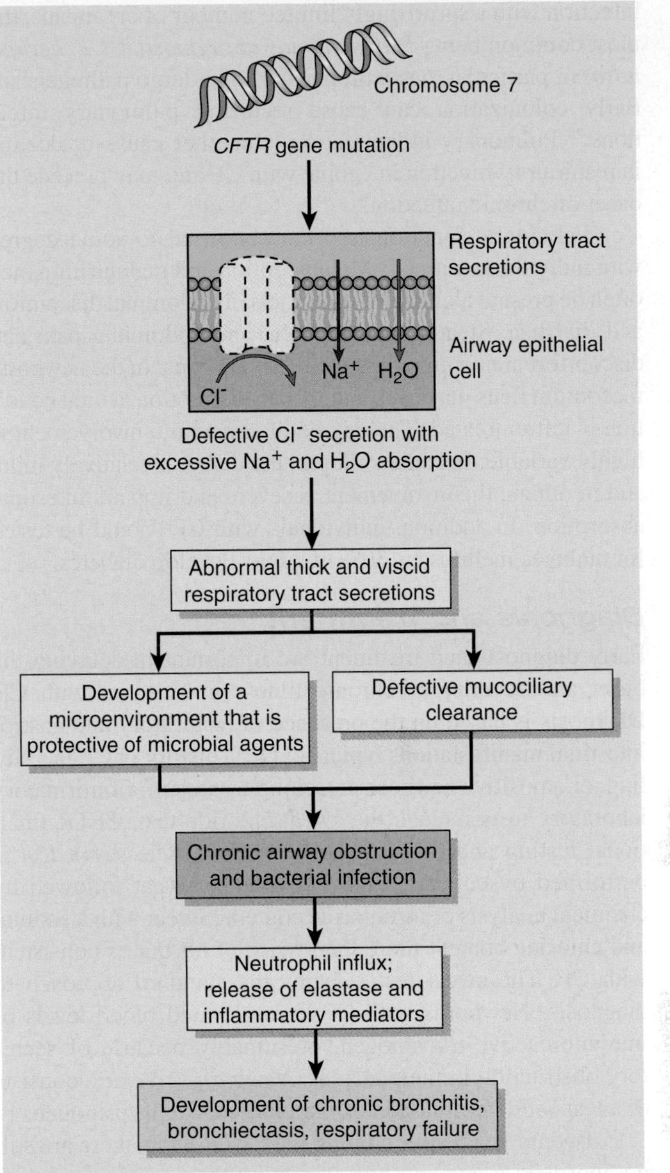

Figure 31.14 • Pathogenesis of CF.

This lowers the water content of the mucociliary blanket coating the respiratory epithelium, causing it to become more viscid. The resulting dehydration of the mucous layer leads to defective mucociliary function and accumulation of viscid secretions that obstruct the airways and predispose to recurrent pulmonary infections. Similar transport abnormalities and pathophysiologic events take place in the pancreatic and biliary ducts and in the vas deferens in boys.

Clinical Manifestations

Respiratory manifestations of CF are caused by an accumulation of viscid mucus in the bronchi, impaired mucociliary clearance, and lung infections. Chronic bronchiolitis and bronchitis are the initial lung manifestations. However, after months and years, structural changes in the bronchial wall lead to bronchiectasis. In addition to airway obstruction, the basic genetic defect that occurs with CF predisposes to chronic infection with a surprisingly limited number of organisms, the most common being *Pseudomonas aeruginosa*.[28,41] *P. aeruginosa*, in particular, has a propensity to undergo pathogenesis. Early colonization can cause recurring pulmonary infections.[28] Pulmonary inflammation is another cause of decline in respiratory function in people with CF and may precede the onset of chronic infection.

Pancreatic function is often abnormal to some degree with individuals with CF. Malabsorption and malnutrition may often be present along with symptoms of abdominal discomfort and diarrhea. Steatorrhea, diarrhea, and abdominal pain and discomfort are common associated symptoms. In the newborn, meconium ileus may cause intestinal obstruction, a fatal condition if left untreated. The degree of pancreatic involvement is highly variable. In some children, the defect is relatively mild, and in others, the involvement is severe and impairs intestinal absorption. In addition, individuals with CF should be tested for diabetes mellitus, as 30% of adults develop diabetes.[28,42]

Diagnosis and Treatment

Early diagnosis and treatment are important in delaying the onset and severity of chronic illness in children with CF. Diagnosis is based on the presence of respiratory and gastrointestinal manifestations typical of CF, a history of CF in a sibling, or a positive newborn screening test result. Confirmatory laboratory tests include the sweat chloride test, CFTR functional testing and CFTR genetic analysis. The *sweat test* is performed by collecting the individual's sweat followed by chemical analysis of its chloride content. Sweat with a sodium and chloride content more than twice of normal is consistent with CF. The sweat test remains the standard approach to diagnosis. Newborns with CF have elevated blood levels of immunoreactive trypsinogen, presumably because of secretory obstruction in the pancreas. *Newborn screening* consists of a test for determination of immunoreactive trypsinogen.[43]

Twenty years after cloning the CFTR gene, there are still no approved treatments for correcting the genetic defects in CF or to reverse the ion transport abnormalities associated with the dysfunctional CFTR. Thus, treatment measures are directed toward slowing the progression of secondary organ dysfunction and sequelae such as chronic lung infection and pancreatic insufficiency. They include the use of oral and inhaled antibiotics to prevent and manage infections, bronchodilators, anti-inflammatory medications, the use of chest physical therapy (chest percussion and postural drainage) and mucolytic agents to prevent airway obstruction, and nutritional therapy.[44]

Appropriate antibiotic therapy directed against bacterial pathogens isolated from the respiratory tract is an essential component in the management of CF lung disease. Indications for oral antibiotics include the presence of respiratory tract symptoms and identification of pathogenic organisms in respiratory tract cultures. Intravenous antibiotics are used for progressive and unrelenting symptoms.

People with CF who have complete loss of exocrine pancreas function and have inadequate digestion of fats and proteins require diet adjustment, pancreatic enzyme replacement, and supplemental vitamins and minerals. Many people with CF have a higher-than-normal caloric need because of the increased WOB and perhaps because of the increased metabolic activity related to the basic defect. Pancreatic enzyme dosage and product type are individualized for each person.

Progression of the disease is variable. Improved medical management has led to longer survival. Lung transplantation is being used as a treatment for people with end-stage lung disease. Pulmonary rehabilitation is also used in medical management of CF.[44] Current hopes reside in research that would make gene therapy a feasible alternative for people with the disease

IN SUMMARY

Obstructive ventilatory disorders are characterized by airway obstruction and limitation in expiratory airflow. Asthma is a chronic inflammatory disorder of the airways characterized by airway hyperreactivity, airway narrowing, and airway remodeling. T_1H cells differentiate in response to microbes and stimulate the differentiation of B cells into IgM– and IgG-producing plasma cells. Whereas, T_2H cells respond to allergens by stimulating B cells to differentiate into IgE-producing plasma cells, produce growth factors for mast cells, and recruit and activate eosinophils. In people with allergic asthma, T-cell differentiation appears to be skewed toward a proinflammatory T_2H response. It appears that both genetic and environmental factors play a role in the development of asthma or reactive airway disease.

COPD describes a group of conditions characterized by obstruction to airflow in the lungs. Among the conditions associated with COPD are emphysema, chronic bronchitis, and bronchiectasis. Emphysema is characterized by a loss of lung elasticity, abnormal, permanent enlargement of the airspaces distal to the terminal bronchioles, and hyperinflation of the lungs. Chronic bronchitis is caused by inflammation of major and small airways and is characterized by edema and hyperplasia of submucosal glands and excess mucus secretion into the bronchial tree. A history of a chronic productive cough that has persisted for at least 3 months and for at least 2 consecutive years in the absence of other disease is necessary for the diagnosis of chronic bronchitis. Emphysema and chronic bronchitis are manifested by eventual mismatching of ventilation and perfusion. As the condition advances, signs of respiratory distress and impaired gas exchange become evident, with development of hypercapnia and hypoxemia. Bronchiectasis is a less common form of COPD that is characterized by an abnormal dilation of the large bronchi associated with infection and destruction of the bronchial walls.

CF is an autosomal recessive genetic disorder manifested by chronic lung disease, pancreatic exocrine deficiency, and elevation of sodium chloride in the sweat. The disorder is caused by a mutation of a single gene on the long arm of chromosome 7 that codes for the CFTR, which functions in the transepithelial transport of the chloride ion. The defect causes exocrine gland secretions to become exceedingly viscid, and it promotes colonization of the respiratory tract with *P. aeruginosa* and other organisms such as *Staphylococcus aureus*. Accumulation of viscid mucus in the bronchi, impaired mucociliary function, and infection contribute to the development of chronic lung disease and a decreased life expectancy.

CHRONIC INTERSTITIAL (RESTRICTIVE) LUNG DISEASES

After completing this section of the chapter, the learner will be able to meet the following objectives:

- State the difference between COPDs and interstitial lung diseases (ILDs) in terms of their pathology and manifestations.
- Cite the characteristics of occupational dusts that determine their pathogenicity in terms of the production of pneumoconiosis.
- Describe the pathophysiology of idiopathic pulmonary fibrosis.
- Describe the causes of hypersensitivity pneumonitis.
- Describe the systemic pathophysiology of organ involvement in sarcoidosis.

The diffuse ILDs are a diverse group of lung disorders that produce similar inflammatory and fibrotic changes in the interstitium or interalveolar septa of the lung. Because the ILDs result in a stiff and noncompliant lung, they are commonly classified as restrictive lung disorders. In contrast to obstructive lung diseases, the lungs are stiff and difficult to expand, despite normally functioning airways.

Etiology and Pathogenesis of Interstitial Lung Diseases

The ILDs may be acute or insidious in onset. They may be rapidly progressive, slowly progressive, or static in their course. They include occupational lung diseases such as the pneumoconioses, which are caused by the inhalation of dusts, gases, fumes and asbestos; hypersensitivity pneumonitis; lung diseases caused by exposure to toxic drugs (*e.g.,* methotrexate, bleomycin, phenytoin, amiodarone); and granulomatous disorders such as sarcoidosis (Chart 31.2). Some of the most common ILDs are caused by exposure to inhaled dust and particles and, in others, no specific cause can be found.

In contrast to the obstructive lung diseases, which primarily involve the airways of the lung, the interstitial lung disorders exert their effects on the collagen and elastic connective tissue found in the delicate interstitium of the alveolar walls. Certain ILDs affect the distal part of the alveoli and this causes physiologic restrictions and decreased lung volumes.[45] Other ILDs impact the interstitium closer to the proximal aspect of the acinus near the bronchioles, which causes physiologic obstruction but does not impact the lung volumes.[8] Many of these diseases also involve the airways, arteries, and veins. In general, these lung diseases share a pattern of lung dysfunction that includes diminished lung volumes, reduced diffusing capacity of the lung, and varying degrees of hypoxemia.

It is thought that these disorders are initiated by some type of injury to the alveolar epithelium, followed by an inflammatory process that involves the alveoli and interstitium of the lung. An accumulation of inflammatory and immune cells causes continued damage to lung tissue and replacement of normally functioning lung tissue with fibrous scar tissue.

CHART 31.2 CAUSES OF INTERSTITIAL LUNG DISEASE

Occupational and Environmental Inhalants
Pneumoconioses
- Coal miner's pneumoconiosis
- Silicosis
- Asbestosis

Hypersensitivity pneumonitis
- Farmer's lung
- Pigeon breeder's lung

Drugs and Therapeutic Agents
Cancer drugs
- Bleomycin
- Busulfan
- Cyclophosphamide
- Methotrexate

Amiodarone

Immunologic Lung Disease
Sarcoidosis
Collagen vascular disease
- Systemic lupus erythematosus
- Rheumatoid arthritis
- Scleroderma

*This list is not intended to be inclusive.

Clinical Manifestations

In general, the ILDs are characterized by clinical changes consistent with restrictive rather than obstructive changes in the lung, although some people have both components. People with ILDs have dyspnea, tachypnea, and eventual cyanosis, without evidence of wheezing or signs of airway obstruction. Usually, there is an insidious onset of breathlessness that initially occurs during exercise and may progress to the point at which the person is totally incapacitated. Typically, a person with a restrictive lung disease breathes with a tachypneic pattern of breathing, in which the respiratory rate is increased and the tidal volume is decreased. This pattern of breathing serves to maintain minute volume yet reduces the WOB because it takes less work to move air through the airways at an increased rate than it does to stretch a stiff lung to accommodate a larger tidal volume. A nonproductive cough may develop, particularly with continued exposure to the inhaled irritant, along with clubbing of the fingers and toes.

Lung volumes, including vital capacity and TLC, are reduced in ILD. In contrast to COPD, in which expiratory flow rates are reduced, the $FEV_{1.0}$ usually is preserved, even though the ratio of $FEV_{1.0}$ to FVC may increase. Although resting arterial blood gases usually are normal early in the course of the disease, arterial PO_2 levels may fall during exercise. In persons with advanced disease, hypoxemia often is present, even at rest. In the late stages of the disease, hypercapnia and respiratory acidosis develop. Alterations in the alveolar–capillary membrane, as well as an increase in shunt resulting from unventilated regions of the lung, are thought to cause the impaired diffusion of gases in people with ILD.

Diagnosis and Treatment

The diagnosis of ILD requires a comprehensive personal and family history, with particular emphasis on exposure to environmental, occupational, and other injurious agents. Chest radiographs and other imaging may be used as an initial diagnostic method, and serial chest films often are used to follow the progress of the disease. A surgical lung biopsy specimen for histologic study and culture is the preferred diagnostic examination.[45]

The treatment goals for people with ILD focus on identifying and removing the injurious agent, suppressing the inflammatory response, preventing progression of the disease, and providing supportive therapy for people with advanced disease. In general, the treatment measures vary with the type of lung disease. Immunosuppressants and corticosteroid drugs frequently are used. Many of the supportive treatment measures used in the late stages of the disease, such as oxygen therapy and measures to prevent infection, are similar to those discussed for people with COPD. For some people a lung transplant may be the only potentially effective treatment.

KEY POINTS

INTERSTITIAL LUNG DISEASES

- ILDs result from inflammatory conditions that affect the interalveolar structures of the lung and produce lung fibrosis and a stiff lung.
- A stiff and noncompliant lung is difficult to inflate, increasing the WOB and causing decreased exercise tolerance due to hypoxemia.
- Because of the increased effort needed for lung expansion, people with ILD tend to take small but more frequent breaths.

Occupational and Environmental Interstitial Lung Diseases

The occupational and environmental ILDs include the pneumoconioses, drug-induced ILD, and the hypersensitivity diseases. The *pneumoconioses* are caused by the inhalation of inorganic dusts and particulate matter. The *hypersensitivity diseases* result from the inhalation of organic dusts and related occupational antigens. A third type of occupational lung disease, byssinosis, a disease that affects cotton workers, has characteristics of the pneumoconioses and hypersensitivity lung diseases.

Among the pneumoconioses are silicosis, found in hard-rock miners, foundry workers, sandblasters, pottery makers, and workers in the slate industry; coal miner's pneumoconiosis; asbestosis, found in asbestos miners, manufacturers of asbestos products, and installers and removers of asbestos insulation; talcosis, found in talc miners, millers, or drug abusers and in infants or small children who accidentally inhale powder containing talc; and berylliosis, found in ore extraction workers and alloy production workers. The danger of exposure to asbestos dust is not confined to the workplace. The dust pervades the general environment because it was used in the construction of buildings and in other applications before its health hazards were realized. It has been mixed into paints and plaster, wrapped around water and heating pipes, used to insulate hair dryers, and woven into theater curtains, hot pads, and ironing board covers.

Important etiologic determinants in the development of the pneumoconioses are the size of the dust particle, its chemical nature and ability to incite lung destruction, and the concentration of dust and the length of exposure to it. Particles that are deposited below the larynx are less than 10 μm in size and are divided into three categories bases on their source and size.[46] Coarse particles (2.5 to 10 μm) are elements such as iron, silica, and aluminum. Fine-mode fraction (<2.5 μm) are products of gases, fumes and vapors. Finally, ultrafine particles, also known as nanoparticles (<0.1 μm), make up the largest category of particles.[46]

All particles in the alveoli must be cleared by the lung macrophages. Macrophages are thought to transport engulfed particles from the small bronchioles and the alveoli, which have neither cilia nor mucus-secreting cells, to the mucociliary escalator or to the lymphatic channels for removal from the lung. This clearing function is hampered when the function of the macrophage is impaired by factors such as cigarette smoking, consumption of alcohol, and hypersensitivity reactions. This helps to explain the increased incidence of lung disease among smokers exposed to asbestos. In silicosis, the ingestion of silica particles leads to the destruction of the lung macrophages and the release of substances resulting in inflammation and fibrosis.[46] Tuberculosis and other diseases caused by mycobacteria are common in people with silicosis. Because the macrophages are responsible for protecting the lungs from tuberculosis, the destruction of macrophages accounts for an increased susceptibility to tuberculosis in people with silicosis.

The concentration of some dusts in the environment strongly influences their effects on the lung. For example, acute silicosis is seen only in people whose occupations entail intense exposure to silica dust over a short period. It is seen in sandblasters, who use a high-speed jet of sand to clean and polish bricks and the insides of corroded tanks; in tunnelers; and in rock drillers, particularly if they drill through sandstone. Acute silicosis is a rapidly progressive disease, usually leading to severe disability and death within 5 years of diagnosis. In contrast to acute silicosis, which is caused by exposure to extremely high concentrations of silica dust, the symptoms related to chronic, low-level exposure to silica dust usually do not begin to develop until after many years of exposure, and then the symptoms often are insidious in onset and slow to progress.

Drug-Induced Interstitial Lung Disease

Drugs can cause a variety of both acute and chronic alterations in lung function. For example, some of the cytotoxic drugs (*e.g.,* bleomycin, busulfan, methotrexate, cyclophosphamide) used in treatment of cancer cause pulmonary damage as a result of direct toxicity of the drug and by stimulating the influx of inflammatory cells into the alveoli.[45] Amiodarone, a drug used to treat cardiac arrhythmias, is preferentially sequestered in the lung and can cause significant pneumonitis in individuals receiving more than 400 mg per day.[45]

Hypersensitivity Pneumonitis

The hypersensitivity occupational lung disorders (*e.g.,* hypersensitivity pneumonitis or also termed extrinsic allergic alveolitis) are caused by intense and often prolonged exposure to inhaled organic dusts and related occupational antigens.[46] Those affected have a heightened sensitivity to the antigen. The most common forms of hypersensitivity pneumonitis are farmer's lung, which results from exposure to moldy hay; pigeon breeder's lung, provoked by exposure to the serum, excreta, or feathers of birds; bagassosis, from contaminated sugar cane; and humidifier or air conditioner lung, caused by mold in the water reservoirs of these appliances. Unlike asthma, this type of hypersensitivity reaction involves primarily the alveoli. These disorders cause progressive fibrotic lung disease, which can be prevented by the removal of the environmental agent.

Sarcoidosis

Sarcoidosis is a systemic disorder in which granulomas are found in affected tissues and organ systems, particularly the lung and lymphatic system.[45] An important qualification is that these granulomas occur in the absence of exogenous (infection or environmental) agents known to cause granulomatous inflammation. The disorder predominantly affects people between 10 and 40 years of age, although it can occur in older people. The incidence of sarcoidosis in the United States is approximately 10.9 of 100,000 persons per year for whites and 35.5 of 100,000 persons per year for blacks.[45]

Etiology and Pathogenesis

The characteristic lesion of sarcoidosis is the noncaseating granuloma. Unlike the granulomatous lesions that develop in tuberculosis and histoplasmosis, the collection of tissue macrophages composing the granulomas in sarcoidosis do not show evidence of necrosis or caseation. In addition to granulomas, in which multinuclear giant cells are frequently seen, there is often alveolitis or inflammation of the alveoli.

The cause of sarcoidosis remains obscure. It is thought that the disorder may result from exposure of genetically predisposed persons to specific environmental agents.[45] Support for a genetic influence comes from epidemiologic studies that have demonstrated the higher incidence in American Blacks and Scandinavian populations. Additional evidence comes from familial clustering of the disease. Analysis of human leukocyte antigen (HLA) genes located in the major histocompatibility complex also suggests that unique HLA genes can be linked to disease susceptibility and prognosis. Despite advances, including the identification of sarcoidosis genetic factors, a specific etiologic agent has yet to be identified.

Clinical Manifestations

Sarcoidosis has variable manifestations and an unpredictable course of progression in which any organ system can be affected. Routine chest screenings detect 20% to 30% of pulmonary cases in asymptomatic individuals.[45] The most commonly manifested symptoms occur in the lungs skin, eyes, and neurologic system. People with sarcoidosis frequently seek health care either as a result of abnormalities detected on an incidental chest film or because of insidious onset of respiratory symptoms (shortness of breath, nonproductive cough, chest pain) or constitutional signs and symptoms (*e.g.,* fever, sweating, anorexia, weight loss, fatigue, myalgia).[45] Eye involvement (anterior uveitis) and skin involvement (skin papules and plaques) are particularly common extrathoracic manifestations. However, symptoms of sarcoidosis may affect any organ system and there may be cardiac, neuromuscular, hematologic, hepatic, endocrine, or lymph node findings.[45]

Sarcoidosis follows an unpredictable course characterized by either progressive chronicity or periods of activity interspersed with remissions, sometimes permanent, that may be spontaneous or induced by corticosteroid therapy. The disease is thought to be connected to abnormal immunologic function since there is an increase in ratio of $CD4^+$ and $CD8^+$ lymphocytes and increased proinflammatory cytokines.[45] Although there is low risk of death or disability, the course of the disease varies. Approximately one third of individuals diagnosed with sarcoidosis have the progressive disease.[45]

Diagnosis and Treatment

The diagnosis of sarcoidosis is based on history and physical examination, tests to exclude other diseases, chest radiography, and biopsy to obtain confirmation of noncaseating granulomas. The use of CT scans and magnetic resonance imaging (MRI) as routine methods for diagnosis of sarcoidosis remains controversial. For example, increased angiotensin-converting enzyme (ACE) is commonly seen with sarcoidosis; however, it is not specific so is deemed controversial.[45]

Treatment is directed at interrupting the granulomatous inflammatory process that is characteristic of the disease and managing the associated complications. When treatment is indicated, corticosteroid drugs are used. These agents produce clearing of the lung, as seen on the chest radiograph, and improve pulmonary function, but it is not known whether they affect the long-term outcome of the disease.

IN SUMMARY

The ILDs are characterized by fibrosis and decreased compliance of the lung. They include the occupational and environmental lung diseases and granulomatous disorders, such as sarcoidosis. These disorders are thought to result from an inflammatory process that begins in the alveoli and extends to involve the interstitial tissues of the lung. Unlike COPD, which affects the airways, ILDs affect the supporting collagen and elastic tissues that lie between the airways and blood vessels. These lung diseases generally decrease lung volumes, reduce the diffusing capacity of the lung, and cause various degrees of hypoxemia. Because lung compliance is reduced, people with this form of lung disease tend to maintain their minute volume by a rapid, shallow breathing pattern.

DISORDERS OF THE PULMONARY CIRCULATION

After completing this section of the chapter, the learner will be able to meet the following objectives:

- Describe the cause of pulmonary embolism and the clinical manifestations of the disorder.
- Describe the pathophysiology of pulmonary hypertensive disorders.
- Describe the rationale for right ventricular hypertrophy with cor pulmonale.

As blood moves through the pulmonary capillaries, oxygen content increases and carbon dioxide decreases. These processes depend on the matching of ventilation (*i.e.*, gas exchange) and perfusion (*i.e.*, blood flow). This section discusses two major problems of the pulmonary circulation: pulmonary embolism and pulmonary hypertension.

KEY POINTS

DISORDERS OF THE PULMONARY CIRCULATION

- Pulmonary thromboemboli are blood clots that originate in the systemic venous system and become lodged in a pulmonary blood vessel as they move from the right heart into and through the pulmonary circulation.
- Pulmonary hypertension is an elevated pulmonary arterial pressure. It may arise as a primary disorder of the pulmonary arteries in which an abnormal thickening of the vessel wall increases the resistance to blood flow, or as a secondary disorder due to chronic lung disorders or environmental conditions that produce hypoxemia and a resultant constriction of small pulmonary arteries, cardiac disorders that increase pulmonary venous pressure, or thromboembolic disorders that occlude pulmonary blood vessels.

Pulmonary Embolism

Pulmonary embolism develops when a blood-borne substance lodges in a branch of the pulmonary artery and obstructs blood flow. The embolism may consist of a thrombus (Fig. 31.15), air that has accidentally been injected during intravenous infusion, fat that has been mobilized from the bone marrow after a fracture or from a traumatized fat depot, or amniotic fluid that has entered the maternal circulation after rupture of the membranes at the time of delivery. When a pulmonary embolism occurs during the setting of a malignancy, the fatality rate is 25%.[45]

Etiology and Pathogenesis

Pulmonary emboli are thrombi that generally occur from deep vein thrombosis (DVT) in the lower and upper extremities.[45] The presence of thrombosis in the deep veins of the legs or pelvis often is unsuspected until embolism occurs. The effects of emboli on the pulmonary circulation are related to mechanical obstruction of the pulmonary circulation and neurohumoral reflexes causing vasoconstriction. Obstruction of pulmonary blood flow causes reflex bronchoconstriction in the affected area of the lung, wasted ventilation and impaired gas exchange, and loss of alveolar surfactant. Pulmonary hypertension and right heart failure may develop when there is massive vasoconstriction because of a large embolus. Although small areas of infarction may occur, frank pulmonary infarction is uncommon.

Among the physiologic factors that contribute to venous thrombosis is Virchow's triad, which consists of venous stasis, venous endothelial injury, and hypercoagulability states. The thrombophilias (*e.g.*, antithrombin III deficiency, protein C and S deficiencies, factor V Leiden mutation) are a group of inherited disorders affecting coagulation that make

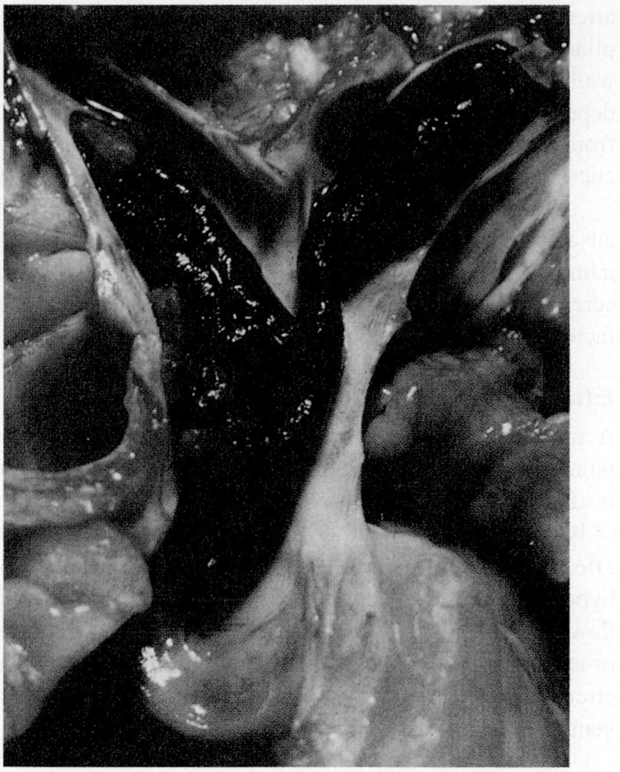

Figure 31.15 • Pulmonary embolism. The main pulmonary artery and its bifurcation have been opened to reveal a large saddle embolus. (From Strayer D., Rubin R. (Eds.) (2015). *Rubin's pathology: Clinicopathologic foundations of medicine* (7th ed., Fig. 7-16, p. 308). Philadelphia, PA: Lippincott Williams & Wilkins.)

an individual prone to development of venous thromboemboli.[45] Venous stasis and venous endothelial injury can result from prolonged bed rest, trauma, surgery, childbirth, fractures of the hip and femur, myocardial infarction and congestive heart failure, and spinal cord injury. People undergoing orthopedic surgery and gynecologic cancer surgery are at particular risk, as are immobilized persons. Hypercoagulability is related to various factors. Cancer cells can produce thrombin and synthesize procoagulation factors, increasing the risk for thromboembolism. Use of oral contraceptives, pregnancy, and hormone replacement therapy are thought to increase the resistance to endogenous anticoagulants.

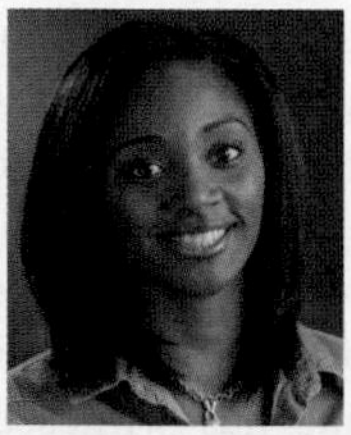

Refer back to Ms. French in discussion about pulmonary embolism etiology. Ms. French, who was introduced at the beginning of the unit, presented to the emergency department with soreness in her right calf. This was because the embolus originated in the saphenous vein of her right leg and then broke free and traveled to the pulmonary circulation. Ms. French's history of cigarette smoking and use of estrogen-based oral contraceptives increased her risk for thrombus development, because these agents cause vasoconstriction and inflammation.

Clinical Manifestations

The manifestations of pulmonary embolism depend on the size and location of the obstruction. Chest pain, dyspnea, and increased respiratory rate are the most frequent signs and symptoms of pulmonary embolism. Pulmonary infarction often causes pleuritic pain that changes with respiration; it is more severe on inspiration and less severe on expiration. Moderate hypoxemia without carbon dioxide retention occurs as a result of impaired gas exchange. Small emboli that become lodged in the peripheral branches of the pulmonary artery may go unrecognized unless the person is compromised, such as occurs in the elderly or acutely ill. Repeated small emboli gradually reduce the size of the pulmonary capillary bed, resulting in pulmonary hypertension. People with moderate-sized emboli often present with breathlessness accompanied by pleuritic pain, apprehension, slight fever, and cough productive of blood-streaked sputum. Tachycardia often occurs to compensate for decreased oxygenation, and the breathing pattern is rapid and shallow. People with massive emboli usually present with sudden collapse, crushing substernal chest pain, shock, and sometimes loss of consciousness. The pulse is rapid and weak, the blood pressure is low, the neck veins are distended, and the skin is cyanotic and diaphoretic. Massive pulmonary emboli often are fatal.

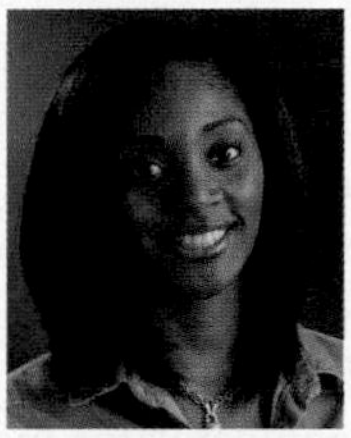

Refer back to Ms. French in discussion about pulmonary embolism clinical features. On presentation, Ms. French's heart rate was elevated (132 beats/minute) and the electrocardiogram (ECG) showed sinus tachycardia. Her breathing was rapid and shallow. In a person with pulmonary embolism, tachycardia and tachypnea often occur to compensate for decreased oxygenation.

Diagnosis

The diagnosis of pulmonary embolism is based on clinical signs and symptoms, blood gas determinations, venous thrombosis studies, troponin, D-dimer testing, lung scans, and helical CT scans of the chest. Laboratory studies and radiologic films are useful in ruling out other conditions that might give rise to similar symptoms. Because emboli can cause an increase in pulmonary vascular resistance, the ECG may be used to detect signs of right heart strain.

Because most pulmonary emboli originate from DVT, venous studies such as *lower limb compression ultrasonography*, *impedance plethysmography,* and *contrast venography* are often used as initial diagnostic procedures. Of these, lower limb compression ultrasonography has become an important noninvasive means for detecting DVT. *D-dimer testing* involves the measurement of plasma D-dimer, a degradation product of coagulation factors that have been activated as the result of a thromboembolic event. Troponin levels may be increased due to stretching of the right ventricle by a large pulmonary infarction. The *ventilation–perfusion scan* uses radiolabeled albumin, which is injected intravenously, and a radiolabeled gas, which is inhaled. A scintillation (gamma) camera is used to scan the various lung segments for blood flow and distribution of the radiolabeled gas. Ventilation–perfusion scans are useful only when their results are either normal or indicate a high probability of pulmonary embolism. *Helical (spiral) CT angiography* requires administration of an intravenous radiocontrast medium. It is sensitive for the detection of emboli in the proximal pulmonary arteries and provides another method of diagnosis. *Pulmonary angiography* involves the passage of a venous catheter through the right heart and into the pulmonary artery under fluoroscopy. Although it remains the most accurate method of diagnosis, it is infrequently done since it is such an invasive procedure. An embolectomy sometimes is performed during this procedure.

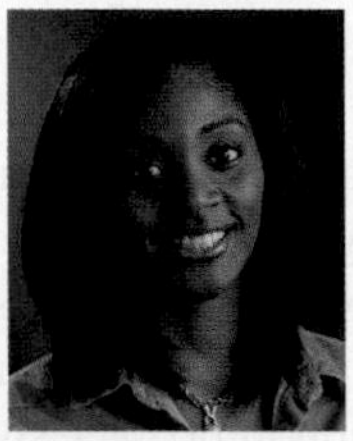

Refer back to Ms. French in discussion about pulmonary embolism diagnostics. D-dimer testing involves the measurement of plasma D-dimer, a degradation product of coagulation factors that have been activated as the result of a thromboembolic event. Recall that Ms. French's D-dimer levels were elevated.

Treatment

The treatment goals for pulmonary emboli focus on preventing DVT and the development of thromboemboli; protecting the lungs from exposure to thromboemboli when they occur; and, in the case of large and life-threatening pulmonary emboli, sustaining life and restoring pulmonary blood flow. Thrombolytic therapy using recombinant tissue plasminogen activator may be indicated in people with multiple or large emboli.

Prevention focuses on identifying people at risk, avoidance of venous stasis and hypercoagulability states, and early detection of venous thrombosis. It is important that people start to become mobile as soon as possible after surgery or illness. For people at risk, graded compression elastic stockings and intermittent pneumatic compression (IPC) boots can be used to prevent venous stasis. Surgical interruption of the vena cava may be indicated when pulmonary embolism poses a life-threatening risk.

Pharmacologic prophylaxis involves the use of anticoagulant drugs. Anticoagulant therapy may be used to decrease the likelihood of DVT, thromboembolism, and fatal pulmonary embolism after major surgical procedures. Low molecular weight heparin, which can be administered subcutaneously on an outpatient basis, often is used. Warfarin, an oral anticoagulation drug, may be used for people with a long-term risk for development of thromboemboli.

Pulmonary Hypertension

The pulmonary circulation is a low-pressure system designed to accommodate varying amounts of blood delivered from the right heart and to facilitate gas exchange. The main pulmonary artery and major branches are relatively thin-walled, compliant vessels. The distal pulmonary arterioles also are thin walled and have the capacity to dilate, collapse, or constrict depending on the presence of vasoactive substances released from the endothelial cells of the vessel, neurohumoral influences, flow velocity, oxygen tension, and alveolar ventilation.

Pulmonary hypertension is a disorder characterized by an elevation of pressure within the pulmonary circulation, namely, the pulmonary arterial system. The elevation in pressure may be acute or chronic, depending on the causative factors.

Etiology and Pathogenesis

A number of factors can contribute to the pathogenesis of pulmonary arterial hypertension (PAH), including a decrease in the cross-sectional area of the pulmonary arteries, a loss of blood vessels from either scarring or destructive processes affecting the alveolar walls, vasoconstriction in response to hypoxia, the need to accommodate excessive inflow of blood flow without any anatomic changes in the pulmonary arteries or arterioles, or the occlusion of outflow from the pulmonary circulation due to elevated pressures within the left atrium or ventricle.

The disorder may be due to changes in the arterial wall, often referred to as *pulmonary arterial hypertension*, or it may occur as a secondary condition related to the occlusion of the pulmonary circulation by pulmonary emboli or to disruption of the pulmonary circulation due to heart or lung disease.

Pulmonary Arterial Hypertension

The term *pulmonary arterial hypertension* (PAH) is used to describe a type of pulmonary hypertension that has its origin in the pulmonary arteries. The World Health Organization categorizes PAH into five groups related to their disease mechanism.[47]

- Group I is pulmonary arterial or idiopathic hypertension.
- Group II is pulmonary venous hypertension.
- Group III is pulmonary hypertension associated with hypoxemia.
- Group IV is pulmonary hypertension due to chronic thrombotic or embolic disease or both.
- Group V comprises miscellaneous disorders that cause PAH.[47]

PAH is a rare and debilitating disorder characterized by abnormal proliferation and contraction of vascular smooth muscle, coagulation abnormalities, and marked intimal fibrosis leading to obliteration or obstruction of the pulmonary arteries and arterioles (Fig. 31.16). The resulting increase in pressure results in progressive right heart failure, low cardiac output, and death if left untreated. The past decade has witnessed dramatic advances in the treatment of PAH, with medical therapies targeting specific pathways that are believed to play pathogenetic roles in development of the disorder. Despite these achievements, PAH remains a serious, life-threatening condition.

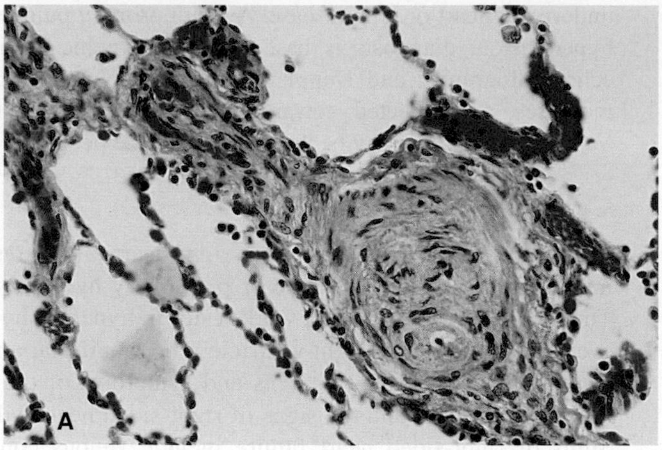

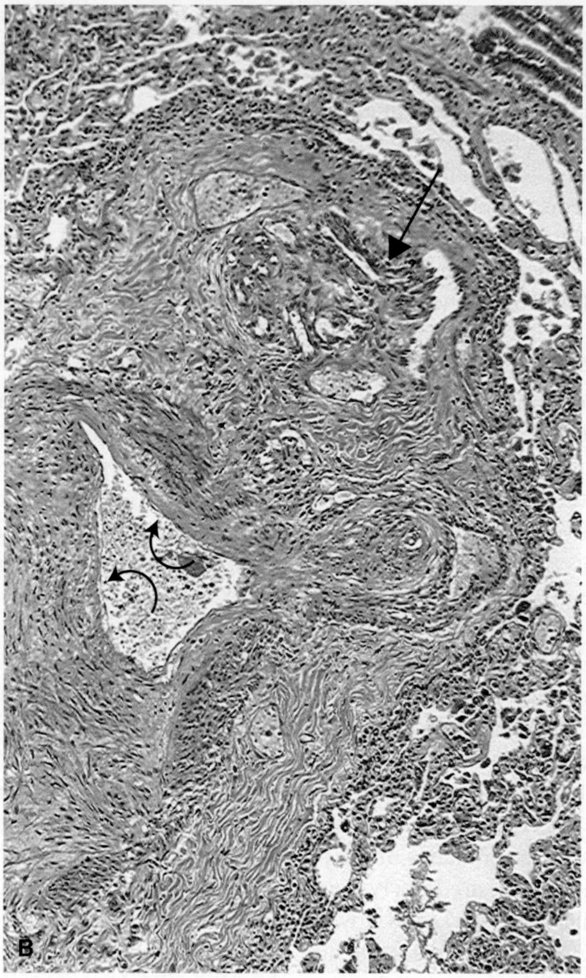

Figure 31.16 • Pulmonary artery hypertension. **(A)** A small pulmonary artery occluded by concentric intimal fibrosis and thickening of the media. **(B)** A plexiform lesion (*arrow*) is characterized by a glomeruloid proliferation of thin-walled vessels adjacent to a parent artery, which shows marked hypertensive changes of intimal fibrosis and medial thickening (*curved arrows*). (From Strayer D., Rubin R. (Eds.) (2015). *Rubin's pathology: Clinicopathologic foundations of medicine* (7th ed., Fig. 18-76, p. 733). Philadelphia, PA: Lippincott Williams & Wilkins.)

Etiology and Pathogenesis. The familial form of PAH appears to be inherited as an autosomal dominant trait with a variable but low penetrance, with some people inheriting the trait without exhibiting the disease. The bone morphogenetic protein receptor type II gene (*BMPR2*), which codes for a member of the transforming growth factor-β (TGF-β) superfamily of receptors, was identified as causative of familial PAH. Mutations in these receptors are thought to prevent TGF-β and related molecules from exerting an inhibitory effect on smooth muscle and endothelial cell proliferation.[48] Other conditions associated with PAH include collagen vascular disorders (*e.g.,* scleroderma), drugs and toxins, human immunodeficiency virus (HIV) infection, portal hypertension, and persistent pulmonary hypertension in the newborn.[47]

Although the specific mechanisms responsible for the vascular changes that occur in PAH remain unknown, a number of mechanisms have been proposed. These include enhanced expression of the serotonin transporter, diminished levels of nitric oxide and prostacyclin, and increased levels of several growth factors, including endothelin, vascular endothelial growth factor, and platelet-derived growth factor. The endothelium-relaxing factor, nitric oxide, is a potent pulmonary vasodilator that is produced locally in the lung and has profound effects on smooth muscle relaxation and proliferation. Endothelin 1 is a peptide produced by the vascular endothelium that has potent vasoconstrictor and paracrine effects on vascular smooth muscle. The endothelium also produces prostacyclin (PGI2), an inhibitor of platelet aggregation and potent vasodilator. Results of studies relating these mechanisms to the structure and function of the pulmonary arterial circulation have already been translated into targeted therapies for PAH, with the probability that more will be investigated in the future.

Clinical Manifestations. PAH is defined by persistent elevation in pulmonary artery pressure with normal left ventricular pressures, differentiating it from left-sided heart failure. Symptoms typically progress from shortness of breath and decreasing exercise tolerance to right heart failure, with marked peripheral edema and functional limitations. Other common symptoms include fatigue, angina, and syncope (fainting) or near-syncope.

Diagnosis and Treatment. The diagnosis of primary pulmonary hypertension is based on an absence of disorders that cause secondary hypertension and mean pulmonary artery pressures greater than 25 mm Hg at rest or 30 mm Hg with exercise.

Treatment consists of measures to improve right heart function as a means of reducing fatigue and peripheral edema. Supplemental oxygen may be used to increase exercise tolerance. This agent often improves symptoms, sometimes dramatically, in people who have not responded to other vasodilators. Sildenafil (*e.g.,* Viagra) a highly selective phosphodiesterase-5 inhibitor, which acts in a manner similar to nitric oxide to produce vasodilation, is another treatment of pulmonary hypertension.[47] Lung transplantation may be an alternative for people who do not respond to other forms of treatment.

Secondary Pulmonary Hypertension

Although pulmonary hypertension can develop as a primary disorder, most cases develop secondary to conditions such as chronic hypoxemia due to COPD, ILD, or sleep-disordered breathing; increased resistance to pulmonary venous drainage due to conditions such as diastolic dysfunction of the left heart or disorders of mitral or aortic valves; or chronic thromboembolic disorders.

Etiology and Pathogenesis. Continued exposure of the pulmonary vessels to hypoxemia is a common cause of pulmonary hypertension. Unlike blood vessels in the systemic circulation, most of which dilate in response to hypoxemia and hypercapnia, the pulmonary vessels constrict. The stimulus for constriction seems to originate in the airspaces near the smaller branches of the pulmonary arteries. In regions of the lung that are poorly ventilated, the response is adaptive in that it diverts blood flow away from the poorly ventilated areas to those areas that are more adequately ventilated. This effect, however, becomes less beneficial as more and more areas of the lung become poorly ventilated. Pulmonary hypertension is a common problem in people with advanced COPD or ILD. It also may develop at high altitudes in people with normal lungs. People who experience marked hypoxemia during sleep (such as those with sleep apnea) often experience marked elevations in pulmonary arterial pressure.

Elevation of pulmonary venous pressure is common in conditions such as mitral valve disorders or left ventricular diastolic dysfunction. In each of these alterations, the elevated left atrial pressure is transmitted to the pulmonary circulation. Continued increases in left atrial pressure can lead to medial hypertrophy and intimal thickening of the small pulmonary arteries, causing sustained hypertension. Another cause of secondary pulmonary hypertension is obstruction of pulmonary blood flow due to pulmonary thromboemboli. People who are promptly treated for acute pulmonary thromboembolism with anticoagulants rarely develop pulmonary hypertension. However, in some people chronic obstruction of the pulmonary vascular bed develops because of impaired resolution of the thromboemboli.

Clinical Manifestations, Diagnosis, and Treatment. The signs and symptoms of secondary pulmonary hypertension reflect both the elevated pulmonary arterial pressure and the underlying heart or lung disease. As with primary pulmonary hypertension, diagnosis is based on radiographic findings, echocardiography, and Doppler ultrasonography. Treatment measures are directed toward the underlying disorder. Vasodilator therapy may be indicated for some people.

Cor Pulmonale

The term *cor pulmonale* refers to right heart failure resulting from primary lung disease or pulmonary hypertension. The increased pressures and work result in hypertrophy and eventual failure of the right ventricle. The manifestations of cor pulmonale include the signs and symptoms of the primary lung disease and the signs of right-sided heart failure. Signs of right-sided heart failure include venous congestion, peripheral edema, shortness of breath, and a productive cough, which becomes worse during periods of heart failure. Plethora (*i.e.,* redness), cyanosis, and warm, moist skin may result from the compensatory polycythemia and desaturation of arterial blood that accompany chronic lung disease. Drowsiness and altered consciousness may occur as the result of carbon dioxide retention. Management of cor pulmonale focuses on the treatment of the lung disease and heart failure (Fig. 31.17). Low-flow oxygen therapy may be used to reduce the pulmonary hypertension and polycythemia associated with severe hypoxemia caused by chronic lung disease.

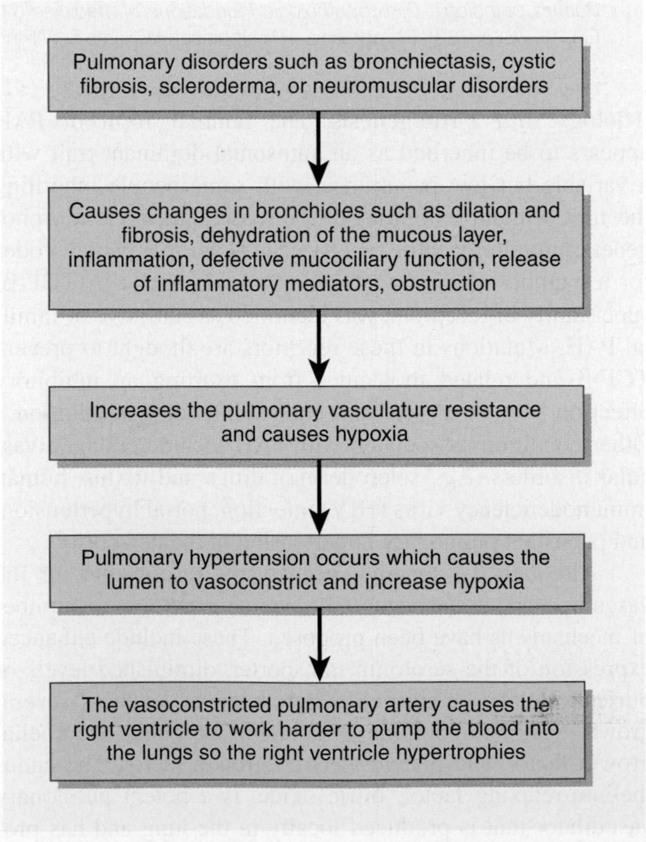

Figure 31.17 • Pathogenesis of cor pulmonale.

IN SUMMARY

Pulmonary vascular disorders include pulmonary embolism and pulmonary hypertension. Pulmonary embolism develops when a blood-borne substance lodges in a branch of the pulmonary artery and obstructs blood flow. The embolus can consist of a thrombus, air, fat, or amniotic fluid. The most common form is thromboemboli arising from the Differentiate between the causes and manifestations of hypoxemic and hypercapnic/hypoxemic respiratory failure. deep venous channels of the lower extremities. Pulmonary hypertension is the elevation of pulmonary arterial pressure. It has been categorized into five groups. *Cor pulmonale* describes right heart failure caused by primary pulmonary disease and long-standing pulmonary hypertension.

ACUTE RESPIRATORY DISORDERS

After completing this section of the chapter, the learner will be able to meet the following objectives:

- Describe the pathologic lung changes that occur in ARDS.
- Describe the clinical manifestations of acute respiratory failure.
- Describe the treatment of respiratory failure.

The function of the respiratory system is to add oxygen to the blood and remove carbon dioxide. Disruptions in this function occur with ALI/respiratory distress syndrome and acute respiratory failure. Although the mechanisms that disrupt gas exchange may vary, both conditions represent a life-threatening situation with high risks of morbidity and mortality.

Acute Lung Injury/Acute Respiratory Distress Syndrome

ARDS is the most severe form of ALI. The symptoms generally manifest with symptoms of diffuse crackles, dyspnea, cyanosis, tachypnea, tachycardia and diaphoresis. The severity of lung dysfunction is evaluated by the PaO_2/FiO_2 ratio.[49] ARDS is a more severe aspect of ALI and is differentiated primarily for early intervention, prevention, and research purposes.

ARDS may result from a number of conditions, including aspiration of gastric contents, major trauma (with or without fat emboli), sepsis secondary to pulmonary or nonpulmonary infections, acute pancreatitis, hematologic disorders, metabolic events, and reactions to drugs and toxins (Chart 31.3).

CHART 31.3 CONDITIONS IN WHICH ARDS CAN DEVELOP*

Aspiration
Near drowning
Aspiration gastric contents

Drugs, Toxins, and Therapeutic Agents
Free-base cocaine smoking
Heroin
Inhaled gases (*e.g.*, smoke, ammonia)
Breathing high concentrations of oxygen
Radiation

Infections
Septicemia

Trauma and Shock
Burns
Fat embolism
Chest trauma

Disseminated Intravascular Coagulation

Multiple Blood Transfusions

*This list is not intended to be inclusive.

Etiology and Pathogenesis

Although a number of conditions may lead to ALI/ARDS, they all produce similar pathologic lung changes that include diffuse epithelial cell injury with increased permeability of the alveolar–capillary membrane (Fig. 31.18). The increased permeability permits fluid, plasma proteins, and blood cells to move out of the vascular compartment into the interstitium and alveoli of the lung.[49] Diffuse alveolar cell damage leads to accumulation of fluid, surfactant inactivation, and formation of a hyaline membrane that is impervious to gas exchange. As the disease progresses, the WOB becomes greatly increased as the lung stiffens and becomes more difficult to inflate. There is increased intrapulmonary shunting of blood, impaired gas exchange, and refractory hypoxemia despite high supplemental oxygen therapy. Gas exchange is further compromised by alveolar collapse resulting from abnormalities in surfactant production. When injury to the alveolar epithelium is severe, disorganized epithelial repair may lead to fibrosis (Fig. 31.19).

The pathogenesis of ALI/ARDS is unclear, although both local and systemic inflammatory responses occur so often when a person has been diagnosed with ARDS they already have leaky capillary syndrome in other organs such as the pancreas. Neutrophils accumulate early in the course of the disorder and are considered to play a role in the pathogenesis of ALI/ARDS. Activated neutrophils synthesize and release a variety of products, including proteolytic enzymes, toxic oxygen species, and phospholipid products that increase the inflammatory response and cause further injury to the capillary endothelium and alveolar epithelium.

Clinical Manifestations and Diagnosis

Clinically, ALI/ARDS is marked by a rapid onset of respiratory distress, usually within 12 to 18 hours of the initiating event, an increase in respiratory rate, and signs of respiratory

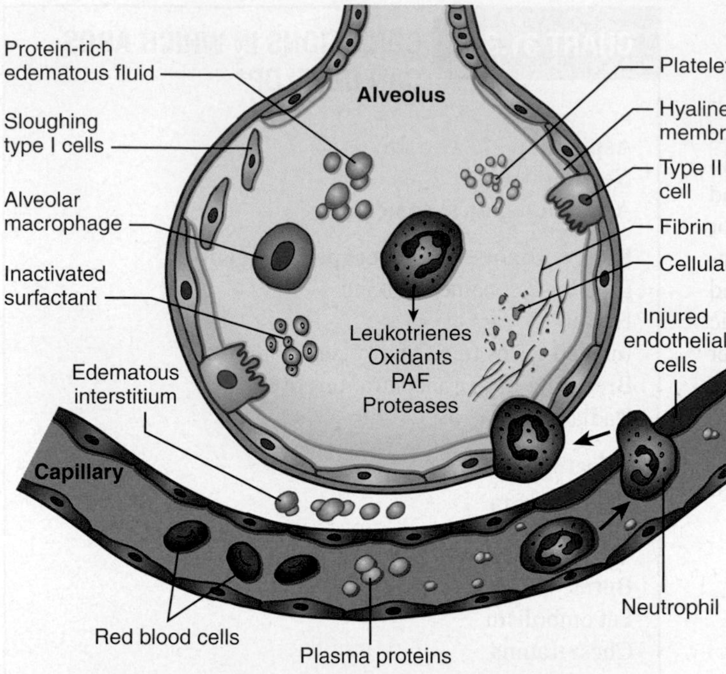

Figure 31.18 • The mechanism of lung changes in ARDS. Injury and increased permeability of the alveolar capillary membrane allow fluid, protein, cellular debris, platelets, and blood cells to move out of the vascular compartment and enter the interstitium and alveoli. Activated neutrophils release a variety of products that damage the alveolar cells and lead to edema, surfactant inactivation, and formation of a hyaline membrane. PAF, platelet-activating factor.

failure. Marked hypoxemia occurs that is refractory to treatment with supplemental oxygen therapy, which results in a decrease in the PF ratio. Many people with ARDS have a systemic response that results in multiple organ failure, particularly of the renal, gastrointestinal, cardiovascular, and CNSs. Chest radiography shows diffuse bilateral infiltrates of the lung tissue in the absence of cardiac dysfunction.

Treatment

The treatment goals in ARDS are to (1) adequately oxygenate the lungs and vital organs, (2) recognize and treat underlying medical and surgical disorders, (3) prevent further lung injury and complications, including but not limited to venous thromboembolism, aspiration, nosocomial infections, and (4) ultimately decrease mortality.[50] Assisted ventilation using high concentrations of oxygen may be required to correct the hypoxemia. Extensive study has been conducted to determine optimal pressures and volumes to correct the hypoxemia yet prevent further lung injury due to the barotrauma often seen with mechanics of ventilation.[50]

Acute Respiratory Failure

Respiratory failure can be viewed as a failure in gas exchange due to either heart or lung failure, or both. It is not a specific disease but can occur in the course of a number of conditions that impair ventilation, compromise the matching of ventilation and perfusion, or impair gas diffusion. Acute respiratory failure may occur in previously healthy people as the result of acute disease or trauma involving the respiratory system, or it may develop in the course of a chronic neuromuscular or lung disease.

Respiratory failure is a condition in which the respiratory system fails in one or both of its gas exchange functions—oxygenation of mixed venous blood and elimination of carbon dioxide. The function of the respiratory system can be said to consist of two aspects: gas exchange (movement of gases across the alveolar–capillary membrane) and ventilation (movement of gases into and out of the alveoli due to the action of the respiratory muscles, respiratory center in the CNS, and the pathways that connect the centers in the CNS with the respiratory muscles). Thus, respiratory failure is commonly divided into two types:

1. Hypoxemic respiratory failure due to failure of the gas exchange function of the lung
2. Hypercapnic/hypoxemic respiratory failure due to ventilatory failure[49]

The classification should not be viewed as rigid since lung disorders that cause impaired gas exchange can be complicated by ventilatory failure. In addition, ventilatory failure can be accompanied by lung disorders that impair gas diffusion. Causes of respiratory failure are summarized in Chart 31.4.

Hypoxemic Respiratory Failure

In people with hypoxemic respiratory failure, two major pathophysiologic factors contribute to the lowering of arterial PO_2—ventilation–perfusion mismatching or impaired diffusion.

Mismatching of Ventilation and Perfusion. The mismatching of ventilation and perfusion occurs when areas of the lung are ventilated but not perfused or when areas are perfused but not ventilated. Usually the hypoxemia seen in situations of ventilation–perfusion mismatching is more severe in relation to hypercapnia than that seen in hypoventilation. Severe mismatching of ventilation and perfusion

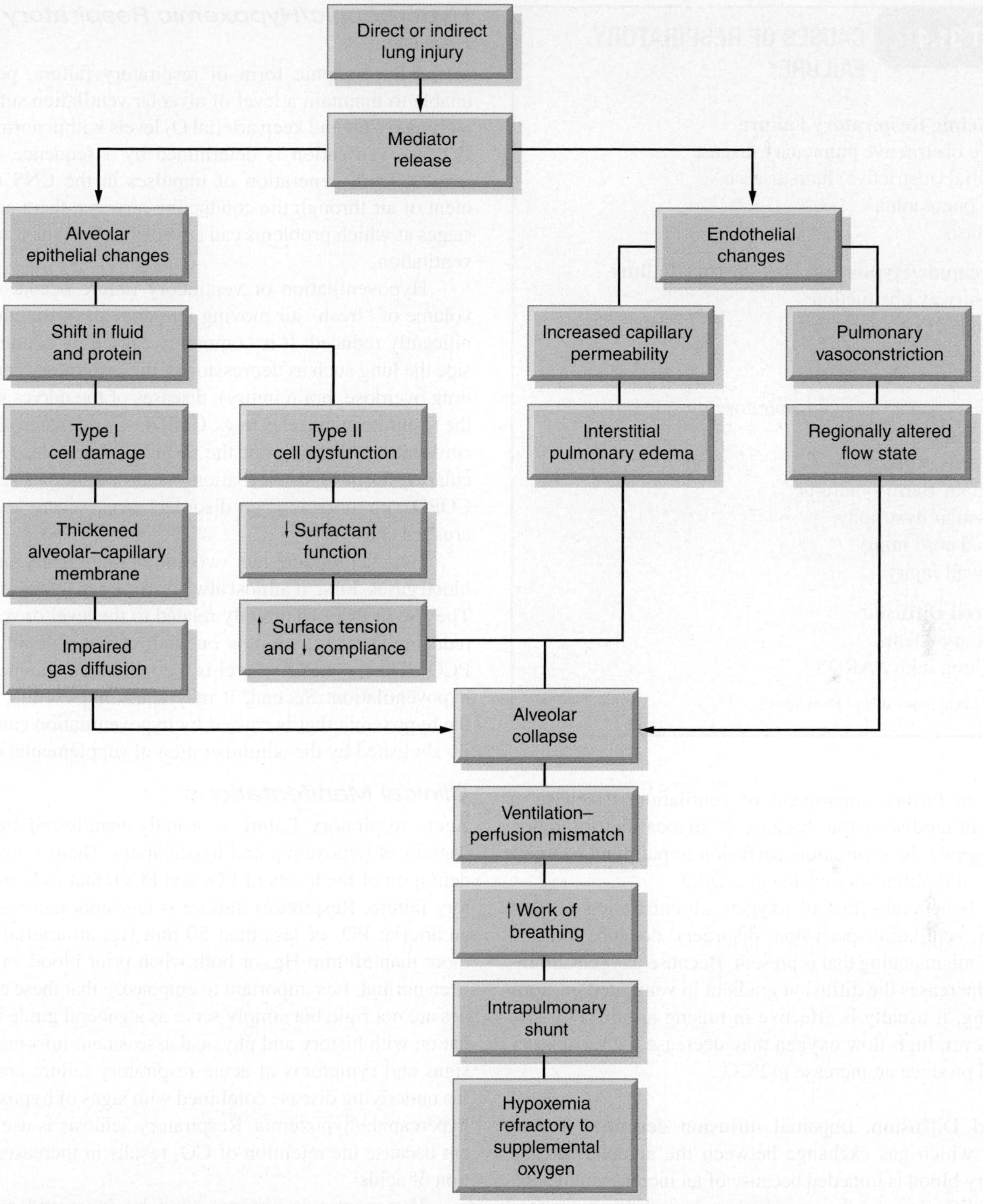

Figure 31.19 • Pathophysiologic cascade is initiated by an injury resulting in mediator release. The multiple effects result in changes to the alveoli, vascular tissue, and bronchi. The ultimate effect is ventilation–perfusion mismatching and refractory hypoxemia. (From Morton P. G., Fontaine D. K. (2018). *Critical care nursing: A holistic approach* (11th ed., Fig. 27-2, p. 522). Philadelphia, PA: Lippincott Williams & Wilkins.)

often is seen in people with advanced COPD. These disorders contribute to the retention of carbon dioxide by reducing the effective alveolar ventilation, even when total ventilation is maintained. This occurs because a region of the lung is not perfused and gas exchange cannot take place or because an area of the lung is not being ventilated. Maintaining a high ventilation rate effectively prevents hypercapnia but also increases the WOB.

The hypoxemia associated with ventilation–perfusion disorders often is exaggerated by conditions such as hypoventilation and decreased cardiac output. For example, sedation can cause hypoventilation in people with severe COPD,

CHART 31.4 CAUSES OF RESPIRATORY FAILURE*

Hypoxemic Respiratory Failure
Chronic obstructive pulmonary disease
Interstitial (restrictive) lung disease
Severe pneumonia
Atelectasis

Hypercapnic/Hypoxemic Respiratory Failure
Upper airway obstruction
- Infection (*e.g.*, epiglottitis)
- Laryngospasm
- Tumors

Weakness or paralysis of respiratory muscles
- Brain injury
- Drug overdose
- Guillain-Barré syndrome
- Muscular dystrophy
- Spinal cord injury

Chest wall injury

Impaired Diffusion
Pulmonary edema
Acute lung injury/ARDS

*This list is not intended to be inclusive.

resulting in further impairment of ventilation. Likewise, a decrease in cardiac output because of myocardial infarction can exaggerate the ventilation–perfusion impairment in a person with mild pulmonary edema or COPD.

The beneficial effect of oxygen administration on PO_2 levels in ventilation–perfusion disorders depends on the degree of mismatching that is present. Because oxygen administration increases the diffusion gradient in ventilated portions of the lung, it usually is effective in raising arterial PO_2 levels. However, high-flow oxygen may decrease the respiratory drive and produce an increase in PCO_2.

Impaired Diffusion. Impaired diffusion describes a condition in which gas exchange between the alveolar air and pulmonary blood is impeded because of an increase in the distance for diffusion or a decrease in the permeability or surface area of the respiratory membranes to the movement of gases. It most commonly occurs in conditions such as ILD, ALI/ARDS, pulmonary edema, and pneumonia.

Conditions that impair diffusion may produce severe hypoxemia but no hypercapnia because of the increase in ventilation and greater diffusion rate of carbon dioxide. Hypoxemia resulting from impaired diffusion can be partially or completely corrected by the administration of high concentrations of oxygen. In this case, the high concentration of oxygen serves to overcome the decrease in diffusion by establishing a larger alveolar-to-capillary diffusion gradient.

Hypercapnic/Hypoxemic Respiratory Failure

In the hypercapnic form of respiratory failure, people are unable to maintain a level of alveolar ventilation sufficient to eliminate CO_2 and keep arterial O_2 levels within normal range. Because ventilation is determined by a sequence of events ranging from generation of impulses in the CNS to movement of air through the conducting airways, there are several stages at which problems can adversely affect the total minute ventilation.

Hypoventilation or ventilatory failure occurs when the volume of "fresh" air moving into and out of the lung is significantly reduced. It is commonly caused by conditions outside the lung such as depression of the respiratory center (*e.g.*, drug overdose, brain injury), diseases of the nerves supplying the respiratory muscles (*e.g.*, Guillain-Barré syndrome, spinal cord injury), disorders of the respiratory muscles (*e.g.*, muscular dystrophy), exacerbation of chronic lung disease (*e.g.*, COPD), or thoracic cage disorders (*e.g.*, severe scoliosis or crushed chest).

Hypoventilation has two important effects on arterial blood gases. First, it almost always causes an increase in PCO_2. The rise in PCO_2 is directly related to the level of ventilation; reducing the ventilation by one half causes a doubling of the PCO_2. Thus, the PCO_2 level is a good diagnostic measure for hypoventilation. Second, it may cause hypoxemia, although the hypoxemia that is caused by hypoventilation can be readily abolished by the administration of supplemental oxygen.

Clinical Manifestations

Acute respiratory failure is usually manifested by varying degrees of hypoxemia and hypercapnia. There is no absolute definition of the levels of PO_2 and PCO_2 that indicate respiratory failure. Respiratory failure is conventionally defined by an arterial PO_2 of less than 50 mm Hg, an arterial PCO_2 of more than 50 mm Hg, or both when prior blood values have been normal. It is important to emphasize that these cutoff values are not rigid but simply serve as a general guide in combination with history and physical assessment information. The signs and symptoms of acute respiratory failure are those of the underlying disease combined with signs of hypoxemia and hypercapnia/hypoxemia. Respiratory acidosis is usually present because the retention of CO_2 results in increased production of acids.

Hypoxemia is accompanied by increased respiratory drive and increased sympathetic tone. Potential signs of hypoxemia include cyanosis, restlessness, confusion, anxiety, delirium, fatigue, tachypnea, hypertension, cardiac arrhythmias, and tremor. The initial cardiovascular effects are tachycardia with increased cardiac output and increased blood pressure. Serious arrhythmias may be triggered. The pulmonary vasculature constricts in response to low alveolar PO_2. If severe, the pulmonary vasoconstriction may result in acute right ventricular failure with manifestations such as jugular vein distention and dependent edema. Profound acute hypoxemia can cause convulsions, retinal hemorrhages, and permanent brain damage. Hypotension and bradycardia often are preterminal events in people with hypoxemic respiratory failure, indicating the failure of compensatory mechanisms.

Many of the adverse consequences of hypercapnia are the result of respiratory acidosis. Direct effects of acidosis include depression of cardiac contractility, decreased respiratory muscle contractility, and arterial vasodilation. Raised levels of PCO_2 greatly increase cerebral blood flow, which may result in headache, increased cerebrospinal fluid pressure, and sometimes papilledema. The headache is due to dilation of the cerebral vessels. Additional indicators of hypercapnia are warm and flushed skin and hyperemic conjunctivae. Hypercapnia has nervous system effects similar to those of an anesthetic—hence the term *carbon dioxide narcosis*. There is progressive somnolence, disorientation, and, if the condition is untreated, coma. Mild to moderate increases in blood pressure are common. Air hunger and rapid breathing occur when alveolar PCO_2 levels rise to approximately 60 to 75 mm Hg; as PCO_2 levels reach 80 to 100 mm Hg, the person becomes lethargic and sometimes semicomatose.

Treatment

The treatment of the person with acute respiratory failure consists of specific therapy directed toward the underlying disease, respiratory supportive care directed toward maintenance of adequate gas exchange, and general supportive care. A number of treatment modalities are available, including the establishment of an airway and the use of anti-inflammatory bronchodilators, mucolytics, and antibiotics for respiratory infections. The main therapeutic goal in acute hypoxemic respiratory failure is to ensure adequate oxygenation of vital organs, which is generally accomplished by mechanical ventilation.

IN SUMMARY

The hallmark of ALI and ARDS is a pronounced inflammatory response that affects the lung and may or may have already resulted in systemic organ failure. In fact, the damage to the lung in ARDS may not be the initial manifestation but part of a multiorgan shutdown due to leaky capillary syndrome. The acute inflammatory response results in damage and dysfunction of the alveolar–capillary membrane of the lung. Classically, there is interstitial edema of lung tissue, an increase in surface tension caused by inactivation of surfactant, collapse of the alveolar structures, a stiff and noncompliant lung that is difficult to inflate, and impaired diffusion of the respiratory gases with severe hypoxia that is totally refractory to oxygen therapy.

Acute respiratory failure is a condition in which the lungs fail to oxygenate the blood adequately (hypoxemic respiratory failure) or prevent undue retention of carbon dioxide (hypercapnic/hypoxemic respiratory failure). The causes of respiratory failure are many. It may arise acutely in people with previously healthy lungs, or it may be superimposed on chronic lung disease. Treatment of acute respiratory failure is directed toward treatment of the underlying disease, maintenance of adequate gas exchange and tissue oxygenation, and general supportive care. When alveolar ventilation is inadequate to maintain PO_2 or PCO_2 levels because of impaired respiratory function or neurologic failure, mechanical ventilation may be necessary. There are multiple problems that can result from the barotraumas caused by the mechanical ventilation to the lung parenchyma. This condition is caused by ventilator-induced lung injury (VILI), which needs to be prevented if at all possible. Lung protective strategies are focused on increasing compliance and decreasing shear stresses, which occur with the frequent alveolar collapse secondary to the high pressure needed to ventilate the lungs.

GERIATRIC Considerations

- Bronchiectasis, heart problems, and higher mortality rates often occur in older asthmatics due to the additional stress that asthma has on the heart.[51]
- Bronchospasms associated with cold damp weather alert the older person that symptoms of chronic bronchitis are worsening.[51]
- The risk of emphysema increases with age, as do mortality rates from the disease. Recurrent lung infections, heart failure and cardiac arrhythmias are serious complications resulting from emphysema.[51]
- Carbon dioxide narcosis is associated with aging and emphysema.[51]

PEDIATRIC Considerations

- ARDS in children can result in residual lung disease in children. Nasal flaring with sternal retractions are common clinical manifestations.[52]
- Asthma impacts over 10 million American children prior to age 18 and accounts for over 3 billion dollars in health care cost annually.[52]
  - The increase in asthma, as well as the severity, is thought to be due to air pollution, more children living in urban areas, and the ability to accurately diagnose the disease.
- CF screening is performed as part of the newborn assessment and is strongly recommended preconception.[52]

REVIEW EXERCISES

1. A 30-year-old man is brought to the emergency department with a knife wound to the chest. On visual inspection, asymmetry of chest movement during inspiration, displacement of the trachea, and absence of breath sounds on the side of the wound are noted. His neck veins are distended, and his pulse is rapid and thready. A rapid diagnosis of tension pneumothorax is made.
   A. *Explain the observed respiratory and cardiovascular function in terms of the impaired lung expansion and the air that has entered the chest as a result of the injury.*
   B. *What type of emergent treatment is necessary to save this man's life?*
2. A 10-year-old boy who is having an acute asthmatic attack is brought to the emergency department by his parents. The boy is observed to be sitting up and struggling to breathe. His breathing is accompanied by use of the accessory muscles, a weak cough, and audible wheezing sounds. His pulse is rapid and weak and both heart and breath sounds are distant on auscultation. His parents relate that his asthma began to worsen after he developed a "cold," and now he doesn't even get relief from his "albuterol" inhaler.
   A. *Explain the changes in physiologic function underlying this boy's signs and symptoms.*
   B. *The boy is treated with a systemic corticosteroid and inhaled anticholinergic and β_2-adrenergic agonist and then transferred to the intensive care unit. Explain the action of each of these medications in terms of relieving this boy's symptoms.*
3. A 62-year-old man with an 8-year history of chronic bronchitis reports to his health care provider with complaints of increasing shortness of breath, ankle swelling, and a feeling of fullness in his upper abdomen. The expiratory phase of his respirations is prolonged and expiratory wheezes and crackles are heard on auscultation. His blood pressure is 160/90 mm Hg, his red blood cell count is 6.0×10^6 mL (normal 4.2 to 5.4 × 10^6 µmL), his hematocrit is 65% (normal male value 40% to 50%), his arterial PO_2 is 55 mm Hg, and his O_2 saturation, which is 85% while he is resting, drops to 55% during walking exercise.
   A. *Explain the physiologic mechanisms responsible for his edema, hypertension, and elevated red blood cell count.*
   B. *His arterial PO_2 and O_2 saturation indicate that he is a candidate for continuous low-flow oxygen. Explain the benefits of this treatment in terms of his activity tolerance, blood pressure, and red blood cell count.*
   C. *Explain why the oxygen flow rate for persons with COPD is normally titrated to maintain the arterial PO_2 between 60 and 65 mm Hg.*
4. An 18-year-old woman is admitted to the emergency department with a suspected drug overdose. Her respiratory rate is slow (4 to 6 breaths/minute) and shallow. Arterial blood gases reveal a PCO_2 of 80 mm Hg and a PO_2 of 60 mm Hg.
   A. *What is the cause of this woman's high PCO_2 and low PO_2?*
   B. *Hypoventilation almost always causes an increase in PCO_2. Explain.*
   C. *Even though her PO_2 increases to 90 mm Hg with institution of oxygen therapy, her PCO_2 remains elevated. Explain.*

References

1. Boron W. F., Boulpaep E. L. (2017). *Ventilation and Perfusion of the Lungs: Medical Physiology.* (2nd ed., pp. 675–699.e1). Philadelphia, PA: Elsevier, Inc.
2. West J. B. (2016). *West's Pulmonary Pathophysiology; The Essentials* (9th ed., pp. 3–44, 61–120). Philadelphia, PA: Wolters Kluwer.
3. Deacon A. J., Pratt O. W. (2017). Measurement of pulse oximetry, capnography and PH. *Anesthesia and Intensive Care Medicine* 18(12), 639–643.
4. Awasthi S., Raka R., Deepak M. (2013). Peripheral venous blood gas analysis: an alternative to arterial blood gas analysis for initial assessment and resuscitation in emergency and intensive care unit patients. *Anesthesia, Essays and Researches* 7(3):355–358.
5. Reske A. W., Costa E. L., Reske V. (2013). Bedside estimation of nonaerated lung tissue using blood gas analysis. *Critical Care Medicine* 41(3), 732–743.
6. Peterson J., Glenny R. W. (2014). Gas exchange and ventilation perfusion-relationships in the lung. *European Respiratory Journal* 44, 1023–1040.
7. Kim S. M., et al. (2017). Successful extubation after weaning failure by noninvasive ventilation in patients with neuromuscular disease: case series. *Annals of Rehabilitation Medicine* 41(3), 450–455.
8. Andreoli T., Benjamin I., Griggs R., et al. (Eds.). (2016). *Disorders of the pleura, mediastinum, and chest wall. Andreoli and Carpenter's Cecil Essentials of Medicine* (9th ed., pp. 248–253). St Louis, MO: Elsevier.
9. Kasper D. L., Fauci A. S. (2015). *W. Disorders of the Pleura. Harrison's Principles of Internal Medicine* (19th ed., ch 316). New York, NY: McGraw-Hill.
10. Sood A. (2015). Evaluation of respiratory impairment and disability. In Elias J. A., Fishman J. A., Kotloff R. M., et al. (Eds.), *Fishman's Pulmonary Diseases and Disorders* (5th ed., ch 38). New York, NY: McGraw-Hill. http://accessmedicine.mhmedical.com/content.aspx?bookid=1344&sectionid=811880
11. Loannidis G., et al. (2015). Barotrauma and pneumothorax. *Journal of Thoracic Disease* 7(Suppl 1), S38–S43. *PMC.* Web. 13 Dec. 2017.
12. Centers for Disease Control and Prevention. (2017). *Asthma FASTSTATS* 2017. Available: https://www.cdc.gov/nchs/fastats/asthma.htm. Accessed November 26, 2017. Retrieved November 26, 2017 from https://www.cdc.gov/nchs/fastats/asthma.htm
13. National Heart Lung Blood Institute. (2017). *National Asthma Education and Prevention Program (NAEP) NHLBI.* Available: https://www.nhlbi.nih.gov/health-topics/asthma. Retrieved December 12, 2017.
14. Barnes PJ. (2014). Asthma. In Kasper D., Fauci A., Hauser S., et al. (Eds.), *Harrison's Principles of Internal Medicine* (19th ed., ch 309). New York, NY: McGraw-Hill.

15. Beigelman A., Bacharier L. B. (2016). Early life respiratory infections and asthma development: Role in disease pathogenesis and potential targets for disease prevention. *Current Opinion in Allergy and Clinical Immunology* 16(2), 172–178. doi:10.1097/ACI.0000000000000244
16. Gelfand E. W., Joetham A., Wang M., et al. (2017). Spectrum of T-lymphocyte activities regulating allergic lung inflammation. *Immunological Reviews* 278, 63–86. https://doi.org/10.1111/imr.12561
17. Kato A., et al. B Lymphocyte lineage cells and the respiratory system. *The Journal of Allergy and Clinical Immunology* 131(4), 933–957. *PMC*. Web. 13 Dec. 2017.B.
18. Yang T., et al. (2017). Characteristics of proinflammatory cytokines and chemokines in airways of asthmatics: Relationships with disease severity and infiltration of inflammatory cells. *Chinese Medical Journal* 130(17), 2033–2040. *PMC*. Web. 13 Dec. 2017.
19. Meyer N., et al. (2017). Safeguarding of fetal growth by mast cells and natural killer cells: Deficiency of one is counterbalanced by the other. *Frontiers in Immunology* 8, 711. *PMC*. Web. 13 Dec. 2017.
20. Kim H., et al. (2017). Asthma biomarkers in the age of biologics. *Allergy, Asthma, and Clinical Immunology: Official Journal of the Canadian Society of Allergy and Clinical Immunology* 13, 48. *PMC*. Web. 13 Dec. 2017.
21. Schauer S. G., Cuenca P. J., Johnson J. J., Ramirez S. (2013). Management of acute asthma in the emergency department. *Emergency Medicine Practice* 15(6), 1–28.
22. Manning B. M., et al. (2015). Single-cell analysis of mast cell degranulation induced by airway smooth muscle-secreted chemokines. *Biochimica et Biophysica Acta* 1850(9), 1862–1868. *PMC*. Web. 13 Dec. 2017.
23. Hong C.-C., et al. (2014). Younger pubertal age is associated with allergy and other atopic conditions in girls. *Pediatric allergy and immunology: Official publication of the European Society of Pediatric Allergy and Immunology* 25(8), 773–780. *PMC*. Web. 13 Dec. 2017.
24. Keselman A., Heller N. (2015). Estrogen signaling modulates allergic inflammation and contributes to sex differences in asthma. *Frontiers in Immunology* 6, 568. *PMC*. Web. 13 Dec. 2017.
25. Kc P., Martin R. J. (2010). Role of central neurotransmission and chemoreception on airway control. *Respiratory Physiology & Neurobiology* 173(3), 213–222. *PMC*. Web. 13 Dec. 2017.
26. Lee E. J., et al. (2017). Alteration of inflammatory mediators in the upper and lower airways under chronic intermittent hypoxia: Preliminary animal study. *Mediators of Inflammation* 2017, 4327237. *PMC*. Web. 13 Dec. 2017.
27. Solidoro P., Bellocchia M., Facchini F. (2016). The immunobiological and clinical role of vitamin D in obstructive lung diseases. *Minerva Medica* 107(3 Suppl 1), 12–19.
28. Loscalzo J. (2017). Chronic obstructive pulmonary disease. In Kasper D. L., Longo D. L., Fauci A. S., et al. (Eds.), *Harrison's Pulmonary and Critical care Medicine* (3rd ed., pp. 191–203). New York, NY: McGraw Hill.
29. Cipriani F., Calamelli E., Ricci G. (2017). Allergen avoidance in allergic asthma; *Frontiers in pediatrics*. Available: https://doi.org/10.3389/fped.2017.00103. Accessed November 28, 2017.
30. Loscalzo J. (2017). Asthma. In *Harrison's Pulmonary and Critical Care Medicine* (3rd ed., pp. 64–82). New York, NY: McGraw Hill.
31. Franklin A. N., et al. (2014). Anti-immunoglobulin E therapy. In *Middleton's Allergy: Principles and Practice* (8th ed., pp. 1480–1490). Philadelphia, PA: Saunders.
32. Al-Alawi M., Hassan T., Chotirmall S. H. (2014). Advances in the diagnosis and management of asthma in older adults. *The American Journal of Medicine* 127(5), 370–378. Available: http://www.sciencedirect.com/science/article/pii/S0002934313011108. Accessed November 28, 2017.
33. Centers for Disease Control and Prevention. (2013). *Asthma-related missed school days among children aged 5–17 years*. Available: http://www.cdc.gov/asthma/asthma_stats/missing_days.htm. Accessed November 28, 2017
34. Global Initiative for Asthma. (2017). Global strategy for asthma management and prevention (report). Available: http://ginasthma.org/2017-gina-report-global-strategy-for-asthma-management-and-prevention/. Accessed November 27, 2017.
35. COPD Foundation. (2017). *COPD statistics across America*. Available: http://www.copdfoundation.org/What-is-COPD/COPD-Facts/Statistics.aspx. Accessed November 28, 2017
36. National Institutes of Health. (2017). *COPD National Action Plan*. Available: https://www.nhlbi.nih.gov/sites/www.nhlbi.nih.gov/files/National%20Action%20Plan_508c_8%2018%2017.pdf. Accessed November 28, 2017
37. Global Initiative for Chronic Obstructive Lung Disease. (2018). Global Strategy for the Diagnosis, Management and Prevention of Chronic Obstructive Pulmonary Disease (2018 Report). Available: http://goldcopd.org/wp-content/uploads/2017/11/GOLD-2018-v6.0-FINAL-revised-20-Nov_WMS.pdf. Accessed November 28, 2017
38. Stoller J. K., Lacbawan F. L., Aboussouan L. S. *Alpha-1 antitrypsin deficiency. 2006 Oct 27 [Updated 2017 Jan 19]. GeneReviews®*. 1993–2017. Available from: https://www-ncbi-nlm-nih-gov.ezproxy.uthsc.edu/books/NBK1519/. Accessed November 29, 2017
39. Mejza F., et al. (2017). Prevalence and burden of chronic bronchitis symptoms: results from the BOLD study. *European Respiratory Journal* 50(5). Available: http://erj.ersjournals.com.ezproxy.uthsc.edu/content/50/5/1700621. Accessed November 29, 2017
40. Cystic Fibrosis Foundation. (2017). *About cystic fibrosis*. Available: http://www.cff.org/AboutCF/. Accessed December 9, 2017
41. U.S. National Library of Medicine. (2017). *CFTR gene, cystic fibrosis transmembrane conductance regulator. Genetics home reference*. Available: ghr.nlm.nih.gov/gene/CFTR#conditions. Accessed December 9, 2017
42. Gemma V., Gemma M., et al. (2017). Diagnosis and management of cystic fibrosis: summary of NICE guidance. *British Medical Journal* 359, j4574. Available: http://www.bmj.com.ezproxy.uthsc.edu/content/359/bmj.j4574.long Accessed December 9, 2017
43. Farell P. M., et al. (2017). Diagnosis of cystic fibrosis: consensus guidelines from the cystic fibrosis foundation. *The Journal of Pediatrics* 181, S4–S15. DOI: org/10.1016/j.jpeds.2016.09.064
44. National Institute of Health. (2013). How is cystic fibrosis treated?. *National Heart Lung and Blood Institute*. Available: www.nhlbi.nih.gov/health/health-topics/topics/cf/treatment. Accessed December 10, 2017
45. Jankowich M. D. (2016). Interstitial lung diseases. In Benjamin I. J., Griggs R. C., Wing E. J., et al. (Eds.), *Andreoli and Carpenter's Cecil Essentials of Medicine* (9th ed., pp. 222–239). PA: Saunders/Elsevier.
46. Kasper D. L., Fauci A. S. (2015). Occupational and environmental lung disease. In Kasper D. L., Longo D. L., Fauci A. S., et al. (Eds.), *Harrison's Principles of Internal Medicine* (19th ed.). New York, NY: McGraw Hill.
47. Kasper D. L., Fauci A. S. (2015). Pulmonary hypertension. *In Harrison's Principles of Internal Medicin* (19th ed.). New York, NY: McGraw Hill.
48. Girerd B., et al. (2017). Genetics of pulmonary hypertension in the clinic. *Current Opinion in Pulmonary Medicine* 23(5), 386–391. DOI: 10.1097/MCP.0000000000000414.
49. Selvakumar N., Casserly B., Rounds S. (2016). Essentials in critical care medicine. In Benjamin I. J., Griggs R. C., Wing E. J., et al. (Eds.), *Andreoli and Carpenter's: Cecil Essentials of Medicine* (9th ed., pp. 259–265). PA: Saunders/Elsevier.
50. Kasper D. L., Fauci A. S. (2015). Acute respiratory distress syndrome. In Kasper D. L., Longo D. L., Fauci A. S., et al. (Eds.), *Harrison's Principles of Internal Medicine* (19th ed.). New York, NY: McGraw Hill.
51. Eliopoulos C. (2018). *Gerontological Nursing*. (9th ed.). Philadelphia, PA: Wolter Kluwers.
52. Kyle T., Carman S. (2015). Essentials of Pediatric Nursing. (3rd ed.). Philadelphia, PA: Wolters Kluwer.

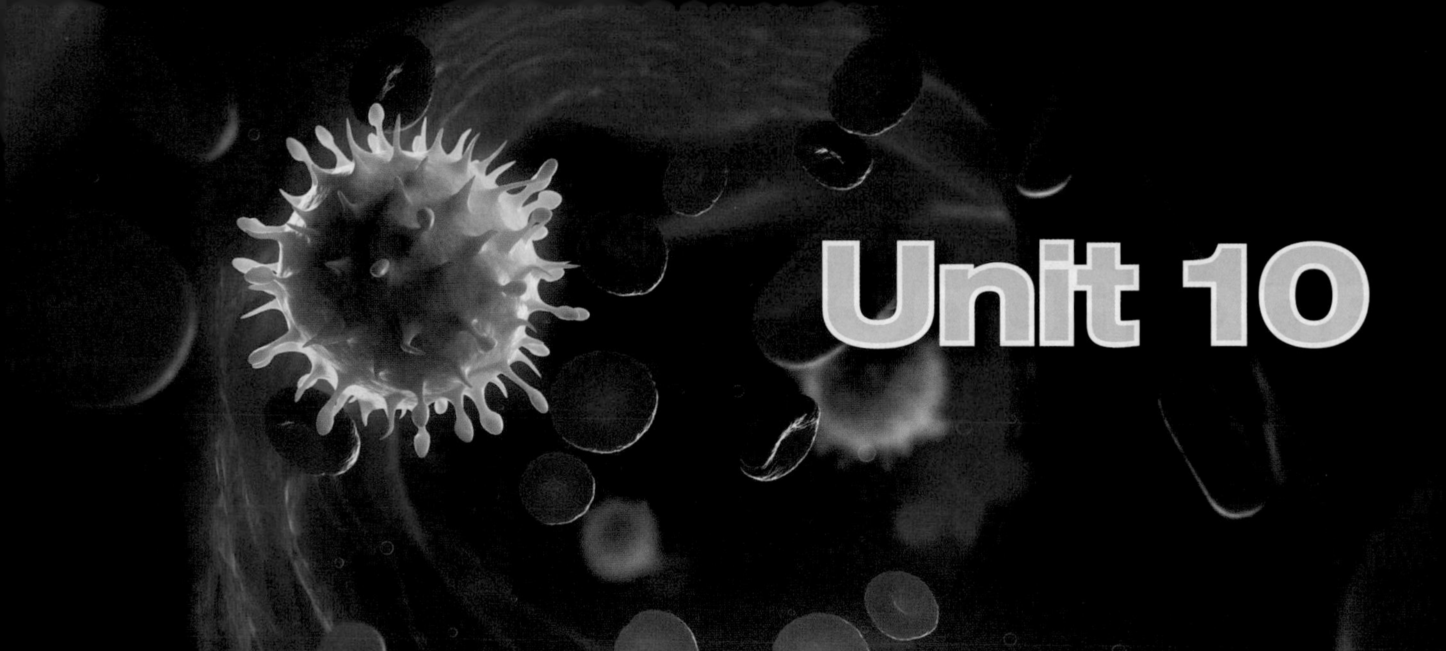

Unit 10

Disorders of Renal Function

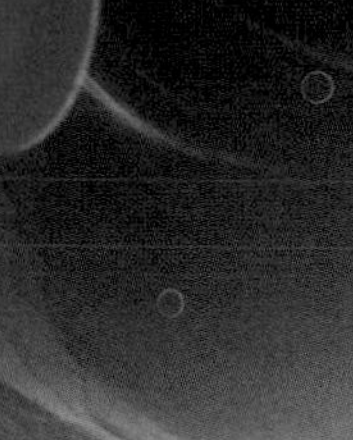

Joseph Reterez, 45 years old, is admitted to the emergency department with abdominal and flank discomfort, distension of the abdomen, anorexia, fatigue, and nausea. He says that his urine is really cloudy, and he thinks there is some blood visible in the urine. His mother, his maternal grandfather, and two maternal uncles died in their late 40s from renal disease, but no one in his family has had genetic testing. His assessment shows an increased abdominal girth, enlarged kidneys, mild (1+) pedal edema, and bilateral flank pain. His vital signs are as follows: temperature, 100.1°F; blood pressure, 145/92 mm Hg (indicative of hypertension); pulse, 92/minute; and respiratory rate, 14/minute. Significant (abnormal) blood chemistry values include the following: blood urea nitrogen (BUN), 45 mg/dL (normal, 8 to 20 mg/dL); creatinine, 2.0 mg/dL (normal, 0.3 to 1.2 mg/dL); and serum sodium, 147 mEq/L (normal, 135 to 145 mEq/L). His urine specimen shows mildly elevated (+1) protein and the presence of RBCs. Genetic testing reveals a mutation in the PKD1 gene, a common cause of adult polycystic kidney disease. Mr. Reterez's diagnosis is discussed in Chapter 33.

Structure and Function of the Kidney

32

KIDNEY STRUCTURE AND FUNCTION
- Gross Structure and Location
- Renal Blood Supply
- The Nephron
  - *The Glomerulus*
  - *Tubular Components of the Nephron*
- Urine Formation
  - *Glomerular Filtration*
  - *Tubular Reabsorption and Secretion*
  - *Regulation of Urine Concentration*
- Regulation of Renal Blood Flow
  - *Neural and Humoral Control Mechanisms*
  - *Autoregulatory Mechanisms*
  - *Effect of Increased Protein and Glucose Load*
- Elimination Functions of the Kidney
  - *Renal Clearance*
  - *Regulation of Electrolytes*
  - *Regulation of pH*
  - *pH-Dependent Elimination of Organic Ions*
  - *Uric Acid Elimination*
  - *Urea Elimination*
  - *Drug Elimination*
- Endocrine Functions of the Kidney
  - *The Renin–Angiotensin–Aldosterone Mechanism*
  - *Erythropoietin*
  - *Vitamin D*
- Action of Diuretics
  - *Diuretics That Block Sodium Reabsorption*
  - *Osmotic Diuretics*

TESTS OF RENAL FUNCTION
- Urine Tests
- Glomerular Filtration Rate
- Blood Tests
  - *Serum Creatinine*
  - *Blood Urea Nitrogen*
- Cystoscopy and Ureteroscopy
- Ultrasonography
- Radiologic and Other Imaging Studies

Linda C. Mefford
Reba A. Umberger

The kidneys are remarkable organs. Each is smaller than a person's fist, but in a single day, the two organs process approximately 22% to 25% of the cardiac output, or 1100 mL/minute.[1,2] A primary function of the kidney is to filter the blood to selectively reabsorb molecules needed for normal body function while excreting unneeded substances through the urine. The kidneys perform both excretory and endocrine functions to regulate the volume and composition of body fluids. This chapter focuses on the structure and function of the kidneys and tests of renal function.

KIDNEY STRUCTURE AND FUNCTION

After completing this section of the chapter, the learner will be able to meet the following objectives:

- Describe the importance of maintaining adequate renal perfusion and the mechanisms for regulating renal blood flow (RBF).
- Describe the structure and function of the nephron and the mechanisms through which renal regulation of extracellular fluid is accomplished.
- Describe how the kidney produces concentrated or dilute urine.

Gross Structure and Location

The kidneys are paired, bean-shaped organs that lie outside the peritoneal cavity in the posterior upper abdomen. One kidney lies on each side of the vertebral column at the level of the 12th thoracic to 3rd lumbar vertebrae (Fig. 32.1).[1] The right kidney is typically situated lower than the left, because of the position of the liver. In the adult, each kidney is approximately 10- to 12-cm long, 5- to 6-cm wide, and 2.5-cm deep and weighs approximately 113 to 170 g.[1] The medial border of the kidney is indented by a deep fissure called the *hilus*, where blood vessels and nerves enter and leave the kidney. The ureters, which connect the kidneys with the bladder, also enter the kidney at the hilus.[2]

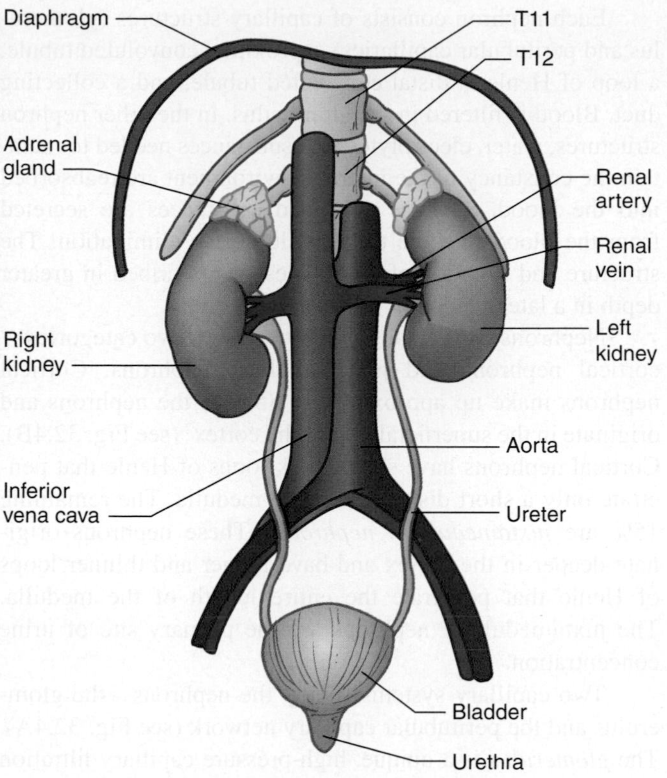

Figure 32.1 • Kidneys, ureters, and bladder. (The right kidney is usually lower than the left.)

The kidney is a multilobular structure, composed of between 8 and 18 lobes.[2] Each lobe is composed of nephrons, the functional units of the kidney. Each kidney contains approximately 800,000 to 1,000,000 nephrons.[2] Each nephron has a glomerulus that filters the blood and a system of tubular structures that selectively reabsorb needed substances back into the blood and secrete unneeded substances into the tubular filtrate that will become urine. On a longitudinal section, a kidney can be divided into an outer cortex and an inner medulla (Fig. 32.2). The cortex, which is reddish–brown, contains the glomeruli and convoluted tubules of the nephron and blood vessels. The medulla consists of light-colored, cone-shaped masses—the renal pyramids. The columns of the cortex that extend into the medulla divide the renal pyramids. Each pyramid, topped by a region of the cortex, forms a lobe of the kidney. The apices of the pyramids form the papillae (with 8 to 18 per kidney, corresponding to the number of lobes), which are perforated by the openings of the collecting ducts.[2] The renal pelvis is a wide, funnel-shaped structure at the upper end of the ureter. It is made up of the calyces or cuplike structures that drain the upper and lower halves of the kidney.[1,2]

The kidney is sheathed in a fibrous external capsule and surrounded by a mass of fatty connective tissue, particularly at the ends and borders. The adipose tissue protects the kidney from mechanical blows and assists the attached blood vessels and fascia to secure the kidney in place.[3,4] Although the kidneys are relatively well protected, they may be bruised by blows to the sides of the body or by compression between the lower ribs and the ileum. Because the kidneys are located outside the peritoneal cavity, injury does not produce the same threat of peritoneal involvement as with intraperitoneal organs, such as the liver or spleen.

Renal Blood Supply

A single renal artery arises on either side of the aorta to supply each kidney. As the renal artery approaches the kidney, it divides into five segmental arteries that enter the hilus. Inside the kidney, each segmental artery branches into several lobular arteries that supply the upper, middle, and lower parts of

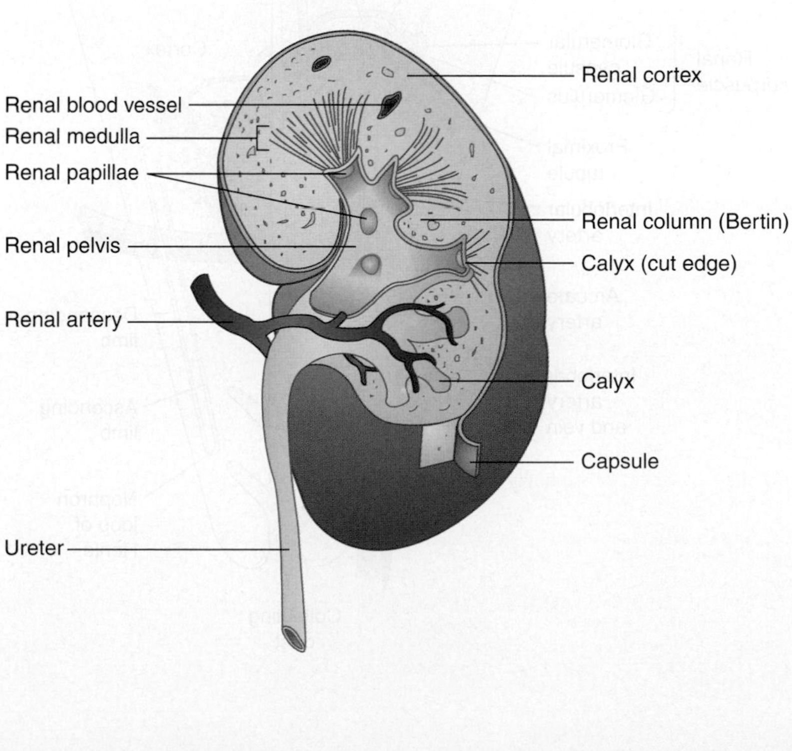

Figure 32.2 • Internal structure of the kidney.

the kidney.[2] The lobular arteries further subdivide to form the interlobular arteries at the level of the corticomedullary junction (Fig. 32.3). These arteries branch into the arcuate arteries, which arch across the top of the pyramids. Small intralobular arteries radiate from the arcuate arteries to supply the cortex of the kidney. The afferent arterioles that supply the glomeruli arise from the intralobular arteries.[5]

Although nearly all the blood flow to the kidneys passes through the cortex, less than 10% is directed to the medulla and only approximately 1% goes to the papillae.[2] Under conditions of decreased perfusion or increased sympathetic nervous system stimulation, blood flow can be redistributed away from the cortex toward the medulla. This redistribution of blood flow decreases glomerular filtration while maintaining the urine-concentrating ability of the kidneys, a factor that is important during conditions such as shock.[2]

The Nephron

Each kidney is composed of more than approximately 1 million tiny, closely packed functional units called *nephrons* (Fig. 32.4A).[2] The kidney has no ability to regenerate nephrons. Therefore, with aging, there is a generalized decrease in functioning nephrons.[2] In fact, adults tend to lose approximately 10% of their nephrons for each decade beginning at 40 years of age.[2]

Each nephron consists of capillary structures (glomerulus and peritubular capillaries), a proximal convoluted tubule, a loop of Henle, a distal convoluted tubule, and a collecting duct. Blood is filtered in the glomerulus. In the other nephron structures, water, electrolytes, and substances needed to maintain the constancy of the internal environment are reabsorbed into the blood, whereas unneeded substances are secreted from the blood into the tubular filtrate for elimination. The structure and function of the tubules are described in greater depth in a later section.

Nephrons can be roughly grouped into two categories—cortical nephrons and juxtamedullary nephrons. Cortical nephrons make up approximately 85% of the nephrons and originate in the superficial part of the cortex[2] (see Fig. 32.4B). Cortical nephrons have short, thick loops of Henle that penetrate only a short distance into the medulla. The remaining 15% are *juxtamedullary nephrons.*[2] These nephrons originate deeper in the cortex and have longer and thinner loops of Henle that penetrate the entire length of the medulla. The juxtamedullary nephrons are the primary site of urine concentration.[2]

Two capillary systems supply the nephrons—the glomerulus and the peritubular capillary network (see Fig. 32.4A). The *glomerulus* is a unique, high-pressure capillary filtration system located between two arterioles, the afferent and the efferent arterioles. Because the arterioles are high-resistant

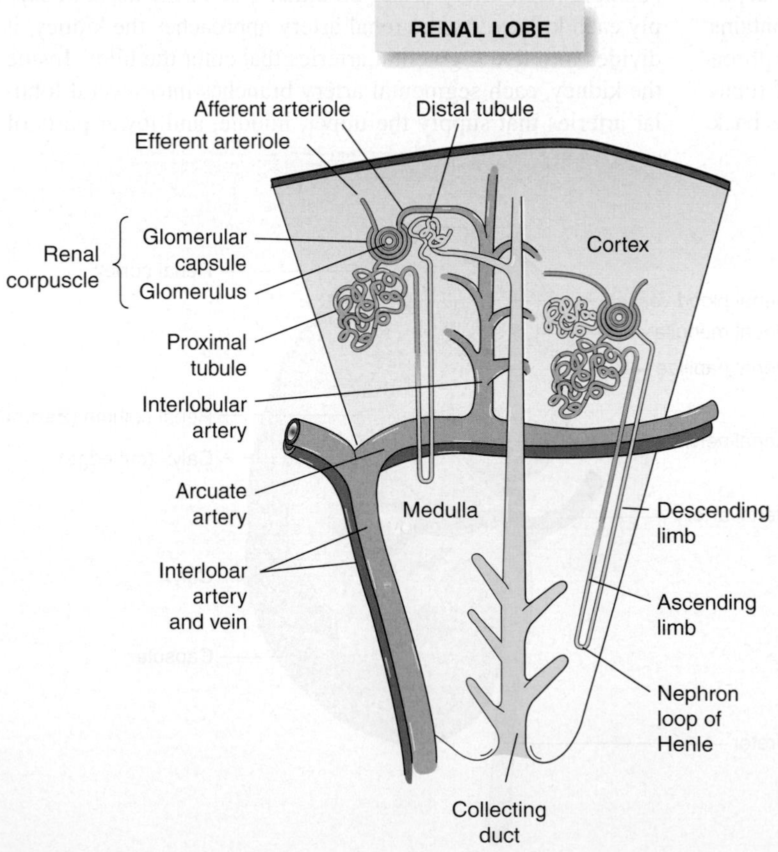

Figure 32.3 • Arterial supply of the kidney. (From Strayer, D., Rubin E. (Eds.) (2015). *Rubin's pathology: Clinicopathologic foundations of medicine* (7th ed., p. 904). Philadelphia, PA: Lippincott Williams & Wilkins.)

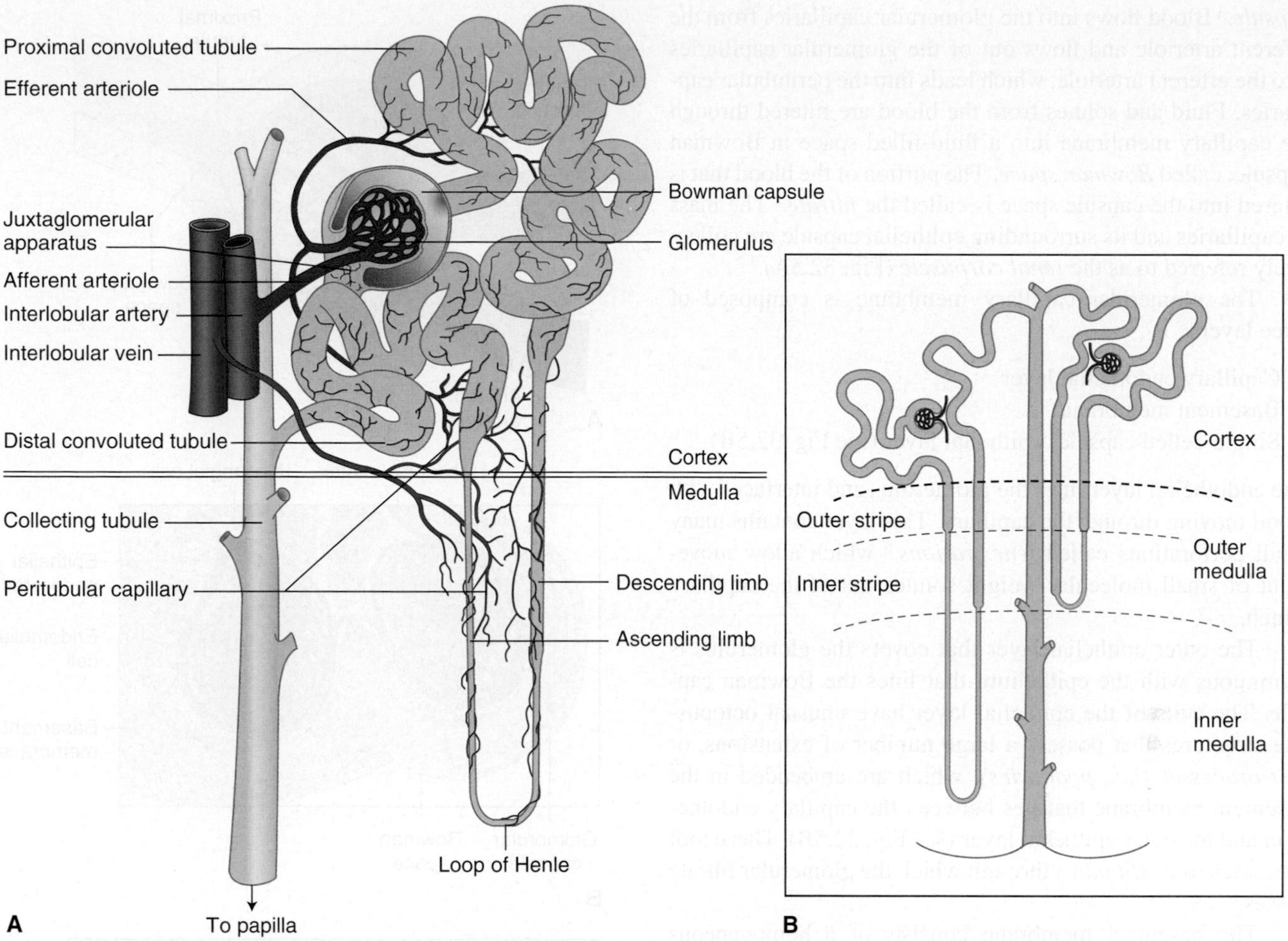

Figure 32.4 • **(A)** Nephron showing the glomerular and tubular structures along with the blood supply. **(B)** Comparison of differences in location of tubular structures of the cortical and juxtamedullary nephrons.

vessels and the afferent arteriole has a larger diameter than the efferent arteriole, the blood pressure in the glomerulus is extraordinarily high for a capillary bed. This elevated capillary hydrostatic pressure easily forces fluid and solutes out of the glomerular capillaries into the surrounding tubular structure, called the Bowman capsule.[2] The structure and function of the glomerulus are described in greater depth in the following section. The *peritubular capillaries* originate from the efferent arteriole. They are low-pressure vessels that are adapted for reabsorption rather than filtration.[2] These peritubular capillaries with low hydrostatic pressure surround all portions of the tubules, facilitating rapid reabsorption of water and solutes from the tubules to the blood. In the deepest part of the renal cortex, the efferent arterioles serving the juxtaglomerular nephron also continue into long, thin-walled looping vessels called the *vasa recta*.[2] The vasa recta surround the long loops of Henle in the medullary portion of the kidney to facilitate exchange of substances in that portion of the nephron.[2] The peritubular capillaries rejoin to form the venous channels through which blood leaves the kidneys and empties into the inferior vena cava.[2]

KEY POINTS

THE NEPHRON

- The nephron, which is the functional unit of the kidney, is composed of vascular components (the glomerulus and peritubular capillaries) and tubular components. Fluid and solutes are filtered from the glomerular capillaries into the tubular structures, in which urine is formed for elimination from the body.
- In the tubular portion of the nephron, substances needed by the body are reabsorbed into the peritubular capillaries, whereas unneeded substances are secreted from the peritubular capillaries into the urine filtrate.

The Glomerulus

The glomerulus consists of a compact tuft of capillaries encased in a thin, double-walled capsule called *Bowman capsule.*[2] Blood flows into the glomerular capillaries from the afferent arteriole and flows out of the glomerular capillaries into the efferent arteriole, which leads into the peritubular capillaries. Fluid and solutes from the blood are filtered through the capillary membrane into a fluid-filled space in Bowman capsule, called *Bowman space.* The portion of the blood that is filtered into the capsule space is called the *filtrate.*[2] The mass of capillaries and its surrounding epithelial capsule are collectively referred to as the *renal corpuscle* (Fig. 32.5A).[2]

The glomerular capillary membrane is composed of three layers:

1. Capillary endothelial layer
2. Basement membrane
3. Single-celled capsular epithelial layer (see Fig. 32.5B)

The endothelial layer lines the glomerulus and interfaces with blood moving through the capillary. This layer contains many small perforations called *fenestrations,*[6] which allow movement of small molecular weight solutes out of the capillary lumen.

The outer epithelial layer that covers the glomerulus is continuous with the epithelium that lines the Bowman capsule. The cells of the epithelial layer have unusual octopus-like structures that possess a large number of extensions, or *foot processes* (*i.e., podocytes*), which are embedded in the basement membrane that lies between the capillary endothelium and the outer epithelial layer (see Fig. 32.5B). These foot processes form *slit pores* through which the glomerular filtrate passes.[6]

The basement membrane consists of a homogeneous acellular meshwork of collagen fibers, glycoproteins, and mucopolysaccharides (see Fig. 32.5C). The endothelial and epithelial layers of the glomerular capillary have porous structures, and thus the basement membrane determines the permeability of the glomerular capillary membrane. The spaces between the fibers that make up the basement membrane act as pores of a filter to create a size-dependent permeability barrier for the glomerulus. The size of the pores in the basement membrane normally prevents red blood cells and plasma proteins from passing through the glomerulus into the filtrate. Evidence indicates that the epithelium plays a major role in producing the basement membrane components, with epithelial cells likely active in forming new basement membrane material throughout life. Alterations in the structure and function of the glomerular basement membrane are responsible for the leakage of proteins and blood cells into the filtrate that occurs in many forms of glomerular disease.[2]

Another important component of the glomerulus is the *mesangium.*[6] In some areas, the capsular epithelium and the basement membrane do not completely surround each capillary. Instead, the mesangial cells, which lie between the capillary tufts, provide support for the glomerulus in these areas (see Fig. 32.5B).[6] The mesangial cells produce an intercellular substance similar to that of the basement membrane. This substance covers the endothelial cells where they are not covered by basement membrane.[6] The mesangial cells possess phagocytic properties and remove macromolecules that enter the intercapillary spaces. Mesangial cells also exhibit contractile properties in response to neurohumoral substances and are thought to contribute to the regulation of blood flow through the glomerulus. In normal glomeruli, the mesangial area is narrow and contains only a small number of cells. Mesangial hyperplasia and increased mesangial matrix occur in a number of glomerular diseases.[6]

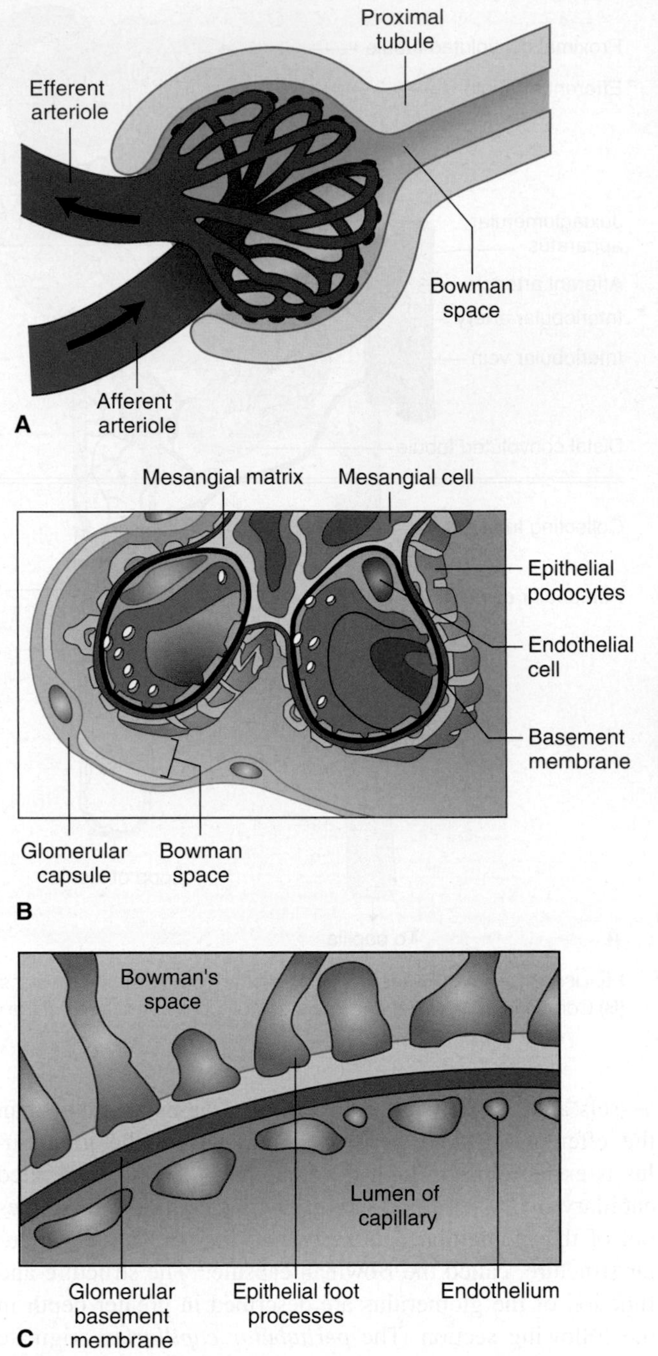

Figure 32.5 • Renal corpuscle. **(A)** Structures of the glomerulus. **(B)** Cross-section of the glomerular membrane showing the position of the endothelium, basement membrane, and epithelial foot processes. **(C)** Position of the mesangial cells in relation to the capillary loops and Bowman capsule.

Tubular Components of the Nephron

The nephron tubule is divided into four segments:

1. A highly coiled segment called the *proximal convoluted tubule*, which drains the Bowman capsule
2. A thin, looped structure called the *loop of Henle*
3. A distal coiled portion called the *distal convoluted tubule*
4. A *collecting tubule* (or *collecting duct*), which joins with several tubules to collect the filtrate[6]

The filtrate passes through each of these segments before reaching the pelvis of the kidney.

The proximal tubule dips toward the renal pelvis to become the descending limb of the loop of Henle. The ascending loop of Henle returns to the region of the renal corpuscle, where it becomes the distal tubule.[6] The distal convoluted tubule begins at the juxtaglomerular complex and is divided into two segments—the *diluting segment* and the *late distal tubule*. The late distal tubule fuses with the collecting tubule (or collecting duct). Like the distal tubule, the collecting duct is divided into two segments—the *cortical collecting tubule* and the *inner medullary collecting tubule*.[6]

Throughout its course, the tubule is composed of a single layer of epithelial cells resting on a basement membrane. The structure of the epithelial cells varies with tubular function. The cells of the proximal tubule have a fine, villous structure that increases the surface area for reabsorption. They also are rich in mitochondria, which support active transport processes. The epithelial layer of the thin segment of the loop of Henle has few mitochondria, indicating minimal metabolic activity and reabsorptive function.[6]

Urine Formation

Urine formation involves (a) the filtration of blood through the glomerulus to form an *ultrafiltrate of urine* and (b) the tubular reabsorption of electrolytes and nutrients needed to maintain the constancy of the internal environment while eliminating waste materials.

Glomerular Filtration

Urine formation begins with the filtration of essentially protein-free plasma through the glomerular capillaries into the Bowman space. The movement of fluid through the glomerular capillaries is determined by the same factors that facilitate fluid movement in all capillary beds: capillary hydrostatic pressure (filtration pressure), capillary colloidal osmotic pressure (reabsorptive pressure), and capillary permeability.[2] The glomerular filtrate has a chemical composition similar to plasma, but it contains almost no proteins because large molecules do not readily cross the glomerular wall. Approximately 125 mL of filtrate is formed each minute.[6] This is called the *glomerular filtration rate (GFR)*. This rate can vary from a few milliliters per minute to as high as 200 mL/minute. The average adult has a GFR of 125 mL/minute or 180 L/day.[2]

The location of the glomerulus between two arterioles allows for maintenance of a high-pressure filtration system. The capillary filtration pressure (approximately 60 mm Hg) in the glomerulus is approximately two to three times higher than that of other capillary beds in the body. The filtration pressure and the GFR are regulated by the constriction and relaxation of the afferent and efferent arterioles. Constriction of the efferent arteriole increases resistance to outflow from the glomeruli and increases the glomerular pressure and the GFR. Constriction of the afferent arteriole causes a reduction in RBF, glomerular filtration pressure, and GFR.[2] The afferent and the efferent arterioles are innervated by the sympathetic nervous system and are sensitive to vasoactive hormones, such as angiotensin II, as well. These neurohormonal mechanisms will be discussed in greater depth later in this chapter.[2]

Tubular Reabsorption and Secretion

From the Bowman capsule, the glomerular filtrate moves into the tubular segments of the nephron. While moving through the lumen of the tubular segments, the chemical composition of glomerular filtrate is changed considerably by the tubular transport of water and solutes. Tubular transport can result in reabsorption of substances from the tubular filtrate into the peritubular capillaries or secretion of substances from the peritubular capillaries into the tubular filtrate[2] (Fig. 32.6).

The basic mechanisms of transport across the tubular epithelial cell membrane are similar to those of other cell membranes in the body (including both active and passive

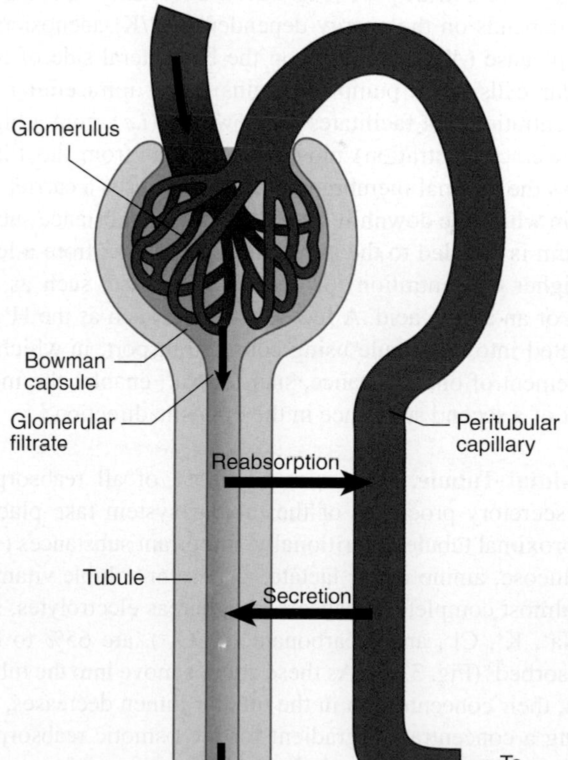

Figure 32.6 • Reabsorption and secretion of substances between the renal tubules and peritubular capillaries.

transport mechanisms). Water and urea are passively absorbed along concentration gradients. Sodium (Na^+), potassium (K^+), chloride (Cl^-), calcium (Ca^{2+}), and phosphate ions, as well as urate, glucose, and amino acids, are reabsorbed across the tubular epithelial cells and into the blood using primary or secondary active transport mechanisms. Some substances, such as hydrogen (H^+), K^+, and urate ions, are secreted from the blood, across the tubular epithelial cells, and into the tubular filtrate. Under normal conditions, only approximately 1 mL of the 125 mL of glomerular filtrate formed each minute is excreted in the urine.[2] The other 124 mL is reabsorbed in the tubules. This means that the average output of urine is approximately 60 mL/hour.

Renal tubular cells have two membrane surfaces through which substances must pass as they are reabsorbed from the tubular fluid. The outside membrane adjacent to the interstitial fluid is called the *basolateral membrane*. The side in contact with the tubular lumen and tubular filtrate is called the *luminal membrane.*[6] In most cases, substances move across the luminal membrane along a concentration gradient but require facilitated transport or active carrier systems to move across the basolateral membrane into the interstitial fluid, where the substances are absorbed into the peritubular capillaries.

The bulk of energy used by the kidney supports active transport mechanisms that facilitate Na^+ reabsorption with cotransport of other electrolytes and substances such as glucose and amino acids. This is called *secondary active transport* or *cotransport* (Fig. 32.7). Secondary active transport depends on the energy-dependent Na^+/K^+-adenosine triphosphatase (ATPase) pump on the basolateral side of renal tubular cells.[2] The pump maintains a low intracellular Na^+ concentration that facilitates the downhill (*i.e.*, from a higher to lower concentration) movement of Na^+ from the filtrate across the luminal membrane. Cotransport uses a carrier system in which the downhill movement of one substance such as sodium is coupled to the uphill movement (*i.e.*, from a lower to higher concentration) of another substance, such as glucose or an amino acid. A few substances, such as the H^+, are secreted into the tubule using countertransport, in which the movement of one substance, such as Na^+, enables the movement of a second substance in the opposite direction.[2]

Proximal Tubule. Approximately 65% of all reabsorptive and secretory processes of the tubular system take place in the proximal tubule. Nutritionally, important substances (such as glucose, amino acids, lactate, and water-soluble vitamins) are almost completely reabsorbed, whereas electrolytes, such as Na^+, K^+, Cl^-, and bicarbonate (HCO_3^-), are 65% to 80% reabsorbed[2] (Fig. 32.8). As these solutes move into the tubular cells, their concentration in the tubular lumen decreases, providing a concentration gradient for the osmotic reabsorption of water. The proximal tubule is highly permeable to water, and the osmotic movement of water occurs so rapidly that the concentration difference of solutes on either side of the membrane seldom is more than a few milliosmoles.[2]

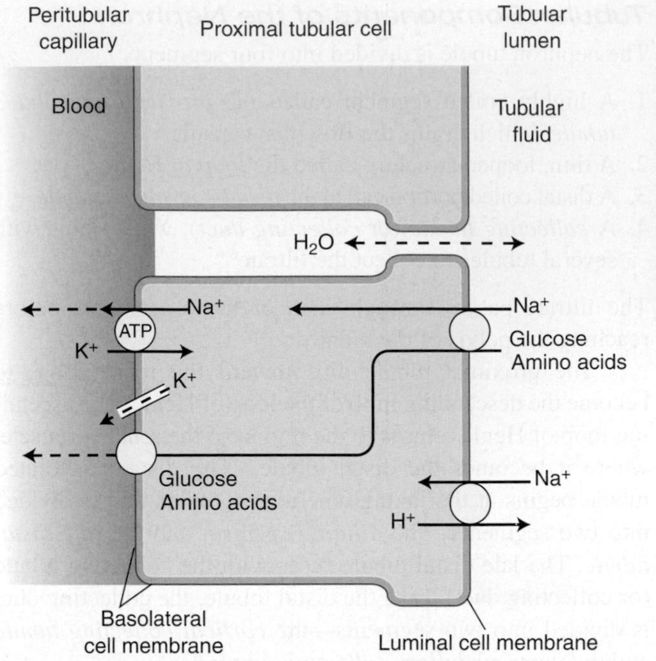

Figure 32.7 • Mechanism for secondary active transport or cotransport of glucose and amino acids in the proximal tubule. The energy-dependent sodium–potassium pump on the basal lateral surface of the cell maintains a low intracellular gradient that facilitates the downhill movement of sodium and glucose or amino acids (cotransport) from the tubular lumen into the tubular cell and then into the peritubular capillary.

Many substances, such as glucose, are freely filtered in the glomerulus and reabsorbed by energy-dependent cotransport carrier mechanisms. The maximum amount of substance that these transport systems can reabsorb per unit time is called the *transport maximum*. The transport maximum is related to the number of carrier proteins that are available for transport and usually is sufficient to ensure that all of a filtered substance such as glucose can be reabsorbed rather than be eliminated in the urine. The plasma level at which the substance appears in the urine is called the *renal threshold.* Under some circumstances, the amount of substance filtered in the glomerulus exceeds the transport maximum. For example, when the blood glucose level is elevated in uncontrolled diabetes mellitus, the amount that is filtered in the glomerulus often exceeds the transport maximum (approximately 320 mg/minute), and glucose spills into the urine.[2]

In addition to *reabsorbing* solutes and water, cells in the proximal tubule also *secrete* organic cations and anions into the urine filtrate (see Figs. 32.6 and 32.8). Many of these organic anions and cations are end products of metabolism (*e.g.*, urate, oxalate) that circulate in the plasma. The proximal tubule also secretes exogenous organic compounds such as penicillin, aspirin, and morphine. Many of these compounds can be bound to plasma proteins and are not freely filtered in the glomerulus. Therefore, excretion by filtration alone eliminates only a small portion of these potentially toxic substances from the body.[2]

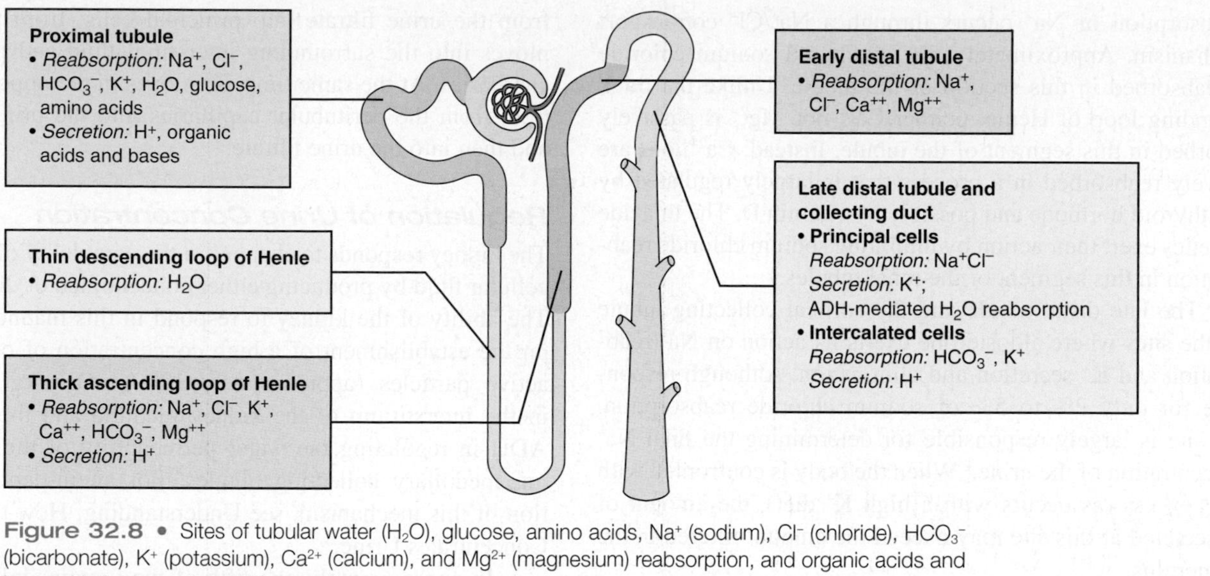

Figure 32.8 • Sites of tubular water (H_2O), glucose, amino acids, Na^+ (sodium), Cl^- (chloride), HCO_3^- (bicarbonate), K^+ (potassium), Ca^{2+} (calcium), and Mg^{2+} (magnesium) reabsorption, and organic acids and bases, H^+ (hydrogen), and K^+ secretion.

The Loop of Henle. The loop of Henle plays an important role in controlling the concentration of the urine. It does this by establishing a high concentration of osmotically active particles in the interstitium surrounding the medullary collecting tubules where the antidiuretic hormone (ADH) exerts its effects.

The loop of Henle is divided into three segments—the thin descending segment, the thin ascending segment, and the thick ascending segment. The loop of Henle, taken as a whole, always reabsorbs more Na^+ and Cl^- than water. This is in contrast to the proximal tubule, which reabsorbs Na^+ and water in equal proportions. The thin descending limb is highly permeable to water and moderately permeable to urea, Na^+, and other ions. As the urine filtrate moves down the descending limb, water moves out of the filtrate into the surrounding interstitium. Thus, the osmolality of the filtrate reaches its highest point at the elbow of the loop of Henle. In contrast to the descending limb, the ascending limb of the loop of Henle is impermeable to water.[2] In this segment, solutes are reabsorbed, but water cannot follow and remains in the filtrate. As a result, the tubular filtrate becomes more and more dilute, often reaching an osmolality of 100 mOsm/kg of water as it enters the distal convoluted tubule, compared with the 285 mOsm/kg of water in plasma.[2] This allows for excretion of free water from the body. For this reason, it is often called the *diluting segment*.[2]

The thick segment of the loop of Henle begins in the ascending limb where the epithelial cells become thickened. As with the thin ascending limb, this segment is impermeable to water. The thick segment contains a $Na^+/K^+/2Cl^-$ cotransport system[6] (Fig. 32.9). This system involves the cotransport of a positively charged Na^+ and a positively charged K^+ ion accompanied by two negatively charged Cl^- ions. The gradient for the operation of this cotransport system is provided by the basolateral Na^+/K^+-ATPase pump, which maintains a low intracellular sodium concentration. Approximately 20% to 25% of the filtered load of Na^+, K^+, and Cl^- is reabsorbed in the thick loop of Henle. Movement of these ions out of the tubule leads to the development of a transmembrane potential that favors the passive reabsorption of small divalent cations such as Ca^{2+} and magnesium (Mg^{2+}).[6] The thick ascending loop of Henle is the site of action for the powerful "loop" diuretics (*e.g.*, furosemide [Lasix]), which exert their action by inhibiting the $Na^+/K^+/2Cl^-$ cotransporters.[7]

Distal and Collecting Tubules. Like the thick ascending loop of Henle, the distal convoluted tubule is relatively impermeable to water, and reabsorption of sodium chloride from this segment further dilutes the tubular fluid.

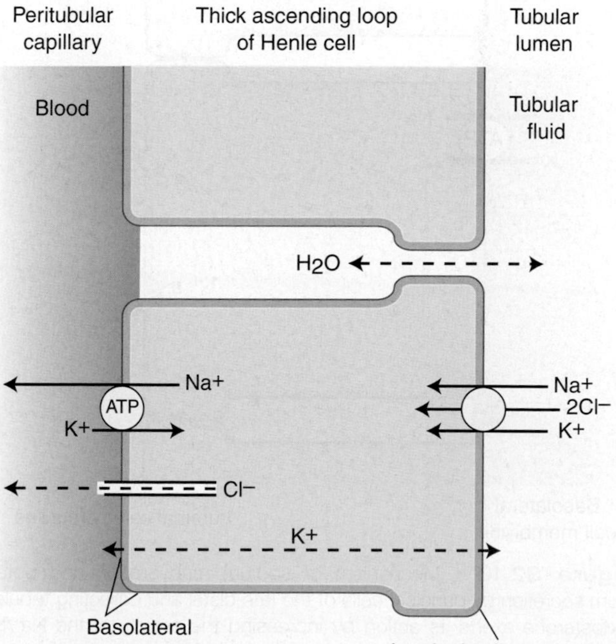

Figure 32.9 • Sodium, chloride, and potassium reabsorption in the thick segment of the loop of Henle.

Reabsorption of Na^+ occurs through a Na^+/Cl^- cotransport mechanism. Approximately 5% of filtered sodium chloride is reabsorbed in this section of the tubule. Unlike the thick ascending loop of Henle, neither Ca^{2+} nor Mg^{2+} is passively absorbed in this segment of the tubule. Instead, Ca^{2+} ions are actively reabsorbed in a process that is largely regulated by parathyroid hormone and possibly by vitamin D. The thiazide diuretics exert their action by inhibiting sodium chloride reabsorption in this segment of the renal tubules.[7]

The late distal tubule and the cortical collecting tubule are the sites where aldosterone exerts its action on Na^+ reabsorption and K^+ secretion and elimination. Although responsible for only 2% to 5% of sodium chloride reabsorption, this site is largely responsible for determining the final Na^+ concentration of the urine.[2] When the body is confronted with a K^+ excess (as occurs with a high K^+ diet), the amount of K^+ secreted at this site may exceed the amount filtered in the glomerulus.

The mechanism for Na^+ reabsorption and K^+ secretion in this section of the nephron is distinct from other tubular segments. This segment is composed of two types of cells, the *intercalated cells*, where K^+ is reabsorbed and H^+ is secreted, and the *principal cells*, where aldosterone exerts its action.[6] The secretion of H^+ into the tubular fluid by the intercalated cells is accompanied by the reabsorption of HCO_3^-. The intercalated cells can also reabsorb K^+. The principal cells reabsorb Na^+ and facilitate the movement of K^+ into the urine filtrate (Fig. 32.10). Under the influence of aldosterone, Na^+ moves from the urine filtrate into principal cells; from there, Na^+ moves into the surrounding interstitial fluid and peritubular capillaries. At the same time, K^+ moves in the opposite direction, from the peritubular capillaries into the principal cells and then into the urine filtrate.[6]

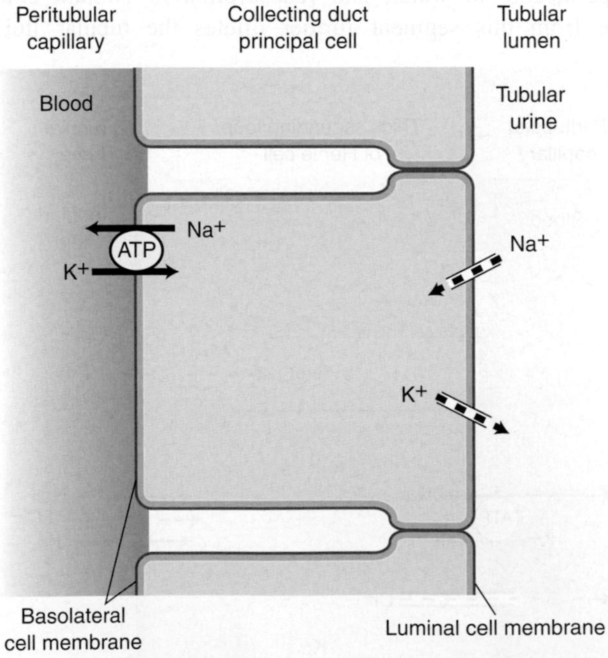

Figure 32.10 • Mechanism of sodium reabsorption and potassium secretion by principal cells of the late distal and collecting tubules. Aldosterone exerts its action by increasing the activity of the Na^+/K^+-ATPase pump that transports sodium outward through the basolateral membrane of the cell and into the blood at the same time it pumps potassium into the cell. Aldosterone also increases the permeability of the luminal membrane for potassium.

Regulation of Urine Concentration

The kidney responds to changes in the osmolality of the extracellular fluid by producing either concentrated or dilute urine. The ability of the kidney to respond in this manner depends on the establishment of a high concentration of osmotically active particles (approximately 1200 mOsm/kg of water) in the interstitium of the kidney medulla and the action of ADH in regulating the water permeability of the surrounding medullary collecting tubules. For an in-depth description of this mechanism, see Understanding: How the Kidney Concentrates Urine.[6]

In approximately one fifth of the juxtamedullary nephrons, the loops of Henle and special hairpin-shaped capillaries called the *vasa recta* descend into the medullary portion of the kidney. There, they form a countercurrent system that controls water and solute movement so that water is kept out of the area surrounding the tubule and solutes are retained.[6] The term *countercurrent* refers to a flow of fluids in opposite directions in adjacent structures. In this case, there is an exchange of solutes between the adjacent descending and ascending loops of Henle and between the ascending and descending sections of the vasa recta. Because of these exchange processes, a high concentration of osmotically active particles (approximately 1200 mOsm/kg of water) collects in the interstitium of the kidney medulla. The presence of these osmotically active particles in the interstitium surrounding the medullary collecting tubules facilitates the ADH-mediated reabsorption of water.[6]

ADH assists in maintenance of the extracellular fluid volume by controlling the permeability of the medullary collecting tubules. Osmoreceptors in the hypothalamus sense an increase in osmolality of extracellular fluids and stimulate the release of ADH from the posterior pituitary gland. In exerting its effect, ADH, also known as *vasopressin*, binds to receptors on the basolateral side of the tubular cells.[6] Binding of ADH to the vasopressin receptors causes water channels, known as *aquaporin-2 channels*, to move into the luminal side of the tubular cell membrane, producing a marked increase in water permeability. At the basolateral side of the membrane, water exits the tubular cell into the hyperosmotic interstitium of the medullary area, where it enters the peritubular capillaries for return to the vascular system.[6]

Regulation of Renal Blood Flow

In the adult, the kidneys are perfused with 1000 to 1300 mL of blood per minute, or 20% to 25% of the cardiac output. This large blood flow is mainly needed to ensure a sufficient GFR for the removal of waste products from the blood, rather than for the metabolic needs of the kidney. Feedback mechanisms,

Understanding How the Kidney Concentrates Urine

The osmolarity of body fluids relies heavily on the ability of the kidney to produce dilute or concentrated urine. Urine concentration depends on three factors: (a) the osmolarity of interstitial fluids in the urine-concentrating part of the kidney, (b) the ADH, and (c) the action of ADH on the cells in the collecting tubules of the kidney.

Osmolarity

In approximately one fifth of the juxtamedullary nephrons, the loops of Henle and special hairpin-shaped capillaries called the *vasa recta* descend into the medullary portion of the kidney to form a countercurrent system—a set of parallel passages in which the contents flow in opposite directions. The countercurrent design serves to increase thc osmolarity in this part of the kidney by promoting the exchange of solutes between the adjacent descending and ascending loops of Henle and between the descending and ascending sections of the vasa recta. Because of these exchange processes, a high concentration of osmotically active particles (approximately 1200 mOsm/kg of water) collects in the interstitium surrounding the collecting tubules where the ADH-mediated reabsorption of water takes place.

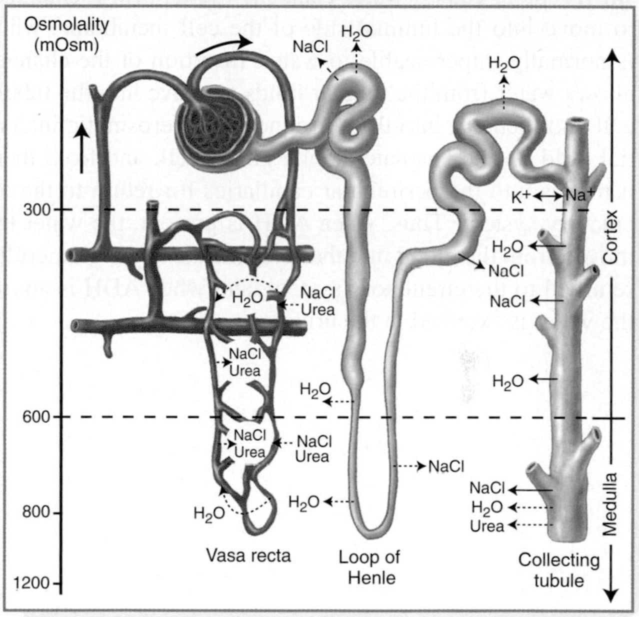

Antidiuretic Hormone

ADH, which regulates the ability of the kidneys to concentrate urine, is synthesized by neurons in the hypothalamus and transported down their axons to the posterior pituitary gland and then released into the circulation. One of the main stimuli for synthesis and release of ADH is an increase in serum osmolarity. ADH release is also controlled by cardiovascular reflexes that respond to changes in blood pressure or blood volume.

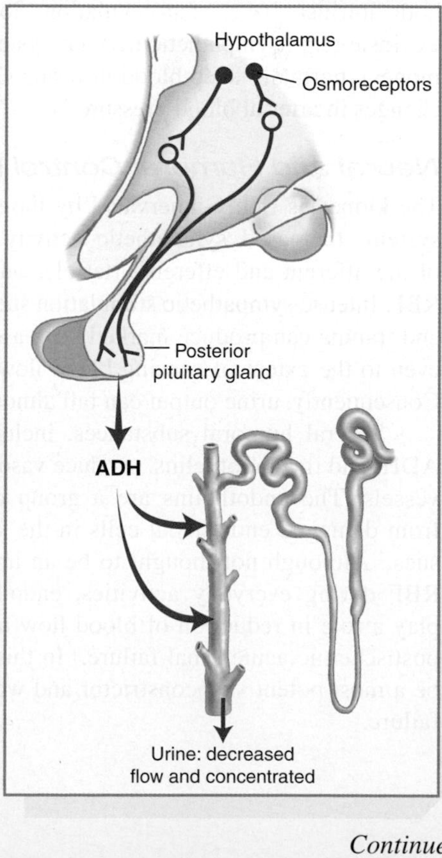

Continued

Understanding How the Kidney Concentrates Urine *(Continued)*

Action of ADH

ADH, also known as vasopressin, acts at the level of the collecting tubule to increase water absorption. It exerts its action by binding to vasopressin receptors on the basolateral membrane of the tubular cell. Binding of ADH to the vasopressin receptors causes water channels (*aquaporin-2 channels*) to move into the luminal side of the cell membrane, which is normally impermeable to water. Insertion of the channels allows water from the tubular fluids to move into the tubular cell and then out into the surrounding hyperosmotic interstitial fluid on the basolateral side of the cell, and from there, it moves into the peritubular capillaries for return to the circulatory system. Thus, when ADH is present, the water that moved from the blood into the urine filtrate in the glomeruli is returned to the circulatory system, and when ADH is absent, the water is excreted in the urine.

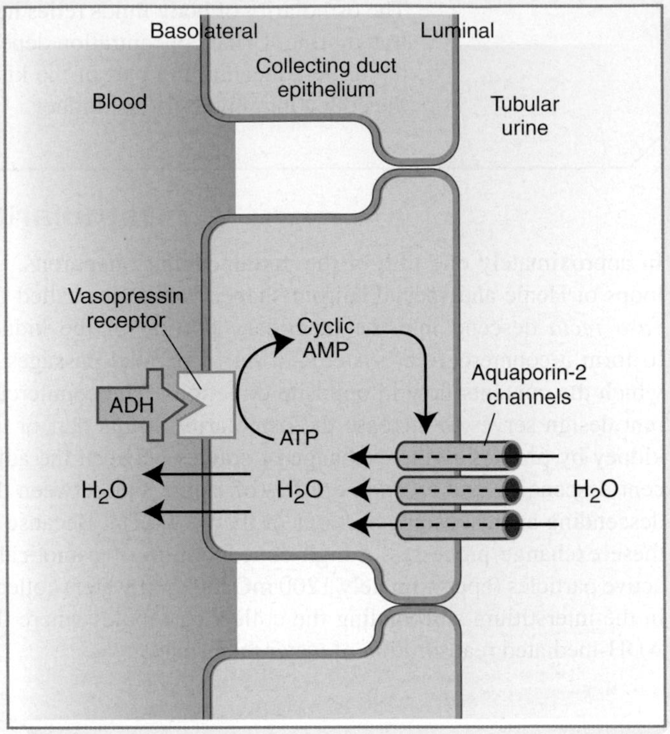

both intrinsic (*e.g.*, autoregulation, local hormones) and extrinsic (*e.g.*, sympathetic nervous system, blood-borne hormones), normally keep blood flow and GFR constant despite changes in arterial blood pressure.[2]

Neural and Humoral Control Mechanisms

The kidney is richly innervated by the sympathetic nervous system. Increased sympathetic activity causes constriction of the afferent and efferent arterioles and thus a decrease in RBF. Intense sympathetic stimulation such as occurs in shock and trauma can produce marked decreases in RBF and GFR, even to the extent of causing blood flow to cease altogether. Consequently, urine output can fall almost to zero.[2]

Several humoral substances, including angiotensin II, ADH, and the endothelins, produce vasoconstriction of renal vessels. The endothelins are a group of peptides released from damaged endothelial cells in the kidney and other tissues.[2] Although not thought to be an important regulator of RBF during everyday activities, endothelin 1 (ET-1) may play a role in reduction of blood flow in conditions such as postischemic acute renal failure.[6] In this situation, ET-1 can be a most potent vasoconstrictor and worsen the acute renal failure.

Other substances such as dopamine, nitric oxide, and prostaglandins (*i.e.*, E_2 and I_2) produce vasodilation. Nitric oxide, a vasodilator produced by the vascular endothelium, appears to be important in preventing excessive vasoconstriction of renal blood vessels and allowing normal excretion of sodium and water. Prostaglandins are a group of mediators of cell function that are produced locally and exert their effects locally. Although prostaglandins do not appear to be of major importance in regulating RBF and GFR under normal conditions, they may protect the kidneys against the vasoconstricting effects of sympathetic stimulation and angiotensin II.[6] Nonsteroidal anti-inflammatory drugs (NSAIDs) that inhibit prostaglandin synthesis may cause reduction in RBF and GFR under certain conditions and should be used cautiously with people who have hypertension or kidney disease.[8]

Autoregulatory Mechanisms

A process called autoregulation maintains the constancy of RBF. Normally, autoregulation of blood flow is designed to maintain blood flow at a level consistent with the metabolic needs of the tissues. In the kidney, autoregulation of blood flow also must allow for precise regulation of solute and water excretion. For autoregulation to occur, the resistance to blood flow through the kidneys must be varied in direct proportion to the arterial pressure. The exact mechanisms responsible for the intrarenal regulation of blood flow are unclear. One of the proposed mechanisms is a direct effect on vascular smooth muscle that causes the blood vessels to relax when there is an increase in blood pressure and to constrict when there is a decrease in pressure. A second proposed mechanism is the juxtaglomerular complex.[2]

The Juxtaglomerular Complex. The juxtaglomerular complex is thought to represent a feedback control system that links changes in GFR with RBF. The juxtaglomerular complex is located at the site where the distal tubule extends back to the glomerulus and then passes between the afferent and efferent arterioles[2] (Fig. 32.11). The distal tubular site that is nearest to the glomerulus is characterized by densely nucleated cells called the *macula densa.*[2] In the adjacent afferent arteriole, the smooth muscle cells of the media are modified as special secretory cells called *juxtaglomerular cells*. These cells contain granules of inactive renin, an enzyme that functions in the conversion of angiotensinogen to angiotensin.[2]

Renin functions by means of angiotensin II to produce vasoconstriction of the efferent arteriole to prevent large decreases in the GFR. Angiotensin II also increases sodium reabsorption indirectly by stimulating aldosterone secretion from the adrenal gland and directly by increasing sodium reabsorption by the proximal tubule cells. The renin–angiotensin–aldosterone mechanism is illustrated in Figure 32.12.

Because of its location between the afferent and efferent arterioles, the juxtaglomerular complex plays an essential role in linking RBF to both GFR and the composition of the distal tubular fluid. Specialized juxtaglomerular cells monitor the systemic arterial blood pressure by sensing the stretch of the afferent arteriole and also monitor the concentration of sodium chloride in the tubular filtrate as it passes through the macula densa. This information is then used in determining how much renin should be released to keep the arterial blood pressure within its normal range and maintain a relatively constant GFR.[2] It is thought that a decrease in the GFR slows the flow rate of the urine filtrate in the ascending loop of Henle, thereby increasing sodium and chloride reabsorption. This, in turn, decreases the delivery of sodium chloride to the macula densa.

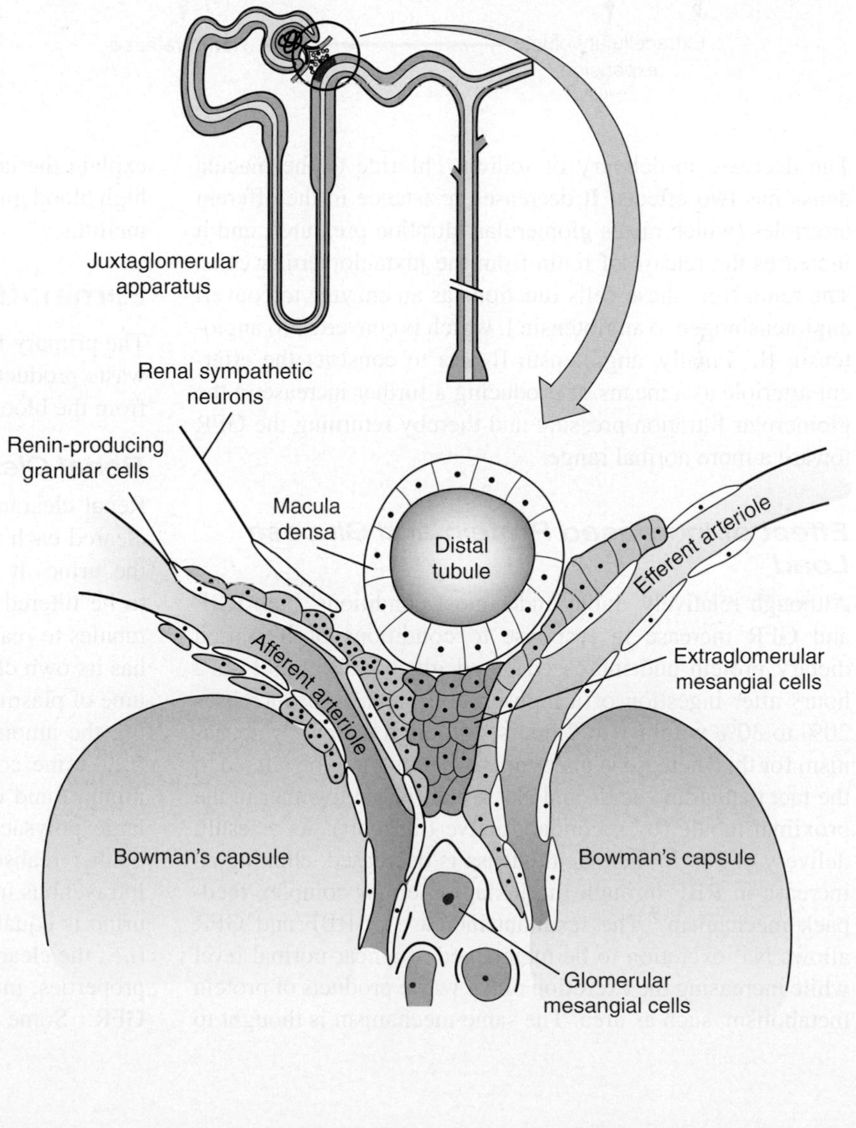

Figure 32.11 • Juxtaglomerular apparatus and macula densa in tubuloglomerular feedback. The juxtaglomerular apparatus and macula densa cells at the beginning of the distal tubule are in close proximity. Chloride delivery is sensed by the N⁺–K⁺–2Cl⁻ cotransporter in the thick ascending limb, and feedback regulates GFR. Renin release is also regulated at this site. (From Rennke H. G., Denker B. M. (2014). *Renal pathophysiology: The essentials* (4th ed., Fig. 1.9, p. 21). Philadelphia, PA: Lippincott Williams & Wilkins.)

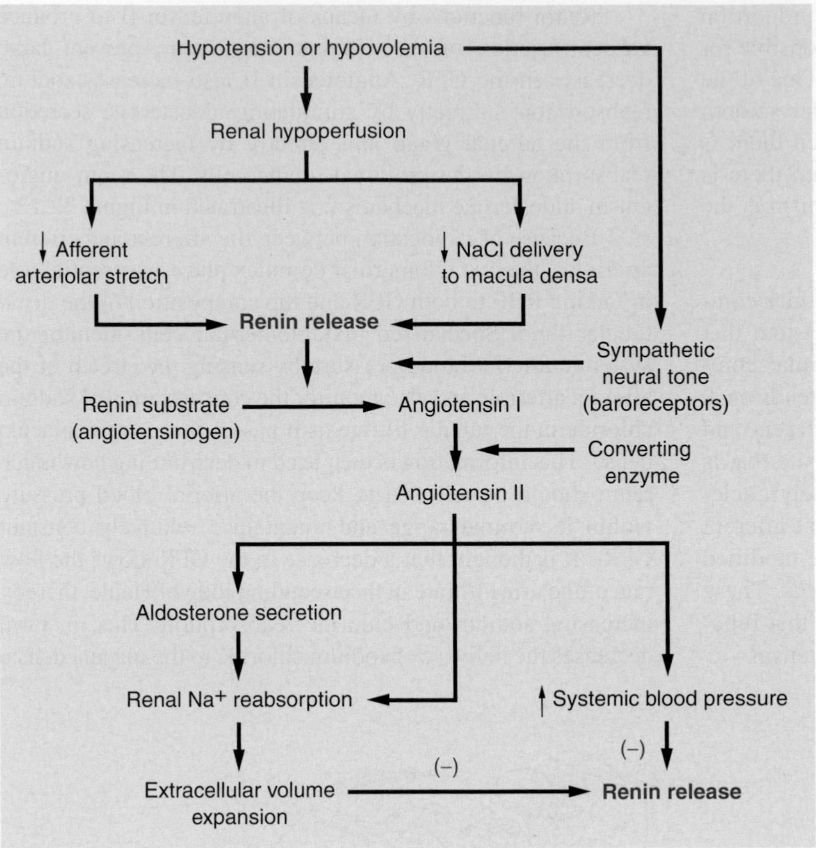

Figure 32.12 • Pathway of angiotensin production. (From Rennke H. G., Denker B. M. (2014). *Renal pathophysiology: The essentials* (4th ed., Fig. 2.6, p. 49). Philadelphia, PA: Lippincott Williams & Wilkins.)

The decrease in delivery of sodium chloride to the macula densa has two effects: It decreases resistance in the afferent arterioles (which raises glomerular filtration pressure), and it increases the release of renin from the juxtaglomerular cells. The renin from these cells functions as an enzyme to convert angiotensinogen to angiotensin I, which is converted to angiotensin II.[2] Finally, angiotensin II acts to constrict the efferent arteriole as a means of producing a further increase in the glomerular filtration pressure and thereby returning the GFR toward a more normal range.

Effect of Increased Protein and Glucose Load

Although relatively stable under most conditions, both RBF and GFR increase in response to conditions of increased dietary protein and increased blood glucose. Within 1 to 2 hours after ingestion of a high-protein meal, RBF increases 20% to 30% within 1 to 2 hours. Although the exact mechanism for this increase is uncertain, it is thought to be related to the fact that amino acids and Na^+ are absorbed together in the proximal tubule (by secondary active transport). As a result, delivery of Na^+ to the macula densa is decreased, eliciting an increase in RBF through the juxtaglomerular complex feedback mechanism.[2] The resultant increase in RBF and GFR allows Na^+ excretion to be maintained at a near-normal level while increasing the excretion of the waste products of protein metabolism, such as urea. The same mechanism is thought to explain the large increases in RBF and GFR that occur with high blood glucose levels in people with uncontrolled diabetes mellitus.[2]

Elimination Functions of the Kidney

The primary functions of the kidney are elimination of water, waste products, excess electrolytes, and unwanted substances from the blood.[2]

Renal Clearance

Renal clearance is the volume of plasma that is completely cleared each minute of any substance that finds its way into the urine. It is determined by the ability of the substance to be filtered in the glomeruli and the capacity of the renal tubules to reabsorb or secrete the substance. Every substance has its own clearance rate, the units of which are always volume of plasma per unit time. It can be determined by measuring the amount of a substance that is excreted in the urine (*i.e.*, urine concentration × urine flow rate in milliliters per minute) and dividing by its plasma concentration.[9] Inulin, a large polysaccharide, is freely filtered in the glomeruli and neither reabsorbed nor secreted by the tubular cells.[2] After intravenous injection, the amount of inulin that appears in the urine is equal to the amount that is filtered in the glomeruli (*i.e.*, the clearance rate is equal to the GFR). Because of these properties, inulin can be used as a laboratory measure of the GFR.[2] Some substances, such as urea, are freely filtered in the glomeruli, but the volume that is cleared from the plasma is less than the GFR, indicating that at least some of the substance is being reabsorbed. At normal plasma levels, glucose has a clearance of zero because it is reabsorbed in the tubules and none appears in the urine.

Regulation of Electrolytes

Elimination of electrolytes, particularly Na^+ and K^+, is regulated by the GFR and by humoral agents that control their reabsorption. Aldosterone functions in the regulation of Na^+ and K^+ elimination. Reabsorption of Na^+ in the distal tubule and collecting duct is highly variable and depends on the presence of aldosterone secretion by the adrenal gland. In the presence of aldosterone, almost all the sodium in the distal tubular fluid is reabsorbed, and the urine essentially becomes sodium-free. In the absence of aldosterone, virtually no sodium is reabsorbed from the distal tubule. The remarkable ability of the distal tubular and collecting duct cells to alter sodium reabsorption in relation to changes in aldosterone allows the kidneys to excrete urine with sodium levels that range from a few tenths of a gram to 40 g/day.[2]

Free filtration of K+ also occurs at the glomerulus; however, K^+ is reabsorbed from and secreted into the tubular fluid. The secretion of K^+ into the tubular fluid occurs in the distal tubule and is also regulated by aldosterone. Only approximately 70 mEq of K^+ is delivered to the distal tubule each day, but the average person consumes this much and more K^+ in the diet. Excess K^+ that is not filtered in the glomerulus and delivered to the collecting tubule therefore must be secreted (*i.e.*, transported from the blood into the tubular filtrate) for elimination from the body.[2] In the absence of aldosterone, as in Addison disease, K^+ secretion becomes minimal. In these circumstances, K^+ reabsorption exceeds secretion, and blood levels of K^+ increase.

Also contributing to the excretion of Na^+ and water by the kidney are the *natriuretic peptides*, a group of peptides secreted by the heart in response to the stretch of cardiac muscle fibers. The primary renal effect of this group of chemicals is to increase the renal excretion of sodium (natriuresis), with a resultant osmotic increase in the excretion of water. This loss of sodium and water leads to a reduction in cardiac preload, which creates a negative feedback loop to decrease cardiac muscle stretch.[2] Atrial muscle cells release *atrial natriuretic peptide (ANP)* in response to muscle stretch. The primary effect of ANP is to inhibit sodium and water reabsorption, with action predominant in the collecting ducts. ANP also acts to disrupt the renin–angiotensin–aldosterone cascade by inhibiting the renal secretion of renin. This disruption of the RAA cascade thus further decreases the reabsorption of sodium and water by the renal tubules.[2] Ventricular muscle cells release a similar natriuretic peptide, the *B-type natriuretic peptide (BNP)* in response to ventricular muscle stretch. BNP and a precursor molecule N-terminal pro-BNP (NT-proBNP) have been demonstrated to be useful markers for the diagnosis and management of heart failure[10] and are showing promise to serve as useful markers for predicting outcomes in myocardial infarction.[11,12]

Regulation of pH

The kidneys regulate body pH by conserving HCO_3^- and eliminating H^+. Most H^+ excreted in the urine is due to tubular secretory mechanisms. The lowest tubular fluid pH that can be achieved is 4.4 to 4.5.[13,14] The ability of the kidneys to excrete H^+ depends on buffers in the urine that combine with the H^+. The three major urine buffers are bicarbonate (HCO_3^-), phosphate, and ammonia. The combination of HCO_3^- and H^+ in the renal tubule results in the formation of carbonic acid, which then dissociates into carbon dioxide and water. The carbon dioxide is then absorbed into the tubular cells, and HCO_3^- is regenerated inside the tubule cells through the action of the enzyme carbonic anhydrase. In the second renal buffering system, phosphate ions (which are produced by cells as end products of metabolic processes) join with H^+ in the renal tubules, and then the resultant compound is eliminated in the urine. In the third renal buffer system, ammonia is synthesized in tubular cells by deamination of the amino acid glutamine (which is produced by the liver during amino acid metabolism and then transported to the kidneys). Ammonia diffuses into the tubular fluid, where it combines with H^+, and the compound molecule is eliminated through the urine.[2]

KEY POINTS

THE FUNCTIONS OF THE KIDNEY

- The kidney regulates the composition and pH of body fluids through the reabsorption and elimination or conservation of water and substances, particularly the electrolytes Na^+, K^+, H^+, Cl^-, and HCO_3^-.
- The kidney regulates the osmolality of the extracellular fluid through the action of ADH.
- The kidney plays a central role in blood pressure regulation through the influences of the renin–angiotensin–aldosterone and ANP mechanisms on Na^+ and water elimination.

pH-Dependent Elimination of Organic Ions

The proximal tubule actively secretes large amounts of different organic anions. Foreign anions (*e.g.*, salicylates, penicillin) and endogenously produced anions (*e.g.*, bile acids, uric acid) are actively secreted into the tubular fluid. Most of the anions that are secreted use the same transport system, allowing the kidneys to rid the body of many different drugs and environmental agents.[2] Because the same transport system is shared by different anions, there is competition for transport such that elevated levels of one substance tend to inhibit the secretion of other anions. The proximal tubules also possess an active transport system for organic cations that is analogous to that for organic anions.

Uric Acid Elimination

Uric acid (an organic anion) is a product of purine metabolism. Excessively high blood levels (*i.e.*, hyperuricemia) can cause gout, and high levels of uric acid in the urine can cause kidney stones. Uric acid is freely filtered in the glomerulus and is reabsorbed and secreted in the proximal tubules.[5] Tubular reabsorption normally exceeds secretion, and the net effect is removal of uric acid from the filtrate. Although the rate of reabsorption exceeds secretion, the secretory process is homeostatically controlled to maintain a constant plasma level. Many people with elevated uric acid levels secrete less uric acid compared to people with normal uric acid levels.[5]

Urea Elimination

Urea is formed in the liver as a by-product of protein metabolism and is eliminated entirely by the kidneys. Healthy adults produce urea in the range of 25 to 30 g/day. Blood urea levels rise with a high-protein diet, excessive tissue breakdown, or gastrointestinal bleeding.[2] In gastrointestinal bleeding, the intestinal flora breaks down the blood to form ammonia, which is then absorbed into the portal venous circulation and transported to the liver, where it is converted to urea before being released into the bloodstream. The kidneys then regulate blood urea nitrogen (BUN) levels, maintaining a normal BUN in the range of 8 to 25 mg/dL (2.9 to 8.9 mmol/L).[2] During periods of dehydration, the blood volume and GFR drop, causing BUN levels to increase. This rise in BUN occurs because when GFR is reduced, the filtrate moves more slowly through the tubules, allowing more time for urea resorption. In contrast, when the GFR is high, only small amounts of urea are reabsorbed into the blood.[2]

Drug Elimination

Many drugs are eliminated in the urine. Only drugs that are not bound to plasma proteins are filtered in the glomerulus and therefore able to be eliminated by the kidneys.[7] Because uric acid competes for the same anion transport systems as some drugs (such as aspirin, sulfinpyrazone, and probenecid), these drugs can affect the blood levels of uric acid and therefore may not be indicated for use in persons with gout. Thiazide and loop diuretics (*i.e.*, furosemide and ethacrynic acid) also can cause hyperuricemia and gout, presumably through a decrease in extracellular fluid volume and enhanced uric acid reabsorption.[6]

Endocrine Functions of the Kidney

In addition to regulating body fluids and electrolytes, the kidneys function as an endocrine organ by producing chemical mediators that travel through the blood to distant sites where they exert their actions. Endocrine functions of the kidneys include:

- Assisting with blood pressure regulation through the renin–angiotensin–aldosterone mechanism
- Regulation of red blood cell production through the synthesis of erythropoietin
- Assisting with calcium homeostasis by activating vitamin D

The Renin–Angiotensin–Aldosterone Mechanism

As introduced earlier, the renin–angiotensin–aldosterone mechanism plays an important part in short- and long-term regulation of blood pressure. Renin is an enzyme that is synthesized and stored in the juxtaglomerular cells of the kidney. This enzyme is thought to be released in response to a decrease in RBF or a change in the composition of the distal tubular fluid or as the result of sympathetic nervous system stimulation. Renin itself has no direct effect on blood pressure. Rather, it acts enzymatically to convert a circulating plasma protein called *angiotensinogen* to angiotensin I. Angiotensin I, which has few vasoconstrictor properties, leaves the kidneys and enters the circulation; as it is circulated through the lungs, *angiotensin-converting enzyme* catalyzes the conversion of angiotensin I to angiotensin II. Angiotensin II is a potent vasoconstrictor, and it acts directly on the kidneys to decrease salt and water excretion. Both mechanisms have relatively short periods of action. Angiotensin II also stimulates aldosterone secretion by the adrenal gland. Aldosterone acts on the distal tubule to increase sodium reabsorption and exerts a longer-term effect on the maintenance of blood pressure. Renin also functions via angiotensin II to produce constriction of the efferent arteriole as a means of preventing a serious decrease in glomerular filtration pressure.[2]

Erythropoietin

Erythropoietin is a glycoprotein hormone that is produced by fibroblasts in the renal interstitium and regulates the production of red blood cells in the bone marrow. The synthesis of erythropoietin is stimulated by tissue hypoxia, which may be brought about by anemia, residence at high altitudes, or impaired oxygenation of tissues because of cardiac or pulmonary disease. Persons with end-stage kidney disease often are anemic because of an inability of the kidneys to produce erythropoietin. This anemia usually is managed by the administration of a recombinant erythropoietin (epoetin alfa) produced through DNA technology to stimulate erythropoiesis.[15]

Vitamin D

Activation of vitamin D occurs in the kidneys. Vitamin D increases calcium absorption from the gastrointestinal tract and helps to regulate calcium deposition in the bone. It also has a weak stimulatory effect on renal calcium absorption. Although vitamin D is not synthesized and released from an endocrine gland, it often is considered as a hormone because of its pathway of molecular activation and mechanism of action.

Vitamin D exists in two forms—natural vitamin D (cholecalciferol), produced in the skin from ultraviolet irradiation, and synthetic vitamin D (ergocalciferol), derived from irradiation of ergosterol. The active form of vitamin D is 1,25-dihydroxycholecalciferol. Cholecalciferol and ergocalciferol must undergo chemical transformation to become active: first to 25-hydroxycholecalciferol in the liver and then to 1,25-dihydroxycholecalciferol in the kidneys. People with end-stage renal disease are unable to transform vitamin D to its active form and may require pharmacologic preparations of the active vitamin (calcitriol) for maintaining mineralization of their bones.[6]

Action of Diuretics

Diuretics are drugs that increase urine volume. Many diuretic agents (loop diuretics, thiazide diuretic, and potassium-sparing diuretics) exert their effects by blocking the reabsorption of sodium in the renal tubules. Others exert osmotic effects that prevent water reabsorption in the water-permeable parts of the nephron.[7]

Diuretics That Block Sodium Reabsorption

Most diuretics share the same mechanism of action—blockade of Na^+ and Cl^- reabsorption. By blocking the reabsorption of these solutes, diuretics create an osmotic pressure gradient within the nephron that prevents the passive reabsorption of water. Thus, diuretics cause both Na^+ and water to be retained in the tubule, thereby promoting the excretion of both. The increase in urine flow that a diuretic produces is related to the amount of Na^+ and Cl^- reabsorption that it blocks. Because the amount of Na^+ becomes progressively less as the urine filtrate flows from the proximal tubule to the collecting ducts, drugs that act early in the nephron have the opportunity to block the greatest amount of Na^+ reabsorption. Approximately 65% of the Na^+ filtered in the glomeruli of the kidney is reabsorbed in the proximal tubule, 20% is reabsorbed in the thick ascending loop of Henle, 10% is reabsorbed in the early distal convoluted tubule, and 2% to 5% is reabsorbed in the late distal and cortical collecting tubules (Fig. 32.13).[6]

The so-called loop diuretics exert their effect in the thick ascending loop of Henle. Because of their site of action, these drugs are the most effective diuretic agents available. These drugs inhibit the coupled $Na^+/K^+/2Cl^-$ transport system on the luminal side of the ascending loop of Henle (see Fig. 32.8). By inhibiting this transport system, they reduce the reabsorption of sodium chloride, decrease K^+ reabsorption, and increase Ca^{2+} and Mg^{2+} elimination.[7] Prolonged use of loop diuretics can cause significant loss of Mg^{2+} in some people. Because Ca^{2+} is actively reabsorbed in the distal convoluted tubule, loop diuretics usually do not cause hypocalcemia. The loop diuretics may also increase uric acid retention and impair glucose tolerance.

The *thiazide diuretics* act by preventing the reabsorption of sodium chloride in the early distal convoluted tubule. Because of their later site of action, the thiazide diuretics are less effective than loop diuretics in terms of effecting diuresis. However, the thiazide diuretics produce increased loss of K^+ in the urine, uric acid retention, and some impairment in glucose tolerance. In contrast to the loop diuretics, which inhibit Ca^{2+} reabsorption, the thiazide diuretics actually enhance Ca^{2+} reabsorption in the distal convoluted tubule.[7]

The *aldosterone antagonists*, also called *potassium-sparing diuretics*, reduce Na^+ reabsorption and decrease K^+ secretion in the late distal tubule and cortical collecting tubule sites regulated by aldosterone (see Fig. 32.8). Because K^+ secretion is linked to K^+ reabsorption in this segment of the tubule, these

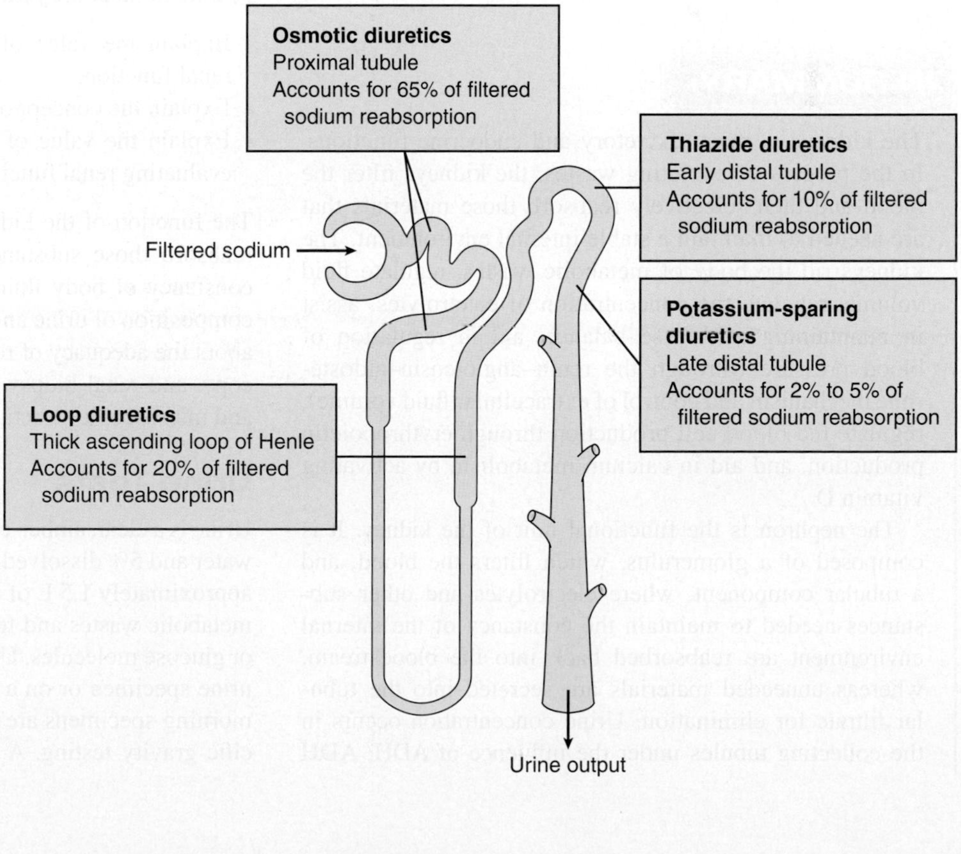

Figure 32.13 • Tubular sites of diuretic action and percentage of sodium reabsorption.

agents may reduce K^+ excretion and cause severe hyperkalemia. These agents may also interfere with secretion of H^+ ions in the collecting duct, contributing to the development of metabolic acidosis.[7]

There are two types of potassium-sparing diuretics—those that act as direct aldosterone antagonists and those that act independently of aldosterone. The first type (*e.g.*, spironolactone) binds to the mineralocorticoid receptor in the tubule, preventing aldosterone from entering the cell and exerting its effects. The second type (*e.g.*, triamterene, amiloride) does not bind to the aldosterone receptor but instead directly interferes with sodium entry through the sodium-selective ion channel. The potassium-sparing diuretics produce only mild diuresis because they inhibit such a small percentage of Na^+ sodium reabsorption. Therefore, their main use is in combination with other diuretics to inhibit K^+ secretion by the principal cells. These diuretics may also be used in treatment of conditions associated with mineralocorticoid (*i.e.*, aldosterone) excess.[7]

Osmotic Diuretics

The osmotic diuretics act in the proximal tubule and ascending loop of Henle, both of which are highly permeable to water. In contrast to the loop, thiazide, and potassium-sparing diuretics that exert their effects by blocking specific tubular Na^+ transport mechanisms, the osmotic diuretics, which are filtered but not reabsorbed, cause water to be retained in the urine filtrate and promote water diuresis. One such agent, mannitol, is used mainly to reduce increased intracranial pressure but is occasionally used to promote prompt removal of toxins. Because it is not absorbed, mannitol must be given parenterally to act as a diuretic. If given orally, it causes osmotic diarrhea.[7]

IN SUMMARY

The kidneys perform excretory and endocrine functions. In the process of excreting wastes, the kidneys filter the blood and then selectively reabsorb those materials that are needed to maintain a stable internal environment. The kidneys rid the body of metabolic wastes, regulate fluid volume, regulate the concentration of electrolytes, assist in maintaining acid–base balance, aid in regulation of blood pressure (through the renin–angiotensin–aldosterone mechanism and control of extracellular fluid volume), regulate red blood cell production through erythropoietin production, and aid in calcium metabolism by activating vitamin D.

The nephron is the functional unit of the kidney. It is composed of a glomerulus, which filters the blood, and a tubular component, where electrolytes and other substances needed to maintain the constancy of the internal environment are reabsorbed back into the bloodstream, whereas unneeded materials are secreted into the tubular filtrate for elimination. Urine concentration occurs in the collecting tubules under the influence of ADH. ADH maintains extracellular volume by returning water to the vascular compartment, producing concentrated urine by removing water from the tubular filtrate.

The GFR is the amount of filtrate that is formed each minute as blood moves through the glomeruli. It is regulated by the arterial blood pressure and RBF in the normally functioning kidney. The juxtaglomerular complex is thought to represent a feedback control system that links changes in the GFR with RBF. Renal clearance is the volume of plasma that is completely cleared each minute of any substance that finds its way into the urine. It is determined by the ability of the substance to be filtered in the glomeruli and the capacity of the renal tubules to reabsorb or secrete the substance.

Diuretics are drugs that increase urine volume. Many diuretic agents (loop diuretics, thiazide diuretics, and potassium-sparing diuretics) exert their effect by blocking the reabsorption of sodium at specific sites in the renal tubules. Others exert osmotic effects that prevent water reabsorption in the water-permeable parts of the nephron. The effectiveness of a diuretic is related to its site of action. Accordingly, diuretics such as the loop diuretics that act in the thick ascending loop of Henle, where approximately 20% of sodium reabsorption takes place, produce the greatest diuresis.

TESTS OF RENAL FUNCTION

After completing this section of the chapter, the learner will be able to meet the following objectives:

- Explain the value of urine specific gravity in evaluating renal function.
- Explain the concept of the GFR.
- Explain the value of serum creatinine and BUN levels in evaluating renal function.

The function of the kidneys is to filter the blood, selectively reabsorb those substances that are needed to maintain the constancy of body fluid, and excrete metabolic wastes. The composition of urine and blood provides valuable information about the adequacy of renal function. Radiologic tests, endoscopy, and renal biopsy provide means for viewing the gross and microscopic structures of the kidneys and urinary system.

Urine Tests

Urine is a clear, amber-colored fluid that is approximately 95% water and 5% dissolved solids. The kidneys normally produce approximately 1.5 L of urine each day. Normal urine contains metabolic wastes and few or no plasma proteins, blood cells, or glucose molecules. Urine tests can be performed on a single urine specimen or on a 24-hour urine specimen. First-voided morning specimens are useful for qualitative protein and specific gravity testing. A freshly voided specimen is the most reliable. Urine specimens that have been left standing may contain lysed red blood cells, disintegrating *casts*, and rapidly multiplying bacteria.[9] Table 32.1 describes urinalysis values for normal urine.

Casts are molds of the distal nephron lumen. A gel-like substance called *Tamm-Horsfall mucoprotein*, which is formed in the tubular epithelium, is the major protein constituent of urinary casts.[6] Casts composed of this gel but devoid of cells are called *hyaline casts*. These casts develop when the protein concentration of the urine is high (as in nephrotic syndrome), urine osmolality is high, and urine pH is low. The inclusion of granules or cells in the matrix of the protein gel leads to the formation of various other types of casts.[6]

Proteinuria is excessive protein excretion in the urine. Because of the glomerular capillary filtration barrier, less than 150 mg/L of protein is excreted in the urine over 24 hours in a healthy person. Urine tests for proteinuria are used to detect abnormal filtering of albumin in the glomeruli or defects in its reabsorption in the renal tubules. A protein reagent dipstick can be used as a rapid screening test for the presence of proteins in the urine. Once the presence of proteinuria has been detected, a 24-hour urine test is often used to quantify the amount of protein that is present.[9]

Albumin, which is the smallest of the plasma proteins, is filtered more readily than globulins or other plasma proteins. Thus, *microalbuminuria* tends to occur long before clinical proteinuria becomes evident. A dipstick test for microalbuminuria is available for screening purposes. The microalbuminuria dipstick method, however, only indicates an increase in urinary albumin that is below the detectable range of the standard proteinuria test. It does not specify the amount of albumin that is present in the urine. Therefore, a 24-hour urine collection is the standard method for detecting microalbuminuria (an albumin excretion >30 mg/day is abnormal).[9]

The *specific gravity* of urine varies with its concentration of solutes. Urine specific gravity provides a valuable index of the hydration status and functional ability of the kidneys. With a normal fluid intake, the usual range of urine specific gravity is 1.010 to 1.025. Healthy kidneys can produce concentrated urine with a specific gravity of 1.030 to 1.040. During periods of marked hydration, the specific gravity can approach 1.000. With diminished renal function, there is a loss of renal concentrating ability, and the urine specific gravity may fall to levels of 1.006 to 1.010.[9] *Urine osmolality*, which depends on the number of particles of solute in a unit of solution, is a more exact measurement of urine concentration than specific gravity.[9] More information concerning renal function can be obtained if the serum and urine osmolality tests are done at the same time. The normal ratio between urine and serum osmolality is 3:1. A high urine-to-serum ratio is seen in concentrated urine. With poor concentrating ability, the ratio is low.[9]

Glomerular Filtration Rate

The GFR can be measured clinically by collecting timed samples of blood and urine. *Creatinine* is produced by muscles as a product of the metabolism of a molecule called creatine. The formation and release of creatinine are relatively constant and proportional to the amount of muscle mass present. Creatinine is freely filtered in the glomeruli, is not reabsorbed from the tubules into the blood, and is only minimally secreted into the tubules from the blood. Therefore, its blood values depend closely on the GFR. The comparison of creatinine levels in the blood and urine can provide a useful measure of GFR. The clearance rate for creatinine is the amount that is completely cleared by the kidneys in 1 minute. The formula is expressed as $C = UV/P$, in which C is the clearance rate (mL/minute), U is the urine concentration (mg/dL), V is the urine volume excreted (mL/minute or 24 hours), and P is plasma concentration (mg/dL).[9]

Normal creatinine clearance is 115 to 125 mL/minute.[9] This value is corrected for body surface area, which reflects the muscle mass where creatinine production takes place. The test may be done on a 24-hour basis, with a blood creatinine level drawn at the completion of a 24-hour urine collection.

TABLE 32.1 NORMAL VALUES FOR ROUTINE URINALYSIS

GENERAL CHARACTERISTICS AND MEASUREMENTS	CHEMICAL DETERMINATIONS	MICROSCOPIC EXAMINATION OF SEDIMENT
Color: yellow amber	Glucose: negative	Casts negative: occasional hyaline casts
Appearance: clear to slightly hazy	Ketones: negative	Red blood cells: negative or rare
Specific gravity: 1.005–1.025 with a normal fluid intake	Blood: negative	Crystals: negative (none)
pH: 4.5–8.0; average person has a pH of about 5–6	Protein: negative	White blood cells: negative or rare
Volume: 600–2500 mL/24 hour; average volume is 1200 mL/24 hour	Bilirubin: negative	Epithelial cells: few; hyaline casts 0–1/1pf (low-power field)
	Urobilinogen: 0.5–4.0 mg/day	
	Nitrate for bacteria: negative	
	Leukocyte esterase: negative	

From Fischbach F., Dunning M. (2014). *A manual of laboratory and diagnostic tests* (9th ed., p. 192). Philadelphia, PA: Lippincott Williams & Wilkins.

In another method, two 1-hour urine specimens are collected, with a blood sample drawn in between.[9]

Although the creatinine clearance test is the traditional method of measuring GFR, most labs are now reporting a calculated "estimated GFR" (or eGFR) as part of various metabolic panels. The eGFR estimates the GFR using a measured plasma creatinine in a mathematical formula accounting for additional factors such as age, sex, and race.[15] Creatinine, which is a waste product of muscle metabolism, is filtered at the glomerulus, which allows serum creatinine levels to provide a good reflection of GFR. However, because creatinine is a molecule produced in the muscle and because muscle mass varies widely among different populations, creatinine levels can be less accurate as a GFR predictor among certain populations. Creatinine levels tend to increase among persons with increased levels of physical activity, higher muscle mass, and diets higher in meat and in persons with better health status.[16]

Additional biologic measures are being introduced into clinical practice to provide better assessment of GFR. The serum protein *cystatin C* has been demonstrated to serve as a useful marker of GFR because it is also filtered at the glomerulus but has a stable production rate across populations. An estimating equation for GFR that combines the effects of creatinine and cystatin C has been developed and has been demonstrated to perform better than eGFR equations based on either creatinine or cystatin C alone.[17] Additional novel biomarkers that are being explored for improving the estimation of GFR are beta-2-microglobulin and beta-trace protein.[17]

Blood Tests

Blood tests can provide valuable information about the kidneys' ability to remove metabolic wastes and maintain normal electrolyte and pH composition of the blood. Normal blood values are listed in Table 32.2. Serum levels of K^+, phosphate, BUN, and creatinine increase in renal failure, whereas serum pH, Ca^{2+}, and HCO_3^- levels decrease in renal failure.[2]

TABLE 32.2 NORMAL BLOOD CHEMISTRY LEVELS

SUBSTANCE	NORMAL VALUE*
BUN	8.0–20.0 mg/dL (2.9–7.1 mmol/L)
Creatinine	0.6–1.2 mg/dL (50–100 mmol/L)
Sodium	135–145 mEq/L (135–145 mmol/L)
Chloride	98–106 mEq/L (98–106 mmol/L)
Potassium	3.5–5 mEq/L (3.5–5 mmol/L)
Carbon dioxide (CO_2 content)	24–29 mEq/L (24–29 mmol/L)
Calcium	8.5–10.5 mg/dL (2.1–2.6 mmol/L)
Phosphate	2.5–4.5 mg/dL (0.77–1.45 mmol/L)
Uric acid	
Male	2.4–7.4 mg/dL (140–440 μmol/L)
Female	1.4–5.8 mg/dL (80–350 μmol/L)
pH	7.35–7.45

*Values may vary among laboratories, depending on the method of analysis used.

Serum Creatinine

As discussed above, serum creatinine levels reflect the GFR. The normal creatinine value is approximately 0.7 mg/dL for a woman with a small frame, approximately 1.0 mg/dL for a normal adult man, and approximately 1.5 mg/dL (60 to 130 mmol/L) for a muscular man.[9] There is an age-related decline in creatinine clearance in many older adults because muscle mass and the GFR decline with age. A normal serum creatinine level usually indicates normal renal function. In addition to its use in calculating the GFR, the serum creatinine level is used in estimating the functional capacity of the kidneys (Fig. 32.14). If the value doubles, the GFR (and renal function) probably has fallen to one half of its normal state. A rise in the serum creatinine level to three times its normal value suggests that there is a 75% loss of renal function, and with creatinine values of 10 mg/dL or more, it can be assumed that approximately 90% of renal function has been lost.[9]

Blood Urea Nitrogen

As discussed above, urea is an end product of protein metabolism, with blood levels regulated by the kidneys. BUN levels are therefore related to the GFR; however, unlike creatinine, BUN is also influenced by protein intake, gastrointestinal bleeding, and hydration status (see earlier discussion of urea elimination for specific mechanisms). Approximately two thirds of renal function must be lost before a significant rise in the BUN level occurs.[9]

Although BUN levels are less specific for renal insufficiency than plasma creatinine levels, the *BUN–creatinine ratio* provides useful diagnostic information. The ratio normally is approximately 10:1. Ratios greater than 15:1 represent prerenal conditions (such as congestive heart failure and upper gastrointestinal tract bleeding) that produce an increase in BUN but not in creatinine. A ratio of less than 10:1 occurs in situations such as liver disease, low-protein diet, or chronic dialysis (because BUN is more readily dialyzable than creatinine).[9]

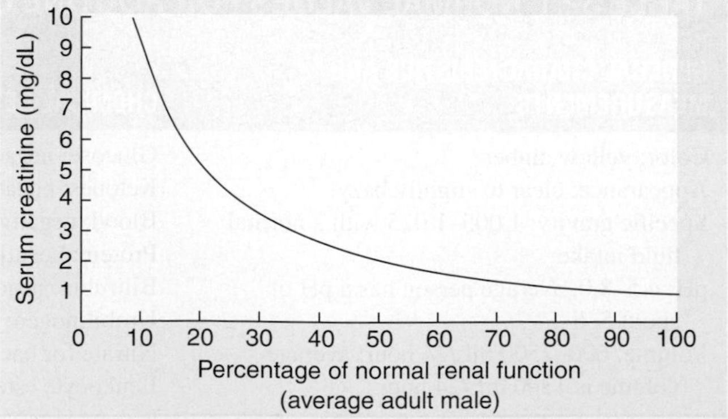

Figure 32.14 • Relation between the percentage of renal function and serum creatinine levels.

Cystoscopy and Ureteroscopy

Cystoscopy is the visualization of the bladder by the insertion of an instrument called a cystoscope through the urethra into the bladder. Cystoscopy provides a means for direct visualization of the urethra, bladder, and ureteral insertion sites. Biopsy specimens, lesions, small stones, and foreign bodies can be removed from the bladder via the cystoscope. Ureteroscopy involves the use of a smaller, thinner scope that may be used to remove stones from the ureter and aid in the treatment of ureteral disorders, such as ureteral strictures.[18]

Ultrasonography

Ultrasonography uses the reflection of ultrasonic waves to visualize the deep structures of the body. The procedure is painless, is noninvasive, and requires no patient preparation. Ultrasonography is used to visualize the structures of the kidneys and has proved useful in the diagnosis of many urinary tract disorders, including congenital anomalies, renal abscesses, hydronephrosis, and kidney stones. It can differentiate a renal cyst from a renal tumor. The use of ultrasonography also enables accurate placement of needles for renal biopsy and catheters for percutaneous nephrostomy.[9]

Radiologic and Other Imaging Studies

Radiologic studies of the kidneys, ureters, and bladder can be used to determine the size, shape, and position of the kidneys and to observe any radiopaque stones that may be in the kidney pelvis or ureters. In excretory urography, or *intravenous pyelography*, a radiopaque dye is injected into a peripheral vein. The dye is then filtered by the glomerulus and excreted into the urine, and x-ray films are taken as the dye moves through the kidneys and ureters.[9]

Urography is used to detect space-occupying lesions of the kidneys, pyelonephritis, hydronephrosis, vesicoureteral reflux, and kidney stones.[9] Some people are allergic to the dye used for urography and may have an anaphylactic reaction after its administration; therefore, every person undergoing urographic studies should be questioned about previous reactions to dyes. If the test is considered essential in a person with a prior allergic reaction, premedication with antihistamines and corticosteroids may be used. The dye also reduces RBF; therefore, acute renal failure can occur, particularly in people with vascular disease or pre-existing renal insufficiency.[9]

Other diagnostic tests include computed tomographic (CT) scans, magnetic resonance imaging (MRI), radionuclide imaging, and renal angiography. CT scans may be used to outline the kidneys and detect renal masses and tumors. MRI is used in imaging the kidneys, retroperitoneum, and urinary bladder. It is particularly useful in evaluating vascular abnormalities in and around the kidneys. Radionuclide imaging involves the injection of a radioactive material that subsequently is detected externally by a scintillation camera, which detects the radioactive emissions. Radionuclide imaging is used to evaluate renal function and the structural integrity of the kidneys and urinary tract. It is particularly useful in evaluating the function of kidney transplants. Renal angiography provides x-ray pictures of the blood vessels that supply the kidneys through the injection of a radiopaque dye directly into the renal artery. Typically, a catheter is introduced through the femoral artery and advanced under fluoroscopic view into the abdominal aorta. The catheter tip then is maneuvered into the renal artery, and the dye is injected.[9] This test is used to evaluate people suspected of having renal artery stenosis, abnormalities of renal blood vessels, or vascular damage to the renal arteries after trauma.

IN SUMMARY

Urinalysis and blood tests that measure serum levels of pH, electrolytes, and by-products of metabolism provide valuable information about renal function. Urine specific gravity is used to assess the kidneys' ability to concentrate urine. Dipstick and 24-hour urine tests for proteinuria and microalbuminuria are used to detect abnormal filtering of albumin in the glomeruli or defects in its reabsorption in the renal tubules. Creatinine is a product of creatine metabolism in muscles that is freely filtered in the glomeruli and neither reabsorbed nor secreted in the tubules; therefore, serum creatinine levels are commonly used to estimate the GFR. Urea is formed in the liver as a by-product of protein metabolism and is eliminated entirely by the kidneys. BUN is therefore related to the GFR but, unlike creatinine, also is influenced by protein intake, gastrointestinal bleeding, and hydration status.

Cystoscopic and ureteroscopic examinations can be used for direct visualization of the urethra, bladder, and ureters. Ultrasonography can be used to determine kidney size, and renal radionuclide imaging can be used to evaluate the kidney structures. Radiologic methods, such as excretory urography, provide a means to examine kidney structures such as the renal calyces, pelvis, ureters, and bladder. Other diagnostic tests include CT scans, MRI, radionuclide imaging, and renal angiography.

GERIATRIC Considerations

- At age 40, renal function begins to decline, but if a person is healthy, the decline has little impact until age 90.[19]
- The following changes are associated with aging and increase the risk for incontinence:
  - Hypertrophy of the bladder muscle and thickening of bladder reduce urine storage.
  - Changes in cortical control of micturition.[20]
- A lower creatinine clearance and specific gravity occur with aging.[20]
- Older adults may be hyperglycemic because of changes in renal threshold for glucose.[20]

PEDIATRIC Considerations

- The bladder empties by reflex mechanisms in the sacral spinal cord during infancy.[21]
- Palpation of the kidneys is not usually possible except in the neonate.[22]
- Young children (less than 2 years) are at increased risk of dehydration because of decreased RBF, reabsorption of amino acids, and inability to fully concentrate urine.[22]
- The kidneys do not reach maturity until about 2 years of age and do not function independently until after birth.[22]
- End-stage renal disease in children is most often attributed to congenital disorders of the kidneys.[22]

REVIEW EXERCISES

1. A 32-year-old woman with diabetes is found to have a positive result on a urine dipstick test for microalbuminuria. A subsequent 24-hour urine specimen reveals an albumin excretion of 50 mg (an albumin excretion >30 mg/day is abnormal).
   A. *Use the structures of the glomerulus in Figure 32.5 to provide a possible explanation for this finding. Why specifically test for the albumin rather than the globulins or other plasma proteins?*
   B. *Strict control of blood sugars and treatment of hypertension have been shown to decrease the progression of kidney disease in persons with diabetes. Explain the physiologic rationale for these two types of treatments.*
2. A 10-year-old boy with bed-wetting was placed on an ADH nasal spray at bedtime as a means of treating the disorder.
   A. *Explain the rationale for using ADH to treat bed-wetting.*
3. A 54-year-old man, seen by his physician for an elevated blood pressure, was found to have a serum creatinine of 2.5 and BUN of 30. He complains that he has been urinating more frequently than usual, and his first morning urine specimen reveals dilute urine with a specific gravity of 1.010.
   A. *Explain the elevation of serum creatinine in terms of renal function.*
   B. *Explain the inability of people with early renal failure to produce concentrated urine as evidenced by the frequency of urination and the low specific gravity of his first morning urine specimen.*
4. A 60-year-old woman with a diagnosis of hypertension is being treated with a thiazide diuretic.
   A. *What diuretic effect would you expect the woman to have based on the percentage of sodium reaching the site where the diuretic exerted its action?*
   B. *What type of effects might be expected in terms of renal losses of potassium and calcium?*

References

1. Ross M., Pawlina W. (2015). *Histology: A text and atlas with correlated cell and molecular biology* (7th ed.). Philadelphia, PA: Lippincott Williams & Wilkins.
2. Hall J. E. (2015). *Guyton and Hall textbook of medical physiology* (13th ed.). Philadelphia, PA: Elsevier Saunders.
3. Saladin K.S. (2015). *Anatomy & physiology: The unity of form and function* (7th ed.). New York: McGraw Hill.
4. McCance K. L., Huether S. E. (2014). *Pathophysiology: The biologic basis of disease in adults and children* (7th ed.). St. Louis, MO: Mosby Elsevier.
5. Rubin R., Strayer D. S. (Eds.) (2014). *Rubin's pathology: Clinicopathologic foundations of medicine* (7th ed.). Philadelphia, PA: Lippincott Williams & Wilkins.
6. Boron W. F., Boulpaep E. L. (2016). *Medical physiology* (3rd ed.). St. Louis, MO: Saunders Elsevier.
7. Lehne R. A. (2016). *Pharmacology for nursing care* (9th ed.). St. Louis, MO: Elsevier.
8. Pham P.C., Khaing K., Sievers T. M., et al. (2017). 2017 updated on pain management in patients with chronic kidney diseases. *Clinical Kidney Journal* 10(5), 688–697.
9. Fischbach F., Dunning M. (2014). *A manual of laboratory and diagnostic tests* (9th ed.). Philadelphia, PA: Lippincott Williams & Wilkins.
10. Ibrahim N. E., Gaggin H. K., Konstam M. A., et al. (2016). Established and emerging roles of biomarkers in heart failure clinical trials. *Circulation Heart Failure* 9, e002598. doi:10.1161/CIRCHEARTFAILURE.115.002528.
11. He P., Duan C., Liu Y., et al. (2016). N-terminal pro-brain natriuretic peptide improves the C-ACS risk score prediction of clinical outcomes in patients with ST-elevation myocardial infarction. *BMC Cardiovascular Disorders* 16, 255. doi 10.1186/s12872-016-0430-0
12. Carvalho L. S. F., Bogniotti L. A. C., Rangel de Almeida O. L., et al. (2018). Change of BNP between admission and discharge after ST-elevation myocardial infarction (Killip I) improves risk prediction of heart failure, death, and recurrent myocardial infarction compared to single isolated measurement in addition to the GRACE score. *European Journal of Acute Cardiovascular Care* doi: 10.1177/2048872617753049
13. Rennke H. G., Denker B. M. (2014). *Renal pathophysiology: The essentials* (4th ed.). Philadelphia, PA: Lippincott Williams & Wilkins.
14. Zeisberg M., Kalluri R. (2015). Physiology of the renal interstitium. *Clinical Journal of the American Society of Nephrology* 10(10), 1831–1840.
15. American Association for Clinical Chemistry (2016). *Estimated glomerular filtration rate (eGFR)*. Available: https://labtestsonline.org/understanding/analytes/gfr/tab/glance
16. Shilpak M. G., Mattes M. D., Peralta C. A. (2013). Update on cystatin C: Incorporation into clinical practice. *American Journal of Kidney Disease* 62(3), 595–603.
17. Karger A. B., Inker L. A., Coresh J., Levey A. S., Eckfeldt J. H. (2017). Novel filtration markers for GFR estimation. *Journal of the International Federation of Clinical Chemistry and Laboratory Medicine* 28(4), 277–288.

18. NIH National Institute of Diabetes and Digestive and Kidney Diseases (2015). Cystoscopy and Ureteroscopy. Downloaded from https://www.niddk.nih.gov/health-information/diagnostic-tests/cystoscopy-ureteroscopy
19. Tabloski P. A. (2013). *Gerontological nursing* (3rd ed.). Boston: Pearson.
20. Eliopoulos C. (2018). *Urinary elimination in gerontological nursing* (9th ed). Philadelphia, PA: Wolters Kluwer.
21. Hogan-Quigley B. (2017). The gastrointestinal and renal systems. In *Bates' nursing guide to physical examination and history* (2nd ed). Philadelphia, PA: Wolters Kluwer Health/Lippincott Williams & Wilkins.
22. Bowden V., Greenberg C. S. (2014). *Children and their families: The continuum of nursing care* (3rd ed). Philadelphia, PA: Wolters Kluwer Health.

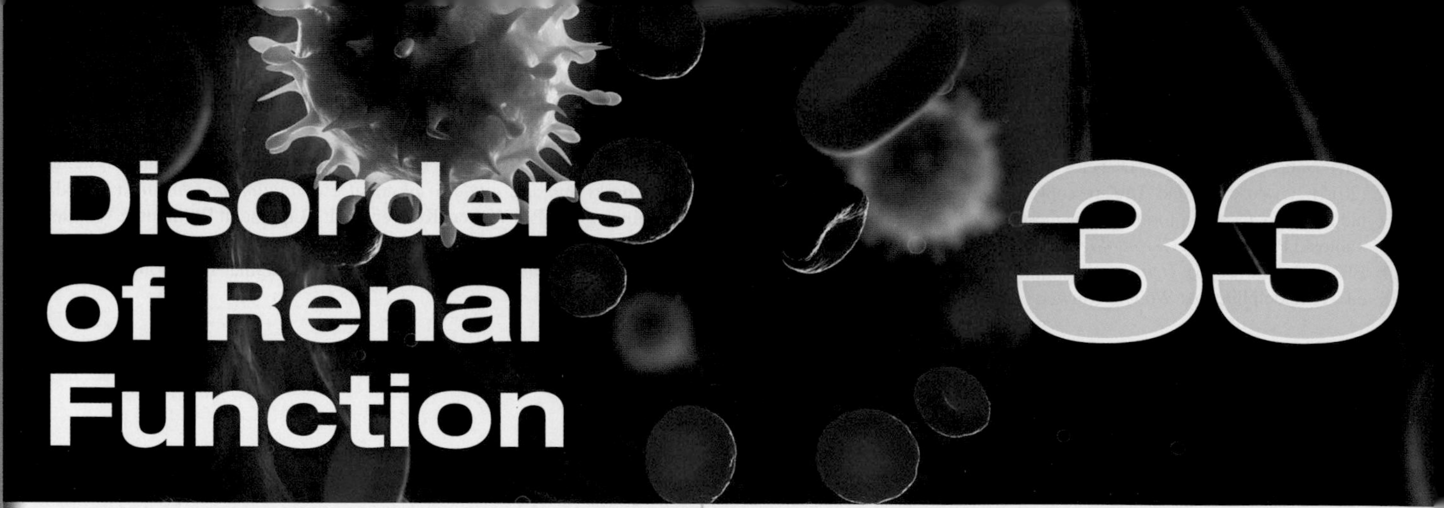

Disorders of Renal Function 33

Reba A. Umberger and
Linda C. Mefford

Kidney disease is a frequent cause of health care utilization and missed work among both men and women. Approximately 30 million people (more than one in seven) in the United States have chronic kidney disease, yet the majority have mild disease and remain unaware.[1] Kidney stones account for about 2.1 million annual emergency department (ED) visits in the United States,[2] whereas urinary tract infections (UTIs) account for about 1 million ED visits and 7 million office visits.[3] Although many forms of kidney disease originate in the kidneys, others develop secondary to disorders such as hypertension, diabetes mellitus, and systemic lupus erythematosus (SLE). The content in this chapter focuses on congenital disorders of the kidneys, obstructive disorders, UTIs, disorders of glomerular function, tubulointerstitial disorders, and neoplasms of the kidneys.

CONGENITAL AND INHERITED DISORDERS OF THE KIDNEYS

After completing this section of the chapter, the learner will be able to meet the following objectives:

- Define the terms *agenesis*, *hypoplasia*, and *dysgenesis*, and discuss them as they refer to the development of the kidney.
- Describe the inheritance, pathology, and manifestations of the different types of polycystic kidney disease.

Congenital Disorders of the Kidneys

The kidneys begin to develop early and begin producing urine by week 13 of gestation.[4] Fetal urine is excreted into the amniotic cavity and is the main constituent of amniotic fluid. Thus, the relative amount of amniotic fluid can provide information about the status of fetal renal function. In pregnancies that involve infants with nonfunctional kidneys or outflow obstruction of urine from the kidneys, the amount of amniotic fluid is small. This condition is called *oligohydramnios*.[5]

Anomalies in shape and position are the most common congenital kidney problems. Less common are disorders involving a decrease in renal mass (*e.g.*, agenesis, hypogenesis) or a change in renal structure (*e.g.*, renal dysplasia). The kidneys can be visualized as early as 12 weeks' gestation by ultrasonography, allowing many fetal urinary abnormalities to be detected before birth.[5,6] Congenital abnormalities represent up to 50% of pediatric and 7% of adult end-stage renal disease. It is now recognized that single-gene mutations with high penetrance rates play a larger role than previously recognized in these abnormalities.[7]

Agenesis and Hypoplasia

The term *dysgenesis* refers to a failure of an organ to develop normally. *Agenesis* refers to failure of an organ to develop at all. Newborns with bilateral renal agenesis—a rare condition—are born stillborn or live for only a few hours.[4,8] Unilateral renal agenesis occurs in about 1 of 1000 to 2000 newborn infants. Boys are affected more often than girls.[4] Detection of unilateral agenesis may be delayed because the healthy kidney usually undergoes compensatory hypertrophy and performs the function of the missing kidney.

Newborns with renal agenesis often have characteristic facial features, previously called *Potter syndrome*, resulting from the effects of oligohydramnios.[4] Without the amniotic fluid to protect and cushion, the uterus may compress the developing fetus. The eyes are widely separated and have epicanthic folds, the ears are low set, the nose is beaklike, the chin is receding, and limb defects are often present.[5]

In *renal hypoplasia*, the kidneys do not develop to normal size and contain fewer renal lobes. Like agenesis, hypoplasia more commonly affects only one kidney. When both kidneys are affected, renal failure progressively develops. In some cases, although the number of nephrons is reduced, the nephrons enlarge in size as the kidneys work harder to compensate, thus increasing the risk for glomerular disease (discussed later in this chapter).[5] The prevalence of renal hypoplasia is unknown because it is often an incidental finding and small kidneys may also result from atrophy and scarring.[6]

Renal Dysplasia

Renal dysplasia is caused by an abnormality in the differentiation of kidney structures during embryonic development. It is characterized by undifferentiated tubular structures surrounded by primitive embryonic tissue and may contain smooth muscle and cartilage.[5] Noncommunicating cysts of varying size may replace normal renal parenchyma. This occurs in approximately 1 of 4300 pregnancies.[6] When cysts are present, the condition is referred to as *cystic dysplasia*. One or both kidneys may be involved, and the affected kidney may be abnormally large or abnormally small. Many forms of dysplasia are accompanied by other urinary tract abnormalities, especially disorders that cause obstruction to urine flow (*e.g.*, ureteral agenesis or atresia, ureteropelvic junction obstruction).

A multicystic kidney is one in which the kidney is replaced by cysts and does not function. The kidney does not have the usual kidney shape, but is rather a mass of cysts. The finding of an abdominal mass in newborns is commonly caused by unilateral multicystic renal dysplasia.[5] The function of the opposite kidney is usually normal, and these children have an excellent prognosis after surgical removal of the affected kidney. Bilateral renal dysplasia causes oligohydramnios, leading to Potter facies, pulmonary hypoplasia, and renal failure.

Alterations in Kidney Position and Form

The development of the kidneys during embryonic life can result in *ectopic kidneys* that lie outside their normal position. One or both kidneys may be in an abnormal position. An ectopic kidney may be located within the pelvic cavity on the same or opposite side of its ureter, or it may be located within the margins of the iliac crest or in the abdominal or chest cavities.[6] Because of the abnormal position, kinking of the ureters and obstruction of urinary flow may occur.

The most common alterations in kidney form—occurring in approximately 1 of every 500 births—is an abnormality called a *horseshoe kidney*.[6] In this disorder, the upper or lower poles of the two kidneys are fused, producing a horseshoe-shaped structure that is continuous along the midline of the body anterior to the great vessels. Most horseshoe kidneys are fused at the lower pole (Fig. 33.1). The condition usually does not cause problems unless there is an associated defect in the renal pelvis or other urinary structures that obstructs urinary flow.

Inherited Cystic Kidney Diseases

The inherited cystic kidney diseases are single-gene disorders transmitted through Mendelian patterns and include autosomal dominant and recessive polycystic kidney disease as well as nephronophthisis–medullary cystic disease. Polycystic kidney diseases are a group of kidney disorders characterized by fluid-filled sacs or segments that have their origins in the tubular structures of the kidney. The cysts may be single or multiple and can vary in size from microscopic to several centimeters in diameter. Although they may arise as a developmental abnormality or be acquired later in life, most forms are hereditary. In the *autosomal dominant polycystic kidney disease (ADPKD)*, thousands of large cysts are derived from every segment of the nephron (Fig. 33.2).[5] The tubule wall (which is lined by a single layer of tubular cells) expands

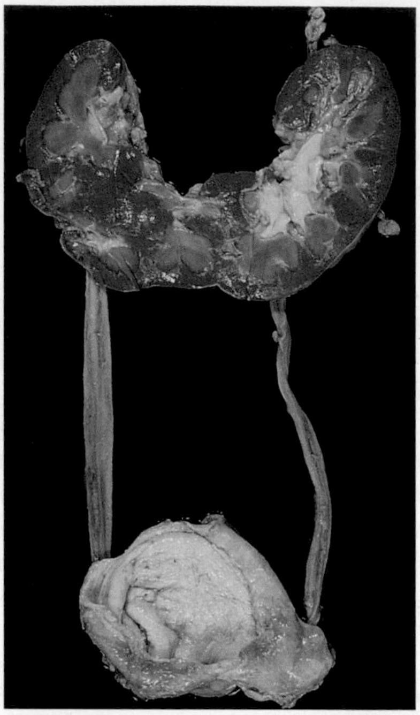

Figure 33.1 • Horseshoe kidney. The kidneys are fused at the lower poles. (From Rubin R., Strayer D. (Eds.) (2015). *Rubin's pathology: Clinicopathologic foundations of medicine* (7th ed., p. 907, Figure 22.7). Philadelphia, PA: Wolters Kluwer Health.)

and then rapidly closes the cyst off from the tubule of origin. In the *autosomal recessive polycystic kidney disease*, small, elongated cysts form in the collecting ducts and maintain contact with the nephron of origin (see Fig. 33.2).[5] In acquired cystic disease, simple cysts develop in the kidney as a consequence of aging, dialysis, or other conditions that affect tubular function.

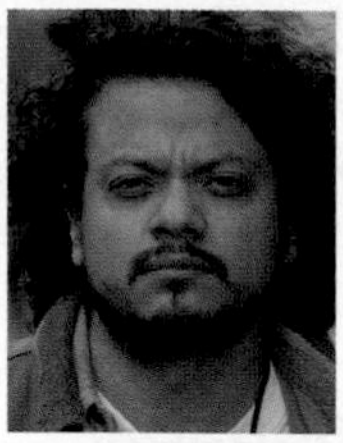

Remember **Mr. Reterez,** the man with the polycystic kidney disease you were introduced to in the unit-opening case study? It is very likely that he has ADPKD because his mother, maternal uncles, and maternal grandfather died from this disease. When so many people in one family die from a similar problem or from multiple problems related to one specific part of the human body, that person, or his or her children, should seek genetic counseling and screening.

Autosomal Dominant Polycystic Kidney Disease

Autosomal dominant polycystic kidney disease (ADPKD), also known as *adult polycystic disease*, is the most common hereditary form of renal cystic disease.[5] ADPKD results in the formation of destructive fluid-filled cysts in the kidney and other organs. This inherited disorder is the fourth leading cause of end-stage renal disease in the United States.

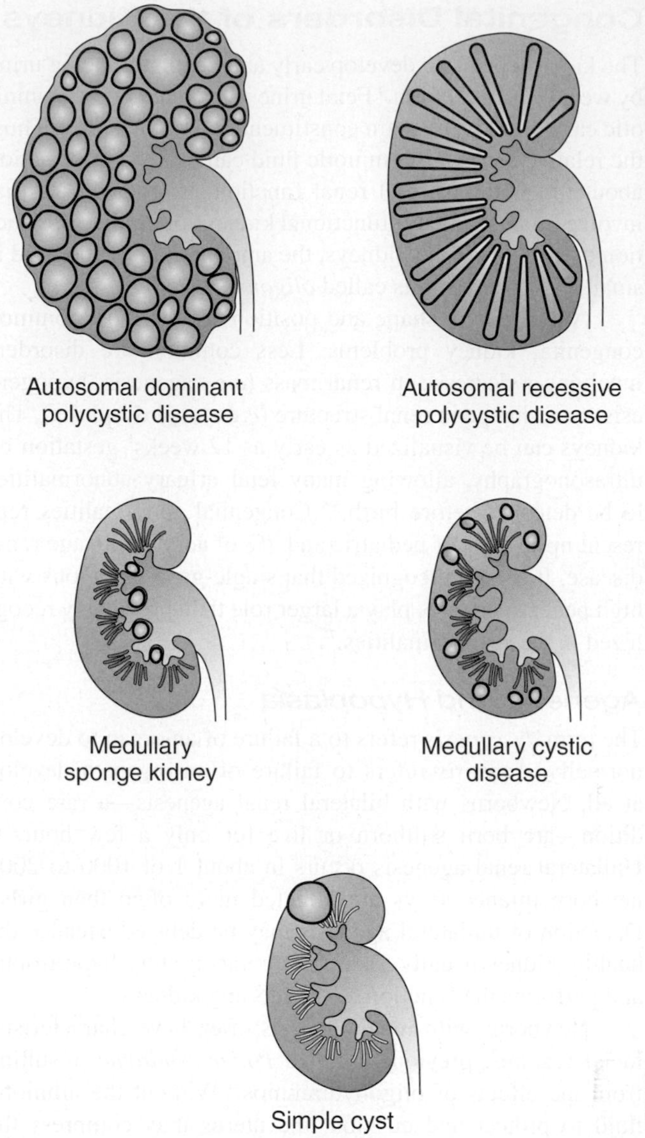

Figure 33.2 • Polycystic kidney diseases. Polycystic kidney diseases include five kidney disorders with fluid-filled segments originating in the tubular structures of the kidney. (From Strayer D. S., Rubin E. (Eds.) (2015). *Rubin's pathology: Clinicopathologic foundations of medicine* (7th ed., p. 909, Figure 22.10). Philadelphia, PA: Wolters Kluwer Health.)

Adoption of consistent standards to define ADPKD provides the basis for accurate reporting to registries and evaluation of future interventions.[9] These standards take into account factors beyond a stable glomerular filtration rate (GFR); they also include total kidney volume (TKV) to measure cyst expansion and development. The disease accounts for 5% of all cases of chronic kidney disease that require dialysis or transplantation.[5]

The cause of ADPKD was originally believed to be mutations in the *PKD1* and *PDK2* genes, thought to account for 85% and 15% or cases, respectively. However, emerging research on cases of AKPKD without these mutations demonstrate mutations in the *GANAB* gene as well as the *PKD1* and *PKD2* genes.[5,10] The products of these genes, polycystin-1 and polycystin-2, are found in the primary cilia that line the apical surface of the tubular epithelium. These primary cilia are thought to act as sensors of urinary flow and as signal transducers for tubular cell proliferation, differentiation, and apoptosis.[5] The *GANAB* gene, which codes for glucosidase, causes a mild form of disease accompanied by polycystic liver disease.[10]

Etiology and Pathogenesis. Although the pathogenesis of ADPKD is not clear, it is thought that the cysts arise in segments of the renal tubules from a few epithelial cells.[5] The epithelial cells lining the cysts of ADPKD have a high proliferation rate and are relatively undifferentiated. Concomitantly, a defective basement membrane immediately underlying the abnormal epithelium allows for dilation and cyst formation. Cysts frequently detach from the tubule and grow by active fluid secretion from the epithelial lining cells. Historically, it was thought that the chronic decline in renal function resulted from pressure exerted by the expanding cysts on the surrounding normal kidney tissue. However, it is now appreciated that cysts arise in less than 2% of nephrons and that factors other than compression by the expanding cysts account for loss of functioning renal tissue.[5] Apoptotic loss of renal tubular cells and accumulation of inflammatory mediators are now thought to contribute to the destruction of normal kidney tissue. Mutations in the *PKD1* and *PKD2* genes produce identical renal and extrarenal disease, but disease progression is typically more rapid in people with type I disease.[5]

Clinical Manifestations. Typically, the progress of the kidney disease is slow, and end-stage renal failure (ESRF) is uncommon for adults before 40 years of age. Initially, the person with renal cysts is generally asymptomatic, with normal kidney and liver function.

As the kidney disease progresses, the manifestations of ADPKD include pain from the enlarging cysts that may reach debilitating levels, episodes of gross hematuria from bleeding into a cyst, infected cysts from ascending UTIs, and hypertension resulting from compression of intrarenal blood vessels with activation of the renin–angiotensin mechanism.

The kidneys are usually enlarged in people with ADPKD and may achieve enormous sizes (Fig. 33.3).[5] The external contours of the kidneys are distorted by numerous cysts, some as large as 5 cm in diameter, which are filled with straw-colored fluid.[5] Cysts also may be found in the liver and, less commonly, in the pancreas and spleen.

As the disease continues to progress, extrarenal manifestations such as aneurysms are frequent, underscoring the systemic nature of the disease. Approximately 10% of people with polycystic kidney disease have an associated intracranial aneurysm, and subarachnoid or intracerebral hemorrhages are the most serious complications, which may lead to death.[11]

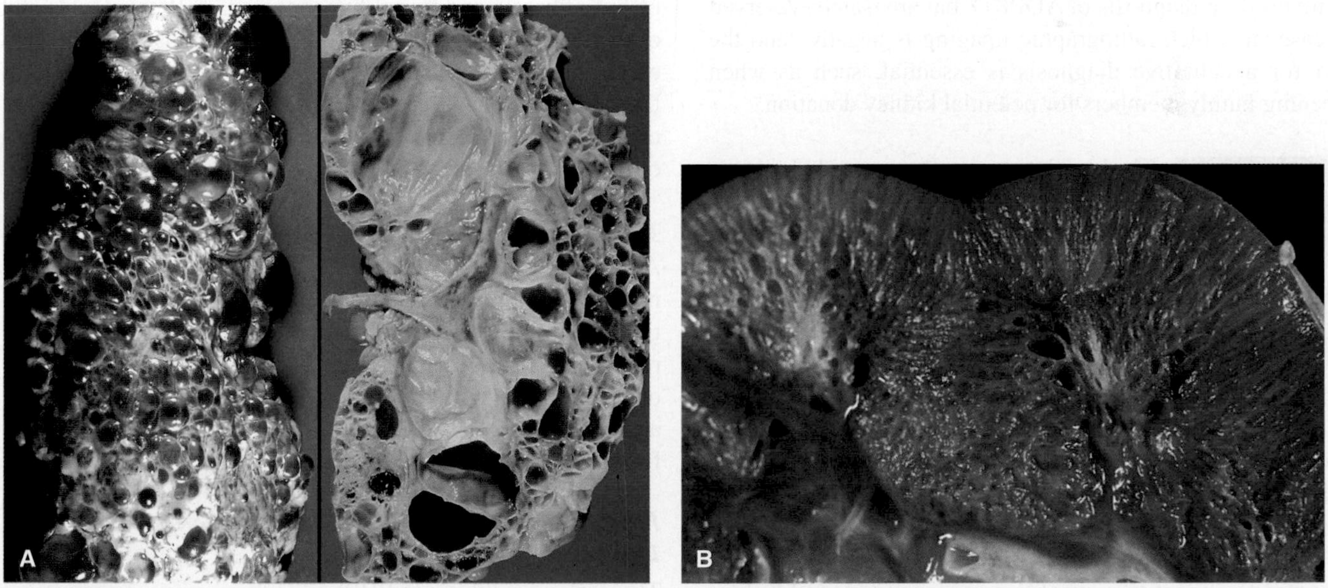

Figure 33.3 • **(A)** Autosomal dominant polycystic disease. The kidneys are enlarged and studded with multiple fluid-filled structures (*left*). The parenchyma is almost entirely replaced by cysts of varying size (*right*). **(B)** Autosomal recessive polycystic kidney disease. The dilated cortical and medullary collecting ducts are arranged radially, and the external surface is smooth. (From Rubin R., Strayer D. (Eds.) (2015). *Rubin's pathology: Clinicopathologic foundations of medicine* (7th ed., p. 909–909, Figure 22.11, 22.12). Philadelphia, PA: Wolters Kluwer Health.)

Screening these people for intracranial aneurysm is particularly important when family history of hemorrhagic stroke or intracranial aneurysms exists.[11]

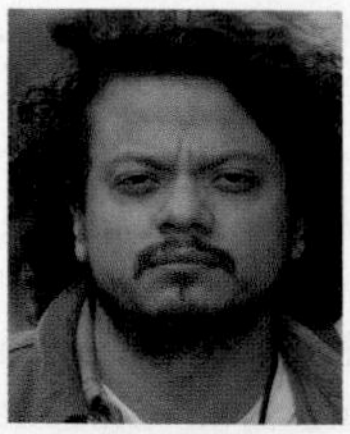

Mr. Reterez is experiencing abdominal and flank discomfort, which could be caused by enlarging or bleeding cysts or by a urinary tract infection. His abdominal girth is abnormally large, reflecting the presence of multiple fluid-filled cysts. He also has evidence of significant renal dysfunction (approaching end-stage failure), including 1+ pedal edema, nausea, anorexia, fatigue, and hypertension (blood pressure, 140/92 mm Hg).

The death of Mr. Reterez's nephrons reduces the production of erythropoietin (EPO) by his kidneys. EPO promotes red blood cell (RBC) production by the bone marrow, so EPO deficiency causes anemia. Mr. Reterez may thus suffer from chronic renal failure anemia, which is characterized by normocytic and normochromic RBCs and a hemoglobin concentration less than 12 g/dL.

Diagnosis and Treatment. Serum creatinine levels have not been found to be an effective predictor marker for worsening ADPKD, but TKV in relation to age is a reliable predictor of increasing cyst burden. Increased TKV is associated with hematuria, proteinuria, and decreased kidney function.[12] Ultrasonography usually is the preferred technique for diagnosis of ADPKD in symptomatic people and for screening of asymptomatic family members. Computed tomography (CT) may be used for detection of small cysts. Genetic linkage studies are used for diagnosis of ADPKD, but are usually reserved for cases in which radiographic imaging is negative and the need for a definitive diagnosis is essential, such as when screening family members for potential kidney donation.

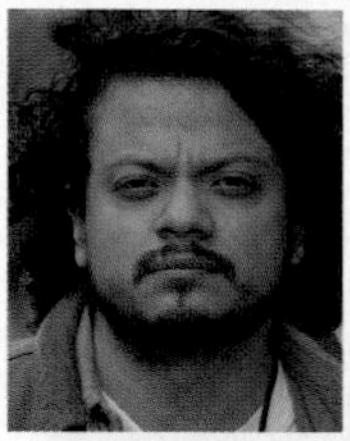

The blood and urine tests provide evidence of the destruction of Mr. Reterez's kidney tissue. He has elevated blood urea nitrogen (BUN) and blood sodium concentrations, with albumin and red blood cells present in his urine. These indicators of kidney function will likely worsen as he moves along the continuum toward complete renal failure. The finding of hematuria (blood in the urine) will need a comprehensive workup, because it can also indicate problems unrelated to his kidney disease.

The treatment of ADPKD has been largely supportive, including treatment to control hypertension and modify lifestyle, as well as targeted prevention of complications through screening (*e.g.*, cerebral aneurysm). Lifestyle interventions include following a low-sodium diet, drinking adequate fluids (2 to 3 L/day), and avoiding smoking and agents such as nonsteroidal anti-inflammatory agents, which can be nephrotoxic.[13] Identification of drugs to delay progression of disease has failed until recently. The drug, Tolvaptan, which is a selective vasopressin V_2 receptor antagonist, has been studied and found to inhibit cyst growth and preserve kidney function. It not currently available for use in all countries, and safety studies are still underway in the United States.[13] Control of hypertension and prevention of ascending UTIs are important. Pain is a common complaint of people with ADPKD. A stepwise approach has been proposed to explore the underlying cause of pain. Pain management begins with nonpharmacologic approaches and can escalate to include complex invasive therapies.[14] Dialysis and kidney transplantation are reserved for those who progress to kidney failure. However, it is important to note that prolonged dialysis will increase cyst formation even in people without ADPKD.[5]

Autosomal Recessive Polycystic Kidney Disease

Autosomal recessive polycystic kidney disease (ARPKD) is characterized by cystic dilation of the cortical and medullary collecting tubules. As shown in Figure 33.2, the surface of the kidney is generally smooth.[5] It is rare in comparison with the autosomal dominant form. There is one case of ARPKD for about every 20,000 live births.[15] ARPKD is caused by mutations in the *PKHD1* gene. The gene product, fibrocystin, is found in the kidney, liver, and pancreas and appears to be involved in the regulation of cell proliferation and adhesion.[5]

Clinical Manifestations. The typical infant with ARPKD presents with bilateral flank masses, accompanied by severe renal failure. The very large size of the kidneys restricts lung development and function. There are also varying degrees of liver fibrosis and portal hypertension.[5,16] Potter facies and other defects associated with oligohydramnios may be present. Hypertension is usually noted within the first few weeks of life and is often severe. Death during the perinatal period often results from pulmonary hypoplasia.[5] Exceptional cases of ARPKD manifest in older children and adults.

Treatment. The treatment of ARPKD is largely supportive. Aggressive ventilatory support is often necessary in the neonatal period because of pulmonary hypoplasia and hypoventilation. Modern neonatal respiratory techniques and renal replacement therapy have increased the 10-year survival rate of children surviving beyond the first year of life. Morbidity and mortality in older children are related to complications from chronic renal failure and liver disease.

Nephronophthisis–Medullary Cystic Disease Complex

The nephronophthisis (NPHP)–medullary cystic disease complex is a group of renal disorders that have their onset in childhood. Common characteristics of this autosomal recessive kidney disease are small, shrunken kidneys and the presence of a variable number of cysts, usually concentrated at the corticomedullary junction.[17] The initial insult involves the distal tubules, with tubular basement membrane disruption followed by chronic and progressive tubular atrophy involving both the medulla and cortex. Although the presence of medullary cysts is important, the cortical and tubular damage is the eventual cause of chronic kidney disease and failure.[17]

NPHP is a progressive form that typically advances to end-stage renal disease prior to adulthood.[18] Affected children present first with polyuria, polydipsia, and enuresis (bed-wetting), which reflect impaired ability of the kidneys to concentrate urine. Other manifestations of the disorders include salt wasting, growth retardation, anemia, and progressive renal insufficiency. The mean age of onset is specific to each of the three clinical variants (infantile, juvenile, and adolescent). Extrarenal complications may occur, including skeletal defects, ocular motor abnormalities, retinitis pigmentosa, liver fibrosis, cardiac septal and valve defects, and cerebellar abnormalities.[18]

Simple and Acquired Renal Cysts

Simple cysts are a common disorder of the kidney. The cysts may be single or multiple, unilateral or bilateral, and they usually are less than 1 cm in diameter, although they may grow larger. Most simple cysts do not produce signs or symptoms or compromise renal function. When symptomatic, the cysts may cause flank pain, hematuria, infection, and hypertension related to ischemia-produced stimulation of the renin–angiotensin system. They are most common in older adults. Although the cysts are benign, they may be confused clinically with renal cell carcinoma.

An acquired form of renal cystic disease occurs in people with ESRF who have undergone prolonged dialysis treatment.[5] Although the condition is largely asymptomatic, the cysts may bleed, causing hematuria. Tumors, usually adenomas but occasionally adenosarcomas, may develop in the walls of these cysts.

IN SUMMARY

Approximately 10% of infants are born with potentially significant malformations of the urinary system. These abnormalities can range from bilateral renal agenesis (which is incompatible with life) to hypogenesis of one kidney (which usually causes no problems unless the function of the remaining kidney is impaired). Renal dysplasia is caused by an abnormality in the differentiation of kidney structures during embryonic development. A multicystic kidney is one in which the kidney is replaced by cysts and does not function. The horseshoe kidney is a common developmental disorder in which the upper or lower poles of the two kidneys are fused, producing a horseshoe-shaped structure.

Renal cystic disease is a condition in which there is dilation of tubular structures with cyst formation. Cysts may be single or multiple. Polycystic kidney disease is an inherited form of renal cystic disease; it can be inherited as an autosomal dominant or recessive trait. The autosomal dominant form of the disease (ADPKD) results in the formation of numerous fluid-filled cysts in the tubular structures of both kidneys with the threat of progression to chronic renal failure. Other manifestations of the disease include hypertension, cardiovascular abnormalities, cerebral aneurysms, and cysts in other organs such as the liver and pancreas (Fig. 41.3). The autosomal recessive form (ARPKD) is characterized by cystic transformation of the collecting ducts (Fig. 33.3). It is rare compared with ADPD and usually presents as severe renal dysfunction during infancy. The nephronophthisis–medullary cystic disease complex is a group of hereditary disorders that usually have their onset during childhood and are characterized by the presence of cysts in the medullary portion of the kidney, renal atrophy, and eventual kidney failure. Single or multiple simple renal cysts most commonly occur in people older than 50 years of age.

OBSTRUCTIVE DISORDERS

After completing this section of the chapter, the learner will be able to meet the following objectives:

- List four common causes of urinary tract obstruction.
- Define the term *hydronephrosis* and relate it to the destructive effects of urinary tract obstruction.
- Describe the role of urine supersaturation, nucleation, and inhibitors of stone formation in the development of kidney stones.

Urinary obstruction can occur in people of any age and can involve any level of the urinary tract, from the urethra to the renal pelvis (Fig. 33.4). Obstruction may be sudden or insidious, partial or complete, and unilateral or bilateral. The

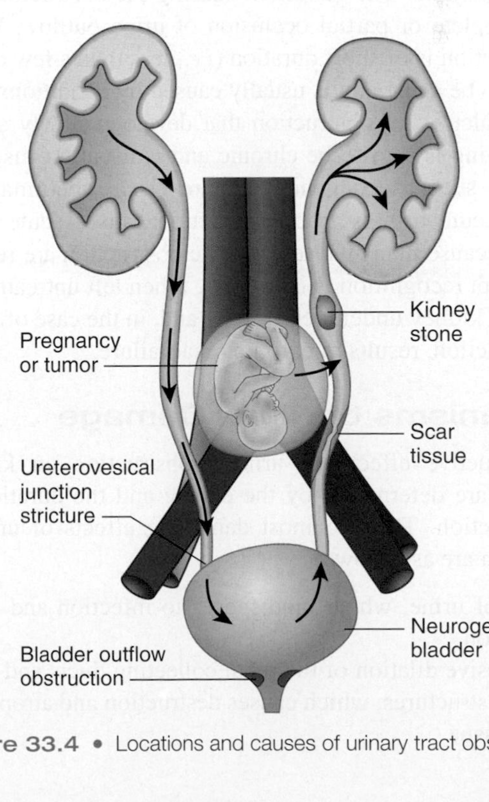

Figure 33.4 • Locations and causes of urinary tract obstruction.

TABLE 33.1 CAUSES OF URINARY TRACT OBSTRUCTION

LEVEL OF OBSTRUCTION	CAUSE
Renal pelvis	Renal calculi
	Papillary necrosis
Ureter	Renal calculi
	Pregnancy
	Tumors that compress the ureter
	Ureteral stricture
	Congenital disorders of the ureterovesical junction and ureteropelvic junction strictures
Bladder and urethra	Bladder cancer
	Neurogenic bladder
	Bladder stones
	Prostatic hyperplasia or cancer
	Urethral strictures
	Congenital urethral defects

conditions that cause urinary tract obstruction include congenital anomalies, urinary calculi (*i.e.*, stones), pregnancy, benign prostatic hyperplasia, scar tissue resulting from infection and inflammation, tumors, and neurologic disorders such as spinal cord injury. The causes of urinary tract obstructions are summarized in Table 33.1.

Obstructive uropathy is usually classified according to site, degree, and duration of obstruction.[19] Lower urinary tract obstructions are located below the ureterovesical junction and are bilateral in nature. Upper urinary tract obstructions are located above the ureterovesical junction and are usually unilateral. The condition causing the obstruction can cause complete or partial occlusion of urine outflow. When the obstruction is of short duration (*i.e.*, less than a few days), it is said to be acute and is usually caused by conditions such as renal calculi. An obstruction that develops slowly and is longer lasting is said to be chronic and is usually caused by conditions such as congenital ureterovesical abnormalities. Bilateral acute urinary tract obstruction causes acute renal failure. Because many causes of acute obstruction are reversible, prompt recognition is important. When left untreated, an obstructed kidney undergoes atrophy and, in the case of bilateral obstruction, results in chronic renal failure.

Mechanisms of Renal Damage

The destructive effects of urinary obstruction on kidney structures are determined by the degree and the duration of the obstruction. The two most damaging effects of urinary obstruction are as follows:

1. Stasis of urine, which predisposes to infection and stone formation
2. Progressive dilation of the renal collecting ducts and renal tubular structures, which causes destruction and atrophy of renal tissue

A common complication of urinary tract obstruction is infection. Stagnation of urine predisposes to infection, which may spread throughout the urinary tract. Once established, the infection is difficult to treat. Urea-splitting organisms (*e.g.*, *Proteus*, staphylococci) that increase ammonia production and cause the urine to become alkaline often cause infection.[5] When present, urinary calculi serve as foreign bodies and contribute to the infection. Calcium salts precipitate more readily in stagnant alkaline urine; thus, urinary tract obstructions also predispose to stone formation.

In situations of severe partial or complete obstruction, the impediment to the outflow of urine causes dilation of the renal pelvis and calices associated with progressive atrophy of the kidney. Even with complete obstruction, glomerular filtration continues for a period of time. Because of the continued filtration, the calices and pelvis of the affected kidney may become markedly dilated. The high pressure in the renal pelvis is transmitted back through the collecting ducts of the kidney, compressing renal vasculature and causing renal atrophy. Initially, the functional alterations are largely tubular, manifested primarily by impaired urine-concentrating ability. Only later does the GFR begin to diminish.

Hydronephrosis

Hydronephrosis refers to urine-filled dilation of the renal pelvis and calices associated with progressive atrophy of the kidney because of obstruction of urine outflow. The degree of hydronephrosis depends on the duration, degree, and level of obstruction. In far-advanced cases, the kidney may be transformed into a thin-walled cystic structure with parenchymal atrophy, total obliteration of the pyramids, and thinning of the cortex (Fig. 33.5).[5] The condition is usually unilateral. Bilateral hydronephrosis occurs only when the obstruction is below the level of the ureterovesical junction. When the obstruction affects the outflow of urine from the distal ureter, the increased pressure dilates the ureter, a condition called

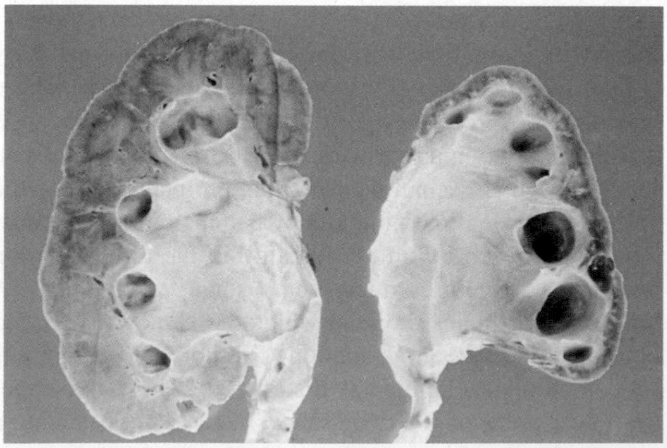

Figure 33.5 • Hydronephrosis. Bilateral urinary tract obstruction has led to conspicuous dilation of the ureters, pelves, and calices. The kidney on the right shows severe cortical atrophy. (From Rubin R., Strayer D. (Eds.) (2015). *Rubin's pathology: Clinicopathologic foundations of medicine* (7th ed., p. 951, Figure 22.83). Philadelphia, PA: Wolters Kluwer Health.)

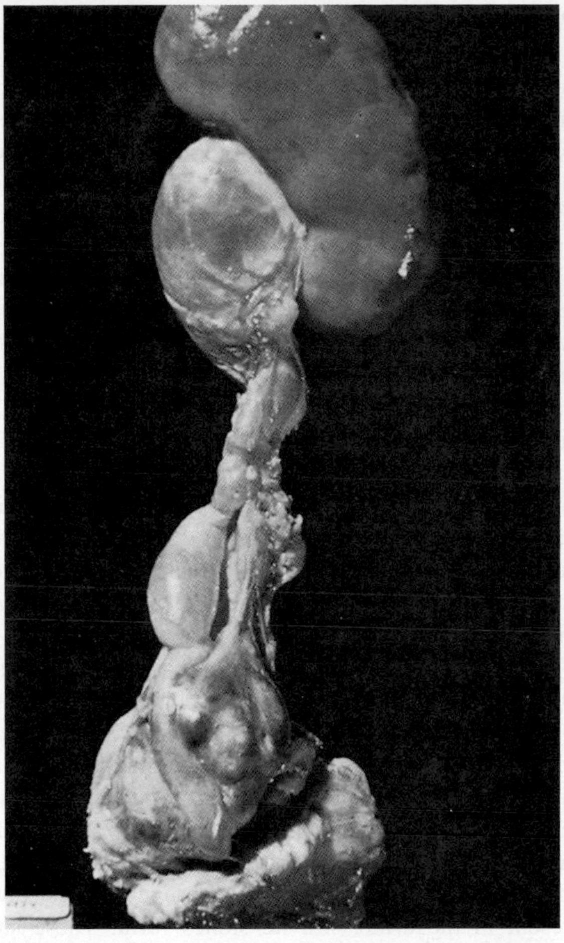

Figure 33.6 • Hydroureter caused by ureteral obstruction in a woman with cancer of the uterus.

hydroureter (Fig. 33.6). Bilateral hydroureter may develop as a complication of bladder outflow obstruction because of prostatic hyperplasia.

Clinical Manifestations

The manifestations of urinary obstruction depend on the site of obstruction, the cause, and the rapidity with which the condition developed. The underlying pathologic process produces most of the early symptoms. Urinary tract obstruction encourages the growth of microorganisms and should be suspected in people with recurrent UTIs.

Complete or partial unilateral hydronephrosis may remain silent for long periods because the unaffected kidney can maintain adequate kidney function. Obstruction may provoke pain because of distention of the collecting system and renal capsule. Acute supravesical obstruction, such as that because of a kidney stone lodged in the ureter, is associated with excruciatingly severe pain. By contrast, more insidious causes of obstruction, such as narrowing of the ureteropelvic junction, generally produce little pain but totally destroy the kidney.

Complete bilateral obstruction results in oliguria, progressing to anuria and renal failure. Acute bilateral obstruction may mimic prerenal failure. With partial bilateral obstruction, the earliest manifestation is an inability to concentrate urine, reflected by polyuria and nocturia. Hypertension is an occasional complication of urinary tract obstruction. It is more common in cases of unilateral obstruction in which renin secretion is enhanced, probably secondary to impaired renal blood flow. In these circumstances, removal of the obstruction often leads to a reduction in BP. When hypertension accompanies bilateral obstruction, it is volume related. The relief of bilateral obstruction leads to a loss of volume and a decrease in BP. In some cases, relieving the obstruction does not correct the hypertension.

Diagnosis and Treatment

Early diagnosis of urinary tract obstruction is important because the condition usually is treatable and a delay in therapy may result in permanent damage to the kidneys. Diagnostic methods vary with the symptoms. Ultrasonography has been shown to be the single most useful noninvasive diagnostic modality for urinary obstruction. Radiologic methods, CT scans, and intravenous urography may also be used.[20] Other diagnostic methods, such as urinalysis, are used to determine the extent of renal involvement and the presence of infection.

Treatment of urinary tract obstruction depends on the cause. Urinary stone removal may be necessary, or surgical treatment of structural defects may be indicated. Treatment of a complicated UTI because of urinary stasis is also important.

Renal Calculi

The most common cause of upper urinary tract obstruction is urinary calculi. Although stones can form in any part of the urinary tract, most develop in the kidneys. Renal calculi, or kidney stones, are a common pathophysiologic condition of the urinary tract, exceeded only by UTIs and prostate disorders. Kidney stones are polycrystalline aggregates composed of materials that the kidneys normally excrete in the urine.

Etiology and Pathogenesis

The etiology of urinary stone formation is complex. It is thought to encompass a number of factors, including increases in blood and urinary levels of stone components and interactions among the components, anatomic changes in urinary tract structures, metabolic and endocrine influences, dietary and intestinal absorption factors, and UTIs.[5] Several factors contribute to stone formation, including a supersaturated urine, presence of a nucleus for crystal formation, and deficiency of inhibitors of stone formation.[5]

Kidney stone formation requires a supersaturated urine and an environment that allows the stone to grow. The risk for stone formation is increased when the urine is supersaturated with stone components (*e.g.*, calcium salts, uric acid, magnesium ammonium phosphate, cystine). Supersaturation depends on urinary pH, temperature, solute concentration, ionic strength, and complexation. The greater the concentration of two ions, the more likely they are to precipitate.

In addition to a supersaturated urine, kidney stone formation requires a nidus or nucleus that facilitates crystal aggregation. In supersaturated urine, stone formation begins with small clusters of crystals such as calcium oxalate. Most small clusters tend to disperse because the internal forces that hold them together are too weak to overcome the random tendency of ions to move apart. Larger ion clusters form nuclei and remain stable because the attraction forces balance surface losses. Once they are stable, nuclei can grow at levels of supersaturation below that needed for their creation.[21]

The fact that many people experience supersaturation of their urine without development of kidney stones is believed to be a result of the presence of natural stone inhibitors, including magnesium and citrate. Citrate supplementation (potassium citrate) may be of benefit in some people with calcium stones, with the increased citrate concentration thought to decrease the calcium crystallization.[20]

KEY POINTS

KIDNEY STONES

- Stones require a nidus to form and a urinary environment that supports continued crystallization of stone components.
- The development of kidney stones is influenced by the concentration of stone components in the urine, the ability of the stone components to complex and form stones, and the presence of substances that inhibit stone formation.

Types of Stones

Four basic types of kidney stones have been identified—calcium stones (*i.e.*, oxalate or phosphate), magnesium ammonium phosphate stones, uric acid stones, and cystine stones.[21,22] The causes and treatment measures for each of these types of renal stones are described in Table 33.2. Most kidney stones (75% to 80%) are calcium stones—calcium oxalate, calcium phosphate, or a combination of the two materials.[21] Calcium stones usually are associated with increased concentrations of calcium in the blood and urine. Excessive bone resorption caused by immobility, bone disease, hyperparathyroidism, and renal tubular acidosis (RTA) all are contributing conditions. High oxalate concentrations in the blood and urine predispose to formation of calcium oxalate stones. Uric acid stones are associated with increased BMI and low urine pH.[22] The prevalence of obesity seems to be contributing to increasing uric acid stones in the population over time.[22] Emerging research indicates that 13% to 44% of calcium oxalate stones are culture positive, with *Escherichia coli* and *Pseudomonas* spp. representing the leading organisms.[23]

Magnesium ammonium phosphate stones, also called *struvite stones*, form only in alkaline urine (pH > 7.0) and in the presence of bacteria that possess an enzyme called *urease*, which splits the urea in the urine into ammonia and carbon dioxide.[21] The ammonia that is formed takes up a hydrogen ion to become an ammonium ion, increasing the pH of the urine so that it becomes more alkaline. Because phosphate levels are increased in alkaline urine and because magnesium always is present in the urine, struvite stones form. These stones enlarge as the bacterial count grows, and they can increase in size until they fill an entire renal pelvis (Fig. 33.7). Because of their shape, they often are called *staghorn stones*.[21] They are

TABLE 33.2 COMPOSITION, CONTRIBUTING FACTORS, AND TREATMENT OF KIDNEY STONES

TYPE OF STONE	CONTRIBUTING FACTORS	TREATMENT
Calcium (oxalate and phosphate)	Hypercalcemia and hypercalciuria Immobilization Hyperparathyroidism Vitamin D intoxication Diffuse bone disease Milk-alkali syndrome Renal tubular acidosis Hyperoxaluria Intestinal bypass surgery	Treatment of underlying conditions Increased fluid intake Thiazide diuretics Dietary restriction of foods high in oxalate
Magnesium ammonium phosphate (struvite)	Urea-splitting UTIs	Treatment of UTI Acidification of the urine Increased fluid intake
Uric acid (urate)	Formed in acid urine with pH of ~5.5 Gout High-purine diet	Increased fluid intake Allopurinol for hyperuricosuria Alkalinization of urine
Cystine	Cystinuria (inherited disorder of amino acid metabolism)	Increased fluid intake Alkalinization of urine

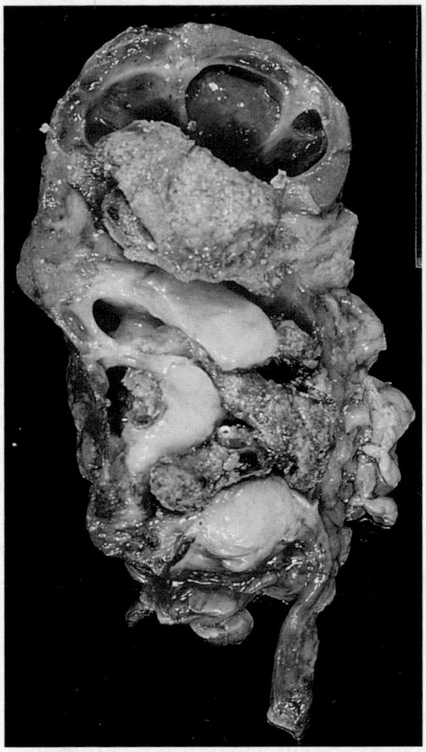

Figure 33.7 • Staghorn stones. The kidney shows hydronephrosis and stones that are casts of the dilated calices. (From Rubin R., Strayer D. (Eds.) (2015). *Rubin's pathology: Clinicopathologic foundations of medicine* (7th ed., p. 951, Figure 22.82). Philadelphia, PA: Wolters Kluwer Health.)

typically associated with UTIs caused by urease-producing bacteria; however, struvite accounts for a small percentage of all kidney stones.[23] Because these stones act as a foreign body, treatment of the infection often is difficult. Struvite stones usually are too large to be passed and require lithotripsy or surgical removal.

Uric acid stones develop in conditions of gout and high concentrations of uric acid in the urine and account for about 7% of all stones.[21] Hyperuricosuria also may contribute to calcium stone formation by acting as a nucleus for calcium oxalate stone formation. Unlike radiopaque calcium stones, uric acid stones are not visible on x-ray films. Uric acid stones form most readily in acidic urine.[24] Thus, these stones can be treated by raising the urinary pH from 6 to 6.5 with potassium alkali salts.

Cystine stones account for less than 1% to 3% of kidney stones overall but represent a significant proportion of childhood calculi.[24] They are seen in cystinuria, which results from an autosomal recessive genetic defect in renal transport of cystine so there is a decrease in cystine tubular absorption. These stones resemble struvite stones except that infection is unlikely to be present.

Clinical Manifestations

One of the major manifestations of kidney stones is pain. Depending on location, there are two types of pain associated with kidney stones: renal colic and noncolicky renal pain.[24] *Renal colic* is the term used to describe the colicky pain that accompanies stretching of the collecting system or ureter. The symptoms of renal colic are caused by stones 1 to 5 mm in diameter that can move into the ureter and obstruct flow. Classic ureteral colic is manifested by acute, intermittent, and excruciating pain in the flank and upper outer quadrant of the abdomen on the affected side. The pain may radiate to the lower abdominal quadrant, bladder area, perineum, or scrotum in the man. The skin may be cool and clammy, and nausea and vomiting are common. Noncolicky pain is caused by stones that produce distention of the renal calyces or renal pelvis. The pain usually is a dull, deep ache in the flank or back that can vary in intensity from mild to severe. The pain is often exaggerated by drinking large amounts of fluid.

Diagnosis and Treatment

People with kidney stones often present with acute renal colic, and the diagnosis is based on symptomatology and diagnostic tests, which include urinalysis, plain film radiography, intravenous pyelography (IVP), and abdominal ultrasonography.[25] Urinalysis provides information related to hematuria, infection, the presence of stone-forming crystals, and urine pH. Most stones are radiopaque and readily visible on a plain radiograph of the abdomen. The noncontrast spiral CT scan is the imaging modality of choice in people with acute renal colic.[25] IVP uses an intravenously injected contrast medium that is filtered in the glomeruli to visualize the collecting system of the kidneys and ureters. Abdominal ultrasonography is highly sensitive to hydronephrosis, which may be a manifestation of ureteral obstruction. A new imaging technique called *nuclear scintigraphy* uses bisphosphonate markers as a means of imaging stones.[25] The method has been credited with identifying stones that are too small to be detected by other methods.

Treatment of acute renal colic usually is supportive. Pain relief may be needed during acute phases of obstruction, and antibiotic therapy may be necessary to treat UTIs. Most stones that are less than 5 mm in diameter pass spontaneously. All urine should be strained during an attack in the hope of retrieving the stone for chemical analysis and determination of type. This information, along with a careful history and laboratory tests, provides the basis for long-term preventive measures.

A major goal of treatment in people who have passed kidney stones or have had them removed is to prevent their recurrence. Prevention requires investigation into the cause of stone formation using urine tests, blood chemistries, and stone analysis. Underlying disease conditions, such as hyperparathyroidism, are treated. Adequate fluid intake reduces the concentration of stone-forming crystals in the urine and needs to be encouraged. Depending on the type of stone that is formed, dietary changes, medications, or both may be used to alter the concentration of stone-forming elements in the urine. For example, people who form calcium oxalate stones may need to decrease their intake of foods that are high in oxalate (*e.g.*, spinach, Swiss chard, cocoa, chocolate, pecans, peanuts).

Dietary recommendations to prevent stones have been mixed; however, increased fluid intake has been recommended by the American College of Physicians to prevent recurrent stones.[26]

Calcium supplementation with calcium salts such as calcium carbonate and calcium phosphate also may be used to bind oxalate in the intestine and decrease its absorption. Thiazide diuretics lower urinary calcium by increasing tubular reabsorption so that less remains in the urine. Drugs that bind calcium in the gut (*e.g.*, cellulose phosphate) may be used to inhibit calcium absorption and urinary excretion.

Measures to change the pH of the urine also can influence kidney stone formation. In people who lose the ability to lower the pH of (or acidify) their urine, there is an increase in the divalent and trivalent forms of urine phosphate that combine with calcium to form calcium phosphate stones. The formation of uric acid stones is increased in acid urine; stone formation can be reduced by raising the pH of urine to 6.0 to 6.5 with potassium alkali (*e.g.*, potassium citrate) salts. Table 33.2 summarizes measures for preventing the recurrence of different types of kidney stones.

In some cases, stone removal may be necessary. Several methods are available for removing kidney stones—ureteroscopic removal, percutaneous removal, and extracorporeal lithotripsy.[20] All these procedures eliminate the need for an open surgical procedure, which is another form of treatment. Open stone surgery may be required to remove large calculi or those that are resistant to other forms of removal.

Ureteroscopic removal involves the passage of an instrument through the urethra into the bladder and then into the ureter. The development of high-quality optics has improved the ease with which this procedure is performed and its outcome. The procedure, which is performed under fluoroscopic guidance, involves the use of various instruments for dilating the ureter and for grasping, fragmenting, and removing the stone. Preprocedure radiologic studies using a contrast medium (*i.e.*, excretory urography) are done to determine the position of the stone and direct the placement of the ureteroscope.[25]

Percutaneous nephrolithotomy is the treatment of choice for removal of renal or proximal ureteral calculi.[25] It involves the insertion through the flank of a small-gauge needle into the collecting system of the kidney. The needle tract is then dilated, and an instrument called a *nephroscope* is inserted into the renal pelvis. The procedure is performed under fluoroscopic guidance. Preprocedure radiologic and ultrasonographic examinations of the kidney and ureter are used to determine the placement of the nephroscope. Stones up to 1 cm in diameter can be removed through this method. Larger stones must be broken up with an ultrasonic lithotripter (*i.e.*, stone breaker).

A nonsurgical treatment, called *extracorporeal shock wave lithotripsy*, uses acoustic shock waves to fragment calculi into sandlike particles that are passed in the urine over the next few days. Because of the large amount of stone particles that are generated during the procedure, a ureteral stent (*i.e.*, a tubelike device used to hold the ureter open) may be inserted to ensure adequate urine drainage.

IN SUMMARY

Obstruction of urine flow can occur at any level of the urinary tract. Among the causes of urinary tract obstruction are developmental defects, pregnancy, infection and inflammation, kidney stones, neurologic defects, and prostatic hypertrophy. Obstructive disorders produce stasis of urine, increase the risk for infection and calculi formation, and produce progressive dilation of the renal collecting ducts and renal tubular structures, which causes renal atrophy.

Hydronephrosis refers to urine-filled dilation of the renal pelvis and calices associated with progressive atrophy of the kidney because of obstruction of urine outflow. Unilateral hydronephrosis may remain silent for long periods because the unaffected kidney can maintain adequate kidney function. With partial bilateral obstruction, the earliest manifestation is an inability to concentrate urine, reflected by polyuria and nocturia. Complete bilateral obstruction results in oliguria, anuria, and renal failure.

Kidney stones are a major cause of upper urinary tract obstruction. There are four types of kidney stones: calcium (*i.e.*, oxalate and phosphate) stones, which are associated with increased serum calcium levels; magnesium ammonium phosphate (*i.e.*, struvite) stones, which are associated with UTIs; uric acid stones, which are related to elevated uric acid levels; and cystine stones, which are seen in cystinuria. A major goal of treatment for people who have passed kidney stones or have had them removed is to identify stone composition and prevent their recurrence. Treatment measures depend on stone type and include adequate fluid intake to prevent urine saturation, dietary modification to decrease intake of stone-forming constituents, treatment of UTI, measures to change urine pH, and the use of diuretics that decrease the calcium concentration of urine.

URINARY TRACT INFECTIONS

After completing this section of the chapter, the learner will be able to meet the following objectives:

- List three physiologic mechanisms that protect against UTIs.
- Describe factors that predispose to UTIs in children, sexually active women, pregnant women, and older adults.
- Cite measures used in the diagnosis and treatment of UTIs.

UTIs are a frequent type of bacterial infection seen by health care providers. UTIs include several distinct entities, including asymptomatic bacteriuria, symptomatic infections, lower UTIs such as cystitis, and upper UTIs such as pyelonephritis. Because of their ability to cause renal damage, upper UTIs are considered more serious than lower UTIs. Acute pyelonephritis represents an infection of the renal parenchyma and renal pelvis. Improperly treated, it can lead to sepsis, renal abscesses, chronic pyelonephritis, and chronic renal failure. Approximately 7 million visits to a primary care provider are made each year for treatment of lower UTIs.[3]

KEY POINTS

URINARY TRACT INFECTIONS

- Infection is facilitated by host conditions that disrupt washout of the agent from the urinary tract through urine flow, change the protective properties of the mucin lining of the urinary tract, disrupt the protective function of the normal bacterial flora, or impair the function of the immune system.
- Virulence of the agent is derived from its ability to gain access to and thrive in the environment, adhere to the tissues of the lower or upper urinary tract, evade the destructive effects of the host's immune system, and develop resistance to antimicrobial agents.

Etiology and Pathogenesis

Most uncomplicated lower UTIs are caused by *E. coli*,[5] and complicated UTIs are caused by a number of pathogens such as *Klebsiella pneumoniae*, *Enterococcus faecalis*, *Enterobacter* spp., *Proteus mirabilis*, and *Pseudomonas aeruginosa*.[27] Most UTIs are caused by bacteria that enter through the urethra. Bacteria can also enter through the bloodstream usually in immunocompromised people and neonates. Although the distal portion of the urethra often contains pathogens, the urine formed in the kidneys and found in the bladder normally is sterile or free of bacteria. This is because of the *washout phenomenon*, in which urine from the bladder normally washes bacteria out of the urethra. When a UTI occurs, it is usually from bacteria that have colonized the urethra, vagina, or perianal area. Thus, factors that impact colonization (*e.g.*, having a prior UTI, sexual activity with a new partner, and changes in vaginal flora via pH changes) are risk factors for UTI.[28]

There is an increased risk for UTIs in people with urinary obstruction and reflux, in people with neurogenic disorders that impair bladder emptying, in women who are sexually active, in postmenopausal women, in men with diseases of the prostate, and in older adults.[29] Instrumentation and urinary catheterization are the most common predisposing factors for nosocomial UTIs because they bypass protective mechanisms.[20] People with diabetes are at increased risk for complications associated with UTIs, including pyelonephritis, and they are more susceptible to fungal infections (particularly *Candida* species).[30]

Host–Agent Interactions

Because certain people tend to be predisposed to development of UTIs, considerable interest has been focused on host–pathogen interactions and factors that increase the risk for UTI.[29] UTIs are more common in women than men; specifically, young sexually active women are at higher risk. Every year in the United States, about 10% of all females experience a symptomatic UTI, with 60% of all females having a symptomatic UTI during their lifetime.[29] In males, the longer length of the urethra and the antibacterial properties of the prostatic fluid, which contains immunoglobulins (IgA and IgG), provide some protection from ascending UTIs.[31] When UTIs occur in males, they typically develop complicated UTI related to acute prostatitis.[29] In older men, prostatic hypertrophy becomes more common and with it may come obstruction and increased risk for UTI. For older adults with indwelling urinary catheters, a biofilm builds up and promotes more bacterial growth. Therefore, older adults, who already have decreased immunologic function related to aging, need meticulous surveillance for signs of infection.[21,32]

Host Defenses. In the development of a UTI, host defenses are matched against the virulence of the pathogen. The host defenses of the bladder include:

- The washout phenomenon, whereby bacteria are removed from the bladder and urethra during voiding
- The bladder lining, which assists in providing a barrier to protect against bacterial invasion
- The body's immune response

In the ureters, peristaltic movements facilitate the movement of urine from the renal pelvis through the ureters and into the bladder. Immune mechanisms, particularly secretory immunoglobulin (Ig) A, appear to provide an important antibacterial defense. Phagocytic blood cells further assist in the removal of bacteria from the urinary tract.

Other important host factors include the normal flora of the periurethral area in women and prostate secretions in men.[5] In women, the normal flora of the periurethral area, which consists of organisms such as *Lactobacillus*, provides defense against the colonization of uropathic bacteria. Alterations in the periurethral environment, such as that occurring with a decrease in estrogen levels during menopause or the use of antibiotics, can alter the protective periurethral flora, allowing uropathogens to colonize and enter the urinary tract. In men, the prostatic fluid has antimicrobial properties that protect the urethra from colonization.

Pathogen Virulence. Virulence factors help microorganisms to evade the host defenses and produce disease.[29] Not all bacteria are capable of adhering to and infecting the urinary tract; only those with increased ability to adhere to the epithelial cells of the urinary tract are able to produce UTIs. Of the many strains of *E. coli*, some serogroups produce more infections with a higher clinical severity. For example, serotypes O, K, and H are associated with development of pyelonephritis.[29] *E. coli* strains capable of causing UTI are known as uropathogenic *E. coli* (EPEC). These bacteria have fine protein filaments, called pili or *fimbriae*, that enhance colonization by helping these bacteria adhere to receptors on the lining of urinary tract structures.[29] The two main types of pili (types 1 and P) found on *E. coli* that cause UTIs are morphologically similar, but they differ in their ability to mediate hemagglutination in the presence of mannose. Type P pili are mannose resistant and were named because of their increased presence in *E. coli* that cause pyelonephritis and because of their association with the P blood group system.[29] Neutrophils do not have receptors for P pili, so bacteria with P pili are resistant to phagocytosis. The host response to P pili via toll-like receptor 4 (TLR-4) is enhanced, resulting in release of inflammatory cytokines. These P pili strains of *E. coli* are a frequent cause of urosepsis (bacteremia caused from UTI). P pili have also been observed in over 90% of *E. coli* strains causing pyelonephritis. Although *E. coli* with P pili enhance colonization of the colon, *E. coli* with type I pili are more likely to colonize the bladder and cause cystitis. Type I pili strains have a higher affinity to adhere and can form biofilm-like inclusions.[29]

Obstruction and Reflux

Obstruction and reflux are other contributing factors in the development of UTIs. Any microorganisms that enter the bladder normally are washed out during voiding. When outflow is obstructed, urine remains in the bladder and acts as a medium for microbial growth. The microorganisms in the contaminated urine can then ascend along the ureters to infect the kidneys. The presence of residual urine correlates closely with bacteriuria and with its recurrence after treatment. Another aspect of bladder outflow obstruction and bladder distention is increased intravesical pressure, which compresses blood vessels in the bladder wall, leading to a decrease in the mucosal defenses of the bladder.

In UTIs associated with stasis of urine flow, the obstruction may be anatomic or functional. Anatomic obstructions include urinary tract stones, prostatic hyperplasia, pregnancy, and malformations of the ureterovesical junction. Functional obstructions include neurogenic bladder, infrequent voiding, detrusor (bladder) muscle instability, and constipation.

Reflux occurs when urine from the urethra moves into the bladder (*i.e.*, urethrovesical reflux).[5] In women, *urethrovesical reflux* can occur during activities such as coughing or squatting, in which an increase in intra-abdominal pressure causes the urine to be squeezed into the urethra and then to flow back into the bladder as the pressure decreases. This also can happen when voiding is abruptly interrupted. Because the urethral orifice frequently is contaminated with bacteria, the reflux mechanism may cause bacteria to be drawn back into the bladder.

A second type of reflux mechanism, *vesicoureteral reflux*, occurs at the level of the bladder and ureter. Normally, the distal portion of the ureter courses between the muscle layer and the mucosal surface of the bladder wall, forming a flap (Fig. 33.8). The flap is compressed against the bladder wall during micturition, preventing urine from being forced into the ureter. In people with vesicoureteral reflux, the ureter enters the bladder at an approximate right angle such that urine is forced into the ureter during micturition.[5] It is seen most commonly in children with UTIs and is believed to result from congenital defects in length, diameter, muscle structure, or innervation of the submucosal segment of the ureter. The concave shape of the peripheral papilla may contribute to reflux. Vesicoureteral reflux also is seen in adults with obstruction to bladder outflow, primarily because of increased bladder volume and pressure.

Catheter-Induced Infection

Urinary catheters are tubes made of latex or plastic. They are inserted through the urethra into the bladder for the purpose of draining urine. They are a source of urethral irritation and provide a means for entry of microorganisms into the urinary tract.[21]

Catheter-associated bacteriuria remains the most frequent cause of gram-negative infections in hospitalized people. Bacteria adhere to the surface of the catheter and initiate the growth of a biofilm that then covers the surface of the catheter.[21] The biofilm tends to protect the bacteria from the host's response and action of antibiotics, which makes treatment difficult. A closed drainage system (*i.e.*, closed to air and other sources of contamination) and careful attention to perineal hygiene (*i.e.*, cleaning the area around the urethral meatus) help to prevent infections in people who require an indwelling catheter. Careful handwashing and early detection and treatment of UTIs also are essential.

Clinical Manifestations

The manifestations of UTI depend on whether the infection involves the lower (bladder) or upper (kidney) urinary tract and whether the infection is acute or chronic. The majority of UTIs are acute uncomplicated bladder infections that occur in women. Upper UTIs affect the parenchyma and pelvis of the kidney (pyelonephritis).[24] They are less common and occur more frequently in children and adults with urinary tract obstructions or other predisposing conditions such as diabetes.

An acute episode of cystitis (bladder infection) is characterized by frequency of urination, lower abdominal or back discomfort, and burning and pain on urination (*i.e.*, dysuria).[20,24] Occasionally, the urine is cloudy and foul smelling. Manifestations in children younger than two are typically nonspecific, whereas children over five tend to have the localized symptoms of cystitis mentioned above.[29] In adults, fever and other signs of infection usually are absent. If there are no complications, the symptoms disappear within 48 hours of treatment. The symptoms of cystitis also may represent urethritis caused by *Chlamydia trachomatis*, *Neisseria gonorrhoeae*, or herpes simplex virus or vaginitis attributable to *Trichomonas vaginalis* or *Candida* species.[5]

Diagnosis and Treatment

The diagnosis of UTI usually is based on symptoms and on examination of the urine for the presence of microorganisms. When necessary, x-ray films, ultrasonography, and CT and renal scans are used to identify contributing factors, such as obstruction.

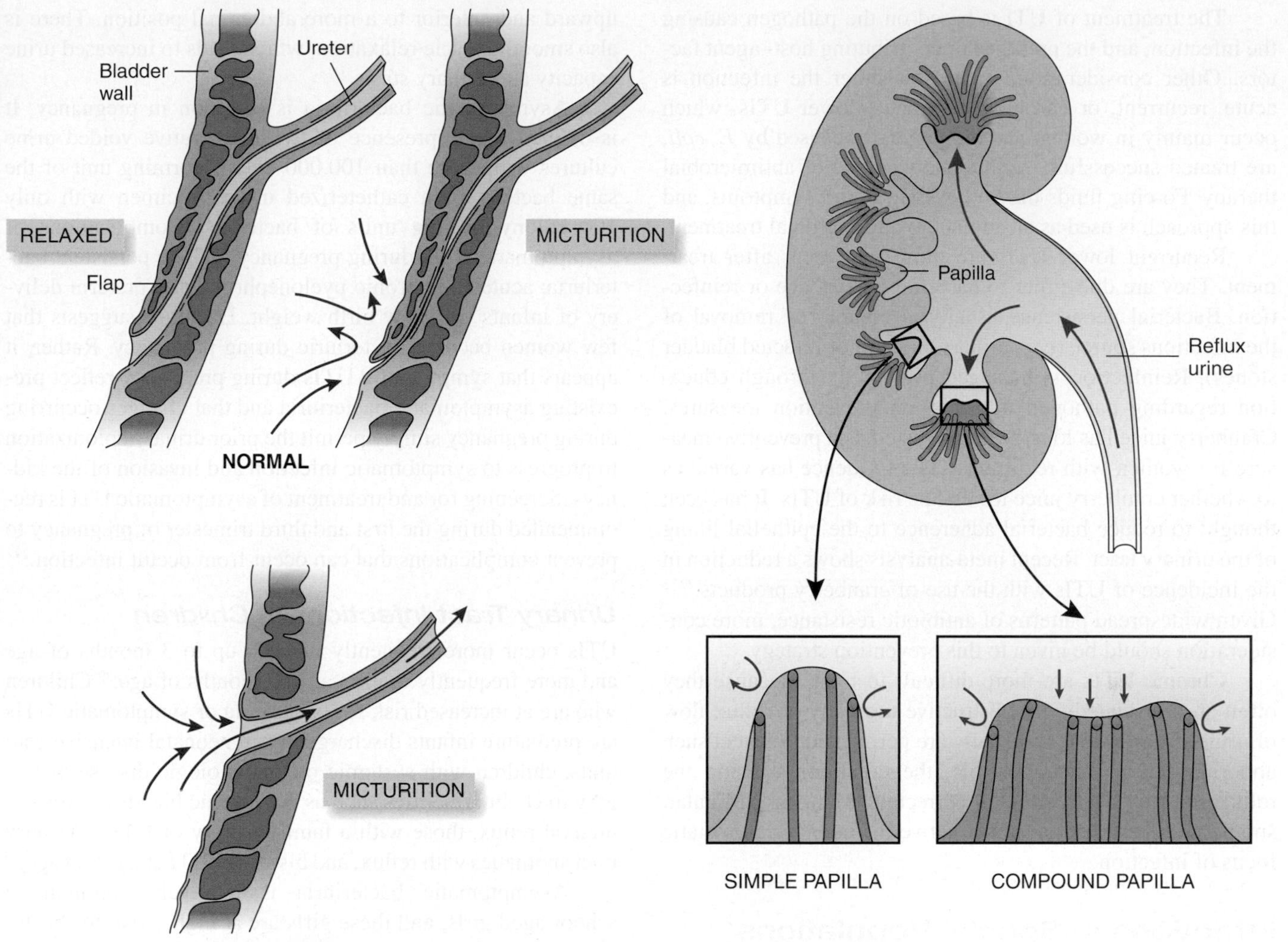

Figure 33.8 • Anatomic features of the bladder and kidney in pyelonephritis caused by ureterovesical reflux. In the normal bladder, the distal portion of the intravesical ureter courses between the mucosa and the muscularis, forming a mucosal flap. On micturition, the elevated intravesicular pressure compresses the flap against the bladder wall, occluding the lumen. People with congenital short intravesical ureter have no mucosal flap, because the angle of entry of the ureter into the bladder approaches a right angle. Thus, micturition forces urine into the ureter. In the renal pelvis, simple papillae of the central calyces are convex and do not readily allow reflux of urine. By contrast, the peripheral compound papillae are concave and permit entry of the refluxed urine. (From Rubin R., Strayer D. (Eds.) (2015). *Rubin's pathology: Clinicopathologic foundations of medicine* (7th ed., p. 945, Figure 22.72). Philadelphia, PA: Wolters Kluwer Health.)

Urine tests are used to establish the presence of bacteria in the urine and for a diagnosis of UTI. A commonly accepted criterion for diagnosis of a UTI is the presence of 100,000 colony-forming units (CFU) or more bacteria per milliliter (mL) of urine.[25] Colonization usually is defined as the multiplication of microorganisms in or on a host without apparent evidence of invasiveness or tissue injury. Pyuria (the presence of less than five to eight leukocytes per high-power field) indicates a host response to infection rather than asymptomatic bacterial colonization.[25] A Gram stain may be done to determine the type (gram positive or gram negative) of organism that is present. A urine culture may be done to confirm the presence of pathogenic bacteria in urine specimens, allow for their identification, and permit the determination of their sensitivity to specific antibiotics.

Urine may be screened using a simple dipstick method or via urinalysis to chemically screen urine for biomarkers of infection. Two simple tests are the nitrite and leukocyte esterase test.[25] These tests are relatively inexpensive, easy to perform, and can be done in the clinic setting or even in the home. Bacteria reduce nitrates in the urine to nitrites, providing a means for chemical analysis. Similarly, activated leukocytes secrete leukocyte esterase, which can be detected chemically.[25] Nitrite tests may be negative if the causative organism is not nitrate producing (*e.g.*, enterococci, *Staphylococcus saprophyticus*). The nitrite test can also be negative if the urine specimen is too diluted.

The treatment of UTI is based on the pathogen causing the infection, and the presence of contributing host–agent factors. Other considerations include whether the infection is acute, recurrent, or chronic. Most acute lower UTIs, which occur mainly in women and are generally caused by *E. coli*, are treated successfully with a short course of antimicrobial therapy. Forcing fluids may relieve signs and symptoms, and this approach is used as an adjunct to antimicrobial treatment.

Recurrent lower UTIs are those that recur after treatment. They are due either to bacterial persistence or reinfection. Bacterial persistence usually is curable by removal of the infectious source (*e.g.*, urinary catheter or infected bladder stones). Reinfection is managed principally through education regarding pathogen transmission prevention measures. Cranberry juice has long been suggested as a preventive measure for women with recurrent UTIs. Evidence has varied as to whether cranberry juice lowers the risk of UTIs. It has been thought to reduce bacterial adherence to the epithelial lining of the urinary tract. Recent meta-analysis shows a reduction in the incidence of UTIs with the use of cranberry products.[27,33] Given widespread patterns of antibiotic resistance, more consideration should be given to this prevention strategy.

Chronic UTIs are more difficult to treat. Because they often are associated with obstructive uropathy or reflux flow of urine, diagnostic tests usually are performed to detect such abnormalities.[20] When possible, the condition causing the reflux flow or obstruction is corrected. Men, in particular, should be investigated for obstructive disorders or a prostatic focus of infection.

Infections in Special Populations

UTIs affect people of all ages. In infants, they occur more often in boys than in girls. After the first year of life, UTIs occur more often in girls. This is because of the shorter length of the female urethra and because the vaginal vestibule can be easily contaminated with fecal flora. Approximately 60% of all adult women have at least one UTI during their lifetime.[32] The major risk factors for young women are related to sexual intercourse and use of spermicidal agents.[29,32] The anterior urethra usually is colonized with bacteria; urethral massage or sexual intercourse can force these bacteria back into the bladder.[29]

Urinary Tract Infections in Pregnant Women

Pregnant women are at increased risk for UTIs. Normal anatomic and physiologic changes in the functioning of the urinary tract that occur during pregnancy predispose to UTIs.[34] These changes involve the collecting system of the kidneys and include dilation of the renal calyces, pelvis, and ureters that begin during the first trimester and become most pronounced during the third trimester. This dilation of the upper urinary system is accompanied by a reduction in the peristaltic activity of the ureters that is thought to result from the muscle-relaxing effects of progesterone-like hormones and mechanical obstruction from the enlarging uterus. In addition to the changes in the kidneys and ureters, the bladder becomes displaced from its normal pelvic position to be displaced upward and anterior to a more abdominal position. There is also smooth muscle relaxation, which leads to increased urine capacity and urinary stasis.[34]

Asymptomatic bacteriuria is common in pregnancy. It is defined as the presence of two consecutive voided urine cultures with more than 100,000 colony-forming unit of the same bacteria or a catheterized urine specimen with only 100 colony-forming units of bacteria.[34] Complications of asymptomatic UTIs during pregnancy include persistent bacteriuria, acute and chronic pyelonephritis, and preterm delivery of infants with low birth weight. Evidence suggests that few women become bacteriuric during pregnancy. Rather, it appears that symptomatic UTIs during pregnancy reflect preexisting asymptomatic bacteriuria and that changes occurring during pregnancy simply permit the prior urinary colonization to progress to symptomatic infection and invasion of the kidneys. Screening for and treatment of asymptomatic UTI is recommended during the first and third trimester of pregnancy to prevent complications that can occur from occult infection.[29]

Urinary Tract Infections in Children

UTIs occur more frequently in boys up to 3 months of age and more frequently in girls after 3 months of age.[29] Children who are at increased risk for bacteriuria or symptomatic UTIs are premature infants discharged from neonatal intensive care units, children with systemic or immunologic disease or urinary tract abnormalities such as neurogenic bladder or vesicoureteral reflux, those with a family history of UTI or urinary tract anomalies with reflux, and history of UTI at a young age.[29]

Asymptomatic bacteriuria is relatively common in school-aged girls, and these girls are at higher risk for bacteriuria later in life. Prognosis is good when there are no structural or functional abnormalities.[29] Reflux is present in up to 50% of young children with symptomatic UTI.

UTIs in children frequently involve the upper urinary tract (pyelonephritis). In children in whom renal development is not complete, pyelonephritis can lead to hypertension, renal scarring, and permanent kidney damage.[29] The incidence of scarring is greatest in children with gross vesicoureteral reflux or obstruction, in children with recurrent UTIs, and in those with a delay in treatment.

Clinical Manifestations. Unlike adults, children frequently do not present with the typical signs of a UTI.[29,35] Many neonates with UTIs have bacteremia and may show signs and symptoms of septicemia, including fever, hypothermia, apneic spells, poor skin perfusion, abdominal distention, diarrhea, vomiting, lethargy, and irritability. Older infants may present with feeding problems, failure to thrive, diarrhea, vomiting, fever, and foul-smelling urine. Toddlers often present with abdominal pain, vomiting, diarrhea, abnormal voiding patterns, foul-smelling urine, fever, and poor growth. In older children with lower UTIs, the classic features—enuresis, frequency, dysuria, and suprapubic discomfort—are more common. Fever is a common sign of UTI in children, and the possibility of UTI should be considered in any child with unexplained fever.[36] Delayed diagnosis in young children increased the risk of permanent kidney scaring; yet, about 60% of pediatricians reported that delays in detection of febrile UTIs were common in practice.[35] The nature of symptoms in children may be inconsistent and vague, which contributes to the delay.

Diagnosis and Treatment Physical exam and urinalysis and urine culture are required for diagnosis and treatment.[36] Diagnosis is based on a careful history of voiding patterns and symptomatology; physical examination to determine fever, hypertension, abdominal or suprapubic tenderness, and other manifestations of UTI; and urinalysis to determine bacteriuria, pyuria, proteinuria, and hematuria. A positive urine culture that is obtained correctly is essential for proper diagnosis.[36] Additional diagnostic methods may be needed to determine the cause of the disorder. Vesicoureteral reflux is the most commonly associated abnormality in UTIs, and reflux nephropathy is an important cause of end-stage renal disease in children and adolescents. Children with a relatively uncomplicated first UTI may turn out to have significant reflux. Therefore, even a single documented UTI in a child requires careful diagnosis. Urinary symptoms in the absence of bacteriuria suggest vaginitis, urethritis, sexual molestation, the use of irritating bubble baths, pinworms, or viral cystitis. In adolescent girls, a history of dysuria and vaginal discharge makes vaginitis or vulvitis a consideration. Studies have shown that uncircumcised males are at higher risk of UTI.[29]

The approach to treatment is based on the clinical severity of the infection (*e.g.*, location of the infection, risk for sepsis, and the presence of structural abnormalities).[29,36] The immediate treatment of infants and young children is essential. Most infants with symptomatic UTIs and many children with clinical evidence of acute upper UTIs require hospitalization, rehydration, and intravenous antibiotic therapy. Follow-up is essential for children with febrile UTIs to ensure resolution of the infection. Follow-up urine cultures often are done at the end of treatment to ensure the antibiotic was effective. Imaging studies often are recommended for all children after their first UTI to detect renal scarring, vesicoureteral reflux, or other abnormalities.

Urinary Tract Infections in Older Adults

UTIs are the second most common cause of infection, after pneumonia, in older adults. UTIs cause about 11% of infections among healthy community-dwelling older adults and up to 50% of infections among those in long-term care facilities.[37]

Normal age-related changes associated with immune function increase the risk of infection in older adults. In addition, the risk of infection is increased by several predisposing factors, including immobility resulting in poor bladder emptying, bladder outflow obstruction caused by prostatic hyperplasia or kidney stones, bladder ischemia caused by urine retention, constipation, senile vaginitis, and diminished bactericidal activity of urine and prostatic secretions. Added to these risks are other health problems that necessitate instrumentation of the urinary tract. Having a history of a UTI is an important predictor for subsequent UTIs in older adults.[38]

Older adults with bacteriuria have varying symptoms, ranging from the absence of symptoms to the presence of typical UTI symptoms. Even when symptoms of lower UTIs are present, they may be difficult to interpret because older adults without UTIs commonly experience urgency, frequency, and incontinence. Alternatively, older adults may have vague symptoms such as anorexia, fatigue, weakness, or change in mental status.[37] Even with more serious upper UTIs (*e.g.*, pyelonephritis), the classic signs of infection such as fever, chills, flank pain, and tenderness may be altered or absent in older adults. Sometimes, no symptoms occur until the infection is far advanced.

IN SUMMARY

UTI is the second most common type of bacterial infection seen by health care professionals. Infections can range from asymptomatic bacteriuria to severe kidney infections that cause irreversible kidney damage. Predisposition to infection is determined by host defenses and pathogen virulence. Host defenses include the washout phenomenon associated with voiding, the protective mucin lining of the bladder, and the local immune defenses. Pathogen virulence is enhanced by the presence of pili that facilitate adherence to structures in the urinary tract, lipopolysaccharides that bind to host cells and elicit an inflammatory reaction, and cnzymes that break down RBCs and make iron available for bacterial metabolism and multiplication.

Most UTIs ascend from the urethra and bladder. A number of factors interact in determining the predisposition to development of UTIs, including urinary tract obstruction, urine stasis and reflux, pregnancy-induced changes in urinary tract function, age-related changes in the urinary tract, changes in the protective mechanisms of the bladder and ureters, impaired immune function, and virulence of the pathogen. Urinary tract catheters and urinary instrumentation contribute to the incidence of UTIs. Early diagnosis and treatment of UTI are essential to preventing permanent kidney damage.

DISORDERS OF GLOMERULAR FUNCTION

After completing this section of the chapter, the learner will be able to meet the following objectives:

- Describe the two types of immune mechanisms involved in glomerular disorders.
- Use the terms proliferation, sclerosis, *membranous*, *diffuse*, focal, *segmental*, and *mesangial* to explain changes in glomerular structure that occur with glomerulonephritis.
- Briefly describe the difference among the nephritic syndromes, rapidly progressive glomerulonephritis, nephrotic syndrome, asymptomatic glomerular disorders, and chronic glomerulonephritis.

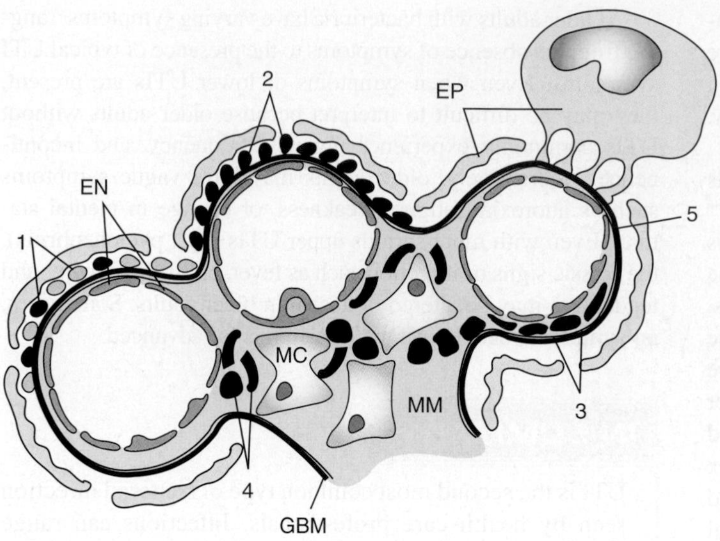

Figure 33.9 • Schematic representation of three glomerular capillaries depicting the sites of immune complex formation. Subepithelial deposits are seen in postinfectious glomerulonephritis (*1*) and membranous nephropathy (*2*) and are likely to be assembled locally by an in situ mechanism. Subendothelial deposits (*3*) and mesangial deposits (*4*) may also form locally but are more often the result of passive entrapment of preformed circulating immune complexes. Anti-GBM antibodies bind in a linear pattern to the GBM (*5*), and because the specific antigen is part of the heavily cross-linked basement membrane, electron-dense deposits at the ultrastructural level are missing. EN, endothelial cell; EP, visceral epithelial cell or podocyte; MC, mesangial cell; MM, mesangial matrix. (From Rennke H. G., Denker B. M. (2014). *Renal pathophysiology: The essentials* (4th ed., p. 242). Philadelphia, PA: Lippincott Williams & Wilkins.)

The glomeruli are tufts of capillaries that lie between the afferent and efferent arterioles. The capillaries of the glomeruli are arranged in lobules and supported by a stalk consisting of mesangial cells and a basement membrane–like extracellular matrix (Fig. 33.9). The glomerular capillary membrane is composed of three structural layers: an endothelial cell layer that lines the inner surface of the capillary, a basement membrane made up of a network of matrix proteins, and a layer of epithelial cells that surrounds the outer surface of the capillary and lines the inner surface of the Bowman capsule. The epithelial cells are attached to the basement membrane by long, footlike processes (*podocytes*) that encircle the outer surface of the capillaries. The glomerular capillary membrane is selectively permeable, allowing water and small particles (*e.g.*, electrolytes and dissolved particles, such as glucose and amino acids) to leave the blood and enter the Bowman space and preventing larger particles (*e.g.*, plasma proteins and blood cells) from leaving the blood.[6]

Glomerulonephritis is an inflammatory process that involves glomerular structures. It is the second leading cause of kidney failure worldwide and ranks third, after diabetes and hypertension, as a cause of chronic kidney disease in the United States.[5] There are many causes of glomerular disease. The disease may occur as a primary condition in which the glomerular abnormality is the only disease present, or it may occur as a secondary condition in which the glomerular abnormality results from another disease, such as diabetes mellitus or SLE. See Figure 33.10 for an algorithm regarding primary versus secondary glomerulonephritis.

Etiology and Pathogenesis of Glomerular Injury

The causative agents or triggering events that produce glomerular injury include immunologic, nonimmunologic, and hereditary mechanisms. Most cases of primary and many cases of secondary glomerular disease probably have an immune origin.[5] Although many glomerular diseases are driven by immunologic events, a variety of nonimmunologic metabolic (*e.g.*, diabetes), hemodynamic (*e.g.*, hypertension), and toxic (*e.g.*, drugs, chemicals) stresses can induce glomerular injury, either alone or along with immunologic mechanisms. Hereditary glomerular diseases such as Alport syndrome, although relatively rare, are an important category of glomerular disease because of their association with progressive loss of renal function and transmission to future generations.

Two types of immune mechanisms have been implicated in the development of glomerular disease:

1. Injury resulting from antibodies reacting with fixed glomerular antigens or antigens planted within the glomerulus
2. Injury resulting from circulating antigen–antibody complexes that become trapped in the glomerular membrane (Fig. 33.11)

Antigens responsible for development of the immune response may be of endogenous origin, such as autoantibodies to deoxyribonucleic acid (DNA) in SLE, or they may be of exogenous origin, such as streptococcal membrane antigens in poststreptococcal glomerulonephritis. Frequently, the source of the antigen is unknown.

The cellular changes that occur with glomerular disease include increases in glomerular or inflammatory cell number (proliferative or hypercellular), basement membrane thickening (membranous), and changes in noncellular glomerular components (sclerosis and fibrosis).[5,6] An increase in cell numbers is characterized by one or more of the following: proliferation of endothelial and mesangial cells, leukocyte infiltration (neutrophils, monocytes, and, in some cases, lymphocytes), and formation of crescents (half-moon–shaped collections of proliferating epithelial cells and infiltrating leukocytes) in the Bowman space.[5,6] *Basement membrane thickening* involves deposition of dense, noncellular material on the endothelial and epithelial sides of the basement membrane

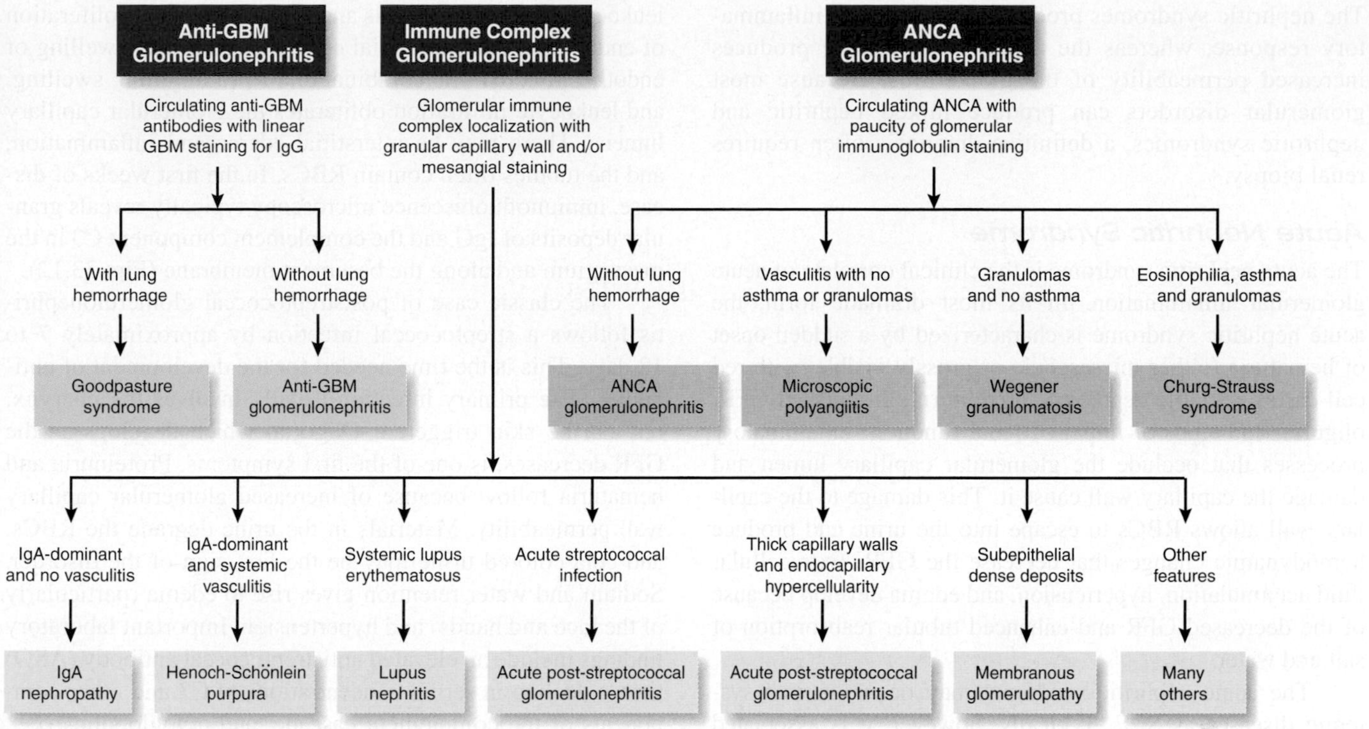

Figure 33.10 • Algorithm demonstrating the integration of pathologic findings with clinical data to make a diagnosis of a specific form of primary or secondary glomerulonephritis. An important initial categorization is an anti-GBM immune complex or antineutrophil cytoplasmic autoantibody (ANCA) glomerulonephritis. Once this determination is made, more specific diagnoses depend on additional clinical or pathologic observations. (From Rubin R., Strayer D. (Eds.) (2015). *Rubin's pathology: Clinicopathologic foundations of medicine* (7th ed., p. 915, Figure 22.15). Philadelphia, PA: Wolters Kluwer Health.)

or within the membrane itself. Sclerosis refers to an increased amount of extracellular material in the mesangial, subendothelial, or subepithelial tissue of the glomerulus. Fibrosis refers to the deposition of collagen fibers. Glomerular changes can be *diffuse*, involving all glomeruli and all parts of the glomeruli; focal, in which only some glomeruli are affected and others are essentially normal; *segmental*, involving only a certain segment of each glomerulus; or *mesangial*, affecting only mesangial cells.[5,6] Figure 33.9B illustrates the location of lesions associated with various types of glomerular disease.

Types of Glomerular Disease

The clinical manifestations of glomerular disorders generally fall into one of five categories:

1. Nephritic syndromes
2. Rapidly progressive glomerulonephritis
3. The nephrotic syndrome
4. Asymptomatic disorders of urinary sediment (*i.e.*, hematuria, proteinuria)
5. Chronic glomerulonephritis[5]

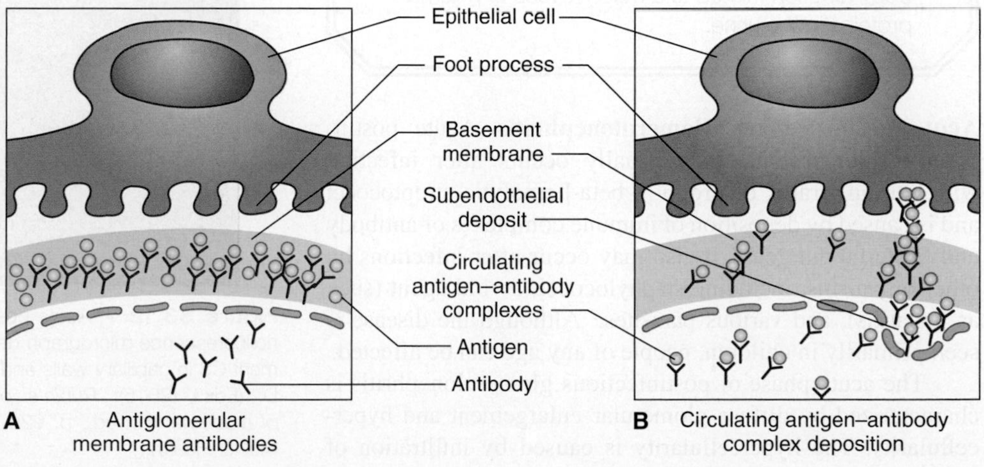

Figure 33.11 • Immune mechanisms of glomerular disease. **(A)** Antiglomerular membrane antibodies leave the circulation and interact with antigens that are present in the basement membrane of the glomerulus. **(B)** Antigen–antibody complexes circulating in the blood become trapped as they are filtered in the glomerulus.

The nephritic syndromes produce a proliferative inflammatory response, whereas the nephrotic syndrome produces increased permeability of the glomerulus. Because most glomerular disorders can produce mixed nephritic and nephrotic syndromes, a definitive diagnosis often requires renal biopsy.

Acute Nephritic Syndrome

The acute nephritic syndrome is the clinical correlate of acute glomerular inflammation. In its most dramatic form, the acute nephritic syndrome is characterized by a sudden onset of hematuria (either microscopic or grossly visible, with red cell casts), variable degrees of proteinuria, diminished GFR, oliguria, and signs of impaired renal function. Inflammatory processes that occlude the glomerular capillary lumen and damage the capillary wall cause it. This damage to the capillary wall allows RBCs to escape into the urine and produce hemodynamic changes that decrease the GFR. Extracellular fluid accumulation, hypertension, and edema develop because of the decreased GFR and enhanced tubular reabsorption of salt and water.

The acute nephritic syndrome may occur in such systemic diseases as SLE. Typically, however, it is associated with acute proliferative glomerulonephritis such as postinfectious glomerulonephritis.

> **KEY POINTS**
>
> **GLOMERULAR DISORDERS**
>
> - Glomerular disorders affect the semipermeable properties of the glomerular capillary membrane that allow water and small particles to move from the blood into the urine filtrate while preventing blood cells and plasma proteins from leaving the circulation.
> - The nephritic syndromes produce a decrease in glomerular permeability and manifestations related to a decrease in GFR, fluid retention, and nitrogenous waste accumulation.
> - The nephrotic syndrome produces an increase in glomerular permeability and manifestations of altered body function related to a massive loss of plasma proteins in the urine.

Acute Postinfectious Glomerulonephritis. Acute postinfectious glomerulonephritis usually occurs after infection with certain strains of group A beta-hemolytic streptococci and is caused by deposition of immune complexes of antibody and bacterial antigens.[5] It also may occur after infections by other organisms, including staphylococci, a viral agent (such as hepatitis), and various parasites.[3] Although the disease is seen primarily in children, people of any age can be affected.

The acute phase of postinfectious glomerulonephritis is characterized by diffuse glomerular enlargement and hypercellularity. The hypercellularity is caused by infiltration of leukocytes, both neutrophils and monocytes, and proliferation of endothelial and mesangial cells.[5] There is also swelling of endothelial cells. The combination of proliferation, swelling, and leukocyte infiltration obliterates the glomerular capillary lumens. There may be interstitial edema and inflammation, and the tubules often contain RBCs. In the first weeks of disease, immunofluorescence microscopy typically reveals granular deposits of IgG and the complement component C3 in the mesangium and along the basement membrane (Fig. 33.12).

The classic case of poststreptococcal glomerulonephritis follows a streptococcal infection by approximately 7 to 12 days. This is the time needed for the development of antibodies. The primary infection usually involves the pharynx, but can be skin triggered. Oliguria, which develops as the GFR decreases, is one of the first symptoms. Proteinuria and hematuria follow because of increased glomerular capillary wall permeability. Materials in the urine degrade the RBCs, and cola-colored urine may be the first sign of the disorder. Sodium and water retention gives rise to edema (particularly of the face and hands) and hypertension. Important laboratory findings include an elevated antistreptococcal antibody (ASO) titer, a decline in serum concentrations of C3 and other components of the complement cascade, and cryoglobulins (*i.e.*, large immune complexes) in the serum.

Treatment of acute poststreptococcal glomerulonephritis includes elimination of the streptococcal infection with antibiotics and providing supportive care. The disorder carries an excellent prognosis and rarely causes chronic kidney disease.[5]

Rapidly Progressive Glomerulonephritis

Rapidly progressive glomerulonephritis is a clinical syndrome characterized by signs of severe glomerular injury that do not have a specific cause. As its name indicates, this type

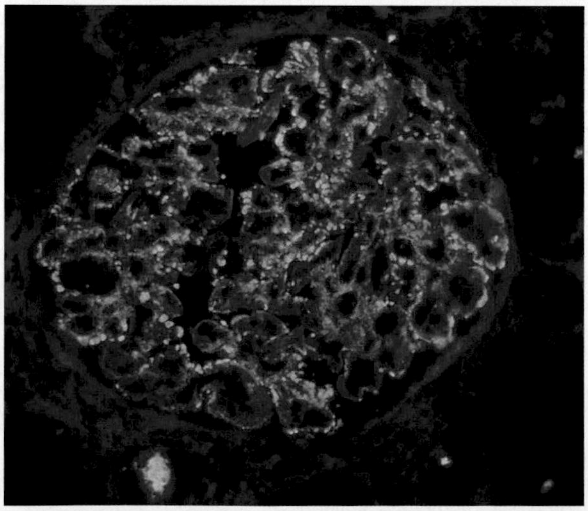

Figure 33.12 • Acute postinfectious glomerulonephritis. An immunofluorescence micrograph demonstrates granular staining for complement C3 in capillary walls and the mesangium. (From Rubin R., Strayer D. (Eds.) (2015). *Rubin's pathology: Clinicopathologic foundations of medicine* (7th ed., p. 926, Figure 22.37). Philadelphia, PA: Wolters Kluwer Health.)

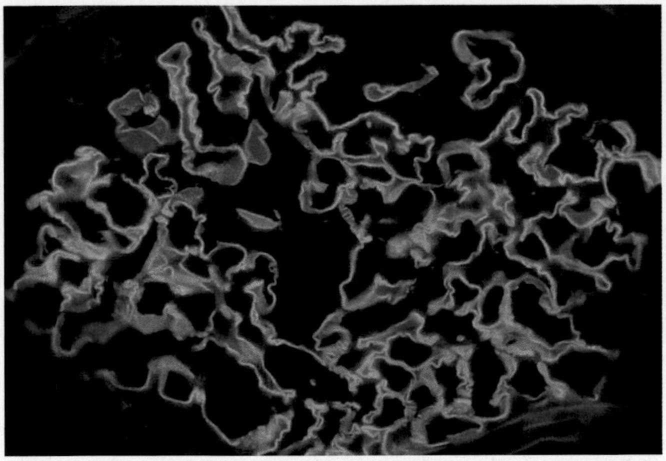

Figure 33.13 • Anti-GBM glomerulonephritis. Linear immunofluorescence for IgG is seen along the GBM. Contrast this with the granular pattern of immunofluorescence typical of most types of immune complex deposition within the capillary wall. (From Rubin R., Strayer D. (Eds.) (2015). *Rubin's pathology: Clinicopathologic foundations of medicine* (7th ed., p. 933, Figure 22.52). Philadelphia, PA: Wolters Kluwer Health.)

of glomerulonephritis is rapidly progressive, often within a matter of months. The disorder involves focal and segmental proliferation of glomerular cells and recruitment of monocytes and macrophages with formation of crescent-shaped structures that obliterate the Bowman space.[39] Rapidly proliferative glomerulonephritis may be caused by a number of immunologic disorders, some systemic and others restricted to the kidney. Among the diseases associated with this form of glomerulonephritis are immune complex disorders such as SLE, small-vessel vasculitides (*e.g.*, microscopic polyangiitis), and an immune disorder called *Goodpasture syndrome.*

Goodpasture Syndrome. Goodpasture syndrome is an uncommon and aggressive form of glomerulonephritis that is caused by antibodies to the alveolar and glomerular basement membrane (GBM). The anti-GBM antibodies cross-react with the pulmonary alveolar basement membrane to produce the syndrome of pulmonary hemorrhage associated with renal failure. The pathologic hallmark of anti-GBM glomerulonephritis is diffuse linear staining of GBMs for IgG (Fig. 33.13). The cause of the disorder is unknown, although influenza infection, exposure to hydrocarbon solvent (found in paints and dyes), various drugs, and cancer have been implicated in some people. There is some thought that Goodpasture syndrome has a genetic predisposition, but this is not conclusive.

Treatment includes plasmapheresis to remove circulating anti-GBM antibodies and immunosuppressive therapy (*i.e.*, corticosteroids and cyclophosphamide) to inhibit antibody production.[31]

Nephrotic Syndrome

The nephrotic syndrome is characterized by massive proteinuria (>3.5 g/day) and lipiduria (*e.g.*, free fat, oval bodies, fatty casts) along with an associated hypoalbuminemia (<3 g/dL), generalized edema, and hyperlipidemia (cholesterol > 300 mg/dL).[3] The nephrotic syndrome is not a specific glomerular disease but a constellation of clinical findings that result from an increase in glomerular permeability and loss of plasma proteins in the urine[5] (Fig. 33.14).

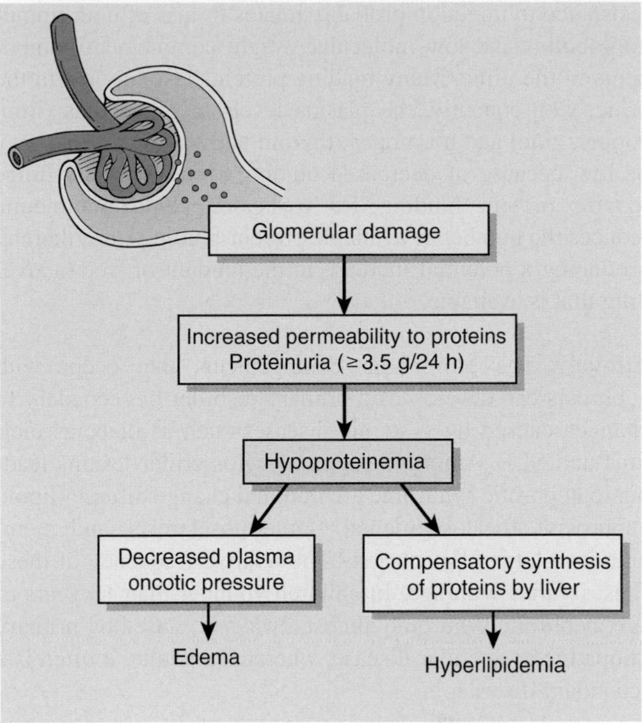

Figure 33.14 • Pathophysiology of the nephrotic syndrome.

Pathogenesis. Any increase in glomerular membrane permeability allows proteins to escape from the plasma into the glomerular filtrate. Massive proteinuria results, leading to hypoalbuminemia. Generalized edema, which is a hallmark of the nephrotic syndrome, results from the loss of colloidal osmotic pressure of the blood with subsequent accumulation of fluid in the interstitial tissues.[5] There is also salt and water retention, which aggravates the edema. This appears to be due to several factors, including a compensatory increase in aldosterone, stimulation of the sympathetic nervous system, and a reduction in secretion of natriuretic factors. Initially, the edema presents in dependent parts of the body such as the lower extremities but becomes more generalized as the disease progresses. Dyspnea because of pulmonary edema, pleural effusions, and diaphragmatic compromise because of ascites can develop in people with nephrotic syndrome.

The hyperlipidemia that occurs in people with nephrosis is characterized by elevated levels of triglycerides and low-density lipoproteins (LDLs). Levels of high-density lipoproteins (HDLs) usually are normal. Because of the elevated LDL levels, people with nephrotic syndrome are at increased risk for development of atherosclerosis.

The largest proportion of protein lost in the urine is albumin, but globulins also may be lost. As a result, people with nephrosis may be vulnerable to infections, particularly those caused by staphylococci and pneumococci.[5] This decreased resistance to infection probably relates to loss of both immunoglobulins and low molecular weight complement components in the urine. Many binding proteins also are lost in the urine. Consequently, the plasma levels of many ions (iron, copper, zinc) and hormones (thyroid and sex hormones) may be low because of decreased binding proteins. Many drugs require protein binding for transport. Hypoalbuminemia reduces the number of available protein-binding sites, thereby producing a potential increase in the amount of free (active) drug that is available.

Etiology. The glomerular derangements that occur with nephrosis can develop as a primary disorder or secondary to changes caused by systemic diseases such as diabetes mellitus and SLE. Among the primary glomerular lesions leading to nephrotic syndrome are minimal change disease (lipoid nephrosis), focal segmental glomerulosclerosis, and membranous glomerulonephritis.[5] The relative frequency of these causes varies with age. In children younger than 15 years of age, nephrotic syndrome almost always is caused by primary idiopathic glomerular disease, whereas in adults, it often is a secondary disorder.[5]

Minimal Change Disease (Lipoid Nephrosis). Minimal change disease is characterized by diffuse loss (through fusion) of the foot processes of cells in the epithelial layer of the glomerular membrane. It is most commonly seen in children but may occasionally occur in adults. The cause of minimal change nephrosis is unknown. Although minimal change disease does not progress to renal failure, it can cause significant complications, including predisposition to infection with gram-positive organisms, a tendency toward thromboembolic events, hyperlipidemia, and protein malnutrition.

Membranous Glomerulonephritis. Membranous glomerulonephritis is the most common cause of primary nephrosis in adults, most commonly those in the fifth and sixth decades of life and almost always after 30 years of age.[5] The disorder is caused by diffuse thickening of the GBM because of deposition of immune complexes. The disorder may be idiopathic or associated with a number of disorders, including autoimmune diseases such as SLE, infections such as chronic hepatitis B, and metabolic disorders such as diabetes mellitus. The presence of immunoglobulins and complement in the subendothelial deposits suggests that the disease represents a chronic immune complex–mediated disorder.

The disorder usually begins with an insidious onset of the nephrotic syndrome or, in a small percentage of people, with nonnephrotic proteinuria. Hematuria and mild hypertension may be present. The progress of the disease is variable. Some people experience a complete remission, others have repeated remissions and relapses, and still others progress to complete renal failure and even death. Spontaneous remissions and a relatively benign outcome occur more commonly in women and those with proteinuria in the nonnephrotic range. Treatment is controversial.

Focal Segmental Glomerulosclerosis. Focal segmental glomerulosclerosis is characterized by sclerosis (*i.e.*, increased collagen deposition) of some, but not all glomeruli, and in the affected glomeruli, only a portion of the glomerular tuft is involved.[5] It is a particularly common cause of nephrotic syndrome in Hispanic and African Americans.

Although focal segmental sclerosis often is an idiopathic syndrome, it may be associated with reduced oxygen in the blood (*e.g.*, sickle cell disease and cyanotic congenital heart disease), human immunodeficiency virus (HIV) infection, or intravenous drug abuse, or it may occur as a secondary event reflecting glomerular scarring because of other forms of glomerulonephritis.[5] Impairment of autophagy (a repair process necessary to maintain homeostasis post cell injury) may be responsible for limited regenerative capacity of podocytes.[40]

The presence of hypertension and decreased renal function distinguishes focal sclerosis from minimal change disease. In addition, research indicates that people with minimal change disease (MCD) (a manifestation of nephrotic syndrome diagnosed by renal biopsy) may later progress to focal segmental glomerulosclerosis.[41] The protein nephrin seems to be a marker for podocyte injury. People with MCD respond to varying degrees to corticosteroids. People who were treated and did not experience nephrin loss had a 96% remission rate compared with a 61% remission rate among those who experienced nephron loss.[41] Most people with the disorder progress to kidney failure within 5 to 10 years.

Asymptomatic Hematuria or Proteinuria

Many cases of glomerulonephritis result in mild asymptomatic illness that is not recognized or brought to the attention of a health care professional and therefore remains undiagnosed. Population-based screening studies have shown that kidney damage as evidenced by proteinuria, hematuria, low GFR, or a combination of these features is present in the population. Disorders such as Henoch-Schönlein purpura often resolve without permanent kidney damage, whereas others, such as IgA nephropathy and Alport syndrome, can progress to chronic kidney disease and renal failure.

Immunoglobulin A Nephropathy. Immunoglobulin A nephropathy (*i.e.*, Berger disease) is a primary glomerulonephritis characterized by the presence of glomerular IgA immune complex deposits. It can occur at any age, but most commonly, the peak age of diagnosis is between 15 and 30 years of age.[5] The disease occurs more commonly in men than women and is the most common cause of glomerular nephritis in Asians.

The disorder is characterized by the deposition of IgA-containing immune complexes in the mesangium of the glomerulus. Once deposited in the kidney, the immune complexes are associated with glomerular inflammation. The cause of the disorder is unknown, and there is a need for more specific classifications of the stages of IgA nephropathy so more information can be interpreted. Therefore, the International IgA Nephropathy Network is developing IgAN classifications to assist providers in diagnosing this disease. The classification system is based on biopsy findings in a minimum of eight glomeruli to yield a MEST-C score.[42] Some people with the disorder have elevated serum IgA levels.

Early in the disease, many people with the disorder have no obvious symptoms and are unaware of the problem. In these people, IgA nephropathy is suspected during routine screening or examination for another condition. In other people, the disorder presents with gross hematuria that is preceded by upper respiratory tract infection, gastrointestinal tract symptoms, or a flulike illness. The hematuria usually lasts 2 to 6 days. Approximately one-half of the people with gross hematuria have a single episode, whereas the remainder experience a gradual progression in the disease with recurrent episodes of hematuria and mild proteinuria. Progression usually is slow, extending over several decades.

Immunofluorescence microscopy is essential for diagnosis of IgA nephropathy.[5] The diagnostic finding is mesangial staining for IgA more intense than staining for IgG or IgM (Fig. 33.15). At present, there are no satisfactory treatment measures for IgA nephropathy. The role of immunosuppressive drugs such as steroids and cytotoxic drugs is not clear. There has been recent interest in the use of omega-3 fatty acids in delaying the progression of the disease.

Henoch-Schönlein Purpura Nephritis. Henoch-Schönlein purpura is a small-vessel vasculitis that causes a purpuric rash largely of the lower extremities, arthritis or arthralgia, abdominal pain, and renal involvement identical to that of IgA nephropathy. Incidence has seasonal variation, with twice as many cases in the winter and fall.[43] The disease is seen most commonly in children but can also occur in adults. Renal involvement is not always present initially, but its incidence increases with time and is more common in older children, who have associated abdominal pain and a persistent rash. Although hematuria and proteinuria are the most common presentation, some people present with manifestations of acute nephritis, and others may present with combined nephritis

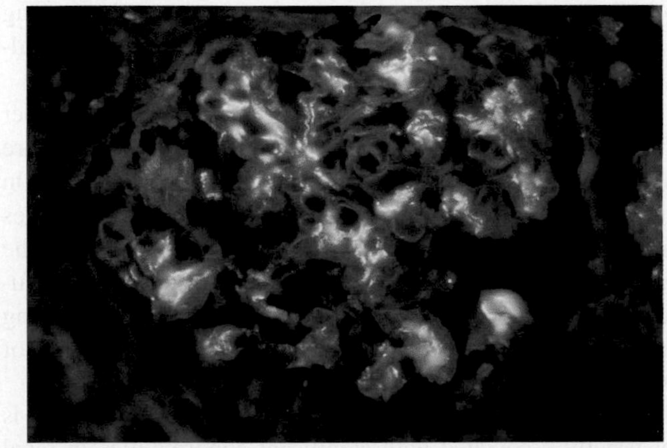

Figure 33.15 • IgA nephropathy. An immunofluorescence micrograph shows deposits of IgA in the mesangial areas. (From Rubin R., Strayer D. (Eds.) (2015). *Rubin's pathology: Clinicopathologic foundations of medicine* (7th ed., p. 931, Figure 22.48). Philadelphia, PA: Wolters Kluwer Health.)

and nephrotic manifestations. Most people recover fully over a period of several weeks. Some cases progress to end-stage renal disease. Corticosteroids are the most effective treatment and have been found to decrease the duration and intensity of abdominal and joint pain.[43]

Alport Syndrome

Alport syndrome represents a hereditary defect of the GBM that results in hematuria and may progress to chronic renal failure. It tends to be associated with defects in the ears or eyes.[5] The syndrome is caused by type IV collagen mutations. Approximately 85% of cases are inherited as an X-linked autosomal dominant trait, whereas others have autosomal dominant and recessive patterns of inheritance.[5] In X-linked pedigrees, boys are usually affected more seriously than girls. Affected boys usually progress to renal failure as adults, but progression may occur during adolescence. Although many girls never have more than mild hematuria with or without mild proteinuria, some have more significant disease and may even progress to kidney failure.

Diagnosis of Alport syndrome is often made after examination of the urine of a child from a family with multiple cases of hereditary nephritis. Children may initially present with heavy microscopic hematuria, followed by the development of proteinuria. Many, but not all, people with Alport syndrome have sensorineural deafness and various eye disorders, including lens dislocation, posterior cataracts, and corneal dystrophy. The hearing loss is bilateral and often is first detected during adolescence.

Chronic Glomerulonephritis

Chronic glomerulonephritis represents the chronic phase of a number of specific types of glomerulonephritis.[5] Some forms of acute glomerulonephritis (*e.g.*, poststreptococcal glomerulonephritis) undergo complete resolution, whereas others progress at variable rates to chronic glomerulonephritis. Some people who present with chronic glomerulonephritis have no history of glomerular disease. These cases may represent the end result of relatively asymptomatic forms of glomerulonephritis. Histologically, the condition is characterized by small kidneys with sclerosed glomeruli. In most cases, chronic glomerulonephritis develops insidiously and slowly progresses to chronic kidney disease over a period of years.

Glomerular Lesions Associated with Systemic Disease

Many immunologic, metabolic, or hereditary systemic diseases are associated with glomerular injury. In some diseases, such as SLE, diabetes mellitus, and hypertension, the glomerular involvement may be a major clinical manifestation.

Systemic Lupus Erythematosus Glomerulonephritis

Renal involvement is clinically evident in 40% to 85% of people with SLE and is seen more commonly in black women.[5] The pathogenesis of SLE is uncertain but seems to be related to dysregulated B-cell immunity with production of autoantibodies to a variety of nuclear, cytoplasmic, extracellular matrix, and cell membrane components.[5] It also involves dysregulated T-cell function, with the ratios of T-cell subpopulation playing an important role in SLE pathogenesis.[44] Most glomerular injury is triggered by the formation of immune complexes within the glomerular capillary wall.

Clinical Manifestations. The clinical manifestations of lupus nephritis depend on the site of immune complex–mediated injury. Immune complexes confined to the mesangium cause less inflammation than subendothelial immune complexes, which have greater exposure to inflammatory cells and mediators in the blood, and which therefore are more likely to produce inflammation.[5] The World Health Organization (WHO) classified the renal glomerular lesions of SLE as class I, normal; class II, mesangial proliferation; class III, focal and segmental proliferation; class IV, diffuse proliferation; and class V, membranous proliferation. Classification has been further refined to enhance communication between the pathologists and clinicians as well as to improve reproducibility and uniformity in reports.[45]

Diagnosis and Treatment. Because of the high risk for kidney disease, all people with SLE should undergo routine urinalysis to monitor for the appearance of hematuria or proteinuria. If urinary abnormalities are noted, renal biopsy is often performed. Treatment depends on the extent of glomerular involvement. People with class I or II glomerulonephritis usually require no treatment. Progression to higher classes is usually accompanied by an increase in lupus serology activity and evidence of deteriorating renal function (*i.e.*, rising serum creatinine and a decrease in calculated GFR). Oral corticosteroids and angiotensin-converting enzyme (ACE) inhibitors are the mainstays of treatment. People with more advanced disease may require treatment with immunosuppressive agents (*e.g.*, intravenous cyclophosphamide or oral mycophenolate mofetil). Clinical trials using other immunosuppressant agents are ongoing.

Diabetic Glomerulosclerosis

Diabetic nephropathy is a major cause of chronic kidney disease and the most common cause of kidney failure treated by renal replacement therapy in the United States.[5] It occurs in both type 1 and type 2 diabetes mellitus. It is more prevalent among African Americans, Asians, and Native Americans than whites.

Pathophysiology. The lesions of diabetic nephropathy most commonly involve the glomeruli. Widespread thickening of the glomerular capillary basement membrane occurs in almost all people with diabetes and can occur without evidence of proteinuria. This is followed by a diffuse increase in mesangial matrix, with mild proliferation of mesangial cells. As the disease progresses, the mesangial cells impinge on the capillary lumen, reducing the surface area for glomerular filtration. In nodular glomerulosclerosis, also known as *Kimmelstiel-Wilson syndrome*, there is nodular deposition of hyaline in the mesangial portion of the glomerulus.[5] As the sclerotic process progresses in the diffuse and nodular forms of glomerulosclerosis, there is complete obliteration of the glomerulus, with impairment of renal function.

Although the mechanisms of glomerular change in diabetes are uncertain, they are thought to represent enhanced or defective synthesis of the GBM and mesangial matrix with an inappropriate incorporation of glucose into the noncellular components of these glomerular structures.[5] Alternatively, hemodynamic changes that occur secondary to elevated blood glucose levels may contribute to the initiation and progression of diabetic glomerulosclerosis.[5] It has been hypothesized that elevations in blood glucose produce an increase in GFR and glomerular pressure that leads to enlargement of glomerular capillary pores by a mechanism that is, at least partly, mediated by angiotensin II. This enlargement results in an increase in the protein content of the glomerular filtrate, which in turn requires increased endocytosis of the filtered proteins by tubular endothelial cells, a process that ultimately leads to nephron destruction and progressive deterioration of renal function.

Clinical Manifestations and Treatment. The clinical manifestations of diabetic glomerulosclerosis are closely linked to those of diabetes. The increased GFR that occurs in people with early alterations in renal function is associated with *microalbuminuria*, which is defined as urinary albumin excretion of 30 to 300 mg in 24 hours.[25,46] Microalbuminuria is an important predictor of future diabetic nephropathies. In many cases, these early changes in glomerular function can be reversed by careful control of blood glucose levels. Inhibition of angiotensin by ACE inhibitors or angiotensin receptor blockers (ARBs) has been shown to have a beneficial effect, possibly by reversing increased glomerular pressure.[47] Hypertension and cigarette smoking have been implicated in the progression of diabetic nephropathy.

Hypertensive Glomerular Disease

Mild to moderate hypertension causes sclerotic changes in renal arterioles and small arteries, referred to as *benign nephrosclerosis*.[5] It is most prevalent and most aggressive among blacks. Among African Americans, hypertension is the leading cause of end-stage renal disease.

Hypertensive nephropathy is associated with a number of changes in kidney structure and function. The kidneys are smaller than normal and are usually affected bilaterally. On histologic examination, there is narrowing of the arterioles and small arteries, caused by thickening and scarring of the vessel walls. As the vascular structures thicken and perfusion diminishes, blood flow to the nephron decreases, causing patchy tubular atrophy, interstitial fibrosis, and a variety of changes in glomerular structure and function.

Although uncomplicated hypertensive nephrosclerosis is not usually associated with significant abnormalities in renal function, a few people may progress to end-stage renal disease. Three groups of people are at particular risk for development of renal failure—blacks, people with more severe BP elevations, and people with a second underlying disease, such as diabetes.

IN SUMMARY

Glomerulonephritis, an inflammatory process that involves glomerular structures, is the second leading cause of kidney failure worldwide and ranks third, after diabetes and hypertension, as a cause of chronic kidney disease in the United States. The disease may occur as a primary condition in which the glomerular abnormality is the only disease present, or it may occur as a secondary condition in which the glomerular abnormality results from another disease, such as diabetes mellitus or SLE. Most cases of primary and many cases of secondary glomerular disease probably have an immune origin.

The clinical manifestations of glomerular disorders generally fall into one of five categories: the nephritic syndromes, rapidly progressive glomerulonephritis, nephrotic syndrome, asymptomatic disorders (*i.e.*, hematuria, proteinuria), and chronic glomerulonephritis. The nephritic syndrome evokes an inflammatory response in the glomeruli and is characterized by hematuria with red cell casts in the urine, a diminished GFR, azotemia, oliguria, and hypertension. The nephrotic syndrome affects the integrity of the glomerular capillary membrane and is characterized by massive proteinuria, hypoalbuminemia, generalized edema, lipiduria, and hyperlipidemia. Asymptomatic hematuria and proteinuria represent glomerular disorders that are not recognized or brought to the attention of a health care professional and therefore remain undiagnosed. Chronic glomerulonephritis represents the chronic phase of a number of specific types of glomerulonephritis. Secondary causes of glomerular kidney disease include SLE, diabetes mellitus, and hypertension.

TUBULOINTERSTITIAL DISORDERS

After completing this section of the chapter, the learner will be able to meet the following objectives:

- Differentiate between the defects in tubular function that occur in proximal and distal tubular acidosis.
- Explain the pathogenesis of kidney damage in acute and chronic pyelonephritis.

Several disorders affect renal tubular structures, including the proximal and distal tubules. Most of these disorders also affect the interstitial tissue that surrounds the tubules. These disorders, sometimes referred to as *tubulointerstitial disorders*, include acute tubular necrosis, renal tubular acidosis, acute and chronic pyelonephritis, and the effects of drugs and toxins.

Tubulointerstitial renal diseases may be divided into acute and chronic disorders. The acute disorders are characterized by their sudden onset and by signs and symptoms of interstitial edema. They include acute pyelonephritis and acute hypersensitivity reaction to drugs. The chronic disorders produce interstitial fibrosis, atrophy, and mononuclear infiltrates. Most people with chronic disorders are asymptomatic until late in the course of the disease. In the early stages, tubulointerstitial diseases commonly are manifested by fluid and electrolyte imbalances that reflect subtle changes in tubular function. These clinical manifestations can include inability to concentrate urine, as evidenced by polyuria and nocturia; interference with acidification of urine, resulting in metabolic acidosis; and diminished tubular reabsorption.[5]

Renal Tubular Acidosis

Renal tubular acidosis (RTA) refers to a group of tubular defects in reabsorption of bicarbonate ions (HCO_3^-) or excretion of hydrogen ions (H^+) that result in metabolic acidosis and its subsequent complications, including metabolic bone disease, kidney stones, and growth failure in children. Proximal tubular disorders that affect bicarbonate reabsorption, and distal tubular defects that affect the secretion of fixed metabolic acids are the two major types of RTA. A third type of RTA results from aldosterone deficiency or resistance to its action that leads to impaired reabsorption of sodium ions (Na^+) with decreased elimination of H^+ and potassium ions (K^+). Renal acidosis also occurs in kidney failure.

Proximal Renal Tubular Acidosis

Proximal RTA involves a defect in proximal tubular reabsorption, the nephron site where 85% of filtered HCO_3^- is reabsorbed. With the onset of impaired tubular HCO_3^- reabsorption, there is a loss of HCO_3^- in the urine that reduces plasma HCO_3^- levels. The concomitant loss of Na^+ in the urine leads to contraction of the extracellular fluid volume with increased aldosterone secretion and a resultant decrease in serum K^+ levels. With proximal tubular defects in acid–base regulation, the distal tubular sites for secretion of the fixed acids into the urine continue to function, and the reabsorption of HCO_3^- eventually resumes, albeit at a lower level of serum HCO_3^-. Whenever serum levels rise above this decreased level, HCO_3^- is lost in the urine. People with proximal RTA generally have plasma HCO_3^- levels greater than 15 mEq/L and seldom develop severe acidosis.

Proximal RTA may occur as a hereditary or acquired disorder and may involve an isolated defect in HCO_3^- reabsorption or accompany other defects in proximal tubular function (Fanconi syndrome). Isolated defects in HCO_3^- reabsorption are relatively rare. The term *Fanconi syndrome* is used to describe a generalized proximal tubular dysfunction in which the RTA is accompanied by impaired reabsorption of glucose, amino acids, phosphate, and uric acid. Children with Fanconi syndrome are likely to have growth retardation, rickets, osteomalacia, and abnormal vitamin D metabolism in addition to mild acidosis associated with proximal RTA.

Children and infants with proximal RTA require alkali therapy because of the high incidence of growth retardation because of acidemia. Potassium supplements are also needed because of increased loss of potassium that occurs with alkali therapy. Adults may also require alkali therapy. Vitamin D and phosphate are appropriate treatments for rickets and hypophosphatemia.

Distal Renal Tubular Acidosis

Distal RTA has its origin in the distal convoluted tubule and the collecting duct, where about 15% of the filtered bicarbonate is reabsorbed. The clinical syndrome of distal RTA includes hypokalemia, hyperchloremic metabolic acidosis, inability to acidify the urine, nephrocalcinosis, and nephrolithiasis. Additional features include osteomalacia or rickets.

Distal RTA results from a distal tubular defect in H^+ secretion with failure to acidify the urine. Because the secretion of H^+ in the distal tubules is linked to sodium reabsorption, failure to secrete H^+ results in a net loss of sodium bicarbonate in the urine. This results in contraction of fluids in the extracellular fluid compartment, a compensatory increase in aldosterone levels, and development of hypokalemia. The persistent acidosis, which requires buffering by the skeletal system, causes calcium to be released from bone. Increased losses of calcium in the urine lead to increased levels of parathyroid hormone, osteomalacia, bone pain, impaired growth in children, and development of kidney stones and nephrocalcinosis.

Long-term treatment of distal RTA requires alkali supplementation. Greater amounts are needed for children because of the need for base deposition in growing bone and because bicarbonate wastage is greater in children than in adults. Alkali therapy generally allows for correction of potassium wasting and hypokalemia.

Pyelonephritis

Pyelonephritis refers to infection of the kidney parenchyma and renal pelvis. There are two forms of pyelonephritis—acute and chronic.

Acute Pyelonephritis

Acute pyelonephritis represents an upper UTI, specifically the renal parenchyma and renal pelvis. Risk factors for complicated acute pyelonephritis are those that increase the host's susceptibility or reduce the host response to infection. People with diabetes mellitus are at increased risk. A less frequent and more serious type of acute pyelonephritis, called *necrotizing pyelonephritis*, is characterized by necrosis of the renal papillae. It is particularly common in people with diabetes and may also be a complication of acute pyelonephritis when there is significant urinary tract obstruction.

Etiology. Gram-negative bacteria, including *E. coli* and *Proteus*, *Klebsiella*, *Enterobacter*, and *Pseudomonas* species, are the most common causative agents. The infection usually ascends from the lower urinary tract, with the exception of *Staphylococcus aureus*, which is usually spread through the bloodstream. Factors that contribute to the development of acute pyelonephritis are catheterization and urinary instrumentation, vesicoureteral reflux, pregnancy, and neurogenic bladder.

Hematogenous acute pyelonephritis occurs most often in debilitated, chronically ill people and those receiving immunosuppressive therapy. Immunosuppression favors the development of subclinical (silent) pyelonephritis and infections caused by nonenteric, aerobic, gram-negative rods, and *Candida*.

Clinical Manifestations Acute pyelonephritis tends to present with an abrupt onset of chills, high fever, and an ache or tenderness in the costovertebral angle (flank area of the back) that is unilateral or bilateral.[15] Lower urinary tract symptoms, including dysuria, frequency, and urgency, also are common. Nausea and vomiting may occur along with abdominal pain. Palpation or percussion over the costovertebral angle on the affected side usually causes pain. Pyuria occurs but is not diagnostic because it also occurs in lower UTIs. The development of necrotizing papillitis is associated with a much poorer prognosis.

Treatment. Acute pyelonephritis is treated with appropriate antimicrobial drugs and may also require intravenous hydration. Unless obstruction or other complications occur, the symptoms usually disappear within several days. Treatment with an appropriate antimicrobial agent usually is continued for 10 to 14 days. People with complicated acute pyelonephritis and those who do not respond to outpatient treatment may require hospitalization.

Chronic Pyelonephritis

Chronic pyelonephritis represents a progressive process. There is scarring and deformation of the renal calyces and pelvis[5] (Fig. 33.16). The disorder appears to involve a bacterial infection superimposed on obstructive abnormalities or vesicoureteral reflux. Chronic obstructive pyelonephritis is associated with recurrent bouts of inflammation and scarring, which eventually lead to chronic pyelonephritis. Reflux, which is the most common cause of chronic pyelonephritis, results from superimposition of infection on congenital vesicoureteral reflux or intrarenal reflux. Reflux may be unilateral with involvement of a single kidney or bilateral, leading to scarring and atrophy of both kidneys with the eventual development of chronic renal insufficiency.

Clinical Manifestations. Chronic pyelonephritis may cause many of the same symptoms as acute pyelonephritis, or its onset may be insidious. Often, there is a history of recurrent episodes of UTI or acute pyelonephritis. Loss of tubular function and the ability to concentrate urine give rise to polyuria, nocturia, and mild proteinuria. Severe hypertension often is a contributing factor in the progress of the disease. Chronic pyelonephritis is a significant cause of renal failure

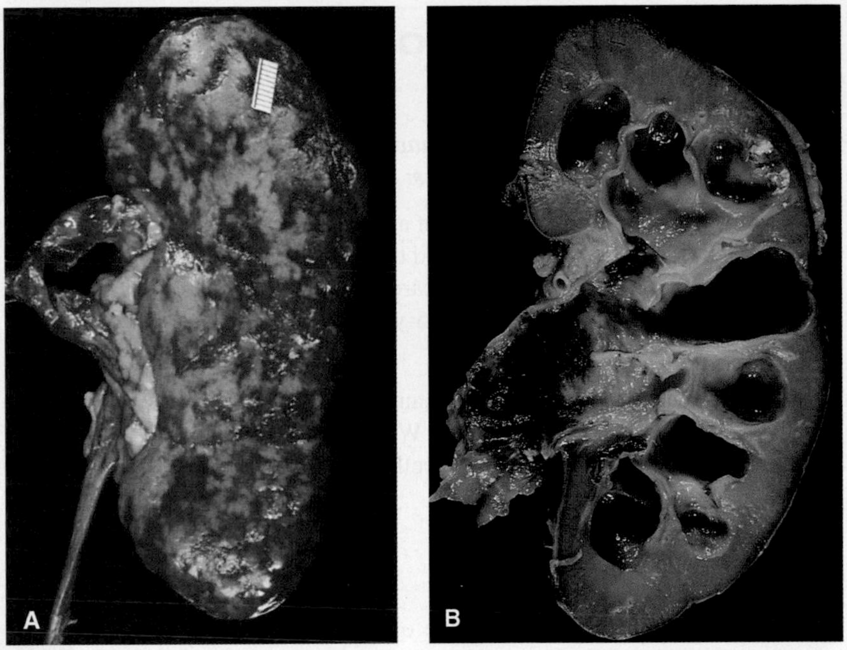

Figure 33.16 • Chronic pyelonephritis. **(A)** The cortical surface contains many irregular, depressed scars (*reddish* areas). **(B)** There is marked dilation of calices caused by inflammatory destruction of papillae, with atrophy and scarring of the overlying cortex. (From Rubin R., Strayer D. (Eds.) (2015). *Rubin's pathology: Clinicopathologic foundations of medicine* (7th ed., p. 947, Figure 22.76). Philadelphia, PA: Wolters Kluwer Health.)

Drug-Related Nephropathies

Drug-related nephropathies involve functional or structural changes in the kidneys that occur after exposure to a drug. Because of their large blood flow and high filtration pressure, the kidneys are exposed to any substance that is in the blood. The kidneys also are active in the metabolic transformation of drugs and therefore are exposed to a number of toxic metabolites. The tolerance to drugs varies with age and depends on renal function, state of hydration, BP, and the pH of the urine. Older adults are particularly susceptible to kidney damage caused by drugs and toxins. The dangers of nephrotoxicity are increased when two or more drugs capable of producing kidney damage are given at the same time.

Drugs and toxic substances can damage the kidneys by causing a decrease in renal blood flow, obstructing urine flow, directly damaging tubulointerstitial structures, or producing hypersensitivity reactions.[5] Some drugs, such as diuretics, high molecular weight radiocontrast media, the immunosuppressive drugs cyclosporine and tacrolimus, and the nonsteroidal anti-inflammatory drugs (NSAIDs), can cause acute prerenal failure by decreasing renal blood flow. People at particular risk are those who already have compromised renal blood flow. Other drugs such as sulfonamides and vitamin C (because of oxalate crystals) can form crystals that cause kidney damage by obstructing urinary flow in the tubules.

Acute drug-related hypersensitivity reactions produce tubulointerstitial nephritis, with damage to the tubules and interstitium. This condition was observed initially in people who were sensitive to the sulfonamide drugs; currently, it is observed most often with the use of methicillin and other synthetic antibiotics and with the use of furosemide and the thiazide diuretics in people sensitive to these drugs. At the onset, there is fever, eosinophilia, hematuria, mild proteinuria, and, in approximately one fourth of cases, a rash. In approximately 50% of cases, signs and symptoms of acute renal failure develop. Withdrawal of the drug commonly is followed by complete recovery, but there may be permanent damage in some people, usually in older people. Drug nephritis may not be recognized in its early stage because it is relatively uncommon.

NSAIDs also have the potential for damaging renal structures, including medullary interstitial cells. Prostaglandins (particularly PGI_2 and PGE_2) contribute to the regulation of tubular blood flow.[5] The deleterious effects of NSAIDs on the kidney are thought to result from their ability to inhibit prostaglandin synthesis. People particularly at risk are older adults because of age-related changes in renal function, people who are dehydrated or have a decrease in blood volume, and those with preexisting hypertension and kidney disease or renal insufficiency.

IN SUMMARY

Tubulointerstitial diseases affect the tubules and the surrounding interstitium of the kidneys. These disorders include RTA, acute and chronic pyelonephritis, and the effects of drugs and toxins. RTA describes a form of systemic acidosis that results from tubular defects in bicarbonate reabsorption or hydrogen ion secretion. Pyelonephritis, or infection of the kidney and kidney pelvis, can occur as an acute or a chronic condition. Acute pyelonephritis typically is caused by ascending bladder infections or infections that come from the bloodstream; it usually is successfully treated with appropriate antimicrobial drugs. Chronic pyelonephritis is a progressive disease that produces scarring and deformation of the renal calyces and pelvis. Drug-induced impairment of tubulointerstitial structure and function usually is the result of direct toxic injury, decreased blood flow, or hypersensitivity reactions.

MALIGNANT TUMORS OF THE KIDNEY

After completing this section of the chapter, the learner will be able to meet the following objectives:

- Characterize Wilms tumor in terms of age of onset, possible oncogenic origin, manifestations, and treatment.
- Cite the risk factors for renal cell carcinoma, describe its manifestations, and explain why the 5-year survival rate has been so low.

There are two major groups of malignant tumors of the kidney—embryonic kidney tumors (*i.e.*, Wilms tumor), which occur during childhood, and renal cell carcinoma, which occurs in adults.

Wilms Tumor

Wilms tumor (nephroblastoma) is one of the most common primary neoplasms of young children. It usually presents between 3 and 5 years of age and is the most common malignant abdominal tumor in children. It may occur in one or both kidneys. The incidence of bilateral Wilms tumor is 5% in sporadic cases and up to 20% in familial cases.[5]

Histologically, the tumor is composed of elements that resemble normal fetal tissue—blastemic, stromal, and epithelial. An important feature of Wilms tumor is its association with other congenital anomalies, including aniridia (absence of the iris), hemihypertrophy (enlargement of one side of the face or body), and other congenital anomalies, usually of the genitourinary system. Several chromosomal abnormalities have been associated with Wilms tumor. One Wilms tumor gene, *WT1*, which is located on chromosome 11, encodes a transcription factor that is critical for normal kidney development.[5] Although genetic and epigenetic associations with Wilms tumor are known, they explain only 5% of the cases.[48]

Wilms tumor usually is a solitary mass that occurs in any part of the kidney. It usually is sharply demarcated and variably encapsulated (Fig. 33.17). The tumors grow to a large size, distorting kidney structure. The tumors usually are staged using the National Wilms Tumor Study Group classification[49]:

- Stage I tumors are limited to the kidney and can be excised with the capsular surface intact.
- Stage II tumors extend into the renal capsule, but can be excised.
- Stage III tumors extend to the abdomen, but not beyond.
- Stage IV tumors have undergone hematogenous metastasis, most commonly involving the lung.
- Stage V tumors have bilateral involvement when diagnosed.

The common presenting signs are a large asymptomatic abdominal mass and hypertension.[49] The tumor is often discovered inadvertently, and it is not uncommon for the mother to discover it while bathing the child. Some children may present with abdominal pain, vomiting, or both.

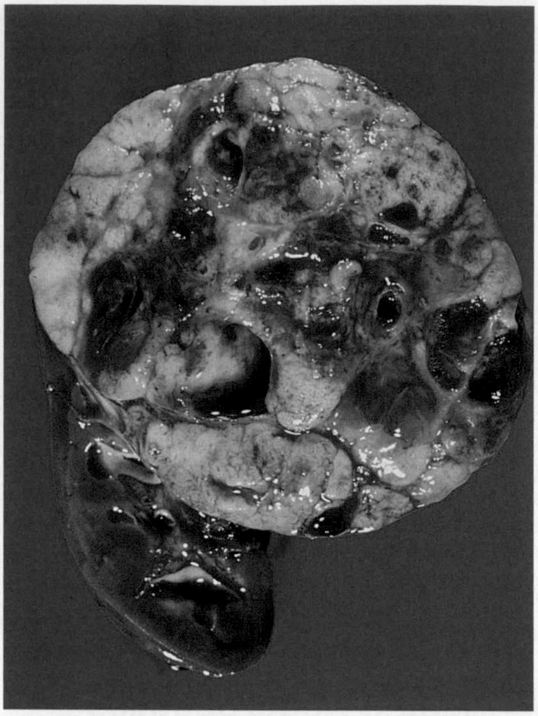

Figure 33.17 • Wilms tumor. A cross-section of a pale tan neoplasm attached to a residual portion of the kidney. (From Rubin R., Strayer D. (Eds.) (2015). *Rubin's pathology: Clinicopathologic foundations of medicine* (7th ed., p. 956, Figure 22.90). Philadelphia, PA: Wolters Kluwer Health.)

Treatment involves surgery, chemotherapy, and sometimes radiation therapy. Once diagnosed, care should be taken during physical exam to avoid vigorous physical exam, which could rupture the tumor capsule.[49] Prognosis is dependent on the findings at the time of diagnosis (*e.g.*, histology, stage, molecular markers, and age). The 5-year survival rate is 90%.

Renal Cell Carcinoma

Renal cell carcinoma is an often malignant tumor that accounts for up to 90% of all primary renal cancers.[5] Cancer of the kidney incidence peaks in people in their sixties and seventies. The increased use of imaging procedures such as ultrasonography, CT scanning, and magnetic resonance imaging (MRI) has contributed significantly to earlier diagnosis and more accurate staging of kidney cancers. The tumor usually arises from the renal tubular or ductal epithelial cells.[5]

Etiology and Pathogenesis

The cause of renal cell carcinoma remains unclear. Epidemiologic evidence suggests a correlation between heavy smoking and kidney cancer. Obesity also is a risk factor,

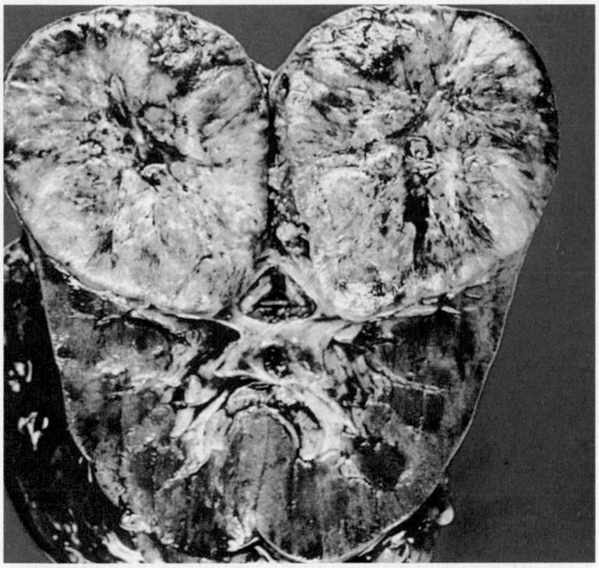

Figure 33.18 • Clear cell renal cell carcinoma. The kidney contains a large irregular neoplasm with a variegated cut surface. *Yellow* areas correspond to lipid-containing cells. (From Rubin R., Strayer D. (Eds.) (2015). *Rubin's pathology: Clinicopathologic foundations of medicine* (7th ed., p. 957, Figure 22.92). Philadelphia, PA: Wolters Kluwer Health.)

particularly in women. The risk for renal cell carcinoma also is increased in people with acquired cystic kidney disease associated with chronic renal insufficiency.

There are pathologic variants of renal cell carcinoma that reflect differences in cellular pathology, genetic profile, and clinical features ranging from benign to highly malignant. Clear cell carcinoma represents the majority of cases (70% to 75% of cases) (Fig. 33.18), with non–clear cell tumors (papillary or chromophilic tumors and chromophobic tumors) representing the remaining cases.[50] Clear cell tumors have a clear cytoplasm, usually show chromosome 3 deletions, and arise from proximal tubular epithelial cells. Papillary renal cell tumors tend to be bilateral and multifocal; show trisomies 7, 16, and 17; and arise from proximal tubular cells.[5] Collecting duct tumors arise from the collecting ducts within the renal medulla, are very rare, affect younger people, and are very aggressive.

Clinical Manifestations

Kidney cancer is largely a silent disorder during its early stages, and symptoms usually denote advanced disease. Presenting features include hematuria, flank pain, and presence of a palpable flank mass. Gross or microscopic hematuria, which occurs in the majority of cases, is an important clinical clue. It is, however, intermittent and may be microscopic. As a result, the tumor may reach considerable size before it is detected. Because of the widespread use of ultrasonography and CT scanning for diverse indications, renal tumors are being detected incidentally in people with no urologic symptoms.

Diagnosis and Treatment

Kidney cancer is suspected when there are findings of hematuria and a renal mass. Ultrasonography and CT scanning are used to confirm the diagnosis. MRI may be used when involvement of the inferior vena cava is suspected. Renal cancer is commonly staged using the American Joint Committee on Cancer staging system (Tumor, Node, Metastasis system).[50]

As with other forms of cancer, prognosis is based on staging at the time of diagnosis. Surgery (radical nephrectomy with lymph node dissection) is the treatment of choice for all resectable tumors. People are further classified based on models to predict postoperative outcomes. Nephron-sparing surgery may be done when both kidneys are involved or when an associated disease such as hypertension or diabetes mellitus threatens the contralateral kidney. There have been major advances in chemotherapy over the past decade, from nonspecific therapy to a more targeted approach using next-generation vascular endothelial growth factor (VEGF)-targeted therapies, immunotherapy agents, and combinations. It is anticipated that sequencing of the various subtypes of RCC will lead to specific genomic signatures that will guide therapy in the future.[50]

IN SUMMARY

There are two major groups of renal neoplasms—embryonic kidney tumors (*i.e.*, Wilms tumor) that occur during childhood and adult renal cell carcinomas. Wilms tumor is one of the most common malignant tumors of children. The most common presenting signs are a large abdominal mass and hypertension. Treatment is surgery, chemotherapy, and sometimes radiation therapy. The long-term survival rate for children with Wilms tumor is approximately 90%, with an aggressive plan of treatment.

Renal cancer accounts for about 3% of all cancers, with a peak incidence in people in their sixties and seventies. Renal cell carcinoma accounts for 80% to 90% of kidney tumors. These tumors are characterized by a lack of early warning signs, diverse clinical manifestations, and resistance to chemotherapy and radiation therapy. Because of the widespread use of ultrasonography and CT scanning for diverse indications, renal tumors are being detected incidentally in people with no urologic symptoms. Diagnostic methods include ultrasonography and CT scans. The treatment of choice is surgical resection. Prognosis depends on the stage of the cancer. The 5-year survival rate is 90% if the tumor has not extended beyond the renal capsule but drops considerably if metastasis has occurred.[5]

GERIATRIC Considerations

- UTIs increase in prevalence with age; however, the gap between the genders is diminished because of decreased sexual intercourse in women and benign prostatic hyperplasia in men.[51]
- UTIs are the single most common type of health care–associated infection in the elderly.
- Older men are three times more likely to develop bladder cancer than older women, with 90% of all bladder cancer occur after age 55.[51]
- The clinical manifestations of glomerulonephritis in the elderly are nonspecific and initially unnoticed; it is thought that glomerulonephritis already exists with the onset of an acute condition.[51]

PEDIATRIC Considerations

- Bilateral hypoplastic kidneys are a leading cause of end-stage renal disease in children younger than 10 years.[52]
- Biliary dysgenesis and hepatic fibrosis in some form are always found in children with autosomal recessive polycystic kidney disease.[52]
- In children, edema is the first symptom of nephrotic syndrome in the triad of proteinuria, hypercholesterolemia, and hypoalbuminemia.[52]
- Proteinuria (up to 100 mg/m^2 BSA daily) is not uncommon in healthy children.[52]

REVIEW EXERCISES

1. A 36-year-old man is admitted to the emergency department with a sudden onset of severe, intermittent, cramping pain that makes him feel nauseated. He describes the pain as originating in the left groin and radiating toward the flank. Microscopic examination of his urine reveals the presence of RBCs. His temperature is normal, and he does not exhibit signs of sepsis.
   A. *What is the probable cause of this man's pain?*
   B. *What diagnostic measure could be used to confirm the cause of his pain?*
   C. *A plain film radiograph reveals a 4- to 5-mm kidney stone in the left ureter. What are the chances that this man will pass the stone spontaneously?*
   D. *What type of medications and other treatments should this man receive?*
   E. *Once the stone has been passed, what type of measures can he use to prevent stone recurrence?*
2. A 6-year-old boy is diagnosed with acute glomerulonephritis that developed after a streptococcal throat infection. At this time, the following manifestations are noted: a decrease in urine output, increasing lethargy, hyperventilation, and generalized edema. Trace amounts of protein are detected in his urine. Blood analysis reveals the following: pH = 7.35, HCO_3 = 18 mEq/L, hematocrit = 29%, Na = 132 mEq/L, K = 5.6 mEq/L, BUN = 62 mg/dL, creatinine = 4.1 mg/dL, and albumin = 2 g/dL.
   A. *What is the probable cause of this boy's glomerular disease?*
   B. *Use the laboratory values in the Appendix to interpret his laboratory test results. Which values are significant and why?*
   C. *Is he progressing to uremia? How can you tell?*
3. A 26-year-old woman makes an appointment with her health care provider, complaining of urinary frequency, urgency, and burning. She reports that her urine is cloudy and smells abnormal. Her urine is cultured, and she is given a prescription for antibiotics.
   A. *What is the most likely cause of the woman's symptoms?*
   B. *What microorganism is most likely responsible for the infection?*
   C. *What factors may have predisposed her to this disorder?*
   D. *What could this woman do to prevent future infection?*

References

1. Centers for Disease Control and Prevention. (2017) *National Chronic Kidney Disease Fact Sheet, 2017*. Atlanta, GA: US Department of Health and Human Services, Centers for Disease Control and Prevention. Available: https://www.cdc.gov/diabetes/pubs/pdf/kidney_factsheet.pdf
2. Daniels B., Gross C. P., Molinaro A., et al. (2016). STONE PLUS: Evaluation of emergency department patients with suspected renal colic, using a clinical prediction tool combined with point-of-care limited ultrasonography. *Annals of Emergency Medicine* 67(4), 439–448. doi:10.1016/j.annemergmed.2015.10.020
3. Simmering J. E., Tang F., Cavanaugh J. E., et al. (2017). The increase in hospitalizations for urinary tract infections and the associated costs in the United States, 1998-2011. *Open Forum Infectious Diseases* 4(1), ofw281. doi:10.1093/ofid/ofw281.
4. Children and Youth with Special Health Needs. (2017). *Renal agenesis/hypoplasia fact sheet*. Minnesoto Department of Health. Available: http://www.health.state.mn.us/divs/cfh/topic/diseasesconds/renalagenesis.cfm
5. Strayer D. S., Rubin R. (Eds.) (2015). *Rubin's pathology: Clinicopathologic foundations of medicine* (7th ed.). Philadelphia, PA: Wolters Kluwer Health.
6. Ramanathan S., Kumar D., Khanna M., et al. (2016). Multi-modality imaging review of congenital abnormalities of kidney and upper urinary tract. *World Journal of Radiology* 8(2), 132–141. doi:10.4329/wjr.v8.i2.132.
7. Capone V. P., Morello W., Taroni F., et al. (2017). Genetics of congenital anomalies of the kidney and urinary tract: The current state of play. *International Journal of Molecular Sciences* 18(4). doi:10.3390/ijms18040796

8. National Organization for Rare Disorders. (2017). *Renal agenesis, bilateral*. Available: https://rarediseases.org/rare-diseases/renal-agenesis-bilateral/
9. Perrone R. D., Neville J., Chapman A. B., et al. (2015). Therapeutic area data standards for autosomal dominant polycystic kidney disease: A report from the Polycystic Kidney Disease Outcomes Consortium (PKDOC). *American Journal of Kidney Diseases* 66(4), 583–590. doi:10.1053/j.ajkd.2015.04.044.
10. Sweeney W. E. Jr, Avner E. D. (2017). Emerging therapies for childhood polycystic kidney disease. *Frontiers in Pediatrics* 5, 77. doi:10.3389/fped.2017.00077.
11. Zhou Z., Xu Y., Delcourt C., et al. (2017). Is regular screening for intracranial aneurysm necessary in patients with autosomal dominant polycystic kidney disease? A systematic review and meta-analysis. *Cerebrovascular Diseases* 44(1-2), 75-82. doi:10.1159/000476073
12. Chapman A. B., Devuyst O., Eckardt K. U., et al. (2015). Autosomal-dominant polycystic kidney disease (ADPKD): executive summary from a Kidney Disease: Improving Global Outcomes (KDIGO) Controversies Conference. *Kidney International* 88(1), 17–27. doi:10.1038/ki.2015.59
13. Sommerer C., Zeier, M. (2016). Clinical manifestation and management of ADPKD in Western Countries. *Kidney Diseases (Basel, Switzerland)* 2(3), 120–127. doi:10.1159/000449394.
14. Casteleijn N. F., Visser F. W., Drenth J. P., et al. (2014). A stepwise approach for effective management of chronic pain in autosomal-dominant polycystic kidney disease. *Nephrology, Dialysis, Transplantation* 29(Suppl 4), iv142–iv153. doi:10.1093/ndt/gfu073.
15. Guay-Woodford L. M., Bissler J. J., Braun M. C., et al. (2014). Consensus expert recommendations for the diagnosis and management of autosomal recessive polycystic kidney disease: report of an international conference. *The Journal of Pediatrics* 165(3), 611–617. doi:10.1016/j.jpeds.2014.06.015.
16. Hartung E. A., Guay-Woodford L. M. (2014). Autosomal recessive polycystic kidney disease: a hepatorenal fibrocystic disorder with pleiotropic effects. *Pediatrics* 134(3), e833–e845. doi:10.1542/peds.2013-3646.
17. Srivastava S., Sayer J. A. (2014). Nephronophthisis. *Journal of Pediatric Genetics* 3(2), 103–114. doi:10.3233/PGE-14086.
18. Niaudet, P. (2017). Clinical manifestations, diagnosis, and treatment of nephronophthisis. *UpToDate*. Available: http://www.uptodate.com.
19. Frokiaer J. (2017). Urinary tract obstruction. In Skerecki K, Chertow G. M., Marsden P. A., et al. (Eds.) *Brenner and Rector's The Kidney* (10th ed.). Philadelphia, PA: Elsevier Health.
20. Goroll A. H., Mulley A. G. (2014). *Primary care medicine: Office evaluation and management of the adult patient* (7th ed.). Philadelphia, PA: Lippincott Williams & Wilkins.
21. Heuther S. E., McCance K. L. (Eds.) (2017). *Understanding Pathophysiology*. St. Louis, MO: Elsevier.
22. Xu L. H. R., Adams-Huet B., Poindexter J. R., et al. (2017). Temporal changes in kidney stone composition and in risk factors predisposing to stone formation. *Journal of Urology* 197(6), 1465–1471. doi:10.1016/j.juro.2017.01.057.
23. Schwaderer A. L., Wolfe A. J. (2017). The association between bacteria and urinary stones. *Annals of Translational Medicine* 5(2), 32, 1–6. doi:10.21037/atm.2016.11.73.
24. Dunphy L. M., Winland–Brown J. E., Porter B., et al. (2015). *Primary care: The art and science of advanced practice nursing* (4th ed.). Philadelphia, PA: Lippincott Williams & Wilkins.
25. Panga K., Panga T., & Panga T. (2017). *Mosby's Diagnostic and Laboratory Test Reference* (13th ed.). St. Louis, MO: Elsevier.
26. Qaseem A., Dallas P., Forciea M. A., et al., & Clinical Guidelines Committee of the American College of Physicians. (2014). Dietary and pharmacologic management to prevent recurrent nephrolithiasis in adults: a clinical practice guideline from the American College of Physicians. *Annals of Internal Medicine* 161(9), 659–667. doi:10.7326/M13-2908.
27. Bader M. S., Loeb M., Brooks A. A. (2017). An update on the management of urinary tract infections in the era of antimicrobial resistance. *Postgraduate Medicine* 129(2), 242–258. doi:10.1080/00325481.2017.1246055.
28. Center for Disease Control and Prevention. (2015). *Urinary tract infection*. Available: https://www.cdc.gov/antibiotic-use/community/for-patients/common-illnesses/uti.html
29. Sobel J. D., Kaye D. (2015). Urinary tract infections. In Bennet J. E., Dolin R., Blaser M. J. (Eds.) *Mandell, Douglas, and Bennett's Principles and Practice of Infectious Disease* (Updated ed.). Philadelphia, PA: Elsevier.
30. Thomas L., & Tracy C. R. (2015). Treatment of fungal urinary tract infection. *The Urology Clinics of North America* 42(4), 473–483. doi:10.1016/j.ucl.2015.05.010.
31. Silva J. A. F., Biancardi M. F., Stach-Machado D. R., et al. (2017). The origin of prostate gland-secreted IgA and IgG. *Scientific Reports* 7(1), 16488. doi:10.1038/s41598-017-16717-3.
32. Flores-Mireles A. L., Walker J. N., Caparon M., et al. (2015). Urinary tract infections: epidemiology, mechanisms of infection and treatment options. *Nature Reviews Microbiology* 13(5), 269–284. doi:10.1038/nrmicro3432.
33. Luis A., Domingues F., Pereira L. (2017). Can cranberries contribute to reduce the incidence of urinary tract infections? A systematic review with meta-analysis and trial sequential analysis of clinical trials. *Journal of Urology* 198(3), 614–621. doi:10.1016/j.juro.2017.03.078.
34. Glaser A. P., Schaeffer A. J. (2015). Urinary tract infection and bacteriuria in pregnancy. *The Urology Clinics of North America* 42(4), 547–560. doi:10.1016/j.ucl.2015.05.004.
35. Bunting-Early T. E., Shaikh N., Woo L., et al. (2017). The need for improved detection of urinary tract infections in young children. *Frontiers in Pediatrics* 5, 24. doi:10.3389/fped.2017.00024.
36. Becknell B., Schober M., Korbel L., et al. (2015). The diagnosis, evaluation and treatment of acute and recurrent pediatric urinary tract infections. *Expert Review of Anti-Infective Therapy* 13(1), 81–90. doi:10.1586/14787210.2015.986097.
37. Umberger R., Callen B., Brown M. L. (2015). Severe sepsis in older adults. *Critical Care Nursing Quarterly* 38(3), 259–270. doi:10.1097/CNQ.0000000000000078.
38. Rowe T. A., Juthani-Mehta M. (2014). Diagnosis and management of urinary tract infection in older adults. *Infectious Disease Clinics of North America* 28(1), 75–89. doi:10.1016/j.idc.2013.10.004.
39. Rennke H. G., Denker B. M. (2014). *Renal pathophysiology: The essentials* (4th ed.). Philadelphia, PA: Lippincott Williams & Wilkins.
40. Fogo A. B. (2015). Causes and pathogenesis of focal segmental glomerulosclerosis. *Nature Reviews Nephrology* 11(2), 76–87. doi:10.1038/nrneph.2014.216.
41. van de Lest N. A., Zandbergen M., IJpelaar DHT, et al. (2018). Nephrin Loss can be used to predict remission and long-term renal outcome in patients with minimal change disease. *Kidney International Reports* 3(1), 168–177. doi:10.1016/j.ekir.2017.09.011.
42. Trimarchi H., Barratt J., Cattran D. C., et al. (2017). Oxford Classification of IgA nephropathy 2016: an update from the IgA Nephropathy Classification Working Group. *Kidney International* 91(5), 1014–1021. doi:10.1016/j.kint.2017.02.003.
43. Heineke M. H., Ballering A. V., Jamin A., et al. (2017). New insights in the pathogenesis of immunoglobulin A vasculitis (Henoch-Schonlein purpura). *Autoimmunity Reviews* 16(12), 1246–1253. doi:10.1016/j.autrev.2017.10.009.
44. Suarez-Fueyo A., Bradley S. J., Tsokos G. C. (2016). T cells in systemic lupus erythematosus. *Current Opinion in Immunology* 43, 32–38. doi:10.1016/j.coi.2016.09.001.
45. Kiremitci S., Ensari A. (2014). Classifying lupus nephritis: an ongoing story. *Scientific World Journal* 2014, 580620. doi:10.1155/2014/580620.
46. Fischbach F., Dunning M. B. (2015). *A manual of laboratory and diagnostic tests* (9th ed.). Philadelphia, PA: Lippincott Williams & Wilkins.

47. Burchum J. R., Rosenthal L. D. (2016). *Lehne's pharmacology for nursing care* (9th ed.). St. Louis, MO: Elsevier.
48. Bahrami A., Joodi M., Maftooh M., et al. (2018). The genetic factors contributing to the development of Wilm's tumor and their clinical utility in its diagnosis and prognosis. *Journal of Cellular Physiology* 233(4), 2882–2888. doi:10.1002/jcp.26021.
49. Chintagumpala M., Muscal J. A. (2017). Treatment and prognosis of Wilms tumor. In Pappo A. S. (Ed.) *UpToDate*. Available: https://www-uptodate-com.ezproxy.uthsc.edu/contents/treatment-and-prognosis-of-wilms-tumor
50. Barata P. C., Rini B. I. (2017). Treatment of renal cell carcinoma: Current status and future directions. *CA: a Cancer Journal for Clinicians* 67(6), 507–524. doi:10.3322/caac.21411.
51. Eliopoulos C. (2018). *Urinary elimination in gerontological nursing* (9th ed.). Philadelphia, PA: Wolters Kluwer.
52. Bowden V., Greenberg C. S. (2014). The child with altered genitourinary status. In *Children and their families: The continuum of nursing care* (3rd ed.). Philadelphia, PA: Wolters Kluwer Health.
53. Pawlina W. (2016). *Histology: A text and atlas with correlated cell and molecular biology* (7th ed.). Philadelphia, PA: Lippincott Williams & Wilkins.

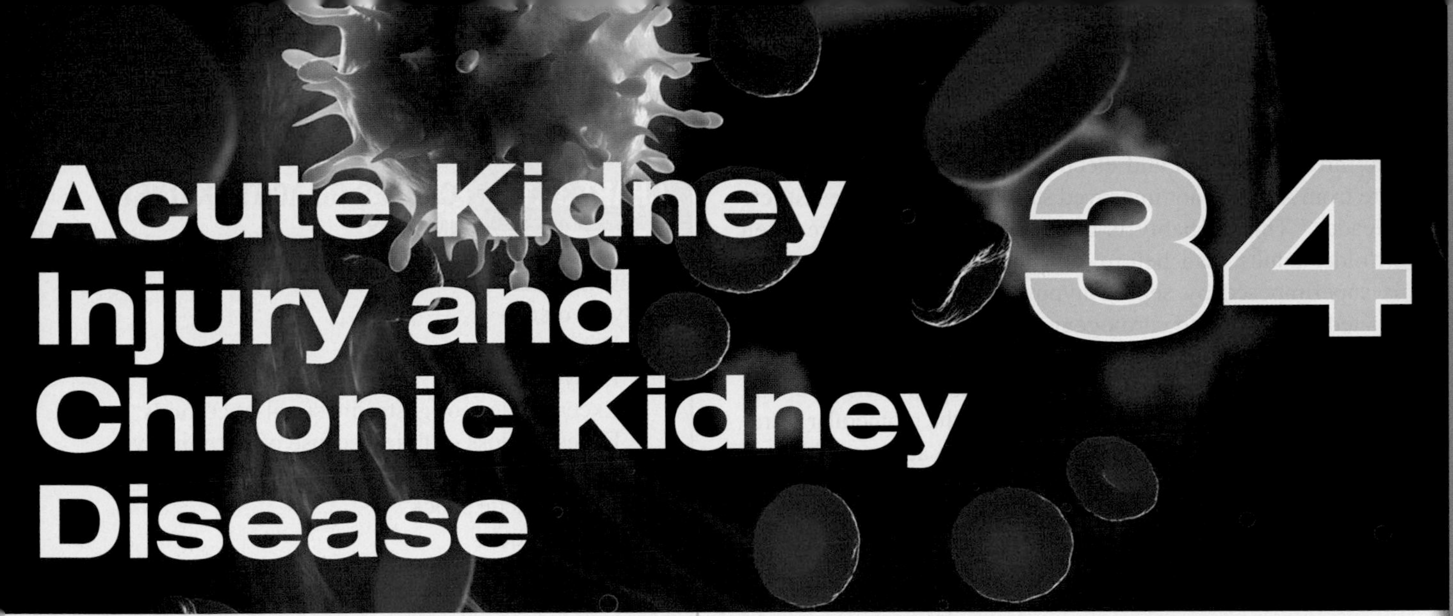

Acute Kidney Injury and Chronic Kidney Disease

34

Jami S. Brown

Renal failure is a condition in which the kidneys fail to remove metabolic end products from the blood and regulate the fluid, electrolyte, and pH balance of the extracellular fluids. The underlying cause may be renal disease, systemic disease, or urologic defects of nonrenal origin. Renal failure can occur as an acute or a chronic disorder. Acute kidney injury is abrupt in onset and often is reversible if recognized early and treated appropriately. In contrast, chronic kidney disease is the end result of irreparable damage to the kidneys. It develops slowly, usually over the course of a number of years. In fact, 80% of the nephrons need to be nonfunctioning before the symptoms of chronic kidney disease are manifested. Approximately 30 million American adults have some form of renal disease.[1]

ACUTE KIDNEY INJURY

After completing this section of the chapter, the learner will be able to meet the following objectives:

- Describe acute kidney injury in terms of its causes, treatment, and outcome.
- Differentiate the prerenal, intrarenal, and postrenal forms of acute kidney injury in terms of the mechanisms of development and manifestations.

Acute kidney injury (AKI) represents a rapid decline in kidney function that happens within a few hours or within a day. AKI causes a buildup of nitrogenous waste products and impairs fluid and electrolyte balance.[1] Unlike chronic kidney disease (CKD) and failure, acute renal injury is potentially reversible if the precipitating factors can be corrected or removed before permanent kidney damage has occurred.

AKI is a common threat to seriously ill people in intensive care units, with a mortality rate ranging from 15% to 60%.[2,3] Although treatment methods such as dialysis and renal replacement therapies are effective in correcting life-threatening fluid and electrolyte disorders, the mortality rate from AKI has not improved substantially over the last few decades.[4] This probably is because AKI is seen more often in older adults than before, and because it most frequently is superimposed by sepsis, hypovolemia, drug-/medication-related problems and cardiogenic shock.[4]

The most common indicator of AKI is *azotemia*, an accumulation of nitrogenous wastes (urea nitrogen, uric acid, and creatinine) in the blood and a decrease in the glomerular filtration rate (GFR). New biomarkers for more accurate diagnosing of AKI are discussed. As a result, excretion of nitrogenous wastes is reduced, and fluid and electrolyte balance cannot be maintained.

KEY POINTS

ACUTE KIDNEY INJURY

- AKI is caused by conditions that produce an acute shutdown in renal function.
- It can result from decreased blood flow to the kidney (prerenal AKI), disorders that disrupt the structures in the kidney (intrarenal AKI), or disorders that interfere with the elimination of urine from the kidney (postrenal AKI).
- AKI, although it causes an accumulation of products normally cleared by the kidney, is a potentially reversible process if the factors causing the condition can be corrected.

CHART 34.1 CAUSES OF ACUTE KIDNEY INJURY

Prerenal AKI
- Hypovolemia
  - Hemorrhage
  - Dehydration
  - Excessive loss of gastrointestinal tract fluids
  - Excessive loss of fluid because of burn injury
- Decreased vascular filling
  - Anaphylactic shock
  - Septic shock
- Heart failure and cardiogenic shock
- Decreased renal perfusion because of sepsis, vasoactive mediators, drugs, and diagnostic agents

Intrarenal AKI
- Acute tubular necrosis/acute renal injury
  - Prolonged renal ischemia
  - Exposure to nephrotoxic drugs, heavy metals, and organic solvents
  - Intratubular obstruction resulting from hemoglobinuria, myoglobinuria, myeloma light chains, or uric acid casts
  - Acute renal disease (acute glomerulonephritis, pyelonephritis)

Postrenal AKI
- Bilateral ureteral obstruction
- Bladder outlet obstruction

Types of AKI

AKI can be caused by several types of conditions, including a decrease in blood flow without ischemic injury; ischemic, toxic, or obstructive tubular injury; and obstruction of urinary tract outflow. The causes of AKI commonly are categorized as prerenal, intrarenal, and postrenal[2] (Fig. 34.1). Collectively, prerenal and intrarenal causes account for 80% to 95% of AKI cases.[3] Causes of AKI within these categories are summarized in Chart 34.1.

Prerenal AKI

Prerenal AKI, the most common form of AKI, is characterized by a marked decrease in renal blood flow. It is reversible if the cause of the decreased renal blood flow can be identified and corrected before kidney damage occurs. Causes of prerenal AKI include profound depletion of vascular volume (*e.g.*, hemorrhage, loss of extracellular fluid volume), impaired perfusion because of heart failure and cardiogenic shock, and decreased vascular filling because of increased vascular capacity (*e.g.*, anaphylaxis or sepsis). Older adults are particularly at risk because of their predisposition to hypovolemia and their high prevalence of renal vascular disorders.

Some vasoactive mediators, drugs, and diagnostic agents stimulate intense intrarenal vasoconstriction and can induce glomerular hypoperfusion and prerenal AKI. Examples include endotoxins, radiocontrast agents such as those used for cardiac

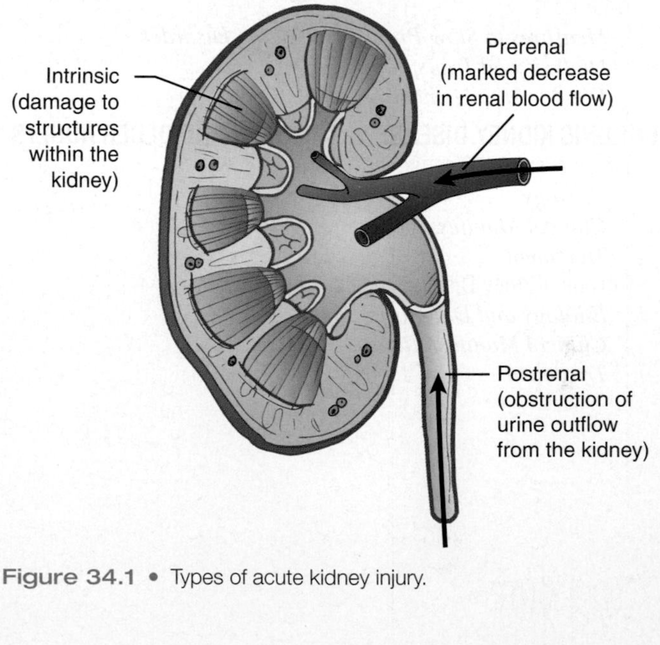

Figure 34.1 • Types of acute kidney injury.

catheterization, cyclosporine (an immunosuppressant drug that is used to prevent transplant rejection), and nonsteroidal anti-inflammatory drugs (NSAIDs).[2] Many of these drugs also cause acute tubular necrosis (ATN; discussed later). In addition, several commonly used classes of drugs can impair renal adaptive mechanisms and can convert compensated renal hypoperfusion into prerenal failure. Angiotensin-converting enzyme (ACE) inhibitors and angiotensin receptor blockers (ARBs) reduce the effects of renin on renal blood flow; when combined with diuretics, they may cause prerenal AKI in people with decreased blood flow because of large-vessel or small-vessel kidney disease. Prostaglandins have a vasodilatory effect on renal blood vessels. NSAIDs can reduce renal blood flow through inhibition of prostaglandin synthesis. In some people with diminished renal perfusion, NSAIDs can precipitate prerenal AKI.

Normally, the kidneys receive 20% to 25% of the cardiac output.[5] This large blood supply is required for the glomeruli to remove metabolic wastes and regulate body fluids and electrolytes. Fortunately, the normal kidney can tolerate relatively large reductions in blood flow before renal damage occurs. As renal blood flow is reduced, the GFR decreases, the amount of sodium and other substances that are filtered by the glomeruli is reduced, and the need for energy-dependent mechanisms to reabsorb these substances is reduced.[5] As the GFR and urine output approach zero, oxygen consumption by the kidney approximates that required to keep renal tubular cells alive. When blood flow falls below this level, which is about 20% to 25% of normal, ischemic changes occur.[5] Because of their high metabolic rate, the tubular epithelial cells are most vulnerable to ischemic injury. Improperly treated, prolonged renal hypoperfusion can lead to ischemic tubular necrosis with significant morbidity and mortality. However, the majority of people who experience the prolonged renal hypoperfusion do not have tubular epithelial necrosis, so the term ATN is being used less frequently and AKI refers to this intrarenal pathology.[6]

Prerenal AKI is manifested by a sharp decrease in urine output and a disproportionate elevation of blood urea nitrogen (BUN) in relation to serum creatinine levels. The kidney normally responds to a decrease in the GFR with a decrease in urine output. Thus, an early sign of prerenal AKI is a sharp decrease in urine output. A low fractional excretion of sodium (<1%) suggests that oliguria is due to decreased renal perfusion and that the nephrons are responding appropriately by decreasing the excretion of filtered sodium in an attempt to preserve vascular volume.[2] BUN levels also depend on the GFR. A low GFR allows more time for small particles such as urea to be reabsorbed into the blood. Creatinine, which is larger and nondiffusible, remains in the tubular fluid, and the total amount of creatinine that is filtered, although small, is excreted in the urine. Consequently, there also is a disproportionate elevation in the ratio of BUN to serum creatinine, from a normal value of 10:1 to a ratio greater than 15:1 to 20:1.[2]

Intrarenal AKI

Intrarenal AKI results from conditions that cause damage to structures within the kidney. The most frequent etiology of intrarenal AKI causes damage to the parenchyma in the glomeruli, vessels, tubules, or interstitium.[6] The major causes of intrarenal failure are ischemia associated with prerenal AKI, toxic insult to the tubular structures of the nephron, and intratubular obstruction. Acute glomerulonephritis and acute pyelonephritis also are intrarenal causes of acute renal failure. The decreased glomerular filtration and epithelial injury are due to many causes such as intrarenal vasoconstriction, decreased hydrostatic pressure in the glomeruli, changes in arterial tone by tubuloglomerular feedback, decreased capillary permeability in the glomeruli, increased tubular hydrostatic pressure secondary to obstruction, and backflow of glomerular filtrate into the interstitium.[6] Injury to the tubular structures of the nephron is the most common cause and often is ischemic or toxic in origin.

Acute Tubular Injury or Necrosis. Acute tubular injury or necrosis is characterized by the destruction of tubular epithelial cells with acute suppression of renal function (Fig. 34.2). This acute injury can be caused by a variety of conditions, including acute tubular damage because of ischemia, sepsis, nephrotoxic effects of drugs, tubular obstruction, and toxins from a massive infection.[2] Tubular epithelial cells are particularly sensitive to ischemia and also are vulnerable to toxins. The tubular injury that occurs frequently is reversible.

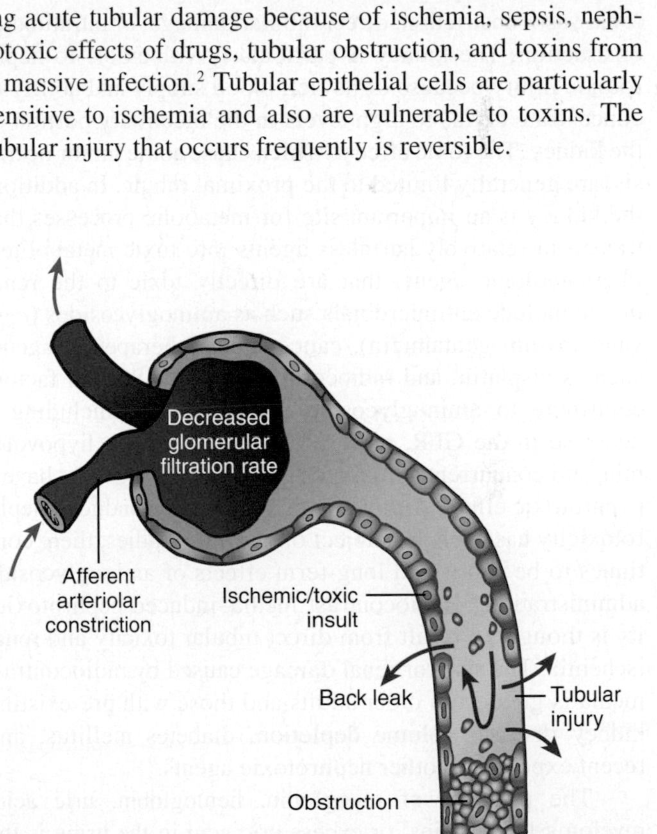

Figure 34.2 • Pathogenesis of acute renal failure caused by acute tubular injury (acute tubular necrosis). Sloughing and necrosis of tubular epithelial cells lead to obstruction and increased intraluminal pressure, which reduce glomerular filtration. Afferent arteriolar vasoconstriction caused in part by tubuloglomerular feedback mechanisms results in decreased glomerular capillary filtration pressure. Tubular injury and increased intraluminal pressure cause fluid to move from the tubular lumen into the interstitium (back leak). (From Strayer D., Rubin E. (Eds.). (2015). *Rubin's pathology: Clinicopathologic foundations of medicine* (7th ed., p. 943). Philadelphia, PA: Wolters Kluwer Health/Lippincott Williams & Wilkins.)

Ischemic ATN or acute tubular injury occurs most frequently in people who have extensive surgery, severe hypovolemia, or overwhelming sepsis, trauma, or burns.[4] Sepsis produces ischemia by provoking a combination of systemic vasodilation and intrarenal hypoperfusion. In addition, sepsis results in the generation of toxins that sensitize renal tubular cells to the damaging effects of ischemia. ATN complicating trauma and burns frequently is multifactorial in origin, resulting from the combined effects of hypovolemia, myoglobinuria, and other toxins released from damaged tissue. Acute tubular injury is a complication of intravascular hemolysis associated with many forms of hemolytic disease, such as sickle cell disease and mechanical trauma from artificial heart valves.[7] In contrast to prerenal AKI, the GFR does not improve with the restoration of renal blood flow in AKI caused by ischemic ATN or acute tubular injury.

Nephrotoxic ATN or acute tubular injury complicates the administration of or exposure to many structurally diverse drugs and other nephrotoxic agents. These agents cause tubular injury by inducing varying combinations of renal vasoconstriction, direct tubular damage, or intratubular obstruction. The kidney is particularly vulnerable to nephrotoxic injury because of its rich blood supply and ability to concentrate toxins to high levels in the medullary portion of the kidney. The toxic effects, which cause some minor necrosis, are generally limited to the proximal tubule. In addition, the kidney is an important site for metabolic processes that transform relatively harmless agents into toxic metabolites. Pharmacologic agents that are directly toxic to the renal tubule include antimicrobials such as aminoglycosides (*e.g.*, vancomycin, gentamicin), cancer chemotherapeutic agents such as cisplatin, and radiocontrast agents.[2] Several factors contribute to aminoglycoside nephrotoxicity, including a decrease in the GFR, pre-existing renal disease, hypovolemia, and concurrent administration of other drugs that have a nephrotoxic effect. Although aminoglycoside-induced nephrotoxicity has been the subject of multiple studies, there continues to be short- and long-term effects of aminoglycoside administration.[8] Radiocontrast media–induced nephrotoxicity is thought to result from direct tubular toxicity and renal ischemia. The risk for renal damage caused by radiocontrast media is greatest in older adults and those with pre-existing kidney disease, volume depletion, diabetes mellitus, and recent exposure to other nephrotoxic agents.[9]

The presence of myoglobin, hemoglobin, uric acid, myeloma light chains, or excess uric acid in the urine is the most frequent cause of ATN because of intratubular obstruction.[2,4] Hemoglobinuria results from blood transfusion reactions and other hemolytic crises.[7] Skeletal and cardiac muscles contain myoglobin, which corresponds to hemoglobin in function, serving as an oxygen reservoir in the muscle fibers. Myoglobin normally is not found in the serum or urine. Myoglobinuria most commonly results from muscle trauma, but may result from extreme exertion, hyperthermia, sepsis, prolonged seizures, potassium or phosphate depletion, and alcoholism or drug abuse. Both myoglobin and hemoglobin discolor the urine, which may range from the color of tea to red, brown, or black. "Dirty brown" granular casts and epithelial cells in the urine are correlated with acute tubular injury, red blood cell casts and protein in the urine are reflected by glomerulonephritis, and white blood cell casts and pyuria relate to acute tubulointerstitial nephritis.[6,9]

Postrenal AKI

Postrenal AKI results from obstruction of urine outflow from the kidneys. The obstruction can occur in the ureter (*i.e.*, calculi and strictures), bladder (*i.e.*, tumors or neurogenic bladder), or urethra (*i.e.*, prostatic hyperplasia). Because of the increased urine not being able to be excreted due to the obstruction, retrograde pressure occurs throughout the tubules and nephrons, which ultimately damages the nephrons.[2] Prostatic hyperplasia is the most common underlying problem. Because both ureters must be occluded to produce renal failure, obstruction of the bladder rarely causes acute renal failure unless one of the kidneys already is damaged or a person has only one kidney. The treatment of postrenal AKI consists of treating the underlying cause of obstruction so that urine flow can be reestablished before permanent nephron damage occurs.

The course of AKI can be divided into four phases[10]:

1. Onset phase
2. Oliguric (anuric) phase
3. Diuretic phase
4. Recovery phase

The *onset phase*, which lasts hours or days, is the time from the onset of the precipitating event (*e.g.*, ischemic phase of prerenal failure or toxin exposure) until tubular injury occurs.

The *oliguric (anuric) phase* lasts 8 to 14 days or longer depending on the nature of AKI. It is characterized by a marked decrease in the GFR, causing sudden retention of endogenous metabolites, such as urea, potassium, sulfate, and creatinine, which normally are cleared by the kidneys. The urine output usually is lowest at this point. Fluid retention gives rise to edema, water intoxication, and pulmonary congestion. If the period of oliguria is prolonged, hypertension frequently develops and with it signs of uremia. When untreated, the neurologic manifestations of uremia progress from neuromuscular irritability to seizures, somnolence, coma, and death. Hyperkalemia usually is asymptomatic until the serum potassium level rises above 6 to 6.5 mEq/L, at which point characteristic electrocardiographic changes and symptoms of muscle weakness are seen.

The *diuretic phase* occurs when the kidneys try to heal and urine output increases, but tubule scarring and damage occur. Diuresis often occurs before renal function has fully returned to normal. Consequently, the BUN, serum creatinine, potassium, and phosphate levels may remain elevated or continue to rise even though urine output is increased. During this phase, the GFR increases, urine output increases to 400 mL/day, and electrolytes are possibly depleted from excretion of more water and osmotic effects of a high BUN.

The *recovery phase* is the period during which tubular edema resolves and renal function improves. During this phase, there is normalization of fluid and electrolyte balance. Eventually, renal tubular function is restored with improvement in concentrating ability. At about the same time, the BUN and creatinine begin to return to normal and the GFR returns to 70% to 80% normal. In some cases, mild to moderate kidney damage persists.

Diagnosis and Treatment

Given the high morbidity and mortality rates associated with AKI, attention should be focused on prevention and early diagnosis. This includes assessment measures to identify people at risk for development of AKI, including those with pre-existing renal insufficiency and diabetes. These people are particularly at risk for development of AKI because of nephrotoxic drugs (*e.g.*, aminoglycosides and radiocontrast agents) or drugs such as the NSAIDs that alter intrarenal hemodynamics. Older adults are susceptible to all forms of acute renal failure because of the effects of aging on renal reserve.[9]

Careful observation of urine output is essential for people at risk for development of acute AKI. Urine tests that measure urine osmolality, urinary sodium concentration, and fractional excretion of sodium help differentiate prerenal azotemia, in which the reabsorptive capacity of the tubular cells is maintained, from tubular necrosis, in which these functions are lost. One of the earliest manifestations of tubular damage is the inability to concentrate the urine.

Further diagnostic information that can be obtained from the urinalysis includes evidence of proteinuria, hemoglobinuria, and casts or crystals in the urine. Blood tests for BUN and creatinine provide information regarding the ability to remove nitrogenous wastes from the blood. It also is important to exclude urinary obstruction. However, these conventional markers of serum creatinine and urea nitrogen, fractional secretion of sodium to assess GFR, and urine output do not manifest for 1 to 2 days after the acute renal failure has begun. For example, when assessing serum creatinine in critically ill people, one cannot assume the person is in a steady hemodynamic state. Therefore, an increase in the creatinine level lags behind the renal injury. Also, the person's age, gender, muscle mass, and medications influence the creatinine levels. Urea is also not produced consistently, and the amount of urea is increased by diet, medications, and infection and also affected by liver disease.

Urea is formed by the hepatic metabolism of amino acids and excreted primarily by glomerular filtration. Serum concentrations of urea may vary as a result of changes in urea production, such as in a gastrointestinal bleed and tubular urea reabsorption during hypovolemic states without changes in GFR. This makes urea an unreliable marker of renal function.[11] Lastly, fractional excretion of sodium is impacted by diuretics, specific diseases, and infection and is not an accurate predictor of decreased GFR. In situations associated with hypovolemia or hypoperfusion, healthy kidneys respond by increasing urine osmolarity and reducing sodium and/or urea or uric acid excretion. This physiologic response may be variable by interventions such as diuretic therapy, aminoglycosides, and cardiopulmonary bypass.[12]

Some new biomarkers for assessing AKI earlier than the conventional parameters are being trialed. Interleukin (IL)-18 is produced in the proximal tubule after AKI and is an inflammatory cytokine.[4] This marker increases with ischemic AKI and is easily measured in the urine.[13,14] Neutrophil gelatinase–associated lipocalin (NGAL) is normally present in several organs including the kidneys.[13,14] NGAL is measured in the blood and urine, and increased levels have been found to be predictive of graft dysfunction in renal transplants.[13,14] Kidney injury molecule-1 is increased with acute renal injury in the proximal tubular cells.[13,14]

A major concern in the treatment of AKI is identifying and correcting the cause (*e.g.*, improving renal perfusion, discontinuing nephrotoxic drugs). Fluids are carefully regulated in an effort to maintain normal fluid volume and electrolyte concentrations. Because secondary infections are a major cause of death in people with acute renal failure, constant effort is needed to prevent and treat such infections.

Hemodialysis or continuous renal replacement therapy (CRRT) may be indicated when nitrogenous wastes and the water and electrolyte balance cannot be kept under control by other means.[2] CRRT has emerged as a method for treating acute renal failure in people too hemodynamically unstable to tolerate hemodialysis. An associated advantage of the CRRTs is the ability to administer nutritional support. The disadvantages are the need for prolonged anticoagulation and continuous sophisticated monitoring.

IN SUMMARY

AKI is an acute, potentially reversible suppression of kidney function. It is a common threat to seriously ill people in intensive care units, with a high mortality rate. AKI is characterized by a decrease in GFR, accumulation of nitrogenous wastes in the blood (*i.e.*, azotemia), and alterations in body fluids and electrolytes. AKI is classified as prerenal, intrinsic or intrarenal, or postrenal in origin. Prerenal AKI is caused by decreased blood flow to the kidneys, intrarenal AKI by disorders in the kidney itself, and postrenal AKI by obstruction to urine output. The main cause of AKI is ischemia, sepsis, or nephrotoxic agents. ATN typically progresses through four phases: the onset phase, which is the time from the onset of the precipitating event until tubular injury occurs; the oliguric/anuric phase, during which there is marked decrease in the GFR, causing sudden retention of endogenous metabolites; the diuretic phase, in which the kidneys try to heal and urine output increases, but tubule scarring and damage occur; and the recovery phase, during which the GFR, urine output, and blood levels of nitrogenous wastes return to normal.

Because of the high morbidity and mortality rates associated with AKI, identification of people at risk is important to clinical decision-making. New biomarkers such as IL-18, NGAL, and kidney injury molecule-1 are in various trial stages, which should be helpful in earlier assessment of AKI in the future. AKI often is reversible, making early identification and correction of the underlying cause (*e.g.*, improving renal perfusion, discontinuing nephrotoxic drugs) important. Treatment includes the judicious administration of fluids and hemodialysis or CRRT.

CHRONIC KIDNEY DISEASE

After completing this section of the chapter, the learner will be able to meet the following objectives:

- State the most common causes of chronic kidney disease.
- Explain the physiologic mechanisms underlying the common problems associated with chronic kidney disease, including alterations in fluid and electrolyte balance and disorders of skeletal, hematologic, cardiovascular, immune system, neurologic, skin, and sexual function.
- State the basis for adverse drug reactions in people with chronic kidney disease.
- Cite the possible complications of kidney transplantation.

Chronic kidney disease (CKD) is a worldwide problem that affects people of all ages, races, and economic groups. The prevalence and incidence of the disease, which mirror those of conditions such as diabetes, hypertension, and obesity, are rising. In the United States alone, more than 20 million people, or 1 in 9 adults, have CKD. Another 20 million people are at increased risk for development of the disorder.[1]

Definition and Classification

In 2002, the Kidney Disease Outcome Quality Initiative (K/DOQI) of the National Kidney Foundation (NKF) published clinical practice guidelines for CKD.[15] The goals of the Work Group that developed the guidelines were to define CKD and classify its stages, to evaluate laboratory measures used for assessment of kidney disease, and to associate the level of kidney function with the complications of CKD. The guidelines use the GFR to classify CKD into five stages, beginning with kidney damage with normal or elevated GFR, progressing to CKD and, potentially, to kidney failure. It is anticipated that early detection of kidney damage along with implementation of aggressive measures to decrease its progression can delay or prevent the onset of kidney failure.[2]

According to the NKF guidelines, people with a GFR of 60 to 89 mL/min/1.73 m^2 (corrected for body surface area) without kidney damage are classified as "decreased GFR."[15] Decreased GFR without recognized markers of kidney damage can occur in infants and older adults and is usually considered to be "normal for age." Other causes of chronically decreased GFR without kidney damage in adults include removal of one kidney, extracellular fluid volume depletion, and systemic illnesses associated with reduced kidney perfusion, such as heart failure and cirrhosis.[15] Even at this stage, there is often a characteristic loss of renal reserve.

CKD is defined as either kidney damage or a GFR less than 60 mL/min/1.73 m^2 for 3 months or longer.[15] CKD can result from a number of conditions that cause permanent loss of nephrons, including diabetes, hypertension, glomerulonephritis, systemic lupus erythematosus, and polycystic kidney disease.

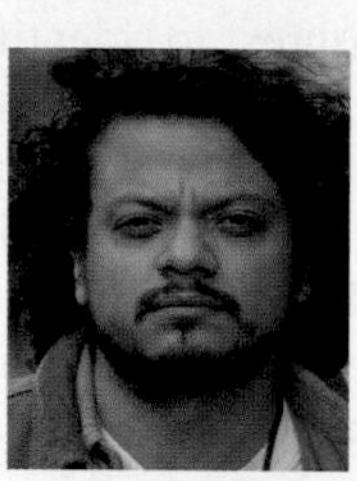

Remember Mr. Reterez who was introduced to you at the beginning of this unit? He had been diagnosed with polycystic kidney disease. With this genetic disorder, a person manifests symptoms in his or her fourth decade. Mr. Reterez is 45 years of age. His GFR is most likely less than 60 mL/minute, which indicates that he is retaining nitrogenous waste. In addition, his BUN is rising as well as his creatinine (BUN = 45, creatinine = 2.0 at emergency department visit). His symptoms are all due to CKD.

Hypertension and diabetic kidney disease are the two main causes of CKD in the United States.[2]

The NKF practice guidelines define kidney failure "as either

1. A GFR of less than 15 mL/min/1.73 m^2, usually accompanied by most of the signs and symptoms of uremia, or
2. A need to start renal replacement therapy (dialysis or transplantation)"[15]

These guidelines point out that kidney failure is not synonymous with end-stage renal disease (ESRD).

Regardless of cause, CKD represents a loss of functioning kidney nephrons with progressive deterioration of glomerular filtration, tubular reabsorptive capacity, and endocrine functions of the kidneys (Fig. 34.3). All forms of CKD are characterized by a reduction in the GFR, reflecting a corresponding reduction in the number of functional nephrons. The rate of nephron destruction differs from case to case, ranging from several months to many years. Typically, the signs and symptoms of CKD occur gradually and do not become evident until the disease is far advanced. This is because of the amazing compensatory ability of the kidneys. As kidney structures are destroyed, the remaining nephrons undergo structural and functional hypertrophy, each increasing its function as a means of compensating for those that have been lost. In the process, each of the remaining nephrons must filter more solute particles from the blood. It is only when the few remaining nephrons are destroyed that the manifestations of kidney failure become evident.[2]

KEY POINTS

CHRONIC KIDNEY DISEASE

- CKD represents the progressive decline in kidney function because of the permanent loss of nephrons.
- CKD can result from a number of conditions, including diabetes, hypertension, glomerulonephritis, and other kidney diseases.
- The GFR is considered the best measure of kidney function.

Assessment of Glomerular Filtration Rate and Other Indicators of Renal Function

The GFR is considered the best measure of overall function of the kidney. The normal GFR, which varies with age, sex, and body size, is approximately 120 to 130 mL/min/1.73 mL/m^2 for normal young healthy adults.[15] In clinical practice, GFR is usually estimated using the serum creatinine concentration. Although the GFR can be obtained from measurements of creatinine clearance using timed (*e.g.*, 24-hour) urine collection methods, the levels gathered are reportedly no more reliable than the estimated levels obtained by using serum creatinine levels.[15] Because GFR varies with age, sex, ethnicity, and body size, the Cockroft and Gault or Modification of Diet in Renal Diseases (MDRD) equations that take these factors into account are used for estimating the GFR based on serum creatinine levels[15–17] (Chart 34.2).

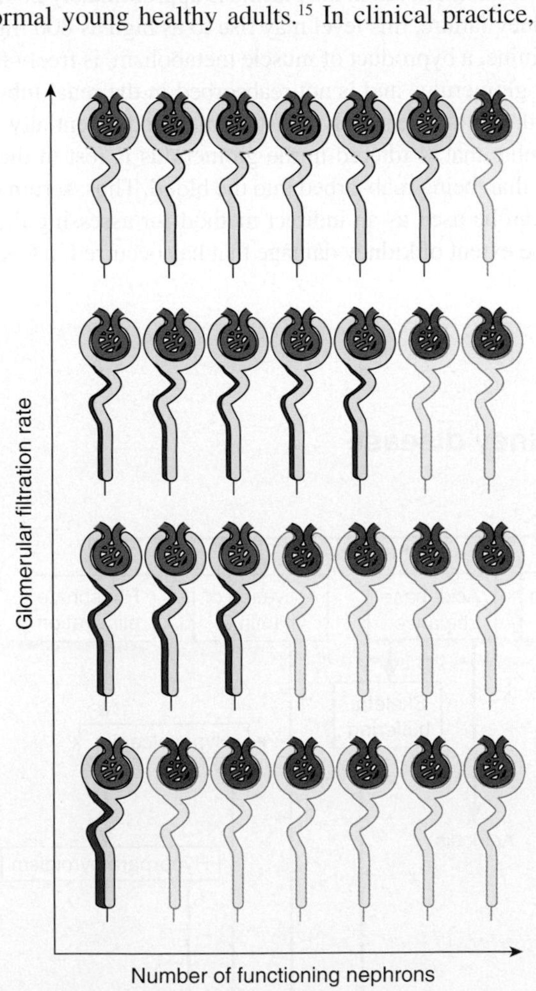

Figure 34.3 • Relation of renal function and nephron mass. Each kidney contains about 1 million tiny nephrons. A proportional relation exists between the number of nephrons affected by a disease process and the resulting GFR.

Albuminuria serves as a key marker of kidney damage.[18] Urine normally contains small amounts of protein. However, if the kidneys are damaged, protein can "leak" out of the kidneys into the urine. The type of protein (*e.g.*, low molecular weight globulins or albumin) depends on the type of kidney disease. Increased excretion of low molecular weight globulins is a marker of tubulointerstitial disease, and excretion of albumin a marker of CKD, resulting from hypertension or diabetes mellitus.[19] For the diagnosis of CKD in adults and postpubertal children with diabetes, measurement of urinary albumin is preferred.[19] In most cases, urine dipstick tests are acceptable for detecting albuminuria. If the urine dipstick test is positive (1+ or greater), albuminuria is usually confirmed by quantitative measurement of the albumin-to-creatinine ratio in a spot (untimed) urine specimen. The NKF classifies microalbuminuria as urine albumin to creatinine ratio (UACR) 30 to 300 mg/g and macroalbuminuria as >300 mg/g (nearly equivalent to positive protein dipstick).[19,20] Microalbuminuria, which is an early sign of diabetic kidney disease, refers to albumin excretion that is above the normal range, but below the range normally detected by tests of total protein excretion in the urine.[20] Populations at risk for CKD (*i.e.*, those with diabetes mellitus, hypertension, or family history of kidney disease) should be screened for microalbuminuria, at least annually, as part of their health examination.[19]

Albuminuria and estimated glomerular filtration rate (eGFR) are the classical guideline-endorsed biomarkers for the classification of CKD.[4] These biomarkers are strong

CHART 34.2 PREDICTION OF CREATININE CLEARANCE USING SERUM CREATININE

- The Modification of Diet in Renal Diseases (MDRD) equation can be used to calculate adult creatinine clearance. Use the following Web site: http://nkdep.nih.gov/professionals/gfr_calculators/idms_con.htm.
- The Cockroft and Gault equation can be used to calculate older adults' creatinine clearance. Use the following Web site: http://www.mdcalc.com/creatinine-clearance-cockcroft-gault-equation. The equation result should be multiplied by a factor of 0.85 for women.

predictors of renal disease progression as well as CVD and mortality, but the search for novel biomarkers to improve the early identification of people with high-risk continues.[20]

Other markers of kidney damage include abnormalities in urine sediment (red and white blood cells) and abnormal findings on imaging studies.[20] Also, the biomarker amino acid, cystatin C also known as cystatin 3, which has been used for predicting new-onset cardiovascular disease, has also been found to predict kidney disease.[21] Ultrasonography is particularly useful for detecting a number of kidney disorders, including urinary tract obstructions, infections, stones, and polycystic kidney disease.

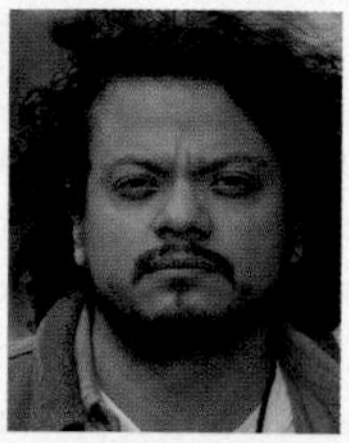

Mr. Reterez has a + urine dipstick for albumin/protein and blood. If he had been screened a few years ago, his microalbumin would most likely have tested positive. It would have been very helpful if his family members had told him more information regarding the family's genetic disorder, which has seemingly been passed down through the generations. It is essential to know whether or not one carries the polycystic kidney gene for two reasons. First, a person can be screened carefully for any signs of renal disease and, second, a person can be put on a list for a renal transplant early before the systemic symptoms and multisystem disease manifest. Both of Mr. Reterez's kidneys are involved with polycystic kidney disease. Therefore, he is in urgent need of dialysis or a bilateral renal transplant.

Clinical Manifestations

The manifestations of CKD include an accumulation of nitrogenous wastes; alterations in water, electrolyte, and acid–base balance; mineral and skeletal disorders; anemia and coagulation disorders; hypertension and alterations in cardiovascular function; gastrointestinal disorders; neurologic complications; disorders of skin integrity; and disorders of immunologic function[18,22] (Fig. 34.4). The point at which these disorders make their appearance and the severity of the manifestations are determined largely by the extent of renal function that is present and the coexisting disease conditions. Many of them make their appearance before the GFR has reached the kidney failure stage.

Accumulation of Nitrogenous Wastes

The accumulation of nitrogenous wastes in the blood, or azotemia, is an early sign of kidney failure, usually occurring before other symptoms become evident. Urea is one of the first nitrogenous wastes to accumulate in the blood, and the BUN level becomes increasingly elevated as CKD progresses. The normal concentration of urea in the plasma is approximately 20 mg/dL. In kidney failure, this level may rise to as high as 800 mg/dL.[18] Creatinine, a byproduct of muscle metabolism, is freely filtered in the glomerulus and is not reabsorbed in the renal tubules. It is produced at a relatively constant rate, and essentially all the creatinine that is filtered in the glomerulus is lost in the urine rather than being reabsorbed into the blood. Thus, serum creatinine can be used as an indirect method for assessing the GFR and the extent of kidney damage that has occurred in CKD.[18]

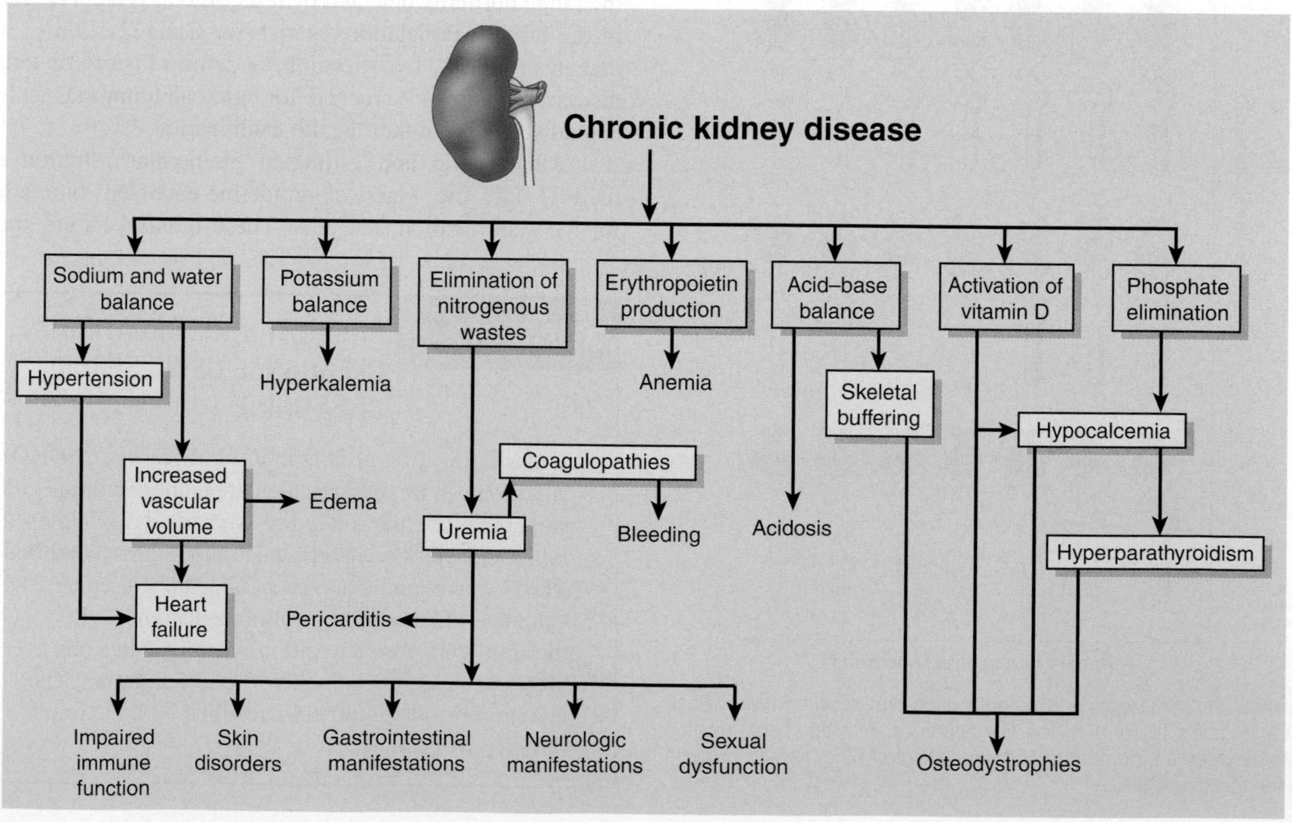

Figure 34.4 • Mechanisms and manifestations of CKD.

Uremia, which literally means "urine in the blood," is the term used to describe the clinical manifestations of kidney failure. Few symptoms of uremia appear until at least two thirds of the kidney's nephrons have been destroyed. Uremia differs from azotemia, which merely indicates the accumulation of nitrogenous wastes in the blood and can occur without symptoms. The uremic state includes signs and symptoms of altered fluid, electrolyte, and acid–base balance; alterations in regulatory functions (*e.g.*, blood pressure control, production of red blood cells, and impaired vitamin D synthesis); and the effects of uremia on body function (*e.g.*, uremic encephalopathy, peripheral neuropathy, pruritus). At this stage, virtually every organ and structure in the body is affected. The symptoms at the onset of uremia (*e.g.*, weakness, fatigue, nausea, apathy) often are subtle. More severe symptoms include extreme weakness, frequent vomiting, lethargy, and confusion. Without treatment of dialysis or a renal transplant, coma and death follow.

Fluid, Electrolyte, and Acid–Base Disorders

The kidneys function in the regulation of extracellular fluid volume. They do this by either eliminating or conserving sodium and water. Chronic renal failure can produce dehydration or fluid overload, depending on the pathologic process of the kidney disease. In addition to volume regulation, the ability of the kidneys to concentrate the urine is diminished. One of the earliest symptoms of kidney damage is polyuria with urine that is almost isotonic with plasma (*i.e.*, specific gravity of 1.008 to 1.012) and varies little from voiding to voiding.

As renal function declines further, the ability to regulate sodium excretion is reduced. The kidneys normally tolerate large variations in sodium intake while maintaining normal serum sodium levels. In chronic renal failure, they lose the ability to regulate sodium excretion. There is impaired ability to adjust to a sudden reduction in sodium intake and poor tolerance of an acute sodium overload. Volume depletion with an accompanying decrease in the GFR can occur with a restricted sodium intake or excess sodium loss caused by diarrhea or vomiting. Abnormal serum sodium levels have been associated with increased mortality in numerous observational studies. And those with CKD represent a group with a high prevalence of comorbid conditions that could predispose one to dysnatremias. Salt wasting is a common problem in advanced kidney failure because of impaired tubular reabsorption of sodium.[23] Increasing sodium intake in people with kidney failure often improves the GFR and whatever renal function remains. In people with associated hypertension, the possibility of increasing blood pressure or producing congestive heart failure often excludes supplemental sodium intake.

Approximately, 90% of potassium excretion is through the kidneys.[5] In kidney failure, potassium excretion by each nephron increases as the kidneys adapt to a decrease in the GFR. In addition, excretion in the gastrointestinal tract is increased. As a result, hyperkalemia usually does not develop until kidney function is severely compromised. Because of this adaptive mechanism, it usually is not necessary to restrict potassium intake in people with CKD until the GFR has dropped below 5 to 10 mL/min/1.73 m^2.[5] In people with kidney failure, hyperkalemia often results from failure to follow dietary potassium restrictions; constipation; acute acidosis that causes the release of intracellular potassium into the extracellular fluid; trauma or infection that causes release of potassium from body tissues; or exposure to medications that contain potassium, prevent its entry into cells, or block its secretion in distal nephrons.

The kidneys normally regulate blood pH by eliminating hydrogen ions produced in metabolic processes and regenerating bicarbonate. This is achieved through hydrogen ion secretion, sodium and bicarbonate reabsorption, and the production of ammonia, which acts as a buffer for titratable acids. With a decline in kidney function, these mechanisms become impaired, and metabolic acidosis may occur when the person is challenged with an excessive acid load or loses excessive alkali, as in diarrhea. The acidosis that occurs in people with kidney failure seems to stabilize as the disease progresses, probably as a result of the tremendous buffering capacity of the bone. However, this buffering action is thought to increase bone resorption and contribute to the skeletal disorders that occur in people with CKD.

Disorders of Calcium and Phosphorus Metabolism and Bone Disease

Abnormalities of calcium and phosphorus metabolism occur early in the course of CKD.[18] The regulation of serum phosphate levels requires a daily urinary excretion of an amount equal to that ingested in the diet. With deteriorating renal function, phosphate excretion is impaired, and as a result, serum phosphate levels rise. At the same time, serum calcium levels, which are inversely regulated in relation to serum phosphate levels, fall. The drop in serum calcium, in turn, stimulates parathyroid hormone (PTH) release, with a resultant increase in calcium resorption from the bone. Although serum calcium levels are maintained through increased PTH function, this adjustment is accomplished at the expense of the skeletal system and other body organs.

Vitamin D synthesis also is impaired in CKD. The kidneys regulate vitamin D activity by converting the inactive form of vitamin D (25[OH] vitamin D_3) to calcitriol (1,25[OH] vitamin D_3), the active form of vitamin D.[24] Calcitriol is known to have a direct suppressive effect on PTH production; therefore, reduced levels of calcitriol cause elevated levels of PTH. In addition, reduced calcitriol levels lead to impaired calcium absorption from the gastrointestinal tract. Vitamin D also regulates osteoblast differentiation, thereby affecting bone replacement.

Most people with CKD develop a secondary hyperparathyroidism, the result of down-regulation of parathyroid receptors on the parathyroid gland. Both vitamin D and calcium receptors are down-regulated, causing an elevation in the PTHs and decreased serum calcium and vitamin D levels. Vitamin D works in conjunction with PTH to mobilize calcium and phosphate from the bone to maintain serum calcium and phosphate levels.[25,26] Over the past two to three decades, the principal biochemical marker for diagnosis of CKD has been the measurement of PTH function using an immunoreactive technique called *intact PTH*.

Skeletal Disorders. The term *renal osteodystrophy* or *CKD–mineral bone disorder (CKD–MBD)* is used to describe the skeletal complications of CKD.[18] The skeletal changes that occur with CKD have been divided into two major types of disorders: high–bone-turnover and low–bone-turnover osteodystrophy. Some people may have predominantly one type of bone disorder, whereas others may have a mixed type of bone disease. Inherent to both of these conditions are abnormal reabsorption and defective remodeling of the bone. Mild forms of defective bone metabolism may be observed in early stages of CKD (stage 2), and they become more severe as kidney function deteriorates as in stage 5.

High–bone-turnover osteodystrophy, sometimes referred to as *osteitis fibrosa*, is characterized by increased bone resorption and formation, with bone resorption predominating. The disorder is associated with secondary hyperparathyroidism; altered vitamin D metabolism, along with resistance to the action of vitamin D; and impaired regulation of locally produced growth factors and inhibitors. There is an increase in both osteoblast and osteoclast numbers and activity. Although the osteoblasts produce excessive amounts of bone matrix, mineralization fails to keep pace, and there is a decrease in bone density and formation of porous and coarse-fibered bone. Cortical bone is affected more severely than cancellous bone.[6] Bone marrow fibrosis is another component of osteitis fibrosa; it occurs in areas of increased bone cell activity. In advanced stages of the disorder, cysts may develop in the bone, a condition called *osteitis fibrosa cystica*.

Low–bone-turnover osteodystrophy is characterized by decreased numbers of osteoblasts and low or reduced numbers of osteoclasts, a low rate of bone turnover, and an accumulation of unmineralized bone matrix. There are two forms of low–bone-turnover osteodystrophy: osteomalacia and adynamic osteodystrophy. *Osteomalacia* is characterized by a slow rate of bone formation and defects in bone mineralization, which may be caused by vitamin D deficiency, excess aluminum deposition, or metabolic acidosis. Metabolic acidosis is thought to have a direct effect on both osteoblastic and osteoclastic activities, as well as on the mineralization process, by decreasing the availability of trivalent phosphate. Until the 1980s, the osteomalacia seen in CKD resulted mainly from aluminum intoxication. Aluminum intoxication causes decreased and defective mineralization of the bone by existing osteoblasts and more long-term inhibition of osteoblast differentiation.[6] During the 1970s and 1980s, it was discovered that accumulation of aluminum from water used in dialysis and aluminum salts used as phosphate binders caused osteomalacia and adynamic bone disease. This discovery led to a change in the composition of dialysis solutions and the substitution of calcium carbonate for aluminum salts as phosphate binders. As a result, the prevalence of osteomalacia in people with CKD has declined.

The second type of low–bone-turnover osteodystrophy, *adynamic osteodystrophy*, is characterized by a low number of osteoblasts, with the osteoclast number being normal or reduced. It is now recognized as being as common as high–bone-turnover osteodystrophy and is especially common among people with diabetes. Adynamic bone disease is characterized by reduced bone volume and mineralization that may result, in part, from excessive suppression of PTH production with calcitriol. The high prevalence of adynamic osteodystrophy has been attributed to many factors, such as diabetes, use of drugs down-regulating parathormone release, high calcium intake, and advanced age.[27]

Regardless of the cause of skeletal abnormalities in CKD, bone disease can lead to bone tenderness and muscle weakness. Bone fractures complicate both high- and low-turnover types of bone disease. However, it is now recognized that people with adynamic bone disease may be more predisposed to fractures than those with osteitis fibrosa cystica. In the latter disorder, however, PTH-associated proximal muscle weakness in the lower extremities often coexists, giving rise to gait abnormalities and making it difficult to get out of a chair or climb stairs.

Early treatment of hyperphosphatemia and hypocalcemia is important to prevent or slow the development of skeletal complications. Milk products and other foods high in phosphorus content are restricted in the diet. Phosphate-binding antacids (aluminum salts, calcium carbonate, or calcium acetate) may be prescribed to decrease absorption of phosphate from the gastrointestinal tract. Calcium-containing phosphate binders can lead to hypercalcemia, thus worsening soft tissue calcification, especially in people receiving vitamin D therapy. Aluminum-containing antacids can contribute to the development of osteodystrophy or CKD–mineral and bone disorder.

Activated pharmacologic forms of vitamin D (*e.g.*, calcitriol) often are used to increase serum calcium levels and, at least partially, reverse the secondary hyperparathyroidism and osteitis fibrosis that occur with CKD. Although calcitriol is effective in controlling PTH overproduction, its stimulatory effects on intestinal absorption of calcium and phosphorus, along with its suppressive effects on bone turnover, predispose to hypercalcemia and hyperphosphatemia and to an increase in the calcium–phosphate ($Ca \times P$) product. Among people with CKD, there is a prevalence of cardiac arrest and CKD–MBD risk factors, such as electrolyte imbalance, defect in mineral metabolism, anemia, and diabetes.[28] Yet, there is more to osteodystrophy and chronic renal disease than skeletal bone dysfunction, because people with this condition also have a higher cardiovascular risk and have been found to have left ventricular hypertrophy and arterial stiffness secondary to vascular calcification.[28]

Secondary hyperparathyroidism in CKD may also be treated by activating the calcium-sensing receptor on the parathyroid gland with medication such as the calcimimetic agent cinacalcet. Cinacalcet is used to lower elevated serum PTH levels in people with CKD stage 5. Cinacalcet mimics the action of calcium on calcium-sensing receptors in the parathyroid glands to suppress PTH secretion.[29] However, because adynamic bone disease is often a consequence of overzealous treatment of secondary hyperthyroidism, these agents require careful use.

Hematologic Disorders

Anemia. Chronic anemia (hemoglobin levels <13.0 g/dL in adult men and <12 g/dL in adult women) is the most profound hematologic alteration that accompanies CKD.[22] African Americans and people with diabetes have even higher rates of anemia for each advanced stage of CKD.[26] The NKF guidelines recommend that those people with a GFR less than 60 mL/min/1.73 m^2 should be evaluated for anemia. Assessment for anemia and its causes includes measures of hemoglobin, hematocrit, and iron stores.

The anemia of CKD is due to several factors, including chronic blood loss, hemolysis, bone marrow suppression because of retained uremic factors, and decreased red cell production because of impaired production of erythropoietin and iron deficiency. The kidneys are the primary site for the production of the hormone *erythropoietin*, which controls red blood cell production.[22] In renal failure, erythropoietin production usually is insufficient to stimulate adequate red blood cell production by the bone marrow. Among the causes of iron deficiency in people with CKD are anorexia and dietary restrictions that limit intake and the blood loss that occurs during dialysis.[22]

When untreated, anemia causes or contributes to weakness, fatigue, headache, irritability, depression, insomnia, and decreased cognitive function. There also is an increasing concern regarding the physiologic effects of anemia on cardiovascular function.[22] The anemia of renal failure produces a decrease in blood viscosity and a compensatory increase in heart rate. The decreased blood viscosity also exacerbates peripheral vasodilation and contributes to decreased vascular resistance. Cardiac output increases in a compensatory fashion to maintain tissue perfusion. Anemia also limits myocardial oxygen supply, particularly in people with coronary heart disease, leading to angina pectoris and other ischemic events.[30]

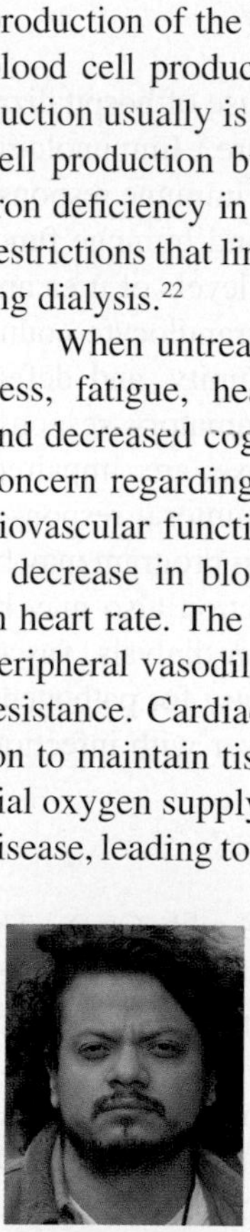

Mr. Reterez has severe fatigue, probably because of a low hematocrit and hemoglobin secondary to his CKD, which occurred due to his polycystic kidney disease. This is anemia of chronic disease. Most likely, Mr. Reterez will be put on an erythropoietin supplement to assist in triggering his bone marrow to reproduce more red blood cells. He will also be carefully checked by his primary care provider for signs of cardiovascular disease and also managed for hypertension because his blood pressure is 145/92 and his pulse is 92.

Iron and erythropoietin-stimulating agents (ESAs) are used to treat anemia and to decrease red cell transfusions and their risks. A significant advance in medical management of CKD was realized when recombinant human erythropoietin (rhEPO) and ESA became available in 1989 to help maintain hematocrit levels in people with kidney failure.[2] Darbepoetin alfa, a hyperglycosylated analog of rhEPO, is an erythropoiesis-stimulating protein with a prolonged half-life that was introduced for treatment of anemia in CKD. However, evidence suggests it is no more effective, but is more expensive for people with CKD on dialysis than epoetin alfa.[31] Secondary benefits of treating anemia with rhEPO, previously attributed to the correction of uremia, include improvement in appetite, energy level, sexual function, skin color, and hair and nail growth, and reduced cold intolerance. Because worsening of hypertension and seizures have occurred when the hematocrit was raised too suddenly, frequent measurements of hematocrit are necessary. The effect of ESAs on dialysis initiation in people with advanced CKD is not clear. More evidence is needed to validate whether the erythropoietin-stimulating agents should be used or not.[32]

Coagulopathies. Bleeding disorders are manifested by epistaxis, menorrhagia, gastrointestinal bleeding, and bruising of the skin and subcutaneous tissues. Although platelet production often is normal in CKD, platelet function is impaired.[6,18] Coagulative function improves with dialysis but does not completely normalize, suggesting that uremia contributes to the problem. People with CKD also have greater susceptibility to thrombotic disorders.

Cardiovascular Disorders

The overall mortality rate from cardiovascular disease in people with CKD is many times that of the general population.[30] Even after stratification for age, the incidence of cardiovascular disease remains 10 to 20 times higher in people with CKD than in the general population.[30]

Hypertension. Hypertension commonly is an early manifestation of CKD. The mechanisms that produce hypertension in CKD are multifactorial. They include an increased vascular volume, elevation of peripheral vascular resistance, decreased levels of renal vasodilator prostaglandins, and increased activity of the renin–angiotensin system.

Early identification and aggressive treatment of hypertension have been shown to slow the progression of renal impairment in many types of kidney disease.[2] Controlling blood pressure through lifestyle and pharmacologic interventions is an essential component of slowing the progression of kidney disease. Treatment involves salt and water restriction and the use of antihypertensive medications to control blood pressure. Many people with CKD need to take several antihypertensive medications to control blood pressure. There is a new class of hypertension drugs called endothelin blockers. These drugs are being trialed in people with difficult-to-manage hypertension.[33]

Heart Disease. The spectrum of cardiovascular disease because of CKD includes left ventricular hypertrophy and ischemic heart disease. People with CKD tend to have an increased prevalence of left ventricular dysfunction, with both depressed left ventricular ejection fraction, as in systolic dysfunction, and impaired ventricular filling, as in diastolic failure.[2] Multiple factors lead to development of left ventricular dysfunction, including extracellular fluid overload, shunting of blood through an arteriovenous fistula for dialysis, and anemia. Anemia, in particular, has been correlated with the presence of left ventricular hypertrophy.[22] These abnormalities, coupled with the hypertension that often is present, cause increased myocardial work and oxygen demand, with eventual development of heart failure.

Congestive heart failure and pulmonary edema tend to occur in the late stages of kidney failure. Coexisting conditions that have been identified as contributing to the burden of cardiovascular disease include hypertension, anemia, diabetes mellitus, dyslipidemia, and coagulopathies. PTH also may play a role in the pathogenesis of cardiomyopathy in renal failure.[28]

Pericarditis. Pericarditis occurs in many people with stage five CKD because of the uremia and prolonged dialysis.[2] The manifestations of uremic pericarditis resemble those of viral pericarditis, with all its potential complications, including cardiac tamponade. The presenting signs include mild to severe chest pain with respiratory accentuation and a pericardial friction rub. Fever is variable in the absence of infection and is more common in dialysis than uremic pericarditis.[2]

Gastrointestinal Disorders

Anorexia, nausea, and vomiting are common in people with uremia, along with a metallic taste in the mouth that further depresses the appetite.[2] Early morning nausea is common. Ulceration and bleeding of the gastrointestinal mucosa may develop, and hiccups are common. A possible cause of nausea and vomiting is the decomposition of urea by intestinal flora, resulting in a high concentration of ammonia. PTH increases gastric acid secretion and contributes to gastrointestinal problems. Nausea and vomiting often improve with restriction of dietary protein and after initiation of dialysis and disappear after kidney transplantation.

Neuromuscular Disorders

Many people with CKD have alterations in peripheral and central nervous system function.[2] Peripheral neuropathy, or involvement of the peripheral nerves, affects the lower limbs more frequently than the upper limbs. It is symmetric and affects both sensory and motor function. Neuropathy is caused by atrophy and demyelination of nerve fibers, possibly caused by uremic toxins. Restless legs syndrome is a manifestation of peripheral nerve involvement and can be seen in as many as two thirds of people on dialysis. This syndrome is characterized by creeping, prickling, and itching sensations that typically are more intense at rest. Temporary relief is obtained by moving the legs. A burning sensation of the feet, which may be followed by muscle weakness and atrophy, is a manifestation of uremia.

The central nervous system disturbances in uremia are similar to those caused by other metabolic and toxic disorders. Sometimes referred to as *uremic encephalopathy*, the condition is poorly understood and may result, at least in part, from an excess of toxic organic acids that alter neural function. Electrolyte abnormalities, such as sodium shifts, also may contribute. The manifestations are more closely related to the progress of the uremic disorder than to the level of the metabolic end products. Reductions in alertness and awareness are the earliest and most significant indications of uremic encephalopathy. These often are followed by an inability to fix attention, loss of recent memory, and perceptual errors in identifying people and objects. Delirium and coma occur late in the disease course. Seizures are the preterminal event.

Disorders of motor function commonly accompany the neurologic manifestations of uremic encephalopathy. During the early stages, there often is difficulty in performing fine movements of the extremities. The person's gait becomes unsteady and clumsy with tremulousness of movement. Asterixis (dorsiflexion movements of the hands and feet) typically occurs as the disease progresses. It can be elicited by having the person hyperextend his or her arms at the elbow and wrist with the fingers spread apart. If asterixis is present, this position causes side-to-side flapping movements of the fingers.

Altered Immune Function

Infection is a common complication and cause of hospitalization and death for people with kidney failure.[2] Immunologic abnormalities decrease the efficiency of the immune response to infection.[2] All aspects of inflammation and immune function may be affected adversely by the high levels of urea and metabolic wastes, including a decreased granulocyte count, impaired humoral and cell-mediated immunity, and defective phagocyte function. The acute inflammatory response and delayed-type hypersensitivity response are impaired. Although people with CKD have normal humoral responses to vaccines, a more aggressive immunization program may be needed. Skin and mucosal barriers to infection also may be defective. In people who are maintained on dialysis, vascular access devices are common portals of entry for pathogens. Many people with CKD fail to mount a fever with infection, making the diagnosis more difficult.

Disorders of Skin Integrity

Skin manifestations are common in people with CKD.[2] The skin often is pale owing to anemia and may have a sallow, yellow–brown hue. The skin and mucous membranes often are dry, and subcutaneous bruising is common. Skin dryness or xerosis is caused by a reduction in perspiration owing to the decreased size of sweat glands and the diminished activity of oil glands. Pruritus is common; it results from the high serum phosphate levels and the development of phosphate crystals that occur with hyperparathyroidism. Severe scratching and repeated needle sticks, especially with hemodialysis, break the skin integrity and increase the risk for infection. In the advanced stages of untreated kidney failure, urea crystals may precipitate on the skin as a result of the high urea concentration in body fluids. The fingernails may also become thin and brittle.

Sexual Dysfunction

The cause of sexual dysfunction in men and women with CKD is unclear. The cause probably is multifactorial and may result from high levels of uremic toxins, neuropathy, hormonal disturbances, anemia, MBD, comorbidities, altered endocrine function, psychological factors (*e.g.*, anxiety, depression, low self-esteem, social withdrawal, and body image), and medications (*e.g.*, antihypertensive drugs, antidepressants). Alterations in physiologic sexual responses, reproductive ability, and libido are common.[34]

Impotence occurs in many men on dialysis.[34] Derangements of the pituitary and gonadal hormones, such as decreases in testosterone levels, chronic physical illness, social pressures (*e.g.*, stress, infertility), and increases in prolactin and luteinizing hormone levels, are common and cause erectile difficulties and decreased spermatocyte counts. Loss of libido may result from chronic anemia and decreased testosterone levels. Several drugs, such as exogenous testosterone and bromocriptine, have been used in an attempt to return hormone levels to normal. Sildenafil citrate has been shown in small trials of people on long-term hemodialysis to be effective and safe.[34]

Impaired sexual function in women is manifested by abnormal levels of progesterone, luteinizing hormone, and prolactin. Hypofertility, menstrual abnormalities, decreased vaginal lubrication, and various orgasmic problems have been described.

Elimination of Drugs

The kidneys are responsible for the elimination of many drugs and their metabolites. CKD and its treatment can interfere with the absorption, distribution, and elimination of drugs.[2] The administration of large quantities of phosphate-binding antacids to control hyperphosphatemia and hypocalcemia in people with advanced renal failure interferes with the absorption of some drugs.[2] Many drugs are bound to plasma proteins, such as albumin, for transport in the body; the unbound portion of the drug is available to act at the various receptor sites and is free to be metabolized. A decrease in plasma proteins, particularly albumin, that occurs in many people with CKD results in less protein-bound drug and greater amounts of free drug.

In the process of metabolism, some drugs form intermediate metabolites that are toxic if not eliminated. Some pathways of drug metabolism, such as hydrolysis, are slowed with uremia. In people with diabetes, for example, insulin requirements may be reduced as renal function deteriorates. Decreased elimination by the kidneys allows drugs or their metabolites to accumulate in the body and requires that drug dosages be adjusted accordingly. Some drugs contain unwanted nitrogen, sodium, potassium, and magnesium and must be avoided in people with CKD. Penicillin, for example, contains potassium. Nitrofurantoin and ammonium chloride add to the body's nitrogen pool. Many antacids contain magnesium. Because of problems with drug dosing and elimination, people with CKD should be cautioned against the use of over-the-counter remedies.

Treatment

CKD is treated by conservative management to prevent or slow the rate of nephron destruction and, when necessary, by renal replacement therapy with dialysis or transplantation.

Measures to Slow Progression of the Disorder

Conservative treatment can often delay the progression of CKD.[18] It includes measures to retard deterioration of renal function and assist the body in managing the effects of impaired function. Urinary tract infections should be treated promptly and medication with renal damaging potential should be avoided. It should be noted that these strategies are complementary to the treatment of the original cause of the renal disorder, which is of the utmost importance and needs to be continually addressed.

Blood pressure control is important, as is control of blood sugar in people with diabetes mellitus. Intensive glycemic control in people with diabetes helps to prevent the development of microalbuminuria and retards the progression of diabetic nephropathy. In addition to reduction in cardiovascular risk, antihypertensive therapy in people with CKD aims to slow the progression of nephron loss by lowering intraglomerular hypertension and hypertrophy.[32] Elevated blood pressure also increases proteinuria because of transmission of the elevated pressure to the glomeruli. The ACE inhibitors and ARBs, which have a unique effect on the glomerular microcirculation (*i.e.*, dilation of the efferent arteriole), are increasingly being used in the treatment of hypertension and proteinuria, particularly in people with diabetes.[33]

Smoking has a negative impact on kidney function, and it is one of the most remedial risk factors for CKD.[35,36] The mechanisms of smoking-induced renal damage appear to include both acute hemodynamic effects (*i.e.*, increase in blood pressure, intraglomerular pressure, and urinary albumin excretion) and chronic effects (endothelial cell dysfunction).[35,36] Smoking is nephrotoxic in older adults with hypertension and those with diabetes. Importantly, the adverse effects of smoking appear to be independent of the underlying kidney disease.

Dialysis and Transplantation

Dialysis or renal replacement therapy is indicated when advanced uremia or serious electrolyte imbalances are present. Just 50 years ago, many people with CKD progressed to the final stages of kidney failure and then died. The high mortality rate was associated with limitations in the treatment of kidney disease and with the tremendous cost of ongoing treatment. In 1972, federal support began for dialysis and transplantation through a Medicare entitlement program in the United States.[37] During the past several decades, an increasing number of people have required renal replacement therapy with dialysis or transplantation. The number of people beginning hemodialysis has grown substantially. In 2008, greater than half a million people in the United States started on dialysis or received a renal transplant.[38] In 2016, 100,791 people were awaiting kidney transplants. In 2014, 17,107 kidney transplants took place in the United States. Of these, 11,570 came from deceased donors, and 5537 came from living donors.[38]

The choice between dialysis and transplantation is dictated by age, related health problems, donor availability, and personal preference. Although transplantation often is the preferred treatment, dialysis plays a critical role as a treatment method for kidney failure. It is life sustaining for people who are not candidates for transplantation or who are awaiting transplantation. There are two broad categories of dialysis: hemodialysis and peritoneal dialysis.

Hemodialysis. The basic principles of hemodialysis have remained unchanged over the years, although new technology has improved the efficiency and speed of dialysis. A hemodialysis system, or artificial kidney, consists of three parts: a blood delivery system, a dialyzer, and a dialysis fluid delivery system. The dialyzer is usually a hollow cylinder composed of bundles of capillary tubes through which blood circulates, while the dialysate travels on the outside of the tubes.[2] The walls of the capillary tubes in the dialysis chamber are made up of a semipermeable membrane material that allows all molecules except blood cells and plasma proteins to move freely in both directions—from the blood into the dialyzing solution and from the dialyzing solution into the blood. The direction of flow is determined by the concentration of the substances contained in the two solutions. The waste products and excess electrolytes in the blood normally diffuse into the dialyzing solution. If there is a need to replace or add substances, such as bicarbonate, to the blood, these can be added to the dialyzing solution (Fig. 34.5).

During dialysis, blood moves from an artery through the tubing and blood chamber in the dialysis machine and then back into the body through a vein. Access to the vascular system is accomplished through a synthetic graft or an external arteriovenous shunt (*i.e.*, tubing implanted into an artery and a vein) or, more commonly, through an internal arteriovenous fistula (*i.e.*, anastomosis of a vein to an artery, usually in the forearm). Heparin is used to prevent clotting during the dialysis treatment; it can be administered continuously or intermittently. Problems that may occur during dialysis, depending on the rates of blood flow and solute removal, include hypotension, nausea, vomiting, muscle cramps, headache, chest pain, and disequilibrium syndrome.

The most prominent complications, which can occur with any type of access, are recognized as being thrombosis or stenosis, infection, and formation of an aneurysm. To successfully care for a patient with a graft, shunt, or fistula, the nurses needs to follow these guidelines:[39]

- Palpate for a thrill and auscultate for a bruit prior to cannulation.
- Do not take blood pressure readings on an extremity in which the vascular access is placed.
- Do not start an intravenous (IV) line or perform a venipuncture in the extremity in which vascular access is placed.
- Assess the patient's distal pulses and circulation in the extremity with the vascular access.
- Assess for manifestations of infection such as fever, tachycardia, redness, and drainage at the needle site.
- Check for bleeding at needle insertion sites.

Most people undergo dialysis three times each week for 3 to 4 hours. Treatment is determined by kinetic profiles, referred to as *Kt/V* values, which consider dialyzer size, dialysate, flow rate, time of dialysis, and body size. Many dialysis centers provide the option for people to learn how to perform hemodialysis at home.

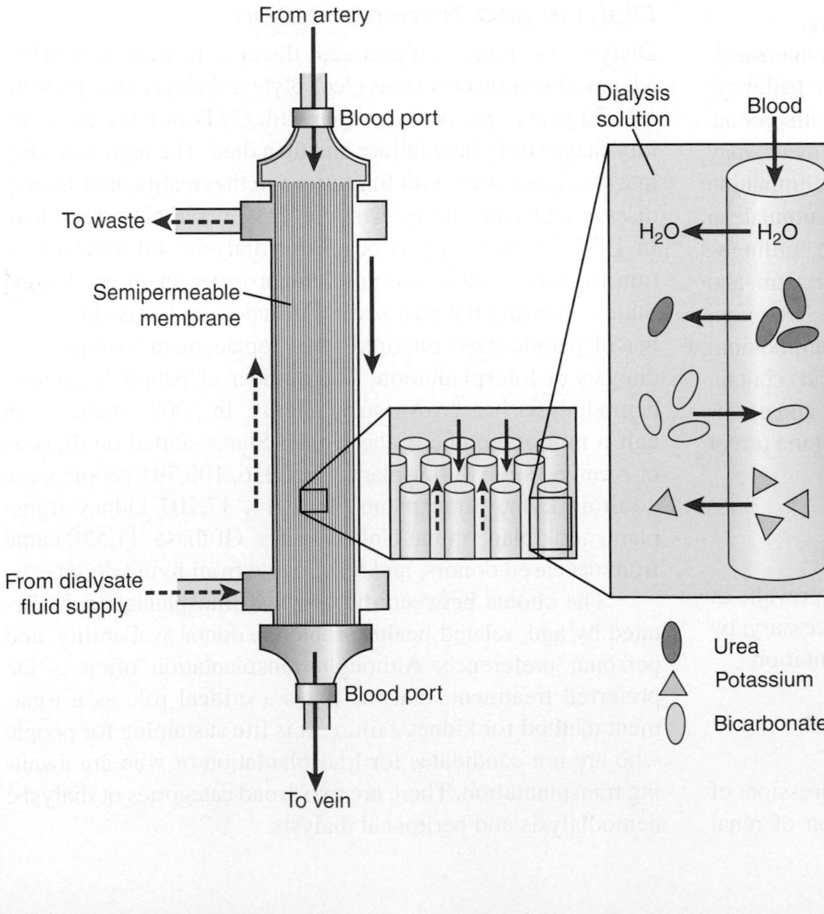

Figure 34.5 • Schematic diagram of a hemodialysis system. The blood compartment and dialysis solution compartment are separated by a semipermeable membrane. This membrane is porous enough to allow all the constituents, except the plasma proteins and blood cells, to diffuse between the two compartments.

Peritoneal Dialysis. Peritoneal dialysis was introduced in the mid-1970s. Improvements in technology and the ability to deliver adequate dialysis resulted in improved outcomes and the acceptance of peritoneal dialysis as a renal replacement therapy.

The same principles of diffusion, osmosis, and ultrafiltration that apply to hemodialysis apply to peritoneal dialysis.[2] The thin serous membrane of the peritoneal cavity serves as the dialyzing membrane. A Silastic catheter is surgically implanted in the peritoneal cavity below the umbilicus to provide access. The catheter is tunneled through subcutaneous tissue and exits on the side of the abdomen (Fig. 34.6). The dialysis process involves instilling a sterile dialyzing solution (usually 1 to 3 L) through the catheter over a period of approximately 10 minutes. The solution then is allowed to remain, or *dwell*, in the peritoneal cavity for a prescribed amount of time, during which the metabolic end products and extracellular fluid diffuse into the dialysis solution. At the end of the dwell time, the dialysis fluid is drained out of the peritoneal cavity by gravity into a sterile bag. Glucose in the dialysis solution accounts for water removal. Commercial dialysis solution is available in 1.5%, 2.5%, and 4.25% dextrose concentrations. Solutions with higher dextrose levels increase osmosis, causing more fluid to be removed. As with hemodialysis, *Kt/V* values are used to evaluate adequacy of peritoneal dialysis.

Peritoneal dialysis can be performed at home or in a dialysis center and can be carried out by continuous ambulatory peritoneal dialysis (CAPD), continuous cyclic peritoneal dialysis (CCPD), or nocturnal intermittent peritoneal dialysis (NIPD)—all with variations in the number of exchanges and dwell times.[2] Individual preference, manual ability, lifestyle, knowledge of the procedure, and physiologic response to treatment are used to determine the type of dialysis that is used. The most common method is CAPD, a self-care procedure in which the person manages the dialysis procedure at home. CAPD involves instilling the dialysate into the peritoneal cavity and rolling up the bag and tubing and securing them under clothing during the dwell. After the dwell time is completed (usually 4 to 6 hours during the day), the bag is unrolled and lowered, allowing the waste-containing dialysis solution to drain from the peritoneal cavity into the bag. Each exchange, which involves draining the solution and infusing a new solution, requires approximately 30 to 45 minutes. Four exchanges usually are performed each day. In CCPD, exchanges are performed in an automated manner, usually at night, with the person connected to an automatic cycler, which then performs four or five cycles, while the person sleeps. In the morning, the person, with the last exchange remaining in the abdomen, is disconnected from the cycler and goes about his or her usual activities. In NIPD, the person is given approximately 10 hours of automatic cycling each night, with the abdomen left dry during the day.

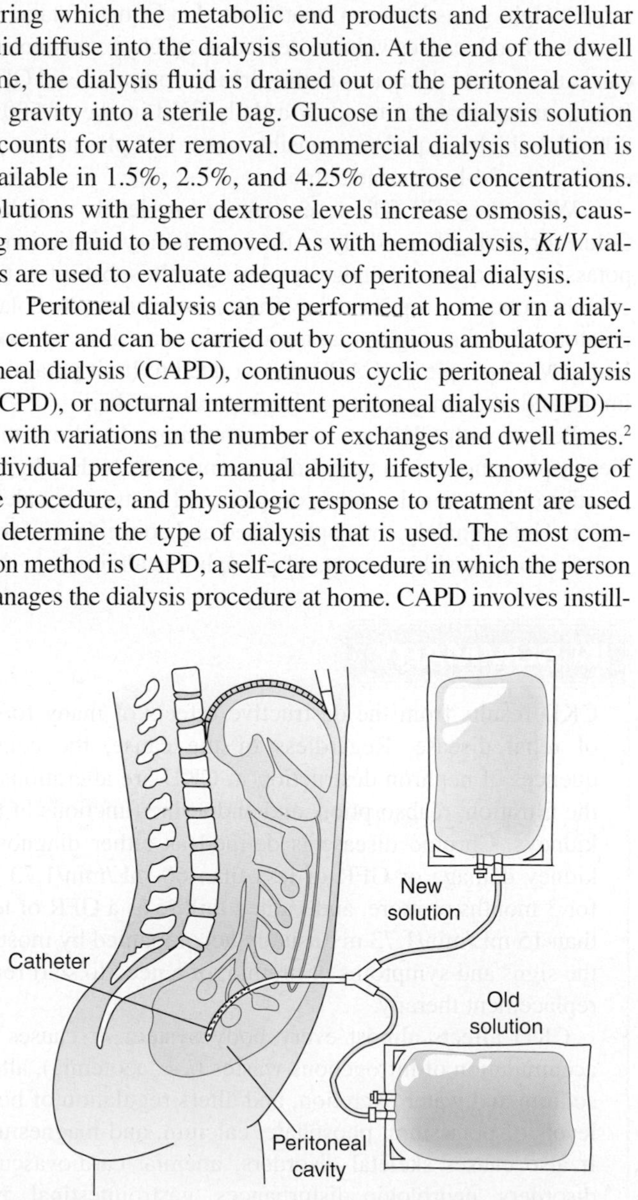

Figure 34.6 • Peritoneal dialysis. A semipermeable membrane, richly supplied with small blood vessels, lines the peritoneal cavity. With dialysate dwelling in the peritoneal cavity, waste products diffuse from the network of blood vessels into the dialysate.

Potential problems with peritoneal dialysis include infection, catheter malfunction, dehydration caused by excessive fluid removal, hyperglycemia, and hernia. The most serious complication is infection, which can occur at the catheter exit site, in the subcutaneous tunnel, or in the peritoneal cavity (*i.e.*, peritonitis).

Transplantation. Greatly improved success rates have made kidney transplantation the treatment of choice for many people with CKD. The availability of donor organs continues to limit the number of transplantations performed each year. Donor organs are obtained from cadavers and living related donors (*e.g.*, parent, sibling). Transplants from living unrelated donors (*e.g.*, spouse) have been used in cases of suitable ABO blood type and tissue compatibility.

The success of transplantation depends on multiple variables such as the general health of the person, the degree of histocompatibility with the donor, the degree of end-organ disease the person may have, and how well the immunologic response is managed. Maintenance immunosuppressive therapy typically consists of prednisone, azathioprine, and cyclosporine (or tacrolimus). IL-2, a cytokine, plays an essential role in T- and B-cell activation. Cyclosporine and tacrolimus, calcineurin inhibitors, inhibit IL-2 synthesis. IL-2 receptor antagonists such as basiliximab and daclizumab are more frequently being used.[40] Monoclonal antibodies such as alemtuzumab are starting to be used.[40] OKT-3 (directed against the CD3 T-cell receptor) and ATGAM, which is a polyclonal antibody, are used rarely such as when the person is experiencing steroid resistance and allograft rejection. The Janus kinase (JAK) 3 inhibitors are a new classification of immunosuppressive therapy that are also starting to be in use and have effective results.[40] Two examples of this drug category include AEB-071, which inhibits protein kinase, and LEA29Y or belatacept, which have both improved transplant people' rate of rejection. However, most of these immunosuppressive drugs have serious side effects such as cardiovascular problems, metabolic dysfunction, and cancer.[40]

Rejection, which is categorized as acute and chronic, can occur at any time. Acute rejection most commonly occurs during the first several months after transplantation and involves a cellular response with the proliferation of T lymphocytes. Chronic rejection can occur months to years after transplantation. Because chronic rejection is caused by both cellular and humoral immunities, it does not respond well to increased immunosuppressive therapy.

Maintenance immunosuppressive therapy and increased use of immunosuppression to treat rejection predispose the person to a spectrum of infectious complications. Prophylactic antimicrobials may be prescribed to decrease the incidence of common infections, such as candidiasis, herpesvirus infections, and *Pneumocystis jiroveci* (formerly *P. carinii*) pneumonia. Other infections, such as cytomegalovirus infection and aspergillosis, are seen with chronic immunosuppression.

Dietary Management

A major component in the treatment of CKD is nutritional management. The goal of dietary treatment is to provide optimum nutrition while maintaining tolerable levels of metabolic wastes. The specific diet prescription depends on the type and severity of renal disease and on the dialysis modality. Because of the severe restrictions placed on food and fluid intake, these diets may be complicated and unappetizing. After kidney transplantation, some dietary restrictions still may be necessary, even when renal function is normal, to control the adverse effects from immunosuppressive medication.

Protein. Restriction of dietary proteins may decrease the progress of renal impairment in people with advanced renal disease. Proteins are broken down to form nitrogenous wastes, and reducing the amount of protein in the diet lowers the BUN and reduces symptoms.

Considerable controversy exists over the degree of protein restriction needed. If the diet is too low in protein, protein malnutrition can occur, with a loss of strength, muscle mass, and body weight. People on hemodialysis usually require a higher dietary protein intake to prevent protein and energy malnutrition because of anorexia from uremia itself, the dialysis procedure, intercurrent illness, and acidemia. People on peritoneal dialysis also have significant protein losses and require a higher dietary protein intake. At least 50% of the protein intake should consist of proteins of high biologic value, such as those in eggs, lean meat, and milk, which are rich in essential amino acids. Proteins with a high biologic value are believed to promote the reuse of endogenous nitrogen, decreasing the amount of nitrogenous wastes that are produced and ameliorating the symptoms of uremia. In reusing nitrogen, the proteins ingested in the diet are broken down into their constituent amino acids and recycled in the synthesis of protein required by the body. In contrast to proteins with a high biologic value, fewer than half of the amino acids in cereal proteins are reused. Amino acids that are not reused to build body proteins are broken down and form the end products of protein metabolism, such as urea.

Carbohydrates, Fat, and Calories. With CKD, adequate calories in the form of carbohydrates and fat are required to meet energy needs. This is particularly important when the protein content of the diet is severely restricted. If sufficient calories are not available, the limited protein in the diet goes into energy production, or body tissue itself is used for energy purposes. Caloric intake for people on CAPD includes food intake and calories absorbed from the dialysis solution.

Fluid and Electrolytes. The sodium and fluid restrictions depend on the kidneys' ability to excrete sodium and water and must be individually determined. Renal disease of glomerular origin is more likely to contribute to sodium retention, whereas tubular dysfunction causes salt wasting. Fluid intake in excess of what the kidneys can excrete causes circulatory overload, edema, and water intoxication. Thirst is a common problem among people on hemodialysis, often resulting in large weight gains between treatments. Inadequate intake, on the other hand, causes volume depletion and hypotension and can cause further decreases in the already compromised GFR. It is common practice to allow a daily fluid intake of 500 to 800 mL, which is equal to insensible water loss plus a quantity equal to the 24-hour urine output.

When the GFR falls to extremely low levels in kidney failure or during hemodialysis therapy, dietary restriction of potassium becomes mandatory. Using salt substitutes that contain potassium or ingesting fruits, fruit juice, chocolate, potatoes, or other high-potassium foods can cause hyperkalemia. Most people on CAPD do not need to limit potassium intake and often may even need to increase intake.

People with CKD are usually encouraged to limit their dietary phosphorus as a means of preventing secondary hyperparathyroidism, renal osteodystrophy, and metastatic calcification. Unfortunately, many processed and convenience foods contain considerable amounts of phosphorus additives.

IN SUMMARY

CKD results from the destructive effects of many forms of renal disease. Regardless of the cause, the consequences of nephron destruction in CKD are alterations in the filtration, reabsorption, and endocrine functions of the kidneys. Chronic disease is defined as either diagnosed kidney damage or GFR of less than 60 mL/min/1.73 m^2 for 3 months or more, and kidney failure as a GFR of less than 15 mL/min/1.73 m^2, usually accompanied by most of the signs and symptoms of uremia, or a need to start renal replacement therapy.

CKD affects almost every body system. It causes an accumulation of nitrogenous wastes (*i.e.*, azotemia), alters sodium and water excretion, and alters regulation of body levels of potassium, phosphate, calcium, and magnesium. It also causes skeletal disorders, anemia, cardiovascular disorders, neurologic disturbances, gastrointestinal dysfunction, and discomforting skin changes.

The treatment measures for CKD can be divided into two types: conservative treatment measures and renal replacement therapy. Conservative treatment consists of measures to prevent or retard deterioration in remaining renal function and assist the body in compensating for the existing impairment. Interventions that have been shown to retard the progression of CKD include blood pressure normalization and control of blood glucose in people with diabetes. Activated vitamin D can be used to increase calcium absorption and control secondary hyperparathyroidism. rhEPO is being assessed as to whether it should be used to treat the profound anemia that occurs in people with CKD. Renal replacement therapy (dialysis or kidney transplantation) is indicated when advanced uremia and serious electrolyte problems are present.

CHRONIC KIDNEY DISEASE IN CHILDREN AND OLDER ADULTS

After completing this section of the chapter, the learner will be able to meet the following objectives:

- List the causes of CKD in children and describe the special problems of children with kidney failure.
- State why CKD is more common in older adults and describe measures to prevent or delay the onset of kidney failure in this population.

Although the spectrum of CKD among children and older adults is similar to that of adults, several unique issues affecting these groups warrant further discussion.

Chronic Kidney Disease in Children

The true incidence of CKD in infants and children is unknown. CKD has a prevalence of 1.5 to 3.0 per 1,000,000 among children younger than the age of 16 years. Yet, the pediatric incidence of ESRD has been stable over the past 30 years worldwide, but prevalence has increased along with incidence of dialysis and renal transplant recipients.[41]

Etiology

The causes of CKD in children include congenital malformations, inherited disorders, acquired diseases, and metabolic syndromes. The cause of CKD differs between pediatric and adult people. Diabetic nephropathy, hypertension, and autosomal dominant polycystic kidney disease are prevalent diseases in adults, whereas in children, the congenital anomalies of the kidney and urinary tract (CAKUT) are the most common pathology, followed by the hereditary nephropathies and glomerulonephritis.[42] In children younger than 5 years of age, CKD is commonly the result of congenital malformations such as renal dysplasia or obstructive uropathy. After 5 years of age, acquired diseases (*e.g.*, glomerulonephritis) and inherited disorders (*e.g.*, familial juvenile nephronophthisis) predominate. CKD related to metabolic disorders, such as hyperoxaluria and inherited disorders, such as polycystic kidney disease may present throughout childhood.[42–44]

The stages for progression of CKD in children are similar to those for adults, but apply only to children who are older than 2 years of age. This is because of the extremely small body size of infants and toddlers in addition to their very low GFR.[43]

Clinical Manifestations

The manifestations of CKD in children are quite varied and depend on the underlying disease condition. Features of CKD that are marked during childhood include severe growth impairment, developmental delay, delay in sexual maturation, bone abnormalities, and development of psychosocial problems. Critical growth periods occur during the first 2 years of life and during adolescence. Physical growth and cognitive development are slowed in children with CKD. Puberty usually occurs at a later age in children with CKD, partly because of endocrine abnormalities. Renal osteodystrophies are more common and extensive in children than in adults. The most common condition seen in children is high–bone-turnover bone disease caused by secondary hyperparathyroidism. Some hereditary renal diseases, such as medullary cystic disease, have patterns of skeletal involvement that further complicate the problems of renal osteodystrophy. Clinical manifestations of renal osteodystrophy include muscle weakness, bone pain, and fractures with minor trauma.[45] In growing children, rachitic changes, varus and valgus deformities of long bones, and slipped capital femoral epiphysis may be seen. Additionally, any child with CKD will have the potential to develop ectopic vascular calcification, which begins in the early stages of CKD before dialysis is initiated.[43] Once the child reaches ESRD and is on dialysis three times a week, cardiovascular dysfunction progresses very quickly.[43]

Factors related to impaired growth include deficient nutrition, anemia, renal osteodystrophy, chronic acidosis, and cases of nephrotic syndrome that require high-dose corticosteroid therapy. Nutrition is believed to be one of the most important determinants during infancy.[45] For many children, catch-up growth is important because a growth deficit frequently is established during the first months of life.

Treatment

All forms of renal replacement, or more appropriately named supportive therapy, can be safely and reliably used for children. Age is a defining factor in dialysis modality selection. More children between birth and 5 years of age receive peritoneal dialysis. A substantial percentage of children develop CKD early in life, with congenital renal disorders such as obstructive uropathy and aplasia, hypoplasia, or dysplasia being responsible for almost one half of all cases. Those older than 12 years of age are more apt to receive hemodialysis.[45] The most favored ESRD treatment modality in children is an early renal transplantation.[44] Immunosuppressive therapy in children is similar to that used in adults. All of these immunosuppressive agents have side effects, including increased risk for infection. Corticosteroids, which have been the mainstay of chronic immunosuppressive therapy for decades, carry the risk for hypertension, orthopedic complications (especially aseptic necrosis), cataracts, and growth retardation.

Chronic Kidney Disease in Older Adults

Today, there are an increasing number of people over 65 years of age presenting with CKD, particularly in the more advanced stages.[46] However, the true prevalence or outcomes of CKD in older adults have not been systematically studied. The presentation and course of CKD may be altered because of age-related changes in the kidneys and concurrent medical conditions. More research needs to be conducted that includes older adults with CKD who may have the problem secondary to aging versus diabetes mellitus.[47] It seems most older adults (>65 years) do not have CKD because of proteinuria or diabetes.[47]

Etiology and Diagnosis

Aging is associated with a steady decline in kidney function, a decreasing GFR, and subsequently with reduced homeostatic regulation under stressful conditions.[46] This reduction in GFR makes older adults more susceptible to the detrimental effects of nephrotoxic drugs, such as radiographic contrast compounds. The reduction in GFR related to aging is not accompanied by a parallel rise in the serum creatinine level because the serum creatinine level, which results from muscle metabolism, is significantly reduced in older adults because of diminished muscle mass and other age-related changes. The NKF guidelines suggest that the same criteria for establishing the presence of CKD in younger adults (*i.e.*, GFR < 60 mL/min/1.73 m^2) should be used for the older adults.[48] Evaluation of older adults with a GFR of 60 to 89 mL/min/1.73 m^2 should include age-adjusted measurements of creatinine clearance, along with assessment of CKD risks, and a blood pressure reading.

Clinical Manifestations

The prevalence of cerebrovascular, cardiovascular, and skeletal system chronic disease is frequently seen with older adults. Because of concurrent disease, the presenting symptoms of kidney disease in older adults may be less typical than those observed in younger adults. For example, congestive heart failure and hypertension may be the dominant clinical features with the onset of acute glomerulonephritis, whereas oliguria and discolored urine more often are the first signs in younger adults. The course of CKD may be more complicated in older people with numerous chronic diseases.

Treatment

The NKF guidelines indicate that clinical interventions for older adults with CKD should be based on diagnosis, severity of kidney function impairment, and stratification of risk for progression to renal failure and cardiovascular disease.[48] People with low risk may require only modification of dosages of medications excreted by the kidney, monitoring of blood pressure, avoidance of drugs and procedures that increase the risk of acute renal failure, and lifestyle modification to reduce the risk of cardiovascular disease.

Older adults with more severe impairment of kidney function may require renal replacement therapy. Treatment options for CKD in older adults include hemodialysis, peritoneal dialysis, transplantation, and acceptance of death from uremia. Neither hemodialysis nor peritoneal dialysis has proved to be superior in older adults. The mode of renal replacement therapy should be individualized, taking into account underlying medical and psychosocial factors. Age alone should not determine renal transplantation.[48] With increasing experience, many transplantation centers have increased the age for acceptance on transplant waiting lists. Reluctance to provide transplantation as an alternative may have been due, at least in part, to the scarcity of available organs and the view that younger people are more likely to benefit for a longer time. The general reduction in T-lymphocyte function that occurs with aging has been suggested as a beneficial effect that increases transplant graft survival.

IN SUMMARY

Available data suggest that approximately 1% of people with CKD are in the pediatric age range. The causes of CKD include congenital malformations (*e.g.*, renal dysplasia and obstructive uropathy), inherited disorders (*e.g.*, polycystic kidney disease), acquired diseases (*e.g.*, glomerulonephritis), and metabolic syndromes (*e.g.*, hyperoxaluria). Problems associated with CKD in children include growth impairment, delay in sexual maturation, and more extensive bone abnormalities than in adults. Although all forms of renal replacement therapy can be safely and reliably used in children, CCPD, NIPD, or transplantation optimizes growth and development.

Currently, it is common practice to accept older adults for renal replacement therapy programs if it is assessed that this will increase their quality of life. Normal aging is associated with a decline in the GFR, which makes elderly people more susceptible to the detrimental effects of nephrotoxic drugs and other conditions that compromise renal function. Current guidelines for diagnosis of CKD and stratification of risk for progression to kidney failure are the same as for younger adults. Treatment options for failure in older adults are also similar to those for younger adults.

GERIATRIC Considerations

- Common causes of AKI in older adults include prerenal factors such as dehydration, intrarenal factors such as nephrotoxic agents including certain medications, and complications of major surgery.[45]
- Older adults are at higher risk for renal disease because of the decrease in glomeruli and the glomerular filtration rate.[46]
- Postural hypotension is a common finding in prerenal acute renal failure in older adults.[46]
- Acute renal failure is often due to dehydration in the older adult.[46]

PEDIATRIC Considerations

- The most common cause of AKI in children is decreased renal perfusion, which can result from septic shock or hypovolemia.[47]
- Infants are at risk for renal failure because of their immature kidneys and large body surface area (BSA).[48]
- The most common causes of chronic renal failure in children are uropathies (31%) and glomerular disease (27%).[48]
- Renal failure decreases the child's ability to form clots, placing the child at risk for prolonged bleeding.[48]
- Infection is a consequence of decreased renal function. Failure to thrive and short stature are findings in young children, whereas delayed puberty is found in older children and adolescents.[48]
- Oliguria is a common finding in prerenal acute renal failure in children.[46]

REVIEW EXERCISES

1. A 55-year-old man with diabetes and coronary heart disease, who had undergone cardiac catheterization with the use of a radiocontrast agent 2 days ago, is admitted to the emergency department with a flulike syndrome including chills, nausea, vomiting, abdominal pain, fatigue, and pulmonary congestion. His serum creatinine is elevated, and he has protein in his urine. He is admitted to the intensive care unit with a tentative diagnosis of AKI because of radiocontrast nephropathy.
   A. *Radiocontrast agents are thought to exert their effects through decreased renal perfusion and through direct toxic effects on renal tubular structures. Explain how each of these phenomena contributes to the development of AKI.*
   B. *Explain the elevated serum creatinine, proteinuria, and presence of pulmonary congestion.*
2. A 35-year-old, 70-kg white man with diabetes mellitus is seen in the diabetic clinic for his 6-month check-up. His serum creatinine, which was slightly elevated at his last visit, is now 1.6 mg/dL. Use the following Web site to estimate his GFR: http://www.mdcalc.com/creatinine-clearance-cockcroft-gault-equation.
   A. *Would he be classified as having CKD? If so, what stage? What might be done to delay or prevent further deterioration of his kidney function?*
3. CKD is accompanied by hyperphosphatemia, hypocalcemia, impaired activation of vitamin D, hyperparathyroidism, and skeletal complications.
   A. *Explain the impaired activation of vitamin D and its consequences on calcium and phosphate homeostasis, parathyroid function, and mineralization of the bone in people with CKD.*
   B. *Explain the possible complications of the administration of activated forms of vitamin D on parathyroid function and calcium and phosphate homeostasis (e.g., calcium × phosphate product).*

References

1. National Kidney Foundation. (2017). Kidney disease. [Online]. Available: http://www.kidney.org/kidneyDisease/. Accessed September 23, 2017.
2. Morton P. G., Fontaine D. (2018). Critical care nursing: A holistic approach (11th ed.). Philadelphia, PA: Wolters Kluwer.
3. Singhartl K., Kellum J. A. (2012). AKI in the ICU: Definition, epidemiology, risk stratification, and outcomes. *Kidney International* 81(9), 819.
4. Urden L., Stacy K., Lough M. (2017). Critical care nursing (8th ed.). St. Louis, MO: Mosby.
5. Hall J. E. (2013). Guyton and Hall textbook of medical physiology (13th ed.). Philadelphia, PA: Saunders.
6. Strayer D. (2012). Rubin's pathology: Clinicopathologic foundations of medicine (7th ed.). Philadelphia, PA: Wolters Kluwer.
7. Khalighi M., Henriksen K., Chang A. M., et al. (2014). Intratubular hemoglobin casts in hemolysis-associated acute kidney injury. *American Journal of Kidney Diseases* 65(2), 337–341.
8. Wargo K., Edwards J. (2014), Aminoglycoside-induced nephrotoxicity. *Journal of Pharmacy Practice* 27(6), 573–577.
9. Tanagho E. A., McAninch J. W. (2012). Smith's general urology (18th ed.). New York, NY: McGraw Hill.
10. Dirkes S. (2015). Acute kidney injury: Causes, phases, and early detection. *American Nurse Today.* 10(7). [Online]. Available: https://www.americannursetoday.com/acute-kidney-injury/ Accessed October 4, 2017.
11. Ostermann M., Philips B., Forni G. (2012). Clinical review: Biomarkers of acute kidney injury: Where are we now?. *Critical Care* 15(233). [Online]. Available https://doi.org/10.1186/cc11380. Accessed October 9, 2017.
12. Prowle J., Bagshaw S., Bellomo R. (2012). Renal blood flow, fractional excretion of sodium and acute kidney injury: Time for a new paradigm? *Current Opinion in Critical Care* 18(6), 585–592.
13. Alge J., Arthur J. (2015). Biomarkers of AKI: A review of mechanistic relevance and potential therapeutic implications. *Clinical Journal of the American Society of Nephrology* 10, 147–155.
14. National Kidney Foundation. (2017). About chronic kidney disease. [Online]. Available: https://www.kidney.org/atoz/content/about-chronic-kidney-disease. Accessed October 2, 2017.
15. Van Gelder V., Scherpbier-De Haan N., De Grauw W., et al. (2016). Quality of chronic kidney disease management in primary care: A retrospective study. *Scandinavian Journal of Primary Health Care* 34(1), 73–80. Available: http://doi.org/10.3109/02813432.2015.1132885. Accessed January 25, 2018.
16. National Kidney Disease Educational Program. (2017). GFR calculator for adults. [Online]. Available: https://www.niddk.nih.gov/health-information/communication-programs/nkdep/laboratory-evaluation/glomerular-filtration-rate-calculators. Accessed October 2, 2017.
17. Kidney Disease: Improving Global Outcomes CKD 2012 Work Group. (2013). Clinical practice guidelines for the evaluation and management of chronic kidney disease. *Kidney International Supplements* 3, 20.
18. Wu M., Lam K., Lee W., et al. (2012). Albuminuria, proteinuria, and urinary albumin to protein ratio in chronic kidney disease. *Journal of Clinical Laboratory Analysis* 26, 82–92.

19. Pena M., Zeeuw D., Mischak H., et al. (2015). Prognostic clinical and molecular biomarkers of renal disease in type 2 diabetes. *Nephrology Dialysis Transplantation* 30(4), iv86–iv95. Available: https://doi.org/10.1093/ndt/gfv252. Accessed January 25, 2018.
20. Lopez-Giacoman S., Madero M. (2015). Biomarkers in chronic kidney disease, from kidney function to kidney damage. *World Journal of Nephrology* 4(1), 57–73. http://doi.org/10.5527/wjn.v4.i1.57
21. Headley C., Doss-McQuitty S., Dutka P., et al. (2015). Chapter 1: The kidney in health and disease. In Counts C. (Ed.), Core curriculum for nephrology nursing: Physiologic and psychosocial basics for nephrology nursing practice. Pittman, NJ: American Nephrology Nurses Association.
22. Kovesdy C. (2012). Significance of hypo- and hypernatremia in chronic kidney disease. *Nephrology Dialysis Transplantation* 27(3), 891–898.
23. Cuppari L., Garcia Lopes M. G., Kaminura M. A. (2012). Vitamin D biology: From the discovery to its significance in CKD. *Journal of Renal Nutrition* 21(1), 113–116.
24. Cunningham J., Locatelli F., Rodriguez M. (2012). Secondary hyperparathyroidism: Pathogenesis, disease progression, and therapeutic options. *Clinical Journal of the American Society of Nephrology* 6(4), 913–921.
25. Brommage D., Clement L., Cotton A., et al. (2015). Chapter 4: Foundation in nutrition and clinical applications in nephrology nursing. In C. Counts (Ed.), Core curriculum for nephrology nursing: Physiologic and psychosocial basics for nephrology nursing practice. Pittman, NJ: American Nephrology Nurses Association.
26. Giamalis P., Economidou D., Dimitriadis C., et al. (2015). Treatment of adynamic bone disease in a haemodialysis patient with teriparatide. *Clinical Kidney Journal* 8(2), 188–190.
27. Azab A., Elsayed A. (2017). Chronic kidney disease-mineral bone disease (CKD-MBD and cardiac arrest risk factors among renal failure patients. *Journal of Applied Biotechnology and Bioengineering* 3(5).
28. Palmer S., Nistor I., Craig J., et al. (2013). Cinacalcet in patients with chronic kidney disease: A cumulative meta-analysis of randomized controlled trials. *PLoS Medicine* 10(4), e1001436.
29. Kidney International Supplements. (2013). KDIGO clinical practice guidelines for anemia in chronic kidney disease. *Kidney International Supplements* 2(4), 279–335. [Online]. Available: http://www.kdigo.org/clinical_practice_guidelines/pdf/KDIGO-Anemia%20GL.pdf. Accessed October 11, 2017.
30. Wish J. (2014). Anemia and other hematological complications of chronic kidney disease. In S. J. Gilbert, D. E. Weiner (Eds.), National Kidney Foundation Primer on Kidney Disease (6th ed.). Philadelphia, PA: Elsevier Saunders.
31. Pan S., Chiang W., Chen P., et al. (2017). Restricted use of erythropoiesis-stimulating agent is safe and associated with deferred dialysis initiation in Stage 5 chronic kidney disease. *Scientific Reports* 7, 44013.
32. Weber M., Schiffrin E., White W., et al. (2014). Clinical practice guidelines for the management of antihypertension in the community. *The Journal of Clinical Hypertension* 16(1), 12–26.
33. National Kidney Foundation. (2017). Sexuality and kidney disease. [Online]. Available: https://www.kidney.org/atoz/content/sexuality. Accessed October 12, 2017.
34. Hain D., Haras M. (2015). Chapter 2: Chronic kidney disease. In C. Counts (Ed.) Core curriculum for nephrology nursing: Physiologic and psychosocial basics for nephrology nursing practice. Pittman, NJ: American Nephrology Nurses Association.
35. National Kidney Foundation. (2017). Smoking and your health. [Online]. Available: https://www.kidney.org/atoz/content/smoking. Accessed January 25, 2018.
36. National Kidney Foundation. (2017). Organ donation and transplants. [Online]. Available: https://www.kidney.org/news/newsroom/factsheets/Organ-Donation-and-Transplantation-Stats Accessed October 12, 2017.
37. Kaspar C., Bholah R., Bunchman T. (2016). A review of pediatric chronic kidney disease. *Blood Purification* 41, 211–217.
38. Tasic V., Janchevska A., Emini N., et al. (2016). Chronic kidney disease: Pediatric risk factors. [Online]. Available: https://www.degruyter.com/downloadpdf/j/prilozi.2016.37.issue-1/prilozi-2016-0003/prilozi-2016-0003.pdf. Accessed October 12, 2017.
39. Gilliland M., Brown J. S., Pryor L. (2017). Nursing care for patients with synthetic arteriovenous grafts. *Nephrology Nursing Journal* 44(5), 391–399.
40. National Institute of Diabetes and Digestive and Kidney Diseases. (2017). Kidney disease in children. [Online]. Available: https://www.niddk.nih.gov/health-information/kidney-disease/children. Accessed October 12, 2017.
41. Saeed B. (2012). Pediatric renal transplantation. *International Journal of Organ Transplantation Medicine* 3(2), 62–73.
42. National Institute of Diabetes and Digestive and Kidney Diseases. (2017). Slow progression and reduce complications. [Online]. Available: https://www.niddk.nih.gov/health-information/communication-programs/nkdep/identify-manage-patients/manage-ckd/slow-progression-reduce-complications. Accessed October 12, 2017.
43. Fassett R. G. (2014). Current and emerging treatment options for the elderly patient with chronic kidney disease. *Clinical Interventions in Aging* 9, 191–199.
44. Mallappallil M., Friedman E. A., Delano B. G., et al. (2014). Chronic kidney disease in the elderly: Evaluation and management. *Clinical Practice* 11(5), 525–535.
45. Elliott, R. W. (2012). Demographics of the older adult and chronic kidney disease: A literature review. *Nephrology Nursing Journal* 39(6), 491–496.
46. Zurakowski T. L. (2013). The genitourinary & renal systems. In P. A. Tabloski (Ed.), Gerontological nursing (3rd ed., pp. 445–475). Upper Saddle River, NJ: Pearson.
47. Kyle T., Carman S. (2017). Essentials of pediatric nursing (3rd ed.). PA: Wolters Kluwer.
48. Bowden V., Greenberg C. S. (2014). Children and their families: The continuum of nursing care (3rd ed.). Philadelphia, PA: Lippincott Williams & Wilkins.

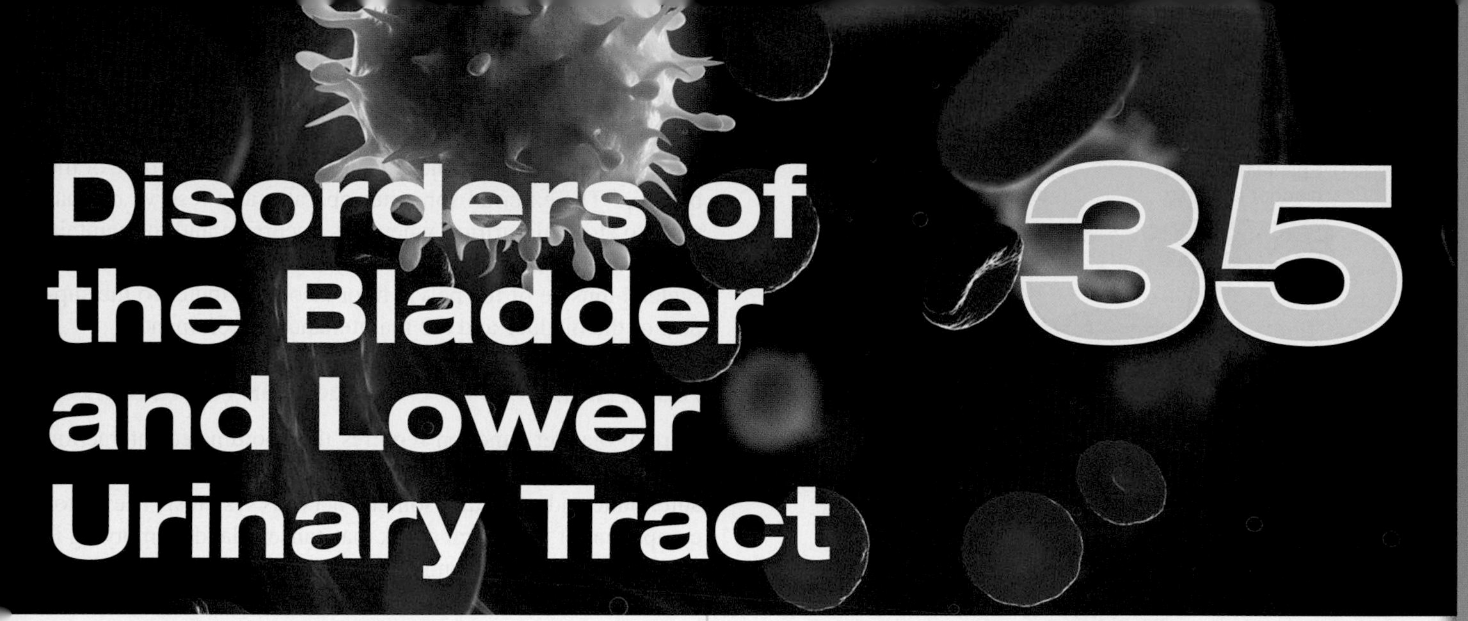

Disorders of the Bladder and Lower Urinary Tract

35

Keevia Porter

CONTROL OF URINE ELIMINATION
- Bladder Structure
- Neural Control of Bladder Function
  - *Spinal Cord Centers*
  - *Pontine Micturition Center*
  - *Cortical and Subcortical Centers*
  - *Micturition and Maintenance of Continence*
  - *Pharmacology of Micturition*
  - *Continence in Children*
- Diagnostic Methods of Evaluating Bladder Structure and Function
  - *Physical Examination*
  - *Laboratory and Radiologic Studies*
  - *Urodynamic Studies*

ALTERATIONS IN BLADDER FUNCTION
- Lower Urinary Tract Obstruction and Stasis
  - *Compensatory and Decompensatory Changes*
  - *Treatment of Lower Urinary Tract Obstruction*
- Neurogenic Bladder Disorders
  - *Spastic Bladder: Failure to Store Urine*
  - *Flaccid Bladder: Failure to Empty Urine*
  - *Nonrelaxing External Sphincter*
  - *Treatment of Neurogenic Bladder Disorders*
- Urinary Incontinence
  - *Stress Incontinence*
  - *Overactive Bladder/Urge Incontinence*
  - *Overflow Incontinence*
  - *Functional Incontinence*
  - *Other Causes of Incontinence*
  - *Diagnosis*
  - *Treatment*
  - *Special Needs of Older Adults*

CANCER OF THE BLADDER
- Etiology and Pathophysiology
- Clinical Manifestations
- Diagnosis and Treatment

Although the kidneys control the formation of urine and regulate the composition of body fluids, the bladder stores urine and controls its elimination from the body. Alterations in the storage and expulsion functions of the bladder can result in incontinence, with its accompanying social and hygienic problems, or obstruction of urinary flow, which has detrimental effects on ureteral and, ultimately, renal function. The discussion in this chapter focuses on the normal control of urine elimination, urinary obstruction and stasis, neurogenic bladder, incontinence, and bladder cancer.

CONTROL OF URINE ELIMINATION

After completing this section of the chapter, the learner will be able to meet the following objectives:

- Trace the ascending sensory and descending motor impulses between the detrusor muscle and external urinary sphincter and the spinal cord, pontine micturition center, and cerebral cortex.
- Describe at least three urodynamic studies that can be used to assess bladder function.

Bladder Structure

The bladder, also known as the *urinary vesicle*, is a freely movable organ located retroperitoneally on the pelvic floor, just posterior to the pubic symphysis. It consists of two main components: the body, in which urine collects, and the neck, which is a funnel-shaped extension of the body that connects with the urethra.[1] In the male, the urethra continues anteriorly through the penis, with the prostate gland surrounding the neck of the bladder where it empties into the urethra. In the female, the bladder is located anterior to the vagina and uterus.

Urine passes from the kidneys to the bladder through the ureters. The interior of the bladder has openings for both the ureters and the urethra. The smooth triangular area that

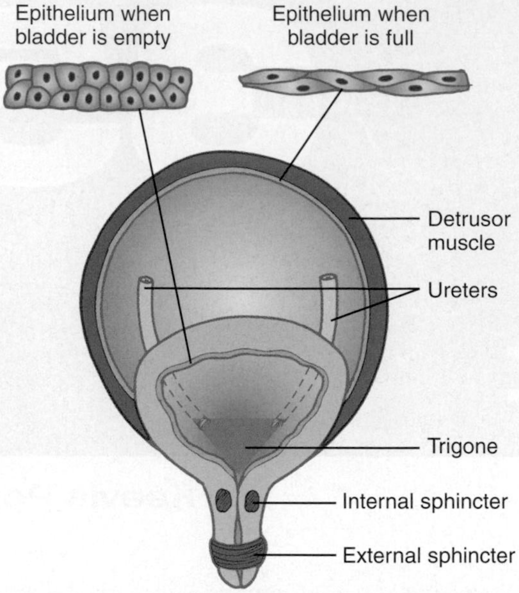

Figure 35.1 • Diagram of the bladder, showing the detrusor muscle, ureters, trigone area, and urethral orifice. Note the flattening of epithelial cells when the bladder is full and the wall is stretched.

is bounded by these three openings is called the trigone[1] (Fig. 35.1). There are no valves at the ureteral openings, but as the pressure of the urine in the bladder rises, the ends of the ureters are compressed against the bladder wall to prevent the backflow of urine.[1]

The bladder is composed of four layers. The first is an outer serosal layer, which covers the upper surface and is continuous with the peritoneum. The second is a network of smooth muscle fibers called the *detrusor muscle*. The third is a submucosal layer of loose connective tissue, and the fourth is an inner mucosal lining of transitional epithelium (urothelium).[1] This stratified epithelium is essentially impermeable to salts and water. The tonicity and composition of the urine often are quite different from that of the blood, and the epithelial lining of the bladder acts as an effective barrier to prevent the passage of water and other urine elements between the bladder and the blood. The epithelial lining of the bladder is several layers thick in the empty bladder. However, when the bladder is distended, as few as two or three layers are seen. This change reflects the ability of these cells to flatten and unfold to accommodate the increased surface area of a distended bladder (see Fig. 35.1).[2]

The detrusor muscle is the muscle of micturition (passage of urine). When it contracts, urine is expelled from the bladder. Muscles in the bladder neck, sometimes referred to as the *internal urethral sphincter*, are a continuation of the detrusor muscle.[2] They run down obliquely behind the proximal urethra, forming the posterior urethra in males and the entire urethra in females.[1] In the female, the urethra (4 cm) is shorter than in the male (20 cm) and usually is less resistant to urine outflow.[2]

Another muscle important to bladder function is the *external sphincter*, a circular muscle composed of striated muscle fibers that surrounds the urethra distal to the base of the bladder.[1] The external sphincter operates as a reserve mechanism to stop micturition when it is occurring and to maintain continence in the face of unusually high bladder pressure. The skeletal muscle of the pelvic floor also contributes to the support of the bladder and the maintenance of continence.

Neural Control of Bladder Function

Normal bladder function requires the coordinated interaction between the sensory and motor components of the involuntary autonomic and voluntary somatic nervous systems.[1] The motor component of the neural reflex that causes bladder emptying is controlled by the parasympathetic nervous system, whereas the relaxation and storage function of the bladder is controlled by the sympathetic nervous system.[1] The somatic nervous system provides for the voluntary control of the external sphincter and pelvic floor muscles. These functions are controlled by three neurologic centers: the spinal cord reflex centers, the micturition center in the pons, and cortical and subcortical centers.[1]

Spinal Cord Centers

The centers for reflex control of bladder function are located in the sacral (S1 through S4) and thoracolumbar (T11 through L2) segments of the spinal cord[1] (Fig. 35.2). The parasympathetic lower motor neurons (LMNs) for the detrusor muscle of the bladder are located in the sacral segments of the spinal cord; their axons travel to the bladder by way of the *pelvic nerve*.[1] LMNs for the external sphincter also are located in the sacral segments of the spinal cord. These LMNs receive their control from the motor cortex through the corticospinal

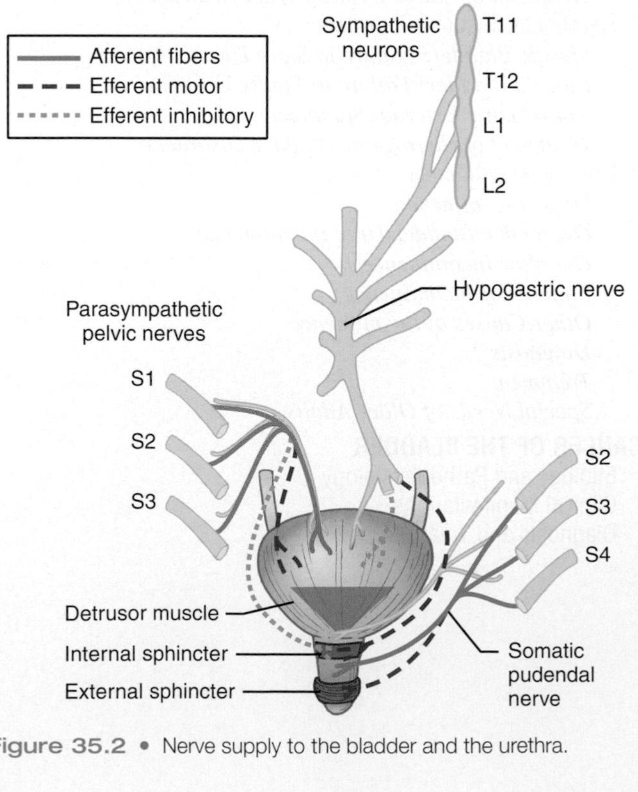

Figure 35.2 • Nerve supply to the bladder and the urethra.

tract and send impulses to the external sphincter through the *pudendal nerve.*[1] The bladder neck and trigone area of the bladder, because of their different embryonic origins, receive sympathetic outflow from the thoracolumbar (T11 to L2) segments of the spinal cord. In the male, the seminal vesicles, ampulla, and vas deferens also receive sympathetic innervation from the thoracolumbar segments of the cord.[1]

The afferent input from the bladder and urethra is carried to the central nervous system (CNS) by fibers that travel with the parasympathetic (pelvic), somatic (pudendal), and sympathetic (hypogastric) nerves.[1] The pelvic nerve carries sensory fibers from the stretch receptors in the bladder wall, the pudendal nerve carries sensory fibers from the external sphincter and pelvic muscles, and the hypogastric nerve carries sensory fibers from the trigone area.[1]

Pontine Micturition Center

The immediate coordination of the normal micturition reflex occurs in the micturition center in the pons, facilitated by descending input from the forebrain and ascending input from the reflex centers in the spinal cord[1–3] (Fig. 35.3). This center is thought to coordinate the activity of the detrusor muscle and the external sphincter. As bladder filling occurs, ascending spinal afferents relay this information to the micturition center, which also receives important descending information from the forebrain concerning behavioral cues for bladder emptying and urine storage. Descending pathways from the pontine micturition center produce coordinated inhibition or relaxation of the external sphincter. Disruption of pontine control of micturition, as in spinal cord injury, results in uninhibited spinal reflex–controlled contraction of the bladder without relaxation of the external sphincter, a condition known as *detrusor–sphincter dyssynergia.*[1]

Cortical and Subcortical Centers

Cortical brain centers enable inhibition of the micturition center in the pons and conscious control of urination. Neural influences from the subcortical centers in the basal ganglia modulate the contractile response. They modify and delay the detrusor contractile response during filling and then modulate the expulsive activity of the bladder to facilitate complete emptying.

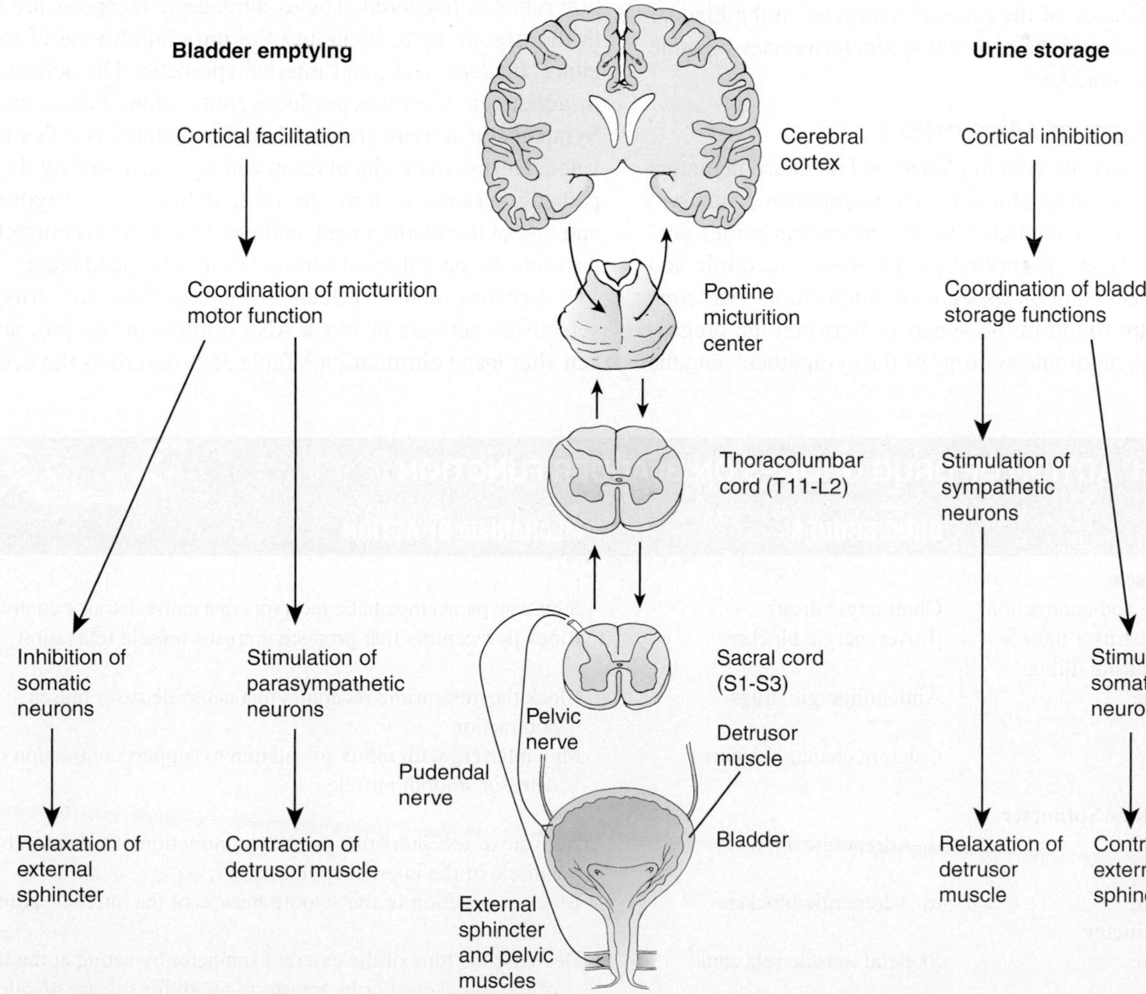

Figure 35.3 • Pathways and CNS centers involved in the control of bladder emptying **(left)** and storage **(right)** functions. Efferent pathways for micturition **(left)** and urine storage **(right)** also are shown.

Micturition and Maintenance of Continence

To maintain continence, or retention of urine, the bladder must function as a low-pressure storage system, with the pressure in the bladder being lower than that in the urethra. To ensure that this condition is met, the increase in intravesical pressure (internal bladder pressure) that accompanies bladder filling is almost imperceptible. Abnormal sustained elevations in intravesical pressures (>40 to 50 cm H_2O) often are associated with vesicoureteral reflux (*i.e.*, backflow of urine from the bladder into the ureter) and the development of ureteral dilation. Although the pressure in the bladder is maintained at low levels, sphincter pressure remains high (45 to 65 cm H_2O) as a means of preventing loss of urine as the bladder fills.

Micturition, or the act of bladder emptying, involves both sensory and motor functions associated with bladder emptying.[1] When the bladder is distended to 150 to 250 mL in the adult, the sensation of fullness is transmitted to the spinal cord and then to the cerebral cortex.[3] At approximately 400 to 500 mL, the person will sense fullness of the bladder.[3] During the act of micturition, the detrusor muscle of the bladder fundus and bladder neck contract down on the urine; the ureteral orifices are forced shut; the bladder neck is widened and shortened as it is pulled up by the globular muscles in the bladder fundus; the resistance of the internal sphincter in the bladder neck is decreased; and the external sphincter relaxes as urine moves out of the bladder.[3]

Pharmacology of Micturition

The autonomic nervous system (ANS) and its neuromediators play a central role in micturition. Parasympathetic innervation of the bladder is mediated by the neurotransmitter acetylcholine. Two types of cholinergic receptors, nicotinic and muscarinic, affect various aspects of micturition. *Nicotinic* (N) receptors are found in the synapses between the preganglionic and postganglionic neurons of the sympathetic and the parasympathetic system, as well as in the neuromuscular end plates of the striated muscle fibers of the external sphincter and pelvic muscles. *Muscarinic* (M) receptors are found in the postganglionic parasympathetic endings of the detrusor muscle. Several subtypes of M receptors have been identified. Both M_2 and M_3 receptors appear to mediate detrusor muscle activity, with the M_3 subtype mediating direct activation of detrusor muscle contraction. The M_2 subtype appears to act indirectly by inhibiting sympathetically mediated detrusor muscle relaxation.[4] The identification of muscarinic receptor subtypes has facilitated the development of medications, muscarinic agonists, that selectively target only the bladder structures while minimizing undesired side effects.[5] However, many people still experience side effects from some of the muscarinic agonists, including dry mouth and constipation.[6]

Although sympathetic innervation is not essential to the act of micturition, it allows the bladder to store a large volume without the involuntary escape of urine—a mechanism that is consistent with the fight-or-flight function served by the sympathetic nervous system. The bladder is supplied with α_1- and β_2-adrenergic receptors. The β_2-adrenergic receptors are found in the detrusor muscle. They produce relaxation of the detrusor muscle, increasing the bladder volume at which the micturition reflex is triggered. The α_1-adrenergic receptors are found in the trigone area, including the intramural ureteral musculature, bladder neck, and internal sphincter. The activation of α_1-adrenergic receptors produces contraction of these muscles. Sympathetic activity ceases when the micturition reflex is activated. During male ejaculation, which is mediated by the sympathetic nervous system, the musculature of the trigone area and that of the bladder neck and prostatic urethra contracts and prevents the backflow of seminal fluid into the bladder.

Because of their effects on bladder function, drugs that selectively activate or block ANS outflow or receptor activity can alter urine elimination.[5] Table 35.1 describes the action of

TABLE 35.1 ACTION OF DRUG GROUPS ON BLADDER FUNCTION

FUNCTION	DRUG GROUPS	MECHANISM OF ACTION
Detrusor Muscle		
Increased tone and contraction	Cholinergic drugs	Stimulate parasympathetic receptors that cause detrusor contraction
Inhibition of detrusor muscle relaxation during filling	β_2-Adrenergic blockers	Block β_2 receptors that produce detrusor muscle relaxation
Decreased tone	Anticholinergic drugs	Block the muscarinic receptors that cause detrusor muscle contraction
	Calcium channel blockers	May interfere with influx of calcium to support contraction of detrusor smooth muscle
Internal Bladder Sphincter		
Increased tone	α_1-Adrenergic agonists	Activate α_1 receptors that produce contraction of the smooth muscle of the internal sphincter
Decreased tone	α_1-Adrenergic blockers	Block contraction of the smooth muscle of the internal sphincter
External Sphincter		
Decreased tone	Skeletal muscle relaxants	Decrease the tone of the external sphincter by acting at the level of the spinal cord or by interfering with the release of calcium in the muscle fibers

drug groups that can impair bladder function or can be used in the treatment of micturition disorders. Many of the nonprescription cold preparations contain α-adrenergic agonists, and many antihistamine agents have anticholinergic properties. These drugs can cause urinary retention. In addition, many antidepressant and antipsychotic drugs also have anticholinergic actions that frequently cause urine retention, which puts people at risk for urinary infections.[5]

Continence in Children

In infants and young children, micturition is an involuntary act that is triggered by a spinal cord reflex; when the bladder fills to a given capacity, the detrusor muscle contracts, and the external sphincter relaxes. As the child grows, the bladder gradually enlarges, with an increase in capacity, in ounces, that approximates the age of the child plus 2.[7,8] This formula applies up to age 12 to 14 years.[8] As the bladder grows and increases in capacity, the tone of the external sphincter muscle increases. Toilet training begins at about 2 to 3 years of age when the child becomes conscious of the need to urinate. Conscious control of bladder function depends on (1) normal bladder growth, (2) myelination of the ascending afferents that signal awareness of bladder filling, (3) development of cortical control and descending communication with the sacral micturition center, (4) ability to consciously tighten the external sphincter to prevent incontinence, and (5) motivation of the child to stay dry. Females typically achieve continence before males, and bowel control is typically achieved before bladder control.

KEY POINTS

BLADDER FUNCTION

- The control of the storage and emptying functions of the bladder involves both the involuntary autonomic nervous system (ANS) and voluntary (somatic nervous system) control.
- The striated muscles in the external sphincter and pelvic floor, which are innervated by the somatic nervous system, provide for the voluntary control of urination and maintenance of continence.

Diagnostic Methods of Evaluating Bladder Structure and Function

Bladder structure and function can be assessed by a number of methods.[9] Reports or observations of frequency, hesitancy, straining to urinate or void, and a weak or interrupted stream are suggestive of outflow obstruction. Palpation and percussion provide information about bladder distention.

Physical Examination

Postvoid residual (PVR) urine volume provides information about bladder emptying. It can be estimated by abdominal palpation and percussion. Catheterization and ultrasonography can be used to obtain specific measurements of PVR. A PVR value of less than 50 mL is considered adequate bladder emptying, and more than 200 mL indicates inadequate bladder emptying.[9]

Pelvic examination is used in females to assess perineal skin condition, perivaginal muscle tone, genital atrophy, pelvic prolapse (*e.g.*, cystocele, rectocele, uterine prolapse), pelvic mass, or other conditions that may impair bladder function. Bimanual examination (*i.e.*, pelvic and abdominal palpation) can be used to assess PVR volume. Rectal examination is used to test for perineal sensation, sphincter tone, fecal impaction, and rectal mass. It is also used to assess the contour of the prostate in males.

Laboratory and Radiologic Studies

Urine tests provide information about kidney function and urinary tract infections. The presence of bacteriuria or pyuria suggests urinary tract infection and the possibility of urinary tract obstruction. Blood tests (*i.e.*, blood urea nitrogen and creatinine) provide information about renal function.

Bladder structures can be visualized indirectly by taking x-ray films of the abdomen and by using excretory urography, which involves the use of a radiopaque dye, computed tomographic (CT) scanning, magnetic resonance imaging (MRI), or ultrasonography. Cystoscopy enables direct visualization of the urethra, bladder, and ureteral orifices.[9]

Ultrasonographic Bladder Scan. The ultrasonographic bladder scan provides a noninvasive method for estimating bladder volume, such as the PVR.[9] The device uses ultrasonic reflections to differentiate the urinary bladder from the surrounding tissue. A computer system calculates and displays bladder volume. The device can be used to determine the need for catheterization, for evaluation and diagnosis of urinary retention, to measure PVR volumes, and for facilitating volume-dependent or time-dependent catheterization or toileting programs.

Urodynamic Studies

Urodynamic studies are used to study bladder function and voiding problems. Three aspects of bladder function can be assessed by urodynamic studies: bladder, urethral, and intra-abdominal pressure changes, characteristics of urine flow, and the activity of the striated muscles of the external sphincter and pelvic floor.[10] Specific urodynamic tests include uroflowmetry, cystometry, urethral pressure profile, and sphincter electromyography (EMG). It often is advantageous to evaluate several components of bladder function simultaneously.

Uroflowmetry. Uroflowmetry measures the flow rate (milliliters per minute) during urination.[10] It commonly is done using a weight-recording device located at the bottom of a commode receptacle unit. As the person being tested voids, the weight of the commode receptacle unit increases. This weight change is electronically recorded and then analyzed as volume (weight converted to milliliters) versus time.

Cystometry. Cystometry is used to measure bladder pressure during filling and voiding. It provides valuable information about total bladder capacity, intravesical pressures during bladder filling, the ability to perceive bladder fullness and the desire to urinate, the ability of the bladder to contract and sustain a contraction, uninhibited bladder contractions, and the ability to inhibit urination.[10] The test can be done by allowing physiologic filling of the bladder with urine and recording intravesical pressure throughout a voiding cycle or by using a catheter to fill the bladder with water and measuring intravesical pressure against the volume of water instilled into the bladder.[10]

In a normally functioning bladder, the sensation of bladder fullness is first perceived when the bladder contains 100 to 200 mL of urine while bladder pressure remains constant at approximately 8 to 15 cm H_2O. The desire to void occurs when the bladder is full (normal capacity is approximately 400 to 500 mL). At this point, a definite sensation of fullness occurs, the pressure rises sharply to 40 to 100 cm H_2O, and voiding occurs around the catheter.[9] Urinary continence requires that urethral pressure exceed bladder pressure. If the urethral resistance is high because of obstruction, greater pressure is required, a condition that can be detected by cystometry.

Urethral Pressure Profile. The urethral pressure profile is used to evaluate the intraluminal pressure changes along the length of the urethra with the bladder at rest.[10] It provides information about smooth muscle activity along the length of the urethra. This test can be done using the infusion method, the membrane catheter method, or the microtip transducer. The infusion method involves the insertion of a small double-lumen urethral catheter, followed by the infusion of water into the bladder and measurement of the changes in urethral pressure as the catheter is slowly withdrawn.

Sphincter Electromyography. Sphincter EMG allows the activity of the striated (voluntary) muscles of the perineal area to be studied.[10] Activity is recorded using an anal plug electrode, a catheter electrode, adhesive skin electrodes, or needle electrodes.[9] Electrode placement is based on the muscle groups that need to be tested. The test usually is done along with urodynamic tests such as cystometry and uroflowmetry.

IN SUMMARY

Although the kidneys function in the formation of urine and the regulation of body fluids, it is the bladder that stores and controls the elimination of urine. Micturition is a function of the peripheral ANS, subject to facilitation or inhibition from higher neurologic centers. The parasympathetic nervous system controls the function of the detrusor muscle and internal sphincter; its cell bodies are located in S1 through S3 of the spinal cord and communicate with the bladder through the pelvic nerve. Efferent sympathetic control originates at the thoracolumbar level (T11 through L2) of the spinal cord and produces relaxation of the detrusor muscle and contraction of the internal sphincter. Skeletal muscle found in the external sphincter and the pelvic muscles that support the bladder are supplied by the pudendal nerve, which exits the spinal cord at the sacral level (S2 through S4) of the spinal cord. The pontine micturition center coordinates the action of the detrusor muscle and the external sphincter, whereas cortical centers permit conscious control of micturition.

Bladder structure and function can be evaluated using physical examination; laboratory and radiologic studies; urodynamic studies that measure bladder, urethral, and abdominal pressures; urine flow characteristics; and skeletal muscle activity of the external sphincter.

ALTERATIONS IN BLADDER FUNCTION

After completing this section of the chapter, the learner will be able to meet the following objectives:

- Describe the causes of, and compensatory changes that occur with, urinary tract obstruction.
- Differentiate lesions that produce storage dysfunction associated with spastic bladder from those that produce emptying dysfunction associated with flaccid bladder in terms of the level of the lesions and their effects on bladder function.
- Define *incontinence* and differentiate between stress incontinence, overactive bladder/urge incontinence, and overflow incontinence.

Alterations in bladder function include urinary obstruction with retention or stasis of urine and urinary incontinence with involuntary loss of urine. Although the two conditions have almost opposite effects on urination, they can have similar causes. Both can result from structural changes in the bladder, urethra, or surrounding organs or from impairment of neurologic control of bladder function.

Lower Urinary Tract Obstruction and Stasis

Urinary tract obstructions are classified according to cause (congenital or acquired), degree (partial or complete), duration (acute or chronic), and level (upper or lower urinary tract).[11] In lower urinary tract obstruction and stasis, urine is produced normally by the kidneys but is retained in the bladder. Because it has the potential to produce vesicoureteral reflux and cause kidney damage, lower urinary tract obstruction and stasis are serious disorders.

The common sites of congenital obstructions are the external meatus (*i.e.*, meatal stenosis) in boys and just inside the external urinary meatus in girls. Another congenital cause of urinary stasis is the damage to sacral nerves that is seen in spina bifida and meningomyelocele.

The acquired causes of lower urinary tract obstruction and stasis are numerous. In males, the most important acquired cause of urinary obstruction is external compression of the urethra caused by the enlargement of the prostate gland. In males and females, gonorrhea and other sexually transmitted infections contribute to the incidence of infection-produced urethral strictures. Bladder tumors and secondary invasion of the bladder by tumors arising in structures that surround the bladder and urethra can compress the bladder neck or urethra and cause obstruction. Because of the proximity of the involved structures, constipation and fecal impaction can compress the urethra and produce urethral obstruction.

Compensatory and Decompensatory Changes

The body compensates for the obstruction of urine outflow with mechanisms designed to prevent urine retention. These mechanisms can be divided into two stages: a compensatory stage and a decompensatory stage.[10] The degree to which these changes occur and their effect on bladder structure and urinary function depend on the extent of the obstruction, the rapidity with which it occurs, and the presence of other contributing factors, such as neurologic impairment and infection.

During the early stage of obstruction, the bladder begins to hypertrophy and becomes hypersensitive to afferent stimuli arising from stretch receptors in the bladder wall. The ability to suppress urination is diminished, and bladder contraction can become so strong that it produces bladder spasm. There is urgency, sometimes to the point of incontinence, and frequency during the day and at night.[10]

With continuation and progression of the obstruction, compensatory changes begin to occur. There is further hypertrophy of the bladder muscle, the thickness of the bladder wall may double, and the pressure generated by detrusor contraction can increase from a normal 20 to 40 cm H_2O to 50 to 100 cm H_2O to overcome the resistance from the obstruction. As the force needed to expel urine from the bladder increases, compensatory mechanisms may become ineffective, causing muscle fatigue before complete emptying can be accomplished. After a few minutes, voiding can again be initiated and completed, accounting for the frequency of urination.

The inner bladder surface forms smooth folds. With continued outflow obstruction, this smooth surface is replaced with coarsely woven structures (*i.e.*, hypertrophied smooth muscle fibers) called *trabeculae*. Small pockets of mucosal tissue, called *cellules*, commonly develop between the trabecular ridges.[10] These pockets form diverticula when they extend between the actual fibers of the bladder muscle (Fig. 35.4). Because the diverticula have no muscle, they are unable to contract and expel their urine into the bladder, and secondary infections caused by stasis are common.

Along with hypertrophy of the bladder wall, there is hypertrophy of the trigone area and the interureteric ridge, which is located between the two ureters. This causes back pressure on the ureters, the development of hydroureters (*i.e.*, dilated, urine-filled ureters), and, eventually, kidney damage.

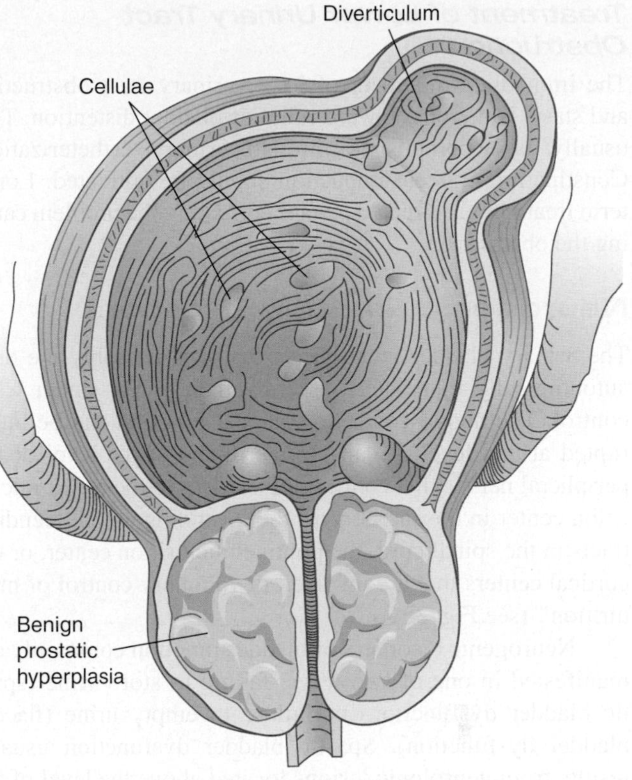

Figure 35.4 • Destructive changes of the bladder wall with development of diverticulum caused by benign prostatic hypertrophy.

Stasis of urine predisposes an individual to urinary tract infections.[10]

When compensatory mechanisms no longer are effective, signs of decompensation begin to appear. The period of detrusor muscle contraction becomes too short to expel the urine completely, and residual urine remains in the bladder. At this point, the symptoms of obstruction—frequency of urination, hesitancy, need to strain to initiate urination, a weak and small stream, and termination of the stream before the bladder is completely emptied—become pronounced. With progressive decompensation, the bladder may become severely overstretched, with a residual urine volume of 1000 to 3000 mL.[10] At this point, it loses its power of contraction and overflow incontinence occurs. The signs of outflow obstruction and urine retention are summarized in Chart 35.1.

CHART 35.1 SIGNS OF OUTFLOW OBSTRUCTION AND URINE RETENTION

- Bladder distention
- Hesitancy
- Straining when initiating urination
- Small and weak stream
- Frequency
- Feeling of incomplete bladder emptying
- Overflow incontinence

Treatment of Lower Urinary Tract Obstruction

The immediate treatment of lower urinary tract obstruction and stasis is directed toward relief of bladder distention. This usually is accomplished through urinary catheterization. Constipation or fecal impaction should be corrected. Long-term treatment is directed toward correcting the problem causing the obstruction.

Neurogenic Bladder Disorders

The urinary bladder is unique in that it is probably the only autonomically innervated visceral organ that is under CNS control. The neural control of bladder function can be interrupted at any level. It can be interrupted at the level of the peripheral nerves that connect the bladder to the reflex micturition center in the sacral cord, the ascending and descending tracts in the spinal cord, the pontine micturition center, or the cortical centers that are involved in voluntary control of micturition[10] (see Fig. 35.3).

Neurogenic disorders of bladder function commonly are manifested in one of two ways: failure to store urine (spastic bladder dysfunction) or failure to empty urine (flaccid bladder dysfunction). Spastic bladder dysfunction usually results from neurologic lesions located above the level of the sacral micturition reflexes, whereas flaccid bladder dysfunction results from lesions at the level of the sacral micturition reflexes or the peripheral nerves that innervate the bladder. In addition to disorders of detrusor muscle function, disruption of micturition occurs when the neurologic control of external sphincter function is disrupted. Some disorders, such as stroke and Parkinson disease, may affect both the storage and emptying functions of the bladder. Table 35.2 describes the characteristics of neurogenic bladder according to the level of the lesion.

Spastic Bladder: Failure to Store Urine

Failure to store urine results from conditions that cause reflex bladder spasm and a decrease in bladder volume. It commonly is caused by conditions that produce partial or extensive neural damage above the micturition reflex center in the sacral cord (see Fig. 35.3). As a result, segmental reflexes regulate bladder function, without control from higher brain centers.[10] The degree of bladder spasticity and dysfunction depends on the level and extent of neurologic dysfunction. Usually, both the ANS neurons controlling bladder function and the somatic neurons controlling the function of the striated muscles in the external sphincter are affected. In some cases, there is a detrusor–sphincter dyssynergia with uncoordinated contraction and relaxation of the detrusor and external sphincter muscles. The most common causes of spastic bladder dysfunction are spinal cord disorders such as spinal cord injury, herniated intervertebral disk, vascular lesions, tumors, and myelitis.[10] Other neurologic conditions that affect voiding are stroke, multiple sclerosis, and brain tumors.

Bladder Dysfunction Caused by Spinal Cord Injury. The immediate and early effects of spinal cord injury on bladder function are quite different from those that follow recovery from the initial injury. During the period immediately after spinal cord injury, a state of spinal shock develops, during which all the reflexes, including the micturition reflex, are depressed. During this stage, the bladder becomes atonic and cannot contract. Catheterization is necessary to prevent injury to urinary structures associated with overdistention of the

TABLE 35.2 TYPES AND CHARACTERISTICS OF NEUROGENIC BLADDER

LEVEL OF LESION	CHANGE IN BLADDER FUNCTION	COMMON CAUSES
Sensory cortex, motor cortex, or corticospinal tract	Loss of the ability to perceive bladder filling; low-volume, physiologically normal micturition that occurs suddenly and is difficult to inhibit	Stroke and advanced age
Basal ganglia or extrapyramidal tract	Detrusor contractions are elicited suddenly without warning and are difficult to control; bladder contraction is shorter than normal and does not produce full bladder emptying	Parkinson disease
Pontine micturition center or communicating tracts in the spinal cord	Storage reflexes are provoked during filling, and external sphincter responses are heightened; uninhibited bladder contractions occur at a lower volume than normal and do not continue until the bladder is emptied; antagonistic activity occurs between the detrusor muscle and the external sphincter	Spinal cord injury
Sacral cord or nerve roots	Areflexic bladder fills but does not contract; loss of external sphincter tone occurs when the lesion affects the α-adrenergic motor neurons or pudendal nerve	Injury to sacral cord or spinal roots
Pelvic nerve	Increased filling and impaired sphincter control cause increased intravesicular pressure	Radical pelvic surgery
Autonomic peripheral sensory pathways	Bladder overfilling occurs owing to a loss of the ability to perceive bladder filling	Diabetic neuropathies, multiple sclerosis

bladder. Intermittent catheterization is the preferred method of catheterization.

After the acute stage of spinal cord injury, the micturition response changes from a long-tract reflex to a segmental reflex. Because the sacral reflex arc remains intact, stimuli generated by bladder stretch receptors during filling produce frequent spontaneous contractions of the detrusor muscle. This creates a small, hyperactive bladder subject to high-pressure and short-duration uninhibited bladder contractions. Voiding is interrupted, involuntary, or incomplete. Dilation of the internal sphincter and spasticity of the external sphincter and perineal muscles innervated by upper motor neurons occur, producing resistance to bladder emptying. Hypertrophy of the trigone develops, often leading to vesicoureteral reflux and risk for renal damage.

Spastic bladder because of spinal cord injuries at the cervical level is often accompanied by a condition known as *autonomic hyperreflexia*. Because the injury interrupts CNS control of sympathetic reflexes in the spinal cord, severe hypertension, bradycardia, and sweating can be triggered by insertion of a catheter or mild overdistention of the bladder.[11]

Uninhibited Neurogenic Bladder. A mild form of reflex neurogenic bladder, sometimes called *uninhibited bladder*, can develop after a stroke, during the early stages of multiple sclerosis, or as a result of lesions located in the inhibitory centers of the cortex or the pyramidal tract. With this type of disorder, the sacral reflex arc and sensation are retained, the urine stream is normal, and there is no residual urine. Bladder capacity is diminished, however, because of increased detrusor muscle tone and spasticity.

Detrusor–Sphincter Dyssynergia. Depending on the level of the lesion, the coordinated activity of the detrusor muscle and the external sphincter may be affected. Lesions that affect the micturition center in the pons or impair communication between the micturition center and spinal cord centers interrupt the coordinated activity of the detrusor muscle and the external sphincter. This is called *detrusor–sphincter dyssynergia*. Instead of relaxing during micturition, the external sphincter becomes more constricted. This condition can lead to elevated intravesical pressures, vesicoureteral reflux, and kidney damage.

Treatment of Spastic Bladder. Among the methods used to treat spastic bladder and detrusor–sphincter dyssynergia are the administration of anticholinergic medications to decrease bladder hyperactivity and urinary catheterization to produce bladder emptying. A sphincterotomy (surgical resection of the external sphincter) or implantable urethral stent may be used to decrease outflow resistance in a person who cannot be managed with medications and catheterization procedures. An alternative to surgical resection of the external sphincter is the injection of botulinum toxin type A (BTX-A) to produce paralysis of the striated muscles in the external sphincter.

KEY POINTS

NEUROGENIC BLADDER DISORDERS

- Spastic bladder dysfunction results from neurologic lesions above the level of the sacral cord that allow neurons in the micturition center to function reflexively without control from higher CNS centers.
- Flaccid bladder dysfunction results from neurologic disorders affecting the motor neurons in the sacral cord or peripheral nerves that control detrusor muscle contraction and bladder emptying.

Flaccid Bladder: Failure to Empty Urine

Failure to empty the bladder can be due to flaccid bladder dysfunction, peripheral neuropathies that interrupt afferent or efferent communication between the bladder and the spinal cord, or conditions that prevent relaxation of the external sphincter (see Fig. 35.3).

Flaccid Bladder Dysfunction. Detrusor muscle areflexia, or flaccid neurogenic bladder, occurs when there is injury to the micturition center of the sacral cord, the cauda equina, or the sacral nerves that supply the bladder.[10] Atony of the detrusor muscle and loss of the perception of bladder fullness permit the overstretching of the detrusor muscle that contributes to weak and ineffective bladder contractions. External sphincter tone and perineal muscle tone are diminished. Voluntary urination does not occur, but increasing the intra-abdominal pressure or applying manual suprapubic pressure can achieve fairly efficient emptying. Among the causes of flaccid neurogenic bladder are trauma, tumors, and congenital anomalies (*e.g.*, spina bifida, meningomyelocele).

Bladder Dysfunction Caused by Peripheral Neuropathies. In addition to CNS lesions and conditions that disrupt bladder function, disorders of the peripheral (pelvic, pudendal, and hypogastric) nerves that supply the muscles of micturition can occur. These neuropathies can selectively interrupt sensory or motor pathways for the bladder or involve both pathways.

Bladder atony with dysfunction is a frequent complication of diabetes mellitus.[10] The disorder initially affects the sensory axons of the urinary bladder without involvement of the pudendal nerve. This leads to large residual volumes after micturition, sometimes complicated by infection. There frequently is a need for straining, accompanied by hesitation, weakness of the stream, dribbling, and a sensation of incomplete bladder emptying.[10] The chief complications are vesicoureteral reflux and ascending urinary tract infection. Because people with diabetes are already at risk for development of kidney disease, urinary stasis and reflux can have serious effects on renal function. Treatment consists of client education, including the need for frequent voiding (*e.g.*, every 3 to 4 hours while awake), use of abdominal compression to achieve more complete bladder emptying, and intermittent catheterization when necessary.

Nonrelaxing External Sphincter

Another condition that affects micturition and bladder function is the nonrelaxing external sphincter. This condition usually is related to a delay in maturation, developmental regression, psychomotor disorders, or locally irritative lesions. Inadequate relaxation of the external sphincter can be the result of anxiety or depression. Any local irritation can produce spasms of the sphincter through afferent sensory input from the pudendal nerve, including vaginitis, perineal inflammation, and inflammation or irritation of the urethra. In men, chronic prostatitis contributes to impaired relaxation of the external sphincter.

Treatment of Neurogenic Bladder Disorders

The goals of treatment for neurogenic bladder disorders focus on preventing bladder overdistention, urinary tract infections, and potentially life-threatening kidney damage and reducing the undesirable social and psychological effects of the disorder. The methods used in the treatment of neurogenic bladder disorders are individualized based on the type of neurologic lesion that is involved; information obtained through the health history, including fluid intake; report or observation of voiding patterns; presence of other health problems; urodynamic studies when indicated; and the ability of the person to participate in the treatment. Treatment methods include catheterization, bladder training, pharmacologic manipulation of bladder function, and surgery.

Catheterization. Catheterization involves the insertion of a small diameter latex or silicone tube into the bladder through the urethra. The catheter may be inserted on a one-time basis to relieve temporary bladder distention, left indwelling (*i.e.*, retention catheter), or inserted intermittently. With acute overdistention of the bladder, usually no more than 1000 mL of urine is removed from the bladder at one time. The theory behind this limitation is that removing more than this amount at one time releases pressure on the pelvic blood vessels and predisposes to alterations in circulatory function.

Permanent indwelling catheters sometimes are used when there is urine retention or incontinence in people who are ill or debilitated or when conservative or surgical methods for the correction of incontinence are not feasible. The use of permanent indwelling bladder catheters in people with spinal cord injury has been shown to produce a number of complications, including urinary tract infections, pyelonephritis, and kidney stones. Because urethral catheters often produce urethral irritation and injury, a suprapubic catheter may be inserted in people requiring long-term catheter drainage.[12,13]

Intermittent catheterization is used to treat urine retention or incomplete emptying secondary to various neurologic or obstructive disorders.[10] Properly used, it prevents bladder overdistention and urethral irritation, allows more freedom of activity, and provides periodic distention of the bladder to prevent muscle atony. It often is used with pharmacologic manipulation to achieve continence. When possible, it is learned and managed as a self-care procedure (*i.e.*, intermittent self-catheterization).

The clean procedure typically is used for self-catheterization. It is performed at 3- to 4-hour intervals to prevent overdistention of the bladder. The best results are obtained if only 300 to 400 mL is allowed to collect in the bladder between catheterizations. Following this plan, it would be less likely for autonomic dysreflexia to occur.

Bladder Retraining. Bladder retraining differs with the type of disorder.[13] Methods used to supplement bladder retraining include monitoring fluid intake to prevent urinary tract infections and control urine volume and osmolality, developing scheduled times for urination, and using body positions that facilitate micturition. Adequate fluid intake also is needed to prevent urinary tract infections, the irritating effects of which increase bladder irritability and the risk for urinary incontinence and renal damage. Fluid intake must be balanced to prevent bladder overdistention from occurring during the night. Developing scheduled times for urinating prevents overdistention of the bladder.

The methods used for bladder retraining depend on the type of lesion causing the disorder.[13] In spastic neurogenic bladder, methods designed to trigger the sacral micturition reflex are used; in flaccid neurogenic bladder, manual methods that increase intravesical pressure are used. Credé maneuvers, which are used with the person in a sitting position, consist of applying pressure with four fingers of one hand or both hands to the suprapubic area as a means of increasing intravesical pressure. The Valsalva maneuver (*i.e.*, bearing down by exhaling against a closed glottis) increases intra-abdominal pressure and aids in bladder emptying. This maneuver is repeated until the bladder is empty. For the best results, the person must cooperate fully with the procedures and, if possible, learn to perform them independently.

Biofeedback methods have been useful for teaching some aspects of bladder control. They involve the use of EMG or cystometry as a feedback signal for training a person to control the function of the external sphincter or raise intravesical pressure enough to overcome outflow resistance.

Pharmacologic Manipulation. Pharmacologic manipulation includes the use of drugs to alter the contractile properties of the bladder, decrease the outflow resistance of the internal sphincter, and relax the external sphincter. The usefulness of drug therapy often is evaluated during cystometric studies. Antimuscarinic drugs, such as oxybutynin, tolterodine, and propantheline, decrease detrusor muscle tone and increase bladder capacity in people with spastic bladder dysfunction.[5] Cholinergic drugs that stimulate parasympathetic receptors, such as bethanechol, provide increased bladder tonus and may prove helpful in the symptomatic treatment of milder forms of flaccid neurogenic bladder.[5] Muscle relaxants, such as diazepam and baclofen, may be used to decrease the tone of the external sphincter.

Surgical Procedures. Among the surgical procedures used in the management of neurogenic bladder are sphincterectomy, reconstruction of the sphincter, nerve resection of the sacral reflex nerves that cause spasticity or the pudendal nerve that controls the external sphincter, and urinary diversion.[10] Urinary diversion can be done by creating an ileal or a colon loop into which the ureters are anastomosed; the distal end of the loop is brought out and attached to the abdominal wall. Extensive research is being conducted on methods of restoring voluntary control of the storage and evacuation functions of the bladder through the use of implanted electrodes.

Urinary Incontinence

Urinary incontinence is defined as the involuntary loss or leakage of urine. Urinary incontinence is a common problem, particularly in older adults, with women being affected twice as often as men.[14,15]

Incontinence can be caused by a number of conditions. It can occur without the person's knowledge or the person may be aware of the condition but be unable to prevent it. Several types and causes of urinary incontinence have been identified. These include stress urinary incontinence, overactive bladder, urge incontinence, and overflow incontinence.[16] Recently, the term *urge incontinence* has been expanded to include *overactive bladder* (*i.e.*, overactive bladder/urge incontinence). One other category, functional incontinence, must also be considered. This type of incontinence includes those people who cognitively are not capable of knowing they need to urinate and so just urinate whenever the bladder is full. Table 35.3 summarizes the characteristics of stress incontinence, overactive bladder/urge incontinence, overflow incontinence, and functional incontinence.

TABLE 35.3 TYPES AND CHARACTERISTICS OF URINARY INCONTINENCE

TYPE	CHARACTERISTICS
Stress	Involuntary loss of urine associated with activities, such as coughing, that increase intra-abdominal pressure
Overactive bladder/ urge incontinence	Urgency and frequency associated with hyperactivity of the detrusor muscle; may or may not involve involuntary loss of urine
Overflow	Involuntary loss of urine when intravesicular pressure exceeds maximal urethral pressure in the absence of detrusor activity
Functional	Lack of cognitive function to go to the bathroom, commode, or urinal/bedpan resulting in spontaneous urination

Stress Incontinence

Stress incontinence is the involuntary loss of urine during coughing, laughing, sneezing, or lifting that increases intra-abdominal pressure commonly because of pelvic floor muscle dysfunction.[10,16] With severe urinary stress incontinence, any strain or increase in bladder pressure leads to urinary leakage.

In women, the angle between the bladder and the posterior proximal urethra (*i.e.*, urethrovesical junction) is important to continence (Fig. 35.5). During the first stage of voiding, this angle is lost as the bladder descends. In women, diminution of muscle tone associated with normal aging, childbirth, or surgical procedures can cause weakness of the pelvic floor muscles and result in stress incontinence by obliterating the critical posterior urethrovesical angle. In these women, loss of the posterior urethrovesical angle, descent and funneling of the bladder neck, and backward and downward rotation of the bladder occur, so that the bladder and urethra are already in an anatomic position for the first stage of voiding. Any activity that causes downward pressure on the bladder is sufficient to allow the urine to escape involuntarily.

Another cause of stress incontinence is intrinsic urethral deficiency, which may result from congenital conditions that may occur with epispadias or meningomyelocele. It also may be acquired as a result of trauma or irradiation. Stress incontinence in men may result from previous prostate disease or surgery.[17] Neurologic dysfunction, as occurs with impaired sympathetic innervation of the bladder neck, impaired pelvic nerve innervation to the intrinsic sphincter, or impaired pudendal nerve innervation to the external sphincter, may also be contributing factors.[18]

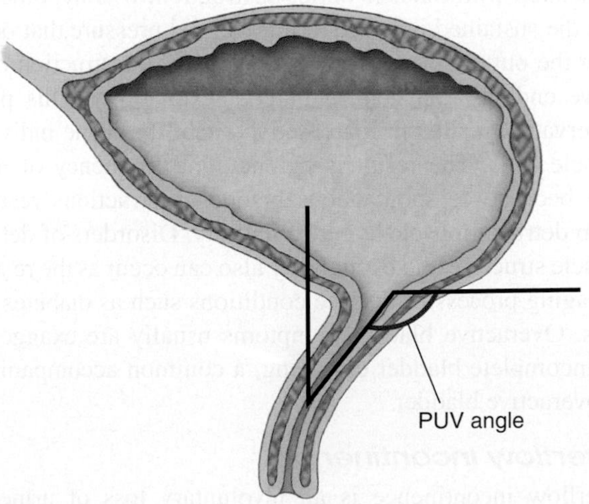

Figure 35.5 • Normal 90- to 100-degree posterior urethrovesical (PUV) angle. In the presence of a normal PUV angle, sudden changes in intra-abdominal pressure are transmitted optimally to all sides of the proximal urethra, ensuring that intraurethral pressure remains higher than intravesical pressure. Loss of the PUV angle results in displacement of the vesicle neck to the most dependent portion of the bladder, preventing the equal transmission of sudden increases in intra-abdominal pressure.

Overactive Bladder/Urge Incontinence

Urge incontinence is defined as the involuntary loss of urine associated with a strong desire to void (urgency).[16] *Overactive bladder* is used to describe the clinical syndrome that describes not only urge incontinence but frequency, dysuria, and nocturia.[14,15] Although overactive bladder often is associated with urge incontinence, it can occur without incontinence. Approximately 16% of women and 17% of men over 40 years of age in the United States have OAB.[19] Despite media coverage of overactive bladder and advances in treatment, many people continue to suffer in silence, probably because they are embarrassed or think it is an inevitable consequence of aging.

The symptoms of overactive bladder, which are caused by involuntary bladder contractions during filling, may occur alone or in any combination, and they constitute overactive bladder when they occur in the absence of other pathologic processes. Regardless of the primary cause of overactive bladder, two types of mechanisms are thought to contribute to its symptomatology: those involving CNS and neural control of bladder sensation and emptying (neurogenic) and those involving the smooth muscle of the bladder itself (myogenic).[20]

The neurogenic theory for overactive bladder postulates that the CNS functions as an on–off switching circuit for voluntary control of bladder function. Therefore, damage to the CNS inhibitory pathways may trigger bladder overactivity owing to uncontrolled voiding reflexes.[20,21] Neurogenic causes of overactive bladder include stroke, Parkinson disease, and multiple sclerosis. Other neurogenic causes of overactive bladder include increased sensitization of the afferent nerves that sense bladder filling or increased sensitivity to efferent nerves that produce bladder emptying.[20]

The myogenic causes of overactive bladder are thought to result from changes in the properties of the smooth muscle of the bladder itself. One example is overactive bladder associated with bladder outlet obstruction. It is hypothesized that the sustained increase in intravesical pressure that occurs with the outlet obstruction causes a partial destruction of the nerve endings that control bladder excitability. This partial denervation results in increased excitability of the individual muscle cells. The result is urgency and frequency of urination because of spontaneous bladder contractions resulting from detrusor muscle hyperexcitability. Disorders of detrusor muscle structure and excitability also can occur as the result of the aging process or disease conditions such as diabetes mellitus. Overactive bladder symptoms usually are exaggerated by incomplete bladder emptying, a common accompaniment of overactive bladder.[20]

Overflow Incontinence

Overflow incontinence is an involuntary loss of urine that occurs when intravesical pressure exceeds the maximal urethral pressure because of bladder distention in the absence of detrusor activity.[10] It can occur with retention of urine owing to nervous system lesions or obstruction of the bladder neck. With this type of incontinence, the bladder is distended, and small amounts of urine are passed, particularly at night. In men, one of the most common causes of obstructive incontinence is enlargement of the prostate gland. Another cause that commonly is overlooked is fecal impaction (*i.e.*, dry, hard feces in the rectum). When a large bolus of stool forms in the rectum, it can push against the urethra and block the flow of urine.

Functional Incontinence

Functional incontinence is often the term given to the type of incontinence that causes problems for a person attempting to use the toilet when they feel they need to urinate.

This type of incontinence may be caused by factors outside the lower urinary tract, such as the inability to locate, reach, or receive assistance in reaching an appropriate place to void. This may be a particular problem for older adults, who may have problems with mobility and manual dexterity or find themselves in unfamiliar surroundings. It occurs when a person cannot find or reach the bathroom or manipulate clothing quickly enough. Failing vision may contribute to the problem. Embarrassment in front of other people at having to use the bathroom, particularly if the timing seems inappropriate, may cause a person to delay emptying the bladder and may lead to incontinence. Treatment with drugs such as diuretics may cause the bladder to fill more rapidly than usual, making it difficult to reach the bathroom in time if there are problems with mobility or if a bathroom is not readily available. Night sedation may cause a person to sleep through the signal that normally would awaken a person so that he or she could get up and empty the bladder and avoid wetting the bed.

Other Causes of Incontinence

Other causes of incontinence include decreased bladder compliance or distensibility. This abnormal bladder condition may result from radiation therapy, radical pelvic surgery, or interstitial cystitis. Many people with this disorder have severe urgency related to bladder hypersensitivity that results in loss of bladder elasticity, such that any small increase in bladder volume or detrusor function causes a sharp rise in bladder pressure and severe urgency.

Incontinence may occur as a transient and correctable phenomenon, or it may not be totally correctable and occur with various degrees of frequency. Among the transient causes of urinary incontinence are recurrent urinary tract infections, medications that alter bladder function or perception of bladder filling and the need to urinate, diuretics and conditions that increase bladder filling, stool impaction, restricted mobility, and confusional and cognitive dysfunction states.

Diagnosis

Urinary incontinence is not a single disease but a symptom with many possible causes. As a symptom, it requires full investigation to establish its cause.[10] This usually is accomplished through a careful history, physical examination, blood tests, and urinalysis. A voiding record (*i.e.*, diary) may be used to determine the frequency, timing, and amount of voiding, as well as other factors associated with the incontinence. Because many drugs affect bladder function, a full drug history is essential.

Estimation of PVR volume is recommended for all people with incontinence. Provocative stress testing is done when stress incontinence is suspected. This test is done by having the person relax and then cough vigorously while the examiner observes for urine loss. The test usually is done in the lithotomy position; if no leakage is observed, it is repeated in the standing position. Urodynamic studies may be needed to provide information about urinary pressures and urine flow rates.[22]

Treatment

Treatment or management depends on the type of incontinence, accompanying health problems, and the person's age. It includes behavioral (*e.g.*, pelvic floor exercises) measures, pharmacologic measures, surgical correction of pelvic relaxation disorders associated with stress incontinence, and, when urine flow cannot be controlled, noncatheter devices to obstruct urine flow or collect urine as it is passed.[10,23] Indwelling catheters, although a solution to the problem of urinary incontinence, usually are considered only after all other treatment methods have failed. In some types of incontinence, such as that associated with spinal cord injury or meningomyelocele, self-catheterization may provide the best means for controlling urine elimination.

Behavioral Measures. Behavioral methods include fluid management, timed/prompted voiding, pelvic floor exercises, bladder retraining, and toileting assistance. Bladder retraining and biofeedback techniques seek to re-establish cortical control over bladder function by having the person ignore urgency and respond only to cortical signals during waking hours.[23] Toileting assistance techniques are caregiver-dependent techniques used to treat people with cognitive and motor dysfunction.

Muscle-tensing exercises of the pelvic muscles may prove effective in the treatment of stress incontinence. These pelvic floor muscle exercises were first advocated by Kegel, and they commonly are called *Kegel exercises*.[24] Two groups of muscles are strengthened: those of the back part of the pelvic floor (*i.e.*, muscles used to contract the anus and control the passing of stool) and the front muscles of the pelvic floor (*i.e.*, muscles used to stop the flow of urine during voiding). In learning the exercises, a woman concentrates on identifying the muscle groups and learning how to control contraction. After this has been accomplished, she can start an exercise program that consists of slowly contracting the muscles, beginning at the front and working to the back while counting to four and then releasing. The exercises can be done while sitting or standing and usually are performed in repetitions of 10, three times each day. A vaginal cone, a tampon-like device, may be used to enhance the benefits of the exercise. The cone is placed in the vagina, and the woman is instructed to hold it in place by contracting the proper inner muscles.[24–26]

Pharmacologic Treatment. Pharmacologic treatment is aimed at using drugs to alter the physiologic mechanisms that contribute to the neurogenic or myogenic causes of incontinence.[5] They include the use of drugs that increase sphincter tone in stress incontinence, decrease hyperreactivity of the detrusor muscle in overactive bladder/urge incontinence, or relieve outflow obstruction in overflow incontinence.

The α-adrenergic agonist drugs, such as pseudoephedrine, increase sympathetic relaxation of the detrusor muscle and internal sphincter tone and may be used in treating stress incontinence. The tricyclic antidepressants (particularly imipramine hydrochloride) are useful in facilitating urine storage because they decrease bladder contractility and increase outlet resistance. Although these drugs have a weak anticholinergic effect on the smooth muscle, it has recently been postulated that their beneficial effects may be caused by increased serotonin activity (because of reuptake blockade) in the CNS. This may involve a direct inhibition of normal excitatory pathways or depression of afferent ascending neural activity. Duloxetine, a selective serotonin and norepinephrine reuptake inhibitor, is thought to increase external sphincter tone by stimulation of the pudendal motor α_1-adrenergic receptors and serotonin-2 receptors.[5] Because serious side effects (*e.g.*, CNS effects, postural hypotension, cardiac arrhythmias) can occur with imipramine and other tricyclic antidepressants, these agents need to be used with caution.

Acetylcholine is the neurotransmitter that mediates detrusor contraction in overactive bladder. Therefore, anticholinergic medications are used to suppress these contractions. Some of the antimuscarinic drugs (*e.g.*, oxybutynin, tolterodine, trospium, darifenacin, solifenacin) have greater selectivity for the M_3 muscarinic receptors and produce fewer side effects than some of the older agents (*e.g.*, hyoscyamine, propantheline).[5] All anticholinergic drugs can have bothersome side effects. Although dry mouth is the most common, constipation, gastroesophageal reflux, blurred vision, urinary retention, and cognitive effects can occur.[5] The use of controlled-release (*e.g.*, oxybutynin, tolterodine) or transdermal drug delivery (*e.g.*, oxybutynin) can reduce but not completely eliminate side effects. Botulinum toxin type A (BTX-A) injection into the bladder was recently introduced as an alternative treatment for people with overactive bladder who do not respond to anticholinergic agents or cannot tolerate their side effects.[27]

The primary treatment of overflow incontinence that results from benign prostatic hypertrophy is relief of outflow obstruction. α-Adrenergic blocker therapy is based on the hypothesis that clinical manifestations of prostatic hyperplasia are caused partly by α_1-adrenergic–mediated contraction of prostatic smooth muscle, resulting in bladder outlet obstruction. Bladder outlet obstruction contributes to overfilling of the bladder and large-volume contraction or frequency of urination resulting from incomplete bladder emptying. α-Adrenergic antagonists such as alfuzosin, doxazosin, tamsulosin, and terazosin are treatment options for men with symptomatic prostatic hyperplasia.[5] The primary adverse effects of α-adrenergic blocker therapy are orthostatic hypotension, dizziness, fatigue, ejaculatory problems, and nasal congestion.

Surgical Treatment of Stress Incontinence. Surgical intervention may be considered when other treatment methods have proved ineffective. Three types of surgical procedures are used: procedures that increase outlet resistance, decrease detrusor muscle instability, or remove outflow obstruction to reduce overflow incontinence and detrusor muscle instability. A minimally invasive procedure for the treatment of stress incontinence is the periurethral injection of a bulking agent.[28] Both of these agents typically require multiple treatment sessions to achieve a cure.[28]

Noncatheter Device Management Measures. Two types of noncatheter devices commonly are used in the management of urinary incontinence: One obstructs flow, and the other collects urine as it is passed. Obstruction of urine flow is achieved by compressing the urethra or stimulating contraction of the pelvic floor muscles. Penile clamps are available that occlude the urethra without obstructing blood circulation to the penis. Clamps must be removed at 3-hour intervals to empty the bladder. Complications such as penile and urethral erosion can occur if clamps are used incorrectly. In women, compression of the urethra usually is accomplished by intravaginal devices.

Surgically implanted artificial sphincters are available for use in men and women. These devices consist of an inflatable cuff that surrounds the proximal urethra. The cuff is connected by tubing to an implanted fluid reservoir and an inflation bulb. Pressing the bulb, which is placed in the scrotum in men, inflates the cuff. It is emptied in a similar manner.

When urinary incontinence cannot be prevented, various types of urine collection devices or protective pads are used. Men can be fitted with collection devices (*i.e.*, condom or sheath urinals) that are worn over the penis and attached to a container at the bedside or fastened to the body. There are no effective external collection devices for women. Pants and pads usually are used. Dribbling bags (men) and pads (women) in which the urine changes to a nonpourable gel are available for occasional dribbling but are unsuitable for considerable wetting.

KEY POINTS

INCONTINENCE

- Incontinence represents the involuntary loss of urine because of increased bladder pressures (overactive bladder with urge incontinence or overflow incontinence) or decreased ability of the vesicourethral sphincter to prevent the escape of urine (stress incontinence).

Special Needs of Older Adults

Urinary incontinence is a common problem in older adults, both male and female.[29] Incontinence increases social isolation, frequently leads to institutionalization of older adults, and predisposes to infections and skin breakdown. The economic and social costs of incontinence are staggering.

Many factors contribute to incontinence in older adults, a number of which can be altered. The overall capacity of the bladder is reduced, as is the urethral closing pressure.[10] Detrusor muscle function also tends to decline with aging. Thus, there is a trend toward a reduction in the strength of bladder contraction and impairment in emptying that leads to larger PVR volumes.[10] It has been proposed that many of these changes are due to degenerative detrusor muscle changes rather than neurologic changes, as was once thought. The combination of involuntary detrusor contraction (detrusor hyperactivity) leading to urge incontinence with impaired contractile function leads to incomplete bladder emptying. Urge incontinence is the most frequent type of incontinence in older men. In about 50% of these men, detrusor overactivity is found. The urge to urinate comes on suddenly, without warning, accompanied by an uncontrolled detrusor contraction causing incontinence.[29]

Furthermore, immobility, changes in mental status, lack of easy access for toileting, and neurologic issues can precipitate urinary incontinence.[29] Many older adults experience nocturia and also have difficulty getting to the toilet in time. This can be caused by arthritis that makes walking or removing clothing difficult or by failing vision that makes trips to the bathroom precarious, especially in new and unfamiliar surroundings.

Medication prescribed for other health problems may prevent a healthy bladder from functioning normally.[5] Potent, fast-acting diuretics are known for their ability to cause urge incontinence. Impaired thirst or limited access to fluids predisposes to constipation with urethral obstruction and overflow incontinence and to concentrated and infected urine, which increases bladder excitability. Drugs such as hypnotics, tranquilizers, and sedatives can interfere with the conscious inhibition of voiding, leading to urge incontinence. Diuretics, particularly in older adults, increase the flow of urine and may contribute to incontinence, particularly in people with diminished bladder capacity and in those who have difficulty reaching the toilet.

Diagnosis and Treatment. As with urinary incontinence in younger people, incontinence in older adults requires a thorough history and physical examination to determine the cause of the problem. A voiding history is important. A voiding diary provides a means for the person to provide objective information about the number of bathroom visits, the number of protective pads used, and even the volume of urine voided. A medication history is also important because medications can affect bladder function.[5]

There are many neurologic conditions that predispose to urinary incontinence. The transient and often treatable causes of urinary incontinence in older adults may best be remembered with the acronym DIAPPERS, in which *D* stands for dementia/dementias, *I* for infection (urinary or vaginal), *A* for atrophic vaginitis, *P* for pharmaceutical agents, *P* for psychological causes, *E* for endocrine conditions (diabetes), *R* for restricted mobility, and *S* for stool impaction.[30] These eight transient causes of incontinence should be identified and treated before other treatment options are considered.

Treatment may involve changes in the physical environment so that the older adult can reach the bathroom more easily or remove clothing more quickly. Habit training with regularly scheduled toileting—usually every 2 to 4 hours—often is effective. Many older adults who void on a regular schedule can gradually increase the interval between toileting while improving their ability to suppress bladder instability. The treatment plan may require dietary changes to prevent constipation or a plan to promote adequate fluid intake to ensure adequate bladder filling and prevent urinary stasis and symptomatic urinary tract infections.

IN SUMMARY

Alterations in bladder function include urinary obstruction with retention of urine, neurogenic bladder, and urinary incontinence with involuntary loss of urine. Urine retention occurs when the outflow of urine from the bladder is obstructed because of urethral obstruction or impaired bladder innervation. Urethral obstruction causes bladder irritability, detrusor muscle hypertrophy, formation of trabeculae and diverticula, development of hydroureters, and eventual renal failure.

Neurogenic bladder is caused by interruption in the innervation of the bladder. It can result in spastic bladder dysfunction caused by failure of the bladder to fill or flaccid bladder dysfunction caused by failure of the bladder to empty. Spastic bladder dysfunction usually results from neurologic lesions that are above the level of the sacral micturition reflex center; flaccid bladder dysfunction results from lesions at the level of the sacral micturition reflexes or peripheral innervation of the bladder. A third type of neurogenic disorder involves a nonrelaxing external sphincter.

Urinary incontinence is the involuntary loss of urine in amounts sufficient to be a problem. It may manifest as stress incontinence, in which the loss of urine occurs as a result of coughing, sneezing, laughing, or lifting; overactive bladder/urge incontinence, characterized by urgency, frequency, and nocturia associated with hyperactive bladder contractions; or overflow incontinence, which results when intravesical pressure exceeds the maximal urethral pressure because of bladder distention. Other causes of incontinence include a small, contracted bladder or external environmental conditions that make it difficult to access proper toileting facilities, which is called functional incontinence.

Diagnosis usually is accomplished through a careful history (including a voiding record and full drug history), physical examination, blood tests and urinalysis, and in some cases urodynamic studies. Treatment methods include correction of the underlying cause, such as the removal of obstruction because of prostatic hyperplasia, behavioral methods that focus on bladder and habit training and exercises to improve pelvic floor function, pharmacologic methods to improve bladder and external sphincter tone, surgical treatment, noncatheter device management measures, and the use of catheters and urine collection devices.

Urinary incontinence is a common problem in older adults. Many factors, including health problems, medications, and changes in bladder structure and function, contribute to incontinence in elderly people. The acronym DIAPPERS—*D* dementia, *I* infection, *A* atrophic vaginitis, *P* pharmaceutical, *P* psychological, *E* endocrine, *R* restricted mobility, and *S* stool impaction—emphasizes the transient and often treatable causes of incontinence in the elderly.

CANCER OF THE BLADDER

After completing this section of the chapter, the learner will be able to meet the following objectives:

- Discuss the difference between superficial and invasive bladder cancer in terms of bladder involvement, extension of the disease, and prognosis.
- State the most common sign of bladder cancer.

Bladder cancer is the most frequent form of urinary tract cancer in the United States, accounting for more than 79,030 new cases and 16,870 deaths each year.[31] African Americans have only half the risk of white European Americans of getting bladder cancer, and men are more commonly diagnosed than women. Approximately 90% of people with bladder cancer are older than 55 years of age.[31]

The most common bladder cancer is derived from the transitional (urothelium) cells that line the bladder, so it is sometimes referred to as urothelial carcinoma.[31] These tumors can range from low-grade noninvasive tumors to high-grade tumors that invade the bladder wall and metastasize frequently.[31] The low-grade tumors, which may recur after resection, have an excellent prognosis, with only a small number progressing to higher-grade tumors.[31] There are three other types of bladder cancer: squamous cell carcinoma, which is rare and generally invasive; adenocarcinoma, which is also rare and highly metastatic; and small cell carcinoma, which is the most rare of all types.[31]

Etiology and Pathophysiology

Although the cause of bladder cancer is unknown, evidence suggests that its origin is related to local influences, such as carcinogens that are excreted in the urine and stored in the bladder. These include the breakdown products of aromatic amines used in the dye industry and products used in the manufacture of rubber, textiles, paint, chemicals, and petroleum.[31,32] Smoking also deserves attention, and cigarette smoking is highly correlated with bladder cancer. Chronic bladder infections and bladder stones also increase the risk for bladder cancer.

Clinical Manifestations

The most common sign of bladder cancer is painless hematuria.[33,34] Gross hematuria is a presenting sign in the majority of people with the disease, and microscopic hematuria is present in most others. Frequency, urgency, and dysuria occasionally accompany the hematuria. Because hematuria often is intermittent, the diagnosis may be delayed. Periodic urine cytology is recommended for all people who are at high risk for the development of bladder cancer because of exposure to urinary tract carcinogens. Ureteral invasion leading to bacterial and obstructive renal disease and dissemination of the cancer are potential complications and ultimate causes of death. The prognosis depends on the histologic grade of the cancer and the stage of the disease at the time of diagnosis.

Diagnosis and Treatment

Given the fact that bladder cancer is one of the ten most frequently diagnosed cancers in the United States, it is reasonable to understand the need for earlier screening of hematuria for bladder cancer, especially with people who have high risk factors such as history of cigarette smoking, family history of bladder cancer, exposure to chemicals, male gender, and age greater than 55 years.[33]

Diagnostic methods include cytologic studies, excretory urography, cystoscopy, and biopsy. Ultrasonography, CT scans, and MRI are used as aids for staging the tumor. Cytologic studies performed on biopsy tissues or cells obtained from bladder washings may be used to detect the presence of malignant cells.[10] A technique called *flow cytometry* is helpful in screening people at high risk for the disease and for monitoring the results of therapy. In flow cytometry, the interaction between fluorochromes or dyes with deoxyribonucleic acid (DNA) causes the emission of high-intensity light similar to that produced by a laser.[31] Flow cytometry can be carried out on biopsy specimens, bladder washings, or cytologic preparations.[10]

The treatment of bladder cancer depends on the extent of the lesion and the health of the person. Endoscopic resection usually is done for diagnostic purposes and may be used as a treatment for superficial lesions. Diathermy (*i.e.*, electrocautery) may be used to remove the tumors. Segmental surgical resection may be used for removing a large single lesion. When the tumor is invasive, cystectomy with resection of the pelvic lymph nodes frequently is the treatment of choice. In men, the prostate and seminal vesicles often are removed as well. Cystectomy requires urinary diversion, an alternative reservoir, usually created from the ileum (*e.g.*, an ileal loop) that is designed to collect the urine. Traditionally, the ileostomy reservoir drains urine continuously into an external collecting device.

Although a number of chemotherapeutic drugs have been used in the treatment of bladder cancer, no chemotherapeutic regimens for the disease have been established. A primary protocol for early-diagnosed bladder cancer has been initially successful, but there is no proven secondary protocol at this time.[33] Perhaps of more importance is the increasing use of intravesical chemotherapy, in which the cytotoxic drug is instilled directly into the bladder, thereby avoiding the side effects of systemic therapy. These drugs can be instilled prophylactically, after surgical resection of all the demonstrable tumor tissue, or therapeutically, in the presence of residual disease. Among the chemotherapeutic drugs that have been used for this purpose are thiotepa, mitomycin C, and doxorubicin (Adriamycin).[5] The intervesicular administration of bacille Calmette-Guérin (BCG) vaccine, made from a strain of *Mycobacterium bovis* that formerly was used to protect against tuberculosis, causes a significant reduction in the rate of relapse and prolongs relapse-free intervals in people with cancer in situ.[34] The vaccine is thought to act as a nonspecific stimulator of cell-mediated immunity. It is not known whether the effects of BCG are immunologic or include a component of direct toxicity. Several strains of this agent exist, and it is not known which strains are the most active and least toxic. There are also inhibitors of tumor angiogenesis and inhibitors of epidermal growth factor drugs that are proving effective with bladder cancer.[34]

IN SUMMARY

Cancer of the bladder is the most common cause of urinary tract cancer in the United States. Bladder cancers fall into two major groups: low-grade noninvasive tumors and high-grade invasive tumors that are associated with metastasis and a worse prognosis. Although the cause of cancer of the bladder is unknown, evidence suggests that carcinogens excreted in the urine may play a role. Microscopic and gross, painless hematuria are the most frequent presenting signs of bladder cancer. The methods used in treatment of bladder cancer depend on the cytologic grade of the tumor and the lesion's degree of invasiveness. The methods include surgical removal of the tumor, radiation therapy, and chemotherapy. In many cases, chemotherapeutic or immunotherapeutic agents can be instilled directly into the bladder, thereby avoiding the side effects of systemic therapy.

GERIATRIC Considerations

- High voiding pressures because of an enlarging prostate gland contributes to difficulty with initiating and maintaining urine flow in men after age 45; the pressure increases with age and hypertrophy of the prostate gland.[35] Similarly, females are prone to incomplete emptying of the bladder and urinary stasis, which increase bladder pressure and overflow incontinence.[35]
- Residual voiding amounts increase to 50 to 100 mL with aging compared to less than 50 mL in middle-age adults.[35]
- The decrease in estrogen in elderly women contributes to urinary incontinence because of urethral irritation.[35]

PEDIATRIC Considerations

- Parents should be educated to report any abnormal colored or cloudy urine because this is an early indication of a urinary tract infection.[36]
- A clear drainage from the base of the umbilical cord may indicate a fistula between the bladder and umbilicus (patent urachus).[36]
- Exstrophy of the bladder is a defect that occurs in utero during week 10 of development, resulting in the bladder being openly exposed to the environment and constantly draining urine from the open surface.[36]
- A urinary tract infection should be suspected when the child presents with a fever that has no other cause.[36]
- Vesicoureteral reflux in children causes retrograde flow of urine from the bladder to the ureters and is a cause of recurrent urinary tract infections.[36]

REVIEW EXERCISES

1. A 23-year-old man is recovering after the acute phase of a cervical (C6) spinal cord injury with complete loss of motor and sensory function below the level of injury. He is now experiencing spastic bladder contractions with involuntary and incomplete urination. Urodynamic studies reveal spastic contraction of the external sphincter with urine retention and high bladder pressures.
   A. *Explain the reason for the involuntary urination and incomplete emptying of the bladder despite high bladder pressures.*
   B. *What are possible complications associated with overdistention and high pressure within the bladder?*
2. A 66-year-old woman complains of leakage of urine during coughing, sneezing, laughing, or squatting down.
   A. *Explain the source of this woman's problem.*
   B. *One of the recommended treatments for stress incontinence is the use of Kegel exercises, which focus on strengthening the muscles of the pelvic floor. Explain how these exercises contribute to the control of urine leakage in women with stress incontinence.*

References

1. Hall J. E. (2016). *Guyton and Hall textbook of medical physiology* (13th ed.). Philadelphia, PA: Elsevier Saunders.
2. Tortora G. J., Derrickson B. (2014). *Principles of anatomy and physiology*. Danvers, MA: Wiley.
3. Boron W. F., Boulpaep E. L. (2016). *Medical physiology* (3rd ed.). Philadelphia, PA: Saunders Elsevier.
4. Sellers D. J., Chess-Williams R. (2012). *Muscarinic agonists and antagonists: Effects on the urinary bladder*. Muscarinic Receptors (pp. 375–400). Springer Berlin Heidelberg.
5. Woo T. M., Wynne A. L. (2015). *Pharmacotherapeutics for nurse practitioner prescribers* (4th ed.). Philadelphia, PA: F A Davis.
6. Igawa Y., Michel M. (2012). Pharmacological profile of β3-adenocepter agonists in clinical development for the treatment of overactive bladder syndrome. *Naunyn-Schmeideberg's Archives of Pharmacology* 356, 1–7.
7. Vermandel A., Van Hal G., De Wachter S., et al. (2015). The voiding pattern in healthy pre- and term infants and toddlers: a literature review. *European Journal of Pediatrics* 174(9), 1129–1142.
8. Elder J. S. (2015). Enuresis and Voiding dysfunction. In Behrman R. E., Kliegman R. M., Jenson H. B., et al. (Eds.), *Nelson textbook of pediatrics* (20th ed., pp. 2581–2586). Philadelphia, PA: Elsevier Saunders.
9. Goroll A. H., Mulley A. G. (2014). *Primary care medicine: Office evaluation and management of the adult patient*. Philadelphia, PA: Wolters Kluwer/Lippincott Williams & Wilkins Health.
10. Tanagho E. A., McAninch J. W. (Eds.). (2013). *Smith &Tanagho's general urology* (18th ed.). New York: McGraw Hill.
11. Bauman C. A., Milligan J. D., Lee F. J.,et al. (2012). Autonomic dysreflexia in spinal cord injury patients: An overview. *Journal of the Canadian Chiropractic Association* 56(4), 247–250.
12. Maeda S., Takiuti T., Komastu T., et al. (2013). Current status of long-term indwelling catheter management by visiting nurses. *International Journal of Urological Nursing* 7(2), 76–84.
13. Woodward S. (2013). Managing urological incontinence in people with neurological disorders. Part 2: Interventions. *British Journal of Neuroscience Nursing* 9(2), 63–70.
14. Starr J. A. (2016). Pelvic floor biofeedback via a smartphone app for treatment of stress urinary incontinence. *Urologic Nursing* 36(2), 88–91. doi:10.7257/1053-816X.2016.36.2.88.
15. Bettez M., Tu L. M., Carlson K., et al. (2012). 2012 Update: Guidelines for adult urinary incontinence collaborative consensus document for the Canadian Urological Association. *Canadian Urological Association Journal* 6(5), 354–363. Available: http://doi.org/10.5489/cuaj.12248
16. Rai J., Parkinson R. (2014). Urinary incontinence in adults. *Surgery (United Kingdom)* 32(6), 286–291. doi:10.1016/j.mpsur.2014.05.004.
17. Winkleman C. (2016). Care of patients with urinary problems. In Ignatavicius D., Workman M. (Eds.), *Medical-surgical nursing: Patient-centered collaborative care* (8th ed., pp. 1366–1393).
18. National Clinical Guideline Centre (UK). (2012). Urinary incontinence in neurological disease: Management of lower urinary tract dysfunction in neurological disease. *London: Royal College of Physicians (UK)* 148, 1–368.
19. Lee U. J., Scott V., Rashid R., et al. (2013). Defining and managing overactive bladder: Disagreement among the experts. *Urology* 81, 257–262.

20. Meng E., Lin W, Lee W., et al. (2012). Pathophysiology of overactive bladder. *Luts: Lower Urinary Tract Symptoms* 4(1), 448–455. doi:10.1111/j.1757-5672.2011.00122.x.
21. Linsenmeyer T., Stone J., Steins S. (2012). Neurogenic bladder and bowel. In Frontera W. R. (Ed.) *DeLisa's physical medicine and rehabilitation: Principles and Practice* (5th ed., pp. 1345–1392).
22. The American College of Obstetrics and Gynecology. (2014). Evaluation of uncomplicated stress urinary incontinence in women before surgical treatment, Committee Opinion No. 633m. *Obstetrics & Gynecology* 123, 1403–1407. Accessed August 31, 2017.
23. Zeren M. F., Yüksel M. B., Temeltas G. (2014). The comparison of urinary findings in women with various types of urinary incontinence. *International Brazilian Journal of Nursing* 40(2), 232–239. doi:10.1590/S1677-5538.INJU.2014.02.14.
24. Bali P., Mahalingam G., Bala K. (2016). Effectiveness of Kegel exercise on women with urinary incontinence. *International Journal of Nursing Education* 8(3), 155–162. doi:10.5958/0974-9357.2016.00109.4.
25. Herbison G. P. (2013). Weighted vaginal cones for urinary incontinence. *Cochrane Database of Systematic Reviews* (7), CD002114. doi:10.1002/14651858.CD002114.pub2.
26. Ferreira M., Santos P. C., Duarte J. A., et al. (2012). Exercise programmes for women with stress urinary incontinence. *Primary Health Care* 22(3), 24–27.
27. Bardsley A. (2016). An overview of urinary incontinence. *British Journal of Nursing* 25(18), S14.
28. Leone Roberti Maggiore U., Bogani G., Meschia M., et al. (2015). Urethral bulking agents versus other surgical procedures for the treatment of stress urinary incontinence: A systematic review and meta-analysis. *European Journal of Obstetrics & Gynecology & Reproductive Biology* 189, 48–54. doi:10.1016/ejogrb.2015.03.025.
29. Neki N. (2016). Urinary incontinence in elderly. *Journal of Krishna Institute of Medical Science University* 5(1), 5–13.
30. Time of Care Medicine Notebook. (2017). *DIAPPERS: Treatable causes of urinary tract infections*. Available: https://www.timeofcare.com/diappers-treatable-causes-of-urinary-incontinence/. Accessed February 1, 2018.
31. American Cancer Society. (2016). *Bladder cancer overview*. Available: http://www.cancer.org/Cancer/BladderCancer/OverviewGuide/bladder-cancer-overview-key-statistics. Accessed October 16, 2017.
32. Yaxley J. (2016). Urinary tract cancers: An overview for general practice. *Journal of Family Medicine Primary Care* 5(3), 533–538.
33. Feber A., Dhami P., Dong L., et al. (2017). Uro Mark-a urinary biomarker assay for the detection of bladder cancer. *Clinical Epigenetics* 9(1), 8. doi:10.1186/s13148-016-0303-5.
34. Secci D., Gentile V., Cristini C., et al. (2012). Current and emerging strategies in bladder cancer. *Anti-Cancer Agents in Medicinal Cancer* 12(6), 589–603.
35. Hinkle, J. (2018). *Brunner & Suddarth's textbook of medical-surgical nursing* (14th ed., pp. 1554). Philadelphia, PA: Wolters Kluwer.
36. Silbert-Flagg J. (2018). *Maternal and child health nursing* (8th ed.). Philadelphia, PA: Wolters Kluwers.

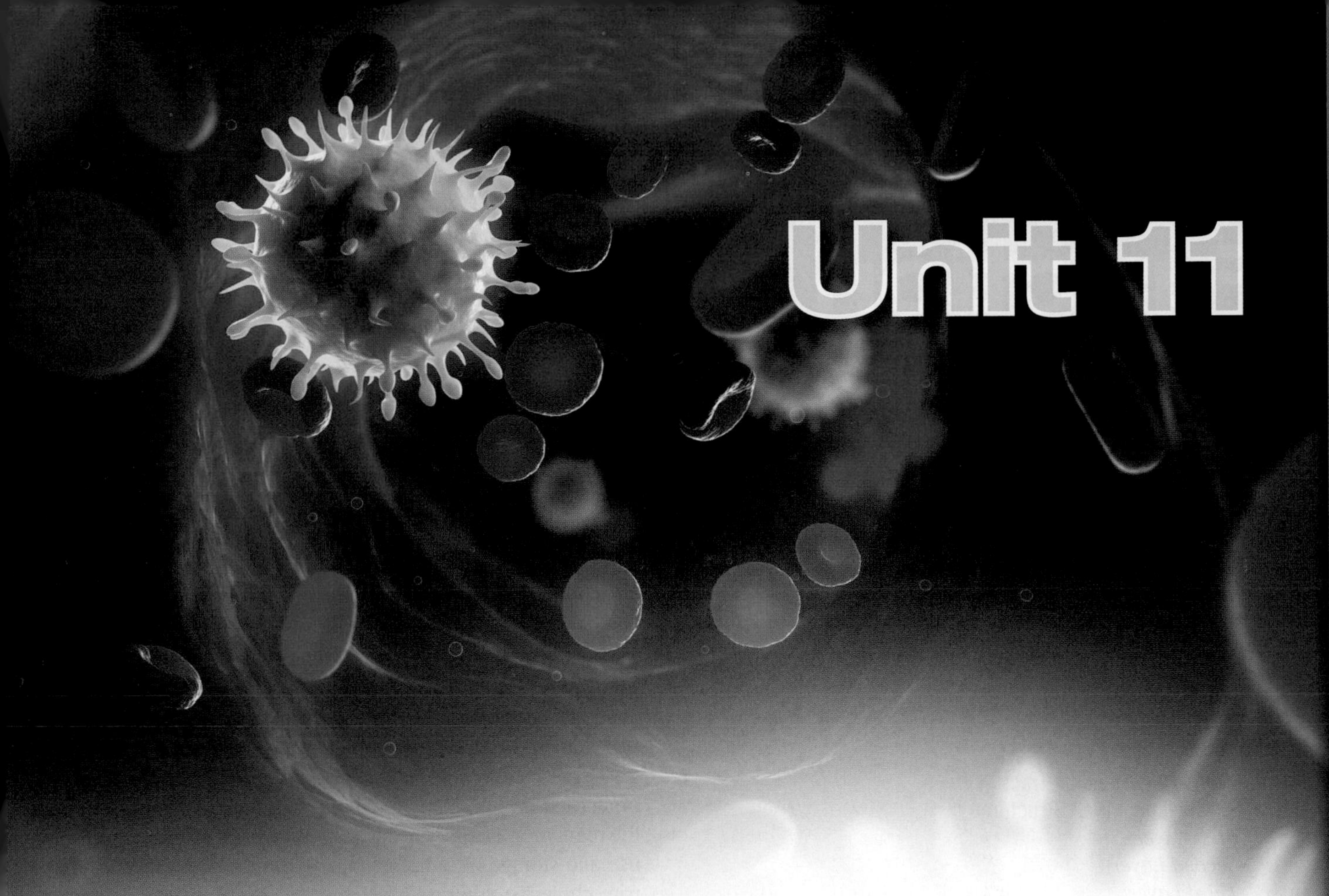

Unit 11

Disorders of Gastrointestinal Function

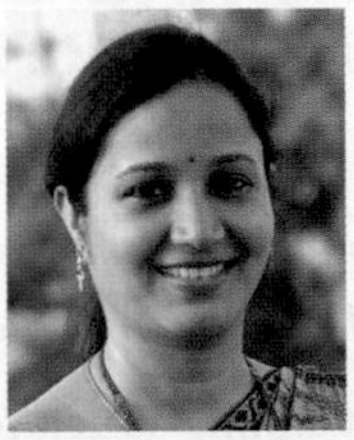

Ms. Rytel, 26 years old, presents with a 36-hour history of vomiting and abdominal pain. She has never experienced these symptoms before; however, she has a history of multiple abdominal surgeries, including lysis of adhesions, because of a motor vehicle crash that occurred 12 months ago. On examination, Ms. Rytel's abdomen is distended and slightly tender with hypoactive sounds. She cannot recall the last time she had a bowel movement and is presently not passing gas. She has pallor and is diaphoretic. Her vital signs are as follows: heart rate, 99 per minute; blood pressure, 134/76 mm Hg; respiratory rate, 25 bpm/minute; SpO_2, 98% on room air; and temperature 99.0°F. Her WBC count is 18,000 per μL (normal, 4.8 to 10.8 × 10^3 per μL), and an abdominal x-ray is pending.

Structure and Function of the Gastrointestinal System

36

Freddy W. Cao

In the digestive system, food is broken down and its nutrients are absorbed, wastes are collected and eliminated, vitamins are synthesized, and enzymes are produced. The gastrointestinal (GI) tract is also becoming increasingly recognized as an endocrine organ that produces and augments hormones that contribute to the regulation of appetite and nutrient intake and function in the use and storage of nutrients. Three groups of hormones—gastrin, cholecystokinin (CCK), and secretins—can affect the GI tract in multiple ways consistent with endocrine, paracrine, and neurocrine substances.[1] The GI tract has multiple collections of specialized cells interspersed throughout GI tissue that secrete these types of hormones. This differs from the thyroid, which is primarily composed of dense collections of specialized cells.

The GI tract also is referred to as the *digestive tract*, the *alimentary canal*, and, at times, the *gut*. The intestinal portion also may be called the *bowel*. For the purposes of this text, the liver and pancreas, which produce secretions that aid in digestion, are considered *accessory organs*.

STRUCTURE AND ORGANIZATION OF THE GASTROINTESTINAL TRACT

After completing this section of the chapter, the learner will be able to meet the following objectives:

- Describe the anatomic structures of the upper, middle, and lower gastrointestinal tract.
- Describe the four layers of the gastrointestinal tract wall.
- Describe the structure and function of the peritoneum and how it attaches to the abdominal wall.

The major physiologic functions of the GI system are to digest food and absorb nutrients into the bloodstream. It carries out these functions by motility, secretion, digestion, and absorption. In the digestive tract, food and other materials move slowly along its length as they are systematically broken down into ions and molecules that can be absorbed into the body. In the large intestine, unabsorbed nutrients and wastes are collected for later elimination.

Structurally, the GI tract is a long tube with a lumen (*i.e.*, hollow center) beginning at the esophagus and ending at the rectum (Fig. 36.1). Nutrients do not become part of the internal environment until they have passed through the intestinal wall and have entered the blood or lymph channels. The GI tract can be divided into three parts:

1. The upper part—the mouth, esophagus, and stomach—acts as an intake source and receptacle through which food passes and in which initial digestive processes take place.
2. The middle portion—the duodenum, jejunum, and ileum—is where most digestive and absorptive processes occur.
3. The lower segment—the cecum, colon, and rectum—serves as a storage channel for the efficient elimination of waste.

The accessory organs, which include the salivary glands, liver, and pancreas, produce secretions that aid in digestion.

Upper Gastrointestinal Tract

The mouth forms the entryway for food to pass into the GI tract. It contains the teeth, used in the mastication of food, and the tongue and other structures needed to direct food toward the pharyngeal structures and the esophagus. The mouth also serves as a receptacle for saliva produced by the salivary glands. Saliva moistens and lubricates food, so it is easier to swallow. It also contains enzymes involved in the initial digestion of lipids and starches.

Esophagus

The esophagus is a straight, collapsible tube, about 25 cm (10 inches) in length. It lies behind the trachea and connects the oropharynx with the stomach. The esophagus functions

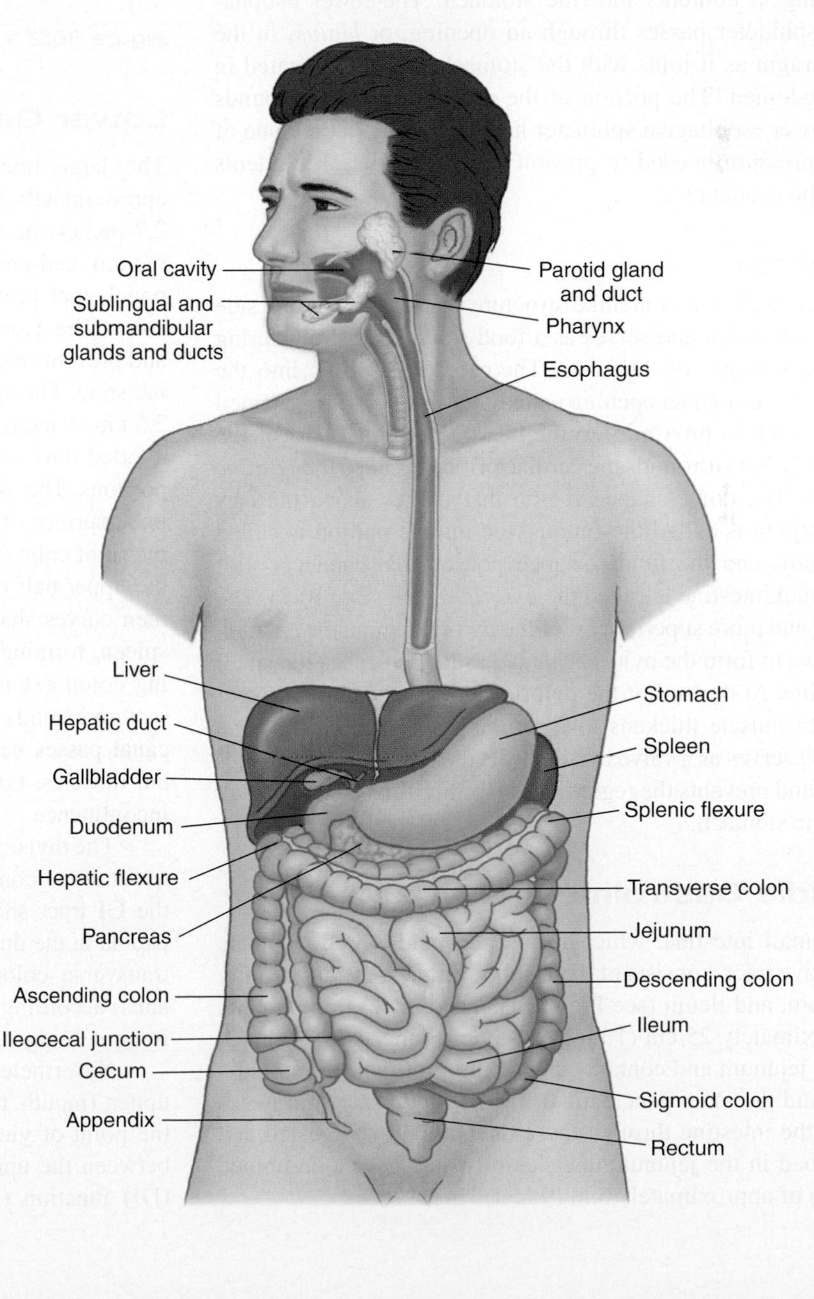

Figure 36.1 • The digestive system.

primarily as a conduit for the passage of food from the pharynx to the stomach. Its structure is uniquely designed for this purpose. The smooth muscle layers provide the peristaltic movements needed to move food along its length. In addition, the mucosal and submucosal glands secrete mucus, which protects its surface and aids in lubricating food.

There are sphincters at either end of the esophagus—an upper esophageal sphincter and a lower esophageal sphincter. The upper sphincter, the *pharyngoesophageal sphincter*, consists of a circular layer of striated muscle. It keeps air from entering the esophagus and stomach during breathing. The lower sphincter, the *gastroesophageal sphincter*, lies just above the area where the esophagus joins the stomach. The circular muscle in this area normally remains tonically contracted, creating a zone of high pressure that serves to prevent reflux of gastric contents into the esophagus. During swallowing, there is "receptive relaxation" of the lower esophageal sphincter, which allows easy propulsion of the esophageal contents into the stomach. The lower esophageal sphincter passes through an opening, or *hiatus*, in the diaphragm as it joins with the stomach, which is located in the abdomen. The portion of the diaphragm that surrounds the lower esophageal sphincter helps to maintain the zone of high pressure needed to prevent reflux of stomach contents into the esophagus.

Stomach

The stomach is a pouchlike structure that lies in the left side of the abdomen and serves as a food storage reservoir during the early stages of digestion. The esophagus opens into the stomach through an opening called the *cardiac orifice* (named because of its proximity to the heart). The small part of the stomach that surrounds the cardiac orifice is called the *cardiac region*. The dome-shaped region that bulges above the cardiac region is called the fundus, the middle portion is called the *body*, and the funnel-shaped portion that connects with the small intestine is called the *pyloric region* (Fig. 36.2). The wider and more superior part of the pyloric region, the *antrum*, narrows to form the pyloric channel as it approaches the small intestine. At the end of the pyloric channel, the circular layer smooth muscle thickens to form the *pyloric sphincter*. This muscle serves as a valve that controls the rate of stomach emptying and prevents the regurgitation of intestinal contents back into the stomach.

Middle Gastrointestinal Tract

The small intestine, which forms the middle portion of the digestive tract, consists of three subdivisions—the duodenum, jejunum, and ileum (see Fig. 36.1). The duodenum, which is approximately 25 cm (10 inches) long, connects the stomach to the jejunum and contains the opening for the common bile duct and the main pancreatic duct. Bile and pancreatic juices enter the intestine through these ducts. Food is digested and absorbed in the jejunum and ileum, which have a combined length of approximately 3 m (9 feet).[2]

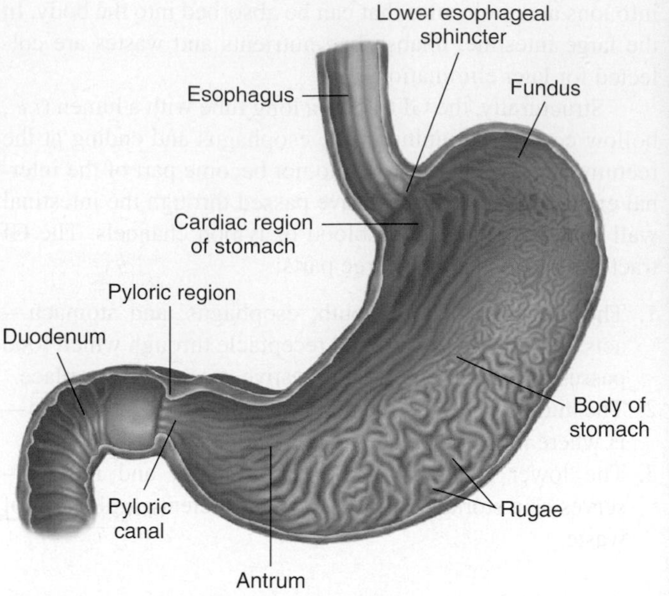

Figure 36.2 • Structures of the stomach.

Lower Gastrointestinal Tract

The large intestine, which forms the lower GI tract, is approximately 1.5 m (4.5 to 5 feet) long and 6 to 7 cm (2.4 to 2.7 inches) in diameter.[2] It is divided into the cecum, colon, rectum, and anal canal (see Fig. 36.1). The cecum is a blind pouch that projects down at the junction of the ileum and colon. The ileocecal valve lies at the upper border of the cecum and prevents the return of feces from the cecum into the small intestine. The appendix arises from the cecum approximately 2.5 cm (1 inch) from the ileocecal valve. The colon is further divided into ascending, transverse, descending, and sigmoid portions. The ascending colon extends from the cecum to the undersurface of the liver. From here, it turns abruptly to form the right colic (hepatic) flexure. The transverse colon crosses the upper half of the abdominal cavity from right to left and then curves sharply downward beneath the lower end of the spleen, forming the left colic (splenic) flexure. The descending colon extends from the colic flexure to the rectum. The rectum extends from the sigmoid colon to the anus. The anal canal passes between the two medial borders of the levator ani muscles. Powerful sphincter muscles guard against fecal incontinence.

The division of the GI tract into upper and lower is a matter of some confusion and debate. On embryologic grounds, the GI tract should be divided into upper (mouth to major papilla in the duodenum), middle (duodenal papilla to the mid-transverse colon), and lower (mid-transverse colon to the anus) according to the derivation of these three areas from the foregut, midgut, and hindgut, respectively.

Nevertheless, the GI tract is conventionally divided into upper (mouth to ileum) and lower (cecum to anus). From the point of view of GI bleeding, however, the demarcation between the upper and lower GI tract is the duodenojejunal (DJ) junction (ligament of Treitz); bleeding above the DJ junction is called upper GI bleeding and that below the DJ junction is called lower GI bleeding.[3]

Gastrointestinal Wall Structure

The digestive tract, below the upper third of the esophagus, is essentially a four-layered tube (Fig. 36.3).

First Layer

The inner *mucosal* (first) *layer* is made up of a lining epithelium, an underlying connective tissue called the *lamina propria*, and the muscularis mucosae, composed of smooth muscle cells that can contract and change the shape and surface area of the mucosal layer.[4]

The mucosal layer performs numerous functions in its role as an interface between the body and environment, including

- Production of the mucus that lubricates and protects the inner surface of the alimentary canal
- Secretion of the digestive enzymes and substances that break down food
- Absorption of the breakdown products of digestion
- Maintenance of a barrier to prevent the entry of noxious substances and pathogenic organisms (This barrier includes lymphatics within the mucosa, which serve as the body's first line of immune defense.)

The epithelial cells in the mucosal layer are constantly turning over and move from the outside of the wall structure to the luminal face every 5 days.[5] Because of the regenerative capabilities of the mucosal layer, injury to this layer heals rapidly without leaving scar tissue.

Second Layer

The *submucosal* (second) *layer* consists of dense connective tissue and aggregates of adipose tissue. It contains the blood vessels, nerves, and structures responsible for secreting digestive enzymes. The submucosal glands deliver their secretions either directly to the lumen of the mucosal glands or via ducts that pass through the mucosa to the luminal surface.

Third Layer

The third layer, the *muscularis externa*, consists of an inner layer of circularly arranged smooth muscle cells and an outer layer of longitudinally arranged smooth muscle layers, which facilitate movement of contents of the GI tract.

Fourth Layer

The fourth or *serosal layer* is a serous membrane consisting of the mesothelium, which is composed of a layer of simple squamous epithelium, and underlying connective tissue. This is the outermost layer (also known as the visceral peritoneum) of organs that are suspended in the peritoneal cavity. It is continuous with the parietal peritoneum and the mesenteries that make up the ventral and dorsal abdominal wall.[5]

The peritoneum is the largest serous membrane in the body, having a surface area approximately equal to that of the skin. The peritoneum consists of two continuous layers—the *visceral peritoneum* and the *parietal peritoneum* (which lines the wall of the abdominopelvic cavity). Between the two layers is the *peritoneal cavity*, a potential space containing fluid secreted by the serous membranes. This serous fluid forms a moist and slippery surface that prevents friction between the continuously moving abdominal structures.

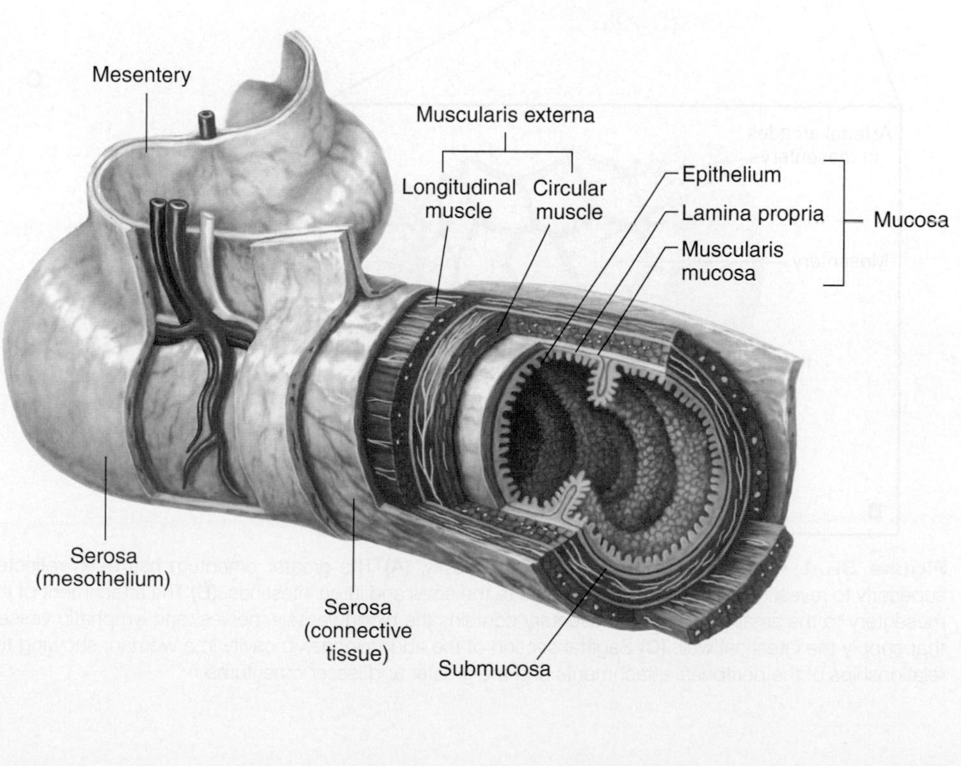

Figure 36.3 • Transverse section of the digestive system.

A *mesentery* is the double layer of the peritoneum that encloses a portion or all of one of the abdominal viscera and attaches it to the abdominal wall (Fig. 36.4A). The mesentery contains the blood vessels, nerves, and lymphatic vessels that supply the intestinal wall (see Fig. 36.4B). It also holds the organs in place and stores fat. There are dorsal as well as ventral mesenteries. However, in most places, the mesentery is dorsal and attaches to the posterior abdominal wall. The mesentery that attaches to the jejunum and ileum is gathered in folds that attach to the dorsal abdominal wall along a short line of insertion. This gives the mesentery a fan-shaped appearance, with the intestines at the edge.

An *omentum* is a double-layered extension or fold of the peritoneum that passes from the stomach or proximal part of the duodenum to adjacent organs in the abdominal cavity or abdominal wall. The *greater omentum* extends from the stomach to cover the transverse colon and the folds of the intestine. The *lesser omentum* extends between the transverse fissure of the liver and the lesser curvature of the stomach (see Fig. 36.4C). The greater omentum always contains some fat, which can be a considerable amount in some obese people. The greater omentum has considerable mobility and moves around in the peritoneal cavity with the peristaltic movements of the intestines. It often forms adhesions (*i.e.*, bands of fibrous

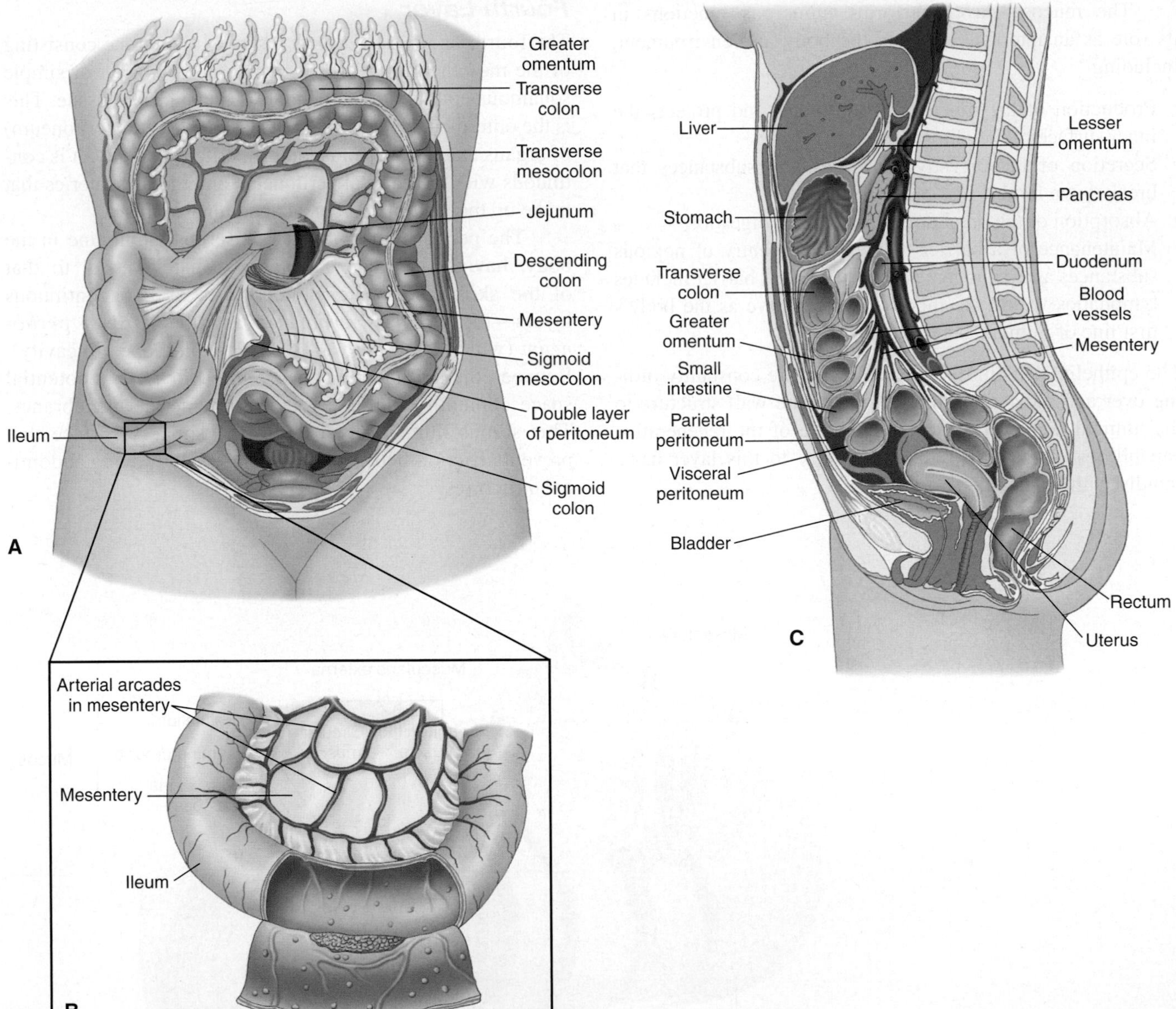

Figure 36.4 • Mesenteries of the abdominal cavity. **(A)** The greater omentum has been reflected superiorly to reveal the mesentery attachments to the small and large intestines. **(B)** The attachment of the mesentery to the small bowel. The mesentery contains the blood vessels, nerves, and lymphatic vessels that supply the intestinal wall. **(C)** Sagittal section of the abdominopelvic cavity in a woman, showing the relationships of the peritoneal attachments and the greater and lesser omentums.

scar tissue) adjacent to inflamed organs such as the appendix, walling off the infection and thereby preventing its spread. The greater omentum also cushions the abdominal organs against injury and provides insulation against the loss of body heat.

KEY POINTS

STRUCTURE AND FUNCTION OF THE GASTROINTESTINAL TRACT

- The GI tract is a long, hollow tube that extends from the mouth to the anus. Food and fluids that enter the GI tract do not become part of the internal environment until they have been broken down and absorbed into the blood or lymph channels.
- The nutrients contained in ingested foods and fluids must be broken down into molecules that can be absorbed across the wall of the intestine. Gastric acids and pepsin from the stomach begin the digestive process. Bile from the liver, digestive enzymes from the pancreas, and brush border enzymes break carbohydrates, fats, and proteins into molecules that can be absorbed from the intestine.

IN SUMMARY

The GI tract is a long tube, with a lumen (*i.e.*, hollow center) beginning at the esophagus and ending at the rectum. The functioning of the GI tract is dependent upon the release and regulation of hormones that occur in response to the consumption of food. The digestive tract can be divided into three parts—an upper part, consisting of the mouth, esophagus, and stomach; a middle part, consisting of the duodenum, jejunum, and ileum; and a lower part, consisting of the cecum, colon, and rectum. The accessory organs of the GI system consist of the salivary glands, liver, and pancreas. These organs produce secretions that aid in digestion.

Throughout its length, except for the mouth, throat, and upper esophagus, the GI tract is composed of four layers: an inner mucosal layer, a submucosal layer, a layer of circular and longitudinal smooth muscle fibers, and an outer serosal layer that forms the peritoneum and is continuous with the mesentery.

MOTILITY

After completing this section of the chapter, the learner will be able to meet the following objectives:

- Describe the properties of the interstitial smooth muscle cells that act as pacemakers for the GI tract.
- Compare the actions of the enteric system and autonomic nervous system (ANS) as they relate to motility of the GI tract.
- Differentiate tonic and peristaltic movements in the GI tract.

Control of Gastrointestinal Motility

The motility of the GI tract propels food and fluids along its length, from the mouth to anus, in a manner that facilitates digestion and absorption. The movements of the GI tract can be either rhythmic or tonic. The *rhythmic movements* consist of intermittent contractions that are responsible for mixing and moving food along the digestive tract. Rhythmic movements are found in the esophagus, antrum of the stomach, and small intestine. The *tonic movements* consist of a constant level of contraction or tone without regular periods of relaxation. They are found in the lower esophagus, upper region of the stomach, ileocecal valve, and internal anal sphincter.

Pacemaker-Generated Slow-Wave Activity

All of the contractile tissue in the GI tract is smooth muscle, except for that in the pharynx, upper third of the esophagus, and external anal sphincter. Although the smooth muscle found in each region of the GI tract exhibits structural and functional differences, certain basic properties are common to all of the muscle cells. All of the smooth muscle of the GI tract is unitary smooth muscle. Low-resistance pathways, called gap junctions, electrically couple the cells. This allows the electrical signals initiating muscle contractions to move rapidly from one fiber to the next within each bundle.[6]

Like the self-excitable cardiac muscle cells in the heart, some smooth muscle cells of the GI tract function as pacemaker cells. The interstitial cells of Cajal that are found in groups between the layers of smooth muscle tissue are hypothesized to function as the pacemakers. These cells display rhythmic, spontaneous oscillations in membrane potentials, called *slow waves*, ranging in frequency from about 3 per minute in the stomach to 12 per minute in the duodenum.[6]

The amplitude and, to a lesser extent, the frequency of the slow waves can be modulated by the enteric nervous system, which lies entirely within the wall of the GI tract, and by the parasympathetic and sympathetic divisions of the ANS. In addition, a number of peptides, including neurotransmitters and GI hormones, assist in regulating GI motility. In general, the activity of the sympathetic nervous system decreases the amplitude of the slow waves or abolishes them altogether. In contrast, activation of the parasympathetic nervous system increases the amplitude of the slow waves.

Enteric Nervous System

The enteric nervous system consists of the myenteric and submucosal plexuses in the wall of the GI tract. These two plexuses are networks of nerve fibers and ganglion cell bodies. Interneurons in the plexuses connect afferent sensory fibers, efferent motor neurons, and secretory cells to form reflex circuits that are located entirely in the GI tract wall.[7]

The *myenteric* (Auerbach) *plexus* consists mainly of a linear chain of interconnecting neurons that is located between the circular and longitudinal muscle layers.[2] Because it lies between the two muscle layers and extends all the way down the intestinal wall, it is concerned mainly with motility along the length of the gut. The *submucosal* (Meissner) *plexus*, which lies between the mucosal and muscle layers of the intestinal wall, is mainly concerned with controlling the secretions, absorption, and contraction of each segment of the intestinal tract.[6]

The activity of the neurons in the myenteric and submucosal plexuses is regulated by local influences, by input from the ANS, and by interconnecting fibers that transmit information between the two plexuses. Mechanoreceptors monitor the stretch and distention of the GI tract wall, and chemoreceptors monitor the chemical composition (*i.e.*, osmolality, pH, and digestive products of protein and fat metabolism) of its contents. These receptors can communicate directly with ganglionic cells in the intramural plexuses or with visceral afferent fibers that influence ANS control of GI function.

Autonomic Nervous System Innervation

The autonomic innervation of the GI system is mediated by both the sympathetic and parasympathetic nervous systems (Fig. 36.5). Parasympathetic innervation to the stomach, small intestine, cecum, ascending colon, and transverse colon occurs through the vagus nerve. The remainder of the colon is innervated by parasympathetic fibers that exit the sacral segments of the spinal cord by way of the pelvic nerves. Preganglionic parasympathetic fibers can synapse with intramural plexus neurons, or they can act directly on intestinal smooth muscle.[1] In addition, these same nerve bundles provide many afferent nerves whose receptors lie within the various tissues of the gut. Their nerves project to the spinal cord and brain to provide sensory input for integration. Most parasympathetic innervation is excitatory. Numerous vagovagal reflexes influence motility and secretions of the digestive tract.

Sympathetic innervation occurs through the thoracic chain of sympathetic ganglia and the celiac, superior mesenteric, and inferior mesenteric ganglia. The sympathetic nervous system exerts several effects on GI function. It controls the extent of mucous secretion by the mucosal glands, reduces motility by inhibiting the activity of intramural plexus neurons, enhances sphincter function, and increases the vascular smooth muscle tone of the blood vessels that supply the GI tract.[7] The effect of sympathetic stimulation is to block the release of the excitatory neuromediators in the intramural plexuses, inhibiting GI motility. Sympathetic control of GI function is largely mediated by activity in the intramural plexuses.[8] For example, when GI motility is enhanced because of increased vagal activity, stimulation of sympathetic centers in the hypothalamus promptly, and often completely, inhibits motility.

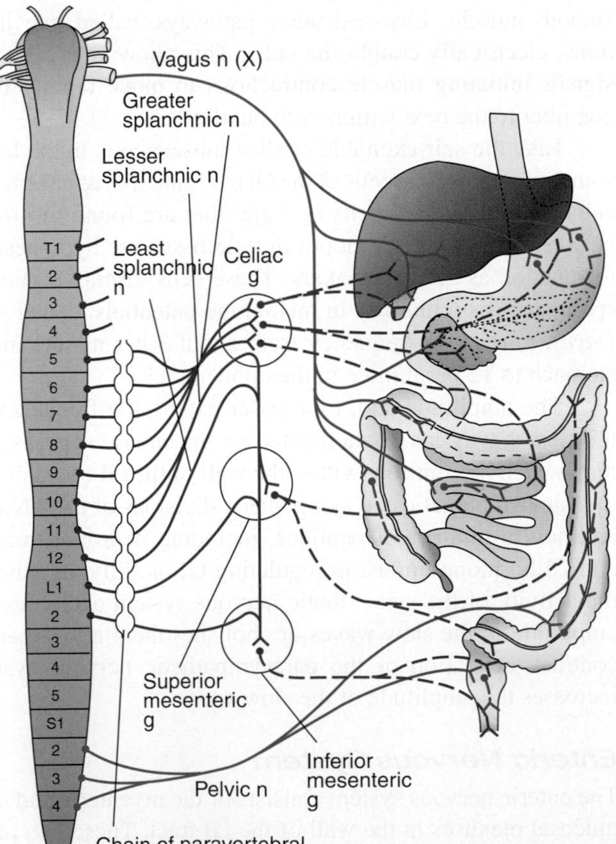

Figure 36.5 • Autonomic innervation of the gastrointestinal tract (g, ganglion; n, nerve). Parasympathetic innervation is indicated in *blue* and sympathetic in *red*.

Swallowing and Esophageal Motility

Mastication begins the digestive process. Mastication (chewing) breaks food down into smaller pieces that can be easily swallowed. During this process, food is also lubricated with saliva and exposed to salivary amylase, which breaks down starch-containing foods. Although chewing usually is considered a voluntary act, it can be carried out involuntarily by a person who has lost the function of the cerebral cortex.

The swallowing reflex is a rigidly ordered sequence of events that results in the propulsion of food from the mouth to the stomach through the esophagus. Although swallowing is initiated as a voluntary activity, it becomes involuntary as food or fluid reaches the pharynx. Sensory impulses for the reflex begin at tactile receptors in the pharynx and esophagus and are integrated with the motor components of the response in an area of the reticular formation of the medulla and lower pons called the *swallowing center*. The motor impulses for the oral and pharyngeal phases of swallowing are carried in the trigeminal (V), glossopharyngeal (IX), vagus (X), and hypoglossal (XII) cranial nerves, and impulses for the esophageal phase are carried by the vagus nerve. Diseases that disrupt these brain centers or their cranial nerves disrupt the coordination of swallowing and predispose a person to food and fluid lodging in the trachea and bronchi, which leads to risk of asphyxiation or aspiration pneumonia.

Understanding Intestinal Motility

Motility of the small intestine is organized to optimize the digestion and absorption of nutrients and the propulsion of undigested material toward the colon. Peristaltic movements mix the ingested foodstuffs with digestive enzymes and secretions and circulate the intestinal contents to facilitate contact with the intestinal mucosa. The regulation of motility results from an interplay of input from the (1) enteric and (2) ANSs and the intrinsic pacemaker activity of the (3) intestinal smooth muscle cells.

Enteric Nervous System Innervation

The GI system has its own nervous system, called the *enteric nervous system*. The enteric nervous system is composed mainly of two plexuses: (1) the outer *myenteric (Auerbach) plexus* that is located between the longitudinal and circular layers of smooth muscle cells and (2) an inner *submucosal* (Meissner) *plexus* that lies between the mucosal and circular muscle layers. The myenteric plexus controls mainly intestinal movements along the length of the gut, whereas the submucosal plexus is concerned mainly with controlling the function within each segment of the intestine. Fibers in the submucosal plexus also use signals originating from the intestinal epithelium to control intestinal secretion and local blood flow.

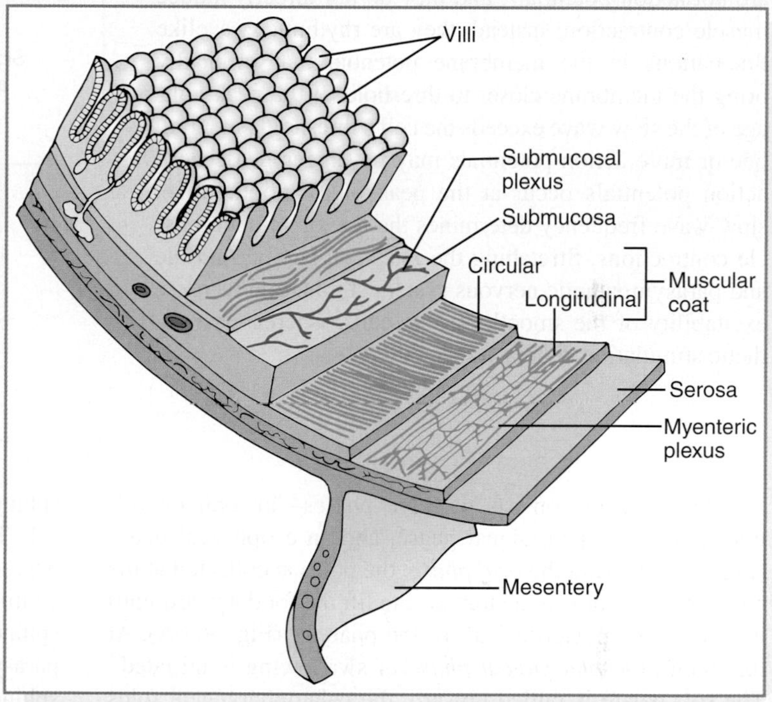

ANS Innervation

The intestine is also innervated by the parasympathetic and sympathetic branches of the ANS (see Fig. 36.5). *Parasympathetic innervation* is supplied mainly by the vagus nerve with postganglionic neurons located primarily in the myenteric and submucosal plexuses. Stimulation of these parasympathetic nerves causes a general increase in both intestinal motility and secretory activity. *Sympathetic innervation* is supplied by nerves that run between the spinal cord and the prevertebral ganglia and between these ganglia and the intestine. Stimulation of the sympathetic nervous system is largely inhibitory, producing a decrease in intestinal motility and secretory activity.

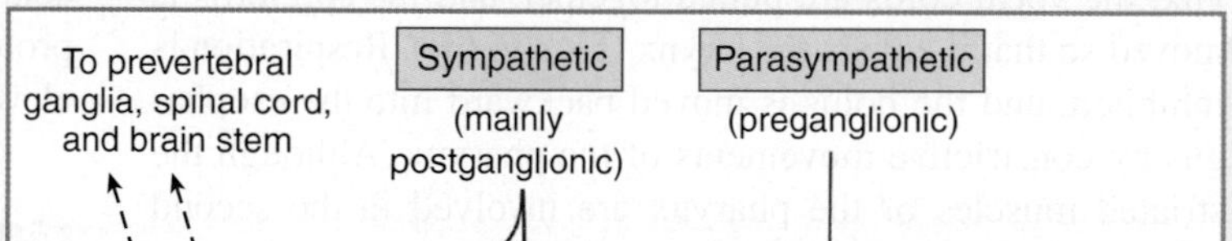

Continued

Understanding Intestinal Motility *(Continued)*

Intestinal Smooth Muscle

Intestinal smooth muscle has its own intrinsic slow-wave activity, which varies from about 12 per minute in the duodenum to 8 or 9 per minute in the ileum. This slow-wave activity is thought to reside in a network of specialized pacemaker cells, the *interstitial cells of Cajal*, that are interposed between the smooth muscle cells. Slow waves are not action potentials, and they do not directly induce muscle contraction; instead, they are rhythmic, wavelike fluctuations in the membrane potential that cyclically bring the membrane closer to threshold. If the peak voltage of the slow wave exceeds the cell's threshold potential, one or more action potentials may be triggered. Because action potentials occur at the peak of a smooth wave, slow-wave frequency determines the rate of smooth muscle contractions. Stretching the intestinal smooth muscle and parasympathetic nervous system stimulation increase excitability of the smooth muscle cells, whereas sympathetic stimulation decreases excitability.

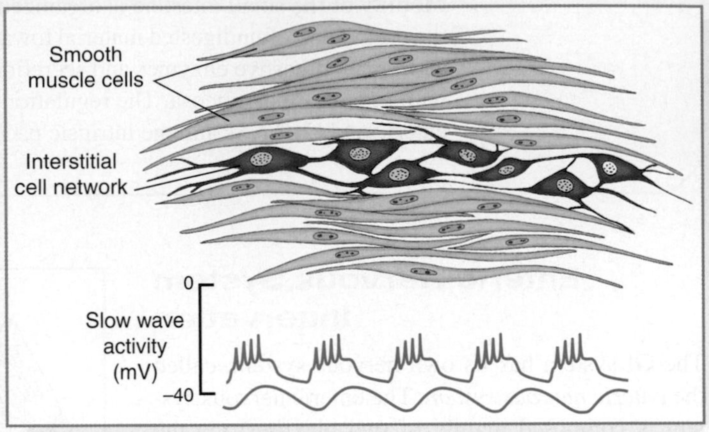

Swallowing consists of three phases—an oral or voluntary phase, a pharyngeal phase, and an esophageal phase (Fig 36.6). During the *oral phase*, the bolus is collected at the back of the mouth so the tongue can lift the food upward until it touches the posterior wall of the pharynx (Fig. 36.6A). At this point, the *pharyngeal phase* of swallowing is initiated.[9] The soft palate is pulled upward, the palatopharyngeal folds are pulled together so that food does not enter the nasopharynx, the vocal cords are pulled together, and the epiglottis is moved so that it covers the larynx (Fig. 36.6B). Respiration is inhibited, and the bolus is moved backward into the esophagus by constrictive movements of the pharynx. Although the striated muscles of the pharynx are involved in the second stage of swallowing, it is an involuntary stage.

The third phase of swallowing is the *esophageal stage* (Fig. 36.6C).[9] As food enters the esophagus and stretches its walls, local and central nervous system (CNS) reflexes that initiate peristalsis are triggered.

There are two types of peristalsis—primary and secondary. Primary peristalsis is controlled by the swallowing center in the brain stem and begins when food enters the esophagus. Secondary peristalsis is partially mediated by smooth muscle fibers in the esophagus and occurs when primary peristalsis is inadequate to move food through the esophagus. Peristalsis begins at the site of distention and moves downward. Before the peristaltic wave reaches the stomach, the lower esophageal sphincter relaxes to allow the bolus of food to enter the stomach. The pressure in the lower esophageal sphincter normally is greater than that in the stomach, an important factor in preventing the reflux of gastric contents. The lower esophageal sphincter is innervated by the vagus nerve. Increased levels of parasympathetic stimulation increase the constriction of the sphincter. The hormone gastrin also increases constriction of the sphincter. Gastrin provides the major stimulus for gastric acid production. Its action on the lower esophageal sphincter protects the esophageal mucosa when gastric acid levels are elevated.

Gastric Motility

The stomach serves as a food storage reservoir. The stomach has the ability to expand and contract in size in response to the amount of food or gas within it; in some cases, it may hold up to 1 to 1.5 L of volume.[3] The chemical breakdown of protein begins in the stomach where food is converted to a creamy mixture called *chyme*.

Motility of the stomach results in the churning and mixing of solid foods and regulates the emptying of the gastric contents, or chyme, into the duodenum. Peristaltic mixing and churning contractions begin in a pacemaker area in the middle of the stomach and move toward the antrum. They occur at a frequency of three to five contractions per minute, each

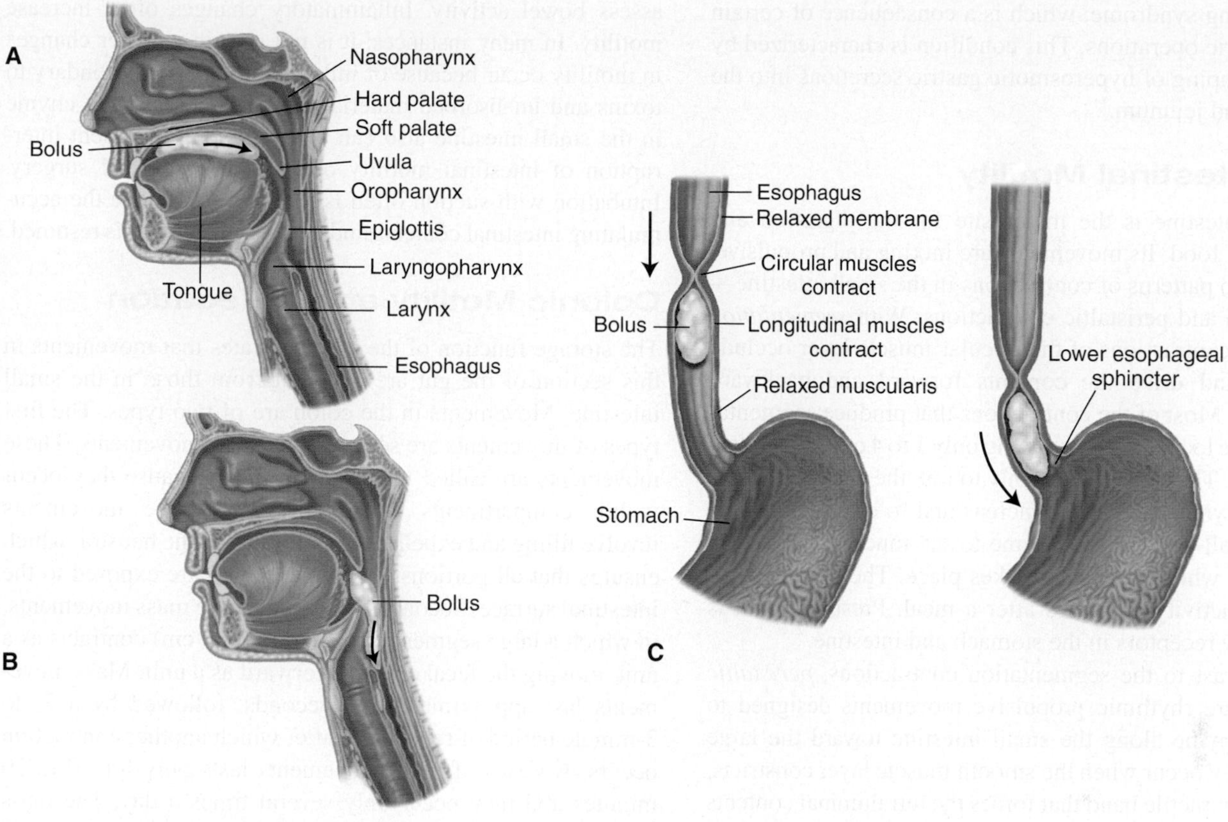

Figure 36.6 • Steps in the swallowing reflex. **(A)** The *oral* or *voluntary phase* during which the bolus is collected at the back of the mouth so the tongue can lift the food upward and into the pharynx. **(B)** The *pharyngeal phase* during which food movement into the respiratory passages is prevented as the tongue is elevated and pressed against the soft palate closing the epiglottis, the upper esophageal sphincter relaxes, and the superior constrictor muscle contracts forcing food into the esophagus. **(C)** The *esophageal phase* during which peristalsis moves food through the esophagus and into the stomach.

lasting 2 to 20 seconds. As the peristaltic wave approaches the antrum, it pushes the bolus of food toward the closed pylorus. Contraction of the antrum reverses the movement of the chyme, returning the larger particles to the body of the stomach for further churning and kneading. Because the pylorus is contracted during antral contraction, the gastric contents are emptied into the duodenum between contractions.[1]

The pyloric sphincter prevents the backflow of gastric contents and allows them to flow into the duodenum at a rate commensurate with the ability of the duodenum to accept them. This is important because the regurgitation of bile salts and duodenal contents can damage the mucosal surface of the antrum and lead to gastric ulcers. Likewise, the duodenal mucosa can be damaged by the rapid influx of highly acid gastric contents.

Like other parts of the GI tract, the stomach is richly innervated by the enteric nervous system and its connections with the sympathetic and parasympathetic nervous systems. Axons from the intramural plexuses innervate the smooth muscles and glands of the stomach. Parasympathetic innervation is provided by the vagus nerve and sympathetic innervation by the celiac ganglia. The emptying of the stomach is regulated by hormonal and neural mechanisms.[9] The hormones CCK and glucose-dependent insulinotropic polypeptide (GIP) (formerly known as *gastric inhibitory peptide*), which are thought in part to control gastric emptying, are released in response to the pH, osmolality, and fatty acid composition of the chyme.[10] Both local and central circuitries are involved in the neural control of gastric emptying. Afferent receptor fibers synapse with the neurons in the intramural plexus or trigger intrinsic reflexes through vagal or sympathetic pathways that participate in extrinsic reflexes.

Disorders of gastric motility can occur when the rate is too slow or too fast. A rate that is too slow leads to gastric retention. It can be caused by obstruction or gastric atony. Obstruction can result from the formation of scar tissue in the pyloric area after a peptic ulcer. Another example of obstruction is *hypertrophic pyloric stenosis*, which can occur in infants with an abnormally thick muscularis layer in the terminal pylorus. Myotomy, or surgical incision of the muscular ring, may be done to relieve the obstruction. Gastric atony can occur as a complication of visceral neuropathies in diabetes mellitus. Surgical procedures that disrupt vagal activity also can result in gastric atony. Abnormally fast emptying occurs in the dumping syndrome, which is a consequence of certain types of gastric operations. This condition is characterized by the rapid dumping of hyperosmotic gastric secretions into the duodenum and jejunum.[11]

Small Intestinal Motility

The small intestine is the major site for the digestion and absorption of food. Its movements are mixing and propulsive. There are two patterns of contractions in the small intestine—segmentation and peristaltic contractions. With *segmentation waves*, slow contractions of the circular muscle layer occlude the lumen and drive the contents forward and backward (Fig. 36.7A). Most of the contractions that produce segmentation waves are local events involving only 1 to 4 cm of the intestine at a time. They function mainly to mix the chyme with the digestive enzymes from the pancreas and to ensure adequate exposure of all parts of the chyme to the mucosal surface of the intestine, where absorption takes place. The frequency of segmenting activity increases after a meal. Presumably, it is stimulated by receptors in the stomach and intestine.

In contrast to the segmentation contractions, *peristaltic movements* are rhythmic propulsive movements designed to propel the chyme along the small intestine toward the large intestine. They occur when the smooth muscle layer constricts, forming a contractile band that forces the intraluminal contents forward. Normal peristalsis always moves in the direction from the mouth toward the anus. Regular peristaltic movements begin in the duodenum near the entry sites of the common duct and the main hepatic duct. They are accomplished by contraction of the proximal portion of the intestine with the sequential relaxation of its distal, or caudal, portion (see Fig. 36.7B). After material has been propelled to the ileocecal junction by peristaltic movement, stretching of the distal ileum produces a local reflex that relaxes the sphincter and allows fluid to squirt into the cecum. Motility disturbances of the small bowel are common, and auscultation of the abdomen can be used to assess bowel activity. Inflammatory changes often increase motility. In many instances, it is not certain whether changes in motility occur because of inflammation or are secondary to toxins and unabsorbed materials. Delayed passage of chyme in the small intestine also can be a problem. Transient interruption of intestinal motility often occurs after GI surgery. Intubation with suction often is required to remove the accumulating intestinal contents and gases until activity is resumed.

Colonic Motility and Defecation

The storage function of the colon dictates that movements in this section of the gut are different from those in the small intestine. Movements in the colon are of two types. The first types of movements are segmental mixing movements. These movements are called *haustral churning* because they occur within compartments called haustra.[2] These movements involve filling and expelling the contents of the haustra, which ensures that all portions of the fecal mass are exposed to the intestinal surface. Second are the propulsive mass movements, in which a large segment of the colon (≥20 cm) contracts as a unit, moving the fecal contents forward as a unit. Mass movements last approximately 30 seconds, followed by a 2- to 3-minute period of relaxation, after which another contraction occurs. A series of mass movements lasts only for 10 to 30 minutes and may occur only several times a day. The mass movements normally initiate defecation. The normal colonic transit time is 24 to 48 hours, and normal stool is composed of 75% water and 25% solid matter.[6]

Defecation is controlled by the action of two sphincters—the internal and external anal sphincters (Fig. 36.8). The internal sphincter is a several-centimeters-long, circular thickening of smooth muscle that lies inside the anus. The external sphincter, which is composed of striated voluntary muscle, surrounds the internal sphincter. The external sphincter is controlled by nerve fibers in the pudendal nerve, which is part of the somatic nervous system and therefore under voluntary

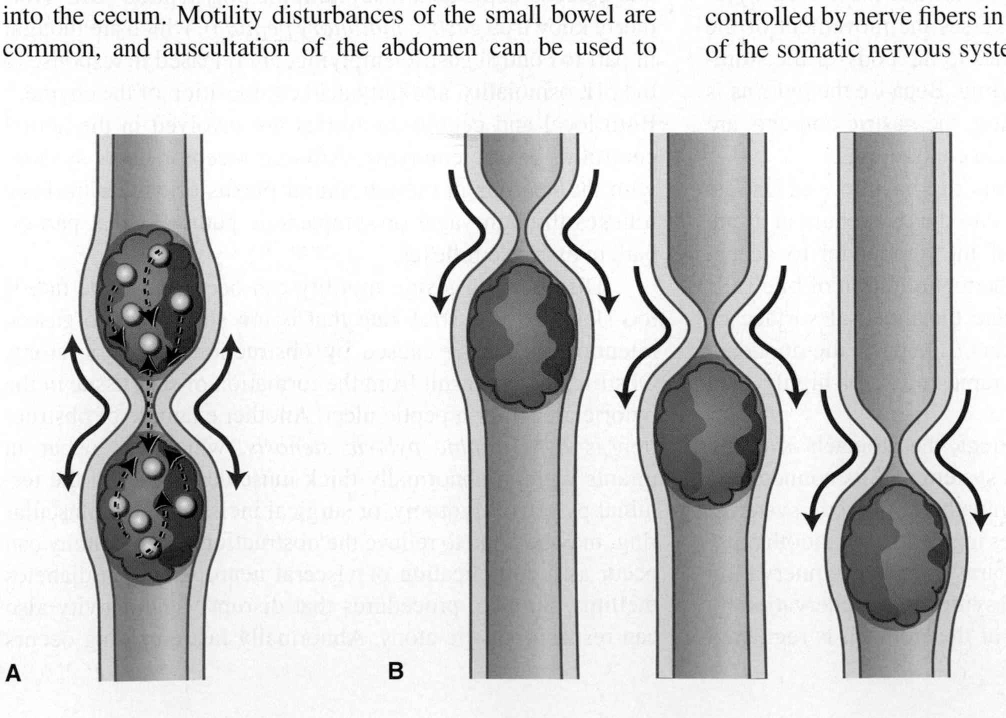

Figure 36.7 • Two types of small intestine movements. **(A)** Mixing *segmentation waves* in which slow contractions of the circular muscle layer occlude the lumen and drive the contents forward and backward. **(B)** Propulsive *peristaltic movements* in which segmental contractions followed by sequential relaxation moves the contents forward.

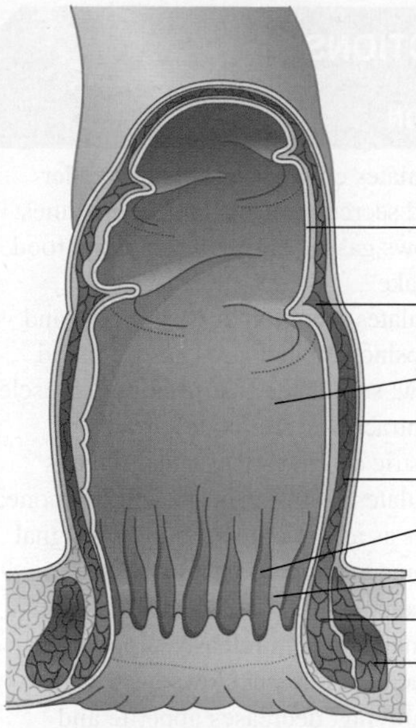

Figure 36.8 • Interior of the rectum and anal canal.

control. Defecation reflexes control defecation. One of these reflexes is the intrinsic myenteric reflex mediated by the local enteric nervous system. It is initiated by distention of the rectal wall, with initiation of reflex peristaltic waves that spread through the descending colon, sigmoid colon, and rectum. A second defecation reflex, the parasympathetic reflex, is integrated at the level of the sacral cord. When the nerve endings in the rectum are stimulated, signals are transmitted first to the sacral cord and then reflexively back to the descending colon, sigmoid colon, rectum, and anus by the pelvic nerves. These impulses greatly increase peristaltic movements as well as relax the internal sphincter.

To prevent involuntary defecation from occurring, the external anal sphincter is under the conscious control of the cortex. As afferent impulses arrive at the sacral cord, signaling the presence of a distended rectum, messages are transmitted to the cortex. If defecation is inappropriate, the cortex initiates impulses that constrict the external sphincter and inhibit efferent parasympathetic activity. Normally, the afferent impulses in this reflex loop fatigue easily, and the urge to defecate soon ceases. At a more convenient time, contraction of the abdominal muscles compresses the contents in the large bowel, reinitiating afferent impulses to the cord.

IN SUMMARY

Motility of the GI tract propels food products and fluids along its length from the mouth to anus. The activity of GI smooth muscle is self-propagating and can continue without input from the nervous system. However, a network of intramural neurons that receive input from the ANS and local receptors that monitor wall stretch and the chemical composition of luminal contents regulate the rate and strength of contractions. Parasympathetic innervation occurs through the vagus nerve and nerve fibers from sacral segments of the spinal cord. This innervation increases GI motility. Sympathetic activity occurs through thoracolumbar output from the spinal cord, its paravertebral ganglia, and celiac, superior mesenteric, and inferior mesenteric ganglia. Sympathetic stimulation enhances sphincter function and reduces motility by inhibiting the activity of intramural plexus neurons.

HORMONAL, SECRETORY, AND DIGESTIVE FUNCTIONS

After completing this section of the chapter, the learner will be able to meet the following objectives:

- Explain the protective function of saliva.
- Describe the function of the gastric mucosal barrier.
- Discuss the function of gut flora in terms of metabolic activities, trophic effects, and protection against invasion by pathogenic microorganisms.

Gastrointestinal Hormones

The GI tract is the largest endocrine organ in the body. It produces hormones that are involved in endocrine and paracrine regulation. Endocrine regulation involves an activated cell releasing a protein or hormone into the bloodstream. This hormone then reaches a target cell, which responds by releasing another hormone or chemical (*e.g.*, when stomach acid in chyme enters the intestine and stimulates the release of secretin). Paracrine regulation is a local event. For example, it occurs when a hormone reaches a target cell by simply crossing a cell membrane.

In addition, GI hormones can also interact with the CNS through the enteric and ANSs. Among the hormones produced by the GI tract are gastrin, ghrelin, secretin, CCK, and incretin hormones (glucagon-like peptide 1 [GLP-1] and GIP).[8] These hormones influence appetite, GI motility, enzyme activity, electrolyte levels, and the secretion and actions of hormones such as growth hormone, insulin, and glucagon. A variety of factors stimulate them, including pH, quantity and type of macronutrient intake, nervous stimulation, and a deficit or excess of present hormone level. The actions of many of these hormones overlap. For example, two or more GI hormones may affect the same process in the same direction, or they may inhibit each other. The GI tract hormones and their functions are summarized in Table 36.1.

The stomach is the source of two important GI hormones—gastrin and ghrelin. G cells, located predominantly in the antrum of the stomach, produce gastrin. The primary function of *gastrin* is the stimulation of gastric acid secretion. Gastrin also has a trophic, or growth-producing, effect on the mucosa of the small intestine, colon, and acid-secreting area of the stomach. *Ghrelin* is another peptide hormone synthesized and secreted by gastric oxyntic cells. Blood levels of

TABLE 36.1 SELECTED GASTROINTESTINAL HORMONES AND THEIR ACTIONS

HORMONE	SITE OF SECRETION	STIMULUS FOR SECRETION	ACTION
Cholecystokinin	Duodenum, jejunum	Products of protein digestion and long-chain fatty acids	Stimulates contraction of gallbladder and secretion of pancreatic enzymes; slows gastric emptying; inhibits food intake
Gastrin	Antrum of stomach, duodenum	Vagal stimulation; epinephrine; neutral amino acids; calcium-containing foods such as milk; alcohol Secretion inhibited by acid content of stomach antrum (pH < 2.5)	Stimulates secretion of gastric acid and pepsinogen; increases gastric blood flow; stimulates gastric smooth muscle contractions; stimulates growth of gastric and intestinal mucosal cells
Ghrelin	Fundus of stomach	Nutritional (fasting) and hormonal (decreased levels of growth hormone)	Stimulates secretion of growth hormone; acts as an appetite-stimulating signal from stomach when an increase in metabolic efficiency is necessary
Glucagon-like peptide-1 (GLP-1)	Distal small intestine	High-carbohydrate meal	Augments insulin release; suppresses glucagon release; slows gastric emptying; decreases appetite and body weight
Glucose-dependent insulinotropic polypeptide (GIP)	Small intestine, mainly jejunum	High-carbohydrate meal	Augments insulin release
Secretin	Duodenum	Acid pH or chyme entering duodenum (pH < 3.0)	

this hormone exhibit circadian fluctuation, which are aligned with mealtimes, spiking preprandially followed by rapid postprandial reductions. These have positioned ghrelin as a key regulator of meal initiation, stimulating a cascade of events to prepare the body for an impending meal. All of the above has led to the designation of ghrelin as the "hunger hormone." To date, however, it remains the only known peripheral hormone with orexigenic effects via a centrally mediated mechanism. Furthermore, ghrelin contributes to the regulation of body weight by potently stimulating growth hormone secretion from the pituitary, increasing adiposity and reducing energy expenditure. Ghrelin has also been shown to be involved in reward processes, mood, memory and learning, and stress response, while peripheral functions span gastric motility, glucose homeostasis, immune function, cardiac output, and bone formation.[12]

The intestine is the source of secretin, CCK, and incretin hormones. *Secretin*, which is secreted by S cells in the mucosa of the duodenum and jejunum, inhibits gastric acid secretion. The entry of an acid chyme into the intestine stimulates the release of secretin, which inhibits the release of gastrin. Secretin is released in response to duodenal pH, which stimulates the pancreas to secrete large quantities of fluid with a high bicarbonate concentration.[13] The primary function of CCK, secreted by I cells in the intestinal mucosa, is the stimulation of pancreatic enzyme secretion. It potentiates the action of secretin, increasing the pancreatic bicarbonate response to low circulating levels of secretin, stimulates biliary secretion of fluid and bicarbonate, and regulates gallbladder contraction and gastric emptying. In a recent study, CCK has also been shown to inhibit food intake and to be an important mediator for appetite and the control of meal size.[14]

Several gut-derived hormones have been identified as having what is termed an *incretin* effect. This means that they increase insulin release after an oral glucose load. This suggests that gut-derived factors can stimulate insulin secretion after a predominantly carbohydrate meal. The two hormones that account for about 90% of the incretin effect are GLP-1, which is released from L cells in the distal small bowel, and GIP, which is released by K cells in the upper gut (mainly the jejunum). Because increased levels of GLP-1 and GIP can lower blood glucose levels by augmenting insulin release in a glucose-dependent manner (*i.e.*, at low blood glucose levels no further insulin is secreted, minimizing the risk of hypoglycemia), these hormones have been targeted as possible antidiabetic drugs. Moreover, GLP-1 can exert other metabolically beneficial effects, including suppression of glucagon release, slowing of gastric emptying, augmenting of net glucose clearance, and decreasing appetite and body weight.[15,16]

Gastrointestinal Secretions

Throughout the GI tract, secretory glands serve two basic functions:

1. Production of mucus to lubricate and protect the mucosal layer of the GI tract wall
2. Secretion of fluids and enzymes to aid in the digestion and absorption of nutrients

TABLE 36.2 SECRETIONS OF THE GASTROINTESTINAL TRACT

SECRETIONS	AMOUNT DAILY (ML)
Salivary	1200
Gastric	2000
Pancreatic	1200
Biliary	700
Intestinal	2000
Total	**7100**

Each day, approximately 7000 mL of fluid is secreted into the GI tract (Table 36.2). Approximately 100 to 200 mL of this fluid leaves the body in the stool. The remainder is reabsorbed in the small and large intestines.[9] These secretions are mainly water and have sodium and potassium concentrations similar to those of extracellular fluid. Because water and electrolytes for digestive tract secretions are derived from the extracellular fluid compartment, excessive secretion or impaired absorption can lead to extracellular fluid deficit.

The secretory and digestive functions of the gut are influenced by local, humoral, and neural influences. Neural control of GI secretory activity is mediated through the ANS. Secretory activity, like motility, is increased with parasympathetic stimulation and inhibited with sympathetic activity. Many of the local influences, including pH, osmolality, and chyme, consistently act as stimuli for neural and humoral mechanisms.

Salivary Secretions

Saliva is secreted by the salivary glands. The salivary glands consist of the parotid, submaxillary, sublingual, and buccal glands. Saliva has three functions. The first is protection and lubrication. Saliva is rich in mucus, which protects the oral mucosa and coats the food as it passes through the mouth, pharynx, and esophagus. The sublingual and buccal glands produce only mucus-type secretions. The second function of saliva is its protective antimicrobial action. The saliva cleans the mouth and contains the enzyme lysozyme, which has an antibacterial action. Third, saliva contains ptyalin and amylase, which initiate the digestion of dietary starches. The ANS primarily regulates secretions from the salivary glands. Parasympathetic stimulation increases flow and sympathetic stimulation decreases flow. The dry mouth that accompanies anxiety attests to the effects of sympathetic activity on salivary secretions.

Gastric Secretions

Mucus-secreting epithelial cells line the luminal surface and gastric pits of the stomach and serve as a protective barrier for the entire surface of the stomach (Fig. 36.9). In addition, the stomach mucosa has several other types of cells that secrete substances necessary for digestion. These include the parietal (or oxyntic) cells, chief cells, and G cells.

The parietal and chief cells are located in the proximal 80% (body and fundus) of the stomach and situated in the bases of the gastric pits (see Fig. 36.9). There are approximately 1 billion parietal cells in the stomach, which secrete hydrochloric acid (HCl) and intrinsic factor. The two major functions of gastric acid are to chemically breakdown and disinfect ingested food. Intrinsic factor is necessary for the

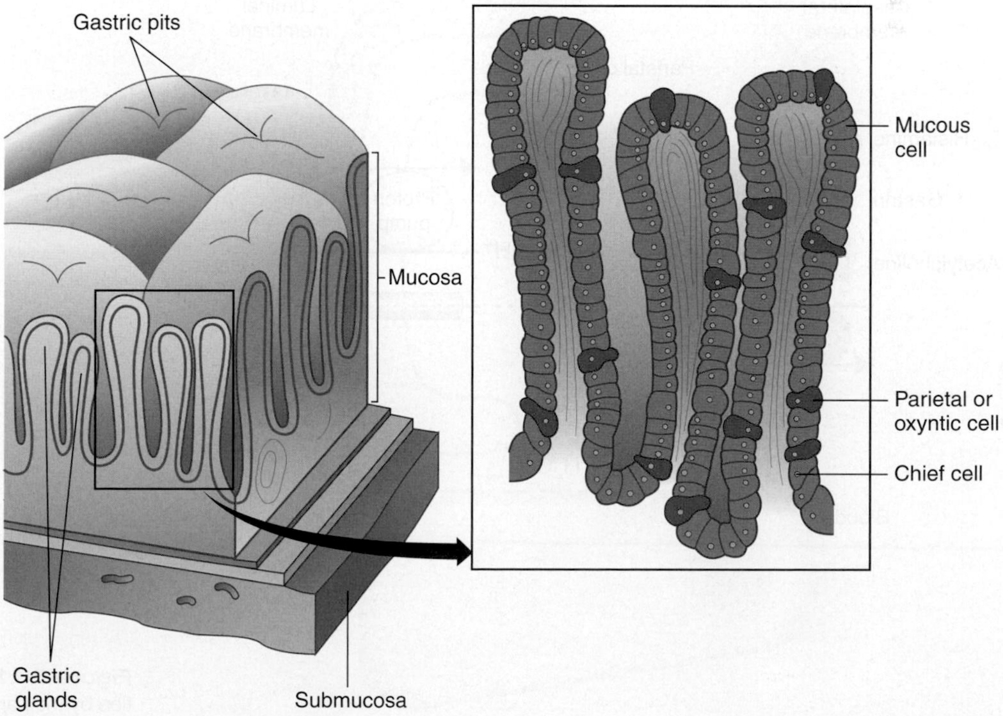

Figure 36.9 • Gastric pit from body of the stomach.

absorption of vitamin B_{12}.[1] The chief cells secrete pepsinogen, which is converted rapidly to pepsin when exposed to the low pH of the gastric juices. Pepsin is an enzyme that initiates proteolysis or breakdown of proteins. The antrum is located in the distal 20% of the stomach. This area contains the G cells, which secrete gastrin.[1]

Together, the epithelial, parietal, chief, and G cells within the stomach mucosa produce and secrete approximately 20 mEq of HCl in several hundred milliliters of gastric secretions (or gastric juices) each hour.

Gastric Acid Secretion. The cellular mechanism for HCl secretion by the parietal cells in the stomach involves the hydrogen (H^+)/potassium (K^+) adenosine triphosphatase (ATPase) transporter and chloride (Cl^-) channels located on their luminal membrane[1] (Fig. 36.10). During the process of HCl secretion, carbon dioxide (CO_2) produced by aerobic metabolism combines with water (H_2O), catalyzed by carbonic anhydrase, to form carbonic acid (H_2CO_3), which dissociates into H^+ and bicarbonate (HCO_3^-). The H^+ is secreted with Cl^- into the stomach, and the HCO_3^- moves out of the cell and into blood from the basolateral membrane. The absorbed HCO_3^- is responsible for the alkaline tide (increased pH) that occurs after a meal. At the luminal side of the membrane, H^+ is secreted into the stomach by the H^+/K^+-ATPase transporter (also known as the *proton pump*). Chloride follows H^+ into the stomach by diffusing through Cl^- channels in the luminal membrane. The proton pump inhibitors (*e.g.*, omeprazole), which are used in the treatment of acid reflux and peptic ulcer, inhibit gastric acid secretion by binding irreversibly to the sulfhydryl groups of the H^+/K^+-ATPase transporter.[1]

Three substances stimulate HCl secretion by the parietal cells: acetylcholine, gastrin, and histamine. Although each substance binds to different receptors on the parietal cell and has a different mechanism of action, they all serve to stimulate an increase in H^+ secretion through the H^+/K^+-ATPase transporter. Acetylcholine is released from vagal nerves innervating the stomach and binds to acetylcholine receptors on the parietal cells. Gastrin is secreted by G cells in the antrum of the stomach and reaches the parietal cells through the circulation. It binds to cholecystokinin type 2 (CCK2) receptors on the parietal cells.[9] Histamine is released from special endocrine cells in the gastric mucosa and diffuses to nearby parietal cells, where it binds to histamine-2 (H_2) receptors. H_2 receptor blockers (*e.g.*, cimetidine), used in the treatment of peptic ulcer and gastroesophageal reflux, bind to H_2 receptors and block the action of histamine on parietal cells.

Mucosal Barrier. One of the important characteristics of the gastric mucosa is resistance to the highly acidic secretions

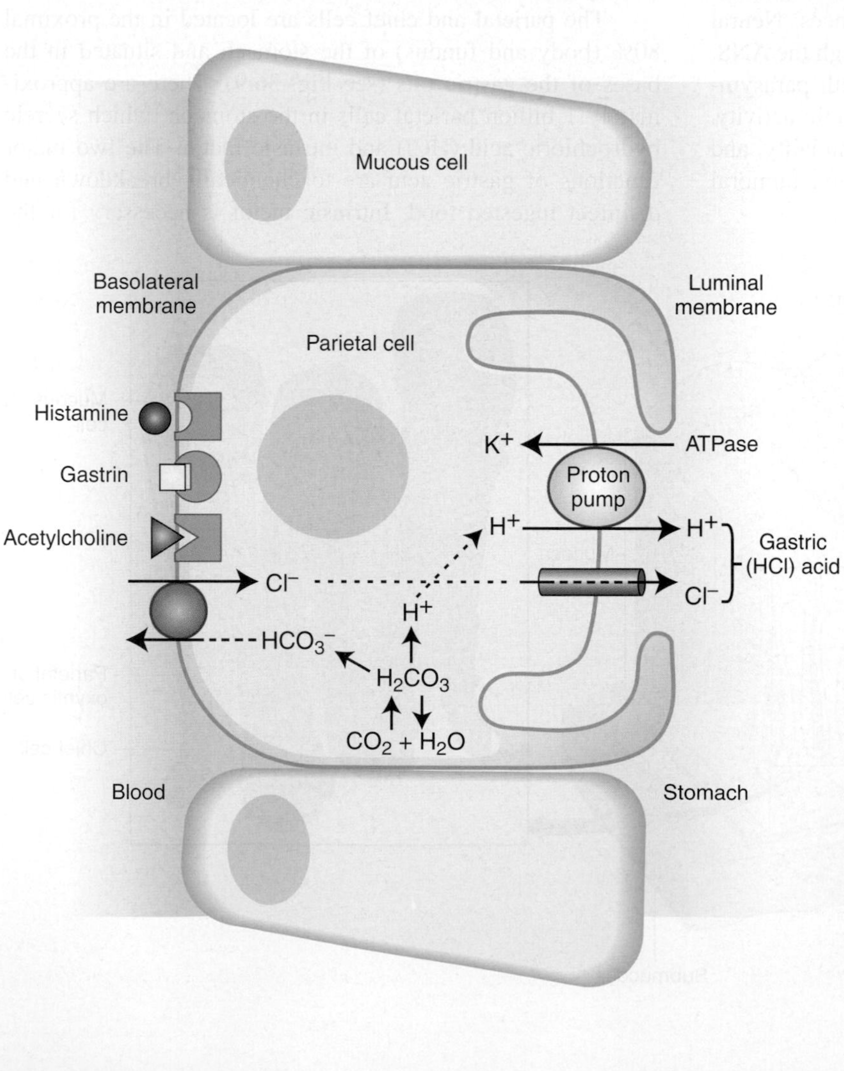

Figure 36.10 • Mechanism of gastric acid secretion by the parietal cells in the stomach.

that it produces. In contrast to the acid-stimulatory factors discussed previously, prostaglandin E_2 (after binding to its receptor) inhibits acid secretion and stimulates mucous production. Hence, it is an important factor in the maintenance of the gastric mucosal barrier.[13]

However, when aspirin, nonsteroidal anti-inflammatory drugs (NSAIDs), *Helicobacter pylori*, ethyl alcohol, or bile salts damage the gastric mucosa, this barrier is disrupted and hydrogen ions move into the tissue. As the hydrogen ions accumulate in the mucosal cells, intracellular pH decreases, enzymatic reactions become impaired, and cellular structures are disrupted. The result is local ischemia, vascular stasis, hypoxia, and tissue necrosis. The mucosal surface is further protected by prostaglandins. However, aspirin and NSAIDs inhibit prostaglandin synthesis by inhibition of cyclooxygenase (known as COX; hence, these agents are also known as COX inhibitors), which also impairs the integrity of the mucosal surface.

Intestinal Secretions

The small intestine secretes digestive juices and receives secretions from the liver and pancreas. An extensive array of mucous-producing glands, called *Brunner glands*, is concentrated at the site where the contents from the stomach and secretions from the liver and pancreas enter the duodenum. These glands secrete large amounts of alkaline mucus that protect the duodenum from the acid content in the gastric chyme and from the action of the digestive enzymes. The activity of Brunner glands is strongly influenced by ANS activity. For example, sympathetic stimulation causes a marked decrease in mucous production, leaving this area more susceptible to irritation. As a result, ulcers are four times more likely to occur in the duodenum than in the stomach.[17]

In addition to mucus, the intestinal mucosa produces two other types of secretions. The first is a serous fluid (pH 6.5 to 7.5) secreted by specialized cells (*i.e.*, crypts of Lieberkühn) in the intestinal mucosal layer. This fluid, which is produced at the rate of 2000 mL/day, acts as a vehicle for absorption.[1] The second type of secretion consists of surface enzymes that aid absorption. These enzymes are the peptidases, or enzymes that separate amino acids, and the disaccharidases, or enzymes that split sugars.

The large intestine usually secretes only mucus. ANS activity strongly influences mucous production in the bowel, as in other parts of the digestive tract. During intense parasympathetic stimulation, mucous secretion may increase to the point that the stool contains large amounts of obvious mucus. Although the bowel normally does not secrete water or electrolytes, these substances are lost in large quantities when the bowel becomes irritated or inflamed.

Intestinal Flora

The gut is the natural habitat of a large and diverse bacterial community. The major functions of the gut microflora include metabolic activities that salvage energy and absorbable nutrients, trophic effects on intestinal epithelial cells, and protection of the colonized host against invasion by pathogenic organisms.

The stomach and small intestine contain only a few species of bacteria. This is probably because of the composition of luminal contents (*i.e.*, acids, bile, pancreatic secretions), which kills most ingested microorganisms, and the propulsive movements of this area, which impedes their colonization. The large intestine, on the other hand, contains a large and complex microbial ecosystem. It has been estimated that each individual has 300 to 500 different species of intestinal bacteria, with anaerobic bacteria outnumbering aerobic bacteria by a large percentage.

Colonization of the GI tract begins shortly after birth and is influenced by passage through the birth canal and the type of diet (breast milk versus formula) the infant receives. Other environmental factors such as neonatal care, stress, pH, and immunologic status also can have an effect on the flora of infants.

The major metabolic function of colonic microflora is the fermentation of undigestible dietary residue and endogenous mucus produced by the epithelial cells. The genetic diversity of the microorganisms in the gut provides various enzymes and biochemical pathways that are distinct from those of the host. Fermentation of nondigestible carbohydrates, including resistant starches, cellulose, pectins, and unabsorbed sugars, is a major source of energy in the colon.

Colonic microorganisms also play a role in vitamin synthesis and in absorption of calcium, magnesium, and iron. The colonic flora, for example, synthesizes vitamin K. The newborn infant does not synthesize an adequate amount of vitamin K for the first week or so of life until the normal colonic bacterial flora becomes established.

The resident gut flora also provides a crucial line of resistance to colonization by exogenous microbes. Therefore, it is highly protective against invasion of tissues by pathogens. Colonization resistance also applies to opportunistic bacteria that are present in the gut but whose growth is restricted. The administration of broad-spectrum antibiotics can disrupt the microbial balance and allow overgrowth of species with potential pathogenicity, such as *Clostridium difficile*.[18]

The role of probiotics as a supplement to the normal diet and as a treatment for several disease states has become increasingly recognized. Probiotics are live microorganisms that, when ingested, can modify the composition of enteric microflora. Commonly used probiotics are lactobacilli, bifidobacteria, and nonpathogenic *Escherichia coli*.[19] Probiotics have shown value in several diseases, such as maintaining remission in ulcerative colitis.[20]

IN SUMMARY

The secretions of the GI tract include saliva, gastric juices, bile, and pancreatic and intestinal secretions. Each day, more than 7000 mL of fluid is secreted into the digestive tract. All but 50 to 200 mL of this fluid is reabsorbed.

Water, derived from the extracellular fluid compartment, is the major component of GI tract secretions. Neural, humoral, and local mechanisms contribute to the control of these secretions. The parasympathetic nervous system increases secretion, and sympathetic activity exerts an inhibitory effect. In addition to secreting fluids containing digestive enzymes, the GI tract produces and secretes hormones, such as gastrin, ghrelin, secretin, CCK, and the incretin hormones (GLP-1 and GIP), that influence appetite, GI motility, enzyme activity, and the secretions as actions of hormones such as growth hormone, insulin, and glucagon.

The gut is also the natural habitat of a large and diverse bacterial community. The major functions of the gut microflora include metabolic activities that salvage energy and absorbable nutrients, impart trophic effects on intestinal epithelial cells, and protect the colonized host against invasion by pathogenic organisms.

DIGESTION AND ABSORPTION

After completing this section of the chapter, the learner will be able to meet the following objectives:

- Differentiate digestion from absorption.
- Relate the characteristics of the small intestine to its absorptive function.
- Compare the digestion and absorption of carbohydrates, fats, and proteins.

Digestion is the process of dismantling foods into their constituent parts. Digestion requires hydrolysis, enzyme cleavage, and fat emulsification. Hydrolysis is the breakdown of a compound that involves a chemical reaction with water. The importance of hydrolysis to digestion is evidenced by the amount of water (7 to 8 L) that is secreted into the GI tract daily.[8] The intestinal mucosa is impermeable to most large molecules. Therefore, most proteins, fats, and carbohydrates must be broken down into smaller particles before they can be absorbed. Although some digestion of carbohydrates and proteins begins in the stomach, digestion takes place mainly in the small intestine. The breakdown of fats to free fatty acids and monoglycerides takes place entirely in the small intestine.[8] The liver, with its production of bile, and the pancreas, which supplies a number of digestive enzymes, play important roles in digestion.

Absorption is the process of moving nutrients and other materials from the external environment in the lumen of the GI tract into the internal environment. Absorption is accomplished by active transport and diffusion. The absorptive function of the large intestine focuses mainly on water reabsorption. A number of substances require a specific carrier or transport system. For example, vitamin B_{12} is not absorbed in the absence of intrinsic factor, which is secreted by the parietal cells of the stomach. Transport of amino acids and glucose occurs mainly in the presence of sodium. Water is absorbed passively along an osmotic gradient.

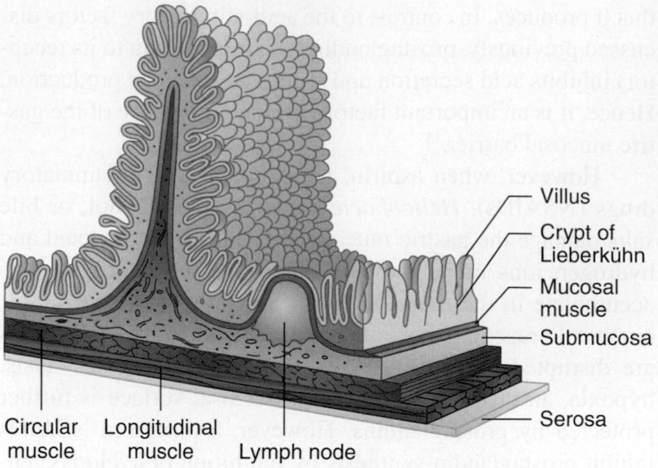

Figure 36.11 • The mucous membrane of the small intestine. Note the numerous villi on a circular fold.

The distinguishing characteristic of the small intestine is its large surface area, which in the adult is estimated to be approximately 250 m^2. Anatomic features that contribute to this enlarged surface area are the circular folds that extend into the lumen of the intestine and the villi. Villi are finger-like projections of mucous membrane, numbering as many as 25,000, which line the entire small intestine (Fig. 36.11). Each villus is equipped with an artery, vein, and lymph vessel (*i.e.*, lacteal), which bring blood to the surface of the intestine and transport the nutrients and other materials that have passed into the blood from the lumen of the intestine (Fig. 36.12). Fats rely largely on the lymphatics for absorption.

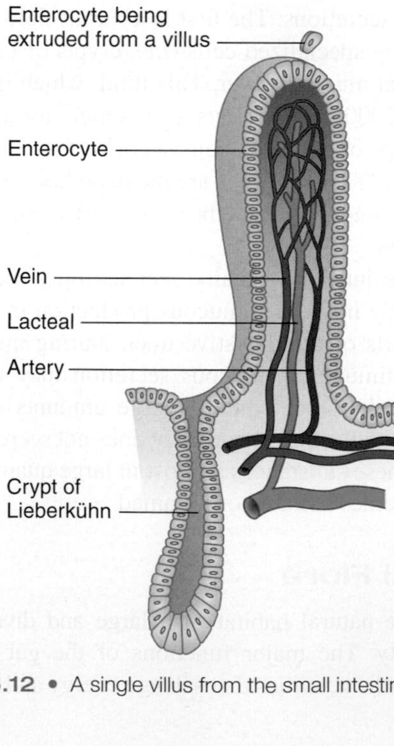

Figure 36.12 • A single villus from the small intestine.

TABLE 36.3 ENZYMES USED IN DIGESTION OF CARBOHYDRATES

DIETARY CARBOHYDRATES	ENZYME	MONOSACCHARIDES PRODUCED
Lactose	Lactase	Glucose and galactose
Sucrose	Sucrase	Fructose and glucose
Starch	Amylase	Maltose, maltotriose, and α-dextrins
Maltose and maltotriose	Maltase	Glucose and glucose
α-Dextrins	α-Dextrinase	Glucose and glucose

Each villus is covered with cells called *enterocytes* that contribute to the absorptive and digestive functions of the small bowel and goblet cells that provide mucus. The crypts of Lieberkühn are glandular structures that open into the spaces between the villi. The enterocytes have a life span of approximately 3 to 5 days.[5] It is believed that replacement cells differentiate from progenitor cells located in the area of the crypts. The maturing enterocytes migrate up the villus and eventually are extruded from the tip.

The enterocytes secrete enzymes that aid in the digestion of carbohydrates and proteins. These enzymes are called *brush border enzymes* because they adhere to the border of the villus structures. In this way, they have access to the carbohydrates and protein molecules as they come in contact with the absorptive surface of the intestine. This mechanism of secretion places the enzymes where they are needed and eliminates the need to produce enough enzymes to mix with the entire contents filling the lumen of the small bowel. The digested molecules diffuse through the membrane or are actively transported across the mucosal surface to enter the blood or, in the case of fatty acids, the lacteal. These molecules are then transported through the portal vein or lymphatics into the systemic circulation.

Carbohydrate Absorption

Carbohydrates must be broken down into monosaccharides, or single sugars, before they can be absorbed from the small intestine. The average daily intake of carbohydrate in the American diet is approximately 350 to 400 g. Starch makes up approximately 60% of this total, sucrose (*i.e.*, table sugar) approximately 30%, lactose (*i.e.*, milk sugar) approximately 10%, and maltose less than 1%.[21]

Digestion of starch begins in the mouth with the action of amylase. Pancreatic secretions also contain an amylase. Amylase breaks down starch into several disaccharides, including maltose, isomaltose, and α-dextrins. The brush border enzymes convert the disaccharides into monosaccharides that can be absorbed (Table 36.3). Sucrose yields glucose and fructose, lactose is converted to glucose and galactose, and maltose is converted to two glucose molecules. When the disaccharides are not broken down to monosaccharides, they cannot be absorbed but remain as osmotically active particles in the contents of the digestive system, causing diarrhea. People with a deficiency of lactase, the enzyme that breaks down lactose, experience diarrhea when they drink milk or eat dairy products.[8]

Fructose is transported across the intestinal mucosa by facilitated diffusion, which does not require energy expenditure. Glucose and galactose move from the intestinal lumen into the intestinal cells by way of a sodium–glucose cotransporter (SGLT-1), against a chemical gradient. The energy for this step does not come directly from adenosine triphosphate (ATP), but from the sodium gradient created by the Na^+/K^+-ATPase pump located on the basolateral side of the membrane (Fig. 36.13). Glucose and galactose are transported from

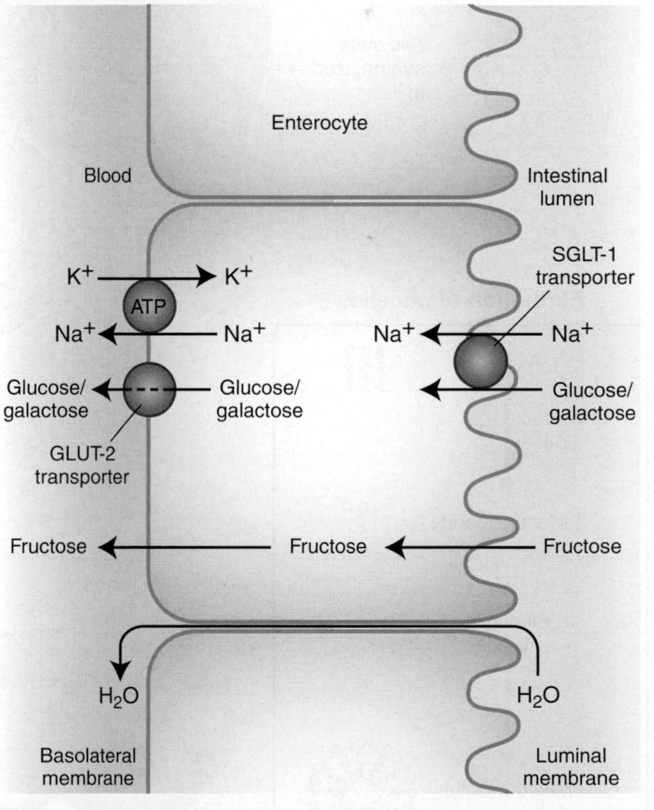

Figure 36.13 • Intestinal transport of glucose, galactose, and fructose. Glucose and galactose are transported across the apical membrane by the sodium–glucose cotransporter (SGLT-1). Glucose moves out of the intestinal cell and into the blood using a glucose transporter-2 (GLUT-2) protein. Sodium is transported out of the cell by the Na^+/K^+-ATPase sodium pump. This creates the gradient needed to operate the transport system. Fructose is passively transported across the apical and basolateral membranes of the intestinal cell.

the cell into the blood across the basolateral membrane by facilitated diffusion using a glucose transporter-2 (GLUT-2) protein. Water absorption from the intestine is linked to absorption of osmotically active particles, such as glucose and sodium.[4] It follows that an important consideration in facilitating the transport of water across the intestine (and decreasing diarrhea) after temporary disruption in bowel function is to include sodium and glucose in the fluids that are consumed.

Fat Absorption

The average adult eating a Western diet consumes approximately 120 to 140 g of fat daily, principally as triglycerides. The first step in digestion of lipids is to break the large globules of dietary fat into smaller sizes so that water-soluble digestive enzymes can act on the surface molecules. This process, which is called *emulsification*, begins in the stomach with agitation of the globules and continues in the duodenum under the influence of bile from the liver (Fig. 36.14). Emulsification greatly increases the number of triglyceride molecules exposed to pancreatic lipase, which splits triglycerides into free fatty acids and monoglycerides. Bile salts play an additional role by forming micelles that transport these substances to the surface of the intestinal villi. Here, they are taken into the epithelial cells and used to form new triglycerides. Water-soluble triglycerides, called chylomicrons, are formed and then released into the lymphatic system.[4] Small quantities of short- and medium-chain fatty acids are absorbed directly into the portal blood rather than being converted into triglycerides and absorbed by way of the lymphatics.

Fat that is not absorbed in the intestine is excreted in the stool. *Steatorrhea* is the term used to describe fatty stools. Laboratory tests involve measuring the amount of fat contained in a 72-hour stool collection during which time the person is instructed to consume 50 to 150 g of fat per day. More than 6 g of fat per 24 hours is significant for poor absorption.[22]

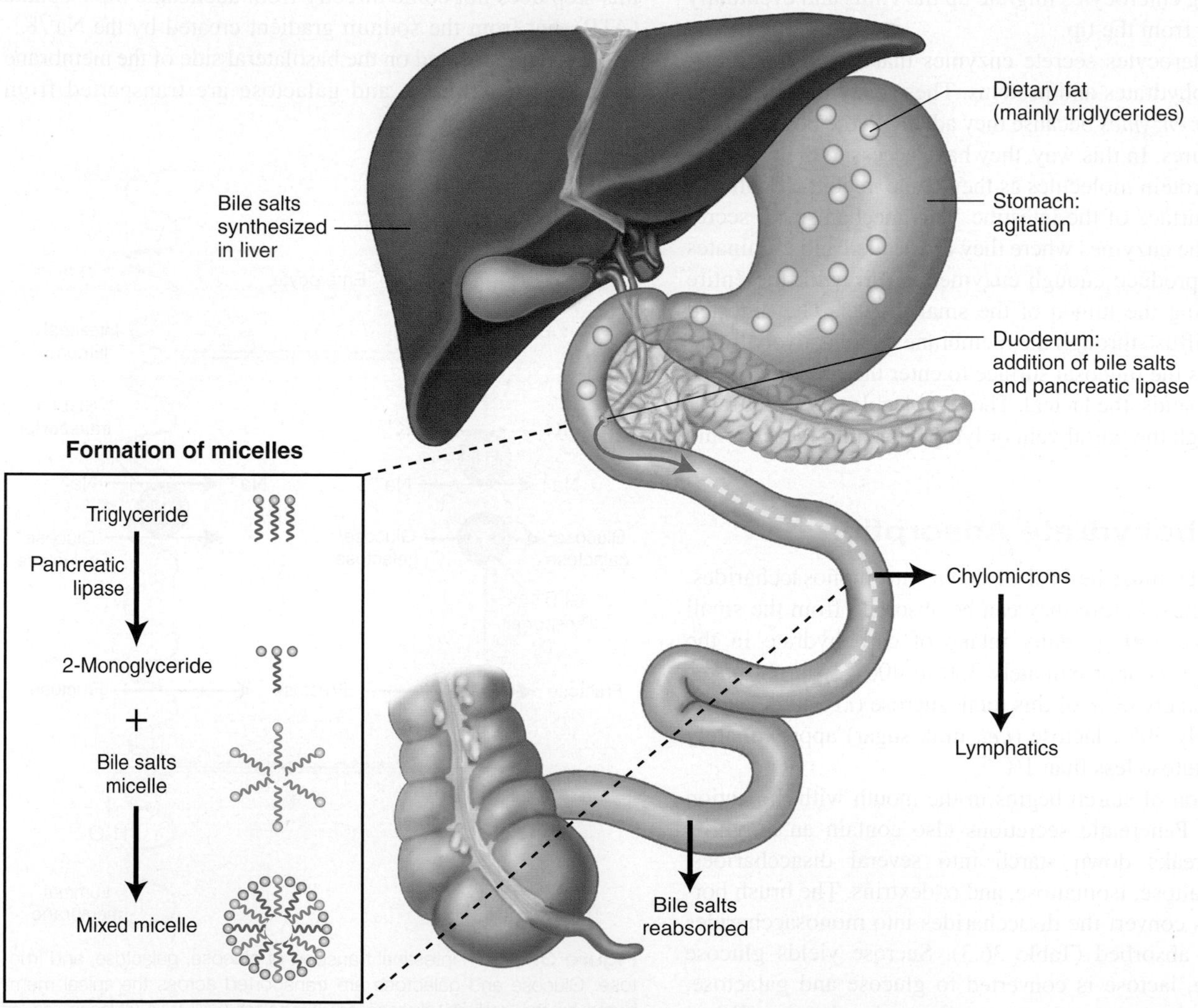

Figure 36.14 • Mechanisms of dietary fat absorption. During digestion, agitation in the stomach and bile from the liver break large globules of dietary fat into small sizes that facilitate the action of pancreatic lipase in splitting triglycerides into free fatty acids and monoglycerides (glycerol with one fatty acid chain attached). Bile salts also facilitate formation of micelles that transport the monoglycerides and free acids to the intestinal mucosa, where they are absorbed and converted to chylomicrons for transport in the lymphatic channels.

Protein Absorption

Protein digestion begins in the stomach with the action of pepsin. In response to a meal and acid pH, the chief cells secrete pepsinogen, the enzyme precursor of pepsin. Pepsin is inactivated when it enters the intestine by the alkaline pH.

Proteins are broken down further by pancreatic enzymes, such as trypsin, chymotrypsin, carboxypeptidase, and elastase. As with pepsin, the pancreatic enzymes are secreted as precursor molecules. An enzyme located on the brush border cells of the duodenal enterocytes activates trypsinogen, which lacks enzymatic activity. Activated trypsin activates additional trypsinogen molecules and other pancreatic precursor proteolytic enzymes. The amino acids are then liberated on the surface of the mucosal surface of the intestine by brush border enzymes that degrade proteins into peptides that are one, two, or three amino acids long. Similar to glucose, many amino acids are transported across the mucosal membrane in a sodium-linked process that uses ATP as an energy source. Facilitated diffusion processes that do not require sodium absorb some amino acids.[4]

IN SUMMARY

The digestion and absorption of foods take place mainly in the small intestine. Digestion is the process of dismantling foods into their constituent parts. Digestion requires hydrolysis, enzyme cleavage, and fat emulsification. Proteins, fats, carbohydrates, and other components of the diet are broken down into molecules that can be transported from the intestinal lumen into the body fluids. Absorption is the process of moving nutrients and other materials from the external environment of the GI tract into the internal environment. Brush border enzymes break carbohydrates into monosaccharides that can be transported across the intestine into the bloodstream. The digestion of proteins begins in the stomach with the action of pepsin and is further facilitated in the intestine by the pancreatic enzymes, such as trypsin, chymotrypsin, carboxypeptidase, and elastase. Enzymes that break down proteins are released as proenzymes that are activated in the GI tract. The absorption of glucose and amino acids is facilitated by a sodium-dependent transport system. Fat in the diet is broken down by pancreatic lipase into triglycerides containing medium- and long-chain fatty acids. Bile salts form micelles that transport these substances to the surface of intestinal villi, where they are absorbed.

THE GASTROINTESTINAL IMMUNITY

After completing this section of the chapter, the learner will be able to meet the following objectives:

- Describe the role of the gastrointestinal system in immunity.
- Compare the contribution of each immune cell located in the gastrointestinal system.

The GI system plays a central role in immune system homeostasis.[23] It is the main route of contact with the external environment and is overloaded every day with external stimuli. These stimuli are sometimes dangerous—pathogens (bacteria, protozoa, fungi, viruses) or toxic substances—and, in other cases very useful—food or commensal flora. The crucial position of the GI system is testified by the huge amount of immune cells that reside within it.[24]

Immune Barrier

The surface area of the GI tract is estimated to be about 32 m^2, or about half a badminton court.[25] With such a large exposure, these immune components function to prevent pathogens from entering the blood and lymph circulatory systems.[26] Fundamental components of this protection are provided by the intestinal mucosal barrier, which is composed of physical, biochemical, and immune elements elaborated by the intestinal mucosa.[27] Low pH (ranging from 1 to 4) of the stomach is fatal for many microorganisms that enter it.[28] Similarly, mucus (containing IgA antibodies) neutralizes many pathogenic microorganisms.[29]

Gut-associated lymphoid tissue (GALT) is a component of the mucosa-associated lymphoid tissue (MALT), which works in the immune system to protect the body from invasion in the gut.[30] The GALT lies throughout the intestine, covering an area of approximately 260 to 300 m^2,[25] and consists of isolated or aggregated lymphoid follicles forming Peyer patches.[31] The number of lymphocytes in the GALT is roughly equivalent to those in the spleen, and based on location, these cells are distributed in three basic populations.

Peyer Patches

These are lymphoid follicles similar in many ways to lymph nodes, located in the mucosa and extending into the submucosa of the small intestine, especially the ileum. In adults, B lymphocytes predominate in Peyer patches. Smaller lymphoid nodules can be found throughout the intestinal tract (see Fig. 36.15).

Lamina Propria Lymphocytes

The lamina propria is a thin layer of connective tissue that forms part of the moist linings known as mucous membranes or mucosa. The normal intestinal lamina propria contains B cells, T cells, and numerous innate immune cells, including dendritic cells, macrophages, eosinophils, and mast cells. IgA-producing plasma cells predominate throughout the length of the intestine.[32]

Intraepithelial Lymphocytes

These are lymphocytes that are positioned in the basolateral spaces between luminal epithelial cells, beneath the tight junctions. Unlike other T cells, intraepithelial lymphocytes do not need priming. Upon encountering antigens, they

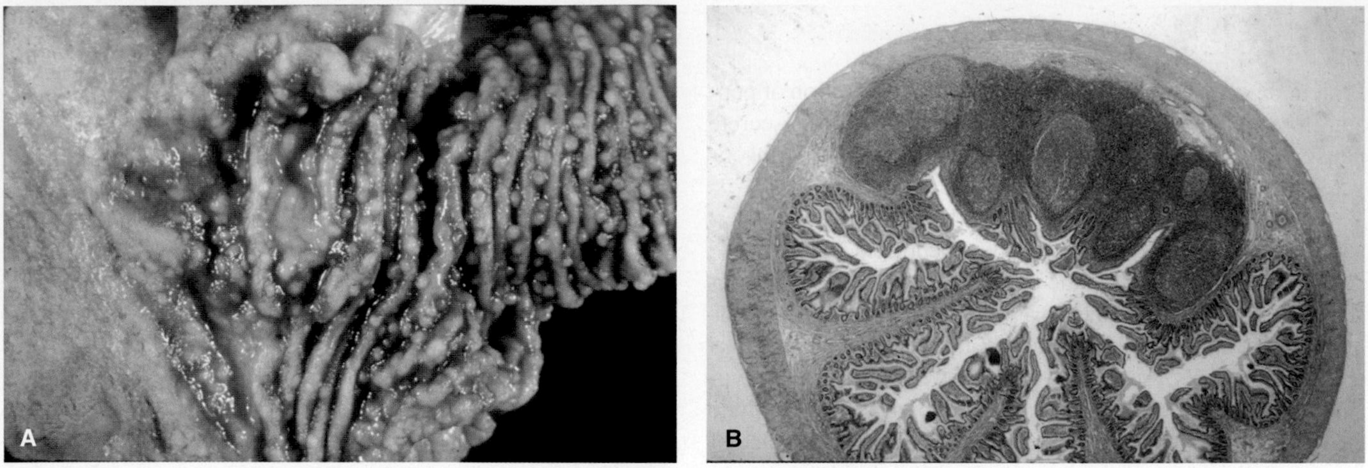

Figure 36.15 • **(A) Peyer patches** are particularly prominent in the terminal ileum; they are small dome-shaped mucosal mounds. **(B)** The Peyer patch is composed of lymphoid tissue, often with prominent germinal centers, displacing the epithelial structure. (From Strayer D. S., Rubin E. (2015). *Rubin's pathology: Clinicopathologic foundations of medicine* (7th ed.). Philadelphia: Wolters Kluwer (Fig. 19.38, p. 778).)

immediately release cytokines and cause killing of infected target cells.[33]

Microfold Cells

Another important component of the GI immune system is the M or microfold cell. M cells are a specific cell type in the intestinal epithelium over lymphoid follicles that endocytose a variety of protein and peptide antigens. Unlike their neighbor cells, M cells have the unique ability to take up antigen from the lumen of the small intestine via endocytosis, phagocytosis, or transcytosis and transport them into the underlying tissue, where they are taken up by local delivered to antigen-presenting cells (APCs), such as dendritic cells, B lymphocytes, and macrophages.[34]

Antigen-Presenting Cells

APCs, such as dendritic cells and macrophages, that receive antigens from M cells present them to T cells in the GALT, leading ultimately to appearance of IgA-secreting plasma cells in the mucosa. These antibodies are released into the gut mucosa, salivary glands, and lymph nodes. In females who are lactating, M cells recognize antigen and IgA is directed from the gut to the mammary gland. IgA traveling from the gut to breast milk supply is controlled by hormones, chemokines, and cytokines. Thus, the mammary gland and breast milk have critical roles alongside M cells in mucosal immune system.[35]

T Cells

T cells exposed to antigen in Peyer patches also migrate into the lamina propria and the epithelium, where they mature to cytotoxic T cells, providing another mechanism for containing microbial assaults. In addition, lymph nodes that receive lymph draining from the mesenteric lymph nodes and intestinal macrophages play important roles in protecting the body against invasion.[23]

IN SUMMARY

The gastrointestinal immunity system plays a vital role in protection against a host of pathogens. The size of the GI tract alone allows the pathogens to be exposed to a large area that serves as a barrier along with a vast number of immune cells. The Peyer patch, which is part of the lymphatic system formed by the GALT, has the ability to monitor and destroy pathogens. M cells have the ability to take up antigens from the small intestines, where they can be delivered to immune cells, producing an immune response. The T cell is another important cell type found in the Peyer patches; these mature into cytotoxic T cells and T helper cells, signaling the immune system to attack pathogens.

GERIATRIC Considerations

- Slower motility in the large intestine associated with aging contributes to indigestion and constipation.[36]
- A decrease in vitamin B_{12} absorption increases the risk for pernicious anemia.[36]
- A reduction in saliva, ptyalin, and amylase, along with tooth loss and injury, makes swallowing and chewing difficult.[36]

PEDIATRIC Considerations

- The submucosal lymphoid tissue in the appendix is exceptionally dynamic in children.[37]
- When the normal sequencing of innervation of the colon is disrupted, distal obstruction results in Hirschsprung disease.[37]
- The muscle tone of the lower esophageal sphincter is not fully developed until 1 month of age, resulting in regurgitation of stomach contents in infants.[38]
- Stomach capacity increases from 10 to 20 ml in the newborn to 200 ml by 2 months of age.[38]
- HCl, which aids in digestion, reaches adult levels by 6 months of age.[38]
- The liver is easily palpated in infancy because of its large size at birth.[38]

REVIEW EXERCISES

1. People receiving chemotherapeutic agents, which interfere with mitosis of cancer cells as well as the cells of other rapidly proliferating tissues in the body, often experience disorders such as ulcerations in the mucosal tissues of the mouth and other parts of the GI tract. These disorders are resolved once the chemotherapy treatment has been completed.
   A. *Explain.*
2. People with gastroesophageal reflux (movement of gastric contents into the esophagus) often complain of heartburn that becomes worse as the pressure in the stomach increases.
   A. *Use information on hormonal control of gastric emptying to explain why eating a meal that is high in fat content often exaggerates the problem.*
3. Infections of the GI tract often cause profound diarrhea.
   A. *Describe the neural mechanisms involved in the increase in GI motility that produces the diarrhea.*
   B. *Explain the rationale for using a "drink" that contains both glucose and sodium to treat the fluid deficit that often occurs with diarrhea.*
4. Explain the physiologic mechanisms associated with the occurrence of diarrhea in people with:
   A. *Lactase deficiency*
   B. *Obstruction of bile flow into the intestine*
   C. *Disruption of the normal intestinal flora because of antibiotic therapy*

References

1. Binder H. J. (2016). Gastric function. In Boron F. W., Boulpaep E. L. (Eds.) *Medical physiology* (3rd ed., pp. 863–878). Philadelphia, PA: Saunders Elsevier.
2. Tortora G. J., Derrickson B. (2013). *Principles of anatomy and physiology* (14th ed., pp. 1004–1013). Hoboken, NJ: Wiley.
3. Kapoor V. K. (2016). Gest. In Thomas R. (Ed.) *Upper GI tract anatomy*. Available: Medscape. WebMD LLC. Accessed June 26, 2016.
4. Patton K. T., Thibodeau G. A. (2015). *Anatomy & physiology* (9th ed., pp. 848–856). St. Louis, MO: Mosby Elsevier.
5. Ross M. H., Pawlina W. (2015). *Histology: A text and atlas* (7th ed., pp. 568–624). Philadelphia, PA: Lippincott Williams & Wilkins.
6. Hall J. E. (2015). *Guyton and Hall: Textbook of medical physiology* (13th ed., pp. 753–772). Philadelphia, PA: Saunders Elsevier.
7. Richerson G. B. (2016). The autonomic nervous system. In Boron F. W., Boulpaep E. L. (Eds.) *Medical physiology* (3rd ed., pp. 356–359). Philadelphia, PA: Saunders Elsevier.
8. Barrett K. M., Barman S. M., Boitano S., et al. (2015). *Ganong's review of medical physiology* (25th ed.). New York, NY: McGraw Hill. Available: http://www.accessmedicine.com. Accessed Jan 8, 2018.
9. Koeppen B. M., Stanton B. (Eds.) (2017). *Berne & Levy: Physiology* (7th ed., pp. 511–519). St. Louis, MO: Mosby.
10. Hasler W. L. (2015). The physiology of gastric motility and gastric emptying. In Yamada T. (Ed.) *Textbook of gastroenterology* (6th ed., pp. 207–230). Hoboken, NJ: Wiley-Blackwell.
11. Glasgow R. E., Mulvihill S. J. (2015). Surgery for peptic ulcer disease and postgastrectomy syndromes. In Yamada T. (Ed.) *Textbook of gastroenterology* (6th ed., pp. 1060–1063). Hoboken, NJ: Wiley-Blackwell.
12. Howick K., Griffin B., Cryan J., et al. (2017). From belly to brain: Targeting the ghrelin receptor in appetite and food intake regulation. *International Journal of Molecular Sciences* 18, 273.
13. Del Valle J., Todisco A. (2015). Gastric secretion. In Yamada T. (Ed.) *Textbook of gastroenterology* (6th ed., pp. 284–329). Hoboken, NJ: Wiley-Blackwell.
14. Irwin N., Flatt P. R. (2013). Enteroendocrine hormone mimetics for the treatment of obesity and diabetes. *Current Opinion in Pharmacology* 13(6), 989–995.
15. Keely S. J., Montrose M. H., Barrett K. E. (2015). Electrolyte secretion and absorption: Small intestine and colon. In Yamada T. (Ed.) *Textbook of gastroenterology* (6th ed., pp. 330–367). Hoboken, NJ: Wiley-Blackwell.
16. de Graaf C., Donnelly C., Wootten D., et al. (2016). Glucagon-like peptide-1 and its class B G protein-coupled receptors: A long march to therapeutic successes. *Pharmacological Reviews* 68(4), 954–1013. doi:10.1124/pr.115.011395.
17. Turner J. R. (2014). The gastrointestinal tract. In Kumar V., Abbas A. K., Fausto N., et al. (Eds.) *Robbins and Cotran pathologic basis of disease* (9th ed., pp. 780–781). Philadelphia, PA: Saunders Elsevier.
18. Elena P. C. A., Andrés M., José G. M., et al. (2015). Colonization resistance of the gut microbiota against Clostridium difficile. *Antibiotics* 4(3), 337.
19. McClain C. J., Dryden G. W., Krueger K. (2015). In Yamada T. (Ed.) *Textbook of gastroenterology* (6th ed., pp. 2844–2862). Hoboken, NJ: Wiley-Blackwell.
20. Shen J., Zuo Z. X., Mao A. P. (2014). Effect of probiotics on inducing remission and maintaining therapy in ulcerative colitis, Crohn's disease, and pouchitis: Meta-analysis of randomized controlled trials. *Inflammatory Bowel Diseases* 20(1), 21–35.
21. Keim N. L., Levin R. L., Havel P. J. (2012). Carbohydrates. In Shils M. E., Shike M., Ross A. K., et al. (Eds.) *Modern nutrition in health and disease* (12th ed., pp. 62–82). Baltimore, MD: Lippincott Williams & Wilkins.
22. Chernecky C. C., Berger B. J. (2012). *Laboratory test and diagnostic procedures* (6th ed.). Philadelphia, PA: Saunders Elsevier.
23. Mowat A. M., Agace W. W. (2014). Regional specialization within the intestinal immune system. *Nature Reviews Immunology* 14(10), 667–685.

24. Peterson L. W., Artis D. (2014) Intestinal epithelial cells: Regulators of barrier function and immune homeostasis. *Nature Reviews Immunology* 14, 141–153.
25. Helander H. F., Fändriks L. (2014). Surface area of the digestive tract-revisited. *Scandinavian Journal of Gastroenterology* 49(6), 681–689.
26. Flannigan K. L., Geem D., Harusato A., et al. (2015). Intestinal antigen-presenting cells: Key regulators of immune homeostasis and inflammation. *The American Journal of Pathology* 185(7), 1809–1819.
27. Sánchez de Medina F., Romero-Calvo I., Mascaraque C., et al. (2014). Intestinal inflammation and mucosal barrier function. *Inflammatory Bowel Diseases* 20(12), 2394–2404.
28. Schubert M. L. (2014). Gastric secretion. *Current Opinion in Gastroenterology* 30(6), 578–582.
29. Márquez M., Fernández Gutiérrez Del Álamo C., Girón-González J. A. (2016). Gut epithelial barrier dysfunction in human immunodeficiency virus-hepatitis C virus coinfected patients: Influence on innate and acquired immunity. *World Journal of Gastroenterology* 22(4), 1433–1448.
30. McGhee J. R., Fujihashi K. (2012). Inside the mucosal immune system. *PLoS Biology* 10(9), e1001397. doi: 10.1371/journal.pbio.1001397.
31. Bonnardel J., et al. (2015). Innate and adaptive immune functions of Peyer's patch monocyte-derived cells. *Cell Reports* 11, 770–784. doi: 10.1016/j.celrep.2015.03.067.
32. Society for Mucosal Immunology. (2012). Lymphocyte populations within the Lamina Propria. In Smith P. D., MacDonald T. T., Blumberg R. S. (Eds.) *Principles of mucosal immunology* (1st ed., Chapter 7, pp. 87–101). London/New York: Garland Science.
33. Schuppan D., Dieterich W. (2016). Pathogenesis, epidemiology, and clinical manifestations of celiac disease in adults. In Gorver S. (Ed.), *UpToDate*. Available: https://www-uptodate-com./contents/pathogenesis-epidemiology-and-clinical-manifestations-of-celiac-disease-in-adults?source=history_widget. Accessed March 5, 2018.
34. Mabbott N. A., Donaldson D. S., Ohno H., et al. (2013). Microfold (M) cells: Important immunosurveillance posts in the intestinal epithelium. *Mucosal Immunology* 6, 666–677. doi: 10.1038/mi.2013.30.
35. Milligan L. (2013). From mother's gut to milk. SPLASH! Milk science update. Available: http://milkgenomics.org/issue/splash-milk-science-update-september-2017. Accessed September 2017.
36. Hinkle J. L., Cheever K. H. (2018). *Brunner & Suddarth's textbook of medical-surgical nursing* (14th ed.). Philadelphia: Wolters Kluwer.
37. Strayer D. S., Rubin E. (2015). *Rubin's pathology: Clinicopathologic foundations of medicine* (7th ed.). Philadelphia: Wolters Kluwer.
38. Kyle T., Carman S. (2017). *Essentials of pediatric nursing* (3rd ed.). Philadelphia: Wolters Kluwer.

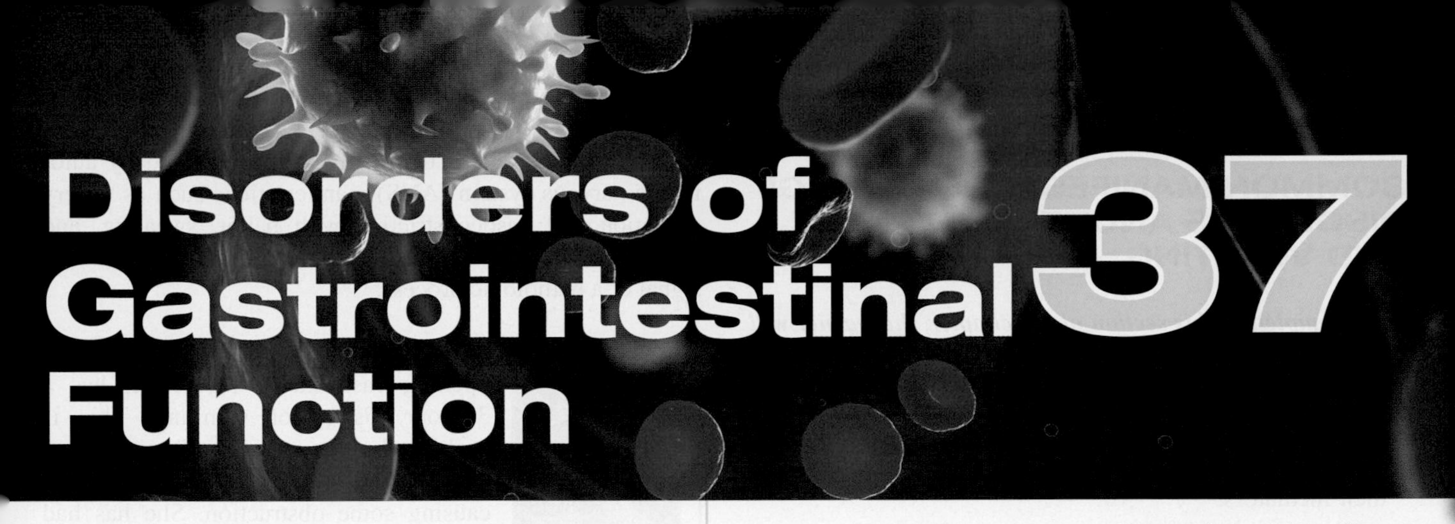

Disorders of Gastrointestinal Function

37

Freddy W. Cao

Gastrointestinal (GI) disorders do not receive the same publicity in the health-related media as heart disease, cancer, and cerebrovascular disease. In 2014, GI disease was not among the top 10 causes of death in the United States.[1] However, GI disease has a profound effect on those who suffer from it. According to government reports, digestive diseases rank third in the total economic burden of illness, resulting in considerable human suffering, personal expenditures for treatment, and lost working hours, as well as a drain on the nation's economy. It has been estimated that 60 to 70 million people in the United States have a digestive disease. Spending on GI diseases in the United States has been estimated at $142 billion per year in direct and indirect costs.[2] Even more important is the fact that proper nutrition or a change in health practices could prevent or minimize many of these disorders.

Disruption in structure and function can occur at any level of the GI tract, from the esophagus to the colon and rectum. This chapter is divided into four sections:

1. Common manifestations of GI disorders
2. Disorders of the esophagus
3. Disorders of the stomach
4. Disorders of the small and large intestines

Disorders of the hepatobiliary system and exocrine pancreas are discussed in Chapter 38.

COMMON MANIFESTATIONS OF GI DISORDERS ANOREXIA, NAUSEA, AND VOMITING

After completing this section of the chapter, the learner will be able to meet the following objectives:

- Characterize the relationship among anorexia, nausea, retching, and vomiting.
- Describe the neural structures involved in vomiting and their mediators.

Anorexia, nausea, and vomiting are physiologic responses that are common to many GI disorders. These responses are protective to the extent that they signal the presence of disease and, in the case of vomiting, remove noxious agents from the GI tract. However, they also can contribute to impaired intake or loss of fluids and nutrients.

Anorexia

Anorexia represents a loss of appetite. Several factors influence appetite. One is hunger, which is stimulated by contractions of the empty stomach. The hypothalamus and other associated centers in the brain regulate appetite or the desire for food intake. Smell plays an important role, as evidenced by the fact that appetite can be stimulated or suppressed by the smell of food. Loss of appetite is associated with emotional factors, such as fear, depression, frustration, and anxiety. Many drugs and disease states cause anorexia. For example, in uremia, the accumulation of nitrogenous wastes in the blood contributes to the development of anorexia. Anorexia often is a forerunner of nausea, and most conditions that cause nausea and vomiting also produce anorexia.

Many people refer to anorexia as anorexia nervosa, which is an eating disorder characterized by low weight, fear of gaining weight, and a strong desire to be thin, resulting in food restriction. People with anorexia nervosa perceive themselves as overweight even though they are underweight. They usually deny that they have a problem with low weight.[3]

Nausea

Nausea is an ill-defined and unpleasant subjective sensation. It is the conscious sensation resulting from stimulation of the medullary vomiting center that often precedes or accompanies vomiting. Nausea is a nonspecific symptom, which means that it has many possible causes. Some common causes of nausea are motion sickness, dizziness, migraine, fainting, low blood sugar, gastroenteritis (stomach infection), food poisoning, or severe pain. Nausea is a side effect of many medications, including chemotherapy, and morning sickness in early pregnancy.

Nausea usually is preceded by anorexia, and stimuli such as foods and drugs that cause anorexia in small doses usually produce nausea when given in larger doses. A common cause of nausea is distention of the duodenum or upper small intestinal tract. Nausea frequently is accompanied by autonomic nervous system (ANS) manifestations such as watery salivation and vasoconstriction with pallor, sweating, and tachycardia. Nausea also may function as an early warning signal of a pathologic process.

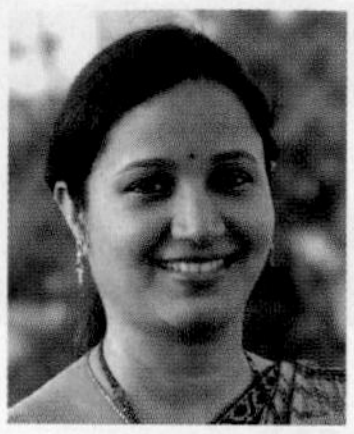

Remember **Ms. Rytel** from the unit-opening case study? Ms. Rytel has a 36-hour history of vomiting. This is probably because of some adhesions from her multiple surgeries, which may be causing some obstruction. She has had nausea and experienced tachycardia and tachypnea and her color is very pale, which are all ANS manifestations.

Retching and Vomiting

Retching consists of the rhythmic spasmodic movements of the diaphragm, chest wall, and abdominal muscles. It usually precedes or alternates with periods of vomiting. Vomiting or emesis is the sudden and forceful oral expulsion of the contents of the stomach. It usually is preceded by nausea. The contents that are vomited are called *vomitus*. Vomiting, as a basic physiologic protective mechanism, limits the possibility of damage from ingested noxious agents by emptying the contents of the stomach and portions of the small intestine. Nausea and vomiting may represent a total-body response to drug therapy, including overdose, cumulative effects, toxicity, and side effects.

Vomiting involves two functionally distinct medullary centers—the *vomiting center* and the *chemoreceptor trigger zone*.[4] The act of vomiting is thought to be a reflex that is integrated in the vomiting center, which is located in the dorsal portion of the reticular formation of the medulla near the sensory nuclei of the vagus (Fig. 37.1). The chemoreceptor trigger zone is located in a small area on the floor of the fourth ventricle, where it is exposed to both blood and cerebrospinal fluid. It is thought to mediate the emetic effects of blood-borne drugs and toxins.

The act of vomiting consists of taking a deep breath, closing the airways, and producing a strong, forceful contraction of the diaphragm and abdominal muscles along with relaxation of the gastroesophageal sphincter. Respiration ceases during the act of vomiting. Vomiting may be accompanied by dizziness, light-headedness, a decrease in blood pressure, and bradycardia.

The vomiting center receives input from the GI tract and other organs; from the cerebral cortex; from the vestibular apparatus, which is responsible for motion sickness; and from the chemoreceptor trigger zone, which is activated by many drugs and endogenous and exogenous toxins (see Fig. 37.1). Hypoxia exerts a direct effect on the vomiting center, producing nausea and vomiting. This direct effect probably accounts for the vomiting that occurs during periods of decreased cardiac output, shock, environmental hypoxia, and brain ischemia

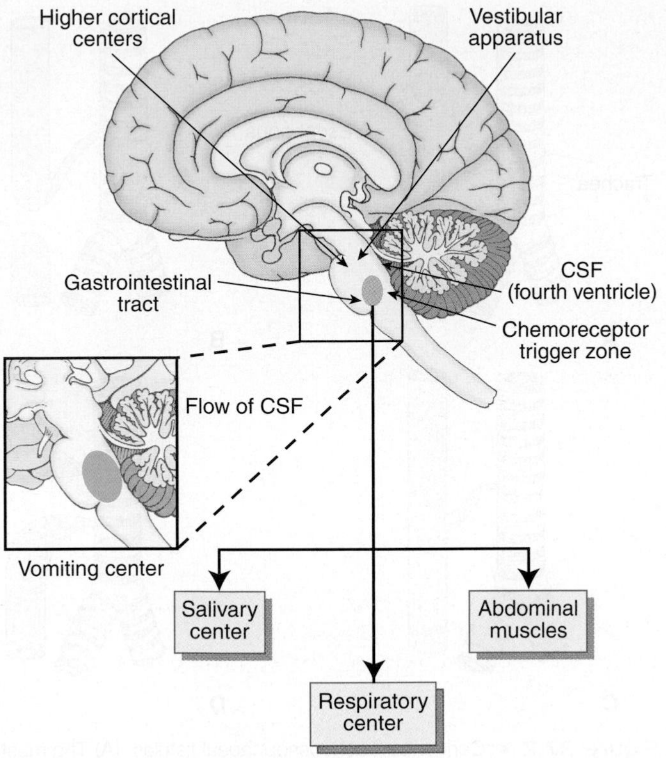

Figure 37.1 • Physiologic events involved in vomiting. CSF, cerebrospinal fluid.

caused by increased intracranial pressure. Inflammation of any of the intra-abdominal organs, including the liver, gallbladder, or urinary tract, can cause vomiting because of the stimulation of the visceral afferent pathways that communicate with the vomiting center. Distention or irritation of the GI tract also causes vomiting through the stimulation of visceral afferent neurons.

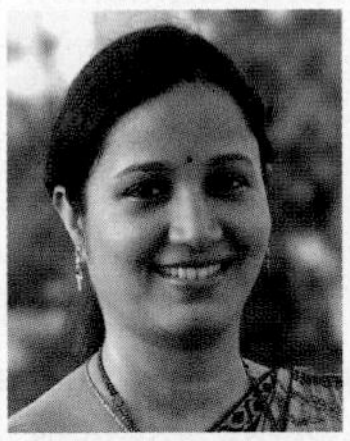

Refer back to **Ms. Rytel.** Ms. Rytel has been vomiting for 36 hours. This is most likely due to distention and irritation of the bowel caused by adhesions, which resulted from multiple surgeries. The irritation is causing persistent stimulation of the visceral afferent pathways, which are linked with the vomiting center.

Several neurotransmitters and receptor subtypes are implicated as neuromediators in nausea and vomiting. Dopamine, serotonin, and opioid receptors are found in the GI tract and in the vomiting center and chemoreceptor trigger zone. Dopamine antagonists, such as prochlorperazine, depress vomiting caused by stimulation of the chemoreceptor trigger zone. Serotonin is believed to be involved in the nausea and emesis associated with cancer chemotherapy and radiation therapy. Serotonin antagonists (*e.g.*, granisetron, ondansetron) are effective in treating the nausea and vomiting associated with these stimuli. Motion sickness appears to be a central nervous system (CNS) response to vestibular stimuli. Norepinephrine and acetylcholine receptors are located in the vestibular center. The acetylcholine receptors are thought to mediate the impulses responsible for exciting the vomiting center. Norepinephrine receptors may have a stabilizing influence that resists motion sickness. Many of the motion sickness drugs (*e.g.*, dimenhydrinate) have a strong CNS anticholinergic effect and act on the receptors in the vomiting center and areas related to the vestibular system.

IN SUMMARY

The signs and symptoms of many GI tract disorders are manifested by anorexia, nausea, and vomiting. Anorexia, or loss of appetite, may occur alone or may accompany nausea and vomiting. Nausea, which is an ill-defined, unpleasant sensation, signals the stimulation of the medullary vomiting center. It often precedes vomiting and frequently is accompanied by autonomic responses, such as salivation and vasoconstriction with pallor, sweating, and tachycardia. The act of vomiting, which is integrated by the vomiting center, involves the forceful oral expulsion of the gastric contents. It is a basic physiologic mechanism that rids the GI tract of noxious agents.

DISORDERS OF THE ESOPHAGUS

After completing this section of the chapter, the learner will be able to meet the following objectives:

- Define and cite the causes of dysphagia, odynophagia, and achalasia.
- Relate the pathophysiology of gastroesophageal reflux (GER) to measures used in the diagnosis and treatment of the disorder in adults and children.
- State the reason for the poor prognosis associated with esophageal cancer.

The esophagus is a tube that connects the oropharynx with the stomach. It lies posterior to the trachea and larynx and extends through the mediastinum, intersecting the diaphragm at the level of the 11th thoracic vertebra.

The esophagus functions primarily as a conduit for passage of food and liquid from the pharynx to the stomach. The walls of the esophagus consist of a mucosal, submucosal, muscularis externa, and adventitial layer, reflecting the general structural organization of the GI tract. The inner mucosal layer contains nonkeratinized stratified epithelium. At the esophageal–stomach junction, the abrasion-resistant epithelium changes abruptly to the simple columnar epithelium of the stomach. The submucosal layer contains mucus-secreting glands that provide the mucin-containing fluids that lubricate the esophageal wall and aid in the passage of food. The muscularis externa layer consists of skeletal muscle in the superior third of the esophagus, a mixture of skeletal and smooth muscle in its middle third, and entirely smooth muscle in its lower third. The outer fibrous adventitial layer of the esophagus is composed entirely of connective tissue, which blends with surrounding structures along its route.

There are sphincters at either end of the esophagus: an upper esophageal sphincter and a lower esophageal sphincter. The upper esophageal, or pharyngoesophageal, sphincter consists of a circular layer of striated muscle, the cricopharyngeal muscle. The lower esophageal, or gastroesophageal, sphincter is an area approximately 3 cm above the junction with the stomach. The gastroesophageal sphincter is a physiologic rather than a true anatomic sphincter. That is, it acts as a valve, but the only structural evidence of a sphincter is a slight thickening of the circular smooth muscle. The smooth muscle in this portion of the esophagus normally remains tonically constricted, creating an intraluminal pressure of about 30 mm Hg, in contrast to the midportion of the esophagus, which normally remains relaxed.[5] The lower esophageal sphincter passes through an opening, or *hiatus*, in the diaphragm as it joins with the stomach, which is located in the abdomen. The portion of the diaphragm that surrounds the lower esophageal sphincter helps to maintain the zone of high pressure needed to prevent reflux of stomach contents.

Congenital Anomalies

Congenital anomalies of the esophagus require early detection and correction because they are incompatible with life. Esophageal atresia (EA) and tracheoesophageal fistula (TEF) are very common congenital anomalies of the esophagus, affecting approximately 1 in 45,000 neonates.[6] In the most common form of EA, representing 85% of cases,[7] the upper esophagus ends in a blind pouch and the TEF is connected to the trachea (Fig. 37.2). This defect now has a survival rate greater than 90% owing largely to early recognition and improved neonatal intensive care units. Infants weighing less than 1500 g have the greatest risk for mortality, especially when combined with a cardiac anomaly.[7]

The newborn infant with EA/TEF typically has frothing and bubbling at the mouth and nose and episodes of coughing, vomiting, cyanosis, and respiratory distress. Feeding exacerbates these manifestations, causes regurgitation, and precipitates aspiration. The inability to pass a catheter into the stomach provides further evidence of the disorder. The infant with isolated TEF may develop respiratory symptoms at a later age.

Treatment of EA and TEF is surgical. Surgical ligation of the TEF and end-to-end anastomosis of the esophagus is performed when possible. Temporary ligation of the TEF and insertion of a gastrostomy tube may be used to delay the need for primary closure in preterm infants and those with more complicated lesions. The main goal of preoperative management is to maintain the airway and prevent lung damage from aspiration of gastric contents. Prone positioning minimizes movement of gastric secretions into a distal fistula, and esophageal suctioning minimizes the risk of aspiration from a blind pouch.

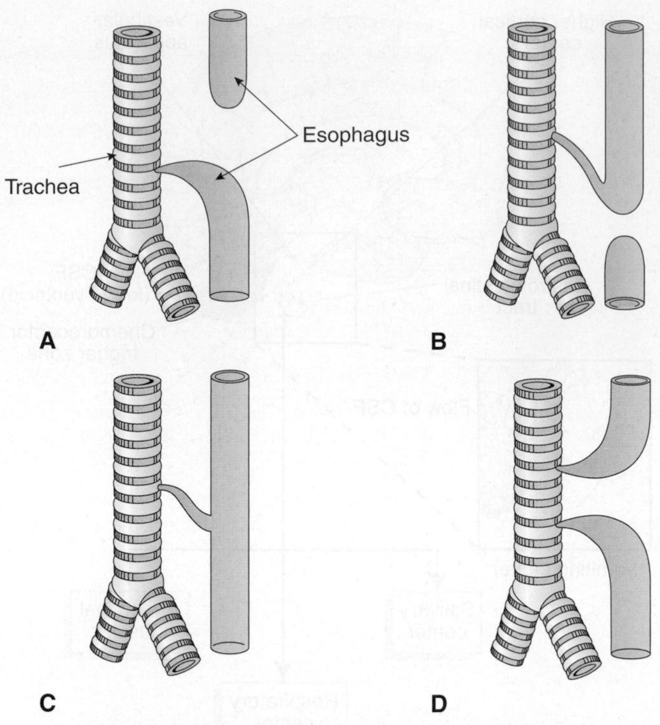

Figure 37.2 • Congenital tracheoesophageal fistulas. **(A)** The most common type (85% of cases) is a communication between the trachea and the lower portion of the esophagus. The upper segment of the esophagus ends in a blind sac. **(B)** In a few cases, the proximal esophagus communicates with the trachea. **(C)** H-type fistula without esophageal atresia, and **(D)** tracheal fistulas to both a proximal esophageal pouch and distal esophagus. (From Strayer D. S., Rubin R. (Eds.) (2015). *Rubin's pathophysiology: Clinicopathologic foundations of medicine* (7th ed., Figure 19-1, p. 753). Philadelphia, PA: Lippincott Williams & Wilkins.)

Dysphagia

The act of swallowing depends on the coordinated action of the tongue and pharynx. These structures are innervated by cranial nerves V, IX, X, and XII. Dysphagia refers to difficulty in swallowing. If swallowing is painful, it is referred to as *odynophagia*. Dysphagia can result from neuromuscular or structural causes. These disorders can produce narrowing of the esophagus, lack of salivary secretion, weakness of the muscular structures that propel the food bolus toward the stomach, or disruption of the neural networks coordinating the swallowing mechanism.[8] An example of a neuromuscular cause involves lesions of the CNS, such as a stroke, which often involve the cranial nerves that control swallowing. Cancer of the esophagus and strictures resulting from scarring, a structural cause, can reduce the size of the esophageal lumen and make swallowing difficult. Scleroderma, an autoimmune disease that causes fibrous replacement of tissues throughout the body and in the GI tract, is another important cause of dysphagia.[9] People with dysphagia usually complain of choking, coughing, or an abnormal sensation of food sticking in the back of the throat or upper chest when they swallow.

In a condition called *achalasia*, the lower esophageal sphincter fails to relax because of a disruption in the input from the enteric neural plexus and the vagus nerve.[10] This results in difficulty passing food into the stomach, and the esophagus above the lower esophageal sphincter becomes enlarged. One or several meals may lodge in the esophagus and pass slowly into the stomach over time. There is danger of aspiration of esophageal contents into the lungs when the person lies down.

Endoscopy, barium esophagoscopy, and videoradiography may be used to determine the site and extent of a swallowing disorder. Esophageal manometry, a procedure in which a small pressure-sensing catheter is inserted into the esophagus, may be done to measure pressures in different parts of the esophagus. Treatment of swallowing disorders depends on the cause and type of altered function that is present. Treatment of dysphagia often involves a multidisciplinary team of health professionals, including a speech pathologist. Mechanical dilation or surgical procedures may be done to enlarge the lower esophageal sphincter in people with esophageal strictures.

Esophageal Diverticulum

A diverticulum of the esophagus is a herniation of the esophageal wall caused by a weakness of the muscularis layer.[11] An esophageal diverticulum tends to retain food. Complaints that the food stops before it reaches the stomach are common, as are reports of gurgling, belching, coughing, and foul-smelling breath. The trapped food may cause esophagitis and ulceration. Because the condition usually is progressive, correction of the defect requires surgical intervention.

Tears (Mallory-Weiss Syndrome)

Longitudinal tears in the esophagus at the esophagogastric junction that often extend distally are termed *Mallory-Weiss tears*.[12] They are most often encountered in people with chronic alcoholism after a bout of severe retching or vomiting but may also occur during acute illness with severe vomiting. The presumed pathogenesis is inadequate relaxation of the esophageal sphincter during vomiting, with stretching and tearing of the esophageal junction at the moment of propulsive expulsion of gastric contents. Tears may involve only the mucosa or may penetrate the wall of the esophagus. Infection may lead to inflammatory ulcer or mediastinitis.

Most often bleeding is not severe and does not require surgical intervention. Severe bleeding usually responds to vasoconstrictive medications, transfusions, and balloon compression. Healing is usually prompt, with minimal or no residual effects.

Hiatal Hernia

Hiatal hernia is characterized by a protrusion or herniation of the stomach through the esophageal hiatus of the diaphragm. There are two anatomic patterns of hiatal herniation: axial, or sliding, and nonaxial, or paraesophageal.[13] The sliding hiatal hernia is characterized by a bell-shaped protrusion of the stomach above the diaphragm (Fig. 37.3). Small sliding hiatal hernias are common and considered to be of no significance in asymptomatic people. However, in cases of severe erosive esophagitis where GER and a large hiatal hernia coexist, the hernia may retard esophageal acid clearance and contribute to the more severe esophagitis, especially Barrett esophagus (to be discussed). In paraesophageal hiatal hernias, a separate portion of the stomach, usually along the greater portion of the stomach, enters the thorax through a widened opening and then progressively enlarges. In extreme cases, most of the stomach herniates into the thorax. Large paraesophageal hiatal hernias may require surgical treatment.

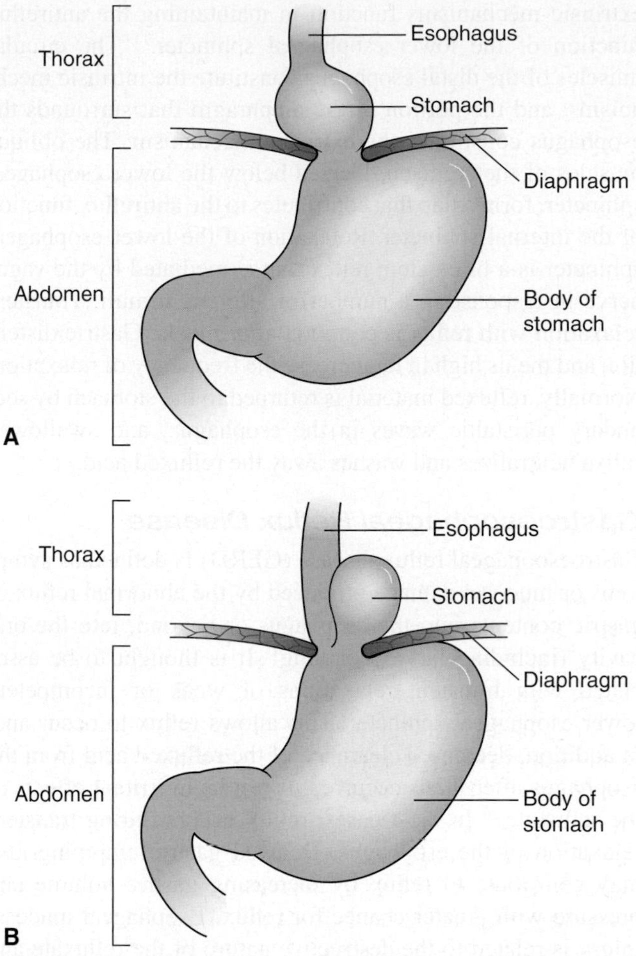

Figure 37.3 • Hiatal hernia. **(A)** Sliding hiatal hernia. **(B)** Paraesophageal hiatal hernia.

Gastroesophageal Reflux

The term reflux refers to backward or return movement. In the context of GER, it refers to the backward movement of gastric contents into the esophagus, a condition that causes heartburn or pyrosis. It probably is the most common disorder originating in the GI tract. The associated symptoms usually occur soon after eating, are short lived, and seldom cause more serious problems.

The lower esophageal sphincter regulates the flow of food from the esophagus into the stomach. Both intrinsic and extrinsic mechanisms function in maintaining the antireflux function of the lower esophageal sphincter.[14] The circular muscles of the distal esophagus constitute the intrinsic mechanisms, and the portion of the diaphragm that surrounds the esophagus constitutes the extrinsic mechanism. The oblique muscles of the stomach, located below the lower esophageal sphincter, form a flap that contributes to the antireflux function of the internal sphincter. Relaxation of the lower esophageal sphincter is a brain stem reflex that is mediated by the vagus nerve in response to a number of afferent stimuli. Transient relaxation with reflux is common after meals. Gastric distention and meals high in fat increase the frequency of relaxation. Normally, refluxed material is returned to the stomach by secondary peristaltic waves in the esophagus, and swallowed saliva neutralizes and washes away the refluxed acid.

Gastroesophageal Reflux Disease

Gastroesophageal reflux disease (GERD) is defined as symptoms or mucosal damage produced by the abnormal reflux of gastric contents into the esophagus or beyond, into the oral cavity (including larynx) or lung[15] It is thought to be associated with transient relaxations of weak or incompetent lower esophageal sphincter. This allows reflux to occur and, in addition, decreased clearance of the refluxed acid from the esophagus after it has occurred. It results in irritant effects of the refluxate.[16] In most cases, reflux occurs during transient relaxation of the esophagus. Delayed gastric emptying also may contribute to reflux by increasing gastric volume and pressure with greater chance for reflux. Esophageal mucosal injury is related to the destructive nature of the refluxate and the amount of time it is in contact with mucosa. Acidic gastric fluids ($pH < 4.0$) are particularly damaging. The GER normally is cleared and neutralized by esophageal peristalsis and salivary bicarbonate. Decreased salivation and salivary buffering capacity may contribute to impaired clearing of acid reflux from the esophagus.

GERD is a more serious and long-lasting form of GER. GER that occurs more than twice a week for a few weeks could be GERD. GERD can lead to more serious health problems over time.[17] In the Western world, between 10 and 20% of the population are affected by GERD. GERD is broadly classified into two groups on the basis of endoscopy findings: having esophageal mucosal damage (erosive esophagitis and Barrett esophagus) and no mucosal damage (endoscopy-negative reflux disease or nonerosive reflux disease, NERD).[18]

Clinical Manifestations. Heartburn and regurgitation are the characteristic symptoms of GERD. Heartburn is defined as a burning sensation in the retrosternal area. Regurgitation is defined as the perception of flow of refluxed gastric contents into the mouth or hypopharynx. It frequently is severe, occurring 30 to 60 minutes after eating. It often is made worse by bending at the waist and recumbency and usually is relieved by sitting upright. The severity of heartburn is not indicative of the extent of mucosal injury. Only a small percentage of people who complain of heartburn have mucosal injury. Often, the heartburn occurs during the night. Antacids give prompt, although transient, relief. Other symptoms include belching and chest pain. The pain usually is located in the epigastric or retrosternal area and often radiates to the throat, shoulder, or back. Because of its location, the pain may be confused with angina. The reflux of gastric contents also may produce respiratory symptoms such as asthma, chronic cough, and laryngitis, but it is important to note that the presence of these symptoms is often multifactorial in addition to the diagnosis or GERD.[18] The proposed mechanisms of reflux-associated asthma and chronic cough include microaspiration and macroaspiration, laryngeal injury, and vagal-mediated bronchospasm.

Reflux esophagitis involves mucosal injury to the esophagus, hyperemia, and inflammation. Complications, such as strictures and *Barrett esophagus*, can result from persistent reflux, which produces a cycle of mucosal damage that causes hyperemia, edema, and erosion of the luminal surface. Strictures are caused by a combination of scar tissue, spasm, and edema. They produce narrowing of the esophagus and cause dysphagia when the lumen becomes sufficiently constricted. Barrett esophagus (Fig. 37.4) refers to an abnormal change (metaplasia) in the cells of the lower portion of the esophagus characterized by a reparative process in which the squamous mucosa that normally lines the esophagus gradually is replaced by abnormal columnar epithelium resembling that in the stomach or intestines.[19] It is associated with increased risk for development of esophageal adenocarcinoma.

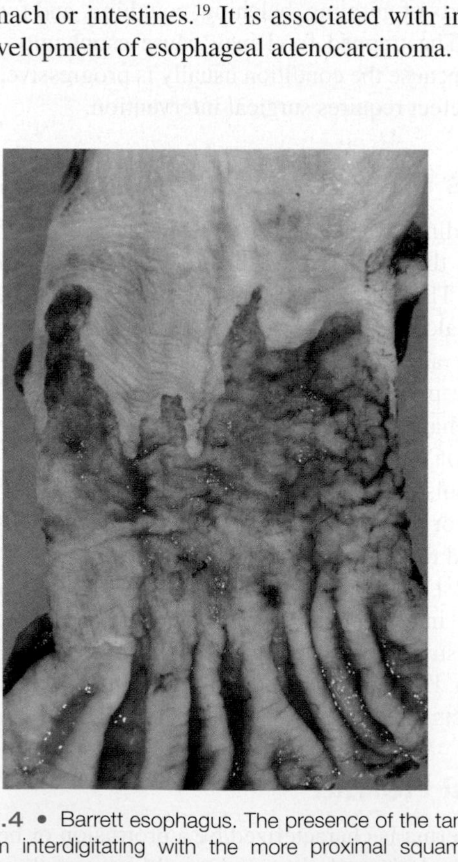

Figure 37.4 • Barrett esophagus. The presence of the tan tongues of epithelium interdigitating with the more proximal squamous epithelium is typical of Barrett esophagus. (From Strayer D. S., Rubin R. (Eds.) (2015). *Rubin's pathophysiology: Clinicopathologic foundations of medicine* (7th ed., Figure 19-6A, p. 757). Philadelphia, PA: Lippincott Williams & Wilkins.)

Diagnosis. Diagnosis of GER depends primarily on a history of reflux symptomatology and the use of optional diagnostic methods, including acid suppression trials, esophagoscopy, and ambulatory esophageal pH monitoring.[16] Acid suppression trials involve administering a proton pump inhibitor (PPI) medication for 7 to 14 days to determine if the symptoms are alleviated. Esophagoscopy involves the passage of a flexible fiberoptic endoscope into the esophagus for the purpose of visualizing the lumen of the upper GI tract. It also permits performance of a biopsy, if indicated. For 24-hour pH monitoring, a small tube with a pH electrode is passed through the nose and down into the esophagus. Data from the electrode are recorded in a small, lightweight box worn on a belt around the waist and later are analyzed by computer. The device allows the person to indicate position changes, meals, heartburn, or pain, which then can be correlated with episodes of acid reflux.

Treatment. The treatment of GER usually focuses on conservative measures. These measures include avoidance of positions and conditions that increase gastric reflux.[16] Avoidance of large meals and foods that reduce lower esophageal sphincter tone (*e.g.*, caffeine, fats, chocolate), alcohol, and smoking is recommended. It is recommended that meals be eaten sitting up and that the recumbent position be avoided for several hours after a meal. Bending for long periods should be avoided because it tends to increase intra-abdominal pressure and cause gastric reflux. Sleeping with the head elevated helps to prevent reflux during the night. This is best accomplished by placing blocks under the head of the bed or by using a wedge-shaped bolster to elevate the head and shoulders by at least 6 inches. Weight loss usually is recommended in overweight people.

Antacids or a combination of antacids and alginic acid also are recommended for mild disease. Alginic acid produces a foam when it comes in contact with gastric acid; if reflux occurs, the foam rather than acid rises into the esophagus. Histamine-2 receptor (H_2)–blocking antagonists, which inhibit gastric acid production, is another recommended treatment. The PPIs act by inhibiting the gastric proton pump, which regulates the final pathway for acid secretion. These agents may be used for people who continue to have daytime symptoms, recurrent strictures, or large esophageal ulcerations. Surgical treatment may be indicated in some people.

Gastroesophageal Reflux in Children

GER, defined as the passage of gastric contents into the esophagus, is distinguished from GERD, which includes troublesome symptoms or complications associated with GER. GER occurs in more than two thirds of otherwise healthy infants and is a topic of discussion with pediatricians at one quarter of all routine 6-month infant visits. GER is considered a normal physiologic process that occurs several times a day in healthy infants, children, and adults. GER is generally associated with transient relaxations of the lower esophageal sphincter independent of swallowing, which permits gastric contents to enter the esophagus. Less is known about the normal physiology of GER in infants and children, but regurgitation or spitting up, the most visible symptom, is reported to occur daily in 50% of all infants.[20]

The small reservoir capacity of an infant's esophagus coupled with frequent spontaneous reductions in sphincter pressure contributes to reflux. At least one episode of regurgitation a day occurs in as much as half of infants aged 0 to 3 months.[21] By 8 months of age, it becomes less frequent, and it abates by 2 years of age[21] as the child's diet naturally advances and they are able to maintain a more upright posture. Although many infants have minor degrees of reflux, complications can occur in children with more frequent or persistent episodes. The condition occurs more frequently in children with cerebral palsy, Down syndrome, cystic fibrosis, and other neurologic disorders.

In most cases, infants with simple reflux are thriving and healthy, and symptoms resolve between 9 and 24 months of age. Pathologic reflux is classified into three categories:

1. Regurgitation and malnutrition
2. Esophagitis
3. Respiratory problems

Clinical Manifestations. Symptoms of reflux vary depending on the child's age. Preadolescent children often experience heartburn, epigastric pain, abdominal pain, regurgitation, and intermittent vomiting. Infants and toddlers, however, more commonly experience regurgitation and feeding difficulties. If recurrent vomiting is accompanied by symptoms of poor weight gain, excessive crying, irritability, disturbed sleep, feeding, or respiratory problems, or if symptoms are persistent despite using a hypoallergenic formula or empirical acid suppression, then additional diagnostic tests may be required.[22] Tilting of the head to one side and arching of the back may be noted in children with severe reflux. The head positioning is thought to represent an attempt to protect the airway or reduce the pain-associated reflux. Sometimes regurgitation is associated with dental caries and recurrent otalgia. The ear pain is thought to occur through referral from the vagus nerve in the esophagus to the ear.

A variety of respiratory symptoms are caused by damage to the respiratory mucosa when gastric reflux enters the esophagus. Reflux may cause laryngospasm, apnea, and bradycardia. Asthma may co-occur with GERD in about 50% of asthmatic children.[21] Asthmatic children who are particularly likely to have GERD as a provocative factor are those with symptoms of reflux, those with refractory or steroid-dependent asthma, and those with nocturnal worsening of symptoms.[21]

Diagnosis and Treatment. Diagnosis of GER in infants and children often is based on parental and clinical observations.

Diagnostic testing is generally not necessary because it has not been found to be more reliable than the history and physical examination for diagnosing GER or GERD. Tests should be reserved for situations with atypical symptoms, warning signs, or doubts about the diagnosis; suspected complications of GERD or other conditions; or failure of initial therapies. The diagnosis may be confirmed by esophageal pH probe studies, barium fluoroscopic esophagography, and nuclear scintigraphy. In some cases, esophagoscopy may be used to demonstrate reflux and obtain a biopsy.[23]

Various treatment methods are available for infants and children with GER. Most infants, children, and adolescents who have reflux improve with conservative measures. In infants, feeding changes may reduce symptoms. For formula-fed infants, reducing feeding volumes in overfed infants, or offering smaller and more frequent feeds, may decrease reflux episodes and should be tried first. Adding thickening agents decreases observed regurgitation but does not reduce the reflux index (percentage of time the esophageal pH is <4) and can lead to excess weight gain.[23] Changing the infant's body position while awake can be effective. The prone and left-side-down positions are associated with fewer reflux episodes but should be recommended only in awake, observed infants during the postprandial period. In older infants and children, raising the head of the bed and keeping the child upright may help. Medications usually are not added to the treatment regimen until pathologic reflux has been documented by diagnostic testing. Antacids are the most commonly used antireflux therapy and are readily available over the counter. H_2-receptor antagonists and PPIs may be used in children with persistent reflux. Prokinetic agents (*e.g.*, metoclopramide, a dopamine-2 and 5-hydroxytryptamine [$5\text{-}HT_3$] receptor antagonist; bethanechol, a cholinergic agonist) are associated with significant side effects, and their use in treatment is not recommended.[23]

Cancer of the Esophagus

Carcinoma of the esophagus accounts for approximately 1% of all diagnosed cancers.[24] It is more common in adults over the age of 65 years. It occurs three times more frequently in men than women, and its occurrence is equal between African Americans and whites.[24]

There are two types of esophageal cancer: squamous cell carcinoma and adenocarcinoma. Most squamous cell esophageal carcinomas are attributable to alcohol and tobacco use. Worldwide, squamous cell carcinomas are the most common type of esophageal cancers, but in the United States, there has been a significant increase in adenocarcinomas.[25] Barrett esophagus and GERD are the two most common risk factors for esophageal adenocarcinoma.[26]

Progressive dysphagia is by far the most frequent complaint of people with esophageal cancer. It is apparent first with ingestion of bulky food, later with soft food, and finally with liquids. Unfortunately, it is a late manifestation of the disease. Unintentional weight loss, anorexia, fatigue, and pain on swallowing also may occur.

Treatment of esophageal cancer depends on tumor stage. Surgical resection provides a means of cure when done in early disease and palliation when done in late disease. Radiation may be used as an alternative to surgery. Chemotherapy may be used before surgery to decrease the size of the tumor, or it may be used along with irradiation and surgery in an effort to increase survival.[27]

The prognosis for people with cancer of the esophagus, although poor, has improved. Even with modern forms of therapy, however, the long-term survival is limited because, in many cases, the disease has already metastasized by the time the diagnosis is made.

IN SUMMARY

The esophagus is a tube that connects the oropharynx with the stomach; it functions primarily as a conduit for passage of food from the pharynx to the stomach. Although relatively uncommon, congenital anomalies (*i.e.*, EA and TEFs) must be corrected early because they cause aspiration of gastric and oral secretions and are incompatible with life. Dysphagia refers to difficulty in swallowing; it can result from altered nerve function or from disorders that produce narrowing of the esophagus. A diverticulum of the esophagus is an outpouching of the esophageal wall caused by a weakness of the muscularis layer. Longitudinal tears (Mallory-Weiss tears) at the esophagogastric junction can occur with severe bouts of retching or vomiting. They are most often encountered in people with chronic alcoholism, but may also occur during acute illness with severe vomiting. Hiatal hernia is characterized by a protrusion or herniation of the stomach through the esophageal hiatus of the diaphragm. There are two anatomic patterns of herniation: (1) the axial or sliding hiatal hernia, which is the most common type and is characterized by bell-shaped protrusion of the stomach above the diaphragm and (2) the nonaxial or paraesophageal hernia, in which a portion of the stomach enters the thorax through a widened opening.

GER refers to the backward movement of gastric contents into the esophagus, a condition that causes heartburn. Although most people experience occasional GER and heartburn, persistent reflux can result in a cycle of mucosal damage that causes hyperemia, edema, erosion luminal surface, and Barrett esophagus. Reflux can cause respiratory symptoms, including chronic cough, and serve as a potential trigger for asthma. GER is a common problem in infants and children. Reflux commonly corrects itself with age, and symptoms abate in most children by 2 years of age. Although many infants have minor degrees of reflux, some infants and small children have significant reflux that interferes with feeding, causes esophagitis, and results in respiratory symptoms and other complications.

Carcinoma of the esophagus is more common in older adults and occurs more frequently in men than women. There are two types of esophageal cancer: squamous cell carcinoma and adenocarcinoma. Most squamous cell carcinomas are attributable to alcohol and tobacco use. Adenocarcinomas are more closely linked to GER and Barrett esophagus.

DISORDERS OF THE STOMACH

After completing this section of the chapter, the learner will be able to meet the following objectives:

- Differentiate between the causes and manifestations of acute and chronic gastritis.
- Characterize the proposed role of *Helicobacter pylori* in the development of chronic gastritis and peptic ulcer and cite methods for diagnosis and treatment of the infection.
- Cite the etiologic factors in ulcer formation related to Zollinger-Ellison syndrome and stress ulcer.

The stomach is a reservoir for contents entering the digestive tract. It lies in the upper abdomen, anterior to the pancreas, splenic vessels, and left kidney. Anteriorly, the stomach is bounded by the anterior abdominal wall and the left inferior lobe of the liver. While in the stomach, food is churned and mixed with hydrochloric acid and pepsin before being released into the small intestine. Normally, the mucosal surface of the stomach provides a barrier that protects it from the hydrochloric acid and pepsin contained in gastric secretions. Disorders of the stomach include gastritis, peptic ulcer, and gastric carcinoma.

Gastric Mucosal Barrier

The stomach lining usually is impermeable to the acid it secretes, a property that allows the stomach to contain acid and pepsin without having its walls digested. Several factors contribute to the protection of the gastric mucosa, including an exceptionally tight fitting and therefore impermeable epithelial cell surface covering. This is coupled with the tenacious, thick mucus that is secreted by cells, which creates a protective covering for the inner stomach wall that also contains bicarbonates that serve to maintain a neutral pH.[5,28] These mechanisms are collectively referred to as the *gastric mucosal barrier*.

The cells of the gastric epithelia are connected by tight junctions that prevent acid penetration, and they are covered with an impermeable hydrophobic lipid layer that prevents diffusion of ionized water-soluble molecules. Aspirin is able to cross the lipid layer and cause damage to the superficial cells, which can result in acute erosions.[29] Gastric irritation and occult bleeding due to gastric irritation occur in a significant number of people who take aspirin on a regular basis. Alcohol, which like aspirin is lipid soluble, also disrupts the mucosal barrier. When aspirin and alcohol are taken in combination, the permeability of the gastric mucosal barrier is significantly increased and cellular damage occurs.[30] Bile acids also attack the lipid components of the mucosal barrier and afford the potential for gastric irritation when there is reflux of duodenal contents into the stomach.

Normally, the secretion of hydrochloric acid by the parietal cells of the stomach is accompanied by secretion of bicarbonate ions (HCO_3^-). For every hydrogen ion (H^+) that is secreted, an HCO_3^- is produced, and as long as HCO_3^- production is equal to H^+ secretion, mucosal injury does not occur. Changes in gastric blood flow, as in shock, tend to decrease HCO_3^- production. This is particularly true in situations in which decreased blood flow is accompanied by acidosis. Aspirin and the nonsteroidal anti-inflammatory drugs (NSAIDs), also impair HCO_3^- secretion by way of inhibiting gastric COX-1, a fatty acid enzyme that synthesizes prostaglandins that mediate bicarbonate secretion.[31,32]

The mucus that protects the gastric mucosa is of two types: water insoluble and water soluble.[27] Water-insoluble mucus forms a thin, stable gel that adheres to the gastric mucosal surface and provides protection from the proteolytic (protein-digesting) actions of pepsin. It also forms an unstirred layer that traps bicarbonate, forming an alkaline interface between the luminal contents of the stomach and its mucosal surface. The water-soluble mucus is washed from the mucosal surface and mixes with the luminal contents; its viscid nature makes it a lubricant that prevents mechanical damage to the mucosal surface.

Prostaglandins, chemical messengers derived from cell membrane lipids, play an important role in protecting the gastric mucosa from injury.[31] The prostaglandins are thought to exert their effect through improved mucosal blood flow, decreased acid secretion, increased bicarbonate ion secretion, and enhanced mucus production.

KEY POINTS

DISRUPTION OF THE GASTRIC MUCOSA AND ULCER DEVELOPMENT

- The stomach is protected by a mucosal barrier that prevents gastric secretions and other destructive agents from injuring the epithelial and deeper layers of the stomach wall.
- Two of the major causes of gastric irritation and ulcer formation are aspirin or NSAIDs and infection with *H. pylori*.

Gastritis

Gastritis refers to inflammation of the gastric mucosa. There are many causes of gastritis, most of which can be grouped as either acute or chronic gastritis.

Acute Gastritis

Acute gastritis is characterized by an acute mucosal inflammatory process, usually transient in nature. The inflammation may be accompanied by emesis, pain, and, in severe cases, hemorrhage and ulceration.[33] This erosive form is an important cause of acute GI bleeding. The condition is most commonly associated with local irritants such aspirin or other NSAIDs, alcohol, or bacterial toxins. Oral administration of corticosteroids may also be complicated by acute hemorrhagic gastritis. Any serious illness or trauma that is accompanied by profound physiologic stress that requires substantial medical or surgical treatment renders the gastric mucosa more vulnerable to acute hemorrhagic gastritis because of mucosal injury (discussed under stress ulcers).[13] Uremia, treatment with cancer chemotherapy drugs, and gastric radiation are other causes of acute gastritis.

The complaints of people with acute gastritis vary. People with aspirin-related gastritis can be totally unaware of the condition or may complain only of heartburn or sour stomach. Gastritis associated with excessive alcohol consumption is often a different situation; it often causes transient gastric distress, which may lead to vomiting and, in more severe situations, to bleeding and hematemesis. Gastritis caused by the toxins of infectious organisms, such as the staphylococcal enterotoxins, usually has an abrupt and violent onset, with gastric distress and vomiting ensuing approximately 5 hours after the ingestion of a contaminated food source. Acute gastritis usually is a self-limiting disorder, with complete regeneration and healing occurring within several days of removal of the inciting agent.

Chronic Gastritis

Chronic gastritis is a separate entity from acute gastritis. It is characterized by the absence of grossly visible erosions and the presence of chronic inflammatory changes, leading eventually to atrophy of the glandular epithelium of the stomach. There are types of chronic gastritis: *H. pylori*, metaplastic atrophic gastritis and chemical gastropathy.[13]

Helicobacter pylori **Gastritis.** *Helicobacter pylori* infection is the most common cause of chronic gastritis. The prevalence in the United States is associated with socioeconomic status, increased age, and Hispanic and African American ethnicity.[34] *H. pylori* is present in two thirds of the world's population.[34] It has been suggested that transmission in industrialized countries is largely person to person by vomitus, saliva, or feces, whereas additional transmission routes such as water may be important in developing countries. In industrialized countries, the rate of infection with *H. pylori* has decreased substantially over the past several decades owing to improved sanitation.

Helicobacter pylori gastritis is a chronic inflammatory disease of the antrum and body of the stomach. Chronic infection with *H. pylori* can lead to gastric atrophy and peptic ulcer and is associated with increased risk of gastric adenocarcinoma and the creation of mucosa-associated lymphoid tissue, which can progress to lymphoma.[33]

Pathogenesis. *Helicobacter pylori* are small, curved, or spiral shaped, gram-negative rods (proteobacteria) that can colonize the mucus-secreting epithelial cells of the stomach.[33] (Fig. 37.5). *H. pylori* have multiple flagella, which allow them to move through the mucous layer of the stomach, and they secrete urease, which enables them to produce sufficient ammonia to buffer the acidity of their immediate environment. These properties help to explain why the organism is able to survive in the acidic environment of the stomach. *H. pylori* produce enzymes and toxins that have the capacity to interfere with the local protection of the gastric mucosa against acid, produce intense inflammation, and elicit an immune response. There is increased production of proinflammatory cytokines (IL-6, IL-8) that serve to recruit and activate neutrophils.[35] Several *H. pylori* proteins are immunogenic, and they evoke an intense immune response in the mucosa. Both T and B cells can be seen in the chronic gastritis caused by *H. pylori*. T cells may be responsible for decreasing the constant inflammatory response caused by the cytokines, allowing *H. pylori* to maintain its colonization of the stomach for long periods of time. Although the role of T and B cells in causing epithelial injury has not been established, T-cell–driven activation of B cells may be involved in the pathogenesis of gastric lymphomas.[13]

Why some people with *H. pylori* infection develop clinical disease and others do not is unclear. Scientists are

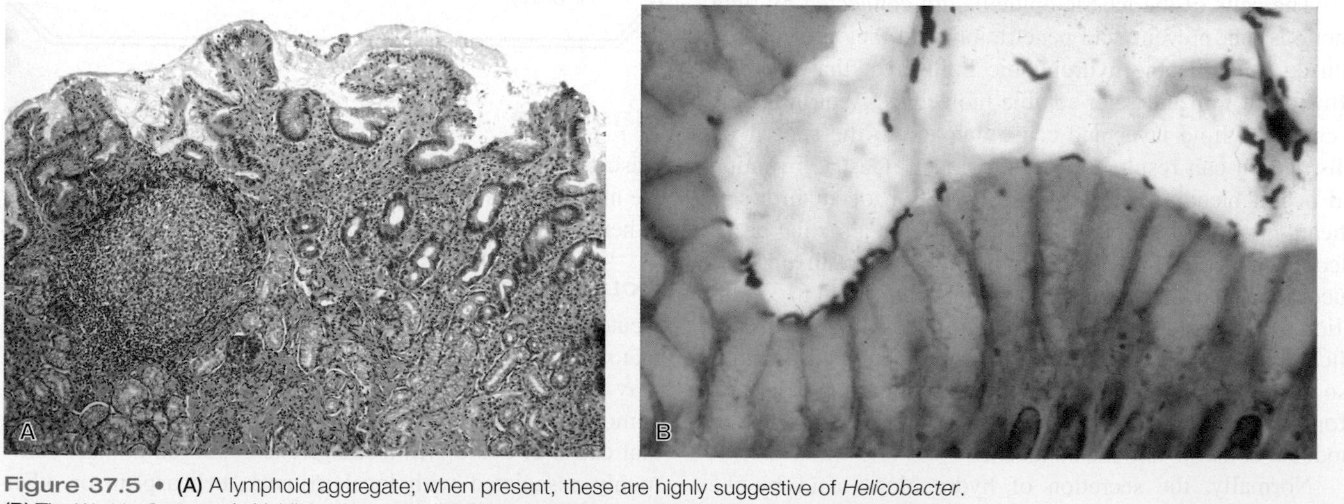

Figure 37.5 • **(A)** A lymphoid aggregate; when present, these are highly suggestive of *Helicobacter*. **(B)** The Warhin-Starry stain highlights the small curvilinear organisms at the foveolar surface. (From Strayer D. S., Rubin R. (Eds.) (2015). *Rubin's pathophysiology: Clinicopathologic foundations of medicine* (7th ed., Figure 19-16B and D, p. 764). Philadelphia, PA: Lippincott Williams & Wilkins.)

studying the different strains of the bacteria in an attempt to establish whether certain strains are more virulent than others and whether host and environmental factors contribute to the development of clinical disease.[13]

Diagnosis and Treatment. Methods for establishing the presence of *H. pylori* infection include the carbon (C) urea breath test using a radioactive carbon isotope (^{13}C- or ^{14}C-urea), serologic tests, the stool antigen test, and endoscopic biopsy for urease testing.[36] Serologic titers of *H. pylori* antibodies specifically isolate immunoglobulin (Ig) G and A.

Achieving optimal eradication of *H. pylori* has proven difficult. Combination regimens that use two or three antibiotics with a PPI or bismuth are necessary to achieve adequate rates of eradication and to reduce the number of failures because of antibiotic resistance. Standard first-line triple therapy with a PPI (omeprazole or lansoprazole), amoxicillin, and clarithromycin remains the most commonly prescribed *H. pylori* eradication regimen. Treatment duration from 7 to 10 or from 10 to 14 days is associated with a significantly higher eradication rate, with the optimal duration of therapy being of at least 14 days.[37] Second-line therapy, a 14-day course of "quadruple therapy" with a PPI, bismuth, tetracycline, and metronidazole or tinidazole is a more complicated but also more effective regimen.[38]

Eradication of *H. pylori* has proved difficult. Treatment requires combination therapy that includes the use of antibiotics such as amoxicillin, tetracycline, aminoglycoside, or bismuth salts in combination with PPIs such as lansoprazole and omeprazole.[36] Treatment is usually continued for 10 to 14 days. *H. pylori* mutate rapidly to develop antibiotic-resistant strains. The combination of two or more antimicrobial agents increases the rates of cure and reduces the risk of resistant strains developing. The PPIs have direct antimicrobial properties against *H. pylori*, and by raising the intragastric pH, they suppress bacterial growth and optimize antibiotic efficacy. Bismuth has a direct antibacterial effect against *H. pylori*.

Chronic Atrophic Gastritis. According to the Updated Sydney System Classification, atrophic gastritis is categorized into multifocal (*H. pylori*, environmental factors, specific diet) and corpus-predominant (autoimmune). Because metaplasia is a key histologic characteristic in people with atrophic gastritis, it has been recommended to use the word "metaplastic" in both variants of atrophic gastritis: autoimmune metaplastic atrophic gastritis (AMAG) and environmental metaplastic atrophic gastritis.[39]

Autoimmune atrophic gastritis, which accounts for less than 10% of cases of chronic gastritis, is a diffuse form of gastritis that is limited to the body and fundus of the stomach, with a lack or minimal involvement of the antrum.[33] The disorder results from the presence of autoantibodies to components of gastric gland parietal cells and intrinsic factor. Gastric gland and mucosal atrophy lead to a loss of acid production. In the most severe cases, production of intrinsic factor is lost, leading to a vitamin B_{12} deficiency and pernicious anemia. This type of chronic gastritis frequently is associated with other autoimmune disorders such as Hashimoto thyroiditis, Addison disease, and Graves disease.

Multifocal atrophic gastritis is a disorder of uncertain etiology that affects the antrum and adjacent areas of the stomach. It is more common than autoimmune gastritis and is seen more frequently in whites than in other races. It is particularly common in Asia, Scandinavia, and parts of Europe and Latin America.[13] As with autoimmune gastritis, it is associated with reduced gastric acid secretion, but achlorhydria and pernicious anemia are uncommon.

Chronic autoimmune gastritis and multifocal atrophic gastritis usually cause few symptoms related directly to gastric changes. When severe parietal cell loss occurs in the presence of autoimmune gastritis, hypochlorhydria or achlorhydria and hypergastrinemia are characteristically present. More important is the relationship of chronic gastritis to the development of peptic ulcer and gastric carcinoma. The long-term risk of gastric cancer in people with autoimmune gastritis is miniscule.[33]

Chemical Gastropathy. Chemical gastropathy is a chronic gastric injury resulting from reflux of alkaline duodenal contents, pancreatic secretions, and bile into the stomach. It is most commonly seen in people who have had gastroduodenostomy or gastrojejunostomy surgery. A milder form may occur in people with gastric ulcer, gallbladder disease, or various motility disorders of the distal stomach.

Peptic Ulcer Disease

Peptic ulcer disease is a term used to describe a group of ulcerative disorders that occur in areas of the upper GI tract that are exposed to acid–pepsin secretions. It is related to variety of causes, such as medication use and *H. pylori* infection.[40] Peptic ulcer disease, with its remissions and exacerbations, is a chronic health problem.

Peptic Ulcers

The most common forms of peptic ulcer are duodenal and gastric ulcers. Approximately 10% of the population have or will develop a peptic ulcer.[13] Duodenal ulcers occur five times more commonly than gastric ulcers. The peak age for peptic ulcer has progressively increased in the last 50 years and is now between 30 and 60 years of age for duodenal ulcers, although the disorder can occur in people of any age. Gastric ulcers are more prevalent among middle-aged and older adults. For duodenal ulcers, there is a male predominance, whereas the incidence of gastric ulcers is more equally distributed between men and women.[13]

A peptic ulcer can affect one or all layers of the stomach or duodenum (Fig. 37.6). The ulcer may penetrate only the mucosal surface, or it may extend into the smooth muscle layers. Occasionally, an ulcer penetrates the outer wall of the stomach or duodenum. Spontaneous remissions and

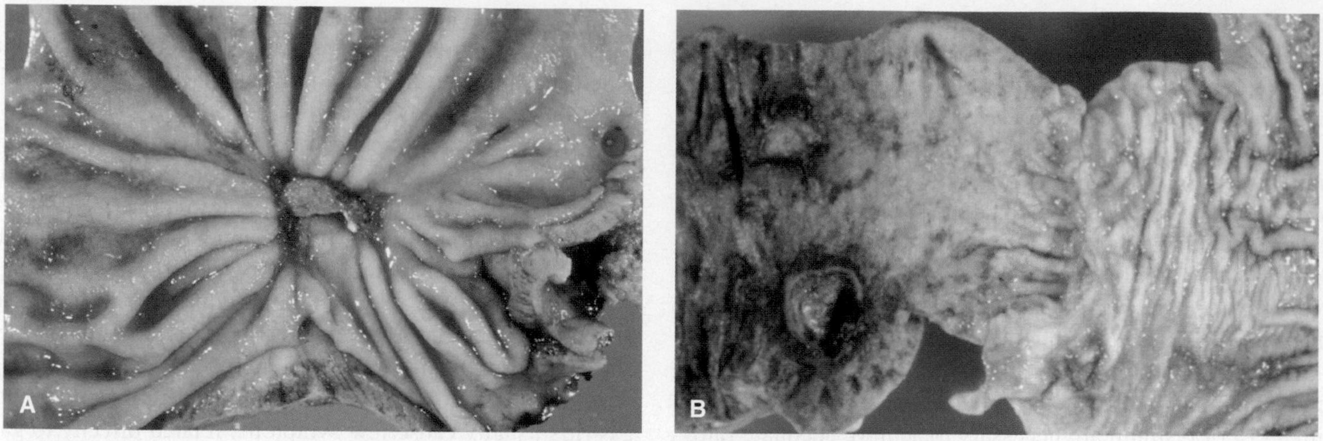

Figure 37.6 • Gastric and duodenal ulcers. **(A)** Gastric ulcer—there is a characteristic sharp demarcation from the surrounding mucosa, with radiating gastric folds. The base of the ulcer is gray owing to fibrin deposition. **(B)** Duodenal ulcer—there are two sharply demarcated duodenal ulcers surrounded by inflamed duodenal mucosa. The gastroduodenal junction is in the midportion of the photograph. (From Rubin R., Strayer D. S. (Eds.) (2012). *Rubin's pathophysiology: Clinicopathologic foundations of medicine* (6th ed., p. 625). Philadelphia, PA: Lippincott Williams & Wilkins.)

exacerbations are common. Healing of the muscularis layer involves replacement with scar tissue. Although the mucosal layers that cover the scarred muscle layer regenerate, the regeneration often is less than perfect, which contributes to repeated episodes of ulceration.

Etiology and Pathogenesis. A variety of risk factors have been shown to have an association with peptic ulcer disease. The two most important are infection with the bacteria *H. pylori* and use of aspirin and other NSAIDs.[40] Both *H. pylori* infection and exposure to NSAIDs have been shown to impair the mechanisms that protect the gastric mucosa from the destructive effects of the corrosive acid that is continually challenging the upper GI tract mucosa, and ulceration reflects a failure of these mechanisms.

The exact mechanism by which *H. pylori* promotes the development of peptic ulcer has not been fully elucidated. *H. pylori*'s ability to induce inflammation and stimulate the release of cytokines and other mediators of inflammation contributes to mucosal damage. Infection, predominantly in the antrum of the stomach, leads to hypergastrinemia and an increased acid production. Acid injury to the duodenum is thought to promote the development of gastric metaplasia, allowing the organism to colonize these areas and promote the development of duodenal ulcers.

The pathogenesis of NSAID-induced ulcers is thought to involve mucosal injury and inhibition of prostaglandin synthesis.[33] Aspirin appears to be the most ulcerogenic of the NSAIDs. Ulcer development in NSAID users is dose dependent, but some risk occurs even with aspirin doses of 81 mg/day.[41] In contrast to peptic ulcer from other causes, NSAID-induced gastric injury often is without symptoms, and life-threatening complications can occur without warning. There is reportedly less gastric irritation with the newer class of NSAIDs that selectively inhibit cylcooxygenase-2 (COX-2–selective NSAIDs), the principal enzyme involved in prostaglandin synthesis at the site of inflammation, than with the nonselective NSAIDs that also inhibit COX-1, the enzyme involved in prostaglandin production in the gastric mucosa.

Epidemiologic studies have identified independent factors that augment the effect of *H. pylori* infection and NSAID-produced peptic ulcer disease. These factors include advancing age, a prior history of peptic ulcer, multiple NSAID use, and concurrent use of warfarin (an anticoagulant) and corticosteroid drugs. Smoking may augment the risk of peptic ulcer by impairing healing. Alcohol use may cause increased acid production.[40] There is no convincing evidence that dietary factors play a role in development of peptic ulcer. There is increased incidence of peptic ulcer in families. This finding is likely due to familial clustering of *H. pylori* infection, and inherited genetic factors reflecting responses to the organism likely play a secondary role.

Clinical Manifestations. The clinical manifestations of uncomplicated peptic ulcer focus on discomfort and pain. The pain, which is described as burning, gnawing, or cramplike, usually is rhythmic and frequently occurs when the stomach is empty—between meals and at 1 or 2 o'clock in the morning. The pain usually is located over a small area near the midline in the epigastrium near the xiphoid and may radiate below the costal margins, into the back, or, rarely, to the right shoulder. Superficial and deep epigastric tenderness and voluntary muscle guarding may occur with more extensive lesions. An additional characteristic of ulcer pain is periodicity. The pain tends to recur at intervals of weeks or months. During an exacerbation, it occurs daily for a period of several weeks and then remits until the next recurrence. Characteristically, the pain is relieved by food or antacids.

The most common complications of peptic ulcer are hemorrhage, perforation and penetration, and gastric outlet obstruction. Hemorrhage is caused by bleeding from granulation tissue or from erosion of an ulcer into an artery or vein. Acute post hemorrhagic anemia is the second most common secondary diagnosis, when people are admitted to the hospital with peptic ulcer disease.[42] Evidence of bleeding may consist of hematemesis or melena. Bleeding may be sudden, severe, and without warning, or it may be insidious, producing only occult blood in the stool. Up to 20% of people with bleeding ulcers have no antecedent symptoms of pain; this is particularly true in people using NSAIDs. Acute hemorrhage is evidenced by the sudden onset of weakness; dizziness; thirst; cold, moist skin; the desire to defecate; and the passage of loose, tarry, or even red stools and coffee-ground emesis. Signs of circulatory shock develop depending on the amount of blood lost.

Perforation occurs when an ulcer erodes through all the layers of the stomach or duodenum wall. When perforation occurs in older adults, their mortality is significantly increased. With perforation, GI contents enter the peritoneum and cause peritonitis. Radiation of the pain into the back, severe night distress, and inadequate pain relief from eating foods or taking antacids in people with a long history of peptic ulcer may signify perforation. Penetration is a process similar to perforation, but with penetration the ulcer crater erodes into adjacent organs, including the pancreas, liver, or biliary tree.[40] Typically it has a subtle presentation marked by a gradual increase in severity and frequency of pain.

Outlet obstruction is caused by edema, spasm, or contraction of scar tissue and interference with the free passage of gastric contents through the pylorus or adjacent areas. The presentation of an obstruction is typically insidious, with symptoms of early satiety, feeling of epigastric fullness and heaviness after meals, GER, weight loss, and abdominal pain. With severe obstruction, there is vomiting of undigested food.

Diagnosis and Treatment. Diagnostic procedures for peptic ulcer include history taking, laboratory tests, radiologic imaging, and endoscopic examination. The history should include careful attention to aspirin and NSAID use. Peptic ulcer should be differentiated from other causes of epigastric pain. Laboratory findings of hypochromic anemia and occult blood in the stools indicate bleeding. Endoscopy (*i.e.*, gastroscopy and duodenoscopy) can be used to visualize the ulcer area and obtain biopsy specimens to test for *H. pylori* and exclude malignant disease. X-ray studies with a contrast medium such as barium are used to detect the presence of an ulcer crater and to exclude gastric carcinoma.

The treatment of peptic ulcer has changed dramatically over the past several decades and now aims to eradicate the cause and promote a permanent cure for the disease. Pharmacologic treatment focuses on eradicating *H. pylori*, relieving ulcer symptoms, and healing the ulcer crater. Acid-neutralizing, acid-inhibiting drugs and mucosa-protective agents are used to relieve symptoms and promote healing of the ulcer crater. There is no evidence that special diets are beneficial in treating peptic ulcer. Aspirin and NSAID use should be avoided when possible.

There are two pharmacologic methods for reducing gastric acid content. The first involves the neutralization of gastric acid through the use of antacids, and the second a decrease in gastric acid production through the use of H_2-receptor antagonists or PPIs. Essentially three types of antacids are used to relieve gastric acidity: calcium carbonate, aluminum hydroxide, and magnesium hydroxide. Many antacids contain a combination of ingredients, such as magnesium-aluminum hydroxide. *Calcium preparations* are constipating and may cause hypercalcemia and the milk-alkali syndrome. This syndrome is the third leading cause for hypercalcemia hospital admissions.[43] *Magnesium hydroxide* is a potent antacid that also has laxative effects. Approximately 5% to 10% of the magnesium in this preparation is absorbed from the intestine; because magnesium is excreted through the kidneys, this formulation should not be used in people with renal failure. *Aluminum hydroxide* reacts with hydrochloric acid to form aluminum chloride. It combines with phosphate in the intestine, and prolonged use may lead to phosphate depletion and osteoporosis. Because antacids can decrease the absorption, bioavailability, and renal elimination of a number of drugs, this should be considered when antacids are administered with other medications.

Histamine is the major physiologic mediator for hydrochloric acid secretion. The H_2-receptor antagonists block gastric acid secretion stimulated by histamine, gastrin, and acetylcholine. The absorption of the drug is not altered by the presence or absence of food in the stomach.[44] The volume of gastric secretion and the concentration of pepsin also are reduced. The PPIs block the final stage of hydrogen ion secretion by blocking the action of the gastric parietal cell proton pump.

Among the agents that enhance mucosal defenses are sucralfate and prostaglandin analogs. The drug sucralfate, which is a complex salt of sucrose containing aluminum and sulfate, selectively binds to damaged ulcer tissue and serves as a barrier to acid, pepsin, and bile. Sucralfate also can directly absorb bile salts and initiate the secretion of bicarbonate and mucus.[44] The drug is not absorbed systemically. The drug requires an acid pH for activation and should not be administered with antacids or an H_2 antagonist. Misoprostol, a prostaglandin E derivative, promotes ulcer healing by stimulating mucus and bicarbonate secretion and by modestly inhibiting acid secretion. It is the only drug in this class approved by the U.S. Food and Drug Administration (FDA) for clinical use in the prevention of NSAID-induced peptic ulcers. The drug causes dose-dependent diarrhea, and because of its stimulant effect on the uterus, it is contraindicated in women of childbearing age.

The current surgical management of peptic ulcer disease is largely limited to treatment of complications. When surgery is needed, it usually is performed using minimally invasive methods. With bleeding ulcers, hemostasis often can be achieved by endoscopic methods, and endoscopic balloon dilation often is effective in relieving outflow obstruction.

Zollinger-Ellison Syndrome

The Zollinger-Ellison syndrome is a rare condition caused by a gastrin-secreting tumor (gastrinoma). In people with this disorder, increased gastric acid secretion results in GERD or severe peptic ulcer disease.[45] The tumors may be single or multiple; duodenal tumors account for 40% to 50% of this type of gastrinoma.[46] Approximately 50% of gastrin-producing tumors are malignant.[47] The increased gastric secretions cause symptoms related to peptic ulcer. Diarrhea may result from hypersecretion or from the inactivation of intestinal lipase and impaired fat digestion that occur with a decrease in intestinal pH.

Hypergastrinemia may also occur in an autosomal dominant disorder called the *multiple endocrine neoplasia type 1 (MEN 1) syndrome*, which is characterized by multiple endocrine neoplasms. The syndrome is characterized by hyperparathyroidism and multiple endocrine tumors, including gastrinomas. Approximately 20% to 25% of gastrinomas are due to MEN 1.[45]

The diagnosis of the Zollinger-Ellison syndrome is based on elevated serum gastrin and basal gastric acid levels and elimination of the MEN 1 syndrome as a cause of the disorder. Computed tomography (CT), abdominal ultrasonography, and selective angiography are used to localize the tumor and determine if metastatic disease is present.

Treatment of Zollinger-Ellison syndrome involves control of gastric acid secretion by PPIs and treatment of the malignant neoplasm.[47] Surgical removal is indicated when the tumor is malignant and has not metastasized.

Stress Ulcers

A stress ulcer refers to GI ulcerations that develop in relation to major physiologic stress.[13] People at high risk for development of stress ulcers include those with large surface area burns (Curling ulcer),[48] trauma, sepsis, acute respiratory distress syndrome, severe liver failure, and major surgical procedures. These lesions occur most often in the fundus and body of the stomach and are thought to result from ischemia to the mucosal tissue and alterations in the gastric mucosal barrier.[48]Another form of stress ulcer, called *Cushing ulcer*, consists of gastric, duodenal, and esophageal ulcers arising in people with intracranial injury, operations, or tumors. They are thought to be caused by hypersecretion of gastric acid resulting from stimulation of vagal nuclei by increased intracranial pressure.

People admitted to hospital intensive care units are at particular risk for development of stress ulcers.[49] PPIs are the first line of medications used in the prevention of stress ulcers.[48]

Cancer of the Stomach

According to the International Agency for Research in Cancer, in 2014, stomach cancer is the fifth most common cancer worldwide, with an estimated 952,000 new cases (7% of total cancer incidence) and 723,000 deaths (9% of total cancer mortality) in 2014. Almost three quarters of the new cases occurred in Asia, and more than two fifths occurred in China.[50] Stomach cancer occurs most commonly in East Asia and Eastern Europe. It occurs twice as often in males as in females. In 2017, about 28,000 new diagnoses of stomach cancer (17,750 in men and 10,250 in women) were predicted in the United States, and almost 11,000 people were predicted to die because of the disease.[51]

Etiology and Pathogenesis

Factors thought to increase the risk of gastric cancer include genetic factors, carcinogenic factors in the diet (*e.g.*, *N*-nitroso compounds and benzopyrene found in smoked and preserved foods), autoimmune gastritis, and gastric adenomas or polyps. The incidence of stomach cancer in the United States has significantly decreased since 1930, presumably because of improved storage of food with decreased consumption of salted, smoked, and preserved foods.[51] Chronic infection with *H. pylori* appears to serve as a cofactor in some types of gastric carcinomas. The bacterial infection causes gastritis, followed by atrophy, intestinal metaplasia, and carcinoma. This sequence of cellular events depends on both the presence of the bacterial proteins and the host immune response, with the latter being influenced by the host genetic background. In addition to genetics, the likelihood of developing gastric cancer from an *H. pylori* infection is related to strain of *H. pylori* infection, environmental factors, and the duration of infection.[52] Autoimmune gastritis, like *H. pylori* infection, increases the risk of gastric cancer, presumably due to chronic inflammation and intestinal metaplasia.[53]

Between 50% and 60% of gastric cancers occur in the pyloric region or adjacent to the antrum. Compared with a benign ulcer, which has smooth margins and is concentrically shaped, gastric cancers tend to be larger, are irregularly shaped, and have irregular margins.

Clinical Manifestations

Unfortunately, stomach cancer is often either asymptomatic or may cause only nonspecific symptoms in its early stages. By the time symptoms occur, the cancer has often reached an advanced stage and may have metastasized. Stomach cancer can cause the following signs and symptoms:

Early cancers may be associated with indigestion or a burning sensation. However, less than 1 in every 50 people referred for endoscopy because of indigestion has cancer. Abdominal discomfort and loss of appetite, especially for meat, can occur.

Stomach cancers that have enlarged and invaded normal tissue can cause weakness, fatigue, bloating of the stomach after meals, abdominal pain in the upper abdomen, nausea and occasional vomiting, diarrhea, or constipation. Further enlargement may cause weight loss or bleeding with vomiting blood or having blood in the stool, the latter apparent as black discoloration (melena) and sometimes leading to anemia. Dysphagia suggests a tumor in the cardia or extension of the gastric tumor into the esophagus.

Because symptoms of stomach cancer often do not appear until the disease is advanced, only about 1 in 5 stomach cancers in the United States is found at an early stage, before it has spread to other areas of the body.

Diagnosis and Treatment

Diagnosis of gastric cancer is accomplished by a variety of techniques, including barium x-ray studies, endoscopic studies with biopsy, and cytologic studies (*e.g.*, Papanicolaou smear) of gastric secretions.[54] Cytologic studies can prove particularly useful as routine screening tests for people with atrophic gastritis or gastric polyps. CT and endoscopic ultrasonography often are used to delineate the spread of a diagnosed stomach cancer.

In 2013, Chinese and Israeli scientists reported a successful pilot study of a breathalyzer-style breath test intended to diagnose stomach cancer by analyzing exhaled chemicals without the need for an intrusive endoscopy.[55] A larger-scale clinical trial of this technology was completed in 2014.[56]

Depending on the location and extent of the lesion, surgery in the form of radical subtotal gastrectomy usually is the treatment of choice. Irradiation and chemotherapy have not proved particularly useful as primary treatment modalities in stomach cancer. These methods usually are used for palliative purposes or to control metastatic spread of the disease. The short overall life expectancy and lack of a standard chemotherapy regimen make it important to identify novel treatment modalities for gastric cancer. Molecular targeted therapy has attracted substantial attention to improve the specificity of anticancer efficacy and significantly reduce nonselective resistance and toxicity. Multiple clinical studies have confirmed that molecular targeted therapy acts on various mechanisms of gastric cancer, such as the regulation of epidermal growth factor, angiogenesis, immuno-checkpoint blockade, the cell cycle, cell apoptosis, key enzymes, and insulin-like growth factor receptors, to exert a stronger antitumor effect. An in-depth understanding of the mechanisms that underlie molecular targeted therapies will provide new insights into gastric cancer treatment.[57]

IN SUMMARY

Disorders of the stomach include gastritis, peptic ulcer, and cancer of the stomach. Gastritis refers to inflammation of the gastric mucosa. Acute gastritis refers to a transient inflammation of the gastric mucosa; it is associated most commonly with local irritants such as bacterial endotoxins, caffeine, alcohol, and aspirin. Chronic gastritis is characterized by the absence of grossly visible erosions and the presence of chronic inflammatory changes leading eventually to atrophy of the glandular epithelium of the stomach. There are three main types of chronic gastritis: *H. pylori* gastritis, autoimmune gastritis and multifocal atrophic gastritis, and chemical gastropathy. *H. pylori* is an "S"-shaped bacterium that colonizes the mucus-secreting epithelial cells of the stomach. Infection increases the risk of chronic gastritis, peptic ulcer, gastric carcinoma, and low-grade B-cell lymphoma. Treatment of *H. pylori* infection involves the use of multidrug therapy aimed at increasing the pH of gastric secretions and antimicrobial agents designed to eradicate the organism.

Peptic ulcer is a term used to describe a group of ulcerative disorders that occur in areas of the upper GI tract that are exposed to acid–pepsin secretions, most commonly the duodenum and stomach. There are two main causes of peptic ulcer: *H. pylori* infection and aspirin or NSAID use. The treatment of peptic ulcer focuses on eradication of *H. pylori*, avoidance of gastric irritation from NSAIDs, and conventional pharmacologic treatment directed at symptom relief and ulcer healing.

The Zollinger-Ellison syndrome is a rare condition caused by a gastrin-secreting tumor in which gastric acid secretion reaches such levels that ulceration becomes inevitable. Stress ulcers, also called *Curling ulcers*, occur in relation to major physiologic stresses such as burns and trauma and are thought to result from ischemia, tissue acidosis, and bile salts entering the stomach in critically ill people with decreased GI tract motility. Another form of stress ulcer, Cushing ulcer, occurs in people with intracranial trauma or surgery and is thought to be caused by hypersecretion of gastric acid resulting from stimulation of vagal nuclei by increased intracranial pressure.

Although the incidence of cancer of the stomach has declined over the past 50 years in the United States, it remains the third (8.8%) leading cause of cancer death worldwide after lung cancer and liver cancer.[50] Because there are few early symptoms with this form of cancer, the disease often is far advanced at the time of diagnosis.

DISORDERS OF THE SMALL AND LARGE INTESTINES

After completing this section of the chapter, the learner will be able to meet the following objectives:

- Compare the characteristics of Crohn disease and ulcerative colitis.
- Describe the pathogenesis of the symptoms associated with appendicitis.

There are many similarities in conditions that disrupt the integrity and function of the small and large intestines. The walls of the small and large intestines consist of five layers:

1. An inner mucosal layer, which lines the lumen of the intestine
2. A submucosal layer
3. A circular muscularis layer
4. A layer of longitudinal muscle fibers
5. An outer serosal layer

Among the conditions that cause altered intestinal function are irritable bowel syndrome (IBS), inflammatory bowel disease (IBD), diverticulitis, appendicitis, disorders of bowel motility (*i.e.*, diarrhea, constipation, and bowel obstruction), malabsorption syndrome, and cancers of the colon and rectum.

Irritable Bowel Syndrome

The term *irritable bowel syndrome* is used to describe a functional GI disorder characterized by a variable combination of chronic and recurrent intestinal symptoms not explained by structural or biochemical abnormalities. There is evidence to suggest that 10% to 15% of the U.S. population have the disorder and one in four people worldwide.[58]

IBS is characterized by persistent or recurrent symptoms of abdominal pain; altered bowel function; and varying complaints of flatulence, bloating, nausea and anorexia, constipation or diarrhea, and anxiety or depression. A hallmark of IBS is abdominal pain that is relieved by defecation and associated with a change in consistency or frequency of stools. Abdominal pain usually is intermittent, cramping, and in the lower abdomen. It does not usually occur at night or interfere with sleep. The condition is believed to result from dysregulation of intestinal motor activity and central neural functions modulated by the CNS.[59] People with IBS tend to experience increased motility and abnormal intestinal contractions in response to psychological and physiologic stresses. The role that psychological factors play in the disease is uncertain. Although changes in intestinal activity are normal responses to stress, these responses appear to be exaggerated in people with IBS. Women tend to be affected more often than men. Menarche often is associated with onset of the disorder. Women frequently notice an exacerbation of symptoms during the premenstrual period, suggesting a hormonal component.

Clinical Manifestations and Diagnosis

Because IBS lacks anatomic or physiologic markers, diagnosis is usually based on signs and symptoms of abdominal pain or discomfort, bloating, and constipation or diarrhea, or alternating bouts of constipation and diarrhea. A commonly used set of diagnostic criteria require continuous or recurrent symptoms of at least 12 weeks' duration (which may be nonconsecutive) of abdominal discomfort or pain in the preceding 12 months, with two of three accompanying features: relief with defecation, onset associated with a change in bowel frequency, and onset associated with a change in form (appearance) of stool.[60]

Other symptoms that support the diagnosis of IBS include abnormal stool frequency (more than three times per day or less than three times per week), abnormal stool form (lumpy/hard or loose/watery), abnormal stool passage (straining, urgency, or feeling of incomplete evacuation), passage of mucus, and bloating or feeling of abdominal distention.[60] A history of lactose intolerance should be considered because intolerance to lactose and other sugars may be a precipitating factor in some people. The acute onset of symptoms raises the likelihood of organic disease, as does weight loss, anemia, fever, occult blood in the stool, nighttime symptoms, or signs and symptoms of malabsorption. These signs and symptoms require additional investigation of differential diagnoses.[61]

Treatment

The treatment of IBS focuses on methods of stress management, particularly those related to symptom production. Reassurance is important. Usually, no special diet is indicated, although adequate fiber intake usually is recommended. Avoidance of offending dietary substances by following specific elimination diets that omit such foods as fatty and gas-producing foods, alcohol, and caffeine-containing beverages may be beneficial.[62] Various pharmacologic agents, including antispasmodic and anticholinergic drugs, have been used with varying success in treatment of the disorder. Alosetron, a 5-HT_3 antagonist, was the first specific drug to be approved by the FDA for the treatment of irritable bowel disease. It acts by reducing intestinal secretion, decreasing visceral afferent nerve activity (thereby reducing abdominal pain), and reducing intestinal motility. The drug, which was indicated for treatment of women with the severe diarrheal form of the disease, was removed from the market in late 2000 because of serious side effects involving ischemic colitis and severe constipation and then reintroduced in 2002 under a restricted prescribing program.[63]

Inflammatory Bowel Disease

The term *inflammatory bowel disease* is used to designate two related inflammatory intestinal disorders: Crohn disease and ulcerative colitis. Over 1 million residents in the United States and 2.5 million in Europe are estimated to have IBD. Currently, the prevalence of IBD in the Western world is up to 0.5% of the general population.[64] Although the two diseases differ sufficiently to be distinguishable, they have many features in common. Both diseases produce inflammation of the bowel, both lack confirming evidence of a proven causative agent, both have a pattern of familial occurrence, and both can be accompanied by systemic manifestations. Crohn disease most commonly affects the distal small intestine and proximal colon, but can affect any area of the GI tract from the esophagus to the anus, whereas ulcerative colitis is confined to the colon and rectum (Fig. 37.7). The distinguishing characteristics of Crohn disease and ulcerative colitis are summarized in Table 37.1.

Etiology and Pathogenesis

A remarkable feature of the GI tract is that the mucosal immune system is always ready to respond against ingested pathogens but is unresponsive to the normal intestinal microflora. According to the currently accepted hypothesis, this normal state of homeostasis is disrupted in IBD, leading to unregulated and exaggerated immune responses. The question remains if the response is an appropriate defense mechanism to a pathogen or is the immune system responding in

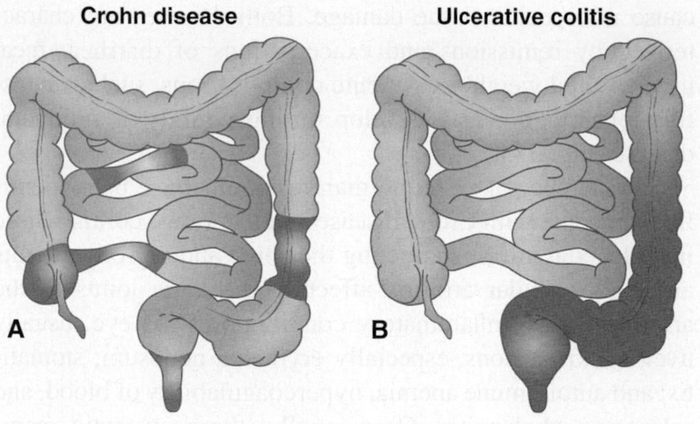

Figure 37.7 • Distribution patterns of disease with **(A)** skip lesions in Crohn disease and **(B)** continuous involvement of the colon, beginning with the rectum, in ulcerative colitis.

an inappropriate manner. Thus, as in many other autoimmune disorders, the pathogenesis of Crohn disease and ulcerative colitis involves a failure of immune regulation, genetic predisposition, and an environmental trigger, especially microbial flora.[65]

Genetic Susceptibility. The genetic basis of IBD has long been suspected. First-degree relatives of people diagnosed with IBD have a 30 to 100 times greater incidence of IBD.[66] Genome-wide association studies (GWAS) have identified 163 distinct loci that confer risk of, or protection from, the development of Crohn disease and ulcerative colitis, with a substantial portion of these loci common to both diseases.[67] The concordance rate in monozygotic twins is 30% to 35% for Crohn disease compared to only 10% to 15% for ulcerative colitis. Nevertheless, family history remains the strongest predictor of IBD, although only 10% of people have an affected first-degree relative.[68] These associations clearly indicate that genetic susceptibility plays an important role in the development of IBD. However, classic mendelian inheritance patterns are not seen, and IBD therefore cannot be attributed to a single gene. Many candidate genes are known to be associated with, and likely to contribute to, the development of IBD. These include the human leukocyte antigen (HLA) associations. Accumulating evidence also suggests that both Crohn disease and ulcerative colitis are associated with profound disorders of mucosal immunity. Nucleotide-binding oligomerization domain-containing protein 2 (NOD2), also known as caspase recruitment domain-containing protein 15 (CARD15) or inflammatory bowel disease protein 1 (IBD1), is a protein that in humans is encoded by the NOD2 gene located on chromosome 16.[67] The NOD2 protein is expressed in many types of leukocytes as well as epithelial cells and is thought to act as an intracellular receptor for lipopolysaccharides on microbes. On binding microbial products, it may trigger the NFκβ pathway, which leads to the production of cytokines and other proteins involved in the innate immune defense against microorganisms. The NOD2 mutations that are associated with Crohn disease may reduce the activity of the protein, resulting in persistence of intracellular microbes and prolonged immune responses. Another region studied extensively is IBD3 on chromosome 6. This is the area that includes the HLA complex that has been linked to Crohn disease and ulcerative colitis. Another area linked specifically to Crohn disease is on chromosome 5q (IBD5). This area is rich in genes encoding several cytokines that may contribute to the disease.

The most recent and largest genetic association study, which employed genome-wide association data for over 75,000 people with IBD and controls, identified 163 susceptibility loci for IBD, encompassing approximately 300 potential candidate genes. Of these 163 loci, 110 conferred risk to both IBD subtypes, whereas 30 loci where unique to Crohn disease and 23 loci were unique to ulcerative colitis. More recently, a trans-ethnic analysis, including over 20,000 people of European and non-European ancestry, identified an additional 38 new IBD loci, highlighting shared genetic risk across populations and increasing the number of known IBD risk loci to 200.[69,70] Identified genetic factors account for only a small proportion of the disease variance: 13.1% for Crohn disease

TABLE 37.1 DIFFERENTIATING CHARACTERISTICS OF CROHN DISEASE AND ULCERATIVE COLITIS

CHARACTERISTIC	CROHN DISEASE	ULCERATIVE COLITIS
Types of inflammation	Granulomatous	Ulcerative and exudative
Level of involvement	Primarily submucosal	Primarily mucosal
Extent of involvement	Skip lesions	Continuous
Areas of involvement	Primarily ileum, secondarily colon	Primarily rectum and left colon
Diarrhea	Common	Common
Rectal bleeding	Rare	Common
Fistulas	Common	Rare
Strictures	Common	Rare
Perianal abscesses	Common	Rare
Development of cancer	Uncommon	Relatively common

and 8.2% for ulcerative colitis. Overall, explainable susceptibility loci and genetic risk factors discovered so far account for only 20% to 25% of the heritability (genetic risk).[69,71]

Role of Environmental Factors. Although family history is the strongest risk factor for IBD, and genes play an important role, as demonstrated by the identification of the 163 distinct genetic risk alleles, considerable epidemiologic data supports a key role for the environment. The earliest and most consistently described environmental factor impacting Crohn disease and ulcerative colitis incidence is smoking.[72] Current smokers have a twofold increase in risk of Crohn disease, with a more modest association in former smokers. In contrast, former smoking is associated with substantial increase in risk of ulcerative colitis within 1 year of quitting, whereas current smoking appears to be protective.[73] The precise reason for this divergent effect is unclear. Smoking might contribute to the development of IBD by influencing the intestinal microbiome, as people with Crohn disease who smoke show a dysbiosis within their intestinal microbiota.[74]

Animal studies have definitively established the importance of the gut flora in IBD. The sites affected by IBD, the distal ileum and the colon, are awash with bacteria. Recent antibiotic use within 2 to 5 years of diagnosis was also associated with increased risk of adult-onset IBD, with increasing effect seen with greater number of antibiotic courses and exposure earlier in life.[75] Although it is unlikely that IBD is directly caused by microbes, it seems likely that microbes may provide the antigen trigger for an unregulated immune response.

Clinical Manifestations

The clinical manifestations of both Crohn disease and ulcerative colitis are ultimately the result of activation of inflammatory cells with elaboration of inflammatory mediators that cause nonspecific tissue damage. Both diseases are characterized by remissions and exacerbations of diarrhea, fecal urgency, and weight loss. Acute complications, such as intestinal obstruction, may develop during periods of fulminant disease (Fig. 37.8).

A number of systemic manifestations have been identified in people with Crohn disease and ulcerative colitis. These include axial arthritis affecting the spine and sacroiliac joints and oligoarticular arthritis affecting the large joints of the arms and legs; inflammatory conditions of the eye, usually uveitis; skin lesions, especially erythema nodosum; stomatitis; and autoimmune anemia, hypercoagulability of blood, and sclerosing cholangitis. Occasionally, these systemic manifestations may herald the recurrence of intestinal disease. In children, growth retardation may occur, particularly if the symptoms are prolonged and nutrient intake has been poor.

Crohn Disease

Crohn disease is a recurrent, granulomatous type of inflammatory response that can affect any area of the GI tract. The terminal ileum or cecum is the most common portion of the bowel where inflammation occurs.[66,76] It is a slowly progressive, relentless, and often disabling disease. The disease usually strikes people in their twenties or thirties, with women being affected slightly more often than men.

A characteristic feature of Crohn disease is the sharply demarcated, granulomatous lesions that are surrounded by normal-appearing mucosal tissue. When the lesions are multiple, they often are referred to as *skip lesions* because they are interspersed between what appear to be normal segments of the bowel. All the layers of the bowel are involved, with the submucosal layer affected to the greatest extent. The surface of the inflamed bowel usually has a characteristic "cobblestone" appearance resulting from the fissures and crevices that develop, surrounded by areas of submucosal edema[13,76]

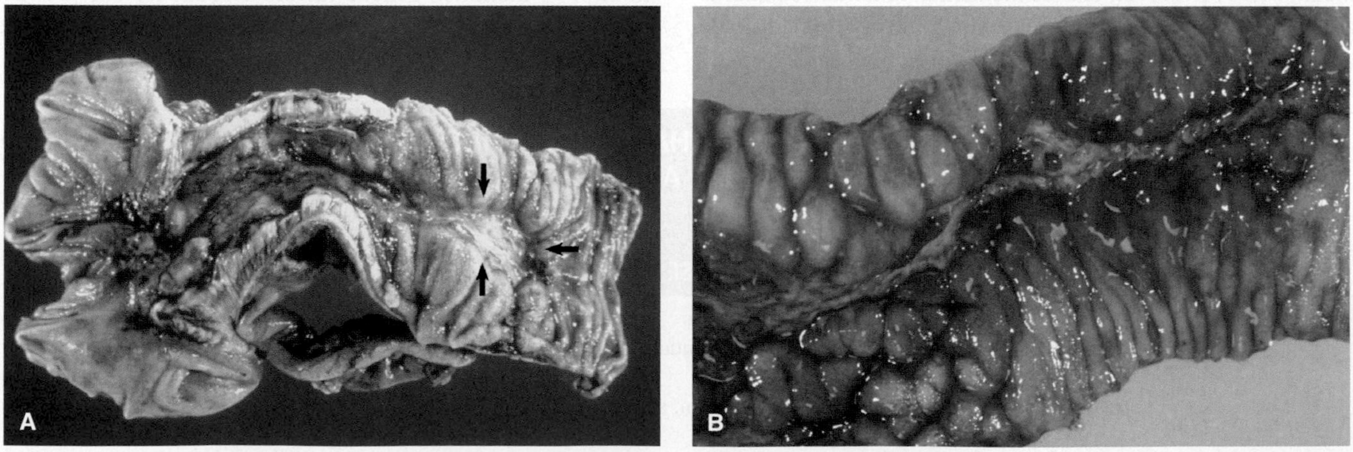

Figure 37.8 • Crohn disease. **(A)** The terminal ileum shows striking thickening of the wall of the distal portion with distortion of the ileocecal valve. A longitudinal ulcer is present (*arrows*). **(B)** Another longitudinal ulcer is seen in this segment of the ileum. The large rounded areas of edematous damaged mucosa give a "cobblestone" appearance to the involved mucosa. A portion of the mucosa to the lower right is uninvolved. (From Rubin R., Strayer D. S. (Eds.) (2015). *Rubin's pathophysiology: Clinicopathologic foundations of medicine* (6th ed., Figure 19-52, p. 803). Philadelphia, PA: Lippincott Williams & Wilkins.)

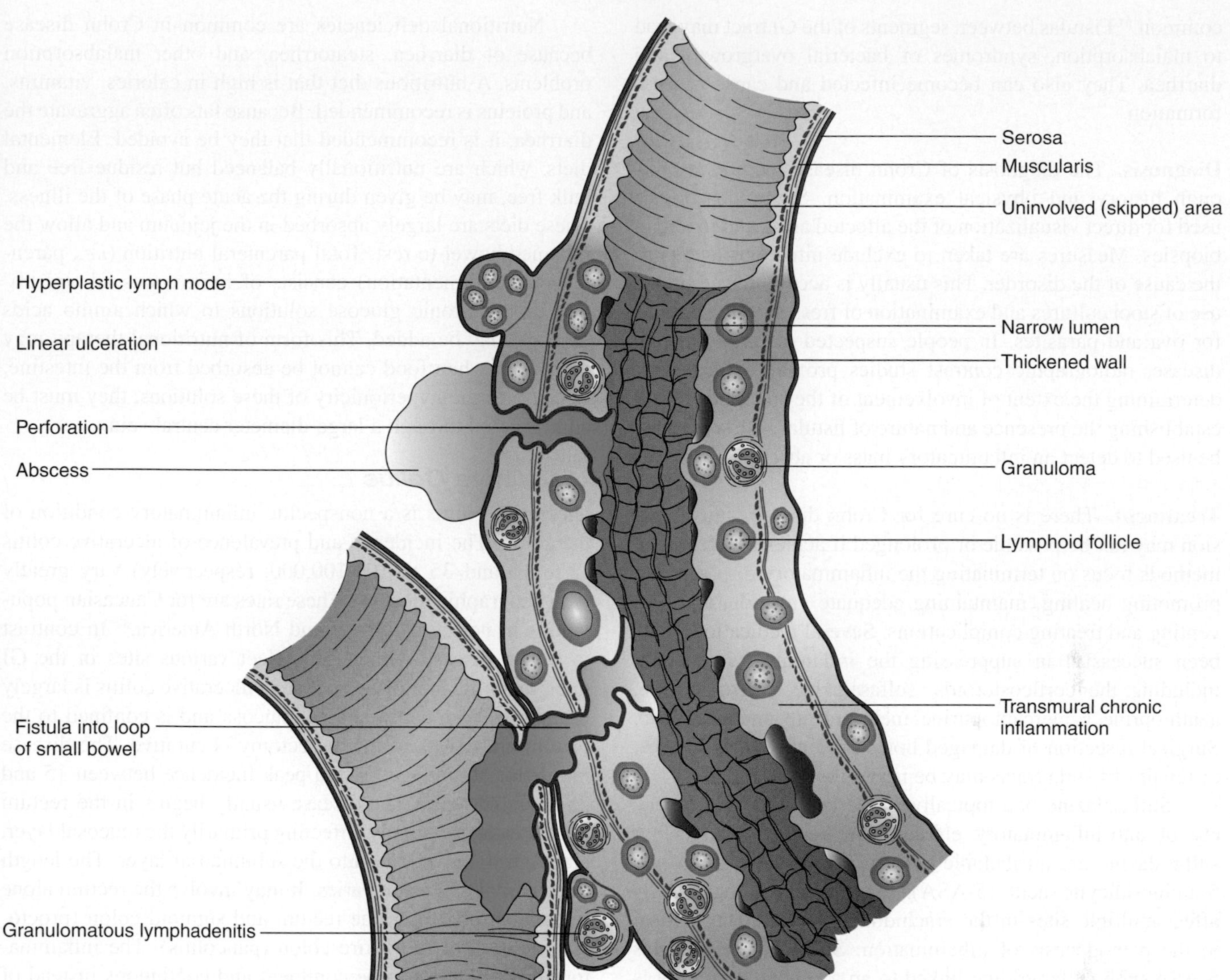

Figure 37.9 • Crohn disease. A schematic representation of the major features of Crohn disease in the small intestines. (From Rubin R., Strayer D. S. (Eds.) (2015). *Rubin's pathophysiology: Clinicopathologic foundations of medicine* (7th ed., Figure 19-73, p. 805). Philadelphia, PA: Lippincott Williams & Wilkins.)

(Fig. 37.9). There usually is a relative sparing of the smooth muscle layers of the bowel, with marked inflammatory and fibrotic changes of the submucosal layer. The bowel wall, after a time, often becomes thickened and inflexible; its appearance has been likened to a lead pipe or rubber hose. The adjacent mesentery may become inflamed, and the regional lymph nodes and channels may become enlarged.

Clinical Manifestations. The clinical course of Crohn disease is variable; often, there are periods of exacerbations and remissions, with symptoms being related to the location of the lesions. The principal symptoms, which are dependent upon the area of the GI system that is affected, include diarrhea, abdominal pain, weight loss, fluid and electrolyte disorders, malaise, and low-grade fever.[76] Because Crohn disease affects the submucosal layer to a greater extent than the mucosal layer, there is less bloody diarrhea than with ulcerative colitis. Ulceration of the perianal skin is common, largely because of the severity of the diarrhea. The absorptive surface of the intestine may be disrupted; nutritional deficiencies may occur, related to the specific segment of the intestine involved. When Crohn disease occurs in childhood, one of its major manifestations may be retardation of growth and significant malnutrition.[77]

Complications of Crohn disease include fistula formation, abdominal abscess formation, and intestinal obstruction. Fistulas are tubelike passages that form connections between different sites in the GI tract. They also may develop between other sites, including the bladder, vagina, urethra, and skin. Perineal fistulas that originate in the ileum are relatively common.[64] Fistulas between segments of the GI tract may lead to malabsorption, syndromes of bacterial overgrowth, and diarrhea. They also can become infected and cause abscess formation.

Diagnosis. The diagnosis of Crohn disease requires a thorough history and physical examination. Sigmoidoscopy is used for direct visualization of the affected areas and to obtain biopsies. Measures are taken to exclude infectious agents as the cause of the disorder. This usually is accomplished by the use of stool cultures and examination of fresh stool specimens for ova and parasites. In people suspected of having Crohn disease, radiographic contrast studies provide a means for determining the extent of involvement of the small bowel and establishing the presence and nature of fistulas. CT scans may be used to detect an inflammatory mass or abscess.

Treatment. There is no cure for Crohn disease, and remission may not be possible or prolonged if achieved. Treatment methods focus on terminating the inflammatory response and promoting healing, maintaining adequate nutrition, and preventing and treating complications. Several medications have been successful in suppressing the inflammatory reaction, including the corticosteroids, sulfasalazine, metronidazole, azathioprine, 6-mercaptopurine, methotrexate, and infliximab. Surgical resection of damaged bowel, drainage of abscesses, or repair of fistula tracts may be necessary.

Sulfasalazine is a topically active agent that has a variety of anti-inflammatory effects. The beneficial effects of sulfasalazine are attributable to one component of the drug, 5-aminosalicylic acid (5-ASA). Agents containing 5-ASA affect multiple sites in the arachidonic acid pathway critical to the pathogenesis of inflammation. Sulfasalazine contains 5-ASA with sulfapyridine linked to an azo bond. The drug is poorly absorbed from the intestine, and the azo linkage is broken down by the bacterial flora in the ileum and colon to release 5-ASA. Metronidazole is an antibiotic used to treat bacterial overgrowth in the small intestine. A recent meta-analysis found two thiopurine drugs, azathioprine and 6-mercaptopurine, to be effective in reducing the reoccurrence of Crohn disease.[78] The use of methotrexate is another option for clinicians to choose instead of the thiopurine drugs, although the studies regarding its use are limited.[65] Infliximab is a monoclonal antibody that targets the destruction of tumor necrosis factor (TNF), a mediator of the inflammatory response, whose expression is increased in inflammatory processes such as Crohn disease.[76] It is the first drug approved specifically for Crohn disease and is used in the treatment of people with active moderate-to-severe Crohn disease who have had an inadequate response to corticosteroids or other immune modulators. Subsequently, two additional anti-TNF agents, adalimumab and certolizumab pegol, have been approved for Crohn disease. The monoclonal antibody ustekinumab appears to be a safe treatment option and may help people with moderate to severe active Crohn disease.[79] The long-term safety and effectiveness of monoclonal antibody treatment is not known.

Nutritional deficiencies are common in Crohn disease because of diarrhea, steatorrhea, and other malabsorption problems. A nutritious diet that is high in calories, vitamins, and proteins is recommended. Because fats often aggravate the diarrhea, it is recommended that they be avoided. Elemental diets, which are nutritionally balanced but residue free and bulk free, may be given during the acute phase of the illness. These diets are largely absorbed in the jejunum and allow the inflamed bowel to rest. Total parenteral nutrition (*i.e.*, parenteral hyperalimentation) consists of intravenous administration of hypertonic glucose solutions to which amino acids and fats may be added. This form of nutritional therapy may be needed when food cannot be absorbed from the intestine. Because of the hypertonicity of these solutions, they must be administered through a large-diameter central vein.

Ulcerative Colitis

Ulcerative colitis is a nonspecific inflammatory condition of the colon. The incidence and prevalence of ulcerative colitis (2 to 10 and 35 to 100/100,000, respectively) vary greatly with geographic location. These rates are for Caucasian populations in northern Europe and North America.[80] In contrast to Crohn disease, which can affect various sites in the GI tract, the inflammatory response in ulcerative colitis is largely limited to the mucosa and submucosa and is confined to the rectum and colon so that colectomy is curative. The disease may arise at any age, with a peak incidence between 15 and 25 years of age.[66] The disease usually begins in the rectum and spreads proximally, affecting primarily the mucosal layer, although it can extend into the submucosal layer. The length of proximal extension varies. It may involve the rectum alone (ulcerative proctitis), the rectum and sigmoid colon (proctosigmoiditis), or the entire colon (pancolitis). The inflammatory process tends to be confluent and continuous instead of skipping areas, as it does in Crohn disease.

The cause of ulcerative colitis is unknown.[81] Theories involve immune system dysfunction, genetics, changes in the normal gut bacteria, and environmental factors. Characteristic of the disease are the lesions that form in the crypts of Lieberkühn in the base of the mucosal layer. The inflammatory process leads to the formation of pinpoint mucosal hemorrhages, which in time suppurate and develop into *crypt abscesses*. These inflammatory lesions may become necrotic and ulcerate. Although the ulcerations usually are superficial, they often extend, causing large denuded areas (Fig. 37.10). As a result of the inflammatory process, the mucosal layer often develops tonguelike projections that resemble polyps and therefore are called *pseudopolyps*. The bowel wall thickens in response to repeated episodes of colitis.

Clinical Manifestations. Ulcerative colitis typically presents as a relapsing disorder marked by attacks of diarrhea. The diarrhea may persist for days, weeks, or months and then subside, only to recur after an asymptomatic interval of several months to years or even decades. Because ulcerative colitis affects the mucosal layer of the bowel, the stools typically contain blood

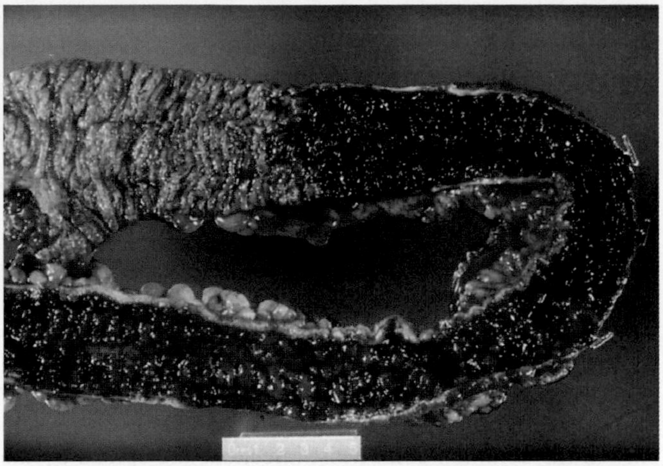

Figure 37.10 • Ulcerative colitis. Prominent erythema and ulceration of the colon begin in and are the most severe in the rectosigmoid area and extend into the ascending colon. (From Strayer D. S., Rubin R. (Eds.) (2015). *Rubin's pathophysiology: Clinicopathologic foundations of medicine* (7th ed., Figure 19-74, p. 806). Philadelphia, PA: Lippincott Williams & Wilkins.)

and mucus. Nocturnal diarrhea usually occurs when daytime symptoms are severe. There may be mild abdominal cramping and fecal incontinence. Anorexia, weakness, and fatigability are common.

Based on clinical and endoscopic findings, the disease is characterized by how much of the colon is affected and the extent of the inflammation. Severity is defined as mild, moderate, severe, or fulminant.[66] The most common form of the disease is the mild form, in which the person has less than four stools daily, with or without blood, no systemic signs of toxicity, and a normal erythrocyte sedimentation rate (ESR). People with moderate disease have more than four stools daily, but have minimal signs of toxicity. Severe disease is manifested by more than six bloody stools daily, and evidence of toxicity as demonstrated by fever, tachycardia, anemia, and elevated ESR (Fig. 37.11). People with fulminant disease have features that include more than 10 bowel movements a day, continuous bleeding, fever and other signs of toxicity, abdominal tenderness and distention, need for blood transfusions, and colonic dilation on abdominal radiographs. These people are at risk

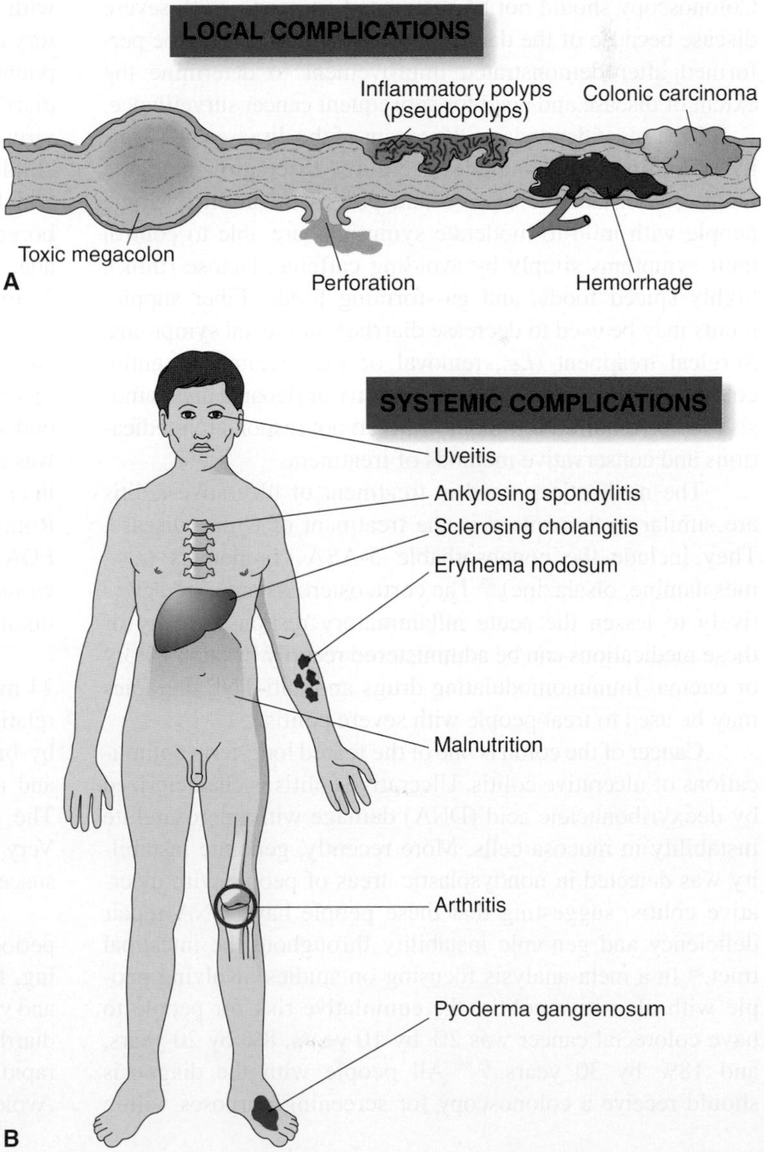

Figure 37.11 • Complications of ulcerative colitis. **(A)** A schematic representation of the major features of ulcerative colitis in the colon. **(B)** Systemic complications. (A: From Strayer D. S., Rubin R. (Eds.) (2012). *Rubin's pathophysiology: Clinicopathologic Foundations of Medicine* (6th ed., Figure 19-77, p. 807). Philadelphia, PA: Lippincott Williams & Wilkins; B: From Rubin R., Strayer D. S. (Eds.) (2012). *Rubin's pathophysiology: Clinicopathologic foundations of medicine* (6th ed., p. 658). Philadelphia, PA: Lippincott Williams & Wilkins.)

for development of toxic megacolon, which is characterized by dilation of the colon and signs of systemic toxicity. It results from extension of the inflammatory response, with involvement of neural and vascular components of the bowel.

Ulcerative colitis is believed to have a systemic (*i.e.*, autoimmune) origin, so people may present with comorbidities leading to symptoms and complications outside the colon. The frequency of such extraintestinal manifestations has been reported as anywhere between 6% and 47% (Fig. 37.11).[82] The extraintestinal manifestations may include arthritis, uveitis, deep venous thrombosis, primary sclerosing cholangitis, or ankylosing spondylitis, etc. The most common extraintestinal manifestation of IBD is arthritis. For some people, especially those with primary sclerosing cholangitis or ankylosing spondylitis, the extraintestinal manifestations may be more problematic than the bowel disease.[66]

Diagnosis and Treatment. Diagnosis of ulcerative colitis is based on history and physical examination. The diagnosis usually is confirmed by sigmoidoscopy, colonoscopy, biopsy, and by negative stool examinations for infectious or other causes. Colonoscopy should not be performed on people with severe disease because of the danger of perforation, but may be performed after demonstrated improvement to determine the extent of disease and need for subsequent cancer surveillance.

Treatment depends on the extent of the disease and severity of symptoms. It includes measures to control the acute manifestations of the disease and prevent recurrence. Some people with mild-to-moderate symptoms are able to control their symptoms simply by avoiding caffeine, lactose (milk), highly spiced foods, and gas-forming foods. Fiber supplements may be used to decrease diarrhea and rectal symptoms. Surgical treatment (*i.e.*, removal of the rectum and entire colon) with the creation of an ileostomy or ileoanal anastomosis may be required for people who do not respond to medications and conservative methods of treatment.

The medications used in treatment of ulcerative colitis are similar to those used in the treatment of Crohn disease. They include the nonabsorbable 5-ASA compounds (*e.g.*, mesalamine, olsalazine).[83] The corticosteroids are used selectively to lessen the acute inflammatory response. Many of these medications can be administered rectally by suppository or enema. Immunomodulating drugs and anti-TNF therapies may be used to treat people with severe colitis.

Cancer of the colon is one of the feared long-term complications of ulcerative colitis. Ulcerative colitis is characterized by deoxyribonucleic acid (DNA) damage with microsatellite instability in mucosa cells. More recently, genomic instability was detected in nondysplastic areas of people with ulcerative colitis, suggesting that these people have DNA repair deficiency and genomic instability throughout the intestinal tract.[84] In a meta-analysis focusing on studies involving people with ulcerative colitis, the cumulative risk for people to have colorectal cancer was 2% by 10 years, 8% by 20 years, and 18% by 30 years..[85,86] All people with the diagnosis should receive a colonoscopy for screening purposes within 8 years after they begin to have symptoms. The frequency of surveillance colonoscopies is often every 1 to 2 years and is dependent upon the results of the examinations and biopsies obtained.[87]

Infectious Enterocolitis

A number of microbial agents, including viruses, bacteria, and protozoa, can infect the GI tract, causing diarrhea and sometimes ulcerative and inflammatory changes in the small or large intestine. Infectious enterocolitis is a global problem, causing more than 12,000 deaths per day among children in developing countries. Although far less common in industrialized countries, these disorders still have infection rates second only to the common cold. Most infections are spread by the oral–fecal route, often through contaminated water or food.

Viral Infection

Most viral infections affect the superficial epithelium of the small intestine, destroying these cells and disrupting their absorptive function. Repopulation of the small intestinal villi with immature enterocytes and preservation of crypt secretory cells leads to net secretion of water and electrolytes compounded by incomplete absorption of nutrients and osmotic diarrhea. Symptomatic disease is caused by several distinct viruses, including the rotavirus, which most commonly affects children 6 to 24 months of age; the norovirus (or Norwalk), which is responsible for the majority of nonbacterial foodborne epidemic gastroenteritis in all age groups; and enteric adenoviruses, which primarily affect children younger than 24 months.[88]

Rotavirus. Worldwide, rotavirus is the leading cause of severe diarrhea and is estimated to cause 527,000 children under the age of 5 to die each year.[89] Prior to 2006, the disease was responsible for 400,000 doctor visits and 20 to 60 deaths in children below the age of 5 in the United States.[90] In 2006, RotaTeq, a live oral vaccine for rotavirus was approved by the FDA. A different live vaccine was approved in 1998 but was withdrawn from the market less than a year later when several infants developed intussusception after receiving the vaccine.

The disease tended to be most severe in children 3 to 24 months of age. Infants younger than 3 months of age are relatively protected by transplacental antibodies and possibly by breast-feeding. The virus spreads via a fecal–oral route, and outbreaks are common in children in day care centers. The virus is shed before and for days after clinical illness. Very few infectious virions are needed to cause disease in a susceptible host.

Rotavirus infection typically begins after an incubation period of 1 to 3 days, with mild-to-moderate fever and vomiting, followed by onset of frequent watery stools.[88] The fever and vomiting usually disappear on about the second day, but the diarrhea continues for 5 to 7 days. Dehydration may develop rapidly, particularly in infants. Treatment is largely supportive. Avoiding and treating dehydration are the main goals.

Bacterial Infection

Infectious enterocolitis can be caused by a number of bacteria. There are several pathogenic mechanisms for bacterial enterocolitis: ingestion of preformed toxins that are present in contaminated food; infection by toxigenic organisms that proliferate in the gut lumen and produce an enterotoxin; and infection by enteroinvasive organisms, which proliferate in the lumen and invade and destroy mucosal epithelial cells. The pathogenic effects of bacterial infections depend on the ability of the organism to adhere to the mucosal epithelial cells, elaborate enterotoxins, and then invade the mucosal epithelial cells.

In general, bacterial infections produce more severe effects than viral infections. The complications of bacterial enterocolitis result from massive fluid loss or destruction of intestinal mucosa and include dehydration, sepsis, and perforation. Among the organisms that cause bacterial enterocolitis are *Staphylococcus aureus* (toxins associated with "food poisoning"), *Escherichia coli*, *Shigella* species, *Salmonella*, and *Campylobacter*.[91] Two particularly serious forms of bacterial enterocolitis are caused by *Clostridium difficile* and *E. coli* O157:H7.

***Clostridium difficile* Colitis.** *Clostridium difficile* colitis is associated with antibiotic therapy.[92–94] *C. difficile* is a gram-positive, spore-forming bacillus that is part of the normal flora in 1% to 3% of humans.[59] The spores are resistant to the acid environment of the stomach and convert to vegetative forms in the colon. Treatment with broad-spectrum antibiotics predisposes to disruption of the normal protective bacterial flora of the colon, leading to colonization by *C. difficile* along with the release of toxins that cause mucosal damage and inflammation. Almost any antibiotic may cause *C. difficile* colitis, but broad-spectrum antibiotics with activity against gram-negative enteric bacteria are the most frequent agents. After antibiotic therapy has made the bowel susceptible to infection, colonization by *C. difficile* occurs by the oral–fecal route. *C. difficile* infection usually is acquired in the hospital, where the organism is commonly encountered.

In general, *C. difficile* is noninvasive. Development of *C. difficile* colitis and diarrhea requires an alteration in the normal gut flora, acquisition and germination of the spores, overgrowth of *C. difficile*, and toxin production. The toxins bind to and damage the intestinal mucosa, causing hemorrhage, inflammation, and necrosis. The toxins also interfere with protein synthesis, attract inflammatory cells, increase capillary permeability, and stimulate intestinal peristalsis. The infection commonly manifests with diarrhea that is mild to moderate and sometimes is accompanied by lower abdominal cramping. Typically symptoms begin within 4 to 9 days after an antibiotic treatment has been started and, in most cases, systemic manifestations are absent, and the symptoms subside after the antibiotic has been discontinued.[95]

A more severe form of colitis, *Pseudomembranous colitis*, is characterized by an adherent inflammatory membrane overlying the areas of mucosal injury. It is a life-threatening form of the disease. People with the disease are acutely ill, with lethargy, fever, tachycardia, abdominal pain and distention, and dehydration. The smooth muscle tone of the colon may be lost, resulting in toxic dilation of the colon. Prompt therapy is needed to prevent perforation of the bowel.

The diagnosis of *C. difficile*–associated diarrhea requires a careful history, with particular emphasis on antibiotic use. Diagnostic findings include a history of antibiotic use and laboratory tests that confirm the presence of *C. difficile* toxins in the stool. Treatment includes the immediate discontinuation of antibiotic therapy. Specific treatment aimed at eradicating *C. difficile* is used when symptoms are severe or persistent. Metronidazole is the drug of choice, with vancomycin being reserved for people who cannot tolerate metronidazole, do not respond to the drug, or have severe symptoms. Metronidazole can be given intravenously or oral. When given oral, it is absorbed from the upper GI tract and may cause side effects, such as nausea. Vancomycin can be given orally or via an enema. It is poorly absorbed systemically, and its actions are limited to the GI tract, resulting in a smaller number of side effects.[96]

***Escherichia coli* O157:H7 Infection.** *Escherichia coli* O157:H7 has become recognized as an important cause of epidemic and sporadic colitis.[97] *E. coli* O157:H7 is a strain of *E. coli* found in the feces and contaminated milk of healthy dairy and beef cattle, but it also has been found in contaminated pork, poultry, and lamb. Infection usually is by food-borne transmission, often by ingesting undercooked hamburger. The organism also can be transferred to nonmeat products such as fruits and vegetables. Transmission has also been reported in people swimming in a fecally contaminated lake as well as among visitors to farms and petting zoos, where children are in direct contact with animals. Person-to-person transmission may occur, particularly in nursing homes, day care settings, and hospitals. The very young and the very old are particularly at risk for the infection and its complications.

The infection may cause no symptoms or cause a variety of manifestations, including acute, nonbloody diarrhea; hemorrhagic colitis; hemolytic uremic syndrome (HUS); and thrombotic thrombocytopenic purpura. The infection often presents with abdominal cramping and watery diarrhea and subsequently may progress to bloody diarrhea. The diarrhea commonly lasts 5 to 10 days.[98]

Most strains of *E. coli* are harmless. However, enterohemorrhagic *E. coli* can release *Shigella*-like toxins that attach to and damage the mucosal lining of the intestine. Subsequently, the *Shigella*-like toxins gain access to the circulatory system and travel in the plasma and on the surface of platelets and monocytes. The *Shigella*-like toxins bind to high-affinity galactose-containing receptors in the membranes of glomerular, cerebral, or microvascular endothelial cells; renal mesangial and tubular cells; and monocytes and platelets.[99] Two complications of the infection, HUS and thrombotic thrombocytopenic purpura, reflect the effects of the *Shigella*-like toxins. The HUS is characterized by hemolytic anemia, thrombocytopenia, and renal failure. It occurs predominantly in infants and young children and is the most common cause of acute renal failure in children. The prognosis of people with HUS is generally good, and most children recover fully without subsequent relapses The mortality rate in children is less than 5% but higher in adults (25%).[100] Thrombotic thrombocytopenic purpura is manifested by thrombocytopenia, renal failure, fever, and neurologic manifestations. It often is regarded as the severe end of the disease that leads to HUS plus neurologic problems.

No specific therapy is available for *E. coli* O157:H7 infection. Treatment is largely symptomatic and directed toward treating the effects of complications. The use of antibiotics or antimotility/antidiarrheal agents in the early stages of diarrhea has been shown to increase the risk of HUS because the gut is exposed to a greater amount of toxins for a longer time.

Because of the seriousness of the infection and its complications, education of the public about techniques for decreasing primary transmission of the infection from animal sources is important. Undercooked meats and unpasteurized milk are sources of transmission. Food handlers and consumers should be aware of the proper methods for handling uncooked meat to prevent cross-contamination of other foods. Particular attention should be paid to hygiene in day care centers and nursing homes, where the spread of infection to the very young and very old may result in severe complications.

Protozoan Infection

Amebiasis refers to an infection by *Entamoeba histolytica* involving the colon and occasionally the liver.[33] Humans are the only known reservoir for *E. histolytica*, which reproduce in the colon and pass in the feces. Although *E. histolytica* infection occurs worldwide, it is more common and more severe in tropical and subtropical areas, where crowding and poor sanitation prevail. Intestinal amebiasis ranges from completely asymptomatic infection to serious dysenteric disease.

Entamoeba histolytica has two distinct stages: the trophozoites (ameboid form) and cysts.[101] The trophozoites thrive in the colon and feed on bacteria and human cells. They may colonize any portion of the large bowel, but the area of maximum disease is usually the cecum. People with symptomatic disease pass both cysts and trophozoites in their feces, but quickly die when exposed to air outside of the body. Only the cysts are infectious because they survive gastric acidity, which destroys the trophozoites. Once established, the trophozoites invade the crypts of colonic glands and burrow down into the submucosa; the organism then fans out to create a flask-shaped ulcer with a narrow neck and broad base. *Entamoeba histolytica* that have invaded into the submucosal veins of the colon enter the portal vein and embolize to the liver to produce solitary and, less often, multiple discrete hepatic abscesses.[102]

Some people have an acute onset of diarrhea as early as 8 days (commonly 2 to 4 weeks) after infection.[103] Others may be asymptomatic or have only mild intestinal symptoms for months or several years before either intestinal symptoms or liver abscesses appear. Manifestations include abdominal discomfort, tenderness, cramps, and fever, often accompanied by nausea, vomiting, and passage of malodorous flatus. There may be frequent passage of liquid stools containing bloody mucus, but the duration of diarrhea is not usually so prolonged as to cause dehydration. The infection often persists for months or years, causing emaciation and anemia. In severe cases, massive destruction of the colonic mucosa may lead to hemorrhage, perforation, or peritonitis. People with amebic liver abscesses often present with severe right upper quadrant pain, low-grade fever, and weight loss.[102]

Diagnostic methods include microscopic examination of the stool for *E. histolytica*, serum antibody tests, and colonoscopy with specimen collection or biopsy. Treatment includes use of the antimicrobial agents tinidazole and metronidazole, which act against the trophozoites, and diloxanide (not available in the United States), which is effective against the cysts.

Diverticular Disease

A diverticulum (plural: diverticula) is the medical term for an outpouching of a hollow structure in the body. Diverticulosis is the condition of having diverticula in the colon that are not inflamed. Most people with diverticulosis do not have symptoms or problems. Their presence when associated with symptoms such as left iliac fossa pain and alteration of bowel habit is known as diverticular disease.[66] Diverticulosis commonly occurs on the distal descending and sigmoid colon, in which the mucosal layer of the colon herniates through the muscularis layer.[104] There are often multiple diverticula, most of which occur in the sigmoid colon (Fig. 37.12). Diverticular disease is common in Western society, affecting approximately 40% of the population by age 60 and 60% of the population by age 80.[104] Although the disorder is prevalent in the developed countries of the world, it is almost nonexistent in many African nations and underdeveloped countries. This suggests that factors such as lack of fiber in the diet, a decrease in physical activity, and poor bowel habits (*e.g.*, neglecting the urge

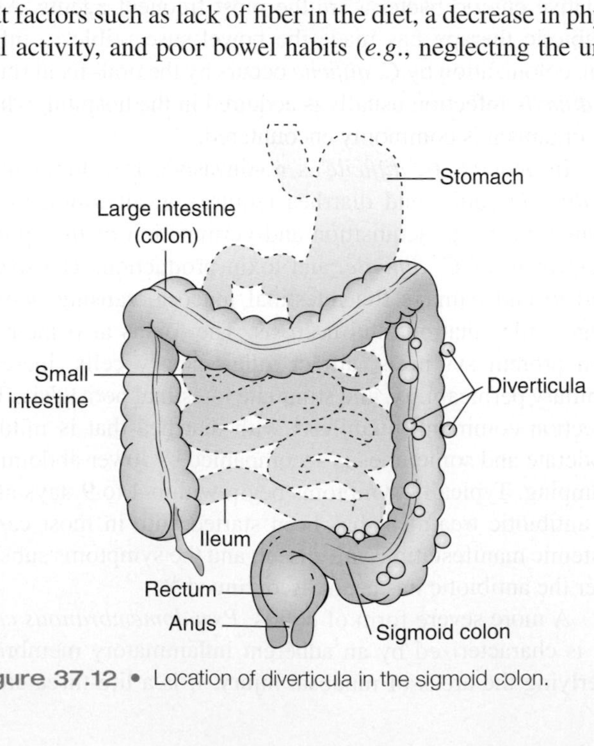

Figure 37.12 • Location of diverticula in the sigmoid colon.

to defecate), along with the effects of aging, contribute to the development of the disease.

In the colon, the longitudinal muscle does not form a continuous layer, as it does in the small bowel. Instead, there are three separate longitudinal bands of muscle called the *teniae coli*. In a manner similar to the small intestine, bands of circular muscle constrict the large intestine. As the circular muscle contracts at each of these points (approximately every 2.5 cm), the lumen of the bowel becomes constricted, so that it is almost occluded. The combined contraction of the circular muscle and the lack of a continuous longitudinal muscle layer cause the intestine to bulge outward into pouches called *haustra*. Diverticula develop between the longitudinal muscle bands of the haustra, in the area where the blood vessels pierce the circular muscle layer to bring blood to the mucosal layer. An increase in intraluminal pressure in the haustra provides the force for creating these herniations. The increase in pressure is thought to be related to the volume of the colonic contents. The scantier the contents, the more vigorous are the contractions and the greater is the pressure in the haustra.

Diverticular disease often is found when x-ray studies are done for other purposes. When symptoms do occur, they often are attributed to IBS or other causes. Ill-defined lower abdominal discomfort, a change in bowel habits (*e.g.*, diarrhea, constipation), bloating, and flatulence are common.

Meckel diverticulum is an outpouching of all layers of the small intestine wall (usually in ileum). It is the most common malformation of the GI tract and is present in approximately 2% of the population.[105]The majority of people with a Meckel diverticulum are asymptomatic.[106] An asymptomatic Meckel diverticulum is called a silent Meckel diverticulum. If symptoms do occur, they typically appear before the age of 2 years. The most common presenting symptom is painless rectal bleeding followed by intestinal obstruction, volvulus, and intussusception. Treatment in those with symptoms is surgical resection.[107]

Diverticulitis is a complication of diverticulosis in which there is inflammation and gross or microscopic perforation of the diverticulum. One of the most common complaints of diverticulitis is pain in the lower left quadrant, accompanied by nausea and vomiting, tenderness in the lower left quadrant, a slight fever, and an elevated white blood cell count.[108] These symptoms usually last for several days, unless complications occur, and usually are caused by localized inflammation of the diverticula with perforation and development of a small, localized abscess. Complications include perforation with peritonitis, hemorrhage, and bowel obstruction. Fistulas can form, involving the bladder (*i.e.*, vesicosigmoid fistula) but sometimes involving the skin, perianal area, vagina or small bowel. Pneumaturia (*i.e.*, air in the urine) is a sign of vesicosigmoid fistula.

The diagnosis of diverticular disease is based on history and presenting clinical manifestations. The disease may be confirmed by CT scans or ultrasonographic studies. CT scans are the safest and most cost-effective method.[108] Although barium enema was used in the past, it is no longer recommended because of the risk of extravasation of contrast material if perforation has occurred.[108] Flat abdominal radiographs may be used to detect complications associated with acute diverticulitis.

The usual treatment for diverticular disease is to prevent symptoms and complications. This includes increasing the bulk in the diet and bowel retraining so that the person has at least one bowel movement each day. The increased bulk promotes regular defecation and increases colonic contents and colon diameter, thereby decreasing intraluminal pressure. Acute diverticulitis is treated by withholding solid food and administering a broad-spectrum antibiotic.[108] Hospitalization may be required for people who show significant inflammation, are unable to tolerate oral fluids, are febrile, or have signs and symptoms that suggest systemic involvement. Immunomodulatory agents such as mesalamine and probiotics are two therapies that are becoming more frequently used to manage diverticular disease.[108,109] Surgical treatment is reserved for people experiencing nonresolving symptoms and complications.[104]

Appendicitis

Acute appendicitis is extremely common. In the United States, there is a 12% risk of developing appendicitis for males and a 25% risk for females.[110] The appendix becomes inflamed, swollen, and gangrenous, and it eventually perforates if not treated. Appendicitis is related to intraluminal obstruction with a fecalith (*i.e.*, hard piece of stool), gallstones, tumors, parasites, or lymphatic tissue.

Appendicitis usually has an abrupt onset, with pain referred to the epigastric or periumbilical area. This pain is caused by stretching of the appendix during the early inflammatory process. At approximately the same time that the pain appears, there are one or two episodes of nausea. Initially, the pain is vague, but over a period of 2 to 12 hours, it gradually increases and may become colicky. When the inflammatory process has extended to involve the serosal layer of the appendix and the peritoneum, the pain becomes localized to the lower right quadrant. There may be an elevated white blood cell count but not in all cases.[111] Palpation of the abdomen usually reveals a deep tenderness in the lower right quadrant, which is confined to a small area approximately the size of the fingertip. It usually is located at approximately the site of the inflamed appendix. The person with appendicitis often is able to place his or her finger directly over the tender area. Rebound tenderness, which is pain that occurs when pressure is applied to the area and then released, and spasm of the overlying abdominal muscles are common.

Diagnosis is usually based on symptoms and findings on physical examination, which can be supported by an elevation of neutrophilic white blood cells. Ultrasonography or CT may be used to confirm the diagnosis in cases where alternative causes of abdominal pain are suspected.[112] Treatment consists of surgical removal of the appendix. Complications include peritonitis, localized periappendiceal abscess formation, and septicemia.

Alterations in Intestinal Motility

The movement of contents through the GI tract is controlled by neurons located in the submucosal and myenteric plexuses of the gut. The axons from the cell bodies in the myenteric plexus innervate the circular and longitudinal smooth muscle layers of the gut. These neurons receive impulses from local receptors located in the mucosal and muscle layers of the gut and extrinsic input from the parasympathetic and sympathetic nervous systems. As a general rule, the parasympathetic nervous system tends to increase the motility of the bowel, whereas sympathetic stimulation tends to slow its activity.

The colon has sphincters at both ends: the ileocecal sphincter, which separates it from the small intestine, and the anal sphincter, which prevents the movement of feces to the outside of the body. The colon acts as a reservoir for fecal material. Normally, approximately 400 mL of water, 55 mEq of sodium, 30 mEq of chloride, and 15 mL of bicarbonate are absorbed each day in the colon. At the same time, approximately 5 mEq of potassium is secreted into the lumen of the colon. The amount of water and electrolytes that remains in the stool reflects the absorption or secretion that occurs in the colon. The average adult ingesting a typical American diet evacuates approximately 100 to 200 g of stool each day.

KEY POINTS

DISORDERS OF GASTROINTESTINAL MOTILITY

- The luminal contents move down the GI tract as a result of peristaltic movements regulated by a complex interaction of electrical, neural, and hormonal control mechanisms.
- Local irritation and the composition and constituents of GI contents influence motility through the submucosal afferent neurons of the enteric nervous system. GI wall distention, chemical irritants, osmotic gradients, and bacterial toxins exert many of their effects on GI motility through these afferent pathways.

Diarrhea

The usual definition of *diarrhea* is excessively frequent passage of loose or unformed stools. The complaint of diarrhea is a general one and can be related to a number of pathologic and nonpathologic factors. Diarrhea can be acute or chronic and can be caused by infectious organisms, food intolerance, drugs, or intestinal disease. Acute diarrheas that last less than 4 days are predominantly caused by infectious agents and follow a self-limited course.[113]

Acute Diarrhea. Diarrhea that is acute in onset and persists for less than 2 weeks is commonly caused by infectious agents (see previous discussion of infectious enterocolitis). Acute diarrhea is commonly divided into noninflammatory (large-volume) and inflammatory (small-volume) diarrhea, based on the characteristics of the diarrheal stool. Enteric organisms cause diarrhea by several ways. Some are noninvasive and do not cause inflammation, but secrete toxins that stimulate fluid secretion.[112] Others invade and destroy intestinal epithelial cells, thereby altering fluid transport so that secretory activity continues while absorption activity is halted.[114]

Noninflammatory diarrhea is associated with large-volume watery and nonbloody stools, periumbilical cramps, bloating, and nausea or vomiting. It is commonly caused by toxin-producing bacteria (*e.g.*, *S. aureus*,[115] enterotoxigenic *E. coli*, *Cryptosporidium parvum*, *Vibrio cholerae*) or other agents (*e.g.*, viruses, *Giardia*) that disrupt the normal absorption or secretory process in the small bowel.[116] Prominent vomiting suggests viral enteritis or *S. aureus* food poisoning. Although typically mild, the diarrhea (which originates in the small intestine) can be voluminous and result in dehydration with hypokalemia and metabolic acidosis (*i.e.*, cholera). Because tissue invasion does not occur, leukocytes are not present in the feces.

Inflammatory diarrhea is usually characterized by the presence of fever and bloody diarrhea (dysentery). It is caused by invasion of intestinal cells (*e.g.*, *Shigella*, *Salmonella*, *Yersinia*, and *Campylobacter*) or the toxins associated with the previously described *C. difficile* or *E. coli* O157:H7 infection. Because infections associated with these organisms predominantly affect the colon, the diarrhea is frequent and small in volume[117] and is associated with left lower quadrant cramps, urgency, and tenesmus. Infectious dysentery must be distinguished from acute ulcerative colitis, which may present with bloody diarrhea, fever, and abdominal pain. Diarrhea that persists for 14 days is not attributable to bacterial pathogens (except for *C. difficile*), and the person should be evaluated for chronic diarrhea.

Chronic Diarrhea. Diarrhea is considered to be chronic when the symptoms persist for 4 weeks or greater.[113] Chronic diarrhea is often associated with conditions such as IBD, IBS, malabsorption syndrome, endocrine disorders (hyperthyroidism, diabetic autonomic neuropathy), or radiation colitis. There are four major causes of chronic diarrhea: presence of hyperosmotic luminal contents, increased intestinal secretory processes, inflammatory conditions, and infectious processes[113] (Chart 37.1). Factitious diarrhea is caused by indiscriminate use of laxatives or excessive intake of laxative-type foods.

In *osmotic diarrhea*, water is pulled into the bowel by the hyperosmotic nature of its contents to such a quantity that the colon is unable to reabsorb the excess fluid. It occurs when osmotically active particles are not absorbed. In people with lactase deficiency, lactose intolerance is due to the lack of enzyme lactase in the small intestines to break lactose down into glucose and galactose.[118] Inadequate lactase activity allows lactose to reach the large intestine. There, the gut flora provides a salvage pathway for lactose digestion by cleaving lactose into short-chain fatty acids (SCFA) and

CHART 37.1 CHRONIC DIARRHEA

- Hyperosmotic diarrhea
  - Saline cathartics
  - Lactase deficiency
- Secretory diarrhea
  - Acute infectious diarrhea
  - Failure to absorb bile salts
  - Fat malabsorption
  - Chronic laxative abuse
  - Carcinoid syndrome
  - Zollinger-Ellison syndrome
  - Fecal impaction
- Inflammatory bowel disease
  - Crohn disease
  - Ulcerative colitis
- Infectious disease
  - Shigellosis
  - Salmonellosis
- Irritable colon

gas, mainly hydrogen (H_2), carbon dioxide (CO_2), and methane (CH_4). Nondigested lactose can cause osmotic diarrhea; products of its bacterial digestion can lead to secretory diarrhea and gas distending the intestines, events that are likely to lead to clinical symptoms. Lactose intolerance is characterized by abdominal symptoms (*e.g.*, nausea, bloating, and pain) after ingestion of dairy products. Magnesium salts, which are contained in milk of magnesia and many antacids, are poorly absorbed and cause diarrhea when taken in sufficient quantities. Another cause of osmotic diarrhea is decreased transit time, which interferes with absorption. Osmotic diarrhea usually disappears with fasting.[118,119]

Secretory diarrhea occurs when the secretory processes of the bowel are increased. Secretory diarrhea also occurs when excess bile acids remain in the intestinal contents as they enter the colon. This often happens with disease processes of the ileum because bile salts are absorbed there. It also may occur with bacterial overgrowth in the small bowel, which interferes with bile absorption. Some tumors, such as those of the Zollinger-Ellison syndrome and carcinoid syndrome, produce hormones that cause increased secretory activity of the bowel.[120]

Inflammatory diarrhea commonly is associated with acute or chronic inflammation or intrinsic disease of the colon, such as ulcerative colitis or Crohn disease. Inflammatory diarrhea usually is evidenced by frequency and urgency and colicky abdominal pain. It commonly is accompanied by tenesmus (*i.e.*, painful straining at stool), fecal soiling of clothing, and awakening during the night with the urge to defecate.

Chronic parasitic infections may cause chronic diarrhea through a number of mechanisms. Pathogens most commonly associated with chronic diarrhea include the protozoans *Giardia*, *E. histolytica*, and *Cyclospora*. People who are immunocompromised are particularly susceptible to infectious organisms that can cause acute and chronic diarrhea, including *Cryptosporidium*, cytomegalovirus (CMV), and *Mycobacterium avium-intracellulare* complex.

Diagnosis and Treatment. The diagnosis of diarrhea is based on complaints of frequent stools and a history of accompanying factors such as concurrent illnesses, medication use, and exposure to potential intestinal pathogens. Disorders such as IBD and celiac disease should be considered.[113] If the onset of diarrhea is related to travel outside the United States, the possibility of traveler's diarrhea must be considered.

Although most acute forms of diarrhea are self-limited and require no treatment, diarrhea can be particularly serious in infants and small children, people with other illnesses, elderly people, and even previously healthy people if it continues for any length of time. Thus, the replacement of fluids and electrolytes is considered to be a primary therapeutic goal in the treatment of diarrhea.

Drugs used in the treatment of diarrhea include diphenoxylate (Lomotil) and loperamide (Imodium), which are opium-like drugs. These drugs decrease GI motility and stimulate water and electrolyte absorption. Adsorbents, such as kaolin and pectin, adsorb irritants and toxins from the bowel. These ingredients are included in many over-the-counter antidiarrheal preparations because they adsorb toxins responsible for certain types of diarrhea. Bismuth subsalicylate (Pepto-Bismol) can be used to reduce the frequency of unformed stools and increase stool consistency, particularly in cases of traveler's diarrhea. The drug is thought to inhibit intestinal secretion caused by enterotoxigenic *E. coli* and cholera toxins. Antidiarrheal medications should not be used in people with bloody diarrhea, high fever, or signs of toxicity because of the risk of worsening the disease. Antibiotics should be reserved for use in people with identified enteric pathogens.

Acute Diarrheal Disease in Children. Despite global success in the reduction of diarrhea-specific mortality in the past 30 years, diarrhea remains the second leading cause of death because of infections among children under 5 years of age worldwide. It is estimated that diarrhea accounted for 9.9% of the 6.9 million deaths among children under 5 in 2011.[121] Although diarrheal diseases are less prevalent in the United States than in other countries, they place a burden on the health care system. Diarrhea is also the leading cause of malnutrition in children and most frequently affects children under the age of 2 years.[121]

The causes of acute diarrhea in children vary with location, time of year, and population studied. There is increasing recognition of a widening array of enteric pathogens that cause acute diarrhea in children. Viruses are the most common pathogen causing diarrheal illness.[122]

Rotaviruses and noroviruses are the frequently observed pathogens. Other viruses that have been observed in the stools of children include astroviruses and enteric adenoviruses. Many of these pathogens are transmitted easily through food and water or from one person to another. Prevention remains the most vital measure in managing diarrheal disease in children. Important measures to prevent spread of pathogens include proper sanitation methods for food processing and preparation, sanitary water supplies, proper hand hygiene, exclusion of infected people from handling food or providing health care, and exclusion of people with diarrhea from using public recreational water (*i.e.*, swimming pools, ponds, and lakes).

The main objectives in the approach to a child with acute diarrhea are to assess the degree of dehydration, prevent spread of the infection, determine the nature of the etiologic agent, and provide specific therapy as needed. The hydration status of children can be assessed on the basis of easily observed signs and symptoms. Questions about oral intake, frequency and volume of stool output, general appearance and activity of the child, and frequency of urination provide essential information about hydration. Thirst, dry mucous membranes, and decreased skin turgor are common symptoms of dehydration.[122] Data should be obtained about day care attendance, recent travel to a diarrhea-endemic area, use of antimicrobial drugs, and exposure to contaminated water, unwashed fruits or vegetables, or improperly cooked meats because they may indicate the cause of the disorder. Fever is suggestive of an inflammatory process but also occurs with dehydration.[122]

Management of dehydration remains the cornerstone of treatment of children with diarrhea. Infants in particular are more susceptible to dehydration because of their greater surface area, higher metabolic rate, and inability effectively to concentrate their urine. Oral replacement therapy (ORT) is usually the method of choice for infants and children with uncomplicated diarrhea that can be treated at home.

First applied to the treatment of diarrhea in developing countries, ORT can be regarded as a case of reverse technology, in which the protocols originally implemented in these countries have changed health care in industrialized countries as well.[123] Complete ORT solutions contain carbohydrate, sodium, potassium, chloride, and base to replace that lost in the diarrheal stool.[123] Commonly used beverages such as apple juice and cola drinks, which have increased osmolarity because of their high carbohydrate content and low electrolyte content, are not recommended. The effectiveness of ORT is based on the coupled transport of sodium and glucose or other actively transported small organic molecules (see Chapter 36). Bottled ORT solutions are available but can be costly, particularly in cases where large amounts of replacement fluids are needed. The cost can represent a sizable burden for socioeconomically disadvantaged families. Less expensive, premeasured packets and recipes for preparing replacement solutions are available. The use of ORT for treatment of diarrhea in infants and small children is often labor intensive, requiring frequent feeding, sometimes using a spoon or a nasogastric feeding tube.[122] More importantly, the diarrhea does not promptly cease after ORT has been instituted; this can be discouraging for parents and caregivers who desire early results from their efforts. Children who are severely dehydrated with changes in vital signs or mental status require emergency intravenous fluid resuscitation. After initial treatment with intravenous fluids, these children can be given ORT.

Evidence suggests that feeding should be continued during diarrheal illness, particularly in children.[123] It has been shown that unrestricted diets do not worsen the course or symptoms of mild diarrhea and can decrease stool output.[124] Starch and simple proteins are thought to provide cotransport molecules with little osmotic activity, increasing fluid and electrolyte uptake by intestinal cells. The luminal contents associated with early refeeding are also a known growth factor for enterocytes and help facilitate repair after injury. It is recommended that children who require rehydration therapy because of diarrhea be fed an age-appropriate diet. Although there is little agreement on which foods are best, fatty foods and foods high in simple sugars are best avoided. Almost all infants with acute gastroenteritis can tolerate breast-feeding. For formula-fed infants, diluted formula does not provide an advantage over full-strength formula.

Constipation

Constipation can be defined as the infrequent, incomplete, or difficult passage of stools.[113] The difficulty with this definition arises from the many individual variations of function that are normal. What is considered normal for one person (*e.g.*, two or three bowel movements per week) may be considered evidence of constipation by another. Constipation can occur as a primary disorder of intestinal motility, as a side effect of drugs, as a problem associated with another disease condition, or as a symptom of obstructing lesions of the GI tract. Some common causes of constipation are failure to respond to the urge to defecate, inadequate fiber in the diet, inadequate fluid intake, weakness of the abdominal muscles, inactivity and bed rest, pregnancy, and hemorrhoids. The pathophysiology of constipation can be classified into three broad categories: normal-transit constipation, slow-transit constipation, and disorders of defecatory or rectal evacuation. Normal-transit constipation (or functional constipation) is characterized by perceived difficulty in defecation and usually responds to increased fluid and fiber intake.[115] Slow-transit constipation, which is characterized by infrequent bowel movements, is often caused by alterations in the motor function of the colon.[125] Hirschsprung disease is an extreme form of slow-transit constipation in which the ganglion cells in the distal bowel are absent because of a defect that occurred during embryonic development; the bowel narrows at the area that lacks ganglionic cells.[126] Although most people with this disorder present in infancy or early childhood, some with a relatively short segment of involved colon do not have symptoms until later in life. Defecatory disorders are most commonly due to deficiencies in muscle coordination involving the pelvic floor or anal sphincter.

Diseases associated with chronic constipation include neurologic diseases such as spinal cord injury, Parkinson disease, and multiple sclerosis; endocrine disorders such as hypothyroidism; and obstructive lesions in the GI tract. Drugs such as narcotics, anticholinergic agents, calcium channel blockers, diuretics, calcium (antacids and supplements), iron supplements, and aluminum antacids tend to cause constipation. Older adults with long-standing constipation and straining with defecation may develop dilation of the rectum, colon, or both. This condition allows large amounts of stool to accumulate with little or no sensation. Constipation, in the context of a change in bowel habits, may be a sign of colorectal cancer.

Diagnosis of constipation usually is based on a history of infrequent stools, straining with defecation, the passing of hard and lumpy stools, or the sense of incomplete evacuation with defecation. Rectal examination is used to determine whether fecal impaction, anal stricture, or rectal masses are present. Constipation as a sign of another disease condition should be ruled out. Tests that measure colon transit time and defecatory function are reserved for refractory cases.

The treatment of constipation usually is directed toward relieving the cause. A conscious effort should be made to respond to the defecation urge. A time should be set aside after a meal, when mass movements in the colon are most likely to occur, for a bowel movement. Mimicking a squatting position while sitting on the toilet by elevating the feet may assist in promoting a bowel movement.[125] Adequate fluid intake and bulk in the diet should be encouraged. Moderate exercise is essential, and people on bed rest benefit from passive and active exercises. Laxatives and enemas should be used judiciously. They should not be used on a regular basis to treat simple constipation because they interfere with the defecation reflex and actually may damage the rectal mucosa.

Fecal Impaction

Fecal impaction is the retention of hardened or putty-like stool in the rectum and colon, which interferes with normal passage of feces. If not removed, it can cause partial or complete bowel obstruction. It may occur in any age group but is more common in incapacitated older adults. Fecal impaction may result from painful anorectal disease, tumors, or neurogenic disease; use of constipating antacids or bulk laxatives; a low-residue diet; drug-induced colonic stasis; or prolonged bed rest and debility. In children, a habitual neglect of the urge to defecate in the school setting because of cleanliness of the facilities,[127] modesty, or play interference may promote impaction.

The manifestations may be those of severe constipation, but frequently there is a history of watery diarrhea, fecal soiling, and fecal incontinence.[128] This is caused by increased secretory activity of the bowel, representing the body's attempt to break up the mass so that it can be evacuated. The abdomen may be distended, and there may be blood and mucus in the stool. The fecal mass may compress the urethra, giving rise to urinary incontinence. Fecal impaction should be considered in an elderly or immobilized person who develops watery stools with fecal or urinary incontinence.

Digital examination of the rectum is done to assess for the presence of a fecal mass. The mass may need to be broken up and dislodged manually or with the use of a sigmoidoscope. Oil enemas often are used to soften the mass before removal. The best treatment is prevention.

Intestinal Obstruction

Intestinal obstruction designates an impairment of movement of intestinal contents in a cephalocaudad direction. The causes can be categorized as mechanical or paralytic. Strangulation with necrosis of the bowel may occur and lead to perforation, peritonitis, and sepsis.

Mechanical obstruction can result from a number of conditions, intrinsic or extrinsic, that encroach on the patency of the bowel lumen (Fig. 37.13). Postoperative causes such as external hernia (*i.e.*, inguinal, femoral, or umbilical) and postoperative adhesions are responsible for 75% of intestinal obstruction occurrences.[129] Less common causes are strictures, tumors, foreign bodies, intussusception, and volvulus.

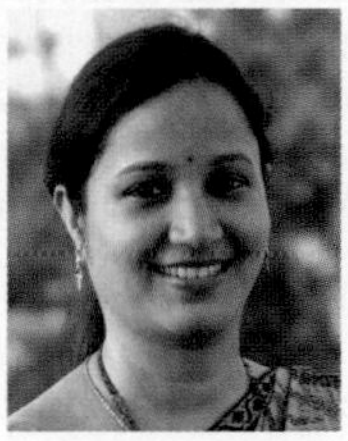

Remember **Ms. Rytel,** from the unit-opening case study? She is most likely experiencing an obstruction related to the adhesions that occurred due to the necessary repairs required after the motor vehicle collision. At this point, she is monitored closely and receives a nasogastric tube to decompress the upper portion of her GI tract. She is also given nothing by mouth, and her nausea is controlled with intravenous antiemetics. If her vitals began to deteriorate, she would be prepped to go to the operating room for an open exploration of her abdomen for possible lysis of adhesions.

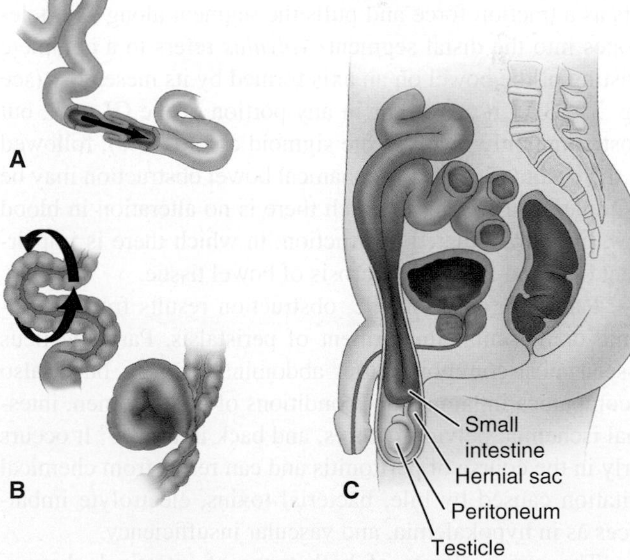

Figure 37.13 • Three causes of intestinal obstruction. **(A)** Intussusception; invagination or shortening of the bowel caused by movement of one segment of the bowel into another. **(B)** Volvulus of the sigmoid colon; the twist is counterclockwise in most cases. Note the edematous section of bowel. **(C)** Hernia (inguinal). The sac of the hernia is a continuation of the peritoneum of the abdomen. The hernial contents are intestine, omentum, or other abdominal contents that pass through the hernial opening into the hernial sac. (From Hinkle J., & Cheever, K. H. (Eds). (2018) *Brunner and Suddarth's textbook of medical-surgical nursing* (14th ed., Figure 47-5, p. 1327). Philadelphia, PA: Lippincott Williams & Wilkins.)

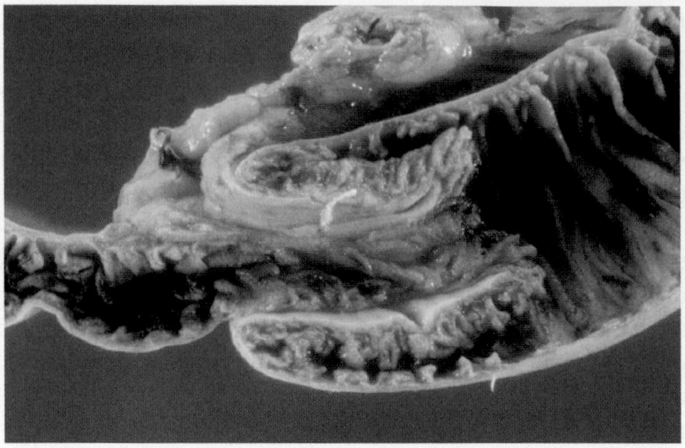

Figure 37.14 • Intussusception. The proximal ileum has telescoped into the distal ileum in this case of intussusception; the anatomy is well seen in the cut section. (From Strayer D. S., Rubin R. (Eds.) (2012). *Rubin's pathophysiology: Clinicopathologic foundations of medicine* (7th ed., Figure 19-42B, p. 781). Philadelphia, PA: Lippincott Williams & Wilkins.)

Intussusception involves the telescoping of bowel into the adjacent segment (Fig. 37.14). It is the most common cause of intestinal obstruction in children younger than 2 years of age.[130] The most common form is intussusception of the terminal ileum into the right colon, but other areas of the bowel may be involved. The condition is diagnosed most often in infancy and early childhood. It strikes about 2000 infants in the United States in the first year of life. In most cases, the cause of the disorder is unknown. The condition can also occur in adults when an intraluminal mass or tumor acts as a traction force and pulls the segment along as it telescopes into the distal segment. *Volvulus* refers to a complete twisting of the bowel on an axis formed by its mesentery (see Fig. 37.13B). It can occur in any portion of the GI tract, but most commonly involves the sigmoid colon (75%), followed by the cecum (22%).[131] Mechanical bowel obstruction may be a simple obstruction, in which there is no alteration in blood flow, or a strangulated obstruction, in which there is impairment of blood flow and necrosis of bowel tissue.

Paralytic, or adynamic, obstruction results from neurogenic or muscular impairment of peristalsis. Paralytic ileus is seen most commonly after abdominal surgery, but it also accompanies inflammatory conditions of the abdomen, intestinal ischemia, pelvic fractures, and back injuries.[132] It occurs early in the course of peritonitis and can result from chemical irritation caused by bile, bacterial toxins, electrolyte imbalances as in hypokalemia, and vascular insufficiency.

The major effects of both types of intestinal obstruction are abdominal distention and loss of fluids and electrolytes (Fig. 37.15). Gases and fluids accumulate in the area; if untreated, the distention resulting from bowel obstruction tends to perpetuate itself by causing atony of the bowel and further distention. Distention is further aggravated by the accumulation of gases. As the process continues, the distention moves proximally (*i.e.*, toward the mouth), involving additional segments of bowel. Either form of obstruction

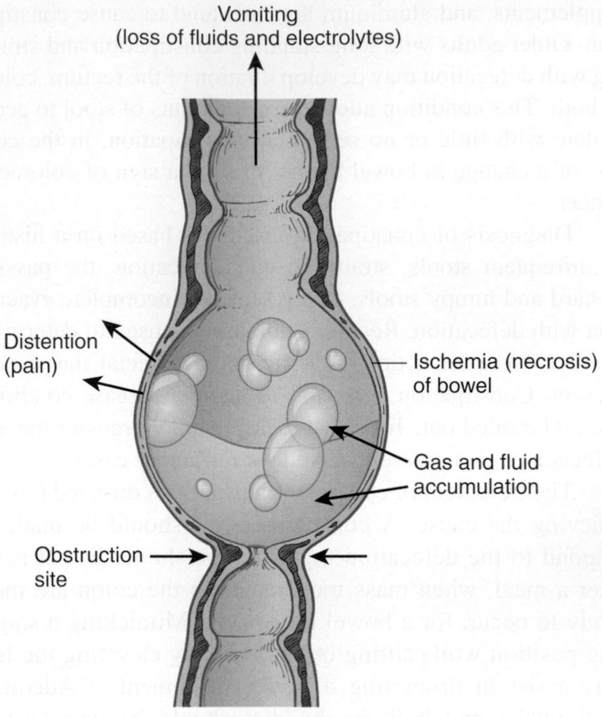

Figure 37.15 • Pathophysiology of intestinal obstruction.

eventually may lead to strangulation (*i.e.*, interruption of blood flow), gangrenous changes, and, ultimately, perforation of the bowel. The increased pressure in the intestine tends to compromise mucosal blood flow, leading to necrosis and movement of blood into the luminal fluids. This promotes rapid growth of bacteria in the obstructed bowel, which has the potential to move into the lymph system and surrounding organs.[131] The movement of the bacteria outside of the digestive tract results in increased inflammation, which can result in further ischemia and organ failure.[131]

The manifestations of intestinal obstruction depend on the degree of obstruction and its duration. With acute obstruction, the onset usually is sudden and dramatic. With chronic conditions, the onset often is more gradual. The cardinal symptoms of intestinal obstruction are pain, absolute constipation, abdominal distention, sign of fluid volume deficit, and vomiting. With mechanical obstruction, the pain is severe and colicky, in contrast with the continuous pain and silent abdomen of paralytic ileus. There also is borborygmi (*i.e.*, rumbling sounds made by propulsion of gas in the intestine); audible, high-pitched peristalsis; and peristaltic rushes that tend to associate with episodes of abdominal pain.[131] Visible peristalsis may appear along the course of the distended intestine. Extreme restlessness and conscious awareness of intestinal movements are experienced along with weakness, perspiration, and anxiety. Should strangulation of the bowel occur, the symptoms change. The character of the pain shifts from the intermittent colicky pain caused by the hyperperistaltic movements of the intestine to a severe and steady type of pain. Vomiting and fluid and electrolyte disorders occur with both types of obstruction.

Diagnosis of intestinal obstruction usually is based on history and physical findings. Plain film radiography of the abdomen may be used to determine the presence of an obstruction as well as differentiate between partial and complete obstruction by analysis of gas patterns within the bowel.[129] CT scans and ultrasonography may also be used to detect the presence of mechanical obstruction.

Treatment depends on the cause and type of obstruction. Correction of fluid and electrolyte imbalances to baseline levels and measurement of output using a Foley catheter are recommended. Most cases of adynamic obstruction respond to decompression of the bowel through nasogastric suction. Strangulation and complete bowel obstruction require surgical intervention. Intraoperatively, the bowel is observed for return of normal color and peristalsis. If necrotic tissue present, it is resected, and an anastomosis is made.

Peritonitis

Peritonitis is an inflammatory response of the serous membrane that lines the abdominal cavity and covers the visceral organs. It can be caused by bacterial invasion or chemical irritation. Most commonly, enteric bacteria enter the peritoneum because of a defect in the wall of one of the abdominal organs. Causes of peritonitis include perforated peptic ulcer, ruptured appendix, perforated diverticulum, gangrenous bowel, pelvic inflammatory disease, and gangrenous gallbladder. Other environmental causes are abdominal trauma, foreign body ingestion, and infected peritoneal dialysis catheters. Generalized peritonitis, although no longer the overwhelming problem it once was, is still a leading cause of death after abdominal surgery.

The peritoneum has several characteristics that increase its vulnerability to or protect it from the effects of peritonitis. One weakness of the peritoneal cavity is that it is a large, unbroken space that favors the dissemination of contaminants. For the same reason, it has a large surface area that permits rapid absorption of bacterial toxins into the blood. The peritoneum is particularly well adapted for producing an inflammatory response as a means of controlling infection. It tends, for example, to exude a thick, sticky, and fibrinous substance that adheres to other structures, such as the mesentery and omentum, and that seals off the perforated viscus and aids in localizing the process. Localization is enhanced by sympathetic stimulation that limits intestinal motility. Although the diminished or absent peristalsis that occurs tends to give rise to associated problems, it does inhibit the movement of contaminants throughout the peritoneal cavity.

One of the most important manifestations of peritonitis is the translocation of extracellular fluid into the peritoneal cavity (through weeping or serous fluid from the inflamed peritoneum) and into the bowel as a result of bowel obstruction. Nausea and vomiting cause further losses of fluid. The fluid loss may encourage development of hypovolemia and shock. The onset of peritonitis may be acute, as with a ruptured appendix, or it may have a more gradual onset, as occurs in pelvic inflammatory disease. Pain and tenderness are common symptoms. The pain usually is more intense over the inflamed area. The person with peritonitis usually lies still because any movement aggravates the pain. Breathing often is shallow to prevent movement of the abdominal muscles. The abdomen usually is rigid and sometimes described as boardlike because of reflex muscle guarding. Vomiting is common. Fever, an elevated white blood cell count, tachycardia, and hypotension are common. Hiccups may develop because of irritation of the phrenic nerve. Paralytic ileus occurs shortly after the onset of widespread peritonitis and is accompanied by abdominal distention. Peritonitis that progresses and is untreated leads to toxemia and shock.

Treatment. Treatment measures for peritonitis are directed toward preventing the extension of the inflammatory response, intravenously correcting the fluid and electrolyte imbalances that develop, and minimizing the effects of paralytic ileus and abdominal distention. Oral resuscitation is avoided because of the potential need for surgical intervention. Surgical intervention may be needed to address the source of the inflammation, for example, removing an acutely inflamed appendix or closing the opening in a perforated peptic ulcer.

Nasogastric suction, which entails the insertion of a tube placed through the nose into the stomach or intestine, is used to decompress the bowel and relieve the abdominal distention. Fluid and electrolyte replacement is essential. These fluids are prescribed on the basis of frequent blood chemistry determinations. Antibiotics are given to combat infection. Narcotics often are needed for pain relief.

Alterations in Intestinal Absorption

Malabsorption is the failure to transport dietary constituents, such as fats, carbohydrates, proteins, vitamins, and minerals, from the lumen of the intestine into the extracellular fluid compartment for transport to the various parts of the body. It can selectively affect a single component, such as vitamin B_{12} or lactose, or its effects can extend to all the substances absorbed in a specific segment of the intestine. When one segment of the intestine is affected, another may compensate. For example, the ileum may compensate for malabsorption in the proximal small intestine by absorbing substantial amounts of fats, carbohydrates, and amino acids. Similarly, the colon, which normally absorbs water, sodium, chloride, and bicarbonate, can compensate for small intestine malabsorption by absorbing additional end products of bacterial carbohydrate metabolism.

The conditions that impair one or more steps involved in digestion and absorption of nutrients can be divided into three broad categories: intraluminal maldigestion, disorders of transepithelial transport, and lymphatic obstruction. Intraluminal maldigestion involves a defect in processing of nutrients in the intestinal lumen. The most common causes are pancreatic insufficiency, hepatobiliary disease, and intraluminal bacterial growth. Disorders of transepithelial transport are caused by mucosal lesions that impair uptake and transport of available intraluminal nutrients across the mucosal surface of the intestine. They include disorders such as celiac disease and Crohn disease. Lymphatic obstruction interferes with the transport of the products of fat digestion to the systemic circulation after they have been absorbed by the intestinal mucosa. The process can be interrupted by congenital defects, neoplasms, trauma, and selected infectious diseases.

Malabsorption Syndrome

People with intestinal malabsorption usually have symptoms directly referable to the GI tract that include diarrhea, flatulence, distention, abdominal pain and/or cramps, and ascites.[133] Weakness, muscle wasting, weight loss, and abdominal distention often are present. Weight loss often occurs despite normal or excessive caloric intake. Steatorrheic stools contain excess fat. The fat content causes bulky, yellow-gray, malodorous stools. In a person consuming a diet containing 80 to 100 g of fat each day, excretion of 7 to 9 g of fat indicates steatorrhea.[133]

Along with loss of fat in the stools, there is failure to absorb the fat-soluble vitamins. This can lead to easy bruising and bleeding (*i.e.*, vitamin K deficiency), bone pain, a predisposition to the development of fractures and tetany (*i.e.*, vitamin D and calcium deficiency), macrocytic anemia,[134] and glossitis (*i.e.*, folic acid deficiency). Neuropathy, atrophy of the skin, and peripheral edema may be present. Table 37.2

TABLE 37.2 SITES OF AND REQUIREMENTS FOR ABSORPTION OF DIETARY CONSTITUENTS AND MANIFESTATIONS OF MALABSORPTION

DIETARY CONSTITUENT	SITE OF ABSORPTION	REQUIREMENTS	MANIFESTATIONS
Water and electrolytes	Mainly small bowel	Osmotic gradient	Diarrhea Dehydration Cramps
Fat	Upper jejunum	Pancreatic lipase Bile salts Functioning lymphatic channels	Weight loss Steatorrhea Fat-soluble vitamin deficiency
Carbohydrates			
Starch	Small intestine	Amylase Maltase Isomaltase α-dextrins	Diarrhea Flatulence Abdominal discomfort
Sucrose	Small intestine	Sucrase	
Lactose	Small intestine	Lactase	
Maltose	Small intestine	Maltase	
Fructose	Small intestine		
Protein	Small intestine	Pancreatic enzymes (*e.g.*, trypsin, chymotrypsin, elastin)	Loss of muscle mass Weakness Edema
Vitamins			
A	Upper jejunum	Bile salts	Night blindness Dry eyes Corneal irritation
Folic acid	Duodenum and jejunum	Absorptive; may be impaired by some drugs (*i.e.*, anticonvulsants)	Cheilosis Glossitis Megaloblastic anemia
B_{12}	Ileum	Intrinsic factor	Glossitis Neuropathy Megaloblastic anemia
D	Upper jejunum	Bile salts	Bone pain Fractures Tetany
E	Upper jejunum	Bile salts	Uncertain
K	Upper jejunum	Bile salts	Easy bruising and bleeding
Calcium	Duodenum	Vitamin D and parathyroid hormone	Bone pain Fractures Tetany
Iron	Duodenum and jejunum	Normal pH (hydrochloric acid secretion)	Iron deficiency anemia Glossitis

describes the signs and symptoms of impaired absorption of dietary constituents.

Celiac Disease

Celiac disease, also known as *Celiac sprue* and *Gluten-sensitive enteropathy*, is an immune-mediated disorder triggered by ingestion of gluten-containing grains (including wheat, barley, and rye).[135,136] Until recently, celiac disease was considered to be a rare malabsorption syndrome that manifested during early childhood, but today it is known to be one of the most common genetic diseases, with a mean prevalence of 1% to 6% in the general population.[137–139]

The disease results from an inappropriate T-cell–mediated immune response against ingested α-gliadin (a component of gluten protein) in genetically predisposed people. Almost all people with the disorder share the major histocompatibility complex class II allele HLA-DQ2 or HLA-DQ8.[140] People with the disease have increased levels of antibodies to a variety of antigens, including transglutaminase, endomysium, and gliadin. The resultant immune response produces an intense inflammatory reaction that results in loss of absorptive villi from the small intestine (Fig. 37.16). When the resulting lesions are extensive, they may impair absorption of macronutrients (*i.e.*, proteins, carbohydrates, fats) and micronutrients (*i.e.*, vitamins and minerals). Small bowel involvement is most prominent in the proximal part of the small intestine, where the exposure to gluten is greatest.

There are a number of populations who are at higher risk for celiac disease. These include people with type 1 diabetes mellitus, other autoimmune endocrinopathies, dermatitis herpetiformis, first- and second-degree relatives of people with celiac disease, and people with Turner syndrome.[141,142] Various malignancies also appear to be a direct result of celiac disease, in that the increased incidence seen in people with celiac disease returns to that of the general population after several years of a gluten-free diet. These malignancies include head and neck squamous cell carcinoma, small intestinal adenocarcinoma, and non-Hodgkin lymphoma.

The classic form of celiac disease presents in infancy and manifests as failure to thrive, diarrhea, muscle wasting, abdominal distention, and, occasionally, severe malnutrition.[143] Beyond infancy, the manifestations tend to be less dramatic. Older children may present with anemia, constitutional short stature, dental enamel defects, and constipation. In adults, GI symptoms may manifest as diarrhea, constipation, or other symptoms of malabsorption such as bloating, flatus, or belching.

The diagnosis of celiac disease is based on clinical manifestations, supported by serologic tests and confirmed by intestinal biopsy.[135,141] Based on very high sensitivities, the best available tests are the Ig A antihuman tissue transglutaminase (TTG) and IgA endomysial antibody immunofluorescence (EMA) tests.[135] Biopsies of the proximal small bowel are indicated in people with a positive celiac disease antibody test.[141] Usually, additional laboratory tests are done

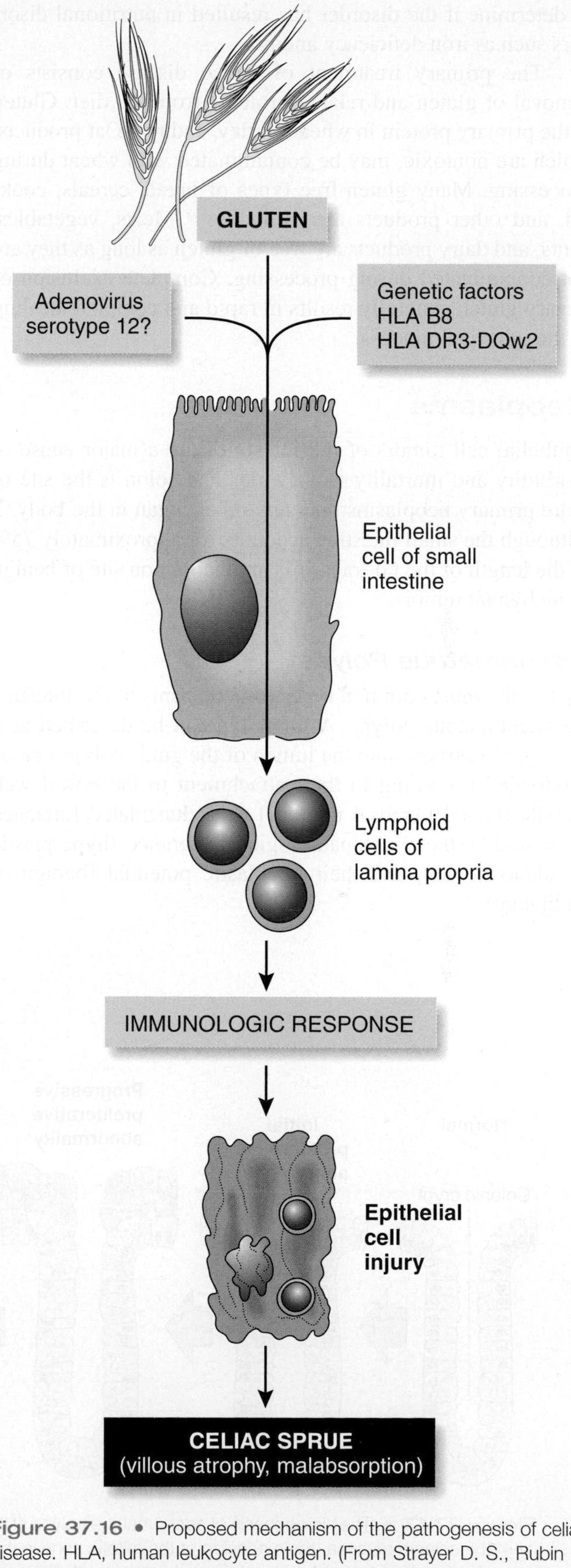

Figure 37.16 • Proposed mechanism of the pathogenesis of celiac disease. HLA, human leukocyte antigen. (From Strayer D. S., Rubin R. (Eds.) (2015). *Rubin's pathophysiology: Clinicopathologic foundations of medicine* (6th ed., Figure 19-44, p. 783). Philadelphia, PA: Lippincott Williams & Wilkins.)

to determine if the disorder has resulted in nutritional disorders such as iron deficiency anemia.

The primary treatment of celiac disease consists of removal of gluten and related proteins from the diet. Gluten is the primary protein in wheat, barley, and rye. Oat products, which are nontoxic, may be contaminated with wheat during processing. Many gluten-free types of bread, cereals, cookies, and other products are available.[136] Meats, vegetables, fruits, and dairy products are free of gluten as long as they are not contaminated during processing. Complete exclusion of dietary gluten generally results in rapid and complete healing of the intestinal mucosa.

Neoplasms

Epithelial cell tumors of the intestines are a major cause of morbidity and mortality worldwide. The colon is the site of more primary neoplasms than any other organ in the body.[144] Although the small intestine accounts for approximately 75% of the length of the GI tract, it is an uncommon site of benign or malignant tumors.

Adenomatous Polyps

By far, the most common types of neoplasms of the intestine are adenomatous polyps. A GI polyp can be described as a mass that protrudes into the lumen of the gut.[13] Polyps can be subdivided according to their attachment to the bowel wall (sessile [raised mucosal nodules] or pedunculated [attached by a stalk]), their histopathologic appearance (hyperplastic or adenomatous), and their neoplastic potential (benign or malignant).[13]

Adenomatous polyps (adenomas) are benign neoplasms that arise from the mucosal epithelium of the intestine. They are composed of neoplastic cells that have proliferated in excess of those needed to replace the cells that normally are shed from the mucosal surface (Fig. 37.17). The pathogenesis of adenoma formation involves neoplastic alteration in the replication of the crypt epithelial cells. There may be diminished apoptosis, persistence of cell replication, and failure of cell maturation and differentiation of the cells that migrate to the surface of the crypts.[10] Normally, DNA synthesis ceases as the cells reach the upper two thirds of the crypts, after which they mature, migrate to the surface, and become senescent. They then become apoptotic and are shed from the surface.[13] Adenomas arise from a disruption in this sequence, such that the epithelial cells retain their proliferative ability throughout the entire length of the crypt. Alterations in cell differentiation can lead to dysplasia and progression to the development of invasive carcinoma.

More than half of all adenomatous polyps are located in the rectosigmoid colon and can be detected by rectal examination or sigmoidoscopy.[13] The remainder are evenly distributed throughout the rest of the colon. Adenomas can range in size from a barely visible nodule to a large, sessile mass. They can be classified as tubular, villous, or tubulovillous adenomas.

Tubular adenomas, which constitute approximately 65% of benign large bowel adenomas, typically are smooth-surfaced spheres, usually less than 2 cm in diameter, that are attached to the mucosal surface by a stalk.[13] Although most tubular adenomas display little epithelial dysplasia, approximately 20% show a range of dysplastic changes, from mild nuclear changes to frank invasive carcinoma. *Villous adenomas*

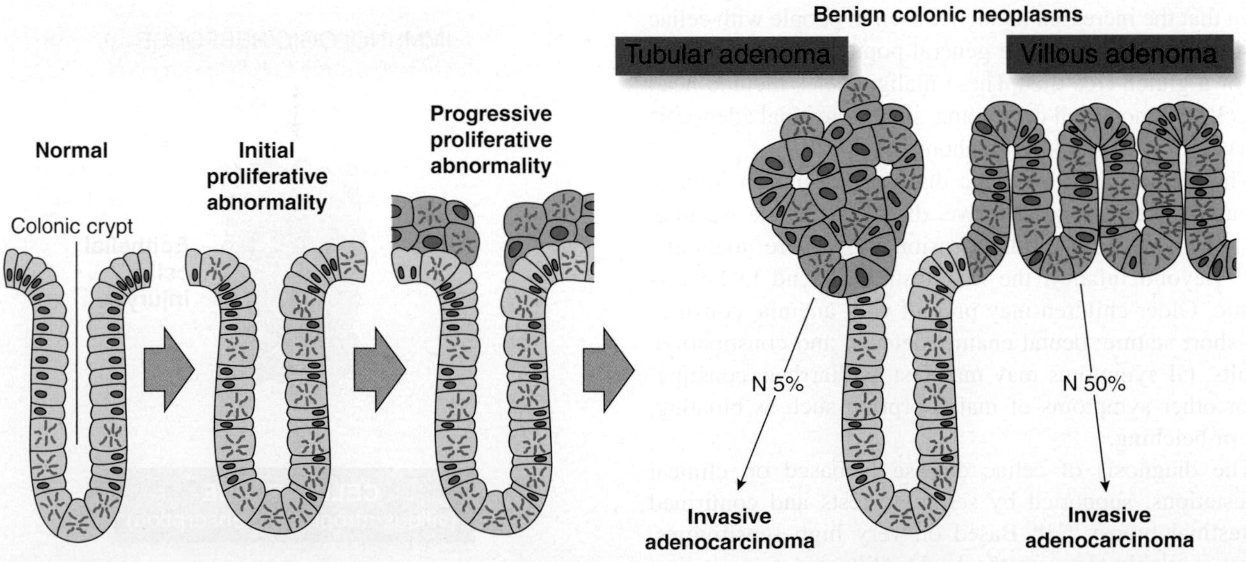

Figure 37.17 • The histogenesis of adenomatous polyps of the colon. The initial proliferative abnormality of the colonic mucosa, the extension of the mitotic zone in the crypts, leads to accumulation of mucosal cells. The formation of adenomas may reflect epithelial–mesenchymal interactions. (From Rubin R., Strayer D. S. (Eds.) (2012). *Rubin's pathophysiology: Clinicopathologic foundations of medicine* (6th ed., p. 663). Philadelphia, PA: Lippincott Williams & Wilkins.)

constitute 10% of adenomas of the colon.[13] They are found predominantly in the rectosigmoid colon. They typically are broad-based, elevated lesions, with a shaggy, cauliflower-like surface. In contrast to tubular adenomas, villous adenomas are more likely to contain malignant cells. When invasive carcinoma develops, there is no stalk to isolate the tumor and invasion is directly into the wall of the colon. *Tubulovillous adenomas* manifest both tubular and villous architecture. They are intermediate between tubular and villous adenomas in terms of invasive carcinoma risk.

Most cases of colorectal cancer begin as benign adenomatous colonic polyps. The frequency of polyps increases with age, and the prevalence of adenomatous polyps significantly increases after 60 years of age.[145] Men and women are equally affected. The peak incidence of adenomatous polyps precedes by some years the peak for colorectal cancer. Programs that provide careful follow-up for people with adenomatous polyps and removal of all suspect lesions have substantially reduced the incidence of colorectal cancer.[13]

Colorectal Cancer

Globally, colorectal cancer is the second most diagnosed cancer, with 1 million new cases worldwide each year.[146] In the United States, colorectal cancer is the third most common cancer in men and women, with 142,820 estimated new cases in 2013.[147] At current rates, approximately 5% of people will develop colorectal cancer within their lifetime. Although colorectal cancer is the second leading cause of cancer death in the United States, accounting for an estimated 50,830 deaths in 2013,[147] the death rate for colorectal cancer has been steadily declining since the early 1980s. This may be due to a decreased number of cases, earlier diagnosis, and improved treatments.[148]

The cause of cancer of the colon and rectum is largely unknown. The risk of colorectal cancer increases with age; the median age at diagnosis for colon cancer is 68 in men and 72 in women. Most cases (72%) occur in people who are in their 40s.[144] Its incidence is increased among people with a family history of cancer, people with Crohn disease or ulcerative colitis, and those with familial adenomatous polyposis of the colon. People with a familial risk—those who have two or more first- or second-degree relatives (or both) with colorectal cancer—make up approximately 20% of all people with colorectal cancer.[149] Familial adenomatous polyposis is a rare autosomal dominant trait linked to a mutation in the long arm of chromosome 5. People with the disorder develop multiple adenomatous polyps of the colon at an early age.[149] Carcinoma of the colon is inevitable, often by 40 years of age, unless a total colectomy is performed.

Diet also is thought to play a role.[144] Attention has focused on dietary fat intake, refined sugar intake, fiber intake, and the adequacy of such protective micronutrients as vitamins A, C, and E in the diet. It has been hypothesized that a high level of fat in the diet increases the synthesis of bile acids in the liver, which may be converted to potential carcinogens by the bacterial flora in the colon. Bacterial organisms in particular are suspected of converting bile acids to carcinogens. Their proliferation is enhanced by a high dietary level of refined sugars. Dietary fiber is thought to increase stool bulk and thereby dilute and remove potential carcinogens. Refined diets often contain reduced amounts of vitamins A, C, and E, which may act as oxygen free radical scavengers.

Reports indicate that aspirin may protect against colorectal cancer.[150,151] Although the mechanism of aspirin's action is unknown, it may be related to its effect on the synthesis of prostaglandins, one or more of which may be involved in signal systems that influence cell proliferation or tumor growth. Aspirin inhibits cyclooxygenase, the enzyme that catalyzes the conversion of arachidonic acid in cell membranes to prostaglandins. One form of cyclooxygenase, COX-2, promotes inflammation and cell proliferation, and colorectal cancers often overexpress this enzyme. Regular use of aspirin appears to reduce the risk of colorectal cancers that overexpress COX-2, but not the risk of colorectal cancers with weak or absent expression of COX-2. Supplemental folate and calcium, selected vitamins.[152]

Usually, cancer of the colon and rectum is present for a long time before it produces symptoms. Bleeding is a highly significant early symptom and usually is the one that causes people to seek medical care. Other symptoms include a change in bowel habits, diarrhea or constipation, and sometimes a sense of urgency or incomplete emptying of the bowel. Pain usually is a late symptom.

The prognosis for people with colorectal cancer depends largely on the extent of bowel involvement and on the presence of metastasis at the time of diagnosis. Colorectal cancer commonly is classified into four TNM (tumor, node, and metastasis) stages. In this system, a stage I tumor is limited to invasion of the mucosal and submucosal layers of the colon and has a 5-year survival rate of 90% to 100%.[15] A stage II (lymph node–negative) tumor infiltrates into, but not through, the muscularis propria and has a 5-year survival rate of 80%.[15] With a stage III (lymph node–positive) tumor, in which there is invasion of the serosal layer and regional lymph node involvement, the 5-year survival rate is 30% to 50%.[14] Stage IV (metastatic) tumors penetrate the serosa or adjacent organs and have a much poorer prognosis.

Screening, Diagnosis, and Treatment. The single most important prognostic indicator of colorectal cancer is the extent (stage) of the tumor at time of diagnosis.[144] Therefore, the challenge is to discover the tumors at their earliest stages. Among the methods used for the detection of colorectal cancers are the digital rectal examination and the fecal occult blood test, usually done during routine physical examinations; x-ray studies using barium (*e.g.*, barium enema); and flexible sigmoidoscopy and colonoscopy.[144] Digital rectal examinations are most helpful in detecting neoplasms of the rectum. Rectal examination should be considered a routine part of a good physical examination. The American Cancer Society recommends that all asymptomatic men and women older than 40 years of age should have a digital rectal examination performed annually as a part of their physical examination. Beginning at 50 years of age, both men and women should follow one of these five screening options: fecal occult blood test every year; flexible sigmoidoscopy examination every 5 years; annual fecal occult blood test for blood and flexible sigmoidoscopy every 5 years; double-contrast barium enema every 5 years; or a colonoscopy every 10 years.[144] People with increased risk for colorectal cancer should be screened earlier and more often. Colonoscopy is recommended whenever a screening test is positive.

Almost all cancers of the colon and rectum bleed intermittently, although the amount of blood is small and usually not apparent in the stools. It therefore is feasible to screen for colorectal cancers using commercially prepared tests for occult blood in the stool.[15,144] Two slides must be prepared from three consecutive bowel movements. To reduce the likelihood of false-positive test results, people are instructed to avoid NSAIDs such as ibuprofen and aspirin for 7 days before testing; to avoid vitamin C in excess of 250 mg from either supplements or citrus fruits for 3 days before testing; and to avoid red meats for 3 days before testing. The most commonly used tests are guaiac-based fecal occult blood tests, which are uncomplicated and can be processed in a health care provider's office. There are also immunochemistry-based tests that may be processed in a laboratory or in the health care provider's office, but they are less commonly used. People with a positive fecal occult blood test should be referred to their physician for further study. Usually, a physical examination, rectal examination, and flexible sigmoidoscopy or colonoscopy are done.

Flexible sigmoidoscopy involves examination of the rectum and sigmoid colon with a hollow, lighted tube that is inserted through the rectum. The procedure is performed without sedation and is well tolerated. Approximately 40% of cancers and polyps are out of the reach of the sigmoidoscope, emphasizing the need for fecal occult blood tests. Polyps can be removed or tissue can be obtained for biopsy during the procedure.

Colonoscopy provides a means for direct visualization of the rectum and colon. The colonoscope consists of a flexible, 4-cm-diameter glass fiber bundle that contains approximately 250,000 glass fibers and has a lens at either end to focus and magnify the image. Light from an external source is transmitted by the fiberoptic-viewing bundle. Instruments are available that afford direct examination of the sigmoid colon or the entire colon. This method is used for screening people at high risk for development of cancer of the colon (*e.g.*, those with ulcerative colitis) and for those with symptoms. Colonoscopy also is useful for obtaining a biopsy and for removing polyps. Although this method is one of the most accurate for detecting early colorectal cancers, it is not suitable for mass screening because it is expensive and time consuming and must be done by a person who is highly trained in the use of the instrument.

The only recognized treatment for cancer of the colon and rectum is surgical removal.[153] Preoperative radiation therapy may be used and has in some cases demonstrated increased 5-year survival rates. Postoperative adjuvant chemotherapy may be used. Radiation therapy and chemotherapy are used as palliative treatment methods.

IN SUMMARY

Disorders of the small and large intestines include IBS, IBD, diverticular disease, disorders of motility (*i.e.*, diarrhea, constipation, fecal impaction, and intestinal obstruction), alterations in intestinal absorption, and colorectal cancer.

IBS is a functional disorder characterized by a variable combination of chronic and recurrent intestinal symptoms not explained by structural or biochemical abnormalities. The term *inflammatory bowel disease* is used to designate two inflammatory conditions: Crohn disease, which affects the small and large bowel, and ulcerative colitis, which affects the colon and rectum. Both are chronic diseases characterized by remissions and exacerbations of diarrhea, weight loss, fluid and electrolyte disorders, and systemic signs of inflammation.

Infectious forms of enterocolitis include viral (*e.g.*, rotavirus), bacterial (*e.g.*, *C. difficile* and *E. coli* O157:H7), and protozoal (*E. histolytica*) infections. Diverticular disease includes diverticulosis, which is a condition in which the mucosal layer of the colon herniates through the muscularis layer, and diverticulitis, in which there is inflammation and gross or microscopic perforation of the diverticulum.

Diarrhea and constipation represent disorders of intestinal motility. Diarrhea is characterized by excessively frequent passage of stools. It can be acute or chronic and can be caused by infectious organisms, food intolerance, drugs, or intestinal disease. Acute diarrheas that last less than 4 days are predominantly caused by infectious agents and follow a self-limited course. Chronic diarrhea persists beyond 3 to 4 weeks and is caused by the presence of hyperosmotic luminal contents, increased intestinal secretory processes, inflammatory conditions, and infectious processes. Constipation can be defined as the infrequent passage of stools; it commonly is caused by failure to respond to the urge to defecate, inadequate fiber or fluid intake, weakness of the abdominal muscles, inactivity and bed rest, pregnancy, hemorrhoids, and GI disease. Fecal impaction is the retention of hardened or putty-like stool in the rectum and colon, which interferes with normal passage of feces. Intestinal obstruction designates an impairment of movement of intestinal contents in a cephalocaudad direction as the result of mechanical or paralytic mechanisms. Peritonitis is an inflammatory response of the serous membrane that lines the abdominal cavity and covers the visceral organs. It can be caused by bacterial invasion or chemical irritation resulting from perforation of the viscera or abdominal organs.

Malabsorption results from the impaired absorption of nutrients and other dietary constituents from the intestine. It can involve a single dietary constituent, such as vitamin B_{12}, or extend to involve all of the substances absorbed in a particular part of the small intestine. Malabsorption can result from disease of the small bowel and disorders that impair digestion and, in some cases, obstruct the lymph flow by which fats are transported to the general circulation. Celiac disease is an immune-mediated disorder triggered by ingestion of gluten-containing grains (including wheat, barley, and rye).

Colorectal cancer, the second most common fatal cancer, is seen most commonly in people older than 50 years of age. Most, if not all, cancers of the colon and rectum arise in preexisting adenomatous polyps. Programs that provide careful follow-up for people with adenomatous polyps and removal of all suspect lesions have substantially reduced the incidence of colorectal cancer.

GERIATRIC Considerations

- Xerostomia (dry mouth) is common in older adults and increases the risk for oral infections and altered communication.[154]
- The dangers of surgery increase with age; however, it is recommended that gastric cancer be removed.[154]
- Hypokalemia and dehydration are serious consequences of diarrhea for the elderly individual.[154]
- Elderly people taking digitalis must be closely monitored for hypokalemia due to risk of toxicity.[154]
- Fatigue associated with colon cancer is tied to iron deficiency in aging adults.[154]
- With age, motility in the colon slows, allowing dietary carcinogens to remain longer, increasing the risk for colon cancer.[154]

PEDIATRIC Considerations

- A maternal history of polyhydramnios is the first indication of EA in the fetus. Polyhydramnios is due to the inability of the fetus to swallow amniotic fluid.[155]
- An increased α-fetoprotein level during pregnancy prompts further investigation of the presence of an omphalocele (evisceration of abdominal content due to anomaly of anterior abdominal wall).[155]
- The incidence of duodenal ulcers in children is greater than for gastric ulcers.
- Encopresis (fecal incontinence beyond expected toilet training age) is often caused by chronic constipation or delaying stooling.[155]
- The absence of meconium within the first 24 hours of life is a common manifestation of Hirschsprung disease (congenital aganglionic megacolon).[155]
- Functional abdominal pain, common in children and adolescents, is recurrent abdominal pain of sufficient severity to interfere with daily activities without any confirmable disease.[155]

REVIEW EXERCISES

1. A 40-year-old man reports to his health care provider complaining of "heartburn" that occurs after eating and also wakes him up at night. He is overweight, admits to enjoying fatty foods, and usually lies down on the sofa and watches TV after dinner. He also complains that lately he has been having a cough and some wheezing. A diagnosis of GERD was made.
   A. *Explain the cause of heartburn and why it becomes worse after eating.*
   B. *People with GERD are advised to lose weight, avoid eating fatty foods, remain sitting after eating, and to sleep with their head slightly elevated. Explain the possible relationship between these situations and the occurrence of reflux.*
   C. *Explain the possible relationship between GERD and the respiratory symptoms this man is having.*
2. A 36-year-old woman who has been taking aspirin for back pain experiences a sudden episode of tachycardia and feeling faint, accompanied by the vomiting of a coffee-ground emesis and the passing of a tarry stool. She relates that she has not had any signs of a "stomach ulcer" such as pain or heartburn.
   A. *Relate the mucosal protective effects of prostaglandins to the development of peptic ulcer associated with aspirin or NSAID use.*
   B. *Explain the apparent suddenness of the bleeding and the fact that the woman did not experience pain as a warning signal.*
   C. *Among the results of her initial laboratory tests is an elevated blood urea nitrogen (BUN) level. Explain the reason for the elevated BUN.*
3. A 29-year-old woman has been diagnosed with Crohn disease. Her medical history reveals that she began having symptoms of the disease at 24 years of age and that her mother died of complications of the disease at 54 years of age. She complains of diarrhea and chronic cramping abdominal pain.
   A. *Define the term inflammatory bowel disease and compare the pathophysiologic processes and manifestations of Crohn disease and ulcerative colitis.*
   B. *One of the recommended treatments for stress incontinence is the use of Kegel exercises, which focus on strengthening the muscles of the pelvic floor. Explain how these exercises contribute to the control of urine leakage in women with stress incontinence.*
   C. *Relate the use of the monoclonal antibody infliximab to the pathogenesis of the inflammatory lesions that occur in Crohn disease.*

References

1. Kochanek M. A., Xu J., Murphy S. L. (2016). Deaths: Preliminary data for 2014. *National Vital Statistics Reports* 65(4), 1. [Online]. Available: https://www.cdc.gov/nchs/data/nvsr/nvsr65/nvsr65_04.pdf. Accessed February 1, 2018
2. Peery A. F., et al. (2012).Burden of gastrointestinal disease in the United States: 2012 update. *Gastroenterology* 143(5), 1179–1187.e3. *PMC.* Web. 20 Jan. 2018.
3. (2013). *Diagnostic and statistical manual of mental disorders: DSM-5* (5th ed., pp. 338–345). Washington, DC: American Psychiatric Publishing. ISBN 978-0-89042-555-8
4. Hasler W. L. (2014). Nausea, vomiting, and indigestion. In: Kasper D., Fauci A., Hauser S., Longo D,, Jameson J., Loscalzo J. (Eds), *Harrison's Principles of Internal Medicine* (19th ed.). New York, NY: McGraw-Hill. http://accessmedicine.mhmedical.com./content.aspx?bookid=1130&sectionid=79726154. Accessed March 08, 2018
5. Hall J. E. (2015). *Guyton and Hall: Textbook of Medical Physiology* (13th ed.). Philadelphia, PA: Saunders Elsevier.
6. Goyal A., Jones M. O., Couriel J. M., et al. (2017). Oesophageal atresia, tracheoesophageal fistula. *Archives of Disease in Childhood. Fetal and Neonatal Edition* 201, 381–384.
7. Teitelbaum J. E. (2017). Congenital abnormalities. In Kleinman R. E., Sanderson I. R., Goulet O., et al. (Eds), *Walker's Pediatric Gastrointestinal Disease: Physiology, Diagnosis, Management* (pp. 1–17). Hamilton, ON: BC Decker.
8. Devault K. R. (2016). Symptoms of esophageal disease. In Feldman M., Feldman L. S., Brandt L. J. (Eds), *Sleisenger and Fordtran's Gastrointestinal and Liver Disease: Pathophysiology, Diagnosis, Management* (10th ed., pp. 185–193). Philadelphia, PA: Saunders Elsevier.
9. Kumar V., Abbas A. K., Fausto N., et al. (Eds). (2014). The gastrointestinal tract. In *Robbins and Cotran: Pathologic Basis of Disease* (9th ed., pp. 749–819). Philadelphia, PA: Saunders Elsevier.
10. Vaezi M. F., Pandolfino J. E., Vela M. F. (2013). ACG Clinical Guideline: Diagnosis and management of achalasia. *American Journal of Gastroenterology* 108, 1238–1249. [Online]. Available: http://gi.org/wp-content/uploads/2013/07/ACG_Guideline_Achalasia_July_2013.pdf
11. Kahrilas P. J., Pandolfino J. E. (2016). Esophageal neuromuscular function and motility disorders. In Feldman M., Feldman L. S., Brandt L. J. (Eds), *Sleisenger and Fordtran's Gastrointestinal and Liver Disease: Pathophysiology, Diagnosis, Management* (10th ed., pp. 701–732). Philadelphia, PA: Saunders Elsevier.
12. Savides T. J., Jensen D. M. (2016). Gastrointestinal bleeding. In Feldman M., Feldman L. S., Brandt L. J. (Eds), *Sleisenger and Fordtran's Gastrointestinal and Liver Disease: Pathophysiology, Diagnosis, Management* (10th ed., pp 297–335). Philadelphia, PA: Saunders Elsevier.
13. Mitos F. A., Rubin E. (2015). The gastrointestinal tract. In Rubin R., Strayer D. S. (Eds), *Rubin's Pathophysiology: Clinicopathologic Foundations of Medicine* (7th ed., pp. 751–824). Philadelphia, PA: Lippincott Williams & Wilkins.
14. Martinucci I., de Bortoli N., Russo S., et al. (2016). Barrett's esophagus in 2016: From pathophysiology to treatment. *World Journal of Gastrointestinal Pharmacology and Therapeutics* 7(2), 190–206. DOI: 10.4292/wjgpt.v7.i2.190.
15. Badillo R., Francis D. (2014). Diagnosis and treatment of gastroesophageal reflux disease. *World Journal of Gastrointestinal Pharmacology and Therapeutics* 5(3), 105–112. http://doi.org/10.4292/wjgpt.v5.i3.105
16. Roman S., Pandolfino J. E., Kahrilas P. J. (2015). Gastroesophageal reflux disease. In Yamada Y. (Ed.), *Textbook of Gastroenterology* (6th ed., pp. 906–928). Oxford, UK: Wiley-Blackwell.
17. Gastroesophageal Reflux (GER) and Gastroesophageal Reflux Disease (GERD) in Adults. NIDDK. November 13, 2014. Archived from the original on 5 October 2016. Retrieved 13 September 2016.
18. Sylvester Chuks Nwokediuko, (2012). Current trends in the management of gastroesophageal reflux disease: A review. *ISRN Gastroenterology* 2012(Article ID 391631), 11. DOI: 10.5402/2012/391631
19. Spechler J. S., Wang D. H., Souza R. F. (2016). Barrett esophagus and esophageal adenocarcinoma. In Yamada Y. (Ed.), *Textbook of Gastroenterology* (6th ed., pp. 949–974). Oxford, UK: Wiley-Blackwell.
20. Wu A. (2015). Gastroesophageal reflux disease management in pediatric patients. *US Pharmacist* 40(12), 28–32.
21. Rudolph C. D. (2011). Gastroesophageal reflux other causes of esophageal inflammation. In Rudolph C. D., Rudolph A. M., Lister G. E., et al. (Eds), *Rudolph's Pediatrics* (22nd ed., pp. 1405–1412). New York, NY: McGraw-Hill.
22. Tolia V., Gilger M. A., Barker P. N., Illueca M. (2015). Healing of erosive esophagitis and improvement of symptoms of gastroesophageal reflux disease after esomeprazole treatment in children 12 to 36 months old. *Journal of Pediatrics Gastroenterology and Nutrition* 60(Suppl 1), S31–S36.
23. Baird D. C., Harker D. J., Karmes A. S., Darnall C. R. (2015) Diagnosis and treatment of gastroesophageal reflux in infants and children. *American Family Physician* 92(8), 705–717.
24. Howlader N., Noone A. M., Krapcho M., et al. (Eds). SEER Cancer Statistics Review, 1975–2014, National Cancer Institute. Bethesda, MD, https://seer.cancer.gov/csr/1975_2014/, based on November 2016 SEER data submission, posted to the SEER web site, updated on April 2017.
25. Gibson M. K., Tanabe K. K., Goldberg R. M., Savarese D. M. F. Epidemiology, pathobiology, and clinical manifestations of esophageal cancer https://www.uptodate.com/contents/epidemiology-pathobiology-and-clinical-manifestations-of-esophageal-cancer, updated on February 10, 2017
26. Wang H.-W., Kuo C.-J., Lin W.-R., et al. (2015). Barrett's esophagus and risk of esophageal adenocarcinoma: A retrospective analysis. *Advances in Digestive Medicine* 2(4), 135–140.
27. Patel N. C., Famirez F. C. (2016). Esophageal tumors. In Feldman M., Feldman L. S., Brandt L. J. (Eds), *Sleisenger and Fordtran's Gastrointestinal and Liver Disease: Pathophysiology, Diagnosis, Management* (10th ed., pp 773–791). Philadelphia, PA: Saunders Elsevier.
28. Ross M. H., Pawlina W. (2015). *Histology: A Text and Atlas: With Correlated Cell and Molecular Biology* (7th ed.). Baltimore, MD: Lippincott Williams & Wilkins.
29. Cryer B., Mahaffey K. W. (2014). Gastrointestinal ulcers, role of aspirin, and clinical outcomes: pathobiology, diagnosis, and treatment. *Journal of Multidisciplinary Healthcare* 7, 137–146. http://doi.org/10.2147/JMDH.S54324
30. Zatorski H. (2017) Pathophysiology and risk factors in peptic ulcer disease. In Fichna J. (Ed.), *Introduction to Gastrointestinal Diseases* (Vol. 2, pp. 7–20). Springer
31. Rang H. P., Dale M. M., Ritter J. M., et al. (2015). *Rang and Dale's Pharmacology* (8th ed.). Philadelphia, PA: Elsevier
32. Kemmerly T., Kaunitz J. D. (2014). Gastroduodenal mucosal defense. *Current Opinion in Gastroenterology* 30(6), 583–588. http://doi.org/10.1097/MOG.0000000000000124.
33. Turner J. R. (2014). The gastrointestinal tract. In Kumar V., Abbas A. K., Fausto N., et al. (Eds), *Robbins and Cotran: Pathologic Basis of Disease* (9th ed., pp. 763–831). Philadelphia, PA: Saunders Elsevier.
34. Santacroce L. (2017). Helicobacter Pylori Infection Medscape Medical News from WebMD. Updated on October 12, 2017. Available at https://emedicine.medscape.com/article/176938-overview. Accessed January 27, 2018.
35. Kumar P., Clark M. (2012). *Clinical Medicine* (8th ed.). Philadelphia, PA: Saunders Elsevier.
36. Cover T. L., Blaser M. J. (2015). *Helicobacter pylori* and other gastric *Helicobacter* species. In Mandell G. L., Bennett J. E., Dolin R. (Eds), *Mandell, Douglas and Bennett's Principles and Practice of Infectious Disease* (8th ed., pp. 2494–2505). Philadelphia, PA: Churchill Livingstone Elsevier.
37. O'Connor A.., et al. (2014) Treatment of Helicobacter pylori infection 2014. *Helicobacter* 19(Suppl 1):38–45.
38. Molina J., et al. (2013). Optimized nonbismuth quadruple therapies cure most patients with helicobacter pylori infection in populations with high rates of antibiotic resistance. *Gastroenterology* 145(1), 121–128.

39. Minalyan A., et al. (2017). Autoimmune atrophic gastritis: Current perspectives. *Clinical and Experimental Gastroenterology* 10, 19–27.
40. Vakil N. (2016). Peptic ulcer disease. In Feldman M., Friedman L. S., Brandt L. J. (Eds), *Sleisenger and Fordtran's Gastrointestinal and Liver Disease: Pathophysiology, Diagnosis and Management* (10th ed., pp. 884–900). Philadelphia, PA: Saunders Elsevier.
41. Lanas A. (2016). *NSAIDs and Aspirin: Recent Advances and Implications for Clinical Management* (1st ed.). Switzerland: Springer International Publishing AG.
42. Lanas A., Chan F. K. L. (2017). Peptic ulcer disease. *The Lancet* 39(10094), 613–624. [Online] Available: https://doi.org/10.1016/S0140-6736(16)32404-7.
43. Scofield R. H., et al. for eMedicine. Updated on September 09, 2017 eMedicine: Milk-Alkali Syndrome. https://emedicine.medscape.com/article/123324-overview. Accessed January 28, 2018
44. Chan F. K., Lau J. Y. (2016). Treatment of peptic ulcer disease. In Feldman M., Friedman L. S., Brandt L. J. (Eds), *Sleisenger and Fordtran's Gastrointestinal and Liver Disease: Pathophysiology, Diagnosis and Management* (10th ed., pp. 888–891). Philadelphia, PA: Saunders Elsevier.
45. Jenson R. T., Norton J. A., Oberg K. (2016). Neuroendocrine tumors. In Feldman M., Friedman L. S., Brandt L. J. (Eds), *Sleisenger and Fordtran's Gastrointestinal and Liver Disease: Pathophysiology, Diagnosis and Management* (10th ed., pp. 501–541). Philadelphia, PA: Saunders Elsevier.
46. Bonheur J. L., et al. for eMedicine, updated on October 24, 2017 eMedicine: Gastrinoma. [Online]. Available: https://emedicine.medscape.com/article/184332-overview. Accessed January 28, 2018
47. Jensen R. T. (2015). Zollinger-Ellison syndrome. In Yamada T. (Ed.), *Textbook of Gastroenterology* (6th ed., pp. 1078–1102). Hoboken, NJ: Wiley-Blackwell.
48. Del Valle J. (2014). Peptic ulcer disease and related disorders. In: Kasper D., Fauci A., Hauser S., Longo D., Jameson J., Loscalzo J. (Eds), *Harrison's Principles of Internal Medicine* (19th ed.). New York, NY: McGraw-Hill. http://accessmedicine.mhmedical.com./content.aspx?bookid=1130&sectionid=79747602. Accessed March 08, 2018
49. Madsen K. R., Lorentzen K., Clausen N., et al. (2014). Guideline for stress ulcer prophylaxis in the intensive care unit. *Danish Medical Journal* 61(3), C4811–C4811.
50. Carneiro F. (2014). Chapter 5.4 stomach cancer. In Stewart B. W., Wild C. P. (Eds). *World Cancer Report 2014* (pp. 383–391). WHO press, ISBN 978-92-832-0443-5
51. American Cancer Society. (2017). What are the key statistics about stomach cancer? Retrieved May 18, 2017. [Online]. Available: http://www.cancer.org
52. Abrams J. A., Wang T. C. (2016). Adenocarcinoma and other gastric tumors. In Feldman M., Friedman L. S., Brandt L. J. (Eds), *Sleisenger and Fordtran's Gastrointestinal and Liver Disease: Pathophysiology, Diagnosis and Management* (10th ed., pp. 901–920). Philadelphia, PA: Saunders Elsevier.
53. Lee E. L., Feldman M. (2016). Gastritis. In Feldman M., Friedman L. S., Brandt L. J. (Eds), *Sleisenger and Fordtran's Gastrointestinal and Liver Disease: Pathophysiology, Diagnosis and Management* (10th ed., pp. 868–883). Philadelphia, PA: Saunders Elsevier.
54. Mayer R. J. (2014). Lower gastrointestinal cancers. In: Kasper D., Fauci A., Hauser S., Longo D., Jameson J., Loscalzo J. (Eds), *Harrison's Principles of Internal Medicine* (19th ed.). New York, NY: McGraw-Hill. http://accessmedicine.mhmedical.com./content.aspx?bookid=1130&sectionid=69857907. Accessed March 08, 2018.
55. Xu Z. Q., Broza Y. Y., Ionsecu R., et al. (2013). A nanomaterial-based breath test for distinguishing gastric cancer from benign gastric conditions. *British Journal of Cancer* 108(4), 941–950.
56. Amal H., et al. (2015). Detection of precancerous gastric lesions and gastric cancer through exhaled breath. *Gut* 65, 400–407. PMID 25869737. DOI: 10.1136/gutjnl-2014-308536
57. Xu W., Yang Z., Lu N. (2016). Molecular targeted therapy for the treatment of gastric cancer. *Journal of Experimental & Clinical Cancer Research* 35, 1–407. [Online] Available: https://doi.org/10.1186/s13046-015-0276-9.
58. Defrees D. N., Bailey J. (2017). Irritable bowel syndrome: Epidemiology, pathophysiology, diagnosis, and treatment. *Primary Care* 44(4), 655–671. DOI: 10.1016/j.pop.2017.07.009
59. Owyang C. (2014). Irritable bowel syndrome. In Kasper D., Fauci A., Hauser S., Longo D., Jameson J., Loscalzo J. (Eds), *Harrison's Principles of Internal Medicine* (19th ed.). New York, NY: McGraw-Hill. http://accessmedicine.mhmedical.com./content.aspx?bookid=1130&sectionid=79748082. Accessed March 08, 2018
60. Drossman D. A. Hasler W. L. (2016). Rome IV-functional GI disorders: Disorders of gut-brain interaction. *Gastroenterology* 150(6), 1257–1261. DOI: 10.1053/j.gastro.2016.03.035
61. Cremonini F., Cheng V., Lembo A. (2013). Diagnosing IBS: No more million dollar workup? *Clinical Gastroenterology and Hepatology the Official Clinical Practice Journal of the American Gastroenterological Association* 11(8).
62. Cozma-Petruţ A., Loghin F., Miere D., Dumitraşcu D. L. (2017). Diet in irritable bowel syndrome: What to recommend, not what to forbid to patients! *World Journal of Gastroenterology* 23(21), 3771–3783. http://doi.org/10.3748/wjg.v23.i21.3771.
63. Nicandro J. P., Shin P., Chuang E. Evaluation of treatment continuation with alosetron by IBS-D severity criteria. *Current Medical Research and Opinion* 2012;28:449.
64. Molodecky N. A., et al. (2012) Increasing incidence and prevalence of the inflammatory bowel diseases with time, based on systematic review. *Gastroenterology* 142, 46–54.
65. Sands B. E., Siegel C. A. (2016). Crohn's disease. In Feldman M., Friedman L. S., Brandt L. J. (Eds), *Sleisenger and Fordtran's Gastrointestinal and Liver Disease: Pathophysiology, Diagnosis and Management* (10th ed., pp. 1990–2022). Philadelphia, PA: Saunders Elsevier.
66. Ananthakrishnan A. N., Xavier R. J. U., Podolsky D. K. (2015). Inflammatory bowel disease. In Yamada T. (Ed.), *Textbook of Gastroenterology* (6th ed., pp. 1364–1377). Hoboken, NJ: Wiley-Blackwell.
67. Jostins L., Ripke S., Weersma R. K., et al. (2012). Host-microbe interactions have shaped the genetic architecture of inflammatory bowel disease. *Nature* 491, 119.
68. Baumgart D. C., Sandborn W. J. (2012). Crohn's disease. *The Lancet* 380(9853), 1590–1605.
69. Liu J. Z., et al. (2015) Association analyses identify 38 susceptibility loci for inflammatory bowel disease and highlight shared genetic risk across populations. *Nature Genetics* 47(9), 979–986.
70. McGovern D., Kugathasan S., Cho J. H. (2015). Genetics of inflammatory bowel diseases. *Gastroenterology* 149(5), 1163–1176.
71. Uhlig H. H. (2013). Monogenic diseases associated with intestinal inflammation: implications for the understanding of inflammatory bowel disease. *Gut* 62, 1795–1805.
72. Ananthakrishnan A. N. (2015). Epidemiology and risk factors for IBD. *Nature Reviews Gastroenterology & Hepatology* 12, 205–217.
73. Higuchi L. M., Khalili H., Chan A. T., et al. (2012). A prospective study of cigarette smoking and the risk of inflammatory bowel disease in women. *American Journal of Gastroenterology* 107, 1399.
74. Benjamin J. L., et al. (2012). Smokers with active Crohn's disease have a clinically relevant dysbiosis of the gastrointestinal microbiota. *Inflammatory Bowel Diseases* 18, 1092–1100.
75. Kronman M. P., Zaoutis T. E., Haynes K., et al. (2012) Antibiotic exposure and IBD development among children: A population-based cohort study. *Pediatrics* 130, e794.
76. Friedman S., Blumberg R. S. (2014). Inflammatory bowel disease. In: Kasper D., Fauci A., Hauser S., Longo D., Jameson J., Loscalzo J. (Eds), *Harrison's Principles of Internal Medicine* (19th ed.). New York, NY: McGraw-Hill. http://accessmedicine.mhmedical.com./content.aspx?bookid=1130&sectionid=79747914. Accessed March 08, 2018
77. Gasparetto M., Guariso G. (2014). Crohn's disease and growth deficiency in children and adolescents. *World Journal of Gastroenterology: WJG* 20(37), 13219–13233. http://doi.org/10.3748/wjg.v20.i37.13219

78. Chande N., Patton P. H., Tsoulis D. J., Thomas B. S., MacDonald J. K. (2015). Azathioprine or 6-mercaptopurine for maintenance of remission in Crohn's disease. *Cochrane Database of Systematic Reviews* (10): CD000067. DOI: 10.1002/14651858.CD000067.pub3
79. Khanna R., et al. (2015). Anti-IL-12/23p40 antibodies for induction of remission in Crohn's disease. *Cochrane Database of Systematic Reviews* (5): CD000067. ISSN 1469-493X. PMID 25942580. DOI: 10.1002/14651858.CD007572.pub2
80. Molodecky N. A., Soon I. S., Rabi D. M., et al. (2012). Increasing incidence and prevalence of the inflammatory bowel diseases with time, based on systematic review. *Gastroenterology* 142, 46.
81. Ulcerative Colitis. NIDDK. September 2014. Archived from the original on 28 July 2016. Retrieved 3 August 2016.
82. Vavricka S. R., Schoepfer A., Scharl M., Lakatos P. L., Navarini A., Rogler G. (2015). Extraintestinal manifestations of inflammatory bowel disease. *Inflammatory Bowel Diseases* 21(8), 1982–1992. http://doi.org/10.1097/MIB.0000000000000392
83. Osterman M. T., Lichtenstein G. R. (2016). Ulcerative colitis. In Feldman M., Friedman L. S., Brandt L. J. (Eds), *Sleisenger and Fordtran's Gastrointestinal and Liver Disease: Pathophysiology, Diagnosis and Management* (10th ed., pp. 2023–2061). Philadelphia, PA: Saunders Elsevier.
84. Bardia A., Tiwari S. K., Vishwakarma S. K., et al. (2014). Haplotype analyses of DNA repair gene polymorphisms and their role in ulcerative colitis. *PLoS ONE* 9(9), e108562. https://doi.org/10.1371/journal.pone.0108562
85. Jess T., Rungoe C., Peyrin–Biroulet L.. (2012). Risk of colorectal cancer in patients with ulcerative colitis: A meta-analysis of population-based cohort studies. *Clinical Gastroenterology and Hepatology* 10(6), 639–645.
86. Wanders L. K., Dekker E., Pullens B., et al. (2014). Cancer risk after resection of polypoid dysplasia in patients with longstanding ulcerative colitis: A meta-analysis. *Clinical Gastroenterology and Hepatology* 12(5):756–764.
87. Castaño-Milla C., Chaparro M., Gisbert J. P. (2014). Systematic review with meta-analysis: the declining risk of colorectal cancer in ulcerative colitis. *Alimentary Pharmacology and Therapeutics* 39, 645–659. DOI: 10.1111/apt.12651
88. Laurens M. B., Donnenburg M. S. (2011). Gastrointestinal Infections. In Rudolph C. D., Rudolph A. M., Lister G. E., et al. (Eds), *Rudolph's Pediatrics* (22nd ed., pp. 945–947). New York, NY: McGraw Hill.
89. John B. M., Devgan A., Mitra B. (2014). Prevalence of rotavirus infection in children below two years presenting with diarrhea. *Medical Journal Armed Forces India* 70(2), 116–119. http://doi.org/10.1016/j.mjafi.2014.02.008
90. The Centers for Disease Control and Prevention. (2016). Rotavirus. [Online]. Available: https://www.cdc.gov/rotavirus/index.html. Accessed January 24, 2018
91. LaRocque R. C., Ryan E. T., Calderwood S. B. (2014). Acute infectious diarrheal diseases and bacterial food poisoning. In: Kasper D., Fauci A., Hauser S., Longo D., Jameson J., Loscalzo J. (Eds), *Harrison's Principles of Internal Medicine* (19th ed.). New York, NY: McGraw-Hill. http://accessmedicine.mhmedical.com./content.aspx?bookid=1130&sectionid=79734063. Accessed March 08, 2018.
92. Khanna S., Pardi D. S., Aronson S. L., et al. (2012). The epidemiology of community-acquired Clostridium difficile infection: A population-based study. *American Journal of Gastroenterology* 107(1), 89–95.
93. Brandt L. J., Aroniadis O. C., Mellow M., et al. (2012). Long-term follow-up of colonoscopic fecal microbiota transplant for recurrent Clostridium difficile infection. *American Journal of Gastroenterology* 107(7), 1079–1087.
94. Laidman J. Fecal transfer proves potent clostridium difficile treatment. [serial online]. Medscape Medical News. January 16, 2013. Available at http://www.medscape.com/viewarticle/777772. Accessed: July 23, 2013
95. Cohen M. B. (2015). Bacterial, viral and toxic causes of diarrhea, gastroenteritis and anorectal infections. In Yamada T. (Ed.), *Textbook of Gastroenterology* (6th ed., pp. 1196–1248). Hoboken, NJ: Wiley-Blackwell.
96. Kelly C. P., Lamont J. T. (2016). Antibiotic-associated diarrhea and clostridium-associated diarrhea and colitis. In Feldman M., Friedman L. S., Brandt L. J. (Eds), *Sleisenger and Fordtran's Gastrointestinal and Liver Disease: Pathophysiology, Diagnosis and Management* (10th ed., pp. 1939–1954). Philadelphia, PA: Saunders Elsevier.
97. Haines C. F., Sears C. L. (2016). Infectious enteritis and proctocolitis. In Feldman M., Friedman L. S., Brandt L. J. (Eds), *Sleisenger and Fordtran's Gastrointestinal and Liver Disease: Pathophysiology, Diagnosis and Management* (10th ed., pp. 1896–1929). Philadelphia, PA: Saunders Elsevier.
98. Russo T. A., Johnson J. R. (2014). Diseases caused by Gram-negative Enteric Bacilli. In: Kasper D., Fauci A., Hauser S., Longo D., Jameson J., Loscalzo J. (Eds), *Harrison's Principles of Internal Medicine* (19the ed.). New York, NY: McGraw-Hill. http://accessmedicine.mhmedical.com./content.aspx?bookid=1130&sectionid=79735990. Accessed March 08, 2018.
99. Mayer C. L., Leibowitz C. S., Kurosawa S., Stearns-Kurosawa D. J. (2012). Shiga toxins and the pathophysiology of hemolytic uremic syndrome in humans and animals. *Toxins* 4(11), 1261–1287. http://doi.org/10.3390/toxins4111261
100. Taylor C. M., Machin S., Wigmore S. J., Goodship T. H., Working Party from the Renal Association, The British Committee for Standards in Haematology and the British Transplantation Society. Working Party from the Renal Association, the British Committee for Standards in Haematology and the British Transplantation Society. (2010). Clinical practice guidelines for the management of atypical haemolytic uraemic syndrome in the United Kingdom. *British Journal of Haematology* 148, 37–47. DOI: 10.1111/j.1365-2141.2009.07916.x
101. Reed S. L. (2015). Amebiasis and infection with free-living amebas. In Fauci A. S., Braunwald E., Kasper D. L., et al. (Eds), *Harrison's Principles of Internal Medicine* (19th ed., pp. 1275–1280). New York, NY: McGraw Hill.
102. Schwartz D. A., Genta R. M., Bennett D. P., et al. (2015). Infectious and parasitic diseases. In Rubin R., Strayer D. S. (Eds), *Rubin's Pathophysiology: Clinicopathologic Foundations of Medicine* (7th ed., pp. 367–474). Philadelphia, PA: Lippincott Williams & Wilkins.
103. Goldsmith R. S. (2017). Infectious diseases: Protozoal and helminthic. In Tierney L. M., McPhee S. J., Papadakis M. (Eds), *Current Medical Diagnosis and Treatment* (56th ed., pp. 1498–1503). New York, NY: McGraw-Hill Medical.
104. McNevin M. S. (2018). Diverticulitis. *American Society of Colon and Rectal Surgeons*. Available: https://www.fascrs.org/patients/disease-condition/diverticular-disease-expanded-version-0. Accessed January 27, 2018
105. Pietrzak J., Obuchowicz A., Majda D., Kiedos A. Meckel's diverticulum – a congenital defect of the gastrointestinal tract underestimated in differential diagnostics. Own experience. *Developmental Period Medicine* 2017, 21(1):38–42.
106. Thorson A. G., Goldberg S. M. (2016). Benign colon: Diverticular disease. In Wolff B. G., Fleshman J. W., Beck D. E., et al. (Eds), *The ASCRS Textbook of Colon and Rectal Surgery.* New York, NY: Springer. Accessed (3rd ed) May 27, 2011
107. Quarrie R., Lindsey D., Bahner D. P. (2014). Review of the incidence and management of Meckel's diverticulum. *Austin Journal of Surgery* 1(3), 1015.
108. Rezapour M., Ali S., Stollman N. (2017). Diverticular disease: An update on pathogenesis and management. *Gut and Liver*. DOI: 10.5009/gnl16552
109. Floch M. H. (2013). Emerging studies in diverticular disease. *Journal of Clinical Gastroenterology* 47(5), 381–382.
110. Jacobs D. O. (2014). Acute Appendicitis and peritonitis. In Kasper D., Fauci A., Hauser S., Longo D., Jameson J., Loscalzo J. (Eds.), *Harrison's Principles of Internal Medicine* (19th ed.). New York, NY: McGraw-Hill. Accessed March 08, 2018.
111. Shogilev D. J., Duus N., Odom S. R., Shapiro N. I. (2014). Diagnosing appendicitis: evidence-based review of the diagnostic approach in 2014. *The Western Journal of Emergency Medicine (Review)* 15(7), 859–871.

DOI: 10.5811/westjem.2014.9.21568. PMC 4251237 Freely accessible. PMID 25493136

112. DeKoning E. P. (2015). Acute appendicitis. In Tintinalli J. E., Stapczynski J. S., Cline D. M., et al. (Eds), *Tintinalli's Emergency Medicine: A Comprehensive Study Guide* (8th ed.). Available: http://www.accessmedicine.com/. Accessed May 27, 2011
113. Camilleri M., Murray J. A. (2014). Diarrhea and constipation. In: Kasper D., Fauci A., Hauser S., Longo D., Jameson J., Loscalzo J. (Eds), *Harrison's Principles of Internal Medicine* (19th ed.). New York, NY: McGraw-Hill. http://accessmedicine.mhmedical.com/content.aspx?bookid=1130&sectionid=79726207. Accessed March 08, 2018
114. Arenas-Hernández M. M., Martínez-Laguna Y., Torres A. G. (2012). Clinical implications of enteroadherent *Escherichia coli*. *Curr Gastroenterol Rep* 14(5), 386–394. DOI: 10.1007/s11894-012-0277-1. PMID: 22798032; PMCID: PMC3448025.
115. Larcombe S., et al. (2016). Involvement of bacteria other than *Clostridium difficile* in antibiotic-associated diarrhoea. *Trends in Microbiology* 24(6), 463–476.
116. Shane A. L., et al. (2017). 2017 Infectious Diseases Society of America Clinical Practice Guidelines for the diagnosis and management of infectious diarrhea. *Clinical Infectious Diseases* 65(12), e45–e80.
117. Schiller L. R., Sellin J. H. (2016). Diarrhea. In Feldman M., Friedman L. S., Brandt L. J. (Eds), *Sleisenger and Fordtran's Gastrointestinal and Liver Disease: Pathophysiology, Diagnosis and Management* (10th ed., pp. 221–241). Philadelphia, PA: Saunders Elsevier.
118. Deng Y., Misselwitz B., Dai N., Fox M. (2015). Lactose intolerance in adults: Biological mechanism and dietary management. *Nutrients (Review)* 7(9), 8020–8035.
119. Banks M. R., Farthing M. J. G. (2012). Diarrhea. In Hawkey C. J., Bosch J., Richter J. E., Garcia-Tsao G., Chan F. K. L. (Eds), *Textbook of Clinical Gastroenterology and Hepatology* (2nd ed.). Oxford, UK: Wiley-Blackwell. DOI: 10.1002/9781118321386.ch6
120. Shinohara E., Millar L. B. (2016). All About Carcinoid and Neuroendocrine Tumors [Online]. Available: https://www.oncolink.org/print/pdf/2001?print_2001.pdf, last modified June 28, 2016. Accessed January 30, 2018
121. Liu L., Johnson H. L., Cousens S., Perin J., Scott S., et al. (2012). Global, regional, and national causes of child mortality: An updated systematic analysis for 2010 with time trends since 2000. *The Lancet* 379, 2151–2161.
122. Caicedo R. A., Hill I. D. (2011). Diarrhea. In Rudolph C. D., Rudolph A. M., Lister G. E., et al. (Eds), *Rudolph's Pediatrics* (22nd ed., pp. 1381–1389). New York, NY: McGraw Hill.
123. Prescilla R. P. , et al. Pediatric Gastroenteritis Treatment & Management, Medscape Medical News. Available at https://emedicine.medscape.com/article/964131-treatment. May 27, 2016. Accessed January 27, 2018
124. Churgay C. A., Aftab Z., (2012). Gastroenteritis in children: Part II. Prevention and management. *Am Fam Physician* 85(11), 1066–1070. [Online]. Available: https://www.aafp.org/afp/2012/0601/p1066.pdfs
125. Lembo A. J., Ullman S. P. (2016). Constipation. In Feldman M., Friedman L. S., Brandt L. J. (Eds), *Sleisenger and Fordtran's Gastrointestinal and Liver Disease: Pathophysiology, Diagnosis and Management* (10th ed., pp. 270–296). Philadelphia, PA: Saunders Elsevier.
126. Hanni Gulwani Hirschsprungs disease. PathologyOutlines.com website. http://www.pathologyoutlines.com/topic/colonhirschsprung.html, updated on December 13, 2016. Accessed January 31, 2018
127. Sood M. R. (2011). Constipation and fecal incontinence. In Rudolph C. D., Rudolph A. M., Lister G. E., et al. (Eds), *Rudolph's Pediatrics* (22nd ed., pp. 1386–1389). New York, NY: McGraw Hill.
128. McQuaid K. R. (2017). Alimentary tract. In Tierney L. M., McPhee S. J., Papadakis M. (Eds), *Current Medical Diagnosis and Treatment* (56th ed., pp. 555, 567–585, 617–623, 652–658). New York, NY: Lange Medical Books/McGraw-Hill.
129. Gearhart S. L., Silen W. (2015). Acute intestinal obstruction. In Fauci A. S., Braunwald E., Kasper D. L., et al. (Eds), *Harrison's Principles of Internal Medicine* (19th ed., pp. 1912–1917). New York, NY: McGraw Hill.
130. Densmore J. C., Lal D. R. (2011). Intussusception. In Rudolph C. D., Rudolph A. M., Lister G. E., et al. (Eds), *Rudolph's Pediatrics* (22nd ed., pp. 1428–1429). New York, NY: McGraw Hill.
131. Turnage R. H., Heldmann M. (2016). Intestinal obstruction. In Feldman M., Friedman L. S., Brandt L. J. (Eds), *Sleisenger and Fordtran's Gastrointestinal and Liver Disease: Pathophysiology, Diagnosis and Management* (10th ed., pp. 2154–2170). Philadelphia, PA: Saunders Elsevier.
132. Allan P., Lal S. Intestinal failure: a review [version 1; referees: 2 approved]. F1000Research 2018, 7(F1000 Faculty Rev):85 (DOI: 10.12688/f1000research.12493.1)
133. Hogenauer C., Hammer H. F. (2016). Maldigestion and malabsorption. In Feldman M., Friedman L. S., Brandt L. J. (Eds), *Sleisenger and Fordtran's Gastrointestinal and Liver Disease: Pathophysiology, Diagnosis and Management* (10th ed., pp. 1788–1823). Philadelphia, PA: Saunders Elsevier.
134. Kannan A., Tilak V., Rai M., Gupta V. (2016). Evaluation of clinical, biochemical and hematological parameters in macrocytic anemia. *International Journal of Research in Medical Sciences* 4(7), 2670–2678.
135. Rubio-Tapia A., Hill I. D., Kelly C. P., Calderwood A. H., Murray J. A. (2013). ACG Clinical Guidelines: diagnosis and management of celiac disease. *American Journal of Gastroenterology* 108, 656–676. DOI: 10.1038/ajg.2013.79
136. Celiac.com. Celiac disease and gluten-free diet information. [Online]. Available: www.celiac.com. Accessed January 29, 2018
137. Gujral N., Freeman H. J., Thomson A. B. (2012). Celiac disease: Prevalence, diagnosis, pathogenesis and treatment. *World Journal of Gastroenterology: WJG* 18(42), 6036–6059. http://doi.org/10.3748/wjg.v18.i42.6036.
138. Fasano A., Catassi C. (2012). Celiac disease. *New England Journal of Medicine* 367, 2419–2426. DOI: 10.1056/NEJMcp1113994
139. Ludvigsson J. F., Card T. R., Kaukinen K., et al. (2015). Screening for celiac disease in the general population and in high-risk groups. *United European Gastroenterology Journal* 3(2), 106–120. http://doi.org/10.1177/2050640614561668
140. Cecilio L. A., Bonatto M. W. (2015). The prevalence of HLA DQ2 and DQ8 in patients with celiac disease, in family and in general population. *Arquivos Brasileiros de Cirurgia Digestiva : ABCD = Brazilian Archives of Digestive Surgery* 28(3), 183–185. http://doi.org/10.1590/S0102-67202015000300009
141. Binder H. J. (2014). Disorders of absorption. In: Kasper D., Fauci A., Hauser S., Longo D., Jameson J., Loscalzo J. (Eds), *Harrison's Principles of Internal Medicine* (19th ed.). New York, NY: McGraw-Hill. http://accessmedicine.mhmedical.com/content.aspx?bookid=1130&sectionid=79747771. Accessed March 08, 2018
142. Farrell R. J., Kelly C. P. (2016). Celiac disease and refractory celiac disease. In Feldman M., Friedman L. S., Brandt L. J. (Eds), *Sleisenger and Fordtran's Gastrointestinal and Liver Disease: Pathophysiology, Diagnosis and Management* (10th ed., pp. 1849–1872). Philadelphia, PA: Saunders Elsevier.
143. Hill I. D., Caicedo R. A. (2011). Disorders of absorption and absorption. In Rudolph C. D., Rudolph A. M., Lister G. E., et al. (Eds), *Rudolph's Pediatrics* (22nd ed., pp. 1438–1453). New York, NY: McGraw Hill.
144. American Cancer Society. (2017). Colorectal cancer facts and figures, 2016–2019. [Online]. Available: http://www.cancer.org. Accessed January 29, 2018
145. Itzkowitz S. H., Potack J. (2016). Colonic polyps and polyposis syndromes. In Feldman M., Friedman L. S., Brandt L. J. (Eds), *Sleisenger and Fordtran's Gastrointestinal and Liver Disease: Pathophysiology, Diagnosis and Management* (10th ed., pp. 2213–2247). Philadelphia, PA: Saunders Elsevier.
146. Ferlay J., Soerjomataram I., Ervik M., et al. (2013). *GLOBOCAN 2012 v1.0, Cancer Incidence and Mortality Worldwide: IARC Cancer Base No. 11*. Lyon, France: International Agency for Research on Cancer.
147. National Cancer Institute. Colon and rectal cancer. Available at: http://www.cancer.gov/cancertopics/types/colon-and-rectal. Accessed June 2014

148. Siegel R., Naishadham D., Jemal A. (2013). Cancer statistics, 2013. *CA: A Cancer Journal for Clinicians* 63, 11–33.
149. American Cancer Society. (2017). American Cancer Society Recommendations for Colorectal Cancer Early Detection. [Online]. Available: https://www.cancer.org/cancer/colon-rectal-cancer/detection-diagnosis-staging/acs-recommendations.html, last revised on July 7, 2017. Accessed January 29, 2018
150. Ananthakrishnan A. N., et al. (2014) Serum inflammatory markers and risk of colorectal cancer in patients with inflammatory bowel diseases. *Clinical Gastroenterology and Hepatology* 12(8), 1342–1348.e1.
151. Friis S., Riis A. H., Erichsen R., Baron J. A., Sørensen H. T. (2015). Low-dose aspirin or nonsteroidal anti-inflammatory drug use and colorectal cancer risk: A population-based, case–control study. *Annals of Internal Medicine* 163, 347–355. DOI: 10.7326/M15-0039
152. Manzano A., Pérez-Segura P. (2012). Colorectal cancer chemoprevention: Is this the future of colorectal cancer prevention? *The Scientific World Journal* 2012(Article ID 327341), 8. DOI: 10.1100/2012/327341
153. Bresalier R. S. (2016). Colorectal cancer. In Feldman M., Friedman L. S., Brandt L. J. (Eds), *Sleisenger and Fordtran's Gastrointestinal and Liver Disease: Pathophysiology, Diagnosis and Management* (10th ed., pp. 2248–2296). Philadelphia, PA: Saunders Elsevier.
154. Bartlett, J. L. (2018). Management of patients with oral esophageal disorders. In J. L. Hinkle J. L., Cheever K. H. (Eds). *Brunner & Suddarth's textbook of medical-surgical nursing* (14th ed, pp. 1264–1290). Philadelphia, PA: Wolters Kluwer.
155. Kyle T., Carman S. (2017). Nursing care of the child with an alteration in bowel elimination/gastrointestinal disorder. In *Essentials of Pediatric Nursing* (3rd ed.). Philadelphia, PA: Wolters Kluwer.

Disorders of Hepatobiliary and Exocrine Pancreas Function

38

Freddy W. Cao

The liver, the gallbladder, and the exocrine pancreas are classified as accessory organs of the gastrointestinal tract. In addition to producing digestive secretions, the liver and the pancreas have other important functions. The endocrine pancreas, for example, supplies the insulin and glucagon needed for cell metabolism, whereas the liver synthesizes glucose, plasma proteins, and blood clotting factors and are responsible for the degradation and elimination of drugs and hormones, among other functions. This chapter focuses on functions and disorders of the liver, the biliary tract and gallbladder, and the exocrine pancreas.

THE LIVER AND HEPATOBILIARY SYSTEM

After completing this section of the chapter, the learner will be able to meet the following objectives:

- Describe the lobular structures of the liver.
- Describe the function of the liver in terms of carbohydrate, protein, and fat metabolism.
- Relate the mechanism of bile formation and elimination to the development of cholestasis.

The liver is the largest visceral organ in the body, weighing approximately 1.3 kg (3 lb) in the adult. It is located below the diaphragm and occupies much of the right hypochondrium (Fig. 38.1). A tough fibroelastic capsule, called the Glisson capsule, surrounds the liver. The liver is anatomically divided into two large lobes (the right and left lobes) and two smaller

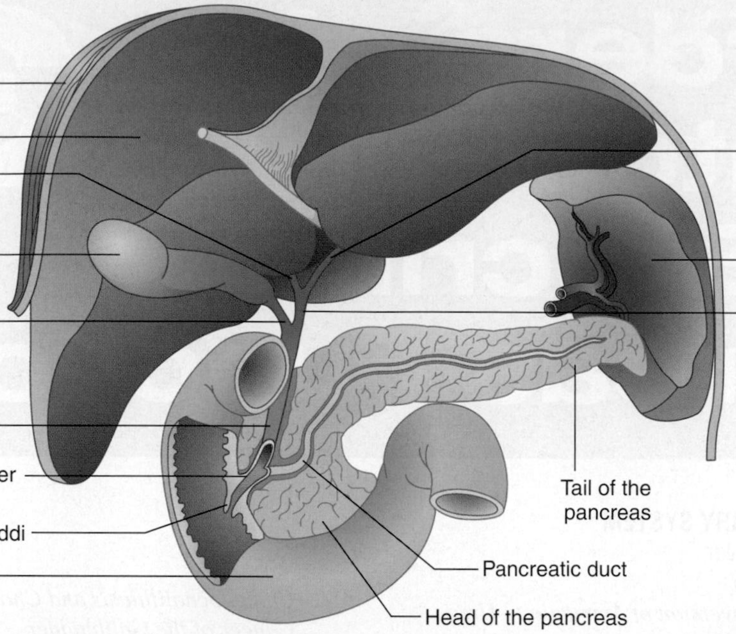

Figure 38.1 • The liver and biliary system, including the gallbladder and bile ducts.

lobes (the caudate and quadrate lobes). Except for the portion that is in the epigastric area, the liver is contained within the rib cage, and cannot normally be palpated in healthy people.

The liver receives 25% of the resting cardiac output.[1] The liver is unique among the abdominal organs in having a dual blood supply consisting of a venous (portal) supply through the hepatic portal vein and an arterial supply through the hepatic artery. Approximately 25% of blood per minute enters the liver through the hepatic artery; the remaining 75% enters by way of the valveless portal vein.[2] The venous blood delivered by the hepatic portal vein comes from the digestive tract and major abdominal organs, including the pancreas and spleen (Fig. 38.2). The portal blood supply carries nutrient and toxic materials absorbed in the intestine, blood cells and their breakdown products from the spleen, and insulin and glucagon from the pancreas. Although the blood from the portal vein is incompletely saturated with oxygen, it supplies approximately 75% of the oxygen needs of the liver.[1]

The venous outflow from the liver is carried by the valveless hepatic veins, which empty into the inferior vena cava just below the level of the diaphragm. The pressure difference between the hepatic vein and the portal vein normally is such that the liver has the ability to store approximately 500 to 1000 mL of blood.[3] This blood can be shifted back into the general circulation during periods of hypovolemia and shock. In right heart failure in which the pressure in the vena cava increases, blood backs up and accumulates in the liver.

The *lobules* are the functional units of the liver. Each lobule is a cylindrical structure that measures approximately 0.8 to 2 mm in diameter and several millimeters in length. There are approximately 50,000 to 100,000 lobules in the liver.[3] Each lobule is organized around a central vein that empties into the hepatic veins and from there into the vena cava. The terminal bile ducts and small branches of the portal vein and hepatic artery are located at the periphery of the lobule. Plates of hepatic cells radiate centrifugally from the central vein like spokes on a wheel (Fig. 38.3). These hepatic plates are separated by wide, thin-walled sinusoidal capillaries, called *sinusoids*, which extend from the periphery of the lobule to its central vein. The sinusoids are supplied by blood from the portal vein and hepatic artery. The sinusoids are in intimate contact with the hepatocytes and provide for the exchange of substances between the blood and liver cells. The sinusoids are lined with two types of cells: the typical capillary endothelial cells and Kupffer cells. *Kupffer cells* are reticuloendothelial cells that are capable of removing and phagocytizing old and defective blood cells, bacteria, and other foreign material from the portal blood as it flows through the sinusoid. This phagocytic action removes enteric bacilli and other harmful substances that filter into the blood from the intestine.

A major exocrine function of the liver is bile secretion. Small tubular channels, called *bile canaliculi*, which lie between the cell membranes of adjacent hepatocytes, also supply the lobules. The bile produced by the hepatocytes flows into the canaliculi and then to the periphery of the lobules, draining into progressively larger ducts, until it reaches the right and left hepatic ducts. The intrahepatic and extrahepatic bile ducts often are collectively referred to as the *hepatobiliary tree*. These ducts unite to form the common duct (see Fig. 38.1). The common duct, which is approximately 10 to 15 cm long, descends and passes behind the pancreas and enters the descending duodenum. The pancreatic duct joins the common duct at a short dilated tube called the *hepatopancreatic ampulla* (ampulla of Vater), which empties into the duodenum through the duodenal papilla. Muscle tissue at the junction of the papilla, sometimes called the *sphincter of Oddi*, regulates the flow of bile into the duodenum. When this sphincter is closed, bile moves back into the common duct and gallbladder.

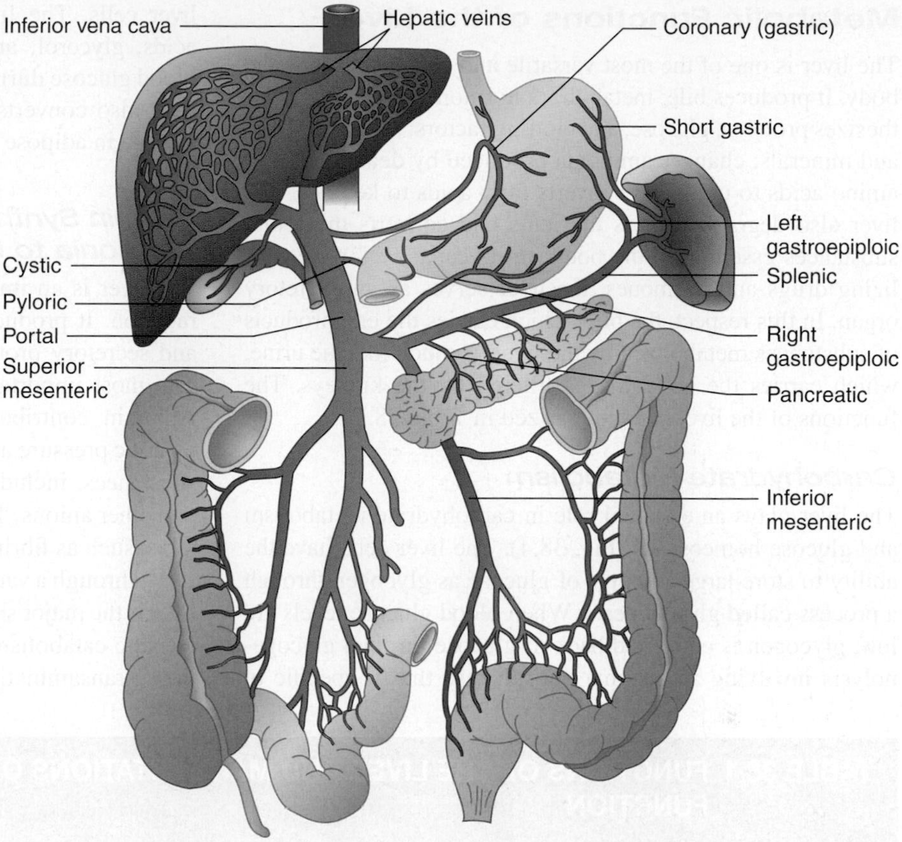

Figure 38.2 • The portal circulation. Blood from the gastrointestinal tract, spleen, and pancreas travels to the liver through the portal vein before moving into the vena cava for return to the heart.

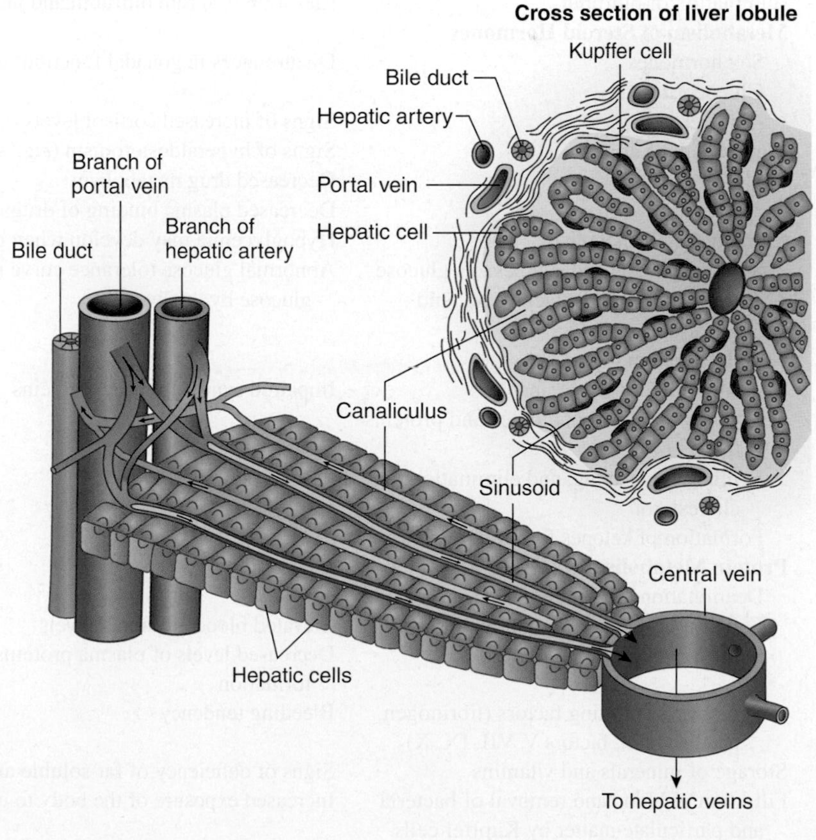

Figure 38.3 • A section of liver lobule showing the location of the hepatic veins, hepatic cells, liver sinusoids, and branches of the portal vein and hepatic artery.

Metabolic Functions of the Liver

The liver is one of the most versatile and active organs in the body. It produces bile; metabolizes hormones and drugs; synthesizes proteins, glucose, and clotting factors; stores vitamins and minerals; changes ammonia produced by deamination of amino acids to urea; and converts fatty acids to ketones. The liver also degrades excess nutrients and converts them into substances essential to the body. In its capacity for metabolizing drugs and hormones, the liver serves as an excretory organ. In this respect, the bile, which carries the end products of substances metabolized by the liver, is much like the urine, which carries the body wastes filtered by the kidneys. The functions of the liver are summarized in Table 38.1.

Carbohydrate Metabolism

The liver plays an essential role in carbohydrate metabolism and glucose homeostasis (Fig. 38.4). The liver cells have the ability to store large amounts of glucose as glycogen through a process called glycogenesis. When blood glucose levels are low, glycogen is converted back to glucose through glycogenolysis involving an enzyme phosphatase that is specific to liver cells. The liver also synthesizes glucose from amino acids, glycerol, and lactic acid as a means of maintaining blood glucose during periods of fasting or increased need. The liver also converts excess carbohydrates to triglycerides for storage in adipose tissue.

Protein Synthesis and Conversion of Ammonia to Urea

The liver is an important site for protein synthesis and degradation. It produces the proteins for its own cellular needs and secretory proteins that are released into the circulation. The most important of these secretory proteins is albumin. Albumin contributes significantly to the plasma colloidal osmotic pressure and to the binding and transport of numerous substances, including some hormones, fatty acids, bilirubin, and other anions. The liver also produces other important proteins, such as fibrinogen and the blood clotting factors.

Through a variety of anabolic and catabolic processes, the liver is the major site of amino acid interconversion (Fig. 38.5). Hepatic catabolism and degradation involve two major reactions: transamination and deamination.[3] In *transamination*, an

TABLE 38.1 FUNCTIONS OF THE LIVER AND MANIFESTATIONS OF ALTERED FUNCTION

FUNCTION	MANIFESTATIONS OF ALTERED FUNCTION
Production of bile salts	Malabsorption of fat and fat-soluble vitamins
Elimination of bilirubin	Elevation in serum bilirubin and jaundice
Metabolism of Steroid Hormones	
Sex hormones	Disturbances in gonadal function, including gynecomastia in the male
Glucocorticoids	
Aldosterone	Signs of increased cortisol levels (*i.e.*, Cushing syndrome)
Metabolism of drugs	Signs of hyperaldosteronism (*e.g.*, sodium retention and hypokalemia)
	Decreased drug metabolism
	Decreased plasma binding of drugs owing to a decrease in albumin production
Carbohydrate metabolism	Hypoglycemia may develop when glycogenolysis and gluconeogenesis are impaired
Stores glycogen and synthesizes glucose from amino acids, lactic acid, and glycerol	Abnormal glucose tolerance curve may occur because of impaired uptake and release of glucose by the liver
Fat Metabolism	
Formation of lipoproteins	Impaired synthesis of lipoproteins
Conversion of carbohydrates and proteins to fat	
Synthesis, recycling, and elimination of cholesterol	Altered cholesterol levels
Formation of ketones from fatty acid	
Protein Metabolism	
Deamination of proteins	
Formation of urea from ammonia	Elevated blood ammonia levels
Synthesis of plasma proteins	Decreased levels of plasma proteins, particularly albumin, which contributes to edema formation
Synthesis of clotting factors (fibrinogen, prothrombin, factors V, VII, IX, X)	Bleeding tendency
Storage of minerals and vitamins	Signs of deficiency of fat-soluble and other vitamins that are stored in the liver
Filtration of blood and removal of bacteria and particulate matter by Kupffer cells	Increased exposure of the body to colonic bacteria and other foreign matter

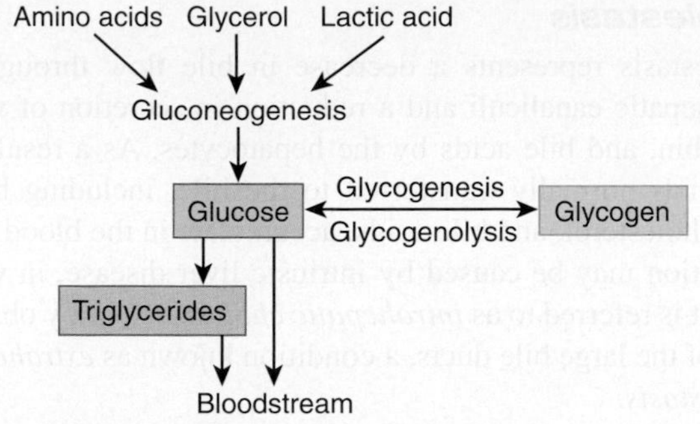

Figure 38.4 • Hepatic pathways for storage and synthesis of glucose and conversion of glucose to fatty acids.

amino group (NH_2) is transferred to an acceptor substance. As a result of transamination, amino acids can participate in the intermediary metabolism of carbohydrates and lipids. During periods of fasting or starvation, amino acids are used for producing glucose (*i.e.*, gluconeogenesis). Most of the nonessential amino acids are synthesized in the liver by transamination. The process of transamination is catalyzed by *aminotransferases*, enzymes that are found in high amounts in the liver.

Oxidative *deamination* involves the removal of the amino groups from amino acids and conversion of amino acids to keto acids and ammonia. This occurs mainly by transamination, in which the amino groups are removed and then transferred to another acceptor substance. The acceptor substance can then transfer the amino group to still another substance or release it as ammonia. Because ammonia is very toxic to body tissues, particularly neurons, the ammonia that is released during deamination is rapidly removed from the blood by the liver and converted to urea. Essentially, all urea formed in the body is synthesized by the urea cycle in the liver and then excreted by the kidneys.[3] Although urea is mostly excreted by the kidneys, some diffuses into the intestine, where it is converted to ammonia by enteric bacteria. The intestinal production of ammonia also results from bacterial deamination of unabsorbed amino acids and proteins derived from the diet, exfoliated cells, or blood in the gastrointestinal tract. Ammonia produced in the intestine is absorbed into the portal circulation and transported to the liver, where it is converted to urea before being released into the systemic circulation. Intestinal production of ammonia is increased after ingestion of high-protein foods and gastrointestinal bleeding. In advanced liver disease, urea synthesis often is impaired, leading to an accumulation of blood ammonia.

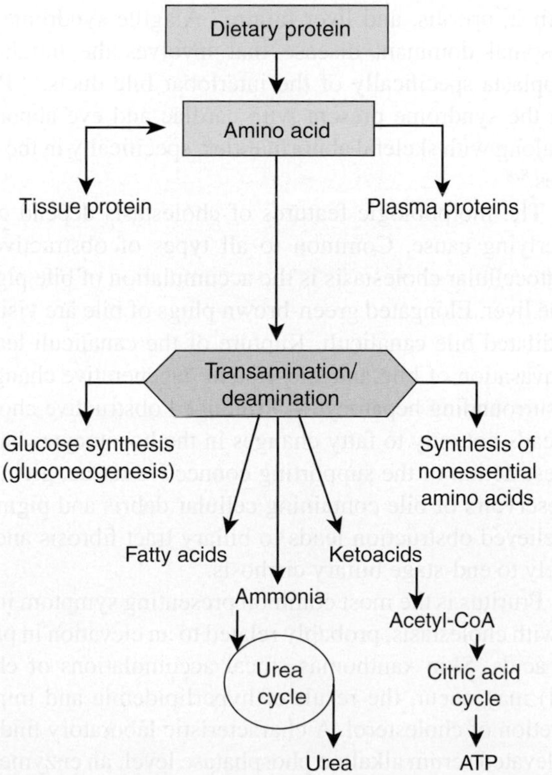

Figure 38.5 • Hepatic pathways for conversion of amino acids to proteins, nucleic acids, keto acids, and glucose. The urea cycle converts ammonia generated by the deamination of amino acids to urea. Acetyl-CoA, acetyl-coenzyme A; ATP, adenosine triphosphate.

Pathways of Lipid Metabolism

Although most cells of the body metabolize fat, certain aspects of lipid metabolism occur mainly in the liver, including the oxidation of free fatty acids to keto acids that supply energy for other body functions; synthesis of cholesterol, phospholipids, and lipoproteins; and formation of triglycerides from carbohydrates and proteins (Fig. 38.6). To derive energy from triglycerides, the molecule must first be split into glycerol and

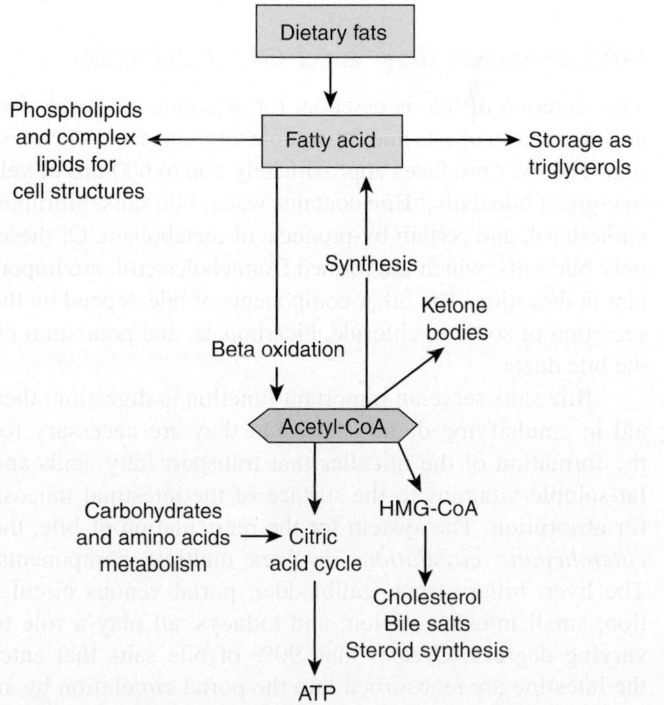

Figure 38.6 • Hepatic pathways for fat metabolism. Beta oxidation breaks fatty acids into two-carbon acetyl-CoA units that are used in the citric acid cycle to generate ATP or are used in the synthesis of cholesterol of keto acids that are released into the blood for use by other tissues as an energy source.

fatty acids, and then the fatty acids must be split into two-carbon acetyl-coenzyme A (acetyl-CoA) units by a process called *beta oxidation*. Acetyl-CoA is readily channeled into the citric acid cycle to produce adenosine triphosphate (ATP). Because the liver cannot use all the acetyl-CoA that is formed, it converts the excess into acetoacetic acid, a highly soluble keto acid that is released into the bloodstream and transported to other tissues, where it is used for energy. During periods of starvation, ketones become a major source of energy as fatty acids released from adipose tissue are converted to ketones by the liver.

Acetyl-CoA units from fat metabolism also are used to synthesize cholesterol and bile acids in the liver. Cholesterol can be used in several ways by the liver. It can be esterified and stored; it can be exported bound to lipoproteins; or it can be converted to bile acids. The rate-limiting step in cholesterol synthesis is that which is catalyzed by 3-hydroxy-3-methylglutaryl-coenzyme A reductase (HMG-CoA reductase). The HMG-CoA reductase inhibitors, or statins (fluvastatin, lovastatin, pravastatin, and atorvastatin), are used to treat high cholesterol levels by inhibiting this step in cholesterol synthesis.

Almost all the fat synthesis in the body from carbohydrates and proteins occurs in the liver. Whenever a greater quantity of carbohydrates enters the body than can be immediately used, the excess is converted to triglycerides in the liver. The triglycerides formed in the liver are transported mainly in low-density lipoproteins (LDLs) to the adipose tissue, where they are stored.

Bile Production and Cholestasis

The secretion of bile is essential for digestion of dietary fats and absorption of fats and fat-soluble vitamins from the intestine. The liver produces approximately 500 to 600 mL of yellow-green bile daily.[4] Bile contains water, bile salts, bilirubin, cholesterol, and certain by-products of metabolism. Of these, only bile salts, which are formed from cholesterol, are important in digestion. The other components of bile depend on the secretion of sodium, chloride, bicarbonate, and potassium by the bile ducts.

Bile salts serve an important function in digestion; they aid in emulsifying dietary fats, and they are necessary for the formation of the micelles that transport fatty acids and fat-soluble vitamins to the surface of the intestinal mucosa for absorption. The system for the recirculation of bile, the *enterohepatic circulation*, involves multiple components. The liver, biliary tract, gallbladder, portal venous circulation, small intestine, colon, and kidneys, all play a role to varying degrees. Greater than 90% of bile salts that enter the intestine are reabsorbed into the portal circulation by an active transport process that takes place in the distal ileum.[4] From the portal circulation, the bile salts move into the liver cells and are recycled. Normally, bile salts travel this entire circuit approximately 17 times before being expelled in the feces.[3]

Cholestasis

Cholestasis represents a decrease in bile flow through the intrahepatic canaliculi and a reduction in secretion of water, bilirubin, and bile acids by the hepatocytes. As a result, the materials normally transferred to the bile, including bilirubin, cholesterol, and bile acids, accumulate in the blood.[5] The condition may be caused by intrinsic liver disease, in which case it is referred to as *intrahepatic cholestasis*, or by obstruction of the large bile ducts, a condition known as *extrahepatic cholestasis*.

A number of mechanisms are implicated in the pathogenesis of cholestasis. Primary biliary cirrhosis (PBC) (an autoimmune disease) and primary sclerosing cholangitis (PSC) are caused by disorders of the small intrahepatic canaliculi and bile ducts. In the case of extrahepatic obstruction, which can be caused by conditions such as cholelithiasis, common duct strictures, or obstructing neoplasms, the effects begin with increased pressure in the large bile ducts. Genetic disorders that can result in cholestasis include benign recurrent cholestasis, Byler syndrome, and Alagille syndrome. Benign recurrent cholestasis involves the transport of bile into the canaliculi.[6] Byler syndrome is also known as progressive familial intrahepatic cholestasis type I (PFIC-1). People with PFIC-1 have mutations in ATP8B1 (encoding ATP8B1 protein), which maps to chromosome 18q21-22. ATP8B1 protein is highly expressed in the small bowel and pancreas, which affects the gastrointestinal and endocrine systems. The ATP8B1gene mutation responsible for the disease results in diarrhea, pruritis, and liver failure.[7] Alagille syndrome is an autosomal dominant disease that involves the intrahepatic hypoplasia specifically of the interlobar bile ducts.[8,9] People with the syndrome present with cardiac and eye abnormalities along with skeletal abnormalities, specifically in the facial bones.[8,9]

The morphologic features of cholestasis depend on the underlying cause. Common to all types of obstructive and hepatocellular cholestasis is the accumulation of bile pigment in the liver. Elongated green-brown plugs of bile are visible in the dilated bile canaliculi. Rupture of the canaliculi leads to extravasation of bile and subsequent degenerative changes in the surrounding hepatocytes. Prolonged obstructive cholestasis leads not only to fatty changes in the hepatocytes but also to destruction of the supporting connective tissue, giving rise to reservoirs of bile containing cellular debris and pigment.[10] Unrelieved obstruction leads to biliary tract fibrosis and ultimately to end-stage biliary cirrhosis.

Pruritus is the most common presenting symptom in people with cholestasis, probably related to an elevation in plasma bile acids. Skin xanthomas (focal accumulations of cholesterol) may occur, the result of hyperlipidemia and impaired excretion of cholesterol. A characteristic laboratory finding is an elevated serum alkaline phosphatase level, an enzyme present in the bile duct epithelium, and canalicular membrane of hepatocytes. Other manifestations of reduced bile flow relate to intestinal absorption, including nutritional deficiencies of the fat-soluble vitamins A, D, and K.

Bilirubin Elimination and Jaundice

Bilirubin is the final product of the breakdown of heme contained in aged red blood cells. Bilirubin is the substance that gives bile its color. In the process of degradation, the hemoglobin from the red blood cell is broken down to form biliverdin, which is rapidly converted to free bilirubin (Fig. 38.7). Free bilirubin, which is insoluble in plasma, is transported in the blood attached to plasma albumin. Even when it is bound to albumin, this bilirubin is still called *free bilirubin*, to distinguish it from conjugated bilirubin. As it passes through the liver, free bilirubin is absorbed through the hepatocytes' cell membrane and released from its albumin carrier molecule. Inside the hepatocytes, free bilirubin is converted to conjugated bilirubin, making it soluble in bile. Conjugated bilirubin is secreted as a constituent of bile, and in this form it passes through the bile ducts into the small intestine. In the intestine, approximately one half of the bilirubin is converted into a highly soluble substance called *urobilinogen* by the intestinal flora. Approximately one fifth of the urobilinogen produced is either absorbed into the portal circulation and the remaining is excreted in the feces.[10] Most of the urobilinogen that is absorbed is returned to the liver to be reexcreted into the bile.

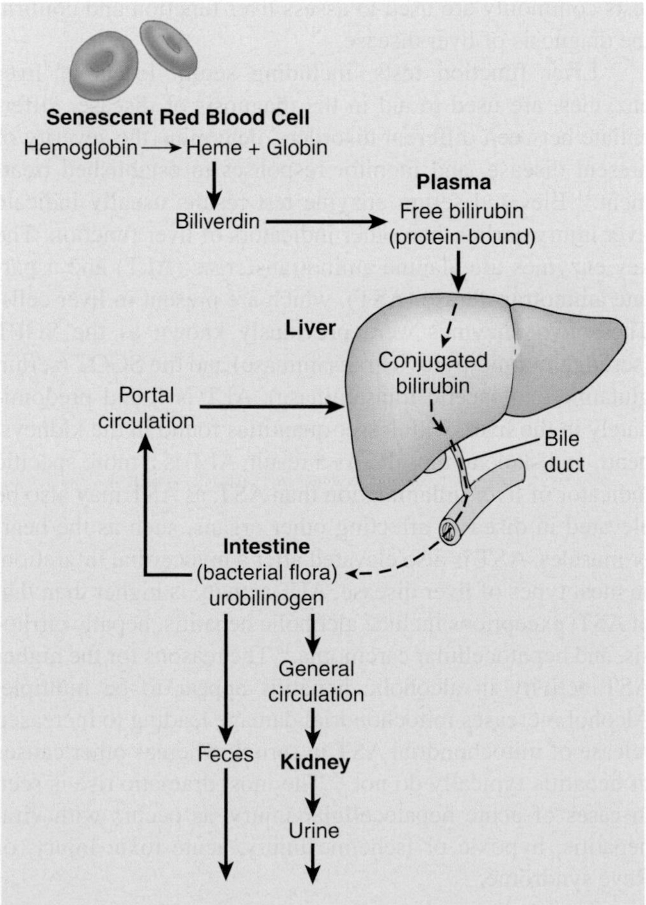

Figure 38.7 • The process of bilirubin formation, circulation, and elimination.

Usually, only a small amount of bilirubin is found in the blood; the normal level of total serum bilirubin is less than 1.5 mg/dL (17 to 20.5 μmol).[11] Laboratory measurements of bilirubin usually measure the free and the conjugated bilirubin as well as the total bilirubin. These are reported as the direct (conjugated) bilirubin and the indirect (unconjugated or free) bilirubin.

Jaundice

Jaundice (*i.e.*, icterus) or a yellowish discoloration of the skin and deep tissues results from abnormally high levels of bilirubin in the blood. Jaundice occurs when there is an imbalance between the synthesis of bilirubin and the clearance of bilirubin. Jaundice becomes evident when the serum bilirubin levels rise above 2 to 2.5 mg/dL (34.2 to 42.8 μmol).[5,10] Because normal skin has a yellow cast, the early signs of jaundice often are difficult to detect, especially in people with dark skin. Bilirubin has a special affinity for elastic tissue. The sclera of the eye, which contains a high proportion of elastic fibers, usually is one of the first structures in which jaundice can be detected (Fig. 38.8).

The five major causes of jaundice are excessive destruction of red blood cells, impaired uptake of bilirubin by the liver cells, decreased conjugation of bilirubin, obstruction of bile flow in the canaliculi of the hepatic lobules or in the intrahepatic or extrahepatic bile ducts, and excessive extrahepatic production of bilirubin.[12] From an anatomic standpoint, jaundice can be categorized as prehepatic, intrahepatic, and posthepatic. Chart 38.1 lists the common causes of prehepatic, hepatic, and posthepatic jaundice.

The major cause of prehepatic jaundice is excessive hemolysis of red blood cells. Hemolytic jaundice occurs when red blood cells are destroyed at a rate in excess of the liver's ability to remove the bilirubin from the blood. It may follow a hemolytic blood transfusion reaction, because of the decreased lifespan of the donated red blood cells, or may occur in diseases such as hereditary spherocytosis, in which the red cell membranes are defective, or in hemolytic disease of the newborn. When internal hemorrhage occurs, there can

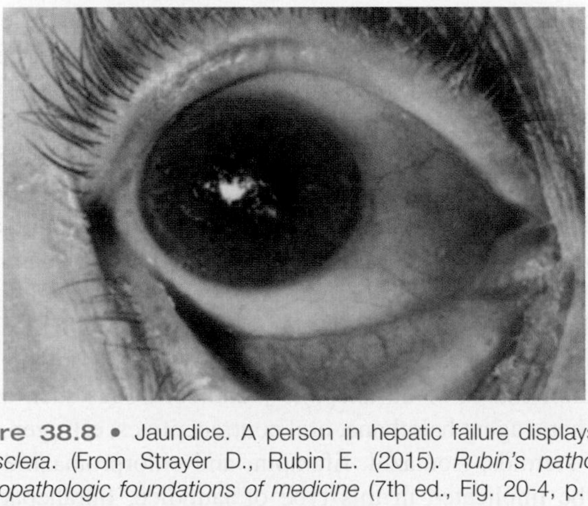

Figure 38.8 • Jaundice. A person in hepatic failure displays *yellow sclera*. (From Strayer D., Rubin E. (2015). *Rubin's pathology: Clinicopathologic foundations of medicine* (7th ed., Fig. 20-4, p. 829). Philadelphia, PA: Lippincott Williams & Wilkins.)

CHART 38.1 CAUSES OF JAUNDICE

Prehepatic (Excessive Red Blood Cell Destruction)
Hemolytic blood transfusion reaction
Hereditary disorders of the red blood cell
- Sickle cell disease
- Thalassemia
- Spherocytosis

Acquired hemolytic disorders
Hemolytic disease of the newborn
Autoimmune hemolytic anemias

Intrahepatic
Decreased bilirubin uptake by the liver
Decreased conjugation of bilirubin
Hepatocellular liver damage
- Hepatitis
- Cirrhosis
- Cancer of the liver

Drug-induced cholestasis

Posthepatic (Obstruction of Bile Flow)
Structural disorders of the bile duct
Cholelithiasis
Congenital atresia of the extrahepatic bile ducts
Bile duct obstruction caused by tumors

also be excess bilirubin production with the reabsorption of the blood. In addition, diseases resulting in ineffective erythropoiesis can also increase bilirubin production.[10] Neonatal hyperbilirubinemia results from increased production of bilirubin in newborn infants and their limited ability to excrete it from 0 to 14 days old.[10] Premature infants are at particular risk because their red cells have a shorter life span and higher turnover rate. In prehepatic jaundice, there is mild jaundice, the unconjugated bilirubin is elevated, the stools are of normal color, and there is no bilirubin in the urine.

Intrahepatic or hepatocellular jaundice is caused by disorders that directly affect the ability of the liver to remove bilirubin from the blood or conjugate it so it can be eliminated in the bile. Gilbert disease is inherited as a dominant trait and results in a reduced, by 66% on average, removal of bilirubin from the blood. The disorder is benign and fairly common with a prevalence rate of approximately 8%.[12] Affected people have no symptoms other than a slightly elevated unconjugated bilirubin and mild jaundice. Conjugation of bilirubin is impaired whenever liver cells are damaged, when transport of bilirubin into liver cells becomes deficient, or when the enzymes needed to conjugate the bile are lacking. Liver diseases such as hepatitis and cirrhosis are the most common causes of intrahepatic jaundice. Drugs such as the anesthetic agent halothane, oral contraceptives, estrogen, anabolic steroids, isoniazid, rifampin, and chlorpromazine may also be implicated in this type of jaundice. Intrahepatic or hepatocellular jaundice usually interferes with all phases of bilirubin metabolism—uptake, conjugation, and excretion. Both conjugated and unconjugated bilirubin are elevated, the urine often is dark because of bilirubin in the urine, and the serum alkaline phosphatase is slightly elevated.

Posthepatic or obstructive jaundice, also called *cholestatic jaundice*, occurs when bile flow is obstructed between the liver and the intestine, with the obstruction located at any point between the junction of the right or left hepatic duct and the point where the bile duct opens into the intestine. Among the causes are strictures of the bile duct, gallstones, and tumors of the bile duct or the pancreas. Conjugated bilirubin levels usually are elevated; the stools are clay colored because of the lack of bilirubin in the bile; the urine is dark; the levels of serum alkaline phosphatase are markedly elevated; and the aminotransferase levels are slightly increased. Blood levels of bile acids often are elevated in obstructive jaundice. As the bile acids accumulate in the blood, pruritus develops. A history of pruritus preceding jaundice is common in obstructive jaundice.

Tests of Hepatobiliary Function

The history and physical examination, in most instances, provide clues about liver function. Diagnostic tests help to evaluate liver function and the extent of liver damage. Laboratory tests commonly are used to assess liver function and confirm the diagnosis of liver disease.

Liver function tests, including serum levels of liver enzymes, are used to aid in the diagnosis of disease, differentiate between different disorders, determine the severity of present disease, and monitor responses to established treatment.[13] Elevated serum enzyme test results usually indicate liver injury earlier than other indicators of liver function. The key enzymes are alanine aminotransferase (ALT) and aspartate aminotransferase (AST), which are present in liver cells. These two enzymes were previously known as the SGPT (serum glutamic-pyruvic transaminase) and the SGOT (serum glutamic-oxaloacetic transaminase). ALT is found predominately in the liver, with lesser quantities found in the kidneys, heart, and skeletal muscle. As a result, ALT is a more specific indicator of liver inflammation than AST, as AST may also be elevated in diseases affecting other organs, such as the heart or muscles. AST is also elevated after a myocardial infarction. In most types of liver disease, ALT activity is higher than that of AST; exceptions include alcoholic hepatitis, hepatic cirrhosis, and hepatocellular carcinoma.[14] The reasons for the higher AST activity in alcoholic hepatitis appear to be multiple. Alcohol increases mitochondrial damage leading to increased release of mitochondrial AST in serum, whereas other causes of hepatitis typically do not.[15] The most dramatic rise is seen in cases of acute hepatocellular injury, as occurs with viral hepatitis, hypoxic or ischemic injury, acute toxic injury, or Reye syndrome.

The liver's synthetic capacity is reflected in measures of serum protein levels and prothrombin time (*i.e.*, synthesis of coagulation factors). Hypoalbuminemia because of depressed synthesis may complicate severe liver disease. Deficiencies of coagulation factor V and vitamin K–dependent factors (II, VII, IX, and X) may occur.

Serum bilirubin, γ-glutamyltransferase (GGT), 5′-nucleotidase, and alkaline phosphatase measure hepatic excretory function. Alkaline phosphatase and 5′-nucleotidase are present in the membranes between liver cells and the bile duct and are released by disorders affecting the bile duct.[13] GGT is located in the endoplasmic reticulum of the hepatocytes and in the bile duct epithelial cells. It is thought to function in the transport of amino acids and peptides into liver cells. Measurement of GGT may be helpful in diagnosing alcohol abuse and is an indicator of hepatobiliary disease.[16]

Ultrasonography provides information about the size, composition, and blood flow of the liver. It has largely replaced cholangiography in detecting stones in the gallbladder or biliary tree. Computed tomography (CT) scanning provides information similar to that obtained by ultrasonography. Magnetic resonance imaging (MRI) has proved to be useful in some disorders. Selective angiography of the celiac, superior mesenteric, or hepatic artery may be used to visualize the hepatic or portal circulation. A liver biopsy affords a means of examining liver tissue without surgery. There are several methods for obtaining liver tissue: percutaneous liver biopsy, which uses a suction, cutting, or spring-loaded cutting needle[11]; laparoscopic liver biopsy; and fine-needle biopsy, which is performed under endoscopic ultrasound guidance.[17] The type of method used is based on the number of specimens needed and the amount of tissue required for evaluation. Laparoscopic liver biopsy provides the means for examining abdominal masses, evaluating ascites of unknown cause, and staging liver cancers.

IN SUMMARY

The hepatobiliary system consists of the liver, gallbladder, and bile ducts. The liver is the largest and, in functions, one of the most versatile organs in the body. It is located between the gastrointestinal tract and the systemic circulation; venous blood from the intestine flows through the liver before it is returned to the heart. In this way, nutrients can be removed for processing and storage, and bacteria and other foreign matter can be removed by Kupffer cells before the blood is returned to the systemic circulation.

The liver synthesizes fats, glucose, and plasma proteins. Other important functions of the liver include the deamination of amino acids, conversion of ammonia to urea, and the interconversion of amino acids and other compounds that are important to the metabolic processes of the body. The liver produces approximately 500 to 600 mL of yellow-green bile daily. Bile serves as an excretory vehicle for bilirubin, cholesterol, and certain products of organic metabolism, and it contains bile salts that are essential for digestion of fats and absorption of fat-soluble vitamins. The liver also removes, conjugates, and secretes bilirubin into the bile. Jaundice occurs when bilirubin accumulates in the blood. It can occur because of excessive red blood cell destruction, failure of the liver to remove and conjugate the bilirubin, or obstructed biliary flow.

Liver function tests, including serum aminotransferase levels, are used to assess injury to liver cells. Serum bilirubin, GGT, 5′-nucleotidase, and alkaline phosphatase are used as measures of hepatic excretory function. Ultrasonography, CT scans, and MRI are used to evaluate liver structures. Angiography may be used to visualize the hepatic or portal circulation, and a liver biopsy obtains tissue specimens for microscopic examination.

DISORDERS OF HEPATIC AND BILIARY FUNCTION

After completing this section of the chapter, the learner will be able to meet the following objectives:

- State the three ways by which drugs and other substances are metabolized or inactivated in the liver and provide examples of liver disease related to the toxic effects of drugs and chemical agents.
- Compare hepatitis A, B, C, D, and E in terms of source of infection, incubation period, acute disease manifestations, development of chronic disease, and the carrier state.
- Describe the physiologic basis for portal hypertension and relate it to the development of ascites, esophageal varices, and splenomegaly.

The structures of the hepatobiliary system are subject to many of the same pathologic conditions that affect other body systems: injury from drugs and toxins; infection, inflammation, and immune responses; metabolic disorders; and neoplasms. This section focuses on alterations in liver function because of drug-induced injury; viral and autoimmune hepatitis (AIH); intrahepatic biliary tract disorders; alcohol-induced liver disease; cirrhosis, portal hypertension, and liver failure; and cancer of the liver.

Hepatotoxic Disorders

By virtue of its many enzyme systems that are involved in biochemical transformations and modifications, the liver has an important role in the metabolism of many drugs and chemical substances. The liver is particularly important in terms of metabolizing lipid-soluble substances that cannot be directly excreted by the kidneys. The liver is central to the metabolic disposition of virtually all drugs and foreign substances. Therefore, drug-induced liver toxicity is a potential complication of many medications.

Drug and Hormone Metabolism

Three major types of reactions are involved in the hepatic detoxification and metabolism of drugs and other chemicals:

1. Phase 1 reactions, which involve chemical modification or inactivation of a substance
2. Phase 2 reactions, which involve conversion of lipid-soluble substances to water-soluble derivatives
3. Phase 3 reactions, which involve the substance, its metabolites, or conjugates being secreted as bile[18]

All three types of reactions may be linked, depending upon the composition of the substance being eliminated. For example, many phase 1 reactants are not water soluble and must therefore undergo a subsequent phase 2 reaction to be eliminated. These reactions, which are called *biotransformations*, are important considerations in drug therapy.

Phase 1 Reactions. *Phase 1 reactions* result in chemical modification of reactive drug groups by oxidation, reduction, hydroxylation, or other chemical reactions. Most drug-metabolizing enzymes are located in the lipophilic membranes of the smooth endoplasmic reticulum of liver cells. When these membranes are broken down and separated in the laboratory, they re-form into vesicles called *microsomes*. The enzymes in these membranes are often referred to as *microsomal enzymes*. The enzymes involved in most phase 1 oxidation–reduction processes are products of a gene superfamily that has nearly 300 members.[19] These genes code for a group of microsomal isoenzymes that make up the cytochrome (CYP) P-450 system. (The name cytochrome *P-450* is derived from the spectral properties [absorb light at 450 nm] of the hemoproteins that participate in oxidation–reduction processes.) The gene products of many of the *CYP* genes have been identified and traced to the metabolism of specific drugs and to potential interactions among drugs. Each family of genes is responsible for certain drug-metabolizing processes, and each member of the family undertakes specific drug-metabolizing functions. For example, the *CYP3* gene family contains an A subfamily and several genes numbered 1, 2, 3, and so forth. For example, the primary enzyme for the metabolism of erythromycin in humans is CYP 3A4.[19]

Many gene members of the *CYP* system can have their activity induced or suppressed as they undergo the task of metabolizing drugs. For example, drugs such as alcohol and barbiturates can induce certain members to increase enzyme production, accelerating drug metabolism and decreasing the pharmacologic action of the drug, and of coadministered drugs that use the same member of the CYP system. In the case of drugs metabolically transformed to reactive intermediates, enzyme induction may exacerbate drug-mediated tissue toxicity. Enzymes in the cytochrome system also can be inhibited by drugs. For example, imidazole-containing drugs such as cimetidine (a histamine type 2 receptor–blocking drug that is used to reduce gastric acid secretion) and ketoconazole (an antifungal agent) effectively inhibit the metabolism of testosterone.[19] Environmental pollutants also are capable of inducing *CYP* gene activity. For example, exposure to benzo[*a*]pyrene, which is present in tobacco smoke, charcoal-broiled meat, and other organic pyrolysis products, is known to induce members of the *CYP* family and alter the rates of metabolism of some drugs.

Phase 2 Reactions. *Phase 2 reactions*, which involve the conversion of lipid-soluble derivatives to water-soluble substances, may follow phase 1 reactions or proceed independently. Conjugation, catalyzed by endoplasmic reticulum enzymes that couple the drug with an activated endogenous compound to render it more water soluble, is one of the most common phase 2 reactions. Although many water-soluble drugs and endogenous substances are excreted unchanged in the urine or bile, lipid-soluble substances tend to accumulate in the body unless they are converted to less active compounds or water-soluble metabolites. In general, the conjugates are more soluble than the parent compound and are pharmacologically inactive. Because the endogenous substrates used in the conjugation process are obtained from the diet, nutrition plays a critical role in phase 2 reactions.

An alternative cytochrome P-450–dependent conjugation pathway is important in detoxifying reactive metabolic intermediates. This pathway uses a thiol, or sulfur-containing substance, called *glutathione*, which is used in conjugating drugs that form potentially harmful electrophilic groups. Glutathione is depleted in the detoxification process and must be constantly replenished by compounds from the diet or by cysteine-containing drugs such as *N*-acetylcysteine.[19] The glutathione pathway is central to the detoxification of a number of compounds, including the over-the-counter pain medication acetaminophen (*e.g.*, Tylenol). Acetaminophen metabolism involves a phase 2 reaction. Normally, the capacity of the phase 2 reactants is much greater than that required for metabolizing recommended doses of the drug. However, in situations of acetaminophen overdose, the capacity of the phase 2 system is exceeded, and the drug is transformed into toxic metabolites that can cause necrosis of the liver if allowed to accumulate. In this situation, the glutathione pathway plays a critical role in the detoxification of these metabolites. Because the glutathione stores are rapidly depleted, the drug *N*-acetylcysteine, which serves as a glutathione substitute, is used as a treatment for acetaminophen overdose.[20] Chronic alcohol ingestion decreases glutathione stores and increases the risk of acetaminophen toxicity.

Phase 3 Reactions. *Phase 3 reactions* involve the secretion of drugs, drug metabolites, or drug conjugates into bile. ATP-binding cassette (ABC) proteins are intricately involved in this process. One example is multidrug resistance proteins 1, 2, and 3, which transport cationic drugs and their conjugates into bile.[18]

In addition to its role in metabolism of drugs and chemicals, the liver also is responsible for hormone inactivation or modification. Insulin and glucagon are inactivated by proteolysis or deamination. Thyroxine and triiodothyronine are metabolized by reactions involving deiodination. Steroid hormones such as the glucocorticoids are first inactivated by a phase 1 reaction and then conjugated by a phase 2 reaction.

Drug-Induced Liver Disease. Drug-induced liver disease, also known as drug-induced hepatotoxicity, drug-induced liver injury, or drug-induced hepatitis, is a frequent cause of acute liver injury. It may be extremely severe and is responsible for more than 50% of all cases of acute liver failure in the United States. As the major drug-metabolizing and detoxifying organ in the body, the liver is subject to potential damage from the enormous array of pharmaceutical and environmental chemicals. Many of the widely used therapeutic drugs, including over-the-counter "natural" products, can cause hepatic injury. In a multicenter study, 10% of 300 cases of drug-induced liver injury were attributed to use of herbal products.[21]

Numerous host factors contribute to the susceptibility to drug-induced liver disease, including genetic predisposition, age differences, underlying chronic liver disease, diet and alcohol consumption, and the use of multiple interacting drugs. In a study examining 1198 people with acute liver failure, drug-induced liver injury was found to be the cause of failure in 11.1% of cases.[22] Early identification of drug-induced liver disease is important because withdrawal of the drug is curative in most cases.

Drugs and chemicals can exert their effects by causing hepatocyte injury and death or by cholestatic liver damage because of injury of biliary drainage structures.[18] Drug reactions can be predictable based on the drug's chemical structure and metabolites or unpredictable (idiosyncratic) based on individual characteristics of the person receiving the drug.

Direct Hepatotoxic Injury. Some drugs are known to have toxic effects on the liver based on their chemical structure and the way they are metabolized in the liver. Direct hepatic damage often is age and dose dependent. Direct hepatotoxic reactions usually are a recognized characteristic of certain drugs. They usually result from drug metabolism and the generation of toxic metabolites. Because of the greater activity of the drug-metabolizing enzymes in the central zones of the liver, these agents typically cause centrilobular necrosis. Acetaminophen, antimicrobials, psychotropic agents, lipid-lowering agents, and nonsteroidal anti-inflammatory drugs (NSAIDs) are most commonly associated with acute liver injury.[23] Acetaminophen toxicity is characterized by marked elevations in ALT and AST values with minimally elevated alkaline phosphatase. Bilirubin levels invariably are increased, and the prognosis often is worse when hepatocellular necrosis is accompanied by jaundice.

Idiosyncratic Reactions. In contrast to direct hepatotoxic drug reactions, idiosyncratic reactions are unpredictable, not related to dose, and sometimes accompanied by features suggesting an allergic reaction. In some cases, the reaction results directly from a metabolite that is produced only in certain people based on a genetic predisposition. For example, certain people are capable of rapid acetylation of isoniazid, an antituberculosis drug.

Cholestatic Reactions. Cholestatic drug reactions result in decreased secretion of bile or obstruction of the biliary tree. Acute intrahepatic cholestasis is one of the most frequent types of idiosyncratic drug reactions. Among the drugs credited with causing cholestatic drug reactions are estradiol; chlorpromazine, an antipsychotic drug; and some of the antibiotics, including amoxicillin/clavulanic acid, erythromycin, and nafcillin. Typically, cholestatic drug reactions are characterized by an early onset of jaundice and pruritus, with little alteration in the person's general feeling of well-being. The symptoms of acute drug-induced cholestasis subside once the drug is withdrawn, but the biliary secretory function returns at a slower rate than does the function of the liver itself.[24]

Chronic Hepatitis. Some drugs produce a more indolent form of liver damage that closely resembles AIH. Early identification of drug-related chronic hepatitis often is difficult. Cirrhosis may develop before the hepatitis is diagnosed. Identifying the responsible drug that caused the liver damage may be difficult retrospectively if the person has been consuming alcohol or taking several drugs.

KEY POINTS

DISEASES OF THE LIVER

- Diseases of hepatocytes impair the metabolic and synthetic functions of the liver, causing disorders in carbohydrate, protein, and fat metabolism; metabolism and removal of drugs, hormones, toxins, ammonia, and bilirubin from the blood; and the interconversion of amino acids and synthesis of proteins. Elevations in serum aminotransferase levels signal the presence of hepatocyte damage.
- Diseases of the biliary drainage system obstruct the flow of bile and interfere with the elimination of bile salts and bilirubin, producing cholestatic liver damage because of the backup of bile into the lobules of the liver. Elevations in bilirubin and alkaline phosphatase signal the presence of cholestatic liver damage.

Viral Hepatitis

Hepatitis refers to inflammation of the liver. It can be caused by hepatotropic viruses that primarily affect liver cells or hepatocytes, autoimmune mechanisms, or reactions to drugs and toxins, or be secondary to other systemic disorders. Viruses causing systemic disease that can involve the liver include Epstein-Barr virus (infectious mononucleosis), which may cause a mild hepatitis during the acute phase; cytomegalovirus (particularly in newborns and people who are immunosuppressed); herpesviruses; and enteroviruses.

The known hepatotropic viruses include hepatitis A virus (HAV), hepatitis B virus (HBV), the hepatitis B–associated delta virus (HDV), hepatitis C virus (HCV), and hepatitis E virus (HEV). Although all of these viruses cause acute hepatitis, they differ in the mode of transmission and incubation period; mechanism, degree, and chronicity of liver damage; and ability to evolve to a carrier state. The presence of viral antigens and their antibodies can be determined through laboratory tests. Epidemiologic studies have indicated that some cases of infectious hepatitis are due to other agents. A viral agent similar to HCV has been cloned and was identified as hepatitis G virus (HGV), also referred to as GBV-C.[25] Evidence of HGV has been found in 2% of blood donors in the United States.[26] However, HGV is not linked to liver disease or exacerbations of liver disease.[25]

Etiology and Pathogenesis

There are two mechanisms of liver injury in viral hepatitis: direct cellular injury and induction of immune responses against the viral antigens. The mechanisms of injury have been most closely studied in HBV. It is thought that the extent of inflammation and necrosis depends on the person's immune response. Accordingly, a prompt immune response during the acute phase of the infection would be expected to cause cell injury but at the same time eliminate the virus. Thus, people who respond with fewer symptoms and a marginal immune response are less likely to eliminate the virus, and hepatocytes expressing the viral antigens persist, leading to the chronic or carrier state. Fulminant hepatitis would be explained in terms of an accelerated immune response with severe liver necrosis.

The clinical course of viral hepatitis involves a number of syndromes, including asymptomatic infection with only serologic evidence of disease; acute hepatitis; the carrier state without clinically apparent disease or with chronic hepatitis; chronic hepatitis with or without progression to cirrhosis; or fulminating disease with rapid onset of liver failure. Not all hepatotoxic viruses provoke each of the clinical syndromes.

Clinical Manifestations

The manifestations of acute viral hepatitis can be divided into three phases: the prodromal or preicterus period, the icterus period, and the recovery period. The manifestations of the prodromal period vary from abrupt to insidious, with general malaise, myalgia, arthralgia, easy fatigability, and anorexia.[27] Gastrointestinal symptoms such as nausea, vomiting, and diarrhea or constipation may also occur.[27] Serum levels of AST and ALT show variable increases during the preicterus phase of acute hepatitis and precede a rise in bilirubin that accompanies the onset of the icterus or jaundice phase of infection. The icterus phase, if it occurs, usually follows the prodromal phase by 7 to 14 days. People have tenderness around the area of the liver, mild weight loss, and spider angiomas.[27] Approximately 80% of people with acute Hepatitis C do not have any symptoms.[28] The recovery phase is characterized by an increased sense of well-being, return of appetite, and disappearance of jaundice. The acute illness usually subsides gradually over 2 to 12 weeks period, with complete clinical recovery in 1 to 4 months depending on the type of hepatitis.[27] Infection with HBV and HCV can produce a *carrier state* in which the person does not have symptoms but harbors the virus and can therefore transmit the disease.[29] Evidence also indicates a carrier state for HDV infection. There is no carrier state for HAV infection. There are two types of carriers: healthy carriers who have few or no ill effects and those with chronic disease who may or may not have symptoms. Factors that increase the risk of becoming a carrier are age at time of infection and immune status. The carrier state for infections that occur early in life, as in infants of HBV-infected mothers, may be as high as 90%.[27] Other people at high risk of becoming carriers are those with impaired immunity, those who have received multiple transfusions or blood products, those who are on hemodialysis, and drug addicts.

Hepatitis A

Hepatitis A is caused by the HAV, a small, unenveloped, single-stranded ribonucleic acid (RNA) virus. It usually is a benign, self-limited disease, although it can cause acute fulminant hepatitis and death or need for transplantation in 0.15% to 0.2% of cases.[30]

Etiology and Pathogenesis. Hepatitis A is contracted primarily by the fecal–oral route.[31] It has a brief incubation period of 14 to 28 days.[32] The virus replicates in the liver, is excreted in the bile, and is shed in the stool. The fecal shedding of HAV occurs during the first 2 weeks of the illness.[31] The disease often occurs sporadically or in epidemics. Drinking contaminated milk or water and eating shellfish from infected waters are fairly common routes of transmission. At special risk are people traveling abroad who have not previously been exposed to the virus. Because young children are asymptomatic, they play an important role in the spread of the disease. Institutions housing large numbers of people (usually children) sometimes are stricken with an epidemic of hepatitis A. Oral behavior and lack of toilet training promote viral infection among children attending preschool day care centers, who then carry the virus home to older siblings and parents. Hepatitis A usually is not transmitted by transfusion of blood or plasma derivatives, presumably because its short period of viremia usually coincides with clinical illness, so that the disease is apparent and blood donations are not accepted.

Clinical Manifestations. The onset of symptoms usually is abrupt and includes fever, malaise, nausea, anorexia, abdominal discomfort, dark urine, and jaundice. The presentation of symptoms is dependent upon age, with the severity of symptoms increasing in older age groups.[33] Children younger than 6 years often are asymptomatic, and few develop jaundice. The illness in older children and adults usually is symptomatic and jaundice occurs in approximately 70% of cases.[33] Symptoms usually last approximately 2 months but can last longer. HAV does not cause chronic hepatitis or induce a carrier state.

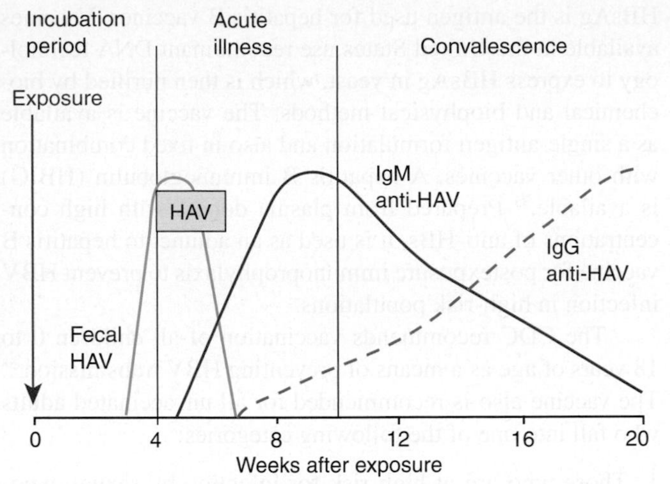

Figure 38.9 • The sequence of fecal shedding of the HAV, HAV viremia, and HAV antibody (IgM and IgG anti-HAV) changes in hepatitis A.

Serologic Markers. Antibodies to HAV (anti-HAV) appear early in the disease and tend to persist in the serum (Fig. 38.9). The IgM antibodies usually appear during the first week of symptomatic disease and slowly decline over a period of 3 to 4 months. Their presence coincides with a decline in fecal shedding of the virus. Peak levels of immunoglobulin G (IgG) antibodies occur after 1 month of illness and may persist for life; they provide long-term protective immunity against reinfection.[31] The presence of IgM anti-HAV is indicative of acute hepatitis A, whereas IgG anti-HAV merely documents past infection.

Immunization. A hepatitis A vaccine is available.[33] Immunization is intended to replace the use of immune globulin in people at high risk for HAV exposure. These include international travelers to regions where sanitation is poor and endemic HAV infections are high, children living in communities with high rates of HAV infection, homosexually active men, and users of illicit drugs. People with preexisting chronic liver disease also may benefit from immunization. A public health benefit also may be derived from vaccinating people with increased potential for transmitting the disease (*e.g.*, food handlers). The Centers for Disease Control and Prevention (CDC) has recently recommended vaccination of children in states, counties, and communities with high rates of infection.[34] Because the vaccine is of little benefit in prevention of hepatitis in people with known HAV exposure, IgG is recommended for these people.

Hepatitis B

Hepatitis B is caused by the HBV, a double-stranded deoxyribonucleic acid (DNA) virus.[35] The complete virion, also called a *Dane particle*, consists of an outer envelope and an inner nucleocapsid that contains HBV DNA and DNA polymerase (Fig. 38.10).[36] HBV infection can produce acute hepatitis, chronic hepatitis, progression of chronic hepatitis to cirrhosis, fulminant hepatitis with massive hepatic necrosis, and the carrier state. It also participates in the development of hepatitis D (delta hepatitis).

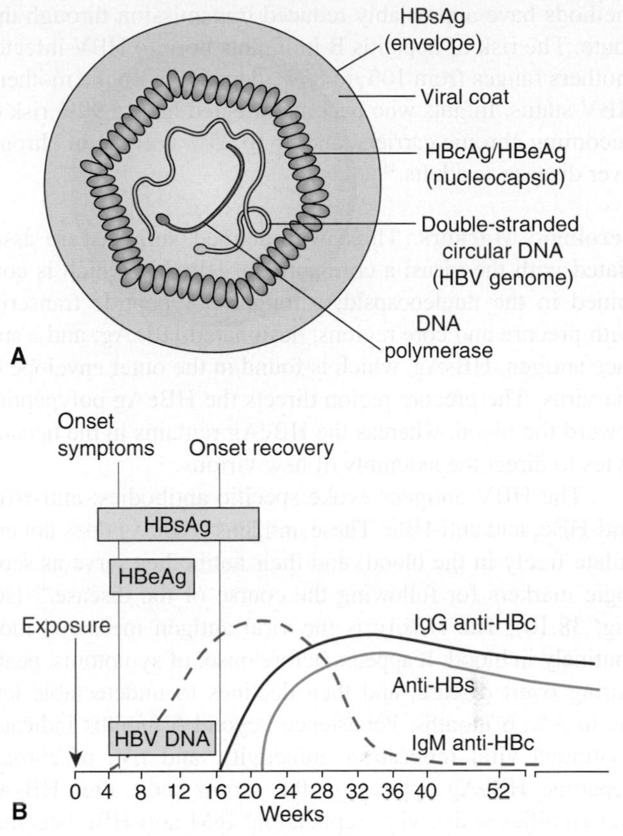

Figure 38.10 • **(A)** The HBV. **(B)** The sequence of HBV viral antigens (HBsAg, HBeAg), HBV DNA, and HBV antibody (IgM, IgG, anti-HBc, and anti-HBs) changes in acute resolving hepatitis B.

Worldwide, 350 million people have long-term hepatitis B infections.[37] In the United States, acute hepatitis B has been declining in incidence since 1990, mainly because of effective vaccination strategies.[38] The number of reported cases of acute hepatitis B has remained relatively stable since 2009. A total of 2791 acute cases were reported in 2014. However, chronic HBV infection remains a major public health challenge; recent CDC investigations report approximately 850,000 people with HBV infection in the United States. In the United States, 850,000–2.2 million people are estimated to be living with HBV infection,[39,40] many of whom are unaware of their infection status.[41] To improve health outcomes for these people, the CDC recommended HBV testing for populations at risk for HBV infection and public health management of people living with chronic HBV infection.[42]

Hepatitis B has a longer incubation period and represents a more serious health problem than hepatitis A. The virus usually is transmitted through inoculation with infected blood or serum. However, the viral antigen can be found in most body secretions and can be spread by oral or sexual contact. In the United States, most people with hepatitis B acquire the infection as adults or adolescents. The disease is highly prevalent among injecting drug users, heterosexuals with multiple sex partners, and men who have sex with men.[43,44] Health care workers are at risk owing to blood exposure and accidental needle injuries. Although the virus can be spread through transfusion or administration of blood products, routine screening methods have appreciably reduced transmission through this route. The risk of hepatitis B in infants born to HBV-infected mothers ranges from 10% to 85%, depending on the mother's HBV status. Infants who become infected have a 90% risk of becoming chronic carriers, and up to 25% will die of chronic liver disease as adults.[44,45]

Serologic Markers. Three well-defined antigens are associated with the virus: a core antigen, HBcAg, which is contained in the nucleocapsid; a longer polypeptide transcript with precore and core regions, designated HBeAg; and a surface antigen, HBsAg, which is found in the outer envelope of the virus. The precore region directs the HBeAg polypeptide toward the blood, whereas the HBcAg remains in the hepatocytes to direct the assembly of new virions.

The HBV antigens evoke specific antibodies: anti-HBs, anti-HBc, and anti-HBe. These antigens (HBcAg does not circulate freely in the blood) and their antibodies serve as serologic markers for following the course of the disease.[46] (see Fig. 38.10). The *HBsAg* is the viral antigen measured most routinely in blood. It appears before onset of symptoms, peaks during overt disease, and then declines to undetectable levels in 3 to 6 months. Persistence beyond 6 months indicates continued viral replication, infectivity, and risk of chronic hepatitis. HBeAg appears in the serum soon after HBsAg and signifies active viral replication. IgM anti-HBc becomes detectable shortly before the onset of symptoms, concurrent with onset of an elevation in serum transaminases. Over the months, the IgM antibody is replaced by IgG anti-HBc. Anti-HBe is detectable shortly after the disappearance of HBeAg, and its appearance signals the onset of resolution of the acute illness. IgG anti-HBs, a specific antibody to HBsAg, occurs in most people after clearance of HBsAg. The time between the removal of the HBsAg and the appearance of anti-HBs is called the *window period.* Development of anti-HBs signals recovery from HBV infection, noninfectivity, and protection from future HBV infection. Anti-HBs is the antibody present in people who have been successfully immunized against HBV.

The presence of HBV DNA in peripheral blood is a reliable marker of active HBV replication.

HBV DNA is detectable within a few days after infection. It generally increases to reach a peak at the time of acute hepatitis, before progressively decreasing and disappearing when the infection resolves spontaneously. In cases of acute viral hepatitis with equivocal HBsAg test results, testing for HBV DNA in serum may be a useful adjunct in the diagnosis of acute HBV infection, because HBV DNA can be detected approximately 21 days before HBsAg typically appears in the serum.[47] Polymerase chain reaction (PCR) tests have been developed to detect and measure the amount of HBV DNA, called the viral load, in clinical specimens. These tests are used to assess a person's infection status and to monitor treatment.[48]

Immunization. Hepatitis B vaccine provides long-term protection (up to 20 years in some cases) against HBV infection.[38] HBsAg is the antigen used for hepatitis B vaccines. Vaccines available in the United States use recombinant DNA technology to express HBsAg in yeast, which is then purified by biochemical and biophysical methods. The vaccine is available as a single-antigen formulation and also in fixed combination with other vaccines. A hepatitis B immunoglobulin (HBIG) is available.[35] Prepared from plasma donors with high concentrations of anti-HBs, it is used as an adjunct to hepatitis B vaccine for postexposure immunoprophylaxis to prevent HBV infection in high-risk populations.

The CDC recommends vaccination of all children 0 to 18 years of age as a means of preventing HBV transmission.[38] The vaccine also is recommended for all unvaccinated adults who fall into one of the following categories:

1. Those who are at high risk for infection by sexual exposure, including sex partners of HBsAg-positive people, sexually active people who are not in a long-term mutually monogamous relationship, people seeking evaluation for treatment of sexually transmitted diseases, and men who have sex with men.
2. Those who are at high risk for infection by percutaneous or mucosal exposure to blood, including current and recent injecting drug abusers, household contacts of HBsAg-positive people, residents, and staff of institutions for the developmentally disabled, health care, and public safety workers with reasonably anticipated risk for exposure to blood or blood-contaminated body fluids, and people with chronic kidney disease (predialysis, hemodialysis, peritoneal dialysis, and home dialysis people).
3. *Others*, including international travelers to regions with high or intermediate levels of endemic HBV infection, people with chronic liver disease, people with human immunodeficiency virus (HIV) infection, and all other people seeking protection from HBV infection.[35] The CDC also recommends that all pregnant women be routinely tested for HBsAg during an early prenatal visit and that infants born to HBsAg-positive mothers receive appropriate doses of HBIG and hepatitis B vaccine.[38]

HBIG may be effective for unvaccinated people who are exposed to the infection if given within 7 days of exposure. Hepatitis vaccination is recommended for preexposure and postexposure prophylaxis.

Hepatitis C

It is estimated that 143 million people (2%) of people globally are living with chronic hepatitis C.[49] About 3 to 4 million people are infected per year, and more than 350,000 people die yearly from hepatitis C-related diseases. In the United States, about 2% of people have chronic hepatitis C.[50] In 2014, an estimated 30,500 new acute hepatitis C cases occurred. After many years of decrease, the incidence of HCV infection doubled between 2010 and 2014. Before 1990, the main route of transmission of HCV was through contaminated blood transfusions or blood products. With implementation of

HCV testing in blood banks, the risk of HCV infection from blood transfusion is almost nonexistent in the United States and other developed countries.[51,52] However, unsafe medical procedures and unscreened blood transfusions may be the most important sources of HCV infections in less developed countries of the world. Currently, recreational injecting drug use is the most common mode of HCV transmission in the United States and Canada.[51,52] High-risk sexual behavior, defined as having sex with multiple sexual partners or sex with an HCV-infected partner, is currently the second most common risk factor in the United States. The rate of transmission to infants born to HCV RNA–positive mothers ranges from 4.6% to 10%.[51] HCV also can be spread through exposure in the health care setting, primarily through needle-stick injuries. There also is concern that transmission of small amounts of blood during tattooing, acupuncture, and body piercing may facilitate the transmission of HCV. Hepatitis C is the leading reason for liver transplantation, though the virus usually recurs after transplantation.[53]

HCV is a single-stranded RNA virus, with properties similar to those of the flaviviruses, a genus of the family of *Flaviviridae* that includes yellow fever and St. Louis encephalitis viruses.[54] The genome contains a single open reading frame that encodes a polyprotein of about 3000 amino acids.[54] The transcript is cleaved into single proteins, including three structural proteins (one core and two envelope proteins) and four nonstructural proteins. The virus is genetically unstable, which leads to multiple genotypes and subtypes. Six different genotypes and more than 70 subtypes of the virus have been recognized.[55] Genotype 1a and b account for the majority of infections in the United States.[56] It is likely that the wide diversity of genotypes contributes to the pathogenicity of the virus, allowing it to escape the actions of host immune mechanisms and antiviral medications, and to difficulties in developing a preventive vaccine.[54] Development of a vaccine and treatment measures has also been hampered by the lack of a reliable, reproducible, and efficient culture system for propagating the virus.[54]

Clinical Manifestations. The incubation period for HCV infection ranges from 2 to 26 weeks (average, 6 to 12 weeks). Most children and adults who acquire the infection usually are asymptomatic. Jaundice is uncommon, and only 10% of symptomatic adults have jaundice.[55] These symptoms usually last for 2 to 12 weeks. Fulminant hepatic failure is rare, and only a few cases have been reported. A minority of people who are newly infected with HCV will clear the infection, but most (80%) go on to develop chronic hepatitis.[57] Factors associated with spontaneous clearing of HCV infection appear to include younger age, female sex, and certain histocompatibility genes. The most serious consequences of chronic HCV infection are progressive liver fibrosis leading to cirrhosis, end-stage liver disease, and hepatocellular cancer. Host factors that may exacerbate the progression of liver disease include older age at onset of infection, male sex, an immunosuppressed state, concurrent HBV infection, alcohol consumption, and hepatotoxic medications.

Serologic Markers. Both antibody and viral tests are available for detecting the presence of HCV infection (Fig. 38.11). False-negative results can occur in immunocompromised people and early in the course of the disease before antibodies develop. Direct measurement of HCV in the serum remains the most accurate test for infection. The viral tests are highly sensitive and specific, but more costly than antibody tests. With newer antibody testing methods, infection often can be detected as early as 6 to 8 weeks after exposure, and as early as 1 to 2 weeks with viral tests that use polymerase chain reaction methods. Unlike hepatitis B, antibodies to HCV are not protective, but they serve as markers for the disease.[55]

Hepatitis D and E

Hepatitis D virus, of the Deltaviridae family, is the sole RNA virus of the genus.[35] Hepatitis D is an incomplete virus, in that it requires the assistance of HBV in order to replicate.[58] It can cause acute or chronic hepatitis. Infection depends on concomitant infection with HBV, specifically the presence of HBsAg.[34] Acute hepatitis D occurs in two forms: co-primary infection that occurs simultaneously with acute hepatitis B and a superinfection in which hepatitis D is imposed on chronic hepatitis B infection.[35] The delta agent often increases the severity of HBV infection. It can convert mild HBV infection into severe, fulminating hepatitis, cause acute hepatitis in asymptomatic carriers, or increase the tendency for progression to chronic hepatitis and cirrhosis.

The routes of transmission of hepatitis D are similar to those for hepatitis B. In the United States, infection is restricted largely to people at high risk for HBV infection, particularly injecting drug users. The greatest risk is in HBV carriers. These people should be informed about the dangers of HDV superinfection.

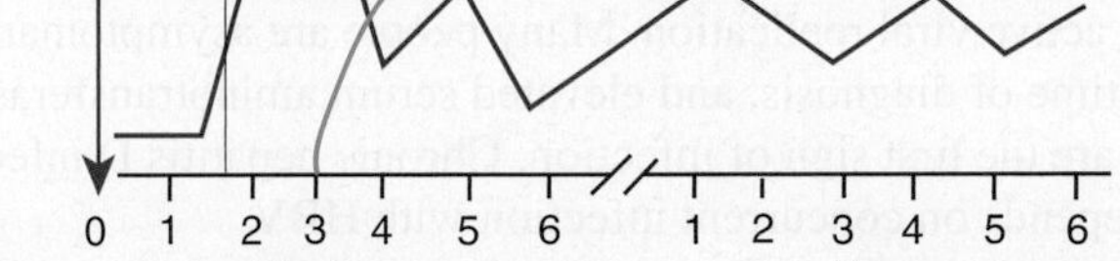

Figure 38.11 • The sequence of serologic changes in chronic hepatitis C, with persistence of HCV RNA and exacerbations and remissions of clinical symptoms indicated by changes in serum ALT levels.

Hepatitis D is diagnosed by detection of antibody to HDV (anti-HDV) in the serum or HDV RNA in the serum. There is no specific treatment for hepatitis D. Because the infection is linked to hepatitis B, prevention of hepatitis D should begin with prevention of hepatitis B through vaccination.

HEV is an unenveloped, single-stranded RNA virus. It is transmitted by the fecal–oral route and causes manifestations of acute hepatitis that are similar to hepatitis A. Genotype 3 of the virus has been linked to chronic HEV infection. Solid organ transplant recipients, HIV infection, chemotherapy, and hematologic conditions have been found with chronic forms of the disease.[59,60] Although Hepatitis E often causes an acute and self-limiting infection with low mortality rates in the western world, it bears a high risk of developing chronic hepatitis in immunocompromised people with substantial mortality rates.[61] Hepatitis E occasionally develops into an acute, severe liver disease, and is fatal in about 2% of all cases. Clinically, it is comparable to hepatitis A, but in pregnant women the disease is more often severe and is associated with a clinical syndrome called fulminant liver failure. Pregnant women, especially those in the third trimester, have an elevated mortality rate from the disease of around 20%.[62] A preventative vaccine (HEV 239) is approved for use in China.[63] Reported cases in the United States involve people who have recently been in an endemic area. People with no history of travel are very rarely affected.[64]

Chronic Viral Hepatitis

Chronic hepatitis is defined as a chronic inflammatory reaction of the liver of more than 3 to 6 months' duration. It is characterized by persistently elevated serum aminotransferase levels and characteristic histologic findings on liver biopsy. The clinical features of chronic viral hepatitis are highly variable and not predictive of outcome. The most common symptoms are fatigue, malaise, loss of appetite, and occasional bouts of jaundice. Elevation of serum aminotransferase concentrations depends on the level of disease activity.

Chronic viral hepatitis is the principal cause of chronic liver disease, cirrhosis, and hepatocellular cancer in the world and now ranks as the chief reason for liver transplantation in adults.[65] Of the hepatotropic viruses, only three are known to cause chronic hepatitis—HBV, HCV, and HDV. Hepatitis B, which is less likely than hepatitis C to progress to chronic infection, accounts for 5% to 10% of chronic liver disease and cirrhosis in the United States.[65] It is characterized by the persistence of HBV DNA and usually by HBeAg in the serum, indicating active viral replication. Many people are asymptomatic at the time of diagnosis, and elevated serum aminotransferase levels are the first sign of infection. Chronic hepatitis D infection depends on concurrent infection with HBV.

Chronic hepatitis C accounts for most cases of chronic viral hepatitis. HCV infection becomes chronic in 60% to 85% of cases.[51] Chronic HCV infection often smolders over a period of years, silently destroying liver cells. Most people with chronic hepatitis C are asymptomatic, and diagnosis usually follows a finding of elevated serum aminotransferase levels or complaints of fatigue or nonspecific weakness. Because the course of acute hepatitis C often is mild, many people do not recall the events of the acute infection.

Treatment. There are no simple and effective treatment methods for chronic viral hepatitis. Drugs used in the treatment of chronic HBV include interferons (recombinant interferon-2α and peginterferon) and the nucleotide and nucleotide analog antiretroviral agents (lamivudine, entecavir, and tenofovir).[35,65] People with active viral replication may be treated with peginterferon (pegylated interferon alfa-2a). Peginterferons have a prolonged serum half-life and are given once a week.[35] Up to 40% of treated people respond with sustained normalization of liver enzyme levels, disappearance of HBeAg and HBV DNA from the serum, appearance of anti-HBe, and improved survival.[65] Nucleoside and nucleotide analogs may be used instead of interferon for treatment of chronic HBV infection and are better tolerated. Lamivudine can be given orally and usually is well tolerated, but has a higher rate of viral resistance, a lower durable rate of response, and a greater need for prolonged therapy compared with interferon. Entecavir, another nucleoside analog, can be used in the treatment of people who are resistant to lamivudine or have cirrhosis. Tenofovir, a drug used for treatment of HIV infection, also has considerable activity against HBV. Other antiviral agents are under study, and strategies using multiple drugs are likely to be investigated. In people with concurrent hepatitis D infection, interferon therapy may lead to normalization of aminotransferase levels, histologic improvement, and elimination of HDV RNA from the serum in approximately 50% of cases, but relapse is common after the therapy is stopped.[65] Lamivudine is not effective in chronic hepatitis D.

Currently, there are 10 FDA-approved direct-acting agents marketed by 8 different companies for HCV treatment. Combining two or more agents targeting different steps in the viral replication process has proven to be the most successful strategy. Many HCV treatment regimens use sofosbuvir, a nucleotide prodrug. The activated form of sofosbuvir acts as a defective substrate for the RNA-dependent viral nonstructural protein 5B (NS5B) RNA polymerase. It is incorporated into viral RNA and terminates synthesis, resulting in disruption of viral replication. Primary therapy is administration of sofosbuvir, an NS5B polymerase inhibitor, combined with either the NS5A inhibitor velpatasvir or ledipasvir, resulting in cure rates of 95% to 100% after 12 to 24 weeks of treatment.[66] Either drug combination can be used regardless of whether the person has cirrhosis. Therefore, a person with chronic HCV without cirrhosis or with compensated cirrhosis of any HCV genotype could be treated with velpatasvir–sofosbuvir.[67] Although most people with HCV infection are candidates for treatment, many have other health problems that are contraindications to therapy.

Liver transplantation is a treatment option for end-stage liver disease because of viral hepatitis. Liver transplantation has been more successful in people with hepatitis C than those with hepatitis B. Although the graft often is reinfected, the disease seems to progress more slowly.

Autoimmune Hepatitis

Autoimmune hepatitis (AIH) is a severe type of chronic hepatitis of unknown origin that is associated with interface hepatitis, circulating autoantibodies, and hypergammaglobulinemia.[68] The worldwide prevalence of AIH is unknown; most reported cases are in people of European Caucasian or Japanese descent. The point prevalence and incidence of AIH in Northern Europeans is approximately 18 per 100,000 people per year and 1.1 per 100,000 people per year, respectively, and it is assumed that this data can be extrapolated to the North American population. Interestingly, the prevalence of AIH in Native Alaskan population is much higher, with a point prevalence of 42 per 100,000 people per year.[68,69] This form of the disease occurs in elderly people who exhibit mild necroinflammatory activity and a good response to immunosuppressive therapy. AIH, like most autoimmune disorders, is more common in female people, with a male:female ratio of roughly 1:4. It can present at any age, but younger people appear to have a more severe form of the disease.[69]

Clinical and laboratory observations have led to the hypothesis that AIH is a multifactorial disorder, with genetic and environmental factors playing important roles. Most knowledge of the genetics of the disease comes from the human leukocyte antigen (HLA) genes that reside in the major histocompatibility complex (MHC), located on the short arm of chromosome 6. In people of European descent, AIH is associated with the HLA A1-B8-DR3 haplotype and particularly with DR3. In Japan, it appears to be primarily associated with the DR4 haplotype.[69] The environmental agents assumed to induce AIH have not been delineated, but include viruses and chemical agents.

Two distinct types of AIH have been identified. Type I AIH, the most common form of the disease, is characterized by increased levels of anti–smooth muscle and antinuclear autoantibodies. Approximately 78% of cases occur in women and 38% have other autoimmune diseases.[69] Susceptibility to type I AIH resides mainly with the *HLA-DRB1* gene.[70] Type II AIH occurs mainly in children 2 to 14 years of age and is characterized by the presence of antibody to liver and kidney microsomes and liver cytosol. The disorder is often accompanied by other autoimmune disorders, especially type 1 diabetes mellitus, vitiligo, and thyroiditis.[70] The genetic component for this type of AIH is less well defined.

Clinical Manifestations

Clinical manifestations of the disorder cover a spectrum that extends from no apparent symptoms to signs of inflammatory liver disease or cirrhosis.[69] Physical examination may reveal no abnormalities, but may also reveal hepatomegaly, splenomegaly, jaundice, and signs and symptoms of chronic liver disease. In asymptomatic cases, the disorder may be discovered when abnormal serum enzyme levels are identified during performance of routine screening tests.

Diagnosis and Treatment

The differential diagnosis includes measures to exclude other causes of liver disease, including hepatitis B and C. A characteristic laboratory finding is that of a marked elevation in serum gamma globulins. A biopsy is used to confirm the diagnosis.

Corticosteroid and immunosuppressant drugs are the treatment of choice for this type of hepatitis. Although some people remain in remission after drug treatment is withdrawn, most require long-term maintenance treatment. Liver transplantation may be required for people who are refractory to or intolerant of immunosuppressive therapy and in whom end-stage liver disease develops.

Intrahepatic Biliary Disorders

Intrahepatic biliary diseases disrupt the flow of bile through the liver, causing cholestasis and biliary cirrhosis. Among the causes of intrahepatic biliary disease are primary biliary cirrhosis and secondary biliary cirrhosis.

Primary Biliary Cirrhosis

Primary biliary cirrhosis (PBC) is a chronic disease of the liver characterized by the autoimmune destruction of intralobar bile ducts causing cholestasis.[71] The disease is seen most commonly in women 40 to 60 years of age. Familial occurrences of the disease are found between parents and children and among siblings. However, unlike other autoimmune disorders, there is little, if any, association with any particular MHC alleles. In addition, with the possible exception of a reportedly higher risk of a polymorphism of the gene for the vitamin D receptor, there are no clear genetic influences for the disorder. As with other autoimmune disorders, possible environmental triggers include infectious and chemical agents.

Clinical Manifestations. The disorder is characterized by an insidious onset and progressive scarring and destruction of liver tissue. The liver becomes enlarged and takes on a green hue because of the accumulated bile. The earliest symptoms are unexplained pruritus or itching, weight loss, and fatigue, followed by dark urine and pale stools. Osteoporosis occurs in 51% of women with the disorder.[72] Jaundice is a late manifestation of the disorder, as are other signs of liver failure. Serum alkaline phosphatase levels are elevated in people with PBC.

Diagnosis and Treatment. Diagnosis of the disease occurs when the person has two of the three following signs and symptoms: destruction of bile ducts and presence of nonsuppurative cholangitis on liver biopsy, cholestasis with alkaline phosphatase elevation for at least 6 months, and presence of antimitochondrial antibodies in blood tests.[73]

Treatment is largely symptomatic. Ursodeoxycholic acid (ursodiol), the only drug approved for treating PBC, increases bile flow, decreases the toxicity of bile contents, and has been shown to decrease the rate of clinical deterioration. Cholestyramine, a bile acid–binding drug, may prove beneficial for treatment of pruritus. Colchicine, which acts to prevent leukocyte migration and phagocytosis, and methotrexate, a drug with immunosuppressive properties, have also resulted in reported benefits in terms of symptom relief. Corticosteroids have been shown to improve liver histology and serum liver function test, but involve serious long-term side effects.[74] Liver transplantation remains the only treatment for advanced disease.[74] PBC does not recur after liver transplantation if appropriate immunosuppression is used.

Secondary Biliary Cirrhosis

Secondary biliary cirrhosis results from prolonged obstruction of the extrabiliary tree. The most common cause is cholelithiasis. Other causes of secondary biliary cirrhosis are malignant neoplasms of the biliary tree or head of the pancreas and strictures of the common duct caused by previous surgical procedures. Extrahepatic biliary cirrhosis may benefit from surgical procedures designed to relieve the obstruction.

Alcohol-Induced Liver Disease

The spectrum of alcoholic liver disease includes fatty liver disease, alcoholic hepatitis, and cirrhosis. Most deaths from alcoholic cirrhosis are attributable to liver failure, bleeding esophageal varices, or kidney failure. It has been estimated that there are 14 million alcoholics in the United States. Approximately 10% of alcoholics develop cirrhosis with continued heavy drinking.[75]

Metabolism of Alcohol

Alcohol is absorbed readily from the gastrointestinal tract; it is one of the few substances that can be absorbed from the stomach. As a substance, alcohol fits somewhere between a food and a drug. It supplies calories but cannot be broken down or stored as protein, fat, or carbohydrate. As a food, the metabolism of alcohol yields 7.1 kcal/g.[76] Between 80% and 90% of the alcohol, a person drinks is metabolized by the liver. The rest is excreted through the lungs, kidneys, and skin.

Alcohol (ethyl alcohol or ethanol) metabolism proceeds simultaneously by two pathways: the alcohol dehydrogenase (ADH) system, located in the cytoplasm of the hepatocytes, and the microsomal ethanol-oxidizing system (MEOS), located in the endoplasmic reticulum.[76] The ADH and MEOS pathways produce specific metabolic and toxic disturbances. A third and minor pathway, the catalase pathway, located in the peroxisomes, can break down ethanol in unusual circumstances.[76]

The major pathway for ethanol metabolism involves ADH, an enzyme that catalyzes the conversion of alcohol to acetaldehyde. In the ADH-mediated oxidation of alcohol, both acetaldehyde and hydrogen are produced. The hydrogen (H^+) is transferred to the cofactor nicotinamide adenine dinucleotide (NAD), which is converted to its reduced form (NADH). The formed acetaldehyde again loses hydrogen and is metabolized to acetate, much of which is released in the bloodstream. As a result, ethanol metabolism generates an excess of NADH, which is thought to contribute to the liver damage that often accompanies excess alcohol consumption.

NAD is also necessary for many other metabolic processes, including the metabolism of pyruvates, urates, and fatty acids. Because alcohol competes for the use of NAD, it tends to disrupt other metabolic functions of the liver. The preferential use of NAD for alcohol metabolism can result in increased production and accumulation of lactic acid in the blood. By reducing the availability of NAD, alcohol also impairs the liver's ability to form glucose from amino acids and other glucose precursors. Alcohol-induced hypoglycemia can develop when excessive alcohol ingestion occurs during periods of depleted liver glycogen stores.

The MEOS pathway, which is located in the smooth endoplasmic reticulum, produces acetaldehyde and free radicals. Prolonged and excessive alcohol ingestion results in enzyme induction and increased activity of the MEOS. One of the most important enzymes of the MEOS, a member of the CYP P-450 system, also oxidizes a number of other compounds, including various drugs (*e.g.*, acetaminophen, isoniazid), toxins (*e.g.*, carbon tetrachloride, halothane), vitamins A and D, and carcinogenic agents (*e.g.*, aflatoxin, nitrosamines). Increased activity of this system enhances the susceptibility of people with heavy alcohol consumption to the hepatotoxic effects of other substances.

The metabolic end products of alcohol metabolism (*e.g.*, acetaldehyde, free radicals) are responsible for a variety of metabolic alterations that can cause liver injury. Acetaldehyde, for example, has multiple toxic effects on liver cells and liver function. Age and sex play a role in metabolism of alcohol and production of harmful metabolites. The ADH system is depressed by testosterone. Thus, women tend to produce greater amounts of acetaldehyde and are more predisposed to alcohol-induced liver damage than men.[76] Age also appears to affect the alcohol-metabolizing abilities of the liver and the resistance to hepatotoxic effects. Furthermore, genetic factors may influence the severity of alcohol-induced liver disease. ADH has multiple isoenzymes, the genetic polymorphism of which is now being studied in terms of possible clinical implications.[76]

Alcoholic Liver Disease

The metabolism of alcohol leads to chemical attack on certain membranes of the liver, but whether the damage is caused by acetaldehyde or other metabolites is unknown. Acetaldehyde is known to impede the mitochondrial electron transport system, which is responsible for oxidative metabolism and generation of ATP; as a result, the hydrogen ions that are generated in the mitochondria are shunted into lipid synthesis and ketogenesis.[76] Abnormal accumulations of these substances are found in hepatocytes (*i.e.*, fatty liver) and blood. Binding of acetaldehyde to other molecules impairs the detoxification of free radicals and synthesis of proteins. Acetaldehyde also promotes collagen synthesis and fibrogenesis. The lesions of hepatocellular injury tend to be most prevalent in the centrilobular area that surrounds the central vein, where the pathways for alcohol metabolism are concentrated. This is the part of the lobule that has the lowest oxygen tension; it is thought that the low oxygen concentration in this area of the liver may contribute to the damage.

The amount of alcohol required to produce chronic liver disease varies widely, depending on body size, age, sex, and ethnicity, but the high end of the range is about 80 g/day for 10 to 12 years.[77] This amount of alcohol can be in the form of 8 oz of 86 proof (41% alcohol) whiskey, two bottles of wine, or six 12-oz bottles of beer. Even after alcohol intake has stopped and all alcohol has been metabolized, the processes that damage liver cells may continue for many weeks and months. Clinical and chemical effects often become worse before the disease resolves. The accumulation of fat usually disappears within a few weeks, and cholestasis and inflammation also subside with time. However, fibrosis and scarring remain. The liver lobules become distorted as new liver cells regenerate and form nodules.

Although the mechanism by which alcohol exerts its toxic effects on liver structures is somewhat uncertain, the changes that develop can be divided into three stages: fatty liver, alcoholic hepatitis, and cirrhosis.[77]

Fatty liver is characterized by the accumulation of fat in hepatocytes, a condition called *steatosis* (Fig. 38.12). The liver becomes yellow and enlarges owing to excessive fat accumulation. The pathogenesis of fatty liver is not completely understood and can depend on the amount of alcohol consumed, dietary fat content, body stores of fat, hormonal status, and other factors. There is evidence that ingestion of large amounts of alcohol can cause fatty liver changes even with an adequate diet. The fatty changes that occur with ingestion of alcohol usually do not produce symptoms and are reversible after the alcohol intake has been discontinued.

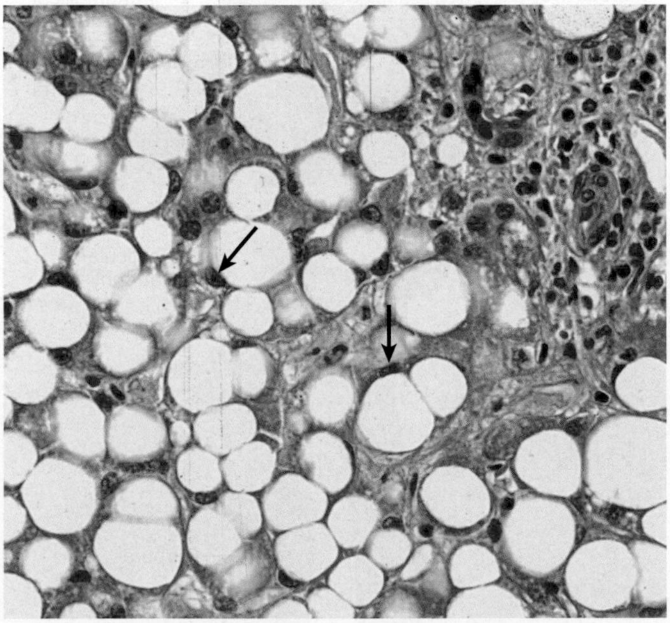

Figure 38.12 • Alcoholic fatty liver. The cytoplasm of almost all the hepatocytes to be distended by fat, which displaces the nucleus to the periphery. (From Rubin E., Strayer D. (2015). *Rubin's pathology: Clinicopathologic foundations of medicine* (7th ed., Fig. 20-34, p. 855). Philadelphia, PA: Lippincott Williams & Wilkins.)

Alcoholic hepatitis is the intermediate stage between fatty changes and cirrhosis. It often is seen after an abrupt increase in alcohol intake and is common in "spree" drinkers. Although it is a treatable form of alcoholic liver disease, there is a high rate of short- and long-term mortalities. The overall inpatient mortality was 6.6% to 6.8% for acute alcoholic hepatitis and 13.6% for chronic alcoholic hepatitis in population-based studies.[78] Alcoholic hepatitis is characterized by inflammation and necrosis of liver cells. This stage usually is characterized by hepatic tenderness, pain, anorexia, nausea, fever, jaundice, ascites, and liver failure, but some people may be asymptomatic. The condition is always serious and sometimes fatal. The immediate prognosis correlates with severity of liver cell injury. In some cases, the disease progresses rapidly to liver failure and death. In people who survive and continue to drink, the acute phase often is followed by persistent alcoholic hepatitis with progression to cirrhosis in a matter of 1 to 2 years.

Alcoholic cirrhosis is the end result of repeated bouts of drinking-related liver injury and designates the onset of end-stage alcoholic liver disease. The gross appearance of the early cirrhotic liver is one of fine, uniform nodules on its surface. The condition has traditionally been called *micronodular* or *Laennec cirrhosis*. With more advanced cirrhosis, regenerative processes cause the nodules to become larger and more irregular in size and shape. As this occurs, the nodules cause the liver to become relobulized through the formation of new portal tracts and venous outflow channels. The nodules may compress the hepatic veins, curtailing blood flow out of the liver and producing portal hypertension, extrahepatic portosystemic shunts, and cholestasis.

Nonalcoholic Fatty Liver Disease

The term *nonalcoholic fatty liver disease* (NAFLD) is caused by metabolic dysfunction that affects the liver. NAFLD is the most common liver disorder in developed countries.[79,80] In the United States, it is the most frequently occurring form of chronic liver disease.[10] The condition can range from simple steatosis (fatty infiltration of the liver) to nonalcoholic steatohepatitis (steatosis with inflammation and hepatocyte necrosis). Although steatosis alone does not appear to be progressive, approximately 10% to 25% of people with nonalcoholic steatohepatitis progress to cirrhosis.[81] Obesity, type 2 diabetes, the metabolic syndrome, and hyperlipidemia are coexisting conditions frequently associated with fatty liver disease. The condition is also associated with other nutritional abnormalities, surgical conditions, drugs, and occupational exposure to toxins. Both rapid weight loss and parenteral nutrition may lead to NAFLD. Jejunoileal bypass, a surgical procedure used for weight loss, has largely been abandoned for this reason.

Pathogenesis. The pathogenesis of NAFLD is thought to involve both lipid accumulation within hepatocytes and formation of free radicals, in a manner similar to that which occurs with alcohol metabolism. The primary metabolic abnormalities leading to lipid accumulation are poorly understood but are thought to include alterations in pathways for uptake, synthesis, degradation, or secretion of hepatic lipids resulting from insulin resistance. Obesity increases the synthesis and reduces the oxidation of free fatty acids. Type 2 diabetes or insulin resistance also increases adipose tissue lipolysis and the subsequent production of free fatty acids.[82] When the capacity of the liver to export triglyceride is exceeded, excess fatty acids contribute to the formation of fatty liver.[82] Both ketones and free fatty acids are inducers of previously described CYP P-450 enzymes of the MEOS pathway, which results in free radical formation, including hydrogen peroxide and superoxide. Abnormal lipid peroxidation ensues, followed by direct hepatocyte injury, release of toxic by-products, inflammation, and fibrosis.

Clinical Manifestations. NAFLD is usually asymptomatic, although fatigue and discomfort in the right upper quadrant of the abdomen may be present. Mildly to moderately elevated serum levels of AST, ALT, or both are the most common and often the only abnormal laboratory findings. Other abnormalities, including hypoalbuminemia, a prolonged prothrombin time, and hyperbilirubinemia, may be present in people with cirrhotic-stage liver disease. The diagnosis of NAFLD requires liver biopsy and exclusion of alcohol as a cause of the disorder.

Treatment. The aim of treatment is to slow progression of NAFLD and to prevent liver-related illness. Both weight loss and exercise improve insulin resistance and are recommended in conjunction with treatment of associated metabolic disturbances. Alcohol use should be avoided. Disease progression is slow and the magnitude of disease-related morbidity and mortality is uncertain. A recent study has shown the use of statins and antioxidants such as vitamin A and E have been effective in reducing the odds of having hepatic steatosis in people with NAFLD.[83] Liver transplantation is an alternative for some people with end-stage liver disease, but NAFLD may reoccur in up to 39% of people post liver transplantation.[84]

Cirrhosis, Portal Hypertension, and Liver Failure

Cirrhosis

Cirrhosis represents the end-stage chronic liver disease, in which much of the functional liver tissue has been replaced by fibrous tissue. Although cirrhosis usually is associated with alcoholism, it can develop in the course of other disorders, including viral hepatitis, toxic reactions to drugs and chemicals, biliary obstruction, and NAFLD. Cirrhosis also accompanies metabolic disorders that cause the deposition of minerals in the liver. Two of these disorders are hemochromatosis (*i.e.*, iron deposition) and Wilson disease (*i.e.*, copper deposition).

Cirrhosis is characterized by diffuse fibrosis and conversion of normal liver architecture into nodules containing proliferating hepatocytes encircled by fibrosis. The formation of nodules, which vary in size from very small (<3 mm, micronodules) to large (several centimeters, macronodules), represents a balance between regenerative activity and constrictive scarring.[10] The fibrous tissue that replaces normally functioning liver tissue forms constrictive bands that disrupt flow in the vascular channels and biliary duct systems of the liver. The disruption of vascular channels predisposes to portal hypertension and its complications; obstruction of biliary channels and exposure to the destructive effects of bile stasis; and loss of liver cells, leading to liver failure.

Clinical Manifestations. The manifestations of cirrhosis are variable, ranging from asymptomatic hepatomegaly to hepatic failure (Fig. 38.13). Often there are no symptoms until

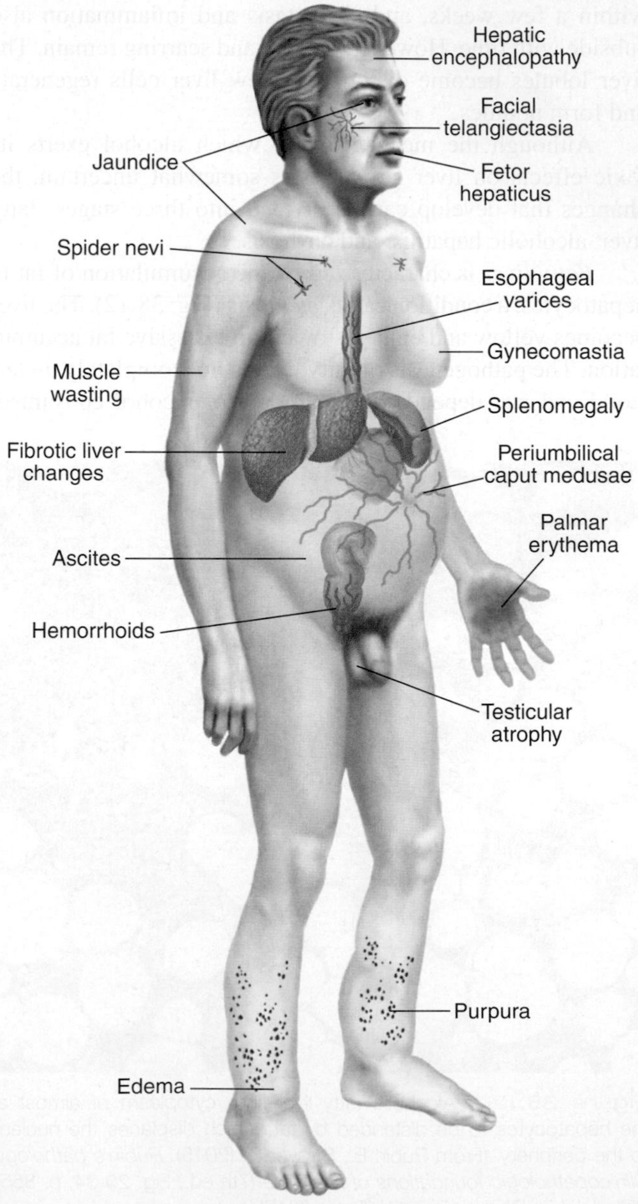

Figure 38.13 • Clinical manifestations of cirrhosis.

the disease is far advanced.[10] The most common signs and symptoms of cirrhosis are weight loss (sometimes masked by ascites), weakness, and anorexia. Diarrhea frequently is present, although some people may complain of constipation. Hepatomegaly and jaundice also are common signs of cirrhosis. There may be abdominal pain because of liver enlargement or stretching of the Glisson capsule. This pain is located in the epigastric area or in the upper right quadrant and is described as dull, aching, and causing a sensation of fullness.

The late manifestations of cirrhosis are related to portal hypertension and liver cell failure. Splenomegaly, ascites, and portosystemic shunts (*i.e.*, esophageal varices, hemorrhoids, and caput medusae) result from portal hypertension.[10] Other complications include bleeding because of decreased clotting factors, thrombocytopenia because of splenomegaly, gynecomastia and a feminizing pattern of pubic hair distribution in men because of testicular atrophy, spider angiomas, palmar erythema, and encephalopathy with asterixis and neurologic signs.

Portal Hypertension

Portal hypertension is characterized by increased resistance to flow in the portal venous system and sustained portal vein pressure. Normally, venous blood returning to the heart from the abdominal organs collects in the portal vein and travels through the liver before entering the vena cava. Portal hypertension can be caused by a variety of conditions that increase resistance to hepatic blood flow, including prehepatic, posthepatic, and intrahepatic obstructions (with *hepatic* referring to the liver lobules rather than the entire liver). Prehepatic causes of portal hypertension include portal vein thrombosis and external compression because of cancer or enlarged lymph nodes that produce obstruction of the portal vein before it enters the liver.

Posthepatic obstruction refers to any obstruction to blood flow through the hepatic veins beyond the liver lobules, either within or distal to the liver. It is caused by conditions such as thrombosis of the hepatic veins, venoocclusive disease, and severe right-sided heart failure that impede the outflow of venous blood from the liver. *Budd-Chiari syndrome* refers to congestive disease of the liver caused by occlusion of multiple hepatic veins or the hepatic portion of the inferior vena cava.[10] The principal cause of the Budd-Chiari syndrome is thrombosis of the hepatic veins, in association with diverse conditions such as polycythemia vera, hypercoagulability states associated with malignant tumors, pregnancy, bacterial infection, metastatic disease of the liver, and trauma. *Sinusoidal obstruction syndrome* or *hepatic venoocclusive disease* is a variant of the Budd-Chiari syndrome seen most commonly in people treated with certain cancer chemotherapeutic drugs, hepatic irradiation, or bone marrow transplantation.[85,86]

Intrahepatic causes of portal hypertension include conditions that cause obstruction of blood flow within the liver. In alcoholic cirrhosis, which is the major cause of portal hypertension, bands of fibrous tissue and fibrous nodules distort the architecture of the liver and increase the resistance to portal blood flow, which leads to portal hypertension.

Complications of portal hypertension arise from the increased pressure and dilation of the venous channels behind the obstruction (Fig. 38.14). In addition, collateral channels open that connect the portal circulation with the systemic circulation. The major complications of the increased portal vein pressure and the opening of collateral channels are ascites, splenomegaly, hepatic encephalopathy, and the formation of portosystemic shunts with bleeding from esophageal varices.[10]

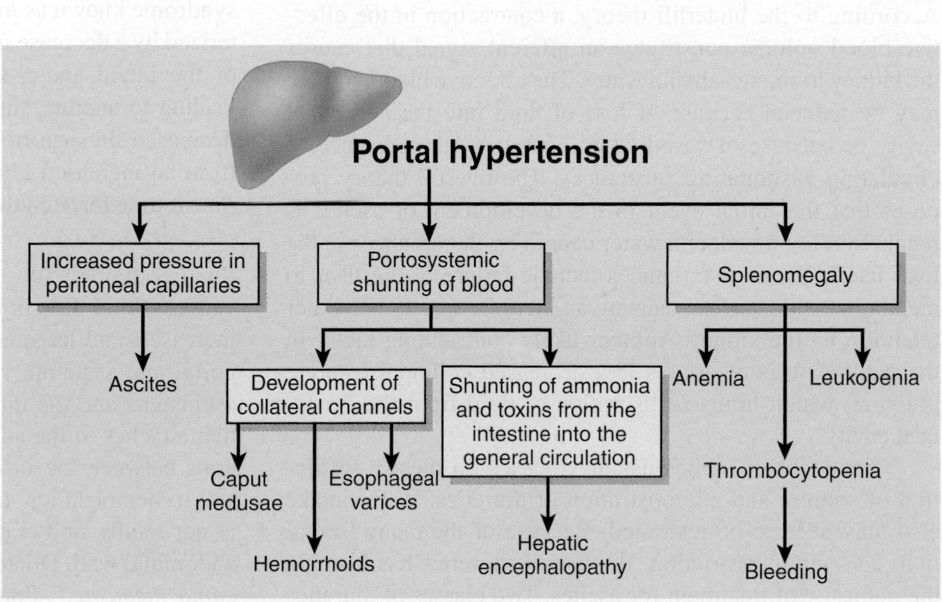

Figure 38.14 • Mechanisms of disturbed liver function related to portal hypertension.

KEY POINTS

PORTAL HYPERTENSION

- Venous blood from the gastrointestinal tract empties into the portal vein and travels through the liver before moving into the general venous circulation.
- Obstruction of blood flow in the portal vein produces an increase in the hydrostatic pressure within the peritoneal capillaries, contributing to the development of ascites, splenic engorgement with sequestration and destruction of blood cells and platelets, and shunting of blood to collateral venous channels causing varicosities of the hemorrhoidal and esophageal veins.

Ascites. Ascites occurs when the amount of fluid in the peritoneal cavity is increased and is a late-stage manifestation of cirrhosis and portal hypertension.[87] It is not uncommon for people with advanced cirrhosis to present with an accumulation of 15 L or more of ascitic fluid. These people often experience abdominal discomfort, dyspnea, and insomnia. They may also have difficulty walking or living independently.

Although the mechanisms responsible for the development of ascites are not completely understood, several factors seem to contribute to fluid accumulation, including an increase in capillary pressure because of portal hypertension and obstruction of venous flow through the liver, salt and water retention by the kidney, and decreased colloidal osmotic pressure because of impaired synthesis of albumin by the liver. Diminished blood volume (*i.e.*, underfill theory) and excessive blood volume (*i.e.*, overfill theory) have been used to explain the increased salt and water retention by the kidney. According to the underfill theory, a contraction in the effective blood volume constitutes an afferent signal that causes the kidney to retain salt and water. The effective blood volume may be reduced because of loss of fluid into the peritoneal cavity or because of vasodilation caused by the presence of circulating vasodilating substances. The overfill theory proposes that the initial event in the development of ascites is renal retention of salt and water caused by disturbances in the liver itself. These disturbances include failure of the liver to metabolize aldosterone, causing an increase in salt and water retention by the kidney. Another likely contributing factor in the pathogenesis of ascites is a decreased colloidal osmotic pressure, which limits reabsorption of fluid from the peritoneal cavity.

Treatment of ascites usually focuses on dietary restriction of sodium and administration of diuretics. Water intake also may need to be restricted. Because of the many limitations in sodium restriction, the use of diuretics has become the mainstay of treatment for ascites. Two classes of diuretics are used: a diuretic that acts in the distal part of the nephron to inhibit aldosterone-dependent sodium reabsorption and a loop diuretic such as furosemide. Oral potassium supplements often are given to prevent hypokalemia. Bed rest has traditionally been recommended for people with ascites on the basis that upright posture increases aldosterone levels, which is associated with sodium retention. Although bed rest has been shown to increase natriuresis in cirrhosis, there are no data available to support improvement in clinically relevant outcomes in ascites. Furthermore, prolonged bed rest is impractical, expensive, and difficult to enforce.[88]

Large-volume paracentesis (removal of 5 L or more of ascitic fluid) may be done in people with massive ascites and pulmonary compromise. Because the removal of fluid produces a decrease in vascular volume along with increased plasma renin activity and aldosterone-mediated sodium and water reabsorption by the kidneys, a volume expander such as albumin usually is administered to maintain the effective circulating volume.[89] A transjugular intrahepatic portosystemic shunt (TIPS) may be inserted in people with refractory ascites.[89]

Spontaneous bacterial peritonitis is a complication in people with both cirrhosis and ascites. The infection is serious and carries a high mortality rate even when treated with antibiotics. Presumably, the peritoneal fluid is seeded with bacteria from the blood or lymph or from passage of bacteria through the bowel wall. Symptoms include fever, altered mental status, and abdominal pain. Other symptoms include worsening of hepatic encephalopathy, diarrhea, hypothermia, and shock. It is diagnosed by a neutrophil count of 250/mm^3 or higher.[90]

Splenomegaly. The spleen enlarges progressively in portal hypertension because of shunting of blood into the splenic vein. The enlarged spleen often gives rise to sequestering of significant numbers of blood elements and development of a syndrome known as *hypersplenism*. Hypersplenism is characterized by a decrease in the lifespan of all the formed elements of the blood and a subsequent decrease in their numbers, leading to anemia, thrombocytopenia, and leukopenia.[90] The decreased lifespan of the blood elements is thought to result from an increased rate of removal because of the prolonged transit time through the enlarged spleen.

Portosystemic Shunts. With the gradual obstruction of venous blood flow in the liver, the pressure in the portal vein increases, and large collateral channels develop between the portal and systemic veins that supply the lower rectum and esophagus and the umbilical veins of the falciform ligament that attaches to the anterior wall of the abdomen. The collaterals between the inferior and internal iliac veins may give rise to hemorrhoids. In some people, the fetal umbilical vein is not totally obliterated; it forms a channel on the anterior abdominal wall. Dilated veins around the umbilicus are called *caput medusae*.[91] Portopulmonary shunts also may develop and cause blood to bypass the pulmonary capillaries, interfering with blood oxygenation and producing cyanosis.

Clinically, the most important collateral channels are those connecting the portal and coronary veins that lead to reversal of flow and formation of thin-walled varicosities in the submucosa of the esophagus[92] (Fig. 38.15). These thin-walled *esophageal varices* are subject to rupture, producing massive and sometimes fatal hemorrhage. Impaired hepatic synthesis of coagulation factors and decreased platelet levels (*i.e.*, thrombocytopenia) because of splenomegaly may further complicate the control of esophageal bleeding. Esophageal varices are present in nearly 30% to 40% of people with compensated cirrhosis and in 60% of those with decompensated cirrhosis. Variceal hemorrhage is perhaps the most devastating portal hypertension-related complication in people with cirrhosis, occurring in up to 30% of such people during the course of their illness. Although mortality rates of variceal hemorrhage in people with cirrhosis have been falling over the last few decades because of the implementation of effective treatments and improvements in general medical care, it still carries a mortality rate of up to 20% within 6 weeks of the bleeding episode.[92]

Treatment of portal hypertension and esophageal varices is directed at prevention of initial hemorrhage, management of acute hemorrhage, and prevention of recurrent hemorrhage. Pharmacologic therapy is used to lower portal venous pressure and prevent initial hemorrhage. β-Adrenergic–blocking drugs (*e.g.*, propranolol) commonly are used for this purpose.

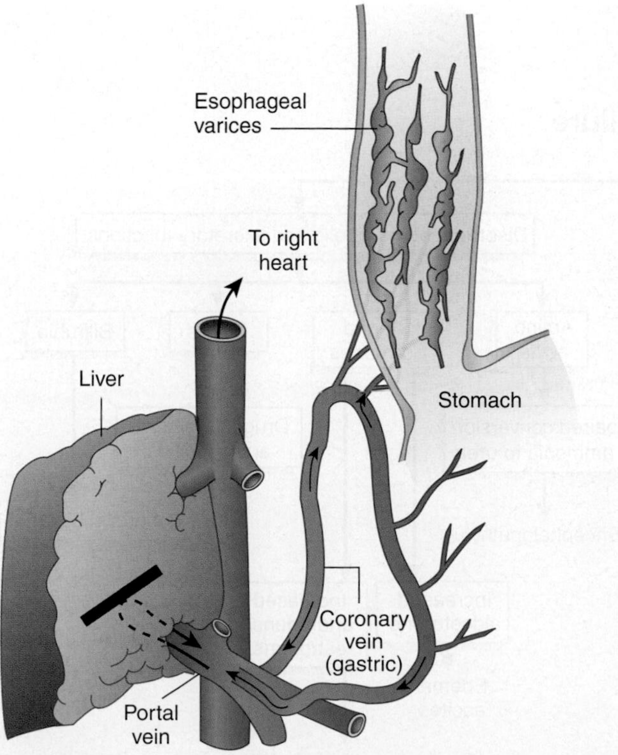

Figure 38.15 • Obstruction of blood flow in the portal circulation, with portal hypertension and diversion of blood flow to other venous channels, including the gastric and esophageal veins.

These agents reduce portal venous pressure by decreasing splanchnic blood flow and thereby decreasing blood flow in collateral channels.

Several methods are used to control acute hemorrhage, including administration of octreotide or vasopressin, balloon tamponade, endoscopic injection sclerotherapy, vessel ligation, or esophageal transection. Octreotide, a long-acting synthetic analog of somatostatin, reduces splanchnic and hepatic blood flow and portal pressures in people with cirrhosis. Vasopressin, a hormone from the posterior pituitary, is a nonselective vasoconstrictor, which can potentially produce unwanted side effects and therefore has limited the use of the drug.[93] Because octreotide has fewer side effects and appears to be more effective than vasopressin, it has become the drug of choice for pharmacologic management of acute variceal bleeding.[93] Balloon tamponade provides compression of the varices and is accomplished through the insertion of a tube with inflatable gastric and esophageal balloons. After the tube has been inserted, the balloons are inflated; the esophageal balloon compresses the bleeding esophageal veins, and the gastric balloon helps to maintain the position of the tube. During endoscopic sclerotherapy, the varices are injected with a sclerosing solution that obliterates the vessel lumen.

Prevention of recurrent hemorrhage focuses on lowering portal venous pressure and diverting blood flow away from the easily ruptured collateral channels. Two procedures may be used for this purpose: the surgical creation of a portosystemic shunt or a TIPS. *Surgical portosystemic shunt* procedures involve the creation of an opening between the portal vein and a systemic vein. These shunts have a considerable complication rate, and TIPS has evolved as the preferred treatment for refractory portal hypertension. The TIPS procedure involves insertion of an expandable metal stent between a branch of the hepatic vein and the portal vein using a catheter inserted through the internal jugular vein. A limitation of the procedure is that stenosis and thrombosis of the stent occur in most cases over time, with consequent risk of rebleeding. A complication that is associated with the creation of a portosystemic shunt is hepatic encephalopathy, which is thought to result when ammonia and other neurotoxic substances from the gut pass directly into the systemic circulation without going through the liver.

Liver Failure

The most severe clinical consequence of liver disease is hepatic failure. It may result from sudden and massive liver destruction, as in fulminant hepatitis, or be the result of progressive damage to the liver, as occurs in alcoholic cirrhosis. Whatever the cause, 80% to 90% of hepatic functional capacity must be lost before liver failure occurs.[10] In many cases, the progressive decompensating effects of the disease are hastened by intercurrent conditions such as gastrointestinal bleeding, systemic infection, electrolyte disturbances, or superimposed diseases such as heart failure.

Clinical Manifestations. The manifestations of liver failure reflect the various synthesis, storage, metabolic, and elimination functions of the liver (Fig. 38.16). *Fetor hepaticus* refers to a characteristic musty, sweetish odor of the breath in the person in advanced liver failure, resulting from the metabolic by-products of the intestinal bacteria.[10]

Hematologic Disorders. Liver failure can cause anemia, thrombocytopenia, coagulation defects, and leukopenia. Anemia may be caused by blood loss, excessive red blood cell destruction, and impaired formation of red blood cells. A folic acid deficiency may lead to severe megaloblastic anemia. Changes in the lipid composition of the red blood cell membrane increase hemolysis. Because factors II, VII, IX, and X, protein C, and protein S are synthesized by the liver, their decline in liver disease contributes to bleeding disorders.[94] Malabsorption of the fat-soluble vitamin K contributes further to the impaired synthesis of these clotting factors. Thrombocytopenia often occurs as the result of splenomegaly. The person with liver failure is subject to purpura, easy bruising, hematuria, and abnormal menstrual bleeding and is vulnerable to bleeding from the esophagus and other segments of the gastrointestinal tract.

Endocrine Disorders. The liver metabolizes the steroid hormones. Endocrine disorders, particularly disturbances in gonadal (sex hormone) function, are common accompaniments of cirrhosis and liver failure. Women may have menstrual irregularities (usually amenorrhea), loss of libido, and sterility. In men, testosterone levels usually fall; the testes atrophy; and loss of libido, impotence, and gynecomastia occur. A decrease in aldosterone metabolism may contribute to salt and water retention by the kidney, along with a lowering of serum potassium resulting from increased elimination of potassium.

Skin Disorders. Liver failure brings on numerous skin disorders. These lesions, called variously *vascular spiders, telangiectases, spider angiomas*, and *spider nevi*, are seen most often in the upper half of the body. They consist of a central pulsating arteriole from which smaller vessels radiate. Palmar erythema is redness of the palms, probably caused by increased blood flow from higher cardiac output. Clubbing of the fingers may be seen in people with cirrhosis. Jaundice usually is a late manifestation of liver failure.

Hepatorenal Syndrome. The hepatorenal syndrome refers to a functional renal failure sometimes seen during the terminal stages of liver failure when no functional causes of renal disease exist.[10] It is characterized by progressive azotemia, increased serum creatinine levels, and oliguria. Although the basic cause is unknown, a decrease in renal blood flow is believed to play a part. Ultimately, when renal failure is superimposed on liver failure, azotemia and elevated levels of blood ammonia occur; this condition is thought to contribute to hepatic encephalopathy and coma.

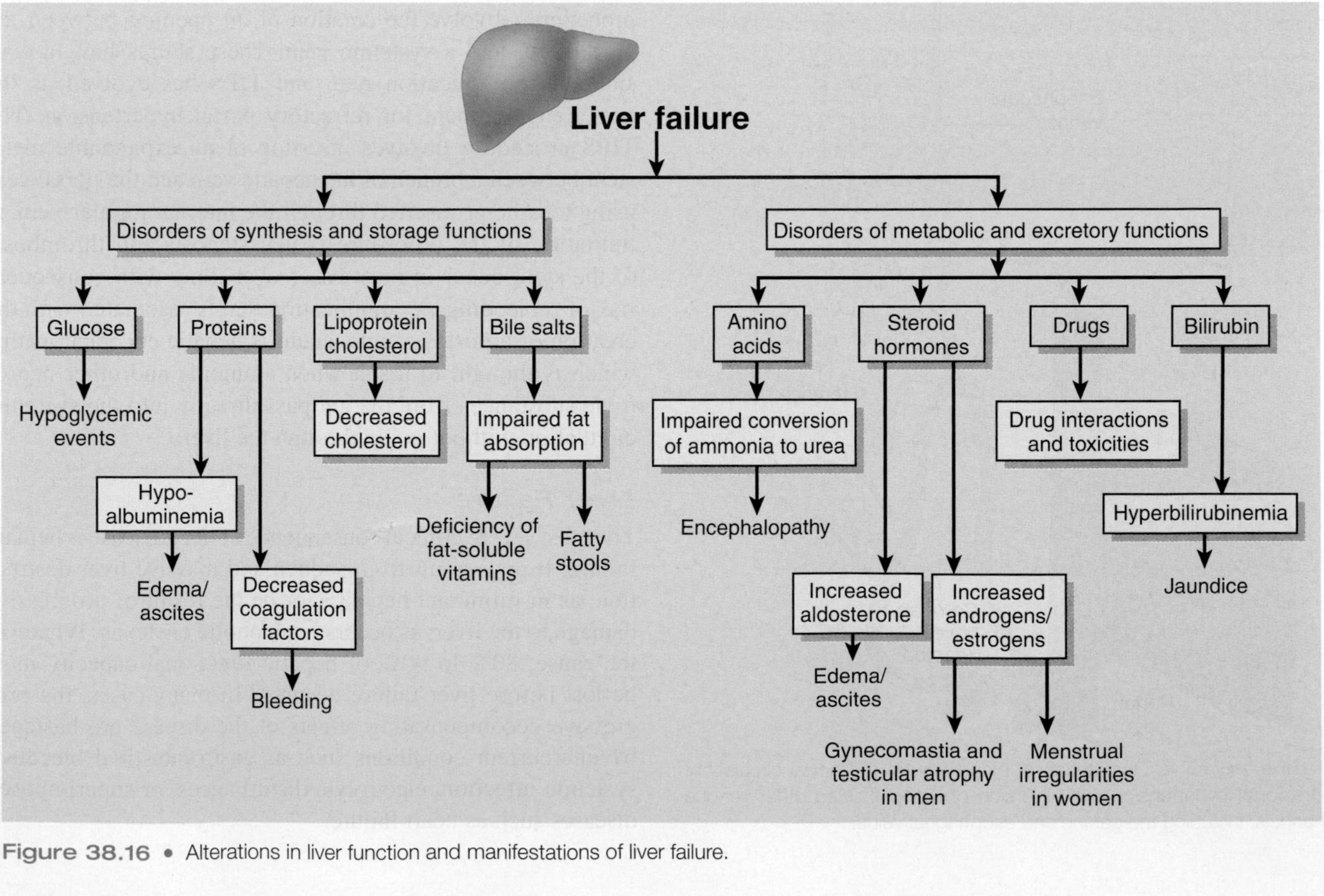

Figure 38.16 • Alterations in liver function and manifestations of liver failure.

Hepatic Encephalopathy. Hepatic encephalopathy refers to the totality of central nervous system manifestations of liver failure. It is characterized by neural disturbances ranging from a lack of mental alertness to confusion, coma, and convulsions. A very early sign of hepatic encephalopathy is a flapping tremor called asterixis. Various degrees of memory loss may occur, coupled with personality changes such as euphoria, irritability, anxiety, and lack of concern about personal appearance and self. Speech may be impaired, and the people may be unable to perform certain purposeful movements. The encephalopathy may progress to decerebrate rigidity and then to a terminal deep coma.

Although the cause of hepatic encephalopathy is unknown, the accumulation of neurotoxins, which appear in the blood because the liver has lost its detoxifying capacity, is believed to be a factor.

One of the suspected neurotoxins is ammonia. A particularly important function of the liver is the conversion of ammonia, a by-product of protein and amino acid metabolism, to urea. The ammonium ion is produced in abundance in the intestinal tract, particularly in the colon, by the bacterial degradation of luminal proteins and amino acids. Normally, these ammonium ions diffuse into the portal blood and are transported to the liver, where they are converted to urea before entering the general circulation. When the blood from the intestine bypasses the liver or the liver is unable to convert ammonia to urea, ammonia moves directly into the general circulation and from there to the cerebral circulation. Hepatic encephalopathy may become worse after a large protein meal or gastrointestinal tract bleeding. Narcotics and tranquilizers are poorly metabolized by the liver, and administration of these drugs may cause central nervous system depression and precipitate hepatic encephalopathy.

A nonabsorbable antibiotic, such as neomycin, may be given to eradicate bacteria from the bowel and thus prevent ammonia production. Another drug that may be given is lactulose. It is not absorbed from the small intestine but moves directly to the large intestine, where it is catabolized by colonic bacteria to small organic acids that cause production of large, loose stools with a low pH. The low pH favors the conversion of ammonia to ammonium ions, which are not absorbed by the blood. The acid pH also inhibits the intestinal degradation of amino acids, proteins, and blood.

Treatment. The treatment of liver failure is directed toward eliminating alcohol intake when the condition is caused by alcoholic cirrhosis; preventing infections; providing sufficient carbohydrates and calories to prevent protein breakdown; correcting fluid and electrolyte imbalances, particularly hypokalemia; and decreasing ammonia production in the gastrointestinal tract by controlling protein intake.

In many cases, liver transplantation remains the only effective treatment. Liver transplantation rapidly is becoming a realistic form of treatment for many people with irreversible chronic liver disease, fulminant liver failure, primary biliary cirrhosis, chronic active hepatitis, sclerosing cholangitis, and certain metabolic disorders that result in end-stage liver disease. In 2012, 6256 liver transplants were performed in the United States. The 5-year survival rate in 2012 for the United States was 70.5%.[95] In addition to longer survival, many liver recipients are now experiencing improved quality of life, including return to active employment. Unfortunately, the shortage of donor organs severely limits the number of transplantations that are done, and many people die each year while waiting for a transplant.[96] During 2012, 10,143 candidates were added to the liver transplant waiting list.[95] During the past several years, a number of innovative methods have been developed to deal with the shortage, including split liver transplantation, in which a cadaver liver is split into two pieces and transplanted into two recipients, and living donor transplantation, in which a segment or lobe from the liver from a living donor is resected and grafted into a recipient.[97]

Cancer of the Liver

Primary Liver Cancers

A cancer that starts in the liver is called primary liver cancer. Cancer that has spread from elsewhere to the liver, known as secondary liver cancer or liver metastasis, is more common than that which starts in the liver.[98] There are two major types of primary liver cancer: hepatocellular carcinoma, which arises from the liver cells, and cholangiocarcinoma, which is a primary cancer of bile duct cells.[10]

Hepatocellular Carcinoma. Hepatocellular carcinoma (HCC) is the most common primary liver tumor[99] and one of the most common tumors worldwide, representing 7.9% of all malignancies. Although final data are not available for 2017, an estimated 40,710 new cases of liver cancer were predicted to be diagnosed in the United States during 2017, approximately three-fourths of which would be HCC.[99] Liver cancer is largely a problem of the less developed regions, where 83% of the estimated 782,000 new cancer cases worldwide occurred in 2012. Most cases of HCC (>80%) occur in Eastern Asia and sub-Saharan Africa, with typical incidence rates of greater than 20 per 100,000 people. Southern European countries, (such as Spain, Italy, and Greece) tend to have mid-incidence levels (10.0 to 20.0 per 100,000 people), whereas North America, South America, Northern Europe, and Oceania have a low incidence of HCC (<5.0 per 100,000 people). Recent decreases in the incidence of HCC were reported among Chinese populations; the incidence in Japan is also decreasing. However, cases of HCC are increasing in low-incidence areas such as the United States and Canada.[100] Although primary tumors of the liver are relatively rare in developed countries of the world, the liver shares with the lung the distinction of being the most common site of metastatic tumors. The most common secondary tumor is a metastasis from colorectal cancer.[101]

Among the factors identified as etiologic agents in liver cancer are chronic viral hepatitis (*i.e.*, HBV, HCV, and HDV), cirrhosis, long-term exposure to environmental agents such as aflatoxin, and drinking water contaminated with arsenic.

Just how these etiologic agents contribute to the development of liver cancer is still unclear. With HBV and HCV, both of which become integrated into the host DNA, repeated cycles of cell death and regeneration afford the potential for development of cancer-producing mutations. Aflatoxins, produced by food spoilage molds, such as *Aspergillus flavus* and *Aspergillus parasiticus*, in certain areas endemic for HCC, are particularly potent carcinogenic agents.[102] They are activated by hepatocytes and their products incorporated into the host DNA with the potential for developing cancer-producing mutations. A particularly susceptible site for aflatoxin mutation is the *p53* tumor suppressor gene.[103]

Clinical Manifestations and Diagnosis. The manifestations of HCC often are insidious in onset and masked by those related to cirrhosis or chronic hepatitis. The initial symptoms include weakness, anorexia, weight loss, fatigue, abdominal swelling, a sensation of abdominal fullness, and a dull, aching abdominal pain.[103,104] Ascites, which often obscures weight loss, is common. Jaundice, if present, usually is mild. There may be a rapid increase in liver size and worsening of ascites in people with preexisting cirrhosis. Usually, the liver is enlarged when these symptoms appear. Various paraneoplastic syndromes (*e.g.*, disturbances because of ectopic hormone or growth factor production by the tumor) have been associated with hepatocellular cancer, including erythrocytosis (erythropoietin), hypoglycemia (insulin-like growth factor), and hypercalcemia (parathyroid-related protein). Serum α-fetoprotein is present during fetal life but barely detectable in the serum after the age of 2 years.[104] α-fetoprotein is often raised in HCC and is used as a tumor marker to aid diagnosis and monitor disease progression.[105] When high levels of α-fetoprotein are found in adults, it is usually indicative of HCC, although not all primary liver cancers produce α-fetoprotein. Because symptoms are often mild or absent, presentation is often late, and people are often unresectable at the time of presentation. As a result, ultrasound surveillance programs are recommended for people who are at risk of developing HCC—namely, cirrhotic people or chronic hepatitis B or C carriers.[106] Additional methods, such as ultrasonography, CT scans, and MRI, are recommended for diagnosis.[104] Liver biopsy may be used to confirm the diagnosis.

Treatment. The curative options for treatment of HCC are liver resection or liver transplantation. Radiofrequency ablation (RFA) or microwave ablation involve burning the HCC and may be curative if the lesion is very small. Primary cancers of the liver usually are far advanced at the time of diagnosis. The treatment of choice is subtotal hepatectomy, if conditions permit. Chemotherapy and radiation therapy are largely palliative. Although liver transplantation may be an option when the underlying liver disease is more advanced and the HCC size and number are high, it often is impractical because of the shortage of donor organs.

Cholangiocarcinoma. Cholangiocarcinoma, which is cancer of the bile ducts, is a relatively rare malignancy accounting for 2% of all malignancies reported worldwide. However, it is important for liver surgeons because it is the second most common primary liver malignancy.[107] Cholangiocarcinoma, with an incidence of 1.2 to 0.5 per 100,000 in North America, occurs much less frequently than HCC.[10] Other risk factors include chronic cholangitis, increasing age, and inflammatory bowel disease. The etiology, clinical features, and prognosis vary considerably with the part of the biliary tree that is the site of origin. Cholangiocarcinoma is not associated with the same risk factors as HCC. Instead, most of the risk factors revolve around long-standing inflammation and injury of the bile duct epithelium. The most common predisposing risk factor for cholangiocarcinoma is PSC. Between 5% and 10% of people with PSC develop cholangiocarcinoma.[107] Cholangiocarcinoma often presents with pain, weight loss, anorexia, and abdominal swelling or awareness of a mass in the right hypochondrium. Tumors affecting the central or distal bile ducts may present with jaundice. The only treatment option for a potential cure is surgical resection, and often a radical surgical approach is required.

Metastatic Tumors

Metastatic tumors of the liver are much more common than primary tumors. Common sources include colorectal cancer and those spread from breast, colon, lung, or urogenital cancer. In addition, tumors of neuroendocrine origin spread to the liver. It often is difficult to distinguish primary from metastatic tumors with the use of CT scans, MRI, or ultrasonography. Usually the diagnosis is confirmed by biopsy.

IN SUMMARY

The liver is subject to most of the disease processes that affect other body structures, such as vascular disorders, inflammation, metabolic diseases, toxic injury, and neoplasms. As the major drug-metabolizing and detoxifying organ in the body, the liver is subject to potential damage from the enormous array of pharmaceutical and environmental chemicals. Drugs and chemicals can exert their effects by causing hepatocyte injury and death or by cholestatic liver damage because of injury of biliary drainage structures. Drug reactions can be predictable based on the drug's chemical structure and metabolites or unpredictable (idiosyncratic) based on individual characteristics of the person receiving the drug. Early identification of drug-induced liver disease is important because withdrawal of the drug is curative in most cases.

Hepatitis is characterized by inflammation of the liver. Acute viral hepatitis is caused by hepatitis viruses A, B, C, D, and E. Although all these viruses cause acute hepatitis, they differ in terms of mode of transmission, incubation period, mechanism, degree and chronicity of liver damage, and the ability to evolve to a carrier state. HBV, HCV, and HDV infections have the potential for progression to the carrier state, chronic hepatitis, and HCC.

Intrahepatic biliary diseases disrupt the flow of bile through the liver, causing cholestasis and biliary cirrhosis.

Among the causes of intrahepatic biliary diseases are PBC, PSC, and secondary biliary cirrhosis. Because alcohol competes for use of intracellular cofactors normally needed by the liver for other metabolic processes, it tends to disrupt the metabolic functions of the liver. The spectrum of alcoholic liver disease includes fatty liver disease, alcoholic hepatitis, and cirrhosis.

Cirrhosis represents the end-stage chronic liver disease in which much of the functional liver tissue has been replaced by fibrous tissue. The fibrous tissue replaces normally functioning liver tissue and forms constrictive bands that disrupt flow in the vascular channels and biliary duct systems of the liver. The disruption of vascular channels predisposes to portal hypertension and its complications, loss of liver cells, and eventual liver failure. Portal hypertension is characterized by increased resistance to flow and increased pressure in the portal venous system; the pathologic consequences of the disorder include ascites, the formation of collateral bypass channels (*e.g.*, esophageal varices) from the portosystemic circulation, and splenomegaly. Liver failure represents the end stage of a number of liver diseases and occurs when less than 10% to 20% of liver tissue is functional. The manifestations of liver failure reflect the various functions of the liver, including hematologic disorders, disruption of endocrine function, skin disorders, hepatorenal syndrome, and hepatic encephalopathy.

There are two types of primary cancers of the liver: hepatocellular (the most common form, derived from hepatocytes and their precursors) and cholangiocarcinoma (bile duct cancer, arising from biliary epithelium). HCC, which is associated with HBV and HCV hepatitis, alcoholic cirrhosis, and food contaminants (*e.g.*, aflatoxins), is the fifth most common cancer and third leading cause of cancer-related mortality worldwide. Cholangiocarcinoma occurs primarily in older adults with a history of chronic disorders of the bile ducts. Although primary tumors of the liver are relatively rare in developed countries of the world, the liver shares with the lung the distinction of being the most common site of metastatic tumors.

DISORDERS OF THE GALLBLADDER AND EXOCRINE PANCREAS

After completing this section of the chapter, the learner will be able to meet the following objectives:

- Explain the function of the gallbladder in regulating the flow of bile into the duodenum and relate to the formation of cholelithiasis (gallstones).
- Describe the clinical manifestations of acute and chronic cholecystitis.
- Cite the possible causes and describe the manifestations and treatment of acute and chronic pancreatitis.

Disorders of the Gallbladder and Extrahepatic Bile Ducts

The hepatobiliary system consists of the gallbladder; the left and right hepatic ducts, which come together to form the common hepatic duct; the cystic duct, which extends to the gallbladder; and the common bile duct, which is formed by the union of the common hepatic duct and the cystic duct (Fig. 38.17). The common bile duct descends posteriorly to the first part of the duodenum, where it comes in contact with the main pancreatic duct. These ducts unite to form the hepatopancreatic ampulla. The circular muscle around the distal end of the bile duct is thickened to form the sphincter of the bile duct.

The gallbladder is a distensible, pear-shaped muscular sac located on the ventral surface of the liver. It has an outer serous peritoneal layer, a middle smooth muscle layer, and an inner mucosal layer that is continuous with the linings of the bile duct. The function of the gallbladder is to store and concentrate bile. Bile contains bile salts, cholesterol, bilirubin, lecithin, fatty acids, and water and the electrolytes normally found in the plasma. The cholesterol found in bile has no known function. It is assumed to be a by-product of bile salt formation, and its presence is linked to the excretory function of bile.[108] Normally insoluble in water, cholesterol is rendered soluble by the action of bile salts and lecithin, which combine with it to form micelles. In the gallbladder, water and electrolytes are absorbed from the liver bile, causing the bile to become more concentrated. Because neither lecithin nor bile salts are absorbed in the gallbladder, their concentration increases along with that of cholesterol; in this way, the solubility of cholesterol is maintained.

Entrance of food into the intestine causes the gallbladder to contract and the sphincter of the bile duct to relax, such that bile stored in the gallbladder moves into the duodenum. The stimulus for gallbladder contraction is primarily hormonal. Products of food digestion, particularly lipids, stimulate the release of a gastrointestinal hormone called *cholecystokinin* from the mucosa of the duodenum. Cholecystokinin provides a strong stimulus for gallbladder contraction. The role of other gastrointestinal hormones in bile release is less clearly understood.

Pressure in the common duct largely is responsible for regulating passage of bile into the intestine. Normally, the gallbladder regulates this pressure. It collects and stores bile as it relaxes and the pressure in the common bile duct decreases, and it empties bile into the intestine as the gallbladder contracts, producing an increase in common duct pressure. After gallbladder surgery, the pressure in the common duct changes, causing the common duct to dilate. The sphincters in the common duct then regulate the flow of bile.

Two common disorders of the biliary system are cholelithiasis (*i.e.*, gallstones) and inflammation of the gallbladder (cholecystitis) or common bile duct (cholangitis). In adult Western populations, 15% of people have gallstones.[109] In both circumstances, hypersecretion of biliary cholesterol appears to play a major role.

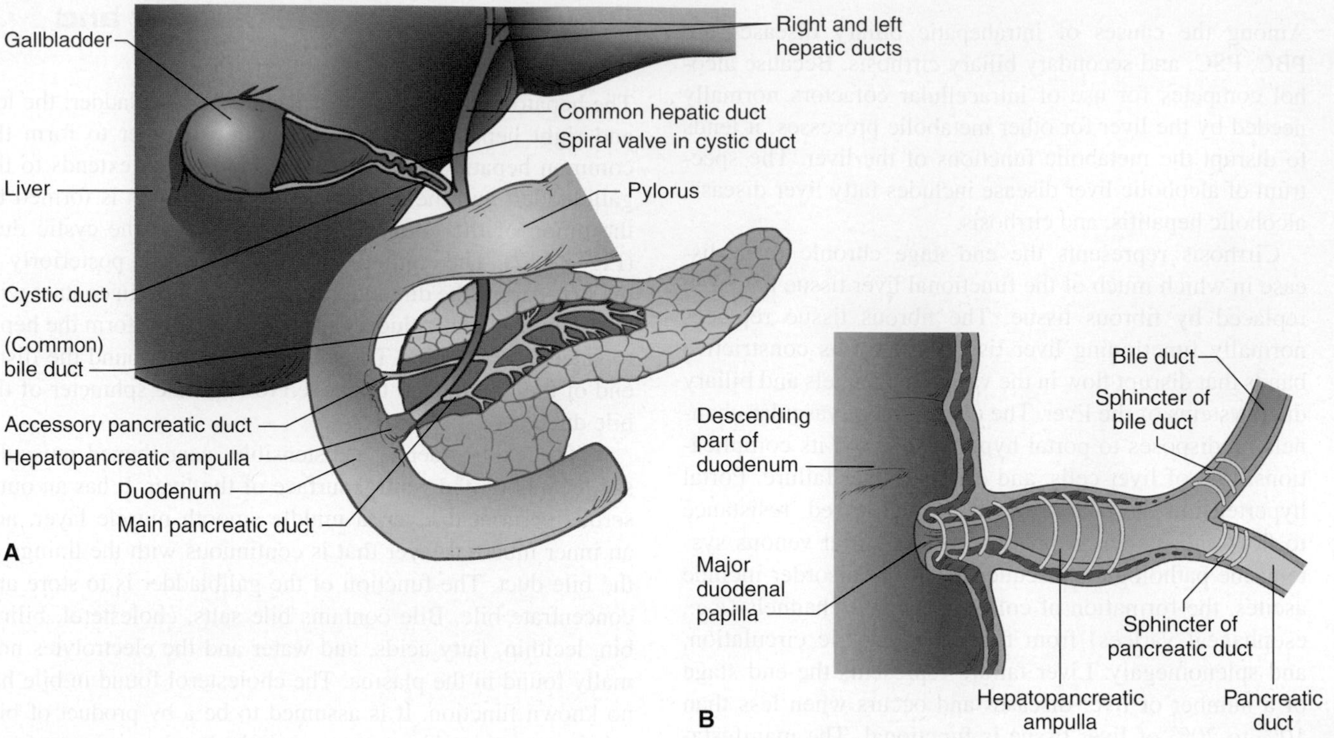

Figure 38.17 • **(A)** Extrahepatic bile passages, gallbladder, and pancreatic ducts. **(B)** Entry of bile duct and pancreatic duct into the hepatopancreatic ampulla, which opens into the duodenum.

Cholelithiasis

Cholelithiasis or gallstones is caused by precipitation of substances contained in bile, mainly cholesterol and bilirubin. Approximately 80% of gallstones are composed primarily of cholesterol; the other 20% are black or brown pigment stones composed of mucin glycoproteins and calcium salts.[110] Many stones have a mixed composition. Figure 38.18 shows a gallbladder with numerous cholesterol gallstones.

Two primary factors contribute to the formation of gallstones: abnormalities in the composition of bile (particularly increased cholesterol) and the stasis of bile.[110] The formation of cholesterol stones is associated with obesity and occurs more frequently in women, especially women who have had multiple pregnancies or who are taking oral contraceptives. All of these factors cause the liver to excrete more cholesterol into the bile. Estrogen reduces the synthesis of bile acid in women. Gallbladder sludge (thickened gallbladder mucoprotein with tiny trapped cholesterol crystals) is thought to be a precursor of gallstones. Sludge frequently occurs with pregnancy, starvation, and rapid weight loss. Drugs that lower serum cholesterol levels, such as clofibrate, also cause increased cholesterol excretion into the bile. Malabsorption disorders stemming from ileal disease or intestinal bypass surgery, for example, tend to interfere with the absorption of bile salts, which are needed to maintain the solubility of cholesterol. Inflammation of the gallbladder alters the absorptive characteristics of the mucosal layer, allowing excessive absorption of water and bile salts. Cholesterol gallstones are extremely common among Native Americans and Chilean Indians and Chilean Hispanics, which suggests that a genetic component may have a role in gallstone formation.[111] Pigment stones containing bilirubin are seen in people with hemolytic disease (*e.g.*, sickle cell disease) and hepatic cirrhosis.

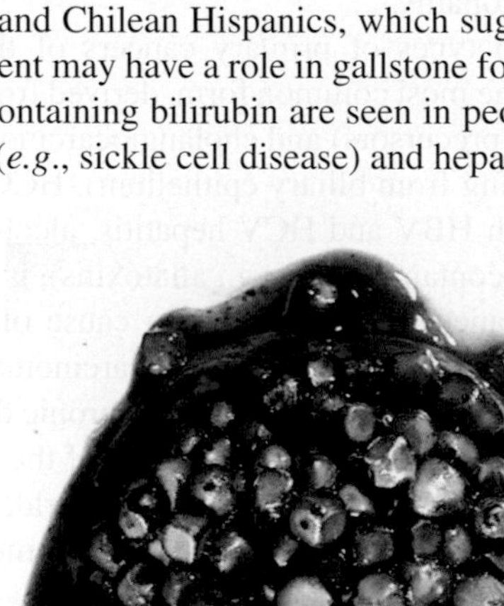

Figure 38.18 • Cholesterol gallstones. The gallbladder has been opened to reveal numerous yellow cholesterol gallstones. (From Rubin R., Strayer D. (2015). *Rubin's pathology: Clinicopathologic foundations of medicine* (7th ed., Fig. 20-71, p. 881). Philadelphia, PA: Lippincott Williams & Wilkins.)

Clinical Manifestations. Many people with gallstones have no symptoms. Gallstones cause symptoms when they obstruct bile flow or cause inflammation.[110] Small stones (*i.e.*, <8 mm in diameter) pass into the common duct, producing symptoms of indigestion and biliary colic. Larger stones are more likely to obstruct flow and cause jaundice. The pain of biliary colic is usually located in the upper right quadrant or epigastric area and may be referred to the upper back, the right shoulder, or midscapular region. Typically the pain is abrupt in onset, increases steadily in intensity, persists for 30 minutes to 5 hours, and is followed by soreness in the upper right quadrant.

Acute and Chronic Cholecystitis

Acute cholecystitis is a diffuse inflammation of the gallbladder, usually secondary to obstruction of the gallbladder outlet. Most cases of acute cholecystitis (85% to 90%) are associated with the presence of gallstones (calculous cholecystitis).[111] The remaining cases (acalculous cholecystitis) are associated with sepsis, severe trauma, or infection of the gallbladder. It has been theorized that obstruction of the cystic duct by a gallstone leads to the release of phospholipase from the epithelium of the gallbladder. In turn, this enzyme may hydrolyze lecithin and release lysolecithin, a membrane-active toxin.[111] At the same time, disruption of the normally protective mucous lining of the epithelium renders the mucosal cells vulnerable to damage by the detergent action of concentrated bile salts. Acute acalculous cholecystitis occurs with no apparent cause in 50% of cases, trauma, burns, biliary sludge and vasculitis have been possible causative factors.[110] Acute acalculous cholecystitis can rapidly progress to gangrene and perforation because the process appears to involve a transmural infarction, rather than inflammatory changes associated with stones.

Chronic cholecystitis results from repeated episodes of acute cholecystitis or chronic irritation of the gallbladder by stones. It is characterized by varying degrees of chronic inflammation. Gallstones almost always are present. Cholelithiasis with chronic cholecystitis may be associated with acute exacerbations of gallbladder inflammation, common duct stone, pancreatitis, and, rarely, carcinoma of the gallbladder.

Clinical Manifestations. People with acute cholecystitis usually experience an acute onset of upper right quadrant or epigastric pain, frequently associated with mild fever, anorexia, nausea, and vomiting. Whereas in biliary colic the cystic duct obstruction is transient, in acute cholecystitis it is persistent. People with calculous cholecystitis usually, but not always, have experienced previous episodes of biliary pain. The pain may appear with remarkable suddenness and constitute a surgical emergency. In the absence of medical attention, the attack usually subsides in 7 to 10 days. In people who recover, recurrence is common. The onset of acalculous cholecystitis tends to be more insidious because the manifestations are obscured by the underlying conditions precipitating the attack. In the severely ill person, early recognition is crucial because a delay in treatment can prove life threatening. People with acute cholecystitis usually have an elevated white blood cell count, and many have mild elevations in AST, ALT, alkaline phosphatase, and bilirubin.

The manifestations of chronic cholecystitis are more vague than those of acute cholecystitis. There may be intolerance to fatty foods, belching, and other indications of discomfort. Often, there are episodes of colicky pain with obstruction of biliary flow caused by gallstones. The gallbladder, which in chronic cholecystitis usually contains stones, may be enlarged, shrunken, or of normal size.

Diagnosis and Treatment. The methods used to diagnose gallbladder disease include ultrasonography, cholescintigraphy (nuclear scanning), and CT scans.[111] Ultrasonography is widely used in diagnosing gallbladder disease and has largely replaced the oral cholecystogram in most medical centers. It can detect stones as small as 1 to 2 cm, and its overall accuracy in detecting gallbladder disease is high. In addition to stones, ultrasonography can detect wall thickening, which indicates inflammation. It also can rule out other causes of right upper quadrant pain such as tumors. Cholescintigraphy, also called a *gallbladder scan*, relies on the ability of the liver to extract a rapidly injected radionuclide, technetium-99m, bound to one of several iminodiacetic acids, that is excreted into the bile ducts. Serial scanning images are obtained within several minutes of the injection of the tracer and every 10 to 15 minutes during the next hour. The gallbladder scan is highly accurate in detecting acute cholecystitis. Although CT is not as accurate as ultrasonography in detecting gallstones, it can show thickening of the gallbladder wall or pericholecystic fluid associated with acute cholecystitis.

Gallbladder disease usually is treated by removing the gallbladder. The gallbladder stores and concentrates bile, and its removal usually does not interfere with digestion. Laparoscopic cholecystectomy has become the treatment of choice for symptomatic gallbladder disease.[112] The procedure involves insertion of a laparoscope through a small incision near the umbilicus, and surgical instruments are inserted through several stab wounds in the upper abdomen. Although the procedure requires more time than the older open surgical procedure, it usually requires only one night in the hospital. A major advantage of the procedure is that people can return to work in 1 to 2 weeks, compared with 4 to 6 weeks after open cholecystectomy.

Choledocholithiasis and Cholangitis

Choledocholithiasis refers to stones in the common duct and *cholangitis* to inflammation of the common duct. Common duct stones usually originate in the gallbladder, but can form spontaneously in the common duct.

Clinical Manifestations. The manifestations of choledocholithiasis are similar to those of gallstones and acute cholecystitis. There is a history of acute biliary colic and right upper abdominal pain, with chills, fever, and jaundice associated with episodes of abdominal pain. Bilirubinuria and an elevated serum bilirubin are present if the common duct is obstructed. Complications include acute suppurative cholangitis accompanied by purulent fluid in the common duct. It is characterized by the presence of an altered sensorium, lethargy, and septic shock.[10] Acute suppurative cholangitis represents an endoscopic or surgical emergency. Common duct stones also can obstruct the outflow of the pancreatic duct, causing a secondary pancreatitis.

Diagnosis and Treatment. Ultrasonography, CT scans, and radionuclide imaging may be used to demonstrate dilation of bile ducts and impaired blood flow. Endoscopic ultrasonography and magnetic resonance cholangiography are used for detecting common duct stones. Both percutaneous transhepatic cholangiography (PTC) and endoscopic retrograde cholangiopancreatography (ERCP) provide a direct means for determining the cause, location, and extent of obstruction. PTC involves the injection of dye directly into the biliary tree. It requires the insertion of a thin, flexible needle through a small incision in the skin with advancement into the biliary tree. ERCP involves the passage of an endoscope into the duodenum and the passage of a catheter into the hepatopancreatic ampulla. ERCP can be used to enlarge the opening of the sphincter of the hepatopancreatic ampulla, which may allow the lodged stone to pass, or an instrument may be inserted into the common duct to remove the stone.

Common duct stones in people with cholelithiasis usually are treated by stone extraction followed by laparoscopic cholecystectomy. Antibiotic therapy, with an agent that penetrates the bile, is used to treat the infection. Emergency decompression of the common duct, usually by ERCP, may be necessary for people who are septic or fail to improve with antibiotic treatment.

Cancer of the Gallbladder

Gallbladder cancers (GBC) are cancers arising from the gallbladder mucosa. The incidence of GBC in the United States is 1 to 2 per 100,000. The incidence of GBC increases with age, with the greatest incidence in people aged 65 or older. GBC affects women three to four times more often than men, and is more common in Caucasians than in African Americans. Risk factors for GBC include genetic characteristics, gallstone disease, bile composition, calcification of the gallbladder wall, congenital biliary cysts or ductal anatomy, some infections, environmental carcinogens, and drugs. People with gallbladder cancer are often asymptomatic, and the diagnosis may be made at the time of imaging or cholecystectomy for other indications. When symptoms are present, they are nonspecific.[113] The onset of symptoms usually is insidious, and they resemble those of cholecystitis. The diagnosis often is made unexpectedly at the time of gallbladder surgery. About 70% to 80% of people with gallbladder cancer have cholelithiasis.[114] Because of its ability to produce chronic irritation of the gallbladder mucosa, it is believed that cholelithiasis plays a role in the development of gallbladder cancer. Gallbladder cancer is generally considered to confer a poor prognosis because this tumor typically remains dormant until an advanced and often noncurative stage. Historically gallbladder cancer had an overall 5-year survival rate of less than 5%.[115] Five-year survival rates are 80% in stage 0 disease, 50% in stage I, 28% in stage II, 7% to 8% in stage III, and 2% to 4% in stage IV.[116]

Disorders of the Exocrine Pancreas

The pancreas lies transversely in the posterior part of the upper abdomen (see Fig. 38.1). The head of the pancreas is at the right of the abdomen; it rests against the curve of the duodenum in the area of the hepatopancreatic ampulla and its entrance into the duodenum. The body of the pancreas lies beneath the stomach. The tail touches the spleen. The pancreas is virtually hidden because of its posterior position; unlike many other organs, it cannot be palpated. Because of the position of the pancreas and its large functional reserve, symptoms from conditions such as cancer of the pancreas do not usually appear until the disorder is far advanced.

The pancreas is both an endocrine and exocrine organ. The exocrine pancreas is made up of lobules that consist of acinar cells, which secrete digestive enzymes into a system of microscopic ducts. These ducts empty into the main pancreatic duct, which extends from left to right through the substance of the pancreas. The main pancreatic duct and the bile duct unite to the form hepatopancreatic ampulla, which empties into the duodenum. The sphincter of the pancreatic duct controls the flow of pancreatic secretions into duodenum (see Fig. 38.17).

The pancreatic secretions contain proteolytic enzymes that break down dietary proteins, including trypsin, chymotrypsin, carboxypolypeptidase, ribonuclease, and deoxyribonuclease. The pancreas also secretes pancreatic amylase, which breaks down starch, and lipases, which hydrolyze neutral fats into glycerol and fatty acids. The pancreatic enzymes are secreted in the inactive form and become activated in the intestine.[117] This is important because the enzymes would digest the tissue of the pancreas itself if they were secreted in the active form. The acinar cells secrete a trypsin inhibitor, which prevents trypsin activation. Because trypsin activates other proteolytic enzymes, the trypsin inhibitor prevents subsequent activation of the other enzymes.

Two types of pancreatic disease are discussed in this chapter: acute and chronic pancreatitis and cancer of the pancreas.

Acute Pancreatitis

Acute pancreatitis represents a reversible inflammatory process of the pancreatic acini brought about by premature activation of pancreatic enzymes.[118,119] Although the disease process may be limited to pancreatic tissue, it also can involve peripancreatic tissues or those of more distant organs. In the United States, up to 220,000 people are admitted to the hospital each year with acute pancreatitis.[119] Acute pancreatitis is best defined clinically by a people presenting with two of the following three criteria[120,121]: (1) symptoms (e.g., epigastric pain) consistent with pancreatitis, (2) a serum amylase or lipase level greater than three times the laboratory's upper limit of normal, and (3) radiologic imaging consistent with pancreatitis, usually using CT or MRI.

The pathogenesis of acute pancreatitis involves the autodigestion of pancreatic tissue by inappropriately activated pancreatic enzymes. The process is thought to begin with the activation of trypsin. Once activated, trypsin can then activate a variety of digestive enzymes that cause pancreatic injury, resulting in an intense inflammatory response. The acute inflammatory response itself causes substantial tissue damage and may progress beyond the pancreas to produce a systemic inflammatory response syndrome and multiorgan failure.[119] Although a number of factors are associated with the development of acute pancreatitis, most cases result from gallstones (stones in the common duct) or alcohol abuse.[119] In the case of biliary tract obstruction because of gallstones, pancreatic duct obstruction or biliary reflux is believed to activate the enzymes in the pancreatic duct system. The precise mechanisms whereby alcohol exerts its action are largely unknown. The capacity for oxidative and nonoxidative metabolism of ethanol by the pancreas and the harmful by-products that result have been related to the disease process.[119] A study, looking at specifically beer, has shown that pancreatic secretions may be stimulated by the nonalcoholic ingredients in the beverage.[122] Acute pancreatitis also is associated with hyperlipidemia, hypercalcemia, infections (particularly viral), abdominal and surgical trauma, and drugs such as thiazide diuretics.[119]

Clinical Manifestations. The manifestations of acute pancreatitis can range from mild with minimal organ dysfunction to severe and life threatening. Overall, about 20% of people with acute pancreatitis have a severe course.[123] Abdominal pain is a cardinal manifestation of acute pancreatitis. The pain is usually located in the epigastric or periumbilical region and may radiate to the back, chest, or flank areas. Physical examination findings are variable and include fever, tachycardia, hypotension, severe abdominal tenderness, respiratory distress, and abdominal distention. Recognized markers of severe disease include laboratory values that measure the inflammatory response (*e.g.*, C-reactive protein), scoring systems that assess inflammation or organ failure, and findings on imaging studies. Clinical findings such as thirst, poor urine output, progressive tachycardia, tachypnea, hypoxemia, agitation, confusion, a rising hematocrit level, and lack of improvement in symptoms within the first 48 hours are warning signs of impending severe disease. Complications include the systemic inflammatory response, acute respiratory distress syndrome, acute tubular necrosis, and organ failure. An important disturbance related to acute pancreatitis is the loss of a large volume of fluid into the retroperitoneal and peripancreatic spaces and the abdominal cavity.

Diagnosis and Treatment. The diagnosis of acute pancreatitis requires two of the following three features: (1) abdominal pain characteristic of acute pancreatitis; (2) serum amylase and/or lipase three or more times the upper limit of normal; and (3) characteristic findings of acute pancreatitis on transabdominal ultrasound, contrast-enhanced computed tomography (CT) scan, or magnetic resonance imaging (MRI). This definition allows for the possibility that an amylase and/or lipase might be less than three times the upper limit of normal in acute pancreatitis. In a person with abdominal pain characteristic of acute pancreatitis and serum enzyme levels that are lower than three times the upper limit of normal, a CT scan must be performed to confirm a diagnosis of acute pancreatitis.

Once the diagnosis of acute pancreatitis is established, people are classified based on disease severity. The Atlanta Criteria revision of 2012[121] classifies severity as mild, moderately severe, or severe. Mild acute pancreatitis, the most common form, has no organ failure, no local or systemic complications, and usually resolves in the first week. Moderately severe acute pancreatitis is defined by the presence of transient organ failure (lasting <48 hours) and/or local complications. Severe acute pancreatitis is defined by persistent organ failure (lasting >48 hours). Local complications include peripancreatic fluid collections, pancreatic and peripancreatic necrosis (sterile or infected), pseudocyst, and walled-off necrosis (sterile or infected). The white blood cell count may be increased, and hyperglycemia and an elevated serum bilirubin level may be present. Determination of the cause is important in guiding the immediate management and preventing recurrence. Abdominal ultrasonography is usually performed to assess for gallstones. CT scans and dynamic contrast-enhanced CT of the pancreas are used to detect necrosis and fluid accumulation. Recent research has focused on potential biomarkers for predicting the severity and prognosis of pancreatitis. One study has examined trypsinogen-2 and pancreatic proteases, enzymes involved in the autodigestive processes.[124] Other investigational serologic markers include tumor necrosis factor, C-reactive protein, procalcitonin, phospholipase A_2, and the cytokines interleukin-6 (IL-6), IL-8, and IL-10.[125]

Treatment measures depend on the severity of the disease. People who present with persistent or severe pain, vomiting, dehydration, or signs of impending severe acute pancreatitis require hospitalization. Treatment measures are directed at pain relief, "putting the pancreas to rest" by withholding oral foods and fluids, and restoration of lost plasma volume. Meperidine rather than morphine usually is given for pain relief because it causes fewer spasms of the sphincter of the pancreatic duct. Gastric suction is instituted to treat distention of the bowel and prevent further stimulation of the secretion of pancreatic enzymes. Intravenous fluids and electrolytes are administered to replace those lost from the circulation and to combat hypotension and shock. Intravenous colloid solutions are given to replace the fluid that has become sequestered in the abdomen and retroperitoneal space.

Complications. Sequelae in people surviving an episode of severe acute pancreatitis include fluid collections and infection.[123] In people with acute necrotizing pancreatitis, the necrotic debris becomes infected, usually by gram-negative organisms from the alimentary canal, further complicating the condition.[126] Fluid collections with a high level of pancreatic enzymes are usually associated with pancreatic duct disruptions and may eventually form pseudocysts (a collection of pancreatic fluid enclosed in a layer of inflammatory tissue). A pseudocyst most often is connected to a pancreatic duct, so that it continues to increase in mass. The symptoms depend on its location; for example, jaundice may occur when a cyst develops near the head of the pancreas, close to the common duct. Pseudocysts may resolve or, if they persist, may require surgical intervention.

Chronic Pancreatitis

Chronic pancreatitis is characterized by progressive destruction of the exocrine pancreas, by fibrosis, and, in the later stages, by destruction of the endocrine pancreas. Most factors that cause acute pancreatitis can also cause chronic pancreatitis. However, the chief distinction between the two conditions is the irreversibility of pancreatic function that is characteristic of chronic pancreatitis.[127] By far the most common cause of chronic pancreatitis in Western countries is long-term alcohol abuse.[123] Less common causes are long-standing obstruction of the pancreatic duct by pseudocysts, calculi, or neoplasms; autoimmune chronic pancreatitis, which occurs in association with autoimmune disorders such as Sjögren syndrome, PSC, and inflammatory bowel disease; idiopathic chronic pancreatitis, associated with cystic fibrosis; and hereditary pancreatitis, a rare autosomal dominant disorder that is associated with both acute and chronic pancreatitis.

Clinical Manifestations. Chronic pancreatitis is manifested in episodes that are similar, albeit of lesser severity, to those of acute pancreatitis. People with chronic pancreatitis have persistent, recurring episodes of epigastric and upper left quadrant pain; the attacks often are precipitated by alcohol abuse or overeating. Anorexia, nausea, vomiting, constipation, and flatulence are common. Eventually, the disease progresses to the extent that endocrine and exocrine pancreatic functions become deficient. At this point, signs of diabetes mellitus and the malabsorption syndrome (*e.g.*, weight loss, fatty stools [steatorrhea]) become apparent.

Treatment. Treatment consists of measures to treat coexisting biliary tract disease. A low-fat diet usually is prescribed. The signs of malabsorption may be treated with pancreatic enzymes. When diabetes is present, it is treated with insulin. Alcohol is forbidden because it frequently precipitates attacks. Because of the frequent episodes of pain, narcotic addiction is a potential problem in people with chronic pancreatitis. Surgical intervention sometimes is needed to relieve the pain and usually focuses on relieving any obstruction that may be present. In advanced cases, a subtotal or total pancreatectomy may be necessary.[123]

Cancer of the Pancreas

There are a number of types of pancreatic cancer. The most common, pancreatic adenocarcinoma, accounts for about 85% of cases, and the term "pancreatic cancer" is sometimes used to refer only to that type.[128] Pancreatic cancer is the second most common GI malignancy in the United States, and approximately 55,440 (29,200 men and 26,240 women) new cases were expected to occur in 2018. It is the cause of 7% of all cancer deaths. It ranks fourth as a cause of cancer death in both men and women in the United States each year. Early stage pancreatic cancer usually has no symptoms and spreads quickly throughout the body, making it difficult to detect and harder to treat when it is found in its later stages.[129] For all stages combined, the 5-year survival rate is about 7% to 8%. The 5-year survival rate for people with stage I, II, III and IV are about 13%, 6%, 3%, and 1%, respectively.[130] One to two percent of cases of pancreatic cancer are neuroendocrine tumors (NETs), which arise from the hormone-producing cells of the pancreas. Pancreatic neuroendocrine tumors (PanNETs) are a diverse group of benign or malignant tumors and are generally less aggressive than pancreatic adenocarcinoma.[128]

Etiology. The cause of pancreatic cancer is unknown. Age, smoking, alcohol, obesity, diabetes mellitus, male gender, chronic pancreatitis, and hereditary factors have been found to be risk factors.[123] Pancreatic cancer rarely occurs in people younger than 50 years of age, and the risk increases with age. The most significant and reproducible environmental risk factor is cigarette smoking.[118,131] The incidence of pancreatic cancer is twice as high among smokers than nonsmokers. Overweight or obesity during early adulthood has been associated with a greater risk of pancreatic cancer. A younger age of disease onset and onset at an older age were associated with lower overall survival in people with pancreatic cancer. As per the SEER 2010-2014 database, the incidence rate of pancreatic cancer in males is 14.2 cases/100,000 people, compared with 11.1/100,000 cases in women. The incidence rate of pancreatic cancer in African Americans is 15.5 cases/100,000 people compared with 12.5/100,000 cases in Caucasians.[132] Hereditary pancreatitis and familial atypical mole multiple melanoma syndrome are two other causes linked to pancreatic cancer.[123]

Clinical Manifestations. Most pancreatic cancers are adenocarcinomas of the ductal epithelium, and symptoms are primarily caused by mass effect rather than disruption of exocrine or endocrine function. The clinical manifestations depend on the size and location of the tumor as well as its metastasis. Pain, jaundice, and weight loss constitute the classic presentation of the disease. The most common pain is a dull epigastric pain often accompanied by back pain, often worse in the supine position, and relieved by sitting forward. Although the tumor can arise anywhere in the pancreas, the most frequent site is the head (60%), followed by the body (10%), and tail (5%). The pancreas is diffusely involved in the remaining 25%.[118] Because of the proximity of the pancreas to the common duct and the hepatopancreatic ampulla, cancer of the head of the pancreas tends to obstruct bile flow. Jaundice frequently is the presenting symptom of a person with cancer of the head of the pancreas, and it usually is accompanied by complaints of pain and pruritus.[133] Cancer of the body of the pancreas usually impinges on the celiac ganglion, causing pain. The pain usually worsens with ingestion of food or assumption of the supine position. Cancer of the tail of the pancreas usually has metastasized before symptoms appear.

Migratory thrombophlebitis (deep vein thrombosis) develops in about 10% of people with pancreatic cancer, particularly when the tumor involves the body or tail of the pancreas.[118] Thrombi develop in multiple veins, including the deep veins of the legs, the subclavian vein, the inferior and superior mesentery veins, and even the vena cava. It is not uncommon for the migratory thrombophlebitis to provide the first evidence of pancreatic cancer, although it may present in other cancers as well. The mechanism responsible for the hypercoagulable state is largely unclear but may relate to activation of clotting factors by proteases released from the tumor cells.[118]

Diagnosis and Treatment. Person history, physical examination, and elevated serum bilirubin and alkaline phosphate levels may suggest the presence of pancreatic cancer, but are not diagnostic.[133] The serum cancer antigen (CA19-9), a Lewis blood group antigen, may help confirm the diagnosis in symptomatic people and may help predict prognosis and recurrence after resection. However, CA 19-9 has a sensitivity and specificity of 80% to 90%, so it does not confirm the diagnosis.[133]

Ultrasonography and CT scanning are the most frequently used diagnostic methods to confirm the disease. Intravenous and oral contrast–enhanced spiral CT is the preferred method for imaging the pancreas. Percutaneous fine-needle aspiration cytology of the pancreas has been one of the major advances in the diagnosis of pancreatic cancer. Unfortunately, the smaller and more curable tumors are most likely to be missed by this procedure. ERCP may be used for evaluation of people with suspected pancreatic cancer and obstructive jaundice.

Surgical resection of the tumor is done when the tumor is localized. However, this only occurs in 15% to 20% of people because most cancers of the pancreas have metastasized by the time of diagnosis.[134] Otherwise, surgical resection is reserved for palliative measures. Radiation therapy may be useful when the disease is not resectable but appears to be localized. The use of irradiation and chemotherapy for pancreatic cancer continues to be investigated. Pain control is one of the most important aspects in the management of people with end-stage pancreatic cancer. Ultimately, prognosis for pancreatic cancer remains poor, even after potentially curative surgery in appropriately selected people. Five-year survival rates after resection remain approximately 25%.[135]

IN SUMMARY

The biliary tract serves as a passageway for the delivery of bile from the liver to the intestine. This tract consists of the bile ducts and gallbladder. The most common causes of biliary tract disease are cholelithiasis and cholecystitis. Three factors contribute to the development of cholelithiasis: abnormalities in the composition of bile, stasis of bile, and inflammation of the gallbladder. Cholelithiasis predisposes to obstruction of bile flow, causing biliary colic and acute or chronic cholecystitis. Cancer of the gallbladder, which has a poor 5-year survival rate, occurs in 2% of people with biliary tract disease.

The pancreas is an endocrine and exocrine organ. The exocrine pancreas produces digestive enzymes that are secreted in an inactive form and transported to the small intestine through the main pancreatic duct, which usually empties into the hepatopancreatic ampulla and then into the duodenum through the sphincter of the pancreatic duct. The most common diseases of the exocrine pancreas are acute and chronic forms of pancreatitis, and cancer. Acute and chronic pancreatitis are associated with biliary reflux and chronic alcoholism. Acute pancreatitis is an inflammatory condition of the pancreas because of inappropriate activation of pancreatic enzymes, with manifestations that can range from mild to severe and life threatening. Chronic pancreatitis causes progressive destruction of the endocrine and exocrine pancreas. It is characterized by episodes of pain and epigastric distress that are similar to but less severe than those that occur with acute pancreatitis. Cancer of the pancreas is the fourth leading cause of cancer death in the United States. It usually is far advanced at the time of diagnosis, and the 5-year survival rate is 5%.

GERIATRIC Considerations

- The risk for gallstone disease increases with age because of a decrease in bile salt synthesis.[136]
- Intolerance to fatty foods is due to the atrophy and fibrosis of the pancreas.[136]
- Symptoms of pancreatic cancer are vague; however, common symptoms include pain relief with leaning forward and worsening pain when lying down.[136]

PEDIATRIC Considerations

- Treatment for pancreatitis in children includes immediate bowel rest and monitoring of serum amylase. Surgery is not usually indicated unless abdominal trauma or ductal abnormalities exist.[137]
- In children, the most common complication of gallstone disease is pancreatitis.[137]
- The cause of biliary atresia (the absence of biliary ducts) is unknown, but ischemia, infection, or autoimmune causes are suspected.[137]
- Children in liver failure manifest hepatic necrosis.[137]
- An increase in nonalcoholic liver disease is associated with childhood obesity.[138]

REVIEW EXERCISES

1. A 24-year-old woman reports to her health care professional with complaints of a yellow discoloration of her skin, loss of appetite, and a feeling of upper gastric discomfort. She denies use of intravenous drugs and has not received blood products. She cannot recall eating uncooked shellfish or drinking water that might have been contaminated. She has a daughter who attends day care.
   A. *What tests could be done to confirm a diagnosis of hepatitis A?*
   B. *What is the most common mode of transmission for hepatitis A? It is suggested that the source might be through the day care center that her daughter attends. Explain.*
   C. *What methods could be used to protect other family members from getting the disease?*
2. A 56-year-old man with a history of heavy alcohol consumption and a previous diagnosis of alcoholic cirrhosis and portal hypertension is admitted to the emergency department with acute gastrointestinal bleeding because of a tentative diagnosis of bleeding esophageal varices and signs of circulatory shock.
   A. *Relate the development of esophageal varices to portal hypertension in people with cirrhosis of the liver.*
   B. *Many people with esophageal varices have blood coagulation problems. Explain.*
   C. *What are the possible treatment measures for this man, in terms of both controlling the current bleeding episode and preventing further bleeding episodes?*
3. A 40-year-old woman presents in the emergency department with a sudden episode of vomiting and severe right epigastric pain that developed after eating a fatty evening meal. Although there is no evidence of jaundice in her skin, the sclera of her eyes is noted to have a yellowish discoloration. Palpation reveals tenderness of the upper right quadrant with muscle splinting and rebound pain. Right upper quadrant abdominal ultrasonography confirms the presence of gallstones. The woman is treated conservatively with pain and antiemetic medications. She is subsequently scheduled for a laparoscopic cholecystectomy.
   A. *Relate this woman's signs and symptoms to gallstones and their effect on gallbladder function.*
   B. *Explain the initial appearance of jaundice in the eyes as opposed to the skin. Which of the two laboratory tests for bilirubin would you expect to be elevated—direct (conjugated) or indirect (unconjugated or free)?*
   C. *What effect will removal of the gallbladder have on the storage and release of bile into the intestine, particularly as it relates to meals?*

References

1. Segal S. S. (2017). Special circulations. In Boron W. F., Boulpaep E. L. (Eds.) *Medical physiology* (3rd ed., pp. 556–571). Philadelphia, PA: Saunders Elsevier.
2. Suchy F. J. (2017). Hepatobiliary function. In Boron W. F., Boulpaep E. L. (Eds.) *Medical physiology* (3rd ed., pp. 944–971). Philadelphia, PA: Saunders Elsevier.
3. Hall J. E. (2015). *Guyton and Hall textbook of medical physiology* (13th ed., pp. 881–886). Philadelphia, PA: Saunders Elsevier.
4. Dawson P. A. (2016). Bile secretion and enterohepatic circulation. In Feldman M., Friedman L. S., Brandt L. J. (Eds.) *Sleisenger and Fordtran's gastrointestinal and liver disease* (10th ed., pp. 1085–1099). Philadelphia, PA: Saunders Elsevier.
5. Rubin R., Rubin E. (2014). The liver and biliary system. In Rubin R., Strayer D. S. (Eds.) *Rubin's pathophysiology: Clinicopathologic foundations of medicine* (7th ed., pp. 825–886). Philadelphia, PA: Lippincott Williams & Wilkins.
6. Savio J., Pratt D. S. (2014). Jaundice. In Kasper D., Fauci A., Hauser S., et al. (Eds.) *Harrison's principles of internal medicine* (19th ed.). New York, NY: McGraw-Hill. Available: http://accessmedicine.mhmedical.com.ezproxy.uthsc.edu/content.aspx?bookid=1130&sectionid=79726384. Accessed March 05, 2018
7. Deng B.-C. et al. (2012). Novel ATP8B1 mutation in an adult male with progressive familial intrahepatic cholestasis. *World Journal of Gastroenterology* 18(44), 6504–6509. doi:10.3748/wjg.v18.i44.6504
8. Patel K. R. *Alagille syndrome. PathologyOutlines.com. [Online]*. Available: http://www.pathologyoutlines.com/topic/liveralagillessyndrome.html. Accessed January 31, 2018
9. Suchy F. J. (2016). Anatomy, histology, embryology, developmental anomalies, and pediatric disorders of the biliary tract. In Feldman M., Friedman L. S., Brandt L. J. (Eds.) *Sleisenger and Fordtran's gastrointestinal and liver disease* (10th ed., pp. 1055–1077). Philadelphia, PA: Saunders Elsevier.
10. Theise N. D., Crawford J. M., Lui C. (2015). The liver and bile ducts. In Kumar V., Abbas A. K., Aster J. C. (Eds.) *Robbins and Cotran pathologic basis of disease* (9th ed., pp. 821–881). Philadelphia, PA: Saunders Elsevier.
11. Chernecky C. C., Berger B. J. (2012). *Laboratory tests and diagnostic procedures* (6th ed.). Philadelphia, PA: Saunders Elsevier.
12. Wolkoff A. W. (2014). The hyperbilirubinemias. In Kasper D., Fauci A., Hauser S., et al. (Eds.) *Harrison's principles of internal medicine* (19th ed.). New York, NY: McGraw-Hill. Available: http://accessmedicine.mhmedical.com.ezproxy.uthsc.edu/content.aspx?bookid=1130&sectionid=79748447. Accessed March 05, 2018
13. Pratt D. S. (2014). Evaluation of liver function. In Kasper D., Fauci A., Hauser S., et al. (Eds.) *Harrison's principles of internal medicine* (19th ed.). New York, NY: McGraw-Hill. Available: http://accessmedicine.mhmedical.com.ezproxy.uthsc.edu/content.aspx?bookid=1130&sectionid=79748389. Accessed March 05, 2018
14. Larson D. (2017). Chapter 8: Enzymes. In *Clinical chemistry: Fundamentals and laboratory techniques.* ISBN 9781455742141
15. Botros M., Sikaris K. A. (2013). The de ritis ratio: The test of time. *The Clinical Biochemist Reviews* 34(3), 117–130.
16. Torruellas C., French S. W., Medici V. (2014). Diagnosis of alcoholic liver disease. *World Journal of Gastroenterology* 20(33), 11684–11699. doi:10.3748/wjg.v20.i33.11684
17. Oh D., Seo D.-W., Hong S.-M., et al. (2017). Endoscopic ultrasound-guided fine-needle aspiration can target right liver mass. *Endoscopic Ultrasound* 6(2), 109–115. doi:10.4103/2303-9027.204813
18. Teoh N. C., Chitturi S., Farrell G. C. (2016). Hepatic drug metabolism and liver disease caused by drugs. In Feldman M., Friedman L. S., Brandt L. J. (Eds.) *Sleisenger and Fordtran's gastrointestinal and liver disease* (10th ed., pp. 1442–1477). Philadelphia, PA: Saunders Elsevier.
19. Katzung B. G. (2014). *Basic and clinical pharmacology* (13th ed., pp. 50–63). New York: McGraw-Hill Medical.
20. Farrell S. E. (2018). Acetaminophen toxicity treatment & management. *Medscape Medical News*. Available: https://emedicine.medscape.com/article/820200-treatment. Accessed January 31, 2018

21. Chalasani N., Ahmad J., et al. (2015). Features and outcomes of 899 patients with drug-induced liver injury: The DILIN prospective study. *Gastroenterology* 148(7):1340–1352.e7
22. Lee W. M. (2013). Drug-induced acute liver failure. *Clinics in Liver Disease* 17(4), 575–586. doi:10.1016/j.cld.2013.07.001.
23. Pandit A., Sachdeva T., Bafna P. (2012). Drug-induced hepatotoxicity: A review. *Journal of Applied Pharmaceutical Science* 02(05), 233–243.
24. Harshad D. (2012). An update on drug-induced liver injury. *Journal of Clinical and Experimental Hepatology* 2(3), 247–259.
25. Feld J. J., Heathcote E. J. (2016). Hepatitis caused by other viruses. In Feldman M., Friedman L. S., Brandt L. J. (Eds.) *Sleisenger and Fordtran's gastrointestinal and liver disease* (10th ed., pp. 1366–1373). Philadelphia, PA: Saunders Elsevier.
26. Stapleton J. T., Williams C. F., Xiang J. (2004). GB virus C: A beneficial infection? *Journal of Clinical Microbiology* 42, 3915–3919.
27. Dienstag J. L. (2014). Acute viral hepatitis. In: Kasper D., Fauci A., Hauser S., et al. (Eds.) *Harrison's principles of internal medicine* (19th ed.). New York, NY: McGraw-Hill. Available: http://accessmedicine.mhmedical.com.ezproxy.uthsc.edu/content.aspx?bookid=1130&sectionid=79748507. Accessed March 05, 2018
28. World Health Organization. (2017). *Hepatitis C: Fact sheet [Online]*. Available: http://www.who.int/mediacentre/factsheets/fs164/en/. Accessed January 31, 2018
29. Dudley T. (2016). Viral hepatitis. In Sargent S. (Ed.) *Liver diseases: An essential guide for nurses and healthcare professionals*. PDF, ePub eBook. Hoboken, NJ: Wiley-Blackwell. http://canadasgreenestschool.ca/pdf-book/liver-diseases-an-essential-guide-for-nurses-and-health-care-professionals
30. Lai M., Chopra S. (2016). Hepatitis A virus infection in adults: Epidemiology, clinical manifestations, and diagnosis. *UpToDate*. Available: https://www.uptodate.com/contents/hepatitis-a-virus-infection-in-adults-epidemiology-clinical-manifestations-and-diagnosis. Accessed January 12, 2018
31. Sjogren M. H., Basssett J. T. (2015). Hepatitis A. In Feldman M., Friedman L. S., Brandt L. J. (Eds.) *Sleisenger and Fordtran's gastrointestinal and liver disease* (10th ed., pp. 1302–1308). Philadelphia, PA: Saunders Elsevier.
32. World Health Organization. (2017). *Hepatitis A: Fact sheet*. Available: http://www.who.int/mediacentre/factsheets/fs328/en/. Accessed January 31, 2018
33. World Health Organization. (2017). *Hepatitis A: Vaccine. [Online]*. Available: http://www.who.int/ith/vaccines/hepatitisA/en/. Accessed January 31, 2018
34. Centers for Disease Control and Prevention. (2015). *[Online]*. Available: https://www.cdc.gov/vaccines/pubs/pinkbook/hepa.html. Accessed January 31, 2018
35. Wells J. T., Perillo R. (2016). Hepatitis B. Hepatitis D. In Feldman M., Friedman L. S., Brandt L. J. (Eds.) *Sleisenger and Fordtran's gastrointestinal and liver disease* (10th ed., pp. 1309-1331; 1353–1359). Philadelphia, PA: Saunders Elsevier.
36. Hu J., Liu K. (2017), Complete and incomplete Hepatitis B virus particles: Formation, function, and application. *Viruses* 9(3), 56. [Online]. Available: http://www.mdpi.com/1999-4915/9/3/56/pdf
37. World Health Organization. (2017). *Hepatitis B: Fact sheet. [Online]*. Available: http://www.who.int/mediacentre/factsheets/fs204/en/. Accessed January 31, 2018
38. Centers for Disease Control and Prevention. (2018). *Hepatitis B FAQs for health professionals. [Online]*. Available: https://www.cdc.gov/hepatitis/hbv/hbvfaq.htm. Accessed January 31, 2018
39. Roberts H., et al. (2016). Prevalence of chronic hepatitis B virus (HBV) infection in U.S. households: National Health and Nutrition Examination Survey (NHANES), 1988–2002. *Hepatology* 63(2), 388–973.
40. Kowdley K. V., et al. (2012). Prevalence of chronic hepatitis B among foreign-born persons living in the United States by country of origin. *Hepatology* 56(2), 422–433.
41. Spradling P. R., et al. (2012). Hepatitis B and C virus infection among 1.2 million persons with access to care: Factors associated with testing and infection prevalence. *Clinical Infectious Diseases* 55(8), 1047–1055.
42. Centers for Disease Control and Prevention. (2018). *Viral hepatitis. [Online]*. Available: https://www.cdc.gov/hepatitis/hbv/testingchronic.htm. Accessed January 31, 2018
43. Centers for Disease Control and Prevention. (2017). *Surveillance for viral hepatitis–United States, 2015. [Online]*. Available: https://www.cdc.gov/hepatitis/statistics/2015surveillance/index.htm. Accessed January 31, 2018
44. Schillie S., Vellozzi C., Reingold A., et al. (2018). Prevention of hepatitis B virus infection in the United States: Recommendations of the Advisory Committee on Immunization Practices. *Morbidity and Mortality Weekly Report. Recommendations and Reports* 67(RR-1), 1–31. doi:10.15585/mmwr.rr6701a1
45. Terrault N. A., Bzowej N. H., Chang K.-M., et al. *AASLD guidelines for treatment of chronic hepatitis B. [Online]*. Available: https://www.aasld.org/sites/default/files/guideline_documents/hep28156.pdf. Accessed January 18, 2018
46. Al-Joudi F. S., Mohd Arif M. B., Mohamed Z. B., et al. (2014). Testing for hepatitis B virus core antigen and e antigen may confer additional safety of donors' blood negative for heptitis B virus surface antigen. *Asian Journal of Transfusion Science* 8, 63–64.
47. Mansouri N., Movafagh A., Sayad A., et al. (2014). Hepatitis B virus infection in patients with blood disorders: A concise review in pediatric study. *Iranian Journal of Pediatric Hematology and Oncology* 4(4), 178–187
48. Hepatitis B Foundation. (2016). *HBV viral load test. [Online]*. Available: http://www.hepb.org/blog/tag/hbv-viral-load-test/. Accessed February 1, 2018
49. GBD 2015 Disease and Injury Incidence and Prevalence, Collaborators. (2016). Global, regional, and national incidence, prevalence, and years lived with disability for 310 diseases and injuries, 1990–2015: A systematic analysis for the Global Burden of Disease Study 2015. *Lancet* 388(10053), 1545–1602.
50. National Academies of Sciences, Engineering, and Medicine. (2016). *Eliminating the public health problem of hepatitis B and C in the United States: Phase one report*. Washington, DC: The National Academies Press. doi:10.17226/23407
51. Lee M.-H., Yang H.-I., Yuan Y., et al. (2014). Epidemiology and natural history of hepatitis C virus infection. *World Journal of Gastroenterology* 20(28), 9270–9280. doi:10.3748/wjg.v20.i28.9270.
52. Huffman M. M., Mounsey A. L. (2014). Hepatitis C for primary care physicians. *Journal of the American Board of Family Medicine* 27, 284–291. doi:10.3122/jabfm.2014.02.130165.
53. Akamatsu N., Sugawara Y. (2012). Liver transplantation and hepatitis C. *International Journal of Hepatology* 2012, 22. Article ID 686135. doi:10.1155/2012/686135
54. Horsley-Silva J. L., Vargas H. E. (2017). New therapies for hepatitis C virus infection. *Gastroenterology & Hepatology* 13(1), 22–31.
55. Wedeyer H. (2016). Hepatitis C. In Feldman M., Friedman L. S., Brandt L. J. (Eds.) *Sleisenger and Fordtran's gastrointestinal and liver disease* (10th ed., pp. 1332–1352). Philadelphia, PA: Saunders Elsevier.
56. Nouroz F, Shaheen S, Mujtaba G, et al. (2015) An overview on hepatitis C virus genotypes and its control. *Egyptian Journal of Medical Human Genetics* 16, 291–298.
57. Centers for Disease Control and Prevention. (2017). *Hepatitis C FAQs for health professionals. [Online]*. Available: https://www.cdc.gov/hepatitis/hcv/hcvfaq.htm. Accessed January 31, 2018
58. Centers for Disease Control and Prevention. (2015). *Hepatitis D. [Online]*. Available: https://www.cdc.gov/hepatitis/hdv/index.htm. Accessed January 31, 2018
59. de Alencar Arrais Guerra J. A., et al. (2017). Hepatitis E: A literature review. *Journal of Clinical and Translational Hepatology* 5(4), 376–383. doi:10.14218/JCTH.2017.00012
60. Patrick B., et al. (2014). The impact of hepatitis E in the liver transplant setting. *Journal of Hepatology.* 61(6), 1418–1429.
61. Zhou X., et al. (2013). Epidemiology and management of chronic hepatitis E infection in solid organ transplantation: A comprehensive literature review. *Reviews in Medical Virology* 23(5), 295–304.
62. WHO. (2012). *Global Alert and Response (GAR); Hepatitis E.* Accessed January 26, 2012

63. Li S.-W., et al. (2015). The development of a recombinant hepatitis E vaccine HEV 239. *Human Vaccines & Immunotherapeutics*. 11(4), 908–914.
64. Centers for Disease Control and Prevention. (2015). *Hepatitis E: FAQs for health professionals. [Online]*. Available: https://www.cdc.gov/hepatitis/hev/hevfaq.htm. Accessed January 31, 2018
65. Friedman L. S. (2018). Liver, biliary tract, & pancreas disorders. In Papadakis M. A., McPhee S. J., Rabow M. W., (Eds.) *Current medical diagnosis & treatment 2017*. New York, NY: McGraw-Hill. Available: http://accessmedicine.mhmedical.com.ezproxy.uthsc.edu/content.aspx?bookid=1843&sectionid=135711381. Accessed March 05, 2018
66. AASLD–IDSA. (2017). *HCV guidance: Recommendations for testing, managing, and treating hepatitis C. [Online]*. Available: http://www.hcvguidelines.org. Accessed February 1, 2018
67. Feld J. J., Jacobson C., Hézode T., et al. (2015). Sofosbuvir and velpatasvir for HCV genotype 1, 2, 4, 5, and 6 infection. *New England Journal of Medicine* 373, 2599–2607.
68. Fialho A., Fialho A., Carey W. D. (2015). *Autoimmune hepatitis. [Online]*. Cleveland Clinic–Center for Continuing Education. Available: http://www.clevelandclinicmeded.com/medicalpubs/diseasemanagement/hepatology/chronic-autoimmune-hepatitis/. Accessed August 2017
69. Hubscher S. G., Burt A. D., Portmann B. C., et al. (2017). *MacSween's pathology of the liver* (e-book, 7th ed.). Philadelphia, PA: Elsevier, [2018].
70. Czaja A. J. (2016). Autoimmune hepatitis. In Feldman M., Friedman L. S., Brandt L. J. (Eds.) *Sleisenger and Fordtran's gastrointestinal and liver disease* (10th ed., pp. 1493–1551). Philadelphia, PA: Saunders Elsevier.
71. Angulo P., Lindor K. D. (2015). Primary biliary cirrhosis. In Feldman M., Friedman L. S., Brandt L. J. (Eds.) *Sleisenger and Fordtran's gastrointestinal and liver disease* (10th ed., pp. 1477–1487). Philadelphia, PA: Saunders Elsevier.
72. Raszeja-Wyszomirska J., Miazgowski T. (2014). Osteoporosis in primary biliary cirrhosis of the liver. *Przegląd Gastroenterologiczny* 9(2), 82–87. doi:10.5114/pg.2014.42502
73. Yamagiwa S., et al. (2014). Autoantibodies in primary biliary cirrhosis: Recent progress in research on the pathogenetic and clinical significance. *World Journal of Gastroenterology* 20(10), 2606–2612. doi:10.3748/wjg.v20.i10.2606.
74. Pietro I., et al. (2017). Primary biliary cholangitis: Advances in management and treatment of the disease. *Digestive and Liver Disease* 49(8), 841–846.
75. Mathurin P., Bataller R. (2015). Trends in the management and burden of alcoholic liver disease. *Journal of Hepatology* 62(1 Suppl), S38–S46. doi:10.1016/j.jhep.2015.03.006
76. Cederbaum A. I. (2012). Alcohol metabolism. *Clinics in Liver Disease* 16(4), 667–685. doi:10.1016/j.cld.2012.08.002.
77. Carithers R. L., McClain C. J. (2016). Alcoholic liver disease. In Feldman M., Friedman L. S., Brandt L. J. (Eds.) *Sleisenger and Fordtran's gastrointestinal and liver disease* (10th ed., pp. 1409–1427). Philadelphia, PA: Saunders Elsevier.
78. Rahimi E., Pan J.-J. (2015). Prognostic models for alcoholic hepatitis. *Biomarker Research* 3, 20. doi:10.1186/s40364-015-0046-z.
79. Shaker M., et al. (2014). Liver transplantation for nonalcoholic fatty liver disease: New challenges and new opportunities. *World Journal of Gastroenterology* 20(18), 5320.
80. Rinella M. E. (2015). Nonalcoholic fatty liver disease: A systematic review. *JAMA* 313(22), 2263–2273.
81. Calzadilla Bertot L., Adams L. A. (2016). The natural course of non-alcoholic fatty liver disease. *International Journal of Molecular Sciences* 17(5), 774. doi:10.3390/ijms17050774
82. Reid A. E. (2016). Nonalcoholic fatty liver disease. In Feldman M., Friedman L. S., Brandt L. J. (Eds.) *Sleisenger and Fordtran's gastrointestinal and liver disease* (10th ed., pp. 1401–1411). Philadelphia, PA: Saunders Elsevier.
83. Pastori D., et al. (2015). The efficacy and safety of statins for the treatment of non-alcoholic fatty liver disease. *Digestive and Liver Disease* 47(1), 4–11.
84. Raluca P., et al. (2016). NAFLD and liver transplantation: Current burden and expected challenges. *Journal of Hepatology* 65(6), 1245–1257.
85. Fan C. Q., Crawford J. M. (2014). Sinusoidal obstruction syndrome (hepatic veno-occlusive disease). *Journal of Clinical and Experimental Hepatology* 4(4), 332–346. doi:10.1016/j.jceh.2014.10.002.
86. Sakumura M., et al. (2017). Hepatic sinusoidal obstruction syndrome induced by non-transplant chemotherapy for non-Hodgkin lymphoma. *Internal Medicine* 56(4), 395–400.
87. Runyon B. A. (2016). Ascites and bacterial peritonitis. In Feldman M., Friedman L. S., Brandt L. J. (Eds.) *Sleisenger and Fordtran's gastrointestinal and liver disease* (10th ed., pp. 1553–1576). Philadelphia, PA: Saunders Elsevier.
88. Tasneem, et al. (2015). Causes, management and complications of ascites: A review. *International Current Pharmaceutical Journal* 4(3), 370–377. Available: http://www.icpjonline.com/documents/Vol4Issue3/02.pdf
89. National Guideline Centre (UK). (2016). *Cirrhosis in over 16s: Assessment and management*. London: National Institute for Health and Care Excellence (UK). (NICE Guideline, No. 50.) 12, Transjugular intrahepatic portosystemic shunt (TIPS) versus large-volume paracentesis (LVP) for ascites. Available: https://www.ncbi.nlm.nih.gov/books/NBK385213/
90. Bacon B. R. (2014). Cirrhosis and its complications. In: Kasper D., Fauci A., Hauser S., et al. (Eds.) *Harrison's principles of internal medicine* (19th ed.). New York, NY: McGraw-Hill. Available: http://accessmedicine.mhmedical.com.ezproxy.uthsc.edu/content.aspx?bookid=1130&sectionid=79748841. Accessed March 05, 2018
91. Philips C. A., Arora A., Shetty R., et al. (2016). A comprehensive review of portosystemic collaterals in cirrhosis: Historical aspects, anatomy, and classifications. *International Journal of Hepatology* 2016, 6170243. doi:10.1155/2016/6170243.
92. Kim D. H., Park J. Y. (2013). Prevention and management of variceal hemorrhage. *International Journal of Hepatology* 2013, 434609. doi:10.1155/2013/434609.
93. Biecker E. (2013). Portal hypertension and gastrointestinal bleeding: Diagnosis, prevention and management. *World Journal of Gastroenterology* 19(31), 5035–5050.
94. Caldwell S. H. (2014). Management of coagulopathy in liver disease. *Gastroenterology & Hepatology* 10(5), 330–332.
95. The U.S. Organ Procurement and Transplantation Network and Scientific Registry of Transplant Recipients. (2012). *2012 OPTN/SRTR Annual Report: Transplant Data. [Online]*. Available: http://optn.transplant.hrsa.gov. Accessed October 11, 2017
96. Organ Procurement and Transplantation Network. (2011). *Overall current patient waiting list by organ*. Available: http://optn.tranplant.hrsa.gov. Accessed July 09, 2011
97. Carrion A. F., Martin P. (2016). Liver transplantation. In Feldman M., Friedman L. S., Brandt L. J. (Eds.) *Sleisenger and Fordtran's gastrointestinal and liver disease* (10th ed., pp. 1628-1646). Philadelphia, PA: Saunders Elsevier.
98. WorldHealthOrganization.(2014).*WorldCancerReport2014.*Chapter5.6. ISBN 9283204298.
99. American Cancer Society. (2017). *Cancer facts & figures*. Available: https://www.cancer.org/content/dam/cancer-org/research/cancer-facts-and-statistics/annual-cancer-facts-and-figures/2017/cancer-facts-and-figures-2017.pdf. Accessed January 31, 2018
100. El-Serag H. B. (2012). Epidemiology of viral hepatitis and hepatocellular carcinoma. *Gastroenterology* 142(6), 1264–1273. doi:10.1053/j.gastro.2011.12.061.
101. Cai G.-X., Cai S.-J. (2012). Multi-modality treatment of colorectal liver metastases. *World Journal of Gastroenterology* 18(1), 16–24. doi:10.3748/wjg.v18.i1.16.
102. Magnussen A., Parsi M. A. (2013). Aflatoxins, hepatocellular carcinoma and public health. *World Journal of Gastroenterology* 19(10), 1508–1512. doi:10.3748/wjg.v19.i10.1508.
103. Hamid A. S., et al. (2013). Aflatoxin B1-induced hepatocellular carcinoma in developing countries: Geographical distribution, mechanism of action and prevention. *Oncology Letters* 5(4), 1087–1092. doi:10.3892/ol.2013.1169.

104. DiBisceglie A. M., Befeler A. S. (2016). Hepatic tumors and cysts. In Feldman M., Friedman L. S., Brandt L. J. (Eds.) *Sleisenger and Fordtran's gastrointestinal and liver disease* (10th ed., pp. 1603-1627). Philadelphia, PA: Saunders Elsevier.
105. Zhao Y. J., Ju Q., Li G. C. (2013). Tumor markers for hepatocellular carcinoma. *Molecular and Clinical Oncology* 1, 593–598.
106. Fitzmorris P., Singal A. K. (2015). Surveillance and diagnosis of hepatocellular carcinoma. *Gastroenterology & Hepatology* 11(1), 38–46.
107. Khan S. A., Davidson B. R., Goldin R. D., et al. (2012). Guidelines for the diagnosis and treatment of cholangiocarcinoma: An update. *Gut* 61, 1657–1669.
108. Boyer J. L. (2013). Bile formation and secretion. *Comprehensive Physiology* 3(3), 1035–1078. doi:10.1002/cphy.c120027.
109. Stinton L. M., Shaffer E. A. (2012). Epidemiology of gallbladder disease: Cholelithiasis and cancer. *Gut and Liver* 6(2), 172–187. doi:10.5009/gnl.2012.6.2.172.
110. Greenberger N. J., Paumgartner G. (2014). Diseases of the gallbladder and bile ducts. In Kasper D., Fauci A., Hauser S., et al. (Eds.) *Harrison's principles of internal medicine* (19th ed.). New York, NY: McGraw-Hill. Available: http://accessmedicine.mhmedical.com.ezproxy.uthsc.edu/content.aspx?bookid=1130&sectionid=79749108. Accessed March 05, 2018
111. Wang D. Q., Afdhal N. H. (2016). Gallstone disease. In Feldman M., Friedman L. S., Brandt L. J. (Eds.) *Sleisenger and Fordtran's gastrointestinal and liver disease* (10th ed., pp. 1100-1133). Philadelphia, PA: Saunders Elsevier.
112. Glasgow R. E., Mulvihill S. J. (2015). Treatment of gallstone disease. In Feldman M., Friedman L. S., Brandt L. J. (Eds.) *Sleisenger and Fordtran's gastrointestinal and liver disease* (10th ed., pp. 1134-1151). Philadelphia, PA: Saunders Elsevier.
113. Patel T. (2016). Tumors of the biliary tract. In Yamada Y. (Ed.) *Textbook of gastroenterology* (6th ed., pp. 1858–1874). Oxford, UK: Wiley-Blackwell.
114. Anstee Q. M., Jones D. E. J. (2014). Liver and biliary tract disease. In Colledge N. R., Walker B. R., Ralston S. H. (Eds.) *Davidson's principles and practice of medicine* (22nd ed., pp. 921-988). New York, NY: Churchill Livingstone Elsevier.
115. Kanthan R., Senger J.L., Ahmed S., et al. (2015). Gallbladder cancer in the 21st century. *Journal of Oncology* 2015, 26. Article ID 967472. doi:10.1155/2015/967472.
116. American Cancer Society. (2014). *Survival statistics for gallbladder cancer by stage. [Online]*. Available: https://www.cancer.org/cancer/gallbladder-cancer/detection-diagnosis-staging/survival-rates.html. Accessed February 3, 2018
117. Patton K. T., Thibodeau G. A. (2015). *Anatomy and physiology* (9th ed., pp. 861–930). St. Louis, MO: Mosby Elsevier.
118. Lauwers G. Y., Mino-Kenudson M., Rubin R. (2012). The pancreas. In Rubin R., Strayer D. S. (Eds.) *Rubin's pathophysiology: Clinicopathologic foundations of medicine* (6th ed., pp. 887-902). Philadelphia, PA: Lippincott Williams & Wilkins.
119. Warren K. R., Murray M. M. (2013). Alcoholic liver disease and pancreatitis: Global health problems being addressed by the US National Institute on Alcohol Abuse and Alcoholism. *Journal of Gastroenterology and Hepatology* 28(S1), 4–6.
120. Tenner S., Baillie J., DeWitt V., et al. (2013). American College of Gastroenterology guideline: Management of acute pancreatitis. *American Journal of Gastroenterology* 108, 1400–1415.
121. Banks P. A., Bollen T. L., Dervenis C., et al. (2013). Classification of acute pancreatitis—2012: Revision of classification and definitions by international consensus. *Gut* 62, 102–111.
122. Gerloff A. (2012). Pancreas-non-Alcohol constituents and its effects. In *Pancreatic diseases—Advances in research and treatment* (2012 ed., Chapter 3).
123. Penman I. D., Lees C. W. (2014). Alimentary tract and pancreatic disease. In Colledge N. R., Walker B. R., Ralston S. H. (Eds.) *Davidson's principles and practice of medicine* (22nd ed., pp. 837–920). New York, NY: Churchill Livingstone Elsevier.
124. Dawra D. A., Dudeja R. K., Saluja V., et al. (2016). Role of trypsinogen activation in genesis of pancreatitis. *Pancreapedia: Exocrine Pancreas Knowledge Base*. doi:10.3998/panc.2016.25
125. Meher S., Mishra T. S., Sasmal P. K., et al. (2015). Role of biomarkers in diagnosis and prognostic evaluation of acute pancreatitis. *Journal of Biomarkers* 2015, 13. doi:10.1155/2015/519534.
126. Dupuis C. S., et al. (2013). Diagnosis and management of acute pancreatitis and its complications. *Gastrointestinal Intervention* 2(1), 36–46. doi:10.1016/j.gii.2013.03.001.
127. Conwell D. L., Banks P., Greenberger N. J. (2014). Acute and chronic pancreatitis. In: Kasper D, Fauci A, Hauser S, et al. (Eds.) *Harrison's principles of internal medicine* (19th ed.). New York, NY: McGraw-Hill. Available: http://accessmedicine.mhmedical.com.ezproxy.uthsc.edu/content.aspx?bookid=1130&sectionid=79749276. Accessed March 05, 2018
128. World Health Organization. (2014). *World Cancer Report 2014* (Chapter 5.7). ISBN 92-832-0429-8
129. American Cancer Society. (2016). *Pancreatic cancer. [Online]*. Available: https://www.cancer.org/cancer/pancreatic-cancer.html. Accessed February 3, 2018
130. American Cancer Society. (2016). *Pancreatic cancer survival rates, by stage. [Online]*. Available: https://www.cancer.org/cancer/pancreatic-cancer/detection-diagnosis-staging/survival-rates.html. Accessed February 3, 2018
131. Fanta P. T., Lowy A. M. (2016). Adenocarcinoma of the pancreas. In Yamada Y., (Ed.) *Textbook of gastroenterology* (6th ed., Chapter 87). Oxford, UK: Wiley-Blackwell.
132. Howlader N., et al. (Eds.) (2017). *SEER cancer statistics review, 1975–2014*. Bethesda, MD: National Cancer Institute. Available: https://seer.cancer.gov/csr/1975_2014/, based on November 2016 SEER data submission, posted to the SEER website
133. Smyth E., Cunningham D. (2014). Pancreatic cancer. In Kasper D., Fauci A., Hauser S., et al. (Eds.) *Harrison's principles of internal medicine* (19th ed.). New York, NY: McGraw-Hill. Available: http://accessmedicine.mhmedical.com.ezproxy.uthsc.edu/content.aspx?bookid=1130&sectionid=69858054. Accessed March 05, 2018
134. De La Cruz M. S., Young A. P., Ruffin M. T. (2014). Diagnosis and management of pancreatic cancer. *American Family Physician* 89(8), 626–632.
135. Lewis R., Drebin J., Callery M., et al. (2013). A contemporary analysis of survival for resected pancreatic ductal adenocarcinoma. *HPB* 15, 49–60.
136. Eliopoulos C. (2018). Digestion and bowel elimination. In *Gerontological nursing*. Philadelphia: Wolters Kluwer.
137. Kyle T., Carman S. (2017). Nursing care of the child with an alteration in bowel elimination/gastrointestinal disorder. In *Essentials of pediatric nursing* (3rd ed.). Philadelphia: Wolters Kluwer.
138. Bowden V. R., Greenberg C. S. (2014). *Children and their families: The continuum of nursing care* (3rd ed.). Philadelphia: Wolters Kluwer.

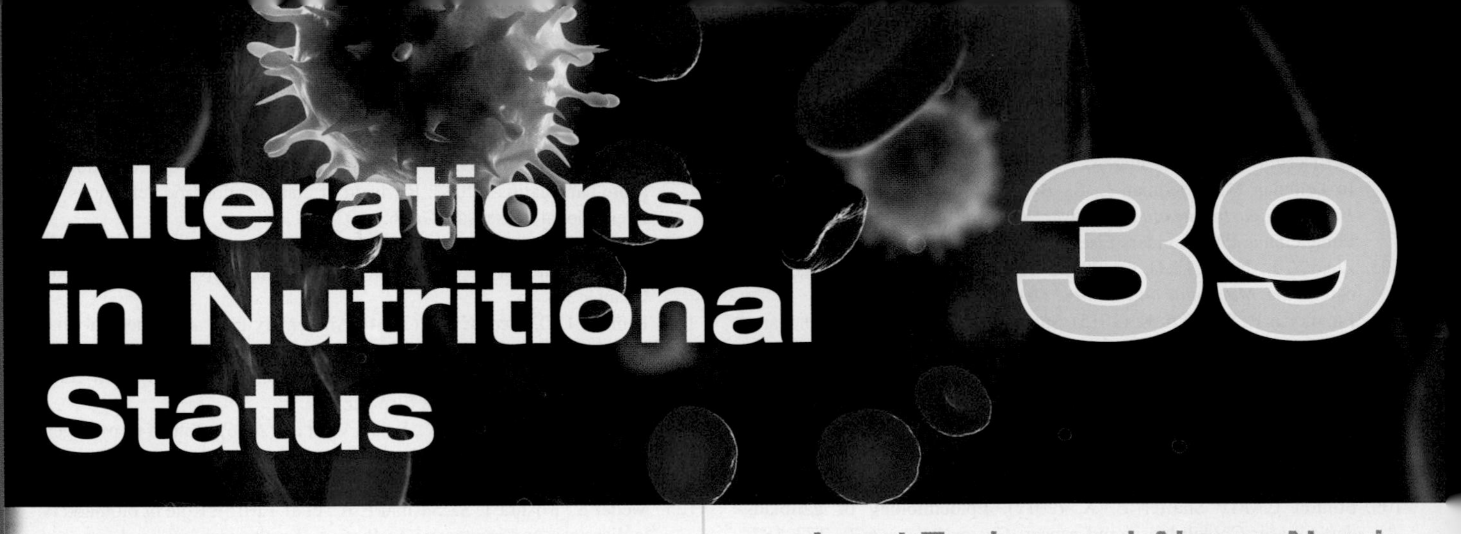

Alterations in Nutritional Status

39

Janet Tucker and Alyssa Norris

Nutritional status describes the condition of the body with respect to the availability and use of nutrients. Nutrients that are taken into the body can be used to provide the energy needed to perform various body functions, or they can be stored for future use. The stability and composition of body weight over time require that a person's energy intake be balanced with energy expenditure. When a person is overfed and nutrient intake consistently exceeds expenditure, most of the nutrients are stored and body weight increases. Conversely, when energy expenditure exceeds nutrient intake, energy stores are lost and body weight decreases.

Also, because different foods contain different amounts of proteins, fats, carbohydrates, vitamins, and minerals, appropriate amounts of these dietary elements must be maintained to ensure that all parts of the body's metabolic systems can be supplied with requisite materials. This chapter discusses the regulation of energy expenditure and storage, nutritional needs, overnutrition and obesity, and undernutrition and eating disorders.

NUTRITIONAL STATUS

After completing this section of the chapter, the learner will be able to meet the following objectives:

- Define *calorie* and state the number of calories derived from the oxidation of 1 g of protein, fat, or carbohydrate.
- Describe four types of energy expenditure.

The nutrients that the body uses to maintain its nutritional status are derived from the digestive tract through the ingestion of foods or, in some cases, through liquid feedings that are delivered directly into the gastrointestinal tract by a synthetic tube (*i.e.*, tube feedings). The exception occurs in people with certain illnesses in which the digestive tract is bypassed and the nutrients are infused directly into the circulatory system. Once inside the body, nutrients are used for energy or as the building blocks for tissue growth and repair. When excess nutrients are available, they frequently are stored for future use. If the required nutrients are unavailable, the body adapts by conserving and using its nutrient stores.

Energy Metabolism

Energy is measured in heat units called *calories*. A calorie, spelled with a small *c* and also called a *gram calorie*, is the amount of heat or energy required to raise the temperature of 1 g of water by 1°C. A *kilocalorie* (kcal) or *large Calorie*, which is equivalent to 1000 calories, is the amount of energy needed to raise the temperature of 1 kg of water by 1°C.[1] Because a gram calorie is so small, the kilocalorie or large Calorie, spelled with a capitol "C," is often used when discussing energy metabolism. The oxidation of proteins provides 4 kcal/g; fats, 9 kcal/g; carbohydrates, 4 kcal/g; and alcohol, 7 kcal/g.

Metabolism is the organized process through which nutrients such as carbohydrates, fats, and proteins are broken down, transformed, or otherwise converted into cellular energy. The process of metabolism is unique in that it enables the continual release of energy, and it couples this energy with physiologic functioning. For example, the energy used for muscle contraction is derived largely from energy sources that are stored in muscle cells and then released as the muscle contracts. Because most of our energy sources come from the nutrients in the food that is eaten, the ability to store energy and control its release is important.

Anabolism and Catabolism

There are two phases of metabolism: anabolism and catabolism. *Anabolism* is the phase of metabolic storage and synthesis of cell constituents. Anabolism does not provide energy for the body; it requires energy. *Catabolism* involves the breakdown of complex molecules into substances that can be used in the production of energy. The chemical intermediates for anabolism and catabolism are called metabolites. Both anabolism and catabolism are catalyzed by enzyme systems located in body cells. A *substrate* is a substance on which an enzyme acts. Enzyme systems selectively transform fuel substrates into cellular energy and facilitate the use of energy.

Because body energy cannot be stored as heat, the cellular oxidative processes that release energy are low-temperature reactions that convert food components to chemical energy that can be stored or dissipated. The body transforms carbohydrates, fats, and proteins into the intermediary compound, *adenosine triphosphate* (ATP).[1] ATP is called the *energy currency of the cell* because almost all body cells store and use ATP as their energy source. The metabolic events involved in ATP formation allow cellular energy to be stored, used, and replenished. However, under some circumstances, decreasing metabolic efficiency can increase energy expenditure. This process may have relevance to obesity (the more energy "wasted" as heat loss, the less weight gain) but is also important in maintaining body warmth in newborns. This is because the increased proportion of *brown fat* found in neonates is much less efficient at generating ATP than white fat, resulting in increased heat production.

Energy Storage

Adipose Tissue

More than 90% of body energy is stored in the adipose tissues of the body. *Adipocytes*, or fat cells, occur singly or in small groups in loose connective tissue. In many parts of the body, they cushion body organs such as the kidneys. In addition to isolated groups of fat cells, entire regions of fat tissue are committed to fat storage. Collectively, fat cells constitute a large body organ that is metabolically active in the uptake, synthesis, storage, and mobilization of lipids, which are the main source of stored fuel for the body. Some tissues, such as liver cells, are able to store small amounts of lipids, but when these lipids accumulate (so-called ectopic deposition, as occurs in fatty liver), they begin to interfere with normal cell function. Adipose tissue not only serves as a storage site for body fuels but also provides insulation for the body, fills body crevices, and protects body organs.

Studies of adipocytes in the laboratory have shown that fully differentiated cells do not divide. However, such cells have a long life span, and anyone born with large numbers of adipocytes runs the risk of becoming obese. Some immature adipocytes (termed *preadipocytes*) capable of division are present in postnatal life.[2] Fat deposition can result from proliferation of these existing immature adipocytes. Some medications can also have an important effect on fat cell numbers. The thiazolidinedione class of antidiabetic drugs can also stimulate the formation of new fat cells from preadipocytes, allowing increased uptake of glucose into these cells (and storage as fat) and resulting in the desired reduction in serum glucose levels, but with unwanted weight gain. In contrast, some drugs can cause loss of fat cells, resulting in lipodystrophy. This occurs in human immunodeficiency virus (HIV)-associated lipodystrophy in people treated with highly active antiretroviral therapy (HAART). The mechanism of fat loss is unknown. However, it may be due to increased programmed cell death of the adipocytes (*i.e.*, increased apoptosis).

There are two types of adipose tissue: white fat and brown fat. White fat, which despite its name is cream colored or yellow, is the prevalent form of adipose tissue in postnatal life. It constitutes 10% to 20% of body weight in adult men and 15% to 25% in adult women. At body temperature, the lipid content of fat cells exists as oil. It consists of triglycerides, which are three molecules of fatty acids esterified to a glycerol molecule. Triglycerides, which contain no water, have the highest caloric content of all nutrients and are an efficient form of energy storage. Fat cells synthesize triglycerides, the major fat storage form, from dietary fats and carbohydrates. Insulin is required for transport of glucose into fat cells. When calorie intake is restricted for any reason, fat cell triglycerides are broken down, and the resultant fatty acids and glycerol are released as energy sources.

Brown fat differs from white fat in terms of its thermogenic capacity or ability to produce heat. Brown fat is found primarily in early neonatal life in humans and in animals that hibernate. The major function of brown fat is to generate heat in animals or humans that do not shiver, and it contains a higher concentration of specialized mitochondria, which enable this process.[2] In humans, brown fat decreases with age but is still detectable in the sixth decade. This small amount of brown fat has a minimal effect on energy expenditure.

Adipose Tissue as an Endocrine Organ

Adipose tissue is now recognized as an endocrine and paracrine organ that secretes a number of important factors.[2] These factors are termed *adipokines* and include leptin, certain cytokines (*e.g.*, tumor necrosis factor-α [TNF-α]), growth factors, and adiponectin (important in insulin resistance). Figure 39.1 identifies many of the substances produced by adipose tissue.

The discovery of leptin (from the Greek meaning "thin"), a peptide released from adipocytes, has led to renewed interest in adipose tissue and its role in energy homeostasis. Recent studies suggest that leptin acts at the level of the hypothalamus to decrease food intake and increase energy expenditure through an increase in thermogenesis and sympathetic nervous system activity. Leptin is also involved in glucose metabolism and normal sexual maturation and reproduction and has interactions with the hypothalamic–pituitary–adrenal, thyroid, and growth hormones axes.

Leptin acts by binding, and activating, specific leptin receptors found in several peripheral tissues and in many areas of the brain, including specific regions of the hypothalamus. Receptors in these hypothalamic regions are known to be involved in appetite, food intake, sympathetic nervous system activity, temperature regulation, and insulin release by the pancreatic beta cells. Leptin levels tend to rise after food intake and fall during fasting. Adipose tissue signals the brain via leptin that sufficient storage of calories has been achieved and increased food intake is not necessary. *Leptin resistance* or a failure to respond to the high levels of leptin may result in obesity.[3]

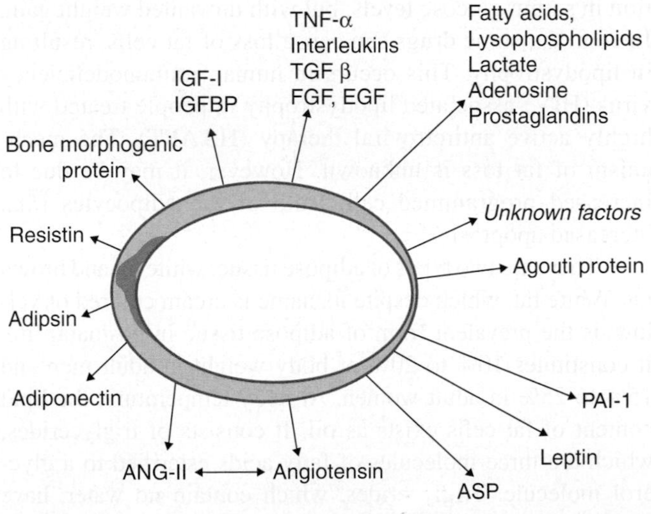

Figure 39.1 • Influence of adipose tissue secretions on other organs. Multiple proteins and metabolites are secreted by adipose tissue and act locally or at a distance in other organs. They have an impact on food intake, insulin signaling, vascular function, energy expenditure, and other homeostatic processes in the body. ANG-II, angiotensin II; ASP, acetylation-stimulating protein; EGF, epidermal growth factor; FGF, fibroblast growth factor; IGF, insulin-like growth factor; IGFBP, insulin-like growth factor-binding protein; PAI-1, plasminogen activating factor 1; TGF, transforming growth factor; TNF, tumor necrosis factor. (From Rubin R., Strayer D. (Ed.) (2012). *Rubin's pathology: Clinicopathologic foundations of medicine* (p. 1085). Philadelphia, PA: Lippincott Williams & Wilkins.)

Energy Expenditure

The expenditure of body energy results from five mechanisms of heat production (*i.e.*, thermogenesis): basal metabolic rate (BMR) or resting energy equivalent (REE), diet-induced thermogenesis, exercise-induced thermogenesis, nonexercise activity thermogenesis (NEAT), and thermogenesis in response to changes in environmental conditions. The amount of energy used varies with age, body size, rate of growth, and state of health.

Basal Metabolic Rate

The BMR refers to the minimum amount of energy expended that is compatible with life.[1] These reactions are necessary to provide energy for maintenance of normal body temperature, cardiovascular and respiratory function, muscle tone, and other essential activities of tissues and cells in the resting body. The BMR constitutes 50% to 70% of body energy needs.[4] The BMR is measured using an instrument called an *indirect calorimeter* that measures a person's rate of oxygen use. Oxygen consumption is measured under basal conditions: after a full night's sleep, after at least 12 hours without food, after no strenuous activity for 1 hour, and while the person is awake and at rest in a warm and comfortable room. Women in general have a 5% to 10% lower BMR than men because of their higher percentage of adipose tissue. Although much of the BMR is accounted for by essential activities of the central nervous system, kidneys, and other body organs, the variations in BMR among different people are related largely to skeletal muscle mass and body size. Under normal resting conditions, skeletal muscle accounts for 20% to 30% of the BMR.[5] For this reason, the BMR is commonly corrected for body size by expressing it as calories per hour per square meter of body surface area. Factors that affect the BMR are age, sex, physical state, and pregnancy. A progressive decline in the normal BMR occurs with aging and is likely related to loss of muscle mass and replacement with adipose tissue.[1] The BMR can be used to predict the calorie needs for maintenance of nutrition.

The REE is used for predicting energy expenditure. The most accurate way to determine REE is by indirect calorimetry. However, this is expensive and requires trained personnel. Multiplying the REE by a factor of 1.2 usually adequately predicts the caloric needs for maintenance of nutrition when the person is in a state of health. A factor of 1.5 usually provides the needed nutrients during repletion and during illnesses such as pneumonia, long bone fractures, cancer, peritonitis, and recovery from most types of surgery.

Diet- and Exercise-Induced Thermogenesis

Diet-induced thermogenesis, or thermic effect of food, describes the energy used by the body for the digestion, absorption, and assimilation of food after its ingestion. It is energy expended over and above the caloric value of the food and accounts for approximately 8% of the total calories expended. When food is eaten, the metabolic rate rises and then returns to normal within a few hours. The ingestion of a high-protein meal increases the normal metabolic rate more significantly, by up to 30%, and lasts 3 to 12 hours.

The type of activity performed, the length of participation, and the person's weight and physical fitness determine the amount of energy expended for physical activity. The most significant increases in metabolic rate come from strenuous activity.

Nonexercise Activity Thermogenesis

Energy expenditure can also be affected by increasing NEAT. NEAT includes the energy expended in maintaining posture and in activities such as fidgeting.[6] Lower percentage levels of NEAT may be related to a propensity to gain weight. People with increased NEAT may have less fat gain than those with decreased NEAT.

Environmentally Related Thermogenesis

Shivering in response to cold also produces heat through increased muscle activity. Nonshivering thermogenesis occurs in response to cold stress as well, caused by sympathetic nervous system activation, with the release of norepinephrine and epinephrine causing increased metabolic activity. Sympathetic stimulation also causes brown fat to generate heat.

Recent studies have shown that obese people with persistent excess caloric intake have increased sympathetic activity. Although the exact mechanism is not known, this appears to be triggered in part by leptin and results in increased thermogenesis. This increase in energy production can help to limit the amount of weight gained. Although clearly not enough to stop or reverse the weight gain process completely, it may contribute to the rate of weight gain or stabilization of overweight at a certain point.

IN SUMMARY

Nutritional status describes the condition of the body related to the availability and use of nutrients. Nutrients provide the energy and materials necessary for performing the activities of daily living and for the growth and repair of body tissues. Metabolism is the organized process whereby nutrients such as carbohydrates, fats, and proteins are broken down, transformed, or otherwise converted to cellular energy. Glucose, fats, and amino acids from proteins serve as fuel sources for cellular metabolism. These fuel sources are ingested during meals and stored for future use. Glucose is stored as glycogen or converted to triglycerides in fat cells for storage. Fats are stored in adipose tissue as triglycerides. Fat also functions as an endocrine organ in producing adipokines such as leptin and cytokines, which affect weight gain. Amino acids are the building blocks of proteins, and most of the stored amino acids are contained in body proteins and as fuel sources for cellular metabolism. Energy is measured in heat units called *calories*.

The expenditure of body energy results from heat production (*i.e.*, thermogenesis) associated with the BMR or basal energy equivalent, diet-induced thermogenesis, exercise-induced thermogenesis, NEAT, and thermogenesis in response to changes in environmental conditions.

NUTRITIONAL NEEDS

After completing this section of the chapter, the learner will be able to meet the following objectives:

- Discuss the different dietary standards that are utilized to formulate uniform diet guidelines for calories, proteins, fats, carbohydrates, fiber, vitamins, and minerals.
- Differentiate between hunger, appetite, and satiety.
- State the interactions between neurohormones in both short-term and long-term mechanisms to control food intake.

Dietary Reference Intakes

The *dietary reference intakes* (DRIs) include a set of nutrient-based reference values—the *recommended dietary allowance* (RDA), the *adequate intake* (AI), the estimated average requirement, the tolerable upper intake level, and the *acceptable macronutrient distribution range* (AMDR), each of which has specific uses.[7,8] The DRIs, which are periodically updated, are published by the National Academy of Sciences. The DRIs are used to advise people about the level of nutrient intake they need to decrease the risk of chronic disease. The current recommended DRIs for selected nutrients, vitamins, and minerals are available on the U.S. Department of Agriculture's (USDA) Food and Nutrition Information Center Web site at: http://fnic.nal.usda.gov/fnic/interactiveDRI/. This site contains an interactive tool that calculates a person's current nutritional needs based on gender, height, weight, age, and activity levels.[9]

The RDA defines the intakes that meet the nutrient needs of almost all healthy people in a specific age and sex group. The most recent guidelines have established RDA levels for carbohydrates but not for fats. Recommended fat intake is outlined in the AMDR and expressed as percentage of overall daily dietary intake, rather than a set level.[8]

The AI is set when there is not enough scientific evidence to estimate an average requirement. The AI is derived from experimental or observational data that show a mean intake that appears to sustain a desired indicator of health. An *estimated average requirement* is the intake that meets the estimated nutrient need of half of the people in a specific group. This figure is used as the basis for developing the RDA. Nutrition policy makers use this when evaluating the adequacy of a nutrient for a specific group and for planning how much of the nutrient the group should consume. The *tolerable upper intake* level is the maximum intake that is judged unlikely to pose a health risk in almost all healthy people in a specified group. It refers to the total intakes from food, fortified food, and nutrient supplements. This value is not intended to be a recommended level of intake, and there are no established benefits for people who consume nutrients at the RDA or AI levels.[8]

Food and supplement labels use *daily values* (DVs), which are set by the U.S. Food and Drug Administration (FDA). However, the DVs are based on data that are older than the data used to determine the DRIs. Percent daily value (%DV) tells the consumer what percentages of the DV one serving of a food or supplement supplies.

Nutritional Needs

Proteins, fats, carbohydrates, vitamins and minerals, and fiber each have their own function in providing the body with what it needs to maintain life and health.

Calories

Energy requirements are greater during growth periods. A person requires approximately 115 kcal/kg of body weight at birth, 105 kcal/kg at 1 year of age, and 80 kcal/kg from 1 to 10 years of age. During adolescence, boys require 45 kcal/kg of body weight and girls require 38 kcal/kg. During pregnancy, a woman needs an extra 300 kcal/day above her usual requirement, and during the first 3 months of breast-feeding, she requires an additional 500 kcal.[7]

Proteins

Proteins are required for growth and maintenance of body tissues, enzymes and antibody formation, fluid and electrolyte balance, and nutrient transport. Proteins are composed of amino acids, nine of which are essential to the body (*i.e.*, these amino acids cannot be synthesized by the body and must be derived from dietary sources). These are leucine, isoleucine, methionine, phenylalanine, threonine, tryptophan, valine, lysine, and histidine. Complete protein foods are those that provide these essential amino acids in adequate amounts. Complete proteins most often are derived from animal sources and include milk, eggs, meat, fish, and poultry. However, there are a few vegetable-derived complete protein sources, including soy and quinoa. Other vegetable proteins, including dried peas and beans, nuts, seeds, and grains, contain all the essential amino acids but in less than adequate proportions. These proteins need to be combined with each other to meet the amino acid requirements for protein synthesis (though combining them at one meal is not necessary). The average daily protein requirement is 30 to 50 g, provided the protein is of good quality, and the diet contains adequate carbohydrates and fats.[9] Diets that are adequate in calories but inadequate in protein can result in kwashiorkor. If both calories and protein are inadequate, protein–calorie malnutrition occurs (see the section, "Protein–Energy Malnutrition").

Fats

Fat is the most concentrated source of energy. The Food and Nutrition Board has set an AMDR for fat of 20% to 35% of daily caloric intake in adults, 25% to 35% in children between 4 and 18 years of age, and 30% to 40% in children between 1 and 3 years of age.[9] The daily dietary recommendation for cholesterol is <300 mg. Cholesterol is a waxy lipid contained in every body cell, which is produced in the liver. It is necessary for numerous body functions, including hormone production, metabolism of many vitamins, nerve function, and cell permeability. Excess cholesterol in the body can cause significant harm to the cardiovascular system and increase risk of serious cardiac disease. Careful monitoring of blood levels and reduction of dietary intake of cholesterol help to keep cholesterol levels in balance.

Dietary fats are composed primarily of triglycerides (*i.e.*, a mixture of fatty acids and glycerol). The fatty acids are saturated (*SFA*), monounsaturated (*MUFA*), or polyunsaturated (*PUFA*). The SFAs elevate blood cholesterol, whereas the monounsaturated and polyunsaturated fats lower blood cholesterol. Saturated fats usually are from animal sources and remain solid at room temperature. With the exception of coconut and palm oils (which are saturated), unsaturated fats are found in plant oils and usually are liquid at room temperature. *Trans fatty acids* (*TFAs*) are produced when unsaturated oils are partially hydrogenated and are called *artificial trans fats*. They are found primarily in vegetable shortenings, some margarines, and in foods containing either of these. Natural sources of TFAs include dairy products, some meats, and other animal-based foods. TFAs increase low-density lipoprotein (LDL) cholesterol ("bad cholesterol") and decrease high-density lipoprotein (HDL) cholesterol ("good cholesterol"). However, the naturally occurring trans fats may have a beneficial effect. Dietary fats provide energy, function as carriers for the fat-soluble vitamins, serve as precursors of prostaglandins, and are a source of fatty acids.

PUFAs, including linoleic acid (an omega-6 fatty acid) and alpha-linolenic acid (an omega-3 fatty acid), are examples of essential fatty acids. This means that they are not synthesized in the body and must be included in the diet. An AI has been set for both linoleic and alpha-linolenic acids.[9] Because certain vegetable oils are rich sources of alpha-linolenic and linoleic acid, the AI can be met by including two teaspoons per day of vegetable oil in the diet. Deficiency of linoleic acid results in dermatitis, and deficiency of alpha-linolenic acid can result in neurologic abnormalities and poor growth.

Omega-3 and omega-6 fatty acids have been found to contribute to both formation and treatment of many disease states. Gamma linolenic acid, a derivative of linoleic acid, may promote inflammation, whereas alpha-linolenic acid has been effective in treating some disease states with inflammatory states but not in others.[1] Much is still unknown about the effects of this group of nutrients. Omega-3 acids are primarily found in cold water fish, walnuts, and flaxseeds. Omega-6 fatty acids are found in seeds and nuts. In general, omega-6 fatty acids promote inflammation, blood clotting, and cell proliferation, whereas omega-3 fatty acids decrease these functions. A diet with a balanced intake of both is often recommended.

Carbohydrates

Dietary carbohydrates are composed of simple sugars, complex carbohydrates, and indigestible carbohydrates (*i.e.*, fiber). Because of their vitamin, mineral, and fiber content, it is recommended that the bulk of the carbohydrate content in the diet be in the complex form rather than as simple sugars that contain few nutrients.

Although some tissues, such as the nervous system, require glucose as an energy source, this need can be met through the conversion of amino acids and the glycerol part of the triglyceride molecule to glucose. The fatty acids from triglycerides are converted to ketones and used for energy by other body tissues. A carbohydrate-deficient diet usually results in the loss of tissue proteins and the development of ketosis. Because protein and fat metabolism increase the production of osmotically active metabolic wastes that must be eliminated through the kidneys, there is a danger of dehydration and electrolyte imbalances. The amount of carbohydrate needed to prevent tissue wasting and ketosis is 50 to 100 g/day.

In practice, carbohydrates should supply most of the daily energy requirement because many protein sources also are high in fat and more expensive. The AMDR indicates that carbohydrate intake should consist of 45% to 65% of the daily calories in the diet.[9]

Carbohydrates should be in the form of whole grains, vegetables, and fruits, which have higher fiber content compared to refined flour and sugar products.

Vitamins and Minerals

Vitamins. Vitamins are a group of organic compounds that act as catalysts in various chemical reactions. A compound cannot be classified as a vitamin unless it is shown that a deficiency of it causes disease. Contrary to popular belief, vitamins do not provide energy directly. As catalysts, they are part of the enzyme systems required for the release of energy from protein, fat, and carbohydrates. Vitamins also are necessary for the formation of red blood cells, hormones, genetic materials, and the nervous system. They are essential for normal growth and development.

There are two types of vitamins: fat soluble and water soluble. The four fat-soluble vitamins are vitamins A, D, E, and K. The nine required water-soluble vitamins are thiamine, riboflavin, niacin, pyridoxine (vitamin B_6), pantothenic acid, vitamin B_{12}, folic acid, biotin, and vitamin C. Fat-soluble vitamins are stored in the body and may reach toxic levels if ingested in amounts greater than what is required by the body. Because the water-soluble vitamins are excreted in the urine, they are less likely to accumulate in the body to toxic levels. Table 39.1 lists major food sources of vitamins.

Minerals. Minerals serve many functions. They are involved in acid–base balance and in the maintenance of osmotic pressure in body compartments. Minerals are components of vitamins, hormones, and enzymes. They maintain normal hemoglobin levels, play a role in nervous system function, and are involved in muscle contraction and skeletal development and maintenance. Minerals that are present in relatively

TABLE 39.1 MAJOR FOOD SOURCES OF VITAMINS

VITAMIN	MAJOR FOOD SOURCES
Vitamin A (retinol, provitamin, carotenoids)	Retinol: liver, butter, whole milk, cheese, egg yolk; provitamin A: carrots, green leafy vegetables, sweet potatoes, pumpkin, winter squash, apricots, cantaloupe, fortified margarine
Vitamin D (calciferol)	Fortified dairy products, fortified margarine, fish oils, egg yolk
Vitamin E (tocopherol)	Vegetable oil, margarine, shortening, green and leafy vegetables, wheat germ, whole-grain products, egg yolk, butter, liver
Vitamin C (ascorbic acid)	Broccoli, sweet and hot peppers, collards, Brussels sprouts, kale, potatoes, spinach, tomatoes, citrus fruits, strawberries
Thiamin (vitamin B_1)	Pork, liver, meat, whole grains, fortified grain products, legumes, nuts
Riboflavin (vitamin B_2)	Liver, milk, yogurt, cottage cheese, meat, fortified grain products
Niacin (nicotinamide, nicotinic acid)	Liver, meat, poultry, fish, peanuts, fortified grain products
Folacin (folic acid)	Liver, legumes, green leafy vegetables
Vitamin B_6 (pyridoxine)	Meat, poultry, fish, shellfish, green and leafy vegetables, whole-grain products, legumes
Vitamin B_{12}	Meat, poultry, fish, shellfish, eggs, dairy products
Biotin	Kidney, liver, milk, egg yolk, most fresh vegetables
Pantothenic acid	Liver, kidney, meats, milk, egg yolk, whole-grain products, legumes

TABLE 39.2 SOURCES AND FUNCTIONS OF MINERALS

MINERAL	MAJOR SOURCES	FUNCTIONS
Calcium	Milk and milk products, fish with bones, greens	Bone formation and maintenance; tooth formation, vitamin B absorption, blood clotting, nerve and muscle function
Chloride	Table salt, meats, milk, eggs	Regulates pH of stomach, acid–base balance, osmotic pressure of extracellular fluids
Cobalt	Organ meats, meats	Aids in maturation of red blood cells (as part of B_{12} molecule)
Copper	Cereals, nuts, legumes, liver, shellfish, grapes, meats	Catalyst for hemoglobin formation, formation of elastin and collagen, energy release (cytochrome oxidase and catalase), formation of melanin, formation of phospholipids for myelin sheath of nerves
Fluoride	Fluorinated water	Strengthens bones and teeth
Iodine	Iodized salt, fish	Thyroid hormone synthesis and its function in maintenance of metabolic rate
Iron	Meats, heart, liver, clams, oysters, lima beans, spinach, dates, dried nuts, enriched and whole-grain cereals	Hemoglobin synthesis, cellular energy release (cytochrome pathway), killing bacteria (myeloperoxidase)
Magnesium	Milk, green vegetables, nuts, bread, cereals	Catalyst of many intracellular nerve impulses, retention of reactions, particularly those related to intracellular enzyme reactions; low magnesium levels produce an increase in irritability of the nervous system, vasodilation, and cardiac arrhythmias
Phosphorus	Meats, poultry, fish, milk and cheese, cereals, legumes, nuts	Bone formation and maintenance; essential component of nucleic acids and energy exchange forms such as ATP
Potassium	Oranges, dried fruits, bananas, meats, potatoes, peanut butter, coffee	Maintenance of intracellular osmolality, acid–base balance, transmission of nerve impulses, catalyst in energy metabolism, formation of proteins, formation of glycogen
Sodium	Table salt, cured meats, meats, milk, olives	Maintenance of osmotic pressure of extracellular fluids, acid–base balance, neuromuscular function; absorption of glucose
Zinc	Whole-wheat cereals, eggs, legumes	Integral part of many enzymes, including carbonic anhydrase, which facilitates combination of carbon dioxide with water in red blood cells; component of lactate dehydrogenase, which is important in cellular metabolism; component of many peptidases; important in digestion of proteins in gastrointestinal tract

large amounts in the body are called *macrominerals*. These include calcium, phosphorus, sodium, chloride, potassium, magnesium, and sulfur. Other minerals are classified as *trace minerals* and include iron, manganese, copper, iodine, zinc, cobalt, fluorine, and selenium. Over- or underingestion of recommended levels of minerals can result in illness or toxicity. Table 39.2 provides a list of mineral sources and their functions.

Fiber

Total fiber, which has physioligic benefits includes dietary fiber, the nondigestible carbohydrates found in plants such as fruits, vegetables, beans, nuts, and whole grains; functional fiber, and isolated nondigestible carbohydrates. Functional fibers are synthetic or extracted from plant sources and added to food. Examples include psyllium and methylcellulose, and they are commonly found in processed foods. Dietary fiber provides increased bulk, viscosity, and fermentation. Bulking slows gastric emptying, therefore increasing satiety, and increases the rate of transport through the gastrointestinal tract, thereby increasing stool bulk and facilitating normal bowel movements. Viscosity thickens the lining of the intestinal track, helps moderate blood glucose levels, and lowers cholesterol levels. Fermentation contributes to growth of healthy intestinal bacteria and to immune system functioning. More studies are needed to establish whether fiber prevents colon cancer and promotes weight loss. In 2002, the Food and Nutrition Board gave its first recommended intake for fiber. Current recommendations for men and women who are young adults are 34 and 28 g, respectively, of fiber daily, whereas those older than 50 years should have 28 and 22 g, respectively, each day.[8,9]

Regulation of Food Intake and Energy Storage

Stability of body weight and composition over time requires that energy intake matches energy utilization. Environmental, cultural, genetic, and psychological factors all influence food intake and energy expenditure. In addition, body weight is tightly controlled by various physiologic feedback control systems that contribute to the regulation of hunger, food intake, and energy expenditure.[1]

Hunger, Appetite, and Control Mechanisms of Food Intake

The sensation of *hunger* is associated with several sensory perceptions, such as the rhythmic contractions of the stomach and that "empty feeling" in the stomach that stimulates a person to seek food. A person's *appetite* is the desire for a particular type of food. It is useful in helping the person determine the type of food that is eaten. *Satiety* is the feeling of fullness or decreased desire for food.

Two centers in the brain interact with various hormones and neurotransmitters to help control food intake and energy output. The arcuate nucleus of the hypothalamus has been identified as the center for hunger and satiety. Other centers in the brainstem also contribute to the mechanisms.[10] These centers receive neural input from the gastrointestinal tract that provides information about stomach filling, chemical signals from nutrients (glucose, amino acids, and fatty acids) in the blood, and input from the cerebral cortex regarding the smell, sight, and taste of the food. Centers in the hypothalamus also control the secretion of several hormones (*e.g.*, thyroid and adrenocortical hormones) that regulate energy balance and metabolism.

The control of food intake is subject to short-term regulation, which is concerned with the amount of food that is consumed at a meal or snack, and intermediate- and long-term regulation, which is concerned with the maintenance of energy stores over time.[11]

Neuro-hormones are responsible for the short-term regulation of food intake either by increasing feeding considered to be orexigenic or decreasing feeding classified as anorexigenic.[11] Figure 39.2 lists several of these neural messengers and the overall effects they promote. Over 30 gastrointestinal hormone genes have been identified that play a role in regulating hunger and satiety.[12] Research is providing additional insights into the complex system; however, much is still unknown.[12,13]

Three main short-term messengers that promote orexigenic effects include ghrelin, produced mainly in the stomach, and neuropeptide Y (NPY) and agouti-related protein (AGRP), both produced in the hypothalamus. Many of the other gut hormones have anorexigenic effects by signaling satiety to the neural centers. All of these messengers send messages of satiety that ultimately help decrease food intake.[10]

The intermediate- and long-term regulation of food intake is determined by the amount of nutrients that are in the blood and in storage sites. It has long been known that a decrease in blood glucose causes hunger. In contrast, an increase in breakdown products of lipids such as ketoacids produces a decrease in appetite. A ketogenic weight-loss diet (*e.g.*, the Atkins diet) relies partly on the appetite-suppressant effects of ketones in the blood.

Adipocytes release leptin in proportion to the amount of fat stores. The stimulation of leptin receptors in the hypothalamus produces a decrease in appetite and food intake as well as an increase in metabolic rate and energy consumption. It also produces a decrease in insulin release from the beta cells, which decreases energy storage in fat cells.[14]

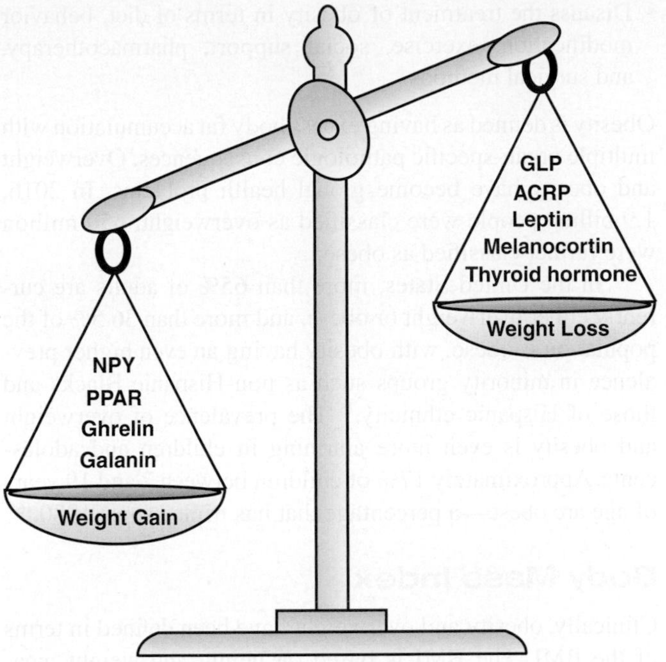

Figure 39.2 • The balance of chemical mediators impacting weight gain and loss. ACRP, adipocyte complement–related protein; GLP, glucagon-like peptide; NPY, neuropeptide Y; PPAR, peroxisome proliferator–activated receptor. (From Strayer D., Rubin R. (Ed.) (2015). *Rubin's pathology: Clinicopathologic foundations of medicine* (7th ed., Figure 13-1, p. 517). Philadelphia, PA: Lippincott Williams & Wilkins.

IN SUMMARY

The body requires more than 40 nutrients on a daily basis. Nutritional status reflects the continued daily intake of nutrients over time and the deposition and use of these nutrients in the body. The DRIs classify the amounts of essential nutrients considered to be adequate to meet the known nutritional needs of healthy people. The DRIs have 22 age and sex classifications and include recommendations for calories, proteins, fats, carbohydrates, vitamins, and minerals. Hunger and satiety are controlled by a complex group of neurohormones, many of which are produced in the gastrointestinal tract. These messengers function to either stimulate hunger or signal satiety to control both short- and long-term effects. Although much information has been revealed through research in recent years, there is still much to be learned in order to effectively manage the complex process more effectively.

OVERWEIGHT AND OBESITY

After completing this section of the chapter, the learner will be able to meet the following objectives:

- Explain the use of body mass index (BMI) in evaluating body weight.
- Define and discuss the causes and types of obesity and health risks associated with obesity.

- Discuss the treatment of obesity in terms of diet, behavior modification, exercise, social support, pharmacotherapy, and surgical methods.

Obesity is defined as having excess body fat accumulation with multiple organ-specific pathologic consequences. Overweight and obesity have become global health problems. In 2016, 1.9 billion people were classified as overweight; 650 million were further classified as obese.

In the United States, more than 65% of adults are currently either overweight or obese, and more than 36.5% of the population is obese, with obesity having an even higher prevalence in minority groups such as non-Hispanic Blacks and those of Hispanic ethnicity.[15] The prevalence of overweight and obesity is even more alarming in children and adolescents. Approximately 17% of children between 2 and 19 years of age are obese—a percentage that has tripled since 1980.[16]

Body Mass Index

Clinically, obesity and overweight have been defined in terms of the BMI. The BMI is based on height and weight measurements (see Fig. 39.3) and has a correlation with body fat. In 1997, the World Health Organization (WHO) defined the various classifications of overweight (BMI ≥ 25) and obesity (BMI ≥ 30). The National Institutes of Health (NIH) subsequently adopted this classification.[17] The use of a BMI cutoff of 25 as a measure of overweight raised some concern that the BMI of some men might be a function of muscle rather than fat weight. However, it has been shown that a BMI cutoff of 25 can sensitively detect most people with overweight and does not erroneously detect people with overlean.

The definition for obesity in children is a BMI at or above the sex- and age-specific 95th percentile, whereas a BMI between the 85th and 95th percentiles is defined as being overweight.[6] These criteria have been selected because they correspond to adult BMIs of 30 and 25, respectively.

Causes of Obesity

The epidemic of obesity results from many causative factors, and research is adding to the body of knowledge almost daily.

Although overweight and obesity ultimately result from an energy imbalance of eating too many calories and not getting enough physical activity, many factors contribute to both the development of obesity and the body's response to attempts to control it. Commonly acknowledged contributing causes include genetics, metabolism, behavior, environment, culture, and socioeconomic status.[13] Medical conditions such as thyroid disorder, Cushing syndrome, and polycystic ovarian syndrome can also contribute to weight gain and obesity, as do many medications.

The relationship between genetics and weight gain is complex and, as yet, not fully understood. The most recent update of the human obesity gene map, completed in 2005, suggests that there are 100 chromosomal locations relevant to obesity.[18] Many of these relate to known brain–gut controls of hunger and satiety, metabolism, and the body's storage mechanisms. Researchers believe that these theories may help to explain differences in obesity levels found in various populations. Identification of these genetic influences may allow for more targeted treatment interventions in the future. It is yet unknown how genes and mutations may directly or indirectly interact with environmental causes of obesity. One description for the complex interaction between environment and genetics is attributed to George Bray, a noted expert on obesity, who stated "the genetic background loads the gun, but the environment pulls the trigger."[19]

There is new evidence that behavior-based interventions may help keep genetic influence in check.[13]

Though genetic research gives new insight into the genesis of obesity, environmental influence remains the major contributor to this worldwide issue.[13,18] Obesity rates have reached epidemic proportions in populations with high availability of calorie-rich foods and few opportunities for physical activity.[18] Influences such as family eating patterns, time spent on the computer, watching television, reliance on the automobile for transportation, easy access to food, higher energy density of food, increased consumption of sugar-sweetened beverages, and increasing portion sizes have all been cited as contributing factors to overweight trends. More recent epidemiologic studies indicate that while decreased physical activity plays a role in increasing rates of overweight and obesity, diet changes because of increased availability of cheap, tasty, highly promoted, obesogenic types of food appear to have caused a much more steep rise in obesity.[20]

Psychological factors are another area of influence on behavior related to weight gain. Eating may be a way to cope with stress, mood, or anxiety.[21] Grazing, emotional eating, and binge eating disorder (BED) have been noted to be predictors for classifying obese patients.[22]

Culture and socioeconomic status are also believed to be contributing factors in the increased rates of overweight and obesity. It is clear that interventions will need to be developed to address the needs of different cultures, as well as to address the socioeconomic barriers to improved dietary choices.[13] Much discussion and debate will continue related to causative factors, especially as effective means to treat and prevent obesity are sought.

$$\textbf{Body Mass Index} = \frac{\text{weight in kilograms}}{\text{height in meters}^2} \quad \text{OR} \quad \frac{\text{weight in pounds}}{\text{height in inches}^2} \times 703$$

Figure 39.3 • Body mass index equation.

Types of Obesity

Two types of obesity based on distribution of fat have been described: upper body and lower body obesity (see Fig. 39.4). *Upper body obesity* is also referred to as *central, abdominal,*

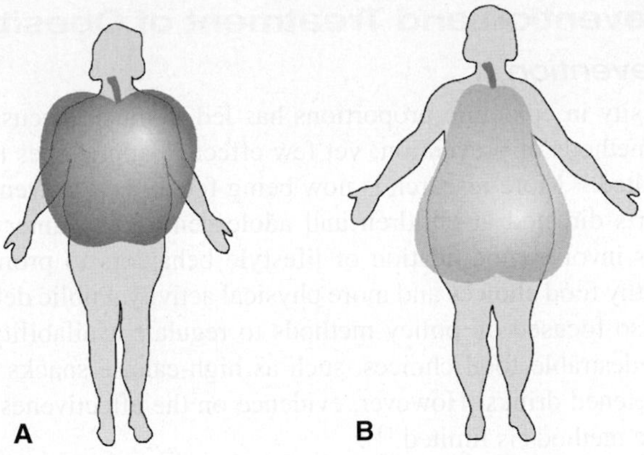

Figure 39.4 • Distribution of adipose tissue in (**A**) upper body or central (visceral) obesity and (**B**) lower body or peripheral (subcutaneous) obesity. People with upper body obesity are often described as having an "apple-shaped" body and those with lower body obesity as having a "pear-shaped" body.

visceral, or *male* ("*android*") obesity. Lower body obesity is also known as *peripheral, gluteal–femoral*, or *female* ("*gynoid*") obesity. Subjects with upper body obesity are often referred to as being shaped like an "apple" compared with lower body obesity, which is more "pear" shaped. In general, men have more intra-abdominal fat and women more subcutaneous fat. As men age, the proportion of intra-abdominal fat to subcutaneous fat increases. After menopause, women tend to acquire more central fat distribution.

The obesity type is determined by dividing the waist by hip circumference. Comparison of the waist measurement and hip measurement can identify the type of obesity. A waist–hip ratio >1.0 in men and 0.8 in women also indicates upper body or central obesity. Central obesity can be further differentiated into intra-abdominal adipose tissue (visceral fat) and subcutaneous abdominal adipose tissue by the use of computed tomography (CT) or magnetic resonance imaging (MRI) scans.[23] Waist circumference, which is a measure of central fat distribution, measures both subcutaneous abdominal adipose tissue and intra-abdominal adipose tissue. One of the characteristics of visceral fat is the release of adipokines (such as TNF-α and adiponectin) and fatty acids directly to the liver before entering the systemic circulation, having a potentially greater impact on hepatic function (*e.g.*, the increased fatty acids are deposited in the liver, causing fatty liver, resulting in insulin resistance in the liver). Higher levels of these adipokines and circulating free fatty acids in people with obese, particularly those with upper body obesity, are thought to be associated with many of the adverse effects of obesity.[24]

The presence of excess fat in the abdomen out of proportion to total body fat is an independent predictor of risk factors and mortality. Both BMI and waist circumference are positively correlated with total body adipose tissue, but waist circumference is a better predictor of abdominal or visceral fat content than BMI.[25] A waist circumference 88 cm (35 in) or greater in women and 102 cm (40 in) or greater in men has been associated with increased health risk[26] (see Table 39.3).

Weight loss causes a preferential loss of visceral fat (because of higher turnover of visceral fat cells than subcutaneous) and can result in improvements in metabolic and hormonal abnormalities. Although peripheral obesity is associated with varicose veins in the legs and mechanical problems, it is not as strongly associated with cardiometabolic risk. In terms of weight reduction, some studies have shown that people with upper body obesity are easier to treat than those with lower body obesity. Other studies have shown no difference in terms of success with weight reduction programs between the two types of obesity.

Health Risks Associated with Obesity

The excess body fat of obesity often significantly impairs health. As a result, obesity puts many people at risk for the some of the leading causes of death in the United States. These

TABLE 39.3 CLASSIFICATION OF OVERWEIGHT AND OBESITY BY BMI, WAIST CIRCUMFERENCE, AND ASSOCIATED DISEASE RISK*

			DISEASE RISK* RELATIVE TO NORMAL WEIGHT AND WAIST CIRCUMFERENCE	
	BMI (KG/M²)	OBESITY CLASS	*MEN ≤ 102 CM (≤40 INCHES) WOMEN ≤ 88 CM (≤35 INCHES)*	*MEN > 102 CM (>40 INCHES) WOMEN > 88 CM (>35 INCHES)*
Underweight	<18.5		–	–
Normal†	18.5–24.9		–	–
Overweight	25.0–29.9		Increased	High
Obesity	30.0–34.9	I	High	Very high
	35.0–39.9	II	Very high	Very high
Extreme obesity	≥40	III	Extremely high	Extremely high

BMI, body mass index.
*Disease risk for type 2 diabetes, hypertension, and cardiovascular disease.
†Increased waist circumference also can be a marker for increased risk, even in people of normal weight.
National Heart, Lung, and Blood Institute. (nd). Clinical guidelines on the identification, evaluation, and treatment of overweight and obesity in adults. Accessed April 16, 2018 from https://www.nhlbi.nih.gov/health/educational/lose_wt/BMI/bmi_dis.htm.

include stroke, cancer, diabetes, kidney disease, heart disease, and respiratory diseases.[27] It has been predicted that the health effects of obesity will result in a shorter life expectancy for today's youth.[28] Adults with a BMI > 40 have a shorter life expectancy by 6 to 13 years.[29]

Obesity affects nearly every body system (see Fig. 39.5). Cardiac disease is increased, as well as hypertension, hypertriglyceridemia, and decreased HDL cholesterol. Significant weight gain increases the risk of developing type 2 diabetes, obstructive sleep apnea, gastric reflux, urinary stress incontinence, and gallbladder disease. Limited mobility and increased joint disorders are functional results of increased weight on the body's skeletal system. In women, obesity can contribute to infertility, higher risk pregnancy, gestational diabetes, maternal hypertension, and difficulty in labor and delivery. Infants who are born to obese mothers are more likely to be high birth weight, contributing to an increased rate of cesarean section delivery. Several types of cancer are seen in higher frequency in people who are obese, including endometrial, colon, gallbladder, prostate, kidney, and postmenopausal breast cancer. Obesity also causes nonalcoholic steatohepatitis and fatty liver disease.[17,19]

In the United States as well as in other countries, there are many negative stereotypes associated with obesity.[30,31] People, especially women, are expected to be thin, and obesity may be seen as a sign of lack of self-control. Obesity may negatively affect employment and educational opportunities, as well as marital status.[31] Obesity may also play a role in a person's treatment by health professionals.[30] Although caregivers, physicians, and other health professionals are aware of the low success rate and difficulty in treating weight problems, they still may place the blame on the person with obesity.[30]

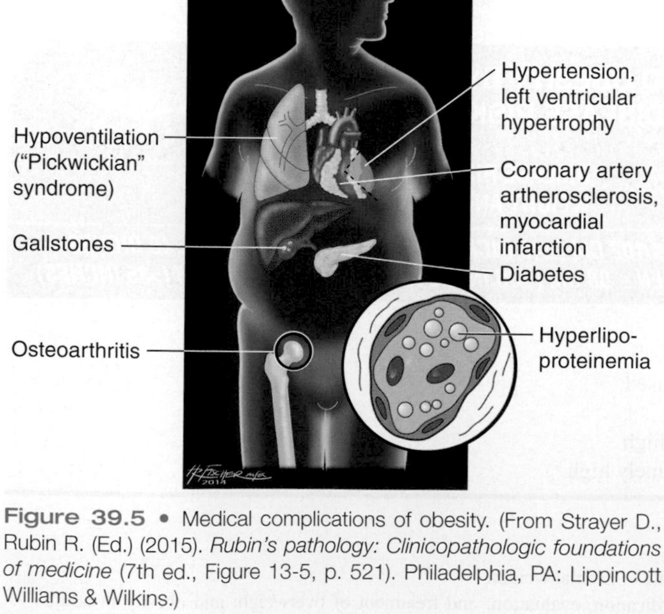

Figure 39.5 • Medical complications of obesity. (From Strayer D., Rubin R. (Ed.) (2015). *Rubin's pathology: Clinicopathologic foundations of medicine* (7th ed., Figure 13-5, p. 521). Philadelphia, PA: Lippincott Williams & Wilkins.)

Prevention and Treatment of Obesity

Prevention

Obesity in epidemic proportions has led to much discussion on methods of prevention; yet few effective approaches have resulted.[13] More research is now being focused on prevention efforts directed at children and adolescents. Most interventions involve modification of lifestyle behaviors to promote healthy food choices and more physical activity. Public debate is also focused on policy methods to regulate availability of less desirable food choices, such as high-calorie snacks and sweetened drinks. However, evidence on the effectiveness of these methods is limited.[13,18]

Major public education and policy efforts are now being undertaken by federal agencies. *We Can*! is a national educational program developed by the NIH to help children between 8 and 13 years old achieve or stay at a healthy weight by encouraging healthy eating, increasing physical activity, and reducing screen time for the family as a whole. Another program, entitled ChooseMyPlate.gov (see Fig. 39.6), developed by the USDA, translates dietary guidelines into demonstrable eating behaviors. Successful prevention measures will utilize not only governmental agency strategies and regulatory measures but also private sector initiatives and communication as well.[20]

Treatment

The current recommendation is that treatment is indicated in all people who have a BMI of 30 or higher and in those who have a BMI of 25 to 29.9 or a high waist circumference and an additional two or more risk factors.[32] Treatment should focus on individualized lifestyle modification through a combination of a reduced calorie diet, increased physical activity, and behavior therapy. These three modes of therapy form the basis of all weight management programs. Pharmacotherapy and surgery are available as adjuncts to lifestyle changes in people who meet specific criteria.

Before treatment begins, an assessment should be made of the degree of overweight and the overall risk status. This

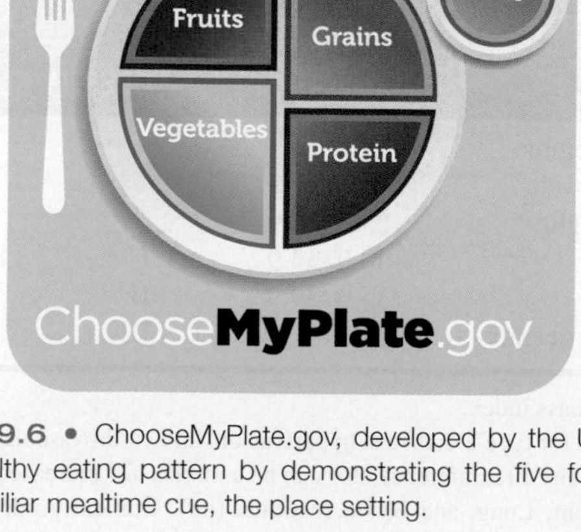

Figure 39.6 • ChooseMyPlate.gov, developed by the USDA, outlines a healthy eating pattern by demonstrating the five food groups using a familiar mealtime cue, the place setting.

should include assessment of the following risk factors or complications: coronary heart disease and other atherosclerotic diseases, sleep apnea, gynecologic abnormalities, osteoarthritis, gallstones, stress incontinence, cigarette smoking, hypertension, high LDL cholesterol levels, reduced HDL cholesterol levels, high triglyceride levels, prediabetes or type 2 diabetes, family history of premature coronary heart disease, and physical inactivity.[32]

It also is advisable to determine the person's barriers and readiness to lose weight. Several factors can be evaluated to make this assessment. These include reasons and motivations for weight loss, previous history of weight loss attempts, social support, attitude toward physical activity, ability to participate in physical activity, time available for attempting intervention, understanding the causes of obesity and its contribution to disease, and, finally, barriers the person has for making changes.

Dietary Therapy. The two major components of all diet therapy are caloric restriction and diet composition. Although diet modification and caloric restriction are important components of weight loss therapy, no one method has been shown to be most effective.[13] Therefore, dietary therapy should be individually prescribed based on the person's overweight status and risk profile. The diet should be a personalized plan with realistic goals.

Caloric restriction may vary from low-calorie diets (LCDs) to very-low-calorie diets (VLCDs). LCDs typically restrict caloric intake to 1200 kcal/day. This results in a variable reduction, depending on the initial dietary intake of the individual. VLCDs restrict calories to approximately 450 kcal/day, primarily made up of protein. This diet has higher risks, including abnormal heart rhythms and cholelithiasis. Anyone on this diet should be under direct supervision of a medical professional.

A more conservative dietary approach is to reduce the current dietary intake by 500 to 1000 kcal/day. Total caloric intake should be distributed in four or five meals or snacks throughout the day. Portion control is an effective technique to help achieve calorie reduction. Many overweight people have not practiced or monitored portion size. Keeping daily diet logs of all food ingested helps to increase awareness of both content and frequency. Meal replacements, such as protein shakes with vitamins and minerals, may also be used as a substitute for solid food meals.

After caloric restriction is determined, diet composition should be addressed. There are many methods of altering dietary content, including low-fat diets and low-carbohydrate/high-protein diets. Low-fat diets strive to limit daily calories from fat to 10% to 15% of total calorie intake. This level may be difficult to achieve and often is less palatable. Low-carbohydrate/high-protein diets became popular in the 1960s and 1970s. Although effective for weight loss, especially in the initial stages, they can contribute to health risks. Higher-protein diets can increase the risk of kidney stones, and the decrease in fiber can also increase risks of cancer and raise cholesterol levels.

Physical Activity. There is convincing evidence that increased physical activity decreases the risk of overweight and obesity. In addition, it reduces cardiovascular and diabetes risk beyond that achieved by weight loss alone. Although physical activity is an important part of weight loss therapy and helps with maintaining weight loss, it does not independently lead to a significant weight loss.[13] It may, however, help reduce abdominal fat, increase cardiorespiratory fitness, and prevent the decrease in muscle mass that often occurs with weight loss. Exercise should be started slowly with the duration and intensity increased independently of each other. The goal for adults should be a minimum of 150 to 300 minutes or more of moderate to vigorous activity per week to achieve and maintain a healthy weight.[9,13]

Behavior Therapy. Lifestyle modification is an essential factor in treating weight loss. Strategies include helping participants learn to self-monitor eating habits, including where and when they eat, and identifying situations that trigger eating behavior. Techniques for changing behavior include stress management, stimulus control, problem solving, contingency management, cognitive restructuring, social support, and relapse prevention.[32] Another important aspect to behavior modification is helping the person to set realistic weight loss goals.

Pharmacotherapy. Drugs approved by the USFDA can be used as an adjunct to the aforementioned regimen in some people with a BMI of 30 or more with no other risk factors or diseases and for people with a BMI of 27 or more with concomitant risk factors or diseases.[32] The risk factors and diseases defined as warranting pharmacotherapy are coronary heart disease, type 2 diabetes, metabolic syndrome, gynecologic abnormalities, osteoarthritis, gallbladder disease, stress incontinence, and sleep apnea.

Medications that have been approved for the treatment of obesity generally fall into one of two categories:

1. Reduction of food intake via the central nervous system
2. Action primarily outside the brain

Medications that primarily act via the central nervous system either block or activate portions of the neurotransmitter systems that are involved in signaling hunger and satiety. Pathways, which may be affected, include norepinephrine, serotonin, dopamine, and histamine. The endocannabinoid system is also known to affect food intake and is the focus of research for effective weight reduction therapy. Many psychoactive drugs have been shown to produce weight loss or weight gain as a side effect of their desired treatment goal, further emphasizing that these complex pathways exist. Drug development in this category, while promising in early stages, has thus far resulted in no effective, safe long-term treatments. Several sympathomimetic drugs have been approved for short-term therapy of 12 weeks or less.

Drugs that act peripherally include those that cause the blockade of lipase absorption in the gastrointestinal track ("fat-blockers") and newer drugs that target areas in the pancreas and intestine as well as the brain to help reduce food intake, increase insulin secretion, and slow gastric emptying.

A growing area of research and drug utilization includes non–FDA-approved usage of medications approved for other indications. Examples include antidepressants such as bupropion and fluoxetine, antiepileptic drugs such as topiramate, and antidiabetic medications such as metformin, pramlintide, and exenatide. With all such applications, use should be carefully monitored for any untoward side effects, as well as for desired weight loss effects.[33]

Weight Loss (Bariatric) Surgery. In people with clinically severe obesity (a BMI > 40) and in those with a BMI > 35 who have comorbid conditions who have failed medical attempts to control weight, surgical therapy is currently the most effective treatment of obesity. Weight loss surgery provides medically significant weight loss sustained for 10 years or more in most people.[32]

There are three types of weight loss surgery: (1) restrictive procedures, which reduce the amount of food that can be taken in; (2) malabsorptive procedures, which bypass sections of the intestine and result in less nutrients being absorbed; and (3) combined restrictive and malabsorptive procedures. Restrictive procedures include the adjustable gastric band and the sleeve gastrectomy, whereas the malabsorptive procedures include the biliopancreatic diversion with duodenal switch. The Roux-en-Y gastric bypass is the combined restrictive and malabsorptive procedure. Each surgery has specific risks and potential complications and requires lifelong nutritional monitoring after surgery. The key to long-term success and maintenance of weight loss after these surgical procedures is participation in a program that provides guidance in nutrition, physical activity, behavioral therapy, and social support.

One major benefit of weight loss surgery is resolution or remission of comorbid disease states. The significant improvement of type 2 diabetes symptoms and reduction of complications has prompted a joint statement by five international diabetes organizations that now include surgery in the treatment algorithm to improve outcomes.[34]

IN SUMMARY

Obesity is defined as having excess body fat accumulation with multiple organ-specific pathologic consequences. Genetic, socioeconomic, cultural, and environmental factors; psychological influences; and activity levels have been implicated as causative factors in the development of obesity. There are two types of obesity—upper body and lower body obesity. Upper body obesity is associated with a higher incidence of health risks. The health risks associated with obesity affect almost every body system. The treatment of obesity focuses on nutritionally adequate weight loss diets, behavior modification, exercise, social support, and, in situations of marked obesity, pharmacotherapy, and surgical methods.

UNDERNUTRITION AND EATING DISORDERS

After completing this section of the chapter, the learner will be able to meet the following objectives:

- State the difference between protein–calorie starvation (*i.e.*, marasmus) and protein malnutrition (*i.e.*, kwashiorkor).
- Explain the effect of malnutrition on muscle mass, respiratory function, acid–base balance, wound healing, immune function, bone mineralization, the menstrual cycle, and testicular function.
- Compare the eating disorders of anorexia and bulimia nervosa (BN) and the complications associated with each.

Undernutrition continues to be a major health problem throughout the world. Globally, undernourished rates have been falling over the past few decades, although they increased to 815 million in 2016, up from 777 million in 2015.[35,36] Developing countries have a prevalence of 12.9% undernourished populations and are responsible for 98% of the overall total.[36] In developed countries, undernutrition is most commonly seen in the pediatric and older adult populations.[37]

Malnutrition and Starvation

Malnutrition and starvation are conditions in which a person does not receive or is unable to use an adequate amount of nutrients for body function. An adequate diet should provide adequate energy in the form of carbohydrates, fats, and proteins; essential amino acids and fatty acids for use as building blocks for synthesis of structural and functional proteins and lipids; and vitamins and minerals, needed to function as coenzymes or hormones in vital metabolic processes, or, as in the case of calcium and phosphate, as important structural components of bone.

Among the many causes of malnutrition are poverty and ignorance, acute and chronic illness, and self-imposed dietary restriction. Homeless people, older adults, and children of the poor often demonstrate the effects of protein and energy malnutrition, as well as vitamin and mineral deficiencies. Even the affluent may fail to recognize that infants, adolescents, and pregnant women have increased nutritional needs. Some types of malnutrition are caused by acute and chronic illnesses, such as occurs in people with Crohn disease who are unable to absorb nutrients from their food. Anorexia nervosa (AN) and less overt eating disorders affect a large population of people who are concerned about body image or athletic performance.

Protein–Energy Malnutrition

Protein and energy (calorie) malnutrition represents a depletion of the body's lean tissues caused by starvation or a combination of starvation and catabolic stress. The lean tissues are the fat-free, metabolically active tissues of the body, namely, the skeletal muscles, viscera, and cells of the blood and immune system. Because lean tissues are the largest body compartment, their rate of loss is the main determinant of total body weight in most cases of protein–energy malnutrition.

Much of the literature on malnutrition and starvation has dealt with infants and children in underdeveloped countries in which food deprivation results in an inadequate intake of protein and calories to meet the body's energy needs. Protein–energy malnutrition in this population commonly is divided into two distinct conditions: marasmus (protein and calorie deficiency) and kwashiorkor (protein deficiency). The pathologic changes for both types of malnutrition include humoral and cellular immunodeficiencies resulting from protein deficiency and lack of immune mediators. There is impaired synthesis of pigments of the hair and skin (*e.g.*, hair color may change and the skin may become hyperpigmented) because of a lack of substrate (tyrosine) and coenzymes.

Marasmus represents a progressive loss of muscle mass and fat stores because of inadequate food intake that is equally deficient in calories and protein.[38] It results in a reduction in body weight adjusted for age and size. The child with marasmus has a wasted appearance, with loss of muscle mass, stunted growth, and loss of subcutaneous fat; a protuberant abdomen (from muscular hypotonia); wrinkled skin; sparse, dry, and dull hair; and depressed heart rate, blood pressure, and body temperature. Diarrhea is common. Because immune function is impaired, concurrent infections occur and place additional stress on an already weakened body. An important characteristic of marasmus is growth failure; if sufficient food is not provided, these children will not reach their full potential stature.[38]

Kwashiorkor results from a deficiency in protein.[38] The term *kwashiorkor* comes from an African word meaning "the disease suffered by the displaced child," because the condition develops soon after a child is displaced from the breast after the arrival of a new infant and placed on a starchy gruel feeding. Kwashiorkor is a more severe form of malnutrition than marasmus. Unlike marasmus, severe protein deficiency is associated with extensive loss of the visceral protein compartment with a resultant hypoalbuminemia that gives rise to generalized or dependent edema. The child with kwashiorkor usually presents with edema, desquamating skin, discolored hair, anorexia, and extreme apathy (Fig. 39.7). There are "flaky paint" lesions of the skin on the face and extremities. In addition, the hair becomes a sandy or reddish color, with linear depigmentation (flag sign).[39,40] There is generalized growth failure and muscle wasting as in marasmus, but subcutaneous fat is normal because calorie intake is adequate. Other manifestations include skin lesions, hepatomegaly and distended abdomen, cold extremities, and decreased cardiac output and tachycardia.

Marasmus–kwashiorkor is an advanced protein–energy deficit coupled with increased protein requirement or loss. This results in a rapid decrease in anthropometric measurements, with obvious edema and wasting and loss of organ mass. One essential aspect of severe protein–energy malnutrition is fatty degeneration of such diverse organs as the heart and liver. This degeneration causes subclinical and overt cardiac dysfunction, especially when malnutrition is accompanied by edema. A second injurious aspect is the loss of subcutaneous fat, which markedly reduces the body's capacity for temperature regulation and water storage. As a consequence, malnourished children become dehydrated and hypothermic more quickly and more severely than normally nourished children. Most children with severe protein–energy malnutrition have asymptomatic infections because their immune system fails to respond appropriately. Their immune system is so depressed that many are unable to produce the fever that is typical of an acute infection.

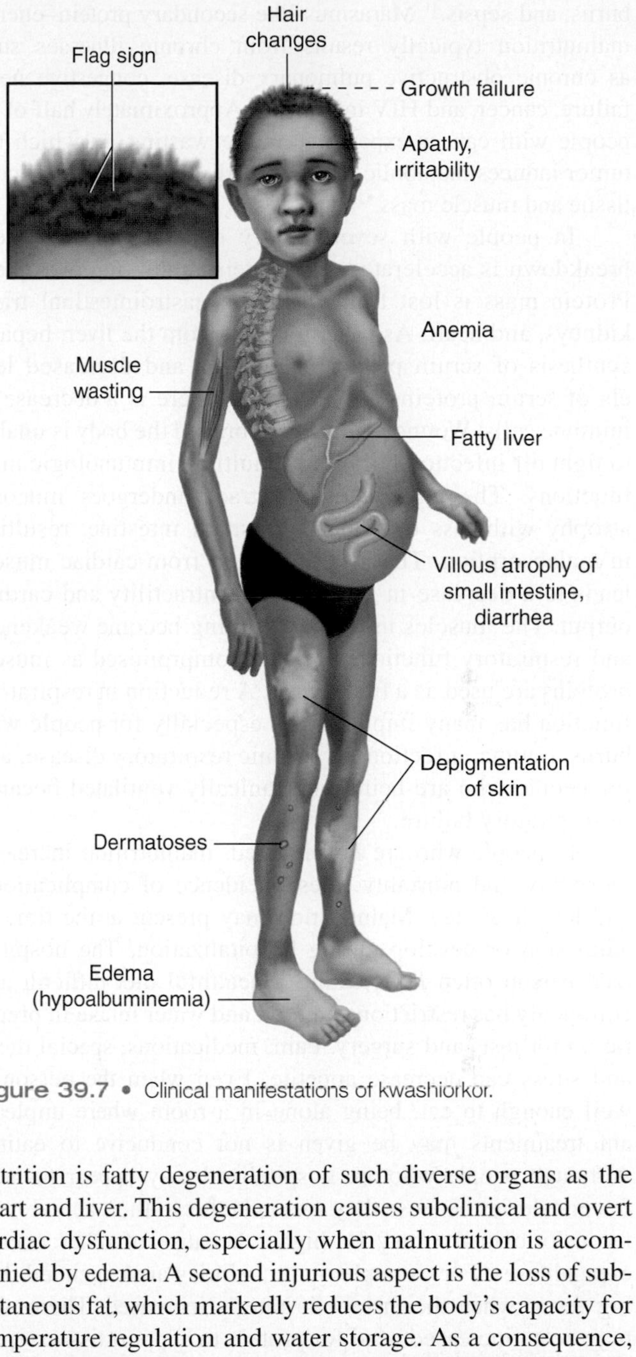

Figure 39.7 • Clinical manifestations of kwashiorkor.

Malnutrition in Trauma and Illness

In industrialized societies, protein–energy malnutrition most often occurs secondary to trauma or illness. Kwashiorkor-like protein malnutrition occurs most commonly in association with hypermetabolic acute illnesses, such as trauma, burns, and sepsis.[41] Marasmus-like secondary protein–energy malnutrition typically results from chronic illnesses such as chronic obstructive pulmonary disease, congestive heart failure, cancer, and HIV infection.[38] Approximately half of all people with cancer experience tissue wasting, in which the tumor induces metabolic changes leading to a loss of adipose tissue and muscle mass.[42]

In people with severe injury or illness, net protein breakdown is accelerated and protein rebuilding disrupted. Protein mass is lost from the liver, gastrointestinal tract, kidneys, and heart. As protein is lost from the liver, hepatic synthesis of serum proteins decreases and decreased levels of serum proteins are observed. There is a decrease in immune cells. Wound healing is poor, and the body is unable to fight off infection because of multiple immunologic malfunctions. The gastrointestinal tract undergoes mucosal atrophy with loss of villi in the small intestine, resulting in malabsorption. The loss of protein from cardiac muscle leads to a decrease in myocardial contractility and cardiac output. The muscles used for breathing become weakened, and respiratory function becomes compromised as muscle proteins are used as a fuel source. A reduction in respiratory function has many implications, especially for people with burns, trauma, infection, or chronic respiratory disease, and for people who are being mechanically ventilated because of respiratory failure.

In people who are hospitalized, malnutrition increases morbidity and mortality rates, incidence of complications, and length of stay. Malnutrition may present at the time of admission or develop during hospitalization. The hospitalized person often finds eating a healthful diet difficult and commonly has restrictions on food and water intake in preparation for tests and surgery. Pain, medications, special diets, and stress can decrease appetite. Even when the person is well enough to eat, being alone in a room where unpleasant treatments may be given is not conducive to eating. Although people who are hospitalized may appear to need fewer calories because they are on bed rest, their actual need for caloric intake may be higher because of other energy expenditures. For example, more calories are expended during fever, when the metabolic rate is increased. There also may be an increased need for protein to support tissue repair after trauma or surgery.

Diagnosis

No single diagnostic measure is sufficiently accurate to serve as a reliable test for malnutrition. Techniques of nutritional assessment include evaluation of dietary intake, anthropometric measurements, nutrition-focused physical examination, and laboratory tests.[43] Evaluation of body composition can be assessed with weight, edema, muscle wasting, and subcutaneous fat loss. Serum albumin and prealbumin are used in the diagnosis of protein–calorie malnutrition. Albumin, which has historically been used as a determinant of nutrition status, has a relatively large body pool and a half-life of 20 days and is less sensitive to changes in nutrition than prealbumin, which has a shorter half-life and a relatively small body pool.[43]

Treatment

The treatment of severe protein–energy malnutrition involves the use of measures to correct fluid and electrolyte abnormalities and replenish proteins, calories, and micronutrients. Treatment is started with modest quantities of proteins and calories based on the person's actual weight. Concurrent administration of vitamins and minerals is needed. Either the enteral or parenteral route can be used. The treatment should be undertaken slowly to avoid complications. The administration of water and sodium with carbohydrates can overload a heart that has been weakened by malnutrition and result in heart failure. Enteral feedings can result in malabsorptive symptoms because of abnormalities in the gastrointestinal tract. Refeeding edema is benign-dependent edema that results from renal sodium reabsorption and poor skin and blood vessel integrity. It is treated by elevation of the dependent area and modest sodium restrictions. Diuretics are ineffective and may aggravate electrolyte deficiencies.

Eating Disorders

Eating disorders affect an estimated 30 million Americans of all ages and gender.[44] These illnesses, which include AN, BN, and BED and their variants, incorporate serious disturbances in eating, such as restriction of intake and binging, with an excessive concern over body shape or body weight.[44] Eating disorders manifest in both men and women, with occurrence in women at slightly higher rates. BED is the most common of the eating disorders in the United States.[45]

Eating disorders are more prevalent in industrialized societies and occur in all socioeconomic and major ethnic groups. A combination of genetic, biologic, behavioral, psychological, and social factors is thought to contribute to the development of the disorders.[45] Preoccupation with weight and excessive self-evaluation of weight and shape are common to all disorders, and people with eating disorders may demonstrate a mixture of symptoms from the disorders.[45] People with eating disorders may require concomitant evaluation for psychiatric illness because eating disorders often are accompanied by mood, anxiety, and personality disorders.

Anorexia Nervosa

AN is an eating disorder that usually begins in adolescence and is characterized by determined dieting, often accompanied by compulsive exercise and, in a subgroup of people, purging behavior with or without binge eating, resulting in sustained low weight. Other features include a disturbed body image, a pervasive fear of becoming obese, and an obsession with severely restricted caloric intake and frequently with excessive physical exercise. AN is more prevalent among young women compared to men.[44,46]

The causes of anorexia appear to be multifactorial, with determinants that include genetic influence; personality traits of perfectionism and compulsiveness; anxiety disorders; family history of depression and obesity; and peer, familial, and cultural pressures with respect to appearance. Diagnostic criteria for AN are (1) a refusal to maintain a minimally normal body weight for age and height (*e.g.*, at least 85% of minimal expected weight or BMI ≥ 17.5); (2) an intense fear of gaining weight or becoming fat; (3) a disturbance in the way one's body size, weight, or shape is perceived; and (4) amenorrhea (in girls and women after menarche).[47] Other psychiatric disorders often coexist with AN, including major depression or dysthymia, and obsessive–compulsive disorder.

Many organ systems are affected by the malnutrition that accompanies AN. The severity of the abnormalities tends to be related to the degree of malnutrition and is reversed by refeeding. The most frequent complication of anorexia is amenorrhea and loss of secondary sex characteristics with decreased levels of estrogen, which can eventually lead to osteoporosis. Bone loss can occur, and symptomatic compression fractures and kyphosis have been reported.[44] Constipation, cold intolerance, and failure to shiver when cold, bradycardia, hypotension, decreased heart size, electrocardiographic changes, blood and electrolyte abnormalities, and increased growth of lanugo (*i.e.*, fine hair) are common. Abnormalities in cognitive function may also occur. The brain loses both white and gray matter during severe weight loss; there is a correlation between gray matter loss and duration of illness.[48] Unexpected sudden deaths have been reported; the risk appears to increase as weight drops to <35% to 40% of ideal weight. It is believed that these deaths are caused by myocardial degeneration and heart failure rather than arrhythmias.

One of the most challenging aspects of the treatment of anorexia is the inability of the person with anorexia to recognize that there is a problem. People with the disorder are usually willing to talk about their preoccupation with weight loss, food refusal and rituals about food, and excessive exercise routines; purging and laxative use; and withdrawal from activities and relationships but have difficulty recognizing this behavior as pathologic.[44] Because anorexia is a form of starvation, it can lead to death if left untreated. A multidisciplinary approach appears to be the most effective method of treating people with the disorder.[49] The goals of treatment are eating and weight gain; resolution of issues with the family; healing of pain from the past; and efforts to work on psychological, relationship, and emotional issues. Specialized eating disorder treatment programs may include inpatient hospitalization, partial hospitalization, or intensive outpatient specialty eating disorder programs, depending on the level of weight loss, medical complications, and availability of family support.

Bulimia Nervosa

BN is defined by recurrent binge eating and activities such as vomiting, fasting, excessive exercise, and use of diuretics, laxatives, or enemas to compensate for that behavior. The criteria for BN are (1) recurrent binge eating (at least two times per week for 3 months); (2) inappropriate compensatory behaviors such as self-induced vomiting, abuse of laxatives or diuretics, fasting, or excessive exercise that follow the binge eating episode; (3) self-evaluation that is unduly influenced by body shape and weight; and (4) a determination that the eating disorder does not occur exclusively during episodes of AN.[46,47] In contrast to AN, which is characterized by a weight that is <85% of the normal value, most people with BN are of normal weight. The diagnostic criteria for BN now include subtypes to distinguish people who compensate by purging (*e.g.*, vomiting or abuse of laxatives or diuretics) and those who use nonpurging behaviors (*e.g.*, fasting or excessive exercise). The disorder may be associated with other psychiatric disorders such as anxiety disorder or depression. There is also an association with substance abuse and risky and self-destructive behaviors.[44]

The complications of BN include those resulting from overeating, self-induced vomiting, and cathartic and diuretic abuse.[44] Among the complications of self-induced vomiting are dental disorders, parotitis, and fluid and electrolyte disorders. Dental abnormalities, such as sensitive teeth, increased dental caries, and periodontal disease, occur with frequent vomiting because the high acid content of the vomitus causes tooth enamel to dissolve. Esophagitis, dysphagia, and esophageal strictures are common. With frequent vomiting, there often is reflux of gastric contents into the lower esophagus because of relaxation of the lower esophageal sphincter. Vomiting may lead to aspiration pneumonia, especially in intoxicated or debilitated people. Potassium, chloride, and hydrogen are lost in the vomitus, and frequent vomiting predisposes to metabolic alkalosis with hypokalemia. An unexplained physical response to vomiting is the development of benign, painless parotid gland enlargement.

The weights of people with BN may fluctuate, although not to the dangerously low levels seen in AN. Their thoughts and feelings range from fear of not being able to stop eating to a concern about gaining too much weight. They also experience feelings of sadness, anger, guilt, shame, and low self-esteem.

Treatment strategies include psychological and pharmacologic treatments. Cognitive–behavioral therapy and interpersonal therapy are predominantly used.[44] These therapies are designed to help the person become aware of other ways to cope with the feelings that precipitate the desire to purge and to try to correct maladaptive beliefs regarding their self-image. Unlike people with AN, people with BN or binge eating are upset by the behaviors practiced and the thoughts and feelings experienced, and they are more willing to accept help. Antidepressants such as serotonin reuptake inhibitors have been found to be useful in treating bulimia and BEDs and one, fluoxetine, has received USFDA approval for treatment.[33]

Eating Disorder Not Otherwise Specified

Eating disorder not otherwise specified (EDNOS) is a diagnostic category for people who have eating disorder symptoms but do not meet the full criteria for either AN or BN. Within this group is the subgroup, BED.

Binge Eating Disorder. Binge eating is characterized by recurrent episodes of binge eating at least 2 days per week for 6 months and at least three of the following: (1) eating rapidly; (2) eating until becoming uncomfortably full; (3) eating large amounts when not hungry; (4) eating alone because of embarrassment; and (5) disgust, depression, or guilt because of eating episodes. The great majority of people with BED are overweight, and, in turn, people with obesity have a higher prevalence of BED than the nonobese population.[44,46]

The primary goal of therapy for BED is to establish a regular, healthful eating pattern. People with BED who have been successfully treated for their eating disorder have reported that making meal plans, eating a balanced diet of three regular meals a day, avoiding high-sugar foods and other binge foods, recording food intake and binge eating episodes, exercising regularly, finding alternative activities, and avoiding alcohol and drugs are helpful in maintaining their more healthful eating behaviors after treatment.

IN SUMMARY

Undernutrition can range from a selective deficiency of a single nutrient to starvation, in which there is deprivation of all nutrients. Malnutrition and starvation are among the most widespread causes of morbidity and mortality in the world. Protein–energy malnutrition in this population commonly is divided into two distinct conditions: marasmus (protein and calorie deficiency) and kwashiorkor (protein deficiency). Malnutrition is common during illness, recovery from trauma, and hospitalization. The effects of malnutrition and starvation on body function are widespread. They include loss of muscle mass, impaired wound healing, impaired immunologic function, decreased appetite, loss of calcium and phosphate from bone, anovulation and amenorrhea in women, and decreased testicular function in men.

AN and BN are eating disorders that result in malnutrition. In AN, distorted attitudes about eating lead to determined dieting, weight loss to below 85% of normal body weight, and malnutrition. BN is characterized by secretive episodes or binges of eating large quantities of easily consumed, high-calorie foods, followed by compensatory behaviors such as fasting, self-induced vomiting, or abuse of laxatives or diuretics. EDNOS is a new diagnostic category for patients who have eating disorders such as BED but do not meet the full criteria for either AN or BN.

GERIATRIC Considerations

- Obesity rates increase after age 60,[50] most likely due to a reduction in lean skeletal muscle and an increase in adipose tissue.[51]
- Basal metabolism (BM rate) decreases by 2% each decade of life; exercise and decreased calorie intake is needed to maintain desired weight with increased age.[51]
- Obesity in older adults increases risk for falls, decreased oxygen saturation at rest, need for indwelling urinary catheters, and risk of admission to long-term care.[51]
- Decreased number of taste buds places aging adult at risk for increased caloric intake of salts and sweets to compensate for loss of taste.[52]
- Loss of teeth and poor condition of remaining teeth in many aging adults contribute to poor nutrition because of pain and inability to properly chew foods.[52]
- Nutritional needs of older adults must take into consideration the decrease in energy expenditure. The Harris-Benedict equation (or resting energy expenditure), shown below, determines the calorie needs to maintain current body weight with no exercise expenditure[52]:

Males : $66 + [13.7 \times \text{weight (kg)}] + [5 \times \text{height (cm)}] - (6.76 \times \text{age in years})$

Females : $655 + [9.6 \times \text{weight (kg)}] + [1.8 \times \text{height (cm)}] - (4.7 \times \text{age in years})$

- Familial hypercholesterolemia results in high levels of LDL and cholesterol deposits in the arteries, tendons, and skin increasing the risk for atherosclosclerosis.[53]

PEDIATRIC Considerations

- Obesity rates are increasing at an earlier age, with almost 9% of 2- to 5-year-old children being considered obese.[50]
- When the child is developing, key nutrients are important and must be balanced with exercise and proper nutrition to prevent obesity and set positive lifelong eating habits.[50]
- Lack of proper nutrition is linked to decreased cognitive ability, lowered mental well-being, increased childhood morbidity, and stunted physical growth.[54]

- Breast milk and commercial infant formulas are fortified to provide adequate nutrition for children up to 12 months of age; cow's or goat's milk may lead to anemia because of decreased amounts of iron. Low- and nonfat milk should be avoided because they do not support the nutritional needs of the growing child.[3]
- Amino acid disorders include PKU (discussed earlier in chapter) and maple syrup urine disease, an inherited autosomal recessive disorder, which causes severe neurologic symptoms because of insufficiency of branched-chain 2-oxoacid dehydrogenase, recognized by a sweet odor of body fluids. Early intervention and dietary management can prevent encephalopathy and developmental delays.[55]
- Mineral disorders include Menkes disease (X-linked recessive) and Wilson disease (autosomal recessive disorder), which are associated with an altered copper metabolism can lead to toxicity and death unless early screening and interventions occur. X-linked hypophosphatemic rickets (X-linked dominant) results in an inability of the renal tubes to absorb phosphate, leading to phosphaturia in the urine and hypophosphatemia in the serum and causing bowing of the legs and dental decay.[55]
- Carbohydrate disorders include galactosemia (inherited autosomal recessive trait), in which galactose can't be metabolized, causing severe and sometimes fatal damage to the neurologic, renal, reproductive, and sensory systems.[55]
- Mucopolysaccharide disorders such as Hurler syndrome (autosomal recessive trait) are the result of lipid and polysaccharide storage defects. This particular disorder is characterized by "gargoyle" facies, with death ensuing in the first decade from respiratory or cardiac failure.[55]

REVIEW EXERCISES

1. A 25-year-old woman is 65 in (165 cm) tall and weighs 300 lb (136 kg). She works as a receptionist in an office, brings her lunch to work with her, spends her evenings watching television, and gets very little exercise. She reports that she has been fat ever since she was a little girl, has tried "every diet under the sun," and when she diets she loses some weight, but gains it all back again.
   A. *Calculate her BMI*
   B. *How would you classify her obesity?*
   C. *What are her risk factors for obesity?*
   D. *What would be one of the first steps in helping her develop a plan to lose weight?*
2. A 16-year-old high school student is brought into the physician's office by her mother, who is worried because her daughter insists on dieting because she thinks she is too fat. The daughter is 67 in (170 cm) tall and weighs 96 lb (43.5 kg). Her history reveals that she is a straight-A student, plays in the orchestra, and is on the track team. Although she had been having regular menstrual periods, she has not had a period in 4 months. She is given a tentative diagnosis of AN.
   A. *What are the criteria for a diagnosis of AN?*
   B. *What is the physiologic reason for her amenorrhea?*
   C. *What are some of the physiologic manifestations associated with malnutrition and severe weight loss?*

References

1. Mahan L., Raymon J. (2017). *Karuse's food and nutrition care process* (14th ed., pp. 31–55, 41, 57–58). St. Louis, MO: Elsevier Saunders.
2. Rosen E. D., Spiegelman B. M. (2014). What we talk about when we talk about fat. *Cell* 156(0), 20–44. http://doi.org/10.1016/j.cell.2013.12.012.
3. Bowden V. R., Greenberg C. S. (2014). *Children and their families: The continuum of nursing care* (3rd ed.). Philadelphia, PA: Wolters Kluwer.
4. Loureiro L. L., Fonseca S., Castro N. G., et al. (2015). Basal metabolic rate of adolescent modern pentathlon athletes: Agreement between indirect calorimetry and predictive equations and the correlation with body parameters. *PLoS ONE* 10(11), e0142859.
5. Smith I. C., Bombardier E., Vigna C., et al. (2013). ATP consumption by sarcoplasmic reticulum Ca^{2+} pumps accounts for 40-50% of resting metabolic rate in mouse fast and slow twitch skeletal muscle. *PLoS ONE* 8(7), e68924.
6. Villablance P., Alegria J., Mookadam F., et al. (2015). Nonexercise activity thermogenesis in obesity management. *Mayo Clinic Proceedings* 90(4), 509–519.
7. Kominiarek M., Rajan P. (2016). Nutrition recommendations in pregnancy and lactation. *Medical Clinics of North America* 100(6), 1199–1215.
8. Panel on Macronutrients, Panel on the Definition of Dietary Fiber, Subcommittee on Upper Reference Levels of Nutrients, Subcommittee on Interpretation and Uses of Dietary Reference Intakes, and the Standing Committee on the Scientific Evaluation of Dietary Reference Intakes. (2005). *Dietary reference intakes for energy, carbohydrate, fiber, fat, fatty acids, cholesterol, protein and amino acids (macronutrients)*. Washington, DC: National Academies Press.
9. U.S. Department of Health and Human Services and U.S. Department of Agriculture. (2015). *Dietary Guidelines for Americans 2015–2020* (8th ed.). Available at: http://health.gov/dietaryguidelines/2015/guidelines/. Accessed March 8, 2018.
10. Adamska E., Ostrowska L., Górska M., et al. (2014). The role of gastrointestinal hormones in the pathogenesis of obesity and type 2 diabetes. *Przegląd Gastroenterologiczny* 9(2), 69–76. http://doi.org/10.5114/pg.2014.42498.
11. Perry B., Wang Y. (2012). Appetite regulation and weight control: The role of gut hormones. *Nutrition & Diabetes* 2(1), e26.
12. Office of Surveillance, Epidemiology, and Laboratory Services, Public Health Genomics. (2010). Obesity and genetics. [Online]. Available: http://www.cdc.gov/genomics/resources/diseases/obesity/index.htm. Accessed March 9, 2018.
13. Hruby A., Hu F. B. (2015). The epidemiology of obesity: A big picture. *PharmacoEconomics* 33(7), 673–689. http://doi.org/10.1007/s40273-014-0243-x 1.

14. Fu Z., Gilbert E. R., Liu D. (2013). Regulation of insulin synthesis and secretion and pancreatic beta-cell dysfunction in diabetes. *Current Diabetes Reviews* 9(1), 25–53.
15. Ogden C. L., Carroll M. D., Fryar C. D., et al. (2015). *Prevalence of obesity among adults and youth: United States, 2011–2014*. NCHS data brief, no 219. Hyattsville, MD: National Center for Health Statistics.
16. Center for Disease Control and Infection. Childhood obesity facts. (2017). (Online). Available: https://www.cdc.gov/obesity/data/childhood.html. Accessed March 25, 2018.
17. World Health Organization. Obesity and overweight. (2018). [Online]. Available: http://www.who.it/mediacentre/factsheets/fs311/en. Accessed March 9, 2018.
18. Rao K. R., Lal N., Giridharan N. V. (2014). Genetic & epigenetic approach to human obesity. *The Indian Journal of Medical Research* 140(5), 589–603.
19. Bray G. A. (2004). The epidemic of obesity and changes in food intake: The fluoride hypothesis. *Physiological Behavior* 82, 115–121.
20. Malik V. S., et al. (2013). *Nature Reviews Endocrinology* 9, 13–27. doi:10.1038/nrendo.2012.199.
21. Singh M. (2014). Mood, food, and obesity. *Frontiers in Psychology* 5, 925.
22. Caroleo M., Primerano A, Rania M, et.al. (2018). A real world study on the genetic, cognitive and psychopathological differences of obese patients clustered according to eating behavours. *European Psychiatriaty* 48, 58–64.
23. Wang H., Chen Y. E., Eitzman D. T. (2014). Imaging body fat: Techniques and cardiometabolic implications. *Arteriosclerosis, Thrombosis, and Vascular Biology* 34(10), 2217–2223.
24. Lee M., Wu Y., Fried S. (2013). Adipose tissue heterogeneity: Implication of depot differences inadipose tissue for obesity complications. *Molecular Aspects of Medicine* 341, 1–11.
25. Barreira T., Staiano A., Harrington D., et al. (2012). Anthropometric correlates of total body fat, abdominal adiposity, and cardiovascular disease risk factors in a biracial sample of men and women. *Mayo Clinic Proceeding* 87(5), 452–460.
26. National Heart, Lung, and Blood Institute. (2018). (Online). Available: https://www.nhlbi.nih.gov/health/educational/lose_wt/BMI/bmi_dis.htm. Accessed March 25, 2018.
27. Center for Disease Control. (2014). (Online). Available: https://www.cdc.gov/healthreport/publications/compendium.pdf. Accessed March 9, 2018.
28. American Heart Association. (2018). (Online). Available: http://www.heart.org/HEARTORG/HealthyLiving/HealthyKids/ChildhoodObesity/Overweight-in-Children_UCM_304054_Article.jsp#.Wr2LLdPwZmA. Accessed March 25, 2018.
29. Kitahara C. M., Flint A. J., Berrington de Gonzalez A., et al. (2014). Association between class III obesity (BMI of 40–59 kg/m^2) and mortality: A pooled analysis of 20 prospective studies. *PLoS Medicine* 11(7), e1001673. http://doi.org/10.1371/journal.pmed.1001673.
30. Phelan S. M., Burgess D. J., Yeazel M. W., et al. (2015). Impact of weight bias and stigma on quality of care and outcomes for patients with obesity. *Obesity Review* 16, 319–326. doi:10.1111/obr.12266.
31. O'Brien K., Latner J., Ebneter D., et al. (2013). Obesity discrimination: The role of physical appearance, personal ideology, and anti-fat prejudice. *International Journal of Obesity* 37, 455–460.
32. O'Brien P., MacDonald L., Anderson M., et al. (2013). Long-term outcomes after bariatric surgery: Fifteen-year follow-up of adjustable gastric banding and a systematic review of the bariatric surgical literature. *Annals of Surgery* 257(1), 87–94.
33. Flament M. F., Bissada H., Spettigue W. (2012). Evidence-based pharmacotherapy of eating disorders. *International Journal of Neuropsychopharmacology* 15(2), 189–207, https://doi.org/10.1017/S1461145711000381.
34. Rubino F., Nathan D., Eckel R., et. al. (2017). Metabolic surgery in the treatment algorithm for type 2 diabetes: A joint statement by international diabetes organizations. *Obesity Surgery* 27(1), 2–21.
35. FAO, IFAD, UNICEF, WFP and WHO. (2017). *2017 The state of food security and nutrition in the world: Building resilience for peace and food security*. Rome: FAO.
36. Roser M., Ritchie H. (2018). Hunger and undernourishment. Available: https://ourworldindata.org/hunger-and-undernourishment. Accessed March 25, 2018.
37. Morley J. (2012). Undernutrition in older adults. *Family Practice* 29, 89–93.
38. Guyton A. C., Hall J. E. (2011). *Textbook of medical physiology* (12th ed., pp. 807–810, 859–866, 880–887). Philadelphia, PA: Elsevier Saunders.
39. Trehan I., Manary M. J. (2015). Management of severe acute malnutrition in low-income and middle-income countries. *Archives of Disease in Childhood* 100, 283–287.
40. Nigam P. K., Nigam P. (2017). Premature greying of hair (premature canities): A concern for parent and child. *Pigmentary Disorders* 4, 261.
41. Mehta N., Corkins M., Lyman B. (2013). Defining pediatric malnutrition: A paradigm shift toward etiology-related definitions. *Journal of Parenteral and Enteral Nutrition* (37)4, 460–481.
42. Rosen E. D., Spiegelman B. M. (2014). What we talk about when we talk about fat. *Cell* 156(0), 20–44. http://doi.org/10.1016/j.cell.2013.12.012.
43. Bharadwaj S., Ginoya S., Tandon P., et al. (2016). Malnutrition: Laboratory markers vs nutritional assessment. *Gastroenterology Report* 4(4), 272–280. http://doi.org/10.1093/gastro/gow013.
44. National Eating Disorders Association. (2018). (Online). Available: https://www.nationaleatingdisorders.org/learn. Accessed March 9, 2018.
45. National Institute of Mental Health. Eating disorders. (2016). (Online). Available: https://www.nimh.nih.gov/health/topics/eating-disorders/index.shtml. Accessed March 9, 2018.
46. National Association of Anorexia Nervosa and Associated Disorders. Statistics on eating disorders. (2016). [Online]. Available: http://www.anad.org/get-information/about-eating-disorders/eating-disorders-statistics/. AccessedMarch 9, 2018.
47. American Psychiatric Association. (2013). *Diagnostic and statistical manual of mental disorders* (5th ed.). Arlington, VA: American Psychiatric Publishing.
48. Fonville L., Giampietro V., Williams S., et al. (2014). Alterations in brain structure in adults with anorexia nervosa and the impact of illness duration. *Psychological Medicine* 44(9), 1965–1975. doi:10.1017/S0033291713002389.
49. American Psychiatric Association. (2012). Guideline watch (August 2012): *Practice guideline for the treatment of patients with eating disorders* (3rd ed.). [Online]. Available: https://psychiatryonline.org/pb/assets/raw/sitewide/practice_guidelines/guidelines/eatingdisorders-watch.pdf. Accessed March 9, 2018.
50. Segal L. M., Rayburn J., Martin A. (2016). *The state of obesity: Better policies for a healthier America: 2016*. Robert Wood Johnson Foundation. Retrieved April 8, 2018. stateofobesity.org/files/stateofobesity2016.pdf.
51. Cheever K. H. (2018). Assessment and management of patients with obesity. In Hinkle J. L., Cheever K. H. (Ed.) *Brunner & Suddarth's textbook of medical-surgical nursing* (14th ed.). Philadelphia, PA: Wolters Kluwer.
52. Epiopoulos C. (2018). *Gerontological nursing*. (9th ed.). Philadelphia, PA: Wolters Kluwer.
53. Strayer D. S., Rubin E. (Eds.) (2015). *Rubin's pathology: Clinicopathologic foundations of medicine* (7th ed). Philadelphia, PA: Wolters Kluwer.
54. Kyle T., Carman S. (2017). *Essentials of pediatric nursing*. Philadelphia, PA: Wolters Kluwer.
55. Goodhue C. J. (2014). The child with an inborn error of metabolism. In Bowden V. R., Greenberg, C. S. (Eds.) *Children and their families the continuum of nursing care*. Philadelphia, PA: Wolters Kluwer.

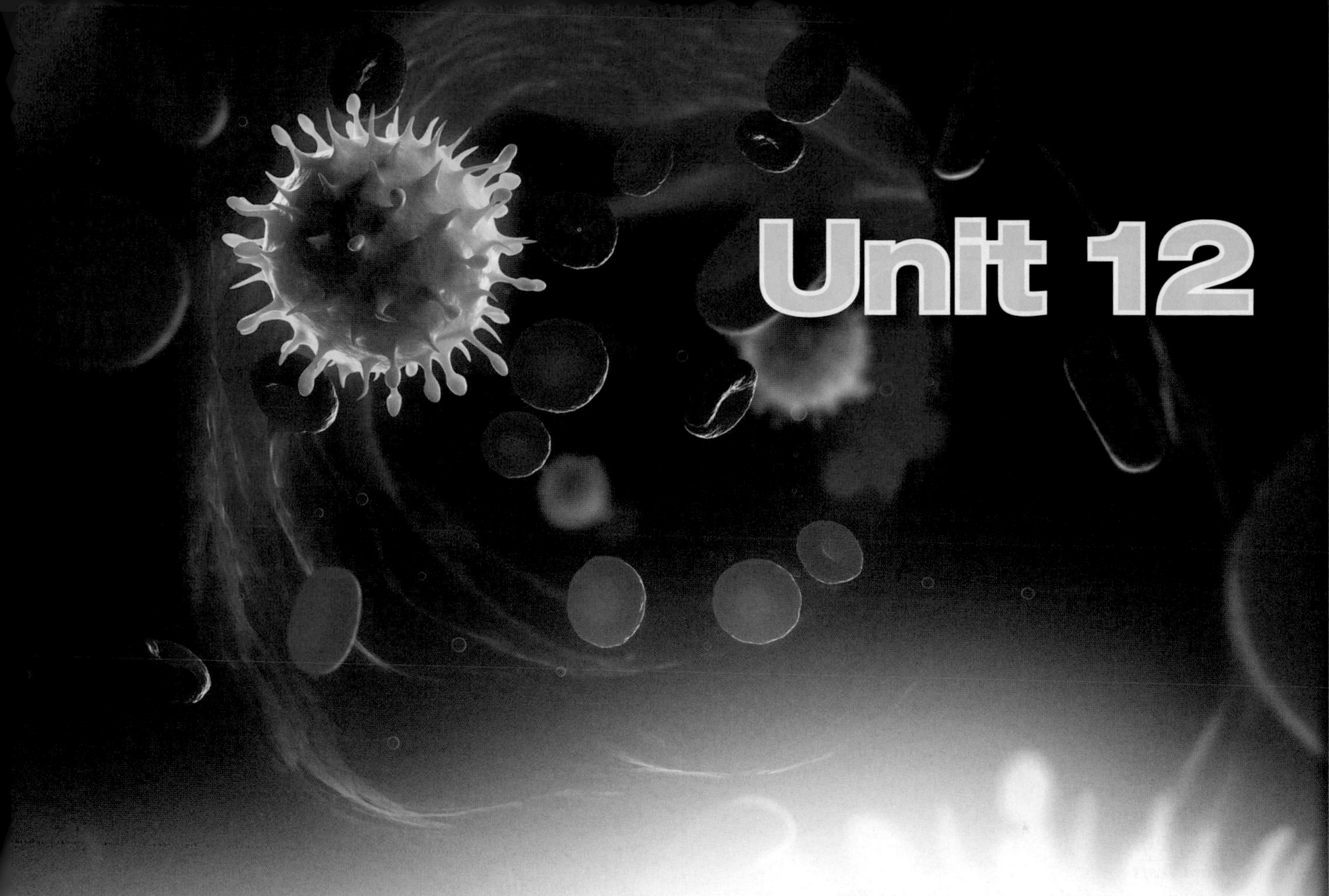

Unit 12

Disorders of Endocrine Function

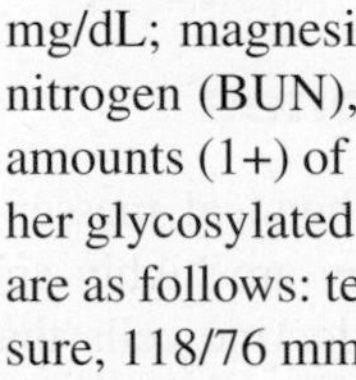

Emily Toronto, 7 years old, has been feeling nauseous for the last few days. Her mother states that she has been very thirsty and urinating frequently over the last 2 months. Today, she has vomited three times and is lethargic. Her mother says her breath smells "fruity," and she seems slightly confused. Emily's past medical history is unremarkable, but her grandfather has type 1 diabetes mellitus. She is admitted to the hospital's pediatric unit. Arterial blood gas analysis indicates that she is in metabolic acidosis (arterial pH, 7.29; $PaCO_2$, 42 mm Hg [normal, 35 to 45 mm Hg]); bicarbonate ($HCO3^-$) 10 mEq/L (normal 21 to 28 mEq/L). Blood chemistry test results include the following: glucose, 650 mg/dL; calcium, 10.4 mg/dL; magnesium, 1.1 mg/dL; phosphate, 3.2 mg/dL (normal, 2.7 to 4.5 mg/dL); blood urea nitrogen (BUN), 44 mg/dL; and creatinine, 2.4 mg/dL. Urinalysis reveals the presence of small amounts (1+) of ketones. Her complete blood count (CBC) with differential is unremarkable, but her glycosylated hemoglobin level (hemoglobin A1c) is 10% (normal, 4% to 7%). Her vital signs are as follows: temperature, 98.3°F; pulse, 126/minute and normal sinus rhythm; and blood pressure, 118/76 mm Hg. Her respiratory rate is fast (46/minute) and irregular. She is diagnosed with diabetic ketoacidosis and type 1 diabetes mellitus.

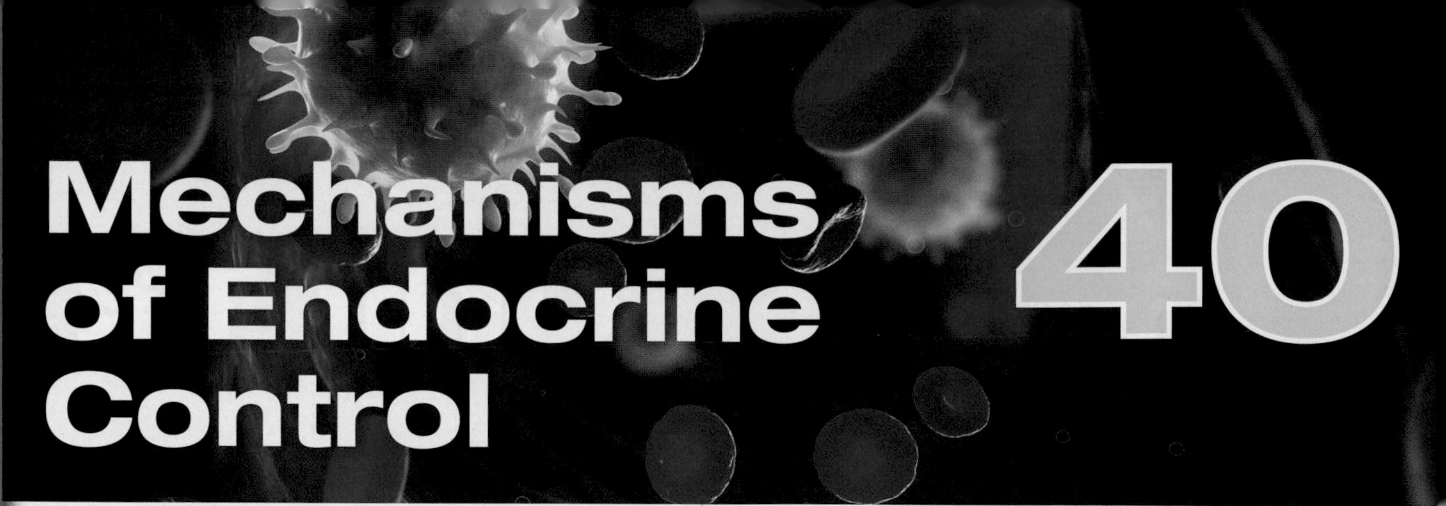

Mechanisms of Endocrine Control

40

Linda C. Mefford

The endocrine system is involved in all of the integrative aspects of life, including growth, sex differentiation, metabolism, and adaptation to an ever-changing environment. This chapter focuses on the general aspects of endocrine function, organization of the endocrine system, hormone receptors and hormone actions, and regulation of hormone levels.

THE ENDOCRINE SYSTEM

After completing this section of the chapter, the learner will be able to meet the following objectives:

- State the function of a hormone receptor and the difference between cell surface hormone receptors and intracellular hormone receptors.
- Describe the role of the hypothalamus in regulating pituitary control of endocrine function.
- State the major difference between positive and negative feedback control mechanisms.

The endocrine system uses chemical substances called *hormones* as a means of regulating and integrating body functions. The endocrine system participates in many essential body functions, including the regulation of digestion, the usage and storage of nutrients, growth and development, electrolyte and water metabolism, and reproductive functions. The endocrine network does not work in isolation. It is closely integrated with the central and peripheral nervous systems as well as with the immune systems. Therefore, the terms "neuroendocrine" or "neuroendocrine–immune" are often used to describe these interactions.[1,2]

Hormones

Hormones are chemical messengers that are transported in body fluids. They are highly specialized organic molecules produced by endocrine cells that exert their action on specific target cells. The word *hormone* is from the Greek word for "arouse to activity."[2] Hormones do not perform reactions themselves, but instead hormones function as modulators of cellular and systemic responses. Most hormones are present in body fluids at all times, in greater or lesser amounts depending on the needs of the body.[3,4] Hormones are released from various organs that are classically considered as "endocrine glands," including the pituitary gland, thyroid gland, adrenal glands, and pancreas. However, it is becoming increasingly evident that many other organs and tissues throughout the body also actively secrete hormonal substances that regulate activities in other areas of the body. These "nonclassical" endocrine tissues include organs such as the heart, kidneys, liver and gastrointestinal tract, as well as lymphocytes and adipose tissue.[2,3]

A characteristic of hormones is that a single hormone can exert a specific effect in distant body tissues. For example, the heart is the principal source of atrial natriuretic peptide, which acts to induce natriuresis in a distant target organ—the kidney. Erythropoietin is produced by the kidney in response to renal hypoxia and then travels through the blood to stimulate erythropoiesis in the bone marrow.[3] In some situations, several different hormones work together to regulate a single function. Lipolysis, which is the release of free fatty acids from adipose tissue, is an example of a single function that is regulated by several hormones. Lipolysis is regulated by the actions of the catecholamines, insulin, and glucagon as well as by a cytokine, tumor necrosis factor-α.[5] Table 40.1 lists the major actions and sources of selected hormones.

Hormonal Actions

Hormonal actions are classified based on the relationship between where the hormone is produced and where the biologic effects occur. Classifications include endocrine, paracrine, autocrine, intracrine, and neuroendocrine (Chart 40.1). The effect is *endocrine* when a hormone is released into the circulation and then travels in the blood to produce a biologic effect on distant target cells.[6] Alternately, some hormones and hormone-like substances never enter the bloodstream but instead act locally in the vicinity in which they are released. When they act locally on cells other than those that produced the hormone, the action is called *paracrine*. The action of sex steroids on the ovary is a paracrine action. The hormone effect is *autocrine* when a hormone produces a biologic effect on the same cell that produced it.[6] For example, the release of insulin from pancreatic beta cells can inhibit the release of additional insulin from the same cells. The final classification of hormone effect, *intracrine*, describes a hormone that is synthesized and acts intracellularly in the same cell.[7] Some hormonal effects are *neuroendocrine*, in which the hormone (a *neurohormone*) is produced and released from neurons and then travels through the blood to exert effects on target cells in the body. Vasopressin (antidiuretic hormone [ADH]) and epinephrine are examples of hormonal substances with neuroendocrine effects.[6] Neurohormones are subtype of signaling molecules known as neurotransmitters, which are released from neurons and traverse the synaptic cleft for a variety of postsynaptic responses.[3]

CHART 40.1 HORMONAL ACTIONS

- Endocrine: Hormones are released to circulation to act on a target organ
- Paracrine: Hormones act locally on cells in the vicinity of where they are released
- Autocrine: Hormones produce a biologic action on the cell that released them
- Intracrine: Hormone action is within the cell that produced it
- Neuroendocrine: Hormone produced within a neuron then travels through circulation to exert effects on target cells

Structural Classification

Hormones have diverse structures, ranging from single amino acids to complex proteins and lipids. Hormones may be classified into four categories based on their chemical structure.[2]

1. Amines and amino acids
2. Peptides proteins, and glycoproteins
3. Steroids
4. Fatty acids

Examples of hormones for each of these structural classifications are shown in Table 40.2.

The first category, the amines, includes norepinephrine and epinephrine, which are derived from a single amino acid (*i.e.*, tyrosine), and the thyroid hormones, which are derived from two iodinated tyrosine amino acid residues.[2] The second category of hormones, the protein-based hormones, constitutes the majority of hormones. These protein hormones can

KEY POINTS

HORMONES

- Hormones function as chemical messengers, moving through the blood to distant target sites of action (endocrine), or acting more locally as paracrine or autocrine messengers to produce more local effects. The term intracrine describes a hormone that is synthesized and acts within the same cell. The term neuroendocrine refers to hormonal substances produced by and secreted from neurons, which then travel through the blood to exert effects on target cells.
- Hormones exert their actions by interacting with high-affinity cellular receptors linked to one or more effector systems in the cell. Some hormone receptors are located on cell surfaces and act through second messenger mechanisms. Others are intracellular receptors, which can act to alter processes within the cell nucleus and thereby modulate the synthesis of proteins.

TABLE 40.1 MAJOR ACTION AND SOURCE OF SELECTED HORMONES

SOURCE	HORMONE	MAJOR ACTION
Hypothalamus	Releasing and inhibiting hormones CRH TRH GHRH GnRH	Controls the release of pituitary hormones
	Somatostatin	Inhibits GH and TSH
	Dopamine	Inhibits prolactin release from the pituitary Inhibits FSH and LH
Anterior pituitary	GH	Stimulates growth of bone and muscle, promotes protein synthesis and fat metabolism, decreases carbohydrate metabolism
	ACTH	Stimulates synthesis and secretion of adrenal cortical hormones
	TSH	Stimulates synthesis and secretion of thyroid hormone
	FSH	Female: stimulates growth of ovarian follicle, ovulation Male: stimulates sperm production
	LH	Female: stimulates development of corpus luteum, release of oocyte, production of estrogen and progesterone Male: stimulates secretion of testosterone, development of interstitial tissue of testes
	Prolactin	Prepares female breast for breast-feeding
Posterior pituitary	ADH (arginine vasopressin, AVP)	Increases water reabsorption by kidney
	Oxytocin	Stimulates contraction of pregnant uterus, milk ejection from breasts after childbirth
Adrenal cortex	Mineralocorticosteroids, mainly aldosterone	Increases sodium absorption, potassium loss by kidney
	Glucocorticoids, mainly cortisol	Affects metabolism of all nutrients; regulates blood glucose levels, affects growth, has anti-inflammatory action, and decreases effects of stress
	Adrenal androgens, mainly dehydroepiandrosterone (DHEA) and androstenedione	Have minimal intrinsic androgenic activity; they are converted to testosterone and dihydrotestosterone (DHT) in the periphery
Adrenal medulla	Epinephrine Norepinephrine	Serve as neurotransmitters for the sympathetic nervous system
Thyroid (follicular cells)	Thyroid hormones: triiodothyronine (T_3), thyroxine (T_4)	Increase the metabolic rate; increase protein and bone turnover; increase responsiveness to catecholamines; necessary for fetal and infant growth and development
	Calcitonin	Lowers blood calcium and phosphate levels
Parathyroid glands	Parathyroid hormone (PTH)	Regulates serum calcium
Pancreatic islet cells	Insulin	Lowers blood glucose by facilitating glucose transport across cell membranes of muscle, liver, and adipose tissue
	Glucagon	Increases blood glucose concentration by stimulation of glycogenolysis and glyconeogenesis
	Somatostatin	Delays intestinal absorption of glucose
Kidney	1,25-Dihydroxyvitamin D	Stimulates calcium absorption from the intestine
Ovaries	Estrogen	Affects development of female sex organs and secondary sex characteristics
	Progesterone	Influences menstrual cycle; stimulates growth of uterine wall; maintains pregnancy
Testes	Androgens, mainly testosterone	Affect development of male sex organs and secondary sex characteristics; aid in sperm production

TABLE 40.2 CLASSES OF HORMONES BASED ON STRUCTURE

AMINES AND AMINO ACIDS	PEPTIDES, PROTEINS, AND GLYCOPROTEINS	STEROIDS	FATTY ACIDS
Dopamine	CRH	Aldosterone	Prostaglandins
Epinephrine	GHRH	Glucocorticoids	Thromboxanes
Norepinephrine	TRH	Estrogens	Leukotrienes
Thyroid hormone	ACTH	Testosterone	Prostacyclins
	FSH	Progesterone	
	LH	Androstenedione	
	TSH	1,25-Dihydroxyvitamin D	
	GH	DHT	
	ADH	DHEA	
	Oxytocin		
	Insulin		
	Glucagon		
	Somatostatin		
	Calcitonin		
	PTH		
	Prolactin		

be as small as thyrotropin-releasing hormone (TRH), which contains three amino acids, and as large and complex as growth hormone (GH), which has approximately 200 amino acids. Glycoproteins are large peptide hormones associated with a carbohydrate (*e.g.*, follicle-stimulating hormone [FSH]). The third category consists of the steroid hormones, which are derivatives of cholesterol.[2–4] Although the structures of most hormonal substances are within these first three categories, there is a fourth category of hormonal messenger molecules derived from fatty acids, including the group of chemicals called the *eicosanoids*. Important among this class are the arachidonic acid derivatives, which include the prostaglandins.[2]

Synthesis and Release

The mechanisms for hormone synthesis and release are not fully understood and vary with hormone structure. Some hormones (such as the protein hormones) are synthesized and stored in vesicles in the cytoplasm of the endocrine cell until secretion is required. These vesicle-mediated hormones are released from the originating endocrine cell in response to some type of stimuli, which is often a negative feedback mechanism (to be discussed later). Stimulation of the endocrine cell causes the vesicles to move to the cell membrane and release their hormones.[3] The protein hormones are typically synthesized in the form of a precursor hormone that contains additional peptide units that ensure proper folding of the molecule and insertion of essential linkages. This type of precursor hormone molecule is called a *prohormone*.[3]

Cholesterol-based hormones are not stored in vesicles; instead, these lipid-soluble molecules, which are often produced in smooth endoplasmic reticulum, typically leave the cell as soon as they are synthesized by diffusing across the cell membrane.[3] Hormones synthesized by these non–vesicle-mediated pathways include the glucocorticoids, androgens, estrogens, and mineralocorticoids, which are all steroid hormones derived from cholesterol. Certain steroids serve as precursors for the production of other hormones. In the adrenal cortex, for example, pregnenolone and other steroid intermediates are enzymatically converted within the adrenal mitochondria into aldosterone, cortisol, or androgens.[3]

Transport

When hormones are released into the bloodstream, they circulate as either free, unbound molecules or as hormones attached to transport carriers (Fig. 40.1). Peptide hormones and protein hormones are water-soluble molecules and usually do not require a transport carrier. Steroid hormones and thyroid hormones are lipophilic molecules and therefore do require a carrier protein for transport through the blood. The liver synthesizes specific carrier proteins for steroid hormones and thyroid hormones.[3] The extent of protein carrier binding influences the rate at which hormones leave the blood and enter the cells. The half-life of a hormone—the time it takes for the body to reduce the concentration of the hormone in the blood by one half—is positively correlated with its percentage of protein binding.[3] Thyroxine, which is more than 99% protein bound, has a half-life as long as 6 days. In contrast, angiotensin II is freely water soluble with a half-life less than 1 minute.[3] Drugs that compete with a hormone for binding with transport carrier molecules increase hormone action by increasing the availability of the active unbound hormone. For example, aspirin competes with thyroid hormone for binding to transport proteins. When aspirin is administered to people with excessive levels of circulating thyroid hormone, such as during thyroid crisis, serious effects may occur because of the increased dissociation of free hormone from the binding proteins.[8]

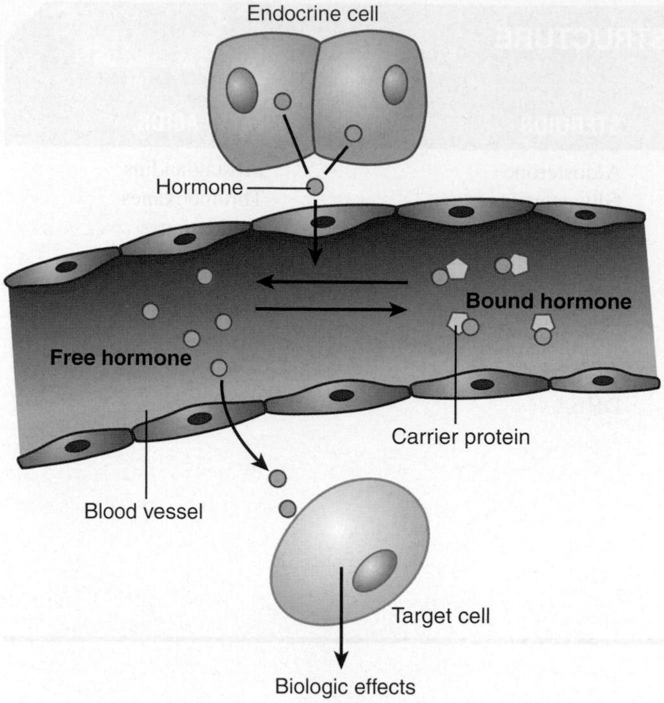

Figure 40.1 • Relationship of free and carrier-bound hormones.

Metabolism and Elimination

Hormones secreted by endocrine cells must be inactivated continuously to prevent their accumulation. Intracellular and extracellular mechanisms participate in the inactivation of hormone function. Most peptide hormones and catecholamines are water soluble and circulate freely in the blood. They are usually degraded by enzymes in the blood or tissues and then excreted by the kidneys and liver. In general, peptide hormones also have a short lifespan in the circulation. Their major mechanism of degradation is through binding to cell surface receptors, with subsequent uptake and degradation by peptide-splitting enzymes in the cell membrane or inside the cell.[2,3] Most steroid hormones are bound to protein carriers for transport and are inactive in the bound state. Their activity depends on the availability of transport carriers. Transport carriers may be specific carrier molecules for the individual hormone, or may be plasma proteins such as albumin. Notable exceptions to the requirement of a protein carrier for steroid hormones are the mineralocorticoids, including aldosterone, which do not require protein carriers.[2]

Mechanisms of Action

Hormones produce their effects through interaction with high-affinity receptors, which in turn are linked to one or more effector systems within the cell. These mechanisms involve many of the cell's metabolic activities, ranging from ion transport at the cell surface to stimulation of nuclear transcription of complex molecules.[2,3] The rate at which hormones react depends on their mechanism of action. Certain neurotransmitters, for example, which control the opening of ion channels have a reaction time of milliseconds. Thyroid hormone, which functions in the control of cell metabolism and synthesis of intracellular signaling molecules, requires days for its full effect to occur.[3]

Receptors. Hormone receptors are complex molecular structures (usually proteins) that are located either on the cell surface or inside target cells.[3] The function of these receptors is to recognize a specific hormone and translate the hormonal signal into a cellular response. The structure of these receptors is specific to a particular hormone, which allows target cells to respond to one hormone and not to others. For example, receptors in the thyroid are specific for thyroid-stimulating hormone (TSH), and receptors on the gonads respond to the gonadotropic hormones.[3]

The degree of responsiveness of a target cell to a hormone varies with the *number* of receptors present and with the *affinity* of these receptors for hormone binding.[3] Receptor number and affinity are influenced by a variety of factors. Antibodies may destroy or block the receptor proteins. Increased or decreased hormone levels often induce changes in the activity of the genes that synthesize hormone receptors. For example, decreased hormone levels often produce an increase in receptor numbers by means of a process called *up-regulation*. This increases the sensitivity of the body to the hormone. Up-regulation of hormone receptors may be an adaptive response when there are low levels of hormone in the body. In contrast, sustained levels of excess hormone often lead to a decrease in receptor numbers through *down-regulation* of the cellular synthesis of receptors, producing a decrease in hormone sensitivity.[3] In some instances, the reverse effect occurs, and an increase in hormone levels appears to recruit its own receptors, thereby increasing the sensitivity of the cell to the hormone. The process of up-regulation and down-regulation of receptors is regulated largely by inducing or repressing the transcription of receptor genes.[3]

As noted previously, some hormone receptors are located on the surface of the cell and act through second messenger mechanisms to influence cellular activity, whereas other receptors are located inside the cell. Whether the receptors are cell surface receptors or intracellular receptors, the ultimate effect of the hormone is usually exerted in the cell nucleus with the modulation of protein synthesis.[2,3] Chart 40.2 lists examples of hormones that act through the two types of receptors.

Cell Surface Receptors. Peptide hormones and catecholamines tend to be water-soluble molecules that are electrically charged (polar) molecules. Because of their low lipid solubility and high electrical charge, peptide hormones and catecholamines cannot readily cross the lipid cellular membrane.[2,3] Instead, these hormones interact with surface receptors to generate an intracellular signal through a *second messenger* signaling system, with the hormone acting as the first messenger. The first messenger hormone signals the need for action; however, the hormone itself never enters the cell. It is the second messenger molecules inside

CHART 40.2 HORMONE–RECEPTOR INTERACTIONS

Second Messenger Interactions
Glucagon
Insulin
Epinephrine
PTH
TSH
ACTH
FSH
LH
ADH
Secretin

Intracellular Interactions
Estrogens
Testosterone
Progesterone
Adrenal cortical hormones
Thyroid hormones

the cell that interact directly with the intracellular control mechanisms to effect the change.[2,3] For example, the first messenger hormone glucagon binds to surface receptors on liver cells to send a second intracellular message for glycogen breakdown.[2,3]

Intracellular Receptors. Lipid-soluble hormones (such as steroid hormones and the thyroid hormones) are typically nonpolar and can pass freely through cell membranes to bind with intracellular receptors.[2,3] The intracellular hormone–receptor complex can then directly exert the hormonal effects by entering the cell nucleus to bind with hormone response elements that activate or suppress intracellular mechanisms of protein synthesis.[2,3]

Control of Hormone Levels

Hormone secretion varies widely over a 24-hour period. Some hormones, such as GH and adrenocorticotropic hormone (ACTH), have diurnal fluctuations that vary with the sleep–wake cycle.[2] Others, such as the female sex hormones, are secreted in a complicated cyclic manner. The levels of hormones such as insulin and antidiuretic hormone (ADH) are regulated by feedback mechanisms that monitor substances such as glucose (insulin) and water (ADH) in the body. The levels of many of the hormones are regulated by feedback mechanisms that involve the hypothalamic–pituitary target cell system.[3]

Hypothalamic–Pituitary Regulation

The hypothalamus and pituitary gland form a functional unit that exerts control over the activities of several endocrine glands, and thus a wide range of physiologic functions. The hypothalamus is located centrally in the brain and serves as the coordinating center of the brain for endocrine, behavioral, and autonomic nervous system function. It is at the level of the hypothalamus that emotion, pain, body temperature, and other neural inputs are communicated to the endocrine system.[3]

The pituitary gland is connected to the floor of the hypothalamus by the pituitary stalk, with the main structural portion of the pituitary gland encased in a bony structure called the sella turcica. The opening to the sella turcica is bridged over by the diaphragma sellae, which protects the pituitary gland from the transmission of the pressures from the cerebrospinal fluid.[6] The pituitary gland is also called the "hypophysis." The pituitary consists of two structurally different sections (Fig. 40.2):

a. The *anterior pituitary*, also called the adenohypophysis because of its glandular structure. The hypothalamus and anterior pituitary are connected by blood flow through the hypophysial portal venous system, which begins in the hypothalamus and drains into the anterior pituitary gland.
b. The *posterior pituitary*, also called the neurohypophysis. The hypothalamus and posterior pituitary are connected through nerve axons from neurons that originate in the hypothalamus and connect the supraoptic and paraventricular nuclei of the hypothalamus with the posterior pituitary gland.

Hypothalamic Hormones. The hypothalamus produces hormones that act upon the anterior pituitary to regulate the synthesis and release of anterior pituitary hormones. These hypothalamic hormones are called releasing or inhibiting hormones, based on the response sent to the anterior pituitary. Releasing hormones (RHs) signal for the anterior pituitary to increase the synthesis and release of a particular hormone, whereas inhibiting hormones have the reverse effect—decreased hormonal release by the anterior pituitary. These releasing and inhibiting hormones travel to the anterior pituitary through a localized portal venous system[2,3] (Fig. 40.2). The hypothalamic hormones that regulate the secretion of anterior pituitary hormones include GH-releasing hormone (GHRH), somatostatin, dopamine, TRH, corticotropin-releasing hormone (CRH), and gonadotropin-releasing hormone (GnRH).[2,3]

The hypothalamus also sends regulatory signals to the posterior pituitary; however, the route through which the message is conducted is through nerve tracts instead of through release of hormones into the blood. The posterior pituitary is called the neurohypophysis because it contains a series of neurons whose cell bodies are located in the hypothalamus and axons extend down into the posterior pituitary. The posterior pituitary can essentially be thought of as an extension of the hypothalamus. The posterior pituitary hormones, ADH and oxytocin, are synthesized in the cell bodies of neurons in the hypothalamus that have axons that travel to the posterior pituitary.[2,3]

The activity of the hypothalamus is regulated by both hormonally mediated signals (*e.g.*, negative feedback signals) and by neuronal input from a number of sources. Neuronal signals are mediated by neurotransmitters such as acetylcholine, dopamine, norepinephrine, serotonin,

Understanding Hormone Receptors

Hormones bring about their effects on cell activity by binding to specific cell receptors. There are two general types of receptors: (1) cell surface receptors that exert their actions through cytoplasmic second messenger systems and (2) intracellular nuclear receptors that modulate gene expression by binding to deoxyribonucleic acid (DNA) or promoters of target genes.

Cell Surface Receptors

Water-soluble peptide hormones (such as parathyroid hormone [PTH] and glucagon) cannot penetrate the lipid layer of the cell plasma membrane and therefore exert their effects through intracellular second messengers. They bind to a portion of a membrane receptor that protrudes through the surface of the cell. This produces a structural change in the receptor molecule itself, causing activation of a hormone-regulated signal system located on the inner aspect of the cell membrane. This system allows the cell to sense extracellular events and pass this information to the intracellular environment. There are several types of cell surface receptors, including G-protein–coupled receptors, which mediate the actions of catecholamines, prostaglandins, TSH, and others. Binding of the hormone to the receptor activates a G protein, which in turn acts on an effector such as adenyl cyclase to generate a second messenger such as cyclic adenosine monophosphate (cAMP). The second messenger, in turn, activates other enzymes that participate in cellular secretion, gene activation, or other target cell responses.

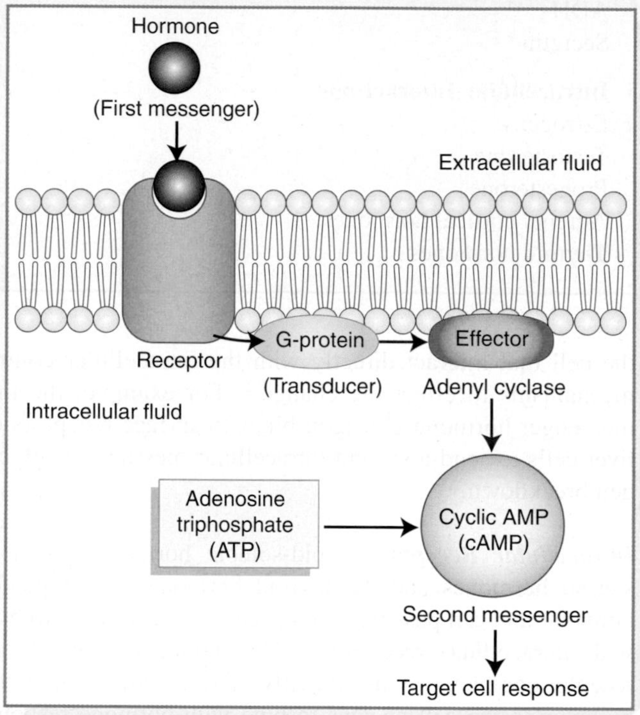

Understanding Hormone Receptors *(Continued)*

Nuclear Receptors

Steroid hormones, vitamin D, thyroid hormones, and other lipid-soluble hormones diffuse across the cell membrane into the cytoplasm of the target cell. Once inside the cell, these hormones bind to an intracellular receptor that is activated by the binding. The activated hormone–receptor complex then moves to the nucleus, where the hormone binds to a hormone response element in the promoters on a target gene or to another transcription factor. This binding results in transcription of a specific mRNA. The mRNA then moves into the cytoplasm, where the "transcribed message" is translated by cytoplasmic ribosomes to produce new cellular proteins or to change the production of existing proteins. This hormone-directed change in protein synthesis leads to cellular responses such as the promotion of a specific intracellular response or the synthesis of specific proteins to be secreted from the cell.

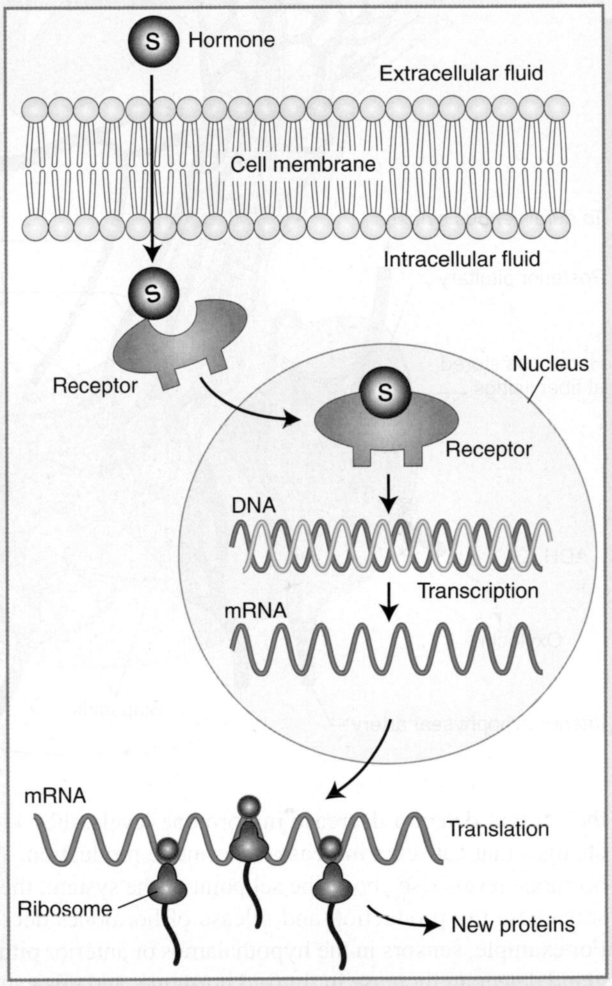

γ-aminobutyric acid (GABA), and opioids. Cytokines that are involved in immune and inflammatory responses, such as the interleukins, also are involved in the regulation of hypothalamic function. This is particularly true of the hormones involved in the hypothalamic–pituitary–adrenal axis. Thus, the hypothalamus can be viewed as a bridge by which signals from multiple systems are relayed to the pituitary gland.[2,3] (Fig. 40.3).

Pituitary Hormones. The pituitary gland has been called the *master gland* because its hormones control the functions of many target glands and cells.[2] Hormones produced by the anterior pituitary control body growth and metabolism (GH), function of the thyroid gland (TSH), glucocorticoid hormone levels (ACTH), function of the gonads (FSH and luteinizing hormone [LH]), and breast growth and milk production (prolactin). Hypothalamic releasing hormones regulate most of the pituitary hormones. GH secretion is stimulated by GHRH; TSH by TRH; ACTH by CRH; and LH and FSH by GnRH.[2,3]

Feedback Regulation

The level of many of the hormones in the body is regulated by negative feedback mechanisms.[2,3] The function of this type of system is similar to that of the thermostat in a heating system. In the endocrine system, sensors detect a change in the hormone level and adjust hormone secretion so that body levels are maintained within an appropriate range. When

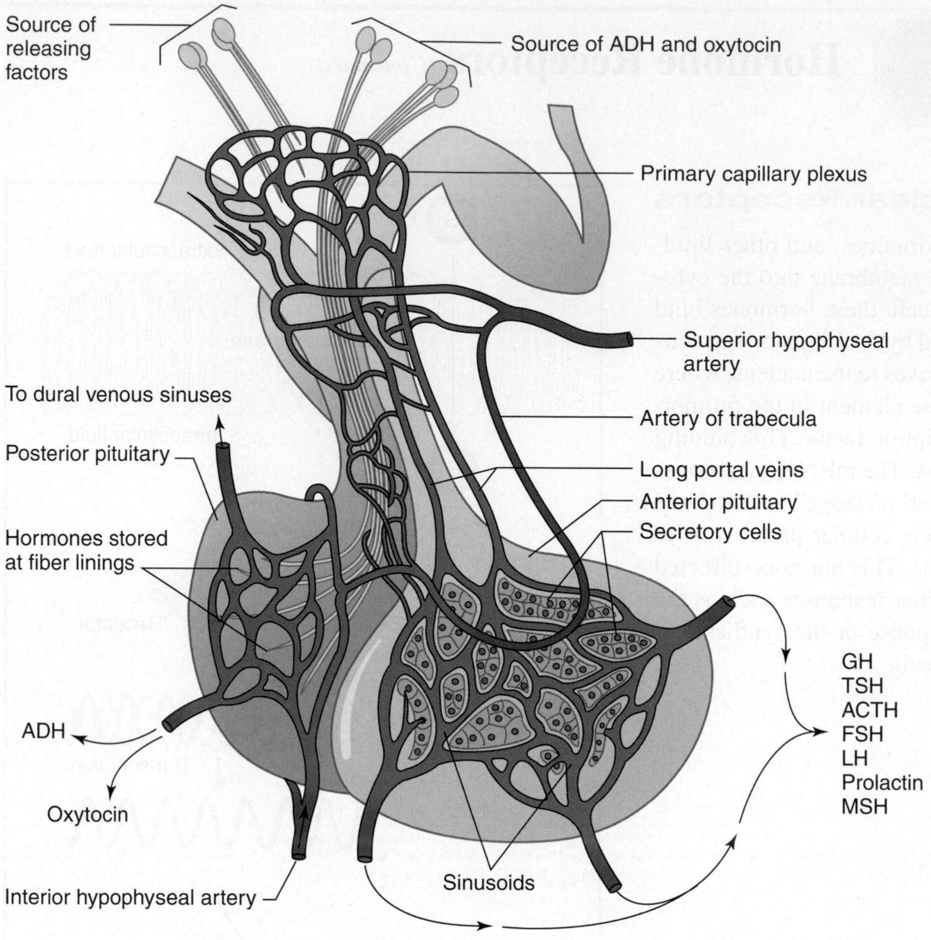

Figure 40.2 • The hypothalamus and the anterior and posterior pituitary. The hypothalamic releasing or inhibiting hormones are transported to the anterior pituitary through the portal vessels. ADH and oxytocin are produced by nerve cells in the supraoptic and paraventricular nuclei of the hypothalamus and then transported through the nerve axon to the posterior pituitary, where they are released into the circulation.

the sensors detect a decrease in hormone levels, they initiate changes that cause an increase in hormone production. When hormone levels rise above the set point of the system, the sensors cause the production and release of hormones decrease. For example, sensors in the hypothalamus or anterior pituitary gland detect an increase in thyroid hormone, and this causes a reduction in the secretion of TSH, with a subsequent decrease in the output of thyroid hormone from the thyroid gland. The feedback loops for the hypothalamic–pituitary feedback mechanisms are illustrated in Figure 40.3.

Positive feedback control also occurs but is not well understood. In positive feedback control, rising levels of a hormone cause another gland to release a hormone that is stimulating to the first.[3] An example of such a system is that of the female ovarian hormone estradiol. Increased estradiol production during the follicular stage of the menstrual cycle causes increased gonadotropin (FSH) production by the anterior pituitary gland. This stimulates further increases in estradiol levels until the demise of the follicle, which is the source of estradiol, results in a fall in gonadotropin levels.[3]

Diagnostic Tests

Many techniques are available for assessing endocrine function and hormone levels. Diagnostic assessments include blood tests, urine tests, hormone stimulation and suppression tests, genetic testing, and diagnostic imaging studies.

Blood Tests

Blood tests for endocrine disorders encompass a wide variety of strategies to assess endocrine function. Hormones can be measured directly or, very commonly, physiologic indicators of hormone function can be measured to indirectly reflect hormone levels. For example, measurement of blood glucose levels indirectly reflects blood levels of insulin. Blood hormone levels provide information about hormone levels at a specific time under specific conditions. For example, blood insulin levels can be measured along with blood glucose at specific time intervals after administration of a challenge dose of glucose to measure the trajectory of change in blood insulin levels.

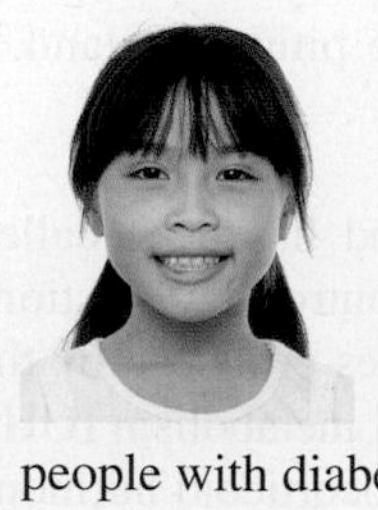

Emily, the young girl who was introduced at the beginning of this unit, presented with a blood glucose of 650 mg/dL, which is far above normal blood glucose levels (70 to 110 mg/dL). Her glycated hemoglobin test (hemoglobin A1c) was also very high at 10% when the normal range for people with diabetes is 6% to 7%.

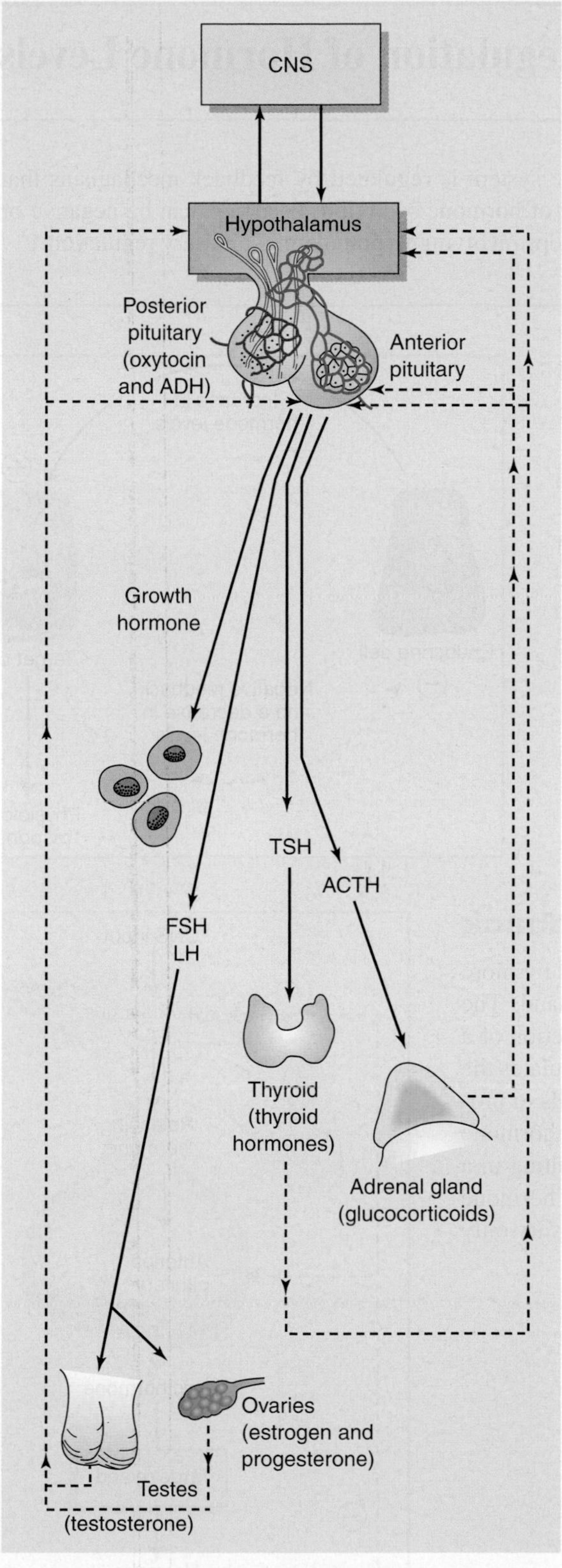

Figure 40.3 • Control of hormone production by the hypothalamic–pituitary target cell feedback mechanism. Hormone levels from the target glands regulate the release of hormones from the anterior pituitary through a negative feedback system. The *dashed line* represents feedback control.

Hormone levels in plasma are measured using radioimmunoassay (RIA) methods based on the competitive binding of hormones.[3] This method uses a radiolabeled form of the hormone and a hormone antibody that has been prepared by a purified form of the hormone. The unlabeled hormone in the sample being tested competes with the radiolabeled hormone for attachment to the binding sites of the antibody.[3] Measurement of the radiolabeled hormone–antibody complex then provides a means of arriving at a measure of the hormone level in the sample. Because hormone binding is competitive, the amount of radiolabeled hormone–antibody complex that is formed decreases as the amount of unlabeled hormone in the sample is increased. The limitations of RIA include a lack of specificity because of cross-reactivity with more than one hormone along with limited shelf life of the radiolabeled hormone and the cost for the disposal of radioactive waste.[3] Newer techniques of RIA have been introduced, including the immunoradiometric assay (IRMA). IRMA uses the same principle of antibody recognition with two antibodies instead of one. These two antibodies are directed against two different parts of the molecule, and therefore IRMA assays are more specific.[9]

Enzyme-linked immunosorbent assays (ELISA) are another newer diagnostic test for assessing endocrine function, which does not require the use of radioisotopes. ELISA testing combines the use of antibody testing using two antibodies that use different antigen binding sites (which allows higher specificity) with an enzyme testing approach (which has high sensitivity). The ELISA test method is widely used and has been demonstrated to be both cost-effective and accurate.[3] Other blood tests that are routinely measured in endocrine disorders include tests for various autoantibodies. For example, antithyroid peroxidase (anti-TPO) antibodies are measured during the initial diagnostic workup and subsequent follow-up of persons with Hashimoto thyroiditis. Other endocrine disorders that use autoantibody testing include type 1 diabetes, Graves disease, autoimmune hypoparathyroidism, and autoimmune Addison disease.[10,11]

Urine Tests

Measurements of urinary hormone or hormone metabolite excretion often are done on a 24-hour urine sample and provide a better measure of hormone levels during that period compared to hormones measured in an isolated blood sample. In particular, a 24-hour urine sample for urinary cortisol levels is frequently performed in the diagnostic workup for Cushing syndrome.[12]

Hormone Stimulation and Suppression Tests

Hormone stimulation tests are used when hypofunction of an endocrine organ is suspected. A tropic or stimulating hormone can be administered to test the capacity of an endocrine organ to increase hormone production. The capacity of the target gland to respond is measured by an increase in the appropriate hormone.[2] For example, the function of the hypothalamic–pituitary–thyroid system can be evaluated through stimulation tests using TRH and measuring TSH response. Failure to increase TSH levels after a TRH stimulation test suggests an

Understanding Feedback Regulation of Hormone Levels

Like many physiologic systems, the endocrine system is regulated by feedback mechanisms that enable the endocrine cells to change their rate of hormone secretion. Feedback can be negative or positive and may involve complex feedback loops involving hypothalamic–pituitary regulation.

Negative Feedback

With negative feedback, the most common mechanism of hormone control, some feature of hormone action directly or indirectly inhibits further hormone secretion so that the hormone level returns to an ideal level or set point. In the simple negative feedback loop, the amount of hormone or its effect on a physiologic mechanism regulates the response of the endocrine gland. After a meal, for example, a rise in blood glucose stimulates the pancreas to secrete insulin; insulin acts on target cells to take up the glucose, thus lowering blood glucose. The lowered glucose levels, in turn, suppress insulin release, causing blood glucose to rise.

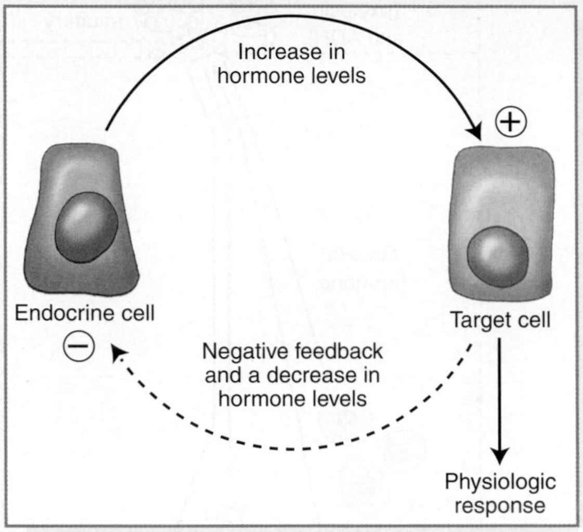

Hypothalamic–Pituitary Target Cell Feedback

Hormones of the thyroid, adrenal cortex, and the gonads are regulated by more complex loops involving the hypothalamus and anterior pituitary gland. The hypothalamus produces a releasing hormone that stimulates the production of a tropic hormone by the anterior pituitary. The tropic hormone then stimulates the peripheral target gland to secrete its hormone, which acts on target cells to produce a physiologic response. A rise in blood levels of the target gland hormone also feeds back to the hypothalamus and anterior pituitary gland, resulting in a decrease in tropic hormone secretion and a subsequent reduction in hormone secretion by the target gland. As a result, blood levels of the hormone vary only within a narrow range.

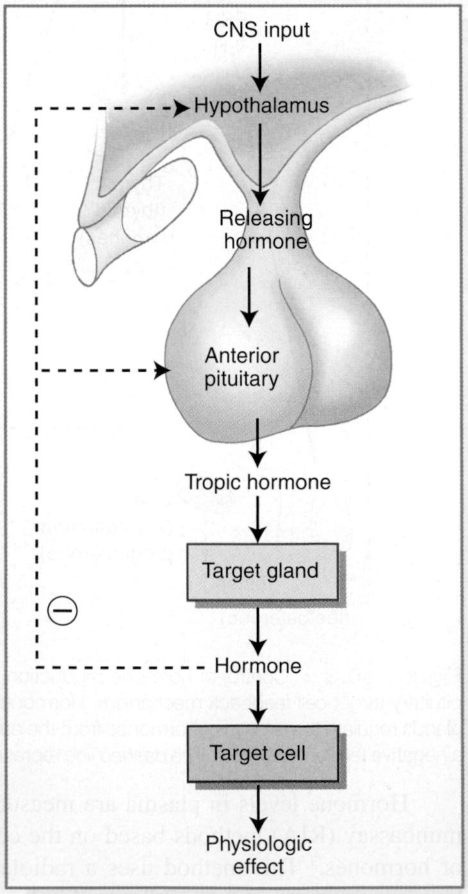

Understanding Feedback Regulation of Hormone Levels *(Continued)*

Positive Feedback

A small number of hormones are regulated by positive feedback. In this type of regulation, a hormone stimulates continued secretion until appropriate levels are reached. An example of positive feedback is the preovulatory surge in LH levels that trigger ovulation. At that time, an increase in estrogen levels exerts a positive feedback effect on the anterior pituitary secretion of LH.

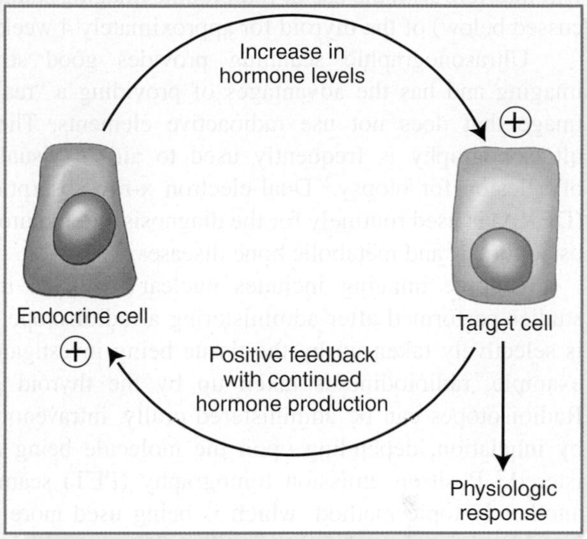

inadequate capacity to produce TSH by the pituitary (*i.e.*, the pituitary is dysfunctional in some way).

Suppression tests are used when hyperfunction of an endocrine organ is suspected. When an organ or tissue is functioning autonomously (*i.e.*, it is not responding to the normal negative feedback control mechanisms and continues to secrete excessive amounts of hormone), a suppression test may be useful to confirm the situation.[2] For example, when a GH-secreting tumor is suspected, the GH response to a glucose load is measured as part of the diagnostic workup. Normally, a glucose load would suppress GH levels. However, in adults with GH-secreting tumors (a condition known as *acromegaly*), GH levels are not suppressed.[13]

Genetic Testing

Genetic testing is rapidly becoming an important approach for diagnosing selected endocrine disorders. Some endocrine-related disorders for which specific genetic pathophysiologic markers have been identified include X-linked hypophosphatemic rickets, epithelial thyroid carcinoma, hypopituitarism, familial pheochromocytoma and paraganglioma, multiple endocrine neoplasia types I and II, and certain disorders of short stature including Turner syndrome.[2] Multiple endocrine neoplasia type II is an example of how genetic testing can be useful in diagnosing endocrine disorders. Development of this disorder has been connected with the RET protooncogene, which is located on the long arm of chromosome 10, at position 10q11.21.[14] Persons who are believed to be at risk for multiple endocrine neoplasia type II can now be tested for the presence of the RET protooncogene. If genetic testing for the RET protooncogene is positive, the person can consider prophylactic treatment for some of the conditions that are characteristic of multiple endocrine neoplasia type II, which include medullary thyroid carcinoma and pheochromocytoma. A drawback to genetic testing is the cost, which at this point in the development of the technology, can still be quite expensive.[2]

Imaging

Imaging studies are important in the diagnosis and follow-up of endocrine disorders. Imaging modalities related to endocrinology can be divided into nonisotopic and isotopic types.

Nonisotopic imaging includes magnetic resonance imaging (MRI) and computed tomography (CT) scanning, both of which provide important information about structural changes within solid tissue. An advantage of MRI is that it does not require the use of ionizing radiation (which is required for CT scanning); disadvantages of MRI scanning include the long time needed to complete the scan. Many MRI scanners require the person to be in an enclosed space for the long scanning time, which some individuals do not tolerate well. Open MRI scanners have been developed to respond to this concern. An issue that must be considered with CT scanning is the use of contrast agents. Nonradioactive iodine is often used as a contrast agent to enhance the quality of CT images. However, these iodine contrast preparations must be used with caution with persons with renal disease and allergies. Additionally, the previous use of nonradioactive iodine contrast material will interfere with the use of radioiodine imaging studies (discussed below) of the thyroid for approximately 4 weeks.[2]

Ultrasonographic scanning provides good structural imaging and has the advantages of providing a "real-time" image that does not use radioactive elements. Therefore, ultrasonography is frequently used to aid in visualization of a lesion for biopsy.[2] Dual-electron x-ray absorptiometry (DEXA) is used routinely for the diagnosis and monitoring of osteoporosis and metabolic bone diseases.[15]

Isotopic imaging includes nuclear medicine imaging studies performed after administering a radioisotope, which is selectively taken up by the tissue being investigated (for example, radioiodine is taken up by the thyroid gland). Radioisotopes can be administered orally, intravenously, or by inhalation, depending upon the molecule being administered.[2] Positron emission tomography (PET) scanning is another isotopic method, which is being used more widely in evaluating selected endocrine disorders, such as detecting the presence of metastatic thyroid cancers. PET scanning involves the administration of a short-lived radionuclide emitter of positrons in a form that is taken up by body tissues.[2] PET scanning has expanded to PET/CT imaging in which both types of images are acquired almost simultaneously for enhanced detail and identification of previously difficult structures. The advantage of PET/CT is that the CT component allows a good examination of the tissue structure, whereas the PET component provides information about tissue function.[16] PET/CT has been demonstrated to be useful in managing thyroid cancers.[17]

IN SUMMARY

The endocrine system acts as a communication system that uses chemical messengers, or hormones, for the transmission of information from cell to cell and from organ to organ. Hormones act by binding to receptors that are specific for the different types of hormones. Many of the endocrine glands are under the regulatory control of other parts of the endocrine system. The hypothalamus and the pituitary gland form a complex integrative network that interconnects the nervous system and the endocrine system; this central network controls the output from many of the other glands in the body.

Endocrine function can be assessed directly by measuring hormone levels or indirectly by assessing the effects that a hormone has on the body (*e.g.*, assessment of insulin function through blood glucose). Imaging techniques are used to visualize endocrine structures, and genetic techniques are used to determine the presence of genetic markers specific for selected endocrine disorders.

GERIATRIC Considerations

- With age, the thyroid gland decreases in size and activity, reducing the basic metabolic rate but still meeting daily needs.[18]
- Age-related hormonal changes may affect sexual function. For example, reduced pituitary ACTH or reduced adrenal gland function lead to atrophy of secondary sex organs because of decreased adrenal production of glucocorticoids, estrogen, progesterone, androgen, and 17-ketosteroids.[18]
- Glucose regulation becomes a challenge with age due to the reduced ability of the *B* cells to produce insulin.[18]

PEDIATRIC Considerations

- At 20 weeks' gestation, the pancreas of the fetus is secreting insulin.[19]
- The thyroid gland is present at day 24 in the embryo and becomes functional at 2 weeks postconceptual age.[19]
- The master gland for all age groups is the pituitary gland.[19]
- Glucocorticoid and mineralocorticoids are secreted by the adrenal cortex in the embryo, and at puberty, the adrenal cortex produces androgenic steroid needed for secondary sex characteristics.[19]
- Ongoing measurement of physical growth parameters and comparison to population norms on pediatric growth curves is important in children with endocrine disorders.[20]
- Because hormone function and control is still developing, infants have difficulty with stabilizing fluid and electrolytes, blood sugars, amino acids, and trace minterals.[20]

REVIEW EXERCISES

1. Thyroid hormones are transported in the serum bound to transport proteins such as thyroid-binding globulin and albumin.
   A. *Explain why free thyroxine (T_4) levels are usually used to assess thyroid function rather than total T_4 levels.*

2. People who are being treated with exogenous forms of corticosteroid hormones often experience diminished levels of ACTH and endogenously produced cortisol.
   A. *Explain, using information regarding the hypothalamic–pituitary feedback control of cortisol production by the adrenal cortex.*

References

1. Verburg-van Kemenade B. M. L., Cohen N., Chadzinska M. (2017). Neuroendocrine-immune interaction: Evolutionarily conserved mechanisms that maintain allostasis in an ever-changing environment. *Developmental and Comparative Immunology* 66, 2–23. doi: http://dx.doi.org/10.1016/j.dci.2016.05.015.
2. Neal, J. M. (2016). *How the endocrine system works* (2nd ed.). West Sussex, UK: John Wiley & Sons.
3. Hall J. E. (2015). *Guyton and Hall textbook of medical physiology* (13th ed.). Philadelphia, PA: Elsevier.
4. Saladin, K. S. (2015). *Anatomy & physiology: The unity of form and function* (7th ed.). New York: McGraw Hill Education.
5. Fruhbeck G., Mendez-Gimenez L., Fernandez-Formoso J. A., et al. (2014). Regulation of adipocyte lipolysis. *Nutrition Research Reviews* 27, 63–93. doi: 10.1017/S095442241400002X.
6. Rubin R., Strayer D. S., Saffitz, J. E., et al. (Ed.), (2015). *Rubin's pathology: Clinicopathologic foundations of medicine* (7th ed.) Philadelphia, PA: Wolters Kluwer.
7. Styne, D. M. (2016). *Pediatric endocrinology: A clinical handbook.* Switzerland: Springer.
8. Ildrose, A. M. (2015). Acute and emergency care for thyrotoxicosis and thyroid storm. *Acute Medicine and Surgery* 2, 147–157. doi: 10.1002/ams2.104.
9. Government of India Department of Atomic Energy Board of Radiation and Isotope Technology. (2016). *Frequently Asked Questions: Medical & Biological Products*. Downloaded from: http://www.britatom.gov.in/htmldocs/faqs_ec3.html
10. American Association for Clinical Chemistry. (2014). *Autoantibodies*. Downloaded from: https://labtestsonline.org/tests/autoantibodies
11. Kemp E. H., Weetman A. P. (2015). Autoimmune hypoparathyroidism. In: Brandi M., Brown E. (Ed.), *Hypoparathyroidism*. Milano: Springer.
12. American Association for Clinical Chemistry. (2016). *Cushing Syndrome*. Downloaded from: https://labtestsonline.org/conditions/cushing-syndrome.
13. Dineen R., Stewart P. M., Sherlock M. (2017). Acromegaly. *QJM: An International Journal of Medicine* 2017, 411–420. doi: 10.1093/qjmed/hcw004.
14. National Institutes of Health, U.S. National Library of Medicine. (2013). *RET Gene*. Downloaded from: https://ghr.nlm.nih.gov/gene/RET#location.
15. The Royal Australian and New Zealand College of Radiologists. (2018). *Bone Mineral Density Scan (Bone Densitometry or DXA Scan)*. Downloaded from: https://www.insideradiology.com.au/bone-mineral-density-scan-hp/.
16. The American Board of Nuclear Medicine. (2017). *What is PET/CT?* Downloaded from: https://www.abnm.org/index.php/sample-page-2/what-is-petct/.
17. Marcus C., Whitworth, P. W., Surasi, D. S., et al. (2014). PET/CT in the management of thyroid cancers. *American Journal of Roentgenology* 202, 1316–1329. doi: 10.2214/AJR.13.11673.
18. Epiopoulos, C. (2018). Endocrine function. In Epiopoulos C. (Ed.), *Gerontological nursing* (9th ed., pp. 378–389). Philadelphia, PA: Wolters Kluwer.
19. Goodhue, C. J. (2014). The child with an inborn error of metabolism. In Bowden, V. R., Greenberg, C. S. (Ed.), *Children and their families the continuum of nursing care* (3rd ed.). Philadelphia, PA: Wolters Kluwer.
20. Aduddel, K. (2017). Essentials of pediatric nursing. In Kyle, T., Carman, S. (Ed.), *Nursing care of the child with an endocrine disorder* (3rd ed.). Philadelphia, PA: Wolters Kluwer.

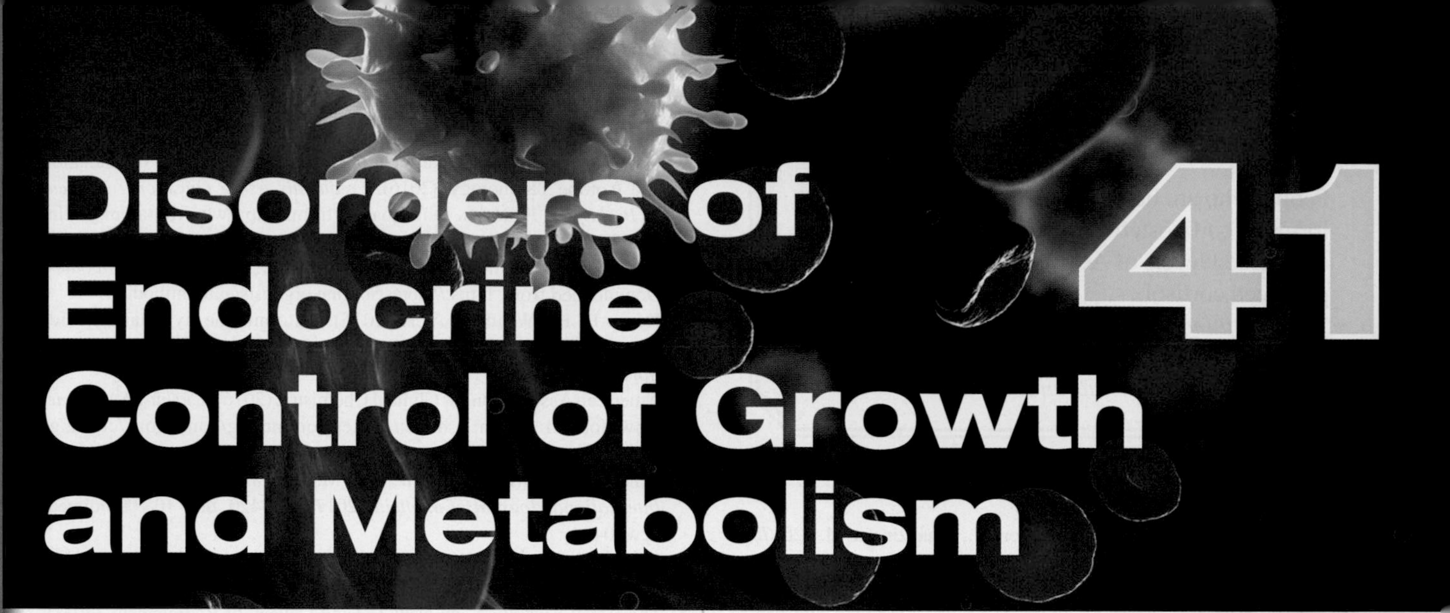

Disorders of Endocrine Control of Growth and Metabolism

41

Linda C. Mefford

The endocrine system affects all aspects of body function, including growth and development, energy metabolism, muscle and adipose tissue distribution, sexual development, fluid and electrolyte balance, and inflammation and immune responses. This chapter focuses on disorders of pituitary function, growth and growth hormone (GH), thyroid function, and adrenal cortical function. This chapter also addresses the increasingly prevalent conditions of diabetes mellitus and the metabolic syndrome.

GENERAL ASPECTS OF ALTERED ENDOCRINE FUNCTION

After completing this section of the chapter, the learner will be able to meet the following objectives:

- Describe the mechanisms of endocrine hypofunction, hyperfunction, and hormone resistance.
- Differentiate among primary, secondary, and tertiary endocrine disorders.

Hypofunction, Hyperfunction, and Hormone Resistance

Disturbances of endocrine function usually are related to either hypofunction or hyperfunction of an endocrine gland or to hormone resistance of the target cells. Hypofunction of an endocrine gland can occur for a variety of reasons, such as the absence or impaired development of a gland or deficiency of an enzyme needed for hormone synthesis. The gland may be destroyed by a disruption in blood flow, infection, inflammation, autoimmune responses, or neoplastic growth. Decline in function may occur with aging, or an endocrine gland may atrophy as a result of drug therapy or for unknown reasons. A gland may produce a biologically inactive hormone, or circulating antibodies may destroy an active hormone before it can exert its action.[1–3]

Endocrine hyperfunction usually is due to excessive hormone production. This can result from excessive stimulation and hyperplasia of the endocrine gland or from a hormone-producing tumor. A tumor can produce hormones that are not normally secreted by the tissue from which the tumor is derived (ectopic hormone production). For example, certain bronchogenic tumors and other cancerous tumors produce hormones such as antidiuretic hormone (ADH) and adrenocorticotropic hormone (ACTH).[1–3]

Endocrine dysfunction because of hormone resistance may be associated with receptor defects at the target cells. Hormone receptors may be absent or the receptor binding of hormones may be defective. Laron syndrome is a type of dwarfism that is caused by abnormalities in the receptors for GH in target tissues. Another mechanism associated with hormone resistance is an impaired intracellular responsiveness to stimulation by the hormone. This impaired cellular responsiveness occurs in congenital adrenal hyperplasia (CAH) in which the adrenal gland is receiving stimulation by ACTH but cannot respond appropriately because of a defect in the intracellular pathways within the adrenal cortex for production of cortisol.[1–3]

Primary, Secondary, and Tertiary Disorders

Endocrine disorders can be considered as primary, secondary, and tertiary disorders, related to the cascade of hormonal responses regulated through the hypothalamic–pituitary–target endocrine gland axis. *Primary disorders* of endocrine function originate in the target endocrine gland responsible for producing the hormone. For example, total thyroidectomy produces a primary deficiency of thyroid hormones. Addison disease is another example of a primary endocrine disorder. In Addison disease, the adrenal cortex is damaged by autoimmune mechanisms, resulting in underproduction of adrenal cortical hormones.[1,2]

In *secondary disorders* of endocrine function, the target endocrine gland is essentially normal; however, the gland is not producing appropriate levels of hormone because it is not receiving appropriate stimulation from the pituitary gland. The actual source of dysfunction is at the level of the pituitary gland. An example of a secondary endocrine disorder is a pituitary adenoma that results in increased secretion of pituitary hormones and excessive stimulation of target endocrine glands such as the adrenal glands and thyroid gland.[1,2] A *tertiary disorder* results from hypothalamic dysfunction (as may occur with craniopharyngiomas or cerebral irradiation). Thus, both the pituitary and target organ are understimulated.[3]

IN SUMMARY

Endocrine disorders typically occur as the result of either hypofunction or hyperfunction of an endocrine gland or as a result of hormone resistance by target cells. Endocrine disorders can be classified as a primary disorder (because of a dysfunction of a target endocrine gland of the hypothalamic–pituitary axis, such as the thyroid gland or the adrenal glands), a secondary disorder (because of dysfunction of the pituitary gland), or a tertiary disorder (resulting from a defect in the hypothalamus).

PITUITARY AND GROWTH DISORDERS

After completing this section of the chapter, the learner will be able to meet the following objectives:

- Describe the clinical features and causes of hypopituitarism.
- Analyze the effects of a deficiency in GH.
- Relate the functions of GH to the manifestations of acromegaly and adult-onset GH deficiency.

The pituitary gland, or *hypophysis*, is a pea-sized gland located at the base of the brain, where it lies in a saddle-shaped depression in the sphenoid bone called the *sella turcica*. A short funnel-shaped stalk, the *infundibulum*, connects the pituitary gland with the hypothalamus. The pituitary gland has two components—a posterior lobe that is the neural component (neurohypophysis) and an anterior glandular lobe (adenohypophysis).[4,5]

The anterior lobe of the pituitary gland produces ACTH, thyroid-stimulating hormone (TSH), GH, the gonadotrophic hormones (follicle stimulating hormone [FSH] and luteinizing hormone [LH]), and prolactin. Four of these, ACTH, TSH, LH, and FSH, control the secretion of hormones from other endocrine glands:

- ACTH controls the release of cortisol from the adrenal gland.
- TSH controls the secretion of thyroid hormone from the thyroid gland.
- LH regulates sex hormones in the ovaries and testes.
- FSH regulates fertility in the ovaries and testes.[4,5]

Assessment of Hypothalamic–Pituitary Function

A general overview of the various strategies available for assessing endocrine function is provided in Chapter 40. Assessment of the baseline status of the hypothalamic–pituitary and target cell hormones may include measuring the following (ideally the laboratory specimens are obtained before 8:00 AM because of circadian variations):

- Serum cortisol
- Serum prolactin
- Serum thyroxine and TSH
- Serum testosterone (male), serum estrogen (female), and serum LH/FSH
- Serum GH and serum insulin-like growth factor-1 (IGF-1, also known as somatomedin C)
- Plasma osmolality and urine osmolality

Imaging studies (*e.g.*, magnetic resonance imaging [MRI] of the hypothalamus/pituitary) should also be performed as indicated. When further information regarding pituitary function is required, combined hypothalamic–pituitary function tests are undertaken using hormone stimulation and/or suppression testing. Additional diagnostic methods include dynamic testing of hypothalamic–pituitary–adrenal (HPA) axis function, as well as the insulin tolerance test, glucagon stimulation test, and short synacthen (corticotropin) test.[6]

Pituitary Tumors

Pituitary tumors can be divided into primary and secondary tumors (*i.e.*, metastatic lesions). Tumors of the pituitary can be further divided into functional tumors that secrete pituitary hormones and nonfunctional tumors that do not secrete hormones. They can range in size from small lesions that do not enlarge the gland (microadenomas, <10 mm) to large, expansive tumors (macroadenomas, >10 mm) that erode the sella turcica and impinge on surrounding cranial structures. Small, nonfunctioning tumors are found in up to 27% of adult autopsies.[1] Benign adenomas account for most of the functioning anterior pituitary tumors. Carcinomas of the pituitary are less common tumors. Functional adenomas can be subdivided according to cell type and the type of hormone secreted (Table 41.1).[1]

Hypopituitarism

Hypopituitarism is characterized by a decreased secretion of pituitary hormones and is associated with increased morbidity and mortality. The cause may be congenital or may result from a variety of acquired abnormalities (Chart 41.1).[2]

Typically, approximately 75% of the anterior pituitary must be destroyed before hypopituitarism becomes clinically evident.[2] The clinical manifestations of hypopituitarism usually occur gradually but can present as an acute and life-threatening condition. People usually complain of being chronically unfit, with weakness, fatigue, loss of appetite, impairment of sexual function, and cold intolerance. ACTH deficiency

TABLE 41.1 FREQUENCY OF ADENOMAS OF THE ANTERIOR PITUITARY

CELL TYPE	HORMONE	FREQUENCY (%)
Lactotrope	Prolactin (PRL)	26
Somatotrope	Growth hormone (GH)	14
Corticotrope	Adrenocorticotropic hormone (ACTH)	15
Gonadotrope	Follicle-stimulating hormone (FSH), Luteinizing hormone (LH)	8
Thyrotrope	Thyroid-stimulating hormone (TSH)	1

Adapted from Strayer D., Rubin E., Saffitz J.E., Schiller A.L. (Eds.) (2015). *Rubin's pathology: Clinicopathologic foundations of medicine* (7th ed., Table 27.1, p. 1177). Philadelphia, PA: Wolters Kluwer, with permission.)

CHART 41.1 CAUSES OF HYPOPITUITARISM

- Tumors and mass lesions—pituitary adenomas, cysts, metastatic cancer, and other lesions
- Pituitary surgery or radiation
- Infiltrative lesions and infections—hemochromatosis and lymphocytic hypophysitis
- Pituitary infarction—infarction of the pituitary gland after substantial blood loss during childbirth (Sheehan syndrome)
- Pituitary apoplexy—sudden hemorrhage into the pituitary gland
- Genetic diseases—rare congenital defects of one or more pituitary hormones
- Empty sella syndrome—an enlarged sella turcica that is not entirely filled with pituitary tissue
- Hypothalamic disorders—tumors and mass lesions (*e.g.*, craniopharyngiomas and metastatic malignancies), hypothalamic radiation, infiltrative lesions (*e.g.*, sarcoidosis), trauma, and infections

(secondary adrenal insufficiency) is the most serious endocrine deficiency, leading to weakness, nausea, anorexia, fever, and postural hypotension.[3]

Anterior pituitary hormone loss tends to follow a typical sequence, especially with progressive loss of pituitary reserve because of tumors or previous pituitary radiation therapy. The sequence of loss of pituitary hormones can be remembered by the mnemonic "*G*o *L*ook *F*or *T*he *A*denoma":

- GH (GH secretion typically is first to be lost)
- LH (results in sex hormone deficiency)
- FSH (causes infertility)
- TSH (leads to secondary hypothyroidism)
- ACTH (usually the last to become deficient, results in secondary adrenal insufficiency)[7]

Treatment of hypopituitarism includes treating any identified underlying cause. Hormone deficiencies should be treated as dictated by baseline hormone levels and more sophisticated pituitary testing where appropriate. Cortisol replacement is started when ACTH deficiency is present; thyroid replacement when TSH deficiency is detected; and sex hormone replacement when LH and FSH are deficient. GH replacement is indicated for pediatric GH deficiency and may also be used to treat GH deficiency in adults.[1–3]

Growth and Growth Hormone Disorders

Several hormones are essential for normal body growth and maturation, including GH, insulin, thyroid hormone, and androgens. In addition to its actions on carbohydrate and fat metabolism, insulin plays an essential role in growth processes. Children with diabetes, particularly those who have difficulty with balancing blood sugar, often fail to grow normally even though GH levels are normal. When levels of thyroid hormone are lower than normal, bone growth and epiphyseal closure are delayed. Androgens such as testosterone and dihydrotestosterone exert anabolic growth effects through their actions on protein synthesis. Glucocorticoids at excessive levels inhibit growth, apparently because of their antagonistic effect on GH secretion.[4,8,9]

Growth Hormone

Growth hormone (GH), also called *somatotropin*, is a 191-amino acid polypeptide hormone synthesized and secreted by special cells in the anterior pituitary called *somatotropes*. It has been a common belief that GH was produced primarily during periods of growth. However, this has proved incorrect because the rate of GH production in adults is almost as great as it is in children. GH is necessary for growth and contributes to the regulation of metabolic functions (Fig. 41.1). GH stimulates all aspects of cartilage growth. One of the most obvious effects of GH is on linear bone growth, resulting from its action on the epiphyseal growth plates of long bones. The width of bone increases because of enhanced periosteal growth. Visceral and endocrine organs, skeletal and cardiac muscle, skin, and connective tissue all undergo increased growth in response to GH.[1,4]

Additionally, GH facilitates the rate of protein synthesis in the body. It enhances fatty acid mobilization, increases the use of fatty acids for fuel, and maintains or increases blood glucose levels by decreasing the use of glucose for fuel.[4] GH has an initial effect of increasing insulin levels. However, the predominant effect of prolonged GH excess is to increase glucose levels despite an insulin increase. This is because GH induces a resistance to insulin in the peripheral tissues, inhibiting the uptake of glucose by muscle and adipose tissues.[4]

Many of the effects of GH depend on *IGFs*, also called *somatomedins*, which are produced mainly by the liver. GH cannot directly cause bone growth. Instead, it acts indirectly by causing the liver to produce IGF. These IGF peptides act on cartilage and bone to promote their growth. At least four IGFs have been identified. Of these, IGF-1 (somatomedin C) appears to be the more important in terms of growth. It is also the most frequently measured IGF in laboratory tests. The IGFs have been sequenced and have structures similar to those of proinsulin. This explains the insulin-like activity of the IGFs and the weak action of insulin on growth. IGF levels are themselves influenced by a family of six-binding factors called *IGF-binding proteins* (IGFBPs).[4]

GH is carried unbound in the plasma and has a half-life of <50 minutes.[4] Two hypothalamic hormones regulate the secretion of GH:

- GH-releasing hormone (GHRH) that increases GH release
- Somatostatin that inhibits GH release

The secretion of GH fluctuates over a 24-hour period, with peak levels occurring 1 to 4 hours after onset of sleep

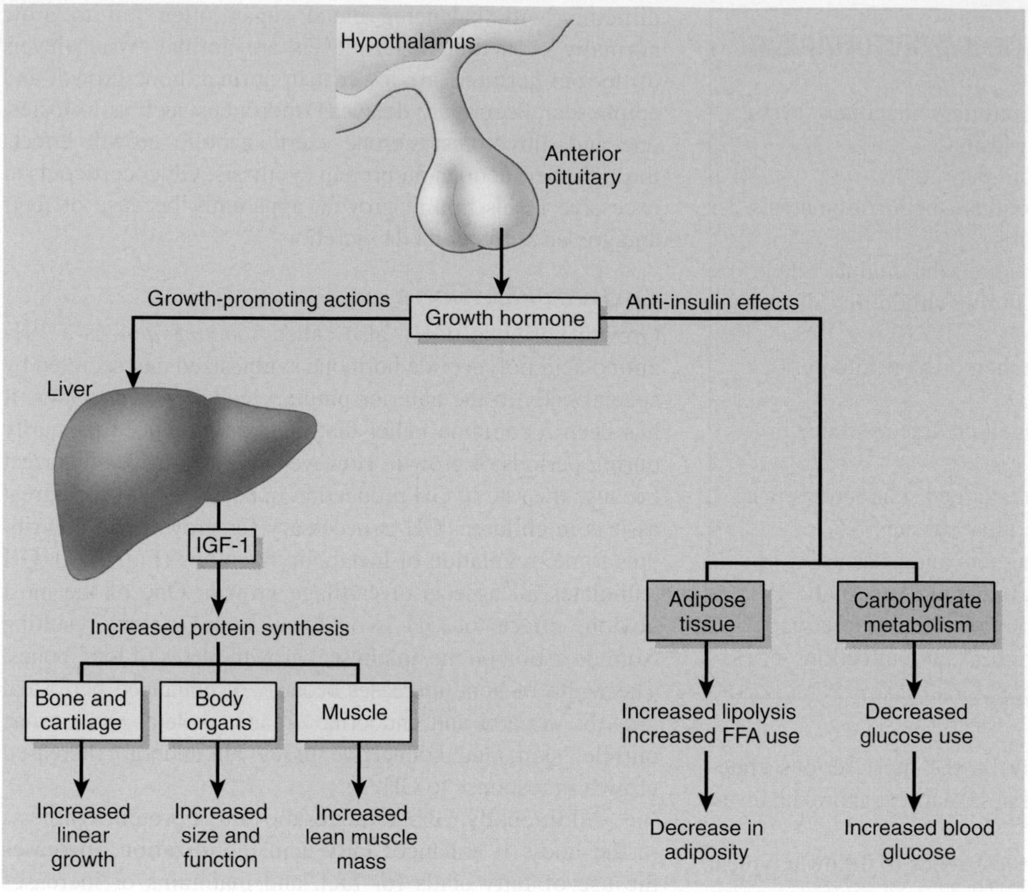

Figure 41.1 • Growth promoting and anti-insulin effects of GH. (FFA, free fatty acids; IGF-1, insulin-like growth factor-1.)

(*i.e.*, during sleep stages 3 and 4). GH secretion is stimulated by hypoglycemia, fasting, starvation, increased blood levels of amino acids (particularly arginine), and decreased blood levels of fatty acids. Stress conditions such as trauma, excitement, emotional stress, and heavy exercise also increase GH, as does secretion of the hormone ghrelin by the stomach and the hormones estrogen and testosterone. GH is inhibited by increased glucose levels, levels of free fatty acids (FFAs) in the blood, cortisol, and obesity. GH levels also decrease with aging.[4]

KEY POINTS

GROWTH HORMONE

- Growth hormone (GH), which is produced by somatotropes in the anterior pituitary, is necessary for linear bone growth in children. It also increases the rate at which cells transport amino acids across their cell membranes, and it increases the rate at which they use fatty acids and decreases the rate at which they use carbohydrates.
- The effects of GH on linear growth are dependent upon IGFs, which are produced mainly by the liver.

Short Stature in Children

Short stature is a condition in which height is less than the third percentile on the appropriate growth curve (which is <2 standard deviations below the population mean for age and sex).[10,11] Short stature, or growth retardation, may have a variety of endocrine causes, including GH deficiency, hypothyroidism, and panhypopituitarism (*i.e.*, deficiency of *all* pituitary-derived hormones). Some of these hormonal deficiencies are now being linked to alterations in specific genes. A variety of other genetic and chromosomal causes of short stature have been noted, including Turner syndrome, Noonan syndrome, achondroplasia, and various types of skeletal dysplasias.[12] Other conditions known to cause short stature include protein–calorie malnutrition, chronic diseases such as chronic kidney disease and poorly controlled diabetes mellitus, malabsorption syndromes (including celiac disease), and certain pharmacologic therapies such as steroids, anticonvulsants, and drugs for attention deficit and hyperactivity. Emotional disturbances can lead to functional endocrine disorders, causing psychosocial dwarfism, which is also referred to as psychosocial short stature. The causes of short stature are summarized in Chart 41.2.[1,2,10,11]

A thorough physical and history, including developmental history, is important in diagnosing growth disorders. Accurate measurement of height and weight is an important part of the physical examination of children, with careful

CHART 41.2 CAUSES OF SHORT STATURE

Variants of Normal
Genetic or "familial" short stature
Constitutional short stature

Low Birth Weight (*e.g.*, Intrauterine Growth Retardation)

Endocrine Disorders
GH deficiency
- Primary GH deficiency
- Idiopathic GH deficiency
- Pituitary agenesis
- Secondary GH deficiency (panhypopituitarism)

Biologically inactive GH production
Deficient IGF-1 production in response to normal or elevated GH (Laron-type dwarfism)
Hypothyroidism
Diabetes mellitus in poor control
Glucocorticoid excess
- Endogenous (Cushing syndrome)
- Exogenous (glucocorticoid drug treatment)

Abnormal mineral metabolism (*e.g.*, pseudohypoparathyroidism)

Chronic Illness and Malnutrition
Chronic organic or systemic disease (*e.g.*, asthma, especially when treated with glucocorticoids; heart or renal disease)
Nutritional deprivation
Malabsorption syndrome (*e.g.*, celiac sprue)

Functional Endocrine Disorders (Psychosocial Dwarfism)

Chromosomal Disorders (*e.g.*, Turner Syndrome)

Skeletal Abnormalities (*e.g.*, Achondroplasia)

evaluation and tracking on growth curves. Diagnosis of short stature is not made on a single measurement but is based on sequential height measurements, velocity of growth, and parental height.[11,13]

The diagnostic procedures for children with short stature include tests to exclude nonendocrine causes. Suggested tests for conditions that may cause short stature include: complete blood count (anemia), comprehensive metabolic panel (renal and hepatic disease), CRP and erythrocyte sedimentation rate (inflammatory bowel disease), FSH and karyotyping (Turner syndrome and other chromosomal abnormalities), IGF 1 (GH deficiency), TSH and free thyroxine (hypothyroidism), tissue transglutaminase and immunoglobulin A (celiac disease), and urinalysis (renal disease).[11] Test for IGFBP-3 may also be useful to assess for GH deficiency and chronic disease.[11] Radiologic films are used to assess bone age, which often is delayed.[14] MRI of the hypothalamic–pituitary area is recommended if a lesion is clinically suspected.[9] After the cause of short stature has been determined, treatment with recombinant DNA GH is approved for certain disorders, including GH deficiency, certain genetic problems (such as Prader-Willi syndrome and Noonan syndrome), chronic renal disease, and idiopathic short stature.[11]

Familial and Constitutional Short Stature. Two forms of short stature, genetic (familial) short stature and constitutional delay of growth and puberty, are not disease states but variations from population norms. These conditions require monitoring but not treatment. Genetically, short children tend to be well proportioned and to have a height close to the midparental height of their parents. The bone age and chronologic age of these children are equivalent. Children who have constitutional delay of growth have bone age that is less than the chronologic age, with the absence of other causes of decreased growth.[11,13]

Psychosocial Dwarfism (Psychosocial Short Stature). Psychosocial dwarfism (psychosocial short stature) involves a functional hypopituitarism and is seen in some emotionally deprived children. These children usually present with poor growth, potbelly, and poor eating and drinking habits. Typically, there is a history of disturbed family relationships in which the child has been severely neglected or disciplined. Often, the neglect is confined to one child in the family. GH function usually returns to normal after the child is removed from the constraining environment. The prognosis depends on improvement in behavior and catch-up growth.[15]

Growth Hormone Deficiency in Children

Several forms of GH deficiency present in childhood. Children with GH deficiency often present with physical findings of short stature (pituitary dwarfism), increased subcutaneous fat in the abdominal area, immature facial features with frontal bossing, delayed dentition, and an underdeveloped nasal bridge.[14] Several genetic mutations have been identified in the gene that codes for GH; however, some children present with idiopathic GH deficiency in which none of the known mutations are found. Childhood GH deficiency can also occur as a result of pituitary tumors. When short stature is caused by a GH deficiency, replacement therapy with GH produced by recombinant DNA technology is the treatment of choice. GH is administered by daily subcutaneous injection during the period of active growth and can be continued into adulthood.[4,11,16]

In a rare condition called *Laron syndrome (or Laron dwarfism)*, the pathophysiologic problem is hormone resistance because of abnormal GH receptors. GH levels are normal or elevated; however, levels of IGF-1 are low. Laron syndrome can be treated with IGF-1 replacement. Transmission of Laron syndrome is through autosomal recessive inheritance, with over 30 different mutations of GH receptors identified.[1]

Growth Hormone Deficiency in Adults

There are two categories of GH deficiency in adults:

1. GH deficiency that was present in childhood
2. GH deficiency that developed during adulthood, mainly as the result of hypopituitarism resulting from a pituitary tumor or its treatment

Some of the differences between childhood and adult-onset GH deficiency are described in Table 41.2.

The diagnosis of GH deficiency in adults is made by finding subnormal serum GH responses to provocative stimuli. A low IGF-1 level in the presence of low levels of three or more pituitary hormones indicates GH deficiency. Either the insulin tolerance test or the combination of the GHRH and arginine test is used as stimulation tests to detect GH deficiency.[17]

Treatment with recombinant GH replacement is indicated for adults with documented GH deficiency, with serum IGF-1 levels used to guide treatment.[17] The risk of atherosclerosis has been shown to be increased in children with GH deficiency. Treatment with GH has been demonstrated to improve the lipid profile and reduce the thickness of the intimal layer of the carotid artery in this population.[18] GH levels can also decline with aging, and there has been interest in the effects of declining GH levels in older adults (described as *somatopause*). GH replacement is obviously important in the growing child. However, the role in adults (especially for somatopause) is being debated, and a consensus decision has not yet been achieved.[19,20]

Tall Stature in Children

Height that is greater than the 97th percentile norms for age and sex is considered tall stature in children (>2 standard deviations above the population mean).[11] As with short stature, normal variants of tall stature include familial tall stature and constitutional advancement of growth. Other causes of tall stature are genetic or chromosomal disorders such as Marfan syndrome, Klinefelter (XXY) syndrome, Fragile X syndrome, and Beckwith-Wiedemann syndrome. Treatment is not usually indicated for these non–GH-related causes of tall stature, or with the normal variants. In the past, treatment with high-dose sex steroids was used to promote early closure of the epiphyseal plates; however, this treatment approach is no longer recommended because of adverse treatment effects.[11]

TABLE 41.2 DIFFERENCES BETWEEN CHILDHOOD AND ADULT-ONSET GH DEFICIENCY

CHARACTERISTIC	CHILDHOOD ONSET	ADULT ONSET
Adult height	↓	NL
Body fat	↑	↑
Lean body mass	↓↓	↓
Bone mineral density	↓	NL, ↓
Insulin-like growth factor (IGF)-1	↓↓	NL, ↓
IGF binding protein-3	↓	NL
Low-density lipoprotein cholesterol	↑	↑
High-density lipoprotein cholesterol	NL, ↓	↓

NL, normal.

Growth Hormone Excess in Children

GH excess occurring before puberty and the fusion of the epiphyses of the long bones results in pituitary *gigantism*. All body tissues grow rapidly, including the bones.[4] Excessive secretion of GH by somatotrope adenomas causes gigantism in the prepubertal child. It occurs when the epiphyses are not fused and high levels of IGF-1 stimulate excessive skeletal growth. The individual often has other complications because of the larger body mass and possible excessive secretion of other pituitary hormones. Fortunately, the condition is rare because of early recognition and treatment of the adenoma.[3] Treatment for GH excess typically consists of administration of the medications octreotide and pegvisomant to decrease GH levels.[11]

Growth Hormone Excess in Adults

When GH excess occurs in adulthood or after the epiphyses of the long bones have fused, the condition is referred to as *acromegaly*. The annual incidence of acromegaly is 3 to 4 cases per 1 million people, with a prevalence of 30 to 60 cases per million.[21]

Etiology and Pathogenesis. Clinical manifestations of acromegaly result from the effects on body cells from excess circulating blood levels of GH and IGF-1.[21] The most common cause of acromegaly is a GH-secreting somatotrope adenoma in the pituitary gland. Approximately 75% of people with acromegaly have a somatotrope macroadenoma at the time of diagnosis, and most of the remainder has microadenomas.[1] The other causes of acromegaly are hypothalamic tumors that result in excess secretion of GHRH, ectopic secretion of GHRH by nonendocrine tumors (such as carcinoid tumors or small cell lung cancers), or, more rarely, GH secretion from nonendocrine tumors. The binding of the excess circulating GH with the GH receptors in hepatic cells triggers an excess secretion of IGF-1 from hepatic cells. Then, it is the circulating IGF-1 molecules that bind with the IGF-1 receptor molecules in peripheral tissues, which directly act to stimulate the tissue growth that produces the clinical manifestations of acromegaly.[21]

Clinical Manifestations. The disorder usually has an insidious onset, with symptoms often present for a considerable period before a diagnosis is made. Because acromegaly is the production of excessive GH in adulthood, after the epiphyses of the long bones have closed, the person cannot grow taller;

however, the soft tissues continue to grow. Enlargement of the small bones of the hands and feet and of the membranous bones of the face and skull results in a pronounced enlargement of the hands and feet, a broad and bulbous nose, a protruding lower jaw, and a slanting forehead (Fig. 41.2). The teeth become splayed, causing a disturbed bite and difficulty in chewing. The cartilaginous structures in the larynx and respiratory tract also become enlarged, resulting in a deepening of the voice and tendency to develop bronchitis. Vertebral changes often lead to kyphosis or hunchback. Bone overgrowth often leads to arthralgias and degenerative arthritis of the spine, hips, and knees. Virtually, every organ of the body is increased in size. Enlargement of the heart, the development of hypertension, and accelerated atherosclerosis can produce significant morbidity and mortality.[1,2,21,22]

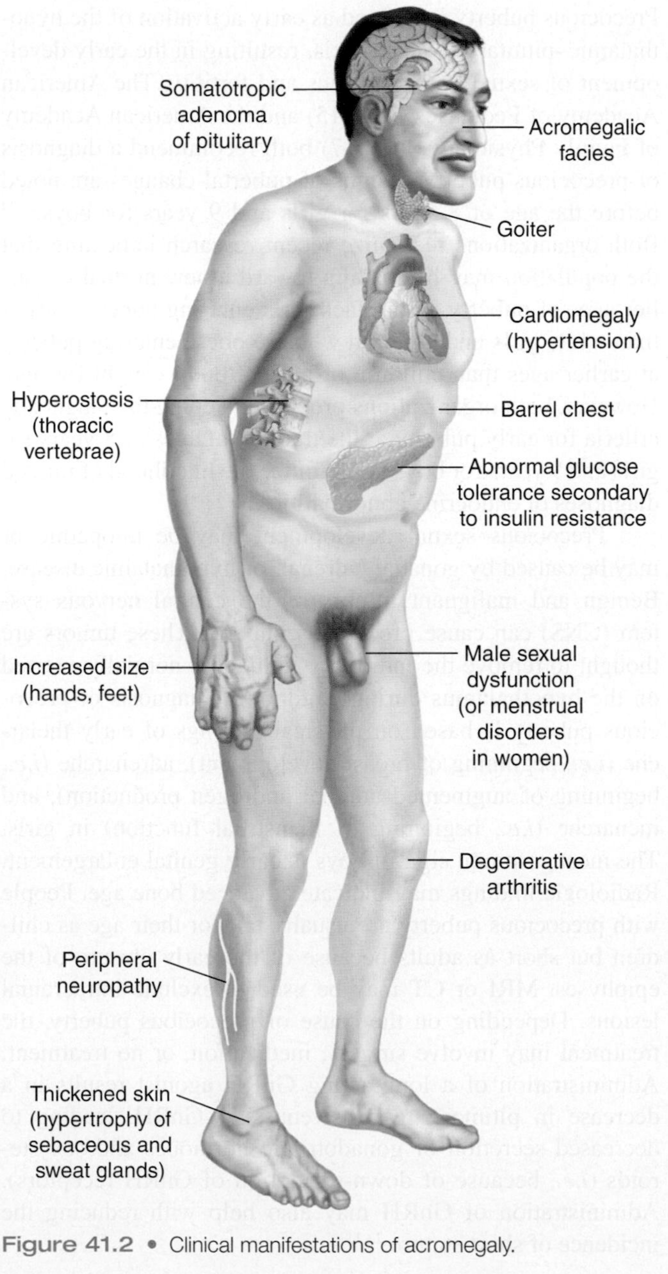

Figure 41.2 • Clinical manifestations of acromegaly.

The metabolic effects of excess levels of GH and IGF-1 include alterations in fat and carbohydrate metabolism. GH causes lipolysis, with the increased release of FFAs from adipose tissue leading to increased concentration of FFAs in body fluids. In addition, GH enhances the formation of ketones and the use of FFAs for energy in preference to use of carbohydrates and proteins. GH exerts multiple effects on carbohydrate metabolism, including decreased glucose uptake by tissues such as skeletal muscle and adipose tissue, increased glucose production by the liver, and increased insulin secretion.[4] Each of these changes results in GH-induced insulin resistance. This leads to glucose intolerance, which stimulates the beta cells of the pancreas to produce additional insulin. Long-term elevation of GH results in overstimulation of the beta cells, which may cause them literally to "burn out." The net result of these metabolic changes is impaired glucose regulation that often leads to the development of diabetes mellitus.[22]

Plasma levels of IGF-1 have been demonstrated to be more predictive of the risk for developing diabetes mellitus than are plasma GH levels. Higher plasma levels of IGF-1 have been associated with an increased risk for the development of diabetes in people with acromegaly; however, plasma concentrations of GH have not demonstrated the same correlation. Reported prevalence of diabetes mellitus in people with acromegaly ranges from 12% to 37.6%. When other forms of glucose dysregulation are considered (such as impaired fasting glucose and impaired glucose tolerance), the reported prevalence rates for glucose dysregulation in people with acromegaly rise to 16% to 54%.[22]

Additional clinical manifestations associated with acromegaly are related to pituitary adenomas, as this is the etiologic cause of most cases of acromegaly. As the pituitary adenoma grows, it causes further dysfunction of the pituitary gland and surrounding brain structures. The pituitary gland is located in the pituitary fossa of the sphenoid bone (*i.e.*, sella turcica), which lies directly below the optic nerve. Enlargement of the pituitary gland eventually causes erosion of the surrounding bone, and because of its location, this can lead to headaches, visual field defects resulting from compression of the optic nerve (classically, bitemporal hemianopia), and palsies of cranial nerves III, IV, and VI. Compression of other pituitary structures can cause secondary hypothyroidism, hypogonadism, and adrenal insufficiency. Hypogonadism can result from direct damage to the hypothalamic or pituitary system or indirectly because of hyperprolactinemia owing to prevention of the prolactin inhibitory factor (dopamine) from reaching pituitary lactotropes (cells that secrete prolactin) because of damage by the pituitary tumor.[1–3]

Other manifestations include excessive sweating with an unpleasant odor, oily skin, heat intolerance, moderate weight gain, muscle weakness and fatigue, menstrual irregularities, and decreased libido. Hypertension is relatively common. Sleep apnea syndrome is present in up to 90% of people. The pathogenesis of sleep apnea syndrome is obstructive in the majority of people because of increased pharyngeal soft tissue accumulation. Paresthesias may develop because of nerve entrapment and compression caused by excess soft tissue and accumulation of subcutaneous fluid (especially carpal tunnel syndrome). Acromegaly is also associated with an increased risk of colonic polyps and colorectal cancer.[1,21,22] The mortality rate of people with acromegaly is higher than the general population; however, advances in treatment have reduced the mortality rate from the previous two to three times the general population, to the current mortality rate that is less than two times the expected rate.[21] Mortality in people with acromegaly is primarily due to cardiovascular disease (60%), respiratory disease (25%), and cancer (15%).[21] The cardiovascular disease results from the combination of cardiomyopathy, hypertension, insulin resistance and hyperinsulinemia, and hyperlipidemia.[21,22]

Diagnosis. Acromegaly often develops insidiously, with an estimated 20% of people already having developed diabetes mellitus at the time of the acromegaly diagnosis.[22] The diagnosis of acromegaly is made via combination of a clinical exam revealing the typical physical features of the disorder (including enlargement of the hands and feet and coarsening of facial features) and diagnostic lab studies. Serum IGF-1 testing is the recommended initial lab test in evaluating a suspected diagnosis of acromegaly, and a finding of normal plasma IGF-1 levels essentially rules out the diagnosis. If the serum IGF-1 is elevated or equivocal, then the confirmatory test is a glucose challenge test. If serum GH levels are not suppressed by a glucose load, then the diagnosis of acromegaly is confirmed. MRI scanning is the recommended first-line imaging approach to detect and localize pituitary lesions, with CT scanning as the alternative if MRI is contraindicated. Visual field testing is also recommended because of the anatomic proximity of the pituitary gland to the optic chiasm.[21]

Treatment. Treatment for acromegaly focuses on the correction of metabolic abnormalities; normalization of IGF-1 levels to age- and sex-matched control levels; removal or reduction of the tumor mass; relieving the central pressure effects; and improvement of adverse clinical features. Pituitary tumors are removed surgically using the transsphenoidal approach. Medical therapy is used in an adjunctive role, or as a primary treatment approach if the pituitary tumor is assessed to be inoperable. Somatostatin is a hormone that has many actions in the body, including inhibiting the release of GH by the pituitary. Somatostatin analog drugs (such as the somatostatin receptor ligand drug octreotide) therefore can be effective in the medical management of acromegaly by producing feedback inhibition of GH secretion. Another drug that has demonstrated efficacy is pegvisomant, which operates through a different mechanism of action as a GH receptor blocker. Pegvisomant is a pegylated recombinant DNA analogue that incorporates nine different mutations, making the drug molecule different than the endogenous GH molecule. Pegvisomant can bind with the GH receptor sites and block GH binding; therefore, although GH levels remain elevated, the GH action on the target cells is reduced. Because the mechanism of action of pegvisomant does not reduce actual GH secretion by the pituitary tumor, a concern with this therapeutic approach is that the tumor may continue to grow. A third class of drugs used in the treatment of acromegaly are the dopamine agonists (such as bromocriptine), which exert their action by binding to dopamine receptors in the pituitary gland, thereby reducing pituitary secretion of both GH and prolactin. Radiotherapy is another option for adjuvant therapy, particularly useful if surgical treatment is not possible and medical therapy is not well tolerated. Radiotherapy has demonstrated success with lowering serum GH levels; however, radiotherapy has not been as effective in lowering serum IGF-1 levels.[21]

Precocious Puberty

Precocious puberty is defined as early activation of the hypothalamic–pituitary–gonadal axis, resulting in the early development of sexual characteristics and fertility. The American Academy of Pediatrics (in 2015) and the American Academy of Family Physicians (in 2017) both recommend a diagnosis of precocious puberty if signs of pubertal changes are noted before the age of 8 years for girls and 9 years for boys.[23,24] Both organizations recognize recent research indicating that the population may be shifting toward a new normal of earlier ages of puberty, with black girls entering puberty earlier than white girls and children who are obese entering puberty at earlier ages than children of normal body weight for age. However, both organizations proposed keeping the diagnostic criteria for early puberty at the traditional ages of 8 years for girls and 9 years for boys to minimize the likelihood of missed diagnoses of endocrine abnormalities.[23,24]

Precocious sexual development may be idiopathic or may be caused by gonadal, adrenal, or hypothalamic disease. Benign and malignant tumors of the central nervous system (CNS) can cause precocious puberty. These tumors are thought to remove the inhibitory influences normally exerted on the hypothalamus during childhood. Diagnosis of precocious puberty is based on physical findings of early thelarche (*i.e.*, beginning of breast development), adrenarche (*i.e.*, beginning of augmented adrenal androgen production), and menarche (*i.e.*, beginning of menstrual function) in girls. The most common sign in boys is early genital enlargement. Radiologic findings may indicate advanced bone age. People with precocious puberty are usually tall for their age as children but short as adults because of the early closure of the epiphyses. MRI or CT may be used to exclude intracranial lesions. Depending on the cause of precocious puberty, the treatment may involve surgery, medication, or no treatment. Administration of a long-acting GnRH agonist results in a decrease in pituitary responsiveness to GnRH, leading to decreased secretion of gonadotropic hormones and sex steroids (*i.e.*, because of down-regulation of GnRH receptors). Administration of GnRH may also help with reducing the incidence of short stature.[23,24]

IN SUMMARY

Pituitary tumors can result in deficiencies or excesses of pituitary hormones. Hypopituitarism, which is characterized by a decreased secretion of pituitary hormones, is a condition that affects many of the other endocrine systems. Depending on the extent of the disorder, it can result in decreased levels of GH, thyroid hormones, adrenal corticosteroid hormones, and testosterone in the male and estrogens and progesterone in the female.

A number of hormones are essential for normal body growth and maturation, including GH, insulin, thyroid hormone, and androgens. GH exerts its growth effects through IGF-1. GH also exerts an effect on metabolism and is produced in the adult and in the child. Its metabolic effects include a decrease in peripheral use of carbohydrates and an increased mobilization and use of fatty acids.

In children, alterations in growth include short stature, tall stature, and precocious puberty. Short stature is a condition in which the attained height is below the third percentile on the appropriate growth curve for a child's age and sex. Short stature can occur as a variant of normal growth (*i.e.*, familial short stature or constitutional delay of growth and puberty) or can occur as the result of endocrine disorders, chronic illness, malnutrition, emotional disturbances, or chromosomal disorders. Short stature resulting from GH deficiency can be treated with human GH preparations. In adults, GH deficiency represents a deficiency carried over from childhood or one that develops during adulthood as the result of a pituitary tumor or its treatment. GH levels also can decline with aging, and there has been interest in the effects of declining GH levels with aging (described as *somatopause*).

Tall stature refers to the condition in which children are tall for their age and gender. It can occur as a variant of normal growth (*i.e.*, familial tall stature or constitutional advancement of growth), as the result of a genetic or chromosomal abnormality or GH excess. GH excess in adults results in acromegaly, which involves proliferation of bone, cartilage, and soft tissue along with the metabolic effects of excessive hormone levels. Precocious puberty defines a condition of early activation of the hypothalamic–pituitary–gonadal axis, resulting in the development of appropriate sexual characteristics and fertility. It is associated with tall stature during childhood but may lead to short stature in adulthood because of the early closure of the epiphyses.

THYROID DISORDERS

After completing this section of the chapter, the learner will be able to meet the following objectives:

- Characterize the synthesis, transport, and regulation of thyroid hormone.
- Describe tests in the diagnosis and management of thyroid disorders.

Control of Thyroid Function

The thyroid gland is a shield-shaped structure located immediately below the larynx in the anterior middle portion of the neck (Fig. 41.3A). It is composed of a large number of tiny, saclike structures called *follicles* (see Fig. 41.3B). These are the functional units of the thyroid. Each follicle is formed by a single layer of epithelial (follicular) cells and is filled with a secretory substance called *colloid*, which consists largely of a glycoprotein–iodine complex called *thyroglobulin*.[4,9]

The thyroglobulin that fills the thyroid follicles is a large glycoprotein molecule that contains about 100 tyrosine amino acid residues.[4] It is these tyrosine molecules to which iodine is attached to create thyroid hormone. This process of thyroid synthesis occurs within the follicles of the thyroid gland.[4]

The thyroid is remarkably efficient in its use of iodide. A yearly absorption of approximately 50 mg of ingested iodine, or about 1 mg/week, is all that is required to form normal quantities of thyroid hormone.[4] In the process of removing the iodine from the blood and storing it for future use, iodide is pumped into the follicular cells against a concentration gradient. Iodide (I^-) is transported across the basement membrane of the thyroid cells by an intrinsic membrane protein called the *Na^+/I symporter* (NIS).[4] At the apical border, a second I^- transport protein called *pendrin* moves iodine into the colloid, where it is involved in hormonogenesis.[4] The NIS derives its energy from Na^+/K^+-ATPase, which drives the process. As a result, the concentration of iodide in the normal thyroid gland is approximately 30 times than that in the blood.[4]

Once inside the follicle, most of the iodide is oxidized by the enzyme thyroid peroxidase (TPO) in a reaction that facilitates combination with a tyrosine molecule to form monoiodotyrosine (MIT) and then diiodotyrosine (DIT).[4] Two DIT residues are coupled to form thyroxine (T_4), or a MIT and a DIT are coupled to form triiodothyronine (T_3).[4] Only T_4 (93%) and T_3 (7%) are released into the circulation[4] (see Fig. 41.3C). Although T_3 is significantly more potent in its activity, T_4 has a much longer half-life in the blood (7 days) than T_3 (1 day); therefore, T_4 serves as an effective storage molecule. The circulating T_4 is converted to T_3 when needed.[9]

Stimulation by TSH from the pituitary gland serves as the stimulus for the thyroid gland to secrete the T_3 and T_4 thyroid hormones into the blood.[9] Thyroid hormones are bound to thyroxine-binding globulin (TBG) and other plasma proteins for transport in the blood. Only the free T_3 or T_4 hormone can enter target cells to exert the hormonal effect; the protein-bound forms cannot enter the cells. Protein-bound thyroid hormone forms a large reservoir that is slowly drawn on as free thyroid hormone is needed. There are three major thyroid-binding proteins: TBG, transthyretin (also known as thyroxine-binding prealbumin [TBPA]), and albumin. More than 99% of T_4 and T_3 is carried in these bound forms.[4,25]

A number of disease conditions and pharmacologic agents can decrease the amount of binding protein in the plasma or influence the binding of hormone. Several genetic alterations of TBG function have been identified, including an X-linked TBG deficiency associated with a gene on the

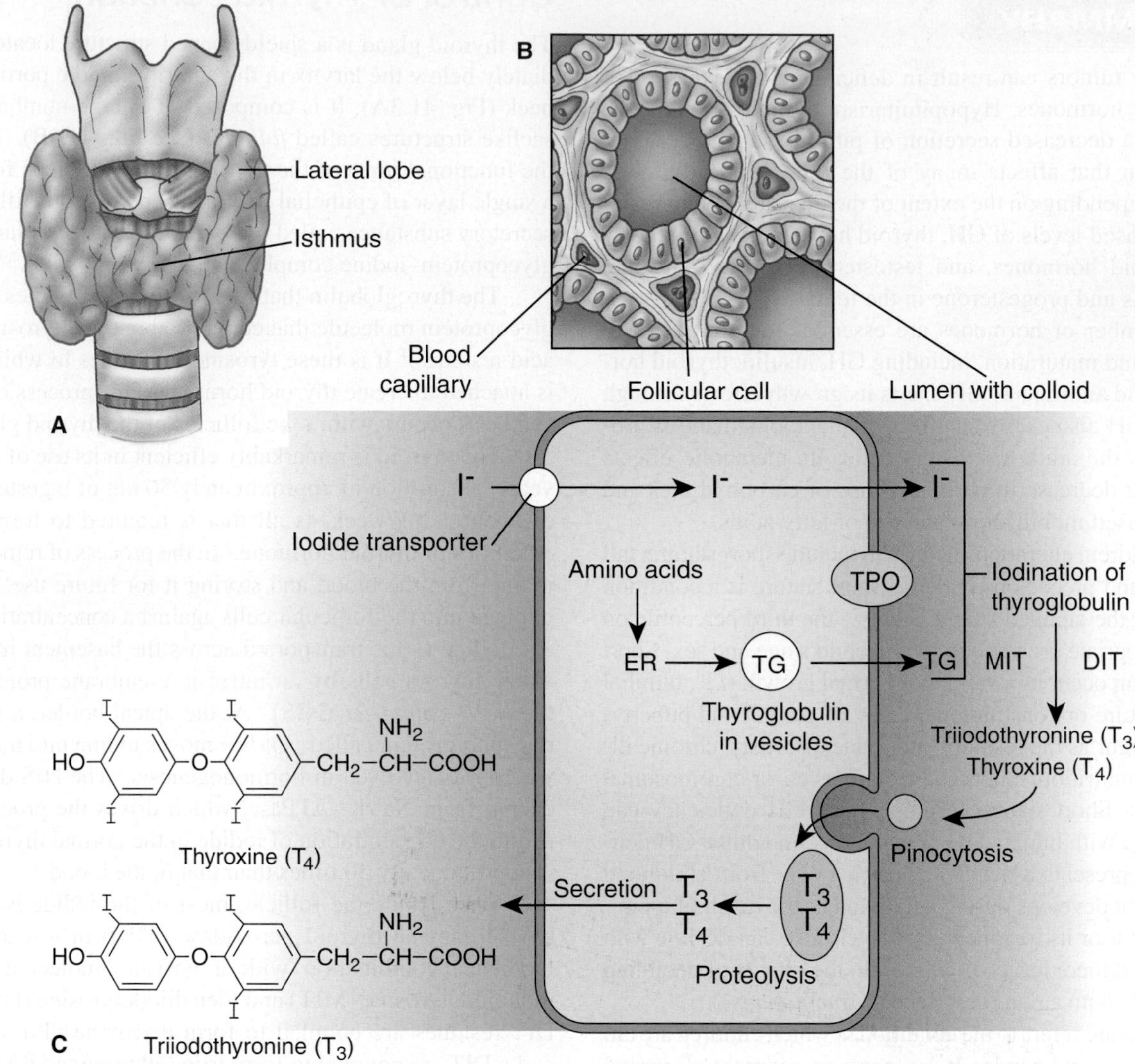

Figure 41.3 • **(A)** The thyroid gland. **(B)** Microscopic structure of thyroid follicles. **(C)** Cellular mechanisms for transport of iodide (I^-), oxidation of I^- by thyroperoxidase (TPO), coupling of oxidized I^- with thyroglobulin to form thyroid hormones, and movement of T_3 and T_4 into the follicular cell by pinocytosis and release into the blood.

long arm of the X chromosome.[25] Glucocorticoid medications and systemic disease conditions such as protein malnutrition, nephrotic syndrome, and cirrhosis can decrease TBG concentrations of the thyroid-binding proteins. A variety of drugs, such as phenytoin, salicylates, and diazepam, can affect the binding of thyroid hormone to normal concentrations of binding proteins or disrupt thyroid metabolism in other ways.[26]

The secretion of thyroid hormone is regulated by the hypothalamic–pituitary–thyroid feedback system (see Chapter 40, Fig. 40.3). In this system, thyrotropin-releasing hormone (TRH), which is produced by the hypothalamus, controls the release of TSH from the anterior pituitary gland. TSH increases the overall activity of the thyroid gland by increasing thyroglobulin breakdown and the release of thyroid hormone from follicles into the bloodstream, activating the iodide pump (by increasing NIS activity), increasing the oxidation of iodide and the coupling of iodide to tyrosine, and increasing the number and the size of the follicle cells.[4,9]

Increased plasma levels of thyroid hormone lead to feedback inhibition of TRH or TSH. High levels of iodide also cause a temporary decrease in thyroid activity that lasts for several weeks, probably through a direct inhibition of TSH on the thyroid. Cold exposure is one of the strongest stimuli for increased thyroid hormone production and probably is mediated through TRH from the hypothalamus. Various emotional reactions can also affect the output of TRH and TSH.[4]

Actions of Thyroid Hormone

Altered levels of thyroid hormone affect all the major organs in the body. Thyroid hormone has two major functions—it increases metabolism and protein synthesis, and it is necessary for growth and development in children, including mental development and attainment of sexual maturity. These actions are mainly mediated by T_3. In the cell, T_3 binds to a nuclear receptor, resulting in transcription of specific thyroid hormone response genes.[4]

Metabolic Rate. Thyroid hormone increases the metabolism of target cells throughout the body. The basal metabolic rate can increase by 60% to 100% above normal when large amounts of T_4 are present.[4] As a result of this higher metabolism, the rate of glucose, fat, and protein use increases. Lipids are mobilized from adipose tissue, and the catabolism of cholesterol by the liver is increased. Blood levels of cholesterol are decreased in hyperthyroidism and increased in hypothyroidism. Muscle proteins are broken down and used as fuel, probably accounting for some of the muscle fatigue that occurs with hyperthyroidism. The absorption of glucose from the gastrointestinal tract is increased.[4]

Cardiovascular Function. Cardiovascular and respiratory functions are strongly affected by thyroid function. With an increase in metabolism, there is a rise in oxygen consumption and production of metabolic end products, with an accompanying increase in vasodilation. Blood flow to the skin, in particular, is augmented as a means of dissipating the body heat that results from the higher metabolic rate. Blood volume, cardiac output, and ventilation are all increased as a means of maintaining blood flow and oxygen delivery to body tissues. Heart rate and cardiac contractility are enhanced as a means of maintaining the needed cardiac output. Blood pressure is likely to change little because the increase in vasodilation tends to offset the increase in cardiac output.[4]

Gastrointestinal Function. Thyroid hormone enhances gastrointestinal function, causing an increase in motility and production of gastrointestinal secretions that often result in diarrhea. An increase in appetite and food intake accompanies the higher metabolic rate that occurs with increased thyroid hormone levels. At the same time, weight loss occurs because of the increased use of calories.[4]

Neuromuscular Effects. Thyroid hormone has marked effects on neural control of muscle function and tone. Slight elevations in hormone levels cause skeletal muscles to react more vigorously, and a drop in hormone levels causes muscles to react more sluggishly. In the hyperthyroid state, a fine muscle tremor is present. The cause of this tremor is unknown, but it may represent an increased sensitivity of the neural synapses in the spinal cord that controls muscle tone. In the infant, thyroid hormone is necessary for normal brain development. The hormone enhances cerebration; in the hyperthyroid state, it causes extreme nervousness, anxiety, and difficulty in sleeping.[4]

Evidence suggests a strong interaction between the thyroid hormone and the sympathetic nervous system.[4] Many of the signs and symptoms of hyperthyroidism suggest over activity of the sympathetic division of the autonomic nervous system, such as tachycardia, palpitations, and sweating. Tremor, restlessness, anxiety, and diarrhea may also reflect autonomic nervous system imbalances. Drugs that block sympathetic activity have proved to be valuable adjuncts in the treatment of hyperthyroidism because of their ability to relieve some of these undesirable symptoms.[2]

KEY POINTS

THYROID HORMONE

- Thyroid hormone increases the metabolism and protein synthesis in nearly all of the tissues of the body.
- When hypothyroidism occurs in older children or adults, it produces a decrease in metabolic rate, an accumulation of a hydrophilic mucopolysaccharide substance (myxedema) in the connective tissues throughout the body, and an elevation in serum cholesterol.
- Hyperthyroidism has an effect opposite to that of hypothyroidism. It produces an increase in metabolic rate and oxygen consumption, increased use of metabolic fuels, and increased sympathetic nervous system responsiveness.

Tests of Thyroid Function

Various tests aid in the diagnosis of thyroid disorders. Measures of T_3 (total and free), T_4 (total and free), and TSH have been made available through immunoassay methods. The total T_3 and T_4 tests measure both the protein-bound and free components of each hormone. The free T_3 and T_4 tests measure the fractions that are not bound to plasma proteins, which are therefore free to enter cells to produce effects. TSH levels are used to differentiate between primary thyroid disorders (which originate at the thyroid gland) and secondary thyroid disorders (which originate at the pituitary gland). T_3 and T_4 levels (bound and free) are low in primary hypothyroidism; however, the TSH level is elevated. The assessment of thyroid autoantibodies (*e.g.*, anti-TPO antibodies in Hashimoto thyroiditis) is also important in the diagnostic workup and follow-up of people with thyroid disorders.[2,9]

The radioiodine (^{123}I) uptake test measures the ability of the thyroid gland to concentrate and retain iodine from the blood. Thyroid scans (^{123}I, ^{99m}Tc-pertechnetate) can be used to detect thyroid nodules and determine the functional activity of the thyroid gland. Ultrasonography can be used to differentiate cystic from solid thyroid lesions, and CT and MRI scans are used to demonstrate tracheal compression or impingement on other neighboring structures. Fine-needle aspiration biopsy of a thyroid nodule has proved to be the best method for differentiation of benign from malignant thyroid disease.[2,9]

Alterations in Thyroid Function

An alteration in thyroid function can represent a hypofunctional or a hyperfunctional state. The manifestations of these two altered states are summarized in Table 41.3. Disorders of

TABLE 41.3 MANIFESTATIONS OF HYPOTHYROID AND HYPERTHYROID STATES

LEVEL OF ORGANIZATION	HYPOTHYROIDISM	HYPERTHYROIDISM
Basal metabolic rate	Decreased	Increased
Sensitivity to catecholamines	Decreased	Increased
General features	Myxedematous features	Exophthalmos (in Graves disease)
	Deep voice	Lid lag
	Impaired growth (child)	Accelerated growth (child)
Blood cholesterol levels	Increased	Decreased
General behavior	Intellectual disability (infant)	Restlessness, irritability, anxiety
	Mental and physical sluggishness	Hyperkinesis
	Somnolence	Wakefulness
Cardiovascular function	Decreased cardiac output	Increased cardiac output
	Bradycardia	Tachycardia and palpitations
Gastrointestinal function	Constipation	Diarrhea
	Decreased appetite	Increased appetite
Respiratory function	Hypoventilation	Dyspnea
Muscle tone and reflexes	Decreased	Increased, with tremor and twitching
Temperature tolerance	Cold intolerance	Heat intolerance
Skin and hair	Decreased sweating	Increased sweating
	Coarse and dry skin and hair	Thin and silky skin and hair
Weight	Gain	Loss

the thyroid may be due to a congenital defect in thyroid development, or they may develop later in life, with a gradual or sudden onset.

Goiter is an increase in the size of the thyroid gland (Fig. 41.4). It can occur in hypothyroid, euthyroid, and hyperthyroid states. Goiters may be diffuse, involving the entire gland without evidence of nodularity, or they may contain nodules. Diffuse goiters usually become nodular. Goiters may be toxic, producing signs of extreme hyperthyroidism, or thyrotoxicosis, or they may be nontoxic. Diffuse nontoxic and multinodular goiters are the result of compensatory hypertrophy and hyperplasia of follicular epithelium from some derangement that impairs thyroid hormone output.[1,2,4]

The degree of thyroid enlargement is usually proportional to the extent and duration of thyroid deficiency. Multinodular goiters produce the largest thyroid enlargements. When sufficiently enlarged, they may compress the esophagus and trachea, causing difficulty in swallowing, a choking sensation, and inspiratory stridor. Such lesions may also compress the superior vena cava, producing distention of the veins of the neck and upper extremities, edema of the eyelids and conjunctiva, and syncope with coughing.[1,2,4]

Hypothyroidism

Hypothyroidism can occur as a congenital or an acquired defect. Congenital hypothyroidism develops prenatally and is present at birth. Acquired hypothyroidism develops because of primary disease of the thyroid gland or secondary to disorders of hypothalamic or pituitary origin.

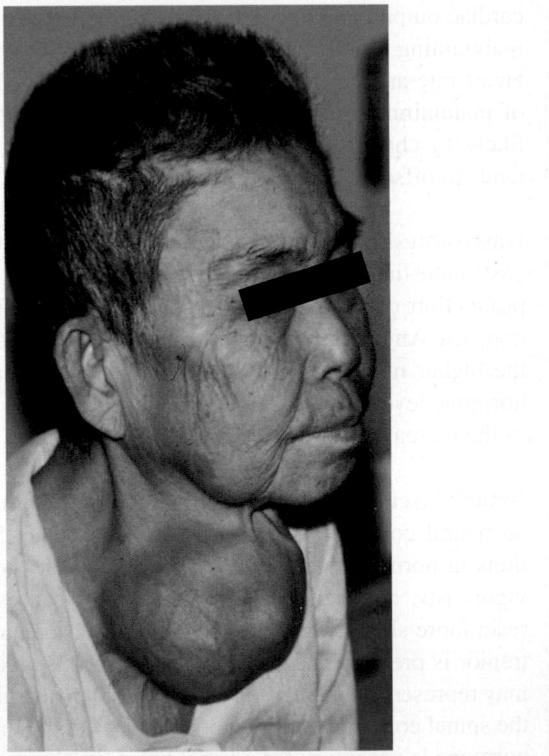

Goiter

Figure 41.4 • Nontoxic goiter. In a middle-aged woman with nontoxic goiter, the thyroid has enlarged to produce a conspicuous neck mass. (From Strayer D., Rubin E. (Eds.) (2015). *Rubin's pathology: Clinicopathologic foundations of medicine* (7th ed., Figure 27-11A, p. 1183). Philadelphia, PA: Wolters Kluwer.)

Congenital Hypothyroidism

Congenital hypothyroidism is a common cause of preventable intellectual disability. Hypothyroidism in the infant may result from a congenital lack of the thyroid gland or from abnormal biosynthesis of thyroid hormone or deficient TSH secretion. With congenital lack of the thyroid gland, the infant usually appears normal and functions normally at birth because hormones have been supplied in utero by the mother.[1,2,4]

Thyroid hormone is essential for normal growth and brain development, almost half of which occurs during the first 6 months of life. If untreated, congenital hypothyroidism causes intellectual disability and impairs physical growth. The manifestations of untreated congenital hypothyroidism are referred to as cretinism. However, the term does not apply to the normally developing infant in whom replacement thyroid hormone therapy was instituted shortly after birth.[1,2,4]

Many countries throughout the world now routinely perform neonatal screening to detect congenital hypothyroidism during early infancy.[27] Premature or sick newborn infants need to be screened with a comprehensive serum thyroid profile to prevent missing primary hypothyroidism in these infants.

Transient congenital hypothyroidism (characterized by high TSH levels with low or normal thyroid hormone levels) has been recognized more frequently since the introduction of neonatal screening. The fetal and infant thyroid gland is sensitive to iodine excess. Iodine can cross the placenta, be excreted in breast milk, and is also readily absorbed by infant skin. Transient hypothyroidism may be caused by maternal or infant exposure to substances such as povidone–iodine used as a disinfectant (*i.e.*, vaginal douche or skin disinfectant). Antithyroid drugs such as propylthiouracil and methimazole can also cross the placenta and block fetal thyroid function.[1,2,4,27]

Congenital hypothyroidism is treated by thyroid hormone replacement. Evidence indicates that it is important to normalize T_4 levels as rapidly as possible because a delay is accompanied by poorer psychomotor and mental development. Dosage levels are adjusted as the child grows. When early and adequate thyroid hormone replacement treatment is implemented for congenital hypothyroidism, the risk of intellectual disability is very low.[1,2,4,27]

Acquired Hypothyroidism and Myxedema

Hypothyroidism in older children and adults causes a general slowing down of metabolic processes and myxedema. Myxedema implies the presence of a nonpitting mucus type of edema caused by an accumulation of a hydrophilic mucopolysaccharide substance in the connective tissues throughout the body. The hypothyroid state may be mild, with only a few signs and symptoms, or it may progress to a life-threatening condition with angioedema.[1,2,4]

Etiology and Pathogenesis. Acquired hypothyroidism can result from destruction or dysfunction of the thyroid gland (*i.e.*, primary hypothyroidism), or it can be a secondary disorder caused by impaired pituitary function or as a tertiary disorder caused by a hypothalamic dysfunction.

Primary hypothyroidism is much more common than secondary (and tertiary) hypothyroidism. It may result from thyroidectomy (*i.e.*, surgical removal) or ablation of the gland with radiation for treatment of hyperthyroidism. Certain goitrogenic agents, such as lithium carbonate (used in the treatment of manic-depressive states), and the antithyroid drugs propylthiouracil and methimazole in continuous dosage can block hormone synthesis and produce hypothyroidism with goiter. Large amounts of iodine (*i.e.*, ingestion of kelp tablets or iodide-containing cough syrups, or administration of iodide-containing radiographic contrast media or the cardiac antiarrhythmic class III drug amiodarone, which contains iodine) can also block thyroid hormone production and cause hypothyroidism, particularly in people with autoimmune thyroid disease. Iodine deficiency, which can cause goiter and hypothyroidism, is uncommon in the United States because of the widespread use of iodized salt and other iodide sources. However, iodine deficiency continues to occur in less developed areas of the world.[1,2,4] Subacute thyroiditis, which can occur in postpartum women (postpartum thyroiditis), is another cause of hypothyroidism.[28]

The most common cause of acquired hypothyroidism is Hashimoto thyroiditis, an autoimmune disorder in which the thyroid gland may be totally destroyed by an immunologic process. It is the major cause of acquired hypothyroidism in children and adults.[1,27] Hashimoto thyroiditis is predominantly a disease of women. The course of the disease varies. At the onset, only a goiter may be present. In time, hypothyroidism usually becomes evident. Although the disorder usually causes hypothyroidism, a hyperthyroid state may develop midcourse in the disease. The transient hyperthyroid state may be related to leakage of preformed thyroid hormone from damaged cells of the gland.[1,2,4]

Clinical Manifestations. Hypothyroidism may affect almost all body functions. The manifestations of the disorder are related largely to two factors: the hypometabolic state resulting from thyroid hormone deficiency and myxedematous involvement of body tissues. The hypometabolic state associated with hypothyroidism is characterized by a gradual onset of weakness and fatigue, a tendency to gain weight despite a loss of appetite, and cold intolerance (Fig. 41.5). As the condition progresses, the skin becomes dry and rough and the hair becomes coarse and brittle. The face becomes puffy with edematous eyelids, and there is thinning of the outer third of the eyebrows. Gastrointestinal motility is decreased, producing constipation, flatulence, and abdominal distention. Delayed relaxation of deep tendon reflexes and bradycardia are sometimes noted. CNS involvement is manifested in mental dullness, lethargy, and impaired memory.[1,2,4]

Although the myxedematous fluid is usually most obvious in the face, it can collect in the interstitial spaces of

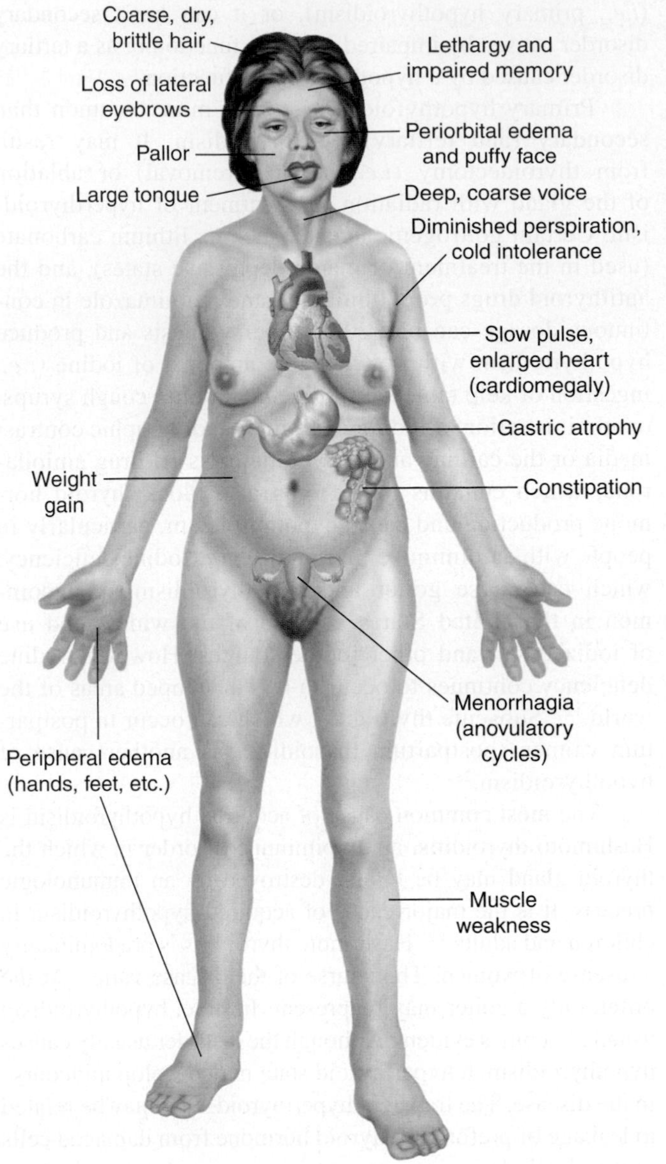

Figure 41.5 • Clinical manifestations of hypothyroidism.

almost any body structure and is responsible for many of the manifestations of the severe hypothyroid state. The tongue is often enlarged, and the voice becomes hoarse and husky. Carpal tunnel and other entrapment syndromes are common, as is impairment of muscle function with stiffness, cramps, and pain. Mucopolysaccharide deposits in the heart cause generalized cardiac dilation, bradycardia, and other signs of altered cardiac function. The signs and symptoms of hypothyroidism are summarized in Table 41.3.[1,2,4]

Diagnosis and Treatment. Diagnosis of hypothyroidism is based on history, physical examination, and laboratory tests. A low serum T_4 and elevated TSH levels are characteristic of primary hypothyroidism. The tests for antithyroid antibodies should be done when Hashimoto thyroiditis is suspected (anti-TPO antibody titers are tested frequently).[1,2,4]

Hypothyroidism is treated by replacement therapy with synthetic preparations of T_3 or T_4. Most people are treated with T_4. Serum TSH levels are used to estimate the adequacy of T_4 replacement therapy. When the TSH level is normalized, the T_4 dosage is considered satisfactory (for primary hypothyroidism only). A "go low and go slow" approach should be considered in the treatment of older people with hypothyroidism because of the risk of inducing acute coronary syndromes in the susceptible individual. It is also important that people consistently take the form of T_4 prescribed, so that their laboratory values are the most representative of their thyroid state. Therefore, people should remain on generic forms of T_4 and, similarly, if people are put on brand names of T_4, they should stay on the same drug.[1,2,4,29]

Myxedematous Coma

Myxedematous coma is a life-threatening, end-stage expression of hypothyroidism. Long-standing hypothyroidism leads to a crisis state with severely reduced cellular metabolism that affects all organ systems throughout the body. Hypothermia also develops and is a strong predictor of mortality. The condition is associated with cardiovascular collapse, hypoventilation, and severe metabolic disorders that include hyponatremia, hypoglycemia, and lactic acidosis.[8,30]

Treatment includes aggressive management of precipitating factors; supportive therapy such as management of cardiorespiratory status, hyponatremia, and hypoglycemia; and thyroid replacement therapy. If hypothermia is present, active rewarming of the body is contraindicated because it may induce vasodilation and vascular collapse. Prevention is preferable to treatment and entails special attention to high-risk populations, such as women with a history of Hashimoto thyroiditis. These people should be informed about the signs and symptoms of severe hypothyroidism and the need for early medical treatment.[8,30]

Hyperthyroidism

Thyrotoxicosis is the clinical syndrome that results when tissues are exposed to high levels of circulating thyroid hormone.[4]

Etiology and Pathogenesis

In most instances, thyrotoxicosis is due to hyperactivity of the thyroid gland, or hyperthyroidism. The most common cause of hyperthyroidism is Graves disease, which is accompanied by ophthalmopathy (or dermopathy) and diffuses goiter. Other causes of hyperthyroidism are multinodular goiter, adenoma of the thyroid, and thyroiditis. Iodine-containing agents can induce hyperthyroidism as well as hypothyroidism. Thyroid crisis, or storm, is an acutely exaggerated manifestation of the thyrotoxic state.[1,8]

Clinical Manifestations

Many of the manifestations of hyperthyroidism are related to the increase in oxygen consumption and use of metabolic fuels associated with the hypermetabolic state, as well as to the increase in sympathetic nervous system activity that occurs. The fact that many of the signs and symptoms of hyperthyroidism resemble those of excessive sympathetic nervous system activity suggests that thyroid hormone may heighten the sensitivity of the body to the catecholamines or that it may act as a pseudocatecholamine. With the hypermetabolic state, there are frequent complaints of nervousness, irritability, and fatigability (Fig. 41.6). Weight loss is common despite a large appetite. Other manifestations include tachycardia, palpitations, shortness of breath, excessive sweating, muscle cramps, and heat intolerance. The person appears restless and has a fine muscle tremor. Even in people without exophthalmos (*i.e.*, bulging of the eyeballs seen in ophthalmopathy), there is an abnormal retraction of the eyelids and infrequent blinking such that they appear to be staring. The hair and skin are usually thin and have a silky appearance.[1,8,31] Atrial fibrillation occurs in 10% to 15% of adults with hyperthyroidism.[32] The signs and symptoms of hyperthyroidism are summarized in Table 41.3.

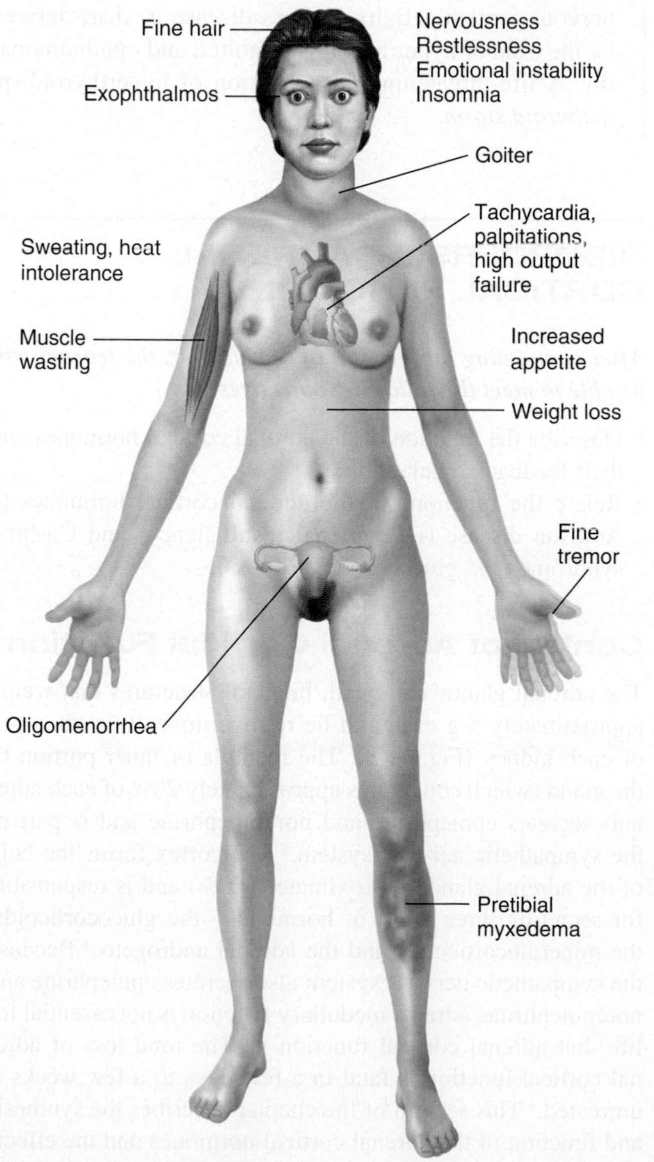

Figure 41.6 • Clinical manifestations of hyperthyroidism.

The treatment of hyperthyroidism is directed toward reducing the level of thyroid hormone. This can be accomplished with eradication of the thyroid gland with radioactive iodine, through surgical removal of part or all of the gland, or the use of drugs that decrease thyroid function and thereby the effect of thyroid hormone on the peripheral tissues. Eradication of the thyroid with radioactive iodine is more frequently undertaken than surgery. The β-adrenergic blocking drugs (propranolol, metoprolol, atenolol, and nadolol are preferred) are administered to block the effects of the hyperthyroid state on sympathetic nervous system function. They are given in conjunction with antithyroid drugs such as propylthiouracil and methimazole. These drugs prevent the thyroid gland from converting iodine to its organic (hormonal) form and block the conversion of T_4 to T_3 in the tissues (propylthiouracil only).[1,8,31,33]

Graves Disease

Graves disease is a state of hyperthyroidism, goiter, and ophthalmopathy. It affects approximately 0.5% to 1% of the population under 40 years of age.[1] Graves disease is an autoimmune disorder characterized by abnormal stimulation of the thyroid gland by thyroid-stimulating antibodies (TSH receptor antibodies) that act through the normal TSH receptors. It may be associated with other autoimmune disorders such as myasthenia gravis. The disease is associated with a major histocompatibility complex class 1 chain–related gene A (MICA), with genotypes MICA A5 correlated with Graves disease and MICA A6/A9 being preventive for Graves disease.[1]

The ophthalmopathy, which occurs in up to one third of people with Graves disease, is thought to result from accumulation of T lymphocytes sensitized to antigens along thyroid follicular cells and orbital fibroblasts that secrete cytokines.[1] The ophthalmopathy of Graves disease can cause severe eye problems, including tethering of the extraocular muscles resulting in diplopia; involvement of the optic nerve, with some visual loss; and corneal ulceration because the lids do not close over the protruding eyeball (because of the exophthalmos). The ophthalmopathy usually tends to stabilize after treatment of the hyperthyroidism. However, ophthalmopathy can worsen acutely after radioiodine treatment. Some physicians prescribe glucocorticoids for several weeks surrounding the radioiodine treatment if the person had signs of ophthalmopathy. Ophthalmopathy can also be aggravated by smoking, which should be strongly discouraged.[34] Figure 41.7 shows a woman with Graves disease.

Thyroid Storm

Thyroid storm, or thyrotoxic crisis, is an extreme and life-threatening form of thyrotoxicosis rarely seen today because

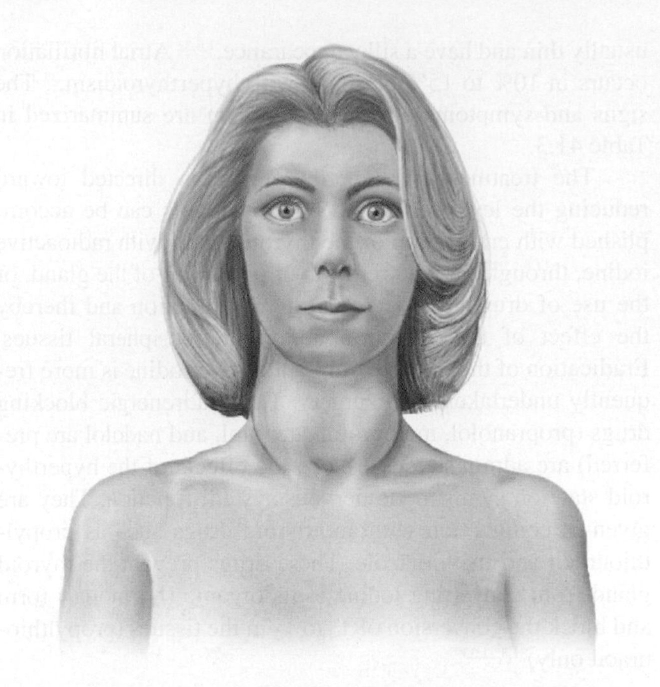

Figure 41.7 • Graves disease. A patient with Graves disease may show symptoms of an enlarged thyroid (goiter) and protrusion of one or both eyeballs (exophthalmos). (Asset provided by Anatomical Chart Co.)

of improved diagnosis and treatment methods. When it does occur, it is seen most often in undiagnosed cases or in people with hyperthyroidism who have not been adequately treated. It is often precipitated by stress, such as an infection, by physical or emotional trauma, or by manipulation of a hyperactive thyroid gland during thyroidectomy. Thyroid storm is manifested by a very high fever, extreme cardiovascular effects (*i.e.*, tachycardia, congestive failure, and angina), and severe CNS effects (*i.e.*, agitation, restlessness, and delirium). The mortality rate is high.[35–37]

Thyroid storm requires rapid diagnosis and implementation of treatment. Initially, the person must be hemodynamically stabilized. The thyroid hormones can be removed by plasmapheresis, dialysis, or hemoperfusion adsorption. Peripheral cooling is initiated with cold packs and a cooling mattress. For cooling to be effective, the shivering response must be prevented. General supportive measures to replace fluids, glucose, and electrolytes are essential during the hypermetabolic state. A β-adrenergic blocking drug, such as propranolol, is given to block the undesirable effects of T_4 on cardiovascular function. Glucocorticoids are used to correct the relative adrenal insufficiency resulting from the stress imposed by the hyperthyroid state and to inhibit the peripheral conversion of T_4 to T_3. Propylthiouracil or methimazole may be given to block thyroid synthesis. Aspirin increases the level of free thyroid hormones by displacing the hormones from their protein carriers and should not be used during thyroid storm.[35–37]

IN SUMMARY

Thyroid hormones play a role in the metabolic process of almost all body cells and are necessary for normal physical and mental growth in the infant and young child. Alterations in thyroid function can manifest as a hypothyroid or a hyperthyroid state. Hypothyroidism can occur as a congenital or an acquired defect. Congenital hypothyroidism leads to intellectual disability and impaired physical growth unless treatment is initiated during the first month of life. Acquired hypothyroidism leads to a decrease in metabolic rate and an accumulation of a mucopolysaccharide substance in the intercellular spaces; this substance attracts water and causes a mucous type of edema called *myxedema*. Hyperthyroidism causes an increase in metabolic rate and alterations in body function similar to those produced by enhanced sympathetic nervous system activity. Graves disease is characterized by the triad of hyperthyroidism, goiter, and ophthalmopathy. A life-threatening complication of hyperthyroidism is *thyroid storm*.

DISORDERS OF ADRENAL CORTICAL FUNCTION

After completing this section of the chapter, the learner will be able to meet the following objectives:

- Describe the function of the adrenal cortical hormones and their feedback regulation.
- Relate the functions of the adrenal cortical hormones to Addison disease (*i.e.*, adrenal insufficiency) and Cushing syndrome (*i.e.*, glucocorticoid excess).

Control of Adrenal Cortical Function

The adrenal glands are small, bilateral structures that weigh approximately 5 g each and lie retroperitoneally at the apex of each kidney (Fig. 41.8). The medulla or inner portion of the gland (which constitutes approximately 20% of each adrenal) secretes epinephrine and norepinephrine and is part of the sympathetic nervous system.[4] The cortex forms the bulk of the adrenal gland (approximately 80%) and is responsible for secreting three types of hormones—the glucocorticoids, the mineralocorticoids, and the adrenal androgens.[4] Because the sympathetic nervous system also secretes epinephrine and norepinephrine, adrenal medullary function is not essential for life, but adrenal cortical function is. The total loss of adrenal cortical function is fatal in a few days to a few weeks if untreated.[4] This section of the chapter describes the synthesis and function of the adrenal cortical hormones and the effects of adrenal cortical insufficiency and excess.

Biosynthesis, Transport, and Metabolism

More than 30 hormones are produced by the adrenal cortex. Of these hormones, aldosterone is the principal mineralocorticoid, cortisol (hydrocortisone) is the major glucocorticoid, and androgens are the chief sex hormones. All of the adrenal cortical hormones have a similar structure in which all are steroids and are synthesized from acetate and cholesterol. Each of the steps involved in the synthesis of the various hormones requires a specific enzyme (see Fig. 41.8). The ACTH secreted by the anterior pituitary gland controls the secretion of the glucocorticoids and the adrenal androgens.[4,9]

Cortisol, aldosterone, and the adrenal androgens are secreted in an unbound state and bind to plasma proteins for transport in the circulatory system. Cortisol binds largely to corticosteroid-binding globulin and to a lesser extent to albumin. Aldosterone and androgens circulate mostly bound to albumin. It has been suggested that the pool of protein-bound hormones may extend the duration of their action by delaying metabolic clearance.[4,9]

The main site for metabolism of the adrenal cortical hormones is the liver, where they undergo a number of metabolic conversions before being conjugated and made water-soluble. They are then eliminated in either the urine or the bile.[4,9]

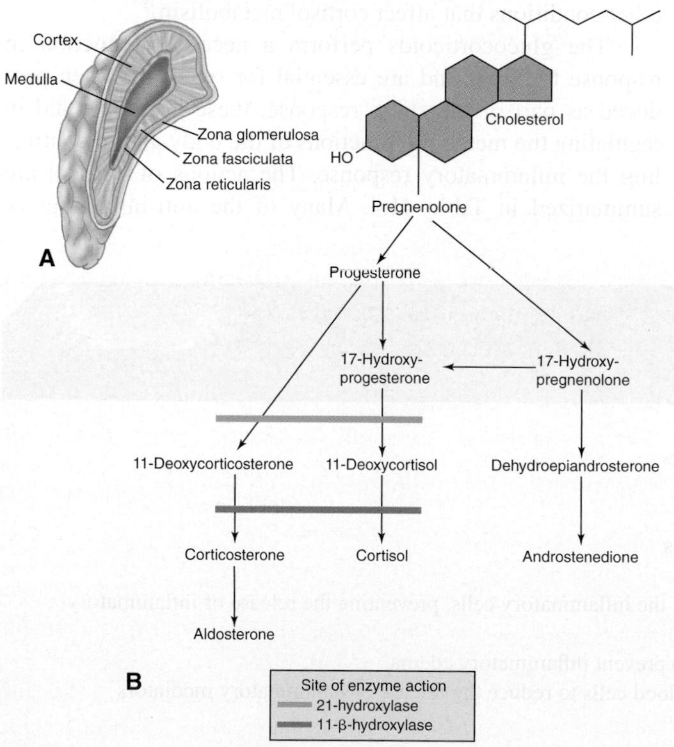

Figure 41.8 • (A) The adrenal gland showing the medulla and the three layers of the cortex. The outer layer of the cortex (zona glomerulosa) is primarily responsible for mineralocorticoid production, and the middle layer (zona fasciculata) and the inner layer (zona reticularis) produce the glucocorticoids and the adrenal androgens. **(B)** Predominant biosynthetic pathways of the adrenal cortex. Critical enzymes in the biosynthetic process include 11-β-hydroxylase and 21-hydroxylase. A deficiency in one of these enzymes blocks the synthesis of hormones dependent on that enzyme and routes the precursors into alternative pathways.

KEY POINTS

ADRENAL CORTICAL HORMONES

- The manifestations of primary adrenal cortical insufficiency are related mainly to mineralocorticoid deficiency (impaired ability to regulate salt and water elimination) and glucocorticoid deficiency (impaired ability to regulate blood glucose and control the effects of the immune and inflammatory responses).
- Adrenal cortical excess results in derangements in glucose metabolism, disorders of sodium and potassium regulation (increased sodium retention and potassium loss), impaired ability to respond to stress because of inhibition of inflammatory and immune responses, and signs of increased androgen levels such as hirsutism.

Adrenal Androgens

The adrenal androgens are synthesized primarily by the zona reticularis and the zona fasciculata of the cortex (see Fig. 41.8A).[4] These sex hormones probably exert little effect on normal sexual function. There is evidence, however, that the adrenal androgens (the most important of which is dehydroepiandrosterone [DHEA] and its sulfate [DHEAS]) contribute to the pubertal growth of body hair, particularly pubic and axillary hair in women. They may also play a role in steroid hormone economy of the pregnant woman and the fetal–placental unit. DHEAS is increasingly being used for treating both Addison disease and adults who have decreased levels of DHEAS. Adrenal androgens are physiologically important in women with Addison disease, and daily replacement of DHEAS should be considered. Because the testes produce these hormones, there is no rationale for using it in men. The levels of DHEAS and other adrenal hormones decline with age, a process referred to as the *adrenopause*. The value of routine replacement of DHEAS in the adrenopause is largely unproven. DHEAS levels may represent another aging marker because it is involved with cardiovascular, immunologic, and endocrine systems and may be a trend indicator for prevention of specific problems with aging.[38–40]

Mineralocorticoids

The mineralocorticoids play an essential role in regulating potassium and sodium levels and water balance. They are produced in the zona glomerulosa, the outer layer of cells of the adrenal cortex. Aldosterone secretion is regulated by the renin–angiotensin mechanism and by blood levels of potassium. Increased levels of aldosterone promote sodium retention by the distal tubules of the kidney while increasing urinary losses of potassium.[4]

Aldosterone is significant for balancing sodium, chloride, and potassium as well as maintaining the total body volume. To understand the importance of aldosterone, consider that both aldosterone and cortisone provide mineralcorticoid

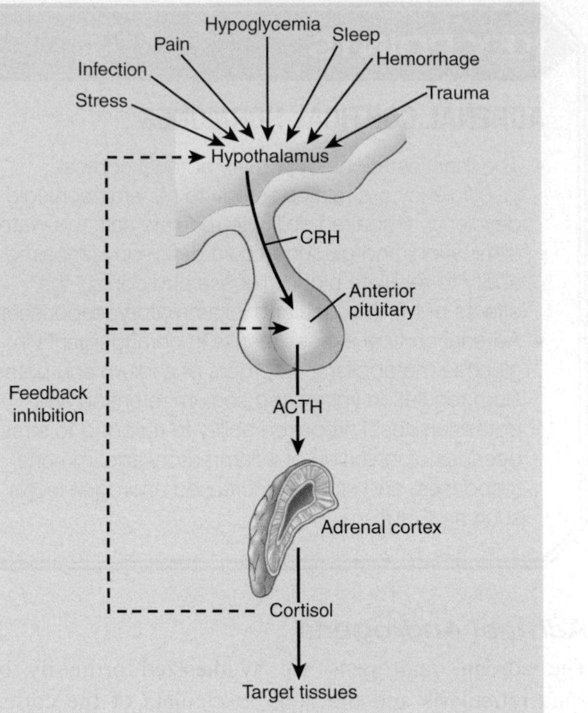

Figure 41.9 • The HPA feedback system that regulates glucocorticoid (cortisol) levels. Cortisol release is regulated by ACTH. Stress exerts its effects on cortisol release through the HPA system and CRH, which controls the release of ACTH from the anterior pituitary gland. Increased cortisol levels incite a negative feedback inhibition of ACTH release.

function; however, approximately 90% of mineralcorticoid function is provided through aldosterone. Although aldosterone is responsible for about 3000 times greater the amount of mineralocorticoid activity than cortisol, there is nearly 2000 times more serum cortisol than aldosterone.[4] Because of the potency of aldosterone, it is crucial that the body does not have excess or deficiency of this potent steroid. The consequences of excess aldosterone are low potassium and muscle weakness, although low amounts of aldosterone cause high potassium and cardiac toxicity.[4]

Glucocorticoids

The glucocorticoid hormones, mainly cortisol, are synthesized in the zona fasciculata and the zona reticularis of the adrenal gland.[4] The blood levels of these hormones are regulated by negative feedback mechanisms of the HPA system (Fig. 41.9). Just as other pituitary hormones are controlled by releasing factors from the hypothalamus, corticotropin-releasing hormone (CRH) is important in controlling the release of ACTH. Cortisol levels increase as ACTH levels rise and decrease as ACTH levels fall. There is considerable diurnal variation in ACTH levels, which reach their peak in the early morning (around 6 to 8 AM) and decline as the day progresses. This appears to be due to rhythmic activity in the CNS, which causes bursts of CRH secretion and, in turn, ACTH secretion. This diurnal pattern is reversed in people who work during the night and sleep during the day. The rhythm may also be changed by physical and psychological stresses, endogenous depression, manic-depressive psychosis, and liver disease or other conditions that affect cortisol metabolism.[4]

The glucocorticoids perform a necessary function in response to stress and are essential for survival. When produced as part of the stress response, these hormones aid in regulating the metabolic functions of the body and in controlling the inflammatory response. The actions of cortisol are summarized in Table 41.4. Many of the anti-inflammatory

TABLE 41.4 ACTIONS OF CORTISOL

MAJOR INFLUENCE	EFFECT ON BODY
Glucose metabolism	Stimulates gluconeogenesis Decreases glucose use by the tissues
Protein metabolism	Increases breakdown of proteins Increases plasma protein levels
Fat metabolism	Increases mobilization of fatty acids Increases use of fatty acids
Anti-inflammatory action (pharmacologic levels)	Stabilizes lysosomal membranes of the inflammatory cells, preventing the release of inflammatory mediators Decreases capillary permeability to prevent inflammatory edema Depresses phagocytosis by white blood cells to reduce the release of inflammatory mediators Suppresses the immune response Causes atrophy of lymphoid tissue Decreases eosinophils Decreases antibody formation Decreases the development of cell-mediated immunity Reduces fever Inhibits fibroblast activity
Psychic effect	May contribute to emotional instability
Permissive effect	Facilitates the response of the tissues to humoral and neural influences, such as that of the catecholamines, during trauma and extreme stress

actions attributed to cortisol result from the administration of pharmacologic levels of the hormone.[4]

Metabolic Effects. Cortisol stimulates glucose production by the liver, promotes protein breakdown, and causes mobilization of fatty acids. As body proteins are broken down, amino acids are mobilized and transported to the liver, where they are used in the production of glucose (*i.e.*, gluconeogenesis). Mobilization of fatty acids converts cell metabolism from the use of glucose for energy to the use of fatty acids instead. As glucose production by the liver rises and peripheral glucose use falls, a moderate resistance to insulin develops. In people with diabetes and those who are diabetes prone, this has the effect of raising the blood glucose level.[4,9]

Psychological Effects. The glucocorticoid hormones appear to be involved directly or indirectly in emotional behavior. Receptors for these hormones have been identified in brain tissue, which suggests that they play a role in the regulation of behavior. People treated with adrenal cortical hormones have been known to display behavior ranging from mildly aberrant to psychotic.[41]

Immunologic and Inflammatory Effects. Cortisol influences multiple aspects of immunologic function and inflammatory responsiveness. Large quantities of cortisol are required for an effective anti-inflammatory action. This is achieved by the administration of pharmacologic rather than physiologic doses of synthetic cortisol. The increased cortisol blocks inflammation at an early stage by decreasing capillary permeability and stabilizing the lysosomal membranes, so that inflammatory mediators are not released. Cortisol suppresses the immune response by reducing humoral and cell-mediated immunity. With this lessened inflammatory response comes a reduction in fever. During the healing phase, cortisol suppresses fibroblast activity and thereby lessens scar formation. Cortisol also inhibits prostaglandin synthesis, which may account in large part for its anti-inflammatory actions.[4]

Pharmacologic Suppression of Adrenal Function

A highly significant aspect of long-term therapy with pharmacologic preparations of the glucocorticoids is adrenal insufficiency on withdrawal of drugs. The deficiency results from suppression of the HPA system. Chronic suppression causes atrophy of the adrenal gland, and the abrupt withdrawal of drugs can cause acute adrenal insufficiency. Recovery to a state of normal adrenal function may be prolonged, requiring 6 to 12 months or more.[42]

Tests of Adrenal Function

Several diagnostic tests can be used to evaluate adrenal cortical function and the HPA system. Blood levels of cortisol, aldosterone, and ACTH can be measured using immunoassay methods. A 24-hour urine specimen measuring the excretion of various metabolic end products of adrenal hormones provides information about alterations in the biosynthesis of the adrenal cortical hormones. The 24-hour urinary free cortisol, late-night (between 11 PM and midnight) serum or salivary cortisol levels, and the overnight 1-mg dexamethasone suppression test are excellent screening tests for Cushing syndrome.[39,43,44]

Suppression and stimulation tests afford a means of assessing the state of the HPA feedback system. For example, a test dose of ACTH can be given to assess the response of the adrenal cortex to stimulation. Similarly, administration of dexamethasone, a synthetic glucocorticoid drug, provides a means of measuring negative feedback suppression of ACTH. Adrenal tumors and ectopic ACTH-producing tumors are usually unresponsive to ACTH suppression by dexamethasone. CRH tests can be used to diagnose a pituitary ACTH-secreting tumor (*i.e.*, Cushing disease). Corticotropin (cosyntropin) stimulation testing is the most frequently used diagnostic test to assess testing responsiveness of the HPA axis.[39,43,44]

Congenital Adrenal Hyperplasia

CAH, or the adrenogenital syndrome, describes a congenital disorder caused by an autosomal recessive trait in which a deficiency exists in any of the enzymes necessary for the synthesis of cortisol (see Fig. 41.8). A common characteristic of all types of CAH is a defect in the synthesis of cortisol that results in increased levels of ACTH and adrenal hyperplasia.[1] The increased levels of ACTH overstimulate the pathways for production of adrenal androgens. Mineralocorticoids may be produced in excessive or insufficient amounts, depending on the precise enzyme deficiency. Infants of both sexes are affected. Boys are seldom diagnosed at birth unless they have enlarged genitalia or lose salt and manifest adrenal crisis.[1] In female infants, an increase in androgens is responsible for creating the virilization syndrome of ambiguous genitalia with an enlarged clitoris, fused labia, and urogenital sinus (Fig. 41.10). In male and female children, other secondary sex characteristics are normal, and fertility is unaffected if appropriate therapy is instituted.[1]

A spectrum of 21-hydroxylase deficiency states exists, ranging from simple virilizing CAH to a complete salt-losing enzyme deficiency. Simple virilizing CAH impairs the synthesis of cortisol, and steroid synthesis is shunted to androgen production. People with these deficiencies usually produce sufficient aldosterone or aldosterone intermediates to prevent signs and symptoms of mineralocorticoid deficiency. The salt-losing form is accompanied by deficient production of aldosterone and its intermediates, resulting in fluid and electrolyte disorders (including hyponatremia, vomiting, dehydration, and shock). Hyperkalemia is not always present, so it should not be considered a major screening diagnostic parameter.[1,45]

The 11-β-hydroxylase deficiency is rare and manifests a spectrum of severity. Affected people have excessive androgen production and impaired conversion of 11-deoxycorticosterone to corticosterone. The overproduction of 11-deoxycorticosterone, which has mineralocorticoid activity, is responsible for the hypertension that accompanies this deficiency. Diagnosis of CAH depends on the precise biochemical

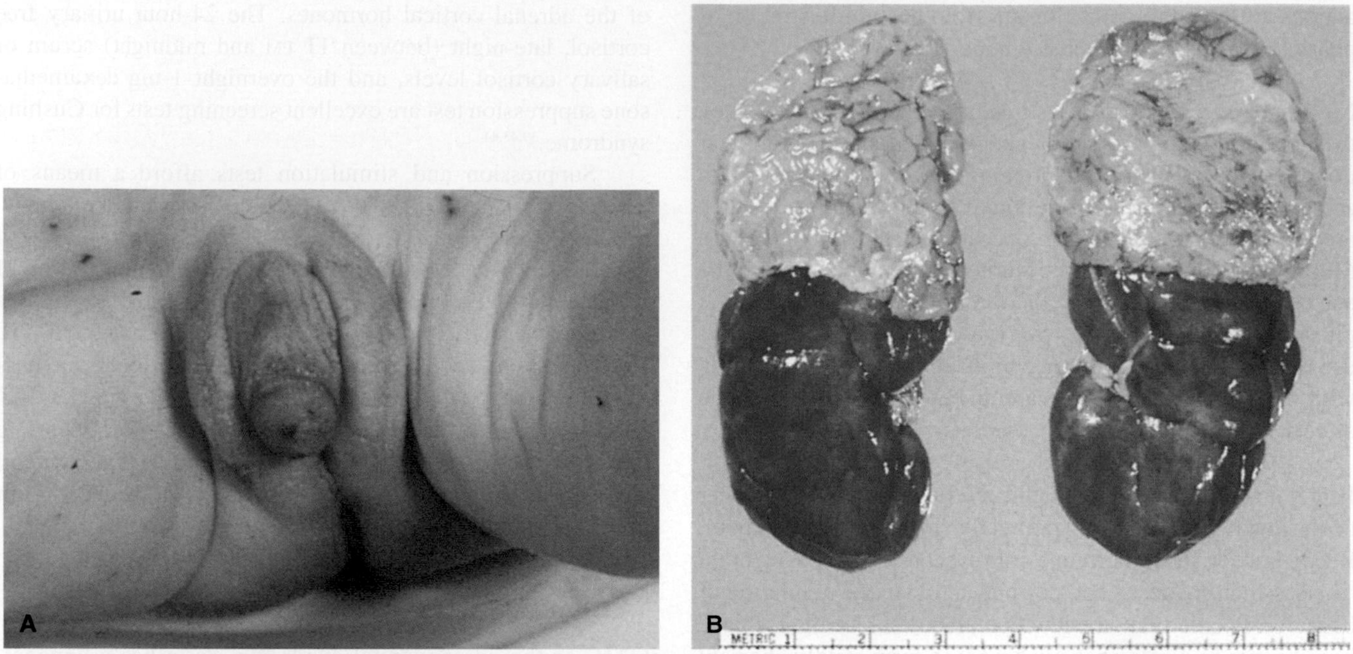

Figure 41.10 • **(A)** A female infant is markedly virilized with hypertrophy of the clitoris and partial fusion of labioscrotal folds with CAH demonstrating virilization of the genitalia with hypertrophy of the clitoris and partial fusion of labioscrotal folds. **(B)** A 7-week-old male died of severe salt-wasting CAH. At autopsy, both adrenal glands were markedly enlarged. (From Strayer D., Rubin E. (Eds.) (2015). *Rubin's pathology: Clinicopathologic foundations of medicine* (7th ed., Figure 27.31, p. 1203). Philadelphia, PA: Wolters Kluwer.)

evaluation of metabolites in the cortisol pathway and on clinical signs and symptoms. Genetic testing is also invaluable. However, correlation between the phenotype and genotype is not always straightforward.[45]

Medical treatment of CAH includes oral or parenteral glucocorticoid replacement. Fludrocortisone acetate, a mineralocorticoid, may also be given to children who are salt losers. Stress dosing of glucocorticoids (increasing the dose) is necessary during periods of illness or other significant stressors, including emotional stress. People with CAH should also wear a medical alert badge or bracelet/medallion. Depending on the degree of virilization, reconstructive surgery during the first year of life may be indicated to reduce the size of the clitoris, separate the labia, and exteriorize the vagina. Women with CAH who are experiencing unwanted hair growth or androgenic hair loss may be prescribed anti-androgen drugs, although the side effects of those drugs must be considered.[45]

Adrenal Cortical Insufficiency

There are two forms of adrenal insufficiency—primary and secondary[1] (see Table 41.5 for distinguishing features). Primary adrenal insufficiency, or Addison disease, is caused by destruction of the adrenal gland. Secondary adrenal insufficiency results from a disorder of the HPA system.

TABLE 41.5 CLINICAL FINDINGS OF ADRENAL INSUFFICIENCY

FINDING	PRIMARY	SECONDARY/TERTIARY
Anorexia and weight loss	Yes (100%)	Yes (100%)
Fatigue and weakness	Yes (100%)	Yes (100%)
Gastrointestinal symptoms, nausea, diarrhea	Yes (50%)	Yes (50%)
Myalgia, arthralgia, abdominal pain	Yes (10%)	Yes (10%)
Orthostatic hypotension	Yes	Yes
Hyponatremia	Yes (85%–90%)	Yes (60%)
Hyperkalemia	Yes (60%–65%)	No
Hyperpigmentation	Yes (>90%)	No
Secondary deficiencies of testosterone, growth hormone, thyroxine, antidiuretic hormone	No	Yes
Associated autoimmune conditions	Yes	No

Primary Adrenal Cortical Insufficiency

Addison disease is a primary adrenal insufficiency (i.e., originating in the adrenal glands) in which adrenal cortical hormones are deficient and ACTH levels are elevated because of lack of feedback inhibition.

Etiology and Pathogenesis. This disease is a relatively rare disorder in which all the layers of the adrenal cortex are destroyed. Autoimmune destruction is the most common cause of Addison disease in western societies, accounting for 75% of cases. When the disease was first described by Thomas Addison in 1855, tuberculosis was the major cause, and it continues to be a major cause of the disease in countries where it is more prevalent.[1] Rare causes include metastatic carcinoma, fungal infection (particularly histoplasmosis), cytomegalovirus infection, amyloid disease, CAH, Waterhouse-Friderichsen Syndrome, and hemochromatosis. Bilateral adrenal hemorrhage may occur in people taking anticoagulants, during open-heart surgery, and during birth or major trauma. Adrenal insufficiency can be caused by acquired immunodeficiency syndrome in which the adrenal gland is destroyed by a variety of opportunistic infectious agents. Drugs that inhibit synthesis or cause excessive breakdown of glucocorticoids can also result in adrenal insufficiency (*e.g.*, ketoconazole).[1,2,46,47]

Clinical Manifestations. The adrenal cortex has a large reserve capacity, and the manifestations of adrenal insufficiency usually do not become apparent until approximately 90% of the gland has been destroyed.[4] These manifestations are related primarily to mineralocorticoid deficiency, glucocorticoid deficiency, and hyperpigmentation resulting from elevated ACTH levels. Although lack of the adrenal androgens (*i.e.*, DHEAS) exerts few effects in men because the testes produce these hormones, women have sparse axillary and pubic hair.[4,48]

Mineralocorticoid deficiency causes increased urinary losses of sodium, chloride, and water, along with decreased excretion of potassium (Fig. 41.11). The result is hyponatremia, loss of extracellular fluid, decreased cardiac output, and hyperkalemia. There may be an abnormal appetite for salt. Orthostatic hypotension is common. Dehydration, weakness, and fatigue are common early symptoms. If loss of sodium and water is extreme, cardiovascular collapse and shock ensue. Because of a lack of glucocorticoids, the person with Addison disease has poor tolerance to stress. This deficiency causes hypoglycemia, lethargy, weakness, fever, and gastrointestinal symptoms such as anorexia, nausea, vomiting, and weight loss.[1,48]

Hyperpigmentation results from elevated levels of ACTH. The skin looks bronzed or suntanned in exposed and unexposed areas, and the normal creases and pressure points tend to become especially dark. The gums and oral mucous membranes may become bluish black. The amino acid sequence of ACTH is strikingly similar to that of melanocyte-stimulating hormone; hyperpigmentation occurs in >90% of people with Addison disease and is helpful in distinguishing the primary and secondary forms of adrenal insufficiency.[1,48]

Treatment. Addison disease, like type 1 diabetes mellitus, is a chronic metabolic disorder that requires lifetime hormone replacement therapy. The daily regulation of the chronic phase of Addison disease is usually accomplished with oral replacement therapy, with higher doses being given during periods of stress. The pharmacologic agent that is used should have both glucocorticoid and mineralocorticoid activities. Mineralocorticoids are needed only in primary adrenal insufficiency. Hydrocortisone is usually the drug of choice. In mild cases, hydrocortisone alone may be adequate. Fludrocortisone (a mineralocorticoid) is used for people who do not obtain a

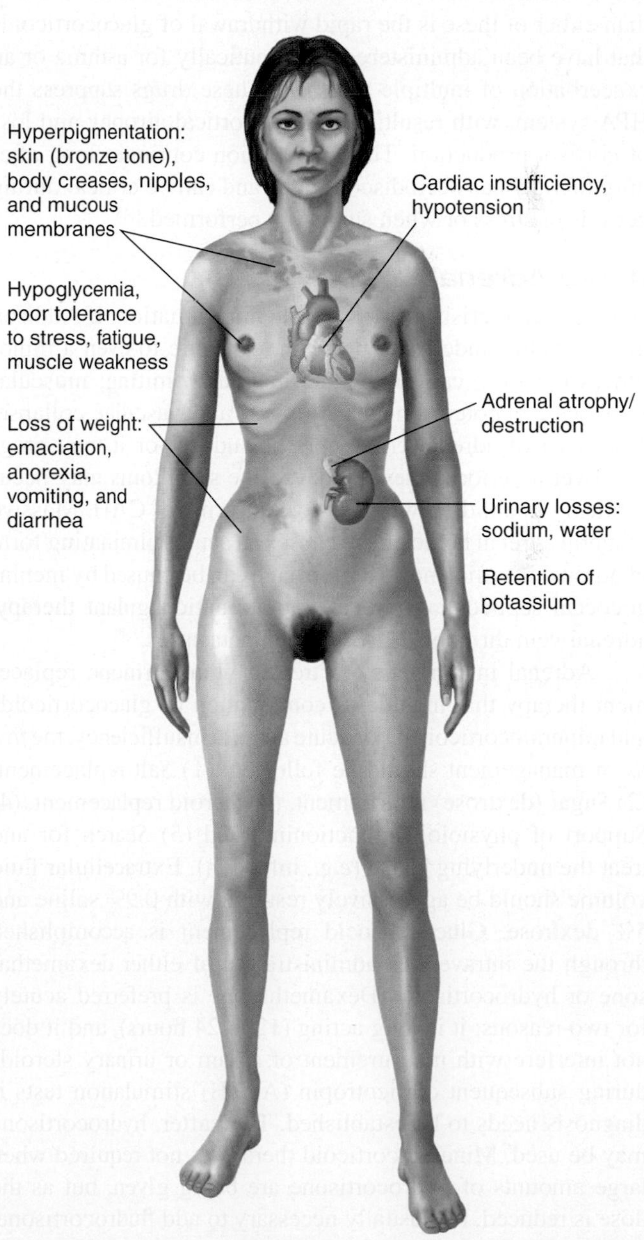

Figure 41.11 • Clinical manifestations of primary (Addison disease) and secondary adrenal insufficiency.

sufficient salt-retaining effect from hydrocortisone. DHEAS replacement may also be helpful in the female patient.[1,48]

Because people with the disorder are likely to have episodes of hyponatremia and hypoglycemia, they need to have a regular schedule for meals and exercise. People with Addison disease also have limited ability to respond to infections, trauma, and other stresses. Such situations require immediate medical attention and treatment. People with Addison disease should be advised to wear a medical alert bracelet or medallion/badge.[1,48]

Secondary Adrenal Cortical Insufficiency

Secondary adrenal insufficiency can occur as the result of hypopituitarism or because the pituitary gland has been surgically removed. Tertiary adrenal insufficiency results from a hypothalamic defect. However, a far more common cause than either of these is the rapid withdrawal of glucocorticoids that have been administered therapeutically for asthma or an exacerbation of multiple sclerosis. These drugs suppress the HPA system, with resulting adrenal cortical atrophy and loss of cortisol production. This suppression continues long after drug therapy has been discontinued and can be critical during periods of stress or when surgery is performed.[1,48]

Acute Adrenal Crisis

Acute adrenal crisis is a life-threatening situation. If Addison disease is the underlying problem, exposure to even a minor illness or stress can precipitate nausea, vomiting, muscular weakness, hypotension, dehydration, and vascular collapse. The onset of adrenal crisis may be sudden, or it may progress over a period of several days. The symptoms may occur suddenly in children with salt-losing forms of CAH. Massive bilateral adrenal hemorrhage causes an acute fulminating form of adrenal insufficiency. Hemorrhage can be caused by meningococcal septicemia, adrenal trauma, anticoagulant therapy, adrenal vein thrombosis, or adrenal metastases.[1,49]

Adrenal insufficiency is treated with hormone replacement therapy that includes a combination of glucocorticoids and mineralocorticoids. For acute adrenal insufficiency, the *five Ss* of management should be followed: (1) *S*alt replacement, (2) *S*ugar (dextrose) replacement, (3) *S*teroid replacement, (4) *S*upport of physiologic functioning, and (5) *S*earch for and treat the underlying cause (*e.g.*, infection). Extracellular fluid volume should be aggressively restored with 0.9% saline and 5% dextrose. Glucocorticoid replacement is accomplished through the intravenous administration of either dexamethasone or hydrocortisone. Dexamethasone is preferred acutely for two reasons: it is long acting (12 to 24 hours), and it does not interfere with measurement of serum or urinary steroids during subsequent corticotropin (ACTH) stimulation tests if diagnosis needs to be established. Thereafter, hydrocortisone may be used. Mineralocorticoid therapy is not required when large amounts of hydrocortisone are being given, but as the dose is reduced, it is usually necessary to add fludrocortisone. Glucocorticoid and mineralocorticoid replacement therapy is monitored using heart rate and blood pressure measurements, serum electrolyte values, and titration of plasma renin activity into the upper-normal range.[1,49]

Glucocorticoid Hormone Excess (Cushing Syndrome)

The term *Cushing syndrome* refers to the manifestations of hypercortisolism from any cause.[1] Three important forms of Cushing syndrome result from excess glucocorticoid production by the body. One is a pituitary form, which results from excessive production of ACTH by a tumor of the pituitary gland. This form of the disease was the one originally described by Cushing. Therefore, it is called *Cushing disease*. The second form is the adrenal form, caused by a benign or malignant adrenal tumor. The third form is ectopic Cushing syndrome, caused by a nonpituitary ACTH-secreting tumor. Certain extrapituitary malignant tumors such as small cell carcinoma of the lung may secrete ACTH or, rarely, CRH and produce Cushing syndrome. Cushing syndrome can also result from long-term therapy with one of the potent pharmacologic preparations of glucocorticoids; this form is called *iatrogenic Cushing syndrome*.[1]

Clinical Manifestations

The major manifestations of Cushing syndrome represent an exaggeration of the many actions of cortisol (see Table 41.4). Altered fat metabolism causes a peculiar deposition of fat characterized by a protruding abdomen; subclavicular fat pads or "buffalo hump" on the back; and a round, plethoric "moon face" (Figs. 41.12 and 41.13). There is muscle weakness, and the extremities are thin because of protein breakdown and muscle wasting. In advanced cases, the skin over the forearms and legs becomes thin, having the appearance of parchment. Purple striae, or stretch marks, from stretching of the catabolically weakened skin and subcutaneous tissues are distributed over the breast, thighs, and abdomen. Osteoporosis may develop because of destruction of bone proteins and alterations in calcium metabolism, resulting in back pain, compression fractures of the vertebrae, and rib fractures. As calcium is mobilized from bone, renal calculi may develop.[1,2,8]

The glucocorticoids possess mineralocorticoid properties. This causes hypokalemia, as a result of excessive potassium excretion, and hypertension, resulting from sodium retention. Inflammatory and immune responses are inhibited, resulting in increased susceptibility to infection. Cortisol increases gastric acid secretion, which may provoke gastric ulceration and bleeding. An accompanying increase in androgen levels causes hirsutism, mild acne, and menstrual irregularities in women. Excess levels of the glucocorticoids may give rise to extreme emotional lability, ranging from mild euphoria and absence of normal fatigue to grossly psychotic behavior.[1,2,8]

Diagnosis and Treatment

Diagnosis of Cushing syndrome is a two-step process: the first step is the diagnosis of hypercortisolism, and the second

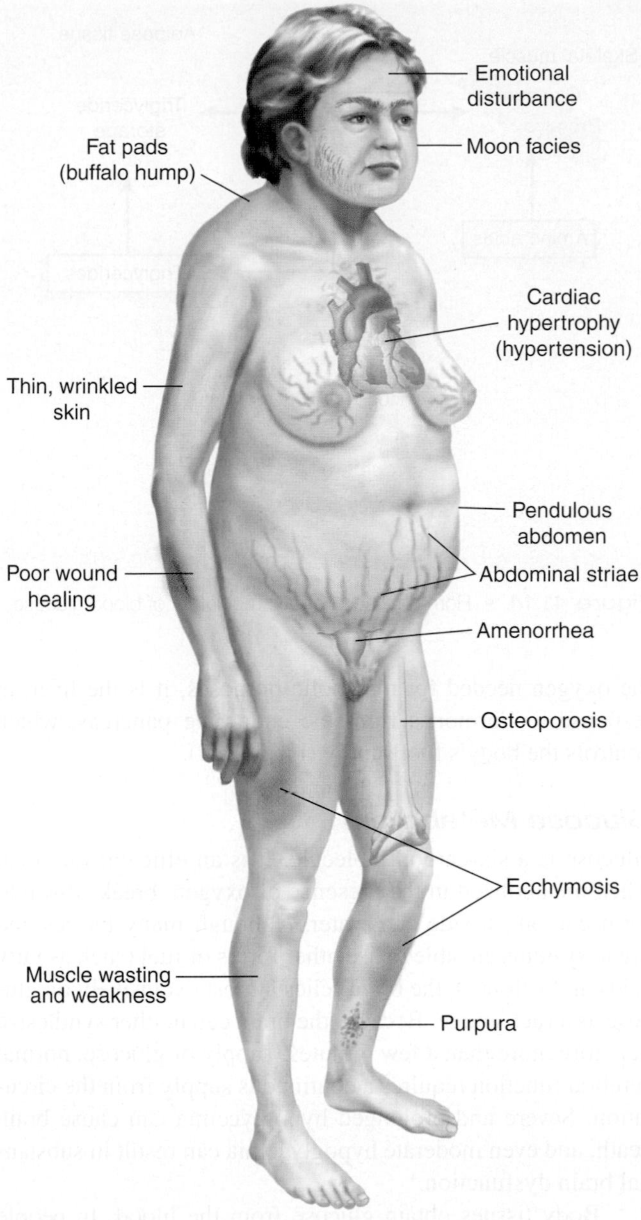

Figure 41.12 • Clinical features of Cushing syndrome.

step is testing to determine the cause of the cortisol hypersecretion. The tests most commonly used for diagnosis are the 24-hour urinary free cortisol level, the midnight plasma and late-night salivary cortisol measurements, and the low-dose dexamethasone suppression test. The dexamethasone-CRH test may also be helpful during the diagnostic workup. After a diagnosis of Cushing syndrome has been made, the following tests can be used to help determine the cause: CRH stimulation test, high-dose dexamethasone suppression test, radiologic imaging of the pituitary and adrenal glands, and petrosal sinus sampling.[50]

Untreated, Cushing syndrome produces serious morbidity and even death. The choice of surgery, irradiation, or pharmacologic treatment is determined largely by the cause of the hypercortisolism. The goal of treatment for Cushing syndrome is to remove or correct the source of hypercortisolism without causing permanent pituitary or adrenal damage. Transsphenoidal removal of a pituitary adenoma or a hemihypophysectomy is the preferred method of treatment for Cushing disease. This allows removal of only the tumor rather than the entire pituitary gland. After successful removal, the person must receive cortisol replacement therapy for 6 to 12 months or until adrenal function returns. People may also receive pituitary radiation therapy. Unilateral or bilateral adrenalectomy may be done in the case of adrenal adenoma. When possible, ectopic ACTH-producing tumors are also removed. Pharmacologic agents that block steroid synthesis (*i.e.*, mitotane, ketoconazole, and metyrapone) may be used to treat people with ectopic tumors or adrenal carcinomas that cannot be resected. Precautions to minimize infections may also be necessary because of the immune suppression caused by hypercortisolism.[50,51]

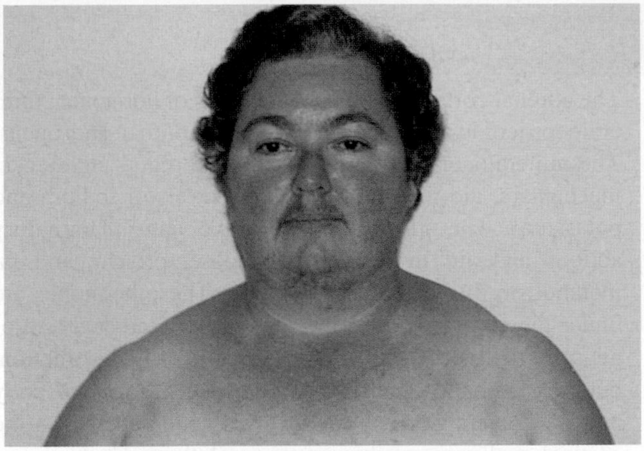

Figure 41.13 • Cushing syndrome. A woman who had a pituitary adenoma that produced adrenocroticotropic hormone (ACTH) exhibits a moon face, buffalo hump, increased facial hair and thinning of the scalp hair. (Strayer D., Rubin E. (Eds.) (2015). *Rubin's pathology: Clinicopathologic foundations of medicine* (7th ed., Figure 27-37, p. 1209). Philadelphia, PA: Wolters Kluwer.)

Incidental Adrenal Mass

An incidentaloma is a mass found unexpectedly in an adrenal gland by an imaging procedure (done for other reasons), most commonly CT (but also MRI and ultrasonography). Incidentalomas can also occur in other organs (*e.g.*, pituitary, thyroid). The two most important points to establish regarding incidentalomas are if they are malignant and if they are hormonally active. Primary adrenal carcinoma is quite rare, but other cancers, particularly lung cancers, commonly metastasize to the adrenal gland (other cancers include breast, stomach, pancreas, colon, kidney, melanomas, and lymphomas). The size and imaging characteristics of the mass may help determine whether the tumor is benign or malignant. Appropriate screening to exclude a hormonally active lesion includes tests to rule out pheochromocytoma, Cushing syndrome, and Conn syndrome (mineralocorticoid excess).[1]

IN SUMMARY

The adrenal cortex produces three types of hormones: mineralocorticoids, glucocorticoids, and adrenal androgens. The mineralocorticoids, along with the renin–angiotensin mechanism, aid in controlling body levels of sodium and potassium. The glucocorticoids have anti-inflammatory actions and aid in regulating glucose, protein, and fat metabolism during periods of stress. These hormones are under the control of the HPA system. The adrenal androgens exert little effect on daily control of body function, but they probably contribute to the development of body hair in women. CAH is caused by a genetic defect in the cortisol pathway resulting from a deficiency of one of the enzymes needed for its synthesis. Depending on the enzyme involved, the disorder causes virilization of female infants and, in some instances, fluid and electrolyte disturbances because of impaired mineralocorticoid synthesis.

Chronic adrenal insufficiency can be caused by destruction of the adrenal gland (Addison disease) or by dysfunction of the HPA system. Adrenal insufficiency requires replacement therapy with adrenal cortical hormones. Acute adrenal insufficiency is a life-threatening situation. Cushing syndrome refers to the manifestations of excessive glucocorticoid levels. This syndrome may be a result of pharmacologic doses of glucocorticoids, a pituitary or adrenal tumor, or an ectopic tumor that produces ACTH. The clinical manifestations of Cushing syndrome reflect the very high level of glucocorticoid that is present.

An incidental adrenal mass is a mass found unexpectedly in an adrenal gland by an imaging procedure done for other reasons. They are being recognized with increasing frequency, emphasizing the need for correct diagnosis and treatment.

GENERAL ASPECTS OF ALTERED GLUCOSE REGULATION

After completing this section of the chapter, the learner will be able to meet the following objectives:

- Discuss the functions of glucose, fats, and proteins in meeting the energy needs of the body.
- Discuss the actions of insulin with respect to glucose, fat, and protein metabolism.
- Explain what is meant by *counter-regulatory hormones*, and describe the actions of glucagon, epinephrine, GH, and the glucocorticoid hormones in regulation of blood glucose levels.

Hormonal Control of Glucose, Fat, and Protein Metabolism

The body uses glucose, fatty acids, and other substrates as fuel to satisfy its energy needs. Although the pulmonary and circulatory systems combine efforts to furnish the body with the oxygen needed for metabolic purposes, it is the liver, in response to hormones from the endocrine pancreas, which controls the body's fuel supply (Fig. 41.14).

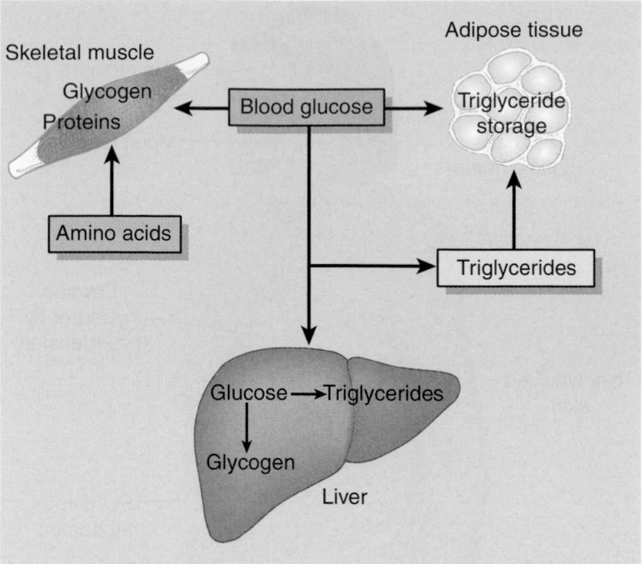

Figure 41.14 • Hormonal and hepatic regulation of blood glucose.

Glucose Metabolism

Glucose is a six-carbon molecule. It is an efficient fuel that, when metabolized in the presence of oxygen, breaks down to form carbon dioxide and water. Although many tissues and organ systems are able to use other forms of fuel (such as fatty acids and ketones), the brain relies almost exclusively on glucose as a fuel source. Because the brain can neither synthesize nor store more than a few minutes' supply of glucose, normal cerebral function requires a continuous supply from the circulation. Severe and prolonged hypoglycemia can cause brain death, and even moderate hypoglycemia can result in substantial brain dysfunction.[4]

Body tissues obtain glucose from the blood. In people without diabetes, fasting blood glucose levels are usually tightly regulated between 80 and 90 mg/dL. After a meal, blood glucose levels rise to 100 to 120 mg/dL, and the normal hormonal regulatory mechanisms return the blood levels to the control range within approximately 2 hours.[4] Insulin is secreted in response to this rise in glucose. The hormone insulin facilitates the entry of glucose into body cells (to be discussed in greater depth later). Most of the glucose that is ingested with a meal is removed from the blood and stored in the liver as glycogen, with the remaining glucose used for cellular metabolic needs. Between meals, the liver releases glucose from the stored glycogen as a means of maintaining the blood glucose within its normal range. Some glycogen can also be stored within muscle for use within muscle cells by energy. The process of breaking down glycogen to release glucose is called *glycogenolysis*.[4] In addition to mobilizing its glycogen stores, the liver can also synthesize new glucose from amino acids, glycerol, and lactic acid in a process called *gluconeogenesis*. This newly formed glucose may be released directly into the circulation or stored as glycogen.[4]

Fat Metabolism

Fat is the most dense form of fuel storage, providing 9 kcal/g of stored energy, compared with the 4 kcal/g provided by carbohydrates and proteins. The metabolism of triglycerides from fats produces a glycerol molecule and three fatty acids. The glycerol molecule can enter the glycolytic pathway and be used along with glucose to produce energy, or it can be used to produce glucose. The fatty acids are transported to tissues where they may also be used for energy by most body cells, with the previously noted exception of the brain.[4]

When fatty acids are used for energy, organic acid molecules called ketones are released into the bloodstream, creating a situation of *ketosis*. During periods of excessive use of fatty acids for fuels, the increased accumulation of these organic keto acids can produce a condition of metabolic acidosis called *ketoacidosis*. Conditions of decreased availability of either glucose or insulin create an increased risk of ketoacidosis.[4]

Protein Metabolism

Proteins are essential for the formation of all body structures, including genes, enzymes, contractile structures in muscle, matrix of bone, and hemoglobin of red blood cells.[4] Amino acids are the building blocks of proteins. Unlike glucose and fatty acids, excess amino acids can be stored in only a limited capacity in the body. Amino acids in excess of those needed for protein synthesis are converted to fatty acids, ketones, or glucose.[4] Because fatty acids cannot be converted to glucose, the body must break down proteins and use the amino acids as a major substrate for gluconeogenesis during periods when the metabolic needs for glucose exceed glucose intake.[4]

Glucose-Regulating Hormones

The hormonal control of blood glucose resides largely with the endocrine pancreas. The pancreas is made up of two major tissue types—the acini and the islets of Langerhans (Fig. 41.15). The acini secrete digestive juices into the duodenum; the islets of Langerhans secrete hormones into the blood.[4] Each islet is composed of beta cells (which secrete insulin and amylin), alpha cells (which secrete glucagon), and a small number of delta cells (which secrete somatostatin).[4]

Insulin

Although several hormones increase blood glucose levels, insulin is the only hormone that acts to lower blood glucose levels. The active form of insulin is produced in the beta cells of the pancreas from a larger molecule called *proinsulin* (Fig. 41.16). Insulin is formed by cleaving away the C-peptide of the proinsulin molecule, leaving the A and B polypeptide chains, which form the active insulin molecule.[4] The insulin molecule itself has a short plasma half-life of approximately 6 minutes, with clearance from the body primarily through

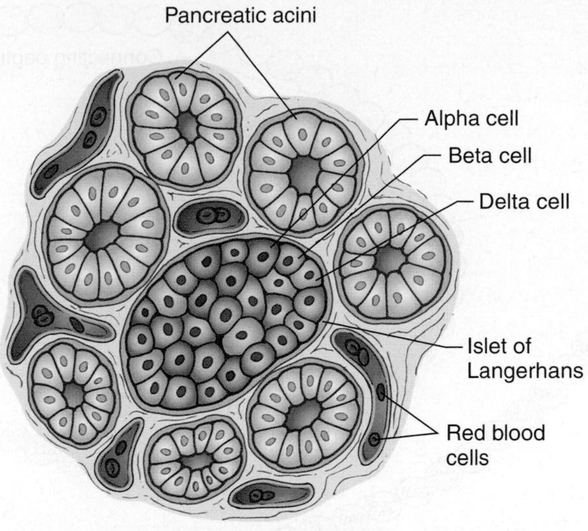

Figure 41.15 • Islet of Langerhans in the pancreas.

hepatic mechanisms and the action of the enzyme *insulinase*.[4] However, circulating blood levels of the C-peptide molecule can be measured and are used as a proxy measure to reflect pancreatic insulin production.[4,52]

The actions of insulin include:

1. Promoting glucose uptake by target cells and storage of glucose as glycogen (in liver and muscles) or fat (in adipose tissue).
2. Inhibiting fat and glycogen breakdown.
3. Inhibiting gluconeogenesis and increasing protein synthesis[1,2,4] (Table 41.6).

Target cells for insulin include fat cells; therefore, insulin acts to promote fat storage by increasing the transport of glucose into fat cells. Within the fat cells, insulin facilitates the synthesis of triglycerides from glucose and inhibits the intracellular breakdown of stored triglycerides. Insulin increases protein synthesis and inhibits protein breakdown by increasing the active transport of amino acids into body cells. When sufficient glucose and insulin are present, protein breakdown is minimal because the body uses glucose and fatty acids for energy.[4]

Blood glucose levels regulate the release of insulin from the pancreatic beta cells. Insulin levels increase as blood glucose levels rise and decrease as blood glucose levels decline. Insulin binds to specific insulin receptor molecules embedded within the plasma membranes of the target cells for insulin. The insulin molecule itself does not enter the target cells; instead, the binding of insulin to its receptor causes several actions to occur within the cell, including the activation of the glucose transport proteins (described below). Other cellular actions triggered by the binding of insulin with its receptor include increasing the cellular permeability to amino acids and to potassium ions and phosphate ions, which increase the rate of transfer of these molecules into the cell.[4]

The binding of insulin with its cell surface receptors triggers the insertion into the cell membrane of specific glucose

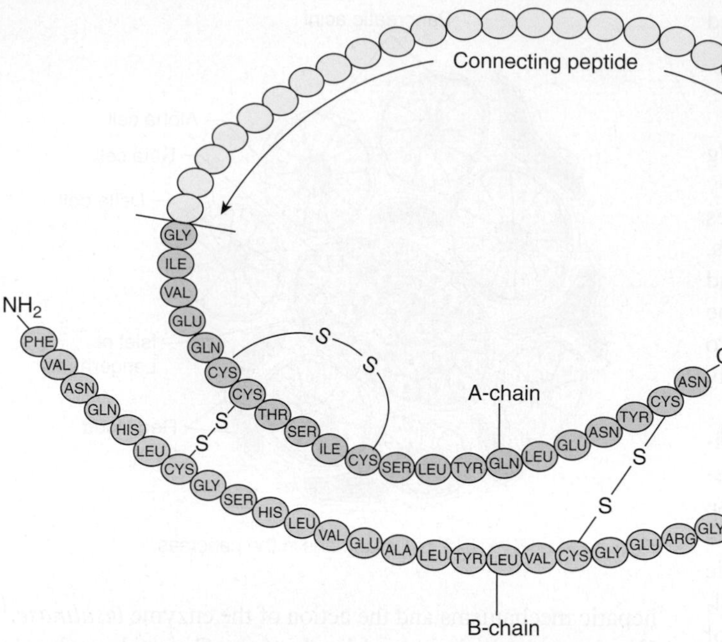

Figure 41.16 • Structure of proinsulin. With removal of the connecting peptide (C-peptide), proinsulin is converted to insulin.

transporter proteins. The liver does most of the processing of glucose. When a glucose molecule enters hepatic cells through the glucose transporter protein, the glucose molecule is phosphorylated by the enzyme *glucokinase*, which creates a molecule that cannot diffuse through the cell membrane, thus effectively "trapping" the glucose inside the liver.[4] Insulin also activates the enzyme *glycogen synthase*, which then catalyzes the intrahepatic process transformation of glucose into glycogen.[4]

Because cell membranes are impermeable to glucose, a family of glucose transporters mediates the movement of glucose from the blood into the cells. These glucose transporters (named *GLUT-1*, *GLUT-2*, etc.) each have their own unique tissue distribution. For example, GLUT-4 is the insulin-responsive glucose transporter for skeletal muscle and adipose tissue. The GLUT-4 protein is sequestered inside the cell membrane and unable to function as a glucose transporter until a signal from insulin-receptor binding causes the GLUT-4 protein to move into the cell membrane, where it can then facilitate glucose entry into the cell.[4] This process is shown in Figure 41.17.

Glucagon

Glucagon is a polypeptide molecule produced in the pancreas by the alpha cells of the islets of Langerhans in response to a decrease in blood glucose. The actions of glucagon maintain blood glucose levels between meals and during periods of fasting. Glucagon levels also increase during strenuous exercise to prevent a decrease in blood glucose. After release from the pancreas, glucagon travels through the portal vein to the liver to initiate hepatic breakdown of glycogen (glycogenolysis), which rapidly raises blood glucose (see Table 41.6). Glucagon also increases the transport of amino acids into the liver and stimulates protein conversion into new glucose through the previously described process of gluconeogenesis. Because liver glycogen stores are limited, gluconeogenesis is important in maintaining blood glucose levels over time.[4]

Somatostatin, Amylin, and Gut-Derived Hormones

Somatostatin is a pancreatic polypeptide hormone containing only 14 amino acids. It has an extremely short plasma half-life of 3 minutes; however, it acts locally in the islets of Langerhans to decrease secretion of insulin and also of glucagon. Somatostatin secretion is triggered by multiple characteristics related to the ingestion of food, including the release of certain gastrointestinal hormones as well as increased blood levels of glucose, fatty acids, and amino acids. In addition to the local pancreatic effects to reduce insulin and glucagon secretion, somatostatin also decreases gastrointestinal motility and slows the absorption of food. The overall role of somatostatin appears to be to increase the time in which nutrients are available in the bloodstream for use by the body cells.[4]

Islet amyloid polypeptide, or *amylin*, is another hormone secreted by the pancreatic beta cells. Plasma levels of amylin increase after a meal or a glucose infusion.[3]Amylin appears to work with insulin to regulate plasma glucose concentrations by suppressing postprandial secretion of glucagon and slowing gastric emptying.[4,53] Several *gut-derived hormones* have been identified as having what is termed an *incretin effect*, meaning that they increase insulin release and decrease glucagon release when the plasma glucose is elevated.[4]

Counter-Regulatory Hormones

Other hormones that can affect blood glucose include the catecholamines, GH, and the glucocorticoids. These hormones, along with glucagon, are sometimes called *counter-regulatory hormones* because they counteract the storage functions of insulin to regulate blood glucose levels during periods of

TABLE 41.6 ACTIONS OF INSULIN AND GLUCAGON ON GLUCOSE, FAT, AND PROTEIN METABOLISM

	INSULIN	GLUCAGON
Glucose		
Glucose transport	Increases glucose transport into skeletal muscle and adipose tissue	
Glycogen synthesis	Increases glycogen synthesis	Promotes glycogen breakdown
Gluconeogenesis	Decreases gluconeogenesis	Increases gluconeogenesis
Fats		
Fatty acid and triglyceride synthesis	Promotes fatty acid and triglyceride synthesis by the liver	
Fat storage in adipose tissue	Increases the transport of fatty acids into adipose cells Increases conversion of fatty acids to triglycerides by increasing the availability of a-glycerol phosphate through increased transport of glucose in adipose cells Maintains fat storage by inhibiting breakdown of stored triglycerides by adipose cell lipase	Activates adipose cell lipase, making increased amounts of fatty acids available to the body for use as energy
Proteins		
Amino acid transport	Increases active transport of amino acids into cells	Increases amino acid uptake by liver cells and their conversion to glucose by gluconeogenesis
Protein synthesis	Increases protein synthesis by increasing transcription of messenger RNA and accelerating protein synthesis by ribosomal RNA	
Protein breakdown	Decreases protein breakdown by enhancing the use of glucose and fatty acids as fuel	

fasting, exercise, and other situations that either limit glucose intake or deplete glucose stores.[1,2,4]

Epinephrine

Epinephrine, a catecholamine from the adrenal medulla, helps to maintain blood glucose levels during periods of stress by stimulating glycogenolysis in the liver, thus causing large quantities of glucose to be released into the blood. Epinephrine also inhibits insulin release from pancreatic beta cells, which decreases movement of glucose into muscle cells and increases the breakdown of muscle glycogen stores. Although the glucose released from muscle glycogen does not enter the blood, the use of these internal energy stores by muscles conserves blood glucose for use by tissues such as the brain. Epinephrine also has a direct lipolytic effect on adipose cells, increasing the availability of fatty acids for use as an energy source. The blood glucose–elevating effect of epinephrine is also an important homeostatic mechanism during periods of hypoglycemia.[1,2,4]

Growth Hormone

In addition to the previously described effects on growth, GH has metabolic effects, which include increasing cellular protein synthesis, stimulating release of fatty acids from adipose tissue, and antagonizing the effects of insulin. Secretion of GH is normally inhibited by insulin and by increased levels of blood glucose. During periods of fasting, when both blood

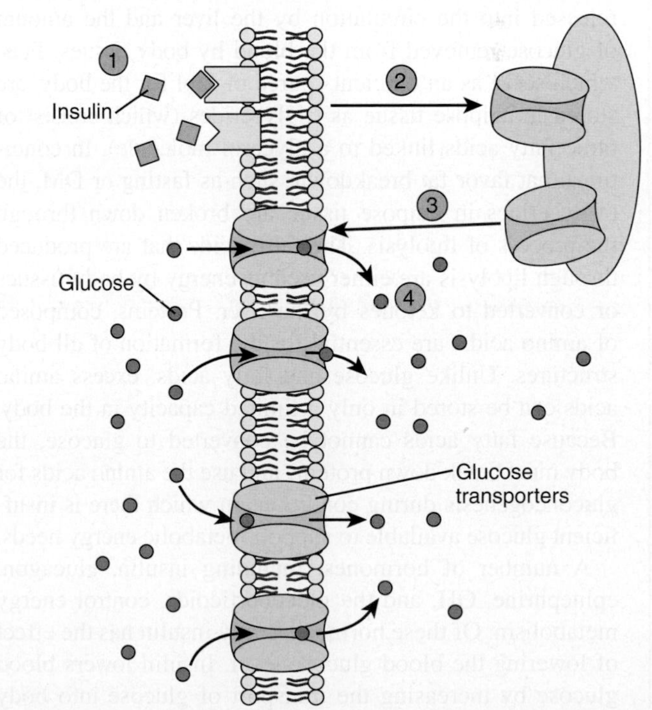

Figure 41.17 • Insulin-dependent glucose transporter (GLUT-4). (*1*) Binding of insulin-to-insulin receptor on the surface of the cell membrane, (*2*) generation of intracellular signal, (*3*) insertion of GLUT-4 receptor from its inactive site into the cell membrane, and (*4*) transport of glucose across the cell membrane.

glucose levels and insulin secretion fall, GH levels increase. Exercise, such as running and cycling, and various stresses, including anesthesia, fever, and trauma, increase GH levels. Chronic hypersecretion of GH, as occurs in acromegaly, can lead to glucose intolerance and the development of DM. The production of GH increases during childhood, peaks at puberty, and decreases with aging.[1,2,4]

Glucocorticoid Hormones

The glucocorticoid hormones, synthesized in the adrenal cortex, are critical to survival during periods of fasting and starvation, with hypoglycemia a potent stimulus of glucocorticoid release. These hormones stimulate gluconeogenesis by the liver, thus increasing hepatic glucose production. Glucocorticoids also suppress the inflammatory phase of the immune response. The pharmacotherapeutic use of glucocorticoids is a common treatment for inflammatory diseases, with hyperglycemia a potential side effect of these drugs.[1,2,4]

IN SUMMARY

The body can use glucose, fatty acids, and proteins as fuel to satisfy its energy needs; however, the brain neurons are exclusively dependent on glucose for energy. The liver stores excess glucose as glycogen and can convert amino acids, lactate, and glycerol into glucose through the process of gluconeogenesis during periods of fasting or when glucose intake does not keep pace with demand. Blood glucose levels reflect the difference between the amount of glucose released into the circulation by the liver and the amount of glucose removed from the blood by body tissues. Fats, which serve as an efficient source of fuel for the body, are stored in adipose tissue as triglycerides (which consist of three fatty acids linked to a glycerol molecule). In conditions that favor fat breakdown, such as fasting or DM, the triglycerides in adipose tissue are broken down through the process of lipolysis. The fatty acids that are produced through lipolysis are either used as energy by body tissues or converted to ketones by the liver. Proteins, composed of amino acids, are essential for the formation of all body structures. Unlike glucose and fatty acids, excess amino acids can be stored in only a limited capacity in the body. Because fatty acids cannot be converted to glucose, the body must break down proteins and use the amino acids for gluconeogenesis during conditions in which there is insufficient glucose available to support metabolic energy needs.

A number of hormones, including insulin, glucagon, epinephrine, GH, and the glucocorticoids, control energy metabolism. Of these hormones, only insulin has the effect of lowering the blood glucose level. Insulin lowers blood glucose by increasing the transport of glucose into body cells and decreasing the hepatic production and release of glucose. Insulin also has the effect of decreasing the use of fats as an energy source by decreasing lipolysis. Other hormones—glucagon, epinephrine, GH, and the glucocorticoids—act to maintain or increase blood glucose concentrations; these hormones are referred to as *counter-regulatory hormones*. Glucagon and epinephrine promote glycogenolysis (the breakdown of glycogen stores). Glucagon and the glucocorticoids increase gluconeogenesis (the production of new glucose from nonglucose substrates, primarily amino acids). GH decreases the peripheral use of glucose. Epinephrine and glucagon also increase the use of fat for energy by increasing the release of fatty acids from adipose cells.

DIABETES MELLITUS AND THE METABOLIC SYNDROME

After completing this section of the chapter, the learner will be able to meet the following objectives:

- Discuss statistics of incidence and prevalence of diabetes mellitus.
- Differentiate the types of blood and urine testing used in the diagnosis and management of diabetes mellitus.
- Differentiate the distinguishing features of the four classifications of diabetes mellitus (type 1, type 2, gestational, and diabetes due to other causes).
- Discuss the metabolic syndrome and its relationship with type 2 diabetes mellitus.

Overview, Incidence, and Prevalence

Diabetes mellitus (DM) refers to a group of common metabolic disorders characterized by hyperglycemia resulting from imbalances between insulin secretion and cellular responsiveness to insulin. A person with uncontrolled diabetes is unable to transport glucose into cells. As a result, body cells are starved, and the breakdown of fat and protein is increased to generate cellular energy.[1,2] DM is classified into 4 types, as described in Chart 41.3.

According to the United States Centers for Disease Control and Prevention (CDC), DM is a chronic health problem, with 2015 statistics reporting 23.1 million adults (aged 18 years or older) with diagnosed diabetes (approximately 7.2% of the U.S. population).[54] Of the total number of adults with diagnosed diabetes, only 5% had type 1 diabetes, with the majority of people having type 2 diabetes. In addition, another 84.1 million adults aged 18 years or older (33.9%) have been classified as having "prediabetes," based on lab findings of elevations in either the fasting glucose or hemoglobin A1C levels (both to be discussed later in this chapter). Prediabetes and diabetes affect people across genders, ages, races, and ethnicity. Among U.S. adults, DM is more prevalent among American Indians/Alaska Natives (14.9% of men; 15.3% of women), non-Hispanic African Americans (12.2% of men; 13.2% of women), and Hispanic Americans (12.6%

CHART 41.3 CLASSIFICATIONS OF DM

Prediabetes
- This classification is used when the blood glucose levels are elevated but do not meet the diagnostic criteria for diabetes.

Type 1 DM
- Characterized by insufficient insulin production, typically because of autoimmune destruction of pancreatic beta cells and frequently leading to absolute insulin deficiency. There is also a subtype that is idiopathic in which no autoimmune antibodies are detected.

Type 2 DM
- Characterized by a state of insulin resistance and progressive decline in pancreatic beta-cell secretion of insulin. Commonly accompanied by co-occurring clinical manifestations called the "metabolic syndrome."

Gestational DM
- Abnormalities of glucose regulation presenting initially during pregnancy, primarily during the second or third trimester.

Diabetes due to other causes
- Includes monogenic diabetic syndromes (such as neonatal diabetes and maturity-onset diabetes of the young [MODY]), as well as diabetes related to conditions such as cystic fibrosis and organ transplantation.

Adapted from American Diabetes Association. (2018). Classification and diagnosis of diabetes: Standards of medical care in diabetes – 2018. *Diabetes Care* 41(Suppl 1), S13–S27.

of men; 11.7% of women).[54] Type 1 diabetes is the more prevalent form in children, with the childhood incidence of new cases of type 1 diabetes highest in non-Hispanic whites. The incidence of type 2 diabetes in children is also increasing, with the incidence of new childhood cases of type 2 diabetes highest in minority populations.[54]

DM, and the resulting impact of short-term and long-term blood glucose fluctuations, can lead to a variety of complications, ranging from acute medical emergencies to disability and death. DM is a significant risk factor in coronary heart disease and stroke, and it is the leading cause of blindness and chronic kidney disease as well as a common cause of lower extremity amputations. Optimizing glycemic control, through a variety of interventions, minimizes the complications associated with diabetes.[1,2]

Testing for Diagnosis and Management

The diagnosis of DM is confirmed through the use of laboratory tests that measure blood glucose levels. The diagnostic criteria for each type of DM are described in

CHART 41.4 CRITERIA FOR THE DIAGNOSIS OF DIABETES

Fasting plasma glucose ≥126 mg/dL (7.0 mmol/L). Fasting is defined as no caloric intake for at least 8 hours.

OR

2-h PG ≥ 200 mg/dL (11.1 mmol/L) during OGTT.

OR

Hemoglobin A1C ≥ 6.5% (48 mmol/L) tested using a laboratory method that is NGSP certified and standardized to the DCCT assay. Repeat testing should be done to confirm the results in the absence of unequivocal hyperglycemia.

OR

A random plasma glucose of ≥200 mg/dL (11.1 mmol/L) in a person with classic symptoms of hyperglycemia or hyperglycemic crisis.

Adapted from American Diabetes Association (2018). Classification and diagnosis of diabetes: Standards of medical care in diabetes – 2018. *Diabetes Care*, 41(Suppl 1), page S15.

Chart 41.4. Both blood glucose measurements and tests for urinary glucose and ketones are useful in the management of diabetes.

Blood Tests

Blood tests that are useful in the diagnosis and management of DM include the fasting blood glucose test, the random (or casual) blood glucose test, the oral glucose tolerance test (OGTT), capillary whole blood glucose testing, and glycated hemoglobin levels.

Fasting Plasma Glucose Test. The fasting plasma glucose (FPG) test is a measure of plasma glucose after a period of at least 8 hours with no caloric intake.[55] An FPG level below 100 mg/dL (5.6 mmol/L) is considered normal (see Chapter 50, Table 50.2). A level between 100 and 125 mg/dL (5.6 and 6.9 mmol/L) is significant and is defined as impaired fasting glucose (IFG). The diagnostic FPG level for diabetes is 126 mg/dL (7.0 mmol/L) or higher.[55]

Random Blood Glucose Test. A random (or casual) plasma glucose is one that is done without regard to the time of the last meal. A random plasma glucose concentration that is unequivocally elevated (≥200 mg/dL [11.1 mmol/L]) in a person with classic symptoms of diabetes (such as polydipsia, polyphagia, polyuria, and blurred vision) or in a person in hyperglycemic crisis is diagnostic of DM.[55]

Oral Glucose Tolerance Test. The OGTT is an important screening test for diabetes, measuring the body's ability to remove glucose from the blood. In both men and women, the test measures the plasma glucose response to 75 g of a concentrated glucose solution at selected intervals, usually 1 and 2 hours. In people with normal glucose tolerance, blood glucose levels return to normal within 2 to 3 hours after ingestion of a glucose load in which case it can be assumed that sufficient insulin is present to allow glucose to leave the blood and enter body cells. Because a person with diabetes lacks the ability to respond to an increase in blood glucose by releasing adequate insulin to facilitate storage, blood glucose levels rise above those observed in people with normal glucose tolerance and remain elevated for longer periods. For diagnostic purposes, the 2-hour plasma glucose (2-h PG) value during an OGTT is used as an indicator, with levels ≥200 mg/dL (11.1 mmol/L) serving as a threshold criteria for diagnosis of DM (see Table 41.7).[55,56]

Capillary Whole Blood Glucose Monitoring. Technologic advances have provided the means for monitoring blood glucose levels by using a drop of capillary blood. This procedure has provided health professionals with a rapid and economical means for monitoring blood glucose and has given people with diabetes a way of maintaining near-normal blood glucose levels through self-monitoring of blood glucose. These methods use a drop of capillary blood obtained by pricking the finger with a special needle or small lancet. The drop of capillary blood is placed on or absorbed by a reagent strip, and glucose levels are determined electronically using a glucose meter. Most monitors approved for home use calibrate blood glucose readings to plasma values for easier comparison to lab values. It is important for testers to know how the meter they are using is calibrated to be able to appropriately interpret results because tests done on whole blood *without* the calibration to plasma glucose would be expected to report whole blood glucose results that are 10% to 15% lower than plasma glucose levels.[57,58]

Continuous glucose monitoring systems are becoming available to fine-tune glucose management. The various systems have small catheters implanted in the subcutaneous tissue to provide frequent samples. Endocrine centers are increasingly using this technology in selected people to achieve optimal glycemic management. The variety and accuracy of these systems are continually improving. However, finger-stick glucose monitoring remains the standard of care.[59]

TABLE 41.7 CORRELATION BETWEEN HEMOGLOBIN A1C LEVEL AND MEAN PLASMA GLUCOSE LEVELS

	MEAN PLASMA GLUCOSE	
HEMOGLOBIN A1C (%)	IN MG/DL	IN MMOL/L
6	126 (100–152)	7.0 (5.5–8.5)
7	154 (123–185)	8.6 (6.8–10.3)
8	183 (147–217)	10.2 (8.1–12.1)
9	212 (170–249)	11.8 (9.4–13.9)
10	240 (193–282)	13.4 (10.7–15.7)
11	269 (217–314)	14.9 (12.0–17.5)
12	298 (240–347)	16.5 (13.3–19.3)

Adapted from American Diabetes Association. (2018). Glycemic targets: Standards of medical care in diabetes – 2018. *Diabetes Care* 48 (Suppl 1), S55–S64.

Glycated Hemoglobin Testing (Hemoglobin A1C). Hemoglobin A1C is a test that measures the quantity of a subtype of hemoglobin that has been glycated, meaning glucose molecules have become bound to the hemoglobin molecule. This process is also sometimes referred to as glycosylation, although glycated is the more accurate term because the process does not require enzyme activity.[60] When red blood cells are released from the bone marrow, hemoglobin normally does not contain glucose; however, during the 120-day life span of the red blood cell, hemoglobin normally becomes glycated. Because glucose entry into red blood cells is not insulin-dependent, the rate at which glucose becomes attached to the hemoglobin molecule reflects blood glucose levels. Glycosylation is essentially irreversible; therefore, the *level of A1C present in the blood provides an index of blood glucose levels over the approximate 120-day lifespan of red blood cells.* In conditions of hyperglycemia, the A1C level is increased. Table 41.7 lists A1C values with correlations of mean plasma glucose levels.

Urine Tests

Urine tests for glucose indicate that the renal threshold for reabsorption of glucose has been exceeded, which is typically accompanied by hyperglycemia. Renal tests for ketones indicate that the body is producing excessive ketone bodies, typically because of the use of nonglucose energy substrates for fuel.[61,62]

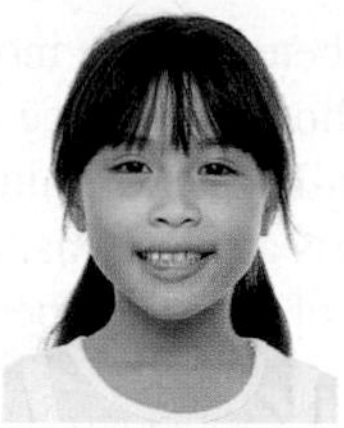

Emily and her family will need to learn how and when to check urine for ketones as well as how to use a blood glucose meter to monitor blood glucose levels.

Classifications and Pathophysiology

An overview of the classification scheme of DM is shown in Chart 41.3. The pathophysiologic characteristics and clinical manifestations of each type are described in the following sections.

Prediabetes

Prediabetes is the diagnostic term used when the blood glucose is elevated but does not yet meet the threshold criteria for the diagnosis of DM. Detection of the prediabetic state is more common in people at risk for type 2 DM. If prediabetes is detected, lifestyle modifications of diet, exercise, and weight loss can help to prevent the progression to type 2 DM.[1,2,52]

Type 1 Diabetes Mellitus

Type 1 DM is characterized by destruction of the pancreatic beta cells. Approximately 5% of the cases of DM are type 1.[55] Most instances of type 1 DM are immune mediated, as reflected by the detection of specific autoantibodies. A small minority of people with type 1 DM are considered to have an idiopathic form of type 1 DM in which no autoantibodies are detected. This idiopathic form is more likely in people of Asian or African ancestry.[55] From a treatment perspective, the types of type 1 diabetes are not differentiated; however, sometimes the immune-mediated form is referred to as type 1A and the idiopathic form as type 1B.[52]

Immune-mediated type 1 DM was formerly called *juvenile-onset diabetes* or *insulin-dependent diabetes.*[55] It occurs more commonly in young people but can occur at any age. The rate of beta-cell destruction is quite variable, being rapid in some people and slow in others. The rapidly progressive form is not only commonly observed in children but also may occur in adults. Adults with type 2 DM sometimes also present with a slowly progressive form of insulin-dependent DM with autoimmune findings similar to type 1 DM. This slowly progressive adult form is sometimes referred to as *latent autoimmune diabetes in adults* (LADAs).[52] Immune-mediated type 1 DM is often related to a genetic predisposition (*i.e.*, diabetogenic genes). Susceptibility to type 1A DM involves multiple genes; however, the major susceptibility gene for type 1A DM is located in the human leukocyte antigen (HLA) gene related to antigen presentation to T cells.[63]

Type 1 diabetes is a catabolic disorder characterized by an absolute lack of insulin, an elevation in blood glucose, and a breakdown of body fats and proteins. The absolute lack of insulin in people with type 1 DM means that they are particularly prone to the development of ketoacidosis. One of the actions of insulin is the inhibition of *lipolysis* (*i.e.*, fat breakdown) and release of FFAs from fat cells. In the absence of insulin, ketosis develops when these fatty acids are released from fat cells and converted to ketones in the liver. Because of the loss of insulin response, *all people with immune-mediated type 1 diabetes require exogenous insulin replacement* to reverse the catabolic state, control blood glucose levels, and prevent ketosis.[1,2,52,55,63]

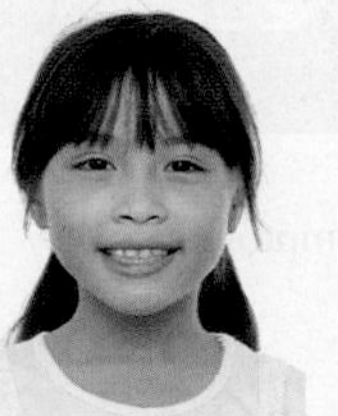

In the unit opener case study, we met **Emily Toronto,** the 7-year-old diagnosed with type 1 diabetes. Emily had classic symptoms of severe hyperglycemia, the associated dehydration (osmotic diuresis), and metabolic acidosis. Because she was at risk for diabetes, because of her family history, she may have had testing for the presence of diabetes autoantibodies. Treatment of her acute needs will be discussed in more detail in the section on diabetic ketoacidosis (DKA).

Type 2 Diabetes Mellitus and the Metabolic Syndrome

Type 2 DM accounts for the majority of cases of diabetes, approximately 90% to 95%.[55] It is a heterogeneous condition that describes the presence of hyperglycemia in association with *relative* insulin deficiency. Many people with type 2 diabetes are adults and overweight; however, recent trends indicate that type 2 diabetes has become a more common occurrence in adolescents and children with obesity, a condition termed *MODY*.[52] Although autoimmune destruction of the beta cells does not occur, people with type 2 diabetes eventually may require insulin. Therefore, the previous terms related to type 2 diabetes, such as *adult-onset diabetes* and *non–insulin-dependent diabetes*, can generate confusion and are thus obsolete.[55] Type 2 diabetes has a strong genetic component. A number of genetic and acquired pathogenic factors have been implicated in the progressive impairment of beta-cell function in people with prediabetes and type 2 diabetes.[52,63]

The metabolic abnormalities associated with type 2 diabetes are illustrated in Figure 41.18. These abnormalities include:

1. Insulin resistance
2. Deranged secretion of insulin by the pancreatic beta cells
3. Increased glucose production by the liver[52,55,63]

In contrast to type 1 diabetes, where *absolute* insulin deficiency is present, people with type 2 diabetes can have high, normal, or low insulin levels. Insulin resistance is the decreased ability of insulin to act effectively on target tissues, especially muscle, liver, and fat. It is the predominate characteristic of type 2 diabetes and results from a combination of factors such as genetic susceptibility and obesity.[52,55,63] Table 41.8 compares the characteristics of type 1 and type 2 DM.

Insulin resistance initially stimulates an increase in insulin secretion, often to a level of modest hyperinsulinemia, as the beta cells attempt to maintain a normal blood glucose level. In time, the increased demand for insulin secretion leads to beta-cell exhaustion and failure. This results in elevated postprandial blood glucose levels and an eventual increase in glucose production by the liver. Because people with type 2 DM do not have an absolute insulin deficiency, they are less prone to ketoacidosis compared to people with type 1 diabetes.[52,55,63]

In type 2 DM, the basal hepatic insulin resistance is manifested by a hepatic overproduction of glucose despite a fasting hyperinsulinemia, with the rate of glucose production being the primary determinant of the elevated FPG in people with type 2 diabetes. Although the insulin resistance seen in people with type 2 diabetes can be caused by a number of factors, it is strongly associated with obesity and physical inactivity.[1,2,52,55,63] Specific causes of beta-cell dysfunction in type 2 DM are unclear; however, it appears that in both type 1 DM and type 2 DM, there may be an increased apoptosis of pancreatic beta cells in response to the stress of hyperglycemia.[63]

Insulin Resistance and the Metabolic Syndrome. Increasing evidence indicates that insulin resistance not only contributes to the hyperglycemia in people with type 2 diabetes, but it also may play a role in other metabolic abnormalities. These include obesity, high levels of plasma triglycerides and low levels of high-density lipoproteins (HDL), hypertension,

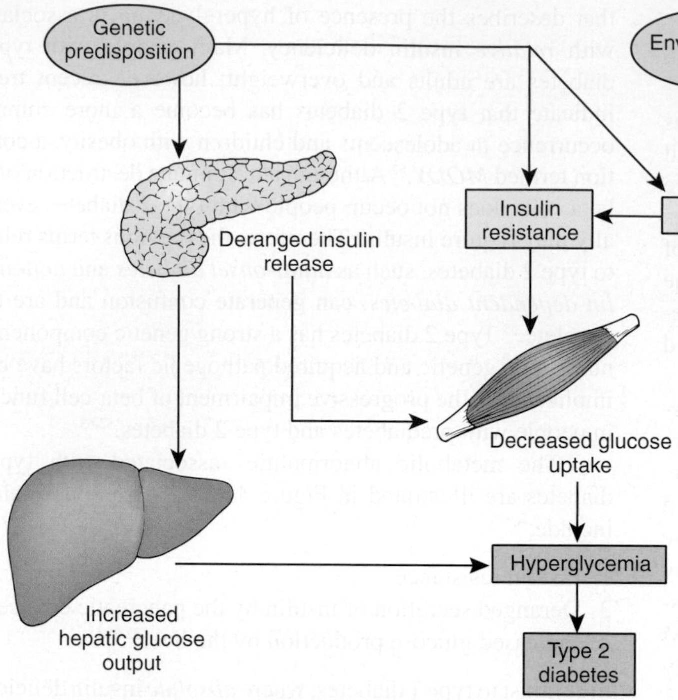

Figure 41.18 • Pathogenesis of type 2 DM.

systemic inflammation (as detected by C-reactive protein [CRP] and other mediators), abnormal fibrinolysis, abnormal function of the vascular endothelium, and macrovascular disease (coronary artery, cerebrovascular, and peripheral arterial disease). This constellation of abnormalities is often referred to as the *insulin resistance syndrome*, *syndrome X*, or, the preferred term, *metabolic syndrome*.[1,2,52,55,63] The clinical signs, laboratory abnormalities, and associated illnesses associated with this syndrome are described in Chart 41.5.

A major factor in people with metabolic syndrome that leads to type 2 diabetes is obesity. People with obesity have increased resistance to the action of insulin and impaired suppression of glucose production by the liver, resulting in both hyperglycemia and hyperinsulinemia. The type of obesity is an important consideration in the development of type 2 diabetes. People with upper body (or central) obesity are at greater risk for developing type 2 diabetes and metabolic disturbances than people with lower body (or peripheral) obesity. Waist circumference and waist–hip ratio (WHR), which are both surrogate measures of central obesity, have been shown to correlate well with insulin resistance. A loss of 5% to 10% of body weight has the potential to improve insulin resistance and lower blood glucose levels.[1,2,55]

The increased adipose tissue and/or dense distribution of central adiposity challenge the vascular perfusion of that tissue, leading to chronic underperfusion with areas of tissue hypoxia and necrosis in the adipose tissue. Tissue macrophages respond to the hypoxic–ischemic cellular damage that induces a condition of chronic inflammation. This inflammatory state begins in the adipose tissue and progresses to other areas of

TABLE 41.8 COMPARISON OF TYPE 1 AND TYPE 2 DM

	TYPE 1 DIABETES	TYPE 2 DIABETES
Age of onset	Usually childhood	Usually adulthood
Type of onset	Abrupt; symptomatic (polyuria, polydipsia, dehydration) often with severe ketoacidosis	Gradual; usually subtle; often asymptomatic
Usual body weight	Normal; recent weight loss is common	Overweight
Family history	Occurs, but less common	Very common
HLA associations	+	No
Islet lesions	Early—inflammation Late—atrophy and fibrosis	Late—fibrosis, amyloid
Beta-cell mass	Markedly reduced	Normal or slightly reduced
Circulating insulin level	Markedly reduced	Elevated or normal
Clinical management	Insulin absolutely required	Insulin usually not needed initially; insulin supplementation may be needed at later stages; weight loss typically improves the condition

HLA, human leukocyte antigen.

CHART 41.5 FREQUENTLY OBSERVED CONCOMITANTS OF THE METABOLIC SYNDROME

Clinical Signs
- Central (upper body) obesity with increased waist circumference
- Acanthosis nigricans (hypertrophic, hyperpigmented skin changes)

Laboratory Abnormalities
- Elevated fasting and/or postprandial glucose
- Insulin resistance with hyperinsulinemia
- Dyslipidemia characterized by increased triglycerides and low HDL cholesterol
- Abnormal thrombolysis
- Hyperuricemia
- Endothelial and vascular smooth muscle dysfunction
- Albuminuria

Comorbid Illnesses
- Hypertension
- Atherosclerosis
- Hyperandrogenism with polycystic ovary syndrome

Adapted from Rubin R., Strayer D. S... (2015). *Rubin's pathology: Clinicopathologic foundations of medicine* (7th ed., Table 13-1, p. 521). Philadelphia, PA: Lippincott Williams & Wilkins.

the body to foster a chronic systemic inflammatory response state with oxidative stress that contributes to the development of atherosclerotic plaque and atherothrombosis.[64]

In type 2 DM, adipose tissues are among the tissues that demonstrate inadequate response to insulin, contributing to the pancreatic response of hyperinsulinemia to attempt to reduce the hyperglycemia. Overexpression of insulin receptors also may occur. Normally, cellular response to insulin binding stimulates two intracellular pathways—the phosphoinositide 3-kinase (P13K) pathway and the mitogen activated protein (MAP) pathway. In type 2 DM, the P13K pathway does not maintain its function; this P13K functional decline contributes to decreased nitric oxide production from endothelial cells and to a decrease in the translocation of the GLUT 4 proteins that facilitate glucose entry into cells.[64] Nitric oxide is a powerful endothelial-derived relaxing factor, which promotes vasodilation.[4] Therefore, the decline in nitric oxide production contributes to vasoconstriction and increased vascular resistance. In type 2 DM, the MAP pathway that is also stimulated by the binding of insulin to cellular insulin receptors continues to function. The actions of stimulation of the MAP pathway include stimulation of the vasoconstriction molecule endothelin-1, along with increased expression of adhesion molecules and smooth muscle stimulation, all of which further contribute to the increased risk of development of atherosclerosis in type 2 DM.[64]

Insulin also normally signals the inhibition of lipolysis; however, the insulin resistance in type 2 DM causes increased lipolysis with increased release of FFAs. The liver transforms these FFAs into triglycerides and very-low-density lipoproteins (VLDLs). The net results of the combined systemic inflammation, increased oxidative stress, endothelial dysfunction, and increased blood lipids all contribute to the constellation of metabolic alterations that are present in the metabolic syndrome—including dyslipidemia, hypertension, vascular pathology, and abnormal coagulation.[64]

KEY POINTS

DIABETES MELLITUS
- DM is a disorder of carbohydrate, fat, and protein metabolism brought about by impaired beta-cell synthesis or release of insulin, or the inability of tissues to use insulin.
- Type 1 DM results from loss of beta-cell function and an absolute insulin deficiency.
- Type 2 DM results from impaired ability of the tissues to use insulin (insulin resistance) accompanied by a relative lack of insulin or impaired release of insulin in relation to blood glucose levels (beta-cell dysfunction).

Gestational Diabetes

Gestational diabetes mellitus (GDM) is any degree of glucose intolerance that occurs initially during pregnancy, particularly presenting during the second and third trimesters. Diagnosis and careful medical management are essential because women with GDM are at higher risk for complications of pregnancy, mortality, and fetal abnormalities. Fetal abnormalities include macrosomia (*i.e.*, large body size), hypoglycemia, hypocalcemia, polycythemia, and hyperbilirubinemia. Women with GDM have an increased risk of developing type 2 DM; therefore, women in whom GDM is diagnosed should be followed after delivery to detect diabetes early in its course.[55,65]

Diabetes due to Other Causes

A small percentage of the overall number of cases of diabetes consist of specific types of diabetes associated with certain other conditions and syndromes. Such diabetes can occur with pancreatic disease or the removal of pancreatic tissue and with endocrine diseases, such as acromegaly, Cushing syndrome, or pheochromocytoma. Endocrine disorders that produce hyperglycemia do so by increasing the hepatic production of glucose or decreasing the cellular use of glucose. Several specific types of diabetes are associated with monogenetic defects in beta-cell function. Other causes for diabetes can be genetic defects in beta-cell function or insulin secretion, drug treatment, or chemicals.[1,2,52,55]

Clinical Manifestations of Diabetes Mellitus

In type 1 DM, signs and symptoms often arise suddenly. Type 2 DM usually develops more insidiously, often existing for years without detection until diagnosed during a routine medical examination or care for other conditions.

The most commonly identified signs and symptoms of diabetes are referred to as the *three polys*:

1. Polyuria (*i.e.*, excessive urination)
2. Polydipsia (*i.e.*, excessive thirst)
3. Polyphagia (*i.e.*, excessive hunger)

These three symptoms are closely related to the hyperglycemia and glycosuria of diabetes. Glucose is a small, osmotically active molecule. When blood glucose levels are sufficiently elevated, the amount of glucose filtered by the glomeruli of the kidney exceeds the amount that can be reabsorbed by the renal tubules. This results in glycosuria accompanied by osmotic large volume losses of water in the urine. Thirst results from the intracellular dehydration that occurs as blood glucose levels rise causing an osmotic movement of water out of body cells, including cells in the hypothalamic thirst center. This early symptom of increased thirst may be easily overlooked in people with type 2 DM, particularly in those who have had a gradual increase in blood glucose levels. Polyphagia is usually not present in people with type 2 diabetes. In type 1 diabetes, polyphagia probably results from cellular starvation and the depletion of cellular stores of carbohydrates, fats, and proteins.[1,2,4,52,63]

Weight loss despite normal or increased appetite is a common occurrence in people with uncontrolled type 1 diabetes. The cause of weight loss is twofold. First, loss of body fluids results from osmotic diuresis. Vomiting may exaggerate fluid loss in ketoacidosis. Second, body tissue is lost because the lack of insulin forces the body to use fat stores and cellular proteins for energy. Although weight loss is a frequent phenomenon in people with uncontrolled type 1 DM, type 2 DM is associated with obesity. However, some people with undiagnosed type 2 DM may experience unexplained weight loss as cellular resistance to circulating insulin reduces energy availability.[1,2,4,52,63]

Other signs and symptoms of hyperglycemia include recurrent blurred vision, fatigue, and skin infections. In type 2 DM, these are often the symptoms that prompt a person to seek medical treatment. Blurred vision develops as the lens and retina are exposed to hyperosmolar fluids. Lowered plasma volume produces weakness and fatigue. Chronic skin infections often occur in people with type 2 DM. Hyperglycemia and glycosuria also favor the growth of yeast organisms. *Candida* infections are common initial complaints in women with diabetes.[1,2,4,52,63]

Treatment

The desired management outcome in both type 1 and type 2 DM is normalization of blood glucose with the goal of preventing short-term and long-term complications. Treatment plans involve medical nutrition therapy, exercise, and antidiabetic agents. People with type 1 diabetes require insulin therapy from the time of diagnosis. Weight loss and dietary management may be sufficient to control blood glucose levels in some people with type 2 diabetes who adopt lifestyle changes long term. However, follow-up care is also important for type 2 diabetes because insulin secretion from the beta cells may decrease or insulin resistance may persist or worsen. If this is the case, medications to treat insulin resistance are prescribed. Pancreas transplantation methods are also increasingly being used as a method of diabetic control.[1,2,55,65]

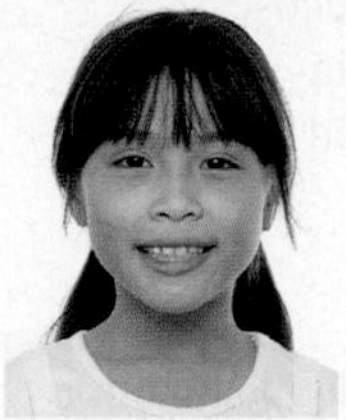

Emily Toronto, the child with type 1 diabetes, will require insulin for the rest of her life. Pediatric insulin regimens are quite individualized, making use of different strategies to maximize glycemic control while considering safety concerns of this age group. When Emily becomes older and more independent with her care, she will likely be independent with an intensive insulin regime. She and her family will also be informed of the use of insulin pumps and make a decision regarding if, or when, Emily may use this therapy. Emily and her family should work closely with a registered dietitian throughout her lifespan to maximize understanding regarding the vital role of nutrition for her health. Today's approach to flexible, individualized meal planning will allow Emily to enjoy a normal healthy diet rather than the need for a specialized and rigid regime, which alienates her from her peers.

IN SUMMARY

DM is a disorder of carbohydrate, protein, and fat metabolism resulting from an imbalance between insulin availability and insulin need. The disease can be classified as type 1 DM in which there is destruction of beta cells and an absolute insulin deficiency, or type 2 DM in which there is a lack of insulin availability or effectiveness. GDM develops during pregnancy, and although glucose tolerance often returns to normal after childbirth, it indicates an increased risk for the development of diabetes. The metabolic syndrome represents a constellation of metabolic abnormalities characterized by obesity, insulin resistance, high triglyceride levels and low HDL levels, hypertension, cardiovascular disease, insulin resistance, and increased risk for development of type 2 DM.

The most commonly identified symptoms of type 1 DM are polyuria, polydipsia, polyphagia, and weight loss despite normal or increased appetite. Although people with type 2 DM may present with one or more of these symptoms, they are often asymptomatic initially. The diagnosis of DM is based on clinical signs of the disease, fasting blood glucose levels, random plasma glucose measurements, and results of the glucose tolerance test. Glycation involves the irreversible attachment of glucose to the hemoglobin molecule; the measurement of A1C provides an index of blood glucose levels over several months. Self-monitoring provides a means of maintaining near-normal blood glucose levels through frequent testing of blood glucose and adjustment of insulin dosage.

COMPLICATIONS OF DIABETES MELLITUS

After completing this section of the chapter, the learner will be able to meet the following objectives:

- Differentiate among the common acute complications of diabetes: DKA, hyperosmolar hyperglycemic state (HHS), and hypoglycemia.
- Discuss complications of diabetes related to counter-regulatory hormones: the Somogyi effect and the dawn phenomenon.
- Differentiate among the common chronic complications of diabetes: microvascular effects, macrovascular effects, diabetic foot ulcers, and infections.

Acute Complications of Diabetes

The three major acute complications of diabetes are DKA, HHS, and hypoglycemia. All are life-threatening conditions that demand immediate recognition and treatment. These complications account for a significant number of hospitalizations and consumption of health care resources.[1,2,4]

Diabetic Ketoacidosis

DKA most commonly occurs in a person with type 1 diabetes in whom the lack of insulin leads to increased release of fatty acids from adipose tissue because of the unsuppressed adipose cell lipase activity that breaks down triglycerides into fatty acids and glycerol. The increase in fatty acid levels leads to ketone production by the liver (Fig. 41.19). DKA can occur at the onset of the disease, often before diagnosis, and can occur as a complication during the course of the disease.

Stress increases the release of gluconeogenic hormones and predisposes the person to the development of ketoacidosis. DKA is often preceded by physical or emotional stress, such as infection or inflammation, pregnancy, or extreme anxiety. In clinical practice, ketoacidosis also occurs with the omission or inadequate use of insulin.[1,2,4]

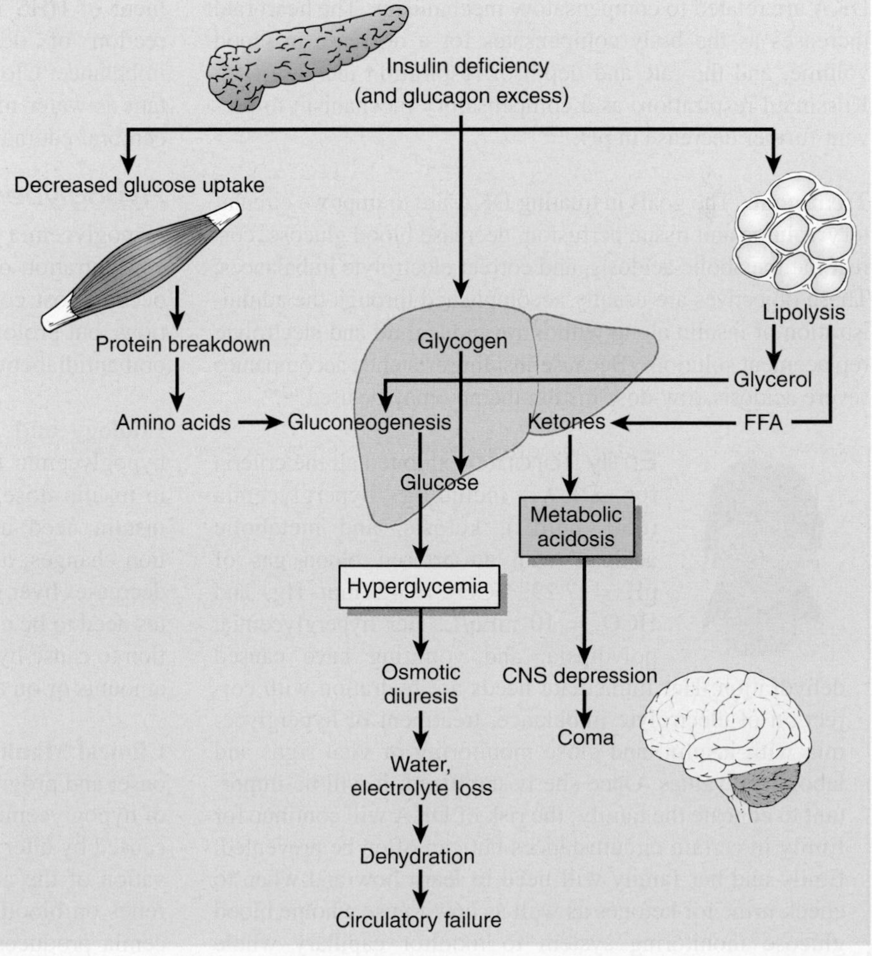

Figure 41.19 • Mechanisms of DKA. DKA is associated with very low insulin levels and extremely high levels of glucagon, catecholamines, and other counter-regulatory hormones. Increased levels of glucagon and the catecholamines lead to mobilization of substrates for gluconeogenesis and ketogenesis by the liver. Gluconeogenesis in excess of that needed to supply glucose for the brain and other glucose-dependent tissues produces a rise in blood glucose levels. Mobilization of FFA from triglyceride stores in adipose tissue leads to accelerated ketone production and ketosis. (CNS, central nervous system.)

Etiology and Pathogenesis. The three major metabolic derangements in DKA are hyperglycemia, ketosis, and metabolic acidosis. Hyperglycemia leads to osmotic diuresis, dehydration, and a critical loss of electrolytes. Hyperosmolality of extracellular fluid because of hyperglycemia leads to a shift of water from the intracellular to the extracellular compartment. Extracellular sodium concentration is frequently low or normal despite increased urinary water losses because of the intracellular–extracellular fluid shift. This dilutional effect is referred to as *pseudohyponatremia*. Serum potassium levels may be normal or elevated despite total potassium depletion resulting from protracted polyuria and vomiting. Metabolic acidosis is caused by the excess keto acids that require buffering by bicarbonate ions. This leads to a marked decrease in serum bicarbonate levels. The severity of DKA is classified on the severity of the metabolic acidosis.[1,2,4]

Clinical Manifestations. A day or more of polyuria, polydipsia, nausea, vomiting, and marked fatigue, with eventual stupor that can progress to coma commonly precedes DKA. Abdominal pain and tenderness may be experienced without abdominal disease. The breath has a characteristic fruity smell because of the presence of the volatile keto acids. Hypotension and tachycardia may be present because of a decrease in blood volume. A number of the signs and symptoms that occur in DKA are related to compensatory mechanisms. The heart rate increases as the body compensates for a decrease in blood volume, and the rate and depth of respiration increase (*i.e.*, Kussmaul respiration) as a compensatory mechanism to prevent further decrease in pH.[1,2,4]

Treatment. The goals in treating DKA are to improve circulatory volume and tissue perfusion, decrease blood glucose, correct the metabolic acidosis, and correct electrolyte imbalances. These objectives are usually accomplished through the administration of insulin along with intravenous fluid and electrolyte replacement solutions. Because insulin resistance accompanies severe acidosis, low-dose insulin therapy may be used.[1,2,65]

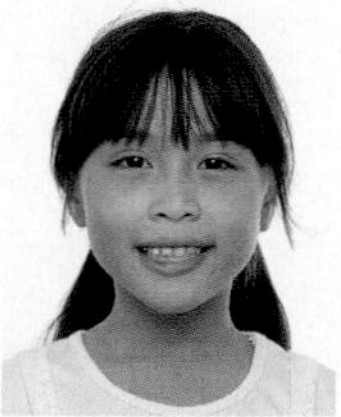

Emily Toronto exhibited all the criteria for DKA, including hyperglycemia (650 mg/dL), ketosis, and metabolic acidosis with an arterial blood gas of pH = 7.29, pCO_2 = 42 mm Hg, and HCO_3 = 10 mEq/L. Her hyperglycemia, polydipsia, and vomiting have caused dehydration. Her immediate needs are hydration with correction of electrolyte imbalance, treatment of hyperglycemia with insulin, and close monitoring of vital signs and laboratory values. Once she is stabilized, it will be important to educate the family; the risk of DKA will continue for Emily in certain circumstances but can often be prevented. Emily and her family will need to learn how and when to check urine for ketones as well as how to use a home blood glucose monitoring system to monitor capillary whole blood glucose levels.

Hyperosmolar Hyperglycemic State

HHS is characterized by hyperglycemia, hyperosmolarity with dehydration, the absence of ketoacidosis, and depression of the sensorium. HHS occurs frequently in people with type 2 diabetes.[1,2,4]

Etiology and Pathogenesis. A partial or relative insulin deficiency may initiate HHS by reducing glucose utilization while increasing glucagon release and hepatic glucose output. The hyperglycemia leads to large volume water loss through osmotic diuresis. Dehydration is usually more severe in HHS than in DKA. As the plasma volume contracts, renal insufficiency develops. The resultant decrease in renal elimination of glucose further elevates blood glucose levels, which increases the severity of the hyperosmolar state. In hyperosmolar states, the increased serum osmolarity has the effect of pulling water out of body cells, including brain cells. HHS may also be complicated by thromboembolic events related to the contraction of plasma volume with increased coagulability because of stasis.[1,2,4]

Clinical Manifestations and Treatment. The most prominent manifestations of HHS are weakness, dehydration, polyuria, neurologic alterations, and excessive thirst. Neurologic alterations include hemiparesis, seizures, and coma; these symptoms may be mistaken for a stroke. Successful treatment of HHS involves careful patient monitoring and correction of dehydration, hyperglycemia, and electrolyte imbalance. Close observation and care is particularly important as water moves back into brain cells, posing a threat of cerebral edema.[1,2,65]

Hypoglycemia

Hypoglycemia is generally defined as any blood glucose concentration of <70 mg/dL, with or without symptoms.[65] It occurs most commonly in people treated with insulin injections, but prolonged hypoglycemia can also result from some oral antidiabetic agents.[1,2,65]

Etiology and Pathogenesis. Many factors can precipitate hypoglycemia in a person with type 1 DM, including error in insulin dose, failure to eat, increased exercise, decreased insulin need after removal of a stress situation, medication changes, and a change in insulin injection site. Alcohol decreases liver gluconeogenesis; therefore, people with diabetes need to be cautioned about the potential for alcohol ingestion to cause hypoglycemia, particularly if consumed in large amounts or on an empty stomach.[1,2,65]

Clinical Manifestations. Hypoglycemia usually has a rapid onset and progression of symptoms. The signs and symptoms of hypoglycemia can be divided into two categories: (a) those caused by altered brain function and (b) those related to activation of the autonomic nervous system. Because the brain relies on blood glucose as its main energy source, hypoglycemia produces behaviors related to altered brain function. Headache, difficulty in problem solving, disturbed or altered behavior, coma, and seizures may occur. At the onset of the hypoglycemic episode, activation of the parasympathetic nervous system often causes hunger. The initial parasympathetic response is followed by activation of the sympathetic nervous system; this causes anxiety, tachycardia, sweating, and constriction of the skin vessels (*i.e.*, the skin is cool and clammy).[1,2,4]

The signs and symptoms of hypoglycemia are highly variable, and not everyone manifests all or even most of the symptoms. The signs and symptoms are particularly variable in children and in older adults. Older adults may not display the typical autonomic responses associated with hypoglycemia but frequently develop signs of impaired function of the CNS, including mental confusion. Some people develop hypoglycemic unawareness. Unawareness of hypoglycemia should be suspected in people who do not report symptoms when their blood glucose concentrations are <50 to 60 mg/dL (2.8 to 3.3 mmol/L). This occurs most commonly in people who have a longer duration of diabetes and A1C levels within the normal range. Some medications, such as β-adrenergic blocking drugs, interfere with the sympathetic response normally seen in hypoglycemia.[1–3,65]

Treatment. Recommended treatment of an insulin reaction is the immediate oral administration of a rapidly absorbed form of glucose, which can be repeated as necessary. For people who are unconscious or unable to swallow, glucagon may be given intramuscularly or subcutaneously, to raise blood glucose through hepatic glycogenolysis.[65]

Diabetic Complications Related to Counter-Regulatory Mechanisms

The counter-regulatory mechanisms described above are associated with several patterns of diabetic complications, known as the Somogyi effect and the dawn phenomenon.

The Somogyi Effect

During the 1930s, Dr. Michael Somogyi theorized the presence of a cyclical pattern of early morning hyperglycemia in response to an insulin-induced hypoglycemia occurring during the previous evening.[66] In people with DM, the insulin-induced hypoglycemia produces a compensatory increase in blood levels of counter-regulatory hormones such as catecholamines, glucagon, cortisol, and GH. These counter-regulatory hormones cause blood glucose to become elevated and produce some degree of insulin resistance. The cycle begins when the increase in blood glucose and insulin resistance is treated with larger insulin doses. The Somogyi phenomenon is less common than the dawn phenomenon, which is described below.[66]

Clinically, high blood glucose levels in the morning can complicate medical treatment of diabetes if not fully understood to be a counter-regulatory result of hypoglycemia. The hypoglycemic episode often occurs during the night or at a time when it is not recognized, rendering the diagnosis of the phenomenon more difficult. Without proper evaluation, an increase in medication can exacerbate the situation. When a Somogyi situation is suspected, people may be asked to test blood sugars in the middle of the night to identify possible hypoglycemia.[66]

The Dawn Phenomenon

The dawn phenomenon is characterized by increased fasting blood glucose and/or insulin requirements during the early morning hours that are *not* triggered by a preceding hypoglycemic event (in contrast with the Somogyi effect described above). The dawn phenomenon is the result of circadian variations in hormone secretion, with glucagon secretion to release energy stores in preparation for the activity of the day. High fasting blood glucose levels are common in people with type 2 DM because of the dawn phenomenon.[67]

Chronic Complications of Diabetes Mellitus

The chronic complications of diabetes include disorders of the microvasculature (*i.e.*, neuropathies, nephropathies, and retinopathies), disorders of gastrointestinal motility, macrovascular complications (*i.e.*, coronary artery, cerebral vascular, and peripheral vascular disease), and foot ulcers (Fig. 41.20). People with diabetes are also more susceptible to infections. The level of chronic hyperglycemia is the best predictive factor for diabetic complications; therefore, glycemic control is a primary goal of diabetic treatment.[55,65,68]

Microvascular Complications

The microvascular complications of DM are related to the production of advanced glycation end products (AGEs), as reflected in the hemoglobin A1C measure. AGEs induce vascular damage by stimulating an increased production of reactive oxygen species (ROS). These ROS are thought to damage endothelial cells by decreasing the production of the vascular endothelial relaxing factor NO, thus leading to endothelial dysfunction.[69]

In type 2 DM, this damage from AGEs may be compounded by the increased oxidative stress, chronic systemic inflammation, and dyslipidemia associated with the metabolic syndrome (as described previously). The types of microvascular complications that occur in DM can include neuropathy, retinopathy, nephropathy, and disorders of gastrointestinal motility. In the United States, diabetes is a leading cause of vision loss and blindness as well as chronic kidney disease.[1,2]

Macrovascular Complications

Because of the previously discussed vascular damage owing to hyperglycemia and the metabolic syndrome, people with DM are at increased risk of macrovascular complications such as coronary artery disease, cerebrovascular disease and stroke, and peripheral vascular disease.

KEY POINTS

CHRONIC COMPLICATIONS OF DIABETES

- The chronic complications of diabetes result from elevated blood glucose levels and associated impairment of lipid and other metabolic pathways.
- Macrovascular disorders such as coronary heart disease, stroke, and peripheral vascular disease reflect the combined effects of unregulated blood glucose levels, elevated blood pressure, and hyperlipidemia.
- The chronic complications of diabetes are best prevented by measures aimed at tight control of blood glucose levels, maintenance of normal lipid levels, and control of hypertension.

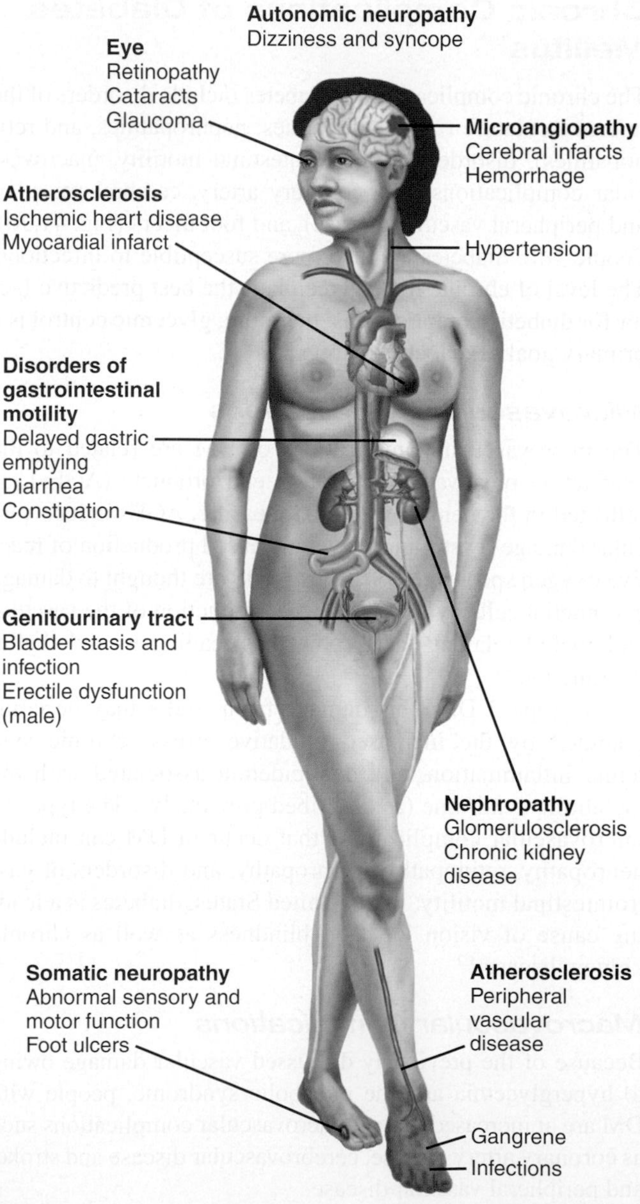

Figure 41.20 • Long-term complications of DM.

Diabetic Foot Ulcers

Foot problems are common among people with diabetes and may become severe enough to cause ulceration, infection, and, eventually, the need for amputation. In people with diabetes, lesions of the feet represent the effects of neuropathy and vascular insufficiency. People with sensory neuropathies have impaired pain sensation and are often unaware of the constant trauma to the feet caused by poorly fitting shoes, improper weight bearing, hard objects or pebbles in the shoes, or infections such as athlete's foot. Neuropathy reduces the perception of pain; thus, injuries and infections often go undetected. Motor neuropathy can lead to weakness of the intrinsic muscles of the foot and may result in foot deformities with focal areas of high pressure. When this abnormal focus of pressure is coupled with loss of sensation, a foot ulcer can occur. Common sites of trauma are the back of the heel, the plantar metatarsal area, or the great toe, where weight is borne during walking.[1,2,55,65] (Fig. 41.21).

Infections

Infections are a primary concern to people with diabetes, with certain types of infections occurring with increased frequency (including soft tissue infections of the extremities, osteomyelitis, urinary tract infections and pyelonephritis, candida infections of the skin and mucous surfaces, dental caries, and periodontal disease). The presence of chronic vascular complications contributes to suboptimal response to infection in a

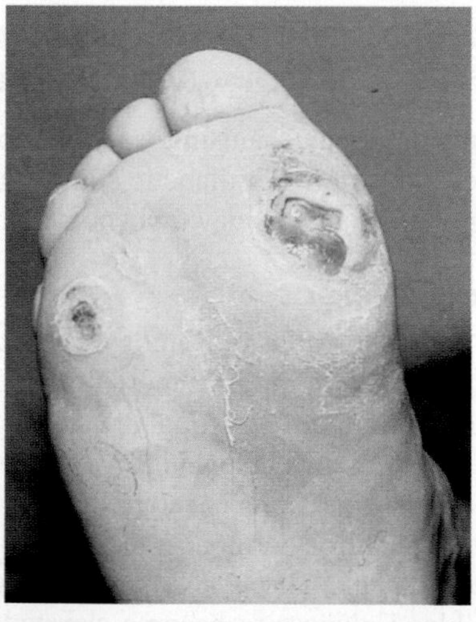

Figure 41.21 • Peripheral neuropathies, most common in people with DM and chronic hyperglycemia, are classified as somatic or autonomic. Somatic neuropathies typically affect lower extremities. Paresthesia, burning sensations, and numbness may occur along with decreased senses of vibration, pain, temperature, and proprioception. These symptoms increase risk for tissue injury and falls. Daily foot assessment is critical because these people may not feel a break in the skin or a burn and develop subsequent foot lesions, which are challenging to heal. For some people, peripheral neuropathies cause chronic lower extremity pain. Pain assessment and management are crucial to their quality of life. A pharmacologic approach to management is often employed. (From Marks R. (1987). *Skin disease in old age*. Philadelphia, PA: JB Lippincott.)

person with diabetes, as do hyperglycemia and altered neutrophil function. Sensory deficits may cause a person with diabetes to ignore minor trauma and infection. Vascular disease may impair circulation and delivery of blood cells and other necessary substances for promotion of adequate inflammatory response and effective healing. Hyperglycemia and glycosuria may influence the growth of microorganisms and increase severity of infections.[1,2,4]

IN SUMMARY

The metabolic disturbances associated with diabetes affect almost every body system. The acute complications of diabetes include DKA, hyperglycemic hyperosmolar state, and hypoglycemia in people with insulin-treated diabetes. Complications also occur because of compensatory changes by counter-regulatory hormones. The chronic complications of diabetes affect the microvascular system (including the retina, kidneys, and peripheral nervous system) and the macrovascular system (coronary, cerebrovascular, and peripheral arteries). Microvascular and macrovascular dysfunctions contribute to diabetic foot ulcers. Infection is a significant concern because of the alterations in the healing process associated with the physiologic changes in diabetes. Chronic hyperglycemia plays a key role in complications, and people should receive significant education and support to learn to control blood sugar and minimize complications.

GERIATRIC Considerations

- The increased rate of hypothyroidism associated with aging is due to altered immune function and comorbidities.[70]
- Older women with hypothyroidism often present with no symptoms or subclinical symptoms such as fatigue, confusion, and muscle aches/tenderness.[71]
- Hyperthyroidism may be misdiagnosed as normal aging. Serum TSH measurement is recommended when symptoms such as muscle weakness or mental decline are present.[71]
- Hypo/hyperthyroidism is more common in older women than in men.[70,71]
- Type 2 DM is the seventh leading cause of death among older adults and affects 20% of older people.[71]
- Screening for diabetes every 3 years is indicated in older adults because classic symptoms are often missing and nonspecific symptoms may delay diagnosis.[71]
- Hypoglycemia in older adults leads to a set of unique symptoms unlike those in younger adults and includes nighttime headaches, slurring of speech, and confusion that may lead to unusual behavior.[71]

PEDIATRIC Considerations

- GH deficiency in the child is often diagnosed when a normal growth pattern at birth declines to less than the third percentile by the third month.[72]
- Congenital hypothyroidism is more common in females and less common among African American children.[73]
- A genetic marker and family history of autoimmune thyroid disease exist in children affected by hyperthyroidism due to Graves disease. Mothers with Graves disease may pass on a congenital form of hyperthyroidism known as neonatal thyrotoxicosis.[73]
- Male children with CAH may enter puberty by age 2 to 3 years.[73]
- The rate of type 2 DM (20% to 40% of children diagnosed with diabetes) has increased in the past few years in both children and adolescents and is thought to be related to obesity and decreased physical activity.
- Normal levels of blood glucose and HbA1C vary considerably with the age of the child. The American Diabetes Association publishes updates and should be used as a reference.[73]

REVIEW EXERCISES

1. A 59-year-old man was referred to a neurologist for evaluation of headaches. Subsequent MRI studies revealed a large suprasellar mass (2.5 × 2.4 cm), consistent with a pituitary tumor. His history is positive for hypertension, and on direct inquiry, he believes that his hands are slightly larger than previously, and he is experiencing increased sweating. Family history is negative, as are weight change, polyuria and polydipsia, visual disturbance, and erectile dysfunction. Subsequent laboratory findings reveal a baseline serum GH of 8.7 ng/mL (normal is 0 to 5 ng/mL), which is unsuppressed after oral glucose tolerance testing; glucose intolerance; and increased insulin-like growth factor-1 (IGF-1) on two occasions (1044 and 1145 μg/L [upper limit of normal is 480 μg/L]). Other indices of pituitary function are within the normal range.
   A. *What diagnosis would this man's clinical features, MRI, and laboratory findings suggest?*
   B. *What is the reason for asking the person about weight change, polyuria and polydipsia, visual disturbance, and erectile dysfunction?*

C. How would you explain his impaired glucose tolerance?
D. What are the possible local effects of a large pituitary tumor?

2. A 76-year-old woman presents with weight gain, subjective memory loss, dry skin, and cold intolerance. On examination, she is found to have a multinodular goiter. Laboratory findings reveal a low serum T_4 and elevated TSH.
   A. What diagnosis would this woman's history, physical, and laboratory tests suggest?
   B. Explain the possible relationship between the diagnosis and her weight gain, dry skin, cold intolerance, and subjective memory loss.
   C. What type of treatment would be indicated?
3. A 45-year-old woman presents with a history of progressive weakness, fatigue, weight loss, nausea, and increased skin pigmentation (especially of creases, pressure areas, and nipples). Her blood pressure is 120/78 mm Hg when supine and 105/52 mm Hg when standing. Laboratory findings reveal a serum sodium of 120 mEq/L (normal is 135 to 145 mEq/L); a potassium level of 5.9 mEq/L (normal is 3.5 to 5 mEq/L); and low plasma cortisol and high ACTH levels.
   A. What diagnosis would this woman's clinical features and laboratory findings suggest?
   B. Would her diagnosis be classified as a primary or secondary endocrine disorder?
   C. What is the significance of her darkened skin?
   D. What type of treatment would be indicated?
4. A 6-year-old boy is admitted to the emergency department with nausea, vomiting, and abdominal pain. He is very lethargic; his skin is warm, dry, and flushed; his pulse is rapid; and he has a sweet smell to his breath. His parents relate that he has been very thirsty during the past several weeks, his appetite has increased, and he has been urinating frequently. His initial plasma glucose is 420 mg/dL (23.1 mmol/L), and a urine test for ketones is strongly positive.
   A. What is the most likely cause of this boy's elevated blood glucose and ketonuria?
   B. Explain his presenting signs and symptoms in terms of the elevated blood glucose and metabolic acidosis.
   C. What are the priorities of treatment?
   D. What associated electrolyte disturbances would you expect and why?
5. A 53-year-old accountant presents for his routine yearly examination. His history indicates that he was found to have a fasting plasma glucose of 120 mg/dL (6.7 mmol/L) on two prior occasions. Currently, he is asymptomatic. He has no other medical problems and does not use any medications. He neither smokes nor drinks alcohol. His father had type 2 diabetes at age 60 years. His physical examination reveals a blood pressure of 125/80 mm Hg, a body mass index (BMI) of 32 kg/m^2, and a waist circumference of 45 inches (114 cm). Laboratory study results are as follows: complete blood count (CBC), TSH, and alanine aminotransferase (ALT) are within normal limits. The lipid panel shows that his HDL cholesterol (30 mg/dL [0.8 mmol/L]) and LDL cholesterol (136 mg/dL [3.5 mmol/L]) are within the normal range, and triglycerides are elevated (290 mg/dL [2.3 mmol/L]; normal is <165 mg/dL [1.9 mmol/L]).
   A. What is this man's probable diagnosis?
   B. Based on this man's blood glucose level and the ADA diabetes classification system, what diabetic status would you place this man in? Does he need a 75-g OGTT for further assessment of his IFG?
   C. His OGTT test result reveals a 2-hour glucose value of 175 mg/dL (9.63 mmol/L). What is the diagnosis? What type of treatment would be appropriate for this man?

References

1. Rubin R., Strayer D. S., Saffitz J. E., et al. (Eds.) (2015). *Rubin's pathology: Clinicopathologic foundations of medicine* (7th ed.). Philadelphia, PA: Wolters Kluwer.
2. Kumar V., Abbas A. K., Aster J. C. (Eds.) (2015). *Robbins and Cotran pathologic basis of disease* (9th ed.). Philadelphia, PA: Elsevier.
3. Capriotti T., Frizzell J. P. (2016). *Pathophysiology: Introductory concepts and clinical perspectives*. Philadelphia, PA: F.A. Davis.
4. Hall J. E. (2015). *Guyton and Hall textbook of medical physiology* (13th ed.). Philadelphia, PA: Elsevier.
5. Saladin K. S. (2015). *Anatomy & physiology: The unity of form and function* (7th ed.). New York, NY: McGraw Hill Education.
6. Garrahy A., Agha A. (2016). How should we interrogate the hypothalamic-pituitary-adrenal axis in patients with suspected hypopituitarism? *BMC Endocrine Disorders* 16(36), 1–8. DOI: 10.1186/s12902-016-0117-7.
7. Skugor M., Hamrahian A. H. (2012). Pituitary disorders. *Cleveland Clinic for Continuing Education*. Available at: http://www.clevelandclinicmeded.com/medicalpubs/diseasemanagement/endocrinology/pituitary-disorders/
8. Hammer G. D., McPhee S. J. (Eds.) (2014). *Pathophysiology of disease: An introduction to clinical medicine* (7th ed.). New York, NY: McGraw Hill Education.
9. Neal J. M. (2016). *How the endocrine system works* (2nd ed.). West Sussex, UK: John Wiley & Sons.
10. Braun L. R., Marino R. Disorders of growth and stature. *Pediatrics in Review* 38(7), 293–304.
11. Barstow C., Rerucha C. (2015). Evaluation of short and tall stature in children. *American Family Physician* 92(1), 43–50.
12. Dauber A., Rosenfeld R. G., Hirschhorn J. N. (2014). Genetic evaluation of short stature. *Journal of Clinical Endocrinology and Metabolism* 99(9), 3080–3092. DOI: 10.1210/jc.2014-1506.

13. Rogol A. D., Hayden G. F. (2014). Etiologies and early diagnosis of short stature and growth failure in children and adolescents. *The Journal of Pediatrics* 164(5 suppl), 1–14. http://dx.doi.org/10.1016/j.jpeds.2014.02.027
14. Cohen L. E. (2014). Idiopathic short stature: A clinical review. *Journal of the American Medical Association* 311(17), 1787–1796. DOI: 10.1001/jama.2014.3970.
15. Sirotnak A. P., Pataki C. (2015). Psychosocial short stature. *Emedicine Medscape*. Available at: https://emedicine.medscape.com/article/913843-overview#a5
16. Calabria A. (2017). Growth hormone deficiency in children (pituitary dwarfism). *Merck Manual Professional*. Available at: https://www.merckmanuals.com/professional/pediatrics/endocrine-disorders-in-children/growth-hormone-deficiency-in-children
17. Eledrisi M. S., Griffing G. T. (2018). Growth hormone deficiency in adults. *Emedicine Medscape*. Available at: https://emedicine.medscape.com/article/120767-overview
18. Binay C., Simsek E., Yıldırım A., et al. (2015) Growth hormone and the risk of atherosclerosis in growth hormone-deficient children. *Growth Hormone and IGF Research* 25(6), 294–297.
19. Sonksken P. (2013). Idiopathic growth hormone deficiency in adults, Ben Johnson, and the somatopause. *The Journal of Clinical Endocrinology and Metabolism* 98(6), 2270–2273.
20. Gentili A., Griffing G. T. (2015). Growth hormone replacement in older men. *Emedicine Medscape*. Available at: https://emedicine.medscape.com/article/126999-overview
21. Dineen R., Stewart P. M., Sherlock M. (2015). Acromegaly. *QJM: An International Journal of Medicine* 110(7), 411–420. DOI: 10.1093/qjmed/hcw004.
22. Hannon A. M., Thompson C. J., Sherlock M. (2017). Diabetes in patients with acromegaly. *Current Diabetes Reports* 17(8), 1–8. DOI: 10.1007/s11892-017-0838-7.
23. Kaplowitz P., Bloch C. (2015). Evaluation and referral of children with signs of early puberty. *Pediatrics*. Originally published online December 14, 2015. Available at: http://pediatrics.aappublications.org/content/early/2015/12/11/peds.2015-3732
24. Klein D. A., Emerick J. E., Sylvester J. E., et al. (2017). Disorders of puberty: An approach to diagnosis and management. *American Family Physician* 96(9), 590–599. Available at: https://www.aafp.org/afp/2017/1101/p590.html
25. Sarlis N. J., Griffing G. T. (2017). Thyroxine-binding globulin deficiency. *Emedicine Medscape*. Available at: https://emedicine.medscape.com/article/125764-overview
26. Procopiou M., Meyer C. A. (2017). Effects of drugs on thyroid function tests. *Renal and Urology News*. Available at: https://www.renalandurologynews.com/endocrinology-metabolism/effects-of-drugs-on-thyroid-function-tests/article/595483/
27. Nierengarten M. B., Bauer A. J. (2016). Hypothyroidism in children. *Contemporary Pediatrics* 33(5), 29–33.
28. American Thyroid Association. (2014). *Postpartum Thyroiditis*. Brochure Available at: https://www.thyroid.org/postpartum-thyroiditis/
29. Orlander P. R., Griffing G. T. (2018). Hypothyroidism. *Emedicine Medscape*. Available at: https://emedicine.medscape.com/article/122393-treatment
30. Eledrisi M. S., Griffing G. T. (2017). Myxedema coma or crisis. *Emedicine Medscape*. Available at: https://emedicine.medscape.com/article/123577-overview#a1
31. Lee S. L., Khardori R. (2017). Hyperthyroidism and thyrotoxicosis. *Emedicine Medscape*. Available at: https://emedicine.medscape.com/article/121865-overview
32. Osuna P. M., Udovcic M., Sharma M. D. (2017). Hyperthyroidism and the heart. *Methodist Debakey Cardiovascular Journal* 13(2), 60–63.
33. Felicilda-Reynaldo R. F. D., Kenneally M. (2016). Antithyroid drugs for hyperthyroidism. *Medsurg Nursing*, 25(1), 50–54.
34. Ing E., Roy H. (2016). Thyroid-associated orbitopathy. *Emedicine Medscape*. Available at: https://emedicine.medscape.com/article/1218444-overview
35. Idrose A. M. (2015). Acute and emergency care for thyrotoxicosis and thyroid storm. *Acute Medicine and Surgery* 2, 147–157.
36. Misra M., Hoffman R. P. (2018). Thyroid storm. *Emedicine Medscape*. Available at: https://emedicine.medscape.com/article/925147-overview
37. Schraga E. D., Khardori R. (2017). Hyperthyroidism, thyroid storm, and Graves disease. *Emedicine Medscape*. Available at: https://emedicine.medscape.com/article/767130-overview
38. Turcu A., Smith J. M., Auchus R., et al. (2014). Adrenal androgens and androgen precursors: Definition, synthesis, regulation, and physiologic actions. *Comprehensive Physiology* 4(4), 1369–1381.
39. National Institute of Diabetes and Digestive and Kidney Diseases. (2014). *Adrenal Insufficiency and Addison's Disease*. Available at: https://www.niddk.nih.gov/health-information/endocrine-diseases/adrenal-insufficiency-addisons-disease
40. Papierska L. (2017). The adrenopause: Does it really exist? *Menopause Review* 16I(2), 57–60.
41. Judd L. L., Schettler P. J., Brown E. S., et al. (2014). Adverse consequences of glucocorticoid medication: Psychological, cognitive, and behavioral effects. *American Journal of Psychiatry* 171(10), 1045–1051. DOI: 10.1176/appi.ajp.2014.13091264.
42. Younes A. J., Younes N. K. (2017). Recovery of steroid induced adrenal insufficiency. *Translational Pediatrics* 6(4), 269–273. DOI: 10.21037/tp.2017.10.01.
43. American Association for Clinical Chemistry. (2017). *Adrenal Insufficiency and Addison Disease*. Available at: https://labtestsonline.org/conditions/adrenal-insufficiency-and-addison-disease
44. Elhomsy G., Staros E. B. (2014). Dexamethasone suppression test. *Emedicine Medscape*. Available at: https://emedicine.medscape.com/article/2114191-overview
45. Witchel S. F. (2017). Congenital adrenal hyperplasia. *Journal of Pediatric and Adolescent Gynecology* 30(2017), 520–534.
46. Charmandari E., Nicolaides N. C., Chrousos G. P. (2014). Adrenal insufficiency. *The Lancet* 383, 2152–2167.
47. Pramano L., Purnamasari D., Tarigan T. J. E., et al. (2015). Generalized hyperpigmentation caused by Addison's disease in a patient with HIV/AIDS and multiple opportunistic infections. *Journal of the ASEAN Federation of Endocrine Societies* 30(2), 169–173.
48. Griffing G. T., Khardori R. (2018). Addison disease. *Emedicine Medscape*. Available at: https://emedicine.medscape.com/article/116467-overview
49. Kirkland L., Griffing G. T. (2018) Adrenal Crisis. *Emedicine Medscape*. Available at: https://emedicine.medscape.com/article/116716-overview
50. National Institute of Diabetes and Digestive and Kidney Diseases. (2012). *Cushing's Syndrome*. Available at: https://www.niddk.nih.gov/health-information/endocrine-diseases/cushings-syndrome
51. Nguyen H. C. T., Khardori R. (2017). Endogenous Cushing syndrome. *Emedicine Medscape*. Available at: https://emedicine.medscape.com/article/2233083-overview
52. Leslie R. D., Palmer J., Schloot N. C., et al. (2016). Diabetes at the crossroads: Relevance of disease classification to pathophysiology and treatment. *Diabetologia* 59, 13–20. DOI: 10.1007/s00125-015-3789-z.
53. Hay D. L., Chen S., Lutz T. A., et al. (2015). Amylin: Pharmacology, physiology, and clinical potential. *Pharmacological Reviews* 67, 564–600. http://dx.doi.org/10.1124/pr.115.010629.
54. Centers for Disease Control and Prevention. (2017). *National Diabetes Statistics Report, 2017*. Atlanta, GA: Centers for Disease Control and Prevention, U.S. Dept of Health and Human Services.
55. American Diabetes Association. (2018). Classification and diagnosis of diabetes: Standards of medical care in diabetes – 2018. *Diabetes Care* 41(Suppl 1), S13–S27.
56. Lin J. L. J., Papantonlou L.G.C., Staros E. B. (2016). Glucose tolerance testing. *Emedicine Medscape*. Available at: https://emedicine.medscape.com/article/2049402-overview#a4
57. Breslin Diabetes Center of Harvard Medical School. (2018). *Plasma glucose meters and whole blood meters*. Available at: http://www.joslin.org/info/plasma_glucose_meters_and_whole_blood_meters.html

58. Breslin Diabetes Center of Harvard Medical School. (2018). *Blood glucose testing delivers tight control*. Available at: http://www.joslin.org/info/blood-glucose-testing-delivers-tight-control.html
59. Breslin Diabetes Center of Harvard Medical School. (2018). *The facts about continuous glucose monitoring*. Available at: http://www.joslin.org/info/the_facts_about_continuous_glucose_monitoring.html
60. Horowitz G. L., Wheeler T. M. (2015). Hemoglobin A1C testing. *Emedicine Medscape*. Available at: https://emedicine.medscape.com/article/2049478-overview#a3
61. American Association of Clinical Chemistry. (2014). Glucose tests. *Lab Tests Online*. Available at: https://labtestsonline.org/tests/glucose-tests
62. Breslin Diabetes Center of Harvard Medical School. (2018). *Ketone testing: What you need to know*. Available at: http://www.joslin.org/info/ketone_testing_what_you_need_to_know.html
63. Skyler J. S., Bakris G. L., Bonifacio E., et al. (2017). Differentiation of diabetes by pathophysiology, natural history, and prognosis. *Diabetes* 66, 241–255.
64. Bokhari A. S., Alshaya M. M., Badghaish M. M. O., et al. (2018). Metabolic syndrome: Pathophysiology and treatment. *The Egyptian Journal of Hospital Medicine* 70(8), 1388–1392. DOI: 10.12816/0044654.
65. Handelsma Y., Bloomgarden Z. T., Grunberger G., et al. (2015). American Association of Clinical Endocrinologists and American College of Endocrinology – Clinical Practice Guidelines for Developing a Diabetes Mellitus Comprehensive Care Plan – 2015 – Executive Summary. *Endocrine Practice* 21(4), 413–437.
66. Cooperman M., Griffing G. (2016). Somogyi phenomenon. *Emedicine Medscape*. Available at: https://emedicine.medscape.com/article/125432-overview
67. American Diabetes Association. (2017). Dawn phenomenon. Available at: http://www.diabetes.org/living-with-diabetes/treatment-and-care/blood-glucose-control/dawn-phenomenon.html
68. American Diabetes Association. (2018). Glycemic targets: Standards of medical care in diabetes – 2018. *Diabetes Care* 48(Suppl 1), S55–S64.
69. Yang S. L., Zhu L., Han R., et al. (2017). Pathophysiology of peripheral arterial disease in diabetes mellitus. *Journal of Diabetes* 9, 133–140. DOI: 10.1111/1753-0407.12474.
70. Hinkle J. L., Cheever K. H. (2018). *Brunner & Suddarth's textbook of medical-surgical nursing* (14th ed.). Philadelphia, PA: Wolters Kluwer.
71. Epiopoulos C. (2018). *Gerontological nursing* (9th ed.). Philadelphia, PA: Wolters Kluwer.
72. Skyler J. S., Bakris G. L., Bonifacio E., et al. (2017). Differentiation of diabetes by pathophysiology, natural history, and prognosis. *Diabetes* 66, 241–255.
73. Kyle T., Carman S. (2017). *Essentials of pediatric nursing* (3rd ed.). Philadelphia, PA: Wolters Kluwer.

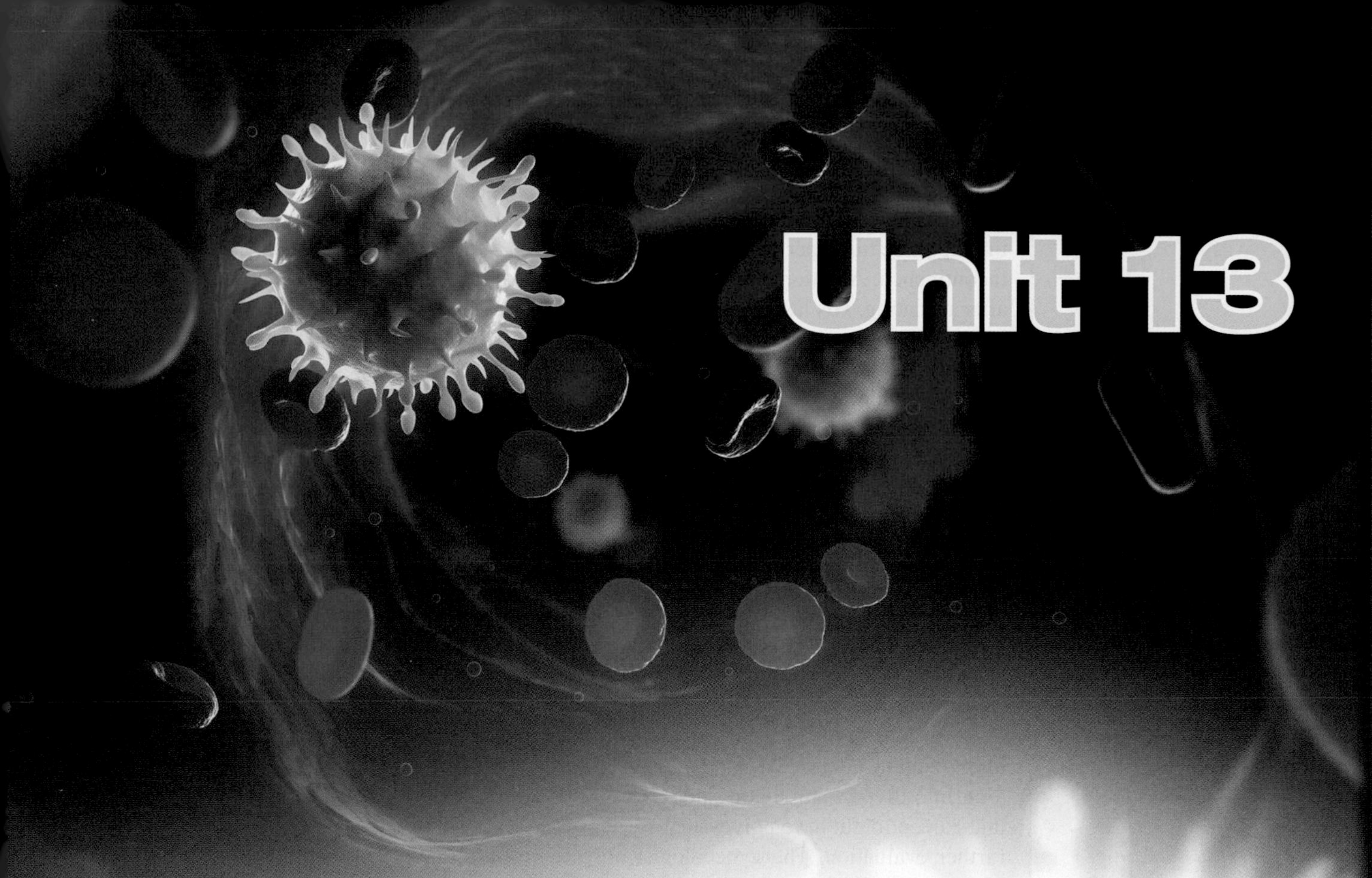

Unit 13

Disorders of Genitourinary and Reproductive Function

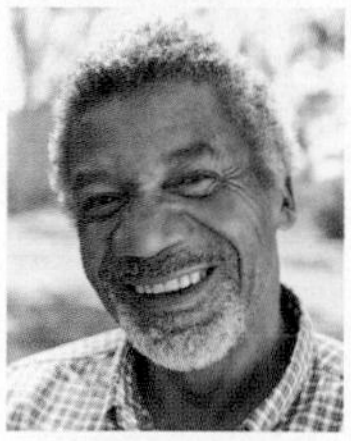

Mr. E. Topers, a 57-year-old African American, has had benign prostate hyperplasia for about 5 years.

His grandfather and one uncle both had prostate cancer. He has a 20-year, pack-a-day cigarette history, which he stopped 15 years ago. He has controlled hypertension, type II diabetes mellitus, and hyperlipidemia. In the past year, his body mass index (BMI, in kg/m^2) decreased to 26 (slightly overweight) from 28 (overweight). He has been taking an α1-adrenergic antagonist to relax the smooth muscle in his prostate and thus improve urine flow. Last year, his score on the American Urologic Association (AUA) Symptom Score Index was 1 or 2, indicating very mild symptoms.

(continued on next page)

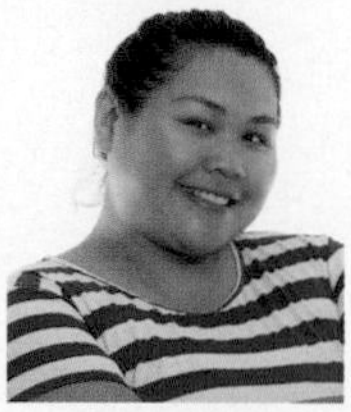

Eileen, aged 19, presents to the local community health center desiring oral contraception. She states that she is sexually active and feels she needs protection. Her periods have been irregular since menarche at age 11, and she cannot remember the last time she had her period. Eileen has not been to a physician since she was about 13 years old. She does not know of any family members who have irregular periods, but her older sister has been trying to get pregnant for the last 4 years. She has a family history of type II diabetes mellitus, obesity, and hypertension. Her physical examination shows abdominal obesity, facial hirsutism, and acne. Given her large body habitus, the ovaries are difficult to palpate. A urine pregnancy test is negative. Her body mass index (BMI) is 29 kg/m^2, which is classified as overweight.

(continued on next page)

Mr. E. Topers *(continued)*

Today, his AUA score is 11, indicating that his symptoms are affecting his quality of life. He is getting up three times per night to void, urinates often during the day, and is experiencing some urge incontinence. Additionally, he frequently feels like he needs to urinate and has some dribbling after urinating. His last prostate-specific antigen (PSA) level was 7 ng/mL (less than 4.0 ng/mL is considered normal), and his other blood work was within normal limits. Today, his PSA is greater than 12 ng/mL, and his blood urea nitrogen (BUN) and creatinine concentrations are elevated significantly. His uroflow examination shows obstruction with a flow of less than 7 mL/second (average normal flow is 12 mL/second). His digital rectal exam (DRE) reveals that his prostate has significantly enlarged (from a previous score of 3+ to a score of 4+) and firmed (from a previous score of 1+ to a score of 2+). He is scheduled for a transrectal ultrasound and biopsy of his prostate. The findings are positive for prostate cancer. However, his Gleason Staging Score is 3, which indicates a slow-growing cancer.

Eileen *(continued)*

A fasting blood test reveals abnormally high concentrations of glucose, insulin, lipids, luteinizing hormone (LH), and total testosterone; a slightly elevated prolactin concentration; and a normal thyroid-stimulating hormone (TSH) concentration. The health care provider suspects that Eileen might have polycystic ovarian syndrome (PCOS) and refers her to a gynecologist for further evaluation. The gynecologist observes multiple bilateral ovarian cysts on transvaginal ultrasound and is able to rule out related disorders, leading to a conclusive diagnosis of PCOS. Eileen is prescribed metformin (an insulin-sensitizing drug) and combined oral contraceptives, referred to a dietician for a low-fat and low-calorie diet, and assigned to work with a personal trainer.

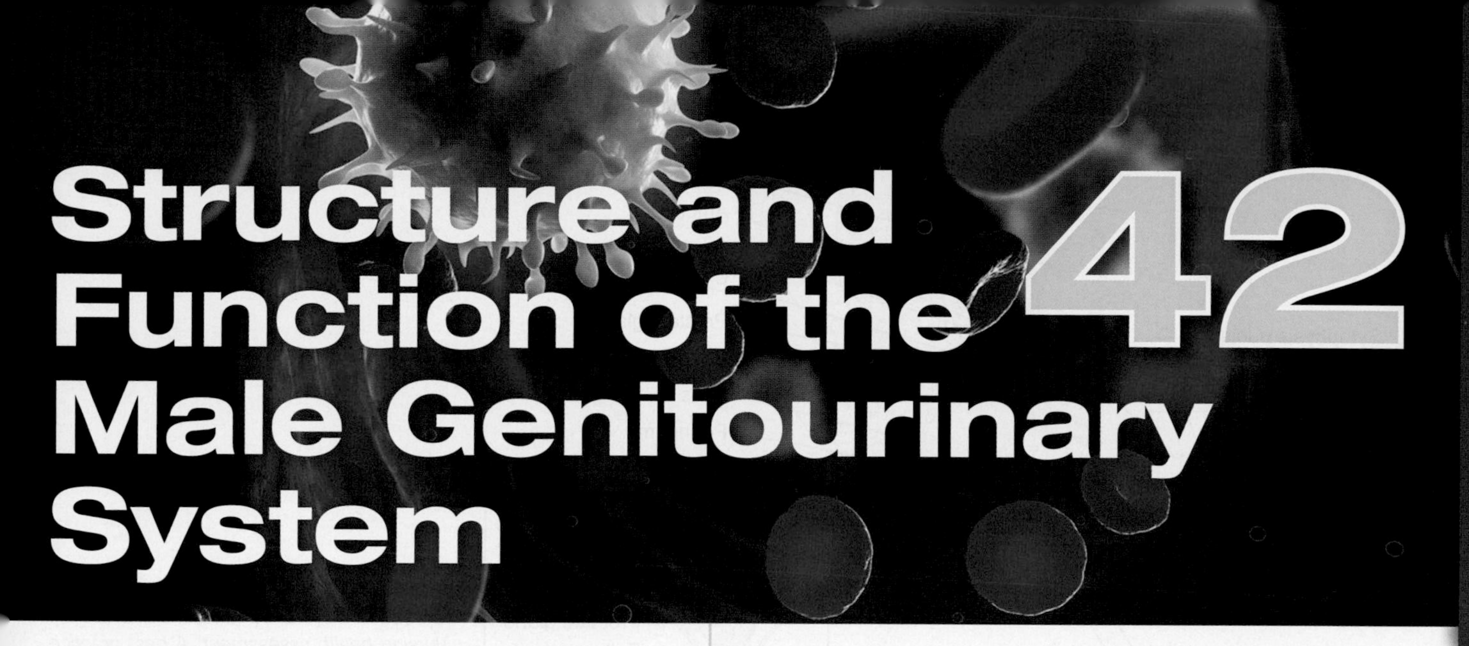

Structure and Function of the Male Genitourinary System 42

Sawsan Abuhammad

The male genitourinary system consists of the paired gonads (the testes), the genital ducts, accessory organs, and penis (Fig. 42.1). The main function of the testes is to produce male sex hormones and male germ cells. The internal accessory organs produce the fluid constituents of semen, and the ductile system facilitates the storage and transport of spermatozoa. The functions of the penis include urine elimination and sexual function. This chapter focuses on the structure of the male reproductive system, spermatogenesis and control of male reproductive function, neural control of sexual function, and changes in function that occur at puberty and as a result of the aging process.

STRUCTURE OF THE MALE REPRODUCTIVE SYSTEM

After completing this section of the chapter, the learner will be able to meet the following objectives:

- Characterize the embryonic development of the male reproductive organs and genitalia.
- Describe the structure and function of the testes and scrotum, the genital ducts, accessory organs, and penis.

Embryonic Development

Sex chromosomes determine the sex of a person at the time of fertilization. The tissues that produce the female and male reproductive systems are undifferentiated at the embryonic stage. A small region in the arm of the Y chromosome determines the sex of the embryo.[1] It is impossible to determine whether an embryo is male or female unless the chromosomes are studied in a karyotype or until approximately the 7th week of gestation. Until this time, the male and female genital tracts both consist of two wolffian ducts, from which the male genitalia develop, and two müllerian ducts, from which the female genital structures develop. During these early weeks of gestation, the gonads (*i.e.*, ovaries and testes) are also undifferentiated.[1]

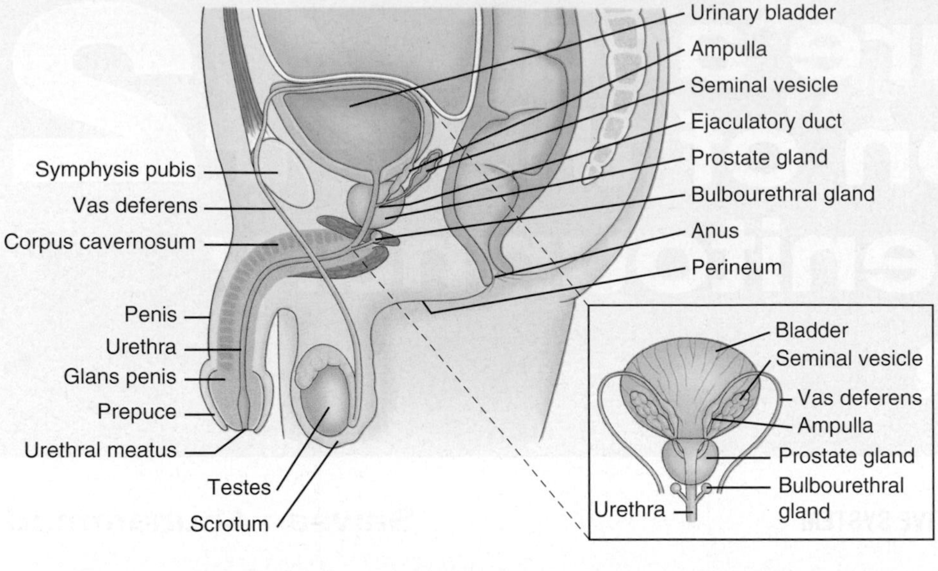

Figure 42.1 • The structures of the male reproductive system. (From Jensen S. (2015). *Nursing health assessment: A best practice approach* (2nd ed., p. 703). Philadelphia, PA: Lippincott Williams & Wilkins.)

Between the 6th and 8th weeks of gestation, the testes begin their development under the influence of the Y chromosome. The action of the *SRY* gene differentiates the undifferentiated gonads into testes. Conversely, if the *SRY* gene is absent, the gonads develop into ovaries.

During gestation, the testicular cells of the male embryo produce two major hormones: anti-müllerian hormone (AMH) and testosterone.[1] AMH suppresses the müllerian ducts and prevents development of the uterus and fallopian tubes in the male. In parallel, testosterone stimulates the wolffian ducts to develop into the epididymis, vas deferens, and seminal vesicles.[1] Testosterone is also the precursor of a third hormone, dihydrotestosterone (DHT), which is responsible for forming the male urethra, prostate, and external genitalia. The enzyme 5α-reductase converts testosterone to DHT, predominantly in the peripheral tissues.[1] Although both testosterone and DHT share the same nuclear androgen receptor, they have marked differences in tissue activity. For example, DHT exerts most of its effects on the external genitalia, including the prostate, and is subsequently important for the development of facial and body hair. If testosterone and DHT are absent in gestation, the development of the müllerian ducts will not be inhibited, and therefore a male embryo with XY chromosomes will develop female external genitalia.[1,2]

Testes and Scrotum

The testes (the male gonads) are located outside the abdominal cavity in the scrotum.[3] The adult male testes are approximately 15 to 25 mL in volume (greater than 4 mL indicates pubertal onset). Approximately 80% of this volume is allotted to cells involved in spermatogenesis, and 20% of this volume is for testosterone production. Embryologically, the testes develop in the abdominal cavity and then descend through the inguinal canal into a pouch of peritoneum (which becomes the tunica vaginalis) in the scrotum.[4] Testicular descent occurs in two stages. The first stage occurs between 7 and 12 weeks of fetal life, with AMH being responsible for descent to the inguinal region. The second stage occurs the 26th week of gestation, with testosterone being responsible for descent into the scrotum.[1] As they descend, the testes pull their arteries, veins, lymphatics, nerves, and conducting excretory ducts with them. These structures are encased by the cremaster muscle and layers of fascia that constitute the spermatic cord.[4] After descent of the testes, the inguinal canal closes almost completely. Failure of this canal to close increases the risk of development of an inguinal hernia later in life. An inguinal hernia or "rupture" is a protrusion of the parietal peritoneum and part of the intestine through an abnormal opening from the abdominal cavity. A loop of small bowel may become incarcerated in an inguinal hernia (strangulated hernia), in which case its lumen may become obstructed and its vascular supply compromised.

The testes consist of a double-layered membrane, the tunica vaginalis, which is derived from the abdominal peritoneum.[4] An outer covering, the tunica albuginea, is a tough, white, fibrous sheath that resembles the sclera of the eye. The tunica albuginea protects the testes and gives them their ovoid shape. The cremaster muscles, which are bands of skeletal muscle arising from the internal oblique muscles of the trunk, elevate the testes. The testes receive their arterial blood supply from the long testicular arteries, which branch from the abdominal artery. The testicular veins, which drain the testes, arise from a venous network called the *pampiniform plexus* that surrounds the testicular artery. Fibers from the autonomic nervous system innervate the testes.[4] Associated sensory nerves transmit pain impulses, resulting in excruciating pain especially when the testes are hit forcibly.

The scrotum houses the testes and is composed of a thin outer layer of skin that forms rugae, or folds, and is continuous with the perineum and outer skin of the groin. Under the outer skin lies a thin layer of fascia and smooth muscle, the dartos muscle. This layer contains a septum that separates the two testes. The dartos muscle responds to changes in temperature[3]: When it is cold, the muscle contracts, bringing the testes closer to the body and the scrotum becomes shorter and heavily wrinkled. When it is warmer, the muscle relaxes, allowing the scrotum to fall away from the body.

The location of the testes in the scrotum is important for sperm production, which is optimal at 2°C to 3°C below body temperature. Two systems maintain the temperature of the testes at a level consistent with sperm production. One system is the pampiniform plexus of testicular veins that surrounds the testicular artery. This plexus absorbs heat from the arterial blood, cooling it as it enters the testes. The second system is the cremaster muscles, which respond to decreases in testicular temperature by moving the testes closer to the body.[4] Prolonged exposure to elevated temperatures, as a result of prolonged fever or dysfunction of thermoregulatory mechanisms, may impair the process of spermatogenesis. Tight-fitting undergarments that hold the testes against the body are thought to contribute to a decrease in sperm counts and increase infertility by interfering with the thermoregulatory function of the scrotum. Cryptorchidism, the failure of the testes to descend into the scrotum, also exposes the testes to the higher temperature of the body.

KEY POINTS

MALE REPRODUCTIVE SYSTEM

- The ductile system (epididymides, vas deferens, and ejaculatory ducts) transports and stores sperm and assists in their maturation, and the accessory glands (seminal vesicles, prostate gland, and bulbourethral glands) prepare the sperm for ejaculation.
- Sperm production requires temperatures that are 2°C to 3°C below body temperature. The position of the testes in the scrotum and the unique blood flow cooling mechanisms provide this environment.

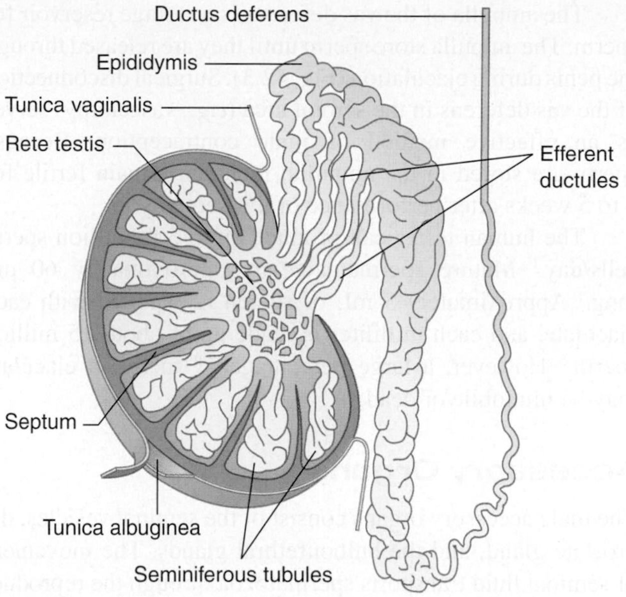

Figure 42.2 • The parts of the testes and epididymis.

Genital Duct System

Internally, the testes consist of several hundred compartments or lobules (Fig. 42.2). Each lobule contains one or more coiled seminiferous tubules. These tubules are the site of sperm production. As the tubules lead into the efferent ducts, the seminiferous tubules become the rete testis, which are multiple interconnecting channels in the mediastinum.[1] From the rete testis, 10,000 to 20,000 efferent ducts emerge to join the epididymis, which is the final site for sperm maturation. Because the spermatozoa are not motile at this stage of development, peristaltic movements of the ductal walls of the epididymis aid in their movement. The spermatozoa continue their migration through the ductus deferens, also called the *vas deferens*.[1]

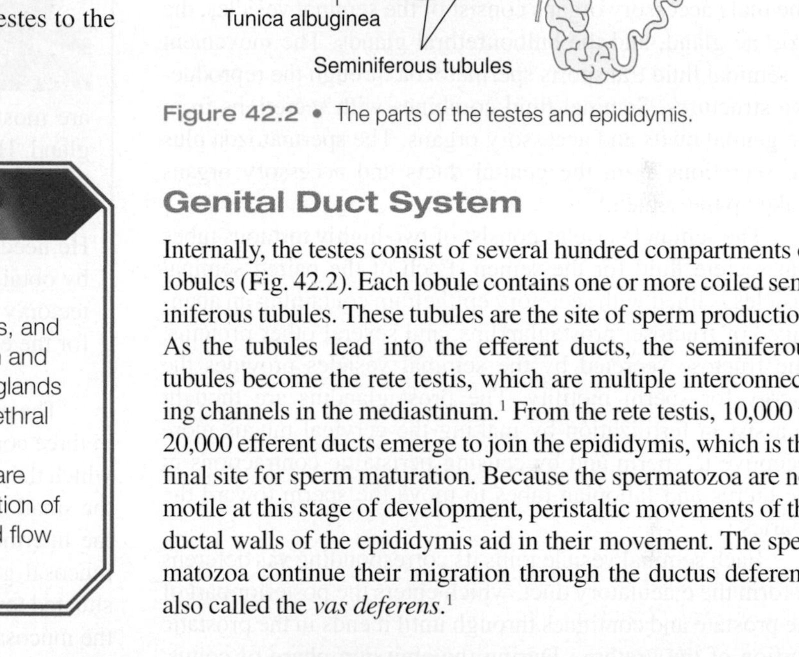

Figure 42.3 • The excretory ducts of the male reproductive system and the path that sperm follows as it leaves the testis and travels to the urethra.

The ampulla of the vas deferens is a storage reservoir for sperm. The ampulla store sperm until they are released through the penis during ejaculation (Fig. 42.3). Surgical disconnection of the vas deferens in the scrotal area (*e.g.*, vasectomy) serves as an effective method of male contraception. Because sperm are stored in the ampulla, men can remain fertile for 4 to 5 weeks after performance of a vasectomy.

The human testes can produce up to 300 million sperm cells/day.[1] Mature spermatozoa are approximately 60 μm long.[1] Approximately 3 mL of semen is expelled with each ejaculate, and each milliliter is made up of about 15 million sperm.[5] However, a large percentage of sperm in ejaculate may be immobile or dead.[1]

Accessory Organs

The male accessory organs consist of the seminal vesicles, the prostate gland, and the bulbourethral glands. The movement of seminal fluid transports spermatozoa through the reproductive structures. Seminal fluid combines with secretions from the genital ducts and accessory organs. The spermatozoa plus the secretions from the genital ducts and accessory organs make up the semen.[1]

The seminal vesicles consist of two highly tortuous tubes that secrete fluid for the semen. Each of the paired seminal vesicles is lined with secretory epithelium containing an abundance of fructose, prostaglandins, and several other proteins. The fructose secreted by the seminal vesicles provides the energy for sperm motility. The prostaglandins are thought to assist in fertilization by making the cervical mucus more receptive to sperm and by causing peristaltic contractions in the uterus and fallopian tubes to move the sperm toward the ovaries.[1]

Each seminal vesicle joins its corresponding vas deferens to form the ejaculatory duct, which enters the posterior part of the prostate and continues through until it ends in the prostatic portion of the urethra.[1] During the emission phase of coitus, each vesicle empties fluid into the ejaculatory duct, adding bulk to the semen. Approximately 70% of the ejaculate originates in the seminal vesicles.

The prostate is a fibromuscular and glandular organ lying just inferior to the bladder. The prostate gland secretes a thin, milky, alkaline fluid containing citric acid, calcium, acid phosphate, a clotting enzyme, and a profibrinolysin. During ejaculation, the capsule of the prostate contracts and the added fluid increases the bulk of the semen.[1] Both vaginal secretions and the fluid from the vas deferens are strongly acidic. Because sperm mobilization occurs at a pH of 6.0 to 6.5, the alkaline nature of the prostatic secretions is essential for successful fertilization of the ovum.[4] The bulbourethral or Cowper glands lie on either side of the membranous urethra and secrete alkaline mucus, which further aids in neutralizing acids from the urine that remain in the urethra.[4]

The prostate gland also eliminates urine through a specialized section of the urethra defined as the *prostatic urethra*. This region of the prostate gland consists of a thin, fibrous capsule that encloses the circularly oriented smooth muscle fibers and collagenous tissue that surround the urethra where it joins the bladder. The prostatic urethra traverses the prostate gland, where it is lined by a thin, longitudinal layer of smooth muscle that is continuous with the bladder wall. The smooth muscle that surrounds the prostate gland is derived primarily from the longitudinal bladder musculature. This smooth muscle represents the true involuntary sphincter of the male posterior urethra. Because the prostate surrounds the urethra, enlargement of the gland can produce urinary obstruction.[1]

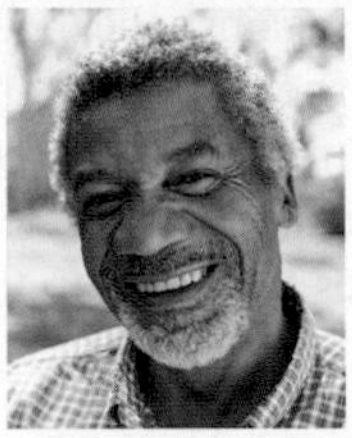

Mr. Topers, who was introduced to you at the beginning of Unit 13, has benign prostate hyperplasia (BPH) and prostate cancer. He is experiencing symptoms of obstruction, including dribbling after urinating and the continuous sensation of having to urinate. These symptoms are most likely due to further enlargement of his prostate gland. His uroflow examination showed obstruction with a flow of less than 7 mL/second so the prostate is pressing on his urethra and narrowing it, causing his urine to back up. He needs to be assessed for a lower urinary tract infection by obtaining a urine culture. He has selected a total prostatectomy because of his family history. Surgery is scheduled for the end of the week.

The prostate gland is made up of secretory glands arranged in three concentric areas surrounding the prostatic urethra, into which they open. The component glands of the prostate include the small mucosal glands associated with the urethral mucosa, the intermediate submucosal glands that lie peripheral to the mucosal glands, and the large main prostatic glands that are situated toward the outside of the gland.[1] It is the overgrowth of the mucosal glands that causes BPH in older men.

Penis

The penis is the external genital organ through which the urethra passes. Anatomically, the external penis consists of a shaft that ends in a tip called the *glans* (Fig. 42.4). The loose skin of the penis shaft folds to cover the glans, forming the prepuce, or foreskin. The glans of the penis contains many sensory nerves, making this the most sensitive portion of the penile shaft. It is the foreskin that is removed during circumcision.

The shaft of the penis (the cylindrical body) consists of three masses of erectile tissue. These three masses are held together by fibrous strands and covered with a thin layer of skin. The first two lateral masses of tissue are called the *corpora cavernosa*. The third ventral mass is called the *corpus spongiosum* where the spongy part of the urethra is found.[1] The corpora cavernosa and corpus spongiosum are cavernous sinuses that are relatively empty but become engorged with blood during penile erection.

IN SUMMARY

The male reproductive system consists of a pair of gonads (*i.e.*, testes), a system of excretory ducts (*i.e.*, seminiferous tubules and efferent ducts), the accessory organs (*i.e.*, epididymis, seminal vesicles, prostate, and Cowper glands), and the penis. During the 7th week of gestation, the XY chromosome pattern and the *SRY* gene in the male embryo are responsible for the development of the testes; the subsequent production of AMH and testosterone results in the development of the internal and external male genital structures. Before this period of embryonic development, the tissues from which the male and female reproductive structures develop are undifferentiated. In the absence of testosterone production and its derivative, DHT, a male embryo with an XY chromosomal pattern will develop female external genitalia.

SPERMATOGENESIS AND HORMONAL CONTROL OF MALE REPRODUCTIVE FUNCTION

After completing this section of the chapter, the learner will be able to meet the following objectives:

- Describe the process of spermatogenesis.
- State the functions of testosterone.
- Draw a diagram illustrating the secretion, site of action, and feedback control of gonadotropin-releasing hormone, luteinizing hormone, follicle-stimulating hormone, and inhibin.

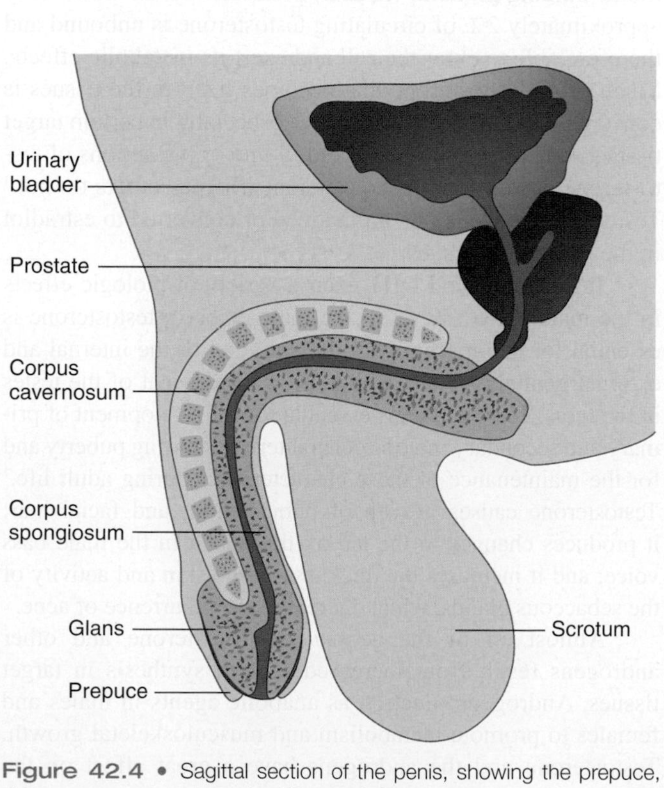

Figure 42.4 • Sagittal section of the penis, showing the prepuce, glans, corpus cavernosum, and corpus spongiosum.

During childhood, the gonads remain essentially quiescent. At puberty, the male gonads and testes begin to mature and to carry out spermatogenesis and hormone production. At approximately 10 or 11 years of age, the anterior pituitary, under the control of the hypothalamus, begins to secrete gonadotropins. The gonadotropins stimulate testicular function and cause the interstitial Leydig cells to begin producing testosterone. At the same time, hormonal stimulation induces mitotic activity of the germ cells that develop into sperm. After cell maturation has begun, the testes begin to enlarge rapidly as the individual tubules grow. Males attain full maturity and spermatogenesis by 15 or 16 years of age.

Spermatogenesis

Spermatogenesis refers to the generation of spermatozoa or sperm. It begins at an average age of 13 years and continues throughout the reproductive years of a man's life. Spermatogenesis occurs in the seminiferous tubules of the testes (see Fig. 42.2). These tubules, if placed end to end, would measure approximately 750 ft. The outer layer of the seminiferous tubules is made up of connective tissue and smooth muscle. The inner lining is composed of Sertoli cells, which are embedded with sperm in various stages of development (Fig. 42.5A). Sertoli cells secrete a special fluid that contains nutrients to bathe and nourish the immature germ cells. They provide digestive enzymes that play a role in spermiation (*i.e.*, converting the spermatocytes to sperm) and they are thought to play a role in shaping the head and tail of the sperm.[1] Sertoli cells also secrete several hormones, including AMH, which is secreted by the testes during fetal life to inhibit development of fallopian tubes; estradiol, the principal feminizing sex hormone, which seems to be required in the male for spermatogenesis; and inhibin, which controls the function of Sertoli cells through feedback inhibition of follicle-stimulating hormone (FSH) from the anterior pituitary gland.[1,4] For spermatogenesis to occur, FSH binds to specific receptors in Sertoli cells. This process also requires a high concentration of intratesticular testosterone.[1]

In the first stage of spermatogenesis, small and unspecialized diploid germinal cells (*spermatogonia*) are located immediately adjacent to the tubular wall. Spermatogonia undergo rapid mitotic division and provide a continuous source of new germinal cells. As these cells multiply, the more mature spermatogonia divide into two daughter cells, which grow and become the primary spermatocytes—the precursors of sperm.[1] Over several weeks, large primary spermatocytes divide by a process called *meiosis* to form two smaller secondary spermatocytes. Meiosis is a unique form of cell division that occurs only in the gonads. It consists of two consecutive nuclear divisions with formation of four daughter cells, each containing a single set of 23 chromosomes rather than a pair of 46 chromosomes, as occurs during mitotic cell division in other somatic cells. In the case of sperm, the secondary spermatocytes divide to form two spermatids, each containing 23 chromosomes.

The spermatid elongates into a spermatozoon (the mature sperm cell) with a head and tail (see Fig. 42.5B). The outside

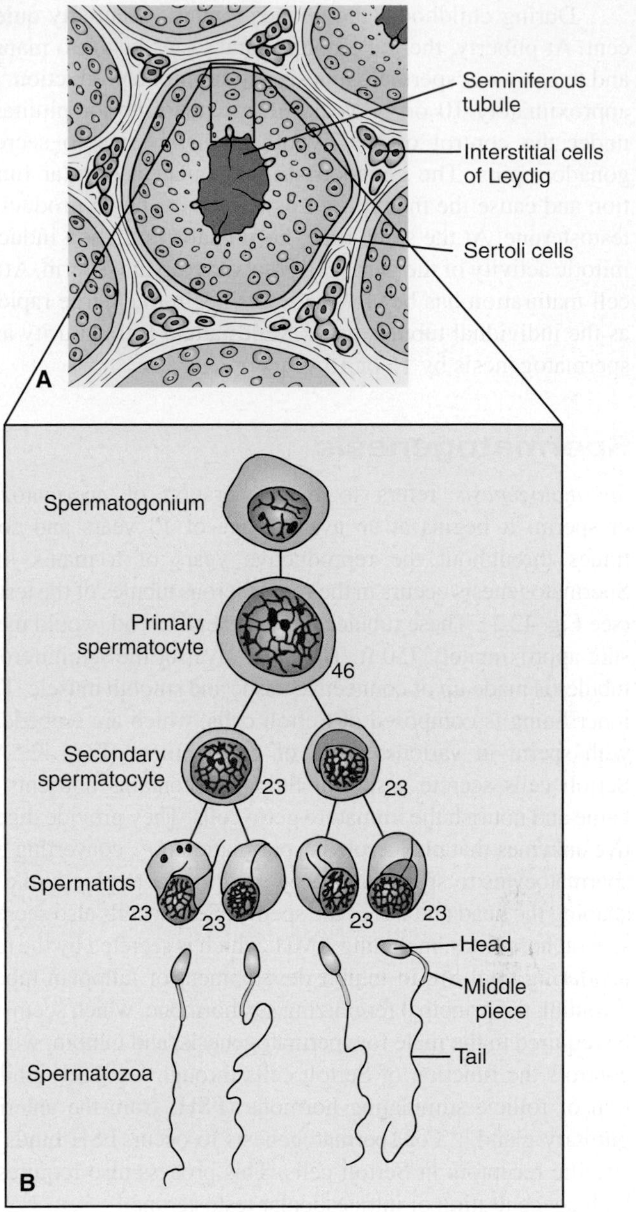

Figure 42.5 • The various stages of spermatogenesis. **(A)** Cross-section of seminiferous tubule. **(B)** Stages of development of spermatozoa.

of the anterior two thirds of the head, called the *acrosome*, contains enzymes necessary for penetration and fertilization of the ovum.[1] The to-and-fro flagellar motion of the tail imparts movement to the sperm. The mitochondria in the midpiece, which connects the sperm tail to the head, supply energy for the movement of sperm. A normal sperm moves in a straight line at a velocity of 1 to 4 mm/minute, which allows it to move through the female genital tract. As the sperm grows to full size, it moves to the epididymis to mature further and gain motility. The epididymis does have the capacity to store a small quantity of sperm, but the ampulla of the vas deferens stores most of the sperm. With excessive sexual activity, storage may not exceed longer than a few days. Sperm can live for many weeks in the male genital tract but can survive in the female genital tract for only 1 to 2 days.[1] Frozen sperm have been preserved for years.

The entire process of spermatogenesis and sperm maturation takes approximately 90 days. Infertility may occur when insufficient numbers of motile, healthy sperm are present. A "fertile sample" on seminal fluid analysis is associated with a count greater than 15 million/mL, greater than 40% motility, normal morphology, and a volume of 1.5 or more.[5] The field of reproductive endocrinology is greatly expanding: Technological advances will eventually make it possible for the majority of people interested in conceiving to be successful.

Hormonal Control of Male Reproductive Function

Testosterone and Other Male Sex Hormones

The testes secrete several male sex hormones (androgens), including *testosterone*, *dihydrotestosterone*, and *androstenedione*. The adrenal cortex also produces androgens, although in much smaller quantities (less than 5% of the total male androgens) than those produced in the testes. Testosterone, which is the most abundant of these hormones, is considered the main testicular hormone.[4] The testes also secrete small quantities of estradiol and estrone.[1,4]

The interstitial Leydig cells in the testes produce and secrete testosterone under the influence of luteinizing hormone (LH). Leydig cells produce approximately 6 mg/day of testosterone.[1] Testosterone is metabolized in the liver and excreted by the kidneys. In the bloodstream, testosterone exists in a free (unbound) or a bound form. The bound form is attached to plasma proteins, including albumin and the sex hormone–binding globulin (SHBG) produced by the liver. Only approximately 2% of circulating testosterone is unbound and therefore able to enter the cell and exert its metabolic effects. Much of the testosterone that becomes fixed to the tissues is converted to DHT by 5α-reductase, especially in certain target tissues such as the prostate gland. Some of the actions of testosterone depend on this conversion, whereas others do not.[1] Testosterone can also be aromatized or converted to estradiol in the peripheral tissues.

Testosterone and DHT exert a variety of biologic effects in the male (Chart 42.1). In the male embryo, testosterone is essential for the appropriate differentiation of the internal and external genitalia, and it is necessary for descent of the testes in the fetus. Testosterone is essential to the development of primary and secondary male sex characteristics during puberty and for the maintenance of these characteristics during adult life.[1] Testosterone causes growth of pubic, chest, and facial hair; it produces changes in the larynx that result in the male bass voice; and it increases the thickness of the skin and activity of the sebaceous glands, which increases the occurrence of acne.

Almost all of the actions of testosterone and other androgens result from increased protein synthesis in target tissues. Androgens function as anabolic agents in males and females to promote metabolism and musculoskeletal growth. Testosterone and the androgens have a great effect on the development of increasing musculature during puberty, with

CHART 42.1 MAIN ACTIONS OF TESTOSTERONE

Induces differentiation of the male genital tract during fetal development
Induces development of primary and secondary sex characteristics
- Gonadal function
- External genitalia and accessory organs
- Male voice timbre
- Male skin characteristics
- Male hair distribution

Anabolic effects
- Promotes protein metabolism
- Promotes musculoskeletal growth
- Influences subcutaneous fat distribution

Promotes spermatogenesis (in FSH-primed tubules) and maturation of sperm
Stimulates erythropoiesis

boys averaging approximately a 50% increase in muscle mass compared with girls. Chart 42.2 describes the abuse of androgens by athletes to enhance athletic performance.

Action of the Hypothalamic and Anterior Pituitary Hormones

The hypothalamus and the anterior pituitary gland play an essential role in promoting spermatogenic activity in the testes and maintaining the endocrine function of the testes by the gonadotropic hormones. Gonadotropin-releasing hormone (GnRH), which is synthesized by the hypothalamus and secreted into the hypophysial portal blood stream, regulates the synthesis and release of gonadotropic hormones from the anterior pituitary (Fig. 42.6).[1]

The anterior pituitary gland secretes two gonadotropic hormones: LH and FSH. LH regulates the production of testosterone by the interstitial Leydig cells (see Fig. 42.6). FSH binds selectively to Sertoli cells surrounding the seminiferous tubules, where it functions in the initiation of spermatogenesis. Under the influence of FSH, Sertoli cells produce androgen-binding protein, plasminogen activator, and inhibin. Androgen-binding protein binds testosterone and serves as a carrier of testosterone in Sertoli cells and as a storage site for testosterone.[1] Although FSH is necessary for the initiation of spermatogenesis, full maturation of the spermatozoa requires testosterone (the intratesticular concentration of testosterone is 100-fold greater than serum levels). Androgen-binding protein also serves as a carrier of testosterone from the testes to the epididymis. Plasminogen activator, which converts plasminogen to plasmin, functions in the final detachment of mature spermatozoa from Sertoli cells.

The negative feedback actions of testosterone regulate circulating levels of the gonadotropic hormones: high levels of testosterone suppress LH secretion through a direct action on the pituitary and an inhibitory effect on the hypothalamus. A substance called *inhibin* that is produced by Sertoli cells inhibits FSH. Inhibin suppresses FSH release from the pituitary gland. The pituitary gonadotropic hormones and Sertoli cells in the testes form a classic negative feedback loop in which FSH stimulates inhibin and inhibin suppresses FSH.[1,4] Unlike the cyclic hormonal pattern in females, in males, FSH, LH, and testosterone secretion and spermatogenesis occur at relatively unchanging rates during adulthood.[1]

CHART 42.2 ABUSE OF ANDROGENS TO ENHANCE ATHLETIC PERFORMANCE

- Athletes use synthetic androgens to improve their skill and endurance by bulking up their muscles.
- Athletes have taken virtually all androgens produced for human and veterinary purposes.
- Occasionally, athletes take several medications simultaneously in an attempt to increase the overall effect on performance, which can cause potentially more deleterious side effects.
- Hormones are frequently taken in doses that far exceed physiologic levels.
- There are potential harmful effects to taking these supplements including acne, decreased testicular size, and azoospermia.
- The detrimental effects may persist for months after use of the agents has ceased, depending on the type and dose administered.
- Because testosterone can be aromatized to estradiol in the peripheral tissues, androgens can also produce gynecomastia (breast enlargement).

Hypogonadism

Hypogonadism results from the reduced function of the gonads. Primary hypogonadism is due to a problem in the testes, secondary hypogonadism is due to the lack of secretion of LH and FSH from the anterior pituitary, and tertiary hypogonadism is due to the lack of stimulation of LH and FSH secretion from the anterior pituitary due to decreased/absent GnRH secretion from the hypothalamus.[1] Scientists describe primary hypogonadism in men as low androgens and sperm count due to lack of negative feedback at the hypothalamic–pituitary level, coupled with high levels of gonadotropins (*i.e.*, low testosterone and high LH and FSH).[6] Secondary and tertiary hypogonadisms are described by low androgens and sperm count resulting from the lack of secretion of gonadotropins at the hypothalamic–pituitary level coupled with low levels of gonadotropins (*i.e.*, low testosterone and low LH and FSH).

Clinical Manifestations. The clinical features of male hypogonadism depend on whether the impairment is primary hypogonadism or secondary hypogonadism. Primary hypogonadism occurs because the testes are not functioning

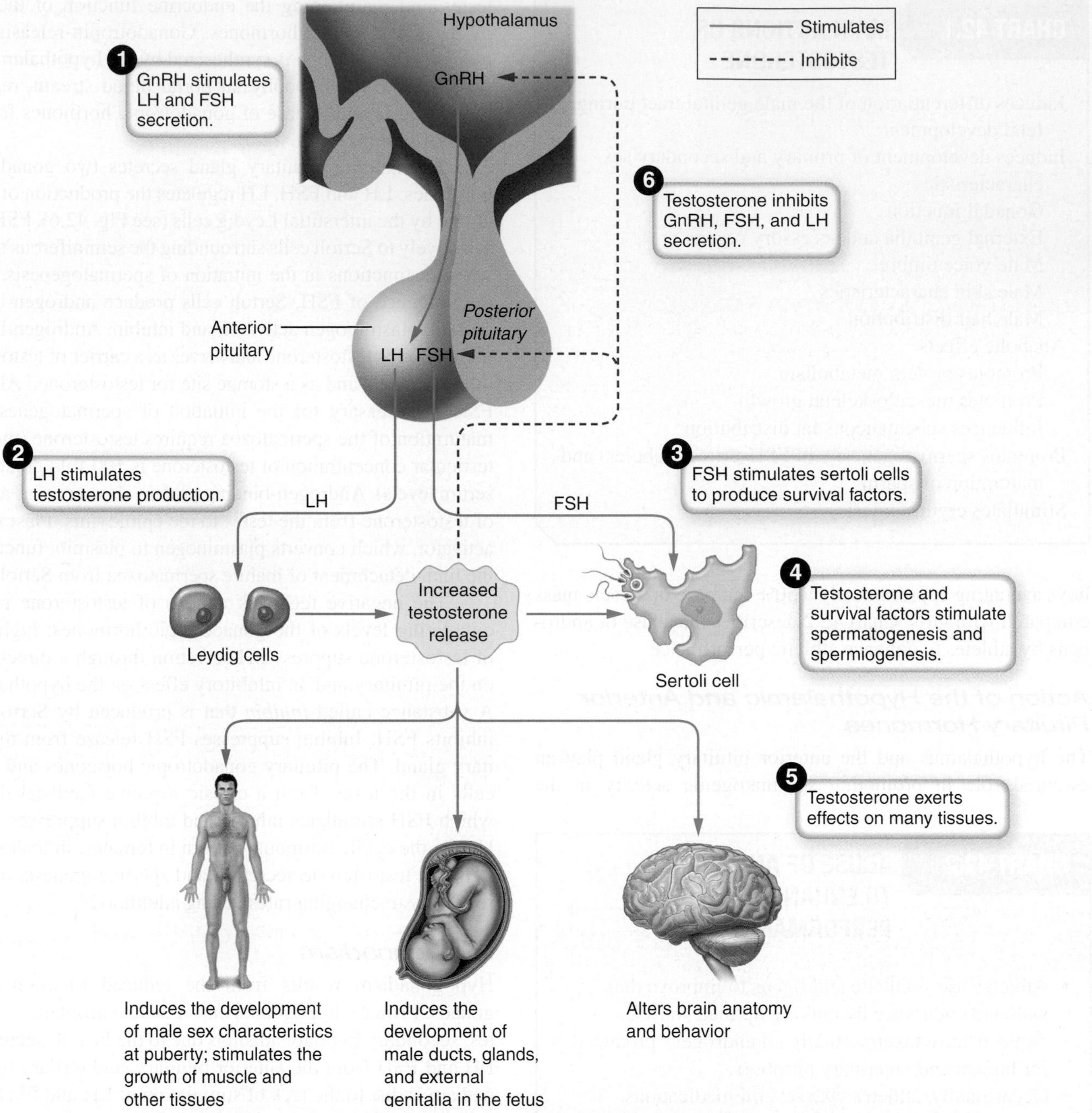

Figure 42.6 • Hypothalamic–pituitary feedback control of spermatogenesis and testosterone levels in the male. FSH, follicle-stimulating hormone; GnRH, gonadotropin-releasing hormone; LH, luteinizing hormone. (From McConnell T., Hull K. (2011). *Human form human function: Essentials of anatomy & physiology* (p. 675). Philadelphia, PA: Lippincott Williams & Wilkins.)

normally. Mumps and Klinefelter syndrome are often the cause. Sperm counts that are lower than normal are often identified. Secondary hypogonadism is caused by the failure of the hypothalamus or pituitary gland, resulting in decreased testosterone levels.[6] Onset occurring in the adult is associated with fatigue, depression, decreased libido, erectile dysfunction, loss of secondary sex characteristics, changes in body composition (including loss of muscle mass and increase in fat mass), and decreased bone density or osteoporosis.[6] When hypogonadism is diagnosed, clinicians should follow up with a comprehensive cardiovascular examination, because hypogonadism, along with erectile dysfunction and type II diabetes mellitus, are predictors of cardiac disease.[7]

It is more challenging to identify the correct etiology and complete pathophysiology of hypogonadism in adolescents. However, there are multiple treatment options to induce puberty and to manage the adolescent's symptoms of hypogonadism.[8]

Diagnosis. Diagnosis of hypogonadism includes measurement of total testosterone levels (ideally between 7 AM and 11 AM, when the testosterone level is usually at its peak) in the ambulatory man. If the initial total testosterone level is low, the clinician should confirm diagnosis of hypogonadism with either a repeat measure of total testosterone or a measure of free (bioavailable) testosterone. Once the clinician establishes a diagnosis of hypogonadism, LH and FSH levels should be measured. A subsequently high LH and FSH indicates a primary hypogonadism (hypergonadotropic hypogonadism), and low or normal LH and FSH indicates a secondary or tertiary hypogonadism (hypogonadotropic hypogonadism). Seminal fluid analyses should be considered in all types of hypogonadism if a person has concerns about fertility. Clinicians should assess pituitary hormones and conduct a pituitary magnetic resonance imaging (MRI) scan in men with hypogonadotropic hypogonadism. In cases of hypergonadotropic hypogonadism, clinicians should conduct a karyotype (chromosome) analysis because Klinefelter syndrome is the most common chromosomal abnormality associated with male hypogonadism. The usual karyotype in Klinefelter syndrome is 47,XXY, although mosaicism or variants can present with a similar phenotype (the normal male is 46,XY and the normal female is 46,XX).[6] Males with Klinefelter syndrome characteristically have small, firm testes (unlike many other cases of hypogonadism, in which the testicular consistency is soft).[9] Other common causes of primary hypogonadism are listed in Chart 42.3.

Treatment. Testosterone therapy is available for treatment of androgen deficiency to men with confirmed hypogonadism (as evidenced by a distinctly subnormal serum testosterone concentration). The principal goal of testosterone therapy is to restore the serum testosterone concentration to the normal range while keeping in mind the risks and benefits especially with men diagnosed or at risk for BPH and/or prostate cancer.

CHART 42.3 COMMON CAUSES OF PRIMARY GONADAL FAILURE

Chromosomal abnormalities (*e.g.*, Klinefelter syndrome)
Disorders of androgen biosynthesis
Cryptorchidism
Alkylating and antineoplastic agents
Other medications (*e.g.*, ketoconazole and glucocorticoids)
Infections—mumps orchitis (gonadal failure is a much more common manifestation when mumps occurs after puberty)
Radiation (direct and indirect testicular radiation)
Environmental toxins
Trauma
Testicular torsion
Autoimmune damage
Chronic systemic diseases (many of these can result in both primary and secondary hypogonadism, *e.g.*, cirrhosis, hemochromatosis, chronic renal failure, and AIDS)
Idiopathic

IN SUMMARY

The function of the male reproductive system is under the negative feedback control of the hypothalamus and the anterior pituitary gonadotropic hormones FSH and LH. FSH initiates spermatogenesis, and LH regulates the production of testosterone. Testosterone is produced by the interstitial Leydig cells in the testes. In addition to its role in the differentiation of the internal and external genitalia in the male embryo, testosterone is essential for the development of secondary male characteristics during puberty, the maintenance of these characteristics during adult life, and spermatozoa maturation.

Hypogonadism refers to a decrease in testicular function. It can present as a primary hypogonadism originating in the testes; a secondary hypogonadism arising from lack of stimulation from the pituitary gonadotropins (LH and FSH); or as a tertiary hypogonadism due to decreased or absent GnRH secretion from the hypothalamus.

NEURAL CONTROL OF SEXUAL FUNCTION AND CHANGES WITH AGING

After completing this section of the chapter, the learner will be able to meet the following objectives:

- Describe the autonomic and peripheral nervous systems' control of erection, emission, and ejaculation.
- Describe changes in the male reproductive system that occur with aging.

In the male, the stages of the sexual act involve erection, emission, ejaculation, and detumescence. The physiology of the sexual act involves a complex interaction between spinal cord reflexes, higher neural centers, the vascular system, and the endocrine system.

Neural Control

The impulse stimulation for initiating the male sexual act is the glans penis, which contains a highly organized sensory system. Afferent impulses from sensory receptors in the glans penis pass through the pudendal nerve to ascending fibers in the spinal cord by way of the sacral plexus. Stimulation of other perineal areas, such as the anal epithelium, the scrotum, and the testes, can transmit signals to higher brain centers, such as the limbic system and cerebral cortex, through the cord, adding to sexual arousal.[1]

The psychological element to sexual stimulation, such as thinking sexual thoughts, can cause erection and ejaculation.[1]

Although psychological involvement and higher-center functions contribute to the sex act, they are not necessary for sexual performance. Genital stimulation can produce erection and ejaculation in some men with complete transection of the spinal cord.

Erection involves the shunting of blood into the corpus cavernosum. It is controlled by the sympathetic, parasympathetic, and nonadrenergic–noncholinergic (NANC) systems. Nitric oxide is the locally released NANC mediator that produces relaxation of vascular smooth muscle. In the flaccid or detumescent state, sympathetic discharge through α-adrenergic receptors maintains contraction of the arteries that supply the penis and vascular sinuses of the corpora cavernosa and corpus spongiosum (Fig. 42.7). Parasympathetic stimulation produces erection by inhibiting sympathetic neurons that cause detumescence and by stimulating the release of nitric oxide to effect a rapid relaxation of the smooth muscle in the sinusoidal spaces of the corpus cavernosum. During sexual stimulation, parasympathetic impulses also cause the urethral and bulbourethral glands to secrete mucus to aid in lubrication. Parasympathetic innervation is effected through the pelvic nerve and sacral segments of the spinal cord. Sympathetic innervation exits the spinal cord at the L1 and L2 levels.

Emission and ejaculation, which constitute the culmination of the male sexual act, are a function of the sympathetic nervous system. Spinal cord reflexes regulate both emission and ejaculation. With increasing intensity of the sexual stimulus, reflex centers of the spinal cord begin to emit sympathetic impulses that leave the cord at the L1 and L2 levels and pass through the hypogastric plexus to the genital organs to initiate emission. Emission is the forerunner of ejaculation and causes the sperm to move from the epididymis to the urethra. Efferent impulses from the spinal cord produce contraction of smooth muscle in the vas deferens and ampulla that move sperm forward and close the internal urethral sphincter to prevent retrograde ejaculation into the bladder.[1]

Ejaculation represents the expulsion of the sperm from the urethra. It involves contraction of the seminal vesicles and prostate gland, which add fluid to the ejaculate and propel it forward. Ejaculation is accompanied by the contraction of the ischiocavernosus and bulbocavernosus muscles located at the base of the penis. The filling of the internal urethra elicits signals that are transmitted through the pudendal nerves from the spinal cord, giving the sudden feeling of fullness of the genital organs. Rhythmic increases in pressure in the urethra cause the semen to be propelled to the exterior, resulting in ejaculation. At the same time, rhythmic contractions of the pelvic and trunk muscles produce thrusting movements of the pelvis and penis, which help propel the ejaculate into the vagina.

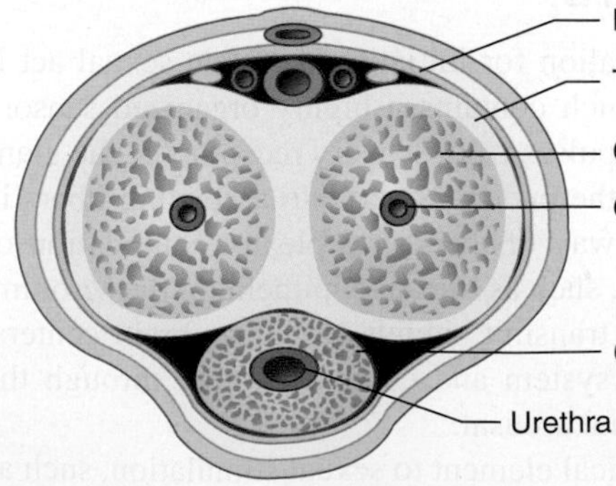

Figure 42.7 • Erectile tissue of the penis.

Together, the period of emission and ejaculation is defined as the male orgasm. After ejaculation, erection ceases within 1 to 2 minutes. A man usually ejaculates approximately 3 mL of semen (though that amount can range from 2 to 5 mL). Ejaculate volume may vary with frequency of intercourse; ejaculate volume may be less with frequent ejaculations and may increase to two to four times its normal amount during periods of abstinence. The ejaculate is approximately 98% fluid and approximately 2% sperm.[1]

Changes with Aging

Like other body systems, the male reproductive system undergoes degenerative changes as a result of the aging process, becoming less efficient with age. The declining physiologic efficiency of male reproductive function occurs gradually and involves the endocrine, circulatory, and neuromuscular systems. Compared with the marked physiologic changes in aging females, the changes in the aging male are more gradual and less drastic. Age does not directly result in gonadal and reproductive failure, so men may remain fertile into advanced age; 80- and 90-year-old men have been known to father children.[1]

As the male ages, his reproductive system becomes measurably different in structure and function from that of the younger male. Male sex hormone levels, particularly of testosterone, decrease with age, but the rate varies in different men and is affected by multiple variables.[10] Beginning at about 25 to 30 years of age in healthy, nonobese men, testosterone levels gradually decrease at approximately 10% per decade. The term *andropause* has been used to describe an ill-defined collection of symptoms in aging men, generally men older than 50 years, who have some degree of hypogonadism associated with aging.[10] The existence and significance of andropause has important public health implications given the current number of men older than 65 years of age, with the number expected to double over the next 30 years.

The sex hormones play a part in the structure and function of the reproductive system and other body systems from conception to old age; they affect protein synthesis, salt and water balance, bone growth, and cardiovascular function. Low testosterone levels have an atherogenic effect that may be part of the etiology of the higher incidence of cardiovascular disease in androgen-deficient men.[7,10] Decreasing levels of testosterone affect sexual energy, muscle strength, and the genital tissues. The testes become smaller and lose their firmness. The seminiferous tubules, which produce spermatozoa, thicken and begin a degenerative process that finally inhibits sperm production, resulting in a decrease in viable spermatozoa. The prostate gland enlarges and its contractions become weaker. The force of ejaculation decreases because of a reduction in the volume and viscosity of the seminal fluid. The seminal vesicle changes little from childhood to puberty. The pubertal increases in the fluid capacity of the gland remain throughout adulthood and decline after 60 years of age. After 60 years of age, the walls of the seminal vesicles thin, the epithelium shrinks, and the muscle layer is replaced by connective tissue. Age-related changes in the penis consist of fibrotic changes in the trabecula in the corpus spongiosum, with progressive sclerotic changes in arteries and veins. Sclerotic changes also follow in the corpora cavernosa, with the condition becoming generalized in 55- to 60-year-old men.

Erectile dysfunction is commonly seen in older men with type II diabetes mellitus, cardiovascular disease and hyperlipidemia.[7] *Erectile dysfunction* has largely replaced the term *impotence*. It is defined as the persistent inability to achieve and maintain an erection sufficient to permit satisfactory sexual intercourse. Aging is a major etiologic factor in this condition. Diseases that accompany aging can have a direct bearing on male reproductive function. Secondary impotence may be related to various cardiovascular, respiratory, hormonal, neurologic, and hematologic disorders. For example, vascular disease affects male potency because it may impair blood flow to the pudendal arteries or their tributaries, resulting in loss of blood volume with subsequent poor distention of the vascular spaces of erectile tissue. Other diseases affecting potency include hypertension, diabetes, cardiac disease, and malignancies of the reproductive organs. In addition, certain medications can have an effect on sexual function.

One of the greatest inhibitors of sexual functioning in older men is the loss of self-esteem and the development of a negative self-image. The emphasis on youth pervades much of our society. The image of success for a man often involves qualities of masculinity and sexual attractiveness. When queried about success, men often mention such things as work, managing money well, participating in sports or other activities, discussing politics or world events, advising younger persons, and being attractive to women. When a man feels good about himself and expresses self-confidence, sexual attractiveness is communicated regardless of age. Many older men live in environments that are not sensitive to the importance of helping them maintain a positive self-image. Premature cessation of esteem-building activities can contribute to loss of libido and zest for life in the older man.

Clinicians may use testosterone and other synthetic androgens in older men with low androgen levels to improve muscle strength and vigor. Preliminary studies of androgen replacement in aging men with low androgen levels show an increase in lean body mass and a decrease in bone turnover. If clinicians initiate testosterone replacement therapy, they should screen for prostate cancer.[7,11] Testosterone is available in several different formulations, including an injectable form, transdermal patch, topical gel, or buccal delivery system. Side effects of replacement therapy may include acne, gynecomastia, and reduced high-density lipoprotein cholesterol levels.[6,7,11]

At present, the routine treatment of older men with testosterone is not recommended. A trial of testosterone administration might be warranted in an older man whose serum testosterone concentration is less than 300 ng/dL (although some believe it should be even lower, *i.e.*, less than 200 ng/dL) and who has manifestations of testosterone deficiency.[7,11] If treatment is undertaken, the man should be screened before treatment and monitored during therapy for evidence of testosterone-dependent diseases.

IN SUMMARY

The sex act involves erection, emission, ejaculation, and detumescence. The physiology of these functions involves a complex interaction between autonomic-mediated spinal cord reflexes, higher neural centers, and the vascular system. Erection is mediated by the parasympathetic nervous system and emission and ejaculation by the sympathetic nervous system. Like other body systems, the male reproductive system undergoes changes as a result of the aging process. The changes occur gradually and involve parallel changes in endocrine, circulatory, and neuromuscular function. Testosterone levels decrease (andropause), the size and firmness of the testes decrease, sperm production declines, and the prostate gland enlarges. There is usually a decrease in frequency of intercourse, intensity of sensation, speed of attaining erection, and force of ejaculation. However, sexual thought, interest, and activity usually continue into old age.

GERIATRIC Considerations

- The number of sperm produced each day diminishes with age.[12]
- The prostate gland, located below the bladder, activates sperm and is often enlarged in older men, resulting in benign prostate hypertrophy.[12]
- Trauma and infection can result in the formation of a hydrocele in aging adults.[12]
- The seminiferous tubules undergo structural changes associated with aging, which include a thinner epithelium, thicker basement membrane, narrow lumen, and fibrosis.[13]
- The testes become smaller (atrophy) and lose mass.[13,14]

PEDIATRIC Considerations

- The testes prepare for sperm production prior to puberty by increasing the number of spermatogonia.[12]
- All of the characteristics that a baby will inherit from its father are found in the chromosomes located in each sperm head.[12]
- Testosterone is responsible for the masculinization of young boys, such as voice change.
- Circumcision in the newborn male is recommended to reduce the spread of some sexually transmitted diseases, such as HIV.[12]
- Failure of the testes to descend can be due to a physical obstruction or hormonal imbalance.[12]

REVIEW EXERCISES

1. In the absence of the *SRY* gene on the Y chromosome, a developing embryo with an XY genotype will develop female genitalia.
   A. Explain.
2. Men who have had a vasectomy often remain fertile for 4 to 5 weeks after the procedure has been done.
   A. Explain.
3. A 55-year-old man presents with various vague symptoms (fatigue, depression). On examination, he is noted to have small testes (8 mL bilaterally), marked gynecomastia, and scanty body hair. He is obese at 122 kg, with a body mass index (BMI) of 34.2. Investigations reveal low testosterone and elevated gonadotropin (LH and FSH) levels.
   A. What endocrine diagnosis is related to this phenotype and these biochemical manifestations?

References

1. Ross M. H., Pawlina W. (2015). *Histology: A text and atlas* (7th ed.). Philadelphia, PA: Lippincott Williams & Wilkins.
2. Rubin R., Strayer D. (2015). *Rubin's pathology: Clinicopathologic foundations of medicine* (6th ed.). Philadelphia, PA: Lippincott Williams & Wilkins.
3. Scanlon V. C., Sanders T. (2014). *Essentials of anatomy and physiology*. FA Davis.
4. Boron W. F., Boulpaep E. L. (2016). *Medical physiology* (3rd ed.). Philadelphia, PA: Elsevier Health Sciences.
5. World Health Organization. (2010). *WHO laboratory manual for the examination and processing of human semen* (5th ed.). Available: http://apps.who.int/iris/bitstream/10665/44261/1/9789241547789_eng.pdf?ua=1.
6. Sandher R. K., Aning J. (2017). Diagnosing and managing androgen deficiency in men. *The Practitioner* 261(1803), 19–22.
7. Phe V., Roupret M. (2012). Erectile dysfunction and diabetes: A review of the current evidence-based medicine and a synthesis of the main available therapies. *Diabetes & Metabolism* 38(1), 1–13.
8. Simoni M., Huhtaniemi I. T. (Eds.) (2017). *Endocrinology of the testis and male reproduction*. Springer International Publishing.
9. NIH U.S. National Library of Medicine. (2017). *Klinefelter syndrome*. Available: https://ghr.nlm.nih.gov/condition/klinefelter-syndrome.
10. Cunningham G. (2013). Andropause or male menopause? Rationale for testosterone replacement therapy in older men with low testosterone levels. *Endocrine Practice* 19(5), 847–852.
11. Lunenfeld B., Arver S., Moncada I., et al. (2012). How to help the aging male? Current approaches to hypogonadism in primary care. *The Aging Male* 15(4), 187–197.
12. Patton K. T., Thibodeau G. A. (2014). *The human body in health and disease*. Maryland Heights, MO: Elsevier.
13. Epiopoulos C. (2018). *Gerontological nursing* (9th ed.). Philadelphia, PA: Wolters Kluwer.
14. Winston L. R. (2013). *Infertility: A sympathetic approach to understanding the causes and options for treatment*. Random House.

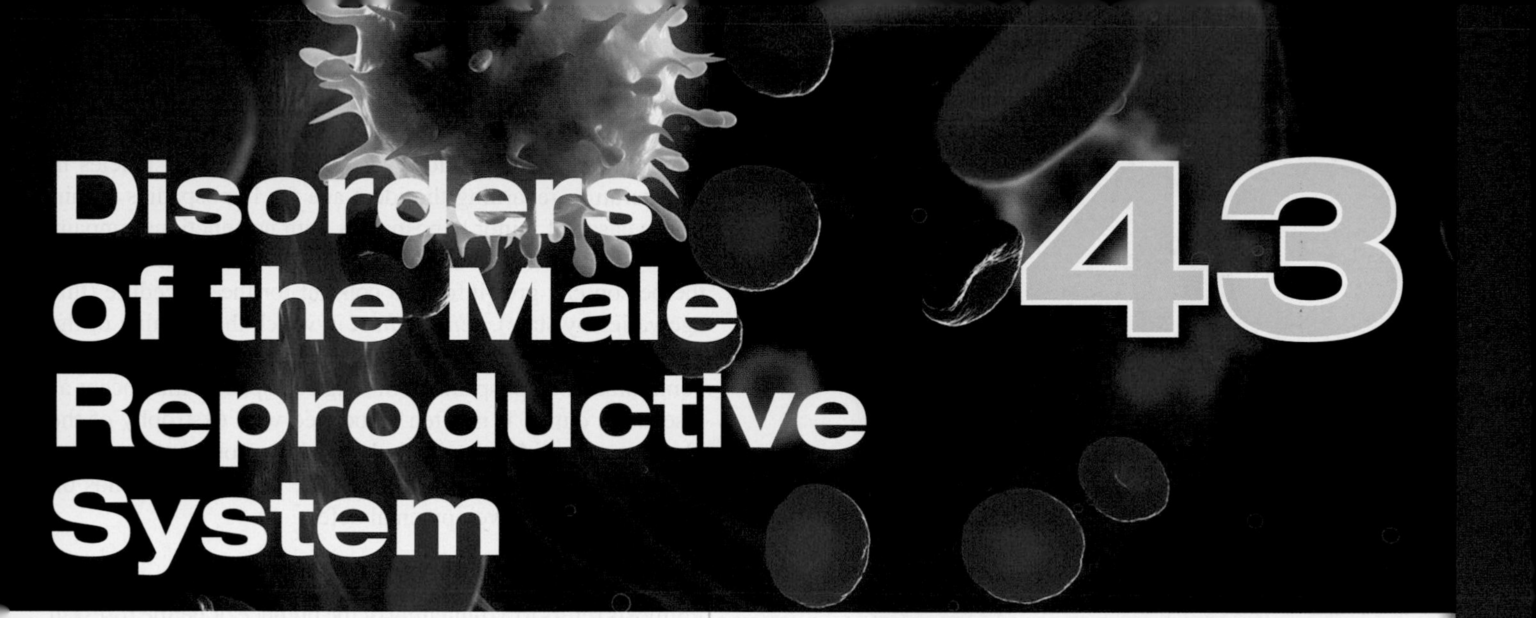

Disorders of the Male Reproductive System

43

Melissa Brown

The male genitourinary system is subject to structural defects, inflammation, and neoplasms, all of which can affect urine elimination, sexual function, and fertility. This chapter discusses disorders of the penis, the scrotum and testes, and the prostate.

DISORDERS OF THE PENIS

After completing this section of the chapter, the learner will be able to meet the following objectives:

- Describe the anatomic changes, signs, and symptoms that occur with various penile disorders, both acquired and congenital.
- Explain the physiology of penile erection and relate it to erectile dysfunction and priapism.
- List the signs of penile cancer.

The penis is the external male genital organ through which the urethra passes to the exterior of the body. It is involved in urinary and sexual function. Disorders of the penis include congenital and acquired defects, inflammatory and infectious conditions, and neoplasms.

Congenital and Acquired Disorders

Hypospadias and Epispadias

Hypospadias and epispadias are congenital disorders of the penis resulting from embryologic defects in the development of the urethral groove and penile urethra (Fig. 43.1). In hypospadias, which affects approximately 1 in 350 male infants, the urethral opening or meatus may be at any location along the underside of the shaft of the penis, the scrotum, or the perineum.[1] Hypospadias is most commonly classified as proximal or distal, with proximal cases being considered more severe and being associated with more negative psychological effects.[2] Hypospadias is a result of abnormal fusion of urethral tissue at the time of organ development. During weeks 8 to 14 of fetal development, fetal testes release hormones

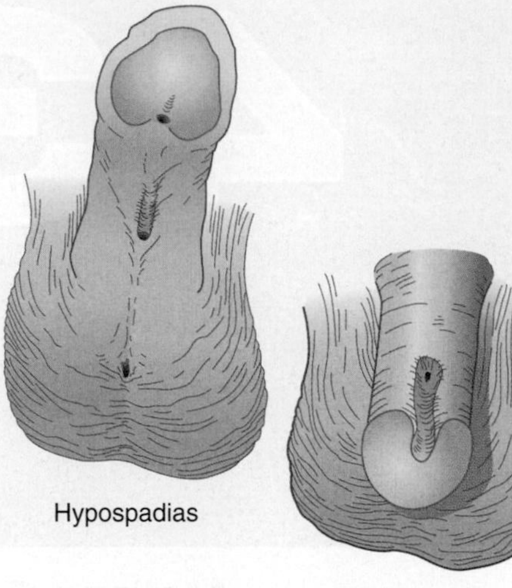

Figure 43.1 • Hypospadias and epispadias.

called androgens that stimulate male sexual differentiation. Inactivity or deficiency of these androgens is believed to be responsible for the development of hypospadias. The majority of cases involve multifactorial causes that include both genetic and environmental components. Risk factors for developing hypospadias include family history of hypospadias and maternal factors (*e.g.*, older maternal age, multiple pregnancies, high body mass index, health conditions such as hypertension or preeclampsia). Prenatal exposure to various medications has also been investigated, with first trimester exposure to valproic acid (antiseizure medication) being consistently associated with hypospadias. The testes are undescended in 10% of males born with hypospadias, and chordee (*i.e.*, ventral bowing of the penis) and inguinal hernia may accompany the disorder.

In the newborn with severe hypospadias and cryptorchidism (undescended testes), the differential diagnosis should consider ambiguous genitalia and masculinization that is seen in females with congenital adrenal hyperplasia. Recently, the term *disorders of sex development* (DSD) has been proposed to define congenital conditions in which development of chromosomal, gonadal, or anatomic sex is altered from normal.[3] In fact, ambiguous genitalia may pose a concern regarding gender assignment for the child.[3]

The most common treatment intervention for hypospadias is surgical repair.[3] In mild cases, the surgery is done for cosmetic reasons only. In more severe cases, repair becomes essential for normal sexual and urinary functioning and to prevent the psychological sequelae of having malformed genitalia. The goal of surgery is the construction of a urethral meatus at the tip of the glans that allows for easy passage of urine and semen. If chordee is present, straightening of the penis is also an indication for surgery. The recommended timing of surgery involving the male genitalia is between 6 and 18 months of age.[4] Surgical and anesthetic risk as well as the psychological impact of surgery on the child are factors that influence the timing of the surgery. However, there are inconsistencies in the literature regarding the ideal age for hypospadias repair, and in cases of minor hypospadias with no functional impairment, there are concerns that surgery should be delayed until the person can give informed consent for the procedure (this age varies by state).[2] *Epispadias*, in which the opening of the urethra is on the dorsal or upper surface of the penis, is less common than hypospadias. Although epispadias may occur as a separate entity, it is often associated with exstrophy of the bladder, a condition in which the bladder protrudes through a weakness in the abdominal wall.[1] The treatment depends on the extent of the developmental defect.

Phimosis and Paraphimosis

Phimosis refers to a tightening of the prepuce or penile foreskin that prevents its retraction over the glans.[4] Embryologically, the foreskin begins to develop during the 8th week of gestation as a fold of skin at the distal edge of the penis that eventually grows forward over the base of the glans.[1] By the 16th week of gestation, the prepuce and the glans are adherent. Only a small percentage of newborns have a fully retractable foreskin. With growth, a space develops between the glans and foreskin, and the majority of males have retractable foreskins.[4]

Because the foreskin of many males cannot be fully retracted in early childhood, it is important that the area be cleaned thoroughly. People with phimosis may seek medical care when signs and symptoms of infection develop, including pain and swelling of the foreskin or purulent discharge from the penile meatus.[5] There is no need to retract the foreskin forcibly because this could lead to infection, scarring, or paraphimosis.[2] As the child grows, the foreskin becomes retractable, and the glans and foreskin should be cleaned routinely. If symptomatic phimosis occurs after childhood, such as with uncircumcised males with multiple infections, it can cause difficulty with voiding or sexual activity. Circumcision is then the treatment of choice. Phimosis is also one of the most important predisposing factors for penile cancer.[2]

In *paraphimosis*, the foreskin is so tight and constricted that it cannot cover the glans. A tight foreskin can constrict the blood supply to the glans and lead to ischemia and necrosis. Many cases of paraphimosis result from the foreskin being retracted for an extended period, as in the case of catheterized uncircumcised males.[2] Paraphimosis can present as a swollen, tender penis with multiple skin folds just under the glans.[5]

Balanitis and Balanoposthitis

Balanitis refers to inflammation, either chronic or acute, of the glans penis, and posthitis is inflammation of the prepuce. Often both the glans penis and prepuce are affected, which results in the condition *balanoposthitis*.[6] The condition may be characterized by erythema of the glans and prepuce, itching, soreness, blisters, ulcers, and painful urination.[7] Foul-smelling discharge may also be present. Males with poor hygiene, immunosuppression, or diabetes are more prone to balanoposthitis.[2] Balanoposthitis is usually encountered in males with phimosis or a large, redundant prepuce that interferes with cleanliness and predisposes to bacterial growth in the accumulated secretions and smegma (*i.e.*, debris from the desquamated epithelia). The condition is uncommon in circumcised males.[7] Potential complications include permanent scarring of the glans and/or prepuce, phimosis, urethral stenosis or narrowing, sexual dysfunction, and malignant transformation.[7] The causes of balanoposthitis include infection, trauma, or irritation. Infective balanoposthitis may be caused by a wide variety of organisms including, but not limited to, *Candida albicans*, *Chlamydia trachomatis*, streptococci, staphylococci, herpes simplex virus, human papillomavirus (HPV), and *Mycoplasma genitalium*.[7] Although inflammation is common across all forms of balanoposthitis, treatment will vary depending on the exact cause.[7] If the suspected cause is a specific microorganism, appropriate treatment requires correct identification of that microorganism through use of microbial smears and cultures. Treatment will then be tailored to the results of those tests. For example, people with balanoposthitis caused by *Candida* are treated commonly with oral and topical antifungal medications. Cases of balanoposthitis caused by Lichen sclerosis, an inflammatory skin condition that may be an autoimmune disease, are treated with topical steroids used to suppress the overactive immune system that is contributing to the balanoposthitis.[7] For some people with balanoposthitis, no causative agent can be identified, yet the person is chronically symptomatic. This is known as *nonspecific balanoposthitis*. Circumcision is curative in these situations.

Because certain causes of balanoposthitis are potentially cancerous or precancerous, biopsy is often included in the care of people with balanoposthitis.[7] The goals of balanoposthitis management are to reduce sexual dysfunction, to minimize urinary dysfunction, to exclude penile cancer, to treat premalignant disease, and to diagnose and treat sexually transmitted infections.[7]

Peyronie Disease

Peyronie disease involves a localized and progressive fibrosis of unknown origin that affects the tunica albuginea (*i.e.*, the tough, fibrous sheath that surrounds the corpora cavernosa) of the penis. Approximately 1% of males are impacted by this disorder.[2] The disorder is characterized initially by an inflammatory process that results in dense fibrous plaque formation. The plaque is usually on the dorsal midline of the shaft, causing upward bowing of the shaft during erection (Fig. 43.2). Some males may develop scarring on both the dorsal and ventral aspects of the shaft, causing the penis to be straight but shortened or have a lateral bend.[2] The fibrous tissue prevents lengthening of the involved area during erection, making intercourse difficult and painful. The disease usually occurs in males older than 40 years of age.[2]

The manifestations of Peyronie disease include painful erection, bent erection, and the presence of a hard mass at the site of fibrosis. Approximately two thirds of males complain of pain as a symptom. Inflammation of the adjacent fascial

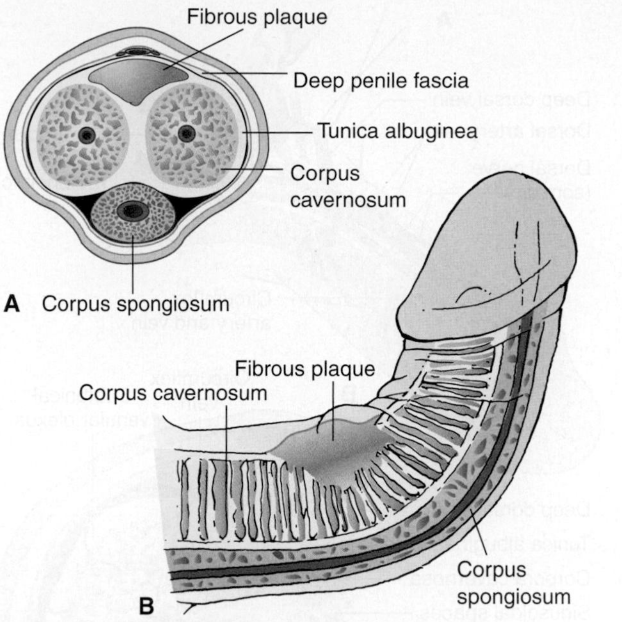

Figure 43.2 • Peyronie disease. **(A)** Penile cross-section showing plaque between the corpora. **(B)** Penile curvature.

tissue is thought to generate the pain. The pain usually disappears as the inflammation resolves. During the first year or so after formation of the plaque, while the scar tissue is undergoing the process of remodeling, penile distortion may increase, remain static, or resolve and disappear completely.[8] In some cases, the scar tissue may progress to calcification and formation of bonelike tissue.

Diagnosis is based on history and physical examination. Doppler ultrasonography may be used to assess causation of the disorder. Surgical intervention can be used to correct the disorder. Indications for surgery include penile shortening, persistent pain, severe curvature, and penile narrowing or indentation.

Disorders of Erectile Function

Erection is a neurovascular process involving the autonomic nervous system, neurotransmitters and endothelial relaxing factors, the vascular smooth muscle of the arteries and veins supplying the penile tissue, and the trabecular smooth muscle of the sinusoids of the corpora cavernosa (Fig. 43.3). The penis is innervated by both the autonomic and somatic nervous systems.[8] In the pelvis, the sympathetic and parasympathetic components of the autonomic nervous systems merge to form what are called the cavernous nerves.[8] Erection is under the control of the parasympathetic nervous system, and ejaculation and detumescence (penile relaxation) are under sympathetic nervous system control.[8] Somatic innervation, which occurs through the pudendal nerve, is responsible for penile sensation and contraction and relaxation of the extracorporeal striated muscles (bulbocavernosus and ischiocavernous).

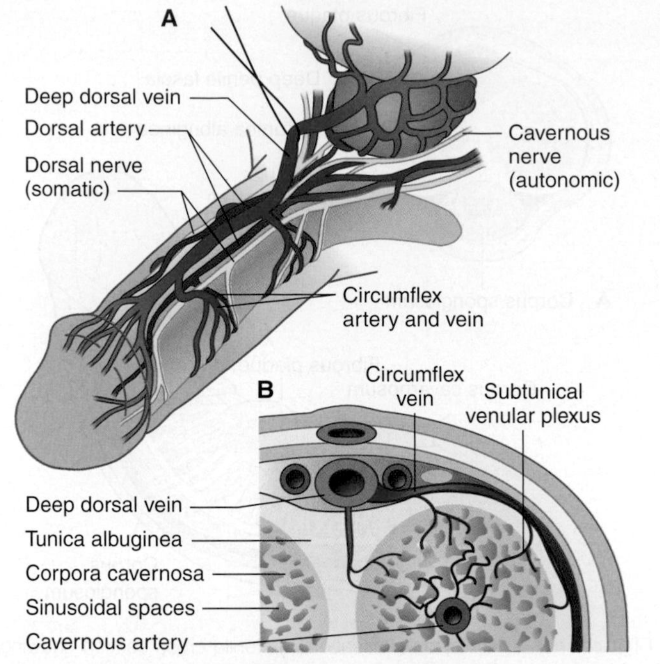

Figure 43.3 • Anatomy and mechanism of penile erection. **(A)** Innervation and arterial and venous blood supply to the penis. **(B)** Cross-section of the sinusoidal system of the corpora cavernosa.

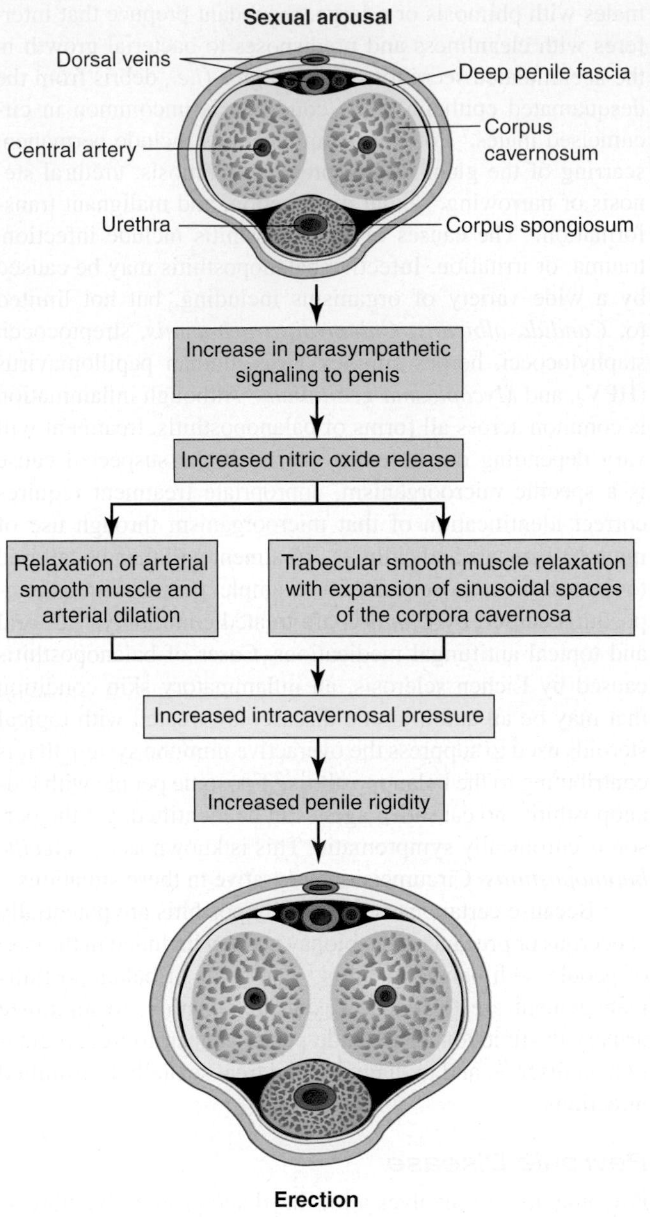

Figure 43.4 • Mechanisms of penile erection and sites of action of drugs, vacuum suction, and penile prosthesis used in treatment of erectile dysfunction.

Penile erection is the first effect of male sexual stimulation, whether psychological or physical (Fig. 43.4). It is a neurovascular phenomenon that requires dilation of penile vasculature, relaxation of smooth muscle, increased intracavernosal blood flow, and normal venoocclusive function. It involves increased inflow of blood into the corpora cavernosa due to relaxation of the trabecular smooth muscle that surrounds the sinusoidal spaces and compression of the veins controlling outflow of blood from the venous plexus. Erection is mediated by parasympathetic impulses that pass from the sacral segments of the spinal cord through the pelvic nerves to the penis. Parasympathetic stimulation results in release of the neurotransmitter nitric oxide, a nonadrenergic–noncholinergic neurotransmitter (NANC), which causes relaxation of trabecular smooth muscle of the corpora cavernosa.[2] This relaxation permits inflow of blood into the sinuses of the cavernosa at pressures approaching those of the arterial system. Because the erectile tissues of the cavernosa are surrounded by a nonelastic fibrous covering, high pressure in the sinusoids causes ballooning of the erectile tissue to such an extent that the penis becomes hard and elongated. At the same time, contraction of the somatically innervated ischiocavernous muscles forcefully compresses the blood-filled corpora cavernosa, producing a further rise in intercavernous pressures. During this phase of erection, inflow and outflow of blood cease.

Parasympathetic innervation must be intact and nitric oxide synthesis must be active for erection to occur. Nitric oxide activates guanyl cyclase, an enzyme that increases the concentration of cyclic guanosine monophosphate (cGMP), which in turn causes smooth muscle relaxation. Other smooth muscle relaxants (*e.g.*, prostaglandin E_1 analogs and α-adrenergic antagonists), if present in high enough concentrations, can independently cause sufficient cavernosal relaxation to result in erection. Many of the drugs that have been developed to treat erectile dysfunction (ED) act at the level of these mediators.[9]

Detumescence or penile relaxation is largely a sympathetic nervous system response. It can result from a cessation of neurotransmitter release, the breakdown of second messengers such as cGMP, or sympathetic discharge during ejaculation. Contraction of the trabecular smooth muscle opens the venous channels so that the trapped blood can be expelled and penile flaccidity can return.

KEY POINTS

DISORDERS OF PENILE ERECTION

- Erection is a neurovascular process involving the autonomic nervous system, the somatic nervous system by way of the pudendal nerve, the vascular system, and the sinusoidal spaces of the corpora cavernosa.
- Erectile failure can result from disorders in one or a combination of the neural, vascular, or chemical pathways that produce an erection.

Erectile Dysfunction

Erectile dysfunction (ED) is defined as the persistent inability to achieve and maintain an erection sufficient to permit satisfactory sexual intercourse.[10]

According to data from the Unites States, ED affects approximately 30 million males aged 40 to 70 years.[11] Thirty million American men have erectile dyfunction.[10] ED was once believed to be solely a psychological condition, and it was frequently grouped with mental health. Today, we know that ED has a physical etiology for most men, commonly involving blood flow to and from the penis.

Psychogenic Causes. Psychogenic causes of ED include performance anxiety, a strained relationship with a sexual partner, depression, and overt psychotic disorders. Psychogenic factors can be further exacerbated by the side effects of many of the therapies used to treat these disorders, which can themselves cause ED.

Organic Causes. Organic causes of ED span a wide range of pathologic processes. They include neurogenic, hormonal, vascular, drug-induced, and penile-related etiologies. The most common cause of ED, especially in older men, is vascular and involves the penile arteries, veins, or both.[11] Arterial issues are usually caused by arteriosclerosis, or hardening of the arteries, although sometimes they are due to trauma to the arteries.[11] Preventable risk factors that predispose people to arteriosclerosis include obesity, physical inactivity, high cholesterol levels, high blood pressure, and cigarette smoking. These risk factors can result in ED before the heart is ever affected.[11] Another proposed vascular cause of ED is a partial or complete wasting or atrophy of smooth muscle in the penis (cavernous smooth muscle) or the growth of excessive smooth muscle tissue (fibrosis). This atrophy or fibrosis can contribute to impaired ability to maintain an erection.

There are many neurologic causes of ED. Parkinson disease, multiple sclerosis, heavy metal poisoning, stroke, cerebral trauma, and spinal cord and nerve injuries can all cause ED. In spinal cord injury, the extent of neural impairment depends on the level, location, and extent of the lesion.

ED is also common in people with diabetes. An estimated 10.9 million adult males in the United States have diabetes, and 35% to 50% of these males have ED. The process involves premature and unusually severe hardening of the arteries. Peripheral neuropathy, with involvement of the nerves controlling erection, is also commonly seen in people with diabetes. A history of extensive pelvic surgery, especially radical prostatectomy, is a common cause of ED, due to both direct and indirect nerve damage.

Endocrine disorders—such as hypogonadism, hyperprolactinemia, and thyroid disease—play a significant role in ED physiology. Testosterone regulates cavernosal nerve structure and function, nitric oxide synthesis, and corporal smooth muscle cell growth and differentiation. Prolactin acts to inhibit the release of gonadotropin-releasing hormone (GnRH) from the hypothalamus in the brain.

For people with hypertension, erectile function is impaired not so much by the increased blood pressure as by the associated arterial lesions caused by the high pressure that narrows the vessel lumen (known as stenosis). Focal stenosis of the common penile artery most often occurs in males who sustained blunt pelvic or perineal trauma (*e.g.*, from bicycling accidents). Failure of the veins to close completely during an erection (venoocclusive dysfunction) may occur in males with large venous channels that drain the corpora cavernosa.

Many drugs are reported to cause ED, including antidepressants, antipsychotics, antiandrogens, glaucoma eye drops, chemotherapy drugs, and antihypertensive medications.[11] Cigarette smoking can induce vasoconstriction and penile venous leakage because of its effects on cavernous smooth muscle and can double the risk of ED.[12] Alcohol in small amounts may increase libido and improve erection. However, in large amounts, it can cause central sedation, decreased libido, and transient ED.

Aging is known to increase the risk of ED.[10] Many of the pathologic processes that contribute to ED, including diabetes, hyperlipidemia, vascular disease, and the long-term effects of cigarette smoking, are more common in older men. Age-related declines in testosterone may also play a role (andropause).

Diagnosis and Treatment. A diagnosis of ED requires a careful history (medical, sexual, and psychosocial), physical examination, and laboratory tests to rule out organic causes of the disorder. Because many medications—including prescribed, over-the-counter, and illicit drugs—can cause ED, an accurate drug history is also needed.

Metabolic syndrome is now understood to have a major association with ED.[12]

Metabolic syndrome is a group of metabolic conditions. When a person presents with multiple metabolic conditions simultaneously, the likelihood of developing cardiovascular disease is greater than if that person had a single metabolic disorder.[13] Examples of measurements included in the diagnosis of metabolic syndrome are abdominal obesity, triglyceride levels of 150 mg/dL of blood or more, and fasting blood

IN SUMMARY

Disorders of the penis can be congenital or acquired. Hypospadias and epispadias are congenital defects in which there is malpositioning of the urethral opening: it is located on the ventral surface in hypospadias and on the dorsal surface in epispadias. Phimosis is the condition in which the opening of the foreskin is too tight to permit retraction over the glans. Balanitis is an acute or chronic inflammation of the glans penis, and balanoposthitis is an inflammation of the glans and prepuce. Peyronie disease is characterized by the growth of a band of fibrous tissue on top of the penile shaft. ED is defined as the inability to achieve and maintain an erection sufficient to permit satisfactory sexual intercourse. It can be caused by psychogenic factors, organic disorders, or mixed psychogenic and organic conditions. Priapism is a prolonged, painful erection that can lead to thrombosis with ischemia and necrosis of penile tissue. Cancer of the penis accounts for less than 1% of male genital cancers in developed countries. Although the tumor is slow growing and highly curable when diagnosed early, the greatest hindrance to successful treatment is a delay in seeking medical attention.

DISORDERS OF THE SCROTUM AND TESTES

After completing this section of the chapter, the learner will be able to meet the following objectives:

- Compare the cause, appearance, and significance of hydrocele, hematocele, spermatocele, and varicocele.
- Describe the symptoms of epididymitis.
- State the cell types involved in seminoma, embryonal carcinoma, teratoma, and choriocarcinoma tumors of the testes.

The scrotum is a skin-covered pouch that contains the testes and their accessory organs. Defects of the scrotum and testes include cryptorchidism, disorders of the scrotal sac, vascular disorders, inflammation of the scrotum and testes, and neoplasms.

Congenital and Acquired Disorders

Cryptorchidism

Cryptorchidism, or undescended testes, occurs when one or both of the testicles fail to move down into the scrotal sac. The condition is usually unilateral, but it may be bilateral in 30% of cases.[2] The undescended testes may remain in the lower abdomen, at a point of descent in the inguinal canal, or in the upper scrotum (Fig. 43.5).[2]

Cryptorchidism is the most common congenital disorder of the genitourinary system affecting male infants.[18] The incidence is 2% to 4%, but as many as one third of premature newborn males are affected.[14] The pathophysiology of cryptorchidism is not fully understood, although several theories have been posed. Clinical research conducted in the 1940s demonstrated that uncorrected cryptorchidism has extreme implications, particularly on fertility potential and malignant transformation of some testicular cell lines.[14] Clinically, the presence of unilateral cryptorchidism is more common than that of bilateral cryptorchidism. Approximately 80% of cases are unilateral, whereas the remaining 20% represent bilateral cryptorchidism.[19]

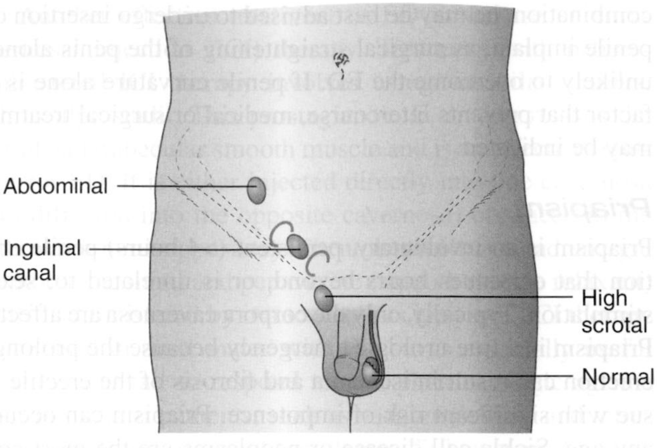

Figure 43.5 • Possible locations of undescended testes.

To understand the occurrence of undescended testes it is helpful to have knowledge of the phases of testicular descent into the scrotum. Chapter 42 describes this process.

Cryptorchidism can be divided into primary or secondary types. In primary cryptorchidism, the testis failed to complete its migration from its pararenal embryologic origin to the scrotum. Instead, it may be located in a nonpalpable intra-abdominal position or may be palpable in an intracanalicular position, suprascrotal position, or an ectopic position (outside of the normal path of descent). In secondary cryptorchidism, a testis that had previously been in a scrotal position can be pulled into a suprascrotal position as a result of scarring, often after surgical repair of an inguinal hernia.[17] Identified risk factors for cryptorchidism remain elusive, although many putative risk factors likely to be associated with cryptorchidism have been investigated, including maternal smoking during pregnancy, small birth weight, family history of cryptorchidism, and rare genetic variants such as INSL3.[18,20] The strongest of these is believed to be prematurity; the incidence of cryptorchidism among premature neonates has been reported to be greater than 30%.[21] Among both term and preterm neonates, many cases of cryptorchidism spontaneously descend postnatally. One study found that of cases with spontaneous descent, 82% descended by 2 months of age, an additional 10% by 6 months of age, and another 8% by 12 months of age.[21] Because spontaneous descent after 6 months is less likely, clinical guidelines recommend referral to a specialist if the testis is not completely descended by 6 months of age.[19]

Clinical Manifestations and Complications. The major clinical manifestation of cryptorchidism is the absence of one or both testes from the scrotum. The testis either is not palpable or can be felt external to the inguinal ring.

In males with cryptorchidism, histologic abnormalities of the testes reflect intrinsic defects in the testicle or adverse effects of the extrascrotal environment. There is a delay in germ cell development, changes in the spermatic tubules, and a reduced number of Leydig cells. These changes are progressive over time if the testes remain undescended.

Diagnosis and Treatment. Diagnosis is based on careful examination of the genitalia in male infants. Undescended testes due to cryptorchidism should be differentiated from retractable testes that retract into the inguinal canal in response to an exaggerated cremasteric muscle reflex (normally elicited by stroking the medial aspect of the thigh and observing testicular retraction). Retractable testes are usually palpable at birth but become nonpalpable later. They can be brought down with careful palpation in a warm room. Retractable testes usually assume a scrotal position during puberty.

Techniques for testicular localization include ultrasonography, gonadal venography and arteriography, and laparoscopy.

The only definitive management for an undescended testis is surgical intervention. Hormonal treatments have been used to encourage descent of the cryptorchidism. Both human chorionic gonadotrophin (hCG) and GnRH have been used, with proposed mechanisms of utilizing androgen influence to encourage descent. These medical therapies appear more appropriate for people with low-level cryptorchidism and retractile testes, but success rates are still poor. One recent systematic review demonstrated that hormonal therapies performed only marginally better than placebo, with maximal success rates of approximately 20%.[22] The consequences of cryptorchidism include infertility, malignancy (20- to 40-fold greater risk), testicular torsion (10-fold increased risk), and the possible psychological effects of an empty scrotum.[1] Given the significant consequences of cryptorchidism on fertility and potential malignancy, definitive and corrective surgical therapy has become the mainstay of treatment for cryptorchidism. Therefore, hormonal therapies are no longer recommended by the most recent American Urological Association guidelines.[19]

Treatment of males with undescended testes should include lifelong follow-up, considering the sequelae of testicular cancer and infertility. Parents need to be aware of the potential issues of infertility and increased risk of testicular cancer. On reaching puberty, males should be instructed on the necessity of testicular self-examination.

Hydrocele

Hydrocele is a collection of fluid in the scrotum without an obvious inguinal hernia. The testes and epididymis are completely surrounded by the tunica vaginalis, a serous pouch derived from the peritoneum during fetal descent of the testes into the scrotum. The tunica vaginalis has an outer parietal layer and a deeper visceral layer that adheres to the dense fibrous covering of the testes, the tunica albuginea. A space exists between these two layers that typically contains a few milliliters of clear fluid. A hydrocele forms when excess fluid collects between the layers of the tunica vaginalis (Fig. 43.6C).[9] The typical hydrocele is seen shortly after birth as a unilateral or bilateral swelling in the scrotum, and it may vary in size. The scrotum appears swollen with fluid and may be bluish in color. The scrotum may be very tense and is usually not tender. Transillumination of the scrotum (*i.e.*, shining a light through the scrotum to visualize its internal structures) or ultrasonography can help to determine whether the mass is solid or cystic and whether the testicle is normal. A dense hydrocele that does not illuminate should be differentiated from a testicular tumor. Management of hydrocele is observation during the first 1 to 2 years of a child's life, unless the diagnosis of a hernia cannot be excluded. Hydroceles that persist or appear beyond that age are unlikely to resolve spontaneously and should therefore undergo surgical repair. The prevalence of congenital hydroceles is approximately 6% at birth and 1% in adulthood.[20] Acute hydrocele may develop after local injury, testicular torsion, epididymitis or orchitis (inflammation of the testis), gonorrhea, lymph obstruction, or germ cell testicular tumor, or as a side effect of radiation therapy. Chronic hydrocele is more common, with fluid collecting around the testis and the mass growing gradually.

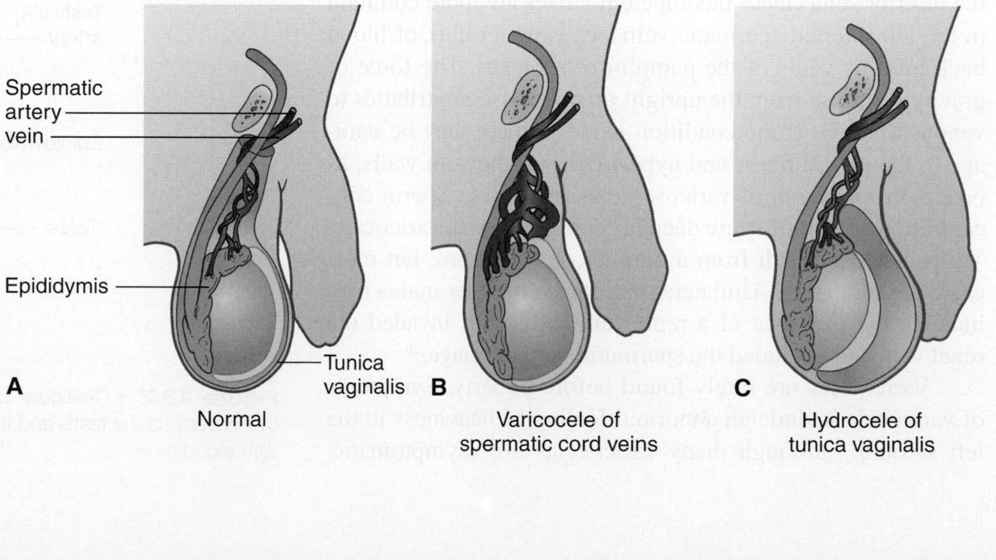

Figure 43.6 • **(A)** Normal testis and appendages, **(B)** varicocele, and **(C)** hydrocele.

Most cases of hydrocele in male infants and children are caused by a patent processus vaginalis, which is continuous with the peritoneal cavity. The processus vaginalis is an outpouching of the peritoneum through the internal inguinal ring, which normally closes spontaneously following testicular descent. Incomplete closure of the processus vaginalis may result in an abnormal communication between the abdominal cavity and the inguinal region.[20] A hydrocele that develops in a young male without apparent cause requires careful evaluation to exclude cancer or infection. In an adult male, a hydrocele is often asymptomatic, and no treatment is necessary. When symptoms do occur, the feeling may be that of heaviness in the scrotum or pain in the lower back. If the hydrocele is painful or cosmetically undesirable, surgical correction is indicated. Surgical repair may be done inguinally or transscrotally.

Hematocele

A hematocele is an accumulation of blood in the space between the parietal and visceral tunica vaginalis, which causes the scrotal skin to become dark red or purple. Hematocele is often associated with hydrocele. It may develop as a result of an abdominal surgical procedure, scrotal trauma, a bleeding disorder, or a testicular tumor.

Spermatocele

A spermatocele is a painless, sperm-containing cyst that forms at the end of the epididymis. It is located above and posterior to the testis, is attached to the epididymis, and is separate from the testes.[2] Spermatoceles may be solitary or multiple and usually are less than 1 cm in diameter. They are freely movable and should transilluminate. Spermatoceles rarely cause problems, but a large one may become painful and require removal.

Varicocele

A varicocele is characterized by varicosities of the pampiniform plexus, a network of veins supplying the testes (see Fig. 43.6B). The left side is more commonly affected because the left internal spermatic vein inserts into the left renal vein at a right angle, whereas the right spermatic vein usually enters the inferior vena cava.[9] Incompetent valves are more common in the left internal spermatic veins, causing a reflux of blood back into the veins of the pampiniform plexus. The force of gravity resulting from the upright position also contributes to venous dilation. If the condition persists, there may be damage to the elastic fibers and hypertrophy of the vein walls, as occurs in formation of varicose veins in the leg. Sperm concentration and motility are decreased in males with varicocele. Varicocele can result from a number of conditions, but most cases are idiopathic. Unilateral varicocele in older males may indicate the presence of a renal tumor that has invaded the renal vein and occluded the spermatic vein drainage.[20]

Varicoceles are rarely found before puberty. Symptoms of varicocele include an abnormal feeling of heaviness in the left scrotum, although many varicoceles are asymptomatic. Usually, the varicocele is readily diagnosed on physical examination with the person in the standing and recumbent positions. Typically, the varicocele disappears in the lying position because of venous decompression into the renal vein.[9] Scrotal palpation of a varicocele has been compared to feeling a "bag of worms."[9] Small varicoceles are sometimes difficult to identify. The Valsalva maneuver (*i.e.*, forced expiration against a closed glottis) may be used to accentuate small varicosities. If the varicocele is present, retrograde blood flow to the scrotum can be detected by Doppler ultrasonography. Other diagnostic aids include radioisotope scanning and spermatic venography.

Treatment options include surgical ligation or sclerosis using a percutaneous transvenous catheter under fluoroscopic guidance. Aside from improving fertility, other reasons for surgery include relief of the sensation of "heaviness" and cosmetic improvement.

Testicular Torsion

Testicular torsion refers to the twisting of the spermatic cord that suspends the testis and subsequent loss of the blood supply to the ipsilateral testicle (Fig. 43.7). Considered a urologic emergency, early diagnosis and treatment are critical to preserving the testicle and future fertility.[23] The rate of testicular viability decreases rapidly after 6 hours from onset of symptoms.[24] It is the most common acute scrotal disorder in the pediatric and young adult population occurring in 1 in 4,000 males younger than 25 years.[9] Testicular torsion can be divided into two distinct clinical entities, depending on the level of spermatic cord involvement: intravaginal and extravaginal torsion.[25]

Intravaginal Torsion. Typically, the tunica vaginalis is attached securely to the posterior lateral side of the testicle, and the spermatic cord is not very mobile. If the attachment of the tunica vaginalis to the testicle is too high, the spermatic cord can rotate within it, which can result in intravaginal torsion. This defect is referred to as the bell clapper deformity,

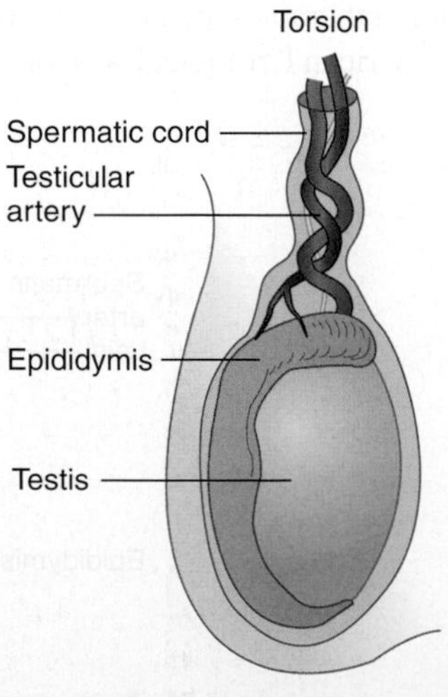

Figure 43.7 • Testicular torsion with twisting of the spermatic cord that suspends the testis and the spermatic vessels that supply the testis with blood.

and it occurs in about 17% of males and is bilateral in 40%.[26] Intravaginal torsion most commonly occurs in adolescents. Increased weight of the testicle after puberty, as well as sudden contraction of the cremaster muscles (which inserts in a spiral fashion into the spermatic cord), are thought to be the catalysts for acute torsion in this population.[26] Intravaginal torsion is considerably more common than extravaginal torsion. People with intravaginal torsion usually present in severe distress within hours of onset and often have nausea, vomiting, and tachycardia. The affected testis is large and tender, with pain radiating to the inguinal area. Intravaginal testicular torsion is a true surgical emergency, and early recognition and treatment are necessary if the testicle is to be saved.

Extravaginal Torsion. Extravaginal torsion, which occurs almost exclusively in neonates, is the less common form of testicular torsion. In neonates, the testicle frequently has not yet descended into the scrotum, where it becomes attached within the tunica vaginalis. This mobility of the testicle predisposes it to torsion. Inadequate fusion of the testicle to the scrotal wall typically is diagnosed within the first 7 to 10 days of life. At birth or shortly thereafter, a firm, smooth, painless scrotal mass is identified. The scrotal skin appears red, and some edema is present. Differential diagnosis is relatively easy because testicular tumors, epididymitis, and orchitis are exceedingly rare in neonates; a hydrocele is softer and can be transilluminated; and physical examination can exclude the presence of hernia. The use of surgical treatment (orchiopexy and orchiectomy) is controversial.[25]

Testicular torsion must be differentiated from epididymitis, orchitis, and trauma to the testis. On physical examination, the testicle is often high in the scrotum and in an abnormal orientation. These changes are caused by the twisting and shortening of the spermatic cord. The degree of scrotal swelling and redness depends on the duration of symptoms. The testes are firm and tender. The cremasteric reflex is frequently absent.[27]

Infection and Inflammation

Epididymitis

Epididymitis is an acute or chronic inflammation of the epididymis, the elongated cordlike structure that lies along the posterior border of the testis, whose function is the storage, transport, and maturation of spermatozoa.[1] The most current published data report that there are approximately 600,000 cases of epididymitis per year in the United States.[28]

People with epididymitis present with gradual onset of posterior testicular pain, usually unilateral, and occasionally, this pain radiates to the lower abdomen.[29] Acute epididymitis usually involves pain, swelling, and inflammation of the epididymis that lasts less than 6 weeks. Chronic epididymitis is characterized by a ≥6-week period of the symptoms described above. Other signs and symptoms such as discharge, dysuria, frequency, urgency, erythema of the scrotal skin, and fever may also be present. Physical elevation of the testicle or scrotum when a patient is standing (known as Prehn sign) decreases the pain of epididymitis but does not decrease pain associated with testicular torsion.

Once a person first presents with testicular pain, a differential diagnosis of testicular torsion must be considered. Torsion usually presents with the acute onset of severe testicular pain. If testicular torsion is the cause of the pain, surgery within 6 hours of presentation is mandatory to prevent infarction, necrosis, atrophy, and loss of the testicle.[29] Fournier gangrene is another possible cause of testicular pain. This disease can present subtly with malaise and scrotal discomfort that transitions to pain with progressing discoloration of the scrotal or perineal skin (erythema and ecchymosis). Eventually, these regions of the body turn black as the tissue becomes necrotic. Fournier gangrene can be a mixed infection with aerobic/anaerobic bacteria resulting from a variety of potential sources including a perirectal abscess, trauma, circumcision, and insect bite, hemorrhoids, or other tissue damage to the perirectal or genital region. Fournier gangrene requires immediate referral to a urologist and/or a surgeon for debridement of the wound along with antibiotic therapy.

Epididymitis is caused by multiple infectious, noninfectious, and even postinfectious microbial sources. In most cases of bacterial epididymitis, retrograde ascent of the organisms is the mechanism of infection. In other cases, such as *Mycobacterium tuberculosis*, hematogenous spread or seeding of the epididymis is the mechanism of infection.[29]

Bacterial agents responsible for epididymitis are highly dependent upon age and sexual practices. Urinary tract pathogens, such as *Escherichia coli*, are responsible for epididymitis in males less than 14 years of age and males greater than 35 years of age.[29] In older men, the epididymis becomes infected in the setting of bacteriuria secondary to bladder outlet obstruction from prostatic hypertrophy, urinary tract instrumentation, prostatic biopsy, or urologic surgery. Anatomic abnormalities also contribute to the etiology of nonspecific bacterial epididymitis caused by a variety of aerobic bacteria. In sexually active males aged 14 to 35 years and in older males who have sex with men, *Neisseria gonorrhoeae* and *C. trachomatis* are the most common offending organisms.

Other bacterial organisms such as *Pseudomonas aeruginosa*, *Klebsiella pneumoniae*, *Haemophilus influenzae*, *Proteus mirabilis*, *Ureaplasma urealyticum*, and *M. genitalium* have also been associated with epididymitis.[29] In children, the most prevalent etiology is viral, with enterovirus and adenovirus being most commonly associated.[29]

Reported causes of noninfectious epididymitis include trauma, postprostatic biopsy, and postvasectomy epididymal inflammation, sarcoidosis, Behçet disease, vasculitis associated with Henoch-Schönlein purpura, and medications such as amiodarone, an antidysrhythmic.[29]

Clinical Manifestations. Epididymitis is characterized by unilateral pain and swelling, accompanied by erythema and edema of the overlying scrotal skin that develops over a period of 24 to 48 hours. Initially, the swelling and induration are limited to the epididymis.[9] However, the distinction between the testis and epididymis becomes less evident as the inflammation progresses, and the testis and epididymis become one mass. In contrast to males with testicular torsion, males with epididymitis usually have a normal cremasteric reflex.[27] There may be tenderness over the groin (spermatic cord) or in the lower abdomen. Fever and complaints of dysuria occur in approximately one half of cases. Whether urethral discharge is present depends on the organism causing the infection; it usually accompanies gonorrheal infections, is common in chlamydial infections, and is less common in infections caused by gram-negative organisms.

Diagnosis and Treatment. Laboratory findings usually reveal an elevated white blood cell count. Urinalysis and urine culture are important in the diagnosis of epididymitis, with bacteriuria and pyuria suggestive of the disorder; however, the urinalysis may be normal. If the diagnosis remains uncertain, color Doppler ultrasonography may be useful, revealing increased blood flow to the affected testis.

The treatment of epididymitis focuses on treating the cause of the infection while reducing adverse symptoms.[28] Empiric antibiotic therapy is indicated before laboratory test results are available. The goals of treatment of acute epididymitis caused by *C. trachomatis* or *N. gonorrhoeae* include curing the infection, limiting signs and symptoms, preventing transmission, and decreasing the potential for complications such as infertility or chronic pain.[29] Bed rest, scrotal elevation, and nonsteroidal anti-inflammatory drugs are recommended until fever and local inflammation have decreased. Complete resolution of discomfort varies and may take weeks after the antibiotic regimen is completed.[28]

Patients should be instructed to return to their health care providers if their symptoms fail to improve within 48 hours of the initiation of treatment.[29] Signs and symptoms of epididymitis that do not subside within 3 days require reevaluation of the diagnosis and therapy.

Men who have acute epididymitis that is confirmed or suspected of being caused by *N. gonorrhoeae* or *C. trachomatis* should be instructed to refer sex partners for evaluation and treatment if contact was within the 60 days preceding onset of their own symptoms.[29] Sexual intercourse should be avoided until antibiotic therapy is completed and the person being treated no longer has any signs or symptoms.

Orchitis

Orchitis involves acute inflammation of the testis secondary to infection. The majority of cases are associated with a viral mumps infection; however, other viruses and bacteria can cause orchitis. The primary infection can be in the genitourinary tract (cystitis, urethritis, prostatitis) and then travel to the epididymis and testis through the vas deferens or the lymphatics of the spermatic cord.[1] Orchitis can develop as a complication of a systematic infection such as mumps, scarlet fever, or pneumonia. Clinical examination of people with orchitis includes enlarged testis, tenderness, scrotal skin erythema, edema of the scrotum, and induration of the testes. If these signs and symptoms are accompanied by an enlarged epididymis, this is concern for epididymo-orchitis. In sexually active males, urethral cultures and Gram stain should be obtained for *C. trachomatis* and *N. gonorrhoeae*. Urinalysis and urine culture should also be obtained. Supportive treatment includes bed rest, hot or cold packs for analgesia, and scrotal elevation. Symptoms of isolated orchitis usually resolve spontaneously in approximately 3 to 10 days, whereas epididymitis will usually resolve in a similar time frame after initiation of antibiotic treatment. Spermatogenesis is irreversibly impaired in approximately 30% of testes damaged by mumps orchitis.

Neoplasms

Tumors can develop in the scrotum or the testes. Benign scrotal tumors are common and often do not require treatment. Carcinoma of the scrotum is rare and is usually associated with exposure to carcinogenic agents. Almost all solid tumors of the testes are malignant.

Scrotal Cancer

Cancer of the scrotum is linked to exposure to tar, soot, and oils.[2] Most squamous cell cancers of the scrotum are linked to poor hygiene and chronic inflammation. Exposure to photochemotherapy or HPV has also been associated with the disease. The mean age of presentation with the disease is 60 years, often preceded by 20 to 30 years of chronic irritation.

In the early stages, cancer of the scrotum may appear as a small tumor or wartlike growth that eventually ulcerates. The thin scrotal wall lacks the tissue reactivity needed to block the malignant process; more than one half of the cases seen involve metastasis to the lymph nodes. Because this tumor does not respond well to chemotherapy or irradiation, the treatment is generally surgery. Prognosis correlates with lymph node involvement.

Testicular Cancer

Testicular cancer accounts for 1% of all male cancers.[2] It is relatively rare. However, testicular cancer is the most common cancer in young men between 15 and 35 years of age. The incidence of testicular tumors has doubled in the past 40 years. The 5-year survival rate exceeds 95%, and after treatment, most survivors can expect a near-normal life expectancy.[30]

Etiology and Pathogenesis. Although the cause of testicular cancer is unknown, there is a possible genetic link and a geographic risk to acquiring this type of cancer.[2] The risk factors include cryptorchidism, genetic factors, and disorders of testicular development.[2] The strongest association has been with cryptorchid testis. Genetic predisposition also appears to be important. Family clustering of the disorder has been described, although a well-defined pattern of inheritance has not been established. An increased incidence of testicular germ cell tumors, particularly seminomas, has been described in human immunodeficiency virus–infected men. Males with disorders of testicular development, including those with Klinefelter syndrome and testicular feminization, have a higher risk of germ cell tumors.

Approximately 90% of malignant tumors arising in the testis are germ cell tumors.[2] Germ cell tumors can be classified as seminomas and nonseminomas based on their origin in primordial germ cells and their ability to differentiate in vivo. Because these tumors derive from germ cells in the testis, they are multipotential (able to differentiate into different tissue types) and often secrete polypeptide hormones or enzymes representing earlier stages of development.

Seminomas account for approximately 40% of germ cell tumors and are most frequent in the fourth decade of life.[2] Seminomas are thought to arise from the seminiferous epithelium of the testes and are the type of germ cell tumor most likely to produce a uniform population of cells.

The nonseminoma tumors include embryonal carcinoma, teratoma, choriocarcinoma, and yolk cell carcinoma derivatives. Nonseminoma tumors usually contain more than one cell type and are less differentiated than seminomas. Embryonal carcinomas are the least differentiated of the tumors, with the totipotential capacity to differentiate into other nonseminomatous cell types. Choriocarcinoma is a rare and highly malignant form of testicular cancer that is identical to tumors that arise in placental tissue. Yolk sac tumors mimic the embryonic yolk sac histologically. Teratomas are composed of somatic cell types from two or more germ-line layers (ectoderm, mesoderm, or endoderm). They are usually benign tumors in children. In adults, they can contain minute foci of cancer cells.

Clinical Manifestations and Diagnosis. Often the first sign of testicular cancer is a slight enlargement of the testicle that may be accompanied by some degree of discomfort. This may be an ache in the abdomen or groin or a sensation of dragging or heaviness in the scrotum.[27] Testicular cancer can spread when the tumor may be barely palpable. Signs of metastatic spread include swelling of the lower extremities, back pain, neck mass, cough, hemoptysis, or dizziness.

The diagnosis of testicular cancer requires a thorough urologic history and physical examination. A painless testicular mass may be cancer. Conditions that produce an intrascrotal mass similar to testicular cancer include epididymitis, orchitis, hydrocele, or hematocele. The examination for masses should include palpation of the testes and surrounding structures, transillumination of the scrotum, and abdominal palpation. Testicular ultrasonography can be used to differentiate testicular masses. CT scans and MRI are used in assessing metastatic spread.

Tumor markers that measure protein antigens produced by malignant cells provide information about the existence of a tumor and the type of tumor present. These markers may detect tumor cells that are too small to be found on physical examination or radiographs. Two tumor markers are useful in evaluating the tumor response to therapy: α-fetoprotein, a glycoprotein that is normally present in fetal serum in large amounts and beta-human chorionic gonadotropin (beta-hCG), a hormone that is normally produced by the placenta in pregnant women.[31] During embryonic development, the totipotential germ cells of the testes travel down normal differentiation pathways and produce different protein products. The reappearance of these protein markers in the adult suggests activity of undifferentiated cells in a testicular germ cell tumor.

The clinical staging (TNM classification) for testicular cancer is as follows: stage I, tumor confined to testes, epididymis, or spermatic cord; stage II, tumor spread to retroperitoneal lymph nodes below the diaphragm; and stage III, metastases outside the retroperitoneal nodes or above the diaphragm.[9] Staging procedures include CT scans of the chest, abdomen, and pelvis; ultrasonography for detection of bulky inferior nodal metastases; and occasionally lymphangiography.

Treatment. The basic treatment of all testicular cancers includes orchiectomy, which is done at the time of diagnostic exploration. Surgical therapy is advantageous because it enables precise staging of the disease. Recommendations for further therapy (*e.g.*, retroperitoneal lymph node dissection, chemotherapy, radiation therapy) are based on the pathologic findings from the surgical procedure.

Treatment after orchiectomy depends on the histologic characteristics of the tumor and the clinical stage of the disease. Testicular cancer is very responsive to treatment. The NCCN practice census guidelines for testicular cancer are used to guide treatment and follow-up.[32] Therapy for testicular cancer can have potentially adverse effects on sexual functioning. Males who have retroperitoneal lymph node dissection may experience retrograde ejaculation or failure to ejaculate because of severing of the sympathetic plexus. Infertility may result from retrograde ejaculation or the toxic effects of chemotherapy or radiation therapy. Sperm banking should be considered for males undergoing these treatments.

IN SUMMARY

The prostate is a firm, glandular structure that surrounds the urethra. Inflammation of the prostate occurs as an acute or a chronic process. Chronic prostatitis probably is the most common cause of relapsing urinary tract infections in men. BPH is a common disorder in males older than 50 years of age. Because the prostate encircles the urethra, BPH exerts its effect through obstruction of urinary outflow from the bladder. Treatment of BPH include laser and robotic surgery, prostatic stents, and pharmacologic treatment using 5α-reductase inhibitors such as finasteride, which reduce prostate size by blocking the effects of androgen on the prostate, and α_1-adrenergic receptor blockers, which inhibit contraction of prostatic smooth muscle.

DISORDERS OF THE PROSTATE

After completing this section of the chapter, the learner will be able to meet the following objectives:

- Compare the pathology and symptoms of acute bacterial prostatitis, chronic bacterial prostatitis, and chronic prostatitis/pelvic pain syndrome.
- Describe the urologic manifestations and treatment of benign prostatic hyperplasia.

The prostate is a firm, glandular structure that surrounds the urethra. It produces a thin, milky, alkaline secretion that aids sperm motility by helping to maintain an optimum pH. The contraction of the smooth muscle in the gland promotes semen expulsion during ejaculation.

Infection and Inflammation

Prostatitis refers to a variety of inflammatory disorders of the prostate gland, some bacterial and some not. It may occur spontaneously, as a result of catheterization or instrumentation, or secondary to other diseases of the male genitourinary system. There are four categories of prostatitis syndromes: acute bacterial prostatitis, chronic bacterial prostatitis, chronic prostatitis/pelvic pain syndrome, and asymptomatic inflammatory prostatitis.[15,17,20–22,33–35] Males with asymptomatic inflammatory prostatitis have no subjective symptoms, and the disorder is detected incidentally on biopsy or examination of prostatic fluid.

Acute Bacterial Prostatitis

Acute bacterial prostatitis is an acute infection of the prostate gland that results in pelvic pain and urinary tract symptoms, such as dysuria, urinary frequency, and urinary retention, and may lead to systemic symptoms, such as fevers, chills, nausea, emesis, and malaise.[36] Acute bacterial prostatitis is estimated to comprise approximately 10% of all cases of prostatitis, and its incidence peaks in persons 20 to 40 years of age and in persons older than 70 years.[36] Most cases of acute bacterial prostatitis are caused by ascending urethral infection or intraprostatic reflux and are facilitated by numerous risk factors including benign prostate hyperplasia, genitourinary infections, history of sexually transmitted diseases, and being immunocompromised (*e.g.*, having human immunodeficiency virus). These infections may occur from direct inoculation after transrectal prostate biopsy and transurethral manipulations (*e.g.*, catheterization and cystoscopy).[36] Direct or lymphatic spread from the rectum, or hematogenous spread via bacterial sepsis, can cause acute bacterial prostatitis.[37] Community-acquired infections are three times more common than hospital-acquired infections. Acute bacterial prostatitis is most frequently caused by *E. coli*, followed by *P. aeruginosa*, and *Klebsiella, Enterococcus, Enterobacter, Proteus*, and *Serratia* species.[36] In sexually active men, *N. gonorrhoeae* and *C. trachomatis* should be considered.[38] People who are immunocompromised are more likely to have uncommon causes of prostatitis, such as *Salmonella, Candida* and *Cryptococcus* species.[36]

People with acute bacterial prostatitis often present with rapid onset of irritative or obstructive voiding symptoms. Whereas irritative symptoms include dysuria, urinary frequency, and urinary urgency, examples of obstructive voiding symptoms are hesitancy, incomplete voiding, straining to urinate, and weak stream. People may report suprapubic, rectal, or perineal pain.[36] Painful ejaculation, hematospermia, and painful defecation may be present. Systemic symptoms—such as fever, chills, nausea, emesis, and malaise—commonly occur, and their presence should prompt physicians to determine if the patient meets the clinical criteria for sepsis.

The physical examination should include an abdominal examination to detect a distended bladder and costovertebral angle tenderness, a genital examination, and a digital rectal examination. A digital rectal examination should be performed gently because vigorous prostatic massage can induce bacteremia and subsequently sepsis.[36] Urine may be cloudy and malodorous because of urinary tract infection. Rectal examination reveals a swollen, tender, warm prostate with scattered soft areas. Prostatic massage produces a thick discharge with white blood cells that grows large numbers of pathogens on culture. The prostate will often be tender, enlarged, or boggy. Because acute prostatitis is often associated with anatomic abnormalities, a thorough urologic examination is usually performed after treatment is completed. If there is concern for obstructed voiding, postvoid residual urine volumes should be measured using ultrasonography.

Treatment of acute bacterial prostatitis depends on the severity of symptoms. It usually includes antibiotics, bed rest, adequate hydration, antipyretics, analgesics (preferably nonsteroidal anti-inflammatory drugs) to alleviate pain, and stool softeners. Acute prostatitis usually responds to appropriate antimicrobial therapy chosen in accordance with the sensitivity of the causative agents in the urethral discharge. Depending on the urine culture results, antibiotic therapy is usually continued for at least 4 weeks. Males who are extremely ill, such as those with sepsis, may require hospitalization. A suprapubic catheter may be indicated if voiding is difficult or painful.

Chronic Bacterial Prostatitis

In contrast to acute bacterial prostatitis, chronic bacterial prostatitis is a subtle disorder that is difficult to treat. Chronic bacterial prostatitis is most often caused by *E. coli* or other gram-negative Enterobacteriaceae and typically affects males 36 to 50 years of age. After an episode of acute bacterial prostatitis, approximately 5% of patients may progress to chronic bacterial prostatitis.[39] Patients may present with a history of relapsing urinary tract infections, which may be episodic or persistent. The urinary tract infections are typically not associated with systemic signs of infection. Other irritative or obstructive urologic symptoms may also be present. Analysis of urine specimens and prostatic fluid is used to confirm the diagnosis. Presenting complaints vary from person to person and may include any of the following: dysuria, urinary urgency and frequency, urinary hesitancy or retention, hematuria, malodorous urine, and urethral discharge. Between episodes of acute infections, some patients are asymptomatic, whereas others may describe a long history of persistent symptoms. Fevers and chills are uncommon; they are typically seen only with acute bacterial prostatitis. The main diagnostic criterion for chronic bacterial prostatitis is positive bacterial cultures of prostatic fluid. There is also often leukocytosis in prostatic fluid, which represents prostatic inflammation but is not specific to chronic bacterial prostatitis.

Even after a diagnosis has been established, treatment of chronic prostatitis is often difficult. Unlike their action in the acutely inflamed prostate, antibacterial drugs penetrate poorly into the chronically inflamed prostate. Long-term therapy (3 to 4 months) with an appropriate low-dose oral antimicrobial agent is often used to treat the infection.[39] Transurethral prostatectomy (TURP) has been used to treat males with refractory disease.

Chronic Prostatitis/Chronic Pelvic Pain Syndrome

Chronic prostatitis/pelvic pain syndrome is both the most common and least understood of the prostatitis syndromes.[39]

Inflammatory Prostatitis. A large group of males with prostatitis have no bacteria in the urinary system, but yet have pain along the penis, testicles, and scrotum; painful ejaculation; low back pain; rectal pain along the inner thighs; urinary symptoms; decreased libido; and ED. Males with nonbacterial prostatitis often have inflammation of the prostate with an elevated leukocyte count and abnormal inflammatory cells in their prostatic secretions. The cause of the disorder is unknown, and efforts to prove the presence of unusual pathogens (*e.g.*, mycoplasmas, *Chlamydia*, trichomonads, viruses) have been largely unsuccessful.

Noninflammatory Prostatitis. Men with noninflammatory prostatitis or prostatodynia have symptoms resembling those of nonbacterial prostatitis but have negative urine culture results and no evidence of prostatic inflammation (*i.e.*, normal leukocyte count). The cause of noninflammatory prostatitis is unknown, but because of the absence of inflammation, the search for the cause of symptoms has been directed toward extraprostatic sources. In some cases, there is an apparent functional obstruction of the bladder neck near the external urethral sphincter. During voiding this results in higher-than-normal pressures in the prostatic urethra that cause intraprostatic urine reflux and chemical irritation of the prostate by urine. In other cases, there is an apparent myalgia (*i.e.*, muscle pain) associated with prolonged tension of the pelvic floor muscles.

Treatment. Treatment methods for chronic prostatitis/pelvic pain syndrome are highly variable and require further study. If the person's urinalysis is normal, the health care provider performs a rectal examination with prostatic massage and evaluation of the expressed prostate fluid.[40] If inflammation is present (≥10 leukocytes per high-power field), a trial of antibiotics is prescribed along with instructions to ejaculate every 3 days.[41] If the prostate fluid culture results are negative for leukocytes, then the same treatment plan is applied with the exception of the antibiotics.[41] Treatment is often directed toward symptom control. Sitz baths and nonsteroidal anti-inflammatory drugs may provide some symptom relief. In males with irritative urination symptoms, anticholinergic agents (*e.g.*, oxybutynin) or α-adrenergic blocking agents may be beneficial.

Hyperplasia and Neoplasms

Benign Prostatic Hyperplasia

Benign prostatic hyperplasia (BPH) is a condition in males in which the prostate gland is enlarged but is not cancerous (Fig. 43.8).[42] BPH is also called benign prostatic hypertrophy or benign prostatic obstruction. The prostate goes through two growth periods during a man's life. The first is early in puberty when the prostate doubles in size.[42] The second phase of growth begins at age 25 and continues during the remainder of a man's life. During the second growth phase, as the prostate enlarges, the gland impinges on the urethra, obstructing urine flow. The bladder wall thickens, and eventually the bladder may weaken and lose the ability to empty completely, leaving some urine in the bladder.[42] The narrowing of the urethra and subsequent urinary retention are associated with many of the signs and symptoms of BPH (*e.g.*, trouble starting urination, an interrupted urine stream, nocturia). BPH is characterized by the formation of large, discrete lesions in the periurethral region of the prostate rather than the peripheral zones, which

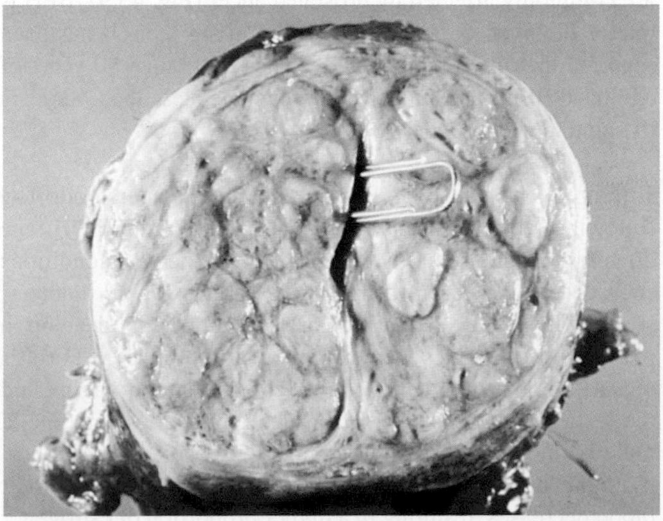

Figure 43.8 • Nodular hyperplasia of the prostate. Cut surface of a prostate enlarged by nodular hyperplasia shows numerous, well-circumscribed nodules of prostatic tissue. The prostatic urethra (*paper clip*) has been compressed to a narrow slit. (From Rubin R., Strayer D. S. (Eds.) (2015). *Rubin's pathology: Clinicopathologic foundations of medicine* (7th ed., p. 989). Philadelphia, PA: Lippincott Williams & Wilkins.)

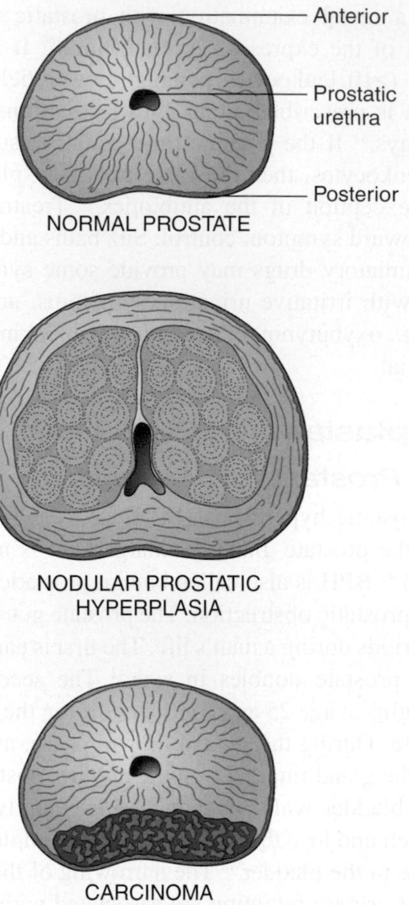

Figure 43.9 • Normal prostate, nodular benign prostatic hypertrophy, and cancer of the prostate. (From Rubin R., Strayer D. S. (Eds.) (2015). *Rubin's pathology: Clinicopathologic foundations of medicine* (7th ed., p. 989). Philadelphia, PA: Lippincott Williams & Wilkins.)

are commonly affected by prostate cancer (Fig. 43.9). BPH is one of the most common diseases of aging men. It has been reported that more than 75% of males older than 80 years of age have BPH.[2] It is uncommon for males less than 40 years of age to develop BPH.

Etiology. The cause of BPH is not well understood. The following factors put males at risk for developing BPH: age 40 years and older; family history of BPH; medical conditions such as obesity, cardiovascular disease, and type 2 diabetes; lack of physical exercise; and ED.[42] BPH does not develop in males whose testicles were removed before puberty. For this reason, some researchers believe factors related to aging and the testicles may cause BPH. Males produce testosterone, a male hormone, and small amounts of estrogen, a female hormone. As males age, the amount of active testosterone in their blood decreases, resulting in a higher proportion of estrogen.[42] Studies have suggested that BPH is a result of this higher proportion of estrogen promoting prostate growth.

Another theory of BPH focuses on dihydrotestosterone (DHT), a male hormone involved in prostate development and growth.[42] DHT research suggests that even with the decline in blood testosterone levels associated with aging, males continue to produce and accumulate high levels of DHT in the prostate. This accumulation of DHT may be responsible for continued prostate growth. In alignment with this theory of BPH, researchers have noted that males who do not produce DHT do not develop BPH. The drug class 5α-reductase inhibitors (*e.g.*, finasteride, dutasteride) has been used to treat BPH. The enzyme 5α-reductase is involved in the metabolic transformation of a number of endogenous steroids. 5α-reductase inhibitors prevent the conversion of testosterone into the more potent DHT.

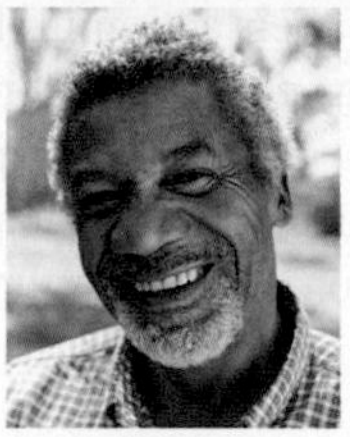

Remember Mr. Topers from the unit-opening case study? Mr. Topers had BPH for approximately 5 years and was just diagnosed with prostate cancer with a Gleason Score of Stage 3. He had risk factors for BPH, including the fact that he is an African American, he has a high BMI (still does at 26), and he is older at 57 years of age.

Pathophysiology and Clinical Manifestations. The anatomic location of the prostate at the bladder neck contributes to the pathophysiology and symptomatology of BPH. There are two prostatic components to the obstructive properties of BPH and development of lower urinary tract symptoms: dynamic and static.[43] The static component of BPH is related to an increase in prostatic size and gives rise to symptoms such as a weak urinary stream, postvoid dribbling, frequency of urination, and nocturia. The dynamic component of BPH is related to prostatic smooth muscle tone. The α_1-adrenergic receptors are the main receptors for the smooth muscle component of the prostate. The recognition of the role of α_1-adrenergic receptors on neuromuscular function in the prostate is the basis for use of α_1-adrenergic receptor blockers in treating BPH. A third component, detrusor instability and impaired bladder contractility, may contribute to the symptoms of BPH independent of the outlet obstruction created by an enlarged prostate.[43]

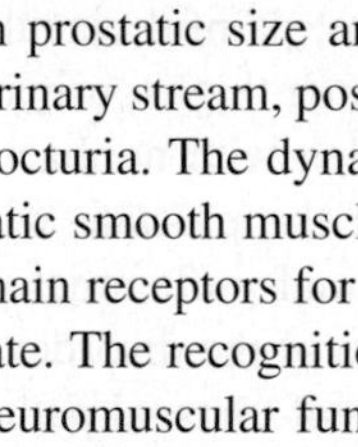

Mr. Topers did experience both the dynamic and static symptoms of postvoid dribbling, frequency of urination, and nocturia, and the dynamic symptoms related to decreased prostatic smooth muscle tone. He was also taking α_1-adrenergic receptor blockers to treat the BPH. Mr. Topers experienced the majority of these symptoms as his prostate gland increased in size and compressed the urethra to cause a partial obstruction of the urine flow. In fact, his urine flow was so compromised that his uroflow test revealed a less than 7 mL/second flow.

Lower urinary tract symptoms suggestive of BPH may include urinary frequency (urination eight or more times a day); urinary urgency (the inability to delay urination; trouble starting a urine stream; a weak or an interrupted urine stream); dribbling at the end of urination; nocturia (frequent urination during periods of sleep); urinary retention; urinary incontinence (the accidental loss of urine); pain after ejaculation or during urination; urine that has an unusual color or smell.[42] Symptoms of BPH most often come from a blocked urethra or a bladder that is overworked from trying to pass urine through the blockage. The size of the prostate does not always determine the degree of the blockage or symptoms.[42] Some males with greatly enlarged prostates have little blockage and few symptoms, whereas other males who have minimally enlarged prostates have greater blockage and more symptoms. Less than half of all males with BPH have lower urinary tract symptoms.[42] Sometimes, males may not know they have a blockage until they cannot urinate at all, a condition called acute urinary retention. This situation can arise from taking over-the-counter cold or allergy medications that contain decongestants, such as pseudoephedrine and oxymetazoline.[42] These medications may prevent the bladder neck from relaxing and allowing urination. Antihistamines such as diphenhydramine can weaken the force of contraction of bladder muscles and cause urinary retention, difficulty urinating, and painful urination. When males have some degree of urethral blockage, urinary retention also can occur as a result of alcohol consumption, cold temperatures, or a long period of inactivity.

Diagnosis. It is now thought that the single most important factor in the evaluation and treatment of BPH is the man's own experiences related to the disorder. The American Urological Association Symptom Index (AUASI) consists of seven questions about symptoms regarding incomplete emptying, frequency, intermittency, urgency, weak stream, straining, and nocturia.[10] Each question is rated with a score of 0 (mild) to 7 (severe). A maximum score of 35 indicates severe symptoms. Total scores below 7 are considered mild; those between 8 and 20 moderate; and scores over 20 severe. A final question relates to quality of life due to urinary problems.

A health care provider may refer males to a urologist, or the health care provider may diagnose BPH on the basis of symptoms and a digital rectal exam. A urologist uses medical tests to help diagnose lower urinary tract problems related to BPH. These tests may include urinalysis, a prostate-specific antigen (PSA) blood test, urodynamic tests (*i.e.*, tests for urine flow), cystoscopy, transrectal ultrasound, and biopsy. PSA is a glycoprotein secreted into the cytoplasm of benign and malignant prostatic cells that is not found in other normal tissues or tumors.

Blood and urine analyses are used as adjuncts to determine BPH complications (*e.g.*, kidney damage, bladder stones, urinary tract infections). Urinalysis is done to detect bacteria, leukocytes, or microscopic hematuria in the presence of infection and inflammation. The PSA test is used to screen for prostate cancer. These evaluation measures, along with the AUASI, are used to describe the extent of obstruction and to determine if other diagnostic tests and/or treatment are needed.

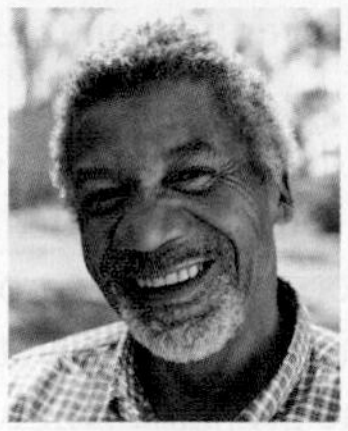

Mr. Topers' International Prostate Symptom Score (IPSS) has increased from between 1 and 2 to 6. He explains that the increased symptoms have negatively influenced his quality of life. His PSA has also had a significant spike from 7 to 12 ng/mL within the last 6 months. Just having an increase in PSA does not warrant a cancer diagnosis by any means, but his digital rectal exam (DRE) showed an increase in prostate size to +3 to +4. Mr. Topers expressed the fear that he may have prostate cancer.

The digital rectal examination is used to examine the external surface of the prostate. Enlargement of the prostate due to BPH usually produces a large, palpable prostate with a smooth, rubbery surface. Hardened areas of the prostate gland suggest cancer and should be sampled for biopsy.

Residual urine measurement may be made by ultrasonography or postvoiding catheterization for residual urine volume. Uroflowmetry provides an objective measure of urine flow rate. The patient is asked to void with a relatively full bladder (at least 150 mL) into a device that electronically measures the force of the stream and urine flow rate. A urinary flow rate of greater than 15 mL/second is considered normal, and less than 10 mL/second is indicative of obstruction.[42]

Transabdominal or transrectal diagnostic ultrasonography can be used to evaluate the kidneys, ureters, and bladder. Urethrocystoscopy is indicated in males with a history of hematuria, stricture disease, urethral injury, or prior lower urinary tract surgery. It is used to evaluate the length and diameter of the urethra, the size and configuration of the prostate, and bladder capacity. CT scans, MRI studies, and radionuclide scans are reserved for rare instances of tumor detection.

Treatment. Until the 1980s, surgery was the mainstay of treatment to alleviate urinary obstruction due to BPH. Currently, there is an emphasis on less invasive methods of treatment, including use of pharmacologic agents. However, when more severe signs of obstruction develop, surgical treatment is indicated to provide comfort and avoid serious kidney damage.

Treatment options for BPH may include lifestyle changes, medications, minimally invasive procedures, and surgery. A health care provider recommends treatment of BPH based on symptom severity, impact on daily life, and personal preferences.[42] Males may not need treatment for a mildly enlarged prostate unless their symptoms are bothersome and affecting their quality of life. In these cases, instead of treatment, a urologist may recommend regular follow-up examinations. Treatment may be recommended if BPH symptoms impact quality of life or present a health risk.[42] Lifestyle changes are often proposed for males whose symptoms are mild. These changes can include reducing liquid intake, especially before sleep; avoiding or reducing intake of caffeinated beverages and alcohol; avoiding or monitoring the use of medications such as decongestants, antihistamines, antidepressants, and diuretics; training the bladder to hold more urine for longer periods; exercising pelvic floor muscles; preventing or treating constipation.[42]

Pharmacologic management includes the use of 5α-reductase inhibitors and α_1-adrenergic blocking drugs.[43] The 5α-reductase inhibitors such as finasteride reduce prostate size by blocking the effect of androgens on the prostate. The presence of α-adrenergic receptors in the prostatic smooth muscle has prompted the use of α_1-adrenergic blocking drugs (*e.g.*, terazosin [Hytrin], doxazosin [Cardura], and tamsulosin [Flomax]) to relieve prostatic obstruction and increase urine flow. Tadalafil (Cialis) is part of the PDE5 inhibitors class of medications that can reduce lower urinary tract symptoms by relaxing smooth muscles in the lower urinary tract. Several studies, such as the Medical Therapy of Prostatic Symptoms (MTOPS) study, have shown that combining two classes of medications instead of using just one can more effectively improve symptoms, urinary flow, and quality of life.

The surgical removal of an enlarged prostate can be accomplished by the transurethral, suprapubic, or perineal approach. Currently, TURP is the most commonly used technique.[43] With this approach, an instrument is introduced through the urethra, and prostate tissue is removed using a resectoscope and electrocautery. Immediate complications of TURP include the inability to urinate, postoperative hemorrhage or clot retention, and urinary tract infection. Late complications of TURP include ED, incontinence, and bladder neck contractures. Retrograde ejaculation is another problem that may occur because of resection of bladder neck tissue.

Many new and experimental techniques have also been used to treat BPH (*e.g.*, transurethral incision of the prostate [TUIP], laser surgery, transurethral vaporization, transurethral microwave therapy, transurethral needle ablation), and each has advantages and disadvantages when considered as an alternative treatment of BPH.

For males who have heart or lung disease or a condition that precludes major surgery, a stent may be used to widen and maintain the patency of the urethra. A stent is a device made of a tubular mesh that is inserted under local or regional anesthesia. Within several months, the lining of the urethra grows to cover the inside of the stent.

KEY POINTS

HYPERPLASIA AND CANCER OF THE PROSTATE

- The prostate gland surrounds the urethra and periurethral enlargement causes manifestations of urinary obstruction.
- BPH is an age-related enlargement of the prostate gland with formation of large, discrete lesions in the periurethral region of the prostate. These lesions compress the urethra and produce symptoms of dysuria or difficulty urinating.

Prostate Cancer

Prostate cancer is the most common nonskin cancer in the United States and is third to lung and colorectal cancer as a cause of cancer-related death in US men.[43] The American Cancer Society estimates that during 2017, approximately 161,360 males in the United States will be diagnosed with prostate cancer, and 26,730 males will die from prostate cancer.[35] The increase in diagnosed cases is thought to reflect earlier diagnosis because of the widespread use of PSA testing. The incidence of prostate cancer varies markedly from country to country and varies among races in the same country.[35] African American and Caribbean males have the highest reported incidence for prostate cancer at all ages.[35] Asians and Native American males have the lowest rate.[35] Prostate cancer is also a disease of aging. The incidence increases rapidly after 50 years of age. In fact, more than 85% of all prostate cancers are diagnosed in males older than 65 years of age.[35]

Etiology and Pathophysiology. The precise cause of prostate cancer is unclear. As with other cancers, it appears that the development of prostate cancer is a multistep process involving genes that control cell differentiation and growth.[35] Several risk factors, such as age, race, heredity, and environmental influences (*e.g.*, a high-fat diet), are suspected of playing a role.[35] Male hormone levels also play a role. There is insufficient evidence linking socioeconomic status, infectious agents, smoking, vasectomy, sexual behavior, or BPH to the pathogenesis of prostate cancer.[35]

The incidence of prostate cancer appears to be higher in relatives of males with prostate cancer. It has been estimated that males who have an affected first-degree relative (*e.g.*, father, brother) and an affected second-degree relative (*e.g.*, grandfather, uncle) have an eightfold increase in risk.[35] It has been suggested that dietary patterns, including increased dietary fats from processed meats and dairy items, may alter the production of sex hormones and growth factors and increase the risk of prostate cancer.[35] Supporting the role of dietary fats as a risk factor for prostate cancer has been the observation that the diet of Japanese men, who have a low rate of prostate cancer, is much lower in fat content than that of US men, who have a much higher incidence.

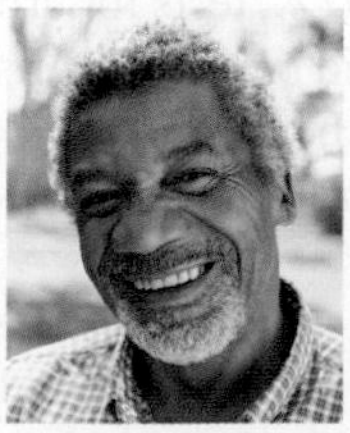

Mr. Topers has a significant risk for prostate cancer given his family history, his obesity, and his history of cigarette smoking.

In terms of hormonal influence, androgens are believed to play a role in the pathogenesis of prostate cancer.[36] Evidence favoring a hormonal influence includes the presence of steroid receptors in the prostate, the requirement of sex hormones for normal growth and development of the prostate, and the fact that prostate cancer almost never develops in males who have been castrated.[36] The response of prostate cancer to estrogen administration or androgen deprivation further supports a correlation between the disease and testosterone levels.

Prostatic adenocarcinomas, which account for 98% of all primary prostate cancers, are commonly multicentric and located in the peripheral zones of the prostate (see Fig. 43.8).[9] The high frequency of invasion of the prostatic capsule by adenocarcinoma relates to its subcapsular location. Invasion of the urinary bladder is less frequent and occurs later in the clinical course. Metastasis to the lung reflects lymphatic spread through the thoracic duct and dissemination from the prostatic venous plexus to the inferior vena cava. Bony metastases, particularly to the vertebral column, ribs, and pelvis, produce pain that often presents as a first sign of the disease.

Most males with early-stage prostate cancer are asymptomatic. The presence of symptoms often suggests locally advanced or metastatic disease. Depending on the size and location of prostate cancer at the time of diagnosis, there may be changes associated with the voiding pattern similar to those found in BPH. These include urgency, frequency, nocturia, hesitancy, dysuria, hematuria, or blood in the ejaculate. On digital rectal examination, the prostate can be nodular and fixed. Bone metastasis is often characterized by low back pain. Pathologic fractures can occur at the site of metastasis. Males with metastatic disease may experience weight loss, anemia, or shortness of breath.

Screening. Because early cancers of the prostate usually are asymptomatic, screening tests are important.[36] The screening tests currently available are digital rectal examination, PSA testing, and transrectal ultrasonography. However, a positive PSA test indicates only the possible presence of prostate cancer. It can also be positive in cases of BPH and prostatitis. In fact, every man who has an elevated PSA will not necessarily have prostate cancer nor will every man with a known prostate cancer diagnosis by biopsy have an elevated PSA. Measures to increase the specificity of PSA testing in terms of predicting prostate cancer are being developed and evaluated. For example, because PSA levels increase with age, age-specific ranges have been established.[36] PSA velocity (a change of PSA level over time) and PSA density (*i.e.*, PSA level/prostate volume as measured by rectal ultrasonography), kallikreins, and other molecular biomarkers are being studied to ascertain if they will be more effective predictors of indolent versus aggressive prostate cancer.[36]

The American Cancer Society and the American Urological Association recommend that males 50 years of age or older should undergo annual measurement of PSA and digital rectal examination for early detection of prostate cancer.[43] Males at high risk for prostate cancer, such as African Americans and those with a strong family history, should undergo annual screening even at an earlier age.[43] However, some controversy regarding the widespread use of PSA for screening remains. Informed decision-making regarding screening with PSA is warranted.

A new approach, transrectal ultrasonography, may detect cancers that are too small to be detected by physical examination. This method is not used for first-line detection because of its expense, but it may benefit males who are at high risk for development of prostate cancer.

Diagnosis. The diagnosis of prostate cancer is based on history and physical examination and confirmed through biopsy methods. Transrectal ultrasonography is used to guide a biopsy needle and document the exact location of the sampled tissue. It is also used for providing staging information. Newly developed small probes for transrectal MRI have been shown to be effective in detecting the presence of cancer in the prostate. Radiologic examination of the bones of the skull, ribs, spine, and pelvis can be used to reveal metastases, although radionuclide bone scans are more sensitive.

Staging. Cancer of the prostate, like other forms of cancer, is graded and staged. Prostatic adenocarcinoma is commonly classified using the Gleason grading system, which grades on a continuum of aggressiveness of prostate cancer with the lower range of 1 and 2 being less aggressive. As the Gleason score increases, this indicates a higher aggressiveness of the prostate cancer.[35] Primary-stage tumors (T1) are asymptomatic and discovered on histologic examination of prostatic tissue specimens; T2 tumors are palpable on digital examination but are confined to the prostate gland; T3 tumors have extended beyond the prostate; and T4 tumors have pushed beyond the prostate to involve adjacent structures (Fig. 43.10). Regional lymph node (N) and distant metastases (M) are described as Nx or Mx (cannot be assessed), N0 or M0 (not present), and N1 or M1 (present).[37]

PSA levels are important in the staging and management of prostate cancer.[44] In untreated cases, the level of PSA tends to correlate with the volume and stage of disease. A rising PSA after treatment is consistent with progressive disease, whether it is locally recurring or metastatic. Measurement of PSA is used to detect recurrence after total prostatectomy. Because the prostate is the source of PSA, levels should drop to zero after surgery; a rising PSA indicates recurring disease.[44]

Treatment. Cancer of the prostate is treated by surgery, radiation therapy, and hormonal manipulations.[35] Chemotherapy has shown limited effectiveness in the treatment of prostate cancer. For some, high-intensity focused ultrasound is used successfully. Treatment decisions are based on tumor grade and stage and on the age and health of the man.

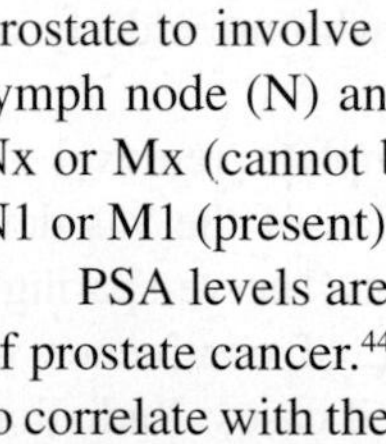

Mr. Topers had a transrectal ultrasound and biopsy that revealed positive prostate cancer with a Gleason Staging Score of 3. This score indicates a relatively early diagnosis, so Mr. Topers has a good prognosis. He does not have metastasis (has a TNM stage of T2) and will undergo surgery, radiation, and hormonal manipulation immediately.

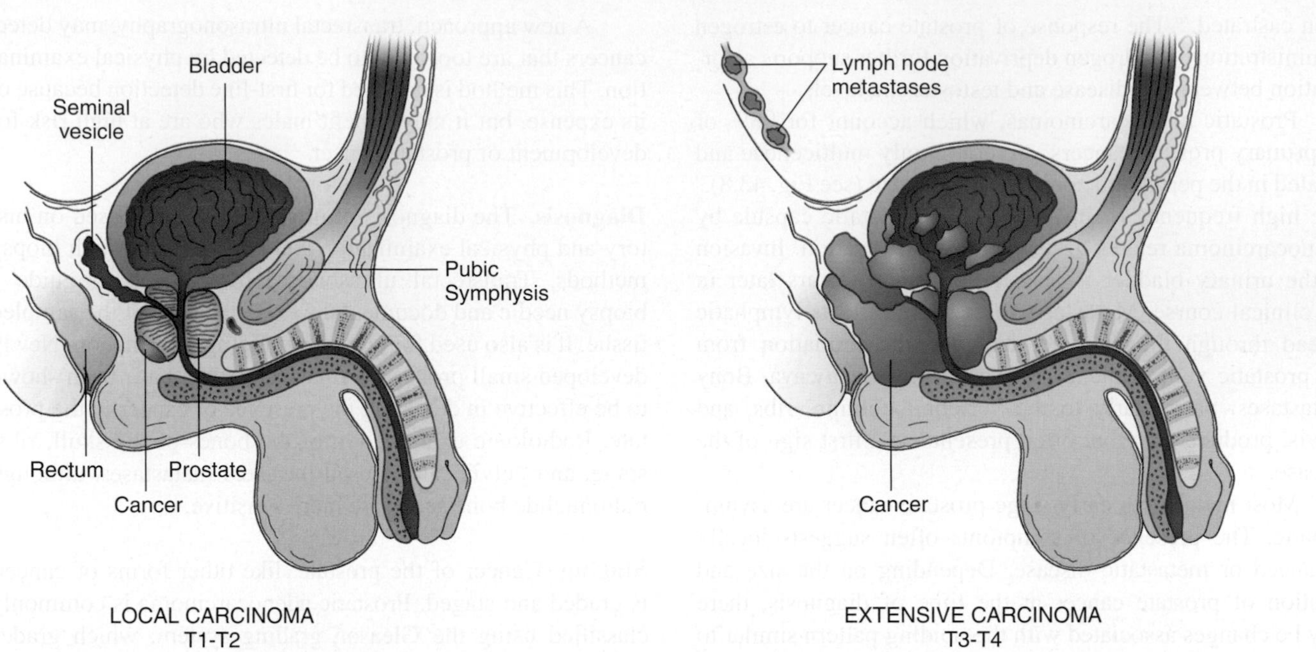

Figure 43.10 • Staging for prostatic carcinoma. Tumor-node-metastasis (TNM) system is most widely used for staging of prostate carcinoma. Stage T1 and T2 are localized to the prostate, whereas stage T3 and T4 tumors have spread outside the prostate. (From Rubin R., Strayer D. S. (Eds.) (2015). *Rubin's pathology: Clinicopathologic foundations of medicine* (7th ed., Fig. 23-47, p. 993). Philadelphia, PA: Wolters Kluwer.)

Expectant therapy (watchful waiting) may be used if the tumor is not producing symptoms, is expected to grow slowly, and is small and contained in one area of the prostate. This approach is particularly suited for males who are elderly or have other health problems.

Radical prostatectomy involves complete removal of the seminal vesicles, prostate, and ampullae of the vas deferens. Refinements in surgical techniques ("nerve-sparing" prostatectomy) have allowed maintenance of continence in most males and erectile function in selected cases. Radiation therapy can be delivered by a variety of techniques, including external-beam radiation therapy and transperineal implantation of radioisotopes (brachytherapy).

Metastatic disease is often treated with androgen deprivation therapy. Androgen deprivation may be induced at several levels along the pituitary–gonadal axis using a variety of methods or agents. Orchiectomy is often effective in reducing symptoms and extending survival. The GnRH analogs (*e.g.*, leuprolide, triptorelin) block LH (and FSH) release from the pituitary and reduce testosterone levels. When given continuously (as opposed to pulsatile, which is the normal physiologic secretory rhythm) and in therapeutic doses, these drugs desensitize GnRH receptors in the pituitary, thereby preventing the release of LH. However, initially, because these agents are GnRH agonists, LH and FSH rise and cause testosterone levels to increase. This can be decreased by pretreatment with antiandrogens. The nonsteroidal antiandrogens (*e.g.*, flutamide, bicalutamide) block the uptake and actions of androgens in the target tissues. Although testosterone is the main circulating androgen, the adrenal gland also secretes androgens. Complete androgen blockade can be achieved by blocking androgens of adrenal origin by combining an antiandrogen with a GnRH agent or orchiectomy. Inhibitors of adrenal androgen synthesis (*i.e.*, ketoconazole and aminoglutethimide) may also be used for treating males with advanced prostate cancer who present with spinal cord compression, bilateral ureteral obstruction, or disseminated intravascular clotting. This is because these males need rapid decreases in their testosterone levels (*i.e.*, ketoconazole can produce chemical castration within 24 hours). Palliative care includes adequate pain control and focal irradiation of symptomatic or unstable bone disease. In males with advanced prostate cancer, the bisphosphonates (*e.g.*, pamidronate, zoledronate), which act mainly by inhibiting osteoclastic activity, have several potential uses in prostate cancer. These include (1) prevention of osteopenia that accompanies the use of androgen deprivation therapy; (2) prevention and delay of skeletal complications (*e.g.*, the need for local radiation treatment, fractures) in patients with metastatic bone involvement; (3) palliation of bone pain; and (4) treatment of hypercalcemia of malignancy.

IN SUMMARY

Disorders of the scrotum and testes include cryptorchidism (*i.e.*, undescended testes), hydrocele, hematocele, spermatocele, varicocele, and testicular torsion. Inflammatory conditions can involve the scrotal sac, epididymis, or testes. Tumors can arise in the scrotum or the testes. Scrotal cancers are usually associated with exposure to petroleum products such as tar, pitch, and soot. Testicular cancers account for 1% of all male cancers. With current treatment methods, a large percentage of males with these tumors can be cured.

Prostate cancer is the most common nonskin cancer in the United States and is third to lung cancer and colon/rectal cancer as a cause of cancer-related death in men. A recent increase in diagnosed cases is thought to reflect earlier diagnosis because of widespread use of PSA testing. The incidence of prostate cancer increases with age and is greater in African American males of all ages. Most prostate cancers are asymptomatic and are incidentally discovered on rectal examination. Screening for prostate cancer has become recognized as a method for early identification of prostate cancer. The American Cancer Society suggests that every man 50 years of age or older should have a digital rectal examination and PSA test done as part of his annual physical examination. Cancer of the prostate, like other forms of cancer, is graded according to the histologic characteristics of the tumor and staged clinically using the TNM system. Treatment, which is based on the extent of the disease, includes surgery, radiation therapy, and hormonal manipulation.

GERIATRIC Considerations

- It is estimated that 25% of men older than 65 have ED[47]; however, when ED is self-reported, it is important to remember that establishing an erection requires more physical stimulation than for younger males and can be lost by a simple noise or interruption.[48]
- In men over age 75, ED has a positive correlation with prostate and urinary problems.[10]
- Testosterone levels decline with increasing age, decreasing libido and sexual function.[47]
- Age is the most important single predictor of overdiagnosis of prostate cancer using PSE screening.[40]
- Testicular tumors are rare in older men and are usually malignant when found.[48]

PEDIATRIC Considerations

- If hypospadias is present, a circumcision may be contraindicated because the foreskin may be used for the reconstructive surgery.[49]
- Children with cryptorchidism should be evaluated on a yearly basis due to the relation of endocrinopathy and malignancy.[49]
- The three types of exstrophy-epispadias (cloacal exstrophy, classic exstrophy, and epispadias) share a mutual precipitating factor: continuance of the cloacal membrane past the point of expected resorption during embryologic development.[49]
- Because children with congenital urologic malformations such as bladder exstrophy are at high risk for the development of latex allergies, use of latex-free products during procedures is recommended.[50]

REVIEW EXERCISES

1. A 64-year-old man presents to his family physician with erectile dysfunction. He is on multiple medications for his "heart disease." An initial physical examination is unremarkable.
   A. *What additional information should be obtained?*
   B. *Given his medical history, what are possible factors contributing to his problem?*
2. A 23-year-old man presents to the emergency department in severe distress. His left testicle is large and tender, and he has pain radiating to the inguinal area.
   A. *What would be a tentative diagnosis for this man?*
   B. *Why would this problem necessitate immediate diagnosis and surgical intervention?*
3. A 72-year-old man had a radical prostatectomy for localized prostate cancer. After surgery, his PSA level was undetectable. He presents 5 years later having been "lost to follow-up." He complains of pain in his hip and lower back. His PSA level is now markedly elevated.
   A. *What initial investigations are warranted?*
   B. *What therapies are available for this complication?*

References

1. Damjanov I., McCue P. A. (2015). The lower urinary tract and male reproductive system. In Strayer D. S., Rubin E. (Eds.), *Rubin's pathology clinicopathologic foundations of medicine* (7th ed., pp. 972–973, 980–981, 993). Philadelphia, PA: Wolters Kluwer.
2. Springer A., Baskin L. (2014). Timing of hypospadias repair in patients with disorders of sex development. *Endocrine Development* 27, 197–202.
3. American Academy of Pediatrics. (2015). Explaining disorders of sex development & intersexuality. Available: https://www.healthychildren.org/English/health-issues/conditions/genitourinary-tract/Pages/Explaining-Disorders-of-Sex-Development-Intersexuality.aspx.
4. Romao R. L., Pippi Salle J. L. (2017). Update on the surgical approach for reconstruction of the male genitalia. *Seminars in Perinatology* 41(4), 218–226. doi:10.1053/j.semperi.2017.03.015.
5. Buttaravoli P., Leffler S. M. (2012). *Minor emergencies* (3rd ed.). Philadelphia, PA: Elsevier Saunders.
6. Pandya I., Shinojia M., Vadukul D., et al. (2014). Approach to balanitis/balanoposthitis: Current guidelines. *Indian Journal of Sexually Transmitted Diseases and AIDS* 35(2), 155–157.
7. Edwards S. K., Bunker C. B., Ziller F., et al. (2014). 2013 European guideline for the management of balanoposthitis. *International Journal of STD & AIDS* 25(9), 615–626.
8. Moore K. L., Dalley A. F., Agur A. M. R. (2018). Pelvis and perineum. In Moore K. L., Dalley A. F., Agur A. M. R. *Clinically orientated anatomy* (8th ed., pp. 650–653). Philadelphia, PA: Wolters Kluwer.
9. Feldman H. A., Goldstein I., Hatzichristou D. G., et al. (1994). Impotence and its medical and psychosocial correlates: Results of the Massachusetts Male Aging Study. *Journal of Urology* 15(1), 54–61.
10. Goroll A. H., Albert G. M. (2014). *Primary care medicine: Office evaluation and management of the adult patient* (7th ed.). Philadelphia, PA: Lippincott Williams & Wilkins.

11. John Hopkins Medicine. (2017). Impotence/Erectile dysfunction. [Online]. Available: http://www.hopkinsmedicine.org/healthlibrary/conditions/kidney_and_urinary_system_disorders/impotenceerectile_dysfunction_85,P01482/. Accessed July 20, 2017.
12. McMahon C. G. (2014). Erectile dysfunction. *Internal Medicine Journal* 44, 18–26.
13. American Heart Association. (2014). About metabolic syndrome. [Online]. Available: http://www.heart.org/HEARTORG/Conditions/More/MetabolicSyndrome/About-Metabolic-Syndrome_UCM_301920_Article.jsp#.WaniEYSpvFI. Accessed July 20, 2017.
14. Ferguson L., Agoulnik A. (2013). Testicular cancer and cryptorchidism. *Frontiers in Endocrinology* 4, 1–9.
15. Erdemir F., Firat F., Markoc F., et al. (2014). *Int Urol Nephrol* 46, 1961. https://doi.org/10.1007/s11255-014-0769-z.
16. National Cancer Institute. (2017). Penile cancer treatment. [Online]. Available: https://www.cancer.gov/types/penile/hp/penile-treatment-pdq. Accessed November 9, 2017.
17. Steinbrecher H. (2014). The undescended testis: Working towards a unified care pathway for 2014. *Archives of Disease in Childhood* 99(5), 397–398.
18. Rodríguez F., Vallejos C., Giraudo F., et al. (2017). Copy number variants of Ras/MAPK pathway genes in patients with isolated cryptorchidism. *Andrology* 5(5), 923. doi:10.1111/andr.12390.
19. Singh R., Hamada A. J., Bukavina L., et al. (2012) Physical deformities relevant to male infertility. *Nature Reviews Urology* 9, 156–174.
20. Bostwick D. G., Cheng L. (2014). *Urologic surgical pathology* (3rd ed.). Philadelphia, PA: Saunders.
21. Kollin C., Granholm T., Nordenskjöld A., et al. (2013). Growth of spontaneously descended and surgically treated testes during early childhood. *Pediatrics* 131(4), e1174–e1180.
22. Penson D., Krishnaswami S., Jules A., et al. (2013). Effectiveness of hormonal and surgical therapies for cryptorchidism: A systematic review. *Pediatrics* 131(6), 1897–1907.
23. Ta A., D'Arcy F. T., Hoag N., et al. (2016). Testicular torsion and the acute scrotum: Current emergency management. *European Journal of Emergency Medicine* 23, 160–165.
24. Barbosa J. A., Denes F. T., Nguyen H. T. (2016). Testicular torsion—Can we improve the management of acute scrotum? *Journal of Urology* 95(6), 1650–1651.
25. Mills S. (2015). Urinary tract and male genital system. In *Sternberg's diagnostic surgical pathology*. Philadelphia, PA: Lippincott Williams & Wilkins.
26. Barthold J. S. (2015). Abnormalities of the testis and scrotum and their surgical management. In McDougal W. S., Kavoussi L. R., Novick A. C., et al., eds. *Campbell-Walsh urology* (11th ed.). Philadelphia, PA: Saunders.
27. Sharp V. J., Kieran K., Arlen A. M. (2013). Testicular torsion: Diagnosis, evaluation, and management. *American Family Physician* 88(12), 835–840.
28. Ghazle H., Bhatt S. (2014). Acute testicular pain. *Journal of the American Osteopathic College of Radiology* 3(4), 25–28.
29. Taylor S. (2015). Epididymitis. *Clinical Infectious Diseases* 61(8), S770–S773.
30. Janssen-Heijnen M., Gondos A., Bray F., et al. (2010). Clinical relevance of conditional survival of cancer patients in Europe: Age-specific analyses of 13 cancers. *Journal of Clinical Oncology* 28(15), 2520–2528. Retrieved from https://doi.org/10.1200/JCO.2009.25.9697.
31. Leman E. S., Gonzalgo M. L. (2010). Prognostic features and markers for testicular cancer management. *Indian Journal of Urology : IJU : Journal of the Urological Society of India* 26(1), 76–81. http://doi.org/10.4103/0970-1591.60450.
32. National Comprehensive Cancer Network (NCCN). (2016). Clinical practice guidelines in oncology: Testicular cancer. Available: www.nccn.org/professionals/default.aspx.
33. Gurney J. K., McGlynn K. A., Stanley J., et al. (2017). Risk factors for cryptorchidism. *Nature Reviews Urology* 14(9), 534–548. doi:10.1038/nrurol.2017.90.
34. Kolon T. F., Herndon C. D., Baker L. A., et al. (2014). Evaluation and treatment of cryptorchidism: AUA guideline. *Journal of Urology* 192(2), 337–345.
35. American Cancer Society. (2017). What are the key statistics about prostate cancer? [Online]. Available: https://www.cancer.org/cancer/prostate-cancer/about/key-statistics.html. Accessed November 9, 2017.
36. Bangma C. H., van Schaik R. H., Blijenberg B. G., et al. (2010). On the use of prostate specific antigen for screening of prostate cancer in European Randomized Study for Screening of Prostate Cancer. *European Journal of Cancer* 46(17), 3109–3119.
37. National Institute of Health Cancer Institute. (2017). Prostate cancer treatment. [Online]. Available: http://www.cancer.gov/cancertopics/pdq/treatment/prostate/HelathProfessionals. Accessed November 9, 2017.
38. Khan F. U., Ihsan A. U., Khan H. U., et al. (2017). Comprehensive overview of prostatitis. *Biomedicine & Pharmacotherapy* 94, 1064–1076.
39. Nickel C. J. (2016). Inflammatory and pain conditions of the male genitourinary tract: Prostatitis and related pain conditions, orchitis, and epididymitis. In *Campbell-Walsh urology* (11th ed.). Philadelphia, PA: Elsevier.
40. Gulati R., Inoue L. Y. T., Gore J. L., Katcher J., et al. (2014). Individualized estimates of overdiagnosis in screen-detected prostate cancer. *JNCI: Journal of the National Cancer Institute* 106(2), djt367, https://doi.org/10.1093/jnci/djt367.
41. Ahuja S. (2016). Nonbacterial prostatitis treatment and management. [Online]. Available: http://emedicine.medscape.com/urology. Accessed July 15, 2017.
42. National Institute of Diabetes and Digestive and Kidney Diseases. (2014). Prostate problems. [Online]. Available: https://www.niddk.nih.gov/health-information/urologic-diseases/prostate-problems/prostate-enlargement-benign-prostatic-hyperplasia. Accessed July 20, 2017.
43. Dunphy L., Winland-Brown J., Porter B., et al. (2012). *Primary care: The art and science of advanced practice nursing*. Philadelphia, PA: FA Davis.
44. American Urological Association. (2013). PSA testing for the pretreatment staging and posttreatment management of prostate cancer. Available: http://www.auanet.org/guidelines/prostate-specific-antigen-(2009-amended-2013). Accessed November 9, 2017.
45. Coker T. J., Dierfeldt D. M. (2016). Acute bacterial prostatitis: Diagnosis and management. *American Family Physician* 93(2), 114–120.
46. Kim S. H., Ha U. S., Yoon B. I., et al. (2014). Microbiological and clinical characteristics in acute bacterial prostatitis according to lower urinary tract manipulation procedure. *Journal of Infection and Chemotherapy* 20(1), 38–42.
47. Jensen S. (2015). *Nursing health assessment*. Philadelphia, PA: Wolters Kluwer.
48. Eliopoulos C. (2018). *Gerontological nursing* (9th ed.). Philadelphia, PA: Wolters Kluwer.
49. Bowden, V. R., Greenberg, C. S. (2014). *Children and their families the continuum of nursing care* (3rd ed.). Philadelphia, PA: Wolters Kluwer.
50. Kyle T., Carman S. (2013). *Essentials of pediatric nursing* (2nd ed.). Philadelphia, PA: Wolters Kluwer.

Structure and Function of the Female Reproductive System

44

REPRODUCTIVE STRUCTURES
- External Genitalia
- Internal Genitalia
  - *Vagina*
  - *Uterus and Cervix*
  - *Fallopian Tubes*
  - *Ovaries*

MENSTRUAL CYCLE
- Hormonal Control of the Menstrual Cycle
  - *Hypothalamic and Pituitary Hormones*
  - *Ovarian Hormones*
- Ovarian Follicle Development and Ovulation
- Endometrial Changes
- Cervical Mucus Changes
- Menopause
  - *Functional Changes*
  - *Hormone Therapy*

BREASTS
- Structure and Function
- Changes During Pregnancy and Lactation

Melody Waller and
Hallie Bensinger

The female genitourinary system consists of internal paired ovaries, fallopian tubes, the uterus, vagina, external mons pubis, labia majora, labia minora, clitoris, urethra, and perineal body. Although the female urinary structures are anatomically separate from the genital structures, their anatomic proximity provides a means for cross-contamination and shared symptomatology between the two systems (Fig. 44.1). This chapter focuses on the internal and external genitalia. It includes a discussion of hormonal and physical changes that occur throughout the life cycle in response to the gonadotropic hormones. The reader is referred to a specialty text for a discussion of pregnancy.

REPRODUCTIVE STRUCTURES

After completing this section of the chapter, the learner will be able to meet the following objectives:

- Name the three layers of the uterus and describe their function.
- Cite the location of the ovaries in relation to the uterus, fallopian tubes, broad ligaments, and ovarian ligaments.
- State the function of endocervical secretions.

External Genitalia

The external genitalia are located at the base of the pelvis in the perineal area and include the mons pubis, labia majora, labia minora, clitoris, and perineal body. The urethra and anus, although not genital structures, are usually considered in a discussion of the external genitalia. The external genitalia, also known collectively as the *vulva*, are diagrammed in Figure 44.2.

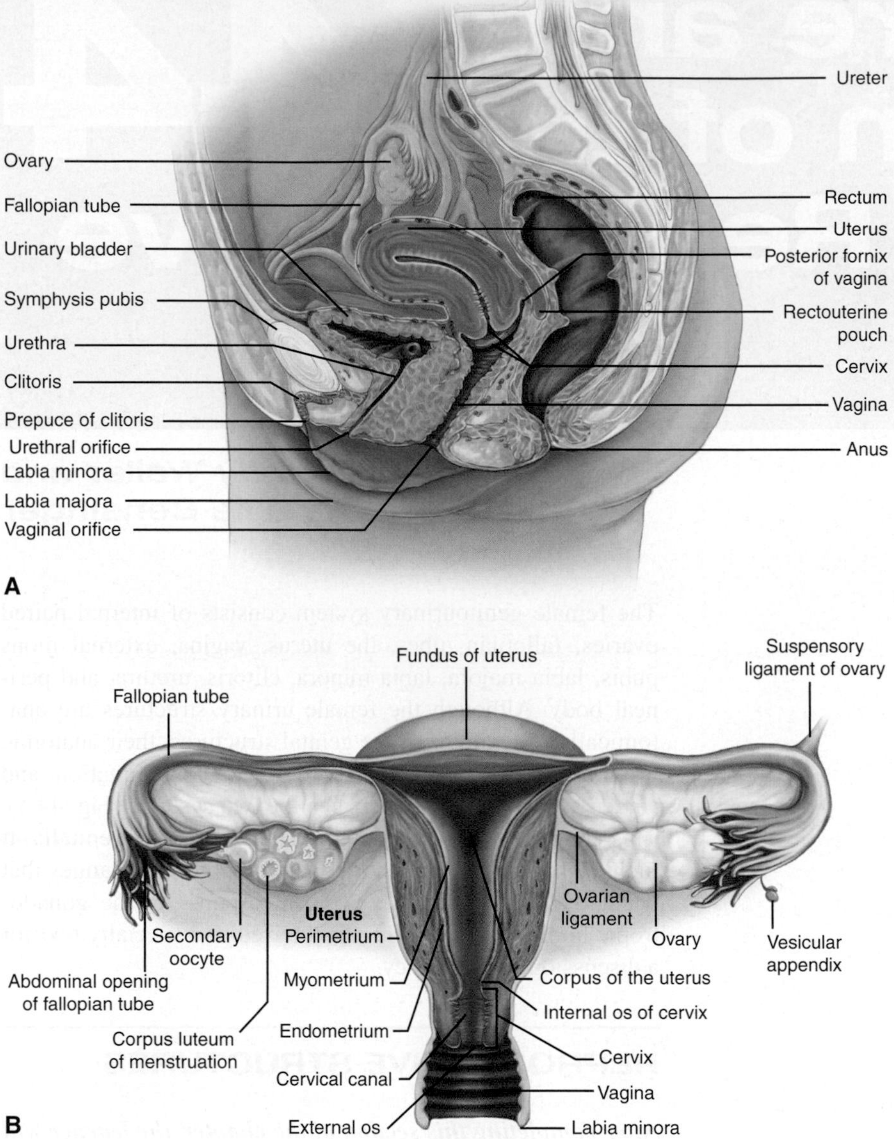

Figure 44.1 • Internal female genitalia. **(A)** Side view. **(B)** Frontal view. (From Jensen S. (2015). *Nursing health assessment: A best practice approach* (2nd ed., Fig. 24.2, p. 739). Philadelphia, PA: Lippincott Williams & Wilkins.)

The *mons pubis* is a rounded, skin-covered fat pad located anterior to the symphysis pubis.[1] Puberty stimulates an increase in the amount of fat and the development of darker and coarser hair over the mons. Normal pubic hair distribution in the female follows an inverted triangle with the base centered over the mons. Hair color and texture varies from person to person and among racial groups. There is an abundance of sebaceous glands in the skin that can become infected owing to normal variations in glandular secretions or poor hygiene. The *labia majora* (singular, labium majus) are analogous to the male scrotum. These structures are the outermost lips of the vulva, beginning anteriorly at the base of the mons pubis and ending posteriorly at the anus. The labia majora are composed of folds of skin and fat and become covered with hair at the onset of puberty. Before puberty, the labia majora have a skin covering similar to that covering the abdomen. With sufficient hormonal stimulation, the labia of a mature woman close over the urethral and vaginal openings; this can change after childbirth or surgery.

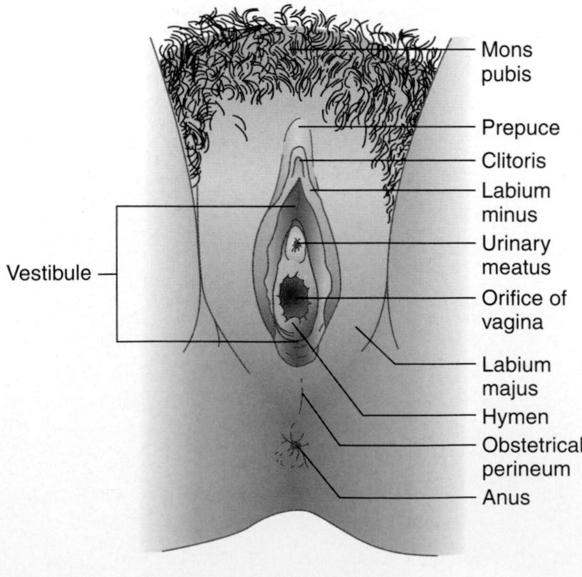

Figure 44.2 • External genitalia of the female.

The *labia minora* (singular, labium minus) are located between the labia majora. These delicate cutaneous structures are smaller than the labia majora and are composed of skin, fat, and some erectile tissue and are similar to the skin of the penis.[1] Unlike the skin of the labia majora, that of the labia minora is hairless and usually light pink. The labia minora begin anteriorly at the hood of the clitoris and end posteriorly at the base of the vagina. During sexual arousal, the labia minora become distended with blood; with resolution, the labia throb and then return to normal size. The clitoris is located below the clitoral hood, or prepuce, which is formed by the joining of the two labia minora. The clitoris is made up of two erectile corpora cavernosa.[1] The female clitoris is an erectile organ, rich in vascular and nervous supply. Analogous to the male penis, it is a highly sensitive organ that becomes distended during sexual stimulation.[1]

The area between labia minora is called the *vestibule* and it is lined with squamous epithelium.[1] Located in the vestibule are the urethral and vaginal openings, and the Bartholin lubricating glands, which are often referred to as the greater vestibular glands.[1] The *urethra*, or urinary meatus, is the external opening of the internal urinary bladder. The urethra is located posterior to the clitoris and is usually closer to the vaginal opening than to the clitoris. The urethral opening is the site of the *Skene glands*, which have a lubricating function and are often referred to as the lesser vestibular glands.[1] The vaginal orifice, commonly known as the *introitus*, is the opening between the external and internal genitalia. The size and shape of the opening are determined by a connective tissue membrane called the *hymen* that surrounds the introitus. The opening may be oval, circular, or sievelike and may be partially or completely occluded. Occlusion may occur because of the presence of an intact or partially intact hymen. Contrary to popular notion, an intact hymen does not indicate virginity because this tissue can be stretched without tearing. At puberty, an intact hymen may require surgical intervention to permit discharge of menstrual fluids.

The *perineal body* is that tissue located posterior to the vaginal opening and anterior to the anus. It is composed of fibrous connective tissue and is the site of insertion of several perineal muscles.

KEY POINTS

FEMALE REPRODUCTIVE STRUCTURES

- The external genitalia (labia majora, labia minora, clitoris, and vestibular glands) surround the openings of the urethra and vagina. Although the female urinary and genital structures are anatomically separate, their close proximity provides a means for cross-contamination and shared symptomatology.
- The internal genitalia of the female reproductive system include the ovaries, fallopian tubes, uterus, cervix, and vagina.

Internal Genitalia

Vagina

Connecting the internal and external genitalia is a fibromuscular tube called the *vagina*. The vagina, which is essentially free of sensory nerve fibers, is located behind the urinary bladder and urethra and anterior to the rectum. It connects the vestibule to the cervix.[1] The uterine cervix projects into the vagina at its upper end, forming recesses called *fornices* (Fig. 44.1). The vagina functions as a route for discharge of menses and other secretions. It also serves as an organ of sexual fulfillment and reproduction.

The membranous vaginal wall forms two longitudinal folds and several transverse folds, or rugae. The vagina is lined with mucus-secreting stratified squamous epithelial cells. Vaginal tissue is usually moist, with a pH maintained within the bacteriostatic range of 3.8 to 4.2.[2,3]

The epithelial cells of the vagina, like other tissues of the reproductive system, respond to changing levels of the ovarian sex hormones. Estrogen stimulates the proliferation and maturation of the vaginal mucosa. This results in a thickening of the vaginal mucosa and an increased glycogen content of the epithelial cells. The glycogen is fermented to lactic acid by the lactobacilli (*i.e.*, Döderlein bacilli) that are part of the normal vaginal flora, accounting for the mildly acid pH of vaginal fluid. The vaginal ecology can be disrupted at many levels, rendering it susceptible to infection. Pregnancy and the use of oral contraceptive agents increase the amount of estrogen in the system. Diabetes or a prediabetic state may increase the glycogen content of the cells.[4] The use of systemic antibiotics may decrease the number of lactobacilli in the vagina.

Decreased estrogen stimulation after menopause causes the vaginal mucosa to become thin and dry, often resulting in dyspareunia (*i.e.*, painful intercourse), atrophic vaginitis, and, occasionally, in vaginal bleeding. Estrogen levels can be estimated by means of vaginal scrapings obtained during a routine pelvic examination. The scrapings are used for a test, the *maturation index*, that examines the cellular structure and configuration of the vaginal epithelial cells.[5,6] The maturation index determines the ratio of parabasal (least mature), intermediate, and superficial (most mature) cells. Typically, this index is 0-40-60 during the reproductive years.[6] With diminished estrogen levels, there is a shift to the left, producing an index of 30-40-30 during the perimenopausal period and an index of 75-25-0 during the postmenopausal period.[6]

Uterus and Cervix

The uterus is a thick-walled, muscular organ. This pear-shaped, hollow structure is located between the bladder and the rectum. The uterus can be divided into three parts: the portion above the insertion of the fallopian tubes, called the *fundus*; the lower constricted part, called the *cervix*; and the portion between the fundus and the cervix, called the *body of the uterus*. The uterus is supported on both sides by four sets of ligaments: the *broad ligaments*, which run laterally from the body of the uterus to the pelvic side walls; the *round ligaments*, which run from the fundus laterally into the mons; the *uterosacral ligaments*, which run from the uterocervical junction to the sacrum; and the *cardinal* or *transverse cervical* ligaments.

The wall of the uterus is composed of three layers: the perimetrium (also known as serosa), the myometrium, and the endometrium. The *perimetrium* is the outer serous covering that is derived from the abdominal peritoneum. This outer layer merges with the peritoneum that covers the broad ligaments. Anteriorly, the perimetrium is reflected over the bladder wall, forming the vesicouterine pouch. Posteriorly, it extends to form the *cul-de-sac*, or *pouch of Douglas*. Because of the proximity of the perimetrium to the urinary bladder, infection of the bladder can cause uterine symptoms, particularly during pregnancy.[1]

The middle muscle layer, the *myometrium*, forms the major portion of the uterine wall. The inner fibers of the myometrium run in various directions, giving it an interwoven appearance. Contractions of these muscle fibers help to expel menstrual flow and the products of conception during miscarriage or childbirth. When pain accompanies the contractions associated with menses, it is called *dysmenorrhea*. The myometrium has an amazing ability to change length during pregnancy and labor to accommodate gestation.[1]

The *endometrium*, the inner layer of the uterus, is made up of a basal and a superficial layer. The superficial layer is shed during menstruation and regenerated by cells of the basal layer. Ciliated cells promote the movement of tubal–uterine secretions out of the uterine cavity into the vagina.[1]

The round *cervix* is the neck of the uterus that projects into the vagina. The cervix is a firm structure, composed of a connective tissue matrix of glands and muscular tissue elements that become soft and pliable under the influence of hormones produced during pregnancy. Glandular tissue provides a rich supply of protective mucus that changes in character and quantity during the menstrual cycle and during pregnancy. The cervix is richly supplied with blood from the uterine artery and can be a site of significant blood loss during delivery.

The opening of the cervix, the os, forms a pathway between the uterus and the vagina. The vaginal opening is called the *cervical os* (see Fig. 44.1). Secretions from the columnar epithelium of the endocervix protect the uterus from infection, alter receptivity to sperm, and form a mucoid "plug" during pregnancy. The endocervical canal provides a route for menstrual discharge and sperm entrance.

Fallopian Tubes

The *fallopian tubes*, or oviducts, are slender, cylindrical structures attached bilaterally to the uterus and supported by the upper folds of the broad ligament.[1,2] The end of the fallopian tube nearest the ovary forms a funnel-like opening with fringed, finger-like projections, called *fimbriae*, that pick up the ovum after its release into the peritoneal cavity after ovulation (Fig. 44.3). The fallopian tubes are formed of smooth muscle and lined with a ciliated, mucus-producing epithelial layer. The beating of the cilia, along with contractile movements of the smooth muscle, propels the nonmotile ovum toward the uterus. If coitus has occurred recently, fertilization normally occurs in the middle to outer portion of the fallopian tube. Besides providing a passageway for ova and sperm, the fallopian tubes provide for drainage of tubal secretions into the uterus.[1]

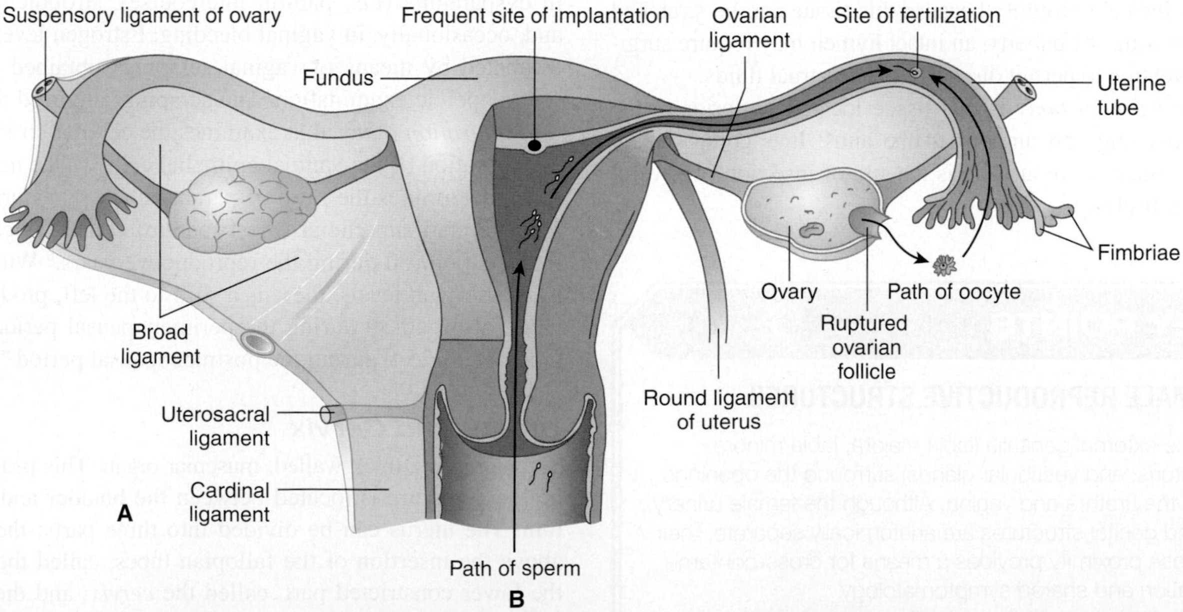

Figure 44.3 • Schematic drawing of female reproductive organs, showing **(A)** suspensory ligament of the ovary and the broad, uterosacral, and cardinal ligaments on the left, and **(B)** the path of the oocyte as it moves from the ovary into the fallopian (uterine) tube; the path of sperm is also shown, as is the usual site of fertilization.

Ovaries

By the third month of fetal life, the *ovaries* have fully developed and descended to their permanent pelvic position. Remnants of the primitive genital system provide lateral supporting attachments to the uterus. In the mature female, these supporting structures evolve into the round and suspensory ligaments. Remnants that do not evolve may form cysts, which may become symptomatic later in life.

Oogenesis is the process of generation of ova by mitotic division that begins at the sixth week of fetal life.[6] These primitive germ cells ultimately provide 1 to 2 million oocytes that are present in the ovaries at birth. At puberty, this number is reduced through cell death to approximately 200,000.[6]

The neonate's ovaries are smooth, pale, and elongated. As the child grows, the ovaries become shorter, thicker, and heavier before the onset of menarche, which is initiated by pituitary influence. The initial hormonal stimulus for this development is believed to come from ovarian rather than systemic estrogen.[1] In the adult, the ovaries are flat, almond-shaped structures that are 3 to 5 cm long, 1.5 cm wide, and 1 cm thick.[1] As the woman matures, the ovaries shrink to approximately one fourth of the size as they were during reproductive years.[1]

The ovaries are located on either side of the uterus below the fimbriated ends of the fallopian tubes.[6] The ovaries are attached to the posterior surface of the broad ligament and to the uterus by the ovarian ligament. They are covered with a thin layer of surface epithelium that is continuous with the lining of the peritoneum. The integrity of this covering is periodically broken at the time of ovulation.

The ovaries, like the male testes, have a dual function: they store the female germ cells, or ova, and produce the female sex hormones, estrogen and progesterone. Unlike the male gonads, which produce sperm throughout a man's reproductive life, the female gonads contain a fixed number of ova at birth that diminishes throughout a woman's life.

Structurally, the mature ovary is divided into a highly vascular inner medulla, which contains supporting connective tissue, and an outer cortex of stroma and epithelial follicles (*i.e.*, vesicles), which contain the primary oocytes, or germ cells.[1] After puberty, the pituitary gonadotropic hormones—follicle-stimulating hormone (FSH) and luteinizing hormone (LH)—stimulate the primordial follicles to develop into *mature graafian follicles*. The graafian follicle produces estrogen, which begins to stimulate the thickening of the endometrium in the uterus.

Although several follicles begin to develop during each ovulatory cycle, only one or two complete the entire developmental process and rupture to release a mature ovum. After ovulation, the follicle becomes luteinized. As the corpus luteum, it produces estrogen and progesterone to support the endometrium until conception occurs or the cycle begins again.[1]

IN SUMMARY

The female reproductive system consists of internal paired ovaries, fallopian or uterine tubes, uterus, vagina, external mons pubis, labia majora, labia minora, clitoris, urethra, and perineal body. The genitourinary system as a whole serves sexual and reproductive functions throughout the life cycle. The uterus is a thick-walled, muscular organ. The wall of the uterus is composed of three layers: the outer perimetrium; the myometrium or muscle layer, which is continuous with the myometrium of the fallopian tubes and the vagina; and the inner lining or endometrium, which is continuous with the lining of the fallopian tubes and vagina. The gonads, or ovaries, which are internal in the female (unlike the testes in the male), have the dual function of storing the female germ cells, or ova, and producing the female sex hormones. Through the regulation and release of sex hormones, the ovaries influence the development of secondary sexual characteristics, regulation of menstrual cycles, maintenance of pregnancy, and advent of menopause.

MENSTRUAL CYCLE

After completing this section of the chapter, the learner will be able to meet the following objectives:

- Describe the feedback control of estrogen and progesterone levels by means of gonadotropin-releasing hormone, LH, FSH, and ovarian follicle function.
- Relate FSH and LH levels to the stages of follicle development and to estrogen and progesterone production.
- Discuss the risks and benefits of hormone replacement therapy in menopausal women.

Between menarche (*i.e.*, first menstrual bleeding) and menopause (*i.e.*, last menstrual bleeding), the female reproductive system undergoes cyclic changes called the *menstrual cycle*. This includes the maturation and release of oocytes from the ovary during ovulation and periodic vaginal bleeding resulting from the shedding of the endometrial lining. It is not necessary for a woman to ovulate to menstruate. Anovulatory cycles do occur, leading to irregular menses. The menstrual cycle produces changes in the breasts, uterus, skin, and ovaries. The maintenance of the cycle affects biologic and sociologic aspects of a woman's life, including fertility, reproduction, sexuality, and femaleness.

Hormonal Control of the Menstrual Cycle

Normal menstrual function results from interactions among the central nervous system, hypothalamus, anterior pituitary, ovaries, and associated target tissues (Fig. 44.4). Although

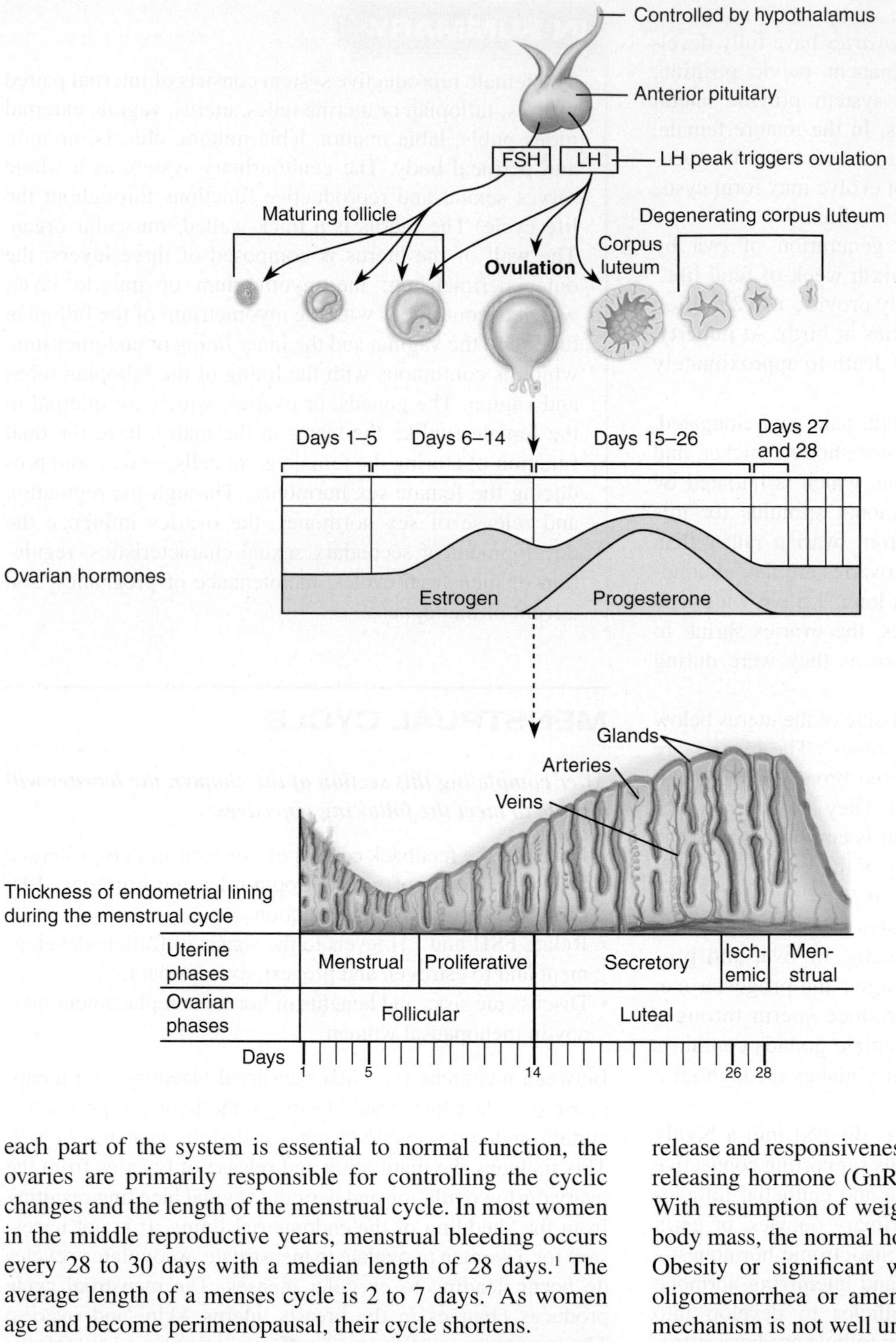

Figure 44.4 • Relationship between hormonal levels (**center**), follicular development (**top**) and the menstrual cycle (**bottom**). (From Jensen S. (2015). *Nursing health assessment: A best practice approach* (2nd ed., Fig. 24.3, p. 740). Philadelphia, PA: Lippincott Williams & Wilkins.)

each part of the system is essential to normal function, the ovaries are primarily responsible for controlling the cyclic changes and the length of the menstrual cycle. In most women in the middle reproductive years, menstrual bleeding occurs every 28 to 30 days with a median length of 28 days.[1] The average length of a menses cycle is 2 to 7 days.[7] As women age and become perimenopausal, their cycle shortens.

The hormonal control of the menstrual cycle is complex. For example, the biosynthesis of estrogens that occurs in adipose tissue may be a significant source of the hormone. There is evidence that a woman must have a minimum body weight and fat content in order for menarche to occur and for the menstrual cycle to be maintained. This is supported by the observation of amenorrhea in women with anorexia nervosa, chronic disease, and malnutrition and in those who are long-distance runners.[8] In women with anorexia nervosa, gonadotropin and estradiol secretion, including LH release and responsiveness to the hypothalamic gonadotropin-releasing hormone (GnRH), can revert to prepubertal levels. With resumption of weight gain and attainment of sufficient body mass, the normal hormonal pattern is usually reinstated. Obesity or significant weight gain is also associated with oligomenorrhea or amenorrhea and infertility, although the mechanism is not well understood.

Hypothalamic and Pituitary Hormones

FSH and LH from the anterior pituitary gland regulate growth, prepubertal maturation, the reproductive cycle, and sex hormone secretion in males and females (Fig. 44.5). Because these hormones promote the growth of cells in the ovaries and testes as a means of stimulating the production of sex hormones, they are called the *gonadotropic hormones*. GnRH from the hypothalamus stimulates the secretion of LH and FSH. In addition to LH and FSH, the anterior pituitary secretes a third

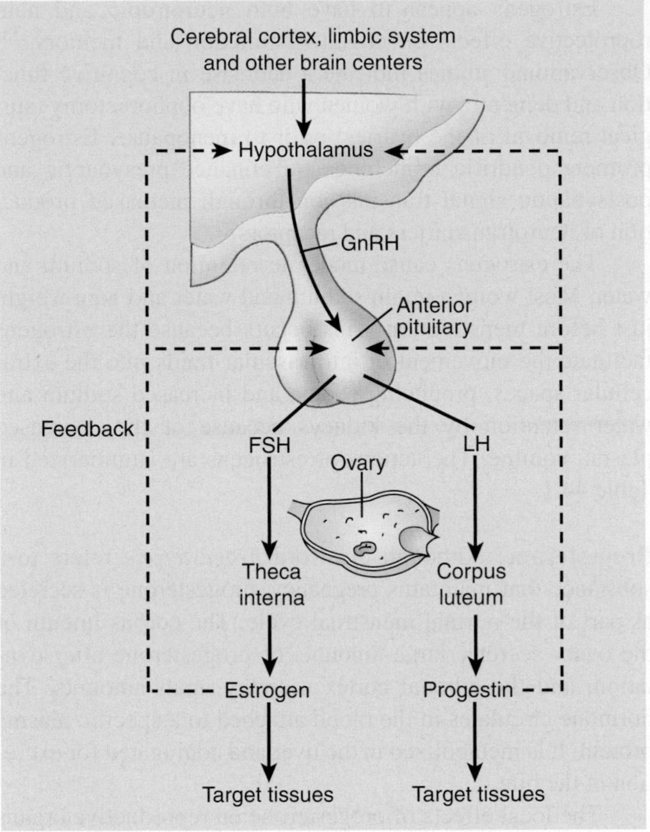

Figure 44.5 • Hypothalamic-pituitary feedback control of estrogen and progesterone levels in the female. The *dashed line* represents negative feedback.

hormone called *prolactin*. The primary function of prolactin is the stimulation of lactation in the postpartum period. During pregnancy, prolactin, along with other hormones such as estrogen, progesterone, insulin, and cortisol, contributes to breast development in preparation for lactation. Although prolactin does not appear to play a physiologic role in ovarian function, hyperprolactinemia leads to hypogonadism. This may include an initial shortening of the luteal phase with subsequent anovulation, oligomenorrhea or amenorrhea, and infertility. The hypothalamic control of prolactin secretion is primarily inhibitory, and dopamine is the most important inhibitory factor. Hyperprolactinemia may occur as an adverse effect of drug treatment using phenothiazine derivatives (*i.e.*, antipsychotic drugs that block dopamine receptors).[1]

Ovarian Hormones

The ovaries produce estrogens, progesterone, and androgens. Ovarian hormones are secreted in a cyclic pattern as a result of the interaction between the hypothalamic GnRH and the pituitary gonadotropic hormones FSH and LH. The steroid sex hormones enter cells by passive diffusion, bind to specific receptor proteins in the cytoplasm, and then move to the nucleus, where they bind to specific sites on the chromosomes. These hormones exert their effects through gene–hormone interactions that stimulate the synthesis of specific messenger ribonucleic acid (mRNA). In addition, estrogen appears to have the ability to influence cell activity through other nongenomic mechanisms. These nongenomic effects take place in cells that have no steroid receptors, possibly mediated by other membrane receptors. This may explain in part some of the nonreproductive effects of estrogen. An example of a nongenomic cardioprotective effect would be the antioxidant activity of estrogen in preventing endothelial injury that can lead to platelet adherence.[2] The number of hormonal receptor sites on a cell is not fixed. Evidence suggests that they are constantly being removed and replaced. An increase or a decrease in the number of receptors can serve as a mechanism for regulating hormonal activity. For example, estrogen may induce the development of an increased number of estrogen receptors in some tissues and may stimulate the synthesis of progesterone receptors in others. In contrast, progesterone may cause a reduction in the number of estrogen and progesterone receptors.

There is a second type of estrogen receptor (ER_2) that is different in structure and tissue distribution, and expression from ER_1 helps to expand our understanding of the mechanism of action of estrogen in the body. ER_2 appears to be an activator of estrogen response, whereas ER_1 appears to modulate or inhibit the action of estrogen.[3] Likewise, the progesterone receptor has two major forms (A and B), expressed by a single gene, but promoted differently in a complex system of transcription regulation.

Estrogens. Estrogens are a family of structurally related female sex hormones synthesized and secreted by cells in the ovaries and, in small amounts, by cells in the adrenal cortex. Androgens can be converted to estrogens peripherally, especially in fat tissue. Three estrogens occur naturally in humans: estrone (E_1), estradiol (E_2), and estriol (E_3). Of these, estradiol is the most biologically potent and the most abundantly secreted product of the ovary. Estrogens are secreted throughout the menstrual cycle. Two peaks occur: one before ovulation and one in the middle of the luteal phase. Estrogens are transported in the blood bound to specific plasma globulins (which can also bind testosterone), inactivated and conjugated in the liver, and then excreted in the bile.

Estrogens are necessary for normal female physical maturation. In concert with other hormones, estrogens provide for the reproductive processes of ovulation, implantation of the products of conception, pregnancy, parturition, and lactation by stimulating the development and maintaining the growth of the accessory organs. In the absence of androgens, estrogens stimulate the intrauterine development of the vagina, uterus, and uterine tubes from the embryonic Müllerian system. They also stimulate the stromal development and ductal growth of the breasts at puberty, are responsible for the accelerated pubertal skeletal growth phase and for closure of the epiphyses of the long bones, contribute to the growth of axillary and pubic hair, and alter the distribution of body fat to produce the typical female body contours, including the accumulation of body fat around the hips and breasts. Larger quantities of estrogen stimulate pigmentation of the skin in the nipple, areolar, and genital regions.

In addition to their effects on the growth of uterine muscle, estrogens play an important role in the development of the endometrial lining. During anovulatory cycles, continued exposure to estrogens for prolonged periods leads to abnormal hyperplasia of the endometrium and abnormal bleeding patterns. When estrogen production is poorly coordinated during the normal menstrual period, inappropriate bleeding and shedding of the endometrium can also occur.

Estrogens have a number of important extragenital metabolic effects. They are responsible for maintaining the normal structure of skin and blood vessels in women. Estrogens decrease the rate of bone resorption by antagonizing the effects of parathyroid hormone on bone. For this reason, osteoporosis is a common problem in estrogen-deficient postmenopausal women. In the liver, estrogens increase the synthesis of transport proteins for thyroxine, estrogen, testosterone, and other hormones. Estrogens also affect the composition of the plasma lipoproteins. They produce an increase in high-density lipoproteins (HDLs), a slight reduction in low-density lipoproteins (LDLs), and a reduction in cholesterol levels.

Estrogens have additional cardioprotective actions, including direct antiatherosclerotic effects on the arterial wall (augmentation of vasodilating and antiplatelet aggregation factors such as nitric oxide and prostacyclin), vasodilation through endothelium-independent mechanisms, antioxidant activity, reduction of levels of angiotensin-converting enzyme and renin, reduction of homocysteine levels, improvement of peripheral glucose metabolism with subsequent decreased circulating insulin levels, and direct effects on cardiac function (*i.e.*, increased left ventricular diastolic filling and stroke volume output). Estrogens increase plasma triglyceride levels and enhance the coagulability of blood by effecting increased circulating levels of plasminogen and factors II, VII, IX, and X.[9–11]

Estrogens appear to have both neurotropic and neuroprotective effects on cognitive function and memory.[12,13] Observational studies indicate a decrease in cognitive function and dementia with women who have oophorectomy (surgical removal of the ovaries) prior to menopause. Estrogens promote dendritic branching and enhance presynaptic and postsynaptic signal transmission through increased production of neurotransmitters and receptors.[12]

The estrogens cause moderate retention of sodium and water. Most women retain sodium and water and gain weight just before menstruation. This occurs because the estrogens facilitate the movement of intravascular fluids into the extracellular spaces, producing edema and increased sodium and water retention by the kidneys because of the decreased plasma volume. The actions of estrogens are summarized in Table 44.1.

Progesterone. Although the word *progesterone* refers to a substance that maintains pregnancy, progesterone is secreted as part of the normal menstrual cycle. The corpus luteum of the ovary secretes large amounts of progesterone after ovulation, and the adrenal cortex secretes small amounts. The hormone circulates in the blood attached to a specific plasma protein. It is metabolized in the liver and conjugated for excretion in the bile.

The local effects of progesterone on reproductive organs include the glandular development of the lobular and alveolar tissue of the breasts and the cyclic glandular development of the endometrium. Progesterone can also compete with aldosterone at the level of the renal tubule, causing a decrease in sodium reabsorption, with a resultant increase in secretion of aldosterone by the adrenal cortex, as occurs in pregnancy. Although the mechanism is uncertain, progesterone is responsible for the increase in basal body temperature that occurs with ovulation. Smooth muscle relaxation under the influence

TABLE 44.1 ACTIONS OF ESTROGENS

GENERAL FUNCTION	SPECIFIC ACTIONS
Growth and Development	
Reproductive organs	Stimulate development of vagina, uterus, and fallopian tubes in utero and of secondary sex characteristics during puberty
Skeleton	Accelerate growth of long bones and closure of epiphyses at puberty
Reproductive Processes	
Ovulation	Promote growth of ovarian follicles
Fertilization	Alter the cervical secretions to favor survival and transport of sperm
	Promote motility of sperm within the fallopian tubes by decreasing mucus viscosity
Implantation	Promote development of endometrial lining in the event of pregnancy
Vagina	Proliferate vaginal mucosa, prevent atrophy
Cervix	Increase mucus consistency
Breasts	Stimulate stromal development and ductal growth
General Metabolic Effects	
Bone resorption	Decrease rate of bone resorption
Plasma proteins	Increase production of thyroid and other binding globulins
Lipoproteins	Increase high-density and slightly decrease low-density lipoproteins

of progesterone plays an important role in maintaining pregnancy by decreasing uterine contractions, and is responsible for many of the common discomforts of pregnancy, such as edema, nausea, constipation, flatulence, and headaches. The increased progesterone present during pregnancy and the luteal phase of the menstrual cycle enhances the ventilatory response to carbon dioxide, leading to a measurable change in arterial and alveolar carbon dioxide (PCO_2) levels.[6]

Androgens. The normal female also produces androgens along with estrogens and progesterone. Approximately 25% of these androgens are secreted from the ovaries, 25% from the adrenal cortex, and 50% from ovarian or adrenal precursors. In the female, androgens contribute to normal hair growth at puberty and may have other important metabolic effects.

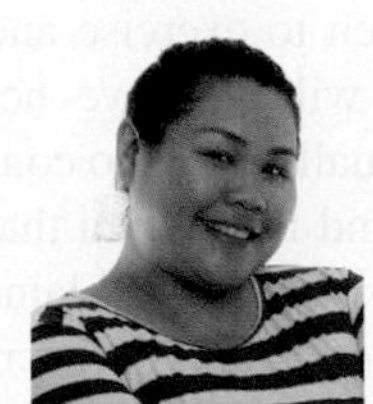

Recall that **Eileen**, who was introduced to you at the beginning of Unit 13, has been diagnosed with polycystic ovarian syndrome (PCOS). As discussed in Chapter 45, previous diagnoses of PCOS require at least two of the three widely accepted Rotterdam Criteria,[14,15] which include

1. Oligo- or anovulation
2. Clinical and/or biochemical signs of hyperandrogenism
3. Polycystic ovaries

Women with PCOS often do not ovulate at all (anovulation) or ovulate infrequently (oligoovulation). A common sign of anovulation or oligoovulation is absent or infrequent menstrual bleeding (periods). Eileen thus meets this first criterion because she cannot recall her last period. Eileen also meets the second criterion because her elevated concentration of testosterone is a biochemical sign of hyperandrogenism (testosterone is an androgen), and her hirsutism and acne are clinical signs. The increased production of testosterone is thought to reflect excess LH production from the anterior pituitary.

Ovarian Follicle Development and Ovulation

The tissues of the adult ovary can be conveniently divided into four compartments, or units: the stroma, or supporting tissue; the interstitial cells; the follicles; and the corpus luteum. The *stroma* is the connective tissue substance of the ovary in which the follicles are distributed. The *interstitial cells* are estrogen-secreting cells that resemble the Leydig cells, or interstitial cells, of the testes.[1]

Beginning at puberty, a cyclic rise in the anterior pituitary hormones FSH and LH stimulates the development of several graafian, or mature, follicles. Follicles at all stages of development can be found in both ovaries, except in menopausal women (see Fig. 44.6). Most follicles exist as primary

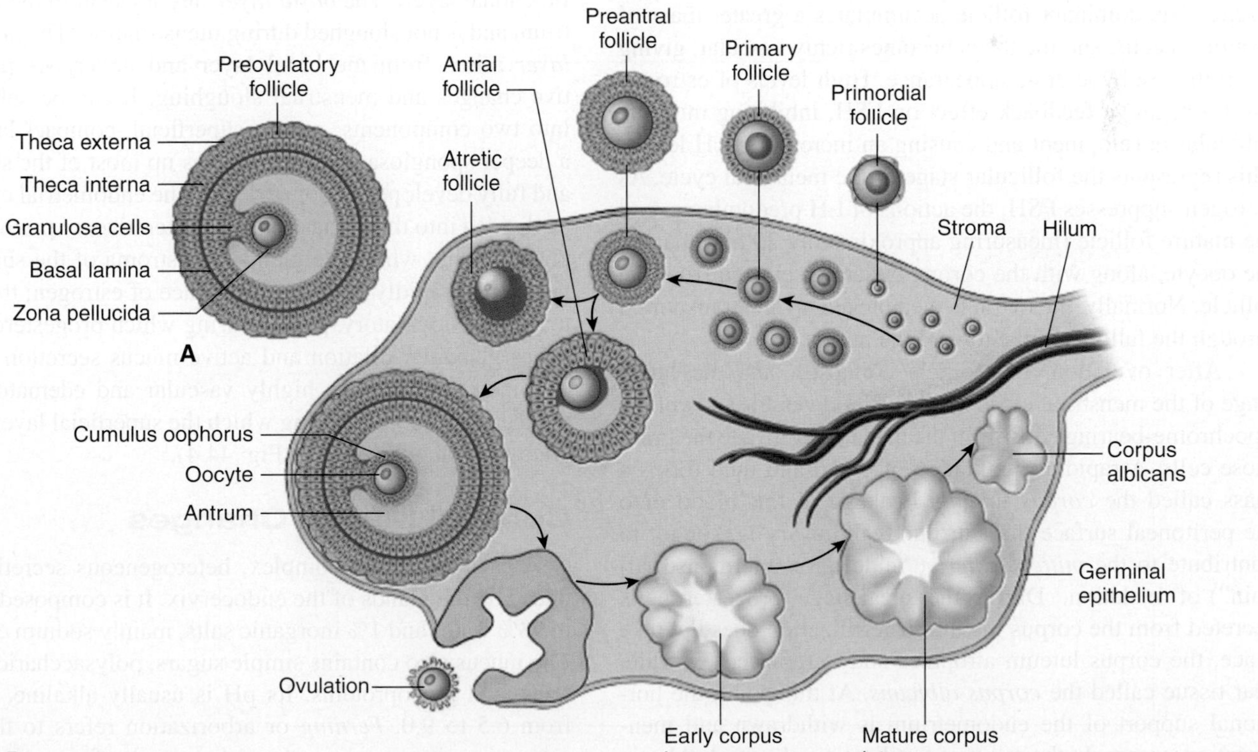

Figure 44.6 • **(A)** Cross-section of preovulatory follicle. **(B)** Schematic diagram of an ovary, showing the sequence of events in the origin, growth, and rupture of an ovarian follicle and the formation and retrogression of a corpus luteum. The atretic follicles are those that show signs of degeneration and death.

follicles, each of which consists of a round oocyte surrounded by a single layer of flattened, epithelium-derived granulosa cells and a basement membrane. The primary follicles constitute an inactive pool of follicles from which all the ovulating follicles develop. Under the influence of endocrine stimulation, 6 to 12 primary follicles develop into secondary follicles once every ovulatory cycle. During the development of the secondary follicle, the primary oocyte increases in size, and the granulosa cells proliferate to form a multilayered wall around it. During this time, a membrane called the *zona pellucida* develops and surrounds the oocyte and small pockets of fluid begin to appear between the granulosa cells. Blood vessels, however, do not penetrate the basement membrane; the granulosa cell layer remains avascular until after ovulation has occurred.

As the follicles mature, FSH stimulates the development of the cell layers. Cells from the surrounding stromal tissue align themselves to form a cellular wall called the *theca*. The cells of the theca become differentiated into two layers: an inner theca interna, which lies adjacent to the follicular cells, and an outer theca externa. As the follicle enlarges, a single large cavity, or *antrum*, is formed, and a portion of the granulosa cells and the oocyte are displaced to one side of the follicle by the fluid that accumulates. The secondary oocyte remains surrounded by a crown of granulosa cells, the corona radiata. As the follicle ripens, granulose cells produce ovarian estrogen. Selection of a dominant follicle occurs with the conversion to an estrogen microenvironment. The lesser follicles, although continuing to produce some estrogen, atrophy or become atretic. The dominant follicle accumulates a greater mass of granulosa cells, and the theca becomes richly vascular, giving the follicle a hyperemic appearance. High levels of estrogen exert a negative feedback effect on FSH, inhibiting multiple follicular development and causing an increase in LH levels. This represents the follicular stage of the menstrual cycle. As estrogen suppresses FSH, the actions of LH predominate, and the mature follicle (measuring approximately 20 mm) bursts; the oocyte, along with the corona radiata, is ejected from the follicle. Normally, the ovum is then picked up and transported through the fallopian tube toward the uterus.

After ovulation, the follicle collapses, and the luteal stage of the menstrual cycle begins. Blood vessels and yellow lipochrome-bearing cells from the theca layer invade the granulose cells. A rapid accumulation of blood and fluid forms a mass called the *corpus luteum*. Leakage of this blood onto the peritoneal surface that surrounds the ovary is thought to contribute to the *mittelschmerz* ("middle [or intermenstrual] pain") of ovulation.[1] During the luteal stage, progesterone is secreted from the corpus luteum. If fertilization does not take place, the corpus luteum atrophies and is replaced by white scar tissue called the *corpus albicans*. At this point, the hormonal support of the endometrium is withdrawn and menstruation occurs. In the event of fertilization, the trophoblastic cells in the blastocyst produce a hormone called human chorionic gonadotropin. This hormone prevents luteal regression. The corpus luteum remains functional for 7 to 10 weeks and provides hormonal support for pregnancy until the placenta is fully functional.[20] Figure 44.6B shows the hormonal changes that occur during the development of the ovarian follicle and ovulation.

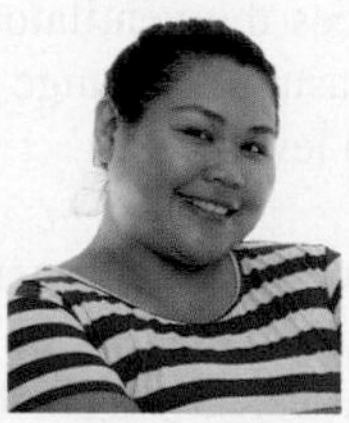

Eileen is requesting an oral contraceptive pill (OCP) to prevent pregnancy. An OCP will have the added benefit of alleviating PCOS symptoms. Combination OCPs contain both estrogen and progestin (a modified progesterone). These two steroids have antiandrogenic (testosterone-opposing) effects and will thus reduce Eileen's acne and hirsutism. The OCP will also give Eileen regular periods and help maintain a healthy uterine lining.

Eileen also expresses anxiety about her ability to have children. The caregiver encourages Eileen to exercise and modify her diet, because weight loss will improve her reproductive function. When she is eventually ready to conceive, Eileen can stop taking the OCP and might find that her cycles are regular and ovulatory. The caregiver explains that there are also pharmacologic options to address her fertility problems if the lifestyle changes are not sufficient.

Endometrial Changes

The endometrium consists of two distinct layers, or zones, that are responsive to hormonal stimulation: a basal layer and a functional layer.[1] The *basal layer* lies adjacent to the myometrium and is not sloughed during menstruation. The *functional layer* arises from the basal layer and undergoes proliferative changes and menstrual sloughing. It can be subdivided into two components: a thin, superficial, compact layer and a deeper spongiosa layer that makes up most of the secretory and fully developed endometrium.[1] The endometrial cycle can be divided into three phases: the proliferative, or preovulatory, phase, during which the glands and stroma of the superficial layer grow rapidly under the influence of estrogen; the secretory, or postovulatory, phase, during which progesterone produces glandular dilation and active mucus secretion and the endometrium becomes highly vascular and edematous; and the menstrual phase, during which the superficial layer degenerates and sloughs off (see Fig. 44.4).[1]

Cervical Mucus Changes

Cervical mucus is a complex, heterogeneous secretion produced by the glands of the endocervix. It is composed of 92% to 98% water and 1% inorganic salts, mainly sodium chloride. The mucus also contains simple sugars, polysaccharides, proteins, and glycoproteins. Its pH is usually alkaline, ranging from 6.5 to 9.0. *Ferning* or arborization refers to the characteristic microscopic pattern that results from the crystallization of the inorganic salts in the cervical mucus when it is dried. Its characteristics are strongly influenced by serum levels of estrogen and progesterone. Estrogen stimulates the production of large amounts of clear, watery mucus through which sperm can penetrate most easily. During ovulation cervical mucous is thin and stretchy. *Spinnbarkeit* is the property that allows cervical mucus to be stretched or drawn into a thread. Spinnbarkeit can be estimated by stretching a sample of cervical mucus between two glass slides and measuring the maximum length of the thread before it breaks. At midcycle, spinnbarkeit usually exceeds 10 cm. Progesterone, even in the presence of estrogen, reduces the secretion of mucus. During the luteal phase of the menstrual cycle, mucus is scant, viscous, and cellular.[20]

KEY POINTS

MENSTRUAL CYCLE

- The menstrual cycle involves the maturation and release of oocytes from the ovary during ovulation and periodic vaginal bleeding resulting from the shedding of the endometrial lining.
- The menstrual cycle is controlled by rhythmic synthesis and release of ovarian hormones (the estrogens and progesterone) under feedback control from the hypothalamic GnRH and the anterior pituitary gonadotropic FSH and LHs.
- Menopause marks the end of a woman's menstrual cycle and is accompanied by a variety of physiologic changes. Hormone replacement therapy can be considered after an individualized risk–benefit analysis is done, taking into account findings from studies such as the Women's Health Initiative.

Menopause

Menopause is the cessation of menstrual cycles. Like menarche, it is more of a process than a single event. Most women stop menstruating between 48 and 55 years of age. *Perimenopause* (the years immediately surrounding menopause) precedes menopause by approximately 4 years and is characterized by menstrual irregularity and other menopausal symptoms. *Climacteric* is a more encompassing term that refers to the entire transition to the nonreproductive period of life. Premature ovarian failure describes approximately 1% of women who experience menopause before the age of 40 years. A woman who has not menstruated for a full year or who has a persistently elevated FSH level (>20 mIU/mL) is considered menopausal.[4]

Functional Changes

Menopause results from the gradual cessation of ovarian function and the resultant diminished levels of estrogen. Although estrogens derived from the adrenal cortex continue to circulate in a woman's body, they are insufficient to maintain the secondary sexual characteristics in the same manner as ovarian estrogens. As a result, body hair, skin elasticity, and subcutaneous fat decrease. The breasts become pendulous with a decrease in tissue mass, leaving only the ducts, fat, and connective tissue. The ovaries and uterus diminish in size; and the cervix and vagina become pale and friable.[16] Vaginal pH increases; a pH greater than 4.5 is usually associated with estrogen deficiency.[20]

Problems that can arise as a result of urogenital atrophy include vaginal dryness, urinary stress incontinence, urgency, nocturia, vaginitis, and urinary tract infection (UTI). Women may find intercourse painful and traumatic, although some type of vaginal lubrication may be helpful. Vaginal estrogen cream may be recommended for vaginal dryness and atrophy. It remains controversial as to the advantages and disadvantages of taking a small amount of transdermal (more likely a gel or spray) estrogen to decrease the vulvovaginal symptoms.[17] Many believe the transdermal gel or spray is more effective than the patch and has less risk for health problems.[1]

Systemically, a woman may experience significant vasomotor instability secondary to the decrease in estrogens and the relative increase in other hormones, including FSH, LH, GnRH, dehydroepiandrosterone, androstenedione, epinephrine, corticotropin, β-endorphin, growth hormone, and calcitonin gene-related peptide.[18] This instability may give rise to "hot flashes," palpitations, dizziness, and headaches as the blood vessels dilate. Despite the association with these biochemical changes, the underlying cause of hot flashes is unknown.[18] Tremendous variation exists in the onset, frequency, severity, and length of time that women experience hot flashes. When they occur at night and are accompanied by significant perspiration, they are referred to as *night sweats*. Insomnia as well as frequent awakening because of vasomotor symptoms can lead to sleep deprivation. A woman may experience irritability, anxiety, and depression as a result of these uncontrollable and unpredictable events.

In addition to changes that closely follow the cessation of ovarian function, there are changes that over many years influence the health and well-being of postmenopausal women. Consequences of long-term estrogen deprivation include osteoporosis because of an imbalance in bone remodeling (*i.e.*, bone resorption occurs at a faster rate than bone formation), and an increased risk for cardiovascular disease (atherosclerosis is accelerated), which is the leading cause of death for women after menopause.[16] Other potential health threats, which reflect both aging and cessation of ovarian function, are loss of vision because of macular degeneration, and cognitive impairment.

Hormone Therapy

Over the past four to five decades, hormone therapy (HT) became increasingly prescribed for postmenopausal women. Initially, HT was used only for symptom management, and later for prevention of osteoporosis. During the 1990s, HT evolved to the status of *replacement* for a vital hormone lost because of an endocrine organ failure (menopause). It was routinely offered to all postmenopausal women based on mounting evidence of preventive benefits in numerous areas.

During this time, data from observational studies demonstrated a 50% reduction in coronary heart disease (CHD) mortality rates in women using HT.[19,20] Other reported advantages to HT included a reduced risk of neurocognitive loss, bone density, and periodontal disease.

The type of HT prescribed was determined by whether the woman had an intact uterus. Women with an intact uterus received a combination of estrogen and progesterone (EPT), and those who had previously had their uterus removed received estrogen (ET) only. The addition of progesterone to HT was the established protocol for women with an intact uterus because the association between unopposed estrogen and the development of endometrial cancer was noted in the 1970s. Unopposed estrogen can lead to the development of endometrial hyperplasia, which in some cases can increase a woman's risk for endometrial cancer. HT that involves the use of both estrogen and progesterone is not associated with endometrial cancer. When used cyclically (continuous sequential estrogen–progesterone therapy [CSEPT]), progesterone is added for 12 to 14 days to mature any endometrium that has developed in response to the estrogen. Progesterone withdrawal results in endometrial shedding (*i.e.*, a cyclic bleeding episode). When used continuously, a small amount of progesterone is added to the daily estrogen regimen. This continuous exposure to progesterone inhibits endometrial development. Eventually, the combined continuous estrogen–progesterone therapy (CCEPT) results in no bleeding. However, it can be associated with irregular bleeding and spotting until the lining becomes atrophic. Prevention of endometrial hyperplasia either by shedding the endometrial build-up or by preventing its development minimizes the risk of endometrial cancer. This protection must now be considered when weighing the risks and benefits of HT.

Women's Health Initiative and Other Studies. With the current shift to evidence-based practice, randomized control trials were undertaken to confirm the reported benefits of HT using an experimental model to demonstrate that the intervention (HT), and not other variables, was in fact responsible for the outcome. Several randomized control trials have now demonstrated that HT does not prevent and can increase the likelihood of a cardiovascular event in women with established heart disease.[10,11] Other studies looking at the effect of HT on cognition and Alzheimer disease have failed to show benefit.[10,16]

The Women's Health Initiative (WHI) was planned as an 8- to 10-year nationwide research effort with an observational study component (93,700 women) and a multicenter, prospective, randomized, double-blind, placebo-controlled clinical trial component (68,000 women) to define the risks and benefits of strategies that could reduce the incidence of heart disease, breast and colorectal cancer, and fractures in postmenopausal women. Between 1993 and 1998, the WHI enrolled 161,809 mostly healthy postmenopausal women (50 to 79 years of age) into a set of clinical trials (trials of low-fat diet, calcium and vitamin D supplementation, and two parallel trials of postmenopausal HT).[21–23]

The two parallel trials of HT were undertaken to determine whether estrogen plus progestin (CCEPT; for women with an intact uterus) or estrogen alone (ET; for women with prior hysterectomy) would reduce the incidence of cardiovascular disease and lead to any change in risk for breast or colorectal cancer in postmenopausal women. A total of 16,608 women with an intact uterus were enrolled in the estrogen plus progestin arm (CCEPT). The study was stopped prematurely in 2002 after 5.2 years of data analysis when it was determined that the risks of HT outweighed its benefits. The study found that the risk of breast cancer crossed the predetermined safety boundary and incidences of CHD, stroke, and venous thromboembolic disease were all increased. On the positive side, there was a reduction in colorectal cancer and hip fractures among the women using HT.[21] The ET-only clinical trial was also stopped prematurely, after 6.8 years.[22,23] The ET-only study demonstrated no increased risk of breast cancer or heart disease, but there was a similar increased risk of stroke and venous thromboembolic disease.

Results from a 3-year follow-up study of women in the CCEPT arm of the WHI trial indicate that the increased cardiovascular risks observed at the time the intervention was stopped were not maintained, but a greater risk of fatal and nonfatal malignancies occurred (global risk index was 12% higher in women from the CCEPT group as compared with the placebo group).[22,23] The follow-up study also found that the positive effects of CCEPT, such as decreased risk of colorectal cancer and hip fractures, also stopped when therapy ended.[22,23]

Cardiovascular Risk. Subsequent critical reassessment and subgroup analyses of the WHI, as well as findings from other studies, have led to a reevaluation of some of the conclusions that were made. A complete review of the literature surrounding HT is beyond the scope of this chapter. However, the following summary statements represent some of the current thinking.

First, the average age (63.7 years) and length of time since menopause (18 years) have been identified as indications that the women in WHI were already potentially predisposed to CHD and that the WHI may, in truth, have been a secondary prevention trial. Analyses of risk by age[24] and time since menopause[25] in the CCEPT trial reveal that the younger women (younger than 60 years of age) and those who started HT within 10 years of menopause demonstrated a trend toward lower rates of CHD. It has been hypothesized that HT, given during a "critical window" after menopause, may continue the cardioprotective actions provided by premenopausal levels of estrogen. However, when HT is started beyond this window period (when women may already have preexisting subclinical atherosclerosis), it may stimulate inflammatory cytokines that predispose to atherosclerotic plaque rupture and development of symptomatic CHD.[26] The majority (70%) of the women in the WHI were in the age group that could be expected to have subclinical changes at the start of the study and therefore would be less likely to benefit from HT.

Second, data from the Nurses' Health Study[27] suggest that women starting HT near the onset of menopause had a significantly reduced risk (30%) of CHD.

Third, a narrative review[27] described a decrease in CHD in younger postmenopausal women undergoing HT. Although there was a reported initial increase in incidence of CHD during the first year in older postmenopausal women (those who started HT after age 60 years), there was a reduced incidence after 2 years. It is still a matter of debate whether the presence of the daily progestin contributed to the higher levels of CHD in the CCEPT group compared with the ET group.

The increased risk of venous thromboembolism does appear to be consistently associated with the use of HT. The absolute risk is low, appears to be greatest in the first 2 years of HT use, and declines thereafter. Women with a history of venous thromboembolism or who have a predisposition to clot formation as a result of coagulation defects such as factor V Leiden are generally advised to avoid the use of HT.

Breast Cancer Risk. The association with breast cancer has long been the other area of concern with HT. In studies reporting estimated risks of breast cancer associated with HT, most of the confidence intervals cross the relative risk of 1 and therefore are not statistically significant.[28] The WHI added to the breast cancer concern by reporting a 26% increased risk of invasive breast cancer in the women using CCEPT.[29] Results from a 3-year WHI follow-up study revealed that the breast cancer risk of women who stopped taking CCEPT continued at a rate similar to that observed during the intervention.[22,23] The use of ET alone did not increase breast cancer risk in the WHI, but it did appear to increase the need for additional follow-up mammograms because of the added density of the breasts in women using estrogen HT.[30]

An update from the Nurses' Health Study showed no increased risk of invasive breast cancer with estrogen HT until 20 years of use.[27,31] In contrast, another large European study recruited over 1 million women aged 50 to 64 years and analyzed the 80% who were postmenopausal for breast cancer incidence (2.6 years average follow-up) and mortality (4.1 years average follow-up). Approximately half the women had used HT at some time. Results of this observational study revealed increased risk among current users of HT. The largest increase in risk was associated with CCEPT, was slightly less with ET, and declined after discontinuation and returned to baseline within 5 years.[32]

Current thinking postulates that these studies may, in fact, constitute detection studies rather than incidence studies, because it is known that breast cancer cells can be present in the body for 8 to 10 years before the cancer can be detected by any currently available means. Estrogen may accelerate the growth of these cells to a point where the cancer can then be detected, which may explain why some studies show a positive correlation between estrogen and breast cancer and others do not. In this case, the increase in breast cancer detection may in fact be a positive outcome because it can be discovered while the cancer is still curable. At present there is insufficient evidence to support estrogen as the cause (initiator) of breast cancer.[33,34] In fact, studies conducted to determine if women with a history of breast cancer who experienced some of the aggravating symptoms of menopause could take HT safely do not have clear answers.[35] Some physicians feel that if the woman is aware of the possible risks of breast cancer or other health problems that can be the result of HT and want to eradicate the symptoms of menopause, they should be able to take HT.[35] Thus, a more reasonable approach may involve identifying predisposing factors for breast cancer and finding better ways for early detection. This would assist women in assessing their own risk–benefit ratio, taking into account their individual circumstances, when making decisions about HT.

Hip Fracture and Other Risks. The release of data from the other two clinical trials within the WHI (low-fat dietary patterns, calcium and vitamin D supplementation) has challenged conventional wisdom in other areas. The use of calcium (1000 mg/day) plus vitamin D (200 IU/day) was shown to result in a small but significant improvement in hip bone density, but failed to reduce the risk of hip fractures.[36] The Institute of Medicine (2010) recommends that all adults take 600 IU/day to maintain healthy bones but could not make any causal relationships with taking vitamin D and any other health outcomes.[37,38]

Final Analysis: Current Recommendations for HT. Although the average age of menopause has not changed substantially since 1900, life expectancy has increased dramatically. Today, the average woman will live almost one third of her life after menopause. Menopause now represents only the end of reproductive capability. Estrogen's role in many other bodily functions has been well documented, but its replacement after the ovary ceases production has become highly controversial. Although the U.S. Preventive Services Task Force has recommended against the routine use of HT for preventing chronic conditions in general,[19] statements of practice recommendations from the North American Menopause Society (NAMS),[39] the American Society for Reproductive Medicine (ASRM),[40] the American College of Obstetricians and Gynecologists (ACOG),[41] and the National Institutes of Health (NIH) State-of-the-Science Conference Statement on Management of Menopause-Related Symptoms[42,43] all indicate that estrogen is the most consistently effective therapy for treating menopausal symptoms. Use of HT in younger, recently menopausal women appears less likely to result in the increased risks reported in the WHI and Heart and Estrogen/Progestin Replacement Study (HERS), which studied predominantly older, asymptomatic women who were on average 10 or more years beyond menopause.

Current recommendations for HT, in light of the findings of the WHI and other clinical trials, are as follows:

- Avoid HT for primary or secondary prevention of CHD
- Develop an individual risk profile for every woman contemplating HT and provide information regarding known risks

- Use HT only in those women who require relief from menopausal symptoms that affect quality of life
- Consider lower-than-standard doses and alternative routes of administration
- Limit the use of HT to the shortest duration consistent with goals, benefits, and risks of treatment for each woman
- Consider alternative therapies if the woman is not symptomatic because of the potential risks associated with HT products that are FDA-approved for the prevention of postmenopausal osteoporosis.[42]

Owing to the mixed results of the WHI, there has been increased interest in alternative methods for management of postmenopausal symptoms, specifically vasomotor symptoms. "Natural" substances derived from plant oils that are similar in structure to human steroid hormones,[39] and "phytoestrogens," substances occurring in nature with estrogen-like properties such as isoflavones (soy, red clover), have all been studied, with various results. SSRIs, gabapentin, and clonidine have been studied for prevention of hot flashes, showing some improvement over placebo in randomized control trials.[20] The use of botanicals and pharmaceuticals for treatment of menopausal symptoms provides another option for women and their providers.[44] However, continued studies are needed to further evaluate efficacy.

IN SUMMARY

Between menarche and menopause, the female reproductive system undergoes cyclic changes called the *menstrual cycle*. The normal menstrual cycle results from complex interactions among the hypothalamus, which produces GnRH; the anterior pituitary gland, which synthesizes and releases FSH, LH, and prolactin; the ovaries, which synthesize and release estrogens, progesterone, and androgens; and associated target tissues, such as the endometrium and the vaginal mucosa. Although each component of the system is essential for normal functioning, the ovarian hormones are largely responsible for controlling the cyclic changes and length of the menstrual cycle. Estrogens are necessary for normal female physical maturation, for growth of ovarian follicles, for generation of a climate that is favorable to fertilization and implantation of the ovum, and for promoting the development of the endometrium in the event of pregnancy. Estrogens also have a number of extragenital effects, including prevention of bone resorption and regulation of the composition of cholesterol-carrying lipoproteins (HDL and LDL) in the blood. The functions of progesterone include the glandular development of the lobular and alveolar tissue of the breasts, the cyclic glandular development of the endometrium, and maintenance of pregnancy. Androgens contribute to hair distribution in the female and may have important metabolic effects.

Menopause is the cessation of menstrual cycles. Systemically, a woman may experience significant vasomotor instability and "hot flashes" secondary to the decrease in estrogens and the relative increase in other hormones, including FSH, LH, GnRH, dehydroepiandrosterone, and androstenedione. The long-term effects of estrogen deprivation include osteoporosis because of an imbalance in bone remodeling (*i.e.*, bone resorption occurs at a faster rate than bone formation) and an increased risk for cardiovascular disease (atherosclerosis is accelerated), which is the leading cause of death in women after menopause. HT, which was regarded as a hormone replacement therapy for postmenopausal women during the late 20th century, has come under scrutiny as a result of the WHI study, which indicates that CCEPT (continuous combined estrogen and progestin) may increase the risk for cardiovascular disease and breast cancer. At this time, careful assessment of a woman's individual history must be undertaken and then an individual risk–benefit analysis that weighs the risk factors versus symptoms should be completed. For women who are placed on hormone replacement therapy, a low dose for a short interval in earlier menopause is preferred.

BREASTS

After completing this section of the chapter, the learner will be able to meet the following objectives:

- Describe the influence of hormones on breast development.
- Characterize the changes in breast structure that occur with pregnancy and lactation.

Although anatomically separate, the breasts are functionally related to the female genitourinary system in that they respond to the cyclic changes in sex hormones and produce milk for infant nourishment. The breasts are also important for their sexual function and for cosmetic appearance. Breast cancer represents the most common malignancy among women in the United States. A high rate of breast cancer has drawn even greater attention to the importance of breast health throughout the life span.

Structure and Function

The breasts, or mammary tissues, are located between the third and seventh ribs of the anterior chest wall and are supported by the pectoral muscles and superficial fascia.[6] They are specialized glandular structures that have an abundant shared nervous, vascular, and lymphatic supply (Fig. 44.7). What are commonly called "breasts" are two parts of a single anatomic breast. This contiguous nature of breast tissue is important in health and illness. Men and women alike are born with rudimentary breast tissue, with the ducts lined with epithelium. In women, the pituitary release of FSH, LH, and prolactin at puberty stimulates the ovary to produce and release estrogen. This estrogen stimulates

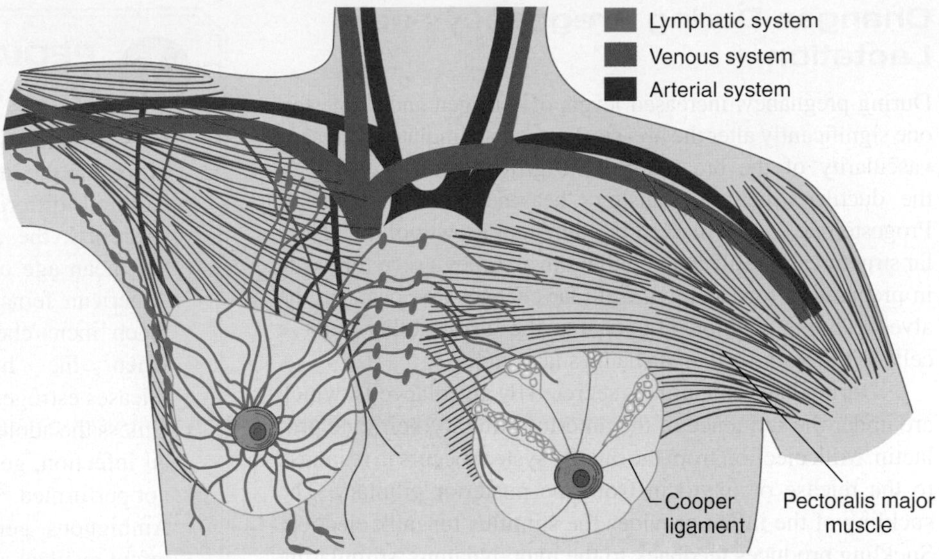

Figure 44.7 • The breasts, showing the shared vascular and lymphatic supply as well as the pectoral muscles.

the growth and proliferation of the ductile system. With the onset of ovulatory cycles, progesterone release stimulates the growth and development of ductile and alveolar secretory epithelium. By adolescence, the breasts have developed characteristic fat deposition patterns and contours.

Structurally, the breast consists of fat, fibrous connective tissue, and glandular tissue.[6] The superficial fibrous connective tissue is attached to the skin, a fact that is important in the visual observation of skin movement over the breast during breast self-examination. The breast mass is supported by the fascia of the pectoralis major and minor muscles and by the fibrous connective tissue of the breast. Fibrous tissue ligaments, called *Cooper ligaments*, extend from the outer boundaries of the breast to the nipple area in a radial manner, like the spokes on a wheel (see Fig. 44.8). These ligaments further support the breast and form septa that divide the breast into about 20 lobes.[6] Each lobe consists of grapelike clusters—alveoli or glands—that are interconnected by ducts. The alveoli are lined with secretory cells capable of producing milk or fluid under the proper hormonal conditions (Fig. 44.8). The route of descent of milk and other breast secretions is from alveoli to duct, to intralobar duct, to lactiferous duct and reservoir, to nipple.[6] Breast milk is produced secondary to complex hormonal changes associated with pregnancy. Fluid is produced and reabsorbed during the menstrual cycle. The breasts respond to the cyclic changes in the menstrual cycle with fullness and discomfort.

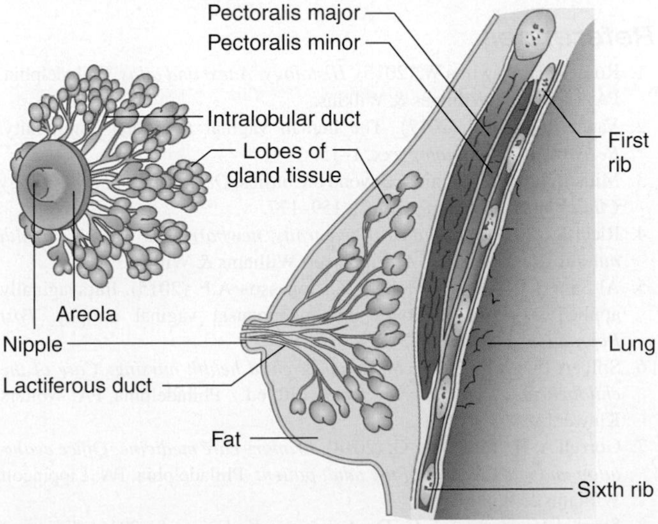

Figure 44.8 • The breast, showing the glandular tissue and ducts of the mammary glands.

The nipple is made up of epithelial, glandular, erectile, and nervous tissue. Areolar tissue surrounds the nipple and is recognized as the darker, smooth skin between the nipple and the breast. The small bumps or projections on the areolar surface known as *Montgomery tubercles* are sebaceous glands that keep the nipple area soft and elastic. At puberty and during pregnancy, increased levels of estrogen and progesterone cause the areola and nipple to become darker and more prominent and the Montgomery glands to become more active.[20] The erectile tissue of the nipple is responsive to psychological and tactile stimuli, which contributes to the sexual function of the breasts.

There are many individual variations in breast size and shape. The shape and texture vary with hormonal, genetic, nutritional, and endocrine factors and with muscle tone, age, and pregnancy. A well-developed set of pectoralis muscles supports the breast mass higher on the chest wall. Poor posture, significant weight loss, and lack of support may cause the breasts to droop.

KEY POINTS

BREASTS

- Structure and function are affected by hormonal changes throughout a woman's lifetime, such as during pregnancy and lactation.

Changes During Pregnancy and Lactation

During pregnancy, increased levels of estrogen and progesterone significantly alter the breasts. Estrogen stimulates increased vascularity of the breasts and the growth and extension of the ductile structures, causing "heaviness" of the breasts. Progesterone causes marked budding and growth of the alveolar structures. The alveolar epithelium assumes a secretory state in preparation for lactation. Cellular changes that occur in the alveolar lining are thought to change the susceptibility of these cells to estrogen-mediated changes later in life.

During lactation, milk is secreted by alveolar cells, which are under the influence of the anterior pituitary hormone prolactin. Milk ejection from the ductile system occurs in response to the release of oxytocin from the posterior pituitary. The suckling of the infant provides the stimulus for milk ejection. Suckling produces feedback to the hypothalamus, stimulating the release of oxytocin from the posterior pituitary. Oxytocin causes contraction of the myoepithelial cells lining the alveoli and ejection of milk into the ductal system.[6] A woman may have breast leakage for 3 months to 1 year after the termination of breast-feeding as breast tissue and hormones regress to the nonlactating state. Overzealous breast stimulation with or without pregnancy can likewise cause breast leakage.

It is important to follow safe guidelines for drug use, including optimal dosing, when a woman is pregnant or lactating because many drugs cross the placenta and enter breast milk.[45] There is controversy over how much vitamin D is best for pregnant woman. Pregnant and lactating women need to follow the current guidelines regarding maternal vitamin D status in order to prevent possible maternal and fetal adverse events because the amount of vitamin D needs to be individualized for each pregnant woman.[46,47]

IN SUMMARY

The breast is a complex structure of variable size, consistency, and composition. Although anatomically distinct, the breasts are functionally related to the female genitourinary system in that they respond to cyclic changes in sex hormones and produce milk for infant nourishment.

GERIATRIC Considerations

- The changes in the genitourinary tract associated with aging are due to decreased or no estrogen secretion.[48]
- The uterus begins to sag and the cervix begins to atrophy because of decreased estrogen.
- Thinning of genital hair and atrophy of fat pads of the labia and clitoris occur.[48,49]
- Sexual intercourse is often painful in the older female because of lack of elasticity of the vaginal mucosa and decreased vaginal secretions as estrogen levels drop.[48,49]

PEDIATRIC Considerations

- Pink discharge at the vagina introitus (entrance) is normal in the infant because of maternal estrogen.[48]
- Cultural differences account for age of puberty. Currently, the age of menarche is declining, with the mean age of menarche being 12.4 years for all American females except African Americans, who reach menarche at age 8 years. Menarche begins when the hypothalamic-pituitary-ovarian axis releases estrogen.[48]
- Unless the adolescent is sexually active or has a genital infection, genital assessment of the adolescent is not performed.[48]
- Ambiguous genitalia (where the anatomy of the infant may not clearly be male or female) is the result of hypersecretion of the adrenal glands, causing increased androgen.[48]

REVIEW EXERCISES

1. Diabetes mellitus and treatment with broad-spectrum antibiotics increase the risk of vaginal infections.
   A. *Explain how these two conditions change the vaginal ecology, making it more susceptible to infection.*
2. Most oral contraceptive agents use low doses of estrogen and progestin to prevent conception.
   A. *Use Figure 44.3 to explain how these oral agents prevent ovulation and pregnancy.*

References

1. Ross M. H., Pawlina W. (2015). *Histology: A text and atlas*. Philadelphia, PA: Lippincott Williams & Wilkins.
2. Vaneechoutte M. (2017). The human vaginal microbial community. *Research in Microbiology* xx, 1–15.
3. Mills B. (2017). Vaginitis: Beyond the basics. *Obstetrics and Gynecology Clinics of North America* 44(2), 159–177.
4. Ricci S. (2017). *Essentials of maternity, newborn, and women's health nursing*. Philadelphia, PA: Lippincott Williams & Wilkins.
5. Al-Saqi S. H., Uvnäs-Moberg K., Jonasson A.F. (2015). Intravaginally applied oxytocin improves post-menopausal vaginal atrophy. *Post Reproductive Health* 21(3), 89–97
6. Sillbert-Flagg J. (2018). *Maternal & child health nursing: Care of the childbearing & childbearing family* (8th ed.). Philadelphia, PA: Wolters Kluwer.
7. Gorroll A. H., Mulley A. G. (2014). *Primary care medicine: Office evaluation and management of the adult patient*. Philadelphia, PA: Lippincott Williams & Wilkins.
8. Singhal V., Maffazioli G. D., Ackerman K. E., et al. (2016). Effect of chronic athletic activity on brown fat in young women. *PLoS One* 11(5), e0156353.
9. Hall J. E. (2015). *Guyton and Hall textbook of medical physiology* (13th ed.). Philadelphia, PA: Elsevier.

10. Howard, B.V., Rossouw, J.E. (2013). Estrogens and cardiovascular disease risk revisited: The Women's Health Initiative. *Current Opinion in Lipidology*, 24(6), 493–499.
11. Vashishta S., Gahlot S., Goyal R. (2017). Effect of menstrual cycle phases on plasma lipid and lipoprotein levels in regularly menstruating women. *Journal of Clinical and Diagnostic Research* 11(5), CC05–CC07.
12. Engler-Chiurazzi E. B., Singh M., Simpkins J. W. (2016). Reprint of: From the 90's to now: A brief historical perspective on more than *two* decades of estrogen neuroprotection. *Brain Research* 1645, 79–82.
13. McCarrey A. C., Resnick S. M. (2015). Postmenopausal hormone therapy and cognition. *Hormones and Behavior* 74, 167–172.
14. Rotterdam ESHRE/ASRM-Sponsored PCOS Consensus Workshop Group. (2004). Revised 2003 consensus on diagnostic criteria and long-term health risks related to polycystic ovary syndrome. *Fertility and Sterility* 81, 19–25.
15. Amsterdam ESHRE/ASRM-Sponsored 3rd PCOS Consensus Workshop Group. (2012). Consensus on women's health aspects of polycystic ovary syndrome (PCOS). *Human Reproduction* 27, 14–24.
16. Panay N., Hamoda H., Arya R., Savvas M. (2013). The 2013 British Menopause Society & Women's Health Concern recommendations on hormone replacement therapy. *Post Reproductive Health* 22(4), 165–183.
17. Beck K. L., Anderson M. C., Kirk J. K. (2017). Transdermal estrogens in the changing landscape of hormone replacement therapy. *Postgraduate Medicine* 129(6), 632–636.
18. Takahashi T. A., Johnson K. M. (2015). Menopause. *Medical Clinics of North America* 99(3), 521–534.
19. Kreatsoulas C., Anand S. S. (2013). Menopausal hormone therapy for the primary prevention of chronic conditions U.S. Preventive Services Task Force recommendation statement. *Polish Archives of Internal Medicine* 123(3), 112–117.
20. Genazzani A., Brincat M. (2014). *Frontiers in gynecological endocrinology: Volume 1: From symptoms to therapies*. New York, NY: Springer International Publishing.
21. Writing Group for the WHI Investigators. (2002). Risks and benefits of estrogen and progestin in healthy postmenopausal women: Principal results from the WHI randomized controlled trial. *Journal of the American Medical Association* 288, 321–333.
22. Anderson G. L., Limacher M., Assaf A. R., et al. (2004). The effects of conjugated equine estrogen in postmenopausal women with hysterectomy. The WHI randomized control trail. *Journal of the American Medical Association* 291, 1702–1712.
23. Chlebowski R. T., Rohan T. E., Manson J. E., et al. (2015). Breast cancer after use of estrogen plus progestin and estrogen alone analyses of data from 2 Women's Health Initiative randomized clinical trials. *JAMA Oncology* 3(1), 296–305.
24. Heiss G., Wallace R., Anderson G. L. (2008). Health risks and benefits 3 years after stopping randomized treatment with estrogen and progestin. *Journal of the American Medical Association* 299(9), 1036–1044.
25. Bolton L. (2016). Menopausal hormone therapy, age, and chronic diseases: Perspectives on statistical trends. *Chemical Research in Toxicology* 29(10), 1583–1590.
26. Hall P. S., Nah G., Howard B. V., et al. (2017). Reproductive factors and incidence of heart failure hospitalization in the Women's Health Initiative. *Journal of the American College of Cardiology* 69(20), 2517–2526.
27. Bassuk S. S., Manson J. E. (2016). The timing hypothesis: Do coronary risks of menopausal hormone therapy vary by age or time since menopause onset? *Metabolism* 65(5), 794–803.
28. Bhupathiraju S.N., Grodstein F., Stampfer M. J., et al. (2016). Exogenous hormone use: Oral contraceptives, postmenopausal hormone therapy, and health outcomes in the Nurses' Health Study. *American Journal of Public Health* 106(9), 1631–1637.
29. Nichols H. B., Trentham-Dietz A., Newcomb P. A., et al. (2012). Postoophorectomy estrogen use and breast cancer risk. *Obstetrics & Gynecology* 120(1), 27–36.
30. Chlebowski R. T., Anderson G. L. (2015). Menopausal hormone therapy and breast cancer mortality: Clinical implications. *Therapeutic Advances in Drug Safety* 6(2), 45–56.
31. Chebowski R. T., Rohan T. E., Manson J. E., et al. (2015). Brest cancer after use of estrogen plus progestin and estrogen alone: Analyses of data from 2 Women's Health Initiative randomized clinical trials. *Journal of the American Medical Association Oncology* 1(3), 296–305.
32. Tamimi R. M., Spiegelman D., Smith-Warner S. A., et al. (2016). Population attributable risk of modifiable and nonmodifiable breast cancer risk factors in postmenopausal breast cancer. *American Journal of Epidemiology* 184(12), 884–893.
33. Beral V.; Million Women Study Collaborators. (2003). Breast cancer and hormone-replacement therapy in the Million Women Study. *Lancet* 362, 419–427.
34. Shapiro S., Farmer R. D., Stevenson J. C., et al. (2013). Does hormonal replacement therapy (HRT) cause breast cancer? An application of causal principles to three studies. *Journal of Family Planning and Reproductive Health Care* 39(2), 80–88.
35. Akram M., Iqbal M., Daniyal M., et al. (2017). Awareness and current knowledge of breast cancer. *Biological Research* 50(1), 33.
36. Garrido Oyarzún M. F., Castelo-Branco C. (2017). Use of hormone therapy for menopausal symptoms and quality of life in breast cancer survivors. Safe and ethical? *Gynecological Endocrinology* 33(1), 10–15.
37. Cauley J. A., Chlebowski R. T., Wactawski-Wende J., et al. (2013). Calcium plus vitamin D supplementation and health outcomes five years after active intervention ended: the Women's Health Initiative. *Journal of Women's Health* 22(11), 915–929.
38. Friedman P. A., Brunton L. L. (2018). Updated vitamin D and calcium recommendations. [Online]. Available: https://www.medscape.com/viewarticle/738275. Accessed March 12, 2018.
39. Moyer V. A.; U.S. Preventive Services Task Force. (2013). Medications to decrease the risk for breast cancer in women: U.S. Preventive Services Task Force recommendation statement. *Annals of Internal Medicine* 159(10), 698–708.
40. North American Menopause Society 2017 Hormone Therapy Position Statement Advisory Panel. (2017). The 2017 hormone therapy position statement of The North American Menopause Society. *Menopause* 24(7), 728–753.
41. Committee on Gynecologic Practice and the American Society for the Reproductive Medicine Practice Committee. (2012). Committee opinion No. 532: Compounded bioidentical menopausal hormone therapy. *Obstetrics & Gynecology* 120(2 Pt 1), 411–415.
42. American College of Obstetricians and Gynecologists. (2014). ACOG practice bulletin no. 141: Management of menopausal symptoms. *Obstetrics & Gynecology* 123(1), 202–216.
43. Institutes of Health State-of-the-Science Conference. (2005). National Institutes of Health State-of-the-Science Consensus Statement: Management of menopause-related symptoms [Online]. Available: http://consensus.nih.gov/2005/menopause.htm. Accessed August 15, 2011.
44. Chew F., Wu X. (2017). Sources of information influencing the state-of-the-science gap in hormone replacement therapy usage. *PLoS One* 12(2), e0171189.
45. Kaunitz A. M., Manson J. E. (2015). Management of menopausal symptoms. *Obstetrics & Gynecology* 126(4), 859–876.
46. Temming T. A., Cahill A. G., Riley L. E. (2016). Clinical management of medications in pregnancy and lactation. *American Journal of Obstetrics and Gynecology* 214(6), 698–702.
47. Schoenmakers I., Pettifor J. M., Peña-Rosas J. P., et al. (2016). Prevention and consequences of vitamin D deficiency in pregnant and lactating women and children: A symposium to prioritise vitamin D on the global agenda. *Journal of Steroid Biochemistry and Molecular Biology* 164, 156–164.
48. Jensen S. (2015). *Nursing health assessment* (2nd ed., pp. 737–769). Philadelphia, PA: Wolters Kluwer.
49. Eliopoulos C. (2018). Reproductive system. In McIntyre N., Brittain, M. L. (Eds.), *Gerontological nursing* (9th ed.). Philadelphia, PA: Wolters Kluwer.

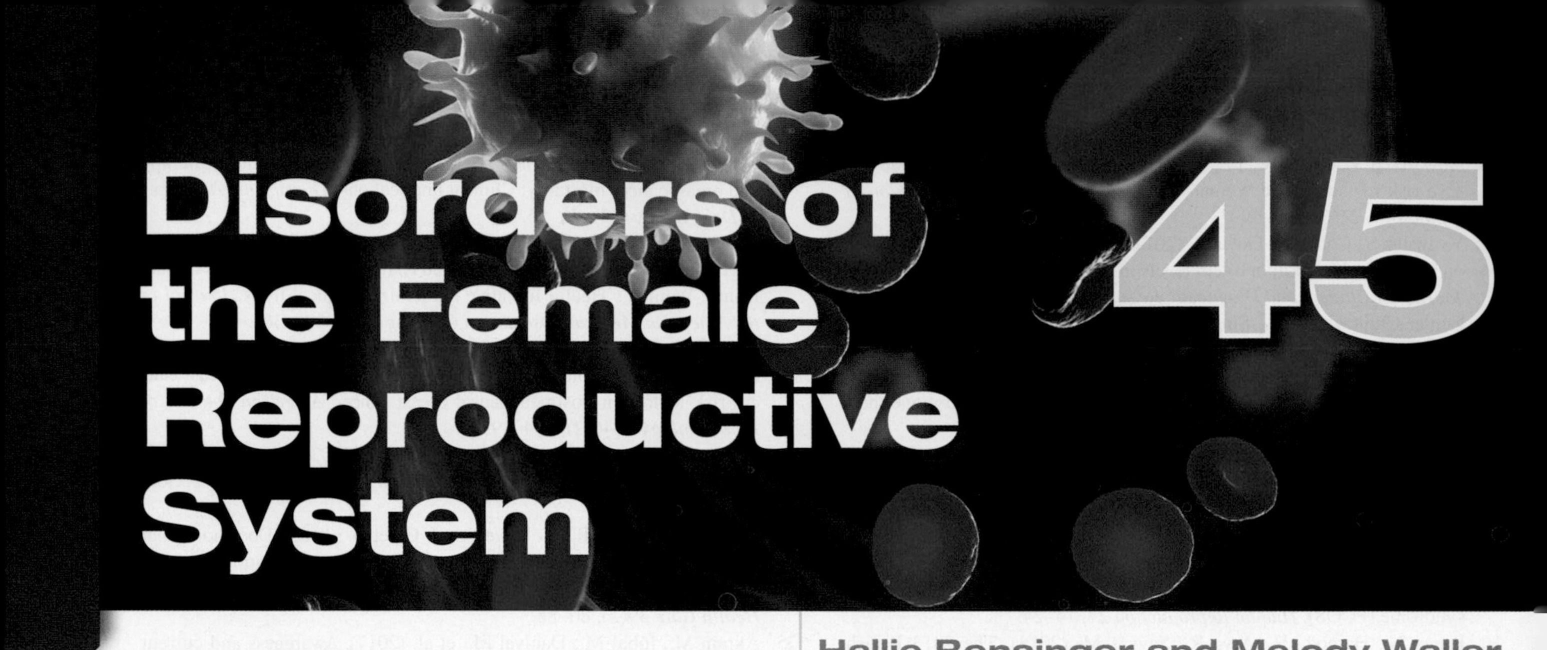

Disorders of the Female Reproductive System

45

Hallie Bensinger and Melody Waller

Disorders of the female genitourinary system have widespread effects on physical and psychological function, including general health status, sexuality, and reproductive potential. The reproductive structures are located close to other pelvic structures, particularly those of the urinary system, and disorders of the reproductive system may affect urinary function. This chapter focuses on infection and inflammation, benign conditions, and neoplasms (benign and malignant) of the female reproductive structures; disorders of pelvic support and uterine position; and alterations in menstruation. An overview of infertility is also included.

DISORDERS OF THE EXTERNAL GENITALIA AND VAGINA

After completing this section of the chapter, the learner will be able to meet the following objectives:

- Discuss the abnormalities associated with Bartholin cysts, nonneoplastic epithelial disorders, vulvodynia, and cancer of the vulva.
- Describe the conditions that predispose to vaginal infections and the methods used to prevent and treat these infections.

Disorders of the External Genitalia

Diseases of the external genitalia are similar to those that affect hair-bearing skin elsewhere in the body. Most skin cysts, nevi, and malignant neoplasms can occur on the skin of the external genitalia as well as on the skin in other parts of the body. The vulva (composed of the mons pubis, labia majora and minora, clitoris, and vestibule) is particularly prone to skin infections because it is constantly exposed to secretions and moisture. Nonspecific vulvitis is particularly common in women with diabetes, chronic kidney disease, blood dyscrasias, and malnutrition.

Bartholin Gland Cyst and Abscess

A Bartholin gland cyst is a fluid-filled sac that results from occlusion of the duct system in the Bartholin gland (Fig. 45.1).[1] If the cyst becomes infected, an abscess may develop in the gland and is commonly caused by staphylococcal, chlamydial, and anaerobic infections.[1–3]

Acute symptoms are usually the result of infection and include pain, tenderness, and dyspareunia (pain with intercourse). The treatment of symptomatic cysts consists of the administration of appropriate antibiotics, local application of moist heat, and incision and drainage. A Word catheter may be inserted to continue to drain the cyst for a few weeks. Frequently reoccurring cysts may require surgical intervention. Because the Bartholin glands usually shrink during menopause, a vulvar growth in postmenopausal women is suspicious and should be evaluated for malignancy.[4]

Nonneoplastic Epithelial Disorders

The term *nonneoplastic epithelial disorders* refers to nonmalignant atrophic and hyperplastic changes of the vulvar skin

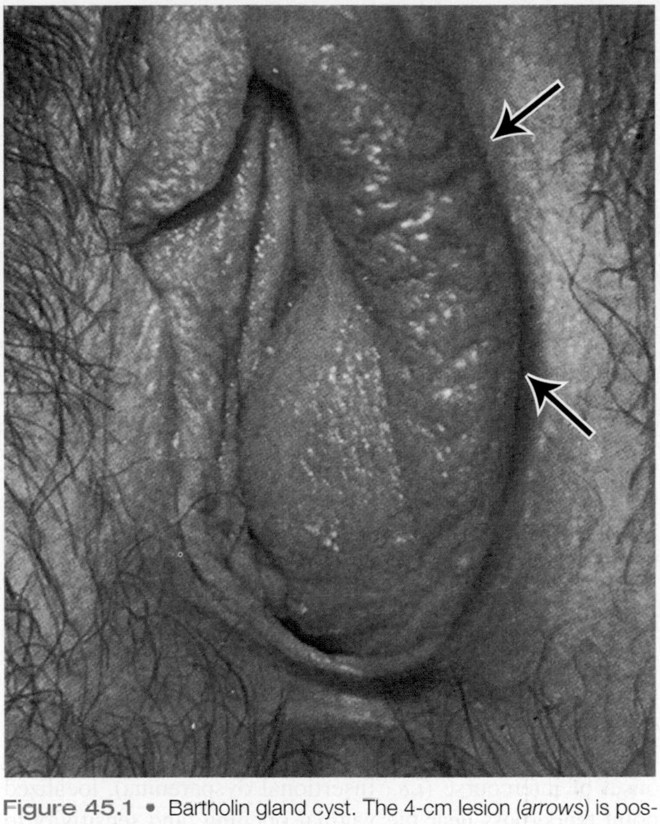

Figure 45.1 • Bartholin gland cyst. The 4-cm lesion (*arrows*) is posterior to the vaginal introitus. (From Strayer D., Rubin R. (Eds.) (2015). *Rubin's pathology: Clinicopathologic foundations of medicine* (7th ed., Fig. 24-3, p. 1001). Philadelphia, PA: Lippincott Williams & Wilkins.)

and mucosa that can develop at any age and can progress to malignancy. Depending on clinical and histologic characteristics, the lesions can be categorized as lichen simplex chronicus, lichen sclerosus, or lichen planus.[5,6] These precursor lesions can progress to differentiated vulvar intraepithelial neoplasia (VIN) or VIN simplex.[1] There is evidence that VIN, invasive squamous cell carcinoma, and lichen sclerosus have the identical p53 gene mutation.[1] Vulvar carcinoma is rare.[1]

Lichen simplex chronicus presents as thickened, gray-white plaques with an irregular surface. Presumed to be a response of the genital skin to some type of irritant, this diagnosis is used only when human papillomavirus (HPV) infection, fungal infections, or other known causative conditions have been ruled out. Vulvar pruritus is the most common presenting complaint. Treatment is aimed at reducing itching and preventing further irritation to the skin.

Lichen sclerosus is an inflammatory disease of the vulva characterized by plaquelike areas that may progress to parchment-thin epithelium with focal areas of ecchymosis and superficial ulceration secondary to scratching.[4] Atrophy and contracture of the vulvar tissues with eventual stenosis of the introitus are common when this condition becomes chronic. Itching is common and dyspareunia is frequent. The condition develops insidiously and has a high risk associated with developing vulvar malignancy.[1] Lichen sclerosus is also seen with autoimmune disorders such as thyroiditis and vitiligo.[1] Current treatment measures for lichen sclerosus favor the use of potent topical corticosteroids.[6,7] Lichen sclerosus frequently recurs, and lifetime maintenance therapy may be required. Hyperplastic areas that occur in the field of lichen sclerosus may be sites of malignant change and warrant close follow-up and possible biopsy.

Lichen planus is thought to have an autoimmune component and is more rarely seen. There are three types of lichen planus including erosive, which is the most common, papulosquamous, and hypertrophic.[4] Generally, a mild topical steroid is the treatment.

Vulvodynia

Vulvodynia is a multifactorial chronic vulvar pain disorder of at least 3 months' duration[8,9]; previously it was referred to as *vulvar pain syndrome* or *burning vulva syndrome*. The International Society for the Study of Vulvovaginal Disorders (ISSVD) defines it as a condition characterized by vulvar pain in the absence of relevant visible findings or a clinically identifiable disorder.[9] It may be primary or secondary. Vulvodynia is further classified as localized or generalized, and as to whether it is provoked, unprovoked, or of mixed origin.[9]

Localized Vulvodynia. *Localized vulvodynia* or *vestibulodynia*, formerly referred to as *vulvar vestibulitis syndrome*, is characterized by often stinging, burning or cutting pain at onset of intercourse (*i.e.*, insertional dyspareunia), localized point tenderness near the vaginal opening, and sensitivity to tampon placement.[10,11] The pain can be primary (present from first contact) or secondary (developing after a period of comfortable sexual relations). The exact etiology is unknown, but evidence suggests that it may involve the brain and spinal cord pain circuits becoming sensitized.[10] Comorbid conditions such as a history of severe dysmenorrhea, interstitial cystitis, and irritable bowel syndrome may be associated with this disorder. Furthermore, women who have anxiety and mood disorders may be predisposed to developing vestibulodynia.[10] Surgical vestibulectomy may be recommended for symptom relief when medical management fails. Because there is no known specific etiology of vestibulodynia and no single treatment with high evidence of efficacy, it is important to individualize treatment. In addition to medical management, biofeedback, sexual counseling, and psychological and emotional support may be beneficial.[11]

Generalized Vulvodynia. *Generalized vulvodynia* involves severe, constant, widespread pain or burning that interferes with daily activities.[8,12] No abnormalities are found on examination, but there is diffuse and variable hypersensitivity and altered sensation to light touch. The quality of this unprovoked pain shares many of the features of other neuropathic pain disorders, particularly complex regional pain syndrome or pudendal neuralgia. Although the cause of the neuropathic pain is unknown, it has been suggested that it may result from myofascial restrictions affecting the sacral and pelvic floor nerves. Surface electromyography-assisted pelvic floor muscle rehabilitation has been shown to be an effective primary therapy or adjunct to medical or surgical therapy for generalized vulvodynia.[8,9]

There are many proposed triggers for vulvodynia, including chronic recurrent vaginal infections; chemical irritation or drug effects, especially prolonged use of topical steroid creams; the irritating effects of elevated urinary levels of calcium oxalate; and immunoglobulin A deficiency or other disorders of immune regulation.[8,9]

Careful history taking and physical assessment are essential for differential diagnosis and treatment. *Vulvodynia* is a diagnosis of exclusion after ruling out infections, such as candidiasis and genital herpes; inflammatory conditions, such as lichen simplex chronicus and lichen sclerosus; vulvar cancer; or neurologic disorders, such as herpes neuralgia or spinal nerve compression, as causes for the pain.

Treatment for this chronic, often debilitating problem is aimed at symptom relief, is frequently long term, and often needs to be managed from a multidimensional, chronic pain perspective.[8,9] Regimens can include a long-term vaginal or oral antifungal therapy, avoidance of potential irritants, sitz baths with baking soda, emollients such as vitamin E or vegetable oil for lubrication, anesthetic or steroid ointments, capsaicin cream (topical analgesic), physical therapy, and surgery. Oral medications, including tricyclic antidepressants, other antidepressants (*e.g.*, selective serotonin receptor uptake inhibitors [SSRIs]), or gabapentin (an antiepileptic drug), are often used to treat the neuropathic pain associated with vulvodynia.[11] Because this condition can cause strain in sexual, family, and work relationships, psychosocial support often is needed.

Cancer of the Vulva

Estimates of carcinoma of the vulva for 2017 in the United States are approximately 6020 new cases per year with 1150 predicted deaths.[13] There is a lifetime risk of 0.3% of women being diagnosed with vulvar carcinoma at some time in their life.[13] Vulvar cancer accounts for about 3% of all of the female genital malignancies occurring in women 60 years of age or older.[1]

In terms of etiology, pathogenesis, and clinical presentation, vulvar carcinoma can be divided into two general groups: human papillomavirus (HPV)-associated usual vulvar intraepithelial neoplasm (uVIN) and HPV-independent VIN (dVIN). uVIN is commonly found in younger women. By contrast, dVIN more commonly occurs in postmenopausal women with a history of lichen sclerosus or lichen simplex chronicus.[14]

One third to one half of uVIN cases appear to be caused by the cancer-promoting potential of certain strains (subtype 16) of HPV that are sexually transmitted and are associated with the type of vulvar cancer found in younger women (*i.e.*, younger than 40 years of age).[1] VIN lesions may take many forms. They may be singular or multicentric, macular or papular, red or white and plaquelike. Microscopically, uVIN presents as a proliferative process and is characterized by epithelial cells with hyperchromatic nuclei, increased mitosis, and a larger nucleus to cytoplasm ratio. The risk of progression to invasive cancer increases in older women and in women with suppressed immune function.[14]

The second form of vulvar cancer, which is seen more often in older women, is generally preceded by vulvar nonneoplastic disorders such as chronic vulvar irritation or lichen sclerosus. The etiology of this group of vulvar cancers is unclear, but they are not typically associated with HPV. Neoplastic changes may arise from lichen sclerosus lesions or hyperplasia, leading directly to malignancy.[14]

The initial lesion of squamous cell vulvar carcinoma may appear as an inconspicuous thickening of the skin, a small raised area or lump, or an ulceration that fails to heal. It may be single or multiple and vary in color from white to velvety red or black.[15] The lesions may resemble eczema or dermatitis and may produce few symptoms other than pruritus, local discomfort, and exudation. The lesion may become secondarily infected, causing pain and discomfort. The malignant lesion gradually spreads superficially or as a deep furrow involving all of one labial side. Because there are many lymph channels around the vulva, the cancer metastasizes freely to the regional lymph nodes. The most common extension is to the superficial inguinal, and then to deep femoral, inguinal, and pelvic lymph nodes.[16] The system developed by the 2009 International Federation of Gynecology and Obstetrics (FIGO) grades vulvar cancer using four stages based on where it has spread.[17]

Early diagnosis is important in the treatment of vulvar carcinoma. Because malignant lesions can vary in appearance and commonly are mistaken for other conditions, biopsy and treatment often are delayed. Treatment is primarily wide surgical excision of the lesion for noninvasive cancer and radical excision or vulvectomy with node resection for invasive cancer. Postoperative groin and pelvic radiation is recommended when groin lymph nodes are involved.[18]

Disorders of the Vagina

The normal vaginal ecology depends on the delicate balance of hormones and bacterial flora. Normal estrogen levels maintain a thick, protective squamous epithelium that contains glycogen. The vaginal flora consists of various bacteria, mostly from the *Lactobacillus* genus that metabolizes glycogen, and in the process produce the lactic acid that normally maintains the vaginal pH of 4.0 to 4.5.[19] Disruptions in these environmental conditions, such as changes in the normal flora by antibiotic use, predispose to infection.

Vaginitis

Vaginitis represents an inflammation of the vagina that is characterized by vaginal discharge and burning, itching, redness, and swelling of vaginal tissues. Pain often occurs with urination and sexual intercourse. Chemical irritants, foreign bodies, or infectious agents may cause vaginitis. The causes of vaginitis differ in various age-groups. In premenarchal girls, most vaginal infections have nonspecific causes, such as poor hygiene, intestinal parasites, or the presence of foreign bodies. *Candida albicans*, *Trichomonas vaginalis*, and bacterial vaginosis are the most common causes of vaginitis in the childbearing years, and some of these organisms can be transmitted sexually.[1]

In postmenopausal women, atrophic vaginitis is the most common form. Atrophic vaginitis is an inflammation of the vagina that occurs after menopause or removal of the ovaries (causing estrogen deficiency). Estrogen deficiency results in a lack of regenerative growth of the vaginal epithelium, rendering these tissues more susceptible to infection and irritation. These changes lead to a decrease in the vaginal flora, causing vaginal secretions to become less acidic. The symptoms of atrophic vaginitis include itching, burning, and painful intercourse. Extreme symptoms can sometimes be reversed by local application of estrogen cream.

Every woman normally experiences vaginal discharge during the menstrual cycle, but it should not cause burning, itching, or have an unpleasant odor. These symptoms suggest inflammation or infection. Because these symptoms are common to the different types of vaginitis, precise identification of the organism is essential for proper treatment. A careful history should include information about systemic disease conditions, the use of drugs such as antibiotics that foster the growth of yeast, dietary habits, stress, and other factors that alter the resistance of vaginal tissue to infections. A physical examination usually is done to evaluate the nature of the discharge and its effects on the genital structures. Microscopic examination of a saline wet-mount smear (prepared by placing a sample of vaginal mucus in one or two drops of normal saline) is the primary means of identifying the organism responsible for the infection. In order to identify candidiasis, potassium hydroxide (KOH) is used with the wet mount instead of the saline.[19]

The prevention and treatment of vaginal infections depend on proper health habits and accurate diagnosis and treatment of ongoing infections. It is important for women to see their providers regarding any problem they may be experiencing in order for the earliest possible diagnosis to be made. An earlier diagnosis may lead to more effective treatment.

Cancer of the Vagina

Primary cancers of the vagina are extremely rare. Approximately 1% of women will develop vaginal cancer in their lifetime.[20] Like vulvar carcinoma, carcinoma of the vagina is largely a disease of older women. Most women are 60 years of age or older at the time of diagnosis. The exception to that is the clear cell adenocarcinoma associated with diethylstilbestrol (DES) exposure in utero, which is still, although rarely, seen in offspring of women who were treated with DES.[1] Vaginal cancers may result from local extension of cervical cancer, from exposure to sexually transmitted HPV, or, rarely, from local irritation such as occurs with prolonged use of a pessary.

Concept Mastery Alert

The most significant risk factor for vaginal cancer is aging. It is a rare cancer, but typically occurs in those over 60 years of age.

Squamous cell carcinomas begin in the epithelium and progress over many years from precancerous lesions called *vaginal intraepithelial neoplasia* (VAIN), 65% to 80% of which contain HPV.[21] The most common symptom of vaginal carcinoma is abnormal bleeding. Other symptoms include an abnormal vaginal discharge, a palpable mass, or dyspareunia. Most women with preinvasive vaginal carcinoma are asymptomatic, with the cancer being discovered during a routine pelvic examination. The anatomic proximity of the vagina to other pelvic structures (urethra, bladder, and rectum) permits early spread to these areas. Therefore, the majority of vaginal cancer, about 80%, is due to metastasis.[1]

Treatment of vaginal cancer must take into consideration the type of cancer, the size, location, and spread of the lesion, and the woman's age. Local excision, laser vaporization, or a loop electrosurgical excision procedure (LEEP) can be considered as treatment with stage 0 squamous cell cancers. Radical surgery and radiation therapy are both curative with more advanced cancers. When there is upper vaginal involvement, radical surgery may be required. This includes a total hysterectomy, pelvic lymph node dissection, and partial vaginectomy. The ovaries usually are preserved unless they are diseased. Extensive lesions and those located in the middle or lower vaginal area usually are treated by radiation therapy, which can be intracavitary, interstitial, or external beam. The prognosis depends on the stage of the disease, involvement of lymph nodes, and the degree of mitotic activity of the tumor.[22]

IN SUMMARY

The surface of the vulva is affected by disorders that affect skin on other parts of the body. Bartholin cysts are the result of occluded ducts in Bartholin glands. They often are painful and can become infected. Nonneoplastic epithelial disorders are characterized by thinning or hyperplastic thickening of vulvar tissues. Vulvodynia is a chronic vulvar pain syndrome with several classifications and variable treatment results. Cancer of the vulva is associated with HPV infections in younger women and lichen sclerosus in older women.

The normal vaginal ecology depends on the delicate balance of hormones and bacterial flora. Disruptions in these normal environmental conditions predispose to vaginal infections. Vaginitis or inflammation of the vagina is characterized by vaginal discharge and burning, itching, redness, and swelling of vaginal tissues. It may be caused by chemical irritants, foreign bodies, or infectious agents. Primary cancers of the vagina are relatively uncommon, accounting for about 1% of all cancers of the female reproductive system. Daughters of women treated with DES to prevent miscarriage are at increased risk for development of adenocarcinoma of the vagina.

DISORDERS OF THE CERVIX AND UTERUS

After completing this section of the chapter, the learner will be able to meet the following objectives:

- Describe the importance of the cervical transformation zone in the pathogenesis of cervical cancer.
- Describe the development of cervical cancer from the appearance of atypical cells to the development of invasive cervical cancer and relate to the importance of the Pap smear in early detection of cervical cancer.
- Compare the pathology and manifestations of endometriosis and adenomyosis.

Disorders of the Uterine Cervix

The cervix is composed of two distinct types of tissue. The exocervix, or visible portion, is covered with stratified squamous epithelium, which also lines the vagina.[1] The endocervix is the canal that leads to the endometrial cavity. It is lined with columnar epithelium that contains large, branched mucus-secreting glands.[1] During each menstrual cycle, the cervical glands undergo important functional changes related to the transport of spermatozoa within the cervical canal. The amount and properties of the mucus secreted by the gland cells vary during the menstrual cycle under the influence of the ovarian hormones. Blockage of the mucosal glands results in trapping of mucus in the deeper glands, leading to the formation of dilated cysts in the cervix called *nabothian cysts*. These benign cysts may grow as large as one centimeter or more.[6]

The junction of the squamous epithelium of the exocervix and mucus-secreting columnar epithelium of the endocervix (*i.e.*, squamocolumnar junction) appears at various locations on the cervix at different points in a woman's life (Fig. 45.2).[6] During a woman's reproductive years, the cervix everts or turns

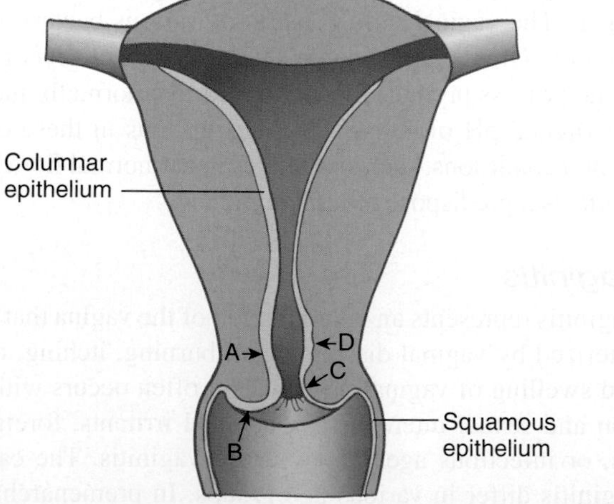

Figure 45.2 • Location of the squamocolumnar junction (transformation zone) in menarchial, menstruating, menopausal, and postmenopausal women. (*A*, menarchial; *B*, menstruating; *C*, menopausal; *D*, postmenopausal.)

outward, exposing the columnar epithelium to the vaginal environment. The combination of hormonal and pH changes, long-term inflammation, and mechanical irritation lead to a gradual transformation from columnar to squamous epithelium—a process called *metaplasia*. This area of continuous change, or process of repair, is called the *transformation zone*.[6]

The transformation zone is a critical area for the development of cervical cancer. During metaplasia, the newly developed squamous epithelial cells are vulnerable to development of dysplasia and genetic change if exposed to cancer-producing agents. *Dysplasia* means disordered growth or development of the cells. Although initially a reversible cell change, untreated dysplasia can develop into carcinoma. The transformation zone is the area of the cervix that must be sampled to have an adequate Pap smear and the area most carefully examined during colposcopy. Colposcopy is a vaginal examination using an instrument called a *colposcope* that affords a well-lit and magnified stereoscopic view of the cervix. A colposcopy is often done when there is an abnormal PAP smear result. During colposcopy, acetic acid solution and sometimes an iodine-based solution called Lugol's are used to accentuate topographic or vascular changes that can differentiate normal from abnormal tissue.[6] A biopsy sample may be obtained from suspect areas and examined microscopically, as is discussed later in the chapter.

Cervicitis and Cervical Polyps

Cervicitis is an acute or chronic inflammation of the cervix. Acute cervicitis may result from the direct infection of the cervix or may be secondary to a vaginal or uterine infection. It may be caused by a variety of infective agents, including *Streptococcus, Staphylococcus, Enterococcus, C. albicans, T. vaginalis, Neisseria gonorrhoeae, Gardnerella vaginalis, Chlamydia trachomatis, Ureaplasma urealyticum*, and herpes simplex virus type 2.[1] *C. trachomatis* is the organism most commonly associated with mucopurulent cervicitis. With acute cervicitis, the cervix becomes reddened and edematous. Irritation from the infection results in copious mucopurulent drainage and leukorrhea.[1] Depending on the causative agent, acute cervicitis is treated with appropriate antibiotic therapy. Untreated cervicitis may extend to include the development of pelvic cellulitis, dyspareunia, cervical stenosis, and ascending infection of the uterus or fallopian tubes as is discussed later in the chapter.

Polyps are the most common lesions of the cervix. They can be found in women of all ages, but their incidence is higher during the reproductive years.[1] Polyps are soft, velvety, red lesions; they usually are pedunculated and often are found protruding through the cervical os. They usually develop as a result of inflammatory hyperplasia of the endocervical mucosa. Polyps typically are asymptomatic, but may be associated with postcoital bleeding. Most are benign, but they should be removed and examined by a pathologist to exclude the possibility of malignant change.[23]

Cancer of the Cervix

Cervical cancer is readily detected and, if detected early, is the most easily cured of all the cancers of the female reproductive system. According to the American Cancer Society, an estimated 13,240 new cases of invasive cervical cancer will be diagnosed in the United States in 2018, with approximately 4170 deaths predicted from cervical cancer during the same period.[24] Over the past 40 years, deaths due to cervical cancer have decreased by 50%, indicating that a large number of potentially invasive cancers are cured by early detection and effective treatment.[24]

Risk Factors. Risk factors for cervical cancer include early age at first intercourse, multiple sexual partners, smoking, and a history of sexually transmitted infections (STIs). Women who have sex with women may have a higher incidence of abnormal Pap smears as they often delay screening. Women who have sex with women should follow the same guidelines for Pap smear screening that heterosexual women follow.[23] HPV is an STI passed through genital or skin-to-skin contact. HPV is highly prevalent; at least 50% of people will contract HPV in their life.[24] Specific strains, HPV type 16 and HPV type 18, have been associated with cervical cancer.[1] Other HPV types that are linked with cervical cancer include HPV types 31, 33, 35, 39,45, 51, 52, 56, 58, 59, and 68.[1] Other factors such as smoking, nutrition, and coexisting sexual infections such as *C. trachomatis*, herpes simplex virus type 2, and HIV may play a contributing role in determining whether a woman with HPV infection develops cervical cancer.[24]

Preventing Cervical Cancer. The HPV vaccine has decreased the risk of cervical cancer by 97%.[1] Gardasil is one type of HPV vaccine to prevent infection with the HPV subtypes 16, 18, 6, and 11. This vaccine has been approved for girls and boys between 9 and 26 years of age (prior to them becoming sexually active) to prevent HPV 6 and HPV 11 genital warts. The vaccine targets the two strains of HPV (HPV 16 and 18) responsible for 70% of cervical cancer, and the two most common benign strains (HPV 6 and 11), which account for up to 90% of genital warts. Clinical studies have confirmed that the vaccine appears safe and effective in inducing a sustained immunity response to HPV.[24,25]

Gardasil 9 vaccine offers the same protection against the HPV strains that Gardasil does, but additionally, this vaccine protects against five more high risk strains: 31, 33, 45, 52, and 58. These nine strains contribute to 90% of cervical cancers.[24] The other FDA approved HPV vaccine is Cervarix, which is recommended to be given to girls between 9 and 25 years of age, prior to becoming sexually active. Cervarix protects against HPV 16 and 18.[26]

Pathogenesis. With Pap smear cytological screening, precancerous lesions can be detected and treated before cancer develops. Pap smears may note atypical cells. Atypical cells differ from normal cervical squamous epithelium. There are changes in the nuclear and cytoplasmic parts of the cell and more variation in cell size and shape (*i.e.*, dysplasia). These precancerous changes represent a continuum of morphologic changes with indistinct boundaries that may gradually progress to cancer in situ and then to invasive cancer, or they may spontaneously regress.[1]

A system of grading devised to describe the histopathological findings of dysplastic changes of cancer precursors uses the term *cervical intraepithelial neoplasia* (CIN).(18a) This term describes premalignant changes in the epithelial tissue. CIN is categorized as:

- CIN I (dysplasia or atypical changes in the cervical epithelium)
- CIN II (moderate dysplasia)
- CIN III (severe dysplasia)[25]

Diagnosis. As discussed earlier, abnormal cells can be detected on a PAP smear. Abnormal Pap smear results will return as: atypical squamous cells of undetermined origin (ASC-US); atypical squamous cells of undetermined origin, cannot exclude high-grade squamous intraepithelial lesion (ASC-H); low-grade squamous intraepithelial lesion (LGSIL); high-grade squamous intraepithelial lesion (HGSIL); or squamous cell cancer. If abnormal results are detected, a colposcopy may be done to look for abnormal lesions on the cervix. Biopsies are taken of these potential abnormal lesions or areas of increased vascularity, as well as a curettage of the endocervical canal that may not be fully seen on colposcopy, and sent to pathology. The abnormal PAP smear finding of LGSIL is often CIN I on biopsy, whereas HGSIL on a PAP smear is more likely CIN II or CIN III on a biopsy[27] (Fig. 45.3).

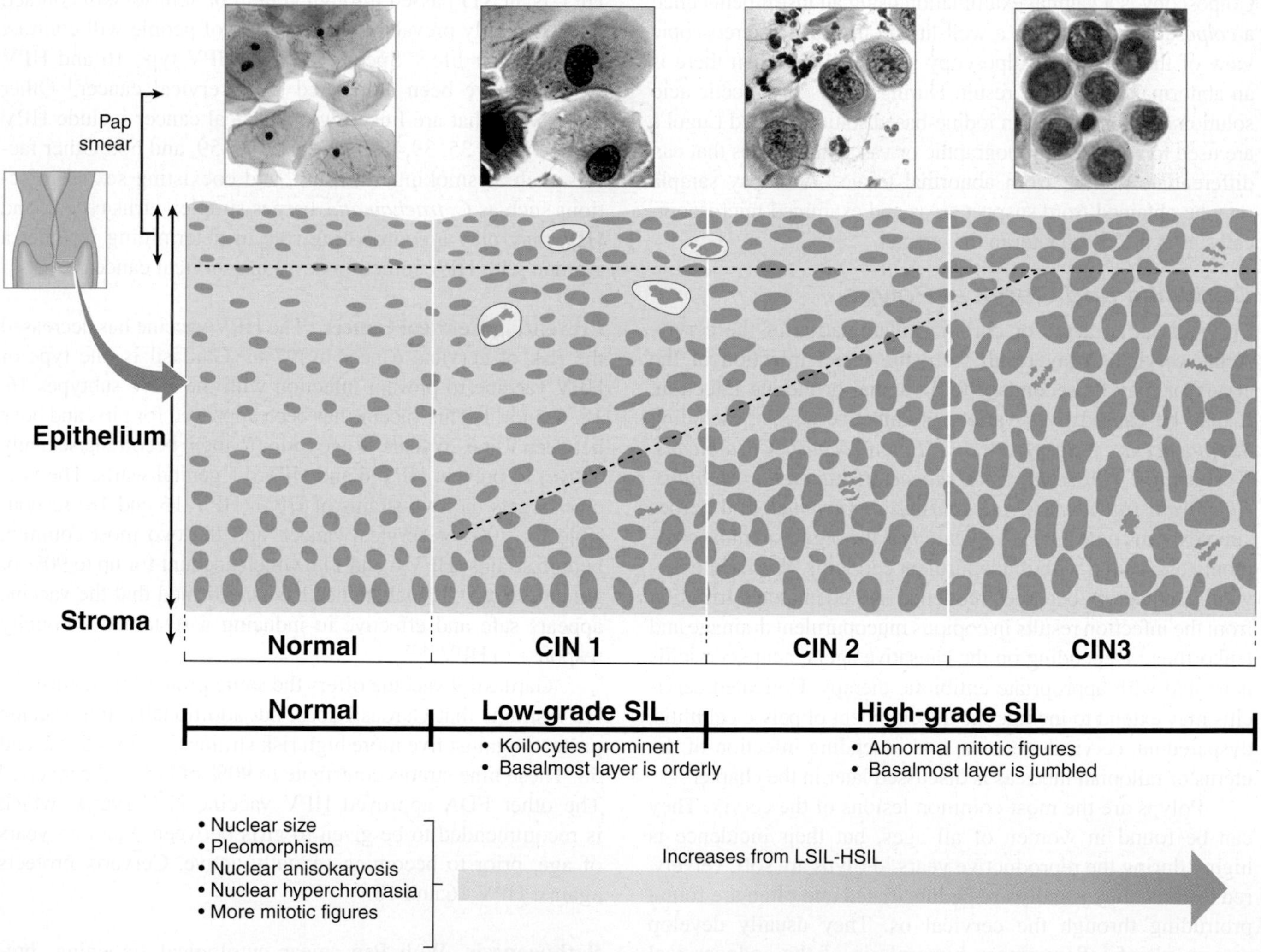

Figure 45.3 • The Bethesda system for designation of premalignant cervical disease as squamous intraepithelial lesions (SILs). This chart integrates multiple aspects across the normal-LGSIL (low-grade squamous intraepithelial lesion), and LIIL-HSIL (high-grade squamous intraepithelial lesion) interfaces, which correspond to therapeutic thresholds. It lists the qualitative and quantitative features that distinguish low-cancer-risk (LSIL) from high-cancer-risk (HSIL) lesions, which are generally caused by different subtypes of HPV. It also illustrates approximate counterparts for the legacy cervical intraepithelial neoplasia (CIN) system, which was based on a model of continuous progression rather than dichotomous viral subtypes. Finally, the scheme illustrates the corresponding cytologic smear resulting from exfoliation of the most superficial cells, indicating that even in the mildest disease state, abnormal cells reach the surface and are shed. (From Strayer D. S., Rubin R., (Eds.) (2015). *Rubin's pathology: Clinicopathologic foundations of medicine* (7th ed., Fig. 24-18, p. 1012). Philadelphia, PA: Lippincott Williams & Wilkins.)

With the discovery that HPV plays a significant role in causing cervical cancer, current recommendations for screening include HPV testing along with cytology in women 30 years of age and older. Results of this co-testing will dictate the next steps in management of the disease. Because of these advances in screening, the American Cancer Society no longer recommends annual Pap smears in women at low risk of getting cervical cancer. Cytology (Pap smear) alone is recommended beginning at the age of 21 years and then every 3 years through the age of 29 years. For women 30 years and older, a Pap smear alone should be performed every 3 years or co-testing can be performed every 5 years.[25]

False negative Pap smears occur,[28] indicating that care must be taken to obtain an adequate smear from the transformation zone that includes endocervical cells and to ensure that the cytologic examination is done by a competent laboratory. The presence of normal endometrial cells in a cervical cytologic sample during the luteal phase of the menstrual cycle or during the postmenopausal period has been associated with endometrial disease and warrants further evaluation with endometrial biopsy. This demonstrates that shedding of even normal cells at an inappropriate time may indicate disease. Because adenocarcinoma of the cervix is being detected more frequently, especially in women younger than 35 years of age, a Pap smear result of atypical glandular cells warrants further evaluation by endocervical or endometrial curettage, hysteroscopy, or, ultimately, a cone biopsy if the abnormality cannot be located or identified through other means.[21]

Before the availability of colposcopy, many women with abnormal Pap smear results required surgical cone biopsy for further evaluation. Cone biopsy involves the removal of a cone-shaped wedge of cervix, including the entire transformation zone and at least 50% of the endocervical canal. Postoperative hemorrhage, infection, cervical stenosis, infertility, and incompetent cervix are possible sequelae that warrant avoidance of this procedure unless it is truly necessary. LEEP (loop electrosurgical excision procedure) has taken the place of cone biopsies in most situations and is now the first-line management for CIN II/III.[21] This outpatient procedure allows for the simultaneous diagnosis and treatment of dysplastic lesions found on colposcopy. It uses a thin, rigid, wire loop electrode attached to a generator that blends high-frequency, low-voltage current for cutting and a modulated higher voltage for coagulation. In skilled hands, this wire can remove the entire transformation zone, providing adequate treatment for the lesion while obtaining a specimen for further histologic evaluation.

Clinical Manifestations and Treatment. In its early stages, cervical cancer often manifests as a poorly defined lesion of the endocervix. Frequently, women with cervical cancer present with abnormal vaginal bleeding, spotting, and discharge. Although bleeding may assume any course, it is reported most frequently after intercourse. Women with more advanced disease may present with pelvic or back pain that may radiate down the leg, hematuria, fistulas (rectovaginal or vesicovaginal), or evidence of metastatic disease to supraclavicular or inguinal lymph node areas.

Early treatment of cervical cancer involves removal of the lesion by one of various techniques. Biopsy or local cautery may be therapeutic in and of itself. Electrocautery, cryosurgery, or carbon dioxide laser therapy may be used to treat moderate to severe dysplasia that is limited to the exocervix (*i.e.*, squamocolumnar junction clearly visible). Therapeutic conization becomes necessary if the lesion extends into the endocervical canal and can be done surgically or with LEEP in the physician's office.

Depending on the stage of involvement of the cervix, invasive cancer is treated with radiation therapy, surgery, or both. External-beam irradiation and intracavitary irradiation or *brachytherapy* (*i.e.*, insertion of radioactive materials into the body) can be used in the treatment of cervical cancer.[29,30] Intracavitary radiation provides direct access to the central lesion and increases the tolerance of the cervix and surrounding tissues, permitting curative levels of radiation to be used. External-beam radiation eliminates metastatic disease in pelvic lymph nodes and other structures, as well as shrinks the cervical lesion to optimize the effects of intracavitary radiation. Surgery can include trachelectomy (removal of the cervix) in women with early stage cancer desiring fertility, radical hysterectomy (includes uterus, cervix, parametria, and upper portion of the vagina) with pelvic lymph node dissection,[29] or pelvic exenteration (*i.e.*, removal of all pelvic organs, including the bladder, rectum, vulva, and vagina).

Disorders of the Uterus

Common disorders of the uterus include endometritis, endometriosis, and endometrial cancer. Additionally, there is a high frequency of leiomyomas, which include uterine fibroid tumors that are benign neoplasms occurring in many women at some time during their life and adenomyosis, which is uterine thickening due to tissue from the endometrium being displaced in the outer muscular wall of the uterus.

Endometritis

The endometrium and myometrium are relatively resistant to infections, primarily because the endocervix normally forms a barrier to ascending infections. Endometritis is inflammation of the endometrium. Acute endometritis can occur as a result of an abortion or after delivery of a newborn when the cervical barrier is compromised.[1] Prophylactic antibiotics are given before and after an abortion to prevent this. There is an increased risk of endometritis after delivery of a newborn if the woman had chorioamnionitis during labor, had a cesarean section, or needed manual or instrumented removal of the placenta. Treatment includes antibiotics, and in cases where there are retained products of conception or placenta, a curettage may be necessary.[1]

Chronic inflammation of the endometrium can occur with pelvic inflammatory disease (PID), after instrumentation of the uterus (*e.g.*, after endometrial biopsy or intrauterine device [IUD] insertion), and with unrecognized retained products of conception after delivery or abortion. The presence of plasma cells (which are not present in the normal endometrium) is required for diagnosis.[1] The clinical picture is variable, but often includes mild to severe uterine tenderness, fever, malaise, and foul-smelling discharge. Treatment involves oral or intravenous antibiotic therapy, depending on the severity of the condition.

Endometriosis

Endometriosis is the condition in which functional endometrial tissue is found in ectopic sites outside the uterus. It is estrogen dependent. Currently, the question of whether endometriosis is an inflammatory disease or an immune disorder is being debated. Because implants of endometriosis are functional, they can lead to scarring, adhesions, and ovarian cysts called endometriomas.[31] The sites where endometriosis may occur include the ovaries, posterior broad ligaments, uterosacral ligaments, pouch of Douglas (cul-de-sac), pelvis, vagina, vulva, perineum, or intestines[32] (Fig. 45.4).

Etiology and Pathogenesis. The cause of endometriosis is unknown. There appears to have been an increase in its incidence in developed Western countries during the past four to five decades. Approximately, 10% of premenopausal women have some degree of endometriosis, causing infertility and chronic pain. Evidence supports that approximately 24% to 50% of infertile women have some degree of endometriosis.[33]

Several theories attempt to explain the origin of the dispersed endometrial lesions that occur in women with endometriosis. One theory, the *regurgitation/implantation theory*, (also known as Sampson's theory) suggests that menstrual blood containing fragments of endometrium is forced upward through the fallopian tubes into the peritoneal cavity. Retrograde menstruation is not an uncommon phenomenon, and it is unknown why endometrial cells implant and grow in some women but not in others. A second theory, the *metaplastic theory*, proposes that dormant, immature cellular elements, spread over a wide area during embryonic development, persist into adult life and then differentiate into endometrial tissue.[31] Another theory, the *vascular* or *lymphatic theory*, suggests that the endometrial tissue may metastasize through the lymphatics or vascular system. Genetic and immune factors also have been studied as contributing factors to the development of endometriosis.[31]

Clinical Manifestations. Endometriosis usually becomes apparent in the reproductive years when ovarian hormones stimulate the lesions in the same way as normal endometrium. The lesions then become proliferative, then secretory, and finally undergo menstrual breakdown. Bleeding into the surrounding structures can cause pain and the development of significant pelvic adhesions. Symptoms tend to be strongest premenstrually, subsiding after cessation of menstruation. Pelvic pain is the most common presenting symptom. Other symptoms include back pain, dyspareunia, and pain on defecation and micturition. Endometriosis is associated with infertility because of adhesions that distort the pelvic anatomy and cause impaired ovum release and transport.[33]

The gross pathologic changes that occur in endometriosis differ with location and duration. In the ovary, the endometrial tissue may form cysts known as endometriomas. These cysts are filled with old blood resembling chocolate syrup, for which they are sometimes referred to as chocolate cysts. Rupture of these cysts can cause peritonitis and adhesions. Elsewhere in the pelvis, the tissue may take the form of

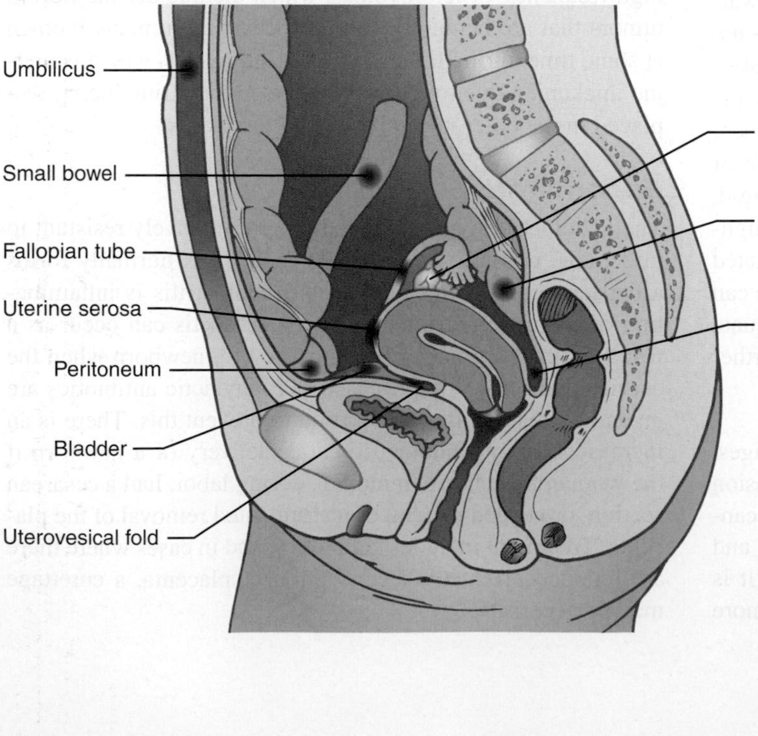

Figure 45.4 • Common locations of endometriosis in the pelvis and abdomen.

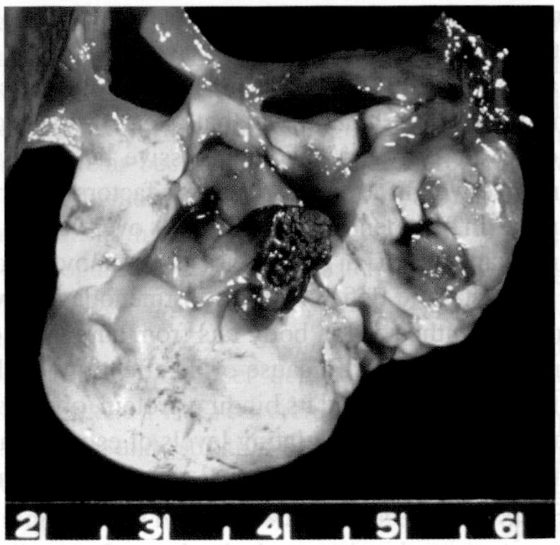

Figure 45.5 • Endometriosis. Implants of endometrium on the ovary appear as red-blue nodules. (From Strayer D. S., Rubin R. (Eds.) (2015). *Rubin's pathology: Clinicopathologic foundations of medicine* (7th ed., Figure 24-73A, p. 1049). Philadelphia, PA: Lippincott Williams & Wilkins.)

small hemorrhagic lesions that may be in a variety of colors, but mostly appearing as red-blue nodules (Fig. 45.5). Some lesions may be surrounded by scar tissue.[31,33]

Diagnosis and Treatment. Endometriosis may be difficult to diagnose because its symptoms mimic those of other pelvic disorders and the severity of the symptoms does not always reflect the extent of the disease. Treatment may be initiated based on clinical presentation alone because definitive diagnosis can be accomplished only through laparoscopy and then confirmed with histological testing.[34,35] This minimally invasive surgery allows direct visualization of pelvic organs to determine the presence and extent of endometrial lesions. Imaging techniques, including ultrasonography and magnetic resonance imaging (MRI), are useful tools in evaluating endometriomas and deep endometriosis.[33]

Treatment modalities fall into three categories: pain relief, endometrial suppression, and surgery. In young women, simple observation and analgesics (nonsteroidal anti-inflammatory drugs [NSAIDs]) may be sufficient treatment. The use of hormones to induce physiologic amenorrhea is based on the observation that pregnancy and menopause afford pain relief by inducing atrophy of the endometrial tissue. This can be accomplished through administration of oral contraceptive pills (OCPs) or continuous progestogen agents (medroxyprogesterone acetate [oral or depot injection] or the levonorgestrel intrauterine system). Danazol (a synthetic androgen) is less commonly used now given the increased side effect profile. In women with severe endometriosis, long-acting gonadotropin-releasing hormone (GnRH) analogs that inhibit the pituitary gonadotropins and suppress ovulation may be used for short-term treatment, but is limited in its time course because of the side effects of prolonged artificial menopause, such as decreased bone density.[36]

Surgery may offer more definitive therapy for women with large or symptomatic endometriomas, or those who have failed medical therapy for endometriosis. The goal of surgical treatment is to restore normal anatomic relationships, remove all visible lesions, and slow progression of the disease—all done in a way that minimizes development of pelvic adhesions and avoids injury to normal surrounding structures. Laparoscopy is the preferred surgical approach aimed at repairing adhesions and ablation of endometrial implants. Laparoscopic treatment options include the use of cautery, laser ablation, and excision techniques. Advantages of laser surgery include better hemostasis, more precision in vaporizing lesions with less damage to surrounding tissue, and better access to areas that are not well visualized or would be difficult to reach with cautery. Electrosurgical, thermal, and ultrasonic ablation techniques are under investigation. Yet, even with extensive surgery, the risk of continued symptoms and disease recurrence is great. Hormone suppression with OCPs or other suppressive therapy before and after surgery can aid in suppression of the disease.[36] Definitive treatment involves total hysterectomy and bilateral salpingo-oophorectomy when the symptoms are unbearable or the woman's childbearing is completed.

Adenomyosis

Adenomyosis is the condition in which endometrial glands and stroma are found within the myometrium, interspersed between the smooth muscle fibers.[1] In contrast to endometriosis, which usually is a problem of young, infertile women, adenomyosis typically is found in multiparous women.[1] It is thought that events associated with repeated pregnancies, deliveries, and uterine involution may cause the endometrium to be displaced throughout the myometrium, However, there is no known cause.[1] Adenomyosis frequently coexists with uterine myomas or endometrial hyperplasia. The diagnosis of adenomyosis often occurs as an incidental finding in a uterus removed for symptoms suggestive of myoma or hyperplasia. Heavy, painful periods with clots and painful intercourse are common complaints of women with adenomyosis. Although in the past the diagnosis was made primarily through careful history and the pelvic examination findings of an enlarged, boggy uterus, MRI is now considered the diagnostic tool for confirming this condition. Conservative medical therapy using oral contraceptives and NSAIDs is the first choice for treatment. However, women with severe adenomyosis will ultimately require a hysterectomy (with preservation of the ovaries in premenopausal women) for full resolution of symptoms.

Endometrial Cancer

Endometrial cancer is the most common cancer found in the female pelvis, occurring more than twice as often as cervical cancer. Most cases of endometrial cancer are adenocarcinomas, with fewer than 1% being sarcomas.[37] In 2017, the American Cancer Society estimated that approximately 61,380 women were diagnosed with endometrial cancer and 10,920 died of the disorder. Endometrial cancer occurs more frequently in older women (average age of 60) and less commonly in women under 45 years of age.[38]

Although the proportion of cases of endometrial cancer with a background of familial risk is low, 5% of endometrial

replacement therapy). Interference with pregnancy is rare unless the tumor is submucosal and interferes with implantation or obstructs the cervical outlet. These tumors may outgrow their blood supply, become infarcted, and undergo degenerative changes.

Most leiomyomas regress with menopause, but if bleeding, pressure on the bladder, pain, or other problems persist, hysterectomy may be required. Myomectomy (removal of just the tumors) can be done to preserve the uterus for future childbearing. Cesarean section is recommended if the uterine cavity is entered during myomectomy. Hypothalamic GnRH agonists (*e.g.*, leuprolide) may be used to suppress leiomyoma growth before surgery. Data suggests uterine artery embolization is a nonsurgical therapy that has demonstrated short-term advantages, but generated higher frequency of reintervention over surgery.[41]

IN SUMMARY

Disorders of the cervix and uterus include inflammatory conditions (*i.e.*, cervicitis and endometritis), cancer (*i.e.*, cervical and endometrial cancer), endometriosis, and leiomyomas. Cervicitis is an acute or chronic inflammation of the cervix. Acute cervicitis may result from the direct infection of the cervix or may be secondary to a vaginal or uterine infection. It may be caused by a variety of infectious agents. Chronic cervicitis represents a low-grade inflammatory process resulting from trauma or nonspecific infectious agents. Cervical cancer arises from precursor lesions that can be detected on a Pap smear, and, if detected early, is the most easily cured of all the cancers of the female reproductive system. Evidence suggests a causal link between HPV infection and cervical cancer. Vaccines against several strains of the HPV are available and show promise for the prevention of cervical cancer.

Endometritis represents an ill-defined inflammation or infection of the endometrium that produces variable symptoms. Endometriosis is the condition in which functional endometrial tissue is found in ectopic sites outside the uterus, particularly in dependent parts of the pelvis and in the ovaries. It causes dysmenorrhea, dyspareunia, and infertility. Adenomyosis is the condition in which endometrial glands and stroma are found in the myometrium, interspersed between the smooth muscle fibers. Endometrial cancer is the most common cancer found in the female pelvis, occurring more than twice as often as cervical cancer. Prolonged estrogen stimulation with hyperplasia of the endometrium has been identified as a major risk factor for endometrial cancer.

Leiomyomas are benign uterine wall neoplasms of smooth muscle origin. They can develop in the corpus of the uterus and can be submucosal, subserosal, or intramural. Submucosal fibroids displace endometrial tissue and are more likely to cause bleeding, necrosis, and infection than either of the other types.

DISORDERS OF THE FALLOPIAN TUBES AND OVARIES

After completing this section of the chapter, the learner will be able to meet the following objectives:

- List the common causes and symptoms of pelvic inflammatory disease.
- Describe the risk factors and symptoms of ectopic pregnancy.
- List the hormones produced by the three types of functioning ovarian tumors.

Pelvic Inflammatory Disease

PID is a polymicrobial infection of the upper reproductive tract (uterus, fallopian tubes, or ovaries) associated with the sexually transmitted organisms such as *N. gonorrhoeae* or *C. trachomatis* as well as endogenous organisms, including anaerobes, such as *Haemophilus influenzae*, enteric Gram-negative rods, and streptococci.[1,42] The organisms ascend through the endocervical canal to the endometrial cavity, and then to the tubes and ovaries. The endocervical canal is slightly dilated during menstruation, allowing bacteria to gain entrance to the uterus and other pelvic structures. After entering the upper reproductive tract, the organisms multiply rapidly in the favorable environment of the sloughing endometrium and ascend to the fallopian tube (Fig. 45.7).

Factors that predispose women to the development of PID include an age of 16 to 24 years, nulliparity, history of multiple sexual partners, and previous history of PID.[42] Although the use of an IUD has been associated with a three- to fivefold increased risk for development of PID, studies have shown that women with only one sexual partner who are at low risk of acquiring STIs have no significant risk for development of PID from using an IUD.

Clinical Manifestations

The symptoms of PID include lower abdominal pain, dyspareunia, back pain, purulent cervical discharge, and the presence of adnexal tenderness and exquisitely painful cervix on bimanual pelvic examination. Fever (>101°F), increased erythrocyte sedimentation rate, multiple leukocytes on wet mount vaginal microscopy, and coinfection with chlamydia and/or gonorrhea are commonly seen and further support the diagnosis of PID. Elevated C-reactive protein levels equate with inflammation and can be used as another diagnostic tool.[42]

Diagnosis and Treatment

Laparoscopy, which allows for direct visualization of the ovaries, fallopian tubes, and uterus, is one of the most specific procedures for diagnosing PID, but is costly and carries the inherent risks of surgery and anesthesia.[12] Minimal criteria for a presumptive diagnosis of PID require the presence of lower abdominal pain, adnexal tenderness, and cervical motion tenderness on bimanual examination with no other apparent cause.[43]

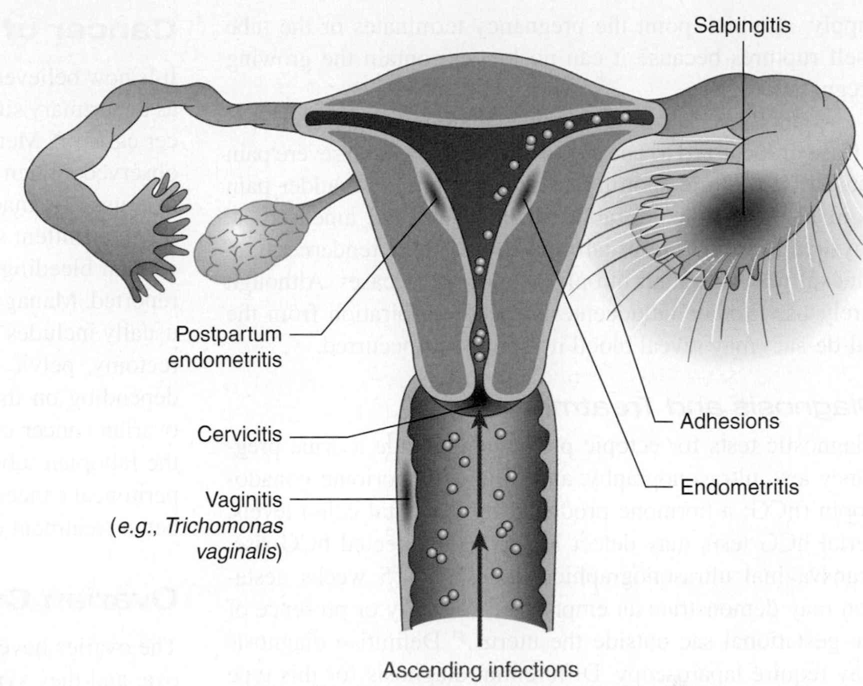

Figure 45.7 • Pelvic inflammatory disease. Microbial agents enter through the vagina and ascend to involve the uterus, fallopian tubes, and pelvic structures.

Outpatient antibiotic therapy is usually sufficient. However, treatment may involve hospitalization with intravenous administration of antibiotics in some cases. Antibiotic regimens should be selected according to STI treatment guidelines, which are published every 4 years by the Centers for Disease Control and Prevention (CDC). Treatment is aimed at preventing complications, which can include pelvic adhesions, infertility, ectopic pregnancy, chronic abdominal pain, and tubo-ovarian abscesses. Accurate diagnosis and appropriate antibiotic therapy may decrease the severity and frequency of PID sequelae. The CDC recommends empiric treatment with a presumptive diagnosis of PID, while waiting for confirmation by culture or other definitive test results.[42]

Ectopic Pregnancy

Although pregnancy is not discussed in detail in this text, it is reasonable to mention ectopic pregnancy because it represents a true gynecologic emergency and should be considered when a woman of reproductive age presents with the complaint of pelvic pain. Ectopic pregnancy occurs when a fertilized ovum implants outside the uterine cavity, the most common site being the fallopian tube (Fig. 45.8). Updated estimates for ectopic pregnancy incidence rates are difficult to determine because many women are now treated on an outpatient basis, so data from hospital discharge records are no longer representative of the scope of the problem. Although ectopic pregnancy is the leading cause of maternal mortality in the first trimester, the death rate has steadily declined as a result of improved diagnostic methods.

The cause of ectopic pregnancy is delayed ovum transport, which may result from decreased tubal motility or distorted tubal anatomy (*i.e.*, narrowed lumen, convolutions, or diverticula). Risk factors most strongly associated with ectopic pregnancy include previous tubal surgery, tubal ligation or reversal, previous ectopic pregnancy, and a tubal lesion or abnormality.[44] Smoking, current IUD use, history of PID or therapeutic abortion, and the use of fertility drugs to induce ovulation have also been associated with an increased risk for ectopic pregnancy.

Clinical Manifestations

The site of implantation in the tube (*e.g.*, isthmus, ampulla) may determine the onset of symptoms and the timing of diagnosis. As the tubal pregnancy progresses, the surrounding tissue is stretched. The pregnancy eventually outgrows its blood

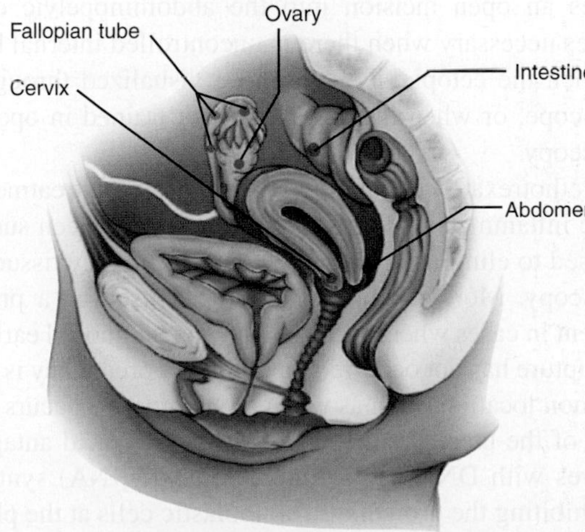

Figure 45.8 • Ectopic pregnancy. (From Jensen S. (2015). *Nursing health assessment: A best practice approach* (2nd ed., p. 778). Philadelphia, PA: Lippincott Williams & Wilkins.)

supply, at which point the pregnancy terminates or the tube itself ruptures because it can no longer contain the growing pregnancy.

Symptoms can include lower abdominal discomfort—diffuse or localized to one side—that progresses to severe pain caused by rupture, spotting, syncope, referred shoulder pain from bleeding into the abdominal cavity, and amenorrhea. Physical examination usually reveals adnexal tenderness; an adnexal mass is found in only about half of cases. Although rarely used today, culdocentesis (needle aspiration from the cul-de-sac) may reveal blood if rupture has occurred.

Diagnosis and Treatment

Diagnostic tests for ectopic pregnancy include a urine pregnancy test, ultrasonography, and β-human chorionic gonadotropin (hCG; a hormone produced by placental cells) levels. Serial hCG tests may detect lower than expected hCG rise. Transvaginal ultrasonographic studies after 5 weeks gestation may demonstrate an empty uterine cavity or presence of the gestational sac outside the uterus.[44] Definitive diagnosis may require laparoscopy. Differential diagnosis for this type of pelvic pain includes ruptured ovarian cyst, threatened or incomplete abortion, PID, acute appendicitis, and degenerating fibroid.

Treatment is aimed at resolving the problem with minimal morbidity and protecting future fertility where possible. Advances in detection now make it possible to treat early ectopic pregnancies medically with methotrexate to stop the pregnancy followed by serial hCG to be assured the ectopic pregnancy has been effectively treated. Surgical removal of the pregnancy is required when it is unlikely medical management will be effective (*e.g.*, large ectopic pregnancy, presence of a fetal heart beat, noncompliance of the client), rupture is imminent or has already occurred, or when the woman is hemodynamically unstable.[12,44,45] Laparoscopic treatment of ectopic pregnancy is well tolerated and more cost-effective than laparotomy because of shorter convalescence and the reduced need for postoperative analgesia. Laparotomy, which involves an open incision into the abdominopelvic cavity, becomes necessary when there is uncontrolled internal bleeding, when the ectopic site cannot be visualized through the laparoscope, or when the surgeon is not trained in operative laparoscopy.

Methotrexate (an antimetabolite used in treatment of chronic inflammatory diseases and cancer) has been successfully used to eliminate residual ectopic pregnancy tissue after laparoscopy. More recently, it has been used as a primary treatment in cases where the pregnancy is diagnosed early and tubal rupture has not occurred, or when the pregnancy is not in a common location, such as when the pregnancy occurs in the cornua of the uterus or the cervix. This folic acid antagonist interferes with DNA and ribonucleic acid (RNA) synthesis, thus inhibiting the growth of trophoblastic cells at the placental implantation site. Adverse effects can include bone marrow depression, transient elevation of liver enzymes, anemia, and stomatitis.[44]

Cancer of the Fallopian Tube

It is now believed that cancer of the fallopian tube contributes as the primary site of cancer in a large majority of ovarian cancer cases.[1,46] Metastasis from the uterus and/or ovaries is also observed. When primary fallopian tube cancer is diagnosed, it is usually anadenocarcinoma.[1] Symptoms are uncommon, but intermittent serosanguineous vaginal discharge, abnormal vaginal bleeding, and colicky low abdominal pain have been reported. Management is similar to that for ovarian cancer and usually includes total hysterectomy, bilateral salpingo-oophorectomy, pelvic lymph node dissection, and chemotherapy, depending on the type of cancer cells. With the finding that ovarian cancer commonly originates from primary lesions in the fallopian tubes, the staging of ovarian, fallopian tube and peritoneal cancer has been integrated, potentially allowing for better treatment options.[1,46]

Ovarian Cysts and Tumors

The ovaries have a dual function: they produce germ cells, or ova, and they synthesize the female sex hormones. Disorders of the ovaries frequently cause menstrual and fertility problems. Benign conditions of the ovaries can present as primary lesions of the ovarian structures or as secondary disorders related to hypothalamic, pituitary, or adrenal dysfunction.

Ovarian Cysts

Cysts are the most common form of ovarian tumor. Many are benign. A follicular cyst is one that results from occlusion of the duct of the follicle. Each month, several follicles begin to develop and are blighted at various stages of development. These follicles form cavities that fill with fluid, producing a cyst. The dominant follicle normally ruptures to release the egg (*i.e.*, ovulation), but occasionally persists and continues growing. Likewise, a luteal cyst is a persistent cystic enlargement of the corpus luteum that is formed after ovulation and does not regress in the absence of pregnancy. Functional cysts are asymptomatic unless there is substantial enlargement or bleeding into the cyst. This can cause considerable discomfort or a dull, aching sensation on the affected side. These cysts usually regress spontaneously. Occasionally, a cyst may become twisted or may rupture into the intra-abdominal cavity (Fig. 45.9).

Polycystic Ovary Syndrome

Polycystic ovary syndrome (PCOS) is a common endocrine disorder affecting 6% to 15% of women of reproductive age, and is a frequent source of chronic anovulation. The diagnosis of PCOS is made after other endocrine diseases are ruled out and the person has some of the following symptoms:

- Oligomenorrhea (irregular infrequent periods)
- Signs of hyperandrogenism (acne and excess body hair [hirsutism])
- Elevated testosterone levels on blood testing
- Polycystic appearing ovaries in which there are numerous small cysts at the periphery of the ovary.[47]

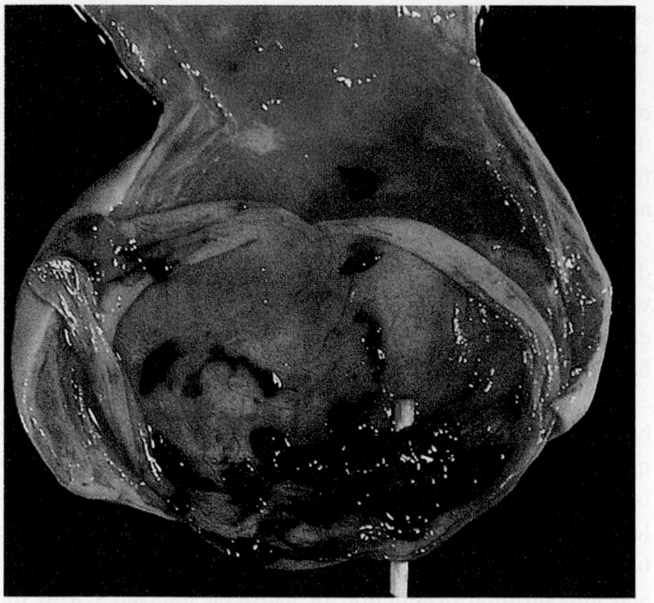

Figure 45.9 • Follicular cyst of the ovary. The rupture of this thin-walled follicular cyst (*dowel stick*) led to intra-abdominal hemorrhage. (From Strayer D. S., Rubin R. (Eds.) (2015). *Rubin's pathology: Clinicopathologic foundations of medicine* (7th ed., Fig. 24-44, p. 1033). Philadelphia, PA: Lippincott Williams & Wilkins.)

Etiology and Pathogenesis. About 50% of women who are diagnosed with PCOS are obese. Hyperinsulinemia and insulin resistance are thought to play a role in the pathogenesis of the disorder. People with PCOS will have irregular menses due to anovulation that can lead to infertility. Because of the hyperandrogenism associated with PCOS, many women with PCOS will suffer from hirsutism and acne.[47]

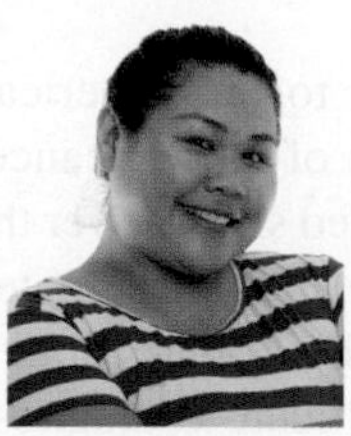

Remember **Eileen**, who was worked up for PCOS. Her periods have been irregular (oligomenorrhea) since age 11. She shows multiple signs of hyperandrogenism, including hirsutism and acne, and she has elevated blood levels of testosterone. Finally, the ultrasound reveals bilateral polycystic ovaries. Eileen thus meets all of the criteria for PCOS, once related disorders are ruled out. Eileen also has increased blood levels of both insulin and glucose, indicating that she is experiencing insulin resistance, and she is overweight. Eileen's hyperinsulinemia and insulin resistance are probably involved in the development of her disease.

The precise etiology of PCOS is still being debated, but it is probably multifactorial. A possible genetic basis has been suggested with an autosomal dominant mode of inheritance. There is increasing evidence that the disorder may begin before adolescence and that many of the manifestations of PCOS begin to make their appearance at that time.[48] Because many of the symptoms common to PCOS, such as excess hair, acne, and obesity, can be detrimental to a teenage girl's health and self-esteem, early detection and treatment of PCOS in adolescents are essential.

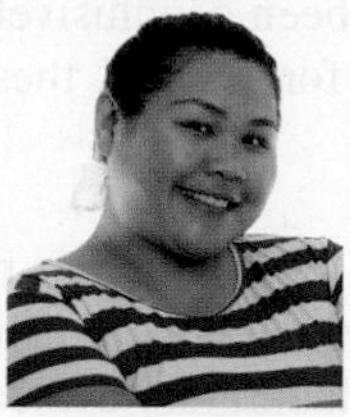

Unfortunately, **Eileen** was just diagnosed with PCOS at 19 years of age. Her irregular periods since menarche (age 11) suggest that she may have suffered from this disorder throughout her adolescence. Because PCOS is hereditary, Eileen's younger female siblings and cousins should be evaluated for PCOS so that if positive, they can benefit from early treatment and avoid some of the systemic pathologic problems experienced by Eileen.

Although this syndrome has been the subject of considerable research, the underlying mechanisms remain unclear. Chronic anovulation is thought to be the underlying cause of the amenorrhea or irregular menses, and enlarged, "polycystic" ovaries associated with this condition. Most women with PCOS have elevated luteinizing hormone (LH) levels with normal estrogen and follicle-stimulating hormone (FSH) production. Elevated levels of circulating total testosterone, free testosterone, and dehydroepiandrosterone sulfate (DHEAS) are not uncommon, and these women occasionally have hyperprolactinemia or hypothyroidism. Persistent anovulation results in an estrogen environment that alters the hypothalamic release of GnRH with a resultant increase in LH secretion and suppression of FSH release by the pituitary gland. This altered LH/FSH ratio often is used as a diagnostic criterion for this condition, but it is not universally present. Although the presence of some FSH allows for new follicular development, full maturation is not attained, and ovulation does not occur. The elevated LH level results in increased androgen production, which in turn prevents normal follicular development and contributes to the vicious cycle of anovulation.[49]

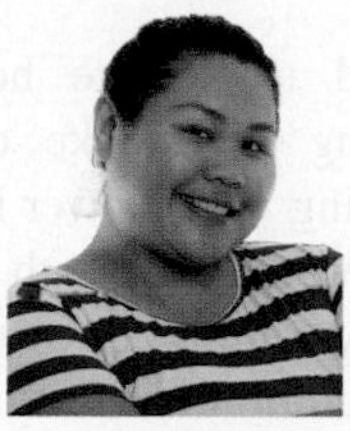

Eileen cannot remember her last menstrual period, and she has hirsutism and acne. These problems are caused, at least partially, by excess testosterone activity (hyperandrogenism). Eileen's hyperandrogenism results from excess LH production.

The association between hyperandrogenism and hyperinsulinemia has been recognized. It has been shown that the cause of hyperinsulinemia is insulin resistance. The frequency and degree of hyperinsulinemia in women with PCOS are often amplified by the presence of obesity. Insulin may cause hyperandrogenism in several ways, although the exact mechanism has not been well defined. It has been shown that the ovary possesses insulin receptors and there is evidence that insulin may act directly on the ovary.[50]

In addition to its clinical manifestations, long-term health problems including cardiovascular disease and diabetes have been linked to PCOS. There is also concern that women with PCOS who are anovulatory do not produce progesterone. Although there is a reported association with breast, endometrial, and ovarian cancer, PCOS has not been conclusively shown to be an independent risk factor for any of these malignancies.[47]

Diagnosis and Treatment. The diagnosis of PCOS can be suspected from the clinical presentation. Although there is no consensus as to which tests should be used, laboratory evaluation to exclude hyperprolactinemia, late-onset adrenal hyperplasia, and androgen-secreting tumors of the ovary and adrenal gland is commonly done. Although a fasting blood glucose, 2-hour oral glucose tolerance test, and insulin levels are often measured to evaluate for hyperinsulinemia, this testing is not required prior to treatment as insulin resistance is almost universal in women with PCOS. Confirmation with ultrasonography of the ovaries is often done, but not required.[51]

The overall goal of treatment should be directed toward symptom relief, prevention of potential malignant endometrial sequelae, and reduction in risk for development of diabetes and cardiovascular disease. The preferred and most effective treatment for PCOS is lifestyle modification. Weight loss may be beneficial in restoring normal ovulation when obesity is present. Although numerous medications and protocols are available, the choice depends on the manifestations that are most bothersome to the woman and her stage in reproductive life. Combined oral contraceptive agents ameliorate menstrual irregularities and improve hirsutism and acne.

Metformin, an insulin-sensitizing drug, used with or without ovulation-inducing medications, is emerging as an important component of PCOS treatment.[51] In addition to expected improvements in insulin sensitivity and glucose metabolism, it has been associated with reductions in androgen and LH levels and is highly effective in restoring normal menstrual regularity and ovulatory cycles.

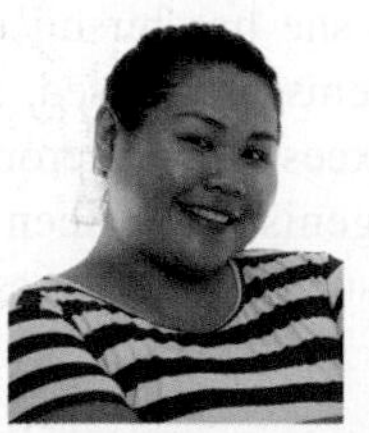

Eileen is encouraged to change her dietary habits, lowering her intake of overall calories and eating foods lower in fat. She is also assigned to work with a personal trainer at a gym affiliated with the medical clinic. In addition to lifestyle modifications, Eileen is prescribed a combined contraceptive agent and metformin.

When fertility is desired, PCOS usually is treated by the administration of the hypothalamic-pituitary–stimulating drug clomiphene citrate or injectable gonadotropins to induce ovulation. These drugs must be used carefully because they can induce extreme enlargement of the ovaries.

Benign and Functioning/Endocrine Active Ovarian Tumors

Ovarian tumors are extremely common with most being benign. Ovarian tumors can arise from any of the ovarian tissue types—serosal epithelium, germ cell layers, or gonadal stroma tissue[21] (Fig. 45.10).

Serous and mucinous cystadenomas are common benign ovarian neoplasms. Endometriomas are the "chocolate cysts" that develop secondary to ovarian endometriosis. Ovarian fibromas are connective tissue tumors composed of varying amounts of collagen. They range in size from 15 to 30 cm. Cystic teratomas, or dermoid cysts, are derived from primordial germ cells and are composed of various combinations of well-differentiated ectodermal, mesodermal, and endodermal elements. Not uncommonly, they contain sebaceous material, hair, or teeth.[1]

The hormonally active tumors can impact the entire body either with an excess or decrease in reproductive hormone excretion. One such tumor, the granulosa cell tumor, is associated with excess estrogen production. Most granulosa cell tumors occur after menopause; however, when these tumors develop during the reproductive period, the persistent and uncontrolled production of estrogen interferes with the normal menstrual cycle. In addition, when present in young females, early puberty and an associated loss of oocytes occur.[1] Androgen-secreting tumors (*i.e.*, Sertoli-Leydig cell tumor or androblastoma) inhibit ovulation and estrogen production. They tend to cause hirsutism and development of masculine characteristics, such as baldness, acne, oily skin, breast atrophy, and deepening of the voice.[1]

Treatment for all ovarian tumors includes surgical excision, chemotherapy, and/or radiation therapy. Tissue, lymph nodes, and fluid is analyzed to determine if the cancer has metastasized. If metastasis has occurred, the goal is to remove as much of the cancer as possible and when combined with chemotherapy provides the best results,[46]

Ovarian Cancer

Ovarian cancer is often lethal. According to the American Cancer Society, it is the fifth leading cause of female cancer deaths. The rate of ovarian cancer has declined slowly over the last 20 years. However, in 2017, there were still an estimated 22,440 new cases of ovarian cancer in the United States, with 14,080 deaths.[52] Ovarian cancer is difficult to diagnose because symptoms mimic many other benign health issues. Because of this, the disease has often spread before the time of discovery.[53]

Risk Factors. The most significant risk factor for ovarian cancer appears to be ovulatory age—the length of time during a woman's life when her ovarian cycle is not suppressed by pregnancy, lactation, or oral contraceptive use. The incidence of ovarian cancer is much lower in parous versus nulliparous women.[54] Family history also is a significant risk factor for ovarian cancer. Women with two or more first- or second-degree relatives who have had *site-specific ovarian cancer* have up to a 50% risk for development of the disease. There are two other types of inherited risk for ovarian cancer: *breast–ovarian cancer syndrome*, where both breast and ovarian cancer occur among first- and second-degree relatives,

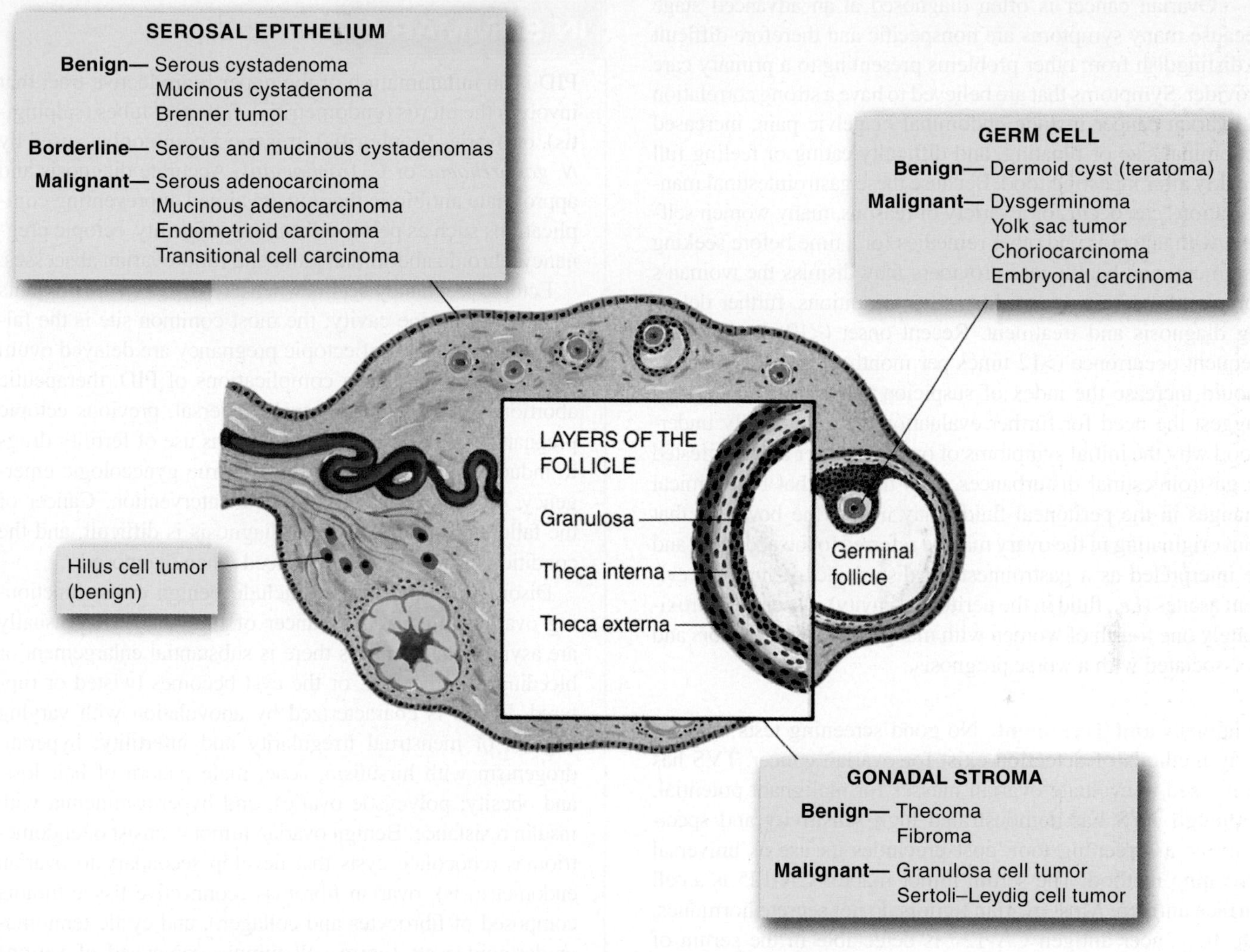

Figure 45.10 • Classification of ovarian neoplasms based on cell of origin. (From Strayer D. S., Rubin R. (Eds.) (2015). *Rubin's pathology: Clinicopathologic foundations of medicine* (7th ed., Fig. 24-48, p. 1035). Philadelphia, PA: Lippincott Williams & Wilkins.)

and *family cancer syndrome* or *Lynch syndrome II* (a subtype of hereditary nonpolyposis colon cancer), in which male or female relatives have a history of colorectal, endometrial, ovarian, pancreatic, or other types of cancer.[21] The breast cancer susceptibility genes, *BRCA1* and *BRCA2*, which are tumor suppressor genes, are incriminated in approximately 10% of hereditary ovarian cancers despite being identified as "breast cancer genes."[29] Susceptibility to ovarian cancer is transmitted as an autosomal dominant characteristic. Therefore, a mutated gene from either parent is sufficient to cause the problem. A high-fat Western diet and use of powders containing talc in the genital area are other factors that have been linked to the development of ovarian cancer.

Prevention. Chemoprevention strategies that have been suggested include long-term oral contraceptive use, acetaminophen and aspirin. In studies with analgesics, findings regarding effectiveness have been inconsistent. Additional clinical trials are needed to support the effectiveness of these chemoprevention agents. Surgical strategies that have reduced the risk of developing ovarian cancer include prophylactic removal of both fallopian tubes and ovaries.[55]

Types of Ovarian Cancer. Cancer of the ovary is a complex neoplasm because of the diversity of tissue types that originate in the ovary. As a result of this diversity, there are several types of ovarian cancers. Malignant neoplasms of the ovary can be divided into three categories: epithelial tumors, germ cell tumors, and gonadal stromal tumors (see Fig. 45.10). Epithelial tumors account for approximately 90% of cases.[21]

Clinical Manifestations. The different types of ovarian cancers display various degrees of virulence, depending on the type of tumor and degree of differentiation involved. A well-differentiated cancer of the ovary may have produced symptoms for many months and still be found to be operable at the time of surgery. A poorly differentiated tumor may have been clinically evident for only a few days but be found to be widespread and inoperable. Often, no correlation exists between the duration of symptoms and the extent of the disease.

Ovarian cancer is often diagnosed at an advanced stage because many symptoms are nonspecific and therefore difficult to distinguish from other problems presenting to a primary care provider. Symptoms that are believed to have a strong correlation to ovarian cancer include abdominal or pelvic pain, increased abdominal size or bloating, and difficulty eating or feeling full quickly after ingesting food. Because these gastrointestinal manifestations can occur for a variety of reasons, many women self-treat with antacids and other remedies for a time before seeking treatment, and health care providers may dismiss the woman's complaints as being caused by other conditions, further delaying diagnosis and treatment. Recent onset (<12 months) and frequent occurrence (>12 times per month) of these symptoms should increase the index of suspicion for ovarian cancer and suggest the need for further evaluation.[21] It is not fully understood why the initial symptoms of ovarian cancer are manifested as gastrointestinal disturbances. It is thought that biochemical changes in the peritoneal fluids may irritate the bowel or that pain originating in the ovary may be referred to the abdomen and be interpreted as a gastrointestinal disturbance. Clinically evident ascites (*i.e.*, fluid in the peritoneal cavity) is seen in approximately one fourth of women with malignant ovarian tumors and is associated with a worse prognosis.

Diagnosis and Treatment. No good screening tests or other early methods of detection exist for ovarian cancer. TVS has been used to evaluate ovarian masses for malignant potential. Although TVS has demonstrated high sensitivity and specificity as a screening tool, cost precludes its use as universal screening method. The serum tumor marker CA-125 is a cell surface antigen. Most ovarian tumors do not secrete hormones, but the cancer antigen CA-125 is detectable in the serum of about half of epithelial tumors confined to the ovary and 90% of those that have spread. The specificity of this test is highest when combined with TVS.[1] Screening with CA-125 is not recommended for screening asymptomatic women. It can be used in monitoring therapy and recurrences when preoperative levels have been elevated. Despite its role in diagnostic evaluation and follow-up, CA-125 is not cancer or tissue specific for ovarian cancer. Levels also are elevated in other cancers and some benign conditions. Because it lacks sensitivity and specificity, CA-125 has limited value as a single screening test.[56]

When ovarian cancer is suspected, surgical evaluation is required for diagnosis, complete and accurate staging, and cytoreduction and debulking procedures to reduce the size of the tumor. The most common surgery involves removal of the uterus, fallopian tubes, ovaries, and omentum. The liver, diaphragm, retroperitoneal and aortic lymph nodes, and peritoneal surface are examined and biopsies are taken as needed. Cytologic washings are done to test for cancerous cells in the peritoneal fluid. Women with very early cancer who may wish to become pregnant will sometimes have only the affected ovary removed. Recommendations regarding treatment beyond surgery and prognosis depend on the stage of the disease.[21] The lack of accurate screening tools and the resistant nature of ovarian cancers significantly affect the success of treatment and survival.

IN SUMMARY

PID is an inflammation of the upper reproductive tract that involves the uterus (endometritis), fallopian tubes (salpingitis), or ovaries (oophoritis). It is most commonly caused by *N. gonorrhoeae* or *C. trachomatis*. Accurate diagnosis and appropriate antibiotic therapy are aimed at preventing complications such as pelvic adhesions, infertility, ectopic pregnancy, chronic abdominal pain, and tubo-ovarian abscesses.

Ectopic pregnancy occurs when a fertilized ovum implants outside the uterine cavity; the most common site is the fallopian tube. Causes of ectopic pregnancy are delayed ovum transport resulting from complications of PID, therapeutic abortion, tubal ligation or tubal reversal, previous ectopic pregnancy, or other conditions such as use of fertility drugs to induce ovulation. It represents a true gynecologic emergency, often necessitating surgical intervention. Cancer of the fallopian tube is rare; the diagnosis is difficult, and the condition usually is well advanced when diagnosed.

Disorders of the ovaries include benign cysts, functioning ovarian tumors, and cancer of the ovary; they usually are asymptomatic unless there is substantial enlargement or bleeding into the cyst, or the cyst becomes twisted or ruptured. PCOS is characterized by anovulation with varying degrees of menstrual irregularity and infertility; hyperandrogenism with hirsutism, acne, male pattern of hair loss, and obesity; polycystic ovaries; and hyperinsulinemia with insulin resistance. Benign ovarian tumors consist of endometriomas (chocolate cysts that develop secondary to ovarian endometriosis), ovarian fibromas (connective tissue tumors composed of fibrocytes and collagen), and cystic teratomas or dermoid cysts (germ cell tumors composed of various combinations of ectodermal, mesodermal, and endodermal elements). Functioning ovarian tumors may be benign or malignant and are of three types: estrogen secreting, androgen secreting, and mixed estrogen–androgen secreting. Because ovarian cancer has vague symptoms until the disease has progressed, it is among the most lethal of female cancers. It can be divided into three categories: epithelial tumors, germ cell tumors, and gonadal stromal tumors. There are no effective screening methods for ovarian cancer, and often the disease is well advanced at the time of diagnosis.

KEY POINTS

GYNECOLOGIC CANCERS

- Cancers of the vulva, cervix, endometrium, and ovaries represent a spectrum of malignancies.
- Ovarian cancer often goes undiagnosed until in advanced stages; therefore, it is often lethal. The most significant risk factors for ovarian cancer are the length of time that a woman's ovarian cycles are not suppressed by pregnancy, lactation, or oral contraceptive use, and family history.

DISORDERS OF PELVIC SUPPORT AND UTERINE POSITION

After completing this section of the chapter, the learner will be able to meet the following objectives:

- Characterize the function of the supporting ligaments and pelvic floor muscles in maintaining the position of the pelvic organs, including the uterus, bladder, and rectum.
- Describe the cause of cystocele, rectocele, enterocele, and uterine prolapse.

Disorders of Pelvic Support

The uterus and the pelvic structures are maintained in proper position by the uterosacral ligaments, round ligaments, broad ligament, and cardinal ligaments. The two cardinal ligaments maintain the cervix in its normal position. The uterosacral ligaments hold the uterus in a forward position and the broad ligaments suspend the uterus, fallopian tubes, and ovaries in the pelvis. The vagina is encased in the semirigid structure of the strong supporting fascia (Fig. 45.11A). The muscular floor of the pelvis is a strong, slinglike structure that supports the uterus, vagina, urinary bladder, and rectum (Fig. 45.12). In the female anatomy, nature is faced with the problems of supporting the pelvic viscera against the force of gravity and increases in intra-abdominal pressure associated with coughing, sneezing, defecation, and laughing while at the same time allowing for urination, defecation, and normal reproductive tract function, especially the delivery of an infant. Three supporting structures are provided for the abdominal pelvic diaphragm. The bony pelvis provides support and protection for parts of the digestive tract and genitourinary structures, and the peritoneum holds the pelvic viscera in place. The main support for the viscera, however, is the pelvic diaphragm, made up of muscles and connective tissue that stretch across the bones of the pelvic outlet. The openings that must exist for the urethra, rectum, and vagina cause an inherent weakness in the pelvic diaphragm. Congenital or acquired weakness of the pelvic diaphragm results in widening of these openings, particularly the vagina, with the possible herniation of pelvic viscera through the pelvic floor (*i.e.*, prolapse).[57]

Relaxation of the pelvic outlet usually comes about because of overstretching of the perineal supporting tissues during pregnancy and childbirth. Although the tissues are stretched only during these times, there may be no difficulty

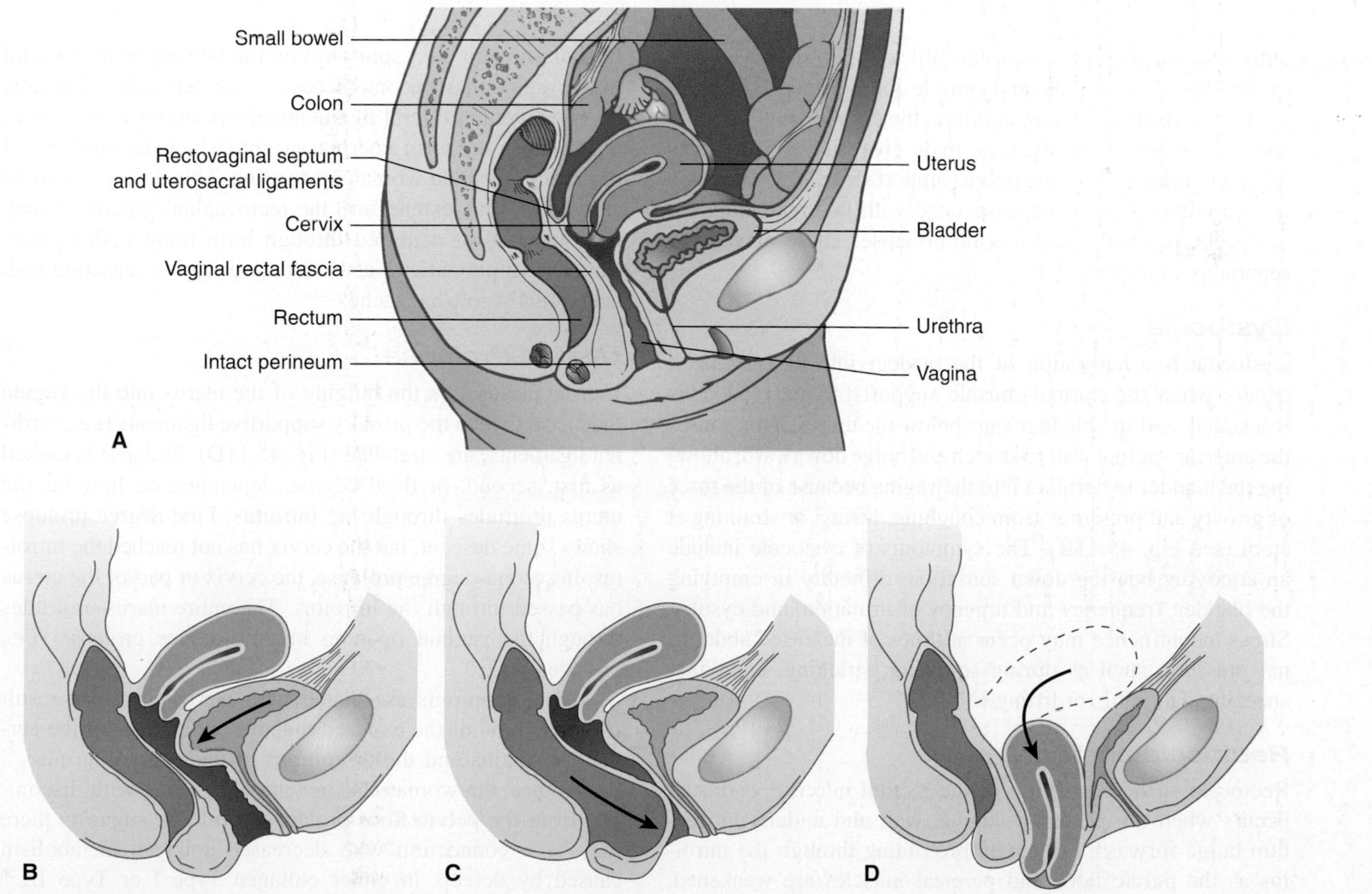

Figure 45.11 • (**A**) Normal support of the uterus and vagina, (**B**) cystocele, (**C**) rectocele, and (**D**) uterine prolapse.

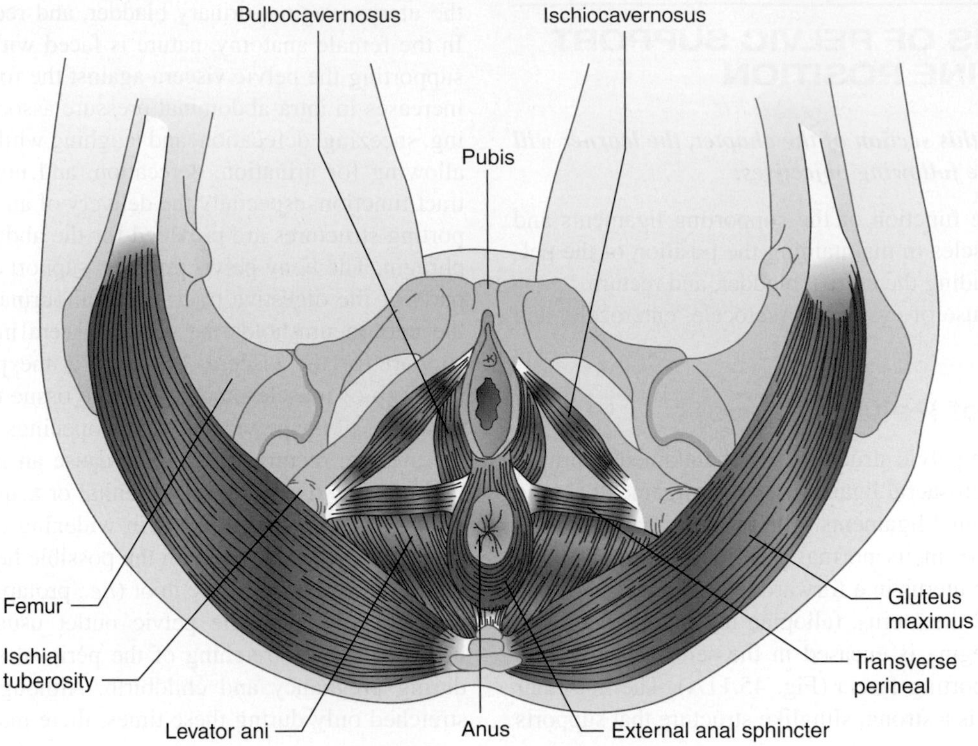

Figure 45.12 • Muscles of the pelvic floor (female perineum).

until later in life, such as in the fifth or sixth decade, when further loss of elasticity and muscle tone occurs. Even in a woman who has not borne children, the combination of aging and postmenopausal changes may give rise to problems related to relaxation of the pelvic support structures. The three most common conditions associated with this relaxation are cystocele, rectocele, and uterine prolapse. These may occur separately or together.[58,59]

Cystocele

Cystocele is a herniation of the bladder into the vagina. It occurs when the normal muscle support for the bladder is weakened, and the bladder sags below the uterus. This causes the anterior vaginal wall to stretch and bulge downward, allowing the bladder to herniate into the vagina because of the force of gravity and pressures from coughing, lifting, or straining at stool (see Fig. 45.11B). The symptoms of cystocele include an annoying bearing-down sensation, difficulty in emptying the bladder, frequency and urgency of urination, and cystitis. Stress incontinence may occur at times of increased abdominal pressure, such as during squatting, straining, coughing, sneezing, laughing, or lifting.[57–59]

Rectocele and Enterocele

Rectocele is the herniation of the rectum into the vagina. It occurs when the posterior vaginal wall and underlying rectum bulge forward, ultimately protruding through the introitus as the pelvic floor and perineal muscles are weakened. The symptoms include discomfort because of the protrusion of the rectum and difficulty in defecation (see Fig. 45.11C). Digital pressure (*i.e.*, splinting) on the bulging posterior wall of the vagina may become necessary for defecation. The area between the uterosacral ligaments just posterior to the cervix may weaken and form a hernial sac into which the small bowel protrudes when the woman is standing. This defect, called an *enterocele*, may extend into the rectovaginal septum. It may be congenital or acquired through birth trauma. Enterocele can be asymptomatic or cause a dull, dragging sensation and, occasionally, low backache.[57–59]

Uterine Prolapse

Uterine prolapse is the bulging of the uterus into the vagina that occurs when the primary supportive ligaments (*i.e.*, cardinal ligaments) are stretched (Fig. 45.11D). Prolapse is ranked as first, second, or third degree, depending on how far the uterus protrudes through the introitus. First-degree prolapse shows some descent, but the cervix has not reached the introitus. In second-degree prolapse, the cervix or part of the uterus has passed through the introitus. The entire uterus protrudes through the vaginal opening in third-degree prolapse (*i.e.*, procidentia).[57,59]

The symptoms associated with uterine prolapse result from irritation of the exposed mucous membranes of the cervix and vagina and the discomfort of the protruding mass.[56] Sometimes, the woman has incontinence along with discomfort from the pelvic floor prolapse. Evidence suggests there may be a connection with decreased collagen metabolism caused by defects in either collagen Type I or Type III.[58] Prolapse often is accompanied by perineal relaxation, cystocele, or rectocele. Like cystocele, rectocele, and enterocele, it occurs most commonly in multiparous women because childbearing is accompanied by injuries to pelvic structures and uterine ligaments. It also may result from pelvic tumors and neurologic conditions, such as spina bifida and diabetic neuropathy, which interrupt the innervation of pelvic muscles. Generally, it is a benign condition, but problems can arise with infection, obstruction, and skin irritation, sometimes leading to skin breakdown.[59]

A pessary may be inserted to hold the uterus in place and may stave off surgical intervention in women who want to have children or in older women for whom the surgery may pose a significant health risk. Pelvic floor physical therapy is another noninvasive treatment suitable for women who wish to preserve their uterus.[60]

Treatment of Pelvic Support Disorders

Kegel exercises, which strengthen the pubococcygeus muscle, may be helpful in cases of mild cystocele or rectocele (or after surgical repair to help maintain the improved function).[58] However, most of the disorders of pelvic relaxation will eventually require surgical correction. Most commonly, surgery is elective and deferred until after the childbearing years, so only one repair will be necessary. Additionally, the symptoms associated with the disorders often are not severe enough to warrant surgical correction, so the risk/benefit ratio needs to carefully be considered. In other cases, the stress of surgery is contraindicated because of other physical disorders. This is particularly true of older women, in whom many of these disorders occur and other nonsurgical interventions may be successful.[58]

There are a number of surgical procedures for the conditions that result from relaxation of pelvic support structures. Removal of the uterus through the vagina (vaginal hysterectomy) with appropriate repair of the vaginal wall (colporrhaphy) often is done when uterine prolapse is accompanied by cystocele or rectocele. A vesicourethral suspension may be done to alleviate the symptoms of stress incontinence. Repair may involve abdominal hysterectomy along with anteroposterior repair.[58,59]

Variations in Uterine Position

Variations in the position of the uterus are common. Some variations are innocuous. Others, which may be the result of weakness and relaxation of the perineum, give rise to various problems that compromise the structural integrity of the pelvic floor, particularly after childbirth.

The uterus usually is flexed approximately 45 degrees anteriorly, with the cervix positioned posteriorly and downward in the anteverted position. When the woman is standing, the angle of the uterus is such that it lies practically horizontal, resting lightly on the bladder.

Asymptomatic, normal variations in the axis of the uterus in relation to the cervix and physiologic displacements that arise after pregnancy or with pathology of the cul-de-sac include anteflexion, retroflexion, and retroversion (Fig. 45.13). An anteflexed uterus is flexed forward on itself.

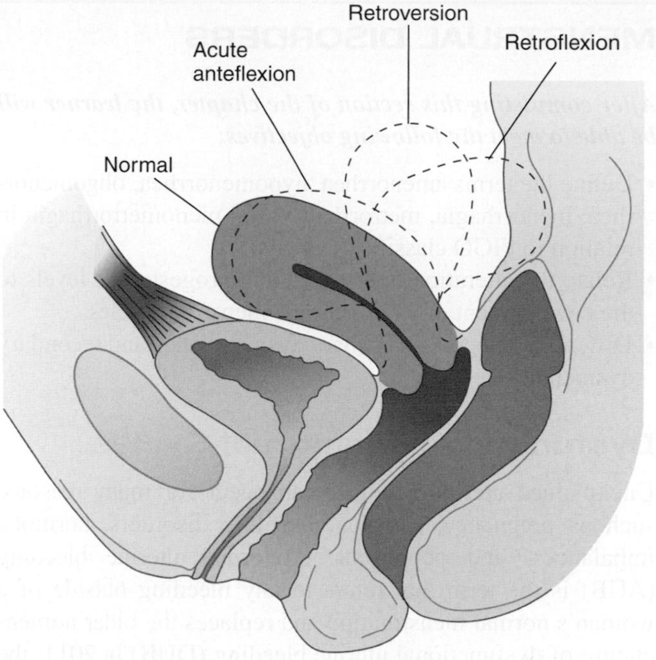

Figure 45.13 • Variations in uterine position.

Retroflexion is flexion backward at the isthmus. Retroversion describes the condition in which the uterus inclines posteriorly while the cervix remains tilted forward. Simple retroversion of the uterus is the most common displacement, found in 30% of normal women. It usually is a congenital condition caused by a short anterior vaginal wall and relaxed uterosacral ligaments; together, these force the uterus to fall back into the cul-de-sac[61]. Retroversion also can follow certain diseases, such as endometriosis and PID, which produce fibrous tissue adherence with retraction of the fundus posteriorly. Large leiomyomas also may cause the uterus to move into a posterior position. Dyspareunia with deep penetration or low back pain with menses can also be associated with retroversion.

IN SUMMARY

Alterations in pelvic support frequently occur because of weaknesses and relaxation of the pelvic floor and perineum. Cystocele and rectocele involve herniation of the bladder or rectum into the vagina. Uterine prolapse occurs when the uterus bulges into the vagina. Pelvic relaxation disorders typically result from overstretching of the perineal supporting muscles during pregnancy and childbirth. The loss of elasticity in these structures that is a normal accompaniment of aging contributes to these problems. Variations in uterine position include anteflexion, retroflexion, and retroversion. These disorders, which often are innocuous, can be the result of a congenital shortness of the vaginal wall, development of fibrous adhesions secondary to endometriosis or PID, or displacement caused by large uterine leiomyomas.

MENSTRUAL DISORDERS

After completing this section of the chapter, the learner will be able to meet the following objectives:

- Define the terms amenorrhea, hypomenorrhea, oligomenorrhea, menorrhagia, metrorrhagia, and menometrorrhagia in relation to FIGO classification.
- Relate the alteration in estrogen and progesterone levels to the development of dysfunctional menstrual cycles.
- Differentiate between primary dysmenorrhea and secondary dysmenorrhea.

Dysfunctional Menstrual Cycles

Unexplained uterine bleeding can occur for many reasons, such as pregnancy, abortion, bleeding disorders, hormone imbalances, and neoplasms. Abnormal uterine bleeding (AUB) is the term that refers to any bleeding outside of a woman's normal menstruation and replaces the older nomenclature of dysfunctional uterine bleeding (DUB).In 2011, the FIGO suggested a new classification for AUB based on bleeding pattern and etiology of the bleeding in an effort to simplify terms, (Callahan) new terms are as follows:

- *Heavy menstrual bleeding* (HMB) (previously referred to as menorrhagia) is defined as regular menses, lasting a week or more, or bleeding that is greater than 80 mL per cycle.
- *Light menstrual bleeding* (previously hypomenorrhea) is defined as a regular period but flow is light.
- *Intermenstrual bleeding* (previously metrorrhagia) is defined as any bleeding between periods. Flow is usually light.
- *Heavy irregular bleeding* (previously menometrorrhea) is defined as prolonged or heavy bleeding that occurs at irregular times.
- *Infrequent cycles* (previously oligomenorrhea) refer to cycles that are irregular and occur greater than 35 days apart.
- *Polymenorrhea*—cycles occur on a regular basis less than 21 days apart.
- *Primary amenorrhea*—no menses and no secondary sexual characteristics by age 14 OR no menses by age 16 with secondary sexual characteristics evident.
- *Secondary amenorrhea*—the woman has had menstrual cycles and then no cycle for a period of at least 6 months.

To classify by etiology, FIGO coined the phrase "PALM-COEIN"—PALM outlining mechanical causes of bleeding and COEIN outlining other causes:

- P=polyps
- A=adenomyosis
- L=leiomyomas
- M=malignancy and hyperplasia
- C=coagulopathy
- O=ovulatory dysfunction
- E=endometrial
- I= iatrogenic causes
- N=not yet classified

Once the etiology has been determined, documentation of AUB will be written accordingly. For example, AUB-P would be bleeding related to polyps, AUB-C might be due to coagulopathy, etc. Treatment is then based on the underlying cause.[62]

Etiology and Pathogenesis

Dysfunctional menstrual cycles are related to alterations in the hormones that support normal cyclic endometrial changes. Estrogen deprivation causes retrogression of a previously built-up endometrium and bleeding. Such bleeding often is irregular in amount and duration, with the flow varying with the time and degree of estrogen stimulation and with the degree of estrogen withdrawal. A lack of progesterone can cause abnormal menstrual bleeding. In its absence, estrogen induces development of a much thicker endometrial layer with a richer blood supply. The absence of progesterone results from the failure of any of the developing ovarian follicles to mature to the point of ovulation, with the subsequent formation of the corpus luteum and production and secretion of progesterone.

Periodic bleeding episodes alternating with amenorrhea are caused by variations in the number of functioning ovarian follicles present. If sufficient follicles are present and active and if new follicles assume functional capacity, high levels of estrogen develop, causing the endometrium to proliferate for weeks or even months. In time, estrogen withdrawal and bleeding develop. This can occur for two reasons: an absolute estrogen deficiency may develop when several follicles simultaneously degenerate, or a relative deficiency may develop as the needs of the enlarged endometrial tissue mass exceed the capabilities of the existing follicles, even though estrogen levels remain constant. Estrogen and progesterone deficiencies are associated with the absence of ovulation, hence the term *anovulatory bleeding*. Because the vasoconstriction and myometrial contractions that normally accompany menstruation are caused by progesterone, anovulatory bleeding seldom is accompanied by cramps, and the flow frequently is heavy. Anovulatory cycles are common among adolescents during the first several years after menarche, when ovarian function is becoming established, among perimenopausal women whose ovarian function is beginning to decline, and, commonly, in obese women with PCOS.

Dysfunctional menstrual cycles can originate as a primary disorder of the ovaries or as a secondary defect in ovarian function related to hypothalamic–pituitary stimulation. The latter can be initiated by emotional stress, marked variation in weight (*i.e.*, sudden gain or loss), or nonspecific endocrine or metabolic disturbances. Nonhormonal causes of irregular menstrual bleeding include endometrial polyps, submucosal myoma (*i.e.*, fibroid), bleeding disorder (*e.g.*, von Willebrand disease, platelet dysfunction), infection, endometrial cancer, and pregnancy.[62]

Treatment

The treatment of dysfunctional bleeding depends on what is identified as the probable cause. The minimum evaluation should include a detailed history with emphasis on bleeding pattern and a physical examination. Endocrine studies (*e.g.*, FSH/LH ratio, prolactin, testosterone, DHEAS levels), β-hCG pregnancy test, ultrasonography of the endometrium, endometrial biopsy, D&C with or without hysteroscopy, and progesterone withdrawal tests may be needed for diagnosis. Nonhormonal causes generally require surgical intervention. D&C can be therapeutic as well as diagnostic. Endometrial ablation (thinning or elimination of the basal layer of the endometrium from which the monthly buildup generates) has become a primary treatment strategy for heavy bleeding. It can be accomplished using heat, cold, microwave, chemicals, or radiofrequency energy sources.[55] If nonhormonal problems have been excluded and alterations in hormone levels are the primary cause, treatment may include the use of oral contraceptives, cyclic progesterone therapy, or long-acting progesterone via injection or an IUD.

Amenorrhea

There are two types of amenorrhea: primary and secondary. Primary amenorrhea is the failure to menstruate by 15 years of age, or by 13 years of age if failure to menstruate is accompanied by absence of secondary sex characteristics. Secondary amenorrhea is the cessation of menses for at least 6 months in a woman who has established normal menstrual cycles.[62]

Etiology

Primary amenorrhea usually is caused by gonadal dysgenesis, congenital müllerian agenesis, testicular feminization, or a hypothalamic–pituitary–ovarian axis disorder. Causes of secondary amenorrhea include pregnancy; ovarian, pituitary, or hypothalamic dysfunction; intrauterine adhesions; chronic conditions or infections (*e.g.*, tuberculosis, syphilis); pituitary tumor; anorexia nervosa; or strenuous physical exercise, which can alter the critical body fat–muscle ratio needed for menses to occur.[63]

Diagnosis and Treatment

Diagnostic evaluation resembles that for AUB, with the possible addition of a computed tomographic scan or MRI to exclude a pituitary tumor. Treatment is based on correcting the underlying cause and inducing menstruation with cyclic progesterone or combined estrogen–progesterone regimens.[62]

KEY POINTS

DYSFUNCTIONAL MENSTRUAL CYCLES

- The pattern of menstrual bleeding tends to be fairly consistent in most healthy women with regard to frequency, duration, and amount of flow.
- Abnormal uterine bleeding in postpubertal women can take the form of absent or scanty periods, infrequent periods, excessive and irregular periods, excessive bleeding during periods, and bleeding between periods.

Dysmenorrhea

Dysmenorrhea is pain or discomfort with menstruation. Although not usually a serious medical problem, it causes some degree of monthly disability for a significant number of women. There are two forms of dysmenorrhea: primary and secondary. Primary dysmenorrhea is menstrual pain that is not associated with a physical abnormality or pathologic process.[64] It usually occurs with ovulatory menstruation beginning 6 months to 2 years after menarche. Symptoms may begin 1 to 2 days before menses, peak on the first day of flow, and subside within several hours to several days. Severe dysmenorrhea may be associated with systemic symptoms such as headache, nausea, vomiting, diarrhea, fatigue, irritability, dizziness, and syncope.[65]The pain typically is described as dull, lower abdominal aching or cramping, spasmodic or colicky in nature, often radiating to the lower back, labia majora, or upper thighs.

Secondary dysmenorrhea is menstrual pain caused by specific organic conditions, such as endometriosis, uterine fibroids, adenomyosis, pelvic adhesions, IUDs, or PID. Laparoscopy often is required for diagnosis of secondary dysmenorrhea if medication for primary dysmenorrhea is ineffective.

Treatment for primary dysmenorrhea is directed at symptom control. Although analgesic agents such as aspirin and acetaminophen may relieve minor uterine cramping or low back pain, prostaglandin synthetase inhibitors (*e.g.*, ibuprofen, naproxen, mefenamic acid, indomethacin) are more specific for dysmenorrhea and the treatment of choice if contraception is not desired. Ovulation suppression and symptomatic relief of dysmenorrhea can be instituted simultaneously with the use of oral contraceptives. Relief of secondary dysmenorrhea depends on identifying the cause of the problem. Medical or surgical intervention may be needed to eliminate the problem.[57]

Premenstrual Symptom Disorders

According to surveys, 80% of women experience some type of premenstrual emotional or physical changes. In addition, 20% of the adult female population indicate that these mild to moderate monthly symptoms cause some difficulty, sometimes enough difficulty to present for medical assistance in treating.[66] Exactly how many of these women have symptoms that are severe enough to warrant treatment is unknown because of the multiple symptoms associated with PMS.[61]

There exists a spectrum of premenstrual symptom disorders, ranging from mild to severe. These disorders include:

- *Premenstrual syndrome* (PMS), which is characterized by mild to moderate physical and psychological symptoms limited to within 14 days preceding menstruation and relieved by onset of the menses
- *Premenstrual dysphoric disorder* (PMDD), which is the most severe form of premenstrual distress and generally is associated with mood disorders.

The incidence of PMS seems to increase with age. It is less common in women in their teens and twenties. Most of the women seeking help for the problem are in their mid-thirties. The disorder is not culturally distinct; it affects both Westerners and non-Westerners.[62]

Etiology

The exact causes of PMS and PMDD remain a mystery; however, they are probably multifactorial. Like dysmenorrhea, PMS has only recently been recognized as a bona fide disorder rather than merely a psychosomatic illness. There has been a tendency to link the disorder with endocrine imbalances such as hyperprolactinemia, estrogen excess, and alteration in the estrogen–progesterone ratio. More recent studies now lead researchers to understand that women may have normal hormone levels but react abnormally to changes in the levels. Other hypotheses suggest that alterations in the renin–angiotensin–aldosterone system and/or prostaglandin excess may also contribute to symptoms.[62]

The most recent theory to emerge suggests a relationship between normal gonadal fluctuations and central neurotransmitter activity, particularly serotonin. There is confusion as to whether decreased levels of serotonin are present during the luteal phase, and only susceptible women respond with varying degrees of premenstrual symptoms, or if women with PMDD have a neurotransmitter abnormality.[67–69]

Clinical Manifestations

Physical symptoms of PMS include painful and swollen breasts, bloating, abdominal pain, headache, and backache. Psychologically, there may be depression, anxiety, irritability, and behavioral changes. Women with PMS may report one or several symptoms, with symptoms varying from woman to woman and from month to month in the same woman.[67,68] Signs and symptoms associated with this disorder are summarized in Table 45.1. PMS can significantly affect a woman's ability to perform at normal levels.

Diagnosis

A complete history and physical examination are necessary to exclude other physical causes of the symptoms. Depending on the symptom pattern, blood studies, including thyroid hormones, glucose, and prolactin assays, may be done. Psychosocial evaluation is helpful to exclude emotional illness that is merely exacerbated premenstrually. The American College of Obstetricians and Gynecologists (ACOG) published clinical management guidelines for PMS that included diagnostic criteria similar to what the American Psychiatric Association did for PMDD in the DSM-V.[61] Diagnosis focuses on identification of symptoms by means of a daily calendar on which the woman records her symptoms for 2 to 3 consecutive months. PMDD is a psychiatric diagnosis that has been developed to distinguish those women whose symptoms are severe enough to interfere significantly with activities of daily living. It requires prospective symptom charting, and a minimum of 5 of the 11 symptom groups as described in the fifth edition of the *Diagnostic and Statistical Manual of Mental Disorders* (*DSM-IV*) to establish a diagnosis of PMDD. Presence of a single symptom is sufficient for the diagnosis of PMS.[66]

Treatment

Management of PMS/PMDD has been largely symptomatic and includes education and support directed toward lifestyle changes for women with mild symptoms. Treatment includes diuretics to reduce fluid retention, analgesics for pain, and anxiolytic drugs to treat mood changes. An integrated program of personal assessment by diary, regular exercise, avoidance of caffeine, and a diet low in simple sugars and high in lean proteins is often beneficial. Additional therapeutic regimens that have been used include vitamin or mineral supplements (particularly pyridoxine, vitamin E, and magnesium), evening primrose oil (which contains linoleic acid, a precursor of prostaglandin E_1), natural progesterone supplements, low-dose oral monophasic contraceptives, GnRH agonists, bromocriptine for prolactin suppression, danazol (a synthetic

TABLE 45.1 SYMPTOMS OF PREMENSTRUAL SYNDROME BY SYSTEM

BODY SYSTEM	SYMPTOMS
Cerebral	Irritability, anxiety, nervousness, fatigue, exhaustion, increased physical and mental activity, lability, crying spells, depression, inability to concentrate
Gastrointestinal	Craving for sweets or salt, lower abdominal pain, bloating, nausea, vomiting, diarrhea, constipation
Vascular	Headache, edema, weakness, fainting
Reproductive	Swelling and tenderness of the breasts, pelvic congestion, ovarian pain, altered libido
Neuromuscular	Trembling of the extremities, changes in coordination, clumsiness, backache, leg aches
General	Weight gain, insomnia, dizziness, acne

androgen), and spironolactone (an aldosterone antagonist and inhibitor of adrenal androgen synthesis).[66] Although a body of knowledge has evolved that offers a variety of therapeutic choices, few treatments have been adequately evaluated in randomized, controlled clinical trials. The SSRI antidepressants, however, have demonstrated significant improvement in overall symptoms compared with placebo, whether used continuously or only in the luteal phase, and are recommended by ACOG as first-line therapy for severe PMS or PMDD.[61,68]

IN SUMMARY

Menstrual disorders include dysfunctional menstrual cycles, dysmenorrhea, and PMS. Dysfunctional menstrual cycles, which involve amenorrhea, oligomenorrhea, metrorrhagia, or menorrhagia, occur when the hormonal support of the endometrium is altered. Estrogen deprivation causes retrogression of a previously built-up endometrium and bleeding. A lack of progesterone can cause abnormal menstrual bleeding; in its absence, estrogen induces development of a much thicker endometrial layer with a richer blood supply. The absence of progesterone results from the failure of any of the developing ovarian follicles to mature to the point of ovulation, with subsequent formation of the corpus luteum and production of progesterone.

Dysmenorrhea is characterized by pain or discomfort during menses. It can occur as a primary or secondary disorder. Primary dysmenorrhea is not associated with other disorders and begins soon after menarche. Secondary dysmenorrhea is caused by a specific organic condition, such as endometriosis or pelvic adhesions. It occurs in women with previously painless menses.

Premenstrual symptom disorders represent a spectrum from molimina, which is present to some degree in most ovulatory women, to PMS and PMDD. PMS represents a cluster of physical and psychological symptoms that precede menstruation by 1 to 2 weeks. PMDD describes the most severe, disabling form of PMS. The true incidence and nature of PMS has been recognized only recently, and its cause and methods for treatment are still under study.

DISORDERS OF THE BREAST

After completing this section of the chapter, the learner will be able to meet the following objectives:

- Describe changes in breast function that occur with galactorrhea, mastitis, and ductal ectasia.
- Describe the methods used in the diagnosis and treatment of breast cancer.

Most breast disease may be described as either benign or cancerous. Breast tissue is never static; the breast is constantly responding to changes in hormonal, nutritional, psychological, and environmental stimuli that cause continual cellular changes. Benign breast conditions are nonprogressive. However, some forms of benign disease increase the risk of malignant disease. In light of this, strict adherence to a dichotomy of benign versus malignant disease may not always be appropriate. However, it is useful for the sake of simplicity and clarity.

Galactorrhea

Galactorrhea is the secretion of breast milk in a nonlactating breast. Galactorrhea may result from vigorous nipple stimulation, exogenous hormones, internal hormonal imbalance, or local chest infection or trauma. A pituitary tumor, such as a prolactinoma, may produce large amounts of prolactin and cause galactorrhea. Galactorrhea occurs in men and women and usually is benign. Observation may be continued for several months before diagnostic hormonal screening. Spontaneous leaking from the breast (occurring without any type of stimulation) is pathologic and warrants a complete workup.[70,71]

Mastitis

Mastitis is inflammation of the breast. It most frequently occurs during lactation but may also result from other conditions in nonlactating women.[72] In the lactating woman, inflammation results from an ascending infection that travels from the nipple to the ductile structures. The most common organisms isolated are *Staphylococcus*.[70] The offending organisms originate from the suckling infant's nasopharynx or the mother's hands. During the early weeks of nursing, the breast is particularly vulnerable to bacterial invasion because of minor cracks and fissures that occur with vigorous suckling. Infection and inflammation cause obstruction of the ductile system. The breast area becomes hard, inflamed, and tender if not treated early. Without treatment, the area becomes walled off and may abscess, requiring incision and drainage. It is advisable for the mother to continue breast-feeding during antibiotic therapy to prevent this.[72]

Mastitis is not confined to the postpartum period; it can occur as a result of hormonal fluctuations, tumors, trauma, or skin infection. Cyclic inflammation of the breast occurs most frequently in adolescents, who commonly have fluctuating hormone levels. Tumors may cause mastitis secondary to skin involvement or lymphatic obstruction. Local trauma or infection may develop into mastitis because of ductal blockage of trapped blood, cellular debris, or the extension of superficial inflammation.[1] Treatment for mastitis symptoms includes application of heat or cold, excision, aspiration, mild analgesics, antibiotics, and a supportive brassiere or breast binder.

Ductal Disorders

Ductal ectasia manifests in older women as a spontaneous, intermittent, usually unilateral, grayish-green nipple discharge. Palpation of the breast increases the discharge. Ectasia occurs during or after menopause and is symptomatically associated with burning, itching, pain, and a pulling sensation of the nipple and areola. The disease results in inflammation of the ducts and subsequent thickening. The treatment requires removal of the involved ductal mass.[73]

Intraductal papillomas are benign epithelial tissue tumors that range in size from 2 mm to 5 cm. A very small percentage of these lesions will have atypical cells that can progress to cancer and excision is recommended. Papillomas usually manifest with a bloody nipple discharge.[71]The tumor may be palpated in the areolar area. *Galactography*, a radiograph taken after dye is injected into the affected duct, is used for diagnosis. The papilloma is probed through the nipple, and the involved duct is removed. It has been argued that MRI may be as effective, and in some cases more effective, in identifying disease.[71,74]

Fibroadenoma and Fibrocystic Changes

Fibroadenomas are seen in premenopausal women, most commonly in the third and fourth decades. The clinical findings include a firm, rubbery, sharply defined round mass. On palpation, the mass "slides" between the fingers and is easily movable. These masses usually are singular; only 15% are multiple or bilateral. Fibroadenomas are asymptomatic and usually found by accident. They are not thought to be precancerous. Treatment involves simple excision.[75]

Fibrocystic changes are the most frequent lesion of the breast. These changes are most common in women between 20 and 50 years of age and are rare in postmenopausal women not receiving hormone replacement.[1] Fibrocystic changes usually present as nodular (*i.e.*, "shotty"), granular breast masses that are more prominent and painful during the luteal or progesterone-dominant portion of the menstrual cycle. Discomfort ranges from heaviness to exquisite tenderness, depending on the degree of vascular engorgement and cystic distention.

Fibrocystic changes encompass a wide variety of lesions and breast changes. Microscopically, fibrocystic changes refer to a constellation of morphologic changes manifested by (a) microscopic cysts, (b) apocrine metaplasia, (c) mild epithelial hyperplasia, and (d) increase in fibrous stroma.[1] Although fibrocystic changes have been thought to increase the risk of breast cancer, only certain variants in which proliferation of the epithelial components is demonstrated represent a true risk. Presence of large cysts and proliferative epithelial lesions with atypia are more common in women who are at increased risk for invasive breast cancer. The nonproliferative form of fibrocystic changes, which does not carry an increased risk for development of cancer, is more common.

Diagnosis of fibrocystic changes is made by physical examination, mammography, ultrasonography, and biopsy (*i.e.*, aspiration or tissue sample). The use of mammography for diagnosis in high-risk groups of women younger than 35 years of age on a routine basis remains controversial. Mammography may be helpful in establishing the diagnosis, but increased breast tissue density in women with fibrocystic changes may make an abnormal or cancerous mass difficult to discern among the other structures and requires MRI. Ultrasonography is useful in differentiating a cystic from a solid mass. Because a mass caused by fibrocystic changes may be indistinguishable from carcinoma on the basis of clinical findings, suspect lesions should undergo biopsy. Fine-needle aspiration may be used, but if a suspect mass that was nonmalignant on cytologic examination does not resolve over several months, it should be removed surgically. Any discrete mass or lump on the breast should be viewed as possible carcinoma, and cancer should be excluded before instituting the conservative measures used to treat fibrocystic changes.

Treatment for fibrocystic changes is usually symptomatic. Mild analgesics (*e.g.*, aspirin, acetaminophen, or NSAIDs), and local application of heat or cold may be used for pain relief. Prominent or persistent cysts may be aspirated and any fluid obtained sent to the laboratory for cytologic analysis.[76]

Breast Cancer

Cancer of the breast is the most common female cancer. One in eight women in the United States will have breast cancer in her lifetime. In 2017, invasive breast cancer affected an estimated 252,710 American women and killed an estimated 40,610 women. Although the breast cancer mortality rate has shown a slight decline, it is second only to lung cancer as a cause of cancer-related deaths in women. An additional 63,410 American women were diagnosed with cancer in situ or precancer.[77] Incidence rates for carcinoma in situ have increased dramatically since the mid-1970s because of recommendations regarding mammography screening. Death rates have decreased, particularly in women younger than 50 years of age. The decline in the breast cancer mortality rate since 1989 is due to earlier diagnosis through screening programs and increased awareness, as well as improvements in cancer treatments.[78]

Risk Factors

Risk factors for breast cancer include sex, increasing age, personal or family history of breast cancer (*i.e.*, at highest risk are those with multiple affected first-order relatives), history of benign breast disease (*i.e.*, primary "atypical" hyperplasia), and hormonal influences that promote breast maturation and may increase the chance of cell mutation (*i.e.*, early menarche, late menopause, no term pregnancies or first child after 30 years of age, and no breastfeeding). Modifiable risk factors include obesity (particularly after menopause), physical inactivity, and alcohol intake greater than one drink per day.[78] However, most women with breast cancer have no identifiable risk factors.

Approximately, 5% to 10% of all breast cancers are hereditary, with genetic mutations causing up to 80% of breast cancers in women younger than 50 years of age.[79] Two breast cancer susceptibility genes—*BRCA1* on chromosome 17 and *BRCA2* on chromosome 13—may account for most inherited forms of breast cancer. *BRCA1* is known to be involved in tumor suppression. A woman with known mutations in *BRCA1* has a lifetime risk of 60% to 85% for breast cancer and an increased risk of ovarian cancer. *BRCA2* is another susceptibility gene that carries an elevated cancer risk similar to that with *BRCA1*.[22,79] Guidelines have been established for when genetic counseling and testing should be offered.[80] Breast cancer risk reduction options available to known carriers of *BRCA1* and *BRCA2* mutations include surveillance, chemoprevention, and surgery. Breast evaluation using MRI is generally preferred over standard mammography for these women because of its enhanced sensitivity and lack of radiation exposure, which may be safer for them. Prophylactic surgery, in the form of bilateral mastectomy, bilateral oophorectomy, or both, has been shown to decrease the risk of developing cancer. These controversial surgeries can have physical and psychological side effects that warrant careful consideration before proceeding. The use of aromatase inhibitors for prevention of breast cancer in women with + BRCA1 and/or 2 gene mutations is dependent on the type of breast cancer.

Detection

Cancer of the breast may manifest clinically as a mass, a puckering, nipple retraction, or unusual discharge. Many cancers are found by women themselves—sometimes when only a thickening or subtle change in breast contour is noticed. The variety of symptoms and potential for self-discovery underscore the need for all women to have an awareness of what their normal breast appearance and texture are like. The American Cancer Society has dropped its recommendation that all women perform regular, systematic self-examination. Research has indicated that most women who discover their own cancer do so outside of a scheduled breast self-examination (BSE). American Cancer Society screening guidelines now place primary emphasis for breast cancer diagnosis on mammography, while encouraging women in the area of self-awareness.[81] Premenopausal women who do perform BSE should conduct the examination right after menses. This time is most appropriate in relation to cyclic breast changes that occur in response to fluctuations in hormone levels. Postmenopausal women and women who have had a hysterectomy can perform the examination any day of the month. Examination may be done in the shower or bath or at bedtime. The most important aspect of BSE is to devise a systematic, convenient, and consistent method of examination. Women should have a clinical examination by a trained health professional at least every 3 years between 20 and 40 years of age, and annually after 40 years of age.

Mammography is the only effective screening technique for the early detection of clinically unapparent lesions. A generally slow-growing form of cancer, breast cancer may have been present for 2 to 9 years before it reaches 1 cm, the smallest mass normally detected by palpation. Mammography can disclose lesions as small as 1 mm and the clustering of calcifications that may warrant biopsy to exclude cancer. Mammography has a sensitivity of 80% to 90% for the detection of breast cancer even when performed by the most capable institutions. Therefore, even if the mammogram is negative, a palpable mass requires further evaluation. Approximately, 40% of breast cancers can be detected only by palpation and another 40% only by mammography.[22] The most comprehensive approach to screening is a combination of individual self-awareness, clinical breast evaluation by a health professional, and mammography.

Diagnosis and Classification

Procedures used in the diagnosis of breast cancer include physical examination, mammography, ultrasonography, percutaneous needle aspiration, stereotactic needle biopsy (*i.e.*, core biopsy), and excisional biopsy. Figure 45.14 illustrates the appearance of breast cancer on mammography. Breast cancer often manifests as a solitary, painless, firm, fixed

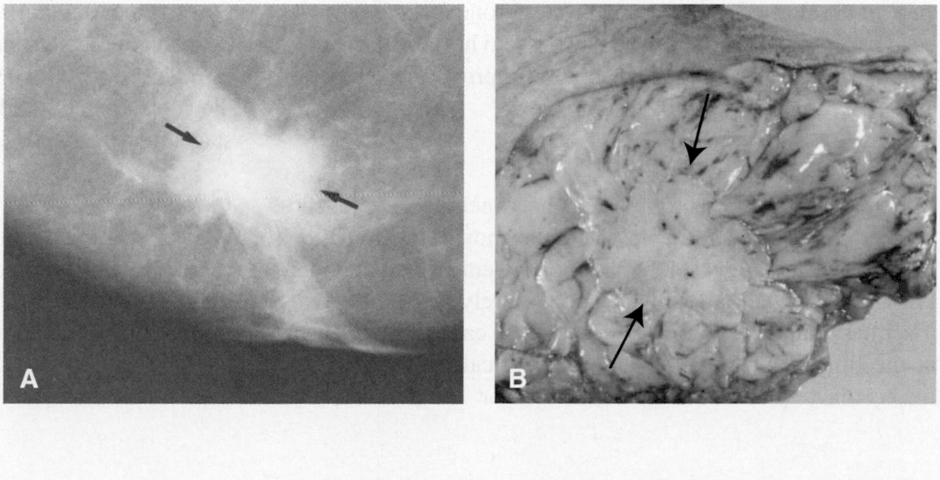

Figure 45.14 • Carcinoma of the breast. **(A)** Mammogram. An irregularly shaped, dense mass (*arrows*) is seen in this otherwise fatty breast. **(B)** Mastectomy specimen. The irregular white, firm mass in the center is surrounded by fatty tissue. (From Strayer D. S., Rubin R. (Eds.) (2015). *Rubin's pathology: Clinicopathologic foundations of medicine* (7th ed., Fig. 25-35A and B, p. 1071). Philadelphia, PA: Lippincott Williams & Wilkins.)

lesion with poorly defined borders. It can be found anywhere in the breast but is most common in the upper outer quadrant. Because of the variability in presentation, any suspect change in breast tissue warrants further investigation. The diagnostic use of mammography enables additional definition of the clinically suspect area (*e.g.*, appearance, character, calcification) and may lead to early detection of cancer. Placement of a wire marker under radiographic guidance can ensure accurate surgical biopsy of nonpalpable suspect areas. Ultrasonography is useful as a diagnostic adjunct to differentiate cystic from solid tissue in women with nonspecific thickening.[82]

Fine-needle aspiration is a simple in-office procedure that can be performed repeatedly in multiple sites and with minimal discomfort. It can be accomplished by stabilizing a palpable mass between two fingers or in conjunction with handheld sonography to define cystic masses or fibrocystic changes and to provide specimens for cytologic examination. Fine needle aspiration can identify the presence of malignant cells, but it cannot differentiate in situ from infiltrating cancers. Stereotactic needle biopsy is an outpatient procedure done with the guidance of a mammography machine. After the lesion is localized radiologically, a large-bore needle is mechanically thrust quickly into the area, removing a core of tissue. Discomfort is similar to that with ear piercing, and even when multiple cores are obtained, healing occurs quite rapidly. Cells are available for histologic evaluation with 96% accuracy in detecting cancer. This procedure is less costly than excisional biopsy. However, excisional biopsy to remove the entire lump provides the only definitive diagnosis of breast cancer, and often is therapeutic without additional surgery. MRI, positron emission tomography (PET), and computer-based or digital mammography are available as additional diagnostic modalities for breast cancer, and may be recommended to supplement conventional mammography in women with radiographically dense breasts or a strong family history of cancer, or who are known carriers of *BRCA1* or *BRCA2*.[83]

Tumors are classified histologically according to tissue characteristics and staged clinically according to tumor size, nodal involvement, and presence of metastasis. It is recommended that estrogen and progesterone receptor analysis be performed on surgical specimens. Information about the presence or absence of estrogen and progesterone receptors can be used in predicting tumor responsiveness to hormonal manipulation. High levels of both receptors improve the prognosis and increase the likelihood of remission.

Treatment

The treatment methods for breast cancer include surgery, chemotherapy, radiation therapy, and hormonal manipulation. Radical mastectomy (*i.e.*, removal of the entire breast, underlying muscles, and all axillary nodes) rarely is used today as a primary surgical therapy unless breast cancer is advanced at the time of diagnosis. Modified surgical techniques (*i.e.*, mastectomy plus axillary dissection or lumpectomy for breast conservation) accompanied by chemotherapy or radiation therapy have achieved outcomes comparable with those obtained with radical surgical methods and constitute the preferred treatment methods.

The prognosis is related more to the extent of nodal involvement than to the extent of breast involvement. Greater nodal involvement requires more aggressive postsurgical treatment, and many cancer specialists believe that a diagnosis of breast cancer is not complete until dissection and testing of the axillary lymph nodes has been accomplished. A newer technique for evaluating lymph node involvement is a sentinel lymph node (SLN) biopsy. A radioactive substance or dye is injected into the region of the tumor. In theory, the dye is carried to the first (sentinel) node to receive lymph from the tumor.[82] This would therefore be the node most likely to contain cancer cells if the cancer has spread. If the sentinel node biopsy is positive, more nodes are removed. If it is negative, further lymph node evaluation may not be needed.

Systemic therapy refers to the administration of chemotherapy, biologic therapy, or hormonal therapy. Neoadjuvant therapy is given before surgery to shrink the tumor and make surgical removal more effective. Adjuvant therapy is given after surgery to women with and without detectable metastatic disease. The goal of this therapy depends on nodal involvement, menopausal status, and hormone receptor status. Systemic adjuvant therapy has been widely studied and has demonstrated benefits in reducing rates of recurrence and death from breast cancer.[83] Biologic therapy, using the drug trastuzumab (Herceptin), is used to stop the growth of breast tumors that express the HER2/neu receptor on their cell surface. The HER2/neu receptor binds an epidermal growth factor that contributes to cancer cell growth. Trastuzumab is a recombinant DNA-derived monoclonal antibody that binds to the HER2/neu receptor.

Hormone therapy is used to block the effects of estrogen on the growth of breast cancer cells. Tamoxifen is a nonsteroidal antiestrogen that binds to estrogen receptors and blocks the effects of estrogens on the growth of malignant cells in the breast. Decreased cancer recurrence, decreased mortality rates, and increased 5-year survival rates have been found in women with estrogen receptor–positive tissue samples who have been treated with Tamoxifen. Aromatase inhibitors block the enzyme that converts androstenedione and testosterone to estrogen in the peripheral tissues. This reduces the circulating estrogen levels in postmenopausal women and is becoming the most effective adjuvant therapy for women with early-stage breast cancer.[84]

Paget Disease

Paget disease accounts for 1% of all breast cancers. The disease presents as an eczematoid lesion of the nipple and areola (Fig. 45.15). Paget disease usually is associated with an infiltrating, intraductal carcinoma. Complete examination is required and includes a mammogram and biopsy. Treatment depends on the extent of spread.[85]

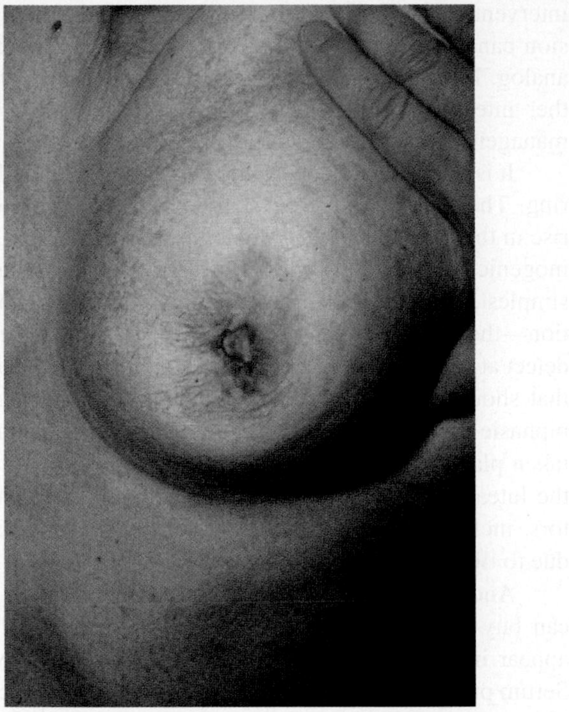

Figure 45.15 • Paget disease of the nipple. (From Strayer D. S., Rubin R. (Eds.) (2015). *Rubin's pathology: Clinicopathologic foundations of medicine* (7th ed., Fig. 25-30A, p. 1069). Philadelphia, PA: Lippincott Williams & Wilkins.)

IN SUMMARY

The breasts are subject to benign and malignant diseases. Mastitis is inflammation of the breast, occurring most frequently during lactation. Galactorrhea is an abnormal secretion of milk that may occur as a symptom of increased prolactin secretion. Ductal ectasia and intraductal papilloma cause abnormal drainage from the nipple. Fibroadenoma and fibrocystic changes are characterized by abnormal masses in the breast that are benign. By far, the most important disease of the breast is breast cancer, which is a significant cause of death of women. Clinical breast examination and mammography afford a woman the best protection against breast cancer. They provide the means for early detection of breast cancer and, in many cases, allow early treatment and cure.

INFERTILITY

After completing this section of the chapter, the learner will be able to meet the following objectives:

- Provide a definition of infertility.
- List male and female factors that contribute to infertility.
- List basic treatments of infertility

Infertility is the inability to conceive a child after 1 year of unprotected intercourse. Primary infertility refers to situations in which there has been no prior conception. Secondary infertility is infertility that occurs after one or more previous pregnancies. Sterility is the inability to father a child or to become pregnant because of congenital anomalies, disease, or surgical intervention. In the United States, approximately 6% to 12% of women ages 15 to 44 are affected by infertility.[86]

In order for pregnancy to occur, three things must be available: (a) oocytes or eggs; (b) spermatazoa or sperm; and (c) a place for oocytes and spermatazoa to fertilize and then implant. Anything that adversely affects any or all of these areas may result in infertility. The complexity of the process that must occur to achieve a pregnancy is taken for granted by most couples. For some couples, pregnancy occurs very easily, whereas for others, it does not.

There are several contributing factors to infertility. Male and female factors each make up about one third. Approximately 20% of couples will suffer from unexplained infertility when a workup finds no definable cause for the inability to conceive. Roughly 10% of infertility is caused by a combination of both male and female factors.[87] Although a full discussion of the diagnosis and treatment of infertility is beyond the scope of this book, an overview of the areas in which problems can occur is presented.

Male Factors

For pregnancy to occur, the man must be able to provide sperm in sufficient quantity, delivered to the upper end of the vagina, with adequate motility to traverse the female reproductive tract. The male contribution to this process is assessed by means of a semen analysis, which evaluates volume of semen (normally 1.5 mL), sperm density (15 to 39 million/mL), motility (>32% good progressive), viability (58%), morphology (4% normal), and viscosity (full liquefaction within 20 minutes).[88] The specimen is best collected by masturbation into a sterile container after 3 days of abstinence. Because of variability in specimens, abnormal results should lead to a repeat test before the need for treatment is presumed. *Azoospermia* is the absence of sperm, *oligospermia* refers to decreased numbers of sperm, and *asthenospermia* refers to poor motility of sperm.[89]

The causes of male infertility include varicocele, ejaculatory dysfunction, hyperprolactinemia, hypogonadotropic hypogonadism, infection, immunologic problems (*i.e.*, antisperm antibodies), obstruction, and congenital anomalies. There are some male risk factors for sperm problems including a history of mumps orchitis, cryptorchidism (*i.e.*, undescended testes), testicular torsion, hypospadias, previous urologic surgery, and history of STIs. Treatment depends on the cause and may include surgery, medication, or the use of artificial insemination to deliver a more concentrated specimen directly to the cervical canal or uterine fundus.[87]

Female Factors

The female contribution to pregnancy is more complex, requiring production and release of a mature ovum capable of being fertilized, production of cervical mucus that assists in sperm transport and maintains sperm viability in the female reproductive tract, patent fallopian tubes with the motility potential to pick up and transfer the ovum to the uterine cavity, development of an endometrium that is suitable for the implantation and nourishment of a fertilized ovum, and a uterine cavity that allows for growth and development of a fetus. Each of these factors is discussed briefly, along with an overview of diagnostic tests and treatment.

Diminished Ovarian Reserve

Conception cannot occur without an oocyte. Important things to consider in reproduction in regards to oocytes are quality, ability to be fertilized, and ovulation. Women are born with their lifetime cache of oocytes; this is in contrast to men, who continue to make spermatozoa throughout their lifetime. As women age, fertility declines. Oocyte quality and quantity also declines (diminished ovarian reserve or DOR), contributing to difficulty getting pregnant. Women with DOR also have a higher rate of miscarriage if they do conceive; this may be related to the quality of the oocytes resulting in poor quality embryos.

Assessment for DOR is generally done early in the menstrual cycle. FSH, LH, and estradiol levels should be lowest days of 1 to 3 when they are measured. FSH levels >10, and/or an estradiol >80 may indicate DOR. Anti-mullerian hormone (AMH) levels should be between 1 and 3.5. Lower levels are indicative of DOR. Ultrasound measurement of the number of antral (primordial) ovarian follicles on day 3 of the menstrual cycle can also be used to detect DOR. An antral follicle count of 3 to 10 on both ovaries and low ovarian volume may indicate DOR. (Gordon)[90] This is not to say that a woman with DOR cannot conceive. It is predictive of chances of successful treatment using the woman's own oocytes. In cases of DOR that use donor oocytes, the quality of oocytes is taken out of the equation. Chances of conception are high as ovum donors are usually young women with proven fertility.

Ovulatory Dysfunction

Ovulatory dysfunction is a common cause of infertility. Ovulatory dysfunction, including anovulation (no ovulation) and oligo-ovulation (irregular ovulation), can be due to primary problems of the ovary or secondary problems related to endocrine dysfunction. When disturbances in ovulation are confirmed, it is reasonable to rule out other endocrine system problems before initiating treatment. If the results of tests for pituitary hormones (*e.g.*, FSH, LH, prolactin), thyroid studies, and tests of adrenal function (*e.g.*, DHEAS, androstenedione) are normal, ovulatory dysfunction is primary and should respond to treatment. Abnormalities in any of the other endocrine areas should be further evaluated as needed and treated appropriately. Hyperprolactinemia requires workup for pituitary lesions or associated endocrinopathies (such as thyroid dysfunction). Continued hyperprolactinemia can be treated with bromocriptine or cabergoline (Dostinex). Hypothyroidism requires thyroid replacement, and hyperthyroidism requires suppressive therapy and, sometimes, surgical intervention with thyroid replacement later. Adrenal suppression can be instituted with dexamethasone, a glucocorticoid analog. Normal ovulatory function may resume without further intervention. If not, treatment can be concurrent with management of other endocrine problems.[90]

It is important to determine if ovulation is actually occurring. The presence of progesterone after ovulation causes a rise in the woman's basal body temperature (BBT). This thermogenic property of progesterone provides the basis for the simplest, most inexpensive beginning test of ovulatory function—the measurement of BBT. Women should be able to detect at least a 0.4°F rise in their BBT (at rest) after ovulation that should be maintained throughout the luteal phase. This biphasic temperature pattern demonstrates that ovulation has taken place, where in the cycle it occurred, and the length of the luteal phase. BBT can be influenced by many other factors, including restless sleep, alcohol intake, drug use, fever due to illness, and change in usual rising time.

Another test for ovulation is with LH predictor kits one can buy at the pharmacy. These test for LH, which should appear in the urine after the LH surge indicating ovulation. Serum progesterone can also be measured after expected ovulation to confirm if ovulation occurred. Finally, endometrial biopsy can also give information on the current phase of a woman's cycle. However, given the invasiveness of the procedure, this is not usually done.

Cervical Mucus Problems

High preovulatory levels of estradiol stimulate the production of large amounts of clear, stretchy cervical mucus that aids the transport of sperm into the uterine cavity and helps to maintain an environment that keeps the sperm viable for up to 72 hours. Insufficient estrogen production (*i.e.*, inherent or secondary to treatment with clomiphene citrate, an antiestrogen), cervical abnormalities from disease or invasive procedures (*e.g.*, DES exposure, stenosis, conization), and cervical infection (*e.g.*, chlamydial infection, mycoplasmal infection, gonorrhea) can adversely affect the production of healthy cervical mucus.

A postcoital test (Sims-Huhner) involves evaluation of the cervical mucus 1 to 8 hours after intercourse within the 48 hours before ovulation. A sample of cervical mucus is obtained using a special syringe and evaluated grossly for amount, clarity, and stretch (*i.e.*, spinnbarkeit) and microscopically for cellularity, number and quality of motile sperm, and the presence of ferning after the sample has air dried on the slide. Intrauterine insemination (IUI) with the husband's sperm can bypass the cervical mucus if issues are noted. Cervical cultures for gonorrhea, chlamydial infection, and mycoplasmal infection should be obtained and treatment instituted as needed.

Uterine Cavity Abnormalities

Alterations in the uterine cavity can occur because of DES exposure, submucosal fibroids, cervical polyps, bands of scar tissue, or congenital anomalies (*e.g.*, bicornuate uterus, uterine septum, single horn). These defects may be suspected from the person's history or pelvic examination but require hysterosalpingography (*i.e.*, x-ray study in which dye is placed through the cervix to outline the uterine cavity and demonstrate tubal patency) or hysteroscopy (*i.e.*, study in which a lighted fiberoptic endoscope placed through the cervix under general anesthesia allows direct visualization of the uterine cavity) for confirmation. Treatment is surgical when possible.

Tubal Factors

Tubal patency is required for fertilization and can be disrupted secondary to PID, ectopic pregnancy, large myomas, endometriosis, pelvic adhesions, and previous tubal ligation. Hysterosalpingography can reveal the location and type of any blockage, such as fimbrial, cornual, or hydrosalpinx. Microsurgical repair sometimes is possible.[90]

Even when tubal patency is demonstrated, tubal disease may make ovum pickup impossible. Contrary to popular belief, the ovum is not extruded directly into the fallopian tube. The tube must be free to move to engulf the ovum after release. Pelvic adhesions from previous infection, surgery, or endometriosis can interfere with the tube's mobility. Laparoscopic evaluation of the pelvis is needed for diagnosis. Laser ablation or cautery can be used to lyse adhesions and remove endometriosis through the laparoscope or, if severe, by means of laparotomy. If tubal damage cannot be repaired through surgery, assisted reproductive technology (ART) may be recommended.

Assisted Reproductive Technology

The number of ART cycles performed annually in the United States has increased from 138,198 cycles in 2006 to 182,154 performed in reporting fertility clinics in 2015.[91] These techniques include in vitro fertilization (IVF) using nondonor and donor oocytes, oocyte and embryo cryopreservation, and donor and nondonor frozen embryo transfers. Future research will focus on improving the implantation process in an effort to decrease the risk of multiple births while providing an optimal chance for pregnancy.

IVF was developed in 1978 for women with significantly damaged or absent tubes to provide them with an opportunity for pregnancy, where none normally exists. Conception occurs in a laboratory. The process involves stimulation of the ovaries to produce multiple follicles in an effort to produce multiple oocytes. To stimulate the ovaries, the woman injects gonadotropin medications of FSH and LH daily. During this time, the woman is carefully monitored with vaginal ultrasounds and blood tests to avoid overstimulation of the ovaries. When the follicles are mature as evidenced by the monitoring, a transvaginal oocyte retrieval is performed. With the woman sedated, a needle, guided by ultrasound, is placed through the vaginal wall into each ovary to remove the oocytes. Sperm is provided by a male partner or a donor. Conception takes place after mixing the oocytes and sperm together in a Petri dish. In some instances, such as severe oligospermia, a single sperm may be injected into each oocyte. This procedure is known as intracytoplasmic sperm injection (ICSI). Once fertilization occurs, the embryo(s) is/are allowed to grow in the dish over 3 to 5 days. Embryos are then transferred back to the woman by passing the catheter through the cervix and into the uterus and gently injecting the embryo(s).

Success is not guaranteed and depends on many factors. In 2015, 91,090 IVF fresh nondonor cycles were initiated resulting in 59,336 embryo transfers and 21,771 live births. Success with donor oocytes is high. Of the 7,331cycles that used fresh donor oocytes, 55.6% had a live birth. This is attributable to the fact that most donors are 20 to 30 years old.[86]

Indications for IVF have been expanded to include male factors (*i.e.*, severe oligospermia or asthenospermia), ovulatory dysfunction, uterine factors, endometriosis, and idiopathic infertility (*i.e.*, infertility of unknown cause). As more is learned about implantation, the substantial risk of multiple pregnancy via IVF is decreasing. Cryopreservation of excess embryos gives the couple another attempt at conception, which gives them the confidence to transfer fewer embryos.

An outgrowth of IVF technology is gamete intrafallopian transfer (GIFT), which uses similar ovarian stimulation protocols and egg retrieval procedures but uses laparoscopy to place ovum and sperm directly into the fallopian tube. Alternatively, zygote intrafallopian transfer (ZIFT) proceeds like an IVF cycle through egg retrieval and fertilization in the laboratory, but the resulting embryo (zygote) is placed directly into the fallopian tube during laparoscopy. Both GIFT and ZIFT are rarely done anymore.

The use of donor gametes (eggs, sperm, embryos) provides an alternative for achieving pregnancy for those couples who are unable to use their own gametes and are comfortable raising a child that is not genetically related to them. Donor eggs provide a much higher likelihood of success for women older than 40 years of age, when both egg numbers and egg quality decline.

IN SUMMARY

Infertility is the inability to conceive a child after 1 year of unprotected intercourse. Male factors are related to number and motility of sperm and their ability to penetrate the cervical mucus and the ovum. Causes of male infertility include varicocele, ejaculatory dysfunction, hyperprolactinemia, hypogonadotropic hypogonadism, infection, immunologic problems (*i.e.*, antisperm antibodies), obstruction, and congenital anomalies. Risk factors for sperm disorders include a history of mumps orchitis, cryptorchidism, testicular torsion, hypospadias, previous urologic surgery, infection, and exposure to known gonadotoxins.

The female contribution to pregnancy is more complex, requiring production and release of a mature ovum capable of being fertilized, production of cervical mucus that assists in sperm transport and maintains sperm viability in the female reproductive tract, patent fallopian tubes with the mobility potential to pick up and transfer the ovum to the uterine cavity, development of an endometrium that is suitable for the implantation and nourishment of a fertilized ovum, and a uterine cavity that allows for growth and development of a fetus.

Evaluation and treatment of infertility can be lengthy and highly stressful for the couple. Options for therapy continue to expand, but newer ART modalities are expensive, and financial resources can be strained while couples seek to fulfill their, sometimes elusive, dream of having a child.

GERIATRIC Considerations

- Senile vulvitis is a vulvar infection associated with hypertrophy or atrophy of the vulvar tissue and is often caused by incontinence and poor hygienic practices. Itching and scratching of the area are common manifestations.[92]
- Cancer of the vulva is often located on the clitoris; a radical vulvectomy is the most common treatment, but radiation therapy is also used.[92]
- Vaginal tissue is more fragile in postmenopausal women, leading to irritation and vaginitis manifested by itching, burning, and soreness along with foul smelling discharge.[92]
- Cancer of the cervix is uncommon in older women (less than 20%) but death due to cervical cancer is high (one third).[92]
- Dyspareunia is more common with aging because of a decrease in hormones and an increase in infections in reproductive organs such as vulvitis and vaginitis.[92]
- Breast cancer increases with age, but older women are less likely to participate in preventative measures such as self-breast exams and mammography. Women should have annual mammograms until age 75, then every 2 to 3 years unless otherwise indicated.[92]

PEDIATRIC Considerations

- Cystic fibrosis causes the mucus normally found in the reproductive systems to be thick resulting in blocked ducts.[93]
- Adhesions or fusion of the labia in children can cause urinary tract infections due to stagnant urine behind the labia.[94]
- Itching and scratching in the perineal area may indicate vulvovaginitis, inflammation of the vulva and vagina, caused by poor hygiene, heat rash, bacterial or yeast infection, or irritation from use of perfumes or chemicals found in some soaps and bubble bath.[94]
- Adolescents with dysmenorrhea or HMB should be encouraged to keep a diary of the timing and description of symptoms, including severity, to discuss with the health care provider. If HMB is severe, iron may be prescribed to prevent/treat anemia. NSAIDS at the first onset of menstrual pain is recommended.[94]
- Ovarian tumors are rare and can be benign (teratoma or epithelial cysts) or malignant (germ cell). A salpingo-oophorectomy is the most common treatment when malignancy is present.[95]

REVIEW EXERCISES

1. A 32-year-old woman has been told that the report of her annual Pap test revealed the presence of mild dysplasia.
   A. *What questions should this woman ask as a means of becoming informed about the significance of these findings?*
   B. *In obtaining additional information about the results of her Pap test, the woman is informed that dysplastic changes are consistent with a CIN 1 classification.*
      1. *Does this mean that the woman has cervical cancer?*
      2. *Cervical cancer is often referred to as a sexually transmitted infection. Explain.*
      3. *What type of follow-up care would be indicated?*
2. A 30-year-old woman consults her gynecologist because of amenorrhea and an inability to become pregnant. Physical examination reveals an obese woman with hirsutism. The physician tells the woman that she might have a condition known as polycystic ovary syndrome and that further laboratory tests are indicated.
   A. *Among the tests ordered were fasting blood glucose, LH, FSH, and dehydroepiandrosterone levels. What information can these tests provide that would help in establishing a diagnosis of polycystic ovary syndrome?*
   B. *What is the probable cause of this woman's amenorrhea, hirsutism, and failure to become pregnant?*
   C. *What type of treatment might be used to help this woman become pregnant?*
3. A 45-year-old woman makes an appointment to see her physician because of a painless lump in her breast that she discovered while doing her routine monthly BSE.

A. What tests should be done to confirm the presence or absence of breast cancer?
B. During the removal of breast cancer, a SLN biopsy is often done to determine whether the cancer has spread to the lymph nodes. Explain how this procedure is done and its value in determining lymph node spread.
C. After surgical removal of breast cancer, an aromatase inhibitor may be used as an adjuvant systemic therapy for women without detectable metastatic disease. The presence or absence of estrogen receptors in the cytoplasm of tumor cells is important in determining the selection of an agent for use in adjuvant therapy. Explain.

References

1. Strayer D., Rubin R. (Eds.), (2015). *Rubin's pathology: Clinicopathologic foundations of medicine* (7th ed.) Philadelphia, PA: Lippincott Williams & Wilkins.
2. Gorrol A. H., Mulley A. G. (2014). *Primary care medicine: Office evaluation and management of the adult patient* (7th ed.) Philadelphia, PA: Lippincott Williams & Wilkins.
3. Krissi H., Shmuely A., Aviram A., et al. (2016). Acute Bartholin's abscess: Microbial spectrum, patient characteristics, clinical manifestation, and surgical outcomes. *European Journal Clinical Microbial Infectious Disease* 35, 443–446.
4. Cash J. C., Glass C. A. (2014). *Family practice guidelines* (3rd ed.) New York, NY: Springer Publishing Company, LLC.
5. Chan M. P., Zimarowski M. J. (2015). *Vulvar dermatoses: A histopathologic review and classification of 183 cases. Journal of Cutaneous Pathology* 42, 510–518.
6. Girardi F., Reich O., Tamussino K. et al. (2015). *Burghardt's colposcopy and cervical pathology: Textbook and atlas* (4th ed.) Stuttgart, New York, Delhi, Rio de Janeiro: Thieme.
7. Lee A., Bradford J., Fischer G. (2015). Long-term management of adult vulvar lichen sclerosus a prospective cohort study of 507 women. *Journal of American Medical Association Dermatology* 151(10), 1061–1067.
8. De Andres J., Sanchis-Lopez N., Marcos Ansensio-Samper J. M., et al. (2016). Vulvodynia—an evidence-based literature review and proposed treatment algorithm. *World Institute of Pain* 16(2), 204-236.
9. International Society for the Study of Vulvovaginal Disorders. (2015). Vulvovaginal disorders. [Online]. Available: https://www.issvd.org/issvd-terminology-classification-of-vulvar-diseases/. Retrieved October 26, 2017
10. Basson R., Driscoll M., Correia S. (2016). When sex is always painful: Provoked vestibulodynia. *British Columbia Medical Journal* 58(2), 77–81.
11. CerVigni M., Natale F. (2014). Gynecological disorders in bladder pain syndrome/interstitial cystitis patients. *International Journal of Urology* 21(suppl 1), 85–88.
12. IsHak W. W. (Ed.), (2017). *The textbook of clinical sexual medicine* (1st ed.). New York, NY: Springer Publishing Company, LLC.
13. National Cancer Institute. (2017). Surveillance, epidemiology, and end results cancer statistics review: Vulva cancer. [Online]. Available: http://seer.cancer.gov/statfacts/html/vulva.html. Retrieved October 27, 2017
14. Reyes M. C., Cooper K. (2014). An update on vulvar intraepithelial neoplasia: terminology and a practical approach to diagnosis. [abstract] *Journal of Clinical Pathology* 67(4), 290–294
15. American College of Obstetrics and Gynecology and American Society for Colposcopy and Cervical Pathology. (2017). Management of vulvar intraepithelial lesions. Committee opinion. [Online]. Available: https://www.acog.org/-/media/Committee-Opinions/Committee-on-Gynecologic-Practice/co675.pdf?dmc=1&ts=20180312T0238240039. Retrieved: March 11, 2018
16. Ramirez P. D., Gershenson D. M., Salvo G. (2018). Vulvar cancer. Merck Manual Professional. [Online]. Available: https://www.merckmanuals.com/professional/gynecology-and-obstetrics/gynecologic-tumors/vulvar-cancer. Retrieved March 4, 2018
17. International Federation of Gynecology and Obstetrics. (2009). Vulvar cancer. [Online]. Available: http://www.ncbi.nlm.nih.gov/pmc/articles/PMC2757555/. Retrieved November 6, 2017
18. Khanna N., Raug L. A., Lachiewicz M. P., et al. (2016). Margins for cervical and vulvar cancer. *Journal of Surgical Oncology* 113, 304–309.
19. Rhoads J., Murphy M. (2014). *Differential diagnosis for the advanced practice nurse*. New York, NY: Springer Publishing Company, LLC.
20. American Cancer Society (2017). What are the key statistics about vaginal cancer? Retrieved from https://www.cancer.org/cancer/vaginal-cancer/about/key-statistics.html
21. Yarbro C. H., Wujcik D., Gobel B. H. (2018). *Cancer nursing: Principles and practice* (8th ed.) Burlington, MA: Jones & Bartlett.
22. Jentschke M., Hoffmeister V., Soergel P., et al. (2016). Clinical presentation, treatment and outcome of vaginal intraepithelial neoplasia. *Archives of Gynecology and Obstetrics* 293, 415–419. doi:10:1007/s0040-015-3835-6.
23. Carcio H. N., Secor M. (2015). *Advanced health assessment of women: Clinical skills and procedures* (3rd ed). New York, NY: Springer Publishing Company, LLC.
24. American Cancer Society. (2018). Cervical cancer [Online]. Available: https://www.cancer.org/content/dam/cancer-org/research/cancer-facts-and-statistics/annual-cancer-facts-and-figures/2018/cancer-facts-and-figures-2018.pdf Retrieved May 5, 2018
25. American Cancer Society (2016). Tests for cervical cancer. [Online]. Available: https://www.cancer.org/cancer/cervical-cancer/detection-diagnosis-staging/how-diagnosed.html. Retrieved October 29, 2017
26. United States Federal Drug Administration. (2017). Cervarix. [Online]. Available: https://www.fda.gov/BiologicsBloodVaccines/Vaccines/ApprovedProducts/ucm186957.htm. Retrieved October 29, 2017
27. Nayar R., Wilbur D. C. (2015). The pap test and Bethesda 2014. *Acta Cytologica* 59, 121–132. doi:10.1159/000381842.
28. Baker E. (2013). HPV and Pap: Shifting roles in cervical cancer screening. [Online]. Medical Laboratory Observer. Available: https://www.mlo-online.com/hpv-and-pap-shifting-roles-in-cervical-screening.php. Retrieved October 29, 2017
29. Medlin E. E., Kushner D.M., Barroilhet L. (2016). Robotic surgery for early stage cervical cancer: evolution and current trends. *Journal of Surgical Oncology* 112, 772–781.
30. Marnitz S., Budach V., Weiber F, et al. (2012). Rectum separation in patients with cervical cancer for treatment planning in primary chemoradiation. *Radiation Oncology* 7, 109.
31. Ahn S. H., Monsanto S. P., Miller C. et al. (2015). Pathophysiology and Immune dysfunction in endometriosis. *Biomed Research International* 2015, 795976. doi:10.1155/2015/795976.
32. Morotti M., Vincent K, Brawn J. et al. (2014). Peripheral changes in endometriosis-associated pain. *Human Reproduction Update* 20(5), 717–736.
33. American Society for Reproductive Medicine. (2012). *Endometriosis a guide for patients [pamphlet]*. Birmingham, AL: American Society for Reproductive Medicine under the direction of the Patient Education Committee and the Publications Committee.
34. Sinervo K. R. (2015). The case for surgery for endometriosis. *Contemporary OB/GYN* 60(10), 51–54.
35. Mishra V. V., Gaddagi R. A., Aggarwal R., et al. (2015). Prevalence; characteristics and management of endometriosis amongst infertile women: a one year retrospective study. *Journal of Clinical and Diagnostic Research* 9(6), 1-3.

36. Fraser I. (2016). Current trends in the medical management of endometriosis "available therapies in perspective". *Indian Obstetrics and Gynaecology* 6(1), 8-17.
37. American Cancer Society. (2017). Endometrial cancer. [Online]. Available: https://www.cancer.org/cancer/endometrial-cancer/about/key-statistics.html. Retrieved October 29, 2017
38. American Cancer Society. (2017). What are key statistics about uterine sarcoma? [Online]. Available: https://www.cancer.org/cancer/uterine-sarcoma/about/key-statistics.html. Retrieved October 31, 2017
39. Folkins A. K., Longmore T. A. (2013). Hereditary gynaecological malignancies: advances in screening and treatment. *Histopathology* 62(2), 2-30.
40. American Cancer Society. (2017). What is endometrial cancer. [Online]. Available: https://www.cancer.org/cancer/endometrial-cancer/about/what-is-endometrial-cancer.html. Retrieved October 29, 2017
41. Tang Y., Chen C., Duan H., et al. (2015). Low vascularity predicts favourable outcomes in leiomyoma patients treated with uterine artery embolization. *European Radiology* 26, 3571–3579.
42. Centers for Disease Control and Prevention. (2015). STI pelvic inflammatory disease. [Online]. Available: https://www.cdc.gov/std/tg2015/pid.htm. Retrieved November 1, 2017
43. Gradison M. (2012). Pelvic inflammatory disease. *American Family Physician*. 85(8), 791–796.
44. Taran F. A., Kagan K. O., Hubner M., et al. (2015). The diagnosis and treatment of ectopic pregnancy. *Deutsches Aerzteblatt International* 112, 693–704.
45. Epee-Bekima M., Overton C. (2013). Diagnosis and treatment of ectopic pregnancy. *The Practitioner* 257(1759), 15–17.
46. American Society of Clinical Oncology (2017). Ovarian, fallopian tube, and peritoneal cancer: statistics. Available: https://www.cancer.net/cancer-types/ovarian-fallopian-tube-and-peritoneal-cancer/statistics. Retrieved April 17, 2018
47. Fauser B. C., Tarlatzis B.C., Rebar, R.W., et al. (2012). Consensus on women's health aspects of polycystic ovary syndrome (PCOS): the Amsterdam ESHRE/ASRM-sponsored 3rd PCOS consensus workshop group. *Fertility and Sterility* 97(1), 28.e25–36.e25. doi:http://dx.doi.org/10.1016/j.fertnstert.2011.09.024
48. Franks S., Berga S. L. (2012). Does PCOS have developmental origins? *Fertility and Sterility* 97(1), 1–6.
49. Tsai Y., Wang T., Wei H., et al. (2013). Dietary intake, glucose metabolism and sex hormones in women with polycystic ovary syndrome (PCOS) compared with women with non-PCOS-related infertility. *British Journal of Nutrition* 109(12), 2190–2198.
50. Dumitrescu R., Mehedintu C., Briceag I., et al. (2015). The polycystic ovary syndrome: an update on metabolic and hormonal mechanisms. *Journal of Medicine and Life* 8(2), 142–145.
51. Legro R. S., Arsianian S. A., Ehrmann D. A., et al. (2013). Diagnosis and treatment of polycystic ovary syndrome: an endocrine society clinical practice guideline. *Journal of Clinical Endocrinology & Metabolism* 98(12), 4565–4592.
52. American Cancer Society. (2017). Ovarian cancer. [Online]. Available: https://www.cancer.org/cancer/ovarian-cancer/about/key-statistics.html. Retrieved October 31, 2017
53. American Cancer Society. (2016). *Can ovarian cancer be found early? [Online].* Available: https://www.cancer.org/cancer/ovarian-cancer/detection-diagnosis-staging/detection.html. Retrieved October 31, 2017
54. Wentzensen N., Poole E. M., Trabert B., et al. (2016). Ovarian cancer risk factors by histologic subtype: an analysis from the ovarian cancer cohort consortium. *Journal of Clinical Oncology* 34(24), 2888–2897.
55. American Cancer Society (2018). *What are the risk factors for ovarian cancer?* Available: https://www.cancer.org/cancer/ovarian-cancer/causes-risks-prevention/risk-factors.html. Retrieved April 17, 2018
56. King G. G. T., Leighton J. C. (2015). CA 125. Medscape Drugs and Diseases/Laboratory Medicine. Available: https://emedicine.medscape.com/article/2087557-overview#a2. Retrieved March 5, 2018
57. Hacker N. F., Gambone J. C., Moore C. J. (2016). *Hacker and Moore's essentials of obstetrics and gynecology* (6th ed.) Philadelphia, PA: Elsevier.
58. McNeely S. G. (2017). Cystoceles, urethroceles, enteroceles, and rectoceles. Merck Manual Professional version. [Online]. Available: https://www.merckmanuals.com/professional/gynecology-and-obstetrice/pelvic-relaxation-syndromes/cystoceles-urethroceles-enteroceles-and-rectoceles. Retrieved March 5, 2018
59. McNeely S. G. (2018). Uterine and vaginal prolapse. Merck manual professional version. [Online]. Available: https://www.merckmanuals.com/professional/gynecology-and-obstetrics/pelvic-relaxation-syndromes/uterine-and-vaginal-prolapse#v1064484. Retrieved March 17, 2018
60. Kow N., Goldman H. B., Ridgeway B. (2013). Management options for women with uterine prolapse interested in uterine preservation. *Current Urology Reports* 14, 395–402.
61. U.S. National Library of Medicine (2017). Premenstrual syndrome: overview. PubMed Health. [Online]. Available: https://www.ncbi.nlm.nih.gov/pubmedhealth/PMH0072449/. Retrieved March 4, 2018
62. Callahan T. (2018). *Blueprints obstetrics gynecology* (7th ed.) Philadelphia, PA: Wolters Kluwer.
63. Fothergill D. (2012). Causes of primary and secondary amenorrhea. *Practice Nursing* 23(9), 465–469.
64. American Congress of Obstetrics and Gynecology (2015). Dysmenorrhea, painful periods. [Online]. Available: https://www.acog.org/Patients/FAQs/Dysmenorrhea-Painful-Periods#are. Retrieved November 1, 2017
65. Hawkins J. W., Roberto-Nichols D. M., Stanley-Haney J. L. (2016). *Guidelines for nurse practitioners in gynecological settings* (11th ed). New York, NY: Springer Publishing Company, LLC.
66. Hantsoo, L. & Epperson, C.N. (2015). Premenstrual dysphoric disorder: epidemiology and treatment. *Current Psychiatry*; 17:87. doi 10.1007/s11920-015-0628-3.
67. Patient education: Premenstrual syndrome (PMS) and premenstrual dysphoric disorder (PMDD) (beyond the basics). [Online]. Available: https://www.uptodate.com/contents/premenstrual-syndrome-pms-and-premenstrual-dysphoric-disorder-pmdd-beyond-the-basics
68. American College of Obstetrics and Gynecology (2015). Frequently asked questions gynecological problems premenstrual syndrome. [Online]. Available: https://www.acog.org/Patients/FAQs/Premenstrual-Syndrome-PMS. Retrieved: March 11, 2018
69. Benjamin I. J., Griggs R. C., Wing E. J., et al. (2016). *Andreoli and Carpenter's Cecil essentials of medicine* (9th ed.) Philadelphia, PA: Saunders.
70. Cullinane M., Amor L. H., Donath S. M., et al. (2015). Determinants of mastitis in women in the CASTLE study: a cohort study. *BMC Family Practice* 16, 181. doi:10.1186/s12875-015-0396-5.
71. Yi W., Xu F., Zou Q., et al. (2013). Completely removing solitary intraductal papillomas using the mammotome system guided by ultrasonography is feasible and safe. *World Journal of Surgery* 37, 2613–2617.
72. American Cancer Society (2017). *Non-cancerous breast conditions mastitis*. Available: https://www.cancer.org/cancer/breast-cancer/non-cancerous-breast-conditions/mastitis.html. Retrieved April 18, 2018
73. American Cancer Society (2018). *Non-cancerous breast conditions duct ectasia*. Available: https://www.cancer.org/cancer/breast-cancer/non-cancerous-breast-conditions/duct-ectasia.html. Retrieved April 17, 2018
74. Manganaro L., D'Ambrosio I., Gigli, S., et al. (2015). Breast MRI in patients with unilateral bloody and serous-bloody nipple discharge: A comparison with galactography. *BioMed Research International*. [Online]. Available: http://dx.doi.org/10.1155/2015/806368. Retrieved November 2, 2017
75. American Cancer Society (2018). *Non-cancerous breast conditions*. Available: https://www.cancer.org/cancer/breast-cancer/non-cancerous-breast-conditions.html. Retrieved April 17, 2018
76. American Cancer Society (2017). Fibrosis and simple cysts in the breast. [Online]. Available: https://www.cancer.org/cancer/breast-cancer/non-cancerous-breast-conditions/fibrosis-and-simple-cysts-in-the-breast.html. Retrieved: March 17, 2018
77. American Cancer Society (2017). Breast cancer. [Online]. Available: https://www.cancer.org/cancer/breast-cancer/about/how-common-is-breast-cancer.html. Retrieved October 31, 2017

78. NIH National Cancer Institute. (2012). Breast cancer risk in American women. Online]. Available: https://www.cancer.gov/types/breast/risk-fact-sheet. Retrieved March 18, 2018
79. Breastcancer.org (2018). U.S. breast cancer statistics. [Online]. Available: http://www.breastcancer.org/symptoms/understand_bc/statistics. Retrieved: March 18, 2018
80. NIH National Cancer Institute (2018). BRCA mutations: cancer risk and genetic counseling.[Online]. Available: https://www.cancer.gov/about-cancer/causes-prevention/genetics/brca-fact-sheet. Retrieved March 9, 2018
81. Oeffinger K. C., Fontham, E.T., Etzioni, R., et al. (2015). Breast cancer screening for women at average risk 2015 guideline update from the American cancer society. *Journal of the American Medical Academy* 314(15):1599–1614. doi:10.1001/jama.2015.12783.
82. Breastcancer.org (2014). What can you tell me about sentinel node biopsy? [Online]. Available: http://www.breastcancer.org/questions/sentinel_node. Retrieved March 11, 2018
83. Odle T. G. (2017). Precision medicine in breast cancer. *Radiologic Technology* 88(40), 401–424.
84. Breastcancer.org (2016). Aromatase inhibitors. [Online]. Available: http://www.breastcancer.org/treatment/hormonal/aromatase_inhibitors. Retrieved November 1, 2017
85. American Cancer Society (2018). Types of breast cancer. Available: https://www.cancer.org/cancer/breast-cancer/understanding-a-breast-cancer-diagnosis/types-of-breast-cancer.html. Retrieved April 17, 2018
86. Center for Disease Control (2017). 2015 Assisted reproductive technology national summary report. [Online]. Available: https://www.cdc.gov/art/pdf/2015-report/ART-2015-National-Summary-Report.pdf. Retrieved March 8, 2018
87. American Society for Reproductive Medicine (2017). Quick facts about infertility. ReproductiveFacts.Org. [Online]. Retrieved March 5, 2018 from: http://www.reproductivefacts.org/faqs/quick-facts-about-infertility/
88. Cooper T. G., Noonan E., Eckardstein S., et al. (2010). World Health Organization reference values for human semen characteristics. *Human Reproduction Update* 16(3), 231–245. Available: http://www.who.int/reproductivehealth/topics/infertility/cooper_et_al_hru.pdf. Retrieved April 17, 2018. [landmark study that has not changed]
89. Ochando I. (2014). Semen quality parameters according to the World Health Organisation (WHO). Available: https://www.institutobernabeu.com/foro/en/2014/02/17/semen-quality-parameters-according-to-the-world-health-organisation-who/. Retrieved April 17, 2018
90. Gordon, J.D., Rydfors, J.T. (2017). *Obstetrics, gynecology and infertility (pocket size) handbook for clinicians*. Philadelphia, PA: Scrub Hill Press.
91. Sunderam S, Kissin D. M., Crawford S. B., et al. (2015). Assisted reproductive technology surveillance—United States, 2013. [Online]. Available: https://www.cdc.gov/mmwr/preview/mmwrhtml/ss6411a1.htm?s_cid=ss6411a1_w Retrieved November 1, 2017
92. Epiopoulos C. (2018). *Gerontological nursing* (9th ed.). Philadelphia: Wolters Kluwer
93. Bowden V. R., Greenberg C. S. (Eds.) (2014). *Children and their families the continuum of nursing care*. (3rd ed.). Philadelphia, PA: Wolters Kluwer
94. Kyle T., Carman S. (Eds.) (2017). *Essentials of pediatric nursing* (3rd ed.). Philadelphia, PA: Wolters Kluwer.
95. Al-Salem A. (2014). Ovarian cysts and tumors. In: *An illustrated guide to pediatric surgery*. Cham: Springer International Publishing. doi:https://doi.org/10.1007/978-3-319-06665 3_60)

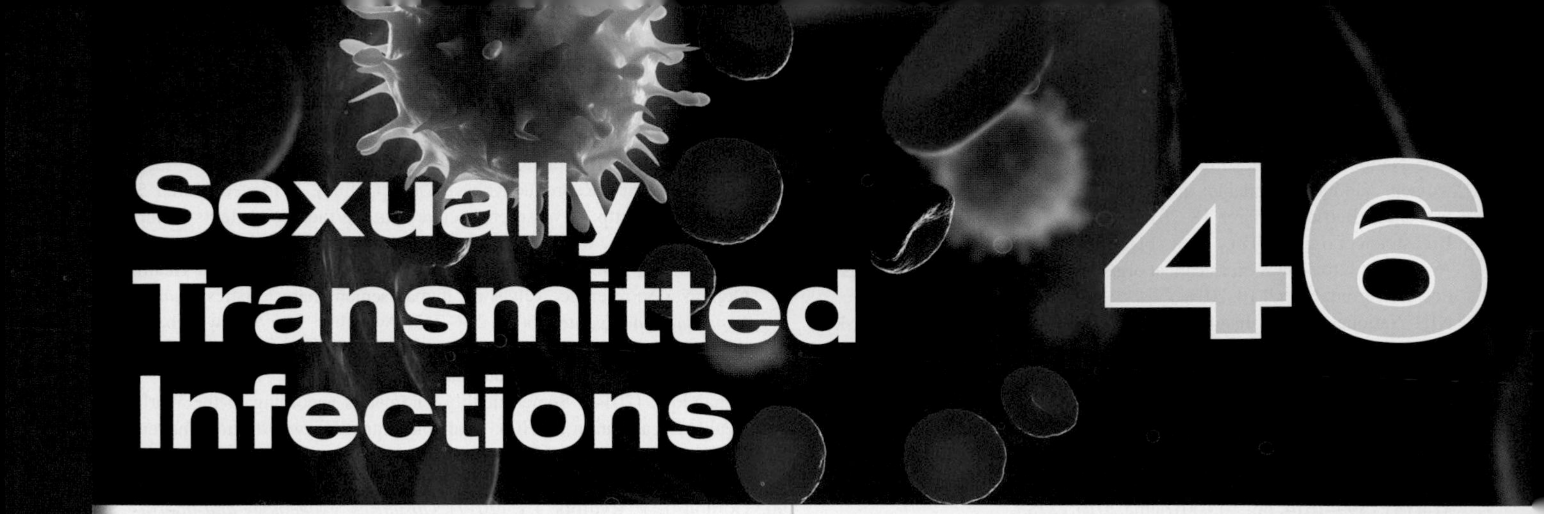

Sexually Transmitted Infections

46

Deborah L. Hopla

Sexually transmitted infections (STIs) encompass a broad range of infectious diseases that are spread by sexual contact. The incidence of STIs is increasing as is the technology's ability to screen STIs.[1] The Centers for Disease Control and Prevention (CDC) (2014) requires reporting of chlamydia, syphilis, and gonorrhea and, therefore, tracks these three STIs most specifically.[1] However, the actual figures of total STIs are probably much higher because many STIs are not reportable or not reported.

There are many factors that contribute to the increased prevalence and the continued spread of STIs. One key factor is that STIs are frequently asymptomatic, which promotes the spread of infection by people who are unaware they are carrying the infection.[2] Furthermore, partners of infected people are often difficult to notify and treat. In addition, there currently are no cures for viral STIs (*e.g.*, human immunodeficiency virus [HIV], herpes simplex virus [HSV]). Although there are drugs available that may help to manage the infections, they do not entirely control the spread.[3] Also, drug-resistant microorganisms are rapidly emerging, making treatment of many STIs more difficult.

Sexual contact transmission has been identified in over 30 bacteria.[2] There are currently four curable infections: trichomoniasis, syphilis, gonorrhea, and chlamydia. Four of the infections are viral and considered incurable: hepatitis B, HSV, HIV, and human papillomavirus (HPV).[2] Portals of entry include the mouth, genitalia, urinary meatus, rectum, and skin. The rates of many STIs are highest among adolescents. All STIs are more common in people who have more than one sexual partner. Furthermore, it is not uncommon for a person to be concurrently infected with more than one type of STI.[2] STIs can result in stillbirth, death of the neonate, prematurity and low-birth weight, sepsis, pneumonia, and congenital deformities.[2]

This chapter discusses the manifestations of STIs in men and women in terms of infections of the external genitalia, vaginal infections, and infections that have genitourinary as well as systemic manifestations.

INFECTIONS OF THE EXTERNAL GENITALIA

After completing this section of the chapter, the learner will be able to meet the following objectives:

- Name the organisms responsible for condylomata acuminata, genital herpes, molluscum contagiosum, chancroid, granuloma inguinale, and lymphogranuloma venereum.
- State the significance of being infected with high-risk strains of the human papillomavirus.
- Explain the pathogenesis of recurrent genital herpes infections.

STIs can selectively infect the mucocutaneous tissues of the external genitalia, cause vaginitis in women, or produce both genitourinary and systemic effects. Some STIs may be transmitted by an infected mother to a fetus or newborn, causing congenital defects or death of the child.[2] The discussion in this section of the chapter focuses on STIs that affect the mucocutaneous tissues of the oropharynx and external genitalia and anorectal tissues. These infections include condylomata acuminata, genital herpes, molluscum contagiosum, chancroid, granuloma inguinale, and lymphogranuloma venereum.

Condylomata Acuminata (Genital Warts)

Condylomata acuminata, or genital warts, are caused by the HPV (Fig. 46.1). Although recognized for centuries, HPV-induced genital warts have become the most common STI, and there are over 40 different types of the HPV virus. The CDC estimates that 20 million Americans carry the virus and up to 6 million new cases are diagnosed each year.[4] Risk factors for acquiring HPV include young age (<25 years), early age of first intercourse (<16 years), increased numbers of sex partners, and having a male partner with multiple sex partners. HPV infection can occur with any type of vaginal or anal penetration and is common in men having sex with men and women having sex with women.

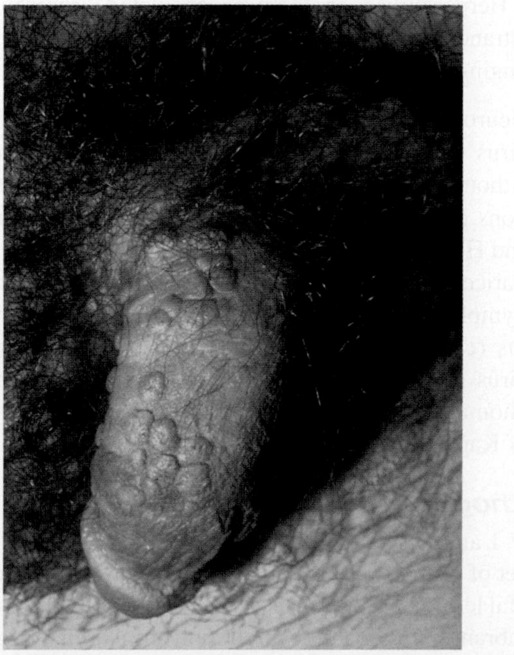

Figure 46.1 • Condylomata of the penis. Raised circumscribed lesions are seen on the shaft of the penis. (From Rubin R., Strayer D. (Eds.) (2015). *Rubin's pathology: Clinicopathologic foundations of medicine* (7th ed., p. 975). Philadelphia, PA: Lippincott Williams & Wilkins.)

Most HPV infections are asymptomatic and transient and resolve spontaneously within 2 years without treatment if the person has an intact immunologic system.[4] However, infection with some HPV types results in genital warts, cervical dysplasia, and cervical cancer.[4]

Types of Human Papillomavirus

HPVs are **nonenveloped**, double-stranded deoxyribonucleic acid (DNA) viruses that cause proliferative lesions of the squamous epithelium.[5] More than 100 distinct HPV subtypes have been identified with some affecting the mouth and throat.[5] These subtypes have been divided into three categories based on their likelihood of inducing dysplasia and carcinoma. For example, HPV types 16 and 18 are strongly associated with cervical dysplasia and anogenital cancers and are considered high risk.[5] However, only a small percentage of women infected with HPV go on to develop cervical cancer. Over 90% of infections clear within 2 years.[5] This suggests that even the most virulent HPV strains may vary in terms of their oncogenic potential. Cofactors that may increase the risk for cervical cancer include smoking, immunosuppression, and exposure to hormonal alteration (*e.g.*, pregnancy, oral contraceptives).[5]

Pathogenesis and Clinical Manifestations

HPV infection begins with viral inoculation into a stratified squamous epithelium, where infection stimulates replication of the squamous epithelium, producing the various HPV-proliferative lesions.[5] The incubation period for HPV-induced genital warts ranges from 3 weeks to several months; for cervical abnormalities, the incubation period is several months, and for cervical cancer, the incubation period is decades.[5] Genital warts typically present as soft, raised, fleshy lesions on the external genitalia, including the penis (Fig. 46.2), vulva, scrotum, perineum, and perianal skin. External warts may appear as small bumps, or they may be flat, rough surfaced, or pedunculated. Less commonly, they can appear as smooth reddish or brown raised papules or as dome-shaped lesions on keratinized skin. Internal warts are cauliflower-shaped lesions that affect the mucous membranes of the vagina, urethra, anus, or mouth.

Subclinical infection occurs more frequently than visible genital warts. Both spontaneous resolution and infection with new HPV types are common. Approximately, 70% of women with HPV become HPV DNA negative within 1 year, and as much as 90% become negative within 2 years.[5] Many women with transient HPV infections develop atypical squamous cells of undetermined significance (ASC-US) or low-grade squamous intraepithelial lesions (LSILs) of the cervix as detected on a Pap test, colposcopy, or biopsy. In men, transient HPV infection may be associated with intraepithelial neoplasia of the penis and anus. Development of an effective immune response helps clear the infection, but the virus can remain dormant for years and reactivate at a later time.

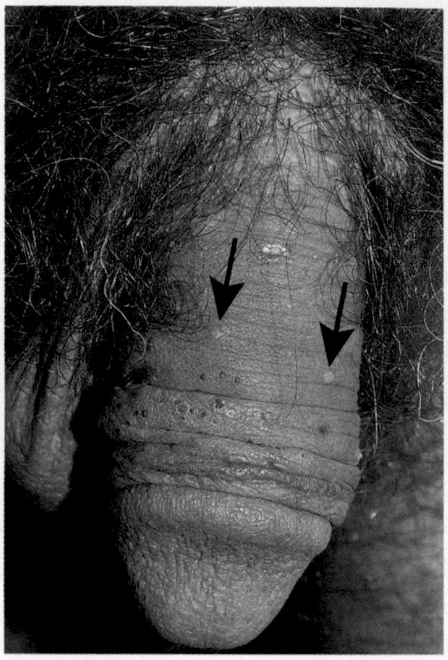

Figure 46.2 • Herpes simplex virus type 1 and 2—HSV 1 (infection of lips, face, buccal mucosa, and throat) and HSV 2 (genitalia) are epidermotropic viruses. Transmission is only by direct contact with active lesions or virus-containing fluid such as saliva. (From Jensen S. (2015). *Nursing health assessment: A best practice approach* (2nd ed., p. 730). Philadelphia, PA: Lippincott Williams & Wilkins.

Diagnosis

The association with premalignant and malignant changes has increased the concern regarding the diagnosis and treatment of this viral infection. Lack of regular cervical cancer screening (Pap test) is the primary risk factor for development of invasive cervical cancer.[5] There are no approved serologic tests for HPV or routine methods for culturing the virus. The only test that is currently approved by the US Food and Drug Administration (FDA) is a solution hybridization method to test for high-risk HPV DNA.[5] The HPV DNA test detects whether one or more of the high-risk types of HPV are present. It does not identify the individual HPV type. HPV DNA testing is warranted with equivocal (ASC-US) Pap test results and is now recommended to determine which women older than 30 years of age need annual Pap smear screening.

Genital condylomata should be considered in any woman who presents with the primary complaint of vulvar pruritus or who has had an abnormal Pap smear result. Microscopic examination of a wet-mount slide preparation and cultures are used to exclude associated vaginitis. Careful inspection of the vulva, with magnification as needed, generally reveals the characteristic lesions, and specimens for biopsy can be taken from questionable areas. Colposcopic examination of the cervix and vagina may be advised as a follow-up measure when there is an abnormal Pap smear result or when HPV lesions are identified on the vulva.

Prevention and Treatment

There are three vaccines currently available to protect against specific HPV strains: Gardasil, Gardasil 9, and Cervarix.[6] In 2016, the CDC changed the vaccine recommendation to two doses if given before the adolescent's 15 birthday and spaced out by 6 to 12 months.[6] The recommendation at age 15 to 26 is still three doses. Both protect against types 16 and 18, which cause 70% of cervical cancers[6] and Gardasil also protects against types 6 and 11, which are known to lead to genital warts. Currently, however, there is no treatment to eradicate the virus once a person has become infected. Prevention of HPV transmission through condom use has not been adequately demonstrated, but circumcision has been shown to decrease acquisition of some STIs, including HPV.[7] Treatment goals are aimed at elimination of symptomatic warts, surveillance for malignancy and premalignant changes, and education and counseling to decrease psychosocial distress.

The choice of treatment is based on the number, size, site, and morphology of the lesions, as well as the person's preference. Genital warts can resolve spontaneously, so expectant management is acceptable if the person is comfortable with this approach. Evaluation and treatment of sexual partners may be suggested, although this may be difficult considering that warts often do not become clinically apparent for several years after exposure.

Genital Herpes

Genital herpes is one of the most common causes of genital ulcers in the United States. Because herpesvirus infection is not reportable in all states, reliable data on its true incidence (estimated number of new cases every year) and prevalence (estimated number of people currently infected) are lacking. Recent estimates in the United States indicate a 16.2% prevalence of genital Herpes.[8] Women have a greater mucosal surface area exposed in the genital area and therefore are at greater risk of acquiring the infection.[8]

Herpes viruses are large, encapsulated viruses with a double-stranded genome.[8] There are nine types of herpesviruses, belonging to three groups, which cause infections in humans:

1. Neurotropic α-group viruses, including herpes simplex virus type 1 (HSV-1; usually associated with cold sores although an increasing number of anogenital herpetic infections caused by HSV 1 are now becoming documented[3]) and HSV-2 (usually associated with genital herpes)
2. Varicella-zoster virus (causes chickenpox and shingles)
3. Lymphotropic β-group viruses, including cytomegalovirus (causes cytomegalic inclusion disease), Epstein-Barr virus (causes infectious mononucleosis and Burkitt lymphoma), and human herpesvirus type 8 (the apparent cause of Kaposi sarcoma)[8]

Pathogenesis

HSV-1 and HSV-2 are genetically similar. Both cause a similar set of primary and recurrent infections, and both can cause genital lesions.[3] These viruses replicate in the skin and mucous membranes at the site of infection (oropharynx or genitalia), where they cause vesicular lesions of the epidermis and infect the neurons that innervate the area.[2] HSV-1 and HSV-2 are *neurotropic* viruses, meaning that they grow in neurons and share the biologic property of latency. Latency refers to the ability to maintain disease potential in the absence of clinical signs and symptoms. In genital herpes, the virus ascends through the peripheral nerves to the sacral dorsal root ganglia (Fig. 46.3). The virus can remain dormant in the dorsal root ganglia, or it can reactivate, in which case the viral particles are transported back down the nerve root to the skin, where they multiply and cause a lesion to develop. During the dormant or latent period, the virus replicates in a different manner so that the immune system or available treatments have no effect on it. It is not known what reactivates the virus. It may be that the body's defense mechanisms are altered. Numerous studies have shown that host responses to infection influence initial development of the disease, severity of infection, development and maintenance of latency, and frequency of HSV recurrences.

HSV is transmitted by contact with infectious lesions or secretions. HSV-1 is transmitted by oral secretions, and infections frequently occur in childhood. HSV-1 may be spread to the genital area by autoinoculation after poor handwashing or through oral–genital contact. It has been estimated that among sexually active adults, new genital HSV-1 infections are almost as common as new HSV-2 infections.[3] HSV-2 usually is transmitted by sexual contact but can be passed to an infant during childbirth if the virus is actively being shed from the genital tract. Most cases of HSV-2 infection are subclinical, manifesting as truly asymptomatic or symptomatic but unrecognized infections. These subclinical infections can occur in people who have never had a symptomatic outbreak or they can occur between recognized clinical recurrences. Genital herpes is spread through asymptomatic shedding by people who do not realize they have the infection. This "unknown" transmission of the virus to sex partners explains why this infection has reached epidemic proportions throughout the world. The incubation period for HSV is 2 to 10 days.

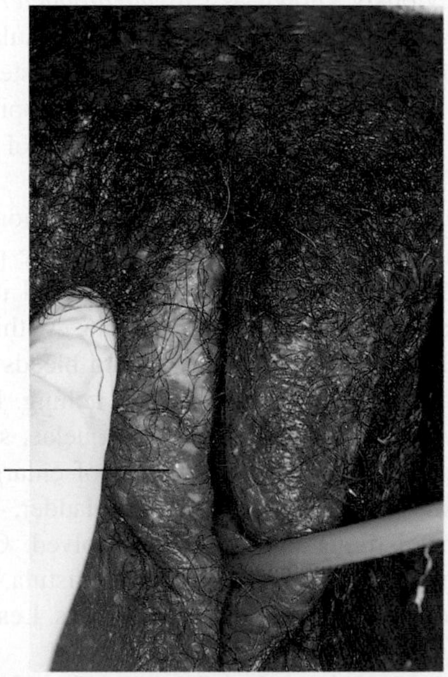

Figure 46.3 • Herpes simplex type 2—There are vesicles on the vulva. (From Jensen S. (2015). *Nursing health assessment: A best practice approach* (2nd ed., p. 772). Philadelphia, PA: Lippincott Williams & Wilkins.)

Clinical Manifestations

Genital HSV infection may manifest as a first episode or recurrent infection.[8] Usually one's first episode is the most painful with an obvious lesion. However, some people may test positive for HSV and not have had any symptoms. Recurrent infections refer to the second or subsequent outbreak because of the same virus type. First-episode infections have more numerous and scattered vesicles and more systemic manifestations. Viral shedding lasts longer with first-episode infections (10 to 15 days) and new lesions continue to form for about 10 days after the initial infection. Many "severe" presumed primary cases are actually first-recognized recurrences in people with long-standing infection.

The initial symptoms of primary genital herpes infections include tingling, itching, and pain in the genital area, followed by eruption of small pustules and vesicles. These lesions rupture on approximately the 5th day to form wet ulcers that are excruciatingly painful to touch and can be associated with dysuria, dyspareunia, and urine retention. This period is followed by a 10- to 12-day interval during which the lesions crust over and gradually heal.[8] Involvement of the cervix, vagina, urethra, and inguinal lymph nodes is common in women with primary infections. In men, the infection can cause urethritis and lesions of the penis and scrotum. Rectal and perianal infections are possible with anal contact. Systemic symptoms associated with primary infections include fever, headache, malaise, muscle ache, and lymphadenopathy.

Recurrent HSV episodes are usually milder than the initial episode. There typically are fewer lesions, and viral shedding occurs at a lower concentration and for a shorter duration (about 3 days).[8] However, the prodromal symptoms of itching, burning, and tingling at the lesion site are similar. Except for the greater tendency of HSV-2 to recur, the clinical manifestations of HSV-2 and genital HSV-1 infection are similar. The frequency and severity of recurrence vary from person to person. Numerous factors, including emotional stress, lack of sleep, overexertion, other infections, vigorous or prolonged coitus, and premenstrual or menstrual distress, have been identified as triggering mechanisms.

Diagnosis

Diagnosis of genital herpes is based on the symptoms, appearance of the lesions, and identification of the virus from swab tests taken from the lesions for cell culture. The likelihood of obtaining a positive culture decreases with each day that has elapsed after a lesion develops. The chance of obtaining a positive culture from a crusted lesion is slight, and people suspected of having genital herpes should be instructed to have a culture as soon as possible after development of new lesions. Polymerase chain reaction (PCR) testing for HSV DNA is more sensitive than culture. Although PCR is more expensive than culture, even small amounts of the virus will result in a positive test, the results can be obtained more quickly, and the method can distinguish between HSV-1 and HSV-2. In many clinics, PCR testing has become the preferred method of testing when active lesions are present.

Type-specific (HSV-1 and HSV-2) serologic tests are available for determining past infection. Because almost all HSV-2 infections are sexually acquired, the presence of type-specific HSV-2 antibodies usually indicates anogenital infection, whereas the presence of HSV-1 antibodies does not distinguish between anogenital and orolabial infections. HSV-1 is generally an oral infection and HSV-2 tends to be an anal–genital infection; however, one can have HSV-1 in the anal–genital region and HSV-2 in the oral area.

Treatment

There is no known cure for genital herpes, and the methods of treatment are largely symptomatic. The antiviral drug valacyclovir has become the cornerstone for management of genital herpes. By interfering with viral DNA replication, this antiviral drug decreases the frequency of recurrences, shortens the duration of active lesions, reduces the number of new lesions formed, and decreases viral shedding with primary infections. Continuous antiviral suppressive therapy may be advised when more than six outbreaks occur within 1 year.[3]

Good hygiene is essential during HSV outbreaks to prevent secondary infections. Sometimes, symptomatic relief can be obtained with cool compresses, sitz baths, topical anesthetic agents, and oral analgesic drugs. Loose-fitting clothing and cotton undergarments are helpful. To prevent spread of the infection, intimate contact should be avoided until lesions are completely healed.

Pregnant women with a history of genital herpes are started on valacyclovir suppression at 36 weeks' gestation. If a woman has an outbreak of herpes when she presents in labor, a cesarean section is recommended. Disseminated neonatal infection carries high mortality and morbidity rates.

Molluscum Contagiosum

Molluscum contagiosum is a common poxvirus that gives rise to multiple umbilicated papules. The infection is mildly contagious. It is transmitted by skin-to-skin contact, fomites, and autoinoculation. Lesions are domelike and have a dimpled appearance. A curdlike material can be expressed from the center of the lesion. Necrosis and secondary infection are possible. Diagnosis is based on the appearance of the lesion and microscopic identification of intracytoplasmic molluscum bodies. Molluscum is a benign and self-limited disease.

Spontaneous regression of mature lesions followed by continued emergence of new lesions is common with molluscum. In the absence of therapy, this cycle may persist for 6 months to a few years.[9] When indicated, treatment consists of removing the top of the papule with a sterile needle or scalpel, expressing the contents of each lesion, and applying alcohol or silver nitrate to the base. Electrodesiccation, cryosurgery, laser ablation, and surgical biopsy are alternative treatments, but seldom are needed unless lesions are large or extend over a wide area. Another approach to therapy is the application of imiquimod 1% cream to lesions.[9] This self-applied therapy is the first to show efficacy in people with immunosuppressive diseases, such as acquired immunodeficiency syndrome (AIDS).

Chancroid

Chancroid (*i.e.*, soft chancre) is a disease of the external genitalia and lymph nodes. The causative organism is the gram-negative bacterium *Haemophilus ducreyi*, which causes acute ulcerative lesions with profuse discharge.[10] This disease has become uncommon in the United States, with most outbreaks occurring in Africa and the Caribbean.[10] It typically occurs in discrete outbreaks rather than as an endemic disease in this country. As a highly infectious disease, chancroid usually is transmitted by sexual intercourse or through skin and mucous membrane abrasions. Autoinoculation may lead to multiple chancres.

Lesions begin as macules, progress to pustules, and then rupture. This painful ulcer has a necrotic base and jagged edges. In contrast, the syphilitic chancre is nontender and indurated. Subsequent discharge can lead to further infection of self or others. On physical examination, lesions and regional lymphadenopathy may be found. Secondary infection may cause significant tissue destruction. Diagnosis usually is made clinically, but may be confirmed through culture. Gram stain rarely is used today because it is insensitive and nonspecific.

Granuloma Inguinale

Granuloma inguinale (*i.e.*, donovanosis, granuloma venereum) is caused by a gram-negative bacillus, *Klebsiella granulomatis* (previously known as *Calymmatobacterium* [*Donovania*] *granulomatis*), which is a tiny, encapsulated intracellular parasite. This disease is almost nonexistent in the United States. It is found most frequently in tropical areas such as India, Brazil, the West Indies, and parts of China, Australia, and Africa.[10]

Granuloma inguinale causes ulceration of the genitalia, beginning with an innocuous papule. The papule progresses through nodular or vesicular stages until it begins to break down as pink, granulomatous tissue. At this final stage, the tissue becomes thin and friable and bleeds easily. There are complaints of swelling, pain, and itching. Extensive inflammatory scarring may cause late sequelae, such as lymphatic obstruction with the development of enlarged and elephantoid external genitalia. The liver, bladder, bone, joint, lung, and bowel tissue may become involved. Genital complications include tubo-ovarian abscess, fistula, vaginal stenosis, and occlusion of vaginal or anal orifices. Lesions may become neoplastic.

Diagnosis is made through the identification of Donovan bodies (*i.e.*, large mononuclear cells filled with intracytoplasmic gram-negative rods) in tissue smears, biopsy samples, or culture.[10] A minimum 3-week period of treatment with doxycycline, azithromycin, ciprofloxacin, or erythromycin is used in treating the disorder.[10]

Lymphogranuloma Venereum

Lymphogranuloma venereum (LGV) is an acute and chronic venereal disease caused by *Chlamydia trachomatis* types L1, L2, and L3.[10,11] The disease, although found worldwide, has a low incidence outside the tropics. Most cases reported in the United States are in men.

The lesions of LGV can incubate for a few days to several weeks and thereafter cause small, painless papules or vesicles that may go undetected. An important characteristic of the infection is the early (1 to 4 weeks later) development of large, tender, and sometimes fluctuant inguinal lymph nodes called *buboes*.[10,11] There may be flulike symptoms with joint pain, rash, weight loss, pneumonitis, tachycardia, splenomegaly, and proctitis.[10,11] In later stages of the disease, a small percentage of affected people develop elephantiasis of the external genitalia, caused by lymphatic obstruction or fibrous strictures of the rectum or urethra from inflammation and scarring. Urethral involvement may cause pyuria and dysuria. Cervicitis is a common manifestation of primary LGV and could extend to perimetritis or salpingitis, which are known to occur in other chlamydial infections.[12] Anorectal structures may be compromised to the point of incontinence. Complications of LGV may be minor or extensive, involving compromise of whole systems or progression to a cancerous state.

Diagnosis usually is accomplished by a complement fixation test for LGV-specific *Chlamydia* antibodies. High titers for this antibody differentiate this group from other chlamydial subgroups.[10,11] Treatment involves 3 weeks of doxycycline or erythromycin.[10,11] Surgery may be required to correct sequelae such as strictures or fistulas or to drain fluctuant lymph nodes.

IN SUMMARY

STIs that primarily affect the external genitalia include HPV-induced genital warts, genital herpes, molluscum contagiosum, chancroid, granuloma inguinale, and LGV. The lesions of these infections occur on the external genitalia of male and female sexual partners. Of concern is the relation between HPV and genital neoplasms. Genital herpes is caused by a neurotropic HSV (HSV-2 and, sometimes, HSV-1) that ascends through the peripheral nerves to reside in the sacral dorsal root ganglia. The herpesvirus can be reactivated, producing recurrent lesions in genital structures that are supplied by the peripheral nerves of the affected ganglia. There is no permanent cure for herpes infections. Molluscum contagiosum is a benign and self-limited infection that is contagious. Chancroid, granuloma inguinale, and LGV produce external genital lesions with various degrees of inguinal lymph node involvement. These last three diseases are uncommon in the United States.

KEY POINTS

SEXUALLY TRANSMITTED INFECTIONS

- In general, STIs because of bacterial pathogens can be successfully treated and the pathogen eliminated by antimicrobial therapy. However, many of these pathogens are developing antibiotic resistance.
- STIs because of viral pathogens such as genital herpes simplex virus infections (HSV-1 and HSV-2) are not eliminated by current treatment modalities and persist with risk of recurrence (HSV infections).

VAGINAL INFECTIONS

After completing this section of the chapter, the learner will be able to meet the following objectives:

- State the difference between wet-mount slide and culture methods of diagnosis of STIs.
- Compare the signs and symptoms of infections caused by *Candida albicans*, *Trichomonas vaginalis*, and bacterial vaginosis.

Candidiasis, trichomoniasis, and bacterial vaginosis are vaginal infections that may be associated with sexual activity. Trichomoniasis is the only form of vaginitis that is known to be sexually transmitted and requires partner treatment. The male partner usually is asymptomatic.

Candidiasis

Also called *yeast infection*, *thrush*, and *moniliasis*, *candidiasis* is the second leading cause of vulvovaginitis in the United States. Approximately, 75% of reproductive age women in the United States experience one episode in their lifetime: 40% to 45% experience two or more infections.[13]

Candida albicans is the most commonly identified organism in vaginal yeast infections. However, other *Candida* species, such as *Candida glabrata* and *Candida tropicalis*, may also be present and be responsible for complicated candidiasis.[13] Although vulvovaginal candidiasis usually is not transmitted sexually, it is included in the CDC STI treatment guidelines because it often is diagnosed in women being evaluated for STIs.[3] The possibility of sexual transmission has been recognized for many years. However, candidiasis requires a favorable environment for growth of the organism. The gastrointestinal tract also serves as a reservoir for this organism, and candidiasis can develop through autoinoculation in women who are not sexually active. Although studies have documented the presence of *Candida* on the penis of male partners of women with vulvovaginal candidiasis (Fig. 46.4), few men develop balanoposthitis that requires treatment.[13]

Etiology and Clinical Manifestations

Reported risk factors for the overgrowth of *C. albicans* include recent antibiotic therapy, which suppresses the normal

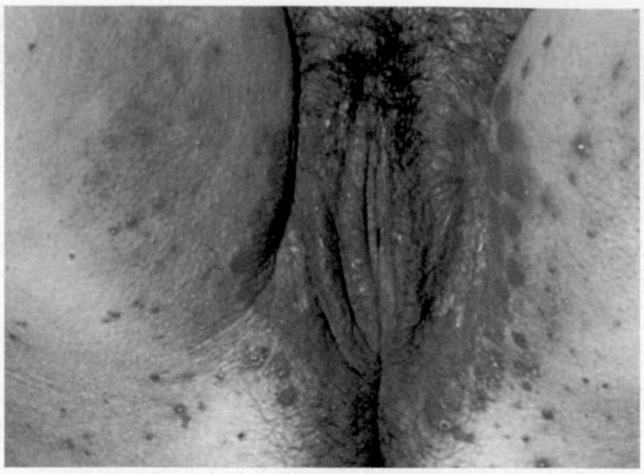

Figure 46.4 • Candidiasis—Women will have vaginal pruritus and usually thick, white, curdlike secretions, but the secretions could be thin. (From Jensen S. (2015). *Nursing health assessment: A best practice approach* (2nd ed., p. 770). Philadelphia, PA: Lippincott Williams & Wilkins.)

protective bacterial flora; high hormone levels owing to pregnancy or the use of oral contraceptives, which cause an increase in vaginal glycogen stores; and uncontrolled diabetes mellitus or HIV infection, because they compromise the immune system.[2] Women with vulvovaginal candidiasis commonly complain of vulvovaginal pruritus accompanied by irritation, erythema, swelling, dysuria, and dyspareunia. The characteristic discharge, when present, is usually thick, white, and odorless. In obese people, *Candida* may grow in skin folds underneath the breast tissue, the abdominal flap, and the inguinal folds.

Concept Mastery Alert

The person with vulvovaginal candidiasis will have redness, swelling, and painful urination. Discharge will be thick and white because of yeast overgrowth and will be odorless.

Diagnosis and Treatment

Accurate diagnosis is made by identification of budding yeast filaments (*i.e.*, hyphae) or spores on a wet-mount slide using 20% potassium hydroxide. The pH of the discharge, which is checked with litmus paper, typically is less than 4.5. When the wet-mount technique is negative but the clinical manifestations are suggestive of candidiasis, a culture may be necessary.

Antifungal agents such as clotrimazole, miconazole, butoconazole, and terconazole, in various forms, are effective in treating candidiasis. These drugs, with the exception of terconazole, are available without prescription for use by women who have had a previously confirmed diagnosis of candidiasis. Oral fluconazole has been shown to be as safe and effective as the standard intravaginal regimen.[3] Chronic vulvovaginal candidiasis, defined as four or more mycologically confirmed episodes within 1 year, affects approximately 5% of women and is difficult to manage.[13] Subsequent prophylaxis (maintenance therapy) often is required for long-term management of this problem.[13]

Trichomoniasis

Trichomoniasis is credited with being a far more prevalent STI than gonorrhea infection, and almost as common as chlamydia.[13–15] In the United States, it has been estimated that 7.4 million new cases of trichomoniasis appear annually.[14] Epidemiologically, *Trichomonas vaginalis* infections are commonly associated with other STIs and are therefore a marker for high-risk sexual behavior. An anaerobic protozoan that can be transmitted sexually, *T. vaginalis*, is shaped like a turnip and has three or four anterior flagella (see Fig. 46.5). Trichomonads can reside in the paraurethral glands of both sexes.

Clinical Manifestations and Complications

Men harbor the organism in the urethra and prostate and are asymptomatic. Although 10% to 25% of women are asymptomatic, trichomoniasis is a common cause of vaginitis when some imbalance allows the protozoan to proliferate.[15] This extracellular parasite feeds on the vaginal mucosa and ingests bacteria and leukocytes. The infection causes a copious, frothy, malodorous, green or yellow discharge. There commonly is erythema and edema of the affected mucosa, with occasional itching and irritation. Sometimes, small hemorrhagic areas, called *strawberry spots*, appear on the cervix.

Trichomoniasis can cause a number of complications.[13] It is a risk factor for HIV transmission and infectivity in both men and women. In women, it increases the risk of tubal infertility and atypical pelvic inflammatory disease (PID), and it is associated with adverse outcomes such as premature birth in pregnant women.[13] Trichomonads attach easily to mucous membranes. They may serve as vectors for the spread of other organisms, carrying pathogens attached to their surface into the fallopian tubes. In men, it is a common cause of nongonococcal urethritis and is a risk factor for infertility.[14]

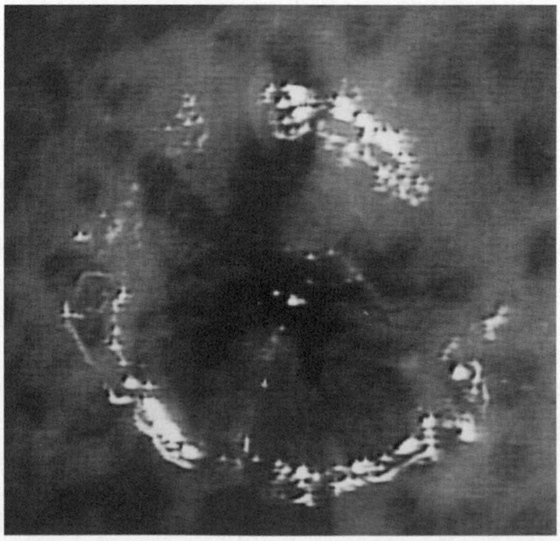

Figure 46.5 • Trichomoniasis—Women will have vaginal pruritus, thin or thick secretions, a foul vaginal odor, and possibly dysuria. (From Jensen S. (2015). *Nursing health assessment: A best practice approach* (2nd ed., p. 771, Table 24.3). Philadelphia, PA: Lippincott Williams & Wilkins.)

Diagnosis and Treatment

Diagnosis is made microscopically by identification of the motile protozoan on a wet-mount slide preparation. The pH of the discharge usually is greater than 6.0. Because the organism resides in other urogenital structures besides the vagina, systemic treatment is recommended. The treatment of choice is oral metronidazole or tinidazole, medications that are effective against anaerobic protozoans.[13] Both drugs are chemically similar to disulfiram (Antabuse), a drug used in the treatment of alcohol addiction that causes nausea, vomiting, flushing of the skin, headache, palpitations, and lowering of the blood pressure when alcohol is ingested. Gastrointestinal disturbances and a metallic taste in the mouth are potential adverse effects of the drugs. Although metronidazole is considered safe for use during pregnancy, data on tinidazole use in pregnancy are limited.[13] Sexual partners should be treated to avoid reinfection, and abstinence is recommended until the full course of therapy is completed.

Bacterial Vaginosis

Bacterial vaginosis is the most prevalent form of vaginal infection seen by health care professionals.[16] The prevalence for bacterial vaginosis is approximately 21.2 million people per year in the 14 to 49 age group.[16] The disorder is associated with having multiple sex partners, a new sex partner, douching, and a lack of vaginal lactobacilli. Its relation to sexual activity is not clear. Sexual activity is believed to be a catalyst rather than a primary mode of transmission, and endogenous factors may play a role in the development of symptoms.

Pathogenesis

The pathogenesis of bacterial vaginosis is poorly understood. It is a complex polymicrobial disorder characterized by a shift in the vaginal flora from one dominated by hydrogen peroxide–producing lactobacilli to one with greatly reduced numbers of *Lactobacillus* species and an overgrowth of other organisms, including *Gardnerella vaginalis*, *Mobiluncus* species, *Mycoplasma hominis*, and numerous anaerobes.[16,17] The massive overgrowth of vaginal anaerobes is associated with increased conversion of vaginal peptides to a variety of amines that, in high pH, become volatile and malodorous. The amines are associated with increased vaginal transudation and squamous epithelial cell exfoliation, creating the typical discharge. In conditions of elevated pH, *G. vaginalis* more efficiently adhere to the exfoliating epithelial cells, creating clue cells (squamous epithelial cells covered with masses of coccobacilli, often with large clumps of organisms floating free from the cell). Amines further provide a suitable substrate for *M. hominis* growth.

Clinical Manifestations

The predominant symptom of bacterial vaginosis is a thin, grayish-white discharge that has a foul, fishy odor. Burning, itching, and erythema usually are absent because the bacteria have only minimal inflammatory potential. Because of the lack of inflammation, the term *vaginosis* rather than *vaginitis* is used to describe the condition. The organisms associated with bacterial vaginosis may be carried asymptomatically by men and women.

In addition to causing bothersome symptoms, bacterial vaginosis is associated with an increased risk of PID, preterm labor, premature rupture of membranes, chorioamnionitis, and postpartum endometritis linked to the organisms associated with bacterial vaginosis. Postoperative infections, including postabortion PID, posthysterectomy cuff cellulitis, and postcesarean endometritis, have been shown to be associated with asymptomatic bacterial vaginosis.

Diagnosis and Treatment

The diagnosis of bacterial vaginosis is made when at least three of the following characteristics are present:

- Homogeneous, thin, white discharge
- Production of a fishy, amine odor when a saline solution is dropped onto the secretions
- Vaginal pH above 4.5 (usually 5.0 to 6.0)
- Appearance of characteristic "clue cells" on wet-mount microscopic studies

When indicated, treatment is aimed at relieving the vaginal symptoms and signs of infection and reducing the risk of infectious complications after abortion or hysterectomy. All women who have symptomatic disease should be treated. Other potential benefits might include a reduction in the risk of other STIs. The CDC recommends treatment by oral metronidazole, metronidazole vaginal gel, or clindamycin vaginal cream.[16] The same treatment regimens used for nonpregnant women can be used in pregnancy. Routine screening for bacterial vaginosis is not advocated, but all pregnant women with bacterial vaginosis should be treated. In addition, women at increased risk for preterm labor should be screened during the first trimester.[16]

IN SUMMARY

Candidiasis, trichomoniasis, and bacterial vaginosis are common vaginal infections that become symptomatic because of changes in the vaginal ecosystem. Only trichomoniasis is spread through sexual contact. Candidiasis, also called a *yeast infection*, is a frequent cause of vulvovaginitis. *Candida* can be present without producing symptoms; usually some host factor, such as altered immune status, contributes to the development of vulvovaginitis. It can be treated with over-the-counter medications. The infection, which is caused by the anaerobic protozoan *T. vaginalis*, incites the production of a copious, frothy, yellow or green, malodorous discharge. It is a risk factor for HIV transmission and infectivity in both men and women. In women, it increases the risk of tubal infertility and atypical PID and it is associated with adverse outcomes such as premature birth in pregnant women. Bacterial vaginosis is the most common cause of vaginal discharge. It is a complex polymicrobial disorder characterized by a shift in the vaginal flora from one dominated by hydrogen peroxide–producing lactobacilli to one with greatly reduced numbers of lactobacilli and an overgrowth of other organisms, including *G. vaginalis*, *Mobiluncus* species, *M. hominis*, and numerous anaerobes. The predominant symptom of bacterial vaginosis is a thin, grayish-white discharge that has a foul, fishy odor. Because it does not produce inflammation, it is referred to as *vaginosis* rather than *vaginitis*.

VAGINAL–UROGENITAL–SYSTEMIC INFECTIONS

After completing this section of the chapter, the learner will be able to meet the following objectives:

- State the genital and nongenital complications that can occur with chlamydial infections, gonorrhea, and syphilis.
- Describe the three stages of syphilis.

Some STIs infect male and female genital and extragenital structures. Among the infections of this type are chlamydial infections, gonorrhea, and syphilis. Many of these infections also pose a risk to infants born to infected mothers. Some infections, such as syphilis, may be spread to the infant while in utero, whereas others, such as chlamydial and gonorrheal infections, can be spread to the infant during the birth process.

Chlamydial Infections

Chlamydial infection is the most prevalent STI in the United States, with an incidence estimated to be more than twice that of gonorrhea. As of 2015, chlamydial infections are reportable in all 50 states and the District of Columbia. According to CDC estimates, chlamydial infections reported from each of the 50 states and the District of Columbia equalled approximately 1.3 million new cases in 2015, predominantly among people younger than 25 years of age.[18] There was an increase of 5.1% of cases since 2009.[18] The CDC estimates about twice the reported rate of people actually are infected with chlamydia.[18] Rates for chlamydial infections have risen significantly over the past 15 years because of an increase in screening programs, improved sensitivity of diagnostic tests, and improved surveillance and reporting systems.

Chlamydia trachomatis is an obligate intracellular bacterial pathogen that tends to be much smaller than most bacteria.[18] It resembles a virus in that it requires tissue culture for isolation, but like bacteria, it has ribonucleic acid (RNA) and DNA and is susceptible to some antibiotics. *C. trachomatis* causes a wide variety of genitourinary infections, including nongonococcal urethritis in men and PID in women. The closely related organisms *Chlamydia pneumoniae* and *Chlamydia psittaci* cause mild and severe pneumonia, respectively. *C. trachomatis* is the most common sexually transmitted disease in North America.[18] It can be serologically subdivided into types A, B, and C, which are associated with trachoma and chronic keratoconjunctivitis; types D through K, which are associated with genital infections and their complications; and types L1, L2, and L3, which are associated with LGV. *C. trachomatis* can cause significant ocular disease in neonates. It is a leading cause of blindness in underdeveloped countries. In these countries, the organism is spread primarily by flies, fomites, and nonsexual personal contact. In industrial countries, the organism is spread almost exclusively by sexual contact and therefore affects primarily the genitourinary structures.

Chlamydiae exist in two forms: elementary and reticulate bodies.[18] The 48-hour growth cycle starts with attachment of the elementary body to the susceptible host cell, after which it is ingested by a process that resembles phagocytosis. Once inside the cell, the elementary body is organized into the reticulate body, the metabolically active form of the organism that is capable of reproduction. The reticulate body is not infectious and cannot survive outside the body. The reticulate bodies divide in the cell for up to 36 hours and then condense to form new elementary bodies, which are released when the infected cell bursts.

Clinical Manifestations

The signs and symptoms of chlamydial infection resemble those produced by gonorrhea. The most significant difference between chlamydial and gonococcal salpingitis is that chlamydial infections may be asymptomatic or clinically nonspecific. If there are symptoms in women, the most common symptom is a mucopurulent cervical discharge (Fig. 46.6). The cervix itself frequently hypertrophies and becomes erythematous, edematous, and extremely friable. This can lead to greater fallopian tube damage and increase the reservoir for further chlamydial infections.

In men, chlamydial infections, if there are symptoms, cause urethritis, including meatal erythema and tenderness, a purulent penile discharge, and urethral itching[18] (Fig. 46.7). Prostatitis and epididymitis with subsequent infertility may develop.

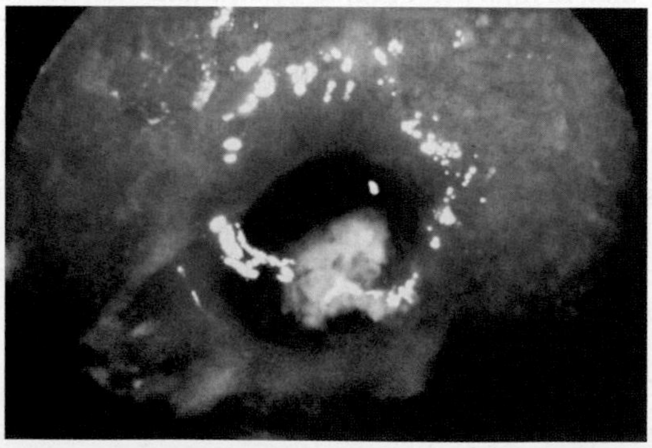

Figure 46.6 • Chlamydia—In women there may be no symptoms or manifestation. Occasionally there are clear or white secretions. (From Jensen S. (2015). *Nursing health assessment: A best practice approach* (2nd ed., p. 770). Philadelphia, PA: Lippincott Williams & Wilkins.)

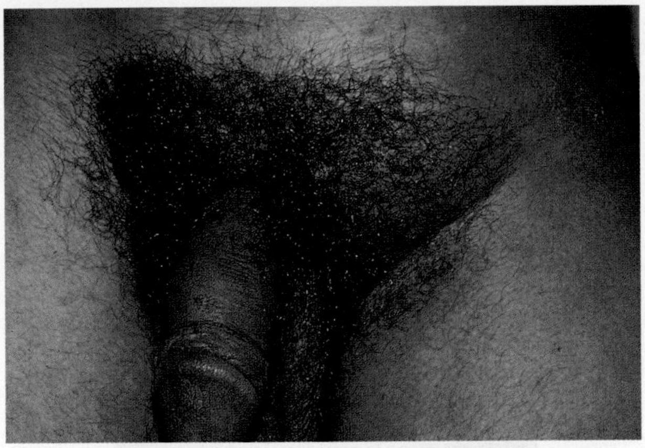

Figure 46.7 • Chlamydia—*Chlamydomonas trachomatis* is a bacterium with a variable incubation period, usually 1 week of exposure. There is a mucopurulent discharge in men. (From Jensen S. (2015). *Nursing health assessment: A best practice approach* (2nd ed., p. 728). Philadelphia, PA: Lippincott Williams & Wilkins.)

The most serious complication of untreated chlamydial infection is the development of Reiter syndrome. This triad of symptoms includes urethritis, conjunctivitis, and arthritis of weight-bearing joints, such as the knees, sacroiliac and vertebral joints.[18] Women can also develop reactive arthritis, but the male-to-female ratio for this complication is 5:1. The arthritis begins 1 to 3 weeks after the onset of chlamydial infection. The joint involvement is asymmetric, with multiple affected joints and a predilection for the lower extremities. Mucocutaneous lesions also occur and are papulosquamous eruptions that tend to be located on the palms of the hands and soles of the feet of both genders. The US Preventive Services Task Force (USPSTF) has suggested annual screening for sexually active adolescents and young female adults in an effort to minimize infection.[19]

Diagnosis and Treatment

Diagnosis of chlamydial infections takes several forms. The identification of polymorphonuclear leukocytes on Gram stain of penile discharge in the man or cervical discharge in the woman provides presumptive evidence. The direct fluorescent antibody test and the enzyme-linked immunosorbent assay that use antibodies against an antigen in the *Chlamydia* cell wall are rapid tests that are highly sensitive and specific. The positive predictive value of these tests is excellent among high-risk groups, but false-positive results occur more often in low-risk groups. The methodologic challenges of culturing this organism have led to the development of non–culture-based tests that amplify and detect *C. trachomatis*–specific DNA and RNA sequences.[18] One of the newest sets of nonculture techniques, the nucleic acid amplification tests (NAATs), does not require viable organisms for detection and can produce a positive signal from as little as a single copy of the target DNA or RNA.[18] The amplification procedures that are now commercially available for chlamydial testing are PCR, transcription-mediated amplification (TMA) of RNA, and strand displacement amplification (SDA). These amplification methods are highly sensitive and, if properly monitored, very specific. NAATs can be performed on urine or self-collected swab specimens from the distal vagina as well as the traditional endocervical and urethral specimens. Most NAATs in use today detect both *C. trachomatis* and *Neisseria gonorrhoeae* in a single test.

The CDC recommends the use of azithromycin or doxycycline in the treatment of chlamydial infection. Penicillin is ineffective. Azithromycin is the preferred choice in pregnancy.[3] Simultaneous antibiotic treatment of both sexual partners is recommended. Abstinence from sexual activity is encouraged to facilitate cure.

Gonorrhea

Gonorrhea is a reportable STI caused by the bacterium *N. gonorrhoeae*. In 2015, 395,216 cases were reported for a rate of 123.9 gonorrhea cases per 100,000 population in the United States.[20] Like chlamydial infection, gonorrhea is frequently underdiagnosed. The CDC estimates there are 600,000 new cases every year.[20] Improved screening efforts as well as greater use of more sensitive nonculture methods of testing may have contributed to this trend.

The gonococcus is a pyogenic (*i.e.*, pus-forming), gram-negative diplococcus.[20] Humans are the only natural host for *N. gonorrhoeae*. The organism grows best in warm, mucus-secreting epithelia. The portal of entry can be the genitourinary tract, eyes, oropharynx, anorectum, or skin.

Transmission usually is by sexual intercourse except for perinatal transmission.[2] Autoinoculation of the organism to the conjunctiva is possible. Neonates born to infected mothers can acquire the infection during passage through the birth canal and are in danger of developing gonorrheal conjunctivitis, with resultant blindness unless treated promptly. An amniotic infection syndrome characterized by premature rupture of the membranes, premature delivery, and increased risk of infant morbidity and mortality has been identified as an additional complication of gonococcal infections in pregnancy. Genital gonorrhea in young children should raise the possibility of sexual abuse.

The infection commonly manifests 2 to 7 days after exposure. It typically begins in the anterior urethra, accessory urethral glands, Bartholin or Skene glands, and the cervix. If untreated, gonorrhea spreads from its initial sites upward into the genital tract. In men, it spreads to the prostate and epididymis. In women, it commonly produces endometritis, salpingitis, and PID.[2] Pharyngitis may follow oral–genital contact. The organism also can invade the bloodstream (*i.e.*, disseminated gonococcal infection), causing serious sequelae such as bacteremic involvement of joint spaces, heart valves, meninges, and other body organs and tissues.[2]

Clinical Manifestations

People with gonorrhea may be asymptomatic and may unwittingly spread the disease to their sexual partners. In men, the initial symptoms include urethral pain and a creamy yellow,

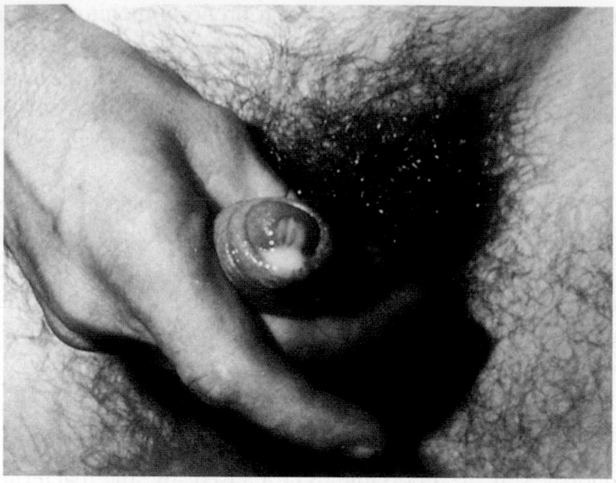

Figure 46.8 • Purulent penile discharge because of gonorrhea. (From Jensen S. (2015). *Nursing health assessment: A best practice approach* (2nd ed., p. 728). Philadelphia, PA: Lippincott Williams & Wilkins.)

sometimes bloody, discharge (Fig. 46.8). The disorder may become chronic and affect the prostate, epididymis, and periurethral glands.[2] Rectal infections are common in homosexual men. In women, recognizable symptoms include unusual genital or urinary discharge, dysuria, dyspareunia, pelvic pain or tenderness, unusual vaginal bleeding (including bleeding after intercourse), fever, and proctitis (Fig. 46.9).[2] Symptoms may occur or increase during or immediately after menses because the bacterium is an intracellular diplococcus that thrives in menstrual blood but cannot survive long outside the human

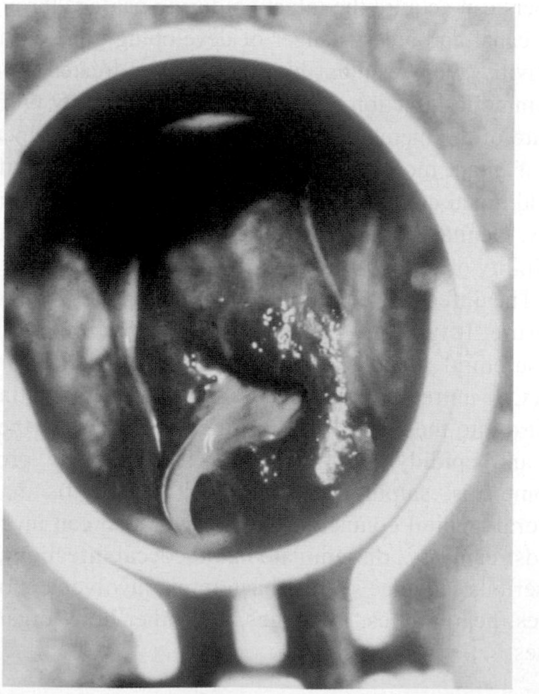

Figure 46.9 • Gonorrhea—Secretions are yellow and the women report dyspareunia and dysuria. (From Jensen S. (2015). *Nursing health assessment: A best practice approach* (2nd ed., p. 771). Philadelphia, PA: Lippincott Williams & Wilkins.)

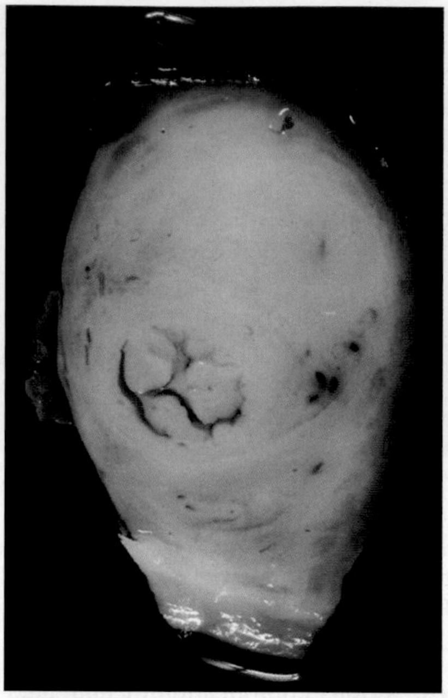

Figure 46.10 • Gonorrhea of the fallopian tube. Cross-section of a "pus tube" shows thickening of the wall and lumen swollen with pus. (From Rubin R., Strayer D. (Eds.) (2015). *Rubin's pathology: Clinicopathologic foundations of medicine* (7th ed., p. 394). Philadelphia, PA: Lippincott Williams & Wilkins.)

body. There may be infections of the uterus and development of acute or chronic infection of the fallopian tubes (*i.e.*, salpingitis), with ultimate scarring and sterility (Fig. 46.10).

Diagnosis

Diagnosis is based on the history of sexual exposure and symptoms. It is confirmed by identification of the organism on Gram stain or culture. A Gram stain usually is an effective means of diagnosis in symptomatic men (*i.e.*, those with discharge). In women and asymptomatic men, a culture usually is preferred because the Gram stain often is unreliable. Culture has been the gold standard, particularly when the Gram stain is negative. A specimen should be collected from the appropriate site (*i.e.*, endocervix, urethra, anal canal, or oropharynx), inoculated onto a suitable medium, and transported under appropriate conditions. *N. gonorrhoeae* is a fastidious organism with specific nutrient and environmental needs. Detection by NAATs (PCR) is generally done. The sensitivity of these tests is similar to that of culture. Men are often more willing to provide a urine specimen than to have a urethral swab done, and NAAT can be offered to women in locations where pelvic examination is not possible.

Updated recommendations from the USPSTF suggest that clinicians screen all sexually active women for gonorrhea who are at increased risk for infection (*i.e.*, younger than 25 years of age, new or multiple sexual partners, inconsistent condom use, sex work, or drug use).[21] Testing for other STIs, particularly syphilis and chlamydial infection, is suggested at the time of examination. Pregnant women are routinely screened at the time of their first prenatal visit. High-risk populations should have repeat cultures during the third trimester. Neonates are routinely treated with various antibacterial agents applied to the conjunctiva within 1 hour of birth to protect against undiagnosed gonorrhea and other diseases.

Treatment

Penicillin-resistant strains of *N. gonorrhoeae* are prevalent worldwide and strains with other kinds of antibiotic resistance continue to evolve and spread. The current treatment recommendation to combat tetracycline- and penicillin-resistant strains of *N. gonorrhoeae* has progressively developed resistance to each of the antimicrobials used for treatment of gonorrhea.[20] Most recently, declining susceptibility to cefixime (an oral cephalosporin antibiotic) resulted in a change to the CDC treatment guidelines (2015) so that dual therapy with ceftriaxone (an injectable cephalosporin) and azithromycin is now the only CDC-recommended treatment regimen for gonorrhea.[20] Cephalosporin resistance highlights the need for continued surveillance of *N. gonorrhoeae* antimicrobial susceptibility.

The combination of persistently high gonorrhea morbidity in some populations and the threat of cephalosporin-resistant gonorrhea reinforces the need to better understand the epidemiology of gonorrhea.

All are equally effective and should be followed with azithromycin for chlamydiae. Quinolone-resistant strains are now common in Asia, the Pacific islands (including Hawaii), and California, so the CDC recommends avoiding the use of fluoroquinolones in those areas for infections in men who have sex with men or for people with a history of recent foreign travel. All sex partners within 60 days prior to discovery of the infection should be contacted, tested, and treated. Test of cure is not required with observed single-dose therapy.

Syphilis

Syphilis is a reportable systemic STI caused by a spirochete, *Treponema pallidum*. In 2015, there were 23,872 primary and secondary cases of syphilis and 26,170 late and late latent cases of syphilis reported in the United States.[22] A total of 50,042 cases of syphilis were reported to the CDC in the United States.[22] Nationally, the highest rates of primary and secondary syphilis cases were among men aged 25 to 29 and 20 to 24 years, among men in the West, and in the South, and among Black men.[22]

T. pallidum is spread by direct contact with an infectious moist lesion, usually through sexual intercourse. Bacteria-laden secretions may transfer the organism during any type of intimate contact. Skin abrasions provide another possible portal of entry. There is rapid transplacental transmission of the organism from the mother to the fetus after 16 weeks' gestation, so that active infection in the mother during pregnancy can produce congenital syphilis in the fetus. Untreated syphilis can cause prematurity, stillbirth, and congenital defects and active infection in the infant. Because the manifestations of maternal syphilis may be subtle, testing for syphilis is mandatory in all pregnancies. Once treated for syphilis, a pregnant woman usually is followed throughout pregnancy by repeat testing of serum titers.

Clinical Manifestations

The clinical disease is divided into three stages: primary, secondary, and tertiary. Primary syphilis is characterized by the appearance of a chancre at the site of exposure, such as on the penis, vulva, anus, or mouth.[2] Chancres typically appear within an average of 3 weeks of exposure but may incubate up to 3 months.[2] The primary chancre begins as a single, indurated, papule up to several centimeters in diameter that erodes to create a clean-based ulcerated lesion on an elevated base. They also are solitary and have discrete raised borders.[2] These lesions usually are painless and located at the site of sexual contact. Primary syphilis is readily apparent in the male, where the lesion is on the scrotum or penis (Fig. 46.11). Although chancres can develop on the external genitalia in females, they are more common on the vagina or cervix, and primary syphilis therefore may go untreated since they are not visible without a speculum examination. Often there is an accompanying inguinal lymphadenopathy.[2] The infection is highly contagious at this stage, but because the symptoms are mild, it frequently goes unnoticed. The chancre usually heals within 3 to 12 weeks, with or without treatment.

The timing of the second stage of syphilis varies even more than that of the first, lasting from 1 week to 6 months. The symptoms of a rash (especially on the palms, mucous membranes, meninges, lymph nodes, stomach, soles, and liver)[2] (Fig. 46.12), fever, sore throat, stomatitis, nausea, loss of appetite, and inflamed eyes may come and go for a year but usually last for 3 to 6 months. Secondary manifestations may include some loss of hair and condylomata lata. These lesions are elevated, red-brown lesions that may ulcerate and produce a foul discharge. They are 2 to 3 cm in diameter, contain many spirochetes, and are highly infectious.

After the second stage, syphilis frequently enters a latent phase that may last the lifetime of the person or progress to tertiary syphilis at some point. Persons can be infective during the first 1 to 2 years of latency.

Tertiary syphilis is a delayed response to the untreated disease. It can occur decades after the initial infection.[2]

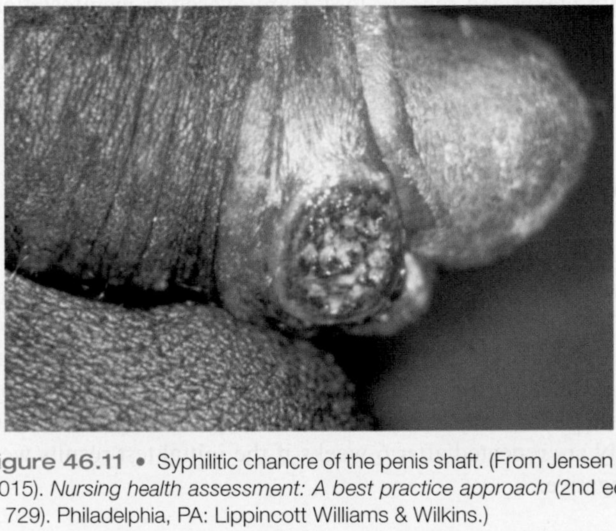

Figure 46.11 • Syphilitic chancre of the penis shaft. (From Jensen S. (2015). *Nursing health assessment: A best practice approach* (2nd ed., p. 729). Philadelphia, PA: Lippincott Williams & Wilkins.)

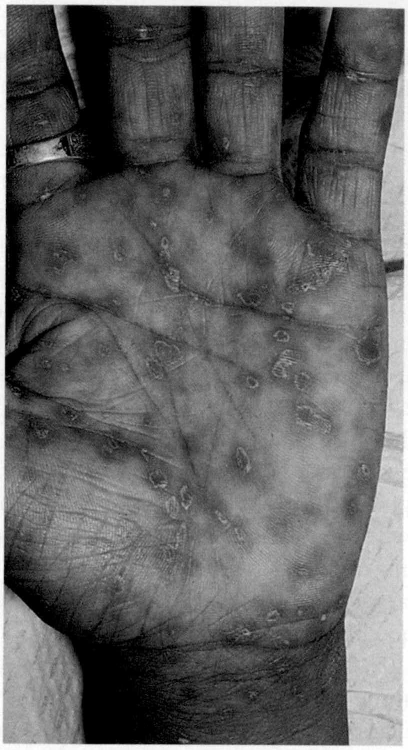

Figure 46.12 • Secondary syphilis. A maculopapular rash is present on the palm. (From Rubin E., Gorstein F., Rubin R., et al. (Eds.) (2015). *Rubin's pathology: Clinicopathologic foundations of medicine* (7th ed., p. 414). Philadelphia, PA: Lippincott Williams & Wilkins.)

When syphilis does progress to the symptomatic tertiary stage, it commonly takes one of three forms: development of localized destructive granuloma-like lesions called *gummas*, development of cardiovascular lesions, or development of central nervous system lesions. The syphilitic gumma is a peculiar, rubbery, necrotic lesion that is caused by noninflammatory tissue necrosis. Gummas can occur singly or multiply and vary in size from microscopic lesions to large, tumorous masses. They most commonly are found in the liver, testes, and bone. Central nervous system lesions can produce dementia, blindness, or injury to the spinal cord, with ataxia and sensory loss. Cardiovascular manifestations usually result from scarring of the medial layer of the thoracic aorta with aneurysm formation. These aneurysms produce enlargement of the aortic valve ring with aortic valve insufficiency.[2]

Diagnosis

T. pallidum is difficult to culture and requires special dark field microscopy to adequately detect the organism. As it evokes a humoral immune response leading to production of antibodies, serologic testing can be done. Although PCR tests have now been developed for syphilis, serology remains the mainstay for diagnosis.[22] Because the disease's incubation period may delay test sensitivity, serologic tests usually are repeated after 6 weeks if the initial test results were negative.

The nontreponemal tests identify the presence of regain, which is an autoantibody directed against cardiolipin antigens. These antibodies are detected by flocculation tests such as the Venereal Disease Research Laboratory (VDRL) test or the rapid plasma reagin (RPR) test.[22] Because these tests are nonspecific, positive results can occur with diseases other than syphilis. The tests are easy to perform, rapid, and inexpensive and frequently are used as screening tests for syphilis. Results become positive 4 to 6 weeks after infection or 1 to 3 weeks after the appearance of the primary lesion. Because these tests are quantitative, they can be used to measure the degree of disease activity or treatment effectiveness. The VDRL titer usually is high during the secondary stage of the disease and becomes less so during the tertiary stage. A falling titer during treatment suggests a favorable response. The fluorescent treponemal antibody absorption test is used to detect specific antibodies to *T. pallidum*. These qualitative tests are used to determine whether a positive result on a nonspecific test such as the VDRL or RPR is attributable to syphilis.

Treatment

The treatment of choice for syphilis is penicillin.[3] Because of the spirochetes' long generation time, effective tissue levels of penicillin must be maintained for several weeks. Long-acting injectable forms of penicillin are used. Tetracycline or doxycycline is used for treatment in people who are sensitive to penicillin. Pregnant women should be desensitized and treated with penicillin because erythromycin does not treat fetal infection. Sexual partners should be evaluated and treated prophylactically even though they may show no sign of infection.

IN SUMMARY

The vaginal–urogenital–systemic STIs—chlamydial infections, gonorrhea, and syphilis—can severely involve the genital structures and manifest as systemic infections. Gonorrheal and chlamydial infections can cause a wide variety of genitourinary complications in men and women, and both can cause ocular disease and blindness in neonates born to infected mothers. Syphilis is caused by a spirochete, *T. pallidum*. It can produce widespread systemic effects and is transferred to the fetus of infected mothers through the placenta.

OTHER INFECTIONS

After completing this section of the chapter, the learner will be able to meet the following objectives:

- State the complications that can occur with infection of the Zika virus.
- Describe the spread of Zika virus.
- Describe the symptoms of Zika infection.

Zika

Zika is a virus that was discovered in 1947 in the Zika Forest of Uganda and was initially spread by the bite of an infected *Aedes* species mosquito (*A. Aegypti and A. Albopictus*).[23,24] The first human cases of Zika were detected in 1952. Zika infection can occur in any of the following ways:

- From a bite from this species of mosquito.[23,24]
- From exposure to an infected sexual partner, including sex (oral, vaginal, or anal sex, or the sharing of sex toys) without a condom.[23,24] (Note that having sex with a partner who traveled to or lives in an area with Zika puts a person at risk of infection.)[23,24]
- This virus can be passed on by a pregnant woman to her fetus, and this infection during pregnancy can cause certain birth defects.[23,24]

Clinical Manifestations

People infected with the Zika virus show few symptoms.[23] Symptoms reported have included fever, rash, joint pain, conjunctivitis, muscle pain, and headache.[23] Zika infection symptoms can last for several days to a week.

Risk

If a woman is infected by Zika during pregnancy, severe birth defects can occur, such as microcephaly, brain defects, hearing and eye defects, and impaired growth.[23] There have also been reports of Guillain-Barré syndrome.[23]

Diagnosis

A blood or urine test can confirm a Zika infection. Collect serum or cerebrospinal fluid (CSF) and send to the CDC, where RNA NAT (nucleic acid testing) and antibody testing are performed. The RNA NAT and virus isolation can be performed on other body fluids for diagnostic testing (*e.g.*, urine and amniotic fluid, or for research purposes (*e.g.*, semen).

Treatment

Currently there is no vaccine or treatment available for infection.[23]

Prevention

Use an insect repellent containing one or more of the following ingredients: DEET, picaridin, IR3535, oil of lemon eucalyptus, para-menthane-diol, or 2-undecanone.[25] Always follow the manufacturer's directions. These products are safe for pregnant and breastfeeding women but should not be used on babies younger than 2 months old.[25] Prevent exposure to mosquitoes by using screens and bed netting.[25] Prevent sexual transmission by using condoms or abstinence.[25]

IN SUMMARY

The Zika virus has been documented for over 70 years but has recently gained attention following an outbreak of the virus and its link to birth defects for the unborn fetus. Transmission is possible through a bite from an infected Aedes species mosquito, through unprotected sex with an infected partner, and from a pregnant woman to her fetus. Although the virus typically causes mild symptoms, pregnant women or those planning to become pregnant should be tested for the Zika antibody. Prevention is key since there is no treatment currently available.

GERIATRIC Considerations

- "At the end of 2014, an estimated 428,724 people aged 50 and over were living with diagnosed HIV in the United States."[21]
- Older people remain sexually active and have the same HIV risk factors as young adults but are less likely to discuss their sexual habits or drug use with their health care provider.[21]
- Misdiagnosis of early symptoms of HIV infection (fatigue, weakness, and memory changes) occurs due to these symptoms being seen as normal signs of aging.[22]

PEDIATRIC Considerations

- Although sexual abuse is of epidemic proportions in the United States, sexually transmitted infections (STIs) are rare (5%) in children who have been sexually abused.[23]
- The first (or on occasion only) indicator of sexual abuse is the presence of an STI in children.[26]
- The rate of reported congenital syphilis cases has increased each year since 2012. From 2011 to 2015, there was a 36.3% increase.[26]

STIs can be passed from a pregnant woman to the baby before and during the birth process; syphilis and HIV can cross the placenta during pregnancy.

REVIEW EXERCISES

1. A 25-year-old woman has been told that her Pap test indicates infection with HPV type 16.
   A. *What are the possible implications of infection with HPV 16?*
   B. *How might she have acquired this infection?*
   C. *What treatments are currently available for treatment of this infection?*
2. A 35-year-old woman presents with vulvar pruritus, dysuria, dyspareunia, and an odorless, thick, cheesy vaginal discharge. She has diabetes mellitus and has recently recovered from a respiratory tract infection, which required antibiotic treatment.
   A. *Given that these manifestations are consistent with a Candida infection, what tests might be used to confirm the diagnosis?*
   B. *What risk factors does this woman have that predispose to this type of vaginitis?*
   C. *How might this infection be treated?*
3. A 21-year-old woman has recently been to Miami, Florida and is complaining of a low-grade fever, rash, and joint pain. Her last menstrual period was 3 months ago. She is sexually active and her pregnancy test is positive.
   A. *Given these symptoms are consistent with Zika virus, what test could be done to confirm the Diagnosis?*
   B. *What is the risk for this woman and her baby?*
   C. *What can be done to prevent this infection in other childbearing women?*

References

1. Centers for Disease Control and Prevention. (2014). Sexually transmitted disease surveillance. [Online]. Available: https://www.cdc.gov/std/stats14/. Accessed January 31, 2017.
2. World Health Organization (WHO). (2016). Sexually transmitted infections. Fact sheet. [Online]. Available: http://www.who.int/mediacentre/factsheets/fs110/en/. Accessed January 31, 2017.
3. Centers for Disease Control and Prevention. (2015). Sexually transmitted disease guidelines. [Online]. Available: https://www.cdc.gov/std/tg2015/. Accessed January 31, 2017.
4. Center for Disease Control and Prevention. (2013). Self-study STD modules for clinicians: genital human papillomavirus (HPV) infection. Pathogenesis and microbiology. [Online]. Available: https://www2a.cdc.gov/stdtraining/self-study/hpv/cdc_self_study_hpv_pathogenesis.html. Accessed February 1, 2017.
5. Centers for Disease Control and Prevention. (2016). Questions and answers about HPV. [Online]. Available: https://www.cdc.gov/hpv/parents/questions-answers.html. Accessed February 1, 2017.
6. Morris B. J. et al. (2017). Effect of male circumcision on risk of sexually transmitted infections and cervical cancer in women. *The Lancet Global Health* 5(11), e1054–e1055. Available: http://www.thelancet.com/journals/langlo/article/PIIS2214-109X%2817%2930386-8/fulltext.
7. Centers for Disease Control and Prevention. (2015). Molluscum Contagiosum. [Online]. Available: https://www.cdc.gov/poxvirus/molluscum-contagiosum/index.html. Accessed February 2, 2017.
8. Centers for Disease Control and Prevention. (2016). Genital herpes: CDC fact sheet. [Online]. Available: https://www.cdc.gov/std/herpes/stdfact-herpes.htm. Accessed February 1, 2017.
9. Centers for Disease Control and Prevention. (2015). Candidiasis. [Online]. Available: https://www.cdc.gov/fungal/diseases/candidiasis/index.html. Accessed February 2, 2017.
10. Center for Disease Control and Prevention. (2015). Trichomoniasis: Fact sheet. [Online]. Available: https://www.cdc.gov/std/trichomonas/STDFact-Trichomoniasis.htm. Accessed February 2, 2017.
11. Centers for Disease Control and Prevention. (2015). Lymphogranuloma Venereum. [Online]. Available: https://www.cdc.gov/std/tg2015/lgv.htm. Accessed February 2, 2017.
12. Afsar F., Seremet S., Afsar I., et al. (2017). A case of scrofuloderma complicated with genital elephantiasis and saxophone penis. *Reviews in Medical Microbiology* 28(1), 5–8.
13. Centers for Disease Control and Prevention. (2015). Bacterial Vaginosis: CDC fact sheet. [Online]. Available: https://www.cdc.gov/std/bv/stdfact-bacterial-vaginosis.htm. Accessed February 2, 2017.
14. Centers for Disease Control and Prevention. (2015). Chlamydia: CDC fact sheet. [Online]. Available: https://www.cdc.gov/std/chlamydia/STDFact-Chlamydia.htm. Accessed February 2, 2017.
15. Centers for Disease Control and Prevention. (2015). [Online]. Available: https://www.cdc.gov/std/tg2015/chlamydia.htm. Accessed February 2, 2017.
16. USPSTF Recommendations for STI Screening. (2016). USPSTF recommendations for STU screening. [Online]. Available: https://www.uspreventiveservicestaskforce.org/Page/Name/uspstf-recommendations-for-sti-screening. Accessed February 2, 2017.
17. Centers for Disease Control and Prevention. (2015). Gonorrhea. [Online]. Available: https://www.cdc.gov/std/stats15/gonorrhea.htm. Accessed February 2, 2017.
18. U.S. Preventive Services Task Force. (2016). Screening for gonorrhea. [Online]. Available: https://www.uspreventiveservicestaskforce.org/Page/Name/uspstf-recommendations-for-sti-screening. Accessed February 2, 2017.
19. Centers for Disease Control and Prevention. (2016). Syphilis. [Online]. Available: https://www.cdc.gov/std/stats15/syphilis.htm. Accessed February 24, 2017.
20. Centers for Disease Control and Prevention. (2017). Collecting and submitting fluid specimens for Zika virus testing. [Online]. Available: https://www.cdc.gov/zika/laboratories/test-specimens-bodyfluids.html. Accessed February 24, 2017.
21. Centers for Disease Control and Prevention. (2017). CDC Prevention. [Online]. Available: https://www.cdc.gov/zika/prevention/prevent-mosquito-bites.html. Accessed February 24, 2017.
22. Center for Disease Control and Prevention. (2017). HIV among people aged 50 and over. Available: https://www.cdc.gov/hiv/group/age/olderamericans/index.html.
23. Stewart A., Graham S. (2013). Sexual risk behavior among older adults. *Clinical Advisor* 16(4), 28–38.
24. Centers for Disease Control and Prevention. (2017). Zika. [Online]. Available: https://www.cdc.gov/zika/about/index.html. Accessed February 24, 2017.
25. Office of Women's Health, U.S. Department of Health and Human Services. (2014). STIs, pregnancy, and breastfeeding. Available: https://www.womenshealth.gov/a-z-topics/stis-pregnancy-and-breast feeding.
26. Hornor G., (2017). Sexually transmitted infections and children: What the PNP should know. *Journal of Pediatric Health Care* 31(2), 222–229.

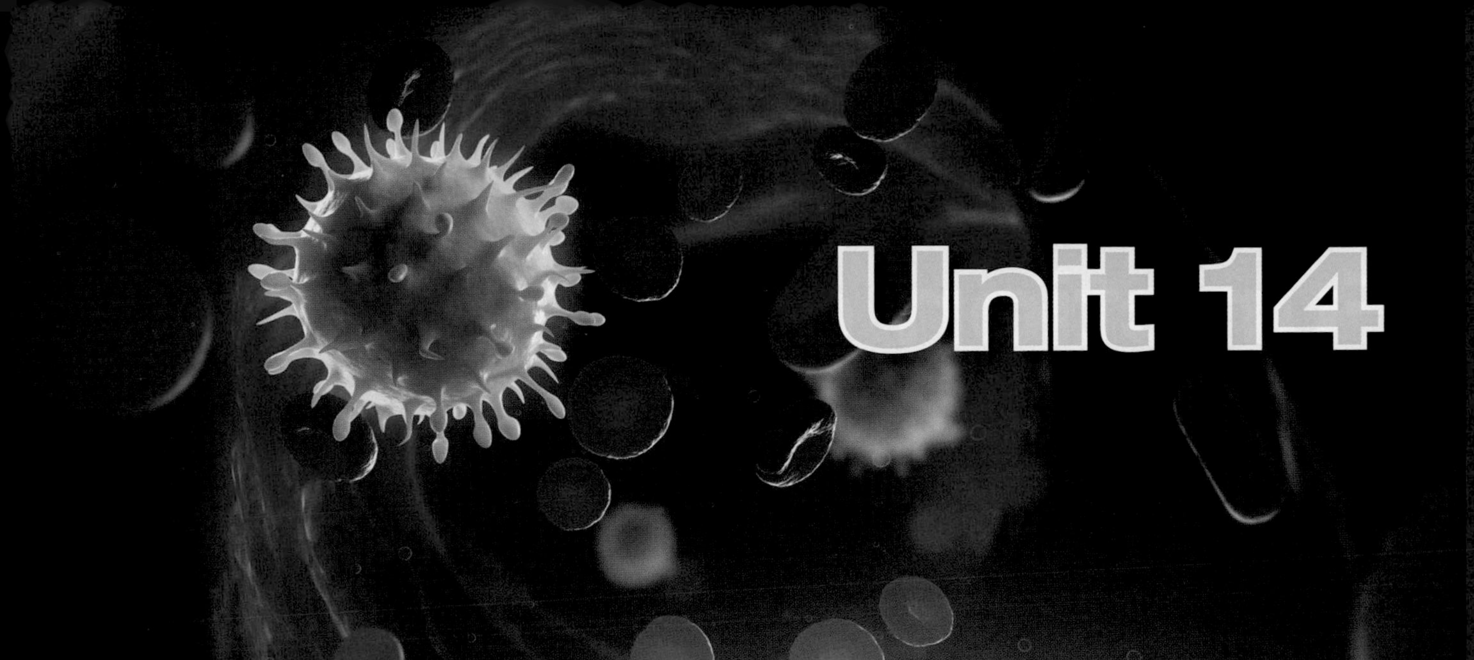

Unit 14

Disorders of Musculoskeletal Function

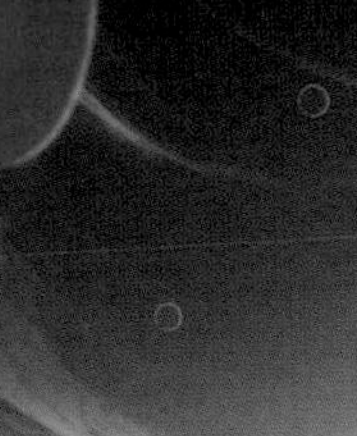

Mrs. Tukey, 68 years of age, presents at a walk-in clinic with worsening lower back pain that has increased over the last 2 weeks. She has had no medical care for 8 years. She does not recall any recent falls or trauma, but she moved several large boxes in her attic over the last couple of weeks. Eight years ago, she had her left hip pinned after a fracture. She has mild kyphosis, has smoked 1.5 packs of cigarettes per day for 40 years, and takes no medications. She states that "her mother had the bone disease that older women get." Mrs. Tukey's diet consists primarily of cereal and biscuits. She does not eat meat and rarely performs aerobic exercise. Her neurologic examination is normal, but she has decreased range of motion in multiple joints and pain and tenderness upon palpation of her lower back muscles. She ranks her back pain as 6/10. Clinical findings include the following: temperature, 99°F; heart rate, 88/minute and regular; respiration rate, 14/minute; blood pressure, 110/64 mm Hg; and BMI, 23 (normal). Her bone density is significantly reduced (T score = −3.0) and the lumbar x-ray shows a fracture of the fifth lumbar vertebra (L5). Her serum calcium concentration is high (12.8 mg/dL) and her serum magnesium concentration is low (1.0 mg/dL). The diagnosis is a pathologic fracture secondary to osteoporosis. She is referred to a nutritionist and a free meal service for senior citizens to address her nutritional issues, the Visiting Nurses Association for follow-up care, the YMCA for a monitored exercise regimen involving swimming and light resistance exercise, and smoking cessation classes. She also is prescribed a bisphosphonate medication to inhibit bone resorption.

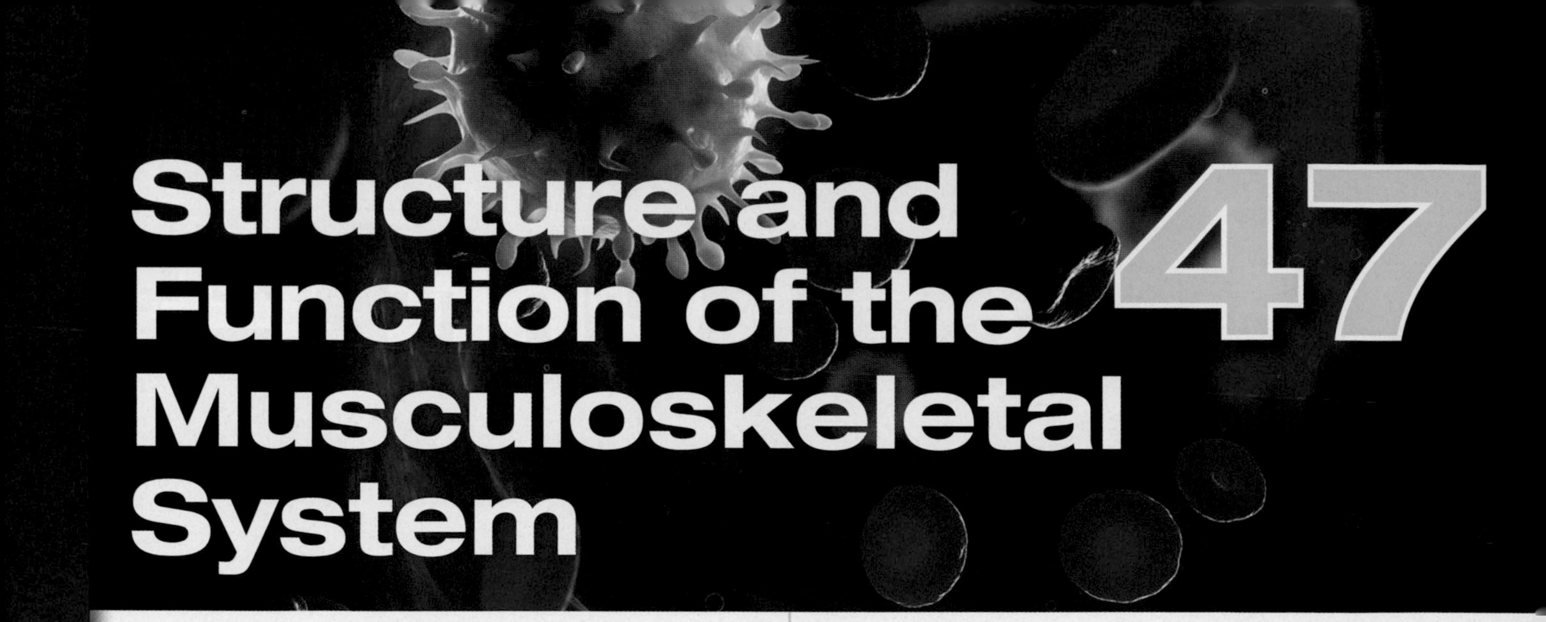

Structure and Function of the Musculoskeletal System

47

Sarah Morgan

The bones of the skeletal system are a framework for the attachment of muscles, tendons, and ligaments. The skeletal system protects soft tissues and maintains them in their proper position, provides stability for the body, and maintains the body's shape. Bones act as a storage reservoir for calcium, and the central cavity of some bones contains the hematopoietic connective tissue in which blood cells are formed. Coordinated movement of the skeleton is made possible by the tendons and ligaments that join bones at joints.

For our purposes, the skeletal system is considered to include the bones and cartilage of the skeletal system, as well as the connective tissue structures (*i.e.*, ligaments and tendons) that connect the bones and join muscles to bone.

BONY STRUCTURES OF THE SKELETAL SYSTEM

After completing this section of the chapter, the learner will be able to meet the following objectives:

- Cite the characteristics and at least one location of, elastic cartilage, hyaline cartilage, and fibrocartilage.
- Name and characterize the function of the four types of bone cells.
- State the function of parathyroid hormone, calcitonin, and vitamin D in terms of bone formation and metabolism.

The skeletal system consists of the axial and appendicular skeleton. The *axial skeleton*, which is composed of the bones of the skull, thorax, and vertebral column, forms the axis of the body. The *appendicular skeleton* consists of the bones of the upper and lower extremities, including the shoulder and hip. The skeletal system contains both bone and cartilage tissue. Bones provide protection for internal organs and rigid support for the extremities. Cartilage provides flexibility for and cushioning of bony structures and for prenatal and postnatal skeletal development.

Bone Structures

There are two types of mature bones: cortical and cancellous bone (Fig. 47.1). Cortical (compact) bone comprises 80% of the skeleton and forms the outer shell of a bone; it has a densely packed, calcified intercellular matrix that makes it more rigid than cancellous bone.[1] Cancellous (spongy) bone is found in the interior of bones and is composed of *trabeculae* and *spicules*, of bone that form a lattice-like pattern.[1] These lattice-like structures are lined with osteogenic cells and filled with red or yellow bone marrow. Cancellous bone is relatively light, but its structure is such that it has considerable tensile strength and weight-bearing properties. Although bones contain both cancellous and cortical elements, their proportions vary in different bones throughout the body and in different parts of the same bone, depending on the relative needs for strength and lightness. Cortical bone is the major component of tubular bones. It is also found along the lines of stress on long bones and forms an outer protective shell on other bones.

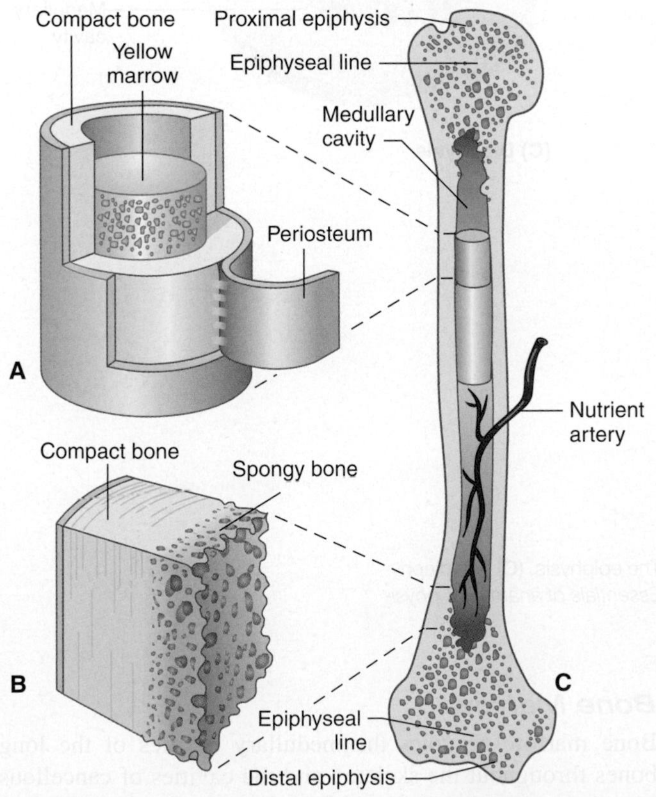

Figure 47.1 • A long bone shown in longitudinal section. **(A)** Periosteum and bone marrow. **(B)** Compact and cancellous bone. **(C)** Epiphysis and source of blood supply from epiphyseal and nutrient arteries.

> **KEY POINTS**
>
> **THE SKELETAL SYSTEM**
>
> - Two types of connective tissue are found in the skeletal system: (1) cartilage, a semirigid and slightly flexible structure that plays an essential role in prenatal and childhood skeletal development and as a surface for the articulating ends of skeletal joints and (2) bone, which provides for the firm structure of the skeleton and serves as a reservoir for calcium and phosphate storage.
> - Bone matrix is maintained by four types of cells: osteoblasts, which synthesize and secrete the constituents of bone; osteoclasts, which resorb surplus bone and are required for bone remodeling; osteocytes, which make up the osteoid tissue of bone; and osteoprogenitor cells, which are the source of all bone cells, except osteoclasts.

Types of Bones

Bones are classified by shape as long, short, flat, or irregular. *Long bones* are found in the upper and lower extremities. *Short bones* are irregularly shaped bones located in the ankle and the wrist. Except for their surface, which is compact bone, these bones are spongy throughout. *Flat bones* are composed of a layer of cancellous bone between two layers of compact bone.[2] They are found in areas such as the skull and rib cage, where extensive protection of underlying structures is needed, or, as in the scapula, where a broad surface for muscle attachment must be provided. *Irregular bones*, because of their shapes, cannot be classified in any of the previous groups. This group includes bones such as the vertebrae and ethmoid bone.[2]

A typical long bone has a shaft, or *diaphysis*, and two ends, called *epiphyses* (Fig. 47.2). Long bones usually are narrow in the midportion and broad at the ends so weight can be distributed over a wider surface. The shaft of a long bone is formed mainly of compact bone roughly hollowed out to form a marrow-filled medullary canal.[2] The ends of long bones are covered with articular cartilage.[2]

In growing bones, the part of the bone shaft that funnels out as it approaches the epiphysis is called the *metaphysis*.[2] It is composed of bony trabeculae that have cores of cartilage.[2] In the child, the epiphysis is separated from the metaphysis by the cartilaginous growth plate. After puberty, the metaphysis and epiphysis merge, and the growth plate is obliterated.[2]

Periosteum and Endosteum

The *periosteum* covers the bones, except at their articular ends (see Fig. 47.1). The periosteum has an outer fibrous layer and an inner layer that contains the osteoprogenitor cells needed for bone growth and development.[3] The periosteum contains

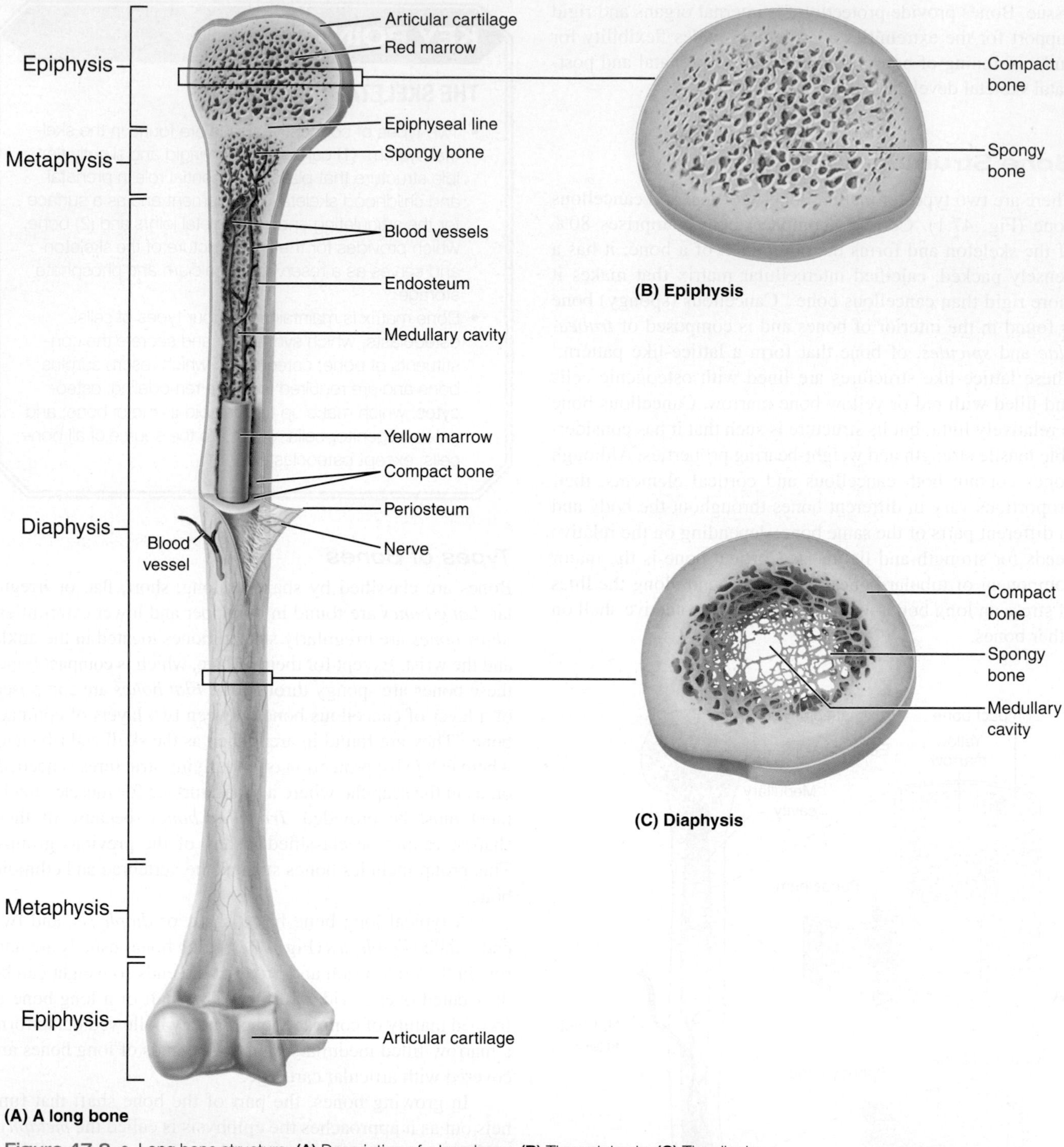

Figure 47.2 • Long bone structure. **(A)** Description of a long bone. **(B)** The epiphysis. **(C)** The diaphysis. (From McConnell T. H., Hull K. L. (2011). *Human form, human function: Essentials of anatomy & physiology* (p. 169, Figure 6–3). Philadelphia, PA: Lippincott Williams & Wilkins.)

blood vessels and acts as an anchor for vessels as they enter and exit the bone. The endosteum is the membrane that lines the spaces of spongy bone, the marrow cavities, and the Haversian canals of cortical bone. It is composed mainly of osteoprogenitor cells that contribute to the growth and remodeling of bone and are necessary for bone repair.[2]

Bone Marrow

Bone marrow occupies the medullary cavities of the long bones throughout the skeleton and the cavities of cancellous bone in the vertebrae, ribs, sternum, and flat bones of the pelvis. The cellular composition of the bone marrow varies with age and skeletal location. Red bone marrow contains developing red blood cells and is the site of blood cell formation. Yellow bone marrow is composed largely of adipose cells.[3] At birth, nearly all marrow is red and hematopoietically active. As the need for red blood cell production decreases during postnatal life, red marrow is gradually replaced with yellow bone marrow in most of the bones.

Concept Mastery Alert

In the adult, red marrow persists in the vertebrae, ribs, sternum, and ilia.

Blood Supply

The cortical bone of long tubular bones receives blood supply from two sources, nutrient and perforating arteries. The nutrient arteries enter the bone through a nutrient foramen and supply the marrow space and the internal one half of the cortex.[4] The perforating arteries are small arteries that extend inward from the periosteal arteries on the external surface of the periosteum and anastomose in the cortex with branches of the nutrient arteries coming from the bone marrow.[4] The distribution of blood in the cortex occurs through the Haversian and Volkmann canals (Fig. 47.3). Haversian canals are spaces in the bone of the cortex that move parallel through the long axis of the bone for a short distance and then branch and communicate with other, similar canals. Each canal carries one or two blood vessels, lymphatics, and some nerve fibers.[4] Volkmann canals, which also contain blood vessels, are spaces in the cortex that run perpendicular to the long axis of the cortex to connect adjacent Haversian canals.[4]

Cancellous bone is usually not penetrated by blood vessels. Instead, the bone cells of cancellous bone are nourished by diffusion from the endosteal surface through canaliculi, which interconnect their surrounding fluid-filled lacunae and extend to the bone surface.

Bone Tissue

Bone is connective tissue in which the intercellular matrix has been impregnated with inorganic calcium salts so that it has great tensile and compressive strength but is light enough to be moved by coordinated muscle contractions. The intercellular matrix is composed of two types of substances—organic matter, which includes bone cells, blood vessels, and nerves, and inorganic salts.

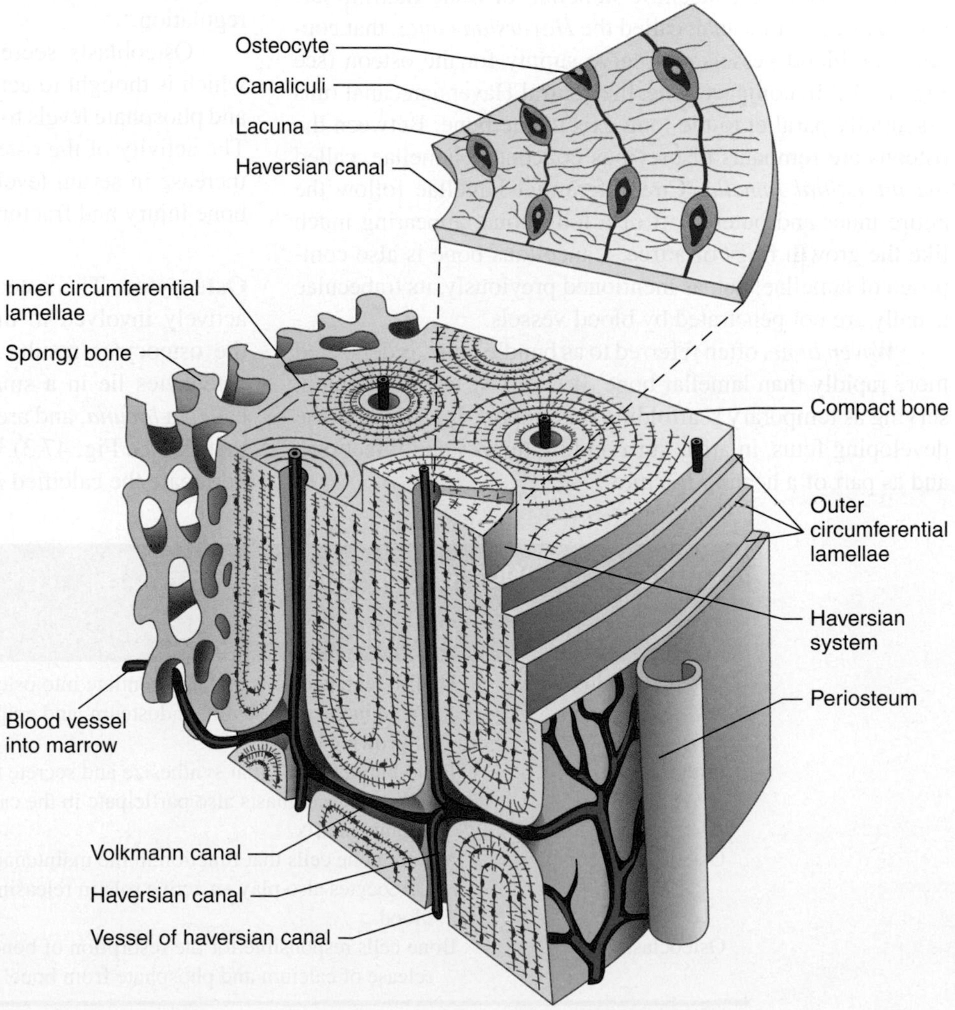

Figure 47.3 • Haversian systems as seen in a wedge of compact bone tissue. The periosteum has been peeled back to show a blood vessel entering a Volkmann canal. **Top,** Osteocytes lying within lacunae; canaliculi permit interstitial fluid to reach each lacuna.

The organic matter consists of 88% type I collagen, 10% other proteins, and 1% to 2% lipids and glycosaminoglycans.[4] The inorganic matter consists of hydroxyapatite, an insoluble macrocrystalline structure of calcium phosphate salts [$Ca_{10}(PO_4)_6(OH)_2$], and small amounts of calcium carbonate and calcium fluoride.[5] Bone may also take up lead and other heavy metals, thereby removing these toxic substances from the circulation. This can be viewed as a protective mechanism. An example of this would be the antibiotic tetracycline being readily bound to calcium deposited in newly formed bones and teeth. When tetracycline is given during pregnancy, it can be deposited in the teeth of the fetus, causing discoloration and deformity. Similar changes can occur if the drug is given for long periods to children younger than 6 years of age.

Lamellar and Woven Bone

There are two types of bone tissue: lamellar bone and woven bone. Both forms of bone can be mineralized or unmineralized, the latter being referred to as *osteoid*.[4] *Lamellar bone* is a strong, mature form of bone that is formed slowly and is highly organized. It is the mature bone found in the adult skeleton. In the adult skeleton, it would be abnormal to observe anything other than lamellar bone.[4] Lamellar bone is composed largely of cylindrical units called *osteons* or *Haversian systems*.[4] The osteons consist of concentric lamellae of bone matrix, surrounding a central canal, called the *Haversian canal*, that contains the blood vessels and nerve supply for the osteon (see Fig. 47.3).[4] In compact bone, the central Haversian canal runs essentially parallel to the long axis of the bone. Between the osteons are remnants of previous concentric lamellae, called the *interstitial lamella*. Circumferential lamellae follow the entire inner and outer shaft of a long bone, appearing much like the growth rings of a tree. Cancellous bone is also composed of lamellae, but, as mentioned previously, its trabeculae usually are not penetrated by blood vessels.

Woven bone, often referred to as bundle bone, is deposited more rapidly than lamellar bone. It is of low tensile strength, serving as temporary scaffolding for support. It is found in the developing fetus, in areas surrounding tumors and infections, and as part of a healing fracture.[4]

Bone Cells

Four types of bone cells participate in the formation and maintenance of bone tissue: osteoprogenitor cells, osteoblasts, osteocytes, and osteoclasts (Table 47.1).

Osteoprogenitor Cells. The undifferentiated osteoprogenitor cells are found in the periosteum, endosteum, and epiphyseal plate of growing bone.[4] These cells differentiate into osteoblasts and are active during normal growth. They may also be activated in adult life during healing of fractures and other injuries. Osteoprogenitor cells also participate in the continual replacement of worn-out bone tissue.[4]

Osteoblasts. The osteoblasts, or bone-building cells, are responsible for the formation of the bone matrix. Bone formation occurs in two stages: ossification and calcification. Ossification involves the formation of osteoid, or prebone. Calcification of bone involves the deposition of calcium salts in the osteoid tissue. The osteoblasts synthesize collagen and other proteins that make up osteoid tissue. They also participate in the calcification process of the osteoid tissue, probably by controlling the availability of calcium and phosphate. In addition, the osteoblasts secrete many growth factors and tumor necrosis factor, which are needed for bone growth regulation.[4]

Osteoblasts secrete the enzyme *alkaline phosphatase*, which is thought to act locally in bone tissue to raise calcium and phosphate levels to the point at which precipitation occurs. The activity of the osteoblasts undoubtedly contributes to the increase in serum levels of alkaline phosphatase that follows bone injury and fractures.

Osteocytes. The osteocytes are mature bone cells that are actively involved in maintaining the bony matrix. Death of the osteocytes results in the resorption of this matrix. The osteocytes lie in a small lake filled with extracellular fluid, called a *lacuna*, and are surrounded by a calcified intercellular matrix (see Fig. 47.3).[2] Extracellular fluid-filled passageways permeate the calcified matrix and connect with the lacunae of

TABLE 47.1 FUNCTION OF BONE CELLS

TYPE OF BONE CELL	FUNCTION
Osteoprogenitor cells	Undifferentiated cells that differentiate into osteoblasts. They are found in the periosteum, endosteum, and epiphyseal growth plate of growing bones.
Osteoblasts	Bone-building cells that synthesize and secrete the organic matrix of bone. Osteoblasts also participate in the calcification of the organic matrix.
Osteocytes	Mature bone cells that function in the maintenance of bone matrix. Osteocytes also play an active role in releasing calcium into the blood.
Osteoclasts	Bone cells responsible for the resorption of bone matrix and the release of calcium and phosphate from bone.

adjacent osteocytes. These passageways are called *canaliculi*. Because diffusion does not occur through the calcified matrix of bone, the canaliculi serve as communicating channels for the exchange of nutrients and metabolites between the osteocytes and the blood vessels on the surface of the bone layer.

Osteoclasts. Osteoclasts are "bone-chewing" cells that function in the resorption of bone, removing the mineral content and the organic matrix. They are large phagocytic cells of monocyte/macrophage lineage. Although the mechanism of osteoclast formation and activation remains elusive, it is known that parathyroid hormone (PTH) increases the number and resorptive function of the osteoclasts. Calcitonin is thought to reduce the number and resorptive function of the osteoclasts. Estrogen also reduces the number and function of the osteoclasts. Thus, the decrease in estrogen levels that occurs at menopause results in increased resorption of bone. The mechanism whereby osteoclasts exert their resorptive effect on bone is unclear.

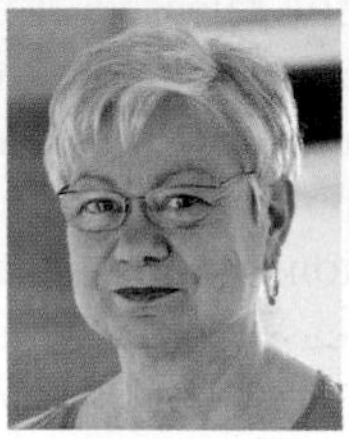

Remember **Mrs. Tukey** from the unit opener case study? At 68 years of age and postmenopausal, Mrs. Tukey more than likely has little to no estrogen left; she has been diagnosed with osteoporosis. She is experiencing an increase in bone resorption to the point where she has actually experienced a lumbar vertebral 5 fracture.

These cells may secrete an acid that removes calcium from the bone matrix, releasing the collagenic fibers for digestion by osteoclasts or mononuclear cells. Osteoclasts, by virtue of their phagocytic lineage, also ingest minute particles of bone matrix and crystals, eventually dissolving and releasing them into the blood.

Cartilage

Cartilage is an essential part of the skeletal system. It constitutes the articular cartilage of joints. It is found in the tendinous and ligamentous insertions, menisci, the symphysis pubis, and insertions of joint capsules. It is also essential for growth before and after birth. In the embryo, most of the axial and appendicular skeleton is formed first as a cartilage model and then replaced by bone. In postnatal life, cartilage continues to play an essential role in the growth of long bones and persists as articular cartilage in the adult.

As a tissue, cartilage both resembles and differs from bone. Both of these connective tissue types consist of living cells, nonliving intercellular fibers, and an amorphous ground substance. The tissue cells are responsible for secreting and maintaining the intercellular substances in which they are housed. However, cartilage consists of more extracellular substance than bone, and its fibers are embedded in a firm gel rather than a calcified cement-like substance.[2] Hence, cartilage has the flexibility of a firm plastic material rather than the rigid characteristics of bone. In fact, articular cartilage has many advantageous characteristics and is considered resilient. Although resilient, it has poor healing properties and is challenging to repair when injured.[6]

There are three types of cartilage: elastic cartilage, hyaline cartilage, and fibrocartilage.[4] *Elastic cartilage* contains some elastin in its intercellular substance. It is found in areas, such as the ear, where some flexibility is important. Pure cartilage is called *hyaline cartilage* (from a Greek word meaning "glass") and is pearly white. It is opaque and seen on the articulating ends of fresh soup bones found in the supermarket. *Fibrocartilage* has characteristics that are between dense connective tissue and hyaline cartilage. It is found in the intervertebral disks, areas where tendons are connected to bone, and the symphysis pubis.[4] In pregnancy, the flexibility of the fibrocartilage allows the symphysis pubis to widen.[7]

Hyaline cartilage is the most abundant type of cartilage. It forms much of the cartilage of the fetal skeleton. In the adult, hyaline cartilage forms the costal cartilages that join the ribs to the sternum and vertebrae, many of the cartilages of the respiratory tract, the articular cartilages, and the epiphyseal plates.

Cartilage cells, which are called *chondrocytes*, are located in lacunae. The lacunae are surrounded by an uncalcified, gellike intercellular matrix of collagen fibers and ground substance. Cartilage is devoid of blood vessels and nerves.[3] The free surfaces of most hyaline cartilage, with the exception of articular cartilage, are covered by a layer of fibrous connective tissue called the *perichondrium*.

It has been estimated that approximately 80% of the wet weight of cartilage is water held in its gel structure. Because cartilage has no blood vessels, this tissue fluid allows the diffusion of gases, nutrients, and wastes between the chondrocytes and blood vessels outside the cartilage.[4] Diffusion cannot take place if the cartilage matrix becomes impregnated with calcium salts, and cartilage dies if it becomes calcified. The other 20% of cartilage consists of two types of macromolecules: type II collagen and proteoglycans.[4]

Hormonal Control of Bone Formation and Metabolism

The process of bone formation and mineral metabolism is complex. It involves the interplay among the actions of PTH, calcitonin, and vitamin D. Other hormones, such as cortisol, growth hormone, thyroid hormone, and the sex hormones, also influence bone formation directly or indirectly (Table 47.2).

Parathyroid Hormone

PTH is an important regulator of calcium and phosphate levels in the blood.[5] Additionally, PTH has been found to be advantageous in fracture healing and prevention of further deterioration of osteoporosis if given as a supplement.[8,9] PTH prevents serum calcium levels from falling below and serum phosphate levels from rising above normal physiologic

TABLE 47.2 ACTIONS OF PARATHYROID HORMONE, CALCITONIN, AND VITAMIN D

ACTIONS	PARATHYROID HORMONE	CALCITONIN	VITAMIN D
Intestinal absorption of calcium	Increases indirectly through increased activation of vitamin D	Probably not affected	Increases
Intestinal absorption of phosphate	Increases	Probably not affected	Increases
Renal excretion of calcium	Decreases	Increases	Probably increases, but less effective than PTH
Renal excretion of phosphate	Increases	Increases	Increases
Bone resorption	Increases	Decreases	1,25-$(OH)_2D_3$ increases
Bone formation	Decreases	Uncertain	24,25-$(OH)_2D_3$ increases (?)
Serum calcium levels	Produces a prompt increase	Decreases with pharmacologic doses	No effect
Serum phosphate levels	Prevents an increase	Decreases with pharmacologic doses	No effect

concentrations.[5] The secretion of PTH is regulated by negative feedback; increased serum levels of ionized calcium inhibit PTH release. PTH maintains serum calcium levels by initiation of calcium release from bone, by conservation of calcium by the kidney, by enhanced intestinal absorption of calcium through activation of vitamin D, and by reduction of serum phosphate levels (Fig. 47.4).[2,4] PTH also increases the movement of calcium and phosphate from bone into the extracellular fluid. Calcium is immediately released from the canaliculi and bone cells. A more prolonged release of calcium and phosphate is mediated by increased osteoclast activity. In the kidney, PTH stimulates tubular reabsorption of calcium while reducing the reabsorption of phosphate. The latter effect ensures that increased release of phosphate from bone during mobilization of calcium does not produce an elevation in serum phosphate levels. This is important because an increase in calcium and phosphate levels could lead to crystallization in soft tissues. PTH increases intestinal absorption of calcium because of its ability to stimulate activation of vitamin D by the kidney.

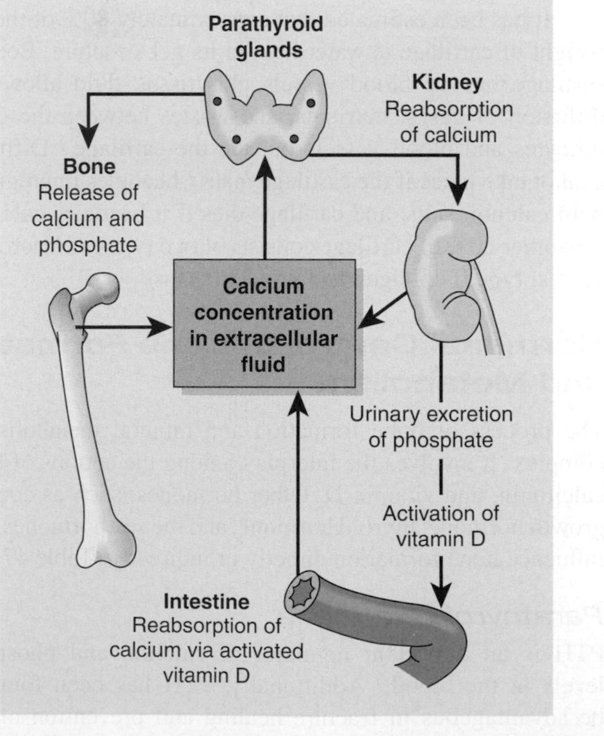

Figure 47.4 • Regulation and actions of PTH. The PTH drives the serum calcium level by triggering release of calcium from the bone, appropriately conserving calcium by the kidney, and by further increasing calcium in the intestine by activating vitamin D.

Calcitonin

Whereas PTH increases blood calcium levels, the hormone calcitonin lowers blood calcium levels.[5] Calcitonin, sometimes called *thyrocalcitonin*, is secreted by the parafollicular, or C cells of the thyroid gland. Calcitonin inhibits the release of calcium from bone into the extracellular fluid.[5] It is thought to act by causing calcium to sequester in bone cells and inhibiting osteoclast activity. Calcitonin also reduces the renal tubular reabsorption of calcium and phosphate; the decrease in serum calcium level that follows administration of pharmacologic doses of calcitonin may be related to this action.[2]

The major stimulus for calcitonin synthesis and release is an increase in serum calcium.[5] The role of calcitonin in overall mineral homeostasis is uncertain. There are no clearly definable syndromes of calcitonin deficiency or excess, which suggests that calcitonin does not directly alter calcium metabolism. It has been suggested that the physiologic actions of calcitonin are related to the postprandial handling and processing of dietary calcium. This theory proposes that after meals, calcitonin maintains PTH secretion at a time when it normally would be reduced by calcium entering the blood from the digestive tract. Although states of excess or deficiency associated with alterations in physiologic levels of calcitonin have not been observed, it has been shown that pharmacologic doses of the hormone reduce osteoclastic activity. Because of this action, calcitonin has proved effective in the treatment of Paget disease. The hormone is also used to reduce serum calcium levels during hypercalcemic crises.

Vitamin D

Vitamin D and its metabolites are not true vitamins but steroid hormones. There are two forms of vitamin D: vitamin D_2 (ergocalciferol) and vitamin D_3 (cholecalciferol).[5] The two forms differ by the presence of a double bond, but they have identical biologic activity. The term *vitamin D* is used to indicate both forms. Vitamin D is an important hormone, and its role in the body, beyond Vitamin D deficiency diseases such as rickets and osteomalacia, is being researched extensively.[10]

Vitamin D has little or no activity until it has been converted to be physiologically active and metabolized to compounds that mediate its activity. Figure 47.5 depicts sources of vitamin D and pathways for activation. The first step of the activation process occurs in the liver, where vitamin D is hydroxylated to form the metabolite 25-hydroxyvitamin D_3 [25-(OH)D_3].[5] From the liver, 25-(OH)D_3 is transported to the kidneys, where it undergoes conversion to 1,25-dihydroxyvitamin D_3 [1,25-$(OH)_2D_3$] or 24,25-dihydroxyvitamin D_3 [24,25-$(OH)_2D_3$].[5] Other metabolites of vitamin D have been and still are being discovered.

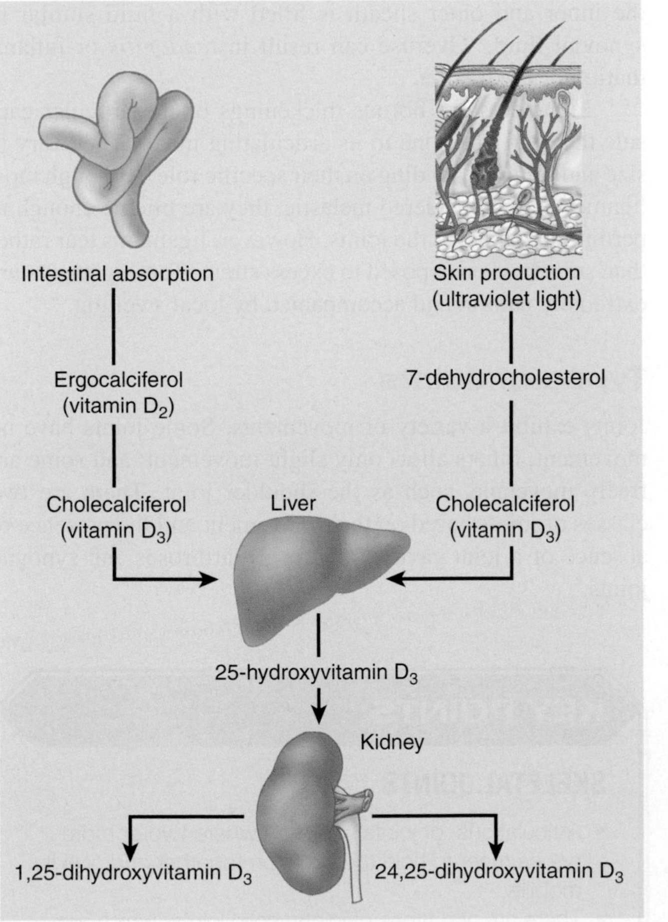

Figure 47.5 • Sources and pathways for activation of vitamin D. The vitamin D source comes from the skin and the intestine. Vitamin D is then hydroxylated into 25-hydroxyvitamin D_3 in the liver and then goes to the kidneys where it is converted into 24,25-dihydroxyvitamin D_3.

The two sources of vitamin D are intestinal absorption and skin production. Intestinal absorption occurs mainly in the jejunum and includes vitamin D_2 and vitamin D_3. The most important dietary sources of vitamin D are fish, liver, and irradiated milk. Because vitamin D is fat soluble, its absorption is mediated by bile salts and occurs by means of the lymphatic vessels.[5] In the skin, ultraviolet radiation from sunlight spontaneously converts 7-dehydrocholesterol D_3 to vitamin D_3. A circulating vitamin D–binding protein provides a mechanism to remove vitamin D from the skin and make it available to the rest of the body.

With adequate exposure to sunlight, the amount of vitamin D that can be produced by the skin is usually sufficient to meet physiologic requirements. The importance of sunlight exposure is evidenced by population studies that report lower vitamin D levels in countries such as England, that have less sunlight than the United States. Older adults who are housebound or institutionalized frequently have low vitamin D levels. The deficiency often goes undetected until there are problems such as pseudofractures or electrolyte imbalances. Seasonal variations in vitamin D levels probably reflect changes in sunlight exposure.

The most potent of the vitamin D metabolites is 1,25-$(OH)_2D_3$.[5] This metabolite increases intestinal absorption of calcium and promotes the actions of PTH on resorption of calcium and phosphate from bone.[5] Bone resorption by the osteoclasts is increased, and bone formation by the osteoblasts is decreased. There is also an increase in acid phosphatase and a decrease in alkaline phosphatase. Intestinal absorption and bone resorption increase the amount of calcium and phosphorus available to the mineralizing surface of the bone. The role of 24,25-$(OH)_2D_3$ is less clear. There is evidence that 24,25-$(OH)_2D_3$, in conjunction with 1,25-$(OH)_2D_3$, may be involved in normal bone mineralization.

Several hormones influence the regulation of vitamin D activity. PTH and prolactin stimulate 1,25-$(OH)_2D_3$ production by the kidney. States of hyperparathyroidism are associated with increased levels of 1,25-$(OH)_2D_3$, and hypoparathyroidism leads to lowered levels of this metabolite.[5] Prolactin may have an ancillary role in regulating vitamin D metabolism during pregnancy and lactation. Calcitonin inhibits 1,25-$(OH)_2D_3$ production by the kidneys. In addition to hormonal influences, changes in the concentration of ions such as calcium, phosphate, hydrogen, and potassium exert an effect on 1,25-$(OH)_2D_3$ and 24,25-$(OH)_2D_3$ production. Under conditions of phosphate and calcium deprivation, 1,25-$(OH)_2D_3$ levels are increased, whereas hyperphosphatemia and hypercalcemia decrease the levels of metabolite.

IN SUMMARY

Skeletal tissue consists of the bones and cartilage that form the appendicular and axial skeleton. There are two types of bone: cortical or compact bone, which forms the outer shell of a bone, and cancellous or spongy bone that forms the interior. The endosteum is the membrane that lines the spaces of spongy bone, the marrow cavities, and the Haversian canals of cortical bone. The periosteum, the membrane that covers bones, contains blood vessels and acts as an anchor for vessels as they enter and leave the bone. Mature bone is largely made up of cylindrical units called *osteons*, formed from concentric layers or lamellae of bone matrix and surrounding a central *Haversian canal*. The Haversian canals contain the blood vessels and nerve supply for the osteon. There are four types of bone cells: osteocytes, or mature bone cells; osteoblasts, or bone-building cells; osteoclasts, which function in bone resorption; and osteoprogenitor cells, which differentiate into osteoblasts.

Cartilage is a firm, flexible type of skeletal tissue that is essential for growth before and after birth. There are three types of cartilage: elastic, hyaline, and fibrocartilage. Hyaline cartilage, the most abundant type, forms the costal cartilages that join the ribs to the sternum and vertebrae, many of the cartilages of the respiratory tract, and the articular cartilages.

The process of bone formation and mineral metabolism involves the interplay of PTH, calcitonin, and vitamin D. PTH acts to maintain serum levels of ionized calcium; it increases the release of calcium and phosphate from bone; the conservation of calcium and elimination of phosphate by the kidney; and the intestinal reabsorption of calcium through vitamin D. Calcitonin inhibits the release of calcium from bone and increases renal elimination of calcium and phosphate, thereby serving to lower serum calcium levels. Vitamin D functions as a hormone in regulating body calcium. It increases absorption of calcium from the intestine and promotes the actions of PTH on bone.

ARTICULATIONS AND JOINTS

After completing this section of the chapter, the learner will be able to meet the following objectives:

- Describe the source of blood supply to a synovial joint.
- Explain why pain is often experienced in all the joints of an extremity when a disease process affects only a single joint.

Articulations, or joints, are areas where two or more bones meet. The term *arthro* is the prefix used to designate a joint; for example, *arthrology* is the study of joints, and *arthroplasty* is the repair of a joint.

Tendons and Ligaments

In the skeletal system, tendons and ligaments are dense connective tissue structures that connect muscles and bones. The dense connective tissue found in tendons and ligaments has a limited blood supply and is composed largely of intercellular bundles of collagen fibers arranged in the same direction and plane (Fig. 47.6). Collagen is a strong, flexible protein.[2] Because of its molecular configuration, collagen has great tensile strength; the breaking point of collagenous fibers found in human tendons is reached with a force of several hundred kilograms per square centimeter. Fresh collagen is colorless, and tissues that contain large numbers of collagenous fibers generally appear white.

Tendons, which attach skeletal muscles to bone, are relatively inextensible because of their richness in collagen fibers. The collagen bundles of tendons aggregate into bundles that are enveloped by loose connective tissue, blood vessels, and nerves. Tendons that may rub against bone or other friction-generating surfaces are enclosed in double-layered sheaths. An outer connective tissue tube is attached to the structures surrounding the tendon, and an inner sheath encloses the tendon and is attached to it.[3] The space between the inner and outer sheath is filled with a fluid similar to synovial fluid.[3] Overuse can result in *tendonitis* or inflammation of the tendon.

Ligaments are fibrous thickenings of the articular capsule that join one bone to its articulating mate.[3] They vary in size and shape depending on their specific role. Although most ligaments are considered inelastic, they are pliable enough to permit movement at the joints. However, ligaments tear rather than stretch when exposed to excess stress. Torn ligaments are extremely painful and accompanied by local swelling.

Types of Joints

Joints exhibit a variety of movements. Some joints have no movement; others allow only slight movement; and some are freely moveable, such as the shoulder joint. There are two classes of joints based on their movement and the presence or absence of a joint cavity: solid or synarthroses and synovial joints.[4]

KEY POINTS

SKELETAL JOINTS

- Articulations, or joints, are sites where two or more bones meet to hold the skeleton together and give it mobility.
- There are two types of joints: solid joints, which are immovable, have no cavity, and are bound by connective tissue or cartilage, and synovial joints, which are freely movable and contain a cavity.[11]

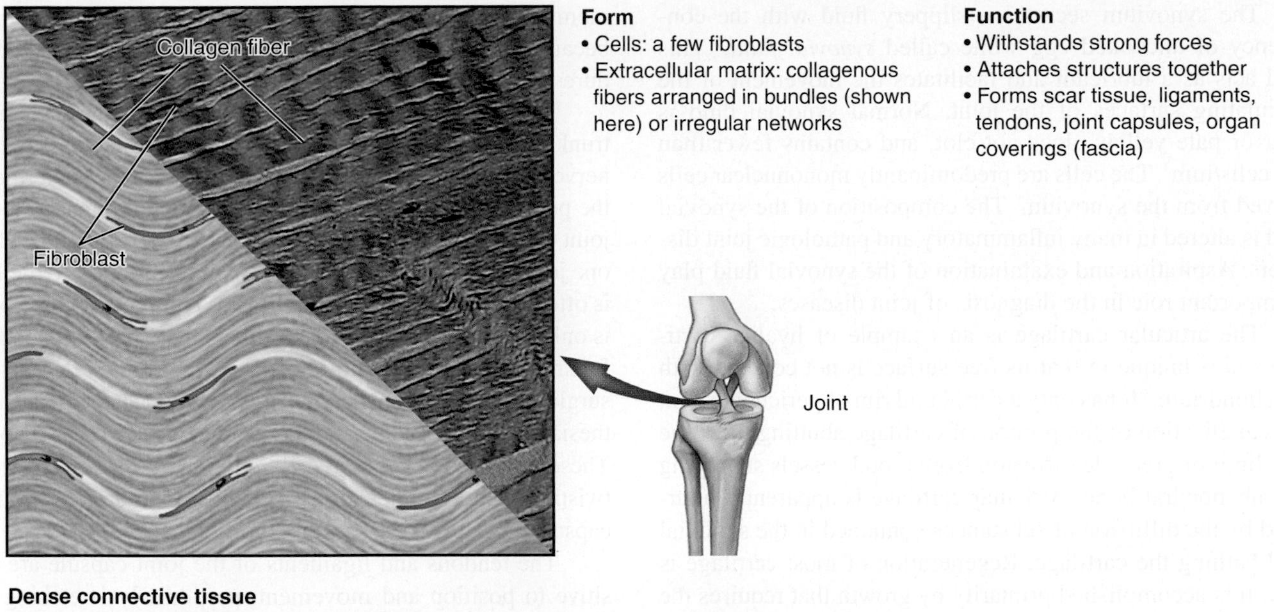

Figure 47.6 • Dense connective tissue in tendons and ligaments. This dense connective tissue shows the collagen fibrous tissue and the fibroblasts. Both of these types of cells withstand strong forces and are found in tendons and ligaments. (From McConnell T. H., Hull K. (2011). *Human form, human function: Essentials of anatomy & physiology* (p. 104). Philadelphia, PA: Lippincott Williams & Wilkins.)

Solid or Synarthroses Joints

Solid joints, also called synarthroses, are either fibrous or cartilaginous.[12] The fibrous joints are divided into sutures, gomphoses, and syndesmoses. Sutures are only found in the skull. Gomphoses connect teeth to the jaw. Syndesmoses are where a ligament connects two adjacent bones. These include the ligamentum flavum, which connect vertebral laminae, and the interosseous membrane that connect the radius and ulna in the forearm. Cartilaginous joints can be divided into synchondroses and symphyses. Synchondroses are where a layer of cartilage separates two ossification centers in a developing bone such as the growth plate found in developing long bone. These are designed for bone growth and eventually ossify. Symphyses are joints in which two separate bones are connected by cartilage. These include the pubic symphysis intervertebral discs.[13]

Synovial (Diarthrodial) Joints

Synovial or diarthrodial joints are freely movable.[3] Most joints in the body are of this type. Although they are classified as freely movable, their movement ranges from almost none (*e.g.*, sacroiliac joint), to simple hinge movement (*e.g.*, interphalangeal joint), to movement in many planes (*e.g.*, shoulder or hip joint). The bony surfaces of these joints are covered with thin layers of articular cartilage, and the cartilaginous surfaces of these joints slide past each other during movement. Diarthrodial joints are the joints most frequently affected by rheumatic disorders.

In a diarthrodial joint, the articulating ends of the bones are not connected directly but are indirectly linked by a strong fibrous capsule (*i.e.*, joint capsule) that surrounds the joint and is continuous with the periosteum (Fig. 47.7). This capsule supports the joint and helps to hold the bones in place. Additional support may be provided by ligaments that extend between the bones of the joint.

The joint capsule consists of two layers: an outer fibrous layer and an inner membrane, the synovium.[3] The synovium surrounds the tendons that pass through the joints and the free margins of other intra-articular structures such as ligaments and menisci. The synovium forms folds that surround the margins of articulations but do not cover the weight-bearing articular cartilage. These folds permit stretching of the synovium so that movement can occur without tissue damage.

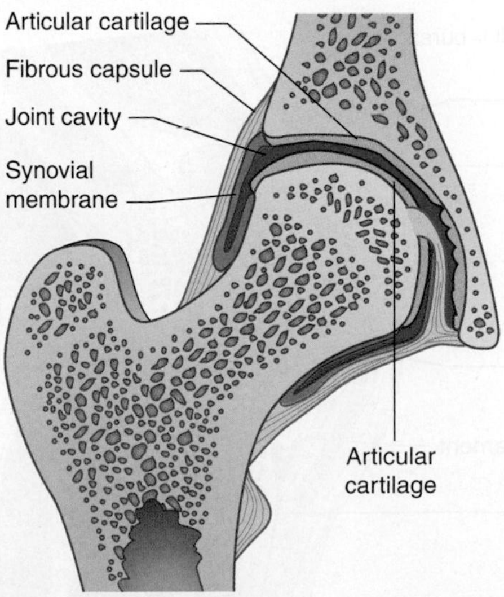

Figure 47.7 • Synovial (diarthrodial) joint, showing the articular cartilage, fibrous joint capsule, joint cavity, and synovial membrane.

The synovium secretes a slippery fluid with the consistency of uncooked egg white called *synovial fluid*.[3] This fluid acts as a lubricant and facilitates the movement of the articulating surfaces of the joint. Normal synovial fluid is clear or pale yellow, does not clot, and contains fewer than 100 cells/mm^3. The cells are predominantly mononuclear cells derived from the synovium. The composition of the synovial fluid is altered in many inflammatory and pathologic joint disorders. Aspiration and examination of the synovial fluid play an important role in the diagnosis of joint diseases.

The articular cartilage is an example of hyaline cartilage and is unique in that its free surface is not covered with perichondrium.[3] It has only a peripheral rim of perichondrium, and calcification of the portion of cartilage abutting the bone may limit or preclude diffusion from blood vessels supplying the subchondral bone. Articular cartilage is apparently nourished by the diffusion of substances contained in the synovial fluid bathing the cartilage. Regeneration of most cartilage is slow. It is accomplished primarily by growth that requires the activity of perichondrium cells. In articular cartilage, which has no perichondrium, superficial injuries heal slowly.

Blood Supply and Innervation

All the tissues of synovial joints, except the articulating surfaces of the articulating cartilage, receive nourishment either directly or indirectly from blood vessels.[14] The articulating areas are nourished indirectly by the synovial fluid that is distributed over the surface of the articular cartilage.

The blood supply to a joint arises from blood vessels that enter the subchondral bone at or near the attachment of the joint capsule and form an arterial circle around the joint. The synovial membrane has a rich blood supply, and constituents of plasma diffuse rapidly between these vessels and the joint cavity. Because many of the capillaries are near the surface of the synovium, blood may escape into the synovial fluid after relatively minor injuries. Healing and repair of the synovial membrane are usually rapid and complete. This is important because synovial tissue is often injured during surgical procedures that involve the joint.

The nerve supply to joints is provided by the same nerve trunks that supply the muscles that move the joints. These nerve trunks also supply the skin over the joints. As a rule, all the peripheral nerves that cross the articulation innervate each joint of an extremity. This accounts for the referral of pain from one joint to another. For example, pain from injury to the knee is often experienced as pain in the hip. The synovial membrane is only innervated by autonomic fibers that control blood flow. It is relatively free of pain fibers, as evidenced by the fact that surgical procedures on the joint are often done under local anesthesia. The joint capsule and the ligaments have pain receptors. These receptors are more easily stimulated by stretching and twisting than are other joint structures. Pain arising from the capsule tends to be diffuse and poorly localized.

The tendons and ligaments of the joint capsule are sensitive to position and movement, particularly stretching and twisting.[14] These structures are supplied by the large sensory nerve fibers that form proprioceptor endings. The proprioceptors function reflexively to adjust the tension of the muscles that support the joint and are particularly important in maintaining muscular support for the joint. For example, when a weight is lifted, there is a proprioceptor-mediated reflex contraction and relaxation of appropriate muscle groups to support the joint and protect the joint capsule and other joint structures. Loss of proprioception and reflex control of muscular support leads to destructive changes in the joint.

Bursae

In some diarthrotic joints, the synovial membrane forms closed sacs that are not part of the joint. These sacs, called *bursae*, contain synovial fluid.[3] Their purpose is to prevent friction on a tendon. Bursae occur in areas where pressure is exerted because of close approximation of joint structures (Fig. 47.8).

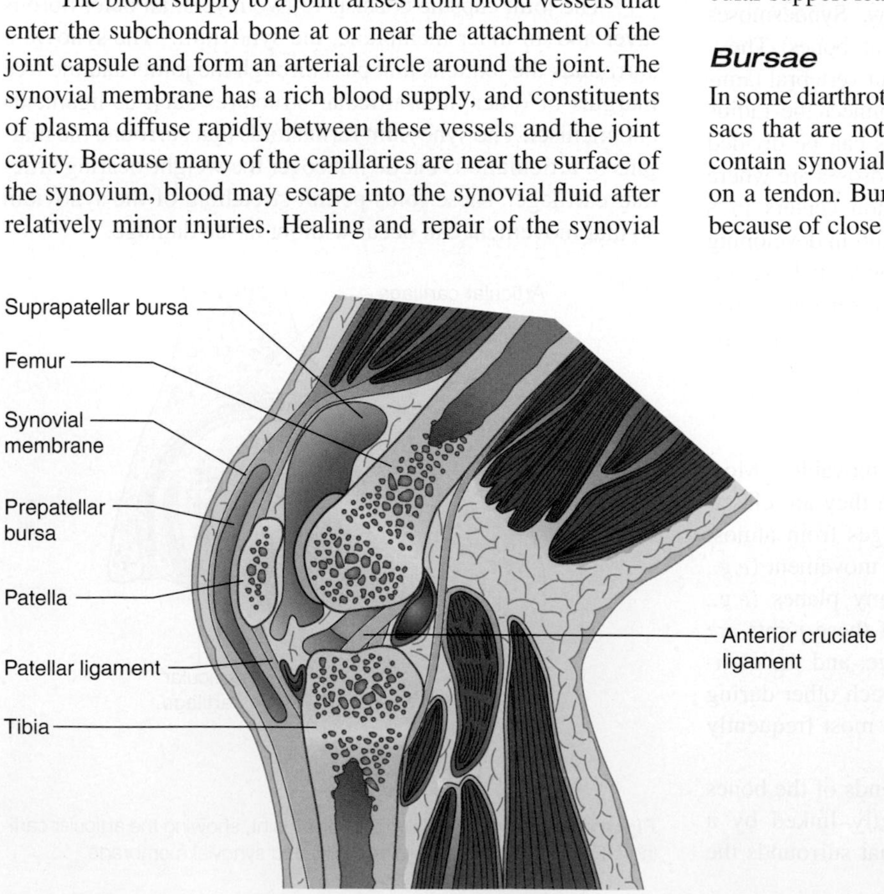

Figure 47.8 • Sagittal section of knee joint, showing prepatellar and suprapatellar bursae.

Such conditions occur when tendons are deflected over bone or where skin must move freely over bony tissue. Bursae may become injured or inflamed, causing discomfort, swelling, and limitation in movement of the involved area.[3] A bunion is an inflamed bursa of the metatarsophalangeal joint of the great toe.

Intra-Articular Menisci

Intra-articular menisci are fibrocartilage structures that occur in some synovial joints. In the joint capsule, fibrocartilage grows inward to create a pad between articulating bones.[3] Menisci may extend part way through the joint and have a free inner border, as at the lateral and medial articular surfaces of the knee, or they may extend through the joint, separating it into two separate cavities, as in the sternoclavicular joint. The menisci of the knee joint may be torn as the result of an injury.

IN SUMMARY

Articulations or joints are areas where two or more bones meet. Tendons and ligaments are dense connective tissue structures that connect muscles and bones. Tendons connect muscles to bones and ligaments connect the movable bones of joints.

Synarthroses are joints in which bones are joined together by fibrous tissue, cartilage, or bone; they lack a joint cavity and have little or no movement. Synovial or diarthrodial joints are freely movable. The surfaces of the articulating ends of bones in synovial joints are covered with a thin layer of articular cartilage, and they are enclosed in a fibrous joint capsule. The joint capsule consists of two layers: an outer fibrous layer and an inner membrane, the synovium. The synovial fluid, which is secreted by the synovium into the joint capsule, acts as a lubricant and facilitates movement of the joint's articulating surfaces. Bursae, which are closed sacs containing synovial fluid, prevent friction in areas where tendons are deflected over bone or where skin must move freely over bony tissue.

Menisci are fibrocartilaginous structures that develop from portions of the articular disk that occupied the space between articular cartilage surfaces during fetal development. The menisci may have a free inner border, or they may extend through the joint, separating it into two cavities.

GERIATRIC Considerations

- Sarcopenia, a decrease in muscle strength/mass associated with normal aging, is a leading cause of loss of independence and can lead to frailty.[15]
  - Exercise or physical activity can slow the rate of sarcopenia by increasing muscle strength and flexibility while also decreasing bone loss.[15]
- Degenerative pain in tendons associated with aging is a common cause of musculoskeletal pain. Drying of joints because of biochemical changes causes decreased movement and increased pain.[16]
- Demineralization of bone and deterioration of connective tissue and joints reduce flexibility.[16]
- Posture changes and a loss in height associated with aging are because of thinning of vertebral disks and curving of the cervical vertebrae.[16]
- Bone mineral density reduces with age causing bones to become brittle and fracture.[16]

PEDIATRIC Considerations

- Closure of the growth plate, which occurs at a unique age for each bone, is stimulated by sex hormones earlier in females than males.[4]
- Bone formation (osteogenesis) begins prior to birth.[17] Tendons, ligaments, and cartilage also develop early in the embryonic stage. All muscles, tendons, ligaments, and cartilage are functional at birth.[18]
- The skeleton of infants and children contains increased amounts of cartilage and undergoes ossification (conversion to bone) at adolescence. Fractures in children younger than 1 are unusual and may indicate need for further investigation of abuse or serious musculoskeletal disorder.[18]
- In children, new bone is added at a faster rate than old bone is removed causing bones to enlarge and become more dense.[17]
- Muscle is 25% of total weight in children compared to 40% in adults.[18]

REVIEW EXERCISES

1. Often pain from injury to the knee is experienced as pain in the hip.
   A. *Explain why this might occur.*
2. Persons with end-stage kidney disease have a deficiency of activated vitamin D.
   A. *Explain why this occurs and what effect it would have on their bones.*
3. Recent studies have revealed that estrogen deficiency as well as normal aging may produce a decrease in osteoblast activity.
   A. *Explain how this would contribute to the development of osteoporosis.*

References

1. Selitz I. A., Teven C. M., Reid R. R. (2018). Repair and grafting of bone. In Gurtner G. C., Neligan P. C. (Ed.), *Plastic surgery: Volume 1: Principles* (4th ed., pp. 18, 284–314.e.10). London/New York/Philadelphia/St. Louis/Sydney: Elsevier.
2. Ross M. H., Pawlina W. (2016). *Histology: A text and atlas: With correlated cell and molecular biology*. Philadelphia, PA: Lippincott Williams & Wilkins.
3. Saladin K. S. (2015). *Anatomy & physiology: The unity of form and function* (7th ed.). New York, NY: McGraw Hill Education.
4. Rubin R., Strayer D. (Ed.), (2012). *Rubin's pathology: Clinicopathologic foundations of medicine* (6th ed.). Philadelphia, PA: Lippincott Williams & Wilkins.
5. Hall J. E. (2016). *Guyton and Hall textbook of medical physiology* (13th ed.). Philadelphia, PA: Saunders.
6. Vinatier C., Guicheux J. (2016). Cartilage tissue engineering: From biomaterials and stem cells to osteoarthritis treatments. *Annals of Physical and Rehabilitation Medicine* 59(3), 139–144.
7. Eickmeyer S. M. (2017). Anatomy and physiology of the pelvic floor. *Physical Medicine and Rehabilitation Clinics of North America* 28, 455–460.
8. Chan K. Y., Mason A., Cooper C., et al. (2016). Novel advances in the treatment of osteoporosis. *British Medical Bulletin* 119(1), 129–142.
9. Collinge C., Favela J. (2016). Use of teriparatide in osteoporotic fracture patients. *Injury* 47(S1), s36–s38.
10. Deluca H. F., Plum L. (Ed.), (2012). The many faces of vitamin D. *Archives of Biochemistry and Biophysics* 523(1), 1–134.
11. Drake R. L., Vogl A. W., Mitchell A. W. M. (2015). *Gray's anatomy for students* (3rd ed.). Philadelphia, PA: Churchill Livingstone.
12. Kumar V., Abbas A. K., Aster J. C. (2015). *Robbins and Cotran pathologic basis of disease* (9th ed.). Philadelphia, PA: Elsevier Saunders.
13. Drake R. L., Vogl A. W., Mitchell A. W. M. (2015). *Gray's basic anatomy*. Philadelphia, PA: Churchill Livingstone.
14. Moore K. L., Dalley A. F., Agur A. M. R. (2017). *Clinically oriented anatomy* (8th ed.). Baltimore, MD: Lippincott Williams & Wilkins.
15. Eliopoulos C. (2018). *Gerontological nursing* (9th ed.). Philadelphia, PA: Wolters Kluwer.
16. Touhy T. A., Jett K. (2016). *Ebersole & Hess' toward healthy aging human needs and nursing response* (9th ed.). St. Louis, MO: Elsevier.
17. Doodolf D. (2018). Assessment of musculoskeletal function. In Hinkle J. L., Cheever K. H. (Ed.), *Brunner & Sudddarth's textbook of medical-surgical nursing*. (14th ed.). Philadelphia, PA: Wolters Kluwer.
18. Kyle T., Carman S. (2017). *Essentials of pediatric nursing* (3rd ed.). Philadelphia, PA: Wolters Kluwer.

Disorders of Musculoskeletal Function: Trauma, Infection, Neoplasms

48

Sarah Morgan

The musculoskeletal system includes the bones, joints, and muscles as well as associated structures such as ligaments and tendons. A human infant is born with over 300 bones. As humans age, some bones fuse, leaving an adult with approximately 206 bones.[1] The musculoskeletal system is subject to a large number of disorders. These disorders affect people in all age groups and walks of life, causing pain and disability. The discussion in this chapter focuses on the effects of trauma, infection, ischemia, and neoplasms on the musculoskeletal structures of the body.

INJURY AND TRAUMA OF MUSCULOSKELETAL STRUCTURES

After completing this section of the chapter, the learner will be able to meet the following objectives:

- Describe the healing process of soft tissue injuries.
- Describe the fracture healing process.
- Differentiate the early complications of fractures from later complications of fracture healing.

A broad spectrum of musculoskeletal injuries result from physical forces, including blunt tissue trauma, disruption of tendons and ligaments, and fractures of bony structures. Many of the forces that cause injury to the musculoskeletal system are typical for a particular environmental setting, activity, or age group. In the United States, the number one cause of death for those between the ages of 1 and 44 is injury[2]; motor vehicle crashes are a leading cause of death for those ages 1 to 30.[3]

Unintentional falls are the number one cause of nonfatal injuries in children and adolescents between 0 and 14 years of age in the United States.[4] Childhood falls cause approximately 2.8 million emergency department visits each year.[4] Sports- and recreation-related injuries send 2.6 million children between the ages of 0 and 19 to the ER each year.[5]

Falls are the most common cause of injury in people 65 years of age and older. In 2014, about 28.7% of older adults reported a fall.[6] Falls among older adults are often due to physiologic changes such as alteration in balance, vision and hearing decline, and unsteady gait. Environmental risks such as inadequate lighting, spills, or even the use of stools or ladders to reach objects in high places can increase the number of falls. Osteoporosis is also a known risk for injury with falls.[7,8] Fall prevention in older adults should focus on strength and balance exercises and vitamin D supplements to improve mobility and bone strength. Polypharmacy, another risk factor for falls, can be mitigated by review of medications. Although most injuries associated with a fall are not serious, mortality following a hip fracture ranges from 18% to 33%.[8]

Athletic Injuries

Athletic injuries are either acute injuries or overuse injuries. Acute injuries are caused by sudden trauma and include injuries to soft tissues (contusion, strains, and sprains) and to bone (fractures). Overuse injuries occur when physical activity applies ongoing and excessive stress to normal musculoskeletal tissue, which fails to adapt.[9] Overuse injuries represent the majority of sports-related injuries among children and adolescents.[9] They commonly occur in the elbow and in tissue where tendons attach to the bone; particularly vulnerable are the apophyses and cartilaginous growth plates in sites such as the heel, elbow, and knee.[10] Because of the vulnerability of growing bones, the consequences of overuse injury are much greater among children and adolescents than adults.[10] Many factors contribute to the potential for injury among adolescent athletes including height and weight, muscle growth and strength, motor skills and performance, body composition, flexibility, growth plate bone structure, and psychological maturity.[9] The treatment of overuse injuries is focused on rest and modification of activities prevention, and education and early diagnosis are essential.[10]

Soft Tissue Injuries

Most skeletal injuries are accompanied by soft tissue (muscle, tendon, or ligament) injuries. These injuries include contusions, hematomas, and lacerations. They are discussed here because of their association with musculoskeletal injuries.

A *contusion* is an injury to soft tissue that results from direct trauma and is usually caused by striking a body part against a hard object. With a contusion, the skin overlying the injury remains intact. Initially, the area becomes ecchymotic (*i.e.*, black and blue) because of local hemorrhage; later, the discoloration gradually changes to brown and then to yellow as the blood is reabsorbed. A large area of local hemorrhage is called a *hematoma*. Hematomas cause pain as blood accumulates and exerts pressure on nerve endings. The pain increases with movement or when pressure is applied to the area. The pain and swelling of a hematoma take longer to subside than those accompanying a contusion. A hematoma may become infected because of bacterial growth. Unlike a contusion, which does not drain, a hematoma may eventually split the skin because of increased pressures and produce drainage. Treatment of a contusion or hematoma consists of elevating the affected part and applying cold every 4 hours for about 20 minutes at a time to reduce the bleeding into the area. A hematoma may need to be aspirated.

A *laceration* is an injury in which the skin is torn or its continuity is disrupted. The seriousness of a laceration depends on the size and depth of the wound and on whether there is contamination from the object that caused the injury. Puncture wounds from nails or rusted material provide the setting for growth of anaerobic bacteria such as those that cause tetanus and gas gangrene.

Lacerations are usually treated by wound closure, which is done after the area is sufficiently cleaned. The closed wound is then covered with a sterile dressing. It is important to minimize contamination of the wound and control bleeding. Contaminated wounds and open fractures are copiously irrigated and debrided, and the skin usually is left open to heal to prevent the development of an anaerobic infection or a sinus tract. Antimicrobial agents are selectively used based on the suspected nature of the contaminants.

Joint (Musculotendinous) Injuries

Joints, or articulations, are sites where two or more bones meet. Joints (*i.e.*, diarthrodial joints) are supported by tough bundles of collagenous fibers called *ligaments* that attach to the joint capsule and bind the articular ends of bones together, and by *tendons* that join muscles to the periosteum of the articulating bones.[11] Joint injuries involve mechanical overloading or forcible twisting or stretching.

Strains and Sprains

Strains. A *strain* is a stretching injury to a muscle or a musculotendinous unit caused by mechanical overloading. This type of injury may result from an unusual muscle contraction or an excessive forcible stretch. Although there usually is no external evidence of a specific injury, pain, stiffness, and swelling exist. The most common sites for muscle strains are the lower back and the cervical region of the spine. The elbow and the shoulder are also supported by musculotendinous units, which are subject to strains. Foot strain is associated with the weight-bearing stresses of the feet. It may be caused by inadequate muscular and ligamentous support, being overweight, or excessive standing, walking, or running.

In the lumbar and cervical spine regions, muscle strains are more common than sprains. Mechanical low back pain is becoming increasingly common in the adolescent athlete.[12] Overuse, especially hyperextension of the lumbar spine in such sports as track, wrestling, gymnastics, and diving, can tear the muscles, fascia, and ligaments. Careful diagnosis is necessary because chronic low back pain may indicate spondylolysis (stress fracture of the pars intra-articularis) or spondylolisthesis (vertebral displacement), which are the most commonly occurring causes.[13] Determining the location of the pain during motion helps in diagnosis and treatment.[14] Fractures near the top and bottom surface of the vertebrae can occur when the growing lumbar spine is overstressed, causing the disks to push into the spinal nerve roots. Early detection and treatment are important to prevent complications and disability. Treatment of back strains consists of a short period of rest and mild analgesics followed by a gradual return to activities. Cold packs or ice should be used to reduce pain and swelling of the affected area. Exercises, correct posture, and good body mechanics help to reduce the risk for reinjury.

Sprains. A *sprain*, which involves the ligamentous structures (strong bands of connective tissue) surrounding the joint, resembles a strain, but the pain and swelling subside more slowly. It usually is caused by abnormal or excessive movement of the joint. With a sprain, the ligaments may be incompletely torn or, as in a severe sprain, completely torn or ruptured (Fig. 48.1).[15] Occasionally, a chip of bone is evident when the entire ligament, including part of its bony attachment, has been ruptured or torn from the bone. The signs of sprain are pain, rapid swelling, heat, disability, discoloration, and limitation of function.

Any joint may be sprained, but the ankle joint is most commonly involved, especially in fast-moving injuries in which an ankle or knee can be suddenly twisted.[15] Most ankle sprains occur in the lateral ankle when the foot is turned inward under a person, forcing the ankle into inversion beyond the structural limits.[15] Other common sites of sprain are the knee (the collateral ligament and anterior cruciate ligament [ACL]) and elbow (the ulnar side). As with a strain, the soft tissue injury that occurs with a sprain is not evident on the radiograph. Wrist sprains most often occur with a fall on an outstretched hand.

Healing. If properly treated, musculotendinous injuries usually heal with the restoration of the original tensile strength. Repair is accomplished by fibroblasts from the inner tendon sheath or, if the tendon has no sheath, from the loose connective tissue that surrounds the tendon. Capillaries infiltrate the injured area during the initial healing process and supply the fibroblasts with the materials they need to produce large amounts of collagen. Formation of the long collagen bundles occurs within the first 2 weeks, and although tensile strength increases steadily thereafter, it is not sufficient to permit strong tendon pulls for approximately 2 months. During the healing process, there is a danger that muscle contraction will pull the injured ends apart, causing the tendon to heal in the lengthened position. There is also a danger that adhesions will develop in areas where tendons pass through fibrous channels, such as in the distal palm of the hands, rendering the tendon useless.

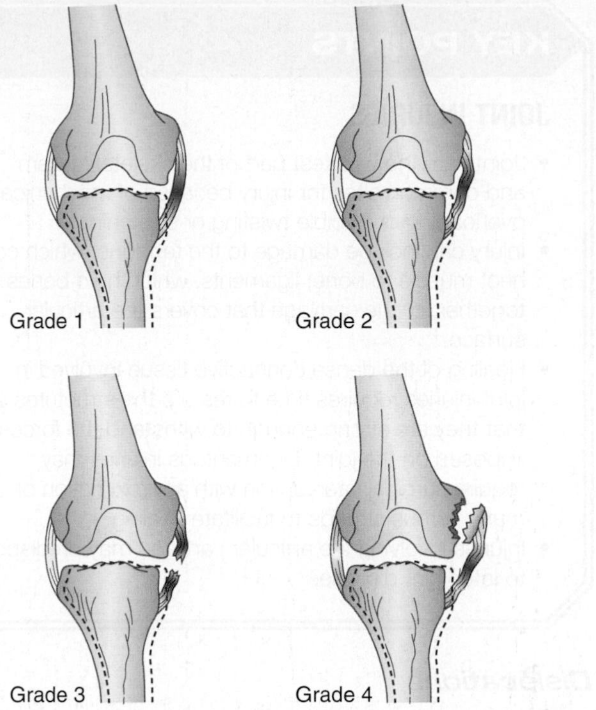

Figure 48.1 • Degrees of sprain on the medial side of the right knee: grade 1, mild sprain of the medial collateral ligament; grade 2, moderate sprain with hematoma formation; grade 3, severe sprain with total disruption of the ligament; and grade 4, severe sprain with avulsion of the medial femoral condyle at the insertion of the medial collateral ligament.

Treatment. The treatment of muscle strains and ligamentous sprains is similar in several ways. For an injured extremity, elevation of the part followed by local application of cold may be sufficient. Compression, accomplished using adhesive wraps or a removable splint, helps reduce swelling and provides support. A cast is applied for severe sprains, especially those severe enough to warrant surgical repair. Immobilization for a muscle strain is continued until the pain and swelling have subsided. In a sprain, the affected joint is immobilized for several weeks. Immobilization may be followed by graded active exercises. Early diagnosis, treatment, and rehabilitation are essential in preventing chronic ligamentous instability.

KEY POINTS

JOINT INJURIES

- Joints are the weakest part of the skeletal system and common sites for injury because of mechanical overloading or forcible twisting or stretching.
- Injury can include damage to the tendons, which connect muscle to bone; ligaments, which hold bones together; or the cartilage that covers the articular surface.
- Healing of the dense connective tissue involved in joint injuries requires time to restore the structures so that they are strong enough to withstand the forces imposed on the joint. Ligamentous injuries may require surgical intervention with approximation of many fibrous strands to facilitate healing.
- Injuries involving the articular cartilage may predispose to later joint disease.

Dislocations

A *dislocation* involves the displacement or separation of the bone ends of a joint with loss of articulation. It usually follows a severe trauma that disrupts the holding ligaments. Dislocations are seen most often in the shoulder and acromioclavicular joints. The shoulder is a complex and unstable joint.[16,17] Most traumatic shoulder dislocations are anterior or are recurrent episodes of a previous injury: either a dislocation or a subluxation.[18] A *subluxation* is a partial dislocation in which the bone ends in the joint are still in partial contact with each other. The first occurrence of an anterior dislocation happens most often in young males and as a result of contact, with recurrence being common.[16,17]

Dislocations can be congenital, traumatic, or pathologic. Congenital dislocations occur in the hip and knee. Traumatic dislocations occur after falls, blows, or rotational injuries. For example, car accidents often cause dislocations of the hip and accompanying acetabular fractures because of the direction of impact. This is true of people wearing seat belts and those who are unrestrained. In the shoulder and patella, dislocations may become recurrent, especially in athletes. They recur with the same motion but require less and less force each time to cause the damage.

Pathologic dislocation in the hip is a late complication of infection, rheumatoid arthritis, paralysis, and neuromuscular diseases. Dislocations of the phalangeal joints are not serious and are usually reduced by manipulation. Less common sites of dislocation, seen mainly in young adults, are the wrist and midtarsal region. They usually are the result of direct force, such as a fall on an outstretched hand. Diagnosis of a dislocation is based on history, physical examination, and radiologic findings. The symptoms are pain, deformity, and limited movement.

The treatment depends on the site, mechanism of injury, and associated injuries such as fractures. Dislocations that do not reduce spontaneously usually require manipulation or surgical repair. Various surgical procedures also can be used to prevent redislocation of the patella, shoulder, or acromioclavicular joints. Immobilization is necessary for several weeks after reduction of a dislocation to allow healing of the joint structures. In dislocations affecting the knee, closed reduction with knee immobilization may be prescribed although open reduction may be required in the case of vascular or soft tissue damage.[19]

Loose Bodies

Loose bodies are small pieces of bone or cartilage within a joint space. These can result from trauma to the joint or may occur when cartilage has worn away from the articular surface, causing a necrotic piece of bone to separate and become free floating. The symptoms are painful and often cause catching and locking of the joint. Loose bodies are commonly seen in the knee, elbow, hip, and ankle. The loose body repeatedly gets caught in the crevice of a joint, pinching the underlying healthy cartilage. Unless the loose body is removed, it may cause osteoarthritis and restricted movement. The treatment consists of removal using operative arthroscopy.

Shoulder and Rotator Cuff Injuries

The shoulder is a complex series of joints that produce extraordinary range of motion. The extreme mobility is accomplished at the expense of relative instability. This instability, combined with its relatively exposed position, makes the shoulder extremely vulnerable to injuries such as sprains and dislocations and degenerative processes such as rotator cuff disorders.

The shoulder is composed of three bones: the scapula, the clavicle, and the humerus. The scapula articulates with the humerus by way of the glenoid cavity and with the clavicle at the acromion process as well as closely with the chest wall. Clavicle fractures are among the most common fractures of childhood. The typical mechanism of fracture is a fall on the point of the shoulder.

Four articulations form the shoulder joint—the acromioclavicular joint that joins the clavicle to the acromion of the scapula, the sternoclavicular joint that joins the sternum to the clavicle, the glenohumeral joint that connects the head of the humerus to the relatively shallow glenoid cavity in the scapula, and the thoracoscapular joint that joins the posterior thoracic cage and the anterior scapula.[18] The stability of these joints is provided by a series of muscles and tendons. Sprains of the acromioclavicular joint can occur as a result of direct or indirect forces such as contact sports or a fall.[20] The most common site of shoulder dislocation is the glenohumeral joint.[21] Most acute dislocations involve anterior displacement of the humeral head with respect to the glenoid cavity, the result of the shoulder being abducted and forcefully extended and rotated. Other mechanisms include a fall on an outstretched arm or a blow to the posterior shoulder.

Motion of the arm involves the coordinated movement of muscles of the rotator cuff (supraspinatus, teres minor, infraspinatus, subscapularis) and their musculotendinous attachments.[19,22] These muscles are separated from the overlying coracoacromial arch by two bursae, the subdeltoid and subcoracoid. These two bursae, sometimes referred to as the *subacromial bursae*, often communicate and are affected by lesions of the rotator cuff.

The rotator cuff (Fig. 48.2) is like other muscle groups of the body in that its risk for injury increases when it is required to perform a high-stress function in an unconditioned state. Rotator cuff injuries and impingement disorders can result from many causes, including excessive use, a direct blow, or stretch injury, usually involving throwing or swinging, as with baseball pitchers or tennis players. Researchers noted that rotator cuff injury in young people is a different disease than that in older adults.[23]

Overuse and degenerative disorders have a slower onset and are seen in older adults with minor or no trauma. The tendons of the rotator cuff fuse together near their insertions into the tuberosities of the humerus to form the musculotendinous cuff. Degeneration of these tendons can result from a number of factors, including repetitive microtrauma, impairment of vascularity as a result of aging, or shoulder instability with secondary overload of the cuff, but incidence does significantly increase with age.[24] Degeneration is most severe near the tendon insertion, with the supraspinous being affected most often. Thickening of the musculotendinous unit decreases the distance between the cuff and the overlying coracoacromial arch. Pain and impingement may be noted when motions of the arm squeeze and pinch these tissues between the humerus and the overlying arch. Overall, rotator cuff injury is caused

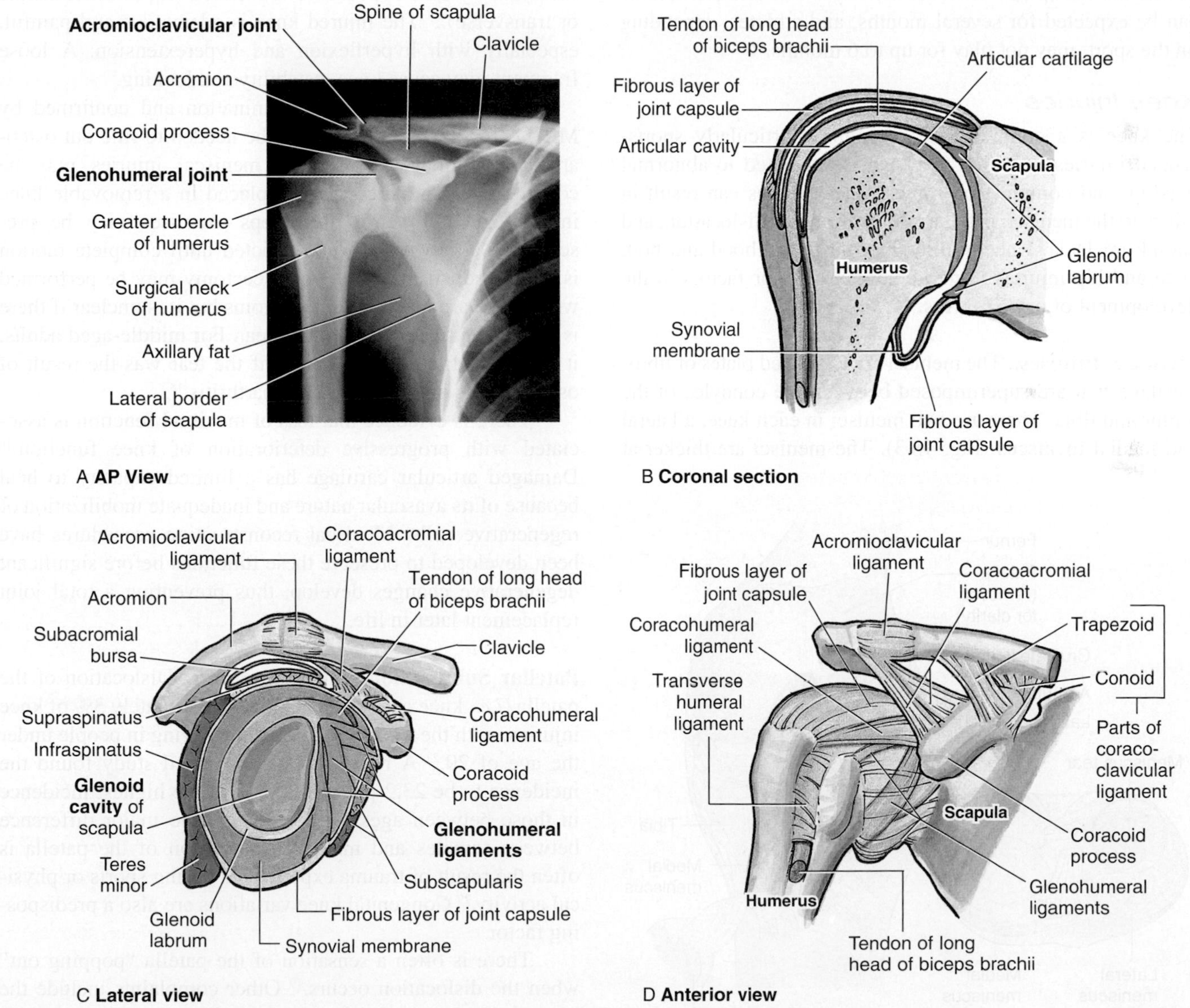

Figure 48.2 • The rotator cuff injury. **(A)** Radiograph. **(B)** Coronal section of the shoulder's acromioclavicular joint and glenohumeral joint. **(C)** Lateral view of glenoid cavity. **(D)** Anterior view of ligaments. (From Moore K. L., Agur A. M., Dalley A. F. (2011). *Essential clinical anatomy* (4th ed., p. 478). Philadelphia, PA: Wolters Kluwer/Lippincott Williams & Wilkins.)

by a multitude of factors—extrinsic and intrinsic—with the weight of each factor being unclear.[19,24]

Several physical examination maneuvers are used to define shoulder pathologic processes.[21,24,25] The history and mechanism of injury are important. In addition to standard radiographs, arthrography, computed tomography (CT), or MRI may be used. Because of the number of rotator cuff injuries, shoulder ultrasound is the most common of the musculoskeletal ultrasound applications.[22] Arthroscopic examination under anesthesia may be used for diagnostic purposes, and operative arthroscopy may be done to repair severe tears. Conservative treatment with anti-inflammatory agents, corticosteroid injections, and physical therapy often is undertaken. A period of rest is followed by a customized exercise and rehabilitation program to improve strength, flexibility, and endurance. After surgery for rotator cuff tears, physical therapy may be needed for up to 3 months, activity limits and restrictions can be expected for several months, and athletes, depending on the sport, may not play for up to 6 months.[19]

Knee Injuries

The knee is a common site of injury, particularly sports-related injuries in which the knee is subjected to abnormal twisting and compression forces. These forces can result in injury to the menisci, patellar subluxation and dislocation, and chondromalacia. Knee injuries in young adulthood and both knee and hip injuries in middle age are major factors in the development of osteoarthritis.[26]

Meniscus Injuries. The menisci are C-shaped plates of fibrocartilage that are superimposed between the condyles of the femur and tibia. There are two menisci in each knee, a lateral and medial meniscus (Fig. 48.3). The menisci are thicker at their external margins and taper to thin, unattached edges at their interior margin. They are firmly attached at their ends to the intercondylar area of the tibia and are supported by the coronary and transverse ligaments of the knee. The menisci play a major role in load bearing and shock absorption. They also help to stabilize the knee by deepening the tibial socket and maintaining the femur and tibia in proper position. In addition, the meniscus assists in joint lubrication and serves as source of nutrition for articular cartilage in the knee.

Meniscus injury commonly occurs as the result of a rotational injury from a sudden or sharp pivot or a direct blow to the knee, as in hockey, basketball, or football. It is often associated with other injuries, such as a torn ACL. The type and location of the meniscal tear are determined by the magnitude and direction of the force that acts on the knee and the position of the knee at the time of injury. Meniscus tears can be described by their appearance or location (*e.g.*, bucket handle or transverse).[19] The injured knee is edematous and painful, especially with hyperflexion and hyperextension. A loose fragment may cause knee instability and locking.

Diagnosis is made by examination and confirmed by MRI. A regular radiograph may be needed to rule out osteoarthritis.[18] Initial treatment of meniscal injuries may be conservative. The knee may be placed in a removable knee immobilizer. Isometric quadriceps exercises may be prescribed. Activity usually is restricted until complete motion is recovered. Arthroscopic meniscectomy may be performed when there are mechanical symptoms but it is unclear if there is a degenerative or a traumatic tear. For middle-aged adults, it may be difficult to determine if the tear was the result of osteoarthritis or will lead to osteoarthritis.[18]

There is evidence that loss of meniscal function is associated with progressive deterioration of knee function.[18] Damaged articular cartilage has a limited capacity to heal because of its avascular nature and inadequate mobilization of regenerative cells. Meniscal reconstruction procedures have been developed to preserve these functions before significant degenerative changes develop, thus preventing a total joint replacement later in life.

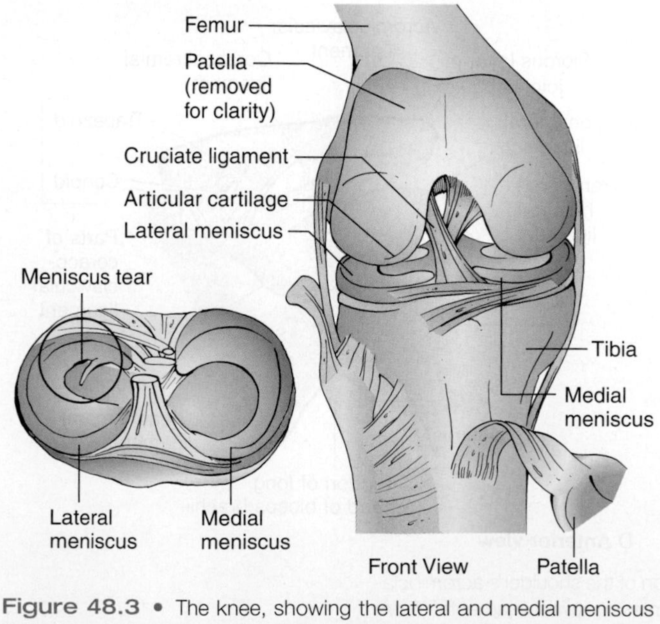

Figure 48.3 • The knee, showing the lateral and medial meniscus (with the patella removed for clarity). **Inset** (*lower left*) shows meniscus tear.

Patellar Subluxation and Dislocations. Dislocation of the patella (*i.e.*, knee cap) accounts for approximately 3% of knee injuries, with the first episode often occurring in people under the age of 20.[27] A recent population-based study found the incidence to be 23.2 per 100,000, with the highest incidence in those between ages 14 and 18, and no major difference between females and males.[28] Dislocation of the patella is often the result of trauma experienced during sports or physical activity.[29] Congenital knee variations are also a predisposing factor.

There is often a sensation of the patella "popping out" when the dislocation occurs.[19] Other complaints include the knee giving out, swelling, crepitus, stiffness, and loss of range of motion. Treatment can be difficult, but nonsurgical methods are used first. They include immobilization with the knee extended, bracing, administration of anti-inflammatory agents, and isometric quadriceps-strengthening exercises. Surgical intervention often is necessary, with numerous options available.[30] Some evidence supports surgical intervention over nonsurgical treatments but is not yet conclusive.[31]

Chondromalacia. Chondromalacia, or degeneration of the articular cartilage, is seen most commonly on the undersurface of the patella.[15] It can be the result of recurrent subluxation of the patella or overuse in strenuous athletic activities. People with this disorder typically complain of pain, particularly when climbing stairs or sitting with the knees bent. Occasionally, the person experiences weakness of the knee.

Treatment consists of rest, isometric exercises, and application of ice after exercise. Part of the patella may be surgically removed in severe cases. In less severe cases, the soft portion is shaved using a saw inserted through an arthroscope. Articular cartilage maintenance and repair is a complex process. Polypeptide growth factors that direct cells to divide, differentiate, migrate, and produce matrix appear to have a role in the preservation and degradation of the articular cartilage matrix.

Hip Injuries

The hip is a ball-and-socket joint in which the femoral head articulates deeply in the acetabulum (Fig. 48.4).[11] The proximal part of the femur consists of a head, neck, and greater trochanter. The vascular anatomy of the femoral head is of critical importance in any disorder of the hip. The main sources of blood supply are the intramedullary vessels and the retinacular arteries arising from the circumflex femoral arteries, both of which course from the intertrochanteric region proximally to nourish the femoral head. Disease or injuries that compromise the circulation may damage the viability of the femoral head and lead to avascular necrosis or osteonecrosis. Disorders of the hip include dislocations and fractures of the hip.

Dislocations of the Hip. Dislocations of the hip are the result of severe trauma and can be anterior or posterior, with posterior being more common.[32] Associated injuries will also impact the outcome of the dislocation.[32]

Hip dislocation is an emergency.[32] In the dislocated position, great tension is placed on the blood supply to the femoral head and avascular necrosis may result.[19,32] Hip osteoarthritis is also a potential long-term complication. To prevent these complications, early reduction is indicated.[32] Weight bearing is usually limited after reduction to prevent dislocation from reoccurring and allow healing to occur.

Fractures of the Hip. Hip fracture is a major public health problem in the Western world, particularly among older adults. It is accompanied by risks for death and impact on function and quality of life.[33] The incidence of hip fractures increases with age. The incidence is also higher in white women as compared to nonwhite women. Risk factors for hip fracture vary with age and sex. For those under the age of 80, greater risk is associated with skeletal issues, whereas for those over

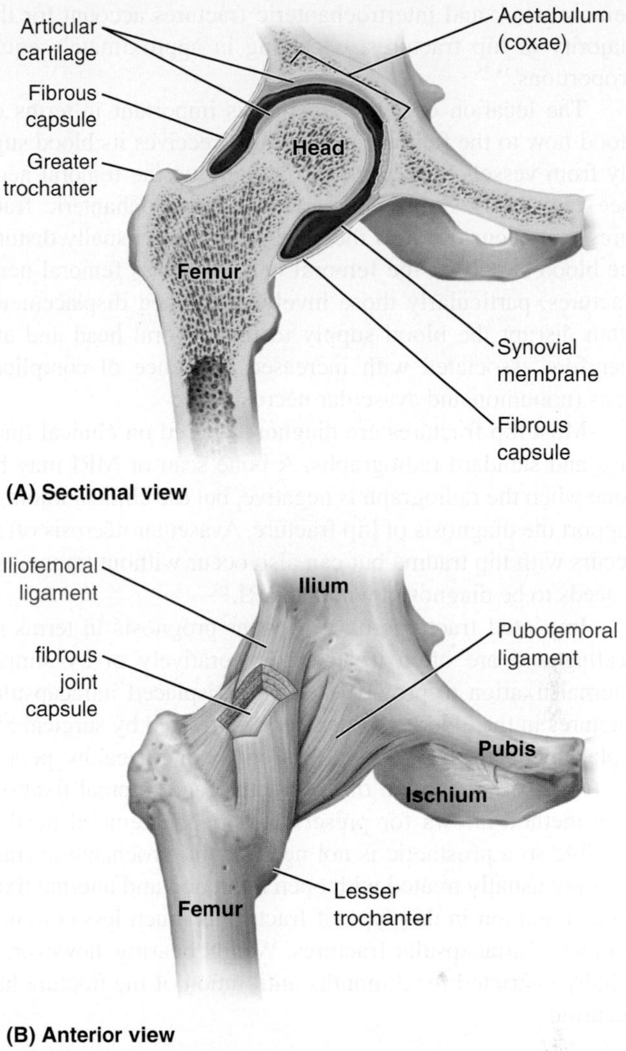

Figure 48.4 • Right hip joint. **(A)** Sectional view. **(B)** Anterior view. (From McConnell T. H., Hull K. L. (2011). *Human form, human function: Essentials of anatomy & physiology* (p. 218). Philadelphia, PA: Lippincott Williams & Wilkins.)

the age of 80, falls are the greatest risk factor.[34] Osteoporosis and osteopenia are also important contributing factors.

Most hip fractures result from falls. Occasionally, the person may actually fracture the hip before falling, the fracture being caused by twisting or excessive force on a femur that has been weakened by osteoporosis or neoplasms. The characteristics of the fall (the direction, site of impact, and protective response) and environmental factors are important factors influencing the risk of hip fracture from a fall.

A hip fracture is classified according to the anatomic part of the hip where the fracture occurs. Generally, it is a fracture of the proximal femur. Femoral neck fractures are located in the area distal to the femoral head but proximal to the greater and lesser trochanters and are considered intracapsular because they are located within the capsule of the hip joint. Intertrochanteric fractures occur in the metaphyseal region between the greater and lesser trochanter. Subtrochanteric fractures are those that occur just below the greater trochanter.

Femoral neck and intertrochanteric fractures account for the majority of hip fractures, occurring in approximately equal proportions.[18,35]

The location of a hip fracture is important in terms of blood flow to the femoral head, which receives its blood supply from vessels that course proximally up the femoral neck (see Fig. 48.4). Subtrochanteric and intertrochanteric fractures that occur distal to these vessels do not usually disturb the blood supply to the femoral head, whereas femoral neck fractures, particularly those involving marked displacement, often disrupt the blood supply to the femoral head and are therefore associated with increased incidence of complications (nonunion and avascular necrosis).[36,37]

Most hip fractures are diagnosed based on clinical findings and standard radiographs. A bone scan or MRI may be done when the radiograph is negative, but the clinical findings support the diagnosis of hip fracture. Avascular necrosis often occurs with hip trauma but can also occur without trauma, so it needs to be diagnosed with an MRI.[18]

Impacted fractures have a better prognosis in terms of healing and are often treated nonoperatively or by simple internal fixation to provide stability. Displaced intracapsular fractures in the elderly are usually best treated by surgical hip replacement and early mobilization. Young, healthy people are treated by reduction of the fracture and internal fixation. This method allows for preservation of the femoral head if possible so a prosthetic is not needed. Intertrochanteric fractures are usually treated with open reduction and internal fixation. Nonunion in this type of fracture is much less common than with intracapsular fractures. Weight bearing, however, is usually restricted for 3 months until union of the fracture has occurred.

Fractures

Fracture, or discontinuity of the bone, is the most common type of bone lesion.[36] Normal bone can withstand considerable compression and shearing forces and, to a lesser extent, tension forces. A fracture occurs when more stress is placed on the bone than it can absorb. Grouped according to cause, fractures can be divided into three major categories: fractures caused by sudden injury, fatigue or stress fractures, and pathologic fractures.[36] The most common fractures are those resulting from sudden injury. The force causing the fracture may be direct, such as a fall or blow, or indirect, such as a massive muscle contraction or trauma transmitted along the bone. For example, the head of the radius or clavicle can be fractured by the indirect forces that result from falling on an outstretched hand. A fatigue fracture results from repeated wear on a bone. Pain associated with overuse injuries of the lower extremities, especially posterior medial tibial pain, is one of the most common symptoms that physically active people, such as runners, experience. Stress fractures in the tibia may be confused with "shin splints," a nonspecific term for pain in the lower leg from overuse in walking and running, because they frequently do not appear on x-ray until 2 weeks after the onset of symptoms.

A pathologic fracture occurs in bones that already are weakened by disease or tumors. Fractures of this type may occur spontaneously with little or no stress. The underlying disease state can be local, as with infections, cysts, or tumors, or generalized, as in osteoporosis, Paget disease, or cancer metastasis.[36]

Classification

Fractures usually are classified according to location, type, and direction or pattern of the fracture line (Fig. 48.5). A long bone is divided into three parts: proximal, midshaft, and distal. A fracture of the long bone is described in relation to its position in the bone. Other descriptions are used when the fracture affects the head or neck of a bone, involves a joint, or is near a prominence such as a condyle or malleolus.

The type of fracture is determined by its communication with the external environment, the degree of break in continuity of the bone, and the character of the fracture pieces. A fracture can be classified as open or closed. When the bone fragments have broken through the skin, the fracture is called an *open* or *compound fracture*.[38] Open fractures often are complicated by infection, osteomyelitis, delayed union, or nonunion. In a closed fracture, there is no communication with the outside skin.

Concept Mastery Alert

People with compound fractures are more likely to experience complications in bone healing than those with other types of fractures.

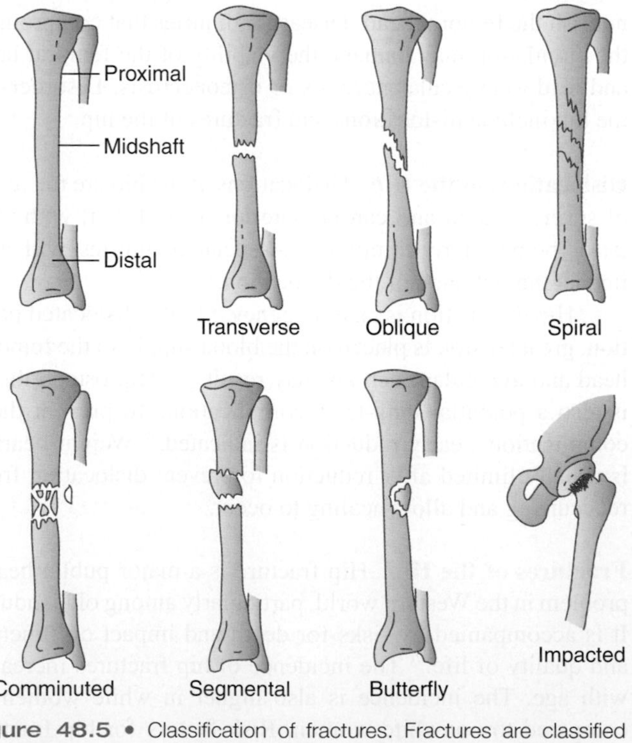

Figure 48.5 • Classification of fractures. Fractures are classified according to location (proximal, midshaft, or distal), the direction of fracture line (transverse, oblique, spiral), and type (comminuted, segmental, butterfly, or impacted).

The degree of a fracture is described in terms of a partial or complete break in the continuity of bone. A *greenstick fracture*, which is seen in children, is an example of a partial break in bone continuity and resembles that seen when a young sapling is broken. This kind of break occurs because children's bones, especially until approximately 10 years of age, are more resilient than the bones of adults.

The character of a fracture is determined by its pieces. A *comminuted fracture* has more than two pieces. A *compression fracture*, as occurs in the vertebral body, involves two bones that are crushed or squeezed together. A fracture is called *impacted* when the fracture fragments are wedged together. This type usually occurs in the humerus, is less serious, and is treated without surgery.

The direction of the trauma or mechanism of injury produces a certain configuration or pattern of fracture. The pattern of a fracture indicates the nature of the trauma and provides information about the easiest method for reduction. *Reduction* is the restoration of a fractured bone to its normal anatomic position. *Transverse fractures* are caused by simple angular forces. A *spiral fracture* results from a twisting motion, or torque. A transverse fracture is not likely to become displaced or lose its position after it is reduced. On the other hand, spiral, oblique, and comminuted fractures often are unstable and may change position after reduction.

Clinical Manifestations

The signs and symptoms of a fracture include pain, tenderness at the site of bone disruption, swelling, loss of function, deformity of the affected part, and abnormal mobility. The deformity varies according to the type of force applied, the area of the bone involved, the type of fracture produced, and the strength and balance of the surrounding muscles.

In long bones, three types of deformities—angulation, shortening, and rotation—are seen. Severely angulated fracture fragments may be felt at the fracture site and often push up against the soft tissue to cause a tenting effect on the skin. Bending forces and unequal muscle pulls cause angulation. Shortening of the extremity occurs as the bone fragments slide and override each other because of the pull of the muscles on the long axis of the extremity (Fig. 48.6).

Rotational deformity occurs when the fracture fragments rotate out of their normal longitudinal axis; this can result from rotational strain produced by the fracture or unequal pull by the muscles that are attached to the fracture fragments. A crepitus or grating may be felt as the bone fragments rub against each other. In the case of an open fracture, there is bleeding from the wound where the bone protrudes. Blood loss from a pelvic fracture or multiple long bone fractures can cause hypovolemic shock in a person who has had a trauma.

Shortly after the fracture has occurred, nerve function at the fracture site may be temporarily lost. The area may become numb, and the surrounding muscles flaccid. This condition has been called *local shock*. During this period, which may last for a few minutes to half an hour, fractured bones may be reduced with little or no pain. After this brief period, the pain returns and, with it, muscle spasms and contractions occur in the surrounding muscles.

The early complications of fractures are associated with loss of skeletal continuity, injury from bone fragments, pressure from swelling and hemorrhage, involvement of nerve fibers, or development of fat emboli. The extent of early complications depends on the severity of the fracture and the area of the body that is involved. For example, bone fragments from a skull fracture may cause injury to brain tissue, or multiple rib fractures may lead to a flail chest and respiratory insufficiency. With flail chest, the chest wall on the fractured side becomes so unstable that it may move in the opposite direction as the person breathes (*i.e.*, in during inspiration and out during expiration).

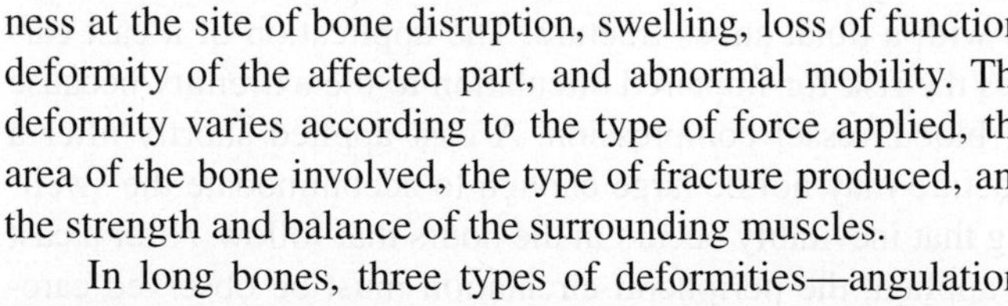

Figure 48.6 • Displacement and overriding of fracture fragments of a long bone (femur) caused by severe muscle spasm.

Diagnosis

Diagnosis is the first step in the care of fractures and is based on history and physical manifestations. X-ray examination is used to confirm the diagnosis and direct the treatment. The ease of diagnosis varies with the location and severity of the fracture. In a person who has had a trauma, the presence of other, more serious injuries may make diagnosis more difficult. A thorough history includes the mechanism, time, and place of the injury; first recognition of symptoms; and any treatment initiated. A complete history is important because a delay in seeking treatment or a period of weight bearing on a fracture may cause further injury or displacement of the fracture.

Determination of the severity of injury to soft tissue is an important component of assessment and management of closed fractures. The response of the soft tissue to blunt injury involves microvascular and inflammatory responses that produce localized tissue hypoxia and acidosis. Incisions placed through such compromised tissue can lead to wound breakdown and infections. Therefore, recognizing the signs of soft tissue injury is the foundation for successful management of closed fractures. The classification of Oestern and Tscherne can be used to characterize the severity of closed fractures[39,40] (Table 48.1). This system remains the only published classification system for the soft tissue injury associated with closed fractures. Fractures are assigned one of four grades, from 0 to 3. The presence of deep skin abrasions, muscle contusion, fracture blisters, and massive soft tissue swelling suggests the need to use external fixation methods to limit further soft tissue injury and facilitate rapid recovery before surgical intervention.

TABLE 48.1 OESTERN AND TSCHERNE CLASSIFICATION OF CLOSED FRACTURES

GRADE	SOFT TISSUE INJURY	BONY INJURY
Grade 0	Minimal soft tissue damage Indirect injury to limb	Simple fracture pattern
Grade 1	Superficial abrasion/contusion	Mild fracture pattern
Grade 2	Deep abrasion with skin or muscle contusion Direct trauma to limb	Severe fracture pattern
Grade 3	Extensive skin contusion or crush Severe damage to underlying muscle Subcutaneous avulsion Compartmental syndrome may be present	Severe fracture pattern

From Bucholz R. W., Heckman J. D. (2010). *Rockwood & Green's fractures in adults* (7th ed., Table 2-2, p. 45). Philadelphia, PA: Lippincott Williams & Wilkins.

Treatment

There are three objectives for treatment of fractures: reduction of the fracture, immobilization, and preservation and restoration of the function of the injured part. Also, it is important to prevent complications during the management of the fracture treatment. Preventive care is vital to avoiding fracture complications.

Reduction and Internal Fixation. When bones are realigned to restore their original structure, it is referred to as reduction. This can be accomplished by closed manipulation or surgical (open) reduction. Closed manipulation uses methods such as manual pressure and traction. Fractures are held in reduction by external or internal fixation devices. The benefits of internal fixation must be balanced against its associated risks. The advantages are precise restoration of the osseous anatomy and early mobilization with at least partial weight bearing. The principal disadvantages are the increased risk of infection and the fact that healing may be impaired if a technique is not used properly. Surgical reduction involves the use of various types of hardware to accomplish internal fixation of the fracture fragments.

Immobilization and External Fixation. Immobilization prevents movement of the injured parts and is the single most important element in obtaining union of the fracture fragments. Immobilization can be accomplished using external devices, such as splints, casts, traction, or external fixation devices, or by internal fixation devices inserted during surgical reduction of the fracture.

Splints are made from many different materials. Metal splints or air splints may be used during transport to a health care facility as a temporary measure until the fracture has been reduced and another form of immobilization instituted. Plaster of Paris splints, which are molded to fit the extremity, work well. Splinting should be done if there is any suspicion of a fracture because motion of the fracture site can cause pain, bleeding, more soft tissue damage, and nerve or blood vessel compression. If the fracture has sharp fragments, movement can cause perforation of the skin and conversion of a closed fracture into an open one. When a splint is applied to an extremity, it should extend from the joint above the fracture site to the joint below it.

Casts, which are made of plaster or synthetic material such as fiberglass, are commonly used to immobilize fractures of the extremities. They often are applied with a joint in partial flexion to prevent rotation of the fracture fragments. Without this flexion, the extremity, which is essentially a cylinder, tends to rotate within the cylindrical structure of the cast. A brace may be used after a cast is removed or instead of a cast, as with a tibial stress fracture. The application of a cast carries the risk for impaired circulation to the extremity because of blood vessel compression. A cast applied shortly after a fracture may not be large enough to accommodate the swelling that inevitably occurs in the hours that follow. After a cast is applied, the peripheral circulation must be observed carefully until this danger has passed. If the circulation becomes inadequate, the parts that are exposed at the distal end of the cast (*i.e.*, the toes with a leg cast and the fingers with an arm cast) usually become cold and cyanotic or pale. An increase in pain may occur initially, followed by paresthesia (*i.e.*, tingling or abnormal sensation) or anesthesia as the sensory neurons that supply the area are affected. There is a decrease in the amplitude or absence of the pulse in areas where the arteries can be palpated. Capillary refill time, which is assessed by applying pressure to the fingernail and observing the rate of blood return, is prolonged to longer than 3 seconds. Signs of impaired circulation demand immediate measures, such as splitting the cast, to restore the circulation and prevent permanent damage to the extremity. A casted extremity should be elevated above the level of the heart for the first 24 hours to minimize swelling.

Traction is another method for achieving immobility, maintaining alignment of the bone ends, and maintaining the reduction, particularly if the fracture is unstable or comminuted. Traction is a pulling force applied to an extremity or part of the body while a counterforce, or countertraction, pulls in the opposite direction. The five goals of traction therapy are to correct and maintain the skeletal alignment of entire bones or joints; reduce pressure on a joint surface; correct, lessen, or prevent deformities such as contractures and dislocations; decrease muscle spasm; and immobilize the fracture site to promote healing. Traction may be used as a temporary measure before surgery or as a primary treatment method. There are three types of traction: manual traction, skin traction, and skeletal traction. *Manual traction* consists of a steady, firm pull that is exerted by the hands. It is a temporary measure used to manipulate a fracture during closed reduction, for support of a neck injury during transport when a cervical spine fracture is suspected, or for reduction of a dislocated joint. *Skin traction* is a pulling force applied to the skin and soft tissue. It is accomplished by strips of adhesive flannel or foam secured to the injured part. *Skeletal traction* is a pulling force applied directly to the bone. Pins, wires, or tongs are inserted through the skin and subcutaneous tissue into the bone distal to the fracture site. Skeletal traction provides an excellent pull and can be used for long periods with large amounts of weight. It is commonly used for fractures of the femur, the humerus, and the cervical spine (*e.g.*, Crutchfield tongs applied to the skull) (Fig. 48.7).

With *external fixation devices*, pins or screws are inserted directly into the bone above and below the fracture site. They are secured to a metal frame and adjusted to align the fracture. This method of treatment is used primarily for open fractures, infections such as osteomyelitis and septic joints, unstable closed fractures, and limb lengthening.

Limb-Lengthening Systems. Limb-lengthening systems, such as the Ilizarov external fixator (Fig. 48.8), are used to lengthen or widen bones, correct angular or rotational defects, or immobilize fractures.[38] The apparatus is applied with a surgical technique, which consists of a percutaneous osteotomy that preserves the periosteal and endosteal tissues. A circular external apparatus is attached to bone by tensioned wires.[38] The continuous pulling activates regeneration of bone, soft tissue, nerves, and blood vessels. Newly formed bone fills the posttraumatic defects and eliminates the need for bone

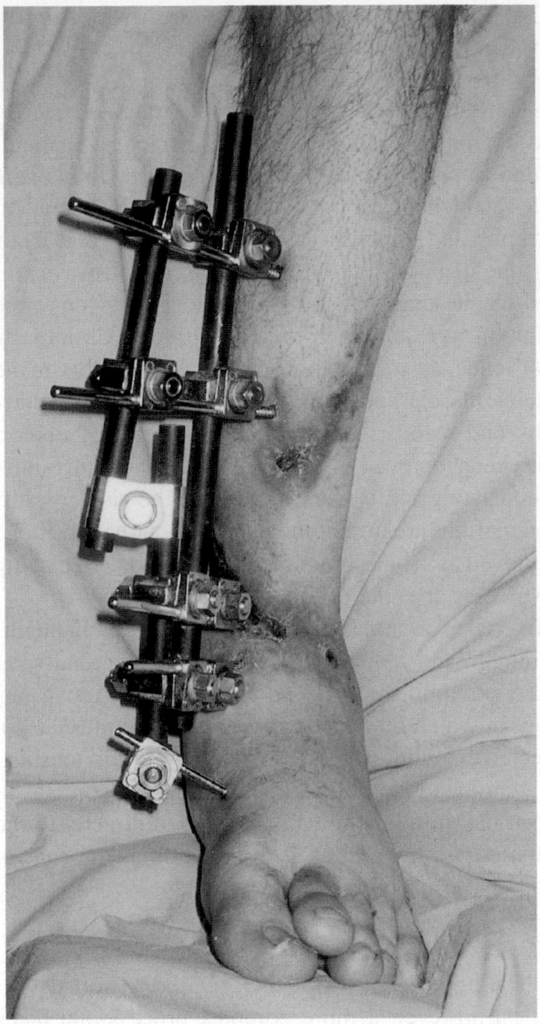

Figure 48.8 • External fixation device. Pins are inserted into bone. The fracture is reduced and aligned and then stabilized by attaching the pins to a rigid portable frame. The device facilitates treatment of soft tissue damaged in complex fractures. (From Hinkle J. L., Cheever, K. H. (2018). *Brunner & Suddarth's textbook of medical-surgical nursing* (14th ed., Figure 40-3, p. 1138). Philadelphia, PA: Lippincott Williams & Wilkins.)

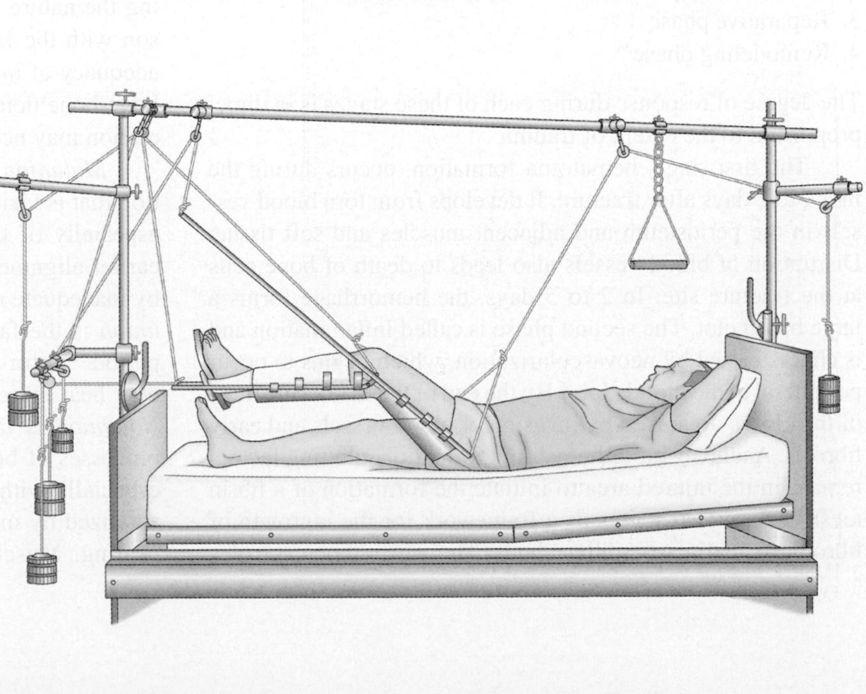

Figure 48.7 • Balanced suspension skeletal traction with Thomas leg splint. The person can move vertically as long as the resultant line of pull is maintained. Note the use of the overhead trapeze. (From Hinkle J. L., Cheever, K. H. (2018). *Brunner & Suddarth's textbook of medical-surgical nursing* (14th ed., Figure 40-6, p. 1140). Philadelphia, PA: Lippincott Williams & Wilkins.)

grafting. The apparatus is left on until the desired length is achieved and consolidation is complete.

Preservation and Restoration of Function. During the period of immobilization required for fracture healing, muscles tend to atrophy because of lack of use. Joints stiffen as muscles and tendons contract and shorten. The degree of muscle atrophy and joint stiffness depends on several factors. In adults, the degree of atrophy and muscle stiffness is directly related to the length of immobilization, with longer periods of immobility resulting in greater stiffness. Children have a natural tendency to move on their own, and this movement maintains muscle and joint function. They usually have less atrophy and recover sooner after the source of immobilization has been removed. Associated soft tissue injury, infection, and preexisting joint disease increase the risk for stiffness. Although limbs are immobilized in a functional position, casts are removed as soon as fracture healing has taken place so that joint stiffness does not occur.

Exercises designed to preserve function, maintain muscle strength, and reduce joint stiffness in the unaffected and affected extremities should be started early. Active range of motion, in which the person moves the extremity, is done on unaffected extremities, and isometric, or muscle-tensing, exercises are done on the affected extremities. In some instances, an electrical muscle stimulator is applied directly to the skin to stimulate isometric muscle contraction as a means of preventing disuse atrophy.

Bone Healing

Bone healing occurs in a manner similar to soft tissue healing. It is, however, a more complex process and takes longer. Although the exact mechanisms of bone healing are open to controversy, four stages of the healing process have been identified:

1. Hematoma formation
2. Inflammatory phase
3. Reparative phase
4. Remodeling phase[36]

The degree of response during each of these stages is in direct proportion to the extent of trauma.

The first stage, hematoma formation, occurs during the first 1 to 2 days after fracture. It develops from torn blood vessels in the periosteum and adjacent muscles and soft tissue. Disruption of blood vessels also leads to death of bone cells at the fracture site. In 2 to 5 days, the hemorrhage forms a large blood clot. The second phase is called inflammation and is characterized by neovascularization, which begins to occur peripheral to the blood clot.[36] By the end of the first week, most of the clot is organized by invasion of blood vessels and early fibrosis. As the result of hematoma formation, clotting factors remain in the injured area to initiate the formation of a fibrin meshwork, which serves as a framework for the ingrowth of fibroblasts and new capillary buds. The woven bone spicules start to appear around the clot and osteoblasts begin to synthesize the bone.[36] There is granulation tissue forming and this is referred to as the beginning of the callus.[36] The reparative phase follows the inflammatory phase and allows the continued formation of the callus of cartilage and woven bone near the fracture site.[36] The final phase is remodeling, which gives the cortex time to be reestablished. The osteoclastic and osteoblastic functions continue at a rapid rate until the fracture site is healed and bone is reconstructed.[36]

Healing Time. Healing time depends on the site of the fracture, the condition of the fracture fragments, hematoma formation, and other local and host factors. In general, fractures of long bones, displaced fractures, and fractures with less surface area heal more slowly. Function usually returns within 6 months after union is complete. However, return to complete function may take longer. Stress fractures usually require less time to heal, usually 2 to 4 weeks, during which time a reduction in activity and protection of the area are needed.

Union of a fracture has occurred when the fracture is solid enough to withstand normal stresses and it is clinically and radiologically safe to remove the external fixation. In children, fractures usually heal quicker than in adults. The increased rate of healing among children compared with adults may be related to the increased cellularity and vascularity of the child's periosteum.

Factors that influence bone healing are specific to the person, the type of injury sustained, and local factors that disrupt healing. Individual factors that may delay bone healing are the person's age; current medications; debilitating diseases, such as diabetes and rheumatoid arthritis; level of immunocompetency, local stress around the fracture site; circulatory problems and coagulation disorders; and poor nutrition.

Impaired Healing

Many factors can contribute to impaired bone healing, including the nature and extent of the injury, the health of the person with the fracture and his or her responses to injury, the adequacy of initial treatment, and pharmacologic factors. For large bone defects caused by trauma or a tumor, bone regeneration may need enhancement.

Malunion is healing with deformity, angulation, or rotation that is visible on x-ray films. Early, aggressive treatment, especially of the hand, can prevent malunion and result in earlier alignment and return of function. Malunion is caused by inadequate reduction or alignment of the fracture. *Delayed union* is the failure of a fracture to unite within the normal period.[38] Intra-articular fractures (*i.e.*, those through a joint) may heal more slowly and may eventually produce arthritis. *Nonunion* is failure to produce union and cessation of the processes of bone repair.[38] It is seen most often in the tibia, especially with open fractures or crushing injuries. It is characterized by mobility of the fracture site and pain on weight bearing. Muscle atrophy and loss of range of motion may

TABLE 48.2 COMPLICATIONS OF FRACTURE HEALING

COMPLICATION	MANIFESTATIONS	CONTRIBUTING FACTORS
Delayed union	Failure of fracture to heal within predicted time as determined by x-ray	Large displaced fracture
		Inadequate immobilization
		Large hematoma
		Infection at fracture site
		Excessive loss of bone
		Inadequate circulation
Malunion	Deformity at fracture site	Inadequate reduction
	Deformity or angulation on x-ray	Malalignment of fracture at time of immobilization
Nonunion	Failure of bone to heal before the process of bone repair stops	Inadequate reduction
	Evidence on x-ray	Mobility at fracture site
	Motion at fracture site	Severe trauma
	Pain on weight bearing	Bone fragment separation
		Soft tissue between bone fragments
		Infection
		Extensive loss of bone
		Inadequate circulation
		Malignancy
		Bone necrosis
		Noncompliance with restrictions

occur. Nonunion usually is established 6 to 12 months after the time of the fracture. The complications of fracture healing are summarized in Table 48.2.

Treatment methods for impaired bone healing include surgical interventions, such as bone grafts, bracing, external fixation, or electrical stimulation of the bone ends. The treatment for delayed union consists of determining and correcting the cause of the delay. Electrical stimulation is thought to stimulate the osteoblasts to lay down a network of bone. Three types of commercial bone growth stimulators are available: a noninvasive model, which is placed outside the cast; a seminoninvasive model, in which pins are inserted around the fracture site; and a totally implantable type, in which a cathode coil is wound around the bone at the fracture site and operated by a battery pack implanted under the skin. The Ilizarov method of circular external fixation is used to treat nonunions, especially those that are infected.

Complications of Fractures and Other Musculoskeletal Injuries

The complications of fractures and other orthopedic injuries are associated with loss of skeletal continuity, injury from bone fragments, pressure from swelling and hemorrhage (*e.g.*, fracture blisters, compartment syndrome), involvement of nerve fibers (*e.g.*, complex regional pain syndrome [CRPS]), or development of venous thromboembolism and fat embolism syndrome (FES).

Fracture Blisters

Fracture blisters are skin bullae and blisters representing areas of epidermal necrosis with separation of the epidermis from the underlying dermis by edema fluid. They occur when the intracompartmental pressure is too high to be relieved through normal means. They are seen with more severe, twisting types of injuries (*e.g.*, motor vehicle accidents and falls from heights) but can also occur after excessive joint manipulation, dependent positioning, and heat application, or from peripheral vascular disease. They can be solitary, multiple, or massive depending on the extent of injury. Most fracture blisters occur in the ankle, elbow, foot, knee, or areas where there is little soft tissue between the bone and the skin. Prevention of fracture blisters is important because they pose an additional risk for infection. They also constitute a warning sign of compartment syndrome.

Compartment Syndrome

Compartment syndrome has been described as a condition of increased pressure within a limited space (*e.g.*, abdominal and limb compartments) that compromises the circulation and function of the tissues in the space. Abdominal compartment syndrome alters cardiovascular hemodynamics, respiratory mechanics, and renal function. The discussion in this chapter is limited to a discussion of limb compartment syndromes.

Etiology and Pathogenesis. The muscles and nerves of an extremity are enclosed in tough, inelastic fascia often termed

Understanding Fracture Healing

A fracture, which is any break in a bone, undergoes a healing process to reestablish bone continuity and strength. The repair of simple fractures is commonly divided into four phases: (1) hematoma formation, (2) inflammation, (3) reparative phase, and (4) remodeling.

Hematoma Formation

When a bone breaks, blood vessels in the bone and surrounding tissues are torn and bleed into and around the fragments of the fractured bone, forming a blood clot, or hematoma. The hematoma facilitates the formation of the fibrin meshwork that seals off the fracture site and serves as a framework for the influx of inflammatory cells, the ingrowth of fibroblasts, and the development of new capillary buds (vessels). It is also the source of signaling molecules that initiate the cellular events that are critical to the healing process.

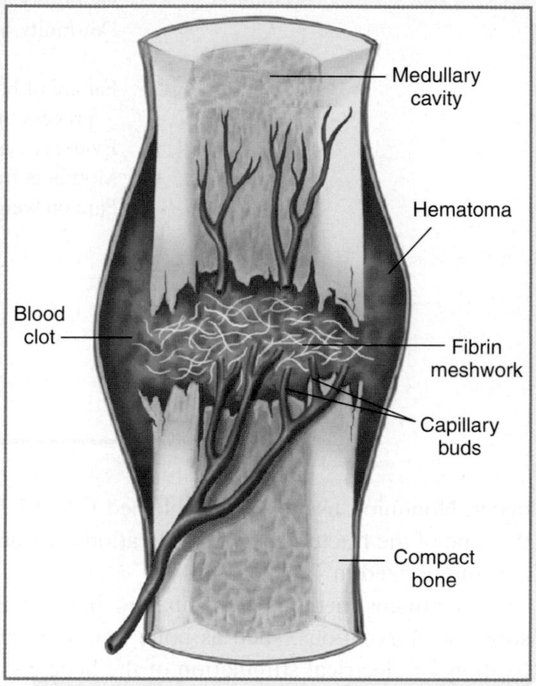

Fibrocartilaginous Callus Formation

As new capillaries infiltrate the hematoma at the fracture site, it becomes organized into a form of granulation tissue called *procallus*. Fibroblasts from the periosteum, endosteum, and red bone marrow proliferate and invade the procallus. The fibroblasts produce a fibrocartilaginous soft callus bridge that connects the bone fragments. Although this repair tissue usually reaches its maximum girth at the end of the 2nd or 3rd week, it is not strong enough for weight bearing.

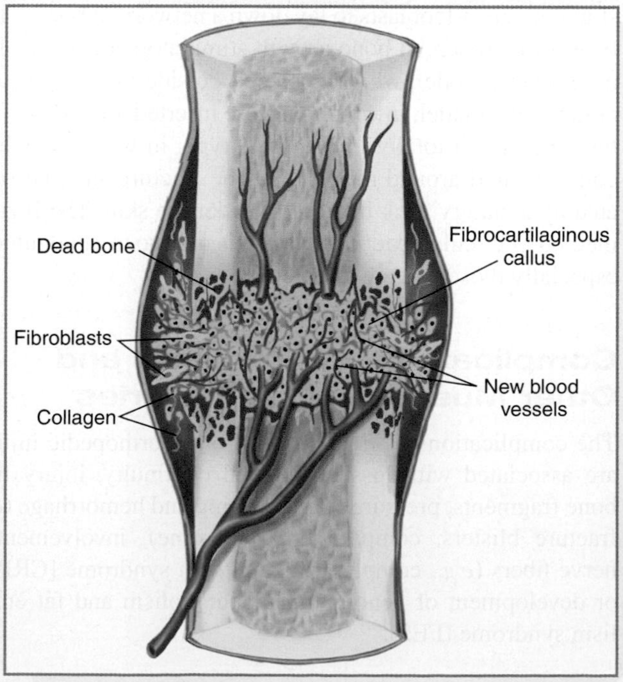

Understanding Fracture Healing *(Continued)*

Bony Callus Formation

Ossification represents the conversion of the fibrocartilaginous cartilage to bony callus. In areas close to well-vascularized bone tissue, osteogenic cells develop into osteoblasts, or bone-building cells, which produce spongy bone trabeculae. The newly formed osteoblasts first deposit bone on the outer surface of the bone some distance from the fracture site. The formation of bone progresses toward the fracture site until a new bony sheath covers the fibrocartilaginous callus. In time, the fibrocartilage is converted to spongy bone, and the callus is then referred to as bony callus. Gradually, the bony callus calcifies and is replaced by mature bone. Bony callus formation begins 3 to 4 weeks after injury and continues until a firm bony union is formed months later.

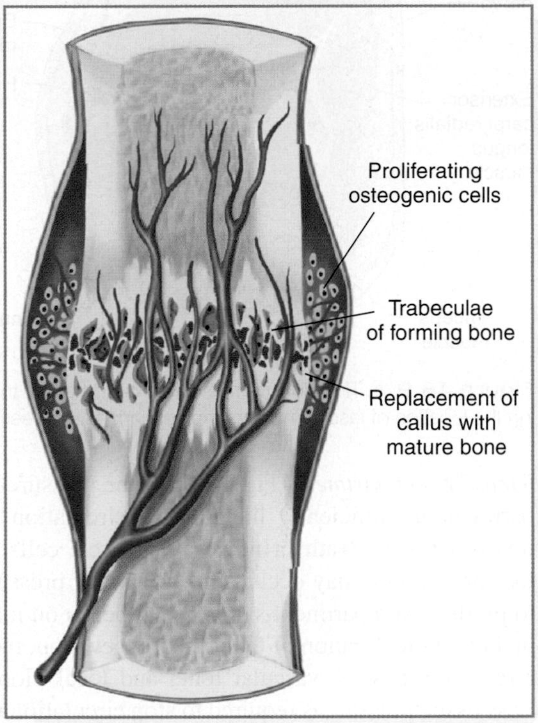

Remodeling

During remodeling of the bony callus, dead portions of the bone are gradually removed by osteoclasts. Compact bone replaces spongy bone around the periphery of the fracture, and there is reorganization of mineralized bone along the lines of mechanical stress. During this period, the excess material on the outside of the bone shaft and within the medullary cavity is removed and compact bone is laid down to reconstruct the shaft. The final structure of the remodeled area resembles that of the original unbroken bone; however, a thickened area on the surface of the bone may remain as evidence of a healed fracture.

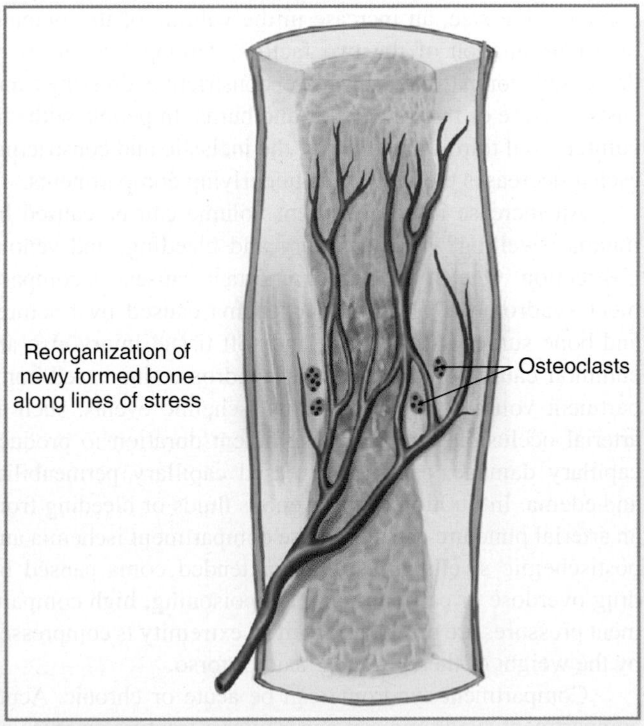

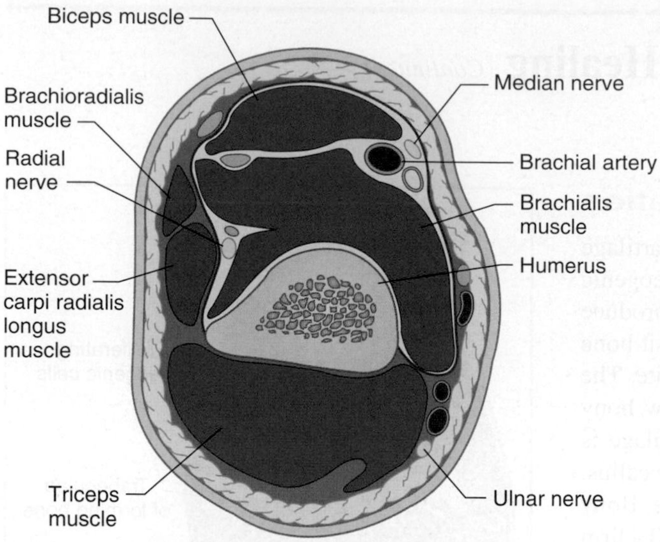

Figure 48.9 • The proximal muscle compartment of the arm, showing the location of fascia, muscles, nerves, and blood vessels.

a *muscle compartment* (Fig. 48.9). If the pressure in the compartment is sufficiently high, tissue circulation is compromised, causing death of nerve and muscle cells. Permanent loss of function may occur. The amount of pressure required to produce compartment syndrome depends on many factors, including the duration of the pressure elevation, the metabolic rate of the tissues, vascular tone, and local blood pressure. Less tissue pressure is required to stop circulation when hypotension or vasoconstriction is present.

Compartment syndrome can result from a decrease in compartment size, an increase in the volume of its contents, or a combination of the two factors. Among the causes of decreased compartment size are constrictive dressings and casts, closure of fascial defects, and burns. In people with circumferential third-degree burns, the inelastic and constricting eschar decreases the size of the underlying compartments.

An increase in compartment volume can be caused by trauma, swelling, vascular injury and bleeding, and venous obstruction. One of the most important causes of compartment syndrome is bleeding and edema caused by fractures and bone surgery. Contusions and soft tissue injury also are common causes of compartment syndrome. Increased compartment volume may also follow ischemic events, such as arterial occlusion, that are of sufficient duration to produce capillary damage, causing increased capillary permeability and edema. Infiltration of intravenous fluids or bleeding from an arterial puncture can also cause compartment ischemia and postischemic swelling. During unattended coma caused by drug overdose or carbon monoxide poisoning, high compartment pressures are produced when an extremity is compressed by the weight of the overlying head or torso.

Compartment syndrome can be acute or chronic. Acute compartment syndrome can occur after a fracture or crushing injury, when excessive swelling around the site of injury results in increased pressure in a closed compartment. This increase in pressure occurs because fascia, which covers and separates muscles, is inelastic and unable to stretch and compensate for the extreme swelling. Chronic compartment syndrome may develop from exertion in long-distance runners and others involved in a major change in activity level. Exertional compartment syndrome is an increase in compartment size and intramuscular pressure during exercise that causes ischemia, pain, and, rarely, neurologic symptoms and signs.

Clinical Manifestations and Diagnosis. The hallmark symptom of an acute compartment syndrome is severe pain that is out of proportion to the original injury or physical findings. Nerve compression may cause changes in sensation (*e.g.*, paresthesias such as burning or tingling or loss of sensation), diminished reflexes, and eventually the loss of motor function. These symptoms generally begin quickly after injury but can also occur in a few days.

Because muscle necrosis can occur quickly, anyone at risk for compartment syndrome needs close surveillance. Assessment should include pain assessment, examination of sensory (*i.e.*, light touch and two-point discrimination) and motor function (*i.e.*, movement and muscle strength), as well as tests of passive stretch and palpation of the muscle compartments. Peripheral pulses frequently are normal in the presence of compartment syndrome because the major arteries are located outside the muscle compartments. Although edema may make it difficult to palpate the pulse, the increased compartment pressure seldom is sufficient to occlude flow in a major artery. Doppler methods usually confirm the existence of a pulse. Disagreement exists regarding the pressure at which ischemic damage occurs; it should not be the only factor in diagnosis.[41,42] A recommended measure is pulse pressure (diastolic blood pressure–tissue pressure), where inadequate perfusion occurs at less than 30 mm Hg.[42]

Treatment. Treatment consists of reducing compartmental pressures. This entails cast splitting or removal of restrictive dressings. These procedures often are sufficient to relieve most of the underlying pressure and symptoms. Elevating the extremity on pillows can help to reduce edema. However, excessive elevation should be avoided because the effects of gravity can lower the arterial pressure in the limb, thereby decreasing compartment perfusion. Sometimes, a fasciotomy may be needed to relieve the pressure in an acute situation. During this procedure, the fascia is incised longitudinally and separated so that the compartment volume can expand and blood flow can be reestablished. Because of potential problems with wound infection and closure, this procedure is usually performed as a last resort.

Complex Regional Pain Syndrome

CRPS, previously referred to as *reflex sympathetic dystrophy* and *causalgia*, is a neurologic condition that impacts limbs and results from surgery or injury.[43–45] The classic complaint is pain that seems out of proportion to the injury, increased sweating, and vasomotor instability.

Pain, which is the prominent symptom of the disorder, is described as severe, aching, or burning. It usually increases in intensity with movement and with noxious and nonnoxious stimuli. The pathophysiologic cause of the pain is unclear, but it is thought to have a sympathetic nervous system component. Muscle wasting, thin and shiny skin, and abnormalities of the nails and bone can occur. Decreased muscle strength and disuse can lead to contractures and osteoporosis. Treatment focuses on pain management, prevention of disability, and improving quality of life with physical and occupational therapy considered to be first-line treatment.[43]

Thromboemboli

The person with a lower extremity fracture is at risk for the development of venous thromboembolic disorders, which include pulmonary embolism and deep vein thrombosis. Age and surgery increase these risks.[46,47] Recommended thromboprophylaxis with pharmacologic and mechanical interventions depends on the type of surgery and risk factors.[47]

The majority of symptomatic venous thromboemboli associated with hospital admissions occur at least 2 months after hospital discharge. Venous Doppler ultrasonography is the accepted test for the diagnosis of lower extremity deep vein thrombosis. A lung scan may be used in the diagnosis of a pulmonary embolus, but it may not differentiate between a thrombus and a fat embolus, especially in an individual with a long bone fracture.

Fat Embolism Syndrome

The FES refers to multiple life-threatening manifestations resulting from the presence of fat droplets in the small blood vessels of the lung, kidneys, brain, and other organs after a long bone or pelvic fracture.[38] The fat emboli are thought to be released from the bone marrow or adipose tissue at the fracture site into the venous system through torn veins.

Pathogenesis. The pathophysiologic process of FES is unclear. Fat embolization involves the presence of fat emboli in the circulation, and FES, an identifiable clinical pattern of organ dysfunction associated with fat emboli in the circulation. One suggestion is that, when a bone is fractured, disruption of the venous sinusoids and fat cells allows fat globules to gain access to the venous circulation. The larger particles then become lodged in and block small pulmonary capillaries, whereas the smaller particles may pass through the lung capillaries and enter the systemic circulation.

Clinical Manifestations. The main clinical features of FES are respiratory failure, cerebral dysfunction, and skin and mucosal petechiae. Cerebral manifestations include encephalopathy, seizures, and focal neurologic deficits unrelated to head injury. Usually, initial symptoms of FES begin to develop within 12 to 72 hours after the injury.[48] The first symptoms include a subtle change in behavior and signs of disorientation resulting from emboli in the cerebral circulation combined with respiratory depression. There may be complaints of substernal chest pain and dyspnea accompanied by tachycardia and a low-grade fever. Diaphoresis, pallor, and cyanosis become evident as respiratory function deteriorates. A petechial rash that does not blanch with pressure often occurs 2 to 3 days after the injury. This rash usually is found on the anterior chest, axillae, neck, and shoulders. It also may appear on the soft palate and conjunctiva. The rash is thought to be related to embolization of the skin capillaries or thrombocytopenia.

Diagnosis and Treatment. An important part of the treatment of FES is early diagnosis. Arterial blood gases should be assayed immediately after recognition of clinical manifestations. Treatment is directed toward correcting hypoxemia and maintaining adequate fluid balance. Mechanical ventilation may be required. Corticosteroid drugs are administered to decrease the inflammatory response of lung tissues, decrease the edema, stabilize the lipid membranes to reduce lipolysis, and combat bronchospasm. Corticosteroids are also given prophylactically to high-risk people. The only preventive approach to FES is early stabilization of the fracture.

IN SUMMARY

Many external physical agents can cause trauma to the musculoskeletal system. Factors such as environment, activity, or age can place a person at greater risk for injury. Some soft tissue injuries, such as contusions, hematomas, and lacerations, are relatively minor and easily treated. Muscle strains and ligamentous sprains are caused by mechanical overload on the connective tissue. They heal more slowly than the minor soft tissue injuries and require some degree of immobilization. Healing of soft tissue begins within 4 to 5 days of the injury and is primarily the function of fibroblasts, which produce collagen. Joint dislocation is caused by trauma to the supporting structures. Repeated trauma to the joint can cause articular softening (*i.e.*, chondromalacia) or the separation of small pieces of bone or cartilage, called *loose bodies*, in the joint.

Fractures occur when more stress is placed on a bone than the bone can absorb. The nature of the stress determines the type of fracture and the character of the resulting bone fragments. Healing of fractures is a complex process that takes place in four stages: hematoma formation, inflammatory phase, reparative process, and the remodeling stage.[36] For satisfactory healing to take place, the affected bone has to be reduced and immobilized. Immobilization is accomplished with the use of external devices, such as splints, casts, traction, or an external fixation apparatus, or with a surgically implanted internal fixation device. The complications associated with fractures can occur early because of soft tissue and nerve damage, or later when the healing process of the fracture is interrupted. The early complications of fractures and other orthopedic injuries are associated with swelling and hemorrhage (fracture blisters and compartment syndrome), involvement of nerve fibers (reflex sympathetic dystrophy and causalgia), and development of fat emboli. Impaired healing of a fracture can cause malunion with deformity, angulation, or rotation; delayed union, in which the healing process is prolonged; or nonunion, in which the fracture fails to heal.

BONE INFECTIONS

After completing this section of the chapter, the learner will be able to meet the following objectives:

- Explain the implications of bone infection.
- Differentiate among osteomyelitis due to spread from a contaminated wound, hematogenous osteomyelitis, and osteomyelitis due to vascular insufficiency in terms of etiologies, manifestations, and treatment.
- Describe the most common sites of tuberculosis of the bone.

Bone infections, including acute and chronic osteomyelitis, are known for their ability to cause pain, disability, and deformity. Despite the common use of antibiotics, they remain difficult to treat and eradicate. A resurgence of tubercular bone infections is occurring in industrialized parts of the world, attributed in part to immigration from developing countries and greater numbers of immunocompromised people.

KEY POINTS

BONE INFECTIONS

- Bone infections may be caused by a wide variety of microorganisms introduced during injury or operative procedures, or through the bloodstream.
- Once localized in bone, the microorganisms proliferate, produce cell death, and spread within the bone shaft, inciting a chronic inflammatory response with further destruction of bone.
- Bone infections are difficult to treat and eradicate. Measures to prevent infection include careful cleaning and debridement of skeletal injuries and strict operating room protocols.

Osteomyelitis

Osteomyelitis represents an acute or chronic infection of the bone. *Osteo* refers to bone, and *myelo* refers to the marrow cavity, both of which are involved in this disease. The infection can be caused by:

- Direct penetration or contamination of an open fracture or wound (exogenous origin)
- Seeding through the bloodstream (hematogenous spread)
- Extension from a contiguous site
- Skin infections in people with vascular insufficiency

Osteomyelitis can occur as an acute, subacute, or chronic condition. All types of organisms, including viruses, parasites, fungi, and bacteria, can produce osteomyelitis, but infections caused by certain pyogenic bacteria and mycobacteria are the most common.

The specific agents isolated in pyogenic bacterial osteomyelitis are often associated with the age of the person or the inciting condition (*e.g.*, trauma or surgery). *Staphylococcus aureus* is the most common cause, but organisms such as *Escherichia coli*, *Neisseria gonorrhoeae*, *Haemophilus influenzae*, and *Salmonella* species are also seen.[36,49]

Hematogenous Osteomyelitis

Hematogenous osteomyelitis originates with infectious organisms that reach the bone through the bloodstream. Acute hematogenous osteomyelitis occurs predominantly in children.[50] In adults, it is seen most commonly in debilitated people and in those with a history of chronic skin infections, chronic urinary tract infections, and intravenous drug use and in those who are immunologically suppressed. Intravenous drug users are at risk for infections with *Streptococcus* and *Pseudomonas*.[36]

Pathogenesis. The pathogenesis of hematogenous osteomyelitis differs in children and adults. In children, the infection usually affects the long bones of the appendicular skeleton. It starts in the metaphyseal region close to the growth plate, where termination of nutrient blood vessels and sluggish blood flow favor the attachment of blood-borne bacteria (Fig. 48.10). With advancement of the infection, purulent exudate collects in the rigidly enclosed bony tissue. Because of the bone's rigid structure, there is little room for swelling and the purulent exudate finds its way beneath the periosteum, shearing off the perforating arteries that supply the cortex with blood, thereby leading to necrosis of cortical bone. Eventually, the purulent drainage may penetrate the periosteum and skin to form a draining sinus. In children 1 year of age and younger, the adjacent joint is often involved because the periosteum is not firmly attached to the cortex.[36] From 1 year of age to puberty, subperiosteal abscesses are more common.[36] As the process continues, periosteal new bone formation and reactive bone formation in the marrow tend to wall in the infection. *Involucrum* refers to a lesion in which bone formation forms a sheath around the necrotic sequestrum. It is seen most commonly in cases of chronic osteomyelitis.

In adults, the long bone microvasculature no longer favors seeding, and hematogenous infection rarely affects the appendicular skeleton. Instead, vertebrae, sternoclavicular and sacroiliac joints, and the symphysis pubis are involved. Infection typically first involves subchondral bone, then spreads to the joint space.[36] With vertebral osteomyelitis, this causes sequential destruction of the endplate, adjoining disk, and contiguous vertebral body. Infection less commonly begins in the joint and spreads to the adjacent bone.

Clinical Manifestations. The signs and symptoms of acute hematogenous osteomyelitis are those of bacteremia accompanied by symptoms referable to the site of the bone lesion. Bacteremia is characterized by chills, fever, and malaise. There often is pain on movement of the affected extremity, loss of movement, and local tenderness followed by redness and swelling. X-ray studies may appear normal initially, but they show evidence of periosteal elevation and increased osteoclast activity after an abscess has formed.

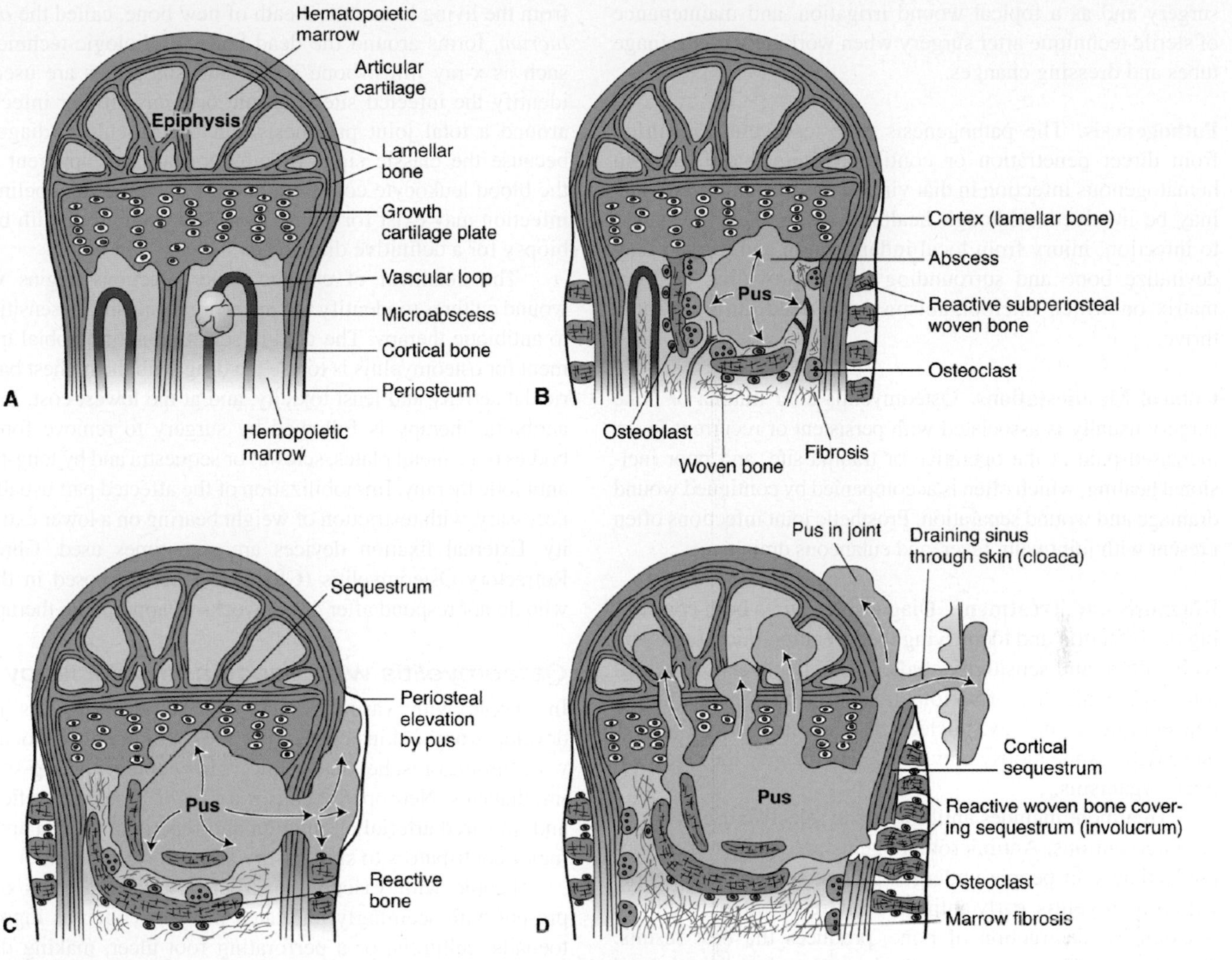

Figure 48.10 • Pathogenesis of hematogenous osteomyelitis. **(A)** This epiphysis, metaphysis, and growth plate are normal. A small, septic microabscess is developing at the capillary loop. **(B)** Expansion of the septic focus stimulates resorption of adjacent bony trabeculae. Woven bone begins to surround this focus. The abscess expands into the cartilage and stimulates reactive bone formation by the periosteum. **(C)** The abscess, which continues to expand through the cortex into the subperiosteal tissue, shears off the perforating arteries that supply the cortex with blood, thereby leading to necrosis of the cortex. **(D)** The extension of this process into the joint space, the epiphysis, and the skin produces a draining sinus. The necrotic bone is called a sequestrum. The viable bone surrounding a sequestrum is termed the involucrum. (From Strayer D. S., Rubin R. (Eds.) (2015). *Rubin's pathology: Clinicopathologic foundations of medicine* (7th ed., Figure 30-17, p. 1325). Philadelphia, PA: Lippincott Williams & Wilkins.)

Treatment. The treatment of hematogenous osteomyelitis begins with identification of the causative organism through blood and bone aspiration cultures.[36,50] Antimicrobial agents are given first parenterally and then orally. The length of time the affected limb needs to be rested and pain control measures used are based on symptoms. Debridement and surgical drainage also may be necessary.

Direct Penetration and Contiguous Spread Osteomyelitis

Direct penetration or extension of bacteria from an outside (exogenous) source is now the most common cause of osteomyelitis in the United States.[36] Bacteria may be introduced directly into the bone by a penetrating wound, an open fracture, or surgery. Inadequate irrigation or debridement, introduction of foreign material into the wound, and extensive tissue injury increase the bone's susceptibility to infection.

Iatrogenic bone infections are those inadvertently brought about by surgery or other treatments. These complications include pin tract infection in skeletal traction, septic (infected) joints in joint replacement surgery, and wound infections after surgery. Staphylococci and streptococci are still commonly implicated, but in 25% of postoperative infections, gram-negative organisms are detected.[36] Measures to prevent these infections include preparation of the skin to reduce bacterial growth before surgery or insertion of traction devices or wires, strict operating room protocols, prophylactic use of antibiotics immediately before and for 24 hours after surgery and as a topical wound irrigation, and maintenance of sterile technique after surgery when working with drainage tubes and dressing changes.

Pathogenesis. The pathogenesis of osteomyelitis resulting from direct penetration or contiguous spread differs from hematogenous infection in that virtually any traumatized bone may be involved. Although healthy bone is highly resistant to infection, injury from local inflammation and trauma may devitalize bone and surrounding tissue, providing an inert matrix on which microorganisms introduced during trauma thrive.

Clinical Manifestations. Osteomyelitis after trauma or bone surgery usually is associated with persistent or recurrent fever, increased pain at the operative or trauma site, and poor incisional healing, which often is accompanied by continued wound drainage and wound separation. Prosthetic joint infections often present with joint pain, fever, and cutaneous drainage.

Diagnosis and Treatment. Diagnosis requires both confirming the infection and identifying the offending microorganism with culture and sensitivity studies. The diagnosis of skeletal infection entails use of various imaging strategies, including conventional radiology, nuclear imaging studies, CT scans, and MRI.[50] Bone biopsy may be used to identify the causative microorganisms.

Treatment includes antibiotics and selective use of surgical interventions. Antimicrobial agents are usually used prophylactically in people undergoing bone surgery. For people with osteomyelitis, early antimicrobial treatment, before there is extensive destruction of bone, produces the best results. The choice of agents and method of administration depend on the microorganisms causing the infection. In acute osteomyelitis that does not respond to antibiotic therapy, surgical decompression is used to release intramedullary pressure and remove drainage from the periosteal area. Prosthesis removal may be necessary in cases of an infected prosthetic joint.

Chronic Osteomyelitis

Chronic osteomyelitis usually occurs in adults. Generally, these infections occur secondary to an open wound, most often to the bone or surrounding tissue. Chronic osteomyelitis has long been recognized as a disease. However, the incidence has decreased in the past century because of improvements in surgical techniques and the advent of broad-spectrum antibiotic therapy. Chronic osteomyelitis includes all inflammatory processes of bone, excluding those in rheumatic diseases that are caused by microorganisms. It may be the result of delayed or inadequate treatment of acute hematogenous osteomyelitis or osteomyelitis caused by direct contamination of bone by exogenous organisms. Chronic osteomyelitis can persist for years; it may appear spontaneously, after a minor trauma, or when resistance is lowered.

The hallmark feature of chronic osteomyelitis is the presence of infected dead bone, a *sequestrum*, that has separated from the living bone.[36] A sheath of new bone, called the *involucrum*, forms around the dead bone. Radiologic techniques such as x-ray films, bone scans, and sinograms are used to identify the infected site. Chronic osteomyelitis or infection around a total joint prosthesis can be difficult to diagnose because the classic signs of infection are not apparent and the blood leukocyte count may not be elevated. A subclinical infection may exist for years. Bone scans are used with bone biopsy for a definitive diagnosis.

The treatment of chronic bone infections begins with wound cultures to identify the microorganism and its sensitivity to antibiotic therapy. The goal in selecting antimicrobial treatment for osteomyelitis is to use the drug with the highest bactericidal activity and least toxicity, and at the lowest cost. Initial antibiotic therapy is followed by surgery to remove foreign bodies (*e.g.*, metal plates, screws) or sequestra and by long-term antibiotic therapy. Immobilization of the affected part usually is necessary, with restriction of weight bearing on a lower extremity. External fixation devices are sometimes used. Chronic Refractory Osteomyelitis (CRO) may be diagnosed in those who do not respond after 4 to 6 weeks of appropriate therapy.[51]

Osteomyelitis with Vascular Insufficiency

In people with vascular insufficiency, osteomyelitis may develop from a skin lesion. It is most commonly associated with chronic or ischemic foot ulcers in people with long-standing diabetes. Neuropathy causes a loss of protective reflexes, and impaired arterial circulation and repetitive trauma are the major contributors to skin fissure and ulcer formation.

People with vascular insufficiency osteomyelitis often present with seemingly unrelated problems such as ingrown toenails, cellulitis, or a perforating foot ulcer, making diagnosis difficult. Furthermore, pain is often muted by peripheral neuropathy. Osteomyelitis is confirmed when bone is exposed in the ulcer bed or after debridement. Radiologic evidence is a late sign.

Treatment depends on the oxygen tension of the involved tissues. Debridement and antibiotic therapy may benefit people who have good oxygen tension in the infected site. Hyperbaric oxygen therapy may be used as an adjunctive treatment.

Tuberculosis of the Bone or Joint

For those at risk, the spread of tuberculosis to the bone occurs through a variety of means but generally through the bloodstream. Although it may occur during primary infection, it is more likely to occur through reactivated latent bacilli.[52]

Tuberculosis can spread from one part of the body, such as the lungs or the lymph nodes, to the musculoskeletal system. Tubercular osteomyelitis tends to be more destructive and difficult to control than pyogenic osteomyelitis. The infection spreads through large areas of the medullary cavity and causes extensive necrosis. In tuberculosis of the spine, also known as *Pott disease or tuberculous spondylitis*, the infection spreads through the intervertebral disks to involve multiple vertebrae and extends into the soft tissue, forming abscesses.

Local symptoms include pain, immobility, and muscle atrophy; joint swelling, mild fever, and leukocytosis also may occur. The most feared complication of spinal tuberculosis is neurologic compromise because of spinal deformity and epidural abscess formation. Because there are no specific radiographic findings in tubercular osteomyelitis, the diagnosis is usually made by tissue biopsy or culture findings. In spinal tuberculosis, a CT-guided biopsy is often used. The mainstay of treatment for tubercular osteomyelitis is similar to the guidelines for respiratory tuberculosis.

IN SUMMARY

Bone infections occur because of the direct or indirect invasion of the musculoskeletal system by microorganisms, most commonly *S. aureus*. Osteomyelitis, or infection of the bone and marrow, can be an acute or chronic disease. Acute osteomyelitis is seen most often as a result of the direct contamination of bone by a foreign object. Chronic osteomyelitis represents an infection that continues beyond 6 to 8 weeks and may persist for years. The incidence of all types of bone infection has been dramatically reduced since the advent of antibiotic therapy. Iatrogenic infections are those inadvertently brought about by surgery or other treatments. Tuberculosis of the bone, which is characterized by bone destruction and abscess formation, is caused by spread of the infection from the lungs or lymph nodes.

OSTEONECROSIS

After completing this section of the chapter, the learner will be able to meet the following objectives:

- Cite four major causes of osteonecrosis.
- Characterize the blood supply of bone and relate it to the pathologic features of the condition.

Osteonecrosis, or death of a segment of bone, is a condition caused by the interruption of blood supply to the marrow, medullary bone, or cortex in the absence of infection[36] (Fig. 48.11). It is a relatively common disorder and can occur in the medullary cavity of the metaphysis and the subchondral region of the epiphysis, especially in the proximal femur, distal femur, and proximal humerus. It is a common complicating disorder of Legg-Calvé-Perthes disease, slipped capital femoral epiphysis, sickle cell disease, steroid therapy, alcohol abuse, and hip trauma, fracture, or surgery. People treated with corticosteroids and/or bisphosphonates are more vulnerable to developing osteonecrosis.[53,54]

Etiology and Pathogenesis

Although bone necrosis results from ischemia, the mechanisms producing the ischemia are varied and include mechanical vascular interruption such as occurs with trauma or a

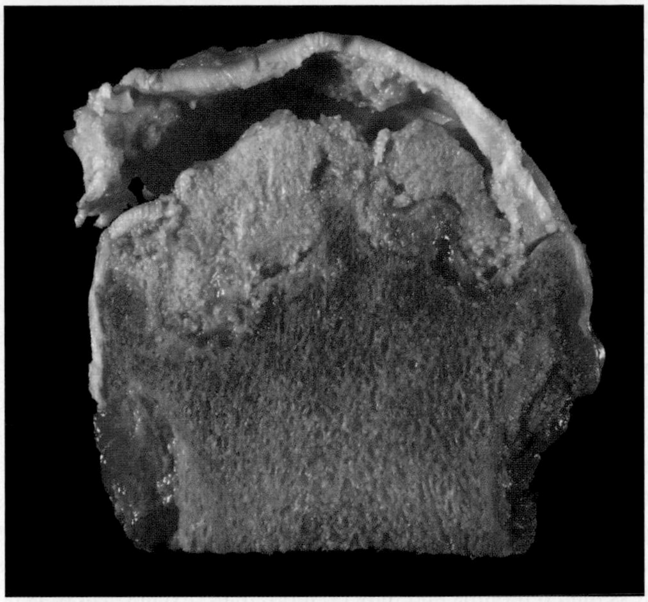

Figure 48.11 • Osteonecrosis of the head of the femur. A coronal section shows a circumscribed area of subchondral infarction with partial detachment of the overlying articular cartilage and subarticular bone. (From Strayer D. S., Rubin R. (Eds.) (2015). *Rubin's pathology: Clinicopathologic foundations of medicine* (7th ed., Figure 30-14A, p. 1321. Philadelphia, PA: Lippincott Williams & Wilkins.)

fracture; thrombosis and embolism (*e.g.*, sickle cell disease, nitrogen bubbles caused by inadequate decompression during deep sea diving); and vessel injury (*e.g.*, vasculitis, radiation therapy). In many cases, the cause of the necrosis is uncertain. Other than fracture, the most common causes of bone necrosis are idiopathic (*i.e.*, those of unknown cause) and prior steroid therapy. Chart 48.1 lists disorders associated with osteonecrosis.

Bone has a rich blood supply that varies from site to site.[36] The flow in the medullary portion of bone originates in

CHART 48.1 CAUSES OF OSTEONECROSIS

Mechanical disruption of blood vessels
- Fractures
- Legg-Calvé-Perthes disease
- Blount disease

Thrombosis and embolism
- Sickle cell disease
- Nitrogen bubbles in decompression sickness

Vessel injury
- Vasculitis
- Connective tissue disease
- Systemic lupus erythematosus
- Rheumatoid arthritis
- Radiation therapy
- Gaucher disease

Corticosteroid therapy

nutrient vessels from an interconnecting plexus that supplies the marrow, trabecular bone, and endosteal half of the cortex. The outer cortex receives its blood supply from periosteal, muscular, metaphyseal, and epiphyseal vessels that surround the bone. Some bony sites, such as the head of the femur, have only limited collateral circulation, so that interruption of the flow, such as with a hip fracture, can cause necrosis of a substantial portion of medullary and cortical bone and irreversible damage.

One of the most frequent causes of osteonecrosis is that associated with administration of corticosteroids.[36] Despite numerous studies, the mechanism of steroid-induced osteonecrosis remains unclear. The condition may develop after the administration of very high, short-term doses; during long-term treatment; or even from intra-articular injection. Although the risk increases with the dose and duration of treatment, it is difficult to predict who will be affected. The interval between corticosteroid administration and onset of symptoms rarely is less than 6 months and may be more than 3 years. There is no satisfactory method for preventing progression of the disease. Osteonecrosis of the jaw has been reported after long-term use of bisphosphonates.[53]

The pathologic features of bone necrosis are the same, regardless of cause. The site of the lesion is related to the vessels involved. There is necrosis of cancellous bone and marrow. The cortex usually is not involved because of collateral blood flow. In subchondral infarcts (*i.e.*, ischemia below the cartilage), a triangular or wedge-shaped segment of tissue that has the subchondral bone plate as its base and the center of the epiphysis as its apex undergoes necrosis. When medullary infarcts occur in fatty bone marrow, the death of bone cells causes calcium release and necrosis of fat cells, with the formation of free fatty acids. Released calcium forms an insoluble "soap" with free fatty acids. Because bone lacks mechanisms for resolving the infarct, the lesions remain for life.

Clinical Manifestations, Diagnosis, and Treatment

The symptoms associated with osteonecrosis are varied and depend on the extent of infarction. Typically, subchondral infarcts cause chronic pain that is initially associated with activity but that gradually becomes more progressive until it is experienced at rest. Subchondral infarcts often collapse and predispose the person to severe secondary osteoarthritis.

Diagnosis of osteonecrosis is based on history, physical findings, radiographic findings, and results of special imaging studies, including CT scans and technetium-99 m bone scans. Treatment of osteonecrosis depends on the underlying pathologic process. In some cases, only short-term immobilization, nonsteroidal anti-inflammatory drugs, exercises, and limitation in weight bearing are used. Osteonecrosis of the hip is particularly difficult to treat. In people with early disease, limitation of weight bearing using crutches may allow the condition to stabilize. Although several surgical approaches have been used, the most definitive treatment of advanced osteonecrosis of the knee or hip is total joint replacement.

IN SUMMARY

Osteonecrosis is a common condition that has long been recognized but is not fully understood. Death of bone is caused by disruption of the blood supply from intravascular or extravascular processes. Sites with poor collateral circulation, such as the femoral head, are most seriously affected. Causative factors include corticosteroid therapy. Symptoms include pain that varies in severity, depending on the extent of infarction. Total joint replacement is the most frequently used treatment for advanced osteonecrosis.

NEOPLASMS

After completing this section of the chapter, the learner will be able to meet the following objectives:

- Differentiate between the properties of benign and malignant bone tumors.
- Contrast osteogenic sarcoma, Ewing sarcoma, and chondrosarcoma in terms of the most common age groups and anatomic sites that are affected.
- List the primary sites of tumors that frequently metastasize to the bone.

Neoplasms in the skeletal system are referred to as *bone tumors*. Primary malignant tumors of the bone are uncommon, constituting less than 0.2% of all cancers.[55] The American Cancer Society projected 3450 new cases of bone cancer and approximately 1590 deaths in 2018.[55] Metastatic disease of the bone, however, is relatively common. Primary bone tumors may arise from any of the skeletal components, including osseous bone tissue, cartilage, and bone marrow. The discussion in this section focuses on primary benign and malignant bone tumors of osseous or cartilaginous origin and metastatic bone disease.

Like other types of neoplasms, bone tumors may be benign or malignant. Benign tumors far outnumber malignant tumors. The benign types, such as osteochondromas, tend to grow rather slowly and usually do not destroy the supporting or surrounding tissue or spread to other parts of the body. Malignant tumors, such as osteosarcoma, grow rapidly and can spread to other parts of the body through the bloodstream or lymphatics. The two major forms of bone cancer in children and young adults are osteosarcoma and Ewing sarcoma.[55] Chondrosarcomas tend to occur during adulthood, with 51 being the average age of diagnosis.[55] The classification of benign and malignant bone tumors is described in Table 48.3.

TABLE 48.3 CLASSIFICATION OF PRIMARY BONE NEOPLASMS

TISSUE TYPE	BENIGN NEOPLASM	MALIGNANT NEOPLASM
Bone	Osteoid osteoma Benign osteoblastoma	Osteosarcoma Parosteal osteogenic sarcoma
Cartilage	Osteochondroma Chondroma Chondroblastoma Chondromyxoid fibroma	Chondrosarcoma
Lipid	Lipoma	Liposarcoma
Fibrous and fibro-osseous tissue	Fibrous dysplasia	Fibrosarcoma Malignant fibrous histiocytoma
Miscellaneous	Giant cell tumor	Malignant giant cell Ewing sarcoma
Bone marrow		Multiple myeloma Reticulum cell sarcoma

Characteristics of Bone Tumors

There are three major manifestations of bone tumors: pain, presence of a mass, and impairment of function. Pain is a feature common to almost all malignant tumors but may or may not occur with benign tumors. For example, a benign bone cyst usually is asymptomatic until a fracture occurs. Pain that persists at night and is not relieved by rest suggests malignancy. A mass or hard lump may be the first sign of a bone tumor. A malignant tumor is suspected when a painful mass exists that is enlarging or eroding the cortex of the bone. The ease of discovery of a mass depends on the location of the tumor; a small lump arising on the surface of the tibia is easy to detect, whereas a tumor that is deep in the medial portion of the thigh may grow to a considerable size before it is noticed. Benign and malignant tumors may cause the bone to erode to the point at which it cannot withstand the strain of ordinary use. In such cases, even a small amount of bone stress or trauma precipitates a pathologic fracture. A tumor may produce pressure on a peripheral nerve, causing decreased sensation, numbness, a limp, or limitation of movement.

KEY POINTS

BONE NEOPLASMS

- Neoplasms of the skeletal system can affect bone tissue, cartilage, or bone marrow.
- Benign tumors tend to grow slowly, do not spread to other parts of the body, and exert their effects through the space-occupying nature of the tumor and their ability to weaken bone structures.
- Malignant bone tumors are rare before 10 years of age, have their peak incidence in the teenage years, tend to grow rapidly, and have a high mortality rate.

Benign Neoplasms

Benign bone tumors usually are limited to the confines of the bone, have well-demarcated edges, and are surrounded by a thin rim of sclerotic bone. An *osteoma* is a small bony tumor found on the surface of a long bone, flat bone, or the skull. It usually is composed of hard, compact (ivory osteoma), or spongy (cancellous) bone. It may be excised or left alone.

A *chondroma* is a tumor composed of hyaline cartilage. It may arise on the surface of the bone (*i.e.*, ecchondroma) or in the medullary cavity (*i.e.*, endochondroma). These tumors may become large and are especially common in the hands and feet. A chondroma may persist for many years and then take on the attributes of a malignant chondrosarcoma. A chondroma usually is not treated unless it becomes unsightly or uncomfortable.

An *osteochondroma* is the most common form of benign tumor in the skeletal system, representing 50% of all benign bone tumors and approximately 15% of all primary skeletal lesions. It grows only during periods of skeletal growth, originating in the epiphyseal cartilage plate and growing out of the bone like a mushroom. An osteochondroma is composed of cartilage and bone and usually occurs singly but may affect several bones in a condition called *multiple exostoses*. Malignant changes are rare, and excision of the tumor is done only when necessary.

A *giant cell tumor*, or *osteoclastoma*, is an aggressive tumor of multinucleated cells that often behaves like a malignant tumor, metastasizing through the bloodstream and recurring locally after excision. It arises most often in people in their 20s to 40s and is found most commonly in the knee, wrist, or shoulder. The tumor begins in the metaphyseal region, grows into the epiphysis, and may extend into the joint surface. Pathologic fractures are common because the tumor destroys the bone substance. Clinically, pain may occur at the tumor site, with gradually increasing swelling. X-ray films show destruction of the bone with expansion of the cortex.

The treatment of giant cell tumors depends on their location. If the affected bone can be eliminated without loss of function, such as the clavicle or fibula, the entire bone or part of it may be removed. When the tumor is near a major joint, such as the knee or shoulder, a local excision is done. Irradiation may be used to prevent recurrence of the tumor.

Malignant Bone Tumors

In contrast to benign tumors, primary malignant tumors tend to be ill defined, lack sharp borders, and extend beyond the confines of the bone. Primary bone tumors occur in all age groups and may arise in any part of the body. However, certain types of tumors tend to target certain age groups and anatomic sites (Fig. 48.12). For example, most osteogenic sarcomas

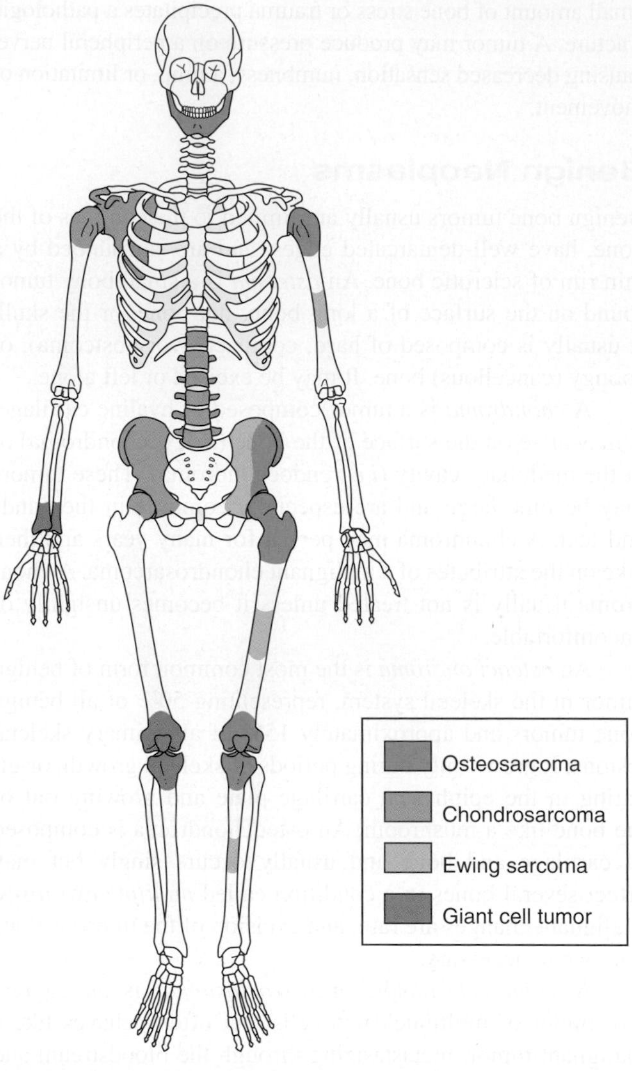

Figure 48.12 • Common sites of primary malignant bone tumors (chondrosarcoma, osteosarcoma, and Ewing sarcoma) and giant cell tumor, a locally aggressive benign tumor.

occur in adolescents and are particularly common around the knee joint. Also, people with certain conditions such as Paget disease are at increased risk for development of bone cancer.

The diagnosis of bone tumors includes radiologic staging and biopsy.[56] Radiographs give the most general diagnostic information, such as malignant versus benign and primary versus metastatic status. The radiograph demonstrates the region of bone involvement, extent of destruction, and amount of reactive bone formed. Radioisotope scans are used to estimate the local intramedullary extent of the tumor and screen for other skeletal areas of involvement. CT scans further aid diagnosis and anatomic localization and can identify small pulmonary metastases not seen by conventional radiographs. MRI is the most accurate method of evaluating the intramedullary extent of bone tumor and can demarcate the soft structures in relation to neurovascular structures without the use of contrast media. It is best used in conjunction with a CT scan. Radionuclide bone scans are used to assess for metastasis. A biopsy also is done because the definitive treatment of most bone tumors is based on pathologic interpretation of the biopsy specimen.

Osteosarcoma

Osteosarcoma is an aggressive and highly malignant bone tumor. It is the most common primary malignant bone tumor, and most often occurs in children.[57] Osteosarcoma affects boys more than girls and accounts for about 56% of cases.[36,57] Although osteosarcomas can develop in any bone, they most commonly arise in the vicinity of bone growth such as the knee, distal femur, or proximal humerus.[36,57]

Etiology. The cause of osteosarcoma is unknown. The tumor is most likely to occur in people younger than 20 years of age and in older adults. The correlation of age and location of most of the tumors with the period of maximum growth suggests some relation to increased osteoblastic activity. In younger people, the primary tumor most often is located at the anatomic sites associated with maximum growth velocity—the distal femur, proximal tibia, and proximal humerus.[36,57] Bone tumors in older adults are more common in the humerus, pelvis, and proximal femur.[36] Paget disease, which is linked to osteosarcoma in adults, also is associated with increased osteoblastic activity. Irradiation from an internal source, such as the radioactive pharmaceutical technetium used in bone scans, or an external source, such as x-ray films, also has been associated with osteosarcoma. There are known genetic factors associated with osteosarcoma. Mutations in two genes are reported to increase the susceptibility to the development of osteosarcoma: the retinoblastoma gene (*RB*) and the *TP53* tumor suppressor gene.[36]

Pathogenesis. Osteosarcomas are aggressive tumors that grow rapidly in a circular, balllike mass in the bone tissue. They often are eccentrically placed in the bone and move from the metaphysis of the bone out into the periosteal surface, with subsequent spread to adjacent soft tissues (Fig. 48.13). The tumor infrequently metastasizes to the lymph nodes because the cells

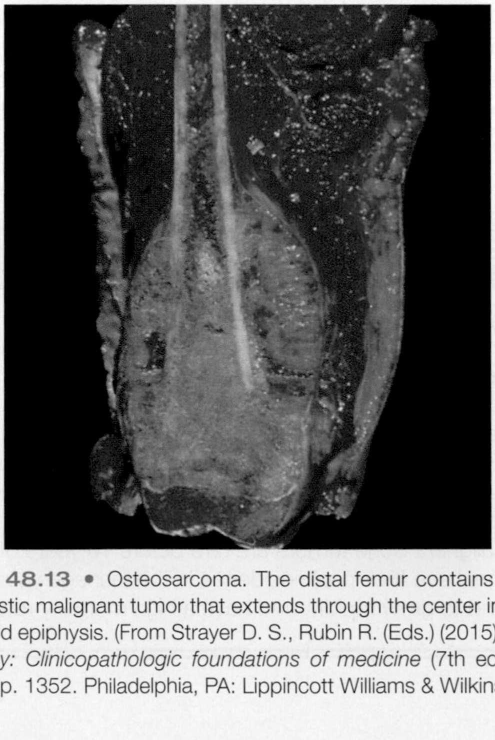

Figure 48.13 • Osteosarcoma. The distal femur contains a dense osteoblastic malignant tumor that extends through the center in the soft tissue and epiphysis. (From Strayer D. S., Rubin R. (Eds.) (2015). *Rubin's pathology: Clinicopathologic foundations of medicine* (7th ed., Figure 30-46A, p. 1352. Philadelphia, PA: Lippincott Williams & Wilkins.)

are unable to grow in the node. Nodal metastases usually occur only in the late course of disseminated disease. Most often, the tumor cells exit the primary tumor through the venous end of the capillary, and early metastasis to the lung is common. Lung metastases, even if massive, usually are relatively asymptomatic. The prognosis for a person with osteosarcoma depends on the aggressiveness of the disease, presence or absence of pathologic fractures, size of the tumor, and rapidity of tumor growth.

Clinical Manifestations and Diagnosis. The primary clinical feature of osteosarcoma is deep, localized pain with nighttime awakening and swelling in the affected bone, which tends to be of a sudden nature. The skin overlying the tumor may be warm, shiny, and stretched, with prominent superficial veins. The range of motion of the adjacent joint may be restricted.

History, physical examination, and radiographic studies are all part of the evaluation of a person with osteosarcoma. Plain films of the primary site and of the chest are first obtained. MRI, CT scan, and full-body scan are required to evaluate the extent of the local disease and to determine the extent of metastasis if present. Radionuclide bone scans are done to evaluate for lung and bone metastasis. An open biopsy is required to confirm the diagnosis and to determine the histologic features and cell type of the tumor.

Treatment. Osteosarcoma is treated by surgery and chemotherapy.[58] In the past, treatment usually entailed amputation above the level of the tumor.[55] Limb salvage surgical procedures, using a metal prosthesis or cadaver allograft, are now a standard alternative. Studies have shown that limb salvage surgery has no adverse effects on the long-term survival or function of people with osteosarcoma.[59] Interestingly, quality of life was found to be similar between the two, and limb salvage shows some difference in local recurrence and complications.[60,61] Although limb sparing surgery is now more common, success depends on many factors such as achieving wide margins; an exact measure of what that entails, however, is not clearly defined. Also, although chemotherapy has had a significant effect on survival, those results have reached a plateau and there has been little development in chemotherapy treatments since the 1980s.[62] Advanced imaging techniques, including serum thallium scans, and the use of angiography assist the surgeon in determining the best type of treatment. Age seems to be a factor in prognosis when comparing young adult to pediatric people, with young adults having less favorable outcomes.[63]

Amputation is also an option. It involves either the removal of expendable bones such as the fibula, ribs, toes, or ulna, or the complete removal of the tumor and the affected limb. The primary objective of overall treatment of people with osteosarcoma is long-term disease-free survival or cure. Preserving limb function is a secondary objective. In cases in which adequate limb salvage surgery cannot be achieved, limb amputation may be necessary.

Ewing Sarcoma

Ewing sarcoma is a member of a group of small round cell, undifferentiated tumors thought to be of neural crest origin.[36] The family of tumors includes Ewing sarcoma of the bone and soft tissue, extraosseous Ewing sarcoma, Askin tumor, and peripheral primitive neuroectodermal tumor (PPNET). Of the tumors in this family, Ewing sarcoma accounts for most cases. Ewing sarcoma and osteosarcoma occur in the same gender and age groups, but they can usually be distinguished radiographically and histologically. About 2% of childhood cancers can be attributed to Ewing sarcoma; it can occur at any age but is most often seen in those under age 20 and is rarely seen after age 30.[64,65] Males are affected slightly more frequently than females.

Pathogenesis. The most frequent site of Ewing sarcoma is the femur, usually in the diaphysis. The pelvis represents the second most common site; other sites include the pubis, sacrum, humerus, vertebrae, ribs, skull, and other flat bones.[36] The characteristic pathologic findings of Ewing sarcoma include densely packed, regularly shaped, small cells with round or oval nuclei. A specific reciprocal translocation of chromosomes 11 and 22, or a variant thereof, is found in most of the Ewing sarcoma family of tumors.[36] Detection of the translocation by routine cytogenetic or polymerase chain reaction analysis can be helpful in confirming the diagnosis in highly undifferentiated tumors.[36]

Clinical Manifestations. Common manifestations of Ewing sarcoma include nonspecific joint pain and dull pain not necessarily related to movement, which late in illness leads to restrictions in movement and swelling.[65] In some children, it is accompanied by systemic manifestations such as fever or weight loss, which may serve to confuse the diagnosis. There may be a delay in diagnosis when the pain and swelling associated with the tumor are attributed to a sports injury or when the tumor is located in the pelvis and the pain is not localized and the mass is not apparent. Pathologic fractures are common because of bone destruction. The most common sites of metastasis are the lungs, bone marrow, and other bones.

Diagnosis and Treatment. Because Ewing sarcoma is a difficult diagnosis to establish, the diagnostic biopsy is very important. Clinical evaluations include MRI and CT scans of the primary tumor, chest radiographs, CT of the chest, bone scan, bilateral bone marrow aspiration, and biopsy of the primary tumor site.[36] The extent of disease at diagnosis is the most important prognostic factor. The presence of metastatic disease at diagnosis is a poor prognostic factor regardless of the site of the primary lesion.

Treatment methods incorporate a combination of multiagent chemotherapy, surgery, and radiation therapy. Chemotherapy is generally given before local control measures are initiated. Ewing sarcoma is considered to be a radiosensitive tumor, and local control may be achieved through radiation or surgery. People with small, nonmetastatic, distally located tumors generally have the best prognosis.

Chondrosarcoma

Chondrosarcoma, a malignant tumor of cartilage, is the most common bone sarcoma among adults and the second most common primary malignant bone cancer overall.[38,66] It occurs primarily in middle or later life and slightly more often in men. The tumor arises from points of muscle attachment to bone, particularly the knee, shoulder, hip, and pelvis. Chondrosarcomas can arise from underlying benign lesions. There are three types of chondrosarcoma including peripheral, central, and juxtacortical; all three affect cartilage.[36]

Chondrosarcomas are slow growing and metastasize late, and often are painless. They can remain hidden in an area such as the pelvis for a long time. This type of tumor, like many primary malignancies, tends to destroy bone and extend into the soft tissues beyond the confines of the bone of origin. Chondrosarcomas mainly affect the bones of the trunk, pelvis, or proximal femur and rarely develop in the distal portion of a bone. Irregular flecks and ringlets of calcification often are prominent radiographic findings.

Early diagnosis is important because chondrosarcoma responds well to early radical surgical excision. It usually is resistant to radiation therapy and available chemotherapeutic agents. Not infrequently, these tumors transform into a highly malignant tumor, mesenchymal chondrosarcoma, which requires a more aggressive treatment, including combination chemotherapy.

Metastatic Bone Disease

Skeletal metastases, or secondary tumors, are more common than primary tumors.[67,68] Approximately half of all people with cancer have bone metastasis at some point in their disease. Metastatic lesions are seen most often in the spine, femur, pelvis, ribs, sternum, proximal humerus, and skull and are less common in anatomic sites more distant from the trunk of the body. Predominant primary tumor sites with bone metastasis include prostate, colorectal, lung, and breast.[69,70] The incidence of metastatic bone disease is highest in people older than 40 years of age.

Clinical Manifestations and Diagnosis

The major symptom of bone metastasis is pain in a specific bone area, and this is validated with evidence of an impending pathologic fracture. It usually develops gradually, over weeks, and is more severe at night. Pain is caused by stretching of the periosteum of the involved bone or by nerve entrapment, as when the nerve roots of the spinal cord are compressed by the vertebral body. The affected bone of the pathologic fracture appears to be eaten away on x-ray images; in severe cases, it crumbles on impact, much like dried toast. Many pathologic fractures occur in the femur, humerus, and vertebrae.

Radiographic examinations are used along with CT, PET-CT, and bone scans to detect, diagnose, and localize metastatic bone lesions.[71] Approximately, one third of people with skeletal metastases have positive bone scans without radiologic findings.

Arteriography using radiopaque contrast media may be helpful in outlining the tumor margins. A bone biopsy usually is done when there is a question regarding the diagnosis or treatment. A closed-needle biopsy with CT localization is particularly useful with spine lesions. Serum levels of alkaline phosphatase and calcium often are elevated in people with metastatic bone disease.

Treatment

The primary goals in treatment of metastatic bone disease are to prevent pathologic fractures and promote survival with maximum functioning, allowing the person to maintain as much mobility and pain control as possible. Standard treatment methods include chemotherapy, irradiation, and surgical stabilization. Radiation therapy is primarily used as a palliative treatment to alleviate pain and prevent pathologic fractures. After a pathologic fracture has occurred, bracing, intramedullary nailing of the femur, or spine stabilization may be done. Because adequate fixation often is difficult in diseased bone, cement (*i.e.*, methyl methacrylate) often is used with internal fixation devices to stabilize the bone.

Recent research has focused on the role of osteoclastic and osteoblastic activity in the pathogenesis of metastatic bone disease and on the use of the COX-2 inhibitors, carbon ion therapy, bisphosphonates (*e.g.*, pamidronate disodium, zoledronic acid), and denosumab, an anti-RANKL, for its treatment.[38,72,73] Bone tissue contains a rich environment of growth factors and cells of various embryonic origins, including hematopoietic, stromal, endothelial, and other cell types. The osteoclasts and osteoblasts, in particular, appear to play a dominant role in the pathogenesis of bone metastasis.

The bisphosphonates, which are now well-established agents for the prevention and treatment of osteoporosis, have recently been shown to decrease symptoms associated with bone metastasis secondary to breast and prostate cancer. These agents bind preferentially to bone at sites of active bone metabolism, are released from the bone matrix during bone resorption, and potentially inhibit osteoclast activity and survival, thereby reducing osteoclast-mediated bone resorption.

IN SUMMARY

Bone tumors, like any other type of neoplasm, may be benign or malignant. Benign bone tumors grow slowly and usually do not destroy the surrounding tissues. Malignant tumors can be primary or metastatic. Primary bone tumors are rare, grow rapidly, metastasize to the lungs and other parts of the body through the bloodstream, and have a high mortality rate. Metastatic bone tumors usually are multiple, originating primarily from cancers of the breast, lung, and prostate. The incidence of metastatic bone disease probably is increasing because improved treatment methods enable people with cancer to live longer. Advances in chemotherapy, radiation therapy, and surgical procedures have substantially increased the survival and cure rates for many types of bone cancers. A primary goal in metastatic bone disease is the prevention of pathologic fractures.

GERIATRIC Considerations

- The risk for vertebral fractures is five times higher for people who have a prior fracture, and women who sustain a vertebral fracture are 20% more likely to have another fracture within a year.[38]
- Balancing calcium intake in older adults is difficult; they need more calcium because it is not absorbed as readily, but too much can lead to renal stones or heart disease.[38]
- Men have a higher mortality rate associated with hip fractures; however, women over age 80 have a 50% risk of osteoporosis, leading to high risk for bone fracture.[38]
- Fracture of the distal radius is common among older adults and typically occurs when they reach out with their hand to stop a fall.[74]

PEDIATRIC Considerations

- *Staphylococcus aureus* is the most common cause of acute hematogenous osteomyelitis causing osteomyelitis in children.[75]
- Spiral fractures in children are rare and when they occur are often the result of physical abuse from twisting of the extremity.[75]
- Ankle and wrist sprains are more common as the growth plate begins to close.[75]
- A dislocation of the knee or hip is rare in children because of the extreme force required; it is considered an emergency. Dislocation of the knee places the child at risk for peroneal nerve and popliteal artery damage.[75]

REVIEW EXERCISES

1. A 39-year-old man is in intensive care after a motorcycle crash in which he skidded across the pavement on his right side. He has fractures of his right femur, pelvis, and several ribs on the right side. His leg was crushed beneath the motorcycle. He is beginning to lose movement in his leg.
   A. *What are the priorities in treating his orthopedic injuries? What are the options for stabilizing his leg?*
   B. *What risk factors for complications of fractures are present?*
   C. *What are the symptoms of compartment syndrome, and how is it treated?*
2. A 73-year-old woman sustained a comminuted fracture in the middiaphysis of her left humerus when her husband lifted her up in bed. She has multiple lucent lesions scattered throughout her proximal humerus, radius, and ulna. She was recently hospitalized for confusion and was found to have diffuse bone metastases. Her bone marrow biopsy showed adenocarcinoma. She has a history of breast cancer 30 years ago, but her most recent mammogram was negative.
   A. *What would you consider to be the most likely cause of her fracture?*
   B. *What are the most common sites for bone metastasis?*
   C. *Explain the treatment goals for people with pathologic fractures.*
3. A 14-year-old boy has complained of recent pain and swelling of his knee, with some restriction in movement. Although he thinks he may have injured his knee playing football, his mother insists that he be seen by an orthopedic specialist, who raises the possibility that the boy may have an osteosarcoma.
   A. *Use the theory that osteosarcoma has its origin in sites of maximal growth velocity to explain the site of this boy's possible tumor.*
   B. *What diagnostic tests could be used to establish a diagnosis of osteosarcoma?*
   C. *The boy and his family are concerned that he will require radical surgery with amputation of the leg. How would you explain possible treatment options to him?*

References

1. Horvai A. (2015). Bones, joints, and soft tissue tumors. In Kumar V., Abbas A., Aster J. (Eds.), *Robbins & Cotran Pathologic Basis of Disease* (9th ed., pp. 1179–1226). Philadelphia, PA: Elsevier/Saunders; Chapter 26.
2. National Centers for Disease Control and Prevention. (2017). *Key Injury and Violence Data.* Available: https://www.cdc.gov/injury/wisqars/overview/key_data.html. Retrieved October 28, 2017.
3. Centers for Disease Control and Prevention Winnable Battles Motor Vehicle Injuries. Available at: https://www.cdc.gov/winnablebattles/report/motor.html. Retrieved on October 28, 2017
4. Centers for Disease Control and Prevention Protect the Ones You Love: Child Injuries are Preventable CDC Childhood Injury Report. Available at: https://www.cdc.gov/safechild/child_injury_data.html. Retrieved October 28, 2017
5. Centers for Disease Control and Prevention Protect the Ones You Love: Child Injuries are Preventable. Available at: https://www.cdc.gov/safechild/sports_injuries/index.html Retrieved October 28, 2017.
6. Bergen G., Stevens M. R., Burns E. R. (2016). Falls and fall injuries among adults aged ≥65 years – united states, 2014. *Morbidity and Mortality Weekly Report* 65(37), 993–998.
7. Vieira L. S., Gomes A. P., Bierhals I. O., et al. (2018). Falls among older adults in the South of Brazil: prevalence and determinants. *Revista de Saúde Pública* 52, 22. http://doi.org.ezproxy.uthsc.edu/10.11606/S1518-8787.2018052000103

8. Rubenstein L. Z. (2016). *Falls in the elderly.* Available: https://www.merckmanuals.com/professional/geriatrics/falls-in-the-elderly/falls-in-the-elderly. Accessed May 5, 2018
9. Patel D., Yamaski A., Brown K. (2017). Epidemiology of sports-related musculoskeletal injuries in young athletes in United States. *Translational Pediatrics* 6(3), 160–166.
10. Hoang Q., Mortazavi M. (2012). Pediatric overuse injuries in sports. *Advances in Pediatrics* 59(1), 359–393.
11. Saladin K. S. (2015) *Anatomy & physiology: The unity of form and function* (7th ed.). New York, NY: McGraw Hill Education.
12. Patel D., Kinsella E. (2017). Evaluation and management of lower back pain in young athletes. *Translational Pediatrics* 6(3), 225–235.
13. Mataliotakis G., Tsirikos A. (2017). Spondylolysis and spondylolisthesis in children and adolescents: Current concepts and treatment. *Spine* 31(6), 395–401.
14. Sairyo K., Nagamachi A. (2016). State-of-the-art management of low back pain in athletes: Instructional lecture. *Journal of Orthopaedic Science* 21(3), 263–272.
15. Gorroll A. H., Mulley A. G. (2014). *Primary Care medicine: Office evaluation and management of the adult patient* (7th ed.). Philadelphia, PA: Lippincott Williams & Wilkins.
16. Rosa J., Checchia C., Miyazaki A. (2017). Traumatic instability of the shoulder. *Revista Brasileira de Ortopedia* 52(5), 513–520.
17. Carpinteiro E., Barros A. (2017) Natural history of anterior shoulder instability. *The Open Orthapaedics Journal* 11(suppl-6, M9), 909–918.
18. Dunphy L. M., Windland-Brown J. E., Porter B. O., et al. (2015). *Primary care: The art and science of advanced practice nursing* (4th ed.). Philadelphia, PA: FA Davis.
19. National Association of Orthopedic Nurses (NAON). (2013). *Core curriculum for orthopaedic nursing* (7th ed.). Boston, MA: Pearson.
20. Hibberd E. E., Kerr Z. Y., Roos K. G., et al. (2016). Epidemiology of acromioclavicular joint sprains in 25 national collegiate association sports: 2009–2020 to 2014–2015 academic years. *The American Journal of Sports Medicine* 44(10), 2667–2674.
21. Monica J., Vredenburgh Z., et al.. (2016) Acute shoulder injuries in adults. *American Family Physician* 94(2), 119–127.
22. Gupta H., Robinson P. Normal shoulder ultrasound: Anatomy and technique. (2015). *Seminars in Musculoskeletal Radiology* 19(3), 203–211.
23. Lazarides A., Alentorn E., Choi J., et al. (2015). Rotator cuff tears in young patients: A different disease than rotator cuff tears in elderly patients. *Journal of Shoulder and Elbow Surgery* 24, 1834–1843.
24. Oliva F., Piccirilli E., Bossa M., et al. (2015). I.S.Mu.L.T. Rotator cuff tears guidelines. *Muscles, Ligaments and Tendons Journal* 5(4), 227–263.
25. Jensen S. (2015). *Nursing health assessment: A best practice approach* (2nd ed.). Philadelphia, PA: Wolters Kluwer Health.
26. Antonelli M., Starz T. (2012). Assessing for risk and progression of osteoarthritis: The nurse's role. *American Journal of Nursing* 112(3), S26–S31.
27. Vetrano M., Oliva F., Bisschia S., et al. (2017). I.S.Mu.L.T. first-time patellar dislocation guidelines. *Muscles, Ligaments and Tendons Journal* 7(1), 1–10.
28. Sanders T., Pareek A., Hewett T., Stuart M., Dahm D., Krych A. (2018). Incidence of first-time lateral patellar dislocation: A 21-year population-based study. *Sports Health* 10(2), 146–151. DOI: 10.1177/1941738117725055
29. Duthon V. (2015). Acute traumatic patellar dislocation. *Orthopaedics & Traumatology: Surgery & Research* 101, S59–S67.
30. Laidlaw M., Diduch D. (2017). Current concepts in the management of patellar instability. *Indian Journal of Orthopaedics* (serial online) (cited March 7 2017) 51, 493–504. Available from http://www.ijoonline.com/text.asp?2017/51/5/493/214211
31. Smith T., Donell S., Song F., et al. (2015) Surgical versus non-surgical interventions for treating patellar dislocation. *Cochrane Database of Systematic Reviews* Issue 2.
32. Dortaj H., Emamifar A. (2015). Case report: Traumatic hip dislocation with associated femoral head fracture. *Case Reports in Orthopedics* 2015(865786), 1–3.
33. Dyer S., Crotty M., Fairhill N., et al. (2016). A critical review of the long-term disability outcomes following hip fracture. *BMC Geriatrics* 16(158), 1–18.
34. Anpalahan M., Morrison S. G., Gibson S. J. (2014). Hip fracture risk factors and the discriminability of hip fracture risk vary by age: A case–control study. *Geriatrics & Gerontology International* 14, 413–419. DOI: 10.1111/ggi.12117
35. Mangram A., Moeser P., Corneille M. G., et al. (2014) Geriatric hip trauma hip fractures: Is there a difference in outcomes based on fracture patterns? *World Journal of Emergency Surgery* 9(59), 1–8.
36. Rubin R., Strayer D. (Eds.). (2012). *Rubin's pathology: Clinicopathologic foundations of medicine* (6th ed.). Philadelphia, PA: Lippincott Williams & Wilkins.
37. Drake R. L., Vogl A. W., Mitchell A. W. M. (2015). *Gray's anatomy for students* (3rd ed.). Philadelphia, PA: Churchill Livingstone.
38. Hinkle J. L., Cheever K. H. (2018). *Brunner & Suddarth's textbook of medical-surgical nursing* (14th ed.). Philadelphia, PA: Lippincott Williams & Wilkins.
39. Browner B. Jupiter J., Krettek K., et al. (2015). *Skeletal trauma: Basic science, management and reconstruction* (5th ed.). Philadelphia, PA: Elsevier Saunders.
40. Valderama-Molina C. O., Estrada-Castrillón M., Hincapie J. A., et al. (2014). Intra- and interobserver agreement on the Oestern and Tscherne classification of soft tissue injury in periarticular lower-limb closed fractures. *Colombia Médica* 45(4), 173–178.
41. Lollo L., Grabinsky A. (2016). Clinical and functional outcomes of acute lower extremity compartment syndrome at a major trauma hospital. *International Journal of Critical Illness and Injury Science* 6(3), 133–142.
42. Garner M. R., Taylor S. A., Gausden E., et al. (2014). Compartment syndrome: Diagnosis, management, and unique concerns in the twenty-first century. *The Musculoskeletal Journal of Hospital for Special Surgery* 10, 143–152.
43. Goh E. L., Chidambaram S., Daqing M. (2017). Complex regional pain syndrome: A recent update. *Burns & Trauma* 5(2), 1–11. DOI: 10.1186/s41038-016-0066-4
44. Tajerian M., Clark J. D. (2016). New concepts in complex regional pain syndrome. *Hand Clinics* 32(1), 41–49.
45. Pons T., Shipton E. A., Williman J., et al. (2015). Potential risk factors for the onset of complex regional pain syndrome type 1: A systematic literature review. *Anesthesiology Research and Practice* 2015(956539), 1–15.
46. Whiting P. S., Jahangir A. A. (2016). Thromboembolic disease after orthopedic trauma. *Orthopedic Clinics of North America* 47, 335–344.
47. Falck-Ytter Y., Francis C. W., Johanson N. A., et al. (2012). Prevention of VTE in orthopedic surgery patients: Antithrombotic therapy and prevention of thrombosis, 9th ed: American College of Chest Physicians Evidence-based Clinical Practice Guidelines. *Chest* 141(2 suppl), e278S–e325S.
48. Kosova E., Bergmark B., Piazza G. (2015). Fat embolism syndrome. *Circulation* 131, 317–320.
49. Tyagi R. (2016) Spinal infections in children: A review. *Journal of Orthopaedics* 13, 254–258.
50. Schmitt S. K. (2017). Osteomyelitis. *Infectious Disease Clinics of North America* 31, 325–338.
51. Hanley M. E., Cooper J. S. (2017). *Hyperbaric, chronic refractory osteomyelitis.* Available https://www.ncbi.nlm.nih.gov/books/NBK430785/. Accessed April 22, 2018
52. Hogan J. I., Hurtado R. M., Nelson S. B. (2017). Mycobacterial musculoskeletal infections. *Infectious Disease Clinics of North America* 31, 369–382.
53. Brown J. P., Morin S., Leslie W., et al. (2014). Bisphosphonates for the treatment of osteoporosis: Expected benefits, potential harms, and drug holidays. *Canadian Family Physician* 60, 324–333.
54. Liu L. H., Zhang Q. Y., Sun W., et al. (2017). Corticosteroid-induced osteonecrosis of the femoral head: Detection, diagnosis, and treatment in earlier stages. *Chinese Medical Journal* 130, 2601–2607.
55. American Cancer Society. (2018). Bone cancer. [Online]. Available: http://www.cancer.org/cancer/bonecancer/detailedguide/bone-cancer-key-statistics. Accessed March 4, 2018

56. American Cancer Society. (2018). Bone cancer. [Online]. Available: https://www.cancer.org/cancer/bone-cancer/detection-diagnosis-staging/how-diagnosed.html. Accessed March 4, 2018
57. American Cancer Society. (2018). Bone cancer. [Online]. Available: https://www.cancer.org/cancer/osteosarcoma/about/what-is-osteosarcoma.html. Accessed March 4, 2018
58. Cronin K., Bui M., Caracciolo J. T. (2015) Osteoblastic osteosarcoma. *Applied Radiology* 44(7), 38–41.
59. He X., Gao Z., Xu H., et al. (2017). A meta-analysis of randomized control trials of surgical methods with osteosarcoma outcomes. *Journal of Orthopaedic Surgery and Research* 12(5), 1–6.
60. Mavrogenis A. F., Novella C., Romagnoli C., et al. (2012). Similar survival but better function for patients after limb salvage versus amputation for distal tibia osteosarcoma. *Clinical Orthopaedics and Related Research* 470, 1735–1748.
61. Mei J., Zhu Z. Wang Z., et al. (2014). Functional outcomes and quality of life in patients with osteosarcoma treated with amputation versus limb-salvage surgery: A systematic review and meta-analysis. *Archives of Orthopaedic and Trauma Surgery* 134, 1507–1516.
62. Anderson M. E. (2016). Update on survival in osteosarcoma. *Orthopedic Clinics of North America* 47, 283–292.
63. Haddox C. L., Han G., Anijar L., et al. (2014). Osteosarcoma in pediatric patients and young adults: a single institution retrospective review of presentation, therapy, and outcome. *Sarcoma* Article ID 402509, 1–10.
64. Brown H. K., Schiavone K., Gouin F., et al. (2018). Biology of bone sarcomas and new therapeutic developments. *Calcified Tissue International* 102, 174–195.
65. Freeman A. K., Sumathis V., Jeys L. (2014). Primary malignant tumors of the bone. *Orthopaedics 1: General Principles Surgery* 33(1), 26–33.
66. The ESMO/European Sarcoma Network Working Group. (2014). Bone sarcomas: ESMO clinical practice guidelines for diagnosis, treatment and follow-up. *Annals of Oncology* 25(suppl 3), iii13–iii123.
67. Bharma J. S., Malik A. A., Aresti N. A., et al. (2012). The perioperative management of skeletal metastases. *Journal of Perioperative Practice* 22(1), 24–29.
68. American Cancer Society. (2018). Bone cancer. [Online]. Available: https://www.cancer.org/treatment/understanding-your-diagnosis/advanced-cancer/what-is.html. Accessed March 4, 2018
69. Hernandez R. K., Wade S. W., Reich A., et al. (2018). Incidence of bone metastases in patients with solid tumors: Analysis of oncology electronic medical records in the United States. *BMC Cancer* 18(44), 1–11.
70. Li S., Peng Y., Weinhandl E. D., et al. (2012), Estimated number of prevalent cases of metastatic bone disease on the US adult population. *Clinical Epidemiology* 4, 87–93.
71. American Cancer Society. (2018). Bone cancer. [Online]. Available: https://www.cancer.org/treatment/understanding-your-diagnosis/advanced-cancer/finding-bone-metastases.html. Accessed March 4, 2018
72. American Cancer Society. (2018). Bone cancer. [Online]. Available: https://www.cancer.org/treatment/understanding-your-diagnosis/advanced-cancer/treating-bone-metastases.html. Accessed March 4, 2018
73. Fujita Y., Inoue K. (2013). A discussion of several approaches for the future based on previous studies of metastatic bone tumors. *International Medical Journal* 20(5), 532–534.
74. Eliopoulos C. (2018). *Gerontological nursing* (9th ed.). Philadelphia, PA: Wolters Kluwer.
75. Bowden V., Greenberg C. S. (2014). *Children and their families: The continuum of nursing care* (3rd ed.). Philadelphia, PA: Wolters Kluwer.

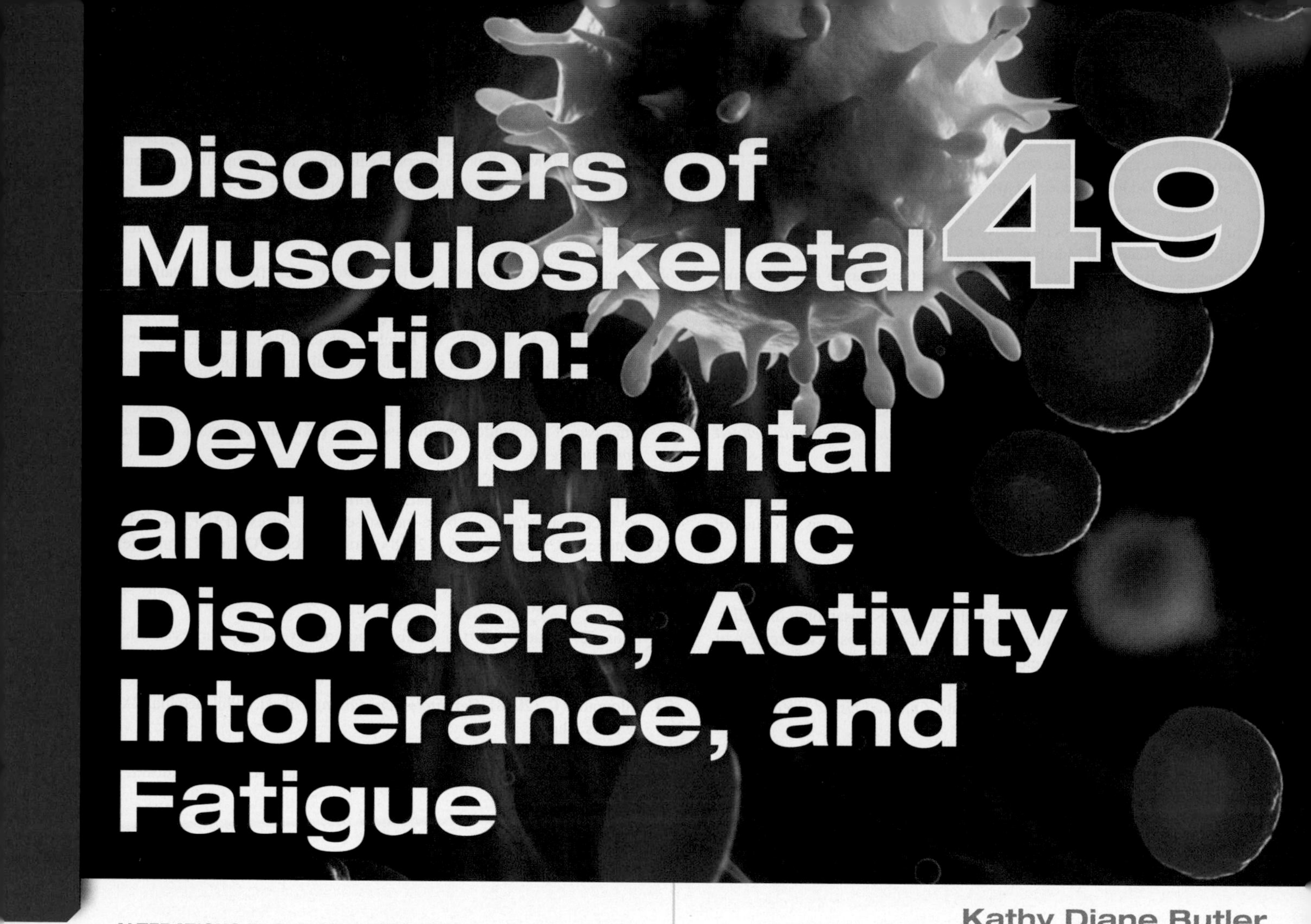

49 Disorders of Musculoskeletal Function: Developmental and Metabolic Disorders, Activity Intolerance, and Fatigue

Kathy Diane Butler

The development of skeletal structures begins in utero and continues to change throughout life. During childhood, skeletal structures grow in length and diameter and sustain a large increase in bone mass. The term *modeling* refers to the formation of the macroscopic skeleton, which ceases at maturity, usually between 18 and 20 years of age. Once skeletal growth has attained its adult size, the process of bone remodeling is responsible for skeletal maintenance. It involves bone resorption and formation and is responsible for skeletal maintenance at sites that require replacement or repair. With aging, bone resorption and formation are no longer perfectly coupled, and there is loss of bone.

Skeletal disorders may develop because of abnormal growth and developmental processes because of hereditary or congenital influences. Other skeletal disorders can occur later in life because of nutritional deficiencies, metabolic disorders, hormonal influences, or the aging process. This chapter is divided into two parts including altered skeletal growth and development and metabolic bone diseases.

ALTERATIONS IN SKELETAL GROWTH AND DEVELOPMENT

After completing this section of the chapter, the learner will be able to meet the following objectives:

- Describe the function of the epiphyseal growth plate in skeletal growth.
- Characterize the abnormalities associated with developmental dysplasia of the hip and methods of diagnosis and treatment.
- Differentiate between congenital, idiopathic, and neuromuscular scoliosis.

Bone Growth and Remodeling

Embryonic and Fetal Development

The skeletal system is generated from the mesodermal and neural crest cells of the developing embryo.[1] Development of the vertebrae of the axial skeleton begins at approximately the 4th week in utero. During the 9th week, ossification begins with the appearance of ossification centers in the lower thoracic and upper lumbar vertebrae. The paddle-shaped limb buds of the lower extremities make their appearance late in the 4th week of development; the hand pads are developed by days 33 to 36; and the finger rays are evident on days 41 to 43.[1]

Abnormalities originating from the embryonic stage of development are relatively uncommon. When they do occur, they are usually limited to defined embryonic structures (*e.g.*, congenital absence of a phalanx; formation of extra bones [supernumerary digits], or fusion of adjacent digits [syndactylism]). In utero positioning during fetal development causes the more common problems. In the newborn, the imprint of in utero positioning may be evident and confused with an abnormality. The effects of in utero positioning are usually physiologic in origin, rather than anatomic.

Bone Growth in Childhood

During the first two decades of life, the skeleton undergoes general overall growth. The long bones of the skeleton, which grow at a relatively rapid rate, are provided with a specialized structure called the *epiphyseal growth plate*[2] (Fig. 49.1). The chondrocytes are involved in synthesizing cartilage of the epiphyseal plate.[2] As long bones grow in length, the deeper layers of cartilage cells in the growth plate multiply and enlarge and ultimately calcify. The embedded cartilage cells then die attracting the osteoblasts to migrate into the area. Osteoid is secreted from the osteoblasts, which assists the mature bone in forming. Therefore, in the epiphyseal plates, there is continuous cartilage synthesis, calcification, erosion, and osteoblast invasion so that there is always active bone formation[2] (Fig. 49.2). This process allows bone growth to proceed without changing the shape of the bone or causing disruption of the articular cartilage. The cells in the growth plate stop dividing at puberty, at which time the epiphysis and metaphysis fuse.

Several factors can influence the growth of cells in the epiphyseal growth plate. Epiphyseal separation can occur in children because of trauma. The separation usually occurs in the zone of the mature enlarged cartilage cells, which is the weakest part of the growth plate. The blood vessels that nourish the epiphysis pass through the growth plate. These vessels are ruptured when the growth plate separates. This can cause cessation of growth and a shortened extremity. The growth plate also is sensitive to nutritional and metabolic changes. Scurvy (*i.e.*, vitamin C deficiency) impairs the formation of the organic matrix of bone, causing slowing of growth at the epiphyseal plate and decreased diaphyseal growth. In rickets (*i.e.*, vitamin D deficiency), calcification of the newly developed bone on the metaphyseal side of the growth plate is impaired. Thyroid hormone, insulin-like growth factor, and insulin are required for normal growth. Alterations in these and other hormones can also affect growth. A few years after reaching puberty, the epiphyseal plates in the long bones become less responsive to the hormones and then become totally unresponsive.[2] Generally, people reach the end of bone growth by the age of 20 as the epiphyseal plate closes. However, some bones remain responsive to hormones and continue to grow. Examples include the skull, fingers, feet, and jaw.[2]

Growth in the diameter of bones occurs as new bone is added to the outer surface of existing bone along with an accompanying resorption of bone on the endosteal or inner surface. Such oppositional growth allows for widening of the marrow cavity while preventing the cortex from becoming too thick and heavy. In this way, the shape of the bone is maintained. As a bone grows in diameter, concentric rings are added to the bone surface, much as rings are added to a tree trunk. These rings form the lamellar structure of mature bone. Osteocytes, which develop from osteoblasts, become buried in the rings. Haversian canals form as periosteal vessels running along the long axis become surrounded by bone.[3]

Alterations During Normal Growth Periods

Infants and children undergo changes in muscle tone and joint motion during growth and development. Toeing-in,

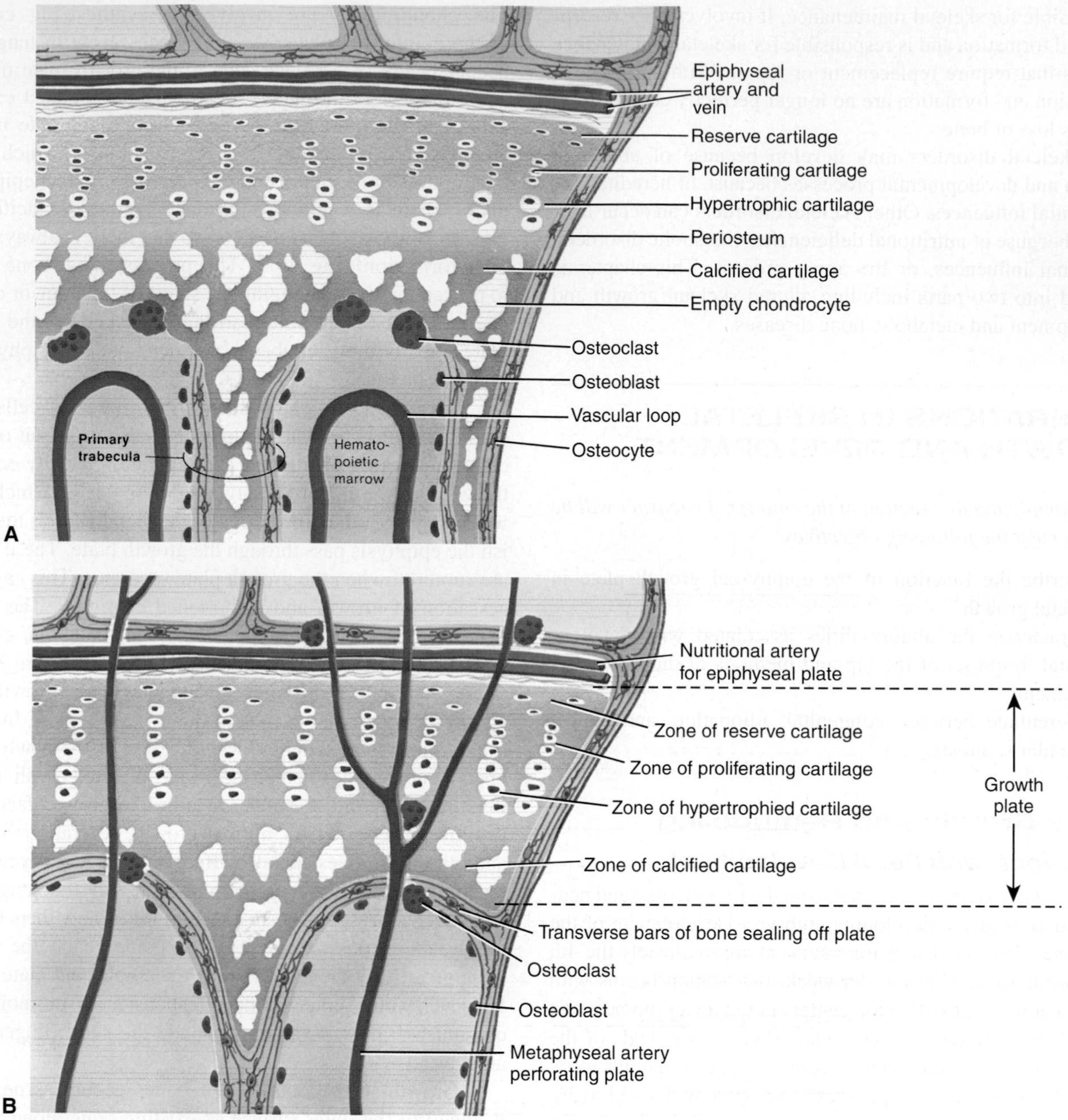

Figure 49.1 • Anatomy of the epiphyseal growth plate. **(A)** Normal growing epiphyseal plate. The epiphysis is separated from the plate by transverse plates of bone that seal the plate so that it grows only toward the metaphysis. There are multiple zones of cartilage. **(B)** Normal closure. The epiphyseal cartilage has stopped growing. There are metaphyseal vessels penetrating the cartilage plate. Transverse bars of bone separate the plate from the metaphysis. (From Rubin R., Strayer D. S. (Eds.) (2015). *Rubin's pathology: Clinicopathologic foundations of medicine* (7th ed., p. 1314). Philadelphia, PA: Lippincott Williams & Wilkins.)

toeing-out, bowlegs, and knock-knees occur frequently in infancy and childhood.[4] They usually cause few problems and are corrected during normal growth processes. There may be physiologic flexion contractures of the hips, which tend to be externally rotated and the patellae point outward, whereas the feet appear to point forward because of the internal pulling force of the tibiae. During the first year of life, the lower extremities begin to straighten out in preparation for walking. Internal and external rotations become equal, and the hips extend.

Musculoskeletal assessment of the newborn is important to identify abnormalities that require early intervention, facilitate treatment, establish baselines for future reference, and educate and counsel parents.[5,6] There are many clinical deviations that are easily correctable in a newborn and others that correct spontaneously as the child grows.

KEY POINTS

DEVELOPMENTAL SKELETAL DISORDERS

- Many disorders of early infancy are caused by intrauterine positions and resolve as the child grows.
- Nutritional and metabolic disorders can impair the formation of the organic matrix of bone, causing slowing of growth at the epiphyseal plate.

Torsional Deformities

All infants and toddlers have lax ligaments that become tighter with age and assumption of the weight-bearing posture. The hypermobility that accompanies joint laxity, coupled with the torsional (*i.e.*, rotational) forces exerted on the limbs during growth, is responsible for many variants seen in young children. Torsional forces caused by intrauterine positions or sleeping and sitting patterns twist the growing bones and can produce the deformities as a child grows and develops.

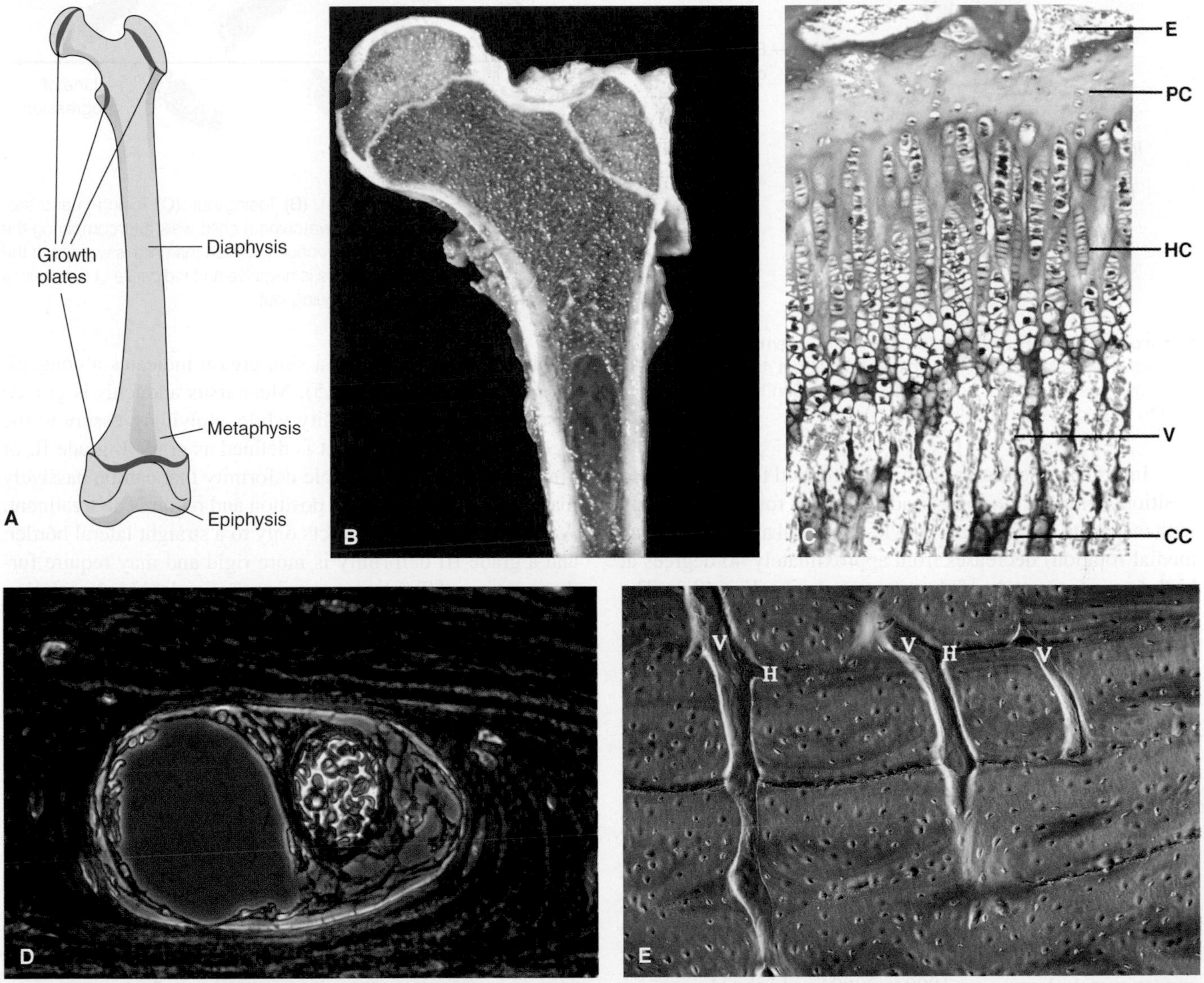

Figure 49.2 • Anatomy of the long bone. **(A)** Diagram of femur illustrating the various compartments. **(B)** Coronal section of the proximal femur illustrates the various anatomic parts of a long bone. The epiphysis of the femoral head and the apophysis of the greater trochanter are separated from the metaphysis by their respective growth plates. The cortex and medullary cavity are well visualized. The medullary cavity contains cancellous bone until the metaphysis narrows into the diaphysis (shaft) of the bone, at which point the medullary cavity is completely devoid of bone and filled with marrow. **(C)** A section of the epiphysis with a zone of proliferating cartilage cells. Beneath this zone, the hypertrophic cartilage cells are arranged in columns. At the bottom, the calcifying matrix is invaded by blood vessels. **(D)** Haversian canal has a venule (thin-walled wider vessel on left) and an arteriole (thicker-walled narrow vessel on the right). **(E)** Volkmann canals. There are three Volkmann canals visible running parallel to each other and perpendicular to the cortex. The openings of two of the haversian canals are also visible. CC, calcified cartilage; E, epiphysis; HC, hypertrophic cartilage; PC, proliferative cartilage; V, vascular invasion. (From Rubin R., Strayer D. S. (Eds.) (2015). *Rubin's pathology: Clinicopathologic foundations of medicine* (7th ed., p. 1308). Philadelphia, PA: Lippincott Williams & Wilkins.)

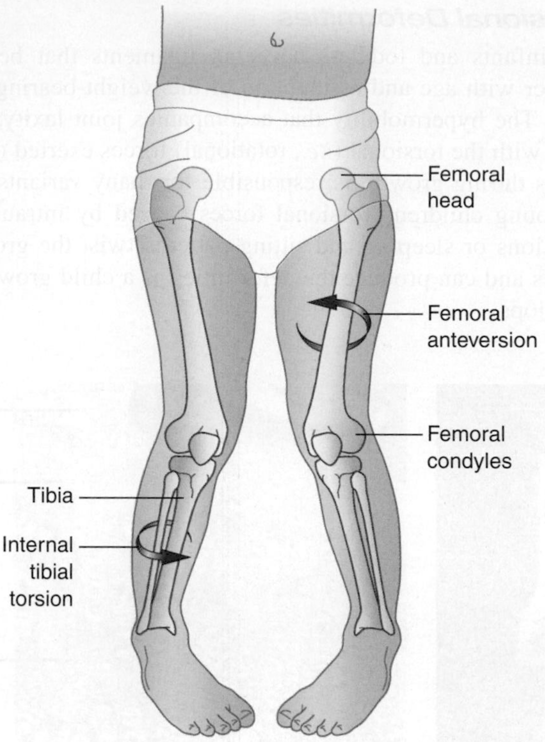

Figure 49.3 • Femoral anteversion and internal tibial rotation. Femoral anteversion normally decreases from about 40 degrees at birth to 15 degrees at maturity, and internal tibial rotation from 5 degrees at birth to 15 degrees at maturity.

In infants, the femur normally is rotated to an anteverted position, with the femoral head and neck rotated anteriorly with respect to the femoral condyles. Femoral anteversion (*i.e.*, medial rotation) decreases from approximately 40 degrees at birth to approximately 15 degrees at maturity (Fig. 49.3). The normal tibia is externally rotated approximately 5 degrees at birth and approximately 15 degrees at maturity. Torsional abnormalities frequently demonstrate a familial tendency.[5]

The foot progression angle describes the angle between the axis of the foot and the line of progression.[4,5] It is determined by watching the child walking and running, although it is usually less noticeable when the child is running or barefoot. Figure 49.4 illustrates the position of the foot in toeing-in and toeing-out, and the line of progression, when a child is walking.

Toeing-In. Toeing-in (*i.e.*, metatarsus adductus) is the most common congenital foot deformity, with an incidence of approximately 1 per every 1000 to 2000 live births.[5] It is sometimes called pigeon toe. The forefoot commonly is adducted and gives the foot a kidney-shaped appearance, whereas the hindfoot is normal[6] (Fig. 49.5). It can be caused by torsion in the foot, lower leg, or entire leg. Toeing-in because of adduction of the forefoot (*i.e.*, congenital metatarsus adductus) usually is the result of the fetal position maintained in utero. It may occur in one foot or both feet. Diagnostic methods include examination of the plantar aspect of the foot, noting the overall shape of the foot and the presence or absence of

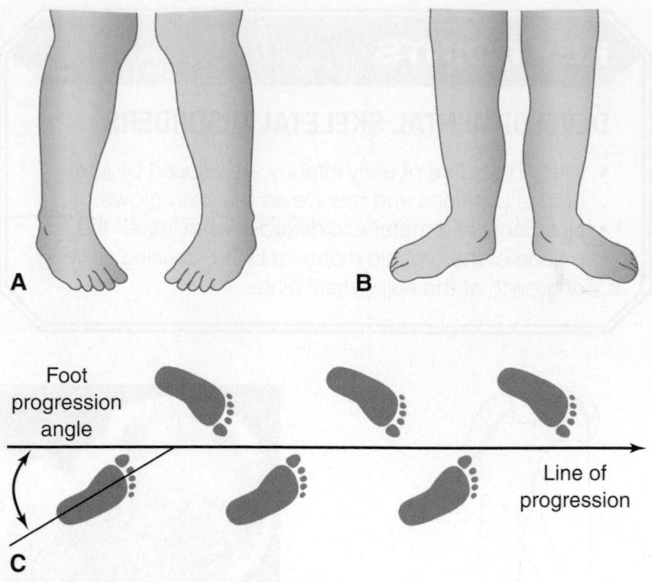

Figure 49.4 • **(A)** Toeing-in. **(B)** Toeing-out. **(C)** Toeing-in and toeing-out can be determined by watching a child walk and comparing the long axis of the foot with the direction in which the child is walking. If the foot is directed inward, the angle is negative and indicative of toeing-in; if it is positive, it is indicative of toeing-out.

an arch.[6] The presence of a skin crease indicates a congenital deformity (see Fig. 49.5). Metatarsus adductus is graded based on the foot's flexibility while applying pressure to the medial forefoot. The defect is defined as grade I, grade II, or grade III. Grade I is a supple deformity that can be passively manipulated into a straight position and requires no treatment. A grade II deformity corrects only to a straight lateral border, and a grade III deformity is more rigid and may require further treatment.[6] Treatment consisting of serial long leg casting or a brace that pushes the metatarsals (not the hindfoot) into abduction usually is required in a fixed (rigid) deformity (*i.e.*, one in which the forefoot cannot be passively manipulated into a straight position).[6]

Toeing-Out. Toeing-out (slew foot) is a common problem in children and is caused by external femoral torsion. It is less common than toeing-in and occurs sometimes with calcaneovalgus and pes planovalgus.[5] This occurs when the femur can

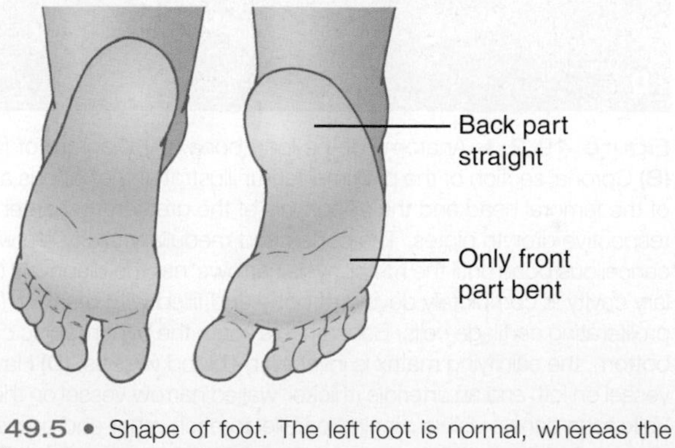

Figure 49.5 • Shape of foot. The left foot is normal, whereas the right foot has metatarsus adductus.

Understanding Bone Remodeling

Bone remodeling constitutes a process of skeletal maintenance once skeletal growth is complete. Significant progress has been made in understanding the phenomenon of bone remodeling as it relates to the coupling of bone resorption with bone formation.

Bone Remodeling Cycle

Mature bone is made up of units called *osteons* in which concentric lamellae (bone layers) surround a central, *haversian* canal. Bone remodeling consists of a sequence of bone resorption within an osteon by osteoclasts, followed by new bone formation by osteoblasts. In the adult, the length of one sequence (*i.e.*, bone resorption and formation) is approximately 4 months. Ideally, the replaced bone should equal the resorbed bone. If it does not, there is net loss of bone. In the elderly, for example, bone resorption and formation no longer are perfectly coupled, and bone mass is lost.

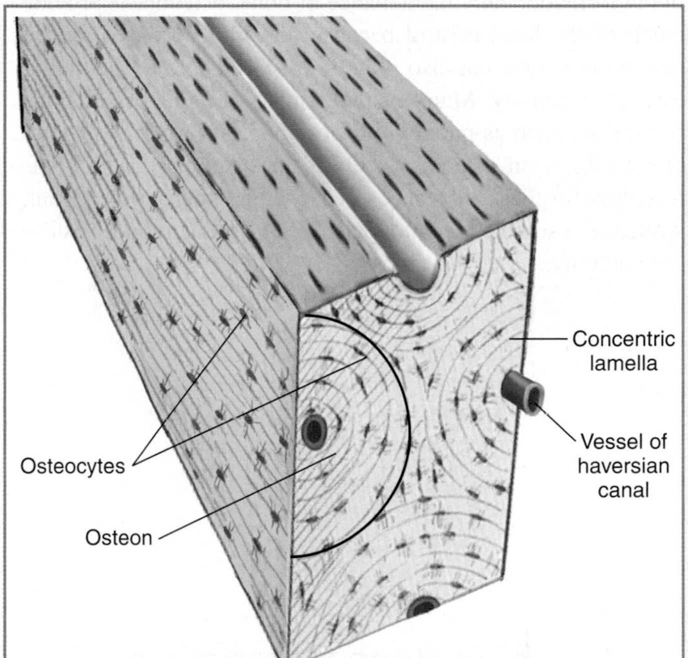

Bone Resorption

The osteoclasts, which are bone-resorbing cells derived from monocyte/macrophage precursors, are the cells involved in the initiation of bone remodeling. The sequence of bone resorption and bone formation is activated by many stimuli, including the action of parathyroid hormone and calcitonin. It begins with osteoclastic resorption of existing bone, during which the organic (protein matrix) and inorganic (mineral) components are removed, creating a tunnel-like space in the osteon. Soluble factors released during resorption aid in the recruitment of osteoblasts to the site, thereby linking bone resorption to bone formation.

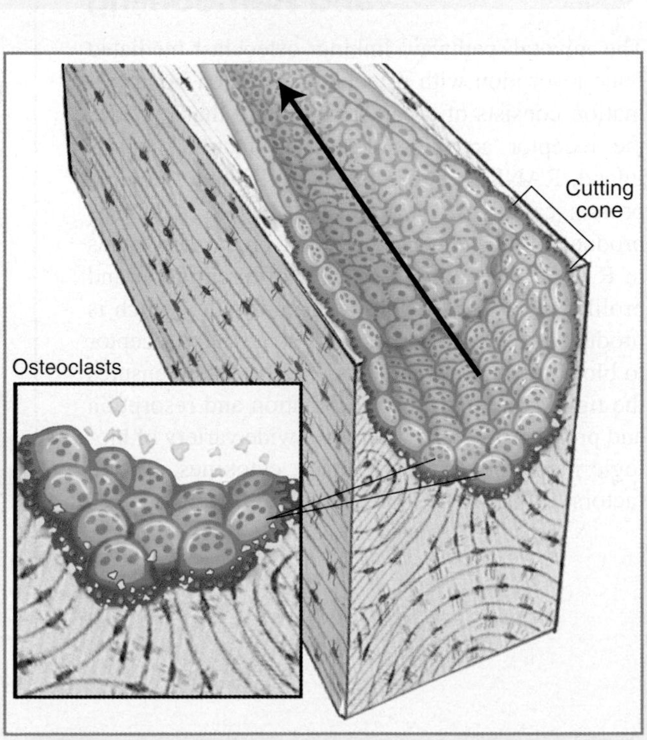

Continued

Understanding Bone Remodeling *(Continued)*

Bone Formation

After osteoclastic activity has ceased, osteoblasts begin to deposit the organic matrix (osteoid) on the wall of the osteon canal. As successive lamellae of bone are deposited, the canal ultimately attains the relative proportions of the original osteon. In the formation and maintenance of bone, osteoblasts provide much of the local control because not only do they produce new bone matrix but also play an essential role in mediating osteoclast activity. Many of the primary stimulators of bone resorption, such as parathyroid hormone, have minimal or no direct effects on osteoclasts. Once the osteoblast, which has receptors for these substances, receives the appropriate signal, it releases a soluble mediator called *RANKL* that induces osteoclast activity.

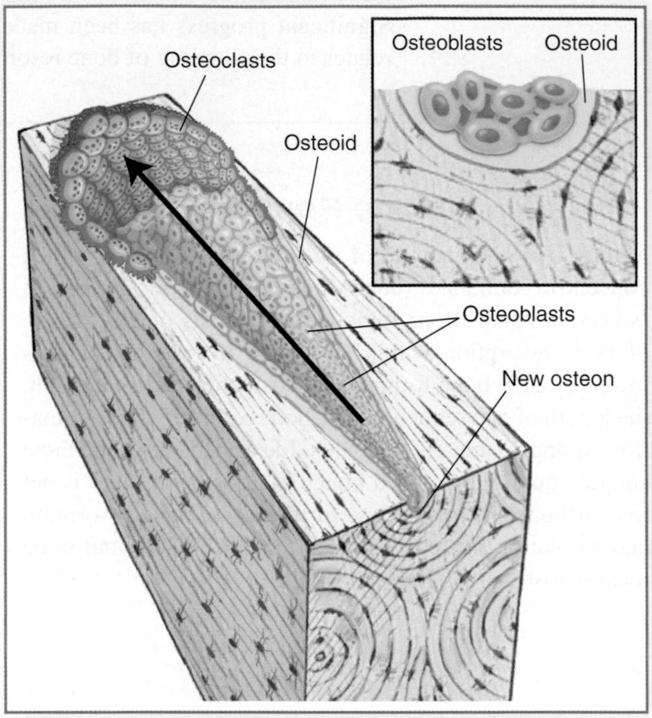

Control of Bone Metabolism and Remodeling

The pivotal pathway linking osteoclast-mediated bone resorption with osteoblast-mediated bone formation consists of a paracrine system that includes the receptor activator of nuclear factor kappa-B ligand, RANKL, its receptor RANK, and a soluble protein called *osteoprotegerin*. RANKL, which is produced by osteoblasts and their precursors, binds to RANK, promoting osteoclast differentiation and proliferation. The soluble OPG molecule, which is produced by many tissues, acts as a decoy receptor to block the action of RANKL. This system ensures the tight coupling of bone formation and resorption and provides a means whereby a wide variety of biologic mediators (*e.g.*, hormones, cytokines, growth factors) influence the homeostasis of bone.

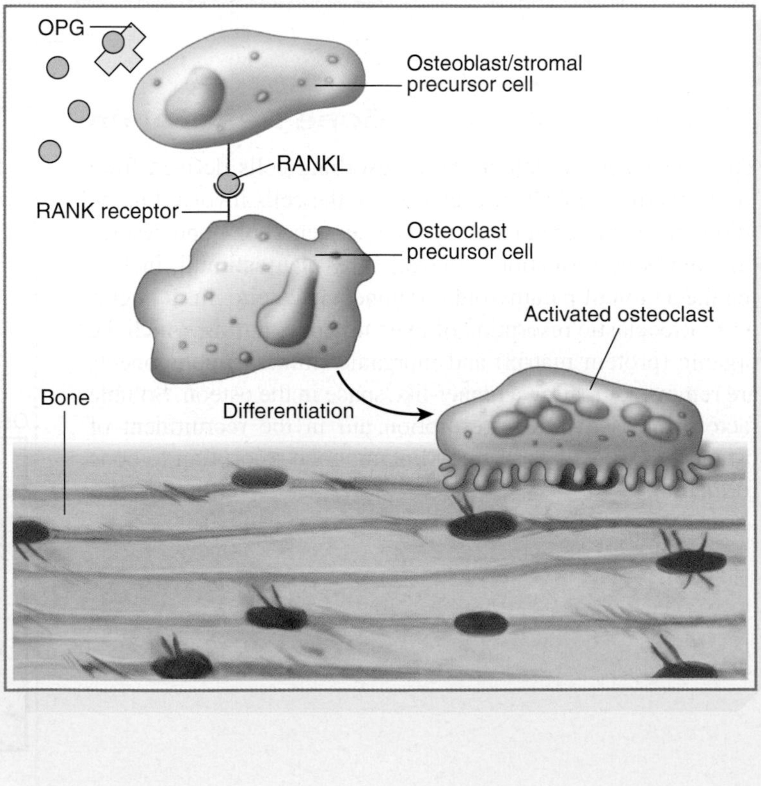

be externally rotated to approximately 90 degrees but internally rotated only to a neutral position or slightly beyond. Because the femoral torsion persists when a child habitually sleeps in the prone position, an external tibial torsion also may develop. If external tibial torsion is present, the feet point lateral to the midline of the medial plane. External tibial torsion rarely causes toeing-out; it only intensifies the condition. Toeing-out usually corrects itself as the child becomes proficient in walking. Occasionally, a night splint is used.

Tibial Torsion. Tibial torsion is determined by measuring the thigh–foot angle, which is done with the ankle and knee positioned at 90 degrees. In this position, the foot normally rotates outward. *Internal tibial torsion* (*i.e.*, bowing of the tibia) is a rotation of the tibia that makes the feet appear to turn inward (see Fig. 49.3). It is the most common cause of toeing-in in children younger than 2 years of age. It is present at birth and may fail to correct itself if children sleep on their knees with the feet turned in or sit on in-turned feet.[5] It is thought to be caused by genetic factors and intrauterine compression, such as an unstretched uterus during a first pregnancy or intrauterine crowding with twins or multiple fetuses. Tibial torsion generally improves naturally with growth, but this may take years.

External tibial torsion, a much less common disorder, is associated with calcaneovalgus foot and is caused by a normal variation of intrauterine positioning or a neuromuscular disorder. It is characterized by an abnormally positive thigh–foot angle of 30 to 50 degrees.[5] The condition corrects itself naturally, and treatment is observational. Significant improvement begins during the first year with the onset of ambulation and usually is complete by 2 to 3 years of age.[5] The normal adult exhibits about 20 degrees of tibial torsion.

Femoral Torsion. *Femoral torsion* refers to abnormal variations in hip rotation. Hip rotation is measured at the pelvic level with the child in the prone position and the knees flexed at a 90-degree angle. In this position, the hip is in a neutral position. Rotating the lower leg outward produces internal or medial femoral rotation; rotating it inward produces external or lateral rotation. During measurement of hip rotation, the legs are allowed to fall to full internal rotation by gravity alone; lateral rotation is measured by allowing the legs to fall inward and cross. Hip rotation in flexion and extension also can be measured with computed tomography (CT). By 1 year of age, there is normally approximately 45 degrees of internal rotation and 45 degrees of external rotation.

Internal femoral torsion, also called *femoral anteversion* (see Fig. 49.3), is a normal variant commonly seen during the first 6 years of life, especially in 3- and 4-year-old girls.[6] Characteristically, there is 80 to 90 degrees of internal rotation of the hip in the prone position. The condition is thought to be related to increased laxity of the anterior capsule of the hip such that it does not provide the stable pressure needed to correct the anteversion that is present at birth. Children are most comfortable sitting in the "W" position, with their hips between their knees. It is believed that this position allows the lower leg to act as a lever, producing torsional changes in the femur. When the child stands, the knees turn in and the feet appear to point straight ahead. When the child walks, the knees and toes point in. Children with this problem are encouraged to sit cross-legged or in the so-called *tailor position*. If left untreated, the tibiae compensate by becoming externally rotated so that by 8 to 12 years of age, the knees may turn in but the feet no longer do so. This can result in patellofemoral malalignment with patellar subluxation or dislocation and pain.[6] A derotational osteotomy may be done in severe cases or if there is functional disability.

External femoral torsion is an uncommon disorder characterized by excessive external rotation of the hip. Bilateral external torsion is usually a benign condition, and treatment is observational. When the disorder is unilateral, slipped capital femoral epiphysis should be ruled out.

Genu Varum and Genu Valgum

Genu varum, or *bowlegs*, is an outward bowing of the knees greater than 1 inch when the medial malleoli of the ankles are touching (Fig. 49.6). As children grow, lower limb alignment usually follows a predicable pattern (Fig. 49.7). Most infants and toddlers have some bowing of their legs up to 18 months of age. If there is a large separation between the knees (>15 degrees) after 2 years of age, the child may require bracing. The child also should be evaluated for diseases such as rickets or tibia vara[6] (Fig. 49.8).

Genu valgum, or *knock-knees*, is a deformity in which there is decreased space between the knees (Fig. 49.6). The medial malleoli in the ankles cannot be brought in contact with each other when the knees are touching. Valgus gradually develops after age 24 months and is most apparent between 3 and 4 years of age. The condition usually is the result of lax

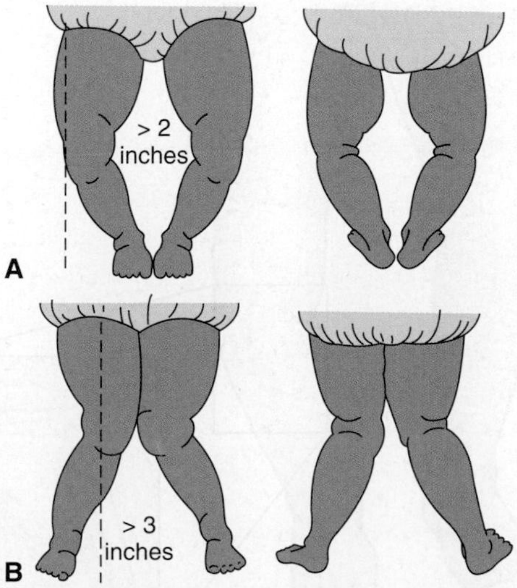

Figure 49.6 • **(A)** Genu varum. **(B)** Genu valgum. (From Silbert-Flagg J., Pillitteri A. (2018). *Maternal and child health nursing: Care of the childbearing and child rearing family* (8th ed., Fig. 51.9, p. 1444). Philadelphia, PA: Lippincott Williams & Wilkins.)

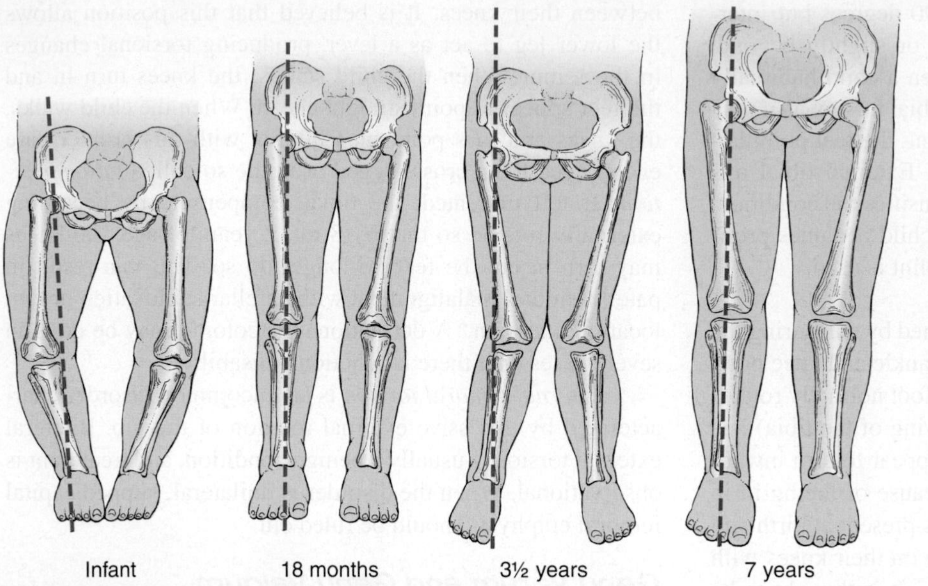

Figure 49.7 • Lower limb alignment follows a predictable pattern. Infants typically have a gentle varus bow throughout the femur and tibia. By 18 to 24 months, the lower leg is nearly straight, with a neutral mechanical axis. Valgus gradually develops and is most apparent between 3 and 4 years of age. By 7 years of age, the lower limb is in slight valgus and changes very little thereafter. Varus should not recur, nor should valgus increase. (From Morissy R. T., Weinstein S. L. (Eds.) (2006). *Lovell & Winter's pediatric orthopaedics* (6th ed.). Philadelphia, PA: Lippincott Williams & Wilkins.)

medial collateral ligaments of the knee. Obesity is also associated with the development of genu valgum and is becoming almost epidemic in the United States.[7] By 7 years of age, the lower limb is in slight valgus and changes very little thereafter. Genu valgum can be ignored up to 7 years of age, unless it is a larger angle, one sided, or associated with short stature. It usually resolves spontaneously and rarely requires treatment. If genu varum or genu valgum persists and is not corrected, osteoarthritis may develop in adulthood as a result of abnormal intra-articular stress. There is a new surgical treatment of both knock-knees and bowlegs, which includes the use of extraphyseal tension band plates that manipulate the angle of the growth plate.[8] Genu varum can cause gait awkwardness and increased risk for sprains and fractures. Uncorrected genu valgum may cause subluxation and recurrent dislocation of the patella, with a predisposition to chondromalacia and joint pain and fatigue. Therefore, new challenges such as obesity need to become a priority management outcome in pediatric orthopedics.[7,9]

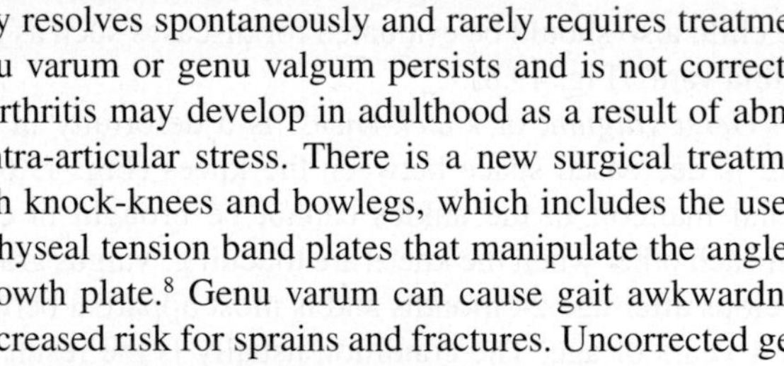

Figure 49.8 • Rotational deformity of the proximal tibia, especially when unilateral, suggests tibia vara (Blount disease).

Flatfoot

Flatfoot (*i.e.*, pes planus) is a deformity characterized by the absence of the longitudinal arch of the foot. Infants normally have a wider and fatter foot than adults. The fat pads that normally are accentuated by pliable muscles with young children create the appearance of fullness often mistaken for flatfoot.[10,11] Until the longitudinal arch develops around 2 years of age, most children appear to have flat feet. The true criterion for flatfoot is that with weightbearing, the talus points medially and downward, so that the heel is everted and the forefoot is inverted.

Obesity, ligament laxity (which is genetically linked), and the wearing of nonsupportive shoes over time are other possible etiologies of pes planus.[10,11] Overweight children have lower plantar arch height because of the excessive body weight putting increased pressure on the child's feet.[10,11]

There are two types of flatfoot—flexible and rigid. Most children with flexible flatfoot have loose ligaments, allowing the feet to sag when they gain weight. With this type of flatfoot, the arch disappears only with weightbearing. No special treatment is needed for flexible flatfoot. People with flexible flatfoot are less prone to pain and injury than those with normal or high arches. The rigid flatfoot is fixed with no apparent arch in any position. It is seen in conjunction with neuromuscular diseases such as cerebral palsy.

In the adult, treatment of flatfoot is conservative and aimed at relieving fatigue and discomfort. Supportive, well-fitting shoes with arch supports may be helpful and prevent ligaments from becoming overstretched. Surgery may be done in cases of severe and persistent symptoms.

Hereditary and Congenital Deformities

Congenital deformities are abnormalities that are present at birth. They range in severity from mild limb deformities, which are relatively common, to major limb malformations, which are relatively rare. The most common anomaly of the toes or fingers is *polydactyly* or the presence of an extra digit on the hand or foot. Macrodactyly occurs when one or more toes or fingers are hypertrophied and are significantly larger than the surrounding toes or fingers.

There may also be a simple webbing of the fingers or toes (syndactyly) or the absence of a bone such as the phalanx, rib, or clavicle. Joint contractures and dislocations produce more severe deformity, as does the absence of entire bones, joints, or limbs. Surgery is done to relieve functional symptoms, such as pain or difficulty in fitting shoes. The cosmetic goal is to alter the grotesque appearance of the hand or foot and to achieve a similar size to the opposite extremity.

Congenital deformities are caused by many factors, some unknown. These factors include hereditary influences, external agents that injure the fetus (*e.g.*, radiation, alcohol, drugs, such as thalidomide taken by pregnant women with morning sickness in the 60s, and viruses), and intrauterine environmental factors. Many of the organic bone matrix components have been identified only recently, and their interactions were found to be more complex than originally thought. Hand and foot disorders associated with abnormalities in bone matrix include those with deficient collagen synthesis and decreased bone mass.[12]

Osteogenesis Imperfecta

Osteogenesis imperfecta (OI) is a hereditary disease characterized by defective synthesis of type I collagen[13,14] (Fig. 49.9). It is one of the most common hereditary bone diseases, with an estimated 20,00 to 50,000 people with OI in the United States.[13] OI is usually transmitted as an autosomal dominant trait. However, the type III form of OI, which is the most progressively deforming type with multiple life-threatening defects, is sometimes, although rarely, inherited as an autosomal recessive trait.[14]

Mutations in the genes connected with type I collagen, which impacts the development of bones, joints, ears, ligaments, teeth, sclerae, and skin, cause the problems.[14] The genes are COL1A1 and COL1A2, which encode the alpha$_1$ and alpha$_2$ chains of type I procollagen.[14] These genes are found in chromosome 17 and 7 and cause different structural and clinical changes in the types of OI.

Clinical Manifestations. The clinical manifestations of OI include a spectrum of disorders marked by extreme skeletal fragility. Four major subtypes of the disorder have been identified each with their specific manifestations[14] (Table 49.1).

The disorder is characterized by thin and poorly developed bones that are prone to multiple fractures. These children have short limbs and a soft, thin cranium with bifrontal prominences that give a triangular appearance to the face. Other problems associated with defective connective tissue synthesis include wormian bone in the skull, thin skin, blue or gray sclera, abnormal tooth development, hypotonic muscles, loose-jointedness, and scoliosis.[15] Hearing loss because of otosclerosis of the tiny bones in the middle ear is common in affected adults. The most serious defects occur with type II. Severely affected fetuses have multiple intrauterine fractures and bowing and shortening of the extremities. Many of these infants are stillborn or die during infancy.

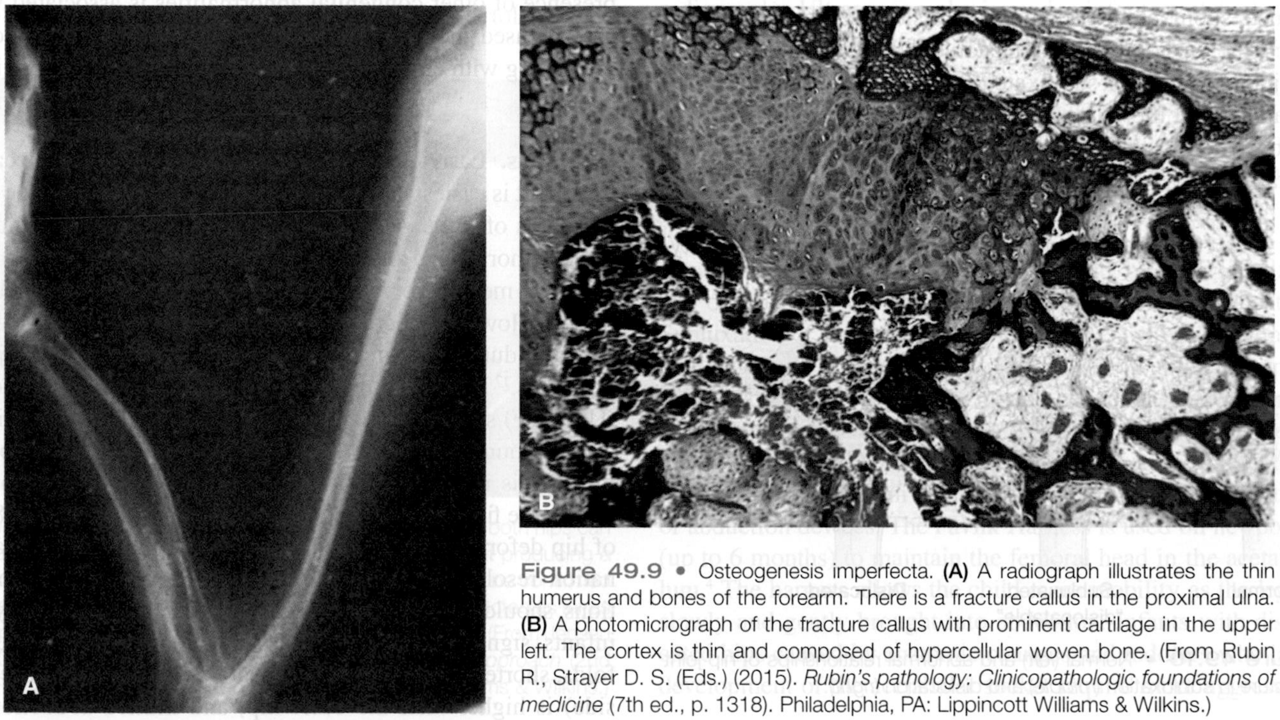

Figure 49.9 • Osteogenesis imperfecta. **(A)** A radiograph illustrates the thin humerus and bones of the forearm. There is a fracture callus in the proximal ulna. **(B)** A photomicrograph of the fracture callus with prominent cartilage in the upper left. The cortex is thin and composed of hypercellular woven bone. (From Rubin R., Strayer D. S. (Eds.) (2015). *Rubin's pathology: Clinicopathologic foundations of medicine* (7th ed., p. 1318). Philadelphia, PA: Lippincott Williams & Wilkins.)

treatment, such as open reduction and joint reconstruction. Treatment at any age includes reduction of the dislocation and immobilization of the legs in an abducted position. The most serious complication of any treatment is avascular necrosis of the femoral head as a result of the forced abduction.[4] This most often occurs as a complication of a closed or open reduction in an older child. In addition, hyperflexion has the potential to cause femoral nerve palsies. With children younger than 3 years of age, skin traction is used when reduction cannot be easily obtained. This treatment is followed by several months of immobilization in a hip spica cast, plaster splints, or an abduction splint. Older children or adults with an unreduced dislocatable hip may require hip surgery because of damage to the articulating surface of the joint. These people have considerable problems after surgery because of soft tissue contractures.

Congenital Clubfoot

Clubfoot, or talipes, is one of the most common pediatric orthopedic conditions. It has an incidence of approximately 1 to 2 cases per 1000 live births, is bilateral in about 50% of cases, and affects boys more often than girls.[20] Like congenital dislocation of the hip, its occurrence follows a multifactorial inheritance pattern. Clubfoot may be associated with chromosomal abnormalities or congenital syndromes that are transmitted by Mendelian inheritance patterns (Fig. 49.14). However, it is most commonly idiopathic and found in normal infants in whom no genetic or chromosomal abnormality or other extrinsic cause can be found.

In forefoot adduction, which accounts for approximately 95% of idiopathic cases, the foot is plantar flexed and inverted. This is the so-called *equinovarus type* in which the foot resembles a horse's hoof. The other 5% of cases are of the calcaneovalgus type, or reverse clubfoot, in which the foot is dorsiflexed and everted. The reverse clubfoot can occur as an isolated condition or in association with multiple congenital defects. At birth, the feet of many infants assume one of these two positions, but they can be passively overcorrected or brought back into the opposite position. If the foot cannot be overcorrected, some type of correction may be necessary.

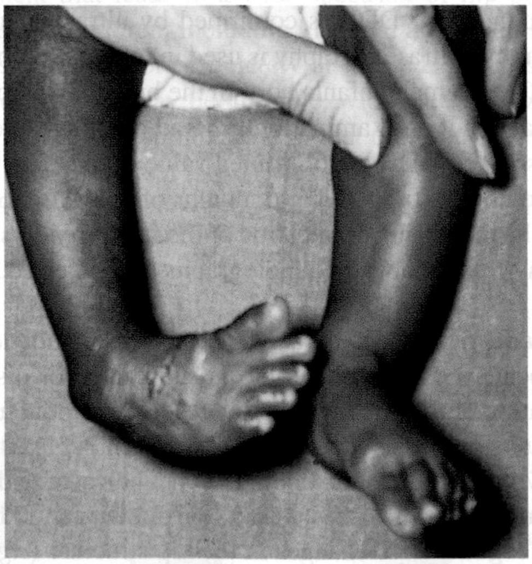

Figure 49.14 • Talipes or clubbing of the right foot. The foot is turned to the side, and the involved foot, calf, and leg are smaller and shorter than the normal side. One or both feet may be affected. This condition is not painful; however, if left untreated, significant discomfort and disability will develop. Treatment ranges from braces or casts to surgery. (From Jensen S. (2015). *Nursing health assessment: A best practice approach* (2nd ed., Fig. 21.3, p. 648). Philadelphia, PA: Lippincott Williams & Wilkins.)

Treatment of clubfoot is begun as soon as the diagnosis is made. One screening tool for equinovarus type clubfoot is the clubfoot assessment protocol, which is also helpful in developing a management plan.[20] When treatment is initiated during the first few weeks of life, a nonoperative procedure may be effective. Serial manipulations and casting are used gently to correct each component of the deformity. One method, called the *Ponseti method*, involves weekly gentle stretching and manipulation of the misaligned bones followed by application of a well-molded long leg plaster cast with the knee held at a right angle.[20] The cast maintains the correction and allows for further relaxation of tight structures in anticipation of the next week's casting. Correction of the deformity is usually obtained within 6 to 8 weeks. Frequently, a percutaneous Achilles tendon lengthening is performed using a topical anesthetic cream before application of the final cast to allow for complete correction of the equinus deformity. The correction is maintained by full-time wear of a Denis Browne splint for 3 months and part-time night and nap wear for approximately 2 to 3 years.[20] Surgery may be required for severe deformities or when nonoperative treatment methods are unsuccessful.

Juvenile Osteochondroses

The term *juvenile osteochondroses* is used to describe a group of children's diseases in which one or more growth ossification centers undergo a period of degeneration, necrosis, or inactivity that is followed by regeneration and usually deformity. The osteochondroses are separated into two groups according to their causes. The first group consists of the true osteonecrotic osteochondroses, so-called because the diseases are caused by localized osteonecrosis of an apophyseal or epiphyseal center (*e.g.*, Legg–Calvé–Perthes disease, Freiberg infraction, Panner disease, Kienböck disease). The second group of juvenile osteochondroses is caused by abnormalities in ossification of cartilaginous tissue resulting from a genetically determined normal variation or from trauma (*e.g.*, Osgood-Schlatter disease, Blount disease, Sever disease, Scheuermann disease). The discussion in this section focuses on Legg-Calvé-Perthes disease from the first group and Osgood-Schlatter disease from the second group. Slipped capital femoral epiphysis is a disorder of the growth plate.

Legg–Calvé–Perthes Disease

Legg-Calvé-Perthes disease is an idiopathic osteonecrotic disease of the proximal (capital) femoral epiphysis.[21] It occurs in 1 of 1200 children, affecting primarily those, mostly boys, between ages 3 and 12 years, with a median age of 7 years.[22] It occurs primarily in boys and is much more common in whites than in African Americans. Although no definite genetic pattern has been established, it occasionally affects more than one family member.

Etiology and Pathogenesis. The cause of Legg-Calvé-Perthes disease is unknown. The disorder is usually insidious at onset and occurs in otherwise healthy children. It may, however, be associated with acute trauma. Evidence suggests a correlation between acquiring Legg-Calvé-Perthes disease and some procoagulation parameters with boys.[22] Affected children usually have a shorter stature. Undernutrition has been suggested as a causative factor. When girls are affected, they usually have a poorer prognosis than boys because they are skeletally more mature and have a shorter period for growth and remodeling than boys of the same age.[22]

The primary pathologic feature of Legg-Calvé-Perthes disease is an avascular necrosis of the bone and marrow involving the epiphyseal growth center in the femoral head.[21] The disorder may be confined to part of the epiphysis, or it may involve the entire epiphysis. In severe cases, there is a disturbance in the growth pattern that leads to a broad, short femoral neck. The necrosis is followed by slow absorption of the dead bone over 2 to 3 years. Although the necrotic trabeculae eventually are replaced by healthy new bone, the epiphysis rarely regains its normal shape. The process occurs in four predictable stages.[21,22] The *first stage*, which lasts for 6 to 12 months, is the avascular stage when the ossification center is becoming necrotic. Damage to the femoral head is determined by the amount of necrosis occurring during this stage. The *second stage*, lasting about 1 to 3 years, is the revascularization stage, during which resorption of the necrotic bone takes place. The *third stage* is the reossification stage, during which radiolucent areas become dense, whereas the shape of the femoral head improves. The *fourth stage*, which is the healed stage, involves the forming of immature bone cells by normal bone cells and the resulting femoral head.[21,22]

Clinical Manifestations. The main symptoms of Legg-Calvé-Perthes disease are pain in the thigh or knee and difficulty in walking. The child may have a painless limp with limited abduction and internal rotation and a flexion contracture of the affected hip. The age of onset is important because young children have a greater capability for remodeling of the femoral head and acetabulum, and thus, less flattening of the femoral head occurs.

Diagnosis and Treatment. Early diagnosis is important and is based on correlating physical symptoms with radiographic findings (*e.g.*, magnetic resonance imaging [MRI], CT scan, ultrasound, arthrography, bone scintigraphy, and radiography), which are related to the stage of the disease.[21]

The goal of treatment is to reduce deformity and preserve the integrity of the femoral head while the necrotic bone is resorbed.[21]

Conservative and surgical interventions are used in the treatment of Legg-Calvé-Perthes disease. Children younger than 4 years of age with little or no involvement of the femoral head may require only periodic observation. In all other children, some intervention is needed to relieve the force of weightbearing, muscular tension, and subluxation of the femoral head. It is important to maintain the femur in a well-seated position in the concave acetabulum to prevent deformity. This is done by keeping the hip in abduction and mild internal rotation. Treatment involves periods of rest, use of assistive devices for walking, nonweightbearing, and abduction braces to keep the legs separated in abduction with mild internal rotation.

Surgery may be done to contain the femoral head in the acetabulum. This treatment usually is reserved for children older than 6 years of age who at the time of diagnosis have more serious involvement of the femoral head. The best surgical results are obtained when surgery is done early, before the epiphysis becomes necrotic. One method, creeping substitution, is the process by which the necrotic marrow is removed and replaced by neurovascular tissue with pluripotent cells.[21,22] Some children with Legg-Calvé-Perthes disease may require total hip replacement surgery at some point in time depending on the degree of avascular necrosis.[22]

Osgood-Schlatter Disease

Osgood-Schlatter disease involves microfractures in the area where the patellar tendon inserts into the tibial tubercle, which is an extension of the proximal tibial epiphysis.[23] This area is particularly vulnerable to injury caused by sudden or continued strain from the patellar tendon during periods of growth, particularly in athletic adolescents.

The patellar tendon is inflamed and thickened from the continuous inflammation and causes pain in front of the knee. There is swelling, tenderness, and increased prominence of the tibial tubercle. The symptoms usually are self-limiting. They may recur during growth periods but usually resolve after closure of the tibial growth plate. In some cases, limitations on activity, tibial bands, or braces to immobilize the knee; anti-inflammatory agents; and application of cold are necessary to relieve the pain.[23] The objective of treatment is to release tension on the quadriceps to permit revascularization and reossification of the tibial tubercle. Complete resolution of symptoms through healing (physical closure) of the tibial tubercle can extend to a year or even 2 years.[23]

Concept Mastery Alert

Osgood-Schlatter disease is characterized by thickening of the patellar tendon. Pain occurs during activity and is focused in the front of the knee.

Slipped Capital Femoral Epiphysis

Slipped capital femoral epiphysis, or coxa vara, is a disorder of the growth plate that occurs near the age of skeletal maturity. It involves a three-dimensional displacement of the epiphysis (posteriorly, medially, inferiorly), meaning that the femur is rotated externally from under the epiphysis. The condition is rare, with an estimated frequency of 10 in 10,000.[24]

The cause of slipped capital femoral epiphysis is obscure, but it may be related to the child's susceptibility to stress on the femoral neck as a result of genetics or structural abnormalities.[24] Boys are affected twice as often as girls, and in approximately half the cases the condition is bilateral. Affected children often are overweight with poorly developed secondary sex characteristics or, in some instances, are extremely tall and thin. In many cases, there is a history of rapid skeletal growth preceding displacement of the epiphysis. The condition also may be affected by nutritional deficiencies or endocrine disorders such as hypothyroidism, hypopituitarism, and hypogonadism.[24]

Children with the condition often complain of referred knee pain accompanied by difficulty in walking, fatigue, and stiffness.[24] The diagnosis is confirmed by radiographic studies in which the degree of slipping is determined and graded according to severity (mild, <33%; moderate, 33% to 50%; and severe, >50%).[9] Early treatment is imperative to prevent lifelong crippling. In situ fixation is recommended.[24] Avoidance of weightbearing on the femur and bed rest are essential parts of the treatment. Traction or gentle manipulation under anesthesia is used to reduce the slip. Surgical insertion of pins to keep the femoral neck and head of the femur aligned is a common method of treatment for children with moderate or severe slips. Crutches are used for several months after surgical correction to prevent full weightbearing until the growth plate closes.

Children with the disorder must be followed closely until the epiphyseal plate closes. Long-term prognosis depends on the amount of displacement that occurs. Complications include avascular necrosis, leg shortening, malunion, and problems with the internal fixation.[24] Degenerative arthritis may develop, requiring joint replacement later in life.

Scoliosis

Scoliosis is a lateral deviation of the spinal column commonly in the coronal or frontal plane that may or may not include rotation or deformity of the vertebrae.[25] Scoliosis, a three-dimensional deformity of the spine, often affects the entire skeletal torso.[25] It can be classified with regard to age of onset and etiology. Generally, girls are affected.[14] The majority of scoliotic deformities are idiopathic.[25] Others can be congenital, associated with neuromuscular disorders (cerebral palsy or muscular dystrophy), a result of intraspinal deformities, or caused by uneven lower limb length.[25]

Idiopathic Scoliosis

Idiopathic scoliosis is classified into three types:

1. Infantile: When the deformity curve is manifested before 3 years of age. This type is rare.
2. Juvenile: When the curve(s) presents between 4 and 9 years of age. This type is uncommon.
3. Adolescent: When the deformity manifests after 10 years of age until the end of growth. This type represents approximately 80% of scoliosis cases.[26]

Idiopathic scoliosis is a structural spinal curvature for which no cause has been established. It occurs in healthy, neurologically normal children. The cause is most likely complex and multifactorial. It seems likely that heredity is involved because mother–daughter pairings are common, but identical twins are not uniformly affected. The magnitude of the curvature in an affected child is not related to magnitude of curvature in relatives. A recent study of the melatonin receptor 1B (*MTNR1B*) gene in people with adolescent idiopathic scoliosis suggests that *MTNR1B* may serve as a susceptibility gene for adolescent idiopathic scoliosis.[27] Also, evidence suggests that many people with neurofibromatosis type 1 (NF-1) have some type of scoliosis.[28] One new screening tool available for diagnosis and determination of treatment especially with adolescent idiopathic scoliosis is the ScoliScore assessment (a collection of genetic markers correlated with scoliosis), which is a genetic testing that studies the person's DNA sample and predicts the curve progression risk for people with scoliosis.[25]

Although a scoliotic curve may be present in any area of the spine, the most common curve is a right thoracic curve, which produces a rib prominence on the convex side and hypokyphosis from rotation of the vertebral column around its long axis as the spine begins to curve.

Congenital Scoliosis

Congenital scoliosis is caused by disturbances in vertebral development during the 6th to 8th weeks of embryologic development.[28] Congenital scoliosis may be divided into failures of formation and failures of segmentation. Failures of formation indicate the absence of a portion of the vertebra, such as hemivertebra (absence of a whole side of the vertebra) and wedge vertebra (missing only a portion of the vertebra). Failure of segmentation is the absence of the normal separation between the vertebrae.[25] The child may have other anomalies and neurologic complications if the spine is involved. Early diagnosis and treatment of progressive curves are essential for children with congenital scoliosis. Surgical intervention is the treatment of choice for progressive congenital scoliosis.[6,25]

Neuromuscular Scoliosis

Neuromuscular scoliosis develops from neuropathic or myopathic diseases. It is seen with cerebral palsy, muscular dystrophy, myelodysplasia, and poliomyelitis. There is often a long, C-shaped curve from the cervical to the sacral region. In children with cerebral palsy, severe deformity may make treatment difficult. Myopathic neuromuscular scoliosis develops with Duchenne muscular dystrophy and usually is not severe.

Clinical Manifestations

Scoliosis is usually first noticed because of the deformity it causes. A high shoulder, prominent hip, or projecting scapula may be noticed by a parent or in a school-based screening program. In girls, difficulty in hemming or fitting a dress may call attention to the deformity. Idiopathic scoliosis usually is a painless process, although pain may be present in severe cases, usually in the lumbar region. The pain may be caused by pressure on the ribs or on the crest of the ilium. There may be shortness of breath because of diminished chest expansion and gastrointestinal disturbances from crowding of the abdominal organs. Adults with less severe deformity may experience mild backache. If scoliosis is left untreated, the curve may progress to an extent that compromises cardiopulmonary function and creates a risk for neurologic complications.

Diagnosis

Early diagnosis of scoliosis can be important in the prevention of severe spinal deformity. The cardinal signs of scoliosis are uneven shoulders or iliac crest, prominent scapula on the convex side of the curve, malalignment of spinous processes, asymmetry of the flanks, asymmetry of the thoracic cage, and rib hump or paraspinal muscle prominence when bending forward. A complete physical examination is necessary for children with scoliosis because the defect may be indicative of other, underlying pathologic processes.

Diagnosis of scoliosis is made by physical examination and confirmed by radiography. A scoliometer should be used at the apex of the curvature to quantify a prominence; a scoliometer reading of greater than 5 degrees requires referral to a physician.[25] The curve is measured by determining the amount of lateral deviation present on radiographs and is labeled "right" or "left" for the convex portion of the curve. Other radiographic procedures may be done, including CT scanning, MRI, and myelography.

Although school screening continues to be mandated in a number of states, the *United States Preventive Services Task Force (USPSTF)* recommends against the routine screening of asymptomatic adolescents for idiopathic scoliosis, indicating that the potential harms from screening include unnecessary follow-up visits and evaluations because of false-positive results, and adverse psychological effects, especially related to brace wear.[25,26] Although routine screening is not recommended, health care professionals should be prepared to evaluate idiopathic scoliosis when it is discovered incidentally or when the adolescent or parent expresses concern about scoliosis.[25]

Treatment

The treatment of scoliosis depends on the severity of the deformity and the likelihood of progression. Larger curves are more likely to progress. Age of presentation also is important. Curves that are detected before menarche are more likely to progress than those detected after menarche. For people with lesser degrees of curvature (10 to 20 degrees), the trend has been away from aggressive treatment and toward a "wait and see" approach, taking advantage of the more sophisticated diagnostic methods that now are available.[25] Treatment is considered for physically immature children with curves between 20 and 30 degrees. Curves between 30 and 40 degrees usually are considered for bracing, and those greater than 40 to 45 degrees are considered for surgery.[25]

IN SUMMARY

Skeletal disorders can result from congenital or hereditary influences or from factors that occur during normal periods of skeletal growth and development. Newborn infants undergo normal changes in muscle tone and joint motion, causing torsional conditions of the femur or tibia. Many of these conditions are corrected as skeletal growth and development take place. OI is a rare autosomal hereditary disorder characterized by defective synthesis of connective tissue, including bone matrix. It results in poorly developed bones that fracture easily. DDH includes a range of structural abnormalities. Dislocated hips are always treated to prevent changes in the anatomic structure. Other childhood skeletal disorders, such as the osteochondroses, slipped capital femoral epiphysis, and scoliosis, are not corrected by the growth process. These disorders are progressive, can cause permanent disability, and require treatment. Disorders such as DDH and congenital clubfoot are present at birth. Both disorders are best treated during infancy. Regular examinations during the first year of life are recommended as a means of achieving early diagnosis of such disorders.

METABOLIC BONE DISEASE

After completing this section of the chapter, the learner will be able to meet the following objectives:

- Describe risk factors that contribute to the development of osteopenia, osteoporosis, osteomalacia, rickets, and Paget disease, and relate them to the prevention of the disorder.

Metabolic bone disease refers to a group of diseases that cause bone demineralization or dysmineralization, usually because of a defect in bone absorption that interferes with the parathyroid hormone, calcium, and vitamin D leading to bone fragility, rickets, or osteoarthritis. As discussed earlier in this chapter, metabolic bone diseases have their origin in the bone remodeling process, which involves an orderly sequence of osteoclastic bone reabsorption, the formation of new bone by the osteoblasts, and mineralization of the newly formed osteoid tissue.

Osteopenia

Osteopenia is a condition that is common to all metabolic bone diseases. It is characterized by a reduction in bone mass greater than expected for age, race, or sex that occurs because of a decrease in bone formation, inadequate bone mineralization, or excessive bone deossification.

Remember Mrs. Tukey who presented to the walk-in clinic with lower back pain and had a family history of osteoporosis? Her x-ray results revealed a fractured L-5 and she was diagnosed with osteoporosis. Mrs. Tukey had a history of a fractured hip at 60 years of age. She probably had osteopenia prior to her hip fracture, but did not know it.

Osteopenia is not a diagnosis but a term used to describe an apparent lack of bone seen on x-ray studies. The major causes of osteopenia are osteoporosis, osteomalacia, malignancies such as multiple myeloma, and endocrine disorders such as hyperparathyroidism and hyperthyroidism. Approximately 44 million people in the United States have osteopenia or osteoporosis.[29]

Osteoporosis

Osteoporosis is a metabolic bone disease characterized by a loss of mineralized bone mass causing increased porosity of the skeleton and susceptibility to fractures.[30] According to World Health Organization, bone density is reported using a T score. This score compares the bone density of a healthy 30-year-old adult to the patient's bone density.[30] The World Health Organization Osteoporosis Guidelines recommends that postmenopausal women and men over 50 years of age be treated according to the following guidelines:

- Those who have a hip or vertebral fracture.
- Those who have T scores less than −2.5 at the neck of the femur or spine after appropriate evaluation to exclude secondary causes.
- Those who have a 10-year probability of a hip fracture greater than 3% and a T score between −1.0 and −2.5 at the spine or neck of the femur.
- Those who have a 10-year probability of a major osteoporosis-related fracture greater than 20%.[30]

Although osteoporosis can occur as the result of several disorders, it most often is associated with the aging process. Because bone loss is positively associated with age, the prevalence of osteoporosis and low bone mass is expected to increase.

Pathogenesis

The pathogenesis of osteoporosis is unclear, but most data suggest an imbalance between bone resorption and formation such that bone resorption exceeds bone formation. Although both of these factors play a role in most cases of osteoporosis, their relative contribution to bone loss may vary depending on age, gender, genetic predisposition, activity level, and nutritional status. Exercise may prevent or delay the onset of osteoporosis by increasing peak bone mass density (BMD) during periods of growth. Poor nutrition or an age-related decrease in intestinal absorption of calcium because of deficient activation of vitamin D may contribute to the development of osteoporosis, particularly in older adults.

Under normal conditions, bone mass increases steadily during childhood, reaching a peak in the young adult years. The peak bone mass, or BMD, is an important determinant of the subsequent risk for osteoporosis. It is determined in part by genetic factors, estrogen levels, exercise, calcium intake and absorption, and environmental factors. Genetic factors are linked, in large part, to the maximal amount of bone in each person, referred to as *peak bone mass*. Race is a key determinant of BMD and the risk of fractures. Incidence rates obtained from studies among racial and ethnic groups demonstrate that although women have higher fracture rates compared with men overall, these differences vary by race and age. White and Asian women had higher rates for all age groups older than 50 years.[30] The highest BMD values and lowest fracture rates have been reported for black women.[30] Body size is another factor affecting the risk of osteoporosis and risk of fractures. Women with smaller body builds are at increased risk of hip fracture because of lower hip BMD.

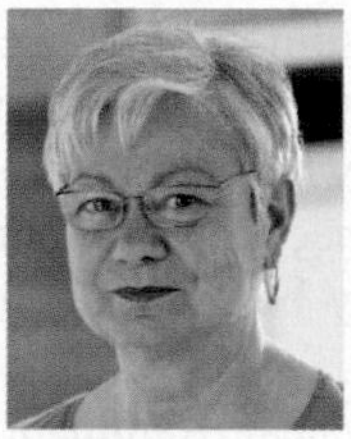

Mrs. Tukey is Caucasian and weighs 128 lb and is 5 foot 3 inches tall. Given her family history, she is a good example of the part that genetics plays in a person's peak bone mass. Being 68 years of age and postmenopausal also puts her at higher risk for osteoporosis.

Hormonal factors play a significant role in the development of osteoporosis, which leads to an imbalance in osteoclast and osteoblast activity, particularly in postmenopausal women.[31,32] Postmenopausal osteoporosis, which is caused by an estrogen deficiency, is manifested by a loss of cancellous bone and a predisposition to fractures of the vertebrae and distal radius. The loss of bone mass is greatest during early menopause, when estrogen levels are withdrawing. Several factors appear to influence the increased loss of bone mass associated with an estrogen deficiency. Decreased estrogen levels are associated with an increase in cytokines (*e.g.*, interleukin-1, interleukin-6, and TNF) that stimulate the production of osteoclast precursors. Estrogen deficiency also influences osteoclast differentiation through the RANK receptor pathways.[32] Estrogen stimulates the production of OPG and thus inhibits the formation of osteoclasts; it also blunts the responsiveness of osteoclast precursors to RANKL.[32] With menopause and its accompanying estrogen deficiency, this inhibition of osteoclast production is lost.[32] Compensatory osteoblastic activity and new bone formation occurs, but it does not keep pace with the bone that is lost.

Sex hormone deficiency may contribute to bone loss in men with senile osteoporosis, although the effect is not of the same magnitude as that caused by estrogen deficiency. Unlike women, men do not have a midlife loss of sex hormone production.[33] Another factor that provides relative protection for men is the fact that they achieve 8% to 10% more peak bone mass than women. Although androgens have long been assumed to be critical for growth and maintenance of the male skeleton, estrogens obtained from peripheral conversion of testicular and adrenal hormone precursors may be even more important than androgens in the maintenance of bone mass in men.

Age-related changes in bone density occur in all people and contribute to the development of osteoporosis in both genders.[33] Age-related changes in bone cells and matrix have a strong impact on bone metabolism. Osteoblasts from older adults have reduced replicative and biosynthetic potential compared with those of younger people. Growth factors that stimulate osteoblastic activity also lose their potential over time. The result is a skeleton that has decreased ability to make bone. Reduced physical activity increases the rate of bone loss because mechanical forces are important stimuli for normal bone remodeling. Thus, the decreased physical activity that often accompanies aging may also contribute to the loss of bone mass in older adults.

Secondary osteoporosis is associated with many conditions, including endocrine disorders, malabsorption disorders, malignancies, alcoholism, and certain medications.[34] People with endocrine disorders such as hyperthyroidism, hyperparathyroidism, Cushing syndrome, or diabetes mellitus are at high risk for development of osteoporosis. Hyperthyroidism causes an acceleration of bone turnover. Some malignancies (*e.g.*, multiple myeloma) secrete the osteoclast-activating factor, causing significant bone loss. Alcohol is a direct inhibitor of osteoblasts and may also inhibit calcium absorption. Corticosteroid use is the most common cause of drug-related osteoporosis, and long-term corticosteroid use in the treatment of disorders such as rheumatoid arthritis and chronic obstructive lung disease is associated with a high rate of fractures. With the increased use of prednisone and other drugs that act like cortisol for the treatment of many inflammatory and autoimmune diseases, this form of bone loss has become a major clinical concern. The prolonged use of medications that increase calcium excretion, such as aluminum-containing antacids, corticosteroids, and anticonvulsants, also is associated with bone loss.

Several groups of children and adolescents are at increased risk for decreased bone mass, including premature infants and those with low birth weight who have lower than expected bone mass in the early weeks of life, children who require treatment with corticosteroid drugs (*e.g.*, those with asthma, inflammatory diseases, and transplant recipients), children with cystic fibrosis, and those with hypogonadal states (*e.g.*, anorexia nervosa and the female athlete triad).[35] Children with cystic fibrosis often have impaired gastrointestinal function that reduces the absorption of calcium and other nutrients, and many also require the frequent use of corticosteroid drugs.

Premature osteoporosis is increasingly being seen in female athletes owing to an increased prevalence of eating disorders and amenorrhea.[35] It most frequently affects women engaged in endurance sports, such as running and swimming; in activities where appearance is important, such as figure skating, diving, and gymnastics; or in sports with weight categories, such as horse racing, martial arts, and rowing. The *female athlete triad* refers to a pattern of disordered eating that leads to amenorrhea and eventually osteoporosis. Poor nutrition, combined with intense training, can decrease the critical body fat-to-muscle ratio needed for normal menses and estrogen production by the ovary. The decreased levels of estrogen combined with the lack of calcium and vitamin D from dietary deficiencies result in a loss of bone density and increased risk for fractures. There is a concern that athletes with low BMD will be at increased risk for fractures during their competitive years. It is unclear whether osteoporosis induced by amenorrhea is reversible. Data are emerging that confirm that having only one or two elements of the triad greatly increases the risk of long-term morbidity in these women.[35]

Clinical Manifestations

Osteoporotic changes occur in the diaphysis and metaphysis of bone. In severe osteoporosis, the bones begin to resemble the fragile structure of a fine porcelain vase. There is loss of trabeculae from cancellous bone and thinning of the cortex to such an extent that minimal stress causes fractures. The changes that occur with osteoporosis have been explained by two distinct disease processes: postmenopausal and senile osteoporosis. In postmenopausal women, the increase in osteoclastic activity affects mainly bones or portions of bone that have increased surface area, such as the cancellous compartment of the vertebral bodies. The osteoporotic trabeculae become thinned and lose their interconnections, leading to microfractures and eventual vertebral collapse. In senile osteoporosis, the osteoporotic cortex is thinned by subperiosteal and endosteal resorption and the haversian systems are widened. In severe cases, the haversian systems are so enlarged that the cortex resembles cancellous bone (Fig. 49.15). Hip fractures, which are seen later in life, are more commonly associated with senile osteoporosis.

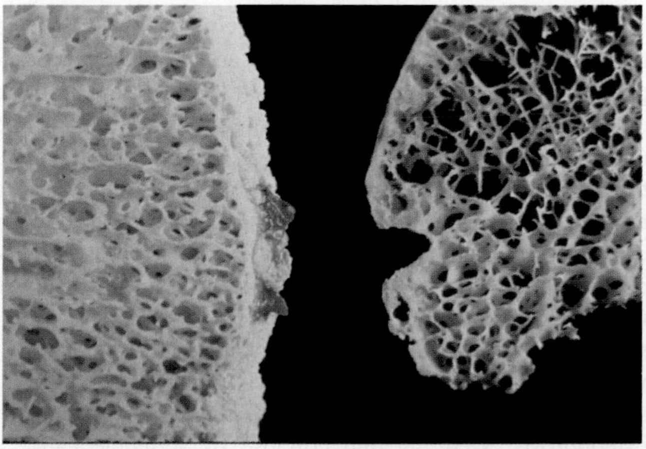

Figure 49.15 • Osteoporosis. Femoral head of an 82-year-old woman with osteoporosis and femoral neck fracture (*right*), compared with a normal control bone cut to the same thickness (*left*). (From Rubin R., Strayer D. S. (Eds.) (2015). *Rubin's pathology: Clinicopathologic foundations of medicine* (7th ed., Fig. 30.24A, p. 1331). Philadelphia, PA: Lippincott Williams & Wilkins.)

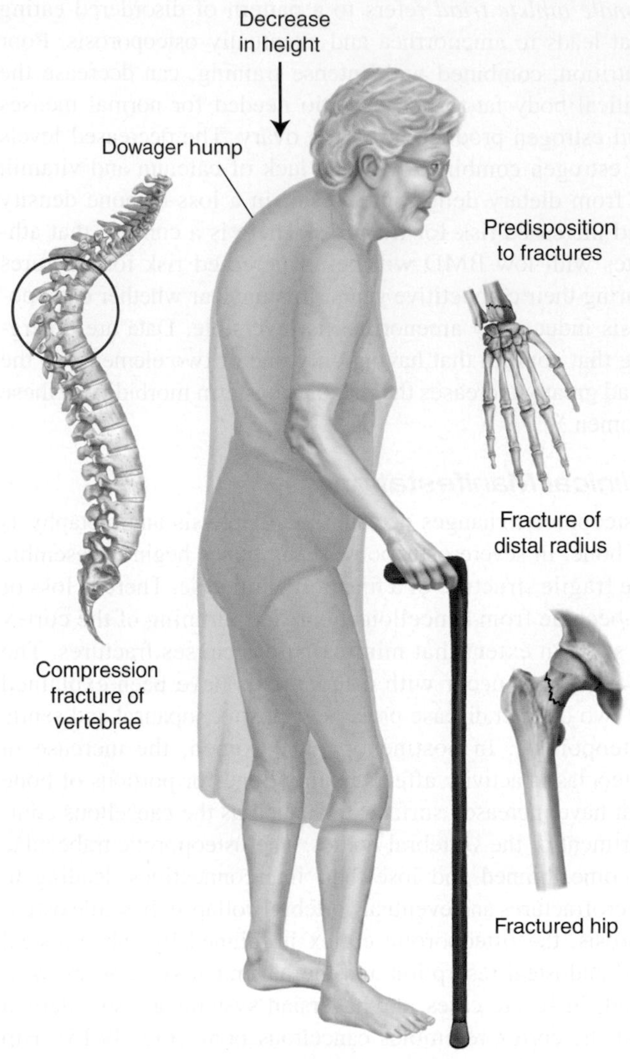

Figure 49.16 • Clinical manifestations of osteoporosis.

Osteoporosis is usually a silent disorder. Often, the first manifestations of the disorder are those that accompany a skeletal fracture—a vertebral compression fracture or fractures of the hip, pelvis, humerus, or any other bone (Fig. 49.16). Typically, the fractures occur with less force than usual, such as when a postmenopausal woman is in a crowded area such as a subway and is pushed slightly by the crowd. If the pushing occurs several times such as by someone brushing up alongside the woman as the crowd moves from the door and to the door of the subway enough pressure could cause the woman to sustain a fracture. Women who present with fractures are much more likely to sustain another fracture than are women of the same age without osteoporosis. Wedging and collapse of vertebrae cause a loss of height in the vertebral column and kyphosis, a condition commonly referred to as *dowager hump*. Usually, there is no generalized bone tenderness. When pain occurs, it is related to fractures. Systemic symptoms such as weakness and weight loss suggest that the osteoporosis may be caused by underlying disease.

Diagnosis

The National Osteoporosis Foundation (NOF) and the World Health Organization (WHO) adapted the WHO Working Group on Osteoporosis Screening Tool, Fracture Risk Assessment Algorithm (FRAX), to identify future hip fracture possibility depending on a person's risk possibility.[30] BMD assessment is most commonly undertaken with dual-energy x-ray absorptiometry (DXA) of the spine and hip. Current practice is to perform DXA on the total hip, the femoral neck, and the anterior lumbar spine (L1 to L4). The site with the lowest score should be used to make a diagnosis. Measurement of BMD has become increasingly common for early detection and fracture prevention. Measurement of serial heights in older adults is another simple way to screen for osteoporosis. A further advance in the diagnosis of osteoporosis is the refinement of risk factors. Testing for BMD should be performed based on the individual person's risk. The NOF have recommended that all women should have a measurement of BMD at 65 years of age unless they have risk factors, which means earlier screening should be performed.[30] Risk factors that may indicate a need for testing women at a younger age include:

- A delayed menarche (*i.e.*, age 15 years or later)
- Low body weight (*i.e.*, <21 kg/m^2, or 127 lb at menopause)
- Current smoker
- History of fractures after menopause (other than skull, facial bone, ankle, finger, or toe)
- History of a hip fracture in a parent[30]

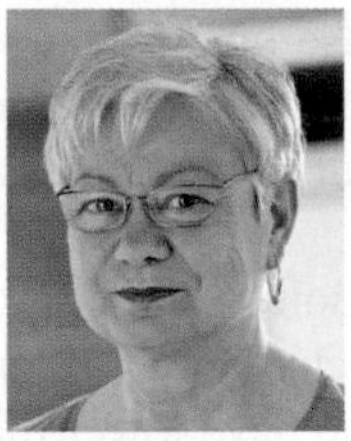

Mrs. Tukey's BMD screening shows a T score of 3.0, which puts her in the osteoporosis range. It is unfortunate that Mrs. Tukey's physician did not perform a BMD screening at the time of her hip fracture 8 years ago. According to the guidelines from the NOF, she should have been considered high risk (hip fracture after menopause, family history, and 1.5 pack/day cigarette smoking history). If she had been screened, it is possible that her osteopenia or osteoporosis could have been slowed down with the use of bisphosphonate therapy.

Treatment

Prevention and early detection of osteoporosis are essential to the prevention of associated deformities and fractures. It is important to identify people in high-risk groups so that treatment can begin early (Chart 49.1). Regular exercise and adequate calcium intake are important factors in preventing osteoporosis. Weight-bearing exercises such as walking, jogging, rowing, and weight lifting are important in the maintenance of bone mass.

CHART 49.1 RISK FACTORS ASSOCIATED WITH OSTEOPOROSIS

Personal Characteristics
Advanced age
Female
White (fair, thin skin)
Small bone structure
Postmenopausal
Family history

Lifestyle
Sedentary
Calcium deficiency (long-term)
High-protein diet
Excessive alcohol intake
Excessive caffeine intake
Smoking

Drug and Disease Related
Aluminum-containing antacids
Anticonvulsants
Heparin
Corticosteroids or Cushing disease
Gastrectomy
Diabetes mellitus
Chronic obstructive lung disease
Malignancy
Hyperthyroidism
Hyperparathyroidism
Rheumatoid arthritis

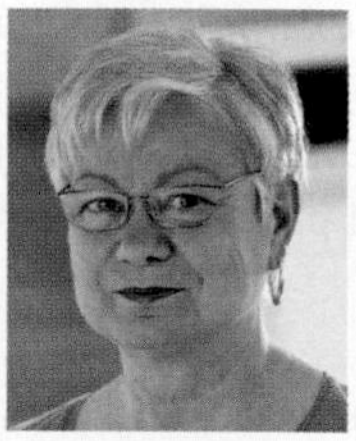

Mrs. Tukey has not been doing any exercises and has now been referred to the YMCA for aerobic exercises, which should assist her in managing the osteoporosis along with her prescribed bisphosphonate therapy and calcium and vitamin supplements. She also needs to quit her cigarette smoking habit. In addition, she has been referred to a nutritionist who will be able to assist her with planning a more balanced diet.

Studies have indicated that premenopausal women need more than 1000 mg/day of calcium, and postmenopausal women should take 1500 mg of calcium daily. Because most older American women do not consume a sufficient quantity of dairy products to meet their calcium needs, calcium supplementation is recommended. Calcium tablets vary in content of elemental calcium. Vitamin D deficiency may be an important factor in the impaired intestinal absorption of calcium in the older adult. On the basis of this evidence, 1,25-dihydroxyvitamin D_3 is being studied as a treatment for osteoporosis.[36] A daily intake of 400 to 800 IU of vitamin D is recommended because vitamin D optimizes calcium absorption and inhibits parathyroid secretion.[36]

Pharmacologic treatment of osteoporosis includes antiresorptive drugs and anabolic agents. There are three main types of antiresorptive agent: estrogens and SERMs, bisphosphonates, and calcitonin. Although estrogen is one of the most effective interventions for reducing the incidence and progression of osteoporosis in postmenopausal women, the use of hormone therapy (estrogen plus progestin) has come under scrutiny since the Women's Health Initiative.[37] Raloxifene, a SERM that acts only on specific estrogen receptors, is effective in the prevention and treatment of osteoporosis in postmenopausal women.

Bisphosphonates are effective inhibitors of bone resorption and the most effective agents for prevention and treatment of osteoporosis. The bisphosphonates (*e.g.*, alendronate, risedronate, ibandronate) are analogs of endogenous inorganic pyrophosphate that the body cannot break down. In bone, they bind to hydroxyapatite and prevent bone resorption by inhibiting osteoclast activity. Bisphosphonates have been shown to be effective in reducing the risk of hip, vertebral, and nonvertebral fractures; however, they also have adverse effects such as causing hip fractures although very rarely.[37] The most dramatic impact has been in the reduction of multiple spine fractures, showing that treatment can decrease progression of the disease.

Calcitonin is an endogenous peptide that partially inhibits osteoclastic activity. Nasal calcitonin and subcutaneous calcitonin have been approved for the treatment of postmenopausal osteoporosis. Teriparatide is a recombinant form of parathyroid hormone for the treatment of osteoporosis. Unlike the antiresorptive drugs, parathyroid hormone stimulates bone remodeling by increasing osteoblast-mediated bone formation.

In men, testosterone appears to play an important role in bone homeostasis by stimulating osteoblasts and inhibiting osteoclasts. The use of testosterone is contraindicated in men with prostate cancer. Men with osteoporosis may also benefit from bisphosphonate, calcitonin, or parathyroid hormone therapy. Like women, they have the same need for calcium and vitamin D supplementation.

People with osteoporosis have many special needs. Walking and swimming are encouraged. Surgical intervention is done for stable fracture fixation that allows early restoration of mobility and function; for fractures of the lower extremities, this means early weightbearing. Vertebral fractures are treated symptomatically. Vertebroplasty and kyphoplasty are minimally invasive spinal procedures that use bone cement to restore vertebral height and relieve pain. Bone cement is instilled directly into the fractured vertebral body to restore height and shape. The procedure for kyphoplasty involves the use of a balloon as a tamp to create a void for the cement. Kyphoplasty seems to be associated with less cement extravasation and better restoration of vertebral height than vertebroplasty.[38]

Osteomalacia and Rickets

In contrast to osteoporosis, which causes a loss of total bone mass and results in brittle bones, osteomalacia and rickets produce a softening of the bones but do not involve a loss of bone matrix.[39,40] Approximately 60% of bone is mineral content, approximately 30% is organic matrix, and the remainder is living bone cells. The organic matrix and the inorganic mineral salts are needed for normal bone consistency. The term *rickets* refers to the disorder in children in which changes in bone growth produce characteristic skeletal abnormalities, and *osteomalacia* is used in adults because the bone that forms during the remodeling process is undermineralized.[14]

Osteomalacia

Osteomalacia is a generalized bone condition in which there is inadequate mineralization of bone. There are two main causes of osteomalacia:

1. Insufficient calcium absorption from the intestine because of a lack of dietary calcium or a deficiency of or resistance to the action of vitamin D.
2. Phosphate deficiency caused by increased renal losses or decreased intestinal absorption.

Vitamin D deficiency is caused most commonly by reduced vitamin D absorption as a result of biliary tract or intestinal diseases that impair fat and fat-soluble vitamin absorption. Lack of vitamin D in the diet is rare in the United States because many foods are fortified with the vitamin. Anticonvulsant medications, such as phenobarbital and phenytoin, induce hepatic hydroxylases that accelerate breakdown of the active forms of vitamin D.

The incidence of osteomalacia is high among older adults because of diets deficient in calcium and vitamin D, a problem often compounded by the intestinal malabsorption that accompanies aging. Osteomalacia often is seen in cultures in which the diet is deficient in vitamin D, such as in northern China, Japan, and northern India. Women in these areas have a higher incidence of the disorder than do men because of the combined effects of pregnancy, lactation, and more indoor confinement. Osteomalacia occasionally is seen in strict vegetarians, people who have had a gastrectomy, and those on long-term anticonvulsants, tranquilizers, sedatives, muscle relaxants, or diuretic drugs. There also is a greater incidence of osteomalacia in the colder regions of the world, particularly during the winter months, probably because of lessened exposure to sunlight.

A form of osteomalacia called *renal rickets* occurs in people with chronic renal failure.[39] It is caused by the inability of the kidney to activate vitamin D and excrete phosphate and is accompanied by hyperparathyroidism, increased bone turnover, and increased bone resorption. Long-standing primary hyperparathyroidism causes increased calcium resorption from bone and hypophosphatemia, which can lead to rickets in children and osteomalacia in adults.

Clinical Manifestations. The clinical manifestations of osteomalacia are bone pain, tenderness, and fractures as the disease progresses. In severe cases, muscle weakness often is an early sign. The cause of muscle weakness is unclear. Osteomalacia predisposes a person to pathologic fractures in the weakened areas, especially in the distal radius and proximal femur. In contrast to osteoporosis, it is not a significant cause of hip fractures. There may be delayed healing and poor retention of internal fixation devices. Osteomalacia usually is accompanied by a compensatory or secondary hyperparathyroidism stimulated by low serum calcium levels. Parathyroid hormone reduces renal absorption of phosphate and removes calcium from the bone. Serum calcium levels are only slightly reduced in osteomalacia.

Diagnosis and Treatment. Diagnostic measures are directed toward identifying osteomalacia and establishing its cause. Diagnostic methods include x-ray studies, laboratory tests, bone scan, and bone biopsy. X-ray findings typical of osteomalacia are the development of transverse lines or pseudofractures. These apparently are caused by stress fractures that are inadequately healed. A bone biopsy may be done to confirm the diagnosis of osteomalacia in a person with nonspecific osteopenia who shows no improvement after treatment with exercise, vitamin D, and calcium.

The treatment of osteomalacia is directed at the underlying cause.[39,40] If the problem is nutritional, restoring adequate amounts of calcium and vitamin D to the diet may be sufficient. The elderly with intestinal malabsorption also may benefit from vitamin D. The least expensive and most effective long-term treatment is a diet rich in vitamin D (*i.e.*, fish, dairy products, and margarine) along with careful exposure to the midday sun. Vitamin D is specific for adult osteomalacia and vitamin D–resistant rickets, but large doses usually are needed to overcome the resistance to calcium absorption action and to prevent renal loss of phosphate. The biologically active forms of vitamin D, 25-OH vitamin D (calciferol) or 1,25-$(OH)_2$ vitamin D (calcitriol), are available for use in the treatment of osteomalacia resistant to vitamin D (*i.e.*, osteomalacia resulting from chronic liver disease and kidney failure). If osteomalacia is caused by malabsorption, the treatment is directed toward correcting the primary disease. For example, adequate replacement of pancreatic enzymes is of paramount importance in pancreatic insufficiency. In renal tubular disorders, the treatment is directed at the altered renal physiology.

Rickets

Rickets is a metabolic bone disease characterized by a failure or delay in calcification of the cartilaginous growth plate in children whose epiphyses have not yet fused.[40] It is also manifested by widening and deformation of the metaphyseal regions of long bones and a delay in the mineralization of trabecular, endosteal, and periosteal bone surfaces. There are several forms of rickets, including nutritional rickets, vitamin D–dependent rickets, and vitamin D–resistant rickets.

Etiology. As with osteomalacia in the adult, rickets can result from kidney failure; malabsorptive syndromes such as celiac disease and cystic fibrosis; and medications such as anticonvulsants, which cause target organ resistance to vitamin D, and aluminum-containing antacids, which bind phosphorus and prevent its absorption.

Nutritional rickets results from inadequate sunlight exposure or inadequate intake of vitamin D, calcium, or phosphate.

Nutritional rickets occurs primarily in underdeveloped areas of the world and among immigrants to developed countries. The causes are inadequate exposure to sunlight (*e.g.*, children are often kept clothed and indoors) and prolonged breast-feeding without vitamin D supplementation. Although the vitamin D content of human milk is low, the combination of breast milk and sunlight exposure usually provides sufficient vitamin D. Another cause of rickets is the use of commercial alternative milks (*e.g.*, soy or rice beverages) that are not fortified with vitamin D. Vitamin D–dependent rickets can result from abnormalities in the gene coding for the enzyme that converts inactive vitamin D to the active vitamin D–resistant rickets and involves hypophosphatemia or a decrease in serum phosphate levels, the most common form being caused by mutations of the phosphate-regulating gene on the X chromosome.[40] Gene mutation causes renal wasting of phosphate at the proximal tubular level of the kidney.

Clinical Manifestations. Rickets is characterized by changes in the growing bones of children with overgrowth of the epiphyseal cartilage because of inadequate provisional calcification and failure of the cartilage cells to disintegrate. Bones become deformed; ossification at the epiphyseal plates is delayed and disordered, resulting in widening of the epiphyseal cartilage plate. Any new bone that does grow is unmineralized. During the nonmobile stage of infancy, the head and chest undergo the greatest stresses. The skull is enlarged and soft, and closure of the fontanels is delayed. Teeth are slow to develop, and the child may have difficulty standing. When an ambulating child develops rickets, deformities are likely to affect the spine, pelvis, and long bones (*i.e.*, tibia), causing, most notably, lumbar lordosis and bowing of the legs. The ends of long bones and ribs are enlarged. The thorax may be abnormally shaped, with prominent rib cartilage (*i.e.*, rachitic rosary). The child usually has stunted growth, with a height sometimes far below the normal range. Weight often is not affected so that the children, many of whom present with a protruding abdomen (*i.e.*, rachitic potbelly), have been described as presenting a Buddha-like appearance when sitting.

Treatment. Nutritional rickets is treated with a balanced diet sufficient in calcium, phosphorus, and vitamin D. Exposure to sunlight also is important, especially for premature infants and those on artificial milk feedings. Supplemental vitamin D exceeding normal daily requirements is given for several months. Maintenance of good posture, positioning, and bracing in older children are used to prevent deformities. After the disease is controlled, deformities may have to be surgically corrected as the child grows.

Children with vitamin D–dependent and vitamin D–independent rickets require special treatment measures. Children with vitamin D–dependent rickets caused by lack of the enzyme needed to convert vitamin D to its active form are treated with calcitriol, the active form of vitamin D.[40] Vitamin D–resistant forms of rickets are treated with oral phosphorus or oral phosphorus and calcitriol.

Paget Disease

Paget disease (*i.e.*, osteitis deformans) is the second most common bone disease after osteoporosis.[14,40,41] The disease tends to occur in people in their fourth decade and is characterized by local areas of excessive bone turnover and disorganized osteoid formation. The disease is more common in people of Northern European heritage.

Paget disease is a focal process with considerable variation in its stage of development in separate sites. At the onset, the disease is marked by regions of rapidly occurring osteoclastic bone resorption, followed by a period of hectic bone formation with increased numbers of osteoblasts rapidly depositing bone in a chaotic fashion such that the newly formed bone is of poor quality and is disorganized rather than lamellar. The poor quality of bone accounts for the bowing and fractures that occur in bones affected by the disease. The bone marrow adjacent to the bone-forming surface is replaced by loose connective tissue that contains osteoprogenitor cells and numerous blood vessels, which transport blood to and from these metabolically active sites.[40] The lesions of Paget disease may be solitary or may occur in multiple sites. They tend to localize to the bones of the axial skeleton, including the spine, skull, hips, and pelvis. The proximal femur and tibia may be involved in more widespread forms of the disease. Histologically, Paget lesions show increased vascularity and bone marrow fibrosis with intense cellular activity. The bone has a somewhat mosaic-like pattern caused by areas of density outlined by heavy blue lines, called *cement lines* (Fig. 49.17).

Etiology

Although the cause of Paget disease remains unclear, there is evidence of both genetic and environmental influences. It has been reported that 15% to 40% of people with the disease have a first-degree relative with Paget disease, and numerous studies have described extended family members with the disease.[40,41] Additionally, evidence supports that people with Paget disease have been found to have a mutation of the SQSM1/p62 gene in their diseased bone and tumor samples.[40,41] It is possible that factors other than genetics are also involved in the pathogenesis of the disease such as a paramyxovirus.[40] This has been supported by the observation of viral particles resembling the paramyxovirus nucleocapsid in the cytoplasm of osteoclasts in people with Paget disease.

In children, hyperostosis corticalis deformans juvenilis (a rare autosomal recessive disorder), hyperphosphatemia, and diseases that cause diaphyseal stenosis may mimic Paget disease and sometimes are referred to as *juvenile Paget disease.*[40] The disorder presents in infancy or early childhood with pain from debilitating fractures and deformities because of a markedly accelerated rate of bone remodeling throughout the skeleton.

Clinical Manifestations

The disease varies in severity from a simple lesion to involvement of many bones. It may be present long before it is

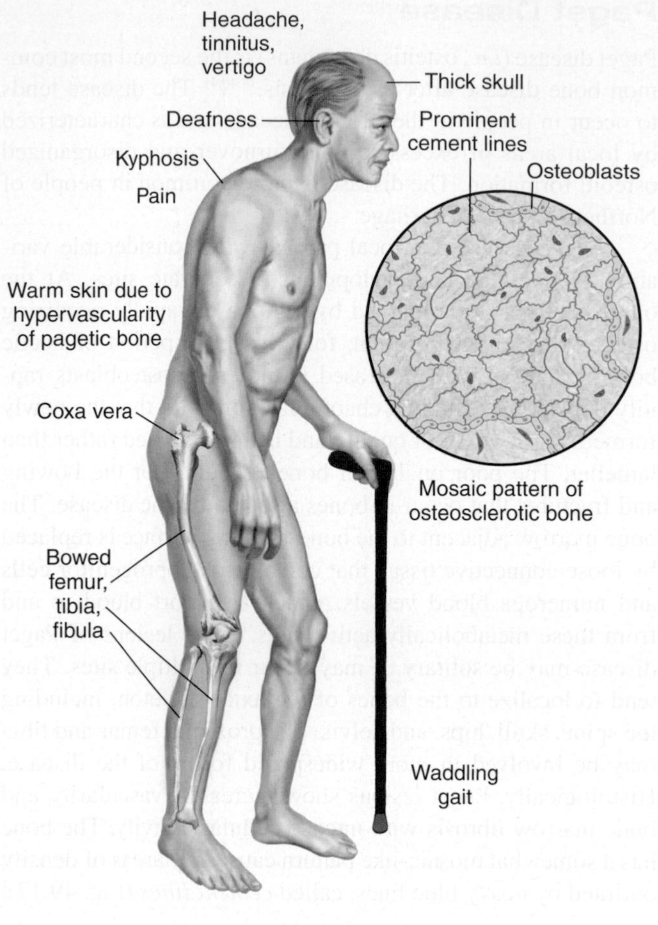

Figure 49.17 • Clinical manifestations of Paget disease.

detected clinically. In fact, many people have no symptoms and their disease is found when managing another health problem. The clinical manifestations of Paget disease depend on the specific area involved (see Fig. 49.17). Involvement of the skull can cause headaches, intermittent tinnitus, vertigo, and eventual hearing loss. In the spine, collapse of the anterior vertebrae causes kyphosis of the thoracic spine. The femur and tibia become bowed. Softening of the femoral neck can cause coxa vara (*i.e.*, reduced angle of the femoral neck). Coxa vara, in combination with softening of the sacral and iliac bones, causes a waddling gait. When the lesion affects only one bone, it may cause only mild pain and stiffness. Progressive deossification weakens and distorts the bone structure. The deossification process begins along the inner cortical surfaces and continues until the substance of the bone disappears. Pathologic fractures may occur, especially in the bones subjected to the greatest stress (*e.g.*, upper femur, lower spine, pelvic bones). These fractures often heal poorly, with excessive and poorly distributed callus.

Other manifestations of Paget disease include nerve palsy syndromes from lesions in the upper extremities, mental deterioration, and cardiovascular disease because of high-output heart failure. Cardiovascular disease is the most serious complication and the most common cause of death in those with advanced generalized Paget disease. Calcific aortic stenosis may occur in severe cases. Ventilatory capacity may be limited by rib and spine involvement.

Osteogenic sarcomas have also been found to occur in people with Paget disease. The bones most often affected, in order of frequency, are the femur, pelvis, humerus, and tibia.

Diagnosis and Treatment

Diagnosis of Paget disease is based on characteristic bone deformities and x-ray changes. Elevated levels of serum alkaline phosphatase and urinary hydroxyproline support the diagnosis and continued surveillance of these levels may be used to monitor the effectiveness of treatment. Bone scans are used to detect the rapid bone turnover indicative of active disease and to monitor the response to treatment. The scan cannot identify bone activity resulting from malignant lesions. Bone biopsy may be done to differentiate the lesion from osteomyelitis or a primary or metastatic bone tumor.

The treatment of Paget disease is based on the degree of pain and the extent of the disease. Pain can be reduced with nonsteroidal or other anti-inflammatory agents. Suppressive agents such as the bisphosphonates and calcitonin are used to manage pain and prevent further spread of the disease and neurologic defects. Early diagnosis and bisphosphonate therapy are the most effective ways to manage Paget disease because of the ability to decrease bone resorption.[40,41] Parenteral bisphosphonates are particularly useful in people who cannot tolerate oral preparations, which have a specific administration protocol. Calcitonin also inhibits bone resorption. It is available in injectable and nasal spray forms, but only the injectable form is approved by the FDA for treatment of Paget disease. Nasal-spray calcitonin, which is approved for other uses, is being studied for use in Paget disease. People with Paget disease should receive adequate doses of calcium and vitamin D. A recombinant form of OPG is also being used to inhibit osteoclastogenesis in children, slowing the osteoclast activity. Juvenile Paget disease is being described as an OPG deficiency.[40,41]

IN SUMMARY

In addition to its structural function, the skeleton is a homeostatic organ. Metabolic bone diseases such as osteoporosis, osteomalacia, rickets, and Paget disease are the result of a disruption in the equilibrium of bone formation and resorption. Osteoporosis, which is the most common of the metabolic bone diseases, occurs when the rate of bone resorption is greater than that of bone formation. It is seen frequently in postmenopausal women and is the major cause of fractures in people older than 45 years of age. Osteomalacia and rickets are caused by inadequate mineralization of bone matrix, primarily because of a deficiency of vitamin D. Paget disease results from excessive osteoclastic activity and is characterized by the formation of poor-quality bone. The success rate of the various drugs and hormones that are used to treat metabolic bone diseases varies. Further research is needed to clarify the cause, pathologic process, and treatment of these diseases.

ACTIVITY INTOLERANCE AND FATIGUE

After completing this section of the chapter, the learner will be able to meet the following objectives:

- Define fatigue, and describe its manifestations.
- Differentiate acute from chronic fatigue.
- Define myalgic encephalomyelitis/chronic fatigue syndrome and describe assessment findings, presenting symptoms, and laboratory values associated with the disorder.

Activity tolerance is the amount of physical activity a person can perform without injury or excessive exertion. Activity tolerance can be measured by having the person describe his or her normal activities, perceived activity tolerance, or level of fatigue. One method of assessing activity tolerance involves the administration of a screening tool in which participants describe their normal activities, their perceived level of activity tolerance, or their level of fatigue. An example of such a tool is the Human Activity Profile (HAP).[42] The HAP originally was developed to assess the quality of life for the people participating in a rehabilitation program for chronic obstructive pulmonary disease. After investigating numerous physiologic and psychological measures, it was noted that the most important aspect of quality of life was the amount of daily activity the person was able to perform. The HAP consists of 94 items representing common activities that require known amounts of average energy expenditure. The person marks each item based on whether he or she is still able to perform the activity or has stopped performing the activity.

Activity intolerance can be viewed as not having sufficient physical or psychological energy reserves to endure or complete required or desired daily activities. Fatigue is the sensation that comes with having exhausted those energy reserves. It is a state experienced by everyone at some time in life. Fatigue can be a normal physical response, such as that following extreme exercise in healthy people, or it can be a symptom experienced by people with limited energy reserve, such as people with cardiac or respiratory disease, anemia, or malnutrition, or those on certain types of drug therapy. Fatigue also may be related to lack of sleep or mental stress.

Like dyspnea and pain, fatigue is a subjective symptom. It often is described as a feeling of just not feeling right and having a lack of energy and motivation to do anything. Fatigue is different from the normal tiredness that people experience at the end of the day. Tiredness is relieved by a good night's sleep, whereas fatigue persists despite sufficient or adequate sleep. Although fatigue is one of the most common symptoms reported to health care professionals, it is one of the least understood of all health problems. Fatigue cannot be explained using a measurement such as amount of activity or exercise.[43]

The physiologic basis of fatigue includes factors such as diaphragmatic, motor, and neurologic mechanisms. Diaphragmatic fatigue occurs in both acute and chronic respiratory conditions where the force and duration of muscle work exceeds muscle energy stores. Neuromuscular fatigue involves the loss of maximal capacity to generate force during exercise.

KEY POINTS

- Acute fatigue is fatigue with a rapid onset resulting from short-term sleep loss or heavy exercise. Adequate sleep and nutrition allow for recovery from acute fatigue.
- Myalgic encephalomyelitis/chronic fatigue syndrome (CFS) is characterized by disabling fatigue and many nonspecific symptoms, including cognitive impairments, sleep disturbances, and musculoskeletal pain. The etiology of CFS is unknown, but it is associated with several chronic diseases such as fibromyalgia, depression, and irritable bowel syndrome.

Mechanisms of Fatigue

The origin or cause of fatigue can be physiologic, psychological, pathologic, or unknown (*e.g.*, CFS or myalgic encephalomyelitis [ME]). It can be caused by environmental factors (*e.g.*, excessive noise, temperature extremes, changes in weather), drug-related incidents (*e.g.*, use of tranquilizers, alcohol, toxic chemical exposure), treatment-related causes (*e.g.*, chemotherapy, radiation therapy, surgery, anesthesia, diagnostic testing), physical exertion (*e.g.*, exercise), and psychological factors (*e.g.*, stress, monotony).

Clinically, fatigue can be described by how it begins, what seems to trigger it, and how it is managed. This information can sometimes assist in determining the etiology of the pain. It is thought that both acute and chronic fatigue can exist in the same person, similar to acute and chronic pain.

Acute Physical Fatigue

Acute fatigue has a rapid onset and is often defined as muscle fatigue associated with increased activity, or exercise, that is carried out to the point of exhaustion. It also is frequently associated with a viral or bacterial infection and may present with other systemic symptoms such as fever or malaise.[43]

If it is associated with muscle fatigue, it is relieved shortly after the activity ceases and serves as a protective mechanism. Physical conditioning can influence the onset of acute fatigue. People who engage in regular exercise compared with sedentary people can perform an activity for longer periods before acute fatigue develops. They can do so in part because their muscles use oxygen and nutrients more efficiently, and their circulatory and respiratory systems are better able to deliver oxygen and nutrients to the exercising muscles.

Acute physical fatigue occurs more rapidly in deconditioned muscle. For example, acute fatigue often is seen in people who have been on bed rest because of a surgical procedure or in people who have had their activity curtailed because of chronic illness, such as heart or respiratory disease (see Fig. 49.18). In such cases, the acute fatigue often is out of proportion to the activity that is being performed (*e.g.*, dangling at the bedside, sitting in a chair for the first time). When resuming activity after a prolonged period of bed rest or inactivity, the person may experience tachycardia and hypotension. Unless these parameters are changed by medications such as β-adrenergic blocking drugs, heart rate and blood pressure become particularly sensitive indicators of activity tolerance or intolerance.

Another example of acute fatigue is that which occurs in people who require the use of assistive devices such as wheelchairs, walkers, or crutches. The upper arm muscles are less well adapted to prolonged exercise than the leg muscles. This is because arm muscles are primarily composed of type II muscle fibers. Type II muscle fibers, which are used when the body requires short bursts of energy, fatigue quickly. As a result, people who use wheelchairs or crutches may quickly experience fatigue until their arms become conditioned to the increased activity.

Chronic Fatigue

Chronic fatigue differs from acute fatigue in terms of onset, intensity, perception, duration, and relief. Chronic fatigue is much more complex and difficult to diagnose. There are several possible causes such as hypothyroidism, anemia, heart disease, Lyme disease, fibromyalgia, lung disease, electrolyte dysfunction, tuberculosis, hepatitis, and cancer.[43] It is a common problem experienced by people with chronic health problems (Table 49.2). In the primary care setting, many people complain of chronic fatigue. Chronic fatigue with HF or emphysema is accepted given the pathophysiology of these conditions. Others may have a transient fatigue that can be managed with vitamin or other medication supplementation.

Although acute fatigue often serves a protective function, chronic fatigue does not. It limits the amount of activity that

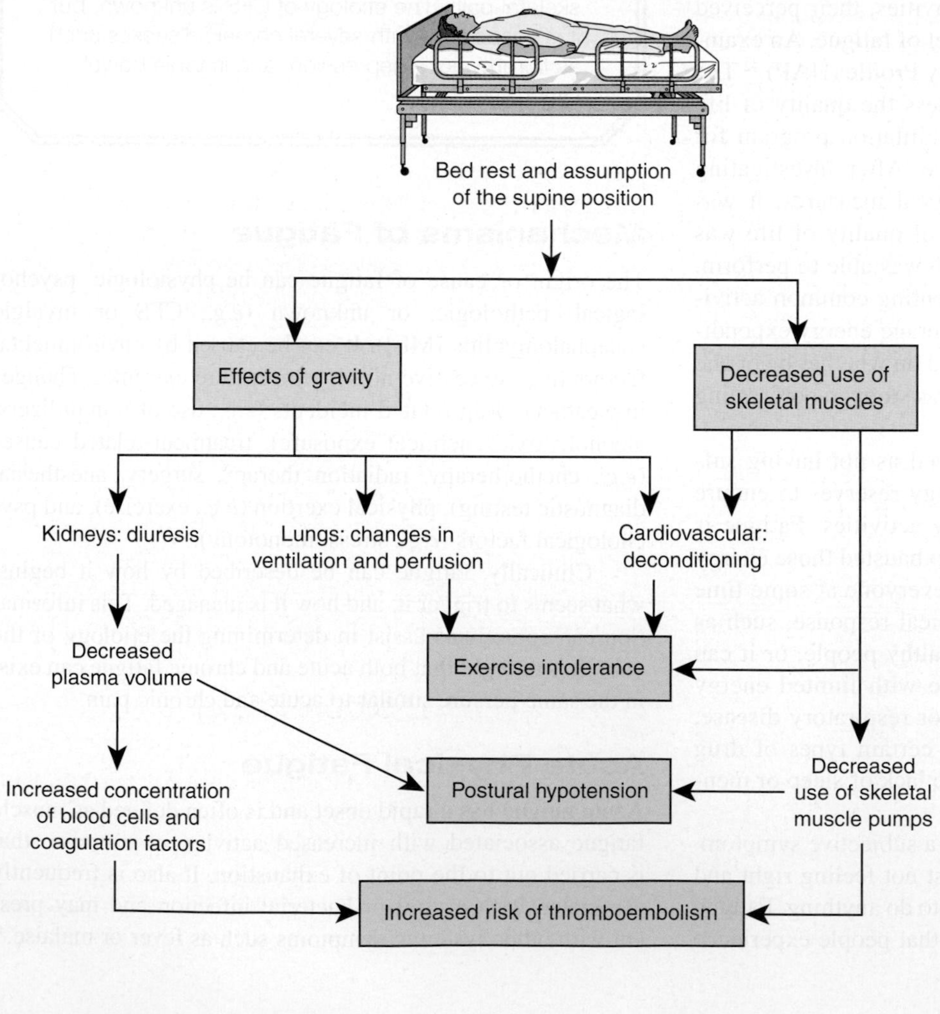

Figure 49.18 • The effects of gravity and decreased use of the skeletal muscles during bed rest and assumption of the supine position on cardiovascular, respiratory, and renal function and their impact on exercise tolerance and the risk of complications such as thromboembolism and postural hypotension.

TABLE 49.2 CHRONIC ILLNESSES AND CAUSES OF CHRONIC FATIGUE

CHRONIC ILLNESS	CAUSE OF FATIGUE
Acquired immunodeficiency syndrome	Impaired immune function, anorexia, muscle weakness, and psychosocial factors associated with the disease
Anemia	Decreased oxygen-carrying capacity of blood
Arthritis	Pain and joint dysfunction lead to impaired mobility, loss of sleep, and emotional factors
Cancer	Presence of chemical products and catabolic processes associated with tumor growth; anorexia and difficulty eating; effects of chemotherapy and radiation therapy; and psychosocial factors such as depression, grieving, hopelessness, and fear
Cardiac Disease	
Myocardial infarction	Death of myocardial tissue results in decreased cardiac output, poor tissue perfusion, and impaired delivery of oxygen and nutrients to vital organs
Congestive HF	Impaired pumping ability of the heart results in poor perfusion of muscle tissue and vital organs
Neurologic Disorders	
Multiple sclerosis	Demyelinating disease of CNS characterized by slowing of nerve conduction, resulting in lower extremity weakness and fatigue
Myasthenia gravis	Disorder of postsynaptic acetylcholine receptors of the myoneural junction, resulting in muscle weakness and fatigue
Chronic lung disease	Increased work of breathing and impaired gas exchange
Chronic renal failure	Accumulation of metabolic wastes; fluid, electrolyte, and acid–base disorders; decreased red blood cell count and oxygen-carrying capacity because of impaired erythropoietin production
Metabolic Disorders	
Hypothyroidism	Decrease in basal metabolic rate manifested by fatigue
Diabetes mellitus	Impaired cellular use of glucose by muscle cells
Obesity	Imbalance in nutritional intake and energy expenditure; increased workload because of excess weight
Steroid myopathy	Glucocorticosteroids interfere with protein and glycogen synthesis, which leads to muscle wasting

a person can perform and may interfere with employment, performance of activities of daily living, and quality of life. Although fatigue often is viewed as a symptom of anxiety and depression, it is important to recognize that the anxiety and depression may instead be symptoms of the fatigue. For example, people with persistent fatigue because of a chronic illness may have to curtail their work schedules, decrease social activities, and limit their usual family responsibilities. These lifestyle changes may be the reasons for the depression rather than the depression being a cause of the fatigue.

Chronic fatigue occurs across a broad spectrum of disease states. It is a common complaint of people with cancer, cardiac disease, end-stage renal disease, chronic lung disease, hepatitis C, arthritis, human immunodeficiency virus (HIV) infection and acquired immunodeficiency syndrome (AIDS), and neurologic disorders such as multiple sclerosis, postpolio syndrome, and Parkinson disease.

Chronic fatigue is an almost universal phenomenon in people with cancer. Of people undergoing treatment for cancer, 14% to 96% percent experience fatigue.[44] Additionally, post treatment, 19% to 82% of people experience fatigue.[44] Cancer-related fatigue may be caused by the disease itself or by the treatment. Cancer-related fatigue involves a number of physiologic, sensory, affective, and cognitive dimensions. There is often a sensation of feeling unusually tired, with generalized weakness and a greater need for rest. There may also be a disturbing lack of motivation, anxiety, and sadness, as well as an inability to concentrate or difficulty in thinking.

There are several types of cancer-related factors that may cause fatigue, the most prominent of which are factors related to energy imbalance from the following disorders: anemia, cachexia, stress, pain, infection, medications, and metabolic disorders. The cytokine theory of cancer-related fatigue is based in part on the observation that people receiving agents such as interferon-α as part of their treatment plan experienced devastating fatigue that appears dose limited. Interferon-α and other agents used to treat cancer also influence the release of other cytokines that are related to fatigue. Cancer cells and the immune system appear to produce or express a number of cytokines with the potential for manufacturing many of the factors that contribute to fatigue, particularly interleukin-1 beta and tumor necrosis factor alpha (TNF-α).[45] One of these cytokines, TNF-α, is thought to be associated with morning fatigue and sleep disturbances.[45,46] Another study demonstrates that the performance of specific skeletal exercises by people with cancer results in the release of interleukin-6, which can decrease the levels of TNF-α and interleukin–1 beta.[45,46]

Management of Chronic Fatigue

Many of the pathologic factors associated with fatigue, including insomnia, anemia, psychological stress, and weakness, respond to appropriate treatment measures. Anemia, which is common among people with HIV/AIDS, people with end-stage renal disease, and people with cancer receiving chemotherapy, causes fatigue by interfering with the oxygen-carrying capacity of the blood. It is sometimes treated with recombinant forms of erythropoietin (epoetin alfa), an endogenous hormone normally produced by the kidney. Insomnia—which occurs for several reasons including anxiety and depression, hot flashes, nocturia, and pain—is treatable with nonpharmacologic and pharmacologic methods. Psychological disturbances, such as anxiety and depression, which are frequently associated with fatigue, can be treated with selected pharmacologic agents. Another cause of fatigue is loss of muscle mass, muscle strength, and endurance. It may be that the person needs to have a thorough physical examination with laboratory studies to determine if there are any musculoskeletal or neurologic problems that may be impacting the person's stamina, such as myositis, Guillain-Barré, or polymyalgia, or if the person needs to build endurance with a consistent exercise program.

Myalgic Encephalomyelitis/Chronic Fatigue Syndrome

ME/CFS is a condition of disabling fatigue of at least 6 months' duration that is typically accompanied by an array of self-reported, nonspecific symptoms such as cognitive impairments, sleep disturbances, and musculoskeletal pain. In the late 20th century and now into the 21st century, the disorder continues to be a relatively common problem.

Definition. Because the etiology of CFS is unknown, there are no biologic markers for the diagnosis of CFS and there are no definitive treatments. Furthermore, the overlap of symptoms of CFS with other functional disorders such as fibromyalgia, multiple chemical sensitivities, depression, and irritable bowel syndrome, which also are characterized by fatigue, complicates the ability to define the syndrome with any degree of certainty. In fact, CFS may describe a group of similar symptoms that develop with different pathophysiologic disturbances.

Because of the need for diagnostic criteria, the case definition for CFS was established in 1988 by the CDC and revised through its International Chronic Fatigue Syndrome Study Group in 1994.[47] To be classified as CFS, the fatigue must be clinically evaluated, cause severe mental and physical exhaustion, and result in a significant reduction in the individual's premorbid activity level. Table 49.3 illustrates examples of conditions that may mimic CFS. Chart 49.2 outlines the CDC's symptoms of CFS and the criteria for diagnosis of CFS.[47,48]

TABLE 49.3 EXAMPLES OF CONDITIONS THAT MAY PRESENT AS CHRONIC FATIGUE

Psychological	Depression Anxiety Somatization disorder
Pharmacologic	Hypnotics Antihypertensives Tranquilizers Drug abuse and drug withdrawal
Endocrine—Metabolic	Hypothyroidism Diabetes mellitus Apathetic hyperthyroidism of the elderly Pituitary insufficiency Hyperparathyroidism of hypercalcemia of any origin Addison disease Chronic renal failure Hepatocellular failure
Neoplastic—Hematologic	Occult malignancy (*e.g.*, pancreatic cancer) Severe anemia
Infectious	Endocarditis Tuberculosis Mononucleosis Hepatitis Parasitic disease HIV infection Cytomegalovirus infection
Cardiopulmonary	Chronic congestive heart failure Chronic obstructive pulmonary disease
Connective tissue disease—immune	Rheumatoid disease
Hyperreactivity	Myalgic encephalomyelitis/ chronic fatigue syndrome
Disturbed sleep	Sleep apnea Esophageal reflux Allergic rhinitis Psychological etiologies (see earlier entries)

Pathophysiology. Theories of the pathogenesis of CFS include genetic expression, infections, stress and prior psychological disorders, a dysfunction in the hypothalamic–pituitary–adrenal axis, nutritional deficiencies, or increased oxidative and nitrosative stress.[48] Despite much research and the development of several theories, the underlying pathophysiology of CFS remains elusive. Many people with CFS attribute the onset of their disease to an influenza-like infection. Thus, the link between infectious agents such as Epstein-Barr virus, human herpesvirus 6, Candida yeast, Borrelia bacteria, and others has been extensively studied. To date, however, none of these agents has been conclusively linked in a cause-and-effect relationship with the development of CFS.[48] It is hypothesized that the immune system may overreact to an environmental agent (most likely an infectious agent) or internal stimuli and be unable to self-regulate after the infectious insult is over.

Psychological disorders often are associated with CFS, especially anxiety and depression, but this is difficult to evaluate. People with CFS are more likely than the general population to have experienced a psychological disorder such as major depression or panic disorder before the development of CFS. However, it also is true that a significant proportion of those people with CFS have not had such episodes, either before or after the development of CFS.[48]

CHART 49.2 CDC SYMPTOMS OF MYALGIC ENCEPHALOMYELITIS/CHRONIC FATIGUE SYNDROME

ME/CFS has three primary symptoms required for diagnosis, with additional common symptoms, which may or may not be experienced with all people with ME/CFS. The primary symptoms include:

1. Decreased ability to participate in activities that were common before the disease, accompanied by fatigue lasting 6 months or longer. The fatigue associated with ME/CFS is severe, does not improve with sleep/rest, was not present prior to the disease, and is not related to performing difficult activities.
2. Increased symptoms following physical or mental activity that were not present prior to the disease; this "postexertional malaise" may last days, weeks, or longer.
3. Alterations in sleep, such as being tired after a full night of sleep.

In addition to the above primary symptoms, *one* of the following must be present for a diagnosis of ME/CFS:

- Difficulty thinking/remembering
- Orthostatic intolerance, in which symptoms become worse when standing or sitting upright.

Other common symptoms:

- Aches and pain in muscles
- Pain in the joints without swelling or erythema
- New or more severe headaches
- Recurring sore throat
- Night sweats/chills
- New sensitivities/allergies to substances such as food or noise
- Tenderness in neck/armpit lymph nodes

Adapted from CDC. (2017). Myalgic encephalomyelitis/chronic fatigue syndrome. [Online]. Available: https://www.cdc.gov/me-cfs/symptoms-diagnosis/symptoms.html. Retrieved February 20, 2018.

Abnormalities of the hypothalamic–pituitary–adrenal axis, such as attenuated activity of corticotropin-releasing hormone and changes in the circadian rhythm of cortisol secretion, have been documented. Although low thyroid hormones, dehydroepiandrosterone (DHEA), and cortisol levels have been found in people with CFS, these parameters are not decreased in all people with CFS.[48]

Genetic links with CFS include a gene associated with Huntington disease neurodegenerative protein, abnormalities in the way genes affect mitochondrial-cell energy production, and connections to depression and anxiety.[47] Additionally, connections with CFS people and a persistent inflammatory state have been determined.[49]

Clinical Manifestations. One of the most important findings in people with CFS is the complaint of fatigue. Often, the symptom of fatigue is preceded by a cold or flulike illness. Frequently, the person describes the illness as recurring, with periods of exacerbations and remissions. With each subsequent episode of the illness, the fatigue increases.

Physical findings include low-grade fever. The fever is intermittent and occurs only when the illness recurs. Other findings include nonexudative pharyngitis, palpable and tender cervical lymph nodes, a mildly enlarged thyroid gland, wheezing, splenomegaly, myalgia, arthralgia, and heme-positive stool with subsequent negative sigmoidoscopy.

Psychological problems include impaired cognition, which the person describes as an inability to concentrate and perform previously mundane tasks. There are reports of mood and sleep disturbances, balance problems, visual disturbances, and various degrees of anxiety and depression.

Diagnosis and Treatment. The diagnosis of CFS is based on integration of the entire clinical picture of the person's symptoms, physical assessment findings, and the results of diagnostic tests. Laboratory investigations are used to detect other disorders. Usually, the final diagnosis is based on the definition of CFS provided by the CDC[48] (see Chart 49.2). There is some discussion that people with less associated symptoms of CFS may be able to be accurately diagnosed with CFS at an earlier state.[48]

Because there is no known cause of CFS, current treatment tends to remain symptomatic, with a focus on management rather than cure. It centers on education, emotional support, treatment of symptoms, and overall management of general health. Symptom management includes development of an exercise program that helps the person regain strength. Along with a structured activity program, people should be encouraged to be as active as possible as they resume their activities of daily living.

A holistic approach to the treatment of CFS is essential. With proper treatment and support, most people with CFS demonstrate improvement. However, relapses can occur. People diagnosed with CFS must continue to receive follow-up care and treatment on a regular basis. Local and national support groups are available for people who experience CFS.

IN SUMMARY

Fatigue is a nonspecific, self-recognized state of physical and psychological exhaustion. It results in the person's not being able to perform routine activities and is not relieved with sleep or rest. Acute fatigue results from excessive use of the body or specific muscle groups and often is related to depletion of energy sources. Chronic fatigue often is associated with a specific disease or chronic illness and may be relieved when the effects of the disease are corrected. CFS is a complex illness that has physiologic and psychological manifestations. It is characterized by debilitating fatigue. Diagnosis often is made by a process of elimination, and treatment requires a holistic approach.

GERIATRIC Considerations

- Spinal pain in the lumbar region may indicate osteoporosis.[50]
- Fatigue can be related to loss of family or friends, which is common in the elderly.[51]

PEDIATRIC Considerations

- Toeing-in (metatarsus adductus) has an increased rate of hip dysplasia.[52]
- Of all children born with clubfoot, 80% live in developing countries.[52]
- Detection of osteogenesis imperfecta may not occur until the child is active and has frequent fractures.[52]

REVIEW EXERCISES

1. A newborn girl was found to have DDH during a routine screening examination.
   A. Describe the anatomic abnormalities that are present in the disorder.
   B. Explain the need for early treatment of DDH.
2. A 12-year-old girl was noted to have asymmetry of the shoulders, scapular height, and pelvic height during routine physical examination. On x-ray examination, she is found to have a 30-degree curvature of the spine.
   A. What possible treatments are available for this girl?
   B. Describe the physical problems associated with progressive scoliosis.
3. A 60-year-old postmenopausal woman presents with a compression fracture of the vertebrae. She has also noticed increased backache and loss of height over the past few years.
   A. Explain how the lack of estrogen and aging contribute to the development of osteoporosis.
   B. What other factors should be considered when assessing the risk for development of osteoporosis?
   C. What is one way to measure bone density?
   D. Name the two most important factors in preventing osteoporosis.
   E. What medications might be used to treat this woman's condition?
4. A 40-year-old woman who is being treated with chemotherapy for breast cancer complains of excessive fatigue and activity intolerance. She claims she has so little energy she can hardly get up in the morning and has difficulty concentrating and doing such simple activities as shopping.
   A. What are some explanations for this woman's excessive fatigue?
   B. What independent interventions might be used to decrease her fatigue?

References

1. Sadler T. (2015). *Langman's medical embryology* (3rd ed.). Philadelphia, PA: Wolters Kluwer.
2. Rhoades R. A., Bell D. R. (2012). *Medical physiology: Principles for clinical medicine* (4th ed.). Philadelphia, PA: Lippincott Williams & Wilkins.
3. Ross M. H., Pawlina W. (2015). *Histology: A text and atlas* (7th ed.). Philadelphia, PA: Lippincott Williams & Wilkins.
4. Hockenberry M., Wilson D., Rodgers C. (2016). *Wong's essentials of pediatric nursing* (10th ed.). St. Louis, MO: Mosby.
5. Staheli L. (2015). *Fundamentals of pediatric orthopedics* (5th ed.). Philadelphia, PA: Lippincott Williams & Wilkins.
6. Cramer K., Scherl S., Tornetta P., et al. (Eds.) (2003). *Pediatrics (orthopedic surgery essential series)*. Philadelphia, PA: Lippincott Williams & Wilkins.
7. Gilbert S. (2013). Obesity in pediatric orthopedics. *Current Orthopaedic Practice* 24(6), 576–580. Available: http://www.medscape.com/viewarticle/813428. Retrieved August 1, 2017.
8. Whitaker A., Vuillermin C. (2016). Lower extremity growth and deformity. *Current Reviews in Musculoskeletal Medicine* 9(4), 454–461.
9. Carr J., Yang S., Lather L. (2016). Pediatric pes planus: A state-of-the-art review. *Pediatrics* 137(3), 1–10. Available: http://pediatrics.aappublications.org/content/137/3/e20151230. Retrieved August 1, 2017.
10. Stoltzman S., Irby M., Callahan A., et al (2015). Pes planus and paediatric obesity: A systematic review of the literature. *Clinical Obesity* 5(2), 52–59.
11. Malik, S. (2013). Polydactyly: Phenotypes, genetics and classification. *Clinical Genetics*, 85(3), 203–212.
12. National Institutes of Health. (2014). What is osteogenesis imperfecta? [Online]. Available: http://www.niams.nih.gov/Health_Info/bone/Osteogenesis_Imperfecta/osteogenesis_imperfecta_ff.asp. Retrieved August 1, 2017.
13. Rubin R., Strayer D. S. (Eds.) (2014). *Rubin's pathology: Clinicopathologic foundations of medicine* (7th ed.). Philadelphia, PA: Lippincott Williams & Wilkins.
14. Van Dijk, F., Sillence, D. (2014). Osteogenesis imperfecta: Clinical diagnosis, nomenclature and severity assessment. *American Journal of Medical Genetics* 164(6), 1470–1481.
15. Wright J., James K. (2016). Developmental dysplasia of the hip. In: Aresti N., Ramachandran M., Paterson M., Barry M. (Eds.) *Paediatric orthopaedics in clinical practice*. London, UK: Springer.
16. U.S. Preventive Services Task Force. (2015). Developmental hip dysplasia: Screening. [Online]. Available: https://www.uspreventiveservicestaskforce.org/Page/Document/UpdateSummaryFinal/developmental-hip-dysplasia-screening. Retrieved February 11, 2018.
17. Jensen S. (2014). *Nursing health assessment: A best practice approach* (2nd ed.). Philadelphia, PA: Lippincott Williams & Wilkins.
18. Delaney L. R., Karmazyn B. (2011). Developmental dysplasia of the hip: Background and the utility of ultrasound. *Seminars in Ultrasound, CT, and MR* 32(2), 151–156.
19. Hossain M., Davis N. (2017). Evidence-based treatment for clubfoot. In: Alshryda S., Huntley J., Banaszkiewicz P. (Eds.) *Paediatric orthopaedics*. Cham: Springer.

20. Hernandez J. (2015). Legg-Calve-Perthes disease in emergency medicine treatment and management. Available: http://emedicine.medscape.com/article/826935-overview. Retrieved August 1, 2017.
21. Chaudhry S., Phillips D., Feldman D. (2014). Legg-Calvé-Perthes disease: An overview with recent literature. *Bulletin of the Hospital for Joint Diseases* 72(1), 18–27. Available: http://presentationgrafix.com/_dev/cake/files/archive/pdfs/2.pdf. Retrieved August 1, 2017.
22. Gregory J. (2017). Osgood Schlatter disease. Available: http://emedicine.medscape.com/article/1993268-overview. Retrieved August 1, 2017.
23. Makhni M. C., Makhni E. C., Swart E. F., et al. (2017). Slipped capital femoral epiphysis. In: Makhni M., Makhni E., Swart E., Day C. (Eds.) *Orthopedic emergencies*. Springer International Publishing.
24. El-Hawary R., Chukwunyerenwa C. (2014). Update on evaluation and treatment of scoliosis. *Pediatric Clinics of North America* 61(6), 1223–1241.
25. Mehlman C. T. (2016). *Idiopathic scoliosis*. Available: http://emedicine.medscape.com/article/1265794-overview. Retrieved August 1, 2017.
26. Morningstar M. W., Strauchman M. N., Stitzel C. J., et al. (2016). Methylenetetrahydrofolate reductase (MTHFR) gene mutations in patients with idiopathic scoliosis: A clinical chart review. Available: http://file.scirp.org/pdf/OJGen_2017033015113499.pdf. Retrieved September 1, 2017.
27. Weinstein S. (2005). The thoracolumbar spine. In Weinstein S. L., Buckwalter J. A. (Eds.) *Turek's orthopaedics: Principles and their application* (6th ed., pp. 477–518). Philadelphia, PA: Lippincott Williams & Wilkins.
28. Looker A., Frenk S. (2015). Percentage of adults aged 65 and over with osteoporosis or low bone mass at the femur neck or lumbar spine: United States, 2005–2010. Available: https://www.cdc.gov/nchs/data/hestat/osteoporsis/osteoporosis2005_2010.pdf
29. Sigl V., Penninger J. (2014). RANKL/RANK—From bone physiology to breast cancer. *Cytokine & Growth Factor Reviews* 25(2), 205–214.
30. Cosman F., de Beur S., LeBoff M., et al. (2014). Clinician's guide to prevention and treatment of osteoporosis. *Osteoporosis International* 25(10), 2359–2381.
31. Naylor K. (2016). Response of bone turnover markers to raloxifene treatment in postmenopausal women with osteopenia. *Osteoporosis International* 27(8), 2585–2592.
32. Martin T.J., Sims N.A. (2016). RANKL/OPG: Critical role in bone physiology. *Reviews in Endocrine & Metabolic Disorders* 16(2), 131–139.
33. Willson T., Nelson S., Newbold J., et al. (2015). The clinical epidemiology of male osteoporosis: A review of the recent literature. *Clinical Epidemiology* 7, 65–76.
34. Bethel M., Carbone L., Lohr K., et al. (2017). Osteoporosis. Available: http://emedicine.medscape.com/article/330598-overview. Retrieved August 2, 2017.
35. Thralls K., Nichols J., Barrack M., et al. (2016). Body mass-related predictors of the female athlete triad among adolescent athletes. *International Journal of Sport Nutrition and Exercise Metabolism* 26(1), 17–25.
36. Aspray T. J., Bowring C., Fraser W., et al. (2014). National Osteoporosis Society Vitamin D guideline summary. *Age and Ageing* 43(5), 592–595.
37. Seton M. (2017). Review: Breaking from bisphosphonates. *Arthritis and Rheumatology* 69(3), 494–498.
38. McDonald R., Lane J., Diehn F., et al. (2016). Percutaneous vertebroplasty: Overview, clinical applications, and current state. *Applied Radiology* 46(1), 24–30.
39. Plotkin H., Finberg L. (2017). Disorders of bone mineralization. Available: http://emedicine.medscape.com/article/985766-overview. Retrieved August 2, 2017.
40. Alikhan M., Driver K., Lohr K.. (2016). Paget disease. Available: http://emedicine.medscape.com/article/334607-overview Retrieved August 2, 2017.
41. Grasemann C., Unger N., Hövel M., et al. (2017). Loss of functional osteoprotegerin: More than a skeletal problem. *Journal of Clinical Endocrinology and Metabolism* 102(1), 210–219.
42. Davidson M., Morton N. (2007). A systematic review of the Human Activity Profile. *Clinical Rehabilitation* 21(2), 151–162.
43. Dunphy L. M., Winland-Brown J. E., Porter B. O., et al. (2015). *Primary care: The art and science of advanced practice nursing* (4th ed.). Philadelphia, PA: Lippincott Williams & Wilkins.
44. National Cancer Institute. (2015). Fatigue. [Online]. Available: http://www.cancer.gov/cancertopics/pdq/supportivecare/fatigue/HealthProfessional/page1. Retrieved September 29, 2017.
45. Kwak S., Choi Y., Yoon H., et al. (2012). The relationship between interleukin-6, tumor necrosis factor-α, and fatigue in terminally ill cancer patients. *Palliative Medicine* 26(3), 275–282.
46. Doong S., Dhruva A., Dunn L. B., et al. (2014). Associations between cytokine genes and a symptom cluster of pain, fatigue, sleep disturbance, and depression in patients prior to breast cancer surgery. *Biological Research for Nursing* 17(3), 237–247.
47. Centers for Disease Control and Prevention. (2015). Chronic fatigue syndrome. [Online]. Available: http://www.cdc.gov/cfs/general/index.html. Retrieved September 19, 2017.
48. Yancey J. R., Thomas S. A. (2012). Chronic fatigue syndrome: Diagnosis and treatment. *American Family Physician* 86(8), 741–746. Available: http://www.aafp.org/afp/2012/1015/p741.pdf. Retrieved September 19, 2017.
49. Centers for Disease Control and Prevention. (2017). Evidence of inflammatory immune signaling in chronic fatigue syndrome: A pilot study of gene expression in peripheral blood. [Online]. Available: https://www.cdc.gov/me-cfs/about/possible-causes.html. Retrieved September 19, 2017.
50. Eliopoulos C. (2018). *Gerontological nursing* (9th ed.). Philadelphia, PA: Wolters Kluwer.
51. National Institute on Aging. (2016). Fatigue in older adults. Available: https://www.nia.nih.gov/health/fatigue-older-adults. Retrieved February 12, 2018.
52. Bowden V. R., Greenberg V. S. (2014). *Children and their families: The continuum of nursing care*. Philadelphia, PA: Wolters Kluwer.

Disorders of Musculoskeletal Function: Rheumatic Disorders

50

Sarah Morgan

Arthritis is a descriptive term applied to more than 100 rheumatic diseases, ranging from localized, self-limiting conditions to those that are systemic autoimmune processes. More than 30 million Americans have osteoarthritis (OA).[1] This type of arthritis impacts people in all age groups and is the leading cause of disability in the United States. Approximately 1.5 million Americans have rheumatoid arthritis and about 300,000 children under 18 years of age have juvenile arthritis or some type of rheumatic condition.[1]

The common use of the term *arthritis* can oversimplify the nature of the varied disease processes, the difficulty in differentiating one form of arthritis or rheumatic disease from another, and the complexity of treatment of these usually chronic conditions. These conditions share inflammation of the joint as a prominent or accompanying symptom. In the systemic rheumatic diseases—those affecting body systems in addition to the musculoskeletal system—the inflammation is primary, resulting from an immune response. In rheumatic conditions limited to a single or few diarthrodial joints, the inflammation is secondary, resulting from a degenerative process and the resulting joint irregularities that occur as the bone attempts to remodel itself. Although arthritis cannot be cured, much can be done to control its progress.

This chapter focuses on systemic autoimmune rheumatic diseases, arthritis associated with spondylitis, OA syndrome, metabolic diseases associated with arthritis, and rheumatic disease in children and older adults.

SYSTEMIC AUTOIMMUNE RHEUMATIC DISEASES

After completing this section of the chapter, the learner will be able to meet the following objectives:

- Characterize the common characteristics of the different systemic autoimmune rheumatic disorders.
- Describe the pathologic changes that may be found in the joint of a person with rheumatoid arthritis.
- Describe the immunologic process that occurs in systemic lupus erythematosus (SLE).

Systemic autoimmune rheumatic diseases are a group of chronic disorders characterized by diffuse inflammatory lesions and degenerative changes in connective tissue.[2] These disorders share similar clinical features and may affect many of the same organs. Rheumatoid arthritis (RA), SLE, polymyalgia rheumatica, temporal arteritis, and juvenile arthritis and dermatomyositis, which share an autoimmune systemic pathogenesis, are discussed in this section.

Rheumatoid Arthritis

RA is a systemic inflammatory disease that affects 1% to 2% of the population.[2] Females are affected approximately three times more frequently than males.[1,2] Although the disease occurs in all age groups, its prevalence increases with age.[1] RA occurring after age 65 is known as elderly onset rheumatoid. The literature is mixed on whether the outcomes are worse for those who develop RA earlier in life than those who develop it later in life.[3]

Etiology and Pathogenesis

Although the cause of RA remains uncertain, evidence points to a genetic predisposition and the development of joint inflammation that is immunologically mediated. It has been suggested that the disease is initiated in a genetically predisposed person by the activation of a T-cell–mediated response to an immunologic trigger, such as a microbial agent (Fig. 50.1). The importance of genetic factors in the pathogenesis of RA is supported by the increased frequency of the disease among first-degree relatives.[2] In addition, it is generally agreed that certain major histocompatibility complex (MHC) genes are expressed in a nonrandom manner in people with RA. An important genetic locus that predisposes to RA is present on the human leukocyte antigen (HLA) loci on the MHC class II molecules, with a specific focus on the DRB1 locus.[4] This HLA-DRB1 gene, which forms a rheumatoid pocket on the HLA molecule, may influence the types of peptides that can be bound by the RA-associated HLA-DR molecules, thereby affecting the immune response.[2]

The pathogenesis of RA can be viewed as an aberrant immune response that leads to synovial inflammation and destruction of the joint architecture. It has been suggested that the disease is initiated by the activation of helper T cells, release of cytokines (*e.g.*, tumor necrosis factor [TNF], interleukin [IL]-1), and antibody formation. Approximately 70% to 80% of people with the disease have a substance called the *rheumatoid factor* (RF), which is an autologous (self-produced) antibody (Ig RF) that reacts with a fragment of immunoglobulin G (IgG) to form immune complexes.[2] Immune complexes (Ig RF + IgG) and complement components are found in the synovium, synovial fluid, and extra-articular lesions of people with RA. Although people with RA may be seronegative (not have Ig RF in their serum), the presence of a high RF titer is frequently associated with severe and unremitting disease, mainly systemic complications. Across people with RA, the presence of autoantibodies is inconsistent; thus, a multi-marker panel may be more useful for diagnosis and prediction of treatment response.[5]

The role of the autoimmune process in the joint destruction of RA remains obscure. At the cellular level, neutrophils, macrophages, and lymphocytes are attracted to the area. The neutrophils and macrophages phagocytize the immune complexes and, in the process, release lysosomal enzymes capable of causing destructive changes in the joint cartilage (see Fig. 50.1). The inflammatory response that follows attracts additional inflammatory cells, setting into motion a chain of events that perpetuates the condition. As the inflammatory process progresses, the synovial cells and subsynovial tissues undergo reactive hyperplasia. Vasodilation and increased blood flow cause warmth and redness. The joint swelling that occurs is the result of the increased capillary permeability that accompanies the inflammatory process.

Characteristic of RA is the development of an extensive network of new blood vessels in the synovial membrane that contributes to the advancement of the rheumatoid synovitis. This destructive vascular granulation tissue, which is called *pannus*, extends from the synovium to involve a region of unprotected bone at the junction between cartilage and the subchondral bone. Pannus is a feature of RA that differentiates it from other forms of inflammatory arthritis[2] (Fig. 50.2B). The inflammatory cells found in the pannus have a destructive effect on the adjacent cartilage and bone. Eventually, pannus develops between the joint margins, leading to reduced joint motion and the possibility of eventual ankylosis. Evidence points to one of the collagen degrading matrix metalloproteinases (MMPs), MMP type 1, being essential for pannus to invade and destroy joints in RA, and new research is exploring the potential protective effect of parthenolide (PAR) against the inflammatory changes.[6] With progression of the disease, joint inflammation and the resulting structural changes lead to joint instability, muscle atrophy from disuse, stretching of the ligaments, and involvement of the tendons and muscles. The effect of the pathologic changes on joint structure and function is related to the degree of disease activity, which can change at any time. Unfortunately, the destructive changes are irreversible.

Clinical Manifestations

RA often is associated with extra-articular as well as articular manifestations (see Fig. 50.2). It usually has an insidious onset

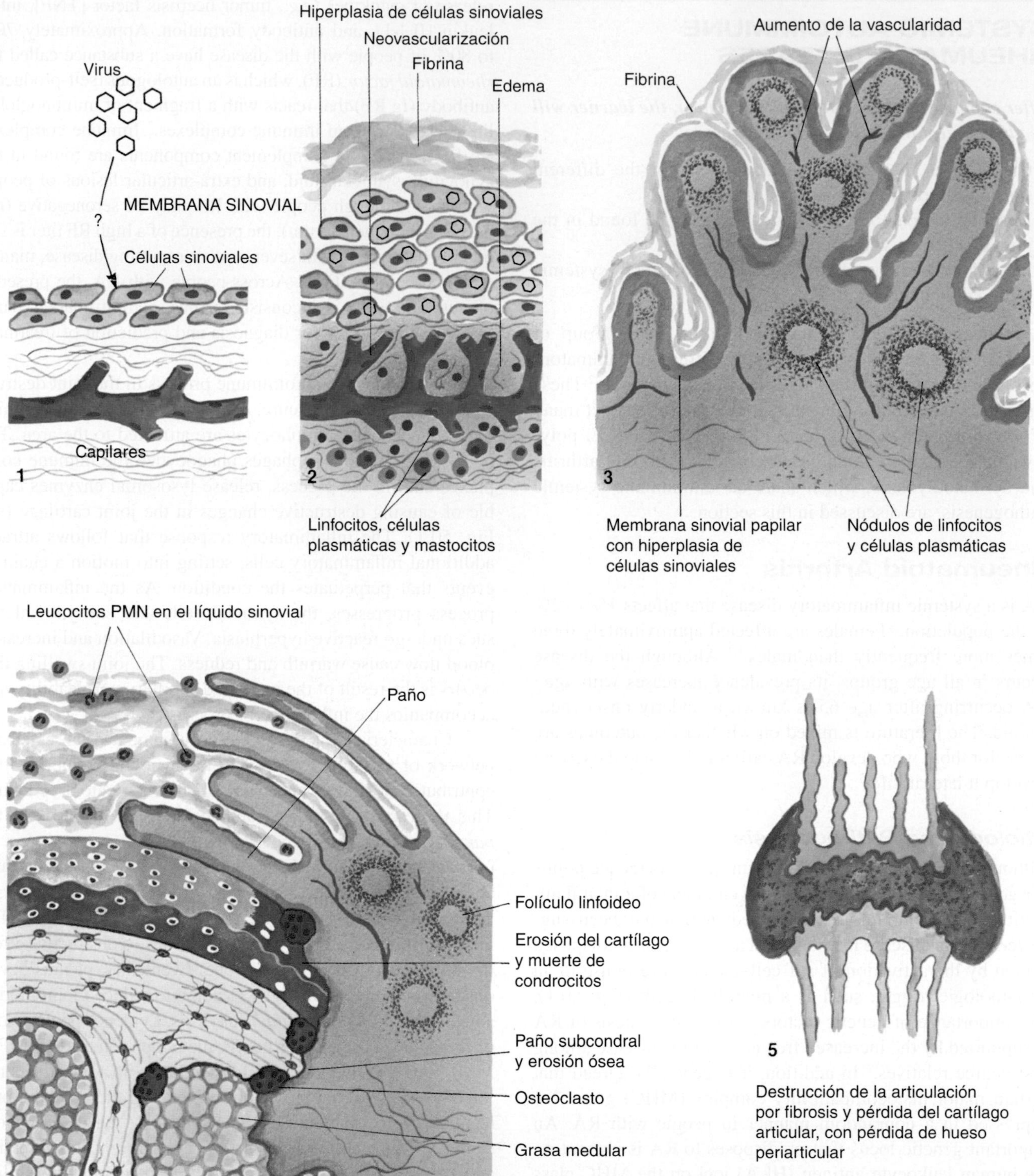

Figure 50.1 • Histogenesis of rheumatoid arthritis. **(1)** A virus or an unknown stress may stimulate the synovial cells to proliferate. **(2)** The influx of lymphocytes, plasma cells, and mast cells, together with neovascularization and edema, leads to hypertrophy and hyperplasia of the synovium. **(3)** Lymphoid nodules are prominent. **(4)** Proliferating synovium extends into the joint space, burrows into the bone beneath the articular cartilage, and covers the cartilage as a pannus. The articular cartilage is eventually destroyed by direct resorption or deprivation of its synovial fluid. The synovial tissue continues to proliferate in the subchondral region as well as in the joint. **(5)** Eventually the joint is destroyed and becomes fused, a condition termed ankylosis. (From Strayer D., Rubin R. (Eds.) (2015). *Rubin's pathology: Clinicopathologic foundations of medicine* (7th ed., Figure 30-55, p. 1363). Philadelphia, PA: Lippincott Williams & Wilkins.)

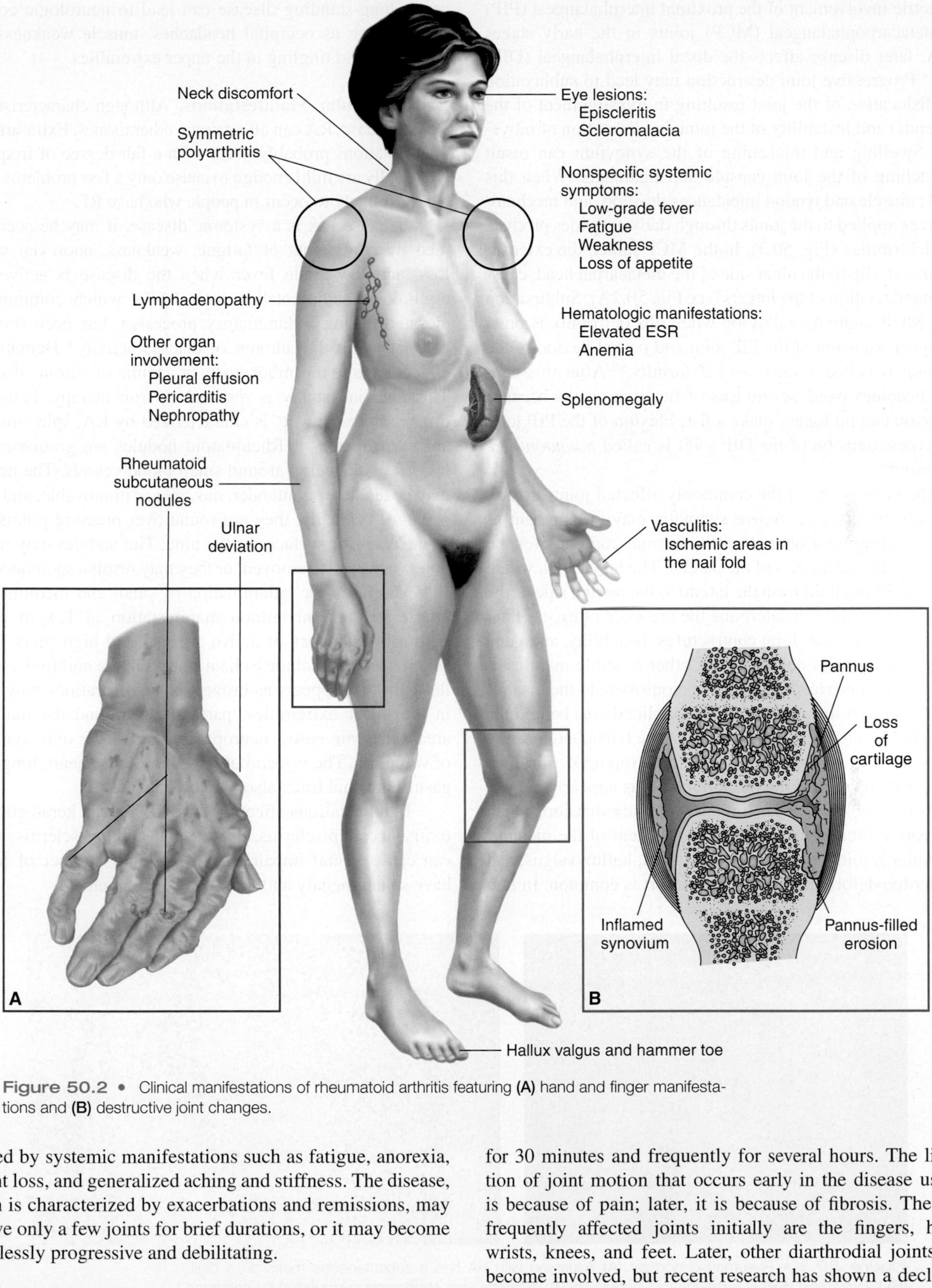

Figure 50.2 • Clinical manifestations of rheumatoid arthritis featuring **(A)** hand and finger manifestations and **(B)** destructive joint changes.

marked by systemic manifestations such as fatigue, anorexia, weight loss, and generalized aching and stiffness. The disease, which is characterized by exacerbations and remissions, may involve only a few joints for brief durations, or it may become relentlessly progressive and debilitating.

Joint Manifestations. Joint involvement usually is symmetric and polyarticular. Any diarthrodial joint can be involved. The person may complain of joint pain and stiffness that lasts for 30 minutes and frequently for several hours. The limitation of joint motion that occurs early in the disease usually is because of pain; later, it is because of fibrosis. The most frequently affected joints initially are the fingers, hands, wrists, knees, and feet. Later, other diarthrodial joints may become involved, but recent research has shown a decline in RA-related joint replacements because of more effective RA drug treatment.[4,7] Spinal involvement usually is limited to the cervical region. In the hands, there usually is bilateral and symmetric involvement of the proximal interphalangeal (PIP) and metacarpophalangeal (MCP) joints in the early stages of RA, later disease affects the distal interphalangeal (DIP) joints.[4] Progressive joint destruction may lead to subluxation (*i.e.*, dislocation of the joint resulting in misalignment of the bone ends) and instability of the joint and limitation of movement. Swelling and thickening of the synovium can result in stretching of the joint capsule and ligaments. When this occurs, muscle and tendon imbalances develop, and mechanical forces applied to the joints through daily activities produce joint deformities (Fig. 50.3). In the MCP joints, the extensor tendons can slip to the ulnar side of the metacarpal head, causing ulnar deviation of the fingers (see Fig. 50.2A). Subluxation of the MCP joints may develop when this deformity is present. Hyperextension of the PIP joint and partial flexion of the DIP joint is called a *swan neck deformity*.[8,9] After this condition becomes fixed, severe loss of function occurs because the person can no longer make a fist. Flexion of the PIP joint with hyperextension of the DIP joint is called a *boutonnière deformity*.[8,9]

The knee is one of the commonly affected joints associated with the disease.[4] Active synovitis may be apparent as visible swelling that obliterates the normal contour over the medial and lateral aspects of the patella. The *bulge sign*, which involves milking fluid from the lateral to the medial side of the patella, may be used to determine the presence of excess fluid when it is not visible. Joint contractures, instability, and genu valgus (knock-knee) deformity are other possible manifestations. Severe quadriceps atrophy can contribute to the disability. A *Baker cyst* may develop in the popliteal area behind the knee. This is caused by enlargement of the bursa but does not usually cause symptoms unless the cyst ruptures, in which case symptoms mimicking thrombophlebitis appear.

Ankle involvement can limit flexion and extension, which can create difficulty in walking. Involvement of the metatarsophalangeal joints can cause subluxation, hallux valgus, and hammer toe deformities. Neck discomfort is common. In rare cases, long-standing disease can lead to neurologic complications such as occipital headaches, muscle weakness, and numbness and tingling in the upper extremities.

Extra-Articular Manifestations. Although characteristically a joint disease, RA can affect many other tissues. Extra-articular manifestations probably occur with a fair degree of frequency but usually are mild enough to cause only a few problems. They are most likely to occur in people who have RF.

Because RA is a systemic disease, it may be accompanied by complaints of fatigue, weakness, anorexia, weight loss, and low-grade fever when the disease is active. The erythrocyte sedimentation rate (ESR), which commonly is elevated during inflammatory processes, has been found to correlate with the amount of disease activity.[4] Hematologic effects include thrombocytosis or anemia of chronic disease.[4] This anemia usually is resistant to iron therapy. Felty syndrome, although rare, is characterized by RA, splenomegaly, and neutropenia.[4,10] Rheumatoid nodules are granulomatous lesions that develop around small blood vessels. The nodules may be tender or nontender, movable or immovable, and small or large. Typically, they are found over pressure points such as the extensor surfaces of the ulna. The nodules may remain unless surgically removed, or they may resolve spontaneously.

Vasculitis, or inflammation of small and medium-sized arteries, is an uncommon manifestation of RA in people with a long history of active arthritis and high titers of RF. Manifestations include ischemic areas in the nail fold and digital pulp that appears as brown spots. Ulcerations may occur in the lower extremities, particularly around the malleolar areas. In some cases, neuropathy may be the only symptom of vasculitis. The visceral organs, such as the heart, lungs, and gastrointestinal tract, also may be affected.

Manifestations affecting the eyes include keratoconjunctivitis sicca, episcleritis, uveitis, and nodular scleritis, which can cause visual impairment.[4,11] A small number of people have splenomegaly and lymph node enlargement.

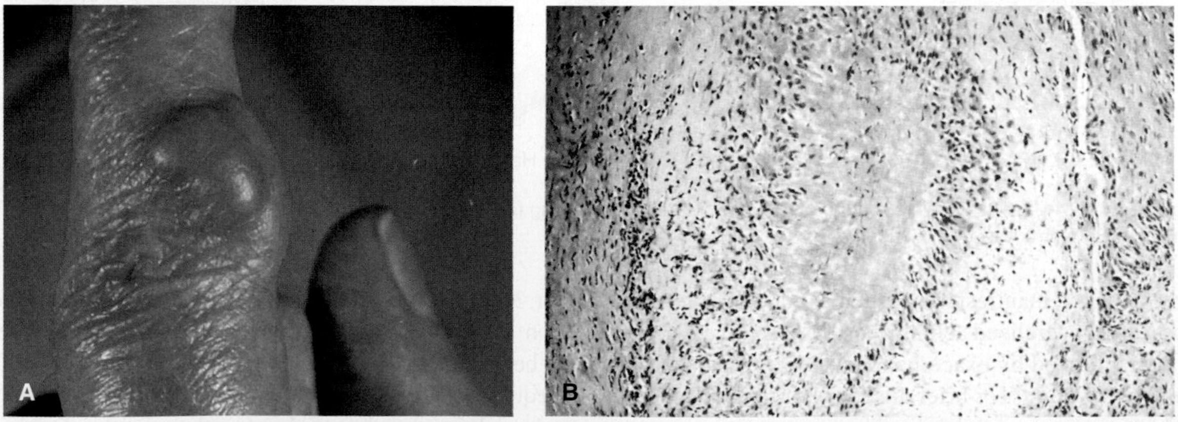

Figure 50.3 • Rheumatoid nodule. **(A)** A person with RA has a subcutaneous mass on a digit. **(B)** Microscopic view of a rheumatoid nodule shows a central area of necrosis surrounded by palisaded macrophages and a chronic inflammatory infiltrate. (From Strayer D., Rubin R. (Eds.) (2015). *Rubin's pathology: Clinicopathologic foundations of medicine* (7th ed., Figure 30-58, p. 1365). Philadelphia, PA: Lippincott Williams & Wilkins.)

KEY POINTS

RHEUMATOID ARTHRITIS

- RA is a chronic systemic inflammatory disease with bilateral involvement of synovial or diarthrodial joints.
- The initial joint changes involve the synovial cells lining the joint. Inflammatory cells accumulate, and angiogenesis and formation of pannus, which proceed to cover the articular cartilage and isolate it from its nutritional synovial fluid, take place.

Diagnosis

The diagnosis of RA is based on findings of the history, physical examination, and laboratory tests. Information should be elicited regarding the duration of symptoms, systemic manifestations, stiffness, and family history. The criteria for RA, updated in 2010 by the American College of Rheumatology (ACR) and the European League Against Rheumatism (EULAR), are useful in establishing the diagnosis of RA earlier than what has been done in the past.[12,13] At least 6 out of 10 possible points must be present to make a diagnosis of RA. These criteria consisting of four categories (joint involvement, serology, acute phase reactants, and duration of symptoms) were developed for use in facilitating earlier recognition of RA so people could begin treatment earlier to prevent recurrences or decrease disease severity.[12,13]

In the early stages, the disease often is difficult to diagnose. On physical examination, the affected joints show signs of inflammation, swelling, tenderness, and possibly warmth and reduced motion. The joints have a soft, spongy feeling because of synovial thickening and inflammation. Body movements may be guarded to prevent pain. Changes in joint structure usually are not visible early in the disease.

The RF test results are not diagnostic for RA, but they can be of value in differentiating RA from other forms of arthritis. A small percentage of healthy people have a positive RF. Also, a person can have RA without the presence of RF. Evidence suggests a stronger linkage of RA and anticitrullinated protein/peptide antibodies (ACPAs), which are measured as anticyclic citrullinated peptide (anti-CCP) autoantibodies.[4] This test has a higher specificity than RF, and identification is possible very early in the RA process but may not be as predictive of disease severity or prognosis.[4] The term citrullination defines the posttranslational change of arginine into citrulline.[14]

RA is linked with the HLA-DRB1 locus,[15] which is thought to be the result of local antigens that trigger an inflammatory response in the joint space leading to joint destruction.[4] T cell response is activated and these cells make up almost half of the immune cells present in an inflamed joint.[4] The challenge has been to understand the antigen specificity of first set of T cells that initiate the immune response.[4]

Radiologic findings also are not diagnostic in RA because joint erosions often are not seen on radiographic images in the early stages of the disorder. Synovial fluid analysis can be helpful in the diagnostic process. The synovial fluid has a cloudy appearance, the white blood cell count is elevated because of inflammation, and the complement components are decreased because of the inflammatory process.

Treatment

The treatment goals for a person with RA are to prevent and/or reduce the pain, decrease stiffness and swelling, maximize mobility, and possibly halt the pathologic process.[4] The treatment plan includes education about the disease and its treatment, rest, therapeutic exercises, and medications. Because of the chronicity of the disease and the need for continuous, long-term adherence to the prescribed treatment modalities, it is important that the treatment be integrated with the person's lifestyle.

Physical rest reduces joint stress. Rest of specific joints is recommended to relieve pain. For example, sitting reduces the weight on an inflamed knee, and the use of lightweight splints reduces undue movement of the hand or wrist. Emotional rest helps muscles relax and is often useful for people who find that emotional stress increases discomfort. Although rest is essential, therapeutic exercises also are important in maintaining joint motion and muscle strength. Range-of-motion exercises involve the active and passive movement of joints. Isometric (muscle-tensing) exercises may be used to strengthen muscles. These exercises are usually taught by a physical therapist and performed daily at home. The difference between normal activity and therapeutic exercise should be emphasized. Acrobic exercise and muscle-strengthening exercises can be an important component of the treatment regimen of selected people.

Instruction in the safe use of hot and cold modalities to relieve discomfort and relaxation techniques also is important. Proper posture, positioning, and body mechanics and the use of supportive shoes can provide further comfort. There often is a need for teaching about the principles of joint protection and work simplification. Some people may need assistive devices to reduce pain and improve their ability to perform activities of daily living.

The goals of pharmacologic therapy for RA are to reduce pain, decrease inflammation, maintain or restore joint function, and prevent bone and cartilage destruction. Medications used to achieve these goals are classified as those that provide relief from arthritis symptoms and those that have the potential for modifying the course of the disease. The trend in RA management is toward a more aggressive pharmacologic approach at an earlier stage in the disease. Ideally, disease-modifying antirheumatic drug (DMARD) therapy should be used when the diagnosis of RA is established and before erosive changes appear on radiography but must be balanced with the potential risks of anti-inflammatory and immunosuppressive interventions.[4,16] Early treatment is based on the theory that T-cell–dependent pathways, which manifest early in the inflammatory process are more responsive to treatment than those that manifest later in the process, when disease progression is controlled by activated fibroblasts and macrophages, and the disease may be more resistant to treatment.

Nonsteroidal anti-inflammatory drugs (NSAIDs) usually are used early in the treatment of RA. The NSAIDs inhibit cyclooxygenase (COX)-mediated synthesis of prostaglandins, which have a damaging effect on joint structures. NSAIDs, including salicylates (*e.g.*, aspirin), provide analgesic and anti-inflammatory effects. Effectiveness, side effects, cost, and dosing schedules are considered when selecting an NSAID. There is a wide range of responses to the various NSAIDs, and the NSAID that works best for any one person is not always predictable. The incidence of adverse reactions to the NSAIDs (*e.g.*, gastric irritation and bleeding, fluid retention, kidney damage) tends to increase with age and long-term use.

Early treatment also includes DMARDs, which are a variety of immunosuppressants and immunomodulators[4] (see Table 50.1). DMARDs include methotrexate, hydroxychloroquine, and sulfasalazine, among others.[16] A therapy that shows more effectiveness uses a combination of DMARDs instead of a single medication.[4] This approach is a generally accepted one, and has been shown to be effective in several studies. Individual drugs with different mechanisms of action are given simultaneously to control the disease. The individual drugs are then tapered as symptoms subside and clinical remission is achieved.[4] All of the DMARDs can be toxic and require close monitoring for adverse effects, especially those related to bone marrow suppression.

Corticosteroid drugs may be used to reduce discomfort. These agents interrupt the inflammatory and immune cascade at several levels, such as interfering with inflammatory cell adhesion and migration, impairing prostaglandin synthesis, and inhibiting neutrophil superoxide production. To avoid long-term side effects, they are used only in specific situations for short-term therapy at a low dose level. They may be used for unremitting disease with extra-articular manifestations. The corticosteroids do not modify the disease and are unable to prevent joint destruction. Intra-articular corticosteroid injections can provide rapid relief of acute or subacute inflammatory synovitis (after infection is excluded) in a few joints. They should not be repeated more than a few times each year.

Other first-line antirheumatic drugs include biologics such as anti-TNFs like etanercept (Enbrel), infliximab (Remicade), and adalimumab (Humira), and non-TNFs such as abatacept, rituximab (Rituxan) and tocilizumab.[4] TNF-α is a cytokine, present in inflammation but overly present in the bloodstream and joints of those with RA.[17] Prescribing DMARDs and biologics involves a careful consideration of factors including indications for use, switching between the two, high-risk people and biologics, screening for TB, and vaccinations.[18] In 2012, updates were made to the 2008 ACR Recommendations for the Use of DMARD and Biologic Agents in the Treatment of Rheumatoid Arthritis to refine this process of RA treatment.[18]

Surgery also may be a part of the treatment of RA. Synovectomy may be indicated to reduce pain and joint damage when synovitis does not respond to medical treatment. The most common soft tissue surgery is tenosynovectomy (*i.e.*, repair of damaged tendons) of the hand to release nerve entrapments. Total joint replacements (*i.e.*, arthroplasty) may be indicated to reduce pain and increase motion. Arthrodesis (*i.e.*, joint fusion) is indicated only in extreme cases when there is so much soft tissue damage and scarring or infection that a replacement is impossible. As noted earlier, joint replacements are on the decline because of more effective and earlier medical treatment.[7]

TABLE 50.1 DMARDS AND BIOLOGIC RESPONSE MODIFIERS

DISEASE MODIFYING ANTIRHEUMATIC DRUGS	SMALL MOLECULE IMMUNOSUPPRESSIVE AGENTS
Synthetic and biologic inactivators (TNF)	First line: methotrexate* (Rheumatrex, Trexall), sulfasalazine, hydroxychloroquine Second line: gold, penicillamine, cyclosporine, leflunomide
Biologic response modifiers	Large molecule drugs that inhibit immunoinflammatory process
TNF inhibitors	Etanercept, infliximab, adalimumab
Non-TNF biologics (shown below)	
IL-1 inhibitors	Anakinra (Kineret)—recombinant form of IL-1 inhibitor
Anti–B-cell agents	Rituximab—chimeric anti-CD20 monoclonal antibody
Costimulation signal modifiers	Abatacept (Orencia)
JAK inhibitors	Tofacitinib (Xeljanz)

*Usually drug of choice for first-line treatment.

Data from Goroll A. H., Mulley A. G. (2014). *Primary care medicine* (7th ed.) Philadelphia, PA: Wolters Kluwer.

Systemic Lupus Erythematosus

SLE is a chronic inflammatory disease that can affect virtually any organ system, including the musculoskeletal system. It is a major rheumatic disease, with approximately 1.5 million Americans and over 5 million people worldwide diagnosed with lupus.[19] Prevalence is related to gender, race, age, and genetics.[4] SLE is more common in females (85% of cases) than males; is more common in African Americans, Hispanics, and Asians than in Caucasians; most cases occur between the ages of 15 and 44[4,19,20]; and it appears to have a genetic component.[4] There are four types of lupus erythematosus: Systemic lupus erythematous (SLE), cutaneous lupus erythematosus, drug-induced lupus erythematous, and neonatal lupus. The most common one is SLE.[16] Cutaneous lupus erythematosus only affects the skin, but 5% to 10% of those who have cutaneous lupus will develop SLE.[19,21] Drug-induced lupus is caused by particular prescription drugs including hydralazine, procainamide and isoniazid, and about 6 months after the drugs are stopped the person's lupus completely resolves.[19,21] Neonatal lupus is the result of mothers (not all of whom have lupus) with particular antibodies, and usually affects the neonate's skin, which clears up during the first few months and rarely lasts until childhood. In a small number of cases (1% to 2%), the infant is born with heart block and requires a pacemaker. Congenital heart block is usually permanent because of altered transfer of conduction of nerve impulses to heart muscles.[19,21]

Etiology and Pathogenesis

The cause of SLE is unknown. It is characterized by the formation of autoantibodies and immune complexes. People with SLE appear to have B-cell hyperreactivity and increased production of antibodies against self (*i.e.*, autoantibodies) and non-self antigens. These B cells are polyclonal, each producing a different type of antibody. The autoantibodies can directly damage tissues or combine with corresponding antigens to form tissue-damaging immune complexes. Autoantibodies have been identified against an array of nuclear and cytoplasmic cell components (*e.g.*, microtubules, ribosomes, RNA). Some autoantibodies that have been identified in SLE are antinuclear antibodies (ANA), including anti-deoxyribonucleic acid (anti-DNA) antibodies, antiphospholipid antibodies, and anti-Smith (Sm) antibodies. In addition to ANAs, people with lupus have a host of other self-autoantibodies including those directed against elements of the blood (red cells, platelets, lymphocytes) and plasma proteins (clotting and complement factors).

The development of autoantibodies can result from a combination of factors, including genetic, hormonal, immunologic, and environmental factors.[4] Genetic predisposition is evidenced by the occurrence of familial cases of SLE, especially among identical twins. The increased incidence among African Americans compared with Caucasians also suggests genetic factors. As many as four genes may be involved in the expression of SLE in humans. Genes linked to the HLA-DR and HLA-DQ loci in the MHC class II molecules show strong support for a genetic link in the development of SLE.[4] Studies also suggest that an imbalance in sex hormone levels may play a role in the development of the disease, especially because the disease is so prevalent among females.[4] Androgens appear to protect against the development of SLE, whereas estrogens seem to favor its development. It has been suggested that an imbalance in sex hormone levels may lead to heightened helper T cell and weakened suppressor T-cell immune responses that could in turn lead to the development of autoantibodies.[4]

Possible environmental triggers include ultraviolet (UV) light, chemicals (*e.g.*, drugs, hair dyes), some foods, and infectious agents (Fig. 50.4).[19] UV light, specifically UVB associated with exposure to the sun or unshielded fluorescent bulbs, may trigger exacerbations. Photosensitivity occurs in approximately one third of people with SLE. Certain drugs may also provoke a lupus-like disorder in susceptible people, particularly in older adults. The most common of these drugs are hydralazine, minocycline, and procainamide.[4] The disease usually recedes when the drug is discontinued.[19,21]

Clinical Manifestations

SLE can manifest in a variety of ways. The disease has been called the *great imitator* because it has the capacity for affecting many different body systems, including the, musculoskeletal system, skin, cardiovascular system, lungs, kidneys, central nervous system (CNS), and red blood cells and platelets (Fig. 50.5). The onset may be acute or insidious, and the course of the disease is characterized by exacerbations and remissions.

Arthralgias and arthritis are among the most commonly occurring early symptoms of SLE. Approximately 90% of all people with the disease complain of joint pain, and this is often the symptom that they present with.[4] The polyarthritis of SLE initially can be confused with other forms of arthritis, especially RA, because of the symmetric arthropathy. However, on radiologic examination, articular destruction rarely is found. Ligaments, tendons, and the joint capsule may be involved, causing varied deformities of people with the disease. Flexion contractures, hyperextension of the interphalangeal joints, and subluxation of the carpometacarpal joints contribute to the deformity and subsequent loss of function in the hands. Other musculoskeletal manifestations of SLE include tenosynovitis, rupture of the intrapatellar and Achilles tendons, and avascular necrosis, frequently of the femoral head.

Skin manifestations can vary greatly and may be classified as acute, subacute, or chronic. The acute skin lesions include the classic malar or "butterfly" rash on the nose and cheeks (see Fig. 50.5). This rash is seen in SLE, but may be associated with other skin lesions, such as hives or livedo reticularis (*i.e.*, reticular cyanotic discoloration of the skin, often precipitated by cold) and fingertip lesions, such as periungual

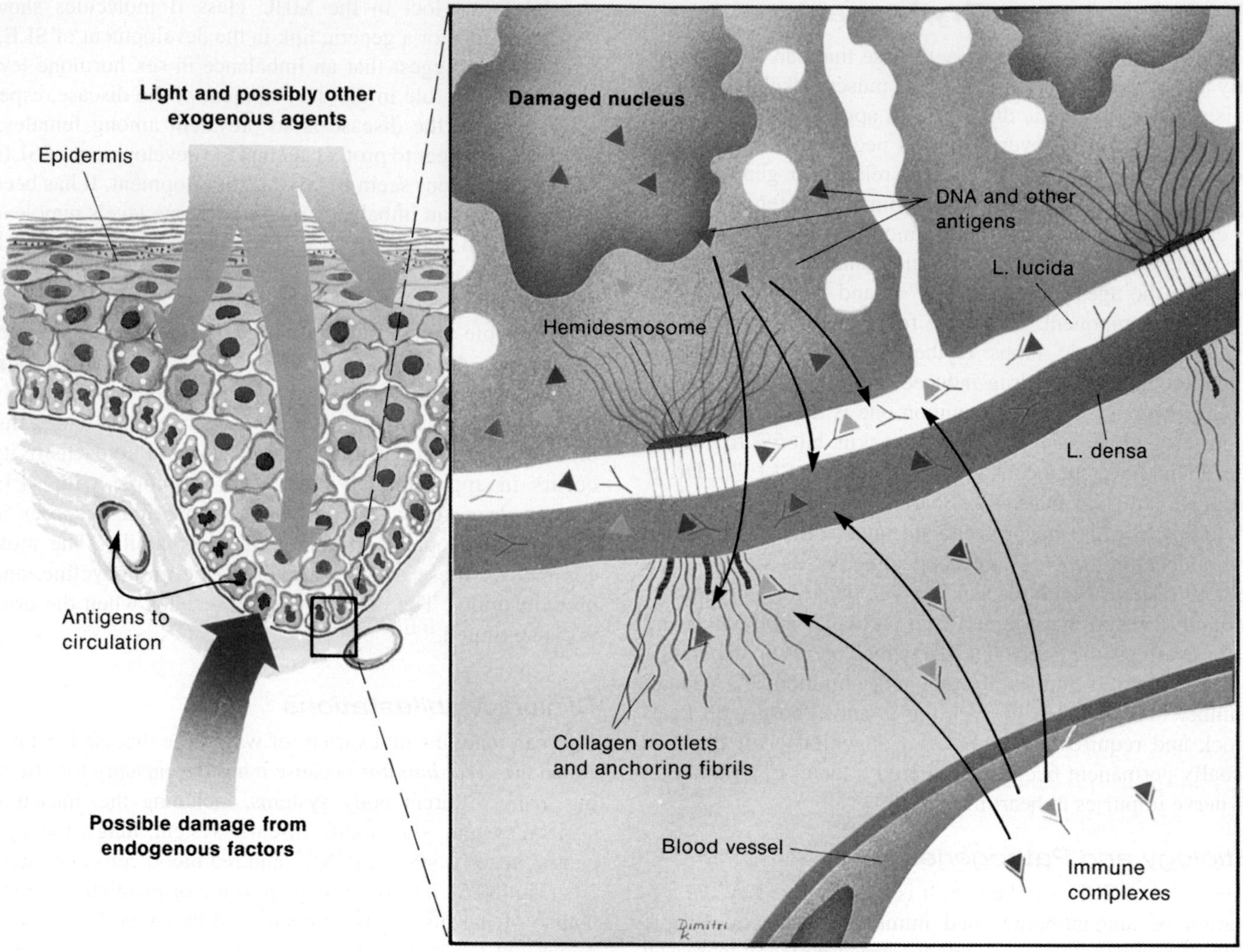

Figure 50.4 • Lupus erythematosus. A cell-mediated immune reaction leads to epidermal cellular damage when initiated by light or other exogenous agents as well as endogenous ones. Such injury releases a large number of antigens, some of which may return to the skin in the form of immune complexes. Immune complexes are also formed in the skin by a reaction of local DNA with antibody that may also be deposited beneath the epidermal basement membrane zone. L = lamina. (From Strayer D., Rubin R. (Eds.) (2015). *Rubin's pathology: Clinicopathologic foundations of medicine* (7th ed., Figure 28-27, p. 1241). Philadelphia, PA: Lippincott Williams & Wilkins.)

erythema, nail fold infarcts, and splinter hemorrhages. Hair loss is common. Mucous membrane lesions tend to occur during periods of exacerbation. Sun sensitivity may occur in SLE even after mild sun exposure.

Renal involvement occurs in close to 50% of people with SLE.[4] Several forms of glomerulonephritis may occur, including mesangial, focal proliferative, diffuse proliferative, and membranous.[4] Of these, diffuse proliferative has the worst prognosis and presents with hypertension and, in up to 50% of cases, can lead to end-stage renal disease (ESRD) or death.[4] Interstitial nephritis also may occur. Nephrotic syndrome causes proteinuria with resultant edema in the legs and abdomen, and around the eyes. Kidney biopsy is the best determinant of renal damage and the extent of treatment needed.

Pulmonary involvement in SLE is manifested primarily by pleural effusions or pleuritis. Less frequently occurring pulmonary problems include acute pneumonitis, pulmonary hemorrhage, chronic interstitial lung disease, and pulmonary embolism.

Pericarditis is the most common of the cardiac manifestations, and is often accompanied by pleural effusions. Myocarditis affects as much as 25% of those with SLE. Secondary heart disease also is a problem in those with SLE. Hypertension may be associated with lupus nephritis and long-term corticosteroid use. Ischemic heart disease can occur in older adults with longer-duration SLE.

The pathologic basis for the CNS symptoms is not entirely clear. It has been related to an acute vasculitis that impedes blood flow, causing strokes or hemorrhage; an

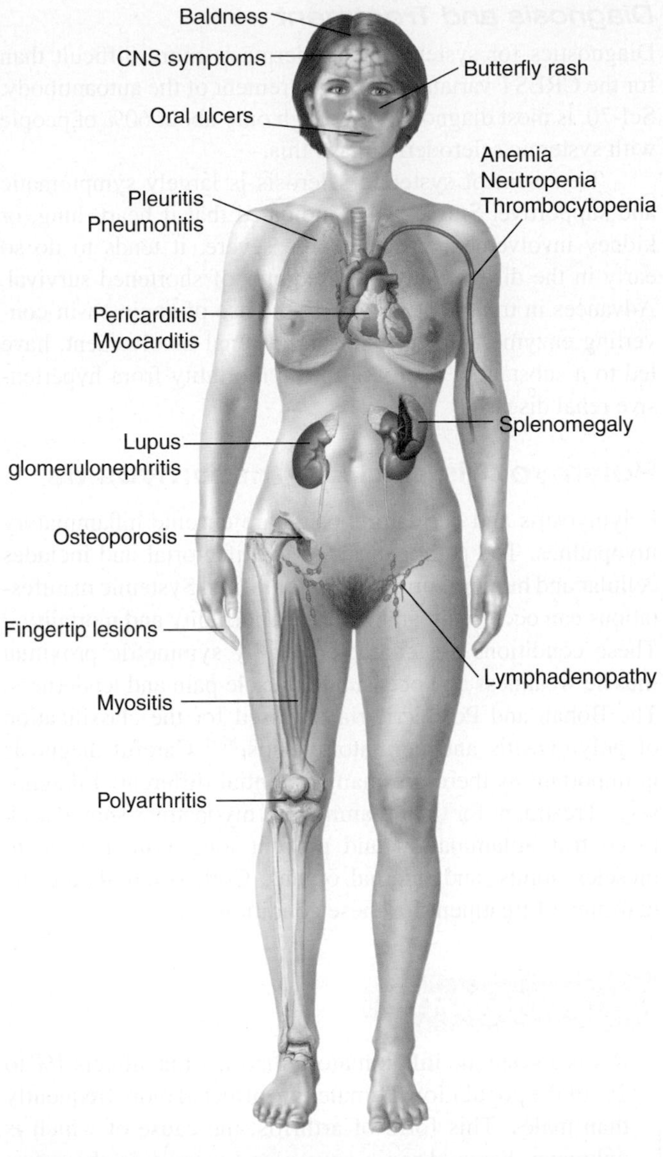

Figure 50.5 • Clinical manifestations of SLE.

immune response involving antineuronal antibodies that attack nerve cells; or production of antiphospholipid antibodies that damage blood vessels and cause blood clots in the brain. Seizures can occur and are more frequent when renal failure is present. Psychotic symptoms, including depression and unnatural euphoria, as well as decreased cognitive functioning, confusion, and altered levels of consciousness, may develop.

Hematologic disorders may manifest as hemolytic anemia, leukopenia, lymphopenia, or thrombocytopenia. Lymphadenopathy also may occur in many people with SLE and is evidence of systemic disease.[4] Discoid SLE involves plaquelike lesions on the head, scalp, and neck. These lesions first appear as red, swollen patches of skin, and later there can be scarring, depigmentation, and plugging of hair follicles. Most people with discoid lupus have disease that involves only the skin.

KEY POINTS

CLINICAL MANIFESTATIONS OF SYSTEMIC LUPUS ERYTHEMATOSUS

- SLE is a chronic autoimmune disorder characterized by production of a wide array of autoantibodies against nuclear and cytoplasmic cell components.
- SLE is often described as the great imitator because it can affect almost any organ system, including the joints of the musculoskeletal system, the skin, kidneys, lungs, nervous system, and the heart.

Diagnosis and Treatment

The diagnosis of SLE can be complicated and difficult. The 1982 ACR (updated in 1997 and currently in review) has defined 11 criteria to be considered in the diagnosis of the disease.[22] If a person has at least 4 of these 11 criteria, the individual has SLE.[22] However, these criteria are intended for use in clinical trials rather than for individual diagnosis.[23] Diagnosis is based on a complete history, physical examination, and analysis of blood work. No single test can diagnose SLE in all people.

The most common laboratory test performed is the immunofluorescence test for ANA. Ninety-five percent of people with untreated SLE have high ANA levels. The ANA test is not specific for SLE, and positive ANA results may be found in healthy people or may be associated with other disorders. The anti-DNA antibody test is more specific for the diagnosis of SLE.[4] Other serum tests may reveal moderate to severe anemia, thrombocytopenia, and leukocytosis or leukopenia. Additional immunologic tests may be done to give support to the diagnosis or to differentiate SLE from other connective tissue diseases.[4]

Treatment of SLE focuses on managing the acute and chronic symptoms of the disease. Communication and trust between health care providers and the person with SLE are the basis for long-term disease management. The goals of treatment include preventing progressive loss of organ function, reducing the possibility of exacerbations, minimizing disability from the disease process, and preventing complications from medication therapy. Treatment with medications may be as simple as a drug to reduce inflammation, such as an NSAID. NSAIDs can control fever, arthritis, and mild pleuritis. An antimalarial drug (*e.g.*, hydroxychloroquine) is generally the next medication considered to treat cutaneous and musculoskeletal manifestations of SLE. Corticosteroids are used to treat more significant symptoms of SLE, such as renal and CNS disorders. High-dose corticosteroids are used for acute symptoms, but although they are effective in delaying organ damage, because the side effects can outweigh the benefits their use must limited.[4] Immunosuppressive drugs are used in cases of severe disease. In the case of diffuse proliferative lupus nephritis, high-dose corticosteroids and immunosuppressants such as cyclophosphamide, azathioprine, and mycophenolate mofetil are indicated.[4] A new drug that has shown positive effects in decreasing inflammatory exacerbations for people with SLE is belimumab, which is a monoclonal antibody that inhibits the B-lymphocyte stimulator.[4]

Systemic Sclerosis/Scleroderma

Systemic sclerosis, sometimes called *scleroderma*, is an autoimmune disease of connective tissue characterized by excessive collagen deposition in the skin and internal organs such as the lungs, gastrointestinal tract, heart, and kidneys. In this disorder, the skin is thickened through fibrosis, with an accompanying fixation of subdermal structures, including the sheaths or fascia covering tendons and muscles.[2] Systemic sclerosis affects females four times as frequently as males, with a peak incidence in the 25- to 50-year-old age group.[2] The cause of this rare disorder is poorly understood. There is correlation between the development of autoantibodies of scleroderma and HLA-DQBI.[2] There is evidence of both humoral and cellular immune system abnormalities.

Clinical Manifestations

Scleroderma presents as two distinct clinical entities: the diffuse or generalized form of the disease and the limited or CREST variant. CREST syndrome is an acronym for several different symptoms that tend to occur with scleroderma:

- C stands for calcinosis.
- R equals Raynaud phenomenon.
- E is esophageal dysmobility.
- S equals sclerodactyly.
- T stands for telangiectasias.

In 2004, another four letters were added to the CREST acronym so that it is known now as ABCDCREST:

- A stands for antibodies to CENP, anti-topo1 or fibrillarin.
- B stands for bibasilar pulmonary fibrosis.
- C stands for contractures of digital joints.
- D stands for dermal thickening proximal to wrists.[24]

Generally, a person would have to have four of these symptoms to be diagnosed with CREST type of scleroderma.

Diffuse scleroderma is characterized by severe and progressive disease of the skin and the early onset of organ involvement. The typical person has "stone facies" because of tightening of the facial skin with restricted motion of the mouth. Involvement of the esophagus leads to hypomotility and difficulty in swallowing. Malabsorption may develop if the submucosal and muscular atrophy affect the intestine. Pulmonary involvement leads to dyspnea and eventually respiratory failure. Vascular involvement of the kidneys is responsible for malignant hypertension and progressive renal insufficiency. Cardiac problems include pericarditis, heart block, and myocardial fibrosis.

Diagnosis and Treatment

Diagnostics for systemic scleroderma is more difficult than for the CREST variant. The measurement of the autoantibody, Scl-70, is most diagnostic, although only about 60% of people with systemic scleroderma have this.

Treatment of systemic sclerosis is largely symptomatic and supportive. Studies have indicated that if heart, lung, or kidney involvement is to become severe, it tends to do so early in the disease and is a predictor of shortened survival. Advances in treatment, primarily the use of angiotensin-converting enzyme (ACE) inhibitors in renal involvement, have led to a substantial decrease in the mortality from hypertensive renal disease.

Polymyositis and Dermatomyositis

Polymyositis and dermatomyositis are chronic inflammatory myopathies. The pathogenesis is multifactorial and includes cellular and humoral immune mechanisms. Systemic manifestations can occur with an impact on morbidity and mortality.[25] These conditions are characterized by symmetric proximal muscle weakness and occasional muscle pain and tenderness. The Bohan and Peter criteria are used for the classification of polymyositis and dermatomyositis.[26,27] Careful diagnosis is important as there are many potential differential diagnoses.[25] Treatment for the inflammatory myopathies should seek to control inflammation and prevent long-term damage to muscles, joints, and internal organs. Corticosteroids are the mainstay of treatment for these conditions.

IN SUMMARY

RA is a systemic inflammatory disorder that affects 1% to 2% of the population. Females are affected more frequently than males. This form of arthritis, the cause of which is unknown, has a chronic course and usually is characterized by remissions and exacerbations. Joint involvement is symmetric and begins with inflammatory changes in the synovial membrane. As joint inflammation progresses, structural changes can occur, leading to joint instability and eventual deformity. Systemic manifestations include weakness, anorexia, weight loss, and low-grade fever. Some extra-articular features include rheumatoid nodules and vasculitis. The treatment goals are to prevent and/or reduce pain, decrease stiffness and swelling, maximize mobility, and possibly halt the pathologic process.

SLE is a chronic autoimmune disorder that affects multiple body systems. There is no known cause of SLE, but the disease may result from an immunoregulatory disturbance brought about by a combination of genetic, hormonal, and environmental factors. Some drugs have been shown to induce SLE, especially in older adults. There is an exaggerated production of autoantibodies, which interact with antigens to produce an immune complex. These immune complexes produce an inflammatory response in affected tissues. Treatment focuses on preventing loss of organ function, controlling inflammation, and minimizing complications of medication therapy.

Systemic sclerosis, often prefixed by the term *progressive*, is sometimes called *scleroderma*. In this disorder, the skin is thickened through fibrosis with an accompanying fixation to the subdermal structures, including the sheaths or fascia covering tendons and muscles. Polymyositis and dermatomyositis are chronic inflammatory myopathies. Its pathogenesis is multifactorial and includes cellular and humoral immune mechanisms.

SERONEGATIVE SPONDYLOARTHROPATHIES

After completing this section of the chapter, the learner will be able to meet the following objectives:

- Cite a definition of the seronegative spondyloarthropathies (SpA).
- Cite the primary features of ankylosing spondylitis (AS).
- Contrast and compare AS, reactive arthritis, and psoriatic arthritis in terms of cause, pathogenesis, and clinical manifestations.

The *SpA* are an interrelated group of multisystem inflammatory disorders that primarily affect the axial skeleton, particularly the spine. Typically, the inflammation begins at sites where tendon and ligament insert into bone rather than in the synovium. Sacroiliitis is a pathologic hallmark of the disorders.[2] People with SpA may also have inflammation and involvement of the peripheral joints, in which case the signs and symptoms overlap with other inflammatory types of arthritis. Because there is an absence of RF, these disorders often are referred to as *seronegative SpA* and are recognized as specific disease entities.[2]

The seronegative SpA include AS, reactive arthritis, arthritis related to inflammatory bowel disease, and psoriatic arthritis.[2] Although they differ in terms of factors such as age and type of onset and extent of joint involvement, there is clinical evidence of overlap between the various seronegative SpA. In none of these disorders is the cause or pathogenesis well understood. There is a striking association with the HLA-B27 antigen, but the presence of the HLA-B27 antigen by itself is neither necessary nor sufficient for the development of any of the diseases.[2]

Ankylosing Spondylitis

AS is a chronic, systemic inflammatory disease of the joints of the vertebral column and sacroiliac joints manifested by pain and progressive stiffening of the spine.[28] Clinical manifestations usually begin in late adolescence or early adulthood and are slightly more common in males than in females. The disease usually evolves more slowly and is less severe in females. AS can occur later in life and, when it does, initial symptoms commonly include more involvement of the cervical spine and arthritis of the upper and lower limbs. The late onset group also demonstrates a higher amount of missed presentations (axial and peripheral joints) as the disease progresses.[29]

AS produces an inflammatory erosion of the sites where tendons and ligaments attach to bone.[28] Typically, the disease process begins with bilateral involvement of the sacroiliac joints and then moves to the smaller joints of the posterior elements of the spine. The result is ultimate destruction of these joints with ankylosis or posterior fusion of the spine. The vertebrae take on a squared appearance and bone bridges fuse one vertebral body to the next across the intervertebral disks. Progressive spinal changes usually follow an ascending pattern beginning with the sacroiliac area and then moving up the spine to involve the costovertebral joints and cervical spine. Occasionally, large synovial joints (*i.e.*, hips, knees, and shoulders) may be involved. The small peripheral joints usually are not affected. The disease spectrum ranges from an asymptomatic sacroiliitis to a progressive disease that can affect many body systems.

Etiology and Pathogenesis

Although the pathogenesis of AS has not been established, the presence of mononuclear cells in the acutely involved tissue suggests an immune response. Epidemiologic findings indicate that genetic and environmental factors play a role in the pathogenesis of the disease. Approximately 90% of those with AS possess the HLA-B27 antigen and nearly 100% of those who also have uveitis or aortitis have the marker; the HLA-B27 antigen also is present in approximately 8% of the normal population.[2] Several theories have been advanced to account for the association between the HLA-B27 antigen and AS. One possibility is that the gene that determines the HLA-B27 antigen may be linked to other genes that determine the pathologic autoimmune phenomena or that lead to increased susceptibility to infections or environmental agents. A second theory postulates molecular mimicry. An autoimmune reaction to an antigenic determinant site in the host's tissues may occur as a consequence of an immunologic response to an identical or closely related antigen of a foreign agent, usually an infectious agent.[30]

Clinical Manifestations

The person with AS typically complains of lower back pain, which may be persistent or intermittent. The pain, which becomes worse when resting, particularly when lying in bed, initially may be attributed to muscle strain or spasm from physical activity. Lumbosacral pain also may be present, with discomfort in the buttocks and hip areas. Sometimes, pain can radiate to the thigh in a manner like that of sciatic pain. Prolonged stiffness is present in the morning and after periods of rest. Walking or exercise may be needed to provide the comfort needed to return to sleep. Loss of motion in the spinal column is characteristic of the disease (Fig. 50.6).

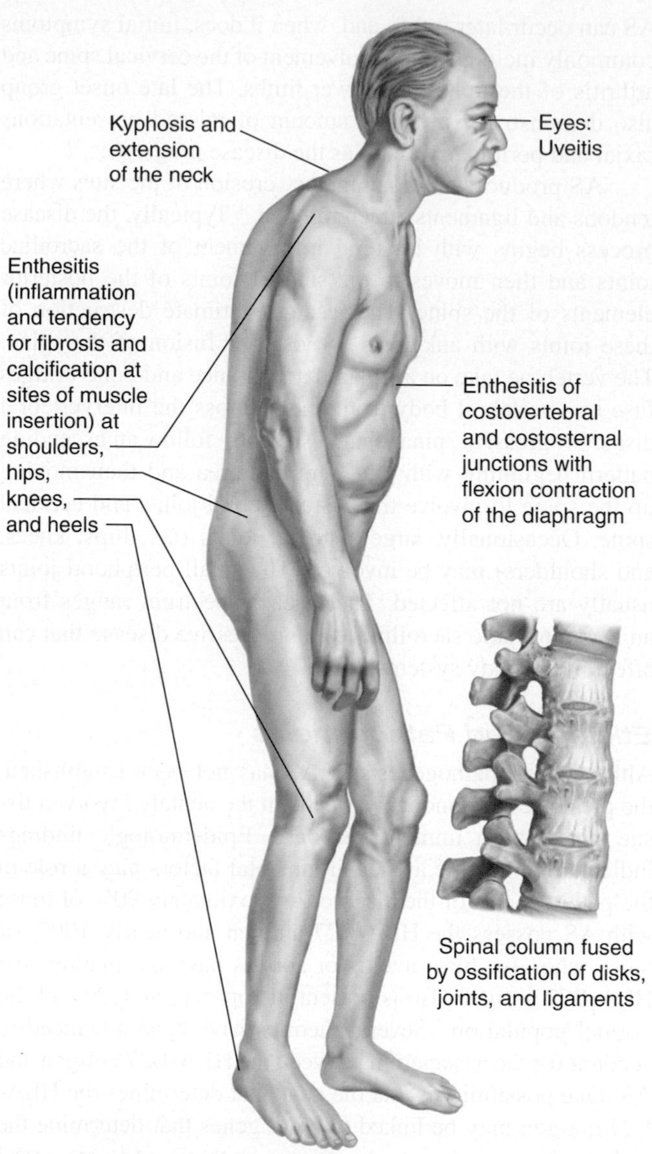

Figure 50.6 • Clinical manifestations of AS.

The severity and duration of disease activity influence the degree of mobility. Loss of lumbar lordosis occurs as the disease progresses, and this is followed by kyphosis of the thoracic spine and extension of the neck. A spine fused in the flexed position is the end result in severe AS. A kyphotic spine makes it difficult for the person to look ahead and to maintain balance while walking. The image is of a person bent over looking at the floor and unable to straighten up. X-ray films show a rigid, bamboo-like spine. The heart and lungs are constricted in the chest cavity. Abnormal weight bearing can lead to degeneration and destruction of the hips, necessitating joint replacement procedures. Peripheral arthritis is more common in the hips and shoulders.

The most common extraskeletal involvement is acute anterior uveitis and may be the first indication of the disease.[28] Systemic features of weight loss, fever, and fatigue may be apparent. Sometimes, the fatigue is a greater problem than pain or stiffness. Osteoporosis can occur, especially in the spine, which contributes to the risk of spinal fracture. Fusion of the costovertebral joints can lead to reduced lung volume.

The disease process varies considerably among people. Exacerbations and remissions are common. The unpredictability of the disease can create uncertainty in planning daily activities and in setting goals. Fortunately, most of those affected can lead productive lives. The prognosis for AS in general is good. The first decade of disease predicts the remainder. Severe disease usually occurs early and is marked by peripheral arthritis, especially of the hip.

Diagnosis

The diagnosis of AS is based on history, physical examination, and x-ray examination. The early and precise diagnosis of AS is closely related to a favorable prognosis. Early recognition allows for implementation of a conservative and usually effective treatment program on a lifelong basis.

Several methods are available to assess spinal mobility, detect sacroiliitis, and diagnose AS. These methods include assessment of sacroiliitis through imaging, spinal flexion as recommended by the Assessment in SpondyloArthritis International Society (ASAS) including chest expansion, modified Schöber test, lateral lumber flexion, cervical rotation and the Bath Ankylosing Spondylitis Metrology Scale (BASMI), and lab values such as C-reactive protein and ESR.[28,31,32] Although these measures alone do not provide a diagnosis of AS or other SpA, they can provide useful measurements for monitoring the disease status. Measurement of chest expansion may be used as an indirect indicator of thoracic involvement, which usually occurs late in the disease course.

Laboratory findings frequently include an elevated ESR. HLA typing is not diagnostic of the disease and should not be used as a routine screening procedure. Radiologic evaluations help differentiate AS from sacroiliitis because of other diseases. However, x-ray images may be negative in early disease. Vertebrae normally are concave on the anterior border. In AS, the vertebrae take on a squared appearance (see Fig. 50.6).

Treatment

Treatment of AS is directed at controlling pain and maintaining mobility by suppressing inflammation. Proper posture and positioning are important. This includes sleeping in a supine position on a firm mattress and using one small pillow or no pillow. A bed board may be used to supply additional firmness. Therapeutic exercises are important to assist in maintaining motion in peripheral joints and in the spine. Muscle-strengthening exercises for extensor muscle groups also are prescribed. Heat applications or a shower or bath may be beneficial before exercise for ease of movement. Swimming is an excellent general conditioning exercise that avoids joint stress and enhances muscle tone. Immobilizing joints is not recommended. Maintaining ideal weight reduces the stress on weight-bearing joints. Smoking should be discouraged because it can exacerbate respiratory problems. Occupational counseling or job evaluation may be warranted because of postural abnormalities.

Pharmacologic treatment includes the use of NSAIDs to reduce inflammation, relieve pain, and reduce muscle spasm. The ASAS-EULAR have recently updated their guidelines for the management of AS to guide practitioners and people. Although DMARDs are used in the treatment of other inflammatory illnesses, they have not been shown to be effective for axial AS; the exception is sulfasalazine, which has shown efficacy for peripheral joint involvement. In high disease activity not responsive to conventional therapy, DMARDs may be considered.

Current practice is to use Anti–TNF-α therapies, including etanercept, infliximab, and adalimumab, which have demonstrated positive effects on disease activity.[28,33]

Reactive Arthropathies

The reactive arthropathies may be defined as sterile inflammatory joint disorders that are distant in time and place from the initial inciting infective process. The infecting agents cannot be cultured and are not viable once they reach the joints. The list of triggering agents is continuously increasing and may be divided into urogenic, enterogenic, and respiratory tract associated, and the idiopathic arthritides.

Reactive arthritis also has been observed in people with acquired immunodeficiency syndrome (AIDS). SpA such as Reiter syndrome and psoriatic arthritis are more severe and frequent in people infected with human immunodeficiency virus (HIV) than in the general population. It is thought that the immune response to HIV infection is selective and largely spares the natural killer cells, which may be quite significant in the pathology of reactive arthritis conditions. This contrasts with RA and SLE, which dramatically improve as immunodeficiency develops. Reactive arthritis may also result from the presence of a foreign substance in the joint tissue, as in silicone implants in the small joints of the hands or feet or after exposure to industrial gases and oils. However, there is no evidence of antigenicity of the causative substance.

Similarities exist between reactive arthritis and bacterial arthritis. Several bacteria cause both diseases. When cultured bacteria are isolated from the synovial fluid, the diagnosis is bacterial arthritis. When they cannot be isolated, even though there has been a preceding infection, the diagnosis of reactive arthritis is made.

Reactive arthritis may follow a self-limited course. It may involve recurrent episodes of arthritis or, in a small number of cases, it may follow a continuous and unremitting course. The treatment is largely symptomatic. NSAIDs are used in treating the arthritic symptoms. Vigorous treatment of possible triggering infections is thought to prevent relapses of reactive arthritis, but in many cases the triggering infection passes unnoticed or is mild, and the person contacts a physician only with the onset of definite arthritis. Short antibiotic courses at this time are not effective.

Reiter Syndrome

Reiter syndrome is considered to be a clinical manifestation of reactive arthritis that may be accompanied by extra-articular symptoms such as uveitis, bowel inflammation, and nonspecific urethritis.[2] The disease often develops in a genetically susceptible host after a bacterial infection (*e.g.*, a sexually transmitted infection).[2]

KEY POINTS

SERONEGATIVE SPONDYLOARTHROPATHIES

- The seronegative SpA represent a group of related multisystem disorders that lack the RF.
- The inflammatory process associated with the disorders commonly affects the axial skeleton, involving areas where ligaments and tendons attach to bone.
- Although the cause of the disorders is unknown, there is a striking association between the HLA-B27 antigen and the development of SpA.

Psoriatic Arthritis

Psoriatic arthritis is a seronegative inflammatory arthropathy that occurs in 7% of people with psoriasis.[2] It is a heterogeneous disease with features of the SpA in some people, RA in others, and features of both coexisting in yet others.

Etiology and Pathogenesis

The etiology of psoriasis and psoriatic arthritis is unknown. Genetic, environmental, and immunologic factors appear to affect susceptibility and play a role in expression of the psoriatic skin disease and the arthritis. Environmental factors that may play a role in the pathogenesis of the disorder include infectious agents and physical trauma. T-cell–mediated immune responses seem to play an important role in the skin and joint manifestations of the disease, as indicated by the observation that there is improvement in disease status after treatment with immunosuppressant agents such as cyclosporine.

Clinical Manifestations and Treatment

Although the arthritis can antedate a detectable skin rash, the definitive diagnosis of psoriatic arthritis cannot be made without evidence of skin or nail changes typical of psoriasis. Psoriatic arthritis falls into five subgroups:

1. Asymmetric—about 35% of cases, often mild
2. Spondylitis—pain and stiffness in the spine and neck
3. Symmetric—about 50% of cases
4. DIP—inflammation and stiffness near the ends of the fingers
5. Mutilans—most severe—only about 5% of cases[34]

This heterogeneous clinical presentation suggests more than one disease is associated with psoriasis or various clinical responses to a common cause. Some with psoriatic arthritis have an elevated serum level of uric acid. The abnormally elevated serum uric acid level is caused by the rapid skin turnover of psoriasis and the subsequent breakdown of nucleic acid followed by its metabolism to uric acid. This finding may lead to a misdiagnosis of gout. Psoriatic arthritis tends to be slowly progressive, but has a more favorable prognosis than RA.

Basic management is similar to the treatment of RA. Suppression of the skin disease may be important in controlling the arthritis. Often, affected joints are surprisingly functional and only minimally symptomatic. If there are musculoskeletal symptoms, NSAIDs may be used.[35] DMARDs such as methotrexate, sulfasalazine, and leflunomide should be considered early in those with active disease.[35] Methotrexate is indicated in psoriatic arthritis and significant psoriasis.[35] TNF inhibitors are indicated when there is an inadequate response to indicated DMARDs, NSAIDs, or steroid injections.[35]

Enteropathic Arthritis

Arthritis that is associated with an inflammatory bowel disease usually is considered an enteropathic arthritis because the intestinal disease is directly involved in the pathogenesis. Most cases of enteropathic arthritis are classified among the SpA. These include cases in which the arthritis is associated with inflammatory bowel disease (*i.e.*, ulcerative colitis and Crohn disease), which is generally 20%, spondylitis (10%), and a few with the reactive arthritides triggered by bacterial infections of the gut, and Whipple disease.[2]

IN SUMMARY

The seronegative arthropathies are a group of rheumatic disorders that lack RF. The *seronegative SpA* affect the axial skeleton, particularly the spine. Inflammation develops at sites where tendons and ligaments insert into bone. They include AS, reactive arthritis, psoriatic arthritis, and enteropathic arthritis. AS is considered a prototype of this classification category. Bilateral sacroiliitis is the primary feature of AS. The disease spectrum ranges from asymptomatic sacroiliitis to a progressive disorder affecting many body systems. The cause remains unknown. However, a strong association between the HLA-B27 antigen and AS has been identified. Loss of motion in the spinal column is characteristic of the disease. Peripheral arthritis may occur in some people. Another form of spondyloarthritis is reactive arthritis. Although there are overlapping features for each of the SpA, identifying etiologic differences and clinical manifestations is important for determining treatment.

Psoriatic arthritis is a seronegative arthropathy that occurs in approximately 7% of people with psoriasis. It is a heterogeneous disease with features of the SpA in some people, RA in others, and features of both coexisting in yet others.

OSTEOARTHRITIS SYNDROME

After completing this section of the chapter, the learner will be able to meet the following objectives:

- Compare RA and OA in terms of joint involvement, level of inflammation, and local and systemic manifestations.
- Describe the pathologic joint changes associated with OA.

Osteoarthritis (OA), formerly called *degenerative joint disease*, is the most prevalent form of arthritis and is a leading cause of disability and pain in older adults. OA is more of a disease process than a specific entity and is considered to have an inflammatory component along with the degenerative aspect. OA is a slowly progressive destruction of articular cartilage of weight-bearing joints and fingers of older adults and the joints of younger people who have experienced trauma.[2] It can occur as a primary disorder or as a secondary disorder, although this distinction is not always clear. Primary variants of OA occur due to intrinsic defects in the articular cartilage that cause joint narrowing, subchondral bone thickening, and ultimately a painful joint.[2] Secondary OA has a known underlying cause such as congenital or acquired defects of joint structures, trauma, infection, endocrinopathies, crystal deposits, osteonecrosis, metabolic disorders, or inflammatory diseases (Chart 50.1).

CHART 50.1 CAUSES OF OSTEOARTHRITIS

Postinflammatory disorders
- Rheumatoid arthritis
- Septic joint

Posttraumatic disorders
- Acute fracture
- Ligament or meniscal injury
- Cumulative occupational or recreational trauma

Anatomic or bony disorders
- Hip dysplasia
- Avascular necrosis
- Paget disease
- Slipped capital femoral epiphysis
- Legg-Calvé-Perthes disease

Metabolic disorders
- Calcium crystal deposition
- Hemochromatosis
- Acromegaly
- Endocrinopathies
- Wilson disease
- Ochronosis

Neuropathic arthritis
- Charcot joint

Hereditary disorders of collagen

Idiopathic or primary variants

The joint changes associated with OA, which include a progressive loss of articular cartilage and synovitis, result from the inflammation caused when cartilage attempts to repair itself, creating osteophytes or spurs. These changes are accompanied by joint pain, stiffness, and limitation of motion, and in some cases by joint instability and deformity.

Epidemiology and Risk Factors

Age, gender, and race interact to influence the time of onset and the pattern of joint involvement in OA. Primary OA affects 4% of people between 18 and 24 years of age; 85% of people with OA are in their seventies.[2] Males are affected more commonly at a younger age, such as 45 years. However, by 55 years of age, females are more frequently affected by OA.[2] Heredity influences the occurrence of hand OA in the DIP joint. Hand OA is more likely to affect Caucasian females, whereas knee OA is more common in African-American females. The incidence of hip OA is lower among the Chinese than Europeans, perhaps representing the influence of other factors such as occupation, obesity, or heredity. Bone mass may also influence the risk of developing OA. In theory, thinner subchondral bone mass may provide a greater shock-absorbing function than denser bone, allowing less direct trauma to the cartilage.

Obesity is a risk factor for OA of the knee in females and a contributory biomechanical factor in the pathogenesis of the disease. Excess fat may have a direct metabolic effect on cartilage beyond the effects of excess joint stress.

Pathogenesis

The pathogenesis of OA resides in the homeostatic mechanisms that maintain the articular cartilage. Articular cartilage plays two essential mechanical roles in joint physiology. First, the articular cartilage serves as a remarkably smooth weight-bearing surface. In combination with synovial fluid, the articular cartilage provides extremely low friction during movement of the joint. Second, the cartilage transmits the load down to the bone, dissipating the mechanical stress.[2] Thus, the subchondral bone protects the overlying articular cartilage, providing it with a pliable bed and absorbing the energy of the force (Fig. 50.7).

Cartilage is a specialized type of connective tissue. As with other types of tissue, it consists of cells (*i.e.*, chondrocytes) nested in an extracellular matrix. In articular cartilage, the extracellular matrix is composed of water, proteoglycans, collagen, and ground substance. The proteoglycans, which are large macromolecules made up of disaccharides and amino acids, afford elasticity and stiffness, permitting articular cartilage to resist compression. The ground substance constitutes a highly hydrated, semisolid gel. Collagen molecules consist of polypeptide chains that form long, fibrous strands. They provide form and tensile strength. The primary function of the collagen fibers is to provide a rigid scaffold to support the chondrocytes and ground substance of cartilage. The hydrated

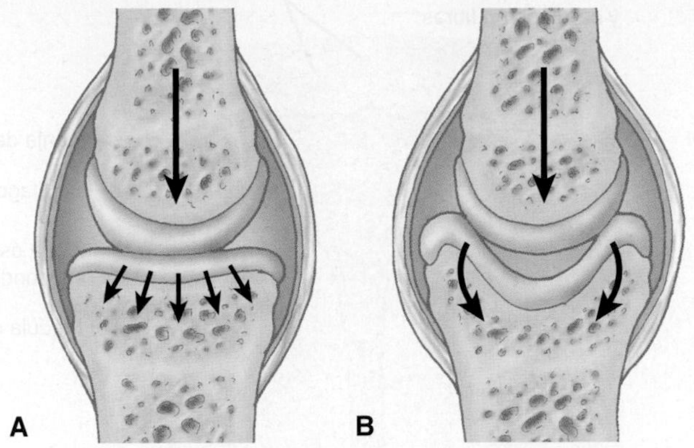

Figure 50.7 • **(A)** A joint normally undergoes deformation of the articular cartilage and the subchondral bone when carrying a load. This maximizes the contact area and spreads the force of the load. **(B)** If the joint does not deform with a load, the stresses are concentrated and the joint breaks down.

proteoglycan molecules, because of their size and charge, are trapped in the collagen meshwork of the extracellular matrix and prevented from expanding to their maximum size. Because of this process, there is high interstitial osmotic pressure and enough fluid available for joint lubrication. As in the case of adult bone, articular cartilage is not static. It undergoes turnover and its "worn out" matrix components are continually degraded and replaced. This turnover is maintained by the chondrocytes, which not only synthesize the matrix but also secrete matrix-degrading enzymes. Thus, the health of the chondrocytes determines joint integrity. In OA, this integrity can be disturbed by many influences.

Popularly known as *wear-and-tear* arthritis, OA is characterized by significant changes in both the composition and mechanical properties of cartilage. Early during the disease, the cartilage contains increased water and decreased concentrations of proteoglycans compared with healthy cartilage. In addition, there appears to be a weakening of the collagen network, presumably caused by a decrease in the local synthesis of new collagen and an increase in the breakdown of existing collagen. It is thought that the injured articular cartilage is due to cytokine release, which triggers destruction of the joint[2] (Fig. 50.8). The resulting damage predisposes the chondrocytes to more injury and impairs their ability to repair the damage by producing new collagen and proteoglycans. The combined effects of inadequate repair mechanisms and imbalances between the proteases and their inhibitors contribute further to disease progression.

The earliest structural changes in OA include enlargement and reorganization of the chondrocytes in the superficial part of the articular cartilage. This is accompanied by edematous changes in the cartilaginous matrix, principally the intermediate layer. The cartilage loses its smooth aspect and surface cracks or microfractures occur, allowing synovial fluid to enter and widen the crack (Fig. 50.9). As the crack deepens and clefts form it eventually extends through the articular surface and into the subchondral aspect of the

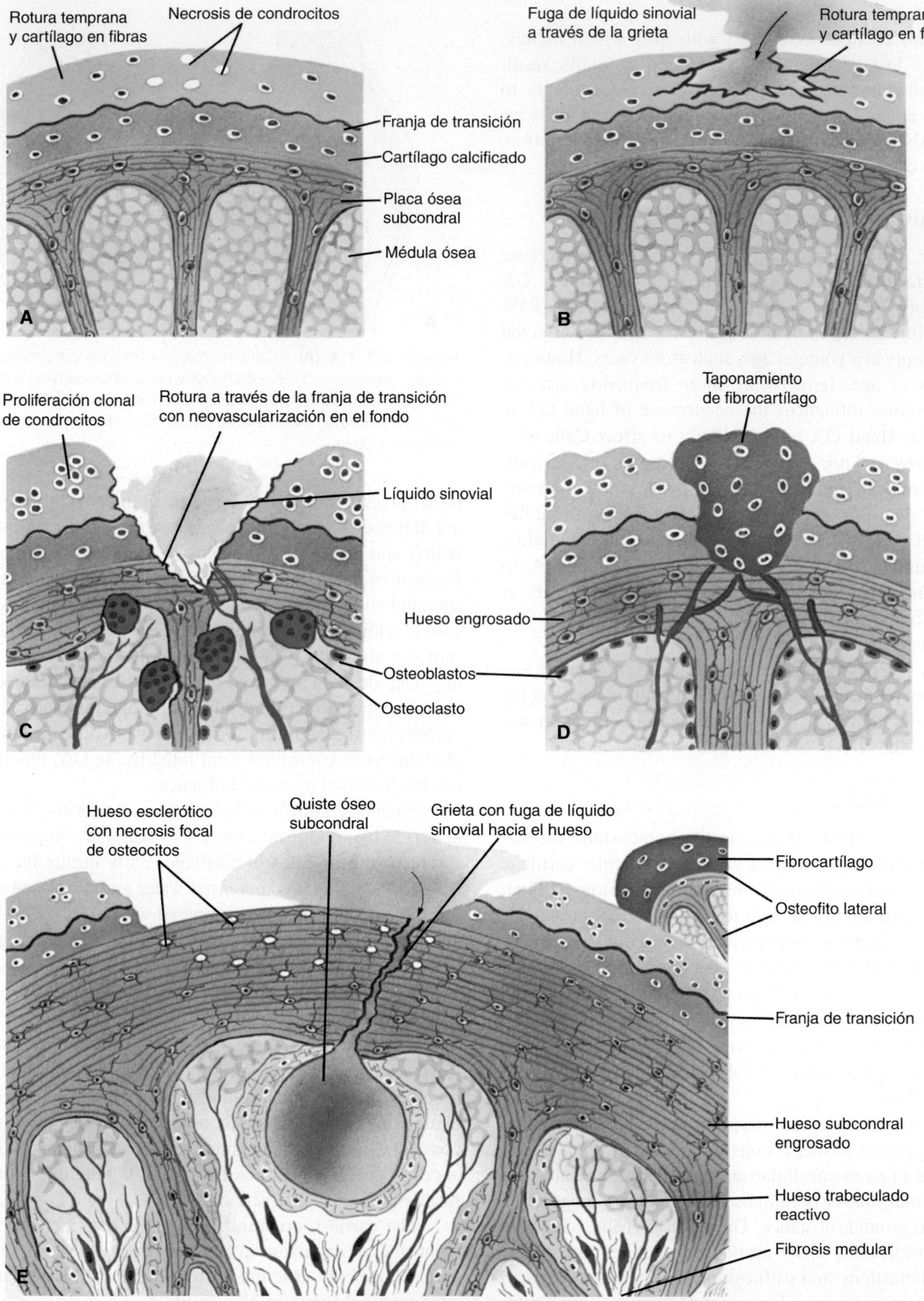

Figure 50.8 • Histogenesis of OA. **(A and B)** The death of chondrocytes leads to a crack in the articular cartilage that is followed by an influx of synovial fluid and further loss of cartilage. **(C)** As a result of this process, cartilage is gradually worn away. Below the tidemark, new vessels grow in from the epiphysis, and fibrocartilage **(D)** is deposited. **(E)** The fibrocartilage plug is not mechanically sufficient and may be worn away, thus exposing the subchondral bone plate, which becomes thickened and eburnated. If there is a crack in this region, synovial fluid leaks into the marrow space and produces a subchondral bone cyst. Focal regrowth of the articular surface leads to the formation of osteophytes. (From Strayer D., Rubin R. (Eds.) (2015). *Rubin's pathology: Clinicopathologic foundations of medicine* (7th ed., Figure 30-53, p. 1361). Philadelphia, PA: Lippincott Williams & Wilkins.)

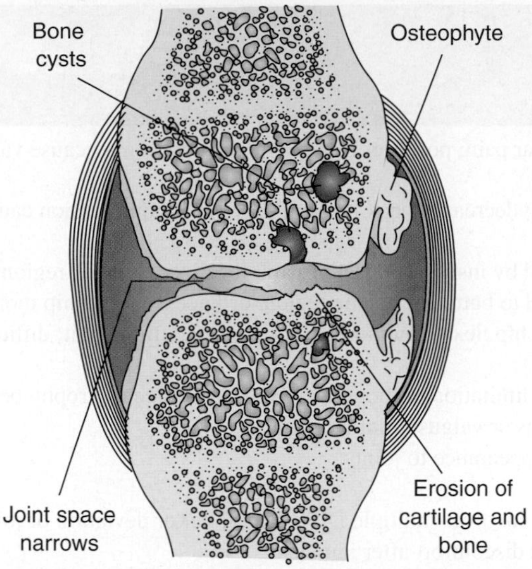

Figure 50.9 • Joint changes in OA. The left side denotes early changes and joint space narrowing with cartilage breakdown. The right side shows more severe disease progression with lost cartilage and osteophyte formation.

bone.[2] Portions of the articular cartilage eventually become completely eroded and the exposed surface of the subchondral bone becomes thickened and polished to an ivory-like consistency. Fragments of cartilage and bone often become dislodged, creating free-floating osteocartilaginous bodies ("joint mice") that enter the joint cavity. As the disease progresses, the underlying trabecular bone becomes sclerotic in response to increased pressure on the surface of the joint, rendering it less effective as a shock absorber. Sclerosis, or formation of new bone and cysts, usually occurs at the joint margins, forming abnormal bony outgrowths called *osteophytes*, or *spurs* (Fig. 50.7). As the joint begins to lose its integrity, there is trauma to the synovial membrane, which results in nonspecific inflammation. Compared with RA, however, the changes in the synovium that occur in OA are not as pronounced, nor do they occur as early.

In secondary forms of OA, repetitive impact loading contributes to joint failure, accounting for the high prevalence of OA specific to vocational or avocational sites, such as the shoulders and elbows of baseball pitchers, ankles of ballet dancers, and knees of basketball players. Immobilization also can produce degenerative changes in articular cartilage. Cartilage degeneration because of immobility may result from loss of the pumping action of lubrication that occurs with joint movement. These changes are more marked and appear earlier in areas of contact but occur also in areas not subject to mechanical compression. Although cartilage atrophy is rapidly reversible with activity after a period of immobilization, impact exercise during the period of remobilization can prevent reversal of the atrophy. Therefore, slow and gradual remobilization may be important in preventing cartilage injury. Clinically, this has implications for instructions concerning the recommended level of physical activity after removal of a cast.

KEY POINTS

OSTEOARTHRITIS

- It can present as a primary disease of unknown etiology or as a secondary disorder related to congenital or acquired defects that affect the distribution of joint stress.
- The pathogenesis of OA includes the progressive disruption of the smooth surface of the articular cartilage with development of surface cracks that deepen to involve the subchondral bone, followed by complete erosion of the articular cartilage with exposure of ivory-like polished subchondral bone, dislodgment of fragments of free-floating osteocartilaginous bodies, development of bone cysts, and formation of abnormal bony spurs at the joint margins.

Clinical Manifestations

The manifestations of OA may arise suddenly or insidiously. Initially, pain may be described as aching and may be somewhat difficult to localize. It usually worsens with use or activity and is relieved by rest. In later stages of disease activity, night pain may be experienced during rest. Pain can occur at rest, several hours after the use of the involved joints. Crepitus and grinding may be evident when the joint is moved. As the disease advances, even minimal activity may cause pain because of the limited range of motion resulting from intra-articular and periarticular structural damage.

The most frequently affected joints are the hips, knees, lumbar and cervical vertebrae, proximal and distal joints of the hands, the first carpometacarpal joint, and the first metatarsophalangeal joints of the feet.[2] Table 50.2 identifies the joints that commonly are affected by OA and the common clinical features correlated with the disease activity of each particular joint. A single joint or several may be affected. Although a single weight-bearing joint may be involved initially, other joints often become affected because of the additional stress placed on them while trying to protect the initial joint. It is not unusual for a person having a knee replacement to discover soon after the surgery is done that the second knee also needs to be replaced. Other clinical features are limitations of joint motion and joint instability. Joint enlargement usually results from new bone formation; the joint feels hard, in contrast to the soft, spongy feeling characteristic of the joint in RA. Sometimes, mild synovitis or increased synovial fluid can cause joint enlargement.

Diagnosis and Treatment

The diagnosis of OA usually is determined by history and physical examination, x-ray studies, and laboratory findings that exclude other diseases. Although OA often is contrasted with RA for diagnostic purposes, the differences are

TABLE 50.2 CLINICAL FEATURES OF OA

JOINT	CLINICAL FEATURES
Cervical spine	Localized stiffness; radicular or nonradicular pain; posterior osteophyte formation may cause vascular compression
Lumbar spine	Low back pain and stiffness; muscle spasm; decreased back motion; nerve root compression causing radicular pain; spinal stenosis
Hip	Most common in older males; characterized by insidious onset of pain, localized to groin region or inner aspect of the thigh; may be referred to buttocks, sciatic region, or knee; reduced hip motion; leg may be held in external rotation with hip flexed and adducted; limp or shuffling gait; difficulty getting in and out of chairs
Knee	Localized discomfort with pain on motion; limitation of motion; crepitus; quadriceps atrophy because of lack of use; joint instability; genu varus or valgus; joint effusion
First carpometacarpal joint	Tenderness at base of the thumb; squared appearance to joint
PIP joint—Bouchard nodes	Same as for DIP joint disease
DIP joint—Heberden nodes	Occurs more frequently in females; usually involves multiple DIPs, lateral flexor deviation of joint, spur formation at joint margins, pain and discomfort after joint use
First metatarsophalangeal joint	Insidious onset; irregular joint contour; pain and swelling aggravated by tight shoes

not always readily apparent. Other rheumatic diseases may be superimposed on OA.

Characteristic radiologic changes initially include medial joint space narrowing, followed by subchondral bony sclerosis, formation of spikes on the tibial eminence, and osteophytes.[2,35] The results of laboratory studies usually are normal because the disorder is not a systemic disease but can be helpful for differential diagnosis.[4] The ESR may be slightly elevated in older adults.[4] If inflammation is present, there may be a slight increase in the white blood cell count. The synovial fluid usually is normal. The ACR (2018) website has guidelines for classification of Hand, Knee, and Hip Criteria for OA.[36]

Because there is no cure, the focus of treatment of OA is symptomatic and includes physical rehabilitative, pharmacologic, and surgical measures. Physical measures are aimed at improving the supporting structures of the joint and strengthening opposing muscle groups involved in cushioning weight-bearing forces. This includes a balance of rest and exercise, use of splints to protect and rest the joint, use of heat and cold to relieve pain and muscle spasm, and adjusting the activities of daily living. Weight reduction is helpful when the knee is involved. The involved joint should not be further abused, and steps should be taken to protect and rest it. These include weight reduction (when weight-bearing surfaces are involved) and the use of a cane or walker if the hips and knees are involved.

Oral medications are aimed at reducing inflammation or providing analgesia. Popular medications used in the treatment of OA are the NSAIDs, many of which are available without a prescription. Ongoing research may confirm that some NSAIDs impede the repair mechanisms in early cartilage lesions. However, studies have shown that the pain of OA may arise from factors other than an inflamed synovium. These factors include stretching of the joint capsule, ligaments, or nerve endings in the periosteum over osteophytes; nontrabecular microfractures; intraosseous hypertension; bursitis or tendinitis; and muscle spasm. In such cases, the analgesic effect of the NSAID may be able to successfully relieve the pain. For many people, acetaminophen may be as effective and less toxic than NSAIDs.

Intra-articular corticosteroid injections may be used when other treatment measures have been unsuccessful in adequately relieving symptoms. They are especially helpful in people who have an effusion of the joint. Injections usually are limited to a total of four and not more than three within 1 year because their use is thought to accelerate joint destruction.

Viscosupplementation is another treatment and is based on the hypothesis that joint lubrication is abnormal in OA.[4] Hyaluronate is injected into the joint weekly for 3 to 5 weeks and may provide relief for six months or longer.[4] Other agents like glucosamine and chondroitin sulfate, which is not FDA-regulated, have been used for relief of OA.[4] Currently, the American Academy of Orthopaedic Surgeons does not recommend the use of glucosamine and chondroitin sulfate for symptomatic arthritis.[37] Disease-modifying agents for OA are also being studied.

Surgery is considered when the person is having severe pain and joint function is severely reduced. Procedures include arthroscopic lavage and debridement, bunion resections, osteotomies to change alignment of the knee and hip joints, and decompression of the spinal roots in osteoarthritic vertebral stenosis. Total hip replacements have provided effective relief of symptoms and improved range of motion for many people, as have total knee replacements. Joint replacement is available for the first carpometacarpal joint. Arthrodesis (surgical stiffening of a joint) is used in advanced disease to reduce pain. However, this results in loss of motion.

Future management of OA lies in the development of techniques to identify and monitor cartilage lesions at an earlier stage. Potential approaches include bone scanning, magnetic resonance imaging, and arthroscopy.

IN SUMMARY

OA, the most common form of arthritis, is a localized condition affecting primarily the weight-bearing joints. Risk factors for OA progression include older age, OA in multiple joints, neuropathy, and, for knees, obesity. The disorder is characterized by degeneration of the articular cartilage and subchondral bone. It has been suggested that the cellular events responsible for the development of OA begin with some type of abnormal mechanical insult or stimulus, including hormones and growth factors, drugs, mechanical stresses, and the extracellular environment. Studies also implicate immunologic factors in the perpetuation and acceleration of the osteoarthritic change. As cartilage ages, biochemical events such as collagen fatigue and fracture occur with less stress. Attempts at repair by increased matrix synthesis and cellular proliferation maintain the integrity of the cartilage until failure of reparative processes allows the degenerative changes to progress. Joint enlargement usually results from new bone formation, which causes the joint to feel hard. Pain and stiffness are primary features of the disease. Inflammatory mediators (*e.g.*, prostaglandins) may increase the inflammatory and degenerative response.

Treatment is directed toward the relief of pain and maintenance of mobility while preserving the articular cartilage. Although there is no known cure for OA, appropriate treatment can reduce pain, maintain or improve joint mobility, and limit functional disability.

CRYSTAL-INDUCED ARTHROPATHIES

After completing this section of the chapter, the learner will be able to meet the following objectives:

- Relate the metabolism and elimination of uric acid to the pathogenesis of crystal-induced arthropathy.
- Describe the clinical manifestations, diagnostic measures, and methods used in the treatment of gouty arthritis.

Metabolic bone and joint disorders result from biochemical and metabolic disorders that affect the joints. Metabolic and endocrine diseases associated with joint symptoms include amyloidosis, osteogenesis imperfecta, diabetes mellitus, hyperparathyroidism, thyroid disease, AIDS, and hypermobility syndromes. The discussion in this chapter is limited to the crystal-induced arthropathy caused by monosodium urate deposition, or gout.

Crystal deposition in joints produces arthritis. In gout, monosodium urate or uric acid crystals are found in the joint cavity. Another condition in which calcium pyrophosphate dihydrate crystals are found in the joints sometimes is referred to as *pseudogout* or *chondrocalcinosis*. A brief discussion of pseudogout is found in the section on rheumatic diseases in older adults.

Gout

Gout is a group of disorders characterized by increased serum uric acid and urate crystal deposits in kidneys and joints.[2] Gout is more prevalent in males (70% of cases), particularly in males of African American descent, and the peak age of occurrence is between ages 40 and 50.[4] High uric acid levels or hyperuricemia (>7 mg/dL in males and 6 mg/dL in females) are present in 5% to 10% of the population of the United States.[4] Asymptomatic hyperuricemia is a laboratory finding and not a disease. About one in five people with hyperuricemia will develop gout.[4] Most people with hyperuricemia do not develop gout. Only one third of people with hyperuricemia have primary gout and the other two thirds have secondary gout.[2]

Gout disorders include acute gouty arthritis with recurrent attacks of severe articular and periarticular inflammation; tophi or the accumulation of crystalline deposits in articular surfaces, bones, soft tissue, and cartilage; gouty nephropathy or renal impairment; and uric acid kidney stones.

The term *primary gout* is used to designate cases in which the cause of the disorder is unknown or caused by an inborn error in metabolism and is characterized primarily by hyperuricemia and gout. Primary gout is predominantly a disease of males, with a peak incidence in the fourth to sixth decade.[2] In secondary gout, the cause of the hyperuricemia is known but the gout is not the main disorder.

Pathogenesis

The pathogenesis of gout resides in an elevation of serum uric acid levels. Uric acid is the end product of purine metabolism.[38] Two pathways are involved in purine synthesis:

1. A de novo pathway in which purines are synthesized from nonpurine precursors.
2. The salvage pathway in which purine bases are recaptured from the breakdown of nucleic acids derived from exogenous (dietary) or endogenous sources.

The elevation of uric acid and the subsequent development of gout can result from overproduction of purines, decreased salvage of free purine bases, augmented breakdown of nucleic acids because of increased cell turnover, or decreased urinary excretion of uric acid (Fig. 50.10). Primary gout, which constitutes 90% of cases, may be a consequence of enzyme defects that result in an overproduction of uric acid or inadequate elimination of uric acid by the kidney.[38] In most cases, the reason is unknown. In secondary gout, the hyperuricemia may be caused by the increased breakdown of nucleic acids, as occurs with rapid tumor cell lysis during treatment for lymphoma or leukemia. Other cases of secondary gout result from chronic renal disease. Some of the diuretics, including the thiazides, can interfere with the excretion of uric acid.

An attack of gout occurs when monosodium urate crystals precipitate in the joint and initiate an inflammatory response. Synovial fluid is a poorer solvent for uric acid than plasma, and uric acid crystals are even less soluble at temperatures below 37 °C. Crystal deposition usually occurs in peripheral areas

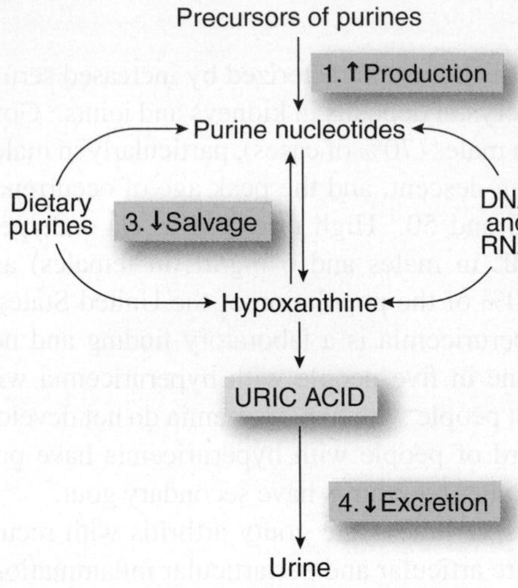

Figure 50.10 • Pathogenesis of hyperuricemia and gout. Purine nucleotides are synthesized de novo from nonpurine precursors or derived from preformed purines in the diet. Purine nucleotides are catabolized to hypoxanthine or incorporated into nucleic acids. The degradation of nucleic acids and dietary purines also produces hypoxanthine. Hypoxanthine is converted into uric acid, which in turn is excreted into the urine. Hyperuricemia and gout from (*1*) increased de novo purine synthesis, (*2*) increased cell turnover, (*3*) decreased salvage of dietary purines and hypoxanthine, and (*4*) decreased uric acid excretion by the kidneys. (From Strayer D., Rubin R. (Eds.) (2015). *Rubin's pathology: Clinicopathologic foundations of medicine* (7th ed., Figure 30-60, p. 1367). Philadelphia, PA: Lippincott Williams & Wilkins.)

of the body, such as the great toe, where the temperatures are cooler than in other parts of the body. With prolonged hyperuricemia, crystals and microtophi (*i.e.*, small, hard nodules with irregular surfaces that contain crystalline deposits of monosodium urate) accumulate in the synovial lining cells and in the joint cartilage.[4] The released crystals are chemotactic to leukocytes and also activate complements. Phagocytosis of urate crystals by polymorphonuclear leukocytes occurs and leads to polymorphonuclear cell death with the release of lysosomal enzymes. As this process continues, the inflammation causes destruction of the cartilage and subchondral bone.

Repeated or untreated attacks of acute arthritis eventually lead to chronic arthritis and the formation of the large, hard nodules called *tophi*[4,38] (Fig. 50.11). They are found most commonly in the synovium, olecranon bursa, Achilles tendon, subchondral bone, and extensor surface of the forearm and may be mistaken for rheumatoid nodules. Tophi usually do not appear until 10 years or more after the first gout attack. This stage of gout, called *chronic tophaceous gout*, is characterized by more frequent and prolonged attacks, which often are polyarticular.

Clinical Manifestations

Gout is categorized into four phases:

1. The asymptomatic hyperuricemia
2. Acute gout arthritis
3. Intercritical gout
4. Chronic tophaceous gout[2]

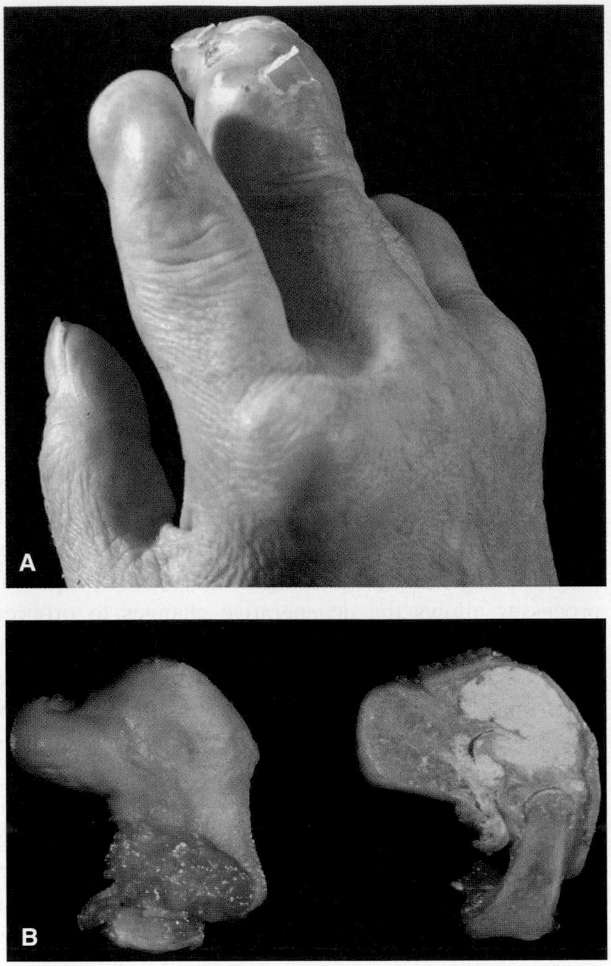

Figure 50.11 • Gout. **(A)** Gouty tophi of the hands appear as multiple rubbery nodules, one of which is ulcerated. **(B)** A cross-section of a digit demonstrates a tophaceous collection of toothpaste-like urate crystals. (From Strayer D., Rubin R. (Eds.) (2015). *Rubin's pathology: Clinicopathologic foundations of medicine* (7th ed., Figure 30-61A and B, p. 1368). Philadelphia, PA: Lippincott Williams & Wilkins.)

The first phase may not even be identified or may be detected during an annual physical examination because the person has no symptoms. The typical acute attack of gout is monoarticular and usually affects the first metatarsophalangeal joint. The tarsal joints, insteps, ankles, heels, knees, wrists, fingers, and elbows also may be initial sites of involvement. Acute gout often begins at night and may be precipitated by excessive exercise, certain medications or foods, alcohol, or dieting. The onset of pain typically is abrupt, and redness and swelling are observed. The attack may last for days or weeks. Pain may be severe enough to be aggravated even by the weight of a bedsheet covering the affected area.

In the early stages of gout after the initial attack has subsided, the person is asymptomatic, and joint abnormalities are not evident. This is the third phase or the *intercritical gout*. After the first attack, it may be months or years before another attack. As attacks recur with increased frequency, joint changes occur and become permanent. This fourth phase is called chronic tophaceous gout.

Gout has been linked with cardiovascular disease, obesity, metabolic syndrome, hyperlipidemia, excessive alcohol use, and renal insufficiency. Therefore, these potential comorbidities need to be ruled out and, if they are ruled out, should be prevented.[39]

Diagnosis and Treatment

Although hyperuricemia is the biochemical hallmark of gout, the presence of hyperuricemia cannot be equated with gout because many people with this condition never develop gout. A definitive diagnosis of gout can be made only when monosodium urate crystals are in the synovial fluid or in tissue sections of tophaceous deposits. Synovial fluid analysis is useful in excluding other conditions, such as septic arthritis, pseudogout, and RA. Diagnostic methods may include measures to determine if the disorder is related to overproduction or to underexcretion of uric acid.[38,39] This is done through measurement of serum uric acid levels and collection of a 24-hour urine sample for determination of urate excretion in the urine.[38,39] The objectives for treatment of gout include the termination and prevention of the acute attacks of gouty arthritis and the correction of hyperuricemia, with consequent inhibition of further precipitation of sodium urate and absorption of urate crystal deposits already in the tissues.

Pharmacologic management of acute gout is directed toward reducing joint inflammation. Hyperuricemia and related problems of tophi, joint destruction, and renal problems are treated after the acute inflammatory process has subsided. NSAIDs, particularly indomethacin and ibuprofen, are used for treating acute gouty arthritis. Alternative therapies include colchicine and intra-articular deposition of corticosteroids. Treatment with colchicine is used early in the acute stage. Colchicine produces its anti-inflammatory effects by inhibition of leukocyte migration and phagocytosis. The acute symptoms of gout usually subside within 48 hours after treatment with oral colchicine has been instituted and within 12 hours after intravenous administration of the drug. The NSAIDs are also effective during the acute stage when used at their maximum dosage and sometimes are preferred to colchicine because they have fewer toxic side effects. The corticosteroid drugs have not been systemically studied, but can be useful in the treatment of acute gout limited to a single joint or bursa.

After the acute attack has been relieved, the hyperuricemia is treated. Treatment of hyperuricemia is aimed at maintaining normal uric acid levels and is lifelong. One method is to reduce hyperuricemia using allopurinol or a uricosuric agent. Allopurinol inhibits xanthine oxidase, an enzyme needed for the conversion of hypoxanthine to xanthine and xanthine to uric acid as does a newer medication, febuxostat (Uloric).[38,39] The uricosuric drugs (*e.g.*, probenecid or sulfinpyrazone, a phenylbutazone derivative) prevent the tubular reabsorption of urate and increase its excretion in the urine. The serum urate concentrations are monitored to determine efficacy and dosage. Prophylactic colchicine or NSAIDs may be used between gout attacks.

Although gout can often be effectively controlled by nonpharmacologic methods, many people with gout have a limited understanding of the disease and therefore a poor compliance with treatment. Thus, education about the disease and its management are fundamental to the treatment and management of gout. Some changes in lifestyle may be needed, such as maintenance of ideal weight, moderation in alcohol consumption, smoking cessation, and avoidance of purine-rich foods (*e.g.*, liver, kidney, sardines, anchovies, and sweetbreads), particularly by people with excessive tophaceous deposits.[38,39]

IN SUMMARY

Crystal-induced arthropathy is characterized by crystal deposition in the joint. Gout is the prototype of this group. Acute attacks of arthritis occur with gout and are characterized by the presence of monosodium urate crystals in the joint. The disorder is accompanied by hyperuricemia, which results from overproduction of uric acid or from the reduced ability of the kidney to rid the body of excess uric acid. Management of acute gout is directed first toward the reduction of joint inflammation, after which the hyperuricemia is treated. Hyperuricemia is treated with uricosuric agents, which prevent the tubular reabsorption of urate, or with medication that inhibits the production of uric acid. Although gout is chronic, most people can control it with appropriate lifestyle changes.

RHEUMATIC DISEASES IN CHILDREN AND OLDER ADULTS

After completing this section of the chapter, the learner will be able to meet the following objectives:

- List three types of juvenile arthritis and differentiate among their major characteristics.
- Name one rheumatic disease that affects only older adults.

Rheumatic Diseases in Children

Children can be affected with almost all the rheumatic diseases. In addition to disease-specific differences, these conditions affect not only the child but also the family. Growth and development require special attention. Adherence to the treatment program requires intervention with the child and parents.

Juvenile Idiopathic Arthritis

Juvenile idiopathic arthritis (JIA), also known as juvenile RA, is characterized by joint inflammation as well as possible impacts on other areas of the body and occurs most frequently among arthritis of childhood.[40,41] In the United States, close to 300,000 children have a type of arthritis.[40] JIA is characterized by synovitis and can influence epiphyseal growth by stimulating growth of the affected side. Generalized stunted growth also may occur. JIA can be regarded not as a single disease, but as a category of diseases with subtypes:

- Systemic JIA
- Oligoarticular JIA
- Polyarticular JIA
- Enthesitis-related JIA
- Juvenile psoriatic arthritis
- Undifferentiated arthritis[4]

The symptoms of systemic JIA include a daily intermittent high fever, which usually is accompanied by a rash, generalized lymphadenopathy, hepatosplenomegaly, leukocytosis, and anemia. Most of these children also have joint involvement, which develops concurrently with fever and rash. Systemic symptoms usually subside in 6 to 12 months. This form of JIA also can make an initial appearance in adulthood. Infections, heart disease, and adrenal insufficiency may cause death. Systemic JIA accounts for about 10% of JIA cases.[40]

Oligoarticular arthritis affects no more than four joints. Uveitis is more common in this subgroup and is seen more often in those with positive ANA results.[40] The third subgroup, accounting for approximately 25% of the total cases of JIA, is polyarticular disease. This third classification affects five or more joints. In this form of arthritis, RF may or may not be present but when it is, the disease process may be more severe and likely to resemble adult RA.[40]

Enthesitis-related JIA is characterized by enthesitis or pain between bones and tendons, ligaments or other connective tissue as well as inflammation in other parts of the body. It may also be called spondyloarthritis and occurs more frequently in boys, beginning between 8 and 15 years of age. Often, the children will present with a positive HLA-B27 gene test.[40]

Juvenile psoriatic arthritis often occurs with psoriasis that may begin long before joint symptoms occur. Undifferentiated arthritis refers to a juvenile arthritis that either spans two or more subtypes or does not fit into any of the listed subtypes.[40]

The prognosis for most children with JIA is variable and dependent on clinical factors. These factors vary based on the subtype and whether the disease is systemic.[41] Treatment also varies based on subtype and clinical factors.[41] NSAIDs generally are the first-line drugs used in treating JIA.[41] Second-line agents are methotrexate, glucocorticoid joint injection, and TNF-α inhibitors.[41] Other aspects of treatment of children with JIA require careful attention to growth and development as well as to nutritional issues.

Systemic Lupus Erythematosus

The features of SLE in children are similar to those in adults. The incidence in children is 0.5 to 0.6 cases per 100,000 in children younger than 15 years.[42] African Americans, especially girls, are the most frequently affected by SLE. Most children who are diagnosed with SLE are 8 years or older, although SLE has been seen from infancy throughout the age cycle.[42] The clinical manifestations of SLE in children reflect the extent and severity of systemic involvement. The best prognostic indicator in children is the extent of renal involvement, which is more common and more severe in children than in adults with SLE.

Children with SLE may present with symptoms including fever, malaise, anorexia, and weight loss. Symptoms of the integumentary, musculoskeletal, central nervous, cardiac, pulmonary, and hematopoietic systems are like those in adults. Endocrine abnormalities include Cushing syndrome from long-term corticosteroid use and autoimmune thyroiditis.

Treatment of SLE in children is like that in adults. The use of NSAIDs, corticosteroids, antimalarial drugs, and immunosuppressive agents depends on the symptoms. Corticosteroids may cause stunting of growth and necrosis of femoral heads and other joints. Immunization schedules should be maintained using attenuated rather than live vaccines. The diversity of the clinical manifestations of SLE in the young requires the establishment of a comprehensive treatment or management program.

Juvenile Dermatomyositis

Juvenile dermatomyositis (JDMS) is a rare inflammatory myopathy primarily involving skin and muscle and associated with a characteristic rash. JDMS is the most frequently occurring disorder among the group of heterogeneous immune-mediated disorders called juvenile idiopathic inflammatory myopathies.[43] JDMS can affect children of all ages, with a mean age at onset of 7.5 years.[43] There is an increased incidence among girls. The cause is not known. Symmetric proximal muscle weakness, elevated muscle enzymes, evidence of vasculitis, and electromyographic changes confirming an inflammatory myopathy are diagnostic for JDMS. Generalized vasculitis is not seen in the adult form of the disease. In children weak proximal muscles, a heliotrope rash around the eyes, Gottron papules, and vasculopathy are characteristic symptoms.[43] The rash may precede or follow the onset of proximal muscle weakness. Periorbital edema, erythema, and eyelid telangiectasia are common. The criteria of Bohan and Pila are used to diagnose this disorder. A child must have three out of the five criteria (progressive proximal symmetrical weakness, increased muscle enzyme levels, abnormal muscle biopsy results, abnormal electromyogram [EMG] results, and compatible cutaneous disease) to be diagnosed with JDMS.[27]

Calcifications can occur in 30% to 50% of children with JDMS and are by far the most debilitating symptom. The calcifications appear at pressure points or sites of previous trauma. JDMS is treated primarily with corticosteroids to reduce inflammation.

Juvenile Spondyloarthropathies

AS, reactive arthritis, psoriatic arthritis, and SpA associated with ulcerative colitis and regional enteritis can affect children as well as adults. In children, spondyloarthropathy manifests in peripheral joints first, mimicking oligoarticular JIA. There is no evidence of sacroiliac or spine involvement until later in the disease, such as months to years after onset. The SpA are more common in boys and commonly occur in children who have a positive family history. HLA-B27 typing is helpful in diagnosing children because of the unusual presentation of the disease.

Management of the disease involves physical therapy, education, and attention to school and growth and development issues. Medication includes the use of salicylates, NSAIDs, and biologic modifiers.

Rheumatic Diseases in Older Adults

Arthritis is the most common complaint of older adults. The pain, stiffness, and muscle weakness affect daily life, often threatening independence and quality of life. Symptoms of the rheumatic diseases can also have an indirect effect on and even threaten the duration of life for older adults. The weakness and gait disturbance that often accompany rheumatic diseases can contribute to the likelihood of falls and fracture, causing suffering, increased health care costs, further loss of independence, and the potential for a decreased life span.

Older adults cope less well with mild to moderately severe disease, which, in younger people, is less likely to lead to serious disability for the same degree of impairment. Unfortunately, older adults, and often their health care providers, think the problems associated with arthritis are an inevitable consequence of aging and fail to take advantage of measures that can improve the quality of life.

Older adults often have multiple problems complicating diagnosis and management. The diagnosis of an older adult with a musculoskeletal problem must consider a wide variety of disorders that usually are regarded as outside the range of typical rheumatic disease. Among these are metastatic malignancy, multiple myeloma, musculoskeletal disorders accompanying endocrine or metabolic disorders, orthopedic conditions, and neurologic disease. The diagnosis may be missed if the assumption is that musculoskeletal problems in the older adult are caused by OA.

There is an increased incidence of false-positive test results for RF and ANA in the older adult population with or without rheumatic disease because older adults are better producers of autoantibodies than younger people. There are differences in the manifestations, diagnosis, and treatment of some of the rheumatic diseases in older adults. The usual presentation of these conditions was discussed earlier in this chapter. One form of rheumatic disease that has a predilection for older adults is polymyalgia rheumatica, which generally affects people greater than 60 years of age.

Rheumatoid Arthritis

The prevalence of RA increases with age.[4] Seropositive people are more likely to have had an acute onset with systemic features and higher disease activity. People with seronegative, elderly onset RA have a disease that usually follows a mild course. It may be that RA in older adults is a broad disorder that includes many distinct subsets with characteristic manifestations, courses, and outcomes.

Systemic Lupus Erythematosus

SLE is another condition with different manifestations in older adults. The disease is accompanied less frequently by renal involvement. However, pleurisy, pericarditis, arthritis, and symptoms closely resembling polymyalgia rheumatica are more common than in younger people. The characteristics of SLE in older adults closely resemble those of drug-induced SLE.

Osteoarthritis

OA is by far the most common form of arthritis among older adults. It is the greatest cause of disability and limitation of activity in older populations worldwide Disease prevention and early intervention is the current focus but has proven difficult because of the multifactorial epidemiology of the disorder including biologic, biomechanical, and genetic factors.[35]

Crystal-Induced Arthropathies

Gout. The incidence of clinical gout increases with advancing age, in part because of the increased involvement of joints after years of continued hyperuricemia. High serum urate levels rarely occur in females, especially before menopause, because of estrogen's uricosuric effects.[38] Gouty attacks in older adults are sometimes precipitated by the use of diuretics. The treatment of gout is often more difficult in older adults.

Pseudogout. As part of the tissue-aging process, OA develops with associated cartilage degeneration and the shedding of calcium pyrophosphate crystals into the joint cavity. These crystals may produce a low-grade chronic inflammation—the chronic pseudogout syndrome. The accumulation of calcium pyrophosphate and related crystalline deposits in articular cartilage is common in the elderly. There are no medications that can remove the crystals from the joints. Although it may be asymptomatic, presence of the crystals may contribute to more rapid cartilage deterioration. This condition may coexist with severe OA.

Polymyalgia Rheumatica

Polymyalgia rheumatica is an inflammatory condition of unknown origin characterized by aching and morning stiffness in the shoulder and pelvic areas.[44,45] Of the forms of arthritis affecting older adults, it is one of the more difficult to diagnose and one of the most important to identify. Older females are especially at risk. Polymyalgia rheumatica is a common syndrome of older adults, rarely occurring before 50 years with a peak between 70 and 79 years of age.[44] The onset can be abrupt, with the person going to bed feeling well and awakening with pain and stiffness in the neck, shoulders, and hips.

Diagnosis is based on the pain and stiffness persisting for at least 1 month and an elevated eosinophil sedimentation rate (ESR). The diagnosis is confirmed when the symptoms respond dramatically to a small dose of prednisone, a corticosteroid. Biopsies have shown that the muscles are normal, despite the name, but that a nonspecific inflammation affecting the synovial tissue is present. It is possible that a number of people are erroneously diagnosed as having RA or OA. For symptomatic people with an elevated ESR, the diagnosis usually is made. Generally, the person is given oral steroids. People with polymyalgia rheumatica typically exhibit striking clinical improvement approximately the 2nd day after beginning the oral steroid, and this response adds to confirmation of the diagnosis.[45] People with RA also show improvement, although usually not as quickly.

Treatment with NSAIDs provides relief for some people, but most require continuing therapy with prednisone, with gradual reduction of the dose over the course of 2 to 6 years, using the person's symptoms as the primary guide. People need close monitoring during the maintenance phase with prednisone therapy. Because their symptoms are relieved, they often quit taking the prednisone and their symptoms recur, or doses are missed and the decreased dosage leads to an increase in symptoms. Unless careful assessment reveals the frequency of missed doses, the physician may be misled into increasing the dosage when it is not needed. Because of the side effects of the corticosteroids, the goal is to use the lowest dose of the drug necessary to control the symptoms. Weaning people off low-dose prednisone therapy after this length of time can be a difficult and extended process.

A certain percentage of people with polymyalgia rheumatica also develop giant cell arteritis (*i.e.*, temporal arteritis) with involvement of the ophthalmic arteries. The two conditions are considered to represent different manifestations of the same disease. Giant cell arteritis, a form of systemic vasculitis, is a systemic inflammatory disease of large and medium-sized arteries.[45] The inflammatory response seems to be a T-cell response to an antigen.

Clinical manifestations of giant cell arteritis usually begin insidiously and may exist for some time before being recognized.[44,45] It is potentially dangerous if missed or mistreated, especially if the temporal artery or other vessels supplying the eye are involved, in which case blindness can ensue quickly without treatment. Initial treatment consists of large doses of prednisone. This dosage is continued for 4 to 6 weeks and then decreased gradually.

Management of Rheumatic Diseases in Older Adults

In addition to diagnosis-specific treatment, older adults require special considerations. Management techniques that rely on modalities other than drugs are particularly important. These include assistive devices, muscle-building exercise, and local heat. Muscle-strengthening and stretching exercises are particularly effective in the older adult with age-related losses in muscle function and should be instituted early.

Joint arthroplasty can also be used for pain relief and increased function. Chronologic age is not a contraindication to surgical treatment of arthritis. In appropriately selected older candidates, survival and functional outcome after surgery are equivalent to those in younger age groups. The more sedentary activity level of the older adult makes them even better candidates for joint replacement because they put less stress and demand on the new joint.

IN SUMMARY

Rheumatic diseases that affect children can be like the adult diseases, but there are also manifestations unique to the younger population. Children with chronic diseases also must be approached with different priorities than adults. Managing rheumatic diseases in children requires a team approach to address issues of the family, school, growth and development, and coping strategies and requires a comprehensive disease management program.

Arthritis is the most common complaint of the older adult population. The pain, stiffness, and muscle weakness affect daily life, often threatening independence and quality of life. There is a difference in the manifestations, diagnosis, and treatment of some of the rheumatic diseases in older adults compared with those in the younger population. OA is the most common form of arthritis among older adults. The prevalence of RA and gout increases with advancing age. One form of rheumatic disease that has a predilection for older adults is polymyalgia rheumatica. A certain percentage of people with polymyalgia rheumatica also have giant cell arteritis, frequently with involvement of the ophthalmic arteries. If this condition is untreated, it carries a serious threat of blindness.

GERIATRIC Considerations

- People with OA report an increase in joint discomfort during damp weather and prolonged use of a particular joint[46] such as with knitting.
- Diets high in essential fatty acids reduce inflammation associated with OA.[46]
- Systemic involvement associated with RA increases with age including weight loss, fatigue, weakness, malaise, and cachexia.[46]
- A decrease in autophagy associated with aging leads to fibrosis in multiple organs such as the heart, lungs, and vasculature.[47]

PEDIATRIC Considerations

- Children with SLE complain of stiffness in the morning along with pain and swelling in the joints—most commonly the hands, wrists, and knees.[48]
- Ibuprofen places children with SLE at risk for aseptic meningitis syndrome and should be avoided[48]
- JIA is the most common chronic inflammatory disorder in children, with females being affected more than males.[48]
- Infants with developmental dysplasia of the hip and femoral anteversion are at risk for early onset OA and must be monitored until the adolescent growth spurt is complete.[48]

REVIEW EXERCISES

1. A 30-year-old woman, recently diagnosed with rheumatoid arthritis (RA), complains of general fatigue and weight loss along with symmetric joint swelling, stiffness, and pain. The stiffness is more prominent in the morning and subsides during the day. Laboratory measures reveal a rheumatoid factor (RF) of 120 IU/mL (nonreactive, 0 to 39 IU/mL; weakly reactive, 40 to 79 IU/mL; reactive, >80 IU/mL) and a positive anti-CCP antibody.
   A. *Describe the immunopathogenesis of the joint changes that occur with RA.*
   B. *How do these changes relate to this woman's symptoms?*
   C. *What is the significance of her RF test results?*
   D. *What is the significance of her + anti-CCP antibody test?*
   E. *How do her complaints of general fatigue and weight loss relate to the RA disease process?*
2. A 65-year-old obese woman with a diagnosis of osteoarthritis (OA) has been having increasing pain in her right knee that worsens with movement and weight bearing and is relieved by rest. Physical examination reveals an enlarged joint with a varus deformity; coarse crepitus is felt over the joint on passive movement.
   A. *Compare the pathogenesis and articular structures involved in OA with those of RA.*
   B. *What is the origin of the enlargement of the affected joint, the varus deformity, and the crepitus that is felt on movement of the affected knee?*
   C. *Explain the predilection for involvement of the knee in people such as this woman.*
   D. *What types of treatment are available for this woman?*
3. A 75-year-old woman is seen by her health care provider because of complaints of fever, malaise, and weight loss. She is having trouble combing her hair, putting on a coat, and getting out of chairs because of the stiffness and pain in her shoulders, hip, and lower back. Because of her symptoms, the health care provider suspects the woman has polymyalgia rheumatica.
   A. *What laboratory test can be used to substantiate the diagnosis?*
   B. *What other diagnostic strategies are used to confirm the diagnosis?*
   C. *How is the disease treated?*

References

1. Arthritis Foundation. (2018). Exercise benefits for hip osteoarthritis. [Online]. Available: https://www.arthritis.org/about-arthritis/types/osteo-arthritis/articles/hip-oa-exercises.php. Accessed March 14, 2018
2. Strayer D., Rubin R. (Eds.). (2015). *Rubin's pathology: Clinicopathologic foundations of medicine* (7th ed.). Philadelphia, PA: Lippincott Williams & Wilkins.
3. Arnold M. B., Bykerk V. P., Boire G., et al. (2014). Are there differences between young- and older-onset early inflammatory arthritis and do these impact outcomes? An analysis from the CATCH cohort. *Rheumatology* 53, 1075–1086.
4. Dunphy L. M., Windland-Brown J. E., Porter B. O., et al. (2015). *Primary Care: The Art and Science of Advanced Practice Nursing* (4th ed.). Philadelphia, PA: FA Davis.
5. Schulte-Pelkum J. S., Schulz-Knappe P. S. (2015). *A Multi-marker Approach to Diagnosing Autoimmune Diseases. MLO: Medical Laboratory Observer* 47(10), 44–46.
6. Liu Q., Zhao J., Zhou H. , et al. (2015). Parthenolide inhibits pro-inflammatory cytokine production and exhibits protective effects on progression of collagen-induced arthritis in a rat model. *Scandinavian Journal of Rheumatology* 44(3), 182–191.
7. Jämsen E., Virta L. J., Hakala M., et al. (2013). The decline in joint replacement surgery in RA is associated with a concomitant increase in the intensity of anti-rheumatic therapy: A nationwide register-based study from 1995–2010. *Acta Orthopaedica* 84(4), 331–337.
8. Jensen S. (2014). *Nursing Health Assessment: A Best Practice Approach* (2nd ed.). Philadelphia, PA: Lippincott Williams & Wilkins.
9. American Academy of Orthopaedic Surgeons; Armstrong A. D., Hubbard M. C. (Eds.). (2016). *Essentials of Musculoskeletal Care* (5th ed.). Rosemont, IL: American Academy of Orthopaedic Surgeons.
10. Woolston W., Connelly L. M.(2017). Felty's syndrome: A qualitative case study. *Medsurg Nursing* 26(2), 105–118.
11. Schuler S., Brunner M. Bernauer W. (2016). Rituximab and acute retinal necrosis in a patient with scleromalacia and rheumatoid arthritis. *Ocular Immunology and Inflammation* 24(1), 96–98.
12. American College of Rheumatology and European League Against Rheumatism Association. (2010). 2010 ACR–EULAR classification criteria of rheumatoid arthritis. [Online]. Available: https://www.rheumatology.org/Portals/0/Files/2010%20Rheumatoid%20Arthritis%20Classification_EXCERPT%202010.pdf. Accessed March 16, 2018
13. Aletaha D., Neogi T., Silman A. J., et al. (2010). 2010 Rheumatoid arthritis classification criteria.: An American college of rheumatology/European league against rheumatism collaborative initiative. *Arthritis and Rheumatism* 62(9), 2569–2581.
14. Mastrangelo A., Colasanti T., Barbati C., et al. (2015). The role of post-translational protein modifications in rheumatological diseases: focus on rheumatoid arthritis. *Journal of Immunology Research* 2015(Article ID: 712490), 1–10.
15. Scally, S.W., Petersen, J., Law, S.C., et al. (2013). A molecular basis for the association of the HLA-DRB1 locus, citrullination, and rheumatoid arthritis. *Journal of Experimental Medicine* 210(12), 2569–2582.
16. Arthritis Foundation. (2018).Rheumatoid arthritis treatment. [Online]. Available: https://www.arthritis.org/about-arthritis/types/rheumatoid-arthritis/treatment.php. Accessed March 17, 2018
17. National Rheumatoid Arthritis Society. (2018). Anti-TNFα treatment in rheumatoid arthritis. [Online]. Available: https://www.nras.org.uk/anti-tnfa-treatment-in-rheumatoid-arthritis. Accessed March 17, 2018
18. Singh J. A., Furst D. E., Bharat A., et al. (2012). 2012 update of the 2008 American College Of Rheumatology recommendations for the use of disease-modifying antirheumatic drugs and biologic agents in the treatment of arthritis. *Arthritis Care and Research* 64(5), 635–639.
19. Lupus Foundation of America. What is lupus? [Online]. Available: https://resources.lupus.org/entry/what-is-lupus?utm_source=lupusorg&utm_medium=answersFAQ. Accessed March 17, 2018
20. American College of Rheumatology. Lupus. [Online]. Available: https://www.rheumatology.org/I-Am-A/Patient-Caregiver/Diseases-Conditions/Lupus. Accessed March 17, 2018

21. The Johns Hopkins Lupus Center. Lupus primer: Types of lupus. [Online]. Available: https://www.hopkinslupus.org/lupus-info/types-lupus/. Accessed March 17, 2018
22. American College of Rheumatology. (2011). Systemic lupus erythematosus. [Online]. Available: https://www.rheumatology.org/Portals/0/Files/1997%20 Update%20of%201982%20Revised.pdf. Accessed March 17, 2018
23. Classification and Response Criteria Subcommittee of the American College of Rheumatology Committee on Quality Measures. (2006). Development of classification and response criteria for rheumatic diseases. *Arthritis and Rheumatism (Arthritis Care and Research)* 55(2), 348–352.
24. Nasdashkevich O., Davis P. Fritzler M. J. (2004). A proposal of criteria for the classification of systemic sclerosis. *Medical Science Monitor* 10, 615–621.
25. Oldroyd A., Lilleker J., Chinoy H. (2017). Idiopathic inflammatory myopathies – a guide to subtypes, diagnostic approach and treatment. *Clinical Medicine* 17(4), 322–328.
26. Bohan A., Peter J. B. (1975). Polymyositis and dermatomyositis (first of two parts). *New England Journal of Medicine* 292, 344–347.
27. Bohan A., Peter J. B. (1975). Polymyositis and dermatomyositis (second of two parts). *New England Journal of Medicine* 292, 403–407.
28. Bond D. (2013). Ankylosing spondylitis: Diagnosis and treatment. *Nursing Standard* 28(16–18), 52–59.
29. Montilla C., Del Pino-Montes J., Collantes-Estevez E., et al. (2012). Clinical features of late-onset ankylosing spondylitis: comparison with early-onset disease. *Journal of Rheumatology* 39(5), 1008–1012.
30. Rashid T., Ebringer A. (2012). Autoimmunity in rheumatic diseases is induced by microbial infections via crossreactivity or molecular mimicry. *Autoimmune Diseases* 2012 (Article ID: 539282), 1–9.
31. Calvo-Gutiérrez J., Garrido-Castro J. L., González-Navas C., et al. (2016). Inter-rater reliability of clinical mobility measures in ankylosing spondylitis. *BMC Musculoskeletal Disorders* 17, 1–6.
32. Rudwaleit M., van der Heijde D., Landewé R., et al. (2009). The development of Assessment of SpondyloArthritis international Society classification criteria for axial spondyloarthritis (part II): Validation and final selection. *Annals of the Rheumatic Diseases* 68(6), 777–783.
33. Van der Heijde D., Ramiro S, Landew R., et al. 2016 Update of the ASAS-EULAR managements recommendations for axial spondyloarthritis. *Annals of the Rheumatic Diseases* 76, 978–991.
34. Arthritis Foundation. (2018). *What is Psoriatic arthritis? [Online].* Available: https://www.arthritis.org/about-arthritis/types/psoriatic-arthritis/what-is-psoriatic-arthritis.php. Accessed March 18, 2018
35. Glyn-Jones S., Palmer A. J. R., Agricola R., et al. (2015). Osteoarthritis. *Lancet* 386, 376–387.
36. American College of Rheumatology. (2018). Osteoarthritis. [Online]. Available: https://www.rheumatology.org/Practice-Quality/Clinical-Support/Clinical-Practice-Guidelines/Osteoarthritis. Accessed March 18, 2018
37. American Academy of Orthopaedics Surgeons. *Choosing Wisely. [Online].* Available: http://www.choosingwisely.org/clinician-lists/american-academy-orthopaedic-surgeons-glucosamine-chondroitin-for-symptomatic-osteoarthritis-of-knee/. Accessed March 18, 2018
38. Abhishek A., Roddy E., Doherty M. (2017). Gout – a guide for the general and acute physicians. *Clinical Medicine* 17(1), 54–59.
39. Khanna D., Fitzgerald J. D., Khanna P. P., et al. (2012) 2012 American College of Rheumatology guidelines for management of gout. Part 1: Systemic nonpharmacologic and pharmacologic therapeutic approaches to hyperuricemia. *Arthritis Care and Research* 64(10), 1431–1446.
40. Arthritis Foundation. (2018). What is juvenile idiopathic arthritis? [Online]. Available: https://www.arthritis.org/about-arthritis/types/juvenile-idiopathic-arthritis-jia/what-is-juvenile-idiopathic-arthritis.php. Accessed March 18, 2018
41. American College of Rheumatology. (2011). 2011 American College of Rheumatology recommendations for the treatment of juvenile idiopathic arthritis: Initiation and safety monitoring of therapeutic agents for the treatment of arthritis and systemic features. *Arthritis Care and Research* 63(4), 465–482.
42. Klein-Gitelman M. S. (2015). Pediatric systemic lupus erythematosus. [Online]. Medscape. Available: http://emedicine.medscape.com/article/1008066-overview#showall. Accessed March 18, 2018
43. Rider, L. G., Katz, J. D., Jones, O.Y. (2013). Developments in the classification and treatment of juvenile idiopathic inflammatory myopathies. *Rheumatic Diseases Clinics of North America* 39(4), 877–904.
44. Kennedy S. (2012). Polymyalgia rheumatica and giant cell arteritis: An in-depth look at diagnosis and treatment. *Journal of the American Academy of Nurse Practitioners* 24(5), 277–285.
45. Werner R. Polymyalgia rheumatica and giant cell arteritis: Common, dangerous, treatable. *Massage & Bodywork* 32(6), 36–39.
46. Eliopoulos C. (2018). Mobility. In *Gerontological Nursing* (9th ed., pp. 328–350). Philadelphia, PA: Wolters Kluwer.
47. Luckhardt T. R., Thannickal V. J. (2015). Systemic sclerosis-associated fibrosis: An accelerated aging phenotype?. *Current Opinion in Rheumatology* 27(6), 571–576. DOI: 10.1097/BOR.0000000000000219
48. Bazner-Chandler J. (2014). The child with altered musculoskeletal status. In Bowden V., Greenberg C. S. (Eds.), *Children and Their Families: The Continuum of Nursing Care*. Philadelphia, PA: Wolters Kluwer.

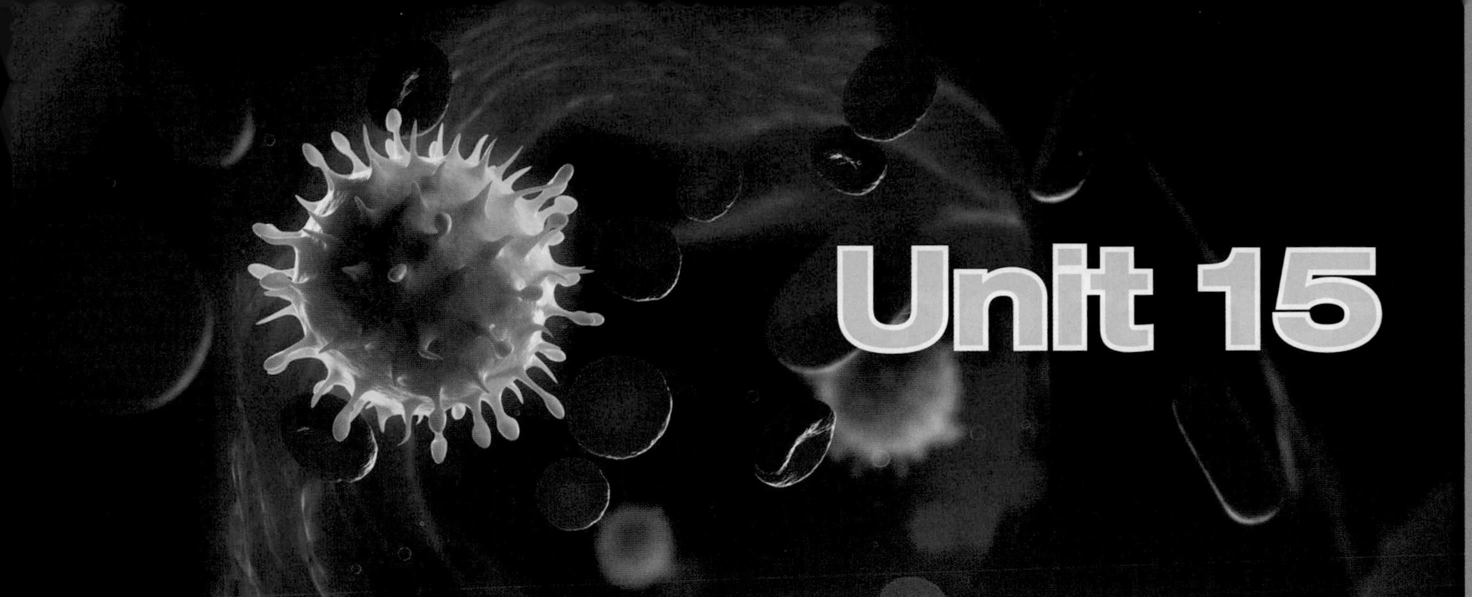

Unit 15

Disorders of Integumentary Function

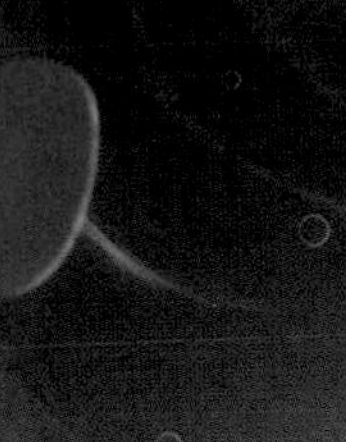

Lauren Ronde, 18 years old, is a college freshman who presents with a growth on her lower right ear lobe and a rash on her fingers that she describes as "very itchy." She explains that the rash started 2 days ago and it is really bothering her. After examining the rash, the caregiver describes the rash as having an erythematous background, slightly swollen, nonpainful to touch, and papular with 1-mm vesicles. It is predominantly on her fingers bilaterally, and a specimen is unable to be obtained for culture. Some of the blisters are intact, but most have erupted and are resolving according to Lauren. After a thorough history and physical examination, the rash is assumed to be a result of a hypersensitivity response to a chemical(s) from just beginning work in her chemistry lab. The rash is presumed to be due to allergic contact dermatitis. She is told to wear gloves at all times in the chemistry lab and apply a slight film of hydrocortisone 1% cream to the rash after her shower every day and upon washing her hands after the lab session each day. A few days later, she calls in to report that after following this process, her rash has almost disappeared and that the hydrocortisone is effective with the itching.

The growth on her right lower ear lobe is irregularly shaped, elevated, and firm to the touch. It is located at the site of her last ear piercing. She is told that this is a keloid and that it was caused by excessive formation of collagen during the repair of dermal tissue after her last ear piercing. It is her first piercing and she was scheduled for three more piercings. After hearing about the etiology of the keloid, she has canceled her piercing appointments. She is told that there is nothing one can do about removing a keloid because doing so would require another incision, which would trigger more keloid formation.

Structure and Function of the Skin

51

Lisa Hight

The skin, also called the *integumentum*, is one of most versatile organs of the body, accounting for roughly 16% of the body's weight. It forms the major interface between the internal organs and the external environment. The thickness of the skin can range from less than 1 to greater than 5 mm.[1] For example, the epidermal thickness on the eyelid is approximately 0.5 mm, whereas the thickness on the sole of the foot is 1.5 mm.[2] As the body's first line of defense, the skin is continuously subjected to potentially harmful environmental agents, including solid matter, liquids, gases, sunlight, and microorganisms. Although it may become bruised, lacerated, burned, or infected, it has remarkable properties that allow for a continuous cycle of shedding, healing, and cell regeneration.

As the outer covering of the body, the skin may demonstrate outwardly what occurs inside the body. A number of systemic diseases are manifested by skin disorders (*e.g.*, malar rash associated with systemic lupus erythematous, bronze skin with Addison disease, and jaundice with liver disease). Thus, it is important to recognize that although skin eruptions are frequently caused by primary disorders of the skin, they may also represent manifestations of systemic disease.

STRUCTURE AND FUNCTION OF THE SKIN

After completing this section of the chapter, the learner will be able to meet the following objectives:

- Characterize the changes in a keratinocyte from its inception in the basal lamina to its arrival on the outer surface of the skin.
- Describe the following skin appendages and their functions: sebaceous gland, eccrine gland, apocrine gland, nails, and hair.
- Characterize the skin in terms of sensory and immune functions.

Skin Structures

There are great variations in skin structure on different parts of the body. Therefore, "normal skin" on any one surface of the body is difficult to describe. Variations are found in the properties of the skin, such as the thickness of skin layers, the distribution of sweat glands, and the number and size of hair follicles. For example, the epidermis is thicker on the palms of the hands and soles of the feet than elsewhere on the body. The dermis, on the other hand, is thickest on the back, whereas the subcutaneous fat layer is thickest on the abdomen and buttocks. Hair follicles are densely distributed on the scalp, axillae, and genitalia, but they are sparse on the inner arms and abdomen. The apocrine sweat glands are confined to the axillae and the anogenital area. Nevertheless, certain structural properties are common to the skin on all areas of the body.

The skin is composed of three layers:

1. Epidermis (outer layer)
2. Dermis (inner layer)
3. Subcutaneous fat layer

The basement membrane divides the first two layers. The subcutaneous tissue, a layer of loose connective and adipose connective tissues, binds the dermis to the underlying tissues of the body (Fig. 51.1).

KEY POINTS

ORGANIZATION OF SKIN STRUCTURES

- The epidermis, which is avascular, is composed of four to five layers of stratified squamous keratinized epithelial cells that are formed in the deepest layer of the epidermis and migrate to the skin surface to replace cells that are lost during normal skin shedding.
- The basement membrane is a thin adhesive layer that cements the epidermis to the dermis. This is the layer involved in blister formation.
- The dermis is a connective tissue layer that separates the epidermis from the underlying subcutaneous fat layer. It contains the blood vessels and nerve fibers that supply the epidermis.

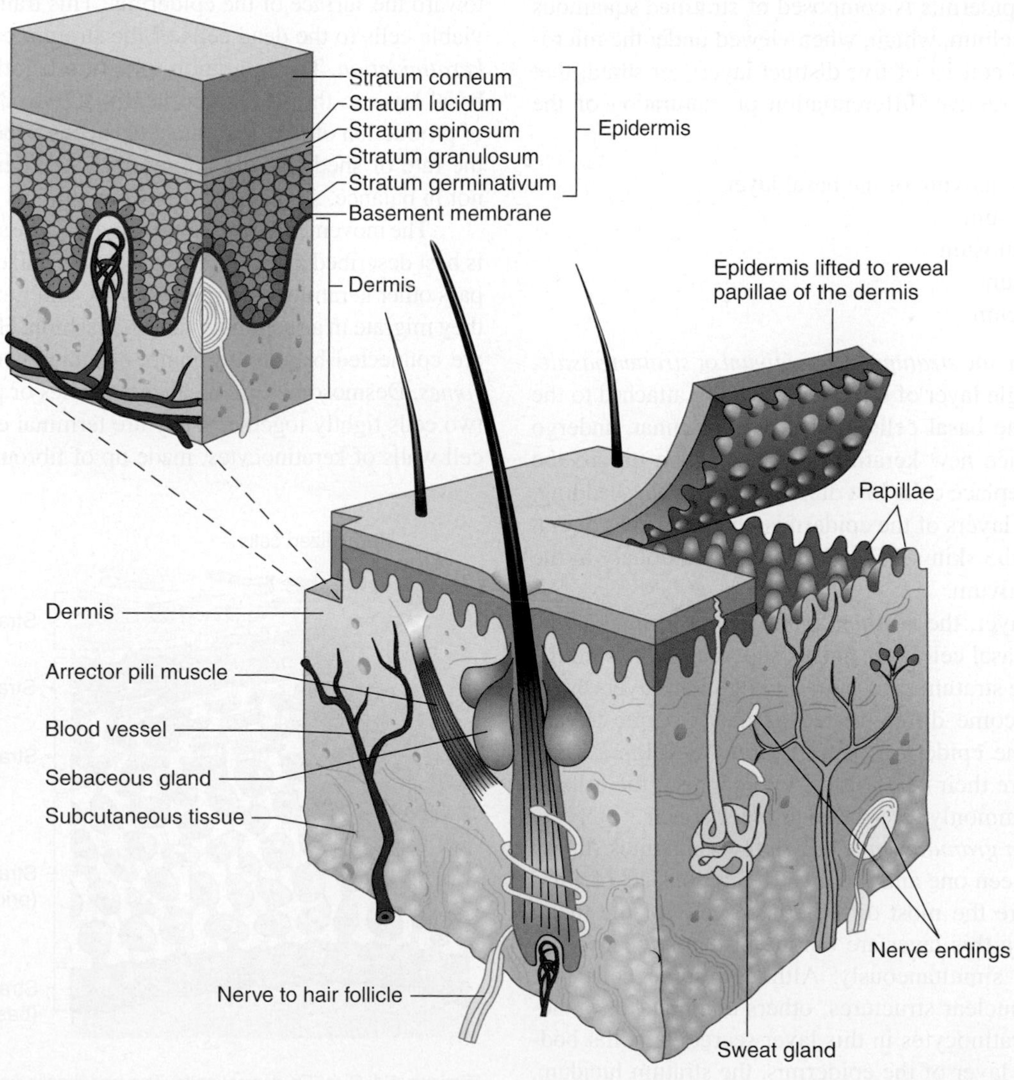

Figure 51.1 • Three-dimensional view of the skin.

Epidermis

The functions of the skin depend on the properties of its outermost layer, the epidermis. The epidermis covers the body. It is specialized in areas to form the various skin appendages, which include the hair, nails, and glandular structures.[3] The keratinocytes of the epidermis produce a fibrous protein called *keratin*, which is essential for the protective function of the skin. In addition to the keratinocytes, the epidermis has three other types of cells that arise from its basal layer—melanocytes, Merkel cells, and Langerhans cells. Melanocytes produce a pigment called *melanin*, which is responsible for skin color, tanning, and protection against ultraviolet radiation. Merkel cells provide sensory information and Langerhans cells link the epidermis to the immune system. The epidermis contains openings for two types of glands—sweat glands, which produce watery secretions, and sebaceous glands, which produce an oily secretion called *sebum*.

Keratinocytes. The *keratinocyte* is the major cell of the epidermis, comprising approximately 85% of the cells of this layer. The epidermis is composed of stratified squamous keratinized epithelium, which, when viewed under the microscope, is seen to consist of five distinct layers, or strata, that represent a progressive differentiation or maturation of the keratinocytes:

1. Stratum germinativum or the basal layer
2. Stratum spinosum
3. Stratum granulosum
4. Stratum lucidum
5. Stratum corneum

The deepest layer, the *stratum germinativum* or *stratum basale*, consists of a single layer of basal cells that are attached to the basal lamina. The basal cells, which are columnar, undergo mitosis to produce new keratinocytes that move toward the skin surface to replace cells lost during normal skin shedding. Unlike the other layers of the epidermis, the basal cells do not migrate toward the skin surface, but remain stationary in the stratum germinativum.

The next layer, the *stratum spinosum*, is formed as the progeny of the basal cell layer moves superficially toward the skin surface. The stratum spinosum is two to four layers thick, and its cells become differentiated as they migrate toward the surface of the epidermis. Because they develop a spiny appearance where their cell borders interconnect, the cells of this layer are commonly referred to as *prickle cells*.[1]

The *stratum granulosum* is only a few cells thick (thickness varies between one and three cells).[1] It consists of granular cells that are the most differentiated cells of the living skin. The cells in this layer are unique in that two opposing functions occur simultaneously. Although some cells lose cytoplasm and nuclear structures, others continue to synthesize keratin. Keratinocytes in this layer secrete lamellar bodies into the next layer of the epidermis, the stratum lucidum, providing the skin with its important water-impermeable properties.

The *stratum lucidum*, which lies just superficial to the stratum granulosum, is a thin, transparent layer found primarily on the thick skin such as over the palms of the hands and soles of the feet.[1] It consists of transitional cells that retain some of the functions of living skin cells from the layers below but otherwise resembles the cells of the stratum corneum.

The most superficial layer, the *stratum corneum*, consists of dead, keratinized cells. This layer contains the most cell layers and the largest cells of the epidermis. It ranges from 15 layers thick in areas such as the face to 25 layers or more on the arm. Specialized areas, such as the palms of the hands or soles of the feet, have 100 or more layers.

The keratinocytes that originate in the basal layer change morphologically as they are pushed toward the outer layer of the epidermis. For example, in the basal layer, keratinocytes are cuboidal to low columnar. As it is pushed into the stratum spinosum, the keratinocyte becomes multisided. It becomes flatter in the granular layer and is flattened and elongated in the stratum corneum (Fig. 51.2). Keratinocytes also change cytoplasmic structure and composition as they are pushed toward the surface of the epidermis. This transformation from viable cells to the dead cells of the stratum corneum is called *keratinization*. The migration time of a keratinocyte from the basal layer to the stratum corneum is 20 to 30 days. The rate of production of new keratinocytes needs to be consistent with the rate of shedding old keratinocytes. When these rates are not in balance, skin anomalies occur.

The movement of the keratinocytes to the surface of the skin is best described as random or nonsynchronized. Keratinocytes pass other keratinocytes, melanocytes, and Langerhans cells as they migrate in a seemingly random fashion. However, the cells are connected by minute points of attachment called *desmosomes*. Desmosomes are localized patches or plaques that hold two cells tightly together. They are terminal end points on the cell walls of keratinocytes, made up of fibrous material that is

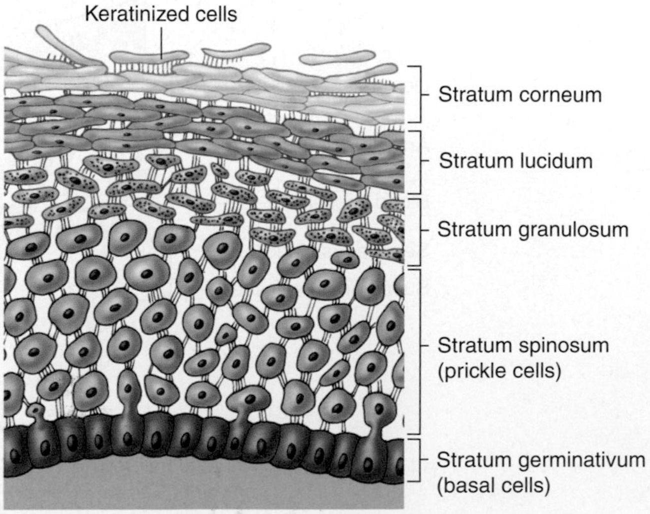

Figure 51.2 • Epidermal cells. The basal cells undergo mitosis, producing keratinocytes that change their size and shape as they move upward, replacing cells that are lost during normal cell shedding.

bound into bundles, called *tonofilaments*. Desmosomes keep the cells from detaching and provide some structure to the skin while it is in perpetual motion. The basal layer provides the underlying structure and stability for the epidermis.

Besides desmosomes, there are three other types of cellular junctions that bind keratinocytes—adherens junctions, gap junctions, and tight junctions. *Adherens junctions* are specialized structures that provide strong mechanical connections between cells. They are responsible for adhesion between cells, communicate about the presence of neighboring cells, and anchor the skin cells. *Gap junctions* are cylindrical channels that permit ions and small molecules to pass between cells. They are composed of proteins called *connexins*. *Tight junctions* are made of transmembrane proteins that function to prevent substances between cells.

Keratinocytes produce keratin, a complex protein that forms the surface of the skin and is also the structural protein of the hair and nails. Once believed to be passive cells passing through epidermal layers while changing morphologically, keratinocytes are now known to be active secretory cells that play an important role in the immunobiology of the skin by communicating and regulating cells of the immune response and secreting cytokines and inflammatory mediators.

Melanocytes. *Melanocytes* are pigment-synthesizing cells that are scattered in the basal layer and are responsible for skin color.[1,2] They function to produce pigment granules called *melanin*, the substance that gives the skin its color. There are two major forms of melanin—*eumelanin* and *pheomelanin*. The two forms of eumelanin are brown and black; pheomelanin is yellow to red. The type of melanin produced depends on the stimulation of specific hormones or proteins and the binding of these substances to receptors on the melanocyte. Eumelanin is the most abundant in humans. Exposure to the sun's ultraviolet rays increases the production of eumelanin, causing tanning to occur. The primary function of such melanin is to protect the skin by absorbing and scattering harmful ultraviolet rays, which are associated with skin cancers. Localized concentrations of eumelanin are also responsible for the formation of freckles and moles.

Pheomelanin, the yellow to red pigment, is found in all humans. It is particularly concentrated in the lips, nipples, glans penis, and vagina. Besides the skin, it is found in the hair, particularly red hair. It has been suggested that the reason fair-haired people are more susceptible to skin cancers may be due to the enhanced photoreactivity of pheomelanin, as compared with eumelanin.

The ability to synthesize melanin depends on the ability of the melanocytes to produce an enzyme called *tyrosinase*, which converts the amino acid tyrosine to a precursor of melanin. A genetic lack of this enzyme results in a clinical condition called *albinism*. People with this disorder lack pigmentation in the skin, hair, and iris of the eye. Tyrosinase is synthesized in the rough endoplasmic reticulum of the melanocytes and then routed to membranous vesicles in the Golgi complex called *melanosomes*. Melanin is subsequently synthesized in

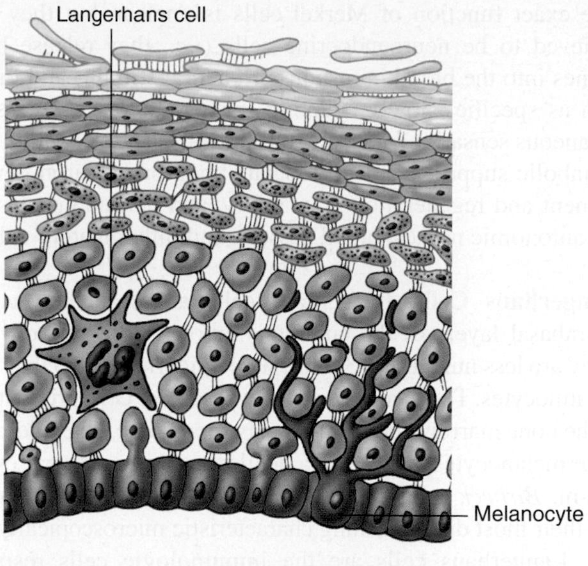

Figure 51.3 • The melanocytes, which are located in the basal layer of the skin, produce melanin pigment granules that give the skin its color. The melanocytes have threadlike, cytoplasm-filled extensions that are used in passing the pigment granules to the keratinocytes.

the melanosomes. Melanocytes have long, cytoplasm-filled dendritic processes that contain accumulated melanosomes and extend between the keratinocytes. Although the melanocytes remain in the basal layer, the melanosomes are transferred to the keratinocytes through their dendritic processes. The dendrite tip containing the melanosome is engulfed by a nearby keratinocyte, and the melanin is transferred (Fig. 51.3).

The amount of melanin in the keratinocytes determines a person's skin color.[2] Dark-skinned and light-skinned people have approximately the same number of melanocytes, but the production and packaging of pigment are different. In dark-skinned people, *larger* melanin-containing melanosomes are produced and transferred individually to the keratinocyte. In light-skinned people, *smaller* melanosomes are produced and then packaged together in a membrane before being transferred to the keratinocyte. All people, regardless of skin color, have relatively few or no melanocytes in the epidermis of the palms of the hands or soles of the feet. In light-skinned people, the number of melanocytes decreases with age, and the skin becomes lighter and is more susceptible to skin cancer when exposed to ultraviolet light. However, people with vitiligo, a skin problem where the melanocytes are destroyed, have a significantly reduced risk of developing nonmelanoma skin cancers, whereas people with albinism have a significantly increased risk.[4]

Merkel Cells. Merkel cells are clear cells found in the stratum basale of the epidermis. They are connected to other skin cells by desmosomes. Each Merkel cell is connected to an afferent nerve terminal, forming a structure known as a *Merkel disk*. They are the sparsest cells of the epidermis and are found over the entire body, but are most plentiful in the basal layer of the fingers, toes, lips, and oral cavity, and in the outermost sheath of hair follicles (*i.e.*, the touch areas).

The exact function of Merkel cells is unclear, but they are believed to be neuroendocrine cells (*i.e.*, they release hormones into the blood in response to neural stimuli) and function as specific, slowly adapting sensory touch receptors in cutaneous sensation.[1] Merkel cells may also be involved in the metabolic support of their associated neurons, neuron development and regeneration after injury, and neurotransmission for autonomic nerves, blood vessels, and inflammatory cells.

Langerhans Cells. Langerhans cells are scattered in the suprabasal layers of the epidermis among the keratinocytes. They are less numerous (3% to 5% of epidermal cells) than the keratinocytes. They are derived from precursor cells originating in the bone marrow and continuously repopulate the epidermis. Like melanocytes, they have a dendritic shape and clear cytoplasm. *Birbeck granules* that often resemble tennis racquets are their most distinguishing characteristic microscopically.[1]

Langerhans cells are the immunologic cells responsible for recognizing foreign antigens harmful to the body (Fig. 51.4). As such, Langerhans cells play an important role in defending the body against foreign antigens. Langerhans cells bind antigen to their surface and process it, and, bearing the processed antigen, migrate from the epidermis into lymphatic vessels and then into regional lymph nodes, where they are known as *dendritic cells*. During their migration in the lymph system, the Langerhans cells become potent antigen-presenting cells.[1] Langerhans cells are innervated by sympathetic nerve fibers, which may explain why the skin's immune system is altered under stress. An example of this is the exacerbations of acne seen in people under stress. Langerhans cells and the keratinocytes produce a number of cytokines that stimulate maturation of skin-localizing T lymphocytes.

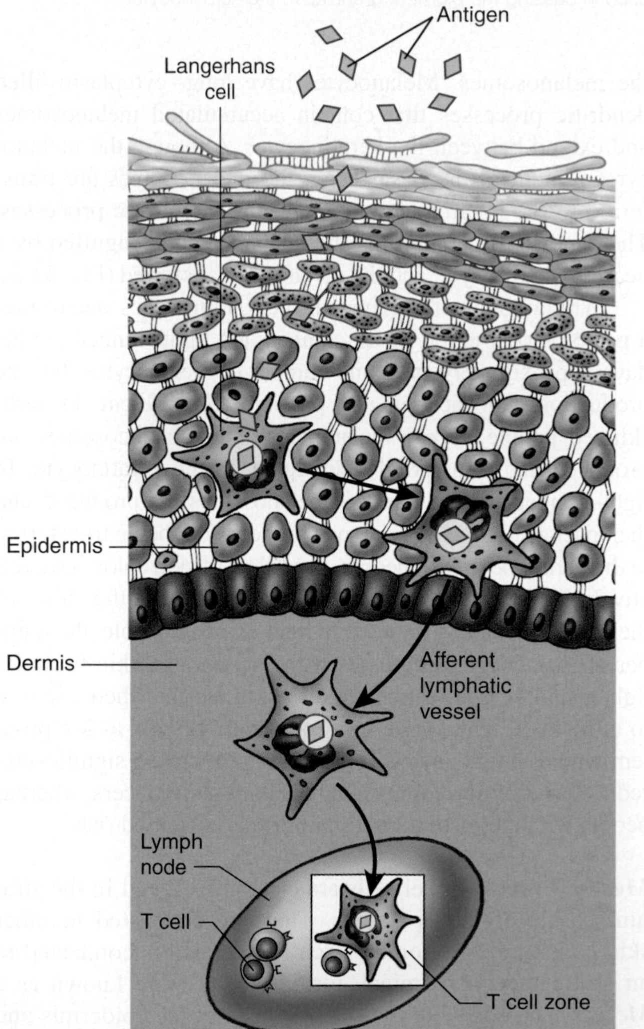

Figure 51.4 • Langerhans cells.

Basement Membrane

The terms *basement membrane* and *basal lamina* are often used interchangeably. Technically, however, the basal lamina is a component of the basement membrane. The basement membrane is a layer of intercellular and extracellular matrices that serves as an interface between the dermis and the epidermis (Fig. 51.5). It separates the epithelium from the underlying connective tissue, it anchors the epithelium to the loose connective tissue underneath, and it serves as a selective filter for molecules moving between the two layers. It is also a major site of immunoglobulin and complement deposition in skin disease. The basement membrane is involved in skin disorders that cause bullae or blister formation.[1]

The basement membrane consists of three distinct zones or layers—lamina lucida, lamina densa, and lamina fibroreticularis—all of which contribute to the adhesion of the two skin layers. The *lamina lucida* is an electron-lucent layer where adherence proteins are located. It consists of fine anchoring filaments and a cell adhesion glycoprotein, called *laminin*, which plays a role in the organization of the macromolecules in the basement membrane zone and promotes attachment of cells to the extracellular matrix. The *lamina densa* contains an adhesive called *type IV collagen* as well as laminin. It is important in dermal–epidermal attachment. Combined, the lamina lucida and the lamina densa comprise what is known as the *basal lamina*. The *lamina fibroreticularis* then completes the basement membrane. This layer contains many anchoring microfibrils. These are short, curved structures that insert into the lamina densa and the superficial dermis, where they are known as *anchoring fibrils*. Type VII collagen, another adherent substance, has been found in the anchoring fibrils and plaques. Another component of the lamina fibroreticularis are elastic fiber bundles that extend to the dermis.[3]

Hemidesmosomes are like half desmosomes in both structure and function. They lie immediately at the basal plasma membrane and form the site or source of tonofilaments, which attach the dermis and epidermis (see Fig. 51.5).[3] Because they form a continuous link between the intracellular keratin filament network and the extracellular basement membrane, they are also involved in relaying signals between the skin layers.

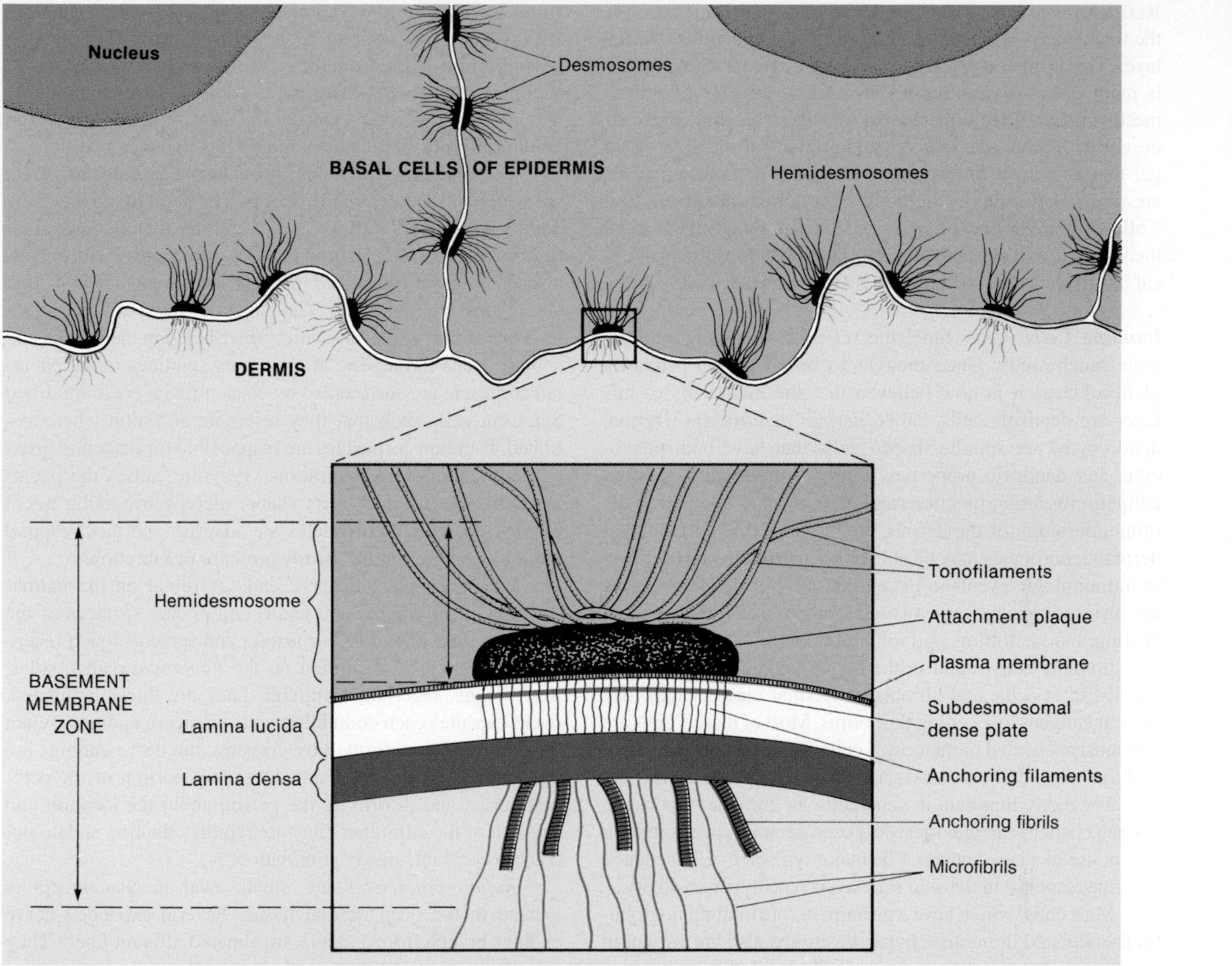

Figure 51.5 • The dermal–epidermal interface and basement membrane zone. The epithelial–mesenchymal interface comprises the basement membrane zone. This structure is mostly synthesized by the basal cells of the epidermis. This is the site of change in most diseases, from tonofilaments and attachment plaques of basal cells to microfibrils and fibrils. (From Strayer D. E., Rubin R. (Eds.) (2015). *Rubin's pathology: Clinicopathologic foundations of medicine* (7th ed., Figure 28-7, p. 1224). Philadelphia, PA: Wolters Kluwer.)

Dermis

The dermis is the connective tissue layer that separates the epidermis from the subcutaneous fat layer (see Fig. 51.1). It supports the epidermis and serves as its primary source of nutrition. The two layers of the dermis, the papillary dermis and the reticular dermis, are composed of cells, fibers, ground substances, nerves, and blood vessels. The main component of the dermis is collagen, a group of fibrous proteins. The collagen is enmeshed in a ground substance called hyaluronic acid.[3] Collagen fibers are loosely arranged in the papillary dermis, but are tightly bundled in the reticular dermis.

The pilar (hair) and glandular structures are embedded in this layer and continue through the epidermis. In general, a dark dermis is more compact than a white dermis, and consequently darker-skinned people show less wrinkling.

Papillary Dermis. The *papillary dermis* (pars papillaris) is a thin, superficial layer that lies adjacent to the epidermis. It consists of collagen fibers and ground substance. This layer is densely covered with conical projections called *dermal papillae* (see Fig. 51.1). The basal cells of the epidermis project into the papillary dermis, forming *rete ridges*. Microscopically, the junction between the epidermis and the dermis appears like undulating ridges and valleys. It is believed that the dense structure of the dermal papillae serves to minimize the separation of the dermis and the epidermis. Dermal papillae contain capillaries, end arterioles, and venules that nourish the epidermal layers of the skin. This layer of the dermis is richly vascularized. Lymph vessels and nerve tissue also are found in this layer.

Reticular Dermis. The *reticular dermis* (pars reticularis) is the thicker area of the dermis and forms the bulk of the dermal layer. This is the tough layer in animal hides from which leather is made. The reticular dermis is characterized by a complex meshwork of three-dimensional collagen bundles interconnected with large elastic fibers and ground substance, a viscid gel that is rich in mucopolysaccharides. The collagen fibers are oriented parallel to the body's surface in any given area. Collagen bundles may be organized lengthwise, as on the abdomen, or in round clusters, as on the heel. The direction of surgical incisions is often determined by this organizational pattern.

Immune Cells. Over time, the reticular dermis has undergone much study. Once thought to be composed primarily of fibroblasts, it is now believed that the main cells of this layer are dendritic cells, called *dermal dendrocytes*. Dermal dendrocytes are spindle-shaped cells that have both phagocytic and dendritic properties. They are believed to possess antigen-presenting functions and play an important part in the immunobiology of the dermis. In addition, it is possible that dermal dendrocytes may be able either to initiate or to respond to immunologic events in the epidermis. Dermal dendrocytes are also thought to be involved in processes such as wound healing, blood clotting, and inflammation.

Immune cells found in the dermis include macrophages, T cells, mast cells, and fibroblasts. Dermal macrophages may present antigens to T cells in the dermis. Most of these T cells are previously activated or memory T cells. T-cell responses to macrophage- or endothelium-associated antigens in the dermis are probably more important in generating an immune response to antigen challenge in previously exposed people than in initiating a response to a new antigen. The major type of T-cell–mediated immune response in the skin is delayed-type hypersensitivity.

Mast cells, which have a prominent role in immunoglobulin E–mediated immediate hypersensitivity, also are present in the dermis. These cells are strategically located at body interfaces such as the skin and mucous membranes and are thought to interact with antigens that come in contact with the skin.

Blood Vessels. The arterial vessels that nourish the skin form two plexuses (*i.e.*, collections of blood vessels), one located between the dermis and the subcutaneous tissue and the other between the papillary and reticular layers of the dermis. The pink color of light skin results primarily from blood in the vessels of this latter plexus. Capillary flow that arises from vessels in this plexus also extends up and nourishes the overlaying epidermis by diffusion. Blood leaves the skin through small veins that accompany the subcutaneous arteries. The lymphatic system of the skin, which aids in combating certain skin infections, also is limited to the dermis.

The skin is richly supplied with arteriovenous anastomoses in which blood flows directly between an artery and a vein, bypassing the capillary circulation. These anastomoses are important for temperature regulation. They can open up, letting blood flow through the skin vessels when there is a need to dissipate body heat, and close off, conserving body heat if the environmental temperature is cold.

Innervation. The innervation of the skin is complex. The skin, with its accessory structures, serves as an organ for receiving sensory information from the environment. The dermis is well supplied with sensory neurons as well as nerves that supply the blood vessels, sweat glands, and arrector pili muscles. The arrector pili muscles connect the dermis to the hair follicles.[1]

The receptors for touch, pressure, heat, cold, and pain are widely distributed in the dermis. The papillary layer of the dermis is supplied with free nerve endings that serve as nociceptors (*i.e.*, pain receptors) and thermoreceptors. The dermis also contains encapsulated pressure-sensitive receptors that detect pressure and touch. The largest of these are the *pacinian corpuscles*, which are widely distributed in the dermis and subcutaneous tissue. The afferent nerve endings of the pacinian corpuscle are surrounded by concentric layers of modified Schwann cells such that they resemble an onion when sectioned. Pacinian corpuscles are responsible for detecting gross pressure changes and vibrations. Pressure causes the pacinian corpuscle to change its shape, thereby triggering nerve impulses. Pacinian corpuscles are adaptive and they respond more to changes than to steady pressure or vibration.

Flat, encapsulated nerve endings found on the palmar surfaces of the fingers and hands and planter surfaces of the feet are called *Meissner corpuscles* and serve as touch receptors.[1] They are concentrated on the fingertips, palms, soles, lips, tongue, face, and genitalia. They are thick, laminated, ovoid capsules each containing up to six nerve endings. When the corpuscle is deformed by pressure, the nerve endings are stimulated, signaling the somatosensory portion of the cerebral cortex and informing the person about the location and strength of the stimulus. They are rapidly adapting and do not react to constant, steady stimulation.

Ruffini corpuscles are small, oval mechanoreceptors located in the deep dermal tissue. Several expanded nerve endings branch from a single, myelinated afferent fiber.[1] They are slowly adapting receptors, responding to heavy pressure and joint movement. They are also believed to detect cold.

Most of the skin's blood vessels are under sympathetic nervous system control. The sweat glands are innervated by cholinergic fibers but controlled by the sympathetic nervous system. Likewise, the sympathetic nervous system controls the arrector pili (pilomotor) muscles that cause elevation of hairs on the skin. Contraction of these muscles tends to cause the skin to dimple, producing "goose bumps or goose flesh."[1]

Subcutaneous Tissue

The subcutaneous tissue layer is the third layer of the skin and consists primarily of fat cells and connective tissues that lend support to the vascular and neural structures supplying the superficial layers of the skin. There is controversy about whether the subcutaneous tissue should be considered an actual layer of the skin. Because the eccrine glands and deep hair follicles extend to this layer and several skin diseases involve the subcutaneous tissue, the subcutaneous tissue may be considered part of the skin.

The subcutaneous layer may have varying levels of thickness depending on its location. The fascia may be thinner over a bony prominence and thicker when covering other organs. Therefore, if there is a break in the skin, which is more likely to occur over a bony prominence, and infection occurs in the subcutaneous tissue, the macrophages will proliferate to fight the infectious agents.[1,3] Hence, the subcutaneous layer of the skin does contribute to the skin's immunologic function.

Skin Appendages

The skin houses a variety of appendages, including sweat glands, sebaceous glands, hair, and nails. The distribution and functions of the appendages vary.

Sweat Glands

There are two types of sweat glands—eccrine and apocrine. *Eccrine sweat glands* are simple tubular structures that originate in the dermis and open directly to the skin surface. They are numerous (several million), vary in density, and are located over the entire body surface except the lips and part of the external genitalia.[1] Their purpose is to transport sweat to the outer skin surface to regulate body temperature. *Apocrine sweat glands* are less numerous than eccrine sweat glands. They are larger and located deep in the dermal layer. They open through a hair follicle, even though a hair may not be present, and are found primarily in the axillae and groin. The major difference between these glands and the eccrine glands is that apocrine glands secrete an oily substance. In animals, apocrine secretions give rise to distinctive odors that enable animals to recognize the presence of others. In humans, apocrine secretions are sterile until mixed with the bacteria on the skin surface. They then produce what is commonly known as "body odor."

Sebaceous Glands

The sebaceous glands are located over the entire skin surface except for the palms, soles, and sides of the feet. They are part of the *pilosebaceous unit*. They secrete a mixture of lipids, including triglycerides, cholesterol, and wax. This mixture is called *sebum*, and it lubricates the hair and skin.[1] Sebum is not the same as the surface lipid film. Sebum prevents undue evaporation of moisture from the stratum corneum during cold weather and helps to conserve body heat. Sebum production is under the control of genetic and hormonal influences. Sebaceous glands are relatively small and inactive until people approach adolescence. The glands then enlarge, stimulated by the rise in sex hormones. Gland size directly influences the amount of sebum produced, and the level of androgens influences gland size. The sebaceous glands are the structures that become inflamed in acne.

Hair

The hair is a structure that originates from hair follicles in the dermis. Most hair follicles are associated with sebaceous glands, and these structures combine to form the pilosebaceous unit. The entire hair structure consists of the hair follicle, sebaceous gland, hair muscle (arrector pili), and, in some instances, the apocrine gland (Fig. 51.6). The hair is a keratinized structure that is pushed upward from the hair follicle. Growth of the hair is centered in the bulb (*i.e.*, base)

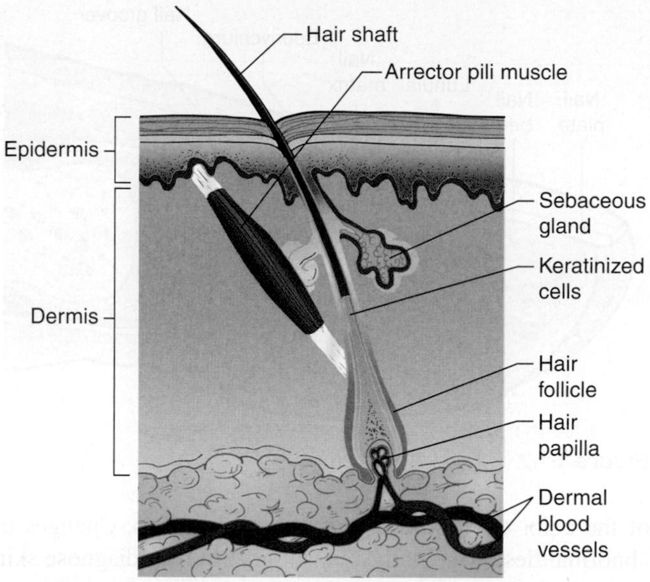

Figure 51.6 • Parts of a hair follicle.

of the hair follicle, and the hair undergoes changes as it is pushed outward. The hair goes through three cyclic phases identified as anagen (the growth phase), catagen (the atrophy phase), and telogen (the resting phase, or no growth). Like most animals, human beings shed hair cyclically. However, human hair follicles work independently and therefore, unlike most animals, humans shed hair asynchronously.

A vascular network at the site of the follicular bulb nourishes and maintains the hair follicle. Melanocytes in the bulb transfer melanosomes to the cells of the bulb matrix in much the same way as in the skin and are therefore responsible for the color of the hair. Similar to the skin, large melanosomes are found in the hair of darker-skinned people. Aggregated and encapsulated melanosomes are found in people with light skin. Red hair has spherical melanosomes, whereas gray hair is the result of a decreased number of melanosome-producing melanocytes. The arrector pili muscle, located deep to the sebaceous gland, provides a thermoregulatory function by contracting the skin to cause goose bumps, thereby reducing the skin surface area that is available for the dissipation of body heat.

Nails

The nails are hardened keratinized plates, called *fingernails* and *toenails*, which protect the fingers and toes and enhance dexterity. The nails grow out from a curved transverse groove called the *nail groove*. The floor of this groove, called the *nail matrix*, is the germinal region of the nail plate (Fig. 51.7). The underlying epidermis, attached to the nail plate, is called the *nail bed*. Like hair, nails are the end product of dead matrix cells that are pushed outward from the nail matrix. Unlike hair, nails grow continuously rather than cyclically, unless permanently damaged or diseased. The epithelium of the fold of the skin that surrounds the nail consists of the usual layers of the skin. The stratum corneum forms the *eponychium* or cuticle. The nearly transparent nail plate provides a useful window for viewing the amount of oxygen in the blood, providing a view

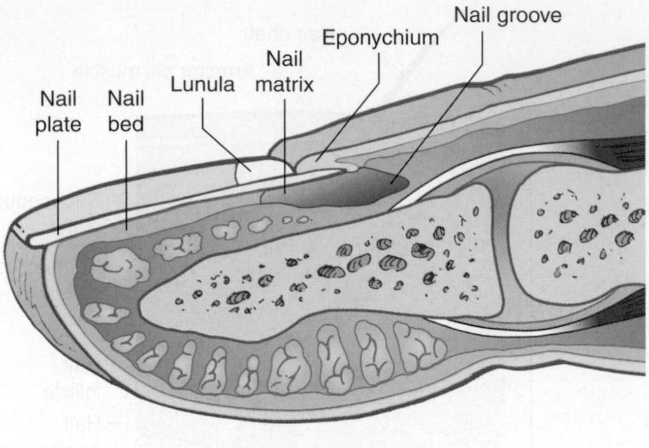

Figure 51.7 • Parts of a fingernail.

of the color of the blood in the dermal vessels. Changes or abnormalities of the nail can also serve to help diagnose skin or systemic diseases.

Functions of the Skin

The skin and its derivatives constitute a complex organ with many cell types. The diversity of cell types and their ability to work together provide a number of ways of protecting a person from the elements in the external environment. Microorganisms find it almost impossible to penetrate the skin from the outside, and water loss is limited from the inside. The skin surface is covered with a thin lipid film containing bactericidal fatty acids that protect against the entry of harmful microorganisms, and it harbors a constant flora of relatively harmless strains of microorganisms that protect against other, more virulent strains. The skin also plays an important role in immune regulation through skin-associated lymphoid tissues, including Langerhans cells, mast cells, and lymphocytes. Langerhans cells, the antigen-presenting cells of the epidermal skin, not only protect against harmful pathogens but also play an important role in the development of allergic skin conditions. As the antigen is phagocytized, it is evident on the Langerhans cell surface, and the cell moves to a regional lymph node where it interacts with T lymphoctyes.[1]

KEY POINTS

FUNCTIONS OF THE SKIN

- The skin prevents body fluids from leaving the body, protects the body from potentially damaging environmental agents, and serves as an area for heat exchange. In addition, cells of the skin immune system provide protection against invading microorganisms.
- Receptors in the skin relay touch, pressure, temperature, and pain sensation to the central nervous system for localization and discrimination.

The skin serves several other vital functions, including somatosensory function, temperature regulation, and vitamin D synthesis. The skin is richly innervated with pain, temperature, and touch receptors. Skin receptors relay the numerous qualities of touch, such as pressure, sharpness, dullness, and pleasure to the central nervous system for localization and fine discrimination. Most of the heat produced in the body is generated by deep organs, such as the liver, heart, and skeletal muscles, and then transferred to the skin, where it is lost to the surrounding environment. The rate at which heat is dissipated from the body is determined by constriction or dilation of the arterioles that supply blood to the skin and through evaporation of moisture and sweat from the skin surface. The skin also functions as an endocrine organ, in which 7-dehydrocholesterol, a substance normally found in epidermal cells, is converted to cholecalciferol (an inactive form of vitamin D), by ultraviolet rays from the sun. The skin is increasingly being understood as a complex and dynamic system involving neuroendocrine, immunologic, and cutaneous interactions.

IN SUMMARY

The skin is primarily an organ of protection. It is the largest organ of the body and forms the major barrier between the internal organs and the external environment. The pigment melanin absorbs harmful ultraviolet light. The skin is richly innervated with pain, temperature, and touch receptors. It synthesizes vitamin D and plays an essential role in fluid and electrolyte balance. It contributes to glucose metabolism through its glycogen stores. Sweat is a means of excreting salt, carbon dioxide, ammonia, and urea. The skin absorbs lipid-soluble materials, toxic substances (such as mercury and lead, and substances in poison ivy and poison oak), fat-soluble vitamins, and certain drugs administered through transdermal patches.

The skin is composed of two layers, the epidermis and the dermis, separated by a basement membrane. A layer of subcutaneous tissue binds the dermis to the underlying organs and tissues of the body. The epidermis, the outermost layer of the skin, contains four to five layers, or strata. The major cells of the epidermis are the keratinocytes, melanocytes, Langerhans cells, and Merkel cells. The stratum germinativum, or basal layer, is the source of the cells in all five layers of the epidermis. The keratinocytes, which are the major cells of the epidermis, are transformed from viable keratinocytes to dead keratin as they move from the innermost layer of the epidermis (*i.e.*, stratum germinativum) to the outermost layer (*i.e.*, stratum corneum). The melanocytes are pigment-synthesizing cells that give the skin its color. The dermis provides the epidermis with support and nutrition and is the source of blood vessels, nerves, and skin appendages (*i.e.*, hair follicles, sebaceous glands, nails, and sweat glands). Sensory receptors for touch, pressure, heat, cold, and pain are widely distributed in the dermis. The skin serves as a first line of defense against microorganisms and other harmful agents. The epidermis contains Langerhans cells, which process foreign antigens for presentation to T cells, and the dermis contains macrophages, T cells, mast cells, and fibroblasts, all contributing to the body's immune defenses.

MANIFESTATIONS OF SKIN DISORDERS

After completing this section of the chapter, the learner will be able to meet the following objectives:

- Describe the following skin rashes and lesions—macule, patch, papule, plaque, nodule, tumor, wheal, vesicle, bulla, and pustule.
- Cite two physiologic explanations for pruritus.
- Describe the causes and treatment of dry skin.

No two skin disorders look exactly alike, nor do the same agents necessarily cause them. Excessive itching, infection, or the effects of self-treatment may further influence the appearance of many skin disorders. Skin color also may influence the appearance. Nevertheless, most skin disorders have some common characteristics that can be used to describe them. This section of the chapter covers lesions and rashes, dry skin, pruritus, skin disorders because of mechanical forces, and variations in dark skin.

Lesions and Rashes

Rashes are temporary eruptions of the skin, such as those associated with childhood diseases, heat, diaper irritation, or drug-induced reactions. The term *lesion* refers to a traumatic or pathologic loss of normal tissue continuity, structure, or function. The components of a rash often are referred to as *lesions*. Rashes and lesions may range in size from a fraction of a millimeter (*e.g.*, the pinpoint spots of petechiae) to many centimeters (*e.g.*, pressure ulcer). They may be blanched (white), erythematous (reddened), hemorrhagic or purpuric (containing blood), or pigmented (colored). Repeated rubbing and scratching can lead to lichenification (thickened, leathery, and roughened skin characterized by prominent markings) or excoriation (a raw, denuded area caused by breakage of the epidermis). Skin lesions may occur as primary lesions arising in previously normal skin, or they may develop as secondary lesions resulting from other disease conditions. Table 51.1 illustrates various types of skin lesions.

TABLE 51.1 PRIMARY AND SECONDARY SKIN LESIONS

LESION	DESCRIPTION	EXAMPLES
Primary Lesions		
MACULE, PATCH 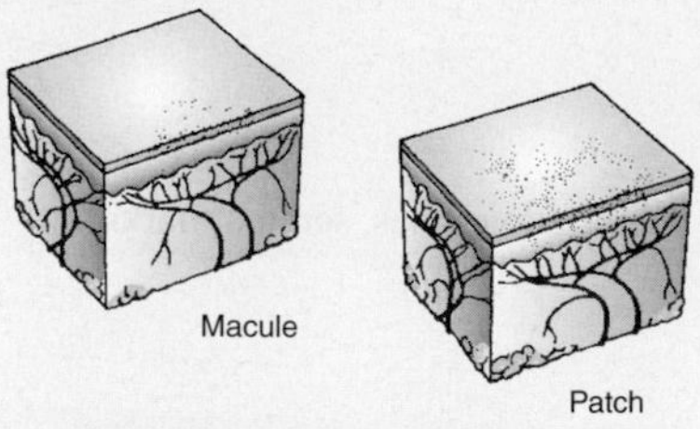	Flat, nonpalpable skin color change (color may be brown, white, tan, purple, red) • *Macule:* <1 cm; circumscribed border • *Patch:* >1 cm; may have irregular border	Freckles, flat moles, petechiae, rubella, vitiligo, port-wine stains, ecchymosis
PAPULE, PLAQUE 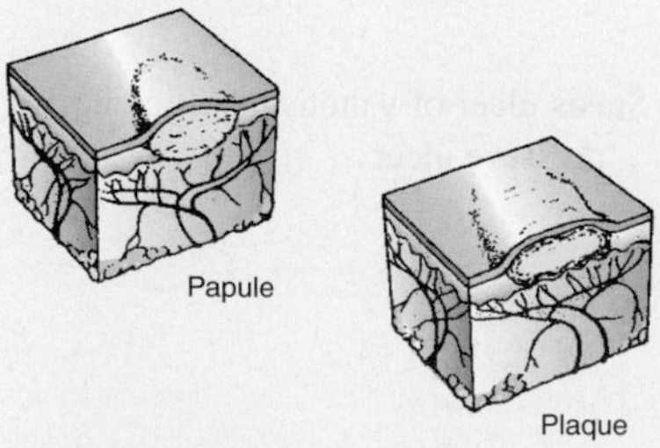	Elevated, palpable, solid mass with a circumscribed border Plaque may be coalesced papules with flat top. • *Papule:* <0.5 cm • *Plaque:* >0.5 cm	*Papules:* Elevated nevi, warts, lichen planus *Plaques:* Psoriasis, actinic keratosis
NODULE, TUMOR 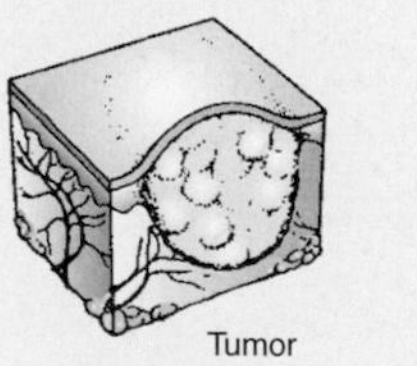	Elevated, palpable, solid mass that extends deeper into the dermis than a papule • *Nodule:* 0.5–2 cm; circumscribed • *Tumor:* >1–2 cm; tumors do not always have sharp borders	*Nodules:* Lipoma, squamous cell carcinoma, poorly absorbed injection, dermatofibroma *Tumors:* Larger lipoma, carcinoma

(*Continued*)

TABLE 51.1 PRIMARY AND SECONDARY SKIN LESIONS *(Continued)*

LESION	DESCRIPTION	EXAMPLES
VESICLE, BULLA 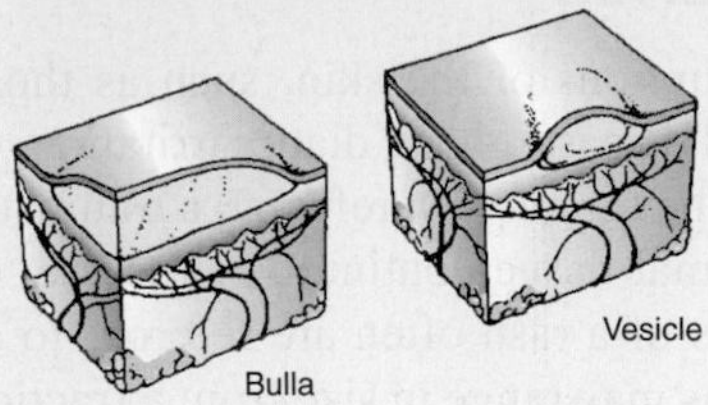	Circumscribed, elevated, palpable mass containing serous fluid • *Vesicle:* <0.5 cm • *Bulla:* >0.5 cm	*Vesicles:* Herpes simplex/zoster, varicella, poison ivy, second-degree burn (blister) *Bulla:* Pemphigus, contact dermatitis, large burn blisters, poison ivy, bullous impetigo
WHEAL 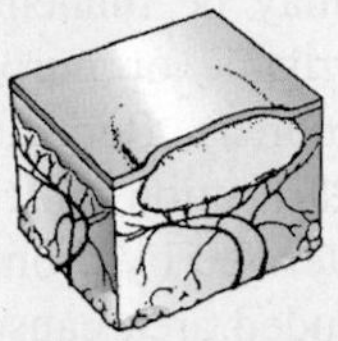	Elevated mass with transient borders; often irregular; size and color vary. Caused by movement of serous fluid into the dermis; does not contain free fluid in a cavity (*e.g.*, as a vesicle does)	Urticaria (hives), insect bites
PUSTULE 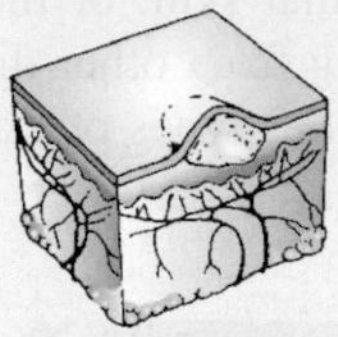	Pus-filled vesicle or bulla	Acne, impetigo, furuncles, carbuncles
CYST 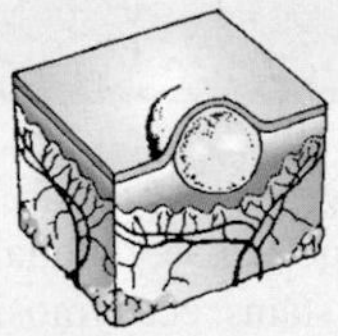	Encapsulated fluid-filled or semisolid mass in the subcutaneous tissue or dermis	Sebaceous cyst, epidermoid cysts
Secondary Lesions		
EROSION 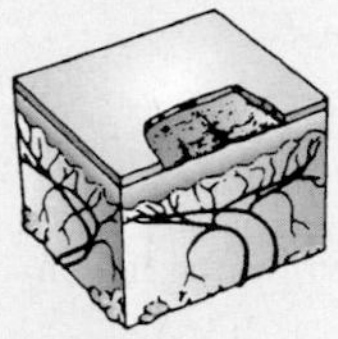	Loss of superficial epidermis that does not extend to dermis; depressed, moist area	Ruptured vesicles, scratch marks
ULCER 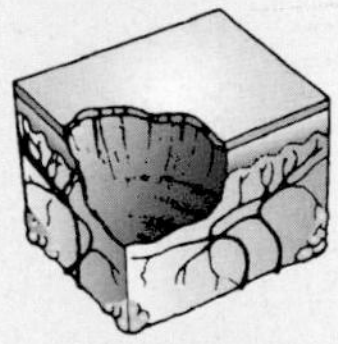	Skin loss extending past epidermis; necrotic tissue loss; bleeding and scarring possible	Stasis ulcer of venous insufficiency, pressure ulcer
FISSURE 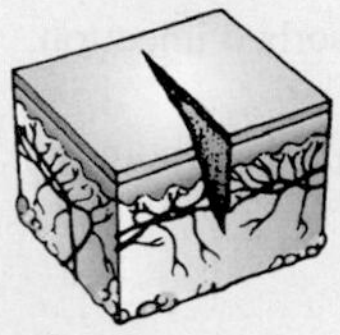	Linear crack in the skin that may extend to dermis	Chapped lips or hands, tinea pedis

TABLE 51.1 PRIMARY AND SECONDARY SKIN LESIONS *(Continued)*

LESION	DESCRIPTION	EXAMPLES
SCALES 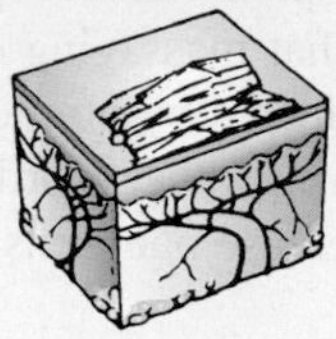	Flakes secondary to desquamated, dead epithelium that may adhere to skin surface; color varies (silvery, white); texture varies (thick, fine).	Dandruff, psoriasis, dry skin, pityriasis rosea
CRUST 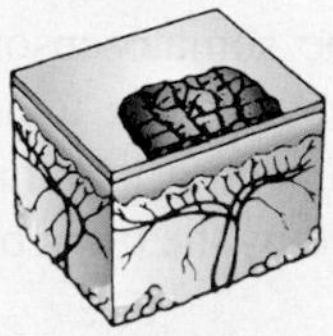	Dried residue of serum, blood, or pus on skin surface Large, adherent crust is a scab.	Residue left after vesicle rupture: impetigo, herpes, eczema
SCAR (CICATRIX) 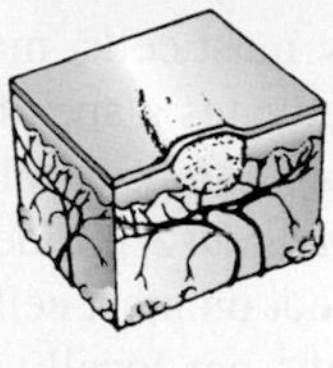	Skin mark left after healing of a wound or lesion; represents replacement by connective tissue of the injured tissue • *Young scars:* Red or purple • *Mature scars:* White or glistening	Healed wound or surgical incision
KELOID 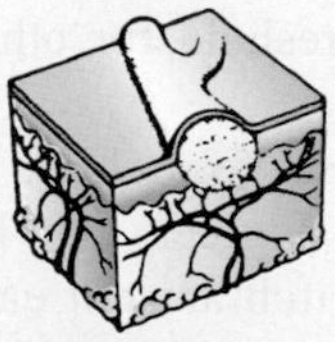	Hypertrophied scar tissue secondary to excessive collagen formation during healing; elevated, irregular, red Greater incidence among African Americans	Keloid of ear piercing or surgical incision
ATROPHY 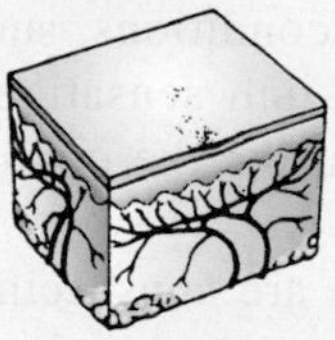	Thin, dry, transparent appearance of the epidermis; loss of surface markings; secondary to loss of collagen and elastin; underlying vessels may be visible.	Aged skin, arterial insufficiency
LICHENIFICATION 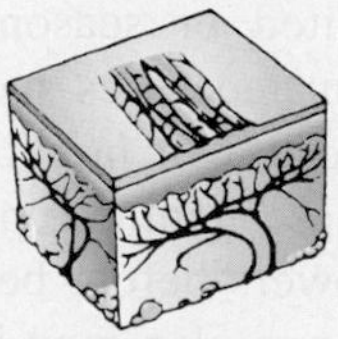	Thickening and roughening of the skin or accentuated skin markings that may be secondary to repeated rubbing, irritation, scratching	Contact dermatitis

Reprinted from Hinkle J. L., Cheever K. H. (2018). *Brunner and Suddarth's textbook of medical-surgical nursing* (14th ed., pp. 1798–1799). Philadelphia, PA: Wolters Kluwer, with permission; Adapted from Bickley L. S. (2013). *Bates' guide to physical examination and history taking* (11th ed.). Philadelphia, PA: Lippincott Williams & Wilkins; Weber J. W., Kelley J. (2014). *Health assessment in nursing* (5th ed.). Philadelphia, PA: Lippincott Williams & Wilkins.

A *blister* is a vesicle or fluid-filled papule. Blisters of mechanical origin are caused by friction from repeated rubbing on a single area of the skin. Friction blisters most commonly occur on the palmar and plantar surfaces of the hands and feet where the skin is constantly exposed to mechanical trauma, such as from shoes and household tools and appliances. Blisters also develop in bullous skin disorders and from burns. Histologically, there is degeneration of the epidermal cells and a disruption of the intercellular junctions, causing the layers of the skin to separate. As a result, fluid accumulates and a noticeable bleb forms on the skin surface. Adhesive bandages and gauze can be used to protect friction blisters and prevent further irritation and rubbing. Breaking the skin of a blister to remove the fluid is inadvisable because of the risk of secondary infection.

A *callus* is a hyperkeratotic plaque of the skin because of chronic pressure or friction. It represents hyperplasia of the dead, keratinized cells that make up the cornified or horny layer of the skin. Increased cohesion between cells results in hyperkeratosis and decreased skin shedding. A callus may be filed down but is likely to recur if pressure continues in the localized area.

Corns (helomas) are small, well-circumscribed, conical, keratinous thickenings of the skin. They usually appear on the toes from rubbing or ill-fitting shoes. The corn may be either hard (heloma durum) with a central hard, horny core or soft (heloma molle), as commonly seen between the toes. They may appear on the hands as an occupational hazard. The hard tissue at the center of the corn looks like a funnel with a broad top and a pointed bottom, hence the name "corn." Corns on the feet often are painful, whereas corns on the hands may be asymptomatic. Corns may be abraded or surgically removed, but they recur if the causative agent is not removed.

Pruritus

Pruritus, or the sensation of itch, is a common symptom of skin disorders. Symptoms of pruritus range from mild to severe. In some people, the condition may be so severe that it interrupts sleep and the general quality of life. Although itching commonly occurs with skin disorders, it can also provide a valuable clue to internal disorders, such as chronic renal disease, diabetes, or biliary disease.

Despite the fact almost all skin diseases manifest in pruritus, very little is known about it. It is generally agreed that itch is a sensation that originates in free nerve endings in the skin, is carried by small myelinated type C nerve fibers to the dorsal horn of the spinal cord, and is then transmitted to the somatosensory cortex through the spinothalamic tract. Until recently, it was believed that pain and itch traveled along the same nerve pathways and that itch was a low-level pain response. It has now been demonstrated through micrographic recordings that there are itch-specific neuronal pathways in the spinothalamic tract and central nervous system that process peripheral itch stimuli.[5,6] Evidence over the years has supported this finding. For example, it has been shown that itch and pain are antagonistic—pain and peripheral inflammation suppress itch, whereas opioids often provoke itch. Further, itch induces scratching, whereas pain induces withdrawal, and itch and pain can be simultaneously perceived. Finally, the belief in polymodal pain–itch receptors may be discounted by the knowledge that massaging or rubbing the skin, which are sensations conducted by nonitch fibers, often results in the sensation of itch. In other words, although rubbing a painful area tends to decrease pain sensations, it increases itch sensations.

Given these new findings, it has been postulated that itch exists both locally and centrally. That is, that in addition to localized itch, an "itch center" exists in the somatosensory cortex. For example, a mosquito bite on most people itches momentarily and then subsides. However, a central itch may be similar to central pain in that it is perceived by the brain but does not exist locally.

Advances have also been made in understanding peripheral mediators (*i.e.*, substances that cause itch) other than histamine. Tryptase, an enzyme released by mast cells, may be an important itch mediator because it activates a specific receptor in the sensory nerves. Opioids operate centrally and peripherally in producing itch, whereas neuropeptides, such as substance P, induce itch by their effect on mast cells. Substances such as bradykinin and bile salts act locally to stimulate the itch sensation. Prostaglandins are modulators of the itch response, lowering the threshold for other mediators.

Scratching, the well-known response to itch, is a spinal reflex response that to varying degrees can be controlled by the person. Many types of itch are not easily localized or relieved by scratching. Excoriations and thickened papular areas develop at the site of repeated scratching or rubbing, and in some skin conditions, such as dry skin, scratching further activates itch sensations. Chronic forms of pruritus can severely affect the quality of a person's life.

Most treatment measures for pruritus are nonspecific. Measures such as using the entire hand to rub over large areas and keeping the fingernails trimmed often can relieve itch and prevent skin damage. Self-limited or seasonal cases of pruritus may respond to treatment measures such as moisturizing lotions, bath oils, and the use of humidifiers. Because vasodilation tends to increase itching, cold applications may provide relief. Cool showers before bed, light sleepwear, and cool home temperatures also may be helpful. Topical corticosteroids may be helpful in some cases, such as itch related to allergy-mediated urticaria. However, unlike for some other skin problems, there is no armamentarium of effective antipruritic drugs available. Another alternative method that has been effective in the treatment of pruritus occurring in atopic dermatitis is the use of Herbavita, which is a combination of oil extracts from plants.[7]

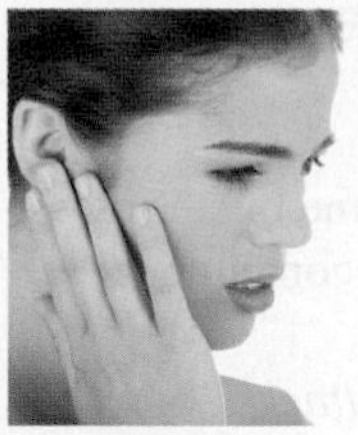

Remember Lauren from the unit opener case study? She complained of her fingers being "very itchy" (pruritus) where the rash is. It seems she has a contact dermatitis secondary to the chemicals she has recently been working with in the chemistry laboratory. She readily offered, "I hardly ever wear gloves in the lab." After using the steroid hydrocortisone 1% (which has anti-inflammatory properties) on her fingers for 24 hours, her pruritus was relieved.

Mild cutaneous disorders, such as bug bites, are mediated by histamine. Therefore, nonsedating antihistamines tend to be the treatment of choice. However, because most cases of pruritus are not histamine related, their management should be directed at the underlying cause. For example, systemic antihistamines and corticosteroids may be indicated for people with severe pruritus or atopic dermatitis. Naltrexone, an opioid receptor antagonist, has been shown to be an effective antipruritic medication for people with jaundice.[6]

Additionally, 80% to 100% of people experience severe pruritus post burn and generally use an antihistamine and emollient for pruritus management. However, studies have documented effective pruritus management can be obtained by using gabapentin, a derivative of the inhibitory neurotransmitter GABA, without an antihistamine.[8] Therefore, more studies need to be conducted to determine the best practices for managing pruritus. Topical capsaicin cream and topical aspirin have been used for localized chronic pruritic disorders. Opioid antagonists may be used for pruritus caused by opioid medications such as morphine. Other modalities that have been used for all cases of pruritus with varying degrees of success are phototherapy, acupuncture, antidepressant medications, behavior modification, and alternative therapies (herbal, nutritional, and reflex therapies). In people with pruritus because of a systemic cause, itching gradually recedes as the primary condition improves.

Given the recent advances in the science of pruritus, health care professionals have new, effective, and disease-specific antipruritic drugs available. Currently, drugs targeting specific pathways of chronic pruritus are being developed with special attention to biologics, which may revamp the treatment of pruritus. Such substances include antinerve growth factor antibodies, kappa opioid receptor agonists, histamine 4 receptor antagonists, antagonists to neuropeptide and cytokine receptors, bile acid transporter inhibitors, and sequestrants. The International Forum for the Study of Itch has developed a classification system dividing chronic pruritus into six major groups based on its underlying cause: dermatologic, systemic, neurologic, psychiatric, multifactorial, or unknown origin.[9] Similar to pain scales, visual analog scales are being developed and used in the diagnosis and treatment of pruritus.[10]

Dry Skin

Dry skin, also called *xerosis*, may be a natural occurrence, as in the drying of the skin associated with aging, or it may be symptomatic of an underlying systemic disease or skin disorder such as contact dermatitis or diabetes mellitus. People with diabetes mellitus often experience xerosis especially on the extremities.[11] Most cases of dry skin are caused by dehydration of the stratum corneum. The effects of aging on skin dryness include a change in the composition of sebaceous gland secretions and a decrease in the secretion of moisture from the sweat glands. Aging is also accompanied by a decrease in skin capillaries as well as a flattening of the dermal rete ridges, resulting in less surface area for exchange of fluids between the dermis, epidermis, and skin surface.[12]

People with dry skin often experience severe pruritus and discomfort, most commonly of the extremities. Other commonly involved areas include the back, abdomen, and waist. Dry skin appears rough and scaly and there may be increased wrinkles or lines. Skin drying also predisposes the skin to scratching, resulting in cracking, fissuring, and a number of other skin maladies.

Some drugs used for other comorbidities can cause dry skin. For example, it has recently been found that epidermal growth factor receptor inhibitors (EGFRIs) frequently cause dermatologic adverse events such as xerosis more so than systemic effects.[13]

Moisturizing agents are the cornerstone of treatment for dry skin. These agents exert their effects by repairing the skin barrier, increasing the water content of the skin, reducing transepidermal water loss, and restoring the lipid barrier's ability to attract, hold, and redistribute water. *Emollients* are fatty acid–containing lotions that replenish the oils on the skin surface, but usually do not leave a residue on the skin. They have a short duration of action and need to be applied frequently. *Humectants* are the additives in lotions, such as alpha hydroxy acids and urea, that draw out water from the deeper skin layers and hold it on the skin surface. However, the water that is drawn to the skin is transepidermal water, not atmospheric water. Thus, continued evaporation from the skin can actually exacerbate dryness. Alpha hydroxy acids are derived from fruits, hence the abundance of fruit additives in shampoos and lotions in over-the-counter preparations. Urea is a nitrogenous substance that has been quite effective in reducing xerosis when combined with lotions. It is a humectant at lower concentrations (10%), but in higher concentrations (20% to 30%), it is mildly keratolytic. *Occlusives* are thick creams that contain petroleum or some other moisture-proof material that can form a barrier. They prevent water loss from the skin. They are the most effective agents for relieving skin dryness, but because of their greasiness and lack of cosmetic appeal, some people do not wish to use them.

Lotion or cream additives include corticosteroids or mild anesthetics, such as camphor, menthol, lidocaine, or benzocaine. These agents work by suppressing itching while moisturizing the skin. Using room humidifiers and keeping room temperatures as low as possible to prevent water loss from the skin also may be helpful. Glycerine soaps, although popular and visually appealing, are drying and can exacerbate the symptoms.

Skin Variations

Skin color is determined by the melanin produced by the melanocytes. Although the number of melanosomes in dark and light skin is the same, dark skin produces more melanin more quickly than light skin. People with darker skin are better protected against skin cancer, premature wrinkling, and aging of the skin that occurs with sun exposure.

Some skin disorders common to people of African, Hispanic, or East Indian descent are not commonly found in people of European descent. Similarly, some skin disorders, such as skin cancers, affect light-skinned people more commonly than dark-skinned people. Because of these differences, serious skin disorders may be overlooked, and normal variations in darker skin may be mistaken for anomalies.

A condition common in people with dark skin is increased or reduced color. Areas of the skin may darken after injury, such as a cut or scrape, or after disease conditions such as acne. These darkened areas may take many months or years to fade. Areas of the skin may lighten because of decreased pigment or melanin, resulting in vitiligo. Dry skin is caused by a reduction in moisture and oils, which can be a problem for people with dark complexions. It can be very noticeable giving skin an ashen appearance. Because of dryness, the skin may feel tight or uncomfortable. Although using a moisturizer may help relieve the discomfort, it may cause a worsening of acne in predisposed people.

Normal variations in skin structure and skin tones often make evaluation of dark skin difficult. The darker pigmentation can make skin pallor, cyanosis, and erythema more difficult to observe. Therefore, verbal histories must be relied on to assess skin changes. The verbal history should include the person's description of her or his normal skin tones. Changes in skin color, in particular hypopigmentation and hyperpigmentation, often accompany disorders of dark skin and are very important signs to observe when diagnosing skin conditions.

IN SUMMARY

Skin lesions and rashes are the most common manifestations of skin disorders. Rashes are temporary skin eruptions. Lesions result from traumatic or pathologic loss of the normal continuity, structure, or function of the skin. Lesions may be vascular in origin. They may occur as primary lesions in previously normal skin or they may develop as secondary lesions resulting from primary lesions. Blisters, calluses, and corns result from rubbing, pressure, and frictional forces applied to the skin. Pruritus and dry skin are symptoms common to many skin disorders. Scratching because of pruritus can lead to excoriation, infection, and other complications. Normal variations in dark skin often make evaluation difficult and result in some disorders being overlooked. Changes in color, especially hypopigmentation or hyperpigmentation, often accompany the skin disorders of dark-skinned people.

REVIEW EXERCISES

1. Bullous pemphigoid is an autoimmune blistering disease caused by autoantibodies to constituents of the dermal–epidermal junction.
   A. *Explain how antibodies, which attack glycoproteins in the lamina lucida and their attachment to the hemidesmosomes, can cause blisters to form (hint: see Fig. 51.5).*
2. "Allergy tests" involve the application of an antigen to the skin, either through a small scratch or by intradermal injection.
   A. *Explain how the body's immune system is able to detect and react to these antigens.*

GERIATRIC Considerations

- Photoaging, caused by sun exposure without protection over many years, causes wrinkling, increased pigmentation, atrophy of cutaneous, and lesions, which are either benign or malignant.[14]
- Slowing of hair growth on lower extremities is normal.[14]
- Many benign skin lesions are part of the aging process; it is critical that providers be able to differentiate these from malignant lesions.[14]
- The loss of anchoring between the skin layers places the aging person at risk for shearing injuries and trauma. There is also delayed wound healing associated with vascular changes.[14]
- The skin atrophies, and cellular replacement is decreased, making the skin thin and transparent.[14]

PEDIATRIC Considerations

- Erythema toxicum, a red splotchy rash with yellow/white bumps that can appear for the first few days of life, is normal.[15]
- Water blisters are evident in newborns who sucked a body part while in utero.[15]
- Sweat glands are immature in the newborn causing milia, tiny white/yellow spots, to appear on the cheeks, nose, or chin, which disappear at about age 3 months.[15]
- Acne in newborns is due to maternal hormones that stimulate the sebaceous glands, disappearing after the first few months of life.[15]
- Biologic differences are more evident in the integumentary system than any other area of the body.[15]
- The fetus is able to repair wounds with scar formation during the second and third trimesters.[15]

References

1. Pawlina W. (2016). *Histology: A text and atlas* (7th ed.). Philadelphia, PA: Wolters Kluwer Health.
2. Habif T. P. (2016). *Clinical dermatology: A color guide to diagnosis and therapy* (6th ed.). St. Louis, MO: Elsevier.
3. Rubin R., Strayer D. E. (Eds.) (2015). *Rubin's pathology: Clinicopathologic foundations of medicine* (7th ed.). Philadelphia, PA: Wolters Kluwer Health.
4. Paradisi A., Tabolli S., Didona B., et al. (2014). Marked by reduced incidence of melanoma and nonmelanoma skin cancer in a nonconcurrent cohort of 10,040 patients with vitiligo. *Journal of American Academy of Dermatology* 71(6), 1110–1116.
5. Mochiezuki H., Ruyusuke K. (2015). Central mechanisms of itch. *Clinical Neurophysiology* 126(9), 1650–1660.
6. Bassari R., Koea J. (2015). Jaundice associated pruritus: A review of pathophysiology and treatment. *World Journal of Gastroenterology* 21(5), 1404–1413.
7. Kim S., Hyun J., Kim H., et al. (2016). Evaluation of anti-pruritic and anti-inflammatory effects of Korean red ginseng extract on atopic dermatitis murine model. *World Allergy Organization Journal* 9(1), 17–18.
8. Lau T., Leung S., Lau W. (2016). Gabapentin for uremic pruritus in hemodialysis patients: A qualitative systematic review. *Canadian Journal of Kidney Health and Disease* 3(2016), 14.
9. Pereira M., Ständer S. (2017). Chronic pruritus: Current and emerging treatment options. *Drugs* 77, 999–1007.
10. Reich A., Riepe C., Anastasiadou Z., et al. (2016). Itch assessment with visual analogue scale and numerical rating scale: Determination of minimal clinically important difference in chronic itch. *Acta Dermato-Venereologica* 96(7), 978–980.
11. Lima A., Illing T., Schliemann S., et al. (2017). Cutaneous manifestations of diabetes mellitus: A review. *American Journal of Clinical Dermatology* 18, 541–553.
12. Greaney J., Stanhewicz A., Kenney W., et al. (2015). Impaired increases in skin sympathetic nerve activity contribute to age-related decrements in reflex cutaneous vasoconstriction. *Journal of Physiology* 543(9), 2199–2211.
13. Chanprapaph K., Vachiramon V., Rattanakamakorn P. (2014). Epidermal growth factor receptor inhibitors: A review of cutaneous adverse events and management. *Dermatology Research and Practice* 2014, 1–8.
14. Hinkle J. L., Cheever K. H. (2018). *Brunner & Suddarth's textbook of medical-surgical nursing* (14th ed., p. 1974). Philadelphia, PA: Wolters Kluwer.
15. Bowden V. R., Greenberg C. S. (2014). *Children and their families the continuum of nursing care* (3rd ed.). Philadelphia, PA: Wolters Kluwer.

Disorders of Skin Integrity and Function

52

Lisa Hight

The skin is a unique organ in that numerous signs of disease or injury are immediately observable on the skin. The skin serves as the interface between the body's internal organs and the external environment. Therefore, skin disorders represent the culmination of environmental forces and the internal functioning of the body. Sunlight, insects, other arthropods, infectious organisms, chemicals, and physical agents all play a role in the pathogenesis of skin diseases. Although most disorders are intrinsic to skin, many are external manifestations of systemic disease. Thus, skin provides a valuable window for the recognition of many systemic disorders. It is through the skin that warmth and other responses are given and received. The skin conveys a sense of health, beauty, integrity, and even emotion.

PRIMARY DISORDERS OF THE SKIN

After completing this section of the chapter, the learner will be able to meet the following objectives:

- Describe the pathogenesis of acne vulgaris and relate it to measures used in treating the disorder.
- Differentiate allergic and contact dermatitis and atopic and nummular eczema.
- Define the term *papulosquamous* and use the term to describe the lesions associated with psoriasis, pityriasis rosea, and lichen planus.

Primary skin disorders are those originating in the skin. They include pigmentary skin disorders, infectious processes, acne, rosacea, papulosquamous dermatoses, allergic disorders and drug reactions, and arthropod infestations. Although most of these disorders are not life threatening, they can affect the quality of life.

KEY POINTS

PRIMARY SKIN DISORDERS

- Infectious skin disorders are caused by viruses, bacteria, and fungi that invade the skin, incite inflammatory responses, and otherwise cause rashes and lesions that disrupt the skin surface.
- Allergic and hypersensitivity responses are caused by antigen–antibody responses resulting from sensitization to topical or systemic antigens.

Pigmentary Skin Disorders

Pigmentary skin disorders involve the melanocytes. In some cases, there is an absence of melanin production, as in vitiligo or albinism. In other cases, there is an increase in melanin or some other pigment, as in mongolian spots or melasma. In either case, the emotional impact can cause much worry and anxiety.

Vitiligo

Vitiligo is a pigmentary problem of concern to darkly pigmented people of all races. It also affects white-skinned people, but not as often, and the effects usually are not as socially problematic. Vitiligo appears at any age. However, roughly half of cases begin before the age of 20 years.[1] Worldwide, it affects people of all races regardless of gender.

Etiology. The cause of vitiligo is not known. However, there are many possible rationales for its etiology including genetics and autoimmunity.[1] In some cases, vitiligo has been reportedly precipitated by emotional stress or physical trauma, such as sunburn. Oxidative stress is responsible for initiating melanocyte destruction and the development of vitiligo.[2] Additionally, vitiligo is associated with concurrent disease such as hypothyroidism, Graves disease, Addison disease, pernicious anemia, type 2 diabetes mellitus, and melanoma.[3–5]

Clinical Manifestations. The classic manifestation of vitiligo is the sudden appearance of white patches on the skin.[1] The lesion is a depigmented macule with definite smooth borders on the face, axillae, neck, or extremities. The patches vary in size from small macules to ones involving large skin surfaces. The large macular type is more common. Depigmented areas appear white, pale colored, or sometimes grayish-blue. The depigmented sites may have melanocytes that no longer produce melanin or may not have any functioning melanocytes or very few.[1] These areas sunburn easily, and they enlarge over time. Vitiligo often is asymptomatic, although pruritus may occur.

There are two types of vitiligo: Vitiligo A and Vitiligo B. Vitiligo A is seen more frequently, and the white patches are symmetrical with discrete borders.[4] Vitiligo A progresses slowly over years to cover first the backs of the hands, the face, and body folds.[4] Vitiligo B is the segmental type, which means that the white patches are not symmetrical but rather randomly disseminated anywhere on the body. The onset of Vitiligo B occurs earlier in life than Vitiligo A.[4]

Treatment. Although there are many treatment regimens for vitiligo, none is curative. Self-tanning lotions, skin stains, and cosmetics are used for camouflage. Corticosteroids administered topically, intralesionally, and orally have been used successfully. Broadband (large area) and narrowband (focused) ultraviolet B (UVB) irradiation has also been used successfully in the treatment of vitiligo.

A variety of skin grafting techniques have been used in people unresponsive to other therapies. Successful skin grafting techniques vary from minigrafting (2-mm full-thickness punch grafts transplanted to involved areas) to grafting melanocytes into involved areas. Micropigmentation (tattooing) has been done on smaller, recalcitrant areas, but it is often difficult to attain a correct color match.

If extensive skin surfaces are involved, the treatment may be reversed and the pigmented areas bleached to match the remainder of the skin color. A melanocytotoxic agent is used to remove remaining melanocytes from skin areas. This process, which is called *depigmentation*, is permanent and irreversible. People need to be apprised of this and their need to avoid the sun and use sunscreens for the remainder of their lives.

Albinism

Albinism, a genetic disorder in which there is complete or partial congenital absence of pigment in the skin, hair, and eyes, is found in all races. Although there are over 10 different types of albinism, the most common type is recessively inherited oculocutaneous albinism, in which there is a normal number of melanocytes, but they have little to no tyrosinase, the enzyme needed for synthesis of melanin.[5] It affects the skin, hair, and eyes. People have pale or pink skin, white or yellow hair, and light-colored or sometimes pink eyes. People with albinism have ocular problems, such as extreme sensitivity to light, refractive errors, foveal hypoplasia, and nystagmus.[5] The most severe form is OCA1A, which is tyrosinase negative since these people have a complete lack of tyrosinase.[5] There is no cure for albinism. Treatment efforts for people with albinism are aimed at reducing their risk for skin cancer through protection from solar radiation and screening for malignant skin changes.

Melasma

Melasma is characterized by darkened facial macules.[6,7] It is common in all skin types but most prominent in brown-skinned people from Asia, India, and South America. It occurs in men but is more common in women, particularly during pregnancy or while using oral contraceptives.[6,8] It may or may not resolve after giving birth or discontinuing hormonal birth control. Melasma is exacerbated by sun exposure.[6–8] Treatment measures are palliative, mostly consisting of limiting exposure to the sun and using sunscreens. Bleaching agents, containing 2% to 4% hydroquinone, are standard treatments. Tretinoin cream and azelaic acid have been useful in treating severe cases.

Infectious Processes

The skin is subject to invasion by a number of microorganisms, including fungi, bacteria, and viruses. Normally, the skin flora, sebum, immune responses, and other protective mechanisms guard the skin against infection. Depending on the virulence of the infecting agent and the competence of the host's resistance, infections may result.

Superficial Fungal Infections

Fungi are free-living, saprophytic plantlike organisms, certain strains of which are considered part of the normal skin flora. Some fungi cause deep infections and others are superficial. There are two types of fungi, yeasts, and molds. Yeasts, such as *Candida albicans*, grow as single cells and reproduce asexually[9] (see Fig. 52.1). Molds grow in long filaments, called *hyphae*.[9] There are thousands of known species of yeasts and molds, but only about 100 of them cause disease in humans and animals.[9] Fungal or mycotic infections of the skin are traditionally classified as superficial or deep. The superficial mycoses, more commonly known as *tinea* or *ringworm*, invade only the superficial keratinized tissue (skin, hair, and nails). Deep fungal infections involve the epidermis, dermis, and subcutaneous tissue. Infections that typically are superficial may exhibit deep involvement in people who are immunosuppressed.[5]

Most of the superficial mycoses, also called *dermatophytoses*, are caused by the dermatophytes, a group of closely related fungi. These fungi are classified into three genera:

- *Microsporum (M. audouinii, M. canis, M. gypseum)*
- *Epidermophyton (E. floccosum)*
- *Trichophyton (T. schoenleinii, T. violaceum, T. tonsurans)*[5]

Two of these, *Microsporum* and *Trichophyton*, affect the hair.[5]

Another way of classifying the dermatophytes is according to their ecologic origin—human, animal, or soil.

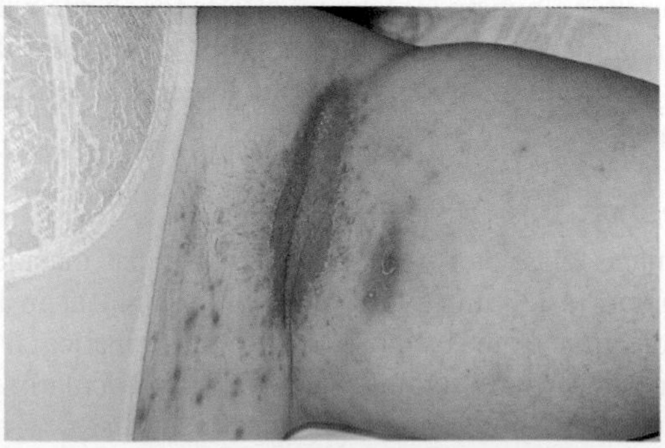

Figure 52.1 • Superficial fungal infection. *Candida* in skin fold. (From Jensen S. (2015). *Nursing health assessment: A best practice approach* (2nd ed., p. 275). Philadelphia, PA: Wolters Kluwer.)

Anthropophilic species (*M. audouinii, M. tonsurans, T. violaceum*) are parasitic on humans and are spread by other infected humans. Zoophilic species (*M. canis* and *T. mentagrophytes*) cause parasitic infections in animals, some of which can be spread to humans. Geophilic species originate in the soil but may infect animals, which in turn serve to infect humans.

Pathogenesis and Clinical Manifestations. The fungi that cause superficial mycoses live on the dead keratinized cells of the epidermis. They emit an enzyme that enables them to digest keratin, which results in superficial skin scaling, nail disintegration, or hair breakage, depending on the location of the infection.[5] An exception to this is the invading fungus of tinea versicolor, which does not produce a keratolytic enzyme. Deeper reactions involving vesicles, erythema, and infiltration are caused by the inflammation that results from exotoxins liberated by the fungus. Fungi also are capable of producing an allergic or immune response.[5] Superficial fungal infections affect various parts of the body, with the lesions varying according to site and fungal species. Tinea can affect the body (tinea corporis), face and neck (tinea faciale), scalp (tinea capitis), hands (tinea manus), feet (tinea pedis), nails (tinea unguium), or genitalia (tinea cruris).[5]

Diagnosis and Treatment. Diagnosis of superficial fungal infections is primarily done by microscopic examination of skin scrapings for fungal spores, the reproducing bodies of fungi. Potassium hydroxide (KOH) preparations are used to prepare slides of skin scrapings. KOH disintegrates human tissue and leaves behind the threadlike filaments or hyphae that grow from the fungal spores. Cultures also may be done using a dermatophyte test medium or a microculture slide that produces color changes and allows for direct microscopic identification. The Wood light (UV light) is another method that can assist with the diagnosis of tinea. Some types of fungi (*e.g., M. canis* and *M. audouinii*) fluoresce yellow-green when the light is directed onto the affected area.[5]

Superficial fungal infections may be treated with topical or systemic antifungal agents. Treatment usually follows diagnosis confirmed by KOH preparation or culture, particularly if a systemic agent is to be used. Topical agents, both prescription and over-the-counter preparations, are commonly used in the treatment of tinea infections. However, success often is limited because of the lengthy duration of treatment, poor compliance, and high rates of relapse at specific body sites.

The oral systemic antifungal agents include griseofulvin, the azoles, and the allylamines. Griseofulvin is a fungicidal agent derived from a species of *Penicillium* that is used only in the treatment of dermatophytoses. It acts by binding to the keratin of newly forming skin, protecting the skin from new infection. Because its action is to prevent new infection, it must be administered for 2 to 6 weeks to allow for skin replacement. The azoles are a group of synthetic antifungal drugs that act by inhibiting the fungal enzymes needed for the synthesis of ergosterol, which is an essential part of fungal cell membranes. The azoles are classified as either imidazoles or triazoles. The imidazoles consist of ketoconazole, miconazole, and clotrimazole. The latter two drugs are used only in topical therapy. The triazoles include itraconazole and fluconazole, both of which are used for the systemic treatment of fungal infections. Terbinafine, a synthetic allylamine, acts by interrupting ergosterol synthesis, causing the accumulation of a metabolite that is toxic to the fungus. In contrast to griseofulvin, the synthetic agents are fungicidal (*i.e.*, kill the fungus) and therefore are more effective over shorter treatment periods. Some of the oral agents can produce serious side effects, such as hepatic toxicity, or interact adversely with other medications. A number of the synthetic fungicides (*e.g.*, ketoconazole, miconazole, clotrimazole, and terbinafine) are available as topical preparations that produce less severe side effects. Topical corticosteroids may be used in conjunction with antifungal agents to relieve itching and erythema secondary to inflammation.

Tinea of the Body or Face. *Tinea corporis* (ringworm of the body) can be caused by any of the fungi but is most frequently caused by *M. canis* in the United States and by *T. rubrum* worldwide (Fig. 52.2). There has been an increase in *T. tonsurans* as the causative agent of tinea corporis as well. Although tinea corporis affects all ages, children seem most prone to infection. Transmission is most commonly from kittens, puppies, and other children who have infections.

The lesions vary, depending on the fungal agent. The most common types of lesions are oval or circular patches on exposed skin surfaces and the trunk, back, or buttocks. Less common are foot and groin infections. The lesion begins as a red papule and enlarges, often with a central clearing. Patches have raised red borders consisting of vesicles, papules, or pustules. The borders are sharply defined, but lesions may coalesce (see Fig. 52.3). Pruritus, a mild burning sensation, and erythema frequently accompany the skin lesion.

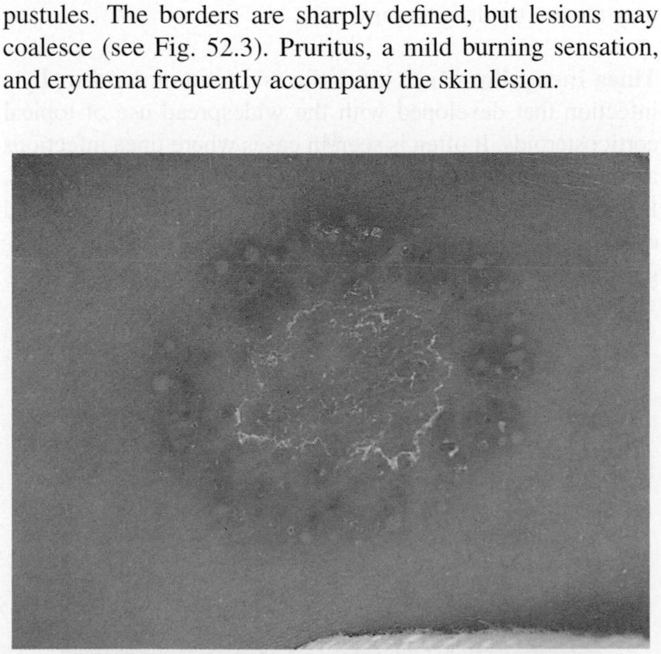

Figure 52.2 • Dermatophytosis—this fungal infection is superficial. Tinea corporis. (From Jensen S. (2015). *Nursing health assessment: A best practice approach* (2nd ed., p. 846). Philadelphia, PA: Wolters Kluwer.)

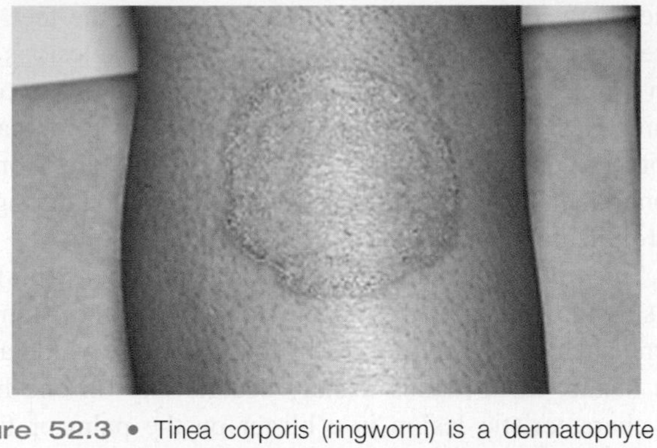

Figure 52.3 • Tinea corporis (ringworm) is a dermatophyte skin infection that is depicted as an annular lesion with a raised border and a central clearing. (From Jensen S. (2015). *Nursing health assessment: A best practice approach* (2nd ed., p. 276). Philadelphia, PA: Wolters Kluwer.)

Tinea faciale, or ringworm of the face, is an infection caused by *T. mentagrophytes* or *T. rubrum*. Tinea faciale may mimic the annular, erythematous, scaling, pruritic lesions characteristic of tinea corporis. It also may appear as flat erythematous patches. Topical antifungal agents usually are effective in treating tinea corporis and tinea faciale. Oral antifungal agents may be used in resistant cases.

Tinea of the Scalp. There are two common types of *tinea capitis* (ringworm of the scalp): primary (noninflammatory) and secondary (inflammatory). In the United States, most of the cases of noninflammatory tinea capitis are caused by *T. tonsurans*, which does not fluorescent green with a Wood lamp. The infection is spread most often among household members who share combs and brushes on which the spores are shed and remain viable for long periods. Depending on the invading fungus, the lesions of the noninflammatory type can vary from grayish, round, hairless patches to balding spots, with or without black dots on the head. The lesions vary in size and are most commonly seen on the back of the head. Mild erythema, crust, or scale may be present. The individual usually is asymptomatic, although pruritus may exist.

The inflammatory type of tinea capitis is caused by virulent strains of *T. mentagrophytes*, *T. verrucosum*, and *M. gypseum*. The onset is rapid, and inflamed lesions usually are localized to one area of the head. The inflammation is believed to be a delayed hypersensitivity reaction to the invading fungus. The initial lesion consists of a pustular, scaly, round patch with broken hairs. A secondary bacterial infection is common and may lead to a painful, circumscribed, boggy, and indurated lesion called a *kerion*.

The treatment for both noninflammatory and inflammatory forms of tinea capitis is oral griseofulvin or synthetic antifungals. Griseofulvin has been the primary treatment for children because it was believed to have fewer side effects than the synthetic antifungals.

Tinea of the Foot and Hand. *Tinea pedis* (athlete's foot) is the most common fungal dermatosis, primarily affecting the spaces between the toes, the soles, or sides of the feet. It is caused by *T. mentagrophytes* and *T. rubrum*. The lesions vary from a mildly scaling lesion to a painful, exudative, erosive, inflamed lesion with fissuring. Lesions often are accompanied by pruritus, pain, and foul odor. Some people are prone to chronic tinea pedis. Mild forms are more common during dry environmental conditions.

Tinea manus usually is a secondary infection with tinea pedis as the primary infection. In contrast to other skin disorders, such as contact dermatitis and psoriasis, which affect both hands, tinea manus usually occurs only on one hand. The characteristic lesion is a blister on the palm or finger surrounded by erythema. Chronic lesions are scaly and dry. Cracking and fissuring may occur. The lesions may spread to the plantar surfaces of the hand. If chronic, tinea manus may lead to tinea of the fingernails. Simple forms of tinea pedis and tinea manus are treated with topical applications of antifungals.

Tinea of the Nail. *Tinea unguium* is a dermatophyte infection of the nails. It is a subset of *onychomycosis*, which includes dermatophyte, nondermatophyte, and candidal infections of the nails. There is an increased incidence of fungal nail infections in recent years, probably reflecting better diagnostics, increased numbers of immunocompromised people who have greater susceptibility, increased use of immunosuppressive drugs, increasing numbers of older adults, worldwide travel, and increased use of communal bathing facilities.

Distal and lateral subungual onychomycosis, the most common form of tinea unguium, usually is caused by *T. rubrum* or *T. mentagrophytes*. Toenails are involved more commonly than fingernails because fingernails are more exposed to air. The infection often begins at the tip of the nail, where the fungus digests the nail keratin. In some cases, the infection may begin from a crushing injury to a toenail or from the spread of tinea pedis. Initially, the nail appears opaque, white, or silver. The nail then turns yellow or brown. The condition often remains unchanged for years. During this time, it may involve only one or two nails and may produce little or no discomfort. Gradually, the nail thickens and cracks as the infection spreads and includes the nail plate. Permanent discoloration and distortion result as the nail plate separates from the nail bed. Less common forms of tinea unguium are superficial white onychomycosis, in which areas of the nails become powdery white and erode, and proximal subungual onychomycosis, in which there is rapid invasion of the nail, leaving it white with no additional thickening of the nail. Although it is one of the less common forms of tinea unguium, proximal subungual onychomycosis has increased among people with human immunodeficiency virus (HIV) infection.

Treatment of tinea unguium usually requires oral antifungal therapy. Toenail infections are usually treated with itraconazole and terbinafine. Fluconazole has been effective, particularly if *Candida* is involved. Itraconazole is administered in pulses (intermittent weeks of therapy), whereas terbinafine or fluconazole is administered without interruption for 12 to 15 weeks. Fingernail infections are more easily treated, in part because the fingernails are more exposed to air. Itraconazole, terbinafine, and, to a lesser extent, griseofulvin have been effective in treating fingernail infections. All of the oral agents require careful monitoring for side effects. A new nail may require 3 to 12 months to grow. Thus, people being treated with antifungal agents need to be reminded that the resolution of the infection requires 4 to 6 months for fingernails and longer for toenails.

Although there has been an increase in the cure rate of toenail fungal infections, primarily because of the synthetic antifungals, recalcitrant cases remain. Some authorities recommend removal of the infected toenails. Many cases of tinea unguium would be prevented if primary infections of tinea pedis were diagnosed and treated promptly.

Tinea Versicolor. Tinea versicolor is a fungal infection involving the upper chest, the back, and sometimes the arms. It is caused by the dimorphic–lipophilic yeasts *Pityrosporum orbiculare* (round form) and *P. ovale* (oval form).[4] The yeast lives within the stratum corneum and hair follicles in areas with sebaceous glands where it is easy to obtain triglycerides and free fatty acids.[4] The characteristic lesion is a yellow, pink, or brown sheet of scaling skin (see Fig. 52.4). The name *versicolor* is derived from the multicolored variations of the lesion. The patches are depigmented and do not tan when exposed to UV light.

Selenium sulfide, found in several shampoo preparations, has been an effective fungistatic treatment measure. Miconazole or ketoconazole creams or shampoos, because of their fungicidal properties, have become the drugs of choice. Oral antifungals are used for extensive cases. The infection may recur after drug therapy.

Tinea Incognito. Tinea incognito is a form of dermatophyte infection that developed with the widespread use of topical corticosteroids. It often is seen in cases where tinea infections are misdiagnosed as eczema and treated with corticosteroids. Because corticosteroids suppress inflammation, scaling and erythema may not be present or it may not resemble a fungal infection at all after several rounds of cortisone therapy.

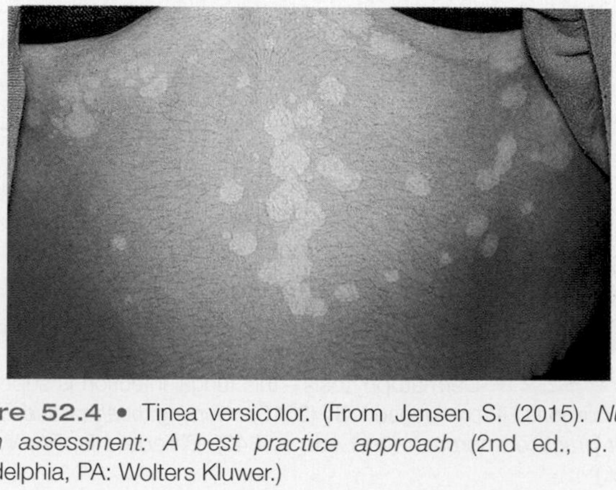

Figure 52.4 • Tinea versicolor. (From Jensen S. (2015). *Nursing health assessment: A best practice approach* (2nd ed., p. 276). Philadelphia, PA: Wolters Kluwer.)

There has been an increased incidence of tinea incognito in people with HIV infection. People with the disorder often present with thickened plaques with lichenification, papules, pustules, and nodules. Telangiectases, atrophy, and striae may be present. Tinea incognito is seen most often on the groin, the palms, or the dorsal aspect of the hand.

Treatment measures include discontinuing topical corticosteroids while using low-dose oral corticosteroids to prevent the flare-up associated with discontinuing potent topical steroids. Topical or oral antifungal agents are used, depending on the severity of the infection.

Dermatophytid Reaction. A secondary skin eruption may occur in people allergic to the fungus responsible for the dermatophytosis. This dermatophytid or allergic reaction may occur during an acute episode of a fungal infection. The most common reaction occurs on the hands in response to tinea pedis. The lesions are vesicles with erythema extending over the palms and fingers, sometimes extending to other areas. Less commonly, a more generalized reaction occurs, in which papules or vesicles erupt on the trunk or extremities. These eruptions may resemble tinea corporis. Lesions may become excoriated and infected with bacteria. Treatment is directed at the primary site of infection. The intradermal reaction resolves in most cases without intervention if the primary site is cleared.

Candidal Infections. Candidiasis (moniliasis) is a fungal infection caused by *C. albicans* and occasionally by a few other *Candida* species. This yeastlike fungus is a normal inhabitant of the gastrointestinal tract, mouth, and vagina. The skin problems result from the release of irritating toxins on the skin surface. *C. albicans* is found almost always on the surface of the skin. It rarely penetrates to the deeper layers of the skin. Some people are predisposed to candidal infections by conditions such as diabetes mellitus, antibiotic therapy, pregnancy, oral contraceptive use, poor nutrition, and immunosuppressive diseases. Oral candidiasis may be the first sign of infection with HIV.

C. albicans thrives on warm, moist, intertriginous areas of the body. The rash is red with well-defined borders. Patches erode the epidermis, and there is scaling. Mild to severe itching and burning often accompany the infection. Severe forms of infection may involve pustules or vesiculopustules. In addition to microscopy, a candidal infection often can be differentiated from a tinea infection by the presence of satellite lesions. These satellite lesions are maculopapular and are found outside the clearly demarcated borders of the candidal infection. Satellite lesions often are diagnostic of diaper rash complicated by *Candida*. The appearance of candidal infections varies according to the site.

Diagnosis usually is based on microscopic examination of the skin or mucous membrane scrapings placed in a KOH solution. Treatment measures vary according to the location. Preventive measures such as wearing rubber gloves are encouraged for people with infections of the hands. Intertriginous areas often are separated with clean cotton cloth and allowed to air dry as a means of decreasing the macerating effects of heat and moisture. Topical and oral antifungal agents, such as clotrimazole, econazole, and miconazole, are used in treatment depending on the site and extent of involvement.

Bacterial Infections

Bacteria are considered normal flora of the skin. Most bacteria are not pathogenic, but when pathogenic bacteria invade the skin, superficial or systemic infections may develop. Bacterial skin infections are commonly classified as primary or secondary infections. Primary infections are superficial skin infections such as impetigo or ecthyma. Secondary infections consist of deeper cutaneous infections, such as infected ulcers. Diagnosis usually is based on cultures taken from the infected site. Treatment measures include antibiotic therapy and measures to promote comfort and prevent the spread of infection.

Impetigo. Impetigo is a common, superficial bacterial infection caused by staphylococci or group A beta-hemolytic streptococci, or both.[4] Impetigo is common among infants and young children, although older children and adults occasionally contract the disease. Its occurrence is highest during warm summer months or in warm, moist climates.

Impetigo initially appears as a small vesicle or pustule or as a large bulla on the face or elsewhere on the body. As the primary lesion ruptures, it leaves a denuded area that discharges a honey-colored serous liquid that hardens on the skin surface and dries as a honey-colored crust (Fig. 52.5). New vesicles erupt within hours. Pruritus often accompanies the lesions, and skin excoriations that result from scratching multiply the infection sites. Although a very low risk, a possible complication of untreated streptococcal impetigo is poststreptococcal glomerulonephritis. Topical mupirocin (Bactroban) is effective in treating impetigo and has few side effects. In most instances, it is the first choice but if a larger area is involved then a systemic antibiotic may be necessary.[10]

Another form of impetigo exists, *bullous impetigo*, which is usually caused by *Staphylococcus aureus*.[4] Bullous impetigo is common among children. It is due to the epidermolytic toxin and is not generally contaminated by streptococci.[4,11]

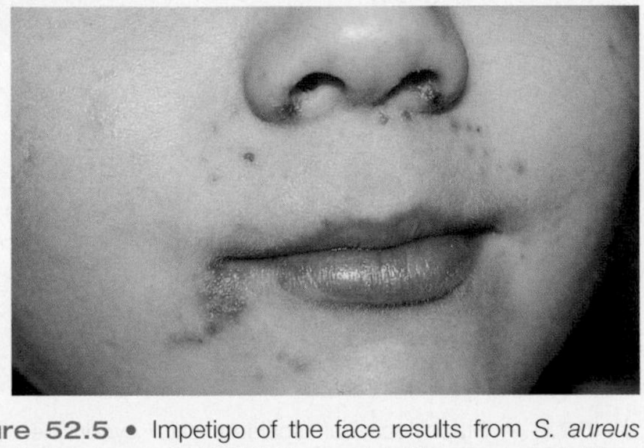

Figure 52.5 • Impetigo of the face results from *S. aureus* commonly. (From Jensen S. (2015). *Nursing health assessment: A best practice approach* (2nd ed., p. 274). Philadelphia, PA: Wolters Kluwer.)

Thin bullae erupt that appear clear to cloudy and coalesce. The bullae open, leaving the original bullous rim with central thin, flat, honey-colored crusts, or in some cases denuded areas. The face is often affected, but bullous impetigo may occur anywhere on the body. The treatment measures are the same as for nonbullous impetigo.

Ecthyma is an ulcerative form of impetigo, usually secondary to minor trauma. It is caused by group A beta-hemolytic streptococci, *S. aureus*, or *Pseudomonas* species. It frequently occurs on the buttocks and thighs of children. The lesions are similar to those of impetigo. A vesicle or pustule ruptures, leaving a skin erosion or ulcer that weeps and dries to a crusted patch, often resulting in scar formation. With extensive ecthyma, there is a low-grade fever and extension of the infection to other organs. Treatment usually involves the use of systemic antibiotics.

A less common form of *S. aureus* infection, called *Ritter disease*, manifests with a diffuse, scarlet fever–like rash, followed by skin separation and sloughing. It is also called *staphylococcal scalded skin syndrome* because the skin looks scalded (Fig. 52.6). Ritter disease usually affects children younger than 5 years of age. However, immunosuppressed adults also are at risk. The disorder, which is considered a deeper skin infection because the superficial layers of the epidermis are separated and shed in sheets, is caused by the hematologic spread of toxins from a focal infection, such as the nasopharynx or a superficial skin abrasion. The onset of the rash may be preceded by malaise, fever, irritability, and extreme tenderness over the skin. The conjunctiva often is inflamed, with purulent drainage. Although the fluid in the unbroken bullae is sterile, cultures usually are obtained from suspected sites of local infection and from the blood. Systemic antibiotics, either oral or parenteral, are used to treat the disorder. Healing usually occurs in 10 to 14 days without scarring.

Cellulitis is a deeper infection affecting the dermis and subcutaneous tissues. It is usually caused by group A beta-hemolytic streptococci or *S. aureus*, but can be caused by bacteria specific to certain activities, such as fish handling, swimming in fresh water, or swimming in salt water, or from animal bites or scratches. Preexisting wounds (*e.g.*, ulcers, erosions) and tinea pedis are often portals of entry. Legs are the most common sites, followed by the hands and pinnae of the ears, but cellulitis may be seen on many body parts. The lesion consists of an expanding red, swollen, tender plaque with an indefinite border, covering a small to wide area (Fig. 52.7). Cellulitis is frequently accompanied by fever, erythema, heat, edema, and pain. Cellulitis often involves the lymph system, and, once compromised, repeat infections may impair lymphatic drainage, leading to chronically swollen legs, and eventually dermal fibrosis and lymphedema. Incorrectly treated, it may result in septicemia, nephritis, or death. Treatment measures (oral and intravenous antibiotics) are aimed at the invasive organisms and the extent of the infection.

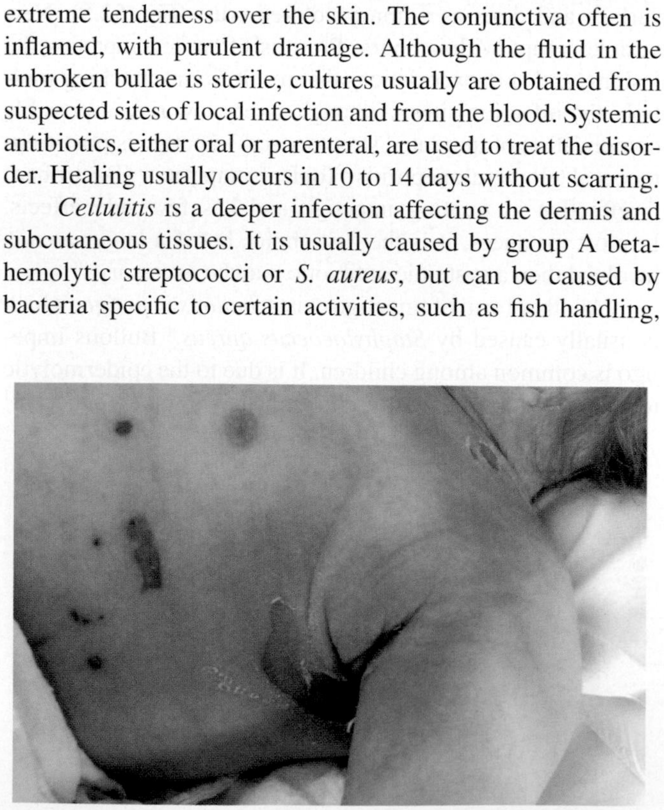

Figure 52.6 • Staphylococcal scalded skin syndrome. (From Jensen S. (2015). *Nursing health assessment: A best practice approach* (2nd ed., p. 846). Philadelphia, PA: Wolters Kluwer.)

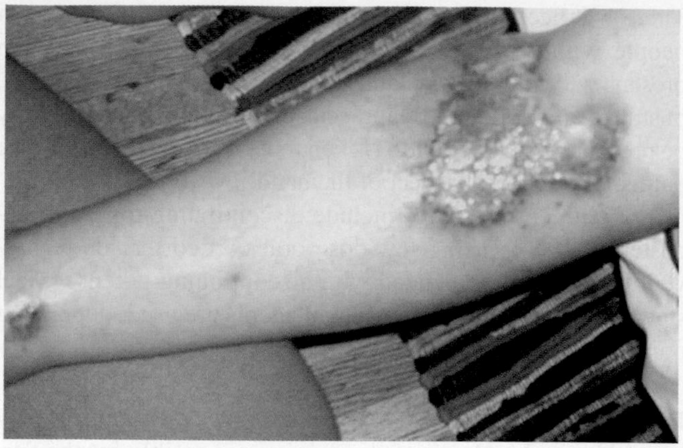

Figure 52.7 • Cellulitis on leg infected with *S. aureus* and *Pseudomonas*.

Viral Infections

Viruses are intracellular pathogens that rely on live cells of the host for reproduction. They have no organized cell structure but consist of a deoxyribonucleic acid (DNA) or ribonucleic acid (RNA) core surrounded by a protein coat. The viruses seen in skin lesion disorders tend to be DNA-containing viruses. Viruses invade the keratinocyte, begin to reproduce, and cause cellular proliferation or cellular death. The rapid increase in viral skin diseases has been attributed to the use of corticosteroid drugs, which have immunosuppressive qualities, and the use of antibiotics, which alter the bacterial flora of the skin. As the number of bacterial infections has decreased, there has been a proportional rise in viral skin diseases.

Verrucae. Verrucae, or warts, are common benign papillomas caused by the DNA-containing human papillomavirus (HPV). Transmission of HPV infection is largely by direct contact between people or by autoinoculation. As benign papillomas, warts represent an exaggeration of the normal skin structures. There is an irregular thickening of the stratum spinosum and greatly increased thickening of the stratum corneum. The classification of warts is based largely on morphology and location.

Although warts vary in appearance depending on their location, it is now recognized that the clinically distinct types of warts result not simply because of the anatomic sites in which they arise but also because of the distinct types of HPV. There are almost 90 types of HPV found on humans that cause several different kinds of warts, including skin warts and genital warts.[4] Many of the HPV types that cause genital warts are sexually transmitted, some of which (types 6, 11, 16, and 18) may increase the risk of cervical cancer.[4,12,13]

Nongenital warts often occur on the hands and feet. They are commonly caused by HPV types 1, 2, 3, 4, 27, and 57 and are not considered precancerous lesions. They are classified as common warts, flat warts, and plantar or palmar warts. Common warts, or verrucae vulgaris, are the most common type. The lesions can occur anywhere but most frequently occur on dorsal surfaces of hands, especially the periungual area, where they appear as small, grayish-white to tan, flat to convex papules with a rough, pebble-like surface. Verrucae plana, or flat warts, are common on the face or dorsal surfaces of the hands. The warts are slightly elevated, flat, smooth, tan papules that are slightly larger than verrucae vulgaris (Fig. 52.8). Verrucae plantaris and verrucae palmaris (*i.e.*, plantar and palmar warts, respectively) occur on the soles of the feet and palms of the hands, respectively. They appear as rough, scaly lesions that may reach 1 to 2 cm in diameter, coalesce, and be confused with ordinary calluses. HPV transmission usually occurs through breaks in skin integrity.

Treatment is usually directed at inducing a "wart-free" period without producing scarring. Warts resolve spontaneously when immunity to the virus develops. The immune response, however, may be delayed for years. Because of their appearance or discomfort, people usually desire their removal, rather than waiting for immunity to develop. Removal is usually done by applying a keratolytic agent, such as salicylic acid gel or plaster that breaks down the wart tissue, or by freezing with liquid nitrogen. Salicylic acid works by dissolving intercellular cement and producing desquamation of the horny layer of skin without affecting normal epidermal cells. Various types of laser surgery, electrosurgery, cryotherapy, immunotherapy (*e.g.*, oral zinc sulfate), and antiviral therapy (*e.g.*, cidofovir) also have been successful in wart eradication.

Herpes Simplex. Herpes simplex virus (HSV) infections of the skin and mucous membrane (*i.e.*, cold sore or fever blister) are common. Two types of HSV infect humans: type 1 and type 2. HSV-1 is usually associated with oropharynx infections, and the organism is spread by respiratory droplets or by direct contact with infected saliva. HSV-1 may also be transmitted to other parts of the body through occupational hazards, such as skin contact athletics, dentistry, and medicine. Genital herpes usually is caused by HSV-2. HSV-1 genital infections and HSV-2 oral infections are becoming more common.

Infection with HSV-1 may present as a primary or recurrent infection. Primary HSV-1 symptoms include fever; sore throat; painful vesicles; and ulcers of the tongue, palate, gingiva, buccal mucosa, and lips. Primary infection results in the production of antibodies to the virus so that recurrent infections are more localized and less severe. After an initial infection, the herpesvirus persists in the trigeminal and other dorsal root ganglia in the latent state, periodically reactivating in recurrent infections. It may be that reactivation of a herpes infection occurs both in the dorsal root ganglion and locally, where it has been found to exist in the epidermis and other organs. The symptoms of a primary HSV-1 infection most often occur in young children (1 to 5 years of age). It is likely that many adults were exposed to HSV-1 during childhood and therefore have antibodies to the virus.

The recurrent lesions of HSV-1 usually begin with a burning or tingling sensation. Umbilicated vesicles and erythema follow and progress to pustules, ulcers, and crusts before healing (Fig. 52.9). Lesions are most common on the lips, face, mouth, nasal septum, and nose. When a lesion is active,

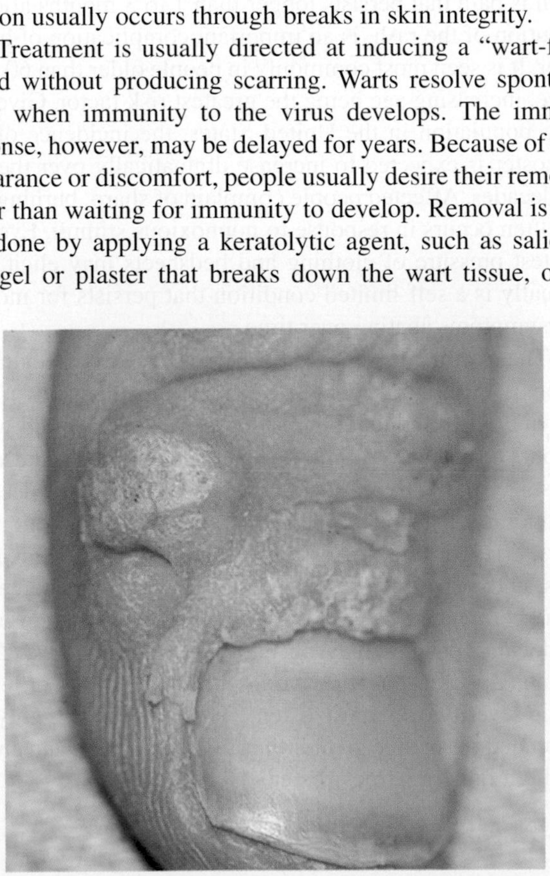

Figure 52.8 • Common warts. (From Jensen S. (2015). *Nursing health assessment: A best practice approach* (2nd ed., p. 273). Philadelphia, PA: Wolters Kluwer.)

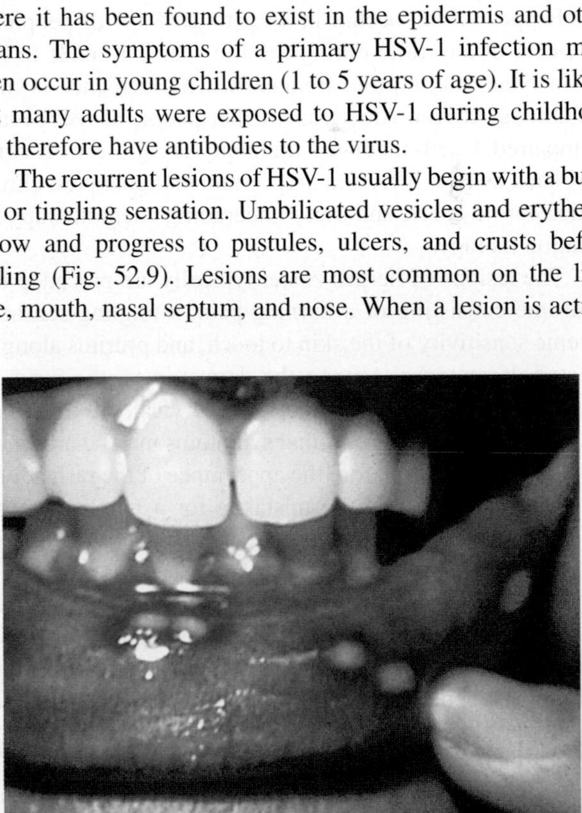

Figure 52.9 • Herpes simplex 1 of the oral mucosa. (From Jensen S. (2015). *Nursing health assessment: A best practice approach* (2nd ed., p. 407). Philadelphia, PA: Wolters Kluwer.)

HSV-1 is shed, and there is risk of transmitting the virus to others. Pain is common, and healing takes place within 10 to 14 days. Precipitating factors may be stress, menses, or injury. In particular, UVB exposure seems to be a frequent trigger for recurrence. There is no cure for oropharyngeal herpes. Most treatment measures are palliative. Penciclovir cream or docosanol cream, topical antiviral agents, applied at the first symptom and then several times daily, reduces the duration of an attack. Application of over-the-counter topical preparations containing antihistamines, antipruritics, and anesthetic agents along with aspirin or acetaminophen may be used to relieve pain. Oral acyclovir, an antiviral drug that inhibits herpesvirus replication, may be used prophylactically to prevent recurrences. The antiviral drugs valacyclovir and famciclovir also may be used for prophylaxis.

Herpes Zoster. Herpes zoster (shingles) is an acute, localized vesicular eruption distributed over a dermatomal segment of the skin. It is caused by the same herpesvirus, varicella–zoster, which causes chickenpox. It is believed to be the result of reactivation of a latent varicella–zoster virus infection that was dormant in the sensory dorsal root ganglia since a primary childhood infection. During an episode of herpes zoster, the reactivated virus travels from the ganglia to the skin of the corresponding dermatome. Although herpes zoster is not as contagious as chickenpox, the reactivated virus can be transmitted to nonimmune contacts.

Herpes zoster occurs in 10% to 20% of all people.[4] It can occur at any time during the life span but tends to happen in older adults more frequently. The incidence is much less among African Americans. Other people at risk because of impaired T-cell–mediated immunity are those with conditions such as HIV infection and certain malignancies, chronic corticosteroid users, and those undergoing chemotherapy and radiation therapy.

The lesions of herpes zoster typically are preceded by a prodrome consisting of a burning pain, a tingling sensation, extreme sensitivity of the skin to touch, and pruritus along the affected dermatome. Among the dermatomes, the most frequently involved are the thoracic, the cervical, the trigeminal, and the lumbosacral. Prodromal symptoms may be present for 1 to 3 days or longer before the appearance of the rash. During this time, the pain may be mistaken for a number of other conditions, such as heart disease, pleurisy, musculoskeletal disorders, or gastrointestinal disorders.

The lesions appear as an eruption of vesicles with erythematous bases that are restricted to skin areas supplied by sensory neurons of a single or associated group of dorsal root ganglia. In immunosuppressed people, the lesions may extend beyond the dermatome. Eruptions usually are unilateral in the thoracic region, trunk, or face. New groups of vesicles erupt for 3 to 5 days along the nerve pathway. The vesicles dry, form crusts, and eventually fall off. The lesions usually clear in 2 to 3 weeks, although they can persist up to 6 weeks in some older adults.

Serious complications can accompany eruptions. Eye involvement can result in permanent blindness and occurs in a large percentage of cases involving the ophthalmic division of the trigeminal nerve (Fig. 52.10). *Postherpetic neuralgia*, which is pain that persists longer than 1 to 3 months after the resolution of the rash, is an important complication of herpes zoster. It is seen most commonly in people older than 60 years of age, increasing age being the greatest risk factor. Given the aging population in the United States, the incidence of herpes zoster is expected to increase dramatically over the next two decades. Affected people complain of sharp, burning pain that often occurs in response to nonnoxious stimuli. Even the slightest pressure of clothing and bedsheets may elicit pain. It usually is a self-limited condition that persists for months, with symptoms abating over time.

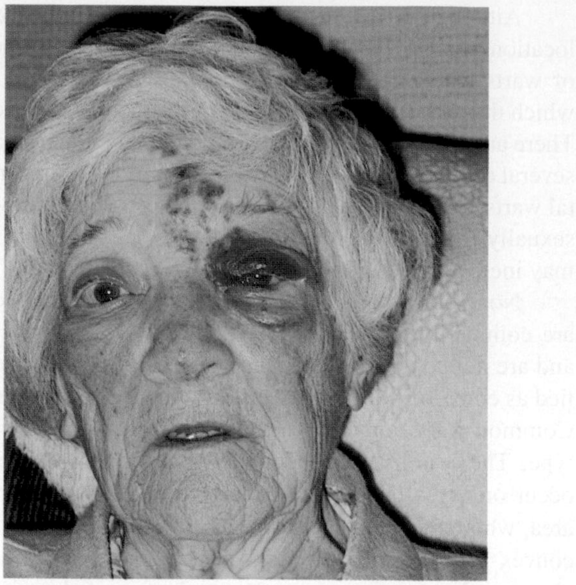

Figure 52.10 • Dermatomal distribution of herpes zoster rash due to varicella–zoster virus. (From Hinkle J. L., Cheever K. H. (2018). *Brunner & Suddarth's Textbook of medical–surgical nursing* (14th ed., p. 1819). Philadelphia, PA: Wolters Kluwer.)

The treatment of choice for herpes zoster is the administration of an antiviral agent (*e.g.*, acyclovir, valacyclovir, famciclovir). The treatment is most effective when started within 72 hours of rash development. When given in the acute vesicular stage, the antiviral drugs have been shown to decrease the amount of lesion development and pain. Narcotic analgesics, tricyclic antidepressants, gabapentin, anticonvulsant drugs, and nerve blocks have been used for management of postherpetic neuralgia. Local application of capsaicin cream or lidocaine patches may be used in selected cases. Zoster vaccine (Zostavax) is effective in either preventing or lessening the severity of herpes zoster.[14] This vaccine is highly recommended for people greater than 50 years of age and anyone with high risk for herpes zoster.[15]

Acne and Rosacea

Acne is a disorder of the pilosebaceous unit, which comprises a tiny vellus hair, hair follicle, and sebaceous gland.[16,17] The hair follicle is a tubular invagination of the epidermis in which hair is produced. The sebaceous glands empty into the hair follicle, and the pilosebaceous unit opens to the skin surface through a widely dilated opening called a *pore*. The sebaceous glands produce a complex lipid mixture called *sebum*. Sebum consists of a mixture of free fatty acids, triglycerides, diglycerides, monoglycerides, sterol esters, wax esters, and squalene. Sebum production occurs through what is called a *holocrine process*, in which the sebaceous gland cells that produce the sebum are completely broken down and their lipid contents emptied through the sebaceous duct into the hair follicle. The amount of sebum produced depends on two factors: the size of the sebaceous gland and the rate of sebaceous cell proliferation. The sebaceous glands are largest on the face, scalp, and scrotum but are present in all areas of the skin except for the soles and palms. Sebaceous cell proliferation and sebum production are uniquely responsive to direct hormonal stimulation by androgens. In men, testicular androgens are the main stimulus for sebaceous activity; in women, adrenal and ovarian androgens maintain sebaceous activity.

Acne lesions are divided into noninflammatory and inflammatory lesions.[18]

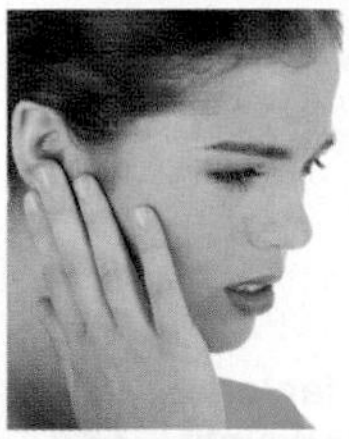

Remember **Lauren** from the unit opener case study who had presented with a "growth on the lower right ear lobe" and an itchy rash on her hands? She seems to think she may have an acne problem with this growth. She asks, "What exactly is this growth on my ear? They said it was a keloid, but I have never heard of anything like that before." She is educated about the keloid that formed after her piercing and says, "Well, I guess it is not acne, but do you think it could be skin cancer?"

Noninflammatory lesions consist of *comedones* (whiteheads and blackheads). *Blackheads* are plugs of material that accumulate in sebaceous glands that open to the skin surface. The color of blackheads results from melanin that has moved into the sebaceous glands from adjoining epidermal cells. *Whiteheads* are pale, slightly elevated papules with no visible orifice. Inflammatory lesions consist of papules, pustules, nodules, and, in severe cases, cysts.[18] *Papules* are raised areas less than 5 mm in diameter. *Pustules* have a central core of purulent material. *Nodules* are larger than 5 mm in diameter and may become suppurative or hemorrhagic. Suppurative nodules often are referred to as *cysts* because of their resemblance to inflamed epidermal cysts. The inflammatory lesions are believed to develop from the escape of sebum into the dermis and the irritating effects of the fatty acids contained in the sebum.

Two types of acne occur during different stages of the life cycle: acne vulgaris, which is the most common form among adolescents and young adults, and acne conglobata, which develops later in life. Other types of acne occur in association with various etiologic agents such as drugs (*e.g.*, steroids, iodides), occupational compounds, cosmetics, and other irritating agents. Treatment measures for these acnes depend on the precipitating agent and the extent of the lesions.

Acne Vulgaris

Acne vulgaris is considered a chronic inflammatory disease of the pilosebaceous unit. It is a disorder of adolescents and young adults, affecting over 80% of people between the ages of 11 and 30 years in westernized countries.[19] In women, acne may begin earlier and persist longer. However, overall, the incidence and severity of acne vulgaris is greater in men. Acne vulgaris lesions form primarily on the face and neck and, to a lesser extent, on the back, chest, and shoulders (Fig. 52.11). The lesions may consist of comedones (whiteheads and blackheads) or inflammatory lesions (pustules, nodules, and cysts).

Etiology. The cause of acne vulgaris remains unknown. However, there is a genetic factor. Multiple generations of family members often experience the disease. Several factors are believed to contribute to acne, including:

- Increased sebum production
- Increased proliferation of the keratinizing epidermal cells that form the sebaceous cells
- The colonization and proliferation of *Propionibacterium acnes*
- Inflammation

These factors are probably interrelated. Increased androgen production results in increased sebaceous cell activity, with resultant plugging of the pilosebaceous ducts. The excessive sebum provides a medium for the growth of *P. acnes*. The *P. acnes* organism contains lipases that break down the free fatty acids that produce the acne inflammation. In addition, there have been new findings regarding the physiology of acne (Fig. 52.12). One example is that *P. acnes* form a biofilm

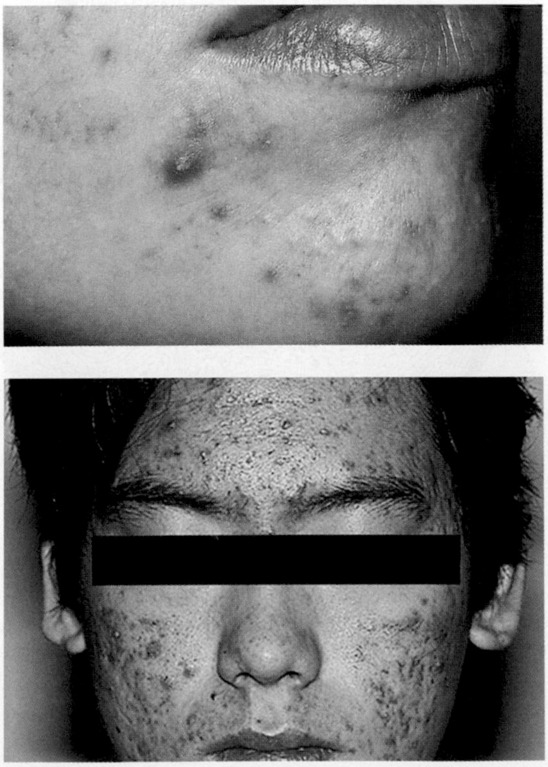

A

B

Figure 52.11 • Pustular acne **(A)** and cystic acne **(B)**. (From Jensen S. (2015). *Nursing health assessment: A best practice approach* (2nd ed., p. 273). Philadelphia, PA: Wolters Kluwer.)

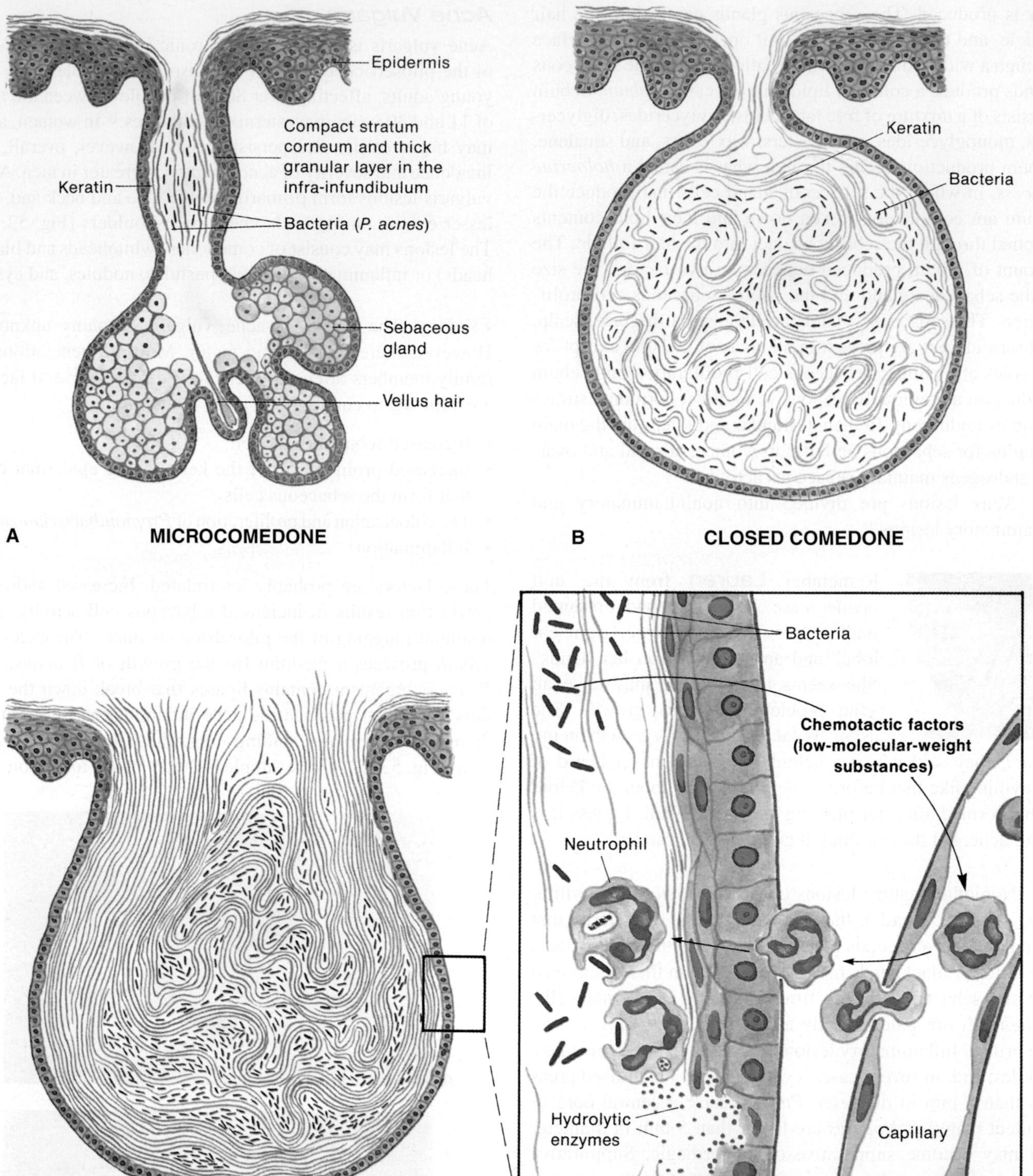

Figure 52.12 • Acne vulgaris. The pathogenesis of follicular distention, rupture, and inflammation is illustrated. Microcomedones **(A)** and closed **(B)** and open **(C)** comedones form. Excessive sebum can be secreted, and the *P. acnes* proliferates. Neutrophilic enzymes are released, and the comedone ruptures causing a cycle of intense inflammation **(D,E)**. (From Strayer D., Rubin R. (2015). *Rubin's pathology: Clinicopathologic foundations of medicine* (7th ed., p. 1250). Philadelphia, PA: Wolters Kluwer.)

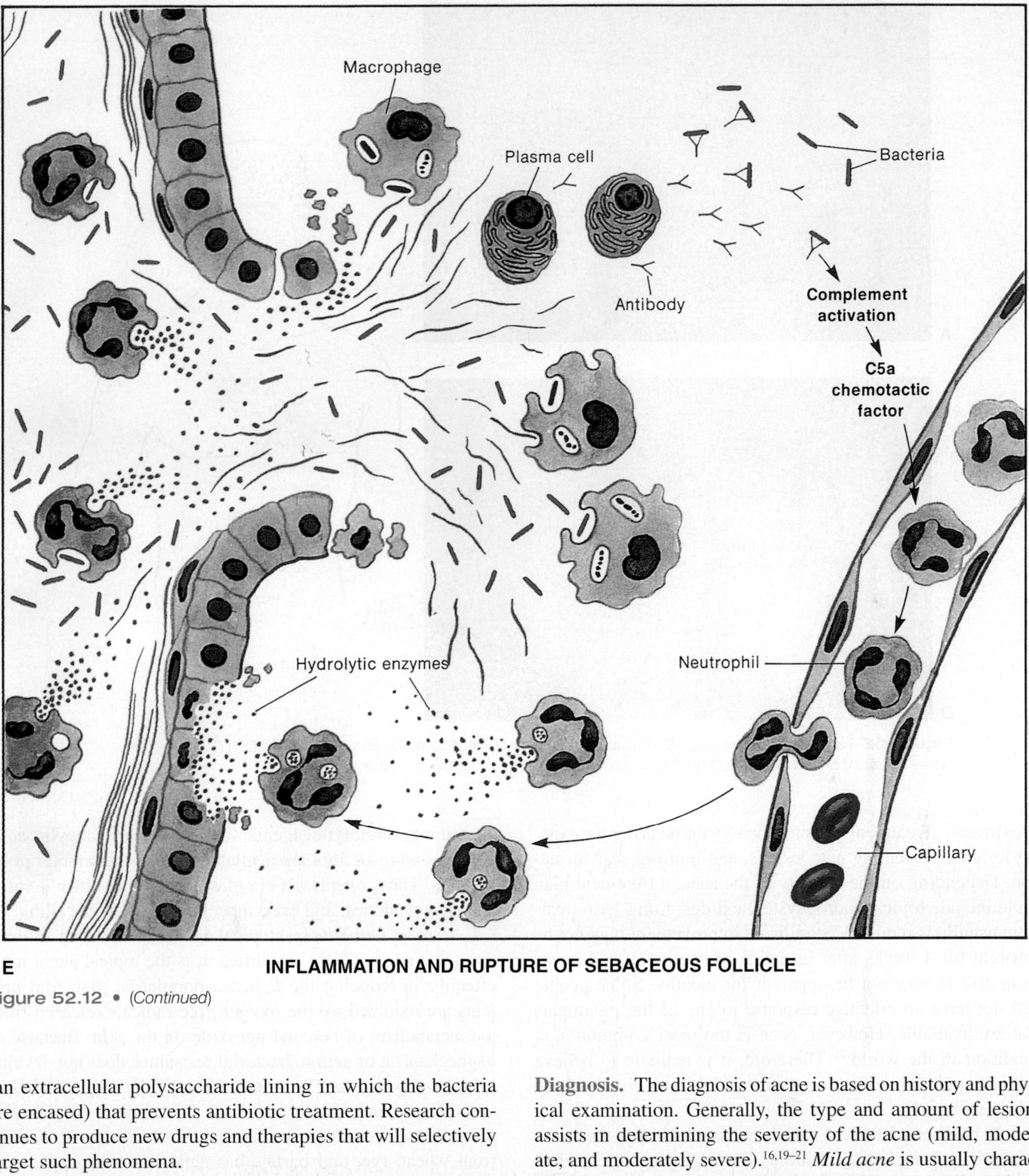

E INFLAMMATION AND RUPTURE OF SEBACEOUS FOLLICLE

Figure 52.12 • (Continued)

(an extracellular polysaccharide lining in which the bacteria are encased) that prevents antibiotic treatment. Research continues to produce new drugs and therapies that will selectively target such phenomena.

Over the years, several factors, such as poor hygiene, acne as an infectious process, diets high in fatty content, and certain foods (*e.g.*, chocolate, fried foods) have been studied empirically and rejected as causal factors in the development of acne. Although general hygienic measures are important, obsessive scrubbing can traumatize the skin and worsen the condition. Instead, it is recommended that the affected areas be washed gently and patted dry.

Diagnosis. The diagnosis of acne is based on history and physical examination. Generally, the type and amount of lesions assists in determining the severity of the acne (mild, moderate, and moderately severe).[16,19–21] *Mild acne* is usually characterized by the presence of a small number (generally <10) of open and closed comedones, with a few inflammatory papules. *Moderate acne* is characterized by the presence of a moderate number (10 to 40) of erythematous papules and pustules, usually limited to the face. Moderately severe acne is characterized by the presence of numerous papules and pustules (40 to 100) and occasionally larger, deeper, nodular inflamed lesions involving the face, chest, and back (see Fig. 52.13).

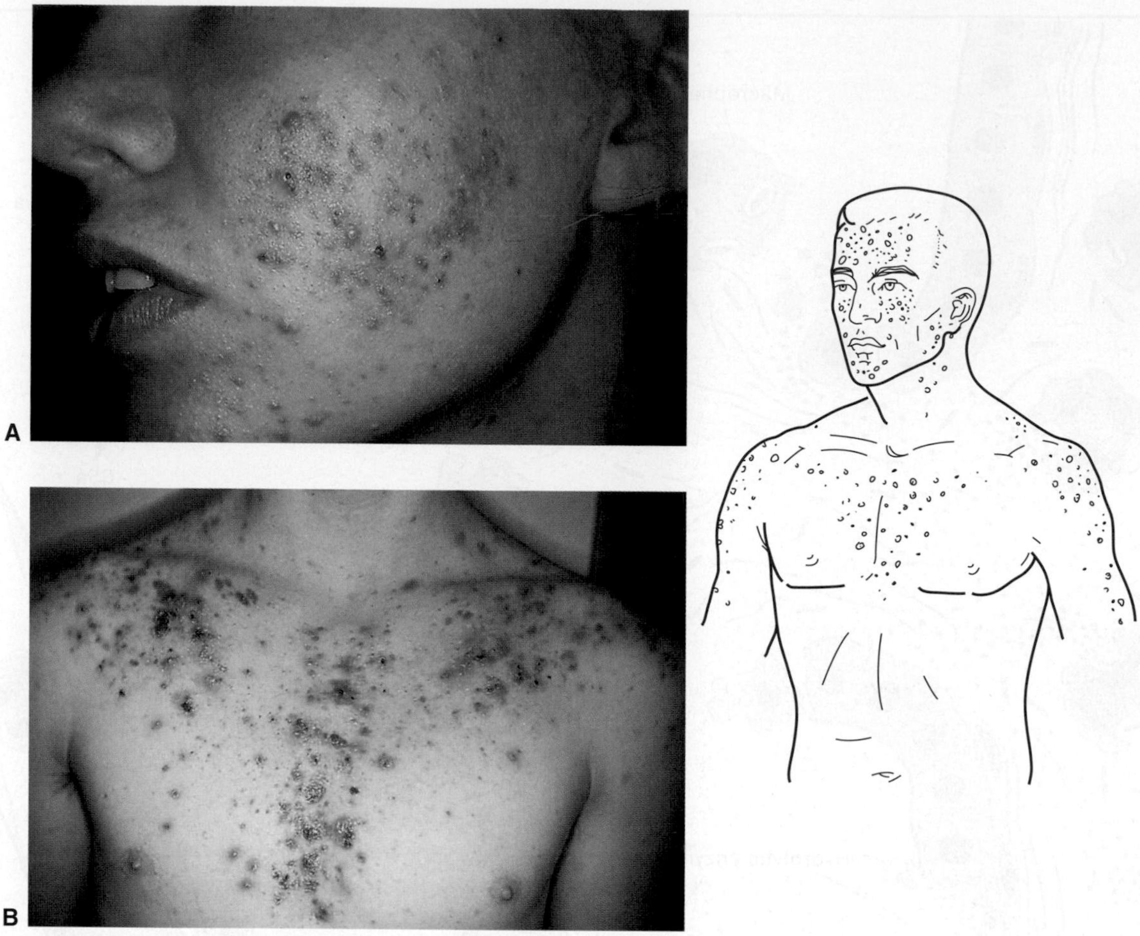

Figure 52.13 • Acne of the face **(A)** and acne of the chest **(B)**. (From Hall B. J., Hall J. C. (2017). *Sauer's manual of skin diseases* (11th ed., p. 180). Philadelphia, PA: Wolters Kluwer.)

Treatment. Treatment of acne focuses on clearing up existing lesions, preventing new lesions, and limiting scar formation. Depending on the severity of the acne, a treatment plan could include topical and/or systemic drugs. Long-term treatment usually is required. Significant improvement may not be apparent for 4 weeks after initiation of treatment, and maximum effects may not be apparent for months. Some people will not have an effective response to any of the treatments that are available. However, acne is the most common skin condition in the world.[21] Therefore, it is realistic to believe that new and more effective treatment measures will continue to be developed.

A number of topical agents are available for the treatment of acne, including retinoids, benzoyl peroxide, azelaic acid, and antibiotics. Topical retinoids, benzoyl peroxide, and azelaic acid are effective treatments for mild acne. Moderate to severe acne often requires combination therapy with a topical agent and systemic antibiotics. The type of topical (cream, gel, or lotion) may be an important consideration in the selection of an agent. People with drier skin may benefit from creams, whereas people with oily skin may have better results using a gel or lotion. Many acne creams and lotions containing keratolytic agents such as sulfur, salicylic acid, phenol, and resorcinol are available as over-the-counter preparations. These agents act chemically to break down keratin, loosen comedones, and exert a peeling effect on the skin.[16,18]

Benzoyl peroxide is a topical agent that has both antibacterial and comedolytic properties. It is the topical agent most effective in reducing the *P. acnes* population. Bacterial proteins are oxidized by the oxygen-free radicals released from the metabolism of benzoyl peroxide on the skin. Because of its mechanism of action, bacterial resistance does not develop to benzoyl peroxide. The irritant effect of the drug also causes vasodilation and increased blood flow, which may hasten resolution of the inflammatory lesions. *Azelaic acid*, derived from wheat, rye, and barley, has actions similar to benzoyl peroxide. It decreases the proliferation of keratinocytes and has antibacterial actions against *P. acnes*. Azelaic cream is moisturizing and causes only minimal skin irritation.

Topical tretinoin (Retin-A), an acid derivative of vitamin A, acts locally to decrease the cohesiveness of epidermal cells and increase epidermal cell turnover. This is thought to result in an increased extrusion of open comedones and a transformation of closed comedones into open ones. Tretinoin is inactivated by UV light and oxidized to benzoyl peroxide and should be applied only at night and not with benzoyl peroxide. All tretinoin formulations are irritating to the skin, an effect that is increased with sun exposure. Another form of tretinoin, Retin-A Micro, works by entrapping the drug in microspheres that move into the follicle and serve as reservoirs for drug release. Other retinoid drugs, such as adapalene and tazarotene, have actions similar to tretinoin. Adapalene appears to be as effective as tretinoin but may be less irritating to the skin.

Topical antibiotics also are effective in treating mild to moderate acne. Topical tetracycline, erythromycin, and clindamycin are used most commonly. They do not affect existing lesions but prevent future lesions by decreasing the amount of *P. acnes* on the skin, thereby reducing subsequent inflammation formed from the presence of sebaceous fatty acid metabolites. Treatment failure can result from development of antibiotic resistance. Combination drugs such as benzoyl peroxide and erythromycin or minocycline also have been effective.

Oral antibiotics are indicated for moderate to severe disease and for the treatment of acne on the chest, back, or shoulders. Low-dose tetracycline has been used effectively for many years. Tetracycline has no effect on sebum production, but it decreases bacterial growth and the amount of free fatty acids produced. Tetracycline requires a sufficient treatment period to establish effective blood levels. Side effects are minimal, which is why the drug has remained so useful. However, it does have teratogenic effects on skeletal and tooth development and should not be given to those who are pregnant or lactating or to children. The tetracycline derivatives, minocycline and doxycycline, are better tolerated than tetracycline. Doxycycline may cause photosensitivity reactions. Erythromycin also is effective in acne treatment, especially when tetracycline and its derivatives cannot be used.

Isotretinoin (Accutane), an orally administered synthetic retinoid or acid form of vitamin A, revolutionized the treatment of recalcitrant cases of acne and cystic acnes. In carefully planned doses, oral isotretinoin has cleared major cases of acne and initiated long-term remissions of the disease. It is administered for 3- to 4-month treatment periods. Although the exact mode of action is unknown, it decreases sebaceous gland activity, prevents new comedones from forming, reduces the *P. acnes* count through sebum reduction, and has an anti-inflammatory effect. However, because of its many side effects, it is used only in people with severe acne and only when no other treatment is effective. Side effects include dryness of the mouth and other mucous membranes, conjunctivitis, and musculoskeletal system abnormalities. Various population-based studies have yielded inconclusive evidence as to whether depression and suicide ideation increases in people taking isotretinoin.[22,23] Careful clinical and laboratory monitoring is necessary because the drug can produce elevated serum lipid levels, abnormal liver enzyme test results, and hematologic disorders. Isotretinoin is a teratogen that causes brain, heart, and ear malformations. Women taking isotretinoin are strongly advised not to become pregnant.

Estrogens reduce the size and secretion of the sebaceous gland, but because of the high dosages required, they are contraindicated in men. In women, oral contraceptive agents that combine estrogen with a progestin that has low androgenic activity may be used.

Other treatment measures for acne include surgery, UV irradiation, cryotherapy (*e.g.*, freezing with carbon dioxide slushes, liquid nitrogen), laser therapy, and intralesional corticosteroid injection. Intralesional injection of corticosteroids using a syringe or needleless injector is limited to severe nodulocystic forms of acne. It has been effective in promoting cyst healing but usually has to be repeated frequently.

Acne Conglobata

Acne conglobata occurs later in life and is a chronic form of severe cystic acne.[5] Comedones, papules, pustules, nodules, abscesses, cysts, and scars occur on the back, buttocks, and chest. Lesions occur to a lesser extent on the abdomen, shoulders, neck, face, upper arms, and thighs. The comedones or cysts have multiple openings, large abscesses, and interconnecting sinuses. Inflammatory nodules are not uncommon. Their discharge is odoriferous, serous or mucoid, and purulent. Healing often leaves deep keloidal lesions. Affected people have anemia with elevated white blood cell counts, erythrocyte sedimentation rates, and neutrophil counts. When people with acne conglobata also have leukocytosis, fever, and arthralgia, this type of acne is diagnosed as acne fulminans.[5] The treatment often includes debridement, systemic corticosteroid therapy, oral retinoids, and systemic antibiotics.

Rosacea

Rosacea is a chronic inflammatory process that occurs in adults between the ages of 30 and 50 years of age.[5] It is easily confused with acne and may coexist with it. Rosacea is more common in fair-skinned people. Rosacea affects an estimated 14 million people in the United States.[24] Most people with rosacea are white women older than 30 years of age.

Etiology. The cause of rosacea is unknown. However, it is believed to be an inflammatory process accompanied by vascular instability with leakage of fluid and inflammatory mediators into the dermis.[25,26] It often is accompanied by gastrointestinal symptoms. *Helicobacter pylori* infection has been implicated as a possible cause, with studies showing an improvement in rosacea after eradication of *H. pylori*. Experts hypothesize that this result occurs because of the anti-inflammatory effects of the antibiotics used in treatment.[26] In addition to microorganisms, other causes postulated have been genetic, environmental, and vascular.

Types and Clinical Manifestations. Rosacea is classified into four types:

1. Erythematotelangiectatic (flushing and persistent central facial erythema)
2. Papulopustular (inflammatory)

3. Phymatous (thickening of the skin with irregular surface nodularities and enlargement)
4. Ocular (involving the eyes)[26]

In the early stage of rosacea development, there are repeated episodes of blushing. The blush eventually becomes a permanent dark red erythema on the nose and cheeks that sometimes extends to the forehead and chin. This stage often occurs before 20 years of age. Ocular problems occur in at least 50% of people with rosacea, which may lead to visual losses.[26–29] Prominent symptoms include eyes that are itchy, burning, or dry; a gritty or foreign body sensation; and erythema and swelling of the eyelid.[26] As the person ages, the erythema persists, and telangiectases with or without acne components (*e.g.*, comedones, papules, pustules, nodules, erythema, edema) develop. After years of affliction, acne rosacea may develop into an irregular bullous hyperplasia (thickening of the skin) of the nose, known as *rhinophyma*.[17] The sebaceous follicles and openings of the nose enlarge, and the skin color changes to a purple-red, resulting in hypertrophy of the nose and impaired breathing. Although rosacea is more common in women, rhinophyma is more common in men. People with rosacea are heat sensitive. They are instructed to avoid vascular stimulating agents such as heat, sunlight, hot liquids, foods, and alcohol.

Treatment. Treatment measures are similar to those used for acne vulgaris. Topical metronidazole and azelaic acid have been effective. Topical antibiotics (*e.g.*, clindamycin, erythromycin) have been useful, as well as systemic antibiotics (*e.g.*, tetracycline and its derivatives). Rhinophyma can be treated by a number of surgical methods, including electrosurgery, laser ablation, dermabrasion, cryosurgery, and excision.

Allergic and Hypersensitivity Dermatoses

Allergic and hypersensitivity dermatoses involve the inflammatory response to multiple exogenous and endogenous agents. The disorders, which are usually characterized by epidermal edema with separation of epidermal cells, include irritant contact dermatitis, allergy contact dermatitis, atopic and nummular eczema, urticaria, and drug-induced skin eruptions.

Contact and Allergic Dermatitis

Contact dermatitis is a common inflammation of the skin. There are two types of contact dermatitis: allergic and irritant contact dermatitis.

Allergic Contact Dermatitis. Allergic contact dermatitis results from a cell-mediated, type IV hypersensitivity response brought about by sensitization to an allergen such as the toxin in poison ivy. More than 2000 allergens have been identified as capable of producing an inflammatory skin response. Crude forms of many naturally occurring substances are in general less allergenic than alloys and synthetic products. Additives such as dyes and perfumes account for the major sources of known allergens. Some of the common topical agents causing allergic rashes are antimicrobial agents (especially neomycin), antihistamines, local anesthetic agents (benzocaine), preservatives (*e.g.*, parabens), and adhesive tape. Additional examples are poison ivy, poison oak, and metal alloys found in jewelry. Also of concern is the increased incidence of contact dermatitis from the heavy use of synthetic latex products, specifically latex gloves and condoms used to prevent communicable diseases.

Common causes of allergic contact dermatitis are paraphenylenediamine base (in hair dyes), nickel, balsam of Peru (perfume fragrance), thimerosal (preservative in cosmetics), neomycin sulfate, fragrance mix, formaldehyde (preservative in paper, paint, medications, fabrics), cobalt chloride (metal in medical products, hair dyes), rubber additives, and colophony (adhesives in fabric dressings).[30,31]

The lesions of allergic contact dermatitis range from a mild erythema with edema to vesicles or large bullae (Fig. 52.14). Secondary lesions from bacterial infection may occur. Lesions can occur almost anywhere on the body, and the many variations of eczema are often classified according to their location (*e.g.*, ear eczema, hand eczema). The location and pattern often help in identifying causative agents. For example, the typical poison ivy lesion consists of vesicles or bullae in a linear pattern (from swiping the plant) on exposed areas. The vesicles and bullae break and weep, leaving an excoriated area.

Irritant Contact Dermatitis. Chemicals (soaps, detergents, organic solvents) that irritate the skin cause irritant contact dermatitis. It can occur from mechanical means such as rubbing (*e.g.*, wool, fiberglass), chemical irritants (*e.g.*, household cleaning products), or environmental irritants (*e.g.*, plants, urine). In contrast to allergic contact dermatitis, no allergens can be identified.

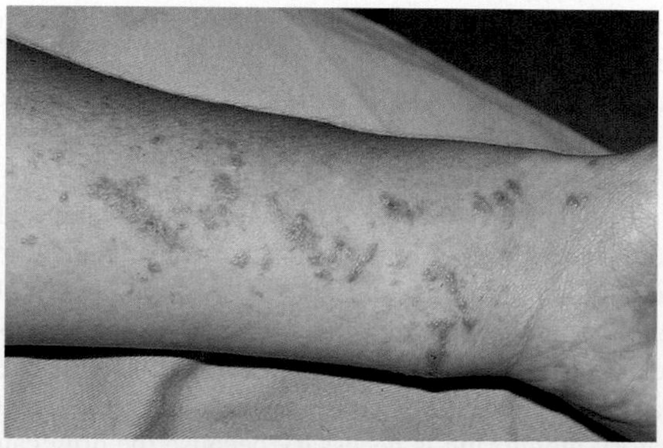

Figure 52.14 • Contact dermatitis. A classic erythematous and pruritic rash on the arm due to an inflammatory response to an antigen that had contact with the skin of the arm. (From Jensen S. (2015). *Nursing health assessment: A best practice approach* (2nd ed., p. 270). Philadelphia, PA: Wolters Kluwer.)

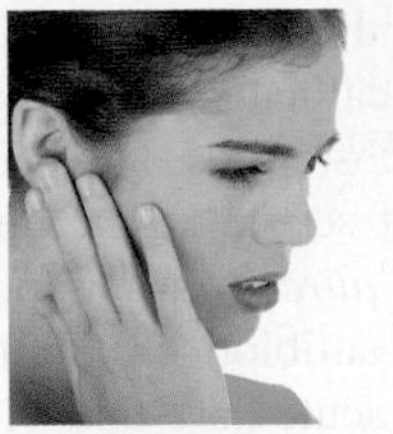

Lauren's itchy rash fits the description of irritant contact dermatitis well. Her rash was first evident after an exposure to a chemical she had worked with in her Chemistry laboratory course.

A history of atopic dermatitis, either in the past or concurrent, is a major risk for the development of irritant contact dermatitis. Four types of irritant contact dermatitis exist: subjective, acute, chronic, and chemical burns. Subjective cases have no clinical manifestation, but the person reports burning or stinging sensations when exposed to the irritant, and the effect can be reproduced. Acute episodes are often due to single exposures to the irritant. There may be dryness and erythema or edema, inflammation, and vesicles.

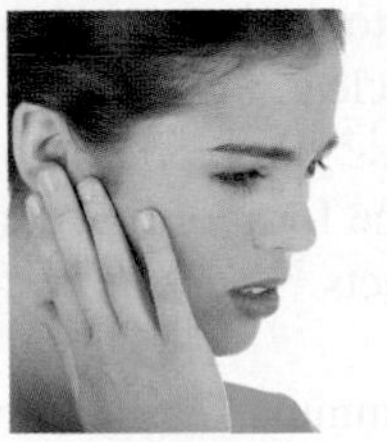

Lauren's irritant contact dermatitis seems to be a result of an acute episode triggered by the chemical. Her rash has an erythematous background, is slightly swollen, is not painful to touch, and has approximately 1 mm papules that are vesicular in origin. She had never worked with this chemical before and had never had this response previously to any other chemical or irritant. She finds the hydrocortisone 1% to be effective, and the rash resolves without further recurrence (as long as she does not have exposure to the chemical again).

Chronic irritant dermatitis results from continued exposure to the irritant. Even when the irritant is removed, the reaction may continue for several years. In addition to dryness and erythema, there may be scales, fissures, and vesicles (Fig. 52.15).

Diagnosis and Treatment. With both allergic and irritant contact dermatitis, the location of the lesions is of great benefit in diagnosing the causative agent. Patch testing, in which a small amount of the suspected antigen is applied to the skin, is used to identify the allergens.[30,32,33]

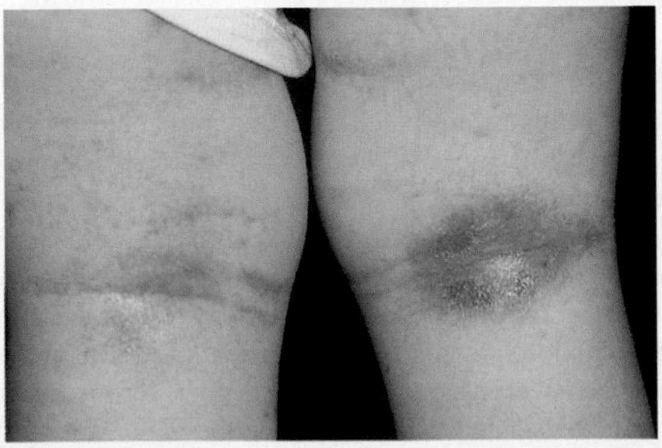

Figure 52.15 • Eczema—also called atopic dermatitis. Eczema can occur anywhere on the body. (From Jensen S. (2015). *Nursing health assessment: A best practice approach* (2nd ed., p. 276). Philadelphia, PA: Wolters Kluwer.)

Treatment measures for both types of contact dermatitis are aimed at removing the source of the irritant or allergen. Minor cases are treated by washing the affected areas to remove further contamination by the irritant or allergen, applying antipruritic creams or lotions, and bandaging the exposed areas. Topical corticosteroids may be helpful in these cases. Systemic treatment regimens differ according to the type of irritant or allergen and the severity of the reaction. Moderate to extreme cases are treated with wet dressings, oral antihistamines, and systemic corticosteroids.

Atopic Dermatitis and Nummular Eczema

Atopic Dermatitis. Atopic dermatitis (atopic eczema) is an itchy, inflammatory skin disorder that is characterized by poorly defined erythema with edema, vesicles, and weeping at the acute stage and skin thickening (lichenification) in the chronic stage.[34] Although often described as an immunoglobulin E (IgE)-mediated hypersensitivity (atopic) disease, allergic causation is difficult to document, and the disorder is increasingly viewed as a skin disease that predisposes to allergies.[34] Approximately 30% of children with atopic dermatitis develop asthma, and 35% will develop allergies in adolescence and adulthood.[34]

Atopic dermatitis presents differently at different ages (infantile and adult) and in people of different races. Approximately 70% of cases of atopic allergy start in children younger than 5 years of age.[34] The infantile form of atopic dermatitis is characterized by vesicle formation, oozing, and crusting with excoriations. It usually begins on the cheeks and may progress to involve the scalp, arms, trunk, and legs (Fig. 52.16). The skin of the cheeks may be paler, with extra

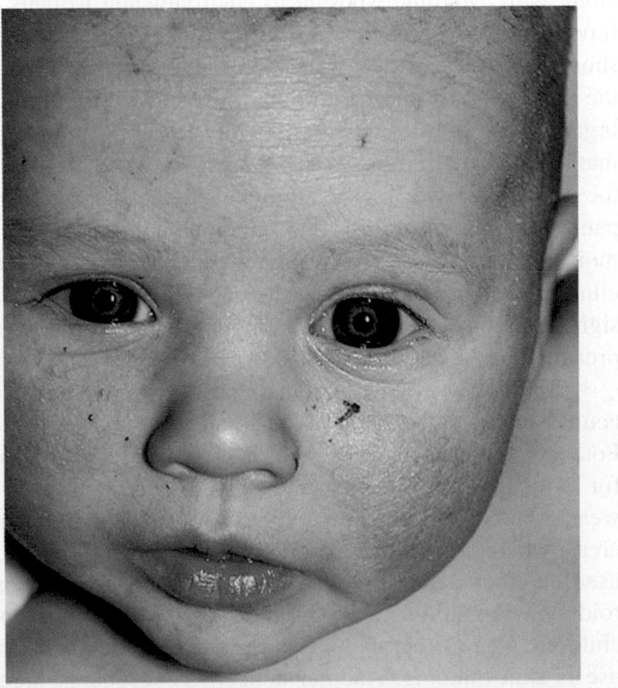

Figure 52.16 • Atopic eczema on an infant's face. (From Jensen S. (2015). *Nursing health assessment: A best practice approach* (2nd ed., p. 848). Philadelphia, PA: Wolters Kluwer.)

creases under the eyes, called *Dennie-Morgan folds*. The infantile form may become milder as the child ages, often disappearing by the age of 15 years. However, many people have resultant eczematous disorders and rhinitis symptoms throughout life.

Adolescents and adults usually have dry, red patches affecting the face, neck, and upper trunk, but without the thickening and discrete demarcation associated with psoriasis. The bends of the elbows and knees are usually involved. In chronic cases, the skin is dry, leathery, and lichenified. People with dark skin may have a papular eruption and poorly demarcated hypopigmentation patches on the cheeks and extremities. In people with black skin, pigmentation may be lost from lichenified skin. Acute flares may present with red patches that are weepy, shiny, or lichenified (*i.e.*, thickened, with more prominent markings) and with plaques and papules. Itching may be severe and prolonged with both childhood and adults forms of atopic dermatitis. Secondary infections are common.

Treatment of atopic eczema is designed to target the underlying abnormalities: dryness, pruritus, infection, and inflammation. The guidelines derived from a combined review of the American Academy of Allergy, Asthma, and Immunology; American College of Allergy, Asthma, and Immunology Joint Task Force 2012; Atopic Dermatitis Practice Parameter; and the American Academy of Dermatology highlight therapies and outline basic principles of atopic dermatitis management.[35] Underlying all treatment measures is a comprehensive education program regarding the cause of the disorder, treatment measures, and avoidance of temperature changes and stress to minimize vascular and sweat responses. Basic therapy begins with optimal skin care, addressing the skin barrier defect with continuous use of emollients and skin hydration, along with avoiding exposure to environmental irritants and foods that cause exacerbations of the symptoms. The person should bathe with warm water and mild soap. Bathing dries the skin, yet it is important to maintain a low level of microorganisms to prevent infection. A key feature of atopic dermatitis is severe dryness of the skin caused by dysfunction of the skin barrier with transepidermal water loss. This is accompanied by intense pruritus and inflammation. Application of moisturizers increases hydration of the skin.[36] A number of clinical trials have shown that they lessen the symptoms and signs of atopic dermatitis, including erythema, fissuring, and pruritus.[35]

Topical corticosteroids remain an important treatment for acute flare-ups but can cause local and systemic side effects. Potency of topical corticosteroids is classified by the potential for vasoconstriction. In general, only preparations that have weak or moderate potency are used on the face and genital areas, whereas those that have moderate or high potency are used on other areas of the body.[34] Lower-potency corticosteroids may be sufficient on all areas of the body in younger children. One of the main concerns of topical corticosteroid use is skin thinning. Another concern is secondary adrenal suppression and the suppression of growth in children resulting from systemic absorption.[34,36]

Wet-wrap therapy, in which a wet dressing is applied over emollients in combination with topical antiseptics (*e.g.*, triclosan, chlorhexidine) or topical corticosteroids, has been shown to be beneficial in some cases of severe atopic dermatitis.[36,37] Secondary infection with *S. aureus* is common and usually treated with short courses of antibiotics.[34] Short-term corticosteroids are also used during acute flare-ups with adult people. Cyclosporine and azathioprine, both immunosuppressive agents, may also be used, keeping in mind their potentially harmful effects. Antihistamines are useful for their sedative effects and may be helpful during severe pruritus episodes. Phototherapy alone or in combination with corticosteroids during acute flares is often practiced, with beneficial results.

Studies have examined the use of *probiotics*, foods containing live microorganisms, such as *Lactobacillus acidophilus* or *Bifidobacterium bifidum*. There is sufficient data to document the role of probiotics in preventing atopic dermatitis, but their effect on atopic dermatitis is not as clear. Probiotics are believed to reduce IgE-mediated reactions.[38] Probiotic preparations are available to the consumer in the form of powders, tablets, drinks, and fermented dairy products.[38]

Nummular Eczema. The lesions of nummular eczema are coin shaped (hence its other name, *discoid eczema*), papulovesicular patches mainly involving the arms and legs. Lichenification and secondary bacterial infections are common. It is not unusual for the initial lesions seemingly to heal, followed by a secondary outbreak of mirror-image lesions on the opposite side of the body. Nummular eczema is mostly chronic, with weeks to years between exacerbations. Exacerbations are more frequent in the cold winter months. The exact cause of nummular eczema is unknown, although many people have a history of atopy (allergy-related disorders), and there is heavy colonization of lesions with staphylococci. Ingestion of iodides and bromides usually aggravates the condition and should be avoided. Treatment is similar to that for other types of dermatitis. Frequent bathing and stress should be reduced, whereas environmental humidity should be increased. Topical emollients, corticosteroids, coal tar preparations, and UV light treatments may be prescribed as necessary.

Urticaria

Urticaria, or hives, are pale, raised, itchy papules or plaques that occur in the most superficial aspect of the dermis anywhere on the skin.[17] These small wheals blanch with pressure and vary in size from a few millimeters to centimeters (Fig. 52.17). They occur as either an immunologic reaction to an antigen in an IgE hypersensitivity response or a nonimmunologic reaction to something that is not known. Angioedema is when the swelling occurs in the deeper dermis and result in large wheals.[17] Occasionally, there may be swelling of the tongue and upper airways. Both urticaria and angioedema can range from an irritation to a life-threatening anaphylactic situation.

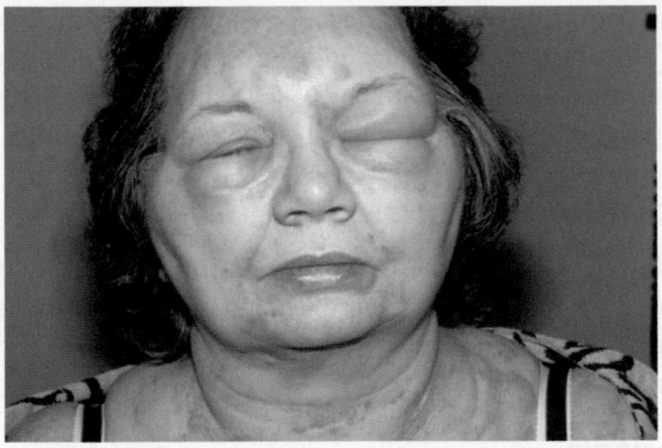

Figure 52.17 • Urticaria—also called hives. This shows the swelling of fluid, which is a result of histamine release. (From Jensen S. (2015). *Nursing health assessment: A best practice approach* (2nd ed., p. 277). Philadelphia, PA: Wolters Kluwer.)

Etiology and Pathogenesis. Urticaria can be acute or chronic and due to known or unknown causes. Numerous factors, both immunologic and nonimmunologic, can be involved in its pathogenesis. The urticarial wheal results from liberation of histamine from mast cells and basophils. Histamine causes hyperpermeability of the microvessels of the skin and surrounding tissue, allowing fluid to leak into the tissues, causing edema and wheal formation.

The most common causes of acute urticaria are foods or drinks, medications (most notably penicillin and cephalosporin), insect stings, viral infections, dust mites, and exposure to pollens or chemicals. Food is the most common cause of acute urticaria in children.

Chronic urticaria affects primarily adults and is twice as common in women as in men. Usually, its cause cannot be determined despite extensive laboratory tests. It appears to be an autoimmune disorder in a substantial number of people. Approximately one half of people with chronic urticaria have circulating IgG antibodies, which trigger the release of histamine by mast cells. In rare cases, urticaria is a manifestation of underlying disease, such as certain cancers, collagen diseases, and hepatitis. It is thought there may be a connection between urticaria and having an autoimmune disease of the thyroid gland.[39] Additionally, a genetic deficiency of a C1 (complement 1) inhibitor also can cause urticaria and angioedema.

The physical urticarias constitute another form of chronic urticaria.[40,41] Physical urticarias are intermittent; usually last less than 2 hours; are produced by exercise, cold, sunlight, vibration, heat, or delayed pressure; have distinctive appearances and locations; and are seen most frequently in young adults.

Diagnosis and Treatment. Appropriate challenge tests (*e.g.*, application of an ice cube to the skin to initiate development of cold urticaria) are used to differentiate physical urticaria from chronic urticaria due to other causes.

Most types of urticaria are treated with second-generation antihistamines that block histamine type 1 (H_1) receptors. These drugs do not cause drowsiness so they are recommended over the first generation. They control urticaria by inhibiting vasodilation and the escape of fluid into the surrounding tissues. They also relieve the pruritis. If the antihistamines are not effective, leukotriene receptor blockers (zafirlukast and montelukast) are used.[41] Colloid-type (*e.g.*, Aveeno) baths may be used as comfort measures. People who experience angioedema of the larynx and pharynx are strongly encouraged to carry an EpiPen. Oral corticosteroids may be used in the treatment of refractory urticaria.

Drug-Induced Skin Eruptions

Most drugs can cause a localized or generalized skin eruption. Topical drugs are usually responsible for localized contact dermatitis types of rashes, whereas systemic drugs cause generalized skin lesions. Although many drug-induced skin eruptions are morbilliform (*i.e.*, measles-like) or exanthematous, they may mimic most of the skin disorders described in this chapter. Because the lesions vary greatly, the diagnosis depends almost entirely on an accurate person history. Management of mild cases is aimed at eliminating the offending drug while treating the symptoms. Severe cases require prompt medical attention and treatment with systemic corticosteroids and antihistamines.

Some drug reactions result in epidermal skin detachment and formation of bullous lesions. Three types of drug reactions that result in bullous skin lesions are *erythema multiforme minor* (Fig. 52.18), *Stevens-Johnson syndrome*, and *toxic epidermal necrolysis* (TEN).

Etiology and Pathogenesis. Erythema multiforme minor is usually self-limiting, and manifestations vary from a few ringlike erythematous macules and blisters. If the reaction involves a systemic ulceration of all mucous membranes and skin, it is called erythema multiforme major, or *Stevens-Johnson syndrome*, which may be a reaction to either a drug or a virus such as HSV.[17,42] The third disease-causing bullous skin lesions triggered by a medication adverse reaction is TEN or Lyell disease, which is life threatening.[17]

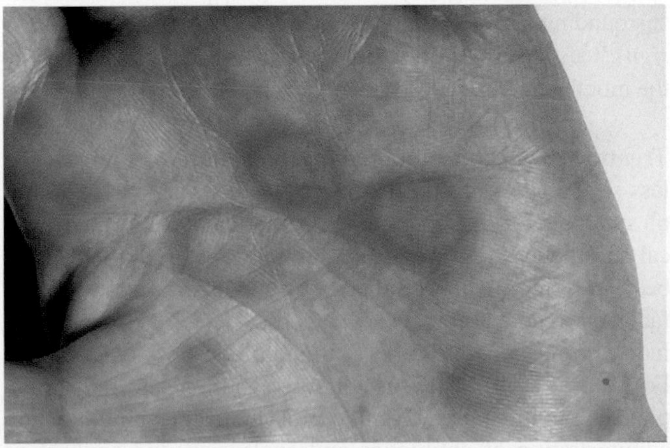

Figure 52.18 • Erythema multiforme of the hand. This "target" rash depicts the central bullae with surrounding erythema, which appeared after antibiotic treatment. (From Strayer D., Rubin R. (Eds.) (2015). *Rubin's pathology: Clinicopathologic foundations of medicine* (7th ed., p. 1240). Philadelphia, PA: Wolters Kluwer.)

Erythema multiforme minor is self-limiting, with a small amount of skin detachment at the lesion sites. Stevens-Johnson syndrome and TEN are caused by hypersensitivity reaction to drugs, the most common being sulfonamides, anticonvulsants, nonsteroidal anti-inflammatory drugs, antimalarials, and allopurinol. Recovery is based on the severity and quick, aggressive treatment.

The skin detachment seen with bullous skin lesions is different from the desquamation (*i.e.*, peeling) that occurs with other skin disorders. For example, with scarlet fever, there is peeling of the dead keratinized layer of the stratum corneum. In the bullous disorders, there is full-thickness detachment of the entire epidermis from the dermis. This leaves the person vulnerable to multiple problems, including loss of body fluids and electrolytes, impaired body temperature control, and a greatly increased risk of infection.

Clinical Manifestations. The lesions of erythema multiforme minor and Stevens-Johnson syndrome are similar. The primary lesion of both is a round, erythematous papule, resembling an insect bite. Within hours to days, these lesions change into several different patterns. The individual lesions may enlarge and coalesce, producing small plaques, or they may change to concentric zones of color appearing as "target" or "iris" lesions. The outermost rings of the target lesions usually are erythematous; the central portion usually is opaque white, yellow, or gray (dusky). In the center, small blisters on the dusky purpuric macules may form, giving them their characteristic target-like appearance. Although there is wide distribution of lesions over the body surface area, there is a propensity for them to occur on the face and trunk.

TEN is the most serious drug reaction. The person experiences a prodromal period of malaise, low-grade fever, and sore throat. Within a few days, widespread erythema and large, flaccid bullae appear, followed by the loss of the epidermis, leaving a denuded and painful dermis. The skin surrounding the large denuded areas may have the typical target-like lesions seen with Stevens-Johnson syndrome. Lateral pressure causes the surrounding skin to separate easily from the dermis (*Nikolsky sign*).[42] Usually, the epithelium of mucosal surfaces, especially the mouth and eyes, is also involved and may lead to blindness.

Treatment. Treatment of erythema multiforme minor and less severe cases of Stevens-Johnson syndrome includes relief of symptoms using compresses, antipruritic drugs, and topical anesthetics. Recurrent cases of erythema multiforme have been prevented with continuous acyclovir therapy, given the fact it is triggered often by HSV. Corticosteroid therapy may be indicated in moderate cases, although its use is controversial. For severe cases of Stevens-Johnson syndrome and TEN, hospitalization is required for fluid replacement, respiratory care, administration of antibiotics and analgesics, and application of moist dressings. When large areas of skin are detached, the care is similar to that for people with thermal burn injuries. Intravenous immunoglobulin may hasten the healing response of the skin. Generally, healing is a slow process, taking 6 weeks or more to regenerate skin. The mucous membranes heal slowly, and follow-up treatment is often needed for ophthalmologic and mucous membrane sequelae.[42] Avoidance of the responsible drug and chemically related compounds is essential.

Papulosquamous Dermatoses

Papulosquamous dermatoses are a group of skin disorders characterized by scaling papules and plaques. Among the major papulosquamous diseases are psoriasis, pityriasis rosea, and lichen planus.

Psoriasis

Psoriasis is a common, chronic inflammatory skin disease characterized by circumscribed, red, thickened plaques with an overlying silvery-white scale. Psoriasis occurs worldwide, although the incidence is lower in warmer, sunnier climates. In the United States and England, it affects 2% to 3% of the population.[43] The average age of onset is in the third decade, and its prevalence increases with age.

Etiology. Approximately one third of people have a genetic history, indicating a hereditary factor. Childhood onset of the disease is more strongly associated with a family history than psoriasis occurring in adults older than 30 years of age. The disease, which can persist throughout life and become exacerbated at unpredictable times, is classified as a chronic ailment. A few cases, however, have been known to clear and not recur. There appears to be an association between psoriasis and arthritis.

The primary cause of psoriasis is uncertain. It is thought that activated T lymphocytes (mainly $CD4^+$ helper cells) produce chemical messengers that stimulate abnormal growth of keratinocytes and dermal blood vessels.[43] Accompanying inflammatory changes are caused by infiltration of neutrophils and monocytes. Skin trauma is a common precipitating factor in people predisposed to the disease. The reaction of the skin to an original trauma of any type is called the *Köbner reaction*. Stress, infections, trauma, xerosis, and use of medications such as angiotensin-converting enzyme inhibitors, β-adrenergic blocking drugs, lithium, and the antimalarial agent, hydroxychloroquine (Plaquenil), may precipitate or exacerbate the condition.[43]

Pathogenesis. Histologically, psoriasis is characterized by increased epidermal cell turnover with marked epidermal thickening, a process called *hyperkeratosis*. The granular layer (stratum granulosum) of the epidermis is thinned or absent, and neutrophils are found in the stratum corneum. There also is an accompanying thinning of the epidermal cell layer that overlies the tips of the dermal papillae (suprapapillary plate), and the blood vessels in the dermal papillae become tortuous and dilated. These capillary beds show permanent damage even when the disease is in remission or resolved. The close proximity of the vessels in the dermal papillae to the hyperkeratotic scale accounts for multiple, minute bleeding points that are seen when the scale is lifted.

Types of Psoriasis. There are several variants or types of psoriasis, including plaque-type psoriasis, guttate psoriasis, pustular psoriasis (localized and generalized), and erythrodermic psoriasis.[43] *Plaque-type psoriasis (psoriasis vulgaris)*, which is the most common type, is a chronic stationary form of psoriasis. The lesions may occur anywhere on the skin, but most often involve the elbows, knees, and scalp (Fig. 52.19). The primary lesions are sharply demarcated, thick, red plaques with a silvery scale that vary in size and shape. In darker-skinned people, the plaques may appear purple. There may be excoriation, thickening, or oozing from the lesions. A differential diagnostic finding is that the plaques bleed from minute points when removed, which is known as the *Auspitz sign*.

Guttate psoriasis occurs in children and young adults and is characterized by teardrop-shaped, pink to salmon, scaly lesions. Its lesions are usually limited to the upper trunk and extremities. This form of psoriasis usually is brought on by a streptococcal infection.[43] It generally responds to treatments such as UVB phototherapy, only to return with recurrent streptococcal infections. *Pustular psoriasis* is characterized by papules or plaques studded with pustules (Fig. 52.20). Localized pustular psoriasis usually is limited to the palms of the hands and soles of the feet. Generalized pustular psoriasis is characterized by more general involvement and may be associated with systemic symptoms such as fever, malaise, and diarrhea. The person may or may not have had preexisting psoriasis.

Erythrodermic psoriasis is a rare form of psoriasis affecting all body surfaces, including the hands, feet, nails, trunk, and extremities. It is characterized by a process in which the lesions scale and become confluent, leaving much of the body surface bright red, with continuous skin shedding. Severe itching and pain often accompany it. Severe complications may develop related to loss of body fluids, proteins, and electrolytes and disturbances in temperature regulation.

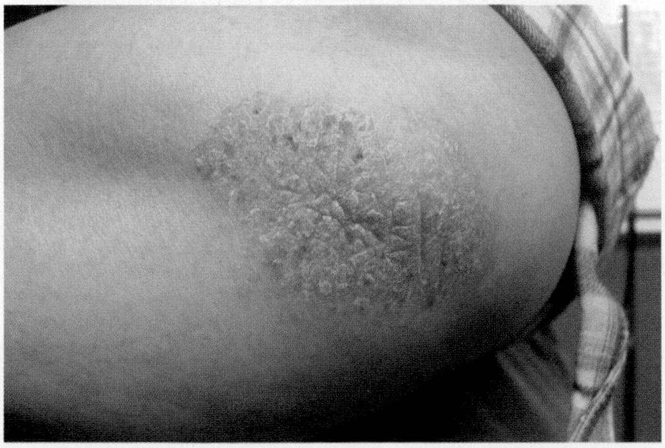

Figure 52.19 • Silvery-white psoriasiform, well-demarcated plaque with imbricated scale on the elbow. (From Hall B. J., Hall J. C. (2017). *Sauer's manual of skin diseases* (11th ed., Figure 16-1, p. 189). Philadelphia, PA: Wolters Kluwer.)

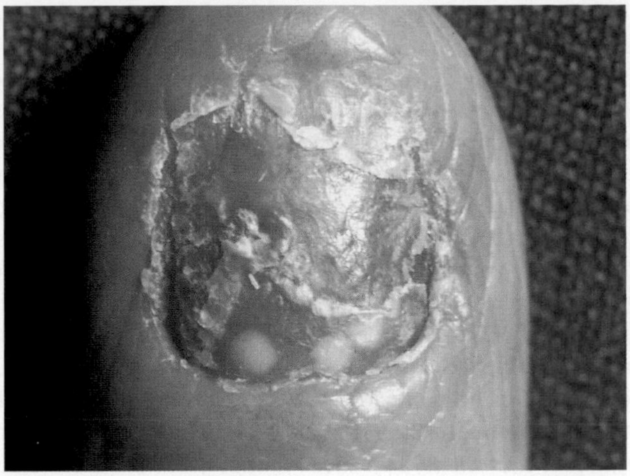

Figure 52.20 • Pustular nail psoriasis. (From Hall B. J., Hall J. C. (2017). *Sauer's manual of skin diseases* (11th ed., p. 404). Philadelphia, PA: Wolters Kluwer.)

Treatment. There is no cure for psoriasis. The goal of treatment is to suppress the signs and symptoms of the disease: hyperkeratosis, epidermal inflammation, and abnormal keratinocyte differentiation. Treatment depends on the severity of the disease, as well as on the person's age, sex, treatment history, and level of treatment compliance. There is no standardized tool to assess severity of psoriasis.[43] Treatment measures are divided into topical and systemic approaches. Usually, topical agents are used first in any treatment regimen and when less than 5% of the body surface is involved.[43] Combination therapies tailored to the needs of the client are most effective. Also, rotating various therapies may decrease the side effects of any one therapy.

Topical agents include emollients, keratolytic agents, coal tar products, anthralin, corticosteroids, and calcipotriene. Emollients hydrate and soften the psoriatic plaques. Petroleum-based products are more effective than water-based, but they are often less acceptable cosmetically to persons with psoriasis. Keratolytic agents are peeling agents. Salicylic acid is the most widely used. It softens and removes plaques. It has been used alone or in conjunction with other topical agents. Coal tar, the byproduct of the processing of coke and gas from coal, is one of the oldest yet more effective forms of treatment. The skin is covered with a film of coal tar for up to several weeks. The exact mechanism of action of tar products is unknown, but side effects of the treatment are few.

Anthralin, a synthesized product of Goa powder from Brazilian araroba tree bark, has remained a topical treatment of choice. It has been effective in resolving lesions in approximately 2 weeks. A disadvantage to anthralin is that it stains the uninvolved skin and clothes brown or purple. A treatment variation, called the *Ingram method*, involves coal tar applications and UVB radiation, followed by anthralin paste application.

Topical corticosteroids, such as keratolytic agents, are widely used and relatively effective. They are generally more acceptable because they do not stain and are easy to use.

Topical corticosteroids are available as low-, medium-, and high-potency preparations. Treatment usually is started with a medium-potency agent. Low-potency drugs usually are used on the face and areas of the body, such as the groin and axillary areas, where the skin tends to be thinner. High-potency preparations are reserved for treatment of thick chronic plaques that do not respond to less potent preparations. Although the corticosteroids are rapidly effective in the treatment of psoriasis, they are associated with flare-ups after discontinuation and they have many potential side effects. Their effectiveness is increased when used under occlusive dressings, but there is an increase in side effects. *Calcipotriene*, a topical vitamin D derivative, has been effective for the treatment of psoriasis. It inhibits epidermal cell proliferation and enhances cell differentiation. *Tazarotene*, a synthetic retinoid, also has been effective, but it is teratogenic and should be avoided in women of childbearing age.

Systemic treatments include phototherapy, photochemotherapy, methotrexate, retinoids, corticosteroids, and cyclosporine. The positive effects of sunlight have long been established. Phototherapy with UVB is a widely used treatment. Photochemotherapy involves using a light-activated form of the drug methoxsalen.

Systemic corticosteroids have been effective in treating severe or pustular psoriasis. However, they cause severe side effects, including Cushing syndrome. Intralesional injection of triamcinolone has proved effective in resistant lesions. The retinoids are another class of systemic psoriasis therapy. These drugs, which are derivatives of vitamin A, are only moderately effective as a monotherapy and are associated with numerous mucocutaneous side effects such as hair loss, cheilitis, and thinning of the nails. Teratogenicity limits use of retinoids in women of childbearing potential.

Methotrexate, which is used for cancer treatment, is an antimetabolite that inhibits DNA synthesis and prevents cell mitosis. Oral methotrexate has been effective in treating psoriasis when other approaches have failed. The drug has many side effects, including nausea, malaise, leukopenia, thrombocytopenia, and liver function abnormalities. Cyclosporine is a potent immunosuppressive drug used to prevent rejection of organ transplants. It suppresses inflammation and the proliferation of T cells in people with psoriasis. Its use is limited to severe psoriasis because of serious side effects, including nephrotoxicity, hypertension, and increased risk of cancers. Intralesional cyclosporine also has been effective. Biologic agents (*e.g.*, infliximab, etanercept, efalizumab, and alefacept) that target the activity of T lymphocytes and cytokines responsible for the inflammatory nature of psoriasis have proven effective, not only with the skin lesions, but in halting the effects of the associated arthritis of psoriasis.[43]

Concept Mastery Alert

Phototherapy, methotrexate, corticosteroids, and cyclosporine are all systemic treatments for psoriasis. Keratolytic agents are topical treatments for psoriasis.

Pityriasis Rosea

Pityriasis rosea is a rash that primarily affects children and young adults. The origin of the rash is unknown but is hypothesized to be triggered by a viral infection.[44] Numerous viruses have been investigated, thus far with no conclusive evidence except for some support for human herpes virus 6 (HHV-6) or 7 (HHV-7).[5,44] The incidence is highest in spring and fall.[4] Cases occur in clusters and among people who live or work closely together, indicating an infectious spread. However, there are no data to support communicability. It may be an immune response to any number of agents.

The characteristic lesion is an oval macule or papule with surrounding erythema (Fig. 52.21). The lesion spreads with central clearing, much like tinea corporis. This initial lesion is a solitary lesion called the *herald patch* and is usually on the trunk or neck. However, there is not always a herald patch.[5] As the lesion enlarges and begins to fade (2 to 10 days), successive crops of lesions appear on the trunk and neck over the next 2 to 3 weeks.[5] The lesions on the back have a characteristic "Christmas tree branch" pattern over the back.[5] The extremities, face, and scalp may be involved more so with children and people of color.[5] Mild to severe pruritus may occur. The disease is self-limited and usually disappears within 6 to 8 weeks.[5] Treatment measures are palliative and include topical steroids, antihistamines, and colloid baths. Systemic corticosteroids may be indicated in severe cases.

Lichen Planus

Lichen planus is a skin disorder characterized by small (2 to 10 mm), flat-topped, violaceous papules with irregular,

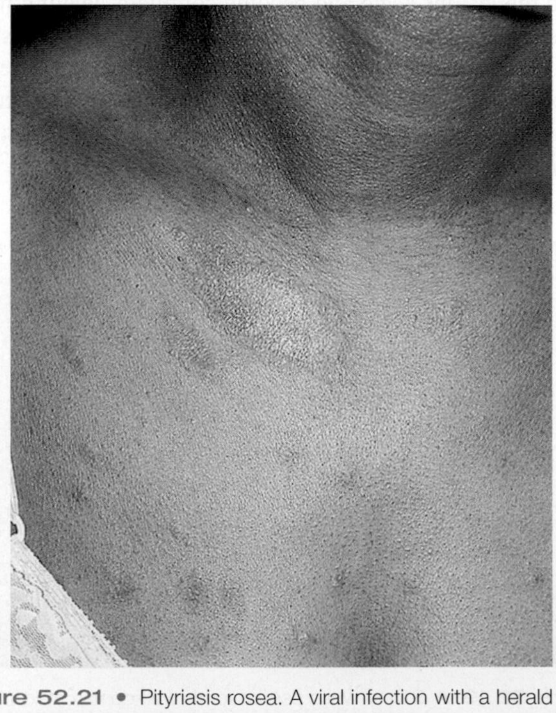

Figure 52.21 • Pityriasis rosea. A viral infection with a herald patch that can be visualized on upper right chest inferior to clavicle. (From Jensen S. (2015). *Nursing health assessment: A best practice approach* (2nd ed., p. 275). Philadelphia, PA: Wolters Kluwer.)

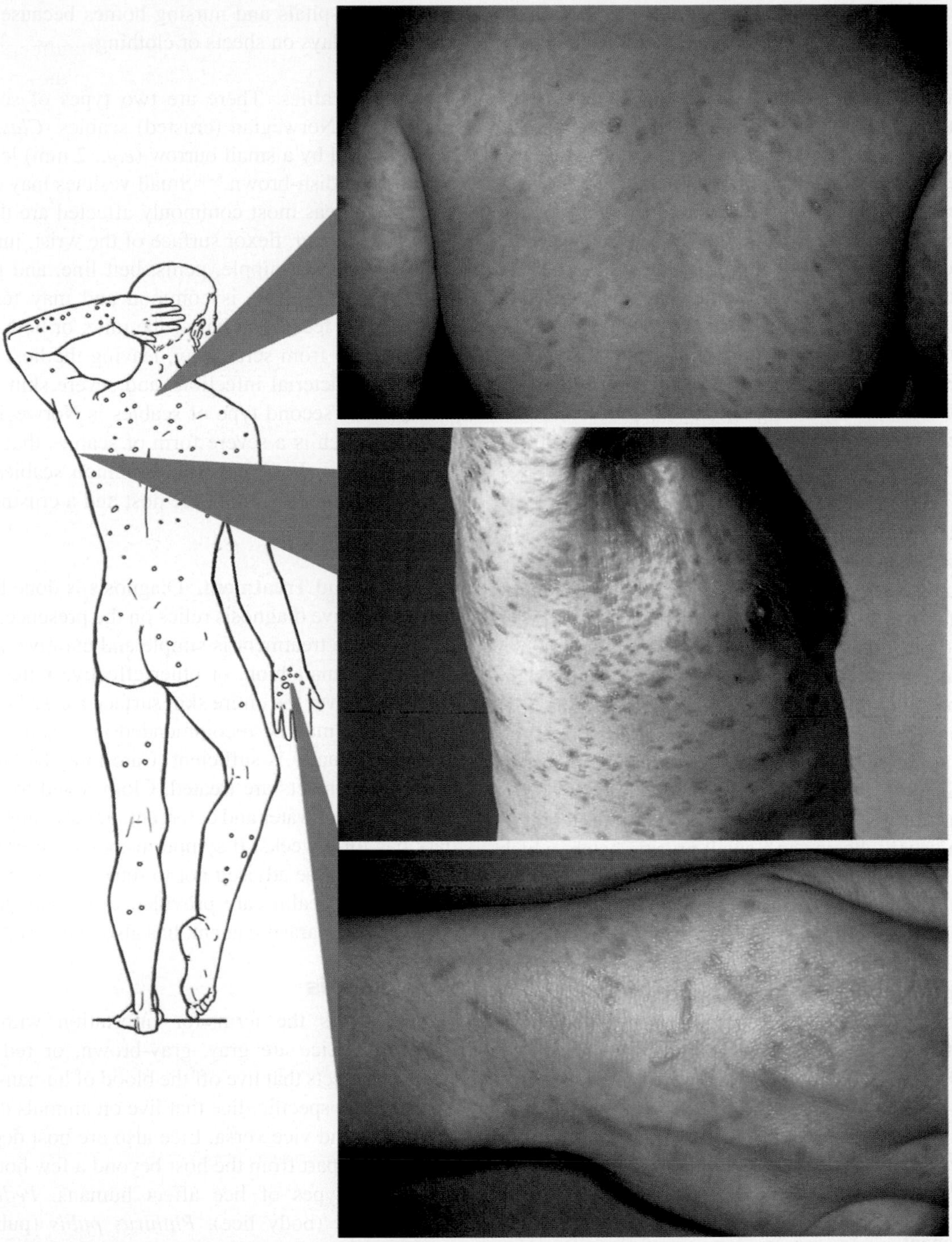

Figure 52.22 • Lichen planus of the back, torso, and hand. (From Hall B. J., Hall J. C. (2017). *Sauer's manual of skin diseases* (10th ed., p. 171). Philadelphia, PA: Wolters Kluwer.)

angulated borders[5] (Fig. 52.22). Lichen planus is an uncommon chronic pruritic disease. It involves inflammation and papular eruption of the skin and mucous membranes. There are variations in the pattern of lesions (*e.g.*, annular, linear) and differences in the sites (*e.g.*, mucous membranes, genitalia, nails, scalp). The characteristic lesion is a purple, polygonal papule covered with a shiny, white, lacelike pattern. The lesions appear most frequently on the wrist, ankles, and trunk of the body. Most people who have skin lesions also have oral lesions, appearing as milky white lacework on the buccal mucosa or tongue.[4] Other mucosal surfaces, such as the genital, nasal, laryngeal, otic, gastric, and anal areas, may also be affected. As with psoriasis, lichen planus lesions can develop on scratches or skin injuries and so can be secondary or primary lesions.

The etiology of lichen planus is unknown, but it is believed to be an autoimmune response in which epithelial cells are recognized as foreign. The disorder involves the epidermal–dermal junction, with damage to the basal cell layer. Some cases of lichen planus have been linked to hepatitis C or B virus infections.[5]

Diagnosis is based on the clinical appearance of the lesions and the histopathologic findings from a punch biopsy. For most people, lichen planus is a self-limited disease. Treatment measures include discontinuation of all medications, followed by treatment with topical corticosteroids and occlusive dressings. Occlusion may be used to enhance the effect of topical medications. Antipruritic agents are helpful in reducing itch. Systemic corticosteroids may be indicated in severe cases. Intralesional corticosteroid injections also may be used. Acitretin, an orally administered retinoid agent, also may be effective. Because retinoids are teratogenic, they should be avoided in women of childbearing age. Cyclosporine, tacrolimus, and other immunosuppressive agents have been helpful.

Lichen Simplex Chronicus

Lichen simplex chronicus or circumscribed neurodermatitis is a localized lichenoid pruritic dermatitis resulting from repeated rubbing and scratching.[4] The term *lichen simplex* denotes the absence of a known predisposing skin disorder in the affected person. It is characterized by the occurrence of itchy, reddened, thickened, and scaly patches of dry skin. People with the condition may have a single or, less frequently, multiple lesions. The lesions are seen most commonly at the nape of the neck, wrists, ankles, or anal area. Women can experience this dermatosis on the vulva and complain of distressing vulvar pruritis that they worsen by constant itching.[45] The condition usually begins as a small pruritic patch, which after a repetitive cycle of itching and scratching develops into a chronic dermatosis. Because of the chronic itching and scratching, excoriations and lichenification with thickening of the skin develops, often giving the appearance of tree bark. Treatment consists of measures to decrease scratching of the area. A moderate-potency corticosteroid is often prescribed to decrease the itching and subsequent inflammatory process.

Arthropod Infestations

The skin is susceptible to a variety of disorders as a result of an invasion or infestation by arthropods, including mites and lice. The type of rash or sometimes singular lesion depends on the causative agent.

Scabies

A mite, *Sarcoptes scabiei*, which burrows into the epidermis, causes scabies. After a female mite is impregnated, she burrows into the skin and lays two to three eggs each day for 4 or 5 weeks. The eggs hatch after 3 to 4 days, and the larvae migrate to the skin surface. At this point, they burrow into the skin only for food or protection. The larvae molt and become nymphs; they molt once more to become adults. After the new adult females are impregnated, the cycle is repeated. Scabies is transmitted by person-to-person contact, including sexual contact. It also is transmitted by contact with mite-infested sheets in hospitals and nursing homes because the mite can live up to 2 days on sheets or clothing.

Types of Scabies. There are two types of scabies: classic scabies and Norwegian (crusted) scabies. *Classic scabies* is characterized by a small burrow (*e.g.*, 2 mm) lesion that may be red to reddish-brown.[5,46] Small vesicles may cover the burrows. The areas most commonly affected are the interdigital web of the finger, flexor surface of the wrist, inner surface of the elbow, axilla, nipple, penis, belt line, and gluteal crease (Fig. 52.23). Pruritus is common and may result from the burrows, the fecal material of the mite, or both. Excoriations may develop from scratching, leaving the host vulnerable to secondary bacterial infections and severe skin lesions if left untreated. A second type of scabies is Norwegian or crusted scabies, which is a severe form of scabies that involves millions of mites. It differs from common scabies in the large number of mites living on the host and a crusting over of the infested region.[46]

Diagnosis and Treatment. Diagnosis is done by skin scrapings. A positive diagnosis relies on the presence of mites, ova, or feces. The treatment is simple and curative. After bathing, permethrin, malathion, or other effective mite-killing agents are applied over the entire skin surface for 12 hours. Repeated applications may be recommended in certain cases, but one treatment usually is sufficient. Care must be taken to ensure that close contacts are treated. Clothes and towels are disinfected with hot water and detergent, or they can be isolated in a dark bag for 2 weeks. If symptoms persist after treatment, the person should be advised not to retreat the condition without consulting a health care provider. Oral ivermectin, a broad-spectrum antiparasitic agent, has also been used successfully.

Pediculosis

Pediculosis is the term for infestation with lice (genus *Pediculus*). Lice are gray, gray-brown, or red-brown, oval, wingless insects that live off the blood of humans and animals. Lice are host specific; lice that live on animals do not transfer to humans and vice versa. Lice also are host dependent; they cannot live apart from the host beyond a few hours.

Three types of lice affect humans: *Pediculus humanus corporis* (body lice), *Phthirus pubis* (pubic lice), and *Pediculus humanus capitis* (head lice).[5] Although these three types differ biologically, they have similar life cycles. The life cycle of a louse consists of a "nit" or unhatched egg, three molt stages, an adult reproductive stage, and death. Before adulthood, lice live off the host and are incapable of reproduction. After fertilization, the female louse lays her eggs along hair shafts. The nits appear pearl-gray to brown. Depending on the site, a female louse can lay between 150 and 300 units in her life. The life span of a feeding louse is 30 to 50 days.[5] Lice are equipped with stylets that pierce the skin. Their saliva contains an anticoagulant that prevents the host's blood from clotting while the louse is feeding. A louse takes up to 1 mL of blood during a feeding.

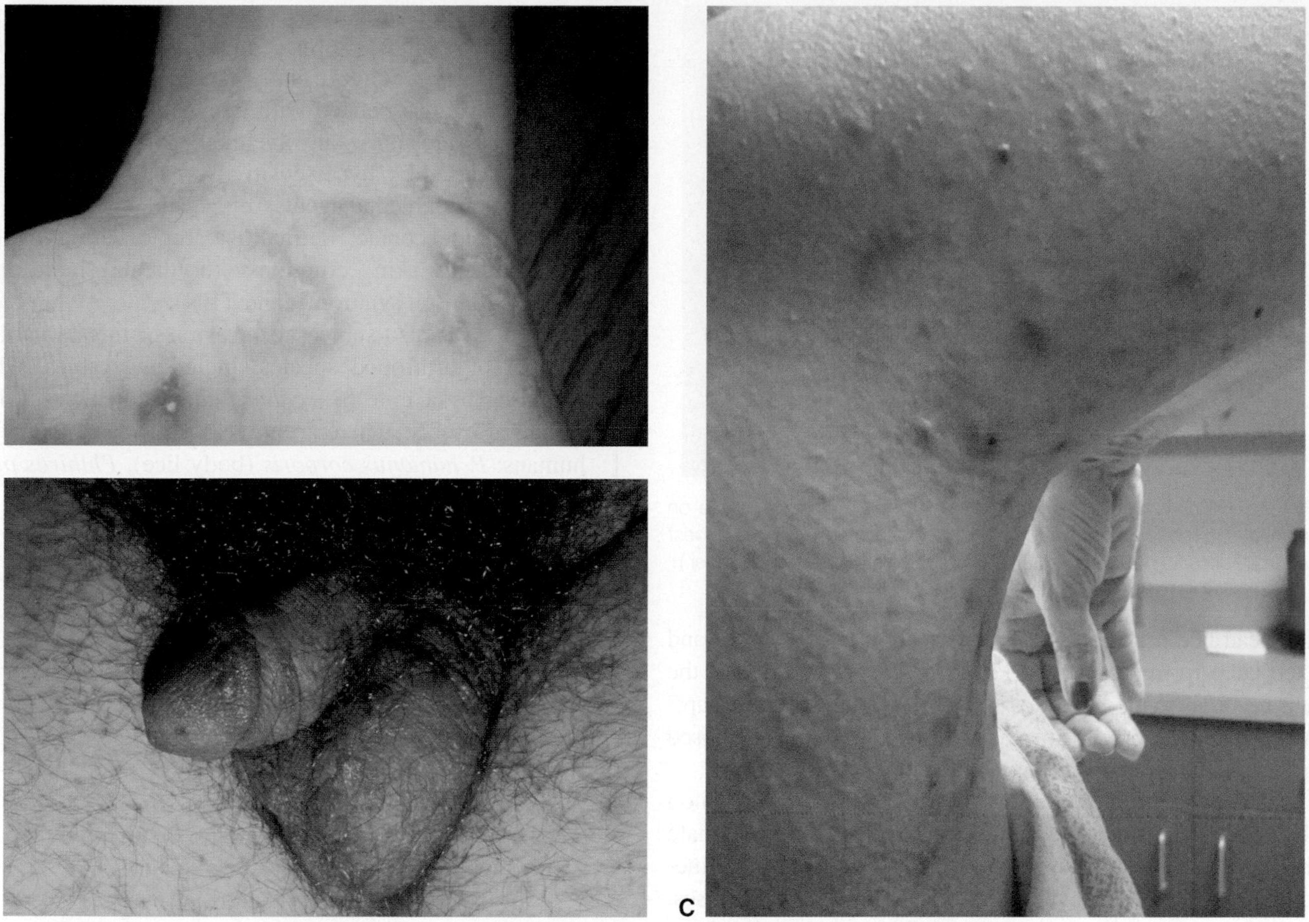

Figure 52.23 • Scabies. **(A)** Base of the palm and flexor wrist with white threadlike burrows with some surrounding erythema. This is a common location to see scabies burrows. **(B)** Inflammatory papules on the penis and scrotum quite characteristic of scabies. **(C)** Inflammatory papules and nodules on the posterior axillary fold typical of nodular scabies. No organisms are found in this probable immune reaction. (From Hall B. J., Hall J. C. (2017). *Sauer's manual of skin diseases* (11th ed., p. 210). Philadelphia, PA: Wolters Kluwer.)

Pediculosis Corporis. Pediculosis corporis is infestation with *P. humanus corporis* or body lice. The lice are transferred chiefly through contact with an infested person, clothing, or bedding. The lice live in clothes fibers, coming out only to feed—usually at night, causing nocturnal pruritus. Unlike pubic and head lice, the body louse can survive 10 to 14 days without the host.

The typical lesion is a macule at the site of the bite. Papules and wheals may develop. The infestation is pruritic and evokes scratching that brings about a characteristic linear excoriation. Eczematous patches are found frequently. Secondary lesions may become scaly and hyperpigmented and leave scars. Areas typically affected are the shoulders, trunk, and buttocks. The presence of nits in the seams of clothes confirms a diagnosis of body lice.

Treatment measures consist of eradicating the louse and nits on the body and on clothing. Dry cleaning, washing in hot water, or steam pressing clothes are recommended methods. Merely storing clothing in plastic bags for 2 weeks also rids clothes of lice. Many health care providers prefer not to treat the body unless nits are in evidence on hair shafts. If treatment is indicated, shampoos or topical preparations containing malathion or other pediculicides are recommended.

Pediculosis Pubis. Pediculosis pubis, the infestation known as crabs or pubic lice, is a disease spread by intimate contact with someone harboring *P. pubis*. The lice and nits are usually found in the pubic area of men and women, where their bites produce itching and erythematous lesions. Occasionally, they may be found in sites of secondary sex characteristics, such as the beard in men or the axillae in both sexes. Symptoms include intense itching and irritation of the skin. Diagnosis is made on the basis of symptoms and microscopic examination. The treatment is the same as for head lice.

Pediculosis Capitis. The incidence of pediculosis capitis, or infestation with head lice, is higher among girls, although hair length has not been indicated as a contributing factor. Infestations of head lice usually are confined to the nape of the neck and behind the ears. Less frequently, head lice are found on the beard, pubic areas, eyebrows, and body hairs. Although head lice can be transmitted by sharing combs and hats, they usually are spread from hair shaft to hair shaft through close personal contact. A positive diagnosis depends on the presence of firmly attached nits or live adult lice on hair shafts. Pruritus and scratching of the head are the primary indicators

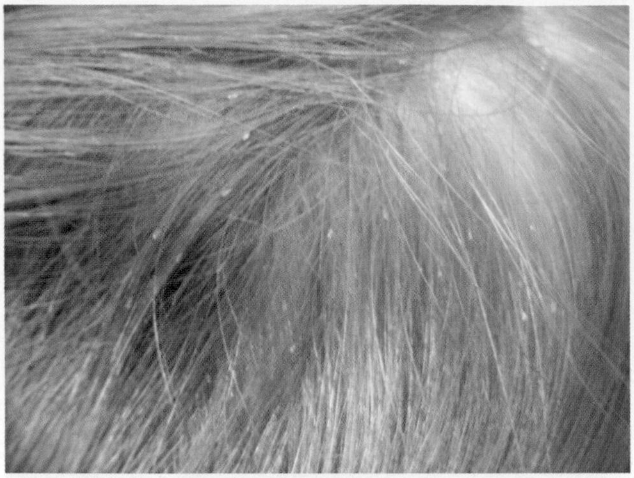

Figure 52.24 • Pediculosis capitis (head lice). Lice are visible on hair shafts. (From Jensen S. (2015). *Nursing health assessment: A best practice approach* (2nd ed., p. 278). Philadelphia, PA: Wolters Kluwer.)

that head lice may be present. The scalp may appear red and excoriated from scratching (Fig. 52.24). In severe cases, the hair becomes matted together in a crusty, foul-smelling "cap." An occasional morbilliform rash, which may be misdiagnosed as rubella, may occur with lymphadenopathy.

Head lice are treated with permethrin or malathion shampoos. Repeated treatments may be needed to eliminate the hatching nits. Dead nits may be removed with a fine-toothed comb or over-the-counter nit removal hair rinses. Over the years, permethrin- and malathion-resistant lice have evolved.

IN SUMMARY

Primary disorders of the skin include pigmentary skin disorders, infectious processes, inflammatory conditions, immune disorders, allergic reactions, and arthropod infestations. Pigmentary skin disorders include vitiligo, albinism, and melasma. Although the causes of the disorders vary, all involve changes in the amount of melanin produced by the melanocytes. These disorders appear in people of every skin type. However, the manifestations of the disorders vary among light-skinned and dark-skinned people.

Superficial fungal infections are called *dermatophytoses* and are commonly known as *tinea* or *ringworm*. Tinea can affect the whole body (tinea corporis), face and neck (tinea faciale), scalp (tinea capitis), hands (tinea manus), feet (tinea pedis), or nails (tinea unguium). The deep fungal infections invade the skin more deeply and go into living tissue and are also capable of involving other organs. Impetigo, which is caused by staphylococci or beta-hemolytic streptococci, is the most common superficial bacterial infection. Viruses are responsible for verrucae (warts), herpes simplex type 1 lesions (cold sores or fever blisters), and herpes zoster (shingles).

Noninfectious inflammatory skin conditions, such as acne, lichen planus, psoriasis, and pityriasis rosea, are of unknown origin. They usually are localized to the skin and are rarely associated with a specific internal disease. Allergic skin responses involve the body's immune system and are caused by hypersensitivity reactions to allergens such as environmental agents, drugs, and other substances. They include contact dermatitis, atopic dermatitis, and drug-induced skin eruptions (erythema multiforme, Stevens-Johnson syndrome, and TEN).

The skin is also subject to invasion or infestation by a number of arthropod species, including scabies, which is caused by a mite (*S. scabiei*), and pediculosis, which is caused by lice. There are three types of lice that affect humans: *P. humanus corporis* (body lice), *Phthirus pubis* (pubic lice), and *P. humanus capitis* (head lice).

ULTRAVIOLET RADIATION, THERMAL, AND PRESSURE INJURY

After completing this section of the chapter, the learner will be able to meet the following objectives:

- Compare the tissue involvement in first-degree, second-degree full-thickness, and third-degree burns.
- Describe the systemic complications of burns.
- Cite two causes of pressure ulcers.

Skin Damage Caused by Ultraviolet Radiation

The skin is the protective shield against harmful UV rays from the sun. Skin cancers and other skin disorders such as early wrinkling and aging of the skin have been attributed to the damaging effects of sunlight.

Sunlight is measured in wavelengths of nanometers (nm; one billionth of a meter) ranging from approximately 290 nm in the UV region up to approximately 2500 nm in the infrared region. UV radiation (UVR) is divided into three types: UVC, UVB, and UVA.[4] UVC rays are short (100 to 290 nm) and do not pass through the earth's atmosphere. However, they can be produced artificially and are damaging to the eyes. UVB rays are 290 to 320 nm. Commonly referred to as *sunburn rays*, they are responsible for nearly all the skin effects of sunlight, including *photoaging*—the wrinkles, pigmentary changes, dryness, and loss of skin tone that occur with and are enhanced by exposure to sunlight. UVA rays are 320 to 400 nm and can pass through window glass. They are further divided into short-wave UVAII (320 to 339 nm) and long-wave UVAI (340 to 400 nm).[4] Nonetheless, UVA, particularly UVAII, contributes greatly to skin alterations. Artificial sources of UVA, such as tanning salons and therapeutic solar interventions (PUVA) for certain skin conditions, also produce the same effects as UVB radiation.

The acute effects of UVA and UVB are short-lived and reversible. They include erythema, pigmentation, and injury to Langerhans cells and keratinocytes in the epidermis. These reactions differ depending on whether the inciting agent is UVA or UVB. For example, UVA-induced erythema occurs immediately, fades within 2 hours, and is believed to be due to the "heat load." UVB-induced erythema has a delayed response, peaking within 6 to 24 hours after exposure to sunlight and fading over 1 or 2 days. Pigmentation or tanning induced by UVA and UVB is due to a delayed increase in the number of melanocytes, elongation and extension of the dendritic processes, and transfer of melanin to keratinocytes. For tanning to occur, there must be UVB-induced erythema. Tanning induced by UVB is protective against subsequent exposures, whereas tanning induced by UVA provides limited protection.

Skin damage induced by UVB is believed to be caused by the generation of reactive oxygen species and by damage to melanin. This type of damage is referred to as photoaging.[3] Solar elastosis is due to a large amount of abnormal, elastotic material in the upper dermis, which causes epidermal thickening and loss of elasticity.[4] This causes deep and coarse wrinkles that never disappear.[4] Cellular proteins and DNA are primarily damaged because of their abundance and ability to absorb UVR. Both UVA and UVB also deplete Langerhans cells and immune cells. Both UVA and UVB are now considered causes of cancer.[4] UVA may actually be more carcinogenic than UVB. Although it causes less sunburn, UVA is present during all daylight hours, year-round. UVB, on the other hand, varies by season, location, and time of day. UVA penetrates deeply and causes greater damage in the keratinocytes, where most skin cancers arise.[4]

KEY POINTS

ULTRAVIOLET RADIATION, THERMAL, AND PRESSURE INJURY

- The ultraviolet rays of sunlight have the potential for directly damaging skin cells, accelerating the effect of aging on the skin, and predisposing to the development of skin cancer.
- Thermal injury can damage skin and subcutaneous tissue and destroy the barrier function of the skin in terms of preventing the loss of body fluids and protecting against the entry of infectious organisms.

Drug-Induced Photosensitivity

Some drugs are classified as photosensitive drugs because they produce an exaggerated response to UVR when the drug is taken in combination with sun exposure. Examples include some of the anti-infective agents (sulfonamides, tetracyclines, nalidixic acid), antihistamines (cyproheptadine, diphenhydramine), antipsychotic agents (phenothiazines, haloperidol), diuretics (thiazides, acetazolamide, amiloride), hypoglycemic agents (sulfonylureas), and nonsteroidal anti-inflammatory drugs (phenylbutazone, ketoprofen, naproxen).

Stopping the drug and switching to a non–photosensitivity-inducing drug can generally manage drug-induced sun damage.[4] However, in some cases, the photosensitivity can continue for months to years even after the medication has been discontinued.[4]

Sunburn

Sunburn is caused by excessive exposure of the epidermal and dermal layers of the skin to UVR, resulting in an erythematous inflammatory reaction. Sunburn ranges from mild to severe. Mild sunburn consists of various degrees of skin redness. The burn can continue to develop for another 1 or 2 days, occasionally followed by peeling skin.[4] Some peeling and itching may continue for several weeks. Inflammation, blistering, weakness, chills, fever, malaise, and pain often accompany severe forms of sunburn. Scaling and peeling follow any overexposure to sunlight. Dark skin also burns and may appear grayish or gray-black. Severe sunburns are those that cover large portions of the body with blisters or are accompanied by a high fever or intense pain.

Mild to moderate sunburns are treated with anti-inflammatory medications, such as aspirin or ibuprofen, until redness and pain subside. Cold compresses, cool baths, and applying a moisturizing cream, such as aloe, to affected skin help treat the symptoms. Blisters should not be broken to preserve the protective layer of the skin, hasten the healing process, and decrease the risk of infection. Extensive second- and third-degree burns may require hospitalization and specialized burn care techniques.

Preventing Skin Damage Caused by Ultraviolet Radiation

The UV rays of sunlight or other sources can be completely or partially blocked from the skin by sunscreens. There are three primary types of sunscreens available on the market: those that reduce or prevent UV erythema chemically, which causes the chemicals in the sunscreen to absorb the UVR; those that work physically by reflecting the UVR; and those that work biologically to block the inflammatory reaction.[4]

Sunscreen products no longer contain para-aminobenzoic acid (PABA), a chemical blocking agent that protects against UVB, because of its allergenic and staining properties. However, PABA derivatives are used widely, but protect only against UVB. Broad-spectrum sunscreen products protect against both UVA and UVB. Sunscreen should be used diligently and according to the person's tendency to burn rather than tan. Sunless suntan creams, such as dihydroxyacetone, produce a tan without exposure to the sun. They come in various tones, with emollients or humectants added for moisturizing or gel or alcohol-based products for drying.

Thermal Injury

About 490,000 people in the United States require medical care for burns each year, with 40,000 requiring hospitalization.[47] The effects and complications of burns fully illustrate the essential function that the skin performs as it protects the body from the damaging elements in the environment while serving to maintain the constancy of the body's internal environment. The massive loss of skin tissue not only predisposes a person to invasion from microbes that are present in the environment but also allows for a substantial loss of body fluids leading to interference with temperature regulation, challenges for the immune system, and excessive demands imposed on the metabolic and reparative processes that are needed to restore the body's interface with the environment.

Burns are caused by a number of sources. Flame burns occur because of exposure to direct fire. Scald burns result from hot liquids spilled or poured on the skin surface. In a child, a scald burn may be indicative of child abuse. Chemical burns occur from industrial agents used in occupational sites. Electrical burns occur from contact with live electrical wires in fields or in the home. Electrical burns are usually more extensive because of internal tissue injury and the presence of entrance and exit wounds. Lightning, electromagnetic radiation, and ionizing radiation also can cause skin burns.

Classification of Burns

Burns are typically classified according to the depth of involvement as first-degree, second-degree, and third-degree burns. The depth of a burn is largely influenced by the duration of exposure to the heat source and the temperature of the heating agent.

First-Degree Burns. *First-degree burns* (superficial partial-thickness burns) involve only the outer layers of the epidermis. They are red or pink, dry, and painful. There usually is no blister formation. A mild sunburn is an example. The skin maintains its ability to function as a water vapor and bacterial barrier and heals in 3 to 10 days. First-degree burns usually require only palliative treatment, such as pain relief measures and adequate fluid intake. Extensive first-degree burns on infants, older adults, and people who receive radiation therapy for cancer may require more care.

Second-Degree Burns. *Second-degree burns* involve both the epidermis and dermis. *Second-degree partial-thickness burns* involve the epidermis and various degrees of the dermis. They are painful, moist, red, and blistered. Underneath the blisters is weeping, bright pink or red skin that is sensitive to temperature changes, air exposure, and touch. The blisters prevent the loss of body water and superficial dermal cells. Excluding excision of large burn areas, it is important to maintain intact blisters after injury because they serve as a good bandage and may promote wound healing. These burns heal in approximately 1 to 2 weeks.

Second-degree full-thickness burns involve the entire epidermis and dermis. Structures that originate in the subcutaneous layer, such as hair follicles and sweat glands, remain intact. These burns can be very painful because the pain sensors remain intact. Tactile sensation may be absent or greatly diminished in the areas of deepest destruction. These burns appear as mottled pink, red, or waxy white areas with blisters and edema. The blisters resemble flat, dry tissue paper, rather than the bullous blisters seen with superficial partial-thickness injury. After healing, in approximately 1 month, these burns maintain their softness and elasticity, but there may be the loss of some sensation. Scar formation is usual. These burns heal with supportive medical care aimed at preventing further tissue damage, providing adequate hydration, and ensuring that the granular bed is adequate to support reepithelialization.

Third-Degree Burns. *Third-degree full-thickness burns* extend into the subcutaneous tissue and may involve muscle and bone. Thrombosed vessels can be seen under the burned skin, indicating that the underlying vasculature is involved. Third-degree burns vary in color from waxy white or yellow to tan, brown, deep red, or black. These burns are hard, dry, and leathery. Edema is extensive in the burn area and surrounding tissues. There is no pain because the nerve sensors have been destroyed. However, there is no such thing as a "pure" third-degree burn. Third-degree burns are almost always surrounded by second-degree burns, which are surrounded by an area of first-degree burns. The injury sometimes has an almost target-like appearance because of the various degrees of burn. Full-thickness burns wider than 1.5 inches usually require skin grafts because all the regenerative (*i.e.*, dermal) elements have been destroyed. Smaller injuries usually heal from the margins inward toward the center, the dermal elements regenerating from the healthier margins. However, regeneration may take many weeks and leave a permanent scar, even in smaller burns (Table 52.1, Fig. 52.25).

TABLE 52.1 BURN CLASSIFICATION

DEPTH OF BURN	BLEEDING	SENSATION	APPEARANCE	BLANCHING
Superficial	Brisk	Pain	Rapid capillary refill	Moist, red
Superficial-dermal	Brisk	Pain	Slowed capillary refill	Dry, pale pink
Dermal	Delayed	No pain	No capillary refill	Mottled cherry red color
Full thickness	None	No pain	No blanching	Dry, leathery, or waxy hard wound surface

Reprinted from Jensen S. (2015). *Nursing health assessment: A best practice approach* (2nd ed., Table 11.6, p. 253). Philadelphia, PA: Wolters Kluwer, with permission.

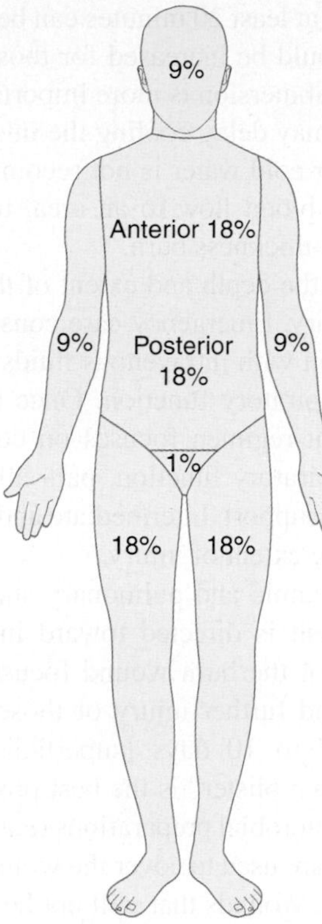

Figure 52.25 • The rule of nines. Estimated percentage of total body surface area (TBSA) in the adult is calculated by sectioning the body surface areas with a numerical value related to nine. (Note: The anterior and posterior head total 9% of TBSA.) (From Hinkle J. L., Cheever K. H. (2018). *Brunner & Suddarth's textbook of medical–surgical nursing* (14th ed., p. 1849). Philadelphia, PA: Wolters Kluwer.)

Extent of the Burn. In addition to the depth of the wound, the extent of the burn also is important. Extent is measured by estimating the amount of total body surface area (TBSA) involved. Several tools exist for estimating the TBSA. For example, the *rule of nines* counts anatomic body parts as multiples of 9% (the head is 9%, each arm 9%, each leg 18%, anterior trunk 18%, posterior trunk 18%), with the perineum 1%[48] (see Fig. 52.24). Other factors, such as age, location, other injuries, and preexisting conditions, must be assessed in order to manage best practice of the burn injury. These factors can increase the assessed severity of the burn and the length of treatment. For example, a first-degree burn is reclassified as a more severe burn if other factors are present, such as burns to the hands, face, and feet; inhalation injury; electrical burns; other trauma; or existence of psychosocial problems. Genital burns almost always require hospitalization because edema may cause difficulty urinating and the location complicates maintenance of a bacteria-free environment.

Systemic Complications

People with burns often experience multiple life-threatening complications such as hemodynamic instability, respiratory failure, infection, and even multiple-organ dysfunction (MOD). The magnitude of the response is proportional to the extent of injury, usually reaching a plateau when approximately 60% of the body is burned. In addition to loss of skin, people with burns often have associated injuries or illnesses. The treatment challenge is to provide immediate resuscitation efforts and long-term maintenance of physiologic function. Pain and emotional problems are additional challenges faced by people with burns.

Hemodynamic Instability. Hemodynamic instability begins almost immediately with injury to capillaries in the burned area and surrounding tissue. Fluid is lost from the vascular, interstitial, and cellular compartments. Because of a loss of vascular volume, people with major burns often present in the emergency department in a form of hypovolemic shock known as *burn shock*. Evidence suggests that lactate serum level at admission can predict, which people in burn shock are going to benefit from therapeutic plasma exchange (TPE).[49] The person has a decrease in cardiac output, increased peripheral vascular resistance, and impaired perfusion of vital organs. Electrical injuries that cause burns can produce cardiac arrhythmias that require immediate attention.

Respiratory System Dysfunction. Another injury commonly associated with burns is smoke inhalation and postburn lung injury. People often are trapped in a burning structure and inhale significant amounts of smoke, carbon monoxide, and other toxic fumes. Water-soluble gases, such as ammonia, sulfur dioxide, and chlorine that are found in smoke from burning plastics and rubber react with mucous membranes to form strong acids and alkalis that induce ulceration of the mucous membrane, bronchospasm, and edema. Lipid-soluble gases, such as nitrous oxide and hydrogen chloride, are transported to the lower airways, where they damage lung tissue. There also may be thermal injury to the respiratory passages. Manifestations of inhalation injury include hoarseness, drooling, an inability to handle secretions, hacking cough, and labored and shallow breathing. Serial blood gases show a fall in the partial pressure of arterial oxygen (PO_2). Signs of mucosal injury and airway obstruction often are delayed for 24 to 48 hours after a burn. It is necessary continually to monitor the person for early signs of respiratory distress. Other pulmonary conditions, such as pneumonia, pulmonary embolism, or pneumothorax, may occur secondarily to the burn.

Hypermetabolic Response. The stress of burn injury increases metabolic and nutritional requirements. Secretion of stress-related hormones such as catecholamines and cortisol is increased in an effort to maintain homeostasis. Heat production is increased in an effort to balance heat losses from the burned area. Hypermetabolism, characterized by increased oxygen consumption, increased glucose use, and protein and fat wasting, is a characteristic response to burn trauma and infection. The hypermetabolic state peaks at approximately 7 to 17 days after the burn, and tissue breakdown diminishes as the wounds heal. Nutritional support is essential to recovery from burn injury. Enteral and parenteral hyperalimentation may be used during this time to deliver sufficient nutrients to prevent tissue breakdown and postburn weight loss.

Dysfunction of Other Organ Systems. Burn shock results in impaired perfusion of vital organs. The person may have impaired function of the kidneys, the gastrointestinal tract, the nervous system, and musculoskeletal tissues. Although the initial insult often is one of hypovolemic shock and impaired organ perfusion, sepsis may contribute to impaired organ function after the initial resuscitation period.

Renal insufficiency can occur in people with burns as a result of the hypovolemic state, damage to the kidneys at the time of the burn, or drugs that are administered. Immediately after the burn, a person goes into a short period of relative anuria, followed by a phase of hypermetabolism characterized by increased urine output and nitrogen loss.

The effects of burn injury on the gastrointestinal tract include gastric dilation and decreased peristalsis. These effects are compounded by immobility and narcotic analgesics. People with burns are observed carefully for vomiting and fecal impaction. Acute ulceration of the stomach and duodenum (called *Curling ulcer*) is a potential complication in people with burns and is thought to be the result of stress and gastric ischemia. It is largely controlled by the prophylactic administration of proton pump inhibitors. Enteral feeding tubes are inserted almost immediately. Tube feeding is intended to mitigate ulcer formation, maintain the integrity of the intestinal mucosa, and provide sufficient calories and protein for the hypermetabolic state.

Neurologic changes can occur from periods of hypoxia. Neurologic damage may result from head injuries, drug or alcohol abuse, carbon monoxide poisoning, fluid volume deficits, and hypovolemia. With an electrical burn, the brain or spine can be directly injured. The responses to neurologic damage may include confusion, memory loss, insomnia, lethargy, and combativeness.

Musculoskeletal effects include fractures that occur at the time of the accident, deep burns extending to the muscles and bone, hypertrophic scarring, and contractures. The hypermetabolic state increases tissue catabolism and produces severe protein and fat wasting.

Sepsis. A significant complication of the acute phase of burn injury is sepsis. It may arise from the burn wound, pneumonia, urinary tract infection, infection elsewhere in the body, or the use of invasive procedures or monitoring devices. Immunologically, the skin is the body's first line of defense. When the skin is no longer intact, the body is open to bacterial infection. Destruction of the skin also prevents the delivery of cellular components of the immune system to the site of injury. There also is loss of normal protective skin flora and a shift to colonization by more pathogenic flora.

Emergency and Long-Term Treatment

Regardless of the type of burn, it is first priority to stop the fire and provide relief to the people affected. The heat source should be removed, and flames should be doused with water or smothered with a blanket. Active cooling removes the heat and prevents progression of the burn. Immersion or irrigation with lukewarm water for at least 20 minutes can be extremely helpful. This period should be increased for those with chemical burns. Immediate submersion is more important than removal of clothing, which may delay cooling the involved areas. The application of ice or cold water is not recommended because it can further limit blood flow to an area, turning a partial-thickness into a full-thickness burn.

Depending on the depth and extent of the burn, medical treatment is necessary. Emergency care consists of resuscitation and stabilization with intravenous fluids while maintaining cardiac and respiratory function. Once hospitalized, the immediate treatment regimen focuses on continued maintenance of cardiorespiratory function, pain alleviation, wound care, and emotional support. Intermediate and long-term treatments depend on the extent of injury.

After hemodynamic and pulmonary stability have been established, treatment is directed toward initial care of the wound. Treatment of the burn wound focuses on protection from desiccation and further injury of those burn areas that reepithelialize in 7 to 10 days (superficial second-degree burns). "Nature's own blister" is the best protection for these burns. Topical antimicrobial preparations (*e.g.*, silver sulfadiazine) and dressings are used to cover the wound when the blister has been broken. Wounds that will not heal spontaneously in 7 to 10 days (deep second-degree and third-degree burns) are usually treated by excision and skin grafts. The sloughed tissue, or *eschar*, produced by the burn is excised as soon as possible. This decreases the chance of infection and allows the skin to regenerate faster.

Burns that encircle the entire surface of the body or a body part (*e.g.*, arms, legs, torso) act like tourniquets and can cause major tissue damage to the muscles, tendons, and vasculature under the area of the leathery eschar skin. These burns are called *circumferential burns*. The eschar is incised longitudinally (escharotomy), and sometimes a fasciotomy (surgical incision through the fascia of the muscle) is performed. The timing of these incisions is important. Incision is done after the person's circulatory condition stabilizes to some degree, thereby limiting some of the massive fluid loss. However, the incisions must be done before eschar formation can cause hypoxia and necrosis of the underlying tissues and organs. This is extremely important when torso burns occur because the pressure placed on the chest can result in an inability to breathe and decreased blood return to the heart.

Systemic infection remains a leading cause of morbidity among persons with extensive burns. Continuous microbiologic surveillance is necessary; protective isolation measures are often instituted. There is an increasing trend toward use of prophylactic antibiotic treatment in persons with major burns.

Skin grafts are surgically implanted as soon as possible, often at the same time the burn tissue is excised, to promote new skin growth, limit fluid loss, and act as a dressing. Skin grafts can be permanent or temporary and split thickness or full thickness. Permanent skin grafts are used over newly excised tissue. Temporary skin grafts are used to cover a burned area until the tissue underneath it has healed.

Various sources of skin grafts exist: *autograft* (skin obtained from the person's own body), *homograft* (skin obtained from another human being, alive or recently dead), and *heterograft* (skin obtained from another species, such as pigs). The best choice is autografting when there is enough uninterrupted skin on the person's body. The thickness of these grafts depends on the donor site and the needs of the burn person. A *split-thickness skin graft* is one that includes the epidermis and part of the dermis. A split-thickness skin graft can be sent through a skin mesher that cuts tiny slits into the skin, allowing it to expand up to nine times its original size. These grafts are used frequently because they can cover large surface areas and there is less autorejection. *Full-thickness skin grafts* include the entire thickness of the dermal layer. They are used primarily for reconstructive surgery or for deep, small areas. The donor site of a full-thickness skin graft requires a split-thickness skin graft to help it heal.

Synthetic skin grafts generally are composed of a layer of silicone, mimicking the properties of the epidermis, and a layer or matrix of fibers. Skin cells attach to the fibers, enabling dermal skin growth. Once the dermal skin has regenerated, the silicone layer is removed and a thin epidermal skin graft is applied, thus requiring less skin grafting overall.

Other treatment measures include positioning, splinting, and physical therapy to prevent contractures and maintain muscle tone. Because the normal body response to disuse is flexion, the contractures that occur with a burn are disfiguring and cause loss of limb or appendage use. Once the wounds have healed sufficiently, elastic pressure garments, sometimes for the full body, often are used to prevent hypertrophic scarring.

Pressure Ulcers

Pressure ulcers are ischemic lesions of the skin and underlying structures caused by unrelieved pressure that impairs the flow of blood and lymph. Pressure ulcers often are referred to as *decubitus ulcers* or *bedsores*. Pressure ulcers are most likely to develop over a bony prominence, but they may occur on any part of the body that is subjected to external pressure, friction, or shearing forces. Several subpopulations are at particular risk, including people with quadriplegia, older adults with restricted activity and hip fractures, and people in the critical care setting. The Agency for Healthcare Research and Quality developed a tool kit to assist hospital health care workers to decrease pressure ulcers.[50] Over 2.5 million people in the United States develop a pressure ulcer every year.[50] The work of multidisciplinary teams has proven successful in reducing the frequency of pressure ulcer occurrence. Development of handbooks covering the prevention of pressure ulcers has led to the implementation of effective protocols responsible for reducing the instances of pressure ulcers.[51] The prevention and treatment of pressure ulcers is a public health issue and is addressed in *Healthy People 2020*, a national public health policy statement.[52]

Mechanisms of Development

Multiple factors contribute to the development of pressure ulcers including other comorbidities such as type 2 diabetes, pressure from positioning and body weight, sweating and/or incontinence are just to name a few. External pressures that exceed capillary pressure interrupt blood flow in the capillary beds. When the pressure between a bony prominence and a support surface exceeds the normal capillary filling pressure, capillary flow essentially is obstructed. If this pressure is applied constantly for 2 hours, oxygen deprivation coupled with an accumulation of metabolic end products leads to irreversible tissue damage. People with impaired circulation will require less pressure to interrupt circulation so they are at even higher risk of developing a pressure ulcer. The same amount of pressure causes more damage when it is distributed over a small area than over a larger area.

Whether a person is sitting or lying down, the weight of the body is borne by tissues covering the bony prominences. Most pressure ulcers are located on the lower part of the body, most often over the sacrum and on bony prominences. Pressure over a bony area is transmitted from the surface to the underlying dense bone, compressing all of the intervening tissue. As a result, the greatest pressure occurs at the surface of the bone and dissipates outward in a conelike manner toward the surface of the skin. Thus, extensive underlying tissue damage can be present when a small superficial skin lesion is first noticed.

Altering the distribution of pressure from one skin area to another prevents tissue injury. Pressure ulcers most commonly occur in people with conditions such as spinal cord injury in which normal sensation and movement to effect redistribution of body weight are impaired. Normally, people unconsciously shift their weight to redistribute pressure on the skin and underlying tissues. For example, during the night, people turn in their sleep, preventing ischemic injury of tissues that overlie the bony prominences that support the weight of the body; the same is true for sitting for any length of time. The movements needed to shift the body weight are made unconsciously, and only when movement is restricted do people become aware of discomfort.

Shearing forces are caused by the sliding of one tissue layer over another with stretching and angulation of blood vessels, causing injury and thrombosis. Shear occurs when the skeleton moves, but the skin remains fixed to an external surface, such as occurs with transfer from a stretcher to a bed or pulling a person up in bed. The same thing happens when the head of the bed is elevated, causing the torso to move toward the foot of the bed while friction and moisture cause the skin to remain fixed to the bed linens. *Friction* contributes to pressure ulceration by damaging the skin at the epidermal–dermal interface. It occurs as persons who are bedridden use their elbows and heels to aid in movement. *Moisture* contributes to pressure ulcer formation by weakening the cell wall of individual skin cells and by changing the protective pH of the skin. This makes the skin more susceptible to pressure, shear, and friction injury.

Prevention

The prevention of pressure ulcers is preferable to their treatment. The Agency for Healthcare Research and Quality is firm in its conviction that using the Prevention of Pressure Ulcers Tool Kit will be effective in decreasing the number of decubitus ulcers.[50]

Risk factors identified as contributing to the development of pressure ulcers were those related to sensory perception (*i.e.*, ability to respond meaningfully to pressure-related discomfort), level of skin moisture, urine and fecal continence, nutrition and hydration status, mobility, circulatory status, and presence of shear and friction forces.

Methods for preventing pressure ulcers include frequent position change, meticulous skin care, and frequent and careful observation to detect early signs of skin breakdown. Moisture macerates and injures skin. Sources of moisture include sweat, wound drainage, urine, and feces. Both urinary and fecal incontinence increase the risk of pressure ulcers. Food crumbs, intravenous tubing, and other debris in the bed can greatly increase local skin pressure points. The prevention of dehydration improves the circulation. It also decreases the concentration of urine, thereby minimizing skin irritation in people who are incontinent, and it reduces urinary problems that contribute to incontinence. Maintenance of adequate nutrition is important (see Table 52.2). Anemia and malnutrition contribute to tissue breakdown and delay healing after tissue injury has occurred.

Staging and Treatment

Pressure ulcers can be staged using four categories.[53] *Stage I ulcers* are characterized by a defined area of persistent redness in lightly pigmented skin or an area of persistent redness with

TABLE 52.2 NECESSARY NUTRIENTS FOR WOUND HEALING

NUTRIENT	FUNCTION	RESULTS OF DEFICIENCY
Proteins	Wound repair	Poor wound healing
	Clotting factor production	Hypoalbuminemia and generalized edema, which slows oxygen diffusion and metabolic transport mechanisms from the capillaries and cell membranes
	White blood cell production and migration	
	Cell-mediated phagocytosis	
	Fibroblast proliferation	Lymphopenia
	Neovascularization	Impaired cellular immunity
	Collagen synthesis	
	Epithelial cell proliferation	
	Wound remodeling	
Carbohydrates	Supply cellular energy	Body uses visceral and muscle proteins for energy
	Spare protein	
Fats	Supply cellular energy	Inhibited tissue repair
	Supply essential fatty acids	Use of visceral and muscle proteins for energy
	Cell membrane structure	
	Prostaglandin production	
Vitamin A	Collagen synthesis	Poor wound healing
	Epithelialization	Impaired immunity
Vitamin C	Membrane integrity	Impaired immunity
	Antioxidant	Poor wound healing
		Capillary fragility
Vitamin K	Normal blood clotting	Increased risk for hemorrhage and hematoma formation
Iron	Collagen synthesis	Anemia, leading to increased risk for local tissue ischemia
	Enhances leukocytic bacterial activity	Impaired tensile strength
	Hemoglobin synthesis	
Zinc	Cell proliferation	Impaired collagen cross-linkage
	Cofactor for enzymes	Slow healing
	Vitamin A utilization	Alteration in taste
		Anorexia
		Impaired immunity
Copper	Collagen cross-linkage	Decreased collagen synthesis
	Red blood cell synthesis	Anemia
Pyridoxine, riboflavin, and thiamine	Energy production	Decreased resistance to infection
	Cellular immunity	Impaired wound healing
	Red blood cell synthesis	
Arginine	Increases local wound immune system	Decreased local wound immune system
	Nitrogen-rich (32% nitrogen, whereas the average amino acid is 16% nitrogen)	
	Precursor to proline, which is converted to hydroxyproline and then to collagen	
Glutamine	Primary fuel for fibroblasts	Less fuel for fibroblasts
	Preservation of lean body mass	

Reprinted from Hess C. T. (2012). *Clinical guide: Wound care* (7th ed.). Ambler, PA: Wolters Kluwer, with permission.

blue or purple hues in darker skin. *Stage II ulcers* represent a partial-thickness loss of skin involving the epidermis or dermis or both. The ulcer is superficial and presents clinically as an abrasion, a blister, or a shallow crater. *Stage III ulcers* represent a full-thickness skin loss involving damage and necrosis of subcutaneous tissue that may extend down to but not through underlying fascia. The ulcer manifests as a deep crater with or without undermining of adjacent tissue. *Stage IV ulcers* involve full-thickness skin loss and necrosis with extensive destruction or damage to the underlying subcutaneous tissues that may extend to involve muscle, bone, and supporting structures (*e.g.*, tendon or joint capsule) (Chart 52.1).

After skin breakdown has occurred, special treatment measures are needed to prevent further ischemic damage, reduce bacterial contamination and infection, and promote healing. Stage I ulcers usually are treated with frequent turning and measures to remove pressure. Stage II or III ulcers with little exudate are treated with semipermeable or occlusive dressings. The occlusive dressing can assist with epithelial cell migration by keeping the wound fluid. Wound fluid is thought to contain a variety of growth factors that enhance wound healing. Occlusive dressings may also relieve wound pain and prevent bacterial contamination. There are several types of occlusive dressings available, including polymer films, hydrogels, hydrocolloids, biomembranes, and absorbing granules. The available products differ in their permeability to water vapor and wound protection, and each has advantages and disadvantages.

Necrotic debris increases the possibility of bacterial infection and delays wound healing. Stage III ulcers with exudate and necrotic debris and stage IV ulcers usually require debridement (*i.e.*, removal of necrotic tissue and eschar). This can be done surgically, with wet-to-dry dressings, or through the use of proteolytic enzymes. Stage IV wounds often require packing to obliterate dead space and are covered with nonadherent dressings. Stage IV ulcers may require surgical interventions, such as skin grafts or myocutaneous flaps.

CHART 52.1 STAGES OF PRESSURE INJURY

Deep Tissue Injury
A purple or maroon area of intact skin or a blood-filled blister due to damage of underlying tissue. Area can be painful, firm or mushy, warm, or cool. Can progress quickly and expose additional layers of tissue.

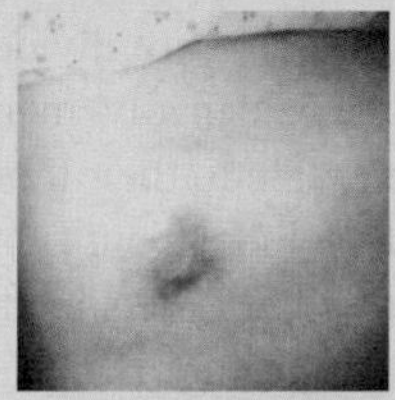

Stage 1
A persistent area of skin redness (without a break in the skin) that does not disappear when pressure is relieved. Usually over a bony prominence.

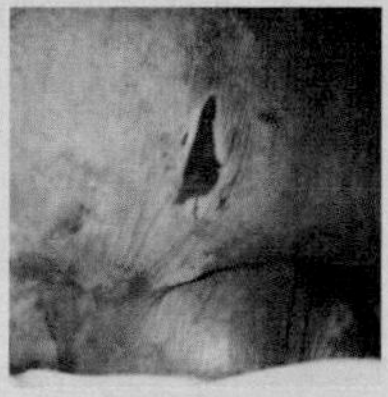

Stage 2
A partial-thickness loss of skin layers involving the epidermis that presents clinically as an intact or open/ruptured blister, or open shallow crater.

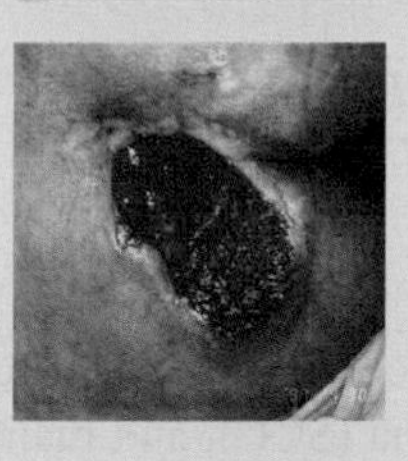

Stage 3
A full thickness of skin is lost extending through the epidermis and exposing the subcutaneous tissues; presents as a deep crater with or without tunneling and undermining adjacent tissue.

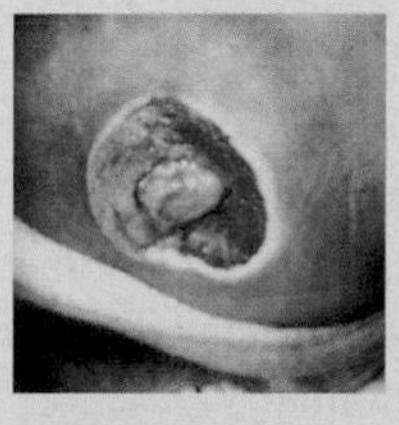

Stage 4
A full thickness of skin and subcutaneous tissue is lost, exposing muscle, bone, or both; presents as a deep crater that may include necrotic tissue, slough, or eschar. Tunneling and undermining often are present.

Unstageable
Full-thickness loss of tissue with base covered by slough and/or eschar. Stage cannot be determined until slough or eschar is removed to expose base and actual depth of wound.

Deep Tissure Pressure Injury
Localized area of nonblanchable deep red or purple discoloration with a dark wound bed or blood-filled blister due to intense or prolonged pressure or shearing force. Skin may be intact or nonintact.

Reprinted from Eliopoulos C. (2018). Skin care. In *Gerontological nursing* (9th ed., Box 27-1, p. 397). Philadelphia, PA: Wolters Kluwer, with permission.

IN SUMMARY

Repeated exposure to the UV rays of the sun predisposes to sunburn, premature aging of the skin (wrinkling, solar elastosis, and irregularities in pigmentation), and skin cancer. Solar and artificial sources of UVR, such as from a tanning parlor, contribute to the amount of radiation to which human beings are exposed. Sunburn, which is caused by excessive exposure to UVR, is an erythematous inflammatory reaction, ranging from mild to severe. Photosensitive drugs can also produce an exaggerated response to UVR when they are taken in combination with sun exposure. Sunscreens are protective agents that work by either reflecting sunlight or preventing its absorption.

Burns cause damage to skin structures, ranging from first-degree burns, which damage the epidermis, to third-degree full-thickness burns, which extend into the subcutaneous tissue and may involve muscle and bone. The extent of injury is determined by the thickness of the burn and the TBSA involved. In addition to skin involvement, burn injury can cause hemodynamic instability with hypovolemic shock, inhalation injury with respiratory involvement, a hypermetabolic state, organ dysfunction, immune suppression and sepsis, pain, and emotional trauma. Treatment methods vary with the severity of injury and include immediate resuscitation and maintenance of physiologic function, wound cleaning and debridement, application of antimicrobial agents and dressings, and skin grafting. Efforts are directed toward preventing or limiting disfigurement and disability.

Pressure ulcers are caused by ischemia of the skin and underlying tissues. They result from external pressure, which disrupts blood flow, or shearing forces, which cause stretching and injury to blood vessels. Pressure ulcers are divided into four stages, according to the depth of tissue involvement. The prevention of pressure ulcers is preferable to their treatment. The goals of prevention should include identifying at-risk persons who need prevention along with the specific factors placing them at risk; maintaining and improving tissue tolerance to pressure to prevent injury; and protecting against the adverse effects of external mechanical forces (*i.e.*, pressure, friction, and shear).

NEVI AND SKIN CANCERS

After completing this section of the chapter, the learner will be able to meet the following objectives:

- Describe the origin of nevi and state their relationship to skin cancers.
- Compare the appearance and outcome of basal cell carcinoma (BCC), squamous cell carcinoma (SCC), and malignant melanoma.

Nevi

Nevi, or moles, are common congenital or acquired tumors of the skin that are benign. Almost all adults have nevi, some in greater numbers than others. Nevi can be pigmented or nonpigmented, flat or elevated, and hairy or nonhairy.

Nevocellular nevi are pigmented skin lesions resulting from proliferation of melanocytes in the epidermis or dermis.[54] Nevocellular nevi are tan to deep brown, uniformly pigmented, small papules with well-defined, rounded borders (Fig. 52.26). They are formed initially by melanocytes with their long dendritic extensions that are normally interspersed among the basal keratinocytes. The melanocytes are transformed into round or oval melanin-containing cells that grow in nests or clusters along the dermal–epidermal junction. Because of their location, these lesions are called *junctional nevi* or active nevi.[5] Eventually, most junctional nevi grow into the surrounding dermis as nests or cords of cells. *Compound nevi* contain epidermal and dermal components.[5] In older lesions, the epidermal nests may disappear entirely, leaving a *dermal nevi*. Compound and dermal nevi usually are more elevated than junctional nevi.

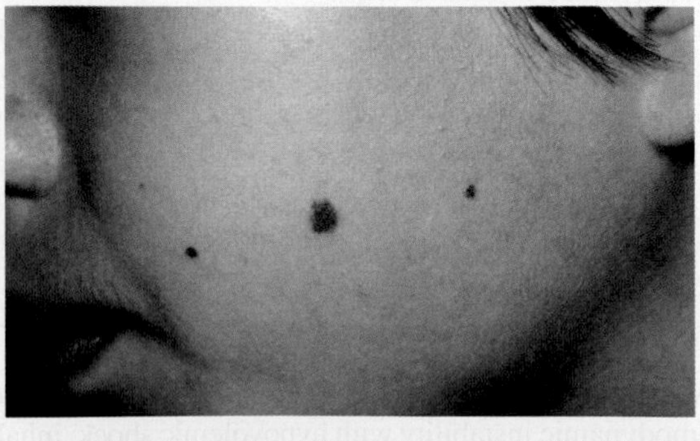

Figure 52.26 • Normal nevi. (From Jensen S. (2015). *Nursing health assessment: A best practice approach* (2nd ed., p. 279). Philadelphia, PA: Wolters Kluwer.)

Another form of nevus is *nevus with architectural disorder with or without cytologic atypia*. (The formerly used term is *dysplastic nevus*; however, an effort is being made to eliminate this term because research reveals that the risk for melanoma is as likely to arise in a common nevus as in a dysplastic nevus.) There are two criteria that correlate nevi with melanoma risk: (1) a high nevus count correlates with a higher risk of melanoma and (2) the presence of large nevi increases the relative risk of melanoma.[55]

Because of the possibility of malignant transformation, any mole that undergoes a change warrants immediate medical attention.[56] The changes to observe and report are changes in size, thickness, or color, itching, and bleeding.

Skin Cancer

There has been an alarming increase in skin cancers over the past several decades. In the United States in 2017, there were approximately 87,110 new cases of melanoma, with 52,170 in men and 34,940 in women.[56] There were also approximately 5.4 million cases per year of highly curable nonmelanoma (basal cell and squamous cell) cancers.[57]

The rising incidence of skin cancer has been attributed to increased sun exposure associated with social and lifestyle changes. The thinning of the ozone layer in the earth's stratosphere is thought to be another factor in this increased incidence. Society's emphasis on sun tanning also is implicated. People tend to have more leisure time and spend increasing amounts of time in the sun with uncovered skin.

Although the factors linking sun exposure to skin cancer are not completely understood, both total cumulative exposure

KEY POINTS

SKIN CANCERS

- The melanocytes, which protect against sunburn through increased production of melanin and sun tanning, are particularly vulnerable to the adverse effects of unprotected exposure to ultraviolet light. Malignant melanoma, which is a malignant tumor of melanocytes, is a rapidly progressive and metastatic form of skin cancer.
- BCC and SCC, which also reflect the effects of increased sun exposure, are less aggressive forms of skin cancer and are more easily cured.

and altered patterns of exposure are strongly implicated. Basal cell carcinoma (BCC) and squamous cell carcinoma (SCC) are often associated with total cumulative exposure to UVR. Thus, BCC and SCC occur more commonly on maximally sun-exposed parts of the body, such as the face and back of the hands and forearms.[5] Melanomas occur most commonly on areas of the body that are exposed to the sun intermittently, such as the back in men and the lower legs in women.

Malignant Melanoma

Malignant melanoma is a malignant tumor of the melanocytes.[5] It is a rapidly progressing, metastatic form of cancer. The dramatic increase in the incidence of malignant melanoma over the past several decades has been credited to increased UVR exposure, including tanning salons. Public health screening measures, early diagnosis, increased knowledge of precursor lesions, and greater public knowledge of the disease may account for earlier intervention.

The risk is greatest in fair-skinned people, particularly those with blond or red hair who sunburn and freckle easily. Other risk factors include a family history of malignant melanoma, presence of marked freckling on the upper back, history of three or more blistering sunburns before 20 years of age, and presence of actinic keratoses. Still other significant risk factors for melanoma are atypical mole/dysplastic nevus syndrome, immunosuppression, and prior photochemotherapy (psoralen and ultraviolet A [PUVA] therapy).

Severe, blistering sunburns in early childhood and intermittent intense sun exposures contribute to increased susceptibility to melanoma in young- and middle-aged adults. Roughly 90% of malignant melanomas in whites occur on sun-exposed skin. However, in darker-skinned people, melanomas often occur on non–sun-exposed areas, such as the mucous membranes and subungual, palmar, and plantar surfaces.[5]

Clinical Manifestations. Malignant melanomas differ in size and shape. Usually, they are slightly raised and black or brown. Borders are irregular and surfaces are uneven. Most seem to arise from preexisting nevi or new molelike growths.[56] There may be surrounding erythema, inflammation, and tenderness. Periodically, melanomas ulcerate and bleed. Dark melanomas are often mottled with shades of red, blue, and white. These three colors represent three concurrent processes: melanoma growth (blue), inflammation and the body's attempt to localize and destroy the tumor (red), and scar tissue formation (white).

There are four types of melanomas including superficial spreading, nodular, lentigo maligna, and acral lentiginous.[5] *Superficial spreading melanoma* is characterized by a raised-edged nevus with lateral growth. It has a disorderly appearance in color and outline. This lesion tends to have biphasic growth, horizontally and vertically. It typically ulcerates and bleeds with growth. These lesions account for two thirds of all melanomas and are most prevalent in people who sunburn easily and have intermittent sun exposure.[5] *Nodular melanomas*, which account for 15% of melanomas, are raised, dome-shaped lesions that can occur anywhere on the body, but most frequently on the trunk, head, and neck.[5] They are commonly a uniform blue-black color and tend to look like blood blisters. Nodular melanomas tend to rapidly invade the dermis from the start, with no apparent horizontal growth phase. *Lentigo maligna melanomas*, which account for 4% to 15% of all invasive melanomas, are slow-growing, flat nevi that occur primarily on sun-exposed areas of older adults.[58] Untreated lentigo maligna tends to exhibit horizontal and radial growth for many years before it invades the dermis to become lentigo maligna melanoma. *Acral lentiginous melanoma*, which accounts for 2% of melanomas, occurs primarily on the palms, soles, nail beds, and mucous membranes. This melanoma has the worse prognosis of all of the melanomas but is not frequently seen.[59] It has the appearance of lentigo maligna.

Detection and Diagnosis. Early detection is critical with malignant melanoma. Regular self-examination of the total skin surface in front of a well-lighted mirror provides a method for early detection. It requires that a person undress completely and examine all areas of the body using a full mirror, handheld mirror, and handheld hair dryer (to examine the scalp). An *ABCD* rule has been developed to aid in early diagnosis and timely treatment of malignant melanoma (Fig. 52.27) This acronym represents *a*symmetry, *b*order irregularity, *c*olor variegation, and *d*iameter greater than 6 mm (14 inch or pencil eraser size).[56] People should be taught to watch for these changes in existing nevi or the development of new nevi, as well as other alterations such as bleeding or itching.

Diagnosis of melanoma is based on biopsy findings from a lesion. Consistent with other cancerous tumors, melanoma is commonly staged using the TNM (tumor, lymph node, and metastasis) staging system or the 2001 American Joint Committee on Cancer Staging System for Cutaneous Melanoma, in which the tumor is rated 0 to 4, with further subclassifications depending on numerous factors, including the tumor thickness, ulceration, sentinel lymph node status, and mitotic rate for stratifying people at low and high risk.[60] The sentinel lymph node is a regional lymph node that receives lymphatic drainage from tumor sites. Ulceration and presence in sentinel lymph node result in a poorer prognosis.[60]

Treatment. Treatment is usually surgical excision, the extent of which is determined by the thickness of the lesion, invasion into the deeper skin layers, and spread to the regional lymph nodes. When diagnosed in a premetastatic phase, melanoma is now treated in ambulatory settings, lessening the cost and inconvenience of care. Current capability allows for mapping lymph flow to a *sentinel lymph node*. The sentinel lymph node is then sampled for biopsy. If tumor cells have spread from the primary tumor to the regional lymph nodes, the sentinel node will be the first node in which tumor cells appear. Therefore, sentinel node biopsy can be used to test for the presence of melanoma cells and determine if radical lymph node dissection is necessary.

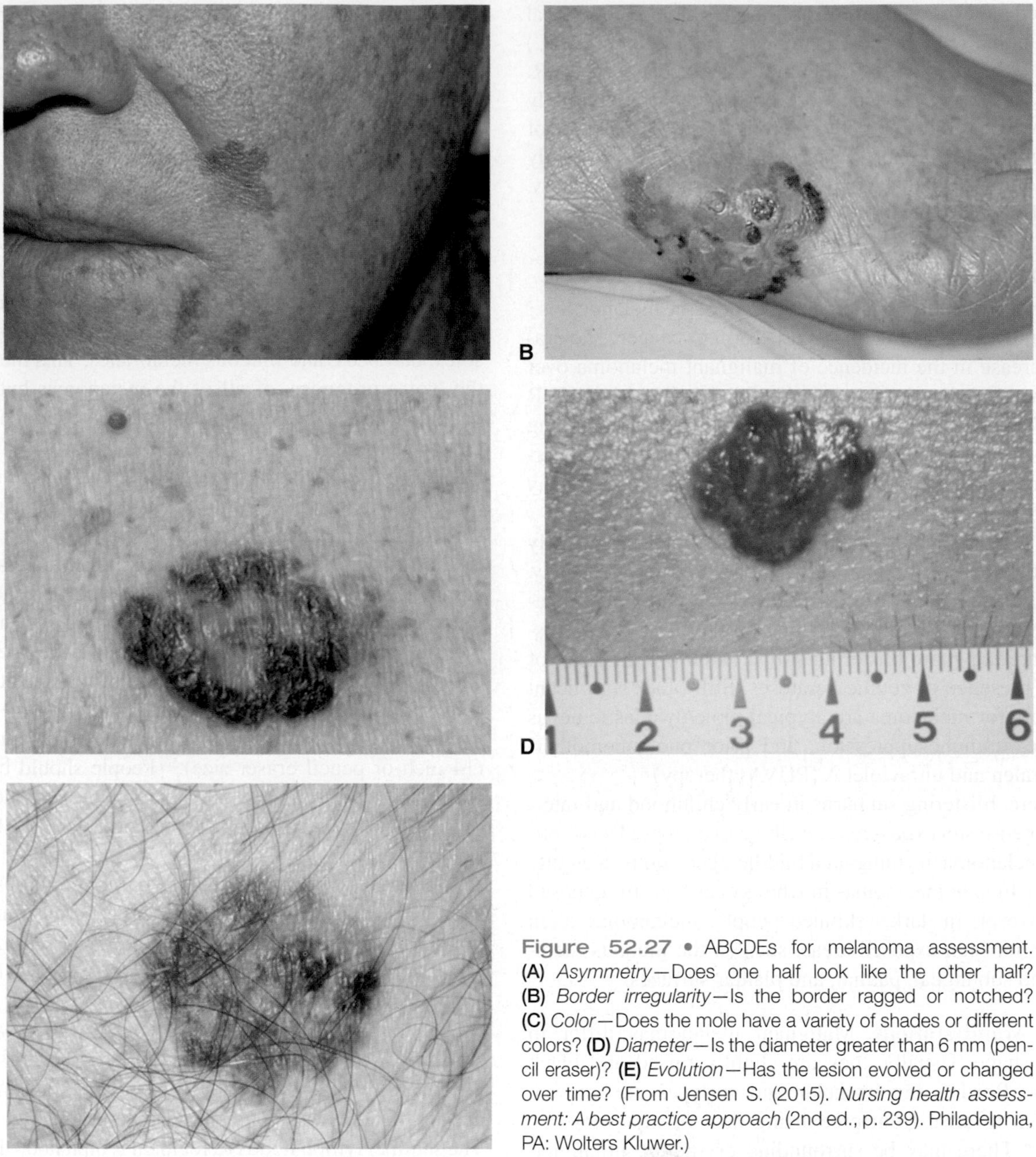

Figure 52.27 • ABCDEs for melanoma assessment. **(A)** *Asymmetry*—Does one half look like the other half? **(B)** *Border irregularity*—Is the border ragged or notched? **(C)** *Color*—Does the mole have a variety of shades or different colors? **(D)** *Diameter*—Is the diameter greater than 6 mm (pencil eraser)? **(E)** *Evolution*—Has the lesion evolved or changed over time? (From Jensen S. (2015). *Nursing health assessment: A best practice approach* (2nd ed., p. 239). Philadelphia, PA: Wolters Kluwer.)

Routine cancer treatment, such as chemotherapy, is indicated when the disease becomes systemic. Despite many interventions used over the years, efforts to cure melanoma in its later stages have been disappointing. However, there is promise in vaccine development or immunotherapy. Vaccines are targeted to prevent the recurrence of melanoma, especially in stages II and III.

Basal Cell Carcinoma

BCC, which is a neoplasm of the nonkeratinizing cells of the basal layer of the epidermis, is the most common skin cancer in light-skinned people (Fig. 52.28). Like other skin cancers, BCC has increased in incidence over the past several decades.

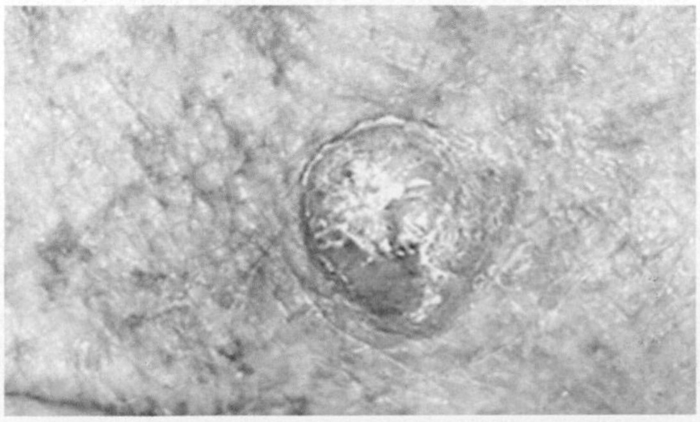

Figure 52.28 • Basal cell carcinoma. The most frequent skin cancer. (From Jensen S. (2015). *Nursing health assessment: A best practice approach* (2nd ed., p. 279). Philadelphia, PA: Wolters Kluwer.)

Fair-skinned people with a history of significant long-term sun exposure are more susceptible. Black- and brown-skinned people are affected occasionally. BCC usually occurs in people who were exposed to great amounts of sunlight. Of the 5.4 million annually diagnosed skin cancers, the majority are BCCs.[56]

BCC usually is a nonmetastasizing tumor that extends wide and deep if left untreated.[5] These tumors are most frequently seen on the head and neck, most often occurring on the skin that has hair. They also occur on skin surfaces unexposed to the sun, although less frequently. There are several histologic types of BCC, with many types being slow growing and many fast growing.[5] Some of the more aggressive BCCs are called sclerosing, morpheaform, micronodular, and infiltrative BCC.[4] Nodular ulcerative and superficial BCCs are the two most frequently occurring types. *Nodular ulcerative BCC* is the most common BCC and has a nodulocystic structure that manifests as a pinkish translucent papule, which grows larger over time. Telangiectatic vessels are often associated with nodular BCC. Over the years, a central depression forms that progresses to an ulcer surrounded by the original shiny, waxy border. BCC in darker-skinned people usually is darkly pigmented and frequently misdiagnosed as other skin diseases, including melanoma.

The second-most common form and less aggressive BCC is *superficial BCC*, which is seen most often on the chest or back.[4] It begins as a flat, nonpalpable, erythematous plaque. The red, scaly areas slowly enlarge, with nodular borders and telangiectatic bases. Generally, there is a thin, raised, white border that surrounds the BCC.[4] This type of skin cancer is difficult to diagnose because it mimics other skin problems.

BCCs develop from basal keratinocytes of the epidermis.[4] With the DNA damage from the UVB, the immunologic response can be triggered to cause cancerous changes in the cells.[4] Although the BCC does not usually metastasize via blood vessels or the lymph system, the BCC can enlarge slowly or rapidly, solely by extension.[4]

Biopsies are obtained from all suspected BCCs for diagnosis. It is highly curable if detected and treated early. The treatment depends on the site and extent of the lesion. The most important treatment goal is complete elimination of the lesion. Also important is the maintenance of function and optimal cosmetic effect. Curettage with electrodesiccation, surgical excision, irradiation, laser, cryosurgery, and chemosurgery are effective in removing all cancerous cells. Immune therapy, gene therapy, and photodynamic therapy are emerging treatments. People should be checked at regular intervals for recurrences.

Squamous Cell Carcinoma

SCCs are the second-most common malignant tumors of the outer epidermis and account for 10% to 20% of all skin cancers.[4,57] The increase in the incidence of SCCs is consistent with increased UVR exposure. There is also a strong occupational hazard link to the development of SCC.

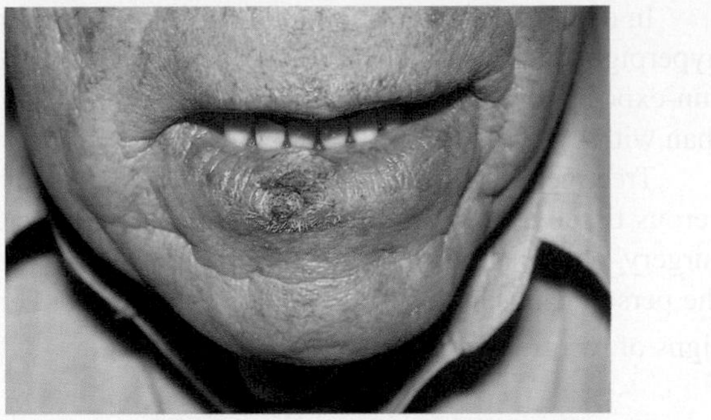

Figure 52.29 • Squamous cell carcinoma. This is the second-most frequent skin cancer and generally is found on sun-exposed surfaces. (From Jensen S. (2015). *Nursing health assessment: A best practice approach* (2nd ed., p. 280). Philadelphia, PA: Wolters Kluwer.)

People exposed to arsenic (*i.e.*, Bowen disease, which is also called SCC in situ), industrial tars, coal, and paraffin have an increased likelihood of contracting SCC. Men are twice as likely as women to have SCC. Dark-skinned people are rarely affected.

There are two types of SCC: intraepidermal and invasive. *Intraepidermal SCC* remains confined to the epidermis for a long time. However, at some unpredictable time, it penetrates the basement membrane to the dermis and metastasizes to the regional lymph nodes (Fig. 52.29). SCC has a significant risk for metastasis in contrast to BCC. It then converts to *invasive SCC*. The invasive type can develop from intraepidermal carcinoma or from a premalignant lesion (*e.g.*, actinic keratoses). It may be slow growing or fast growing with metastasis.

SCC is a red-scaling, keratotic, slightly elevated lesion with an irregular border, usually with a shallow chronic ulcer. The lesions usually lack the pearly rolled border and superficial telangiectases found on BCCs. Later, lesions grow outward, show large ulcerations, and have persistent crusts and raised, erythematous borders. The SCC lesions occur on sun-exposed areas of the skin, particularly the nose, forehead, helix of the ear, lower lip, and back of the hand.

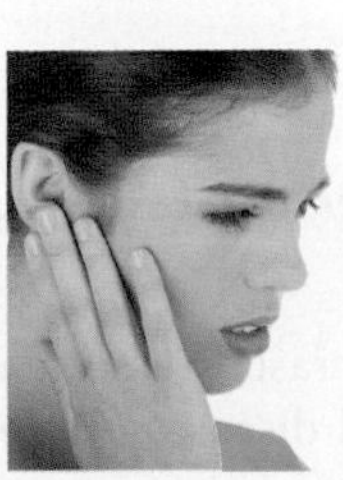

Lauren requests to see a physician regarding her keloid. She wants to be sure it is not skin cancer since she feels it might have been mistakenly diagnosed as a keloid. She feels it should be checked out and that a biopsy should be taken. She says it looks like a type of skin cancer she has seen on the Internet, and she is also worried because she has had previous sunburns on her face, including her ear. The physician reassures her it is a keloid and is a direct result of excessive formation of collagen corneum secondary to the ear piercing. Lauren finally accepts the diagnosis and vows never to have a piercing again. She also vows to always use sunscreen and to stay out of the sun as much as she can.

In dark-skinned black people, the lesions may appear as hyperpigmented nodules and occur more frequently on non–sun-exposed areas. Metastasis is more common with SCC than with BCC.[57]

Treatment measures are aimed at the removal of all cancerous tissue using methods such as electrosurgery, excision surgery, chemosurgery, or radiation therapy. After treatment, the person is observed for the remainder of his or her life for signs of recurrence.

IN SUMMARY

Nevi or moles usually are benign. Because they may undergo cancerous transformation, any mole that undergoes a change warrants immediate medical attention. There has been an alarming increase in skin cancers over the past few decades. Repeated exposure to the UV rays of the sun has been implicated as the principal cause of skin cancer. Neoplasms of the skin include malignant melanoma, BCC, and SCC.

Malignant melanoma is a malignant tumor of the melanocytes. It is a rapidly progressing, metastatic form of cancer. Clinically, malignant melanoma of the skin usually is asymptomatic. The most important clinical sign is the change in size, shape, and color of pigmented skin lesions, such as moles. As the result of increased public awareness, melanomas are being diagnosed earlier, when they can be cured surgically. SCC and BCC are of epidermal origin.

BCCs are the most common form of skin cancer among whites. They are slow-growing tumors that rarely metastasize. The two types of SCC are intraepidermal and invasive. Intraepidermal SCC remains confined to the epidermis for a long time. Invasive SCC can develop from intraepidermal carcinoma or from premalignant lesions such as actinic keratoses.

AGE-RELATED SKIN MANIFESTATIONS

After completing this section of the chapter, the learner will be able to meet the following objectives:

- Describe the distinguishing features of rashes associated with the following infectious childhood diseases: roseola infantum, rubeola, rubella, and varicella.
- Characterize the physiologic changes of aging skin.
- Describe the appearance of skin tags, keratoses, lentigines, and vascular lesions that are commonly seen in older adults.

Many skin problems occur more commonly in certain age groups. Because of aging changes, infants, children, and older adults tend to have different skin problems.

Skin Manifestations of Infancy and Childhood

Skin Disorders of Infancy

Infancy connotes the image of perfect, unblemished skin. For the most part, this is true. However, several congenital skin lesions, such as mongolian spots, hemangiomas, and nevi, are associated with the early neonatal period. There are also several acquired skin conditions, including diaper dermatitis, prickly heat, and cradle cap, that are relatively common in infants.

Pigmented and Vascular Birthmarks. Pigmented and vascular lesions comprise most birthmarks. Pigmented birthmarks represent abnormal migration or proliferation of melanocytes. For example, *mongolian spots* are caused by selective pigmentation. They usually occur on the buttocks or sacral area and are seen commonly in Asian and dark-skinned people. *Nevi* or moles are small, tan to brown, uniformly pigmented solid macules. *Nevocellular nevi* are formed initially from aggregates of melanocytes and keratinocytes along the dermal–epidermal border. *Congenital melanocytic nevi* are collections of melanocytes that are present at birth or develop within the first year of life. They present as macular, papular, or plaquelike pigmented lesions of various shades of brown, with a black or blue focus. The texture of the lesions varies and they may be with or without hair. They usually are found on the hands, shoulders, buttocks, entire arm, or trunk of the body. Some involve large areas of the body in garment-like fashion. They usually grow proportionately with the child. Congenital melanocytic nevi are clinically significant because of their association with malignant melanoma.

Vascular birthmarks are cutaneous anomalies of angiogenesis and vascular development. Two types of vascular birthmarks commonly are seen in infants and small children: bright red, raised hemangiomas of infancy and flat, reddish-purple port-wine stains.

Hemangiomas of infancy are small, red lesions that are noticed shortly after birth. Hemangiomas of infancy are generally benign vascular tumors produced by proliferation of vascular endothelial cells[5] (Fig. 52.30). A small proportion of these lesions are present at birth, and the remainder develop within a few weeks after birth.[4] Girls are three times more likely to have hemangiomas than boys.[4]

Hemangiomas of infancy typically undergo an early period of a proliferation during which they enlarge, followed by a period of slow involution where the growth is reversed until complete resolution generally by 5 or 8 years of age.[4] Hemangiomas of infancy can occur anywhere on the body. However, when they occur in the airway, they can be life threatening. Ulceration, the most frequent complication, can be painful and carries the risk of infection, hemorrhage, and scarring. A small percentage of hemangiomas of infancy develop complications, such as infection or ulceration.[5] Some hemangiomas of infancy are located in anatomic regions associated with other anomalies requiring careful monitoring and early intervention.

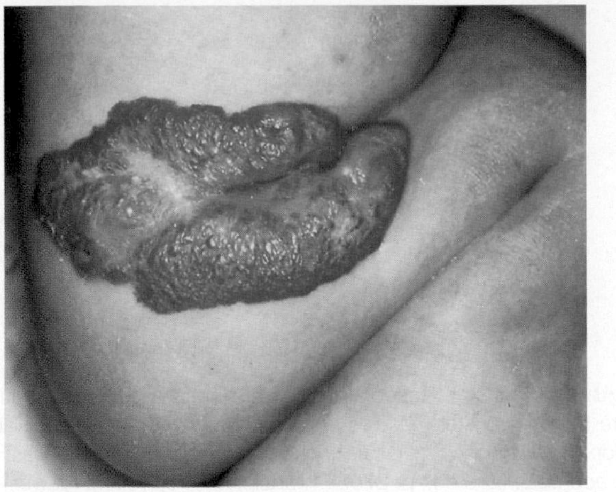

Figure 52.30 • Hemangioma of infancy. (From Hall B. J., Hall J. C. (2017). *Sauer's manual of skin diseases* (11th ed., p. 494). Philadelphia, PA: Wolters Kluwer.)

Port-wine stains are pink or red patches that can occur anywhere on the body and are very noticeable (Fig. 52.31). They represent slow-growing capillary malformations that grow proportionately with the child and persist throughout life. There is progressive dilation of the dermal capillaries, which initially is confined to the immediate epidermis, with gradual involvement of deeper dermal blood vessels, although the greater number is always in the upper dermis.[5] Distribution of lesions on the face roughly corresponds to the sensory branches of the trigeminal nerve. The development of a port-wine stain may follow trauma. Port-wine stains usually are confined to the skin, but may be associated with vascular malformations of the eye, resulting primarily in glaucoma, and other neurologic deficits (Sturge-Weber syndrome).[5] Laser surgery has revolutionized the treatment of port-wine stains.

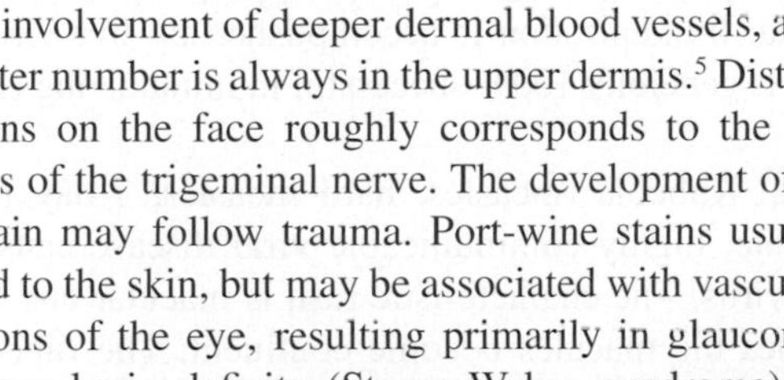

Figure 52.31 • Nevus flammeus (port-wine stain) on the arm and hand. (From Hall B. J., Hall J. C. (2017). *Sauer's manual of skin diseases* (11th ed., p. 494, Figure 45-11). Philadelphia, PA: Wolters Kluwer.)

Diaper Dermatitis. Irritant diaper dermatitis, or *diaper rash*, is a form of contact dermatitis that results from an increased contact with a wet or soiled diaper. The wearing of diapers causes an increase in skin wetness and pH because of ammonia from urine. Prolonged wetness leads to softening and maceration of the skin, making it more susceptible to damage by friction from the surface of the diaper and local irritants. The contents of soiled diapers, if not changed frequently, can lead to contact dermatitis, bacterial infections, or other skin conditions. The proteases and lipases contained in feces are particularly irritating.

The appearance of diaper rash ranges from simple (*i.e.*, widely distributed macules on the buttocks and anogenital areas) to severe (*i.e.*, beefy, red, excoriated skin surfaces in the diaper area). Secondary infections with bacteria and yeasts are common; discomfort may be marked because of intense inflammation. Such conditions as contact dermatitis, seborrheic dermatitis, candidiasis, and atopic dermatitis should be considered when the eruption is persistent and recalcitrant to simple therapeutic measures.

Diaper dermatitis often responds to simple measures, including frequent diaper changes with careful cleansing of the irritated area to remove all waste products. Exposing the irritated area to air is helpful. It has been shown that application of a barrier ointment after each diaper change is a valuable component of therapy.

Selection of a barrier preparation is important. It is now clear that the barrier function of the skin is provided by the stratum corneum, whose main function is to minimize water loss and prevent inward penetration of toxic substances and microorganisms. Ideally, a barrier should mimic the skin's natural function by forming a long-lasting barrier to increase protection against irritants and microorganisms and to maintain optimum moisture levels. Preparations should contain lipids similar to those naturally present in the stratum corneum.

Intractable and severe cases of diaper dermatitis should be seen by a health care provider for treatment of any secondary infections. Secondary candidal (*i.e.*, yeast; Fig. 52.32) or other skin manifestations discussed in this chapter may occur in the diaper area. It is important to differentiate between normal diaper dermatitis and more serious skin problems.

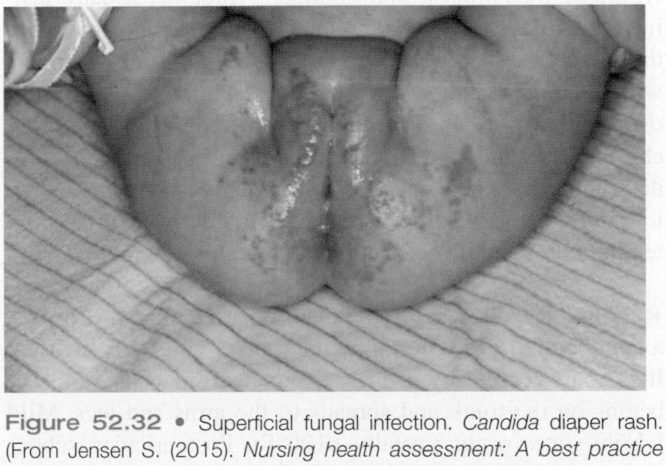

Figure 52.32 • Superficial fungal infection. *Candida* diaper rash. (From Jensen S. (2015). *Nursing health assessment: A best practice approach* (2nd ed., p. 847). Philadelphia, PA: Wolters Kluwer.)

Prickly Heat. Prickly heat or miliaria results from constant maceration of the skin because of prolonged exposure to a warm, humid environment. Maceration leads to midepidermal obstruction by blocking the eccrine glands and possible rupture of these sweat glands. It is possible that an infant could develop a fatal hyperpyrexia if the eccrine glands are congenitally absent.[5] Although commonly seen during infancy, prickly heat may occur at any age. The treatment includes removing excessive clothing, cooling the skin with warm water baths, drying the skin with powders, and avoiding hot, humid environments.

Cradle Cap. Cradle cap is a greasy crust or scale formation on the scalp. It usually is attributed to infrequent and inadequate washing of the scalp. Cradle cap is treated using mild shampoo and gentle combing to remove the scales. Sometimes oil can be left on the head for minutes to several hours, softening the scales before scrubbing. Other emulsifying ointments or creams may be helpful in difficult cases. The scalp may need to be rubbed firmly to remove the buildup of keratinized cells. Recalcitrant cases need to be seen by a health care practitioner. Serious or chronic forms of seborrheic dermatitis may exist.

Skin Manifestations of Common Infectious Diseases

Infectious childhood diseases that produce rashes include exanthem subitum, rubella, rubeola, varicella, and scarlet fever. Although these diseases are seen less frequently because of successful immunization programs and the use of antibiotics, they still occur.

Roseola Infantum. Roseola infantum (exanthem subitum or sixth disease) is a contagious disease caused by HHV-6. Because HHV-6 is the etiologic agent, the condition is often referred to as *sixth disease*. Primary HHV-6 infection occurs early in life. The majority of cases of roseola occur in children between 6 months and 4 years of age.[4] Transplacental antibodies likely protect most infants until 6 months of age.[4] Roseola produces a characteristic maculopapular rash covering the trunk and spreading to the appendages. The rash is preceded by a high fever (≤105°F) that occurs very suddenly, inflamed tympanic membranes, and coldlike symptoms usually lasting 3 to 4 days.[4] These symptoms improve at approximately the same time the rash appears (Fig. 52.33). Because infants with roseola exhibit a unique constellation of symptoms over a short time, the infection may be confused with other childhood exanthems. Blood antibody titers may be taken to determine the actual diagnosis. In most cases, there are no long-term effects from this disease. Infants who spike high temperatures should be seen by their health care providers.

Rubella. Rubella (*i.e.*, 3-day measles or German measles) is a childhood disease caused by the rubella virus (a togavirus). It is characterized by a diffuse, punctate, macular rash that begins on the trunk and spreads to the arms and legs. Mild febrile states occur (usually <100°F). Postauricular, suboccipital, and cervical lymph node adenopathy is common.

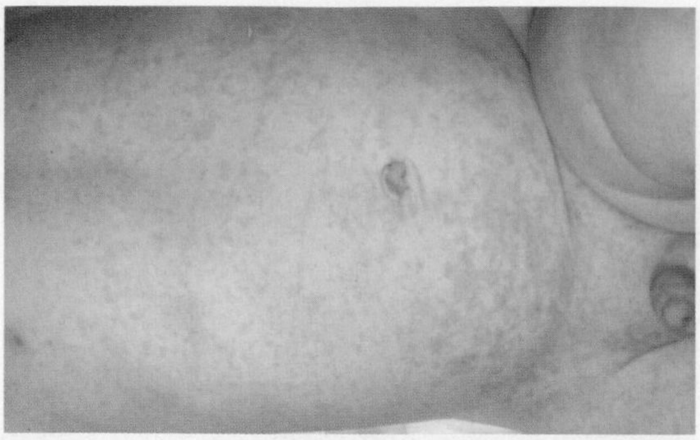

Figure 52.33 • Roseola. This viral illness has a combination of 1- to 5-mm-diameter macules and papules with a surrounding area of pallor. (From Jensen S. (2015). *Nursing health assessment: A best practice approach* (2nd ed., p. 275). Philadelphia, PA: Wolters Kluwer.)

Coldlike symptoms usually accompany the disease in the form of cough, congestion, and coryza (*i.e.*, nasal discharge).

Rubella usually has no long-lasting sequelae. However, the transmission of the disease to pregnant women early in their gestation periods may result in congenital rubella syndrome. Among the clinical signs of congenital rubella syndrome are cataracts, microcephaly, mental retardation, deafness, patent ductus arteriosus, glaucoma, purpura, and bone defects. Most states have laws requiring immunization to prevent transmission of rubella. Immunization is accomplished by live-virus injection and is generally 100% successful in immunizing children.

Rubeola. Rubeola (measles, hard measles, 7-day measles) is an acute, highly communicable viral disease caused by a morbillivirus. The characteristic rash is macular and blotchy; sometimes the macules become confluent. The rubeola rash usually begins on the face and spreads to the appendages. There are several accompanying symptoms: a fever of 100°F or greater, *Koplik spots* (*i.e.*, small, irregular red spots with a bluish-white speck in the center) on the buccal mucosa, and mild to severe photosensitivity (Fig. 52.34). The person

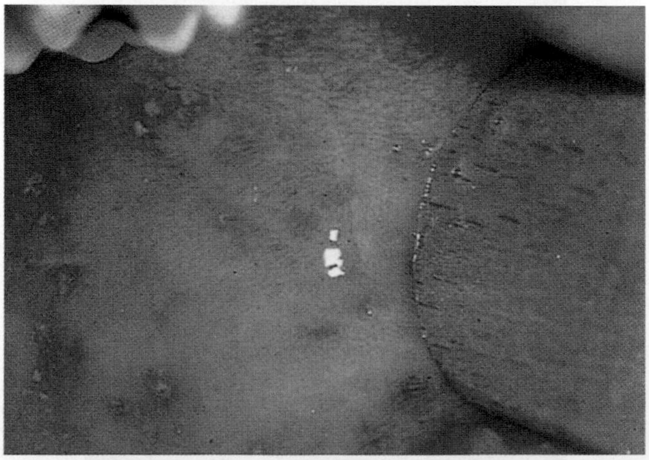

Figure 52.34 • Koplik spots. The rashes of measles. Koplik spots appear as red spots along the inside of the cheek. (From SPL/Custom Medical Stock Photo. Reprinted with permission. Bowden V. R., Greenberg C. S. (2014). *Children and their families: The continuum of nursing care* (3rd ed., p. 1263, Figure 24-8). Philadelphia, PA: Wolters Kluwer.)

commonly has coldlike symptoms, general malaise, and myalgia. In severe cases, the macules may hemorrhage into the skin tissue or onto the outer body surface. This form is called *hemorrhagic measles*. The course of measles is more severe in infants, adults, and malnourished children. There may be severe complications, including otitis media, pneumonia, and encephalitis. Antibody titers are determined for a conclusive diagnosis of rubeola.

Measles is a disease preventable by vaccine, and law in the United States requires immunization. Immunization is accomplished by the injection of a live-virus vaccine. Measles vaccination is generally 100% successful.

Varicella. Varicella (chickenpox) is a common communicable childhood disease. It is caused by the varicella–zoster virus, which also is the agent in herpes zoster (shingles). The characteristic skin lesion occurs in three stages: macule, vesicle, and granular scab. The macular stage is characterized by development within hours of macules over the trunk, spreading to the limbs, buccal mucosa, scalp, axillae, upper respiratory tract, and conjunctiva. During the second stage, the macules form vesicles with depressed centers. The vesicles break open and a scab forms during the third stage. Crops of lesions occur successively, so that all three forms of the lesion usually are visible by the 3rd day of the illness.

Mild to extreme pruritus accompanies the lesions, which can lead to scratching and subsequent development of secondary bacterial infections. Chickenpox also is accompanied by coldlike symptoms, including cough, coryza, and sometimes photosensitivity. Mild febrile states usually occur, typically beginning 24 hours before lesion outbreak. Side effects, such as pneumonia, septic complications, and encephalitis, are rare.

Varicella in adults may be more severe, with a prolonged recovery rate and greater chances for development of varicella pneumonitis or encephalitis. Immunocompromised people may experience a chronic, painful form of the infection.

Skin Manifestations and Disorders in Older Adults

Older adults experience a variety of age-related skin disorders and exacerbations of earlier skin problems. Aging skin is believed to involve a complex process of actinic (solar) damage, normal aging, and hormonal influences. Actinic changes primarily involve increased occurrence of lesions on sun-exposed surfaces of the body.

Normal Age-Related Changes

Normal skin changes associated with aging are seen on areas of the body that have not been exposed to the sun. They include thinning of the dermis and the epidermis, diminution in subcutaneous tissue, a decrease in blood perfusion, and a decrease in the number of melanocytes, Langerhans cells, and Merkel cells.[61] The keratinocytes shrink, but the number of dead keratinized cells at the surface increases. This results in less padding and thinner skin, with color and elasticity changes.[61] The skin also loses its resistance to environmental and mechanical trauma. Tissue repair takes longer.

With aging, there is also less hair and nail growth, and there is permanent hair pigment loss. Hormonally, there is less sebaceous gland activity, although the glands in the facial skin may increase in size. Hair growth reduction also may be hormonally influenced. Although the reason is poorly understood, the skin in most older adults becomes dry, rough, scaly, and itchy. When there is no underlying pathologic process, it is called *senile pruritus*.[62] Itching and dryness become worse during the winter, when the need for home heating lowers the humidity.

The aging of skin, however, is not just a manifestation of age itself. Most skin changes associated with older adults are the result of cumulative actinic or environmental damage. For example, the wrinkled, leathery look of aged skin, as well as odd scars and ecchymotic spots, are due to solar elastotic degenerative change.

Skin Lesions Common among Older Adults

The most common skin lesions in older adults are skin tags, keratoses, lentigines, and vascular lesions. Most are actinic manifestations, which means they occur as a result of exposure to sun and weather over the years.

Skin Tags. Skin tags are soft, brown or flesh-colored papules commonly seen in 25% of adults.[4] They occur on any skin surface, but most frequently the neck, axilla, and intertriginous areas. They range in size from a pinhead to the size of a pea. Skin tags have the normal texture of the skin. They are benign and can be removed with scissors or electrodesiccation for cosmetic purposes.

Keratoses. A *keratosis* is a horny growth or an abnormal growth of the keratinocytes. A *seborrheic keratosis* (*i.e.*, seborrheic wart) is a benign, sharply circumscribed, wartlike lesion that has a stuck-on appearance (Fig. 52.35). They vary in size up to several centimeters. They are usually round or oval, tan, brown, or black lesions. Less pigmented ones may appear yellow or pink. Keratoses can be found on the face or trunk, as a solitary lesion or sometimes by the hundreds. Seborrheic keratoses are benign, but they must be watched for changes in color, texture, or size, which may indicate malignant transformation.

Actinic keratoses are the most common premalignant skin lesions that develop on sun-exposed areas.[4] The lesions usually are less than 1 cm in diameter and appear as dry, brown, scaly areas, often with a reddish tinge. Actinic keratoses often are multiple and more easily felt than seen. They often are indistinguishable from SCC without biopsy. Actinic keratoses may accumulate dense scale on the surface of the skin and become hyperkeratotic (*i.e.*, developing cutaneous growths of fingernail-type tissue that grow into hornlike appendages). This form is more prominent and palpable. Often, there is a weathered appearance to the surrounding skin. Slight changes, such as enlargement or ulceration, may indicate malignant

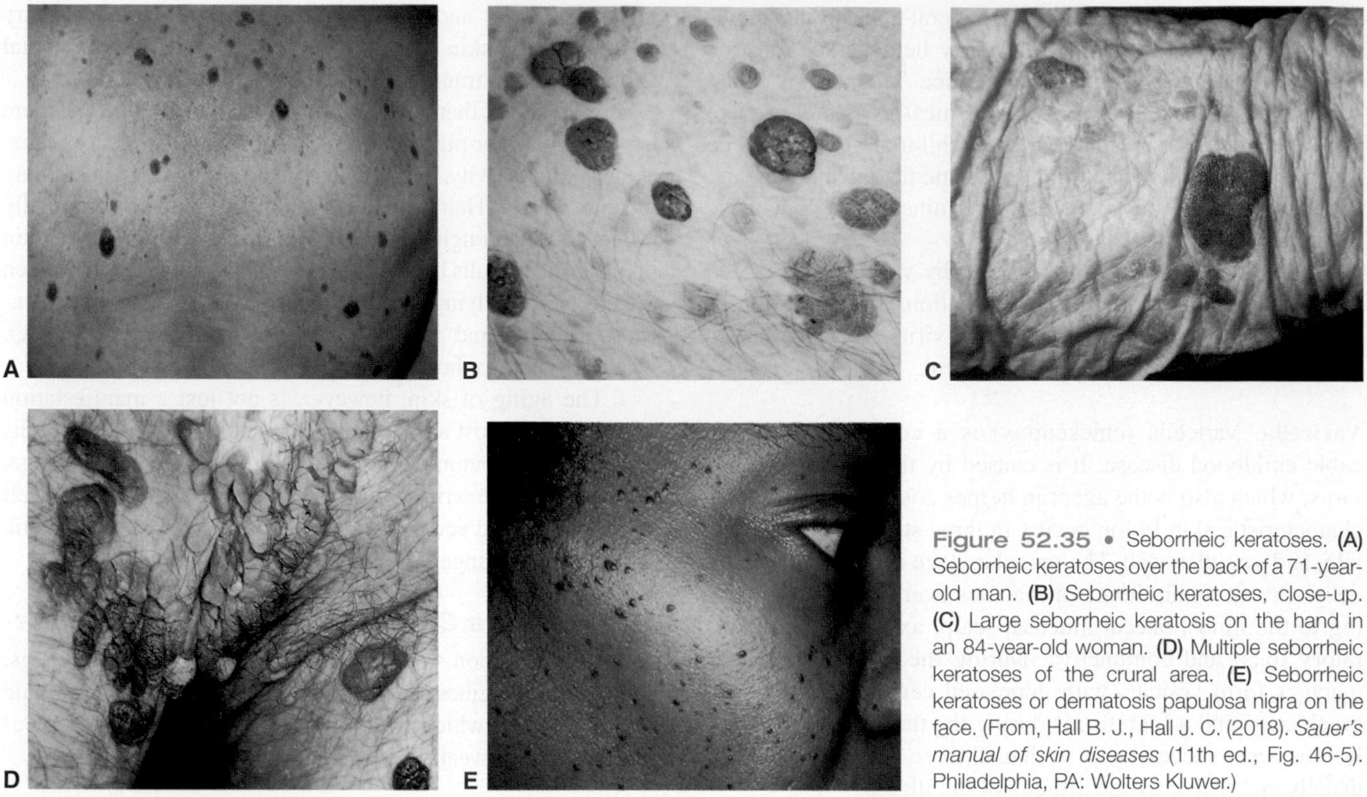

Figure 52.35 • Seborrheic keratoses. **(A)** Seborrheic keratoses over the back of a 71-year-old man. **(B)** Seborrheic keratoses, close-up. **(C)** Large seborrheic keratosis on the hand in an 84-year-old woman. **(D)** Multiple seborrheic keratoses of the crural area. **(E)** Seborrheic keratoses or dermatosis papulosa nigra on the face. (From, Hall B. J., Hall J. C. (2018). *Sauer's manual of skin diseases* (11th ed., Fig. 46-5). Philadelphia, PA: Wolters Kluwer.)

transformation. Actinic keratoses are SCCs confined to the epidermis.[4] Actinic keratoses are removed with cryosurgery, electrodesiccation, or lasers. When surgery is not indicated, they are treated with topical chemotherapy agents, like 5-fluorouracil or imiquimod creams, which erode the lesions.

Lentigines. A *lentigo* is a well-bordered, brown to black macule, usually less than 1 cm in diameter. *Solar lentigines* are tan to brown, benign spots on sun-exposed areas. Commonly referred to as *liver spots*, these lesions are considered risks for the development of skin cancers. Lentigines can be removed surgically (cryotherapy, laser therapy, liquid nitrogen). Topical creams and lotions containing adapalene or tretinoin have been used. Successful treatment depends on avoiding sun exposure and consistently using sunscreens.

Lentigo maligna (*i.e.*, Hutchinson freckle) is a slowly progressive (≤20 years) preneoplastic disorder of melanocytes. It occurs on sun-exposed areas, particularly the face. The lesion is a pigmented macule with a well-defined border and grows to 5 cm or sometimes larger. As it grows over the years, it may become slightly raised and wartlike. If untreated, a true malignant melanoma often develops. Surgery, curettage, and cryotherapy have been effective at removing the lentigines. Careful monitoring for conversion to melanoma is important.

Vascular Lesions. Vascular lesions include angiomas, telangiectases, and venous lakes. *Cherry angiomas* are smooth, cherry-red or purple, dome-shaped papules that occur in nearly all people older than 30 years of age. They usually are found on the trunk and are generally benign unless there is a sudden appearance of many cherry angiomas. *Telangiectases* are single dilated blood vessels, capillaries, or terminal arteries that appear on areas exposed to sun or harsh weather, such as the cheeks and the nose. They occur individually or in clusters, measure 1 cm or less, are nonpalpable, and easily blanch. They can become large and disfiguring. Pulsed dye lasers have been effective in removing them. *Venous lakes* are small, dark blue, slightly raised papules that have a lakelike appearance. They occur on exposed body parts, particularly the backs of the hands, ears, and lips. They are smooth and compressible. Venous lakes can be removed by electrosurgery, laser therapy, or surgical excision if a person desires.

IN SUMMARY

Some skin problems occur in specific age groups. Common in infants are diaper rash, prickly heat, and cradle cap. Infectious childhood diseases that are characterized by rashes include roseola infantum, rubella, rubeola, varicella, and scarlet fever. Vaccines are available to protect against rubella, rubeola, and varicella.

With aging, there is thinning of the dermis and the epidermis, diminution in subcutaneous tissue, loss and thickening of blood vessels, and slowing of hair and nail growth. Dry skin is common among the elderly, becoming worse during the winter months. Among the skin lesions seen in older adults are skin tags, keratoses, lentigines, and vascular lesions.

GERIATRIC Considerations

- Dry skin is common as the eccrine and apocrine gland reduce function.[62,63]
- Rough skin, longer wound heal time, and risk for hypothermia and heat stroke are common with aging due to a slower replication rate of epidermal cells.[62,63]
- Vitamin D synthesis is altered with sun-exposed aged skin.[4]
- The reduced number of Langerhans cells weakens the immune system of the skin.[4]
- Basal cell carcinoma is the most common skin cancer, and the risk increases with age.[4]
- The prevalence of stasis dermatitis increases from 6% to7% over age 50 and to 20% after age 70.[4]
- As we live longer, the risk of chronic venous leg ulcers, pressure ulcers, and diabetic ulcers after age 65 is increased.[4]

PEDIATRIC Considerations

- The neonate is at risk for altered fluid balance due to the thin dermis.[15]
- A child's dry and brittle hair signals a nutritional imbalance.[15]
- Children with recurring impetigo should be cultured for *S. aureus*.[15]
- The risk for atopic dermatitis often occurs along with other genetic-predisposed atopic diseases such as asthma.[4]
- Scalded skin syndrome, caused by infection with *S. aureus*, produces a toxin that causes exfoliation. It is most common during infancy.[64]

REVIEW EXERCISES

1. The mother of a 7-year-old boy notices that he is scratching his head frequently. On close examination, she notices a grayish, round, and roughened area, where the hair has broken off. Examination by the child's pediatrician produces a diagnosis of tinea capitis.
   A. *Explain the cause of the infection and propose possible mechanisms for spread of this infection in school-age children, particularly during winter months.*
   B. *Explain the preference of the superficial mycoses (dermatophytoses) for the skin-covered areas of the body.*
   C. *What methods are commonly used in the diagnosis of superficial fungal infections?*
2. A 75-year-old woman presents with severe burning pain and a vesicular rash covering a strip over the rib cage on one side of the chest. She is diagnosed with herpes zoster or shingles.
   A. *What is the source of this woman's rash and pain?*
   B. *Explain the dermatomal distribution of the lesions.*
3. Psoriasis is a chronically recurring papulosquamous skin disorder, characterized by circumscribed red, thickened plaques with an overlying silvery-white scale.
   A. *Explain the development of the plaques in terms of epidermal cell turnover.*
   B. *Persons with psoriasis are instructed to refrain from rubbing or scratching the lesions. Explain the rationale for these instructions.*
   C. *Among the methods used in the treatment of psoriasis are the use of topical keratolytic agents and corticosteroid skin preparations. Explain how these two different types of agents exert their effect on the plaque lesions.*
4. During the past several decades, there has been an alarming increase in the incidence of skin cancers, including malignant melanoma, that has been attributed to increased sun exposure.
   A. *Explain the possible mechanisms whereby ultraviolet radiation promotes the development of malignant skin lesions.*
   B. *Cite two important clinical signs that aid in distinguishing a dysplastic nevus from a malignant melanoma.*

References

1. Manga P., Elbuluk N., Orlow S. (2016). Recent advances in understanding vitiligo. *F1000 Research* 5, 1–9.
2. Gupta S., et al. (2016). Serum homocysteine and total antioxidant status in vitiligo: A case control study in Indian population. *Indian Journal of Dermatology* 61(2), 131–136.
3. Sahraian M., Owji M., Moghadasi A. (2016). Concomitant multiple sclerosis and another autoimmune disease: Does the clinical course change? *Clinical Neurology and Neurosurgery* 150(2016), 92–95.
4. Habif T., et al. (2017). *Skin disease: Diagnosis and treatment* (4th ed.). Atlanta, GA: Elsevier.
5. Hall J., Hall B. (2017). *Sauer's manual of skin diseases* (11th ed.). Baltimore, MD: Wolters Kluwer.
6. Passeron T. (2013). Melasma pathogenesis and influencing factors—An overview of the latest research. *Journal of the European Academy of Dermatology* 27, 5–6.
7. Lee A. (2014). An updated review of melisma pathogenesis. *Dermatologica Sinica* 32(4), 233–239.
8. Snyder A., Schiecherf R., Zaiac M. (2017). Melasma associated with topical estrogen cream. *Journal of Clinical Aesthetic Dermatology* 10(2), 57–58.

9. Cowan M. (2016). *Microbiology fundamentals: A clinical approach.* (2nd ed.). New York, NY: Mc-Graw-Hill Education.
10. Koning S., et al. (2012). Interventions for impetigo. *Cochrane Database System Review* 1, 1–65.
11. Botka T., et al. (2017). Two highly divergent lineages of exfoliative toxin B-encoding plasmids revealed in impetigo strains of *Staphylococcus aureus*. *International Journal of Medical Microbiology* 307(6), 291–296
12. Cuzick J., et al. (2012). New technologies and procedures for cervical cancer screening. *Vaccine* 305(2012), F107–F116.
13. Osazuwa-Peters N., et al. (2017). Not just a woman's business! Understanding men and women's knowledge of HPV, the HPV vaccine and HPV-associated cancers. *Preventive Medicine* 99(2017), 299–304.
14. Leung J., Broder K., Marin M. (2017). Severe varicella in persons vaccinated with varicella vaccine (breakthrough varicella): A systematic literature review. *Expert Review Vaccines* 16(4), 391–400.
15. Chlibek R., et al. (2016). Long-term immunogenicity and safety of an investigational herpes zoster subunit vaccine in older adults. *Vaccine* 34(6), 863–868.
16. Mahto A. (2017). Acne vulgaris. *Medicine* 45(6), 386–389.
17. Strayer D., Rubin R. (Eds.) (2015). *Rubin's pathology: Clinicopathologic foundations of medicine* (7th ed.). Philadelphia, PA: Wolters Kluwer.
18. Qidwai A., et al. (2017). The emerging principles for acne biogenesis: A dermatological problem of puberty. *Human Microbiome Journal* 4(2017), 7–13.
19. Morris-Jones R. (Ed.) (2014). *ABC of dermatology* (6th ed.). Oxford, UK: Wiley-Blackwell.
20. Pommerville J. C. (2013). *Alcamo's fundamentals of microbiology* (10th ed.). Burlington, MA: Jones & Bartlett Publishers.
21. Que S., Whitaker-Worth D., Chang M. (2016). Acne: Kids are not just little people. *Clinics in Dermatology* 34, 710–716.
22. Gupta M., et al. (2017). Suicidal behaviors in the dermatology patient. *Clinics in Dermatology* 35(3), 302–311.
23. Huang Y., Cheng Y. (2017). Isotretinoin treatment for acne and risk for depression: A systematic review and meta-analysis. *Journal of American Academy of Dermatology* 76(6), 1068–1076.
24. Adams H., Coven C., Grippe K. (2016). An overview of rosacea and its challenges. *Physician Assistant Clinics* 1(2), 255–264.
25. Two A., et al. (2015). Rosacea: Part II—Topical and systemic therapies in the treatment of rosacea. *Journal of American Academy of Dermatology* 72(5), 761–770.
26. Tan J., Berg M. (2013). Rosacea: Current state of epidemiology. *Journal of American Academy of Dermatology* 69(6), s27–s35.
27. Wladis E., Adam A. (2018). Treatment of ocular rosacea. *Survey of Ophthalmology*, 63(3), 340–346.
28. Viera A., Mannis M. (2013). Ocular rosacea: Common and commonly missed. *Journal of American Academy of Dermatology* 69(6), s36–s41.
29. Webster G., Schaller M. (2013). Ocular rosacea: A dermatologic perspective. *Journal of American Academy of Dermatology* 69(6), s42–s45.
30. Lee H., et al. (2016). Patch tests with commercial hair dye products in patients with allergic contact dermatitis to para-phenylenediamine. *Indian Journal of Dermatology, Venereology and Leprology* 82(6), 645–650.
31. Jone R., Horn H. (2014). Identifying the causes of contact dermatitis. *The Practitioner* 258(1772), 27–31.
32. Mowad C., et al. (2016). Allergic contact dermatitis: Patient diagnosis and evaluation. *Journal of American Academy of Dermatology* 74(6), 1029–1040.
33. Kostner L., et al. (2017). Allergic contact dermatitis. *Immunology and Allergy Clinics of North America* 37(1), 141–152.
34. Archer C. (2017). Atopic dermatitis. *Medicine* 45(6), 379–382.
35. Eichenfield L., et al. (2017). Current guidelines for the evaluation and management of atopic dermatitis: A comparison of the Joint Task Force Practice Parameter and American Academy of Dermatology guidelines. *Journal of Allergy and Clinical Immunology* 139(4), s49–s57.
36. Eichenfield L., et al. (2014). Guidelines of care for the management of atopic dermatitis: Section 2—Management and treatment of atopic dermatitis with topic therapies. *Journal of American Academy of Dermatology* 71(1), 116–132.
37. Garnacho-Saucedo G., Salido-Vallejo R., Moreno-Gimenez J. (2013). Atopic dermatitis: Update and proposed management algorithm. *Actas Dermo-Sifiliográficas* 104(1), 4–16.
38. Fuchs-Tarlovsky V., Marquez-Barba M., Srlran K. (2016). Probiotics in dermatologic practice. *Nutrition* 32(2016), 289–295.
39. Kolkhir P., et al. (2017). Autoimmune chronic spontaneous urticarial: What we know and what we do not know. *Journal of Allergy and Clinical Immunology* 139(6), 1772–1781.
40. Sanchez J., et al. (2017). Prevalence of inducible urticarial in patients with chronic spontaneous urticarial: Associated risk factors. *Journal of Allergy and Clinical Immunology: In Practice* 5(2), 464–470.
41. Curto-Barredo L., Silvestre J., Gimenez-Arnau A. (2014). Update on treatment of chronic urticarial. *Actas Dermo-Sifiliográficas* 105(5), 469–482.
42. Creamer D., et al. (2016). UK guidelines for the management of Steven-Johnson syndrome/toxic epidermal necrolysis in adults 2016. *Journal of Plastic Reconstructive and Aesthetic Surgery* 69(2016), e119–e153.
43. Higgins E. (2017). Psoriasis. *Medicine* 45(6), 368–378.
44. Pancar G., Eyupoglu O. (2016). Red cell distribution width and mean platelet volume in patients with pityriasis rosea. *Journal of Clinical Medicine Research* 8(6), 445–448.
45. Fruchter R., Melnick L., Pomeranz M. (2017). Lichenoid vulvar disease: A review. *International Journal of Women's Dermatology* 3(1), 58–64.
46. Korycinska J., Dzika E., Lepczynska M. (2015). Scabies: Clinical manifestations and diagnosis. *Polish Annals of Medicine* 22(1), 63–66.
47. American Burn Association. (2017). Burn statistics. Online. Available: http://www.ameriburn.org/resources_factsheet.php. Accessed August 10, 2017.
48. Tortora G., Derrickson B. (2017). *Principles of anatomy and physiology*. (15th ed.) Hoboken, NJ: John Wiley and Sons.
49. Rae L., Fidler P., Gibran N. (2016). The physiologic basis of burn shock and the need for aggressive fluid resuscitation. *Critical Care Clinics* 32(4), 491–505.
50. Agency for Healthcare Research and Quality. (2017). Preventing pressure ulcers in hospitals: A toolkit for improving quality of care. Online. Available: https://www.ahrq.gov/professionals/systems/hospital/qitoolkit/index.html. Accessed August 14, 2017.
51. Fletcher J., et al. (2012). With a national focus on prevention, how well do we treat pressure ulcers? *Wounds, UK* 13(2), 10–16.
52. Healthy People 2020. (2017). Pressure ulcers. Online. Available: https://www.healthypeople.gov/2020/topics-objectives/topic/older-adults/objectives. Accessed August 14, 2017.
53. Guillen-Sola M., et al. (2013). A multi-center, randomized, clinical trial comparing adhesive polyurethane foam dressing and adhesive hydrocolloid dressing in patients with grade II pressure ulcers in primary care and nursing homes. *BMC Family Practice* 14, 196–213.
54. Patricio da Silva E., et al. (2015). An extensive palate nevus combining intramucosal and blue nevi aspects. *Oral Surgery, Oral Medicine, Oral Pathology, and Oral Radiology* 120(2), e77.
55. Rosendahl C., Grant-Kels J., Que K. (2015). Dysplastic nevus: Fact and fiction. *Journal of American Academy of Dermatology* 73(3), 507–512.
56. American Cancer Society. (2017). Melanoma. Online. Available: https://www.cancer.org/cancer/melanoma-skin-cancer/about/key-statistics.html. Accessed August 15, 2017.
57. American Cancer Society. (2017). Basal and squamous cell carcinoma. Available: https://www.cancer.org/cancer/basal-and-squamous-cell-skin-cancer/about/key-statistics.html. Accessed August 15, 2017.
58. Greveling K., et al. (2016). Epidemiology of lentigo maligna and lentigo maligna melanoma in the Netherlands, 1989–2013. *Journal of Investigative Dermatology* 136(10), 1955–1960.
59. Carrasco P., et al. (2017). RF-acral melanoma and repetitive injury to the sole of the foot. *Actas Dermo-Sifiliográficas.* 108(7):669–670.
60. Ferris L., et al. (2017). Identification of high-risk cutaneous melanoma tumors is improved when combining the online American Joint Committee on cancer individualized melanoma patient outcome prediction tool with a 31-gene expression profile-based classification. *Journal of American Academy of Dermatology* 76(5), 818–825.
61. Tobin D. (2017). Introduction to skin aging. *Journal of Tissue Viability* 26(1), 37–46.
62. Leslie T. (2013). Itch. *Medicine* 41(7), 367–371.
63. Jensen S. (2015). *Nursing health assessment: A best practice approach* (2nd ed., p. 274). Philadelphia, PA: Wolters Kluwer.
64. Kyle T., Carman S. (2013). *Essentials of pediatric nursing* (2nd ed.). Philadelphia, PA: Wolters Kluwer.

Appendix Lab Values

TABLE A.1 PREFIXES DENOTING DECIMAL FACTORS

PREFIX	SYMBOL	FACTOR	PREFIX	SYMBOL	FACTOR
deka	da	10^{1}	deci	d	10^{-1}
hecto	h	10^{2}	centi	c	10^{-2}
kilo	k	10^{3}	milli	m	10^{-3}
mega	M	10^{6}	micro	μ	10^{-6}
giga	G	10^{9}	nano	n	10^{-9}
tera	T	10^{12}	pico	p	10^{-12}
peta	P	10^{15}	femto	f	10^{-15}
exa	E	10^{18}	atto	a	10^{-18}
zetta	Z	10^{21}	zepto	z	10^{-21}
yotta	Y	10^{24}	yocto	y	10^{-24}

TABLE A.2 HEMATOLOGY

TEST	CONVENTIONAL UNITS	SI UNITS
Erythrocyte count (RBC count)	Male: $4.2–5.4 \times 10^{6}/mm^{3}$	Male: $4.2–5.4 \times 10^{12}/L$
	Female: $3.6–5.0 \times 10^{6}/mm^{3}$	Female: $3.6–5.0 \times 10^{12}/L$
Hematocrit (Hct)	Male: 42%–52%	Male: 0.42–0.52
	Female: 36%–48%	Female: 0.36–0.48
Hemoglobin (Hb)	Male: 14.0–17.4 g/dL	Male: 140–174 g/L
	Female: 12.0–16.0 g/dL	Female: 120–160 g/L
Mean corpuscular hemoglobin (MCH)	26–34 pg/cell	0.40–0.53 fmol/cell
Mean corpuscular hemoglobin concentration (MCHC)	32–36 g/dL or 4.9–5.5 mmol/L	
Mean corpuscular volume (MCV)	82–98 mm^{3} or 82–98 fL/cell	
Reticulocyte count	0.5%–1.5% total RBC (women may be slightly higher)	
Platelet count	$140–400 \times 10^{3}/\mu L$	$140–400 \times 10^{9}/L$
Leukocyte count (WBC count)	$4.5–10.5 \times 10^{3}$ cells/mm^{3} or $4.5–10.5 \times 10^{9}/L$	4500–10,500 cells/mm^{3}
	Black adults: $3.2–10.0 \times 10^{3}$ or $\times 10^{9}$	3200–10,000 cells/mm^{3}
Basophils	15–50/mm^{3}	$0.02–0.05 \times 10^{9}/L$
	Differential: 0%–1.0% of total WBC	
Eosinophils	Differential: 0%–3% of total W B C	$0.07 \times 10^{9}/L$
Lymphocytes	24%–40% of total leukocytes count or 1500–4000 cells/mm^{3}	$1.5–4.0 \times 10^{9}/L$
Monocytes	100–500 mm^{3}	0.03–0.07 of total WBC count
	Differential: 3%–7% of total WBC	
Neutrophils (segmented [Segs])	3000–7000/mm^{3}	$3–7 \times 10^{9}/L$
Polymorphonuclear neutrophils (PMN)	Differential: 50% of total of WBC	Black adults: $1.2–6.6 \times 10^{9}/L$*
Neutrophils (bands)	0%–3% of total PMN	

*Ethnic difference occurs for neutrophils only.

TABLE A.3 BLOOD CHEMISTRY*

TEST	CONVENTIONAL UNITS	SI UNITS
Alanine aminotransferase (ALT)	Males: 10–40 U/L Females: 7–35 U/L	Males: 0.17–0.68 µkat/L Females: 0.12–0.60 µkat/L
Albumin	3.9–5.0 g/dL	39–50 g/L
Alkaline phosphatase	52–142 U/L[†,‡]	
Ammonia	15–60 µg/dL	11–35 µmol/L
Amylase	25–125 units/L[†]	0.4–2.1 µkat/L[†]
Arterial blood gas	pH 7.35–7.45 $PaCO_2$ 35–45 mm Hg PaO_2 > 80 mm Hg Base excess > 2 mEq/L Base deficit < −2 mEq/L HCO_3 22–26 mEq/L	
Aspartase aminotransferase (AST)	Males: 14–20 U/L Females: 10–36 U/L[†]	Males: 0.23–0.33 µkat/L[†] Females: 0.17–0.60 µkat/L[†]
Bilirubin (total)	0.3–1.0 mg/dL	5–17 µmol/L
Bilirubin (direct or conjugated)	0.0–0.2 mg/dL	0.0–3.4 µmol/L
Blood urea nitrogen (BUN)	6–20 mg/dL	2.1–7.1 mmol/L
Calcium (Ca^{2+}) (total)	8.8–10.4 mg/dL	2.20–2.60 mmol/L
Chloride	96–106 mEq/L	96–106 mmol/L
Creatine kinase (CK, CPK)	Males: 38–174 units/L[†] Females: 26–140 U/L	Males: 0.63–2.90 µkat/L[†] Females: 0.46–2.38
Creatine kinase isoenzymes:		
MB (CK_2)	0%–6%	0.00–0.06
MM (CK_3)	96% or 100%	0.96–1.0
BB (CK_1)	0%	0.00
Creatinine (serum)	Males: 0.6–1.2 Females: 0.4–1.0 mg/dL[‡]	Males: 71–106 µmol/L Females: 39–90 µmol/L[‡]
Gamma-glutamyl-transpeptidase (GGT)	Males: 7–47 U/L Females: 5–25 U/L	Males: 0.12–1.80 µkat/L[†] Females: 0.08–0.42 µkat/L
Glucose (plasma, fasting)	<100 mg/dL	<5.6 mmol/L
Glycosylated hemoglobin (HbA_{1c})	5.0%–7.0%	5.5–9.3 mmol/L
Lactate dehydrogenase (LDH)	140–280 U/L	2.34–4.68 µkat/L[†]
Lipids		
Cholesterol (fasting)	140–199 mg/dL (desirable) 200–239 mg/dL (borderline high) ≥240 mg/dL (high)	3.63–5.15 mmol/L (optimal) 5.18–6.19 mmol/L (borderline) >6.20 mmol/L (high)
LDL cholesterol	<100 mg/dL (optimal) 100–129 mg/dL (near optimal) 130–159 mg/dL (borderline high) 160–189 mg/dL (high) >190 mg/dL	<2.6 mmol/L 2.6–3.3 mmol/L 3.4–4.1 mmol/L 4.2–4.9 mmol/L >5.0 mmol/L
HDL cholesterol	Male: 35–65 mg/dL Female: 35–80 mg/dL	Male: 0. 91–1.68 mmol/L Female: 0.91–2.07 mmol/L
Triglycerides	<150 mg/dL (desirable) 150–199 mg/dL (borderline high) 200–499 mg/dL ≥500 mg/d:	<1.70 mmol/L (desirable) 1.70–2.25 mmol/L 2.26–5.64 mmol/L ≥5.65 mmol/L
Lipase	10–140 U/L[†]	0.17–2.3 µkat/L[†]
Magnesium	1.8–2.6 mg/dL	0.74–1.07 mmol/L
Osmolality (24-hour urine specimen)	300–900 mOsm/kg H_2O	
Osmolality (serum)	280–303 mOsm/kg H_2O	
Phosphorus (inorganic)	2.7–4.5 mg/dL	0.87–1.45 mmol/L
Potassium	3.5–5.2 mEq/L	3.5–5.2 mmol/L
Prostate-specific antigen (PSA)	<2.5 ng/mL	<2.5 µg/L
Protein total	6.0–8.0 g/dL	60–80 g/L

TABLE A.3 BLOOD CHEMISTRY *(Continued)*

TEST	CONVENTIONAL UNITS	SI UNITS
Immunoglobulin		
IgG	700–1500 mg/dL	7.0–15.0 g/L
IgA	60–400 mg/dL	600–4000 mg/dL
IgM	60–300 mg/d:	600–3000 mg/dL
IgE	3–423 IU/mL	3–423 kIU/L
Thyroid tests		
Thyroxine (T_4) total	5.4–11.5 μg/dL	57–148 nmol/L
Thyroxine, free (FT_4)	0.7–2.0 ng/dL	10–26 pmol/L†
Triiodothyronine (T_3) total	80–200 ng/dL	1.2–3.1 nmol/L
Thyroid stimulating hormone (TSH)	0.45–4.5 μU/mL	0.45–4.5 mU/L
Thyroglobin	2–55 ng/mL	2–55 μg/L
Sodium	136–145 mEq/L	136–145 mmol/L
Uric acid	Male: 3.4–7.0 mg/dL Female: 2.4–6.0 mg/dL	Male: 202–416 μmol/L Female: 143–357 μmol/L

*Values provided are for adults unless otherwise specified. Values may vary with laboratory. The values supplied by the laboratory performing the test should always be used since the ranges may be method specific.

†Laboratory and/or method specific.

‡Varies with pregnancy, puberty, age, and muscle mass.

Values obtained from Fischbach F. T., Fischbach, M. A. (2018). *Fischbach's manual of laboratory and diagnostic tests* (10th ed.). Philadelphia, PA: Lippincott Williams & Wilkins.

Glossary

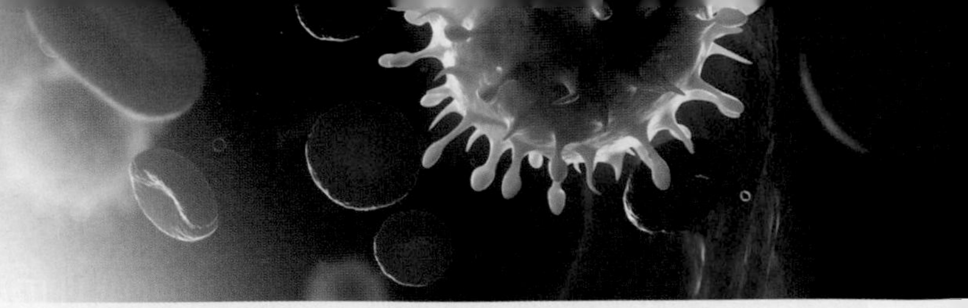

Abduction The act of abducting (moving or spreading away from a position near the midline of the body or the axial line of a limb) or the state of being abducted.

Abrasion The wearing or scraping away of a substance or structure, such as the skin, through an unusual or abnormal mechanical process.

Abscess A collection of pus that is restricted to a specific area in tissues, organs, or confined spaces.

Accommodation The adjustment of the lens (eye) to variations in distance.

Acromion The lateral extension of the spine of the scapula, forming the highest point of the shoulder. (Adjective: acromial)

Active transport The movement of molecules from an area of lower concentration to higher concentration (opposite of diffusion).

Acuity The clearness or sharpness of perception, especially of vision.

Adaptation The adjustment of an organism to its environment, physical or psychological, through changes and responses to stress of any kind.

Adduction The act of adducting (moving or drawing toward a position near the midline of the body or the axial line of a limb) or the state of being adducted.

Adenylyl cyclase An enzyme that converts AMP from ATP.

Adhesin The molecular components of the bacterial cell wall that are involved in adhesion processes.

Adrenergic Activated by or characteristic of the sympathetic nervous system or its neurotransmitters (*i.e.*, epinephrine and norepinephrine).

Aerobic Growing, living, or occurring only in the presence of air or oxygen.

Afferent Bearing or conducting inward or toward a center, as an afferent neuron.

Agglutination The clumping together of particles, microorganisms, or blood cells in response to an antigen–antibody reaction.

Agonist A muscle whose action is opposed by another muscle (antagonist) with which it is paired, or a drug or other chemical substance that has affinity for or stimulates a predictable physiologic function.

Akinesia An abnormal state in which there is an absence or poverty of movement.

Allele One of two or more different forms of a gene that can occupy a particular locus on a chromosome.

Alveolus A small saclike structure, as in the alveolus of the lung.

Amblyopia A condition of vision impairment without a detectable organic lesion of the eye.

Amine An organic compound containing nitrogen.

Amorphous Without a definite form; shapeless.

Amphoteric Capable of reacting chemically as an acid or a base.

Ampulla A saclike dilatation of a duct, canal, or any other tubular structure.

Anabolism A constructive metabolic process characterized by the conversion of simple substances into larger, complex molecules.

Anaerobic Growing, living, or occurring only in the absence of air or oxygen.

Analog A part, organ, or chemical having the same function or appearance but differing in respect to a certain component, such as origin or development.

Anaplasia A change in the structure of cells and in their orientation to each other that is characterized by a loss of cell differentiation, as in cancerous cell growth.

Anastomose The joining of normally separate parts, which occurs during embryonic development.

Anastomosis The connection or joining between two vessels; or an opening created by surgical, traumatic, or pathologic means.

Androgen Any substance, such as a male sex hormone, that increases male characteristics.

Anergy A state of absent or diminished reaction to an antigen or group of antigens.

Aneuploidy A variation in the number of chromosomes within a cell involving one or more missing chromosomes rather than entire sets.

Aneurysm An outpouching or dilation in the wall of a blood vessel or the heart.

Ankylosis Stiffness or fixation of separate bones of a joint, resulting from disease, injury, or surgical procedure. (Verb: ankylose)

Anorexia Lack or loss of appetite for food. (Adjective: anorexic)

Anoxia An abnormal condition characterized by the total lack of oxygen.

Antagonist A muscle whose action directly opposes that of another muscle (agonist) with which it is paired, or a drug or other chemical substance that can diminish or nullify the action of a neuromediator or body function.

Anterior Pertaining to a surface or part that is situated near or toward the front.

Antigen A substance that generates an immune response by causing the formation of an antibody or reacting with antibodies or T-cell receptors.

Antiport Movement of two different molecules across a membrane by a common carrier.

Apex The uppermost point, the narrowed or pointed end, or the highest point of a structure, such as an organ.
Aphagia A condition characterized by the refusal or the loss of ability to swallow.
Aplasia The absence of an organ or tissue due to a developmental failure.
Apnea The absence of spontaneous respiration.
Apoptosis A mechanism of programmed cell death, marked by shrinkage of the cell, condensation of chromatin, formation of cytoplasmic blebs, and fragmentation of the cell into membrane-bound bodies eliminated by phagocytosis.
Apraxia Loss of the ability to carry out familiar, purposeful acts or to manipulate objects in the absence of paralysis or other motor or sensory impairment.
Aquaporins A water channel that forms pores in membranes of cells allowing water to pass.
Articulation The place of connection or junction between two or more bones of a skeletal joint.
Ascites An abnormal accumulation of serous fluid in the peritoneal cavity.
Asepsis The condition of being free or freed from pathogenic microorganisms.
Astereognosis A neurologic disorder characterized by an inability to identify objects by touch.
Asterixis A motor disturbance characterized by a hand-flapping tremor, which results when the prolonged contraction of groups of muscles lapses intermittently.
Ataxia An abnormal condition characterized by an inability to coordinate voluntary muscular movement.
Athetosis A neuromuscular condition characterized by the continuous occurrence of slow, sinuous, writhing movements that are performed involuntarily. (Adjective: athetoid)
Atopy Genetic predisposition toward the development of a hypersensitivity or an allergic reaction to common environmental allergens.
Atresia The absence or closure of a normal body orifice or tubular organ, such as the esophagus.
Atrophy A wasting or diminution of size, often accompanied by a decrease in function, of a cell, tissue, or organ.
Autocrine A mode of hormone action in which a chemical messenger acts on the same cell that secretes it.
Autophagy Segregation of part of the cell's own damaged cytoplasmic material within a vacuole and its disposal.
Autosome Any chromosome other than a sex chromosome.
Avascular The lack of blood vessels.
Axillary Of or pertaining to the axilla, or armpit.
Bacteremia The presence of bacteria in the blood.
Bactericide An agent that destroys bacteria. (Adjective: bactericidal)
Bacteriostat An agent that inhibits bacterial growth. (Adjective: bacteriostatic)
Ballismus An abnormal condition characterized by violent flailing motions of the arms and, occasionally, the head, resulting from injury to or destruction of the subthalamic nucleus or its fiber connections.
Baroreceptor A type of sensory nerve ending such as those found in the aorta and the carotid sinus that is stimulated by changes in pressure.
Basal Pertaining to, situated at, or forming the base, or the fundamental or the basic.
Basal lamina The basement membrane.
Basement membrane Keeps the epithelium in place and separates the epithelial cells from the underlying tissue.
Benign Not malignant or of the character that does not threaten health or life.
Bipolar neuron A nerve cell that has a process at each end—an afferent process and an efferent process.
Bolus A rounded mass of food ready to swallow or such a mass passing through the gastrointestinal tract, or a concentrated mass of medicinal material or other pharmaceutical preparation injected all at once intravenously for diagnostic purposes.
Borborygmus The rumbling, gurgling, or tinkling noise produced by the propulsion of gas through the intestine.
Bronchiectasis Damage to the bronchial tubes due to inflammation.
Bruit A sound or murmur heard while auscultating an organ or blood vessel, especially an abnormal one.
Buccal Pertaining to or directed toward the inside of the cheek.
Buffer A substance or group of substances that prevents change in the concentration of another chemical substance.
Bulla A thin-walled blister of the skin or mucous membranes greater than 5 mm in diameter containing serous or seropurulent fluid.
Bursa A fluid-filled sac or saclike cavity situated in places in the tissues at which friction would otherwise develop, such as between certain tendons and the bones beneath them.
Cachexia A condition of general ill health and malnutrition, marked by weakness and emaciation.
Calculus A stony mass formed within body tissues, usually composed of mineral salts.
Capsid The protein shell that envelops and protects the nucleic acid of a virus.
Carcinogen Any substance or agent that causes the development or increases the incidence of cancer.
Carpal Of or pertaining to the carpus, or wrist.
Caseation A form of tissue necrosis in which the tissue is changed into a dry, amorphous mass resembling crumbly cheese.
Caspase pathway Involved in apoptosis or programmed cell death.
Catabolism A metabolic process through which living organisms break down complex substances to simple compounds, liberating energy for use in work, energy storage, or heat production.
Catalyst A substance that increases the velocity of a chemical reaction without being consumed by the process.

Catecholamines Any one of a group of biogenic amines having a sympathomimetic action and composed of a catechol molecule and the aliphatic portion of an amine.

Caudal Signifying an inferior position, toward the distal end of the spine.

Cell The smallest basic unit of any living organism surrounded by a membrane, which contains a nucleus and cytoplasm.

Cell cycle The stages that cells undergo to divide and produce new cells.

Cell differentiation The process by which cells become specialized.

Cellular respiration Metabolic reactions that take place in cells to generate energy by converting biochemical energy into adenosine triphosphate (ATP).

Cellulitis An acute, diffuse, spreading, edematous inflammation of the deep subcutaneous tissues and sometimes muscle, characterized most commonly by an area of heat, redness, pain, and swelling, and occasionally by fever, malaise, chills, and headache.

Cephalic Of or pertaining to the head, or to the head end of the body.

Cerumen The waxlike secretion produced by vestigial apocrine sweat glands in the external ear canal.

Channelopathies Diseases due to a malfunction of an ion channel.

Cheilosis A noninflammatory disorder of the lips and mouth characterized by chapping and fissuring.

Chelate A chemical compound composed of a central metal ion and an organic molecule with multiple bonds, arranged in ring formation, used especially in treatment of metal poisoning.

Chemoreceptor A sensory nerve cell activated by chemical stimuli, as a chemoreceptor in the carotid artery that is sensitive to changes in the oxygen content in the blood and reflexly increases or decreases respiration and blood pressure.

Chemotaxis A response involving cell orientation or cell movement that is either toward (positive chemotaxis) or away from (negative chemotaxis) a chemical stimulus.

Chimeric Relating to, derived from, or being an individual possessing one's own immunologic characteristics and that of another individual; a phenomenon that can occur as the result of procedures such as a bone marrow graft.

Chondrocyte Any one of the mature polymorphic cells that form the cartilage of the body.

Chromatid One of the paired threadlike chromosome filaments, joined at the centromere, that makes up a metaphase chromosome.

Chromosome Any one of the structures in the nucleus of a cell containing a linear thread of DNA, which functions in the transmission of genetic information.

Chyme The creamy, viscous, semifluid material produced during digestion of a meal that is expelled by the stomach into the duodenum.

Cilia A minute, hairlike process projecting from a cell, composed of nine microtubules arrayed around a single pair. Cilia beat rhythmically to move the cell around in its environment, or they move mucus or fluids over the surface.

Circadian Being, having, pertaining to, or occurring in a period or cycle of approximately 24 hours.

Circumduction The active or passive circular movement of a limb or of the eye.

Cisterna An enclosed space, such as a cavity, that serves as a reservoir for lymph or other body fluids.

Clone One or a group of genetically identical cells or organisms derived from a single parent.

Coagulation The process of transforming a liquid into a semisolid mass, especially of blood clot formation.

Coarctation A condition of stricture or contraction of the walls of a vessel.

Cofactor A substance that must unite with another substance in order to function.

Colic Sharp, intermittent abdominal pain localized in a hollow or tubular organ, resulting from torsion, obstruction, or smooth muscle spasm. (Adjective: colicky)

Collagen The protein substance of the white, glistening, inelastic fibers of the skin, tendons, bone, cartilage, and all other connective tissue.

Collateral Secondary or accessory rather than direct or immediate, or a small branch, as of a blood vessel or nerve.

Columnar cells Tall thin epithelial cells.

Complement Any one of the complex, enzymatic serum proteins that are involved in physiologic reactions, including antigen–antibody reaction and anaphylaxis.

Confluent Flowing or coming together, not discrete.

Congenital Present at, and usually before, birth.

Conjugate To pair and fuse in conjugation, or a form of sexual reproduction seen in unicellular organisms in which genetic material is exchanged during the temporary fusion of two cells.

Contiguous In contact or nearly so in an unbroken sequence along a boundary or at a point.

Contralateral Affecting, pertaining to, or originating in the opposite side of a point or reference.

Cotransport The process by which two substances are transported across a membrane at the same time.

Contusion An injury of a part without a break in the skin, characterized by swelling, discoloration, and pain.

Convolution An elevation or tortuous winding, such as one of the irregular ridges on the surface of the brain, formed by a structure being infolded upon itself.

Corpuscle Any small mass, cell, or body, such as a red or white blood cell.

Costal Pertaining to a rib or ribs.

Countertransport The process by which a substance moves across a membrane in opposite directions.

Crepitus A sound or sensation that resembles a crackling or grating noise.

Cristae The infolding of the inner membrane of the mitochondria.

Cuboidal cells The closely packed cells of the epidermis.

Cutaneous Pertaining to the skin.

Cyanosis A bluish discoloration, especially of the skin and mucous membranes, caused by an excess of deoxygenated hemoglobin in the blood.

Cystic fibrosis An inherited disease causing thick mucus to develop in the lung and other organs.

Cytochromes Hemoproteins which transports electrons.

Cytokine Any of a class of polypeptide immunoregulatory substances that are secreted by cells, usually of the immune system, that affect other cells.

Cytology The study of cells, including their origin, structure, function, and pathology.

Cytoplasm The fluid contained within the cell membrane.

Cytosol Cytoplasm exclusive of membranous components (*e.g.*, mitochondria, endoplasmic reticulum) and nonmembranous insoluble components.

Decibel A unit for expressing the relative power intensity of electric or acoustic signal power that is equal to one tenth of a bel.

Defecation The evacuation of feces from the digestive tract through the rectum.

Deformation The process of adapting in form or shape; also the product of such alteration.

Degeneration The deterioration of a normal cell, tissue, or organ to a less functionally active form. (Adjective: degenerative)

Deglutition The act or process of swallowing.

Degradation The reduction of a chemical compound to a compound less complex, usually by splitting off one or more groups.

Dehydration The condition that results from excessive loss of water from the body tissues.

Delirium An acute, reversible organic mental syndrome characterized by confusion, disorientation, restlessness, incoherence, fear, and often illusions.

Dendrite One of the branching processes that extends and transmits impulses toward a cell body of a neuron. (Adjective: dendritic)

Depolarization The reduction of a cell membrane potential to a less negative value than that of the potential outside the cell.

Dermatome The area of the skin supplied with afferent nerve fibers of a single dorsal root of a spinal nerve.

Desmosome A small, circular, dense area within the intercellular bridge that forms the site of adhesion between intermediate filaments and cell membranes.

Desquamation A normal process in which the cornified layer of the epidermis is shed in fine scales or sheets.

Dialysis The process of separating colloids and crystalline substances in solution, which involves the two distinct physical processes of diffusion and ultrafiltration, or a medical procedure for the removal of urea and other elements from the blood or lymph.

Diapedesis The outward passage of red or white blood corpuscles through the intact walls of the vessels.

Diaphoresis Perspiration, especially the profuse perspiration associated with an elevated body temperature, physical exertion, exposure to heat, and mental or emotional stress.

Diarthrosis A specialized articulation that permits, to some extent, free joint movement. (Adjective: diarthrodial)

Diastole The dilatation of the heart, or the period of dilatation, which is the interval between the second and the first heart sound and is the time during which blood enters the relaxed chambers of the heart from the systemic circulation and the lungs.

Differentiation The act or process in development in which unspecialized cells or tissues acquire more specialized characteristics, including those of physical form, physiologic function, and chemical properties.

Diffusion The process of becoming widely spread, as in the spontaneous movement of molecules or other particles in solution from an area of higher concentration to an area of lower concentration, resulting in an even distribution of the particles in the fluid.

Dimer A compound or unit formed by the combination of two identical molecules or radicals of a simpler compound. (Adjective: dimeric)

Diopter A unit of measurement of the refractive power of lenses equal to the reciprocal of the focal length in meters.

Diploid Pertaining to an individual, organism, strain, or cell that has two full sets of homologous chromosomes.

Disseminate To scatter or distribute over a considerable area.

Distal Away from or being the farthest from a point of reference.

Diurnal Of, relating to, or occurring in the daytime.

Diverticulum A pouch or sac of variable size occurring naturally or through herniation of the muscular wall of a tubular organ.

Dorsum The back or posterior. (Adjective: dorsal)

Down-regulation Depressing the response to a stimuli due to a fewer numbers of receptors.

Dysgenesis Defective or abnormal development of an organ or part, typically occurring during embryonic development. (Also called dysgenesia.)

Dyslexia A disturbance in the ability to read, spell, and write words.

Dyspepsia The impairment of the power or function of digestion, especially epigastric discomfort following eating.

Dysphagia A difficulty in swallowing.

Dysphonia Any impairment of the voice that is experienced as a difficulty in speaking.

Dysplasia The alteration in size, shape, and organization of adult cell types.

Eburnation The conversion of bone or cartilage, through thinning or loss, into a hard and dense mass with a worn, polished, ivory-like surface.

Ecchymosis A small hemorrhagic spot, larger than a petechia, in the skin or mucous membrane caused by the extravasation of blood into the subcutaneous tissues.

Ectoderm The outermost of the three primary germ layers of the embryo, and from which the epidermis and epidermal tissues, such as nails, hair, and glands of the skin, develop.

Ectopic Relating to or characterized by an object or organ being situated in an unusual place, away from its normal location.

Edema The presence of an abnormal accumulation of fluid in interstitial spaces of tissues. (Adjective: edematous)

Efferent Conveyed or directed away from a center.

Effusion The escape of fluid from blood vessels into a part or tissue, as an exudation or a transudation.

Elastin A protein that has the ability to coil and uncoil giving many structures such as the skin elasticity.

Embolus A mass of clotted blood or other formed elements, such as bubbles of air, calcium fragments, or a bit of tissue or tumor, that circulates in the bloodstream until it becomes lodged in a vessel, obstructing the circulation. (Plural: emboli)

Empyema An accumulation of pus in a cavity of the body, especially the pleural space.

Emulsify To disperse one liquid throughout the body of another liquid, making a colloidal suspension, or emulsion.

Endocrine glands Release substances into the blood or tissues of the body.

Endocytosis The uptake or incorporation of substances into a cell by invagination of its plasma membrane, as in the processes of phagocytosis and pinocytosis.

Endoderm The innermost of the three primary germ layers of the embryo, and from which epithelium arises.

Endogenous Growing within the body, or developing or originating from within the body or produced from internal causes.

Endoscopy The visualization of any cavity of the body with an endoscope.

Endothelium The inner most layer of cells in blood and lymphatic vessels.

Enteropathic Relating to any disease of the intestinal tract.

Enzyme A protein molecule produced by living cells that catalyzes chemical reactions of other organic substances without itself being destroyed or altered.

Epiphysis The expanded articular end of a long bone (head) that is separated from the shaft of the bone by the epiphyseal plate until the bone stops growing, the plate is obliterated, and the shaft and the head become united.

Epithelium The covering of the internal and the external surfaces of the body, including the lining of vessels and other small cavities.

Epitope The simplest form of an antigenic determinant that combines with an antibody or a T-cell receptor to cause a specific reaction by an immunoglobulin.

Erectile Capable of being erected or raised to an erect position.

Erythema The redness or inflammation of the skin or mucous membranes produced by the congestion of superficial capillaries. (Adjective: erythematous)

Etiology The study or theory of all factors that may be involved in the development of a disease, including susceptibility of an individual, the nature of the disease agent, and the way in which an individual's body is invaded by the agent, or the cause of a disease.

Eukaryotic Pertaining to an organism with cells having a true nucleus; that is, a highly complex, organized nucleus surrounded by a nuclear membrane containing organelles and exhibiting mitosis.

Euploid Pertaining to an individual, organism, strain, or cell with a balanced set or sets of chromosomes, in any number, that is an exact multiple of the normal, basic haploid number characteristic of the species; or such an individual, organism, strain, or cell.

Evisceration The removal of the viscera from the abdominal cavity or disembowelment, or the extrusion of an internal organ through a wound or surgical incision.

Exacerbation An increase in the severity of a disease as marked by greater intensity in any of its signs and symptoms.

Exfoliation Peeling and sloughing off of tissue cells in scales or layers. (Adjective: exfoliative)

Exocrine glands Release substances such as digestive enzymes to the outside of the body or another surface in the body.

Exocytosis The discharge of cell particles, which are packaged in membrane-bound vesicles, by fusion of the vesicular membrane with the plasma membrane and subsequent release of the particles to the exterior of the cell.

Exogenous Developed or originating outside the body, as a disease caused by a bacterial or viral agent foreign to the body.

Exophthalmos A marked or abnormal protrusion of the eyeball.

Extension A movement that allows the two elements of any jointed part to be drawn apart, increasing the angle between them, as extending the leg increases the angle between the femur and the tibia.

Extrapyramidal Pertaining to motor systems supplied by fibers outside the corticospinal or pyramidal tracts.

Extravasation A discharge or escape, usually of blood, serum, or lymph, from a vessel into the tissues.

Extubation The process of withdrawing a previously inserted tube from an orifice or cavity of the body.

Exudate Fluid, cells, or other substances that have been slowly exuded or have escaped from blood vessels and have been deposited in tissues or on tissue surfaces.

Fascia A sheet or band of fibrous connective tissue that may be separated from other specifically organized structures, as the tendons, the aponeuroses, and the ligaments.

Febrile Pertaining to or characterized by an elevated body temperature, or fever.

Fibrillation A small, local, involuntary contraction of muscle, resulting from spontaneous activation of a single muscle fiber or of an isolated bundle of nerve fibers.

Fibrin A stringy, insoluble protein formed by the action of thrombin on fibrinogen during the clotting process.

Fibrosis The formation of fibrous connective tissue, as in the repair or replacement of parenchymatous elements.

Filtration The process of passing a liquid through or as if through a filter, which is accomplished by gravity, pressure, or vacuum.

Fimbria Any structure that forms a fringe, border, or edge or the processes that resemble such a structure.

Fissure A cleft or a groove, normal or otherwise, on the surface of an organ or a bony structure.

First messengers Extracellular factors that can cause a response within a cell.

Fistula An abnormal passage or communication from an internal organ to the body surface or between two internal organs.

Flaccid Weak, soft, and lax; lacking normal muscle tone.

Flagella and cilia Thin threadlike structures that allow cells to move.

Flatus Air or gas in the intestinal tract that is expelled through the anus. (Adjective: flatulent)

Flexion A movement that allows the two elements of any jointed part to be brought together, decreasing the angle between them, as bending the elbow.

Flora The microorganisms, such as bacteria and fungi, both normally occurring and pathologic, found in or on an organ.

Focal Relating to, having, or occupying a focus.

Follicle A sac or pouchlike depression or cavity.

Fontanelle A membrane-covered opening in bones or between bones, such as the soft spot covered by tough membranes between the bones of an infant's incompletely ossified skull.

Foramen A natural opening or aperture in a membranous structure or bone.

Fossa A hollow or depressed area, especially on the surface of the end of a bone.

Fovea A small pit or depression in the surface of a structure or an organ.

Fundus The base or bottom of an organ or the portion farthest from the mouth of an organ.

G-proteins Bind guanine nucleotides and interact with cell surface receptors to transmit stimuli to inside the cell.

Ganglion One of the nerve cell bodies, chiefly collected in groups outside the central nervous system. (Plural: ganglia)

Genotype The entire genetic constitution of an individual, as determined by the particular combination and location of the genes on the chromosomes, or the alleles present at one or more sites on homologous chromosomes.

Glia The neuroglia, or supporting structure of nervous tissue.

Globulin One of a broad group of proteins classified by solubility, electrophoretic mobility, and size.

Gluconeogenesis The formation of glucose from any of the substances of glycolysis other than carbohydrates.

Glycolysis A series of enzymatically catalyzed reactions, occurring within cells, by which glucose is converted to adenosine triphosphate (ATP) and pyruvic acid during aerobic metabolism.

Glycosaminoglycans Polysaccharides that contain amino acids and attract water serving as a lubricant.

Goblet cells They have the primary role of mucus secretion.

Gonad A gamete-producing gland, as an ovary or a testis.

Gradient The rate of increase or decrease of a measurable phenomenon expressed as a function of a second, or the visual representation of such a change.

Granuloma A small mass of nodular granulation tissue resulting from chronic inflammation, injury, or infection. (Adjective: granulomatous)

GTPase cycle Occurs when hydrolase enzymes break down guanosine triphosphate.

Hapten A small, nonproteinaceous substance that is not antigenic by itself but that can act as an antigen when combined with a larger molecule.

Haustrum A structure resembling a recess or sacculation. (Plural: haustra)

Hematoma A localized collection of extravasated blood trapped in an organ, space, or tissue, resulting from a break in the wall of a blood vessel.

Hematopoiesis The normal formation and development of blood cells.

Hemianopia Defective vision or blindness in half of the visual field of one or both eyes.

Heterogeneous Consisting of or composed of dissimilar elements or parts, or not having a uniform quality throughout. (Noun: heterogeneity)

Heterophagy The taking into the cell of an exogenous substance by phagocytosis or pinocytosis and the subsequent digestion of the newly formed vacuole by a lysosome.

Heterozygous Having two different alleles at corresponding loci on homologous chromosomes.

Histology The branch of anatomy that deals with the minute (microscopic) structure, composition, and function of cells and tissue. (Adjective: histologic)

Homolog Any organ or part corresponding in function, position, origin, and structure to another organ or part, as the flippers of a seal that correspond to human hands. (Adjective: homologous)

Homozygous Having two identical alleles at corresponding loci on homologous chromosomes.

Humoral Relating to elements dissolved in the blood or body fluids.

Hybridoma A tumor of hybrid cells produced by fusion of normal lymphocytes and tumor cells.

Hydrolysis The chemical alteration or decomposition of a compound into fragments by the addition of water.

Hypercapnia Excess amount of carbon dioxide in the blood.

Hyperemia An excess or engorgement of blood in a part of the body.

Hyperesthesia An unusual or pathologic increase in sensitivity of a part, especially the skin, or of a particular sense.

Hyperglycemia High blood sugar or excess of glucose in the blood.

Hyperplasia An abnormal multiplication or increase in the number of normal cells of a body part.

Hypertonic A solution having a greater concentration of solute than another solution with which it is compared, hence exerting more osmotic pressure than that solution.

Hypertrophy The enlargement or overgrowth of an organ that is due to an increase in the size of its cells rather than the number of its cells.

Hypesthesia An abnormal decrease of sensation in response to stimulation of the sensory nerves. (Also called hypoesthesia.)

Hypocapnia A deficiency of carbon dioxide in the blood.

Hypotonic A solution having a lesser concentration of solute than another solution with which it is compared, hence exerting less osmotic pressure than that solution.

Hypoxia An inadequate supply of oxygen to tissue that is below physiologic levels despite adequate perfusion of the tissue by blood.

Iatrogenic Induced inadvertently through the activity of a physician or by medical treatment or diagnostic procedures.

Idiopathic Arising spontaneously or from an unknown cause.

Idiosyncrasy A physical or behavioral characteristic or manner that is unique to an individual or to a group. (Adjective: idiosyncratic)

Immotile cilia syndrome Also known as Kartagener syndrome is a rare autosomal recessive genetic disorder that results in the inability of the cilia of the respiratory track to move.

Incidence The rate at which a certain event occurs (*e.g.*, the number of new cases of a specific disease during a particular period of time in a population at risk).

Inclusion The act of enclosing or the condition of being enclosed, or anything that is enclosed.

Indigenous Native, or natural, to the particular country or region where found.

Infarction Necrosis or death of tissues due to local ischemia resulting from obstruction of blood flow.

Inotropic Influencing the force or energy of muscular contractions.

In situ In the natural or normal place, or something, such as cancer, that is confined to its place of origin and has not invaded neighboring tissues.

Interferon Any one of a group of small glycoproteins (cytokines) produced in response to viral infection and which inhibit viral replication.

Integral proteins Proteins that are permanently attached to the cell membrane.

Interleukin Any of several multifunctional cytokines produced by a variety of lymphoid and nonlymphoid cells, including immune cells, that stimulate or otherwise affect the function of lymphopoietic and other cells and systems in the body.

Interstitial Relating to or situated between parts or in the interspaces of a tissue.

Intermembrane space The space between the inner and outer membrane of a mitochondrion.

Intramural Situated or occurring within the wall of an organ.

Intrinsic Pertaining exclusively to a part or situated entirely within an organ or tissue.

In vitro A biologic reaction occurring in an artificial environment, such as a test tube.

In vivo A biologic reaction occurring within the living body.

Involuntary muscle An automatic response to a stimulus.

Involution The act or instance of enfolding, entangling, or turning inward.

Ionize To separate or change into ions.

Ipsilateral Situated on, pertaining to, or affecting the same side of the body.

Ischemia Decreased blood supply to a body organ or part, usually due to functional constriction or actual obstruction of a blood vessel.

Juxta-articular Situated near a joint or in the region of a joint.

Juxtaglomerular Near to or adjoining a glomerulus of the kidney.

Karyoplasm (nucleoplasm) Also known as nucleoplasm is enveloped by the nuclear membrane and includes chromosomes and the nucleus.

Karyotype The total chromosomal characteristics of a cell, or the micrograph of chromosomes arranged in pairs in descending order of size.

Keratin A fibrous, sulfur-containing protein that is the primary component of the epidermis, hair, and horny tissues. (Adjective: keratinous)

Keratinocytes The most common cell in the epidermis and produces keratin.

Keratosis Any skin condition in which there is overgrowth and thickening of the cornified epithelium.

Ketosis A condition characterized by the abnormal accumulation of ketones (organic compounds with a carboxyl group attached to two carbon atoms) in the body tissues and fluid.

Kinesthesia The sense of movement, weight, tension, and position of body parts mediated by input from joint and muscle receptors and hair cells. (Adjective: kinesthetic)

Krebs cycle The process by which living cells release energy through aerobic respiration.

Kyphosis An abnormal condition of the vertebral column, characterized by increased convexity in the curvature of the thoracic spine as viewed from the side.

Lacuna A small pit or cavity within a structure, especially bony tissue, or a defect or gap, as in the field of vision.

Lateral A position farther from the median plane or midline of the body or a structure, or situated on, coming from, or directed toward the side.

Lesion Any wound, injury, or pathologic change in body tissue.

Lethargy The lowered level of consciousness characterized by listlessness, drowsiness, and apathy, or a state of indifference.

Ligament One of many predominantly white, shiny, flexible bands of fibrous tissue that binds joints together and connects bones or cartilages.

Ligand A group, ion, or molecule that binds to the central atom or molecule in a chemical complex.

Lipid Any of the group of fats and fatlike substances characterized by being insoluble in water and soluble in nonpolar organic solvents, such as chloroform and ether.

Lipoprotein Any one of the conjugated proteins that is a complex of protein and lipid.

Lobule A small lobe.

Lordosis The anterior concavity in the curvature of the lumbar and cervical spine as observed from the side.

Lumen A cavity or the channel within a tube or tubular organ of the body.

Luteal Of or pertaining to or having the properties of the corpus luteum.

Lysis Destruction or dissolution of a cell or molecule through the action of a specific agent.

Lysosomal storage disorders Inherited metabolic diseases due to lysomal dysfunction allowing sugars, fats, and toxic materials to accumulate.

Maceration Softening of tissue by soaking, especially in acidic solutions.

Macroscopic Large enough to be visible with the unaided eye or without the microscope.

Macula A small, flat blemish, thickening, or discoloration that is flush with the skin surface. (Adjective: macular)

Malaise A vague feeling of bodily fatigue and discomfort.

Manometry The measurement of tension or pressure of a liquid or gas using a device called a manometer.

Marasmus A condition of extreme protein-calorie malnutrition that is characterized by growth retardation and progressive wasting of subcutaneous tissue and muscle and occurs chiefly during the first year of life.

Matrix The intracellular substance of a tissue or the basic substance from which a specific organ or kind of tissue develops.

Matrix space The material in which specialized structures are implanted.

Meatus An opening or passage through any body part.

Medial Pertaining to the middle, or situated or oriented toward the midline of the body.

Mediastinum The mass of tissues and organs in the middle of the thorax, separating the pleural sacs containing the two lungs.

Meiosis The division of a sex cell as it matures, so that each daughter nucleus receives one half of the number of chromosomes characteristic of the somatic cells of the species.

Membrane potentials The voltage generated by the differences of ions on opposite side of the cell membrane.

Mesoderm The middle layer of the three primary germ layers of the developing embryo, lying between the ectoderm and the endoderm.

Mesothelium Flat cells derived from the mesoderm and line body cavities such s the thoracic and abdominal cavity.

Metabolism The sum of all the physical and chemical processes by which living organisms are produced and maintained, and also the transformation by which energy is provided for vital processes and activities.

Metaplasia Change in type of adult cells in a tissue to a form that is not normal for that tissue.

Metastasis The transfer of disease (*e.g.*, cancer) from one organ or part to another not directly connected with it. (Adjective: metastatic)

Miosis Contraction of the pupil of the eye.

Mitosis A type of indirect cell division that occurs in somatic cells and results in the formation of two daughter nuclei containing the identical complements of the number of chromosomes characteristic of the somatic cells of the species.

Molecule The smallest mass of matter that exhibits the properties of an element or compound.

Morbidity A diseased condition or state; the relative incidence of a disease or of all diseases in a population.

Morphology The study of the physical form and structure of an organism, or the form and structure of a particular organism. (Adjective: morphologic)

Mosaicism In genetics, the presence in an individual or in an organism of cell cultures having two or more cell lines that differ in genetic constitution but are derived from a single zygote.

Multiunit smooth muscle Muscle fibers not closely jointed and contract as separate units.

Mutagen Any chemical or physical agent that induces a genetic mutation (an unusual change in form, quality, or some other characteristic) or increases the mutation rate by causing changes in DNA.

Mydriasis Physiologic dilatation of the pupil of the eye.

Myoclonus A spasm of a portion of a muscle, an entire muscle, or a group of muscles.

Myofibrils Fine threads in striated muscle cells and can contract.

Myoglobin The oxygen-transporting pigment of muscle consisting of one heme molecule containing one iron molecule attached to a single globin chain.

Myopathy Any disease or abnormal condition of skeletal muscle, usually characterized by muscle weakness, wasting, and histologic changes within muscle tissue.

Myotome The muscle plate or portion of an embryonic somite that develops into a voluntary muscle, or a group of muscles innervated by a single spinal segment.

Necrosis Localized tissue death that occurs in groups of cells or part of a structure or an organ in response to disease or injury.

Neurofibrillary tangles Formed of tau protein and are an indicator of Alzheimer disease and tauopathies.

Neutropenia An abnormal decrease in the number of neutrophilic leukocytes in the blood.

Nidus The point where a morbid process originates, develops, or is located.

Nociception The reception of painful stimuli from the physical or mechanical injury to body tissues by nociceptors (receptors usually found in either the skin or the walls of the viscera).

Nonenveloped Nonenveloped viruses have an outer cover made of proteins. These viruses are more virulent and resistant producing antibodies in the host.

Nosocomial Pertaining to or originating in a hospital, such as a nosocomial infection: an infection acquired during hospitalization.

Nuclear envelope A double-layered membrane that surrounds the nucleus and controls passage of substances into and out of the nucleus.

Nystagmus Involuntary, rapid, rhythmic movements of the eyeball.

Oncogene A gene that is capable of causing the initial and continuing conversion of normal cells into cancer cells.

Oncotic Relating to, caused by, or marked by edema or any swelling.

Oocyte A primordial or incompletely developed ovum.

Oogenesis The process of the growth and maturation of the female gametes or ova.

Opsonization The process of making cells, such as bacteria, more susceptible to the action of phagocytes.

Organelle Any one of the various membrane-bound particles of distinctive morphology and function present within most cells, as the mitochondria, the Golgi complex, and the lysosomes.

Orthopnea An abnormal condition in which a person must be in an upright position in order to breathe deeply or comfortably.

Orthosis An external orthopedic appliance or apparatus, as a brace or splint, used to support, align, prevent or correct deformities, or to improve the function of movable parts of the body.

Osmolality The concentration of osmotically active particles in solution expressed in osmols or milliosmols per kilogram of solvent.

Osmolarity The concentration of osmotically active particles in solution expressed in osmols or milliosmols per liter of solution.

Osmosis The movement or passage of a pure solvent, such as water, through a semipermeable membrane from a solution that has a lower solute concentration to one that has a higher solute concentration.

Osmotic pressure The pressure required to prevent osmosis into a solution.

Osteophyte A bony project or outgrowth.

Oxidative phosphorylation The biochemical process by which ATP is formed in the mitochondria from phosphate and ADP.

Palpable Perceptible by touch.

Papilla A small nipple-shaped projection, elevation, or structure, as the conoid papillae of the tongue.

Papule A small, circumscribed, solid elevation of the skin less than 1 cm in diameter. (Adjective: papular)

Paracrine A mode of hormone action in which a chemical messenger that is synthesized and released from a cell acts on nearby cells of a different type and affects their function.

Paralysis An abnormal condition characterized by the impairment or loss of motor function due to a lesion of the neural or muscular mechanism.

Paraneoplastic Relating to alterations produced in tissue remote from a tumor or its metastases.

Parenchyma The basic tissue or elements of an organ as distinguished from supporting or connective tissue or elements. (Adjective: parenchymal)

Paresis Slight or partial paralysis.

Paresthesia Any abnormal touch sensation, which can be experienced as numbness, tingling, or a "pins and needles" feeling, often in the absence of external stimuli.

Parietal Pertaining to the outer wall of a cavity or organ, or pertaining to the parietal bone of the skull or the parietal lobe of the brain.

Parous Having borne one or more viable offspring.

Passive transport The movement of substances across a cell membrane with the need for energy.

Pathogen Any microorganism capable of producing disease.

Pedigree A systematic presentation, such as in a table, chart, or list, of an individual's ancestors that is used in human genetics in the analysis of inheritance.

Peptide Any of a class of molecular chain compounds composed of two or more amino acids joined by peptide bonds.

Perfusion The process or act of pouring over or through, especially the passage of a fluid through a specific organ or an area of the body.

Peripheral Pertaining to the outside, surface, or surrounding area of an organ or other structure, or located away from a center or central structure.

Peripheral proteins Proteins found on the membrane, which can easily disconnect.

Permeable A condition of being pervious or permitting passage, so that fluids and certain other substances can pass through, as a permeable membrane.

Peroxisomes Found in cytoplasm are responsible for carrying out oxidative reactions.

Pervasive Pertaining to something that becomes diffused throughout every part.

Petechia A tiny, perfectly round, purplish red spot that appears on the skin as a result of minute intradermal or submucous hemorrhage. (Plural: petechiae)

Phagocytosis The process by which certain cells engulf and consume foreign material and cell debris.

Phagocytosis The ingestion of other cells.

Phagosome A vacuole that contains engulfed or ingested particles.

Phalanx Any one of the bones composing the fingers of each hand and the toes of each foot.

Phenotype The complete physical, biochemical, and physiologic makeup of an individual, as determined by the interaction of both genetic makeup and environmental factors.

Pheresis A procedure in which blood is withdrawn from a donor, a portion (plasma, leukocytes, etc.) is separated and retained, and the remainder is reperfused into the donor. It includes plasmapheresis and leukapheresis.

Pili Hair, or in microbiology, the minute filamentous appendages of certain bacteria. (Singular: pilus)

Pinocytosis The process by which cells ingest liquid.

Plasma membrane or cell membrane A thin membrane made of fats and proteins that separate the cell's cytoplasm from the external environment.

Plethoric Relating to an excess of any of the body fluids, especially blood; the term used to describe the beefy red coloration of a newborn.

Plexus A network of intersecting nerves, blood vessels, or lymphatic vessels.

Polycystic kidney disease An inherited disease in which many cysts grow in the kidneys causing hypertrophy and leads to kidney failure.

Polygene Any of a group of nonallelic genes that interact to influence the same character in the same way so that the effect is cumulative, usually of a quantitative nature, as size, weight, or skin pigmentation. (Adjective: polygenic)

Polymorph One of several, or many, forms of an organism or cell. (Adjective: polymorphic)

Polyp A small, tumor-like growth that protrudes from a mucous membrane surface.

Polypeptide A molecular chain of more than two amino acids joined by peptide bonds.

Presbyopia A visual condition (farsightedness) that commonly develops with advancing years or old age in which the lens loses elasticity causing defective accommodation and inability to focus sharply for near vision.

Prevalence The number of new and old cases of a disease that is present in a population at a given time, or occurrences of an event during a particular period of time.

Primary active transport The energy needed to move molecules are derived from the breakdown of ATP.

Primary lysosomes Produced by the Golgi complex and fuse with phagosomes or pinosomes and become **secondary lysosomes** where lysis occurs due to hydrolytic enzymes.

Prodrome An early symptom indicating the onset of a condition or disease. (Adjective: prodromal)

Prokaryotic Pertaining to an organism, such as bacterium, with cells lacking a true nucleus and nuclear membrane that reproduces through simple fission.

Prolapse The falling down, sinking, or sliding of an organ from its normal position or location in the body.

Proliferation The reproduction or multiplication of similar forms, especially cells.

Pronation Assumption of a position in which the ventral, or front, surface of the body or part of the body faces downward. (Adjective: prone)

Propagation The act or action of reproduction.

Proprioception The reception of stimuli originating from within the body regarding body position and muscular activity by proprioceptors (sensory nerve endings found in muscles, tendons, joints).

Prosthesis An artificial replacement for a missing body part, or a device designed and applied to improve function, such as a hearing aid.

Proteasome Breaks down protein especially when not needed.

Protein kinases Modify proteins by adding phosphate groups causing a function change.

Proteoglycans Any one of a group of polysaccharide–protein conjugates occurring primarily in the matrix of connective tissue and cartilage.

Proteolysis The breakdown of proteins such as during digestion.

Proto-oncogene A normal cellular gene that with alteration, such as by mutation, becomes an active oncogene.

Protoplasm The liquid substances of the interior of living cells, which contains both organic and inorganic substances.

Proximal Closer to a point of reference, usually the trunk of the body, than other parts of the body.

Pruritus The symptom of itching, an uncomfortable sensation leading to the urge to rub or scratch the skin to obtain relief. (Adjective: pruritic)

Pseudostratified A layer of epithelial cells in direct contact with the basement membrane.

Pseudostratified epithelium A single layer of epithelial cells that give the appearance of being stratified.

Purpura A small hemorrhage, up to about 1 cm in diameter, in the skin, mucous membrane, or serosal surface, or any of several bleeding disorders characterized by the presence of purpuric lesions.

Purulent Producing or containing pus.

Quiescent Quiet, causing no disturbance, activity, or symptoms.

Receptor-mediated endocytosis The process by which the cells absorbs, get nutrients and other materials into the cell through invagination.

Reflux An abnormal backward or return flow of a fluid, such as stomach contents, blood, or urine.

Regurgitation A flow of material that is in the opposite direction from normal, as in the return of swallowed food into the mouth or the backward flow of blood through a defective heart valve.

Remission The partial or complete disappearance of the symptoms of a chronic or malignant disease, or the period of time during which the abatement of symptoms occurs.

Residual bodies Cytoplasmic vacuoles contain undigestable substances.

Resorption The loss of substance or bone by physiologic or pathologic means, for example, the loss of dentin and cementum of a tooth.

Retrograde Moving backward or against the usual direction of flow, reverting to an earlier state or worse condition (degenerating), catabolic.

Retroversion A condition in which an entire organ is tipped backward or in a posterior direction, usually without flexion or other distortion.

Rhabdomyolysis Destruction or degeneration of muscle, associated with myoglobinuria (excretion of myoglobin in the urine).

Rigor mortis The stiffening of the muscles and joints postmortem due to chemic changes primarily in the muscles.

Rostral Situated near a beak (oral or nasal region).

Rough endoplasmic reticulum A tubular membrane studded with ribosomes giving the uneven appearance and plays a role in synthesizing and storing proteins.

Sacroiliitis Inflammation in the sacroiliac joint.

Sarcolemma The cell membrane that covers striated muscle fiber cells.

Sarcomeres The foundational unit of striated muscle tissue.

Sarcoplasm The cytoplasm of a muscle fiber.

Sarcoplasmic reticulum The storage unit in muscle cells for calcium.

Sclerosis A condition characterized by induration or hardening of tissue resulting from any of several causes, including inflammation, diseases of the interstitial substance, and increased formation of connective tissues.

Scotopic vision Describes vision, especially night vision, when the eye is dark adapted.

Second messengers Intracellular substances released by the cell in response to a first messenger.

Secondary active transport The energy needed to move molecules is derived from stored energy rather than the breakdown of ATP.

Secretory granules A vesicle in which neuropeptides and hormones are stored for secretion.

Semipermeable Partially but not wholly permeable, especially a membrane that permits the passage of some (usually small) molecules but not of other (usually larger) particles.

Senescence The process or condition of aging or growing old.

Sepsis The presence in the blood or other tissues of pathogenic microorganisms or their toxins, or the condition resulting from the spread of microorganisms or their products. (Adjective: septic)

Serous Relating to or resembling serum, or containing or producing serum, such as a serous gland.

Shunt To divert or bypass bodily fluid from one channel, path, or part to another; a passage or anastomosis between two natural channels, especially between blood vessels, established by surgery or occurring as an abnormality.

Signal transduction A chemical reaction that occurs when a signal such as a hormone interacts with a receptor.

Simple cell Converts chemical energy into electrical energy.

Simple columnar epithelium Cells that are taller than wide and are one layer. They line most organs of the digestive track and some other organs such as the respiratory bronchioles and their primary function is secretion and absorption.

Simple cuboidal epithelium A single layer of cuboidal epithelium cells and specializes in secretion.

Single-unit smooth muscle A large number of cells that contract as a unit.

Skeletal muscle Striated muscle connected to the skeleton and under voluntary control.

Smooth endoplasmic reticulum Serves as a storage unit and plays a role in the creating and storage of lipids and steroids.

Smooth muscle Muscle tissue that contracts involuntarily.

Soma The body of an organism as distinguished from the mind; all of an organism, excluding germ cells; the body of a cell.

Spasticity The condition characterized by spasms or other uncontrolled contractions of the skeletal muscles. (Adjective: spastic)

Spatial Relating to, having the character of, or occupying space.

Sphincter A ringlike band of muscle fibers that constricts a passage or closes a natural orifice of the body.

Squamous cells They are flat and make up most of the cells of the epidermis, respiratory, and digestive tract.

Stem cells Undifferentiated cells that are able to become specialized cells.

Stenosis An abnormal condition characterized by the narrowing or stricture of a duct or canal.

Stochastic Involving a random process.

Stratified epithelium Flat cells arranged in layers with only one being in contract with the basement membrane.

Stratified squamous keratinized Dead squamous cells.

Stria A streak or a linear scarlike lesion that often results from rapidly developing tension in the skin, or a narrow bandlike structure, especially the longitudinal collections of nerve fibers in the brain.

Stricture An abnormal temporary or permanent narrowing of the lumen of a duct, canal, or other passage, as the esophagus, because of inflammation, external pressure, or scarring.

Stroma The supporting tissue or the matrix of an organ as distinguished from its functional element or parenchyma.

Stupor A lowered level of consciousness characterized by lethargy and unresponsiveness in which a person seems unaware of his or her surroundings.

Subchondral Beneath a cartilage.

Subcutaneous Beneath the skin.

Subluxation An incomplete or partial dislocation in which the relationship between joint surfaces is altered, but contact remains.

Sulcus A shallow groove, depression, or furrow on the surface of an organ, as a sulcus on the surface of the brain, separating the gyri.

Supination Assuming the position of lying horizontally on the back or with the face upward. (Adjective: supine)

Suppuration The formation of pus or purulent matter.

Symbiosis Mode of living characterized by close association between organisms of different species, usually in a mutually beneficial relationship.

Sympathomimetic An agent or substance that produces stimulating effects on organs and structures similar to those produced by the sympathetic nervous system.

Symport The process by which two molecules move through a membrane by a common carrier or cotransporter.

Synapses Gaps between two nerve cells allowing an electrical or chemic impulse to pass.

Syncope A brief lapse of consciousness due to generalized cerebral ischemia.

Syncytium A multinucleate mass of protoplasm produced by the merging of a group of cells.

Syndrome A complex of signs and symptoms that occur together to present a clinical picture of a disease or inherited abnormality.

Synergist An organ, agent, or substance that aids or cooperates with another organ, agent, or substance.

Synthesis An integration or combination of various parts or elements to create a unified whole.

Systemic Pertaining to the whole body rather than to a localized area or regional portion of the body.

Systole The contraction, or period of contraction, of the heart that drives the blood onward into the aorta and pulmonary arteries.

T tubules The small tubules that run across striated muscle fiber and conduct electrical impulses.

Tamponade Stoppage of the flow of blood to an organ or a part of the body by pathologic compression, such as the compression of the heart by an accumulation of pericardial fluid.

Teratogen Any agent or factor that induces or increases the incidence of developmental abnormalities in the fetus.

Thrombus A stationary mass of clotted blood or other formed elements that remains attached to its place of origin along the wall of a blood vessel, frequently obstructing the circulation. (Plural: thrombi)

Tinnitus A tinkling, buzzing, or ringing noise heard in one or both ears.

Tissue Composed of similar cells performing a specific function.

Tophus A chalky deposit containing sodium urate that most often develops in periarticular fibrous tissue, typically in individuals with gout. (Plural: tophi)

Torsion The act or process of twisting in either a positive (clockwise) or negative (counterclockwise) direction.

Trabecula A supporting or anchoring stand of connective tissue, such as the delicate fibrous threads connecting the inner surface of the arachnoid to the pia mater.

Transitional epithelium Epithelial cells that can contract and expand.

Transmembrane proteins A type of integral membrane proteins and cover the cell membrane.

Transmural Situated or occurring through the wall of an organ.

Transudate A fluid substance passed through a membrane or extruded from the blood.

Transverse A right angle to the long axis of the body or lying across.

Tremor Involuntary quivering or trembling movements caused by the alternating contraction and relaxation of opposing groups of skeletal muscles.

Tricarboxylic acid Known as the citric acid cycle are chemical reactions allowing cells to break down energy in the presence of oxygen.

Trigone A triangular-shaped area.

Tropomyosin A muscle protein that controls muscle contraction and prevents muscle contraction when not needed.

Troponin A protein in skeletal and cardiac muscle causing contraction. When elevated, heart muscle damage has most likely occurred.

Tubulin A protein found in cell cytoplasm that serves as the building block for microtubules.

Ubiquitous The condition or state of existing or being everywhere at the same time.

Ulcer A circumscribed excavation of the surface of an organ or tissue, which results from necrosis that accompanies some inflammatory, infectious, or malignant processes. (Adjective: ulcerative)

Up-regulation An increase response to a stimuli due to an increased number of receptors.

Urticaria A pruritic skin eruption of the upper dermis, usually transient, characterized by wheals (hives) of various shapes and sizes.

Uveitis An inflammation of all or part of the uveal tract of the eye.

Vector An invertebrate animal (*e.g.*, tick, mite, mosquito) that serves as a carrier, transferring an infective agent from one vertebrate host to another.

Ventral Pertaining to a position toward the belly of the body, or situated or oriented toward the front or anterior of the body.

Vertigo An illusory sensation that the environment or one's own body is revolving.

Vesicle A small bladder or sac, as a small, thin-walled, raised skin lesion, containing liquid.

Visceral Pertaining to the viscera or internal organs of the body.

Viscosity Pertaining to the physical property of fluids, caused by the adhesion of adjacent molecules, that determines the internal resistance to shear forces.

Zoonosis A disease of animals that may be transmitted to humans from its primary animal host under natural conditions.

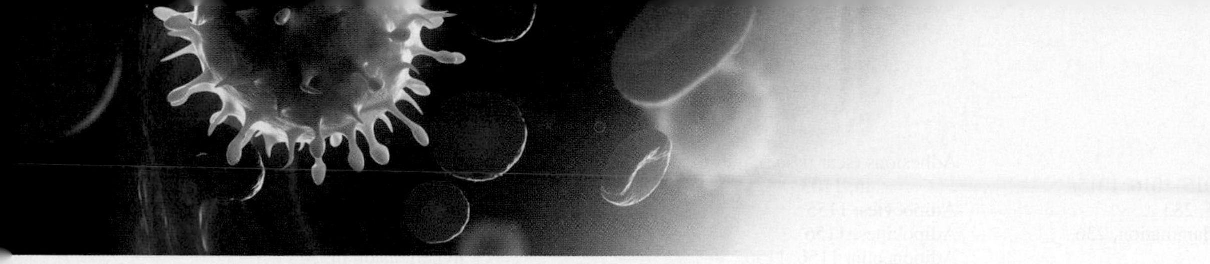

Index

Note: Page numbers followed by the letter "*f*" refer to figures; those followed by the letter "*t*" refer to tables; and those followed by the letter "c" refer to charts.

A

C

D

G

H

I

J

K

N

O

P

Q

R

S

T

U

V

W

X

Y

Z